Obstetrics

Normal and Problem Pregnancies

Obstetrics

Normal and Problem Pregnancies

FIFTH EDITION

STEVEN G. GABBE, MD
Dean, Vanderbilt University School of Medicine
Professor of Obstetrics and Gynecology
Vanderbilt University Medical Center
Nashville, Tennessee

JENNIFER R. NIEBYL, MD
Professor and Head
Department of Obstetrics and Gynecology
University of Iowa Hospitals and Clinics
University of Iowa College of Medicine
Iowa City, Iowa

JOE LEIGH SIMPSON, MD
Executive Associate Dean for Academic Affairs
Professor of Obstetrics and Gynecology
Professor of Human and Molecular Genetics
Florida International University College of Medicine
Miami, Florida

Associate Editors

HENRY GALAN, MD
Professor and Chief
Section of Maternal-Fetal Medicine
Director, Maternal-Fetal Medicine
Fellowship Program
Department of Obstetrics and Gynecology
University of Colorado at Denver
Health Sciences Center
Denver, Colorado

LAURA GOETZL, MD, MPH
Assistant Professor
Department of Obstetrics-Gynecology
Medical University of South Carolina
Charleston, South Carolina

ERIC R. M. JAUNIAUX, MD, PHD
(INTERNATIONAL EDITOR)
Professor and Honorary Consultant
Academic Department of Obstetrics and Gynecology
Institute of Women's Health
Royal Free and University College London
Medical School
London, United Kingdom

MARK B. LANDON, MD
Professor and Vice Chairman
Director of Maternal-Fetal Medicine
Department of Obstetrics and Gynecology
The Ohio State University College of Medicine
Columbus, Ohio

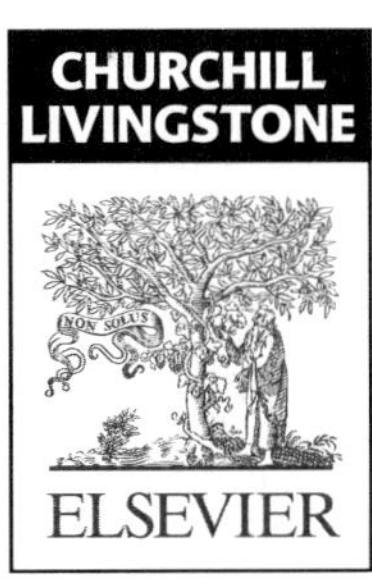

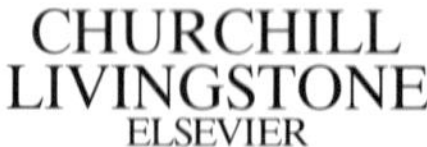

1600 John F. Kennedy Blvd.
Suite 1800
Philadelphia, PA 19103-2899

OBSTETRICS: NORMAL AND PROBLEM PREGNANCIES, 5/E 978-0-443-06930-7

Notice

Knowledge and best practice in this field are constantly changing. As new research and experience broaden our knowledge, changes in practice, treatment and drug therapy may become necessary or appropriate. Readers are advised to check the most current information provided (i) on procedures featured or (ii) by the manufacturer of each product to be administered, to verify the recommended dose or formula, the method and duration of administration, and contraindications. It is the responsibility of the practitioner, relying on their own experience and knowledge of the patient, to make diagnoses, to determine dosages and the best treatment for each individual patient, and to take all appropriate safety precautions. To the fullest extent of the law, neither the Publisher nor the Authors assumes any liability for any injury and/or damage to persons or property arising out or related to any use of the material contained in this book.

The Publisher

Previous editions copyrighted 2002, 1996, 1991, 1986 by Elsevier, Inc.

Library of Congress Cataloging-in-Publication Data
Obstetrics : normal and problem pregnancies / [edited by] Steven G. Gabbe, Jennifer R. Niebyl, Joe Leigh Simpson ; associate editors, Henry Galan . . . [et al.]. – 5th ed.
p. ; cm.
Includes bibliographical references and index.
ISBN 978-0-443-06930-7
1. Obstetrics. 2. Pregnancy–Complications. I. Gabbe, Steven G. II. Niebyl, Jennifer R. III. Simpson, Joe Leigh.
[DNLM: 1. Obstetrics–methods. 2. Pregnancy Complications. 3. Pregnancy. WQ 100 O165 2007] I. Title.
RG524.O3 2007
618.2–dc22 2007013138

Acquisitions Editor: Rebecca Gaertner
Developmental Editor: Melissa Dudlick
Project Manager: David Saltzberg
Design Direction: Steve Stave

Printed in China

Last digit is the print number: 9 8 7 6 5 4 3 2 1

To all who have taught us, supported us, and guided us during the past four decades—and to our patients.

Steven G. Gabbe, MD
Jennifer R. Niebyl, MD
Joe Leigh Simpson, MD

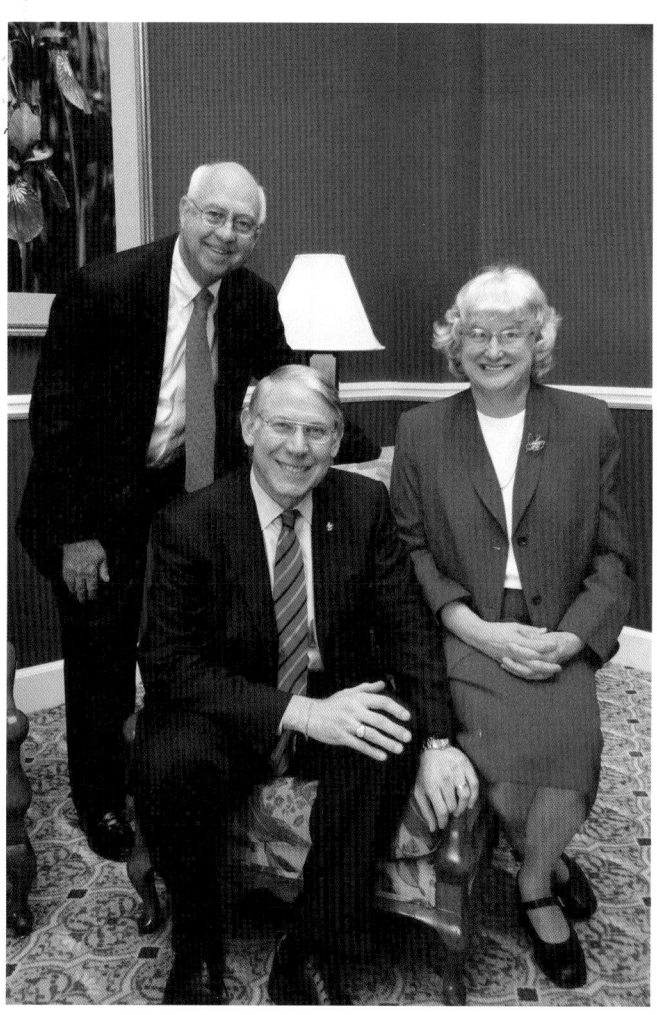

(*Left to right*) Joe Leigh Simpson, Steven G. Gabbe, and Jennifer R. Niebyl

Contributors

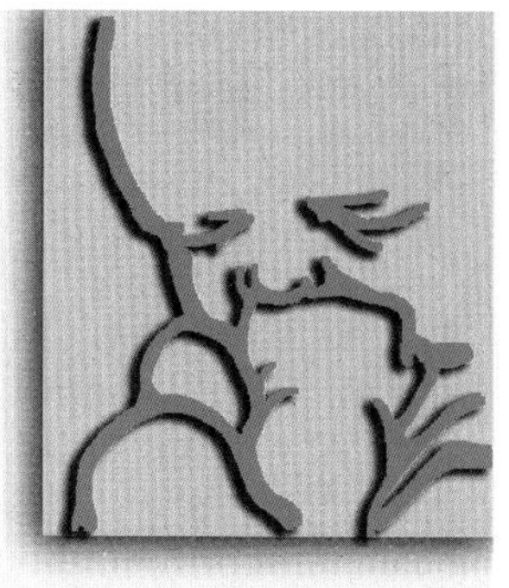

KRISTINA M. ADAMS, MD
Assistant Professor, University of Washington, Seattle, Washington
Maternal-Fetal Immunology

MARGARET ALTEMUS, MD
Associate Professor, Weill Medical College, Cornell University; Associate Attending Physician, New York Presbyterian Hospital, Weill Cornell Medical Center, New York, New York
Psychiatric Disorders

GEORGE J. ANNAS, JD, MPH
Edward R. Utley Professor and Chair, Department of Health Law, Bioethics, and Human Rights, Boston University School of Public Health, Boston, Massachusetts
Legal and Ethical Issues in Obstetric Practice

AHMET ALEXANDER BASCHAT, MD
Associate Professor, and Director, Fetal Surgery Program, University of Maryland, Baltimore, and University of Maryland Medical Center, Baltimore, Maryland
Intrauterine Growth Restriction

LEAH R. BATTISTA, MD
Clinical Instructor, University of California, Irvine, School of Medicine, Irvine; Southern California Permanente Medical Group, Baldwin Park, California
Abnormal Labor and Induction of Labor

RICHARD L. BERKOWITZ, MD
Professor of Obstetrics and Gynecology, Columbia Presbyterian Medical Center, New York, New York
Multiple Gestations

HELENE BERNSTEIN, MD, PHD
Assistant Professor of Obstetrics and Gynecology, David Geffen School of Medicine at UCLA, Los Angeles, California
Maternal and Perinatal Infection—Viral

DEBRA L. BOGEN, MD
Assistant Professor of Pediatrics, University of Pittsburgh School of Medicine; Children's Hospital of Pittsburgh, Pittsburgh, Pennsylvania
Psychiatric Disorders

D. WARE BRANCH, MD
Professor, Department of Obstetrics and Gynecology, and H.A. and Edna Benning Presidential Chair, University of Utah Health Sciences; University of Utah LDS Hospital, Salt Lake City, Utah
Collagen Vascular Diseases

GRAHAM J. BURTON, MA, MD, DSC
Professor of Reproductive Biology, Department of Physiology, Development and Neuroscience, University of Cambridge, Cambridge, United Kingdom
Placental Anatomy and Physiology

MITCHELL S. CAPPELL, MD, PHD
Chief, Division of Gastroenterology, William Beaumont Hospital, Royal Oak, Michigan
Gastrointestinal Disorders

PATRICK M. CATALANO, MD
Professor, Department of Reproductive Biology, Case Western Reserve University; Chairman, Department of Obstetrics and Gynecology, MetroHealth Medical Center, Cleveland, Ohio
Diabetes Mellitus Complicating Pregnancy

DAVID H. CHESTNUT, MD
Director of Medical Education, Gundersen Lutheran Health System; Professor of Anesthesiology, University of Wisconsin School of Medicine and Public Health, La Crosse, Wisconsin
Obstetric Anesthesia

USHA CHITKARA, MD
Professor of Obstetrics and Gynecology, Stanford University School of Medicine, Stanford, California
Multiple Gestations

JANE CLEARY-GOLDMAN, MD
Assistant Clinical Professor of Obstetrics and Gynecology, Columbia Presbyterian Medical Center, New York, New York
Multiple Gestations

DAVID F. COLOMBO, MD
Assistant Professor, Division of Maternal-Fetal Medicine, Department of Obstetrics and Gynecology, The Ohio State University College of Medicine, Columbus, Ohio
Renal Disease

LARRY J. COPELAND, MD
Professor and Chair, William Greenville Pace III and Joann Norris Collins-Pace Chair, Department of Obstetrics and Gynecology, The Ohio State University College of Medicine, Columbus, Ohio
Malignant Diseases and Pregnancy

MYRIAM J. CURET, MD
Associate Professor of Surgery, Stanford University; Stanford Hospital, Stanford, California
Surgical Procedures in Pregnancy

JAN DEPREST, MD, PHD
Director, Center for Surgical Technologies, and Professor of Obstetrics and Gynaecology, Katholieke Universiteit Leuven, Leuven, Belgium
Fetal Therapy

MICHAEL Y. DIVON, MD
Chairman, Department of Obstetrics and Gynecology, Lenox Hill Hospital, New York, New York
Prolonged Pregnancy

MITCHELL P. DOMBROWSKI, MD
Professor and Chair, Department of Obstetrics and Gynecology, St. John Hospital, Detroit, Michigan
Respiratory Diseases in Pregnancy

MAURICE L. DRUZIN, MD
Professor of Gynecology and Obstetrics, and Chief, Division of Maternal-Fetal Medicine, Department of Gynecology and Obstetrics, Stanford University Medical Center, Stanford, California
Antepartum Fetal Evaluation

PATRICK DUFF, MD
Professor, Residency Program Director, Department of Obstetrics and Gynecology, and Associate Dean for Student Affairs, University of Florida, Gainesville, Florida
Maternal and Perinatal Infection—Bacterial

THOMAS R. EASTERLING, MD
Professor, Obstetrics and Gynecology, University of Washington Medical Center, Seattle, Washington
Heart Disease

SHERMAN ELIAS, MD
John J. Sciarra Professor and Chair, Department of Obstetrics and Gynecology, Feinberg School of Medicine, Northwestern University; Chair, Department of Obstetrics and Gynecology, Northwestern Memorial Hospital, Chicago, Illinois
Legal and Ethical Issues in Obstetric Practice

M. GORE ERVIN, PHD
Professor and Graduate Coordinator, Department of Biology, Middle Tennessee State University, Murfreesboro, Tennessee
Fetal Physiology

MARK I. EVANS, MD
Professor of Obstetrics and Gynecology, Mount Sinai School of Medicine; President, Fetal Medicine Foundation of America, and Director, Comprehensive Genetics, New York, New York
Fetal Therapy

ALAN W. FLAKE, MD
Professor of Surgery and Obstetrics and Gynecology, University of Pennsylvania School of Medicine; Director, Children's Institute for Surgical Science, and Pediatric Surgery Residency Training Program, Children's Hospital of Philadelphia, Philadelphia, Pennsylvania
Fetal Therapy

MICHAEL R. FOLEY, MD
Clinical Professor, University of Arizona, Tucson; Medical Director of Academic Affairs, Scottsdale Healthcare, Scottsdale, Arizona
Antepartum and Postpartum Hemorrhage

KARRIE E. FRANCOIS, MD
Clinical Assistant Professor, University of Arizona, Phoenix; Perinatal Medical Director, Scottsdale Healthcare, Scottsdale, Arizona
Antepartum and Postpartum Hemorrhage

STEVEN G. GABBE, MD
Dean, Vanderbilt University School of Medicine; Professor of Obstetrics and Gynecology, Vanderbilt University Medical Center, Nashville, Tennessee
Antepartum Fetal Evaluation; Intrauterine Growth Restriction; Diabetes Mellitus Complicating Pregnancy

HENRY GALAN, MD
Professor and Chief, Section of Maternal-Fetal Medicine, and Director, Maternal-Fetal Medicine Fellowship Program, Department of Obstetrics and Gynecology, University of Colorado at Denver Health Sciences Center, Denver, Colorado
Operative Vaginal Delivery; Intrauterine Growth Restriction

THOMAS J. GARITE, MD
Professor Emeritus, University of California, Irvine; Director of Research and Education, Pediatrix Medical Group, Orange, California
Intrapartum Fetal Evaluation

ETOI GARRISON, MD, PHD
Assistant Professor of Obstetrics and Gynecology, Vanderbilt University Medical Center, Nashville, Tennessee
Normal Labor and Delivery; Operative Vaginal Delivery

WILLIAM M. GILBERT, MD
Professor of Obstetrics and Gynecology, University of California, Davis; Regional Medical Director, Women's Services, Sutter Health, Sac-Sierra Region, Sutter Medical Center, Sacramento, California
Amniotic Fluid Disorders

LAURA GOETZL, MD, MPH
Assistant Professor, Department of Obstetrics-Gynecology, Medical University of South Carolina, Charleston, South Carolina
Obstetric Anesthesia

MICHAEL C. GORDON, MD
Associate Professor, University of Texas Health Science Center at San Antonio, San Antonio, Texas
Maternal Physiology

KIMBERLY D. GREGORY, MD, MPH
Vice Chair, Women's Healthcare Quality and Performance Improvement, Cedars-Sinai Medical Center, Los Angeles, California
Preconception and Prenatal Care: Part of the Continuum

MICHAEL R. HARRISON, MD
Professor of Surgery, Pediatrics, Obstetrics, Gynecology and Reproductive Sciences, and Director, Fetal Treatment Center, University of California, San Francisco, San Francisco, California
Fetal Therapy

JOY L. HAWKINS, MD
Professor of Anesthesiology, University of Colorado School of Medicine; Director of Obstetric Anesthesia, University of Colorado Hospital, Denver, Colorado
Obstetric Anesthesia

CALLA HOLMGREN, MD
Fellow, University of Utah; LDS Hospital, Salt Lake City, Utah
Collagen Vascular Diseases

WOLFGANG HOLZGREVE, MD
Chairman and Chief of Service, Department of Obstetrics and Gynecology, University of Basel, Basel, Switzerland
Genetic Counseling and Genetic Screening

JAY D. IAMS, MD
Frederick P. Zuspan Professor and Endowed Chair, Division of Maternal-Fetal Medicine, Vice-Chair, Department of Obstetrics and Gynecology, The Ohio State University, Columbus, Ohio
Preterm Birth

ERIC R. M. JAUNIAUX, MD, PHD
Professor and Honorary Consultant, Academic Department of Obstetrics and Gynecology, Institute of Women's Health, Royal Free and University College London Medical School, London, United Kingdom
Placental Anatomy and Physiology; Pregnancy Loss

TIMOTHY R. B. JOHNSON, MD
Chair and Bates Professor of Diseases of Women and Children, Arthur F. Thurnau Professor, and Professor, Women's Studies, Department of Obstetrics and Gynecology, University of Michigan Health System, Ann Arbor, Michigan
Preconception and Prenatal Care: Part of the Continuum

VERN L. KATZ, MD
Clinical Professor of Obstetrics and Gynecology, Oregon Health Science University, Portland; Adjunct Professor of Physiology, University of Oregon, Eugene; Medical Director, Obstetric Services, Sacred Heart Medical Center, Eugene, Oregon
Postpartum Care

SARAH KILPATRICK, MD, PHD
Professor, and Chief of Service/Physician Surgeon, University of Illinois at Chicago, Chicago, Illinois
Normal Labor and Delivery; Operative Vaginal Delivery

CHARLES KLEINMAN, MD
Adjunct Professor of Clinical Pediatrics, and Attending Physician, New York Presbyterian Hospital; Professor of Clinical Pediatrics, Columbia University College of Physicians and Surgeons, New York, New York
Fetal Therapy

GEORGE KROUMPOUZOS, MD, PHD
Clinical Assistant Professor of Dermatology, Brown Medical School, Providence, Rhode Island
Hepatic Disorders; Dermatologic Disorders of Pregnancy

DANIEL V. LANDERS, MD
Former Director, Maternal-Fetal Medicine, University of Minnesota Medical School; Maternal-Fetal Medicine Specialist, San Diego Perinatal Center, Sharp Mary Birch Hospital for Women, San Diego, California
Maternal and Perinatal Infection: The Sexually Transmitted Diseases Chlamydia, Gonorrhea, and Syphilis

MARK B. LANDON, MD
Professor and Vice Chairman, and Director of Maternal-Fetal Medicine, Department of Obstetrics and Gynecology, The Ohio State University College of Medicine, Columbus, Ohio
Cesarean Delivery; Diabetes Mellitus Complicating Pregnancy; Malignant Diseases and Pregnancy

SUSAN M. LANNI, MD
Associate Professor of Obstetrics and Gynecology and Maternal-Fetal Medicine, and Director, Labor and Delivery, Virginia Commonwealth University Medical Center, Richmond, Virginia
Malpresentations

CHARLES J. LOCKWOOD, MD
The Anita O'Keefe Young Professor and Chair, Department of Obstetrics, Gynecology and Reproductive Sciences, Yale University School of Medicine; Chief of Obstetrics and Gynecology, Yale-New Haven Hospital, New Haven, Connecticut
Thromboembolic Disorders

ERIKA J. LU, MD
Resident, Department of Surgery, Stanford University and Stanford Hospital, Stanford, California
Surgical Procedures in Pregnancy

JACK LUDMIR, MD
Professor, Obstetrics and Gynecology, University of Pennsylvania School of Medicine; Chief, Department of Obstetrics and Gynecology, Pennsylvania Hospital, University of Pennsylvania Health System, Philadelphia, Pennsylvania
Cervical Incompetence

MAUREEN P. MALEE, PHD, MD
Director, Division of Maternal-Fetal Medicine, Department of Obstetrics and Gynecology, Vanderbilt University Medical Center, Vanderbilt University School of Medicine, Nashville, Tennessee
Pituitary and Adrenal Disorders in Pregnancy

BRIAN M. MERCER, MD, FRCSC, FACOG
Professor, Reproductive Biology, Case Western Reserve University; Vice Chair, Director of Obstetrics and Maternal-Fetal Medicine, Department of Obstetrics and Gynecology, MetroHealth Medical Center, Cleveland, Ohio
Premature Rupture of the Membranes

JORGE H. MESTMAN, MD
Professor of Medicine and Obstetrics and Gynecology, Keck School of Medicine, University of Southern California, Los Angeles, California
Thyroid and Parathyroid Diseases in Pregnancy

DAWN MISRA, MHS, PHD
Associate Professor, University of Michigan School of Public Health, Ann Arbor, Michigan
Psychiatric Disorders

KENNETH J. MOISE, JR., MD
Professor of Obstetrics and Gynecology, Baylor College of Medicine, Houston, Texas
Red Cell Alloimmunization

EDWARD R. NEWTON, MD
Professor and Chairman, Department of Obstetrics and Gynecology, Brody School of Medicine, East Carolina University, Greenville, North Carolina
Breast-Feeding

JENNIFER R. NIEBYL, MD
Professor and Head, Department of Obstetrics and Gynecology, University of Iowa Hospitals and Clinics, University of Iowa College of Medicine, Iowa City, Iowa
Preconception and Prenatal Care: Part of the Continuum; Drugs and Environmental Agents in Pregnancy and Lactation: Embryology, Teratology, Epidemiology; Neurologic Disorders

PETER E. NIELSEN, MD
Adjunct Associate Professor of Obstetrics and Gynecology, F. Edward Hébert School of Medicine, Uniformed Services University of the Health Sciences, Bethesda, Maryland; Clinical Associate Professor of Obstetrics and Gynecology, University of Washington School of Medicine, Seattle, Washington; Chairman, Department of Obstetrics and Gynecology, Madigan Army Medical Center, and Obstetrics/Gynecology Consultant to The Surgeon General, United States Army Medical Command, Madigan Army Medical Center, Tacoma, Washington
Operative Vaginal Delivery

DONALD NOVAK, MD
Professor of Pediatrics, University of Florida; Vice Chair of Clinical Affairs, Shands Children's Hospital, Gainesville, Florida
Fetal Physiology

LUCAS OTAÑO, MD
Professor, Division of Obstetrics and Gynecology, Hospital Italiano de Buenos Aires, Buenos Aires, Argentina
Prenatal Genetic Diagnosis

JOHN OWEN, MD
Professor of Obstetrics and Gynecology, University of Alabama at Birmingham, Birmingham, Alabama
Cervical Imcompetence

JOHN PAPOUTSIS, PHD
Professor, School of Administration of Health Units and Welfare, TEI of Antikalamos, Messinia, Greece
Dermatologic Disorders of Pregnancy

JAMES M. PEREL, PHD
Professor Emeritus of Psychiatry, Professor of Pharmacology and Graduate Neuroscience, University of Pittsburgh; Director of Clinical Pharmacology, Western Psychiatric Institute and Clinic, Pittsburgh, Pennsylvania
Psychiatric Disorders

CHRISTIAN M. PETTKER, MD
Instructor, Yale University School of Medicine; Clinical Fellow, Division of Maternal-Fetal Medicine, Department of Obstetrics, Gynecology and Reproductive Sciences, Yale-New Haven Hospital, New Haven, Connecticut
Thromboembolic Disorders

KIRK D. RAMIN, MD
Professor, Department of Obstetrics and Gynecology, and Interim Director, Maternal-Fetal Medicine, University of Minnesota Medical School; Interim Director, Maternal-Fetal Medicine, University of Minnesota Medical Center, Minneapolis, Minnesota
Maternal and Perinatal Infection: The Sexually Transmitted Diseases Chlamydia, Gonorrhea, and Syphilis

KATHRYN L. REED, MD
Professor and Head of Obstetrics and Gynecology, University of Arizona College of Medicine, Tucson, Arizona
Antepartum Fetal Evaluation

SARAH K. REYNOLDS, PHD
Assistant Professor of Psychiatry, Western Psychiatric Institute and Clinic, University of Pittsburgh Medical Center, Pittsburgh, Pennsylvania
Psychiatric Disorders

DOUGLAS S. RICHARDS, MD
Professor, Obstetrics and Gynecology, University of Florida College of Medicine; Director of Ultrasound Section, Department of Obstetrics, University of Florida College of Medicine, Gainesville, Florida
Ultrasound for Pregnancy Dating, Growth, and the Diagnosis of Fetal Malformations

ROBERTO ROMERO, MD
Chief, Perinatology Research Branch, and Program Director of Obstetrics and Perinatology, National Institute of Clinical Health and Human Development, National Institutes of Health/Department of Health and Human Services, Bethesda, Maryland; Professor, Molecular Obstetrics and Genetics, Wayne State University School of Medicine, Detroit, Michigan
Preterm Birth

ADAM A. ROSENBERG, MD
Professor of Pediatrics, University of Colorado School of Medicine; Director of Newborn Services, Denver, Colorado
The Neonate

MICHAEL G. ROSS, MD, MPH
Professor of Obstetrics and Gynecology and Public Health, David Geffen School of Medicine at UCLA, Los Angeles; Chairman of Obstetrics and Gynecology, Harbor-UCLA Medical Center, Torrance, California
Fetal Physiology; Intrauterine Growth Restriction

PHILIP SAMUELS, MD
Director, Residency Program, Department of Obstetrics and Gynecology, The Ohio State University/Mount Carmel Health; Associate Professor, Division of Maternal-Fetal Medicine, Department of Obstetrics and Gynecology, The Ohio State University College of Medicine, Columbus, Ohio
Renal Disease; Hematologic Complications of Pregnancy; Neurologic Disorders

JOHN W. SEEDS, MD
Professor and Chairman of Obstetrics and Gynecology, Virginia Commonwealth University Medical Center, Richmond, Virginia
Malpresentations

LAURENCE E. SHIELDS, MD
Former Professor of Obstetrics and Gynecology, University of Washington, Seattle, Washington; Staff Perinatologist, Sierra Vista Medical Center, San Luis Obispo, California
Maternal-Fetal Immunology

BAHA M. SIBAI, MD
Professor, University of Cincinnati College of Medicine; The University Hospital, Cincinnati, Ohio
Hypertension

COLIN P. SIBLEY, PHD
Professor of Child Health and Physiology, Division of Human Development, The Medical School, University of Manchester, Manchester, United Kingdom
Placental Anatomy and Physiology

JOE LEIGH SIMPSON, MD
Executive Associate Dean for Academic Affairs, Professor of Obstetrics and Gynecology, and Professor of Human and Molecular Genetics, Florida International University College of Medicine, Miami, Florida
Genetic Counseling and Genetic Screening; Prenatal Genetic Diagnosis; Drugs and Environmental Agents in Pregnancy and Lactation: Embryology, Teratology, Epidemiology; Pregnancy Loss

DOROTHY K. Y. SIT, MD
Assistant Professor of Psychiatry, Department of Psychiatry, University of Pittsburgh School of Medicine, Western Psychiatric Institute and Clinic, Women's Behavioral Healthcare, Pittsburgh, Pennsylvania
Psychiatric Disorders

JAMES F. SMITH JR., MD
Clinical Associate Professor, Department of Obstetrics and Gynecology, Stanford University School of Medicine, Stanford, California
Antepartum Fetal Evaluation

KAREN STOUT, MD
Assistant Professor, Medicine/Cardiology, University of Washington Medical School, Seattle, Washington
Heart Disease

KEERTHY R. SUNDER, MD
Staff Psychiatrist, City and County of San Francisco, San Francisco, California
Psychiatric Disorders

JANICE E. WHITTY, MD
Professor and Director of Maternal-Fetal Medicine, Department of Obstetrics and Gynecology, Meharry Medical College, Nashville, Tennessee
Respiratory Diseases in Pregnancy

DEBORAH A. WING, MD
Associate Professor of Clinical Obstetrics and Gynecology, University of California, Irvine, School of Medicine, Irvine; Associate Professor and Director, Division of Maternal-Fetal Medicine, Department of Obstetrics and Gynecology, University of California, Irvine, Medical Center, Orange, California
Abnormal Labor and Induction of Labor

KATHERINE L. WISNER, MD, MS
Professor of Psychiatry, Obstetrics and Gynecology \and Reproductive Sciences, and Epidemiology, University of Pittsburgh School of Medicine; Director, Women's Behavioral Healthcare, and Associate Member, Magee Women's Research Institute, Western Psychiatric Institute and Clinic, University of Pittsburgh Medical Center, Pittsburgh, Pennsylvania
Psychiatric Disorders

YUVAL YARON, MD
Director, Prenatal Diagnosis Unit, Genetic Institute, Tel Aviv Sourasky Medical Center, Tel Aviv, Israel
Fetal Therapy

Preface to the Fifth Edition

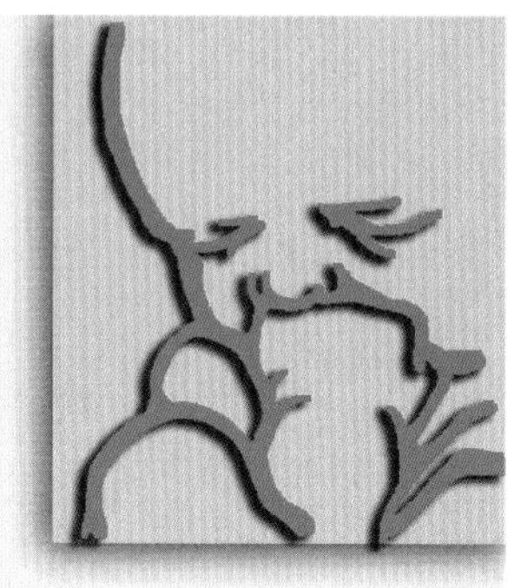

Welcome to the fifth edition of *Obstetrics: Normal and Problem Pregnancies*! For those readers who have included our previous editions in their libraries, we greatly appreciate your continued loyalty and support. For our new readers, we believe you will find this book a valuable resource in your study of normal and high-risk obstetrics.

Like its four predecessors, this book provides an in-depth presentation of the basic science and physiology of normal and complicated obstetrics followed by chapters describing the most updated, evidence-based information on normal obstetrics and high-risk obstetrics. The efforts of a new team of associate editors, the contributions of more than 30 new authors, and a new publisher have enabled us to greatly enhance the content and access to the information in this fifth edition. Four carefully chosen new associate editors, Drs. Henry Galan, Laura Goetzl, Mark Landon, and Eric Jauniaux, each bring their own expertise and insight to this fifth edition. The addition of an international editor from London, Dr. Jauniaux, has enabled us to expand the coverage of this text to include information on clinical care from abroad.

Life-long learning has become essential for the best practice of obstetrics. Our readers will find 14 new chapters, many added to reflect important changes in our knowledge base since the fourth edition in 2001. These new chapters include placental anatomy and physiology, immunology of pregnancy, diagnostic techniques for prenatal diagnosis, management of abnormal labor, operative vaginal delivery, cervical incompetence, preterm premature rupture of the membranes, amniotic fluid disorders, thyroid and parathyroid diseases, adrenal and pituitary disorders, thromboembolic disorders, sexually transmitted diseases, viral infections, and psychiatric disorders. An appendix of normal laboratory values has been added to accompany the appendix on anatomy.

This fifth edition includes more than 30 authors who have joined us for the first time, and we greatly value the new information they have brought to our readers. We also want to recognize the 29 outstanding authors who have continued to contribute. A special tribute is due to 10 leaders in our specialty who have written chapters in every edition of our textbook: Drs. George J. Annas, Richard L. Berkowitz, D. Ware Branch, Sherman Elias, Timothy R. B. Johnson, Mark B. Landon, Adam A. Rosenberg, Phillip Samuels, John W. Seeds, and Baha Sibai.

We greatly appreciate the support of our new publisher, Elsevier, who has joined us for this fifth edition. We have synergistically made significant changes that should benefit our readers. Illustrations are now in full color. Each chapter provides a list of key abbreviations that will facilitate reading. A paginated outline appears at the beginning of each chapter making it easier to locate information on specific topics. The edges of the pages for the two appendices have been colored so that they can be quickly located.

We recognize the outstanding efforts of Melissa Dudlick, Judith Fletcher, Rebecca Gaertner, Stephanie Donley and their team at Elsevier. In addition to the Elsevier staff, the editors have had the invaluable editorial and secretarial support of Robyn Cosby, Nancy Schaapveld, and Belinda Felder. Because this fifth edition will be online and will be continually updated, this entire team will continue to work closely with the editors.

Nearly 25 years ago, the three of us met to discuss our plans for the first edition of *Obstetrics: Normal and Problem Pregnancies*. Like most medical specialties, obstetrics has since become more complex and challenging. Yet, we continue to feel strongly that the practice of normal and high-risk obstetrics remains among the most fascinating and rewarding in medicine and nursing. We believe that this fifth edition will not only serve as an inspiration to those considering a career in obstetrics and gynecology but will also be a valued resource for those who have already joined us in this exciting field.

Steven G. Gabbe, MD
Jennifer R. Niebyl, MD
Joe Leigh Simpson, MD

Contents

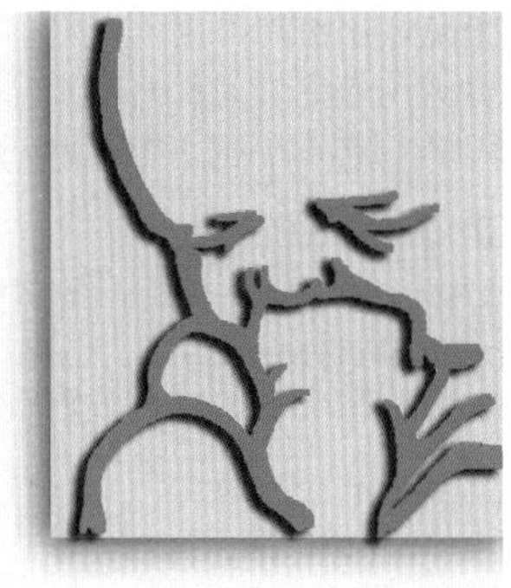

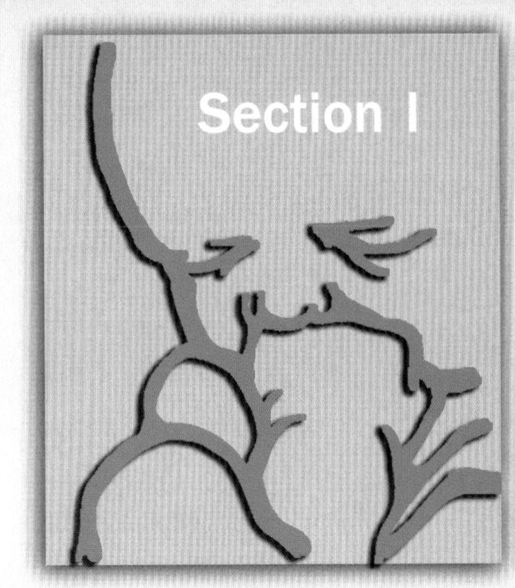

Physiology

Placental Anatomy and Physiology

GRAHAM J. BURTON, COLIN P. SIBLEY, AND ERIC R. M. JAUNIAUX

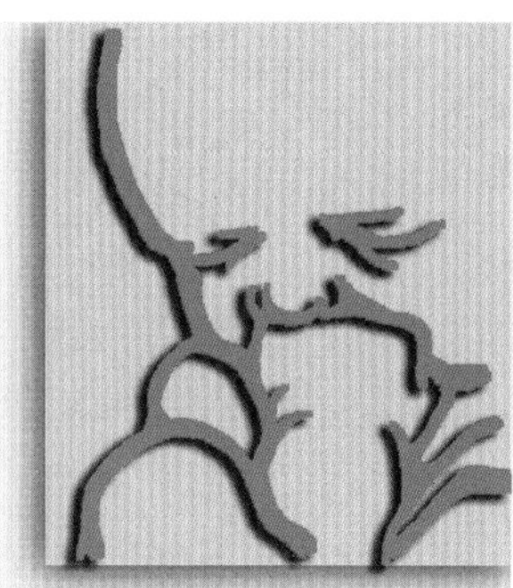

CHAPTER 1

KEY ABBREVIATIONS

Alpha-fetoprotein	AFP
adenosine triphosphate	ATP
Cyclic adenosine monophosphate	cAMP
Cyclic guanosine monophosphate	cGMP
Cytochrome P450scc	P450scc
Dehydroepiandrosterone	DHA
Dehydroepiandrosterone sulfate	DHAS
Epidermal growth factor	EGF
Exocoelomic cavity	ECC
Glucose transporter 1	GLUT1
Human chorionic gonadotropin	hCG
Human chorionic sommatotropin	hCS
Human immunodeficiency virus	HIV
Human placental lactogen	hPL
Insulin-like growth factor	IGF
Immunoglobulin G	IgG
Intervillous space	IVS
Intrauterine growth restriction	IUGR
Luteinizing hormone	LH
Nicotinamide-adenine dinucleotide phosphate	NADPH
P450 cytochrome aromatase	P450arom
Potential difference	PD
Placental growth hormone	PGH
Steroidogenic acute regulatory protein	StAR
Secondary yolk sac	SYS
Type 1 3β-hydroxysteroid dehydrogenase	3β-HSD

INTRODUCTION

The placenta is a remarkable organ. During a relatively short life span, it undergoes rapid growth, differentiation, and maturation. At the same time, it performs diverse functions, including the transport of gases and metabolites, immunologic protection, and the production of steroid and protein hormones. As the interface between the mother and her fetus, the placenta plays a key role in ensuring a successful pregnancy. In this chapter, we review the structure of the human placenta, and relate this to the contrasting functional demands placed on the organ at different stages of gestation. Because many of the morphologic features are best understood through an understanding of the organ's development, and because many complications of pregnancy arise through aberrations in this process, we will approach the subject from this perspective. First, however, for the purposes of orientation and to introduce some basic terminology we provide a brief description of the macroscopic appearance of the delivered organ, with which readers are most likely to be familiar.

OVERVIEW OF THE DELIVERED PLACENTA

At term, the human placenta is usually a discoid organ, 15 to 20 cm in diameter, approximately 3 cm thick at the center, and weighing on average 500 g. These data show considerable individual variation and are also influenced strongly by the mode of delivery.[1,2] Macroscopically, the organ consists of two surfaces or plates; the chorionic

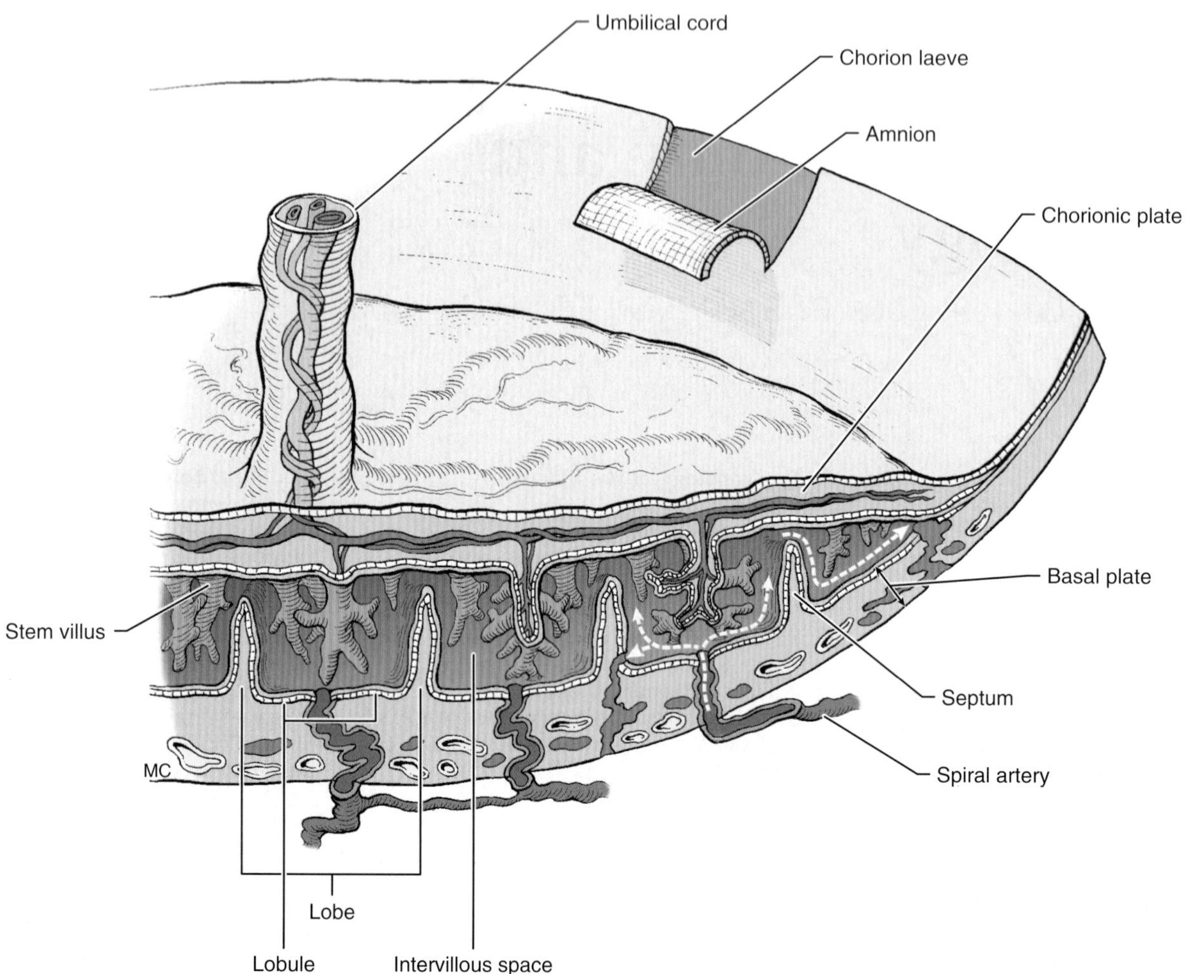

Figure 1-1. Cross-section through a mature placenta showing the chorionic and basal plates bounding the intervillous space. The villous trees arise from stem villi attached to the chorionic plate, and they are arranged as lobules centered over the openings of the maternal spiral arteries.

plate to which the umbilical cord is attached, and the basal plate that abuts the maternal endometrium (Fig. 1-1). Between the two plates is a cavity that is filled with maternal blood, delivered from the endometrial spiral arteries through openings in the basal plate. This cavity is bounded at the margins of the disc by the fusion of the chorionic and basal plates, and the smooth chorion, or chorion laeve, extends from the rim to complete the chorionic sac. The placenta is incompletely divided into 10 to 40 lobes by the presence of septae created by invaginations of the basal plate. The septae are thought to arise from differential resistance of the maternal tissues to trophoblast invasion, and they may help to compartmentalise maternal blood flow through the organ. The fetal component of the placenta comprises a series of elaborately branched villous trees that arise from the inner surface of the chorionic plate and project into the cavity of the placenta. This arrangement is somewhat reminiscent of the fronds of a sea anemone wafting in the seawater of a rock pool. Most commonly, each villous tree originates from a single stem villus that undergoes several generations of branching until the functional units of the placenta, the terminal villi, are created. These consist of an epithelial covering of trophoblast, and a mesodermal core containing branches of the umbilical arteries and tributaries of the umbilical vein. Because of this repeated branching, the tree takes on the topology of an inverted wine glass, often referred to as a lobule, and there may be two to three within a single placental lobe (Fig. 1-1). As is seen later, each lobule represents an individual maternofetal exchange unit. Toward term, the continual elaboration of the villous trees almost fills the cavity of the placenta, which is reduced to a network of narrow spaces collectively referred to as the intervillous space (IVS). The maternal blood percolates through this network of channels, exchanging gases and nutrients with the fetal blood circulating within the villi, before draining through the basal plate into openings of the uterine veins. Therefore, the human placenta is classified in comparative mammalian terms as being of the villous hemochorial type,[3,4] although as we shall see, this arrangement really pertains only to the second and third trimesters of pregnancy.[5]

PLACENTAL DEVELOPMENT

Development of the placenta is initiated morphologically at the time of implantation, when the embryonic pole of the blastocyst establishes contact with the uterine epithelium. At this stage, the wall of the blastocyst comprises an outer layer of unicellular epithelial cells, the trophoblast, and an inner layer of extraembryonic (EE) mesodermal cells derived from the inner cell mass.[6] Together, these layers constitute the chorion. The earliest events have never been observed in vivo for obvious ethical reasons, but are thought to be equivalent to those that take place in the rhesus monkey.[7] Attempts have also been made to replicate the situation in vitro by culturing in vitro fertilized human blastocysts on monolayers of endometrial cells.[8] Although such reductionist systems cannot take into account the possibility of paracrine signals emanating from the underlying endometrial stroma, the profound differences in trophoblast invasiveness displayed by various species are maintained. In the case of the human, the trophoblast in contact with the endometrium undergoes a syncytial transformation, and tongues of syncytiotrophoblast begin to penetrate between the endometrial cells. There is no evidence of cell death being induced as part of this process, but gradually, the conceptus embeds into the stratum compactum of the endometrium. The earliest ex vivo specimens available for study are estimated to be around 7 days postconception, and in these specimens, the conceptus is almost entirely embedded. A plug of fibrin initially seals the defect in the uterine surface, but by Days 10 to 12 the epithelium is restored.[9]

By the time implantation is complete, the conceptus is surrounded entirely by a mantle of syncytiotrophoblast (Fig. 1-2). This multinucleated mantle tends to be thicker beneath the conceptus, in association with the embryonic pole, and rests on a layer of uninucleate cytotrophoblast cells derived from the original wall of the blastocyst. Vacuolar spaces begin to appear within the mantle and gradually coalesce to form larger lacunae, the forerunners of the IVS. As the lacunae enlarge the intervening syncytiotrophoblast is reduced in thickness and forms

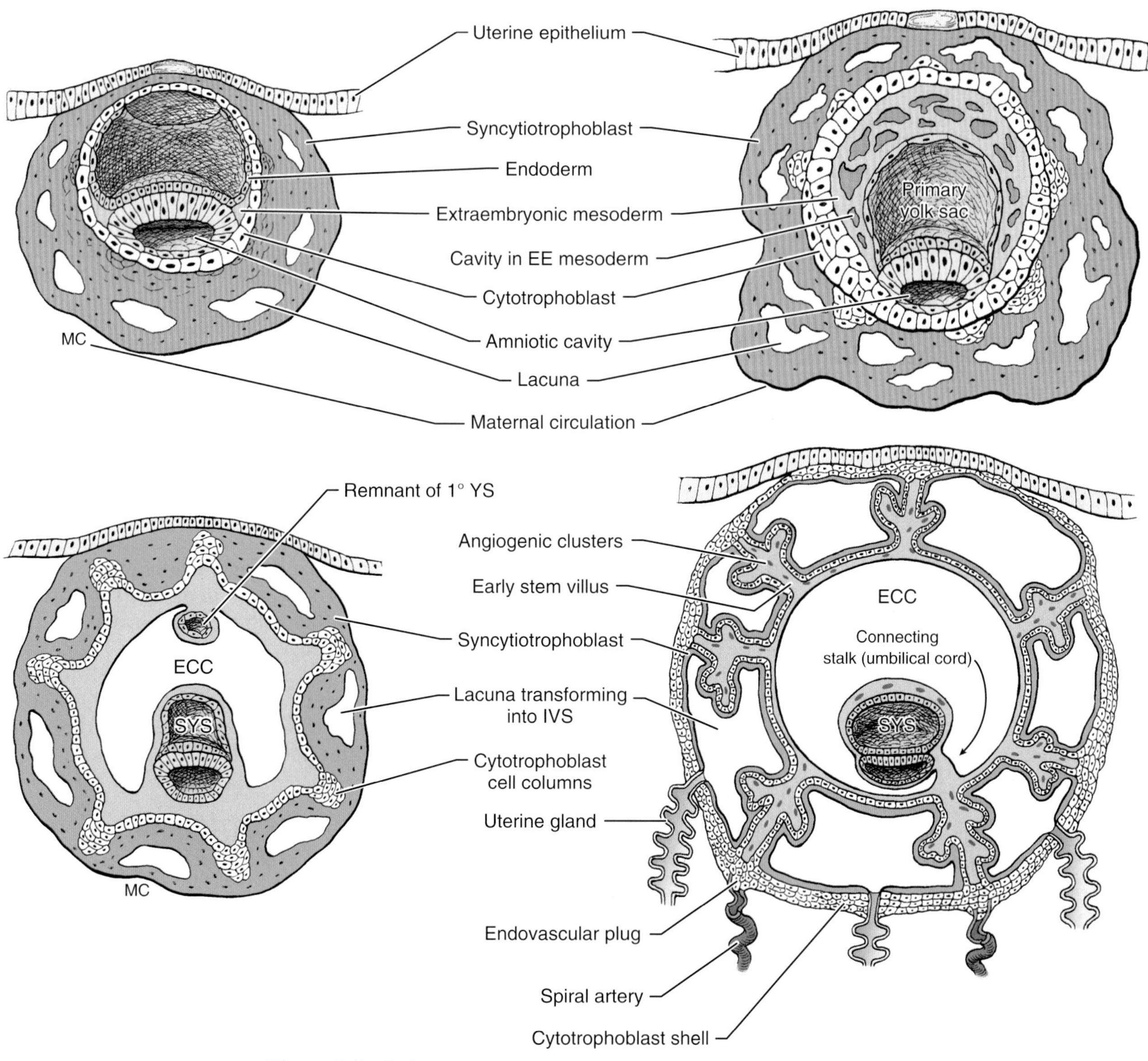

Figure 1-2. Early placental development between Days 9 and 16.

a complex lattice of trabeculae (Fig. 1-2). Soon after, starting around Day 12 postfertilization, the cytotrophoblast cells proliferate and penetrate into the trabeculae. On reaching their tips, approximately 2 days later, the cells spread laterally, establishing contact with those from other trabeculae to form a new layer interposed between the mantle and the endometrium, the cytotrophoblastic shell (Fig. 1-2). Finally, at the start of the third week of development, mesodermal cells derived from the extraembryonic mesoderm invade the trabeculae, bringing with them the hemangioblasts from which the fetal vascular system differentiates. The mesoderm cells do not penetrate right to the tips of the trabeculae, and these remain as an aggregation of cytotrophoblast cells, the cytotrophoblast cell columns, which may or may not have a covering of syncytiotrophoblast (Fig. 1-2). Proliferation of the cells at the proximal ends of the columns, and their subsequent differentiation, contributes to expansion of the cytotrophoblastic shell.[10] Toward the end of the third week, the rudiments of the placenta are therefore in place. The original wall of the blastocyst becomes the chorionic plate, the cytotrophoblastic shell is the precursor of the basal plate, and the lacunae form the IVS. The trabeculae are the forerunners of the villous trees, and repeated lateral branching gradually increases their complexity.

Initially, villi form over the entire chorionic sac, but toward the end of the first trimester, they regress from all except the deep pole, where they remain as the definitive discoid placenta. Abnormalities in this process may account for the persistence of villi at abnormal sites on the chorionic sac, and hence, the presence of accessory or succenturiate lobes.

THE AMNION AND YOLK SAC

While these early stages of placental development are taking place, the inner cell mass also differentiates, giving rise to the amnion, the yolk sac, and the germ disc. The amnion and yolk sac, and the fluid compartment in which they lie, play an important role in the physiology of early pregnancy, and so their development will be described at this point. The initial formation of these sacs has been controversial over the years, due mainly to the small number of specimens available for study. However, there now appears to be consensus that at the time of implantation, the amnion extends from the margins of the epiblast layer over the future dorsal surface of the germ disc, whereas the primary yolk sac extends from the hypoblast layer around the inner surface of the trophoblast, separated from it by a loose reticulum of extraembryonic mesoderm thought to be derived from the hypoblast.[6,11] Over the next few days, considerable remodeling of the yolk sac occurs. This involves three closely interrelated processes. First, formation of the primitive streak, and the subsequent differentiation of definitive endoderm, leads to displacement of the original hypoblast cells into the more peripheral regions of the primary yolk sac. Second, the sac greatly reduces in size, either because the more peripheral portion is nipped off,[6] or because it breaks up into a number of vesicles (Fig. 1-2).[11] Third, the reticulum splits into two layers of mesoderm, except at the future caudal end of the germ disc, where it persists as a mass, the connecting stalk, linking the disc to the trophoblast. One layer lines the inner surface of the trophoblast, so contributing to formation of the chorion, while the other covers the outer surfaces of the amnion and yolk sac. In between these layers is a large fluid-filled space, the exocoelomic cavity (ECC). The net result of this remodeling is the formation of a smaller secondary yolk sac (SYS), which is connected to the embryo by the vitelline duct and floats within the ECC (Fig. 1-2).

The ECC is a conspicuous feature ultrasonographically, and can be clearly visualized using a transvaginal probe toward the end of the third week postfertilization (fifth week of menstrual age). Between 5 and 9 weeks of pregnancy, it represents the largest anatomic space within the chorionic sac. The SYS is the first structure that can be detected ultrasonographically within that space, and its diameter increases slightly between 6 and 10 weeks of gestation, reaching a maximum of 6 to 7 mm, and then decreases slightly.[12,13] Histologically, the secondary yolk sac consists of an inner layer of endodermal cells linked by tight junctions at their apical surface and bearing a few short microvilli.[14,15] Their cytoplasm contains numerous mitochondria, whorls of rough endoplasmic reticulum, Golgi bodies and secretory droplets, giving them the appearance of being highly active synthetic cells. With further development, the epithelium becomes folded to form a series of cyst-like structures or tubules, only some of which communicate with the central cavity. The function of these spaces is not known.[11] On its outer surface, the yolk sac is lined by a layer of mesothelium derived from the extraembryonic mesoderm. This epithelium bears a dense covering of microvilli, and the presence of numerous coated pits and pinocytotic vesicles gives it the appearance of an absorptive epithelium.[14] Although there is no direct evidence of this function in the human as yet, experiments in the rhesus monkey have revealed that the mesothelial layer readily engulfs horseradish peroxidase.[16] Immediately beneath this epithelium lies a well-developed capillary plexus, which drains through the vitelline veins to the developing liver.

By week 9 of pregnancy, however, the secondary yolk sac begins to exhibit morphologic evidence of a decline in function.[17] This appears to be independent of the expansion of the amnion, which is gradually drawn around the ventral surface of the developing embryo. As it does so, it presses the yolk sac remnant against the connecting stalk, forming the umbilical cord. By the end of the third month, the amnion abuts the inner surface of the chorion, and the ECC is obliterated.

THE MATERNOFETAL RELATIONSHIP DURING THE FIRST TRIMESTER

For the placenta to function efficiently as an organ of exchange, it requires adequate and dependable access to the maternal circulation. Establishing that access is arguably one of the most critical aspects of placental development, and, over recent years, has certainly been one of the most controversial. As the syncytiotrophoblastic mantle enlarges, it soon comes into close proximity with superficial veins within the endometrium. These veins undergo dilatation, forming sinusoids, which are subsequently tapped into by the syncytium.[9] As a result, maternal erythrocytes come to lie within the lacunae. Although Hertig and associates[9] commented that surprisingly few erythrocytes were visible within the lacunae, their presence has been taken by modern embryologists as indicating the onset of the maternal circulation to the placenta.[18,19] If this is a circulation, however, it is entirely one of venous ebb and flow, possibly influenced by uterine contractions and other forces.[20] Numerous traditional histologic studies have demonstrated that arterial connections are not established with the lacunae until much later in pregnancy,[21–25] although the exact timing was not known for many years. The advent of high-resolution ultrasound and Doppler imaging appeared to answer this question, because in normal pregnancies, most observers agree that moving echoes indicative of significant fluid flow cannot be detected within the IVS until 10 to 12 weeks of pregnancy.[26–28] These findings have been criticized on the basis of the sensitivity of the equipment used and the precise location within the uterus from which the signals were detected,[29,30] but it is unlikely that these technical points can ever be fully resolved.

There is, however, incontrovertible evidence from other sources that a major change in the maternal circulation to the placenta takes place at the end of the first trimester.[31] First, direct vision into the IVS during the first trimester with a hysterscope reveals the cavity to be filled with a clear fluid rather than maternal blood.[32] Second, perfusion of pregnant hysterectomy specimens with radio-opaque and other media demonstrates that there is little flow into the IVS during the first trimester, except perhaps at the margins of the placental disc.[1,33] Third, the oxygen concentration within the IVS is low (<20 mmHg) before 10 weeks of pregnancy, and rises threefold between weeks 10 and 12.[34] This rise is matched by increases in the activities of, and mRNA concentrations encoding, the principal antioxidant enzymes in the placental tissues, confirming a change in oxygenation at the cellular level.[35]

The mechanism underlying this change in placental perfusion relates to the phenomenon of extravillous trophoblast invasion.

EXTRAVILLOUS TROPHOBLAST INVASION AND PHYSIOLOGIC CONVERSION OF THE SPIRAL ARTERIES

During the early weeks of pregnancy, a subpopulation of trophoblast cells migrate from the deep surface of the cytotrophoblastic shell into the endometrium.[36] Because these cells do not take part in the development of the definitive placenta, they are referred to as extravillous trophoblast. However, their activities are fundamental to the successful functioning of the placenta, for their presence in the endometrium is associated with the physiologic conversion of the maternal spiral arteries. The cell biologic basis of this phenomenon is still not understood, but the net effect is the loss of the smooth muscle cells and elastic fibers from the media of the endometrial segments of the arteries and their replacement by fibrinoid.[37,38] There is some evidence to suggest that this is a two-stage process. Very early in pregnancy, the arteries display endothelial basophilia and vacuolation, disorganization of the smooth muscle cells, and dilatation. Because these changes are observed equally in both the decidua basalis and parietalis, and also within the uterus in cases of ectopic pregnancies, it seems to be independent of local trophoblast invasion. Instead, it has been proposed that it results from activation of decidual renin-angiotensin signalling.[39] Slightly later, during the first few weeks of pregnancy, the invading extravillous trophoblasts become closely associated with the arteries, and infiltrate their walls.[40] Further dilation ensues, and as a result, the arteries are converted from small caliber vasoreactive vessels into funnel-shaped flaccid conduits.

The extravillous trophoblast population itself can be separated into two subgroups; the endovascular trophoblasts, which migrate in a retrograde fashion down the lumens of the spiral arteries replacing the endothelium, and the interstitial trophoblasts, which migrate through the endometrial stroma. In early pregnancy, the volume of the migrating endovascular cells is sufficient to occlude, or plug, the terminal portions of the spiral arteries as they approach the basal plate (Fig. 1-3).[21–23,25] It is the dissipation of these plugs toward the end of the first trimester that establishes the maternal circulation to the placenta. Trophoblast invasion is not equal across the implantation site, being greatest in the central region, where it has presumably been established the longest.[41] It is to be expected, therefore, that the plugging of the spiral arteries will be most extensive in this region, and this may account for the fact that maternal arterial blood flow is most often first detectable ultrasonographically in the peripheral regions of the placental disc.[42] Associated with this blood flow is a high local level of oxidative stress, which can be considered physiologic because it occurs in all normal pregnancies. It has recently been proposed that this stress induces regression of the villi over the superficial pole of the chorionic sac, so forming the chorion laeve (Fig. 1-4).[42]

Under normal conditions the interstitial trophoblast cells invade as far as the inner third of the myometrium, where they appear to fuse and form giant cells.[1,43] The depth of invasion may be determined through their interactions with the uterine natural killer cells.[44] It is essential that the process is correctly regulated, because excessive invasion can result in complete erosion of the endometrium and the condition of placenta accreta, which is associated with a high risk of postpartum hemorrhage.

Physiologic conversion of the spiral arteries is often attributed to ensuring an adequate maternal blood flow to the placenta, but such comments generally oversimplify the phenomenon. By itself, the process cannot increase the volume of blood flow to the placenta because it affects only the most distal portion of the spiral arteries. The most proximal part of the arteries, where they arise from the uterine arcuate arteries, always remains unconverted and so will act as the rate-limiting segment. These segments gradually dilate in conjunction with the rest of the uterine vasculature during early pregnancy, most probably under the effects of estrogen, and as a

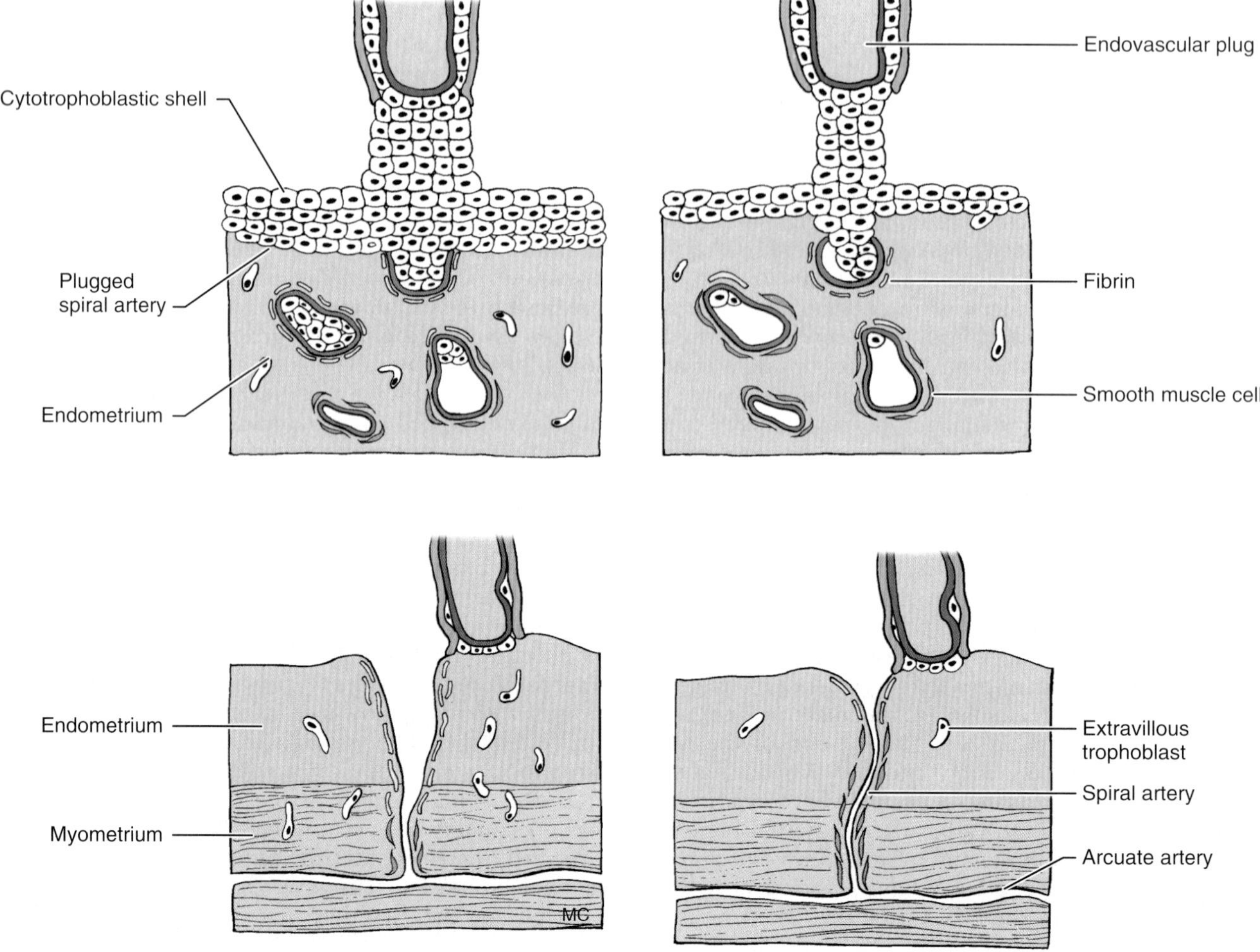

Figure 1-3. During early pregnancy, the tips of the maternal spiral arteries are occluded by invading endovascular trophoblast cells, impeding flow into the IVS. The combination of endovascular and interstitial trophoblast invasion is associated with physiologic conversion of the spiral arteries. Both processes are deficient in preeclampsia, and the retention of vascular smooth muscle may increase the risk of spontaneous vasoconstriction and, hence, an ischemia-reperfusion–type injury to the placenta.

result the resistance of the uterine circulation falls[45] and uterine blood flow increases from approximately 45 ml/min during the menstrual cycle[46] to around 750 ml/min at term.[47] By contrast, the terminal dilatation of the arteries will substantially reduce both the rate and pressure with which that maternal blood flows into the IVS.[48,49] Slowing the rate of blood flow facilitates diffusional exchange, whereas lowering the pressure in the IVS is important to prevent collapse of the fetal capillary network within the villi.[50] Measurements taken in the rhesus monkey indicate that the pressure at the mouth of a spiral artery is only 15 mmHg, and that within the IVS, the pressure is on average 10 mmHg.[48] The pressure within the fetal villous capillaries is estimated to be approximately 20 mmHg, providing a pressure differential favoring their distension of 5–10 mmHg.

Many complications of pregnancy are associated with defects in extravillous trophoblast invasion and failure to establish the maternal circulation correctly. In the most severe cases the cytotrophoblastic shell is thin and fragmented, and this situation is observed in approximately two thirds of spontaneous miscarriages.[51,52] Reduced invasion may reflect defects inherent in the conceptus, such as chromosomal aberrations, or thrombophilia, endometrial dysfunction or other problems in the mother. The net result is that onset of the maternal circulation is both precocious and widespread throughout the developing placenta, consequent upon absent or incomplete plugging of the maternal arteries.[42,53–55] Haemodynamic forces, coupled with excessive oxidative stress within the placental tissues,[56] are likely to be major factors contributing to loss of these pregnancies.

In milder cases, the pregnancy may continue but is complicated by preeclampsia, intrauterine growth restriction, or a combination of the two. The physiologic changes are either restricted in extent to only the superficial endometrial parts of the spiral arteries, or are absent altogether (Fig. 1-3).[57,58] In the most severe cases of preeclampsia associated with major fetal growth restriction, only 10 percent of the arteries may be fully converted compared with 96 percent in normal pregnancies.[41] There is still debate as to whether this is due to an inability of the interstitial trophoblast to invade the endometrium successfully,[59–61] or whether having invaded sufficiently deeply, the trophoblast cells fail to penetrate the walls of the arteries.[62,63] These two possibilities are not mutually

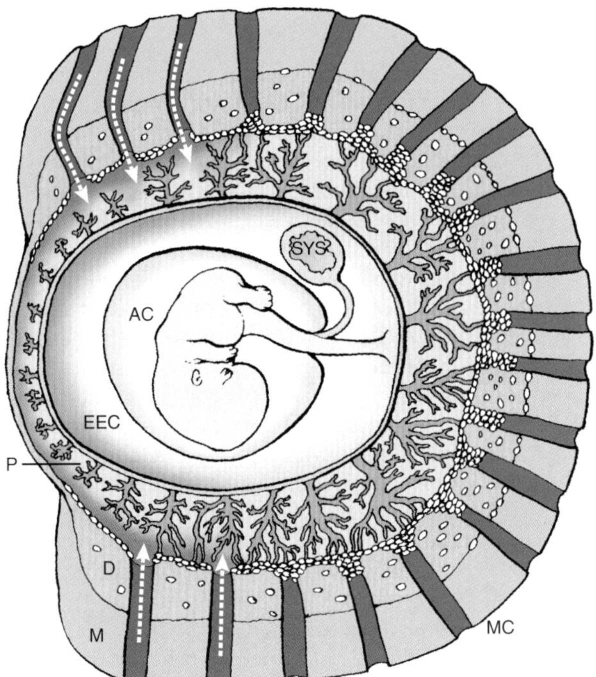

Figure 1-4. Onset of the maternal circulation starts in the periphery of the placenta *(arrows)*, where trophoblast invasion and, hence, plugging of the spiral arteries is least developed. The high local levels of oxidative stress that are induced are thought to induce villous regression and formation of the chorion leave. (Redrawn from Jauniaux E, Cindrova-Davies T, Johns J, et al: Distribution and transfer pathways of antioxidant molecules inside the first trimester human gestational sac. J Clin Endocrinol Metab 89:1452, 2004, with permission.)

exclusive and may reflect different etiologies.[31] Whatever the causation, there are several potential consequences to incomplete conversion of the arteries. First, owing to the absence of the distal dilation, maternal blood enters the IVS with greater velocity than normal, forming jetlike spurts that can be detected ultrasonographically. The villous trees are often disrupted opposite these spurts, leading to the formation of intervillous blood lakes, and the altered hemodynamics within the IVS result in thrombosis and excessive fibrin deposition.[64,65] Second, incomplete conversion allows the spiral arteries to maintain greater vasoreactivity than normal. There is evidence from the rhesus monkey and humans that spiral arteries are not continuously patent but that they undergo periodic constriction independent of uterine contractions.[42,66] It has recently been proposed that exaggeration of this phenomenon due to the retention of smooth muscle in the arterial walls may lead to an hypoxia-reoxygenation–type injury in the placenta, culminating in the development of oxidative stress.[67,68] Placental oxidative stress is a key factor in the pathogenesis of preeclampsia,[69] and clinical evidence suggests that hypoxia-reoxygenation is a more physiologic stimulus for its generation than simply reduced uterine perfusion.[68] The third consequence of incomplete conversion is that the distal segments of the arteries are frequently the site of acute atherotic changes.[58,70] These are likely to be secondary changes, possibly induced by the involvement of these segments in the hypoxia-reoxygenation process, but if the lesions become occlusive, they will further impair blood flow within the IVS, contributing to the growth restriction.[71]

THE ROLE OF THE ENDOMETRIUM DURING THE FIRST TRIMESTER

Signals from the uterine epithelium and secretions from the endometrial glands play a major role in regulating receptivity at the time of implantation,[72] but the potential contribution of the glands to fetal development once implantation is complete has largely been ignored. This has been due to the general assumption that once the conceptus is embedded within the uterine wall, it no longer has access to the secretions in the uterine lumen. However, a recent review of archival placenta-in-situ hysterectomy specimens has revealed that the glands discharge their secretions into the IVS through openings in the basal plate throughout the first trimester (Fig. 1-2).[73] The secretions are a heterogenous mix of maternal proteins; carbohydrates, including glycogen; and lipid droplets. Their phagocytic uptake by the syncytiotrophoblast suggests that they may be used as a source of nutrients, although there is no physiologic evidence to support this claim at present. However, the fact that glycodelin, formerly referred to as PP14 or α_2-PEG, is derived from the glands and yet accumulates within the amniotic fluid, with concentrations peaking at around 10 weeks' gestation[74] indicates that the placenta must be exposed to glandular secretions extensively throughout the first trimester.

Ultrasonographic measurements suggest that an endometrial thickness of 8 mm or more is necessary for successful implantation,[75] although not all studies have found such an association.[76] Nonetheless, these measurements are in line with observations based on placenta-in-situ specimens, in which an endometrial thickness of more than 5 mm was reported beneath the conceptus at 6 weeks of pregnancy.[77] Gradually, over the remainder of the first trimester, the endometrium regresses, so that by 14 weeks, the thickness is reduced to 1 mm. Histologically, there is also a transformation in the glandular epithelial cells over this period. At 6 weeks, they closely resemble those of the secretory phase of the menstrual cycle, being tall and columnar in shape, and their cytoplasm containing abundant organelles and large accumulations of glycogen.[73,77,78] By the end of the first trimester, the cells are more cuboidal and secretory organelles are much less prominent, although the lumens of the glands are still filled with secretions.

The overall picture is that the glands are most prolific and active during the early weeks of pregnancy, with their contribution gradually waning during the first trimester. This would be consistent with a progressive switch from histiotrophic to hemotrophic nutrition as the maternal arterial circulation to the placenta is established. The glands should not be considered solely as a source of nutrients, however, because their secretions are also rich in growth factors such as leukemia inhibitory factor, vascular endothelial growth factor, epidermal growth factor, and transforming growth factor beta.[77] Receptors for these factors are present on the villous tissues, and so the glands may play an important role in modulating placental proliferation and differentiation during early pregnancy, as in other species.[79,80] Attempts to correlate the functional activity of the glands with pregnancy outcome have met with mixed success. Thus, reduced concentrations of mucin 1, glycodelin, and leukemia inhibitory factor have been reported in uterine flushings from women suffering repeated miscarriages.[81,82] However, a recent study has shown no significant association between the expression of these markers within the endometrium and outcome.[83] This difference may reflect impairment in the secretory rather than the synthetic machinery of the gland cells, although further research is required to confirm this point.

From the evidence available, therefore, it would appear that the functional importance of the endometrial glands to a successful pregnancy extends well beyond the time of implantation.

THE TOPOLOGY OF THE VILLOUS TREES

One of the principal functions of the placenta is diffusional exchange, and the physical requirements for this impose the greatest influence on the structure of the organ. The rate of diffusion of an inert molecule is governed by Fick's law, and so is proportional to the surface area for exchange divided by the thickness of the tissue barrier. Therefore, a large surface area will facilitate exchange, and this is achieved by repeated branching of the villous trees.

The villous trees arise from the trabeculae interposed between the lacunae (Fig. 1-2) through a gradual process of remodeling and lateral branching. Initially, the different branches have an almost uniform composition, and the villi can be separated only by their relative size and position in the hierarchical branching pattern. At this stage, the mesodermal core is loosely packed, and at the proximal end of the trees it blends with the extraembryonic mesoderm lining the ECC.[84] The stromal cells possess sail-like processes that often link together to form fluid-filled channels that are oriented parallel to the long axis of the villi. Macrophages are often seen within these channels, and so it is possible they function as a primitive circulatory system prior to vasculogenesis. In this way, proteins derived from the uterine glands could freely diffuse into the coelomic fluid, and it is notable that the macrophages within the channels are strongly immunoreactive for maternal glycodelin.[73]

Toward the end of the first trimester, the villi begin to differentiate into their principal types. The connections to the chorionic plate become remodeled to form stem villi, which represent the supporting framework of each villous tree.[1,85] These progressively develop a compact fibrous stroma, and contain branches of the chorionic arteries and accompanying veins. The arteries are centrally located and are surrounded by a cuff of smooth muscle cells. Although these have the appearance of resistance vessels, physiologic studies indicate that under normal conditions, the fetal placental circulation operates under conditions of full vasodilation.[86] Stem villi contain only a few small-caliber capillaries, and so play little role in placental exchange.

After several generations of branching, stem villi give rise to intermediate villi. These are longer and more slender in form, and can be of two types; immature and mature. Immature villi are seen predominantly in early pregnancy and represent a persistence of the nondifferentiated form as indicated by the presence of fluid-filled stromal channels.[87] Mature intermediate villi provide a distributing framework, and terminal villi arise at intervals from their surface. Within the core are arterioles and venules, but there is also a significant number of capillaries, suggesting a capacity for exchange.

The main functional units of the villous tree are, however, the terminal villi. There is no strict definition as to where a terminal villus starts, but they are most often short stubby branches, up to 100 μm in length and approximately 80 μm in diameter, arising from the intermediate villi.[88] They are highly vascularized, but by capillaries alone and are highly adapted for diffusional exchange, as is seen later.

This differentiation of the villi coincides temporally with the development of the lobular architecture, and the two processes are most likely interlinked. Lobules can be first identified during the early second trimester, following onset of the maternal circulation, when it is thought hemodynamic forces may shape the villous tree.[89] There is convincing radiographic and morphologic evidence that maternal blood is delivered into the center of the lobule, and that it then disperses peripherally, as in the rhesus monkey placenta (Fig. 1-1).[7,90,91] Consequently, it is to be expected that an oxygen gradient will exist across the lobule, and differences in the activities and expression of antioxidant enzymes within the villous tissues suggest strongly that this is the case.[92] Other metabolic gradients, for example, glucose concentration, may also exist, and together these may exert powerful influences on villous differentiation. Villi in the centre of the lobule, where the oxygen concentration is highest, display morphologic and enzymatic evidence of relative immaturity,[93] and so this is considered to be the germinative zone. By contrast, villi in the periphery of the lobule are better adapted for diffusional exchange.[94]

Elaboration of the villous tree is a progressive event that continues at a steady pace throughout pregnancy, and by term, the villi present a surface area of 10 to 14 m^2.[2,95] This may be significantly reduced in cases of intrauterine growth restriction, although this principally reflects an overall reduction in placental volume rather than maldevelopment of the villous tree.[96–99] In cases of preeclampsia alone, villous surface area is normal and is only compromised if there is associated growth restriction.[99–101] Attempts have recently been made to monitor placental growth longitudinally during pregnancy using ultrasound.[102] Although the data show considerable individual variability, they indicate that in cases of growth restriction, placental volume is significantly reduced at 12 to 14 weeks, and that thereafter, placental development continues at a lower trajectory than normal. These findings suggest that the pathology restricting placental growth has its origins firmly in the first trimester.

PLACENTAL HISTOLOGY

The epithelial covering of the villous trees is formed by the syncytiotrophoblast (Fig. 1-5). As its name indicates, this is a true multinucleated syncytium that extends without lateral intercellular clefts over the entire villous surface. In essence, therefore, the syncytiotrophoblast acts as the endothelium of the IVS, and everything passing across the placenta must pass through this layer, either actively or passively. This tissue also performs all hormone synthesis in the placenta, and so a number of potentially conflicting demands are placed upon it.

The syncytiotrophoblast is highly polarized, and one of its most conspicuous features is the presence of a dense covering of microvilli on the apical surface.[1,88] In the first trimester, the microvilli are relatively long (approximately 0.75 to 1.25 μm in length and 0.12 to 0.17 μm in diameter), but as pregnancy advances, they become shorter and more slender, being approximately 0.5 to 0.7 μm in length and 0.08 to 0.14 μm in diameter at term.[103] The microvillous covering is evenly distributed over the villous surface, and measurements of the amplification factor provided vary from 5.2 to 7.7.[103,104] Many receptors and transport proteins have been localized to the microvillous surface by molecular biological and immunohistochemical techniques, as is discussed later. The receptors are thought to reside in lipid rafts, and once bound to their ligand, they migrate to the base of the microvilli, where clathrin-coated pits are present.[105,106] Receptor-ligand complexes are concentrated in the pits, which are then internalized. Disassociation of ligands such as cholesterol may occur in the syncytioplasm, whereas other ligands, such as immunoglobulin G, are exocytosed at the basal surface.[107]

Support for the microvillous architecture is provided by a substantial network of actin filaments and microtubules lying just beneath the apical surface.[108] Also present within the syncytioplasm are numerous pinocytotic vesicles, phagosomes, lysosomes, mitochondria, secretory droplets, strands of endoplasmic reticulum, Golgi bodies, and lipid droplets.[106,109,110] The overall impression is of a highly active epithelium engaged in absorptive, secretory, and synthetic functions. Therefore, it is not surprising that the syncytiotrophoblast should have such a high rate of consumption of oxygen.[111,112]

The syncytiotrophoblast is a terminally differentiated tissue, and consequently mitotic figures are never observed within its nuclei. It has been suggested that this condition, which is frequently observed in the fetal cells at the maternofetal interface in other species, reduces the risk of malignant transformation in the trophoblast and so protects the mother. Whatever the reason, the syncytiotrophoblast is generated by the recruitment of progenitor cytotrophoblast cells. Cytotrophoblast cells are uninucleate and lie on a well-developed basement membrane immediately beneath the syncytium. A proportion represents stem cells that undergo proliferation, with daughter cells undergoing progressive differentiation. Consequently, a range of morphologic appearances are seen, from cuboidal resting cells with a

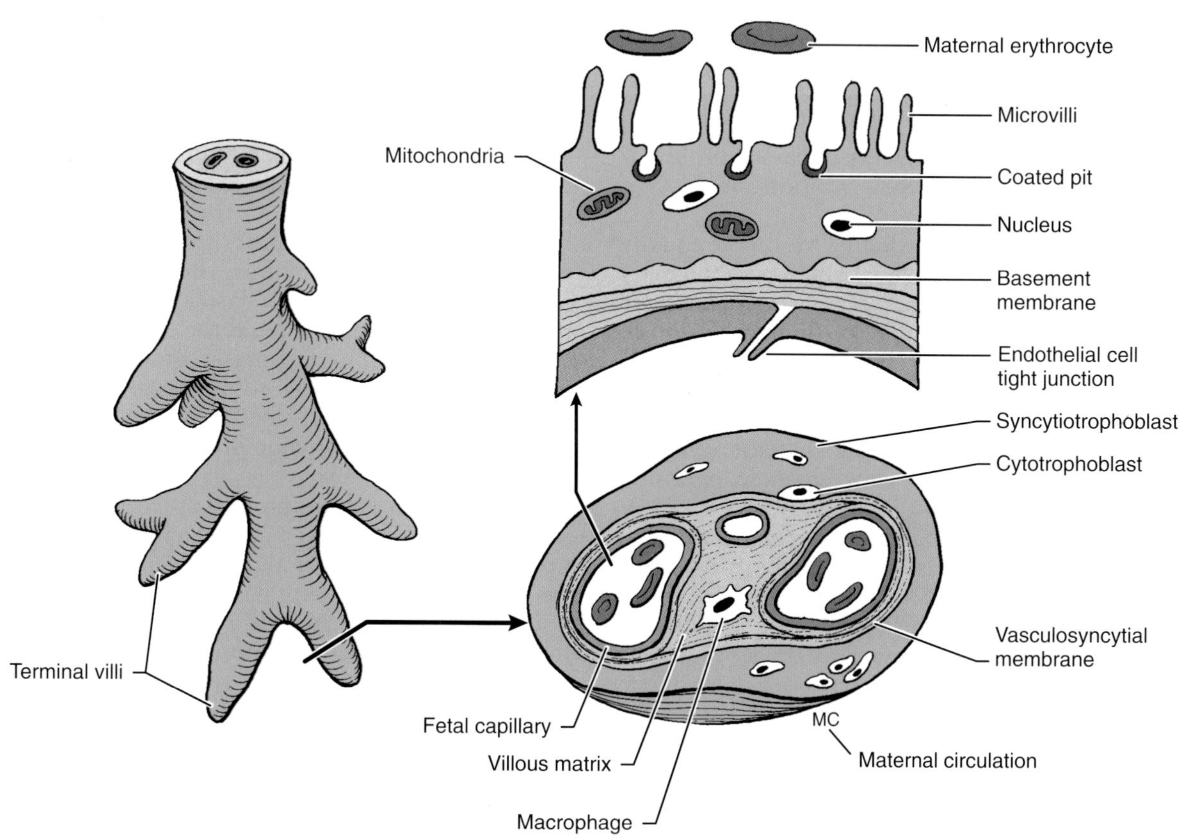

Figure 1-5. An intermediate villus with terminal villi arising from the lateral surface.

general paucity of organelles to fully differentiated cells that closely resemble the overlying syncytium.[106,113] Ultimately, membrane fusion takes place between the two, and the nucleus and cytoplasm are incorporated into the syncytiotrophoblast. Early in pregnancy the cytotrophoblast cells form a complete layer beneath the syncytium, but as pregnancy advances the cells become separated and are seen less frequently in histologic sections. In the past, this observation was interpreted as indicative of a reduction in the number of cytotrophoblast cells, and so a reduction in the proliferative potential of the trophoblast layers. More recent stereologic estimates have revealed a different picture, however, because the total number of these cells increases until term.[114,115] The apparent decline results from the fact that villous surface area increases at a greater rate, and so cytotrophoblast cell profiles are seen less often in any individual histological section.

The stimuli regulating cytotrophoblast cell proliferation are not fully understood. In early pregnancy (before 6 weeks) epidermal growth factor (EGF) may play an important role, because expression of both the factor and its receptor are localized principally to these cells.[116] EGF is also strongly expressed in the epithelium of the uterine glands.[77] In the horse, a tight spatial and temporal correlation exists between glandular expression and proliferation in the overlying trophoblast.[79] Later, during the first trimester, insulin-like growth factor II can be immunolocalized to the cytotrophoblast cells, as can the receptor for hepatocyte growth factor.[117] Hepatocyte growth factor is a powerful mitogen that is expressed by the mesenchymal cells,[118] providing the possibility of paracrine control. Environmental stimuli may also be important, because hypoxia has long been known to stimulate cytotrophoblast proliferation in vitro.[119,120] A greater number of cell profiles is also observed in placentas from high altitude, where they are exposed to hypobaric hypoxia[121] and conditions associated with poor placental perfusion.[122] Whether this represents increased proliferation or decreased fusion with the syncytiotrophoblast is uncertain, however.

The factors regulating and mediating fusion are equally uncertain. Growth factors such as EGF, granulocyte-macrophage colony-stimulating factor and vascular endothelial growth factor are able to stimulate fusion in vitro,[123,124] as are the hormones estradiol and human chorionic gonadotropin (hCG).[125] By contrast, transforming growth factor β, leukemia inhibitory factor, and endothelin inhibit the process, suggesting that the outcome in vivo depends on a balance between these opposing influences. One of the actions of hCG at the molecular level is to promote the formation of gap junctions between cells,[126] and there is strong experimental evidence that communication through gap junctions is an essential prerequisite in the fusion process.[127] Whether membrane fusion is initiated at the sites of gap junctions is not known at present, but there has been much interest recently in other potential mechanisms of fusion. One such is the externalization of phosphatidylserine on the outer leaflet of the cell membrane,[128,129] although whether this represents part of an apoptotic cascade that is completed only in the syncytiotrophoblast,[130,131] or is inherent to cytotrophoblastic differentiation,[129] remains controversial. Another is the expression of the human endogeneous retroviral envelope protein HERV-W, commonly referred to as syncytin. Expression of syncytin appears to be necessary for syncytial transformation of trophoblast cells in vitro, and ectopic expression in other cell types renders them fusigenic.[132,133] Syncytin interacts with the amino acid transporter protein ASCT2, and the expression of both is influenced by hypoxia in trophoblast cell lines in vitro.[134] This could provide an explanation for the increased number of cytotrophoblast cells observed in placentas from hypoxic pregnancies.

Although it is clear that the cascade of events controlling cytotrophoblastic proliferation and fusion has yet to be fully elucidated, it appears to be tightly regulated in vivo. Thus, the ratio of cytotrophoblastic to syncytial nuclei remains at approximately 1:9 throughout pregnancy,[114,115] although it may be perturbed in pathologic cases.

THE INTEGRITY OF THE VILLOUS MEMBRANE

One situation that may alter the balance of the two populations of nuclei is damage to the trophoblast layers and the requirement for repair. Isolated areas of syncytial damage, often referred to as sites of focal syncytial necrosis, are a feature of all placentas, although they are more common in those from pathologic pregnancies.[135,136] Their origin remains obscure, but they could potentially arise from altered hemodynamics within the IVS, or physical interactions between villi.[137] One striking example of the latter is the rupture of syncytial bridges that form between adjacent villi, leading to circular defects on the surface 20 to 40 μm in diameter.[138] Disruption of the microvillous surface leads to the activation of platelets and the deposition of a fibrin plaque on the trophoblastic basement membrane. Apoptosis of syncytial nuclei has been reported in the immediate vicinity of such plaques,[139] but whether this reflects cause or effect has yet to be determined. With time, cytotrophoblast cells migrate over the plaque, differentiate, and fuse to form a new syncytiotrophoblastic layer.[138,140] As a result, the plaque is internalized, and the integrity of the villous surface is restored. In the interim, however, these sites are nonselectively permeable to horseradish peroxidase,[141] although their presence does not seem to be a determinant of vertical transmission of human immunodeficiency virus (HIV).[142]

More widespread apoptosis has been reported in the syncytiotrophoblast layer in pregnancies complicated by preeclampsia,[143] where it may reflect increased turnover of the trophoblast.[144] Placental oxidative stress is considered a key factor in the pathogenesis of preeclampsia,[69] and hypoxia-reoxygenation is a powerful inducer of apoptosis in the syncytiotrophoblast in vitro.[145] The deportation of apoptotic fragments arising from the villous surface has been put forward as one cause of the maternal endothelial activation that characterizes this syndrome.[146]

An even greater degree of trophoblast oxidative stress and damage is seen in cases of missed miscarriage, in which complete degeneration and sloughing of the syncytiotrophoblast layer occurs.[42,56] Although there is increased apoptosis and necrosis among the cytotrophoblast cells, the remaining cells differentiate and fuse to form a new and functional syncytial layer. A similar effect is observed when villi from either first trimester or term placentas are maintained under ambient conditions in vitro.[147,148]

Thus, it is likely that there is considerable turnover of the syncytiotrophoblast over the course of a pregnancy, although in the absence of longitudinal studies, it is impossible to determine how extensive this is. Nonetheless, it is clear that the villous membrane cannot be considered to be an intact physical barrier, and that other elements of the villous trees may play an important role in regulating maternofetal transfer.

PLACENTAL VASCULATURE

The development of the fetal vasculature begins during the third week post conception (5th week of pregnancy) with the de novo formation of capillaries within the villous stromal core. Hemangioblastic cell cords differentiate under the influence of growth factors such as basic fibroblast growth factor and vascular endothelial growth factor.[149,150] By the beginning of the fourth week, the cords have developed lumens and the endothelial cells become flattened. Surrounding mesenchymal cells become closely apposed to the tubes and differentiate to form pericytes.[151] During the next few days, connections form between neighboring tubes to form a plexus, and this ultimately unites with the allantoic vessels developing in the connecting stalk to establish the fetal circulation to the placenta.

Exactly when an effective circulation is established through these vessels is difficult to determine, however. First, the connection between the corporeal and extracorporeal fetal circulations is particularly narrow, suggesting that there can be little flow initially.[152] Second, the narrow caliber of the villous capillaries, coupled with the fact that the fetal erythrocytes are nucleated during the first trimester and hence not readily deformable, will ensure that the circulation presents a high resistance to flow. This is reflected in the Doppler waveform obtained during the first trimester, and the resistance gradually falls as the vessels enlarge over the ensuing weeks.[45]

Early in pregnancy, the capillary network is labile and undergoes considerable remodeling. Angiogenesis continues until term through a series of different phases, which most probably reflect different concentrations and combinations of growth factors induced by the changing intrauterine environment.[149,150] From 25 weeks onward, terminal capillary loops are produced; indeed it is thought that the differential elongation of the capillary network to that of the containing villus causes vascular loops to obtrude from the surface, so creating a new terminal villus.[153]

The caliber of the fetal capillaries is not constant within intermediate and terminal villi, and frequently on the apex of a tight bend the capillaries become greatly dilated, forming sinusoids. These regions may help to reduce vascular resistance and so facilitate distribution of fetal blood flow through the villous trees.[153] Equally important is that the dilations bring the outer wall of the capillaries into close juxtaposition with the overlying trophoblast. The trophoblast is locally thinned, and as a result, the diffusion distance between the maternal and fetal circulations is reduced to a minimum (Fig. 1-5).[154] Because of their morphologic configuration, these specializations are referred to as vasculosyncytial membranes, and are considered the principal sites of gaseous and other diffusional exchange. The arrangement can be considered analagous to that in the alveoli of the lung, where the pulmonary capillaries indent into the alveolar epithelium in order to reduce the thickness of the air-blood diffusion barrier. Thinning of the syncytial layer not only increases the rate of diffusion into the fetal capillaries, it also reduces the amount of oxygen extracted by the trophoblast en route. The syncytiotrophoblast is highly active metabolically owing to the high rates of protein synthesis and ionic pumping, but by having an uneven distribution of the tissue around the villous surface, the oxygen demands of the fetus and the placenta can be separated to a large extent.

It is notable that development of vasculosyncytial membranes is greatest in the peripheral regions of a placental lobule, where the oxygen concentration is lowest,[94,155] and also in placentas from high altitude.[156] In both instances, it is associated with enlargement of the capillary sinusoids and may be viewed as an adaptive response aimed at increasing the diffusing capacity of the placental tissues. Conversely, an increase in the thickness of the villous membrane is often seen in cases of intrauterine growth restriction[99] and in placentas from cigarette smokers.[157] As mentioned earlier, the hydrostatic pressure differential across the villous membrane is an important determinant of the diameter of the capillary dilatations, and hence of the villous membrane thickness.[50] Raising the pressure in the IVS not only compresses the capillaries but also increases the resistance within the umbilical circulation.[158,159] Both effects impair diffusional exchange, highlighting the importance of full conversion of the spiral arteries.

Vascular changes are observed in many complications of pregnancy,[160] where they may underpin changes in the topology of the villous tree. Thus, increased branching of the vascular network is observed in placentas from high altitude, causing the terminal villi to be shorter and more clustered than normal.[161] At present, there are no experimental data indicating that this has any impact on placental exchange, but in theory, shortening the arteriovenous pathway may lead to increased efficiency.

PHYSIOLOGY OF THE SECONDARY YOLK SAC AND EXOCOELOMIC CAVITY

Now that development of the placenta and the extraembryonic membranes has been covered, we turn to their physiologic roles during pregnancy. Phylogenetically, the oldest membrane is the yolk sac, and the SYS plays a major role in the embryonic development of all mammals.[162] The function of the yolk sac has been most extensively studied in laboratory rodents, and it has been demonstrated that the extraembryonic yolk sac is one of the initial sites of hematopoiesis.

The endodermal layer of the human SYS is known to synthesize several serum proteins in common with the fetal liver, such as alpha-fetoprotein (AFP), alpha$_1$-antitrypsin, albumin, prealbumin, and transferrin.[163] With rare exceptions, the secretion of most of these proteins is confined to the embryonic compartments, and the contribution of the SYS to the maternal protein pool is limited.[164,165] This can explain why their concentration is always higher in the ECC than in maternal serum. AFP is also produced by the embryonic liver from 6 weeks until delivery, has a high molecular weight (±70 kDa) and, compared with hCG, is found in similar amounts on both sides of the amniotic membrane. Analysis of concanavalin A affinity molecular variants of AFP have demonstrated that both coelomic and amniotic fluid AFP molecules are mainly of yolk sac origin, whereas maternal serum AFP molecules are mainly derived from the fetal liver.[166] These results suggest that the SYS also has an excretory function and secretes AFP toward the embryonic and extraembryonic compartments. By contrast, AFP molecules from fetal liver origin are probably transferred from the fetal circulation to the maternal circulation, mainly across the placental villous membrane.

The potential absorptive role of the yolk sac membrane has been evaluated by examining the distribution of proteins and enzymes between the ECC and SYS fluids, and by comparing the synthesising capacity of SYS, fetal liver, and placenta for hCG and AFP.[167] The distribution of the trophoblast-specific protein, hCG, in yolk sac and coelomic fluid, together with the absence of hCG mRNA expression in yolk sac tissues, provided the first biologic evidence of its absorptive function. Similarities in the composition of the SYS and coelomic fluids suggest that there is a free transfer for most molecules between the two corresponding compartments. Conversely, an important concentration gradient exists for most proteins between the ECC and amniotic cavity, indicating that transfer of molecules is limited at the level of the amniotic membrane that separates the corresponding fluids.

These findings suggest that the yolk sac membrane is an important zone of transfer between the extraembryonic and embryonic compartments, and that the main flux of molecules occurs from outside the yolk sac, that is, from the ECC in direction to its lumen and subsequently to the embryonic gut and circulation. The recent identification of specific transfer proteins on the mesothelial covering[168] lends further support to this concept. When after 10 weeks of gestation the cellular components of the wall of the SYS start to degenerate, this route of transfer is no longer functional, and most exchanges between the ECC and the fetal circulation must then take place at the level of the chorionic plate.

The development and physiologic roles of the ECC are intimately linked with that of the SYS, for which it provides a stable environment. The higher concentrations of hCG, estriol, and progesterone in the coelomic fluid than in maternal serum[165] strongly suggest the presence of a direct pathway between the trophoblast and the ECC. Morphologically, this may be through the villous stromal channels[87] and the loose mesenchymal tissue of the chorionic plate. Protein electrophoresis has also shown that the coelomic fluid results from an ultrafiltrate of maternal serum with the addition of specific placental and SYS bioproducts. For the duration of the first trimester, the coelomic fluid remains straw colored and more viscous than the amniotic fluid, which is always clear. This is mainly due to the higher protein concentration in the coelomic than in the amniotic cavity. The concentration of almost every protein is higher in coelomic than in amniotic fluid, ranging from 2 to 50 times depending on the corresponding molecular weight of the protein investigated.[165] The coelomic fluid has a very slow turnover, and so the ECC may act as a reservoir for nutrients needed by the developing embryo. These findings suggest that the ECC is a physiologic liquid extension of the early placenta and an important interface in fetal nutritional pathways. Molecules such as vitamin B_{12}, prolactin, and glycodelin (placental protein 14, PP14) are known to be mainly produced by the uterine decidua.[165] They are often found in higher concentrations in coelomic fluid than in maternal serum, suggesting that preferential pathways exist between the decidual tissue and the embryonic fluid cavities through the villous trophoblast. This pathway may be pivotal in providing the developing embryo with sufficient nutrients before the intervillous circulation becomes established.[73]

Some analogies can be drawn between the ECC and the antrum within a developing graafian follicle. It has been suggested that the evolution of the latter was necessary to overcome the problem of oxygen delivery to an increasing large mass of avascular cells.[169] Because the contained fluid has no oxygen consumption, it will permit diffusion more freely than an equivalent thickness of cells. However, because neither follicular nor coelomic fluids contain an oxygen carrier, the total oxygen content must be low. An oxygen gradient will inevitably exist between the source and the target, whether it be an oocyte or an embryo. Measurements in patients undergoing in vitro fertilization have demonstrated that the oxygen tension in follicular fluid falls as follicle diameter, assessed by ultrasound, increases.[170] Thus, diffusion across the ECC may be an important route of oxygen supply to the embryo before the development of a functional placental circulation, but it will maintain the early fetus in a low oxygen environment. This may serve to protect the fetal tissues from damage by oxygen free radicals and prevent disruption of signaling pathways during the crucial stages of embryogenesis and organogenesis.[171] The presence in the ECC of molecules with a well-established antioxidant role as such as taurine, transferrin, Vitamins A and E and selenium[168] support this hypothesis.

PLACENTAL TRANSPORT

For the bulk of pregnancy, the chorioallantoic placenta is the major site of exchange of nutrients (including oxygen) and of waste products of fetal metabolism (including carbon dioxide) between mother and fetus. As described earlier, histiotrophic nutrition most likely occurs in early pregnancy, and the yolk sac probably contributes to this. However, once blood flow to the IVS begins at around 10 weeks' gestation, exchange across the barrier between maternal and fetal circulations within the villi is predominant, although there may be some limited transfer between maternal blood in the endometrium and the fluid of the amniotic sac. As discussed later, many of the transport mechanisms required to effect exchange are present in the placenta by 10 weeks, and these may be up- or down-regulated throughout the rest of pregnancy to meet the requirements of fetal growth and homeostasis.

For a molecule to reach fetal plasma from maternal plasma, and vice versa, it must cross the sycyncytiotrophoblast, the matrix of the villous core, and the endothelium of the fetal capillary. The syncytiotrophoblast is the transporting epithelium and is considered to be the major locus of exchange selectivity and regulation. However, both the matrix and endothelium contribute to the properties of the placenta as an organ of exchange, both because they contribute to the thickness of the barrier and because they may act as a size filter: the finite width of the space between the endothelial cells is likely to restrict the diffusion of larger molecules.[172]

The fact that the syncytiotrophoblast is a true syncytium, with no obvious intercellular water-filled spaces suggests that it forms a tight barrier. However, physiologic data, discussed later, suggest that this is not the case. Nevertheless, exchange most likely occurs predominantly across the two opposing plasma membranes, microvillous (maternal facing) and basal (fetal facing) (Fig. 1-5).

OVERVIEW OF THE EXCHANGE PHYSIOLOGY OF THE PLACENTA AND ITS DEVELOPMENT OVER GESTATION

Maternofetal exchange across the placenta may occur, broadly, by one of four mechanisms: bulk flow/solvent drag, diffusion, transporter-mediated mechanisms, and endocytosis/exocytosis.

Bulk Flow/Solvent Drag

Differences in hydrostatic and osmotic pressures between the maternal and fetal circulations within the exchange barrier will drive water transfer by bulk flow, dragging with it dissolved solutes. These dissolved solutes are filtered as they move through the components of the barrier. Water movement may be through paracellular channels (see later) or across the plasma membranes. The latter may be enhanced by the presence of aquaporins, integral membrane proteins forming water pores in the plasma membrane.[173–175]

Hydrostatic pressure gradients are created by differences in maternal and fetal blood pressure and vascular resistances on the maternal and fetal sides of the placenta. Although the actual pressures are impossible to measure in vivo at this time, evidence suggests that it is lower in the IVS than in the fetal capillaries.[50,176] Because this would drive water from fetus to mother, which is incompatible with fetal growth, there is clearly a deficit here in our knowledge and understanding. The assumptions involved in assessing the hydrostatic pressures could be simply wrong. On the other hand, fetal-maternal water transfer driven by hydrostatic pressures may be opposed and exceeded by maternal-fetal water transfer driven by osmotic pressure gradients created by the active transport of solutes to the fetus across the syncytiotrophoblast.[177,178] These forces may well be altered as gestation proceeds. Altogether, this is an important area where further research is required.

Diffusion

Diffusion of any molecule occurs in both directions across any barrier. When there is a concentration gradient or, for charged species, an electrical gradient, one of these unidirectional fluxes (rates of transfer) is greater in one direction than it is in the other, so that there is a net flux in one direction. Net flux (Jnet) of solute across the placenta for an uncharged molecule may be described by an adaptation of Fick's Law of Diffusion[179]:

$$J_{net} = (AD/l)\,(C_m - C_f) \text{ moles/unit time}$$

where A is the surface area of the barrier available for exchange, D is the diffusion coefficient in water of the molecule (smaller molecules will have larger D), l is the thickness of the exchange barrier across which diffusion is occurring, Cm is the mean concentration of the molecule in maternal plasma, and Cf is the mean concentration of solute in the fetal circulation.

Small, relatively hydrophobic molecules such as oxygen and carbon dioxide diffuse rapidly across the plasma membranes of the barrier, so that their flux is dependent much more on the concentration gradients than on A or l. Because this concentration gradient is affected predominantly by the blood flows in both circulations, the diffusion of such molecules is said to be flow limited. This explains why reductions in uterine and or umbilical flow may result in fetal asphyxia and, consequently, growth restriction.

By contrast, hydrophilic molecules (glucose, amino acids) do not diffuse across plasma membranes easily, and their concentration gradients are maintained and flux is determined predominantly by barrier surface area and thickness. Flux of such membrane-limited molecules is not affected by blood flow unless this is dramatically reduced, but will be altered if abnormal placental development results in reduced A or increased l. There is evidence that this occurs in idiopathic intrauterine growth restriction.[99]

The term (AD/l) in Fick's Law is equivalent to what is described as the permeability of a molecule. Measurements of the passive permeability of the placenta have been made in vivo[180] and in vitro[181] utilizing hydrophilic molecules that would be unlikely to be affected by blood flow and that are not substrates for transporter proteins. These measurements show that there is an indirect relationship between permeability and the molecular size of the hydrophilic tracer. Such a relationship is explained, most simply, by the presence of extracellular water-filled channels or pores across the exchange barrier through which the molecules can diffuse. The existence of this paracellular permeability pathway has been controversial because of the syncytiotrophoblast being syncytial with no obvious paracellular channels. However, there may be transtrophoblastic channels that are not normally visible by electron microscopy.[182] Furthermore, the areas of syncytial denudation that occur in every placenta may themselves provide a route through which molecules may diffuse.[181]

Rates of transfer of hydrophobic molecules by flow-limited diffusion may change over gestation because, as described in previous sections, both uteroplacental and fetoplacental blood flow change over gestation. Changes in concentration and, for charged molecules, electrical gradients between maternal and fetal plasma also affect rates of transfer. Gestational changes do occur in the maternal and fetal plasma concentrations of solutes, so affecting driving forces. For example, glucose and amino acid concentrations in maternal plasma increase over gestation, at least partly due to the effects of insulin resistance in pregnancy and of hormones such as human placental lactogen. A maternal-fetal electrical potential difference (PD), if expressed across the placental exchange barrier, has an effect on the exchange of ions. In humans, there is a small but significant PD between maternal and fetal circulations (PD_{mf}), being -2.7 ± 0.4 mV fetus negative in mid-gestation,[183] and zero or close to it at term.[184] A PD between the mother and coelomic cavity was measured in first-trimester pregnancies.[185] There was no apparent change in the value of this PD (8.7 ± 1 mV fetus negative) between 9 and 13 weeks of gestation, which was somewhat higher than the PD across the syncytiotrophoblast (3 mV) measured using microelectrodes in term placental villi in vitro.[186] The in vitro PD across the microvillous membrane of human syncytiotrophoblast decreases between early (median −32 mV) and late first trimester (median −24 mV), with a small subsequent fall to term (−21 mV).[187] This suggests that the driving force for cation flux into the syncytiotrophoblast decreases and, for anions, increases as pregnancy progresses.

Transporter-Protein–Mediated Processes

Transporter proteins are integral membrane proteins that catalyze transfer of solutes across plasma membranes at faster rates than would occur by diffusion. Transporter proteins are a large and diverse group of molecules but which are generally characterized by showing substrate specificity (i.e. one transporter or class of transporter will predominantly transfer one substrate or class of substrate, for example, amino acids), by having saturation kinetics (i.e., raising the concentration of a substrate solute will not infinitely increase the rate at which it is transferred on transporters), and by being competitively inhibitable (i.e., two structurally similar molecules will compete for transfer by a particular transporter protein). Transporter proteins are found most abundantly in the placenta in the microvillous and basal plasma membranes of the syncytiotrophoblast. A detailed description of all of these elements is beyond the scope of this chapter but may be found in Atkinson et al.[179] In overview, there are channel proteins that form pores in the plasma membrane, allowing diffusion of ions such as K^+ and Ca^{2+}. There are transporters allowing facilitated diffusion down concentration gradients such as the GLUT1 glucose transporter. Exchange transporters, such as the Na^+/H^+ exchanger (involved in pH homeostasis of the syncytiotrophoblast and fetus), and cotransporters such as the System A amino acid transporter (which cotransports small hydrophilic amino acids including alanine, glycine, and serine with Na^+) require the maintenance of an ion gradient through secondary input of energy, often through the Na^+/K^+ATPase. Finally, there are active transporters that transfer against concentration gradients directly utilizing adenosine triphosphate (ATP)—these include the Na^+/K^+ATPase and the Ca^{2+}ATPase, which pumps Ca^{2+} across the basal plasma membrane from syncytiotrophoblast cytosol toward the fetal circulation.

Gestational changes in the flux of solutes through transporter proteins could result from changes in the number of transporters in each plasma membrane, their turnover (i.e., rate of binding to and release from the transporter), or their affinity for solute, as well as from changes in the driving forces acting on them such as electrochemical gradients and ATP availability. There is a variety of evidence that such developmental changes do occur. Using the technique of isolating and purifying microvillous plasma membrane and radioisotopic tracers to measure transport rates in vesicles formed from these membranes, it has been shown that the V_{max} of the Na^+-dependent system A amino acid transporter increases by about 4 fold, per mg membrane protein, between first trimester and term.[188] The activity of the System y^+ cationic amino acid (e.g., arginine, lysine) transporter increases over gestation, whereas the activity of the System y^+L transporter decreases.[189,190] This decrease in System y^+L activity is due to a decrease in the affinity of the transporter for substrate and is accompanied by an increased expression of 4F2hc monomer of the dimer protein.[189,190] The reason for this decline is not known but could well be associated with a specific fetal need. Glucose transporter GLUT1 expression in microvillous membrane increases between first trimester and term.[191] Na^+/H^+ exchanger activity is lower in first-trimester microvillous membrane vesicles as compared with those at term,[188,192] a result borne out by studies on the intrasyncytiotrophoblast pH of isolated placental villi from the two stages in gestation.[193] Interestingly, the expression of the NHE1 isoform of this exchanger in the microvillous membrane does not change across gestation, but the expression of both of its NHE2 and NHE3 isoforms increases between weeks 14 and 18 and term.[192] In contrast, there is no difference in Cl^-/HCO_3^- exchanger activity or, by Western blotting, expression of its AE1 isoform, between first trimester and term.[194] Understanding of how these gestational changes are regulated is currently sparse; studies in knockout mice suggest that hormones such as insulin-like growth factor II (IGF II) from the fetus, signaling demand for the nutrients required for growth, are important,[195] but much more work is needed in this area.

Endocytosis/Exocytosis

Endocytosis is the process by which molecules become entrapped in invaginations of the microvillous plasma membrane of the syncytiotrophoblast, which eventually pinch off and form vesicles within the cytosol. Such vesicles may diffuse through the intracellular compartment and, if they avoid fusion with lysosomes, eventually fuse with the basal plasma membrane and undergo exocytosis, releasing their contents into the fetal milieu. Evidence suggests that immunoglobulin G (IgG) and other large proteins may cross the placenta by this mechanism.[179,196] Specificity and the ability to avoid lysosomal degradation during the endocytosis phase may be provided by the presence of receptors for IgG in the microvillous membrane invaginations and vesicles. However, this mechanism of transfer and its gestational regulation, if any, is still not well understood.

Placental Nutrient Supply and Intrauterine Growth Restriction

The notion that placental insufficiency is a cause of intrauterine growth restriction (IUGR) has been much quoted but little understood until recently. It is often taken as being synonymous with reduced uteroplacental or umbilical blood flow. Doppler measurements of such blood flows have been of assistance in diagnosing and assessing the severity of IUGR but are limited in value.[197] It is now clear that other variables determining the capacity of the placenta to supply nutrients may also contribute to IUGR. For example, the surface area of the exchange barrier is decreased and its thickness decreased in IUGR[99]; such changes are likely to markedly decrease the passive permeability of the placenta. Furthermore, there is now considerable evidence that the activity and expression of transporter proteins in the syncytiotrophoblast is altered in IUGR.[197] The reported data are summarized in Table 1-1. As can be seen, activity of several transporters decrease, at least one increases, and others show no change at all. This variation in response could reflect whether a change in the placenta is causative in IUGR (e.g., the decrease in system A amino acid transporter activity), or is compensatory (e.g., the increase in Ca^{2+} ATPase activity), as well as differential regulation of the transporters. Understanding these placental phenotypes of IUGR may well give clues to novel means of diagnosing and even treating the condition.[197]

Table 1-1. Changes in Activity of Transporter Proteins in the Microvillous (MVM) and Basal (BM) Plasma Membrane of Placentas from IUGR Pregnancies as Compared to Normal Pregnancies

TRANSPORTER	MVM	BM	REFERENCE
System A	Decreased	No change	224–226
System L (leucine)	Decreased	Decreased	227
System y^+/y^+L (arginine/lysine)	No change	Decreased	190, 227
System β	Decreased	No change	228
Na^+-independent Taurine	No change	Decreased	228, 229
GLUT1	No change	No change	191
Na^+/K^+ATPase	Decreased	No change	230
Ca^{2+}ATPase	Not present	Increased	231
Na^+/H^+ Exchanger	Decreased	Activity not present	225, 232
H^+/lactate	No change	Decreased	233

PLACENTAL ENDOCRINOLOGY

The human placenta is an important endocrine organ, signaling the presence of the conceptus to the mother in early pregnancy and optimizing the intrauterine environment and maternal physiology for the benefit of fetal growth. Two major groups of hormones are produced; the steroid hormones, progesterone and the estrogens, and peptide hormones, such as hCG and human placental lactogen (hPL). All are predominantly synthesized in the syncytiotrophoblast, and although the synthetic pathways have been generally elucidated, the factors regulating secretion are still largely unknown.

Progesterone

During the first few weeks of pregnancy, progesterone is mainly derived from the corpus luteum, but gradually as the placental mass increases, this organ's contribution becomes dominant, with the production of around 250 mg/day. The corpus luteum regresses at around 9 weeks, and at that stage it is no longer essential for the maintenance of a pregnancy.

Placental synthesis of progesterone begins with the conversion of cholesterol to pregnenolone, as in other steroid secreting tissues. Placental tissues are poor at synthesizing cholesterol and so use maternal cholesterol derived from low-density lipoproteins taken up in coated pits on the surface of the syncytiotrophoblast. Conversion of the cholesterol to pregnenolone occurs on the inner aspect of the inner mitochondrial membrane, catalyzed by cytochrome P450scc (p450scc; CYP11A1), and in other steroidogenic tissues the delivery of cholesterol to this site is the principal rate-limiting step in progesterone synthesis. There, delivery is facilitated by the steroidogenic acute regulatory (StAR) protein, which binds and transports cholesterol, but this protein is not present in the human placenta.[198,199] Instead, a homologue, MLN64, may carry out a similar function, as freshly isolated cytotrophoblast cells appear to contain concentrations of cholesterol that are near saturating for progesterone synthesis, indicating that supply of the precursor is not rate-limiting.[200] Side-chain cleavage requires molecular oxygen, but it is unclear whether the conditions that prevail during the first trimester are rate-limiting. The rate of production of pregnenolone from radiolabeled cholesterol by placental homogenates in vitro increases across the first trimester,[201] and both the concentration and activity of P450scc increase in placental mitochondria from the first trimester to term.[202] These changes, coupled with the expansion of the syncytiotrophoblast, most likely account for the increase in progesterone synthesis observed.

Side-chain cleavage also requires a supply of electrons, and this is provided by NADPH through a short electron transport chain in the mitochondrial matrix involving adrenodoxin reductase and its redox partner adrenodoxin. Preliminary studies in Tuckey's laboratory suggest that the transport of electrons to P450scc is rate-limiting for the enzyme's activity at midpregnancy,[199] and thus further research on the factors regulating expression and activity of adrenodoxin reductase during gestation is clearly needed.

The resultant pregnenolone is then converted to progesterone by the enzyme type 1 3β-hydroxysteroid dehydrogenase (3β-HSD), principally in the mitochondria. The activity of 3β-HSD in placental tissues is significantly higher than that of cytochrome P450scc, and so this step is unlikely ever to be rate-limiting for the production of progesterone.[203] Once secreted, the principal actions of the hormone are to maintain quiescence of the myometrium, although it may have an immunomodulatory role as well. In addition, our new data on the importance of histiotrophic nutrition during the first few weeks of pregnancy suggest that progesterone may be essential to maintain the secretory activity of the endometrial glands.

Estrogens

The human placenta lacks the enzymes required to synthesize estrogens directly from acetate or cholesterol, and thus uses the precursor dehydroepiandrosterone sulfate (DHAS) supplied by the maternal and fetal adrenal glands in approximately equal proportions near term. Following uptake by the syncytiotrophoblast, DHAS is hydrolyzed by placental sulfatase to dehydroepiandrosterone (DHA), which is further converted to androstenedione by 3β-HSD. Final conversion to estradiol and estrone is achieved by the action of P450 cytochrome aromatase (P450arom) (CYP19), which has been immunolocalized to the endoplasmic reticulum.[204] The syncytiotrophoblast can also use 16-OH DHAS produced by the fetal liver, converting this to 16α-OH androstenedione through the action of 3β-HSD, and thence to estriol through the action of P450arom. Because approximately 90 percent of placental estriol production is reliant on fetal synthesis of the precursor 16-OH DHAS, maternal estriol concentrations have in the past been taken clinically as an index of fetal well-being.[205]

Although the synthesis of estrogens can be detected in placental tissues during the early weeks of gestation, secretion significantly increases toward the end of the first trimester. By 7 weeks of gestation, more than 50 percent of maternal circulating estrogens are of placental origin. Recent analysis of the transcriptional regulation of the P450arom gene has shown it to be oxygen responsive through a novel pathway involving the basic helix-loop-helix transcription factor Mash-2.[206] Production of Mash-2 is increased under physiologically low oxygen conditions, and leads to repression of P450arom gene expression. Hence, the change in oxygenation that occurs at the end of the first trimester[35] may stimulate placental production of estrogens.

Human Chorionic Gonadotropin

hCG is secreted by the trophoblast at the blastocyst stage, and can be detected in the maternal blood and urine approximately 8 to 10 days postfertilization. Its principal function is to maintain the corpus luteum until the placenta is sufficiently developed to take over production of progesterone. hCG is a heterodimeric glycoprotein (approximately 38,000 Da) consisting of α and β subunits that are principally derived from the syncytiotrophoblast. The α subunit is common to that of thyroid-stimulating hormone, luteinizing hormone (LH), and follicle-stimulating hormone, and is encoded by a single gene located at chromosome 6q12-21.[207] It is the β subunit that determines the biologic specificity of hCG, and this evolved by a duplication event at the LHβ gene locus.[208] In humans, there are six copies of the hCGβ gene, located together with a single copy of the LHβ gene at chromosome 19p13.3. Polymerase chain reaction–based techniques have revealed that at least five, possibly all six, of the genes are transcribed in vivo during normal pregnancy. Most of the steady-state hCGβ mRNAs are transcribed from hCGβ genes 5, 3 and 8, however, with the levels of expression being β5 > β3 = β8 > β7, β1/2.[209] The β subunits of LH and hCG share 85 percent amino acid sequence homology, and are functionally interchangeable. One of the principal differences between the two is the presence of a 31-amino acid carboxyl-terminal extension in hCGβ compared with a shorter 7-amino acid stretch in LHβ. This extension is hydrophilic, contains four O-glycosylated serine residues, and is thought to act as a secretory routeing signal targeting release of hCG from the apical membrane of the syncytiotrophoblast.[210]

Assembly of hCG involves a complex process of folding in which a strand of 20 residues of the β subunit is wrapped around the α subunit, and the two are secured by a disulfide bond. Combination of the subunits occurs in the syncytiotrophoblast before the release of intact hCG, and because there is only limited storage in cytoplasmic granules, secretion is largely thought to reflect de novo synthesis. Oxidizing conditions promote combination of the subunits in vitro, most probably through their effects on the disulfide bond,[211] and so the wave of physiologic oxidative stress observed in placental tissues at the transition from the first to second trimester[35] may influence the pattern of secretion in vivo.

Concentrations of the hCG dimer in maternal blood rise rapidly during early pregnancy, peak at 9 to 10 weeks, and subsequently decline to a nadir at approximately 20 weeks. The physiologic role of the hCG peak is unknown, because the serum concentration far exceeds that required to stimulate LH receptors in the corpus luteum. In any case, the corpus luteum is coming to the end of its extended life, and so the peak may therefore merely reflect other physiologic events.[212] Production of the β subunit follows the same pattern, whereas the maternal serum concentration of the α subunit continues to rise during the first and second trimesters. Therefore, synthesis of the β subunit is considered to be the rate-limiting step. Early experiments using primary placental cultures revealed that cyclic adenosine monophosphate (cAMP) plays a key role in the biosynthesis of both subunits, and subsequent work showed it to increase both the transcription and the stability of the α and β mRNAs. The kinetics were different for the two subunits, however, suggesting that the effect occurs through separate pathways or transcription factors. Possible regulatory elements within the α and β genes were extensively reviewed by Jameson and Hollenberg.[213]

Another theory that has been proposed is that intact hCG may modulate its own secretion in an autocrine/paracrine fashion through the LH/hCG receptor.[214] This G protein–coupled receptor has been identified on the syncytiotrophoblast of the mature placenta and contains a large extracellular domain that binds intact hCG with high affinity and specificity. However, during early pregnancy, the receptors in the placenta are truncated and probably functionless until 9 weeks.[215] Hence, in the absence of self-regulation, maternal serum concentrations of hCG may rise steeply until the expression of functional LH/hCG receptors on the syncytiotrophoblast toward the end of the first trimester brings it under control. Reduced synthesis of the functional receptor may underlie the raised serum concentrations of hCG that characterize cases of Down syndrome (trisomy 21).[216]

In addition to changes in the rate of secretion, the hormone also exhibits molecular heterogeneity in both its protein and carbohydrate moieties, and the ratio of the different isoforms secreted changes with gestational age. For the first 5 to 6 weeks of gestation, hyperglycosylated isoforms of the β subunit predominate, resembling the pattern seen in choriocarcinoma.[217] In normal pregnancies, these isoforms then decline and are replaced by those that predominate for the remainder of pregnancy. The rate of decline is greater in pregnancies that go on to spontaneous miscarriage,[218] suggesting there may be some underlying defect in trophoblast differentiation in these cases.

Midtrimester maternal concentrations of hCG were also found to be raised in a retrospective study of early-onset preeclampsia,[219] and recently, a link between the serum concentration and the severity of the maternal oxidative stress has been reported. These data reinforce the putative link between secretion of hCG and the redox status of the trophoblast.

Placental Lactogen

hPL, also known as chorionic sommatotropin or hCS, is a single chain glycoprotein (22,300 Da) that has a high degree of amino acid sequence homology with both human growth hormone (96 percent) and prolactin (67 percent). Therefore, it has been suggested that the genes encoding all three hormones arose from a common ancestral gene through repeated gene duplication. Thus, hPL has both growth-promoting and lactogenic effects, although the former are of rather low activity. The hormone is synthesized exclusively in the syncytiotrophoblast, and is secreted predominantly into the maternal circulation, where it can be detected from the third week of gestation onward. Concentrations rise steadily until they plateau at around 36 weeks of gestation, at which time the daily production rate is approximately 1 g. The magnitude of this effort is reflected by the fact that at term, production of hPL accounts for 5 to 10 percent of total protein synthesis by placental ribosomes, and the encoding mRNA represents 20 percent of the total placental mRNA.

Little is known regarding the control of hPL secretion in vivo, and maternal concentrations correlate most closely with placental mass. There is evidence that calcium influx into the syncytiotrophoblast or an increase in the external concentration in albumin can cause the release of hPL from placental explants in vitro, and this does not appear to be mediated by activation of the inositol phosphate, cAMP, or cGMP pathways.[220]

The hormone has well-defined actions on maternal metabolism, promoting lipolysis and increasing circulating free fatty acid levels, and acting as an insulin antagonist and raising blood glucose concentrations. It also promotes growth and differentiation of the mammary glandular tissue within the breasts in anticipation of lactation.

Placental Growth Hormone

Placental growth hormone (PGH) is expressed from the same gene cluster as hPL, and differs from pituitary growth hormone by only 13 amino acids.[221] It is secreted predominantly by the syncytiotrophoblast into the maternal circulation in a nonpulsatile manner, and cannot be detected in the fetal circulation.[222] Between 10 and 20 weeks of gestation, PGH gradually replaces pituitary growth hormone, which then becomes undetectable until term.[223] In contrast to hPL, PGH has high growth-promoting activities but low lactogenic activities.

Secretion of PGH is not modulated by growth hormone–releasing hormone but appears to be rapidly suppressed by raised glucose concentrations both in vivo and in vitro.[221] Through its actions on maternal metabolism, PGH increases nutrient availability for the fetoplacental unit, promoting lipolysis and also gluconeogenesis. It is also one of the key regulators of maternal insulin-like growth factor 1 (IGF1) concentrations, and circulating levels of PGH are reduced in cases of intrauterine growth restriction.[221]

Key Points

- The mature human placenta is a discoid organ consisting of an elaborately branched fetal villous tree that is bathed directly by maternal blood; the villous hemochorial type.
- Continual development throughout pregnancy leads to progressive enlargement of the surface area for exchange (12 to 14 m^2 at term) and reduction in the mean diffusion distance between the maternal

and fetal circulations (approximately 5 to 6 μm at term).

❑ The maternal circulation to the placenta is not fully established until the end of the first trimester; hence, organogenesis takes place in a low oxygen environment of approximately 20 mmHg that may protect against free radical-mediated teratogenesis.

❑ During the first trimester, the uterine glands discharge their secretions into the placental IVS, and represent an important supply of nutrients, cytokines, and growth factors before the onset of the maternal circulation.

❑ The ECC acts as an important reservoir of nutrients during early pregnancy, and the secondary yolk sac is important in the uptake of nutrients and their transfer to the fetus.

❑ Oxygen is a powerful mediator of trophoblast proliferation and invasion, villous remodeling, and placental angiogenesis.

❑ Ensuring an adequate maternal blood supply to the placenta during the second and third trimesters is an essential aspect of placentation, and is dependent on physiologic conversion of the spiral arteries induced by invasion of the endometrium by extravillous trophoblast during early pregnancy. Many complications of pregnancy, such as preeclampsia, appear to be secondary to deficient invasion.

❑ All transport across the placenta must take place across the syncytial covering of the villous tree, the syncytiotrophoblast, the villous matrix and the fetal endothelium, each of which may impose its own restriction and selectivity. Exchange occurs through one of four basic processes; bulk flow/solvent drag, diffusion, transporter mediated mechanisms, and endocytosis/exocytosis.

❑ The rate of transplacental exchange depends on many factors, such as the surface area available, the concentration gradient, the rates of maternal and fetal blood flows, and the density of transporter proteins. Changes in villous surface area, diffusion distance and transporter expression have been linked with intrauterine growth restriction.

❑ The placenta is an important endocrine gland, producing both steroid and peptide hormones principally from the syncytiotrophoblast. Concentrations of some hormones are altered in pathologic conditions, for example, hCG in trisomy 21, but in general, little is known regarding control of endocrine activity.

REFERENCES

1. Boyd JD, Hamilton WJ: The Human Placenta. Cambridge, Heffer and Sons, 1970, p 365.
2. Bouw GM, Stolte LAM, Baak JPA, et al: Quantitative morphology of the placenta. I. Standardization of sampling. Eur J Obstet Gynecol Repro Biol 6:325, 1976.
3. Mossman HW: Vertebrate fetal membranes: comparative ontogeny and morphology; evolution; phylogenetic significance; basic functions; research opportunities. London, Macmillan, 1987, p 383.
4. Wooding FBP, Flint APF: Placentation. *In* Lamming GE (ed): Marshall's Physiology of Reproduction. London, Chapman & Hall, 1994, p 233.
5. Jauniaux E, Gulbis B, Burton GJ: The human first trimester gestational sac limits rather than facilitates oxygen transfer to the fetus—a review. Placenta 24 Suppl A:S86, 2003.
6. Luckett WP: Origin and differentiation of the yolk sac and extra-embryonic mesoderm in presomite human and rhesus monkey embryos. Am J Anat 152:59, 1978.
7. Ramsey EM, Donner MW: Placental Vasculature and Circulation. Anatomy, Physiology, Radiology, Clinical Aspects, Atlas and Textbook. Stuttgart: Georg Thieme; 1980, p 101.
8. Lindenberg S, Hyttel P, Sjøgren A, et al: A comparative study of attachment of human, bovine and mouse blastocysts to uterine epithelial monolayer. Hum Reprod 4:446, 1989.
9. Hertig AT, Rock J, Adams EC: A description of 34 human ova within the first 17 days of development. Am J Anat 98:435, 1956.
10. Genbacev O, McMaster MT, Fisher SJ: A repertoire of cell cycle regulators whose expression is coordinated with human cytotrophoblast differentiation. Am J Pathol 157:1337, 2000.
11. Enders AC, King BF: Development of the human yolk sac. *In* Nogales FF (ed): The Human Yolk Sac and Yolk Sac Tumors. Berlin, Springer-Verlag, 1993, p 33.
12. Jauniaux E, Jurkovic D, Henriet Y, et al: Development of the secondary human yolk sac: correlation of sonographic and anatomic features. Hum Reprod 6:1160, 1991.
13. Ferrazzi E, Garbo S: Ultrasonography of the human yolk sac. *In* Nogales FF (ed): The Human Yolk Sac and Yolk Sac Tumors. Berlin, Springer-Verlag, 1993, p 161.
14. Gonzalez-Crussi F, Roth LM: The human yolk sac and yolk sac carcinoma. An ultrastructural study. Hum Pathol 7:675, 1976.
15. Jones CJP: The life and death of the embryonic yolk sac. *In* Jauniaux E, Barnea ER,Edwards RG (eds): Embryonic Medicine and Therapy. Oxford, Oxford University Press, 1997, p 180.
16. King BF, Wilson JM: A fine structural and cytochemical study of the rhesus monkey yolk sac: endoderm and mesothelium. Anat Rec 205:143, 1983.
17. Jones CJP, Jauniaux E: Ultrastructure of the materno-embryonic interface in the first trimester of pregnancy. Micron 26:145, 1995.
18. Moore KL, Persaud TVN: The Developing Human. Clinically Orientated Embryology. Philadelphia: W.B. Saunders; 1993, p 493.
19. Larsen WJ: Human Embryology. New York: Churchill Livingstone; 1997, p 512.
20. Enders AC, Carter AM: What can comparative studies of placental structure tell us? A review. Placenta 25 Suppl A:S3, 2004.
21. Hamilton WJ, Boyd JD: Development of the human placenta in the first three months of gestation. J Anat 94:297, 1960.
22. Ramsey EM: Functional anatomy of the primate placenta. Placenta Suppl 1:29, 1981.
23. Hustin J, Schaaps JP: Echographic and anatomic studies of the maternotrophoblastic border during the first trimester of pregnancy. Am J Obstet Gynecol 157:162, 1987.
24. Carter AM: When is the maternal placental circulation established in Man? Placenta 18:83, 1997.
25. Burton GJ, Jauniaux E, Watson AL: Maternal arterial connections to the placental intervillous space during the first trimester of human pregnancy; the Boyd Collection revisited. Am J Obstet Gynecol 181:718, 1999.
26. Jauniaux E, Jurkovic D, Campbell S, et al: Investigation of placental circulations by colour Doppler ultrasound. Am J Obstet Gynecol 164:486, 1991.
27. Jaffe R, Woods JR: Color Doppler imaging and in vivo assessment of the anatomy and physiology of the early uteroplacental circulation. Fertil Steril 60:293, 1993.
28. Coppens M, Loquet P, Kollen F, et al: Longitudinal evaluation of uteroplacental and umbilical blood flow changes in normal early pregnancy. Ultrasound Obstet Gynecol 7:114, 1996.
29. Valentin L, Sladkevicius P, Laurini R, et al: Uteroplacental and luteal circulation in normal first-trimester pregnancies: Doppler ultrasonographic and morphologic study. Am J Obstet Gynecol 174:768, 1996.

30. Kurjak A, Kupesic S, Hafner T, et al: Conflicting data on intervillous circulation in early pregnancy. J Perinat Med 25:225, 1997.
31. Kliman HJ: Uteroplacental blood flow. The story of decidulaisation, menstruation and trophoblast invasion. Am J Pathol 157:1759, 2000.
32. Schaaps JP, Hustin J: In vivo aspect of the maternal-trophoblastic border during the first trimester of gestation. Troph Res 3:39, 1988.
33. Hustin J, Schaaps JP, Lambotte R: Anatomical studies of the utero-placental vascularisation in the first trimester of pregnancy. Troph Res 3:49, 1988.
34. Rodesch F, Simon P, Donner C, et al: Oxygen measurements in endometrial and trophoblastic tissues during early pregnancy. Obstet Gynecol 80:283, 1992.
35. Jauniaux E, Watson AL, Hempstock J, et al: Onset of maternal arterial bloodflow and placental oxidative stress; a possible factor in human early pregnancy failure. Am J Pathol 157:2111, 2000.
36. Pijnenborg R: Trophoblast invasion and placentation in the human: morphological aspects. Troph Res 4:33, 1990.
37. Pijnenborg R, Dixon G, Robertson WB, et al: Trophoblastic invasion of human decidua from 8 to 18 weeks of pregnancy. Placenta 1:3, 1980.
38. Brosens JJ, Pijnenborg R, Brosens IA: The myometrial junctional zone spiral arteries in normal and abnormal pregnancies. Am J Obstet Gynecol 187:1416, 2002.
39. Craven CM, Morgan T, Ward K: Decidual spiral artery remodelling begins before cellular interaction with cytotrophoblasts. Placenta 19:241, 1998.
40. Kam EPY, Gardner L, Loke YW, et al: The role of trophoblast in the physiological change in decidual spiral arteries. Hum Reprod 14:2131, 1999.
41. Brosens IA: The utero-placental vessels at term—the distribution and extent of physiological changes. Troph Res 3:61, 1988.
42. Jauniaux E, Hempstock J, Greenwold N, et al: Trophoblastic oxidative stress in relation to temporal and regional differences in maternal placental blood flow in normal and abnormal early pregnancies. Am J Pathol 162:115, 2003.
43. Al-Lamki RS, Skepper JN, Burton GJ: Are human placental bed giant cells merely aggregates of small mononuclear trophoblast cells? An ultrastructural and immunocytochemical study. Hum Reprod 14:496, 1999.
44. Moffett-King A: Natural killer cells and pregnancy. Nat Rev Immunol 2:656, 2002.
45. Jauniaux E, Jurkovic D, Campbell S, et al: Doppler ultrasound features of the developing placental circulations: correlation with anatomic findings. Am J Obstet Gynecol 166:585, 1992.
46. Ziegler WF, Bernstein I, Badger G, et al: Regional hemodynamic adaptation during the menstrual cycle. Obstet Gynecol 94:695, 1999.
47. Assali NS, Douglass RAJ, Baird WW, et al: Measurement of uterine blood flow and uterine metabolism. IV. Results in normal pregnancy. Am J Obstet Gynecol 66:248, 1953.
48. Moll W, Künzel W, Herberger J: Hemodynamic implications of hemochorial placentation. Eur J Obstet Gynecol Reprod Biol 5:67, 1975.
49. Moll W: Structure adaptation and blood flow control in the uterine arterial system after hemochorial placentation. Eur J Obstet Gynecol Reprod Biol 110:S19, 2003.
50. Karimu AL, Burton GJ: The effects of maternal vascular pressure on the dimensions of the placental capillaries. Br J Obstet Gynaecol 101:57, 1994.
51. Khong TY, Liddell HS, Robertson WB: Defective haemochorial placentation as a cause of miscarriage. A preliminary study. Br J Obstet Gynaecol 94:649, 1987.
52. Hustin J, Jauniaux E, Schaaps JP: Histological study of the materno-embryonic interface in spontaneous abortion. Placenta 11:477, 1990.
53. Jaffe R, Warsof SL: Color Doppler imaging in the assessment of uteroplacental blood flow in abnormal first trimester intrauterine pregnancies: An attempt to define the etiologic mechanisms. J Ultrasound Med 11:41, 1992.
54. Jauniaux E, Zaidi J, Jurkovic D, et al: Comparison of colour Doppler features and pathologic findings in complicated early pregnancy. Hum Reprod 9:243, 1994.
55. Schwärzler P, Holden D, Nielsen S, et al: The conservative management of first trimester miscarriages and the use of colour Doppler sonography for patient selection. Hum Reprod 14:1341, 1999.
56. Hempstock J, Jauniaux E, Greenwold N, et al: The contribution of placental oxidative stress to early pregnancy failure. Hum Pathol 34:1265, 2003.
57. Sheppard BL, Bonnar J: The maternal blood supply to the placenta in pregnancy complicated by intrauterine fetal growth retardation. Troph Res 3:69, 1988.
58. Meekins JW, Pijnenborg R, Hanssens M, et al: A study of placental bed spiral arteries and trophoblast invasion in normal and severe pre-eclamptic pregnancies. Br J Obstet Gynaecol 101:669, 1994.
59. DiFederico E, Genbacev O, Fisher SJ: Preeclampsia is associated with widespread apoptosis of placental cytotrophoblasts within the uterine wall. Am J Pathol 155:293, 1999.
60. Dekker GA, Sibai BM: Etiology and pathogenesis of preeclampsia; current concepts. Am J Obstet Gynecol 179:1358, 1998.
61. Reister F, Frank H-G, Kingdom JCP, et al: Macrophage-induced apoptosis limits endovascular trophoblast invasion in the uterine wall of preeclamptic women. Lab Invest 81:1143, 2001.
62. Kliman HJ: Trophoblast infiltration. Reprod Med Rev 3:137, 1994.
63. Pijnenborg R, Vercruysse L, Verbist L, et al: Interaction of interstitial trophoblast with placental bed capillaries and venules of normotensive and pre-eclamptic pregnancies. Placenta 19:569, 1998.
64. Jauniaux E, Ramsay B, Campbell S: Ultrasonographic investigation of placental morphologic characteristics and size during the second trimester of pregnancy. Am J Obstet Gynecol 170:130, 1994.
65. Jauniaux E, Nicolaides KH: Placental lakes, absent umbilical artery diastolic flow and poor fetal growth in early pregnancy. Ultrasound Obstet Gynecol 7:141, 1996.
66. Martin CB, McGaughey HS, Kaiser IH, et al: Intermittent functioning of the uteroplacental arteries. Am J Obstet Gynecol 90:819, 1964.
67. Hung TH, Skepper JN, Burton GJ: In vitro ischemia-reperfusion injury in term human placenta as a model for oxidative stress in pathological pregnancies. Am J Pathol 159:1031, 2001.
68. Burton GJ, Hung T-H: Hypoxia-reoxygenation; a potential source of placental oxidative stress in normal pregnancy and preeclampsia. Fetal Mat Med Rev 14:97, 2000.
69. Roberts JM, Hubel CA: Is oxidative stress the link in the two-stage model of pre-eclampsia? Lancet 354:788, 1999.
70. De Wolf F, De Wolf-Peeters C, Brosens I: Ultrastructure of the spiral arteries in the human placental bed at the end of normal pregnancy. Am J Obstet Gynecol 117:833, 1973.
71. Burton GJ, Jauniaux E: Placental oxidative stress; from miscarriage to preeclampsia. J Soc Gynecol Invest 11:342, 2004.
72. Beir-Hellwig K, Sterzik K, Bonn B, et al: Contribution to the physiology and pathology of endometrial receptivity: the determination of protein patterns in human uterine secretions. Hum Reprod 4 Suppl:115, 1989.
73. Burton GJ, Watson AL, Hempstock J, et al: Uterine glands provide histiotrophic nutrition for the human fetus during the first trimester of pregnancy. J Clin Endocrinol Metab 87:2954, 2002.
74. Seppälä M, Jukunen M, Riitinen L, et al: Endometrial proteins: a reappraisal. Hum Reprod 7 Suppl. 1:31, 1992.
75. Basir GS, O WS, So WW, et al: Evaluation of cycle-to-cycle variation of endometrial responsiveness using transvaginal sonography in women undergoing assisted reproduction. Ultrasound Obstet Gynaecol 19:484, 2002.
76. Kolibianakis EM, Zikopoulos KA, Fatemi HM, et al: Endometrial thickness cannot predict ongoing pregnancy achievement in cycles stimulated with clomiphene citrate for intrauterine insemination. Reprod Biomed Online 8:115, 2004.
77. Hempstock J, Cindrova-Davies T, Jauniaux E, et al: Endometrial glands as a source of nutrients, growth factors and cytokines during the first trimester of human pregnancy; a morphological and immunohistochemical study. Reprod Biol Endocrinol 2:58, 2004.
78. Demir R, Kayisli UA, Celik-Ozenci C, et al: Structural differentiation of human uterine luminal and glandular epithelium during early pregnancy: an ultrastructural and immunohistochemical study. Placenta 23:672, 2002.

79. Lennard SN, Gerstenberg C, Allen WR, et al: Expression of epidermal growth factor and its receptor in equine placental tissues. J Reprod Fertil 112:49, 1998.
80. Gray CA, Taylor KM, Ramsey WS, et al: Endometrial glands are required for preimplantation conceptus elongation and survival. Biol Reprod 64:1608, 2001.
81. Dalton CF, Laird SM, Estdale SE, et al: Endometrial protein PP14 and CA-125 in recurrent miscarriage patients; correlation with pregnancy outcome. Hum Reprod 13:3197, 1998.
82. Mikolajczyk M, Skrzypczak J, Szymanowski K, et al: The assessment of LIF in uterine flushing—a possible new diagnostic tool in states of impaired infertility. Reprod Biol 3:259, 2003.
83. Tuckerman E, Laird SM, Stewart R, et al: Markers of endometrial function in women with unexplained recurrent pregnancy loss: a comparison between morphologically normal and retarded endometrium. Hum Reprod 19:196, 2004.
84. Burton GJ, Hempstock J, Jauniaux E: Nutrition of the human fetus during the first trimester—review. Placenta 22 Suppl A: S70, 2001.
85. Kaufmann P, Sen DK, Schweikhert G: Classification of human placental villi.1. Histology. Cell Tissue Res 200:409, 1979.
86. Boura ALA, Walter WAW: Autocoids and the control of vascular tone in the human umbilical-placental circulation. Placenta 12:453, 1991.
87. Castellucci M, Kaufmann P: A three-dimensional study of the normal human placental villous core: II. Stromal architecture. Placenta 3:269, 1982.
88. Burton GJ: The fine structure of the human placenta as revealed by scanning electron microscopy. Scanning Microsc 1:1811, 1987.
89. Reynolds SRM: Formation of fetal cotyledons in the hemochorial placenta. A theoretical consideration of the functional implications of such an arrangement. Am J Obstet Gynecol 94:425, 1966.
90. Freese UE: The fetal-maternal circulation of the placenta. 1. Histomorphologic, plastoid injection, and x-ray cinematographic studies on human placentas. Am J Obstet Gynecol 94:354, 1966.
91. Wigglesworth JS: Vascular anatomy of the human placenta and its significance for placental pathology. J Obstet Gynaecol Br Commonw 76:979, 1969.
92. Hempstock J, Bao Y-P, Bar-Issac M, et al: Intralobular differences in antioxidant enzyme expression and activity reflect oxygen gradients within the human placenta. Placenta 24:517, 2003.
93. Schuhmann R, Stoz F, Maier M: Histometric investigations in placentones (materno-fetal circulation units) of human placentae. Troph Res 3:3, 1988.
94. Critchley GR, Burton GJ: Intralobular variations in barrier thichkness in the mature human placenta. Placenta 8:185, 1987.
95. Jackson MR, Mayhew TM, Boyd PA: Quantitative description of the elaboration and maturation of villi from 10 weeks of gestation to term. Placenta 13:357, 1992.
96. Teasdale F: Idiopathic intrauterine growth retardation: histomorphometry of the human placenta. Placenta 5:83, 1984.
97. Jackson MR, Walsh AJ, Morrow RJ, et al: Reduced placental villous tree elaboration in small-for-gestational-age pregnancies: Relationship with umbilical artery Doppler waveforms. Am J Obstet Gynecol 172:518, 1995.
98. Hitschold T, Weiss E, Beck T, et al: Low target birth weight or growth retardation? Umbilical Doppler flow velocity waveforms and histometric analysis of fetoplacental vascular tree. Am J Obstet Gynecol 168:1260, 1993.
99. Mayhew TM, Ohadike C, Baker PN, et al: Stereological investigation of placental morphology in pregnancies complicated by pre-eclampsia with and without intrauterine growth restriction. Placenta 24:219, 2003.
100. Teasdale F: Histomorphometry of the human placenta in maternal preeclampsia. Am J Obstet Gynecol 152:25, 1985.
101. Teasdale F: Histomorphometry of the human placenta in preeclampsia associated with severe intra-uterine growth retardation. Placenta 8:119, 1987.
102. Hafner E, Metzenbauer M, Hofinger D, et al: Placental growth from the first to the second trimester of pregnancy in SGA-foetuses and pre-eclamptic pregnancies compared to normal foetuses. Placenta 24:336, 2003.
103. Teasdale F, Jean-Jacques G: Morphometric evaluation of the microvillus enlargement factor in the human placenta from midgestation to term. Placenta 6:375, 1985.
104. Karimu AL, Burton GJ: The distribution of microvilli over the villous surface of the normal human term placenta is homogenous. Reprod Fertil Dev 7:1269, 1995.
105. Ockleford CD, Whyte A: Differeniated regions of human placental cell surface associated with exchange of materials between maternal and foetal blood: coated vesicles. J Cell Sci 25:293, 1977.
106. Jones CJP, Fox H: Ultrastructure of the normal human placenta. Electron Microsc Rev 4:129, 1991.
107. King BF: Absorption of peroxidase-conjugated immunoglobulin G by human placenta: an in vitro study. Placenta 3:395, 1982.
108. Ockleford CD, Wakely J: The skeleton of the placenta. *In* Harrison RJ, Holmes RL (eds): Progress in Anatomy. London, Cambridge University Press, 1981, p 19.
109. Dearden L, Ockleford CD: Structure of human trophoblast: correlation with function. *In* Loke YW, Whyte A (eds): Biology of Trophoblast. Amsterdam, Elsevier, 1983, p 69.
110. Benirschke K, Kaufmann P: Pathology of the Human Placenta. New York, Springer-Verlag, 2000, p 878.
111. Carter AM: Placental oxygen consumption. Part I: in vivo studies—a review. Placenta 21 Suppl A:S31, 2000.
112. Schneider H: Placental oxygen consumption. Part II: in vitro studies—a review. Placenta 21, Suppl A:S38, 2000.
113. Burton GJ, Skepper JN, Hempstock J, et al: A reappraisal of the contrasting morphological appearances of villous cytotrophoblast cells during early human pregnancy; evidence for both apoptosis and primary necrosis. Placenta 24:297, 2003.
114. Simpson RA, Mayhew TM, Barnes PR: From 13 weeks to term, the trophoblast of human placenta grows by the continuous recruitment of new proliferative units: a study of nuclear number using the disector. Placenta 13:501, 1992.
115. Mayhew TM, Leach L, McGee R, et al: Proliferation, differentiation and apoptosis in villous trophoblast at 13–41 weeks of gestation (including observations on annulate lamellae and nuclear pore complexes. Placenta 20:407, 1999.
116. Maruo T, Matsuo H, Murata K, et al: Gestational age-dependent dual action of epidermal growth factor on human placenta early in gestation. J Clin Endocrinol Metab 75:1362, 1992.
117. Furugori K, Kurauchi O, Itakura A, et al: Levels of hepatocyte growth factor and its messenger ribonucleic acid in uncomplicated pregnancies and those complicated by preeclampsia. J Clin Endocrinol Metab 82:2726, 1997.
118. Uehara Y, Minowa O, Mori C, et al: Placental defect and embryonic lethality in mice lacking hepatocyte growth factor/scatter factor. Nature 373:702, 1995.
119. Fox H: The villous cytotrophoblast as an index of placental ischaemia. J Obstet Gynaecol Br Commonw 71:885, 1964.
120. Huppertz B, Kingdom J, Caniggia I, et al: Hypoxia favours necrotic versus apoptotic shedding of placental syncytiotrophoblast into the maternal circulation. Placenta 24:181, 2003.
121. Ali KZM: Stereological study of the effect of altitude on the trophoblast cell populations of human term placental villi. Placenta 18:447, 1997.
122. Kingdom JCP, Kaufmann P: Oxygen and placental villous development: origins of fetal hypoxia. Placenta 18:613, 1997.
123. Morrish DW, Dakour J, Li H: Functional regulation of human trophoblast differentiation. J Reprod Immunol 39:179, 1998.
124. Dakour J, Li H, Chen H, et al: EGF promotes development of a differentiated trophoblast phenotype having c-myc and junB proto-oncogene activation. Placenta 20:119, 1999.
125. Yang M, Lei ZM, Rao CV: The central role of human chorionic gonadotropin in the formation of human placental syncytium. Endocrinology 144:1108, 2003.
126. Cronier L, Bastide B, Herve JC, et al: Gap junctional communication during human trophoblast differentiation: influence of human chorionic gonadotropin. Endocrinology 135:402, 1994.
127. Frendo JL, Cronier L, Bertin G, et al: Involvement of connexin 43 in human trophoblast cell fusion and differentiation. J Cell Sci 116:3413, 2003.
128. Lyden TW, Ng AK, Rote NS: Modulation of phosphatidylserine epitope expression by BeWo cells during forskolin treatment. Placenta 14:177, 1993.
129. Das M, Xu B, Lin L, et al: Phosphatidylserine efflux and intercellular fusion in a BeWo model of human villous cytotrophoblast. Placenta 25:396, 2004.

130. Huppertz B, Tews DS, Kaufmann P: Apoptosis and syncytial fusion in human placental trophoblast and skeletal muscle. Int Rev Cytol 205:215, 2001.
131. Black S, Kadyrov M, Kaufmann P, et al: Syncytial fusion of human trophoblast depends on caspase 8. Cell Death Differ 11:90, 2004.
132. Mi S, Lee X, Li X, et al: Syncytin is a captive retroviral envelope protein involved in human placental morphogenesis. Nature 403:785, 2000.
133. Frendo JL, Olivier D, Cheynet V, et al: Direct involvement of HERV-W Env glycoprotein in human trophoblast cell fusion and differentiation. Mol Cell Biol 23:3566, 2003.
134. Kudo Y, Boyd CA, Sargent IL, et al: Hypoxia alters expression and function of syncytin and its receptor during trophoblast cell fusion of human placental BeWo cells: implications for impaired trophoblast syncytialisation in pre-eclampsia. Biochim Biophys Acta 1638:63, 2003.
135. Jones CJP, Fox H: Placental changes in gestational diabetes. An ultastructural study. Obstet Gynecol 48:274, 1976.
136. Jones CJP, Fox H: An ultrastructural and ultrahistochemical study of the human placenta in maternal pre-eclampsia. Placenta 1:61, 1980.
137. Burton GJ: On the varied appearances of the human placental villous surface visualised by scanning electron microscopy. Scanning Microsc 4:501, 1990.
138. Burton GJ, Watson AL: The structure of the human placenta: implications for initiating and defending against viral infections. Rev Med Virol 7:219, 1997.
139. Nelson DM: Apoptotic changes occur in syncytiotrophoblast of human placental villi where fibrin type fibrinoid is deposited at discontinuities in the villous trophoblast. Placenta 17:387, 1996.
140. Nelson DM, Crouch EC, Curran EM, et al: Trophoblast interaction with fibrin matrix. Epithelialization of perivillous fibrin deposits as a mechanism for villous repair in the human placenta. Am J Pathol 136:855, 1990.
141. Edwards D, Jones CJP, Sibley CP, et al: Paracellular permeability pathways in the human placenta: a quantitative and morphological study of maternal-fetal transfer of horseradish peroxidase. Placenta 14:63, 1993.
142. Burton GJ, O'Shea S, Rostron T, et al: Significance of placental damage in vertical transmission of human immunodeficiency virus. J Med Virol 50:237, 1996.
143. Leung DN, Smith SC, To KF, et al: Increased placental apoptosis in pregnancies complicated by preeclampsia. Am J Obstet Gynecol 184:1249, 2001.
144. Huppertz B, Kaufmann P, Kingdom J: Trophoblast turnover in health and disease. Fetal and Maternal Med Rev 13:103, 2002.
145. Hung T-H, Skepper JN, Charnock-Jones DS, et al: Hypoxia/reoxygenation: a potent inducer of apoptotic changes in the human placenta and possible etiological factor in preeclampsia. Circ Res 90:1274, 2002.
146. Redman CWG, Sargent IL: Placental debris, oxidative stress and pre-eclampsia. Placenta 21:597, 2000.
147. Palmer ME, Watson AL, Burton GJ: Morphological analysis of degeneration and regeneration of syncytiotrophoblast in first trimester villi during organ culture. Hum Reprod 12:379, 1997.
148. Siman CM, Sibley CP, Jones CJ, et al: The functional regeneration of syncytiotrophoblast in cultured explants of term placenta. Am J Physiol Regul Integr Comp Physiol 280:R1116, 2001,
149. Charnock Jones DS, Kaufmann P, Mayhew TM: Aspects of human fetoplacental vasculogenesis and angiogenesis. I. Molecular recognition. Placenta 25:103, 2004.
150. Kaufmann P, Mayhew TM, Charnock Jones DS: Aspects of human fetoplacental vasculogenesis and angiogenesis. II. Changes during normal pregnancy. Placenta 114, 2004.
151. Dempsey EW: The development of capillaries in the villi of early human placentas. Am J Anat 134:221, 1972.
152. Corner GW: A well-preserved human embryo of 10 somites. Contrib Embryol 20:81, 1929.
153. Kaufmann P, Bruns U, Leiser R, et al: The fetal vascularisation of term placental villi. II. Intermediate and terminal villi. Anat Embryol 173:203, 1985.
154. Burton GJ, Tham SW: The formation of vasculo-syncytial membranes in the human placenta. J Dev Physiol 18:43, 1992.
155. Fox H: The pattern of villous variability in the normal placenta. J Obstet Gynaecol Br Commonw 71:749, 1964.
156. Reshetnikova OS, Burton GJ, Milovanov AP: Effects of hypobaric hypoxia on the feto-placental unit; the morphometric diffusing capacity of the villous membrane at high altitude. Am J Obstet Gynecol 171:1560, 1994.
157. Burton GJ, Palmer ME, Dalton KJ: Morphometric differences between the placental vasculature of nonsmokers, smokers and ex-smokers. Br J Obstet Gynaecol 96:907, 1989.
158. Marx GF, Patel S, Berman JA, et al: Umbilical blood flow velocity waveforms in different maternal positions and with epidural analgesia. Obstet Gynaecol 68:61, 1986.
159. van Katwijk C, Wladimiroff JW: Effect of maternal posture on the umbilical artery flow velocity waveform. Ultrasound Med Biol 17:683, 1991.
160. Mayhew TM, Charnock Jones DS, Kaufmann P: Aspects of human fetoplacental vasculogenesis and angiogenesis. III. Changes in complicated pregnancies. Placenta 25:127, 2004.
161. Ali KZM, Burton GJ, Morad N, et al: Does hypercapillarization influence the branching pattern of terminal villi in the human placenta at high altitude? Placenta 17:677, 1996.
162. Jauniaux E, Moscoso JG: Morphology and significance of the human yolk sac. *In* Barnea ER, Hustin J, Jauniaux E (eds): The First Twelve Weeks of Gestation. Berlin, Springer Verlag, 1992, p 192.
163. Gitlin D, Perricelli A: Synthesis of serum albumin, prealbumin, alphafetoprotein, alpha1-antitrypsin and transferrin by the human yolk sac. Nature 228:995, 1970.
164. Jauniaux E, Lees C, Jurkovic D, et al: Transfer of inulin across the first-trimester human placenta. Am J Obstet Gynecol 176:33, 1997.
165. Jauniaux E, Gulbis B: Fluid compartments of the embryonic environment. Hum Reprod Update 6:268, 2000.
166. Jauniaux E, Gulbis B, Jurkovic D, et al: Protein and steroid levels in embryonic cavities in early human pregnancy. Hum Reprod 8:782, 1993.
167. Gulbis B, Jauniaux E, Cotton F, et al: Protein and enzyme patterns in the fluid cavities of the first trimester gestational sac: relevance to the absorptive role of the secondary yolk sac. Mol Hum Reprod 4:857, 1998.
168. Jauniaux E, Cindrova-Davies T, Johns J, et al: Distribution and transfer pathways of antioxidant molecules inside the first trimester human gestational sac. J Clin Endocrinol Metab 89:1452, 2004.
169. Gosden RG, Byatt-Smith JG: Oxygen concentration gradient across the ovarian follicular epithelium: model, predictions and implications. Hum Reprod 1:65, 1986.
170. Fischer B, Kunzel W, Kleinstein J, et al: Oxygen tension in follicular fluid falls with oocyte maturation. Eur J Obstet Gynecol Reprod Biol 43:39, 1992.
171. Burton GJ, Hempstock J, Jauniaux E: Oxygen, early embryonic metabolism and free radical-mediated embryopathies. Reproductive BioMed Online 6:84, 2003.
172. Firth JA, Leach L: Not trophoblast alone: a review of the contribution of the fetal microvasculature to transplacental exchange. Placenta 17:89, 1996.
173. Wang S, Kallichanda N, Song W, et al: Expression of aquaporin-8 in human placenta and chorioamniotic membranes: evidence of molecular mechanism for intramembranous amniotic fluid resorption. Am J Obstet Gynecol 185:1226, 2001.
174. Damiano A, Zotta E, Goldstein J, et al: Water channel proteins AQP3 and AQP9 are present in syncytiotrophoblast of human term placenta. Placenta 22:776, 2001.
175. Barcroft LC, Offenberg H, Thomsen P, et al: Aquaporin proteins in murine trophectoderm mediate transepithelial water movements during cavitation. Dev Biol 256:342, 2003.
176. Nicolini U, Fisk NM, Talbert DG, et al: Intrauterine manometry: technique and application to fetal pathology. Prenat Diagn 9:243, 1989.
177. Stulc J, Stulcova B: Asymmetrical transfer of inert hydrophilic solutes across rat placenta. Am J Physiol 265:R670, 1993.
178. Stulc J, Stulcova B: Effect of NaCl load administered to the fetus on the bidirectional movement of 51Cr-EDTA across rat placenta. Am J Physiol 270:R984, 1996.
179. Atkinson DE, Boyd RDH, Sibley CP: Placental Transfer. *In* Neill JD (ed): Knobil & Neill's Physiology of Reproduction. Amsterdam, Elsevier, 2006, p 2787.

180. Bain MD, Copas DK, Taylor A, et al: Permeability of the human placenta in vivo to four non-metabolized hydrophilic molecules. J Physiol 431:505, 1990.
181. Brownbill P, Edwards D, Jones C, et al: Mechanisms of alphafetoprotein transfer in the perfused human placental cotyledon from uncomplicated pregnancy. J Clin Invest 96:2220, 1995.
182. Kaufmann P, Schroder H, Leichtweiss HP: Fluid shift across the placenta: II. Fetomaternal transfer of horseradish peroxidase in the guinea pig. Placenta 3:339, 1982.
183. Stulc J, Svihovec J, Drabkova J, et al: Electrical potential difference across the mid-term human placenta. Acta Obstet Gynecol Scand 57:125, 1978.
184. Mellor DJ, Cockburn F, Lees MM, et al: Distribution of ions and electrical potential differences between mother and fetus in the human at term. J Obstet Gynaecol Br Commonw 76:993, 1969.
185. Ward S, Jauniaux E, Shannon C, et al: Electrical potential difference between exocelomic fluid and maternal blood in early pregnancy. Am J Physiol 274:R1492, 1998.
186. Greenwood SL, Boyd RD, Sibley CP: Transtrophoblast and microvillus membrane potential difference in mature intermediate human placental villi. Am J Physiol 265:C460, 1993.
187. Birdsey TJ, Boyd RD, Sibley CP, et al: Microvillous membrane potential (Em) in villi from first trimester human placenta: comparison to Em at term. Am J Physiol 273:R1519, 1997.
188. Mahendran D, Byrne S, Donnai P, et al: Na^+ transport, H^+ concentration gradient dissipation, and system A amino acid transporter activity in purified microvillous plasma membrane isolated from first-trimester human placenta: comparison with the term microvillous membrane. Am J Obstet Gynecol 171:1534, 1994.
189. Ayuk PT, Sibley CP, Donnai P, et al: Development and polarization of cationic amino acid transporters and regulators in the human placenta. Am J Physiol Cell Physiol 278:C1162, 2000.
190. Ayuk PT, Theophanous D, D'Souza SW, et al: L-arginine transport by the microvillous plasma membrane of the syncytiotrophoblast from human placenta in relation to nitric oxide production: effects of gestation, preeclampsia, and intrauterine growth restriction. J Clin Endocrinol Metab 87:747, 2002.
191. Jansson T, Wennergren M, Illsley NP: Glucose transporter protein expression in human placenta throughout gestation and in intrauterine growth retardation. J Clin Endocrinol Metab 77:1554, 1993.
192. Hughes JL, Doughty IM, Glazier JD, et al: Activity and expression of the Na(+)/H(+) exchanger in the microvillous plasma membrane of the syncytiotrophoblast in relation to gestation and small for gestational age birth. Pediatr Res 48:652, 2000.
193. Powell TL, Illsley NP: A novel technique for studying cellular function in human placenta: gestational changes in intracellular pH regulation. Placenta 17:661, 1996.
194. Doughty IM, Glazier JD, Powell TL, et al: Chloride transport across syncytiotrophoblast microvillous membrane of first trimester human placenta. Pediatr Res 44:226, 1998.
195. Reik W, Constancia M, Fowden A, et al: Regulation of supply and demand for maternal nutrients in mammals by imprinted genes. J Physiol 547:35, 2003.
196. Sibley CP, Boyd RDH: Mechanisms of transfer across the human placenta. *In* Polin RA, Fox WW, Abman SH (eds) Fetal and Neonatal Physiology. Philadelphia, Saunders, 2004, p 111.
197. Sibley CP, Turner MA, Cetin I, et al: Placental phenotypes of intrauterine growth. Ped Res 58:827, 2005.
198. Strauss JF, 3rd, Christenson LK, Devoto L, et al: Providing progesterone for pregnancy: control of cholesterol flux to the side-chain cleavage system. J Reprod Fertil Suppl 55:3, 2000.
199. Tuckey RC: Progesterone synthesis by the human placenta. Placenta 26:273, 2005.
200. Tuckey RC, Kostadinovic Z, Cameron KJ: Cytochrome P-450scc activity and substrate supply in human placental trophoblasts. Mol Cell Endocrinol 105:103, 1994.
201. Gunasegaram R, Peh KL, Chew PC, et al: In vitro C-20, 22 desmolase regulation of pregnenolone supply in first trimester human placenta. Acta Endocrinol 90:185, 1979.
202. Simpson ER, Miller DA: Cholesterol side-chain cleavage, cytochrome P450, and iron-sulfur protein in human placental mitochondria. Arch Biochem Biophys 190:800, 1978.
203. Winkel CA, Snyder JM, MacDonald PC, et al: Regulation of cholesterol and progesterone synthesis in human placental cells in culture by serum lipoproteins. Endocrinology 106:1054, 1980.
204. Inkster SE, Brodie AM: Immunocytochemical studies of aromatase in early and full-term human placental tissues: comparison with biochemical assays. Biol Reprod 41:889, 1989.
205. Casey ML, MacDonald PC: Placental Endocrinology. *In* Redman CWG, Sargent IL, Starkey PM (eds): The Human Placenta. A Guide for Clinicians and Scientists. Oxford, Blackwells, 1993, p 237.
206. Mendelson CR, Jiang B, Shelton JM, et al: Transcriptional regulation of aromatase in placenta and ovary. J Steroid Biochem Mol Biol 95:25, 2005.
207. Fiddes JC, Goodman HM: Isolation, cloning and sequence analysis of the cDNA for the α-subunit of the human chorionic gonadotropin. Nature 281:351, 1979.
208. Maston GA, Ruvolo M: Chorionic gonadotropin has a recent origin within primates and an evolutionary history of selection. Mol Biol Evol 19:320, 2002.
209. Bo M, Boime I: Identification of the transcriptionally active genes of the chorionic gonadotropin beta gene cluster in vivo. J Biol Chem 267:3179, 1992.
210. Graham MY, Otani T, Boime I, et al: Cosmid mapping of the human chorionic gonadotropin β genes by field-invasion gel electrophoresis. Nucl Acids Res 15:4437, 1987.
211. Xing Y, Williams C, Campbell RK, et al: Threading a glycosylated protein loop through a protein hole: implications for combination of human chorionic gonadotropin subunits. Protein Sci 10:226, 2001.
212. Nagy AM, Glinoer D, Picelli G, et al: Total amounts of circulating human chorionic gonadotrophin alpha and beta subunits can be assessed throughout human pregnancy using immunoradiometric assays calibrated with the unaltered and thermally dissociated heterodimer. J Endocrinol 140:513, 1994.
213. Jameson JL, Hollenberg AN: Regulation of chorionic gonadotropin gene expression. Endocrine Rev 14:203, 1993.
214. Licht P, Losch A, Dittrich R, et al: Novel insights into human endometrial paracrinology and embryo-maternal communication by intrauterine microdialysis. Hum Reprod Update 4:532, 1998.
215. Rao CV: The beginning of a new era in reproductive biology and medicine: expression of low levels of functional luteinizing hormone/human chorionic gonadotropin receptors in nongonadal tissues. J Physiol Pharmacol 47:41, 1996.
216. Banerjee S, Smallwood A, Chambers AE, et al: A link between high serum levels of human chorionic gonadotrophin and chorionic expression of its mature functional receptor (LHCGR) in Down's syndrome pregnancies. Reprod Biol Endocrinol 3:25, 2005.
217. Kovalevskaya G, Birken S, Kakuma T, et al: Early pregnancy human chorionic gonadotropin (hCG) isoforms measured by an immunometric assay for choriocarcinoma-like hCG. J Endocrinol 161:99, 1999.
218. Kovalevskaya G, Birken S, Kakuma T, et al: Differential expression of human chorionic gonadotropin (hCG) glycosylation isoforms in failing and continuing pregnancies: preliminary characterization of the hyperglycosylated hCG epitope. J Endocrinol 172:497, 2002.
219. Shenhav S, Gemer O, Sassoon E, et al: Mid-trimester triple test levels in early and late onset severe pre-eclampsia. Prenat Diag 22:579, 2002.
220. Lambot N, Lebrun P, Delporte C, et al: Effect of IPs, cAMP, and cGMP on the hPL and hCG secretion from human term placenta. Mol Cell Endocrinol 243:80, 2005.
221. Lacroix MC, Guibourdenche J, Frendo JL, et al: Human placental growth hormone–a review. Placenta 23 Suppl A:S87, 2002.
222. Frankenne F, Closset J, Gomez F, et al: The physiology of growth hormones (GHs) in pregnant women and partial characterization of the placental GH variant. J Clin Endocrinol Metab 66:1171, 1988.
223. Mirlesse V, Frankenne F, Alsat E, et al: Placental growth hormone levels in normal pregnancy and in pregnancies with intrauterine growth retardation. Pediatr Res 34:439, 1993.
224. Mahendran D, Donnai P, Glazier JD, et al: Amino acid (system A) transporter activity in microvillous membrane vesicles from

the placentas of appropriate and small for gestational age babies. Pediatr Res 34:661, 1993.
225. Glazier JD, Cetin I, Perugino G, et al: Association between the activity of the system A amino acid transporter in the microvillous plasma membrane of the human placenta and severity of fetal compromise in intrauterine growth restriction. Pediatr Res 42:514, 1997.
226. Jansson T, Ylven K, Wennergren M, et al: Glucose transport and system A activity in syncytiotrophoblast microvillous and basal plasma membranes in intrauterine growth restriction. Placenta 23:392, 2002.
227. Jansson T, Scholtbach V, Powell TL: Placental transport of leucine and lysine is reduced in intrauterine growth restriction. Pediatr Res 44:532, 1998.
228. Norberg S, Powell TL, Jansson T: Intrauterine growth restriction is associated with a reduced activity of placental taurine transporters. Pediatr Res 44:233, 1998.
229. Roos S, Powell TL, Jansson T: Human placental taurine transporter in uncomplicated and IUGR pregnancies: cellular localization, protein expression and regulation. Am J Physiol Regul Integr Comp Physiol 287:R886, 2004.
230. Johansson M, Karlsson L, Wennergren M, et al: Activity and protein expression of Na+/K+ ATPase are reduced in microvillous syncytiotrophoblast plasma membranes isolated from pregnancies complicated by intrauterine growth restriction. J Clin Endocrinol Metab 88:2831, 2003.
231. Strid H, Bucht E, Jansson T, et al: ATP dependent Ca^{2+} transport across basal membrane of human syncytiotrophoblast in pregnancies complicated by intrauterine growth restriction or diabetes. Placenta 24:445, 2003.
232. Johansson M, Glazier JD, Sibley CP, et al: Activity and protein expression of the Na^+/H^+ exchanger is reduced in syncytiotrophoblast microvillous plasma membranes isolated from preterm intrauterine growth restriction pregnancies. J Clin Endocrinol Metab 87:5686, 2002.
233. Settle P, Mynett K, Speake P, et al: Polarized lactate transporter activity and expression in the syncytiotrophoblast of the term human placenta. Placenta 25:496, 2004.

Fetal Physiology

MICHAEL G. ROSS, M. GORE ERVIN, AND DONALD NOVAK

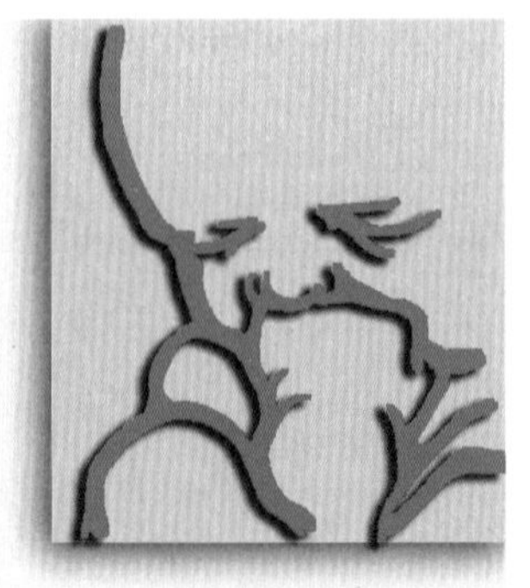

CHAPTER 2

KEY ABBREVIATIONS

2,3-Diphosphoglycerate	2,3-DPG
α-Melanocyte-stimulating hormone	α-MSH
Adenosine triphosphate	ATP
Adrenocorticotropic hormone	ACTH
Angiotension-converting enzyme	ACE
Angiotension II	AII
Arginine vasopressin	AVP
Atrial natriuretic factor	ANF
Carbon dioxide	CO_2
Corticotropin-like intermediate lobe peptide	CLIP
Epidermal growth factor	EGF
Epidermal growth factor receptor	EGF-R
Glomerular filtration rate	GFR
Glucose transporter	GLUT
Human leukocyte antigens	HLA
Immunoglobulin G	IgG
Insulin-like growth factor	IGF
Killer cell immunoglobulin-like receptors	KIR
Low-density lipoproteins	LDLs
Oxygen	O_2
T-helper type 1	Th1
Thyrotropin-releasing hormone	TRH
Thyroid-stimulating hormone	TSH
Thyroxine	T_4
Triiodothyronine	T_3
Uterine natural killer cells	uNK
Vascular endothelial growth factor	VEGF

In obstetric practice, recognition of normal fetal growth, development, and behavior most often allows a conservative management plan. However, abnormalities may require clinical strategies for fetal assessment or intervention, or both. The basic concepts of placental and fetal physiology provide the building blocks necessary for understanding pathophysiology, and thus mechanisms of disease. Throughout this chapter, we have reviewed the essential tenets of fetal physiology and the relevant placental physiology, while relating this information to normal and abnormal clinical conditions.

Much of our knowledge of placental and fetal physiology derives from studies made in mammals other than humans. We have attempted to include only those observations reasonably applicable to the human placenta and fetus and, in most instances, have not detailed the species from which the data were obtained. Should questions arise regarding the species studied, the reader is referred to the extensive bibliography.

PLACENTAL PHYSIOLOGY

The placenta provides the fetus with essential nutrients, water and oxygen (O_2) and a route for clearance of fetal excretory products, and produces a vast array of protein and steroid hormones and factors essential to the maintenance of pregnancy. As a result, it has become increasingly clear that the placenta, far from being a passive conduit, plays a key role in the control of fetal growth.

Placental Metabolism and Growth

Anatomic and histologic aspects of placental growth are detailed in Chapter 1. This section focuses on the physiology of placental metabolism and growth, and its influence on the fetus.

The critical function of the placenta is illustrated by its high metabolic demands. For example, placental O_2 consumption equals that of the fetus, and exceeds the fetal rate when expressed on a weight basis (10 ml/min/kg).[1–3] Between 22 and 36 weeks of gestation, the number of trophoblast nuclei[4] increases four- to fivefold, placing increased metabolic demands on the placenta.[5] Glucose is the principal substrate for oxidative metabolism by placental tissue.[2,6] Of the total glucose leaving the maternal compartment to nourish the uterus and its contents, placental consumption may represent up to 70 percent.[2,7,8] In addition, a significant fraction of placental glucose uptake derives from the fetal circulation[9] and reflects placental oxidative metabolism. Although one third of placental glucose may be converted to the three carbon sugar lactate,[2,4,6,10] placental metabolism is not anaerobic. Instead, placental lactate is thought to be a fetal energetic substrate. The factors regulating short-term changes in placental O_2 and glucose consumption are at present incompletely understood.

The regulation of placental growth is an area of incomplete understanding, although dramatic advances have recently been made in the study of genes as they contribute to placental growth and differentiation. Particular contributions have been made through the use of genetic "knock-out" models.[11,12] Increases in trophoblast numbers exceed increases in fetal placental capillary endothelial cells during the second half of gestation.[4] Whether trophoblast cell proliferation is the primary event or is dependent on endothelial cell growth is not known. Normal term placental weight averages 450 g, representing approximately one seventh, (one sixth with cord and membranes) of fetal weight. Large-appearing placentas, either ultrasonographically or at delivery, may prompt investigation into possible etiologies. Several clinical observations suggest a link between decreased tissue O_2 content and increased placental growth. Thus, increased placental size is associated with maternal anemia,[13–15] fetal anemia associated with erythrocyte isoimmunization, and hydrops fetalis secondary to fetal α-thalassemia with Bart's hemoglobin. The association of a large placenta with maternal diabetes mellitus also has been recognized, possibly a result of insulin-stimulated mitogenic activity or enhanced angiogenesis.[16,17] Enlarged placentas are also found in cloned animals, presumably because of defects in the expression of specific imprinted genes, as well as in the placentas of animals in whom specific gene products have been deleted.[18–21] In humans, increased ratio of placental size to fetal weight is associated with increased morbidity, both in the neonatal period and subsequently.[22,23]

Receptors for growth-promoting peptide hormones (factors) characterized in placental tissue[24] include, among many, the insulin receptor,[25–30] receptors for insulin-like growth factors I and II (IGF-I, IGF-II), epidermal growth factor (EGF),[31–35] leptin, placental growth factor, and a variety of cytokines and chemokines, each of which has been shown to play an important role in fetal/placental development.[36–45] IGF-I and IGF-II are polypeptides with a high degree of homology to human proinsulin.[46] Both IGF-I and IGF-II circulate bound to carrier proteins and are 50 times more potent than insulin in stimulating cell growth.[46] EGF increases RNA and DNA synthesis and cell multiplication in a wide variety of cell types.[24] The observation that placental EGF binding is increased at term, relative to 8 to 18 weeks' gestation, led to a suggested role of EGF in placental growth regulation.[32] The integrated physiologic role of these and other potential placental growth factors[47–49] in regulating placental growth remains to be fully defined. However, the development of null-mutation mouse models for IGF-I, IGF-II, IGF-I receptor and IGF-II receptor as well as for the EGF receptor have provided evidence in this regard.[50–55] Specifically, the EGF receptor appears important in placental development, as does IGF-II. Knockout of IGF-II results in diminished placental size, whereas deletion of the IGF-II receptor results in an increase in placental size. IGF-I does not appear to impact placental growth.

Placental Transfer

General Considerations

In the hemochorial human placenta, maternal blood and solutes are separated from fetal blood by trophoblastic tissue and fetal endothelial cells. Thus, transit from the maternal intervillous space to the fetal capillary lumen takes place across a number of cellular structures (Fig. 2-1). The first step is transport across the microvillus plasma membrane of the syncytiotrophoblast. Because there are no lateral intercellular spaces in the syncytiotrophoblast, all solutes first interact with the placenta at this plasma membrane. The basal (fetal) syncytiotrophoblast membrane represents an additional step in the transport process. The discontinuous nature of the cytotrophoblast cell layer in later gestation suggests that this layer should not limit maternal-to-fetal transfer. However, the presence of anionic sites on the glycoprotein backbone comprising the basal lamina[56] potentially may influence movement of large charged molecules. The fetal capillary endothelial cell imposes two additional plasma membrane surfaces.[57]

A number of specific mechanisms allow transit of the placental membranes, including passive diffusion, facilitated diffusion, active transport, and endocytosis/exocytosis. Solutes lacking specialized transport mechanisms cross by extracellular or transcellular diffusional transport pathways, with permeability determined by size, lipid solubility, ionic charge and maternal serum protein binding. Lipid insoluble (hydrophilic) substances, which cross the trophoblast through extracellular pores, are restricted by molecular size in relation to the extracellular pore size. Up to a molecular weight of at least 5,000 daltons, placental permeability is proportional to the free diffusion of a molecule in water.[58,59] For example, urea (MW = 60) is at least 1,000 times more permeable than inulin (MW = 5,000).[58] Thus, transfer of small solutes will be governed primarily by the maternal-fetal concentration gradient. Because transfer is relatively slow, and the extracellular pore surface area is limited, transfer of these molecules is referred to as "diffusion-limited." In animal models, food restriction enhances the barrier to diffusion, as does placental IGF-II deficiency.[60,61] Con-

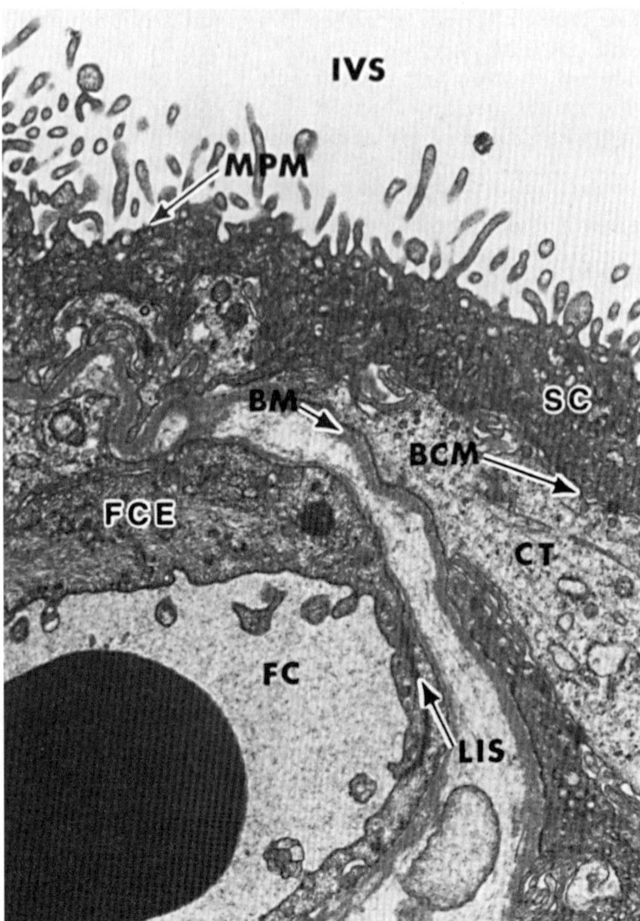

Figure 2-1. Electron micrograph of human placenta demonstrating the cellular and extracellular components with which solutes must interact in moving from the maternal intervillous space (IVS) to the lumen of the fetal capillary (FC). BCM, basal cell membrane of the syncytiotrophoblast; BM, basement membrane; CT, cytotrophoblast cell; FCE, fetal capillary endothelial cell; LIS, lateral intercellular space of fetal endothelial cell; MPM, microvillous plasma membrane of the syncytiotrophoblast; SC, syncytiotrophoblast. (Courtesy of Kent L. Thornburg, PhD, Department of Physiology, Oregon Health Sciences University, Portland, OR.)

versely, highly lipid soluble (lipophilic) substances diffuse readily through the trophoblastic membrane. Thus molecular weight is relatively less important in restricting diffusion. Ethanol, a molecule similar in size to urea, is 500 times more lipid soluble and 10 times more permeable.[62] Because the entire trophoblast surface is available for diffusion and the permeability is high, transfer rates for lipophilic substances to the fetus are limited primarily by placental intervillous and umbilical blood flows ("flow limited"). Both facilitated diffusion and active transport use carrier-mediated transport systems, with the latter requiring energy, either directly or indirectly linked with ionic pump mechanisms. Carrier transport systems are specifically limited to unique classes of molecules (i.e., neutral amino acids). In addition, substances may traverse the placenta through endocytosis (invagination of the cell membrane to form an intracellular vesicle containing extracellular fluids) and exocytosis (release of the vesicle to the extracellular space).

Transfer of Individual Solutes

Respiratory Gases

The exchange or transfer of the primary respiratory gases, O_2 and carbon dioxide (CO_2), is likely "flow limited."[63] Thus, the driving force for placental gas exchange is the partial pressure gradient between the maternal and fetal circulations. Early in gestation, the human embryo develops in a low O_2 environment.[64,65] Such an environment appears to be necessary and is associated with the presence of O_2-sensitive regulatory genes and gene products.[66] After approximately gestation week 10, the placenta becomes important as a respiratory organ. Indeed, estimates of human placental diffusing capacities[67] would predict that the placental efficiency of respiratory gas exchange will allow equilibrium of O_2 and CO_2 tensions at the maternal intervillous space and fetal capillary. However, this prediction varies from the observed 10–mm Hg difference in O_2 tension between the umbilical and uterine veins[68,69] and between the umbilical vein and intervillous space.[70] In addition, even though CO_2 is much more soluble than O_2 in water and tissues and diffuses more readily than O_2, the Pco_2 difference from umbilical to uterine vein is small (3 mm Hg).[71] Po_2 differences could be explained by areas of uneven distribution of maternal-to-fetal blood flows or shunting, limiting fetal and maternal blood exchange, a process that, as in other respiratory organs (i.e., lungs), may be an active one.[72] The most important contribution, however, is likely the high metabolic rate of the placental tissues themselves. Thus, trophoblast cell O_2 consumption and CO_2 production lower umbilical vein O_2 tension and increase uterine vein CO_2 tension to a greater degree than could be explained by an inert barrier for respiratory gas transfer.

The arteriovenous difference in the uterine circulation (and venoarterial difference in the umbilical circulation) widens during periods of lowered blood flow. Proportionate O_2 uptake increases and O_2 consumption remains unchanged over a fairly wide range of blood flows.[73] Thus, both uterine and umbilical blood flows can fall significantly without decreasing fetal O_2 consumption.[74–76] Conversely, unilateral umbilical artery occlusion is associated with significant fetal effects.[77]

CO_2 is carried in the fetal blood both as dissolved CO_2 and as bicarbonate. Owing to its charged nature, fetal-to-maternal bicarbonate transfer is limited. However, CO_2 likely diffuses from fetus to mother in its molecular form, and $[HCO_3^-]$ does not contribute significantly to fetal CO_2 elimination.[78]

Glucose

Placental permeability for D-glucose is at least 50 times the value predicted on the basis of size and lipid solubility.[79] Thus, specialized transport mechanisms must be available on both the microvillous and basal membranes. Membrane proteins facilitating the translocation of molecules across cell membranes are termed transporters. The human placental glucose transporter, originally identified as an approximately 55,000 MW component of the microvillous membrane,[80,81] has subsequently been identified as GLUT1,[82,83] a sodium-independent transporter, as compared with the sodium-dependent transporters found in adult kidney[84] and intestine.[85,86] This transporter, in contrast to that found in human adipocytes (GLUT4)[87–89] is not insulin sensitive.[90,91] The placental D-glucose transporter is saturable at high substrate concentrations; 50 percent saturation is observed at glucose levels of approximately 5 mM (90 mg/dl).[81] Thus, glucose transfer from mother to fetus is not linear, and transfer rates decrease as maternal glucose concentration increases. This effect is reflected in fetal blood glucose levels following maternal sugar loading.[92] Modification of transporter expression within the placenta also occurs in response to maternal diabetes. In this setting, GLUT1 expression is thought to increase on the basolateral membrane, while holding constant on the maternal-facing microvillous membrane.[93] Alterations in transporter expression may also depend on gestational stage, as well as maternal nutrition/placental blood flow.[94,95] A second transporter, GLUT3, has also been noted in the fetal-facing placental endothelium. Its presence within the syncytiotrophoblast remains controversial.[96–98]

Amino acid concentrations are higher in fetal umbilical cord blood than in maternal blood.[99] Like monosaccharides, amino acids enter and exit the syncytiotrophoblast through transport-specific membrane proteins. These transport proteins allow amino acids to be transported against a concentration gradient into the placenta, and subsequently, in most cases, into the fetal circulation. Thus, amino acid transport is considered to be a two-step phenomenon.

Multiple systems mediate neutral, anionic, and cationic amino acid transport into the syncytiotrophoblast. These include both sodium-dependent and sodium-independent transporters. Amino acid entry is, in many cases, coupled to sodium in cotransport systems located at the microvillous membrane facing the maternal intervillous space.[100,101] As long as an inwardly directed sodium gradient is maintained, trophoblast cell amino acid concentrations will exceed maternal blood levels. The sodium gradient is maintained by Na^+-K^+ATPase located on the basal or fetal side of the syncytiotrophoblast.[102] In addition, high trophoblast levels of amino acids transported by sodium-dependent transporters can "drive" uptake of other amino acids through transporters, which function as "exchangers." Examples of these include System ASC and System y^+L.[103–105] Still other transporters function in sodium-independent fashion. Individual amino acids may be transported by single or multiple transport proteins. Transport systems that have been identified in human placenta are defined in Table 2-1 and a general schema may be found in Figure 2-2.

System A, which is responsible for the transport of neutral amino acids with short polar or linear side chains, is a sodium-dependent transport activity localized on both the microvillous and basolateral membranes of the human placenta.[106,107] Other sodium-dependent transport activities localized to the microvillous membrane include that for β-amino acids such as taurine,[108] as well as perhaps glycine transport through System GLY.[109] Sodium-independent transporters mediating neutral amino acid transfer on the microvillous membrane include System L, which exhibits a high affinity for amino acids with bulky side chains such as leucine,[107] and perhaps Systems $b^{o,+}$ and y^+L, capable of transporting both neutral and cationic amino acids such as lysine and arginine.[110,111] Cationic amino acids are also transported by System y^+,[112,113] whereas anionic amino acids (glutamate, aspartate) are transported by the sodium-dependent System X_{AG}^-.[114,115] Basolateral membrane transport activities are similar (Table 2-1); however, a predominance of sodium-independent transporters and exchange (e.g., ASC) allows flow of amino acids down their concentration gradients into the fetal endothelium/fetal blood space. Comparatively little is known regarding transfer into and out of the fetal endothelium,[116] which, for the most part, abuts the syncytiotrophoblast basolateral membrane.

As the proteins responsible for amino acid transport have been identified, it has become clear that more than one protein may mediate each previously defined transport activity within a single tissue. Examples include EAAT 1-5, associated with sodium-dependent anionic amino acid transfer (System X_{AG}^-), CAT 1, 2, 2a, associated with System y^+ activity,[112,117,118] and SNAT1, 2 and 4, associated with System A activity. The reasons underlying

Table 2-1. Placental Neutral Amino Acid Transport Systems

TRANSPORT	A	L	ASC
Representative amino acids	Glycine, proline, alanine, serine, threonine, glutamine	Isoleucine, valine phenylalanine, alanine, serine, threonine, glutamine	Alanine, serine threonine, glutamine
Sodium dependency	+	–	+
Update increased by preincubation	+	–	+
Transinhibition	+	–	–

A, L, ASC: Placental transport systems. See text for details.
Data summarized from Enders et al.,[420] Smith et al.,[121] Smith and Depper,[122] and Steel et al.[421]

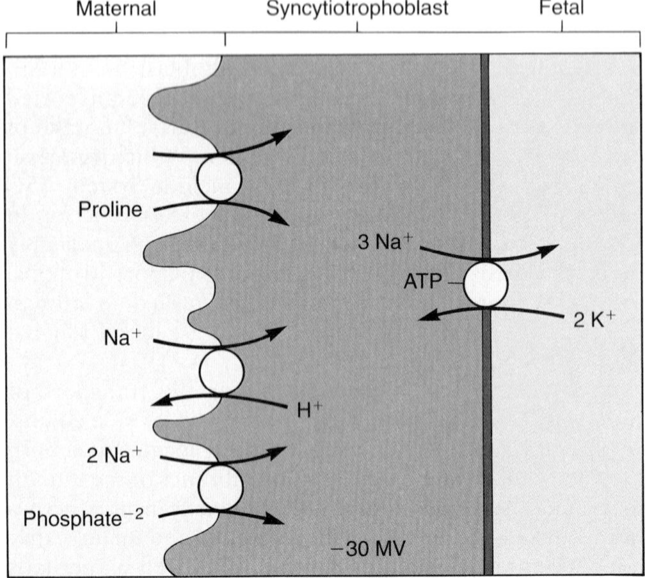

Figure 2-2. Pathways for sodium entry into syncytiotrophoblast and exit to the fetal circulation. (Data from Boyd et al.,[101] Whitsett and Wallick,[102] Lajeunesse and Brunette,[160] Balkovetz et al.,[161] and Bara et al.[166])

this duplication within the placenta, more pronounced than in any other organ with the possible exception of the central nervous system, is unclear. Certainly, as is the case for the anionic amino acid transporters EAAT 1-5, differential distribution within different tissue elements plays a role.[116] Differential regulation within single cell types is another likely reason.[119,120] In isolated trophoblast cells, System A activity is up-regulated by the absence of amino acids,[121–123] partially due to an increase in carrier affinity.[121] Conversely, increases in trophoblast amino acid concentrations may suppress uptake (trans-inhibition). These mechanisms serve to maintain trophoblast cell amino acid levels constant during fluctuations in maternal plasma concentrations. Insulin has also been shown to up-regulate this transport activity,[28,124,125] as has IGF-I. Placental System A activity is down-regulated in intrauterine growth restriction, both in the human and in animal models.[126,127] Conversely, System A activity is up-regulated in the placentas of diabetic mothers, perhaps contributing to the accelerated growth noted in these fetuses.[94] Mechanisms underlying these changes are as of yet unclear.

The coordination between placental/fetal metabolism and amino acid transfer is illustrated by the anionic amino acids glutamate and aspartate, which are poorly transported from mother to fetus.[128,129] Glutamate, however, is produced by the fetal liver from glutamine and then taken up across the basolateral membrane of the placenta through System X_{AG}^-. Within the placenta, the majority of glutamate is metabolized and used as an energy source.[128] As a result, System X_{AG}^- activity is of particular importance on the basolateral membrane, as is System ASC activity, responsible for the uptake of serine, also produced by the fetal liver, into the placenta.[130]

Lipids

Esterified fatty acids (triglycerides) are present in maternal serum as components of chylomicrons and very low-density lipoproteins. Before transfer across the placenta, lipoprotein lipase interacts with these particles, releasing free fatty acids, which, owing to their hydrophobic nature, are relatively insoluble in plasma and circulate bound to albumin. As a result, fatty acid transfer involves dissociation from maternal protein, subsequent association with placental proteins, first at the plasma membrane (FABPpm), then after transfer into the cell (through FAT/CD36 and FATP) with intracytoplasmic binding proteins.[131] Transfer out of the syncytiotrophoblast is thought to occur through interaction with FAT/CD36 and FATP, which are present at both the microvillous and basolateral placental membrane surfaces. Subsequently, interaction with fetal plasma proteins occurs.[132,133] The intracellular fate of transferred fatty acids is less clear. Stable isotope studies suggest differential retention/utilization by the placenta.[134] Recent data also document the presence of adipophilin, a lipid droplet-associated protein, within the human placenta.[135] Although precise interactions and mechanisms remain uncertain, it is clear that lipid uptake is of profound importance to fetal development. Targeted deletion of FABP4, found within the yolk sac placenta, results in fetal lethality.[136]

Early studies documented that placental fatty acid transfer increases logarithmically with decreasing chain length (C16 to C8) and then declines somewhat for C6 and C4.[137] More recent work, however, has clarified the fact that essential fatty acids are, in general, transferred more efficiently than are nonessential fatty acids.[138,139] Of these, docosahexanoic acid seems to be transferred more efficiently than arachidonic acid; oleic acid is transferred least efficiently.[139] Much as in the case of amino acids discussed above, the fetus is significantly enriched in long-chain polyunsaturated fatty acids as compared with the mother.[140] Such selectivity may also relate to the composition of triglycerides in maternal serum, because lipoprotein lipase preferentially cleaves fatty acids in the two positions. In general, fatty acids transferred to the fetus reflect maternal serum lipids and diet.[141] There is also evidence that the placental leptin, a hormone generally secreted by adipocytes, may promote maternal lipolysis, thus providing both placenta and fetus the means by which to ensure an adequate lipid supply.[142] Another possible mechanism by which lipids may be excreted from the placenta involves the synthesis and secretion of apolipoprotein (apo) B–containing lipoproteins.[143] The relative importance of this pathway in the human placenta is at present unclear. Placental uptake and excretion of cholesterol is discussed in the section on receptor-mediated endocytosis.

Water and Ions

Although water transfer across the placenta does not limit fetal water uptake during growth,[144] the factors regulating fetal water acquisition are poorly understood. Water transfer from mother to fetus is determined by a balance of osmotic, hydrostatic, and colloid osmotic forces at the placental interface. Calculation of osmotic pressure from individual solute concentrations is unreliable because osmotic pressure forces depend upon the membrane permeability to each solute. Thus, sodium and chloride, the principal plasma solutes, are relatively permeable across the placenta[145] and would not be expected to contribute important osmotic effects.[146] As a result, although human fetal plasma osmolality is equal to or greater than maternal plasma osmolality,[147,148] these measured values do not reflect the actual osmotic force on either side of the membranes. Coupled with findings that hydrostatic pressure may be greater in the umbilical vein than the intervillous space,[149,150] these data do not explain mechanisms for fetal water accumulation. Alternatively, colloid osmotic pressure differences[151] and active solute transport probably represent the main determinants of net water fluxes—approximately 20 ml/day.[152] It is likely, however, given the large (3.6 L/hr) flux of water between mother and fetus, that more active mechanisms, including perhaps controlled changes in end-vessel resistance, play a significant role.[153,154] In fact, water flux occurs through both transcellular and paracellular pathways. Water channels have been identified within the placenta, but their regulation and relative roles have not been discerned.[155–157]

In comparison to other epithelia, the specialized placental mechanisms for ion transport are incompletely understood.[158] Multiple mechanisms for sodium transport in syncytiotrophoblast membranes exist. The maternal facing microvillous membrane contains, at a minimum, multiple amino acid cotransporters,[159] a sodium phosphate cotransporter in which two sodium ions are transported with each phosphate radical,[160] a sodium-hydrogen ion antiport that exchanges one proton for each sodium ion entering the cell,[161] as well as other nutrient transporters.[162,163] In addition, both sodium and potassium channels have been described.[164,165] A membrane potential with the inside negative (−30 MV) would promote sodium entry from the intervillous space.[166] The fetus-directed basal side of the cell contains the Na,K-ATPase.[102] The microvillous or maternal facing trophoblast membrane has an anion exchanger (AE1)[167] that mediates chloride transit across this membrane, in association with Cl^- conductance pathways (channels), present in both the microvillous and basolateral membranes.[168,169] Paracellular pathways also play an important role. The integration and regulation of these various mechanisms for sodium and chloride transport from mother to fetus is not completely understood; there is accumulating evidence that mineralocorticoids may regulate placental sodium transfer.[170] Furthermore, sodium/hydrogen exchange, mediated by multiple members of the NHE family (NHE1-3), is regulated both over gestation and in response to intrauterine growth restriction,[171] as is expression of the sodium-potassium ATPase.[172]

Calcium

Calcium is an essential nutrient for the developing fetus. Ionized calcium levels are higher in fetal than in maternal blood.[147,173] Higher fetal calcium levels are due to a syncytiotrophoblast basal membrane adenosine triphosphate (ATP)–dependent Ca^{++} transport system[174] exhibiting high affinity (nanomolar range) for calcium.[175] Indeed, analogous to amino acid and sodium/hydrogen exchange proteins, multiple isoforms of the plasma membrane calcium ATPase (PMCA 1-4) are expressed within the placenta.[176] Sodium/calcium exchange proteins are also thought to play a role in extrusion of calcium from the trophoblast—again, multiple isoforms are expressed within the placenta. Calcium transport into the syncytiotrophoblast is mediated by at least one saturable transport process.[177,178] A variety of calcium channels have been identified; CaT1 and CaT2 are thought to play predominant roles in calcium uptake into the syncytiotrophoblast.[176] Intracellular calcium is bound by multiple calcium-binding proteins that have been identified within the placenta; these include CaBP9k, CaBP28k, CaBP57k, oncomodulin, S-100P, S-100alpha, and S-100beta.[179] Calcium transport across the placenta is increased by the calcium-dependent regulatory protein calmodulin[174]; transfer may be regulated by 1,25 dihydroxycholecalciferol, calcitonin, and parathyroid hormone.[158]

Receptor-Mediated Endocytosis/Exocytosis

Endocytosis, through the the clatharin-dependent endocytosis pathway, has long been known to occur within the placenta. Placental endocytosis plays a critical role in cell signaling (examples: insulin[180] and EGF receptors[45]), protein recycling (receptors, transporters), substrate transfer (low-density lipoprotein [LDL] receptor,[181–183] transferrin receptor[184,185]) and transcytosis (immunoglobulin, taken up by endocytosis, and transferred from the maternal to the fetal circulation[184,186,187]). Although the precise steps for each protein-receptor complex are not yet defined, general mechanisms for post-ligand binding, cell entry, and processing can be drawn from available data in other cell types. Following ligand binding, the receptors aggregate on the cell surface and collect in specialized membrane structures termed clatharin-coated pits (Fig. 2-3). These coated pits invaginate, pinch-off, and enter the cell to form vesicles that fuse to form endosomes. The endosomes move deeper into the cytoplasm, where the lower endosome pH facilitates ligand separation from its receptor.

The fate of ligand and receptor differs depending on the specific substrate: Although insulin receptor is probably recycled to the cell surface, maternal insulin does not reach the fetal circulation due to lysosomal degradation. Cholesterol enters with the LDL receptor and may be used for trophoblast pregnenolone/progesterone synthesis or is released into the fetal circulation.[188,189] Immunoglobulin G (IgG) remains complexed to its receptor (the neonatal Fc receptor) and is transferred to the fetus intact through exocytosis at the basal trophoblast membrane.[190] Immunoglobulin that cannot bind to this receptor is degraded within the placenta.[191] Ferrotransferrin carries two ferric ions per molecule and is unique in that it does not separate from the transferrin receptor. Rather, the iron dissociates and binds to ferritin, a

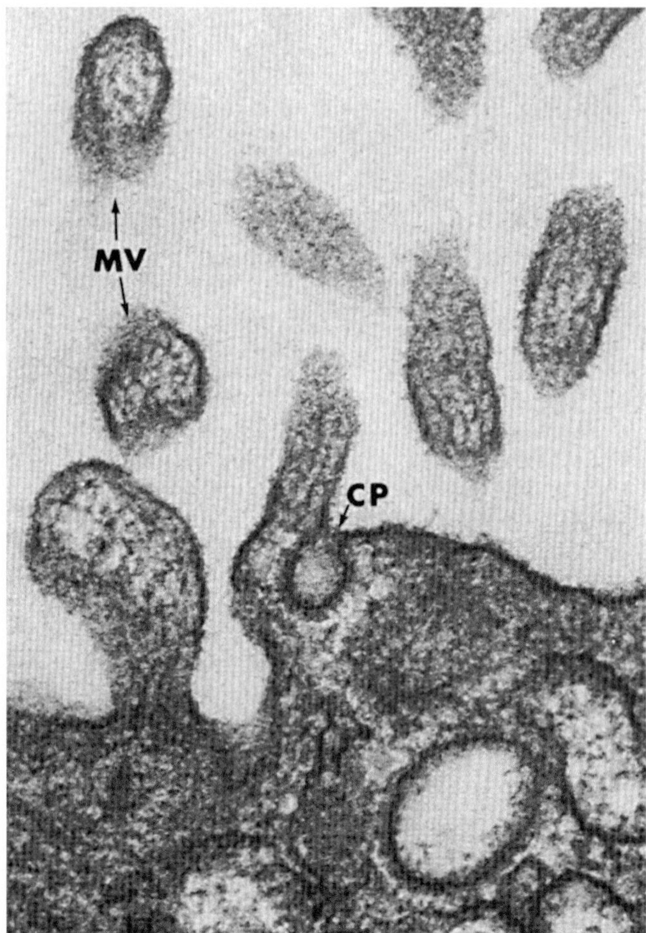

Figure 2-3. Electron micrograph of human placental microvillous plasma membrane demonstrating presence of a coated pit (CP). Note the presence of cytoskeletal components extending into the microvillous space (MV). (Courtesy of Kent L. Thornburg, PhD, Department of Physiology, Oregon Health Sciences University, Portland, OR.)

cytoplasmic iron-storing protein.[192] Iron is then picked up at the basal side of the cell by fetal apotransferrin, whereas the maternal apotransferrin/transferring receptor complex is recycled to the syncytiotrophoblast microvillous membrane.

Endocytosis may also occur through caveolin-dependent and lipid-raft associated mechanisms.[193] The mechanisms within the placenta are not well understood; however, the norepinephrine transporter is recycled by the latter mechanism in trophoblast cells.[194]

Placental Blood Flow

The transport characteristics of the placenta allow respiratory gases and many solutes to reach equal concentration between the maternal intervillous space blood (derived from uterine blood flow) and fetal capillary blood (derived from umbilical blood flow). Thus, the rate of blood flow in these two circulations is an important determinant of fetal O_2 and nutrient supply.

Uterine Blood Flow

Uterine blood flow during pregnancy supplies the myometrium, endometrium, and placenta, with the latter receiving nearly 90 percent of total uterine blood flow near term. Thus, interest has focused primarily on regulation of uteroplacental blood flow. Over the course of a normal singleton ovine gestation, uterine blood flow increases more than 50-fold above nonpregnant values.[195] This long-term increase in uterine blood flow is accompanied by a doubling of maternal cardiac output and a 40 percent increase in blood volume. Two primary factors contribute to this dramatic increase in uterine blood flow: placental growth and maternal arterial vasodilation. Along with fetal and placental growth, placental intervillous space volume almost triples between the 22nd and 36th weeks of gestation. Thus, the marked growth of the maternal placental vascular bed is consistent with the increase in placental diffusing capacity.[196,197] Second, the increase in blood flow is due in part to a direct estrogen-induced vasodilation of the uterine vasculature. This effect is mediated through the release of nitric oxide.[198] These combined effects provide uterine blood flow rates at term of at least 750 ml/min,[199,200] or 10 to 15 percent of maternal cardiac output.

The uterine artery behaves as a nearly maximally dilated system. Still, uterine blood flow is subject to short-term regulatory influences. Systemically administered vasodilator agents preferentially dilate systemic vessels, reducing uterine blood flow.[201] Thus, concerns regarding administration of antihypertensive agents or regional anesthesia with sympathetic blockade are well founded. Although pregnant women display a refractoriness to infused pressor agents,[202] including angiotensin,[203] pressor agent–induced increases in uterine vascular resistance may exceed increases in systemic vascular resistance, reducing uteroplacental blood flow. Thus, elevated maternal plasma catecholamine levels during preeclampsia or pressor agents administered for treatment of maternal hypotension may have adverse effects on uterine blood flow. Although respiratory gases are important regulators of blood flow in a number of organs, there is no indication that either O_2 or CO_2 are responsible for short-term changes in uterine blood flow.[204] During uterine contractions, the relationship between uterine arterial and venous pressures and blood flow no longer holds. Because intrauterine pressures are directly transmitted to the intervillous space,[205] increases in intrauterine pressure are reflected by decreases in placental blood flow. Calcitonin gene–related peptide produces uterine artery relaxation and enhances uterine artery blood flow and improved fetal growth.[206] Conversely, diminished uterine artery blood flow is associated with diminished fetal growth.[207]

Umbilical Blood Flow

Fetal blood flow to the umbilical circulation represents approximately 40 percent of the combined output of both fetal ventricles.[208,209] Over the last third of gestation, increases in umbilical blood flow are proportional to fetal growth,[210] so that umbilical blood flow remains constant when normalized to fetal weight.[211] Human umbilical venous flow can be estimated through the use of triplex mode ultrasonography.[212] Although increases in villous capillary number represent the primary contributor to gestation-dependent increases in umbilical blood flow, the factors that regulate this change are not known. A number of important angiogenic peptides and factors, including vascular endothelial growth factor (VEGF), have been identified.[36,213,214] Short-term changes in umbilical blood flow are primarily regulated by perfusion pressure. The relationship between flow and perfusion pressure is linear in the umbilical circulation.[211,215] As a result, small (2 to 3 mm Hg) increases in umbilical vein pressure evoke proportional decreases in umbilical blood flow.[211,215] Because both the umbilical artery and vein are enclosed in the amniotic cavity, pressure changes due to increases in uterine tone are transmitted equally to these vessels without changes in umbilical blood flow. Relative to the uteroplacental bed, the fetoplacental circulation is resistant to vasoconstrictive effects of infused pressor agents, and umbilical blood flow is preserved unless cardiac output decreases. Thus, despite catecholamine-induced changes in blood flow distribution and increases in blood pressure during acute hypoxia, umbilical blood flow is maintained over a relatively wide range of O_2 tensions.[216–219] Endogenous vasoactive autacoids have been identified; nitric oxide may also be important.[220,221] In particular, Endothelin-1 is associated with diminished fetoplacental blood flow.[222]

Immunologic Properties of the Placenta

The syncytiotrophoblast in contact with maternal blood in the intervillous space and the amniochorion in contact with maternal decidua represent the fetal tissues most prone to immunologic reactions from maternal factors. The rejection of tissue grafts is under genetic control and the genes responsible for this phenomenon are termed histocompatibility genes. Their products at the cell surface–major histocompatibility antigens are integral to the host's recognition of self and non-self. Neither beta-2 microglobulin (which is tightly associated with human leukocyte antigens [HLA]) nor the HLA antigens A, B, C, DR, or DC can be demonstrated on the surface of syncytiotrophoblast.[223–225] This is thought to be the result of the epigenetic silencing of the class II transactivator gene within the trophoblast.[226] Invasive human cytotrophoblasts (extravillous trophoblast) have been shown to express a trophoblast-specific, nonclassic class 1b antigen, HLA-G (reviewed in[227]), in addition to the more widely disseminated HLA-C and HLA-E, each of which serves as a ligand for uterine natural killer cells (uNK), the predominant leukocyte type found within the maternal-fetal junction. These ligands interact with specific killer cell immunoglobulin-like receptors (KIR) on uNK.[228] Postulated roles for HLA-G include protection of invasive cytotrophoblast from uNK, as well as containment of placental infection.[227] HLA-G is also coexpressed with HLA-E, allowing it to be recognized by KIRs, which then induce inhibition of uNK. The interaction of uNK and HLA-C appears to be more complex, in that, depending on the combinatorial pattern of KIRs and HLA-C alleles present, uterine invasion by extravillous trophoblast can be either facilitated of inhibited, leading, perhaps, to the development of preeclampsia.[229] Other postulated "protective" mechanisms include the presence of proteins that "deactivate" the local complement system, alteration of lymphocytes from a T-helper type 1 (Th1) to a T-helper type 2 (Th2) secretory phenotype, associated with a cytokine profile more conducive to fetal survival, as well as mechanisms by which the fetal membranes may facilitate the apoptosis of specific maternal immunoregulatory cells.[230] Others have shown that indoleamine 2,3-dioxygenase, which breaks down tryptophan, may be important in the control of maternal lymphocytes; blocking this enzyme activity is associated with a high rate of fetal abortion.[231] In summary, immunologic aspects of the placenta are difficult to separate from those of the maternal uterus and the mixed deciduas. It is now clear, however, that multiple, elegant, overlapping mechanisms ensure the survival of the placenta and thus the fetus in an immunologically hostile environment.

Amniotic Fluid Volume

Mean amniotic fluid volume increases from 250 to 800 ml between 16 and 32 weeks' gestation. Despite considerable variability, the average volume remains stable up to 39 weeks and then declines to about 500 ml at 42 weeks.[232] The origin of amniotic fluid during the first trimester of pregnancy is uncertain. Possible sources include a transudate of maternal plasma through the chorioamnion or a transudate of fetal plasma through the highly permeable fetal skin, before keratinization.[233] The origin and dynamics of amniotic fluid are better understood beginning in the second trimester, when the fetus becomes the primary determinant. Amniotic fluid volume is maintained by a balance of fetal fluid production (lung liquid and urine) and fluid resorption (fetal swallowing and flow across the amniotic and/or chorionic membranes to the fetus or maternal uterus).

The fetal lung secretes fluid at a rate of 300 to 400 ml/day near term.[234] Chloride is actively transferred from alveolar capillaries to the lung lumen,[235] and water follows the chloride gradient. Thus, lung fluid represents a nearly protein-free transudate with an osmolarity similar to that of fetal plasma.[236] Fetal lung fluid does not appear to regulate fetal body fluid homeostasis, because fetal intravenous volume loading does not increase lung fluid secretion. Rather, lung fluid likely serves to maintain lung expansion and facilitate pulmonary growth. Lung fluid must decrease at parturition to provide for the transition to respiratory ventilation. Notably, several hormones that increase in fetal plasma during labor (i.e, catecholamines, arginine vasopressin [AVP]) also decrease lung fluid production.[237–239] With the reduction of fluid secretion, the colloid osmotic gradient between fetal plasma and lung fluid results in lung fluid resorption across the pulmonary epithelium and clearance through lymphatics. The absence of this process explains the increased incidence of transient tachypnea of the newborn, or "wet lung," in infants delivered by cesarean section in the absence of labor.

Fetal urine is the primary source of amniotic fluid, with outputs at term varying from 400 to 1,200 ml/day.[240,241] Between 20 and 40 weeks' gestation, fetal urine production increases about 10-fold[241] in the presence of marked renal maturation. The urine is normally hypotonic,[242] and the low osmolarity of fetal urine accounts for the hypotonicity of amniotic fluid in late gestation[242] relative to maternal and fetal plasma. Numerous fetal endocrine factors, including AVP, atrial natriuretic factor (ANF), angiotensin II (AII), aldosterone, and prostaglandins alter fetal renal blood flow, glomerular filtration rate, and urine flow rates.[243,244] In response to fetal stress, endocrine-mediated reductions in fetal urine flow may explain the association between fetal hypoxia and oligohydramnios. The regulation of fetal urine production is discussed further in the section Fetal Kidney, later.

Fetal swallowing is believed to be the major route of amniotic fluid resorption,[245–248] although swallowed fluid contains a mixture of amniotic and tracheal fluids.[245] Human fetal swallowing has been demonstrated by 18 weeks' gestation,[249] with daily swallowed volumes of 200 to 500 ml near term.[246,247] Similar to fetal urine flow, daily fetal swallowed volumes (per body weight) are markedly greater than adult values. In observations of fetal neurobehavioral states, fetal swallowing occurs primarily during active sleep states associated with respiratory and eye movements.[249,250] Moderate increases in fetal plasma osmolality increase the number of swallowing episodes and volume swallowed,[251,252] indicating the presence of an intact thirst mechanism in the near-term fetus.

Because amniotic fluid is hypotonic with respect to maternal plasma, there is a potential for bulk water removal at the amniotic-chorionic interface with maternal or fetal plasma. Although fluid resorption to the maternal plasma is likely minimal, intramembranous flow from amniotic fluid to fetal placental vessels may contribute importantly to amniotic fluid resorption.[253] Thus, intramembranous flow may balance fetal urine and lung liquid production with fetal swallowing to maintain normal amniotic fluid volumes.

FETAL PHYSIOLOGY

Growth and Metabolism

SUBSTRATES

Nutrients are uded by the fetus for two primary purposes: oxidation for energy and tissue accretion. Under normal conditions, glucose is an important substrate for fetal oxidative metabolism. The glucose used by the fetus derives from the placenta rather than from endogenous glucose production.[254] However, based on umbilical vein-to-umbilical artery glucose and O_2 concentration differences,[255] glucose alone cannot account for fetal oxidative metabolism. In fact, glucose oxidation accounts for only two thirds of fetal CO_2 production.[256] Thus, fetal oxidative metabolism depends on substrates in addition to glucose. Because a large portion of the amino acids taken up by the umbilical circulation are used by the fetus for aerobic metabolism instead of protein synthesis, amino acids represent one of these substrates. Fetal uptake for a number of amino acids actually exceeds their accretion into fetal tissues.[257] In fetal sheep and likely the human fetus as well, lactate also is a substrate for fetal O_2 consumption.[256] Thus, the combined substrates glucose, amino acids, and lactate essentially provide the approximately 87 kcal/kg/day required by the growing fetus.

Metabolic requirements for new tissue accretion depend on the growth rate and the type of tissue acquired. Although the newborn infant has relatively increased body fat (16 percent),[258] fetal fat content is low at 26 weeks. Fat acquisition increases gradually up to 32 weeks and rapidly thereafter (~82 g [dry weight] of fat per week). Because the necessary enzymes for carbohydrate to lipid conversion are present in the fetus,[259] fat acquisition reflects glucose utilization and not placental fatty acid uptake. In contrast, fetal acquisition of nonfat tissue is linear from 32 to 39 weeks and may decrease to only 30 percent of the fat-acquisition rate in late gestation (~43 g [dry weight] per week).

HORMONES

The role of select hormones in the regulation of placental growth was discussed previously in the section Placental Metabolism and Growth. Fetal hormones influence fetal growth through both metabolic and mitogenic effects. Although growth hormone and growth hormone receptors are present early in fetal life, and growth hormone is essential to postnatal growth,[260] growth hormone appears to have little role in regulating fetal growth. Instead, changes in IGF, IGF-binding proteins, or IGF receptors may explain the apparent reduced role of growth hormone on fetal growth.[261–265] Most if not all tissues of the body produce IGF-I and IGF-II,[266,267] and both IGF-I and IGF-II are present in human fetal tissue extracts after 12 weeks' gestation. Fetal plasma IGF-I and IGF-II levels begin to increase by 32 to 34 weeks' gestation.[268,269] The increase in IGF-I levels directly correlates with increase in fetal size, and a reduction in IGF-I levels is associated with growth restriction. In contrast, there is no correlation between serum IGF-II levels and fetal growth. However, there is a correlation between small offspring and genetic manipulations resulting in only one allele and decreased IGF-II messenger RNA. Thus, tissue IGF-II concentrations and localized IGF-II release may be more important than circulating levels in supporting fetal growth.

A role for insulin in fetal growth is suggested from the increases in body weight, and heart and liver weights in infants of diabetic mothers.[270] Insulin levels within the high physiologic range increase fetal body weight,[271] and increases in endogenous fetal insulin significantly increase fetal glucose uptake.[272,273] In addition, fetal insulin secretion increases in response to elevations in blood glucose, although the normal rapid insulin response phase is absent.[273] Plasma insulin levels sufficient to increase fetal growth[271] also may exert mitogenic effects,[267] perhaps through insulin-induced IGF-II receptor binding.[274] Separate receptors for insulin and IGF-II are expressed in fetal liver cells by the end of the first trimester.[275] Hepatic insulin receptor numbers (per gram tissue) triple by 28 weeks, whereas IGF-II receptor numbers remain constant.[275] The growth patterns of infants of diabetic mothers[276,277] indicate that insulin levels may be most important in late gestation. Although less common, equally dramatically low birth weights are associated with the absence of fetal insulin.[262] Experimentally induced hypoinsulinemia causes a 30-percent decrease in fetal glucose use and decreases fetal growth.[278,279]

As in the adult, β-adrenergic receptor activation increases fetal insulin secretion, whereas β-adrenergic activation inhibits insulin secretion.[280,281] Fetal glucagon secretion also is modulated by the β-adrenergic system.[280] However, the fetal glycemic response to glucagon is blunted, probably caused by a relative reduction in hepatic glucagon receptors.[282]

In addition to the IGFs, a number of other factors including EGF, transforming growth factor, fibroblast growth factor, and nerve growth factor are expressed during embryonic development and appear to exert specific effects during morphogenesis, For example, EGF has specific effects on lung growth and growth, and differentiation of the secondary palate,[283] and normal sympathetic adrenergic system development is dependent on nerve growth factor.[283] However, a specific role of these factors in regulating fetal growth remains to be defined. Similarly, the fetal thyroid also is not important for overall fetal growth but is important for central nervous system development.[261,262]

Substantial evidence now exists to support the view that several cell-specific growth factors and their cognate receptors play an essential role in placental growth and function in a number of species. Growth factors identified to date include family members of EGF,[44,284–290] transforming growth factor-beta,[291–293] nerve growth factor,[294,295] IGF,[296] hematopoietic growth factors,[297–299] VEGF,[300–302] and fibroblast growth factor.[303–305] A number of cytokines also play a role in normal placental development.[306] Limited information is now available on the expression, ontogeny, and regulation of most but not all of the growth factors identified to date. In vitro placental cell culture studies support the concept that growth factors and cytokines exert their functions locally, promoting proliferation and differentiation through their autocrine or paracrine mode of actions, or both. For example, EGF promotes either cell proliferation,[307] invasion,[308] or differentiation,[285,309] depending upon the gestational age. Hepatocyte growth factor[310] and VEGF[311] stimulate trophoblast DNA replication, whereas transforming growth factor beta suppresses cytoplast invasion[312] and endocrine differentiation.[313] In support of local actions, functional receptors for various growth factors have been demonstrated on trophoblast and other cells.[314–317] Various intracellular signal proteins and transcription factors that respond to growth factors also are expressed in placenta.[318–320] A number of elegant studies have identified alterations in growth factors and growth factor receptors in association with placental and fetal growth restriction.[35,55] Developmental regulation of placental growth factor genes and their functions appear to be identical to ones studied in other organs.[308] Transgenic and mutant mice are now aiding the comparison of human and mouse placentas.[55,321,322] Placental defects in growth factor and receptor pathways are now beginning to provide potential mechanisms for explaining complications of human placental development.[323–326]

EGF, a potent mitogen for epidermal and mesodermal cells, is expressed in human placenta.[44,284,285] EGF is involved embryonal implantation,[327] stimulates syncytiotrophoblast differentiation in vitro,[309] and modulates production and secretion of human chorionic gonadotrophin and placental lactogen.[328] EGF also inhibits cytokine-induced apoptosis of human primary trophoblast.[329] The effects of EGF are mediated by EGF receptor (EGF-R), a transmembrane glycoprotein with intrinsic tyrosine kinase activity. EGF-R is expressed on the apical microvillus plasma membrane fractions from early, middle, and term whole placentas.[330] Placental EGF-R expression is regulated by locally expressed parathyroid hormone–related protein.[331] Decreased EGF-R expression has been demonstrated in association with intrauterine growth restriction.[332] Targeted disruption of EGF-R has shown to result in fetal death due to placental defects.[55]

The EGF family now consists of at least 15 members,[333] and five members of EGF family namely, transforming growth factor-alpha, amphiregulin, heparin-binding EGF-like growth factor, betacellulin, and epiregulin have been identified in human placenta.[286–290] Interestingly, different EGF-R family members, including Erb-2-4, have also been identified in placenta.[289,334] Future studies should reveal whether EGF family members play distinct or overlapping roles in mediating placental growth.

Fetal Cardiovascular System

Development

The heart and the vascular system develop from splanchnic mesoderm during the third week after fertilization. The two primordial heart tubes fuse, forming a simple contractile tube early in the fourth week, and the cardiovascular system becomes the first functional organ system. During weeks 5 to 8, this single lumen tube is converted into the definitive four-chambered heart through a process of cardiac looping (folding), remodeling, and partitioning. However, an opening in the interatrial septum, the foramen ovale, is present and serves as an important right to left shunt during fetal life.

During the fourth embryonic week, three primary circulations characterize the vascular system. The aortic/cardinal circulation serves the embryo proper and is the basis for much of the fetal circulatory system. Of note, the left sixth aortic (pulmonary) arch forms a connection between the left pulmonary artery and the aorta as the ductus arteriosus. The ductus arteriosus also functions as a right-to-left shunt by redistributing right ventricular output from the lungs to the aorta and fetal and placental circulations. The vitelline circulation develops in association with the yolk sac, and although it plays a minor role in providing nutrients to the embryo, its rearrangement ultimately provides the circulatory system for the gastro-

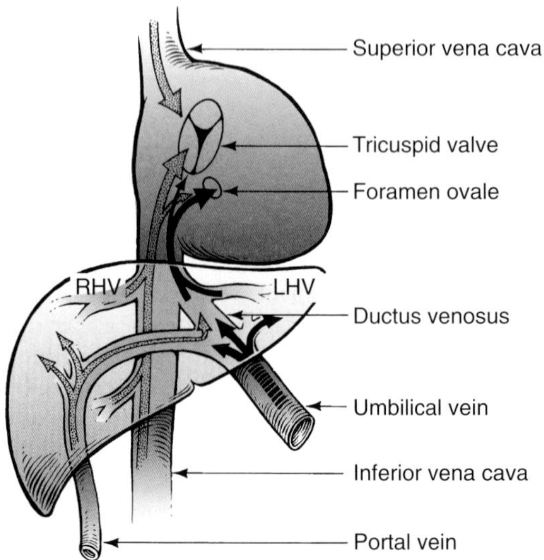

Figure 2-4. Anatomy of the umbilical and hepatic circulation. LHV, left hepatic vein; RHV, right hepatic vein. (From Rudolph AM: Hepatic and ductus venosus blood flows during fetal life. Hepatology 3:254, 1983, with permission.)

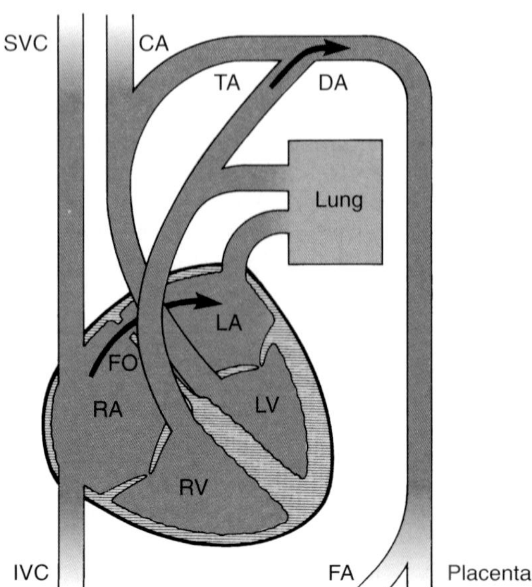

Figure 2-5. Anatomy of fetal heart and central shunts. CA, carotid artery; DA, ductus arteriosus; FA, femoral artery; FO, foramen ovale; IVC, inferior vena cava; LA, left atrium; LV, left ventricle; RA, right atrium; RV, right ventricle; SVC, superior vena cava; TA, thoracic aorta. (From Anderson DF, Bissonnette JM, Faber JJ, Thornburg KL: Central shunt flows and pressures in the mature fetal lamb. Am J Physiol 241:H60, 1981, with permission.)

intestinal tract, spleen, pancreas, and liver. The allantoic circulation develops in association with the chorion and the developing chorionic villi, and forms the placental circulation, composed of two umbilical arteries and two umbilical veins. In humans, the venous pathways are rearranged during embryonic weeks 4 to 8 and only the left umbilical vein is retained. Subsequent rearrangement of the vascular plexus associated with the developing liver forms the ductus venosus, a venous shunt that allows at least half of the estimated umbilical blood flow (70 to 130 ml/min/kg fetal weight[197] after 30 weeks' gestation) to bypass the liver and enter the inferior vena cava.[199]

Placental gas exchange provides well-oxygenated blood that leaves the placenta (Fig. 2-4) through the umbilical vein. In addition to the ductus venosus, small branches into the left lobe of the liver and a major branch to the right lobe account for the remainder of umbilical venous flow. Left hepatic vein blood combines with the well-oxygenated ductus venosus flow as it enters the inferior vena cava. Because right hepatic vein blood combines with the portal vein (only a small fraction of portal vein blood passes through the ductus venosus), right hepatic vein blood is less oxygenated than its counterpart on the left,[199] and the combination of right hepatic/portal drainage with blood returning from the lower trunk and limbs further decreases the O_2 content. Although both ductus venosus blood and hepatic portal/fetal trunk bloods enter the inferior vena cava and the right atrium, little mixing occurs. This stream of well-oxygenated ductus venosus blood is preferentially directed into the foramen ovale by the valve of the inferior vena cava and the crista dividens on the wall of the right atrium. This shunts a portion of the most highly oxygenated ductus venosus blood through the foramen ovale with little opportunity for mixing with superior vena cava/coronary sinus venous return (Figs. 2-4 and 2-5). As a result, left atrial filling results primarily from umbilical vein–ductus venosus blood, with a small contribution from pulmonary venous flow. Thus, blood with the highest O_2 content is delivered to the left atrium, left ventricle, and ultimately, supplies blood to the upper body and limbs, carotid and vertebral circulations, and the brain. Inferior vena cava flow is larger than the volume that can cross the foramen ovale. The remainder of the oxygenated inferior vena cava blood is directed through the tricuspid valve (Fig. 2-4) into the right ventricle (Fig. 2-5) and is accompanied by venous return from the superior vena cava and coronary sinus. However, the very high vascular resistance in the pulmonary circulation maintains mean pulmonary artery pressure 2 to 3 mm Hg above aortic pressure and directs most of right ventricular output through the ductus arteriosus and into the aorta and the fetal and placental circulations.[199]

Fetal Heart

The adult cardiovascular system includes a high-pressure (95–mm Hg) system and a low-pressure (15–mm Hg) pulmonary circuit driven by the left and right ventricles working in series. Although the ejection velocity is greater in the left ventricle than that in the right, equal volumes of blood are delivered into the systemic and pulmonary circulations with contraction of each ventricle. The stroke volume is the volume of blood ejected by the left ventricle with each contraction, and cardiac output is a function of the stroke volume and heart rate (70 ml/beat × 72 beats/min = 5,040 ml/min). For a 70-kg adult man, cardiac output averages 72 ml/min/kg. In addition to heart rate, cardiac output changes with changes in stroke volume, which, in turn, is determined by venous return (preload), pulmonary artery and aortic pressures (afterload), and contractility.

In contrast to the adult heart, in which the two ventricles pump blood in a series circuit, the unique fetal shunts provide an unequal distribution of venous return to the respective atria, and ventricular output represents a mixture of oxygenated and deoxygenated blood. Thus, the fetal right and left ventricles function as two pumps operating in parallel rather than in series, and cardiac output is described as the combined ventricular output. Right ventricular output exceeds 60 percent of biventricular output[199] and is primarily directed through the ductus arteriosus to the descending aorta (Fig. 2-5). As a result, placental blood flow, which represents more than 50 percent of the combined ventricular output, primarily reflects right ventricular output. Owing to the high pulmonary vascular resistance,[199] the pulmonary circulation receives only 5 to 10 percent of the combined ventricular output. Instead, left ventricular output is primarily directed through the ductus arteriosus to the upper body and head. Estimates of fetal left ventricular output average 120 ml/min/kg body weight.[113] If left ventricular output is less than 40 percent of the combined biventricular output,[199] then total fetal cardiac output would be higher than 300 ml/min/kg. The distribution of the cardiac output to fetal organs is summarized in Table 2-2,[112,335] with fetal hepatic distribution reflecting only the portion supplied by the hepatic artery. In fact, hepatic blood flow derives principally from the umbilical vein and to a lesser extent the portal vein,[200] and represents about 25 percent of the total venous return to the heart.

The placenta receives approximately 50 percent of the combined ventricular output, which means that the single umbilical vein also conducts 50 percent of the combined ventricular output. At least half of the umbilical venous blood bypasses the liver through the ductus venosus and the remainder traverses the hepatic circulation. The combination of umbilical vein blood, hepatic portal blood, and blood returning from the lower body contributes approximately 69 percent of the cardiac output that enters the right atrium from the inferior vena cava. Flow across the foramen ovale accounts for approximately one third (27 percent) of the combined cardiac output.[199] Pulmonary venous return to the left atrium is low and represents approximately 7 percent of combined ventricular output. Thus, the left atrium accounts for only about 34 percent (27 percent + 7 percent) of the combined ventricular output. Because a volume of inferior vena cava venous return equivalent to 27 percent of the combined ventricular output is shunted across the foramen ovale, 42 percent remains in the right atrium and contributes to right ventricular output. With another 21 percent from the superior vena cava and 3 percent from the coronary circulation, right ventricular output accounts for 66 percent of the combined ventricular output. However, only 7 percent of right ventricular output enters the pulmonary circulation, leaving 59 percent entering the aorta via the ductus arteriosus. Similarly, 24 percent of the combined ventricular output derived from the left ventricle is distributed to the upper body and brain, with approximately 10 percent combining with right ventricular output in the aorta. Thus, 69 percent of the combined ventricular output reaches the descending aorta and 50 percent of this accounts for placental flow, with the remainder distributed to the fetal abdominal organs and lower body.

Consistent with the greater contribution of the right ventricle to combined ventricular output, coronary blood flow to the myocardium reflects the greater stroke volume of the right side, and right ventricular free wall and septal blood flows are higher than in the left ventricle.[209] It is not surprising then that fetal ventricular wall thickness is greater on the right side relative to the left. As in the adult, fetal ventricular output depends on heart rate, pulmonary artery and aortic pressures, and contractility. The relationship between mean right atrial pressure (the index often used for ventricular volume at the end of diastole) and stroke volume is depicted in Figure 2-6. The steep ascending limb represents the length-active tension relationship for cardiac muscle in the right ventricle.[201] Under normal conditions, fetal right atrial pressure resides at the break point in this ascending limb; increases in pressure do not increase stroke volume. Thus, the contribution of Starling mechanisms to increasing right-sided heart output in the fetus is limited. In contrast, decreases in venous

Table 2-2. Distribution of Fetal Cardiac Output

ORGAN	PERCENTAGE OF BIVENTRICULAR CARDIAC OUTPUT
Placenta	40
Brain	13
Heart	3.5
Lung	7
Liver	2.5 (hepatic artery)
Gastrointestinal tract	5
Adrenal glands	0.5
Kidney	2.5
Spleen	1
Body	25

Data from Rudolph and Heyman,[208] and Paton et al.[422]

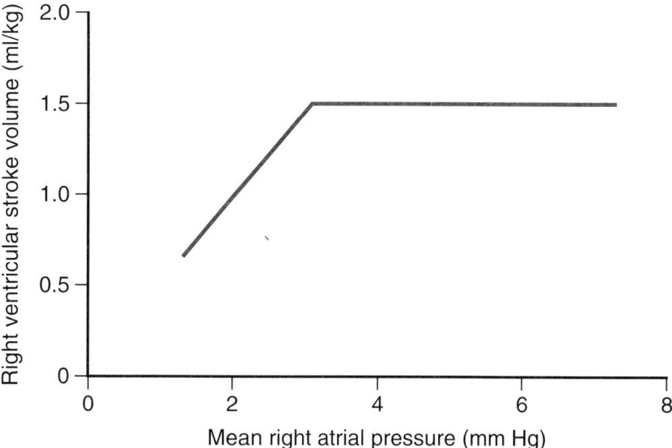

Figure 2-6. Stroke volume of the fetal right ventricle as a function of mean right atrial pressure. (From Thornburg KL, Morton MJ: Filling and arterial pressures as determinants of RV stroke volume in the sheep fetus. Am J Physiol 244:H656, 1983, with permission.)

return and right atrial pressure decrease stroke volume. Compared with the left ventricle, the fetal right ventricle has a greater anteroposterior dimension, increasing both volume and circumferential radius of curvature. This anatomic difference increases the radius/wall thickness ratio for the right ventricle, producing increased wall stress in systole and a decrease in stroke volume when afterload increases.[202] Because the right ventricle is sensitive to afterload, a linear inverse relationship exists between stroke volume and pulmonary artery pressure.[201]

The relationship between atrial pressure and stroke volume in the left ventricle is similar to that shown in Figure 2-6 for the right ventricle. Although the break point occurs near the normal value for left atrial pressure, there is a small amount of preload reserve.[204] In distinction to the fetal right ventricle, the left side is not sensitive to aortic pressure increases. Thus, postnatal increases in systemic blood pressure do not decrease left ventricular stroke volume, and left ventricular output increases to meet the needs of the postnatal systemic circulation. Although Starling mechanism–related increases in stroke volume are limited, especially in the right side of the heart, late-gestation fetal heart β-adrenergic receptor numbers are similar to that of an adult,[205] and circulating catecholamine–induced increases in contractility may increase stroke volume by 50 percent.[208]

Although fetal heart rate decreases during the last half of gestation, particularly between 20 and 30 weeks, fetal heart rate averages more than twofold above resting adult heart rates. If analysis is confined to episodes of low heart rate variability, mean heart rate decreases from 30 weeks to term. However, if all heart rate data are analyzed, mean heart rate is stable at 142 beats per minute over the last 10 weeks of gestation.[336] Variability in mean heart rate over 24 hours includes a nadir between 2 a.m. and 6 a.m., and a peak between 8 a.m. and 10 a.m.[213] Most fetal heart rate accelerations occur simultaneous with limb movement, primarily reflecting central neuronal brain stem output. Also, movement-related decreases in venous return and a reflex tachycardia may contribute to heart rate accelerations.[337] Because ventricular stroke volumes decrease with increasing heart rate, fetal cardiac output remains constant over a heart rate range of 120 to 180 beats per min.[215–217] The major effect of this inverse relationship between heart rate and stroke volume is an alteration in end-diastolic dimension. If end-diastolic dimension is kept constant, there is no fall in stroke volume and cardiac output increases.[216,217]

At birth, major changes in vascular distribution occur with the first breath. Alveolar expansion and the associated increase in alveolar capillary O_2 tension induce a marked decrease in pulmonary microvascular resistance. This decrease in pulmonary vascular resistance has two effects. First, there is an accompanying decrease in right atrial afterload and right atrial pressure. Second, the increase in pulmonary flow increases venous return into the left atrium and, therefore, left atrial pressure. The combined effect of these two events is to increase left atrial pressure above right atrial pressure and provide a physiologic closure of the foramen ovale. The return of the highly oxygenated blood from the lungs to the left atrium, left ventricle, and aorta and the decrease in pulmonary vascular resistance and, hence, pulmonary trunk pressure allow backflow of the O_2-rich blood into the ductus arteriosus. This local increase in ductus arteriosus O_2 tension alters the ductus response to prostaglandins and causes a marked localized vasoconstriction.[338] Concurrent spontaneous constriction (or clamping) of the umbilical cord stops placental blood flow, reducing venous return and perhaps augmenting the decrease in right atrial pressure.

Autonomic Regulation of Cardiovascular Function

Through reflex stimulation of peripheral baroreceptors, chemoreceptors, and central mechanisms, the sympathetic and parasympathetic systems have important roles in the regulation of fetal heart rate, cardiac contractility, and vascular tone. The fetal sympathetic system develops early, whereas the parasympathetic system develops somewhat later.[218–220] Nevertheless, in the third trimester, increasing parasympathetic tone accounts for the characteristic decrease in fetal heart rate with periods of reduced fetal heart rate reactivity. As evidence, fetal heart rate increases in the presence of parasympathetic blockade with atropine.[221] Opposing sympathetic and parasympathetic inputs to the fetal heart contribute to R-R interval variability from one heart cycle to the next, and to basal heart rate variability over periods of a few minutes. However, even when sympathetic and parasympathetic inputs are removed, a level of variability remains.[221]

Fetal sympathetic innervation is not essential for blood pressure maintenance when circulating catecholamines are present.[223] Nevertheless, fine control of blood pressure and fetal heart rate requires an intact sympathetic system.[225] In the absence of functional adrenergic innervation, hypoxia-induced increases in peripheral, renal, and splanchnic bed vascular resistances[130,339] and blood pressure are not seen.[212,227] However, hypoxia-related changes in pulmonary, myocardial, adrenal, and brain blood flows occur in the absence of sympathetic innervation, indicating that both local and endocrine effects contribute to regulation of blood flow in these organs.

Receptors in the carotid body and arch of the aorta respond to pressor or respiratory gas stimulation with afferent modulation of heart rate and vascular tone. Fetal baroreflex sensitivity, in terms of the magnitude of decreases in heart rate per millimeter of mercury increase in blood pressure, is blunted relative to the adult.[340,341] However, fetal baroreflex sensitivity more than doubles in late gestation.[340] Although the set-point for fetal heart rate is not believed to depend on intact baroreceptors, fetal heart rate variability increases when functional arterial baroreceptors are absent.[342] The same observation has been made for fetal blood pressure. Thus, fetal arterial baroreceptors buffer variations in fetal blood pressure during body or breathing movements.[342,343] Changes in baroreceptor tone likely account for the increase in mean fetal blood pressure normally observed in late gestation.[343] In the absence of functional chemoreceptors, mean arterial pressure is maintained[342] whereas peripheral blood flow increases. Thus, peripheral arterial chemoreceptors may be important to maintenance of resting peripheral vascular tone. Peripheral arterial chemoreceptors also are important components in fetal reflex responses to hypoxia; the initial bradycardia is not seen without functional chemoreceptors.[344]

Hormonal Regulation of Cardiovascular Function

Adrenocorticotropic hormone (ACTH) and catecholamines are discussed in the section Fetal Adrenal and Thyroid, later.

Arginine Vasopressin

Significant quantities of AVP are present in the human fetal neurohypophysis by completion of the first trimester.[345] Ovine fetal plasma AVP levels increase appropriately in response to changes in fetal plasma osmolality induced directly in the fetus[346,347] or through changes in maternal osmolality.[348,349] Owing to functional high- and low-pressure baroreceptors and chemoreceptor afferents, decreases in fetal intravascular volume[350,351] or systemic blood pressure[232,352] also increase fetal AVP secretion. Thus, in the late-gestation fetus as in the adult, AVP secretion is regulated by both osmoreceptor and volume/baroreceptor pathways. Hypoxia-induced AVP secretion has been demonstrated beyond midpregnancy of ovine gestation,[353] and reductions in fetal Po_2 of 10 mm Hg (50 percent) evoke profound increases in fetal plasma AVP levels (~2 pg/ml to 200 to 400 pg/ml or more).[233,234] Thus, because fetal AVP responsiveness to hypoxia is augmented relative to the adult (as much as 40-fold), and fetal responsiveness appears to increase during the last half of gestation, hypoxemia is the most potent stimulus known for fetal AVP secretion.[233]

The cardiovascular response pattern to AVP infusion includes dose-dependent increases in fetal mean blood pressure and decreases in heart rate at plasma levels well below those required for similar effects in the adult.[234] Receptors distinct from those mediating AVP antidiuretic effects in the kidney account for AVP contributions to fetal circulatory adjustments during hemorrhage,[235] hypotension,[236] and hypoxia.[237] Corticotropin-releasing factor effects of AVP may contribute to hypoxia-induced increases in plasma ACTH and cortisol levels.[238–241] In addition to effects on fetal heart rate, cardiac output, and arterial blood pressure, AVP-induced changes in peripheral, placental, myocardial, and cerebral blood flows[242–245] directly parallel the cardiovascular changes associated with acute hypoxia. Because many of these responses are attenuated during AVP receptor blockade,[237] AVP effects on cardiac output distribution may serve to facilitate O_2 availability to the fetus during hypoxic challenges. However, other hypoxia-related responses, including decreases in renal and pulmonary blood flows, and increased adrenal blood flow are not seen in response to AVP infusions.[243]

Renin-Angiotensin II

Fetal plasma renin levels are typically elevated during late gestation.[246] A variety of stimuli including changes in tubular sodium concentration,[247] reductions in blood volume,[248] vascular pressure or renal perfusion pressure,[245] and hypoxemia[249] increase fetal plasma renin activity. The relationship between fetal renal perfusion pressure and log plasma renin activity is similar to that of adults.[250] Consistent with the effects of renal nerve activity on renin release in adults,[251] fetal renin gene expression is directly modulated by renal sympathetic nerve activity.[252]

Although fetal plasma AII levels increase in response to small changes in blood volume and hypoxemia,[253] fetal AII and aldosterone levels do not increase in proportion to changes in plasma renin activity.[246] This apparent uncoupling of the fetal renin-angiotensin-aldosterone system and the increase in newborn AII levels may relate to the significant contribution of the placenta to plasma AII clearance in the fetus relative to the adult.[255] Also, limited angiotensin-converting enzyme (ACE) availability due to reduced pulmonary blood flow and direct inhibition of aldosterone secretion by the normally high circulating ANF levels may contribute. Thus, reductions in AII production and aldosterone responses to AII, augmented AII and aldosterone clearances, and the resulting reductions in AII and aldosterone levels and feedback inhibition of rennin, may account for the elevated renin and reduced AII and aldosterone levels typically observed during fetal life.

AII infusion increases fetal mean arterial blood pressure. In contrast to AVP-induced bradycardia, fetal AII infusion increases heat rate (after an initial reflex bradycardia) through both a direct effect on the heart,[256] and decreased baroreflex responsiveness. Both hormones increase fetal blood pressure similar to the levels seen with hypoxemia. However, AII does not reduce peripheral blood flow, perhaps because circulation to muscle, skin, and bone are always under maximum response to AII, thereby limiting increases in resting tone.[256] AII infusions also decrease renal blood flow and increase umbilical vascular resistance, although absolute placental blood flow remains the same. Although the adult kidney contains both AII receptor subtypes (AT_1 and AT_2), the AT_2 subtype is the only form present in the human fetal kidney.[257] Maturational differences in the AII receptor subtype expressed would be consistent with earlier studies demonstrating differing AII effects on fetal renal and peripheral vascular beds.[249] Thus, the receptors mediating AII responses in the renal and peripheral vascular beds differ during fetal life.

Fetal Hemoglobin

The fetus exists in a state of aerobic metabolism, with arterial blood Po_2 values in the 20– to 35–mm Hg range. However, there is no evidence of metabolic acidosis. Adequate fetal tissue oxygenation is achieved by several mechanisms. Of major importance are the higher fetal cardiac output and organ blood flows. A higher hemoglobin concentration (relative to the adult) and an increase in O_2-carrying capacity of fetal hemoglobin also contribute. The resulting leftward shift in the fetal oxygen dissociation curve relative to the adult (Fig. 2-7) increases fetal blood oxygen saturation for any given O_2 tension.

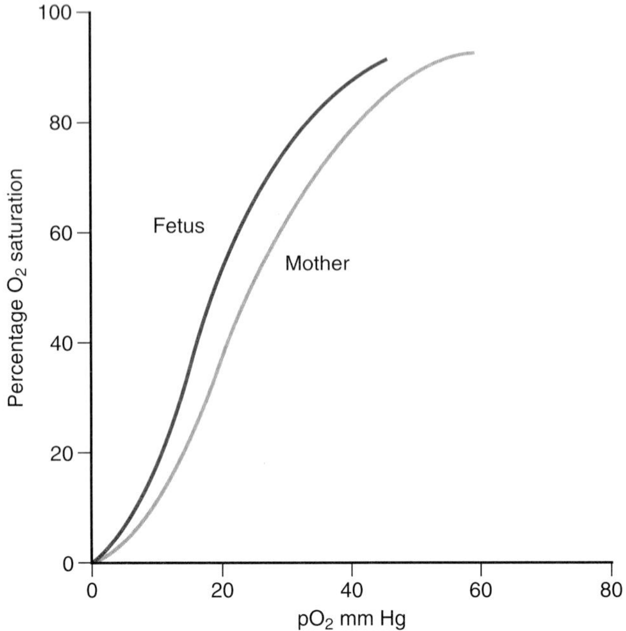

Figure 2-7. Oxyhemoglobin dissociation curves of maternal and fetal human blood at pH 7.4 and 37°C. (Adapted from Hellegers AE, Schruefer JJP: Normograms and empirical equations relating oxygen tension, percentage saturation, and pH in maternal and fetal blood. Am J Obstet Gynecol 81:377, 1961.)

For example, at a partial pressure of 26.5 mm Hg, adult blood oxygen saturation is 50 percent, whereas fetal O_2 saturation is 70 percent. Thus, at a normal fetal Po_2 of 20 mm Hg, fetal whole blood O_2 saturation may be 50 percent.[258]

The basis for increased oxygen affinity of fetal whole blood resides in the interaction of fetal hemoglobin with intracellular organic phosphate 2,3-diphosphoglycerate (2,3-DPG). The fetal hemoglobin (HgbF) tetramer is composed of two α-chains (identical to adult) and two α-chains. The latter differ from the β-chain of adult hemoglobin (HgbA) in 39 of 146 amino acid residues. Among these differences is the substitution of serine in the γ-chain of HgbF for histidine at the β-143 position of HgbA, which is located at the entrance to the central cavity of the hemoglobin tetramer. Owing to a positively charged imidazole group, histidine can bind with the negatively charged 2,3-DPG. Binding of 2,3-DPG to deoxyhemoglobin stabilizes the tetramer in the reduced form. Because serine is nonionized and does not interact with 2,3-DPG to the same extent as histidine,[259] the O_2 affinity of HgbF is increased and the dissociation curve is shifted to the left. If HgbA or HgbF is removed from the erythrocyte and stripped of organic phosphates, the O_2 affinity for both hemoglobins is similar. However, addition of equal amounts of 2,3-DPG to the hemoglobins decreases the O_2 affinity of HgbA (dissociation curve shifts to the right) to a greater extent than for HgbF. Thus, even though overall O_2 affinities are similar, differences in 2,3-DPG interaction result in a higher O_2 affinity for HgbF.

The proportion of HgbF to HgbA changes between 26 and 40 weeks of gestation, HgbF decreases linearly from 100 percent to about 70 percent, so that HgbA accounts for 30 percent of fetal hemoglobin at term.[260] This change in expression from γ- to β-globulin synthesis takes place in erythroid progenitor cells.[261] Although the basis for this switching is not yet known, our understanding of human globin gene regulation has provided important insights into several fetal hemoglobin disorders such as the thalassemias and sickle cell anemia. Duplication of the α-genes on chromosome 16 provides the normal fetus with four gene loci. The genes for the remaining globins are located on chromosome 11 and consist of $^G\gamma$, $^A\gamma$, d and β. The two γ-genes differ in the amino acid in position 36; glycine versus alanine. Hemoglobin A synthesis is dictated by the γ- and β-genes, HgbF by α and γ, and $HgbA_2$ by α and δ. Sequences in the δ region may be responsible for the relative expression of the γ-gene, such that fetal hemoglobin persists when these are absent.[262]

Fetal Kidney

Overall fetal water and electrolyte homeostasis is primarily mediated by fetal-maternal exchange across the placenta. However, urine production by the fetal kidney is essential to maintenance of amniotic fluid volume and composition. Although absolute glomerular filtration rate (GFR) increases during the third trimester, GFR per gram kidney weight does not change[263] because GFR and fetal kidney weight increase in parallel. The genesis of new glomeruli is complete by about 36 weeks.[264] Subsequent increases in GFR reflect increases in glomerular surface area for filtration, effective filtration pressure, and capillary filtration coefficient. Although glomerular filtration is related to hydrostatic pressure, and fetal blood pressure increases in the third trimester, both renal blood flow per gram kidney weight and filtration fraction (GFR/renal plasma flow) remain constant.[263] Newborn increases in filtration fraction parallel increases in arterial pressure, suggesting the lower hydrostatic pressure within the glomerulus contributes to the relatively low filtration fraction and GFR of the intrauterine kidney.[263,265] A mild glomerulotubular imbalance may describe the early-gestation fetus. However, renal tubular sodium and chloride reabsorptions increase in late gestation, such that glomerulotubular balance is maintained in the third-trimester fetus.[265,266]

Although fetal GFR is low, the daily urine production rate is large (equaling 60 to 80 percent of the amniotic fluid volume). The large urine output results from the large portion of the filtered water (20 percent) that is excreted in the form of hypotonic urine. The positive free water clearance characterizing fetal renal function originally led to the hypothesis that the fetal kidney lacked AVP receptors. However, ovine fetal renal collecting duct responses to AVP can be demonstrated in the second trimester,[267] indicating that diminished urine-concentrating ability is not caused by AVP receptor absence. Fetal renal V_2 receptors mediate AVP-induced tubular water reabsorption, and functional V_2 receptors are present in the fetal kidney by the beginning of the last third of gestation.[242,268] In addition, AVP-induced cyclic adenosine monophosphate production is not different from the adult,[269] and AVP-induced apical tubular water channels (aquaporin II) are expressed in the fetal kidney. In fact, the selective AVP V_2 receptor agonist [deamino^1,D-Arg^8]-vasopressin (dDAVP) appropriately increases fetal renal water reabsorption without affecting blood pressure or heart rate.[236] Thus, V_2 receptors mediate AVP effects on fetal urine production and amniotic fluid volume.[236,242] Instead, the reduced concentrating ability of the fetal kidney primarily reflects reductions in proximal tubular sodium reabsorption, short juxtamedullary nephron loops of Henle, and limited medullary interstitial urea concentrations.

Although fetal plasma renin activity levels are high, effective uncoupling of AII production from plasma renin activity and a high placental clearance rate for AII serve to minimize increases in fetal plasma AII levels. Limiting fluctuations in fetal plasma AII levels may be of advantage to the regulation of fetal renal function. For example, fetal AII infusion increases fetal mean arterial pressure, and renal and placental vascular resistances.[270] In contrast, fetal treatment with the ACE inhibitor captopril increases plasma renin activity and decreases arterial blood pressure, renal vascular resistance, and filtration fraction[271]; and urine flow effectively ceases.[272] Given the potential for AII to decrease placental blood flow,[244] uncoupling of renin-induced angiotensin I production, limited ACE activity, and augmented placental AII clearance may protect the fetal cardiovascular system from large increases in plasma AII levels. Collectively, plasma AII levels appear to be regulated within a very narrow range, and this regulation may be important to overall fetal homeostasis.

Atrial natriuretic factor granules are present in the fetal heart, and fetal plasma ANF levels are elevated relative to the adult.[273] Fetal plasma ANF levels increase in response to volume expansion,[274] and ANF infusion evokes limited increases in ovine fetal renal sodium excretion.[275,276] Fetal ANF infusion also decreases fetal plasma volume, with minimal effect on blood pressure.[273] These observations suggest that ANF actions in the fetus are primarily directed at volume homeostasis, with minimal cardiovascular effects.

The ability of the fetal kidney to excrete titratable acid and ammonia is limited relative to the adult. In addition, the threshold for fetal renal bicarbonate excretion (defined as the excretion of a determined amount of bicarbonate per unit GFR) is much lower than in the adult. That is, fetal urine tends to be alkaline at relatively low plasma bicarbonate levels despite the high fetal arterial P_{CO_2}.[277] Because fetal renal tubular mechanisms for glucose reabsorption are qualitatively similar to those of the adult, fetal renal glucose excretion is limited. In fact, the maximum ability of the fetal kidney to reabsorb glucose exceeds that of the adult when expressed as a function of GFR.[278]

Fetal Gastrointestinal System

Gastrointestinal Tract

Amniotic fluid contains measurable glucose, lactate, and amino acid concentrations, raising the possibility that fetal swallowing could serve as a source of nutrient uptake. Fetal swallowing contributes importantly to somatic growth and gastrointestinal development as a result of the large volume of ingested fluid. Ten to fifteen percent of fetal nitrogen requirements may result from swallowing of amniotic fluid protein.[354] Amino acids and glucose are absorbed and used by the fetus if they are administered into the fetal gastrointestinal tract.[355,356] Furthermore, intragastric ovine fetal nutrient administration partially ameliorates fetal growth restriction induced by maternal malnutrition.[357] Further evidence for the role of swallowing in fetal growth results from studies demonstrating that impairment of fetal rabbit swallowing at 24 days gestation (term = 31 days) induces an 8 percent weight decrease (compared with controls) by 28 days.[358] The fetal gastrointestinal tract is directly impacted, because esophageal ligation of fetal rabbit pups results in marked reductions in gastric and intestinal tissue weight and gastric acidity.[1] Reductions in gastrointestinal and somatic growth were reversed by fetal intragastric infusion of amniotic fluid.[1] Similarly, esophageal ligation of 90-day ovine fetuses (term = 145 to 150 days) induces a 30-percent decrease of small intestine villus height[359] and a reduction in liver, pancreas, and intestinal weight.[360] Although ingestion of amniotic fluid nutrients may be necessary for optimal fetal growth, trophic growth factors within the amniotic fluid also importantly contribute. Thus, the reduction in fetal rabbit weight induced by esophageal ligation is reversed by gastric infusion of EGF.[217] Studies in human infants support the association of fetal swallowing and gastrointestinal growth because upper gastrointestinal tract obstructions are associated with a significantly greater rate of human fetal growth restriction as compared with fetuses with lower gastrointestinal obstructions.[361,362]

Blood flow to the fetal intestine does not increase during moderate levels of hypoxemia. The artery-mesenteric vein difference in O_2 content is also unchanged so that at a constant blood flow intestinal O_2 consumption can remain the same during moderate hypoxemia. However, with more pronounced hypoxemia, fetal intestinal O_2 consumption falls as blood flow decreases and the O_2 content difference across the intestine fails to widen. The result is a metabolic acidosis in the blood draining the mesenteric system.[363]

Liver

Near term, the placenta is the major route for bilirubin elimination. Less than 10 percent of an administered bilirubin load is excreted in the fetal biliary tree over a 10-hour period; about 20 percent remains in plasma.[354] Thus, the fetal metabolic pathways for bilirubin and bile salts remain underdeveloped at term. The cholate pool size (normalized to body surface area) is one third and the synthetic rate one half adult levels. In premature infants, cholate pool size and synthesis rates represent less than half and one third, respectively, of term infant values. In fact, premature infant intraluminal duodenal bile acid concentrations are near or below the level required to form lipid micelles.[364] The unique attributes of the fetal hepatic circulation were detailed during the earlier discussion of fetal circulatory anatomy. Notably, the fetal hepatic blood supply primarily derives from the umbilical vein. The left lobe receives its blood supply almost exclusively from the umbilical vein (there is a small contribution from the hepatic artery), whereas the right lobe receives blood from the portal vein as well. The fetal liver under normal conditions accounts for about 20 percent of total fetal O_2 consumption.[365] Because hepatic glucose uptake and release are balanced, net glucose removal by the liver under normal conditions is minimal.[365] During episodes of hypoxemia, β-adrenergic receptor-mediated increases in hepatic glucose release account for the hyperglycemia characteristic of short-term fetal hypoxemia.[281] Hypoxia severe enough to decrease fetal O_2 consumption selectively reduces right hepatic lobe oxygen uptake, which exceeds that of the fetus as a whole. In contrast, O_2 uptake by the left lobe of the liver is unchanged.[365]

Fetal Adrenal and Thyroid

Adrenal

The fetal pituitary secretes ACTH in response to "stress," including hypoxemia.[282] The associated increase in cortisol exerts feedback inhibition of the continued ACTH response.[283] In the fetus and adult, proopiomelanocortin posttranslational processing gives rise to ACTH, corticotropin-like intermediate lobe peptide (CLIP), and α-melanocyte–stimulating hormone (α-MSH). The precursor peptide preproenkephalin is a distinct gene product giving rise to the enkephalins. Fetal proopiomelanocortin processing differs from the adult. For example, although ACTH is present in appreciable amounts, the fetal pituitary contains large amounts of CLIP and α-MSH. The fetal ratio of CLIP plus α-MSH to ACTH decreases from the end of the first trimester to term.[366] Because pituitary corticotropin-releasing hormone expression is relatively low until late gestation, AVP serves as the major corticotrophin-releasing factor in early gestation. With increasing gestational age, fetal cortisol levels progressively increase secondary to hypothalamic-pituitary axis maturation. Cortisol is important to pituitary maturation because it shifts corticotrophs from the fetal to the adult type and to adrenal maturation through regulation of ACTH receptor numbers.[367]

On a body weight basis, the fetal adrenal gland is an order of magnitude larger than in the adult. This increase in size is due to the presence of an adrenal cortical definitive zone and a so-called fetal zone that constitutes 85 percent of the adrenal at birth. Cortisol and mineralocorticoids are the major products of the fetal definitive zone, and fetal cortisol secretion is regulated by ACTH but not human chorionic gonadotropin.[209,368] Low-density lipoprotein–bound cholesterol (see the section entitled Receptor Mediated Endocytosis/Exocytosis) is the major source of steroid precursor in the fetal adrenal.[369,370] Because the enzyme 3α-hydroxysteroid dehydrogenase is lacking in the fetal adrenal, dehydroepiandrosterone sulfate is the major product of the fetal zone. At midgestation, dehydroepiandrosterone sulfate secretion is determined by both ACTH and human chorionic gonadotropin.[209,368] Both fetal ACTH and cortisol levels are relatively low during most of gestation, and there is not a clear correlation between plasma ACTH levels and cortisol production. This apparent dissociation between fetal ACTH levels and cortisol secretion[208] may be explained by (1) differences in ACTH processing and the presence of the large-molecular-weight proopiomelanocortin processing products (CLIP and α-MSH) may suppress ACTH action on the adrenal until late gestation (when ACTH becomes the primary product), (2) fetal adrenal definitive zone ACTH responsiveness may increase, or (3) placental ACTH posttranslational processing intermediates may affect the adrenal response to ACTH.

Resting fetal plasma norepinephrine levels exceed epinephrine levels approximately 10-fold.[371,372] The fetal plasma levels of both catecholamines increase in response to hypoxemia, with norepinephrine levels invariably in excess of the epinephrine levels.[372] Under basal conditions, norepinephrine is secreted at a higher rate than for epinephrine, and this relationship persists during a hypoxemic stimulus.[373] Plasma norepinephrine levels increase in response to acute hypoxemia but decline to remain above basal levels with persistent (>5 minutes) hypoxemia. In contrast, adrenal epinephrine secretion begins gradually but persists during 30 minutes of hypoxemia. These observations are consistent with independent sites of synthesis and regulation of the two catecholamines.[374] Although the initial fetal blood pressure elevation during hypoxemia correlates with increases in norepinephrine, afterward, the correlation between plasma norepinephrine and hypertension is lost.[372]

Thyroid

The normal placenta is impermeable to thyroid-stimulating hormone (TSH), and triiodothyronine (T_3) transfer is minimal.[375] However, appreciable levels of maternal thyroxine (T_4) are seen in infants with congenital hypothyroidism.[376] By the 12th week of gestation, thyrotropin-releasing hormone (TRH) is present in the fetal hypothalamus, and TRH secretion and pituitary sensitivity to TRH increases progressively during gestation. Extrahypothalamic sites including the pancreas also may contribute to the high TRH levels observed in the fetus.[375] Measurable TSH is present in the fetal pituitary and serum, and T_4 is measurable in fetal blood by week 12 of gestation. Thyroid function is low until about 20 weeks, when T_4 levels increase gradually to term. TSH levels increase markedly between 20 and 24 weeks, then slowly decrease until delivery. Fetal liver T_4 metabolism is immature, characterized by low T_3 levels until the 30th week. In contrast, reverse T_3 levels are high until 30 weeks, thereafter declining steadily until term.

Fetal Central Nervous System

Clinically relevant indicators of fetal central nervous system function are body movements and breathing movements. Fetal activity periods in late gestation are often termed active or reactive and quiet or nonreactive. The active cycle is characterized by clustering of gross fetal body movements, a high heart rate variability, heart rate accelerations (often followed by decelerations), and fetal breathing movements. The quiet cycle is noted by absence of fetal body movements and a low variability in the fetal heart rate.[377,378] Fetal heart period variability in this context refers to deviations about the model heart rate period averaged over short (seconds) periods,[379] and is distinct from beat-to-beat variability. In the last 6 weeks of gestation, the fetus is in an active state 60 to 70 percent of total time. The average duration of quiet periods ranges from 15 to 23 minutes (see Table IV in Visser et al.[379] for a review).

The fetal electrocorticogram shows two predominant patterns. Low-voltage (high-frequency) electrocortical activity is associated with bursts of rapid eye movements and fetal breathing movements.[380] Similar to rapid eye movement sleep in the adult, inhibition of skeletal muscle movement is most pronounced in muscle groups having a high percentage of spindles. Thus, the diaphragm, which is relatively spindle free, is not affected. Fetal body movements during low-voltage electrocortical activity are reduced relative to the activity seen during high-voltage (low-frequency) electrocortical activity.[381] Polysynaptic reflexes elicited by stimulation of afferents from limb muscles are relatively suppressed when the fetus is in the low-voltage state.[382] Short-term hypoxia[381] or hypoxemia inhibit reflex limb movements, with the inhibitory neural activity arising in the midbrain area.[382] Fetal cardiovascular and behavioral responses to maternal cocaine use previously have been attributed to reductions in uteroplacental blood flow and resulting fetal hypoxia. However, recent fetal sheep studies indicate that acute fetal cocaine exposure evokes catecholamine, cardiovascular, and neurobehavioral effects in the absence of fetal oxygenation changes.[383] It is not yet clear whether cocaine-induced reductions in fetal low-voltage electrocortical activity reflect changes in cerebral blood flow or a direct cocaine effect on norepinephrine stimulation of central regulatory centers. However, these observations are consistent with the significant neurologic consequences of cocaine use during pregnancy.

Fetal breathing patterns are rapid and irregular in nature, and are not associated with significant fluid movement into the lung.[380] The central medullary respiratory chemoreceptors are stimulated by CO_2,[384] and fetal breathing is maintained only if central hydrogen ion concentrations remain in the physiologic range. That is, central (medullary cerebrospinal fluid) acidosis stimulates respiratory incidence and depth, and alkalosis results in apnea.[385] Paradoxically, hypoxemia markedly decreases breathing activity, possibly due to inhibitory input from centers above the medulla.[386]

Glucose is the principal substrate for oxidative metabolism in the fetal brain under normal conditions.[371] During low-voltage electrocortical activity, cerebral blood flow and O_2 consumption are increased relative to high-voltage values,[387] with an efflux of lactate. During high voltage, the fetal brain shows a net uptake of lactate.[388] The fetal cerebral circulation is sensitive to changes in arterial O_2 content. Despite marked hypoxia-induced increases in cerebral blood flow, cerebral O_2 consumption is maintained without widening of the arteriovenous O_2 content difference across the brain.[389] Increases in CO_2 also cause cerebral vasodilation. However, the response to hypercapnia is reduced relative to the adult.[390]

Gestational Programming

The fetus develops within a complex milieu and is wholly dependent on its mother for nutrients. Disruptions in these processes, whether they are due to genetic, nutritional, or due to underlying or coincident maternal disease, may result in a fetus born smaller than its peers, or in the extreme situation, born with intrauterine growth restriction, a condition long known to be associated with perinatal complications including hypoglycemia, hypocalcemia, and polycythemia (see Chapter 34). Beginning in the late 1980s, however, data gleaned first from population-based epidemiologic studies, later supported by animal research, has provided strong evidence that fetal size at birth is related to a variety of health problems in later life. Furthermore, it has become clear that the risk of these conditions is not limited to those born pathologically small due to intrauterine growth restriction, but rather applies across a continuum of weights. Although a variety of health problems have been linked to size at birth, including stroke,[391] breast cancer,[392] and atopy,[393] the most robust evidence is that correlating size at birth with adult-onset insulin resistance, hypertension, and cardiovascular disease.

In 1986, Barker and Osmond published work linking rates of ischemic heart disease in England and Wales in the decade from 1968 to 1978 with infant mortality rates in the same regions from 1921 to 1925.[394] This work was similar to that performed previously by Rose and Fordahl[395,396] in 1964 and 1977, respectively. Subsequently, however, through the examination of detailed birth records, attributed to Ethel Margaret Burnside, a midwife in Hertfordshire England,[397] spanning the years 1911 to 1948, Barker and colleagues in 1989 made the sentinel observation that weight at birth was inversely related to both mortality from ischemic heart disease[398] and hypertension.[399] These studies were retrospective analyses of adult British men and women who, as infants, had birth measurements meticulously recorded. Data on approximately 16,000 subjects born between 1911 to 1930 revealed that the mortality rate from coronary artery disease was inversely related to birth weight up to 9.5 pounds, after which the risk again began to rise, perhaps because of the presence of infants of diabetic mothers in this group. Data for men is shown in Figure 2-8. The overall increase in mortality was greater if poor growth persisted through 1 year of age. Subsequent work in a variety of populations has supported the observed association between low birth weight and enhanced cardiovascular risk in later life, independent of other lifestyle risk factors.[400,401] Enhanced risk is observed in those exhibiting rapid catch-up growth in subsequent life. Recent data suggest that premature infants may share in theses risks.[402]

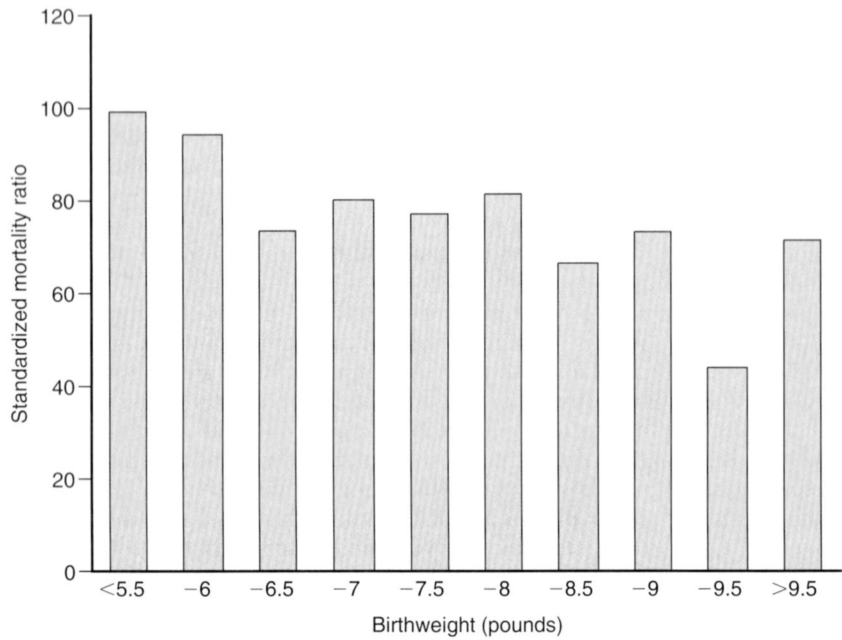

Figure 2-8. Standardized mortality ratio for men by birth weight in a Hertfordshire study.

Perhaps the most studied of all associations with small size at birth is the association with increased blood pressure during later life. Again, this association has been replicated in many different locales and populations. The increase noted in systolic blood pressure during adult life is approximately 3.5 mm Hg per kilogram decrement in weight.[400] Higher rates of postnatal weight gain appear to increase risk, as does advancing age. Twin studies have also been performed and have been broadly supportive of these concepts.[397,401] A few cautions remain; a recent meta-analysis of the association between size at birth and hypertension noted that smaller studies tended to report larger differences in blood pressure between groups, with larger studies often reporting smaller differences.[403] Thus, the possibility of publication bias against the publication of negative results exists. Even so, data supporting this association are plentiful and supported by animal data (see later).

Glucose intolerance and type 2 diabetes mellitus are becoming increasingly common. An association between size at birth (later extended to "thinness" at birth) was first identified in 1991, from review of the Hertfordshire population described earlier.[404,405] As in the earlier examples, these associations have since been confirmed in many other populations, as has the impact of accelerated weight gain, "catch-up" growth upon risk enhancement. The risk of developing glucose intolerance in adulthood increases in an almost linear fashion as birth weight decrease from 9.5 to 5.5 pounds. Thus, no "cutoff" exists, beyond which risk is elevated or eliminated.[406]

The above-mentioned findings have generated what is widely known as the Barker hypothesis or, alternatively, the fetal origins of adult disease hypothesis (see Chapter 34). The Barker hypothesis proposes that alterations in fetal nutrition or endocrine status result in developmental adaptations that may permanently change or "program" an individual's body structure, physiology, and metabolism, thereby predisposing individuals to cardiovascular, metabolic, and endocrine disease in adult life. The related "thrifty hypothesis" posits that suboptimal early nutrition results in fetal/neonatal metabolic adaptations designed to allow the organism to develop efficiently in a nutrient-poor environment. Subsequent exposure to a nutrient-rich environment postnatally then results in untoward consequences, including the development of type 2 diabetes mellitus and the metabolic syndrome.[407]

Both of these hypotheses infer a change or decrement in fetal nutrition as a cause of small size at birth. Evidence garnered from the study of Dutch famine survivors, in particular those in utero during the famine (1944 to 1945), has lent credence to this belief. Exposure to in utero calorie deprivation (400 to 800 kcal/day; baseline 1,800 kcal/day) during the first trimester of pregnancy led to infants born normally sized (maternal intakes normalized abruptly, potentially leading to fetal "catch-up" growth) but with an enhanced risk of coronary artery disease in later life, whereas exposure later in pregnancy led to small infants who, as adults, have had a predisposition to glucose intolerance.[408] These findings were not replicated in the Leningrad famine from 1941 to 1944.[409] The reasons behind the discordance are unclear; possibilities include the longer length of the Leningrad famine, its slow, gradual resolution, and less meticulous record keeping. It is also clear that genetic mechanisms exist by which infants may be predisposed both to small size and glucose intolerance, including abnormalities in the IGF-1 gene.[410] However, such genetic abnormalities thus far appear insufficient to explain the observed linkages between birth size and adult phenotype.

Although the relationship between birth size and hypertension, glucose intolerance, and cardiovascular disease has gained significant acceptance, the mechanisms by which these changes occur remain unclear and can best be explored through animal studies. Many such studies have been performed using models in which the maternal diet has been compromised, either through caloric or protein deprivation. Hypertension has been reliably reproduced in the offspring of laboratory animals deprived of protein, calories, and iron.[411–414] The mechanisms underlying these changes are thought to include programmed alterations in the hypothalamic-pituitary and renin-angiotensin axes, and diminished nephron number with a subsequent decrease in renal mass. In similar fashion, glucose intolerance has been evoked after in utero deprivation, the etiology of which includes diminished pancreatic β-cell mass and subsequent abnormalities in glucose secretion.[415] In addition, hepatic glucokinase activity is decreased, whereas phosphoenolpyruvate carboxykinase activity is increased, contributing to an increase in hepatic gluconeogenesis noted in the offspring of protein deprived mothers.[416]

The impact of infant size at birth, and thus of the fetal in utero milieu, does not end with the first generation. Indeed, mothers themselves born small tend to have smaller than average offspring who suffer higher than average rates of infant mortality.[417] Animal studies support this pattern: When a low-protein diet was administered to a colony of rats over 12 generations, low-protein diet–fed animals decreased to 67 percent of control size. When a regular (high-protein) diet was then introduced at weaning, weights did not "catch up" to control values for three generations. When pregnant animals were switched to a regular diet during pregnancy, however, offspring rapidly caught up to, and indeed surpassed, control weights.[418] These data are strikingly similar to those reported in humans as a result of the Dutch famine and confirm the disparate impact of malnutrition in utero at during different segments of pregnancy. Others have shown, again in animal models, an enhanced propensity to glucose intolerance in the second generation.[419] The mechanisms by which environment-induced alterations in phenotype are propagated generationally remain obscure; however, epigenetic modifications to DNA and DNA associated proteins seems a likely possibility.

Key Points

- Pregnancy-associated cardiovascular changes include a doubling of maternal cardiac output and a 40-percent increase in blood volume.
- Uterine blood flow at term averages 750 ml/min, or 10 to 15 percent of maternal cardiac output.
- Normal term placental weight averages 450 g, representing approximately one seventh (one sixth with cord and membranes) of fetal weight.
- Mean amniotic fluid volume increases from 250 to 800 ml between 16 and 32 weeks, and decreases to 500 ml at term.
- Fetal urine production ranges from 400 to 1,200 ml/day and is the primary source of amniotic fluid.
- The fetal umbilical circulation receives approximately 40 percent of fetal combined ventricular output (300 ml/mg/min).
- Umbilical blood flow is 70 to 130 ml/min after 30 weeks' gestation.
- Fetal cardiac output is constant over a heart rate range of 120 to 180 bpm.
- The fetus exists in a state of aerobic metabolism, with arterial Po_2 values in the 20- to 25-mm Hg range.
- Approximately 20 percent of the fetal O_2 consumption of 8 ml/kg/min is required in the acquisition of new tissue.
- The maternal environment during pregnancy (e.g., undernutrition) may have significant long-term effects, because growth-restricted offspring demonstrate an increased risk of adult metabolic syndrome.

REFERENCES

1. Challier JC, Schneider H, Dancis J: In vitro perfusion of human placenta. V. Oxygen consumption. Am J Obstet Gynecol 126:261, 1976.
2. Meschia G, Battaglia FC, Hay WW, Sparks JW: Utilization of substrates by the ovine placenta in vivo. Fed Proc 39:245, 1980.
3. Hauguel S, Chalier J-C, Cedard L, Olive G: Metabolism of the human placenta perfused in vitro: Glucose transfer and utilization, O2 consumption, lactate and ammomia production. Pediat Res 17:729, 1983.
4. Teasdale F: Gestational changes in the functional structure of the human placenta in relation to fetal growth: A morphometric study. Am J Obstet Gynecol 137:560, 1980.
5. Georgiades P, Ferguson-Smith AC, Burton GJ: Comparative developmental anatomy of the murine and human definitive placentae. Placenta 23:3, 2002.
6. Holzman I, Phillips AF, Battaglia FC: Glucose metabolism, lactate and ammonia production by the human placenta in vitro. Pediat Res 13:117, 1979.
7. Simmons MA, Battaglia FC, Meschia G: Placental transfer of glucose. J Devel Physiol 1:227, 1979.
8. Hay WW Jr, Sparks JW, Wilkening RB, et al: Partition of maternal glucose production between conceptus and maternal tissues in sheep. Am J Physiol 245:E347, 1983.
9. Hay WW Jr, Sparks JW, Wilkening RB, et al: Fetal glucose uptake and utilization as functions of maternal glucose concentration. Am J Physiol 246:E237, 1984.
10. Sparks JW, Hay WW Jr, Bonds D, et al: Simultaneous measurements of lactate turnover rate and umbilical lactate uptake in the fetal lamb. J Clin Invest 70:179, 1982.
11. Cross JC: Genes regulating embryonic and fetal survival. Theriogenology 55:193, 2001.
12. Cross JC: Genetic insights into trophoblast differentiation and placental morphogenesis. Semin Cell Dev Biol 11:105, 2000.
13. Beischer NA, Holsman M, Kitchen WH: Relation of various forms of anemia to placental weight. Am J Obstet Gynecol 101:80, 1968.
14. Beischer NA, Sivasamboo R, Vohras S, et al: Placental hypertrophy in severe pregnancy anaemia. J Obstet Gynaecol Br Comm 77:398, 1970.
15. Agboola A: Placental changes in patients with a low haematocrit. Br J Obstet Gynaecol 82:225, 1975.
16. Mayhew TM: Enhanced fetoplacental angiogenesis in pre-gestational diabetes mellitus: the extra growth is exclusively longitudinal and not accompanied by microvascular remodelling. Diabetologia 45:1434, 2002.

17. Makhseed M, Musini VM, Ahmed MA, Al-Harmi J: Placental pathology in relation to the White's classification of diabetes mellitus. Arch Gynecol Obstet 266:136, 2002.
18. Ogawa H, Ono Y, Shimozawa N, et al: Disruption of imprinting in cloned mouse fetuses from embryonic stem cells. Reproduction 126:549, 2003.
19. Frank D, Fortino W, Clark L, et al: Placental overgrowth in mice lacking the imprinted gene Ipl. Proc Natl Acad Sci U S A 99:7490, 2002.
20. Singh U, Fohn LE, Wakayama T, et al: Different molecular mechanisms underlie placental overgrowth phenotypes caused by interspecies hybridization, cloning, and Esx1 mutation. Dev Dyn 230:149, 2004.
21. Ohgane J, Wakayama T, Senda S, et al: The Sall3 locus is an epigenetic hotspot of aberrant DNA methylation associated with placentomegaly of cloned mice. Genes Cells 9:253, 2004.
22. Lao TT, Wong W: The neonatal implications of a high placental ratio in small-for-gestational age infants. Placenta 20:723, 1999.
23. Barker DJ: The long-term outcome of retarded fetal growth. Schweiz Med Wochenschr 129:189, 1999.
24. Gospodarowicz D: Growth factors and their action in vivo and in vitro. J Pathol 141:201, 1983.
25. Posner B: Insulin receptors in human and animal placental tissue. Diabetes 23:209, 1974.
26. Nelson DM, Smith RM, Jarett L: Nonuniform distribution and grouping of insulin receptors on the surface of human placental syncytiotrophoblast. Diabetes 27:530, 1978.
27. Whitsett JA, Lenard JL: Characteristics of the microvillus brush border of human placenta: Insulin receptor localization in brush border membranes. Endocrinol 103:1458, 1978.
28. Steel RB, Mosley JD, Smith CH: Insulin and placenta: Degradation and stabilization, binding to microvillous membrane receptors, and amnio acid uptake. Am J Obstet Gynecol 135:522, 1979.
29. Deal CL, Guyda HJ: Insulin receptors of human term placental cells and choriocarcinoma (JEG-3) cells: characteristics and regulation. Endocrinology 112:1512, 1983.
30. Harrison LC, Itin A: Purification of the insulin receptor from human placenta by chromatography on immobilized wheat germ and receptor antibody. J Biol Chem 255:12066, 1980.
31. Richards RC, Beardmore JM, Brown PJ, et al: Epidermal growth factor receptors on isolated human placental syncytiotrophoblast plasma membrane. Placenta 4:133, 1983.
32. Lai WH, Guyda HJ: Characterization and regulation of epidermal growth factor receptors in human placental cell cultures. J Clin Endocrinol Metab 58:344, 1984.
33. Zhou J, Bondy CA: Placental glucose transporter gene expression and metabolism in the rat. J Clin Invest 91:845, 1993.
34. Holmes R, Porter H, Newcomb P, et al: An immunohistochemical study of type I insulin-like growth factor receptors in the placentae of pregnancies with appropriately grown or growth restricted fetuses. Placenta 20:325, 1999.
35. Fondacci C, Alsat E, Gabriel R, et al: Alterations of human placental epidermal growth factor receptor in intrauterine growth retardation. J Clin Invest 93:1149, 1994.
36. Costa SC, Ayres dC, da Costa PA, Bernardes J: An interactive web site for research on fetal heart rate monitoring. Obstet Gynecol 95:309, 2000.
37. Peng C: The TGF-beta superfamily and its roles in the human ovary and placenta. J Obstet Gynaecol Can 25:834, 2003.
38. De FS, Gigante B, Persico MG: Structure and function of placental growth factor. Trends Cardiovasc Med 12:241, 2002.
39. Autiero M, Luttun A, Tjwa M, Carmeliet P: Placental growth factor and its receptor, vascular endothelial growth factor receptor-1: novel targets for stimulation of ischemic tissue revascularization and inhibition of angiogenic and inflammatory disorders. J Thromb Haemost 1:1356, 2003.
40. Christou H, Serdy S, Mantzoros CS: Leptin in relation to growth and developmental processes in the fetus. Semin Reprod Medb 20:123, 2002.
41. Bajoria R, Sooranna SR, Ward BS, Chatterjee R: Prospective function of placental leptin at maternal-fetal interface. Placenta 23:103, 2002.
42. Douglas GC, Thirkill TL: Chemokine receptor expression by human syncytiotrophoblast—a review. Placenta 22(Suppl A): S24, 2001.
43. Handwerger S, Freemark M: The roles of placental growth hormone and placental lactogen in the regulation of human fetal growth and development. J Pediatr Endocrinol Metab 13:343, 2000.
44. Maruo T, Matsuo H, Otani T, Mochizuki M: Role of epidermal growth factor (EGF) and its receptor in the development of the human placenta. Reprod Fertil Dev 7:1465, 1995.
45. Evain-Brion D, Alsat E: Epidermal growth factor receptor and human fetoplacental development. J Pediatr Endocrinol 7:295, 1994.
46. Zapf J, Rinderknecht E, Humbel RE, Froesch ER: Nonsupressible insulin-like activity (NSILA) from human serum: recent accomplishments and their physiologic implications. Metab Clin Exp 27:1803, 1978.
47. Cooke NE, Ray J, Emery JG, Liebhaber SA: Two distinct species of human growth hormone–varient mRNA in the human placenta predict the expression of novel growth hormone proteins. J Biol Chem 263:9001, 1988.
48. Eriksson L, Frankenne F, Eden S, et al: Growth hormone secretion during termination of pregnancy. Further evidence of a placental variant. Acta Obstet Gynecol Scand 67:549, 1988.
49. Frankenne F, Closset J, Gomez F: The physiology of growth hormones (GHs) in pregnant women and partial characterization of the placental GH variant. J Clin Endocrinol Metab 66:1171, 1988.
50. Liu JP, Baker J, Perkins AS, et al: Mice carrying null mutations of the genes encoding insulin-like growth factor I (Igf-1) and type 1 IGF receptor (Igf1r). Cell 75:59, 1993.
51. Baker J, Liu JP, Robertson EJ, Efstratiadis A: Role of insulin-like growth factors in embryonic and postnatal growth. Cell 75:73–82, 1993.
52. Lopez MF, Dikkes P, Zurakowski D, Villa-Komaroff L: Insulin-like growth factor II affects the appearance and glycogen content of glycogen cells in the murine placenta. Endocrinology 137:2100, 1996.
53. Wang ZQ, Fung MR, Barlow DP, Wagner EF: Regulation of embryonic growth and lysosomal targeting by the imprinted Igf2/Mpr gene. Nature 372:464, 1994.
54. Sibilia M, Wagner EF: Strain-dependent epithelial defects in mice lacking the EGF receptor. Science 269:234, 1995.
55. Threadgill DW, Dlugosz AA, Hansen LA, et al: Targeted disruption of mouse EGF receptor: effect of genetic background on mutant phenotype. Science 269:230, 1995.
56. King BF: Distribution and characterization of the anionic sites in trophoblast and capillary basal lamina of human placental villi. Anat Record 212:63, 1985.
57. Leach L, Firth JA: Structure and permeability of human placental microvasculature. Microsc Res Tech 38:137, 1997.
58. Thornburg KL, Faber JJ: Transfer of hydrophilic molecules by placenta and yolk sac of the guinea pig. Am J Physiol 233:C111, 1977.
59. Faber JJ: Filtration and diffusion across the immature placenta of the anaesthetized rat embryo. Placenta 20:331, 1999.
60. Sibley CP, Coan PM, Ferguson-Smith AC, et al: Placental-specific insulin-like growth factor 2 (Igf2) regulates the diffusional exchange characteristics of the mouse placenta. Proc Natl Acad Sci U S A 101:8204, 2004.
61. Roberts CT, Sohlstrom A, Kind KL, et al: Altered placental structure induced by maternal food restriction in guinea pigs: a role for circulating IGF-II and IGFBP-2 in the mother? Placenta 22 Suppl A:S77, 2001.
62. Bissonnette JM, Cronan JZ, Richards LL, Wickham WK: Placental transfer of water and nonelectrolytes during a single circulatory passage. Am J Physiol 236:C47, 1979.
63. Faber JJ: Review of flow limited transfer in the placenta. Int J Obstet Anesth 4:230, 1995.
64. Jaffe R, Jauniaux E, Hustin J: Maternal circulation in the first-trimester human placenta—myth or reality? Am J Obstet Gynecol 176:695, 1997.

65. Jauniaux E, Gulbis B, Burton GJ: The human first trimester gestational sac limits rather than facilitates oxygen transfer to the foetus—a review. Placenta 24(Suppl A):S86, 2003.
66. Adelman DM, Gertsenstein M, Nagy A, et al: Placental cell fates are regulated in vivo by HIF-mediated hypoxia responses. Genes Dev 14:3191, 2000.
67. Delivoria-Papadopoulos M, Coburn RF, Forster RE II: The placental diffusing capacity for carbon monixide in pregnant women at term. *In* Longo LD, Bartles H (eds): Respiratory Gas Exchange and Blood Flow in the Placenta. Bethesda, Department of Health, Education, and Welfare, 1972, p 259.
68. Rooth G, Sjostedt S: The placental transfer of gases and fixed acids. Arch Dis Child 37:366, 1962.
69. Bateman DN, Whittingham TA: Measurement of gastric emptying by real-time ultrasound. Gut 23:524, 1982.
70. Sjostedt S, Rooth G, Caligara F: The oxygen tension of the blood in the umbilical cord and intervillous space. Arch Dis Child 35:529, 1960.
71. Wulf H: Der Gasaustausch in der reifen Plazenta des Menschen. Z Geburtsh Gynak 158:117, 1962.
72. Talbert D, Sebire NJ: The dynamic placenta: I. Hypothetical model of a placental mechanism matching local fetal blood flow to local intervillus oxygen delivery. Med Hypotheses 62:511, 2004.
73. Clapp JF III: The relationship between blood flow and oxygen uptake in the uterine and umbilical circulations. Am J Obstet Gynecol 132:410, 1978.
74. Wilkening RB, Meschia G: Fetal oxygen uptake, oxygenations, and acid-base balance as a function of uterine blood flow. Am J Physiol 244:H749, 1983.
75. Itskovitz J, LaGamma EF, Rudolph LAM: The effect of reducing umbilical blood flow on fetal oxygenation. Am J Obstet Gynecol 145:813, 1983.
76. Itskovitz J, LaGamma EF, Rudolph AM: Baroreflex control of the circulation in chronically instrumented fetal lambs. Circ Res 52:589, 1983.
77. Wilkening RB, Meschia G: Effect of occluding one umbilical artery on placental oxygen transport. Am J Physiol 260:H1319, 1991.
78. Longo LD, Delivoria-Papadopoulos M, Foster RE II: Placental Co_2 transfer after fetal carbonic anhydrase inhibition. Am J Physiol 226:703, 1974.
79. Bissonnette JM: Studies in vivo of glucose transfer acorss the guinea-pig placenta. *In* Young M, Boyd RDH, Longo LD, Telegdy G (eds): Placental Transfer: Methods and Interpretations. Philadelphia, W.B. Saunders, 1981, p 155.
80. Johnson LW, Smith CH: Identification of the glucose transport protein of the microvillous membrane of human placenta by photoaffinity labeling. Biochem Biophys Res Comm 109:408, 1982.
81. Ingermann RL, Bissonnette JM, Koch PL: D-glucose-sensitive and -insensitive cytochalasin B binding proteins from microvillous plasma membranes of human placenta: Identification of the D-glucose transporter. Biochim Biophys Acta 730:57, 1983.
82. Illsley NP, Sellers MC, Wright RL: Glycaemic regulation of glucose transporter expression and activity in the human placenta. Placenta 19:517, 1998.
83. Jansson T, Wennergren M, Illsley NP: Glucose transporter protein expression in human placenta throughout gestation and in intrauterine growth retardation. J Clin Endocrinol Metab 77:1554, 1993.
84. Turner RJ, Silverman M: Sugar uptake into brush border vesicles from normal human kidney. Pro Natl Acad Sci U S A 74:2825, 1977.
85. Wright EM, Loo DD, Panayotova-Heiermann M, et al: "Active" sugar transport in eukaryotes. J Exp Biol 196:197, 1994.
86. Heilig CW, Brosius FC, III, Henry DN: Glucose transporters of the glomerulus and the implications for diabetic nephropathy. Kidney Int Suppl 60:S91, 1997.
87. Ciaraldi TP, Kolterman OE, Siegel JA, Olefsky JM: Insulin-stimulated glucose transport in human adipocytes. Am J Physiol 236:E621, 1979.
88. Charron MJ, Katz EB, Olson AL: GLUT4 gene regulation and manipulation. J Biol Chem 274:3253, 1999.
89. Livingstone C, Thomson FJ, Arbuckle MI, et al: Hormonal regulation of the insulin-responsive glucose transporter, GLUT4: some recent advances. Proc Nutr Soc 55:179, 1996.
90. Johnson LW, Smith CH: Monosaccharide transport across microvillous membrane of human placenta. Am J Physiol 236:E621, 1980.
91. Bissonnette JM, Ingermann RL, Thronburg KL: Placental sugar transport. *In* Yudilevich DL, Mann GE (eds): Carrier-mediated transport of solutes from blood to tissue. London, Longman, 1985, p 65.
92. Cordero L Jr, Yeh SY, Grunt JA, Anderson GG: Hypertonic glucose infusion during labor. Am J Obstet Gynecol 407:295, 1970.
93. Baumann MU, Deborde S, Illsley NP: Placental glucose transfer and fetal growth. Endocrine 19:13, 2002.
94. Jansson T, Ekstrand Y, Bjorn C, et al: Alterations in the activity of placental amino acid transporters in pregnancies complicated by diabetes. Diabetes 51:2214, 2002.
95. Jansson T, Ylven K, Wennergren M, Powell TL: Glucose transport and system A activity in syncytiotrophoblast microvillous and basal plasma membranes in intrauterine growth restriction. Placenta 23:392, 2002.
96. Hahn T, Barth S, Graf R, et al: Placental glucose transporter expression is regulated by glucocorticoids. J Clin Endocrinol Metab 84:1445, 1999.
97. Hauguel-de MS, Challier JC, Kacemi A, et al: The GLUT3 glucose transporter isoform is differentially expressed within human placental cell types. J Clin Endocrinol Metab 82:2689, 1997.
98. Lesage J, Hahn D, Leonhardt M, et al: Maternal undernutrition during late gestation-induced intrauterine growth restriction in the rat is associated with impaired placental GLUT3 expression, but does not correlate with endogenous corticosterone levels. J Endocrinol 174:37, 2002.
99. Regnault TR, de VB, Battaglia FC: Transport and metabolism of amino acids in placenta. Endocrine19:23, 2002.
100. Ruzycki SM, Kelly LK, Smith CH: Placental amino acid uptake. IV. Transport by microvillous membrane vesicles. Am J Physiol 234:C27, 1978.
101. Boyd CAR, Lund EK: L-Proline transport by brush border membrane vesicles prepared from human placenta. J Physiol 315:9, 1981.
102. Whitsett JA, Wallick ET; [3H] Oubain binding and Na+-K -ATPase activity in human placenta. Am J Physiol 238:E38, 1980.
103. Zerangue N, Kavanaugh MP: ASCT-1 is a neutral amino acid exchanger with chloride channel activity. J Biol Chem 271:27991, 1996.
104. Chillaron J, Estevez R, Mora C, et al: Obligatory amino acid exchange via systems bo,+-like and y+L-like. A tertiary active transport mechanism for renal reabsorption of cystine and dibasic amino acids. J Biol Chem 271:17761, 1996.
105. Torres-Zamorano V, Leibach FH, Ganapathy V: Amino acid transporter ATB degree. Biochem Biophys Res Commun 245:824, 1998.
106. Hoeltzli SD, Smith CH: Alanine transport systems in isolated basal plasma membrane of human placenta. Am J Physiol 256: C630, 1989.
107. Johnson LW, Smith CH: Neutral amino acid transport systems of microvillous membrane of human placenta. Am J Physiol 254: C773, 1988.
108. Karl PI, Fisher SE: Taurine transport by microvillous membrane vesicles and the perfused cotyledon of the human placenta. Am J Physiol 258:C443, 1990.
109. Liu W, Leibach FH, Ganapathy V: Characterization of the glycine transport system GLYT 1 in human placental choriocarcinoma cells (JAR). Biochim Biophys Acta 1194:176, 1994.
110. Malandro MS, Beveridge MJ, Kilberg MS, Novak DA: Ontogeny of cationic amino acid transport systems in rat placenta. Am J Physiol 267:C804, 1994.
111. Novak DA, Beveridge MJ: Glutamine transport in human and rat placenta. Placenta 18:379, 1997.
112. Kamath SG, Furesz TC, Way BA, Smith CH: Identification of three cationic amino acid transporters in placental trophoblast: cloning, expression, and characterization of hCAT-1. J Membr Biol 171:55, 1999.
113. Furesz TC, Moe AJ, Smith CH: Lysine uptake by human placental microvillous membrane: comparison of system y+ with basal membrane. Am J Physiol 268:C755, 1995.

114. Hoeltzli SD, Kelley LK, Moe AJ, Smith CH: Anionic amino acid transport systems in isolated basal plasma membrane of human placenta. Am J Physiol 259:C47, 1990.
115. Moe AJ, Smith CH: Anionic amino acid uptake by microvillous membrane vesicles from human placenta. Am J Physiol 257: C1005, 1989.
116. Noorlander CW, de Graan PN, Nikkels PG, et al: Distribution of glutamate transporters in the human placenta. Placenta 25:489, 2004.
117. Matthews JC, Beveridge MJ, Malandro MS, et al: Activity and protein localization of multiple glutamate transporters in gestation day 14 vs. day 20 rat placenta. Am J Physiol 274:C603, 1998.
118. Cariappa R, Heath-Monnig E, Smith CH: Isoforms of amino acid transporters in placental syncytiotrophoblast: plasma membrane localization and potential role in maternal/fetal transport. Placenta 24:713, 2003.
119. Novak D, Matthews J: Glutamate transport by Rcho-1 cells derived from rat placenta. Pediatr Res 53:1025, 2003.
120. Novak D, Quiggle F, Artime C, Beveridge M: Regulation of glutamate transport and transport proteins in a placental cell line. Am J Physiol Cell Physiol 281:C1014, 2001.
121. Smith CH, Adcock EW, Teasdale F, et al: Placental amino acid uptake: Tissue preparation, kinetics, and preincubation effect. Am J Physiol 224:558, 1973.
122. Smith CH, Depper R: Placental amino acid uptake. II. Tissue preincubation, fluid distribution and mechanisms of regulation. Pediatr Res 8:697, 1974.
123. Longo LD, Yuen P, Gusseck DJ: Anaerobic glycogen-dependent transport of amnio acids by the placenta. Nature 243:531, 1973.
124. Karl PI, Alpy KL, Fisher SE: Amino acid transport by the cultured human placental trophoblast: effect of insulin on AIB transport. Am J Physiol 262:c834, 1992.
125. Karl PI: Insulin-like growth factor-1 stimulates amino acid uptake by the cultured human placental trophoblast. J Cell Physiol 165:83, 1995.
126. Glazier JD, Sibley CP, Carter AM: Effect of fetal growth restriction on system A amino acid transporter activity in the maternal facing plasma membrane of rat syncytiotrophoblast. Pediatr Res 40:325, 1996.
127. Mahendran D, Donnai P, Glazier JD, et al: Amino acid (system A) transporter activity in microvillous membrane vesicles from the placentas of appropriate and small for gestational age babies. Pediatr Res 34:661, 1993.
128. Moores RR Jr, Vaughn PR, Battaglia FC, et al: Glutamate metabolism in fetus and placenta of late-gestation sheep. Am J Physiol 267:R89, 1994.
129. Vaughn PR, Lobo C, Battaglia FC, et al: Glutamine-glutamate exchange between placenta and fetal liver. Am J Physiol 268: E705, 1995.
130. Cetin I, Fennessey PV, Quick AN Jr, et al: Glycine turnover and oxidation and hepatic serine synthesis from glycine in fetal lambs. Am J Physiol 260:E371, 1991.
131. van der Vusse GJ, van Bilsen M, Glatz JF, et al: Critical steps in cellular fatty acid uptake and utilization. Mol Cell Biochem 239:9, 2002.
132. Campbell FM, Dutta-Roy AK: Plasma membrane fatty acid-binding protein (FABPpm) is exclusively located in the maternal facing membranes of the human placenta. FEBS Lett 375:227, 1995.
133. Campbell FM, Bush PG, Veerkamp JH, Dutta-Roy AK: Detection and cellular localization of plasma membrane–associated and cytoplasmic fatty acid–binding proteins in human placenta. Placenta 19:409, 1998.
134. Larque E, Demmelmair H, Berger B, et al: In vivo investigation of the placental transfer of (13)C-labeled fatty acids in humans. J Lipid Res 44:49, 2003.
135. Bildirici I, Roh CR, Schaiff WT, et al: The lipid droplet-associated protein adipophilin is expressed in human trophoblasts and is regulated by peroxisomal proliferator-activated receptor-gamma/retinoid X receptor. J Clin Endocrinol Metab 88:6056, 2003.
136. Gimeno RE, Hirsch DJ, Punreddy S, et al: Targeted deletion of fatty acid transport protein-4 results in early embryonic lethality. J Biol Chem 278:49512, 2003.
137. Dancis J, Jansen V, Kayden HJ, et al: Transfer across perfused human placenta. 3. Effect of chain length on transfer of free fatty acids. Pediatr Res 8:796, 1974.
138. Honda M, Lowy C, Thomas CR: The effects of maternal diabetes on placental transfer of essential and non-essential fatty acids in the rat. Diabetes Res 15:47, 1990.
139. Haggarty P, Page K, Abramovich DR, et al: Long-chain polyunsaturated fatty acid transport across the perfused human placenta. Placenta 18:635,1997.
140. Haggarty P: Placental regulation of fatty acid delivery and its effect on fetal growth—a review. Placenta 23(Suppl A):S28, 2002.
141. Stammers J, Stephenson T, Colley J, Hull D: Effect on placental transfer of exogenous lipid administered to the pregnant rabbit. Pediatr Res 38:1026, 1995.
142. Hoggard N, Haggarty P, Thomas L, Lea RG: Leptin expression in placental and fetal tissues: does leptin have a functional role? Biochem Soc Trans 29:57, 2001.
143. Madsen EM, Lindegaard ML, Andersen CB, et al: Human placenta secretes apolipoprotein B-100–containing lipoproteins. J Biol Chem 279:55271, 2004.
144. Faber JJ, Thornburg KL: Fetal homeostasis in relation to placental water exchange. Ann Rech Vet 8:353, 1977.
145. Dancis J, Kammerman BS, Jansen V, et al: Transfer of urea, sodium, and chloride across the perfused human placenta. Am J Obstet Gynecol 141:677, 1981.
146. Faber JJ, Thornburg KL: Placental Physiology. New York: Raven Press, 1983. p 95.
147. Faber J, Thornburg K: The forces that drive inert solutes and water across the epitheliochorial placentae of the sheep and the goat and the haemochorial placentae of the rabbit and the guinea pig. Placenta 2:203, 1981.
148. Battaglia F, Prystowsky H, Smisson C, et al: The effect of the administration of fluids intravenously to mothers upon the concentrations of water and electrolytes in plasma of human fetuses. Pediatrics 25:2, 1960.
149. Reynolds SRM: Multiple simultaneous intervillous space pressures recorded in several regions of the hemochorial palcenta in relation to functional anatomy of the fetal cotyledon. Am J Obstet Gynecol 102:1128, 1968.
150. Seeds AE: Water metabolism in the fetus. Am J Obstet Gynecol 92:727, 1965.
151. Anderson DF, Faber JJ: Water flux due to colloid osmotic pressures across the haemochorial placenta of the guinea pig. J Physiol 332:521, 1982.
152. Wilbur WJ, Power GG, Longo LD: Water exchange in the placenta: a mathematical model. Am J Physiol 235:R181, 1978.
153. Sebire NJ, Talbert D: The dynamic placenta: II. Hypothetical model of a fetus driven transplacental water balance mechanism producing low apparent permeability in a highly permeable placenta. Med Hypotheses 62:520, 2004.
154. Brownbill P, Bell NJ, Woods RJ, et al: Neurokinin B is a paracrine vasodilator in the human fetal placental circulation. J Clin Endocrinol Metab 88:2164, 2003.
155. Ma T, Yang B, Verkman AS: Cloning of a novel water and urea-permeable aquaporin from mouse expressed strongly in colon, placenta, liver, and heart. Biochem Biophys Res Commun 240:324, 1997.
156. Hasegawa H, Lian SC, Finkbeiner WE, Verkman AS: Extrarenal tissue distribution of CHIP28 water channels by in situ hybridization and antibody staining. Am J Physiol 266:C893, 1994.
157. Damiano A, Zotta E, Goldstein J, et al: Water channel proteins AQP3 and AQP9 are present in syncytiotrophoblast of human term placenta. Placenta 22:776, 2001.
158. Stulc J: Placental transfer of inorganic ions and water. Physiol Rev 77:805, 1997.
159. Moe AJ: Placental amino acid transport. Am J Physiol 268:C1321, 1995.
160. Lajeunesse D, Brunette MG: Sodium gradient–dependent phosphate transport in placental brush border membrane vesicles. Placenta 9:117, 1988.
161. Balkovetz DF, Leibach FH, Mahesh VB, et al: Na+-H+ exchanager of human placental brush-border membrane: Identification and characterization. Am J Physiol 251:C852, 1986.
162. Wang H, Huang W, Fei YJ, et al: Human placental Na+-dependent multivitamin transporter. Cloning, functional expres-

sion, gene structure, and chromosomal localization. J Biol Chem 274:14875, 1999.
163. Prasad PD, Ramamoorthy S, Leibach FH, Ganapathy V: Characterization of a sodium-dependent vitamin transporter mediating the uptake of pantothenate, biotin and lipoate in human placental choriocarcinoma cells. Placenta 18:527, 1997.
164. Clarson LH, Greenwood SL, Mylona P, Sibley CP: Inwardly rectifying K(+) current and differentiation of human placental cytotrophoblast cells in culture. Placenta 22:328, 2001.
165. Page KR, Ashworth CJ, McArdle HJ, et al: Sodium transport across the chorioallantoic membrane of porcine placenta involves the epithelial sodium channel (ENaC). J Physiol 547:849, 2003.
166. Bara M, Challier JC, Guit-Bara A: Membrane potential and input resistance in syncytiotrophoblast of human term placenta in vitro. Placenta 9:139, 1988.
167. Powell TL, Lundquist C, Doughty IM, et al: Mechanisms of chloride transport across the syncytiotrophoblast basal membrane in the human placenta. Placenta 19:315, 1998.
168. Doughty IM, Glazier JD, Greenwood SL, et al: Mechanisms of maternofetal chloride transfer across the human placenta perfused in vitro. Am J Physiol 271:R1701, 1996.
169. Doughty IM, Glazier JD, Powell TL, et al: Chloride transport across syncytiotrophoblast microvillous membrane of first trimester human placenta. Pediatr Res 44:226, 1998.
170. Driver PM, Rauz S, Walker EA, et al: Characterization of human trophoblast as a mineralocorticoid target tissue. Mol Hum Reprod 9:793, 2003.
171. Sibley CP, Glazier JD, Greenwood SL, et al: Regulation of placental transfer: the Na(+)/H(+) exchanger–a review. Placenta 23(Suppl A):S39, 2002.
172. Persson A, Johansson M, Jansson T, Powell TL: Na(+)/K(+)-ATPase activity and expression in syncytiotrophoblast plasma membranes in pregnancies complicated by diabetes. Placenta 23:386, 2002.
173. Care AD, Ross R, Pickard DW, et al: Calcium homeostasis in the fetal pig. J Devel Physiol 4:85-106, 1982.
174. Fisher GJ, Kelly LK, Smith CH: ATP-dependent calcium transpsort across basal plasma membranes of human placental trophoblast. Am J Physiol 252:C38, 1987.
175. Borke JL, Caride A, Verma AK, et al: Calcium pump epitopes in placental trophoblast basal plasma membranes. Am J Physiol 257:c341, 1989.
176. Belkacemi L, Bedard I, Simoneau L, Lafond J: Calcium channels, transporters and exchangers in placenta: a review. Cell Calcium;37:1–8, 2005.
177. Brunette MG, Leclerc M: Ca2+ transport through the brush border membrane of human placenta syncytiotrophoblasts. Can J Physiol Pharmacol 70:835, 1992.
178. Kamath SG, Kelley LK, Friedman AF, Smith CH: Transport and binding in calcium uptake by microvillous membrane of human placenta. Am J Physiol 262:C789, 1992.
179. Belkacemi L, Simoneau L, Lafond J: Calcium-binding proteins: distribution and implication in mammalian placenta. Endocrine 19:57, 2002.
180. Desoye G, Hartmann M, Jones CJ, et al: Location of insulin receptors in the placenta and its progenitor tissues. Microsc Res Tech 38:63, 1997.
181. Malassine A, Alsat E, Besse C, et al: Acetylated low density lipoprotein endocytosis by human syncytiotrophoblast in culture. Placenta 11:191, 1990.
182. Wittmaack FM, Gafvels ME, Bronner M, et al: Localization and regulation of the human very low density lipoprotein/apolipoprotein-E receptor: trophoblast expression predicts a role for the receptor in placental lipid transport. Endocrinology 136:340, 1995.
183. Wyne KL, Woollett LA: Transport of maternal LDL and HDL to the fetal membranes and placenta of the Golden Syrian hamster is mediated by receptor-dependent and receptor-independent processes. J Lipid Res 39:518, 1998.
184. Fuchs R, Ellinger I: Endocytic and transcytotic processes in villous syncytiotrophoblast: role in nutrient transport to the human fetus. Traffic 5:725, 2004.
185. Loh TT, Higuchi DA, van Bockxmeer FM: Transferrin receptors on the human placental microvillus membrane. J Clin Invest 65:1182, 1980.
186. Ellinger I, Schwab M, Stefanescu A, et al: IgG transport across trophoblast-derived BeWo cells: a model system to study IgG transport in the placenta. Eur J Immunol 29:733, 1999.
187. Bright NA, Ockleford CD, Anwar M: Ontogeny and distribution of Fc gamma receptors in the human placenta. Transport or immune surveillance? J Anat 184(Pt 2):297, 1994.
188. Woollett LA: Origin of cholesterol in the fetal golden Syrian hamster: contribution of de novo sterol synthesis and maternal-derived lipoprotein cholesterol. J Lipid Res 37:1246, 1996.
189. Lin DS, Pitkin RM, Connor WE: Placental transfer of cholesterol into the human fetus. Am J Obstet Gynecol 128:735, 1977.
190. Sooranna SR, Moss J, Contractor SF: Comparison of the intracellular pathways of immunoglobulin-G and low density lipoprotein in cultured human term trophoblast cells. Cell Tissue Res 274:619, 1993.
191. Radulescu L, Antohe F, Jinga V, et al: Neonatal Fc receptors discriminates and monitors the pathway of native and modified immunoglobulin G in placental endothelial cells. Hum Immunol 65:578, 2004.
192. Douglas GC, King BF: Uptake and processing of 125I-labelled transferrin and 59Fe-labelled transferrin by isolated human trophoblast cells. Placenta 11:41, 1990.
193. Liu J, Shapiro JI: Endocytosis and signal transduction: basic science update. Biol Res Nurs 5:117, 2003.
194. Jayanthi LD, Samuvel DJ, Ramamoorthy S: Regulated internalization and phosphorylation of the native norepinephrine transporter in response to phorbol esters. Evidence for localization in lipid rafts and lipid raft-mediated internalization. J Biol Chem 279:19315, 2004.
195. Rosenfeld CR: Circulatory changes in the reproductive tissues of ewes during pregnancy. Gynecol Invest 5:252, 1974.
196. Longo LD, Ching KS: Placental diffusing capacity for carbon monoxide and oxygen in unanesthetized sheep. J Appl Physiol 43:885, 1977.
197. Bissonnette JM, Wickham WK: Placental diffusing capacity for carbon monoxide in unanesthetized guinea pigs. Respir Physiol 31:161, 1977.
198. Rosenfeld CR, Cox BE, Roy T, Magness RR: Nitric oxide contributes to estrogen-induced vasodilation of the ovine uterine circulation. J Clin Invest 98:2158, 1996.
199. Assali NS, Douglas RA, Barid WW, et al: Measurement of uterine blood flow and uterine metabolism. Am J Obstet Gynecol 66:248, 1953.
200. Metcalfe J, Romney SL, Ramsey LH, et al: Estimation of uterine blood flow and uterine metabolism. J Clin Invest 34:1632, 1995.
201. Lumbers ER: Effects of drugs on uteroplacental blood flow and the health of the foetus. Clin Exp Pharmacol Physiol 24:864, 1997.
202. Rosenfeld CR, Naden RP: Responses of uterine and nonuterine tissues to angiotensin II in ovine pregnancy. Am J Physiol 257: H17, 1995.
203. Rosenfeld CR: Mechanisms regulating angiotensin II responsiveness by the uteroplacental circulation. Am J Physiol Regul Integr Comp Physiol 281:R1025, 2001.
204. Meschia G: Circulation to female reproductive organs. *In* Shepherd JT, Abboud FM (eds): Handbook of Physiology—The Cardiovascular System III. Peripheral Circulation and Organ Blood Flow. Bethesda, American Physiological Society, 1983, p 241.
205. Hendricks CH, Quilligan EJ, Tyler CW, Tucker CJ: Pressure relationships between the intervillous space and the amniotic fluid in human term pregnancy. Am J Obstet Gynecol 77:1028, 1959.
206. Gangula PR, Thota C, Wimalawansa SJ, et al: Mechanisms involved in calcitonin gene–related peptide-induced relaxation in pregnant rat uterine artery. Biol Reprod 69:1635, 2003.
207. Lang U, Baker RS, Khoury J, Clark KE: Effects of chronic reduction in uterine blood flow on fetal and placental growth in the sheep. Am J Physiol Regul Integr Comp Physiol 279:R53, 2000.
208. Rudolph AM, Heymann MA: Circulatory changes during growth in the fetal lamb. Circ Res 26:289, 1970.
209. Wladimiroff JW, McGhie J: Ultrasonic assessment of cardiovascular geometry and function in the human fetus. Br J Obstet Gynecol 88:870, 1981.

210. Makowski EL, Meschia G, Droegemueller W, Battaglia FC: Measurement of umbilical arterial blood flow to the sheep placenta and fetus in utero. Circ Res 23:623, 1968.
211. Berman W Jr, Goodlin RC, Heymann MA, Rudolph AM: Relationships between pressure and flow in the umbilical and uterine circulations of the sheep. Cir Res 38:262, 1976.
212. Le Bouteiller P: HLA-G: what's new? Am J Reprod Immunol 38:146, 1997.
213. Athanassiades A, Lala PK: Role of placenta growth factor (PIGF) in human extravillous trophoblast proliferation, migration and invasiveness. Placenta 19:465, 1998.
214. Athanassiades A, Hamilton GS, Lala PK: Vascular endothelial growth factor stimulates proliferation but not migration or invasiveness in human extravillous trophoblast. Biol Reprod 59:643, 1998.
215. Thornburg KL, Bissonnette JM, Faber JJ: Absence of fetal placental waterfall phenomenon in chronically prepared fetal lambs. Am J Physiol 230:886, 1976.
216. Cohn HE, Piasecki GJ, Jackson BT: The effect of fetal heart rate on cardiovascular function during hypoxemia. Am J Obstet Gynecol 138:1190, 1980.
217. Cohn HE, Sacks EJ, Heymann MA, Rudolph AM: Cardiovascular responses to hypoxemia and acidemia in fetal lambs. Am J Obstet Gynecol 120:817, 1974.
218. Parer JT: Fetal oxygen uptake and umbilical circulation during maternal hypoxia in the chronically catheterized sheep. *In* Longo LD, Reneau DD (eds): Fetal and Newborn Cardiovascular Physiology, Vol. 2. New York, Garland STPM Press, 1978, p 231.
219. Peeters LL, Sheldon RE, Jones MD Jr, et al: Blood flow to fetal organs as a function of arterial oxygen content. Am J Obstet Gynecol 135:637, 1979.
220. Gude NM, King RG, Brennecke SP: Autacoid interactions in the regulation of blood flow in the human placenta. Clin Exp Pharmacol Physiol 25:706, 1998.
221. Boura AL, Walters WA, Read MA, Leitch IM: Autacoids and control of human placental blood flow. Clin Exp Pharmacol Physiol 21:737, 1994.
222. Thaete LG, Dewey ER, Neerhof MG: Endothelin and the regulation of uterine and placental perfusion in hypoxia-induced fetal growth restriction. J Soc Gynecol Investig 11:16, 2004.
223. Galbraith RM, Kantor RRS, Ferra GB, et al: Differential anatomical expression of transplantation antigens within the normal human placental chorionic villus. Am J Reprod Immunol 1:331, 1981.
224. Sunderland CA, Naiem M, Mason DY, et al: The expression of major histocompatibility antigens by human chorionic villi. J Reprod Immuol 3:323, 1981.
225. Ober C, van der Ven K: Immunogenetics of reproduction: an overview. Curr Top Microbiol Immunol 222:1, 1997.
226. Murphy SP, Choi JC, Holtz R: Regulation of major histocompatibility complex class II gene expression in trophoblast cells. Reprod Biol Endocrinol 2:52, 2004.
227. Hammer A, Hutter H, Dohr G: HLA class I expression on the materno-fetal interface. Am J Reprod Immunol 38:150, 1997.
228. Moffett-King A: Natural killer cells and pregnancy. Nat Rev Immunol 2:656, 2002.
229. Parham P: NK cells and trophoblasts: partners in pregnancy. J Exp Med 200:951, 2004.
230. Thellin O, Coumans B, Zorzi W, et al: Tolerance to the foeto-placental 'graft': ten ways to support a child for nine months. Curr Opin Immunol 12:731, 2000.
231. Mellor AL, Sivakumar J, Chandler P, et al: Prevention of T cell–driven complement activation and inflammation by tryptophan catabolism during pregnancy. Nat Immunol 2:64, 2001.
232. Brace RA, Wolf EJ: Normal amniotic fluid volume changes throughout pregnancy. Am J Obstet Gynecol 161:382, 1989.
233. Anderson DF, Faber JJ, Parks CM: Extraplacental transfer of water in the sheep. J Physiol 406:75, 1988.
234. Mesher EJ, Platzker AC, Ballard PL, et al: Ontogeny of tracheal fluid, pulmonary surfactant, and plasma corticoids in the fetal lamb. J Appl Physiol 39:1017, 1975.
235. Olver RE, Schneeberger EE, Walters DV: Epithelial solute premeability, ion transport and tight junction morphology in the developing lung of the fetal lamb. J Physiol 315:395, 1981.
236. Adamson TM, Boyd R, Platt H, Strang L: Composition of alveolar liquid in the foetal lamb. J Physiol 204:159, 1969.
237. Walters DV, Olver RE: The role of catecholamines in lung liquid absorption at birth. Pediatr Res 12:239, 1978.
238. Perks AM, Cassin S: The effects of arginine vasopressin on lung fluid secretion in chronic fetal sheep. *In* Jones CT, Nathanielsz PW (eds): The Physiological Development of the Fetus and Newborn. London, Academic Press, 1985, p 252.
239. Castro R, Ervin MG, Ross MG, et al: Ovine fetal lung fluid response to atrial natriuretic factor. Am J Obstet Gynecol 161:1337, 1989.
240. Gresham EL, Rankin JH, Makowski EL, et al: An evaluation of fetal renal function in a chronic sheep preparation. J Clin Invest 51:149, 1972.
241. Rabinowitz R, Peters MT, Vyas S, et al: Measurement of fetal urine production in normal pregnancy by real-time ultrasonography. Am J Obstet Gynecol 161:1264, 1989.
242. Canning JF, Boyd RDH: Mineral and water exchange between mother and fetus. *In* Beard RW, Nathanielsz PW (eds): Fetal Physiology and Medicine. New York, Marcel Dekker; 1984, p 481.
243. Robillard JE, Weitzman RE: Developmental aspects of the fetal renal response to exogenous arginine vasopressin. Am J Physiol 238:F407, 1980.
244. Lingwood B, Hardy KJ, Coghlan JP, Wintour EM: Effect of aldosterone on urine composition in the chronically cannulated ovine foetus. J Endocrinol 76:553, 1978.
245. Harding R, Bocking AD, Sigger JN, Wickham PJ: Composition and volume of fluid swallowed by fetal sheep. Q J Exp Physiol 69:487, 1984.
246. Pritchard JA: Deglutition by normal and anencephalic fetuses. Obstet Gynecol 25:289, 1965.
247. Pritchard JA: Fetal swallowing and amniotic fluid volume. Obstet Gynecol 28:606, 1966.
248. Bradley RM, Mistretta CM: Swallowing in fetal sheep. Science 179:1016, 1973.
249. Abramovich DR: Fetal factors influencing the volume and composition of liquor amnii. J Obstet Gynaecol Br Commonw 77:865, 1970.
250. Harding R, Sigger JN, Poore ER, Johnson P: Ingestion in fetal sheep and its relation to sleep states and breathing movements. Q J Exp Physiol 69:477, 1984.
251. Ross MG, Sherman J, Ervin M, et al: Stimuli for fetal swallowing: Systemic factors. Am J Obstet Gynecol 161:1559, 1989.
252. Abramovich DR, Page KR, Jandial L: Bulk flows through human fetal membranes. Gynecol Invest 7:157, 1976.
253. Gilbert WM, Brace RA: The missing link in amniotic fluid volume regulation: intramembranous absorption. Obstet Gynecol 74:748, 1989.
254. Kalhan SC, D'Angelo LJ, Savin SM, Adam PAJ: Glucose production in pregnant women at term gestation: Sources of glucose for human fetus. J Clin Invest 63:388, 1979.
255. Morris FH Jr, Makowski EL, Meschia G, Battaglia FC: The glucose/oxygen quotient of the term human fetus. Biol Neonate 25:44, 1975.
256. Hay WW Jr, Myers SA, Sparks JW, et al: Glucose and lactate oxidation rates in the fetal lamb. Proc Soc Exp Biol Med 173:553, 1983.
257. Lemons JA, Schreiner RL: Amino acid metabolism in the ovine fetus. Am J Physiol 244:E459, 1983.
258. Widdowson EH, Spray CM: Chemical development in utero. Arch Dis Child 26:205, 1951.
259. Warshaw JB: Fatty acid metabolism during development. Semin Perinatol 3:31, 1979.
260. Schoenle E, Zopf J, Humbel RE, Groesch ER: Insulin-like growth factor I stimulates growth in hypophysectomized rats. Nature 296:252, 1982.
261. Jost A: Fetal hormones and fetal growth. Contr Gynecol Obstet 5:1, 1979.
262. Gluckman PD, Liggins GC: Regulation of fetal growth. *In* Beard RW, Nathanielsz PW (eds): Fetal Physiology and Medicine. New York, Marcel Dekker, 1984, p 511.
263. Gluckman PD: Functional maturation of the neuroendocrine system in the perinatal period: Studies of the somatotrophic axis in the ovine fetus. J Dev Physiol 6:301, 1984.

264. Palmiter RD, Norstedt G, Gelinas RE, et al: Metallothionein-human GH fusion genes stimulate growth of mice. Science 222:809, 1983.
265. Browne CA, Thorburn CA: Endocrine control of fetal growth. Biol Neonate 55:331, 1989.
266. D'Ercole AJ, Stiles AD, Underwood LE: Tissue concentration of somatomedin C: Further evidence for multiple sites of synthesis and paracrine or autocrine mechanism of action. Proc Natl Acad Sci U S A 81:935, 1984.
267. King GL, Kahn CR, Rechler MM, Nissley SP: Direct demonstration of separate receptors for growth and metabolic activities of insulin and multiplication stimulating activity (an insulin-like growth factor) using antibodies to the insulin receptor. J Clin Invest 66:130, 1980.
268. Bennett A, Wilson DM, Liu F, et al: Levels of insulin-like growth factors I and II in human cord blood. J Clin Endocrinol Metab 57:609, 1983.
269. Adams SO, Nissley SP, Handwerger S, Rechler MM: Developmental patterns of insulin-like growth factor I and II synthesis and regulation in rat fibroblasts. Nature 302:150, 1983.
270. Hill DE: Fetal effects of insulin. Obstet Gynecol Ann 11:133, 1982.
271. Susa JG, Gruppuso PA, Widness JA, et al: Chronic hyperinsulinemia in the fetal rhesus monkey: Effects of physiologic hyperinsulinemia on fetal substrates, hormones, and hepatic enzymes. Am J Obstet Gynecol 150:415, 1984.
272. Philips AF, Dubin JW, Raye JR: Fetal metabolic responses to endogenous insulin release. Am J Obstet Gynecol 139:441, 1981.
273. Hay WW, Meznarich HK, Sparks JW, et al: Effect of insulin on glucose uptake in near-term fetal lambs. Proc Soc Exp Biol Med 178:557, 1985.
274. Oppenheimer CL, Pessin JE, Massague J, et al: Insulin action rapidly modulates the apparent affinity of the insulin-like growth factor II receptor. J Biol Chem 258:4824, 1983.
275. Sara VR, Hall K, Misaki M, et al: Ontogenesis of somatomedin and insulin receptors in the human fetus. J Clin Invest 71:1084, 1983.
276. Cardell BS: The infants of diabetic mothers; A morphological study. J Obstet Gynecol Br Comm 60:834, 1953.
277. Siddiqi TA, Miodovnik M, Mimouni F, et al: Biphasic intrauterine growth in insulin-dependent diabetic pregnancies. J Am Coll Nutr 8:225, 1989.
278. Fowden AL, Comline RS: The effects of pancreatectomy on the sheep fetus in utero. Q J Exp Physiol 69:319, 1984.
279. Fowden AL: The role of insulin in fetal growth. J Dev Physiol 12:173, 1989.
280. Sperling MA, Christensen RA, Ganguli S, Anand R: Adrenergic modulation of pancreatic hormone secretion in utero: Studies in fetal sheep. Pediatr Res 14:203, 1980.
281. Jones CT, Ritchie JWK, Walker D: The effects of hypoxia on glucose turnover in the fetal sheep. J Develop Physiol 5:223, 1983.
282. Devaskar SU, Ganuli S, Styer D, et al: Glucagon and glucose dynamics in sheep: Evidence for glucagon resistance in the fetus. Am J Physiol 246:E256, 1984.
283. Gospodarowicz D: Epidermal and nerve growth factors in mammalian development. Ann Rev Physiol 43:251, 1981.
284. Poulsen SS, Kryger-Baggesen N, Nexo E: Immunohistochemical localization of epidermal growth factor in the second-trimester human fetus. Histochem Cell Biol 105:111, 1996.
285. Amemiya K, Kurachi H, Adachi H, et al: Involvement of epidermal growth factor (EGF)/EGF receptor autocrine and paracrine mechanism in human trophoblast cells: functional differentiation in vitro. J Endocrinol 143:291, 1994.
286. Hofmann GE, Horowitz GM, Scott RT Jr, Navot D: Transforming growth factor-alpha in human implantation trophoblast: immunohistochemical evidence for autocrine/paracrine function. J Clin Endocrinol Metab 76:781, 1993.
287. Lysiak JJ, Johnson GR, Lala PK: Localization of amphiregulin in the human placenta and decidua throughout gestation: role in trophoblast growth. Placenta 16:359, 1995.
288. Birdsall MA, Hopkisson JF, Grant KE, et al: Expression of heparin-binding epidermal growth factor messenger RNA in the human endometrium. Mol Hum Reprod 2:31, 1996.
289. Tanimura K, Nakago S, Murakoshi H, et al: Changes in the expression and cytological localization of betacellulin and its receptors (ErbB-1 and ErbB-4) in the trophoblasts in human placenta over the course of pregnancy. Eur J Endocrinol 151:93, 2004.
290. Toyoda H, Komurasaki T, Uchida D, Morimoto S: Distribution of mRNA for human epiregulin, a differentially expressed member of the epidermal growth factor family. Biochem J 326(Pt 1):69, 1997.
291. Schilling B, Yeh J: Transforming growth factor-beta(1), -beta(2), -beta(3) and their type I and II receptors in human term placenta. Gynecol Obstet Invest 50:19, 2000.
292. Schneider-Kolsky ME, Manuelpillai U, Waldron K, et al: The distribution of activin and activin receptors in gestational tissues across human pregnancy and during labour. Placenta 23:294, 2002.
293. Petraglia F: Inhibin, activin and follistatin in the human placenta—a new family of regulatory proteins. Placenta 18:3, 1997.
294. Bigon E, Soranzo C, Minozzi C, et al: Large scale purification and immunological characterization of human placental nerve growth factor. Neurochem Res 15:1197, 1990.
295. Gilmore JH, Jarskog LF, Vadlamudi S: Maternal infection regulates BDNF and NGF expression in fetal and neonatal brain and maternal-fetal unit of the rat. J Neuroimmunol 138:49, 2003.
296. Han VK, Carter AM: Spatial and temporal patterns of expression of messenger RNA for insulin-like growth factors and their binding proteins in the placenta of man and laboratory animals. Placenta 21:289, 2000.
297. Arceci RJ, Shanahan F, Stanley ER, Pollard JW: Temporal expression and location of colony-stimulating factor 1 (CSF-1) and its receptor in the female reproductive tract are consistent with CSF-1–regulated placental development. Proc Natl Acad Sci U S A 86:8818, 1989.
298. Shorter SC, Vince GS, Starkey PM: Production of granulocyte colony–stimulating factor at the materno-foetal interface in human pregnancy. Immunology 75:468, 1992.
299. Dame JB, Christensen RD, Juul SE: The distribution of granulocyte-macrophage colony–stimulating factor and its receptor in the developing human fetus. Pediatr Res 46:358, 1999.
300. Sharkey AM, Charnock-Jones DS, Boocock CA, et al: Expression of mRNA for vascular endothelial growth factor in human placenta. J Reprod Fertil 99:609, 1993.
301. Shiraishi S, Nakagawa K, Kinukawa N, et al: Immunohistochemical localization of vascular endothelial growth factor in the human placenta. Placenta 17:111, 1996.
302. Hauser S, Weich HA: A heparin-binding form of placenta growth factor (PlGF-2) is expressed in human umbilical vein endothelial cells and in placenta. Growth Factors 9:259, 1993.
303. Ferriani RA, Ahmed A, Sharkey A, Smith SK: Colocalization of acidic and basic fibroblast growth factor (FGF) in human placenta and the cellular effects of bFGF in trophoblast cell line JEG-3. Growth Factors 10:259, 1994.
304. Zheng J, Vagnoni KE, Bird IM, Magness RR: Expression of basic fibroblast growth factor, endothelial mitogenic activity, and angiotensin II type-1 receptors in the ovine placenta during the third trimester of pregnancy. Biol Reprod 56:1189, 1997.
305. Arany E, Hill DJ: Fibroblast growth factor-2 and fibroblast growth factor receptor-1 mRNA expression and peptide localization in placentae from normal and diabetic pregnancies. Placenta 19:133, 1998.
306. Bowen JM, Chamley L, Mitchell MD, Keelan JA: Cytokines of the placenta and extra-placental membranes: biosynthesis, secretion and roles in establishment of pregnancy in women. Placenta 23:239, 2002.
307. Maruo T, Matsuo H, Murata K, Mochizuki M: Gestational age–dependent dual action of epidermal growth factor on human placenta early in gestation. J Clin Endocrinol Metab 75:1362, 1992.
308. Bass KE, Morrish D, Roth I, et al: Human cytotrophoblast invasion is up-regulated by epidermal growth factor: evidence that paracrine factors modify this process. Dev Biol 164:550, 1994.
309. Morrish DW, Bhardwaj D, Dabbagh LK, et al: Epidermal growth factor induces differentiation and secretion of human chorionic gonadotropin and placental lactogen in normal human placenta. J Clin Endocrinol Metab 65:1282. 1987.

310. Saito S, Sakakura S, Enomoto M, et al: Hepatocyte growth factor promotes the growth of cytotrophoblasts by the paracrine mechanism. J Biochem (Tokyo) 117:671, 1995.
311. Charnock-Jones DS, Sharkey AM, Boocock CA, et al: Vascular endothelial growth factor receptor localization and activation in human trophoblast and choriocarcinoma cells. Biol Reprod 51:524, 1994.
312. Graham CH, Lala PK: Mechanism of control of trophoblast invasion in situ. J Cell Physiol 148:228, 1991.
313. Morrish DW, Bhardwaj D, Paras MT: Transforming growth factor beta 1 inhibits placental differentiation and human chorionic gonadotropin and human placental lactogen secretion. Endocrinology 129:22, 1991.
314. Regenstreif LJ, Rossant J: Expression of the c-fms proto-oncogene and of the cytokine, CSF-1, during mouse embryogenesis. Dev Biol 133:284, 1989.
315. Uzumaki H, Okabe T, Sasaki N, et al. Identification and characterization of receptors for granulocyte colony–stimulating factor on human placenta and trophoblastic cells. Proc Natl Acad Sci U S A 86:9323, 1989.
316. Fairchild BD, Conrad KP: Expression of the erythropoietin receptor by trophoblast cellsin the human placenta. Biol Reprod 60:861, 1999.
317. Garcia-Lloret MI, Morrish DW, Wegmann TG, et al: Demonstration of functional cytokine-placental interactions: CSF-1 and GM-CSF stimulate human cytotrophoblast differentiation and peptide hormone secretion. Exp Cell Res 214:46, 1994.
318. Peters TJ, Chapman BM, Wolfe MW, Soares MJ: Placental lactogen-I gene activation in differentiating trophoblast cells: extrinsic and intrinsic regulation involving mitogen-activated protein kinase signaling pathways. J Endocrinol 165:443, 2000.
319. Kita N, Mitsushita J, Ohira S, et al: Expression and activation of MAP kinases, ERK1/2, in the human villous trophoblasts. Placenta 24:164, 2003.
320. Corso M, Thomson M: Protein phosphorylation in mitochondria from human placenta. Placenta 22:432, 2001.
321. Fowden AL: The insulin-like growth factors and feto-placental growth. Placenta 24:803, 2003.
322. Yamamoto H, Flannery ML, Kupriyanov S, et al: Defective trophoblast function in mice with a targeted mutation of Ets2. Genes Dev 12:1315, 1998.
323. Johnston DJ, Thompson JM, Hammond K: Additive and nonadditive differences in postweaning growth and carcass characteristics of Devon, Hereford, and reciprocal-cross steers. J Anim Sci 70:2688, 1992.
324. Hill DJ, Petrik J, Arany E: Growth factors and the regulation of fetal growth. Diabetes Care 21(Suppl 2):B60, 1998.
325. Hayashi M, Hamada Y, Ohkura T: Elevation of granulocyte-macrophage colony–stimulating factor in the placenta and blood in preeclampsia. Am J Obstet Gynecol 190:456, 2004.
326. Polliotti BM, Fry AG, Saller DN, et al: Second-trimester maternal serum placental growth factor and vascular endothelial growth factor for predicting severe, early-onset preeclampsia. Obstet Gynecol 101:1266, 2003.
327. Hofmann GE, Drews MR, Scott RT Jr, et al: Epidermal growth factor and its receptor in human implantation trophoblast: immunohistochemical evidence for autocrine/paracrine function. J Clin Endocrinol Metab 74:981, 1992.
328. Maruo T, Matsuo H, Oishi T, et al: Induction of differentiated trophoblast function by epidermal growth factor: relation of immunohistochemically detected cellular epidermal growth factor receptor levels. J Clin Endocrinol Metab 64:744, 1987.
329. Garcia-Lloret MI, Yui J, Winkler-Lowen B, Guilbert LJ: Epidermal growth factor inhibits cytokine-induced apoptosis of primary human trophoblasts. J Cell Physiol 167:324, 1996.
330. Chen CF, Kurachi H, Fujita Y, et al: Changes in epidermal growth factor receptor and its messenger ribonucleic acid levels in human placenta and isolated trophoblast cells during pregnancy. J Clin Endocrinol Metab 67:1171, 1988.
331. Alsat E, Haziza J, Scippo ML, et al: Increase in epidermal growth factor receptor and its mRNA levels by parathyroid hormone (1-34) and parathyroid hormone-related protein (1-34) during differentiation of human trophoblast cells in culture. J Cell Biochem 53:32, 1993.
332. Fujita Y, Kurachi H, Morishige K, et al: Decrease in epidermal growth factor receptor and its messenger ribonucleic acid levels in intrauterine growth–retarded and diabetes mellitus–complicated pregnancies. J Clin Endocrinol Metab 72:1340, 1991.
333. Groenen LC, Nice EC, Burgess AW: Structure-function relationships for the EGF/TGF-alpha family of mitogens. Growth Factors 11:235, 1994.
334. Muhlhauser J, Crescimanno C, Kaufmann P, et al: Differentiation and proliferation patterns in human trophoblast revealed by c-erbB-2 oncogene product and EGF-R. J Histochem Cytochem 41:165, 1993.
335. Bunn HF, Jandl JH: Control of hemoglobin function within the red cell. N Engl J Med 282:1414, 1970.
336. Barbera A, Galan HL, Ferrazzi E, et al: Relationship of umbilical vein blood flow to growth parameters in the human fetus. Am J Obstet Gynecol 181:174, 1999.
337. Cheung CY, Brace RA: Developmental expression of vascular endothelial growth factor and its receptors in ovine placenta and fetal membranes. J Soc Gynecol Investig 6:179, 1999.
338. Nguyen M, Camenisch T, Snouwaert JN, et al: The prostaglandin receptor EP4 triggers remodelling of the cardiovascular system at birth. Nature 390:78, 1997.
339. Harrington B, Glazier J, D'Souza S, Sibley C: System A amino acid transporter activity in human placental microvillous membrane vesicles in relation to various anthropometric measurements in appropriate and small for gestational age babies. Pediatr Res 45:810, 1999.
340. Sunderland CA, Redman CWG, Stirrat GM: HLA A, B, C antigens are expressed on nonvillous trophoblast of the early human placenta. J Immunol 127:2614, 1981.
341. Faulk WP, Hsi B-L: Immunology of human trophoblast membrane antigens. *In* Loke YW, Whyte A (eds): Biology of Trophoblast. New York, Elsevier, 1983, p 535.
342. Szulman AE: The ABH blood groups and development. Curr Top Dev Biol 14:127, 1980.
343. Faulk WP: Immunobiology of human extraembryonic membranes. *In* Wegman TG, Gill TJ (eds): Immunology of Reproduction. New York, Oxford, 1983, p 253.
344. Klopper A: The new placental proteins. Placenta 1:77, 1980.
345. Rocklin RE, Kitzmiller JL, Farvoy MR: Maternal fetal relation. II. Further characterization of an immunologic blocking factor that develops during pregnancy. Clin Immunol Immunopathol 22:305, 1982.
346. Beer AE: Immunologic aspects of normal pregnancy and recurrent spontaneous abortion. Semin Reprod Endocinol 6:163, 1988.
347. Taylor C, Faulk WP: Prevention of recurrent abortions with leukocyte transfusions. Lancet ii:68, 1980.
348. Beer AE, Quebberman JF, Ayers JW, Haines RF: Major histocompatibility antigens maternal and paaternal immune responses and chronic habitual abortion in humans. Am J Obstet Gynecol 141:987, 1981.
349. Komlos L, Zamir R, Joshua H, Halbrecht I: Common HLA antigens in couples with repeated abortions. Clin Immunol Immunopathol 7:330, 1977.
350. Redline RW, Lu CY: Role of local immunosupression in murine fetoplacental listerosis. J Clin Invest 79:1234, 1987.
351. Jacoby DR, Olding LB, Oldstone MD: Immunologic regulation of fetal-maternal balance. Adv Immunol 35:157, 1984.
352. Torry DS, McIntyre JA, Faulk WP: Immunobiology of the trophoblast: mechanisms by which placental tissues evade maternal recognition and rejection. Curr Top Microbiol Immunol;222:127, 1997.
353. Rudolph AM: Homeostasis of the fetal circulation and the part played by hormones. Ann Rech Vet 8:405, 1977.
354. Pitkin RM, Reynolds WA: Fetal ingestion and metabolism of amniotic fluid protein. Am J Obstet Gynecol 123:356, 1975.
355. Charlton V, Reis B: Effects of gastric nutritional supplementation on fetal umbilical uptake of nutrients. Am J Physiol 241: E178, 1981.
356. Charlton VE, Rudolph A: Digestion and absorption of carbohydrates by the fetal lamb in utero. Pediatr Res 13:1018, 1979.
357. Charlton V, Johengen M: Effects of intrauterine nutritional supplementation on fetal growth retardation. Biol Neonate 48:125, 1985.

358. Wesson D, Muraji T, Kent G, et al: The effect of intrauterine esophageal ligation on growth of fetal rabbits. J Pediatr Surg 19:398, 1984.
359. Trahair JF, Harding R, Bocking AD, et al: The role of ingestion in the development of the small intestine in fetal sheep. Q J Exp Physiol 71:99, 1986.
360. Avila C, Harding R, Robinson P: The effects of preventing ingestion on the development of the digestive system in the sheep fetus. Q J Exp Physiol 71:99, 1986.
361. Pierro A, Cozzi F, Colarossi G, et al: Does fetal gut obstruction cause hydramnios and growth retardation? J Pediatr Surg 22:454, 1987.
362. Cozzi F, Wilkinson A: Intrauterine growth rate in relation to anorectal and oesophageal anomalies. Arch Dis Child 44:59, 1969.
363. Edelstone DI, Holzman IR: Fetal intestinal oxygen consumption at various levels of oxygenation. Am J Physiol 242:H50, 1982.
364. Lester R, Jackson BT, Smallwood RA, et al: Fetal and neonatal hepatic function II. Birth Defects 12:307, 1976.
365. Bristow J, Rudolph AM, Itskovitz J, Barnes R: Hepatic oxygen and glucose metabolism in the fetal lamb. Response to hypoxia. J Clin.Invest 71:1047, 1983.
366. Jouppila P, Kirkinen P, Eik-Nes S, Koivula A: Fetal and intervillouos blood flow measurements in late pregnancy. *In* Kurjak A, Kratochwil A (eds): Recent Advances in Ultrasound Diagnosis. Amsterdam, Excerpta Medica, 1981, p 226.
367. Rudolph AM: Hepatic and ductus venosus blood flows during fetal life. Hepatology 3:254, 1983.
368. Anderson DF, Bissonnette JM, Faber JJ, Thornburg KL: Central shunt flows and pressures in the mature fetal lamb. Am J Physiol 241:H60, 1981.
369. Gresores A, Rosenfeld CR, Magness RR, Roy T: Metabolic clearance rate of angiotensin II in fetal and pregnant sheep. Pediatr Res 31:60A, 1992.
370. Thornburg KL, Morton MJ: Filling and arterial pressures as determinants of RV stroke volume in the sheep fetus. Am J Physiol 244:H656, 1983.
371. Pinson CW, Morton MJ, Thornburg KL: An anatomic basis for right ventricular dominance and arterial pressure sensitivity. J Dev Physiol 9:253, 1987.
372. Thornburg KL, Morton MG: Filling and arterial pressures as determinants of left ventricular stroke volume in fetal lambs. Am J Physiol 251:H961, 1986.
373. Cheng JB, Goldfien A, Cornett LE, Roberts JM: Identification of B-adrenergic receptors using [3H] dihydroalprenolol in fetal sheep heart: Direct evidence of qualitative similarity to the receptors in adult sheep heart. Pediatr Res 15:1083, 1981.
374. Andersen PAW, Manning A, Glick KL, Crenshaw CC Jr: Biophysics of the developing heart III. A comparison of the left ventricular dynamics of the fetal and neontal heart. Am J Obstet Gynecol 143:195, 1982.
375. Fisher DJ, Heymann MA, Rudolph AM: Regional myocardial blood flow and oxygen delivery in fetal, newborn and adult sheep. Am J Physiol 243:H729, 1982.
376. Fisher DJ, Heymann MA, Rudolph AM: Myocardial oxygen and carbohydrate consumption in fetal lambs in utero and in adult sheep. Am J Physiol 238:H399, 1980.
377. Timor-Tritsch IE, Dierker LJ, Hertz RH, et al: Studies of antepartum behavioral state in the human fetus at term. Am J Obstet Gynecol 132:524, 1978.
378. Martin CB Jr: Behavioral states in the human fetus. J Reprod Med 26:425, 1981.
379. Visser GHA, Goodman JDS, Levine DH, Dawes GS: Diurnal and other cyclic variations in human fetal heart rate near term. Am J Obstet Gynecol 142:535, 1982.
380. Dawes GS, Fox HE, Leduc BM, et al: Respiratory movements and rapid eye movement sleep in the foetal lamb. J Physiol 220:119, 1972.
381. Natale R, Clewlow F, Dawes GS: Measurement of fetal forelimb movements in the lamb in utero. Am J Obstet Gynecol 140:545, 1981.
382. Blanco CE, Dawes GS, Walker DW: Effect of hypoxia on polysynaptic hindlimb reflexes of unanesthetized foetal and newborn lambs. J Physiol 339:453, 1983.
383. Chan K, Dodd PA, Day L, et al: Fetal catecholamine, cardiovascular, and neurobehavioral responses to cocaine. Am J Obstet Gynecol 167:1616, 1992.
384. Connors G, Hunse C, Carmichal L, et al: Control of fetal breathing in human fetus between 24 and 34 weeks gestation. Am J Obstet Gynecol 160:932, 1989.
385. Hohimer AR, Bissonnette JM, Richardson BS, Machida CM: Central chemical regulation of breathing movements in fetal lambs. Respir Physiol 52:99, 1983.
386. Dawes GS, Gardner WN, Johnson BM, Walker DW: Breathing activity in fetal lambs: The effect of brain stem section. J Physiol 335:535, 1983.
387. Richardson BS, Patrick JE, Abduljabbar H: Cerebral oxidative metabolism in the fetal lamb: Relationship to electrocortical state. Am J Obstet Gynecol 153:426, 1985.
388. Chao CR, Hohimer AR, Bissonnette JM: The effect of electrocortical state on cerebral carbohydrate metabolism in fetal sheep. Brain Res Dev Brain Res 49:1, 1989.
389. Jones MD, Sheldon RE, Peeters LL, et al: Fetal cerebral oxygen consumption at different levels of oxygenation. J Appl Physiol Respirat Envorion Exercise Physiol 43:1080, 1977.
390. Rosenberg AA, Jones MD Jr, Traystman RJ, et al: Response of cerebral blood flow to changes in PCO2 in fetal, newborn, and adult sheep. Am J Physiol 242:H862, 1982.
391. Martyn CN, Barker DJ, Osmond C: Mothers' pelvic size, fetal growth, and death from stroke and coronary heart disease in men in the UK. Lancet 348:1264, 1996.
392. McCormack VA, dos SS, I, De Stavola BL, et al: Fetal growth and subsequent risk of breast cancer: results from long term follow up of Swedish cohort. BMJ 326:248, 2003.
393. Leadbitter P, Pearce N, Cheng S, et al: Relationship between fetal growth and the development of asthma and atopy in childhood. Thorax 54:905, 1999.
394. Barker DJ, Osmond C: Infant mortality, childhood nutrition, and ischaemic heart disease in England and Wales. Lancet;1:1077, 1986.
395. Rose G: Familial patterns in ischaemic heart disease. Br J Prev Soc Med 18:75, 1964.
396. Forsdahl A: Are poor living conditions in childhood and adolescence an important risk factor for arteriosclerotic heart disease? Br J Prev Soc Med 31:91, 1977.
397. Barker D: The midwife, the coincidence, and the hypothesis. BMJ 327:1428, 2003.
398. Barker DJ, Winter PD, Osmond C, et al: Weight in infancy and death from ischaemic heart disease. Lancet 2:577, 1989.
399. Barker DJ, Osmond C, Golding J, et al: Growth in utero, blood pressure in childhood and adult life, and mortality from cardiovascular disease. BMJ 298:564, 1989.
400. Barker DJ: In utero programming of cardiovascular disease. Theriogenology 53:555, 2000.
401. Lau C, Rogers JM: Embryonic and fetal programming of physiological disorders in adulthood. Birth Defects Res C Embryo Today 72:300, 2004.
402. Hofman PL, Regan F, Jackson WE, et al: Premature birth and later insulin resistance. N Engl J Med 351:2179, 2004.
403. Schluchter MD: Publication bias and heterogeneity in the relationship between systolic blood pressure, birth weight, and catch-up growth—a meta analysis. J Hypertens 21:273, 2003.
404. Hales CN, Barker DJ, Clark PM, et al: Fetal and infant growth and impaired glucose tolerance at age 64. BMJ 303:1019, 1991.
405. Barker DJ, Hales CN, Fall CH, et al: Type 2 (non-insulin-dependent) diabetes mellitus, hypertension and hyperlipidaemia (syndrome X): relation to reduced fetal growth. Diabetologia 36:62, 1993.
406. Hales CN, Barker DJ: The thrifty phenotype hypothesis. Br Med Bull 60:5, 2001.
407. Hales CN, Barker DJ: Type 2 (non-insulin-dependent) diabetes mellitus: the thrifty phenotype hypothesis. Diabetologia 35:595, 1992.
408. Ravelli AC, van der Meulen JH, Michels RP, et al: Glucose tolerance in adults after prenatal exposure to famine. Lancet 351:173, 1998.
409. Stanner SA, Bulmer K, Andres C, et al: Does malnutrition in utero determine diabetes and coronary heart disease in adulthood?

Results from the Leningrad siege study, a cross sectional study. BMJ 315:1342, 1997.
410. Jensen RB, Chellakooty M, Vielwerth S, et al: Intrauterine growth retardation and consequences for endocrine and cardiovascular diseases in adult life: does insulin-like growth factor-I play a role? Horm Res 60 (Suppl 3):136, 2003.
411. Lewis RM, Forhead AJ, Petry CJ, et al: Long-term programming of blood pressure by maternal dietary iron restriction in the rat. Br J Nutr 88:283, 2002.
412. Langley SC, Jackson AA: Increased systolic blood pressure in adult rats induced by fetal exposure to maternal low protein diets. Clin Sci (Lond) 86:217, 1994.
413. Kind KL, Simonetta G, Clifton PM, et al: Effect of maternal feed restriction on blood pressure in the adult guinea pig. Exp Physiol 87:469, 2002.
414. Gopalakrishnan GS, Gardner DS, Rhind SM, et al: Programming of adult cardiovascular function after early maternal undernutrition in sheep. Am J Physiol Regul Integr Comp Physiol 287:R12, 2004.
415. Langley-Evans SC, Welham SJ, Jackson AA: Fetal exposure to a maternal low protein diet impairs nephrogenesis and promotes hypertension in the rat. Life Sci 64:965, 1999.
416. Burns SP, Desai M, Cohen RD, et al: Gluconeogenesis, glucose handling, and structural changes in livers of the adult offspring of rats partially deprived of protein during pregnancy and lactation. J Clin Invest 100:1768, 1997.
417. Klebanoff MA, Meirik O, Berendes HW: Second-generation consequences of small-for-dates birth. Pediatrics 84: 343, 1989.
418. Stewart RJ, Preece RF, Sheppard HG: Recovery from long-term protein-energy deficiency. Proc Nutr Soc 32:103A, 1973.
419. Drake AJ, Walker BR, Seckl JR: Intergenerational consequences of fetal programming by in utero exposure to glucocorticoids in rats. Am J Physiol Regul Integr Comp Physiol 288:R34, 2005.
420. Enders RH, Judd RM, Donohue TM, Smith CH: Placental amino acid uptake. III. Transport systems for neutral amino acids. Am J Physiol 230:706, 1976.
421. Steel RB, Smith CH, Kelly LK: Placental amino acid uptake. VI. Regulation by intracellular substrate. Am J Physiol 243:C46, 1982.
422. Paton JB, Fisher DE, Peterson EN: Cardiac output and organ blood flows in the baboon fetus. Biol Neonate 22:50, 1973.

Maternal Physiology

MICHAEL C. GORDON

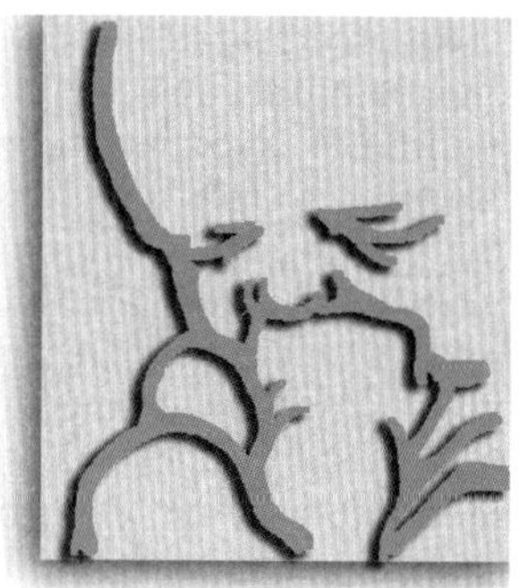

CHAPTER 3

KEY ABBREVIATIONS

Adrenocorticotropic hormone	ACTH
Alanine aminotransferase	ALT
American College of Obstetricians and Gynecologists	ACOG
Arginine vasopressin	AVP
Aspartate aminotransferase	AST
Atrial natriuretic peptide	ANP
Blood pressure	BP
Blood urea nitrogen	BUN
Brain natriuretic peptide	BNP
Carbon dioxide	CO_2
Cardiac output	CO
Colloidal oncotic pressure	COP
Corticosteroid-binding globulin	CBG
Corticotrophin-releasing hormone	CRH
Deoxycorticosterone	DOC
Forced expiratory volume in 1 second	FEV_1
Functional residual capacity	FRC
Glomerular filtration rate	GFR
Heart rate	HR
Human chorionic gonadotropin	hCG
Human placenta lactogen	hPL
Immunoglobulin G	IgG
Mean arterial pressure	MAP
Nitric oxide	NO
Parathyroid hormone	PTH
Premature ventricular contractions	PVCs
Pulmonary capillary wedge pressures	PCWPs
Rapid eye movement	REM
Red blood cell	RBC
Renal blood flow	RBF
Renin-angiotensin-aldosterone system	RAAS
Stroke volume	SV
Systemic vascular resistance	SVR
Thyroid-stimulating hormone	TSH
Thyroxine-binding globulin	TBG
Total thyroxine	TT_4
Total triiodothyronine	TT_3
White blood cell	WBC

Major adaptations in maternal anatomy, physiology, and metabolism are required for a successful pregnancy. Hormonal changes, initiated before conception, significantly alter maternal physiology, and persist through both pregnancy and the initial postpartum period. Although these adaptations are profound and affect nearly every organ system, women return to the nongravid state with minimal residual changes.[1] A full understanding of physiologic changes is necessary to differentiate between normal alternations and those that are abnormal. This chapter describes maternal adaptations in pregnancy and gives specific examples of how they may affect care. Finally, although women may tire of repetitive reassurance that "it is simply normal for pregnancy and of no concern," a complete understanding of physiologic changes allows each obstetrician to provide a more thorough explanation for various changes and symptoms.

BODY WATER METABOLISM

The increase in total body water of 6.5 to 8.5 L by the end of gestation represents one of the most significant adaptations of pregnancy. The water content of the fetus, placenta, and amniotic fluid at term accounts for about 3.5 L. Additional water is accounted for by expansion of the maternal blood volume by 1,500 to 1,600 ml, plasma volume by 1,200 to 1,300 ml, and red blood cells by 300 to 400 ml.[2] The remainder is attributed to extravascular fluid, intracellular fluid in the uterus and breasts, and expanded adipose tissue. As a result, pregnancy is a condition of chronic volume overload with active sodium and water retention secondary to changes in osmoregulation and the renin-angiotensin system. Increase in body water content contributes to maternal weight gain, hemodilution, physiologic anemia of pregnancy, and the elevation in maternal cardiac output (CO). Inadequate plasma volume expansion has been associated with increased risks of preeclampsia and fetal growth restriction.

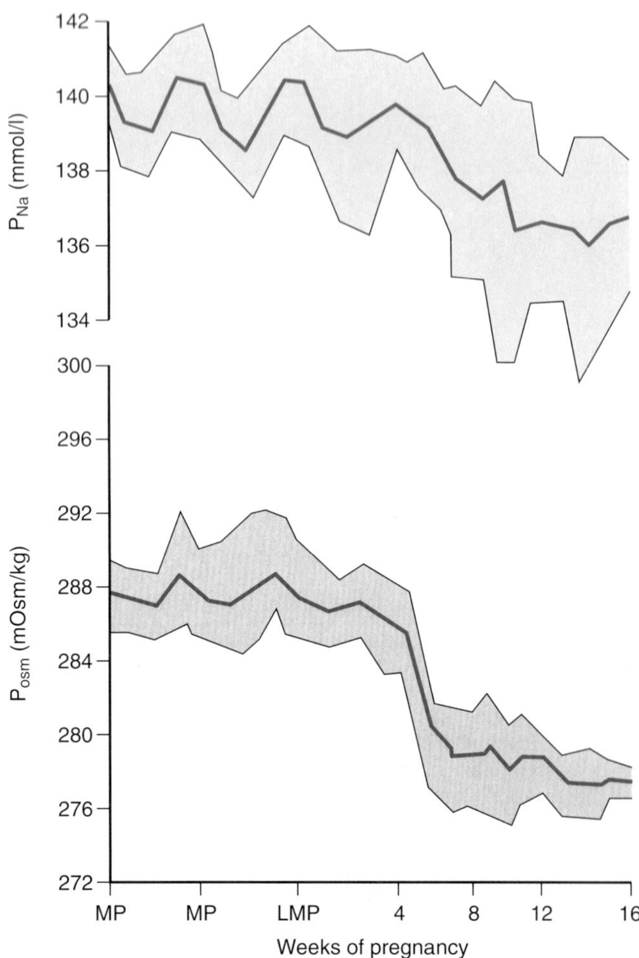

Figure 3-1. Plasma osmolality and plasma sodium during human gestation (n = 9: mean values ± SD). MP, menstrual period; LMP, last menstrual period. (From Davison JM, Vallotton MB, Lindheimer MD: Plasma osmolality and urinary concentration and dilution during and after pregnancy: Evidence that the lateral recumbency inhibits maximal urinary concentration ability. Br J Obstet Gynecol 88:472, 1981, with permission.)

Osmoregulation

Expansion in plasma volume begins shortly after conception, partially mediated by a change in maternal osmoregulation through altered secretion of arginine vasopressin (AVP) by the posterior pituitary. Water retention exceeds sodium retention; although an additional 900 mEq of sodium is retained during pregnancy serum levels of sodium decrease by 3 to 4 mmol/L. This is mirrored by decreases in overall plasma osmolality of 8 to 10 mOsm/kg, a change that is in place by 10 weeks' gestation and continues through 1 to 2 weeks postpartum[3,4] (Fig. 3-1). Similarly, the threshold for thirst changes early in pregnancy; during gestational weeks 5 to 8, an increase in water intake occurs and results in a transient increase in urinary volume but a net increase in total body water.[5] Initial changes in AVP regulation may be due to placental signals involving nitric oxide (NO) and the hormone relaxin.[6,7] After 8 weeks' gestation, the new steady state for osmolality has been established with little subsequent change in water turnover resulting in decreased polyuria. Pregnant women perceive fluid challenges or dehydration normally with changes in thirst and AVP secretion but at a new "osmostat."[6]

Plasma levels of AVP during pregnancy remain relatively unchanged despite heightened production, owing to a three- to fourfold increase in the metabolic clearance. Increased clearance results from a circulating vasopressinase synthesized by the placenta that rapidly inactivates both AVP and oxytocin. This enzyme increases approximately 1,000-fold over the course of gestation proportional to fetal weight with the highest concentrations occurring in multiple gestations. Increased AVP clearance can unmask subclinical forms of diabetes insipidus presumably due to an insufficient pituitary AVP reserve and causes transient diabetes insipidus in pregnancy with an incidence of 2 to 6/1,000.[8] Typically presenting with both polydipsia and polyuria, hyperosmolality is usually mild unless the thirst mechanism is abnormal or access to water is limited.[9]

Salt Metabolism

Sodium metabolism is delicately balanced, facilitating a net accumulation of about 900 mEq of sodium. Sixty percent of the additional sodium is contained within the fetoplacental unit (including amniotic fluid) and is lost at birth. By 2 months postpartum, the serum sodium returns to preconceptional levels.[5] Pregnancy increases the preference for sodium intake, but the primary mechanism is enhanced tubular sodium reabsorption. Increased glomerular filtration raises the total filtered sodium load from 20,000 to about 30,000 mmol/day; sodium reabsorption must increase to prevent sodium loss. However, the adaptive rise in tubular reabsorption surpasses the increase in filtered load resulting in an additional 2 to 6 mEq of sodium reabsorption per day. Alterations in sodium handling represents the largest renal adjustment that occurs in gestation.[10] Hormonal control of sodium balance is under the opposing actions of the renin-angiotensin-aldosterone system (RAAS) and the natriuretic peptides, and both are modified during pregnancy.[11]

Renin-Angiotensin-Aldosterone System

Normal pregnancy is characterized by a marked increase in all components of the RAAS system. In early pregnancy, reduced systemic vascular tone (attributed to gestational hormones and increased NO production) results in decreased mean arterial pressure (MAP). In turn, decreased MAP activates adaptations to preserve intravascular volume through sodium retention.[12] Plasma renin activity, renin substrate (angiotensinogen), and angiotensin levels are all increased a minimum of four- to fivefold over nonpregnant levels. Activation of these components of RAAS leads to twofold elevated levels of aldosterone by the third trimester, increasing sodium reabsorption and preventing sodium loss.[13,14] Despite the elevated aldosterone levels in late pregnancy, normal homeostatic responses still occur to changes in salt balance, fluid loss, and postural stimuli. In addition to aldosterone, other hormones that may contribute to increased tubular sodium retention include deoxycorticosterone and estrogen.

Atrial and Brain Natriuretic Peptide

The myocardium releases neuropeptides that serve to maintain circulatory homeostasis. Atrial natriuretic peptide (ANP) is secreted primarily by the atrial myocytes in response to dilation, and brain natriuretic peptide (BNP) is secreted by the ventricles in response to end-diastolic pressure and volume. Both peptides have similar physiologic actions, acting as diuretics, natriuretics, vasorelaxants, and overall antagonists to the RAAS. Elevated levels of ANP/BNP are found in both physiologic and pathologic conditions of volume overload and can be used to screen for congestive heart failure outside of pregnancy in symptomatic patients.[15–17] Since pregnant women frequently present with dyspnea and since many of the physiologic effects of conception mimic heart disease, whether pregnancy affects the levels of these hormones is clinically important. Gestational alterations in ANP are controversial, because some authors have reported higher plasma levels during different stages of pregnancy, whereas others have reported no change. In a meta-analysis by Castro et al.,[18] ANP levels were 40 percent higher during gestation and 150 percent higher during the first postpartum week. The authors speculate that pregnancy-related expansions in blood volume trigger atrial stretch receptors, potentially triggering ANP/BNP production. Postpartum surges in ANP are consistent with postpartum volume shifts and may contribute to postpartum diuresis.[18] Of interest, although ANP levels may increase with pregnancy, they remain within the normal range, never reaching the pathologic levels associated with heart failure. Alternatively, Sala et al. found that ANP levels increased only in the first trimester, and then only in the supine position. It is possible that differences in body posture dramatically affect ANP production in pregnancy, in part explaining variations in results. Normal ANP levels in later pregnancy may occur in supine women because uterine compression of the vena cava decreases atrial pressure and associated ANP secretion.[17] In contrast, authors that report unchanged ANP levels throughout the gestation, even in the lateral decubitus position, believe that the atrial enlargement during pregnancy results in reduced atrial stretch despite the increased blood volume.[19]

The circulating concentration of BNP is 20% less than that of ANP in normal individuals and has been found to be more useful in the diagnosis of congestive heart failure.[15,16] Levels of BNP are reported to increase largely in the third trimester of pregnancy compared with first-trimester levels (21.5 + 8 pg/ml versus 15.2 + 5 pg/ml) and are highest in pregnancies complicated by preeclampsia (37.1 + 10 pg/ml).[19] In pregnancies with preeclampsia, higher levels of BNP are associated with echocardiographic evidence of left ventricular enlargement.[20] Although the levels of BNP are increased during pregnancy and with preeclampsia, the mean values are still lower than the levels used to screen for cardiac dysfunction (>75 to 100 pg/ml) and, therefore, could potentially still be used to screen for congestive heart failure.[15,16]

CARDIOVASCULAR SYSTEM

Pregnancy causes profound physiologic changes in the cardiovascular system. A series of adaptive mechanisms are activated as early as 5 weeks' gestation in order to maximize oxygen delivery to maternal and fetal tissues.[12] In most women, these physiologic demands are well tolerated. However, in certain cardiac diseases, maternal morbidity and even mortality may occur.[21]

Heart

The combination of displacement of the diaphragm and the effect of pregnancy on the shape of the rib cage (described in the respiratory section below), displaces the heart upward and to the left. In addition, the heart rotates on its long axis, moving the apex somewhat laterally, resulting in an increased cardiac silhouette on radiographic studies, without a true change in the cardiothoracic ratio. Associated radiographic findings include an apparent straightening of the border of the left side of the heart and increased prominence of the pulmonary conus. Therefore, the diagnosis of cardiomegaly by simple radiography should be confirmed by echocardiogram if clinically appropriate.[22]

Although true cardiomegaly is rare, physiologic myocardial hypertrophy of the heart is consistently observed as a result of expanded blood volume in the first half of the pregnancy and progressively increasing afterload in later gestation. These structural changes in the heart are similar to those found in response to physical training and are reversible after pregnancy.[13,23] Most changes begin early in the first trimester and peak by 30 to 34 weeks' gestation. Left ventricular end-diastolic dimension increases 12 percent over preconceptional values by M-mode echocardiography. Concurrently, left ventricular wall mass increases by 52 percent (mild myocardial hypertrophy), and atrial diameters increase bilaterally, peaking at 40 percent above non-pregnant values.[23,24] Pulmonary capillary wedge pressures (PCWPs) are stable, reflecting a combination of decreased pulmonary vascular resistance and increased blood volume. Twin pregnancies increase myocardial hypertrophy, atrial dilation, and end-diastolic ventricular measurements even further.[25]

Within the past decade clinicians and researchers have focused on abnormalities of diastolic function as important contributors to cardiac disease and symptom severity, especially in the setting of normal or near normal systolic function.[26] In a recent review, diastolic dysfunction was pinpointed as a leading causes of cardiac failure in pregnancy.[27] Over the past 5 years, the effects of pregnancy on diastolic function have been thoroughly investigated by using pulsed-wave Doppler echocardiogram.[23,28] In young healthy women, the left ventricle is elastic; therefore, diastolic relaxation is swift and ventricular filling occurs almost completely by early diastole with minimal contribution from the atrial kick. The E/A ratio compares the peak mitral flow velocity in early diastole (E) to the peak atrial kick velocity (A); whereas both velocities increase in pregnancy, the overall ratio falls due to a greater rise in the A-wave velocity. The rise in the A value, which begins in the second trimester and increases throughout the third trimester, indicates the increased importance of the atrial contraction in left ventricular filling during pregnancy.[23,28] Veille et al. determined that in healthy women, pregnancy did not adversely affect baseline diastolic function, but that at maximal exercise, diastolic function was impaired. The reason for the impairment was attributed to increased left ventricular wall stiffness. The authors further speculated that this change maybe the limiting factor for exercise in pregnancy.[29]

Cardiac Output

One of the most remarkable changes in pregnancy is the tremendous increase in CO. Van Oppen et al.[30] reviewed 33 cross-sectional and 19 longitudinal studies and found greatly divergent results on when CO peaked, the magnitude of the rise in CO before labor, and the effect of the third trimester on CO. However, all of the studies agreed that CO increased significantly beginning in early pregnancy, peaking at an average of 30 to 50 percent above preconceptional values. In a longitudinal study by Robson et al. using Doppler echocardiography, CO increased by 50 percent at 34 weeks from a prepregnancy value of 4.88 L/min to 7.34 L/min[30,31] (Fig. 3-2). In twin gestations, CO incrementally increases an addi-

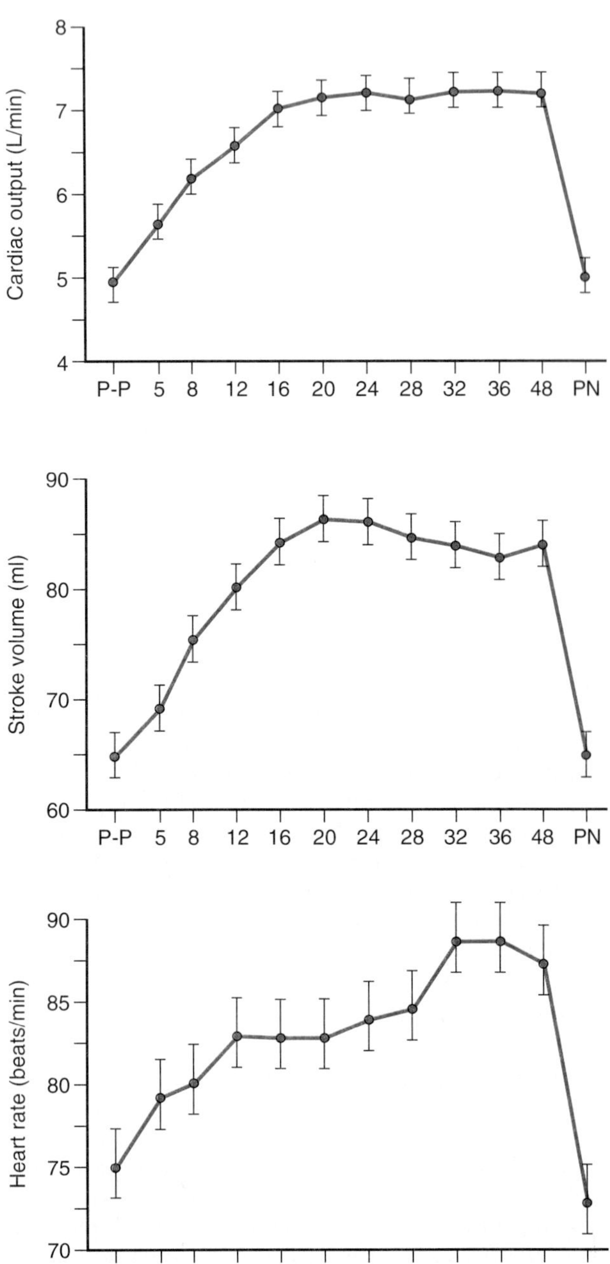

Figure 3-2. Increase in cardiac output from the non-pregnancy state throughout pregnancy, PN, postnatal; P-P, prepregnancy. (From Hunter S, Robson S: Adaptation of the maternal heart in pregnancy. Br Heart J 68:540, 1992, page 541, with permission.)

tional 20 percent above that of singleton pregnancies.[25] Robson et al. demonstrated that, by 5 weeks' gestation, CO has already risen by more than 10 percent. By 12 weeks, the rise in output was 34 to 39 percent above nongravid levels, accounting for about 75 percent of the total increase in CO during pregnancy. Although the literature is not clear regarding the exact gestation when CO peaks, most studies point to a range between 25 and 30 weeks. The data on whether the CO continues to increase in the third trimester are very divergent, with equal numbers of good longitudinal studies showing a mild decrease, a slight increase, or no change.[23,30] The differences in these studies cannot be explained by differences in investigative techniques, position of the women during measurements, or study design. This apparent discrepancy appears to be explained by the small number of individuals in each study and the probability that the course of CO during the third trimester is determined by factors specific to the individual.[30,32] In a recent study, Desai et al. reported that CO in the third trimester is significantly correlated with fetal birth weight and maternal height and weight.[33]

Most of the increase in CO is directed to the uterus, placenta, and breasts. In the first trimester, as in the nongravid state, the uterus receives 2 to 3 percent of CO and the breasts 1 percent. The percentage of CO going to the kidneys (20 percent), skin (10 percent), brain (10 percent), and coronary arteries (5 percent) remains at similar nonpregnant percentages, but because of the overall increase in CO this results in an increase in absolute blood flow of approximately 50 percent.[34] By term, the uterus receives 17 percent (450 to 650 ml/min) and the breasts 2 percent, mostly at the expense of a reduction of the fraction of the CO going to the splanchnic bed and skeletal muscle. The absolute blood flow to the liver is not changed, but the overall percentage of CO is significantly decreased.

CO is the product of stroke volume (SV) and heart rate (HR) (CO = SV × HR), both of which increase during pregnancy and contribute to the overall rise in CO. An initial rise in the HR occurs by 5 weeks' gestation and continues until it peaks at 32 weeks' gestation at 15 to 20 beats above the nongravid rate, an increase of 17 percent. The SV begins to rise by 8 weeks' gestation and reaches its maximum at about 20 weeks, 20 to 30 percent above nonpregnant values. In the third trimester, it is primarily variations in the SV that determine whether CO increases, decreases, or remains stable, as described earlier[32,35] (Fig. 3-2).

CO in pregnancy depends on maternal position. In a study in 10 normal gravid women in the third trimester, using pulmonary artery catheterization, the CO was noted to be highest in the knee-chest position and lateral recumbent position at 6.6 to 6.9 L/min. CO decreased by 22 percent to 5.4 L/min in the standing position[36] (Fig. 3-3). The decrease in CO in the supine position compared with the lateral recumbent position is 10 to 30 percent.[35,37] In both the standing and the supine positions, decreased CO results from a fall in SV secondary to decreased blood return to the heart. In the supine position, the enlarged uterus compresses the inferior vena cava, reducing venous return; before 24 weeks, this effect is not observed. Of note, in late pregnancy, the inferior vena cava is completely occluded in the supine position, with venous return from the lower extremities occurring through the dilated paravertebral collateral circulation.[38,39]

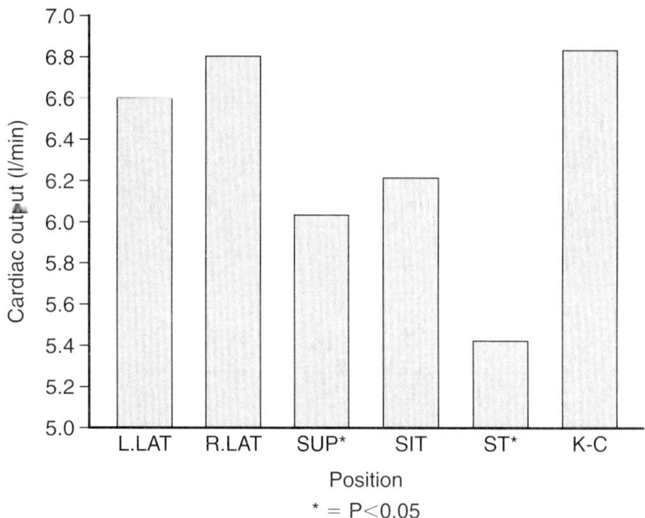

Figure 3-3. Effect of position change on cardiac output during pregnancy. K-C, knee-chest; L.LAT, left lateral; R.LAT, right lateral; SIT, sitting; ST, standing; SUP, supine. (From Clark S, Cotton D, Pivarnik J, et al: Position change and central hemodynamic profile during normal third-trimester pregnancy and postpartum. Am J Obstet Gynecol 164:883, 1991, page 885, with permission.)

Despite decreased CO, the majority of supine women are not hypotensive or symptomatic because of the compensated rise in systemic vascular resistance (SVR). However, 5 to 10 percent of gravidas manifest supine hypotension with symptoms of dizziness, lightheadedness, nausea, and even syncope. The women who become symptomatic have a greater decrease in CO and BP, and a greater increase in HR when in the supine position than do asymptomatic women.[40] Some investigators have proposed that the determination of whether women become symptomatic or not depends on the development of an adequate paravertebral collateral circulation. Interestingly, with engagement of the fetal head, less of an effect on CO is seen.[38] The ability to maintain a normal blood pressure (BP) in the supine position may be lost during epidural or spinal anesthesia because of an inability to increase SVR. Clinically, the effects of maternal position on CO are especially important when the mother is clinically hypotensive or in the setting of a nonreassuring fetal heart rate tracing. The finding of a decreased CO in the standing position may give a physiologic basis for the observation of decreased birth weight and placental infarctions in working women who stand for prolonged periods.[41]

Arterial Blood Pressure and Systemic Vascular Resistance

BP is the product of CO and resistance (BP = CO × SVR). In spite of the large increase in CO, the maternal

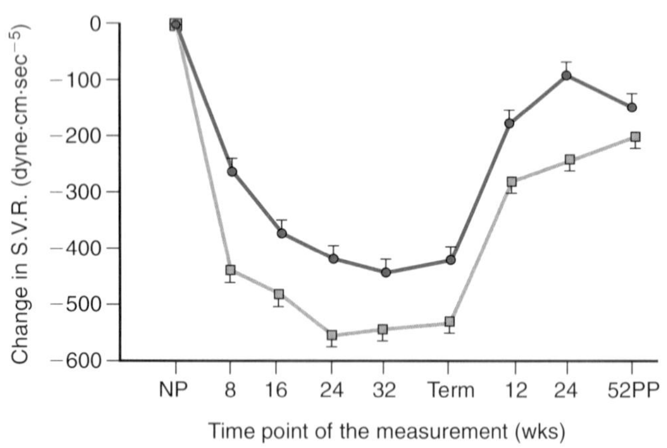

Figure 3-4. Change in systemic vascular resistance (S.V.R.) during normal pregnancy and the first year postpartum in nulliparous and parous women. Open circles (red), 15 nulliparous women; open squares (blue), 15 parous women. Data are presented as mean ± SEM. 52PP, 52 weeks postpartum; NP, nonpregnant. (From Clapp J, Capeless E: Cardiovascular function before, during and after the first and subsequent pregnancies. Am J Cardiol 80:1469, 1997, page 1473, with permission.)

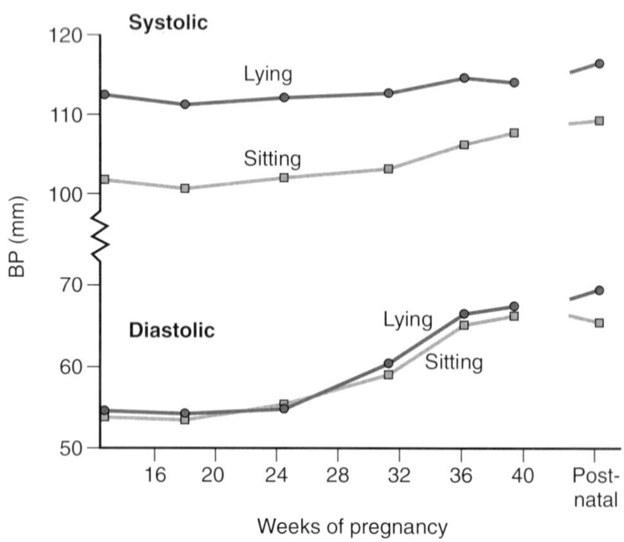

Figure 3-5. Blood pressure trends (sitting and lying) during pregnancy. Postnatal measures performed 6 weeks postpartum. (From MacGillivray I, Rose G, Rowe B: Blood pressure survey in pregnancy. Clin Sci 37:395, 1969, page 399, with permission.)

BP is decreased until later in pregnancy as a result of a decrease in SVR that nadirs midpregnancy and is followed by a gradual rise until term. Even at full term, SVR remains 21 percent lower than prepregnancy values in pregnancies not affected by gestational hypertension or preeclampsia[24,35,42] (Fig. 3-4). The most obvious cause for the decreased SVR is progesterone-mediated smooth muscle relaxation; however, the exact mechanism for the fall in SVR is poorly understood. Earlier theories that uteroplacental circulation acts as an arteriovenous shunt are unlikely. Increased NO also contributes to decreased vascular resistance by direct actions and by blunting the vascular responsiveness to vasoconstrictors such as angiotensin II and norepinephrine. During normal conception, the expression and activity of NO synthase is elevated and the plasma level of cyclic guanosine monophosphate, a second messenger of NO and a mediator of vascular smooth muscle relaxation is also increased.[43] As a result, despite the overall increase in the RAAS in pregnancy, the normal gravid woman is refractory to the vasoconstrictive effects of angiotensin II. Gant et al.[44] showed that nulliparous women who later become preeclamptic retain their response to angiotensin II before the appearance of clinical signs of preeclampsia.

Decreases in maternal BP parallel falling SVR, with initial decreased BP manifesting at 8 weeks' gestation or earlier. Current studies did not include preconception BP or frequent first-trimester BP sampling and, therefore, cannot determine the exact time course of hemodynamic alterations. Because BP fluctuates with menstruation and is decreased in the luteal phase, it seems reasonable that BP drops immediately.[45] The diastolic BP and the mean arterial pressure [MAP = (2 × Diastolic BP + Systolic BP)/3] decrease more than the systolic BP, which changes minimally. The overall decrease in diastolic BP and MAP is 5 to 10 mm Hg[46] (Fig. 3-5). The diastolic BP and the MAP nadir at midpregnancy and return to prepregnancy levels by term and in most studies rarely exceed prepregnancy or postpartum values. However, some investigators have reported that at term, the BP is greater than in matched nonpregnant controls and believe that in the third trimester, BP is higher than pre-pregnant values.[23,28] Current studies are significantly limited by the absence of preconceptional values for comparison within individual patients.

The position when the BP is taken and what Korotkoff sound is used to determine the diastolic BP is important. BP is lowest in the lateral recumbent position, and the BP of the superior arm in this position is 10 to 12 mm Hg lower than the inferior arm. In the clinic, BP should be measured in the sitting position and the Korotkoff 5 sound should be used. This is the diastolic BP when the sound disappears as opposed to the Korotkoff 4, when there is a muffling of the sound. In a study of 250 gravidas, the Korotkoff 4 sound could only be identified in 48 percent of patients, whereas the Korotkoff 5 sound could always be determined. The Korotkoff 4 should only be used when the Korotkoff 5 occurs at 0 mm Hg.[47] Use of automated BP monitors have been compared to mercury sphygmomanometry during pregnancy, and although they tended to overestimate the diastolic BP, the overall results were similar in normotensive women. Of note in patients with suspected preeclampsia, automated monitors appear increasingly inaccurate at higher BPs.[48]

Venous Pressure

Venous pressure in the upper extremities remains unchanged in pregnancy but rises progressively in the lower extremities. Femoral venous pressure increases from values near 10 cm H_2O at 10 weeks' gestation to 25 cm H_2O near term.[49] From a clinical standpoint, this increase in pressure in addition to the obstruction of the inferior vena cava leads to the development of edema, varicose veins, hemorrhoids, and an increased risk of deep venous thrombosis.

Central Hemodynamic Assessment

Clark et al. studied 10 carefully selected normal women at 36 to 38 weeks' gestation and again at 11 to 13 weeks' postpartum with arterial lines and Swan-Ganz catheterization to characterize the central hemodynamics of term pregnancy (Table 3-1). As described earlier CO, HR, SVR and pulmonary vascular resistance change significantly with pregnancy. In addition, clinically significant decreases were noted in colloidal oncotic pressure (COP), and the COP-PCWP difference explaining why gravid women have a greater propensity for developing pulmonary edema with changes in capillary permeability or elevations in cardiac preload. The COP can fall even further after delivery to 17 mm Hg and, if the pregnancy is complicated by preeclampsia, can reach levels as low as 14 mm Hg.[50] When the PCWP is more than 4 mm Hg above the COP, the risk of pulmonary edema increases; therefore, pregnant women can experience pulmonary edema at PCWPs of 18 to 20 mm Hg, which is significantly lower than the typical nonpregnant threshold of 24 mm Hg. No significant gestational changes were found in MAP, PCWP, central venous pressure, or left ventricular stroke work index.[42]

Evaluation of left ventricular function (contractility) is difficult in pregnancy because it is strongly influenced by changes in HR, preload, and after-load. Despite the increase in SV and CO, normal pregnancy is not associated with hyperdynamic left ventricular function during the third trimester as measured by ejection fraction, left ventricular stroke work index, or fractional shortening of the left ventricle. However, some studies have shown that contractility might be slightly increased in the first two trimesters,[32] whereas other articles report no change throughout the pregnancy and some report a decline toward term.[23,28,33]

Normal Changes That Mimic Heart Disease

The physiologic adaptations of pregnancy lead to a number of changes in maternal signs and symptoms that can mimic cardiac disease and make it difficult to determine if true disease is present. Dyspnea is common to both cardiac disease and pregnancy, but certain distinguishing features should be considered. First, the onset of pregnancy-related dyspnea usually occurs before 20 weeks, and 75 percent of women experience it by the third trimester. Unlike cardiac dyspnea, pregnancy-related dyspnea does not worsen significantly with advancing gestation. Second, physiologic dyspnea is usually mild, does not stop women from performing normal daily activities, and does not occur at rest.[51] Other normal symptoms that can mimic cardiac disease include decreased exercise tolerance, fatigue, occasional orthopnea, syncope, and chest discomfort. The reason for this increase in cardiac symptoms is not an increase in catecholamine levels because these levels are either unchanged or decreased in pregnancy. Symptoms that should not be attributed to pregnancy and need a more thorough investigation include hemoptysis, syncope or chest pain with exertion, progressive orthopnea, or paroxysmal nocturnal dyspnea. Normal physical findings that could be mistaken as evidence of cardiac disease include peripheral edema, mild tachycardia, jugular venous distention after midpregnancy, and lateral displacement of the left ventricular apex.

Pregnancy also alters normal heart sounds. At the end of the first trimester, both components of the first heart sound become louder, and there is exaggerated splitting. The second heart sound usually remains normal with only minimal changes. Up to 80 to 90 percent of gravidas demonstrate a third heart sound (S_3) after midpregnancy because of rapid diastolic filling. Rarely, a fourth heart sound may be ausculated, but typically phonocardiography is needed to detect this. Systolic ejection murmurs along the left sternal border develop in 96 percent of pregnancies and are thought to be caused by increased

Table 3-1. Central Hemodynamic Changes

	11–12 WEEKS POSTPARTUM	36–38 WEEKS GESTATION	CHANGE FROM NONPREGNANT STATE
Cardiac output(L/min)	4.3 ± 0.9	6.2 ± 1.0	+43%*
Heart rate (bpm)	71 ± 10.0	83 ± 10.0	+17%*
Systemic vascular resistance (dyne·cm·sec^{-5})	1530 ± 520	1210 ± 266	−21%*
Pulmonary vascular resistance (dyne·cm·sec^{-5})	119 ± 47.0	78 ± 22	−34%*
Colloid oncotic pressure (mm Hg)	20.8 ± 1.0	18 ± 1.5	−14%*
Mean arterial pressure (mm Hg)	86.4 ± 7.5	90.3 ± 5.8	NS
Pulmonary capillary wedge pressure (mm Hg)	3.7 ± 2.6	3.6 ± 2.5	NS
Central venous pressure (mm Hg)	3.7 ± 2.6	3.6 ± 2.5	NS
Left ventricular stroke work index (g·m·m^{-2})	41 ± 8	48 ± 6	NS

Data are presented as mean ± standard deviation
*$P < 0.05$.

NS, not significant.

Although data are not presented, the pulmonary artery pressures were not signigicantly different.

Adapted from Clark S, Cotton D, Lee W, et al: Central hemodynamic assessment of normal term pregnancy. Am J Obstet Gynecol 161:1439, 1989.

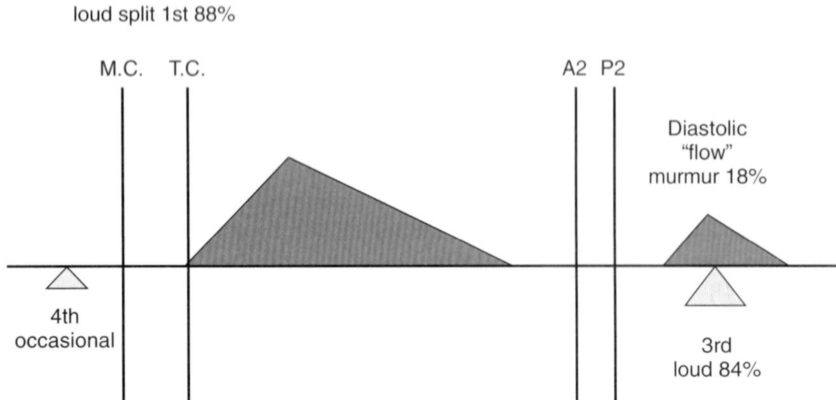

Figure 3-6. Summarization of the findings on auscultation of the heart in pregnancy. MC, mitral closure; TC, tricuspid closure; A2 and P2, Aortic and pulmonary elements of the second sound. (From Cutforth R, MacDonald C: Heart sounds and murmurs in pregnancy. Am Heart J 71:741, 1966, page 747, with permission.)

blood flow across the pulmonic and aortic valves. Most commonly, these are midsystolic and less than grade 3. Diastolic murmurs have been found in up to 18 percent of pregnancies, but their presence is uncommon enough to warrant further evaluation. A continuous murmur in the second to fourth intercostal space may be heard in the second or third trimester of pregnancy due to the so-called mammary souffle caused by increased blood flow in the breast[53,54] (Fig. 3-6).

Effect of Labor and the Immediate Puerperium

The profound anatomic and functional changes on cardiac function reach a crescendo during the labor process. In addition to the dramatic rise in CO with normal pregnancy, even greater increases in CO occur with labor and in the immediate puerperium. In a Doppler echocardiography study by Robson et al. of 15 uncomplicated women without epidural anesthesia, the CO between contractions increased 12 percent during the first stage of labor[31,32] (Fig. 3-7). This increase in CO is caused primarily by an increased SV, but HR may also increase. By the end of the first stage of labor, the CO during contractions is 51 percent above baseline term pregnancy values (6.99 L/min to 10.57 L/min). Increased CO is in part secondary to increased venous return from the 300–500 mL autotransfusion that occurs at the onset of each contraction as blood is expressed from the uterus.[55,56] Paralleling increases in CO, the MAP also rises in the first stage of labor, from 82 mm Hg to 91 mm Hg in early labor to 102 mm Hg by the beginning of the second stage. MAP also increases with uterine contractions.

Much of the increase in CO and MAP is due to pain and anxiety. With epidural anesthesia, the baseline increase in CO is reduced, but the rise observed with contractions persists.[57] Maternal posture also influences hemodynamics during labor. Changing position from supine to lateral recumbent increases CO. This change is greater than the increase seen before labor and suggests that during labor, CO may be more dependent on preload. Therefore, it is important to avoid the supine position in laboring

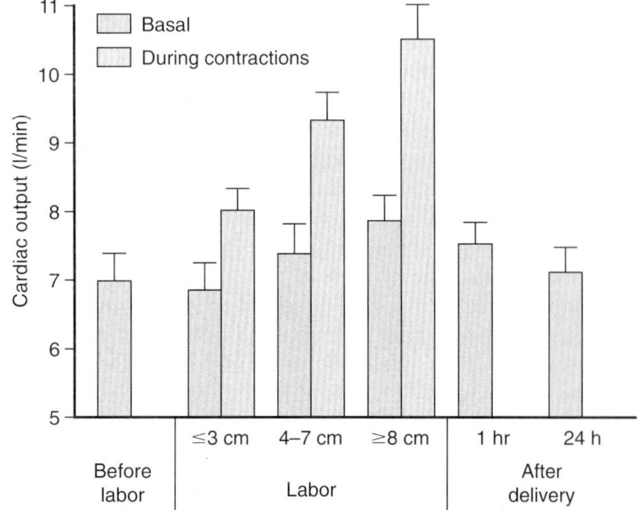

Figure 3-7. Changes in cardiac output and stroke volume during normal labor. (From Hunter S, Robson S: Adaptation of the maternal heart in pregnancy. Br Heart J 68:540, 1992, page 542, with permission.)

women and to give a sufficient fluid bolus before an epidural to maintain an adequate preload.[58]

In the immediate postpartum period (10 to 30 minutes after delivery), CO reaches its maximum, with a further rise of 10 to 20 percent. This increase is accompanied by a fall in the maternal HR that is likely secondary to increased SV. Traditionally, this rise was thought to be the result of uterine autotransfusion as described earlier with contractions, but the validity of this concept is uncertain.[42] In both vaginal and elective cesarean deliveries, the maximal increase in the CO occurs 10 to 30 minutes after delivery, and returns to prelabor baseline 1 hour after delivery.[59] The increase was 37 percent with epidural anesthesia, and 28 percent with general anesthesia. Over the next 2 to 4 postpartum weeks, the cardiac hemodynamic parameters return to near-preconceptional levels.[60]

The effect of pregnancy on cardiac rhythm is limited to an increase in HR and a significant increase in isolated atrial and ventricular contractions. In a Holter monitor study by Shotan et al.,[52] 110 pregnant women referred for evaluation of symptoms of palpitations, dizziness, or syncope were compared with 52 healthy pregnant women. Symptomatic women had similar rates of isolated sinus tachycardia (9 percent), isolated premature atrial complexes (56 percent), and premature ventricular contractions (PVCs) (49 percent), but increased rates of frequent PVCs greater than 10/hour (20 percent versus 2 percent, $p = 0.03$). A subset of patients with frequent premature atrial complexes or PVCs had comparative Holter studies performed postpartum that revealed an 85 percent decrease in arrhythmia frequency ($p < 0.05$). This dramatic decline, with patients acting as their own controls, supports the arrythmogenic effect of pregnancy. In a study of 30 healthy women placed on Holter monitors during labor, a similarly high incidence of benign arrhythmias was found (93 percent). Reassuringly, the prevalence of concerning arrhythmias was no higher than expected. An unexpected finding was a 35 percent rate of asymptomatic bradycardia, defined as a HR of less than 60 bpm, in the immediate postpartum period.[61] Whether labor increases the rate of arrhythmias in women with underlying cardiac disease has not been thoroughly studied, but multiple case reports suggest labor may increase arrhythmias in this subgroup of women.

RESPIRATORY SYSTEM

Upper Respiratory Tract

During pregnancy, the mucosa of the nasopharynx becomes hyperemic and edematous with hypersecretion of mucous due to increased estrogen. These changes often lead to marked nasal stuffiness; epistaxis is also common. Placement of nasogastric tubes may cause excessive bleeding if adequate lubrication is not used.[51] Polyposis of the nose and nasal sinuses develops in some individuals but regresses postpartum. Because of these changes, many gravid women complain of chronic cold symptoms. However, the temptation to use nasal decongestants should be avoided because of risk of hypertension and rebound congestion.[62]

Mechanical Changes

The configuration of the thoracic cage changes early in pregnancy, much earlier than can be accounted for by mechanical pressure from the enlarging uterus. Relaxation of the ligamentous attachments between the ribs and sternum may be responsible. The subcostal angle increases from 68 degrees to 103 degrees, the transverse diameter of the chest expands by 2 cm, and the chest circumference expands by 5 to 7 cm.[63] As gestation progresses, the level of the diaphragm rises 4 cm; however, diaphragmatic excursion is not impeded and actually increases 1 to 2 cm. Respiratory muscle function is not affected by pregnancy, and maximum inspiratory and expiratory pressures are unchanged.[64]

Lung Volume and Pulmonary Function

The described alterations in chest wall configuration and the diaphragm lead to changes in static lung volumes. In a review of studies with at least 15 subjects compared with nonpregnant controls, Crapo compiled the following adaptations (Fig. 3-8 and Table 3-2).[51]

1. The elevation of the diaphragm decreases the volume of the lungs in the resting state, thereby reducing total lung capacity by 5 percent and the functional residual capacity (FRC), the volume of air in the lungs at the end of quiet exhalation, by 20 percent.
2. The FRC can be subdivided into expiratory reserve volume and residual volume and both decrease.
3. The inspiratory capacity, the maximum volume that can be inhaled increases 5 to 10 percent as a result of the reduction in the FRC.
4. The vital capacity does not change.

Spirometric measurements assessing bronchial flow are unaltered in pregnancy. The forced expiratory volume in 1 second (FEV_1) and the ratio of FEV_1 to forced vital capacity are both unchanged, suggesting that airway function remains stable.[65] In addition, peak expiratory flow rates measured using a peak flow meter seem to be unaltered in pregnancy at rates of 450 ± 16 L/min.[66] Harirah et al.[67] performed a longitudinal study of the peak flow in 38 women from the first trimester until 6 weeks postpartum. They reported that the peak flows had a statistically significant decrease as the gestation progressed, but the amount of the decrease was minimal enough to be of questionable clinical significance. Likewise a small decrease in the peak flow was found in the supine position versus the standing or sitting position. Therefore, during gestation, both spirometry and peak flow meters can be used in diagnosing and manag-

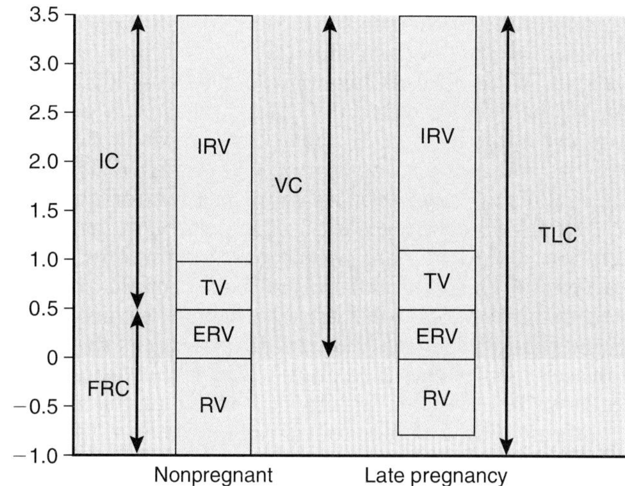

Figure 3-8. Lung volumes in nonpregnant and pregnant women. ERV, expiratory reserve; FRC, functional residual capacity; IC, inspiratory capacity; IRV, inspiratory reserve; RV, residual volume; TLC, total lung capacity; TV, tidal volume; VC, vital capacity. (From Cruickshank DP, Wigton TR, Hays PM: Maternal physiology in pregnancy. In Gabbe SG, Niebyl JR, Simpson JL [eds] Obstetrics: Normal and Problem Pregnancies, 3rd ed. New York, Churchill Livingstone, 1996, p 94, with permission.)

Table 3-2. Lung Volumes and Capacities in Pregnancy

MEASUREMENT	DEFINITION	CHANGE IN PREGNANCY
Respiratory rate (RR)	Number of breaths per minute	Unchanged
Vital capacity (VC)	Maximum amount of air that can be forcibly expired after maximum inspiration (IC + ERV)	Unchanged
Inspiratory capacity (IC)	Maximum amount of air that can be inspired from resting expiratory level (TV + IRV)	Increased 5% to 10%
Tidal volume (TV)	Amount of air inspired and expired with normal breath	Increased 30% to 40%
Inspiratory reserve volume (IRV)	Maximum amount of air that can be inspired at end of normal Inspiration	Unchanged
Functional residual capacity (FRC)	Amount of air in lungs at resting expiratory level (ERV + RV)	Decreased 20%
Expiratory reserve volume (ERV)	Maximum amount of air that can be expired from resting expiratory level	Decreased 15% to 20%
Residual volume (RV)	Amount of air in lungs after maximum expiration	Decreased 20% to 25%
Total lung capacity (TLC)	Total amount of air in lungs at maximal inspiration (VC + RV)	Decreased 5%

From Cruickshank DP, Wigton TR, Hays PM: Maternal physiology in pregnancy. *In* Gabbe SG, Niebyl JR, Simpson JL (eds): Obstetrics: Normal and Problem Pregnancies, 3rd ed. New York, Churchill Livingstone, 1996, p 95, with permission.

ing respiratory illnesses, but the clinician should ensure that measurements are performed in the same maternal position.[67]

Gas Exchange

Increasing progesterone levels drive a state of chronic hyperventilation, as reflected by a 30 to 50 percent increase in tidal volume by 8 weeks' gestation. In turn, increased tidal volume results in an overall parallel rise in minute ventilation, despite a stable respiratory rate. (Minute ventilation = Tidal volume × Respiratory rate). The rise in minute ventilation, combined with a decrease in FRC leads to a larger than expected increase in alveolar ventilation (50 to 70 percent). Chronic mild hyperventilation results in increased alveolar oxygen (PAo_2) and decreased arterial carbon dioxide ($Paco_2$)[68] from normal levels of 37 to 40 mm Hg to 27 to 32 mm Hg.[69] The drop in the $Paco_2$ is especially critical, because it drives a more favorable carbon dioxide (CO_2) gradient between the fetus and mother, facilitating CO_2 transfer. The low maternal $Paco_2$ results in a chronic respiratory alkalosis. Partial renal compensation occurs through increased excretion of bicarbonate, which helps maintain the pH between 7.4 and 7.45 and lowers the serum bicarbonate levels to 18 to 21 mEq/L. Early in pregnancy, the arterial oxygen (Pao_2) increases (106 to 108 mm Hg) as the $Paco_2$ decreases, but by the third trimester, a slight decrease in the Pao_2 (101 to 104) occurs as a result of the enlarging uterus. The alveolar-to-arterial gradient [$P(A\text{-}a)o_2$] increases slightly at the end of gestation from 14 mm Hg to 20 mm Hg. This decrease in the Pao_2 late in pregnancy is even more pronounced in the supine position, with a further drop of 5 to 10 mm Hg and an increase in the $P(A\text{-}a)o_2$ to 26 mm Hg and up to 25 percent of women exhibit a Pao_2 less than 90 mm Hg[51,71,72] (Table 3-3).

As the minute ventilation increases, a simultaneous but smaller increase in oxygen uptake and consumption occurs. Most investigators have found maternal oxygen consumption to be 20 to 40 percent above nonpregnant levels. This increase occurs as a result of the oxygen requirements of the fetus, the placenta, and the increased oxygen requirement of maternal organs. With exercise or during labor, an even greater rise in both minute ventilation and oxygen consumption takes place.[51] During a contraction, oxygen consumption can triple.[68] As a result of the increased oxygen consumption and because the functional residual capacity is decreased, there is a lowering of the maternal oxygen reserve. Therefore, the pregnant patient is more susceptible to the effects of apnea; during intubation, a more rapid onset of hypoxia, hypercapnia, and respiratory acidosis is seen.

Table 3-3. Blood Gas Values in Pregnancy in Third Trimester

	PREGNANT	NONPREGNANT
Pao_2 (mm Hg)*	101.8 ± 1	93.4 ± 2.04
Arterial Hgb saturation (%)†	98.5 ± 0.7%	98 ± 0.8%
$Paco_2$ (mm Hg)*	30.4 ± 0.6	40 ± 2.5
Ph*	7.43 ± 0.006	7.43 ± 0.02
Serum bicarbonate (HCO_3) (mMol/L)	21.7 ± 1.6	25.3 ± 1.2
Base deficit (mmols/l)*	3.1 ± 0.2	1.06 ± 0.6
Alveolar-arterial gradient ($P(A\text{-}a)o_2$ (mm Hg)*	16.1 ± 0.9	15.7 ± 0.6

*Data from Templeton A, Kelman G: Maternal blood-gases, (PAO_2-PaO_2), physiological shunt and VD/VT in normal pregnancy. Br J Anaesth 48:1001, 1976. Data presented as mean ± SEM.

†Data from McAuliffe F, Kametas N, Krampl E: Blood gases in prepregnancy at sea level and at high altitude. Br J Obstet Gynaecol 108:980, 2001. Data presented as mean ± SD.

Intrapulmonary shunting (Qs/Qt) refers to the pulmonary blood flow that does not come into contact with functioning alveoli relative to the total pulmonary blood flow. This value is used to direct and evaluate the efficacy of therapeutic interventions in critically ill patients.

Hankins et al. found that interpulmonary shunting was three times higher during gestation, increasing from a non-pregnant value of 2–5% to 13–15%. This observation is attributed to the combination of the overall decrease in lung volumes with greater ventilation-perfusion mismatches.[73] Interestingly Qs/Qt values of 5–15% are often associated with shortness of breath, particularly on exertion in non-gravid individuals. In a second study, Hankins et al. found no increase in oxygen delivery, oxygen extraction, or the arteriovenous oxygen content difference. Surprisingly, no increase in oxygen consumption was documented during pregnancy in this study, but the results of the study are somewhat limited by a small sample size of 10 women.[74]

Sleep

Pregnancy causes both an increase in sleep disorders and significant changes in sleep profile and pattern that persist into the postpartum period.[75,76] Pregnancy causes such significant changes that the American Sleep Disorder Association has proposed the existence of a new term "pregnancy-associated sleep disorder."[77] It is well known that hormones and physical discomforts affect sleep (Table 3-4). With the dramatic change in hormone levels and the significant mechanical effects that make women more uncomfortable, it is not difficult to understand why sleep is profoundly affected.[76] During the third trimester, multiple discomforts occur that can impair sleep: urinary frequency, backache, general abdominal discomfort and contractions, leg cramps, restless leg syndrome, heartburn, and fetal movement. Interestingly, no changes are seen in melatonin levels, which modulate the body's circadian pacemaker.

The changes in sleep resulting from pregnancy have been investigated by multiple authors using questionnaires, sleep logs, and polysomnographic studies. From these studies, investigators have shown that the vast majority of women (66 to 94 percent) report alterations in sleep, and that the characteristics of sleep change throughout the pregnancy begin as early as the first trimester. In general pregnancy is associated with a decrease in rapid eye movement (REM) sleep and a decrease in stage 3 and 4 non-REM sleep. REM sleep is important for cognitive thinking, and stage 3 and 4 non-REM sleep is the so-called deep sleep and is important for rest. In addition, with advancing gestational age, there is a decrease in sleeping efficiency and increased awake time. By 3 months postpartum, the amount of non-REM and REM sleep recovers but a persistent decrease in sleeping efficiency and nocturnal awakenings occur, presumably due to the newborn.[75,76] Although pregnancy causes changes in sleep, it is important for the clinician to consider other primary sleep disorders unrelated to pregnancy such as sleep apnea. The physiologic changes of pregnancy may predispose to snoring and upper airway obstruction, and may induce obstructive sleep and result in sleep apnea. The prevalence of sleep apnea in pregnancy is unknown, but it appears to increase the risk of intrauterine growth restriction and gestational hypertension if it is associated with hypoxemia.[76] Patients with known sleep apnea may need repeat sleep studies to determine whether changes in treatment are needed to prevent intermittent hypoxia.

Although the majority of gravidas have sleep problems, most do not complain to their providers or ask for treatment. Treatment options include improving sleep habits by avoiding fluids after dinner, establishing regular sleep hours, avoiding naps and caffeine, minimizing bedroom noises, and using pillow support. Other options include relaxation techniques, managing back pain, and use of sleep medications. The best medications include diphenhydramine (Benadryl) and zolpidem (Ambien); both are class B drugs.[76]

Another potential cause of sleep disturbances in pregnancy is due to the development of restless leg syndrome and periodic leg movements during sleep. Restless leg syndrome is a neurosensory disorder that typically begins in the evening and can prevent women from falling asleep. Pregnancy can be a cause of this syndrome and in one study up to 23% of gravidas developed some component of this syndrome in the third trimester although the true prevalence of this disorder during pregnancy is unknown.[77a] Although typically this syndrome is not

Table 3-4. Characteristics of Sleep in Pregnancy

STAGE OF PREGNANCY	SUBJECTIVE SYMPTOMS	OBJECTIVE (POLYSOMNOGRAPHY)
First Trimester	Increased total sleep time: ⇑ naps Increased daytime sleepiness Increased nocturnal insomnia	Increased total sleep time Decreased stage 3 and 4 non-REM sleep
Second Trimester	Normalization of total sleep time Increased awakenings	Normal total sleep time Decreased stage 3 and 4 non-REM sleep Decreased REM sleep
Third Trimester	Decreased total sleep time Increased insomnia Increased nocturnal awakenings Increased daytime sleepiness	Decreased total sleep time Increased awakenings after sleep onset Increased stage 1 non-REM sleep Decreased stage 3 and 4 non-REM sleep Decreased REM sleep

REM: Rapid eye movement sleep, important for cognitive sleep, 20% to 25% of sleep.
Stage 1 and 2 non-REM sleep: Light sleep, 55% of sleep.
Stage 3 and 4 non-REM sleep: Deep sleep, important for rest, 20% of sleep.
Adapted from Santiago J, Nolledo M, Kinzler W: Sleep and sleep disorders in pregnancy. Ann Intern Med 134:396, 2001.

severe enough to warrant treatment, occasionally it is a source of great discomfort to the gravid woman. Treatment options include improving sleep habits, the use of an electric vibrator to the calves, and the use of a benzodiazepine such as clonazepam or a dopaminergic agent such as L-dopa or carbidopa.[76]

HEMATOLOGIC CHANGES

Plasma Volume and Red Blood Cell Mass

Maternal blood volume begins to increase at about 6 weeks' gestation. Thereafter, it increases progressively until 30 to 34 weeks and then plateaus until delivery. The average expansion of blood volume is 40 to 50 percent, although individual increases range from 20 to 100 percent. Women with multiple pregnancies have a larger increase in blood volume than those with singletons.[78] Likewise, volume expansion correlates with infant birth weight, but it is not clear whether this is a cause or an effect. The increase in blood volume results from a combined expansion of both plasma volume and red blood cell (RBC) mass. The plasma volume begins to increase by 6 weeks and expands at a steady pace until it plateaus at 30 weeks' gestation; the overall increase is approximately 50 percent (1,200 to 1,300 ml). The exact etiology for the expansion of the blood volume is unknown, but the hormonal changes of gestation and the increase in NO play important roles.[79]

Erythrocyte mass also begins to increase at about 10 weeks' gestation. Although the initial slope of this increase is slower than that of the plasma volume, erythrocyte mass continues to increase progressively until term without plateauing.[8] Without iron supplementation, RBC mass increases about 18 percent by term, from a mean non-pregnant level of 1,400 ml up to 1,650 ml. Supplemental iron increases RBC mass accumulation to 400 to 450 ml or 30 percent.[78] Because plasma volume increases more than the RBC mass, maternal hematocrit falls. This so-called physiologic anemia of pregnancy reaches a nadir at 30 to 34 weeks. Because the RBC mass continues to increase after 30 weeks when the plasma volume expansion has plateaued, the hematocrit may rise somewhat after 30 weeks[80] (Fig. 3-9). The mean and fifth percentile hemoglobin concentrations for normal iron-supplemented pregnant women are outlined (Table 3-5).[81] In pregnancy, erythropoietin levels increase two- to threefold, starting at 16 weeks and may be responsible for the moderate erythroid hyperplasia found in the bone marrow, and mild elevations in the reticulocyte count.[82] The increased blood volume is protective given the possibility of hemorrhage during pregnancy or at delivery. The larger blood volume also helps fill the expanded vascular system created by vasodilatation and the large low-resistance vascular pool within the uteroplacental unit preventing hypotension.[51]

Vaginal delivery of a singleton infant at term is associated with a mean blood loss of 500 ml; an uncomplicated cesarean birth, about 1,000 ml; and a cesarean hysterectomy, 1,500 ml.[78,83,84] In a normal delivery, almost all of the blood loss occurs in the first hour. Pritchard et al. found that over the subsequent 72 hours, only 80 ml of blood is lost. In the nonpregnant state, blood loss results in an immediate fall in blood volume with a slow re-expansion through volume redistribution; by 24 hours, the blood volume approaches the prehemorrhage level. Isovolemia is maintained with a drop in hematocrit proportional to the blood loss. Gravid women respond to blood loss in a different fashion. In pregnancy, the blood volume drops after postpartum bleeding, but there is no re-expansion to the prelabor level, and there is less of a change in the hematocrit. Indeed, instead of volume redistribution an overall diuresis of the expanded water volume occurs postpartum. After delivery with average blood loss, the hematocrit drops moderately for 3 to 4 days followed by an increase. By days 5 to 7, the postpartum hematocrit is similar to the prelabor hematocrit. If the postpartum hematocrit is lower than the prelabor hematocrit, it suggests either that the blood loss was larger than appreciated or that the hypervolemia of pregnancy was less than normal as in preeclampsia.[78]

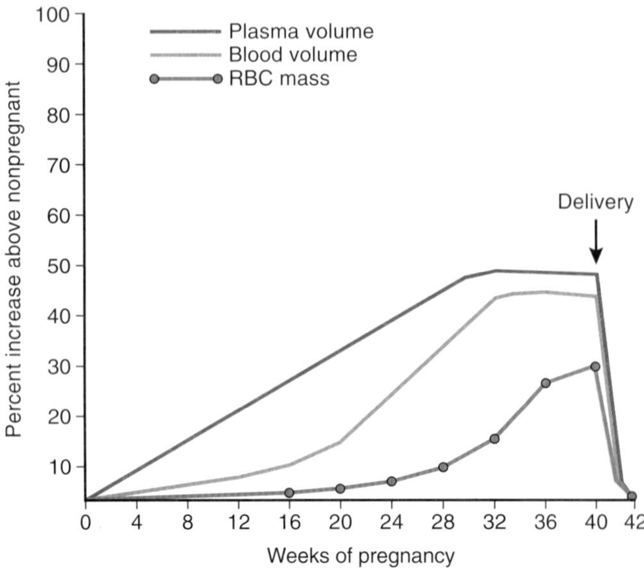

Figure 3-9. Blood volume changes during pregnancy. (From Scott D: Anemia during pregnancy. Obstet Gynecol Ann 1:219, 1972, page 100, with permission.)

Table 3-5. Hemoglobin Values in Pregnancy

WEEKS' GESTATION	MEAN HEMOGLOBIN (G/DL)	FIFTH PERCENTILE HEMOGLOBIN (G/DL)
12	12.2	11.0
16	11.8	10.6
20	11.6	10.5
24	11.6	10.5
28	11.8	10.7
32	12.1	11.0
36	12.5	11.4
40	12.9	11.9

From U.S. Department of Health and Human Services: Recommendations to prevent and control iron deficiency in the United States. MMWR 47:1, 1998.

Iron Metabolism in Pregnancy

Iron absorption from the duodenum is limited to its ferrous (divalent) state, the form found in iron supplements. Ferric (trivalent) iron from vegetable food sources must first be converted to the divalent state by the enzyme ferric reductase. If body iron stores are normal, only about 10 percent of ingested iron is absorbed, most of which remains in the mucosal cells or enterocytes until sloughing leads to excretion in the feces (1 mg/day).[85] Under conditions of increased iron needs, the fraction of iron absorbed increases. After absorption, iron is released from the enterocytes into the circulation, where it is carried bound to transferrin to the liver, spleen, muscle, and bone marrow. In those sites, iron is freed from transferrin and incorporated into hemoglobin (75 percent of iron), and myoglobin, or stored as ferritin and hemosiderin.[85] Menstruating women have about half the iron stores of men, with total body iron of 2 to 2.5 g and iron stores of only 300 mg. Before pregnancy, 8 to 10 percent of women in Western nations have iron deficiency.[85]

The iron requirements of gestation are about 1,000 mg. This includes 500 mg used to increase the maternal RBC mass (1 ml of erythrocytes contains 1.1 mg iron), 300 mg transported to the fetus, and 200 mg to compensate for the normal daily iron losses by the mother.[86] Thus, the normal expectant woman needs to absorb an average of 3.5 mg/day of iron. In actuality, the iron requirements are not constant but increase remarkably during the third trimester to 6 to 7 mg/day. The fetus receives its iron through active transport, primarily during the last trimester. Adequate iron transport to the fetus is maintained despite severe maternal iron deficiency. Thus, there is no correlation between maternal and fetal hemoglobin concentrations.

Currently, whether the nonanemic gravida should receive routine iron supplementation is controversial. Most American obstetricians favor the practice, whereas those in Europe generally consider it unnecessary. A recent Cochrane review concluded the evidence for either a beneficial or harmful effect on pregnancy outcome is inconclusive.[87] With the availability of serum ferritin levels that closely mirror body iron stores, it has become apparent that the unsupplemented patient, although not always anemic, is frequently significantly iron deficient at term. Romslo et al. demonstrated that unsupplemented women who are not anemic at the beginning of gestation have a significant drop in hemoglobin concentration, serum iron, serum ferritin, and transferrin saturation by term.[88] This suggests that the majority of women have insufficient iron stores to meet the demands of pregnancy. The recommended dose for iron supplementation is 30 mg elemental iron daily. More recently Makrides et al.[89] used a lower dose of iron supplementation (20 mg of elemental iron) starting at 20 weeks' gestation and showed similar improvements. Supplemented women were less likely to demonstrate anemia and iron deficiency at delivery and iron deficiency at 6 months postpartum as compared with women not given routine additional iron, unless they were diagnosed with anemia at 28 weeks' gestation (Table 3-6). In addition, the incidence of side effects was not different in this placebo-controlled trial with greater than 80-percent compliance. Still, no differences in pregnancy or neonatal outcomes were found.[89]

Table 3-6. Effect of Iron Supplementation During Pregnancy

	IRON-SUPPLEMENTED GROUP	PLACEBO GROUP
Hemoglobin (g/dl) <20weeks	13.1	13.0
Maternal status @ delivery		
Hemoglobin (g/dl)	12.7	12.0*
Serum ferritin (μg/L)	21	14*
Iron deficiency	35%	58%*
Iron deficiency anemia	3%	11%*
Maternal status @ 6 months		
Hemoglobin (g/dl)	13.5	13.4
Serum ferritin (μg/L)	34	26*
Iron deficiency	16%	29%*
Iron deficiency anemia	2.6%	1.7%

*Significant change between two groups.

Adapted from Makrides M, Crowther C, Gibson R, et al: Efficacy and tolerability of low-dose iron supplements during pregnancy: a randomized controlled trial. Am J Clin Nutr 78:145, 2003.

It is important to remember that the purpose of iron supplementation during pregnancy is not only to raise or even maintain the maternal hemoglobin level, but the goal is also to maintain or restore normal maternal iron levels. Therefore, supplementation is often needed, but rarely needs to be started before 20 to 28 weeks. Taking iron before 20 weeks can worsen the nausea and vomiting of pregnancy. If a woman enters pregnancy with iron deficiency anemia or if diagnosed with anemia, she will need to take additional iron. Available iron supplements include ferrous sulfate 325 mg (65 mg elemental iron), ferrous gluconate 325 mg (35 mg elemental iron), and ferrous fumarate 325 mg (107 mg elemental iron). The usual dose to treat iron deficiency anemia is ferrous sulfate 325 mg bid (130 mg of elemental iron daily), along with a stool softener such as docusate 100 mg bid. Previously, intravenous iron therapy was rarely given due to potential serious side effects associated with intravenous iron dextrans. However, recent studies have shown that intravenous iron sucrose can be given without serious sequalae; but it had limited benefit versus oral administration in reliable patients without abnormalities in iron absorption.[89a]

Platelets

Before the introduction of automated analyzers, studies of platelet counts during pregnancy reported conflicting results, with some showing a decrease, an increase, or no change with gestation. Unfortunately, even with the availability of automated cell counters, the data on the change in platelet count during pregnancy are still somewhat unclear.[90–92] Two studies have used true longitudinal methods with serial measurements in the same women. Pitkin et al.[93] measured platelet counts in 23 women every 4 weeks and found that the counts dropped from $322 \pm 75 \times 10^3/mm^3$ in the first trimester to $278 \pm 75 \times 10^3/mm^3$ in the third trimester. Similarly, O'Brien, in a study of 30 women, found a progressive decline in platelet counts.[94] Therefore, most recent studies show a decline in the platelet count during gestation possibly caused by increased destruction or hemodilution.[91,95] In addition to the mild decrease in the mean platelet count, Burrows and Kelton[96] have demonstrated that in the third trimester, approximately 8 percent of gravidas develop gestational thrombocytopenia, with platelet counts between 70,000 and $150,000/mm^3$. Gestational thrombocytopenia is not associated with an increase in pregnancy complications, and platelet counts return to normal by 1 to 2 weeks postpartum. Gestational thrombocytopenia is thought to be due to accelerated platelet consumption similar to that seen in normal pregnancy, but more marked in this subset of women.[96,97] Consistent with these findings, Boehlen et al.[95] compared platelet counts during the third trimester of pregnancy to nonpregnant controls. They showed a shift to both a lower mean platelet count and an overall shift to the left of the "platelet curve" in the pregnant women (Fig. 3-10). This study found that only 2.5 percent of nonpregnant women have platelet counts less than $150,000/mm^3$ (the traditional value used outside of pregnancy for cutoff for normal) versus 11.5 percent of gravid women. A platelet count of less than $116,000/mm^3$ occurred in 2.5 percent of gravid women, and therefore, these investigators recommended using this value as the lower limit for normal in the third trimester.[95] In addition, they suggested that workups for the etiology of decreased platelet count were unneeded at values above this level.

Immune System and Leukocytes

The peripheral white blood cell (WBC) count rises progressively during pregnancy. During the first trimester, the mean WBC count is $8,000/mm^3$, with a normal range of 5,110 to $9,900/mm^3$. During the second and third trimester, the mean is $8,500/mm^3$, with a range of 5,600 to $12,200/mm^3$.[93] In labor, the count may rise to 20,000 to $30,000/mm^3$, and counts are highly correlated with labor progression as determined by cervical dilation.[98] Because of the normal increase of the WBCs in labor, it should not be used clinically in determining the presence of infection. The increase in the WBC count during pregnancy is largely due to increases in circulating segmented neutrophils and granulocytes whose absolute number is nearly doubled at term. The reason for the increased leukocytosis is unclear, but may be caused by the elevated estrogen and cortisol levels. Naccasha et al. showed that substantial phenotypical and metabolic changes occur in WBCs in normal pregnancy, resulting in an "activated leukocyte." These investigators speculated that the change in the baseline characteristics of the WBCs help explain why during pregnancy women experience the development of the systemic inflammatory response or overwhelming sepsis with infections that clinically do not appear to be severe enough to cause such responses (such as with pyelonephritis) when not pregnant.[99] Leukocyte levels return to normal within 1 to 2 weeks of delivery.

The traditional view of the immunologic system in pregnancy is that the fetus is a semi-allograft and a successful pregnancy is dependent on either evasion of immune surveillance or suppression of the maternal adaptive immune response (see Chapter 4).[100] The immune response can be classified as either innate or adaptive. The innate system is the primary defense

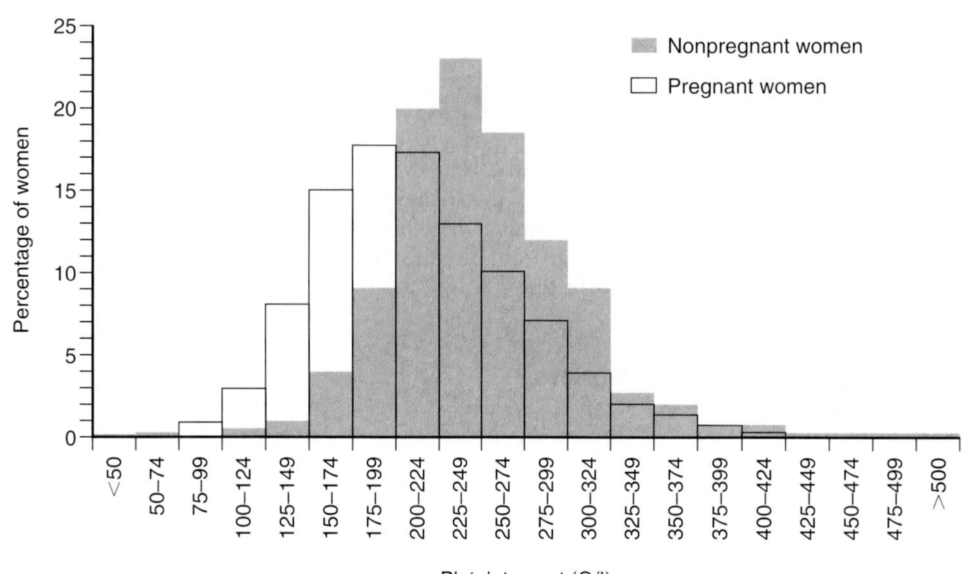

Figure 3-10. Histogram of platelet count of pregnant women in the third trimester (n = 6,770) compared with nonpregnant women (n = 287). (From Boehlen F, Hohlfield P, Extermann P: Platelet count at term pregnancy: a reappraisal of the threshold. Obstet Gynecol 95:29, 2000.)

system and involves granulocytes and phagocytes. The adaptive system is the specific immune recognition system that has memory on repeated exposure. The normal adaptive responses have generally been classified as either cytotoxic (cell destroying or T-helper 1 lymphocytes) or humoral (antibody mediated or T-helper 2 lymphocytes). Although this is a simplistic approach to the immune system, it is helpful in interpreting the changes in immune response in pregnancy. Maternal tolerance appears to be associated with the development of several specific mechanisms that protect the fetus from a maternal cytotoxic immune response.[101] The major change observed is a modulation away from cell-mediated cytotoxic immune responses towards increased humoral and innate immune responses.[100] Such a shift appears to lessen the maternal cytotoxic potential against fetal antigens.[101] Cytotoxic (CD8+) lymphocytes and T-helper cells (CD4+) lymphocytes levels and the CD4+/CD8+ ratio appear to be either unchanged or only insignificantly altered, but natural killer lymphocyte cells (cytotoxic) are decreased 30 percent.[102] Clinically, the decrease in cellular immunity leads to increased susceptibility to intracellular pathogens such as cytomegalovirus virus, herpes simplex virus, varicella, and malaria.[103–105] The decrease in cellular immunity may explain why rheumatoid arthritis frequently improves during gestation, since it is a cell-mediated immunopathologic disease.[106]

In contrast, the humoral immunity characterized by the antibody-mediated immunity, is preserved or even enhanced during gestation. The circulating levels of B-lymphocytes are unchanged, the serum complement level remains normal or is slightly elevated, and the activated lymphocytes produce cytokines that favor antibody production over cytotoxic responses.[1,106–108] However, the level of immunoglobulin G (IgG) decreases and IgM/IgA/IgE levels are unchanged or fall slightly.[102] Clinical examples which demonstrate an intact humoral immunity include appropriate responses to vaccinations, normal IgG stimulation with Staphylococcus aureus, and normal response to PPD testing.[109–111] Therefore, pregnancy is not a state of immunodeficiency but is a state of altered immune functions.[99,106]

The causes of the changes in the pregnant women's immunologic system are complex, but placental hormones appear to play a significant role. Progesterone appears to be the most significant immunoregulatory hormone of pregnancy, but the exact mechanisms by which this hormone mediates its effects are still unclear.[106]

Coagulation System

Pregnancy places women at a 5 to 6 fold increased risk for thromboembolic disease (see Chapter 41). This greater risk is caused by increased venous stasis, vessel wall injury, and changes in the coagulation cascade that lead to hypercoagulability. The overall risk of thromboembolism in pregnancy is estimated to be 1/1,500 and accounts for 25 percent of maternal deaths in the United States.[111,112] In pregnancy, several procoagulant coagulation factors are increased, and changes occur to some of the natural inhibitors of coagulation. In addition, pregnancy causes a decrease in the fibrinolytic system with reduced levels of available circulating plasminogen activator and a two to three-fold increase in plasminogen activator inhibitor (PAI-1).[1] These physiologic changes provide defense against peripartum hemorrhage.

The majority of the procoagulant factors from the coagulation cascade are markedly increased, including factors I, VII, VIII, IX, and X. Factors II, V, and XII are unchanged or mildly increased, and levels of factors XI and XIII decline[1,112,113] (Fig. 3-11). Plasma fibrinogen (factor I) levels begin to increase in the first trimester and peak in the third trimester at levels 50 percent higher than before pregnancy. The rise in fibrinogen is associated with an increase in the erythrocyte sedimentation rate.[114] The prothrombin time, activated partial thromboplastin time, and thrombin time all fall slightly but remain within the limits of normal nonpregnant values, whereas the bleeding time and whole blood clotting times are unchanged. Levels of coagulation factors normalize 2 weeks postpartum.

Pregnancy has been shown to cause a progressive and significant decrease in the levels of total and free protein S from early in pregnancy but to have no effect on the levels of protein C and antithrombin III.[115–117] During gestation, the activated protein C (APC) sensitivity ratio (APC:SR), the ratio of the clotting time in the presence and the absence of APC declines. The APC:SR ratio is considered abnormal if less than 2.6. In a study of 239 women,[115] the APC:SR ratio decreased from a mean of 3.12 in the first trimester to 2.63 by the third trimester. By the third trimester, 38 percent of women were found to have an acquired APC resistance, with APC:SR values below 2.6.[115] Whether the change in the protein S level and the APC:SR ratio are responsible for some of the hypercoagulability of pregnancy is unknown.[118] If a workup for thrombophilias is performed during gestation, the clinician should use caution when attempting to interpret these levels if they are abnormal. Ideally the clinician should order DNA testing for the Leiden mutation instead of testing for APC and a lab value of greater than 45% should be used as normal when measuring free protein S antigen levels during gestation.[117]

During pregnancy, researchers have found evidence to support the theory that a state of low-level intravascular coagulation occurs. Low concentrations of fibrin degradation products (markers of fibrinolysis), elevated levels of fibrinopeptide A (a marker for increased clotting), and increased levels of platelet factor 4 and β-thromboglobulin (markers of increased platelet activity) have been found in maternal blood.[119] The most likely cause for these findings involves localized physiologic changes needed for maintenance of the uterine-placental interface.

URINARY SYSTEM

Anatomic Changes

The kidneys enlarge during pregnancy, with the length as measured by intravenous pyelography increasing about

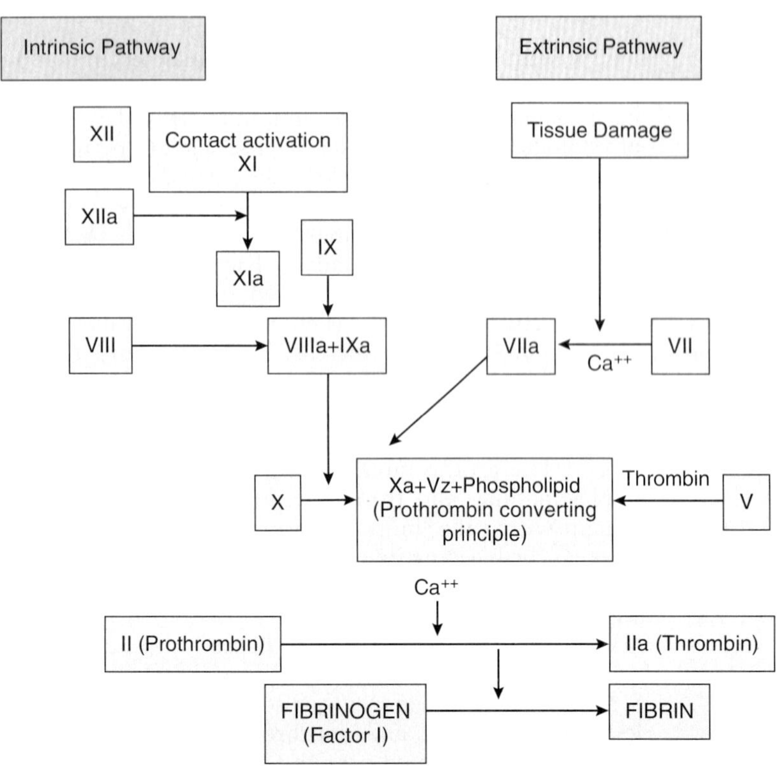

Figure 3-11. The normal components of the coagulation cascade. (From Johnson RL: Thromboembolic disease complicating pregnancy. *In* Foley MR, Strong TH [eds]: Obstetric Intensive Care: A Practical Manual. Philadelphia, WB Saunders Company, 1997, p 91, with permission.)

1 cm. This growth in size and weight is due to increased renal vasculature, interstitial volume, and urinary dead space. The increase in urinary dead space is attributed to dilation of the renal pelvis, calyces, and ureters. Pelvicalyceal dilation by term averages 15 mm (range, 5 to 25 mm) on the right and 5 mm (range, 3 to 8 mm) on the left, with the right greater than the left in most gravid women.[120]

The well-known dilation of the ureters and renal pelves begins by the second month of pregnancy and is maximal by the middle of the second trimester, when ureteric diameter may be as much as 2 cm. The right ureter is almost invariably dilated more than the left, and the dilation usually cannot be demonstrated below the pelvic brim. These findings have led some investigators to argue that the dilation is caused entirely by mechanical compression of the ureters by the enlarging uterus and ovarian venous plexus.[121] However, the early onset of ureteral dilation suggests that smooth muscle relaxation caused by progesterone plays an additional role. Also supporting the role of progesterone is the finding of ureteral dilation in women with renal transplants and pelvic kidneys.[122] By 6 weeks' postpartum, ureteral dilation resolves.[120] A clinical consequence of ureterocalyceal dilatation is an increased incidence of pyelonephritis among gravidas with asymptomatic bacteriuria. In addition, the ureterocalyceal dilatation makes interpretation of urinary radiographs more difficult when evaluating possible urinary tract obstruction or nephrolithiasis.

Anatomic changes are also observed in the bladder. From midpregnancy on, an elevation in the bladder trigone occurs with increased vascular tortuousity throughout the bladder. This can cause an increased incidence of microhematuria. Three percent of gravidas have idiopathic hematuria as defined as greater than 1+ on a urine dipstick, and up to 16 percent have microscopic hematuria.[123] Owing to the increasing size of the fetus and uterus, a decrease in bladder capacity develops, with an increased frequency of urinary incontinence.

Renal Hemodynamics

Renal plasma flow (RPF) increases markedly from early in gestation and may actually initially begin to increase during the luteal phase before implantation.[124] Dunlop showed convincingly that the effective RPF rises 75 percent over nonpregnant levels by 16 weeks' gestation[125] (Table 3-7). The increase is maintained until 34 weeks' gestation, when a decline in RPF of about 25 percent occurs. The fall in RPF has been demonstrated in subjects studied serially in the sitting and the left lateral recumbent positions.[125,126] Like RPF, glomerular filtration rate (GFR) as measured by inulin clearance increases by 5 to 7 weeks. By the end of the first trimester, GFR is 50 percent higher than in the nonpregnant state, and this is maintained until the end of pregnancy. Three months postpartum, GFR values have declined to normal levels.[125,127] Because the RPF increases more than the GFR early in pregnancy, the filtration fraction falls from nonpregnant levels until the late third trimester. At this time, because of the decline in RPF, the filtration fraction returns to preconceptional values of 20 to 21 percent.

Clinically, GFR is not determined by measuring the clearance of infused inulin (inulin is filtered by the glomerulus and is unaffected by the tubules), but rather by measuring endogenous creatinine clearance. This test gives a less precise measure of GFR, because creatinine

Table 3-7. Serial Changes in Renal Hemodynamics

		SEATED POSITION (N = 25)*			LEFT LATERAL RECUMBENT/ POSITION (N = 17)†	
	NONPREGNANT	16 WK	26 WK	36 WK	29 WK	37 WK
Effective renal plasma flow (ml/min)	480 ± 72	840 ± 145	891 ± 279	771 ± 175	748 ± 85	677 ± 82
Glomerular filtration rate (ml/min)	99 ± 18	149 ± 17	152 ± 18	150 ± 32	145 ± 19	138 ± 22
Filtration fraction	0.21	0.18	0.18	0.20	0.19	0.21

*Data from Dunlop W: Serial changes in renal haemodynamics during normal pregnancy. Br J Obstet Gynaecol 88:1, 1981.

†Data from Ezimokhai M, Davison J, Philips P, et al: Nonpostural serial changes in renal function during the third trimester of normal human pregnancy. Br J Obstet Gynaecol 88:465, 1981.

is secreted by the tubules to a variable extent. Therefore, endogenous creatinine clearance is usually higher than the actual GFR. The creatinine clearance in pregnancy is greatly increased to values of 150 to 200 ml/min (normal: 120 ml/min). As with GFR, the increase in creatinine clearance occurs by 5 to 7 weeks' gestation, and normally is maintained until the third trimester.

The increase in the RPF and GFR precede the increase in blood volume and may be induced by a reduction in the pre- and postglomerular arteriolar resistance. Importantly, the increase in hyperfiltration occurs without an increase in glomerular pressure, which if it occurred, could have the potential for injury to a women's kidney with long-term consequences.[124] Recently, the mechanisms underlying the marked increase in RPF and GFR has been carefully studied. Although numerous factors are involved in this process, NO has been demonstrated to play a critical role in the decrease in renal resistance and the subsequent renal hyperemia.[7] During pregnancy, the activation and expression of the NO synthase is enhanced in the kidneys and inhibition of NO synthase isoforms has been shown to attenuate the hemodynamic changes within the gravid kidney.[43,128,129] Finally, the pregnancy hormone relaxin appears to be important by initiating or activating some of the effects of NO within the kidney.[130] Failure of this crucial adaptation to occur is associated with adverse outcomes such as preeclampsia and fetal growth restriction.[7]

The clinical consequences of glomerular hyperfiltration are a reduction in maternal plasma levels of creatinine, blood urea nitrogen (BUN), and uric acid. Serum creatinine falls from a non-pregnant level of 0.8 mg/dl to 0.5 mg/dl by term. Likewise, BUN falls from nonpregnant levels of 13 mg/dl to 9 mg/dl by term.[10] Serum uric acid declines in early pregnancy because of the rise in GFR, reaching a nadir by 24 weeks with levels of 2.0 to 3.0 mg/dl.[131] After 24 weeks, the uric acid level begins to rise, and by the end of pregnancy the levels in most women are essentially the same as before conception. The rise in uric acid levels is caused by increased renal tubular absorption of urate and increased fetal uric acid production. Patients with preeclampsia have elevated uric acid level concentrations; however, because uric acid levels normally rise during the third trimester, overreliance on this test should be avoided in the diagnosis and management of preeclampsia.[131]

During pregnancy, nocturia is more common. In the standing position, sodium and water are retained and, therefore, during the daytime, pregnant women tend to retain an increased amount of water.[132] At night, while in the lateral recumbent position, this added water is excreted, resulting in nocturia.

Renal Tubular Function/Excretion of Nutrients

Despite high levels of aldosterone, which would be expected to result in enhanced urinary excretion of potassium, gravid women retain about 350 mmol of potassium. The majority of the excess potassium is stored in the fetus and placenta. The mean potassium concentrations in maternal blood are just slightly below nonpregnant levels. The kidney's ability to conserve potassium has been attributed to increased progesterone levels.[133] For information on the physiologic changes of sodium in pregnancy, see the section on body water metabolism earlier in this chapter.

Glucose excretion increases in almost all pregnant women, and glycosuria is common. Nonpregnant urinary excretion of glucose is less than 100 mg/day, but 90 percent of gravidas with normal blood glucose levels excrete 1 to 10 g of glucose per day.[134] This glycosuria is intermittent and not necessarily related to blood glucose levels or the stage of gestation. Glucose is freely filtered by the glomerulus, and with the 50 percent increase in GFR, a greater load of glucose is presented to the proximal tubules. There may be a change in the reabsorptive capability of the proximal tubules themselves, but the old concept of pregnancy leading to an overwhelming of the maximum tubular reabsorptive capacity for glucose is misleading and oversimplified.[134,135] The exact mechanisms underlying the altered handling of glucose by the proximal tubules remains obscure. Even though glycosuria is common, gravid women with repetitive glycosuria should be screened for diabetes mellitus if not already tested.

No increase in proteinuria occurs during a normal pregnancy in women without proteinuria before pregnancy. Higby et al.[136] collected 24-hour urine samples on 270 women over the course of pregnancy and determined the amount of proteinuria and albuminuria. These inves-

Table 3-8. Comparison of 24-Hour Urinary Volume Protein and Albumin Excretion for Each Trimester of Pregnancy

	FIRST TRIMESTER (N = 19)	SECOND TRIMESTER (N = 133)	THIRD TRIMESTER (N = 118)	SIGNIFICANCE
Protein (mg/24 h)	80.0 ± 60.6	116.7 ± 69.3	115.3 ± 69.2	p = 0.13
Albumin (mg/24 h)	9.9 ± 5.3	10.8 ± 6.9	12.8 ± 9.5	p = 0.12

Values are expressed as mean ± SD.

From Higby K, Suiter C, Phelps J, et al: Normal values of urinary albumin and total protein excretion during pregnancy. Am J Obstet Gynecol 171:984, 1994.

tigators found that the amount of protein and albumin excreted in urine did not increase significantly by trimester (Table 3-8). They observed that in women without preeclampsia, underlying renal disease, or urinary tract infections, the mean 24-hour urine protein across pregnancy is 116.9 mg, with a 95-percent upper confidence limit of 259.4 mg. They also noted that patients do not normally have microalbuminuria, defined as urinary albumin excretion greater than 30 mg/dl.[136] In women with preexisting proteinuria, the amount of proteinuria increases in both the second and third trimesters, and potentially in the first trimester. In a study of women with diabetic nephropathy, the amount of proteinuria increased from a mean of 1.74 ± 1.33 g/24 h in the first trimester to a mean of 4.82 ± 4.7 g/24 h in the third trimester even in the absence of preeclampsia.[137]

Other changes in tubular function include an increase in the excretion of amino acids in the urine[138] and an increase in calcium excretion (see Calcium Metabolism, later). Also, the kidney responds to the respiratory alkalosis of pregnancy by enhanced excretion of bicarbonate; however, renal handling of acid excretion is unchanged.[139]

ALIMENTARY TRACT

Appetite

Most women experience an increase in appetite throughout pregnancy. In the absence of nausea or "morning sickness," women eating according to appetite will increase food intake by about 200 kcal/day by the end of the first trimester.[140] The recommended dietary allowance calls for an additional 300 kcal/day, although in reality most women make up for this with decreased activity. Energy requirements vary depending on the population studied, and a greater increase may be necessary for pregnant teenagers and women with high levels of physical activity.[141] Extensive folklore exists about dietary cravings and aversions during gestation. Many of these are undoubtedly due to an individual's perception of which foods aggravate or ameliorate such symptoms as nausea and heartburn. The sense of taste may be blunted in some women, leading to an increased desire for highly seasoned food. Pica, a bizarre craving for strange foods, is relatively common among gravid women, and a history of pica should be sought in those with poor weight gain or refractory anemia. Examples of pica include the consumption of clay, starch, toothpaste, and ice.

Mouth

The pH and the production of saliva is probably unchanged during pregnancy.[142] Ptyalism, an unusual complication of pregnancy, most often occurs in women suffering from nausea and may be associated with the loss of 1 to 2 L of saliva per day. Most authorities believe ptyalism actually represents inability of the nauseated woman to swallow normal amounts of saliva rather than a true increase in the production of saliva. A decrease in the ingestion of starchy foods may help decrease the amount of saliva. No evidence exists that pregnancy causes or accelerates the course of dental caries. However, the gums (gingiva) swell and may bleed after tooth brushing, giving rise to the so-called gingivitis of pregnancy.[143] At times, a tumorous gingivitis may occur, presenting as a violaceous pedunculated lesion at the gum line that may bleed profusely.[144] Called either epulis gravidarum or pyogenic granulomas, these lesions consist of granulation tissue and an inflammatory infiltrate (see Chapter 46).

Stomach

The tone and motility of the stomach are decreased during pregnancy, probably because of the smooth muscle–relaxing effects of progesterone and estrogen.[145] Nevertheless, scientific evidence regarding delayed gastric emptying is inconclusive.[146] Davison et al.[147] showed that the mean total emptying time was significantly longer in pregnant women with heartburn versus control women. However, no clear evidence of a delay in emptying was found in gravidas without heartburn. More recently, Macfie and colleagues,[146] using acetaminophen absorption as an indirect measure of gastric emptying, failed to demonstrate a delay in gastric emptying when comparing 15 nonpregnant controls with 15 women in each trimester.[146] However, an increased delay is seen in labor with the etiology ascribed to the pain and stress of labor.[147]

Pregnancy causes a decreased risk of peptic ulcer disease, but at the same time, causes an increase in gastroesophageal reflux disease and dyspepsia in 30 to 50 percent of individuals.[148] This apparent paradox can be partially explained by physiologic changes of the stomach and lower esophagus. The increase in gastroesophageal reflux disease is attributed to esophageal dysmotility caused by gestational hormones and gastric compression from the enlarged uterus. In addition, the decrease in the tone of the gastroesophageal sphincter may lead to increased reflux of stomach acids into the esophagus. Theories proposed to explain the decreased incidence of peptic ulcer disease include increased placental histaminase synthesis with lower maternal histamine levels; increased gastric mucin production leading to protection of the gastric mucosa; reduced gastric acid secretion; and enhanced immunologic tolerance of *Helicobacter pylori,* the infectious agent that causes peptic ulcer disease[148] (see Chapter 43).

Intestines

Perturbations in the motility of the small intestines and colon are common in pregnancy, resulting in an increased incidence of constipation (11 to 38 percent) in some and diarrhea in others. Up to 34 percent of women in one study noted an increased frequency of bowel movements, perhaps related to increased prostaglandin synthesis.[149,150] The motility of the small intestines is reduced in pregnancy, with increased oral-cecal transit times.[151] No studies on the colonic transit time have been performed, but limited information suggests reduced colonic motility.[150] Although progesterone has been thought to be the primary cause of the decrease in gastrointestinal motility, newer studies show the actual etiology may be due to estrogen. Estrogen causes an increased release of NO from nerves that innervate the gastrointestinal tract which then results in relaxation of the gastrointestinal tract musculature.[145] Absorption of nutrients from the small bowel (with the exception of increased iron and calcium absorption) is unchanged, but the decreased transit time allows for more efficient absorption. In the colon, Parry et al.[152] demonstrated an increase in both water and sodium absorption.

The enlarging uterus displaces the intestines and, most importantly, moves the position of the appendix. Thus, the presentation, physical signs, and type of surgical incision are affected in the management of appendicitis. Portal venous pressure is increased, leading to dilation wherever there is portosystemic venous anastomosis. This includes the gastroesophageal junction and the hemorrhoidal veins, which results in the common complaint of hemorrhoids.

Gallbladder

The function of the gallbladder is markedly altered because of the effects of progesterone. After the first trimester, the fasting and residual volumes are twice as great, and the rate at which the gallbladder empties is much slower.[154] In addition, the biliary cholesterol saturation is increased, and the chenodeoxycholic acid level is decreased.[155] This change in the composition of the bile fluid favors the formation of cholesterol crystals, and with incomplete emptying of the gallbladder, the crystals are retained and gallstone formation is enhanced.

Liver

The size and histology of the liver are unchanged in pregnancy.[156] However, many clinical and laboratory signs usually associated with liver disease are present. Spider angiomas and palmar erythema, caused by elevated estrogen levels, are normal and disappear soon after delivery. The serum albumin and total protein levels fall progressively during gestation. By term, albumin levels are 25 percent lower than nonpregnant levels. Despite an overall increase in total body protein, decreases in total protein and albumin concentrations occur as a result of hemodilution. In addition, serum alkaline phosphatase activity rises during the third trimester to levels two to four times that of nongravid women. Most of this increase is caused by placental production of the heat-stable isoenzyme.[1,157] During pregnancy, the serum concentrations of many proteins produced by the liver increase. These include elevations in fibrinogen, ceruloplasmin, and transferrin, and the binding proteins for corticosteroids, sex steroids, thyroid hormones, and vitamin D.[1]

With the exception of alkaline phosphatase, the other "liver function tests" are unaffected by pregnancy, including serum levels of bilirubin, aspartate aminotransferase (AST), alanine aminotransferase (ALT), γ-glutamyltransferase, 5′-nucleotidase, creatinine phosphokinase, and lactate dehydrogenase. In some studies, the mean levels of ALT and AST are mildly elevated but still within normal values.[157,158] Levels of creatinine phosphokinase and lactate dehydrogenase can increase with labor. Finally, pregnancy may cause some changes in bile acid production and secretion. Pregnancy may be associated with mild subclinical cholestasis owing to the high concentrations of estrogen. Reports on serum bile acid concentrations are conflicting, with some studies showing an increase and others no change. The fasting levels are unchanged, and the measurement of a fasting level appears to be the best test for diagnosing cholestasis of pregnancy.[158] Cholestasis of pregnancy results from elevated levels of bile acids and is associated with significant maternal pruritus, usually mild increases of ALT/AST, and an increased risk of poor fetal outcomes.[159] Recently, the extent of genetic variation in 2 different glycoproteins (BSEP and *MDR3*) was studied in a large group of unrelated white women with cholestasis and compared with the extent of genetic variation in healthy pregnant control women. In this group, 47 percent of women with cholestasis had abnormally elevated liver function tests and 77 percent of these patients carried ICP-specific *MDR3* mutations, including three newly detected splicing consensus mutations (intron 21: G(+1)A, intron 25: G(+5)C and C(−3)G) and two nonsynonmous variants in highly conserved regions of the protein (S320F and G762E).[159a]

Nausea and Vomiting of Pregnancy

Nausea and vomiting, or "morning sickness," complicate up to 70 percent of pregnancies. Typical onset is between 4 and 8 weeks' gestation, with improvement before 16 weeks; however, 10 to 25 percent of women still experience symptoms at 20 to 22 weeks' gestation and some women experience this throughout the gestation.[160] Although the symptoms are often distressing, simple morning sickness seldom leads to significant weight loss, ketonemia, or electrolyte disturbances. The cause is not well understood, although relaxation of the smooth muscle of the stomach probably plays a role. Elevated levels of human chorionic gonadotropin (hCG) may be involved, although a good correlation between maternal hCG concentrations and the degree of nausea and vomiting has not been observed.[161] Similarly, minimal data exist to show the etiology is due to higher levels of estrogen or progesterone. Interestingly, pregnancies complicated by nausea and vomiting generally have a more favorable outcome than do those without such symptoms.[160] Treatment is largely supportive, consisting of reassurance, avoidance of foods found to trigger nausea, and frequent small meals. Eating dry toast or crackers before getting out of bed may be beneficial. Recently, the American College of Obstetricians and Gynecologists (ACOG) stated that the use of either vitamin B_6 alone or in combination with doxylamine (Unisom) is safe and effective, and should be considered a first line of medical treatment.[162] A recent review of alternative therapies to antiemetic drugs found that acupressure, wristbands, or treatment with ginger root may be helpful[163] (see Chapter 8).

Hyperemesis gravidarum is a more pernicious form of nausea and vomiting associated with weight loss, ketonemia, electrolyte imbalance, and dehydration. It occurs in 1 to 3 percent of women with persistence often throughout pregnancy and rarely can result in significant complications, including Wernicke's encephalopathy, rhabdomyolysis, acute renal failure, and esophageal rupture.[164] For these patients, the clinician must rule out other diseases such as pancreatitis, cholecystitis, hepatitis, psychiatric disease, and thyroid disease. Hospitalization with intravenous replacement of fluids and electrolytes is often needed. Options of antiemetics include the phenothiazines: promethazine (Phenergan), chlorpromazine (Thorazine), and prochlorperazine (Compazine) or metoclopramide (Reglan), or ondansetron (Zofran). On admission to the hospital, the patient should be given intravenous hydration, and tried on one of the above-mentioned medications (intravenously or intramuscularly initially). Care must be given not to combine the phenothiazines with metoclopramide because of the additive risks of causing extrapyramidal reactions. Chlorpromazine given rectally (25 to 50 mg every 8 hours) may be highly effective in the more refractory cases. Recently, use of oral methylprednisolone, 16 mg three times daily for 3 days and then tapered over 2 weeks, has been shown to be more effective than promethazine,[165] but multiple subsequent studies failed to demonstrate benefit from the use of steroids.[164,166] Unfortunately, no single therapy works in all women, and occasionally, multiple different medications must be tried before finding the one that is effective. Because of potential risks, parenteral caloric replacement should only be used after failure of multiple antiemetic treatments and attempts at enteral tube feedings.[167]

THE SKELETON

Calcium Metabolism

Pregnancy was initially thought to be a state of "physiologic hyperparathyroidism" with maternal skeletal calcium loss needed to supply the fetus with calcium. It was thought that this could result in long-term maternal bone loss. It is now evident that the majority of fetal calcium needs are met through a series of physiologic changes in calcium metabolism without long-term consequences to the maternal skeleton (see later).[168] This allows the fetus to accumulate 21 g (range, 13 to 33) of calcium, 80 percent of this amount during the third trimester, when fetal skeletal mineralization is at its peak.[169,170] Calcium is actively transported across the placenta. Surprisingly, calcium is excreted in greater amounts by the maternal kidneys, so that by term, calciuria is doubled.[171]

Maternal total calcium levels decline throughout pregnancy. The fall in total calcium is caused by the reduced serum albumin levels that result in a decrease in the albumin-bound fraction of calcium. However, the physiologically important fraction, serum ionized calcium, is unchanged and constant[168,172] (Fig. 3-12). Therefore, the maternal serum calcium levels are maintained and the fetal calcium needs are met mainly through increased intestinal calcium absorption. Calcium is absorbed through the small intestines, and its absorption is doubled by 12 weeks' gestation.[168,173,174] The early increase in absorption may allow the maternal skeleton to store calcium in advance of the peak third-trimester fetal demands. Although the majority of the fetal calcium needs are met by increased absorption of calcium, accumulating data confirm that at least some calcium resorption from maternal bone occurs to help meet the increased fetal demands in the third trimester.[175] These data are compatible with the hypothesis that physiologic mechanisms exist to ensure an adequate supply of calcium for fetal growth and milk production without sole reliance on the maternal diet.[174] Maternal serum phosphate levels are likewise unchanged.[168]

Older studies showed an increase in maternal parathyroid hormone (PTH) levels.[176] These studies used less sensitive PTH assays that measured multiple different fragments of PTH, most of which are biologically inactive. In five recent prospective studies, all using newer assays, maternal levels of PTH are not elevated and actually remain in the low-normal range throughout gestation.[168] Therefore, pregnancy is not associated with relative hyperparathyroidism (see Chapter 38). Although, levels of 1,25-dihydroxyvitamin D do increase, doubling in the first trimester, this increase is secondary to increased production by the maternal kidneys and potentially the fetoplacental unit, and is independent of PTH control.[171] The increase in 1,25-dihydroxyvitamin

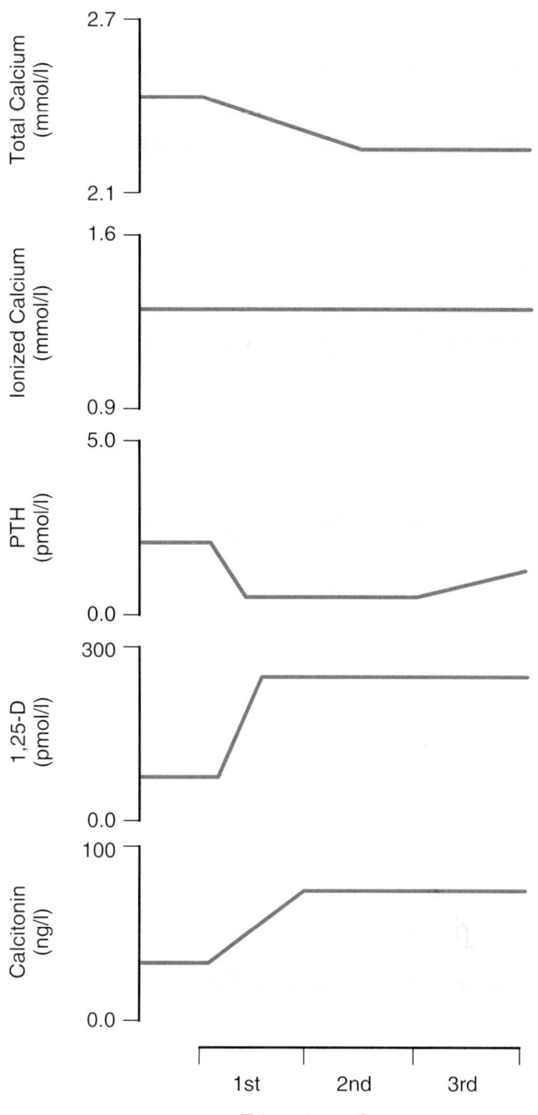

Figure 3-12. The longitudinal changes in calcium and calcitropic hormone levels that occur during human pregnancy. Normal adult ranges are indicated by the shaded areas. (From Kovacs C, Kronenberg H: Maternal-fetal calcium and bone metabolism during pregnancy, puerperium, and lactation. Endocr Rev 18:832, 1997, with permission, page 834.)

D is directly responsible for the increase in intestinal calcium absorption.[168] Calcitonin levels also rise by 20 percent and may help protect the maternal skeleton from excess bone loss.[168,177]

Skeletal and Postural Changes

The effect of pregnancy on bone metabolism is complex, and evidence of maternal bone loss during pregnancy has been inconsistent, with various studies reporting bone loss, no change, and even gain. Whether pregnancy causes bone loss is not the important question; instead, the critical question is whether pregnancy and lactation have a long-term risk of causing osteoporosis later in life.[175,178] In a recent review of 23 studies, Ensom et al.[175] concluded that pregnancy is a period of high bone turnover and remodeling. Both pregnancy and lactation cause reversible bone loss, and this loss is increased in women who breast-feed for longer intervals. Studies do not support an association between parity and osteoporosis later in life. Additionally in a comparison of female twins discordant for parity, pregnancy and lactation were found to have no detrimental effect on long-term bone loss.[179]

Bone turnover appears to be low in the first half of gestation and then increase in the third trimester, corresponding to the peak rate of fetal calcium needs, and may represent turnover of previously stored skeletal calcium.[168] Markers of both bone resorption (hydroxyproline and tartate-resistant acid phosphatase) and bone formation (alkaline phosphatase and procollagen peptides) are increased during gestation.[174] In the only study of bone biopsies performed in pregnancy, Shahtaheri et al. observed a change in the microarchitectural pattern of bone, but no change in overall bone mass was found. This change in the microarchitectural pattern seems to result in a framework more resistant to the bending forces and biomechanical stresses needed to carry a growing fetus.[180] In support of this study, multiple recent studies have shown bone loss occurs only in the trabecular bone and not cortical bone. Promislow et al. measured bone mineral density twice during pregnancies using dual energy x-ray absorptiometry and showed the mean loss of trabecular bone was 1.9 percent per 20 weeks' gestation. However, women placed on bed rest had significantly greater bone loss. In comparison, the mean bone loss in postmenopausal women rarely exceeds 2 percent per year.[178] Older studies indicate that the cortical bone thickness of long bones may even increase with pregnancy.[181]

Although bone loss occurs in pregnancy, the occurrence of osteoporosis during or soon after pregnancy is rare.[175,181] Whether additional calcium intake during pregnancy and lactation prevents bone loss is controversial. The majority of the present studies indicate that calcium supplementation does not decrease the amount of bone loss, but Promislow et al.[178] found that maternal intake of 2 g per day or greater was modestly protective. This is greater than the 1,000 mg/day recommended dietary allowance or the National Institutes of Health consensus panel recommendation of 1,200 to 1,500 mg/day during pregnancy and lactation.[174,178]

Pregnancy results in a progressively increasing anterior convexity of the lumbar spine (lordosis). This compensatory mechanism keeps the woman's center of gravity over her legs, and prevents the enlarging uterus from shifting the center of gravity anteriorly. The unfortunate side effect of this necessary alteration is low back pain, a common complaint during gestation. The ligaments of the pubic symphysis and sacroiliac joints loosen during pregnancy, probably from the effects of the hormone relaxin, the levels of which increase 10-fold in pregnancy.[182] Marked widening of the pubic symphysis occurs by 28 to 32 weeks' gestation, with the width increasing from 3 to 4 mm in 7.7 to 7.9 mm.[183] This commonly results in pain near the symphysis that is referred down the inner thigh with standing and may result in a maternal sensation of snapping or movement of the bones with walking.

ENDOCRINE CHANGES

Thyroid

Thyroid diseases are common in women of childbearing age (see Chapter 38). However, normal pregnancy symptoms mirror those of thyroid disease, making it difficult to know when screening for thyroid disease is appropriate. In addition, the physiologic effects of pregnancy frequently make the interpretation of thyroid tests difficult. Therefore, it is important for the obstetrician to be familiar with the normal changes in thyroid function that occur during pregnancy.[184] Recent data have shown that the correct and timely diagnosis and treatment of thyroid disease is important to prevent both maternal and fetal complications.

Despite alterations in thyroid morphology, histology and laboratory indices, pregnant women remain euthyroid. The thyroid gland increases in size, but not as much as was commonly believed. If adequate iodine intake is maintained, the size of the thyroid gland remains unchanged or undergoes a small increase in size that can be detected only by ultrasound.[185,186] In pregnancy, the World Health Organization recommends that iodine intake be increased from 100 to 150 μg/day to 200 μg/day. In an iodine-deficient state, the thyroid gland is up to 25 percent larger, and goiters may be seen in 10 percent of women.[187] Histologically, during pregnancy an increase in thyroid vascularity occurs with evidence of follicular hyperplasia. The development of a clinically apparent goiter during pregnancy is abnormal and should be evaluated.[188]

During pregnancy, serum iodide levels fall because of increased renal loss. In addition, in the latter half of pregnancy, iodine is also transferred to the fetus, further decreasing maternal levels.[187] However, at least one investigator has reported that in iodine-sufficient regions, the concentration of iodide does not decrease.[189] These alterations cause the thyroid to synthesize and secrete thyroid hormone actively.[187] Although there is increased uptake of iodine by the thyroid, pregnant women remain euthyroid by laboratory evaluation.[190]

Total thyroxine (TT_4) and total triiodothyronine (TT_3) levels begin to increase in the first trimester and peak at midgestation as a result of increased production of thyroid-binding globulin (TBG). The increase in TBG is seen in the first trimester and plateaus at 12 to 14 weeks. The concentration of TT_4 increases in parallel from a normal range of 5 to 12 μg/dl in nonpregnant women to 9 to 16 μg/dl during pregnancy. Only a small amount of TT_4 and TT_3 is unbound, but these free fractions (normally about 0.04 percent for T_4 and 0.5 percent for T_3) are the major determinants of whether an individual is euthyroid. The extent of change in free T_4 and T_3 levels during pregnancy have been controversial, and the discrepancies in past studies have been attributed to the techniques used to measure the free hormone levels.[184] The current best evidence is that the free T_4 levels rise slightly in the first trimester and then decrease so that by delivery, the free T_4 levels are 10 to 15 percent lower than in nonpregnant women. However, these changes are small, and in most pregnant women, free T_4 concentrations remain within the normal nonpregnant range[187,191,192] (Fig. 3-13). Recently Biggio et al.[193] reported that when using newer enzyme immunoassays to measure free T_4 in the second and third trimester, maternal values are more significantly decreased than previously reported, and the mean value was just below the normal range. Free T_3 levels follow a similar pattern.

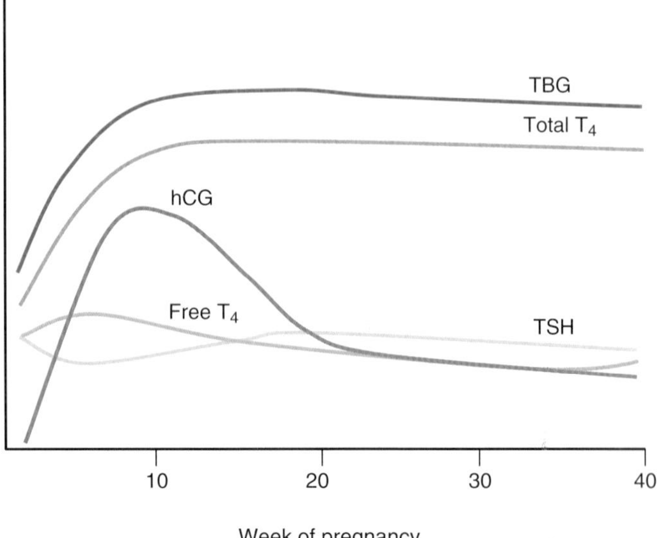

Figure 3-13. Relative changes in maternal thyroid function during pregnancy. (From Burrow G, Fisher D, Larsen P: Maternal and fetal thyroid function. N Engl J Med 331:1072, 1994, page 1072, with permission.)

Thyroid-stimulating hormone (TSH) concentrations decrease transiently in the first trimester and then rise to prepregnant levels by the end of this trimester. TSH levels then remain stable throughout the remainder of gestation.[187,191,192] The transient decrease in TSH coincides with the first-trimester increase in free T_4 levels, and both appear to be caused by the thyrotropic effects of hCG. Women with higher peak hCG levels have more TSH suppression. TSH and hCG are structurally very similar, and they share a common α-subunit and have a similar β-unit. Glinoer et al. estimated that a 10,000 IU/L increment in circulating hCG corresponds to a mean free T_4 increment of 0.6 *p*mol/L (0.1 ng/dL) and, in turn, lowers TSH by 0.1 mIU/L.[187,194] Glinoer et al. measured TSH levels during successive trimesters of pregnancy in a large group of women and found that TSH was suppressed below normal in 18 percent in the first trimester, 5 percent during the second trimester, and 2 percent in the third trimester. In the first two trimesters, the mean hCG level was higher in women with suppressed TSH levels.[194] It clearly appears that hCG has some thyrotropic activity, but conflicting data on the exact role of hCG in maternal thyroid function remain.[187,191,192,195]

The influence of maternal thyroid physiology on the fetus appears much more complex than was previously thought. Whereas the maternal thyroid does not directly control fetal thyroid function, the systems interact by means of the placenta, which regulates the transfer of iodine and a small but important amount of thyroxine to the fetus. It was previously thought that little if any transplacental passage of T_4 and T_3 occurred.[196] It is now recognized that T_4 crosses the placenta and, in fact, in early pregnancy, the fetus is critically dependent on the maternal T_4 supply for normal neurologic development.[197,198] However, as a result of the deiodinase activity of the placenta, a large percentage of T_4 is broken down before transfer to the fetus. The human fetus cannot synthesize thyroid hormones until after 12 weeks' gestation, and any fetal requirement before this time is totally dependent on maternal transfer. Even after the fetal thyroid is functional, the fetus continues to rely to some extent on a maternal supply of thyroxine.[199]

Neonates with thyroid agenesis or a total defect in thyroid hormone synthesis have umbilical cord thyroxine levels between 20 percent and 50 percent of those in normal infants, demonstrating that the placenta is not impermeable to T_4.[200] Further evidence that the fetus is dependent on the maternal thyroid for normal development has recently been published. In women living in iodine-deficient areas, maternal hypothyroidism is associated with neonatal hypothyroidism and defects in long-term neurologic function and mental retardation termed "endemic cretinism." These abnormalities can be prevented if maternal iodine intake is initiated at the beginning of the second trimester.[201,202] Haddow et al.[203] have found that maternal hypothyroidism during pregnancy results in slightly lower IQ scores in children tested at ages 7 to 9. These findings have resulted in controversy over whether all pregnant women should be screened for subclinical hypothyroidism, which occurs in 2 to 5 percent of pregnancies. Position statements from various organizations are currently contradictory. The Endocrine Society recommends universal screening. Currently, ACOG is opposed to this screening in asymptomatic women without a personal history of thyroid disease. In 2004, two separate national meetings in the United States concurred with ACOG that insufficient data are present to recommend such screening.[198] As described earlier, screening in the first trimester will result in an 18-percent screen positive rate, and potential unnecessary treatment. Like T_4, thyrotropin-releasing hormone crosses the placenta, TSH does not.

Because iodine is actively transported across the placenta and the concentration of iodide in the fetal blood is 75 percent that of the maternal blood, the fetus is susceptible to iodine-induced goiters when the mother is given pharmacologic amounts of iodine. Similarly, radioactive iodine crosses the placenta and, if given after 12 weeks' gestation when the fetal thyroid is able to concentrate iodine, profound adverse effects can occur.[190] These include fetal hypothyroidism, mental retardation, attention deficit disorder, and a 1 to 2 percent increase in the lifetime cancer risk.[204]

Adrenal Glands

Pregnancy is associated with marked changes in adrenocortical function, with increased serum levels of aldosterone, deoxycorticosterone, corticosteroid-binding globulin (CBG), cortisol, and free cortisol[205–207] (Table 3-9) (see Chapter 39). Although the combined weight of the adrenal glands does not increase significantly, expansion of the zona fasciculata, which primarily produces glucocorticoids, is observed. The plasma concentration of CBG doubles by the end of the sixth month of gestation when compared with nonpregnant values resulting in elevated levels of total plasma cortisol.[208] The levels of total cortisol rise after the first trimester, and by the end of pregnancy, are nearly three times higher than nonpregnant values (12.5 ± 1.3 μg/dl versus 30.1 ± 6.6 μg/dl).[205] During pregnancy, the diurnal variations in cortisol levels are maintained, with the highest values in the morning.

Only free cortisol, the fraction of cortisol not bound to CBG, is metabolically active, but direct measurements are difficult to perform. However, urinary free cortisol concentrations, the free cortisol index, and salivary cortisol concentrations, all of which reflect active free cortisol levels, are elevated after the first trimester.[205,207,209] In a study of 21 uncomplicated pregnancies, Goland et al.[207] found that the urinary free cortisol concentration doubled from the first to the third trimester (Table 3-9). Although the increase in total cortisol concentrations can be explained by the increase in CBG, this does not explain the higher free cortisol levels.

The elevation in free cortisol levels seems to be caused in part, by a marked increase in corticotropin-releasing hormone (CRH) during pregnancy, which, in turn, stimulates the production of adrenocorticotropic hormone (ACTH) in the pituitary. CRH is produced by the placenta and fetal membranes, and is secreted into the maternal circulation. First-trimester values of CRH are similar to prepregnant levels, followed by an exponential rise in CRH during the third trimester[207] (Table 3-9). Goland

Table 3-9. Sequential Measurements of Plasma CRH, ACTH, Cortisol, Aldosterone, and Urinary Free Cortisol During Pregnancy

WEEKS OF GESTATION	CRH (PG/mL)	ACTH (PG/mL)	CORTISOL (MG/DL)	DHEAS (MG/DL)	ALDOSTERONE (PG/mL)	URINARY FREE CORTISOL (MG/24 H)
11–15	115 ± 45	8.8 ± 2.8	10.5 ± 1.4	102 ± 14	412 ± 63.6	54.8 ± 7.3
21–25	145 ± 30	9.8 ± 1.5	20.0 ± 1.1*	85.1 ± 9.0	487 ± 42.8	84.4 ± 8.4
31–35	1,570 ± 349*	12.1 ± 2.0	22.0 ± 1.2*	62.6 ± 6.8*	766 ± 94	105 ± 8.8*
36–40	4,346 ± 754*	18.6 ± 2.6*	26.0 ± 1.1*	63.8 ± 7.1*	1,150 ± 170*	111 ± 8.7*

ACTH, adrenocorticotropic hormone; CRH, corticotropin-releasing hormone; DHEAS, dehydroepiandrosterone sulfate.
*$p < 0.05$ compared with mean hormone levels at weeks 11 to 15 of pregnancy.
From Goland R, Jozak S, Conwell I: Placental corticotropin-releasing hormone and the hypercortisolism of pregnancy. Am J Obstet Gynecol 171:1287, 1994.

et al. have shown that CRH and ACTH concentrations continue to rise in the third trimester despite the increased levels of total and free cortisol levels, supporting the theory that an increase in CRH drives the increased levels of cortisol seen in pregnancy. Furthermore, significant correlation is observed between the rise in CRH levels and maternal ACTH and urinary free cortisol concentrations.[207,210] Other possible causes for the hypercortisolism of pregnancy include delayed plasma clearance of cortisol as a result of changes in renal clearance and a resetting of the hypothalamic-pituitary sensitivity to cortisol feedback on ACTH production.[205] Although the levels of cortisol are increased to concentrations observed in women who have Cushing's syndrome, little clinical evidence is present for hypercortisolism during pregnancy with the exception of weight gain, striae, and tiredness.[211] In addition, Helal et al.[212] showed that during gestation women have a normal response to a low-dose ACTH stimulation testing and that with maternal steroid administration this testing is suppressed. Both are consistent with an intact pituitary-adrenal axis.

Deoxycorticosterone (DOC), like aldosterone, is a potent mineralocorticoid. Marked elevations in the maternal concentrations of DOC are present by midgestation, reaching peak levels in the third trimester. In contrast to the nonpregnant state, plasma DOC levels in the third trimester do not respond to ACTH stimulation, dexamethasone suppression, or salt intake.[206] These findings suggest that an autonomous source of DOC, specifically the fetoplacental unit, may be responsible for the increased levels. Dehydroepiandrosterone sulfate levels are decreased in gestation because of a marked rise in the metabolic clearance of this adrenal androgenic steroid. Most studies have found a modest decline in circulating levels of dehydroepiandrosterone as well. Maternal concentrations of testosterone and androstenedione are slightly higher; testosterone is increased because of an elevation in sex hormone-binding protein, and androstenedione is increased because of an increase in its synthesis.[213]

Pituitary Gland

The pituitary gland enlarges in pregnancy, principally because of proliferation of prolactin-producing cells in the anterior pituitary (see Chapter 39). Gonzalez et al.[214] recently demonstrated that the mean pituitary volume increased by 36 percent at term. The enlargement of the pituitary makes it more susceptible to alterations in blood supply and increases the risk of postpartum infarction (Sheehan's syndrome) should a large maternal blood loss occur.

Pituitary hormone levels are significantly affected by pregnancy. Serum prolactin levels begin to rise at 5 to 8 weeks' gestation and by term are 10 times higher.[215] Consistent with this, the number of lactotroph (prolactin-producing) cells increases dramatically within the anterior lobe of the pituitary from 20 percent of the cells in nongravid women to 60 percent in the third trimester. Despite the increase, prolactin levels remain suppressible by bromocriptine therapy.[216] The principal function of prolactin in pregnancy is to prepare the breast for lactation. In nonlactating women, the prolactin levels return to normal by 3 months' postpartum. In lactating women, the return to baseline levels takes several months with intermittent episodes of hyperprolactinemia in conjunction with nursing.[217] Maternal follicle-stimulating hormone and luteinizing hormone are decreased to undetectable levels as a result of feedback inhibition from the elevated levels of estrogen, progesterone, and inhibin.[216] Maternal growth hormone levels are also suppressed because of the action of placental growth hormone variant on the hypothalamus and pituitary.[216]

PANCREAS AND FUEL METABOLISM

Glucose

Pregnancy is associated with significant physiologic changes in carbohydrate metabolism. This allows for the continuous transport of energy, in the form of glucose, from the gravid woman to the developing fetus and placenta. Pregnancy taxes maternal insulin and carbohydrate physiology, and in all pregnancies, some deterioration in glucose tolerance occurs. In most, only mild changes take place, whereas in others pregnancy is diabetogenic, with the impairment in glucose metabolism significant enough to result in gestational diabetes mellitus (see Chapter 37). Overall, pregnancy results in fasting hypoglycemia, postprandial hyperglycemia, and hyperinsulinemia.[218,219] To accommodate the increased demand for insulin, hypertrophy and hyperplasia of the β cells (insulin producing) occurs within the islets of Langerhans in the maternal pancreas.[154]

Early in pregnancy, glucose homeostasis is affected by increased insulin release that appears to be caused by increased estrogen stimulation of the β cells. During the first trimester, normal insulin sensitivity is maintained, and this causes a 10-percent lowering of glucose levels because of the heightened peripheral muscle glucose utilization. Because insulin is lipogenic, the increased insulin levels favor enhanced lipogenesis, with storage of fat apparently in preparation for the rise in energy needs later in gestation.[220]

With the accelerated growth of the fetus, changes in maternal maintenance of the fasting state and insulin sensitivity take place. During pregnancy, maternal fasting is characterized by accelerated starvation. The fasting blood glucose level after a 12- to 14-hour fast is 10 mg/dl lower than that observed in a nongravid individual.[221,222] This exaggerated response to fasting is largely a result of the constant drain of maternal glucose by the fetoplacental unit. In the third trimester, glucose uptake by the fetus has been estimated to be approximately 6.0 mg/kg/min.[223] This results in a more rapid conversion from predominantly carbohydrate to predominantly fat utilization because of earlier depletion of liver glycogen stores. In addition, the fetus also withdraws amino acids from the maternal circulation and limits the availability of gluconeogenic amino acids such as alanine. Thus, increased use of fat stores occurs during prolonged fasting in pregnancy. Lipolysis generates glycerol, fatty acids, and ketones for gluconeogenesis and fuel metabolism.[221,222] This produces exaggerated starvation ketosis and preserves the utilization of glucose and amino acids for the maternal central nervous system and fetus. The increased utilization of fat stores is caused by decreased levels of insulin seen during prolonged fasting and the effects of human placental lactogen (hPL).[220] In summary, maternal hypoglycemia, hypoinsulinemia, hyperlipidemia, and hyperketonemia characterize the maternal response to starvation.

By contrast, hyperglycemia, hyperinsulinemia, hyperlipidemia, and reduced tissue sensitivity to insulin characterize the maternal response to feeding.[219] Insulin secretion increases progressively during gestation, with the maximal increase in the third trimester. Insulin resistance occurs after the first trimester,[224,225] with a 50- to 80-percent decline in insulin sensitivity by the third trimester, chiefly in skeletal muscle. In women with type 1 diabetes mellitus, this progressive insulin resistance frequently leads to increased insulin requirements which by the last trimester can more than double.[226] Thus, despite this increase in postprandial hyperinsulinemia, the blood glucose response to the same carbohydrate load is greater in pregnancy.[218] In normal gestation, glucose homeostasis is maintained by the exaggerated response in insulin production and with greater glucose fluctuations from the fasting to the postprandial state. Fasting and postprandial glucose values were determined in 57 nondiabetic gravidas in the third trimester using continuous glucose monitors. The mean fasting (standard deviation) glucose was 83.7 ± 18 mg/dl and the mean values at 1 and 2 hours after a meal were 105.3 ± 12 mg/dl and 97.2 ± 10 mg/dl.[227] If a woman has borderline pancreatic reserve before pregnancy and is unable to increase her insulin production, then gestational diabetes mellitus will be revealed during pregnancy.

The factors responsible for the diabetogenic effects of pregnancy include a variety of hormones secreted by the placenta, especially hPL and placental growth hormone variant.[228] HPL is produced by syncytiotrophoblast cells and has strong lipolytic and antiinsulin actions. HPL secretion is proportional to total placental mass and parallels the development of insulin resistance. Other maternal hormones that contribute to insulin resistance include cortisol, prolactin, estrogen, and progesterone. The diabetogenic effects of pregnancy are advantageous to the growing fetus, providing increased maternal levels of nutrients after a meal.[217,220] Insulin resistance resolves within hours after delivery and consequent removal of the placenta.[226]

The fetus is primarily dependent on maternal glucose for its fuel requirements. The concentration of glucose in the fetus is about 20 mg/dl less than in the maternal serum.[229] Placental glucose transport occurs through a carrier-mediated facilitated transporter that is energy independent.[230] Maternal insulin does not cross the placenta, and hence, the fetus is dependent on its own insulin production. Normal maternal glucose levels are critically important in providing adequate glucose to the fetus. Maternal hyperglycemia can cause birth defects if present in the first trimester and fetal macrosomia if present in the latter half of pregnancy.[231]

Proteins and Fats/Lipids

Amino acids are actively transported across the placenta, where they are used by the fetus for protein synthesis and as an energy source. In late pregnancy, the fetoplacental unit contains approximately 500 mg of protein. During pregnancy, fat stores are preferentially used as a substrate for fuel metabolism, and thus, protein catabolism is decreased.

Plasma lipids and lipoproteins increase in pregnancy. A gradual two- to three-fold rise in triglyceride levels occurs by term and levels of 200 to 300 mg/dl are normal.[232] Total cholesterol and low-density lipoprotein levels are also higher, so that by term, a 50- to 60-percent increase is observed. High-density lipoprotein levels initially rise in the first half of pregnancy and then fall in the second half. By term, high-density lipoprotein concentrations are 15 percent higher than nonpregnant levels. Triglyceride concentrations return to normal by 8 weeks' postpartum even with lactation, but cholesterol and low-density lipoprotein levels remain elevated (Fig. 3-14). The mechanisms for the pregnancy-induced changes in lipids are not completely understood, but appear to be partly caused by

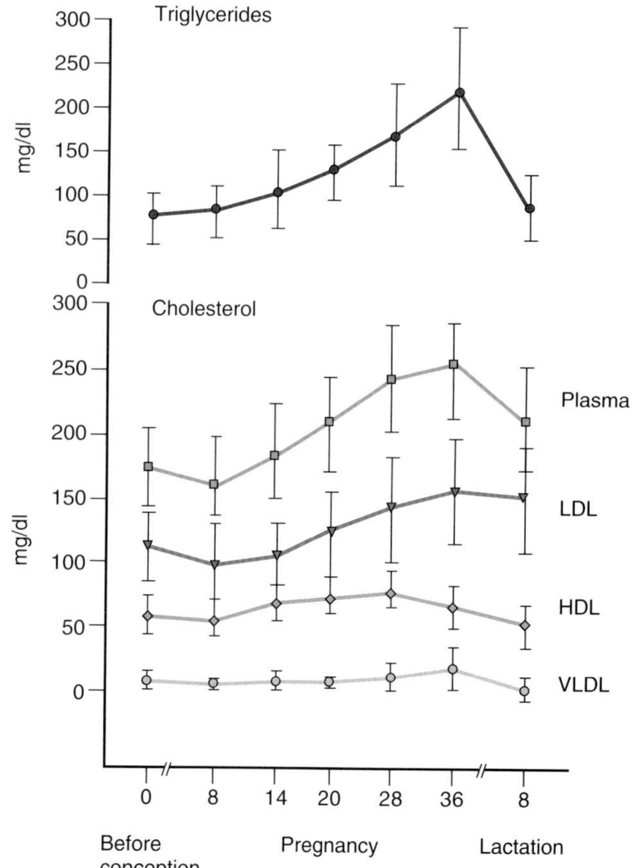

Figure 3-14. Triglycerides (*upper panel*) and cholesterol (*lower panel*) in plasma and in lipoprotein fractions before, during, and after pregnancy. (From Salameh W, Mastrogiannis D: Maternal hyperlipidemia in pregnancy. Clin Obstet Gynecol 37:66, 1994, with permission.)

the elevated levels of estrogen, progesterone, and hPL. The rise in low-density lipoproteins appears to be necessary for placental steroidogenesis. Despite the increase in cholesterol and lipids, no increase in the long-term risk for atherosclerosis has been found.[232] However, women with preexisting hyperlipidemia can have a transient worsening of their lipid profiles that is accentuated by the necessity of discontinuing medications such as Hydroxymethylglutaryl-CoA (HMG-CoA) reductase inhibitors (statins) during pregnancy.

THE EYE

Two consistent and significant ocular changes occur during pregnancy: increased thickness of the cornea and decreased intraocular pressure. Corneal thickening is apparent by 10 weeks' gestation and may cause problems with contact lenses. Corneal changes persist for several weeks postpartum, and patients should be advised to wait before obtaining a new eyeglass or contact prescription.[233] Pizzarello found that 14 percent of women complained of vision changes. All had changes in their visual acuity and refractive error, as well as a myopic shift (became more far-sighted) from pregravid levels, with return to baseline vision postpartum.[234] Owing to these transient alterations in the eye, pregnancy is considered by most to be a contraindication to photorefractive keratectomy, and it has been recommended that pregnancy be avoided for 1 year after such surgery. Intraocular pressure falls by about 10 percent during gestation, and individuals with preexisting glaucoma typically improve. Pregnancy either does not change or minimally decreases visual fields; therefore, any complaints of visual field changes are atypical and need further evaluation.[233]

KEY POINTS

- Plasma osmolality decreases during pregnancy as a result of a reduction in the serum concentration of sodium and associated anions. The osmolality set point for AVP release and thirst is also decreased.
- CO increases 30 to 50 percent during pregnancy. Supine positioning and standing are both associated with a fall in CO. CO is maximal during labor and the immediate postpartum period.
- As a result of the marked fall in systemic vascular resistance and pulmonary vascular resistance, PCWP does not rise, despite an increase in blood volume.
- Maternal BP decreases early in pregnancy. The diastolic BP and the mean arterial pressure nadir at midpregnancy (16 to 20 weeks) and return to prepregnancy levels by term.
- Pa_{O_2} and Pa_{CO_2} fall during pregnancy secondary to increased minute ventilation. This facilitates transfer of CO_2 from the fetus to the mother and results in a mild respiratory alkalosis.
- Maternal plasma volume increases 50 percent during pregnancy. As RBC volume increases approximately 18 to 30 percent, the hematocrit normally decreases during gestation but not below 30 percent.
- Pregnancy is a hypercoagulable state, with increases in the levels of the majority of the procoagulant factors and a decrease in the fibrinolytic system and in some of the natural inhibitors of coagulation.
- BUN and creatinine normally decrease during pregnancy as a result of the increased glomerular filtration rate.
- Despite alterations in thyroid morphology, histology, and laboratory indices, the normal pregnant woman is euthyroid, with the levels of free T_4 within nonpregnant norms.
- Pregnancy is associated with a peripheral resistance to insulin, primarily mediated by human placental lactogen. Insulin resistance increases as pregnancy advances and results in hyperglycemia, hyperinsulinemia, and hyperlipidemia in response to feeding, especially in the third trimester.

REFERENCES

1. Lockitch G: Clinical biochemistry of pregnancy. Crit Rev Clin Lab Sci 34:67, 1997.
2. Theunissen I, Parer J: Fluid and electrolytes in pregnancy. Clin Obstet Gynecol 37:3, 1994.
3. Lindheimer M, Davison J: Osmoregulation, the secretion of arginine vasopressin and its metabolism during pregnancy. Eur J Endocrinol 132:133, 1995.
4. Davison J, Vallotton M, Lindheimer M: Plasma osmolality and urinary concentration and dilution during and after pregnancy: evidence that the lateral recumbency inhibits maximal urinary concentration ability. Br J Obstet Gynaecol 88:472, 1981.
5. Lindheimer M, Barron W, Davison J: Osmoregulation of thirst and vasopressin release in pregnancy. Am J Physiol 257:F225, 1989.
6. Bernstein I, Ziegler W, Badger G: Plasma volume expansion in early pregnancy. Obstet Gynecol 97:669, 2001.
7. Carbillon L, Uzan M, Uzan S: Pregnancy, vascular tone, and maternal hemodynamics: a crucial adaptation. Obstet Gynecol 55:574, 2000.
8. Dürr J: Diabetes insipidus in pregnancy. Am J Kidney Dis 9:276, 1987.
9. El-Hennawy A, Bassi T, Koradia N, et al: Transient gestational diabetes insipidus: report of two cases and review of pathophysiology and treatment. J Matern Fetal Med 14:349, 2003.
10. Schobel H: Pregnancy-induced alterations in renal function. Kidney Blood Press Res 21:276, 1998.
11. Furuhashi N, Kimura H, Nagea H, et al: Brain natriuretic peptide and atrial natriuretic peptide levels in normal pregnancy and preeclampsia. Gynecol Obstet Invest 38:73, 1994.
12. Duvekot J, Cheriex E, Pieters F, et al: Early pregnancy changes in hemodynamics and volume homeostasis are consecutive adjustments triggered by a primary fall in systemic vascular tone. Am J Obstet Gynecol 169:1382, 1993.
13. Chesley LC: Renin, angiotensin, and aldosterone in pregnancy. *In* Chesley LC (ed): Hypertensive Disorders in Pregnancy. New York, Appleton-Century-Crofts, 1978, p 236.
14. Miyamoto S, Shimokawa H, Sumioki H, et al: Circadian rhythm of plasma atrial natriuretic peptide, aldosterone, and blood pres-

sure during the third trimester in normal and preeclamptic pregnancies. Am J Obstet Gynecol 224:393, 1998.
15. Doust J, Glasziou P, Pietrzak E, et al: A systematic review of the diagnostic accuracy of natriuretic peptides for heart failure. Arch Intern Med 164:1978, 2004.
16. Colucci W, Chen, H: Brain and atrial natriuretic peptides in left ventricular dysfunction. UpToDate. 01 Apr 2005 <http://www.uptodateonline.com/application/topic/topicText.>.
17. Sala C, Campise M, Ambroso G, et al: Atrial natriuretic peptide and hemodynamic changes during normal human pregnancy. Hypertension 25:631, 1995.
18. Castro L, Hobel C, Gornbein J: Plasma levels of atrial natriuretic peptide in normal and hypertensive pregnancies: a meta-analysis. Am J Obstet Gynecol 71:1642, 1994.
19. Heenan A, Wolfe L, Davies G, et al: Effects of human pregnancy on fluid regulation responses to short-term exercise. J Appl Physiol 95:2321, 2003.
20. Borghi C, Esposti D, Immordino V, et al: Relationship of systemic hemodynamics, left ventricular structure and function, and plasma natriuretic peptide concentrations during pregnancy complicated by preeclampsia. Am J Obstet Gynecol 183:140, 2000.
21. Siu S, Sermer M, Colman J, et al: Prospective multicenter study of pregnancy outcomes in women with heart disease. Circulation 104: 515, 2001.
22. Bhagwat A, Engel P: Heart disease and pregnancy. Cardiol Clin 13:163, 1995.
23. Kametas N, McAuliffe F, Hancock J, et al: Maternal left ventricular mass and diastolic function during pregnancy. Ultrasound Obstet Gynecol 18:460, 2001.
24. Duvekot J, Peeters L: Maternal cardiovascular hemodynamic adaptation to pregnancy. Obstet Gynecol Surv 49:S1, 1994.
25. Kametas N, McAuliffe F, Krampl E, et al: Maternal cardiac function in twin pregnancy. Obstet Gynecol 102:806, 2003.
26. Labovitz A, Pearson A: Evaluation of left ventricular diastolic function: clinical relevance and recent Doppler echocardiographic insights. Am Heart J 114:836, 1987
27. Desai D, Moodley J, Naidoo D, et al: Cardiac abnormalities in pulmonary oedema associated with hypertensive crises in pregnancy. Br J Obstet Gynaecol 103:523, 1996.
28. Mesa A, Jessum C, Hernandez A, et al: Left ventricular function in normal human pregnancy. Circulation 99:511, 1999.
29. Veille JC, Kitzman D, Millsaps P, et al: Left ventricular diastolic filling response to stationary bicycle exercise during pregnancy and the postpartum period. Am J Obstet Gynecol 185:822, 2001.
30. van Oppen A, Stigter R, Bruinse H: Cardiac output in normal pregnancy: a critical review. Obstet Gynecol 87:310, 1996.
31. Robson S, Hunter S, Boys R, et al: Serial study of factors influencing changes in cardiac output during human pregnancy. Am J Physiol 256:H1061, 1989.
32. Hunter S, Robson S: Adaptation of the maternal heart in pregnancy. Br Heart J 68:540, 1992.
33. Desai K, Moodley J, Naidoo D: Echocardiographic hemodynamics in normal pregnancy. Obstet Gynecol 104:20, 2004.
34. McAnolty J, Metcalfe J, Ueland K: Heart disease and pregnancy. *In* Hurst JN (ed): The Heart, 6th ed. New York, McGraw-Hill, 1985, p. 1383.
35. Clapp J, Capeless E: Cardiovascular function before, during and after the first and subsequent pregnancies. Am J Cardiol 80:1469, 1997.
36. Clark S, Cotton D, Pivarnik J, et al: Position change and central hemodynamic profile during normal third-trimester pregnancy and postpartum. Am J Obstet Gynecol 164:883, 1991.
37. Elkayam U, Gleicher N: Cardiovascular physiology of pregnancy. *In* Elkayam U, Gleicher N (eds): Cardiac Problems in Pregnancy: Diagnosis and Management of Maternal and Fetal Disease. New York, Alan R Liss, 1982, p 5.
38. Kerr M: The mechanical effects of the gravid uterus in late pregnancy. J Obstet Gynaecol Br Commonw 72:513, 1965.
39. Kerr M, Scott D, Samuel E: Studies of the inferior vena cava in late pregnancy. Br Med J 1:532, 1964.
40. Lanni S, Tillinghast J, Silver H: Hemodynamic changes and baroreflex gain in the supine hypotensive syndrome. Am J Obstet Gynecol 187:1636, 2002.
41. Naeye R, Peters E: Working during pregnancy effects on the fetus. Pediatrics 69:724, 1982.
42. Clark S, Cotton D, Lee W, et al: Central hemodynamic assessment of normal term pregnancy. Am J Obstet Gynecol 161:1439, 1989.
43. Granger J: Maternal and fetal adaptations during pregnancy and integrative physiology. Am J Physiol Regul Integr Comp Physiol 283:R1289, 2002.
44. Gant N, Daley G, Chand S, et al: A study of angiotensin II pressor response throughout primigravid pregnancy. J Clin Invest 52:2682, 1973.
45. Dunne F, Barry D, Ferris J, et al: Changes in blood pressure during the normal menstrual cycle. Clin Sci 81:515, 1996.
46. MacGillivray I, Rose G, Rowe B: Blood pressure survey in pregnancy. Clin Sci 37:395, 1969.
47. de Swiet M, Shennan A: Blood pressure measurement in pregnancy. Br J Obstet Gynaecol 103:862, 1996.
48. Lo C, Taylor R, Gamble G, et al: Use of automated home blood pressure monitoring in pregnancy: Is it safe. Am J Obstet Gynecol 187:1321, 2002.
49. McLennan C: Antecubital and femoral venous pressure in normal and toxemia pregnancy. Am J Obstet Gynecol 45:568, 1943.
50. Zinaman M, Rubin J, Lindheimer M: Serial plasma oncotic pressure levels and echoencephalography during and after delivery in severe preeclampsia. Lancet 1:1245, 1985.
51. Crapo R: Normal cardiopulmonary physiology during pregnancy. Clin Obstet Gynecol 39:3, 1996.
52. Shotan A, Ostrzega E, Mehra A, et al: Incidence of arrhythmias in normal pregnancy and relation to palpitations, dizziness, and syncope. Am J Cardiol 79:1061, 1997.
53. Cutforth R, MacDonald C: Heart sounds and murmurs in pregnancy. Am Heart J 71:741, 1966.
54. O'Rourke R, Ewy G, Marcus F, et al: Cardiac auscultation in pregnancy. Med Ann D C 39:92, 1970.
55. Robson S, Dunlop W, Boys R, et al: Cardiac output during labour. BMJ 295:1169, 1987.
56. Kerr M: Cardiovascular dynamics in pregnancy and labour. Br Med Bull 24:19, 1968.
57. Ueland K, Hansen J: Maternal cardiovascular dynamics. III. Labor and delivery under local and caudal analgesia. Am J Obstet Gynecol 103:8, 1969.
58. Danilenko-Dixon D, Tefft L, Cohen R, et al: Positional effects on maternal cardiac output during labor with epidural analgesia. Am J Obstet Gynecol 175:867, 1996.
59. James C, Banner T, Caton D: Cardiac output in women undergoing cesarean section with epidural or general anesthesia. Am J Obstet Gynecol 160:1178, 1989.
60. Robson S, Boys R, Hunter S, et al: Maternal hemodynamics after normal delivery and delivery complicated by postpartum hemorrhage. Obstet Gynecol 74:234, 1989.
61. Romem A, Romem Y, Katz M, Battler A: Incidence and characteristics of maternal cardiac arrhythmias during labor. Am J Cardiol 93:931, 2004.
62. Schatz M, Zieger R: Diagnosis and management of rhinitis during pregnancy. Allergy Proc 9:545, 1988.
63. Thompson K, Cohen M: Studies on the circulation in pregnancy, II: vital capacity in normal pregnant women. Surg Gynecol Obstet 66:591, 1938.
64. Gilroy R, Mangura B, Lavietes M: Rib cage displacement and abdominal volume displacement during breathing in pregnancy. Am Rev Respir Dis 137:668, 1988.
65. Weinberger S, Weiss S, Cohen W, et al: Pregnancy and the lung. Am Rev Respir Dis 121:L559, 1980.
66. Brancazio L, Laifer S, Schwartz T: Peak expiratory flow rate in normal pregnancy. Obstet Gynecol 89:383, 1997.
67. Harirah H, Donia S, Nasrallah F: Effect of gestational age and position on peak expiratory flow rate: A Longitudinal study. Obstet Gynecol 105:372, 2005.
68. Elkus K, Popovich J: Respiratory physiology in pregnancy. Clin Chest Med 13:555, 1992.
69. Lucius H, Gahlenbeck H, Kleine H, et al: Respiratory functions, buffer system, and electrolyte concentration of blood during human pregnancy. Respir Physiol 9:311, 1970.
70. Hankins G, Clark S, Harvey C, et al: Third-trimester arterial blood gases and acid base values in normal pregnancy at moderate altitude. Obstet Gynecol 88:347, 1996.

71. McAuliffe F, Kametas N, Krampl E: Blood gases in prepregnancy at sea level and at high altitude. Br J Obstet Gynaecol 108:980, 2001.
72. Awe R, Nicotra B, Newson T, et al: Arterial oxygenation and alveolar-arterial gradients in term pregnancy. Obstet Gynecol 53:182, 1979.
73. Hankins G, Harvey C, Clark S, et al: The effects of maternal position and cardiac output on intrapulmonary shunt in normal third-trimester pregnancy. Obstet Gynecol 88:327, 1996.
74. Hankins G, Clark S, Uckan E, et al: Maternal oxygen transport variables during the third trimester of normal pregnancy. Am J Obstet Gynecol 180:406, 1999.
75. Lee K, Zaffke M, Mcenany G: Parity and sleep patterns during and after pregnancy. Obstet Gynecol 95:14, 2000.
76. Santiago J, Nolledo M, Kinzler W: Sleep and sleep disorders in pregnancy. Ann Intern Med 134:396, 2001
77. The International Classification of Sleep Disorders, Revised: Diagnostic and Coding Manual. Rochester, MN: American Sleep Disorder Association; 1997: 297.
77a. Sahota P, Jain S, Dhand R: Sleep disorders in pregnancy. Curr Opin Pulm Med 9:477, 2003.
78. Pritchard J: Changes in blood volume during pregnancy and delivery. Anesthesiology 26:393, 1965.
79. Lo F, Kaufman S: Effect of 5α-pregnan-3α-ol-20-one on nitric oxide biosynthesis and plasma volume in rats. Am J Physiol Regul Integr Comp Physiol 280:R1902, 2000.
80. Scott D: Anemia during pregnancy. Obstet Gynecol Ann 1:219, 1972.
81. U. S. Department of Health and Human Services: MMWR Morb Mortal Wkly Rep 38:400, 1989.
82. Ireland R, Abbas A, Thilaganathan B, et al: Fetal and maternal erythropoietin levels in normal pregnancy. Fetal Diagn Ther 7:21, 1992.
83. Pritchard J, Baldwin R, Dickey J, et al: Blood volume changes in pregnancy and the puerperium. II. Red blood cell loss and changes in apparent blood volume during and following vaginal delivery, cesarean section, and cesarean section plus total hysterectomy. Am J Obstet Gynecol 84:1271, 1962.
84. Ueland K: Maternal cardiovascular dynamics. VII. Intrapartum blood volume changes. Am J Obstet Gynecol 126:671, 1976.
85. Andrews N: Disorders of iron metabolism. N Engl J Med 341:1986, 1999.
86. McFee J: Iron metabolism and iron deficiency during pregnancy. Clin Obstet Gynecol 22:799, 1979.
87. Mahomed K: Iron supplementation in pregnancy (Cochrane Review). In: The Cochrane Library. Issue 4. Oxford, United Kingdom: Update Software, 2001.
88. Romslo I, Haram K, Sagen N, et al: Iron requirement in normal pregnancy as assessed by serum ferritin, serum transferrin saturation and erythrocyte protoporphyrin determinations. Br J Obstet Gynaecol 90:101, 1983.
89. Makrides M, Crowther C, Gibson R, et al: Efficacy and tolerability of low-dose iron supplements during pregnancy: a randomized controlled trial. Am J Clin Nutr 78:145;2003.
89a. Bayoumeu F, Subiran-Buisset C, Baka N, et al: Iron therapy in iron deficiency anemia in pregnancy: Intravenous route versus oral route. Am J Obstet Gynecol 186:518, 2002.
90. Tygart S, McRoyan D, Spinnato J, et al: Longitudinal study of platelet indices during normal pregnancy. Am J Obstet Gynecol 154:883, 1986.
91. Fay R, Hughes A, Farron N: Platelets in pregnancy: hyperdestruction in pregnancy. Obstet Gynecol 61:238, 1983.
92. Sejeny S, Eastham R, Baker S: Platelet counts during normal pregnancy. J Clin Pathol 28:812, 1975.
93. Pitkin R, Witte D: Platelet and leukocyte counts in pregnancy. JAMA 242:2696, 1979.
94. O'Brien JR: Platelet count in normal pregnancy. J Clin Pathol 29:174, 1976.
95. Boehlen F, Hohlfeld P, Extermann P, et al: Platelet count at term pregnancy: a reappraisal of the threshold. Obstet Gynecol 95:29, 2000.
96. Burrows R, Kelton J: Incidentally detected thrombocytopenia in healthy mothers and their infants. N Engl J Med 319:142, 1988.
97. American College of Obstetricians and Gynecologists: ACOG practice bulletin. Thrombocytopenia in pregnancy. Number 6, September 1999. Clinical management guidelines for obstetrician-gynecologists. Washington, DC, ACOG-1999.
98. Acker DB, Johnson MP, Sachs BP. Friedman EA, et al: The leukocyte count in labor. Am J Obstet Gynecol 153:737-9, 1985.
99. Naccasha N, Gervasi M, Chaiworapongsa T, et al: Phenotypic and metabolic characteristics of monocytes and granulocytes in normal pregnancy and maternal infection. Am J Obstet Gynecol 185:1118, 2001.
100. Sacks G, Sargent I, Redman C: An innate view of human pregnancy. Immunol Today 20:114,1999.
101. Wegmann T, Lin H, Guibert L, et al: Bidirectional cytokine interactions in the maternal-fetal relationship: is successful pregnancy a TH2 phenomenon? Immunol Today 14:353, 1993.
102. Falkoff R: Maternal immune function during pregnancy. *In* Schatz M, Zeiger R, Claman HN (eds): Asthma and Immunology in Pregnancy and Early Infancy. NY, Marcel Dekker, 1998, p 73.
103. Gehrz R, Christianson W, Linner K, et al: Cytomegalovirus specific humoral and cellular immune response in human pregnancy. J Infect Dis 143:391, 1982.
104. Brown Z, Vontner L, Bendetti J, et al: Genital herpes in pregnancy: risk factors associated with recurrences and asymptomatic viral shedding. Am J Obstet Gynecol 153:24, 1985.
105. Diro M, Beydoun S: Malaria in pregnancy. South Med J 75:959, 1982.
106. Stirrat G: Pregnancy and immunity: changes occur, but pregnancy does not result in immunodeficiency. BMJ 308:1385, 1994.
107. Dodson M, Kerman R, Lange C, et al: T and B cells in pregnancy. Obstet Gynecol 49:299, 1977.
108. Johnson U, Gustavii B: Complement components in normal pregnancy. Acta Pathol Microbiol Scand 95:97, 1987.
109. Bisset L, Fiddes T, Gillet W: Altered humoral immunoregulation during human pregnancy. Am J Reprod Immunol 23:4, 1990.
110. Brabin B: Epidemiology of infection in pregnancy. Rev Infect Dis 7:579, 1985.
111. Present P, Comstock GW: Tuberculin Sensitivity in Pregnancy. Am Rev Respir Dis 112:413, 1975.
112. Johnson RL: Thromboembolic disease complicating pregnancy. *In* Foley MR, Strong TH (eds): Obstetric Intensive Care: A Practical Manual. Philadelphia, WB Saunders Company, 1997, p 91.
113. Hytten F, Lind T: Volume and composition of the blood. *In* Hytten FE, Lind T (eds): Diagnostic Indices in Pregnancy. Basel, Documenta Geigy, 1973, p 36.
114. Ozanne P, Linderkamp O, Miller F, et al: Erythrocyte aggregation during normal pregnancy. Am J Obstet Gynecol 147:576, 1983.
115. Clark P, Brennand J, Conkie J, et al: Activated protein C sensitivity, protein C, protein S, and coagulation in normal pregnancy. Thromb Haemost 79:1166, 1998.
116. Faught W, Garner P, Jones G, et al: Changes in protein C and protein S levels in normal pregnancy. Am J Obstet Gynecol 172(1 Pt 1):147, 1995.
117. Goodwin A, Rosendaal F, Kottke-Marchant K, et al: A review of the technical, diagnostic, and epidemiologic considerations for protein S assays. Arch Pathol Lab Med 126:1349, 2002.
118. Bauer K: Hypercoagulability-a new cofactor in the protein C anticoagulant pathway. N Engl J Med 330:566, 1994.
119. Gerbasi F, Bottoms S, Farag A, et al: Increased intravascular coagulation associated with pregnancy. Obstet Gynecol 75:385, 1990.
120. Fried A, Woodring J, Thompson D: Hydronephrosis of pregnancy: a prospective sequential study of the course of dilatation. J Ultrasound Med 2:255, 1983.
121. Hytten F, Lind T: Indices of renal function. *In* Hytten FE, Lind T (eds): Diagnostic Indices in Pregnancy. Basel, Documenta Geigy, 1973, p 18.
122. Davison J: The effect of pregnancy on kidney function in renal allograft recipients. Kidney Int 27:74, 1985.
123. Stehman-Breen C, Levine R, Qian C, et al: Increased risk of preeclampsia among nulliparous pregnant women with idiopathic hematuria. Am J Obstet Gynecol 187:703, 2002.
124. Lindheimer M, Davison J, Katz A: The kidney and hypertension in pregnancy: Twenty exciting years. Semin Nephrol 21:173, 2001.
125. Dunlop W: Serial changes in renal haemodynamics during normal pregnancy. Br J Obstet Gynaecol 88:1, 1981.

126. Ezimokhai M, Davison J, Philips P, et al: Non-postural serial changes in renal function during the third trimester of normal human pregnancy. Br J Obstet Gynaecol 88:465, 1981.
127. Davison J, Noble F: Glomerular filtration during and after pregnancy. J Obstet Gynaecol Br Commonw 81:588, 1974.
128. Abram S, Alexander B, Bennett W, et al: Role of neuronal nitric oxide synthase in mediating renal hemodynamic changes during pregnancy. Am J Physiol Regul Integr Comp Physiol 281:R1390, 2001.
129. Gandley R, Conrad K, McLaughlin M: Endothelin and nitric oxide mediate reduced myogenic reactivity of small renal arteries from pregnant rats. Am J Physiol Regul Integr Comp Physiol 280:R1, 2001.
130. Jeyabalin A, Novak J, Danielson L, et al: Essential role for vascular gelatinase activity in relaxin-induced renal vasodilation, hyperfiltration, and reduced myogenic reactivity of small arteries. Circ Res 93:1249, 2003.
131. Lind T, Godfrey K, Otun H: Changes in serum uric acid concentrations during normal pregnancy. Br J Obstet Gynaecol 91:128, 1984.
132. Chesley L, Sloan D: The effect of posture on renal function in late pregnancy. Am J Obstet Gynecol 89:754, 1964.
133. Lindheimer M, Richardson D, Ehrlich E, et al: Potassium homeostasis in pregnancy. J Reprod Med 32:517, 1987.
134. Davison J, Hytten F: The effect of pregnancy on the renal handling of glucose. Br J Obstet Gynaecol 82:374, 1975.
135. Kurtzman N, Pillay V: Renal reabsorption of glucose in health and disease. Arch Intern Med 131:901, 1973.
136. Higby K, Suiter C, Phelps J, et al: Normal values of urinary albumin and total protein excretion during pregnancy. Am J Obstet Gynecol 171:984, 1994.
137. Gordon M, London M, Samuels P, et al: Perinatal outcome and long-term follow-up associated with modern management of diabetic nephropathy. Obstet Gynecol 87:401, 1996.
138. Hytten F, Cheyne G: The aminoaciduria of pregnancy. J Obstet Gynaecol Br Commonw 79:424, 1972.
139. Dafnis E, Sabatini S: The effect of pregnancy on renal function: physiology and pathophysiology. Am J Med Sci 303:184, 1992.
140. Hytten F, Lind T: Indices of alimentary function. *In* Hytten FE, Lind T (eds): Diagnostic Indices in Pregnancy. Basel, Documenta Geigy, 1973, p 13.
141. Catalano P, Hollenbeck C: Energy requirements in pregnancy: a review. Obstet Gynecol Surv 47:368, 1992.
142. Kallender D, Sonesson B: Studies on saliva in menstruating, pregnant and postmenopausal women. Acta Endocrinol (Copenh) 48:329, 1965.
143. Parmley T, O'Brien T: Skin changes during pregnancy. Clin Obstet Gynecol 33:713, 1990.
144. Winston G, Lewis C: Dermatosis of pregnancy. J Am Acad Dermatol 6:977, 1982.
145. Shah S, Nathan L, Singh R, et al: E2 and not P4 increases NO release from NANC nerves of the gastrointestinal tract: implications in pregnancy. Am J Physiol Regul Integr Comp Physiol 280: R1554, 2001.
146. Macfie A, Magides A, Richmond M, et al: Gastric emptying in pregnancy. Br J Anaesth 67:54, 1991.
147. Davison J, Davison M, Hay D: Gastric emptying time in late pregnancy and labour. J Obstet Gynaecol Br Commonw 77:37, 1970.
148. Cappell M, Garcia A: Gastric and duodenal ulcers during pregnancy. Gastroenterol Clin North Am 27:169, 1998.
149. Levy N, Lemberg E, Sharf M: Bowel habits in pregnancy. Digestion 4:216, 1977.
150. Bonapace E, Fisher R: Constipation and diarrhea in pregnancy. Gastroenterol Clin North Am 27:197, 1998.
151. Parry E, Shields R, Turnbull A: Transit time in the small intestine in pregnancy. J Obstet Gynaecol Br Commonw 77:900, 1970.
152. Parry E, Shields R, Turnbull A: The effect of pregnancy on the colonic absorption of sodium, potassium and water. J Obstet Gynaecol Br Commonw 77:616, 1970.
153. Braverman D, Johnson M, Kern F: Effects of pregnancy and contraceptive steroids on gallbladder function. N Engl J Med 302:362, 1980.
154. Van Assche F, Aerts L, De Prins F: A morphologic study of the endocrine pancreas in human pregnancy. Br J Obstet Gynaecol 85:818, 1978.
155. Kern F, Everson G, DeMark B, et al: Biliary lipids, bile acids, and gallbladder function in the human female: effects of pregnancy and the ovulatory cycle. J Clin Invest 68:1229, 1981.
156. Combes B, Abarns R: Disorders of the liver in pregnancy. *In* Assali (ed): Pathophysiology of Gestation. San Diego, Academic Press, 1971, p 297.
157. Carter J: Liver function in normal pregnancy. Aust N Z J Obstet Gynaecol 30:296, 1990.
158. Bacq Y, Zarka O, Brechot J-F, et al: Liver function tests in normal pregnancy: a prospective study of 103 pregnant women and 103 matched controls. Hepatology 23:1030, 1996.
159. Mullally B, Hansen W: Intrahepatic cholestasis of pregnancy: Review of the literature. Obstet Gynecol Surv 57:47, 2002.
159a. Pauli-Magnus C, Lang T, Meier Y, et al: Sequence analysis of bile salt export pump (ABCB11) and multidrug resistance p-glycoprotein 3 (ABCB4, *MDR3*) in patients with intrahepatic cholestasis of pregnancy. Pharmacogenetics 14:91, 2004.
160. Furneaux E, Langley-Evans A, Langley-Evans S: Nausea and vomiting of pregnancy: endocrine basis and contribution to pregnancy outcome. Obstet Gynecol Surv 56:775, 2001.
161. Soulos M, Hughes C, Garcia J, et al: Nausea and vomiting of pregnancy: role of human chorionic gonadotropin and 17-hydroxyprogesterone. Obstet Gynecol 55:696, 1980.
162. American College of Obstetricians and Gynecologists: ACOG practice bulletin. Nausea and vomiting of pregnancy, Number 52, April 2004.
163. Murphy A: Alternative therapies for nausea and vomiting of pregnancy. Obstet Gynecol 91:149, 1998.
164. Yost N, McIntire D, Wians F, et al: A randomized, placebo-controlled trial of corticosteroids for hyperemesis due to pregnancy. Obstet Gynecol 102:1250, 2003.
165. Safari H, Fassett M, Souter I, et al: The efficacy of methylprednisolone in the treatment of hyperemesis gravidarum: a randomized, double-blind, controlled study. Am J Obstet Gynecol 179:921, 1998.
166. Magee L, Mazzotta P, Koren G: Evidence-based view of safety and effectiveness of pharmacologic therapy for nausea and vomiting of pregnancy. Am J Obstet Gynecol 186:S256, 2002.
167. Kuscu N, Koyuncu F: Hyperemesis gravidarum: current concepts and management. Postgrad Med J 78:76, 2002.
168. Kovacs C, Kronenberg H: Maternal-fetal calcium and bone metabolism during pregnancy, puerperium, and lactation. Endocr Rev 18:832, 1997.
169. Givens M, Macy I: The chemical composition of the human fetus. J Biol Chem 102:7, 1933.
170. Trotter M, Hixon B: Sequential changes in weight, density, and percentage ash weight of human skeletons from an early fetal period through old age. Anat Rec 179:1, 1974.
171. Hojo M, August P: Calcium metabolism in normal and hypertensive pregnancy. Semin Nephrol 15:504, 1995.
172. Pitkin R, Gebhardt M: Serum calcium concentrations in human pregnancy. Am J Obstet Gynecol 127:775, 1977.
173. Cross N, Hillman L, Allen S, et al: Calcium homeostasis and bone metabolism during pregnancy, lactation, and postweaning: a longitudinal study. Am J Clin Nutr 61:514, 1995.
174. Prentice A: Maternal calcium metabolism and bone mineral status. Ann J Clin Nutr 71:1312S, 2000.
175. Ensom M, Liu P, Stephenson M: Effect of pregnancy on bone mineral density in healthy women. Obstet Gynecol Surv 57:99, 2002.
176. Pitkin R, Reynolds W, Williams G, et al: Calcium metabolism in normal pregnancy, a longitudinal study. Am J Obstet Gynecol 133:781, 1979.
177. Samaan N, Anderson G, Adam-Mayne M: Immunoreactive calcitonin in the mother, neonate, child, and adult. Am J Obstet Gynecol 121:622, 1975.
178. Promislow J, Hertz-Picciotto I, Schramm M, et al: Bed rest and other determinants of bone loss during pregnancy. Am J Obstet Gynecol 191:1077, 2004.
179. Paton L, Alexander J, Nowson C, et al: Pregnancy and lactation have no long-term deleterious effect on measures of bone mineral in healthy women: a twin study. Am J Clin Nutr 77:707, 2003.
180. Shahtaheri S, Aaron J, Johnson D, et al: Changes in trabecular bone architecture in women during pregnancy. Br J Obstet Gynaecol 106:432, 1999.

181. Oliveri B, Parisi M, Zeni S, et al: Mineral and Bone Mass Changes During Pregnancy and Lactation. Nutrition 20:235, 2004.
182. Hall K: Relaxin. J Reprod Fertil 1:369, 1960.
183. Abramson D, Roberts S, Wilson P: Relaxation of the pelvic joints in pregnancy. Surg Gynecol Obstet 58:595, 1934.
184. Fantz C, Dagogo-Jack S, Ladenson J, et al: Thyroid function during pregnancy. Clin Chem 45:2250, 1999.
185. Berghout A, Endert E, Ross A, et al: Thyroid function and thyroid size in normal pregnant women living in an iodine replete area. Clin Endocrinol 42:375, 1994.
186. Nelson M, Wickus G, Caplan R, et al: Thyroid gland size in pregnancy. An ultrasound and clinical study. J Reprod Med 32:888, 1987.
187. Glinoer D: The regulation of thyroid function in pregnancy: pathways of endocrine adaptation from physiology to pathology. Endocr Rev 18:404, 1997.
188. Mazzaferri E: Evaluation and management of common thyroid disorders in women. Am J Obstet Gynecol 176:507, 1997.
189. Lieberman C, Fang S, Braverman L, et al: Circulating iodide concentrations during and after pregnancy. J Clin Endocrinol Metab 83:3545, 1998.
190. Pochin E: The iodine uptake of the human thyroid throughout the menstrual cycle and in pregnancy. Clin Sci 11:441, 1952.
191. Burrow G, Fisher D, Larsen P: Maternal and fetal thyroid function. N Engl J Med 331:1072,1994.
192. Ballabio M, Poshyachinda M, Ekins R: Pregnancy-induced changes in thyroid function: role of human chorionic gonadotropin as putative regulator of maternal thyroid. J Clin Endocrinol Metab 73:824, 1996.
193. Biggio J, Mahan J: Thyroid stimulating hormone and free thyroxine in pregnancy: are levels really unchanged? Am J Obstet Gynecol 191:S89, 2004.
194. Glinoer D, De Nayer P, Robyn C, et al: Serum levels of intact human chorionic gonadotropin (hCG) and its free α and β subunits, in relation to maternal thyroid stimulation during normal pregnancy. J Endocrinol Invest 16:881, 1993.
195. Kennedy R, Darne J, Cohn M, et al: Human chorionic gonadotropin may not be responsible for thyroid-stimulating activity in normal pregnancy serum. J Clin Endocrinol Metab 74:260, 1992.
196. Fisher D, Lehman H, Lackey D: Placental transport of thyroxine. J Clin Endocrinol Metab 24:393, 1964.
197. Ekins R, Sinha A, Ballabio M, et al: Role of the maternal carrier proteins in the supply of thyroid hormones to the feto-placental unit: evidence of a feto-placental requirement for thyroxine. *In* Delange F, Fisher DA, Glinoer D (eds): Research in Congenital Hypothyroidism. New York, Plenum Press, 1989, p. 45.
198. Spong C: Subclinical hypothyroidism: should all pregnant women be screened? Obstet Gynecol 105:235,2005.
199. Blazer S, Moreh-Waterman Y, Miller-Lotan R, et al: Maternal hypothyroidism may affect fetal growth and neonatal thyroid function. Obstet Gynecol 102:232, 2003.
200. Vulsma T, Gons M, de Vijlder J: Maternal-fetal transfer of thyroxine in congenital hypothyroidism due to a total organification defect or thyroid agenesis. N Engl J Med 321:13, 1989.
201. Xue-Yi C, Xin-min J, Zhi-hong D, et al: Timing of vulnerability of the brain to iodine deficiency in endemic cretinism. N Engl J Med 331:1739, 1994.
202. Utiger R: Maternal hypothyroidism and fetal development. N Engl J Med 341:601, 1999.
203. Haddow J, Palomaki G, Allan W, et al: Maternal thyroid deficiency during pregnancy and subsequent neuropsychological development of the child. N Engl J Med 341:549, 1999.
204. Gorman C: Radioiodine and Pregnancy. Thyroid 9:721, 1999.
205. Nolten W, Lindheimer M, Rueckert P, et al: Diurnal patterns and regulation of cortisol secretion in pregnancy. J Clin Endocrinol Metab 51:466, 1980.
206. Nolten W, Lindheimer M, Oparil S, et al: Deoxycorticosterone in normal pregnancy. I. Sequential studies of the secretory patterns of deoxycorticosterone, aldosterone, and cortisol. Am J Obstet Gynecol 132:414, 1978.
207. Goland R, Jozak S, Conwell I: Placental corticotrophin-releasing hormone and the hypercortisolism of pregnancy. Am J Obstet Gynecol 171:1287, 1994.
208. Doe R, Fernandez R, Seal U: Measurements of corticosteroid-binding globulin in man. J Clin Endocrinol Metab 24:1029, 1964.
209. Scott E, McGarrigle H, Lachelin G: The increase in plasma and saliva cortisol levels in pregnancy is not due to the increase in corticosteroid-binding globulin levels. J Clin Endocrinol Metab 71:639, 1990.
210. Goland R, Conwell I, Warren W, et al: Placental corticotrophin-releasing hormone and pituitary-adrenal function during pregnancy. Neuroendocrinology 56:742, 1992.
211. Rainey W, Rehman K, Carr B: Fetal and maternal adrenals in human pregnancy. Obstet Gynecol Clin North Am 31:817, 2004.
212. Helal K, Gordon M, Lightner C, et al: Adrenal suppression induced by betamethasone in women at risk for premature delivery. Obstet Gynecol 96:287, 2000.
213. Belisie S, Osaihanondh R, Tulchinsky D: The effect of constant infusion of unlabelled dehydroepiandrosterone sulfate on maternal plasma androgens and estrogens. J Clin Endocrinol Metab 45:544, 1977.
214. Gonzalez J, Elizondo G, Saldivar D, et al: Pituitary gland growth during normal pregnancy: an in vivo study using magnetic resonance imaging. Am J Med 85:217, 1988.
215. Tyson J, Hwang P, Guyda H, et al: Studies of prolactin secretion in human pregnancy. Am J Obstet Gynecol 113:14, 1972.
216. Prager D, Braunstein G: Pituitary disorders during pregnancy. Endocrinol Metab Clin North Am 24:1, 1995.
217. Bonnar J, Franklin M, Nott P, et al: Effects of breast-feeding on pituitary-ovarian function after childbirth. BMJ 4:82, 1975.
218. Kuhl C: Etiology and pathogenesis of gestational diabetes. Diabetes Care 21:19B, 1998.
219. Phelps R, Metzger B, Freinkel N: Carbohydrate metabolism in pregnancy. Am J Obstet Gynecol 140:730, 1981.
220. Boden G: Fuel metabolism in pregnancy and in gestational diabetes mellitus. Obstet Gynecol Clin North Am 23:1, 1996.
221. Felig P, Lynch V: Starvation in human pregnancy: hypogly-cemia, hypoinsulinemia, and hyperketonemia. Science 170:990, 1970.
222. Tyson J, Austin K, Farinholt J, et al: Endocrine-metabolic response to acute starvation in human gestation. Am J Obstet Gynecol 125:1073, 1976.
223. Page E: Human fetal nutrition and growth. Am J Obstet Gynecol 104:378, 1969.
224. Catalano P, Tyzbir E, Roman N, et al: Longitudinal changes in insulin release and insulin resistance in non-obese pregnant women. Am J Obstet Gynecol 165:1667, 1991.
225. Fisher P, Sutherland H, Bewsher P: The insulin response to glucose infusion in normal human pregnancy. Diabetologia 19:15, 1980.
226. Galerneau F, Inzucchi S: Diabetes mellitus in pregnancy. Obstet Gynecol Clin North Am 31:907, 2004.
227. Yogev Y, Ben-Haroush A, Chen R, et al: Diurnal glycemic profile in obese and normal weight nondiabetic pregnant women. Am J Obstet Gynecol 191:949, 2004.
228. Ryan E: Hormones and insulin resistance in pregnancy. Lancet 362:1777, 2003.
229. Economides D, Nicolaides K: Blood glucose and oxygen tension levels in small-for-gestation fetuses. Am J Obstet Gynecol 160:385, 1989.
230. Bell G, Burant C, Takeda J, et al: Structure and function of mammalian facilitative sugar transporters. J Biol Chem 268:19161, 1993.
231. Cordero L, Landon M: Infant of the diabetic mother. Clin Perinatol 20:635, 1993.
232. Salameh W, Mastrogiannis D: Maternal hyperlipidemia in pregnancy. Clin Obstet Gynecol 37:66, 1994.
233. Dinn R, Harris A, Marcus P: Ocular changes in pregnancy. Obstet Gynecol Surv 58:137, 2003.
234. Pizzarello L: Refractive changes in pregnancy. Graefes Arch Clin Exp Ophthalmol 241:484, 2003.

Maternal-Fetal Immunology

KRISTINA M. ADAMS AND LAURENCE E. SHIELDS

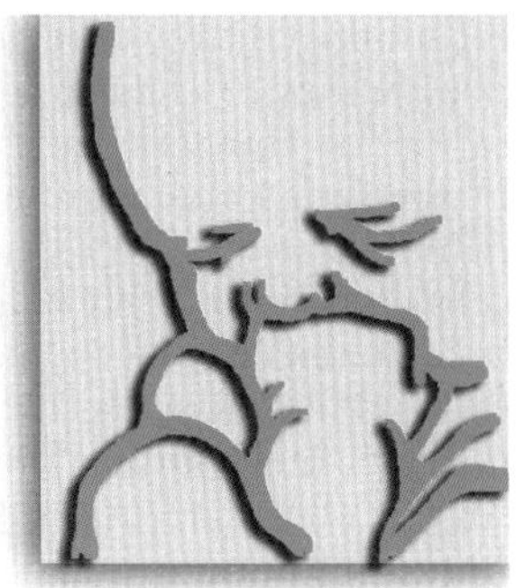

CHAPTER 4

KEY ABBREVIATIONS

Alpha-fetoprotein	AFP
B-cell receptor	BCR
CC receptor	CCR
Class II transactivator	CIITA
CXC receptor	CXCR
Fas ligand	FasL
Graft-versus-host disease	GVHD
Human immunodeficiency virus	HIV
Human leukocyte antigen	HLA
Indoleamine 2,3 dioxygenase	IDO
Immunoglobulin	Ig
Interferon-γ	IFN-γ
Interleukin-1	IL-1
Kilodalton	kDA
Killer cell immunoglobulin-like receptor	KIR
Lipopolysaccharide	LPS
LPS binding protein	LBP
Major histocompatibilty complex	MHC
Membrane attack complex	MAC
Natural killer	NK
Pattern-recognition receptors	PRR
Preterm premature rupture of the membranes	PPROM
T-cell receptor	TCR
T-helper type 1	Th1
T-helper type 2	Th2
TNF-related apoptosis-inducing ligand/Apo-2L	TRAIL
Toll-like receptors	TLR
Transforming growth factor-beta	TGF-β
Tumor necrosis factor-alpha	TNF-α
Uterine NK cells	u-NK

INTRODUCTION

The study of maternal-fetal immunology was initially driven by a desire to understand how a genetically foreign fetus could develop within the mother without immune rejection. Sir Peter Medawar described the immunologic paradox posed by pregnancy by asking, "How does the pregnant mother contrive to nourish within itself, for many weeks or months, a foetus that is an antigenically foreign body?"[1] He suggested several possibilities for fetal tolerance including anatomic separation of the fetus and mother, antigenic immaturity of the fetus, and immunologic inertness of the mother. Although it was later discovered that fetal and maternal cells come into direct contact in the placenta, these ideas became the basis for many early studies of maternal-fetal immunology. In fact, discovery of complex immunologic mechanisms at the maternal-fetal interface suggest that placental immune functions are critical for fetal survival.

The finding of immunologic proteins in blood, amniotic fluid, and vaginal fluid of women with preterm labor and intra-amniotic infection has led to the rapid investigation of maternal-fetal immune responses.[2–7] Discoveries arising from the study of immune responses occuring in infection-associated preterm birth may lead to therapies improving perinatal outcomes.[8,9] Even insight into immunologic events during normal pregnancy may be relevant to improving transplantation outcomes and developing therapies for some autoimmune diseases. It is now known that bidirectional cell trafficking occurs routinely during pregnancy resulting in the persistence of small foreign cell populations, called microchimerism, in the mother and child for decades after birth.[10–13] The role of fetal microchimerism on pregnancy and maternal health is unknown, but is speculated to contribute to fetal tolerance and the pathogenesis of some autoimmune diseases.[11] Understanding basic principles of immunology and new areas of clinically important research will allow the clinician to interpret the rapidly evolving field of maternal-fetal immunology.

IMMUNE SYSTEM OVERVIEW: INNATE AND ADAPTIVE IMMUNITY

The immune system is classically divided into two arms, the innate (Fig. 4-1) and adaptive immune systems (Fig. 4-2). Each system fights infection by a slightly different and complementary method. The innate immune system employs fast, nonspecific methods of pathogen detection to prevent and control an initial infection. Innate immunity consists of immune cells such as macrophages, dendritic cells, natural killer (NK) cells, eosinophils, and basophils. These cells often identify pathogens through pattern-recognition receptors (PRRs), which recognize common pathogen structures and repeating motifs. PRRs include the macrophage mannose receptor and toll-like receptors (TLRs), a large family of PRRs that are likely responsible for the earliest immune responses to a pathogen.[16] Another component of innate immunity is complement, which is a system of plasma proteins that coat pathogen surfaces with protein fragments, targeting them for destruction. In many cases, innate immune defenses are effective in combating pathogens. Sometime pathogens may evolve more rapidly than the hosts they infect or evade innate immune responses. Viruses and encapsulated bacteria avoid being recognized by the innate immune system and require a specific recognition mechanism.

Unlike rapidly acting innate immune responses, there is a delay before adaptive immune responses are activated. Adaptive immunity results in the production of antibodies or lymphocytes against a specific antigen. Although slower to respond, adaptive immunity targets specific components of a pathogen and is capable of eradicating an infection that has overwhelmed the innate immune system. In contrast to the innate immune system, adaptive immunity requires presentation of antigen by specialized antigen-presenting cells, production and secretion of stimulatory cytokines, and ultimately, amplification of antigen-specific lymphocyte clones. These antigen-specific clones provide life-long immunity to the specific antigen.

INNATE IMMUNITY: THE FIRST LINE OF HOST DEFENSE

Epithelial surfaces of the body are the first defenses against infection. Mechanical epithelial barriers to infection include ciliary movement of mucus and epithelial cell tight junctions that prevent microorganisms from easily penetrating intercellular spaces. Chemical mechanisms of defense include enzymes (e.g., lysozyme in saliva, pepsin), low pH in the stomach, and antibacterial peptides (e.g., defensins) that degrade bacteria. Microbiologic mechanisms also exist to prevent bacterial infections. For example, normal flora of the intestine and vagina compete for nutrients and epithelial attachment with other bacteria and can produce antibacterial substances (e.g., lactobacillus regulation of vaginal pH).

After entering the tissues, many pathogens are recognized, ingested, and killed by phagocytes, a process mediated by macrophages and neutrophils. The presence of TLRs, a family of PRRs, on the surface of macrophages and other innate immune cells, represents the primary mechanism of pathogen detection. TLR activation results in secretion of cytokines, which initiate inflammatory responses. Neutrophils are then recruited to sites of inflammation by small immunologic proteins, called chemokines (i.e., interleukin-8 [IL-8]) released by macrophages. Chemokines are a family of structurally related glycoproteins with potent leukocyte activation and chemotactic activity. Chemokines and cytokines are cell-derived polypeptides that regulate cell activation, replication, and differentiation, and are important mediators of cell-mediated immune responses. Cells are attracted to chemokines through chemokine-specific receptors expressed on the surface of the cell. Proinflammatory cytokines have been described in the mother, fetus, and amniotic fluid in women with preterm labor and intra-amniotic infection.[3,4,17]

Antimicrobial Peptides

Antimicrobial peptides are secreted by neutrophils and epithelial cells, and they kill bacteria by damaging pathogen membranes. Defensins are a major family of antimicrobial peptides that protect against bacterial,

INNATE IMMUNITY

- First line of host defense to infection
- Rapid response
- Nonspecific recognition of broad classes of pathogens
- Preexisting effector cell population (*no amplification required*)
- Inability to discriminate self vs. non-self; only recognizes pathogens

A) Cells

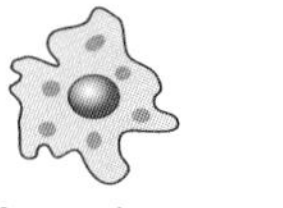

Macrophage

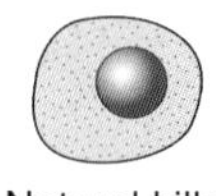

Natural killer (*NK cell*)

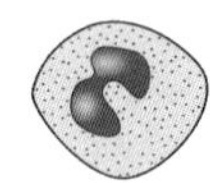

Eosinophil

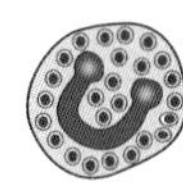

Basophil

B) Pattern Recognition Receptors: Recognize common microbial patterns and structures

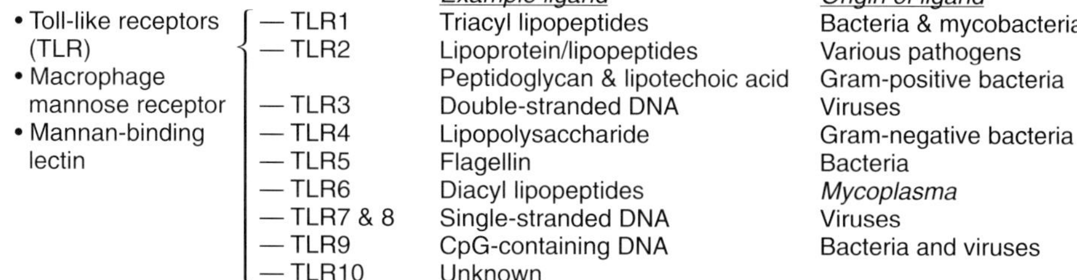

		Example ligand	*Origin of ligand*
• Toll-like receptors (TLR)	— TLR1	Triacyl lipopeptides	Bacteria & mycobacteria
• Macrophage mannose receptor	— TLR2	Lipoprotein/lipopeptides	Various pathogens
• Mannan-binding lectin		Peptidoglycan & lipotechoic acid	Gram-positive bacteria
	— TLR3	Double-stranded DNA	Viruses
	— TLR4	Lipopolysaccharide	Gram-negative bacteria
	— TLR5	Flagellin	Bacteria
	— TLR6	Diacyl lipopeptides	*Mycoplasma*
	— TLR7 & 8	Single-stranded DNA	Viruses
	— TLR9	CpG-containing DNA	Bacteria and viruses
	— TLR10	Unknown	

C) Complement System: Plasma proteins that cooperate to facilitate destruction of pathogens

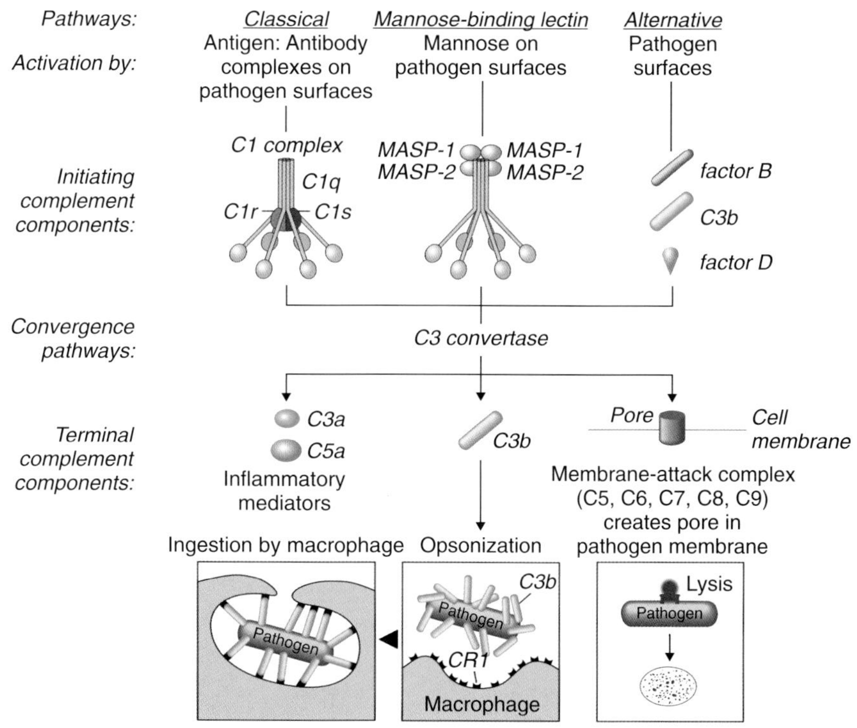

D) Induced Innate Immune Responses

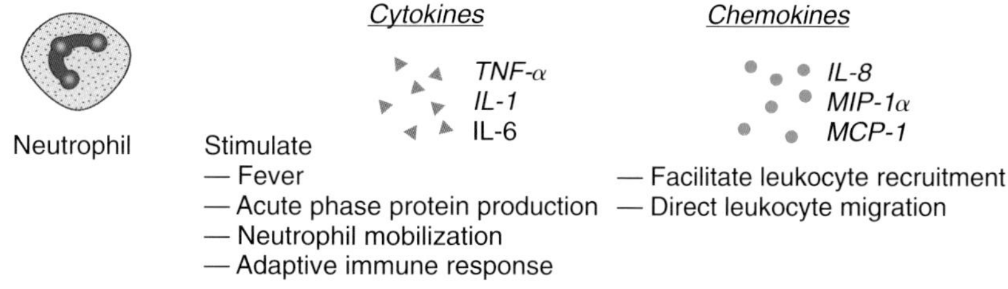

Figure 4-1. The innate immune system. The innate immune system acts as the first line of host defense and consists of immune cells (**1A**), the pattern-recognition receptors that target common pathogen structures (**1B**), the complement system (**1C**), and induced innate immune responses (**1D**). The toll-like receptors and their common ligands are listed because they act as the principal immune sensors of pathogens (**1B**). Complement activation may occur through three different initiating pathways, which converge with production of the C3 convertase and generation of the terminal complement proteins (**1C**). As a result of activation of these components of the innate immune system, neutrophils may be recruited to the site of infection and cytokines/chemokines may be produced (**1D**).

ADAPTIVE IMMUNITY

- Activated when innate immune defenses overwhelmed
- Delayed response
- Specific recognition of small protein peptides
- Requires amplification of lymphocyte clones
- Ability to discriminate self from non-self

A) B Cells Receptors and Antibodies

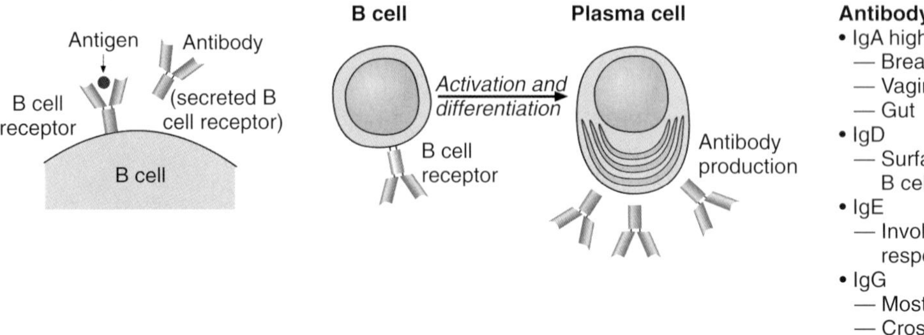

Antibody types

- IgA high in:
  - Breast milk
  - Vaginal fluid
  - Gut
- IgD
  - Surface Ig on naive B cells
- IgE
  - Involved in allergic responses
- IgG
  - Most abundant Ig
  - Crosses placenta
  - Involved in immunologic memory
- IgM
  - Involved in primary B cell responses

B) T Cells and T Cell Receptors

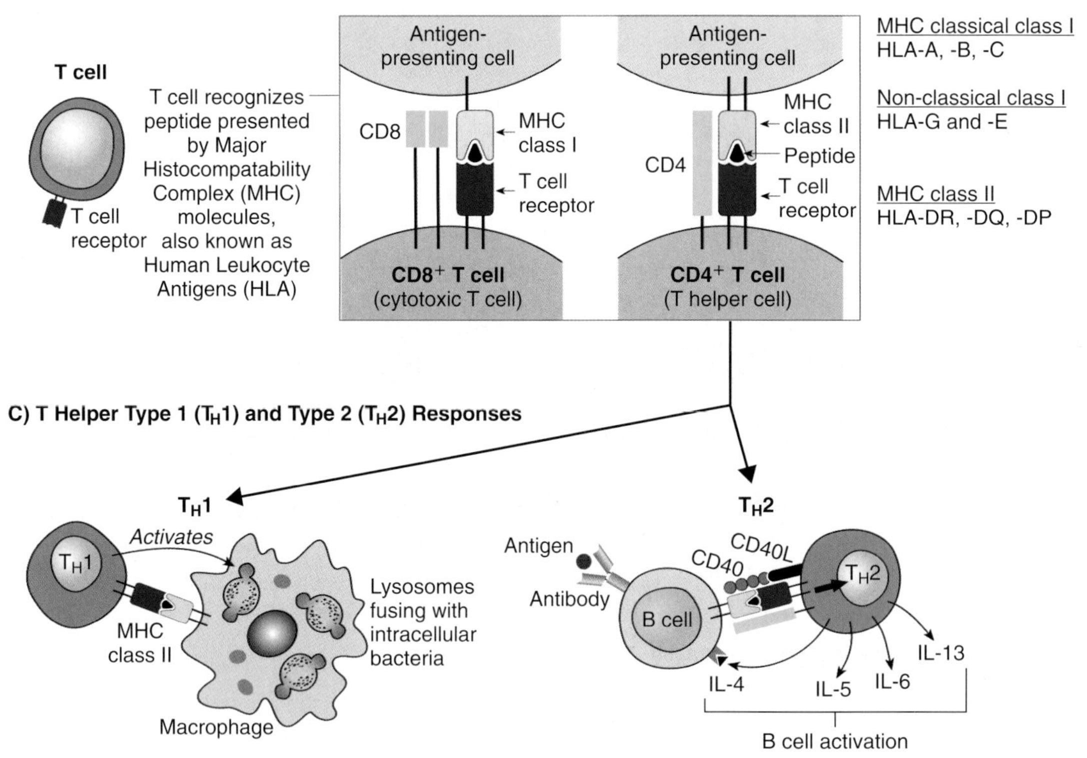

- T helper type 1 response activates macrophages
- Associated cytokines:
  - IFN-γ
  - TNF-α
  - IL-12
  - IL-18
- Induced by *Listeria monocytogenes* and may contribute to intrauterine fetal death

- T helper type 2 response activates B cells
- Associated cytokines:
  - IL-4
  - IL-5
  - IL-6
  - IL-13
- Cytokines with anti-inflammatory properties
  - IL-10
  - TGF-β
- Thought to dominate over Th1 responses in pregnancy

fungal, and viral pathogens. Neutrophils secrete α-defensins and epithelial cells in the gut and lung secrete β-defensins. Both α- and β-defensins are temporally expressed by endometrial epithelial cells during the menstrual cycle.[18–21] Susceptibility to upper genital tract infection may be related in part to the decreased expression of antimicrobial peptides in response to hormonal changes during the menstrual cycle. Many other tissues of the female reproductive tract and placenta secrete defensins, including the vagina, cervix, fallopian tubes, decidua, and chorion.[18,21] Elevated concentrations of vaginal and amniotic fluid defensins have been associated with intra-amniotic infection and preterm birth.[22,23]

Macrophages

Macrophages mature from circulating monocytes that leave the circulation to migrate into tissues throughout the body. Macrophages are an important component of the innate immune system, because they can directly recognize, ingest, and destroy pathogens. Pathogen recognition may occur through PRR, such as TLR, scavenger receptors, and mannose receptors. Macrophages also internalize pathogens or pathogen particles through phagocytosis, macropinocytosis, and receptor-mediated endocytosis. Multiple receptors on the macrophage may induce phagocytosis including the mannose receptor, scavenger receptor, CD14, and complement receptors. Macrophages also produce or release many bactericidal agents after ingesting a pathogen, such as oxygen radicals, nitric oxide, antimicrobial peptides, and lysozyme.

Natural Killer Cells

The NK cell is also a member of the innate immune system with important functions in pregnancy. NK cells represent a lymphoid population that, in contrast to T and B cells, do not develop or express clonally distributed receptors for foreign antigens.[24] They also differ from T cells by their lack of the CD3 T-cell receptor complex. Owing to their early production of cytokines and chemokines, they can lyse target cells without prior sensitization. In adult peripheral blood, NK cells represent about 15 percent of the total circulating lymphoid population. The term NK cells was originally assigned given the ability of these lymphoid cells to directly kill certain tumor cells and virally infected cells in the absence of prior stimulation.[25] These cells also are capable of killing antibody-coated target cells through their CD16 (Fc-receptor complex), a process called antibody-dependent cytoxicity.

The ability of NK cells to recognize and distinguish between normal cells and cells infected with a virus or tumor is based on the concept of "self and non-self" recognition through the expression of MHC class I antigens. During development, NK cells acquire a complex repertoire of activating and inhibitory NK cell receptors. Most of these receptors interact with specific human leukocyte antigen (HLA) families for either an activating or inhibitory effect. The threshold for NK cell activation and killing of target cells is regulated by a fine balance between activating and inhibiting signals (Fig. 4-3).[28] Three major superfamilies of NK cell receptors have been described in humans: the killer cell immunoglobulin-like receptor (KIR), which primarily recognizes HLA-A, -B, -C, -G; the C-type lectin group, which includes

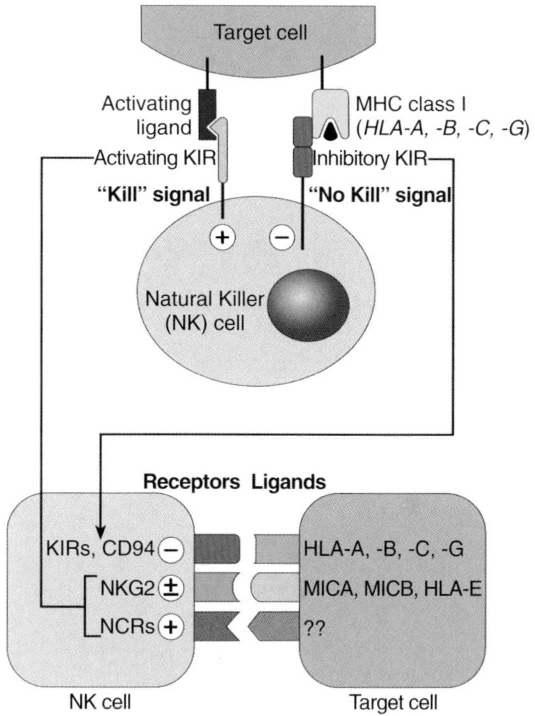

Figure 4-3. Activation and suppression of NK cells. Activation and suppression of NK cell function is carried out through a balance of activating and inhibitory signals. In this figure, a suppressive signal is carried through the interaction of an MHC class I molecule and KIR (killer cell immunoglobulin-like receptor) binding. A tumor or virus-infected cell missing MHC class I molecules may be lysed due to the lack of KIR and MHC class I interaction.

Figure 4-2. The adaptive immune system. The adaptive immune system acts to control infection that has overwhelmed the innate immune system and is also important in immune responses in transplantation rejection and tumor killing. B cells secrete antibodies to protect the extracellular spaces of the body from infection and assist in the activation of T-helper (CD4+) cells (**2A**). Different classes of antibodies reflect structural variations that allow antibodies to be targeted to different bodily compartments and serve slightly different functions. The first step in T-cell activation occurs when the T-cell receptor recognizes a complex of peptide presented by an MHC molecule (**2B**). A CD4+ T cell recognizes peptide presented by MHC class II and a CD8+ T cell interacts with peptides presented by MHC class I. Peptides may be presented by many different types of the listed MHC class I or class II molecules. After activation, the CD4+ T cell (or T-helper cell) may either activate macrophages through a T-helper type 1 response or activate B cells through the T-helper type 2 response (**2C**).

CD94 and NKG2 receptors recognizing HLA-E; and a recently described class of natural cytotoxicity receptors (NCR, Nkp40, Nkp46, Nkp30).[29,30] The specific ligands for NCR are not currently known. NK cells function primarily by killing target cells that have lost or express insufficient amounts of self MHC class I, which is a frequent event in tumor or virus-infected cells that appear to be "missing self."[27]

NK cells can also be differentiated into two populations based on their level of CD56 and CD16 expression. The majority (90 percent) of circulating NK cells are $CD56^{dim}/CD16^{bright}$, whereas the remaining 10 percent of cells are $CD56^{bright}/CD16^{dim}$.[30] The level of CD56 expression also determines if the particular NK cell primarily has cytolytic ($CD56^{dim}$) or cytokine production function ($CD56^{bright}$). In contrast to peripheral blood, the NK cell population that resides in the uterine decidua is primarily $CD56^{bright}$ (see section on uterine leukocytes).

Toll-Like Receptors and Other Pattern-Recognition Receptors of Innate Immunity

Macrophages and neutrophils recognize pathogens by means of cell-surface receptors that discriminate between the surface antigens displayed by pathogens and host cells. These receptors are called PRR and are different from the receptors used by the adaptive immune system. Whereas T or B lymphocytes rearrange gene segments to encode a large repertoire of receptors to recognize an immense variety of antigens, innate immunity depends upon these germ-line encoded receptors to recognize features that are common to many pathogens.

TLR are a recently discovered large family of PRR that play a key role in innate immunity.[6] TLR are now recognized as the principal sensors of pathogens and can activate both the innate and adaptive immune system. At least 11 mammalian Toll homologues have been identified and they recognize a wide range of pathogen ligands (see Fig. 4-1*B*).[31] TLR4 is a TLR that recognizes lipopolysaccharide (LPS), a component of the outermost plasma membrane of gram-negative bacteria (Fig. 4-4).[32,33] LPS from intact or lysed bacteria binds to LPS binding protein (LBP), which is abundant in amniotic fluid and elevated during labor.[34] After LPS binding to LBP, LPS-LBP are then able to bind to the complex involving TLR4, CD14, and MD-2, which initiates a specific intracellular signaling cascade that ultimately leads to translocation of the nuclear transcription factor kappa B (NF-κB) into the cell nucleus. This series of events then leads to cytokine gene expression. TLR4 is expressed on macrophages, dendritic cells, endothelium, and numerous epithelial tissues.

Although an individual TLR recognizes only a subset of all pathogen structures, different types of TLR are thought to collaborate in order to discriminate between common pathogenic microorganisms. TLR2 may associate with either TLR6 or TLR1 to recognize bacterial structures, leading to cytokine induction. TLR also cooperates with many other immune receptors to recognize pathogens including CD14, immunoglobulin receptors, and scavenger receptors.[35]

TLR2 and TLR4 expression have both been demonstrated in the placenta. First trimester trophoblast expresses both TLR2 and TLR4.[36] Activation of TLR2 triggers Fas-mediated apoptosis, whereas TLR4 activation induces cytokine production. The immunologic capability of first-trimester trophoblast to recognize pathogens and induce apoptosis suggests that innate immunity may be an important placental mechanism for triggering spontaneous abortion. TLR4 is also expressed in villous macrophages, villous and extravillous trophoblast, and the amniochorion.[37–39] Expression of TLR4 and TLR2 also increases in the chorioamniotic membranes of women with intraamniotic infection.[39]

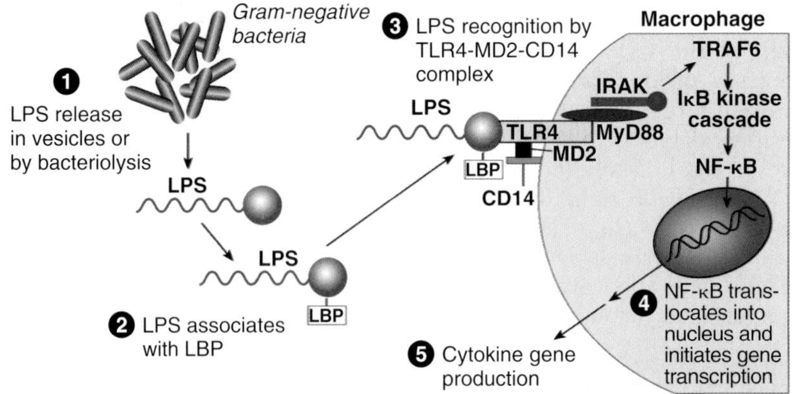

Figure 4-4. Toll-like receptor 4 (TLR4) recognition of liposaccharide (LPS). Recognition of LPS by TLR4 occurs through several steps. (1) LPS is released from intact or lysed bacteria. (2) LPS binds to LPS-binding protein (LBP). (3) The LPS-LBP complex is recognized by a cell surface receptor complex TLR4, CD14, and MD-2. Binding of LPS-LBP to the TLR4, CD14, MD-2 receptor recruits the intracellular adaptor molecule, myeloid differentiation factor 88 (MyD88). Binding of MyD88 promotes the association of IL-1 receptor-associated protein kinase 4 (IRAK). Next, tumor necrosis factor receptor–associated kinase 6 (TRAF6) initiates a signaling cascade resulting in degradation of IkappaB (Iκ-B), which releases nuclear factor kappa B (NF-κB), a transcription factor, into the cytoplasm. (4) NF-κB translocates into the nucleus and activates cytokine gene expression. Although the figure depicts TLR4 activation in a macrophage, many other immunologic and epithelial cells express TLR4 and induce cytokine production through this mechanism.

Although intrauterine injection of LPS induces preterm birth in many murine models, administration of a purified LPS preparation to TLR4 mutant mice does not result in preterm delivery.[40] This finding suggests TLR4 is required for LPS-induced preterm birth in mice and is an important driver of the inflammatory cascade resulting from intra-amniotic infection. There is also a distinct progression in the responsiveness of fetal murine tissue to LPS as a function of gestational age. When fetal lung is exposed to LPS on fetal day 14 (term is 20 days), both the expression of TLR4 and the acute cytokine response are undetectable.[40a] Under the same experimental conditions, TLR4 expression and an acute cytokine response were detected on fetal day 17, with further increases in TLR4 and cytokine production after birth. TLR4 likely controls the magnitude of the LPS-induced cytokine response during the perinatal period, and TLR4 placental expression appears to be dependent on gestational age.[40b]

The Complement System

An important component of the innate immune system is complement, a large number of plasma proteins that cooperate to destroy and facilitate the removal of pathogens (see Fig. 4-1C). Complement is activated by the surface antigens of pathogens. The nature of the initial pathogen trigger determines one of three activation pathways—classical, alternate, and lectin-binding pathways.[41,42] The classical pathway of complement activation is triggered when the complement protein, C1q, binds to antigen-antibody complexes on the surface of pathogens. This binding then results in a series of activation and amplification steps that results in production of the membrane-attack complex (MAC). The MAC is produced from five complement glycoproteins (C5, C6, C7, C8, and C9) that interact to form the multicomponent structure. The primary function of MAC is to form membrane pores or transmembrane channels that result in membrane perturbation and ultimately cell lysis. Formation of the MAC is an important mechanism of host defense against *Neisseria*. Genetic deficiencies in C5-C9 complement proteins have been associated with susceptibility to *Neisseria gonorrhea* and *Neisseria meningitidis*.[41]

The alternate pathway of complement activation is also an essential component of the innate immune system. This system does not require antibody complexes for activation. Low levels of circulating C3b attach directly to the pathogen surface. C3b then catalyzes a series of proteolytic reactions that result in the amplification of C3b and ultimately formation of the MAC. The lectin or mannan-binding pathway is a third pathway of complement activation. In this pathway, mannose-binding protein binds mannose sugar residues on the microbial surface. Mannose-binding protein, a lectin, is markedly elevated during acute phase reactions, and recognizes pathogens expressing the terminal mannose of N-acetylglucosamine. Bacteria or viruses expressing the carbohydrate mannose activate the mannan-binding lectin pathway.

Complement proteins are also detected in the amniotic fluid during intraamniotic infection, and regulation of complement is necessary to protect placental and fetal tissues from inflammation and destruction.[43] Regulatory proteins exist to protect cells from the deleterious effects of complement and are expressed on the placental membranes. Placental tissues at the maternal-fetal interface strongly express several negative regulators of complement activation including CD59 (MAC antagonist), membrane cofactor protein, and decay accelerating factor (inhibitor of C3 and C5 convertases).[44–47]

Cytokines

The release of cytokines and chemokines by macrophages and other immune cells represents an important induced innate immune response (see Fig. 4-1*D* and Table 4-1). Activated macrophages secrete cytokines that

Table 4-1. Cytokines and Their Primary Action

Regulating Immune/Inflammatory Response

CYTOKINE	PRODUCED BY	PRIMARY ACTION
Interferons	Monocytes and macrophages	Produced in response to viruses, bacteria, parasites, and tumor cells. Action includes killing tumor cells and inducing secretion of other inflammatory cytokines. One of the first cytokines that appear during an inflammatory response.
Interleukin-1	Monocytes and macrophages	Induces fever and is an important part of the body's inflammatory response to infection; costimulator of CD4+ T-helper cells
Interleukin-2		Primary growth factor and activation factor for T-cells, NK cells
Interleukin-4	CD4+ T-helper cells	B-cell growth factor for antigen activated B-cells
Interleukin-6	Monocytes and macrophages	Regulates the growth and differentiation of lymphocytes, growth factor for plasma cells, and induces the synthesis of acute phase reactants by the liver
Interleukin-8	Monocytes	Chemoattractant for neutrophils
Interleukin-10	CD4+ T-helper cells	Suppresses the production of interferon, suppresses cell-mediated immunity, enhances humoral immunity
Transforming growth factor-β	T cells and monocytes	Inhibits the proliferation of lymphocytes

initiate inflammatory responses to control infections, which include IL-1, IL-6, IL-12, and tumor necrosis factor alpha (TNF-α). These cytokines are often referred to as proinflammatory, because they mediate fever, lymphocyte activation, tissue destruction, and shock. Pro-inflammatory cytokines have been identified in the amniotic fluid, maternal and fetal blood, and vaginal fluid of women with intraamniotic infection. These cytokines not only serve as a marker of intraamniotic infection, they may also induce preterm labor and neonatal complications.[48,49,49a] The connection between elevated pro-inflammatory cytokines in fetal blood, preterm labor, and increased adverse fetal outcomes has been described as the "fetal inflammatory response syndrome."[49b]

The relative contribution of individual cytokines and chemokines on induction of preterm labor was studied in a unique nonhuman primate model.[49a] Overall, preterm labor was induced by intra-amniotic infusions of IL-1β and TNF-α, but not by IL-6 or IL-8. IL-1β stimulated preterm labor in all cases and an intense contraction pattern. TNF-α induced a variable degree of uterine activity among individual animals characterized as either preterm labor or a uterine contraction pattern of moderate intensity. Despite prolonged elevations in amniotic fluid levels, neither IL-6 nor IL-8 induced an increase in uterine contractions until near term. These results suggested a primary role for IL-1β and TNF-α in the induction of infection-associated preterm birth.

Anti-inflammatory cytokines, like IL-10 and transforming growth factor beta (TGF-β), act to downregulate inflammatory responses. IL-10 has been tested as a potential therapy for infection-induced preterm labor in a nonhuman primate model.[9] In the model, preterm labor was first induced by intraamniotic administration of IL-1 beta (IL-1β). IL-10 inhibited IL-1β-induced uterine contractions and elevations in amniotic fluid TNF-α and prostaglandins. However, other proinflammatory cytokines and hormones involved in labor were not suppressed.

Investigation of the individual effect of a single cytokine on pregnancy or complications of pregnancy in humans has proven challenging for several reasons. Many cytokines tend to be functionally redundant, and the absence of one cytokine can be compensated for by another. Second, there are multiple cytokine receptors (i.e., IL-1 receptor antagonist, IL-18 binding protein) that modulate similar cytokine effects. New families of decoy/silent cytokine receptors and suppressors of cytokine signaling have also been discovered in the placenta and amniotic fluid.[50–52] Finally, molecular variants of cytokines may act as receptor antagonists. Therefore, individual cytokine effects during pregnancy must be interpreted in the context of cytokine receptors, receptor antagonists, and silent cytokine receptors and suppressors of cytokine signaling.

Chemokines

Chemokines represent a class of cytokines that act primarily as chemoattractants and activators of specific types of leukocytes, directing leukocytes to sites of infection. These chemotactic agents constitute a superfamily of small (8 to 10 kilodaltons [kDa]) molecules that can be divided into three groups (C, CC, and CXC) based on the position of either one or two cysteine residues located near the amino terminus of the protein. IL-8, macrophage chemoattract protein-1, and RANTES are a few examples of chemokines. CXC chemokines, like IL-8, bind to CXC receptors (CXCR) and are important for neutrophil activation and mobilization. IL-8 has been described in the amniotic fluid, maternal blood, and vaginal fluid with infection-associated preterm birth.[55a] Other chemokines like RANTES bind to CC receptors (CCR), which are involved in T-lymphocyte trafficking.

Some chemokine receptors are used as a coreceptor for the viral entry of the human immunodeficiency virus (HIV). The two major coreceptors for HIV are CXCR4 and CCR5, both of which are expressed on activated T cells.[56,57] CCR5 is also expressed on dendritic cells and macrophages, which allows HIV to infect these cell types. Rare resistance to HIV infection was discovered to correlate with homozygosity for a nonfunctional variant of CCR5 caused by a gene deletion in the coding region. The gene frequency for this CCR5 variant is highest in Northern Europeans, but has not been detected in many black or Southeast Asian populations, in whom the prevalence of HIV infection is high.[58]

Pathogen Strategies to Avoid the Innate Immune Response

A key feature that distinguishes pathogenic from nonpathogenic microorganisms is their ability to overcome innate immune defenses. Pathogens have developed a variety of strategies to avoid being immediately destroyed by innate immune responses.[59] Preventing phagocytosis is a strategy employed by some bacterial pathogens, like enteropathogenic *Echerichia. coli* and *Pseudomonas aeruginosa.* Both bacteria deliver bacterial proteins into the cell that interfere with signaling downstream from the phagocytic receptor.[60–62] Other intracellular pathogens survive by entering the macrophage and then preventing lysosome fusion with the vesicle that brought them inside the cell. *Mycobacterium tuberculosis,* for example, is able to redirect vesicles entering the macrophage by phagocytosis away from host lysosomes and then alter the vesicle pH to promote virulence of the microbe.[63,64]

ADAPTIVE IMMUNITY

The function of the adaptive immune system is to eliminate infection as the second line of immune defense and provide increased protection against reinfection through "immunologic memory." Adaptive immunity consists of B cells and T cells (lymphocytes), which differ from innate immune cells in several important respects including the mechanism for pathogen recognition and lymphocyte activation. Targeting a specific pathogen component in an immune response is a critical feature of the adaptive immune system and necessary, in most cases, for resolution of the infection. However, achieving this specificity requires generation of an incredible diversity of T-cell receptors (TCR) and B cell receptors (BCR). This creates the potential that self-antigens could be inadvertently targeted, resulting in an autoimmune response. Self-reactive T cells and B cells are thought to either undergo apoptosis in the thymus or be regulated in the periphery. A small population of T cells (regulatory T cells) is now known to contribute to peripheral regulatory mechanisms to prevent autoimmune responses and is discussed specifically in reference to mechanisms of fetal tolerance.

The Major Histocompatibility Complex: Discriminating Self From Non-Self

Unlike macrophages with multiple receptors for different pathogen antigens, each lymphocyte bears antigen receptors specific for a single antigen. The term antigen was originally coined to refer to any molecule that can elicit an antibody response by a B cell. In the context of T lymphocyte activation, antigens are small peptides displayed on host cell surfaces by major histocompatibility complex (MHC) molecules, also called human leukocyte antigens (HLA). Each lymphocyte receptor recognizes a different peptide: MHC complex. The body contains millions of lymphocytes with slightly different antigen receptor specificities, which allows the body to specifically target a wide diversity of pathogens. In order to generate such diversity, complex genetic rearrangements occur during development to produce millions of different genetic variants for lymphocyte receptors. Innate immune cells do not have this capability and their receptors are genetically encoded in the germ line.

The ability of a lymphocyte to recognize self and nonself is based on expression of unique MHC molecules. These highly polymorphic proteins are clustered on the short arm of chromosome 6 and are classically divided into two distinct regions referred to as class I and II. Class I contains classical transplantation HLA genes (HLA-A, -B, and -C) and non-classical HLA genes that are distinguished by their limited polymorphisms (HLA-G -E and -F). Class II molecules include HLA-DR, -DQ, and -DP. The process of graft rejection is beyond the scope of this chapter, but it generally involves recognition of foreign MHC molecules by host T lymphocytes. When confronted with an antigen-presenting cell (APC), in conjunction with self-MHC molecules, host T cells clonally amplify, and if necessary, systematically destroy foreign tissues or cells. Optimizing peripheral blood stem cell and some organ transplants requires matching at multiple HLA class I and II gene loci. This system is significantly different than that of the innate immune system, in which recognition of MHC is not necessary for antigen recognition.

Lymphocyte Activation

Naïve lymphocytes have never encountered their specific antigen. After lymphocyte activation, the cell differentiates and proliferates to create clones of effector lymphocytes, which are capable of removing specific antigen from the body. The effector lymphocytes may then kill the target directly (i.e., CD8+ or cytotoxic T cells) or produce cytokines to kill the pathogen.

Lymphocyte activation is a two-step process that first requires specific binding of the antigen to the lymphocyte receptor. The second activation signal is provided by a "costimulatory" molecule presented by a professional APC. Dendritic cells, macrophages, and B cells are called professional APCs, because they can present the antigen with either MHC class I or II molecules and provide costimulatory signals.

Lymphocyte activation occurs differently for B and T lymphocytes. For B cells, the first signal occurs when a pathogen ligand (i.e., viral coat protein) binds the BCR. The second signal may then be provided by the pathogen itself or by an activated T cell that recognizes degraded pathogen fragments bound to MHC class II molecules on the B-cell surface. The T cell then presents a costimulatory molecule, such as the CD40 ligand (CD40L) to CD40 on the B cell, which provides the critical second signal.

T cells also require two signals for activation. The first occurs when the TCR specifically binds a peptide: MHC complex, usually on the surface of a dendritic cell in a peripheral lymphoid tissue (i.e., spleen, lymph node). The second signal is provided by a professional APC through B7 molecules (B7.1 [CD80] or B7.2 [CD86]) that interact with CD28 on the T cell or by the CD40-CD40L pathway (see Fig. 4-2*C*).

The Humoral Immune Response: B Cells and Antibodies

The function of B cells is to protect the extracellular spaces in the body through which infectious pathogens usually spread (see Fig. 4-2*A*). B cells mainly fight infection by secreting antibodies, also called immunoglobulins (Ig). There are many similarities between B and T lymphocytes. B cells also undergo clonal expansion after antigen stimulation and can be identified by a variety of specific cell surface markers (e.g., CD19, 20, and BCR antigens). Activated B cells may proliferate and differentiate into antibody-secreting plasma cells. Antibodies control infection by several mechanisms including neutralization, opsonization, and complement activation. Neutralization of a pathogen refers to the process of antibody binding, which prevents the pathogen from binding to a cell surface and internalizing. Alternatively, antibodies coating the pathogen may enhance phagocytosis, also referred to as opsonization. Antibodies may also directly activate the classic complement pathway.

Activation of the B cell begins with binding of an antigen by the BCR on the B cell surface. The antigen (e.g., bacterial toxin) is then internalized, degraded, and processed into small peptides that are displayed on the B-cell surface by MHC class II molecules. The second signal for B-cell activation is delivered by a CD4+ T cell that recognizes the antigen presented on the B-cell surface, produces stimulatory cytokines (IL-4) and presents CD40 ligand (CD40L). Binding of the BCR CD40 on the B cell by CD40L, and exposure to IL-4 and other cytokines drives the B cell to proliferate and differentiate into an antibody-secreting plasma cell.[65]

Antibody Isotypes

Antibodies share the same general structure produced by the interaction and binding of four separate polypeptides (Fig. 4-5). These include two identical light (L) chains (molecular weight of 23 kDa), and two identical heavy (H) chains (molecular weight of 55 kDa). The L chains have two domains, variable (V_L) and constant (C_L). The H chains have four domains that consist of three constant regions (C_H1-3) and one variable region (V_H). The composition of the H chain determines the antibody isotype, function, and distribution in the body. In humans, there are five types of H chains designated mu (M), delta (D), gamma (G), alpha (A), and epsilon (E) that correspond to the five major antibody isotypes, (IgM, IgD, IgG, IgA, and IgE). During normal pregnancy, serum concentrations of IgG, IgA, and IgM are unchanged.[66]

In order to effectively combat extracellular pathogens, antibodies must be specialized to cross epithelia into different bodily compartments. In fact, antibodies are made in several distinct classes or isotypes (i.e., IgM and IgG) that vary in their composition. Naïve B cells express only IgM and IgD. B cells must undergo a process called isotype switching to produce different antibody isotypes specialized for different functions and areas of the body. Isotype switching is initiated by the interaction of a B cell with a CD4+ T cell presenting CD40L and cytokines produced in the local milieu.

The first antibody to be produced during an immune response is IgM, because IgM is expressed before isotype switching. The serum concentration of IgM is 50 to 400 mg/dL, with a circulation half-life of 5 days. IgM antibodies are low in affinity but the antibodies form pentamers that compensate by binding at multiple points to the antigen. IgM is highly efficient at activating complement, which is a necessary component during the earliest stages of controlling an infection. IgD is also expressed on naïve B cells, but its function is unknown. Other isotypes dominate in the later stages of antibody responses. IgG represents about 75 percent of serum immunoglobulin in adults with serum concentrations between 500 and 1,500 mg/dL. IgG is further divided into four subclasses (IgG1, IgG2, IgG3, and IgG4). Two subtypes of IgG, IgG1 and IgG3, are efficiently transported across the placenta and are important in conferring humoral immune protection for the fetus after birth. The smaller size of IgG and its monomeric structure allows it to easily diffuse into extravascular sites. IgA is the predominant antibody class in epithelial secretions from the vagina, intestine, and lung, with a serum concentration of 50 to 350 mg/dl. IgA forms dimers and mainly functions as a neutralizing antibody. As a secreted antibody, IgA is not in close contact with either phagocytes or complement and, therefore, is less efficient in opsonization and complement activation. In the vagina, an IgA response mounted against anti–*Gardnerella vaginalis* hemolysin was associated with higher levels of IL-1β.[67] Induction of both an innate and adaptive immune response to lower genital tract infections may be a necessary event in preventing spread to the upper genital tract. IgA is also the predominant antibody in breast milk, which provides the neonate with humoral immunity from the mother. Neonates are particularly susceptible to infectious pathogens through their intestinal mucosa, and IgA is highly effective in neutralizing these bacteria and toxins. Epidemiologic studies indicate that deaths from diarrheal diseases could be reduced between 14- and 24-fold by breast-feeding, owing in part to the maternal-infant transmission of IgA.[68] IgE has the lowest concentration in serum of all the antibodies but is bound efficiently by mast cell receptors. IgE binding of antibody triggers the mast cell to release granules, resulting in an allergic response. Prenatal maternal exposure to allergens may have an effect on IgE in the fetus at birth. In a study of 221 newborns, concentrations of house dust mite allergens correlated in a dose-dependent manner with total IgE measured in heel capillary blood.[69] IgE also plays a prominent role in immune responses to eukaryotic parasites.

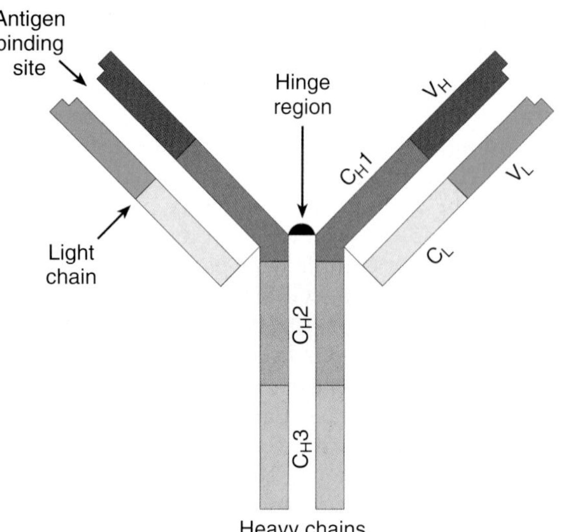

Figure 4-5. Structure of immunoglobulin (IgG).

T CELLS

When pathogens replicate inside cells (all viruses, some bacteria and parasites), they are inaccessible to antibodies and must be destroyed by T cells. T cells are lymphocytes responsible for the cell-mediated immune responses of adaptive immunity, which require direct interactions between T lymphocytes and cells bearing the antigen that the T cells recognize. Common to all mature T cells is the TCR complex. T cells develop the vast array of antigen specificity through a series of TCR gene rearrangements, and many aspects of TCR rearrangements are similar to those producing antibody specificity. For example, during viral replication inside a host cell, viral antigen is expressed on the surface of the infected cell. These foreign antigens are then recognized by T cells along with MHC antigens. In humans, these are referred to as human leukocyte antigens (HLA). MHC class I molecules present peptides from proteins in the cytosol, which may include degraded host or viral proteins. MHC class II molecules bind peptides derived from proteins in intracellular vesicles, and thus display peptides derived from pathogens in macrophage vesicles, internalized by phagocytic cells, and B cells.

A variety of T cells are recognized based on their expression of different cell surface markers (i.e., CD2, CD3, CD4, CD8). Cytotoxic T cells kill infected cells directly and express a variety of cell-surface antigen and specific receptors including CD8. Helper T cells activate B cells and express CD4. Cytotoxic and helper T cells recognize peptides bound to proteins of two different classes of MHC molecules. APCs will present antigen to CD8+ T cells in the context of class I MHC molecules (HLA-A, B, or C). In contrast, APCs that present antigens with MHC class II molecules (HLA-DR, DP, and DQ) interact with T cells bearing CD4.

Each developing T cell generates a unique antigen receptor by rearranging its receptor genes. This process is similar to that which produces diversity in immunoglobulin production where constant region, variable (V), joining (J), and diversity (D) gene rearrangements occur. Lymphocyte development and survival are determined by signals received through their antigen receptors. T cells proliferate in response to antigen in peripheral lymphoid organs, generating effector cells and immunologic memory. T cells can also be divided into two groups based on the type of polypeptide chains forming the TCR. The majority of TCRs are formed by two different polypeptide chains, called alpha and beta (α:β), which function in antigen recognition as previously described. A small number of TCRs are formed instead by gamma and delta polypeptide chains (γ:δ), which may allow the T cell to recognize target antigens directly without the help of an MHC molecule. These T cells represent a minor component of circulating T cells within peripheral blood and migrate into body tissues and epithelia of the intestine, skin, and vagina.

CD4+ T and CD8+ T cells

Early thymic development includes the transition from a CD4-/CD8-/CD3+ prethymocyte that then matures under the influence of IL-7. As maturation and proliferation continue, these cells express both CD4 and CD8. CD4 is a transmembrane glycoprotein of the Ig superfamily and has four extracellular Ig domains. CD8 is made up of two polypeptides designated alpha and beta. CD8+ T cells will be either homodimers (alpha-alpha) or heterodimers (alpha-beta). As maturation continues, cells will express either CD4 or CD8. CD4+ T cells interact with MHC class II alleles, and CD8+ T cells interact with MCH class I alleles.

T-Helper Type 1 and 2 Immune Responses

After a CD4+ T cell encounters its specific antigen presented by MHC Class II, it may differentiate into two main subsets with different functions in the immune response, referred to as T-helper type 1 (Th1) and T-helper type 2 (Th2) (see Fig. 4-2C). The Th1 subset is important in the control of intracellular bacterial infections such as *M. tuberculosis.* Intracellular bacteria survive because the vesicles they occupy do not fuse with intracellular lysosomes, which contain a variety of enzymes and antimicrobial substances. Th1 cells activate macrophages to induce fusion of their lysosomes with vesicles containing the bacteria. Th1 cells also release cytokines and chemokines that attract macrophages to the site of infection, like interferon-γ (IFN-γ), TNF-α, IL-12, and IL-18. Th2 immune responses are mainly responsible for activating B cells by providing a critical "second signal" necessary for B-cell activation. Th2 cells produce cytokines including IL-4, IL-5, IL-6, IL-10, IL-13, and transforming growth factor beta (TGF-β). The signals that trigger differentiation down these two pathways are unknown but are thought to be influenced by cytokines produced in response to the infection.

Adverse effects of Th1 cytokines on murine pregnancy and weakened maternal immunity to intracellular infections requiring Th1 cytokine activity suggest that Th2-type activity predominates in pregnancy.[70–72] IL-10 may be a critical Th2 cytokine in maintaining pregnancy, because it downregulates Th1 cytokine production and prevents fetal resorption in mice genetically predisposed to abortion.[73,74] In a study of women with a history of recurrent spontaneous abortion, maternal cytokine profiles of stimulated peripheral blood mononuclear cells were compared between women with a successful pregnancy and those with a spontaneous abortion. Increased Th2 cytokines were associated with a successful pregnancy, and elevated Th1 cytokines were associted with a spontaneous abortion.[75] Whether Th1 cytokine production causes spontaneous abortion or occurs after fetal death is unknown.[75] Recent evidence suggests that the Th1/Th2 paradigm may be an oversimplification and that cytokine signaling during pregnancy is likely to be a more complicated process.[76]

Pathogen Strategies to Avoid the Adaptive Immune Response

Many pathogens have evolved strategies to evade the adaptive immune response. One approach is to prevent T or B cell activation through interference with cell signaling or T cell activation. *Helicobacter pylori* induces T cells to express Fas ligand, causing T cell apoptosis.[77] *Neisseria gonorrhea* directly inhibits activation of the TCR through expression of the CEACAM1-binding OPA protein on its surface.[78] Mycobacteria induce production of IL-10 and TGF-β, anti-inflammatory cytokines that inhibit T-cell activation.[79,80] *Bordetella pertussis* also induces IL-10 to downregulate the immune response, which may contribute to the production of regulatory T cells that further downregulate T cell activation.[81]

Adaptive immune responses rely upon presentation of pathogen antigens by either MHC class I or class II on the cell surface. Therefore, preventing antigen processing and presentation is a classic strategy employed by pathogens to avoid B and T cell responses. Mycobacteria downregulate the surface expression of class II and interfere with antigen presentation by class II.[82] Specifically, mycobacteria prevent transcription of the main regulator of MHC class II expression, the class II transactivator (CIITA).[83] *Chlamydia trachomatis* also inhibits transcription of the CIITA by degrading an upstream stimulatory factor required for CIITA induction.[84] Degradation of a transcription factor, transcription factor regulatory factor X, by chlamydia also suppresses MHC class I expression.[85]

HIV employs multiple strategies to disable adaptive T cell responses. Targeting viral infection to the CD4+ T cells allows the virus to control and ultimately destroy this important T-cell subset. HIV destroys CD4+ T cells through direct viral killing, lowering the apoptosis threshold of infected cells, and through CD8+ T cells that recognize viral peptides on the CD4+ T cell surface. CD8+ T cells likely contain the infection but are unable to eradicate the virus. Viral mutants produced during one of the earliest steps of viral infection may contribute to escape of virus-infected cells from CD8+ T cell killing. The error-prone reverse transcriptase copies the RNA viral genome into DNA, making "mistakes" that lead to production of these viral variants. The presentation of peptides from HIV variants by CD4+ T cells may also interfere and downregulate the CD8+ T cell response to the original (wild-type) virus. Finally, the HIV negative-regulation factor gene (*nef*) downregulates expression of MHC Class II and CD4, which decreases the presentation of viral antigens on the cell surface.

UTERINE LEUKOCYTES

In the nonpregnant human uterus, many different types of leukocytes are present. Macrophages, uterine NK (u-NK) cells, and mast cells are widely distributed in the uterus, with aggregates of T and B lymphocytes present in the endometrium.[86–88] The role of these leukocytes in immune defense and the menstrual cycle are poorly understood. Mast cells, however, are thought to contribute to the onset of menstruation through the synthesis of proinflammatory cytokines that stimulate endometrial cells to produce matrix metalloproteinases.[89] Matrix metalloproteinases enzymatically degrade the extracellular matrix and may trigger endometrial sloughing. A variety of matrix metalloproteinases are also elevated in amniotic fluid in patients destined to deliver preterm.[90]

Leukocyte populations in the uterus change drastically following implantation and decidualization of the endometrium. Macrophages and u-NK cells then become the most dominant lymphocyte populations. In the first trimester, u-NK cells comprise 30 to 40 percent and macrophages 10 to 15 percent of total decidual cells.[91,92] As gestation advances, there is a dramatic increase in u-NK cells.[93] U-NK cells depend on progesterone for survival, and recruitment of u-NK cells may also be progesterone dependent.[92] Dysregulated migration of u-NK cells occurs in mice genetically defective for the cytokine leukemia inhibitory factor, which has been implicated in implantation failure and early pregnancy loss.[94]

Uterine Macrophages

Uterine macrophages represent up to a third of total leukocytes in pregnancy-associated tissue during the later parts of pregnancy.[95] Macrophages are a major source of inducible nitric oxide synthetase, a rate-limiting enzyme for nitric oxide production. During pregnancy, nitric oxide is thought to relax uterine smooth muscle, and uterine nitric oxide synthetase activity and expression decreases before parturition.[96] Uterine macrophages are also a major source of prostaglandins, inflammatory cytokines, and matrix metalloproteinases that are prominent during term and preterm parturition.[97–99]

Uterine Natural Killer Cells

In contrast to NK cells in peripheral blood, u-NK cells are distinguished by CD56^{bright} expression. U-NK cells also express high levels of CD94/NKG2 that binds to HLA-E and HLA-G on placental trophoblasts. Both of these placental ligands suppress responses by u-NK cells. U-NK cells also have low cytotoxicity against typical NK-cell sensitive targets.[100,101] U-NK cells have the highest expression of CD56, nearly fivefold higher than peripheral blood CD56^{bright} cells, and are also skewed toward cytokine secretion. Analysis of the transcription of 10,000 genes from peripheral blood NK cells (dim and bright) and u-NK cells revealed more than 250 genes in which expression differed at least threefold.[102] At least two of the upregulated proteins, galectin-1 and progestagen-associated protein 14, are known to have immunomodulatory and immunosuppressive functions.

U-NK cells likely contribute to maintenance of the pregnancy and maternal tolerance of the fetus. Mice with genetically defective u-NK cells fail to undergo spiral artery remodeling and normal decidualization, which are critical to normal placentation.[103] This defect is corrected with administration of IFN-γ, a prominent NK cell cytokine, suggesting that uterine leukocytes may play a role in trophoblast invasion.[104] IL-15 is a critical cytokine promoting u-NK differentiation with IL-12 and IL-18 important in later u-NK activation. U-NK cells may also play an important role in complications of pregnancy, such as preeclampsia.[105]

THE FETAL IMMUNE SYSTEM

Descriptions of the development of the fetal immune system are relatively limited, but sufficient information exists to determine that the fetus, even very early in gestation, has innate immune capacity.[106–108] Acquired immunity, particularly the capacity to produce a humoral response, develops more slowly and is not completely functional until well after birth. Many of the immune protective mechanisms that are present to protect the fetus from both pathogen and maternal immune recognition occur at the maternal-fetal interface.

Fetal hematologic development initiates in the fetal yolk sac and aortic-genital ridge.[109,110] The exact contribution of these two sites to hematopoietic development is controversial, with many now favoring the initial site of hematopoietic development for the fetus initiating at the aortic-genital ridge. Hematopoietic stem cells migrate from their site of initial production in the fetal liver, and ultimately reside in the fetal bone marrow, which becomes the major site of hematopoiesis at approximately 28 weeks of gestation.

Fetal thymic development initiates from the third and fourth brachial pouches and cleft. A primordial thymus is present at approximately 7 weeks gestation. The thymus is first colonized with cells from the fetal liver at 8.5 to 9.5 weeks' gestation. These cell express primitive (CD34) and early T cell surface antigen, CD7$^+$.[111,112] Shortly after this, 20 to 50 percent of cells in the fetal thymus express the common T cell surface phenotypes (CD7, CD2). Between 12 and 13 weeks, cells within the fetal liver and spleen express the TCR. By 16 weeks gestation, the fetal thymus has distinct cortical and medullary regions, suggesting functional maturity, and this is confirmed by the brisk response to allogeneic and mitogen stimulation. In the thymus, a multistage developmental process is initiated in the outer cortex by CD7/CD2$^+$ cells. The appearance of CD3$^+$ cells is initially noted in the inner cortex region, followed by the appearance of CD4$^+$ and then CD8$^+$ T cells.[113] This maturational process has also been defined as starting from pro–T-cells bearing CD7/CD45 cell surface phenotypes followed by the appearance of the common T cell marker CD2. The appearance of CD2$^+$/CD7$^+$ thymocytes is then followed by CD3/TCR+ cells, and CD4 and CD8.[114] The majority of intrathymic T cells are thought to be ultimately lost from cell death, as part of the process of self-recognition and self-tolerance. Ultimately, T cells must undergo a process of positive selection, developing the capacity to recognize self MHC class I and II antigens in the context of the T cell receptor-CD3 complex. Functionally, fetal T cells show proliferative capacity very early in gestation. In vitro stimulation by phytohemaglutinin can be demonstrated as early as 10 weeks, and allogeneic responses in mixed lymphocyte culture can be detected in cells obtained from fetal liver as early 9.5 weeks and is consistently seen at 12 weeks of gestation.[115]

The ontogeny of fetal B cell development in many ways parallels the development of T cells, with early pre-B cells (CD19 and CD20) being identified by cell surface markings in the fetal liver by 7 to 8 weeks gestation.[116] Ultimately, these cells are produced in the fetal bone marrow as the marrow becomes the primary hematopoietic organ in the second trimester. Surface expression of IgM can be noted as early as 9 to 10 weeks. Cells in the fetal circulation express the common B cell antigens (CD20) by 14 to 16 weeks gestation, and secretion of IgM has been noted as early as 15 weeks. The level of IgM continues to increase and reaches normal postnatal levels by 1 year of age. The appearance of surface IgG and IgA is noted in fetal B cells at 13 weeks, and secretion of IgG at 20 weeks gestation. Ultimately, cells expressing autoreactive antigens must be eliminated from the B cell repertoire to prevent autoantibody production.[117] Postnatal levels of Ig are not reached until approximately 5 years of age.

NK cells also play an important role in fetal immunity. These cells share a number of antigenic and functional similarities to T cells, but do not rearrange or express T cell antigen receptor genes. Expressed as a percentage of the total lymphocytes, the proportion of NK cells in the fetal circulation is high (30 percent at 13 weeks). Based on their high number, early presence, and the ability to kill cells directly or through antibody mediated toxicity, it is likely that NK cells play a significant role in the fetal innate immune system.

Fortunately, abnormalities of normal immune development are relatively rare. However, when they do occur, they can have profound effects on newborn and child health. Some of the more common immunodeficiencies are listed in Table 4-2.[118,119]

Table 4-2. Common Immune Defects

COMMON NAME	DEFECT	CELLS AFFECTED	COMMENTS
X-SCID	Common gamma chain of IL-2 receptor	T cells and NK cells	X-linked recessive and most common form of SCID accounting for about 45–50% of cases
ADA-SCID	Defect in purine metabolism leading to abnormal accumulation of adenocine	T cells, B cells, and NK cells	Autosomal recessive affecting both male and female infants. Accounts for about 20% of SCID cases.
Jak-3 deficiency	Mutation on chromosome 19 of Jannis kinase-3 that is activated by cytokine binding to the common gamma chain of the IL-2 receptor	T cells and NK cells	Autosomal recessive affecting both male and female infants. Accounts for about 10% of SCID cases.
Hyper-IgM syndrome	Defect in CD40L (T cell) and CD40 (B cell) signaling resulting in the inability of for immunoglobulin class switching	Elevated levels of IgM with switch to IgG	X-linked and autosomal recessive

ADA-SCID, adenosine deaminase severe combined immunodeficiency; IgG, immunoglobulin G; IgM, immunoglobulin M; IL-2, interleukin-2; NK, natural killer; X-SCID, X-linked severe combined immunodeficiency.

MECHANISMS OF FETAL TOLERANCE

Pregnancy is a unique immunologic phenomenon, in which the normal immune rejection of foreign tissues does not occur. The placenta is not a barrier between maternal and fetal cells, and these cells come into direct contact in several locations, which represent the maternal-fetal interface (Fig. 4-6). Syncytiotrophoblast, the outermost layer of chorionic villi, are in direct contact with maternal blood in the intervillous space. Extravillous trophoblast in the decidua are in contact with many different maternal cells, including macrophages, u-NK cells, and T cells. Endovascular trophoblast replace endothelial cells in the maternal spiral arteries and are in direct contact with maternal blood. Finally, fetal and maternal macrophages are in close contact in the chorion layer of the fetal membranes.

Immunologic mechanisms of fetal tolerance must be acting at the maternal-fetal interface to prevent fetal rejection, because the maternal immune system clearly recognizes fetal cells as foreign. Approximately 30 percent of primiparous or multiparous women develop antibodies against the inherited paternal HLA of the fetus.[120,121] Persistence of these antibodies does not appear to be harmful to the fetus.[122,123] Persistent fetal cells in the mother may play a role in the persistence of these antibodies, because in some women the antibodies persist, whereas in others they disappear. Formation of IgG antibodies against inherited paternal HLA antigens is associated with the presence of primed cytotoxic T lymphocytes specific for these HLA antigens.[124] Maternal T lymphocytes specific for fetal antigens do exist during pregnancy, but appear to be hyporesponsive.[125,126] The normal growth and development of the fetus despite maternal immune recognition requires several maternal and fetal adaptations that, in most women, allow pregnancy to be carried uneventfully to term.

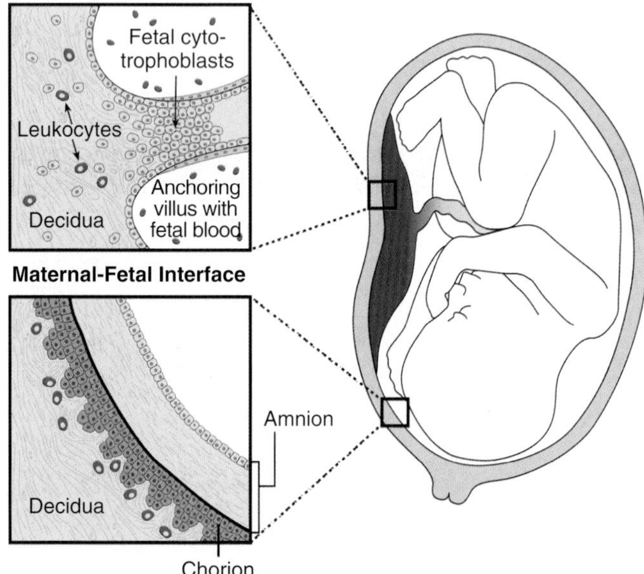

Figure 4-6. The maternal-fetal interface and mechanisms of fetal tolerance. Maternal and fetal cells are in close contact in several sites of the placenta including the decidua and chorion layer of the fetal membranes. The main mechanisms proposed to explain immunologic tolerance of the fetus by the mother are listed.

Tolerance Through Human Leukocyte Antigens

Fetal trophoblast and cells in the placental membranes are in direct contact with maternal blood and cells, and should be at risk for maternal immunologic rejection. The expression of MHC molecules by these fetal cells may at first appear to be an evolutionary disadvantage that could trigger a significant graft rejection immune response. Of the various forms of placental trophoblast, only the extravillous trophoblast cells express MHC class I molecules, and those that are expressed (HLA-C, -E and -G) have identified NK cell–inhibiting receptors. HLA-E, for example, binds CD94/NKG2 KIR receptors on NK cells. Both HLA-C and HLA-E are ubiquitously expressed, whereas HLA-G expression is almost entirely limited to extravillous trophoblast.[127]

Owing to its unique distribution on fetal trophoblastic tissue, HLA-G is thought to be a significant component of fetal tolerance. Although the exact function of HLA-G is unknown, evidence indicates that HLA-G protects the invasive cytotrophoblast from killing by u-NK cells, as well as containment of placental infection.[128,129] HLA-G also inhibits macrophage activation through ILT-4, an inhibitory receptor.[130,131] The presence of a soluble form of HLA-G in high concentration in the amniotic fluid that declines near term suggests a possible role in the initiation of normal labor.[132] HLA-G, through interactions with u-NK cells, likely contributes to maintaining immune tolerance at the maternal-fetal interface and normal pregnancy. However, other mechanisms must also contribute to this process because normal pregnancies in women and fetus lacking a functional HLA-G gene (HLA-G null) have been described.[133]

Tolerance Through Regulation of Maternal T Cells

Maternal T cells acquire a transient state of tolerance for specific paternal alloantigens. This has been most elegantly demonstrated in female mice that were sensitized to known paternal antigens before pregnancy.[125] The female mice became tolerant to the same paternal antigens expressed by the fetus that were previously recognized and destroyed. Several mechanisms must therefore exist to suppress maternal T-cell responses.

A special population of T cells, called regulatory T cells, suppress antigen-specific immune responses and are elevated in the maternal circulation of women and mice during pregnancy.[134–137] Regulatory T cells (CD4+CD25+) act mainly to prevent autoimmune responses from occurring when self-reactive T cells escape from the thymus during normal T cell development. The mechanism of regulatory T cell suppression of T cell responses is unknown but may involve either direct cell contact or production of anti-inflammatory cytokines, like IL-10 and TGF-β. Estrogen has recently been shown to increase proliferation of regulatory T cells, and the higher levels of estrogen in pregnancy may drive expansion of this cell population during pregnancy.[138] In addition, spontaneous abortion could be prevented in a unique murine model by the transfer of regulatory T cells from mice with a normal pregnancy into mice destined to abort.[139]

Another strategy for suppressing maternal T cell responses at the maternal-fetal interface involves tryptophan depletion by indoleamine 2,3 dioxygenase (IDO), an enzyme that catabolizes tryptophan.[140] IDO normally functions as an innate antimicrobial defense mechanism by allowing cells to deplete tryptophan from intracellular pools or local microenvironments. IDO is thought to contribute to T cell hyporesponsiveness during pregnancy, because tryptophan is an essential amino acid for T cell function. IDO-producing cells can be identified in the decidua of human and murine placenta a few days after implantation.[141–143] At this interface, IDO creates a local tissue microenvironment that precludes maternal T-cell activation to fetal alloantigens. Inhibition of IDO leads to rapid rejection and abortion of murine fetuses a few days after implantation.[144] By contrast, mice pregnant with a genetically identical fetus did not reject their fetuses after exposure to an IDO inhibitor.[143] Regulatory T cells may also stimulate IDO expression, which may link these two mechanisms for downregulating T cell responses.[145]

Activated maternal T cells may also be killed through interactions with Fas ligand (FasL) and TNF-related apoptosis-inducing ligand/Apo-2L (TRAIL) expressed on placental trophoblast.[146–151] Both TRAIL and FasL may cooperate to control lymphocyte proliferation after activation and induce apoptotic cell death.

Recently, another mechanism for maternal tolerance of the fetus was proposed that takes into account cell trafficking, which occurs between the mother and fetus.[151a] Fetal cells escape into maternal blood and how the mother tolerates these cells is poorly understood. The hypothesis describes how a significant impact on maternal immunity is expected as a result of continuous shedding of apoptotic synctiotrophoblast debris throughout gestation, a process recently appreciated to result in gram quantities of apoptotic fetal debris entering the maternal circulation daily. Maternal dendritic cells are proposed to present fetal HLA derived from apoptotic synctiotrophoblast under non-inflammatory conditions, leading to tolerogenic signals and tolerance of fetal cells. This novel hypothesis was also suggested to explain the beneficial effects of pregnancy on rheumatoid arthritis, an autoimmune disease that remits or improves in nearly three-quarters of women during pregnancy. Amelioration of RA may occur during pregnancy as a secondary benefit of changes in the maternal peripheral tolerance to fetal cells.

Tolerance Through Regulation of Complement and Cytokines

In the absence of certain autoimmune disorders, serum complement levels are unchanged or elevated during normal pregnancy.[154,155] However, local inhibition of complement in the placenta may be important in preventing certain immunologic-mediated complications of pregnancy. In a murine model of antiphospholipid antibody-induced abortion, antagonism of factor B (alternative complement component) protected against immune-mediated fetal loss.[156] Defects of placental formation were also observed in a murine model associated with activation of the alternative complement pathway and maternal C3.[157] Finally, several negative regulators of complement are expressed by trophoblast, including CD59 (membrane attack complex antagonist), membrane cofactor protein, and decay accelerating factor (inhibitors of C3 and C5 convertases).[46,47] When a negative regulator of murine complement *Crry* was genetically ablated, embryo survival was compromised and placental inflammation observed.[158] C3 activation plays a major role in fetal rejection in this model, because the embryos survived when genetically deficient *Crry* mice were mated to C3-deficient mice. Therefore, complement activation at the maternal-fetal interface may contribute significantly to fetal tolerance.

Although it is speculated that uterine or placental leukocytes regulate trophoblast invasion through cytokine production, many studies in transgenic mouse models have not linked defects in cytokine production with abnormal invasion and pregnancy loss.[92] Among the Th2 cytokines thought to be protective for pregnancy, there is a great deal of functional redundancy. Genetic deficiencies in four of these cytokines (IL-4, IL-5, IL-9, IL-13), did not reduce murine fetal or neonatal survival.[159] Other evidence now implicates IFN-γ in normal placental vascular development, which was previously thought to be detrimental for pregnancy.[160] Whether Th2 cytokines play a major role in fetal tolerance and pregnancy maintenance is unknown.[76]

IMMUNITY IN INFECTION-ASSOCIATED PRETERM BIRTH

Considerable evidence suggests that the immunologic response to infection drives preterm labor in women with intra-amniotic infection. Intrauterine infection is present in most cases of the earliest preterm births and incites an inflammatory response believed to result in preterm labor.[161–168] Proinflammatory cytokines and chemokines likely play a central role in the pathogenesis of preterm labor. These inflammatory mediators include IL-1β, IL-6, IL-8, and tumor necrosis factor (TNF-α). Many placental tissues and immune cells in the placenta produce cytokines/chemokines in response to bacteria or bacterial products including amniotic epithelium, macrophages, decidual cells, and trophoblasts.

A role for proinflammatory cytokines/chemokines in the development of preterm labor is based upon several observations. Amniotic fluid concentrations of IL-1, IL-6, IL-8, and TNF-α are elevated in humans and rabbits with intra-amniotic infection and preterm labor.[2–5,169,170] Bacterial products stimulate the production of IL-1β, IL-6, and TNF-α by human amniotic epithelium, decidua, and trophoblasts.[171] These cytokines stimulate prostaglandin production in decidual explants and amniotic epithelial cell lines in vitro.[2,3,172] Finally, the administration of recombinant IL-1β into the amniotic fluid of pregnant nonhuman primates or systemically in mice induces preterm labor.[49a,173] However, the relative contribution of these proinflammatory cytokines and chemokines to human preterm labor is unknown. Mice that are genetically deficient in the IL-1 receptor remain susceptible to preterm delivery induced by intrauterine injection of heat-killed *E. coli.*[174] IL-6 and IL-8 are also unlikely to be required for infection-induced preterm birth based on data in a mouse and nonhuman primate model.[49a,175,176]

An important immunologic candidate gene linked to preterm labor in genetic association studies is TNF-α. TNF-α is a proinflammatory cytokine present in the amniotic fluid of women with intrauterine infection delivering preterm.[2,177,178] A TNF-α polymorphism that directly affects gene expression is located at nucleotide position -308, and TNF2 (uncommon allele) correlates with enhanced TNF-α production in vitro and in vivo.[177,179] TNF2 homozygosity is associated with an increased susceptibility to cerebral malaria and higher rates of septic shock and death.[180,181] A genetic association study of preterm birth correlated TNF2 homozygosity in 1,048 children with a history of their preterm birth in Western Kenya.[182] Another study associated carriage of TNF2 with a 3-fold increased rate of chorioamnionitis.[183] However, other studies have not linked TNF2 with chorioamnionitis or preterm birth.[184–186] In one study, although there was no significant association between TNF2 carriers (heterozygotes or homozygotes) and preterm delivery, a subgroup analysis revealed an association between TNF2 carriers and preterm premature rupture of the membranes (PPROM).[187] This illustrates a potentially important gene-environment interaction, in which genetic susceptibility may lower the threshold for PPROM, but an environmental factor like subclinical genital tract infection may still be critical to initiate the process. Other genetic association studies have targeted a variety of candidate genes, but the studies have not been repeated or confirmed in different populations.

Several immunomodulators have been successful in inhibiting contractions or delaying infection-induced preterm birth in a nonhuman primate model. Initial studies investigated the efficacy of immunomodulators on preterm labor induced by IL-1β. Dexamethasone (corticosteroid), indomethacin (inhibitor of prostaglandin synthesis), and IL-10 (anti-inflammatory cytokine) were studied. All three inhibited IL-1β–induced uterine contractility but differed in their ability to suppress specific amniotic fluid cytokines and prostaglandins.[8,9] When dexamethasone and indomethacin were used with antibiotics to treat a *Group B Streptococcal* infection in the nonhuman primate model, gestation was significantly longer than in controls treated with antibiotics alone.[187a] This evidence suggests that blockade of the immune response, in combination with antibiotics, may delay infection-induced preterm birth. Whether this approach ultimately proves to reduce preterm birth or neonatal morbidity remains to be demonstrated.

MATERNAL-FETAL HUMAN LEUKOCYTE ANTIGEN COMPATIBILITY AND RECURRENT PREGNANCY LOSS

The hypothesis that maternal-fetal HLA incompatibility is beneficial in mammalian pregnancy was first proposed in the 1960s based on observations of larger placental size with genetically incompatible murine fetuses compared with compatible fetuses.[189] Incompatible murine zygotes were also more likely to implant than compatible zygotes.[190] Several studies began to test the idea that maternal-fetal HLA compatibility in human pregnancy might also result in defective implantation or placentation predisposing to spontaneous abortion. The first studies to evaluate this hypothesis in humans demonstrated significantly more matching at the HLA-A and HLA-B loci among couples with a history of recurrent spontaneous abortion of unknown etiology, compared with fertile control couples.[191,192] However, more than 30 studies of HLA matching in couples with recurrent miscarriage have yielded conflicting results. There is no clear relationship between HLA matching and fetal loss from these retrospective studies.[193] Prospective studies in the Hutterites, one of the most inbred human populations, suggest that HLA matching is a significant risk factor for recurrent spontaneous abortion.[194–196] The overall significance of these findings remains unknown. Randomized immunologic-based therapeutic trials in couples with HLA compatibility and recurrent pregnancy loss have produced conflicting results likely because they preceded a thorough understanding of this phenomenon and the heterogeneity of the populations tested.[197,198]

NATURAL KILLER CELLS, HUMAN LEUKOCYTE ANTIGEN-C, AND PREECLAMPSIA

Although preeclampsia is likely a mutifactorial disorder, there is evidence to suggest that there may be an immunologic component in some cases. In some cases, development of preeclampsia appears to be related to interactions between maternal u-NK cells and KIR.[105] As noted earlier, KIR are a group of NK cell receptors that function to either promote activation or suppression of NK cells function. The KIR gene locus consists of 7 to 15 closely arranged genes.[199] KIR can be generalized to form two groups, designated *A* and *B,* based on the relative content of genes encoding inhibitory and activating KIR. The simpler group, *A* haplotypes, is primarily comprised of inhibitory KIR genes, whereas the more complicated group, *B* haplotypes, has genes encoding both inhibitory and activating KIRs. When polymorphisms of HLA-C were compared with KIR pair haplotypes (AA, AB, BB), it was noted that women lacking most or all activating KIR genotypes (BB) with a fetus expressing HLA-C2 genes were at the highest risk of developing preeclampsia. More important, the risk for development of preeclampsia was related to the relative level of activating KIR. The correlation between HLA and KIR genotype suggests that overly inhibited u-NK cells may be responsible for causing trophoblast to prematurely cease remodeling of maternal blood vessels, thereby increasing the probability for preeclampsia. Studies of pregnant NK cell–defective mice provide further support for this model. Impaired modification of the spiral arteries during murine pregnancy is remedied by administration of IFN-γ, a prominent NK cell cytokine.[160] It is important to note that only a minority of pregnancies with HLA-C2 fetuses and AA mothers developed preeclampsia.

MATERNAL-FETAL CELL TRAFFICKING, MICROCHIMERISM, AND AUTOIMMUNE DISEASE

The application of molecular techniques to the study of human pregnancy has demonstrated that bidirectional cell trafficking occurs routinely between the mother and the fetus.[12] Thus, in nearly every pregnancy, cells that originate from the fetus can be found in the mother, and conversely, cells that originate from the mother can be found in the fetus. The long-term persistence of fetal cells in the mother and maternal cells in her progeny leads to the coexistence of at least two cell populations in a single person and is referred to as microchimerism.[10,13] Other potential sources of foreign cells leading to microchimerism can occur as a result of cell trafficking between twins in utero and after a nonirradiated blood transfusion.[200,201] Substantial levels of fetal cells and DNA have also been detected in the circulation of women undergoing elective termination of pregnancy.[202]

The concept that naturally acquired microchimerism from pregnancy might contribute to autoimmune disease arose in part from observations of iatrogenic chimerism in transplantation.[203] After hematopoietic stem cell transplantation, donor cells may attack the recipient, resulting in graft-versus-host disease (GVHD). Chronic GVHD shares many clinical similarities with autoimmune diseases including systemic sclerosis (i.e., scleroderma), primary biliary cirrhosis, Sjögren's syndrome, and sometimes myositis and systemic lupus erythematosus.[204] Other observations contributing to the hypothesis included the predominance of autoimmune diseases in women in post-childbearing years and the observation that the donor-recipient human leukocyte antigen (HLA) relationship is a critical component of both chronic GVHD and graft rejection.[203] The particular HLA alleles and the HLA relationship between the patient and that of the microchimeric cells also appear to be important factors in determining whether microchimerism has a detrimental, neutral or possibly even beneficial effect on the host. Although beneficial effects of microchimerism have not been specifically shown, it seems likely that fetal and maternal microchimerisms provide benefits to the host because both are commonly found in healthy individuals.

Most studies of fetal microchimerism test for male DNA or male cells as a marker of fetal microchimerism in women with sons. Initial studies of fetal microchimerism in autoimmune disease focused on systemic sclerosis, a disease with clinical similarities to chronic GVHD. The first report described a prospective blinded study of women with systemic sclerosis and healthy women who had given birth to at least one son.[205] This study also reported results of DNA-based HLA typing in which women with systemic sclerosis, healthy control women, and all of their children were studied. Prior birth of a child indistinguishable from the mother for genes encoding HLA-DR molecules was associated with an almost ninefold increased risk of systemic sclerosis.

Fetal microchimerism has also been investigated in diseases such as autoimmune thyroiditis, primary biliary cirrhosis, Sjögren's syndrome, and systemic lupus erythematosus (Fig. 4-7).[11] Maternal microchimerism has been investigated in systemic sclerosis, myositis, and neonatal lupus.[11] Evidence implicating fetal microchimerism is strongest in systemic sclerosis, in which quantitatively higher levels of fetal microchimerism have been found and particular HLA relationships of mother and child are associated with increased risk of subsequent systemic sclerosis in the mother.[205] Maternal microchimerism is implicated in juvenile myositis and neonatal lupus.[206,207,207a] The long-term consequences of naturally acquired microchimerism derived from pregnancy are not yet known. It is likely that microchimerism can have an adverse, neutral, or beneficial effect on the host, depending on other factors with HLA genes and the HLA-relationship among cells probably of key importance. Elucidating the mechanisms by which naturally acquired microchimerism is permitted without detriment to the host may lead to novel strategies with application to prevention and/or treatment of autoimmune diseases.

SUMMARY

During pregnancy, the immunologic adaptations, particularly at the maternal-fetal interface, are remarkable. Although we have gained tremendous insight into how the maternal-fetal interface adapts to the challenge of maintaining the pregnancy and protecting the fetus from immunologic attack, mechanisms that control this aspect of pregnancy are only partially understood. As we gain more knowledge of how pregnancy is maintained in the context of an otherwise normally functioning immune system, we hope to also gain insight into the development and treatment of common complications of pregnancy such as preeclampsia,[105] preterm labor,[208] and maternal autoimmune disorders.[11]

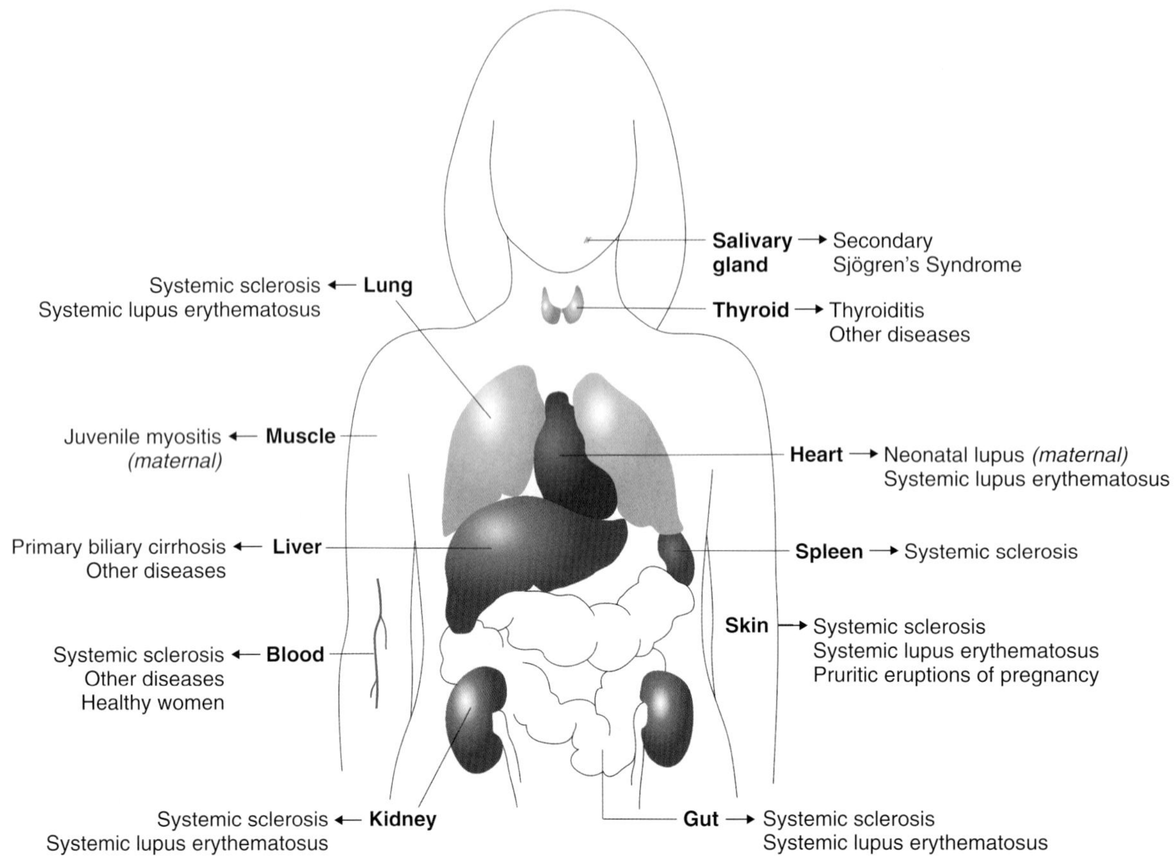

Figure 4-7. Tissues in which fetal (or maternal) microchimerism has been detected and whether detection was in women with aotoimmune disease or healthy women. Bidirectional cell trafficking occurs across the placenta during pregnancy and small populations of fetal and maternal cells persist in mother and child respectively for decades after childbirth. Recent studies examining fetal and maternal microchimerism provide support for the possibility that microchimerism could contribute to the pathogenesis of selected diseases, particularly systemic sclerosis, autoimmune thyroid disease, myositis and neonatal lupus.

Key Points

- Innate immune responses directly attack cells infected by bacteria or viruses. These defense mechanisms include pattern recognition receptors used by immune cells to destroy foreign cells.
- NK cells are important cells of the innate immune system. They also play an important role at the maternal-fetal interface, where they are involved in regulation of trophoblast invasion.
- Maternal concentrations of immunoglobulin do not change during pregnancy.
- $CD4^+$ T cells interact with MHC class II molecules and $CD8^+$ T cells interact with MHC class I molecules.
- Pathogens have developed a variety of mechanisms to avoid detection and destruction by host immune cells. These mechanisms include production of anti-inflammatory cytokines, reducing the expression of MHC Class II, and direct killing of specific host immune cells.
- Fetal immune development occurs early in gestation, and marked activation is frequently seen during intrauterine infection.
- Uterine leukocytes play an important role in the immune acceptance of the fetus, initiation of labor, and the regulation of placental development.
- HLA-G is uniquely distributed on fetal trophoblast cells. There is also a soluble form of HLA-G in high concentration in amniotic fluid.
- Genetic mutations of inflammatory cytokines have been associated with preterm birth.
- Cells can traverse the placenta from either the fetus or the mother. In most women, these cells persist at very low concentrations and have been implicated in a variety of autoimmune diseases.

REFERENCES

1. Medawar PB: The immunology of transplantation. Harvey Lect 4:144, 1956.
2. Romero R, Manogue KR, Mitchell MD, et al: Infection and labor. IV. Cachectin-tumor necrosis factor in the amniotic fluid of women with intraamniotic infection and preterm labor. Am J Obstet Gynecol 161:336, 1989.
3. Romero R, Brody DT, Oyarzun E, et al: Infection and labor. III. Interleukin-1: a signal for the onset of parturition. Am J Obstet Gynecol 160:1117, 1989.
4. Romero R, Avila C, Santhanam U, Sehgal PB: Amniotic fluid interleukin 6 in preterm labor. Association with infection. J Clin Invest 85:1392, 1990.
5. Romero R, Ceska M, Avila C, et al: Neutrophil attractant/activating peptide-1/interleukin-8 in term and preterm parturition. Am J Obstet Gynecol 165:813, 1991.
6. Hitti J, Hillier SL, Agnew KJ, et al: Vaginal indicators of amniotic fluid infection in preterm labor. Obstet Gynecol 97:211, 2001.
7. Romero R, Mazor M, Munoz H, et al: The preterm labor syndrome. Ann N Y Acad Sci 734:414, 1994.
8. Sadowsky DW, Haluska GJ, Gravett MG, et al: Indomethacin blocks interleukin 1 β–induced myometrial contractions in pregnant rhesus monkeys. Am J Obstet Gynecol 183:173, 2000.
9. Sadowsky DW, Novy MJ, Witkin SS, Gravett MG: Dexamethasone or interleukin-10 blocks interleukin-1beta-induced uterine contractions in pregnant rhesus monkeys. Am J Obstet Gynecol 188:252, 2003.
10. Bianchi DW, Zickwolf GK, Weil GJ, et al: Male fetal progenitor cells persist in maternal blood for as long as 27 years postpartum. Proc Natl Acad Sci U S A 93:705, 1996.
11. Adams KM, Nelson JL: Microchimerism: an investigative frontier in autoimmunity and transplantation. JAMA 291:1127, 2004.
12. Lo YM, Lau TK, Chan LY, et al: Quantitative analysis of the bidirectional fetomaternal transfer of nucleated cells and plasma DNA. Clin Chem 46:1301, 2000.
13. Maloney S, Smith A, Furst DE, et al: Microchimerism of maternal origin persists into adult life. J Clin Invest 104:41, 1999.
14. Li Y, Di Naro E, Vitucci A, et al: Detection of paternally inherited fetal point mutations for beta-thalassemia using size-fractionated cell-free DNA in maternal plasma. JAMA 293:843, 2005.
15. Ober C, Van Der Ven K: Immunogenetics of reproduction: an overview. Curr Top Microbiol Immunol 222:1, 1997.
16. Beutler B: Innate immune responses to microbial poisons: discovery and function of the Toll-like receptors. Annu Rev Pharmacol Toxicol 43:609, 2003.
17. Romero R, Avila C, Brekus CA, Morotti R: The role of systemic and intrauterine infection in preterm parturition. Ann N Y Acad Sci 622:355, 1991.
18. Svinarich DM, Gomez R, Romero R: Detection of human defensins in the placenta. Am J Reprod Immunol 38:252, 1997.
19. Quayle AJ: The innate and early immune response to pathogen challenge in the female genital tract and the pivotal role of epithelial cells. J Reprod Immunol 57:61, 2002.
20. Valore EV, Park CH, Quayle AJ, et al: Human beta-defensin-1: an antimicrobial peptide of urogenital tissues. J Clin Invest 101:1633, 1998.
21. King AE, Critchley HO, Kelly RW: Innate immune defences in the human endometrium. Reprod Biol Endocrinol 1:116, 2003.
22. Espinoza J, Chaiworapongsa T, Romero R, et al: Antimicrobial peptides in amniotic fluid: defensins, calprotectin and bacterial/permeability-increasing protein in patients with microbial invasion of the amniotic cavity, intra-amniotic inflammation, preterm labor and premature rupture of membranes. J Matern Fetal Neonatal Med 13:2–21, 2003.
23. Balu RB, Savitz DA, Ananth CV, et al: Bacterial vaginosis, vaginal fluid neutrophil defensins, and preterm birth. Obstet Gynecol 101:862, 2003.
24. Moretta A, Bottino C, Mingari MC, et al: What is a natural killer cell? Nat Immunol 3:6, 2002.
25. Moretta L, Bottino C, Pende D, et al: Human natural killer cells: their origin, receptors and function. Eur J Immunol 32:1205, 2002.
26. Carayol G, Robin C, Bourhis JH, et al: NK cells differentiated from bone marrow, cord blood and peripheral blood stem cells exhibit similar phenotype and functions. Eur J Immunol 28:1991, 1998.
27. Ljunggren HG, Karre K: In search of the "missing self": MHC molecules and NK cell recognition. Immunol Today 11:237–44, 1990.
28. Colucci F, Di Santo JP, Leibson PJ: Natural killer cell activation in mice and men: different triggers for similar weapons? Nat Immunol 3:807, 2002.
29. Natarajan K, Dimasi N, Wang J, et al: Structure and function of natural killer cell receptors: multiple molecular solutions to self, nonself discrimination. Annu Rev Immunol 20:853, 2002.
30. Cooper MA, Fehniger TA, Caligiuri MA: The biology of human natural killer-cell subsets. Trends Immunol 22:633–40, 2001.
31. Takeda K, Kaisho T, Akira S: Toll-like receptors. Annu Rev Immunol 21:335–76, 2003.
32. Poltorak A, He X, Smirnova I, et al: Defective LPS signaling in C3H/HeJ and C57BL/10ScCr mice: mutations in Tlr4 gene. Science 282:2085–8, 1998.
33. Henneke P, Takeuchi O, Van Strijp JA, et al: Novel engagement of CD14 and multiple toll-like receptors by group B streptococci. J Immunol 167:7069, 2001.
34. Gardella C, Hitti J, Martin TR, et al: Amniotic fluid lipopolysaccharide-binding protein and soluble CD14 as mediators of the inflammatory response in preterm labor. Am J Obstet Gynecol 184:1241, 2001.
35. Mukhopadhyay S, Herre J, Brown GD, Gordon S: The potential for toll-like receptors to collaborate with other innate immune receptors. Immunology 112:521–30, 2004.
36. Abrahams VM, Bole-Aldo P, Kim YM, et al: Divergent trophoblast responses to bacterial products mediated by TLRs. J Immunol 173:4286, 2004.
37. Holmlund U, Cebers G, Dahlfors AR, et al: Expression and regulation of the pattern recognition receptors Toll-like receptor-2 and Toll-like receptor-4 in the human placenta. Immunology 107:145, 2002.
38. Kumazaki K, Nakayama M, Yanagihara I, et al: Immunohistochemical distribution of Toll-like receptor 4 in term and preterm human placentas from normal and complicated pregnancy including chorioamnionitis. Hum Pathol 35:47, 2004.
39. Kim YM, Romero R, Chaiworapongsa T, et al: Toll-like receptor-2 and -4 in the chorioamniotic membranes in spontaneous labor at term and in preterm parturition that are associated with chorioamnionitis. Am J Obstet Gynecol 191:1346, 2004.
40. Elovitz MA, Wang Z, Chien EK, et al: A new model for inflammation-induced preterm birth: the role of platelet-activating factor and Toll-like receptor-4. Am J Pathol 163:2103, 2003.

40a. Harju K, Ojaniemi M, Rounioja S, et al: Expression of toll-like receptor 4 and endotoxin responsiveness in mice during perinatal period. Pediatr Res 57:644, 2005.

40b. Adams KM, Lucas J, Kapur RP, Stevens AM: LPS induces translocation of TLR4 in amniotic epithelium. Placenta 2006 Oct 18 [Epub ahead of print].

41. Walport MJ: Complement. Second of two parts. N Engl J Med 344:1140, 2001.
42. Walport MJ. Complement. First of two parts. N Engl J Med 344:1058–66, 2001.
43. Elimian A, Figueroa R, Canterino J, et al: Amniotic fluid complement C3 as a marker of intra-amniotic infection. Obstet Gynecol 92:72, 1998.
44. Vanderpuye OA, Labarrere CA, Mcintyre JA: Expression of CD59, a human complement system regulatory protein, in extra-embryonic membranes. Int Arch Allergy Immunol 101:376, 1993.
45. Vanderpuye OA, Beville CM, Mcintyre JA: Characterization of cofactor activity for factor I: cleavage of complement C4 in human syncytiotrophoblast microvilli. Placenta 15:157, 1994.
46. Cunningham DS, Tichenor JR Jr: Decay-accelerating factor protects human trophoblast from complement-mediated attack. Clin Immunol Immunopathol 74:156, 1995.

47. Holmes CH, Simpson KL, Okada H, et al: Complement regulatory proteins at the feto-maternal interface during human placental development: distribution of CD59 by comparison with membrane cofactor protein (CD46) and decay accelerating factor (CD55). Eur J Immunol 22:1579, 1992.
48. Hitti J, Krohn MA, Patton DL, et al: Amniotic fluid tumor necrosis factor-alpha and the risk of respiratory distress syndrome among preterm infants. Am J Obstet Gynecol 177:50, 1997.
49. Viscardi RM, Muhumuza CK, Rodriguez A, et al: Inflammatory markers in intrauterine and fetal blood and cerebrospinal fluid compartments are associated with adverse pulmonary and neurologic outcomes in preterm infants. Pediatr Res 55:1009, 2004.
49a. Sadowsky DW, Adams KM, Gravett MG, et al: Preterm labor is induced by intraamniotic infusions of interleukin-1 beta and tumor necrosis factor-alpha but not by interleukin-6 or interleukin-8 in a nonhuman primate model. Am J Obstet Gynecol 195:1578, 2006.
49b. Romero R, Gomez R, Ghezzi F, et al: A fetal systemic inflammatory response is followed by the spontaneous onset of preterm parturition. Am J Obstet Gynecol 179:186, 1998.
50. Lonergan M, Aponso D, Marvin KW, et al: Tumor necrosis factor–related apoptosis-inducing ligand (TRAIL), TRAIL receptors, and the soluble receptor osteoprotegerin in human gestational membranes and amniotic fluid during pregnancy and labor at term and preterm. J Clin Endocrinol Metab 88:3835, 2003.
51. Gill RM, Ni J, Hunt JS: Differential expression of LIGHT and its receptors in human placental villi and amniochorion membranes. Am J Pathol 161:2011, 2002.
52. Blumenstein M, Bowen-Shauver JM, Keelan JA, Mitchell MD: Identification of suppressors of cytokine signaling (SOCS) proteins in human gestational tissues: differential regulation is associated with the onset of labor. J Clin Endocrinol Metab 87:1094, 2002.
53. Brombacher F, Kastelein RA, Alber G: Novel IL-12 family members shed light on the orchestration of Th1 responses. Trends Immunol 24:207, 2003.
54. Devergne O, Coulomb-L'Hermine A, Capel F, et al: Expression of Epstein-Barr virus–induced gene 3, an interleukin-12 p40-related molecule, throughout human pregnancy: involvement of syncytiotrophoblasts and extravillous trophoblasts. Am J Pathol 159:1763, 2001.
55. Atamas SP, Choi J, Yurovsky VV, White B: An alternative splice variant of human IL-4, IL-4 delta 2, inhibits IL-4-stimulated T cell proliferation. J Immunol 156:435–41, 1996.
55a. Romero R, Ceska M, Avila C, et al: Neutrophil attractant/activating peptide-1/interleukin-8 in term and preterm parturition. Am J Obstet Gynecol 165:813, 1991.
56. Alkhatib G, Combadiere C, Broder CC, et al: CC CKR5: a RANTES, MIP-1alpha, MIP-1beta receptor as a fusion cofactor for macrophage-tropic HIV-1. Science 272:1955, 1996.
57. Oberlin E, Amara A, Bachelerie F, et al: The CXC chemokine SDF-1 is the ligand for LESTR/fusin and prevents infection by T-cell-line–adapted HIV-1. Nature 382:833, 1996.
58. Su B, Sun G, Lu D, et al: Distribution of three HIV-1 resistance–conferring polymorphisms (SDF1–3'A, CCR2–641, and CCR5-delta32) in global populations. Eur J Hum Genet 8:975, 2000.
59. Coombes BK, Valdez Y, Finlay BB: Evasive maneuvers by secreted bacterial proteins to avoid innate immune responses. Curr Biol 14:R856, 2004.
60. Celli J, Olivier M, Finlay BB: Enteropathogenic *Escherichia coli* mediates antiphagocytosis through the inhibition of PI 3-kinase–dependent pathways. Embo J 20:1245, 2001.
61. Goehring UM, Schmidt G, Pederson KJ, et al: The N-terminal domain of *Pseudomonas aeruginosa* exoenzyme S is a GTPase-activating protein for Rho GTPases. J Biol Chem 274:36369, 1999.
62. Cowell BA, Chen DY, Frank DW, et al: ExoT of cytotoxic *Pseudomonas aeruginosa* prevents uptake by corneal epithelial cells. Infect Immun 68:403, 2000.
63. Cosma CL, Sherman DR, Ramakrishnan L: The secret lives of the pathogenic mycobacteria. Annu Rev Microbiol 57:641, 2003.
64. Hingley-Wilson SM, Sambandamurthy VK, Jacobs WR Jr: Survival perspectives from the world's most successful pathogen, *Mycobacterium tuberculosis*. Nat Immunol 4:949, 2003.
65. Parker DC: T cell–dependent B cell activation. Annu Rev Immunol 11:331, 1993.
66. Marolis GB, Buckley RH, Younger JB: Serum immunoglobulin concentrations during normal pregnancy. Am J Obstet Gynecol 109:971, 1971.
67. Cauci S, Driussi S, Guaschino S, et al: Correlation of local interleukin-1beta levels with specific IgA response against *Gardnerella vaginalis* cytolysin in women with bacterial vaginosis. Am J Reprod Immunol 47:257, 2002.
68. Brandtzaeg P: Mucosal immunity: integration between mother and the breast-fed infant. Vaccine 21:3382, 2003.
69. Schonberger HJ, Dompeling E, Knottnerus JA, et al: Prenatal exposure to mite and pet allergens and total serum IgE at birth in high-risk children. Pediatr Allergy Immunol 16:27, 2005.
70. Wegmann TG, Lin H, Guilbert L, Mosmann TR: Bidirectional cytokine interactions in the maternal-fetal relationship: is successful pregnancy a TH2 phenomenon? Immunol Today 14:353, 1993.
71. Hill JA, Polgar K, Anderson DJ: T-helper 1-type immunity to trophoblast in women with recurrent spontaneous abortion. JAMA 273:1933, 1995.
72. Raghupathy R: Th1-type immunity is incompatible with successful pregnancy. Immunol Today 18:478, 1997.
73. Chaouat G, Assal Meliani A, Martal J, et al: IL-10 prevents naturally occurring fetal loss in the CBA x DBA/2 mating combination, and local defect in IL-10 production in this abortion-prone combination is corrected by in vivo injection of IFN-tau. J Immunol 154:4261, 1995.
74. Chaouat G, Menu E, De Smedt D, et al: The emerging role of IL-10 in pregnancy. Am J Reprod Immunol 35:325, 1996.
75. Makhseed M, Raghupathy R, Azizieh F, et al: Th1 and Th2 cytokine profiles in recurrent aborters with successful pregnancy and with subsequent abortions. Hum Reprod 16:2219, 2001.
76. Chaouat G, Ledee-Bataille N, Dubanchet S, et al: TH1/TH2 paradigm in pregnancy: paradigm lost? Cytokines in pregnancy/early abortion: reexamining the TH1/TH2 paradigm. Int Arch Allergy Immunol 134:93, 2004.
77. Wang J, Brooks EG, Bamford KB, et al: Negative selection of T cells by *Helicobacter pylori* as a model for bacterial strain selection by immune evasion. J Immunol 167:926–34, 2001.
78. Boulton IC, Gray-Owen SD: Neisserial binding to CEACAM1 arrests the activation and proliferation of CD4+ T lymphocytes. Nat Immunol 3:229, 2002.
79. Giacomini E, Iona E, Ferroni L, et al: Infection of human macrophages and dendritic cells with *Mycobacterium tuberculosis* induces a differential cytokine gene expression that modulates T cell response. J Immunol 166:7033, 2001.
80. Toossi Z, Gogate P, Shiratsuchi H, et al: Enhanced production of TGF-beta by blood monocytes from patients with active tuberculosis and presence of TGF-beta in tuberculous granulomatous lung lesions. J Immunol 154:465, 1995.
81. McGuirk P, McCann C, Mills KH: Pathogen-specific T regulatory 1 cells induced in the respiratory tract by a bacterial molecule that stimulates interleukin 10 production by dendritic cells: a novel strategy for evasion of protective T helper type 1 responses by *Bordetella pertussis*. J Exp Med 195:221, 2002.
82. Hmama Z, Gabathuler R, Jefferies WA, et al: Attenuation of HLA-DR expression by mononuclear phagocytes infected with *Mycobacterium tuberculosis* is related to intracellular sequestration of immature class II heterodimers. J Immunol 161:4882, 1998.
83. Wojciechowski W, Desanctis J, Skamene E, Radzioch D: Attenuation of MHC class II expression in macrophages infected with *Mycobacterium bovis* bacillus Calmette-Guerin involves class II transactivator and depends on the Nramp1 gene. J Immunol 163:2688, 1999.
84. Zhong G, Fan T, Liu L: Chlamydia inhibits interferon gamma–inducible major histocompatibility complex class II expression by degradation of upstream stimulatory factor 1. J Exp Med 189:1931, 1999.
85. Zhong G, Liu L, Fan T, et al: Degradation of transcription factor RFX5 during the inhibition of both constitutive and interferon gamma-inducible major histocompatibility complex class I expression in chlamydia-infected cells. J Exp Med 191:1525, 2000.

86. Hunt JS, Pollard JW: Macrophages in the uterus and placenta. *In* Gordon S, Russell S (eds): Current Topics in Microbiology and Immunology, Macrophages and Macrophage Activation. Heidelberg, Springer-Verlag, 1992, p 36.
87. King A, Burrows T, Verma S, et al: Human uterine lymphocytes. Hum Reprod Update 4:480, 1998.
88. Whitelaw PF, Croy BA: Granulated lymphocytes of pregnancy. Placenta 17:533, 1996.
89. Zhang J, Nie G, Jian W, et al: Mast cell regulation of human endometrial matrix metalloproteinases: A mechanism underlying menstruation. Biol Reprod 59:693, 1998.
90. Biggio JR Jr, Ramsey PS, Cliver SP, et al: Midtrimester amniotic fluid matrix metalloproteinase-8 (MMP-8) levels above the 90th percentile are a marker for subsequent preterm premature rupture of membranes. Am J Obstet Gynecol 192:109, 2005.
91. King A, Gardner L, Loke YW: Co-stimulation of human decidual natural killer cells by interleukin-2 and stromal cells. Hum Reprod 14:656, 1999.
92. Hunt JS, Petroff MG, Burnett TG: Uterine leukocytes: key players in pregnancy. Semin Cell Dev Biol 11:127, 2000.
93. Dosiou C, Giudice LC: Natural killer cells in pregnancy and recurrent pregnancy loss: endocrine and immunologic perspectives. Endocr Rev 26:442, 2005.
94. Schofield G, Kimber SJ: Leukocyte subpopulations in the uteri of leukemia inhibitory factor knockout mice during early pregnancy. Biol Reprod 72:872, 2005.
95. Hunt JS: Macrophages in human uteroplacental tissues: a review. Am J Reprod Immunol 21:119, 1989.
96. Natuzzi ES, Ursell PC, Harrison M, et al: Nitric oxide synthase activity in the pregnant uterus decreases at parturition. Biochem Biophys Res Commun 194:1, 1993.
97. Norwitz ER, Starkey PM, Lopez Bernal A, Turnbull AC: Identification by flow cytometry of the prostaglandin-producing cell populations of term human decidua. J Endocrinol 131:327, 1991.
98. Stygar D, Wang H, Vladic YS, et al: Increased level of matrix metalloproteinases 2 and 9 in the ripening process of the human cervix. Biol Reprod 67:889, 2002.
99. Walter I, Boos A: Matrix metalloproteinases (MMP-2 and MMP-9) and tissue inhibitor-2 of matrix metalloproteinases (TIMP-2) in the placenta and interplacental uterine wall in normal cows and in cattle with retention of fetal membranes. Placenta 22:473, 2001.
100. Verma S, King A, Loke YW: Expression of killer cell inhibitory receptors on human uterine natural killer cells. Eur J Immunol 27:979, 1997.
101. Manaseki S, Searle RF: Natural killer (NK) cell activity of first trimester human decidua. Cell Immunol 121:166, 1989.
102. Koopman LA, Kopcow HD, Rybalov B, et al: Human decidual natural killer cells are a unique NK cell subset with immunomodulatory potential. J Exp Med 198:1201, 2003.
103. Croy BA, Esadeg S, Chantakru S, et al: Update on pathways regulating the activation of uterine natural killer cells, their interactions with decidual spiral arteries and homing of their precursors to the uterus. J Reprod Immunol 59:175, 2003.
104. Ashkar AA, Di Santo JP, Croy BA: Interferon gamma contributes to initiation of uterine vascular modification, decidual integrity, and uterine natural killer cell maturation during normal murine pregnancy. J Exp Med 192:259, 2000.
105. Hiby SE, Walker JJ, O'Shaughnessy KM, et al: Combinations of maternal KIR and fetal HLA-C genes influence the risk of preeclampsia and reproductive success. J Exp Med 200:957, 2004.
106. Westgren M, Shields LE: In utero stem cell transplantation in humans. Ernst Schering Res Found Workshop 33:197–221, 2001.
107. Shields LE, Lindton B, Andrews RG, Westgren M: Fetal Hematopoietic stem cell transplantation: A challenge for the twenty-first century. Journal of Hematotherapy and Stem Cell Research 11:617, 2002.
108. Hermann E, Truyens C, Alonso-Vega C, et al: Human fetuses are able to mount an adultlike CD8 T-cell response. Blood 100:2153, 2002.
109. Moore MAS, Metcalf D: Ontogeny of the haemopoietic system: Yolk sac orgin of in vivo colony forming cells in the developing mouse embryo. Br J Haematol 18:279, 1970.
110. Tavassoli M: Embryonic and fetal hematopoiesis: an overview. Blood Cells 17:269, 1991.
111. Lobach DF, Haynes BF: Ontogeny of the human thymus during fetal development. J Clin Immunol 7:81, 1987.
112. Lobach DF, Itoh T, Singer KH, Haynes BF: The thymic microenvironment. Characterization of in vitro differentiation of the IT26R21 rat thymic epithelial cell line. Differentiation 34:50, 1987.
113. Reinherz EL, Schlossman SF: The differentiation and function of human T lymphocytes. Cell 19:821, 1980.
114. Toribio ML, De La Hera A, Borst J, et al: Involvement of the interleukin 2 pathway in the rearrangement and expression of both alpha/beta and gamma/delta T cell receptor genes in human T cell precursors. J Exp Med 168:2231, 1988.
115. Lindton B, Markling L, Ringden O, et al: Mixed lymphocyte culture of human fetal liver cells. Fetal Diagn Ther 15:71, 2000.
116. Gathings WE, Lawton AR, Cooper MD: Immunofluorescent studies of the development of pre-B cells, B lymphocytes and immunoglobulin isotype diversity in humans. Eur J Immunol 7:804, 1977.
117. Van Furth R, Schuit HRE: The immunological development of the human fetus. J Exp Med 122:1173, 1965.
118. Fischer A: Severe combined immunodeficiencies (SCID). Clin Exp Immunol 122:143, 2000.
119. Gulino AV, Notarangelo LDL: Hyper IgM syndromes. Curr Opin Rheumatol 15:422, 2003.
120. Van Rood JJ, Eernisse JG, Van Leeuwen A: Leucocyte antibodies in sera from pregnant women. Nature 181:1735, 1958.
121. Suciu-Foca N, Reed E, Rohowsky C, et al: Anti-idiotypic antibodies to anti-HLA receptors induced by pregnancy. Proc Natl Acad Sci U S A 80:830, 1983.
122. Regan L, Braude PR, Hill DP: A prospective study of the incidence, time of appearance and significance of anti-paternal lymphocytotoxic antibodies in human pregnancy. Hum Reprod 6:294, 1991.
123. Payne R: The development and persistence of leukoagglutinins in parous women. Blood 19:411, 1962.
124. Bouma GJ, Van Caubergh P, Van Bree SP, et al: Pregnancy can induce priming of cytotoxic T lymphocytes specific for paternal HLA antigens that is associated with antibody formation. Transplantation 62:672, 1996.
125. Tafuri A, Alferink J, Moller P, et al: T cell awareness of paternal alloantigens during pregnancy. Science 270:630, 1995.
126. Jiang SP, Vacchio MS: Multiple mechanisms of peripheral T cell tolerance to the fetal "allograft." J Immunol 160:3086, 1998.
127. Le Bouteiller P: HLA-G: what's new? Am J Reprod Immunol 38:146, 1997.
128. Hammer A, Hutter H, Dohr G: HLA class I expression on the materno-fetal interface. Am J Reprod Immunol 38:150, 1997.
129. Rouas-Freiss N, Goncalves RM, Menier C, et al: Direct evidence to support the role of HLA-G in protecting the fetus from maternal uterine natural killer cytolysis. Proc Natl Acad Sci U S A 94:11520, 1997.
130. Braud VM, Allan DS, McMichael AJ: Functions of nonclassical MHC and non-MHC–encoded class I molecules. Curr Opin Immunol 11:100, 1999.
131. Colonna M, Samaridis J, Cella M, et al: Human myelomonocytic cells express an inhibitory receptor for classical and nonclassical MHC class I molecules. J Immunol 160:3096, 1998.
132. Hackmon R, Hallak M, Krup M, et al: HLA-G antigen and parturition: maternal serum, fetal serum and amniotic fluid levels during pregnancy. Fetal Diagn Ther 19:404, 2004.
133. Ober C, Aldrich C, Rosinsky B, et al: HLA-G1 protein expression is not essential for fetal survival. Placenta 19:127, 1998.
134. Sakaguchi S: Regulatory T cells: key controllers of immunologic self-tolerance. Cell 101:455, 2000.
135. Shevach EM: CD4+ CD25+ suppressor T cells: more questions than answers. Nat Rev Immunol 2:389, 2002.
136. Somerset DA, Zheng Y, Kilby MD, et al: Normal human pregnancy is associated with an elevation in the immune suppressive CD25+ CD4+ regulatory T-cell subset. Immunology 112:38, 2004.
137. Aluvihare VR, Kallikourdis M, Betz AG: Regulatory T cells mediate maternal tolerance to the fetus. Nat Immunol 5:266, 2004.

138. Polanczyk MJ, Carson BD, Subramanian S, et al: Cutting edge: estrogen drives expansion of the CD4+ CD25+ regulatory T cell compartment. J Immunol 173:2227–30, 2004.
139. Zenclussen AC, Gerlof K, Zenclussen ML, et al: Abnormal T-cell reactivity against paternal antigens in spontaneous abortion: adoptive transfer of pregnancy-induced CD4+ CD25+ T regulatory cells prevents fetal rejection in a murine abortion model. Am J Pathol 166:811, 2005.
140. Mellor AL, Sivakumar J, Chandler P, et al: Prevention of T cell–driven complement activation and inflammation by tryptophan catabolism during pregnancy. Nat Immunol 2:64, 2001.
141. Munn DH, Shafizadeh E, Attwood JT, et al: Inhibition of T cell proliferation by macrophage tryptophan catabolism. J Exp Med 189:1363, 1999.
142. Kamimura S, Eguchi K, Yonezawa M, Sekiba K: Localization and developmental change of indoleamine 2,3-dioxygenase activity in the human placenta. Acta Med Okayama 45:135–9, 1991.
143. Munn DH, Zhou M, Attwood JT, et al: Prevention of allogeneic fetal rejection by tryptophan catabolism. Science 281:1191–3, 1998.
144. Mellor AL, Munn DH: Tryptophan catabolism and T-cell tolerance: immunosuppression by starvation? Immunol Today 20:469, 1999.
145. Fallarino F, Grohmann U, Hwang KW, et al: Modulation of tryptophan catabolism by regulatory T cells. Nat Immunol 4:1206, 2003.
146. Hunt JS, Vassmer D, Ferguson TA, Miller L: Fas ligand is positioned in mouse uterus and placenta to prevent trafficking of activated leukocytes between the mother and the conceptus. J Immunol 158:4122, 1997.
147. Runic R, Lockwood CJ, Ma Y, et al: Expression of Fas ligand by human cytotrophoblasts: implications in placentation and fetal survival. J Clin Endocrinol Metab 81:3119, 1996.
148. Hammer A, Dohr G: Expression of Fas-ligand in first trimester and term human placental villi. J Reprod Immunol 46:83, 2000.
149. Makrigiannakis A, Zoumakis E, Kalantaridou S, et al: Corticotropin-releasing hormone promotes blastocyst implantation and early maternal tolerance. Nat Immunol 2:1018, 2001.
150. Wiley SR, Schooley K, Smolak PJ, et al: Identification and characterization of a new member of the TNF family that induces apoptosis. Immunity 3:673, 1995.
151. Phillips TA, Ni J, Pan G, et al: TRAIL (Apo-2L) and TRAIL receptors in human placentas: implications for immune privilege. J Immunol 162:6053, 1999.
151a. Adams KM, Yan Z, Stevens AM, Nelson JL: The changing maternal "self" hypothesis: A mechanism for maternal tolerance of the fetus. Placenta 2006 Aug 23 [Epub ahead of print].
152. Murgita RA: The immunosuppressive role of alpha-fetoprotein during pregnancy. Scand J Immunol 5:1003–14, 1976.
153. Murgita RA, Tomasi TB Jr: Suppression of the immune response by alpha-fetoprotein on the primary and secondary antibody response. J Exp Med 141:269, 1975.
154. Kovar IZ, Riches PG: C3 and C4 complement components and acute phase proteins in late pregnancy and parturition. J Clin Pathol 41:650, 1988.
155. Johnson U, Gustavii B: Complement components in normal pregnancy. Acta Pathol Microbiol Immunol Scand [C] 95:97, 1987.
156. Thurman JM, Kraus DM, Girardi G, et al: A novel inhibitor of the alternative complement pathway prevents antiphospholipid antibody-induced pregnancy loss in mice. Mol Immunol 42:87, 2005.
157. Mao D, Wu X, Deppong C, et al: Negligible role of antibodies and C5 in pregnancy loss associated exclusively with C3-dependent mechanisms through complement alternative pathway. Immunity 19:813, 2003.
158. Xu C, Mao D, Holers VM, et al: A critical role for murine complement regulator crry in fetomaternal tolerance. Science 287:498, 2000.
159. Fallon PG, Jolin HE, Smith P, et al: IL-4 induces characteristic Th2 responses even in the combined absence of IL-5, IL-9, and IL-13. Immunity 17:7, 2002.
160. Croy BA, He H, Esadeg S, et al: Uterine natural killer cells: insights into their cellular and molecular biology from mouse modelling. Reproduction 126:149–60, 2003.
161. Chellam VG, Rushton DI: Chorioamnionitis and funiculitis in the placentas of 200 births weighing less than 2.5 kg. Br J Obstet Gynaecol 92:808, 1985.
162. Hillier SL, Martius J, Krohn M, et al: A case-control study of chorioamnionic infection and histologic chorioamnionitis in prematurity. N Engl J Med 319:972, 1988.
163. Watts DH, Krohn MA, Hillier SL, Eschenbach DA: The association of occult amniotic fluid infection with gestational age and neonatal outcome among women in preterm labor. Obstet Gynecol 79:351, 1992.
164. Watterberg KL, Demers LM, Scott SM, Murphy S: Chorioamnionitis and early lung inflammation in infants in whom bronchopulmonary dysplasia develops. Pediatrics 97:210, 1996.
165. Schmidt B, Cao L, Mackensen-Haen S, et al: Chorioamnionitis and inflammation of the fetal lung. Am J Obstet Gynecol 185:173–7, 2001.
166. Munshi UK, Niu JO, Siddiq MM, Parton LA: Elevation of interleukin-8 and interleukin-6 precedes the influx of neutrophils in tracheal aspirates from preterm infants who develop bronchopulmonary dysplasia. Pediatr Pulmonol 24:331, 1997.
167. Lahra MM, Jeffery HE: A fetal response to chorioamnionitis is associated with early survival after preterm birth. Am J Obstet Gynecol 190:147–51, 2004.
168. Horowitz S, Mazor M, Romero R, et al: Infection of the amniotic cavity with *Ureaplasma urealyticum* in the midtrimester of pregnancy. J Reprod Med 40:375, 1995.
169. Hillier SL, Krohn MA, Rabe LK, et al: The normal vaginal flora, H2O2-producing lactobacilli, and bacterial vaginosis in pregnant women. Clin Infect Dis 16(Suppl 4):S273, 1993.
170. McDuffie RS Jr, Sherman MP, Gibbs RS: Amniotic fluid tumor necrosis factor-alpha and interleukin-1 in a rabbit model of bacterially induced preterm pregnancy loss. Am J Obstet Gynecol 167:1583, 1992.
171. Taniguchi T, Matsuzaki N, Kameda T, et al: The enhanced production of placental interleukin-1 during labor and intrauterine infection. Am J Obstet Gynecol 165:131, 1991.
172. Mitchell MD, Dudley DJ, Edwin SS, Schiller SL: Interleukin-6 stimulates prostaglandin production by human amnion and decidual cells. Eur J Pharmacol 192:189, 1991.
173. Romero R, Tartakovsky B: The natural interleukin-1 receptor antagonist prevents interleukin-1–induced preterm delivery in mice. Am J Obstet Gynecol 167:1041, 1992.
174. Hirsch E, Muhle RA, Mussalli GM, Blanchard R: Bacterially induced preterm labor in the mouse does not require maternal interleukin-1 signaling. Am J Obstet Gynecol 186:523, 2002.
175. Yoshimura K, Hirsch E: Interleukin-6 is neither necessary nor sufficient for preterm labor in a murine infection model. J Soc Gynecol Investig 10:423, 2003.
176. Sadowsky DW, Gravett MG, Cook MJ, et al: Repeated intraamniotic infusions of IL-6 or IL-8 do not induce preterm labor in a non-human primate model. (Abstract). J Soc Gynecol Investig 12:258A, 2005.
177. Arntzen KJ, Kjollesdal AM, Halgunset J, et al: TNF, IL-1, IL-6, IL-8 and soluble TNF receptors in relation to chorioamnionitis and premature labor. J Perinat Med 26:17–26, 1998.
178. Wenstrom KD, Andrews WW, Hauth JC, et al: Elevated second-trimester amniotic fluid interleukin-6 levels predict preterm delivery. Am J Obstet Gynecol 178:546, 1998.
179. Wilson AG, De Vries N, Pociot F, et al: An allelic polymorphism within the human tumor necrosis factor alpha promoter region is strongly associated with HLA A1, B8, and DR3 alleles. J Exp Med 177:557–60, 1993.
180. McGuire W, Hill AV, Allsopp CE, et al: Variation in the TNF-alpha promoter region associated with susceptibility to cerebral malaria. Nature 371:508, 1994.
181. Mira JP, Cariou A, Grall F, et al: Association of TNF2, a TNF-alpha promoter polymorphism, with septic shock susceptibility and mortality: a multicenter study. JAMA 282:561, 1999.
182. Aidoo M, McElroy PD, Kolczak MS, et al: Tumor necrosis factor-alpha promoter variant 2 (TNF2) is associated with preterm delivery, infant mortality, and malaria morbidity in western Kenya: Asembo Bay Cohort Project IX. Genet Epidemiol 21:201, 2001.
183. Simhan HN, Krohn MA, Zeevi A, et al: Tumor necrosis factor-alpha promoter gene polymorphism -308 and chorioamnionitis. Obstet Gynecol 102:162, 2003.

184. Dizon-Townson DS, Major H, Varner M, Ward K: A promoter mutation that increases transcription of the tumor necrosis factor-alpha gene is not associated with preterm delivery. Am J Obstet Gynecol 177:810, 1997.
185. Amory JH, Adams KM, Lin MT, et al: Adverse outcomes after preterm labor are associated with tumor necrosis factor-alpha polymorphism -863, but not -308, in mother-infant pairs. Am J Obstet Gynecol 191:1362, 2004.
186. Roberts AK, Monzon-Bordonaba F, Van Deerlin PG, et al: Association of polymorphism within the promoter of the tumor necrosis factor alpha gene with increased risk of preterm premature rupture of the fetal membranes. Am J Obstet Gynecol 180:1297, 1999.
187. Macones GA, Parry S, Elkousy M, et al: A polymorphism in the promoter region of TNF and bacterial vaginosis: preliminary evidence of gene-environment interaction in the etiology of spontaneous preterm birth. Am J Obstet Gynecol 190:1504; discussion 3A, 2004.
187a. Gravett MG, Adams KM, Sadowsky DW, et al: Immunomodulators plus antibiotics delay preterm delivery after experimental intra-amniotic infection in a nonhuman primate model. Am J Obstet Gynecol, in press.
188. Stetzer BP, Mercer BM: Antibiotics and preterm labor. Clin Obstet Gynecol 43:809, 2000.
189. Billington WD: Influence of immunological dissimilarity of mother and foetus on size of placenta in mice. Nature 202:317, 1964.
190. Kirby DR: The egg and immunology. Proc R Soc Med 63:59, 1970.
191. Komlos L, Zamir R, Joshua H, Halbrecht I: Common HLA antigens in couples with repeated abortions. Clin Immunol Immunopathol 7:330, 1977.
192. Schacter B, Muir A, Gyves M, Tasin M: HLA-A,B compatibility in parents of offspring with neural-tube defects or couples experiencing involuntary fetal wastage. Lancet 1:796, 1979.
193. Ober C, Rosinsky B, Grimsley C, et al: Population genetic studies of HLA-G: allele frequencies and linkage disequilibrium with HLA-A1. J Reprod Immunol 32:111, 1996.
194. Ober C, Elias S, O'Brien E, et al: HLA sharing and fertility in Hutterite couples: evidence for prenatal selection against compatible fetuses. Am J Reprod Immunol Microbiol 18:111, 1988.
195. Ober CL, Hauck WW, Kostyu DD, et al: Adverse effects of human leukocyte antigen-DR sharing on fertility: a cohort study in a human isolate. Fertil Steril 44:227, 1985.
196. Ober CL, Martin AO, Simpson JL, et al: Shared HLA antigens and reproductive performance among Hutterites. Am J Hum Genet 35:994, 1983.
197. Coulam CB: Immunotherapy with intravenous immunoglobulin for treatment of recurrent pregnancy loss: American experience. Am J Reprod Immunol 32:286, 1994.
198. Daya S, Gunby J: The effectiveness of allogeneic leukocyte immunization in unexplained primary recurrent spontaneous abortion. Recurrent Miscarriage Immunotherapy Trialists Group. Am J Reprod Immunol 32:294, 1994.
199. Uhrberg M, Valiante NM, Shum BP, et al: Human diversity in killer cell inhibitory receptor genes. Immunity 7:753, 1997.
200. De Moor G, De Bock G, Noens L, De Bie S: A new case of human chimerism detected after pregnancy: 46,XY karyotype in the lymphocytes of a woman. Acta Clin Belg 43:231, 1988.
201. Lee TH, Paglieroni T, Ohto H, et al: Survival of donor leukocyte subpopulations in immunocompetent transfusion recipients: frequent long-term microchimerism in severe trauma patients. Blood 93:3127, 1999.
202. Bianchi DW, Farina A, Weber W, et al: Significant fetal-maternal hemorrhage after termination of pregnancy: implications for development of fetal cell microchimerism. Am J Obstet Gynecol 184:703, 2001.
203. Nelson JL: Maternal-fetal immunology and autoimmune disease: is some autoimmune disease auto-alloimmune or allo-autoimmune? Arthritis Rheum 39:191, 1996.
204. Rouquette-Gally AM, Boyeldieu D, Gluckman E, et al: Autoimmunity in 28 patients after allogeneic bone marrow transplantation: comparison with Sjogren syndrome and scleroderma. Br J Haematol 66:45, 1987.
205. Nelson JL, Furst DE, Maloney S, et al: Microchimerism and HLA-compatible relationships of pregnancy in scleroderma. Lancet 351:559, 1998.
206. Stevens AM: Foreign cells in polymyositis: could stem cell transplantation and pregnancy-derived chimerism lead to the same disease? Curr Rheumatol Rep 5:437, 2003.
207. Reed AM, Picornell YJ, Harwood A, Kredich DW: Chimerism in children with juvenile dermatomyositis. Lancet 356:2156, 2000.
207a. Stevens AM, Hermes HM, Rutledge JC, et al: Myocardial-tissue-specific phenotype of maternal microchimerism in neonatal lupus congenital heart block. Lancet 362:1617, 2003.
208. Li DK, Odouli R, Liu L, et al: Transmission of parentally shared human leukocyte antigen alleles and the risk of preterm delivery. Obstet Gynecol 104:594, 2004.

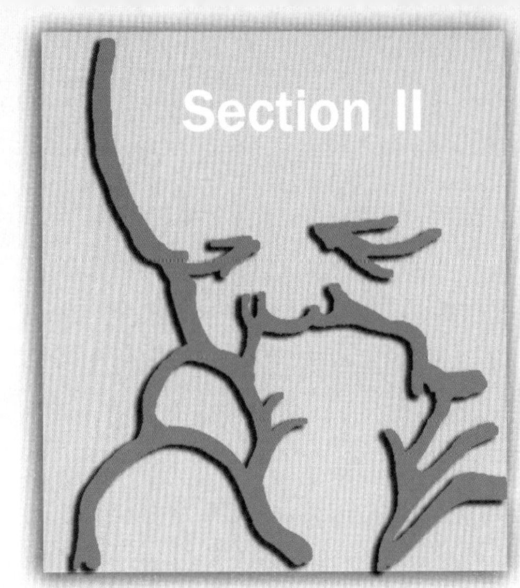

Prenatal Care

Preconception and Prenatal Care: Part of the Continuum

TIMOTHY R. B. JOHNSON, KIMBERLY D. GREGORY, AND JENNIFER R. NIEBYL

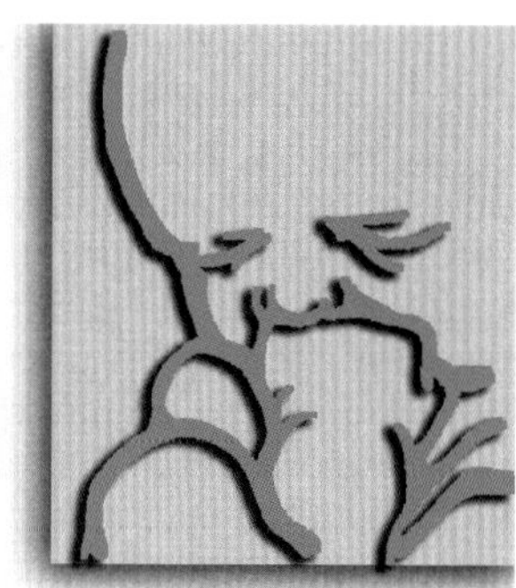

CHAPTER 5

KEY ABBREVIATIONS

American Academy of Pediatrics	AAP
The American College of Obstetricians and Gynecologists	ACOG
Azidothymidine	AZT
The Centers for Disease Control and Prevention	CDC
Cytomegalovirus	CMV
Computed tomography	CT
Diethylstilbestrol	DES
Electronic medical record	EMR
Group B streptococcus	GBS
Human chorionic gonadotropin	hCG
Human immunodeficiency virus	HIV
Last menstrual period	LMP
Magnetic Resonance Imaging	MRI
National Institutes of Health	NIH
Nuchal translucency	NT
Neural tube defect	NTD
Pregnancy-associated placental protein	PAPP-A
Routine antenatal diagnostic imaging with ultrasound study	RADIUS
Recommended dietary allowances	RDA
Rhesus immune globulin	RhIG
Restless legs syndrome	RLS
Rapid plasma reagin test	RPR
Vaginal birth after cesarean delivery	VBAC
Women, infants, and children program	WIC

Pregnancy and child birth are major life events. Preconception and prenatal care are not only part of the pregnancy continuum that culminates in delivery, the postpartum period, and parenthood, but they should also be considered in the context of women's health throughout the life span.[1,2] This chapter reviews pertinent considerations for prenatal care using the broader definitions espoused by The United States Public Health Service and The American College of Obstetricians and Gynecologists (ACOG).[2,3] Specifically prenatal care should consist of a series of interactions that includes three components: (1) early and continuing risk assessment; (2) health promotion; and (3) medical and psychosocial interventions and follow-up.[4] The overarching objective of prenatal care is to promote the health and well-being of the pregnant woman, fetus, and newborn, and also the family. Hence, the breadth of prenatal care does not end with delivery but rather includes preconception care and postpartum care, and extends up to 1 year after the infant's birth.[3] Importantly, this introduces the concept of interconception care, and the notion that almost all health care interactions with reproductive age women are opportunities to assess risk, promote healthy lifestyle behaviors, and identify, treat, and optimize medical and psychosocial issues that could impact pregnancy.

Prenatal care is an excellent example of preventive medicine. In 1929, the Ministry of Health of Great Britain issued a memorandum on the conduct of prenatal clinics. In 1942, vitamin tablets were provided for all British women in the last 6 months of pregnancy. United Kingdom maternal mortality declined from 319 per 100,000 live births in 1936 to 15 per 100,000 live births in 1985. In the United States, the maternal mortality ratio was 13.2/100,000 live births in 1999.[5] The decline in maternal mortality was partly attributed to prenatal care and partly to medical and public policy advances such as maternal mortality reviews with attention to preventable causes of maternal death, shift to hospital births, improvements in anesthesia, widespread availability of blood transfusions and antibiotics, and access to safe and legal abortion services. Recent guidelines addressing the content and efficacy of prenatal care have focused on the medical, psychosocial and educational aspects of prenatal care. Prenatal care satisfies the definition of primary care from the Institute of Medicine as "Integrated, accessible health care services by clinicians who are accountable for addressing a large majority of personal health care needs, developing a sustained partnership with patients, and practicing in the context of family and community."[6] In fact, prenatal care services can be used by obstetricians/gynecologists and other primary care providers as a general model for primary care.[7] Prenatal care satisfies other criteria for primary care in that it is comprehensive and continuous, and provides coordinated health care.[8] Preconception care—planning to ensure the healthiest possible pregnancy outcome—is consistent with this model. We agree that the preconception and prenatal care periods—just as labor, delivery, the puerperium, and postgestation and interconceptional periods—must be seen as episodes in a woman's life and that they provide important opportunities to advance wellness and prevention. It must be recognized that for pregnant women, all of these events are part of a life continuum, with birth leading to the multiple challenges of parenting. They are opportunities to introduce and reinforce habits, knowledge, and lifelong skills in self-care, health education, and wellness, to inculcate principles of routine screening, immunization, and regular assessment for psychological, behavioral, and medical risk factors.[1]

The prenatal record describes in a consistent fashion the comprehensive care that is provided and allows for documentation of coordinated services. The goal of prenatal care is to help the mother maintain her well-being and achieve a healthy outcome for herself and her infant. Education about pregnancy, childbearing, and childrearing is an important part of prenatal care, as are detection and treatment of abnormalities. This process is best realized when begun even before pregnancy. Many services provided traditionally during the intrapartum hospital stay should be provided at prenatal and postpartum outpatient visits.[9] Too often, hospitalization for childbirth has been seen as an opportunity for education about self-care, child-care and parenting, and parenthood rather than as a time to ensure safe passage. Educational interventions have often been targeted for the intrapartum stay, when they can better and more cheaply be performed in the preconceptional, antenatal, or home care environment.[9–11]

MATERNAL MORTALITY

Maternal and neonatal mortality rates are the most widely used indicators of the health of a nation. Maternal death is the demise of any woman from any pregnancy-related cause while pregnant or within 42 days of termination of pregnancy, irrespective of the duration and the site of pregnancy. A direct maternal death is an obstetric death resulting from obstetric complications of the pregnancy state, labor, or puerperium. An indirect maternal death is an obstetric death resulting from a disease previously existing or developing during the pregnancy, labor, or puerperium; death is not directly due to obstetric causes but may be aggravated by the physiologic effects of pregnancy. A nonmaternal death is an obstetric death resulting from accidental or incidental causes unrelated to the pregnancy or its management.

The maternal mortality rate is the number of maternal deaths (direct, indirect, or nonmaternal) per 100,000 women of reproductive age, but because this denominator is difficult to determine precisely, most clinical and research entities use the maternal mortality ratio defined as the number of maternal deaths per 100,000 live births.

Direct obstetric deaths have six major causes: hypertensive diseases of pregnancy, hemorrhage, infections/sepsis, thromboembolism, and in developing countries, obstructed labor and complications from illegal abortion. There are other direct causes of death, such as ectopic pregnancy, complications of anesthesia, and amniotic fluid embolism. The main causes of indirect obstetric deaths are asthma, heart disease, type 1 diabetes, systemic lupus erythematosus, and other conditions that are aggravated by pregnancy to the point of death.[12]

Maternal mortality has been an under-recognized issue worldwide despite an estimated 600,000 maternal deaths per year from pregnancy-related causes.[13,14] Put in numeric perspective, this is equivalent to six jumbo jet crashes per day with the deaths of all 250 passengers on board, all of them women in the reproductive years of life. To put this in a time perspective, every minute of every day, a woman dies from pregnancy-related causes.[15] There is also a marked inequity in geographic distribution, because 95 percent of these deaths occur in developing countries (Fig. 5-1). Maternal mortality is the health indicator with the greatest disparity between wealthy and poor countries (and wealthy and poor women in developed countries). Maternal mortality is highest in Africa, Asia, Latin America, and the Caribbean.[16] The World Health Organization estimates that more than 80 percent of maternal deaths could be prevented though actions that have been proven to be effective and affordable, specifically, providing maternal health services defined

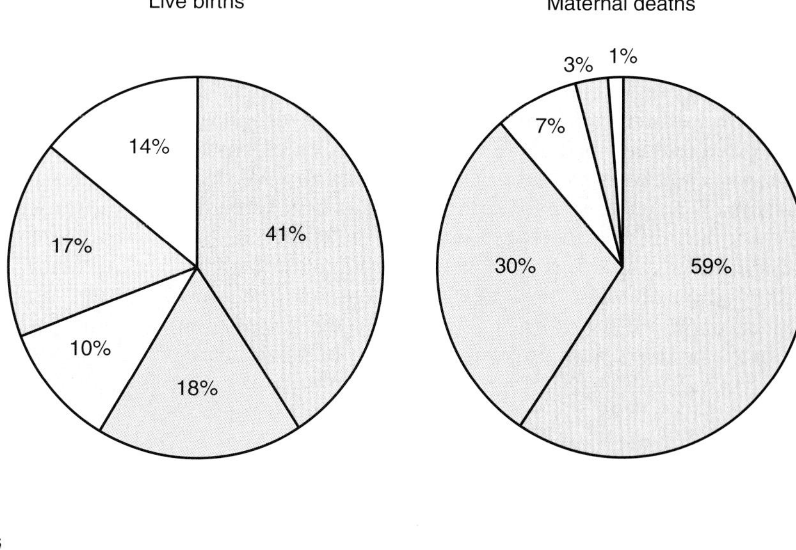

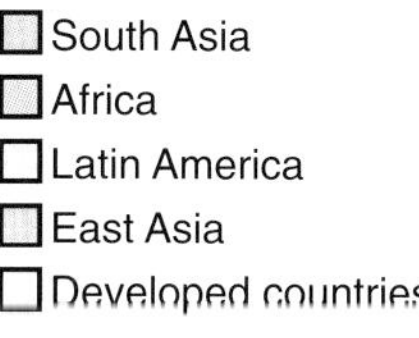

Figure 5-1. Worldwide distribution of live births and maternal deaths by region. (From WHO 861663.)

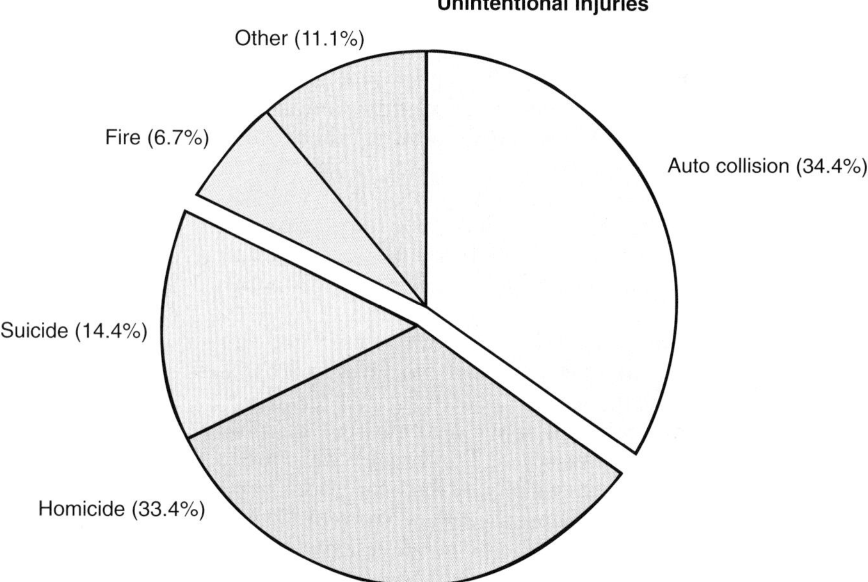

Figure 5-2. Distribution of deaths due to injury in the United States, 1980–1985 (N = 90). (From MMWR Morb Mortal Wkly Rep 37:[SS5]:26, 1988.)

as trained birth attendants, aseptic birth environments, identification of maternal/fetal/neonatal complications and transport to higher level of care when indicated.[15] Even in developed countries, the changing demographic profile of childbearing women (e.g., older women or women with chronic medical conditions) has contributed to an increase in maternal mortality, and many argue that these, too, are preventable—requiring rapid recognition and response to treatable emergency conditions.[15,17–19] Worldwide, we are far from achieving the international Safe Motherhood goal of reducing maternal mortality by 50 percent. Similarly, the United States, will not achieve a reduction in maternal deaths to the Healthy People 2010 goal of 3.3/100,000, emphasizing that it will take an integrated, multifaceted, multidisciplinary public health approach to achieve these goals.

The Centers for Disease Control and Prevention (CDC) and the ACOG have introduced the concept that pregnancy-associated mortality is defined as "the death of a woman, from any cause, while she is pregnant or within one year of termination of pregnancy." Unfortunately, the United States is seeing an increase in nonmaternal deaths of pregnant women resulting from trauma and violence, many of these related to illegal drugs (Fig. 5-2). In North Carolina from 1992 to 1994, 167 deaths to pregnant and postpartum women were identified through an enhanced surveillance system. When all deaths to pregnant women were categorized, direct and indirect obstetric deaths (classically defined maternal deaths) accounted for only 37 percent of deaths to pregnant and postpartum women. Injuries accounted for 38 percent of deaths to pregnant women, with homicide being the most common (36 percent), followed by motor vehicle accidents (32 percent), drug-related death (13 percent), other (11 percent), and suicide (8 percent).[20–24] Acceptance of pregnancy associated mortality as the appropriate measure will lead to increased recognition of these important problems.[25] The prenatal care provider can play a role in preventing these common causes of death in women by advocating use of seat belts and screening for alcohol, drug use, depression, and violence.

Significant disparities exist between the maternal mortality ratios of white and black women. In the United States, maternal mortality occurs four times more often in black women than in white women. In a *Morbidity and Mortality Weekly Report* review of maternal deaths from 1991 to 1999, the pregnancy-related mortality ratio for white women was 8.1; for black women it was 30. On a state by-state basis, maternal mortality ratios for black women were higher in every state.[26,27] Many of the principles espoused to bring about safe motherhood internationally could be applicable to help understand and eradicate the maternal health disparities seen in poor urban and rural environments in the United States. Specifically, they are health education and promotion, identification of maternal/fetal/neonatal complications, transport to a higher level of care, and rapid responses to acute obstetric emergencies. For example, one study demonstrated an inverse relationship between the maternal mortality ratio and the state density of maternal-fetal medicine specialists after controlling for state-level measures of maternal poverty, education, race, age, and interactions.[28] Similarly, regionalization of perinatal services has been a cornerstone for improved neonatal outcomes.[29]

Last, although much attention has been focused nationally and internationally on maternal mortality, perhaps of greater concern is the less well-documented prevalence of severe maternal morbidity, or "near misses" defined as "pregnant women with severe life-threatening conditions who nearly die but, with good luck or good care, survive."[30] Wen et al.[31] found the overall rate of severe maternal morbidity was 4.4/1,000 deliveries, but many feel it is significantly underreported. Severe morbidity was defined as thromboembolism, eclampsia, pulmonary, cardiac or central nervous system complications of anesthesia, cerebrovascular disorders, uterine rupture, adult respiratory distress syndrome, pulmonary edema, myocardial infarction, acute renal failure associated with delivery, cardiac arrest, severe postpartum hemorrhage requiring hysterectomy, and assisted ventilation. Rates of venous thromboembolism, uterine rupture, adult respiratory distress syndrome, pulmonary edema, myocardial infarction, severe postpartum hemorrhage requiring hysterectomy, and assisted ventilation appear to be increasing in incidence since 1991.[31] The presence of preexisting chronic conditions (e.g., systemic lupus erythematosus, cystic fibrosis, chronic renal disease, hypertension, diabetes, pulmonary hypertension, and congenital, rheumatic, and ischemic heart disease) also appears to be increasing among pregnant women, and this is significant since the presence of preexisting conditions increases the risk of both maternal morbidity (6-fold increase) and mortality (158-fold increase).[31–34]

NEONATAL MORTALITY AND MORBIDITY

Historically, in developed countries, when decreased maternal mortality was achieved, attention was then turned to fetal mortality and, later, to fetal morbidity. The stillbirth rate (fetal death rate) is the number of stillborn infants per 1,000 infants born. The neonatal mortality rate is the number of neonatal deaths (deaths in the first 28 days of life) per 1,000 live births. The perinatal mortality combines these two—the number of fetal deaths (stillbirths) plus neonatal deaths per 1,000 total births.

In 1990, the U.S. infant mortality rate was 9.2 per 1,000 live births, ranking the United States 19th internationally.[35] However, there are international differences in the way live births are classified, because some countries exclude infants weighing less than 1 kg and those with fatal anomalies. The United States met the Healthy People 2000 goal of decreasing the infant mortality rate to 7 per 1,000 live births but does not appear to be on course to meet the 2010 goal of 4.5 per 1,000 live births.[36] Infant mortality varies by maternal demographic and health characteristics. Rates are higher in the extreme reproductive ages (young teens and women older than 40 years of age). Other maternal characteristics associated with increased risk for infant mortality include being unmarried or poorly educated, having little or no prenatal care, and engaging in smoking or illicit substance use. Pregnancy-related complications include but are not limited to multiple births and preterm delivery. There are significant racial differences in infant mortality with blacks having a 2.5-fold increased risk.[37] Infant mortality rates in Hispanics are comparable to whites; however, variation exists between country of origin and amount of acculturation.[38–40]

PRENATAL CARE

During the past 30 years, new technology has been introduced to assess the fetus antepartum, including electronic fetal monitoring, sonography, and amniocentesis, with the fetus emerging as a patient in utero. Prevention of morbidity as well as mortality is now the goal. This has made the task of the prenatal clinic more complex, because mother and fetus now require an increasingly sophisticated level of care. At the same time, pregnancy is basically a physiologic process, and the normal pregnant patient may not benefit from application of advanced technology.

Prenatal care is provided at a variety of sites, ranging from the private office, to the public health and county hospital clinics, to the patient's home. Obstetricians must optimize their efforts by resourceful use of other professionals and support groups, including nutritionists, childbirth educators, public health nurses, nurse practitioners, family physicians, nurse midwives, and specialty medical consultants. Most pregnant women are healthy, with normal pregnancies, and can be followed by an obstetric team including nurses, nurse practitioners, and nurse-midwives, with an obstetrician available for consultation. These women can be followed by practitioners who have adequate time to spend on patient education and parenting preparation, whereas physicians can appropriately concentrate on complicated problems requiring their medical skills. This also provides for improved continuity of care, which is recognized as extremely important for patient satisfaction[41,42] (Fig. 5-3).

There have been no prospective controlled trials demonstrating efficacy of prenatal care overall. Documents[2] addressing the content and efficacy of prenatal care have suggested changes in the current prenatal care system.[41,42,44–49] Because of publication of these recommendations, several well-designed randomized clinical trials and cost-benefit analyses have been reported using alternative visit schedules (Table 5-1).[46–49] There was no difference in outcomes for patients undergoing reduced frequency of visits as measured by rates of preterm birth and low birth weight, and the reduced frequency model has been shown to be cost effective. However, fewer visits has been associated with decreased maternal satisfaction with care as well as increased maternal anxiety.[48–50] Recent studies support the concept of reduced antenatal visits for selected women.[11,48,49,51–54]

Efficacy of prenatal care also depends on the quality of care provided by the caretaker. If a blood pressure is recorded as elevated and no therapeutic maneuvers are recommended, this will not change the outcome. Recommendations must be made and must be carried out by the patient, whose compliance is essential to alter outcome. Kogan et al. using national survey data reported that women received only 56 percent of the procedures and 32 percent of the advice recommended as part of prenatal care content, and that poor women and black women received fewer of the recommended interventions. Site of care was also an important determinant, suggesting that infrastructure must be geared to address population-specific needs.[58,59]

RISK ASSESSMENT

The concept of risk in obstetrics can be examined at many levels. All problems that arise in pregnancy, whether common complaints or more hazardous diseases, convey some risk to the pregnancy, depending on how they are managed by the patient and her care provider. Risk assessment has received detailed attention in the past. It has been shown that most women and infants suffering morbidity and mortality will come from a small segment of women with high-risk factors; by reassessing risk factors before pregnancy, during pregnancy, and again in labor, our ability to identify those at highest risk increases.[60] Most of the emphasis for screening, risk assessment, and associated trials for therapeutic interventions have focused primarily on preclampsia and preterm birth prevention.[61–62] Table 5-2 lists representative examples of other clinical conditions that have been proposed to be included as part of routine screening and/or risk assessment during the antepartum period since 1989. Many of these conditions are part of current routine screening programs, but few were implemented as routine care as a result of evidence based criteria. Most have been implemented as a result of expert or consensus opinion, cost/benefit, and/or risk management decisions. Still others have yet to be commonly accepted and await definitive research trials demonstrating efficacy as a screening test, or more importantly, effective treatment options. Cervical length assessment, fetal fibronectin, and salivary estriol determination have been proposed to assess risk of prematurity (see Chapter 26), and prevention programs have been proposed.[63] Definitive trials proving effectiveness of screening and efficacy of treatment have yet to be done.

It is important to individualize patient care and to be thorough. The initial visit includes a detailed history, and physical and laboratory examinations. The initial history requires that the patient be seen in an office setting. She should not be first seen undressed sitting on an examining table.

PRECONCEPTIONAL EDUCATION

We have reached a level of awareness about prenatal care where the optimal time to assess, manage, and treat many pregnancy conditions and complications is before pregnancy occurs.[64–65] The best time to see a woman for prenatal care is when she is considering pregnancy. At routine gynecologic visits and especially infertility visits, patients should be asked about their plans for pregnancy. At that time, much of the risk assessment described later in this chapter can be performed, as well as the basic physical and laboratory evaluations. If there are questions about the history, such as family history of fetal anomaly, or previous cesarean delivery, further details can be obtained from family members or the appropriate medical facility. This is the time to draw a rubella titer and immunize the susceptible patient. Hepatitis B immunization can be given to appropriate patients, and human immunodeficiency virus (HIV) testing can be offered. Varicella titers or immunization is recommended in women with no history of chickenpox. Patients need to use contraception for up to 3 months following immunizations (see Chapter 48). Toxoplasmosis screening based on risk factors may be indicated at this time because approximately one fourth of the U.S. population is infected.[66] Patients who have negative screens are at risk for congenital toxoplasmosis and should be counseled to avoid risks such as contact with wild felines and ingestion of raw or undercooked meat. Immunocompetent patients who screen positive can be reassured of lack of risk with regard to fetal loss, or stillbirth; albeit rare reports of congenital infection after previous infection have been described.[67] A prospective analysis of the population risks and benefits to substantiate routine screening for and/or education about toxoplasmosis has not been done in the United States. However, proponents argue a theoretical benefit based on treatment availability, extrapolated epidemiologic data from European countries where screening is widespread, and the prevalence of congenital infection that is comparable to other congenital diseases that we currently screen for by mandate (e.g., phenylketonuria and congenital hypothyroidism).[68]

Before pregnancy is the time to screen appropriate populations for genetic disease carrier states such as

Pregnancy Information

Both the obstetric patient and her physicians and nurses want the same things for every pregnancy. They are: a comfortable pregnancy free of complications, an easy labor and delivery, and a healthy mother and baby when all is over. In our practice, to a greater or lesser extent, most patients achieve such outcomes. Complications can occur, however, and bad things at times do happen to good people.

The rationale for prenatal care is to prevent complications if possible, to identify complications if they occur, and to manage identified complications so as to minimize their adverse effects. Much of this is our job, but it is your job to keep your appointments, to avoid exposures to chemicals and drugs of abuse including cigarettes, and to use your seatbelts.

Mother Although pregnancy is a stress on you, most women tolerate pregnancy well. Depending on your situation, we may recommend a modification of your activities. Death of the mother during pregnancy is very unusual, but can occur either in mothers with serious underlying illnesses or from rare, but extremely serious obstetric problems. Other risks to the mother include organ injuries (for example, rectum or bladder), infections and hemorrhage. You may require blood transfusions if you have heavy bleeding. Blood is very safe, and the donors are tested for AIDS and hepatitis, but the risk of acquiring infections from blood transfusions is not zero. This is why we are conservative in our use of blood products.

Baby Babies are healthiest if they are full term and appropriately grown. This is why we will instruct you about warning signs of premature labor (cramping, intermittent back pain, vaginal spotting or change in discharge, and pressure in the pelvis), and why we measure the uterus (to get an idea of the size of the baby) at the time of your prenatal visits.

In the latter part of pregnancy, if you are worried about a decrease or lack of the baby's movements, call it to our attention promptly. Do not wait for your next appointment.

All parents fear malformations or birth defects. Although often these can be identified by testing, this is not always so. For example, just because an ultrasound examination does not indicate a particular problem, this does not mean with certainty that it is not there. One in 25 babies is born with a malformation. Many of these are minor or can be successfully corrected.

Cesarean Birth Fifteen to twenty percent of patients in our hospital are delivered by this operation. This is a very safe operation, but is a major operation nonetheless. Cesareans are done for complications in the mother or baby, and are only done with your permission. Risks include injury to normal structures, hemorrhage, infection and anesthetic complications. Most of these can be managed without lasting harm, but occasionally are associated with the need for additional surgery, including hysterectomy, or with continuing difficulties. Rarely, death or severe, permanent problems, including brain damage, may result.

VBAC Most women with previous cesarean births are candidates for attempted vaginal birth after cesarean, or VBAC. Most women successfully complete VBAC trials. If so, the discomforts and risks of cesarean birth are avoided. Approximately one-quarter to one-third of the time, the VBAC attempt will be unsuccessful, and repeat cesarean birth will be required. The most serious complication specifically attributable to VBAC is rupture of the uterus. This occurs less than 1% of the time, but is serious for both mother and baby and emergency surgery is required.

The purpose of the preceding paragraphs is not to frighten you, but to make certain you understand that complications can occur. We will be happy to answer your questions regarding this pregnancy information today or in the future.

I have read the above information and have had opportunity to have my questions answered. I realize that the practice of obstetrics is not an exact science and that no guarantees have been made.

PATIENT: ____

PHYSICIAN: ____

Figure 5-3. Example of prenatal education and consent form. (Courtesy of Dr. Frank Zlatnik.)

Table 5-1. Comparison of Different Recommendations Regarding Visit Frequency and Proposed Clinical Interventions for Prenatal Care for Low-Risk Women

WEEKS' GESTATION	ACOG 1997	EXPERT PANEL NULLIPAROUS WOMAN	EXPERT PANEL MULTIPAROUS WOMAN	CLINICAL INTERVENTION
1–4		X	X	Preconception Dating
5–8	X	X	X	Dating
9–12	X	X		*
13–16	X	X	X	*
17–20	X			AFP/Multiple Marker
21–24	X			Screening*
25–28	X	X	X	Glucose tolerance test
31–32	X	X	X	Childbirth education Risk assessment
35–36	X	X	X	Risk assessment; Growth
37	X	X		Risk assessment
38	X	X		Risk assessment
39	X			
40	X	X		Risk assessment
41	X	X	X	Post term evaluation

ACOG, American College of Obstetricians and Gynecologists.

*Current standard of care would likely include offering first trimester screening and/or some multiple marker screening strategy (integrated or sequential) in the second trimester.

Adapted from Gregory KD, Davidson E: Prenatal Care: Who needs it and why? Clin Obstet Gynecol 42:725–736, 1999.

Tay-Sachs disease, Canavan's disease, cystic fibrosis, or hemoglobinopathies.[69] Resolution of these issues is much easier and less hurried without the time limits placed by an advancing pregnancy. Medical conditions such as anemia or hypothyroidism can be fully evaluated and the woman medically treated before pregnancy. If the patient is obese, weight reduction should be attempted before pregnancy. Patients in whom risks are very serious should be so counseled, and every attempt should be made to let them make a fully informed decision about pregnancy. Often, significant risk factors can be treated or managed so as to reduce risk during pregnancy.

The value of prepregnancy counseling needs to be emphasized to all those who treat women at significant risk for pregnancy problems. Women who are followed by other physicians (family physicians, pediatricians, general internists) for problems such as diabetes, hypertension, or systemic lupus erythematosus should be seen, evaluated, and counseled before pregnancy.

There is evidence that for some conditions, such as diabetes mellitus and phenylketonuria, medical disease management before conception can positively influence pregnancy outcome. Medical management to normalize the biochemical environment should be discussed with the patient and appropriate management plans outlined before conception. This is also the time to review drug usage and other practices, such as alcohol ingestion and smoking (see Chapter 8). Advice can be given about avoiding specific medications in the first trimester (e.g., isotretinoin), and general advice can be given concerning diet, exercise, and occupational exposures.

Periconceptional supplements with folic acid can reduce the incidence of neural tube defects (NTDs), and the use of therapeutic doses to decrease the risk of recurrence has been repeatedly demonstrated. This has resulted in national regulatory mandates for food supplements and national media campaigns to increase public awareness about the importance of this practice.[70–75] The CDC recommends that all women of childbearing age who are capable of becoming pregnant should consume 0.4 mg of folic acid daily, which is most easily achieved by taking a supplement. For women with a previously affected child, the recommendation is that the patient take 4 mg daily from 4 weeks before conception through the first 3 months of pregnancy. The benefits of folic acid supplementation are being investigated with regard to the prevention of other complications of pregnancy as well as chronic maternal disease states (e.g., preterm birth and cardiac disease), further emphasizing the appropriateness of prenatal care as both a model for primary care and a model for the provision of care in the context of a lifespan approach. Care provided at each visit impacts not only pregnancy outcome but ultimately long-term health outcomes for the woman and her family.

The importance of seeking care early for confirmation of pregnancy and gestational age dating can be discussed with the patient. Great precision can be achieved with an accurate menstrual calendar predating pregnancy and provide an opportunity for access to first-trimester screening for aneuploidy and prevent ambiguity about postdatism.

THE INITIAL PRECONCEPTIONAL OR PRENATAL VISIT

Social and Demographic Risks

Extremes of age are obstetric risk factors. The pregnant teenager has particular nutritional and emotional needs.

Table 5-2. Examples of Clinical Conditions Amenable to Antenatal Screening and Risk Assessment

Clinical Condition Screening/Diagnostic Test	Comment	Reference
Post Dates/Multiple Gestation/IUGR		
Early ultrasound	Increased precision of dating; "routine" use has unclear benefit yet used in more than 80% of pregnancies	181, 183, 185
IUGR		
Fundal height	Increased identification of small and large infants; fewer ultrasounds, economic benefit	180, 182
Smoking history	Smoking has demonstrated dose-response association with poor fetal growth; smoking cessation/reduction reverses growth disturbance; likelihood of cessation increased during pregnancy	48–52, 55, 56
Fetal Structural Malformation		
Ultrasound	Ultrasound, MSAFP standard of care for screening for neural tube defects.	199
Maternal serum AFP	See text re: prenatal genetic test	
Drug exposure		
Fetal Chromosomal Aberrations		
Multiple marker screening	Combination of specific maternal serum analytes used to screen for Down's syndrome, Trisomy 13, and 18 with potential detection rate of 60–90% when used with targeted ultrasound, see text	39, 200
Genetic Conditions		
Cystic Fibrosis	Recommended by ACOG	41
Canavan's Disease, "Jewish panel"	Recommended by ACOG	40
Preterm Birth (PTB)		
Cervical length	No benefit from routine screening; Unclear "best practice" and/or benefit of treatment once identified "at risk"	24, 26–28
Fetal fibronectin	No clear benefit as screening test to predict PTB (poor sensitivity and specificity); potential benefit from high negative predictive value	24, 25
Periodontal disease	May be independent risk factor for PTB; treatment reduced risk	29
Bacterial vaginosis	Independent risk factor for PTB; inconclusive if treatment alters risk but shown to be beneficial in selected populations	30–33, 173–175
Preclampsia		
Uterine Doppler	No effective prevention	22, 181
Serum markers	Nonspecific; no effective prevention	23, 191, 201
Thromboembolic Disease		
Pregnancy history Clinical history Laboratory evaluation for hereditary thrombophilias	Clinically relevant topic due to association with adverse pregnancy outcome; potential for life-threatening thromboembolic event; disseminating into practice; inconclusive data re: treatment efficacy	168
Infections		
Group B streptococcus	Screening and treatment prevents neonatal disease	202
HIV	Routine screening and treatment recommended by ACOG, treatment significantly decreases rate of perinatal transmission	34, 35
Bacterial vaginosis	See PTB	203
Psychosocial Risk		

ACOG, American College of Obstetricians and Gynecologists; HIV, human immunodeficiency virus; IUGR, intrauterine growth restriction, MSAFP, maternal serum alpha-fetoprotein.

She is at special risk for sexually transmitted diseases; it has been shown that she benefits particularly from education in areas of childbearing and contraception. The pregnant woman older than 35 years of age is at increased risk for a chromosomally abnormal child,[76] and she must be so advised. Patients should be asked about family histories of Down syndrome, NTDs, hemophilia, hemoglobinopathies, and other birth defects, as well as mental retardation (see Chapter 6). Consultation for genetic counseling and genetic testing, if desired, may be appropriate. Women older than 35 years of age are at increased risk for almost all pregnancy-related morbidities, maternal mortality, and neonatal complications including miscarriage, stillbirth, preterm birth and neonatal mortality. The age of the father is also important, because there may be genetic risks to the fetus when the father is older than 55 years.[77] Certain diseases may be related to race/ethnicity or geographic origin. Patients of African, Asian, or Mediterranean descent should be screened for the various heritable hemoblobinopathies (e.g., sickle cell disease, alpha and beta thalassemia). Patients of Jewish and French Canadian heritage should be screened for Tay-Sachs disease, Canavan's disease, and cystic fibrosis. More recently, it has been suggested that cystic fibrosis screening be offered to all couples planning a pregnancy or seeking prenatal testing.[78]

Low socioeconomic status should be identified and attempts to improve nutritional and hygienic measures undertaken. Appropriate referral to federal programs, such as that for women, infants, and children (WIC), and to public health nurses can have real benefits. If a patient has a history of previous neonatal death or stillbirth, records should be carefully reviewed so that the correct diagnosis is made and recurrence risk appropriately assessed. A history of drug abuse or recent blood transfusion should be elicited. The history of medical illnesses should be detailed and records obtained, if possible. A new rapid procedure for diagnosing mental disorders in primary care may be useful in pregnancy.[79]

Occupational hazards should be identified. If a patient works in a laboratory with chemicals, for example, she should be advised to limit her exposure. Patients whose occupations require heavy physical exercise or excess stress should be informed that they may need to decrease such activity.

Tobacco, alcohol, and recreational drug use can all adversely affect pregnancy and are a critical part of the history. Specific questions concerning smoking, alcohol, and drugs (prescriptive, over-the-counter, and illicit) should be asked.[80] Regular screening for alcohol and substance use should be carried out using such tools as the T-ACE questionnaire (Table 5-3)[81] or other simple screening tools, and appropriate directed therapy should be made available to those women who screen positive. Women should be urged to stop smoking before pregnancy and to drink not at all or minimally once they are pregnant. Studies show smoking cessation counseling by the health care provider works. Pregnancy is an ideal time to initiate this intervention.[82] Drug addiction confers a particularly high risk, and addicted mothers require specialized care throughout pregnancy.

Table 5-3. Alcohol Abuse Screening: The T-ACE Questionnaire*

T	How many drinks does it take to make you feel "high" (can you hold)? (*tolerance;* a positive response consists of two or more drinks)
A	Have people *annoyed* you by criticizing you drinking?
C	Have you ever felt you ought to *cut down* on your drinking?
E	Have you ever had a drink first thing in the morning to steady your nerves or to get rid of a hangover (*eye-opener*)?

Scoring: The tolerance question has substantially more weight (2 points) than the three other questions (1 point each).

*These questions were found to be significant identifiers of risk drinking in pregnancy (i.e., alcohol intake potentially sufficient to damage the embryo/fetus).

From Sokol RJ, Martier SS, Ager JW: The T-ACE questions: practical prenatal detection of risk-drinking. Am J Obstet Gynecol 160:863, 1989, with permission.

Violence against women is increasingly recognized as a problem that should be addressed, with reports suggesting that abuse occurs during 3 to 8 percent of pregnancies. Questions addressing personal safety and violence should be included during the prenatal period, and such tools as the Abuse Assessment Score (Fig. 5-4) are recommended.[83–85]

Medical Risk

A family history of diabetes, hypertension, tuberculosis, seizures, hematologic disorders, multiple pregnancies, congenital abnormalities, and reproductive wastage should be elicited. Often, a family history of mental retardation, birth defect, or genetic trait is difficult to elicit without formal genetic counseling or questionnaires; nonetheless; these areas should be emphasized at the initial history. A better history may be obtained if patients are asked to fill out a preinterview questionnaire or history form. Any significant maternal cardiovascular, renal, or metabolic disease should be defined. Infectious diseases such as urinary tract disease, syphilis, tuberculosis, or herpes genitalis should be identified. Surgical history with special attention to any abdominal or pelvic operations should be noted. A history of previous cesarean delivery should include indication, type of uterine incision, and any complications. A copy of the surgical report may be informative. Allergies, particularly drug allergies, should be prominent on the problem list.

Obstetric Risk

Previous obstetric and reproductive history are essential to optimizing care in subsequent pregnancies. The gravidity and parity should be noted and the outcome

Abuse Assessment Screen (Circle YES or NO for each question)

1. Have you ever been emotionally or physically abused by your partner or someone important to you? . . . . YES NO

2. Within the last year, have you been hit, slapped, kicked, or otherwise physically hurt by someone?. . . . . YES NO

   If YES, by whom (circle all that apply)

   Husband Ex-husband Boyfriend Stranger Other Multiple

   Total No. of times ________

3. Since you've been pregnant, have you been hit, slapped, kicked, or otherwise physically hurt by someone?. . . . . YES NO

   If YES, by whom (circle all that apply)

   Husband Ex-husband Boyfriend Stranger Other Multiple

   Total No. of times ________

   Mark the area of injury on a body map

Score each incident according to the following scale:

1 = Threats of abuse, including use of a weapon
2 = Slapping, pushing; no injuries and/or lasting pain
3 = Punching, kicking, bruises, cuts, and/or continuing pain
4 = Beaten up, severe contusions, burns, broken bones
5 = Head, internal, and/or permanent injury
6 = Use of weapon, wound from weapon

(If any of the descriptions for the higher number apply, use the higher number)

4. Within the last year, has anyone forced you to have sexual activities? . . . YES NO

   If YES, by whom (circle all that apply)

   Husband Ex-husband Boyfriend Stranger Other Multiple

   Total No. of times ________

5. Are you afraid of your partner or anyone you listed above? . . . . YES NO

Figure 5-4. Determination of frequency and severity of physical abuse during pregnancy. (From McFarlane J, Parker B, Soeken K, Bullock L: Assessing for abuse during pregnancy. JAMA 267:3176, 1992, with permission. Copyright 1992, American Medical Association.)

for each prior pregnancy recorded in detail. Previous pregnancy failure (and documentation about the gestational age at the time of the loss) not only confers risk and anxiety for another pregnancy loss but can be associated with an increased risk for genetic disease as well as preterm delivery.[86]

Previous preterm delivery is strongly associated with recurrence; it is important to delineate the events surrounding the preterm birth. Did the membranes rupture before labor? Were there painful uterine contractions? Was there bleeding? Were there fetal abnormalities? What was the neonatal outcome? All of these questions are vital in determining the etiology and prognosis of the condition, although specific recommendations will vary and the efficacy of routine prevention programs is not clear.[63] In patients with a previous premature delivery, progesterone administration may reduce the recurrence of risk.[87,88] Diethylstilbestrol (DES) exposure, incompetent cervix, and uterine anomalies are all conditions that may be known from a previous pregnancy. Previous fetal macrosomia makes glucose screening essential.

After all the specific questions, it is recommended to ask the patient a few general questions: What important items haven't I asked? What else about you and your pregnancy do I need to know? What problems and questions do you have? Leaving time for open-ended questions is the best way to complete the initial visit.

Physical and Laboratory Evaluation

Physical examination should include a general physical examination as well as a pelvic examination. Baseline height and weight as well as prepregnancy weight are recorded. Special attention should be given to the initial vital signs, and cardiac examination, because many healthy young women have not had a physical examination immediately before becoming pregnant. Any physical finding that might have an impact on pregnancy or that might be affected by pregnancy (e.g., mitral valve prolapse) should be defined. It is particularly important to perform and record a complete physical examination at this initial visit, because less emphasis will be placed on nonobstetric portions of the examination as pregnancy progresses in the absence of specific problems or complaints.

The pelvic examination should focus on the uterine size. Before 12 to 14 weeks, size can give a fairly accurate estimate of gestational age in a thin patient. Papanicolaou smear and culture for gonorrhea and chlamydia are done. Bacterial vaginosis should be recognized. The cervix should be carefully palpated, and any deviation from normal should be noted. Clinical pelvimetry should be performed and the clinical impression of adequacy noted. The pelvic examination is limited by examiner and patient variation as well as by obesity. If there is difficulty in examining the uterus, an ultrasound study is indicated.

Basic laboratory studies are routinely performed (Table 5-4). Some studies need not be repeated if recent normal values have been obtained, such as at an initial visit following a preconceptional visit or a recent gynecologic or infertility examination. Blood studies should include Rh type and screening for irregular antibodies, hemoglobin level, or hematocrit and serologic tests for syphilis and rubella. A urine sample should be obtained and tested for abnormal protein and glucose levels. Screening for

Table 5-4. Recommendations for All Women for Prenatal Care

	PRECONCEPTION OR FIRST VISIT	WEEKS								
		6–8*	14–16	24–28	32	36	38	39	40	41
History										
Medical, including genetic	X									
Psychosocial	X									
Update medical and psychosocial		X	X	X	X	X	X	X	X	X
Physical examination										
General	X									
Blood pressure	X	X	X	X	X	X	X	X	X	X
Height	X									
Weight	X	X	X	X	X	X	X	X	X	X
Height and weight profile	X									
Pelvic examination and pelvimetry	X	X								
Breast examination	X	X								
Fundal height			X	X	X	X	X	X	X	X
Fetal position and heart rate			X	X	X	X	X	X	X	X
Cervical examination	X									
Laboratory tests										
Hemoglobin or hematocrit	X	X		X		X				
Rh factor, type blood	X									
Antibody screen	X			X						
Pap smear	X									
Diabetic screen				X						
MSAFP			X							
Urine										
Dipstick	X									
Protein	X									
Sugar	X									
Culture		X								
Infections										
Rubella titer	X									
Syphilis test	X									
Gonococcal culture	X	X				X				
Hepatitis B	X									
HIV (offered)	X	X								
Toxoplasmosis	X									
Illicit drug screen (offered)	X									
Genetic screen	X									

*If preconception care has preceded.
HIV, human immunodeficiency virus; MSAFP, maternal serum α-fetoprotein.

asymptomatic bacteriuria has been traditionally done by urine culture, but screening may be simplified by testing for nitrites and leukocyte esterase.[89] Tuberculosis screening should also be performed in areas of disease prevalence.

First-trimester screening, a multiple marker screen, uses sonographic evaluation of NT (nuchal translucency) and new biochemical markers (pregnancy-associated placental protein [PAPP-A] and free β-hCG) that have been introduced to allow earlier screening for chromosomal aberrations. It is offered between 11 and14 weeks.[90,91] The QUAD test (alpha-fetoprotein, human chorionic gonadotropin [hCG], estriol, and inhibin A)[92] or maternal serum alpha-fetoprotein screening is offered from 15 to 20 weeks' gestation to screen for NTDs and aneuploidy (see Chapter 6). Patients who undergo first trimester screening should also have a maternal serum alpha-fetoprotein level after 15 weeks for NTD screening.

The laboratory evaluations outlined earlier are the standard tests. Specific conditions require further evaluation. A history of thyroid disease leads to thyroid function testing. Anticonvulsant therapy requires blood level studies to determine adequacy of medication. The importance of compliance with dosing and serial evaluation of serum blood levels should be emphasized because both thyroid medications and anticonvulsant levels are sensitive to the physiologic changes in blood volume that occurs during pregnancy. Adequacy of replacement and/or blood levels will need to be monitored throughout pregnancy. Identification of problems on screening (e.g., anemia, abnormal glucose screen) will mandate further testing. Screening for varicella has been suggested for women with no known history of chickenpox. The ACOG has recommended routine screening of all pregnant women for hepatitis B.[93] HIV screening should also be offered, because maternal therapy with azidothymidine (AZT) can reduce vertical transmission (see Chapter 48).[69,93,94] Hepatitis C and cytomegalovirus (CMV) screening should be considered for at risk populations. Recommendations for the content of prenatal care are summarized in Table 5-4.

ASSESSMENT OF GESTATIONAL AGE

During the course of the prenatal interview, assessment of gestational age begins with the question, "What was the first day of the last menstrual period?" From that point, the establishment of an estimated date of delivery and confirmation of that date by accumulation of supportive information remains one of the most important tasks of good prenatal care.

Human pregnancy has a duration of 280 days, measured from the first day of the last menstrual period (LMP) until delivery. The standard deviation is 14 days. It is important to remember that clinicians are measuring menstrual weeks (not conceptional weeks) with an assumption of ovulation and conception based on day 14 of a 28-day cycle. This gives pregnancy the 40-week gestational period in common clinical use. Much confusion exists among patients who try to measure pregnancy in terms of 9 months, when in fact, it is 10 (40/4 = 10) or who try to measure in conceptional weeks. Another problem exists in women whose menstrual cycles do not follow a 28-day cycle and who therefore do not conceive on day 14 of the menstrual cycle. The commonly used term "4 months pregnant" has no meaning (one does not know whether this is 16 or 20 weeks) and has no place on a contemporary prenatal record. It is often helpful to explain to patients and their families that their pregnancy will be described in terms of weeks, rather than months, and that the pregnancy can be broken into three trimesters lasting 1 to 14 weeks, 14 to 28 weeks, and 28 weeks to delivery. Every effort should be made to be consistent in usage to prevent confusion among patients and among clinicians who may assume care of the pregnancy.

Knowledge of gestational age is critical for obstetric decision-making. Generally, in a normal pregnancy, we can extrapolate from gestational age to estimate fetal weight. Throughout pregnancy, these are the two most important determinants of fetal viability and survival. Without accurate knowledge of gestational age, diagnosis of such conditions as prolonged or postterm pregnancy and intrauterine growth restriction is often impossible. Multiple gestation is most often detected early when the size of the uterine fundus is greater than expected for gestation. Appropriate management of preterm labor or a medically complicated pregnancy depends on an accurate estimate of fetal age and weight. Within regional perinatal systems, records of gestational age are important for flow of information, and rapid access to consistent, clear data is vital. In such situations, and during prolonged hospitalization, it is sometimes helpful to define gestational age further by using the notation of fractional weeks (27 4/7 weeks). It must be remembered, however, that we are describing a biologic system and that such precision is being used more for ease of communication and organization than for any ability to date the pregnancy with such a degree of accuracy.

Clinical Dating

The most reliable clinical estimator of gestational age is an accurate LMP. Using Naegele's rule, the estimated date of confinement is calculated by subtracting 3 months and adding 1 week from the first day of the LMP. A careful history must be taken from the patient, verifying that the date given is the first day of the period as well as whether the period was normal, heavy, or light. The date of the previous menstrual period will help ascertain the length of the cycle. History should also be taken about previous use of oral contraceptives, which might influence ovulation.

Other clinical tools can be used to confirm and support LMP data, and in cases in which the LMP is inaccurate or unknown, it has been shown that accumulated clinical information from early pregnancy can predict gestational age with an accuracy approaching that of menstrual dating.[95]

The size of the uterus on early pelvic examination, or by direct measurement of the abdomen from the pubic symphysis to the top of the uterine fundus (over the curve), provides useful information. Experienced practi-

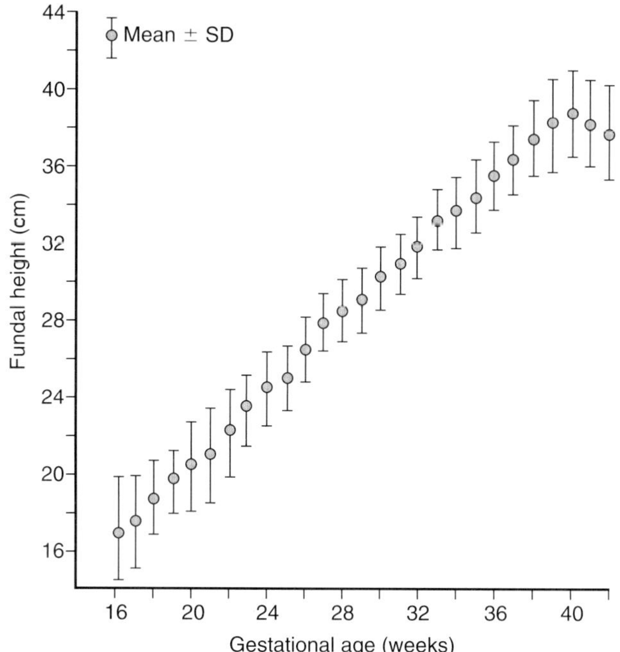

Figure 5-5. Fundal height versus gestational age. (From Knox AJ, Sadler L, Pattison WS, et al: An obstetric scoring system: its development and application in obstetric management. Obstet Gynecol 81:195, 1993, with permission.)

tioners can assess the early pregnancy with reproducibility before 12 to 14 weeks. Fundal height measurement in centimeters using the over-the-curve technique approximates the gestational age from 16 to 38 weeks within 3 cm (Fig. 5-5).

The uterus also tends to reach the umbilicus at about 20 weeks, and this, too, can be assessed when uterine fundal measurements are made. The uterus may be elevated in early pregnancy in a patient with a previous cesarean delivery or with uterine myomas, making the fundal height appear abnormally high. Considerable variations in the level of the umbilicus and in the height of patients make this clinical marker variable. Quickening, the first perception of fetal movement by the mother, occurs at predictable times in gestation. In the first pregnancy, quickening is usually noted at about 19 weeks; in subsequent pregnancies, probably because of the experience of the observer, it tends to occur about 2 weeks earlier.[95] It is helpful to ask the woman to mark on a calendar the first time she feels the baby move and to report this date.

Audible fetal heart tones, in addition to being absolute evidence of pregnancy, are another marker of gestational age. Using an unamplified Hillis-DeLee fetoscope, they are generally audible at 19 to 20 weeks. Observer experience, acuity, and the time spent listening can all affect this number, so this guideline may need to be adapted individually.

Use of the electronic Doppler device is widespread and permits detection of the fetal heart by 11 to 12 weeks. Practitioners can set a standard individualized to their own equipment, which can be used as a gestational age marker. If fetal heart tones are not heard at the expected time, a sonogram is appropriate to look for date/examination discrepancy, fetal viability, twins, or polyhydramnios.

The conversion of a negative urinary pregnancy test to a positive one may be helpful in assessing gestational age, but the sensitivity of the test used must be known in order to interpret the data accurately. These tests may be negative if they are performed too early.

Comparison of the various clinical estimators shows a known LMP date to be the most precise predictor. The clinical estimators can be ranked according to decreasing order of accuracy as follows: (1) LMP; (2) the uterus reaching umbilicus; and (3) fetal heart tone documentation, fundal height measurements, and quickening. Because of inherent biologic variability and differences in the examiner acuity, the estimated date of confinement can be predicted with 90 percent certainty only within ± 3 weeks by even the best single estimator.[96]

Ultrasound

Ultrasound plays a major role in assessment of size and duration of pregnancy. The National Institutes of Health (NIH) consensus conference in 1984 concluded that in a low-risk pregnancy followed from the first trimester, routine ultrasound examination was not justified for determining gestational age. However, a long list of indications justifies an ultrasound examination[97–99] and studies on resource utilization indicate that at least 70 percent of women receive an ultrasound at some point in their pregnancy, and importantly, women have come to expect an ultrasound as part of standard prenatal care.[100] Despite this expectation, a review of the literature regarding women's knowledge about the purpose of the procedure or the limitations of the technology was limited, suggesting that clinicians need to make a greater effort to inform patients about the specific purposes of ultrasound and what it can and cannot achieve, and limit exposure to as low as reasonably achievable.[101]

As previously noted, early prenatal care and clinical assessment facilitates pregnancy dating; however, ultrasound is an accurate means of estimating gestational age in the first half of pregnancy.[102] The crown-rump length, biparietal diameter, and femur length in the first half of pregnancy correlate closely with age. As pregnancy progresses, fetal size varies considerably, and measurement of the fetus is a poor tool for estimation of gestational age, especially in the third trimester (see Chapter 9).

A randomized trial has shown that the risk of being called overdue was reduced from 8 percent to 2 percent for patients who received early ultrasound.[103] Also, twins were detected more often and perinatal mortality was reduced in the ultrasound group. The Routine Antenatal Diagnostic Imaging with Ultrasound (RADIUS) study reported no improvement in perinatal outcome with use of routine ultrasound in normal, low-risk women.[104] However, 61 percent of women were excluded for many reasons such as an uncertain menstrual history, and only 35 percent of anomalies were detected in the ultrasound-screened group (only 17 percent before 24 weeks). The meta-analysis by Bucher and Schmidt[102] indicated that routine scanning can detect many more anomalies. The authors' practice is to perform ultrasound at 16 to 20 weeks for a baseline gestational age measurement and as a screening for fetal abnormality or multiple gestation. If ultrasound is not done routinely, the caregiver must be vigilant in detecting problems that are indications for a scan, and more frequent scans may be necessary.

REPEAT PRENATAL VISITS

A plan of visits is outlined to the patient. This has been traditionally every 4 weeks for the first 28 weeks of pregnancy, every 2 to 3 weeks until 36 weeks, and weekly thereafter, if the pregnancy progresses normally. The Public Health Service[2] suggested that this number of visits can be decreased, especially in parous, healthy women, and studies suggest that this can be done safely (Table 5-5).[105] If there are any complications, the intervals can be increased appropriately. For example, patients with hypertensive disease may require weekly visits. Fetal heart tones can be documented before the 12th week by Doppler devices and generally by the 20th week by Hillis-Delee stethoscope, and this information can be used for gestational dating purposes.

At regular visits, the patient is weighed, the blood pressure is recorded, and the presence of edema is evaluated (see intercurrent problems below). Fundal height is regularly measured with a tape measure, fetal heart tones are recorded, and fetal position is noted. The goal of subsequent pregnancy visits is to assess fetal growth and maternal well-being. In addition, at each prenatal visit, time should be allowed for the following questions: Do you have any problems? Do you have any questions? Family members should be encouraged to come to prenatal visits, ask questions, and participate to the degree that the patient wishes.

A pelvic examination is usually performed only on the first visit. In patients at risk of prematurity or in those with a history of DES exposure, however, frequent cervical checks or sonographic evaluation of cervical length may reveal premature dilation or effacement.

Further laboratory evaluations are routinely performed at 28 weeks, when the hemoglobin or hematocrit and Rh type and the screen for antibodies, as well as the serologic test for syphilis and possibly HIV testing, can be repeated. If the patient is Rh negative and unsensitized, she should receive Rhesus immune globulin (RhIG) prophylaxis at this time. A glucose screening test for diabetes is also appropriately performed at this time (see Chapter 37), and routine fetal movement counting can begin using an organized system.[106] At 36 weeks, a repeat hematocrit, especially in those women with anemia or at risk for peripartum hemorrhage (multipara, repeat cesarean delivery), may be performed. Group B streptococcus (GBS) screening should be performed at 35 to 36 weeks, and results made available for possible intrapartum prophylaxis.[70] Also, appropriate cultures for sexually transmitted disease (gonorrhea, chlamydia) should be obtained as indicated in the third trimester based on geographic prevalence rates, and demographic risk factors.

After 41 weeks from the LMP, the patient should be entered into a screening program for fetal well-being, which may include electronic monitoring tests or ultrasound evaluation (see Chapter 11).

Table 5-5. 1989 Recommended Dietary Allowances

	NONPREGNANT WOMEN				LACTATION (MONTHS)	
	15–18	**19–24**	**25–50**	**PREGNANCY**	**1–6**	**7–1**
Calories (kcal)						
Protein (g)	44	46	50	60	65	62
Vitamin A (μg RE)	800	800	800	800	1,300	1,200
Vitamin D (μg)	10	5	5	10	10	10
Vitamin E (mg TE)	8	8	8	10	12	10
Vitamin C (mg)	60	60	60	70	95	90
Thiamin (mg)	1.1	1.1	1.1	1.5	1.6	
Riboflavin (mg)	1.3	1.3	1.3	1.6	1.8	
Niacin (mg NE)	15	15	15	17	20	2
Vitamin B_6 (mg)	1.5	1.6	1.6	12.2	2.1	
Folate (μg)	180	180	180	400	280	26
Vitamin B_{12} (μg)	2.0	2.0	2.0	2.2	2.6	
Calcium (mg)	1,200	1,200	800	1,200	1,200	1,200
Phosphorus (mg)	1,200	1,200	800	1,200	1,200	1,200
Magnesium (mg)	300	280	280	320	355	340
Iron (mg)	15	15	15	30	15	15
Zinc (mg)	12	12	12	15	19	16
Iodine (μg)	150	150	150	175	200	200
Selenium (μg)	50	55	55	65	75	75

Data from Spitzer RL, Williams JBW, Kroenke K, et al: Utility of a new procedure for diagnosing mental disorders in primary care. JAMA 272:1749, 1994.

INTERCURRENT PROBLEMS

It is the practice in prenatal care to evaluate the pregnant patient for the development of certain complications. Inherent in these checks is surveillance for intervening problems, an important one being preeclampsia. If a patient shows a tendency to blood pressure elevation at 28 weeks, for example, she should be seen again in a week, not a month. Blood pressure changes physiologically in response to pregnancy, but development of hypertension must be recognized and evaluation and hospitalization appropriately instituted.

Weight gain in pregnancy has been shown to be an important correlate of fetal weight gain and, therefore, is closely monitored. Too little weight gain should lead to an evaluation of nutritional factors and an assessment of associated fetal growth. Excess weight gain is one of the first signs of fluid retention, but it may also reflect increased dietary intake or decreased activity. Dependent edema is physiologic in pregnancy, but generalized or facial edema can be a first sign of disease. Periodontal disease may be an independent risk factor for preterm birth,[107] but this has not been confirmed in a randomized trial.[107a] It is critical here, as in all areas, for the practitioner to understand the normal changes associated with pregnancy in order to accept and explain the normal but also to manage aggressively any abnormal changes (see Chapter 3).

Proteinuria reflects urinary tract disease, generally either infection or glomerular dysfunction, possibly the result of preeclampsia. Urinary tract infection should be looked for, and the degree of protein quantitated in a 24-hour urine collection.

Glycosuria is common because of increased glucose filtered through the kidney in pregnancy but warrants evaluation for diabetes with a measurement of capillary glucose when clinical suspicion exists.

Fetal abnormalities are often first detected by deviation from the clinical expectation. In some conditions, risk of fetal anomaly is so high as to prompt some kind of baseline screening or testing (e.g., amniocentesis, sonography, fetal echocardiography). At other times, risk becomes evident only during the course of prenatal care. Growth restriction and macrosomia can often be suspected clinically, usually on the basis of an abnormality in fundal growth. For the patient who has a history of these conditions or other predisposing factors, such as hypertension, renal disease, or diabetes, particular vigilance is in order. Excess amniotic fluid is another condition that can be clinically detected, and an etiology for the hydramnios should be sought. In addition to maternal conditions, hydramnios may be caused by fetal disease that can also be defined using sonography and that may alter management of the pregnancy.

THE PRENATAL RECORD

The prenatal care record describes in a consistent fashion the comprehensive care that is provided and allows for documentation of coordinated services. Prenatal care should be documented by a prenatal record of good quality designed to systematically capture important clinical and psychosocial information over time. One such example is the antepartum record designed by the ACOG. Many of the advances in risk assessment and in regionalization result directly from an improvement in this record and electronic medical records (EMR) are being developed.[108] Technology allows sophisticated recording, display, and retrieval (often computer based) of prenatal care records, but quality relies on accurate consistent compiling and concurrent recording of the information. The record must be complete, yet simple; directive, but flexible; and transmittable, legible, and able to display necessary data rapidly. European nations often have one record for uniform care; many states and regions have adopted records to permit internal consistency.

The commonly used records accurately reflect the following:

1. Demographic data, obstetric history
2. Medical and family history, including genetic screening
3. Baseline physical examination, with emphasis on gynecologic examination
4. Menstrual history, especially last normal menstrual period with documentation of established due date and reference criteria for dating if other than LMP
5. Record of individual visits
6. Routine laboratory data (e.g., Rh, GBS, rapid plasma reagin (RPR), rubella, hepatitis, and HIV)
7. Problem list
8. Space for special notations and plans (e.g., planned vaginal birth after cesarean delivery [VBAC] or repeat cesarean, tubal ligation)

These records must be made available to consultants, and they should be available at the facility where delivery is planned. If transfer is expected, a copy of the prenatal record should accompany the patient.

PRENATAL EDUCATION

Patient education leads to better self-care. As maternal and neonatal outcomes improve, efforts become more sophisticated to improve understanding, involvement, and satisfaction with pregnancy and the perinatal period. In this area, more than any other, the options for paramedical support have expanded. Practitioners and patients have access to a vast array of support persons and groups to assist and advise in the pregnancy and subsequent parenthood. Group prenatal care has recently been proposed and evaluated.[109] The wise practitioner stays abreast of these advances and integrates them into practice. Patients should be educated about care options and participate in decision-making. Although not exhaustive, the following section includes common issues or concerns that the practitioner should address at some point during successive prenatal visits as part of their health education, promotion, and prevention goals with each patient.

Informed Consent and Vaginal Birth After Cesarean Section

During the educational components of prenatal care, there is significant opportunity to accomplish most if not all the informed consent required for the delivery process. There are also advantages to securing documentation of appropriate informed consent for management of labor and associated obstetric procedures, possible interventions, and risks and benefits when they can be thoroughly reviewed and discussed rather than in the throes of labor It is our practice to obtain consent, whenever possible, in the third trimester for "delivery and related procedures including intravenous (IV) fluids, fetal monitoring, labor augmentation, episiotomy, operative vaginal delivery including forceps and vacuum and cesarean delivery," and this is documented on institutional consent forms and signed by the patient. Consent for anesthesia can also be obtained before admission. Risks such as third- and fourth-degree lacerations with episiotomy and operative delivery are appropriate to discuss, as well as the benefits of birth spacing and contraceptive options. Maternal, newborn, and familial benefits have been associated with optimal birth spacing, which is estimated to be approximately 2 to 5 years. Short pregnancy intervals are associated with increased low birth weight, preterm birth, and other adverse pregnancy outcomes attributed to decreased maternal reserves whereas prolonged birth spacing has been associated with increased risk of breast cancer, preeclampsia, and stillbirths. The benefits of intermediate birth spacing needs to be emphasized by health care practitioners and more widely disseminated. It is associated with improved maternal health (decreased risk of uterine rupture, endometritis, antepartum bleeding, anemia, depression), improved child health (decreased childhood illnesses, injuries, death, improved education), and improved family health, functioning, and socioeconomic status.[110–119] Although contraceptive options are numerous, tubal ligation is the most common method in the United States. If tubal ligation is offered, the risks, benefits, and alternatives of postpartum versus interval ligation should be discussed.[120]

The special benefits and risks of vaginal birth after cesarean section are particularly important to discuss before labor, and it is common to document both the components of the informed consent process as well as the patient's choice with respect to route of delivery (Fig. 5-6).

Smoking Cessation

Smoking has a demonstrated dose-response relationship to impaired fetal growth. Smoking cessation or reduction can reverse this growth disturbance. The likelihood of interventions to stop or reduce smoking are increased during pregnancy. Every effort should be made to identify prepregnancy and pregnant smokers and provide both pharmacologic and psychosocial interventions and programs to maximize likelihood of smoking cessation.[121–127]

Drugs and Teratogens

At the preconceptional or first prenatal visit, recommendations for nonpharmacologic remedies for common ailments can be given. This can often be integrated into a discussion of the common side effects of pregnancy. Because of widespread use of over-the-counter drugs, the patient should be warned to take only those drugs specifically approved or prescribed by her practitioner (see Chapter 8). Likewise, the patient should be advised to inform her practitioner about all natural or herbal supplements that are being used. Practitioners should be aware that current studies estimate roughly 40 percent of women have used complementary alternative medicine (including herbal therapy).[128]

Radiologic Studies

Elective radiologic studies can safely be delayed until completion of the pregnancy; however, dental and radiologic diagnostic procedures should be performed during pregnancy when they are indicated with proper shielding of the abdomen. Tests to evaluate life-threatening events such as thromboembolic phenomenon, or as needed for trauma evaluation particularly should not be deferred because this could put the mother's health at undue risk. Judicious use of pulmonary perfusion scans, spiral computed tomography (CT), and magnetic resonance imaging (MRI) have been life-saving for pregnant women with minimal radiation exposure risks.[129] Dental restorative work especially should be performed to allow optimal maternal nutrition. Prevention of periodontal disease may reduce prematurity,[130] but the data are conflicting.[107a]

Nutrition

One of the earliest purposes of prenatal care was to ensure that women received adequate nutrition for pregnancy. The health care provider may be influential in correcting inappropriate dietary habits.[131] Strict vegetarians may need supplemental vitamin B_{12}. Occasionally, consultation with a registered dietitian may be necessary when there is poor compliance or a special medical need such as diabetes mellitus.

Dietary allowances for most substances increase during pregnancy. According to the 1989 recommended dietary allowances (RDAs), only the recommendations for iron, folic acid, and vitamin D double during gestation.[132] The RDA for calcium and phosphorus increase by one half; the RDA for pyridoxine and thiamine increase by about one third. The RDA for protein, zinc, and riboflavin increase by about one fourth. The RDA for all other nutrients except vitamin A increase by less than 20 percent (Tables 5-5 and 5-6) and vitamin A not at all, as that is felt to be stored adequately. All of these nutrients, with the exception of iron, are supplied by a well-balanced diet.

UNIVERSITY OF MICHIGAN HOSPITALS
Department of Obstetrics & Gynecology
Consent Form for
Trial of Labor/Repeat Cesarean Section

Date:__________________________

You have had a previous cesarean section. Although "once a cesarean always a cesarean section" used to be the rule, some women may choose to attempt a vaginal delivery, called a "trial of labor." The American College of Obstetricians and Gynecologists recommend that women with one previous cesarean delivery with a low transverse incision should be encouraged to attempt labor.

Your doctor or nurse-midwife will review the records of your cesarean section to determine whether or not you may safely attempt labor. A safe attempt to deliver vaginally is based on the type of uterine scar that you have. The previous incision in your uterus may have been transverse (back and forth) or vertical (up and down); this may be different from the incision in your skin.

Low transverse (back and forth)

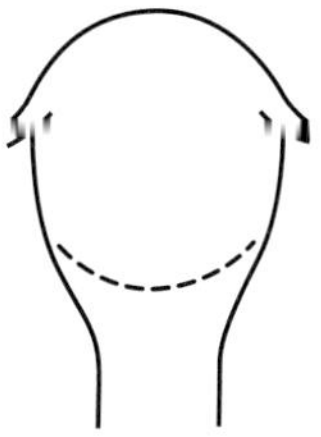

Classic vertical (up and down)

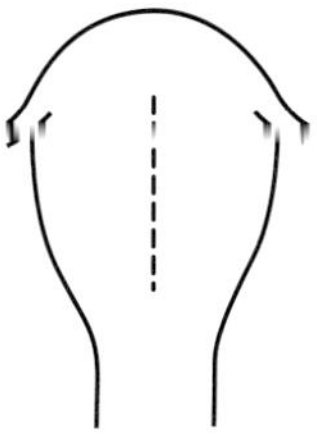

Some vertical incisions are known to be weaker and at greater risk of opening or rupturing during labor. Therefore, women with vertical uterine scars should not be allowed to labor. If you have had more than one cesarean section, it will be necessary to examine the operative note from each of your deliveries.

Large studies have found a success rate of vaginal deliveries in 70%–80% for women who have a trial of labor. The alternative to a trial of labor is to have a repeat cesarean section, without labor. Most obstetricians recommend a repeat cesarean section if the baby is expected to be very large, if the baby is in a breech or transverse position, or for twins.

There are benefits and risks of a trial of labor. The benefits of vaginal delivery after cesarean section include a shorter hospital stay and recovery period for you. A vaginal delivery is considered safer than a cesarean section for the mother, with less blood loss and less risk of infection. The baby may benefit from vaginal birth by less remaining lung fluid after the first breath.

The risks of vaginal delivery after cesarean section should be understood as well. You may require a cesarean section during labor. If you do, you have a higher risk of infection. Cesarean section, however, does not guarantee a healthy/normal baby. Finally, there is a small ($<$1–2%) risk of the uterus opening in the area of the old incision. If this happens, it could cause distress, permanent injury or death to your baby, excessive bleeding, and rarely may require a hysterectomy (removal of the uterus).

If you qualify for a vaginal delivery after cesarean section, then you may choose to either plan a trial of labor or a repeat cesarean section. Your doctor or nurse-midwife will answer any questions that you may have.

________________ Please initial here that you have read and understand the risks and benefits of each procedure.

I have had the opportunity to have my questions answered and I elect:

☐ A trial of labor,

☐ A repeat cesarean section delivery.

____________________________________ ____________________________________
signature date witness signature date

PS2317 7/98 MEDICAL RECORDS University of Michigan Medical Center TRIAL OF LABOR/REPEAT CESAREAN

Figure 5-6. Consent form for trial of labor/repeat cesarean delivery.

Table 5-6. Summary of Recommended Dietary Allowances for Women Aged ≥ 25–50 Years, Changes from Nonpregnant to Pregnant, and Food Sources

NUTRIENT	NONPREGNANT	PREGNANT	PERCENT INCREASE	DIETARY SOURCES
Energy (kcal)	2,200	2,500	+13.6	Proteins, carbohydrates, fats
Protein (g)	50	60	+20	Meats, fish, poultry, dairy
Calcium (mg)	800	1,200	+50	Dairy products
Phosphorus (mg)	800	1,200	+50	Meats
Magnesium (mg)	280	320	+14.3	Seafood, legumes, grains
Iron (mg)	15	30	+100	Meats, eggs, grains
Zinc (mg)	12	15	+25	Meats, seafood, eggs
Iodine (μg)	150	175	+16.7	Iodized salt, seafood
Vitamin A (μg RE)	800	800	0	Dark green, yellow, or orange fruits and vegetables
Vitamin D (IU)	200	400	+100	Fortified dairy products
Thiamin (mg)	1.2	1.5	+36.3	Enriched grains, pork
Riboflavin (mg)	1.3	1.6	+23	Meats, liver, enriched grains
Pyridoxine (mg)	1.6	2.2	+37.5	Meats, liver, enriched grains
Niacin (mg NE)	15	17	+13.3	Meats, nuts, legumes
Vitamin B_{12} (μg)	2.0	2.2	+10	Meats
Folic acid (μg)	180	400	+122	Leafy vegetables, liver
Vitamin C (mg)	60	70	+16.7	Citrus fruits, tomatoes
Selenium (μg)	55	65	+18.2	

From National Academy of Sciences: Recommended Dietary Allowances, 10th ed. Washington, DC, National Academy Press, 1989.

The National Academy of Sciences currently recommends that 30 mg of ferrous iron supplements be given to pregnant women daily, because the iron content of the habitual American diet and the iron stores of many women are not sufficient to provide the increased iron required during pregnancy. For those at high nutritional risk, such as some adolescents, those with multiple gestation, heavy cigarette smokers, and drug and alcohol abusers, a vitamin/mineral supplement should be given. Increased iron is needed both for the fetal needs and for the increased maternal blood volume. Thus, iron-containing foods should also be encouraged. Iron is found in liver, red meats, eggs, dried beans, leafy green vegetables, whole-grain enriched bread and cereal, and dried fruits. The 30-mg iron supplement is contained in approximately 150 mg of ferrous sulfate, 300 mg of ferrous gluconate, or 100 mg of ferrous fumarate. Taking iron between meals on an empty stomach will facilitate its absorption.

Because women of higher socioeconomic status have better reproductive performance and fewer low-birth-weight babies than do women of lower socioeconomic status, and because they also consume more protein, it is probably prudent to continue to recommend a generous amount of dietary protein. However, it has not been documented that protein supplementation will improve pregnancy outcome.[133] Acute caloric restriction in a well-nourished population, such as occurred during the Dutch famine of 1944 to 1945, caused the average birth weight to drop about 250 g, yet no adverse effect on long-term outcome was observed. These mothers ate a calorie-restricted, balanced diet in their second and third trimesters.

Weight Gain

The total weight gain recommended in pregnancy is 25 to 35 lb for normal women.[134] Underweight women may gain up to 40 lb, and overweight women should limit weight gain to 15 lb, although they do not need to gain any weight if they are morbidly obese.[135] About 2 to 3 lb are from increased fluid volume, 3 to 4 lb from increased blood volume, 1 to 2 lb from breast enlargement, 2 lb from enlargement of the uterus, and 2 lb from amniotic fluid. At term, the infant weighs approximately 6 to 8 lb and the placenta 1 to 2 lb. A 4- to 6-lb increase in maternal stores of fat and protein are important for lactation. Usually, 3 to 6 lbs are gained in the first trimester and ½ to 1 lb per week in the last two trimesters of pregnancy.

If the patient does not show a 10-lb weight gain by midpregnancy, her nutritional status should be reviewed. Inadequate weight gain is associated with an increased risk of a low-birth-weight infant (Fig. 5-7). Inadequate weight gain seems to have its greatest effect in women who are of low or normal weight before pregnancy. Underweight mothers must gain more weight during pregnancy to produce infants of normal weight. Patients should be cautioned against weight loss during pregnancy.

When excess weight gain is noted, an assessment for fluid retention is also performed. In the assessment of edema, some dependent edema in the legs is normal as pregnancy advances because of venous compression by the weight of the uterus. Elevation of the feet and bed rest on the left side will help correct this problem. Turning the patient from her back to her left side increases venous return from the legs as the pressure on the vena cava is

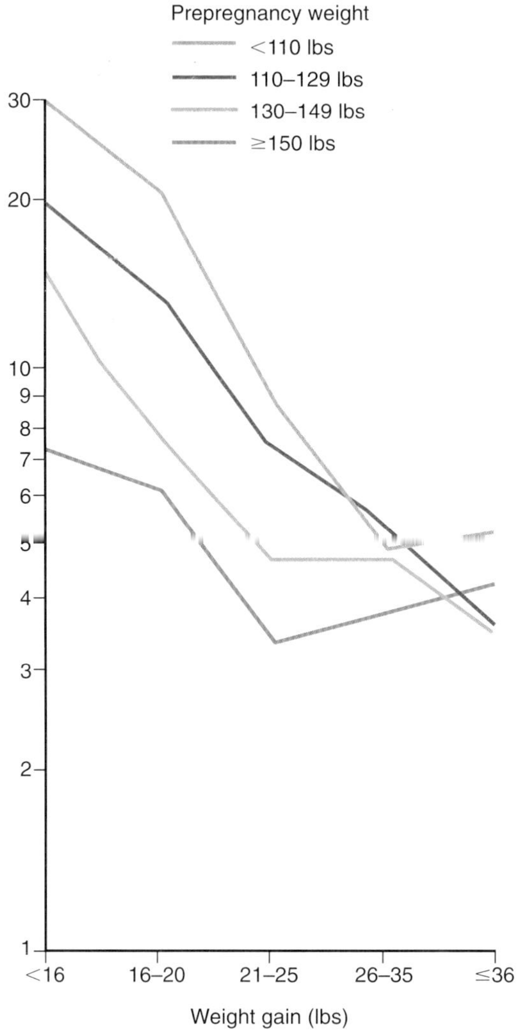

Figure 5-7. Percentage of liveborn infants of low birth weight by maternal weight gain during pregnancy according to the mother's prepregnancy weight. Low birth weight is defined as birth weight of less than 2,500 g or 5 lb, 8 oz. (From the National Natality Survey-United States. DHHS Pub No. [PHS] 86–1922, 1980.)

relieved. This maneuver increases the effective circulating blood volume, cardiac output, and thus the blood flow to the kidney. A diuresis will follow, as well as increased blood flow to the uterus.

Limitation of fluids will neither prevent nor correct fluid retention. Salt is not restricted, although patients with hypertension may be advised to decrease salt load.

Activity and Employment

Most patients are able to maintain their normal activity levels in pregnancy. Mothers tolerate pregnancy with considerable physical activity, such as looking after small children, but heavy lifting and excessive physical activity should be avoided. Modification of activity level as the pregnancy progresses is seldom needed, except if the job involves physical danger. Recreational exercises should be encouraged, such as those available in prenatal exercise classes. Previously sedentary women with no medical contraindications can start with 15 minutes of continuous exercise three times per week and work toward a goal of 30 minutes five times per week. With regard to exercise intensity, a good rule of thumb is the "talk test." If a pregnant, exercising woman cannot maintain a conversation (perceived moderate intensity), she is probably overexercising. Studies suggest that women who engage in regular recreational activity are less likely to develop gestational diabetes and preeclampsia, and have less low back pain/pelvic pain.[136–139] The patient should be counseled to discontinue activity whenever she experiences discomfort.

Healthy pregnant women may work until their delivery, if the job presents hazards no greater than those encountered in daily life. Strenuous physical exercise, standing for prolonged periods, and work on industrial machines as well as other adverse environmental factors may be associated with increased risk of poor pregnancy outcome, and these should be modified as necessary.[140–142]

Travel

The patient should be advised against prolonged sitting during car or airplane travel because of the risk of venous stasis and possible thromboembolism. The usual recommendation is a maximum of 6 hours per day driving, with stopping at least every 2 hours for 10 minutes to allow the patient to walk around and increase venous return from the legs. Hydration and support stockings are also recommended.

The patient should be instructed to wear her seat belt during car travel, but under the abdomen as pregnancy advances. It may also be helpful to take pillows along in a car to increase comfort.

If the patient is traveling a significant distance, it might be helpful for her to carry a copy of her medical record with her in case an emergency arises in a strange environment. She could also check into the medical facilities in the area or perhaps obtain the name of an obstetrician in the event of a problem.

Immunizations

Because of a theoretical risk to the fetus, pregnant women or women likely to become pregnant should not be given live, attenuated-virus vaccines. Influenza vaccination should be given during flu season. Yellow fever and oral polio may be given to women exposed to these infections. Despite theoretical risks, no evidence of congenital rubella syndrome in infants born to mothers inadvertently given rubella vaccine has been reported. Measles, mumps, and rubella viruses are not transmitted by those immunized and can be given to children of pregnant women. There is no evidence of fetal risk from inactivated virus vaccines, bacterial vaccines, toxoids, or tetanus immunoglobulin, which should be administered if appropriate. Post delivery measles, mumps and rubella and varicella vaccinations should be encouraged.

Nausea and Vomiting in Pregnancy

About 50 percent of women have both nausea and vomiting, 25 percent have nausea only, and 25 percent are unaffected. About two thirds of women with severe nausea in a prior pregnancy have similar symptoms in subsequent pregnancies. Research suggests that taking a prenatal vitamin before conception may reduce nausea in pregnancy. Nausea severe enough to cause significant weight loss or hospitalization is seen rarely, affecting 0.5 to 2 of pregnant women. There are four main categories of interventions for nausea: dietary changes, behavior modification, medications and acupressure. Nonpharmacologic measures are usually recommended initially to treat nausea and vomiting in early pregnancy. Behavior modification centers on women avoiding personal triggers for nausea that they identify themselves. Dietary modification with frequent small feedings in order to keep some food in the stomach at all times is helpful. There is some evidence that small, protein rich meals may help reduce nausea. Drug and alternative therapies[143] for nausea in pregnancy are covered in Chapter 8.

Heartburn

Heartburn is a common complaint in pregnancy because of relaxation of the esophageal sphincter. Overeating contributes to this problem. The patient should be advised to save part of her meal for later if she is experiencing postprandial heartburn and also not to eat immediately before lying down. Pillows at bedtime may help. If necessary, antacids may be prescribed. Liquid antacids coat the esophageal lining more effectively than do tablets. In a subset of patients, H-2 blockers may be helpful.

Restless Legs Syndrome

About one in 5 to 10 women will develop restless legs syndrome (RLS) during the second half of pregnancy. RLS usually occurs as women fall asleep and is characterized by tingling or other uncomfortable sensations in the lower legs, resulting in the overwhelming urge to move the legs. Unfortunately, movement, walking around or other measures do not relieve RLS. Iron deficiency anemia has been associated with an increased risk for RLS, and in anemic women, iron supplementation may reduce leg restlessness. Avoidance of caffeine containing drinks like coffee, tea or sodas in the last half of the day should also be recommended, as caffeine may increase symptoms.[144]

Sciatica

Sciatica refers to nerve pain that shoots rapidly down from the buttocks and unilaterally down one leg, usually ending in the foot. True sciatica is rare in pregnancy, affecting less than 1% of pregnancies. True sciatica is caused either by a herniated disc, or less commonly by uterine pressure on the sciatic nerve. In addition to pain, other signs of nerve compression include numbness in the affected leg. True sciatica should prompt referral to an orthopedic surgeon for further evaluation.

Carpal Tunnel Syndrome

The extra fluid retention of pregnancy can exacerbate carpal tunnel syndrome. Higher weight gain during pregnancy is also a risk factor. The most common symptoms of carpal tunnel syndrome are pain and numbness in the thumb, index and middle fingers and weakness in the muscles that move the thumb. Between 25 and 50% of pregnant women will notice some symptoms of carpal tunnel syndrome. Treatment during pregnancy is usually limited to supportive measures such as nighttime splinting that may help reduce increased pressure on the nerve that occurs when the wrist is bent; about 80% of women will notice reduction in symptoms with splinting alone. Severe cases of carpal tunnel syndrome can be treated with steroid injections into the area around the carpal tunnel to reduce swelling and inflammation. Women should be cautioned to avoid non-steroidal anti-inflammatory agents. After delivery, symptoms generally resolve within 4 weeks (see Chapter 44).

Hemorrhoids

Hemorrhoids are varicose veins of the rectum. Since straining during bowel movements contributes to their aggravation, avoidance of constipation is preventive. Prolonged sitting should also be avoided. Hemorrhoids will often regress after delivery but usually will not disappear completely.

Constipation

Constipation is physiologic during pregnancy with decreased bowel transit time, and the stool may be hardened. Dietary modification with increased bulk such as with fresh fruit and vegetables and plenty of water can usually help this problem. Constipation is aggravated by the addition of iron supplementation; if dietary measures are inadequate, patients may require stool softeners. Additional dietary fibers such as Metamucil (psyllium hydrophilic muciloid) or surface-active agents such as Colace (docusate) are recommended. Laxatives are rarely necessary.

Urinary Frequency and Incontinence

Often during the first 3 months of pregnancy, the growing uterus places increased pressure on the bladder. Urinary frequency usually will improve as the uterus rises out of the pelvis by the second trimester. However, as the head engages near the time of delivery, urinary frequency may return as the head presses against the bladder. About 40–50% of women will experience urinary incontinence during their pregnancy. The risk of incontinence of urine is highest in the third trimester. The chances of experiencing incontinence are increased in multiparous women, especially those with a history of incontinence. Incontinence during pregnancy is a risk factor for persistent incontinence. If the patient experiences pain with urination or the new onset of incontinence, it is appropriate to check for infection.

Round Ligament Pain

Frequently, patients will notice sharp groin pains caused by spasm of the round ligaments associated with movement. This is more frequently felt on the right side as a result of the usual dextrorotation of the uterus. The pain may be helped by application of local heat such as with hot soaks or a heating pad. Patients may awaken at night with this pain after having suddenly rolled over in their sleep without realizing it. During the daytime, however, modification of activity with gradual rising and sitting down, as well as avoidance of sudden movement, will decrease problems with this type of pain. Analgesics are rarely necessary.

Syncope

Compression of the veins in the legs from the advancing size of the uterus places patients at risk of venous pooling associated with prolonged standing. This may lead to syncope. Measures to avoid this possibility include wearing support stockings and exercising the calves to increase venous return. In later pregnancy, patients may have problems with supine hypotension, a distinct problem when undergoing a medical evaluation or an ultrasound examination. A left lateral tilt position with wedging below the right hip will help keep the weight of the pregnancy off the inferior vena cava.

Backache

Back pain is a common complaint in pregnancy affecting over 50% of women. Numerous physiologic changes of pregnancy likely contribute to the development of back pain including ligament laxity related to relaxin and estrogen, weight gain, hyperlordosis, and anterior tilt of the pelvis. These altered biomechanics lead to mechanical strain on the lower back.[137] Backache can be prevented to a large degree by avoidance of excessive weight gain, and a regular exercise program before pregnancy. Exercises to strengthen back muscles can also be helpful. Posture is important, and sensible shoes, not high heels, should be worn. Scheduled rest periods with elevation of the feet to flex the hips may be helpful. Other successful treatment modalities that have been described include nonelastic maternity support binders, acupuncture, aquatic exercises, and pharmacologic regimens incorporating acetominophen, narcotics, prednisone, and rarely antiprostaglandins (if remote from term).[137]

Sexual Activity

No restriction need generally be placed on sexual intercourse. The patient is instructed that pregnancy may cause changes in comfort and sexual desire. Frequently, increased uterine activity is noted after sexual intercourse; it is unclear whether this is due to breast stimulation, female orgasm, or prostaglandins in the male ejaculate. For women at risk for preterm labor or with a history of previous pregnancy loss and who note such increased activity, use of a condom or avoidance of sexual activity may be recommended.

Circumcision

Newborn circumcision is a widely practiced elective procedure with significant variation by race/ethnicity, geographic region, education level, and religious belief. While the medical benefits have been widely debated, recent studies suggest circumcision offers protection against urinary tract infection, some sexually transmitted diseases, HIV transmission, cervical cancer, penile cancer and phimosis.[145] Despite these findings, the American Academy of Pediatrics (AAP) does not recommend routine neonatal circumcision.[146] Education about good personal foreskin hygiene offers many of the advantages of circumcision without the risks.

Circumcision in the newborn is an elective procedure and should be performed only if the infant is stable and healthy. If performed, the AAP recommends a multifaceted approach to pain management in order to reduce the observed physiologic response to the newborn's pain.[147]

Breast-Feeding

Breast-feeding as a public policy has been widely endorsed and supported by the Department of Health and Human Services. Healthy People 2000 called for 50% of mothers to breast feed for at least 6 months. Hence, during prenatal visits, the patient should be encouraged to breast-feed her infant (see Chapter 22). Human milk is the most appropriate nutrient for human infants and also provides significant immunologic protection against infection. Infants who are breast-fed have a lower incidence of infection and require fewer sick child office visits and hospitalizations than do infants who are fed formula exclusively.[148,149] A myriad of other infant benefits have been reported, including but not limited to a decreased incidence of sudden infant death syndrome, diabetes, otitis media, respiratory tract disease, tonsillitis, dental caries, and a host of immunologically mediated conditions such as rheumatoid arthritis, Crohn's disease, multiple sclerosis, eczema, and allergic reactions. These benefits are greatest if the infant is exclusively breastfed for 6 months and the protection decreases in proportion to the amount of supplementation.[150]

Maternal advantages of lactation include economy, convenience, more rapid involution of the uterus, and natural child spacing. Breastfeeding protects the mother from infections, cancer (breast, endometrial, and ovarian), osteoporosis, diabetes, and rheumatoid arthritis.[150] The reasons a woman decides to bottle-feed should be explored, as they may be based on a misconception. For example, preterm birth, and/or medical problems are usually not contraindications to breastfeeding. Encouragement from health care providers, liberal use of lactation consultants, and spouse and peer support will sometimes convince a hesitant mother who may then be able to nurse successfully.[150–152] The American Dietetic Association recommends exclusive breastfeeding for the first 6 months and breastfeeding with complementary foods for at least 12 months as the ideal feeding pattern for infants.[153] Studies on incidence and duration of breastfeeding indicate that US women fall far short of that. Based on survey data, American mothers initiate breast feeding at rates ranging from 27–70%, and only 19–33% of women report breastfeeding for at least 6 months.[154] Initiation and duration of breastfeeding are widely influenced by age, race/ethnicity, cultural and peer influences.

Working outside the home need not be a contraindication to breast-feeding. Many women who previously would not have considered nursing an option, such as those with careers, are now finding time to breast-feed their infants. Employer based lactation support programs have contributed to a prolonged duration of breastfeeding as well as specific employer benefits-mothers of breastfed infants were more productive at work, missed fewer days, and used fewer health care benefits because of sick child-care issues.[150] Women should be aware that alternative ways of breast-feeding can be used to correspond with their work schedules. They can decrease the frequency of lactation to a few times a day in most cases and still continue to nurse. Other women may pump their breasts at work, leaving milk for the child's caretaker during the day and thus providing breast milk to the infant even more frequently. The milk may be collected in containers and, if refrigerated, is safe to use for 24 hours. For a longer duration, the milk should be frozen. Because freezing and thawing destroy the cellular content, fresh milk is preferred.

There is no need for specific nipple preparation during pregnancy. In one study, women prepared one nipple and not the other with a variety of techniques, including massage and breast creams, and found no difference in the two.[155] Soap and drying agents should not be used on the nipples, which should be washed only with water.

Preparation for Childbirth

The introduction of childbirth education and consumerism has had significant impact on the practice of obstetrics. The success of obstetric practice in preventing disasters has allowed interest to focus on the quality of the childbirth and of the perinatal experience. Studies have shown that prepared childbirth can have a beneficial effect on labor and delivery.[156,157] The prenatal period should be one in which the patient is exposed to information about pregnancy, normal labor and delivery, anesthesia and analgesia, obstetric complications, and obstetric operations (e.g., episiotomy, cesarean delivery, and forceps or vacuum delivery). The prenatal clinic is an appropriate place to obtain informed consent from the patient for her intrapartum care and management, and to discuss her concerns and preferences about childbirth. Certainly, this affords a more dispassionate, quiet, and pain-free environment than the labor and delivery suite.[158–160]

While the education mentioned above usually can be transmitted by the obstetrician at the initial visit or over a series of shorter return visits, patients have come to expect more personal involvement than to be given a book or handout to read. The appropriate place for such education has evolved to be a series of planned, structured prenatal education classes taught by informed, qualified individuals. These classes can be given in the physician's office, at the hospital, or in free-standing classes. National organizations such as the Childbirth Education Association and the American Society for Psychoprophylaxis in Obstetrics have recognized the need for such instruction and teach prepared childbirth. There are also advantages to office- and hospital-based programs, if the patient volume permits it, since specifics of management and alternatives offered by that practice or hospital can be discussed in these programs. On the other hand, free-standing classes offer the advantage of open-endedness and of presenting many options to the patient, who can then discuss them with her care provider. Group prenatal care also can apparently serve an important education function.[74] Many advances in family-centered practice (e.g., allowing fathers in the delivery room and operating room) have come from consumer requests and demands. A pregnant patient often makes a list of what she would like in the peripartum period, to discuss with her practitioner. Thus, the care provider can understand her needs and desires, better address these needs and desires if labor and delivery do not proceed normally or as planned, and, finally, explain why certain requests are not possible or reasonable.

Signs of Labor

It is important to instruct the patient about certain warning signs that should trigger a call to her care provider or a visit to the hospital. All women should be informed of what to do if contractions become regular, if rupture of the membranes is suspected, or if vaginal bleeding occurs. Patients should be given a number to call where assistance is available 24 hours a day.

Prepared Parenthood and Support Groups

Routine classes on newborn child care and parenting should be part of the prenatal care program. Many parents are completely unprepared for the myriad of changes in their lives, and some idea of what to expect is beneficial. As pregnancy progresses, special needs can arise. Support groups for families with genetic or medical conditions such as Down syndrome, skeletal dysplasias, preterm infants, or maternal support groups for mothers of twins or triplets, and for women who have had cesarean delivery have all shown that they can meet the special needs of these parents. Unsuccessful pregnancies lead to special problems and needs, for which social workers, clergy, and specialized support groups can be invaluable. Miscarriage, stillbirth, and infant death are particularly devastating events, best managed by a team approach, with special attention to the grieving process. Referral to such groups as Compassionate Friends of Miscarriage, Infant Death, and Stillbirth is recommended. Careful evaluation and follow-up for depression should be part of the routine pregnancy and postpartum care.[161]

Postpartum Visit

Most patients should be seen approximately 6 weeks postpartum, sooner for complicated deliveries and/or cesarean deliveries (see Chapter 21). The goal of this visit is to evaluate the physical and psychosocial and mental well being of the mother, provide support and referral for breastfeeding, initiate or encourage compliance with the preferred family planning option, and to initiate preconception care for the next pregnancy.[3] It has been estimated that 77% of managed care enrollees obtain a postpartum visit.[162] Data suggest maternal health after pregnancy is associated with improved child health, and so increasing compliance with postpartum visits has been identified as both a national and international public health priority.[161–165]

SUMMARY

Prenatal care is an effective, if incompletely understood and studied, intervention. It provides a model for primary care services for both obstetricians/gynecologists and other primary care providers. It satisfies the Institute of Medicine criteria for primary care, as it is comprehensive, and continuous, and provides coordinated services. Preconceptional care will introduce necessary changes and can improve pregnancy outcome. Risk assessment, with subsequent elimination or management of risks, health education, advocacy, and disease prevention, as well as appropriate medical management of complications, remain the core of the process. Changes in the number of visits and an improved understanding of the successful components of prenatal care will improve services and efficiency without altering the substance of what has been developed and achieved. Prenatal care should reinforce the importance of lifelong disease surveillance and prevention as well as active participation in personal wellness behaviors for women and their families.

KEY POINTS

- Maternal mortality is the demise of any woman from any pregnancy-related cause while pregnant or within 42 days of termination of a pregnancy. The most frequent causes of maternal death are hemorrhage and embolism. The perinatal mortality combines the number of fetal deaths (stillbirths) plus neonatal deaths per 1,000 total births.
- Preconception evaluation should include rubella, hepatitis B and HIV testing. In selected situations, screening should be extended to varicella, toxoplasmosis, tuberculosis, and hepatitis C. Further tests may be indicated depending on historical genetic risk factors identified.
- Preconception supplementation with folic acid can reduce the incidence of NTDs and other defects. All women of childbearing age should consume 0.4 mg of folic acid daily. Women who have had a child previously affected by an NTD should take 4 mg daily from 4 weeks before conception through the first 3 months of pregnancy.
- There are a number of multiple marker tests available for screening for aneuploidy in the first trimester and/or second trimester. Practitioners should be familiar with the various options and offer them to their patients irrespective of maternal age.
- The number of prenatal visits can be safely decreased in healthy parous women.
- The total weight gain recommended for healthy women is 25 to 35 lb. Underweight women may gain up to 40 lb, and overweight women should limit weight gain to 15 lb.
- Bed rest on the side increases venous return from the legs, as pressure on the vena cava is relieved. This maneuver increases the effective circulating blood volume, cardiac output and, thus, the blood flow to the kidney. A diuresis follows, as well as increased blood flow to the uterus.
- The pregnant woman should be advised against prolonged sitting during car or airplane travel because of the risk of venous stasis and possible thromboembolism.
- Prenatal care should include education of the pregnant woman about labor, delivery, possible operative procedures, obstetric analgesia, breastfeeding, postpartum recovery and contraception.
- For infant nutrition, breastfeeding is best.
- Ultrasound evaluation between 16 and 20 weeks allows accurate assessment of gestational age and a survey for fetal abnormality and multiple gestation.

❑ Postpartum visits, and interconception visits are valuable times for ongoing risk assessment, health promotion and screening about factors likely to impact the health of women and their families (e.g., diet, exercise, breast feeding, family planning, substance use, depression, violence and injury prevention). Practitioners should develop the infrastructure within their practices to provide opportunities for the education of patients about these issues and referral as appropriate.

REFERENCES

1. Misra DP, Guyer B, Allston A: Integrated perinatal health framework. A multiple determinants model with a life span approach. Am J Prev Med 25:65, 2003.
2. Public Health Service: Caring for Our Future: The Content of Prenatal Care—A Report of the Public Health Service Expert Panel on the Content of Prenatal Care. Washington, DC, PHS-DHRS, 1989.
3. American Academy of Pediatrics, American College of Obstetricians and Gynecologists. Guidelines for Perinatal Care, 4th ed. Elk Grove Village, IL, American Academy Pediatrics, 1997.
4. Cochrane A: Foreword. *In* Chalmers I, Enkin M, Keirse M (eds): Effective Care in Pregnancy and Childbirth. Oxford, Oxford University Press, 1989.
5. MMWR Morbidity and Mortality Weekly Report. Pregnancy-related mortality surveillance—United States, 1991–1999, February; 52:1, 2003.
6. Donaldson M, Yordy K, Vanselow N (eds): Defining Primary Care: An Interim Report. Washington, DC, National Academy Press, 1994.
7. American College of Obstetricians and Gynecologists: The Obstetrician-Gynecologist and Primary-Preventive Health Care. Washington, DC, American College of Obstetricians and Gynecologists, 1993.
8. Starfield B: Primary Care: Concept, Evaluation, and Policy. New York, Oxford University Press, 1992.
9. Johnson TRB, Zettelmaier MA, Warner PA, et al: A competency-based approach to comprehensive pregnancy care. Women's Health Issues 10:240, 2000.
10. Johansen KS, Hod M: Quality development in perinatal care-the OBSQID project. Int J Gynecol Obstet 64:167, 1999.
11. Binstock MA, Wolde-Tsadik G: Alternative prenatal care. Impact of reduced visit frequency, focused visits and continuity of care. J Reprod Med 40:507, 1995.
12. Berg CJ, Atrash HK, Koonin LM, Tucker M: Pregnancy related mortality in the United States, 1987–1990. Obstet Gynecol 88:161, 1996.
13. Rosenfield A: Maternal mortality in developing countries. An ongoing but neglected "epidemic." JAMA 262:376, 1989.
14. Revised 1990 Estimates of Maternal Mortality: A new approach by WHO and UNICEF, World Health Organization, April 1996.
15. Callister LC: Global Maternal Mortality: Contributing factors and strategies for change. MCN Am J Matern Child Nurs 30:184, 2005.
16. World Health Organization: Maternal Mortality in 2000. Estimates developed by WHO, UNICEF, and UNFPA. Geneva, 2001.
17. Horon, IL: Underreporing of maternal deaths on death certificates and the magnitude of the problem of maternal mortality. Am J Pub Health 95:478, 2005.
18. Widman K, Bouvier-Colle MH, the MOMS Group: Maternal mortality as an indicator of obstetric care in Europe. Br J Obstet Gynecol 111:164, 2004
19. Minkoff H: Maternal mortality in America: lessons from the developing world. J Am Womens Assoc 57:171, 2002.
20. Frautschi S, Cerulli A, Maine D: Suicide during pregnancy and its neglect as a component of maternal mortality. Int J Gynecol Obstet 47:275, 1994.
21. Center for Disease Control and Prevention: Enhanced maternal mortality surveillance—North Carolina, 1988 and 1989. MMWR Morb Mortal Wkly Rep 40:469, 1996.
22. Harper M, Parsons L: Maternal death due to homicide and other injuries in North Carolina: 1992–1994. Obstet Gynecol 90:920, 1997.
23. Dannenberg AL, Carter DM, Lawson HW, et al: Homicide and other injuries as causes of maternal death in New York City, 1987 through 1991. Am J Obstet Gynecol 172:1557, 1995.
24. Shadigian EM, Bauer ST: Pregnancy-associated death: A qualitative systematic review of homicide and suicide. Obstet Gynecol Survey 60:183, 2005.
25. Deneux-Tharaux, Berg C, Bouvier-Colle MH, et al: Underreporting of pregnancy-related mortality in the United States and Europe. Obstet Gynecol 106:684, 2005.
26. Pregnancy-related mortality surveillance in the United States. MMWR Morb Mort Wkly Rep 52:1, 2003. http://www.cdc.gov/mmwr/pdf/ss/ss5202.pdf.
27. Centers for Disease Control and Prevention: Differences in maternal mortality among black and white women—United States, 1987–1996. MMWR Morb Mortal Wkly Rep 48:492, 1999.
28. Sullivan SA, Hill EG, Newman RB, Menard MK: Maternal-fetal medicine specialist density is inversely associated with maternal mortality ratios. Am J Obstet Gynecol 193:1083, 2005.
29. Yeast JD, Poskin M, Stockbauer JW, Shaffer S: Changing patterns in regionalization of perinatal care and the impact on neonatal mortality. Am J Obstet Gynecol 178(1 Pt 1):131, 1998.
30. Pattinson RC, Hall M: Near misses: a useful adjunct to maternal death enquiries. Br Med Bull 67:231, 2003.
31. Wen SW, Huang L, Liston R, Heaman M, et al and the Maternal Health Study Group, Canadian Perinatal Surveillance System: Severe maternal morbidity in Canada, 1991–2001. CMAJ 173:759, 2005.
32. Berg CJ, Berg CJ, Chang J, et al: Pregnancy-related mortality in the United States, 1991–1997. Obstet Gynecol 101:289, 2003.
33. Danel I, Berg C, Johnson CH, Atrash H: Magnitude of maternal morbidity during labor and delivery: United States, 1993–1997. Am J Pub Health 93:631, 2003.
34. Geller SE, Rosenberg E, Cox SM, et al: The continuum of maternal morbidity and mortality Am J Obstet Gynecol 191:939, 2004
35. Sachs BP, Fretts RC, Gardner R, et al: The impact of extreme prematurity and congenital anomalies on the interpretation of international comparisons of infant mortality. Obstet Gynecol 85:941, 1995.
36. Centers for Disease Control and Prevention (CDC): Racial/ethnic disparities in infant mortality–United States, 1995–2002. MMWR Morb Mortal Wkly Rep 54:553, 2005.
37. Arias E, MacDorman MF, Strobino DM, Guyer B: Annual summary of vital statistics—2002. Pediatrics 112(6 Pt 1):1215, 2003.
38. National Center for Health Statistics: Health United States, 2003. Hyattsville, MD, National Center for Health Statistics, 2003.
39. Martin JA, Hamilton BE, Ventura SJ, et al: Births—Final data for 2000. National Vital Statistics Reports, Vol 50, issue 5. Hyattsville, MD, National Center for Health Statistics, 2002.
40. Singh GK, Miller BA: Health, life expectancy, and mortality patterns among immigrant populations in the United States. Can J Public Health 95:I14, 2004.
41. Stone PW, Zwanziger J, Hinton Walker P, Buenting J: Economic analysis of two models of low-risk maternity care: a freestanding birth center compared to traditional care. Res Nurs Health 23:279, 2000.
42. Tucker JS, Hall MH, Howie PW, et al: Should obstetricians see women with normal pregnancies? A multicentre randomised controlled trial of routine antenatal care by general practitioners and midwives compared with shared care led by obstetricians. BMJ 312:554, 1996.
43. Chalmers I, Enkin M, Keirse M: Effective Care in Pregnancy and Childbirth. Oxford, Oxford University Press, 1989, p 39.

44. Kogan MD, Martin JA, Alexander GR, et al: The changing pattern of prenatal care utilization in the United States, 1981–1995, using different prenatal care indices. JAMA 279:1623, 1998.
45. Misra DP, Guyer B: Benefits and limitations on prenatal care from counting visits to measuring content. JAMA 279:1661, 1998.
46. McDuffie RS, Jr, Beck A, Bischoff K, et al: Effect of frequency of prenatal care visits on perinatal outcome among low-risk women. A randomized controlled trial. JAMA 275:847, 1996.
47. Sikorski J, Wilson J, Clement S, et al: A randomised controlled trial comparing two schedules of antenatal visits: the antenatal care project. BMJ 312:546, 1996.
48. Jewell D, Sharp D, Sanders J, Peters TJ: A randomised controlled trial of flexibility in routine antenatal care. Br J Obstet Gynaecol 107:1241, 2000.
49. Villar J, Ba'aqeel H, Piaggio G, et al: WHO antenatal care randomised trial for the evaluation of a new model of routine antenatal care. Lancet 357:1551, 2001.
50. Henderson J, Roberts T, Sikorski J, et al: An economic evaluation comparing two schedules of antenatal visits. J Health Serv Res Policy 5:69, 2000.
51. Giles W, Collins J, Ong F, MacDonald R: Antenatal care of low risk obstetric patients by midwives. A randomised controlled trial. Med J Aust 157:158, 1992.
52. Clement S, Candy B, Sikorski J, et al: Does reducing the frequency of routine antenatal visits have long term effects? Follow up of participants in a randomised controlled trial. Br J Obstet Gynaecol 106:367, 1999.
53. McDuffie RS, Jr, Bischoff KJ, Beck A, Orleans ML: Does reducing the number of prenatal office visits for low-risk women result in increased use of other medical services? Obstet Gynecol 90:68, 1997.
54. Munjanja SP, Lindmark G, Nystrom L: Randomised controlled trial of a reduced-visits programme of antenatal care in Harare, Zimbabwe. Lancet 348:364, 1996
55. Kogan MD, Alexander GR, Kotelchuck M, et al: Comparing mothers' reports on the content of prenatal care received with recommended national guidelines for care. Pub Health Rep 109:637, 1994.
56. Kogan MD, Kotelchuck M, Alexander GR, et al: Racial disparities in reported prenatal care advice from health care providers. Am J public Health 84:82, 1994.
57. Kogan MD, Alexander GR, Kotelchuck M, Nagey DA: Relathionship of the content of prenatal care to the risk of low birth weight: Maternal reports of health behavior advice and prenatal care procedures. JAMA 271:1130, 1994.
58. Kotelchuck M, Kogan MD, Alexander GR, et al: The influence of site of care on the content of prenatal care for low income women. J Mat Child Health 1:25, 1997.
59. Freda MC, Andersen JF, Damus K, Merkatz IR: Are there differences in information given to private and public prenatal patients. Am J Obstet Gynecol 169:155, 1993.
60. Knox AJ, Sadler L, Pattison NS, et al: An obstetric scoring system: its development and application in obstetric management. Obstet Gynecol 81:195, 1993.
61. Frusca T, Soregaroli M, Platto C, et al: Uterine artery velocimetry in patients with gestational hypertension. Obstet Gynecol 102:136, 2003.
62. Aquilina J, Thompson O, Thilaganathan B, Harrington K: Improved early prediction of pre-eclampsia by combining second-trimester maternal serum inhibin-A and uterine artery Doppler. Ultrasound Obstet Gynecol 17:477, 2001.
63. Carey JC, Klebanoff MA, Hauth JC, et al: Metronidazole to prevent preterm delivery in pregnant women with asymptomatic bacterial vaginosis. N Engl J Med 342:534, 2000.
64. Moos MK, Cefalo RC: Preconceptional health promotion: a focus for obstetric care. Am J Perinatol 4:63, 1987.
65. Adams EM, Bruce C, Shulman MS, et al: The PRAMS Working Group: pregnancy planning and pre-conceptional counseling. Obstet Gynecol 82:955, 1993.
66. Jones JL, Schulkin J, Maquire JH: Therapy for common parasitic diseases in pregnancy in the United States: A review and a survey of obstetrician/gynecologists' level of knowledge about these diseases. Obstet Gynecol Surv 60:386, 2005.
67. Chen KT, Eskild AN, Bresnahan M, et al: Previous maternal infection with *Toxplasma gondii* and the risk of fetal death. Am J Obstet Gynecol 193:443, 2005.
68. Boyer KM, Holfels E, Roisen N, et al: Risk factors for *Toxoplasma gondii* infection in mothers of infants with congenital toxoplasmosis: Implications for prenatal management and screening. Am J Obstet Gynecol 192:564, 2005.
69. American College Obstetrician and Gynecologists Committee Opinion: Number 279, December 2002. Prevention of early-onset group B atreptococcal disease in newborns. ACOG Compendium of Selected Publications, 2005, p 131.
70. Prevention of neural tube defects: results of the Medical Research Council Vitamin Study. MRC Vitamin Study Research Group. Lancet 338:131, 1991.
71. Czeizel AE, Dudas I: Prevention of the first occurrence of neural-tube defects by periconceptional vitamin supplementation. N Engl J Med 327:1832, 1992.
72. Mahomed K: Folate supplementation in pregnancy. Cochrane Database Syst Rev 2:CD000183, 2000.
73. Food standards: amendment of standards of identity for enriched grain products to require addition of folic acid—FDA. Final Rule. Fed Regist 61:9791, 1996.
74. Neill AM: The 'Folic Acid Campaign': has the message got through? A questionnaire study. J Obstet Gynaecol 19:22, 1999.
75. Knowledge and use of folic acid by women of childbearing age—United States, 1995 and 1998. MMWR Morbid Mortal Wkly Rep 48:325, 1999.
76. Hook EB: Rates of chromosome abnormalities at different maternal ages. Obstet Gynecol 58:282, 1981.
77. Stene J, Fischer G, Steve E, et al: Paternal age effect in Down's syndrome. Am J Hum Genet 40:299, 1977.
78. Genetic Testing for Cystic Fibrosis. NIH Consensus Statement Online 15:1, 1997. *www.nih.gov/genetictestingforcysticfibrosis*. Accessed 1/8/06
79. Spitzer RL, Williams JBW, Kroenke K, et al: Utility of a new procedure for diagnosing mental disorders in primary care. JAMA 272:1749, 1994.
80. Moore RD, Bone LR, Geller G, et al: Prevalence detection and treatment of alcoholism in hospitalized patients. JAMA 261:403, 1989.
81. Sokol RJ, Martier SS, Ager JW: The T-ACE questions: practical prenatal detection of risk-drinking. Am J Obstet Gynecol 160:863, 1989.
82. Gregory KD, Johnson CT, Johnson TRB, Entman, SS: Content of Prenatal Care: Update 2005: Women's Health Issues 16:198, 2006.
83. McFarlane J, Parker B, Soeken K, Bullock L: Assessing for abuse during pregnancy. JAMA 267:3176, 1992.
84. Chang G, Wilkins-Haug L, Berman S, et al: Alcohol use and pregnancy: improving identification. Obstet Gynecol 91:892, 1998.
85. Wiist WH, McFarlane J: The effectiveness of an abuse assessment protocol in public health prenatal clinics. Am J Public Health 89:1217, 1999.
86. Creasy RC, Gummer BA, Liggins GC: System for predicting spontaneous preterm birth. Obstet Gynecol 55:692, 1980.
87. Meis PJ, Klebanoff M, Thom E, et al: Prevention of recurrent preterm delivery by 17 α-hydroxyprogesterone caproate. N Engl J Med 348:2379, 2003.
88. da Fonseca EB, Bittar RE, Carvalho MHB, et al: Prophylactic administration of progesterone by vaginal suppository to reduce the incidence of spontaneous preterm birth in women at increased risk: A randomized placebo-controlled double-blind study. Am J Obstet Gynecol 188:419, 2003.
89. Abbasi IA, Hess LW, Johnson TRB Jr, et al: Leukocyte esterase activity in the rapid detection of urinary tract and lower genital tract infection in pregnancy. Am J Perinatol 2:311, 1985.
90. Platt LD, Greene N, Johnson A, et al: Sequential pathways of testing after first-trimester screening for trisomy 21. Obstet Gynecol 104:661, 2004.
91. American College Obstetrician and Gynecologists Committee Opinion. Number 296, July 2004. First trimester screening for fetal aneuploidy. ACOG Compendium of Selected Publications, 2005, p 43.

92. American College Obstetrician and Gynecologists Practice Bulletin. Number 44, July 2003. Neural Tube Defects. ACOG Compendium of Selected Publications, 2005, p 614.
93. ACOG Committee on Obstetric Practice: Scheduled cesarean delivery and the prevention of vertical transmission of HIV infection. ACOG, May, Number 234:158–160, 2000.
94. Wade NA, Birkhead GS, Warren BL, et al: Abbreviated regimens of zidovudine prophylaxis and perinatal transmission of the human immunodeficiency virus. N Engl J Med 339:1409, 1998.
95. Andersen HF, Johnson TRB, Flora JD, et al: Gestational age assessment. II. Prediction from combined clinical observations. Am J Obstet Gynecol 140:770, 1981.
96. Kramer MS, McLean FH, Boyd ME, Usher RH: The validity of gestational age estimation by menstrual dating in term, preterm and postterm gestations. JAMA 260:3306, 1988.
97. Saari-Kemppainen A: Use of antenatal care services in a controlled ultrasound screening trial. Acta Obstet Gynecol Scand 74:12, 1995.
98. Crowther CA, Kornman L, O'Callaghan S, et al: Is an ultrasound assessment of gestational age at the first antenatal visit of value? A randomised clinical trial. Br J Obstet Gynaecol 106:1273, 1999.
99. LeFevre ML, Bain RP, Ewigman BG, et al: A randomized trial of prenatal ultrasonographic screening: impact on maternal management and outcome. RADIUS (Routine Antenatal Diagnostic Imaging with Ultrasound) Study Group. Am J Obstet Gynecol 169:483, 1993.
100. Raynor BD: Routine ultrasound in pregnancy. Clin Obstet Gynecol 46:882, 2003.
101. Garcia J, Brickner L Henderson J, et al: Women's views of pregnancy ultrasound: A systematic review. Birth 29:225, 2002.
102. Bucher HC, Schmidt JG: Does routine ultrasound scanning improve outcome in pregnancy? Meta-analysis of various outcome measures. BMJ 307:13, 1993.
103. Eik-Nes SH, Okland O, Aure JC: Ultrasound screening in pregnancy: a randomized controlled trial. Lancet 1:1347, 1984.
104. Ewigman BG, Crane JP, Frigoletto FD, et al: Effect of prenatal ultrasound screening on perinatal outcome. N Engl J Med 329:821, 1993.
105. Gregory KD, Davidson E: Prenatal Care: Who needs it and why? Clin Obstet Gynecol 42:725, 1999.
106. Grant A, Elbourne D, Valentin L, Alexander S: Routine fetal movement counting and risk of antepartum rate death in normally formed singletons. Lancet 2:345, 1989.
107. Lopez NJ, Smith PC, Gutierrez J: Periodontal therapy may reduce the risk of preterm low birth weight in women with periodontal disease: a randomized controlled trial. J Periodontol 73:911, 2002.
107a. Michalowicz BS, Hodges JS, DiAngelis DMD: Treatment of periodontal disease and the risk of preterm birth. N Engl J Med 335:885, 2006.
108. Miller DW Jr: Prenatal care: a strategic first step toward EMR acceptance. J Healthc Inf Manag 17:47, 2003.
109. Ickovics JR, Kershaw TS, Westdahl C, et al: Group prenatal care and preterm birth weight: Results from a matched cohort study at public clinics. Obstet Gynecol 102:1051, 2003.
110. Smits LJ, Essed GG: Short interpregnancy intervals and unfavorable pregnancy outcome: role of folate depletion. Lancet 358:2074, 2001.
111. King JC: The risk of maternal nutritional depletion and poor outcomes increases in early or closely spaced pregnancies. J Nutr 133:1732S, 2003.
112. Stephansson O, Dickman PW, Cnattingius S: The influence of interpregnancy interval on the subsequent risk of stillbirth and early neonatal death. Obstet Gynecol 102:101, 2003.
113. Zhu BP: Effect of interpregnancy interval on birth outcomes: findings from three recent US studies. Int J Gynecol Obstet 89: S25, 2005.
114. Zhu BP, Le T: Effect of interpregnancy interval on infant low birth weight: a retrospective cohort study using the Michigan Maternally Linked Birth Database. Maternal & Child Health Journal 7:169, 2003.
115. Nathens AB, Neff MJ, Goss CH, Maier RV, et al: Effect of an older sibling and birth interval on the risk of childhood injury. Injury Prevention 6:219, 2000.
116. Shipp TD, Zelop CM, Repke JT, et al: Interdelivery interval and risk of symptomatic uterine rupture. Obstet Gynecol 97:175, 2001.
117. Conde-Agudelo A, Belizan JM: Maternal morbidity and mortality associated with interpregnancy interval: cross sectional study. BMJ 321:1255, 2000.
118. Fuentes-Afflick E, Hessol NA: Interpregnancy interval and the risk of premature infants. Obstet Gynecol 95:383, 2000.
119. Gold R, Connell FA, Heagerty P, et al: Income inequality and pregnancy spacing. Soc Sci Med 59:1117, 2004.
120. American College Obstetricians & Gynecologists Compendium of Selected Publications, 2005. Benefits and Risks of Sterilization Practice Bulletin, Number 46, September 2003.
121. Mayer JP, Hawkins B, Todd R: A randomized evaluation of smoking cessation interventions for pregnant women at a WIC clinic. Am J Public Health 80:76, 1990.
122. Ershoff DH, Mullen PD, Quinn VP: A randomized trial of a serialized self-help smoking cessation program for pregnant women in an HMO. Am J Public Health 79:182, 1989.
123. Mullen P: Smoking Cessation Counseling in Prenatal Care. *In* Merkatz IR, Thompson JE, Mullen PD, Goldenberg RL (eds). New Perspectives in Prenatal Care. New York, Elsevier, 1990, p 161.
124. Ershoff DH, Quinn VP, Boyd NR, et al: The Kaiser Permanente prenatal smoking-cessation trial: when more isn't better, what is enough? Am J Prev Med 17:161, 1999.
125. Windsor RA, Woodby LL, Miller TM, et al: Effectiveness of Agency for Health Care Policy and Research clinical practice guideline and patient education methods for pregnant smokers in medicaid maternity care. Am J Obstet Gynecol 182:68, 2000.
126. Hajek P, Stead L, West R, Jarvis M: Relapse prevention interventions for smoking cessation. Cochrane Database Syst Rev 1: CD003999 2005.
127. Miller DP, Villa KF, Hogue SL, Sivapathasundaram D: Birth and first-year costs for mothers and infants attributable to maternal smoking. Nicotine Tob Res 3:25, 2001.
128. Factor-Litvak P, Cushman LF, Kronenberg F, et al: Use of complementary and alternative medicine among women in New York City: a pilot study. J Altern Complement Med 7:659, 2001.
129. American College Obstetricians & Gynecologists Compendium of Selected Publications, 2005. Guidelines for Diagnostic Imaging During Pregnancy. Number 299, September 2004.
130. Paju S: Periodontal disease as a risk factor for adverse pregnancy outcomes. A systematic review. Ann Periodontol 8:70, 2003.
131. Kulier R, de Onis M, Gulmezoglu AM, Villar J: Nutritional interventions for the prevention of maternal morbidity. Int J Gynecol Obstet 63:231, 1998.
132. National Academy of Sciences: Recommended Dietary Allowances, 10th ed. Washington, DC, National Academy Press, 1989.
133. Zlatnik FJ, Burmeister LF: Dietary protein in pregnancy: effect on anthropometric indices of the newborn infant. Am J Obstet Gynecol 146:199, 1983.
134. Food and Nutrition Board Institute of Medicine, National Academy of Sciences: Nutrition During Pregnancy. Washington, DC, National Academy Press, 1990, p 10.
135. Bianco AT, Smilen SW, Davis Y, et al: Pregnancy outcome and weight gain recommendations for the morbidly obese woman. Obstet Gynecol 91:97, 1998.
136. American College Obstetricians & Gynecologists Committee Opinion #267. Exercise during pregnancy and the postpartum period. ACOG: Washington DC, 2002.
137. Borg-Stein J. Dugan SA, Gruber J: Musculoskeletal aspects of pregnancy. Am J Physic Rehab 84:180, 2005.
138. Dempsey JC, Butler CL, Williams MA: No need for a pregnant pause: physical activity may reduce the occurrence of gestational diabetes mellitus and preeclampsia. Exerc Sport Rev 33:141, 2005.
139. Mogren IM: Previous physical activity decreases the risk of low back pain and pelvic pain during pregnancy. Scand J Pub Health 33:300, 2005.

140. Mamelle N, Laumon B, Lazar P: Prematurity and occupational activity during pregnancy. Am J Epidemiol 119:309, 1984.
141. Luke B, Mamelle N, Keith L, et al: The association between occupational factors and preterm birth: a U.S. nurses' study. Am J Obstet Gynecol 173:849, 1995.
142. Mozurkewich E, Luke B, Avni M, Wolf FM: Working conditions and adverse pregnancy outcome: a meta-analysis. Obstet Gynecol 95:623, 2000.
143. Anderson FWJ, Johnson CT: Complementary and alternative medicine in obstetrics. Int J Gynaecol Obstet 91:116, 2005.
144. Manconi M, Govoni V, DeVito A, et al: Restless legs syndrome and pregnancy. Neurol 63:1065, 2004.
145. Alanis MC, Lucidi RS: Neonatal circumcision: A review of the world's oldest and most controversial operation. Obstet Gynecol Surv 59:379, 2004.
146. American Academy of Pediatrics: Circumcision Policy Statement (RE9850) 103:686, 1999.
147. Maxwell LG, Yaster M, Wetzel RC, et al: Penile nerve block for newborn circumcision. Obstet Gynecol 70:415, 1987.
148. Dermer A: Overcoming medical and social barriers to breast feeding. Am Fam Physician 51:755, 1995.
149. Grugliania ERJ, Calatta WT, Vogelhut J: Effect of breastfeeding support from different sources on mother's decisions to breastfeed. Journal of Human Lactation 10:157, 1994.
150. Wyatt SN: Challenges of the working breastfeeding mother: Workplace solutions. AAOHN J 50:61, 2002.
151. Dermer A: Overcoming medical and social barriers to breast feeding. Am Family Physician 57:755, 1995.
152. Grugliania ERJ, Calatta WT, Vogelhut J: Effect of breastfeeding support form different sources on mothers' decisions to breastfeed. Journal of Human Lactation 10:157, 1994.
153. James DC, Dobson B: Position of the American Dietetic Association: Promoting and supporting breastfeeding. J Am Dietetic Assoc 105:810, 2005.
154. Callen J, Pinelli J: Incidence and duration of breastfeeding for term infants in Canada, United States, Europe, and Australia: A literature review. Birth 31:285, 2004.
155. Brown MS, Hurloch JT: Preparation of the breast for breast feeding. Nurs Res 24:449, 1975.
156. Scott JR, Rose NB: Effect of psychoprophylaxis (Lamaze preparation) on labor and delivery in primiparas. N Engl J Med 294:1205, 1976.
157. Villar J, Farnot U, Barros F, et al: A randomized trial of psychosocial support during high-risk pregnancies. The Latin American Network for Perinatal and Reproductive Biology Research. N Engl J Med 327:1266, 1992.
158. Renkert S, Nutbeam D: Opportunities to improve maternal health literacy through antenatal education: an exploratory study. Health Promot Int 16:381, 2001.
159. Hall RT: Prevention of premature birth: do pediatricians have a role? Pediatrics 105:1137, 2000.
160. Health literacy: report of the Council on Scientific Affairs. Ad Hoc Committee on Health Literacy for the Council on Scientific Affairs, American Medical Association. JAMA 281:552,1999.
161. Marcus SM, Flynn HA, Blow FC, Barry KL: Depressive symptoms among pregnant women screened in obstetrics settings. J Womens Health (Larchmt) 2:373, 2003.
162. National Committee for Quality Assurance. State of managed care quality 2000. Prenatal and postpartum care. Available at: *www.ncqa.org*. Accessed 1/8/06.
163. Lu MC, Prentice J: The postpartum visit: risk factors for nonuse and association with breast-feeding. Am J Obstet Gynecol 187:1329, 2002.
164. Anonymous. Postpartum care of the mother and newborn: a practical guide. Technical Working Group, World Health Organization. Birth 26:255, 1999.
165. Kahn RS, Zuckerman B, Bauchner H, et al: Women's health after pregnancy and child outcomes at age 3 years: a prospective cohort study. Am J Public Health 92:1312, 2002.

Genetic Counseling and Genetic Screening

JOE LEIGH SIMPSON AND WOLFGANG HOLZGREVE

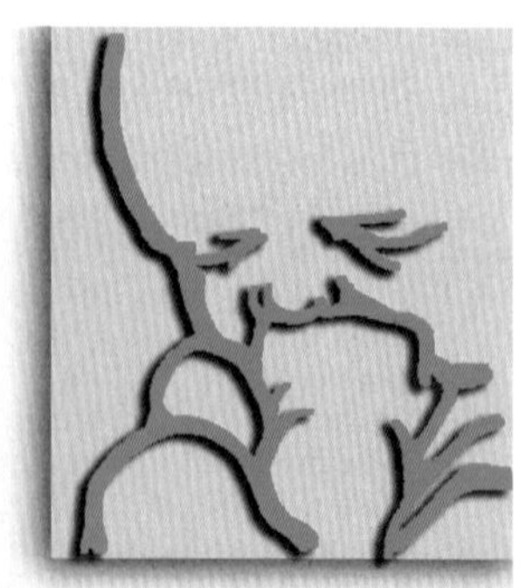

CHAPTER 6

KEY ABBREVIATIONS

American College of Medical Genetics	ACMG
American College of Obstetricians and Gynecologists	ACOG
Congenital bilateral absence of the vas deferens	CBAVD
Cystic fibrosis	CF
Deoxyribosenucleic acid	DNA
Gap Junction B	GJB
Health Resources and Services Administration	HRSA
Intelligence quotient	IQ
Mean corpuscular volume	MCV
Transmembrane conductance regulator	CFTR
Uniparental disomy	UPD

Approximately 3 percent of liveborn infants have a major congenital anomaly. About one half of these anomalies are detected at birth; the remainder becomes evident later in childhood or, less often, adulthood. Although nongenetic factors may cause malformations, genetic factors are usually responsible. In addition, more than 50 percent of first-trimester spontaneous abortions and at least 5 percent of stillborn infants have chromosomal abnormalities (see Chapter 24). Given such a pivotal role for genetic factors, medical genetics becomes integral to the practice of modern obstetrics.

This chapter considers the principles of genetic counseling and genetic screening. Disorders amenable to genetic screening and prenatal diagnosis are enumerated.

FREQUENCY OF GENETIC DISEASE

Phenotypic variation—normal or abnormal—may be considered in terms of several etiologic categories: (1) chromosomal abnormalities, numeric or structural; (2) single-gene or mendelian disorders; (3) polygenic and multifactorial disorders, polygenic implying an etiology resulting from cumulative effects of more than one gene and multifactorial implying interaction as well with environmental factors; and (4) teratogenic disorders, caused by exposure to exogenous factors (e.g., drugs) that deleteriously affect an embryo otherwise destined to develop normally. Principles of these mechanisms are reviewed elsewhere in detail.[1]

Chromosomal Abnormalities

From surveys of liveborn neonates, it is well established that the incidence of chromosomal aberrations is 1 in 160. Table 6-1 shows the incidence of individual abnormalities.[2] The chromosomal abnormality that generates the most attention is autosomal trisomy. Autosomal trisomy usually arises as a result of abnormalities of meiosis, nondisjunction producing a gamete with 24 rather than the expected 23 chromosomes. This results in a zygote having 47 chromosomes. This error most commonly occurs during maternal meiosis, and is associated with the well-known maternal age effect. Table 6-2 shows the year-to-year increase in frequency of Down syndrome and other aneuploidies.[3] Another calculation has shown that the progressive increase with advancing maternal age plateaus around age 45, but this is of relatively little clinical significance.[4] The frequency is about 30 percent higher in midpregnancy than at term, reflecting lethal-

Table 6-1. Chromosomal Abnormalities in Newborn Infants

TYPE OF ABNORMALITY	INCIDENCE
Numeric aberrations	
Sex chromosomes	
47,XYY	1/1,000 MB
47,XXY	1/1,000 MB
Other (men)	1/1,350 MB
47,X	1/10,000 FB
47,XXX	1/1,000 FB
Other (females)	1/2,700 FB
Autosomes	
Trisomies	
13–15 (D group)	1/20,000 LB
16–18 (E group)	1/8,000 LB
21–22 (G group)	1/800 LB
Other	1/50,000 LB
Structural aberrations	
Balanced	
Robertsonian	
t(Dq; Dq)	1/1,500 LB
t(Dq; Gq)	1/5,000 LB
Reciprocal translocations and insertional inversions	1/7,000 LB
Unbalanced	
Robertsonian	1/14,000 LB
Reciprocal translocations and insertional Inversions	1/8,000 LB
Inversions	1/50,000 LB
Deletions	1/10,000 LB
Supernumeraries	1/5,000 LB
Other	1/8,000 LB
Total	1/160 LB

LB, live births; MB, male births; FB, female births.
Pooled data tabulated by Hook and Hamerton.[2]

Table 6-2. Maternal Age and Chromosomal Abnormalities (Live Births)*

MATERNAL AGE	RISK FOR DOWN SYNDROME	RISK FOR ANY CHROMOSOME ABNORMALITIES
20	1/1,667	1/526†
21	1/1,667	1/526†
22	1/1,429	1/500†
23	1/1,429	1/500†
24	1/1,250	1/476†
25	1/1,250	1/476†
26	1/1,176	1/476†
27	1/1,111	1/455†
28	1/1,053	1/435†
29	1/1,100	1/417†
30	1/952	1/384†
31	1/909	1/385†
32	1/769	1/322†
33	1/625	1/317†
34	1/500	1/260
35	1/385	1/204
36	1/294	1/164
37	1/227	1/130
38	1/175	1/103
39	1/137	1/82
40	1/106	1/65
41	1/82	1/51
42	1/64	1/40
43	1/50	1/32
44	1/38	1/25
45	1/30	1/20
46	1/23	1/15
47	1/18	1/12
48	1/14	1/10
49	1/11	1/7

*Because sample size for some intervals is relatively small, confidence limits are sometimes relatively large. Nonetheless, these figures are suitable for genetic counseling.
†47,XXX excluded for ages 20 to 32 (data not available).
Data from Hook[3] and Hook et al.[5]

ity throughout pregnancy.[5] Some trisomies, for example, No. 16, arise almost exclusively in maternal meiosis, usually maternal meiosis I. For a few chromosomes, there is a relatively higher frequency of errors at meiosis II (e.g., trisomy 18), and in yet others, errors in paternal meiosis are not uncommon (e.g., trisomy 2). Autosomal trisomy can also recur, the recurrence risk being approximately 1 percent following either trisomy 18 or 21. This suggests that genetic factors perturb meiosis, a phenomenon that serves as justification for prenatal screening after one aneuploid conception.

In addition to numeric abnormalities, structural chromosomal abnormalities occur. In a balanced interchange (translocation) between 2 or more chromosomes, individuals are phenotypically normal. However, such individuals are at increased risk for offspring with unbalanced gametes. This topic is also discussed in Chapter 24 in the context of repeated pregnancy loss.

Single-Gene Disorders

Approximately 1 percent of liveborn infants are phenotypically abnormal as a result of a single-gene mutation. Mendelian disorders thus account for 40 percent of the congenital defects seen in liveborn infants.

The human genome has now been sequenced and shown to contain approximately 25,000 human genes. In addition, post-transcriptional modifications result in perhaps three times as many proteins (gene products). Perturbation of each gene (deoxyribonucleic acid [DNA] sequence) or protein should theoretically result in a mendelian disorder. However, function is known for only a few thousand genes. Moreover, even the most common single gene (mendelian) disorder is individually rare except in its predominate ethnic group: cystic fibrosis (CF) 1 in 2,500 whites of European or Ashkenazi Jewish origin; sickle cell anemia in blacks; β-thalassemia in Greeks and Italians; α-thalassemia in Southeast Asians; and Tay-Sachs disease, CF, Canavan disease, and familial dysautonomia in Ashkenazi Jews.

Polygenic/Multifactorial Disorders

Another 1 percent of neonates are abnormal but show a normal chromosomal complement and have not ostensibly undergone mutation at a *single* genetic locus. It can be deduced that several different genes are involved (polygenic/multifactorial inheritance).[1]

Disorders in this etiologic category include most common malformations limited to a single organ system. These include hydrocephaly, anencephaly, and spina bifida (neural tube defects); facial clefts (cleft lip and palate); cardiac defects; pyloric stenosis; omphalocele; hip dislocation; uterine fusion defects; and club foot. After the birth of one child with such anomalies, the recurrence risk in subsequent progeny is 1 to 5 percent.[1] This frequency is less than would be expected if only a single gene were responsible but greater than that for the general population. The recurrence risks for malformations are also 1 to 5 percent for offspring of affected parents. That recurrence risks are similar for both siblings and offspring diminishes the likelihood that environmental causes are the exclusive etiologic factor because it is highly unlikely that households in different generations would be exposed to the same teratogen. Further excluding environmental factors as exclusive etiologic agents are observations that monozygotic twins are much more often concordant (similarly affected) than dizygotic twins, despite the fact that both types of twins share a common intrauterine environment.

The above-mentioned observations are best explained on the basis of polygenic/multifactorial inheritance. Although more than one gene is involved, only a few genes are necessary to produce the number of genotypes necessary to explain recurrence risks of 1 to 5 percent. That is, large numbers of genes and complex mechanisms need *not* be invoked. Polygenic/multifactorial etiology can thus plausibly be assumed responsible for liveborn infants having an anomaly of a single organ system without a chromosomal abnormality or a mendelian mutation (Table 6-3).

Table 6-3. Polygenic/Multifactorial Traits*

Hydrocephaly (excepting some forms of aqueductal stenosis and Dandy Walker syndrome)
Neural tube defects (anencephaly, spina bifida, encephalocele)
Cleft lift, with or without cleft plate
Cleft lip (alone)
Cardiac anomalies (most types)
Diaphragmatic hernia
Pyloric stenosis
Omphalocele
Renal agenesis (unilateral or bilateral)
Ureteral anomalies
Posterior urethral values
Hypospadias
Müllerian fusion effects
Müllerian aplasia
Limb reduction defects
Talipes equinovarus (clubfoot)

*Relatively common traits considered to be inherited in polygenic/multifactorial fashion. For each, normal parents have recurrence risks of 1 to 5 percent after one affected child. After two affected offspring, the risk is higher.

Teratogenic Disorders

The perhaps 20 proved teratogens are reviewed in Chapter 8. Although many other agents are suspected teratogens, the quantitative contribution of known teratogens to the incidence of anomalies seems relatively small (with the possible exception of alcohol).

CLINICAL SPECTRUM OF CHROMOSOMAL ABNORMALITIES

Offering a few generalizations concerning chromosomal disorders may be helpful to the obstetrician, who may encounter abnormal fetuses or infants during prenatal genetic studies or at delivery. In this section, we briefly review the clinical and cytogenetic features characteristic of the common numeric chromosomal abnormalities. Standard genetic texts, some geared for the obstetricians-gynecologist,[1] cover the broader spectrum of rare (often mosaic) trisomies and autosomal duplication or deficiency syndromes.

Autosomal Trisomy

TRISOMY 21

Trisomy 21 (Down syndrome, mongolism) is the most frequent autosomal chromosomal syndrome, occurring in 1 of every 800 liveborn infants (Table 6-1). The relationship of Down syndrome to advanced maternal age is well known (Table 6-2). Consistent with this maternal age effect, approximately 95 percent of cases arise in maternal meiosis, usually meiosis I. Characteristic craniofacial features include brachycephaly, oblique palpebral fissures, epicanthal folds, broad nasal bridge, a protruding tongue, and small, low-set ears with an overlapping helix and a prominent antihelix (Fig. 6-1). The mean birth weight in Down syndrome, 2,900 g, is decreased but less so than in other autosomal trisomies. At birth, Down syndrome infants are usually hypotonic. Other features include iridial Brushfield spots, broad short fingers (brachymesophalangia), clinodactyly (incurving deflections resulting from an abnormality of the middle phalanx), a single flexion crease on the fifth digit, and an unusually wide space between the first two toes. A single palmar crease (simian line) is not pathognomonic, being present in only 30 percent of individuals with trisomy 21 and in 5 percent of normal individuals. Relatively common internal anomalies include cardiac lesions and duodenal atresia. Cardiac anomalies and increased susceptibility to both respiratory infections and leukemia contribute to reduced life expectancy. However, mean survival extends into the fifth decade.

Patients with Down syndrome who survive beyond infancy invariably exhibit mental retardation. However, the degree of retardation is not as severe as that of most other chromosomal aberrations. Mean intelligence quotient (IQ) ranges approximately from 25 to 70; 46/47,+21 mosaicism should be suspected if Down syndrome cases show IQs in the 70 to 80 range. Women with Down

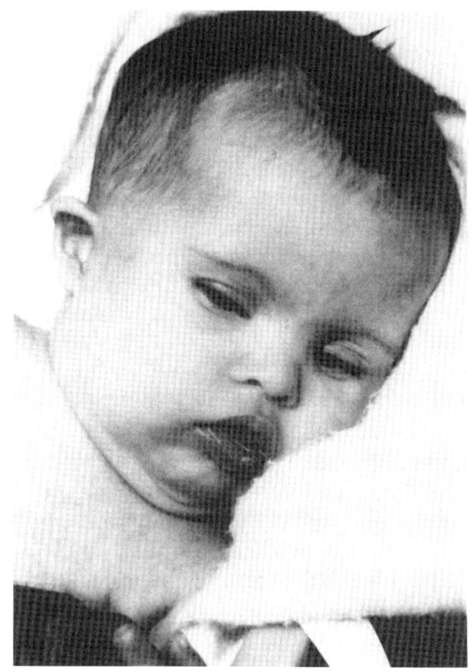

Figure 6-1. An infant with trisomy 21. (From Simpson JL, Elias S: Genetics in Obstetrics and Gynecology, 3rd ed. Philadelphia, WB Saunders Company, p 24, with permission.)

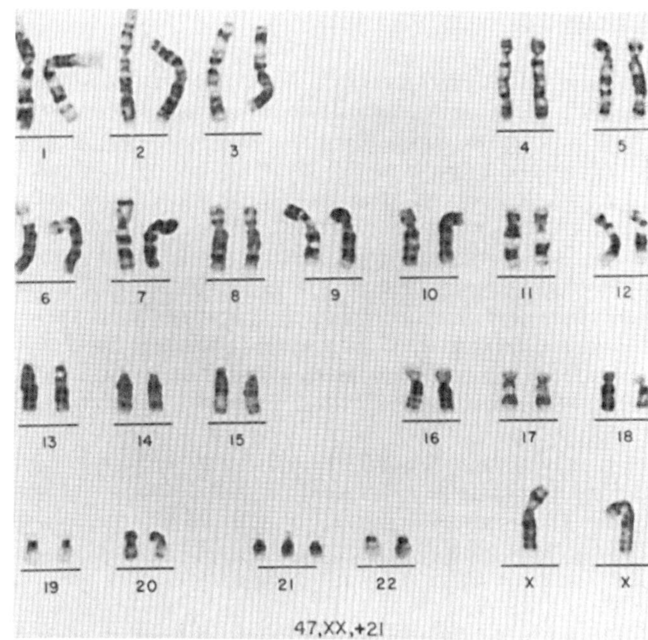

Figure 6-2. Karyotype of a trisomy 21 cell. Trypsin-Giemsa (GTG) banding. (From Simpson JL, Elias S: Genetics in Obstetrics and Gynecology, 3rd ed. Philadelphia, WB Saunders Company, with permission.)

syndrome are fertile. Although relatively few trisomic mothers have reproduced, about 30 percent of their offspring are also trisomic. Men are not considered fertile.

Several cytogenetic mechanisms may be associated with Down syndrome, the actual cause of which involves triplication of a small portion of chromosome 21, namely, band q22. Triplication may be caused either by the presence of an entire additional chromosome 21 or the addition of only band q22. Of all cases of Down syndrome, 95 percent have primary trisomy (47 instead of the normal 46 chromosomes) (Fig. 6-2). It is these cases that show the well-known relationship to both maternal age effect and to errors in maternal meiosis.

Structural chromosomal abnormalities—translocations—show no association to parental age. They may be either sporadic or familial. The translocation most commonly associated with Down syndrome involves chromosomes 14 and 21. With translocation Down syndrome, one parent may have the same translocation (rearrangement), that is, 45,t(14q;21q). Empiric risks are approximately 10 percent for offspring of female robertsonian translocation heterozygotes and 2 percent for offspring of male translocation heterozygotes. A potential concern is that diploid (46,XX or 46,XY) cases actually show uniparental disomy (UPD), both chromosomes originating from the same parent. In 65 Robertsonian translocation carriers [44 t(13q;14q), 11 t(14q;21q), 4 t(14q;22q), 6 others], only 1 UPD case was observed (0.6 percent).[6] The authors also surveyed 357 inherited and 102 de novo published cases, and concluded overall UPD risk for UPD 14 or 15 was 3 percent.

Other structural rearrangements resulting in Down syndrome include t(21q;21q), t(21q;21q), and translocations involving chromosome 21 and other acrocentric chromosomes (13 to 15) or G (21 to 22). In t(21q;21q), normal gametes do not ordinarily form. Thus, only trisomic or monosomic zygotes are produced, the latter presumably appearing as preclinical embryonic losses. Parents having the other translocations have a low empiric risk of having offspring with Down syndrome.

Trisomy 13

Trisomy 13 occurs in about 1 per 20,000 live births. Intrauterine and postnatal growth restrictions are pronounced, and developmental retardation is severe. Nearly 50 percent of affected children die in the first month, and relatively few survive past 3 years of age. Characteristic anomalies include holoprosencephaly, eye anomalies (microphthalmia, anophthalmia, or coloboma), cleft lip and palate, polydactyly, cardiac defects, and low birth weight. Other relatively common features include cutaneous scalp defects, hemangiomata on the face or neck, low-set ears with an abnormal helix, and rocker-bottom feet (convex soles and protruding heels).

Trisomy 13 is usually associated with nondisjunctional (primary) trisomy (47,+13). As in trisomy 21, a maternal age effect exists, and most cases are maternal in origin. Translocations are responsible for less than 20 percent of cases, invariably associated with two group D (13 to 15) chromosomes joining at their centromeric regions (robertsonian translocation). If neither parent has a rearrangement, the risk for subsequent progeny is not increased. If either parent has a balanced 13q;14q translocation, the recurrence risk for an affected offspring is increased but only to 1 to 2 percent. The exception is homologous 13q;13q parental translocation, which carries the same dire prognosis as 21q;21q translocation.

Trisomy 18

Trisomy 18 occurs in 1 per 8,000 live births. Among liveborn infants, girls are affected more often than boys (3:1). Among stillborns and abortuses, however, the sex distribution is more equal.

Facial anomalies characteristic of trisomy 18 include microcephaly, prominent occiput, low-set and pointed "fawn-like" ears, and micrognathia. Skeletal anomalies include overlapping fingers (V over IV, II over III), short sternum, shield chest, narrow pelvis, limited thigh abduction or congenital hip dislocation, rocker-bottom feet with protrusion of the calcaneum, and a short dorsiflexed hallux ("hammer toe"). Cardiac and renal anomalies are common.

Mean birth weight is 2,240 g. Fetal movement is feeble, and approximately 50 percent develop distress during labor. The mean survival is months. Liveborn infants show pronounced developmental and growth retardation. Trisomy 18 is not uncommonly detected among stillborn infants.

Approximately 80 percent of trisomy 18 cases are caused by primary nondisjunction (47,XX,+18 or 47,XY,+18). Errors usually arise in maternal meiosis, frequently meiosis II. Recurrence risk is about 1 percent.

Other Autosomal Trisomies

All autosomes show trisomies, but usually these end in abortuses. In addition to numbers 13, 18, and 21, only a few other trisomies are detected in liveborns (8, 9, 14, 16, and 22), and here often in mosaic forms. All cases show mental retardation, various somatic anomalies, and intrauterine growth restriction. The extent of retardation and the spectrum of anomalies vary.

Monosomy has been claimed for trisomy 21,[7] although undetected mosaicism is always different to exclude.

Autosomal Deletions or Duplications

Deletions or duplications of portions of autosomies also exist. There are numerous types. All are characterized by mental retardation and somatic anomalies, but specific features vary.

In counseling, one should initially exclude parental chromosomal rearrangements like a balanced translocation or inversion (see Chapter 7). If the deletion is sporadic, the recurrence risk is no greater than that for any other couple of comparable parental ages.

Sex Chromosomal Abnormalities

Monosomy X (45,X)

45,X individuals account for approximately 40 percent of gonadal dysgenesis cases ascertained by gynecologists. The incidence of 45,X in liveborn girls is about 1 in 10,000. Because monosomy X accounts for 10 percent of all first-trimester abortions, it can be calculated that more than 99 percent of 45,X conceptuses must end in early pregnancy loss. The error usually (80 percent) involves loss of a paternal sex chromosome.

Gonadal dysgenesis is often associated with an abnormal sex chromosomal constitution. Associated complements include not only monosomy X but structural abnormalities of the X chromosome. Mosaicism is frequent, usually involving a coexisting 45,X cell line. Both the long arm and the short arm of the X chromosome contain determinants necessary for ovarian differentiation and for normal stature, as discussed in detail elsewhere.[1]

45,X individuals not only have streak gonads but invariably are short (<150 cm). Growth hormone treatment increases the final adult height 6 to 8 cm. Various somatic anomalies exist: renal and cardiac defects, skeletal abnormalities like cubitus valgus and clinodactyly, vertebral anomalies, pigmented nevi, nail hypoplasia, and a low posterior hairline. Performance IQ is lower than verbal IQ, but overall IQ should be considered normal. Adult-onset diseases include hypertension and diabetes mellitus. Sybert[8,9] provides guidelines for evaluation and clinical management.

Klinefelter Syndrome

Boys with two or more X chromosomes have small testes, azoospermia, elevated follicle-stimulating hormone and luteinizing hormone levels, and decreased testosterone. The most frequent chromosomal complement associated with this phenotype—Klinefelter syndrome—is 47,XXY; 48,XXXY and 49,XXXXY are less common.

Mental retardation is uncommon in 47,XXY Klinefelter syndrome, but behavioral problems and receptive language difficulties are common. Mental retardation is invariably associated with 48,XXXY and 49,XXXXY. Skeletal, trunk, and craniofacial anomalies occur infrequently in 47,XXY but are commonly observed in 48,XXXY and 49,XXXXY. Regardless of the specific chromosomal complement, patients with Klinefelter syndrome all have unquestioned male phenotypes. The penis may be hypoplastic, but hypospadias is uncommon. With intracytoplasmic sperm injection and other assisted reproductive technologies, siring a pregnancy is now possible. Simpson et al.[10,11] provides guidelines on evaluation and clinical management.

Polysomy X in Girls (47,XXX; 48,XXXX; 49,XXXXX)

About 1 in 800 liveborn girls has a 47,XXX complement. 47,XXX individuals are more likely to show mental retardation than are individuals in the general population, and they show IQs 10 to 15 points lower than their sibs. However, the absolute risk for mental retardation does not exceed 5 to 10 percent, and even then, IQ is usually 60 to 80. Most 47,XXX patients have a normal reproductive system. The theoretical risk of 47,XXX women delivering an infant with an abnormal chromosomal complement is 50 percent, given one half maternal gametes carrying 24 chromosomes (24,XX). Empiric risks are much less. Somatic anomalies are not unusually considered increased in 47,XXX individuals, although anomalies may occur and have been observed in prenatally detected cases.[12] However, 48,XXXX and 49,XXXXX individuals are invariably retarded and more likely to have somatic malformations than 47,XXX individuals.

POLYSOMY Y IN BOYS (47,XYY AND 48,XXYY)

Presence of more than one Y chromosome is another frequent chromosomal abnormality in liveborn boys (1 in 1,000). 47,XYY men seem more likely than 46,XY boys to be tall and display sociopathic behavior. One estimate is that 1 percent of 47,XYY men will be incarcerated compared with 0.1 percent of 46,XY men. 47,XYY men usually have normal male external genitalia.

GENETIC HISTORY

Obstetrician/gynecologists must attempt to determine whether a couple, or anyone in their family, has a heritable disorder or is at increased risk for abnormal offspring. To address this question, some obstetricians find it helpful to elicit genetic information through the use of questionnaires or checklists that are often constructed in a manner that requires action only to positive responses. Figure 6-3 reproduces a form that has been modified from that recommended by the American College of Obstetricians and Gynecologists (ACOG).

One should inquire into the health status of first-degree relatives (siblings, parents, offspring), second-degree relatives (nephews, nieces, aunts, uncles, grandparents), and third-degree relatives (first cousins, especially maternal). Adverse reproductive outcomes such as repetitive spontaneous abortions, stillbirths, and anomalous liveborn infants should be pursued. Couples having such histories should undergo chromosomal studies in order to exclude balanced translocations (see Chapter 24). Genetic counseling may prove sufficiently complex to warrant referral to a clinical geneticist, or it may prove simple enough for the well-informed obstetrician to manage. If a birth defect exists in a second-degree relative (uncle, aunt, grandparent, nephew, niece) or third-degree relative (first cousin), the risk for that anomaly will usually not prove substantially increased over that in the general population. For example, identification of a second- or third-degree relative with an autosomal recessive trait places the couple at little increased risk for an affected offspring, an exception being if the patient and her husband are consanguineous. However, a maternal first cousin with an X-linked recessive disorder could identify a couple at increased risk for a similar occurrence.

Parental ages should also be recorded. Advanced maternal age (Table 6-2) warrants discussion irrespective of a physician's personal convictions regarding pregnancy termination, as knowledge of an abnormality may affect obstetric management. Ethnic origin should be recorded because certain genetic diseases are increased in selected ethnic groups (see below). Such queries apply for both gamete donors as well as couples achieving pregnancy by natural means.

Advanced *maternal* age confers increased risk for aneuploidy. This probably does not hold for advanced *paternal* age. A few studies indicate an increased frequency of aneuploidy in sperm in the sixth and seventh decades. However, risks are only marginally increased above background, and there remains no indication that a liveborn pregnancy risk is increased.

By contrast, a *paternal* age effect exists for single gene mutation, most relevantly de novo autosomal dominant mutations. A pregnancy sired by a man in his sixth decade or beyond carries perhaps a 1 percent increase, owing to the cumulative effects of single gene mutations at many loci. Unfortunately, prenatal testing is not applicable because hundreds of different loci could be involved. There is no evidence of a *maternal* age effect for single gene disorders.

GENETIC COUNSELING

Although genetic counseling may require referral to a clinical geneticist, it is impractical for obstetricians to refer all patients with genetic inquiries. Indeed, obstetricians performing diagnostic procedures such as amniocentesis must counsel their patients before such a procedure. Therefore, salient principles of the genetic counseling process are described.

Communication

Pivotal to counseling is communicating in terms that are readily comprehensible to patients. It is useful to preface remarks with a few sentences recounting the major causes of genetic abnormalities, such as cytogenetic, single-gene, polygenic/multifactorial ("complex"), and environmental (teratogens) causes. Writing unfamiliar words and using tables or diagrams to reinforce important concepts is helpful. Repetition is essential. Allow the couple not only to ask questions but to talk with one another to formulate their concerns.

Written information (letters or brochures) can serve as a couple's permanent record, allaying misunderstanding and assisting in dealing with relatives. Preprinted forms describing common problems (e.g., advanced maternal age) have the additional advantage of emphasizing that the couple's problem is not unique. More complicated scenarios require a letter.

Irrespective of how obvious a diagnosis may seem, confirmation is always obligatory. Accepting a patient's verbal recollection does not suffice, nor would accepting a diagnosis made by a physician not highly knowledgeable about the condition. The anomalous individual may need to be examined by the appropriate authority; examining first-degree relatives may be required as well to detect subtle findings, for example, of an autosomal dominant disorder like neurofibromatosis or Marfan syndrome. If a definitive diagnosis cannot be made, the physician should

Prenatal Genetic Screen

Name ______________________ Patient# ______________ Date __________

1. Will you be 35 years or older when the baby is due? Yes ___ No ___
2. Have you, the baby's father, or anyone in either of your families ever had any of the following disorders?
   Down syndrome (mongolism) Yes ___ No ___
   Other chromosomal abnormality Yes ___ No ___
   Neural tube defect, i.e., spina bifida (meningomyelocele or open spine), anencephaly Yes ___ No ___
   Hemophilia Yes ___ No ___
   Muscular dystrophy Yes ___ No ___
   Cystic fibrosis Yes ___ No ___
   If yes, indicate the relationship of the affected person to you or to the baby's father:
   ____
3. Do you or the baby's father have a birth defect? Yes ___ No ___
   If yes, who has the defect and what is it? ______________________
4. In any previous marriages, have you or the baby's father had a child born, dead or alive, with a birth defect not listed in question 2 above? Yes ___ No ___
5. Do you or the baby's father have any close relatives with mental retardation? Yes ___ No ___
   If yes, indicate the relationship of the affected person to you or to the baby's father:
   ____
   Indicate the cause, if known: ______________________
6. Do you, the baby's father, or a close relative in either of your families have a birth defect, any familial disorder, or a chromosomal abnormality not listed above? Yes ___ No ___
   If yes, indicate the condition and the relationship of the affected person to you or to the baby's father:
   ____
7. In any previous marriage, have you or the baby's father had a stillborn child or three or more first-trimester spontaneous pregnancy losses? Yes ___ No ___
   Have either of you had a chromosomal study? Yes ___ No ___
8. If you or the baby's father is of Jewish ancestry, have either of you been screened for Tay-Sachs disease, Canavan disease, or cystic fibrosis? Yes ___ No ___
   If yes, indicate who and the results: ______________________
9. If you or the baby's father is black, have either of you been screened for sickle cell trait? Yes ___ No ___
   If yes, indicate who and the results: ______________________
10. If you or the baby's father is of Italian, Greek, or Mediterranean background, have either of you been tested for β–thalassemia? Yes ___ No ___
    If yes, indicate who and the results: ______________________
11. If you or the baby's father is of Philippine or Southeast Asian ancestry, have either of you been tested for α–thalassemia? Yes ___ No ___
    If yes, indicate who and the results: ______________________
12. Irrespective of ethnic group, have you or the baby's father been screened for cystic fibrosis? Yes ___ No ___
13. Excluding iron and vitamins, have you taken any medications or recreational drugs since becoming pregnant or since your last menstrual period? (include nonprescription drugs)
    If yes, give name of medication and time taken during pregnancy: ______________________
    ____
14. Have you currently been taking folic acid supplements? Yes ___ No ___

Figure 6-3. Questionnaire for identifying couples having increased risk for offspring with genetic disorders. (Modified from a form recommended by the American College of Obstetricians and Gynecologists: Antenatal Diagnosis of Genetic Disorders. Technical Bulletin No. 108. Washington, DC, ACOG, 1987.)

not hesitate to say so. Proper counseling requires proper diagnosis.

Nondirective Counseling

In genetic counseling, one should provide accurate genetic information yet ideally dictate no particular course of action. Of course, completely nondirective counseling is probably unrealistic. For example, a counselor's unwitting facial expressions may expose his or her unstated opinions. Merely offering antenatal diagnostic services implies approval. Despite the difficulties of remaining truly objective, one should attempt to provide information and then support the couple's decision.

Psychological Defenses

If not appreciated, psychological defenses can impede the entire counseling process. Anxiety is low in couples counseled for advanced maternal age or for an abnormality in a distant relative. So long as anxiety remains low, comprehension of information is usually not impeded. However, couples who have experienced a stillborn infant, an anomalous child, or multiple repetitive abortions are more anxious. Their ability to retain information may be hindered.

Couples experiencing abnormal pregnancy outcomes manifest the same grief reactions that occur after the death of a loved one: denial, anger, guilt, bargaining, and resolution. One should pay deference to this sequence by not attempting definitive counseling immediately after the birth of an abnormal neonate. The obstetrician should avoid discussing specific recurrence risks for fear of adding to the immediate burden. By 4 to 6 weeks, the couple has begun to cope and is more receptive to counseling.

An additional psychological consideration is that of parental guilt. One naturally searches for exogenous factors that might have caused an abnormal outcome. In the process of such a search, guilt may arise. Conversely, a tendency to blame the spouse may be seen. Usually, guilt or blame is not justified, but occasionally the "blame" is realistic (e.g., in autosomal dominant traits). Fortunately, most couples can be assured that nothing could have prevented a given abnormality in their offspring.

Appreciating the psychological defenses described earlier helps one to understand the failure of ostensibly intelligent and well-counseled couples to comprehend genetic information.

GENETIC SCREENING

Genetic screening implies routine monitoring for the presence or absence of a given condition in apparently normal individuals. Screening is now offered routinely for all individuals of certain ethnic groups to identify those individuals heterozygous for a given autosomal recessive disorder (Table 6-4). Ultrasound screening for fetal abnormalities during pregnancy is reviewed in Chapter 9.

Table 6-4. Genetic Screening in Various Ethnic Groups

ETHNIC GROUP	DISORDER	SCREENING TEST
All ethnic groups	Cystic fibrosis	DNA analysis of selected panel of 23 CFTR mutations (alleles present in 0.1 percent of the general U.S. population)
Black	Sickle cell anemia	Mean corpuscular volume <80 percent, followed by hemoglobin electrophoresis
Ashkenazi Jewish	Tay-Sachs disease	Decreased serum hexosaminidase-A or DNA analysis for selected alleles
	Canavan disease	DNA analysis for selected alleles
	Familial dysautonomia	DNA analysis for selected alleles
Cajuns	Tay-Sachs disease	DNA analysis for selected alleles
French-Canadians	Tay-Sachs disease	DNA analysis for selected alleles
Mediterranean people (Italians, Greek)	β-Thalassemia	Mean corpuscular volume (MCV) <80 percent, followed by hemoglobin electrophoresis if iron deficiency excluded
Southeast Asians (Filipinos, Chinese, African, Vietnamese, Laotian, Cambodian, Filipino)	α-Thalassemia	MCV < 80 percent, followed by hemoglobin electrophoresis if iron deficiency excluded

CFTR, cystic fibrosis transmembrane conductance regulator.

Screening Neonates

One could theoretically screen neonates for many other genetic disorders. Screening is actually recommended for relatively few disorders because prerequisites essential for initiating screening programs are not usually met. Widespread testing is ordinarily performed only if an abnormal finding would alter clinical management. In the United States, neonates have long been mandated in all states to be screened for phenylketonuria and hypothyroidism, which are amenable either to dietary or hormonal treatment, respectively. The number of disorders for which neonates are screened varies state by state. In the United States, most commonly mandated are selected inborn errors of metabolism that include galactosemia (diet treatment), sickle cell anemia (early administration of antibiotics), and 21-hydroxylase adrenal hyperplasia (cortisol administration).

Other disorders are mandated less commonly, usually using mass spectrometry. The March of Dimes recommends screening for 30 disorders as well as for deafness. This organization's web site provides state-by-state information *(www.marchofdimes.com/professionals/580.asp)*. Disorders explicitly enumerated by the ACOG and the U.S. Health Resources and Services Administration (HRSA) include not only phenylketonuria, hypothyroidism, galactosemia, sickle cell anemia, and adrenal hyperplasia (see earlier) but also biotinidase deficiency, congenital toxoplasmosis, CF (postnatal), homocystinuria, maple syrup urine disease, and medium chain acyl-CoA dehydrogenase deficiency. The ACOG and HRSA note that although possible, to screen for disorders of fatty acid oxidation, organic acids, and urea cycle, there is less experience.

Considerable recent attention is being given to screening for deafness. More than 70 genes related to hearing are already known. Mutations in gap junction B *(GJB2)*, the gene that codes connexin 26, and the neighboring gene *GJB6* (connexin 30) account for 50 percent of deafness in the newborn.[13] The heterozygote frequency for *GJB2* alone is 3 percent in North American whites.[14]

An accepted principle is that screening is not attempted for neonates with untreatable disorders. Thus, neonatal screening is not recommended for chromosomal abnormalities, Tay-Sachs disease, and Duchenne muscular dystrophy.

Screening Adults

The ACOG recommends population screening for selected disorders, seeking asymptomatic heterozygotes in families in which no affected individual has been born.[15–19] These autosomal recessive disorders are amenable to prenatal diagnosis and are listed in Table 6-4.

Tay Sachs Disease

The prototype for screening is Tay-Sachs disease, an autosomal recessive disorder for which Ashkenazi Jewish individuals are at increased risk. The ACOG cites a heterozygote frequency of 1 in 30.[15] In the United States, Jewish individuals may be uncertain whether they are of Ashkenazic or Sephardic descent (90 percent are Ashkenazi); thus, obstetricians should screen all Jewish couples, as well as couples in which only one partner is Jewish. Other conditions for which genetic screening is recommended in Jewish couples are Canavan disease,[18] familial dysautonomia,[19] and CF (see later). In all of these disorders, the carrier frequency is about 1 in 30. Ashkenazi Jewish individuals may also elect to be screened for other disorders: Gaucher disease, Nieman-Pick disease, Bloom syndrome, Fanconi anemia C, and mucolipidosis.[19] Carrier frequencies for these disorders vary from 1 in 15 (Gaucher disease) to 1 in 127 (mucolipidosis IV). Heterozygote detection rates for each condition are 95 to 99 percent, the efficiency reflecting only a few mutations being responsible for each disorder. In aggregate, the likelihood of an Ashkenazi Jewish individual being heterozygous for one of the autosomal recessive disorders listed in this section is 1 in 4.[19]

Screening usually involves molecular testing for common selected mutations. In Tay Sachs disease, molecular testing in Ashkenazi Jews detects 94 percent of heterozygotes, whereas more laborious biochemical analysis (based on ratio of hexosaminidase A to total hexosaminidase – A plus B) detects 98 percent.[15] If only one partner is Ashkenazi, the ACOG[15,19] suggests screening that individual first. In low-risk populations (e.g., non-Ashkenazi Europeans), carrier frequency is only 1 in 300.[15] Because molecular heterogeneity is so prevalent, biochemical testing is necessary in testing individuals who are not Ashkenazi Jews.

Thalassemias

In Italians and Greeks, screening for β-thalassemia is indicated.[16] This might rely initially on mean corpuscular volume (MCV), which will also screen for α-thalassemia in Southeast Asians, Filipinos, and Africans.[16] MCV of greater than 80 percent excludes heterozygosity for α- or β-thalassemia. Values less than 80 percent are more likely to reflect iron deficiency anemia than thalassemia heterozygosity; thus, tests to exclude the former are indicated. If iron deficiency is not found, hemoglobin electrophoresis showing elevated hemoglobin A2 and hemoglobin F will confirm β-thalassemia. DNA-based testing is necessary to detect α-globin deletions, which cause α-thalassemia.[16]

ACOG has recently recommended that detection of sickle cell trait (heterozygosity) be determined using the same regimen as that for β-thalassemia – MCV <80% followed by hemoglobin electrophoresis if iron deficiency is excluded. Solubility tests previously used to detect sickle cell trait (SA) are now considered less sensitive, and do not detect other abnormal hemoglobins (e.g., hemoglobin C, β-thasassemia).[19a]

Screening for Cystic Fibrosis

Since 2001, screening for CF has been recommended by the ACOG and American College of Medical Genetics (ACMG),[20,21] with guidelines modified by ACOG in late 2005.[22] Severely affected individuals show pulmonary and pancreatic disease. Mean life expectancy is only 30 years and has increased only marginally over the last decades.[23] In the United States a significant portion of lung transplants and heart lung transplants are for CF. The disorder usually is manifested early in childhood, 10 to 20 percent being detected at birth because of meconium ileus. Increasing accumulation of viscous secretions progressively leads to chronic respiratory obstruction. Malnutrition and poor postnatal growth arise secondary to blockage of pancreatic ducts, producing insufficient pancreatic enzymes that interfere with intestinal absorption. Almost all men with CF have azoospermia, the anatomic result of congenital bilateral absence of the vas deferens (CBAVD). Sometimes CBAVD is the only manifestation of CF. In these cases, the mutant alleles are less deleterious than those causing severe (primary and pancreatic CF). Individuals CF who do not show pancreatic insufficiency are said to have mild CF and have a median survival of 56 years.[23] Definitive diagnosis is made by the chloride sweat test, although molecular confirmation is increasingly used. Once a mutation (see later) is recognized in a given family, molecular studies are indicated to detect other heterozygotes and affected relatives.

The CF gene is relatively large (27 exons), and its gene product is a chloride channel. In whites of non-Ashkenazi European descent, about 75 percent of CF mutations are caused by the deletion of three amino acids in codon 508 (ΔF508), resulting in loss of a phenylalanine residue.[24] About 50 percent of couples at risk for CF offspring can be identified by screening solely for this mutation, offering unequivocal prenatal diagnosis. Detecting the remaining couples at risk for CF is more difficult. Screening only for ΔF508 would not infrequently uncover couples in which one parent has the ΔF508 mutation but the other does not. If one parent has ΔF508 but the other does not, the actual risk of that couple having an affected child is low. However, the CF gene product (protein) cannot be assayed per se; thus, prenatal genetic diagnosis could not exclude a fetus who inherited the ΔF508 from the known heterozygous parent and who inherited a deleterious, severe, but unrecognized allele from the other parent. Only molecular methods would distinguish unaffected from affected fetuses. One could exclude fetuses who inherited ΔF508 from their one heterozygous parent of known genotype, but half of the excluded fetuses would be clinically normal (i.e., only heterozygous for a mutant CF allele). Distinguishing compound heterozygosity (affected) from heterozygosity with its only one mutant allele is not possible unless both parental mutations are known.

The obvious solution is to detect all other mutations within the CF locus. In Ashkenazi Jewish individuals, one other mutation (W1282X) quickly proved common,[25] but individual mutations have otherwise been individually rare in all ethnic groups. Figure 6-4 is an early study from the Cystic Fibrosis Foundation showing an increasing detection rate in northern European white and Ashkenazi Jewish populations as increasing numbers of CF-causing alleles are sought.[26] Based on these cases, sensitivity approached but did not exceed 80 or 97 percent in these two ethnic groups, respectively. Differing sensitivities exist using the now-accepted panel of mutations recommended for testing by the ACOG and ACMG in 2001[20,21] and updated in 2005.[22] This is discussed later. Irrespective, not all at-risk pregnancies are identified, a principle applicable in any screening test. Unlike case detection approaches (e.g., Pap smears, invasive testing for aneuploidy), one never expects to detect 100 percent of cases in a screening program. This might be precluded for technical, financial or diagnostic reasons.

Guidelines for Cystic Fibrosis Screening

In 2001, recommendations for CF screening were made jointly by the ACOG, the ACMG, and the National Institutes of Health Genome Center.[20,21] It was recommended that a panethnic mutation panel be used that includes all mutant CF alleles having a frequency of 0.1 percent in the general U.S. population.[21] This was modified in 2004 to encompass 23 mutations (Table 6-5).[27] Screening for other alleles is optional. Vendors offer expanded panels of up to nearly 100 mutations, but this is still only a fraction of the 1,300 reported CF mutations. Even if the entire gene is sequenced, not all CF mutations will be identified. Those not yet identified presumably act in promoter regions or perturb post-translational modification.

The 2001 guidelines stated that one should offer CF heterozygote screening to non-Jewish whites and Ashkenazi Jews, both of which were originally estimated to have carrier frequencies of 1 in 29.[20,21,28] In the most recent tabulation, the frequency was estimated to be 1 in 24 and 1 in 25, respectively.[22] Based on this, the overall heterozygote detection rates in whites and Ashkenazi Jews can now be stated to be 88 and 94 percent, respectively.[22] In other ethnic groups (Asian-Americans, Hispanics, African-Americans), the carrier frequency is lower (Table 6-6). In these ethnic groups, detection rates are also lower (Table 6-7).

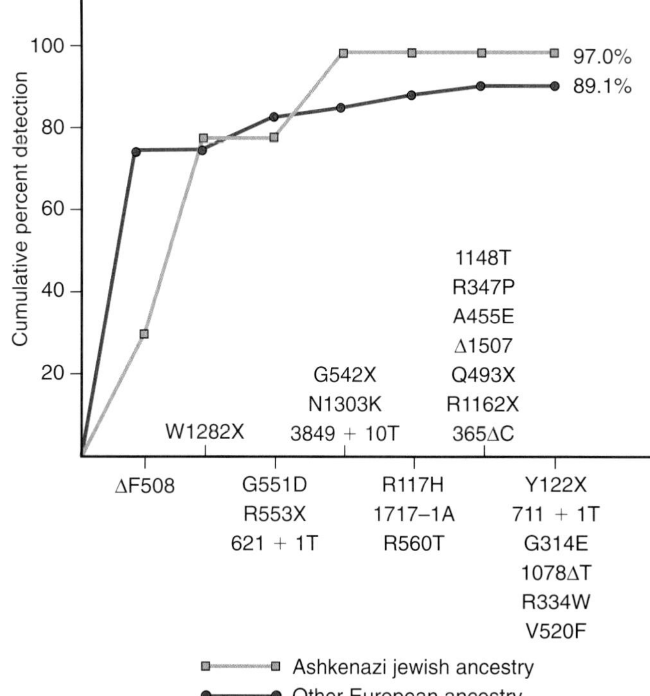

Figure 6-4. Increasing detection rate in northern European white and Ashkenazi Jewish populations as increasing numbers of CF-causing alleles are sought. (From Cystic Fibrosis Foundation Annual Report. New York, 1996.)

Table 6-5. Recommended Panel of 23 Mutations in the Cystic Fibrosis Transmembrane Conductance Regulator (CFTR) Gene That Should Be Sought in Carrier Detection Programs[33*]

ΔF508	ΔI507	G542X	G551D	W1282Z	N1303K
R533X	621 + 1G > T	R117H	1717 − 1G > A	A455E	R560T
R1162X	G85E	R334W	R347P	711 + 1G > T	1898 + 1G > A
2184delA	3120 + 1G > A	3849 + 10kbC > T	2789 + 5G > A	3659delC	

*The panel is applicable in all ethnic groups. If R117H is detected, status of the 5T-7T-9T polymorphism should be determined reflexly. After originally consisting of 25 mutations,[21] two mutations were removed.[27] 1078delT was removed because of its rarity, whereas I148T was removed because the causative gene was actually a second mutation (3199del6) in linkage disequibrium. However, this mutation (3199del6) is too rare to justify screening.

Table 6-6. Detecting Cystic Fibrosis (CF) Heterozygotes (23 Mutation Panel)[27]

ETHNIC GROUP	HETEROZYGOTE CARRIER FREQUENCY	PERCENT OF HETEROZYGOTES DETECTABLE	LIKELIHOOD OF BEING HETEROZYGOUS DESPITE NEGATIVE SCREEN
Ashkenazi Jewish	1/24	94%	1/400
European non-Hispanic White	1/25	88%	1/208
Hispanic-American	1/46	72%	1/164
Black	1/65	65%	1/186
Asian	1/94	49%	1/184

Data of ACOG Committee Opinion 325 (2005).[22] The current panel encompasses 23 mutations,[27] rather than the original 25.[21]

Table 6-7. Likelihood of Affected Fetus after Concurrent versus Sequential Screening for Cystic Fibrosis

	NON-HISPANIC EUROPEAN WHITES	ASHKENAZI JEWISH
No screening	1/2,500	1/2,304
Both partners negative (concurrent)	1/173,056	1/640,000
One partner negative, one untested (sequential)	1/20,800	1/38,400
One partner positive, one negative (concurrent)	1/832	1/1,600
One partner positive, other untested	1/100	1/96
Both partners positive	1/4	1/4

These calculations are based on the frequencies shown in Table 6-6.

Worthy of special comment is allele R117H. This allele is not uncommonly associated with CBAVD, but it is not causative for the classic (severe) CF phenotype as characterized by pulmonary, hepatic, and pancreatic complications. Recall that men with CBAVD usually have two dysfunctional CF alleles.[29] However, in CBAVD only one, *not both* alleles, could be ΔF508 or consist of a CF allele conferring severe phenotype (pancreatic and pulmonary disease). If both alleles were ΔF508 or "severe," the phenotype would not be CBAVD but classic CF. If the other allele were R117H, a compound heterozygous male would have CBAVD (ΔF508/R117H). If his spouse were heterozygous for ΔF508, the likelihood would be 25 percent that any given fetus will have severe CF (ΔF508/ΔF508).

In certain circumstances, however, R117H/ΔF508 compound heterozygotes show severe CF. This arises on the basis of concurrent perturbations involving a polymorphism (5T) in intron 8 of the CF gene.[29] If at that portion of the CF gene there exist 5 thymines (5T), or to a lesser extent seven thymines (7T), splice-junction perturbations occur, deleting exon 8 and, hence, producing a truncated partially dysfunctional transmembrane conductance regulator (CFTR) gene product. With 5T, the CF protein (gene product) is 10 percent of normal. This is more than with ΔF508 and W1282X, in which virtually no CFTR gene product is produced. With 7T, the gene product is 50 percent of normal, and with 9T, it is 100 percent normal. Despite expressing only 10 percent gene product, however, this is enough for a 5T allele not to confer severe CF, that is, pulmonary and pancreatic disease. However, if 5T exists on the same chromosome (i.e., *cis*) as a second similarly mild mutation (specifically R117H), the two alleles in aggregate (on the same chromosome) confer the negligible low levels of CFTR as conferred by a single severe CF mutant allele like ΔF508. If the CF gene (allele) on the other chromosome has a severe CF mutation, the fetus can show severe CF. To clarify:

- If 5T exists on the same chromosome as R117H and the other chromosome has a severe mutation (ΔF508), severe CF will occur.
- If 7T exists on the same chromosome *(cis)* as R117H and the other chromosome has a severe mutation, the fetus is at risk only for mild CF because 7T/R117H still produces sufficient CF gene product. CBAVD can result but not severe CF (pulmonary and pancreatic disease).
- If both chromosomes show 5T (homozygosity) and neither carries another CF mutation, CBAVD may occur but not severe CF.

Given the above-mentioned information, ACOG and ACMG guidelines recommend that laboratories automatically ("reflex") test for 5T whenever R117H is detected.[20,21,27] If R117H is not detected, 5T/ 7T/ 9T status will not be determined. If a physician wishes to know the status of 5T polymorphisms, for example, in excluding CBAVD as a cause for male infertility, a specific request must thus be made for 5T/ 7T/ 9T testing.

Implementing Cystic Fibrosis Screening

How does a practitioner initiate CF screening and comply with guidelines? A few suggestions may be helpful in the office setting.

Recall that if a couple has already had a child with CF, or if there exists an affected relative, genetic screening as will be described above is *not* germane. Rather, case detection strategies then become appropriate. The index case, or the couple if the proband is unavailable, should be screened not just for the panel of 23 mutations alluded to earlier, but if uninformative, a larger panel of CF mutations. If the mutation is still not evident, family studies to identify polymorphic loci informative for linkage analysis should be considered if prenatal genetic diagnosis is planned. Sequencing the entire gene may be desired. Sequencing might also be appropriate in evaluating a man with CBAVD if his spouse is heterozygous for a severe CF allele (e.g., ΔF508) and if the molecular basis is not evident.[22]

Choosing a Panel

Fulfilling ACOG/ACMG guidelines for the 23 mutations is possible through several vendors. Costs are typically \$150 to \$300. Panels screening for more than the 23 mutations are not necessary in the presence of a negative family history; relatively few additional heterozygotes are detected as more alleles are sought. If an extended panel is chosen, it may be prudent to screen every patient in one's practice similarly, or make a special note to justify individual alteration in practice. Analogous reasoning applies to ethnic-specific panels.

Worth emphasizing is that the above-mentioned advice is not applicable when a family member is known to have severe CF. Extended panels or even sequencing should then be undertaken in order to elucidate the molecular basis.

Screening Concurrently or Sequentially

A key decision is whether to screen both the mother and father together (concurrent) or to screen only the mother (sequential); if only the mother is screened, the father would be studied only if the mother were a carrier. Either approach is acceptable. Screening both partners obviously produces the highest detection rate, although not by much (Table 6-7). The downside is that one partner will be a carrier significantly more often (two-fold), thus generating more anxiety and requiring follow-up more often.

"Offering" Cystic Fibrosis Screening

The original (2001) guidelines by the ACOG and ACMG stated that CF screening should be "offered" only to whites of European or Ashkenazi Jewish ancestry.[20,21] It thus seemed reasonable to screen in a fashion analogous to that for Tay-Sachs disease, sickle cell anemia, β- or α-thalassemia. Initiation of a dialogue with the patient is required by the physician or a member of his or her health provider team. One should state that genetic screening is not obligatory. Patient information brochures, such as the ACOG/ACMG publication *Cystic Fibrosis Carrier Testing—The Decision is Yours,*[30] review inheritance of CF, variability of CF symptoms, and likelihood of detecting carrier status. This brochure explicitly states that not all CF mutations are detectable, and hence, not all affected individuals can be detected. That is, false-negative cases are unavoidable. The legal significance of this statement cannot be overemphasized.

In couples of black, Hispanic, and Asian origin, it was originally stated that CF screening should be "made available."[20,21,28] There were no specific recommendations for distinguishing between "offer" and "made available." If applying this, perhaps a brief informative statement about CF could be followed by informing the patient that CF screening exists. Information gained through brochures or other sources could help the undecided patient decide if she wishes to pursue.

More recently, it has become obvious that it was often unwieldy to assign a single ethnicity to a given patient.[31,32] Moreover, ACOG has estimated that two thirds of obstetricians were offering CF screening to all pregnant patients. Thus, it is now considered reasonable to offer CF screening to all pregnant women.

Documenting Compliance

Prudent for litigious protection is adherence to a consistent plan verifying that information on screening was conveyed. This might consist of written notation on the chart. If so, retention of the written informed consent stating the patient's choice is essential. A sample consent form exists in the ACOG/ACMG patient information brochure.[33] However, retaining such a form on every patient might be burdensome, especially in offices using an electronic medical record.

Follow-Up of Cystic Fibrosis Test Results

The following scenarios could arise:

- If CF screening tests on both partners are negative, no further evaluation is required. Recall, however, that detection of 100 percent of carriers is never possible in population screening. Table 6-7 shows frequency of affected fetuses if screening is negative.
- If one partner has a CF mutation, but the other screens negative, no further evaluation is needed. The residual risk of still having a CF fetus is low but finite (Table 6-7).
- If one partner is a CF carrier and the other cannot be tested, the couple has a low but no longer inconsequential risk. In Europeans of non-Ashkenazi white origin, the residual risk is 100 (1 × 1 in 25 × 1 in 4). If Jewish, the risk is 1 in 96. Chorionic villi or amniotic fluid analysis can exclude these fetuses with the maternal mutation, assuring that they will be clinically normal.
- If both couples are heterozygous for the same or for two different deleterious alleles (compound heterozygotes), referral to a geneticist is appropriate. The risk for an unaffected fetus is 25 percent, and options for a definitive diagnosis should be presented. Useful in this regard is the ACOG/ACMG booklet, *Cystic Fibrosis* Testing—*What Happens if Both my Partner and I are Carriers.*[33]

Alerting Relatives

Suppose a patient or her spouse has a severe CF-causing mutation, like ΔF508. Relatives of your patient could well have inherited the same mutation from a common ancestor. The likelihood is 50 percent that any given sib of your patient or her partner will have the same mutation. As caring physicians, we surely wish to alert at-risk individuals; however, we have no authority to contact a relative directly. The solution is using a sample letter, mailed not by the physician but by the patient or her spouse. This letter would inform relatives of the consequence of a CF mutation having been detected. A template for such a letter exists in the ACOG/ACMG booklet *Preconception and Prenatal Carrier Screening for Cystic Fibrosis.*[30]

Key Points

- The frequency of major birth defects is 2 to 3 percent, based on the definition of a defect causing death, a severe dysfunction, or a structural malformation requiring surgery.

- Major etiologic categories include chromosomal abnormalities (1 in 160 live births), single-gene or Mendelian disorders, polygenic/multifactorial disorders, and disorders caused by exogenous factors (teratogens).

- The frequency of autosomal trisomies is higher in midtrimester (30 percent for Down syndrome) than at term, and many trisomies are so lethal that they are found only in abortuses.

- Single-gene disorders in aggregate result in major defects in 1 percent of neonates, and additional disorders are manifested later in life. However, individual disorders are uncommon. CF occurs in 1 per 3,600 whites of northern European or Ashkenazi Jewish origin.

- Principles of genetic counseling include adequate communication, appreciation of psychological defenses, and adherence to nondirective counseling.

- Genetic screening to detect heterozygotes in the nonpregnant and, if not already evaluated, in the pregnant population is appropriate for the following autosomal recessive disorders: Tay-Sachs disease, Canavan disease, familial dysautonomia in Jewish populations; Tay-Sachs disease in Cajun and French-Canadian populations; CF in all populations; α-thalassemia in Asians; β-thalassemia in Mediterranean populations (Greek and Italians); and sickle cell disease in blacks.

- Heterozygosity for β-thalassemia and α-thalassemia can be inexpensively detected on the basis of MCV less than 80 percent followed by hemoglobin electrophoresis, once iron deficiency is excluded.

- CF is found in all ethnic groups, but the heterozygote frequency is higher in non-Hispanic whites of northern European (1 in 25) or Ashkenazi Jewish origin (1 in 24) than in other ethnic groups (black 1/65, Hispanic 1/46, Asian 1/94). The ACOG and the ACMG originally recommended that CF screening be offered to whites and "made available" to other groups. In 2005, the ACOG acknowledged the difficulty in assigning a single ethnicity and stated that it was reasonable to offer screening to all pregnant women.

- The CF gene is large (27 exons), and more than 1,300 disease-causing mutations have been recognized. Screening is obligatory only for a specified panel of 23 mutations.

- In northern European white and Ashkenazi Jewish individuals, the heterozygote detection rate using the specified panel is 84 and 94 percent, respectively. In other ethnic groups detection rates are lower (65 percent blacks, 72 percent Hispanics, 49 percent Asian Americans).

- A couple can either both undergo CF screening simultaneously or the second partner can be screened only if the first proves to be a heterozygote. The former generates the highest detection rate, but the latter method is also acceptable.

- If the 5T polymorphism exists on the same chromosome *(cis)* on which a mild CF mutation exists (e.g., R117H), the effect is the same as if there were a single severe mutation (e.g., ΔF508). Thus, if the other chromosome has a severe mutation (ΔF508), severe CF will result. If both chromosomes show a 5T polymorphism or if 5T exists trans to a chromosome with the ΔF508 mutation, the result is CBAVD.

REFERENCES

1. Simpson JL, Elias S: Genetics in Obstetrics and Gynecology, ed 3. Philadelphia, WB Saunders, 2003.
2. Hook EB, Hamerton JL: The frequency of chromosome abnormalities detected in consecutive newborn studies: Differences between studies-results by sex and by severity of phenotype involvement. *In* Hook EB, Porter IH (eds): Population Cytogenetic Studies in Humans. New York, Academic Press, 1977, p 63.
3. Hook EB: Rates of chromosome abnormalities at different maternal ages. Obstet Gynecol 58:282, 1981.
4. Morris JK, Mutton DE, Alberman E: Revised estimates of the maternal age specific live birth prevalence of Down's syndrome. J Med Screen 9:2, 2002.
5. Hook EB, Cross PK, Schreinemachers DM: Chromosomal abnormality rates at amniocentesis and in live-born infants. JAMA 249:2034, 1983.
6. Ruggeri A, Dulcetti F, Miozzo M, et al: Prenatal search for UPD 14 and UPD 15 in 83 cases of familial and de novo heterologous Robertsonian translocations. Prenat Diagn 24:997, 2004.
7. Mori MA, Lapunzina P, Delicado A, et al: A prenatally diagnosed patient with full monosomy 21: ultrasound, cytogenetic, clinical, molecular, and necropsy findings. Am J Med Genet A 127:69, 2004.
8. Sybert VP, McCauley E: Turner's syndrome. N Engl J Med 351:1227, 2004.
9. Sybert VP: Turner syndrome. *In* Cassidy SB, Allanson J (eds): Management of Genetic Syndromes, ed 2. Hoboken, New Jersey, John Wiley and Sons, Inc., 2005, p 589.
10. Simpson JL, de La Cruz F, Swerdloff RS, et al: Klinefelter syndrome: expanding the phenotype and identifying new research directions. Genet Med 5:460, 2003.
11. Simpson JL, Graham JM, Samango-Sprouse C: Klinefelter syndrome. *In* Cassidy SB, Allanson J (eds): Management of Genetic Syndromes, ed 2, Hoboken, New Jersey, John Wiley and Sons, Inc., 2005, p 323.

12. Haverty CE, Lin AE, Simpson E, et al: 47,XXX associated with malformations. Am J Med Genet A 125:108, 2004.
13. Prasad S, Cucci RA, Green GE, et al: Genetic testing for hereditary hearing loss: connexin 26 (GJB2) allele variants and two novel deafness-causing mutations (R32C and 645–648delTAGA). Hum Mutat 16:502, 2000.
14. Green GE, Scott DA, McDonald JM, et al: Carrier rates in the midwestern United States for GJB2 mutations causing inherited deafness. JAMA 281:2211, 1999.
15. ACOG Committee Opinion: Screening for Tay-Sachs Disease. Washington, DC, American College of Obstetricians and Gynecologists. Report 318, 2005.
16. ACOG Practice Bulletin: Hemoglobinopathies in pregnancy. Washington, DC, American College of Obstetrician and Gynecologists. Report 64, 2005.
17. ACOG Committee Opinion: Genetics in Obstetrics and Gynecology. Washington, DC, American College of Obstetricians and Gynecologists, 2002.
18. ACOG Committee Opinion: Screening for Canavan disease. Washington, DC, American College of Obstetricians and Gynecologists. Report 40, 1998.
19. ACOG Committee Opinion: Prenatal and preconceptional carrier screening for genetic diseases in individuals of eastern European Jewish descent. Washington, DC, American College of Obstetricians and Gynecologists. Report 298:127, 2004.
19a. ACOG Practice Bulletin: Hemoglobinopathies in pregnancy. Number 78, January 2007. Washington, DC, American College of Obstetricians and Gynecologists. Obstet Gynecol 109:229, 2007.
20. ACOG: Preconception and Prenatal Carrier Screening for Cystic Fibrosis. Clinical and Laboratory Guidelines. Washington, DC, Bethesda, MD, ACMG, 2001.
21. Grody WW, Cutting GR, Klinger KW, et al: Laboratory standards and guidelines for population-based cystic fibrosis carrier screening. Genet Med 3:149, 2001.
22. ACOG Committee Opinion. Update on carrier screening for cystic fibrosis. Washington, DC, American College of Obstetricians and Gynecologists. Report 325, 2005.
23. Cutting GR: Cystic Fibrosis. *In* Rimoin DL, Connor JM, Pyeritz RE (eds): Principles and Practices of Medical Genetics, ed 5. Edinburgh, Churchill-Livingstone, 2007, p 1354.
24. Riordan JR, Rommens JM, Kerem B, et al: Identification of the cystic fibrosis gene: cloning and characterization of complementary DNA. Science 245:1066, 1989.
25. Abeliovich D, Lavon IP, Lerer I, et al: Screening for five mutations detects 97% of cystic fibrosis (CF) chromosomes and predicts a carrier frequency of 1:29 in the Jewish Ashkenazi population. Am J Hum Genet 51:951, 1992.
26. Cystic Fibrosis Foundation Annual Report. New York, 1996.
27. Watson MS, Cutting GR, Desnick RJ, et al: Cystic fibrosis population carrier screening: 2004 revision of American College of Medical Genetics mutation panel. Genet Med 6:387, 2004.
28. Mennuti MT, Thomson E, Press N: Screening for cystic fibrosis carrier state. Obstet Gynecol 93:456, 1999.
29. Chillon M, Casals T, Mercier B, et al: Mutations in the cystic fibrosis gene in patients with congenital absence of the vas deferens. N Engl J Med 332:1475, 1995.
30. ACOG, ACMG: Cystic fibrosis carrier testing—the decision is yours. Washington, DC, American College of Obstetricians and Gynecologists/American College of Medical Genetics, 2001.
31. Morgan MA, Driscoll DA, Mennuti MT, et al: Practice patterns of obstetrician-gynecologists regarding preconception and prenatal screening for cystic fibrosis. Genet Med 6:450, 2004.
32. Morgan MA, Driscoll DA, Zinberg S, et al: Impact of self-reported familiarity with guidelines for cystic fibrosis carrier screening. Obstet Gynecol 105:1355, 2005.
33. ACOG/ACMG: Cystic fibrosis testing—What happens if both my partner and I are carriers? Washington, DC, American College of Obstetricians and Gynecologists, 2001.

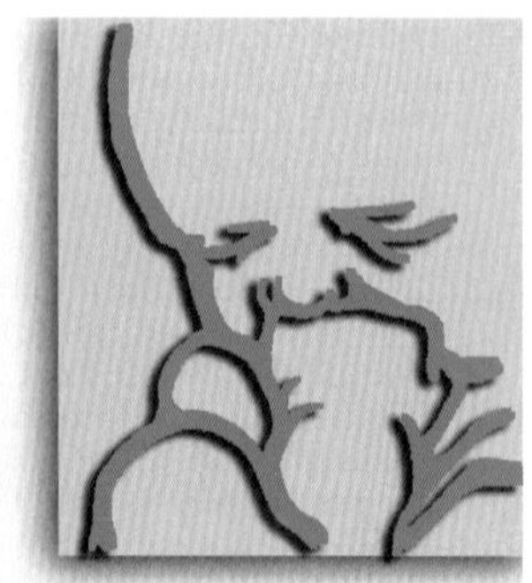

Prenatal Genetic Diagnosis

JOE LEIGH SIMPSON AND LUCAS OTAÑO

CHAPTER 7

KEY ABBREVIATIONS

Acetylcholinesterase	AchE
Allele-specific oligonucleotides	ASO
Alpha-fetoprotein	AFP
American College of Obstetricians and Gynecologists	ACOG
Beta-human chorionic gonadotropin	β-hCG
Blood ultrasound nuchal translucency	BUN
Canadian Early and Mid-Trimester Amniocentesis Trial	CEMAT
Comparative genomic hybridization	CGH
Confidence interval	CI
Confined placental mosaicism	CPM
Chorionic villus sampling	CVS
Chromosomal microarray	CMA
Deoxyribonucleic acid	DNA
Early amniocentesis	EA
First and Second Trimester Evaluation of Risk	FASTER
Fluorescence in situ hybridization	FISH
Human chorionic gonadotropin	hCG
Human leukocyte antigen	HLA
Inhibin A	INHA
Interauterine growth restriction	IUGR
Intracytoplasmic sperm injection	ICSI
Limb reduction deformity	LRD
Maternal serum alpha-fetoprotein	MSAFP
Multiples of the median	MoM
Nasal bone	NB
Neural tube defects	NTDs
Nuchal translucency	NT
Odds ratio	OR
Percutaneous umbilical blood sampling	PUBS
Polymerase chain reaction	PCR
Pregnancy-associated placental protein	PAPP-A
Preimplantation genetic diagnosis	PGD

Restriction fragment length polymorphism	RFLP
Single nucleotide polymorphism	SNP
Talipes equinovarus	TE
Transabdominal chorionic villus sampling	TA-CVS
Transcervical chorionic villus sampling	TC-CVS
Unconjugated estriol	uE_3
Uniparental disomy	UPD
U.S. National Institute of Child Health and Human Development	NICHD
World Health Organization	WHO

Prenatal genetic diagnosis is an important process used to identify some of the 2 to 3 percent liveborn infants who have a congenital abnormality, and has become an integral part of the clinical practice of maternal-fetal medicine. In Chapter 6, we considered etiology (chromosomal, single gene, polygenic/multifactoral) and genetic screening. Detection of many affected fetuses is achievable during pregnancy, usually through analysis of fetal tissue.

In this chapter, we thus identify indications for prenatal testing, for both chromosomal as well as mendelian disorders. We also review those procedures (amniocentesis, chorionic villus sampling) in which fetal cells are obtained, considering both method and safety. Noninvasive screening for aneuploidy and neural tube defects (NTDs) is also discussed. Finally, several new approaches are explored: preimplantation genetic diagnosis (PGD) and recovery of cell-free DNA and intact fetal cells from maternal blood.

DIAGNOSTIC PROCEDURES FOR PRENATAL GENETIC DIAGNOSIS

Analysis of fetal tissue necessitates an invasive procedure, most commonly amniocentesis or chorionic villus sampling (CVS). In this section, we consider common techniques and their safety.

As a common feature of any prenatal invasive procedure, the patient should have a genetic counseling session and must be fully informed about procedures. It is essential in clinical practice to obtain formal consent before an invasive procedure. Written or oral information should include nature, accuracy, and possible results; how, when, and by whom it is performed; safety of the procedure; culture failure rates; reporting time; and post-procedure recommendations.

Amniocentesis

Genetic amniocentesis was first performed in the 1950s.[1,2] A decade later, karyotyping in amniocytes was possible. Since then, almost every genetic condition diagnosable through fetal tissue has been made in amniotic fluid. Overall, amniocentesis is probably the most widely used prenatal diagnostic invasive procedure in medicine.

TECHNIQUE

In genetic amniocentesis, amniotic fluid and cells therein are aspirated. The procedure is applicable from 14 or 15 weeks onward. Ultrasound examination is obligatory in order to determine gestational age, placental position, amniotic fluid location, number of fetuses, fetal status and morphology. The injection of a local anesthetic in the site of puncture is optional. A randomized trial showed that local anesthetic did not reduce pain scores reported by women.[3] The Royal College of Obstetricians and Gynecologists recommends that it is crucially important that amniocentesis not be performed until the operator is certain that the fetus and cord are clear of the intended pool of amniotic fluid.[4]

A 21- or 22-gauge spinal needle with stylet is percutaneously inserted, concurrently with ultrasound, avoiding the fetus, the cord, and the placenta, if possible. Approximately 20 ml of amniotic fluid is aspirated, and the first 1 or 2 ml is usually discarded in order to avoid maternal cell contamination. Rh-immune globulin should be administered to the Rh-negative, Du-negative, unsensitized patient.

Bloody amniotic fluid is occasionally aspirated; however, the blood is almost always maternal in origin and does not adversely affect amniotic cell growth. Continuous visualization of the needle by ultrasound significantly reduces the incidence of bloody amniotic fluid, dry taps and the need for multiple insertions.[5] By contrast, brown, dark red, or wine-colored amniotic fluid is associated with an increased likelihood of poor pregnancy outcome. Dark color indicates that intra-amniotic bleeding has occurred earlier in pregnancy, hemoglobin breakdown products persisting; pregnancy loss eventually occurs in about one third of such cases. If the abnormally colored fluid is characterized by elevated alpha-fetoprotein (AFP), the outcome is almost always unfavorable (fetal demise or fetal abnormality). Greenish amniotic fluid is the result of meconium staining and is apparently not associated with poor pregnancy outcome.

After amniocentesis, the patient may resume all normal activities. Common sense dictates that strenuous exercise such as jogging or aerobic exercise be deferred for a day or so. Deferring sexual activity for 24 to 48 hours seems prudent. The patient should report persistent uterine cramping, vaginal bleeding, leakage of amniotic fluid, or fever; however, physician intervention is almost never required, unless of course overt abortion occurs.

AMNIOCENTESIS IN TWIN PREGNANCIES

In multiple gestations, amniocentesis can usually be performed on all fetuses. It is important to assess chorionicity, fetal viability and anatomy, and sex phenotype, and to carefully identify each sac should selective termination later be required. For this purpose, it is essential to record the locations of each sac, fetal positions, placental locations, cord insertions, and any ultrasound feature that may help to identify the fetuses after results are available. Different techniques have been used to ensure that the same sac is not sampled twice. A simple and reliable technique requires that following aspiration of amniotic fluid from the first sac, 2 to 3 ml of indigo carmine, diluted 1 : 10 in bacteriostatic water, is injected before the needle is withdrawn. A second amniocentesis is then performed at a site determined after visualizing the membranes separating the two sacs. Aspiration of clear fluid confirms that the second (new) sac was entered. Gestations greater than two can be managed similarly, sequentially injecting dye into successive sacs. Cross-contamination of fetal cells in multiple gestations appears rare, but confusion may sometimes arise in interpreting amniotic fluid acetylcholinesterase (AchE) or AFP results. Some obstetricians aspirate the second sac without dye injection, use a single-puncture technique, or perform simultaneous visualization of the two inserted needles in each sac.[6] Elias and Simpson[7] provide additional guidelines on sampling multiple gestations.

If in the second trimester only one fetus in a multiple gestation is abnormal, parents should be prepared to choose between aborting all fetuses or continuing the pregnancy with one or more normal fetuses and one abnormal fetus. Selective termination in the second trimester is possible, but associated with a high rate of complications (fetal loss and prematurity). Success is much greater in the first trimester,[8] for which reason some authors suggest that CVS in the first trimester should be the procedure of choice in twin pregnancies.[3]

SAFETY

Any procedure that involves entering the pregnant uterus logically carries some risk to the fetus. However, the risk of amniocentesis seems very low in experienced hands, at approximately 1 in 400 procedure-related losses, or less. Maternal risks are low, with symptomatic amnionitis occurring only rarely (0.1 percent). Minor maternal complications such as transient vaginal spotting or minimal amniotic fluid leakage occur in 1 percent or less of cases, but these complications are almost always self-limited in nature. Other complications include intra-abdominal viscus injury or hemorrhage. The most serious is fulminant sepsis (*Escherichia coli* or *Clostridia*),[9] extraordinarily with maternal mortality.[10]

Worth recalling for historical perspective are the several large collaborative studies from which the safety of traditional amniocentesis was initially estimated. The 1972 to 1975 prospective study of the U.S. National Institute of Child Health and Human Development (NICHD)[11] encompassed 1,040 subjects and 992 matched controls. Of all women who underwent amniocentesis, 3.5 percent experienced fetal loss between the time of the procedure and delivery compared with 3.2 percent of controls; the small difference was not statistically significant and disappeared completely when corrected for maternal age. The once traditionally cited 1 in 200 (0.5 percent) procedure-related risk of loss following amniocentesis emanated from this report. However, there was actually no statistically significant difference between control and amniocentesis groups. In a Canadian collaborative study conducted at about the same time,[12] 1,223 amniocenteses were performed during 1,020 pregnancies in 900 women. The pregnancy loss rate was 3.2 percent, similar to that reported in the U.S. collaborative study. There was no control group. A 1986 Danish randomized, control study included 4,606 women aged 25 to 34 years, not having risk factors for fetal genetic abnormalities[13]; the control group underwent no procedure. Amniocentesis was performed under real-time ultrasound guidance with a 20-gauge needle. The pregnancy loss rate after 16 weeks was 1.7 percent in the amniocentesis study group compared with 0.7 percent in controls ($p < 0.01$); a 2.6-fold relative risk of spontaneous abortion was observed if the placenta was traversed.

In none of these early collaborative studies, nor others of that era, was high-quality ultrasonography as defined by today's standards available, nor was concurrent ultrasonography ever universally applied.[7] In the collaborative U.S. and Canada studies,[11,12] ultrasound was not used at all. By contrast, studies conducted within the past decade universally employ high-quality ultrasound and have shown no statistical difference between outcomes following amniocentesis groups and controls. In British Columbia, children delivered of women who had second-trimester amniocentesis and were identified by a population-based database of congenital anomalies showed disabilities at the same rate as matched controls (i.e., offspring of women who had not undergone amniocentesis).[14] In Thailand, a randomized study found no statistically significant difference between women undergoing and not undergoing amniocentesis between 15 and 24 weeks; in 2,045 matched pairs, the fetal loss rates were 3.18 and 2.79 percent, respectively.[15] A very low procedure-related rate can be deduced from the work of Armstrong et al.[16] who followed outcomes after 28,613 procedures performed by obstetricians throughout the United States, mostly for advanced maternal age. The total loss rate (background plus procedure-related) was only 1 : 362. In the collaborative NICHD Study (First and Second Trimester Evaluation of Risk [FASTER]), procedure-related loss following amniocentesis was calculated to be 1 in 1,600 cases.[17]

Seeds[18] conducted a systematic review of all reported studies and concluded that the procedure-related loss rate was 0.3 percent (95 percent confidence interval [CI], 0.09, 0.56) over a background rate of 1.08 percent. Among controlled studies reviewed by Seeds,[18] the loss rate was 0.6 percent, although 95 percent confidence limits (CLs) still remained below 1 (0.31, 0.09). Losses were not increased additionally in transplacental amniocentesis. Among other potential complications of mid-trimester amniocentesis, are reports of increased risk preterm delivery and third trimester complications.

In 2007, it seems appropriate to counsel that the risk of pregnancy loss secondary to amniocentesis is low, perhaps 1 in 400 or even much less in experienced hands.[19] It is difficult to be more precise because a sample would have to be very large (perhaps 5,000 or 10,000 in each arm) in order to distinguish between a loss rate of 0.5 percent and 0.2 percent.

Increased risks logically should be increased even further when amniocentesis is performed in twins. However, even this is difficult to prove.

Early Amniocentesis

Amniocentesis before about 14 weeks is not necessarily the same procedure as that performed at 16 to 20 weeks. One problem is membrane "tenting," probably the most common reason for failing to obtain amniotic fluid in early amniocentesis (EA). Membrane tenting becomes increasingly problematic the earlier in gestation one attempts amniocentesis, reflecting incomplete fusion of the chorion and amnion. The American College of Obstetricians and Gynecologists (ACOG) states that amniocentesis before 14 weeks' gestation, especially before 13 weeks' gestation,[20] should not be performed for genetic indications. The basis for this strong statement is four large studies all showing untoward results.

The Canadian Early and Mid-Trimester Amniocentesis Trial (CEMAT)[21,22] comparison involved 1,916 women having an amniocentesis before 13 gestational weeks versus 1,775 having amniocentesis after 15 gestational weeks. Total fetal loss rates were 7.5 percent versus 5.9 percent ($p = 0.012$). Even more troubling, talipes equinovarus occurred in 1.3 percent of offspring in the EA group, compared with the expected population incidence of 0.1 percent in the traditional amniocentesis group.

In 1997, Sundberg et al.[23] reported a randomized cohort study encompassing 581 Swedish women undergoing EA at the 11th to 13th week and 579 women undergoing transabdominal CVS (TA-CVS) at the 10th to 12th week. The most striking difference was in talipes equinovarus (TE) in the CVS group, 1.7 percent of cases being affected. TE occurred when the gestational age at the procedure was 80 to 88 days. AF leakage occurred in 4.4 percent of EA cases but in no CVS cases. The prevalence of TE was almost identical to that observed by Nicolaides et al.[24] in his U.K. study comparing CVS versus EA. Despite CVS being performed earlier in gestation and predictably showing more chromosomal abnormalities (1.6 percent versus 0.7 percent), the total fetal loss rate in the study of Nicolaides et al.[24] was the same or higher (5.4 percent) with EA compared with CVS (4.8 percent).

Virtually identical conclusions were reached by the collaborative study funded by the NICHD, which included 14 centers in the United States, Denmark, and Canada.[25] In all participating centers operators performed at least 25 amniocentesis and 25 CVS procedures in the 11- to 14- week interval of gestation before the trial began. Subjects were randomized and stratified by gestational week. Initially, gestational weeks 11 to 14 were to be studied, but following the report of Sundberg et al.,[23] the study was truncated first to 12 to 14 weeks and then to only 13 to 14 weeks. A total of 3,698 cytogenetically normal subjects were randomized. The sum of all unintended post-procedure losses before 20 weeks (spontaneous abortions plus therapeutic abortions due to complications such as amniotic band disruption or amniotic fluid leakage) was higher with EA than with late CVS. Combined complications totaled 16 of 1,878 in the CVS group versus 27 of 1,820 EA group. At 13 weeks, statistical analysis showed $p = 0.54$ for fetal loss; a larger sample significance might well have shown $p < 0.05$. Three cases of TE occurred following CVS compared with 12 following EA (relative risk, 4.13, 95 percent CI, 1.17 to 14.6 percent; $p = 0.017$).

In conclusion, TE is unequivocally associated with EA.[22–25] This procedure should not be performed before at least 14 weeks' gestation. In exceptional circumstances, if EA is indicated, the mother must be fully informed and made aware of the potential complications.[4]

Amniocentesis in Women with Hepatitis B and Hepatitis C, and HIV

Blood-borne viruses constitute a risk factor for maternal-fetal transmission. Available evidence is limited, but the risk of transmission for hepatitis B seems to be very low.[26] Knowledge of the maternal hepatitis B "e" antigen status is valuable in the counseling of risks associated with amniocentesis. There is less information about hepatitis C, but to date there is no evidence that transmission is increased following amniocentesis.[27]

In HIV-positive women it is suggested that all noninvasive tools should be used prior to considering amniocentesis. Most studies suggest that an invasive test may be a risk factor in transmission and recommend avoiding it, particularly in the third trimester where the relative risk is 4.[27,28] Some authors have suggested that procedures early in pregnancy would carry a very low risk provided that antiretroviral therapy is administered, and the maternal viral load is low.[29]

As a general recommendation, the Society of Obstetricians and Gynaecologists of Canada states that for women infected with hepatitis B, hepatitis C, or HIV, the use of noninvasive methods for prenatal risk screening, (e.g., nuchal translucency [NT], maternal serum screening, and anatomic ultrasound), may help reduce that age-related risk to a level below the threshold for genetic amniocentesis.[27] For those who insist on amniocentesis, every effort should be made to avoid traversing the placenta.[27]

Chorionic Villus Sampling

Chorionic villus sampling (CVS) allows diagnosis in the first trimester of pregnancy. Pregnancy termination can occur early in gestation, when it is much safer for the mother. For example, the maternal death rate is 1 per 100,000 early in pregnancy as compared to 7 to 10 per 100,000 in mid-pregnancy.[30] Early diagnosis also makes feasible selective fetal reduction in multiple gestations, a relatively safe procedure in the first trimester but decidedly less so in the second trimester. Early termination further protects patient privacy. Both chorionic villi analysis and amniotic fluid cell analysis offer the same information concerning chromosomal status, enzyme levels, and DNA patterns. The one major difference is that the few assays requiring amniotic fluid, specifically AFP for neural tube defects, necessitate amniocentesis.

Technique

As described for amniocentesis, before CVS, a comprehensive ultrasound evaluation should be performed in order to determine gestational age, uterine anatomy, chorion morphology and position, number of fetuses, fetal status and anatomy and potential aneuploid markers, especially NT. In cases where abnormal ultrasound findings are detected, it is useful to reevaluate the indication and to discuss it with the patient before performing the invasive procedure.

CVS can be performed by transcervical or transabdominal, approaches. *Transcervical* CVS (TC-CVS) is usually performed with a flexible polyethylene catheter that encircles a metal obturator extending just distal to the catheter tip. The outer diameter is usually about 1.5 mm. Introduced transcervically under simultaneous ultrasonographic visualization (Fig. 7-1), the catheter/obturator is directed toward the trophoblastic tissue surrounding the gestational sac. After withdrawal of the obturator, 10 to 25 mg of villi are aspirated by negative pressure into a 20- or 30-ml syringe containing tissue culture media. The optimal time for transcervical sampling is 10 to 12 completed gestational weeks.

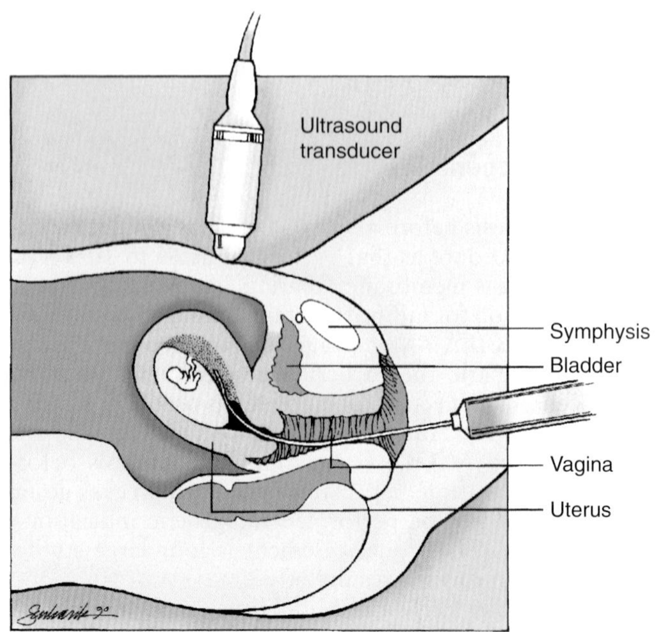

Figure 7-1. Transcervical chorionic villus sampling.

In TA-CVS (Fig. 7-2), concurrent ultrasound is used to direct an 18- or 20-gauge spinal needle into the long axis of the placenta. After removal of the stylet, villi are aspirated into a 20-ml syringe containing tissue culture media, keeping negative pressure and performing a gentle, longitudinal, back and forth movement of the needle. Unlike TC-CVS, TA-CVS can be performed throughout pregnancy. After the first trimester, this procedure is better known as late CVS or placental biopsy. Placental biopsy has now replaced cordocentesis for rapid fetal karyotyping during the second and third trimester in many centers, given that it carries a lower risk, is technically easier, and can yield cytogenetic results within 24 to 48 hours.[31]

In our opinion, the ability to perform both TC-CVS and TA-CVS is very helpful. In many cases, either approach is possible, but in some cases, one or the other approach is greatly preferable. For example, cervical myomas or sharply angulated uteri may preclude transcervical passage of the catheter, whereas TA-CVS would permit sampling. The transabdominal approach is obviously preferable in the presence of genital herpes, cervicitis, or bicornuate uteri. A larger sample can more predictably be obtained with TC-CVS.

With either approach, sampling women sensitized to Rh(D) should probably be deferred until later in gestation. However, Rh-sensitization following CVS is probably no greater than that following amniocentesis.

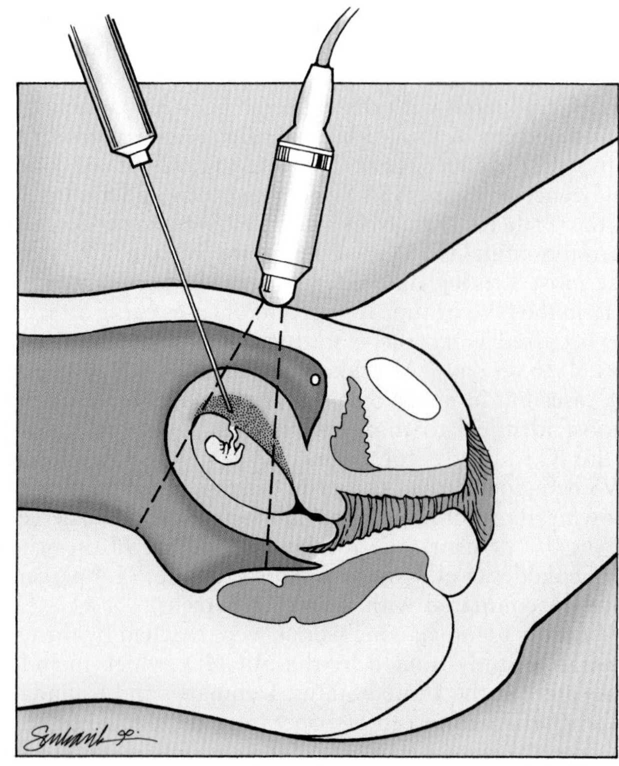

Figure 7-2. Transabdominal chorionic villus sampling.

Safety

Pregnancy Losses

CVS arguably carries no greater risk than amniocentesis, certainly in experienced hands. Both the U.S. Cooperative Clinical Comparison of Chorionic Villus Sampling and Amniocentesis study[32] and the Canadian Collaborative CVS-Amniocentesis Trial Group study[33] reported that pregnancy losses after CVS were no different than loss rates after second-trimester amniocentesis. In the first part of the U.S. study,[32] 2,278 women self-selected TC-CVS; 671 women similarly recruited in the first trimester selected amniocentesis. Excess loss rate in the CVS group was 0.8 percent (80 percent CI, 0.6 to 2.2 percent, not statistically significant). In the near-concurrent Canadian randomized study,[33] 1,391 subjects were assigned to TC-CVS and 1,396 to traditional amniocentesis. The excess loss rate in the former was 0.8 percent, again not statistically different. Variables shown to influence fetal loss rates adversely in CVS include fundal location of the placenta, number of catheter passages, small sample size, and prior bleeding during the current pregnancy. All except the last are presumably surrogates for technical difficulty. Prevalence of intrauterine growth restriction, placental abruption, and premature delivery are also no higher in women undergoing CVS than expected in the general population.[34] A systematic review assessing comparative safety between TA-CVS and TC-CVS, and EA and second-trimester amniocentesis concluded that second-trimester amniocentesis is safer than TC-CVS and EA. Based on that review, TA-CVS would be preferable to EA or TC-CVS.[35]

An important factor in assessing safety is the indication of CVS. If CVS is performed because of an increased NT, a cystic hygroma, or any other anomaly, the risk of miscarriage is increased.[36] Thus, simple comparison to amniocentesis is not always valid.

In U.S. data TC-CVS and TA-CVS appear to be equally safe procedures.[37] In the second phase of the aforementioned U.S. NICHD collaborative study, 1,194 patients were randomized to TC-CVS and 1,929 patients to TA-CVS. Loss rates in cytogenetically normal pregnancies through 28 weeks were 2.5 percent and 2.3 percent, respectively.[38] Of interest, the overall loss rate (i.e., background plus procedure-related) during the randomized trial was 0.8 percent lower than rates observed during the earlier (1985 to 1987) self-selection comparison between TC-CVS and amniocentesis. This decrease in procedure-related loss rate probably reflects increasing operator experience as well as availability of both transcervical and transabdominal approaches. In a randomized trial conducted in Italy, Brambati et al.[39] also found no difference between TA-CVS and TC-CVS. Experience with both approaches seems pivotal.

Differing from most other investigations is the United Kingdom Medical Research Council Study.[40] In this multicenter randomized study, comparison was made between second-trimester amniocentesis and first-trimester CVS, as performed in any fashion deemed suitable by the obstetrician. The outcome assessed was completed pregnancies. The 4.4 percent fewer completed pregnancies in the U.K. CVS cohort reflected both unintended and intended pregnancy terminations. A major pitfall is that operators were considerably less experienced than in the U.S. trials. The only requirement for participation in the U.K. study was 30 "practice" CVS procedures. Greater experience is clearly necessary to become facile with CVS than with amniocentesis. CVS should not be performed by the occasional operator.

Chorionic Villus Sampling in Twin Pregnancies

In experienced hands, CVS is safe in multiple gestations. In a U.S. study from the 1985 to 1989 NICHD trial, the total loss rate of chromosomally normal fetuses (spontaneous abortions, stillborns, neonatal deaths) was 5.0 percent,[41] only slightly higher than the 4.0 percent absolute rate observed in singleton pregnancies.[32] A critical issue in counseling twin pregnancies for prenatal diagnosis is to establish chorionicity. In providing genetic risk figures and considering technical issues, mono- or dichorionic twin pregnancies may imply significant differences. In experienced hands, first trimester ultrasound assessment of chorionicity has almost 100 percent accuracy. All monochorionic twins are monozygotic and, therefore, carry the same genetic constitution, with only a few anecdotal exceptions. Thus, if there are not any significant differences in both fetuses by ultrasound, only one sample need be obtained. For dichorionic twin pregnancies, both chorions must be sampled. With fused chorions, identification of cord insertion and sampling can be helpful. A potential risk of sampling both chorions is the cross-contamination of chorionic tissue, leading to either false-positive or false-negative results.[42] Alternatively, amniocentesis may be the preferred choice. CVS is widely used before selective reduction in multiple gestations. Here, it is especially desirable to sample the inferiorly lying fetus (usually retained in order to minimize risk of ascending infection) as well as at least two or three of their other fetuses potentially slated to be retained.

Limb Reduction Defects

Since the early 1990s, controversy about the safety of CVS has focused less on loss rates than on risk of limb reduction defect. Initially this arose as result of two descriptive reports. In 1991, Firth and colleagues[43] reported that five of 289 (1.7 percent or 17 of 1,000) infants in Oxford, U.K., exposed to CVS between 56 and 66 days of gestation (i.e., 42 to 50 days after fertilization) had severe limb reduction deformities (LRDs). Four of the five infants had oromandibular-limb hypogenesis; the fifth had a terminal transverse limb reduction alone. Reports followed both supporting and refuting such an association.[44–47] In the United States, Burton et al.[48] described a second cluster among 394 infants whose mothers had undergone CVS in Chicago. Thirteen infants (3.3 percent) had major congenital abnormalities, including four with transverse LRD (10 of 1,000 or 1 percent). All four LRDs were transverse distal defects involving hypoplasia or absence of the fingers and toes. Three of these cases followed transcervical sampling, using a device that in the hands of the reporting physicians was associated with an 11 percent fetal loss rate. A publication from Taiwan also reported a number of LRD cases following CVS. Of significance, the procedure was usually performed at less than 9 weeks[49] and apparently by practitioners with relatively little experience.

Frequently cited is the U.S. Centers for Disease Control and Prevention case-control study of Olney et al.[50] Case subjects consisted of 131 infants with nonsyndromic limb deficiency, identified in seven population-based birth defects surveillance programs. Controls consisted of 131 infants with other birth defects, matched to cases by the infant year of birth, mother's age, race, and state of residence. Odds ratio (OR) for all limb deficiencies after CVS during the entire gestational interval 8 to 12 weeks' gestation was only 1.7, not significantly increased given the 95 percent confidence of 0.4 to 6.3. However, the authors then stratified the cases by anatomic subtypes, and now found significant an association for transverse digital deficiency (OR, 6.4; 95 percent CI, 1.1 to 38.6). It was this part of the analysis that led to the frequently stated risk for LRD being 1 in 3,000. Three problems exist with this conclusion: (1) there were only seven exposed cases; (2) procedures were often performed earlier than 10 weeks' gestation, which is the accepted lower limit for gestational age; and (3) the logic is arguable. That is, if there is no association between CVS and *all* types of LRD, yet there is between CVS and *transverse* LRD, is CVS protective against longitudinal limb reduction defects?

Nonetheless, teratogenic mechanisms by which CVS might cause LRDs can be hypothesized. These include (1) decreased blood flow caused by fetomaternal hemorrhage or pressor substances released by disturbing villi or chorion; (2) embolization of chorionic villus material or maternal clots into the fetal circulation; and (3) amniotic puncture and limb entrapment in exocoelomic gel.

In contrast to clusters[43,48] and the conclusion of Olney et al.[50] the consensus of other studies is that LRD is *not* a major concern in experienced hands, at 10 to 13 weeks of gestation.[51,52] The World Health Organization (WHO) Committee on Chorionic Villus Sampling analyzed data collected through its international voluntary registry.[53–55] In its 1998 report,[54] 77 LRD cases were detected among 138,996 infants born after CVS, reported from 63 registering centers. The types of limb reduction defects were compared with those in a population from British Columbia.[56] Defects associated with CVS involved the upper limb in 65 percent, the lower limb in 13 percent, and both in 23 percent; in the general population, frequencies were 68, 23, and 9 percent, respectively. Transverse limb defects occurred in 41 percent of infants in the cohort exposed to CVS, compared with 43 percent in the general population. Longitudinal limb reduction defects were found in 59 percent of cases, compared with 57 percent in the general population. Thus, the pattern analysis of the types of limb defects and calculation of overall incidences failed to reveal a difference between the CVS and background populations. The 1999 WHO[54] report continued to confirm these results. In European registries that in aggregate encompassed over 600,000 births, only 4 of 336 cases (1.2 percent) with limb reduction abnormalities were exposed to CVS compared with 78 of 11,883 (0.66 percent) matched cases having other malformations (OR, 1.8; 95 percent CI, 0.7 to 5.0).[57]

Recently, it has been suggested that the absence of the tip of the third finger would be a distinctive teratogenic effect of CVS. This lesion is similar to as those observed in amniotic bands. Thus, at least of some of the limb reduction defects associated with CVS could result from disruption of the amniotic membrane due to incorrect sampling.[58]

A possible association between late first-trimester CVS (13 to 14 weeks) and a higher risk of hypertension/preeclampsia has been observed. It is hypothesized that focal placental disruption could be the involved mechanism, supporting the theory that disturbances of early placentation lead to maternal hypertension.[59]

In summary, patients may be told that fetal loss rates are comparable in CVS and traditional amniocentesis.[60] This applies in experienced hands. Useful advice in counseling can be derived from the Cochrane Reviews,[35] which concluded that fetal loss following CVS was one third higher than that following traditional amniocentesis. Given that the currently touted loss rates following amniocentesis are 1 in 400[19] to 500 to 1 in 1,600,[17] it is not logical to counsel CVS loss rates as high as some state. In 2001, ACOG[20] stated that when the CVS procedure is performed after 9 menstrual weeks, the risk for limb reduction problems is low and not higher then the general population risk. We follow these guidelines but explicitly state that the rate of limb reduction defects *could* be as high as 1 in 3,000 (3 per 10,000), compared with the background of 6 per 10,000.

Fetal Blood Sampling

Access to the fetal circulation is needed for many diagnostic procedures, including genetic studies. This was initially accomplished by fetoscopy, which allowed direct visualization of the fetus, umbilical cord, and chorionic surface of the placenta using endoscopic instruments.[61] Fetoscopy has now been replaced by ultrasound-directed percutaneous umbilical blood sampling (PUBS), also termed cordocentesis or funipuncture.[62]

Fetal blood sampling is a well-established procedure for rapid karyotyping. It has been used most frequently for fetuses with abnormal ultrasound findings identified during the second and third trimester.[63–66] However, as previously described, placental biopsy, with lower risk, easier technique, and similar or even faster results has replaced fetal blood sampling for rapid karyotyping in many centers. In the same way, the improvements in cytogenetic and molecular diagnosis have decreased the need for fetal blood based diagnosis. For instance, in regions with a high prevalence of hemoglobinopathies, fetal blood sampling was frequently used for this diagnosis. In 1998, Antsaklis and colleagues[67] reported that, of 1981 procedures, 1,437 cordocenteses were done for the detection of hemoglobinopathies. Now, most of those diagnoses are made molecularly during the first trimester by using chorionic villi. Currently, fetal blood chromosome analysis is used most commonly to help clarify chromosome mosaicism detected in cultured amniotic fluid cells or chorionic villi. Fetal blood sampling is also used in the prenatal evaluation of many fetal hematologic abnormalities. The fetal hematocrit can be measured to assess anemia resulting from Rh or other blood antigen isoimmunization states. Fetal blood has been used for the diagnosis of blood factor abnormalities (gene products) like hemophilia A, hemophilia B, or von Willebrand disease. Recovery of fetal blood is important in the assessment of viral, bacterial, or parasitic infections of the fetus. Serum studies of fetal blood permit quantification of antibody titers, and serum can be used to initiate viral, bacterial, or parasitic cultures. However, the ability to apply molecular techniques to more accessible tissues (e.g., amniotic fluid) allows an easier and safer diagnosis. PUBS is also a valuable diagnostic approach in cases of nonimmune hydrops fetalis, because the same procedure yielding fetal blood gives the opportunity to assess different hematologic, genetic, and infectious factors.

Technique

Cordocentesis is usually performed from 18 weeks onward, although successful procedures have been reported as early as 12 weeks.[68,69] Ultrasonographic examination before the procedure is necessary to assess fetal viability, placental and umbilical cord location, fetal position, and presence or absence of fetal or placental anomalies. The use of color flow Doppler imaging is an important tool in evaluating the cord and placenta. Maternal sedation is not usually required, but oral benzodiazepine before the procedure may be of benefit. Although there is no good evidence, many centers use prophylactic antibiotics.

Under continuous ultrasound guidance, a 21- or 22-gauge spinal needle with stylet is percutaneously inserted and directed into the umbilical vein. The needle may be inserted using a freehand technique or using a needle-guiding device fixed to the transducer. Virtually all of the experienced maternal-fetal medicine specialists use the freehand technique.[70] The umbilical vein is preferred over the artery because the former is larger and less likely to be associated with fetal bradycardia and significant hemorrhage when punctured. Of various potential sampling sites, the fixed position of the placental cord root makes this optimal. Free loops of cord or the intrahepatic vein are alternatives.[71] Cardiocentesis has also been described for fetal blood sampling, but obviously it carries a higher fetal loss risk, about 6 percent.[72]

Once the needle is positioned in the umbilical vein, the stylet is removed, and a small amount of blood is aspirated into a heparin-coated syringe. It is crucial to confirm that the sample is fetal in origin; thus, a small amount is used for a complete blood count. Assessment of mean corpuscular volume is the most widely used parameter. Fetal blood cells (140 fl) are larger than maternal cells (80 fl). The mean corpuscular volume of a sample of fetal blood should be higher than 100. A useful alternative when a complete blood analysis cannot be performed at once is the "Apt test" or hemoglobin alkaline denaturation test, especially before 28 weeks of gestation. Based on the ability of fetal hemoglobin to resist denaturation in alkaline conditions, the "Apt test" is a rapid, inexpensive, and simple bedside alternative.[73–75]

Fetal movements can interfere with the procedure and sometimes can dislodge the needle with the risk of complications (bleeding, cord hematoma) and the necessity of further cord punctures.[76] Usually, this is not an issue in procedures for diagnostic purposes. However, in some situations, it may be helpful to perform a fetal neuromuscular blockade as is done in therapeutic cordocentesis. An intravascular injection as part of the cordocentesis or intramuscular administration of pancuronium bromide (0.1 to 0.3 mg/kg of estimated fetal weight) can achieve fetal paralysis.[77]

In at least 1 percent of pregnancies, a single umbilical artery is recognized. Although there would be a higher risk to puncture the only artery (usually it has a larger diameter than normal umbilical cord arteries), the fetal loss risk seems to be no different from that with normal three vessels cords.[76,78] Nevertheless, the use of Doppler color flow mapping to guide the procedure and an experienced operator are recommended.

Safety

Loss rates for patients undergoing PUBS vary greatly by indication and by experience, more so than in amniocentesis or CVS. Thus, no single risk figure is applicable. No randomized clinical trial has been reported, unlike CVS and amniocentesis. The ACOG[20] suggests "less than 2 percent" as the procedure-related loss risk, citing Ghidini et al.[79] Data from several large perinatal centers similarly estimate the risk of in utero death or spontaneous abortion to be 3 percent or less following PUBS.[80–82] Collaborative data from 14 North American centers sampling 1,600 patients at varying gestational ages for a variety of indications found an uncorrected fetal loss rate of 1.6 percent.[83] More recently, Tongsong et al.[83] compared a cohort of 1,281 cordocenteses between 16 and 24 weeks of gestational age with a control group matched one to one by maternal and gestational age, and found that the incremental fetal loss rate associated with cordocentesis at mid-gestation was about 1.4 percent. In selected fetal diagnosis and treatment units in the United States and Japan, the procedure-related fetal loss rate in 1,260 cases was 0.9 percent; excluding diagnoses other than chromosomal abnormalities and severe growth restriction, the procedure-related fetal loss rate was only 0.2 percent. These widely varying complication rates indicate the importance of taking into account the indication (preexisting fetal status) and operator experience.

Other complications associated with cordocentesis include cord hematomas, bleeding from the puncture site in the umbilical cord, transient fetal bradycardia, and fetomaternal hemorrhage. Bleeding from the cord puncture is the most common complication and may be seen in 30 to 41 percent of cases.[84,85] Duration of bleeding is significantly longer after arterial than umbilical vein puncture. However, usually the blood loss is not clinically significant in either case. Van Kamp et al.[76] also describe bleeding from the puncture site significantly more often and of longer duration after transamniotic cord puncture than after transplacental puncture. Transient fetal bradycardia occurs in approximately 10 percent of procedures. Both umbilical artery puncture and severe, early-onset growth restriction were associated with increased rates of bradycardia. Finally, the extent of fetomaternal hemorrhage or transfusion depends on the duration of the procedure, bleeding time, puncture site, and use of a transplacental approach.[86]

Maternal complications are rare, but include amnionitis (less than 1 percent) and transplacental hemorrhage.[83,87] In general, these complications do not significantly compromise maternal health status. However, there are several case reports of severe sepsis.[9,88]

Invasive Prenatal Procedures in Women with Viral Infections

Invasive prenatal testing in the first or second trimester can be carried out in women who carry hepatitis B or C. The limitation of the available data should be explained. Testing in women with HIV should be avoided, particularly in the third trimester.[4]

INDICATIONS FOR PRENATAL GENETIC STUDIES

Indications for prenatal genetic studies arise from those clinical situations associated with an increased risk for a diagnosable prenatal genetic condition. Etiology and risk factors for birth defects have been discussed in Chapter 6. In terms of genetic counseling and potential prenatal procedures, it is important to point out that some of these risk factors are present preconceptionally (e.g., maternal age, parental chromosome rearrangements, heterozygous carriers of mendelian disorders, and so on), and others are detected during the pregnancy (e.g., positive screening tests, fetal structural anomalies, intrauterine growth restriction [IUGR]).[89]

CYTOGENETIC DISORDERS

Every chromosomal disorder is potentially detectable in utero. It is not appropriate, however, to perform amniocentesis or CVS in every pregnancy because for many couples, the risk of an invasive procedure outweighs the diagnostic benefits. Certain indications are considered standard. In addition, couples not having one of the indications mentioned in the following list and, hence, not considered at increased risk may prove to be so after noninvasive screening programs (see later). The most common indications for prenatal diagnosis are

- Advanced maternal age
- Parental chromosome rearrangements
- Previous affected child
- Positive aneuploidy screening test (biochemical and/or ultrasound)
- Abnormal ultrasound findings: fetal structural anomalies, IUGR, amniotic fluid volume anomalies
- Ultrasound markers
- Other indications:
  - Anxiety
  - Syndromes with elevated chromosomal breakage or other cytogenetic aberrations
  - Assisted reproduction through intracytoplasmic sperm injection (ICSI)

Table 7-1. Maternal Age and Chromosomal Abnormalities (Live Births)*

MATERNAL AGE	RISK OF DOWN SYNDROME AT BIRTH	RISK OF ANY CHROMOSOME ABNORMALITY AT BIRTH†
20	1:1667	1:526
21	1:1667	1:526
22	1:1429	1:500
23	1:1429	1:500
24	1:1250	1:476
25	1:1250	1:476
26	1:1176	1:476
27	1:1111	1:455
28	1:1053	1:435
29	1:1000	1:417
30	1:952	1:385
31	1:909	1:385
32	1:769	1:323
33	1:602	1:312
34	1:482	1:253
35	1:375	1:202
36	1:289	1:163
37	1:224	1:129
38	1:173	1:103
39	1:136	1:82
40	1:106	1:65
41	1:82	1:51
42	1:63	1:40
43	1:49	1:32
44	1:38	1:25
45	1:30	1:20
46	1:23	1:16
47	1:18	1:12
48	1:14	1:10
49	1:11	1:8

*Because sample size for some intervals is relatively small, confidence limits are sometimes relatively large. Nonetheless, these figures are suitable for genetic counseling.

†47,XXX excluded for ages 20 to 32 (data not available).

Data from Hook EB, Cross PK, Schreinemachers DM: Chromosomal abnormality rates at amniocentesis and in live-born infants. JAMA 249:2034, 1983 and Schreinemachers DM, Cross PK, Hook EB: Rates of trisomies 21, 18, 13 and other chromosome abnormalities in about 20,000 prenatal studies compared with estimated rates in live births. Hum Genet 61:318, 1982.

ADVANCED MATERNAL AGE

Women most commonly pursue antenatal cytogenetic studies because of advanced maternal age. They may either directly undergo a procedure or do so after noninvasive screening through maternal serum analytes or ultrasound.[90] The overall incidence of trisomy 21 is 1 per 800 liveborn births in the United States. A commonly used table showing age specific risks is Table 7-1.[91] Other calculations exist; Morris et al.[92] showed that the *rate* of increase declines around age 45. Trisomy 13, trisomy 18, 47,XXX, and 47,XXY also increase with advanced age.

In January 2007, ACOG published new recommendations concerning prenatal cytogenetic screening.[92a] Prior to this, it was standard medical practice in the United States to offer invasive chromosomal diagnosis to all women who at their expected delivery date will be 35 years or older and have singleton pregnancies. The choice of age 35 was, however, largely arbitrary, chosen at a time when risk figures were available only in 5-year intervals (i.e., 30 to 34 years, 35 to 39 years, 40 to 44 years) (see Simpson).[93] In twin gestations, it has been recommended for a decade that an invasive procedure be offered at age 32 or 33.[94,95] The rationale was that given most twins being dizygotic, the likelihood that either one of the two will be aneuploid is the sum of the individual risks. At age 33, this combined risk becomes 1 in 347, comparable to the singleton risk at age 35 (1 in 375) (see Table 7-1). The same reasoning applies to all chromosomal aneuploidies: 1 in 176 versus 1 in 202.

Risk figures shown in Table 7-1 are applicable only for liveborn infants. The prevalence of chromosomal abnormalities when amniocentesis is performed is higher by approximately 30 percent.[96] There is a further increase (50 percent) in prevalence at CVS, compared with amniocentesis.[96,97] For example, the risk for a 35-year-old woman is 1 in 270 for Down syndrome at the time of amniocentesis (second trimester) but 1 in 375 at birth. The frequency of aneuploidy in the first trimester is 5 percent higher than in the second trimester. The frequency of chromosomal abnormalities is lower in liveborn infants than in first- or second-trimester fetuses, reflecting the disproportionate likelihood that fetuses lost spontaneously will have chromosomal abnormalities. That is, some abnormal fetuses would have died spontaneously in utero had iatrogenic intervention not occurred in the second trimester. In fact, 5 percent of stillborn infants show chromosomal abnormalities[98] (see Chapter 24).

The 2007 ACOG[92a] guidelines now state that neither age 35 years nor any specific age be used as a threshold for invasive or noninvasive screening. It is stated: "All women, regardless of age, should have the option of invasive testing." ACOG[92a] specifically elaborates that "patients informed of the risks, especially those at increased risk of having an aneuploid fetus, may elect to have diagnostic testing without first having screening." Relatively younger women who elect an invasive procedure directly may do so because of the ability to detect not only trisomies but microdeletions and microduplication syndromes. This is possible through chromosomal microarrays (see below), for which reason a reasonable case can be made for universal invasive testing in women who would exercise reproductive options.

Conversely, first or second trimester noninvasive screening is now considered by ACOG[92a] as appropriate to offer all women who present before 20 weeks of gestation, irrespective of age. For this purpose, a cafeteria of options is available and can be adapted to reflect facilities available. These will be discussed individually later in this chapter. If a noninvasive screening program is applied to a population in which women over maternal age 34 were previously offered an invasive procedure, potential litigious hazard exists if counseling is not lucid. Detection rates for Down syndrome are 80–93% with noninvasive screening, but this is less than the 100 percent previously expected on a direct invasive test. Noninvasive screening in older women is likely to be especially desirable for those who had difficulty especially in achieving a pregnancy. Noninvasive screening is most likely to be applicable for women ages 35 to 37, for after that age the vast majority of women will prove "screen positive" (have abnormal test results) and still require a procedure.

Previous Child with Chromosomal Abnormality

After the occurrence of one child, stillborn, or abortus with autosomal trisomy, the likelihood that subsequent progeny will have autosomal trisomy is increased, even if parental chromosomal complements are normal. Recurrence risks are perhaps 1 percent.[99] Antenatal chromosomal studies should thus be offered for couples having a prior trisomic pregnancy. Recurrence risk data following trisomy 18 are comparable.[99] Describing a risk of 1 percent for either the same or for a differing chromosomal abnormality seems appropriate.

Parental Chromosomal Rearrangements

An uncommon but important indication for prenatal cytogenetic studies is presence of a parental chromosomal abnormality. A balanced translocation is the most common indication, but inversions and other chromosomal rearrangements exist. A mother or father having a balanced translocation is at risk for offspring with an unbalanced translocation and, hence, an abnormal offspring. Given a parental rearrangement (see Chapter 6), empiric data invariably reveal that theoretical risks for abnormal (unbalanced) offspring are greater than empirical risks. The risk of having a liveborn infant with an unbalanced chromosomal complement varies with the particular rearrangement, the sex of the carrier, and the method of ascertainment.[100] Empirical risks at CVS or amniocentesis approximate 12 percent for offspring of either male or female heterozygotes having reciprocal translocations.[101] For robertsonian (centric fusion) translocations, risks vary according to the chromosomes involved. For t(14q;21q), risks are 10 percent for offspring of heterozygous mothers and 2 percent for offspring of heterozygous fathers (Fig. 7-3).[101] For other nonhomologous robertsonian translocations, empirical risks for liveborn infants are less than 1 percent. Later in this chapter, we discuss the different percentages observed at PGD.

For homologous translocations (e.g., 21q;21q), all liveborn offspring should have trisomy 21. For other homologous robertsonian translocations (13q;13q or 22q;22q), almost all pregnancies result in abortions.

Additionally, another genetic issue in a robertsonian translocation is related to the risk of uniparental disomy (UPD).[102] In UPD both homologous chromosomes are derived from a single parent. Several cases of UPD have been observed in carriers (either the parent or the fetus) of balanced robertsonian translocations.[102] Specific evaluation for UPD should be performed in prenatal cases in which a chromosome with known UPD clinical effect is involved (e.g. chromosome 15).[103]

Positive Aneuploidy Screening Test (Biochemical or Ultrasound)

First- and second-trimester noninvasive screening for aneuploidies are discussed later, and it has become one of the most frequent indications for prenatal genetic diagnosis. In fact, this approach may soon become the universal screening procedure with a fetal karyotype used only to evaluate positive screening results.[104] The converse opinion is that invasive procedures (CVS, amniocentesis) in experienced hands are so safe that universal invasive tests constitute a reasonable option.[17,19]

Abnormal Ultrasound Findings

A genetic assessment is recommended whenever a major structural anomaly is detected on ultrasound. There is a high incidence of chromosomal abnormalities, especially in the presence of multiple anomalies or certain anomalies (e.g., cystic hygroma, omphalocele, duodenal atresia, cardiac anomalies) or in association with IUGR and

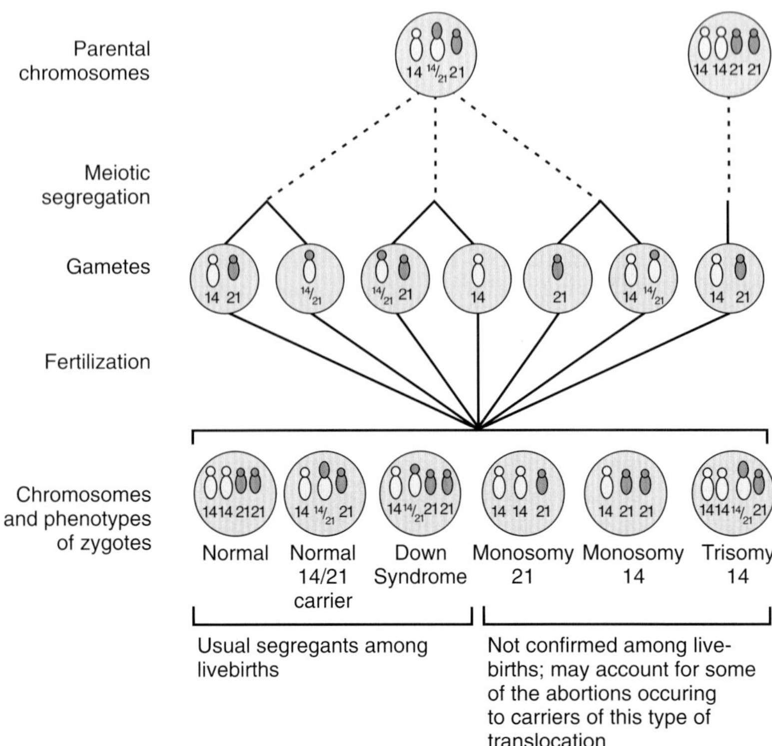

Figure 7-3. Possible gametes and progeny of a phenotypically normal individual heterozygous for a robertsonian translocation between chromosomes 14 and 21 (a form of D/G translocation). Three of the six possible gametes are incompatible with life. The likelihood that an individual with such a translocation would have a child with Down syndrome is theoretically 33 percent. However, the empirical risk is considerably less. (From Gerbie AB, Simpson JL: Antenatal detection of genetic disorders. Postgrad Med 59:129, 1976.).

abnormalities in amniotic fluid volume (oligohydramnios or polyhydramnios).[63,105,106] In cases with cardiac anomalies, especially of the conotruncal type, it is also useful to test for the 22q11 microdeletion by fluorescence in situ by hybridization (FISH).[107,108] More information on ultrasound detection of anomalies is provided in Chapter 9.

Ultrasound Markers

Besides NT, which is an integral part of screening tests to be discussed later, several ultrasound signs, mostly variations of normal fetal anatomy and also known as "minor anomalies" or "soft markers," have been described in association with aneuploidies.[109,110] These markers, like renal pyelectasis, a shortened femur, intracardiac hyperechogenic foci, a choroid plexus cyst, and hyperchogenic bowel, among many others, are not infrequent findings in the second-trimester scan. After identification of a marker, a detailed scan including echocardiography should be offered. With an isolated finding in a young woman, further evaluation is usually not necessary. However, when one of these signs is found in an older woman (>34 years), or is associated with other positive ultrasound or biochemical markers, and of course with another anomaly, an invasive genetic diagnostic study is indicated.

Other Indications

Anxiety

This term has been used in different series when no obvious medical indication or risk factor was present. For instance, a 30-year-old pregnant woman who decides to undergo a prenatal genetic work-up after comprehensive genetic counseling would be classified as having "anxiety" by different authors. However, it is highly questionable to qualify a patient's decision as a result of an unproven psychological condition. It seems more appropriate to refer to this as the "patient's decision." The 2007 ACOG guidelines[92a] actually render this discussion moot.

Syndromes with Elevated Chromosomal Breakage or other Cytogenetic Aberrations

The following genetic mendelian disorders show specific cytogenetic features with the appropriate laboratory technique:

- Fanconi anemia[111]
- Bloom syndrome
- Ataxia-telangiectasia
- Xeroderma pigmentosum
- Robert syndrome

Currently, most of these conditions have a known molecular basis and can be prenatally diagnosed with molecular techniques. However, in Robert syndrome, cytogenetic assessment still plays a role.[112]

Assisted Reproduction Through Intracytoplasmic Sperm Injection

ICSI is an assisted reproductive technology that has allowed men who are subfertile due to different etiologies to reproduce. Empirical data have showed an increased frequency of aneuploidies, mainly sex chromosome anomalies (1 to 2 percent).[113] It seems that this excess risk for aneuploidies is not related to the technique (ICSI) itself, but to the etiology of the male infertility.

COMMON DIAGNOSTIC DILEMMAS IN PRENATAL CYTOGENETIC DIAGNOSIS

The obstetrician-gynecologist should be aware of the common pitfalls associated with the analysis of chorionic villi or amniotic fluid cells. He or she may be called upon to interpret or explain these findings to patients. An obvious problem is that cells may not grow, or growth may be insufficient for proper analysis. Analysis of maternal rather than fetal cells is another problem, which is fortunately uncommon. In amniocentesis, maternal cell contamination can be minimized by discarding the first few drops of aspirated amniotic fluid. In CVS, examination under a dissecting microscope allows one to distinguish villi from maternal decidua.

A more vexing concern is that chromosomal abnormalities detected in villi or amniotic fluid may not reflect fetal status. Chromosomal aberrations may arise in culture (in vitro), or they may may be confined to placental tissue. This possibility should be suspected when mosaicism, more than one cell line, is restricted to only one of the several culture flasks or clones initiated from a single amniotic fluid or CVS specimen, or when an abnormal karyotype with a known severely anomalous phenotype does not correlate with a normal ultrasound.

Numeric

Cells containing at least one additional structurally normal chromosome are detected in 1 to 2 percent of amniotic fluid or CVS specimens.[114] If these abnormal cells are found in a single culture or clone, the phenomenon is termed *pseudomosaicism,* and no clinical significance is attached. Defined by the presence of the same abnormality in more than one clone or culture flask, true fetal mosaicism is rarer but more significant. True mosaicism is confirmed by studies of the abortus or liveborn in 70 to 80 percent of cases[115] and cannot be truly excluded in the remainder because the abnormality could be restricted to a tissue not readily accessible.

Numeric problems are more frequent in short-term cultures, which can be performed on chorionic villi but not on amniotic fluid cells. Metaphases from the trophoblasts or villi can accumulate within hours of sampling, allowing rapid answers. In CVS, discrepancies may also arise between short-term trophoblast cultures and long-term cultures, which are initiated from the mesenchymal core of villi.[116] In turn, discrepancies may further exist between CVS preparations (short-term or long-term) and the embryo, or between amniotic fluid cells and embryo. It is usually possible to recognize these differences, by confirmatory amniocentesis and assessment of the predicted interval growth. The fetus usually proves to be normal at amniocentesis and shows normal interim growth between 10 and 16 weeks. Sometimes mosaicism appears to be present in the placenta but not in the embryo, which is termed confined placental mosaicism (CPM). The likelihood of anomalies is considered low when low-grade mosaicism has been reported.[117]

Although most CPM does not have clinical significance,[118] there are two potential adverse effects associated with CPM that should be considered: UPD and IUGR. UPD, the inheritance of both homologous chromosomes from a single parent, may result from a reduction to disomy from a trisomic embryo, embryo rescue.[119] The phenotypic effect of UPD depends on which chromosome is involved.[103] There is evidence for imprinted genes with phenotypic effects in UPD for chromosome 7 (Russell-Silver syndrome), chromosome 11 (Beckwith-Wiedemann syndrome), chromosome 14 (mental retardation and multiple anomalies) and chromosome 15 (Prader-Willi and Angelman syndromes).

Potential technical problems notwithstanding, both amniotic fluid analysis and chorionic villi analysis are highly accurate. The U.S. NICHD Collaborative Study evaluated 11,473 chorionic villus samples by direct methods, long-term culture, or both. There were no incorrect sex predictions.[116] No diagnostic errors occurred among 148 common autosomal trisomies (+13, +18, +21), 16 sex chromosomal aneuploidies, and 13 structural aberrations; no normal cytogenetic diagnosis with CVS has ever been followed by birth of a trisomic infant. Not confirmed were several rare trisomies (+16, +22, +7), findings consistent with those in other investigations.[120] Overall, accuracy of CVS is comparable to that of amniocentesis; however, additional tests may be necessary before definitive establishment of nonmosaic rare trisomies and, as in amniotic fluid analysis, polyploidies. The U.S. NICHD study observed increased late loss rates (8.6 percent) in pregnancies showing CPM compared with 3.4 percent in pregnancies without mosaicism.

Structural

If a phenotypically normal parent carries the same balanced translocation as the fetus, reassurance is appropriate in the absence of other information (e.g., structural anomalies on ultrasound.) On the other hand, if an ostensibly balanced inversion or translocation is detected in the fetus but is not found in either parent, the rearrangement arose de novo. In this situation, there is increased likelihood that the neonate will be phenotypically abnormal at birth. Presumably, the inversion or translocation is not actually balanced, appearances to the contrary. The risk for the fetus being abnormal has been tabulated at 6 percent for a de novo reciprocal inversion and 10 to 15 percent for a de novo translocation.[121] Risks are not chromosome specific but represent pooled data involving many chromosomes. These risks also apply only to anatomic or developmental abnormalities evident at birth, not taking into account abnormalities that become evident only later in life.

Marker chromosomes, also called supernumerary chromosomes, are those chromosomes that by definition cannot be fully characterized on the basis of standard cytogenetic analyses. These small chromosomes usually contain a centromere, a high proportion derived from the short arms of acrocentric chromosomes (13, 14, 15, 21, and 22). Marker chromosomes are observed in approximately 0.06 percent of the population.[122]

With FISH (see later), the chromosome from which the marker chromosomes originated can often be established. Analogous to translocations and inversions, the risk for phenotypic abnormality in a fetus with a marker chromosome then depends on whether the marker is de novo or familial. Risk is higher when de novo markers are encountered. Studying 15 cases of marker chromosomes ascertained from 12,699 prenatal samples (11,055 amniotic fluids, 1,644 chorionic villus samples), Brondum-Nielsen and Mikkelson[123] found five familial cases, all derived from acrocentric chromosomes (13, 14, 15, 21, and 22); all resulted in phenotypically normal offspring. The other nine cases represented de novo abnormalities. Seven pregnancies were terminated; three showed significant abnormalities at autopsy. In the remaining two cases, pregnancies resulted in phenotypically normal infants at birth; however, in one of the two, minimal psychomotor retardation was evident at age 2 years.

In reviewing 15,522 prenatal diagnostic procedures, Hume et al.[124] ascertained 19 marker chromosomes, five from CVS specimens and 14 from amniotic fluid samples. Monitoring these pregnancies with high-resolution ultrasonography revealed an association between de novo marker chromosomes and anomalies. When ultrasound examination was normal, the likelihood of a phenotypically normal offspring was high.

Ultrasound assessment is an important adjunct tool to cytogenetics in the prenatal genetic counseling of apparently balanced structural "de novo" chromosome anomalies and chromosome markers. NT in the first trimester might be of help in establishing the balanced or unbalanced nature of a "de novo" structural rearrangement.[125]

Newer Cytogenetic Approaches

Fluorescence In Situ Hybridization in Prenatal Diagnosis

FISH merges molecular genetics with cytogenetics. Using DNA sequences unique to the chromosome in question, chromosome-specific probes (e.g., chromosomes 13, 18, 21, the X, or the Y) can be created. The probe is then labeled with a fluorochrome and used to challenge unknown DNA. Disomic cells (metaphase or interphase) should show two separate signals; trisomic cells should show three signals. Because of geometric vicissitudes, not every trisomic cell shows three signals; however, the modal count readily indicates the diagnosis, permitting simultaneous assessment of multiple chromosomes. FISH can be used in interphase cells, thus permitting rapid or same day diagnosis of aneuploidy. This becomes particularly important when a rapid diagnosis is needed to aid in the management of a fetus at risk such as one with ultrasound findings of multiple anomalies.

Quantitative Fluorescent Polymerase Chain Reaction

Quantitative fluorescent polyermase chain reaction (PCR) also allows the rapid and accurate detection of major numeric chromosomal disorders in CVS.[126] This technique can be a powerful adjunct to conventional cytogenetics.

Comparative Genomic Hybridization

Comparative genomic hybridization (CGH) is a molecular cytogenetic technique that allows comprehensive analysis of the entire genome at a finer resolution than banded kayrotypes. The principle is based on single-stranded DNA hybridizing with complementary single standard DNA, whether from the same individual or from different individuals. In CGH as initially devised, normal control DNA in the form of a metaphase was labeled with, for example, a green fluoreschome. Test DNA (e.g., patient) was labeled with a fluorochome different in color (e.g., red). When the denatured, (single-stranded) patient DNA was hybridized to the control metaphase, one would expect regions to be yellow (red and green) if DNA amounts are comparable in control and patient. If the latter has an excess (e.g., trisomy), the relevant chromosome region would be relatively more red.

CGH permits the rapid detection and mapping of DNA sequence copy number differences between a normal and an abnormal genome.[127] CGH is principally applied to cancer cytogenetics. However, it is also a powerful tool for the detection and identification of unbalanced chromosomal abnormalities in prenatal, postnatal, and preimplantation diagnosis.[128] CGH can increase the resolution of analysis by using the microarray-based techniques described below. This will allow the detection of genomic aberrations of less than 1 Mb (million bases) in size.

Chromosomal Microarrays

Chromosomal array (CMA) technology is based on the principle of CGH. In CMAs, small amounts of single-stranded DNA (cDNA) of known sequence are placed by photolithography onto glass slides in ordered fashion. The amount of DNA in each individual is small (i.e., "micro"). The number of sequences is set in advance but can encompass the entire genome. DNA embedded on the slide is labeled with a fluorochrome of one color (e.g., green). Exposure is made to single-stranded test (e.g., patient) DNA, now labeled with a fluorochrome of different color (e.g., red). If control and test DNA are quantitatively equal, the color is yellow. If test DNA is excess, the color is more red; if test DNA is deficient, the color is more green.

Diagnostic microarrays typically contain hundreds of clones (300 to 800). This provides greater resolution than traditional karyotypes.[129–131] This allows detection not only of trisomies, major deletions, or duplications, but also subtle aberrations beyond the scope of high-resolution banded karyotypes. In blinded comparisons, CMAs have detected all abnormalities evident on metaphases, as well as several not detectable by karyotype.[129,130] CMA analysis is applicable in cultured chorionic villi and amniotocytes, as well as uncultured cells subjected to whole genome amplication to produce a sufficient quantity of DNA for analysis.[131,132] Microarray analysis has also been performed on cell-free fetal DNA in amniotic fluid.[133]

Within a decade, chromosomal microarrays may well replace conventional metaphase analysis. The major current impediment is cost, but this should decrease. The ability to detect perhaps 50 to 75 microdeletions syndromes (e.g., di George syndrome) as well as many mendelian disorders should be very attractive. Pitfalls are generally those encountered in traditional cytogenetics analysis: difficulty in detecting mosaicism when the minority line is less than 10 percent, and necessity to exclude polymorphisms that are inherited from parents. One disadvantage is that CMAs cannot distinguish between balanced translocations and normal; unbalanced (duplication; deficiency) rearrangements are readily detected.

MENDELIAN DISORDERS

Increasing numbers of mendelian disorders are now detectable in utero by using DNA analysis. This approach permits diagnoses using any available nucleated cell (chorionic villi, amniotic fluid cells). The nature of the mutant (or absent) gene product need not necessarily even be known, only its chromosomal location. In fact, we can predict confidently that in the foreseeable future all common mendelian disorders should be detectable. The rapid progress and increasing complexity required to diagnose mendelian traits dictate close liaison between the obstetrician-gynecologist and geneticist.

Disorders Detectable Solely by Tissue Sampling

If a gene causing a given disorder is not expressed in amniotic fluid or chorionic villi, enzymatic analysis of such tissues cannot provide information concerning presence or absence of the disorder. However, the morphologic manifestation of the gene might still be evident in other tissues, such as blood, skin, muscle, or liver. Skin biopsy was once obligatory to diagnose certain genodermatoses, initially through fetoscopically directed biopsy and later by ultrasound-directed sampling using smaller (14-gauge) instruments. Procedure-related losses following skin biopsy or other invasive procedures were, not surprisingly, greater than that following CVS or amniocentesis; however, the severity of certain disorders did justify tissue sampling if no other diagnostic method were available. The procedure-related loss rate was usually stated to be 2 to 3 percent.[134]

Skin biopsy or muscle biopsy is now rarely required. Molecular advances have made tissue sampling largely obsolete. Occasionally, histologic and electron microscopic analyses of fetal skin are necessary to diagnose dermatologic or muscle disorders.

Inborn Errors of Metabolism

For the first decade after the introduction of prenatal genetic diagnosis, inborn errors of metabolism (e.g., galactosemia) were the only single-gene disorders for which prenatal genetic diagnosis was available. Antenatal diagnosis is now possible for approximately 100 inborn errors of metabolism, most of which are transmitted in autosomal recessive fashion. Couples at increased risk are usually identified because they have previously had an affected child. Most metabolic disorders are so rare that it is unreasonable to expect obstetricians who are not geneticists to be fully cognizant of diagnostic possibilities.

Until the last few years, enzymatic tests were used to assess gene products such as proteins. Detection of a metabolic defect is now increasingly made by molecular methods, but diagnosis can still be made on the basis of the enzyme being expressed in amniotic fluid cells or chorionic villi. This requirement is fulfilled by most metabolic disorders, a prominent exception being phenylketonuria. Fortunately, phenylketonurea can be detected by the molecular techniques described later. All metabolic disorders detectable in amniotic fluid have proved detectable as well in chorionic villi. Cultured cells are usually used for diagnosis, but one can also arrive at a diagnosis on the basis of a product in amniotic fluid. The most prominent example is 17α-hydroxyprogesterone, elevated concentrations of which indicates adrenal 21-hydroxylase deficiency (congenital adrenal hyperplasia). The spectrum of metabolic and other single gene disorders detectable in utero is beyond the scope of this chapter but is discussed in genetic texts.[135]

Disorders Detectable by Molecular Methods

Molecular approaches can be used on any available nucleated cell. All cells contain the same DNA, and the gene product or enzyme need not be expressed for diagnosis. The obstetrician-gynecologist should be aware of the analytic techniques that make possible diagnosis by molecular methods. These principles are now routinely applied. The reader can find principles of molecular medicine covered in much greater detail elsewhere, ranging from single chapters in volumes intended for obstetrician-gynecologists with no prior knowledge in the field[7] to definitive volumes designed for the investigator. The purpose here is to define briefly the key principles whose understanding is crucial to molecular diagnosis.

Pivotal for these diagnostic procedures was the discovery of *restriction endonucleases*. These bacterial enzymes recognize specific nucleotide sequences five to seven nucleotides in length and cut DNA only at those sites. Use of restriction enzymes permits DNA to be divided into fragments of reproducible lengths.

Pivotal also was development of the PCR procedure. In PCR, a target sequence can be amplified several fold (10^5 to 10^6). Amplification by PCR uses unique DNA primers that flank and are specific for the DNA region in question; thus, the sequence must be known. The region in question may consist of a portion of a gene containing a mutation, a polymorphic DNA sequence closely linked to a given locus, or a repetitive DNA sequence characteristic of a given chromosomal region. In the PCR process, a heat-stable DNA polymerase extracted from *Thermas aquaticus* (*Taq* polymerase) is placed in a single tube with the DNA in question, excess deoxyribonucleoside triphosphates (adenine, thymine, guanine, cytosine), and unique primers specific for the region being studied. DNA synthesis (amplification) is initiated. Raising the temperature denaturates the newly amplified double-stranded DNA back into single-stranded DNA. Upon cooling, amplification occurs again, but this time with twice as many strands. The DNA sequence between primers thus amplifies in geometric fashion with each replication. PCR can be used not only to amplify DNA, but for diagnosis. If PCR results in no DNA sequence being present there must be a deletion of the gene. One can also perform PCR concurrently for multiple sequences (multiplex PCR), an approach that permits assessment of presence or absence of deletions throughout a given region or different regions (genes).

Synthetic oligonucleotides 15 to 18 in length have been constructed called *allele-specific oligonucleotides* (ASO). An ASO is designed to hybridize to an unknown sample if and only if the latter is characterized by all 15 to 18 nucleotides. ASOs can be designed to recognize normal DNA as well as any known mutant sequence. They may be displayed as "dot-blot" DNA or "slot-blot" analysis.

In Southern blotting (Fig. 7-4), agarose gel electrophoresis is used to separate DNA fragments by size, following exposure to restriction endonucleases. DNA is then denatured and transferred from the agarose gel to a nitrocellulose filter, on which specific fragments can be located by hybridization. Labeled strands of known DNA sequences act as probes, hybridizing a specific complementary sequence from among the many DNA fragments on the filter. Fragments containing the sequence that hybridizes with the probe can be detected as bands. Size standards allow one to determine whether a particular-sized fragment is or is not present. *Southern blotting* involves assessment of DNA. The analogous approach involving messenger ribonucleic acid is Northern blotting. Protein (gene product) analysis is termed Western blotting.

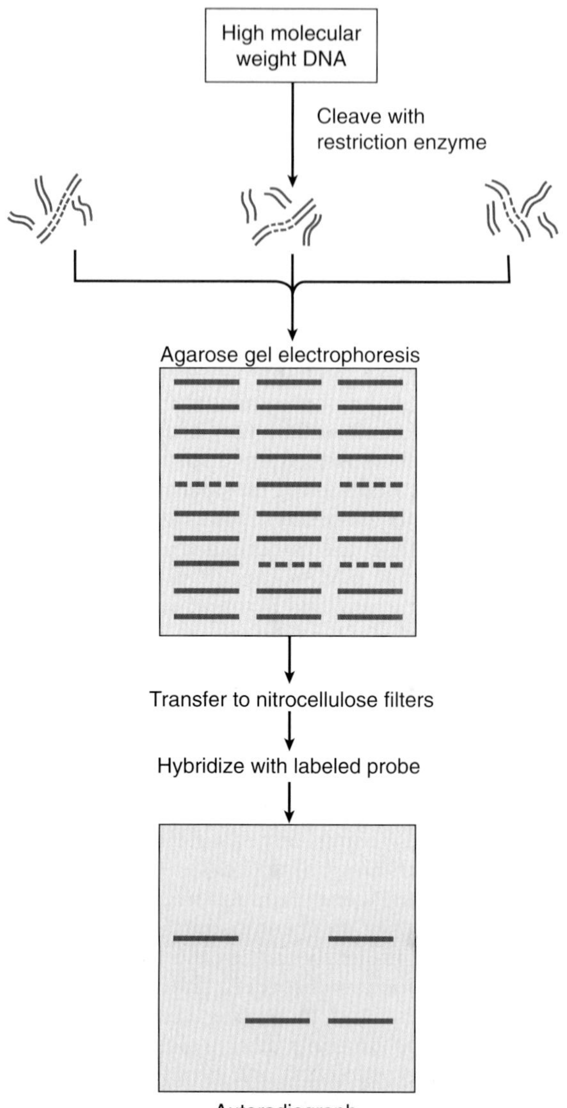

Figure 7-4. Southern blotting cuts DNA at a specific sequence of nucleotides. After DNA is cleaved with restriction enzymes, the cleaved DNA is separated by size using agarose gel electrophoresis. The gel is then laid on a piece of nitrocellulose and buffer allowed to flow through the gel into the nitrocellulose. DNA fragments migrate out of the gel and bind to the filter. A replica of the gel's DNA fragment pattern is thus made on the filter. The filter can then be hybridized to a suitable radioactivity-labeled probe, with DNA fragments hybridizing to the probe identified after autoadiography.

Diagnosis When the Molecular Basis is Known

If a disorder is known to be characterized by absence of DNA, one can determine this by whether a single-stranded, usually labeled, probe does or does not hybridize with the corresponding sequence of denatured DNA from an individual (fetus) of unknown genotype. Failure of hybridization (e.g., using an allele specific oligonucleotide or ASO) indicates that the individual lacks the DNA sequence in question; thus, the disorder is assumed to be present. This approach is used to diagnose α-thalassemia, many cases of Duchenne-Becker muscular dystrophy, β-thalassemia, hemophilia, and other diseases.

In other disorders, DNA is present but the perturbation involves a point mutation. An example is sickle cell anemia, in which the triplet (codon) designating the sixth amino acid has undergone a mutation from adenine to guanine. As a result, codon 6 connotes valine rather than glutamic acid, leading to the abnormal protein (β^S). Several molecular approaches can be exploited to make a diagnosis. For example, restriction enzymes recognize

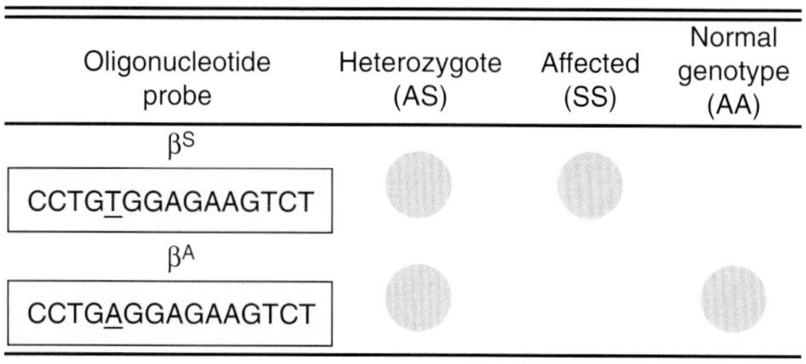

Oligonucleotide probe	Heterozygote (AS)	Affected (SS)	Normal genotype (AA)
β^S			
CCTGTGGAGAAGTCT	●	●	
β^A			
CCTGAGGAGAAGTCT	●		●

Figure 7-5. Dot blot analysis. Oligonucleotides are constructed for sequences complementary to normal DNA (β^A) and mutant DNA (β^S). DNA challenged by the oligonucleotide probe is hybridized if and only if the DNA contains all nucleotides connoted by the probe. Thus, AS individuals will respond to both β^A and β^S probes, whereas AA or SS individuals respond only to one of the two probes (β^A and β^S, respectively). Homozygous individuals respond with a stronger (darker) signal than heterozygous individuals.

the normal but not the mutant DNA sequence at codons 5, 6, and 7. Alternatively, ASOs can be designed to hybridize only if every single nucleotide is present. Once unknown DNA is denatured to become single stranded, a single-stranded β^S oligonucleotide probe will confirm the specific mutant DNA sequence (Fig. 7-5). Numerous diagnostic iterations are now employed, most commonly seeking sequence differences in DNA.

Diagnosis When the Molecular Basis is Not Known

The molecular approaches described earlier are applicable to detecting a disorder only when the precise molecular basis of that disorder is known. This is far from universal. Certain genes are still not cloned or localized. Even if the chromosomal location is known, the exact sequence may not be determined. Furthermore, considerable heterogeneity exists at the molecular level (see cystic fibrosis; Chapter 6). Given that genes are often very large, nucleotide-by-nucleotide assessment may be a daunting task. ASO-like approaches are thus impractical, and sequencing the entire gene for diagnostic purposes may be impractical. Even then, the mutation may not be recognized if it is located in a promoter region or involves translation from messenger ribonucleic acid to gene product.

The necessary diagnostic approach involves linkage analysis. The principle involves taking advantage of the ostensibly innocuous but innumerable differences in DNA that exist among individuals in the general population. These differences are called *polymorphisms,* as illustrated by such well-known polymorphisms as the ABO blood group locus. The initial molecular approach utilized restriction fragment length polymorphisms (RFLPs), differing lengths of DNA fragment lengths arising following exposure to a given restriction endonuclease. More recently, markers have been dinucleotide or trinucleotide polymorphisms. These polymorphisms involve numbers of nucleotide repeats (e.g., the dinucleotides cytosine and adenine at a given locus). Some individuals might have six cysosine and adenine repeats, whereas others might have eight or 10 at a given locus. The almost innumerable number of such polymorphisms forms the scientific basis of DNA analysis for forensic pathology. Widely publicized as well are single nucleotide polymorphisms.

In linkage analysis, diagnosis is made not on the basis of analyzing the mutant gene per se but rather on the basis of the presence or absence of a nearby marker. The marker could be an RFLP variant capable of being recognized following exposure to a given endonuclease, an single nucleotide polymorphism, or a given number of nucleotide repeats.

To illustrate, let us assume that a given RFLP or nucleotide repeat is known to lie close to or preferably within the mutant gene of interest. One next must deduce the relationship between the mutation and the marker. Starting with an individual of known genotype, usually an affected fetus or child, one determines on which parental chromosome a given DNA marker is located, which is the *cis-trans* relationship. Is the marker located on the chromosome carrying the mutant gene, and is it located on the chromosome carrying the normal gene? Figure 7-6 illustrates the use of RFLPs. The principle would be identical using dinucleotide or trinucleotide repeats as the DNA polymorphic marker, or single nucleotide polymorphisms (SNPs).

Pitfalls exist in linkage analysis. First, the marker may or may not be informative in a given family. If all family members show identical DNA fragment patterns at a given locus, that locus is useless because affected and unaffected individuals cannot be distinguished from each other. If a given marker is uninformative, one searches for another informative marker. Fortunately, a nearly limitless number of DNA markers exist. Second, the distance between the mutant gene and the marker is crucial because the likelihood of meiotic recombination is directly related to distance. Recall that during meiosis I recombination can occur between homologous chromosomes. Genes are linked to one another if, after meiosis I, they remain together more often than expected by chance. Recombination can occur even between closely linked loci; thus, prenatal genetic diagnosis based on linkage analysis never achieves 100 percent accuracy. Using polymorphic markers that "flank" (both sides) the mutant can minimize but not exclude the possibility of a recombinational event. Diagnostic reports will reflect these caveats.

Linkage analysis is especially helpful in single-gene (mendelian) disorders showing molecular heterogeneity. These include most forms of Huntington disease; hemophilia A and B; adult-onset polycystic kidney disease; neurofibromatosis, Duchenne-Becker muscular dystrophy, and β-thalassemia.

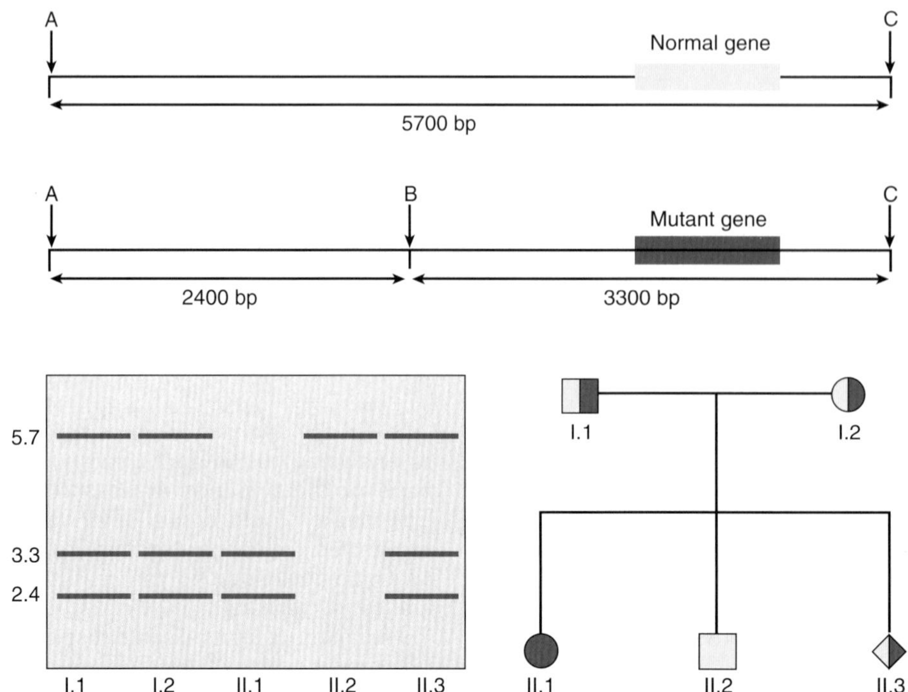

Figure 7-6. Restriction fragment length polymorphisms (RFLPs), which are invaluable for certain prenatal diagnoses. Suppose one mutant gene is linked to another gene (B) that governs whether or not a restriction site *(B)* is present. If the restriction site is present, DNA is cut by a certain restriction enzyme *(arrow)* to produce 3,300- and 2,400-bp–long fragments. If the segment conferring the restriction site is not present, the total fragment is 5,700 bp long. The different lengths can serve as markers to allow genotypes to be deduced. Suppose two obligate heterozygotes I.1 and I.2 have one affected child (II.1). For this autosomal recessive disorder, blue connotes the mutant allele, yellow the normal. Suppose further that a probe for the gene hybridizes to the region *A* to *C*. The probe can thus identify three fragments (2,400, 3,300, and 5,700 bp). If the affected child shows only the 2,400- and 3,300-bp fragments, it can be deduced that the mutant allele is in association (i.e., on the same chromosome) with the gene-conferring restriction site *B* and, thus, is producing both 2,400- and 3,300-bp fragments. In this example this has occurred in both parents. The normal allele must be in association with the allele not conferring restriction *B* and thus is designated by the 5,700-bp fragment. Genotypes can thus be predicted from DNA analysis of chorionic villi and amniotic fluid cells. Fetus II.3 can be assumed to be heterozygous because all three fragments (2,400, 3,300, and 5,700 bp) are present.

NONINVASIVE SCREENING FOLLOWED BY AN INVASIVE PROCEDURE FOR HIGH-RISK PREGNANCIES

Definitive prenatal genetic diagnosis is appropriate for many conditions but not without risk. All procedures (CVS, amniocentesis) incur some risk, even in experienced hands. As a result, many eligible women hesitate to be tested. Yet many would likely do so if they knew their genetic risks were higher. The benefits-risk ratio would then be tilted toward testing, even in younger women. In fact, such an approach is possible. One first uses noninvasive, completely safe, methods. Results then alter a priori risks upward or downward from a given baseline. Women whose newly calculated risk is increased might elect an invasive procedure, whereas those with decreased risk may decide against testing.

NONINVASIVE MATERNAL SERUM ALPHA-FETOPROTEIN SCREENING FOR NEURAL TUBE DEFECTS

Screening for NTDs was the first noninvasive approach.[136] Such screening is still recommended, despite advances in ultrasound. Screening for neural tube defects (NTDs) began because relatively few (5 percent) NTDs occur in families who have had previously affected offspring. Some method other than a positive family history was thus needed to identify couples in the general population at risk for an NTD. Maternal serum alpha-fetoprotein (MSAFP) serves this purpose. Couples with a negative family history who now have elevated MSAFP are at sufficient risk to justify further assessment: targeted ultrasound and an amniotic fluid AFP level.

The initial MSAFP assay should be performed at 15 to 20 weeks' gestation. AFP values are conventionally expressed in multiples of the median (MoM) of non-affected pregnancies, allowing pooling of data obtained from different laboratories, techniques, and commercial kits. Corrections for other significant factors such as gestational age, maternal weight, diabetes, ethnicity and number of fetuses are necessary. MSAFP increases significantly with gestational age. A weight-adjusted MSAFP is needed, because without adjustment, dilutional effects would result in heavier women having a spuriously low value, whereas thinner women would have a spuriously elevated MSAFP. In women with type 1 diabetes mellitus, a population at increased risk for an NTD, the median MSAFP is 15 percent lower than in nondiabetic women.

In women of black ethnicity, who have a lower risk for a fetal NTD, the median MSAFP is higher than in other ethnic groups.

Cutoff Values

Maternal serum values above either 2.0 or 2.5 MoM are usually considered elevated, but exact values are less important than maintaining a consistent policy in the screening program. Values above 2.0 MoM are considered elevated in women with type 1 diabetes, whereas in twin gestations, MSAFP is considered abnormal only at 4.5 to 5.0 MoM or greater.

Approximately 3 to 5 percent of women have an elevated MSAFP, and these are mostly false-positive results. If gestational age assessment is determined accurately, the number of women having an abnormal serum value is lower. If MSAFP is elevated, a repeat sample may or may not be necessary according to the established protocol, usually based on the accessibility to ultrasound evaluation. In our opinion, there is value in repeating the MSAFP if the value lies between 2.50 and 2.99 MoM and if gestational age is 18 weeks or less.

MSAFP is greater than 2.5 multiples of the median (MoM) in 80 to 90 percent of pregnancies in which the fetus has an NTD: 90 percent in anencephaly and 80 percent in open spina bifida.[137] With ultrasound, one should be able to achieve very high detection rates for aneuploidy, as evidenced by major fetal anomalies; however, it would be perilous to assume similar success for spina bifida. Amniocentesis should thus still be offered to all patients, irrespective of ultrasound findings or lack thereof. That considerable overlap exists between MSAFP in normal pregnancies and MSAFP in pregnancies characterized by a fetus with an NTD means that protocols for evaluating elevated MSAFP values are necessary. Elevated MSAFP occurs for reasons other than an NTD: (1) underestimation of gestational age, inasmuch as MSAFP increases as gestation progresses; (2) multiple gestation (60 percent of twins and almost all triplets having MSAFP values that would be elevated if judged on the basis of singleton values); (3) fetal demise, presumably caused by fetal blood extravagating into the maternal circulation; (4) Rh isoimmunization, cystic hygroma, and other conditions associated with fetal edema; and (5) anomalies other than NTD, mainly abdominal wall defects such as gastroschisis and omphalocele.

Ultrasound is obviously necessary to exclude erroneous gestational age, multiple gestations, or fetal demise. Amniocentesis for AFP and AchE becomes necessary if no explanation for elevated MSAFP is evident on ultrasound. Presence of AchE indicates an open NTD or other anomalies. Considered independent of ultrasound, approximately 1 in 15 women having an unexplained elevated serum AFP will have a fetus with a NTD. The sensitivity for detection of a NTD in twin gestations is predictably lower than in singleton gestations, being only about 30 percent for spina bifida given a threshold of 4.5 MoM. The lower sensitivity exists because twins are usually discordant for a NTD. Liberal use of ultrasound is recommended in twin gestations.

If aneuploidy screening is performed in the second trimester, a MSAFP value will be available as part of three (triple) or four (quad) analyte screening for aneuploidy. First-trimester MSAFP is not a sensitive method for detecting NTDs. If first trimester aneuploidy screening alone is performed, second-trimester MSAFP screening is still necessary to detect NTDs.

Some physicians advocate performing an ultrasound after an elevated MSAFP, and will not perform an amniocentesis for AchE in the absence of ultrasound evidence for a NTD. Although logical, the sensitivity of NTD detection cannot be assumed to be as high as with MSAFP followed by amniocentesis.

Unexplained Elevated Maternal Serum Alpha-Fetoprotein

Often, no evident cause is detected after a comprehensive assessment of a patient with an elevated MSAFP. This group of patients has been consistently described to be at higher risk of adverse perinatal outcome: spontaneous abortion, preterm birth, small for gestational age, low birth weight, and infant death. On the other hand, extremely low MSAFP values (<0.25 MoM) has also been associated with an increased morbidity: spontaneous abortion, preterm birth, stillbirth, and infant death.[138,139]

Interestingly, in a large prenatal screening database in western Scotland a direct association between MSAFP and the risk of sudden infant death syndrome (SIDS) has been observed.[140]

NONINVASIVE SCREENING FOR ANEUPLOIDY

Noninvasive screening can identify women whose a priori age-related risk is relatively low for a fetus with Down syndrome, yet who nonetheless are actually at much greater risk than other women of the same age. There are three main approaches: (1) second-trimester screening, (2) first-trimester screening, and (3) sequential screening in both the first and second trimester. Screening for Down syndrome and other aneuploidies is more complex than screening for NTDs in that it involves more than one analyte, and because the risk of Down syndrome is age specific.

Second-Trimester Serum Screening for Trisomy 21

The first analyte identified as useful for noninvasive second trimester screening for Down syndrome was AFP.[141] The median MSAFP in the mid-trimester for a woman carrying a Down syndrome fetus is approximately 0.73 multiples of the median (MoM). That is, MSAFP is on average 27 percent lower in women carrying fetuses with Down syndrome. Although measuring MSAFP provides useful information, a simple threshold cutoff above or below which an invasive procedure can be recommended clearly would not suffice because one must take into account the patient's age given a specific

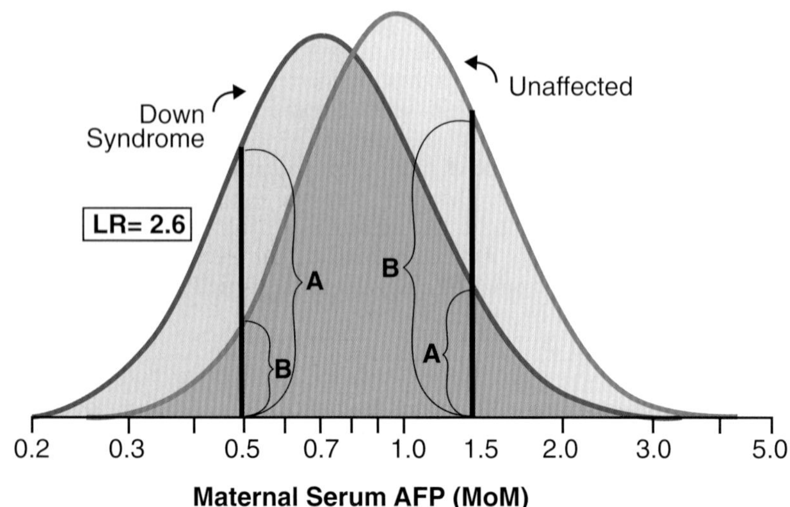

Figure 7-7. Schematic diagram illustrating likelihood ratio, which for Down syndrome at MoM 0.5 is 2.6 (A/B = 2.6) and for MoM 1.5 is 0.4 (A/B = 0.4). (From Simpson JL, Elias S: Prenatal cytogenetic diagnosis and maternal serum analyte screening. *In* Simpson JL, Elias S: Genetics in Obstetrics and Gynecology, 3rd ed. Philadelphia, W.B. Saunders, 2003, p 377.)

MoM. Using a likelihood ratio one can do so.[142] Figure 7-7 shows this approach. Likelihood risks for various informative markers can be taken into account to yield an overall ratio, which is multiplied by the a priori age-related risk. For example, a maternal serum value for AFP of 0.4 MoM carries a likelihood ratio of 3.81 for having a child with Down syndrome. If the a priori (age-specific) risk is 1 in 581 (for a 25-year-old woman), the recalculated risk after taking into account the MSAFP value is 1 in 148. In practice, one calculates likelihood ratios for each analyte tested, using each value to yield the overall likelihood that can be translated into the specific aneuploidy risk for a given patient.

Three other serum analytes progressively increase second-trimester detection rates. The most informative second trimester analyte is human chorionic gonadotropin (hCG). Levels of hCG rise from implantation to 8 weeks' gestation, plateau between 8 and 12 weeks' gestation, decrease from 12 to 18 weeks, and then plateau again until term. Serum hCG levels are increased in women carrying fetuses with Down syndrome.[143] Controversy exists as to whether the free β subunit of hCG is preferable to total hCG in Down syndrome screening, especially in the second trimester.

Unconjugated estriol (uE_3) is synthesized from dehydroepiandrosterone sulfate following conversion to 16 alpha-hydroxydehydroepiandrosteinedione sulfate in the fetal liver and then to uE_3 in the placenta. Levels of uE_3 in maternal serum are lower (25 percent) in pregnancies affected with Down syndrome compared with those in unaffected pregnancies.[144]

Like hCG, inhibin A (INHA) is elevated in Down syndrome pregnancies. This dimeric glycoprotein has an α-subunit and a βA-subunit linked by a disulfide bond. During pregnancy, inhibin is produced by the corpus luteum and then the placenta. Serum inhibin A levels from women carrying fetuses with Down syndrome have a median MoM of about 1.8[145] and do not change significantly with gestational age, unlike most other serum markers. If risk is elevated over background but still is lower than that of a 35-year-old, no action is necessary. When inhibin A is added to the triple screening analytes described, a quadruple test is said to exist.[146,147] At a 5-percent false-positive rate, the combination of serum AFP, hCG, and uE_3 provides approximately 70 percent detection rate for Down syndrome, and with inhibin A approximately 80 percent.[148]

After calculating an overall likelihood ratio, most laboratories report serum screening values as "positive," meaning the risk equals or is greater than the age-specific risk for a fetus with Down syndrome in a 35-year-old woman at 16 weeks' gestation (1 in 270, given a 30 percent loss rate for fetuses with trisomy 21 between 16 weeks at term). For women screening positive, further evaluation (i.e., amniocentesis) is recommended.

In some venues (especially in Europe), serum screening is routinely offered to women of all ages, in lieu of the direct option of an invasive procedure for older women. Through 2006, ACOG bulletins continued to recommend that an invasive procedure be offered to all women aged 35 years or older, without necessity for prior serum screening. The 2007 guideline[92a] states that older women may choose maternal serum screening in lieu of an invasive procedure; they should be told that detection is not 100 percent.

Sensitivity for noninvasive detection of Down syndrome is age dependent. Software is constructed such that the proportion of cases detected at a given age is greater for older women than for younger women; the "false-positive" (procedure) rate also increases with maternal age. Thus, more than 90 percent of cases of Down syndrome will be identified by noninvasive screening in women aged 35 or older, whereas a considerably lower proportion in much younger women. Therefore, women should be given precise answers as to proportion of trisomy 21 cases excluded by screening. In particular, one should not counsel a 25-year-old to expect the same proportion of trisomy 21 fetuses to be detected as in the general population (70 or 80 percent). Although the proportion of cases detected in younger women is lower, the absolute risk remains very low in the screen negative 25 year old.

Detection rates also depend on week (not just trimester) of gestation and on the procedure rate (false-positive rate). If one accepts more procedures (higher false-positive rate), detection rates increases. The converse is also true.

Confounding factors influence serum screening, and adjustments may be necessary. Adjustments for maternal weight and ethnic group are routinely employed. With increased maternal weight, decreased levels of AFP, uE_3, and hCG levels all occur. Type 1 diabetes mellitus is associated with decreased uE_3 and hCG. Maternal smoking increases MSAFP by 3 percent and decreases maternal serum uE_3, and hCG levels by 3 percent and 23 percent, respectively.[149] Maternal serum hCG is higher and MSAFP lower in pregnancies conceived in vitro, compared with pregnancies conceived spontaneously.[150] A recent claim has been made that adjustments should be made for prior aneuploidy; beta-human chorionic gonadotropin (β-hCG) is reported to be 10 percent higher in a pregnancy after aneuploidy, whereas pregnancy-associated placental protein A (PAPP-A) is increased 15 percent in the first trimester.[151]

In summary, using three analytes (AFP, hCG, uE_3), 70 percent of cases of Down syndrome are detected in the entire population. Adding inhibin A increases detection to 80 percent detection. These rates assume a 5 percent false-positive (procedure) rate.

Second-Trimester Screening in Multiple Gestations

Down syndrome occurs 20 percent more often in twin pregnancies than in singleton pregnancies, as expected given the known positive correlation between twinning and maternal age. Unfortunately, Down syndrome screening using multiple serum markers is less sensitive in twin pregnancies than in singleton pregnancies. Using singleton cutoffs, 73 percent of monozygotic twin pregnancies but only 43 percent of dizygotic twin pregnancies with Down syndrome are detected, given a 5-percent false-positive rate.[152] Decreased sensitivity in detecting trisomy 21 in dizygotic twins reflects the blunting effect of the concomitant presence of one normal and one aneuploid fetus. Thus, patients should be informed that the detection rate by serum screening is less than in singleton pregnancies. It may be preferable to perform invasive procedures on both fetuses. The ACOG recommends offering this in twin gestations to women 33 years or older.[94] The noninvasive alternative is first-trimester NT, which will be discussed later.

Second-Trimester Screening for Trisomy 18

Trisomy 18 can be readily detected by maternal serum analyte screening. Decreased levels occur for AFP, uE_3 and hCG. This pattern differs from trisomy 21, in which hCG is elevated. A simple approach is to offer invasive prenatal diagnosis whenever serum screening for each of these three markers falls below certain thresholds (MSAFP 0.6 MoM; hCG 0.55 MoM; uE_3 0.5 MoM).[153] Using these thresholds would detect 60 to 80 percent of trisomy 18 fetuses, with a 0.4 percent amniocentesis rate. Calculating individual risk estimation on the basis of three markers and maternal age, Palomaki and colleagues[154] reported that 60 percent of trisomy 18 pregnancies can be detected with a low false-positive rate of 0.2 percent. The value of individual risk estimates is that one in nine pregnancies identified as being at increased risk for trisomy 18 by serum screening would actually be affected.

First-Trimester Screening for Trisomy 21

Logic dictates that screening in the first trimester is preferable to that in the second trimester.[19] In the first trimester, screening is more private. If necessary, a diagnostic test (CVS) can be performed earlier in pregnancy, and a definitive diagnosis made. This approach avoids the increased risks of late-pregnancy termination should fetal abnormalities exist. The maternal mortality rate with first trimester termination is 1.1 per 100,000, whereas with second-trimester termination, it is 7 to 10 per 100,000.[30]

In the first trimester, PAPP-A and free β-hCG are the most informative biochemical markers for detecting Down syndrome. Down syndrome is associated with low PAPP-A and elevated free β-hCG. Using these two analytes alone can detect perhaps 70 to 75 percent of trisomy 21 cases, equal to second trimester triple screening.[148]

To achieve better first-trimester detection rates, first-trimester PAPP-A, and free β-hCG are usually combined with ultrasound measurement of fetal NT thickening. This reproducible ultrasound measurement was pioneered by Nicolaides, Snijders and colleagues,[155,156] who showed the consistency and usefulness in more than 100,000 pregnancies in London and in surrounding district general hospitals. Trisomy risk was derived by multiplying the background maternal age and gestational age-related risk by a likelihood ratio, reflecting the deviation (in millimeters) of NT measurement from the normal mean for gestation. In an early report involving 96,127 pregnant women of median age 31 years, the calculated risk of 1 in 300 or higher for Down syndrome was observed in 8.3 percent.[156] In 2004, Nicolaides[157] updated information on 200,868 pregnancies from several series. The sample included 871 fetuses with Down syndrome of which 76.8 percent were detected by NT at a false-positive rate of 4.2 percent. Some cases, perhaps 5 percent, may have aborted spontaneously had intervention not occurred, but sensitivity would still have remained well above 70 percent for NT alone. In all of these studies, a critical necessity is the requirement for a robust quality NT assurance program.

In the first U.S. large-scale prospective study, 10,251 women of all ages were screened with PAPP-A and free β-hCG using a dried blood spot method; 5,809 also had a NT measurement.[158] The sample contained 50 cases of Down syndrome and 20 cases with trisomy 18. Using both ultrasound (NT) and serum analytes (PAPP-A, free β-hCG), the detection rate for trisomy 21 was 87.5 percent (7 of 8 cases) in women younger than 35 years of age; in women older than 35 years, the detection rate was 92 percent (23 of 25), albeit with a higher false-positive or invasive procedure rate. For trisomy 18, detection rates were 100 percent in both age groups (n = 4 and n = 9).

Table 7-2. Detection Rates in the NICHD BUN Study of Wapner, Thom, Simpson, et al.[159]*

MATERNAL AGE	DETECTION TRISOMY 21	FALSE-POSITIVE (PROCEDURE) RATE
<35 yr	66.7%	3.7%
≥35 yr	89.8%	15.2%
Total	**85.2%**	**9.4%**
Modeling for U.S		
Population (Mean	78.7%	5%
maternal age 27 yr)	63.9%	1%

*The NICHD first trimester only screening (NT, PAPP-A, free β-hCG) cohort of Wapner, Thom, Simpson, et al.[159]

The sample of 8,515 pregnancies prospectively applied a cut off of 1/270. Detection rate increases with prevalence (increased maternal age), albeit at the cost of more procedures. Because the mean maternal age was 34.5 years, data were than modeled to apply to the U.S. population (whose mean maternal age is 27) at a 5 to 1 percent false-positive rates.

BUN, blood ultrasound nuchal translucency; NICHD, U.S. National Institute of Child Health and Human Development.

Table 7-3. Detection Rates in the NICHD FASTER Trial of Malone, Caneck, Ball, et al.[148]*

TESTS	TRISOMY 21 DETECTION (%)
First Trimester: (free β-hCG, PAPP-A, NT)	
11 wk	87
12 wk	85
13 wk	82
Second Trimester: (15–18 wk)	
AFP, uE$_3$, total hCG ("Triple test")	69
AFP, uE$_3$, total hCG, inhibin A ("Quad test")	81
First plus Second Trimester: (PAPP-A, NT, AFP, uE$_3$, hCG, inhibin A)	
Disclosure of first-trimester results	95
Nondisclosure of first-trimester results	96
Serum screening only	88

*If first trimester ultrasound revealed septated cystic hygromas, intervention was taken (CVS offered). Otherwise results were not disclosed until after second trimester screening. Compiled data were then used to compare detection rates that would have occurred given various approaches, all at 5 percent false-positive (procedure) rates for each.

AFP, alpha-fetoprotein; CVS, chorionic villus sampling; FASTER, First and Second Trimester Evaluation of Risk; hCG, human chorionic gonadotropin; NICHD, U.S. National Institute of Child Health and Human Development; NT, nuchal translucency; PAPP-A, pregnancy-associated placental protein; uE$_3$, unconjugated estriol.

These impressive results validated the application of first-trimester screening for aneuploidy.

In 2003, a NICHD mult-center cohort study—the Blood Ultrasound Nuchal (BUN) Study—reported results in a cohort of 8,514 women screened between 74 and 97 days gestation[159] (Table 7-2). The mean maternal age was 34.5 years. Applying the traditional midtrimester screen positive cutoff of 1:270, 85.2 percent of 61 trisomy 21 pregnancies were identified at a false-positive rate of 9.4 percent. The high false-positive (procedure) rate was predictable, given the higher mean maternal age of the sample. Stratifying by age, the detection rate for trisomy 21 was 66.7 percent for patients younger than age 35 years at a 3.7 percent false-positive rate and 89.8 percent in patients older than age 35 years with a 15.2 percent false-positive rate. The detection rate for trisomy 18 was 90.9 percent. Modeling for the general population (with a lower mean age) and setting a false-positive procedures rate of 5 percent, sensitivity for trisomy 21 would still be 78.7 percent; at a false-positive rate of 1 percent, the sensitivity would be 63.9 percent. These findings were consistent with other studies.

Two other large collaborative studies have also provided results comparable to the NICHD BUN Study,[159] although neither was constructed with the initial intention of providing first-trimester diagnosis. SURUSS (*S*erum *UR*ine and *U*ltrasound *S*creening *S*tudy) was a 25-center European trial[160] in which 47,000 patients were evaluated in both the first and second trimester. Results of first-trimester assays were not disclosed to patients; thus, there could be no intervention. Nonetheless, setting the detection rate at 85 percent and using first trimester PAPP-A, hCG, and NT would have required procedures in 5.6 percent of women screened. To achieve a comparable detection rate in the second-trimester serum screening, the procedure rate or false-positive rate would be 9.9 percent with three second-trimester analytes (AFP, hCG, uE$_3$) or 5.6 percent with four analytes (inhibin-A, AFP, hCG, uE$_3$). Thus, first-trimester screening is preferable.

Nearly the same design was employed by Malone et al.[148] in the NICHD FASTER study which included 38,167 patients in 15 U.S. centers. This study differed from SURUSS in that 134 women having a fetus with a septated cystic hygroma were removed from the cohort, and assumed for analysis to have been detected irrespective of what results for PAPP-A and beta hCG would have been. (Of the 134, 51 percent showed chromosomal abnormalities and 34 percent showed other major abnormalities).[161] Detection rates were 87 percent for Down syndrome at 11 weeks and 85 percent at 12 weeks (Table 7-3). The group[162] later stratified their data and found that NT greater than 4 mm was never associated with a normal noninvasive screen; thus, one should proceed directly to CVS. In fact, only 8 percent of pregnancies with NT greater than 3 mm had a screen negative value.

Nicolaides[157] tabulated that NT, PAPP-A, and hCG detected 87 percent of 215 trisomy fetuses at a false-positive rate of 5 percent. Later results of Avgidou et al.,[163] from the same United Kingdom group, were even better. This group screened 30,564 women with NT, PAPP-A, and hCG, providing results the same day and detecting 93 percent of trisomy 21 cases. These results from the United Kingdom do not even take into account the potential usefulness of nasal bone (NB) assessments, to be discussed below. If NB assessment can be incorporated into first trimester screening, detection rates will increase further. Tricuspid regurgitation has also been proposed as yet another useful marker.

In approximately 5 percent of the screened population, increased NT is associated with a normal karyotype. In these cases, fetal loss rates are increased, and other fetal anomalies are observed.[164] A detailed second-trimester scan and echocardiography are recommended.

First-Trimester Versus Second-Trimester Screening

Using the FASTER protocol,[148] 85 to 87 percent of fetuses with trisomy 21 would have been detected by 11 to 12 weeks if first trimester screening results had been disclosed, given a 5-percent false-positive rate. Screening limited to the second trimester detected fewer cases, 81 percent using four analytes (alpha-fetoprotein, human chorionic gonadotropin, unconjugated estriol, and inhibin A), and 69 percent using the popular "triple screen" (human chorionic gonadotropin, alpha-fetoprotein, and unconjugated estriol). As noted above, various U.K. studies have shown first-trimester detection rates highter than 90 percent. As already noted, results can be even better with NB assessment.

First-trimester screening is thus clearly superior in quantative terms to screening in the second trimester. This is in addition to the obvious advantages to the patient of early detection, such as privacy and safer pregnancy termination. Nicolaides[157] confirmed that pregnant women want results as early as possible. In some locations, first-trimester terminations may be the only readily available reproductive option. The major problem in first-trimester screening is the necessity for a robust quality assurance ultrasound program. In 2006, a NICHD workshop concluded that evidence supports first-trimester screening provided quality control exists for NT and laboratory access, and provided CVS is available.[165]

In 2007 ACOG[92a] stated that first-trimester screening using both nuchal translucency measurement and biochemical markers is "a very effective screening test for Down syndrome" in the general population. ACOG stated that first-trimester screening was superior to triple screening and "comparable to the quadruple screening"; however, sensitivity of first trimester screening (85–87%) was actually better than quadruple screening (81%) in the FASTER trial (see Table 7-3).

First-trimester screening, specifically NT, is the recommended approach in *multiple gestation.* Unlike biochemical markers, NT can be measured separately to assess each fetus individually in twin pregnancies. The distribution of each individual NT measurement in multiple gestations is similar to that in a singleton pregnancy.[166] Thus, in dichorionic or trichorionic pregnancies, it is possible to obtain an independent risk for each fetus. This makes NT the marker of choice for screening in multiple pregnancies.

Sequential First- and Second-Trimester Screening: Nondisclosure (Integrated) and Disclosure (Contingency) Approaches

Sensitivity should theoretically be the highest if the patient is sampled sequentially in both the first trimester as well as in the second trimester. This approach should give the highest possible detection rates, or lowest false-positive rates. This approach has been patented as the "Integrated test," a proprietary designation by Wald and colleages, who in 1999 calculated on the basis of MoMs from existing data sets that the sensitivity should be 93 percent, with a false-positive rate of 5 percent.[167] Alternatively, the detection rate would be 71 percent at a lower (1 percent) rate of amniocentesis.

The algorithm for the sequential screening initially proposed by Wald and colleagues[167] had the major disadvantage of requiring that first-trimester results be withheld (nondisclosure) until second-trimester results were obtained.

In addition to the ethical problems of failing to disclose information in a timely fashion, options for pregnancy termination would be precluded until the second trimester, when maternal risks are 10 times that in the first trimester.[30] If first-trimester information were not withheld, sensitivity was said to be unacceptably decreased. In 2002, Cuckle[168,169] showed that disclosure of first trimester results could be made with little loss in sensitivity. Conversely, detection rates need not be diminished at all if procedure rates were increased only slightly (1 to 2 percent).

Controversy over whether nondisclosure is obligatory in sequential screening was not settled until recently, for neither method had been compared directly until the FASTER trial. As previously mentioned, FASTER was analogous to the previously conducted European SURUSS trial except that septated cystic hygroma cases were removed in the former.

In SURUSS,[160] only the nondisclosure option was available. A total of 25 centers performed *first trimester* NT, PAPP-A, hCG and, without disclosure, *second trimester* inhibin A, free and total hCG, uE_3, and AFP. Detection rates for trisomy 21 were highest with sequential first and second trimester analytes. Conversely, modeling for a Down syndrome detection rate of 85 percent, the false-positive rate (procedure rate) progressively decreased as additional analytes were taken into account. At 85 percent sensitivity, the false-positive rate was 5.6 percent using only first trimester markers (PAPP-A, hCG, NT), 9.9 percent using three second-trimester markers (AFP, hCG, and uE_3 but not inhibin A), and 5.6 percent using four second-trimester serum markers (AFP, hCG, uE_3, and inhibin A). Using both first trimester PAPP-A and the four second-trimester serum analytes (hCG, AFP, uE_3, and inhibin A), the false-positive rate was 2.4 percent. The false-positive rate was 1.3 percent with NT plus first-trimester PAPP-A and hCG, and almost the same (0.9 percent) with NT, first-trimester PAPP-A and four second-trimester serum analytes. In SURUSS, one third of patients failed to return for second-trimester testing, despite being requested to do so. This is a major potential problem with nondisclosure approaches.

Results of the U.S. FASTER trial are shown in Table 7-3.[148] Applying a 5-percent procedure or false-positive rate would have yielded a trisomy 21 detection rate of 96 percent if NT, PAPP-A, and hCG screening had been performed in the first trimester, results not disclosed, and second-trimester screening then performed at 15 weeks for four serum analytes. Another sequential nondisclosure option involves using results only of *serum* values in both the first trimester (PAPP-A) and the second trimester (hCG, MSAFP, uE_3, inhibin-A). With this approach, sensitivity was 88 percent. The "serum integrated test" thus performed slightly better than second-trimester serum testing using four analytes but no better than first-trimester screening (NT, hCG, PAPP-A).

Several studies have addressed the option of disclosing results in the first trimester, followed if normal by testing again in the second trimester as a method of maximizing detection rates. This contengency approach was proposed by Cuckle.[168,169] Platt et al.[171] observed in the BUN NICHD cohort that a sequential program that disclosed first-trimester results for the option of CVS could, if followed by second-trimester testing, detect almost all cases, albeit at a high procedure rate. Among seven first-trimester screen-negative pregnancies that proved to have Down syndrome, six pregnancies showed positive second-trimester screening.

Also realizing the pragmatic difficulty of implementing a nondisclosure model in the United States, Malone et al.[148,170] modeled the NICHD FASTER results into a "comprehensive sequential test." This model assumed that women whose first-trimester screening results (PAPP-A and NT) showed a 1 in 150 risk for Down syndrome would be offered CVS, that is, results disclosed. If risks were lower, quadruple screening using AFP, hCG, uE_3, and INHA would be performed at 15 weeks and results combined with first-trimester NT and PAPP-A. A different cut off (1:300) was then applied in the second trimester to justify a procedure. This method provided a 95-percent detection rate at a 5-percent false-positive rate, only 1 percent less than the nondisclosure approach at the same false-positive rate. Importantly, these results assume patients present at 11 weeks, the optimal time for first trimester screening. If women delay their initial screening until 12 to 13 weeks, sensitivity will drop, as shown in Table 7-3 for first-trimester screening alone.

More recently, Malone et al.[170] compared several different first- plus second-trimester contingent sequential approaches. They concluded that the optimal method was contingency screening, in which patients were divided into three groups: women whose calculated (NT, PAPP-A, hCG) first-trimester risk was greater than 1/30 would undergo CVS; women whose risk was less than 1/1500 would undergo no further testing; all other women would undergo second trimester serum testing. Using this approach, only 21.8 percent of the cohort would need second trimester testing in order to detect 93 percent of trisomy 21 cases at a 4.3 percent false-positive rate; 65 percent would be detected in the first trimester with only 1.5 percent of patients having CVS procedures.

In conclusion, sequential first- plus second-trimester screening predictably increases detection over first-trimester screening alone, but by no more than perhaps 5 percent. Even this difference may shrink if NB assessment can be incorporated (see later). The extent to which one wishes to achieve these small incremental benefits by sequential screening is arguable. If sequential screening is desired, the various sequential calculations of Malone et al.[170] confirm the validity of the contingency (disclosure) screening method developed by Cuckle.[169] There is almost no difference between disclosure and nondisclosure results and, hence, little reason to favor the latter given higher rates of complications for second-trimester pregnancy terminations. Only one option is not recommended by ACOG.[92a] After first trimester screening in which a result is given, ACOG states that "subsequent second trimester screening is not indicated unless it is performed as a component of the Integrated test, stepwise sequential or contingent sequential test."[92a] ACOG finds either nondisclosure (Integrated) or disclosure (contingent sequential) appropriate options.

Incorporating Other Noninvasive Markers

Nasal Bone

In 2001 Cicero et al.[172] reported that ultrasonographic absence of the NB at 10 to 12 weeks correlated with fetal Down syndrome. This measure alone yielded an 82-percent detection rate, with a false-positive rate of 8.3 percent. In a larger cohort of 15,822 pregnancies that included 397 with trisomy 21, Nicolaides et al.[157] reported a detection rate of 69 percent at only a 1.4 percent false-positive rate. Others have confirmed[173,174] the results of Cicero et al.,[172] although less encouraging data were reported by Malone in the FASTER trial.[148,175]

Combining NB and NT, Cicero[172] reported a 92-percent detection rate with a false-positive rate of 3.5 percent in the first trimester.[174] With NT, NB, PAPP-A and hCG, Nicolaides[157] calculated a 97-percent detection rate for trisomy 21 fetuses at a 5-percent false-positive rate, or 91-percent detection at a 0.5-percent false-positive rate. NB assessment clearly has immense promise and, if successfully incorporated, can effectively render sequential screening programs unnecessary, even for those wanting the highest possible noninvasive detection rates. The major difficulty is developing the necessary dexterity for the technique. Even sonologists skilled in NT measurements have experienced difficulties in incorporating NB assessment.

Cell-Free Fetal DNA as an Additional Marker

Cell-Free fetal DNA is present in maternal blood in every pregnancy, beginning early in gestation. Cell-free fetal DNA is especially abundant in maternal plasma. Using nested primer PCR for Y-specific DNA,Y-specific signals were detected in the peripheral blood of pregnant women carrying male fetuses by 33 days' gestation.[176] By 6 weeks' gestation, all pregnancies having a male fetus show Y-specific signals in maternal blood. Presence of Y-DNA could reflect either intact fetal cells or cell-free fetal DNA.

For screening purposes, cell-free fetal DNA is 1.7 times greater in pregnancies with a fetus with Down syndrome than in controls.[177] There is thus considerable potential as a noninvasive aneuploidy marker. Adding DNA to second trimester maternal serum analyte testing (AFP, hCG, uE_3, inhibin A) would increase the detection rate for Down syndrome from 73 to 87 percent, albeit with a slight increase in the false-positive rate (4 to 7 percent).[177]

DEFINITIVE NONINVASIVE PRENATAL DIAGNOSIS

The noninvasive methods discussed earlier are all predicated on the assumption that the results cannot immediately provide a *definitive* answer. An invasive procedure is still necessary to confirm aneuploidy. This need not necessarily be the case. Definitive noninvasive prenatal diagnosis should be achievable.

Cell-Free Fetal DNA

Cell-free fetal DNA analysis readily allows fetal sex to be determined in couples at risk for X-linked recessive traits. If a Y sequence is detected in maternal blood, it can be deduced that its origin must be fetal and, hence, a male fetus. Although alternative confounders potentially exist (e.g., stem cells from a prior male pregnancy, vanishing twin, mosacism), these do not pose practical impediments. Autosomal mutations (mendelian disorders) can also be detected if the father has a DNA sequence that the mother lacks. If the mutant sequence is detected in the mother, it must be of fetal origin. An especially useful application arises when the father is heterozygous (Aa) and the mother homozygous abnormal (aa) for an autosomal recessive trait. The normal allele may or may not be transmitted by thc heterozygous father. If transmitted, its detection in maternal blood should be possible. If blood from the homozygous mother reveals the normal paternal allele (A), the fetus can be deduced to be heterozygous.

The approach is already used widely in Europe to assess fetal rhesus status (D). By analysis of maternal blood, amniocentesis can be avoided. The molecular basis of Rh(D) negativity (dd) is usually a gene deletion, *d* representing lack of the DNA sequence that if present would encode *D*. One can distinguish Rh(D) positive (DD or Dd) from Rh(D) negative (dd) by molecular techniques. If the mother is Rh negative and the father homozygous for Rh(D) (Rh positive), all fetuses must be heterozygous (Dd); every pregnancy would then be at risk for RhD isoimmunization. If the father is heterozygous, however, the likelihood is only 50 percent that the fetus would inherit his RhD gene and, hence, be affected; the other 50 percent of pregnancies would not be at risk for Rh-isoimmunization. If Rh(D) sequences are found in a pregnant Rh-negative woman (dd), their origin must be fetal; thus, the fetus is Dd. This information could be applied early in pregnancy to identify a pregnancy destined to develop isoimmunization. A similar approach can be used at 27 weeks to avoid administering Rh-immunne globulin to an Rh-negative women whose fetus proves to be Rh-negative (despite the father being heterozygous). Interest is increasing in adopting this technology in the United States.[178,179]

Intact Fetal Cells in Maternal Blood

Intact fetal cells circulate in the maternal blood during pregnancy, and their analysis can allow definitive noninvasive prenatal genetic diagnosis. Given the rarity of fetal cells in maternal blood (1 fetal per 10^7 maternal cells), one must enrich the sample for the rare fetal cells. This process first requires targeting a specific fetal cell type: fetal trophoblasts, lymphocytes, granulocytes, or nucleated red blood cells (NRBCs). Analysis for fetal chromosomal complement relies on FISH using chromosome-specific probes.

Analyzing interphase cells by FISH with chromosome-specific probes, Elias, Simpson, and colleagues were the first to detect trisomy 18.[180] This occurred in 1991, followed the next year by noninvasive detection of trisomy 21.[181] Diagnosis was made on the basis of one to three trisomic and, hence, fetal cells recovered from a 20- to 30-ml maternal specimen. One ml of maternal blood is estimated to contain only one intact fetal cell; thus, most fetal cells are lost in processing. Improved sensitivity would be expected with increased fetal cell recovery and especially better cell separation and selection. An NICHD[182] collaborative study had this goal, and assessed the accuracy of intact fetal cell recovery in four centers using different methods. Overall, 74 percent of aneuploidies were detected (32 out of 43) cases. This approach remains highly viable but laborious and hindered by lack of consistent results. With specific antibodies to fetal cells, this detection rate might yield near 100-percent detection.

Fetal Trophoblasts in Cervix

Another attractive approach is isolation and analysis of transcervical trophoblasts in the cervix. Unlike rare fetal cells in maternal blood, fetal cells (trophoblasts) in the cervix are numerous. Thus, fetal cell recovery is more likely to be efficient and amenable to markers that specifically distinguish fetal trophoblasts from surrounding maternal cells.

The early embryo is covered with chorion levae, yet later in gestation, the chorionic surface is smooth. Thus, it has been long assumed that the cervix contains trophoblasts of fetal origin. Shedding is presumed to occur between 7 and 13 weeks' gestation, before fusion of the deciduas basalis and parietalis. Desquamated trophoblasts are believed initially to accumulate behind the cervical mucus at the level of the internal os, later becoming a part of the cervical mucus. In the 1970s, reports suggested that these fetal cells could be recovered for prenatal diagnosis.[183] Later studies reported negative results, leading to skepticism in clinical application. The approach lay fallow for well over a decade, but interest was rekindled following the introduction of CVS.[184–187] Lavage of the endocervical canal or uterus was attempted and said to result in variable detection rates in 40 to 90 percent of specimens examined.[184–193] However, the presumptive fetal cells embedded in mucus did not prove readily amenable for FISH. More recently, novel devices have been developed to recover trophoblasts. Katz-Jaffe et al.[194] used a fine "aspiracath" (Cook, Brisbane, Australia) to aspirate cervical canal mucus from 60 pregnant women between 7 to 10 weeks of gestation, before elective termination of pregnancy. Using immunohistochemistry and DNA allelic profiling of single cells, fetal cells were identified in at least 50 percent of the aspirates. Cioni et al.[195] studied two sampling methods, a cytologic brush and intrauterine lavage, performed serially on 126 pregnant women before pregnancy termination at 7 to 12 weeks' gestation. Recovery was 92.3 percent with uterine lavage and 83.3 percent with endocervical sampling, but biases existed as the former procedure always preceeded the latter. Using transabdominal ultrasound guidance, Ergin et al.[196] reported better recovery from the lower part of the uterus.

The advantages of analysis of trophoblasts is that this permits definitive noninvasive diagnosis. If trophoblasts can indeed be recovered and analyzed, this procedure could easily become the preferred method of definitive noninvasive prenatal diagnosis. A considerable advantage compared with other methods of fetal cell recovery is the relatively large number of fetal cells and, hence, DNA. This higher yield makes feasible the detection of not only trisomies by FISH, but also microarray analysis encompassing microdeletion syndromes and mendelian disorders. A potential problem is sperm contamination.

PREIMPLANTATION GENETIC DIAGNOSIS

In PGD, diagnosis is made before implantation on day 6 by analysis of a single cell blastomere or polar body. PGD can be considered a natural extension of traditional prenatal genetic diagnosis. However, PGD allows novel indications. Foremost is that some couples at risk for an affected offspring will not need to consider pregnancy termination. Without PGD, they have no options for prenatal genetic testing.

Obtaining Cells for Preimplantation Genetic Diagnosis

PGD requires access to gametes (oocytes) or embryos by 6 days after conception or less, the time when implantation occurs. There are three potential approaches: (1) polar body biopsy, (2) blastomere biopsy or aspiration of one to two blastomeres from the six- to eight-cell embryo at 2 to 3 days, and (3) trophectoderm biopsy from the 5- to 6-day blastocyst. The first two are most widely applied. See Verlinsky and Kuliev[197] for technical details.

Blastomere (Six to Eight Cells) Biopsy

Blastomere biopsy involves aspirating one to two of the six to eight cells contained within the zona pellucida, the glycoprotein layer surrounding the oocyte. This can be accomplished by mechanical (razor), laser, or chemical means (pronase, ethylenediaminetetraacetic acid) followed by aspiration with a second pipette. Removal of one or two cells does not affect glucose or pyruvate uptake or delay spontaneous hatching of blastocysts, the traditional indicator of normal embryonic development. By 2004 more than 1,000 and by now perhaps 2,000 babies have been born after PGD, and the rate of anomalies does not seem higher than background.[198] However, much more data are necessary.

Polar Body Biopsy

An alternate approach is analyzing either the first or second polar biopsy, or both.[197,199] Literally, this approach can be preconceptional rather than preimplantation diagnosis. If a woman and her partner were heterozygous for an autosomal recessive disorder, a polar body showing the maternal mutant allele should be complemented by a primary oocyte having the normal allele. The normal oocyte could thus be allowed to fertilize in vitro and be transferred for potential implantation. Conversely, if the polar body were normal, fertilization would not be allowed to proceed because the oocyte would be deduced to contain the mutant allele. Similarly, a polar body containing only one chromosome 21 as determined by FISH using a chromosome-specific probe should be complemented by a primary oocyte that also contains only a single chromosome 21. If the first polar body failed to show a chromosome 21, the oocyte can be presumed to have two 21 chromosomes and would lead to a trisomic zygote.

Polar body biopsy has the theoretical advantage of cell number not being reduced following biopsy. There should also be less likelihood of DNA contamination with sperm. Disadvantages include inability to assess the paternal genotype, precluding application if a father has an autosomal dominant disorder. Inability to obtain information concerning paternal transmission also makes the process less efficient reproductively. If a mutant autosomal recessive allele is deduced to exist in the oocyte (i.e., by its absence in the polar body), that oocyte cannot be fertilized. However, the resulting embryo would actually be affected only if both fertilizing sperm and oocyte contained the same mutant allele.

A major consideration is recombination, the meiotic phenomenon occurring routinely between homologous chromosomes. If crossing over involves the region containing the gene in question, the single chromosome (two chromatids) in the primary oocyte would contain DNA sequences encoding both alleles. That is, the two chromatids of the single chromosome would differ in genotype (heterozygosity). Genotype of the secondary oocyte could thus not be predicted without either biopsy of the second polar body or biopsy of the embryo per se. The "problem" of recombination can actually prove beneficial because presence of two alleles in the first polar body excludes allele dropout (failure of one allele to amplify) at that stage. Thus, one could be confident of the accuracy of a second polar body biopsy showing only one allele.

Diagnostic Accuracy in Preimplantation Genetic Diagnosis

Accuracy is high for both cytogenetic as well as single gene or mendelian disorders. Cytogenetic analysis must rely on FISH, because obtaining a metaphase from only a single cell is not practical. FISH allows detection of not only aneuploidy, but also translocations and other chromosomal rearrangements. Accuracy in blastomeres seems at least as high as in amniotic fluid or chorionic villus cells.

Diagnostic accuracy is also high for mendelian disorders. However, single-cell diagnosis requires specialized technology (nested primer or fluorescent PCR; heteroduplex analysis) that cannot be assumed to exist in a routine genetics or diagnostic laboratory. A major worry is risk of contamination from ambient cells. Failure of amplification (PCR) occurs, but this is less catastrophic than contamination because only the latter would ordinarily lead to a false-negative diagnosis. If in an autosomal recessive disorder the embryo were actually heterozygous and the normal allele failed to amplify, one erroneously would conclude the embryo to be affected; therefore, no transfer would occur. The clinical consequence would be limited to a missed opportunity to achieve a pregnancy. Failing to amplify the abnormal allele would result in transfer of an embryo assumed erroneously to be homozygously normal yet actually heterozygous. In either case, allele-specific PCR failure would not result in a clinically significant error (i.e., false-negative diagnosis).

Choosing Between Preimplantation Genetic Diagnosis and Traditional Prenatal Diagnosis

PGD may be an earlier alternative to traditional prenatal genetic diagnosis for detecting mendelian disorders, aneuploidy, and chromosomal rearrangements. However, PGD is not just an earlier option. That a diagnosis is possible before establishing a clinically recognized pregnancy offers a unique opportunity for couples who wish to avoid a pregnancy termination. PGD also allows embryonic diagnosis without disclosure of parental genotype. Finally, the ability to evaluate multiple embryos makes feasible identification of human leukocyte antigen (HLA)-compatible, unaffected embryos.[200]

Either PGD or traditional prenatal diagnosis could be chosen by couples at increased risk for offspring with an autosomal recessive disorder (25 percent risk). The same holds for those at risk for an unbalanced translocation risk in reciprocal translocation (10 to 15 percent). Some couples might consider these numeric risks dauntingly high and select PGD, whereas others might prefer traditional approaches to prenatal diagnosis.

Preimplantation Genetic Diagnosis is Preferable for Prenatal Diagnosis

PGD is the preferable approach to traditional prenatal genetic diagnosis in other circumstances. PGD seems preferable to CVS or amniocentesis in couples at exceptionally high risk, such as 50 percent, for genetic disorders. Autosomal dominant disorders constitute the obvious paradigm. The risk is equal in a couple in which one partner is homozygous for an autosomal recessive disease and the other is heterozygous for the same condition. In this situation (pseudoautosomal dominant inheritance), 50 percent of offspring will be affected.

If a genetic disorder exists in a husband or wife, the intrafamilial dynamics may favor PGD. Clinical termination of a fetus whose genotype is identical to a partner may be troublesome.

Preimplantation Genetic Diagnosis is Obligatory for Prenatal Diagnosis

In a third set of situations, PGD is the only applicable approach.

Avoiding Clinical Pregnancy Termination

Couples may wish to avoid an abnormal fetus, yet be opposed to pregnancy termination for religious or other reasons. The attraction of PGD for avoiding clinical termination is often underestimated. Despite well-intentioned efforts by providers, considerable disquiet is sometimes unappreciated in couples undergoing pregnancy termination because of a genetically abnormal fetus. Even when there is no religious objection, a couple's ambivalence naturally rises when repeated pregnancy terminations become necessary because consecutive offspring have been affected. In a predominantly European PGD Consortium,[201] 36.2 percent of 1,561 couples stated that their reason for undergoing PGD involved objection to pregnancy termination; another 21.1 percent had a previous termination after traditional prenatal genetic diagnosis.

Nondisclosure of Parental Genotype

PGD is pragmatically essential for prenatal diagnosis if one wishes not to disclose parental genotype. An individual known to be at risk (50 percent) for an autosomal dominant disorder of adult onset may be clinically normal, but unknowingly have the mutant gene and not yet have manifested the disorder. The prototype is

Huntington disease. An at risk adult may wish to avoid transmitting a mutant gene to his/her offspring, but still not learn their own genotype. If a patient's parent has Huntington disease, the risk for any given fetus, a grandchild, is 25 percent. Traditional prenatal genetic diagnosis using CVS or amniocentesis is theoretically applicable, but impractical. Through PGD the at-risk adult can avoid transmitting the potential mutant gene to the offspring and remain unaware of his/her own status. Using PGD, all embryos could be screened. Only those unaffected are transferred, a practical option given that 50 percent should be unaffected per cycle. If the undisclosed parental test reveals the parent to be unaffected, the scenario still must be repeated in subsequent cycles. Otherwise, any at risk patient would readily deduce his or her genotype.

Selecting Human Leukocyte Antigen–Compatible, Unaffected, Embryos

Another unique indication for PGD involves identifying HLA-compatible embryos for transfer. A sibling with a lethal disease may require stem cell transplantation to repopulate his or her bone marrow. The most ready source of stem cells is umbilical cord blood, from the yet to be born younger sibling. Stem cell transplantation with cord blood is highly successful if the cord blood is HLA-compatible; success is far less in absence of HLA-compatibility. Using traditional prenatal diagnosis, it would be possible to identify HLA compatible fetuses through performing amniocentesis or CVS. However, only one of four embryos would be HLA compatible. If the pregnancy were also at risk for an autosomal recessive disorder, even fewer embryos would be acceptable. The likelihood of a genetically normal HLA-compatible embryo would be 3 in 16 (one of four HLA-compatible embryos multiplied by the 3 in 4 likelihood of being unaffected = 3/16).

Transferring only HLA-compatible embryos was first performed by Verlinsky and colleagues.[200] The index couple's older daughter was dying of Fanconi anemia, an autosomal recessive disorder. Bone marrow failure and leukemia necessitated stem cell transplantation to restore hematopoiesis. The couple wanted not only a child devoid of Fanconi anemia, but also concurrently to identify the 25 percent of embryos that were HLA compatible. By 2004, 45 cycles for HLA-typing had been performed[202]; 17.5 percent embryos were genetically suitable for transfer, very near the expected 18.7 percent (3/16). Indications include β-thalassemia, Fanconi anemia, Wiskott-Aldrich syndrome, and leukemia. Aneuploidy can be determined on the same embryos.[203]

Key Points

- All invasive prenatal diagnostic procedures carry risks. Amniocentesis at 15 weeks and later carries a procedure-related risk of perhaps 1 in 400 to 500 or less in experienced hands. Amniocentesis before 13 weeks is not recommended because of an unacceptable risk of clubfoot (talipes equivoques).
- CVS is considered, in experienced hands, equal to amniocentesis in loss rates and diagnostic accuracy. TC-CVS and TA-CVS are equivalent in safety.
- Controversy exists concerning limb reduction defects associated with CVS. Any increased risk appears to exist before 10 weeks' gestation, prior to which the procedure should not generally be performed. The maximum limb reduction risk can be considered to be 1 in 3,000.
- The complication rate associated with fetal blood sampling is uncertain, but the loss rate can be considered 1 to 2 percent. The rate depends greatly on the associated fetal status. No control studies have been conducted.
- Noninvasive screening for trisomies can be offered at any age, providing patient-specific aneuploidy risks (trisomy 21; trisomy 18). If the calculated risk is greater than a given threshold risk (that of a 35-year-old in midgestation), an invasive procedure is offered. Comparing different methods is usually done by assuming a given number of procedures (false-positive rates) (5 percent). Detection rates vary if a different false-positive rate is applied.
- First trimester noninvasive screening uses serum free hCG, PAPP-A, and NT measurements. The detection rate is at least 87 percent at 11 weeks and 85 percent at 12 weeks at a false-positive (procedure) rate of 5 percent. If NB assessments can be incorporated, first trimester detection rates rise to 93 to 97 percent.
- Second-trimester noninvasive screening with three analysts (hCG, AFP, uE_3) has a 70-percent detection rate, whereas screening with four analytes (hCG, AFP uE_3, inhibin A) has an 80-percent detection rate. Thus, second-trimester screening has a lower detection rate than first-trimester screening.
- In sequential screening, one performs both first, followed by second-trimester screening. In contingency screening, one discloses first-trimester results, offering CVS to high-risk women, and performing second-trimester screening only on low-risk women. Alternatively, first-trimester results can be withheld (nondisclosure or integated), with only a single result provided in the second trimester. The two approaches show almost identical detection rates (95 and 96 percent); thus, offering nondisclosure is usually unnecessary. If pursued, nondisclosure screening necessitates rigorous patient follow-up to ensure compliance.

❑ In multiple gestations, each nonidentical twin is at independent risk. Invasive tests should be offered at age 33 years. Noninvasive maternal serum screening is less efficient, with aneuploidy detected in no more than 50 percent for dizygotic twins. It is preferable to use first-trimester NT in twin gestations, and obligatory in higher order gestations.

❑ Many single-gene disorders are detectable by enzymatic analysis, whereas others can be recognized only through molecular methodologies.

❑ Direct molecular analysis is possible whenever the gene sequence is known. Linkage analysis can be applied if the gene has been localized but not yet sequenced, or if the mutation in the family being tested is unknown. Linkage analysis takes advantage of polymorphic DNA markers lying close to the gene in question; accuracy is never 100 percent because recombination can occur between the marker and the mutant gene.

❑ PGD can be performed by removing a single cell (blastomere or polar body) from the embryo. Diagnosis requires special molecular techniques to detect mendelian disorders and single-cell FISH for chromosomal abnormalities (trisomy). Accuracy is 98 to 99 percent, and safety does not seem to be major concern.

❑ PGD is preferable to traditional prenatal diagnosis in certain couples. Indications include avoidance of clinical pregnancy termination, fetal (embryonic) diagnosis without disclosure of parental genotype (e.g., Huntington disease), and desire to select HLA-compatible unaffected embryos. In the latter, cord blood can be used for stem cell transplantation in an older, moribund sibling having a lethal condition.

❑ Fetal cells can be recovered from maternal blood, and fetal trisomies have been detected, with detection rates for autosomal trisomy of approximately 75 percent. However, recovery is laborious and not yet widely applicable. Cell-free DNA in maternal blood also has definitive diagnostic value. Recovery of fetal trophoblasts from the maternal endocervix is a promising method of definitive noninvasive diagnosis.

REFERENCES

1. Serr DM, Sachs L, Danon M: The diagnosis of sex before birth using cells from the amniotic fluid (a preliminary report). Bull Res Counc Isr 5B:137, 1955.
2. Fuchs F, Riis P: Antenatal sex determination. Nature 177:330, 1956.
3. van den Berg C, Braat AP, Van Opstal D, et al: Amniocentesis or chorionic villus sampling in multiple gestations: Experience with 500 cases. Prenat Diagn 19:234, 1999.
4. Royal College of Obstetricians and Gynecologists: Amniocentesis and chorionic villus sampling. London, Royal College of Obstetricians and Gynecologists, 2005. Guideline No. 8.
5. Crandon AJ, Peel KR: Amniocentesis with and without ultrasound guidance. Br J Obstet Gynaecol 86:1, 1979.
6. Bahado-Singh R, Schmitt R, Hobbins JC: New technique for genetic amniocentesis in twins. Obstet Gynecol 79:304, 1992.
7. Elias S, Simpson JL: Amniocentesis and fetal blood sampling. *In* Milunsky A (ed): Genetic Disorders and The Fetus: Diagnosis, Prevention, and Treatment, ed 5. Baltimore, The Johns Hopkins University Press, 2004, p 66.
8. Evans MI, Dommergues M, Timor-Tritsch I, et al: Transabdominal versus transcervical and transvaginal multifetal pregnancy reduction: international collaborative experience of more than one thousand cases. Am J Obstet Gynecol 170:902, 1994.
9. Plachouras N, Sotiriadis A, Dalkalitsis N, et al: Fulminant sepsis after invasive prenatal diagnosis. Obstet Gynecol 104:1244, 2004.
10. Elchalal U, Shachar IB, Peleg D, et al: Maternal mortality following diagnostic 2nd-trimester amniocentesis. Fetal Diagn Ther 19:195, 2004.
11. NICHD National Registry for Amniocentesis Study Group: Midtrimester amniocentesis for prenatal diagnosis. Safety and accuracy. JAMA 236:1471, 1976.
12. Simpson NE, Dallaire L, Miller JR, et al: Prenatal diagnosis of genetic disease in Canada: report of a collaborative study. Can Med Assoc J 115:739, 1976.
13. Tabor A, Philip J, Madsen M, et al: Randomised controlled trial of genetic amniocentesis in 4606 low-risk women. Lancet 1:1287, 1986.
14. Baird PA, Yee IM, Sadovnick AD: Population-based study of long-term outcomes after amniocentesis. Lancet 344:1134, 1994.
15. Tongsong T, Wanapirak C, Sirivatanapa P, et al: Amniocentesis-related fetal loss: a cohort study. Obstet Gynecol 92:64, 1998.
16. Armstrong A, Cohen AW, Bombard AT, et al: Comparison of amniocentesis-related loss rates between obstetrician-gynecologist and perinatologists. Obstet Gynecol 99:65S, 2002.
17. Eddleman K, Malone FD, Sullivan L, et al: Pregnancy loss rates after midtrimester amniocentesis. Obstet Gynecol 108:1067, 2006.
18. Seeds JW: Diagnostic mid trimester amniocentesis: how safe? Am J Obstet Gynecol 191:607, 2004.
19. Simpson JL: Choosing the best prenatal screening protocol. N Engl J Med 353:2068, 2005.
20. ACOG Practice Bulletin: Clinical Management Guidelines for Obstetrician-Gynecologists. Prenatal Diagnosis of Fetal Chromosomal Abnormalities. May 27. ACOG Practice Bulletin, 457, 2001.
21. Johnson JM, Wilson RD, Singer J, et al: Technical factors in EA predict adverse outcome. Results of the Canadian Early (EA) versus Mid-trimester (MA) Amniocentesis Trial. Prenat Diagn 19:732, 1999.
22. CEMAT Group: Randomized trial to assess safety and fetal outcome of early and midtrimester amniocentesis. Lancet 351:242, 1998.
23. Sundberg K, Bang J, Smidt-Jensen S, et al: Randomised study of risk of fetal loss related to early amniocentesis versus chorionic villus sampling. Lancet 350:697, 1997.
24. Nicolaides K, Brizot M, Patel F, et al: Comparison of chorionic villus sampling and amniocentesis for fetal karyotyping at 10–13 weeks' gestation. Lancet 344:435, 1994.
25. Philip J, Silver RK, Wilson RD, et al: Late first-trimester invasive prenatal diagnosis: results of an international randomized trial. Obstet Gynecol 103:1164, 2004.
26. Alexander JM, Ramus R, Jackson G, et al: Risk of hepatitis B transmission after amniocentesis in chronic hepatitis B carriers. Infect Dis Obstet Gynecol 7:283, 1999.
27. Davies G, Wilson RD, Desilets V, et al: Amniocentesis and women with hepatitis B, hepatitis C, or human immunodeficiency virus. J Obstet Gynaecol Can 25:144, 2003.
28. Mandelbrot L, Mayaux MJ, Bongain A, et al: Obstetric factors and mother-to-child transmission of human immunodeficiency virus type 1: the French perinatal cohorts. SEROGEST French Pediatric HIV Infection Study Group. Am J Obstet Gynecol 175:661, 1996.
29. Maiques V, Garcia-Tejedor A, Perales A, et al: HIV detection in amniotic fluid samples. Amniocentesis can be performed in HIV

pregnant women? Eur J Obstet Gynecol Reprod Biol 108:137, 2003.
30. Lawson HW, Frye A, Atrash HK, et al: Abortion mortality, United States, 1972 through 1987. Am J Obstet Gynecol 171:1365, 1994.
31. Carroll SG, Davies T, Kyle PM, et al: Fetal karyotyping by chorionic villus sampling after the first trimester. Br J Obstet Gynaecol 106:1035, 1999.
32. Rhoads GG, Jackson LG, Schlesselman SE, et al: The safety and efficacy of chorionic villus sampling for early prenatal diagnosis of cytogenetic abnormalities. N Engl J Med 320:609, 1989.
33. Canadian Collaborative CVS-Amniocentesis Clinical Trial Group: Multicentre randomized clinical trial of chorionic villus sampling. Lancet 337:1491, 1991.
34. Golbus MS, Simpson JL, Fowler SE, et al: Risk factors associated with transcervical CVS losses. Prenat Diagn 12:373, 1992.
35. Alfirevic Z, Sundberg K, Brigham S: Amniocentesis and chorionic villus sampling for prenatal diagnosis. The Cochrane Database of Systematic Reviews [1], CD003252, 2003.
36. Pajkrt E, Mol BW, Bleker OP, et al: Pregnancy outcome and nuchal translucency measurements in fetuses with a normal karyotype. Prenat Diagn 19:1104, 1999.
37. Jackson L, Wapner R: Chorionic villus sampling. *In* Simpson JL, Elias S (eds): Essentials of Prenatal Diagnosis. New York, Churchill Livingstone, 1993, p 45.
38. Jackson LG, Zachary JM, Fowler SE, et al: A randomized comparison of transcervical and transabdominal chorionic-villus sampling. The U.S. National Institute of Child Health and Human Development Chorionic-Villus Sampling and Amniocentesis Study Group. N Engl J Med 327:594, 1992.
39. Brambati B, Lanzani A, Tului L: Transabdominal and transcervical chorionic villus sampling: efficiency and risk evaluation of 2,411 cases. Am J Med Genet 35:160, 1990.
40. Medical Research Council European Trial of Chorionic Villus Sampling: MRC Working Party on the Evaluation of Chorionic Villus Sampling. Lancet 337:1491, 1991.
41. Pergament E, Schulman JD, Copeland K, et al: The risk and efficacy of chorionic villus sampling in multiple gestations. Prenat Diagn 12:377, 1992.
42. Taylor MJ, Fisk NM: Prenatal diagnosis in multiple pregnancy. Baillieres Best Pract Res Clin Obstet Gynaecol 14:663, 2000.
43. Firth HV, Boyd PA, Chamberlain P, et al: Severe limb abnormalities after chorion villus sampling at 56–66 days' gestation. Lancet 337:762, 1991.
44. Mahoney MJ, USNICHD Collaborators: Limb abnormalities and chorionic villus sampling. Lancet 337:1422, 1991.
45. Jackson LG, Wapner RJ, Brambati B: Limb abnormalities and chorionic villus sampling. Lancet 337:1423, 1991.
46. Mastroiacovo P, Cavalcanti DP: Limb reduction defects and chorion villus sampling. Lancet 337:1091, 1991.
47. Hsieh F-J, Chen D, Tseng L-Heal: Limb-reducation defects and chorionic villus sampling. Lancet 337:1091, 1991.
48. Burton BK, Schulz CJ, Burd LI: Limb anomalies associated with chorionic villus sampling. Obstet Gynecol 79:726, 1992.
49. Hsieh FJ, Shyu MK, Sheu BC, et al: Limb defects after chorionic villus sampling. Obstet Gynecol 85:84, 1995.
50. Olney RS, Khoury MJ, Alo CJ, et al: Increased risk for transverse digital deficiency after chorionic villus sampling: results of the United States Multistate Case-Control Study, 1988–1992. Teratology 51:20, 1995.
51. Simpson JL, Elias S: Techniques for prenatal diagnosis. *In* Simpson JL, Elias S: Genetics in Obstetrics and Gynecology. Philadelphia, W.B. Saunders, 2003, p 345.
52. Brambati B, Tului L: Prenatal genetic diagnosis through chorionic villus sampling. *In* Milunsky A (ed): Genetic Disorders and the Fetus: Diagnosis, Prevention and Treatment, ed 5, Johns Hopkins University Press, 2004, p 179.
53. Kuliev A, Jackson L, Froster U, et al: Chorionic villus sampling safety. Report of World Health Organization/EURO meeting in association with the Seventh International Conference on Early Prenatal Diagnosis of Genetic Diseases, Tel-Aviv, Israel, May 21, 1994. Am J Obstet Gynecol 174:807, 1996.
54. WHO/PAHO Consultation on CVS: Evaluation of chorionic villus sampling safety. Prenat Diagn 19:97, 1999.
55. Froster UG, Jackson L: Limb defects and chorionic villus sampling: results from an international registry, 1992–94. Lancet 347:489, 1996.
56. Froster-Iskenius UG, Baird PA: Limb reduction defects in over one million consecutive livebirths. Teratology 39:127, 1989.
57. Dolk H, Bertrand F, Lechat MF: Chorionic villus sampling and limb abnormalities. The EUROCAT Working Group. Lancet 339:876, 1992.
58. Brambati B, Tului L: Chorionic villus sampling and amniocentesis. Curr Opin Obstet Gynecol 17:197, 2005.
59. Silver RK, Wilson RD, Philip J, et al: Late first-trimester placental disruption and subsequent gestational hypertension/preeclampsia. Obstet Gynecol 105:587, 2005.
60. Shulman LP, Simpson JL, Elias S: Invasive prenatal genetic techniques. *In* Sciarra JJ (ed): Gynecology and Obstetrics, Vol III. Philadelphia, Lippincott, Williams & Wilkins, 2001, p 1.
61. Valenti C: Antenatal detection of hemoglobinopathies. A preliminary report. Am J Obstet Gynecol 115:851, 1973.
62. Daffos F, Capella-Pavlovsky M, Forestier F: A new procedure for fetal blood sampling in utero: preliminary results of fifty-three cases. Am J Obstet Gynecol 146:985, 1983.
63. Nicolaides KH, Snijders RJ, Gosden CM, et al: Ultrasonographically detectable markers of fetal chromosomal abnormalities. Lancet 340:704, 1992.
64. den Hollander NS, Cohen-Overbeek TE, Heydanus R, et al: Cordocentesis for rapid karyotyping in fetuses with congenital anomalies or severe IUGR. Eur J Obstet Gynecol Reprod Biol 53:183, 1994.
65. Donner C, Rypens F, Paquet V, et al: Cordocentesis for rapid karyotype: 421 consecutive cases. Fetal Diagn Ther 10:192, 1995.
66. Costa D, Borrell A, Soler A, et al: Cytogenetic studies in fetal blood. Fetal Diagn Ther 13:169, 1998.
67. Antsaklis A, Daskalakis G, Papantoniou N, et al: Fetal blood sampling–indication-related losses. Prenat Diagn 18:934, 1998.
68. Orlandi F, Damiani G, Jakil C, et al: Clinical results and fetal biochemical data in 140 early second trimester diagnostic cordocenteses. Acta Eur Fertil 18:329, 1987.
69. Orlandi F, Damiani G, Jakil C, et al: The risks of early cordocentesis (12–21 weeks): analysis of 500 procedures. Prenat Diagn 10:425, 1990.
70. Evans MI: Teaching new procedures. Ultrasound Obstet Gynecol 19:436, 2002.
71. Chinnaiya A, Venkat A, Dawn C, et al: Intrahepatic vein fetal blood sampling: current role in prenatal diagnosis. J Obstet Gynaecol Res 24:239, 1998.
72. Antsaklis AI, Papantoniou NE, Mesogitis SA, et al: Cardiocentesis: an alternative method of fetal blood sampling for the prenatal diagnosis of hemoglobinopathies. Obstet Gynecol 79:630, 1992.
73. Moir M, Holbrook RH Jr: Application of the hemoglobin alkaline denaturation test to determine the fetal origin of blood: applicability to funipuncture. Obstet Gynecol 81:793, 1993.
74. Ogur G, Gul D, Ozen S, et al: Application of the 'Apt test' in prenatal diagnosis to evaluate the fetal origin of blood obtained by cordocentesis: results of 30 pregnancies. Prenat Diagn 17:879, 1997.
75. Sepulveda W, Be C, Youlton R, et al: Accuracy of the haemoglobin alkaline denaturation test for detecting maternal blood contamination of fetal blood samples for prenatal karyotyping. Prenat Diagn 19:927, 1999.
76. Van Kamp IL, Klumper FJ, Oepkes D, et al: Complications of intrauterine intravascular transfusion for fetal anemia due to maternal red-cell alloimmunization. Am J Obstet Gynecol 192:171, 2005.
77. Copel JA, Grannum PA, Harrison D, et al: The use of intravenous pancuronium bromide to produce fetal paralysis during intravascular transfusion. Am J Obstet Gynecol 158:170, 1988.
78. Abdel-Fattah SA, Bartha JL, Kyle PM, et al: Safety of fetal blood sampling by cordocentesis in fetuses with single umbilical arteries. Prenat Diagn 24:605, 2004.
79. Ghidini A, Sepulveda W, Lockwood CJ, et al: Complications of fetal blood sampling. Am J Obstet Gynecol 168:1339, 1993.
80. Daffos F: Fetal blood sampling. Annu Rev Med 40:319, 1989.

81. Wilson RD, Farquharson DF, Wittmann BK, et al: Cordocentesis: overall pregnancy loss rate as important as procedure loss rate. Fetal Diagn Ther 9:142, 1994.
82. Weiner CP, Okamura K: Diagnostic fetal blood sampling-technique related losses. Fetal Diagn Ther 11:169, 1996.
83. Tongsong T, Wanapirak C, Kunavikatikul C, et al: Fetal loss rate associated with cordocentesis at midgestation. Am J Obstet Gynecol 184:719, 2001.
84. Daffos F, Capella-Pavlovsky M, Forestier F: Fetal blood sampling during pregnancy with use of a needle guided by ultrasound: a study of 606 consecutive cases. Am J Obstet Gynecol 153:655, 1985.
85. Weiner CP, Wenstrom KD, Sipes SL, et al: Risk factors for cordocentesis and fetal intravascular transfusion. Am J Obstet Gynecol 165:1020, 1991.
86. Sikovanyecz J, Horvath E, Sallay E, et al: Fetomaternal transfusion and pregnancy outcome after cordocentesis. Fetal Diagn Ther 16:83, 2001.
87. Nicolini U, Kochenour NK, Greco P, et al: Consequences of fetomaternal haemorrhage after intrauterine transfusion. BMJ 297:1379, 1988.
88. Li Kim Mui SV, Chitrit Y, Boulanger MC, et al: Sepsis due to *Clostridium perfringens* after pregnancy termination with feticide by cordocentesis: a case report. Fetal Diagn Ther 17:124, 2002.
89. Gadow EC, Otano L, Lippold SE: Congenital malformations. Curr Opin Obstet Gynecol 8:412, 1996.
90. Eucromic. Proceedings of the Eucromic Workshop on Prenatal Diagnosis, Paris, May 23–24, 1996. Eur J Hum Genet 1:1, 1997.
91. Hook EB, Cross PK, Schreinemachers DM: Chromosomal abnormality rates at amniocentesis and in live-born infants. JAMA 249:2034, 1983.
92. Morris JK, Mutton DE, Alberman E: Recurrences of free trisomy 21: analysis of data from the National Down Syndrome Cytogenetic Register. Prenat Diagn 25:1120, 2005.
92a. ACOG: Screening for fetal chromosomal abnormalities. ACOG Practice Bulletin 77 (January 2007). Washington, DC, American College of Obstetricians and Gynecologists. Obstet Gynecol 109:217, 2007.
93. Simpson JL: Maternal serum screening in the United States: Current perspective (1996). *In* Grudzinskas JG, Ward RH (eds): Screening for Down Syndrome in the First Trimester. London, Royal College Ob Gyn, 1997, p 95.
94. ACOG Practice Bulletin: Multiple gestation: Complicated twin, triplet, and high-order multifetal pregnancy. Compendium of Selected Publications. Washington, DC, ACOG, 2005, p 586.
95. Rodis JF, Egan JF, Craffey A, et al: Calculated risk of chromosomal abnormalities in twin gestations. Obstet Gynecol 76:1037, 1990.
96. Hook EB, Cross PK, Jackson L, et al: Maternal age-specific rates of 47,+21 and other cytogenetic abnormalities diagnosed in the first trimester of pregnancy in chorionic villus biopsy specimens: comparison with rates expected from observations at amniocentesis. Am J Hum Genet 42:797, 1988.
97. Hook EB, Cross PK: Maternal age-specific rates of chromosome abnormalities at chorionic villus study: a revision. Am J Hum Genet 45:474, 1989.
98. Kuleshov NP: Chromosome anomalies of infants dying during the perinatal period and premature newborn. Hum Genet 31:151, 1976.
99. Stene J, Stene E, Mikkelsen M: Risk for chromosome abnormality at amniocentesis following a child with a non-inherited chromosome aberration. A European Collaborative Study on Prenatal Diagnoses 1981. Prenat Diagn 4:81, 1984.
100. Boué A, Gallano P: A collaborative study of the segregation of inherited chromosome structural rearrangements in 1356 prenatal diagnoses. Prenat Diagn 4:45, 1984.
101. Daniel A, Hook EB, Wulf G: Risks of unbalanced progeny at amniocentesis to carriers of chromosome rearrangements: data from United States and Canadian laboratories. Am J Med Genet 33:14, 1989.
102. Ledbetter DH, Engel E: Uniparental disomy in humans: development of an imprinting map and its implications for prenatal diagnosis. Hum Mol Genet 4:1757, 1995.
103. Kotzot D: Abnormal phenotypes in uniparental disomy (UPD): fundamental aspects and a critical review with bibliography of UPD other than 15. Am J Med Genet 82:265, 1999.
104. Haddow JE, Palomaki GE, Knight GJ, et al: Reducing the need for amniocentesis in women 35 years of age or older with serum markers for screening. N Engl J Med 330:1114, 1994.
105. Hanna JS, Neu RL, Lockwood DH: Prenatal cytogenetic results from cases referred for 44 different types of abnormal ultrasound findings. Prenat Diagn 16:109, 1996.
106. Ville YG, Nicolaides KH, Campbell S: Prenatal diagnosis of fetal malformations by ultrasound. *In* Milunsky A (ed): Genetic Disorders and the Fetus: Diagnosis, Prevention and Treatment., ed 5, J. Hopkins University Press, 2004, p 836.
107. Manji S, Roberson JR, Wiktor A, et al: Prenatal diagnosis of 22q11.2 deletion when ultrasound examination reveals a heart defect. Genet Med 3:65, 2001.
108. Boudjemline Y, Fermont L, Le Bidois J, et al: Can we predict 22q11 status of fetuses with tetralogy of Fallot? Prenat Diagn 22:231, 2002.
109. Sepulveda W, Lopez-Tenorio J: The value of minor ultrasound markers for fetal aneuploidy. Curr Opin Obstet Gynecol 13:183, 2001.
110. Wellesley D, De Vigan C, Baena N, et al: Contribution of ultrasonographic examination to the prenatal detection of trisomy 21: experience from 19 European registers. Ann Genet 47:373, 2004.
111. Chodirker BN, Davies GAL, Summers AM, et al: Canadian guidelines for prenatal diagnosis. Genetic indications for prenatal diagnosis. J Soc Obstet Gynaecol Can 23:525, 2001.
112. Otano L, Matayoshi T, Gadow EC: Roberts syndrome: first-trimester prenatal diagnosis. Prenat Diagn 16:770, 1996.
113. Simpson JL, Lamb DJ: Genetic effects of intracytoplasmic sperm injection. Semin Reprod Med 19:239, 2001.
114. Simpson JL, Martin AO, Verp MS, et al: Hypermodal cells in amniotic fluid cultures: frequency, interpretation, and clinical significance. Am J Obstet Gynecol 143:250, 1982.
115. Hsu LY: Prenatal diagnosis of chromosome abnormalities through amniocentesis. *In* Milunsky A (ed): Genetic Disorders and the Fetus, 3rd ed. Baltimore, Johns Hopkins Press, 1986, p 155.
116. Ledbetter DH, Zachary JM, Simpson JL, et al: Cytogenetic results from the U.S. Collaborative Study on CVS. Prenat Diagn 12:317, 1992.
117. Stetten G, Escallon CS, South ST, et al: Reevaluating confined placental mosaicism. Am J Med Genet A 131:232, 2004.
118. Wolstenholme J, Rooney DE, Davison EV: Confined placental mosaicism, IUGR, and adverse pregnancy outcome: a controlled retrospective U.K. collaborative survey. Prenat Diagn 14:345, 1994.
119. Hahnemann JM, Vejerslev LO: European collaborative research on mosaicism in CVS (EUCROMIC)—fetal and extrafetal cell lineages in 192 gestations with CVS mosaicism involving single autosomal trisomy. Am J Med Genet 70:179, 1997.
120. Association of Clinical Cytogeneticists Working Party on Chorionic Villi in Prenatal Diagnosis. Cytogenetic analysis of chorionic villi for prenatal diagnosis: an ACC collaborative study of U.K. data. Association of Clinical Cytogeneticists Working Party on Chorionic Villi in Prenatal Diagnosis. Prenat Diagn 14:363, 1994.
121. Warburton D: De novo balanced chromosome rearrangements and extra marker chromosomes identified at prenatal diagnosis: clinical significance and distribution of breakpoints. Am J Hum Genet 49:995, 1991.
122. Sachs ES, Van Hemel JO, Den Hollander JC, et al: Marker chromosomes in a series of 10,000 prenatal diagnoses. Cytogenetic and follow-up studies. Prenat Diagn 7:81, 1987.
123. Brondum-Nielsen K, Mikkelsen M: A 10-year survey, 1980–1990, of prenatally diagnosed small supernumerary marker chromosomes, identified by FISH analysis. Outcome and follow-up of 14 cases diagnosed in a series of 12,699 prenatal samples. Prenat Diagn 15:615, 1995.
124. Hume RF, Jr., Drugan A, Ebrahim SA, et al: Role of ultrasonography in pregnancies with marker chromosome aneuploidy. Fetal Diagn Ther 10:182, 1995.

125. Sepulveda W, Be C, Youlton R, et al: Nuchal translucency thickness and outcome in chromosome translocation diagnosed in the first trimester. Prenat Diagn 21:726, 2001.
126. Pertl B, Kopp S, Kroisel PM, et al: Rapid detection of chromosome aneuploidies by quantitative fluorescence PCR: first application on 247 chorionic villus samples. J Med Genet 36:300, 1999.
127. Kallioniemi A, Kallioniemi OP, Sudar D, et al: Comparative genomic hybridization for molecular cytogenetic analysis of solid tumors. Science 258:818, 1992.
128. Lapierre JM, Tachdjian G: Detection of chromosomal abnormalities by comparative genomic hybridization. Curr Opin Obstet Gynecol 17:171, 2005.
129. Rauch A, Ruschendorf F, Huang J, et al: Molecular karyotyping using an SNP array for genomewide genotyping. J Med Genet 41:916, 2004.
130. Cheung SW, Shaw CA, Yu W, et al: Development and validation of a CGH microarray for clinical cytogenetic diagnosis. Genet Med 7:422, 2005.
131. Sahoo T, Patel A, Ward P, et al: Rapid prenatal diagnosis by microarray-based comparative genomic hybridization: Experience of a pilot program. Abstracts, American Society of Human Genetics 55th Annual Meeting, Salt Lake City, Oct. 25–29, 2005. Abstract 85, p 34, 2005.
132. Richman L, Fiegler H, Carter NP, et al: Prenatal diagnosis by array-CGH. Eur J Med Genet 48:232, 2005.
133. Larrabee PB, Johnson KL, Pestova E, et al: Microarray analysis of cell-free fetal DNA in amniotic fluid: a prenatal molecular karyotype. Am J Hum Genet 75:485, 2004.
134. Elias S, Esterly NB: Prenatal diagnosis of hereditary skin disorders. Clin Obstet Gynecol 24:1069, 1981.
135. Milunsky A: Genetic Disorders and the Fetus: Diagnosis, Prevention, and Treatment, ed 5. Baltimore, John Hopkins University Press, 2004.
136. Brock DJ, Bolton AE, Monaghan JM: Prenatal diagnosis of anencephaly through maternal serum-alphafetoprotein measurement. Lancet 2:923, 1973.
137. American College of Obstetricians and Gynecologists: Maternal serum screening, ACOG Technical Bulletin, Vol 288, Washington DC, 1996.
138. Simpson JL, Palomaki GE, Mercer B, et al: Associations between adverse perinatal outcome and serially obtained serum. Am J Obstet Gynecol 173:1742. 1995.
139. Krause TG, Christens P, Wohlfahrt J, et al: Second-trimester maternal serum alpha-fetoprotein and risk of adverse pregnancy outcome(1). Obstet Gynecol 97:277, 2001.
140. Smith GC, Wood AM, Pell JP, et al: Second-trimester maternal serum levels of alpha-fetoprotein and the subsequent risk of sudden infant death syndrome. N Engl J Med 351:978, 2004.
141. Merkatz IR, Nitowsky HM, Macri JN, et al: An association between low maternal serum alpha-fetoprotein and fetal chromosomal abnormalities. Am J Obstet Gynecol 148:886, 1984.
142. Cuckle HS, Wald NJ, Thompson SG: Estimating a woman's risk of having a pregnancy associated with Down's syndrome using her age and serum alpha-fetoprotein level. Br J Obstet Gynaecol 94:387, 1987.
143. Bogart MH, Pandian MR, Jones OW: Abnormal maternal serum chorionic gonadotropin levels in pregnancies with fetal chromosome abnormalities. Prenat Diagn 7:623, 1987.
144. Canick JA, Knight GJ, Palomaki GE, et al: Low second trimester maternal serum unconjugated oestriol in pregnancies with Down's syndrome. Br J Obstet Gynaecol 95:330, 1988.
145. Wald NJ, Densem JW, George L, et al: Prenatal screening for Down's syndrome using inhibin-A as a serum marker. Prenat Diagn 16:143, 1996.
146. Haddow JE, Palomaki GE, Knight GJ, et al: Second trimester screening for Down's syndrome using maternal serum dimeric inhibin A. J Med Screen 5:115, 1998.
147. Wenstrom KD, Owen J, Chu D, et al: Prospective evaluation of free beta-subunit of human chorionic gonadotropin and dimeric inhibin A for aneuploidy detection. Am J Obstet Gynecol 181:887, 1999.
148. Malone FD, Canick JA, Ball RH, et al: First-trimester or second-trimester screening, or both, for Down's syndrome. N Engl J Med 353:2001, 2005.
149. Palomaki GE, Knight GJ, Haddow JE, et al: Cigarette smoking and levels of maternal serum alpha-fetoprotein, unconjugated estriol, and hCG: impact on Down syndrome screening. Obstet Gynecol 81:675, 1993.
150. Wald NJ, White N, Morris JK, et al: Serum markers for Down's syndrome in women who have had in vitro fertilisation: implications for antenatal screening. Br J Obstet Gynaecol 106:1304, 1999.
151. Cuckle HS, Spencer K, Nicolaides KH: Down syndrome screening marker levels in women with a previous aneuploidy pregnancy. Prenat Diagn 25:47, 2005.
152. Neveux LM, Palomaki GE, Knight GJ, et al: Multiple marker screening for Down syndrome in twin pregnancies. Prenat Diagn 16:29, 1996.
153. Palomaki GE, Knight GJ, Haddow JE, et al: Prospective intervention trial of a screening protocol to identify fetal trisomy 18 using maternal serum alpha-fetoprotein, unconjugated oestriol, and human chorionic gonadotropin. Prenat Diagn 12:925, 1992.
154. Palomaki GE, Haddow JE, Knight GJ, et al: Risk-based prenatal screening for trisomy 18 using alpha-fetoprotein, unconjugated oestriol and human chorionic gonadotropin. Prenat Diagn 15:713, 1995.
155. Nicolaides KH, Brizot ML, Snijders RJ: Fetal nuchal translucency: ultrasound screening for fetal trisomy in the first trimester of pregnancy. Br J Obstet Gynaecol 101:782, 1994.
156. Snijders RJ, Noble P, Sebire N, et al: UK multicentre project on assessment of risk of trisomy 21 by maternal age and fetal nuchal-translucency thickness at 10–14 weeks of gestation. Fetal Medicine Foundation First Trimester Screening Group. Lancet 352:343, 1998.
157. Nicolaides KH: Nuchal translucency and other first-trimester sonographic markers of chromosomal abnormalities. Am J Obstet Gynecol 191:45, 2004.
158. Krantz DA, Hallahan TW, Orlandi F, et al: First-trimester Down syndrome screening using dried blood biochemistry and nuchal translucency. Obstet Gynecol 96:207, 2000.
159. Wapner R, Thom E, Simpson JL, et al: First-trimester screening for trisomies 21 and 18. N Engl J Med 349:1405, 2003.
160. Wald NJ, Rodeck C, Hackshaw AK, et al: First and second trimester antenatal screening for Down's syndrome: the results of the Serum, Urine and Ultrasound Screening Study (SURUSS). J Med Screen 10:56, 2003.
161. Malone FD, Ball RH, Nyberg DA, et al: First-trimester septated cystic hygroma: Prevalence, natural history, and pediatric outcome. Obstet Gynecol 106:288, 2005.
162. Comstock CH, Malone FD, Ball RH, et al: Is there a nuchal translucency millimeter measurement above which there is no added benefit from first trimester serum screening? Am J Obstet Gynecol 195:843, 2006.
163. Avgidou K, Papageorghiou A, Bindra R, et al: Prospective first-trimester screening for trisomy 21 in 30,564 pregnancies. Am J Obstet Gynecol 192:1761, 2005.
164. Souka AP, Krampl E, Bakalis S, et al: Outcome of pregnancy in chromosomally normal fetuses with increased nuchal translucency in the first trimester. Ultrasound Obstet Gynecol 18:9, 2001.
165. Reddy UM, Mennuti MT: Incorporating first-trimester Down syndrome studies into prenatal screening: Executive summary of the National Institute of Child Health and Human Development Workshop. Obstet Gynecol 107:167, 2006.
166. Maymon R, Dreazen E, Tovbin Y, et al: The feasibility of nuchal translucency measurement in higher order multiple gestations achieved by assisted reproduction. Hum Reprod 14:2102, 1999.
167. Wald NJ, Watt HC, Hackshaw AK: Integrated screening for Down's syndrome on the basis of tests performed during the first and second trimesters. N Engl J Med 341:461, 1999.
168. Cuckle H: Integrating antenatal Down's syndrome screening. Curr Opin Obstet Gynecol 13:175, 2001.
169. Cuckle H, Arbuzova S: Multimarker maternal serum screening for chromosomal abnormalities. *In* Milunsky A (ed): Genetic Disorders and the Fetus, ed 5. Baltimore, The Johns Hopkins University Press, 2004, p 795.
170. Malone FD, Cuckle H, Ball RH, et al: Contingent screening for trisomy 21—Results from a general population screening trial. Am J Obstet Gynecol 193:S29, 2005.

171. Platt LD, Greene N, Johnson A, et al: Sequential pathways of testing after first-trimester screening for trisomy 21. Obstet Gynecol 104:661, 2004.
172. Cicero S, Curcio P, Papageorghiou A, et al: Absence of nasal bone in fetuses with trisomy 21 at 11–14 weeks of gestation: an observational study. Lancet 358:1665, 2001.
173. Otaño L, Aiello H, Igarzabal L, et al: Association between first trimester absence of fetal nasal bone on ultrasound and Down syndrome. Prenat Diagn 22:930, 2002.
174. Odibo AO, Sehdev HM, Dunn L, et al: The association between fetal nasal bone hypoplasia and aneuploidy. Obstet Gynecol 104:1229, 2004.
175. Malone FD, Ball RH, Nyberg DA, et al: First-trimester nasal bone evaluation for aneuploidy in the general population. Obstet Gynecol 104:1222, 2004.
176. Thomas MR, Williamson R, Craft I, et al: Y chromosome sequence DNA amplified from peripheral blood of women in early pregnancy. Lancet 343:413, 1994.
177. Lee T, LeShane ES, Messerlian GM, et al: Down syndrome and cell-free fetal DNA in archived maternal serum. Am J Obstet Gynecol 187:1217, 2002.
178. Moise KJ: Fetal RhD typing with free DNA in maternal plasma. Am J Obstet Gynecol 192:663, 2005.
179. Zhou L, Thorson JA, Nugent C, et al: Noninvasive prenatal RHD genotyping by real-time polymerase chain reaction using plasma from D-negative pregnant women. Am J Obstet Gynecol 193:1966, 2005.
180. Price JO, Elias S, Wachtel SS, et al: Prenatal diagnosis with fetal cells isolated from maternal blood by multiparameter flow cytometry. Am J Obstet Gynecol 165:1731, 1991.
181. Elias S, Price J, Dockter M, et al: First trimester prenatal diagnosis of trisomy 21 in fetal cells from maternal blood. Lancet 340:1033, 1992.
182. Bianchi DW, Simpson JL, Jackson LG, et al: Fetal cells in maternal blood: NIFTY clinical trial interim analysis. Prenat Diagn 19:994, 1999.
183. Rhine SA, Cain JL, Cleary RE, et al: Prenatal sex detection with endocervical smears: successful results utilizing Y-body fluoroscence. Am J Obstet Gynecol 122:155, 1975.
184. Adinolfi M, Sherlock J, Soothill P, et al: Molecular evidence of fetal-derived chromosome 21 markers (STRs) in transcervical samples. Prenat Diagn 15:35, 1995.
185. Bulmer JN, Rodeck C, Adinolfi M: Immunohistochemical characterization of cells retrieved by transcervical sampling in early pregnancy. Prenat Diagn 15:1143, 1995.
186. Adinolfi M, Sherlock J, Tutschek B, et al: Detection of fetal cells in transcervical samples and prenatal diagnosis of chromosomal abnormalities. Prenat Diagn 15:943, 1995.
187. Rodeck C, Tutschek B, Sherlock J, et al: Methods for the transcervical collection of fetal cells during the first trimester of pregnancy.Prenat Diagn 15:933, 1995.
188. Tutschek B, Sherlock J, Halder A, et al: Isolation of fetal cells from transcervical samples by micromanipulation: molecular confirmation of their fetal origin and diagnosis of fetal aneuploidy. Prenat Diagn 15:951, 1995.
189. Massari A, Novelli G, Colosimo A, et al: Non-invasive early prenatal molecular diagnosis using retrieved transcervical trophoblast cells. Hum Genet 97:150, 1996.
190. Miller D, Briggs J, Rahman MS, et al: Transcervical recovery of fetal cells from the lower uterine pole: reliability of recovery and histological/immunocytochemical analysis of recovered cell populations. Hum Reprod 14:521, 1999.
191. Fejgin MD, Diukman R, Cotton Y, et al: Fetal cells in the uterine cervix: a source for early non-invasive prenatal diagnosis. Prenat Diagn 21:619, 2001.
192. Bussani C, Cioni R, Scarselli B, et al: Strategies for the isolation and detection of fetal cells in transcervical samples. Prenat Diagn 22:1098, 2002.
193. Cioni R, Bussani C, Scarselli B, et al: Fetal cells in cervical mucus in the first trimester of pregnancy. Prenat Diagn 23:168, 2003.
194. Katz-Jaffe MG, Mantzaris D, Cram DS: DNA identification of fetal cells isolated from cervical mucus: potential for early non-invasive prenatal diagnosis. Br J Obstet Gynaecol 112:595, 2005.
195. Cioni R, Bussani C, Scarselli B, et al: Comparison of two techniques for transcervical cell sampling performed in the same study population. Prenat Diagn 25:198, 2005.
196. Ergin T, Baltaci V, Zeyneloglu HB, et al: Non-invasive early prenatal diagnosis using fluorescent in situ hybridization on transcervical cells: comparison of two different methods for retrieval. Eur J Obstet Gynecol Reprod Biol 95:37, 2001.
197. Verlinsky Y, Kuliev A: Atlas of Preimplantation Genetic Diagnosis, London, Taylor and Francis, 2005.
198. Verlinsky Y, Cohen J, Munné S, et al: Over a decade of experience with preimplantation genetic diagnosis: a multicenter report. Fertil Steril 82:292, 2004.
199. Verlinsky Y, Rechitsky S, Cieslak J, et al: Preimplantation diagnosis of single gene disorders by two-step oocyte genetic analysis using first and second polar body. Biochem Mol Med 62:182, 1997.
200. Verlinsky Y, Rechitsky S, Schoolcraft W, et al: Preimplantation diagnosis for Fanconi anemia combined with HLA matching. JAMA 285:3130, 2001.
201. ESHRE Preimplantation Genetic Diagnosis Consortium: data collection III (May 2001). Hum Reprod 17:233, 2002.
202. Verlinsky Y, Rechitsky S, Sharapova T, et al: Preimplantation HLA testing. JAMA 291:2079, 2004.
203. Rechitsky S, Kuliev A, Sharapova T, et al: Preimplantation HLA typing with aneuploidy testing. Reprod Biomed Online 12:89, 2006.
204. Schreinemachers DM, Cross PK, Hook EB: Rates of trisomies 21, 18, 13 and other chromosome abnormalities in about 20000 prenatal studies compared with estimated rates in live births. Hum Genet 61:318, 1982.
205. Gerbie AB, Simpson JL: Antenatal detection of genetic disorders. Postgrad Med 59:129, 1976.

Drugs and Environmental Agents in Pregnancy and Lactation: Embryology, Teratology, Epidemiology

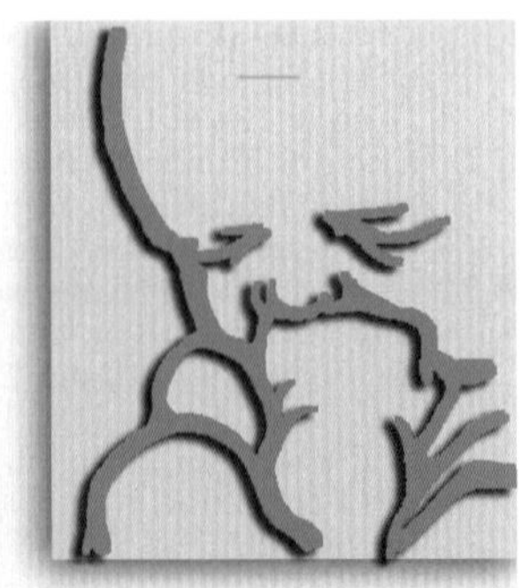

JENNIFER R. NIEBYL AND JOE LEIGH SIMPSON

CHAPTER 8

KEY ABBREVIATIONS

Angiotensin-converting enzyme	ACE
Birth defect surveillance (monitoring) system	BDMS
Diethylstilbestrol	DES
Electroencephalogram	EEG
Fetal alcohol syndrome	FAS
Food and Drug Administration	FDA
Glucose-6-phosphate dehydrogenase	G6PD
Neural tube defect	NTD
Propylthiouracil	PTU
Sudden infant death syndrome	SIDS
Saturated solution of potassium iodide	SSKI
Thyroid-stimulating hormone	TSH
Zidovudine	ZDV

INTRODUCTION

The placenta allows the transfer of many drugs and dietary substances. Lipid-soluble compounds readily cross the placenta, and water-soluble substances pass less well the greater their molecular weight. The degree to which a drug is bound to plasma protein also influences the amount of drug that is free to cross the placenta. Virtually all drugs cross the placenta to some degree, with the exception of large organic ions such as heparin and insulin.

Developmental defects in humans may result from genetic, environmental, or unknown causes. Approximately 25 percent are unequivocally genetic in origin; drug exposure accounts for only 2 to 3 percent of birth defects. Approximately 65 percent of defects are of unknown etiology but may be from combinations of genetic and environmental factors (see Chapter 6).

The incidence of major malformations in the general population is 2 to 3 percent.[1] A major malformation is defined as one that is incompatible with survival, such as anencephaly, or one requiring major surgery for correction, such as cleft palate or congenital heart disease, or one producing major dysfunction, such as mental retardation. If minor malformations are also included, such as ear tags or extra digits, the rate may be as high as 7 to 10 percent. The risk of malformation after exposure to a drug must be compared with this background rate.

There is a marked species specificity in drug teratogenesis.[2] For example, thalidomide was not found to be teratogenic in rats and mice but is a potent human teratogen. Thus, extrapolating from animal studies to humans is hazardous, and of limited applicability clinically.

The Food and Drug Administration (FDA) lists five categories of labeling for drug use in pregnancy. The rating system weighs the degree to which available information has ruled out risk to the fetus against the drug's potential benefit to the patient. The ratings, and their interpretation, are as follows:

A. **Controlled studies show no risk.** Adequate, well-controlled studies in pregnant women have failed to demonstrate a risk to the fetus in any trimester of pregnancy.

B. **No evidence of risk in humans.** Adequate, well-controlled studies in pregnant women have not shown increased risk of fetal abnormalities despite adverse findings in animals, or in the absence of adequate human studies, animal studies show no fetal risk. The chance of fetal harm is remote but remains a possibility.

C. **Risk cannot be ruled out.** Adequate, well-controlled human studies are lacking, and animal studies have shown a risk to the fetus or are lacking as well. There is a chance of fetal harm if the drug is administered during pregnancy; but the potential benefits may outweigh the potential risk.

D. **Positive evidence of risk.** Studies in humans, or investigational or postmarketing data, have demonstrated fetal risk. Nevertheless, potential benefits from the use of the drug may outweigh the potential risk. For example, the drug may be acceptable if needed in a life-threatening situation or serious disease for which safer drugs cannot be used or are ineffective.

X. **Contraindicated in pregnancy.** Studies in animals or humans, or investigational or post-marketing reports, have demonstrated positive evidence of fetal abnormalities or risk which clearly outweighs any possible benefit to the patient.

The Teratology Society suggests abandoning the FDA classification.[3] The categories imply that risk increases from category A to X. However, the drugs in different categories may pose similar risks but be in different categories based on risk/benefit considerations. Second, the categories create the impression that drugs within a category present similar risks, whereas the category definition permits inclusion in the same category drugs that vary in type, degree, or extent of risk, depending on potential benefit.

The categories were designed for prescribing physicians and do not address inadvertent exposure. For example, isotretinoin (Accutane) and oral contraceptives are both category X based on lack of benefit for oral contraceptives during pregnancy, yet oral contraceptives do not have any teratogenic risk with inadvertent exposure. When counseling patients or responding to queries from physicians, we recommend using specific descriptions in teratogen information databases (see Table 8-1).

The classic teratogenic period is from day 31 after the last menstrual period in a 28-day cycle to 71 days from the last period (Fig. 8-1). During this critical period, organs are forming and teratogens may cause malformations that are usually overt at birth. Timing of exposure is important. Administration of drugs early in the period of organogenesis affect the organs developing at that time, such as the heart or neural tube. Closer to the end of the classic teratogenic period, the ear and palate are forming and may be affected by a teratogen.

Before day 31, exposure to a teratogen produces an all-or-none effect. With exposure around conception, the conceptus usually either does not survive or survives without anomalies. Because so few cells exist in the early stages, irreparable damage to some may be lethal to the entire organism. If the organism remains viable, however, organ-specific anomalies are not manifested, because either repair or replacement will occur to permit normal development. A similar insult at a later stage may produce organ-specific defects.

Table 8-1. Teratogen Information Databases

- **MICROMEDEX, Inc.** 6200 South Syracuse Way, Suite 300, Greenwood Village, Colorado 80111-4740, Telephone #800-525-9083 (in US and Canada), http://www.micromedex.com
- Reproductive Toxicology Center, **REPROTOX.** 7831 Woodmont Avenue, Suite 375, Bethesda, MD 20814, Telephone #301-514-3081, http://www.reprotox.org
- **ORGANIZATION OF TERATOLOGY INFORMATION SERVICES (OTIS),** Medical Center, 200 W. Arbor Drive, #8446, San Diego, CA 92103-9981, Telephone #886-626-6847, http://www.otispregnancy.org

EMBRYOLOGY

During the first 3 days after ovulation, development takes place in the fallopian tube. At the time of fertilization, a pronuclear stage exists during which the nuclei from the egg and the sperm retain their integrity within the egg cytoplasm. After the pronuclei fuse, the fertilized egg begins a series of mitotic cell divisions (cleavage). The two-cell stage is reached about 30 hours after fertilization. With continued division, the cells develop into a solid ball of cells (morula), which reaches the endometrial cavity about 3 days after fertilization. Thereafter, a fluid-filled cavity forms within the cell mass, at which time the conceptus is called a *blastocyst.* The number of cells increases from approximately 12 to 32 by the end of the third day to 250 by the sixth day.

Until approximately 3 days after conception, any cell is thought to be totipotential, that is, capable of initiating development of any organ system. For this reason, separation of cells during this period gives rise to monozygotic twins, each normal. At the blastocyst stage, cells first begin to differentiate. By this stage of development, the embryo is located in the uterus, where implantation occurs 6 to 7 days after conception.

One group of cells forms the inner cell mass that will ultimately develop into the fetus. Different tissues arise from each of the three cell layers. Brain, nerves, and skin develop from the ectoderm; lining of the digestive tract, respiratory tract, and part of the bladder, as well as the liver and pancreas from the endoderm, and connective tissue, cartilage, muscle, blood vessels, the heart, kidneys, and gonads develop from the mesoderm. The group of cells forming the periphery of the blastocyst is termed the *trophoblast.* The placenta and the fetal membranes develop from this outer cell layer.

The trophoblast continues to grow, and lacunae form within the previously solid syncytiotrophoblast. The lacunae are the precursors of the intervillous spaces of the placenta, and by 2 weeks after conception, maternal blood is found within them. Meanwhile, the cytotrophoblast is forming cell masses that become chorionic villi.

From the third to the eighth week after conception, the embryonic disk undergoes major developments that lay the foundation for all organ systems. By 4 weeks after conception, the fertilized ovum has progressed from

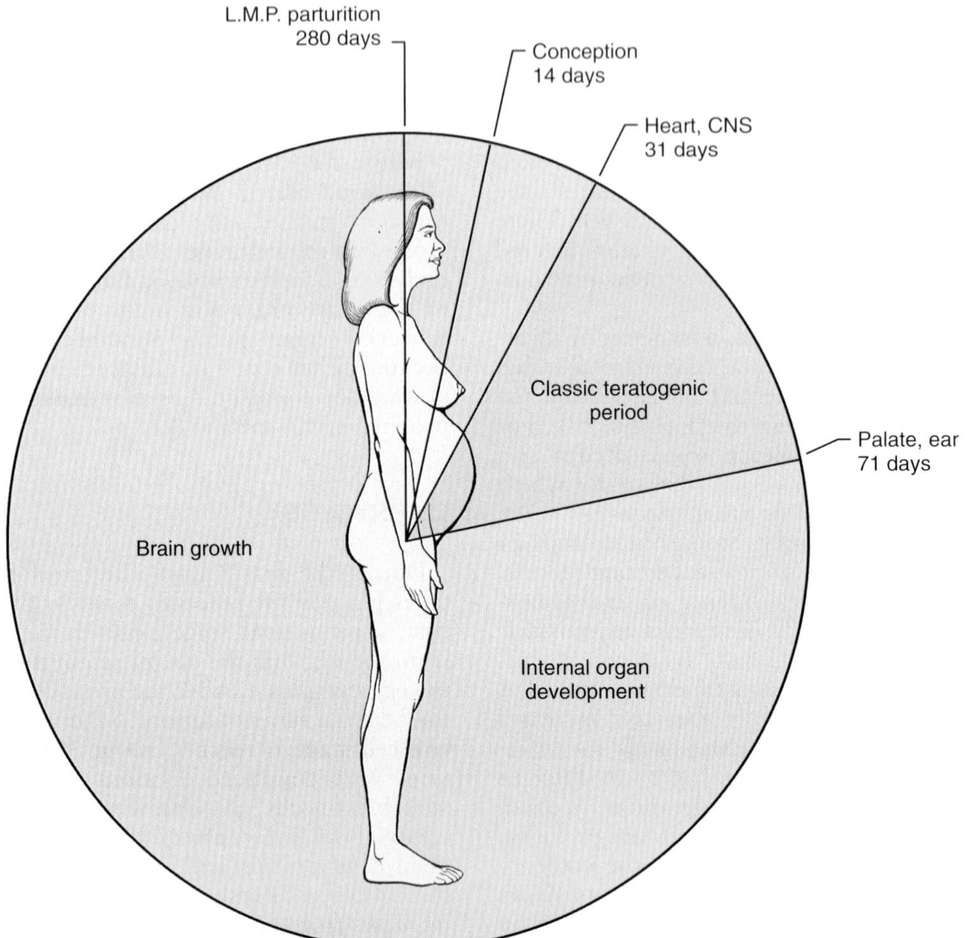

Figure 8-1. Gestational clock showing the classic teratogenic period. (From Blake DA, Niebyl JR: Requirements and limitations in reproductive and teratogenic risk assessment. *In* Niebyl JR [ed]: Drug Use in Pregnancy, 2nd ed. Philadelphia, Lea & Febiger, 1988, p 2, with permission.)

one cell to millions of cells. The rudiments of all major systems have differentiated and blueprints are set for developmental refinements. The embryo has been transformed into a curved tube approximately 6 mm long and isolated from the extraembryonic membranes.

At 5 weeks after conception, the embryo first begins to assume features of human appearance. The face is recognizable, with the formation of discernible eyes, nose, and ears. Limbs emerge from protruding buds; digits, cartilage, and muscles develop. The cerebral hemispheres begin to fill the brain area, and the optic stalk becomes apparent. Nerve connections are established between the retina and the brain. The digestive tract rotates from its prior tubular structure, and the liver starts to produce blood cells and bile. Two tubes emerge from the pharynx to become bronchi, and the lungs have lobes and bronchioles. The heart is beating at 5 weeks and is almost completely developed by 8 weeks after conception. The diaphragm begins to divide the heart and lungs from the abdominal cavity. The kidneys approach their final form at this time. The urogenital and rectal passages separate, and germ cells migrate toward the genital ridges for future transformation into ovaries or testes. Differentiation of internal ducts begins, with persistence of either müllerian or wolffian ducts. Virilization of external genitalia occurs in male embryos. The embryo increases from approximately 6 to 33 mm in length and increases 50 times in weight.

Structurally, the fetus has become straighter, and the tubular neural canal along which the spinal cord develops becomes filled with nerve cells. Ears remain low on the sides of the head. Teeth are forming, and the two bony plates of the palate fuse in the midline. Disruptions during the latter part of the embryonic period lead to various forms of cleft lip and palate. By 10 weeks after the last menstrual period, all major organ systems have become established and integrated.

Development of other organs continues in the second and third trimesters of pregnancy. Therefore, we still need to be concerned about drug use at this time in pregnancy, although the effects may not be recognized until later in life. Some of the uterine anomalies resulting from diethylstilbestrol (DES) occurred with exposure as late as 20 weeks but were not recognized until after puberty. The brain continues to develop throughout pregnancy and the neonatal period. Fetal alcohol syndrome (FAS) may occur with chronic exposure to alcohol in the later stages of pregnancy.

BASIC PRINCIPLES OF TERATOLOGY

To understand the etiology of birth defects, it is important to enumerate the principles of abnormal development (teratogenesis). Wilson's six general principles of teratogenesis[4] provide a framework for understanding how structural or functional teratogens may act.

Genotype and Interaction with Environmental Factors

The first principle is that susceptibility to a teratogen depends on the *genotype of the conceptus* and on the manner in which the genotype interacts with environmental factors. This is perhaps most clearly shown by experiments in which different genetic strains of mice have varied greatly in their susceptibility to teratogens that lead to oral clefts.[5] Some of the variability in responses to human teratogens, such as to anticonvulsant drugs like valproic acid and hydantoin, probably relates to genotype of the embryo. The increasing complexity of these potential interactions is illustrated by a series of elegant studies by Musselman and colleagues.[6]

Timing of Exposure

The second principle is that susceptibility of the conceptus to teratogenic agents varies with the developmental stage at the time of exposure. This concept of *critical stages of development* is particularly applicable to alterations in structure. It is during the second to the eighth weeks of development after conception—the embryonic period—that most structural defects occur. For such defects, it is believed that there is a critical stage in the developmental process, after which abnormal embryogenesis cannot be initiated. For example, most investigators believe that the neural tube defects anencephaly and spina bifida result from the failure of the neural tube to close. Given that this process occurs between 22 and 28 days postconception, any exogenous effect on development must be present at or before this time. Van Allen et al.[7] put forward convincing evidence that the neural tube has five distinct closure sites that may respond differentially to agents and may respond differently in timing. Investigations of thalidomide teratogenicity have clearly shown that the effects of the drug differ as a function of the developmental stage at which the pregnant woman took it.[8]

Mechanisms of Teratogenesis

The third principle is that teratogenic agents act in specific ways (*mechanisms*) on developing cells and tissues in initiating abnormal embryogenesis (pathogenesis). Teratogenic mechanisms are considered separately below.

Manifestations

Irrespective of the specific deleterious agent, the final manifestations of abnormal development are death, malformation, growth restriction, and functional disorder. The manifestation is thought to depend largely on the stage of development at which exposure occurs; a teratogen may have one effect if exposure occurs during embryogenesis and another if the exposure is during the fetal period. Embryonic exposure is likely to lead to structural abnormalities or embryonic death; fetal exposure is likely to lead to functional deficits or growth restriction.

Despite the importance of teratogen timing on specificity of anomalies, a general pattern usually emerges with respect to any given teratogen. This will be evident throughout this chapter as we consider various agents. If no pattern is evident for a purported teratogen, it increases the suspicion that any purported association is spurious, the observation reflecting confounding variables not recognized and, hence, not taken into account.

Agent

The fifth principle is that access of adverse environmental influences to developing tissues depends on the nature of the influence (*agent*). This principle relates to such pharmacologic factors as maternal metabolism and placental passage. Although most clearly understood for chemical agents or drugs, the principle also applies to physical agents such as radiation or heat. For an adverse effect to occur, an agent must reach the conceptus, either transmitted indirectly through maternal tissues or directly traversing the maternal body.

Dose Effect

The final principle is that manifestations of abnormal development increase in degree from the no-effect level to the lethal level as *dosage* increases. This means that the response (e.g., malformation, growth restriction) may be expected to vary according to the dose, duration, or amount of exposure. For most human teratogens, this dose-response is not clearly understood, but along with the principle of critical stages of development, these concepts are important in supporting causal inferences about human reproductive hazards. Data regarding in utero exposure to ionizing radiation clearly show the importance of dose on observed effects.[9] The potential complexity of relationships between dose and observed effects for teratogens has been discussed by Selevan and Lemasters.[10]

EPIDEMIOLOGIC APPROACHES TO BIRTH DEFECTS

Teratogens and reproductive toxicants have been identified and are being sought in various ways. Some are far more robust than others. Here we enumerate most common approaches, their strengths, and their pitfalls.

Case Reports

Many known teratogens and reproductive toxicants were identified initially through case reports of an unusual number of cases or a constellation of abnormalities. These have often come from astute clinicians, who observed something out of the ordinary.[11,12] Although the importance of astute observations of abnormal aggregations of cases or patterns of malformations must be recognized, we cannot rely on such methods for identifying health hazards. Furthermore, etiologic speculations based on case reports or case series usually do not lead to a causal agent and are often false-positive speculations. Whereas case reports may identify a new teratogen, they can never provide an estimate of the risk of disease after exposure.

Descriptive Studies

Descriptive epidemiologic studies provide information about the distribution and frequency of some outcome of interest, resulting in rates of occurrence that can be compared among populations, places, or times. Defining the population at risk is the first step. The population at risk can be defined geographically, such as residents within a state, or medically, such as being a patient at a particular hospital. Definition of the population at risk includes the time period under consideration. The population at risk constitutes the *denominator* for calculating rates of the occurrence of outcomes of interest.

The second step in a descriptive study is to determine the *numerator* for calculating rates for comparison. This involves two important concepts: (1) case definition (what defines a case to be counted) and (2) case ascertainment (how are cases to be identified).

Relevant examples of descriptive studies are surveillance programs. An at-risk population is identified and then followed over time to detect outcomes of interest. Cases are included in the database. Surveillance programs can develop baseline data and subsequently permit early recognition of potential problems, based on ongoing data collection and analysis. Birth defect surveillance (monitoring) systems (BDMSs) are designed to identify cases occurring in a defined population, usually by reviewing vital records or hospital record abstracts or charts. In the past 20 years, there has been a dramatic increase in the number of state-based birth defect surveillance systems. Approximately half the states now have some type of birth defect surveillance system.[13] These programs conduct routine reviews of occurrence rates of specific malformations and attempt to identify increases in rates or clusters of cases.

Case-Control Studies

In a case-control study design, groups of individuals with some outcome or disease of interest (cases) (e.g., a congenital malformation), are compared with controls with regard to a history of one or more exposures. This is the most widely used approach in reproductive outcomes research. Controls are ideally as similar as possible to the cases, except of course lacking the outcome of interest. After cases and controls have been identified, the hypothesis to be tested is whether these two groups differ in exposure as well as outcome. How accurately exposure and its timing are determined may vary greatly among studies, but in any study the same methods must be used to establish the exposure of both cases and controls.[14]

Case-control studies are advantageous in testing outcomes of infrequent occurrence. This can be conducted relatively rapidly and inexpensively. A disadvantage is the potential for several important types of bias, including bias in recalling exposure, in selecting appropriate controls, and in ascertaining cases.

These problems can be addressed in part by use of two control groups, one "normal" and the second "abnormal." Any of several abnormal controls seem equally useful, for example, infants with mendelian or chromosomal disorders as well as infants with no specific malformation.[15] In the former, mothers have incentive to recall but teratogenesis is not the etiology. Ideally, case-control studies of potential teratogens should follow descriptive studies. After suspecting on the basis of case observations that thalidomide was teratogenic, Lenz[16] conducted a case-control study. The association between valproic acid use and spina bifida was verified by case-control studies.[17]

Cohort Studies

In cohort studies, groups are defined by the presence or absence of exposure to a given factor and then are followed over time and compared for rates of occurrence (i.e., incidence rates) of the outcome of interest. Cohort studies have three advantages: (1) the cohort is classified by exposure before the outcome is determined, thereby eliminating exposure recall bias; (2) incidence rates can be calculated among those exposed; and (3) multiple outcomes can be observed simultaneously.

Cohort studies, often called *prospective studies,* require that groups differing in exposure be followed through time, with outcomes observed. Therefore, these studies tend to be time consuming and expensive. In addition, occurrence rates for many adverse reproductive outcomes, such as congenital malformations, are low; thus, large samples must be followed for a considerable period of time. Two main types of cohort studies have been developed: (1) those that identify a cohort and follow it into the future (concurrent cohort study), and (2) those that identify a cohort at some time in the past and follow it to the present (nonconcurrent or historical cohort study). In both cases, risks of adverse outcomes are compared between groups. Cohort studies enable investigators to calculate incidence rates that provide a measure of risk of an outcome after the exposure. Risk in the exposed group can be compared with risk in an unexposed group. Most frequently, ratio of the incidence rate among the exposed to the rate among the unexposed is determined. This ratio, referred to as *relative risk*, is a measure of how much the presence of exposure increases the risk of the outcome.

In *historical prospective studies,* one begins by identifying groups who differ in terms of some past exposure and follow them to the present and determine outcomes; exposure groups are defined before outcomes are known. A major advantage is that although the time frame is prospective, investigators do not have to follow the cohort into the future, waiting for events to occur. A disadvantage is that these studies require the ability to determine exposure status retrospectively.

Clinical Trials

Ideally analytical studies (case control or cohort) are followed by a randomized clinical trial, in which the efficiency of a prevention or treatment regimen is evaluated. That is, subjects are randomly assigned to different treatment groups. The individuals should be as similar as possible in terms of unknown factors that may affect the response before they are randomly assigned to the treatment groups and receive the different regimens.[18]

Clinical trials of both neural tube defect (NTD) recurrence[19] and occurrence[20] have shown a protective effect of periconceptional folic acid supplementation, findings that have led to key public health recommendations regarding the use of folic acid to reduce the risk of these often devastating defects.[21]

MEDICAL DRUG USE

Patients should be educated about avenues other than the use of drugs to cope with tension, aches and pains, and viral illnesses during pregnancy. Drugs should be used only when necessary. The risk/benefit ratio should justify the use of a particular drug, and the minimum effective dose should be employed. Because long-term effects of drug exposure in utero may not be revealed for many years, caution with regard to the use of any drug in pregnancy is warranted.

Effects of Specific Drugs

ESTROGENS AND PROGESTINS

Studies have not confirmed any teratogenic risk for oral contraceptives or progestins.[22,23] A meta-analysis of first-trimester sex hormone exposure revealed no association between exposure and fetal genital malformations.[24] However, because of the medicolegal climate and the conflicting past literature, it is wise to exclude pregnancy before giving progestins to an amenorrheic patient.

ANDROGENIC STEROIDS

Androgens may masculinize a developing female fetus.[25] Danazol (Danocrine) has been reported to produce clitoral enlargement and labial fusion when given inadvertently for the first 9 to 12 weeks after conception[26] (Fig. 8-2) in 23 of 57 female infants exposed.[27]

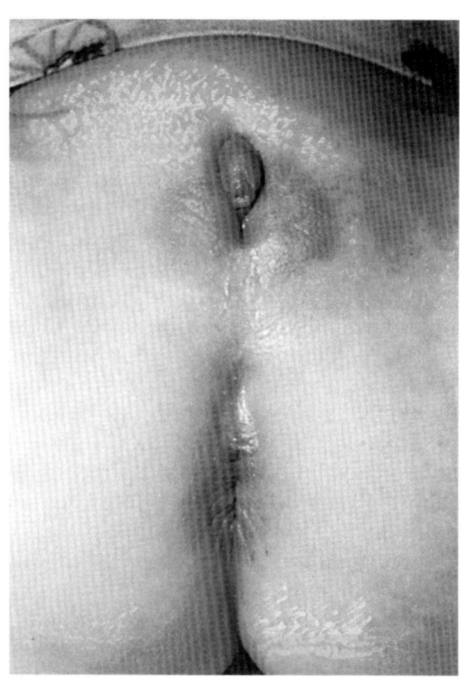

Figure 8-2. Perineum of a female fetus exposed to danazol in utero. (From Duck SC, Katayama KP: Danazol may cause female pseudohermaphroditism. Fertil Steril 35:230, 1981, with permission.)

SPERMICIDES

The once touted increased risk of abnormal offspring in mothers who had used spermicides for contraception has not been confirmed. A meta-analysis of reports of sperimicide exposure concludes that there is no increased risk of birth defects.[28]

ANTICONVULSANTS (see Chapter 50)

Epileptic women taking anticonvulsants during pregnancy have approximately double the general population risk of malformations. Compared with the general risk of 2 to 3 percent, the risk of major malformations in epileptic women on anticonvulsants is about 5 percent, especially cleft lip with or without cleft palate and congenital heart disease. Valproic acid (Depakene) and carbamazepine (Tegretol) each carry approximately a 1 percent risk of NTDs and possibly other anomalies.[29] A high daily dose or a combination of two or three drugs increases the chance of malformations.[30]

Holmes et al.[31] screened 128,049 pregnant women at delivery to identify three groups of infants: those exposed to anticonvulsant drugs, those unexposed to anticonvulsant drugs but with a maternal history of seizures, and those unexposed to anticonvulsant drugs with no maternal history of seizures (control group). The infants were examined systematically for the presence of malformations. The combined frequency of anticonvulsant embryopathy was higher in 223 infants exposed to one anticonvulsant drug than in 508 control infants (20.6 percent vs. 8.5 percent; odds ratio, 2.8; 95 percent confidence interval, 1.1 to 9.7). The frequency was also higher in 93 infants exposed to two or more anticonvulsant drugs than in the controls (28.0 percent vs. 8.5 percent; odds ratio, 4.2; 95 percent confidence interval, 1.1 to 5.1). The greater the number of anticonvulsants, the higher the risk of malformation. The 98 infants whose mothers had a history of epilepsy but who took no anticonvulsant drugs during the pregnancy did not have a higher frequency of those abnormalities than the control infants.

Phenytoin (Dilantin) decreases folate absorption and lowers the serum folate, which has been implicated in birth defects.[32] Therefore, folic acid supplementation should be given to these mothers, but this may require adjustment of the anticonvulsant dose. Although epileptic women were not included in the Medical Research Council study, most authorities would recommend 4 mg/day folic acid for high-risk women[33] (see Chapter 5). One study suggested that folic acid at doses of 2.5 to 5 mg daily could reduce birth defects in women on anticonvulsant drugs.[34]

Fewer than 10 percent of offspring show the fetal hydantoin syndrome,[35] which consists of microcephaly, growth deficiency, developmental delays, mental retardation, and dysmorphic craniofacial features (Fig. 8-3).

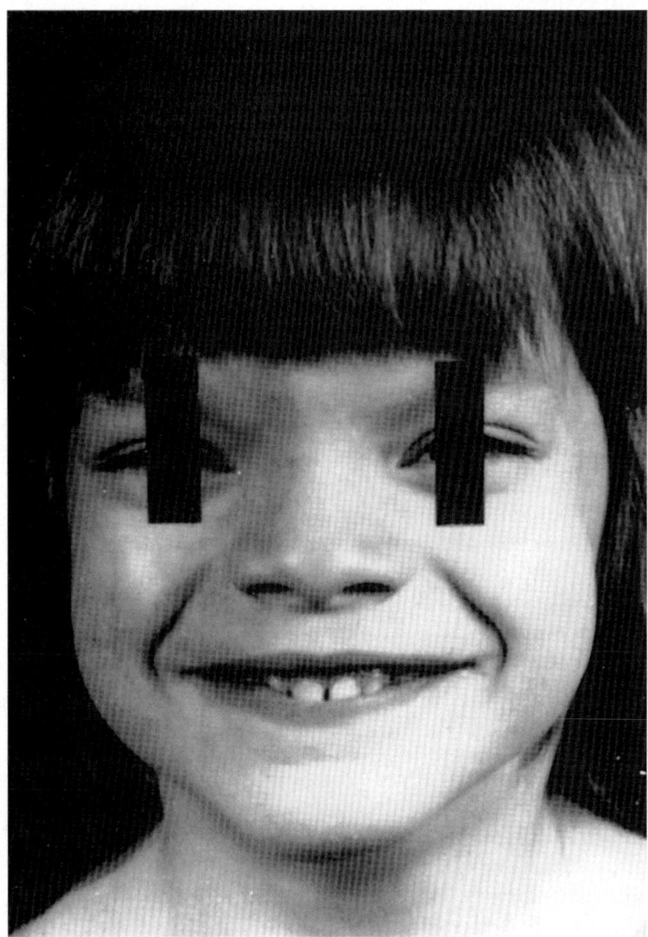

Figure 8-3. Facial features of the fetal hydantoin syndrome. Note broad, flat nasal ridge, epicanthic folds, mild hypertelorism, and wide mouth with prominent upper lip. (Courtesy of Dr. Thaddeus Kelly, Charlottesville, VA.)

In fact, the risk may be as low as 1 to 2 percent above background.[36] Although several of these features are also found in other syndromes, such as FAS, more common in the fetal hydantoin syndrome are hypoplasia of the nails and distal phalanges (Fig. 8-4) and hypertelorism. Carbamazepine (Tegretol) is also associated with an increased risk of a dysmorphic syndrome.[37] A genetically determined metabolic defect in arene oxide detoxification in the infant may increase the risk of a major birth defect.[38] Epoxide hydrolase deficiency may indicate susceptibility to fetal hydantoin syndrome.[39]

In a follow-up study of long-term effects of antenatal exposure to phenobarbital and carbamazepine, there were no neurologic or behavioral differences between the two groups.[40] However, children exposed in utero to phenytoin scored 10 points lower on IQ tests than children exposed to carbamazepine or to nonexposed controls.[41] Also, prenatal exposure to phenobarbital decreased verbal IQ scores in adult men.[42]

Lamotrigine (Lamictal) is an inhibitor of dihydrofolate reductase and decreases embryonic folate levels in experimental animals, so it is theoretically possible that this drug would be associated with an increased malformation risk like the other antiepileptic drugs. Lamotrigine exposures have been compiled in a registry established by the manufacturer, Glaxo Wellcome. Fourteen of 491 infants (2.9%) born to women treated with lamotrigine monotherapy during the first trimester and followed prospectively to birth were found to have congenital anomalies,[43] not significantly increased over the expected rate.

There are no epidemiologic studies of congenital anomalies among children born to women treated with felbamate, gabapentin, oxcarbazepine, tiagabine, topiramate, or vigabatrin,[44] and there is limited information about pregnancy outcomes.

Some women may have taken anticonvulsant drugs for a long period without reevaluation of the need for continuation of the drugs. For patients with idiopathic epilepsy who have been seizure free for 2 years and who have a normal electroencephalogram (EEG), it may be safe to attempt a trial of withdrawal of the drug before pregnancy.[45]

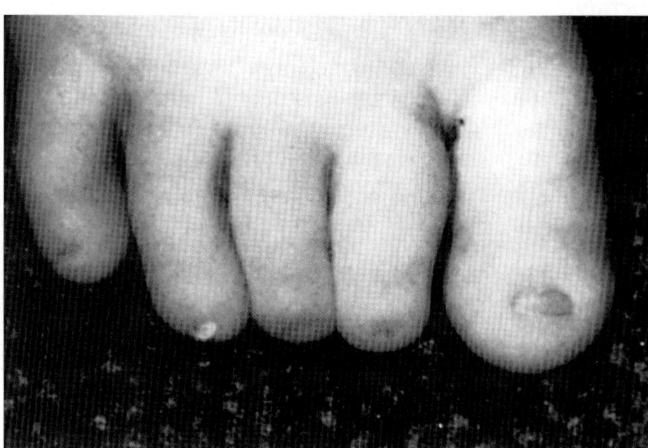

Figure 8-4. Hypoplasia of toenails and distal phalanges. (From Hanson JWM: Fetal hydantoin syndrome. Teratology 13:186, 1976, with permission.)

Most authorities agree that the benefits of anticonvulsant therapy during pregnancy outweigh the risks of discontinuation of the drug if the patient is first seen during pregnancy. The blood level of drug should be monitored to ensure a therapeutic level but minimize the dosage. If the patient has not been taking her drug regularly, a low blood level may demonstrate her lack of compliance and she may not need the drug. Because the albumin concentration falls in pregnancy, the total amount of phenytoin measured is decreased, because it is highly protein bound. However, the level of free phenytoin, which is the pharmacologically active portion, is unchanged.

Pediatric care providers need to be notified at birth when a patient has been on anticonvulsants because this therapy can affect vitamin K–dependent clotting factors in the newborn. Some have recommended vitamin K supplementation at 10 mg daily for these mothers for the last month of pregnancy.[46]

Isotretinoin

Isotretinoin (Accutane) is a significant human teratogen. This drug is marketed for treatment of cystic acne and unfortunately has been taken inadvertently by women who were not planning pregnancy.[47] It is labeled as contraindicated in pregnancy (FDA category X) with appropriate warnings that a negative pregnancy test is required before therapy. Of 154 exposed human pregnancies, there have been 21 reported cases of birth defects, 12 spontaneous abortions, 95 elective abortions, and 26 normal infants in women who took isotretinoin during early pregnancy. The risk of structural anomalies in patients studied prospectively is now estimated to be about 25 percent. An additional 25 percent have mental retardation alone.[48] The malformed infants have a characteristic pattern of craniofacial, cardiac, thymic, and central nervous system anomalies. They include microtia/anotia (small/absent ears) (Fig. 8-5), micrognathia, cleft palate, heart defects, thymic defects, retinal or optic nerve anomalies, and central nervous system malformations including hydrocephalus.[47] Microtia is rare as an isolated anomaly yet appears commonly as part of the retinoic acid embryopathy. Cardiovascular defects include great vessel transposition and ventricular septal defects.

Unlike vitamin A, isotretinoin is not stored in tissue. Therefore, a pregnancy after discontinuation of isotretinoin is not at risk, because the drug is no longer detectable in serum 5 days after its ingestion. In 88 pregnancies prospectively ascertained after discontinuation of isotretinoin, no increased risk of anomalies was noted, in contrast to etretinate (see later).[49] Topical tretinoin (Retin-A) has not been associated with any teratogenic risk.[50]

Etretinate (Tegison)

This drug is marketed for use in psoriasis and may well have a teratogenic risk similar to that of isotretinoin. Case reports of malformation, especially central nervous system,[51] have appeared, but the absolute risk is unknown. The half-life of several months makes levels cumulative, and the drug carries a warning to avoid pregnancy within 6 months of use.

Vitamin A

There is no evidence that vitamin A itself in normal doses is teratogenic, nor is betacarotene. The levels in prenatal vitamins (5,000 IU/day orally) have not been associated with any documented risk. Eighteen cases of birth defects have been reported after exposure to levels of 25,000 IU of vitamin A or greater during pregnancy.

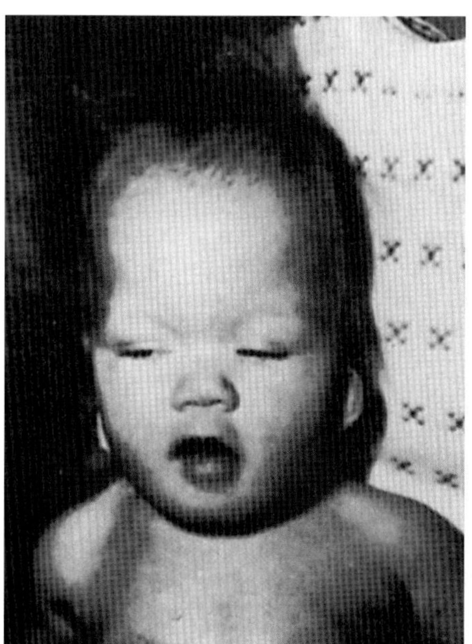

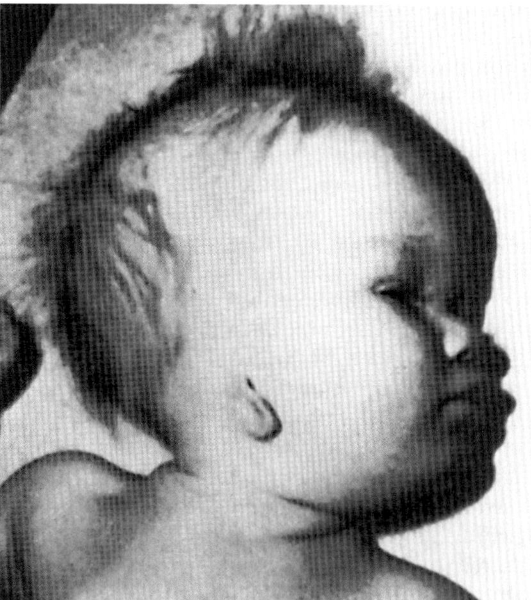

Figure 8-5. Infant exposed to Accutane in utero. Note high forehead, hypoplastic nasal bridge, and abnormal ears. (From Lot IT, Bocian M, Pribam HW, Leitner M: Fetal hydrocephalus and ear anomalies associated with use of isotretinoin. J Pediatr 105:598, 1984, with permission.)

Vitamin A in doses greater than 10,000 IU/day was shown to increase the risk of malformations in one study[51] but not in another.[52]

Psychoactive Drugs

There is no clear risk documented for most psychoactive drugs with respect to overt birth defects. However, effects of chronic use of these agents on the developing brain in humans is difficult to study, and so a conservative attitude is appropriate. Lack of overt defects does not exclude the possibility of behavioral teratogens, and neonatal withdrawal may occurgenes (see Chapter 50).

Tranquilizers

Conflicting reports of the possible teratogenicity of the various tranquilizers, including meprobamate (Miltown) and chlordiazepoxide (Librium), have appeared, but in prospective studies, no increased risk of anomalies has been shown.[53]

A fetal benzodiazepine syndrome has been reported in seven infants of 36 mothers who regularly took benzodiazepines during pregnancy.[54] However, the high rate of abnormality occurred with concomitant alcohol and substance abuse and may not be caused by the benzodiazepine exposure.[55] In most clinical situations, however, the risk/benefit ratio does not justify the use of benzodiazepines in pregnancy. Perinatal use of diazepam (Valium) has been associated with hypotonia, hypothermia, and respiratory depression.

Lithium (Eskalith, Lithobid)

In the International Register of Lithium Babies,[56] 217 infants were listed as exposed at least during the first trimester of pregnancy, and 25 (11.5 percent) were malformed. Eighteen had cardiovascular anomalies, including six cases of the rare Ebstein's anomaly, which occurs in only 1 in 20,000 in the nonexposed population. Of 60 unaffected infants who were followed to age 5 years, no increased mental or physical abnormalities were noted compared with unexposed siblings.[57]

However, two other reports suggest bias of ascertainment in the registry and a risk of anomalies much lower than previously thought. A case-control study of 59 patients with Ebstein's anomaly showed no difference in the rate of lithium exposure in pregnancy from a control group of 168 children with neuroblastoma.[58] A prospective study of 148 women exposed to lithium in the first trimester showed no difference in the incidence of major anomalies compared with controls.[59] One fetus in the lithium-exposed group had Ebstein's anomaly, and one infant in the control group had a ventricular septal defect. The authors concluded that lithium is not a major human teratogen. Nevertheless, we recommend that women exposed to lithium be offered ultrasound and fetal echocardiography.

Lithium is excreted more rapidly during pregnancy; thus, serum lithium levels should be monitored. Perinatal effects of lithium have been noted, including hypotonia, lethargy, and poor feeding in the infant. Also, complications similar to those seen in adults on lithium have been noted in newborns, including goiter and hypothyroidism.

Two cases of polyhydramnios associated with maternal lithium treatment have been reported.[60,61] Because nephrogenic diabetes insipidus has been reported in adults taking lithium, the presumed mechanism of this polyhydramnios is fetal diabetes insipidus. Polyhydramnios may be a sign of fetal lithium toxicity.

It is usually recommended that drug therapy be changed in pregnant women on lithium to avoid fetal drug exposure. Tapering over 10 days delays the risk of relapse.[62] However, discontinuing lithium is associated with a 70-percent chance of relapse of the affective disorder in 1 year as opposed to 20 percent in those who remain on lithium. Discontinuation of lithium may pose an unacceptable risk of increased morbidity in women who have had multiple episodes of affective instability. These women should be offered appropriate prenatal diagnosis with ultrasound, including fetal echocardiography.

Antidepressants

Imipramine (Tofranil) was the original tricyclic antidepressant claimed to be associated with cardiovascular defects, but the number of patients studied remains small. Of 75 newborns exposed in the first trimester, six major defects were observed, three being cardiovascular, and neonatal withdrawal has been observed.[63]

Amitriptyline (Elavil) has been more widely used, and the majority of the evidence supports its safety. In the Michigan Medicaid study, 467 newborns had been exposed during the first trimester, with no increased risk of birth defects.[64]

No increased risk of major malformations has been found after first trimester exposure to fluoxetine (Prozac) in more than 500 pregnancies.[65,66] Nulman and colleagues[67] evaluated the neurobehavioral effects of long-term fluoxetine exposure during pregnancy and found no abnormalities among 228 children aged 16 to 86 months (average age, 3 years). Theoretically, some psychiatric or neurobehavioral abnormality might occur as a result of exposure, but it would be very difficult to ascertain because of all of the confounding variables. In mice, some behavioral effects of paroxetine (Paxil) have been observed.[68]

Chambers and associates[69] found more minor malformations and perinatal complications among infants exposed to fluoxetine throughout pregnancy, but this study is difficult to interpret because the authors did not control for depression. When a group whose mothers received tricyclic agents was used as a control for depression, infants exposed to fluoxetine in utero did not appear to have more minor malformations or perinatal complications.[65] One study suggested an increased risk of low-birth-weight infants with higher doses of fluoxetine (40 to 80 mg) throughout pregnancy.[70]

A study of the newer selective serotonin reuptake inhibitors—fluvoxamine, paroxetine, and sertraline—during the first trimester in 267 women revealed no increased birth defects.[70]

Studies have described neonatal withdrawal in the first 2 days after in utero exposure to these drugs.[72] Infants exposed during pregnancy exhibited more tremulousness and sleep changes at 1 to 2 days of age. However, no abnormalities were found when children were examined at age 16 to 86 months after prolonged exposure during pregnancy.[73]

ANTICOAGULANTS

Warfarin (Coumadin) has been associated with chondrodysplasia punctata, which is similar to the genetically determined Conradi-Hünermann syndrome. Warfarin embryopathy occurs in about 5 percent of exposed pregnancies, includes nasal hypoplasia, bone stippling seen on radiologic examination, ophthalmologic abnormalities including bilateral optic atrophy, and mental retardation (Fig. 8-6). Ophthalmologic abnormalities and mental retardation may occur[74] even with use only beyond the first trimester. The risk for pregnancy complications is higher when the mean daily dose of warfarin is more than 5 mg.[75]

The alternative drug, heparin, does not cross the placenta, because it is a large molecule with a strong negative charge. Because heparin does not have an adverse effect on the fetus when given in pregnancy, it should be the drug of choice for patients requiring anticoagulation except in women with artificial heart valves.[76] However, therapy with 20,000 units/day for greater than 20 weeks has been associated with bone demineralization.[77] Thirty-six percent of patients had more than a 10-percent decrease from baseline bone density to postpartum values.[78] The risk of spine fractures was 0.7 percent with low-dose heparin and 3 percent with a high-dose regimen.[79] Heparin can also cause thrombocytopenia.

Low-molecular-weight heparins may have substantial benefits over standard unfractionated heparin.[80] The molecules are still relatively large and do not cross the placenta.[81] The half-life is longer, allowing for once-daily administration. However, enoxaparin is cleared more rapidly during pregnancy, and so twice-daily dosing is advised. Low-molecular-weight heparins have a much more predictable dose-response relationship, obviating the need for monitoring of partial thromboplastin time. There is less risk of heparin-induced thrombocytopenia and clinical bleeding at delivery, but studies suggesting less risk of osteoporosis are preliminary. However, the cost is substantially higher than standard heparin.[82,83]

Women with mechanical heart valves, especially the first-generation valves, require warfarin anticoagulation,[75] because heparin is not safe or effective.[84] Heparin treatment is associated with more thromboembolic complications and more bleeding complications than warfarin therapy.[76]

The risks of heparin during pregnancy may not be justified in patients with only a single episode of thrombosis in the past.[85,86] Certainly, conservative measures should be recommended, such as elastic stockings and avoidance of prolonged sitting or standing.

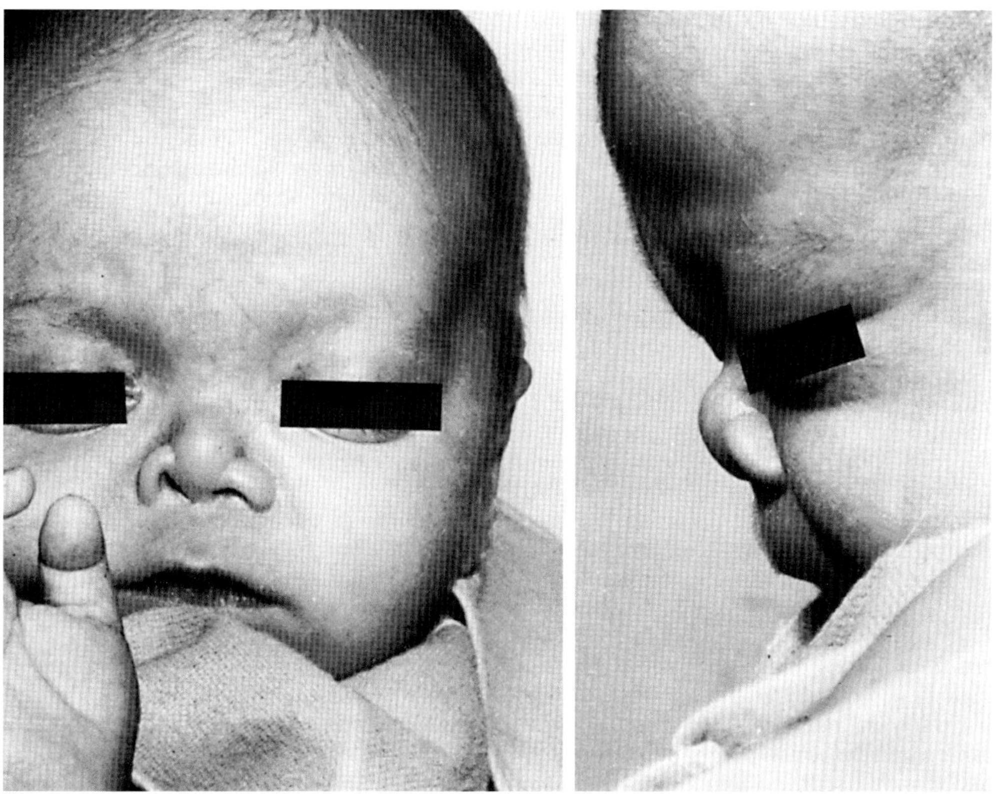

Figure 8-6. Warfarin embryopathy. Note small nose with hypoplastic bridge. (From Shaul W, Hall JG: Multiple congenital anomalies associated with oral anticoagulants. Am J Obstet Gynecol 127:191, 1977, with permission.)

THYROID AND ANTITHYROID DRUGS

Propylthiouracil (PTU) and methimazole (Tapazole) both cross the placenta and may cause some degree of fetal goiter. In contrast, the thyroid hormones triiodothyronine and thyroxine cross the placenta poorly, so that fetal hypothyroidism produced by antithyroid drugs cannot be corrected satisfactorily by administration of thyroid hormone to the mother. Thus, the goal of such therapy during pregnancy is to keep the mother slightly hyperthyroid to minimize fetal drug exposure. By the third trimester, 30 percent of women no longer need antithyroid medication.[87]

Methimazole has been associated with scalp defects in infants and choanal or esophageal atresia,[87] as well as a higher incidence of maternal side effects. However, PTU and methimazole are equally effective and safe for therapy of hyperthyroidism.[88]

Radioactive iodine (^{131}I or ^{125}I) administered for thyroid ablation or for diagnostic studies is not concentrated by the fetal thyroid until after 12 weeks of pregnancy.[89] Thus, with inadvertent exposure before 12 weeks there is no specific risk to the fetal thyroid from ^{131}I or ^{125}I administration.

The need for thyroxine increases in many women with primary hypothyroidism when they are pregnant, as reflected by an increase in serum thyroid-stimulating hormone (TSH) concentrations.[90,91] Because hypothyroidism in pregnancy may adversely affect the fetus,[93] possibly by increasing prematurity,[94] it is prudent to monitor thyroid function throughout pregnancy and to adjust the thyroid dose to maintain a normal TSH level. It is recommended that women with hypothyroidism increase their levothyroxine dose by approximately 30 percent as soon as pregnancy is confirmed (two doses each week) and then have dosing adjustments based on TSH levels.[91]

Topical iodine preparations are readily absorbed through the vagina during pregnancy, and transient hypothyroidism has been demonstrated in the newborn after exposure during labor.[95]

DIGOXIN (LANOXIN)

In 194 exposures, no teratogenicity of digoxin was noted.[96,97] Blood levels should be monitored in pregnancy to ensure adequate therapeutic maternal levels.

Digoxin-like immunoreactive substances may be mistaken in assays for fetal concentrations of digoxin. In one study of fetuses with cardiac anomalies,[98] there was no difference in the immunoreactive digoxin levels whether or not the mother had received digoxin. In hydropic fetuses, digoxin may not easily cross the placenta.[99]

ANTIHYPERTENSIVE DRUGS

α-Methyldopa (Aldomet) has been widely used for the treatment of chronic hypertension in pregnancy. Although postural hypotension may occur, no unusual fetal effects have been noted. Hydralazine (Apresoline) is used frequently in pregnancy, and no teratogenic effect has been observed (see also Chapter 33).

SYMPATHETIC BLOCKING AGENTS

Propranolol (Inderal) is a β-adrenergic blocking agent in widespread use for various indications. Theoretically, propranolol might increase uterine contractility. However, this has not been reported, presumably because the drug is not specific for uterine β_2-receptors. No evidence of teratogenicity has been found. Bradycardia has been reported in the newborn as a direct effect of a dose of the drug given to the mother within 2 hours of delivery.[100]

Several studies of propranolol use in pregnancy show an increased risk of intrauterine growth restriction or at least a skewing of the birth-weight distribution toward the lower range.[101] Ultrasound monitoring of exposed patients is prudent. Studies from Scotland suggest improved outcome with the use of atenolol (Tenormin) to treat chronic hypertension during pregnancy.[102]

ANGIOTENSIN-CONVERTING ENZYME INHIBITORS

Angiotensin-converting enzyme (ACE) inhibitors (e.g., enalapril [Vasotec], captopril [Capoten]) can cause fetal renal tubular dysplasia in the second and third trimesters, leading to oligohydramnios, fetal limb contractures, craniofacial deformities, and hypoplastic lung development.[102] Fetal skull ossification defects have also been described.[104] Fetal exposure in the first trimester is associated with an increased risk of birth defects.[104a] For these reasons, pregnant women on these medications should be switched to other agents.

ANTINEOPLASTIC DRUGS AND IMMUNOSUPPRESSANTS

Methotrexate, a folic acid antagonist, appears to be a human teratogen, although experience is limited. Infants of three women known to receive methotrexate in the first trimester of pregnancy had multiple congenital anomalies, including cranial defects and malformed extremities.[105] Eight normal infants were delivered to seven women treated with methotrexate in combination with other agents after the first trimester. When low-dose oral methotrexate (7.5 mg/week) was used for rheumatoid disease in the first trimester, five full-term infants were normal and three patients experienced spontaneous abortions.[81]

Azathioprine (Imuran) has been used by patients with renal transplants or systemic lupus erythematosus. The frequency of anomalies in 375 total women treated in the first trimester was not increased.[107] Some infants had leukopenia, some were small for gestational age, and the others were normal.

No increased risk of anomalies in fetuses exposed to cyclosporine (Sandimmune) in utero has been reported.[108] An increased rate of prematurity and growth restriction has been noted, but it is difficult to separate the contributions of the underlying disease and the drugs given to these transplant patients. The B-cell line may be depleted more than the T-cell line, and one author recommends that infants exposed to immunosuppressive agents be followed for possible immunodeficiency.[109]

Eight malformed infants have resulted from first-trimester exposure to cyclophosphamide (Cytoxan), but these infants were also exposed to other drugs or radiation.[110] Low birth weight may be associated with use after the first trimester, but this may also reflect the underlying medical problem.

Chloroquine (Aralen) is safe in doses used for malarial prophylaxis, and there was no increased incidence of birth defects among 169 infants exposed to 300 mg once weekly.[111] However, after exposure to larger anti-inflammatory doses (250 to 500 mg/day), two cases of cochleovestibular paresis were reported.[112] No abnormalities were noted in 114 other infants.[113]

When cancer chemotherapy must be used during embryogenesis, there is an increased rate of spontaneous abortion and major birth defects. Later in pregnancy, there is a greater risk of stillbirth and intrauterine growth restriction, and myelosuppression is often present in the infant.[114]

ANTIASTHMATICS

TERBUTALINE (BRETHINE)

Terbutaline has been widely used in the treatment of preterm labor (see Chapter 26). It is more rapid in onset, has a longer duration of action than epinephrine, and is preferred for asthma in the pregnant patient. No risk of birth defects has been reported. Long-term use has been associated with an increased risk of glucose intolerance.[115]

CROMOLYN SODIUM (INTAL)

Cromolyn sodium may be administered in pregnancy, and the systemic absorption is minimal. Teratogenicity has not been reported in humans.[116]

ISOPROTERENOL (ISUPREL) AND METAPROTERENOL (ALUPENT)

When isoproterenol and metaproterenol are given as topical aerosols for the treatment of asthma, the total dose absorbed is usually not significant. With oral or intravenous doses, however, the cardiovascular effects of the agents may result in decreased uterine blood flow. For this reason, they should be used with caution. No teratogenicity has been reported.[117]

CORTICOSTEROIDS

All steroids cross the placenta to some degree, but prednisone (Deltasone) and prednisolone are inactivated by the placenta. When prednisone or prednisolone is maternally administered, the concentration of active compound in the fetus is less than 10 percent of that in the mother. Therefore, these agents are the drugs of choice for treating medical diseases such as asthma. Inhaled corticosteroids are also effective therapy, and very little drug is absorbed. When steroid effects are desired in the fetus to accelerate lung maturity, betamethasone (Celestone) and dexamethasone (Decadron) are preferred, because these are minimally inactivated by the placenta. Corticosteroids may increase the risk of cleft lip and cleft palate threefold perhaps from 1/1000 to 3/1000.[118,119]

IODIDE

Iodide such as found in a saturated solution of potassium iodide (SSKI) expectorant crosses the placenta and may produce a fetal goiter large enough to produce respiratory obstruction in the newborn (Fig. 8-7).[89] Before a pregnant patient is advised to take a cough medicine, one should be sure to ascertain that it does not contain iodide.

ANTIEMETICS

Remedies suggested to help nausea and vomiting in pregnancy without pharmacologic intervention include eating crackers at the bedside on first awakening in the morning (before getting out of bed), getting up very slowly, omitting iron tablets, consuming frequent small meals, and eating protein snacks at night. Faced with a self-limited condition occurring at the time of organogenesis, the clinician is well advised to avoid the use of medications whenever possible and to encourage these supportive measures initially.

VITAMIN B_6

Vitamin B_6 (pyridoxine) 25 mg three times a day has been reported in two randomized placebo-controlled trials to be effective for treating the nausea and vomiting of pregnancy.[120,121] In several other controlled trials, there was no evidence of teratogenicity.

DOXYLAMINE

Doxylamine (Unisom Sleeptabs) is an effective antihistamine for nausea in pregnancy and can be combined with vitamin B_6 to produce a therapy similar to the former preparation Bendectin. Vitamin B_6 (50 mg) and doxylamine (25 mg) at bedtime, and one-half of each tablet in the morning and afternoon, is an effective combination.

MECLIZINE (BONINE)

In one randomized, placebo-controlled study, meclizine gave significantly better results than placebo.[122] Prospective clinical studies have provided no evidence that meclizine is teratogenic in humans.[123] In 1,014 patients in the Collaborative Perinatal Project[96] and an additional 613 patients from the Kaiser Health Plan,[124] no teratogenic risk was found.

DIMENHYDRINATE (DRAMAMINE)

No teratogenicity has been noted with dimenhydrinate, but a 29 percent failure rate and a significant incidence of side effects, especially drowsiness, has been reported.[125]

DIPHENHYDRAMINE (BENADRYL)

In 595 patients treated in the Collaborative Perinatal Project, no teratogenicity was noted with diphenhydramine.[126] Drowsiness can be a problem.

PHENOTHIAZINES

Because of the potential for severe side effects, the phenothiazines have not been used routinely in the treatment of mild or moderate nausea and vomiting but have been reserved for the treatment of hyperemesis gravidarum.

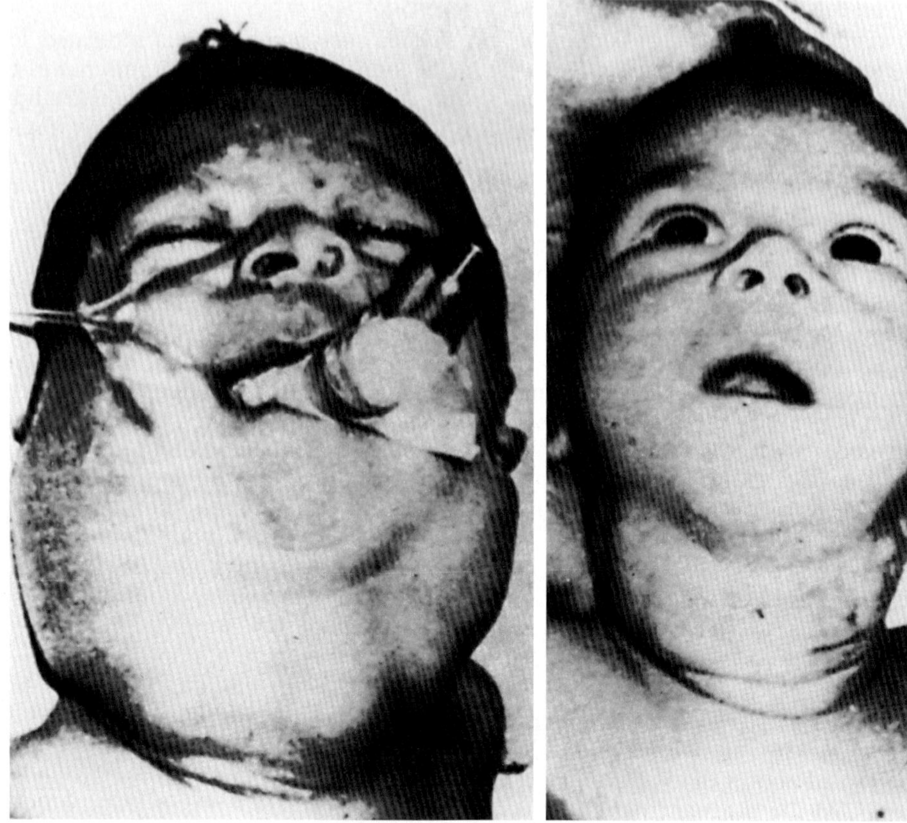

Figure 8-7. Iodide-induced neonatal goiter. *A*, Appearance on the first day of life. *B*, Appearance at 2 months of age. (From Senior B, Chernoff HL: Iodide goiter in the newborn. Pediatrics 47:510, 1971, with permission.)

Chlorpromazine (Thorazine) has been shown to be effective in hyperemesis gravidarum, with the most important side effect being drowsiness.

Teratogenicity does not appear to be a problem with the phenothiazines when evaluated as a group. In the Kaiser Health Plan Study,[124] 976 patients were treated, and in the Collaborative Perinatal Project[96] 1,309 patients were treated; in both studies no evidence of association between these drugs and malformations was noted. In 114 mothers treated with promethazine[128] (Phenergan) and in 877 mothers given prochlorperazine (Compazine),[129] no increased risk of malformations was found.

Ondansetron (Zofran)

Ondansetron is no more effective than promethazine (Phenergan), but less sedating.[130] Ondansetron is considerably more costly, and has not been evaluated in large numbers of patients for teratogenicity.

Methylprednisolone

Forty patients with hyperemesis who were admitted to the hospital were randomized to oral methylprednisolone or oral promethazine, and methylprednisolone was more effective.[131] In a larger study in which all patients received promethazine and metoclopramide as well, methylprednisolone did not reduce the need for rehospitalization.[132] The drug should be used only after 10 weeks of pregnancy due to the potential risk of cleft lip and cleft palate.[118,119]

Ginger

Ginger has been used with success for treating hyperemesis,[133] and nausea and vomiting in the outpatient setting.[134] A significantly greater relief of symptoms was found after ginger treatment than with placebo. Patients took 250-mg capsules containing ginger as powdered root four times a day.

Acid-Suppressing Drugs

The use of cimetidine, omeprazole, and ranitidine has not been found to be associated with any teratogenic risk in 2,261 exposures.[135]

Antihistamines and Decongestants

No increased risk of anomalies has been associated with most of the commonly used antihistamines, such as chlorpheniramine (Chlor-Trimeton).[96,97] However, several reports of note are presented in the following section.

Terfenadine (Seldane) has been associated in one study with an increased risk of polydactyly.[136] Astemizole (Hismanal) did not increase the risk of birth defects in 114 infants exposed in the first trimester.[137]

An association between exposure to antihistamines during the last 2 weeks of pregnancy and retrolental fibroplasia in premature infants has been reported.[138]

In the Collaborative Perinatal Project,[96] an increased risk of birth defects was noted with phenylpropanolamine (Entex LA) exposure in the first trimester. In one retrospective study, an increased risk of gastroschisis was associated with first-trimester pseudoephedrine (Sudafed) use.[139] Although these findings have not been confirmed, use of these drugs for trivial indications should be discouraged, because long-term effects are unknown. If decongestion is necessary, topical nasal sprays will result in a lower dose to the fetus than systemic medication.

Patients should be educated that antihistamines and decongestants are only symptomatic therapy for the common cold and have no influence on the course of the disease. Other remedies should be recommended, such as use of a humidifier, rest, and fluids. If medications are necessary, combinations with two drugs should not be used if only one drug is necessary. If the diagnosis is truly an allergy, an antihistamine alone will suffice.

Antibiotics and Anti-Infective Agents

Because pregnant patients are particularly susceptible to vaginal yeast infections, antibiotics should be used only when clearly indicated. Therapy with antifungal agents may be necessary during or after the course of therapy.

Penicillins

Penicillin, ampicillin, and amoxicillin (Amoxil) are safe in pregnancy. In the Collaborative Perinatal Project,[96] 3,546 mothers took penicillin derivatives in the first trimester of pregnancy, with no increased risk of anomalies. Of 86 infants exposed to dicloxacillin in the first trimester, there was no increase in birth defects.[97]

Clavulanate is added to penicillin derivatives to broaden their antibacterial spectrum. Of 556 infants exposed in the first trimester, no increased risk of birth defects was observed.[140] Amoxicillin/clavulanate was studied in randomized controlled trials as potential therapy for chorioamnionitis in women with preterm premature rupture of membranes.[141] During this trial, amoxicillin/clavulanate was compared with both placebo and erythromycin. An increased incidence of necrotizing enterocolitis was found in the amoxicillin/clavulanate group when compared with both the placebo and erythromycin groups. It has been suggested that amoxicillin/clavulanate selects for specific pathogens, which leads to abnormal microbial colonization of the gastrointestinal tract and ultimately initiation of necrotizing enterocolitis. Therefore, amoxicillin/clavulanate should be avoided in women at risk for preterm delivery.[142]

Cephalosporins

In a study of 5,000 Michigan Medicaid recipients, there was a suggestion of possible teratogenicity (25 percent increased birth defects) with cefaclor, cephalexin, and cephradine, but not other cephalosporins.[143] However, another study of 308 women exposed in the first trimester showed no increase in malformations.[144] The consensus is that these drugs are safe.

Sulfonamides

Among 1,455 human infants exposed to sulfonamides during the first trimester, no teratogenic effects were noted.[96] However, the administration of sulfonamides should be avoided in women deficient in glucose-6-phosphate dehydrogenase (G6PD), because dose-related hemolysis may occur.

Sulfonamides cause no known damage to the fetus in utero, because the fetus can clear free bilirubin through the placenta. These drugs might theoretically have deleterious effects if they are present in the blood of the neonate after birth, however. Sulfonamides compete with bilirubin for binding sites on albumin, thus raising the levels of free bilirubin in the serum and increasing the risk of hyperbilirubinemia in the neonate.[145] Although this toxicity occurs with direct administration to the neonate, kernicterus in the newborn following in utero exposure has not been reported.[146]

Sulfamethoxazole with Trimethoprim (Bactrim, Septra)

Trimethoprim is often given with sulfa to treat urinary tract infections. However, one unpublished study of 2,296 Michigan Medicaid recipients suggested an increased risk of cardiovascular defects after exposure in the first trimester.[147] In one retrospective study of trimethoprim with sulfamethoxazole, the odds ratio for birth defects was 2.3,[148] whereas in another study it was 2.5 to 3.4.[149]

Nitrofurantoin (Macrodantin)

Nitrofurantoin is used in the treatment of acute uncomplicated lower urinary tract infections as well as for long-term suppression in patients with chronic bacteriuria. Nitrofurantoin is capable of inducing hemolytic anemia in patients deficient in G6PD. However, hemolytic anemia in the newborn as a result of in utero exposure to nitrofurantoin has not been reported.

No reports have associated nitrofurantoins with congenital defects. In the Collaborative Perinatal Project,[96] 590 infants were exposed, 83 in the first trimester, with no increased risk of adverse effects. Other studies have confirmed these findings.[150,151]

Tetracyclines

Tetracyclines readily cross the placenta and are firmly bound by chelation to calcium in developing bone and tooth structures. This produces brown discoloration of the deciduous teeth, hypoplasia of the enamel, and inhibition of bone growth.[152] The staining of the teeth takes place in the second or third trimesters of pregnancy, whereas bone incorporation can occur earlier. Depression of skeletal growth was particularly common among premature infants treated with tetracycline. First-trimester exposure to doxycycline is not known to carry any risk.[153] First-trimester exposure to tetracyclines has not been found to have any teratogenic risk in 341 women in the Collaborative Perinatal Project[96] or in 174 women in another study.[97] Overall, alternate antibiotics are currently recommended during pregnancy.

Aminoglycosides

Streptomycin and kanamycin have been associated with congenital deafness in the offspring of mothers who took these drugs during pregnancy. Ototoxicity was reported with doses as low as 1 g of streptomycin twice a week for 8 weeks during the first trimester.[154] Of 391 mothers who had received 50 mg/kg of kanamycin for prolonged periods during pregnancy, nine children (2.3 percent) were found to have hearing loss.[155]

Nephrotoxicity may be greater when aminoglycosides are combined with cephalosporins. Neuromuscular blockade may be potentiated by the combined use of aminoglycosides and curariform drugs. Potentiation of magnesium sulfate–induced neuromuscular weakness has also been reported in a neonate exposed to magnesium sulfate and gentamicin.[156]

No known teratogenic effect other than ototoxicity has been associated with aminoglycosides in the first trimester. In 135 infants exposed to streptomycin in the Collaborative Perinatal Project,[96] no teratogenic effects were observed. Among 1,619 newborns whose mothers were treated for tuberculosis with multiple drugs, including streptomycin, the incidence of congenital defects was the same as in a healthy control group.[157]

Antituberculosis Drugs

There is no evidence of any teratogenic effect of isoniazid, para-aminosalicylic acid, rifampin (Rifadin), or ethambutol (Myambutol).

Erythromycin

No teratogenic risk of erythromycin has been reported. In 79 patients in the Collaborative Perinatal Project[96] and 260 in another study,[97] no increase in birth defects was noted.

Clarithromycin

Of 122 first-trimester exposures, there was no significant risk of birth defects.[158]

Fluoroquinolones

The quinolones (e.g., ciprofloxacin [Cipro], norfloxacin [Noraxin]) have a high affinity for bone tissue and cartilage, and may cause arthralgia in children. However, no malformations or musculoskeletal problems were noted in 38 infants exposed in utero in the first trimester,[159] in 132 newborns exposed in the first trimester in the Michigan Medicaid data,[160] or in 200 other first trimester exposures.[161]

Metronidazole (Flagyl)

Studies have failed to show any increase in the incidence of congenital defects among the newborns of mothers treated with metronidazole during early or late gestation. Among 1,387 prescriptions filled, no increase in birth defects could be determined.[162] A meta-analysis confirmed lack of teratogenic risk.[163]

Acyclovir (Zovirax)

The Acyclovir Registry has recorded 756 first-trimester exposures, with no increased risk of abnormalities in the infants. The Centers for Disease Control and Prevention recommends that pregnant women with disseminated infection (e.g., herpetic encephalitis or hepatitis or varicella pneumonia) be treated with acyclovir.[165]

Lindane (Kwell)

After application of lindane to the skin, about 10 percent of the dose used can be recovered in the urine. Toxicity in humans after use of topical 1 percent lindane has been observed almost exclusively after misuse and overexposure to the agent. Although no evidence of specific fetal damage is attributable to lindane, the agent is a potent neurotoxin, and its use during pregnancy should be limited. Pregnant women should be cautioned about shampooing their children's hair, because absorption could easily occur across the skin of the hands of the mother. An alternate drug for lice is usually recommended, such as pyrethrins with piperonyl butoxide (RID).

Antiretroviral Agents

Zidovudine (ZDV) should be included as a component in the antiretroviral regimen whenever possible because of its record of safety and efficacy. In a prospective cohort study, children exposed to ZDV in the perinatal period through Pediatric AIDS Clinical Trials Group Protocol 076 were studied up to a median age of 4.2 years. No adverse effects were observed in these children.[166] The International Antiretroviral Registry was established in 1989 to detect any major teratogenic effect of the antiretroviral drugs. Through January 2004, more than 1,000 pregnancies had first-trimester exposures to ZDV and lamivudine, and no increase in teratogenity was reported.[167]

Concerns have been raised regarding use of other antiretroviral therapies. Efavirenz is not recommended during pregnancy due to reports of significant malformations in monkeys receiving efavirenz during the first trimester and also three case reports of fetal NTDs in women who received the drug.[168] In 2001, Bristol-Myers Squibb issued a warning advising against the use of didanosine and stavudine in pregnant women due to case reports of lactic acidosis, some of which were fatal.[169] These two drugs should only be used if no other alternatives are available.

Antifungal Agents

Nystatin (Mycostatin) is poorly absorbed from intact skin and mucous membranes, and topical use has not been associated with teratogenesis.[97] Clotrimazole (Lotrimin) or miconazole (Monistat) in pregnancy is not known to be associated with congenital malformations. However, in one study, a statistically significantly increased risk of first-trimester abortion was noted after use of these drugs, but these findings were considered not to be definitive evidence of risk.[170] Of 2,092 newborns exposed in the first trimester in the Michigan Medicaid data, there was no increased risk of anomalies.[171]

Limb deformities were reported in three infants exposed to 400 to 800 mg/day of fluconazole in the first trimester.[172] However, in systematic studies of 460 who received a single 150-mg dose of fluconazole, no increased risk of defects was observed.[173,174]

DRUGS FOR INDUCTION OF OVULATION

In more than 2,000 exposures, no evidence of teratogenic risk of clomiphene (Clomid) has been noted,[175] and the percentage of spontaneous abortions is close to the expected rate. Although infants are often exposed to bromocriptine (Parlodel) in early pregnancy, no teratogenic effects have been observed in more than 1,400 pregnancies.[176]

MILD ANALGESICS

Few pains during pregnancy justify the use of a mild analgesic. Pregnant patients should be encouraged to use nonpharmacologic remedies, such as local heat and rest.

ASPIRIN

There is no evidence of any teratogenic effect of aspirin taken in the first trimester.[96,177] Aspirin does have significant perinatal effects, however, because it inhibits prostaglandin synthesis. Uterine contractility is decreased, and patients taking aspirin in analgesic doses have delayed onset of labor, longer duration of labor, and an increased risk of a prolonged pregnancy.[178]

Aspirin also decreases platelet aggregation, which can increase the risk of bleeding before as well as at delivery. Platelet dysfunction has been described in newborns within 5 days of ingestion of aspirin by the mother.[179] Because aspirin causes permanent inhibition of prostaglandin synthetase in platelets, the only way for adequate clotting to occur is for more platelets to be produced.

Multiple organs may be affected by chronic aspirin use. Of note, prostaglandins mediate the neonatal closure of the ductus arteriosus. In one case report, maternal ingestion of aspirin close to the time of delivery was related to closure of the ductus arteriosus in utero.[180]

ACETAMINOPHEN (TYLENOL, DATRIL)

Acetaminophen has also shown no evidence of teratogenicity.[181] With acetaminophen, inhibition of prostaglandin synthesis is reversible; thus, once the drug has cleared, platelet aggregation returns to normal. Bleeding time is not prolonged with acetaminophen in contrast to aspirin,[182] and the drug is not toxic to the newborn. Thus, if a mild analgesic or antipyretic is indicated, acetaminophen is preferred over aspirin.

OTHER NONSTEROIDAL ANTI-INFLAMMATORY AGENTS

No evidence of teratogenicity has been reported for other nonsteroidal anti-inflammatory drugs (e.g., ibuprofen[183] [Motrin, Advil], naproxen[184] [Naprosyn]), but limited information is available. Chronic use may lead to oligohydramnios, and constriction of the fetal ductus arteriosus or neonatal pulmonary hypertension as has been reported with indomethacin might occur.

PROPOXYPHENE (DARVON)

Propoxyphene is an acceptable alternative mild analgesic with no known teratogenicity.[96] However, it should not be used for trivial indications, because it carries potential for narcotic addiction. Evidence of risk in late pregnancy comes from case reports of infants of mothers who were addicted to propoxyphene and had typical narcotic withdrawal in the neonatal period.[185]

CODEINE

In the Collaborative Perinatal Project, no increased relative risk of malformations was observed in 563 codeine users.[96] Codeine can cause addiction and newborn withdrawal symptoms if used to excess perinatally.

SUMATRIPTAN

Of 264 exposures in the first trimester,[186] seven infants (3.8 percent) had birth defects. This percentage is not significantly different from the nonexposed population.

DRUGS OF ABUSE (see Chapter 50)

Smoking

It is not simple to sort out potential confounding factors when comparing smokers with nonsmokers. However, smoking is associated with a fourfold increase in small size for gestational age as well as an increased prematurity rate.[187] The higher perinatal mortality rate associated with smoking is attributable to an increased risk of abruptio placentae, placenta previa, premature and prolonged rupture of membranes, and intrauterine growth restriction. The risks of complications and of the associated perinatal loss rise with the number of cigarettes smoked. Discontinuation of smoking during pregnancy can reduce the risk of both pregnancy complications and perinatal mortality, especially in women at high risk for other reasons.[189] Maternal passive smoking was also associated with a twofold risk of low birth weight at term in one study.[190]

There is also a positive association between smoking and sudden infant death syndrome (SIDS) and increased respiratory illnesses in children. In such reports, it is not possible to distinguish between apparent effects of maternal smoking during pregnancy and smoking after pregnancy, but both may play a role.

The spontaneous abortion rate may be up to twice that of nonsmokers, and abortions associated with maternal smoking tend to have a higher percentage of normal karyotypes and occur later than those with chromosomal aberrations[188] (see Chapter 24).

Smoking Cessation During Pregnancy

Tobacco smoke contains nicotine, carbon monoxide, and thousands of other compounds. Although nicotine is the mechanism of addiction to cigarettes, other chemicals may contribute to adverse pregnancy outcome. For example, carbon monoxide decreases oxygen delivery to the fetus, whereas nicotine decreases uterine blood flow.

Nicotine withdrawal may first be attempted with nicotine fading, switching to brands of cigarettes with progressively less nicotine over a 3-week period. Exercise may also improve quitting success rates.[191] Nicotine medications are indicated for patients with nicotine dependence. This is defined as smoking greater than one pack per day, smoking within 30 minutes of getting up in the morning, or prior withdrawal symptoms.[192] Nicotine medications are available as patches, gum, or inhalers. Although one might question the propriety of prescribing nicotine during pregnancy, cessation of smoking eliminates many other toxins, including carbon monoxide; nicotine blood levels are not increased over that of smokers.[193]

Congenital anomalies occurred in five of 188 infants of women treated with bupropion (Zyban) during the first trimester of pregnancy, not a significant difference from the number expected.[194]

Alcohol

FAS has been reported in the offspring of alcoholic mothers and includes the features of gross physical retardation with onset prenatally and continuing after birth (Fig. 8-8).[195]

In 1980, the Fetal Alcohol Study Group of the Research Society on Alcoholism proposed criteria for the diagnosis of FAS.[196] At least one characteristic from each of the following three categories had to be present for a valid diagnosis of the syndrome:

1. Growth retardation before and/or after birth
2. Facial anomalies, including small palpebral fissures, indistinct or absent philtrum, epicanthic folds, flattened nasal bridge, short length of nose, thin upper lip, low-set, unparallel ears, and retarded midfacial development
3. Central nervous system dysfunction including microcephaly, varying degrees of mental retardation, or other evidence of abnormal neurobehavioral development, such as attention deficit disorder with hyperactivity.

The full FAS occurs in 6 percent of infants[197] of heavy drinkers, and less severe birth defects and neurocognitive deficits occur in a larger proportion of children whose mothers drink heavily during pregnancy.

Jones et al.,[198] compared 23 chronically alcoholic women with 46 controls and compared the pregnancy outcomes of the two groups. Among the alcoholic mothers, perinatal deaths were about eight times more frequent. Growth restriction, microcephaly, and IQ below 80 were considerably more frequent than among the controls. Overall outcome was abnormal in 43 percent of the offspring of the alcoholic mothers compared with 2 percent of the controls.

Ouellette et al.[199] addressed the risks of smaller amounts of alcohol. Nine percent of infants of abstinent or rare drinkers and 14 percent of infants of moderate drinkers were abnormal, not a significant difference. In heavy drinkers (average daily intake of 3 oz of 100-proof liquor or more), 32 percent of the infants had anomalies. The aggregate pool of anomalies, growth restriction, and an abnormal neurologic examination were found in 71 percent of the children of heavy drinkers, twice the frequency in the moderate and rarely drinking groups. In this study, an increased frequency of abnormality was not found until 45 ml of ethanol (equivalent to three drinks) daily were exceeded. The study of Mills and Graubard[200] also showed that total malformation rates were not significantly higher among offspring of women who had

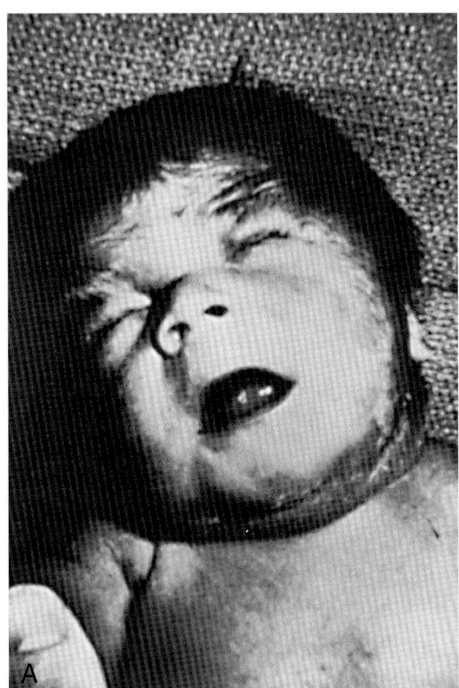

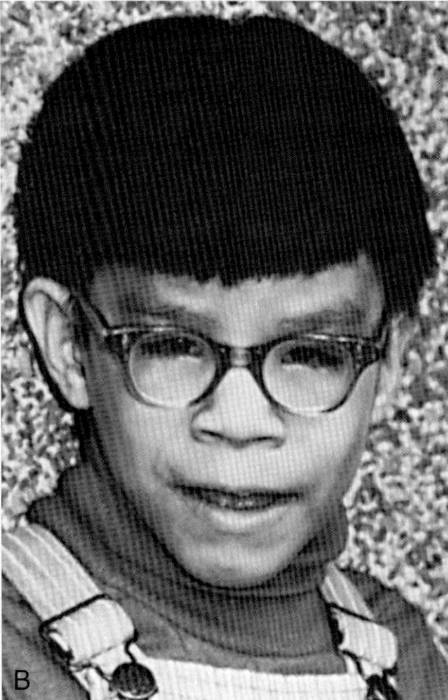

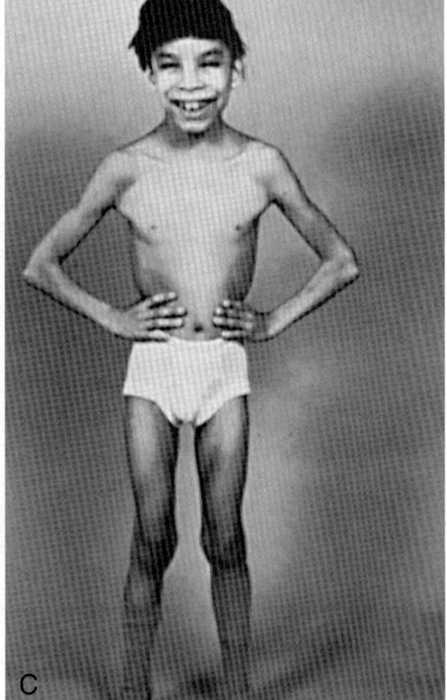

Figure 8-8. Fetal alcohol syndrome. Patient photographed at (*A*) birth, (*B*) 5 years, and (*C*) 8 years. Note short palpebral fissures, short nose, hypoplastic philtrum, thinned upper lip vermilion, and flattened midface. (From Streissguth AP: CIBA Foundation Monograph 105. London, Pitman, 1984, with permission.)

Table 8-2. The T-ACE Questions Found to Identify Women Drinking Sufficiently to Potentially Damage the Fetus*

T	How many drinks does it take to make you feel high (can you hold) (*tolerance*)?
A	Have people *annoyed* you by criticizing your drinking?
C	Have you felt you ought to *cut down* on your drinking?
E	Have you ever had to drink first thing in the morning to steady your nerves or to get rid of a hangover (*eye-opener*)?

*Two points are scored as a positive answer to the tolerance question and one each for the other three. A score of 2 or more correctly identified 69 percent of risk drinkers.

From Sokol RJ, Martier SS, Ager JW: The T-ACE questions: practical prenatal detection of risk-drinking. Am J Obstet Gynecol 160:863, 1989, with permission.

an average of less than one drink per day or one to two drinks per day, than among nondrinkers. Genitourinary malformations increased with increasing alcohol consumption, however, so the possibility remains that for some malformations no safe drinking level exists.

Heavy drinking remains a major risk to the fetus, and reduction even in midpregnancy can benefit the infant. An occasional drink during pregnancy carries no documentable risk, but no level of drinking is known to be safe.

Sokol et al.[201] have addressed history taking for prenatal detection of risk drinking. Four questions help differentiate patients drinking sufficiently to potentially damage the fetus (Table 8-2). The patient is considered at risk if more than two drinks are required to make her feel "high." The probability of "risk drinking" increases to 63 percent for those responding positively to all four questions.

Marijuana

No significant teratogenic effect of marijuana has been documented,[202] but the data are insufficient to say that there is no risk. One study finding a mean 73-g decrease in birth weight associated with marijuana use validated exposure with urine assays rather than relying on self-reporting.[203] Other studies have not shown an effect on birth weight or length.[204,205] Behavioral and developmental alterations have been observed in some studies but not in others.

Cocaine

A serious difficulty in defining the effects of cocaine on the infant is the frequent presence of many confounding variables in the population using cocaine. These mothers often abuse other drugs, smoke, have poor nutrition, fail to seek prenatal care, and live under poor socioeconomic conditions. All of these factors are difficult to take into account in comparison groups. Another difficulty is the choice of outcome measures for infants exposed in utero. The neural systems likely to be affected by cocaine are involved in neurologic and behavioral functions that are not easily quantitated by standard infant development tests.

Cocaine-using women have a higher rate of spontaneous abortion than controls.[206] Three other studies suggested an increased risk of congenital anomalies after first-trimester cocaine use,[207-209] most frequently cardiac and central nervous system. In the study of Bingol et al.,[208] the malformation rate was 10 percent in cocaine users, 4.5 percent in "polydrug users," and 2 percent in controls. MacGregor et al.[209] reported a 6-percent anomaly rate compared with 1 percent for controls.

Cocaine is a central nervous system stimulant and has local anesthetic and marked vasoconstrictive effects. Not surprisingly, abruptio placentae has been reported to occur immediately after nasal or intravenous administration.[206] Several studies have also noted increased stillbirths, preterm labor, premature birth, and small-for-gestational-age infants with cocaine use.[203,206,207,210,211]

The most common brain abnormality in infants exposed to cocaine in utero is impairment of intrauterine brain growth as manifested by microcephaly.[212] In one study, 16 percent of newborns had microcephaly compared with 6 percent of controls.[213] Somatic growth is also impaired, and so the growth restriction may be symmetric or characterized by a relatively low head circumference/abdominal circumference ratio.[214] Multiple other neurologic problems have been reported after cocaine exposure, as well as dysmorphic features and neurobehavioral abnormalities.[211]

Aside from causing congenital anomalies in the first trimester, cocaine has been reported to cause fetal disruption,[215] presumably due to interruption of blood flow to various organs. Bowel infarction has been noted with unusual ileal atresia and bowel perforation. Limb infarction has resulted in missing fingers in a distribution different from the usual congenital limb anomalies. Central nervous system bleeding in utero may result in porencephalic cysts.

Narcotics and Methadone

Menstrual abnormalities, especially amenorrhea, are common in heroin abusers, although they are not associated with the use of methadone. Medical intervention is more likely to involve methadone maintenance, with the goal being a dose of approximately 20 to 40 mg/day. The dose should be individualized at a level sufficient to minimize the use of supplemental illicit drugs, which represent greater risk to the fetus than even the higher doses of methadone required by some patients. Manipulation of the dose in women maintained on methadone should be avoided in the last trimester because of an association with increased fetal complications and in utero deaths attributed to fetal withdrawal in utero.[216] Because management of narcotic addiction during pregnancy requires a host of social, nutritional, educational, and psychiatric interventions, these patients are best managed in specialized programs.

The pregnancy of the narcotic addict is at increased risk for abortion, prematurity, and growth restriction. Withdrawal should be watched for carefully in the neonatal period.[217]

Caffeine

There is no evidence of teratogenic effects of caffeine in humans. The Collaborative Perinatal Project[96] showed no increased incidence of congenital defects in 5,773 women taking caffeine in pregnancy, usually in a fixed-dose analgesic medication. The average cup of coffee contains about 100 mg and a 12 oz can of soda contains about 50 mg of caffeine. Some conflicting evidence exists concerning the association between heavy ingestion of caffeine and increased pregnancy complications. Early studies suggested that the intake of greater than seven to eight cups of coffee per day was associated with low-birth-weight infants, spontaneous abortions, prematurity, and stillbirths.[218] However, these studies were not controlled for the concomitant use of tobacco and alcohol. In one report that controlled for smoking, other habits, demographic characteristics, and medical history, no relationship was found between malformations, low birth weight, or short gestation and heavy coffee consumption.[219] Also, there was no excess of malformations among coffee drinkers. When pregnant women consumed more than 300 mg of caffeine per day, one study suggested an increase in term low-birth-weight infants,[220] less than 2,500 g at greater than 36 weeks.

Concomitant consumption of caffeine with cigarette smoking may increase the risk of low birth weight.[221] Maternal coffee intake decreases iron absorption and may contribute to maternal anemia.[222]

Two other studies have shown conflicting results. One retrospective investigation reporting a higher risk of fetal loss was biased by ascertainment of the patients at the time of fetal loss, because these patients typically have less nausea and would be expected to drink more coffee.[223] A prospective cohort study found no evidence that moderate caffeine use increased the risk of spontaneous abortion or growth restriction.[224] Measurement of serum paraxanthine, a caffeine metabolite, revealed that only extremely high levels are associated with spontaneous abortions.[225]

Thus, up to 300 mg caffeine intake per day can be considered safe in pregnancy.

Aspartame (Nutrasweet)

The major metabolite of aspartame is phenylalanine,[226] which is concentrated in the fetus by active placental transport. Sustained high blood levels of phenylalanine in the fetus as seen in maternal phenylketonuria are associated with mental retardation in the infant. However, within the usual range of aspartame ingestion in normal individuals, peak phenylalanine levels do not exceed normal postprandial levels, and even with high doses, phenylalanine concentrations are still very far below those associated with mental retardation. These responses have also been studied in women who are obligate carriers of phenylketonuria,[227] and their levels are still normal. Thus, it seems unlikely that aspartame during pregnancy would cause any fetal toxicity.

DRUGS IN BREAST MILK

Many drugs can be detected in breast milk at low levels that are not usually of clinical significance to the infant. The rate of transfer into milk depends on the lipid solubility, molecular weight, degree of protein binding, degree of ionization of the drug, and the presence or absence of active secretion. Nonionized molecules of low molecular weight such as ethanol cross easily.[227] If the mother has unusually high blood concentrations such as with increased dosage or decreased renal function, drugs may appear in higher concentrations in the milk.

The amount of drug in breast milk is a variable fraction of the maternal blood level, which itself is proportional to the maternal oral dose. Thus, the dose to the infant is usually subtherapeutic, approximately 1 to 2 percent of the maternal dose on the average. This amount is usually so trivial that no adverse effects are noted. In the case of toxic drugs, however, any exposure may be inappropriate. Allergy may also exist or be initiated. Long-term effects of even small doses of drugs may yet be discovered. Also, drugs are eliminated more slowly in the infant with immature enzyme systems. Short-term effects of most maternal medications on breast-fed infants are mild and pose little risk to the infants. As the benefits of breast-feeding are well known, the risk of drug exposure must be weighed against these benefits.

With respect to drug administration in the immediate few days postpartum before lactation is fully established, the infant receives only a small volume of colostrum; thus, little drug is excreted into the milk. It is also helpful to allay fears of patients undergoing cesarean deliveries that analgesics or other drugs administered at this time have no known adverse effects on the infant. For drugs requiring daily dosing during lactation, knowledge of pharmacokinetics in breast milk may minimize the dose to the infant. For example, dosing immediately after nursing decreases the neonatal exposure, because the blood level will be at it nadir just before the next dose.

Short-term effects, if any, of most maternal medications on breast-fed infants are mild and pose little risk to the infants.[228] Of 838 breast-feeding women, 11.2 percent reported minor infant adverse reactions in the infants, but these reactions did not require medical attention. In 19 percent, antibiotics caused diarrhea; in 11 percent, narcotics caused drowsiness; in 9 percent, antihistamines caused irritability; and in 10 percent, sedatives, antidepressants, or antiepileptics caused drowsiness.[228]

The American Academy of Pediatrics has reviewed drugs in lactation[229] and categorized the drugs as listed below in six categories:

Drugs Commonly Listed as Contraindicated During Breast-Feeding

Cytotoxic Drugs that May Interfere with Cellular Metabolism of the Nursing Infant

Cyclosporine (Sandimmune), doxorubicin (Adriamycin), and cyclophosphamide (Cytoxan) might cause immune suppression in the infant, although data are limited with respect to these drugs. In general, the potential risks of these drugs would outweigh the benefits of continuing nursing.[229]

After oral administration to a lactating patient with choriocarcinoma, methotrexate was found in milk in low but detectable levels. Most individuals would elect to avoid any exposure of the infant to this drug. However, in environments in which bottle feeding is rarely practiced or presents practical and cultural difficulties, therapy with this drug would not in itself appear to constitute a contraindication to breast-feeding.[230]

Drugs of Abuse for which Adverse Effects on the Infant During Breast-Feeding Have Been Reported

Drugs of abuse such as amphetamines, cocaine, heroin, marijuana, and phencyclidine are all contraindicated during breast-feeding because they are hazardous to the nursing infant and to the health of the mother.[229]

Radioactive Compounds that Require Temporary Cessation of Breast-Feeding

The American Academy of Pediatrics[229] suggests consultation with a nuclear medicine physician so that the radionuclide with the shortest excretion time in breast milk be used. The mother can attempt to store breast milk before the study. She should continue to pump to maintain milk production but discard the milk during therapy. Radiopharmaceuticals require variable intervals of interruption of nursing. Recommended intervals are as follows:

1. Gallium-67, 2 weeks.
2. ^{131}I, 2 to 14 days
3. Radioactive sodium, 4 days.
4. Technetium-99, 15 hours to 3 days.

The physician may reassure the patient by counting the radioactivity of the milk before nursing is resumed.

Drugs for which the Effect on Nursing Infants Is Unknown But May Be of Concern

The category includes several classes of psychotrophic drugs, amiodarone (associated with hypothyroidism), lamotrigine (potential for therapeutic serum concentration in the infant), metoclopramide (potential dopaminergic blocking, but no reported detrimental effects), and metronidazole.[229]

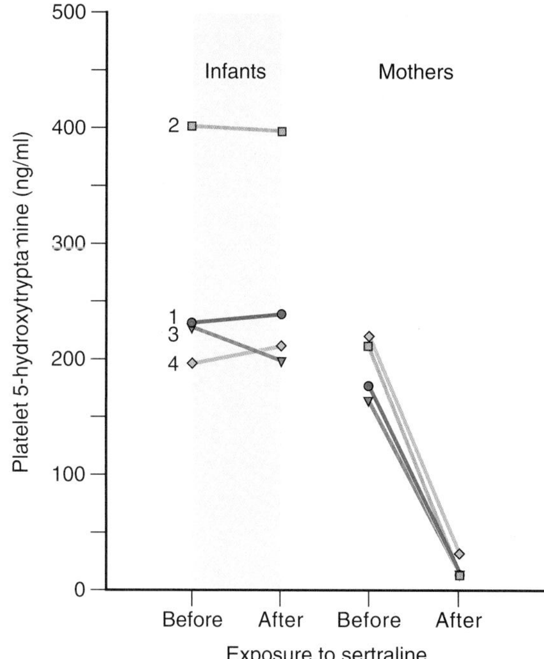

Figure 8-9. Effect of sertraline on platelet 5-hydroxytryptamine levels in four breast-fed infants and their mothers. (From Epperson CN, Anderson GM, McDougle CJ: Sertraline and breast-feeding. N Engl J Med 336:1189, 1997. Copyright 1997 Massachusetts Medical Society, with permission.)

Antianxiety, antidepressant, and antipsychotic agents are sometimes given to nursing mothers. Although there are no data about adverse effects in infants exposed to these drugs through breast milk, they could theoretically alter central nervous system function.[229] Fluoxetine (Prozac) is excreted in breast milk at low levels, so the infant receives approximately 6.7 percent of the maternal dose.[233] The level in the breast-fed newborn is certainly lower than the level during pregnancy.[234]

Sertraline causes a decline in 5-hydroxytryptamine levels in mothers, but not in their breast-fed infants.[235] This implies that the small amount of drug the infant ingests in breast milk is not enough to have a pharmacologic effect (Fig. 8-9). Infants of mothers on psychotropic drugs should be monitored for sedation during use and withdrawal after cessation of the drug.[232]

Perhaps a bigger problem is postpartum depression exacerbated by fatigue, which may be inevitable in the nursing mother. The benefits of nursing should be weighed against the negative effect on bonding resulting from refractory postpartum depression.

Temporary cessation of breast-feeding after a single dose of metronidazole (Flagyl) may be considered. Its half-life is such that interruption of lactation for 12 to 24 hours after single-dose therapy usually results in negligible exposure to the infant. However, no adverse effects in infants have been reported.

Drugs that Have Been Associated With Significant Effects In Some Nursing Infants and Should Be Given To Nursing Mothers With Caution

Bromocriptine

Bromocriptine is an ergot alkaloid derivative. Because it has an inhibitory effect on lactation, it should be avoided unless the mother has taken it during the pregnancy.

Ergotamine

Ergotamine, as used by those with migraine headache, has been associated with vomiting, diarrhea, and convulsions in the infant. Administration of an ergot alkaloid for the treatment of uterine atony does not contraindicate lactation.

Lithium

Breast milk levels of lithium are one-third to one-half maternal serum levels,[237] and the infant's serum levels while nursing are much lower than the fetal levels that occur when the mother takes lithium during pregnancy. The benefits of breast-feeding must be weighed against the theoretical effects of small amounts of the drug on the developing brain.[229] (See comment above about the need to minimize fatigue in order to mitigate against postpartum psychoses.)

Maternal Medication Usually Compatible with Breast-Feeding

Narcotics, Sedatives, and Anticonvulsants

In general, no evidence of adverse effect is noted with most of the sedatives, narcotic analgesics, and anticonvulsants. Patients may be reassured that, in normal doses, carbamazepine (Tegretol),[238] phenytoin (Dilantin),[239] magnesium sulfate, codeine, morphine, and meperidine (Demerol) do not cause any obvious adverse effects in the infants, because the dose detectable in the breast milk is approximately 1 to 2 percent of the mother's dose, which is sufficiently low to have no significant pharmacologic activity.

With diazepam (Valium), the milk/plasma ratio at peak dose is 0.68, with only small amounts detected in the breast milk.[206] In two patients who took carbamazepine (Tegretol) while nursing, the concentration of the drug in breast milk at 4 and 5 weeks postpartum was similar, about 60 percent of the maternal serum level. Accumulation does not seem to occur, and no adverse effects were noted in either infant.[240]

Cold Preparations

No harmful effects of acetaminophen (Tylenol, Datril) have been noted. Although studies are not extensive, no harmful effects have been noted from antihistamines or decongestants. Less than 1 percent of a pseudoephedrine dose or tripolidine dose ingested by the mother is excreted in the breast milk.[241]

Antihypertensives

Thiazides

After a single 500-mg oral dose of chlorothiazide (Diuril), no drug was detected in breast milk.[242] In one mother taking 50 mg of hydrochlorothiazide (HydroDiuril) daily, the drug was not detectable in the nursing infant's serum, and the infant's electrolytes were normal.[243] Thiazide diuretics may decrease milk production in the first month of lactation.[229]

β-Blockers

Propranolol (Inderal) is excreted in breast milk, with milk concentrations after a single 40-mg dose less than 40 percent of peak plasma concentrations.[244] Thus, an infant consuming 500 ml/day of milk would ingest an amount representing approximately 1 percent of a therapeutic dose, which is unlikely to cause any adverse effect.[245]

Atenolol (Tenormin) is concentrated in breast milk to about three times the plasma level.[246] One case has been reported in which a 5-day-old term infant had signs of β-adrenergic blockade with bradycardia (80 bpm) with the breast milk dose calculated to be 9 percent of the maternal dose.[247] Adverse effects in other infants have not been reported. Because milk accumulation occurs with atenolol, infants must be monitored closely for bradycardia. Propranolol is a safer alternative.[248]

Clonidine (Catapres) concentrations in milk are almost twice maternal serum levels.[249] Neurologic and laboratory parameters in the infants of treated mothers are similar to those of controls.

Angiotensin-Converting Energy Inhibitors

Captopril (Capoten) is excreted into breast milk in low levels, and no effects on nursing infants have been observed.[250]

Calcium Channel Blockers

Nifedipine is excreted into breast milk at a concentration of less than 5 percent of the maternal dose,[251] and verapamil at an even lower level. Neither have caused adverse effects in the infant.

Anticoagulants

Most mothers requiring anticoagulation may continue to nurse their infants with no problems. Heparin does not cross into milk and is not active orally.

At a maternal dose of warfarin (Coumadin) of 5 to 12 mg/day in seven patients, no warfarin was detected in infant breast milk or plasma. This low concentration is probably because warfarin is 98-percent protein bound, and the milk would contain insignificant drug to exert an anticoagulant effect.[252] Another report confirmed that warfarin appears only in insignificant quantities in breast milk.[253] The oral anticoagulant bishydroxycoumarin (dicumarol) has been given to 125 nursing mothers with no effect on the infants' prothrombin times and no hemorrhages.[254] Thus, with careful monitoring of maternal prothrombin time so that the dosage is minimized and of neonatal prothrombin times to ensure lack of drug accumulation, warfarin may be safely administered to nursing mothers.

Corticosteroids

Prednisone enters breast milk in an amount not likely to have any deleterious effect.[255] In a study of seven patients,[256] 0.14 percent of a sample was secreted in the milk in the subsequent 60 hours, a negligible quantity. Even at 80 mg/day, the nursing infant would ingest less than 0.1 percent of the dose, less than 10 percent of its endogenous cortisol.[257]

Digoxin (Lanoxin)

Digoxin enters breast milk in small amount due to significant maternal protein binding. In 24 hours, an infant would receive about 1 percent of the maternal dose.[258] No adverse effects in nursing infants have been reported.

Antibiotics

Penicillin derivatives are safe in nursing mothers. Especially at the usual therapeutic doses of penicillin or ampicillin, no adverse effects are noted in the infants. In susceptible individuals or with prolonged therapy, diarrhea and candidiasis are concerns.

Dicloxacillin is 98-percent protein bound. If this drug is used to treat breast infections, very little will get into the breast milk, and nursing may be continued.

Cephalosporins appear only in trace amounts in milk. In one study after cefazolin 500 mg intramuscularly three times a day (Ancef, Kefzol), no drug was detected in breast milk.[259] After 2 g of cefazolin intravenously, the infant was exposed less than 1 percent of the maternal dose.

Tooth staining or delayed bone growth from tetracyclines have not been reported after the drug was taken by a breast-feeding mother. This finding is probably because of the high binding of the drug to calcium and protein, limiting its absorption from the milk. The amount of free tetracycline available is too small to be significant.

Sulfonamides only appear in small amounts in breast milk and are ordinarily not contraindicated during nursing. However, the drug is best avoided in premature, ill, or stressed infants in whom hyperbilirubinemia may be a problem, becasue the drug may displace bilirubin from binding sites on albumin. On the other hand, sulfasalazine was not detected in the breast milk of a mother taking this drug.[260]

Gentamicin (Garamycin) is transferred into breast milk, and half of nursing newborn infants have the drug detectable in their serum. The low levels detected would not be expected to cause clinical effects.[261]

Nitrofurantoin (Macrodantin) is excreted into breast milk in very low concentrations. In one study, the drug could not be detected in 20 samples from mothers receiving 100 mg four times a day.[262]

Erythromycin is excreted into breast milk in small amounts. No reports of adverse effects on infants exposed to erythromycin in breast milk have been noted. Azithromycin (Zithromax) also appears in breast milk in low concentrations.[263] Clindamycin (Cleocin) is excreted into breast milk in low levels, and nursing is usually continued during administration of this drug.

There are no reported adverse effects on the infant of isoniazid administered to nursing mothers, and its use is considered compatible with breast-feeding.[229]

Acyclovir

Acyclovir is compatible with breastfeeding. If a mother takes 1 g/day, the infant receives less than 1 mg/day, a very low dose.[264]

Antifungal Agents

No data are available with nystatin, miconazole, or clotrimazole in breast milk. However, with only small amounts absorbed vaginally, this would not be expected to be a clinical problem. Infant exposure to ketoconazole in human milk was 0.4 percent of the therapeutic dose, again unlikely to cause adverse effects.[265]

Oral Contraceptives

Estrogen and progestin combination oral contraceptives cause dose-related suppression of milk production. Oral contraceptives containing 50 µg and more of estrogen during lactation have been associated with shortened duration of lactation, decreased milk production, decreased infant weight gain, and decreased protein content of the milk. Lactation is inhibited to a lesser degree if the pill is started about 3 weeks postpartum and with lower doses of estrogen than 50 µg. Although the magnitude of the changes is low, the changes may be of nutritional importance, particularly in malnourished mothers.

An infant consuming 600 ml of breast milk daily from a mother using an oral contraceptive containing 50 µg of the ethinylestradiol receives a daily dose in the range of 10 ng of the estrogen.[266] The amount of natural estradiol received by infants who consume a similar volume of milk from mothers not using oral contraceptives is estimated at 3 to 6 ng during anovulatory cycles and 6 to 12 ng during ovulatory cycles. No consistent long-term adverse effects on growth and development have been described.

Evidence indicates that norgestrel (Ovrette) is metabolized rather than accumulated by the infants, and to date, no adverse effects have been identified as a result of progestational agents taken by the mother. Progestin-only contraceptives do not cause alteration of breast milk composition or volume,[267] making them ideal in the breast-feeding mother. When the infant is weaned, the mother should be switched to combined oral contraceptives for maximum contraceptive efficacy.

Alcohol (see Chapter 50)

Alcohol levels in breast milk are similar to those in maternal blood. If a moderate social drinker had two cocktails and had a blood alcohol concentration of 50 mg/dl, the nursing infant would receive about 82 mg of alcohol, which would produce insignificant blood concentrations.[127] There is no evidence that occasional ingestion of alcohol by a mother is harmful to the infant. However, one study showed that ethanol ingested chronically through breast milk might have a detrimental effect on motor development, but not mental development.[268]

Also, alcohol in breast milk has an immediate effect on the odor of the milk, and this may decrease the amount of milk the infant consumes.[269]

PROPYLTHIOURACIL

PTU is found in breast milk in small amounts.[270] If the mother takes 200 mg PTU three times a day, the child would receive 149 µg daily, or the equivalent of a 70-kg adult receiving 3 mg/day. Several infants studied up to 5 months of age show no changes in thyroid parameters. Lactating mothers on PTU can thus continue nursing with close supervision of the infant.[270,271] PTU is preferred over methimazole (Tapazole) because its high protein-binding (80 percent) and lower breast milk concentrations.[272]

H_2-RECEPTOR BLOCKERS

In theory, H_2-receptor antagonists (e.g., ranitidine, cimetidine) might suppress gastric acidity and cause central nervous system stimulation in the infant, but these effects have not been confirmed. The American Academy of Pediatrics now considers H_2-receptor antagonists to be compatible with breast-feeding.[229] Famotidine, nizatidine, and roxatidine are less concentrated in breast milk and may be preferable in nursing mothers.[273]

CAFFEINE

Caffeine has been reported to have no adverse effects on the nursing infant, even after the mother consumes several cups of strong coffee.[274] In one study, the milk level contained 1 percent of the total dose 6 hours after coffee ingestion, which is not enough to affect the infant. In another report, no significant difference in 24-hour heart rate or sleep time was observed in nursing infants when their mothers drank coffee for 5 days or abstained for 5 days.[274]

SMOKING (see Chapter 50)

Nicotine and its metabolite cotinine enter breast milk. Infants of smoking mothers achieve significant serum concentrations of nicotine even if they are not exposed to passive smoking; exposure to passive smoking further raises the levels of nicotine.[275] Women who smoke should be encouraged to stop during lactation as well as during pregnancy.[276]

OCCUPATIONAL AND ENVIRONMENTAL HAZARDS

IONIZING RADIATION

The general hazards of radiation exposure are well known. To provide counseling in specific clinical situations, key variables are dose, timing, and temporal sequence.

Acute Exposure

Systematic studies of atomic bomb survivors in Japan showed conclusively that in utero exposure to high-dose radiation increased the risk of microcephaly and mental and growth restriction in the offspring.[277–280]

Distance from the hypocenter—the area directly beneath the detonated bomb—and gestational age at the time of exposure were directly related to microcephaly, and mental and growth restriction in the infant. The greatest number of children with microcephaly, mental retardation, and growth restriction were in the group exposed at 15 weeks' gestation or earlier. Exposures were calculated by the distance of the victims from the epicenter. Microcephaly and mental retardation were associated with ionizing radiation at doses of 50 rads or greater, with 20 rads being the lowest dose in which microcephaly was observed. It is of note that radiation from the atomic bomb blast differs from the low linear transfer of filtered radiation that is used in diagnostic studies.

Although teratogenic effects have been found in several organ systems of animals exposed to acute, high-dose radiation, the only structural malformations reported among humans exposed prenatally are those mentioned earlier. Using data from animals and from outcomes of reported human exposures at various times during pregnancy, DeKaban[281] constructed a timetable for extrapolating acute, high-dose radiation (>250 rad) to various reproductive outcomes in humans. Similarities between animal and known human effects support DeKaban's proposal.

Effects of chronic low-dose radiation on reproduction have not been identified in animals or humans. Increased risk of adverse outcomes was not detected among animals with continuous low-dose exposure (<5 rad) throughout pregnancy.[282]

The National Council for Radiation Protection[283] concluded that exposures less than 5 rads were not associated with increased risk of malformations. Exposures are expressed as Gray (Gy): 1 Gy equals 1,000 mGy equals 100 rads. Thus 10 mGy equals 1 rad. Fortunately, virtually no single diagnostic test produces a substantive risk. Table 8-3 shows mean and maximum fetal exposure. Only multiple CT scans and fluoroscopies would lead to cumulate exposures of 100 mGy or10 rads. Internal exposures are 50 percent less than maternal surface doses.[284]

Female frequent flyers or crew members may be exposed to radiation during frequent long high-altitude flights. The FAA recommends limiting exposure to 1 mSv (0.1 rad) during the pregnancy.[285]

Therapeutic exposures for maternal thyroid ablation with I^{131} are rare but can cause fetal thyroid damage after 12 weeks of pregnancy.[89]

MUTAGENESIS

Mutagenic effects in the offspring of irradiated women may be manifested years after the birth of the infant. Mutagenic effects presumably explain the 50-percent increased risk of leukemia in children exposed in utero to radiation during maternal pelvimetry examinations[287,288] compared with nonirradiated controls. However, clinical consequence is almost nil. The absolute risk is approximately 1 in 2,000 for exposed versus 1 in 3,000 for unexposed children.

Lowe[283] estimates one additional cancer death per 1,700 10 mGy (1 rad) exposures. If one were to recom-

Table 8-3. Approximate Fetal Doses From Common Diagnostic Procedures

EXAMINATION	MEAN (mGY)	MAXIMUM (mGY)
Conventional X-ray Examinations		
Abdomen	1.4	4.2
Chest	<0.01	<0.01
Intravenous urogram	1.7	10
Lumbar spine	1.7	10
Pelvis	1.1	4
Skull	<0.01	<0.01
Thoracic Spine	<0.01	<0.01
Fluoroscopic Examinations		
Barium meal (UGI)	1.1	5.8
Barium enema	6.8	24
Computed Tomography		
Abdomen	8.0	49
Chest	0.06	0.96
Head	<0.005	<0.005
Lumbar spine	2.4	8.6
Pelvis	25	79

From Lowe SA: Diagnostic radiography in pregnancy: risks and reality. Aust N Z J Obstet Gynaecol 44:191, 2004.

mend that pregnancies be terminated whenever exposure from diagnostic radiation occurred because of the increased probability of leukemia in the offspring, 1,699 exposed pregnancies would have to be terminated to prevent a single case of leukemia. Radiation exposures should be minimized, but fear of radiation should never preclude one from necessary diagnostic procedures. A consent form has been developed for use with pregnant women.[289]

Questions have also been raised about potential risks to children associated with parental (paternal) occupational exposure to low-dose radiation.[290] A case-control study by Gardner et al.[292,293] in the area around the Sellafield Nuclear Facility in the United Kingdom found a statistically significant association between paternal preconception radiation dose and childhood leukemia risk. A similar association had been observed between paternal preconception radiation and risk in workers at the Hanford Nuclear Facility in the United States.[294] The finding regarding childhood leukemia risk is a particularly contentious issue, contradicting studies of the children born to atomic bomb survivors who do not show genetic effects, such as increased risks of childhood cancers.[295] A study in the vicinity of nuclear facilities in Ontario also failed to demonstrate an association between childhood leukemia risk and paternal preconceptional radiation exposure.[296]

Video Display Terminals

Concern about video display terminals linked to adverse reproductive outcomes now seems unwarranted. Early concern grew out of reports of spontaneous abortion clusters among groups of women who used video display terminals at work; some reported clusters included birth defects.[297] Since then numerous reassuring papers have been published on this topic, along with a number of reviews.[297–299] VDT use does not increase the risk of adverse reproductive outcomes.

Lead

Twenty-five years of public health efforts have produced a striking reduction in lead exposure in the United States. The average blood lead level has decreased to less than 20 percent of levels measured in the 1970s. However, elevated blood lead (>20 μg/dl) has a higher incidence among immigrants to Southern California. In Los Angeles, 25 of the 30 cases of elevated blood lead occurred in immigrants.[300]

High lead concentration in maternal blood is associated with an increased risk of delivery of a small-for-gestational-age infant.[301] The frequency of preterm birth was also almost three times higher among women who had umbilical cord levels greater than or equal to 5.1 μg/dl, compared with those who had levels below that cutoff.[302] One study in Norway found an increased risk of low birth weight and also NTDs.[303]

Asking pregnant women about risk factors for lead exposure can aid in assessing prenatal exposure risk. A questionnaire that gathered information on housing conditions, smoking status, and consumption of canned foods had a sensitivity of 89.2 percent and a negative predictive value of 96.4 percent.[304] Consumption of calcium and avoidance of the use of lead-glazed ceramics resulted in lowering of blood lead, especially in pregnant women of low socioeconomic status in Mexico City.[305]

Because the nervous system may be more susceptible to the toxic effects during the embryonic and fetal periods than at any other time of life[306] and because maternal and cord blood lead concentrations are directly correlated,[307] lead concentrations in blood should not exceed 25 μg/dl in women of reproductive age.[308]

Ideally, the maternal blood lead level should be less than 10 μg/dl to ensure that a child begins life with minimal lead exposure. A dose-response relationship is strongly supported by numerous epidemiologic studies of children showing a reduction in IQ with increasing blood lead concentrations above 10 μg/dl. Of note, these studies measured blood lead concentrations over time (often 2 years or more) and reported averaged values. Other neurologic impairments associated with increased blood lead concentrations include attention deficit disorder ("hyperactivity"), hearing deficits, learning disabilities, and shorter stature. Thus, for public health purposes, childhood lead poisoning has been defined as a blood lead level of 10 μg/dl or higher.[309]

In occupational settings, federal standards mandate that women should not work in areas where air lead concentrations can reach 50 μg/cm, because this may result in blood concentrations above 25 to 30 μg/dl.[310] Subtle but permanent neurologic impairment in children may occur at lower blood lead concentrations.[311,312]

Mercury in Fish

Fish and shellfish are an important part of a healthy diet, but some large fish contain significant amounts of mercury. Mercury in high levels may harm the unborn baby or young child's developing nervous system.[313]

Women who may become pregnant, pregnant women, and nursing mothers should avoid shark, swordfish, king mackerel, and tile fish because they contain high levels of mercury. They may eat up to 12 oz a week of shrimp, canned light tuna, salmon, pollock, and catfish, all of which are very low in mercury. Albacore (white) tuna and tuna steaks have more mercury than canned light tuna, but 6 oz per week are allowed.

THE OBSTETRICIAN'S ROLE IN EVALUATING DRUG AND REPRODUCTIVE RISKS IN AND BEYOND THE WORKPLACE

Clinical questions about adverse reproductive outcomes of potential drug teratogens, or environmental or occupational exposures are difficult to answer. Answers are seldom as clear cut as the obstetrician would like. Even if the exposure were known, there is often not a study of similar exposure with a sufficient sample size. Without this, a physician cannot give a reliable estimate of risk.

For drugs and other exposures discussed in this chapter, the threshold is unknown below which no adverse reproductive outcome can be expected. Except for ionizing radiation, maximum recommended exposure levels are difficult to quantify. Epidemiologic studies, when available, often have limitations in design, execution, analysis, or interpretation. Thus, often the questions must be answered on the basis of reasoned judgments in the face of inadequate data.

In addition to traditional genetic referral sources, a variety of teratology information services and computer databases are available to physicians who counsel pregnant women (Table 8-1). The options include personal computer software (Grateful Med, commercial services) and CD-ROM copies in medical libraries or leased from commercial versions. Information is available from a TOXNET representative, National Library of Medicine, Specialized Information Services, 8600 Rockville Pike, Bethesda, MD 20894, (301) 496-6531.

The National Library of Medicine in Bethesda, Maryland, maintains several files on the TOXNET database system, including reproductive and developmental toxicology information in bibliographic or text form. Examples include Developmental and Reproductive Toxicology, GEN-TOX (genetic toxicology), and Environmental Mutagen Information Center. Other very useful sources are Reprotox [http://reprotox.org] and TERIS [depts.washington.edu/%7Eterisweb/teris/index.html].

CONCLUSIONS

Many medical conditions during pregnancy and lactation are best treated initially with nonpharmacologic remedies. Before a drug is administered in pregnancy, the indications should be clear and the risk/benefit ratio should justify drug use. If possible, therapy should be postponed until after the first trimester. In addition, patients should be cautioned about the risks of social drug use such as smoking, alcohol, and cocaine during pregnancy. Most drug therapy does not require cessation of lactation, because the amount excreted into breast milk is sufficiently small to be pharmacologically insignificant.

Key Points

- The critical period of organ development extends from day 31 to day 71 after the first day of the last menstrual period. Infants of epileptic women taking anticonvulsants have double the rate of malformations of unexposed infants; the risk of fetal hydantoin syndrome is less than 10 percent.
- The risk of malformations after in utero exposure to isotretinoin is 25 percent, and an additional 25 percent of infants have mental retardation.
- Heparin is the drug of choice for anticoagulation during pregnancy except for women with artificial heart valves, who should receive coumadin despite the 5 percent risk of warfarin embryopathy.
- ACE inhibitors can cause fetal renal failure in the second and third trimesters, leading to oligohydramnios and hypoplastic lungs.
- Vitamin B_6 25 mg three times a day is a safe and effective therapy for first-trimester nausea and vomiting; doxylamine (Unisom) 12.5 mg three times a day is also effective in combination with B_6.
- Most antibiotics are generally safe in pregnancy. Trimethoprim may carry an increased risk in the first trimester, and tetracyclines taken in the second and third trimesters may cause tooth discoloration. Aminoglycosides can cause fetal ototoxicity.
- Aspirin in analgesic doses inhibits platelet function and prolongs bleeding time, increasing the risk of peripartum hemorrhage.
- FAS occurs in infants of mothers drinking heavily during pregnancy. A safe level of alcohol intake during pregnancy has not been determined.
- Cocaine has been associated with increased risk of spontaneous abortions, abruptio placentae, and congenital malformations, in particular, microcephaly.
- Most drugs are safe during lactation, because subtherapeutic amounts appear in breast milk, approximately 1 to 2 percent of the maternal dose.
- Only a small amount of prednisone crosses the placenta, and so it is the preferred corticosteroid for most medical illnesses. In contrast, betamethasone

and dexamethasone readily cross the placenta and are preferred for acceleration of fetal lung maturity.

❑ Exposure to high-dose ionizing irradiaion during gestation causes microcephaly and mental retardation; however, diagnostic exposures <5 rads do not pose increased teratogenic risks. Mutagenic effects presumably are responsible for the 50-percent increased risk of leukemia in children exposed in utero to radiation during maternal pelvimetry; the absolute risk is very low.

❑ Lead levels in blood have decreased in recent years in all except immigrant populations, making it easier to achieve blood levels less than 25 µg/dl in women of reproductive age; this low level minimizes fetal growth restriction.

❑ Mercury in high levels deleteriously affects the fetal nervous system. For this reason pregnant and nursing women should avoid shark, swordfish, king mackerel, and tile fish; exposures to mercury can further be limited by restricting ingestion of certain other seafood (shrimp, canned tuna, salmon, pollock, catfish) to 12 oz/week.

REFERENCES

1. Wilson JG, Fraser FC: Handbook of Teratology. New York, Plenum, 1979.
2. Blake DA, Niebyl JR: Requirements and limitations in reproductive and teratogenic risk assessment. *In* Niebyl JR (ed): Drug Use in Pregnancy. Philadelphia, Lea & Febiger, 1988.
3. Teratology Society Public Affairs Committee: FDA Classification of drugs for teratogenic risk. Teratol 49:446, 1994.
4. Wilson JG: Current status of teratology—general principles and mechanisms derived from animal studies. *In* Wilson JG, Fraser FC (eds): Handbook of Teratology. New York, Plenum, 1977, p 47.
5. Fraser IS, Shearman RP, Smith A, Russell P: An association among blepharophimosis, resistant ovary syndrome, and true premature menopause. Fertil Steril 50:747, 1988.
6. Musselman AC, Bennett GD, Greer KA, et al: Preliminary evidence of phenytoin-induced alterations in embryonic gene expression in a mouse model. Reprod Toxicol 8:383, 1994.
7. Van Allen MI, Kalousek DK, Chernoff GF, et al: Evidence for multi-site closure of the neural tube in humans. Am J Med Genet 47:723, 1993.
8. Lenz W, Knapp K: Foetal malformation due to thalidomide. Geriatr Med Monthly 7, 253, 1962.
9. Sever LE: Neuroepidemiology of interuterine radiation exposure., *In* Molgaard C (ed): Neuroepidemiology: Theory Method. San Diego, Academic Press, 1993, p 241.
10. Selevan SG, Lemasters GK: The dose-response fallacy in human reproductive studies of toxic exposures. J Occup Med 29:451, 1987.
11. Gregg NM: Congenital cataract following German measles in the mother. Ophthalmol Soc Aust 3:35, 1941.
12. McBride WG: Thalidomide and congenital abnormalities. Lancet 2:1358, 1961.
13. Lynberg MC, Edmonds LD: State use of birth defects surveillance. *In* Wilcox LS, Marks JS (eds): From Data to Action: CDC's Public Health Surveillance for Women, Infants, and Children. Atlanta, Public Health Service, Centers for Disease Control and Prevention, 1994, p 217.
14. Sever LE, Hessol NA: Overall design considerations in male and female occupational reproductive studies. Prog Clin Biol Res 160:15, 1984.
15. Lieff S, Olshan AF, Werler M, et al: Selection bias and the use of controls with malformations in case-control studies of birth defects. Epidemiology 10:238, 1999.
16. Lenz W: Thalidomide and congenital abnormalities. Lancet 1:45, 1962.
17. Lammer EJ, Sever LE, Oakley GP Jr: Teratogen update: valproic acid. Teratology 35:465, 1987.
18. Bracken MB: Design and conduct of randomized clinical trials in perinatal research. *In* Bracken MB (ed): Perinatal Epidemiology, New York, Oxford University Press, 1984, p 397.
19. MRC Vitamin Study Research Group: Prevention of neural tube defects: Results of the Medical Research Council Vitamin Study. Lancet 338:131, 1991.
20. Czeizel AE, Dudas I: Prevention of the first occurrence of neural-tube defects by periconceptional vitamin supplementation. N Engl J Med 327:1832, 1992.
21. Centers for Disease Control and Prevention: Recommendations for the use of folic acid to reduce the number of cases of spina bifida and other neural tube defects. MMWR Morb Mortal Wkly Rep 41:1, 1992.
22. Pardthaisong T, Gray RH, McDaniel EB, Chandacham A: Steroid contraceptive use and exposed to depo-provera during pregnancy or lactation. Contraception 45:313, 1992.
23. Phillips OP, Simpson JL: Contraception and congenital malformations. *In* Sciarra JJ (ed): Gynecology and Obstetrics, Volume VI. Philadelphia, Lippincott, Williams and Wilkins, 2001, p 1.
24. Raman-Wilms L, Tseng AL, Wighardt S, et al: Fetal genital effects of first-trimester sex hormone exposure: A meta-analysis. Obstet Gynecol 85:141, 1995.
25. Wilkins L: Masculinization of female fetus due to use of orally given progestins. JAMA 172:1028, 1960.
26. Duck SC, Katayama KP: Danazol may cause female pseudohermaphroditism. Fertil Steril 35:230, 1981.
27. Brunskill PJ: The effects of fetal exposure to danazol. Br J Obstet Gynaecol 99:212, 1992.
28. Einarson TR, Koren G, Mattice D, et al: Maternal spermicide use and adverse reproductive outcome: A meta-analysis. Am J Obstet Gynecol 162:665, 1990.
29. Rosa FW: Spina bifida in infants of women treated with carbamazepine during pregnancy. N Engl J Med 324:674, 1991.
30. Nakane Y, Okuma T, Tasashashi R, et al: Multi-institutional study on the teratogenicity and fetal toxicity of antiepileptic drugs: A report of a collaborative study group in Japan. Epilepsia 21:663, 1980.
31. Holmes, LB, Harvey EA, Coull BA, et al: The teratogenicity of anticonvulsant drugs. N Engl J Med 344:1132, 2001.
32. Dansky LV, Rosenblatt DS, Andermann E: Mechanisms of teratogenesis: Folic acid and antiepileptic therapy. Neurology 42:32, 1992.
33. Centers for Disease Control: Recommendations for the use of folic acid to reduce the number of cases of spina bifida and other neural tube defects. MMWR Morb Mortal Wkly Rep 41:1, 1992.
34. Biale Y, Lewenthal H: Effect of folic acid supplementation on congenital malformations due to anticonvulsive drugs. Eur J Obstet Gynecol Reprod Biol 18:211, 1984.
35. Hanson JW, Smith DW: The fetal hydantoin syndrome. J Pediatr 87:285, 1975.
36. Gaily E, Granstrom M-L, Hiilesmaa V, et al: Minor anomalies in offspring of epileptic mothers. J Pediatr 112:520, 1988.
37. Jones KL, Lacro RV, Johnson KA, et al: Pattern of malformations in the children of women treated with carbamazepine during pregnancy. N Engl J Med 320:1661, 1989.
38. Strickler SM, Miller MA, Andermann E, et al: Genetic predisposition to phenytoin-induced birth defects. Lancet 2:746, 1985.
39. Buehler BA, Delimont D, VanWaes M, et al: Prenatal prediction of risk of the fetal hydantoin syndrome. N Engl J Med 322:1567, 1990.
40. Van der Pol MC, Hadders-Algra M, Huisjes JH, et al: Antiepileptic medication in pregnancy: late effects on the children's central nervous system development. Am J Obstet Gynecol 164:121, 1991.

41. Scolnik D, Nulman I, Rovet J, et al: Neurodevelopment of children exposed in utero to phenytoin and carbamazepine monotherapy. JAMA 271:767, 1994.
42. Reinisch JM, Sanders SA, Mortensen EL, et al: In utero exposure to phenobarbital and intelligence deficits in adult men. JAMA 274:1518, 1995.
43. GlaxoSmithKline International, Lamotrigine Pregnancy Registry, Interim Report, 1/2005.
44. Morrell MJ: The new antiepileptic drugs and women: efficacy, reproductive health, pregnancy, and fetal outcome. Epilepsia 37: S34, 1996.
45. Callaghan N, Garrett A, Goggin T: Withdrawal of anticonvulsant drugs in patients free of seizures for two years. N Engl J Med 318:942, 1988.
46. Deblay MF, Vert P, Andre M, et al: Transplacental vitamin K prevents haemorrhagic disease of infant of epileptic mother. Lancet 1:1247, 1982.
47. Lammer EJ, Chen DT, Hoar RM, et al: Retinoic acid embryopathy. N Engl J Med 313:837, 1985.
48. Adams J: High incidence of intellectual deficits in 5 year old children exposed to isotretinoin "in utero." Teratology 41:614, 1990.
49. Dai WS, Hsu M-A, Itri L: Safety of pregnancy after discontinuation of isotretinoin. Arch Dermatol 125:362, 1989.
50. Jick SS, Terris BZ, Jick H: First trimester topical tretinoin and congenital disorders. Lancet 341:1181, 1993.
51. Rothman KJ, Moore LL, Singer MR, et al: Teratogenicity of high vitamin A intake. N Engl J Med 333:1369, 1995.
52. Mills JL, Simpson JL, Cunningham GC, et al: Vitamin A and birth defects. Am J Obstet Gynecol 177:31, 1997.
53. Czeizel A: Lack of evidence of teratogenicity of benzodiazepine drugs in Hungary. Reprod Toxicol 3:183, 1988.
54. Laegreid L, Olegard R, Wahlstrom J, et al: Abnormalities in children exposed to benzodiazepines in utero. Lancet 1:108, 1987.
55. Bergman V, Rosa F, Baum C, et al: Effects of exposure to benzodiazepine during fetal life. Lancet 340:694, 1992.
56. Linden S, Rich CL: The use of lithium during pregnancy and lactation. J Clin Psychiatry 44:358, 1983.
57. Weinstein MR, Goldfield MD: Cardiovascular malformations with lithium use during pregnancy. Am J Psychiatry 132:529, 1975.
58. Zalzstein E, Koren G, Einarson T, et al: A case-control study on the association between first trimester exposure to lithium and Ebstein's anomaly. Am J Cardiol 65:817, 1990.
59. Jacobson SJ, Jones K, Johnson K, et al: Prospective multi-centre study of pregnancy outcome after lithium exposure during first trimester. Lancet 339:530, 1992.
60. Krause S, Ebbesen F, Lange AP: Polyhydramnios with maternal lithium treatment. Obstet Gynecol 75:504, 1990.
61. Ang MS, Thorp JA, Parisi VM: Maternal lithium therapy and polyhydramnios. Obstet Gynecol 76:517, 1990.
62. Cohen LS, Friedman MJ, Jefferson JW: A reevaluation of risk of in utero exposure to lithium. JAMA 271:146, 1994.
63. Briggs GG, Freeman RK, Jaffe SJ: Drugs in Pregnancy and Lactation, 6th ed. Philadelphia, Lippincott Williams & Wilkins, 2002, p 693.
64. Briggs GG, Freeman RK, Yaffe SJ: Drugs in Pregnancy and Lactation, 6th ed. Philadelphia, Lippincott Williams & Wilkins, 2002, p 60.
65. Pastuszak A, Schick-Boschetto B, Zuber C, et al: Pregnancy outcome following first-trimester exposure to fluoxetine (Prozac). JAMA 269:2446, 1993.
66. Goldstein DJ, Corbin LA, Sundell KL: Effects of first-trimester fluoxetine exposure on the newborn. Obstet Gynecol 89:713, 1997.
67. Nulman I, Rovert J, Stewart DE, et al: Neurodevelopment of children exposed in utero to antidepressant drugs. N Engl J Med 336:258, 1997.
68. Coleman FH, Christensen HD, Gonzalez CL, et al: Behavioral changes in developing mice after prenatal exposure to paroxetine (Paxil). Am J Obstet Gynecol 181:1166, 1999.
69. Chambers CD, Johnson KA, Dick LM, et al: Birth outcomes in pregnant women taking fluoxetine. N Engl J Med 335:1010, 1996.
70. Hendrick V, Smith LM, Suri R, et al: Birth outcomes after prenatal exposure to antidepressant medication. Am J Obstet Gynecol 188:812, 2003.
71. Kulin NA, Pastuszak A, Sage SR, et al: Pregnancy outcome following maternal use of the new selective serotonin reuptake inhibitors: A prospective controlled multicenter study. JAMA 279:609, 1998.
72. Zeskind PS, Stephens LE: Maternal selective serotonin reuptake inhibitor use during pregnancy and newborn neurobehavior. Pediatrics 113:368, 2004.
73. Nulman I, Rowet J, Stewart DE, et al: Neurodevelopment of children exposed in utero to antidepressant drugs. N Engl J Med 336:258, 1997.
74. Hill RM, Stern L: Drugs in pregnancy: Effects on the fetus and newborn. Drugs 17:182, 1979.
75. Cotrufo M, De Feo M, De Santo LS, et al: Risk of warfarin during pregnancy with mechanical valve prostheses. Obstet Gynecol 99:35, 2002.
76. Sbarouni E, Oakley CM: Outcome of pregnancy in women with valve prostheses. Br Heart J 71:196, 1994.
77. deSwiet M, Ward PD, Fidler J, et al: Prolonged heparin therapy in pregnancy causes bone demineralization. Br J Obstet Gynaecol 90:1129, 1983.
78. Barbour LA, Kick SD, Steiner JF, et al: A prospective study of heparin-induced osteoporosis in pregnancy using bone densitometry. Am J Obstet Gynecol 170:862, 1994.
79. Dahlman TC: Osteoporotic fractures and the recurrence of thromboembolism during pregnancy and the puerperium in 184 women undergoing thromboprophylaxis with heparin. Am J Obstet Gynecol 168:1265, 1993.
80. Nelson-Piercy C, Letsky EA, deSwiet M: Low-molecular-weight heparin for obstetric thromboprophylaxis: experience of sixty-nine pregnancies in sixty-one women at high risk. Am J Obstet Gynecol 176:1062, 1997.
81. Casele HL, Laifer SA, Woelkers DA, et al: Changes in the pharmacokinetics of the low-molecular-weight heparin enoxaparin sodium during pregnancy. Am J Obstet Gynecol 181:1113, 1999.
82. Ginsberg JS, Hirsh J: Use of antithrombotic agents during pregnancy. Chest 114:524S, 1998.
83. Chan WS, Ray JG: Low molecular weight heparin use during pregnancy: issues of safety and practicality. Obstet Gynecol Surv 54:649, 1999.
84. Vitale N, De Feo M, De Santo LS, et al: Dose-dependent fetal complications of warfarin in pregnant women with mechanical heart valves. J Am Coll Cardiol 33:1637, 1999.
85. Tengborn L, Bergqvist D, Matzsch T, et al: Recurrent thromboembolism in pregnancy and puerperium: is there a need for thromboprophylaxis? Am J Obstet Gynecol 160:90, 1989.
86. Brill-Edwards P, Ginsberg JS, Gent M, et al: Safety of withholding heparin in pregnant women with a history of venous thromboembolism. N Engl J Med 343:1439, 2000.
87. Cooper DS: Antithyroid drugs. N Engl J Med 352:905, 2005.
88. Wing DA, Millar LK, Koonings PP, et al: A comparison of propylthiouracil versus methimazole in the treatment of hyperthyroidism in pregnancy. Am J Obstet Gynecol 170:90, 1994.
89. Burrow GN: Thyroid diseases. *In* Burrow GN, Ferris TF (eds): Medical Complications During Pregnancy. Philadelphia, WB Saunders Company, 1988, p 229.
90. Mandel SJ, Larsen PR, Seely EW, et al: Increased need for thyroxine during pregnancy in women with primary hypothyroidism. N Engl J Med 323:91, 1990.
91. Alexander EK, Marqusee E, Lawrence J, et al: Timing and magnitude of increases in levothyroxine requirements during pregnancy in women with hypothyroidism. N Engl J Med 351:241, 2004.
92. Haddow JE, Palomaki GE, Allan WC, et al: Maternal thyroid deficiency during pregnancy and subsequent neuropsychological development of the child. N Engl J Med 341:549, 1999.
93. Blazer S, Moreh-Waterman Y, Miller-Lotan R, et al: Maternal hypothyroidism may affect fetal growth and neonatal thyroid function. Obstet Gynecol 102:232, 2003.
94. Casey BM, Dashe JS, Wells CE, et al: Subclinical hypothyroidism and pregnancy outcomes. Obstet Gynecol 105:239, 2005.

95. l'Allemand D, Gruters A, Heidemann P, et al: Iodine-induced alterations of thyroid function in newborn infants after prenatal and perinatal exposure to povidone iodine. J Pediatr 102:935, 1983.
96. Heinonen OP, Slone S, Shapiro S: Birth Defects and Drugs in Pregnancy. Littleton, MA, Publishing Sciences Group, 1977.
97. Aselton P, Jick H, Milunsky A, et al: First-trimester drug use and congenital disorders. Obstet Gynecol 65:451, 1985.
98. Weiner CP, Landas S, Persoon TJ: Digoxin-like immunoreactive substance in fetuses with and without cardiac pathology. Am J Obstet Gynecol 157:368, 1987.
99. Weiner CP, Thompson MIB: Direct treatment of fetal supraventricular tachycardia after failed transplacental therapy. Am J Obstet Gynecol 158:570, 1988.
100. Pruyn SC, Phelan JP, Buchanan GC: Long-term propranolol therapy in pregnancy: maternal and fetal outcome. Am J Obstet Gynecol 135:485, 1979.
101. Redmond GP: Propranolol and fetal growth retardation. Semin Perinatol 6:142, 1982.
102. Rubin PC, Clark DM, Sumner DJ: Placebo-controlled trial of atenolol in treatment of pregnancy-associated hypertension. Lancet 1:431, 1983.
103. Hanssens M, Keirse MJNC, Vankelecom F, et al: Fetal and neonatal effects of treatment with angiotensin-converting enzyme inhibitors in pregnancy. Obstet Gynecol 78:128, 1991.
104. Piper JM, Ray WA, Rosa FW: Pregnancy outcome following exposure to angiotensin-converting enzyme inhibitors. Obstet Gynecol 80:429, 1992.
104a. Cooper WO, Hernandez-Diaz S, Arbogast PG, et al: Major congenital malformations after first-trimester exposure to ACE inhibitors. N Engl J Med 354:2443, 2006.
105. Basle EV, Conard JV, Weiss L: Adult and two children with fetal methotrexate syndrome. Teratology 57:51, 1998.
106. Kozlowski RD, Steinbrunner JV, MacKenzie AH, et al: Outcome of first-trimester exposure to low-dose methotrexate in eight patients with rheumatic disease. Am J Med 88:589, 1990.
107. Briggs GG, Freeman RK, Yaffe SJ: Drugs in Pregnancy and Lactation, 6th ed. Baltimore, Williams & Wilkins, 2002, p 112.
108. Armenti VT, Ahlswede BA, Ahlswede JR, et al: National transplantation pregnancy registry: analysis of outcome/risks of 394 pregnancies in kidney transplant recipients. Transplant Proc 26:2535, 1994.
109. Takahashi N, Nishida H, Hoshi J: Severe B cell depletion in newborns from renal transplant mothers taking immunosuppressive agents. Transplantation 57:1617, 1994.
110. Briggs GG, Freeman RK, Yaffe SJ: Drugs in Pregnancy and Lactation, 6th ed. Baltimore, Williams & Wilkins, 1998, p 339.
111. Wolfe MS, Cordero JF: Safety of chloroquine in chemosuppression of malaria during pregnancy. Br Med J 290:1466, 1985.
112. Hart CW, Naunton RF: The ototoxicity of chloroquine phosphate. Arch Otolaryngol 80:407, 1964.
113. Levy M, Buskila D, Gladman DD, et al: Pregnancy outcome following first trimester exposure to chloroquine. Am J Perinatol 8:174, 1991.
114. Zemlickis D, Lishner M, Degendorfer P, et al: Fetal outcome after in utero exposure to cancer chemotherapy. Arch Intern Med 152:573, 1992.
115. Main EK, Main DM, Gabbe SG: Chronic oral terbutaline therapy is associated with maternal glucose intolerance. Obstet Gynecol 157:644, 1987.
116. Briggs GG, Freeman RK, Yaffe SJ: Drugs in Pregnancy and Lactation, 6th ed. Baltimore, Williams & Wilkins, 2002, p 334.
117. Briggs GG, Freeman RK, Yaffe SJ: Drugs in Pregnancy and Lactation, 6th ed. Baltimore, Williams & Wilkins, 2002, p 734.
118. Park-Wyllie L, Mazzotta P, Pastuszak A, et al: Birth defects after maternal exposure to corticosteroids: Prospective cohort study and meta-analysis of epidemiological studies. Teratology 62:385, 2000.
119. Carmichael SL, Shaw GM: Maternal corticosteroid use and risk of selected congenital anomalies. Am J Med Genet 86:242, 1999.
120. Sahakian V, Rouse D, Sipes S, et al: Vitamin B_6 is effective therapy for nausea and vomiting of pregnancy: a randomized double-blind, placebo-controlled study. Obstet Gynecol 78:33, 1991.
121. Vutyavanich T, Wongtra-Rjan S, Ruangsri R: Pyridoxine for nausea and vomiting of pregnancy: a randomized double-blind placebo-controlled trial. Am J Obstet Gynecol 173:881, 1995.
122. Diggory PLC, Tomkinson JS: Nausea and vomiting in pregnancy: a trial of meclozine dihydrochloride with and without pyridoxine. Lancet 2:370, 1962.
123. Briggs GG, Freeman RK, Yaffe SJ: Drugs in Pregnancy and Lactation, 6th ed. Baltimore, Williams & Wilkins, 2002, p 845.
124. Milkovich L, Van Den Berg BJ: An evaluation of the teratogenicity of certain antinauseant drugs. Am J Obstet Gynecol 125:244, 1976.
125. Cartwright EW: Dramamine in nausea and vomiting of pregnancy. West J Surg Obstet Gynecol 59:216, 1951.
126. Briggs GG, Freeman RK, Yaffe SJ: Drugs in Pregnancy and Lactation, 6th ed. Baltimore, Williams & Wilkins, 2002, p 425.
127. Briggs GG, Freeman RK, Yaffe SJ: Drugs in Pregnancy and Lactation, 6th ed. Baltimore, Williams & Wilkins, 2002, p 247.
128. Briggs GG, Freeman RK, Yaffe SJ: Drugs in Pregnancy and Lactation, 6th ed. Baltimore, Williams & Wilkins, 2002, p 1168.
129. Briggs GG, Freeman RK, Yaffe SJ: Drugs in Pregnancy and Lactation, 6th ed. Baltimore, Williams & Wilkins, 2002, p 734.
130. Sullivan CA, Johnson CA, Roach H, et al: A pilot study of intravenous ondansetron for hyperemesis gravidarum. Am J Obstet Gynecol 174:2565, 1996.
131. Safari HR, Fassett MJ, Souter IC, et al: The efficacy of methylprednisolone in the treatment of hyperemesis gravidarum: a randomized, double-blind, controlled study. Am J Obstet Gynecol 179:921, 1998.
132. Yost NP, McIntire DD, Wians FH Jr, et al: A randomized, placebo-controlled trial of corticosteroids for hyperemesis due to pregnancy. Obstet Gynecol 102:1250, 2003.
133. Fischer-Rasmussen W, Kjaer SK, Dahl C, et al: Ginger treatment of hyperemesis gravidarum. Eur J Obstet Gynecol Reprod Biol 38:19, 1990.
134. Borrelli F, Caspasso R, Aviello G, et al: Effectiveness and safety of ginger in the treatment of pregnancy-induced nausea and vomiting. Obstet Gynecol 105:849, 2005.
135. Ruigomez A, Garcia Rodriguez LA, Cattaruzzi C, et al: Use of cimetidine, omeprazole, and ranitidine in pregnant women and pregnancy outcomes. Am J Epidemiol 150:476, 1999.
136. Briggs GG, Freeman RK, Yaffe SJ: Drugs in Pregnancy and Lactation, 6th ed. Baltimore, Williams & Wilkins, 2002, p 1322.
137. Pastuszak A, Schick B, D'Alimonte D, et al: The safety of astemizole in pregnancy. J Allergy Clin Immunol 98:748, 1996.
138. Zierler S, Purohit D: Prenatal antihistamine exposure and retrolental fibroplasia. Am J Epidemiol 123:192, 1986.
139. Werler MM, Mitchell AA, Shapiro S: First trimester maternal medication use in relation to gastroschisis. Teratology 45:361, 1992.
140. Briggs GG, Freeman RK, Yaffe SJ: Drugs in Pregnancy and Lactation, 6th ed. Baltimore, Williams & Wilkins, 2002, p 284.
141. Kenyon S, Boulvain M, Neilson J: Antibiotics for preterm rupture of the membranes: A systematic review. Obstet Gynecol 104:1051, 2004.
142. Kenyon SL, Taylor DJ, Tarnow-Mordi W: Broad-spectrum antibiotics for preterm, prelabour rupture of fetal membranes: the ORICLE I randomized trial. ORACLE Collaborative Group. Lancet 357:979, 2001.
143. Briggs GG, Freeman RK, Yaffe SJ: Drugs in Pregnancy and Lactation, 6th ed. Baltimore, Williams & Wilkins, 2002, p 222.
144. Czeizel AE, Rockenbauer M, Sorensen HT, et al: Use of cephalosporins during pregnancy and in the presence of congenital abnormalities: A population-based, case-control study. Am J Obstet Gynecol 184:1289, 2001.
145. Harris RC, Lucey JF, MacLean JR: Kernicterus in premature infants associated with low concentration of billirubin in the plasma. Pediatrics 23:878, 1950.
146. Briggs GG, Freeman RK, Yaffe SJ: Drugs in Pregnancy and Lactation, 6th ed. Baltimore, Williams & Wilkins, 2002, p 1292.
147. Briggs GG, Freeman RK, Yaffe SJ: Drugs in Pregnancy and Lactation, 6th ed. Baltimore, Williams & Wilkins, 2002, p 1393.
148. Czeizel A: A case-control analysis of the teratogenic effects of co-trimoxazole. Reprod Toxicol 4:305, 1990.

149. Hernandez-Diaz S, Werler MM, Walker AM, et al: Folic acid antagonists during pregnancy and the risk of birth defects. N Engl J Med 343:1608, 2000.
150. Hailey FJ, Fort H, Williams JR, et al: Foetal safety of nitrofurantoin macrocrystals therapy during pregnancy: a retrospective analysis. J Int Med Res 11:364, 1983.
151. Lenke RR, VanDorsten JP, Schifrin BS: Pyelonephritis in pregnancy: a prospective randomized trial to prevent recurrent disease evaluating suppressive therapy with nitrofurantoin and close surveillance. Am J Obstet Gynecol 146:953, 1983.
152. Cohlan SQU, Bevelander G, Tiamsic T: Growth inhibition of prematures receiving tetracycline. Am J Dis Child 105:453, 1963.
153. Czeizel AE, Rockenbauer M: Teratogenic study of doxycycline. Obstet Gynecol 89:524, 1997.
154. Robinson GC, Cambon KG: Hearing loss in infants of tuberculous mothers treated with streptomycin during pregnancy. N Engl J Med 271:949, 1964.
155. Nishimura H, Tanimura T: Clinical Aspects of the Teratogenicity of Drugs. Amsterdam, Excerpta Medica, 1976.
156. L'Hommedieu CS, Nicholas D, Armes DA, et al: Potentiation of magnesium sulfate–induced neuromuscular weakness by gentamicin, tobramycin, and amikacin. J Pediatr 102:629, 1983.
157. Marynowski A, Sianozecka E: Comparison of the incidence of congenital malformations in neonates from healthy mothers and from patients treated because of tuberculosis. Ginekol Pol 43:713, 1972.
158. Einarson A, Phillips E, Mawji F, et al: A prospective controlled multicentre study of clarithromycin in pregnancy. Am J Perinatol 15:523, 1998.
159. Berkovitch M, Pastuszak A, Gazarian M, et al: Safety of the new quinolones in pregnancy. Obstet Gynecol 84:535, 1994.
160. Briggs GG, Freeman RK, Yaffe SJ: Drugs in Pregnancy and Lactation, 6th ed. Baltimore, Williams & Wilkins, 2002, p 270.
161. Loebstein R, Addis A, Ho E, et al: Pregnancy outcome following gestational exposure to fluoroquinolones: A multicenter prospective controlled study. Antimicrob Agents Chemother 42:1336, 1998.
162. Piper JM, Mitchel EF, Ray WA: Prenatal use of metronidazole and birth defects: no association. Obstet Gynecol 82:348, 1993.
163. Burtin P, Taddio A, Ariburnu O, et al: Safety of metronidazole in pregnancy: a meta-analysis. Am J Obstet Gynecol 172:525, 1995.
164. Stone KM, Reiff-Eldridge R, White AD, et al: Pregnancy outcomes following systemic prenatal acyclovir exposure: Conclusions from the international acyclovir pregnancy registry, 1984–1999. Birth Defects Res Part A. Clin Mol Teratol 70:201, 2004.
165. Andrews EB, Yankaskas BC, Cordero JF, et al: Acyclovir in pregnancy registry: six years' experience. Obstet Gynecol 79:7, 1992.
166. Culnane M, Fowler MG, Lee SS, et al: Lack of long-term effects of in utero exposure to zidovudine among uninfected children born to HIV-infected women. JAMA 281–151, 1999.
167. Antiretroviral Pregnancy Registry Steering Committee. Antiretroviral pregnancy Registry International Interim Report for 1 January 1989 through 31 January 2004. Wilmington, NC: Registry Coordinating Center; 2004. Available from URL: *www.apregistry.com.*
168. Perinatal HIV Guidelines Working Group. Public Health Service Task Force. Recommendations for use of antiretroviral drugs in pregnant HIV-1-infected women for maternal health and interventions to reduce perinatal HIV-1 transmission in the United States. June 23, 2004, Available from AIDS info Web site: *http://AIDSinfo.nih.gov.*
169. Bristol-Myers Squibb. Important drug warning. Available at: *http://www.fda.gov/medwatch/safety/2001/zerit&videx_letter.htm.*
170. Rosa FW, Baum C, Shaw M: Pregnancy outcomes after first trimester vaginitis drug therapy. Obstet Gynecol 69:751, 1987.
171. Briggs GG, Freeman RK, Yaffe SJ: Drugs in Pregnancy and Lactation, 6th ed. Baltimore, Williams & Wilkins, 2002, p 930.
172. Pursley TJ, Blomquist IK, Abraham J, et al: Fluconazole-induced congenital anomalies in three infants. Clin Infect Dis 22:336, 1996.
173. Jick SS: Pregnancy outcomes after maternal exposure to fluconazole. Pharmacotherapy 19:221, 1999.
174. Mastroiacovo P, Mazzone T, Botto LD, et al: Prospective assessment of pregnancy outcomes after first-trimester exposure to fluconazole. Am J Obstet Gynecol 175:1645, 1996.
175. Asch RH, Greenblatt RB: Update on the safety and efficacy of clomiphene citrate as a therapeutic agent. J Reprod Med 17:175, 1976.
176. Riuz-Velasco V, Tolis G: Pregnancy in hyperprolactinemic women. Fertil Steril 41:793, 1984.
177. Werler MM, Mitchell AA, Shapiro S: The relation of aspirin use during the first trimester of pregnancy to congenital cardiac defects. N Engl J Med 321:1639, 1989.
178. Collins E, Turner G: Salicylates and pregnancy. Lancet 2:1494, 1973.
179. Stuart JJ, Gross SJ, Elrad H, et al: Effects of acetylsalicyclic acid ingestion on maternal and neonatal hemostasis. N Engl J Med 307:909, 1982.
180. Areilla RA, Thilenius OB, Ranniger K: Congestive heart failure from suspected ductal closure in utero. J Pediatr 75:74, 1969.
181. Thulstrup AM, Sorensen HT, Nielsen GL, et al: Fetal growth and adverse birth outcomes in women receiving prescriptions for acetaminophen during pregnancy. Am J Perinatol 16:321, 1999.
182. Waltman T, Tricomi V, Tavakoli FM: Effect of aspirin on bleeding time during elective abortion. Obstet Gynecol 48:108, 1976.
183. Briggs GG, Freeman RK, Yaffe SJ: Drugs in Pregnancy and Lactation, 6th ed. Baltimore, Williams & Wilkins, 2002, p 685.
184. Briggs GG, Freeman RK, Yaffe SJ: Drugs in Pregnancy and Lactation, 6th ed. Baltimore, Williams & Wilkins, 2002, p 974.
185. Tyson HK: Neonatal withdrawal symptoms associated with maternal use of propoxyphene hydrochloride (Darvon). J Pediatr 85:684, 1974.
186. Briggs GG, Freeman RK, Yaffe SJ: Drugs in Pregnancy and Lactation, 6th ed. Baltimore, Williams & Wilkins, 2002, p 1299.
187. Shah NR, Bracken MB: A systematic review and meta-analysis of prospective studies on the association between interval cigarette smoking and preterm delivery. Am J Obstet Gynecol 182:465, 2000.
188. Alberman E, Creasy M, Elliott M, et al: Maternal factors associated with fetal chromosomal anomalies in spontaneous abortions. J Obstet Gynecol 83:621, 1976.
189. Dolan-Mullen P, Ramierez G, Groff JY: A meta-analysis of randomized trials of prenatal smoking cessation interventions. Am J Obstet Gynecol 171:1328, 1994.
190. Martin TR, Bracken MB: Association of low birth weight with passive smoke exposure in pregnancy. Am J Epidemiol 124:633, 1986.
191. Marcus BH, Albrecht AE, King TK, et al: The efficacy of exercise as an aid for smoking cessation in women. Arch Intern Med 159:1229, 1999.
192. Tonnesen P, Norregaard J, Simonsen K, et al: A double-blind trial of a 16-hour transdermal nicotine patch in smoking cessation. N Engl J Med 325:311, 1991.
193. Ogburn PL, Hurt RD, Croghan IT, et al: Nicotine patch use in pregnant smokers: nicotine and cotinine levels and fetal effects. Am J Obstet Gynecol 181:736, 1999.
194. Bupropion Pregnancy Registry: Interim Report: 1 September 1997 through 28 February 2002. Wilmington, NC, PharmaResearch Coproration, June 2002.
195. Jones KL, Smith DW, Ulleland CN, et al: Patterns of malformation in offspring of chronic alcoholic mothers. Lancet 2:1267, 1973.
196. Rosett HL: A clinical perspective of the fetal alcohol syndrome. Alcohol Clin Exp Res 4:119, 1980.
197. Day NL, Richardson GA: Prenatal alcohol exposure: A continuum of effects. Semin Perinatol 15:271, 1991.
198. Jones KL, Smith DW, Streissguth AP, et al: Outcome of offspring of chronic alcoholic women. Lancet 2:1076, 1974.
199. Ouellette EM, Rosett HL. Rosman NP, et al: Adverse effects on offspring of maternal alcohol abuse during pregnancy. N Engl J Med 297:528, 1977.
200. Mills JL, Graubard BI: Is moderate drinking during pregnancy associated with an increased risk of malformations? Pediatrics 80:309, 1987.

201. Sokol RJ, Martier SS, Ager JW: The T-ACE questions: practical prenatal detection of risk-drinking. Am J Obstet Gynecol 160:863, 1989.
202. Linn S, Schoenbaum SC, Monson RR, Rosner R, et al: The association of marijuana use with outcome of pregnancy. Am J Public Health 73:1161, 1983.
203. Zuckerman B, Frank DA, Hingson R, et al: Effects of maternal marijuana and cocaine use on fetal growth. N Engl J Med 320:762, 1989.
204. Visscher WA, Feder M, Burns AM, et al: The impact of smoking and other substance use by urban women on the birthweight of their infants. Subst Use Misuse 38:1063, 2003.
205. Fergusson DM, Horwood LJ, Nortstone K: Maternal use of cannabis and pregnancy outcome. Br J Obstet Gynecol 109:21, 2002.
206. Acker D, Sachs BP, Tracey KJ, et al: Abruptio placentae associated with cocaine use. Am J Obstet Gynecol 146:220, 1983.
207. Little BB, Snell LM, Klein VR, et al: Cocaine abuse during pregnancy: maternal and fetal implications. Obstet Gynecol 73:157, 1989.
208. Bingol N, Fuchs M, Diaz V, et al: Teratogenicity of cocaine in humans. J Pediatr 110:93, 1987.
209. MacGregor SN, Keith LG, Chasnoff IJ, et al: Cocaine use during pregnancy: adverse perinatal outcome. Am J Obstet Gynecol 157:686, 1987.
210. Keith LG, MacGregor S, Friedell S, et al: Substance abuse in pregnant women: recent experience at the perinatal center for chemical dependence of Northwestern Memorial Hospital. Obstet Gynecol 73:715, 1989.
211. Chasnoff IJ, Griffith DR, MacGregor S, et al: Temporal patterns of cocaine use in pregnancy. JAMA 261:1741, 1989.
212. Volpe JJ: Effect of cocaine use on the fetus. N Engl J Med 327:399, 1992.
213. Handler A, Kistin N, Davis F, et al: Cocaine use during pregnancy: perinatal outcomes. Am J Epidemiol 133:818, 1991.
214. Little BB, Snell LM: Brain growth among fetuses exposed to cocaine in utero: asymmetrical growth retardation. Obstet Gynecol 77:361, 1991.
215. Chasnoff IJ, Chisum GM, Kaplan WE: Maternal cocaine use and genitourinary tract malformations. Teratology 37:201, 1988.
216. Finnegan LP, Wapner RJ: Narcotic addiction in pregnancy. *In* Niebyl JR (ed): Drug Use in Pregnancy. Philadelphia, Lea & Febiger, 1988, p 203.
217. Brown HL, Britton KA, Mahaffey D, et al: Methadone maintenance in pregnancy: A reappraisal. Am J Obstet Gynecol 179:459, 1998.
218. Van den Berg BJ: Epidemiologic observations of prematurity: effects of tobacco, coffee and alcohol. *In* Reed DM, Stanley FJ (eds): The Epidemiology of Prematurity. Baltimore, Urban & Schwarzenberg, 1977.
219. Linn S, Schoenbaum SC, Monson RR, et al: No association between coffee consumption and adverse outcomes of pregnancy. N Engl J Med 306:141, 1982.
220. Martin TR, Bracken MB: The association between low birth weight and caffeine consumption during pregnancy. Am J Epidemiol 126:813, 1987.
221. Beaulac-Baillargeon L, Desrosiers C: Caffeine-cigarette interaction on fetal growth. Am J Obstet Gynecol 157:1236, 1987.
222. Munoz LM, Lonnerdal B, Keen CL, et al: Coffee consumption as a factor in iron deficiency anemia among pregnant women and their infants in Costa Rica. Am J Clin Nutr 48:645, 1988.
223. Infante-Rivard C, Fernandez A, Gauthier R, et al: Fetal loss associated with caffeine intake before and during pregnancy. JAMA 270:2940, 1993.
224. Mills JL, Holmes LB, Aarons JH, et al: Moderate caffeine use and the risk of spontaneous abortion and intrauterine growth retardation. JAMA 269:593, 1993.
225. Klebanoff MA, Levine RJ, DerSimonian R, et al: Maternal serum paraxanthine, a caffeine metabolite, and the risk of spontaneous abortion. N Engl J Med 341:1639, 1999.
226. Sturtevant FM: Use of aspartame in pregnancy. Int J Fertil 30:85, 1985.
227. Wilson JT, Brown RD, Cherek DR, et al: Drug excretion in human breast milk: principles of pharmacokinetics and projected consequences. Clin Pharmacokinet 5:1, 1980.
228. Ito S, Blajchman A, Stephenson M, et al: Prospective follow-up of adverse reactions in breast-fed infants exposed to maternal medication. Am J Obstet Gynecol 168:1393, 1993.
229. Committee on Drugs, American Academy of Pediatrics: The transfer of drugs and other chemicals into human milk. Pediatrics 108:776, 2001.
230. Johns BG, Rutherford CD, Laighton RC, et al: Secretion of methotrexate into human milk. Am J Obstet Gynecol 112:978, 1972.
231. Chisolm CA, Kuller JA: A guide to the safety of CNS-active agents during breastfeeding. Drug Safety 17–127–142, 1997.
232. Allaire AD, Kuller JA: Psychotropic drugs in pregnancy and lactation. *In* Yankowitz J, Niebyl JR (eds): Drug Therapy in Pregnancy, 3rd ed. New York, Lippincott Williams & Wilkins, 2001.
233. Nulman I, Koren G: The safety of fluoxetine during pregnancy and lactation. Teratology 53:304, 1996.
234. Burch KJ, Wells BG: Fluoxetine/norfluoxetine concentrations in human milk. Pediatrics 89:676, 1992.
235. Epperson CN, Anderson GM, McDougle CJ: Sertraline and breast-feeding. N Engl J Med 336:1189, 1997.
236. Canales ES, Garcia IC, Ruiz JE, et al: Bromocriptine as prophylactic therapy in prolactinoma during pregnancy. Fertil Steril 36:524, 1981.
237. Linden S, Rich CL: The use of lithium during pregnancy and lactation. J Clin Psychiatry 44:358, 1983.
238. Niebyl JR, Blake DA, Freeman JM, et al: Carbamezapine levels in pregnancy and lactation. Obstet Gynecol 53:139, 1979.
239. Briggs GG, Freeman RK, Yaffe SJ: Drugs in Pregnancy and Lactation, 6th ed. Baltimore, Williams & Wilkins, 2002, p 1124.
240. Pynnonen S, Sillanpaa M: Carbamazepine and mother's milk. Lancet 2:563, 1975.
241. Findlay JWA, Butz RF, Sailstad JM, et al: Pseudoephedrine and triprolidine in plasma and breast milk of nursing mothers. Br J Clin Pharmacol 18:901, 1984.
242. Weithmann MW, Krees SV: Excretion of chlorothiazide in human breast milk. J Pediatr 81:781, 1972.
243. Miller ME, Cohn RD, Burghart PH: Hydrochlorothiazide disposition in a mother and her breast-fed infant. J Pediatr 101:789, 1982.
244. Bauer JH, Pope B, Zajicek J, et al: Propranolol in human plasma and breast milk. Am J Cardiol 43:860, 1979.
245. Anderson PO, Salter FJ: Propranolol therapy during pregnancy and lactation. Am J Cardiol 37:325, 1976.
246. White WB, Andreoli JW, Wong SH, et al: Atenolol in human plasma and breast milk. Obstet Gynecol 63:42S, 1984.
247. Schmimmel MS, Eidelman AJ, Wilschanski MA, et al: Toxic effects of atenolol consumed during breast feeding. J Pediatr 114:476, 1989.
248. Briggs GG, Freeman RK, Yaffe SJ: Drugs in Pregnancy and Lactation, 6th ed. Baltimore, Williams & Wilkins, 2002, p 105.
249. Hartikainen-Sorri AL, Heikkinen JE, Koivisto M: Pharmacokinetics of clonidine during pregnancy and nursing. Obstet Gynecol 69:598, 1987.
250. Devlin RG, Fleiss PM: Selective resistance to the passage of captopril into human milk. Clin Pharmacol Ther 27:250, 1980.
251. Ehrenkranz RA, Ackerman BA, Hulse JD: Nifedipine transfer into human milk. J Pediatr 114:478, 1989.
252. Orme ME, Lewis PJ, deSwiet M, et al: May mothers given warfarin breastfeed their infants? Br Med J 1:1564, 1977.
253. deSwiet M, Lewis PJ: Excretion of anticoagulants in human milk. N Engl J Med 297:1471, 1977.
254. Brambel CE, Hunter RE: Effect of dicumarol on the nursing infant. Am J Obstet Gynecol 59:1153, 1950.
255. Katz FH, Duncan BR: Entry of prednisone into human milk. N Engl J Med 293:1154, 1975.
256. MacKenzie SA, Seeley JA, Agnew JE: Secretion of prednisolone into breast milk. Arch Dis Child 50:894, 1975.
257. Ost L, Wettrell G, Bjorkhem I, et al: Prednisolone excretion in human milk. J Pediatr 106:1008, 1985.
258. Loughnan PM: Digoxin excretion in human breast milk. J Pediatr 92:1019, 1978.
259. Yoshioka H, Cho K, Takimoto M, et al: Transfer of cefazolin into human milk. J Pediatr 94:151, 1979.

260. Berlin CM Jr, Yaffe SJ: Disposition of salicylazosulfapyridine (Azulfidine) and metabolites in human breast milk. Dev Pharmacol Ther 1:31, 1980.
261. Celiloglu M, Celiker S, Guven H, et al: Gentamicin excretion and uptake from breast milk by nursing infants. Obstet Gynecol 84:263, 1994.
262. Hosbach RE, Foster RB: Absence of nitrofurantoin from human milk. JAMA 202:1057, 1967.
263. Kelsey JJ, Moser LR, Jenning JC, et al: Presence of azithromycin breast milk concentrations: a case report. Am J Obstet Gynecol 170:1375, 1994.
264. Meyer LJ, de Miranda P, Sheth N, et al: Acyclovir in human breast milk. Am J Obstet Gynecol 158:586, 1988.
265. Moretti ME, Ito S, Koren G: Disposition of maternal ketoconazole in breast milk. Am J Obstet Gynecol 173:1625, 1995.
266. Nilsson S, Nygren KG, Johansson EDB: Transfer of estradiol to human milk. Am J Obstet Gynecol 132:653, 1978.
267. Grimes DA, Wallach M: Modern Contraception. Totowa, NJ, Emron, 1997, p 249.
268. Little RE, Anderson KW, Ervin CH, et al: Maternal alcohol use during breastfeeding and infant mental and motor development at one year. N Engl J Med 321:425, 1989.
269. Mennella JA, Beauchamp GK: The transfer of alcohol to human milk. Effects on flavor and the infant's behavior. N Engl J Med 325:981, 1991.
270. Kampmann JP, Hansen JM, Johansen K, et al: Propylthiouracil in human milk. Lancet 1:736, 1980.
271. Cooper DS: Antithyroid drugs: to breast-feed or not to breast-feed. Am J Obstet Gynecol 157:234, 1987.
272. Illingsworth RS: Abnormal substances excreted in human milk. Practitioner 171:533, 1953.
273. Anderson PO: Drug use during breast-feeding. Clin Pharm 10:594, 1991.
274. Ryu JE: Effect of maternal caffeine consumption on heart rate and sleep time of breast-fed infants. Dev Pharmacol Ther 8:355, 1985.
275. Luck W, Nau H: Nicotine and cotinine concentrations in serum and urine of infants exposed via passive smoking or milk from smoking mothers. J Pediatr 107:816, 1985.
276. Labrecque M, Marcoux S, Weber J-P, et al: Feeding and urine cotinine values in babies whose mothers smoke. J Pediatr 107:816, 1985.
277. Miller RW: Effects of ionizing radiation from the atomic bomb on Japanese children. Pediatrics 41:257, 1968.
278. Krisch-Volders M: Mutagenicity, Carcinogenicity, and Teratogenicity of Industrial Pollutants. New York, Plenum, 1984.
279. Wood JW, Johnson KG, Omori Y, et al: Mental retardation in children exposed in utero to the atomic bombs in Hiroshima and Nagasaki. Am J Public Health Nations Health 57:1381, 1967.
280. Miller RW: Delayed effects occurring within the first decade after exposure of young individuals to the Hiroshima atomic bomb. Pediatrics 18:1, 1956.
281. Dekaban AS: Abnormalities in children exposed to x-radiation during various stages of gestation: tentative timetable of radiation injury to the human fetus. J Nucl Med 9:471, 1968.
282. Brent RL: The effects of embryonic and fetal exposure to x-ray, microwaves, and ultrasound. Clin Perinatol 13:615, 1986.
283. Lowe SA: Diagnostic radiography in pregnancy: risks and reality. Aust N Z J Obstet Gynaecol 44:191, 2004.
284. Damilakis J, Perisinakis K, Voloudaki A, et al: Estimation of fetal radiation dose from computed tomography scanning in late pregnancy: depth-dose data from routine examinations. Invest Radiol 35:527, 2000.
285. Barish RJ: In-flight radiation exposure during pregnancy. Obstet Gynecol 103:1326, 2004.
286. Stewart A, Kneale GW: Radiation dose effects in relation to obstetric x-rays and childhood cancers. Lancet 1:1185, 1970.
287. Giles D, Hewitt D, Stewart A, et al: Malignant disease in childhood and diagnostic irradiation in utero. Lancet 271:447, 1956.
288. Stewart A, Webb J, Hewett D: A survey of childhood malignancies. Br Med J 30:1495, 1958.
289. El-Khoury GY, Madsen MT, Blake ME, et al: A new pregnancy policy for a new era. Am J Roentgenol 181:335, 2003.
290. Sever LE: Parental radiation exposure and children's health: are there effects on the second generation? Occup Med 6:613, 1991.
291. Gardner MJ, Snee MP, Hall AJ, et al: Results of case-control study of leukaemia and lymphoma among young people near Sellafield nuclear plant in West Cumbria. Br Med J 300:423, 1990.
292. Gardner MJ, Hall AJ, Snee MP, et al: Methods and basic data of case-control study of leukaemia and lymphoma among young people near Sellafield nuclear plant in West Cumbria. Br Med J 300:429, 1990.
293. Sever LE, Gilbert ES, Hessol NA, et al: A case-control study of congenital malformations and occupational exposure to low-level ionizing radiation. Am J Epidemiol 127:226, 1988.
294. Neel JV: Problem of "false positive" conclusions in genetic epidemiology: lessons from the leukemia cluster near the Sellafield nuclear installation. Genet Epidemiol 11:213, 1994.
295. McLaughlin JR, King WD, Anderson TW, et al: Paternal radiation exposure and leukaemia in offspring: the Ontario case-control study. Br Med J 307:959, 1993.
296. Marcus M: Epidemiologic studies of VDT use and pregnancy outcome. Reprod Toxicol 4:51, 1990.
297. Gold EB, Tomich E: Occupational hazards to fertility and pregnancy outcome. Occup Med 9:435, 1994.
298. Blackwell R, Chang A: Video display terminals and pregnancy. A review. Br J Obstet Gynaecol 95:446, 1988.
299. Rothenberg SJ, Manalo M, Jiang J, et al: Maternal blood lead level during pregnancy in South Central Los Angeles. Arch Environ Health 54:151, 1999.
300. Pietrzyk JJ, Nowak A, Mitkowska Z, et al: Prenatal lead exposure and the pregnancy outcome. A case-control study in southern Poland. Przegl Lek 53:342, 1996.
301. Torres-Sanchez LE, Berkowitz G, Lopez-Carrillo L, et al: Intrauterine lead exposure and preterm birth. Environ Res 81:297, 1999.
302. Irgens A, Kruger K, Skorve AH, et al: Reproductive outcome in offspring of parents occupationally exposed to lead in Norway. Am J Ind Med 34:431, 1998.
303. Stefanak MA, Bourguet CC, Benzies-Styka T: Use of the Centers for Disease Control and Prevention childhood lead poisoning risk questionnaire to predict blood lead elevations in pregnant women. Obstet Gynecol 87:209, 1996.
304. Farias P, Borja-Aburto VH, Rios C, et al: Blood lead levels in pregnant women of high and low socioeconomic status in Mexico City. Environ Health Perspect 104:1070, 1996.
305. Sandstead HH, Doherty RA, Mahaffey KA: Effects and metabolism of toxic trace metals in the neonatal period. *In* Clarkson TW, Nordberg GFSRP (eds): Reproductive and Developmental Toxicology of Metals. New York, Plenum, 1983, p 207.
306. Creason JP, Svensgaard DJ, Baumgarner JE: Maternal-fetal tissue levels of sixteen trace elements in eight communities. USEPA Report EPA No. 600, 1:78, 1978.
307. Centers for Disease Control: Preventing lead poisoning in young children—United States. MMWR Morb Mortal Wkly Rep 34:66, 1985.
308. Centers for Disease Control: Preventing lead poisoning in young children. Atlanta, Department of Health and Human Services. Atlanta, Public Health Service, Centers for Disease Control, 1991, p 7.
309. Occupational Safety and Health Administration: Occupational exposure to lead. Fed Reg 43, 52952, 1978.
310. Needleman HL, Schell A, Bellinger D, et al: The long-term effects of exposure to low doses of lead in childhood. An 11-year follow-up report. N Engl J Med 322:83, 1990.
311. Bellinger D, Leviton A, Waternaux C, et al: Longitudinal analyses of prenatal and postnatal lead exposure and early cognitive development. N Engl J Med 316:1037, 1987.
312. U.S. Environmental Protection Agency, March 2004, website: *www.cfsan.fda.gov/*.
313. Harada M: Congenital minamata disease: Intrauterine methylmercury poisoning. Teratology 18:285, 1978.

Ultrasound for Pregnancy Dating, Growth, and the Diagnosis of Fetal Malformations

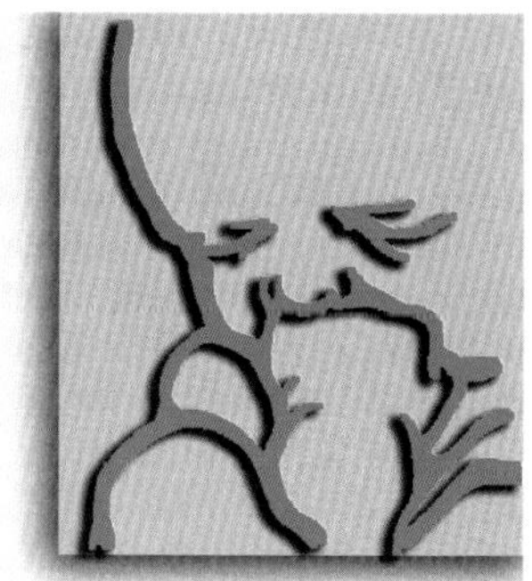

DOUGLAS S. RICHARDS

CHAPTER 9

KEY ABBREVIATIONS

Abdominal circumference	AC
American Institute of Ultrasound in Medicine	AIUM
Biparietal diameter	BPD
Congenital cystic adenomatoid malformation	CCAM
Crown-rump length	CRL
Estimated fetal weight	EFW
Expected date of confinement	EDC
Femur length	FL
Head circumference	HC
Head circumference/abdominal circumference ratio	HC/AC
Intrauterine growth restriction	IUGR
Last menstrual period	LMP
Routine Antenatal Diagnostic Imaging With Ultrasound Study	RADIUS
Sacrococcygeal teratoma	SCT
Small for gestational age	SGA
Ventricular septal defect	VSD

INTRODUCTION

Over the past several decades, the clinical use of ultrasound imaging in obstetrics has expanded remarkably. It is now considered by many to be the most valuable diagnostic tool in the field. Ultrasound was first used clinically in pregnancy in the early 1960s to measure the biparietal diameter as the distance between spikes on an oscilloscope screen. Since then, the technology has progressed to the point that even relatively inexpensive ultrasound machines yield detailed real-time images of the fetus. In this chapter, we begin by discussing how ultrasound is used to determine the gestational age and evaluate fetal growth. Normal and abnormal findings with first-trimester ultrasound are then discussed. Finally, we consider what has become a major use of ultrasound in obstetrics: the diagnosis of birth defects. The use of ultrasound to evaluate many problems in pregnancy, such as multiple gestation, third-trimester bleeding, and incompetent cervix, is covered in other chapters.

ULTRASOUND FOR DETERMINING GESTATIONAL AGE

Determination of the correct gestational age is one of the most important aspects of prenatal care. Making correct management decisions for conditions such as preterm labor, postdates pregnancy, and preeclampsia depends heavily on knowledge of the gestational age of the fetus. Without early confirmation of the expected date of confinement (EDC), it is very difficult to diagnose growth disorders in the fetus. Biochemical screening for open fetal defects and chromosomal anomalies likewise requires accurate dating. For these and other reasons, it has become routine in developed countries to offer at least one ultrasound examination in the first half of pregnancy to accurately establish the gestational age.

Standard Measurements

Ian Donald first demonstrated the clinical use of ultrasound in obstetrics in the early 1960's with the measurement of the biparietal diameter (BPD).[1] Since that time, the plane at which the BPD should be measured has been standardized[2] (Fig. 9-1) and a large number of publications have correlated this parameter with gestational age. The BPD can be measured from 12 to 13 weeks of gestation, when the skull has become ossified.

In the early 1970s, static scanners had advanced to the point that the gestational age could be determined in the first trimester by measuring the crown-rump length (CRL).[3] With modern transvaginal ultrasound, the embryo can be measured when it is only a few millimeters long, between 5 and 6 weeks' gestation.[4] From 6 to 10 weeks' gestation, the maximum length of the embryo is measured. After about 10 weeks, the head, trunk, and extremities are visible, and views of the CRL, such as those shown in Figure 9-2, are obtained. Measurement of the femur length for growth assessment was first described by Queenan in 1980, and was enabled by the development of real-time ultrasound.[5] Using real-time linear array transducers, measurement of the femur length is straightforward after the first trimester (Fig. 9-3). With real-time ultrasound, it is possible to measure

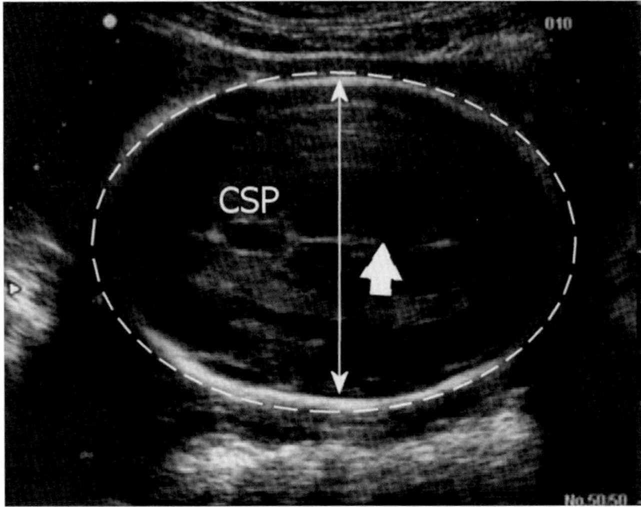

Figure 9-1. Transverse image of the head used for biparietal diameter (*double-headed arrow*) and head circumference (*dashed oval*) measurements. The cursors for the BPD are placed from the leading edge to leading edge of the skull bones. The HC is measured at the outer perimeter of the calvarium. The HC can be calculated from the BPD and occipital frontal diameter rather than measured directly. The image is at the level of the cavum septum pellucidum (CSP), does not include the orbits or brainstem, and has an appropriate oval shape. The fact that the midline echo (*small arrowhead*) is centered indicates that a true axial (not oblique) image is obtained. BPD measurements are most accurate when the head is imaged from the side, not the front or back. BPD, biparietal diameter; HC, head circumference.

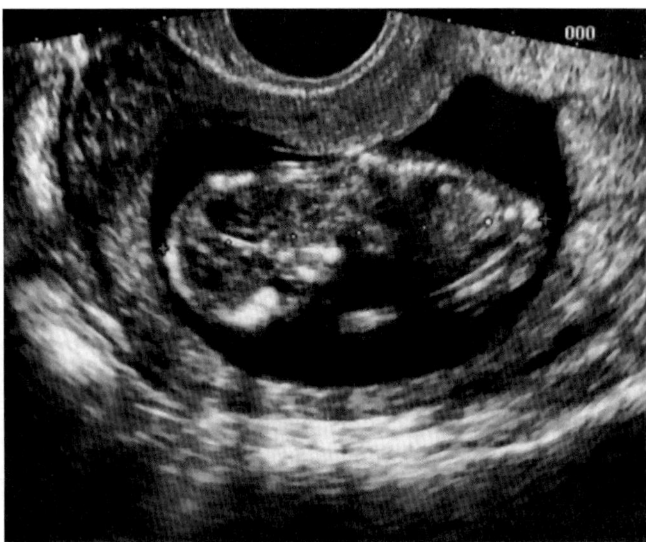

Figure 9-2. Crown rump length (CRL) measurement in an 11-week-old fetus. The CRL should be measured with a sagittal image of the fetus with the head in a neutral position.

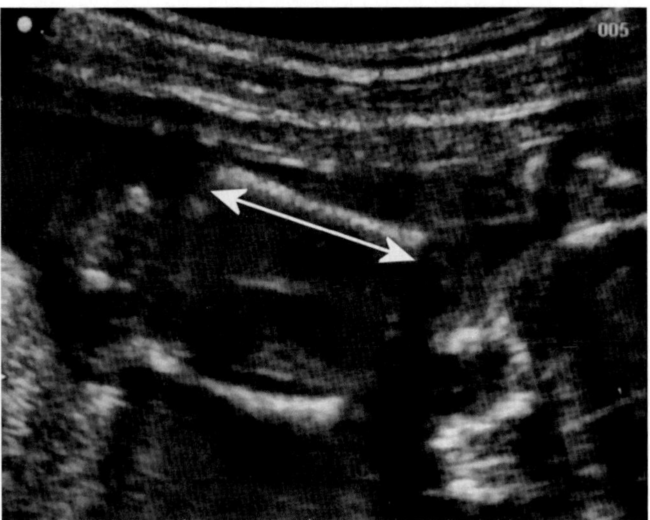

Figure 9-3. Appropriate image for measuring the femur length (*arrow*). Note that the ends of the bone are clearly seen, and the epiphysis in not included in the image. Fuzzy or tapered ends may indicate that the bone is cut obliquely and that the entire femur is not included in the image. It is best if the angle of insonation is perpendicular to the axis of the bone.

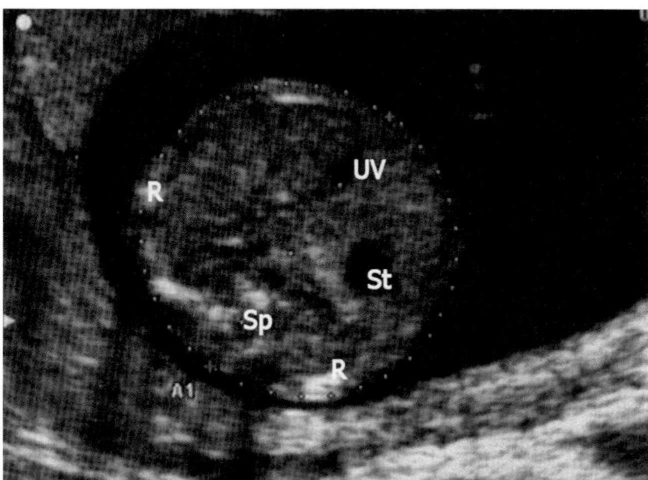

Figure 9-4. Abdominal circumference measurement at the level that the umbilical vein (UV) passes through the liver. Note that the abdominal image is circular, with symmetric rib (R) images, indicating a nonoblique transverse abdominal plane. Note that the abdomen is not flattened by undue pressure from the transducer. The AC measurement is best obtained when the angle of insonation is from the side, not directly through the front or back. The stomach (St) and spine (Sp) are also labeled. AC, abdominal circumference.

virtually any body part of the fetus. Nomograms correlating these measurements with gestational age have been constructed. Over time, however, a standard set of measurements has been accepted as being the most useful for gestational age prediction. In addition to the BPD, CRL, and femur length (FL), the standard set now includes the head circumference (HC) and abdominal circumference (AC) (Fig. 9-4).

Determination of Gestational Age

An intrauterine pregnancy can first be identified with transvaginal ultrasound at 4 weeks from the last menstrual period (LMP). From this time until the embryo can be seen and measured at 5 1/2 to 6 weeks, formulas using the sac diameter can give a fairly close approximation of the gestational age.[6] The mean sac diameter increases by about 1 mm per day during this interval, and the gestational age (in days) can be figured by adding 30 to the mean sac diameter (in mm).[7] Because the range of error in age prediction from sac measurement is significantly greater than for the CRL and other standard measurements, the sac size should not be used as the final gestational age determinant.[8] The measurement of the early embryo, either as the maximum embryo length or CRL, is commonly accepted as the best sonographic method for gestational age determination. Using a static scanner in pregnancies dated by "good" menstrual dates, Robinson found that the 95% confidence intervals for gestational age prediction using the CRL was +4.7 days.[3] Later studies, in which gestational age was determined by in vitro fertilization showed an even smaller random error.[9] The small random dating error found in early embryos is explained by their high weekly percentage change in size and the fact that there is very little variation among early embryos in their growth rates. However, in the late first trimester, flexion and extension of the fetus can significantly alter the CRL, making it less accurate for dating purposes. MacGregor and colleagues found in a study of patients with known ovulation dates that the 95% confidence intervals for CRL gestational age determination reached +9.1 days at 14 weeks gestation.[10] In comparison, Hadlock and others have shown that the 95% confidence intervals for gestational age prediction using the BPD as a single parameter between 14 and 21 weeks is +7 days.[11,12] In a study of pregnancies dated by in vitro fertilization, Chervenak et al.[13] found that in this period of pregnancy, all of the single parameters considered (BPD, HC, FL) performed well, with 95% confidence intervals for the gestational age ranging between +7.5 days for the HC and +8.7 days for the FL. These studies demonstrate that a dating ultrasound performed between 14 and 22 weeks is comparable to one performed in the first trimester, and that the obstetrician need not refer a patient for ultrasound in the first trimester for the sole purpose of establishing optimal dates.

Before the mid-1980s, second- or third-trimester gestational age assignment at the time of ultrasound was typically done by consulting a chart that had BPD or FL as the independent variable and gestational age as the dependent variable. This method did not allow for incorporation of multiple measurements in the gestational age assessment unless ad hoc averaging of the age from different parameters was done. Starting in the late 1980s computer programs that calculated a composite gestational age from multiple measurements became available. These are now routinely used by ultrasound reporting software. Several studies have shown a significant reduction in variability of gestational age estimates when mathematical modeling from multiple parameters (BPD, HC, AC, and FL) is employed.[11,13] This technique reduces the impact of technical errors in measurement and smooths out effects from body part variations. Composite gestational age assessment using mathematical modeling from multiple parameters is now the best-accepted method of ultrasound dating after the first trimester. The studies previously cited show that calculation of gestational age using standard parameters before 22 weeks is accurate to within +7 days, and is comparable to CRL measurement in the first trimester. As pregnancy progress, variability in fetal size grows, and ultrasound prediction of gestational age becomes progressively less accurate.[11] In one study, the composite gestational age assessment had a variability (+2 standard deviations) of 1.8 weeks at 24 to 30 weeks and 2 to 3 weeks beyond 30 weeks.[11]

These calculations of the variability of gestational age represent a statistical description of the variability in the studied population. Assuming a normally growing fetus, it is likely that the gestational age of a pregnancy falls within the bounds described. However, there is no guarantee that the gestational age of a particular fetus is at least or not more than the lower or upper limit of the variability estimate. In the third trimester, growth disorders in fetuses are relatively common and can bring about marked size variation. For this reason, the obstetrician must exercise caution when basing management decisions on gestational age established by ultrasound in the third trimester.

When to Use Ultrasound Dating

Since the time of Nagele in the early 1800s, obstetricians have routinely used menstrual dates to determine the EDC. In pregnancies in which the menstrual dates are unsure or thought to be unreliable because of a history of irregular cycles, recent hormonal contraception use, or an abnormally light LMP, dates derived from ultrasound biometry are always preferred. It is now common practice in many countries for ultrasound to be performed routinely in the first half of all pregnancies, even those with good menstrual dates. In these cases, in which both menstrual dates and ultrasound dates are available, which should be used? Possible strategies would be to always retain the menstrual dates, to use the menstrual dates unless the ultrasound size is out of the expected size range and thus contradicts the menstrual dates, or to ignore the menstrual dates altogether and use the ultrasound dates. A common practice is for ultrasound dates to take precedence over the menstrual dates if an ultrasound performed before approximately 22 weeks' gestation shows a gestational age more than 1 week different from the menstrual dates.[14]

Changing the dates in favor of the ultrasound dates can lead to an incorrect age assignment if the fetus has a significant early-onset growth disorder that accounts for the discrepancy. In the absence of maternal risk factors for early growth restriction or ultrasound signs suggesting a genetic syndrome or placental insufficiency, most sonographers feel safe in changing to ultrasound dates when a discrepancy exists. Delayed ovulation and incorrect recall of the LMP are common, whereas early-onset severe growth disorder is rare; thus, this is usually a good policy. However, in the third trimester, aberrant growth is relatively common, so changing certain menstrual dates in favor of a late ultrasound risks masking the presence of a significant growth disorder. Uncertainties are best avoided by a policy that encourages routine early prenatal care so that firm dates can be established and risk factors for altered fetal growth can be recognized.

There is growing evidence that a dating ultrasound performed before 22 weeks should be used in preference to menstrual dates, regardless of the reliability or closeness of fit with menstrual dates. In 1996, Mongelli and associates evaluated 34,249 patients who had both certain menstrual dates and an ultrasound performed in the first half of pregnancy.[14] Using ultrasound exclusively led to a 70-percent reduction in the number of pregnancies considered post term and more accurately predicted the onset of spontaneous labor. A policy of changing dates only when there was a significant discrepancy between menstrual dates and ultrasound gave inferior results compared with the exclusive use of ultrasound dates. Other studies using the same end points have similarly shown that there is no advantage of taking menstrual dates into account if a relatively early dating sonogram is available.[15] Exclusive use of ultrasound dating has also been shown to improve the predictive accuracy of serum screening for Down syndrome.[16] It has been argued that performing a routine dating ultrasound is not medically indicated because it does not reduce morbidity or mortality in cases in which certain menstrual dates are available.[17] However, in many developed countries, the current practice of performing ultrasound in the first half of almost all pregnancies and the apparent superiority of ultrasound dating make it likely that in the future menstrual dating will become obsolete in these settings.

ASSESSING FETAL GROWTH

The first ultrasound examination is generally considered to be a dating examination, that is, the measurements are used to determine the gestational age. An accurate knowledge of gestational age determined by or confirmed by the first ultrasound examination forms the basis for subsequent clinical and sonographic assessment of fetal growth. Because insufficient or excessive growth can be associated with significant fetal morbidity, recognition of growth abnormalities is one of the primary aims of prenatal care and is an important aspect of ultrasound examinations. In most obstetric practices, ultrasound examinations to assess fetal growth are obtained when abdominal palpation and fundal height measurement raise the suspicion of abnormal growth.[18] A lagging fundal height, combined with the knowledge of clinical risk factors for intrauterine growth restriction (IUGR), is commonly used as a screening test for insufficient fetal growth, whereas ultrasound is considered the diagnostic test. This scheme for the prenatal detection of growth restricted fetuses has met with mixed results. In 1987, Pearce and colleagues showed that fundal height measurement in the third trimester had a sensitivity of 76 percent for detecting small-for-gestational age (SGA) births, with a specificity of 79 percent and a positive predictive value of 36 percent.[19] In contrast, other studies in low- and high-risk pregnancies showed the sensitivity of this stepwise screening for IUGR (defined as birth weight below the 10th percentile) to be 15 to 26 percent, whereas the positive predictive value was only in the range of 50 percent.[20,21] A recent Dutch study reported by Bais and colleagues[21] showed that the sensitivity of schemes for the antenatal diagnosis of small fetuses was significantly better if clinical risk factors were taken into account.

Serial ultrasound examinations have proven to be superior to the physical examinations for diagnosing insufficient growth.[22] For this reason, some European countries have established formal policies requiring a third-trimester ultrasound examination to screen for growth abnormalities, even in low-risk pregnancies. Studies have shown, however, that this policy has little or no impact on perinatal morbidity and mortality.[23,24] Because of the high cost and unproven benefit of such a screening program, routine ultrasound examinations for growth are generally not a part of prenatal care in the United States. Because of the high rates of morbidity associated with growth restriction, it is still accepted that ultrasound should be ordered when the clinical examination is suspicious and when there are significant risk factors for a growth abnormality. Such risk factors include diabetes mellitus, maternal hypertension, previous small or large baby, multiple gestation, or poor maternal weight gain. A risk-based approach is particularly appropriate in cases such as multiple gestation or marked maternal obesity, in which clinical evaluation of fetal size is difficult or impossible.

Diagnosing Abnormal Growth

The best-accepted way of diagnosing abnormal growth in a fetus is to calculate the estimated fetal weight (EFW) using standard ultrasound measurements, then compare the estimated weight with an accepted standard. Some nomograms still in use were based on the birth weight distribution at different gestational ages of children born in the 1960s or 1970s.[25] The reliability of these tables is limited by the fact that the pregnancies in that era did not have ultrasound confirmation of dates. Also, babies born preterm are necessarily from pathologic pregnancies, and these infants tend to be SGA. To overcome these limitations, Hadlock and colleagues derived weight standards from ultrasound estimated weights in pregnancies whose gestational age was confirmed with early ultrasound.[26] Some have found that the normal weight distribution defined by Hadlock is too narrow, possibly because the standards came from a relatively small group of predominately white middle class women. A compromise approach has been to use birth weight data from a heterogeneous mixed-race study population, incorporating only pregnancies with ultrasound confirmation of dates.[27]

The definition of abnormal growth is also a subject of debate. Most commonly, if the EFW is less than the 10th or greater than the 90th percentile the fetus is said to be small or large for the gestational age. Defining abnormal growth using these percentile cutoffs includes many babies who are healthy and are constitutionally large or small. Using a more restrictive definition such as a birth weight less than or greater than the 3rd or 97th percentile is much more predictive of a poor neonatal outcome. Of course, with this approach, many less severely affected fetuses are not detected. Additionally, some infants have birth weights within the normal range but have not grown to their genetic potential. For this reason, some have argued that individual birth weight percentile limits that incorporate such characteristics as maternal weight, height, ethnic group, parity, and fetal sex should be used.[28] Gardosi and colleagues found that with adjusted percentile limits, about a quarter of fetuses judged to be abnormally small using conventional limits were within normal limits. Conversely, a quarter of babies identified as small or large with adjusted percentiles would have been missed by conventional assessment. Another study from the same institution demonstrated that the risk for stillbirth, neonatal death, and low Apgar scores can be better predicted by customized weight percentiles.[29]

In 1977, Campbell described the head to abdomen circumference (HC/AC) ratio as a useful marker for detecting fetal growth restriction.[30] This finding is based on the observation that growth of the soft tissues in the fetal abdomen is more likely to be compromised than the head when there is nutritional deprivation. This understanding led to the concept that asymmetric growth restriction is virtually pathognomonic for nutritional deprivation, whereas symmetric growth restriction signifies an underlying condition such as aneuploidy. This concept has been largely disproven, because there is a great deal of overlap between body ratios of fetuses that are growth restricted from either nutritional or intrinsic factors. However, because a very high HC/AC ratio is uncommon in normal fetuses, this calculation remains useful. For example, in fetuses whose estimated weight is less than the 10th percentile, a high head to abdomen ratio makes it less likely that the small size of a fetus is constitutional.[31] Additionally, it has been shown in newborns that a low weight to length ratio is associated with an increase in several markers of morbidity even if the birth weight is greater than the 10th percentile; perhaps indicating that these infants also experienced growth restriction.[32] Currently, there is no consensus concerning the level of surveillance appropriate for a fetus with a high HC/AC ratio but normal estimated weight.

When a patient presents late for prenatal care and the gestational age is uncertain, diagnosis of a growth disorder is particularly difficult. In these cases, a high or low HC/AC ratio can raise the suspicion of a growth disorder. Other ultrasound findings may be useful to help confirm the suspicion. For example, IUGR is often associated with oligohydramnios, abnormal Doppler flow studies, or an abnormal appearing placenta. Macrosomic fetuses may demonstrate obviously thickened subcutaneous fat pads. In suspected cases, as long as the fetus is stable, serial ultrasound examinations to evaluate growth are appropriate. The rate of growth can be valuable for predicting adverse outcome. Formulas defining rates of normal growth have been published,[33] but most clinicians rely on an observation of progressively increasing or decreasing weight percentiles to evaluate the severity of an ongoing growth disorder.

Estimating Fetal Weight

A large number of formulas for calculating the EFW have been proposed. The most popular of these have been compiled in a recent review by Nyberg and colleagues.[34] All incorporate the abdominal circumference, because this is the standard measurement most susceptible to the variations in fetal soft tissue mass. Although the abdominal circumference alone is a relatively good marker for detecting abnormal fetal growth, the addition of other standard measurements to estimated weight formulas increases their accuracy.[35] It has been shown that the addition of measurements beyond the standard set (BPD, HC, AC, and FL) does not significantly improve weight estimations. It appears that the error inherent in obtaining the basic measurements (especially the AC) is great enough to obscure any refinement in accuracy that might be gained from additional measurements.

Because procedures for standard biometry are well defined and formulas using these measurements yield seemingly precise weight predictions, some clinicians place more confidence in ultrasound weight estimates than is warranted. There have been a large number of studies in which the accuracy of ultrasound for predicting birth weights has been evaluated.[34,36] Published equations applied to a variety of patient populations often show a small systematic error, in the range of 2 to 3 percent, tending to overestimate or underestimate birth weights. It has been claimed in some publications that one formula is better than another when statistically significant differences in accuracy are seen. However, the differences in accuracy are usually of limited clinical significance, and no formula has been consistently shown to be superior to another.[36] When scans are performed by well-trained sonographers, most studies show a mean absolute error in birth weight prediction of about 8 to 10 percent of the birth weight. Perhaps a more telling statistic is that in about 30 percent of cases, the absolute error in estimated weight is greater than 10 percent of the birth weight. In most, but not all, of the remaining cases the error is less than 20 percent of the birth weight. The rate of clinically significant errors is greater if an inexperienced person performs the ultrasound examination.[37]

It is often assumed that ultrasound is more objective than clinical examination and, therefore, that ultrasound estimates of fetal weight are more reliable. Most studies have *not* shown this to be true. In a review of 12 studies by Sherman in which ultrasound was compared to clinical examination for weight estimation, ultrasound was shown to be clearly superior in only one, and this series included a subgroup of patients in which the birth weight was less than 2500 g. In three studies, clinical estimates were superior, and in the remaining eight, the two methods were either equivalent or had mixed results depending on the specific formula used.[36] One small study even showed that the estimate by the patient herself was only marginally less accurate than an ultrasound estimate![37]

There have been several strategies aimed at improving the performance of ultrasound for estimating fetal weights. One is to develop formulas based on subpopulations of fetuses, such as those who are preterm or are thought to be small or large for gestational age. Although this approach seems reasonable, most studies have not shown an improvement in the accuracy of weight estimates compared with traditional one-size-fits-all formulas.[38–40] A more promising approach for improving accuracy of fetal weight estimates is to use equations that incorporate three-dimensional fetal volumes. Lee and colleagues used a simple technique in which the volume of the mid-50 percent of the thigh (the fractional limb volume) was calculated from three-dimensional images by tracing three thigh circumferences at standard locations. A weight equation incorporating this fractional limb volume and abdominal circumference yielded a mean absolute error of only 2 percent, compared with 9 percent using a standard formula.[41] The improved accuracy of this technique was probably due to the fact that the fractional limb volume gave a useful reflection of bone growth of the fetus as well the amount of fat, muscle, and other soft tissues. If the results of additional studies with larger numbers of patients confirm these initial results, this could prove to be the most important clinical use of three-dimensional ultrasound in obstetrics, and this new technology could add significantly to the accuracy of fetal weight estimation.

Macrosomia

It has been hoped by many that ultrasound could aid in the difficult decisions faced by obstetricians when macrosomia is suspected. One of the most feared complications in obstetrics is shoulder dystocia, because it can lead to permanent neurologic injury in the fetus. Unfortunately, ultrasound for fetal weight estimation has proved to be of limited usefulness for the prevention of shoulder dystocia and other complications associated with fetal macrosomia. A study by Gonen and colleagues demonstrated several explanations for this.[42] In a review of 4,480 deliveries, only 17 percent of infants weighing more than 4,500 g were detected by an ultrasound ordered because of a clinical suspicion of macrosomia. Only one of the 23 infants who weighed more than 4,500 g had a brachial plexus injury. Additionally, 93 percent of infants who had shoulder dystocia weighed less than 4,500 g. For these reasons, these and other authors have concluded that most cases of injury resulting from shoulder dystocia cannot be predicted by ultrasound, and that if cesarean delivery were routinely performed when macrosomia was suspected, the cesarean delivery rate would be increased with very little benefit.

FIRST-TRIMESTER ULTRASOUND

Normal Findings

Transvaginal ultrasound is almost always superior to transabdominal ultrasound for first-trimester pregnancy evaluation. Knowledge of the time at which embryonic structures normally appear is important for identifying pathologic pregnancies. The gestational sac can consistently be seen at 4 weeks, the yolk sac at 5 weeks, the fetal pole with cardiac activity at 6 weeks, a single unpartitioned brain ventricle at 7 weeks, the falx cerebri at 9 weeks, and the appearance and disappearance of physiologic gut herniation between 8 and 11 weeks.[43] The stomach can consistently be seen by 11 weeks,[44] and the bladder and kidneys in the majority of fetuses at 11 weeks.[45] The fetal heart rate is initially slow, averaging 100 beats per minute (bpm) at 5 to 6 weeks.[46] It then increases steadily to a peak at a mean of 175 bpm at 9 weeks.[44] Transvaginal ultrasound has the potential to provide good views of the fetal cardiac anatomy in the majority of patients at 13 weeks.[47] As the first trimester advances, the amniotic sac gradually expands until the amnion is fused to the chorion, usually between 13 and 16 weeks' gestation.

Abnormal Findings

Spontaneous abortion occurs in 15 percent of clinically established pregnancies. When cardiac activity has been demonstrated, the miscarriage rate is reduced to 2 to 3 percent in asymptomatic low-risk women.[48] It is important to note, however, that in some groups at very high risk for miscarriage, such as women older than 35 years of age who are undergoing infertility treatments, early

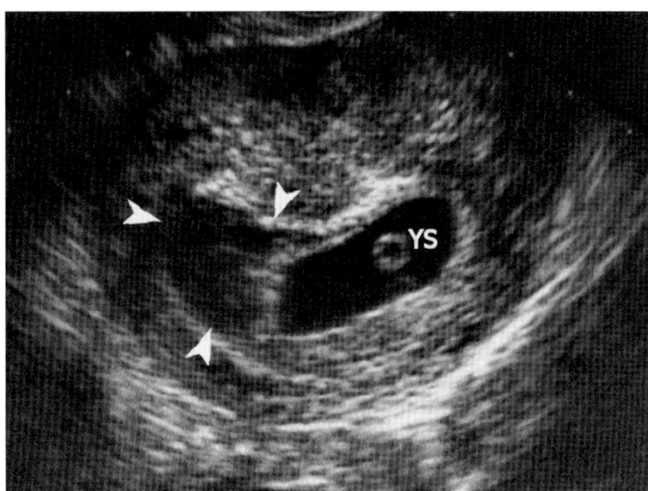

Figure 9-5. An intrauterine hematoma (*arrowheads*) adjacent to a 5-week gestational sac. The yolk sac (YS) is indicated. Sometimes an intrauterine collection of blood is mistakenly thought to represent a second gestational sac.

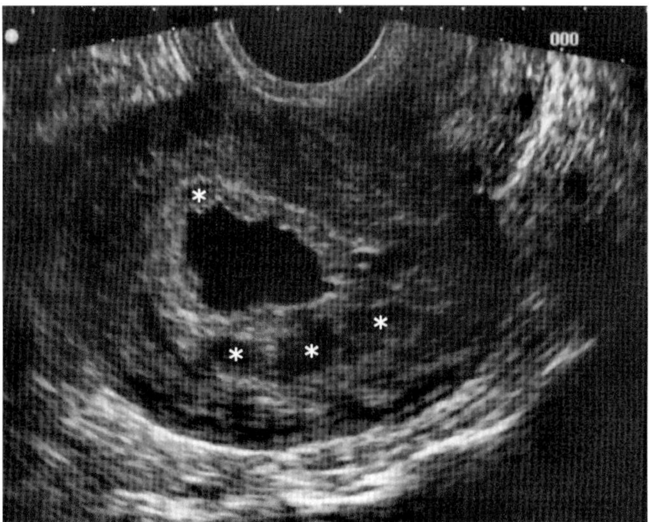

Figure 9-6. Empty gestational sac of an anembryonic gestation. When a nonviable gestational sac is retained for a prolonged period, vascular lacunae (*) develop in the chorionic tissue.

visualization of cardiac activity does not provide as much reassurance. In one study of older women, the miscarriage rate in asymptomatic patients was still 16 percent after a heart beat was documented.[49] In younger women who present with bleeding, only 5 percent miscarry if the ultrasound is normal and shows a live embryo.[50] If there is an intrauterine clot present (Fig. 9-5), coexistent with an otherwise normal appearing pregnancy, the miscarriage rate is 15 percent.[50]

In most pregnancies destined to abort, the embryo does not develop and ultrasound shows an empty gestational sac (Fig. 9-6). Such a pregnancy is termed an anembryonic gestation. When there is no yolk sac seen and the mean sac diameter is at least 13 mm or there is no embryo seen with mean sac diameter of at least 17 mm, it is almost certain that the pregnancy is nonviable.[51] The absence of cardiac activity when the fetal pole measures more than 5 mm is reliably diagnostic for embryonic death.[52] Other findings that are somewhat predictive of spontaneous abortion include a yolk sac that is unusually large or small for the gestational age,[53] a relatively small gestational sac (mean sac diameter/CRL difference of less then 5 mm),[54] or fetal bradycardia.[46] If there are borderline findings and uterine evacuation is being considered, it is prudent to repeat the ultrasound in a week to be absolutely sure that a viable pregnancy is not interrupted.[54]

There is growing evidence that first-trimester ultrasound findings, including thick nuchal translucency, absent nasal bone, abnormally fast or slow fetal heart rate, and some structural malformations can be very useful for predicting the risk of a chromosomal abnormality.[55] The use of ultrasound for aneuploidy screening is discussed in detail in Chapter 7.

The potential for first-trimester ultrasound to diagnose fetal malformations is increasingly being recognized. In one recent study, nearly 5,000 low-risk patients were screened with ultrasound by midwives at 13 to 14 weeks and again at 18 to 22 weeks. Half of the major birth defects were diagnosed at one of the two scans. Of these, one third were detected at the time of the early scan.[56] A partial list of anomalies that can potentially be diagnosed includes amniotic band syndrome, anencephaly, encephalocele, holoprosencephaly, cystic hygroma, major spina bifida, hydrops, abdominal wall defects (after 12 weeks), and bladder outlet obstruction. Conditions involving multiple gestation, including the number of amnions and chorions and the presence of conjoined twins, can also be easily diagnosed in the first trimester.

SECOND- AND THIRD-TRIMESTER ULTRASOUND

Although there are many well-recognized maternal risk factors for congenital anomalies, a sizeable number of birth defects occur in children of low-risk women.[57] For this reason, it is important that anyone who performs obstetric ultrasound have familiarity with the appearance of normal fetal anatomy in order to recognize deviations from normal. A systematic approach to examining the fetus is essential. The American Institute of Ultrasound in Medicine (AIUM), in conjunction with the American College of Obstetrics and Gynecology and the American College of Radiology, have defined a set of criteria for a standard obstetric ultrasound examination performed in the second or third trimesters.[58] Components of a standard obstetric examination are shown in Table 9-1. A complete description of the AIUM guidelines can be found in the listed reference.

All of the aspects of the standard obstetric examination listed in Table 9-1 are important for clinical management and should not be neglected. For example, it is obvious that there could be serious consequences if an ultrasound failed to reveal the presence of placenta previa, multiple gestation, or an ovarian tumor. Ultrasound is often used to answer a pressing clinical question, such as "is this term fetus in a cephalic presentation?" or "is there a placenta previa in this patient with bleeding?" It is sometimes tempting for the practitioner to use ultrasound

Table 9-1. Suggested Components of the Standard Obstetrical Ultrasound Performed in the Second and Third Trimester[58]

Standard biometry
Fetal cardiac activity (present or absent, normal or abnormal)
Number of fetuses (if multiples, document chorionicity, amnionicity, comparison of fetal sizes, estimation of amniotic fluid normality in each sac, fetal genitalia)
Presentation
Qualitative or semiquantitative estimate of amniotic fluid volume
Placental location, especially its relationship to the internal os
Evaluation of the uterus (including fibroids) and adnexal structures
Anatomic survey to include
- Head and neck
  - Cerebellum
  - Choroid plexus
  - Cisterna magna
  - Lateral cerebral ventricles
  - Midline falx
  - Cavum septum pellucidum
- Chest
  - Four-chamber view of the heart
  - Outflow tracts (if possible)
- Abdomen
  - Stomach (presence, size, and location)
  - Kidneys
  - Bladder
  - Umbilical cord insertion into the abdomen
  - Number of umbilical cord vessels
- Spine
- Extremities (presence or absence of legs and arms)

to answer the pressing question at hand and forego the remainder of a complete exam. If this shortcut approach is taken, critically important information is often missed. Limited ultrasound examinations are appropriate when needed to obtain specific information about the pregnancy, but only when a complete examination has been performed in the recent past.[58]

Documentation of ultrasound findings is important, not only for good patient care but also for quality review and legal defense. AIUM guidelines regarding record keeping state: "Adequate documentation of the study is essential for high-quality patient care. This should include a permanent record of the sonographic images, incorporating whenever possible . . . measurement parameters and anatomic findings."[58] Additionally, it is considered standard practice to include a written report in the patient's medical record.

ULTRASOUND DIAGNOSIS OF MALFORMATIONS

Over the past few decades, there have been a large number of publications describing the ultrasound diagnosis of fetal malformations. A catalog of the diseases that are now considered detectable with prenatal ultrasound is beyond the scope of this chapter. However, some of the more common birth defects that have distinctive ultrasound findings are discussed in the following sections. When one of these anomalies or other apparent deviation from normal is suspected, referral to an expert is appropriate.

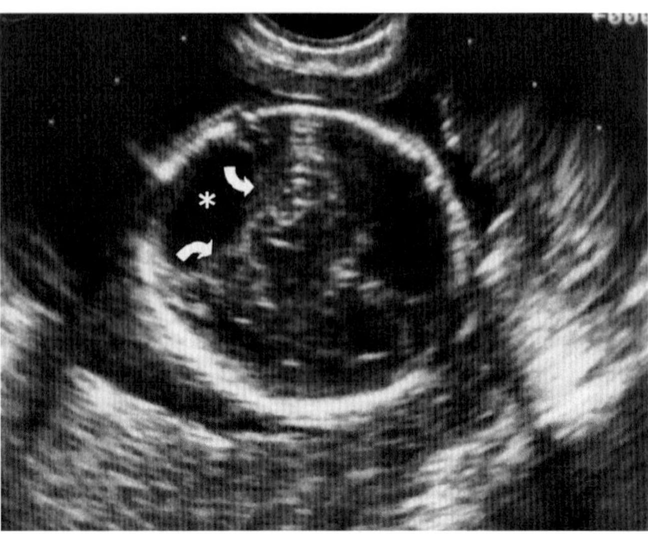

Figure 9-7. Marked brachycephaly. Note the nearly round outline of the calvarium. This fetus has a triploid karyotype with the Dandy-Walker syndrome. There is a posterior fossa cyst (*) and widely separated cerebellar hemispheres (*small arrows*).

HEAD AND SPINE

Abnormal Head Shape

On axial views, the head should have an oval appearance. Elongation of the head (termed dolichocephaly) is often caused by lateral compressive forces associated with oligohydramnios, especially if the fetus is in a breech presentation. An abnormally round shape (termed brachycephaly) can be an important indicator of fetal abnormalities, especially holoprosencephaly and aneuploidies (Fig. 9-7).

Hydrocephalus

Hydrocephalus is a general term used to describe a head in which the cerebral ventricles are dilated. There are many causes, including stenosis of the aqueduct of Sylvius, normal pressure hydrocephalus, agenesis of the corpus callosum, fetal TORCH infections, and other serious developmental malformations of the brain and spine. In some cases, particularly those caused by aqueductal stenosis, the head can be markedly enlarged. The lateral and third ventricles may be very dilated with marked thinning of the cerebral cortex (Fig. 9-8). With atraumatic delivery and appropriate neurosurgical treatment, more than half of infants with aqueductal stenosis survive, but about 75 percent of survivors have moderate to severe developmental delay.[59] The degree of hydroceph-

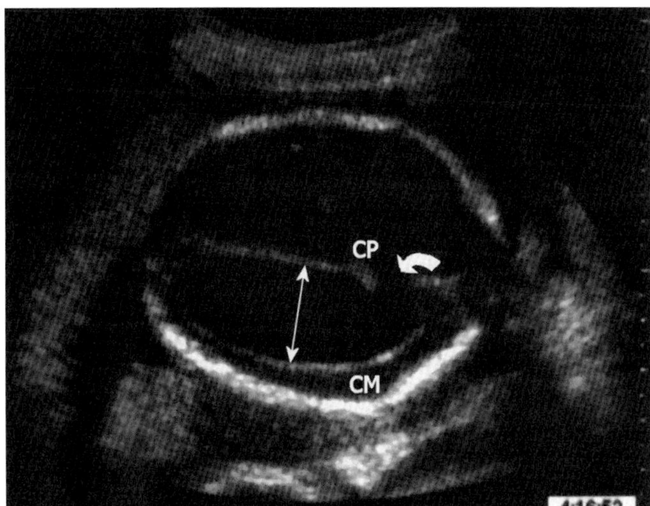

Figure 9-8. Moderate hydrocephalus from aqueductal stenosis. The cortical mantle (CM) is thin, and the lateral ventricles are markedly dilated (*arrow*). The midline echo is absent (*arrowhead*) where the markedly dilated third ventricle is blown out and the choroid plexus (CP) from one side dangles into the ventricle on the opposite, dependent side.

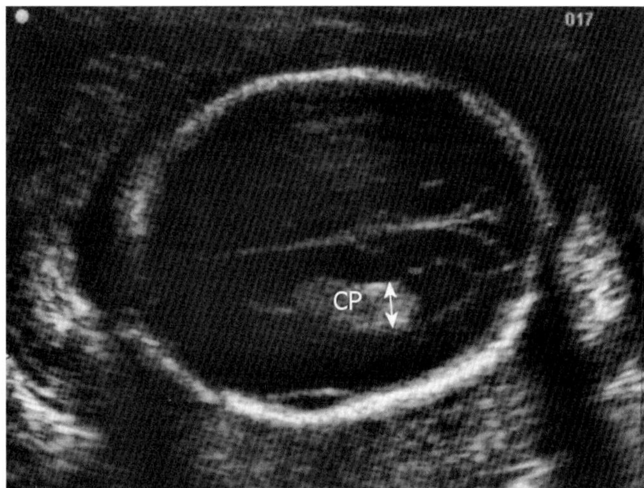

A

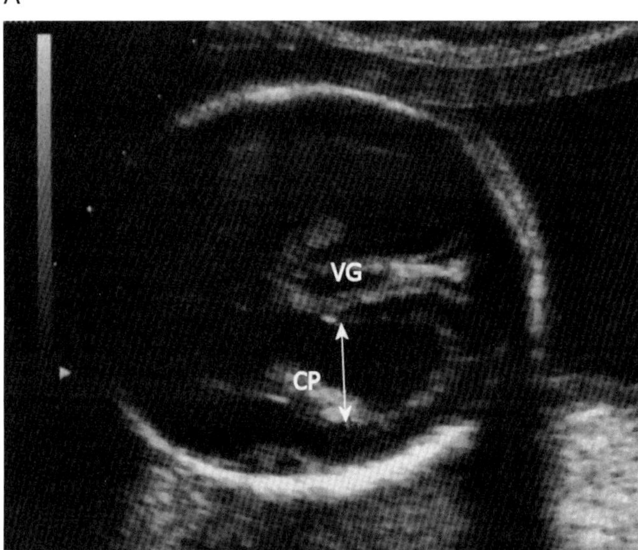

B

Figure 9-9. *A,* Normal lateral ventricles. The width at the atrium (*arrow*) measures less than 10 mm. The choroid plexus (CP) fills the atrium of the ventricle from side to side. *B,* Mild ventriculomegaly. The lateral ventricle measures 14 mm at the atrium (*arrow*) and the choroid plexus (CP) appears compressed. In this case, the hydrocephalus was caused by malformation of the vein of Galen (VG).

alus and the thickness of the remaining cerebral cortex are weak predictors of the neurologic outcome.[59]

Less obvious cases of hydrocephalus are suspected when the diameter of the atrium of the lateral ventricles in an axial view is greater than 10 mm. An associated sign is an abnormal appearance of the choroid plexus. In cases of hydrocephalus, this structure, which usually fills this portion of the lateral ventricle from side to side (Fig. 9-9A), appears compressed and dangling (Fig. 9-9B). Whenever any degree of hydrocephalus is seen, a careful search for other malformations is essential, because their presence strongly influences the prognosis. Isolated mild ventriculomegaly usually has a good prognosis. There is a 96 percent chance of a normal neurologic outcome when the ventricles measure between 10 and 12 mm, and an 86 percent chance with a measurement between 12 and 15 mm.[60] Agenesis of the corpus callosum should be considered when there is modest ventricular dilation that is primarily confined to the posterior horns (Fig. 9-10).

Choroid Plexus Cyst

Cysts within the choroid plexus are noted in about 1 percent of fetuses (Fig. 9-11). They generally are benign and resolve before 26 weeks without sequelae. Because their presence indicates a seven-fold increase in risk that the fetus has trisomy 18, referral for genetic counseling and detailed ultrasound is indicated.[61]

Holoprosencephaly

Holoprosencephaly is characterized by absence or abnormality of midline structures of the brain, resulting from incomplete division of the cerebral hemispheres. With the alobar form of holoprosencephaly, the head is usually small and brachycephalic. There is no midline echo dividing the cerebral cortex, and there is a single crescent-shaped ventricle anterior to the bulbous-appearing thalamus (Fig. 9-12). Many fetuses with holoprosencephaly have facial abnormalities as well, which may include hypotelorism or cyclopia, facial clefts, absent nose or single nostril, and presence of a proboscis above or between the eyes.[62] Chromosomal abnormalities (especially trisomy 13) and other malformations are present in 37 percent of cases. Regardless of the karyotype or presence of other malformations, alobar holoprosencephaly is associated with a dismal neurologic prognosis and death almost always occurs either before or shortly after birth. When there is partial division of the brain, the fetus may have semilobar (Fig. 9-13) or lobar holoprosencephaly, both of which have a somewhat more favorable prognosis.

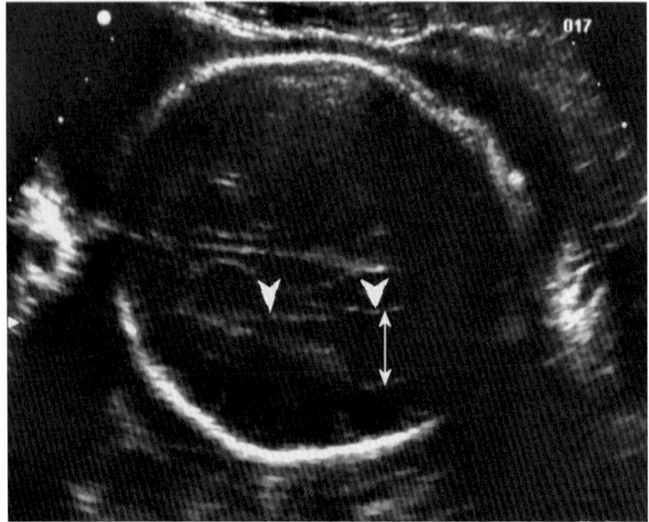

Figure 9-10. Isolated posterior horn dilation (*arrow*), termed colpocephaly. This is a sign of agenesis of the corpus callosum, also indicated by the fact that the medial border of the lateral ventricle is displaced laterally and is nearly parallel to the midline (*arrowheads*).

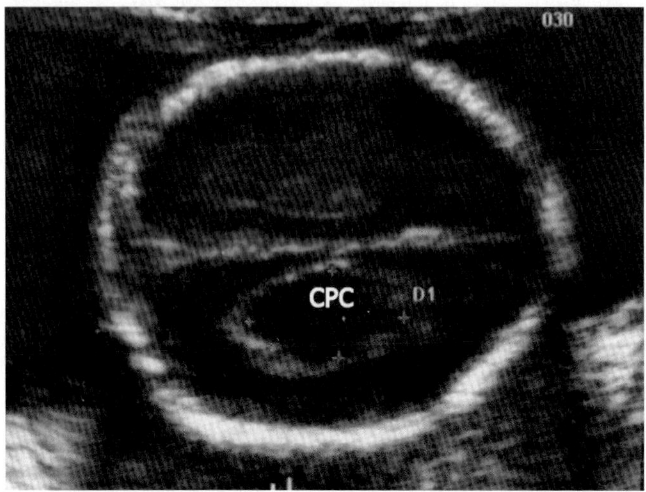

Figure 9-11. Large choroid plexus cyst (CPC), which in this case nearly fills the choroid plexus.

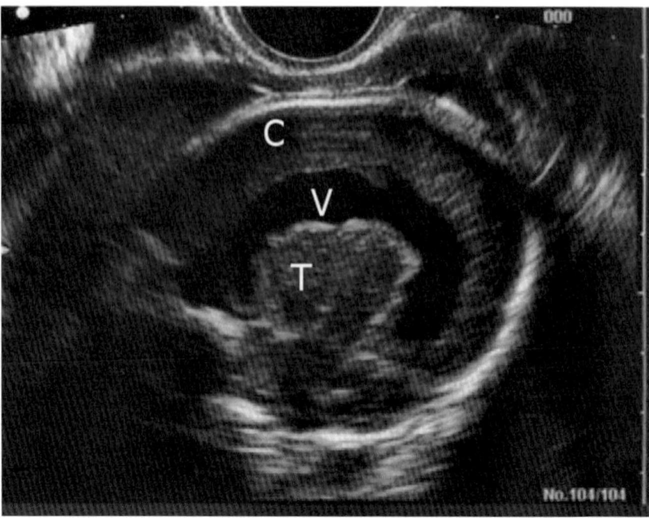

Figure 9-12. Transvaginal coronal view showing alobar holoprosencephaly. Note the undivided cerebral cortex (C) and anterior ventricle (V), and the bulbous appearing undivided thalamus (T).

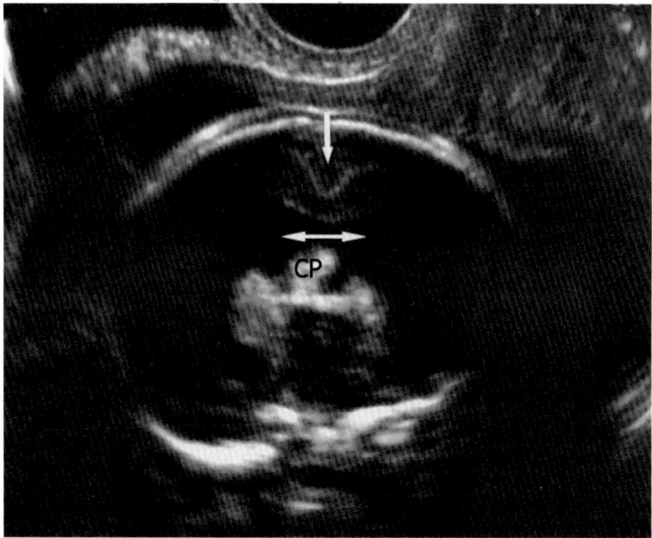

Figure 9-13. Semilobar holoprosencephaly. This is a tranvaginal coronal view of the fetal head. Note that there is partial division of the cortex (*single arrow*), but the falx is not completely formed. Also, the lateral ventricles communicate across the midline (*double arrow*). The choroid plexus (CP) droops across the midline.

Dandy-Walker Syndrome

In the Dandy-Walker syndrome, the anatomy of the normal posterior fossa (Fig. 9-14A) is altered. There is a posterior fossa cyst continuous with the fourth ventricle, complete or partial absence of the cerebellar vermis, and varying degrees of hydrocephalus (Fig. 9-14B). About 50 percent of affected fetuses have other intracranial malformations, 35 percent have extracranial abnormalities, and 15 to 30 percent have aneuploidy.[63,64] Many infants with the Dandy-Walker syndrome die after birth, usually as a result of associated malformations. The majority of survivors have some degree of mental handicap.[65]

Arachnoid Cyst

A unilateral cystic lesion adjacent to the cerebral cortex most likely represents an arachnoid cyst (Fig. 9-15). These lesions generally are associated with a good prognosis but can reach considerable size, causing symptoms such as seizures or hydrocephalus.[66] Postnatal surgical correction is usually successful. Porenecephalic cysts are unilateral cystic lesions in the brain that have a much worse outcome. These arise from intracerebral infarcts or hemorrhages with subsequent liquification of the brain tissue or clot (Fig. 9-16). The resultant cystic cavity within the brain parenchyma may be in communication with the subarachnoid space or a cerebral ventricle.

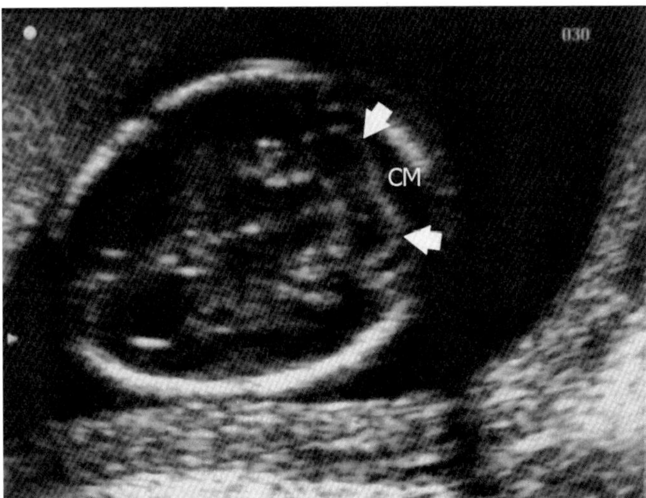

A

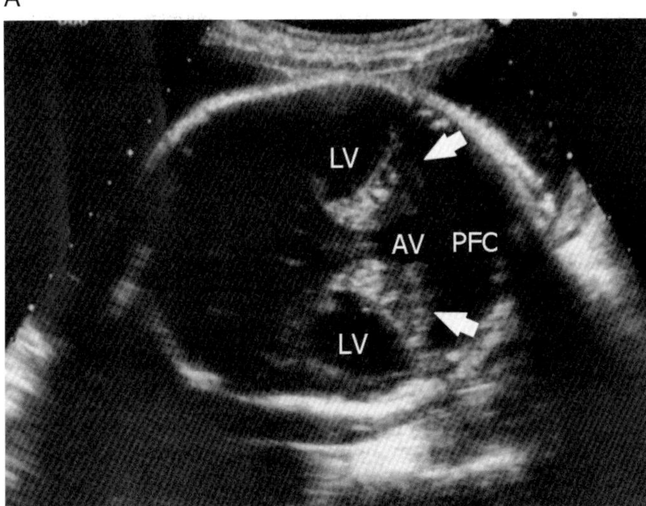

B

Figure 9-14. *A,* Normal cerebellum. The two cerebellar hemispheres are indicated by the arrowheads. The cisterna magna (CM) is the fluid-filled space posterior to the cerebellum. *B,* Dandy-Walker malformation. Note that the cerebellar hemispheres are small and widely separated (*arrowheads*). The vermis is absent (AV), and there is a posterior fossa cyst (PFC). The lateral ventricles (LV) are dilated.

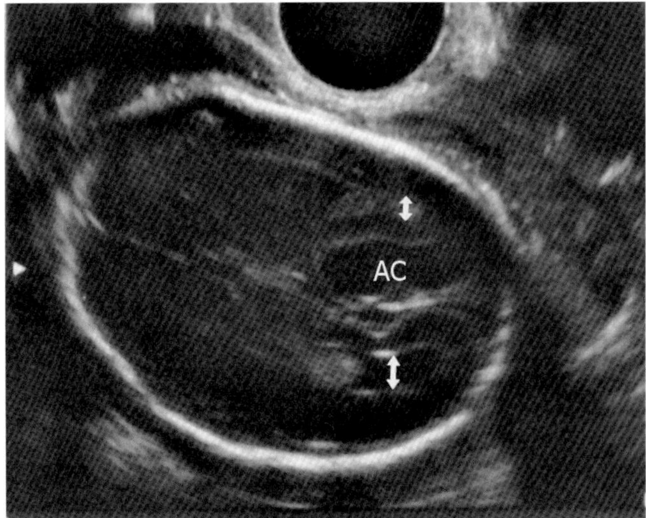

Figure 9-15. Arachnoid cyst. This is a transvaginal axial view of the fetal head showing an arachnoid cyst (AC) medial to the occipital lobe. The posterior horns of the lateral ventricles are indicated by the double arrows.

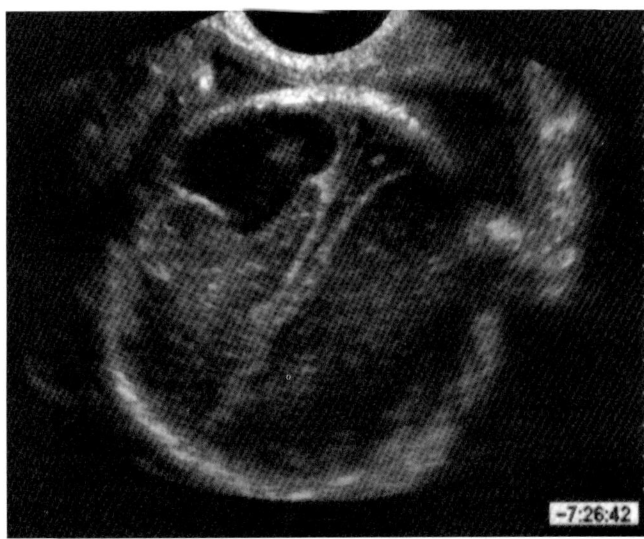

Figure 9-16. Porencephalic cyst. The liquefied space involves much of the lateral aspect of the occipital lobe.

Neural Tube Defects

Anencephaly is often first suspected when a proper image for measuring the BPD cannot be obtained. The absence of the cranial vault can be diagnosed after 10 weeks' gestation.[67] Although the skull is missing, lobulated disorganized brain tissue can be prominent between 9 to 11 weeks (Fig. 9-17). This degenerates by 15 weeks, leaving the characteristic appearance in which there is there is no cortex or cranium and the fetal eyes appear at the top of an intact lower face (Fig. 9-18). Meningomyelocele extending varying distances from the base of the skull down the neck and body may be present along with the anencephaly. Fetuses with anencephaly do not swallow normally, so polyhydramnios usually develops in pregnancies that are allowed to continue.

Whenever anencephaly is seen, especially if there are additional clefts or amputations in the fetus, a careful search should be made for strands of membranes attached to the fetus, which are diagnostic of the amniotic band sequence. There is typically some remaining cerebral cortex with major skull defects caused by amniotic bands. (Fig. 9-19). This is not the case with anencephaly.

Encephalocele is the least common type of neural tube defect, and the condition is manifested by a protrusion of the meninges and sometimes brain tissue through a midline defect in the cranium. Ultrasound shows a midline sac protruding though the skull, most often in the occiput (Fig. 9-20). The outcome with encephalocele is very poor if there is brain tissue within the encephalocele sac or there are other significant associated anomalies. When there is an isolated defect with

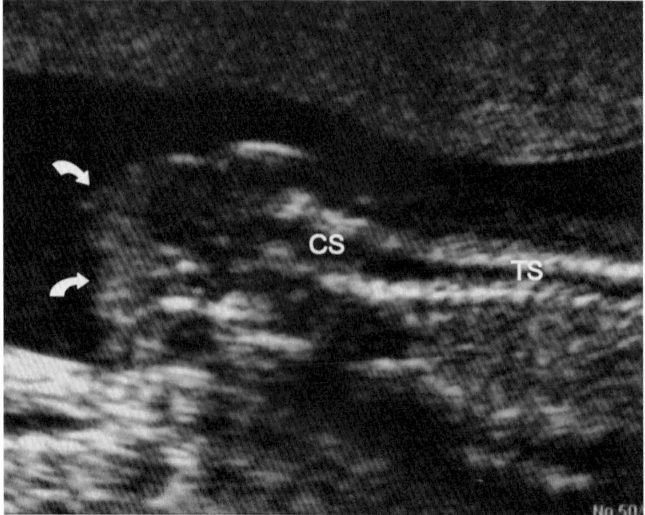

Figure 9-17. Anencephaly. In this coronal view of a 13-week-old fetus, the calvarium is absent, but there is still some abnormal lobulated brain tissue (*curved arrows*). Although this is sometimes referred to as exencephaly, it represents the most common appearance of anencephaly in the first trimester. The cervical spine (CS) and thoracic spine (TS) are indicated.

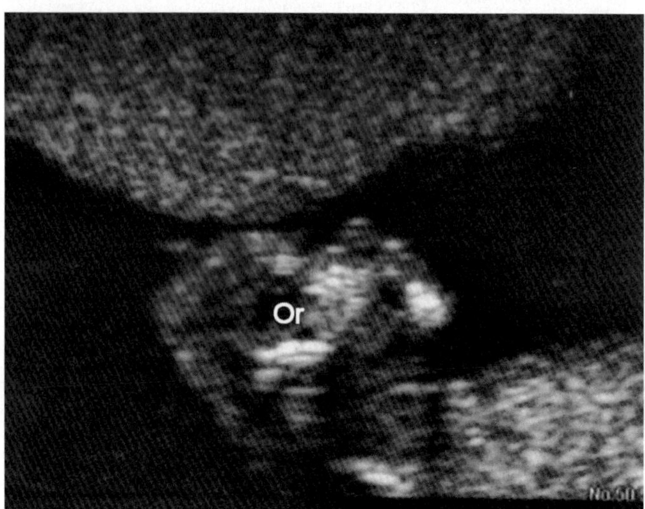

Figure 9-18. Anencephaly. In this sagittal view of a 16-week-old fetus, there is absence of the normal cranial structures above the level of the face and orbits (Or).

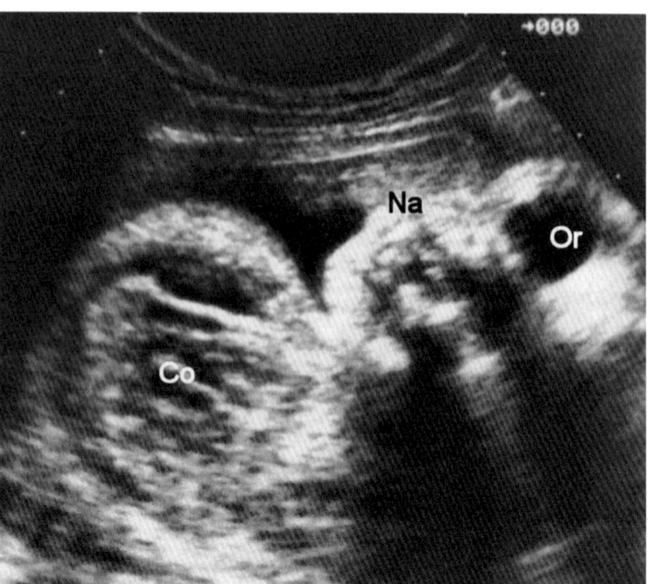

Figure 9-19. Amniotic band syndrome. Transverse view through the head of a 28-week-old fetus at the level of an orbit (Or) and nasal bone (Na). There is a large amount of disorganized cerebral cortex (Co) not covered by calvarium. The finding of uncovered cerebral cortex at this gestational age suggests the diagnosis of amniotic band syndrome. A band was seen running from the brain to the placenta, but is not shown here.

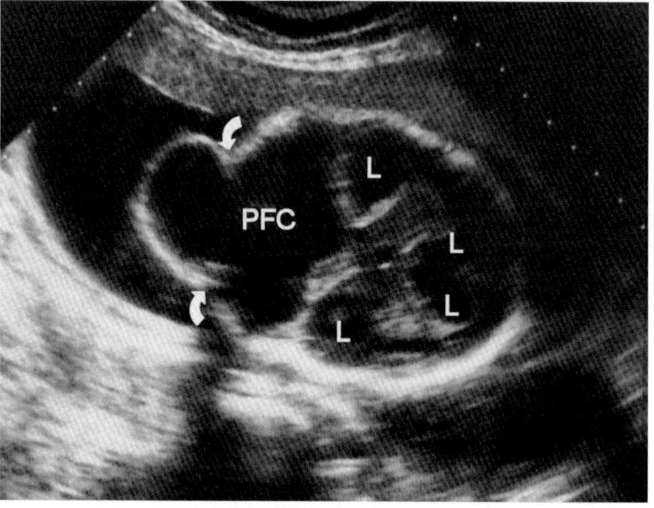

Figure 9-20. Encephalocele protruding through a defect (*curved arrows*) in the occipital bone. This defect was associated with a large posterior fossa cyst (PFC) and dilation of the lateral ventricles (L)

no brain involvement, most children have a good neurologic outcome.[68]

The sensitivity of ultrasound for diagnosing spina bifida increased dramatically in the 1980s when it was discovered that fetuses with this condition have readily apparent secondary changes in the brain and skull.[69] Most consistently, there are changes in the posterior fossa consisting of distortion and crowding of the cerebellar hemispheres with obliteration of the cisterna magna (the banana sign) (Fig. 9-21). Additionally, affected fetuses usually have dilation of the lateral ventricles and frontal narrowing of the skull (the lemon sign) (Fig. 9-22). In spite of the hydrocephalus, the head size is usually not increased.[70] Transverse views of the spine show widening of the lateral echocenters (Fig. 9-23). In longitudinal images, the ossification centers, that usually run a parallel course down the back, are widened in the area of the defect (Fig. 9-24). A meningomyelocele sac is usually present (Fig. 9-25). The presence of clubfeet and absence of movement of the lower extremities signify a poor prognosis for motor function of the lower extremities.

Cleft Lip and Palate

Cleft lip is the most common congenital facial deformity. Approximately two thirds of those with cleft lip also have cleft palate. Frontal scans provide the best views of the face for visualization of clefts (Fig. 9-26).

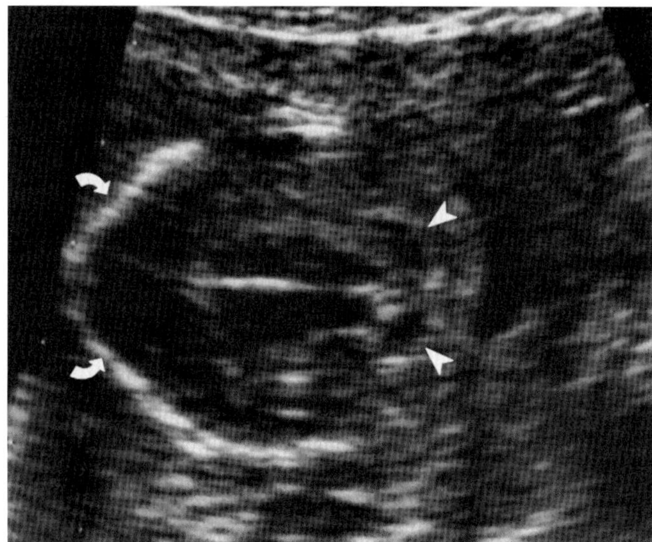

Figure 9-21. Transverse view through the head of a fetus with lumbar spina bifida. This fetus clearly shows the lemon sign, consisting of indentation of the frontal bones (*curved arrows*). Also, an Arnold Chiari type II malformation is present in which the cerebellar hemispheres (*arrowheads*) are elongated and drawn back to fill the posterior fossa (compare with the image of the normal cerebellum and posterior fossa in Figure 9-14A). This distorted appearance of the cerebellum is called the banana sign.

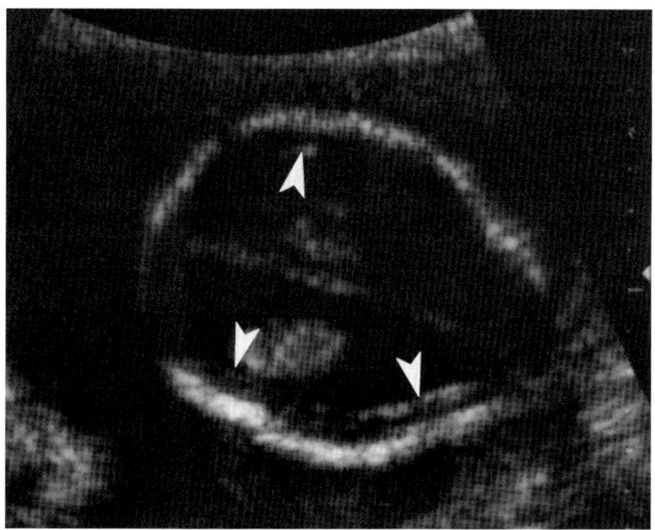

Figure 9-22. Transverse view of the head of another fetus with spina bifida. In addition to the lemon sign, this image also shows hydrocephalus. The *arrowheads* indicate the thinned cerebral cortex.

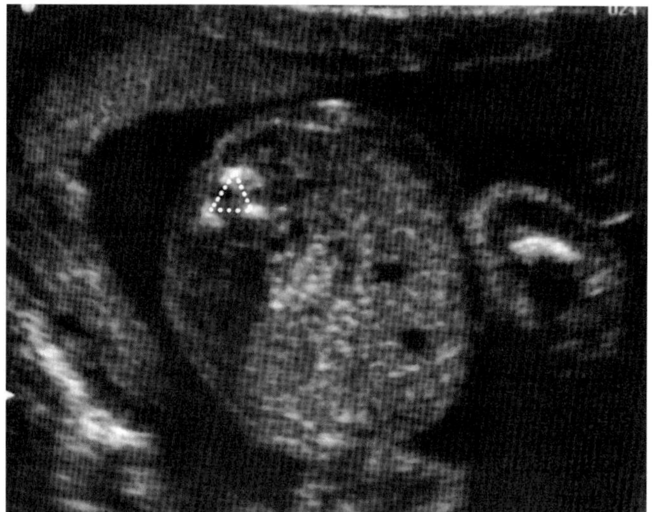

A

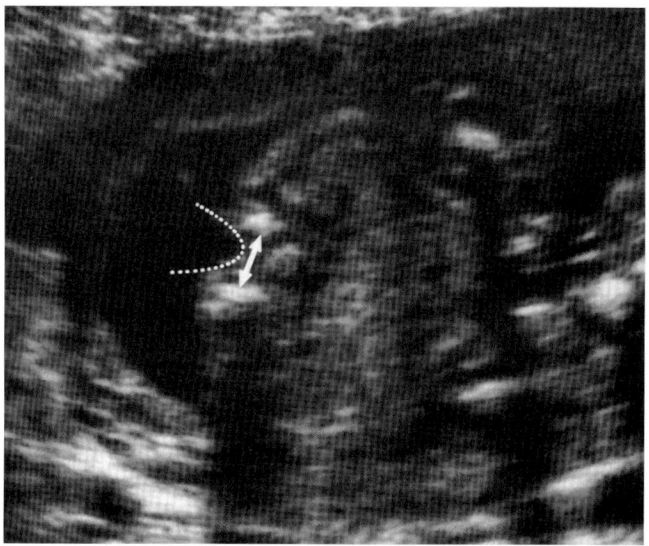

B

Figure 9-23. *A,* Normal transverse abdominal view of a 20-week-old fetus. Note how the echocenters of the spine are at the apices of an equilateral triangle. *B,* Transverse view through the abdomen of a 20-week-old fetus with lumbar spina bifida. Note that the posterior echocenters of the spine are displaced laterally (*double arrow*) so that the three echocenters no longer form an equilateral triangle. Note also the defect in the skin and subcutaneous tissues (*dotted line*).

Oblique axial views may show incomplete formation of the maxillary ridge, indicating cleft palate (Fig. 9-27). An isolated cleft palate is rarely diagnosed with prenatal ultrasound.

Micrognathia

A midsagittal image of the face is the best view for the detection of micrognathia (Fig. 9-28). Micrognathia may be an important marker for a genetic syndrome. Severe hypoplasia of the mandible, such as is seen with Pierre-Robin sequence, can cause breathing difficulties at birth. Therefore, prenatal diagnosis can be invaluable in planning neonatal management.

CHEST AND HEART

Chest Masses

Displacement of the heart away from the midline is often a sign of a lung or chest mass. The most common of these are diaphragmatic hernia, congenital cystic adenomatoid malformation (CCAM) and pulmonary seques-

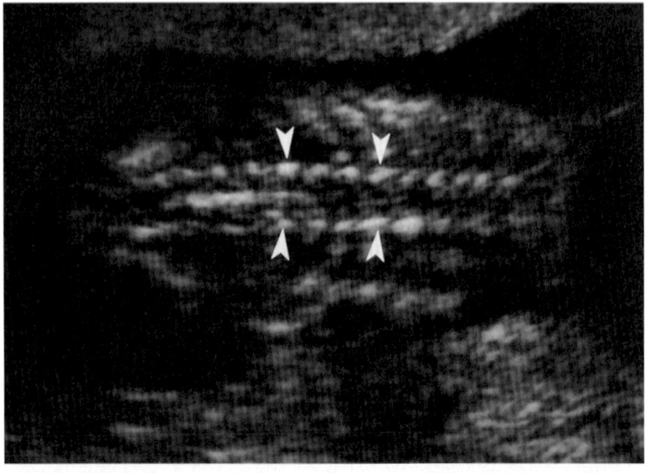

A

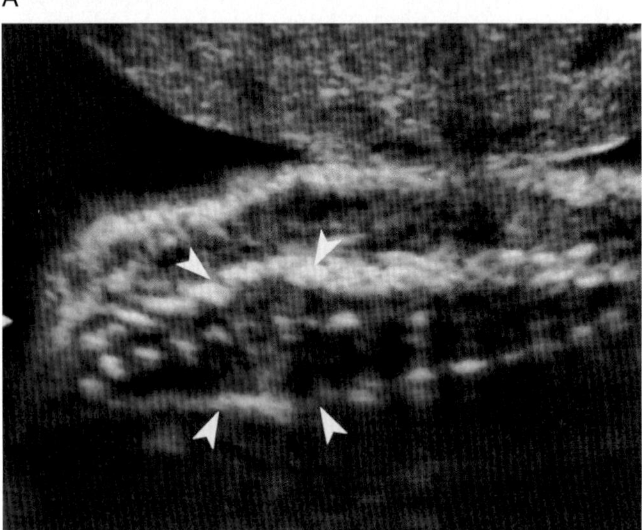

B

Figure 9-24. *A,* Normal coronal view of the fetal spine. Note that the lateral echocenters (*arrowheads*) run in parallel rows down the back. *B,* Coronal view of the spine of a fetus with a lumbar neural tube defect. Note that the lateral echocenters diverge in the area of the defect (indicated by the *arrowheads*).

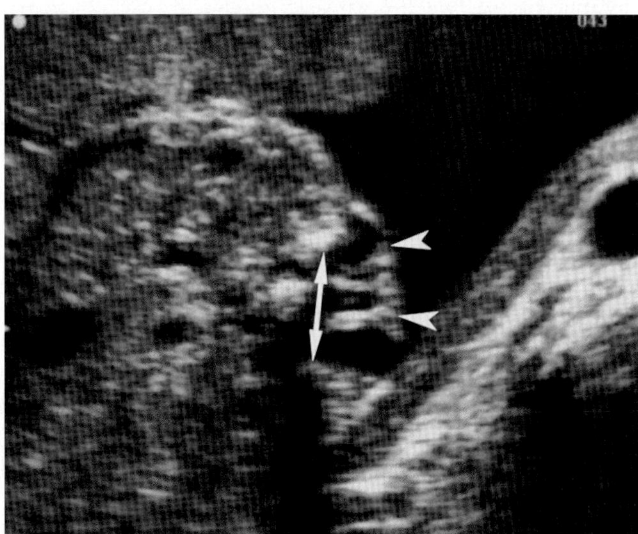

Figure 9-25. Transverse view through the abdomen of another fetus with spina bifida. Note again the lateral displacement of the posterior echocenters (*double arrow*) and, in this case, the presence of a fluid-filled septated meningomyelocele sac (*arrowheads*).

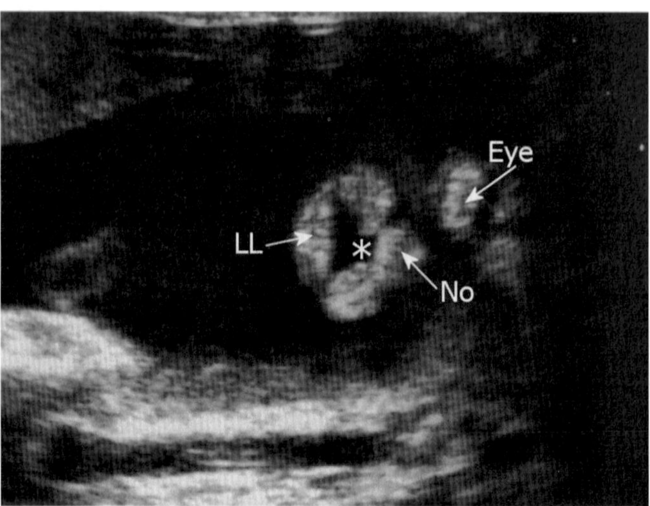

Figure 9-26. Midline cleft lip (*) in a fetus with holoprosencephaly. This is a coronal view through the lower fetal face with the lower lip (LL), tip of the nose (No), and eye indicated. This view is easy to obtain in almost all fetuses by rotating the ultrasound transducer 90 degrees from the plane used to obtain the BPD, then sliding the transducer forward to the face.

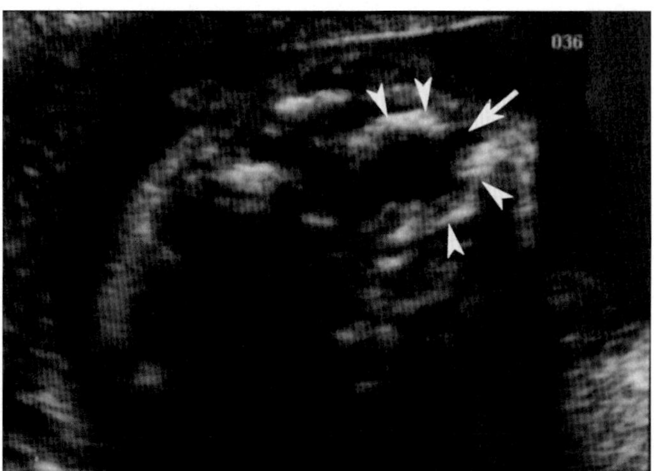

Figure 9-27. This transverse view through the fetal maxilla shows a gap (*arrow*) in the alveolar ridge (*arrowheads*). This indicates that a previously visualized cleft lip extends posteriorly to involve the palate as well.

tration. The presence of these conditions can be life threatening because vital chest structures are compressed or displaced. Space-occupying chest lesions can severely impair lung growth. Compression of the esophagus by a lung mass may cause symptomatic polyhydramnios. Similar pressure on the central veins and lymphatics may cause fetal death from generalized hydrops.

Diaphragmatic Hernia

The most obvious sonographic clue suggesting this diagnosis is the displacement of the heart to the side opposite the location of the defect, which is on the left side in 75 percent of cases. The condition can be distinguished from other chest masses by the appearance of bowel, stomach, and other abdominal organs in the

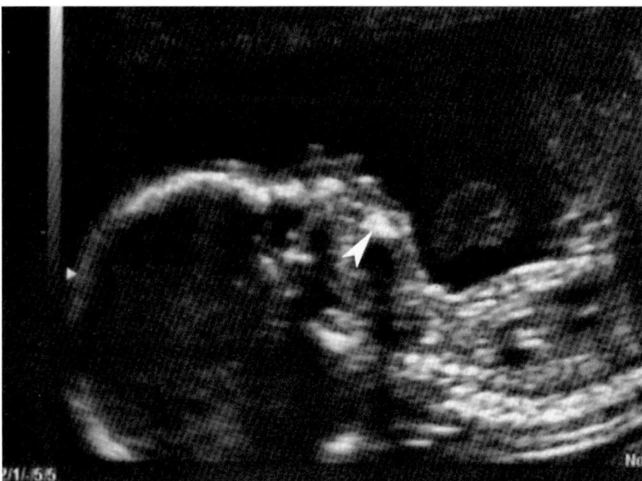

Figure 9-28. Sagittal view of a fetal face showing micrognathia. The small mandible is indicated by the *arrowhead*.

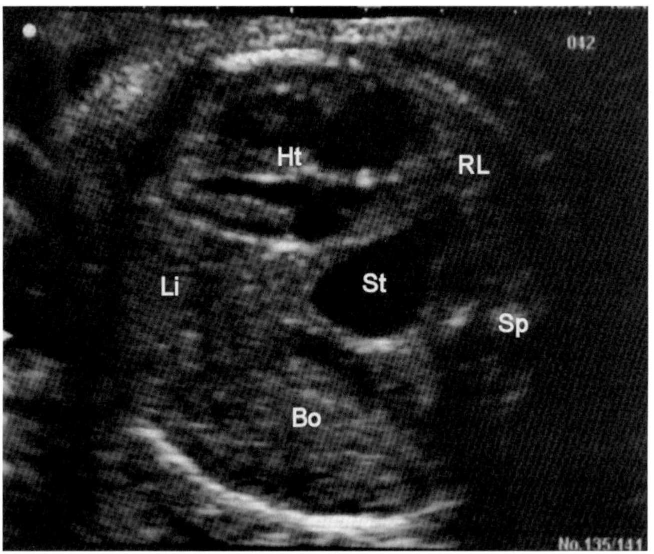

Figure 9-29. Transverse view through the fetal chest showing a left-sided diaphragmatic hernia. The heart (Ht) is displaced to the right side of the chest, the stomach (St) is posterior and to the left of the heart, the left lobe of the liver (Li) is in the anterior left chest, and the posterior left chest is filled with fetal bowel (Bo). The right lung (RL) is very small. The spine (Sp) is also labeled.

chest at the level of the four-chamber view of the heart (Fig. 9-29). In the midabdominal view, the stomach is typically not seen with left-sided hernias, and is shifted toward the right in right-sided lesions. The intrahepatic umbilical vein is usually shifted toward the side of the defect, and variable amounts of liver will sometimes be seen prolapsed into the chest. Ultrasound does not usually demonstrate significant lung tissue on the affected side and the contralateral lung is typically very small. Displacement of the gastrointestinal tract often results in swallowing abnormalities, and half of these cases develop polyhydramnios.

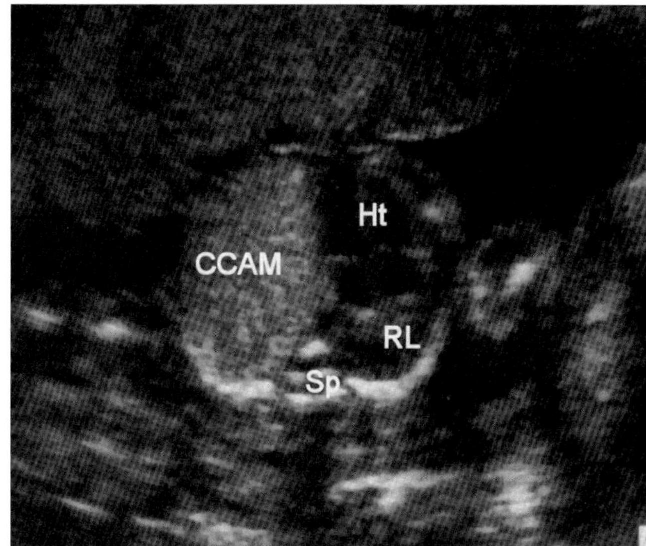

Figure 9-30. Congenital cystic adenomatoid malformation (CCAM) involving the left lung. This is a type III lesion, appearing as a solid tumor which displaces the heart (Ht) to the right. The relatively small right lung (RL) and spine (Sp) are also indicated.

Congenital Cystic Adenomatoid Malformation

CCAM appears as a solid or cystic lung mass that is almost always unilateral and is confined to one lobe. CCAM has been classified according to the size of cysts present. The cysts in type III lesions are not visible sonographically, and the lesion thus has the appearance of an echogenic homogeneous solid tumor (Fig. 9-30). Frequently, there is a shift in the mediastinum with compression of the contralateral lung. Nonimmune hydrops can develop, and this finding is associated with a poor prognosis. Because an apparently very large CCAM can seem to regress as a pregnancy advances, the clinician should be cautious about predicting a poor outcome.[71,72] Most affected children require nonemergent surgical resection.[71]

Pulmonary Sequestration

Pulmonary sequestration is a congenital anomaly in which a mass of lung tissue arises from the foregut independently of the normal lung. It does not communicate with the tracheobronchial tree and receives its blood supply directly from the aorta. Ultrasound shows an echogenic intrathoracic or intraabdominal mass, usually just above or just below the diaphragm. Color Doppler ultrasound can sometimes demonstrate the aberrant blood supply, thus distinguishing a pulmonary sequestration from CCAM (Fig. 9-31). A pulmonary sequestration usually must be removed in childhood but rarely causes prenatal complications.[73]

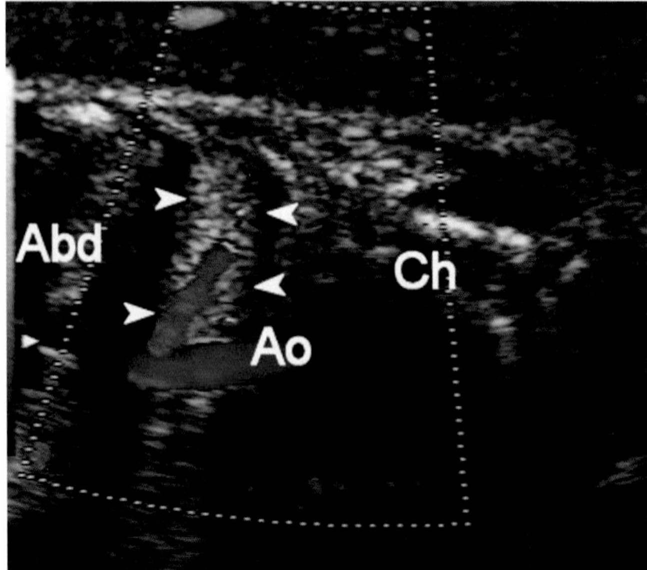

Figure 9-31. Coronal view of a pulmonary sequestration (*outlined by arrowheads*) located at the base of the lung just above the diaphragm. The fetal chest (Ch) is to the right and the abdomen (Abd) to the left. The blood supply to the mass arises directly from the aorta (Ao).

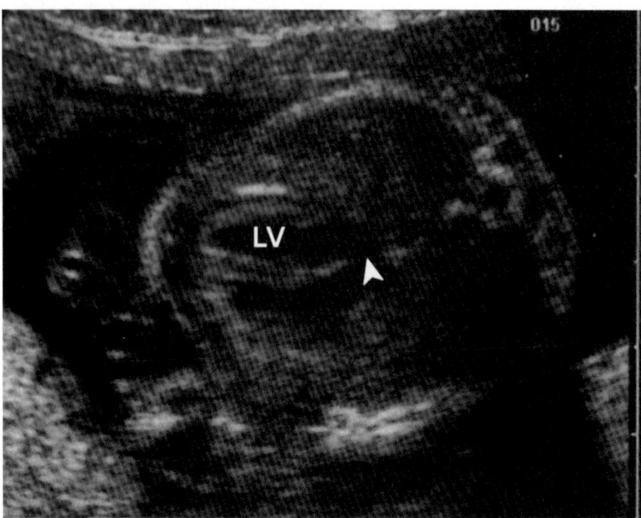

Figure 9-32. Normal four-chamber view of the heart. Note that the position of the heart is central in the chest and the axis is about 45 degrees to the left of the midline. The ventricles are approximately equal in size, whereas the left ventricle (LV) extends further into the apex. The intraventricular septum is intact, and the foramen ovale (*arrowhead*) is seen.

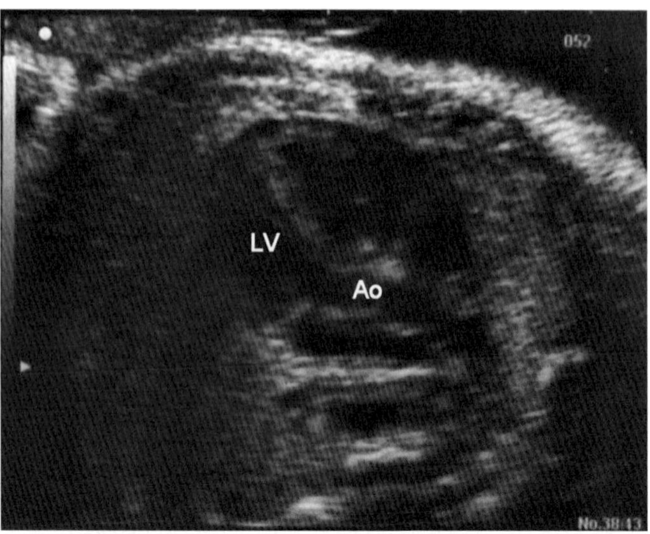

A

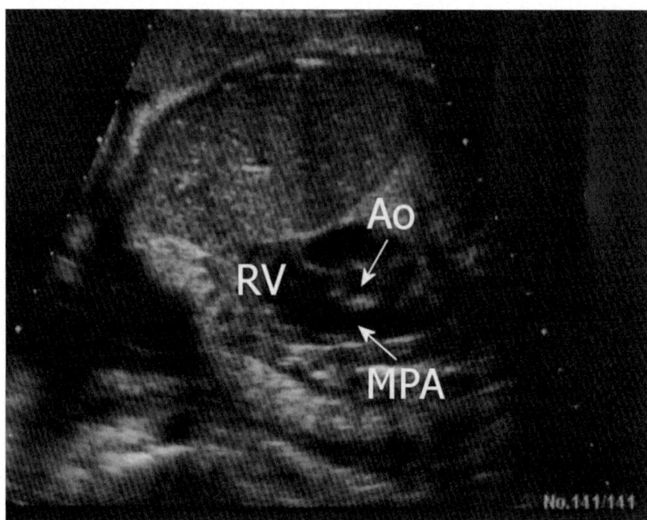

B

Figure 9-33. *A,* Left ventricular outflow tract. A normal aorta (Ao) is seen arising from the left ventricle (LV). *B,* Right ventricular outflow tract. The main pulmonary artery (MPA) arises from the right ventricle (RV) and crosses anterior to the ascending aorta (Ao).

Congenital Heart Disease

As a group, heart defects are the most common form of birth defect, occurring in about 8/1,000 births. The traditional screening method for detecting congenital heart disease, the four-chamber view (Fig. 9-32), has been shown to have a low detection rate. DeVore reviewed three studies from the 1990s in which the four-chamber view was obtained as a part of a screening ultrasound in low-risk populations.[74] Only 8 of 151 cases of congenital heart disease were detected with the four-chamber screening, giving a detection rate of 5 percent. In studies in which the four-chamber view was used by examiners experienced in the detection of heart defects, this view alone demonstrated 55 percent of heart defects. In the same group of patients, visualization of the outflow tracts (Fig. 9-33) in addition to the four-chamber view increased the detection rate to 80 percent.[74] Given the importance of outflow tract visualization for the detection of many heart defects, the AIUM now recommends that an attempt should be made to obtain these views in all second- and third-trimester scans.[58]

Whenever a heart defect is detected, a careful search for other malformations is important, because about 50 to 70 percent of fetuses with heart defects have extracardiac malformations as well.[75] Up to 35 percent of infants with

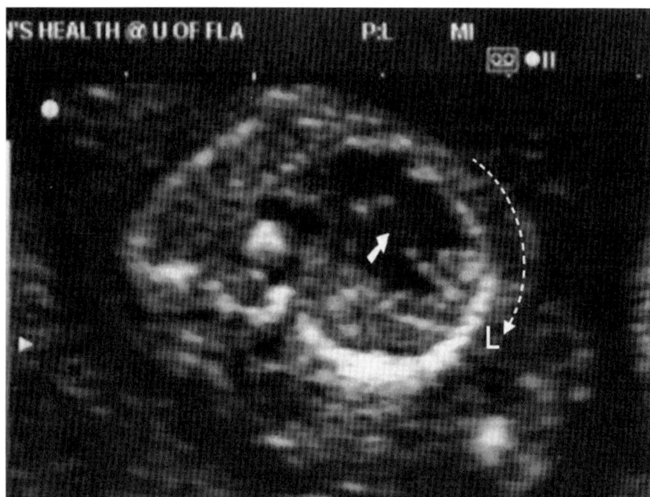

Figure 9-34. Large ventricular septal defect (*arrow*). Note that the axis of the heart is rotated to the left (L). This fetus had multiple anomalies, including transposition of the great vessels and omphalocele.

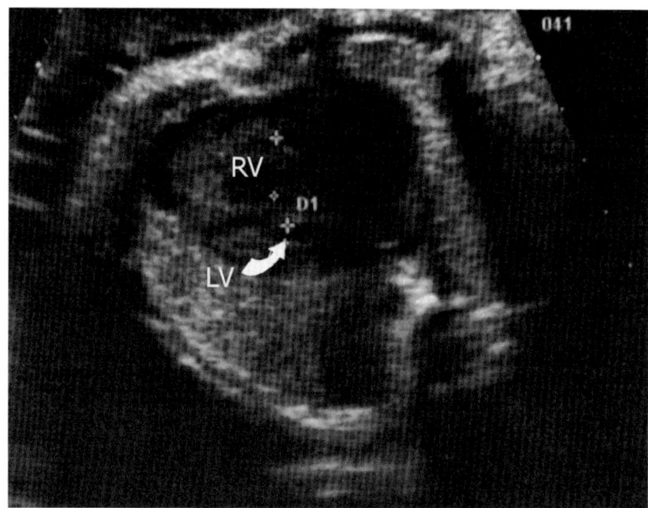

Figure 9-36. Hypoplastic left heart syndrome. Note the very small left ventricular lumen (LV) compared with the right ventricle (RV).

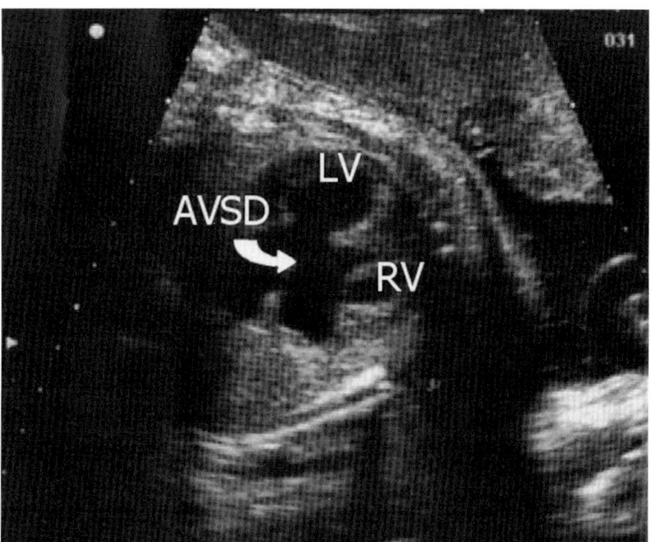

Figure 9-35. Large atrioventricular septal defect (AVSD). The left ventricle (LV) and right ventricle (RV) are indicated.

heart defects diagnosed prenatally have a chromosomal abnormality.[76]

Ventricular Septal Defects

Ventricular septal defects (VSDs) account for 20 to 30 percent of congenital heart defects. Large defects can usually be seen in the four-chamber view (Fig. 9-34), but small defects are commonly missed, even by experienced examiners. In about half of the cases of VSDs, there are other, more complex malformations. One of these, complete atriventricular septal defect, has a large defect in the atrial and ventricular septum and a common atrioventricular valve (Fig. 9-35). This particular lesion has a strong association with Down syndrome, which is present in about half of these cases.

Hypoplastic Left Heart Syndrome

Hypoplastic left heart syndrome is suspected when the left ventricle, which should be similar in size to the right ventricle, appears very narrow on a four-chamber view (Fig. 9-36). When the transducer is rotated to visualize the left ventricular outflow tract, the ascending aorta is seen to be very narrow.

Tetralogy of Fallot

This defect consists of a ventricular septal defect, pulmonary stenosis, and an aorta that overrides the VSD (Fig. 9-37). The fourth part of the tetralogy, hypertrophy of the right ventricle, develops postnatally.

Transposition of the Great Arteries

This disorder is recognized with the outflow tract views when the aorta and pulmonary artery run parallel to each other instead of crossing (Fig. 9-38). The aorta, which can be recognized from the shape of the arch, arises from the right ventricle and runs anterior to the main pulmonary artery, which arises posteriorly from the left ventricle. A ventricular septal defect is found in 40 percent of cases.

ABDOMEN

Esophageal Atresia

The fetal stomach should always be visualized after the first trimester. If the stomach is small or absent and does fill after 30 to 60 minutes of observation, esophageal atresia should be suspected. In most cases, ultrasound also shows polyhydramnios, resulting from an inability of

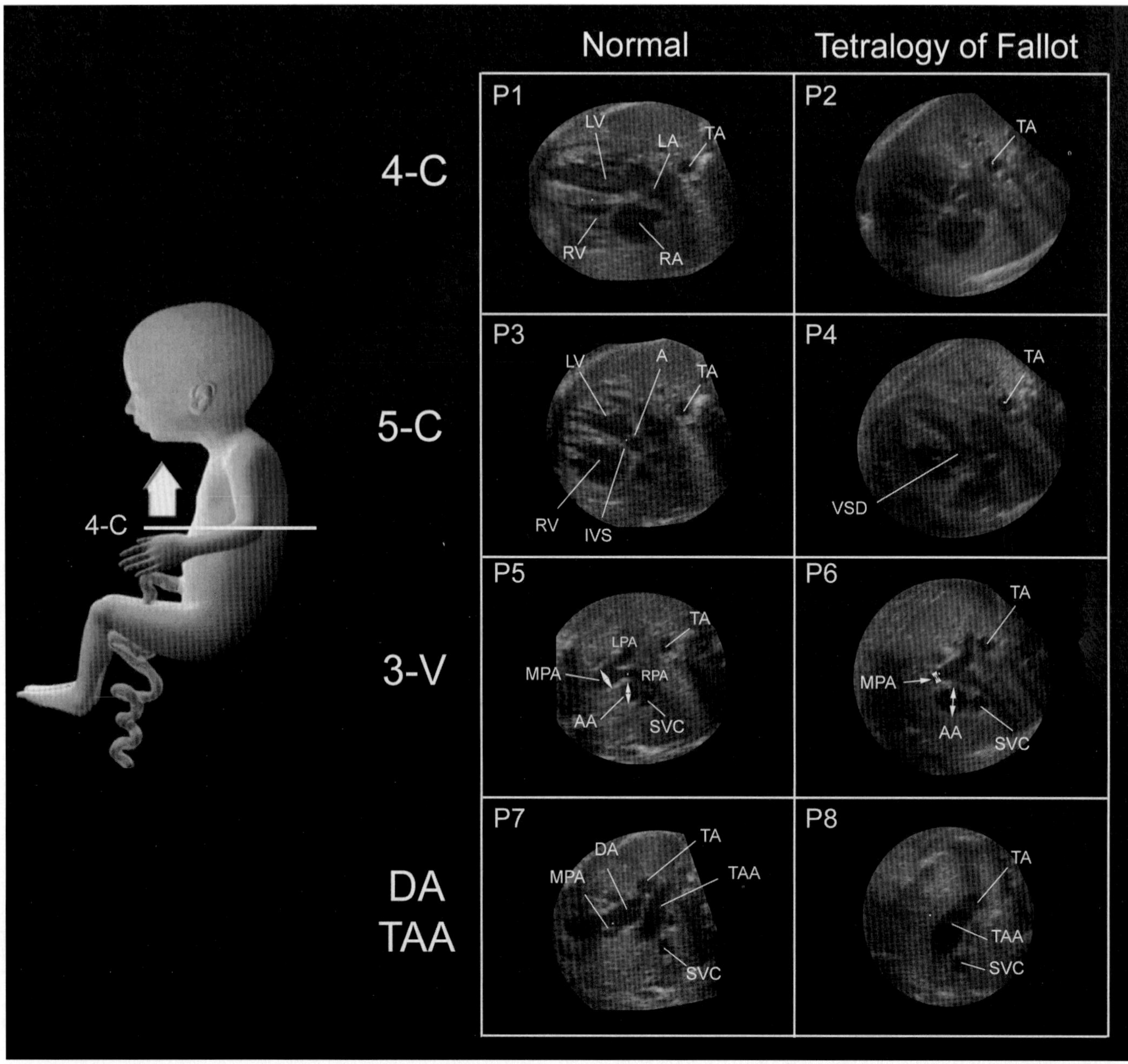

Figure 9-37. Tetralogy of Fallot. The images in panels 1 thru 8 (P1-P8) were obtained by directing the ultrasound beam in a transverse plane from the four-chamber view to the upper chest. This results in four image planes; the four-chamber view (4-C), the five-chamber view (5-C), the 3-vessel view (3-V) and the ductal-transverse aortic arch view (DA-TAA). The four-chamber views are normal (P1, P2). P1, P3, P5, and P7 demonstrate normal anatomy for each of the four levels. P3 illustrates a normal five-chamber view. P5 illustrates a normal main pulmonary artery, normal bifurcating branching pulmonary arteries, and a cross-section of the ascending aorta (AA). In this view, the diameters (*arrowheads*) of the main pulmonary artery (MPA) and the AA are similar. P4 demonstrates the five-chamber view with a ventricular septal defect (VSD) at the level of the ascending aorta as it leaves the left ventricle. P6 demonstrates a small main pulmonary artery (MPA) and an enlarged aorta (AA). P8 demonstrates absence of the ductus arteriosus (DA). AA, ascending aorta; LA, left atrium; LPA, left pulmonary artery; LV, left ventricle; RA, right atrium; RV, right ventricle; RPA, right pulmonary artery; SVC, superior vena cava; TA, thoracic aorta; TAA, transverse aortic arch. (Courtesy of Greggory R. DeVore, M.D., Fetal Diagnostic Centers, Pasadena, CA.)

the fetus to swallow amniotic fluid normally (Fig. 9-39). An empty stomach in a fetus with anhydramnios is not suggestive of gastrointestinal pathology.

Small Bowel Obstruction

Duodenal atresia is usually easily diagnosed by third trimester-fetal ultrasound. The diagnosis is based on the demonstration of the double-bubble sign in which adjacent cysts are seen, representing the fluid-filled dilated stomach and proximal duodenum (Fig. 9-40). Polyhydramnios is a consistent feature in these cases. Trisomy 21 is present in 30 percent of cases of duodenal atresia.

Small bowel obstruction further along the intestinal tract is less common than duodenal atresia. Ultrasound in these cases shows multiple actively peristalsing loops

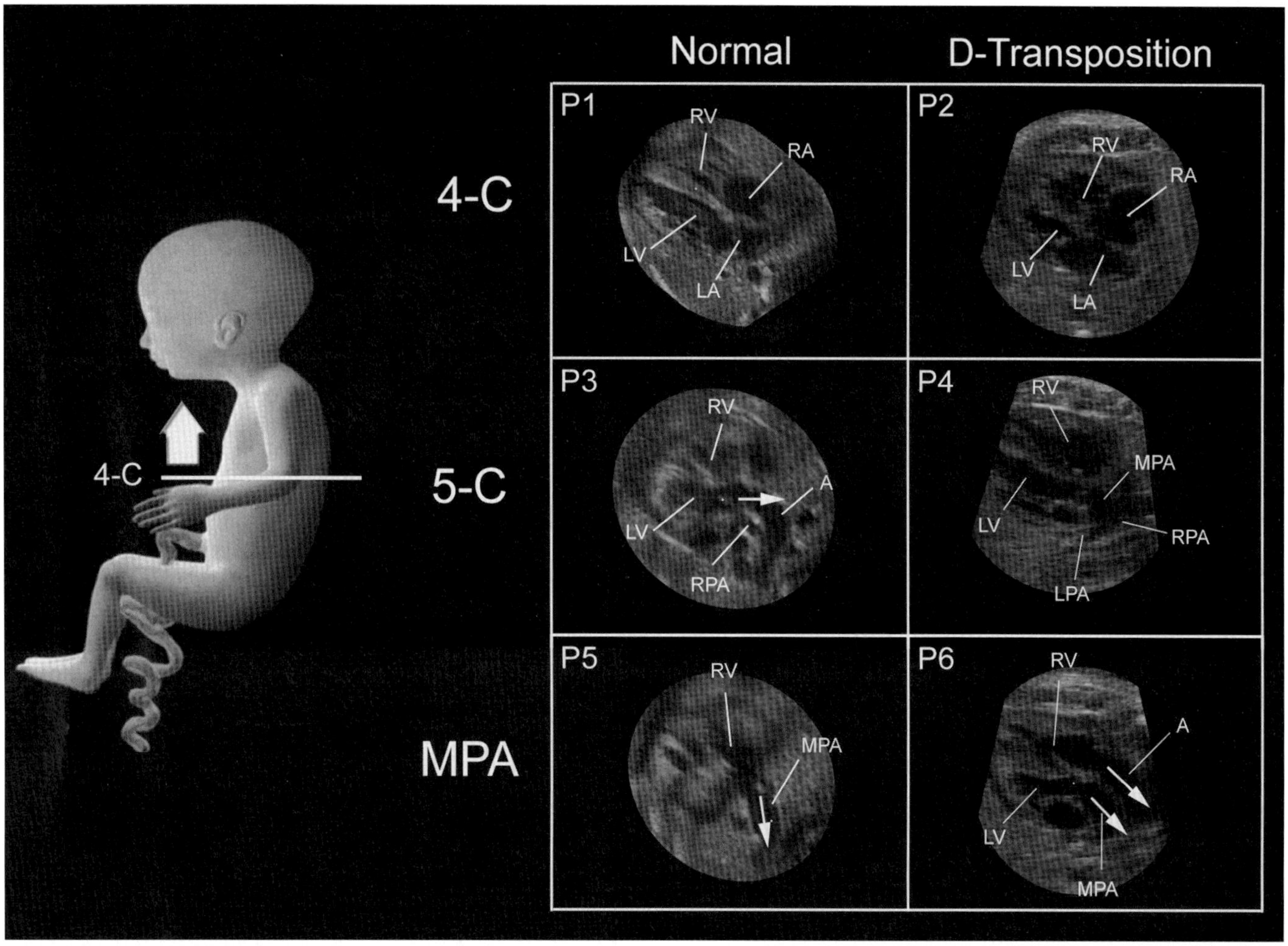

Figure 9-38. Transposition of the great arteries. The images in panels 1 thru 6 (P1 to P6) were obtained by directing the ultrasound beam in a transverse plane from the four-chamber view to the upper chest, with slight rotation to demonstrate the arch of the ascending aorta at the level of the 5-C view. This results in three image planes: the four-chamber view (4-C), the rotated five-chamber view (5-C), and the main pulmonary artery view (MPA). The four-chamber views are normal (P1, P2). P1, P3, and P5 demonstrate normal anatomy for each of the three levels. P3 illustrates a normal rotated five-chamber view illustrating the aortic arch (A). P5 illustrates a normal main pulmonary artery exiting the right ventricle (RV). The arrows in P3 and P5 demonstrate that the outflow tracts (A, MPA) are perpendicular to each other as they exit their respective ventricles. P4 demonstrates the five-chamber view with interruption of what should be the aortic arch. However, this vessel is the main pulmonary artery (MPA) with its bifurcating branches (RPA, LPA). P6 demonstrates parallel outflow tracts that are transposed. LA, left atrium; LV, left ventricle; RA, right atrium; RV, right ventricle. (Courtesy of Greggory R. DeVore, MD, Fetal Diagnostic Centers, Pasadena, CA.)

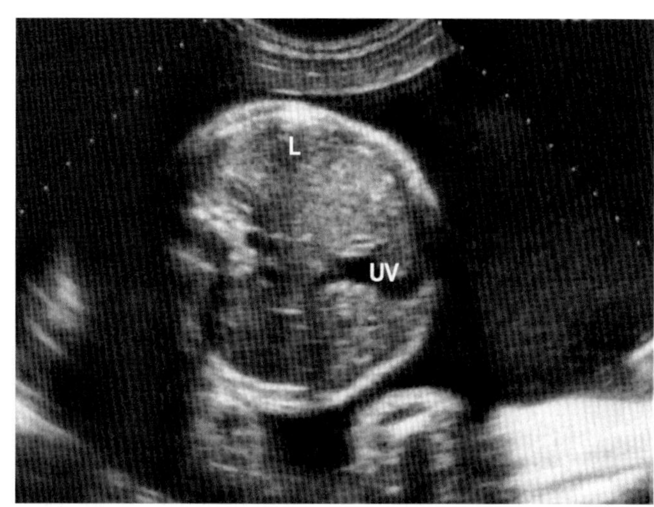

Figure 9-39. Transverse view through the abdomen of a fetus with esophageal atresia. Note the absence of a visible stomach on the left (L) side of the abdomen at the level of the umbilical vein (UV). Note also the presence of polyhydramnios, a result of abnormal fetal swallowing.

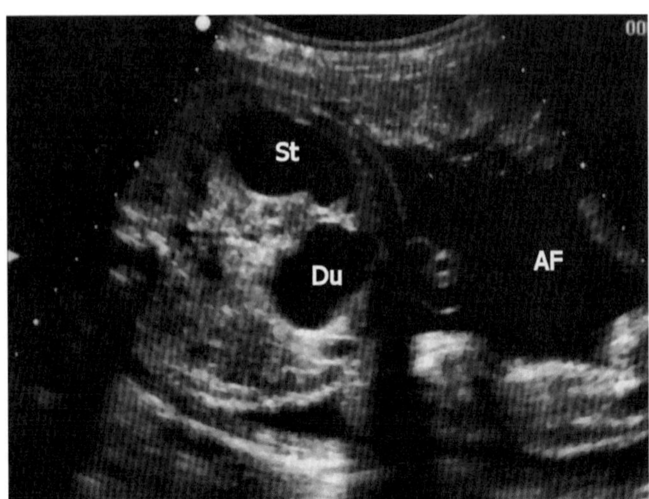

Figure 9-40. Transverse view through the abdomen of a fetus with duodenal atresia. Note the double-bubble sign, a result of the adjacent dilated stomach (St) and proximal duodenum (Du). Note also the presence of increased amniotic fluid (AF).

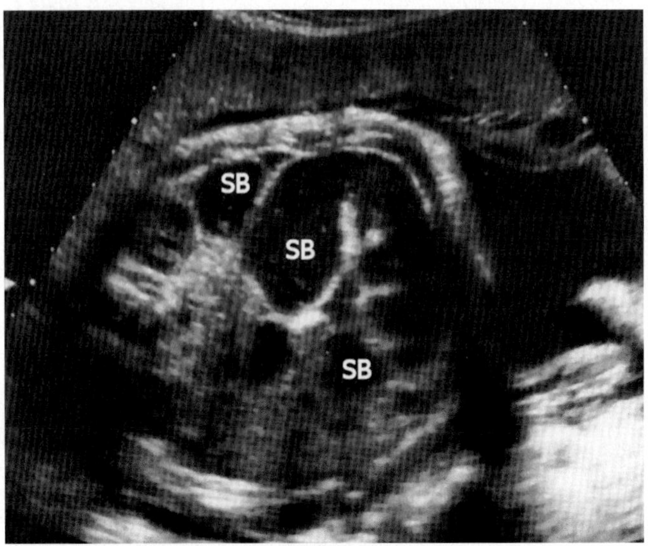

Figure 9-41. Transverse view through the abdomen of a fetus with jejunal atresia. There are multiple loops of dilated small bowel (SB). With real-time ultrasound, these loops were seen to be actively peristalsing.

of distended small bowel (Fig. 9-41). The degree of polyhydramnios depends on the proximity of the obstruction to the stomach.

Omphalocele

Omphalocele is a ventral wall defect characterized by a membrane-covered herniation of the intra-abdominal contents into the base of the umbilical cord. Bowel loops, stomach, and liver are the most frequently herniated organs (Fig. 9-42). With omphalocele, there is a 55- to 75-percent rate of associated birth defects, and the karyotype is abnormal in 20 to 25 percent of cases.[77,78] These

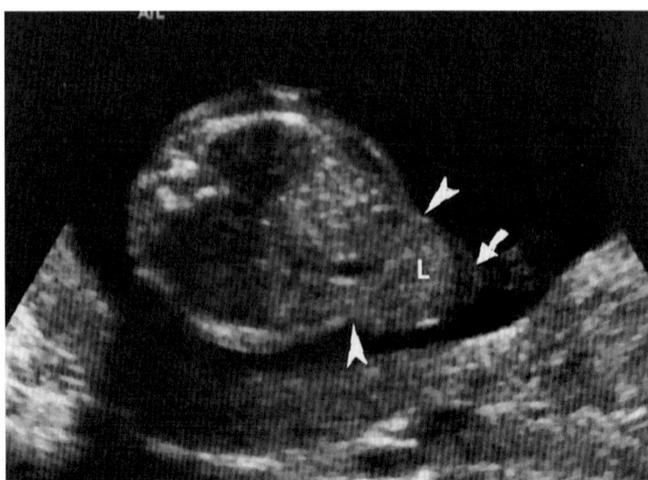

Figure 9-42. Transverse view through the abdomen of a fetus with omphalocele. The abdominal wall defect is demarcated by the *arrowheads*. The umbilical cord is shown entering the omphalocele sac (*arrow*), which contains much of the fetal liver (L).

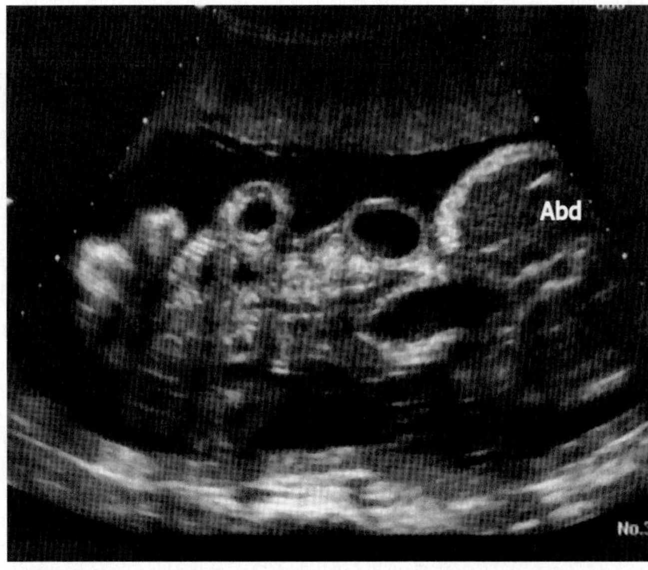

Figure 9-43. Transverse view through the abdomen of a fetus with gastroschisis. The abdomen (Abd) is to the right of the image. The extruded bowel loops, many of which are moderately dilated, are shown. Note that there is no membrane covering the bowel loops, as would be the case with omphalocele.

other problems account for most of the mortality associated with this condition.

Gastroschisis

Gastroschisis is a right paraumbilical defect of the anterior abdominal wall associated with evisceration of the abdominal organs. Gastroschisis is distinguished from omphalocele by the fact that with gastroschisis, the umbilical cord inserts normally into the abdominal wall and there is no membrane covering the herniated viscera (Fig. 9-43). Most commonly, only bowel loops are involved, but liver, stomach, and bladder may be herniated. Because of associated atresias or obstruction at the small abdominal wall ring, bowel loops and the stomach may be dilated inside or outside the abdomen. Gastroschisis is rarely associated with chromosomal abnormalities, and usually does not involve abnormalities outside of the gastrointestinal tract.[77]

URINARY TRACT

Bilateral Renal Agenesis

Bilateral renal agenesis is usually first suspected when there is absent amniotic fluid and nonvisualization of the fetal bladder. The diagnosis is confirmed by the absence of kidneys in the renal fossae. Making a firm diagnosis is sometimes challenging because without amniotic fluid it is difficult to adequately visualize the fetal anatomy and because the discoid-shaped adrenals can be confused with the fetal kidneys (Fig. 9-44). Transvaginal scanning can be helpful, because without amniotic fluid, the fetus is often close to the upper vagina. Bilateral renal agenesis is invariably associated with pulmonary hypoplasia, which is the cause of death in liveborn infants. In this setting, ultrasound shows a small chest, with an increased heart/chest ratio.

Infantile Polycystic Kidney Disease

Infantile polycystic kidney disease is an autosomal recessive disorder characterized by bilateral symmetric enlargement of the kidneys. In this condition, normal parenchyma is replaced by dilated collecting tubules, measuring less than 2 mm in diameter. These cysts are not seen macroscopically with ultrasound but rather give the kidneys a markedly echogenic appearance (Fig. 9-45). In most cases, these kidneys are nonfunctioning, and there is no bladder filling or amniotic fluid production. These neonates die of pulmonary hypoplasia.

Multicystic Dysplastic Kidneys

Multicystic dysplasia occurs sporadically and is characterized by noncommunicating cysts of various sizes scattered randomly through the kidneys. The renal parenchyma between the cysts has an echogenic appearance (Fig. 9-46). The disorder can be bilateral, unilateral, or segmental. The affected kidneys may become large. This

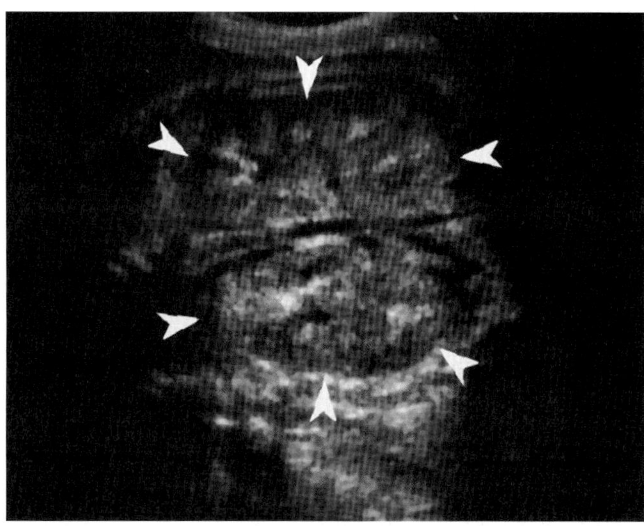

Figure 9-45. Infantile polycystic kidney disease. This coronal view shows the enlarged, echogenic kidneys (outlined with *arrowheads*) characteristic of this condition.

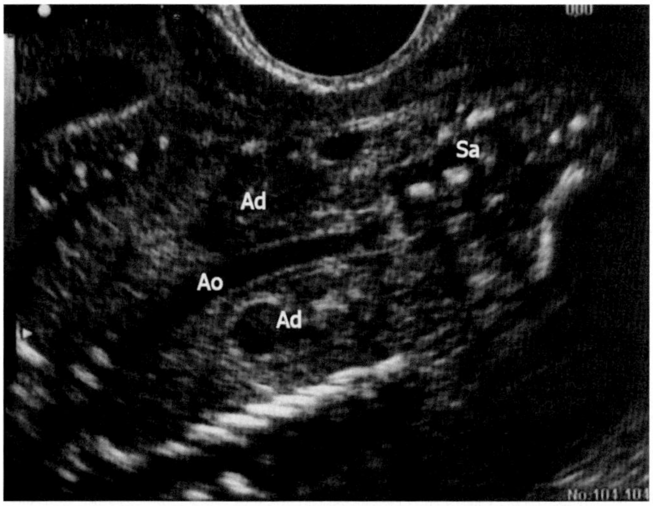

Figure 9-44. Tranvaginal coronal view of the lower abdomen and pelvis of a fetus with bilateral renal agenesis. Note the absence of amniotic fluid and the relatively large adrenal glands (Ad). The aorta (Ao) and sacrum (Sa) are also indicated. No bladder filling was seen, and color Doppler showed no renal arteries.

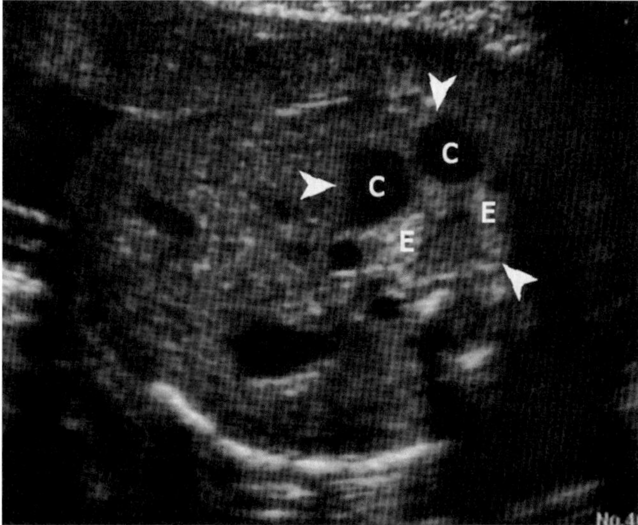

Figure 9-46. Transverse view of the fetal abdomen showing a right unilateral multicystic dysplastic kidney (outlined with *arrowheads*). Note that the cysts (C) do not communicate with one another and do not resemble a dilated renal pelvis or calices. The parenchyma is echogenic (E).

condition should be differentiated from hydronephrosis, in which the parenchyma is normal and a dilated renal pelvis communicates with dilated calyces (Fig. 9-47). In bilateral multicystic dysplasia, urine is not produced. Thus, the bladder is not visualized, there is no amniotic fluid, and the fetus develops pulmonary hypoplasia. Unilateral disease is associated with normal bladder filling and amniotic fluid volume and has an excellent prognosis.

Hydronephrosis

With hydronephrosis, there are varying degrees of dilation of the renal pelvis and calices. Dilated calices (caliectasis) is always considered abnormal and requires follow-up. When only the renal pelvis is dilated (pelviectasis), various criteria have been used to define normality. A simple method involves measuring only the anteroposterior diameter of the renal pelvis (Fig. 9-48). If this measurement is greater than 4 mm up to 32 weeks or greater than 7 mm beyond 32 weeks, follow-up ultrasound is indicated.[79] These cutoffs were set to ensure a sensitivity of nearly 100 percent to identify any postnatal compromise or the need for surgery. Using these cutoffs, 20 to 50 percent of these cases will have normal kidneys at postnatal evaluation. Persistent hydronephrosis is most often caused by ureteropelvic junction obstruction or vesicoureteral reflux.[80] The ureters may be dilated if there is severe vesicoureteral reflux (Fig. 9-49) or ureterovesico junction obstruction. The ureterovesico junction obstruction is often associated with a duplicated collecting system. A ureterocele may form at the point of ureteral implantation into the bladder (Fig. 9-50).

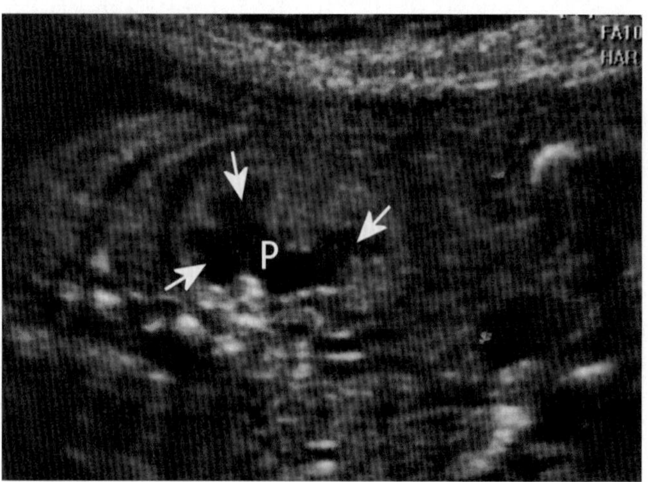

Figure 9-47. Unilateral hydronephrosis. The cystic areas in the kidney all communicate, and consist of dilated calices (*arrows*) draining to a dilated renal pelvis (P).

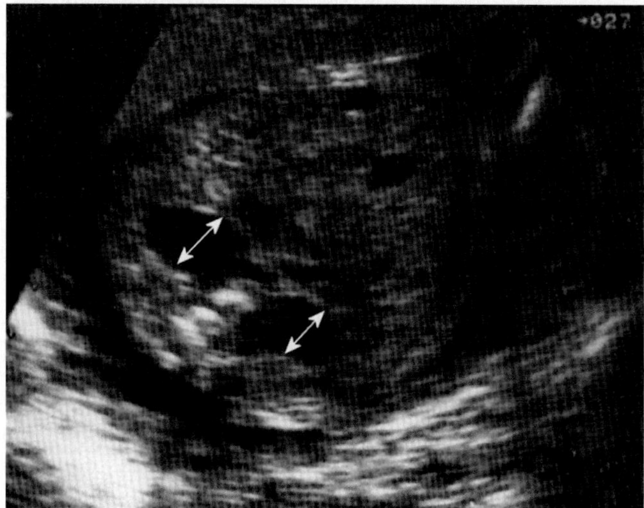

Figure 9-48. Dilated renal pelves (pelviectasis). The anteroposterior measurement of the renal pelvis is used (*arrows*) to define the limits of normal and follow progression.

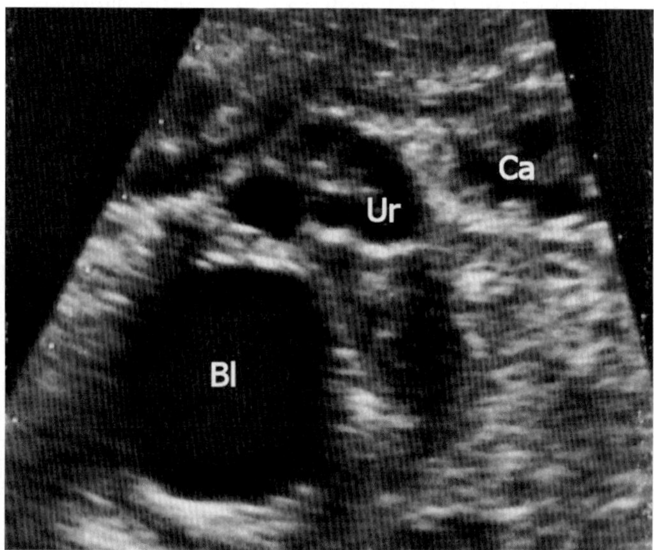

Figure 9-49. Vesicoureteral reflux. The ureter (Ur) and renal calices (Ca) are dilated. The bladder (Bl) is also indicated.

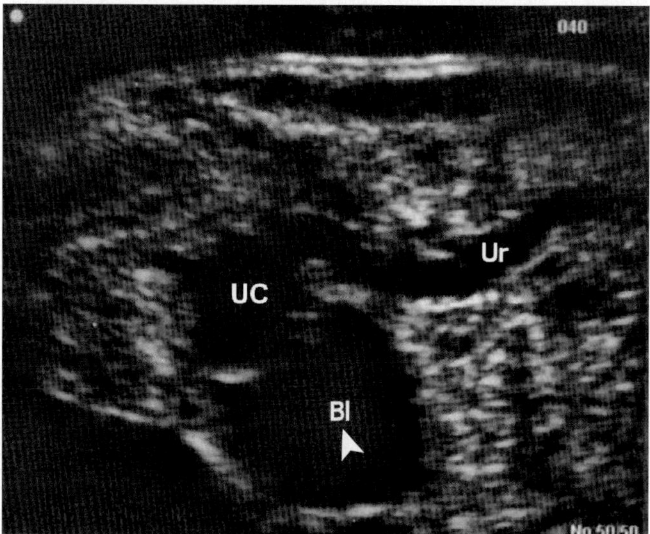

Figure 9-50. Vesicoureteral junction obstruction. The ureter (Ur) is dilated, and there is a ureterocele (UC) at the point the partially obstructed ureter enters the bladder (Bl) (*arrowhead*). The ureters should normally not be visible.

Bladder Outlet Obstruction

Bladder outlet obstruction is most commonly seen in male fetuses and is usually caused by posterior urethral valves. These are membrane-like structures in the posterior urethra that cause varying grades of urethral obstruction. More complex malformations involving the urogenital tract may also cause bladder outlet obstruction, and are more common in the female fetus. Sonographically, bladder outlet obstruction is diagnosed when the bladder is abnormally enlarged, and normal emptying is not seen (Fig. 9-51). When the obstruction is severe, other findings include oligohydramnios, dilated ureters, hydronephrosis, and cystic dysplasia of the kidneys. When complete urethral obstruction has been present from early in pregnancy, anhydramnios causes lethal pulmonary hypolasia and ureteral reflux results in irreversible damage to the kidneys. Prune belly syndrome occurs in male fetuses, and the condition has the same sonographic appearance as bladder outlet obstruction. With this condition, however, the impairment of bladder emptying is thought to result from a neuromuscular defect in the bladder and not physical obstruction of the urethra.

SKELETAL ABNORMALITIES

In most cases of confirmed skeletal dysplasia, the long bones are obviously abnormal, with measurements falling far below the normal range. Concern sometimes arises when routine measurement of the femur gives a result several weeks less than expected for the gestational age. For most long bone nomograms, the lower confidence limit corresponds to 2 weeks behind up to 28 weeks, and 3 weeks behind beyond 28 weeks. For this reason, when the femur is more than 2 or 3 weeks less than expected, a detailed survey of fetal anatomy, especially the long bones, is advisable. A femur/foot ratio close to 1 usually implies that the fetus is normal or merely constitutionally small.[81]

Achondroplasia

Achondroplasia is the most common form of skeletal dysplasia and is associated with a normal life span. Ultrasound shows severe shortening of the long bones, a relatively large head with a protruding forehead, and polyhydramnios. Although this condition has autosomal dominant inheritance, 80 percent of cases result from new mutations. When present in its heterozygous form, bone shortening may be mild enough that the measurements are in the normal range in the first half of pregnancy.

Thanatophoric Dysplasia

Thanatophoric dysplasia is the most common lethal skeletal dysplasia. In this condition, there is extreme shortening of the long bones. The femur is often bowed, resembling a telephone receiver (Fig. 9-52). The fetus has a small, narrow chest that results in lethal pulmonary hypoplasia (Fig. 9-53). The abdomen and head appear relatively enlarged. In about one of six cases, the head has a cloverleaf shape. Hydrocephalus and polyhydramnios are common.

Osteogenesis Imperfecta

There are over a dozen discrete forms of this disease, all characterized by abnormalities of the biochemical composition of the bone matrix. The more severe forms are lethal, manifesting very short limbs and the prenatal

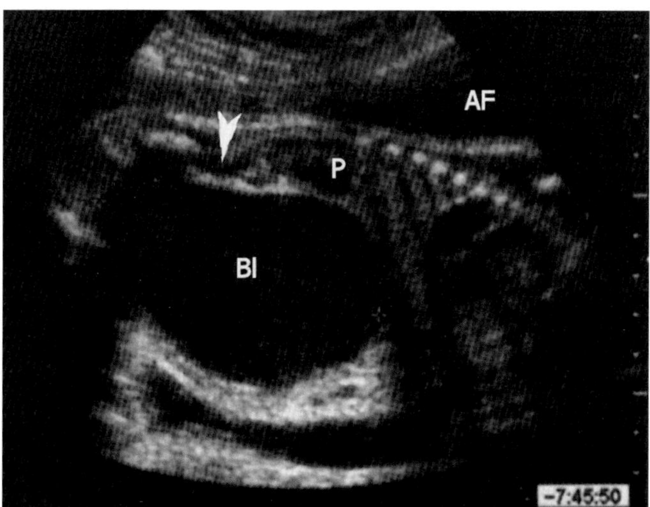

Figure 9-51. Bladder outlet obstruction. The bladder (Bl) is markedly dilated, extending almost all the way to the diaphragm. There is vesicoureteral reflux, as manifested by the dilated ureter (*arrowhead*) and renal pelvis (P). Because there is still amniotic fluid present (AF), the obstruction is not complete.

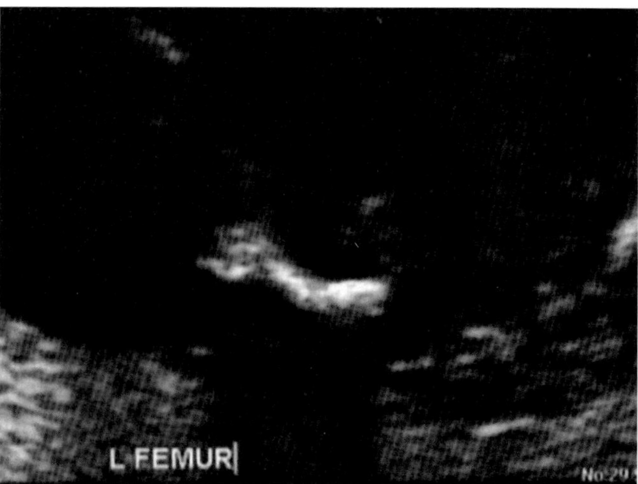

Figure 9-52. Abnormal femur in a fetus with thanatophoric dysplasia. The femur was only one third the normal length and has abnormal morphology. The curved shape and thickened ends characteristic of the femur in this condition has been likened to a telephone receiver in appearance.

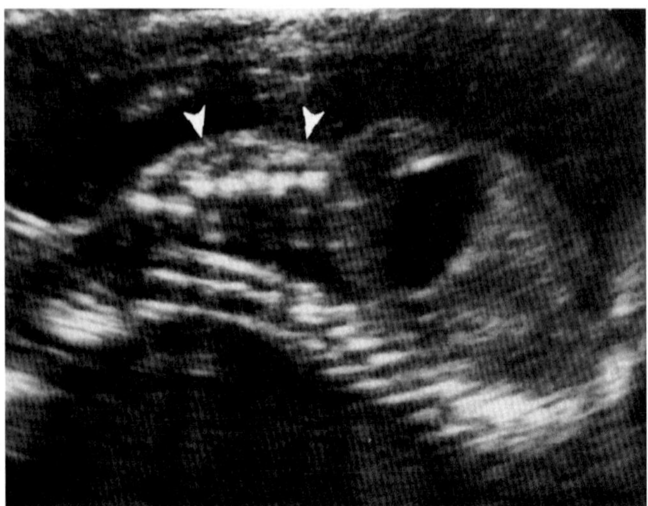

Figure 9-53. Hypoplastic chest (*arrowheads*) in a fetus with thanatophoric dysplasia.

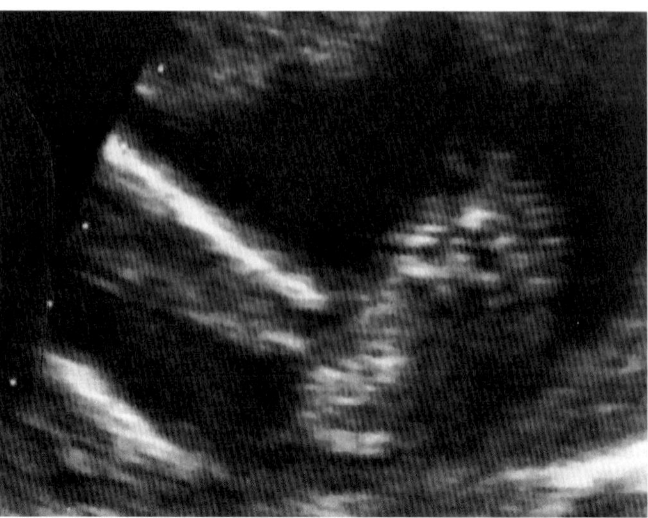

Figure 9-55. Fetal clubfoot. The foot is everted 90 degrees, placing the flat aspect of the foot in the same plane as the lower leg.

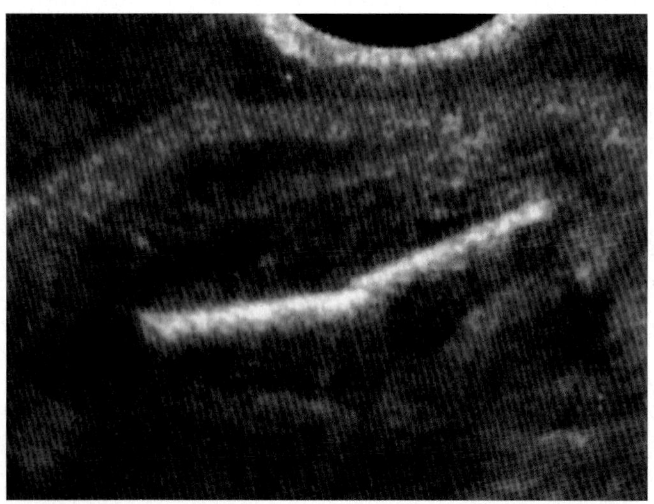

Figure 9-54. Fractured femur in a fetus with osteogenesis imperfecta.

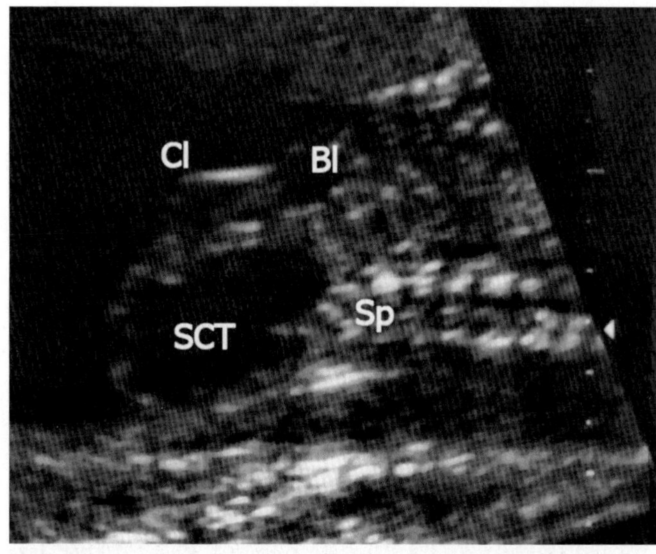

Figure 9-56. Sagittal view through the pelvis of a female fetus showing a sacrococcygeal teratoma (SCT). This tumor is predominantly cystic. The spine (Sp), bladder (Bl), and clitoris (Cl) are also indicated.

occurrence of multiple fractures (Fig. 9-54). More mild forms may show few or no fractures, bowing of the femurs, and limb lengths close to the normal range.

Clubfoot

Clubfoot is best diagnosed with a coronal view of the lower leg, with the tibia and fibula both seen in a lengthwise section. A normal foot is perpendicular to this plane, but a clubfoot is turned down and in, and is seen falling within the coronal plane (Fig. 9-55). It may be very difficult to diagnose clubfoot in the third trimester or in the presence of oligohydramnios.

OTHER ABNORMALITIES

Sacrococcygeal Teratoma

Sacrococcygeal teratoma (SCT) is the most common tumor in the fetus and newborn. Prenatal ultrasound shows a tumor arising from the fetal buttocks (Fig. 9-56) that may be cystic, mixed cystic and solid, or predominantly solid. Benign tumors are usually cystic or calcified. Most sacrococcygeal teratomas present at birth are benign.[82] Resection at birth is usually successful, but is sometimes associated with life-threatening bleeding. Very vascular tumors can also cause high-output fetal heart failure and hydrops. Death can be due to the heart failure itself or polyhydramnios, leading to preterm birth.[83]

Hydrops

Hydrops refers to generalized edema in the neonate, manifested by skin edema and accumulations of fluid in body cavities, including the pleural spaces, pericardium, and peritoneal cavity (Fig. 9-57). Before the introduction of Rh immune prophylaxis, most hydrops resulted from erythrobastosis fetalis. Currently, the great majority of cases of hydrops are from non-immune causes.[84] With improvement in diagnostic methods, the etiology of most cases of nonimmune hydrops can be determined. Table 9-2 lists the more common causes of nonimmune hydrops. In recent years, it has become apparent that parvovirus infection is responsible for many of the cases of hydrops that were previously classified as idiopathic[85] (see Chapter 48).

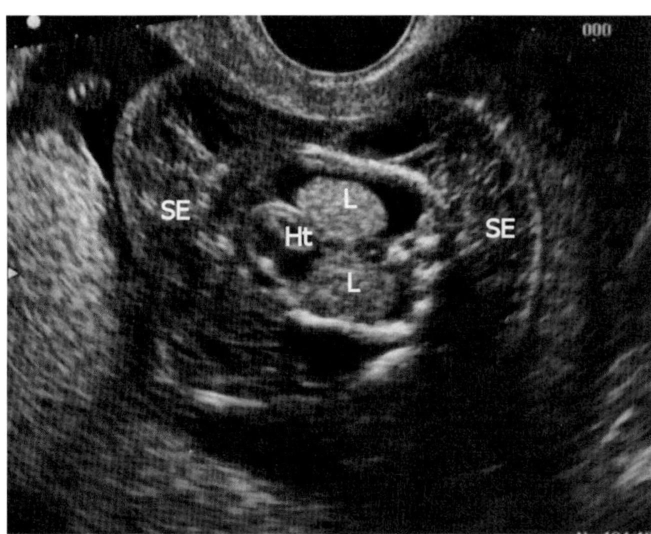

Figure 9-57. Transverse view through the chest of the fetus with generalized hydrops. Severe skin edema (SE) is present as well as bilateral pleural effusions. The heart (Ht) and lungs (L) are labeled.

Table 9-2. Causes of Hydrops Fetalis

Twin-to-twin transfusion
Chromosome abnormalities
Structural heart defects
Cardiac arrhythmia (especially tachyarrhythmia)
Cardiac tumor
High-output failure from vascular malformation or tumor
- Sacrococcygeal teratoma
- Vein of Galen malformation
- Placenta chorangioma
- Twin reverse arterial perfusion sequence

Fetal anemia
- Parvovirus infection
- Alpha-thalassemia
- Fetomaternal hemorrhage

Other infection
- TORCH infection
- Syphilis

Chest mass
- Congenital cystic adenomatoid malformation (CCAM)
- Pulmonary sequestration

Cystic Hygroma

Nuchal cystic hygroma consists of a loculated accumulation of fluid in the posterior neck (Fig. 9-58). Fetal edema may be widespread and is often associated with full-blown hydrops, a finding that precludes survival into the third trimester. A cystic hygroma is associated with a greater than 60 percent likelihood that the fetus has a chromosomal abnormality. Two thirds of these cases have Turner's syndrome, whereas most of the remainder have trisomy 21.[86] Regression of cystic hygroma in fetuses with Turner's syndrome results in the characteristic neck webbing seen after birth.

Molar Pregnancy

With complete mole, there are no recognizable fetal structures seen with ultrasound. Instead, the uterine cavity is filled with small cysts (Fig. 9-59). Color Doppler ultrasound can reveal the highly vascular nature of molar pregnancy. In partial mole, an abnormal fetus with a triploid karyotype coexists with an abnormal placenta. The fetus usually has severe asymmetric growth restriction and a variety of malformations. The placenta has macroscopic cystic spaces, giving it a Swiss cheese appearance.

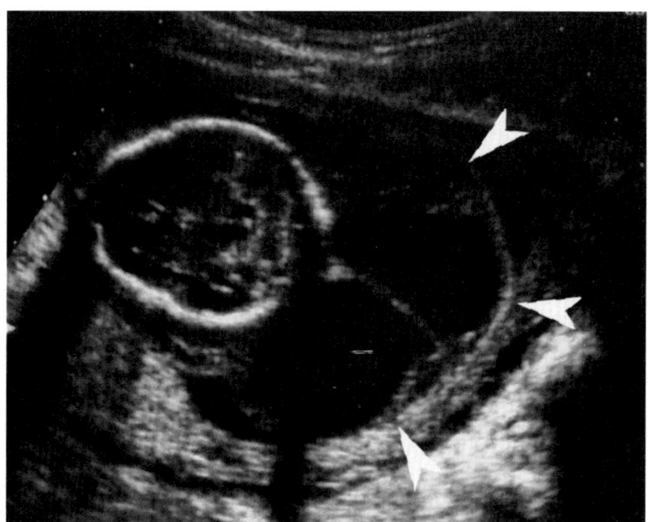

Figure 9-58. Large posterior nuchal cystic hygroma (outlined by *arrowheads*).

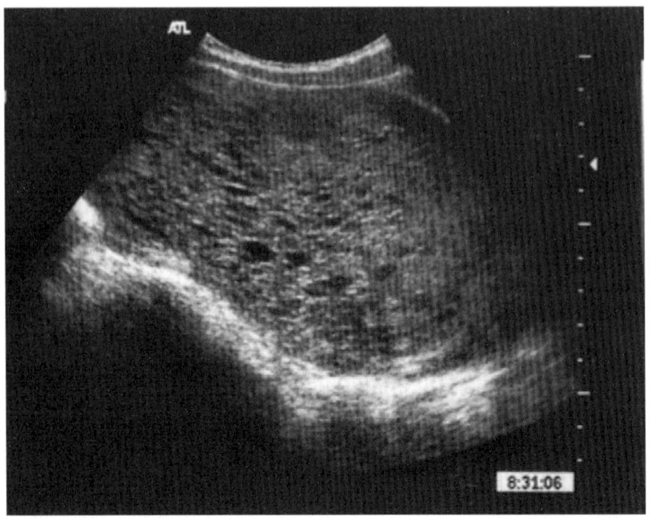

Figure 9-59. Sagittal view of the uterus showing a complete mole. The uterine cavity is filled with innumerable small cysts. Color Doppler ultrasound would show abundant vascularity.

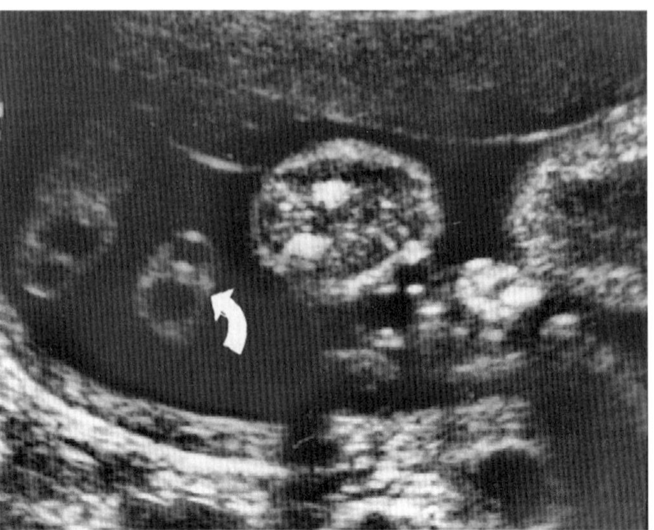

Figure 9-60. A transverse image through the umbilical cord (*arrow*), demonstrating a single umbililcal artery. The artery is the smaller of the two vessels.

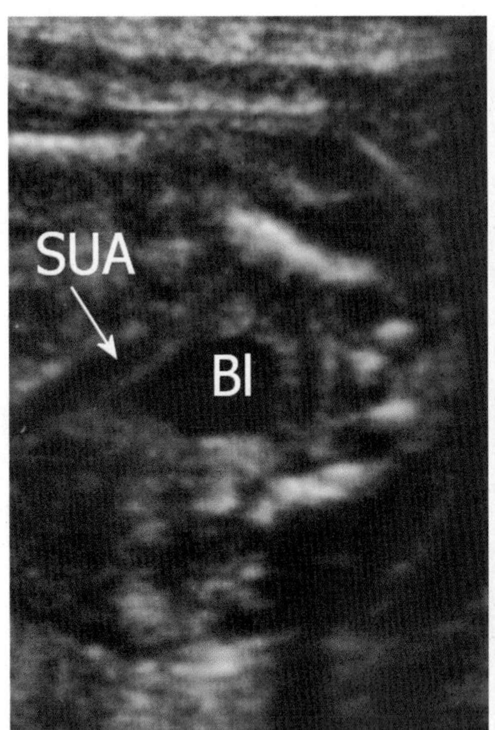

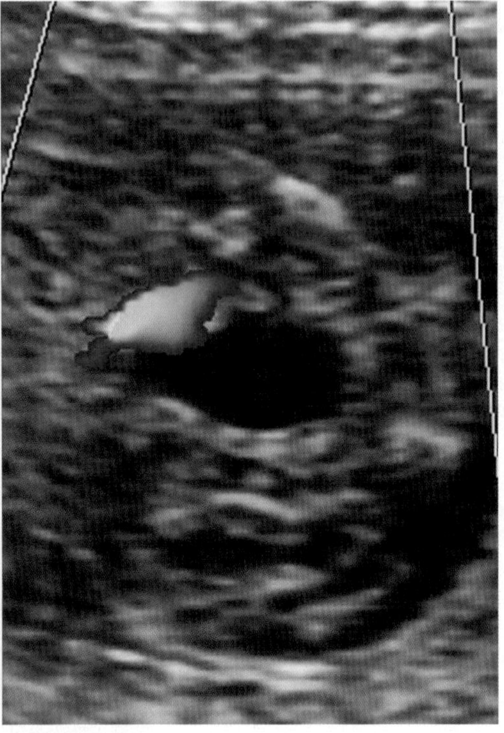

Figure 9-61. Transverse view of the fetal pelvis showing a single umbilical artery (SUA) coursing around the bladder (Bl) in the fetal pelvis. Color Doppler ultrasound makes it easy to confirm that there is no corresponding artery on the opposite side (*right panel*).

Umbilical Cord

An attempt should be made to confirm that there are two arteries and a vein in the umbilical cord.[58] In late pregnancy, this can be easily ascertained by looking at a transverse cut of the cord in a free loop (Fig. 9-60). In the second trimester, two umbilical arteries are most easily confirmed by identifying the vessels as they course around the fetal bladder (Fig. 9-61). These can be seen with gray scale ultrasound but are made much more obvious with color Doppler ultrasound. A single umbilical artery is present in 1 percent of all newborns. Because of the 20-percent incidence of associated malformations, this finding should prompt a detailed fetal survey.

Ultrasound as a Screening Test for Birth Defects

With improvements of ultrasound equipment in the last few decades, many patients and clinicians have come to assume that an ultrasound examination will likely detect any serious fetal anomaly that might be present. Indeed, in the 1980s and early 1990s several individual centers reported detection rates of greater than 75 percent in referral[87] and low-risk[88] patients. However, serious questions regarding the sensitivity of routine ultrasound examinations in more general settings were raised by a large, randomized multicenter trial published in 1993.[17] The RADIUS study (Routine Antenatal Diagnostic Imaging With Ultrasound Study) included standardized ultrasound examinations of more than 15,000 women between 16 and 20 weeks of gestation and then again at 31 to 33 weeks. Patients were selected to be at low risk for pregnancy complications. In this study, only 17 percent of major anomalies were diagnosed by ultrasound before 24 weeks' gestation, and only 35 percent were detected overall. The study's authors concluded that routine ultrasound to screen for birth defects in low-risk women was not efficacious. A subsequent large study of ultrasound screening for birth defects, the Eurofetus study, included more than 200,000 women evaluated with routine ultrasound in 61 hospital units in 14 European countries.[89] In contrast to the low rate of detection of anomalies in the RADIUS trial, 61 percent of malformed fetuses were identified. The sensitivity was higher for major malformations (74 percent), and there was a significant difference in detection rates according to the particular malformation or organ system involved. Defects of the central nervous system and urinary tract were detected 88 percent of the time, whereas only 18 percent of cases of cleft lip and palate were diagnosed. Eighteen percent of minor musculoskeletal malformations and 21 percent of minor cardiac malformations were picked up, whereas sensitivities were 74 percent and 39 percent for major anomalies of these two organ systems.

False-positive results must also be taken into account when considering the effectiveness of ultrasound screening for birth defects. Falsely abnormal results can cause patients and families considerable anguish and result in unnecessary follow-up tests that entail additional risks and costs.[90] Fortunately, in both the RADIUS and the Eurofetus trials, fewer than one in 500 women was erroneously told that her healthy fetus had a malformation. However, of the nearly 3,000 suspected malformations in the Eurofetus study, 10 percent were false-positive diagnoses, and 6 percent involved fetuses in which an initial concern was resolved on a subsequent ultrasound examination.[89] False-positive results are increased considerably when ultrasound is used to screen for Down syndrome markers. These findings, such as thick nuchal skin, do not themselves constitute malformations but indicate an increased risk of chromosomal abnormalities. At least one marker is present in about 14 percent of women who undergo a second-trimester genetic sonogram.[91]

The contrasting detection rates from the RADIUS[17] and Eurofetus[89] trials, and the studies cited by DeVore specifically related to cardiac screening[74] suggest that the expertise of sonographers has a significant impact on the likelihood that anomalies will be detected. It is well recognized that adequate training is essential for the proper performance and interpretation of obstetric ultrasound examinations. In the RADIUS trial, the detection rate for anomalies was almost three times higher when the examinations were performed at a tertiary center compared with a general practice setting (13 versus 35 percent),[17] presumably because of greater experience of sonographers at the tertiary centers. Although qualifications for those performing ultrasound examinations to screen for birth defects have not been standardized, the AIUM has made recommendations regarding the training and experience needed for physicians to perform obstetric ultrasound. These include the completion of an approved training program with the equivalent of 4 months' ultrasound experience and the involvement in the performance of at least 300 examinations, continuing education in the field (at least 30 hours every 3 years), and ongoing practice, consisting of at least 170 obstetric or gynecologic ultrasound examinations performed annually.[92]

It is difficult to prove that prenatal ultrasound reduces morbidity or mortality in newborns with birth defects. The RADIUS study demonstrated similar outcomes in the control group and the group with routine screening.[17] A randomized trial of routine ultrasound conducted in Finland demonstrated a decrease in perinatal mortality when routine ultrasound was used, but this was because most pregnancies with serious malformations were terminated, not because offspring from continued pregnancies did better.[93] Although definitive proof is lacking, it seems self-evident that there are several advantages to prenatal diagnosis: (1) it gives parents the option of pregnancy termination when serious malformations are diagnosed; and (2) it allows families and caregivers time to gather complete information about the fetal problem so the family can be emotionally prepared. Plans can be made for delivery at the proper time at a high-risk perinatal center where the newborn can receive optimal care. When the mother delivers at the tertiary care center, there is then no need to transport a potentially unstable newborn, and the mother and baby can remain together.

Unlike many other diagnostic tests in medicine, prenatal ultrasound is usually viewed as being enjoyable by patients and has not been shown to have any risks.[94] Routine ultrasound to screen for birth defects involves significant costs, but the costs per defect diagnosed are not out of line with other accepted screening tests.[95] It has been shown that the cost/benefit ratio is much more favorable when examinations are performed by sonographers with good detection rates.[95]

Even with the relatively low detection rate demonstrated in the RADIUS study, more than three times as many birth defects were recognized in the routine screening group compared with the group scanned only for clinical indications.[17] Chervenak and colleagues have pointed out that regardless of cost/benefit considerations, respect for a patient's autonomy gives obstetricians the duty to make this diagnostic modality available.[96] Ideally, in offering a screening ultrasound, the obstetrician should inform the patients in general terms of the sensitivity of this test in the setting in which it is to be performed.

Key Points

- A dating ultrasound performed between 14 and 22 weeks is comparable in accuracy to one performed in the first trimester. Beyond that time, variability in fetal size increases, and ultrasound prediction of gestational age becomes progressively less accurate.
- There is growing evidence that a dating ultrasound performed before 22 weeks should be used in preference to menstrual dates, regardless of the reliability or closeness of fit with menstrual dates.
- Customized weight percentiles for each fetus may help identify those with pathologic growth.
- The mean absolute error for ultrasound birth weight prediction is most studies is 8 to 10 percent of the birth weight. In about 30 percent of cases, the absolute error in estimated weight is greater than 10 percent of the birth weight.
- Ultrasound and clinical examinations have similar accuracy for predicting birth weight.
- Ultrasound for weight estimation has a limited potential for predicting or preventing birth injury from shoulder dystocia.
- Knowledge of the normal sequential development of embryonic structures in the first trimester helps predict the likelihood of spontaneous abortion. If there are borderline abnormal findings, it is prudent to perform sequential ultrasound examinations to be absolutely certain that a viable pregnancy will not be interrupted.
- Obstetric ultrasound should be performed by appropriately trained individuals using standard protocols for the content of the examination. Adequate records should document the findings.
- The likelihood that prenatal ultrasound will detect a birth defect varies significantly depending on the expertise of the examiner, the gestational age at which the examination is performed, and the nature and severity of the anomaly.
- Although the cost-effectiveness of ultrasound to screen for birth defects has been debated, the principle of patient autonomy makes it ethically appropriate to offer this test to pregnant women.

REFERENCES

1. Donald I, Abdulla U: Ultrasonics in obstetrics and gynaecology. Br J Radiol 40:604, 1967.
2. Hadlock FP, Deter RL, Harrist RB, et al: Fetal biparietal diameter: Rational choice of plane of section for sonographic measurement. AJR Am J Roentgenol 138:871, 1982.
3. Robinson HP, Fleming JEE: A critical evaluation of sonar "crown-rump length" measurements. Br J Obstet Gynecol 82:702, 1975.
4. Hadlock FP, Shah YP, Kanon DJ, et al: Fetal crown rump length: reevaluation of relation to menstrual age (5–18 weeks) with high-resolution real-time US. Radiology 182:501, 1992
5. Queenan JT, O'Brien GD, Campbell S: Ultrasound measurement of fetal limb bones. Am J Obstet Gynecol 138:297, 1980.
6. Hellman LM, Koboyashi M, Fillisti L, et al: Growth and development of the human fetus prior to the twentieth week of gestation. Am J Obstet Gynecol 103:789, 1969.
7. Nyberg DA, Abuhamad A, Ville Y: Ultrasound assessment of abnormal fetal growth. Semin Perinatol 28:3, 2004.
8. Robinson HP: Gestational age determination: first trimester. *In* Chervenak FA, Isaacson GC, Campbell S (eds): Ultrasound in Obstetrics and Gynecology. Boston, Little, Brown and Company, 1993, p 295.
9. Schats R, Van Os HC, Jansen CA, et al: The crown-rump length in early human pregnancy: a reappraisal. Br J Obstet Gynaecol 98:460, 1991.
10. MacGregor SN, Tamura RK, Sabbagha RE, et al: Underestimation of gestational age by convential crown rump length dating curves. Obstet Gynecol 70:344, 1987.
11. Hadlock FP, Harrist RB, Martinez-Poyer J: How accurate is second trimester fetal dating? J Ultrasound Med 10:557, 1991.
12. Degani S: Fetal biometry: clinical, pathological, and technical considerations. Obstet Gynecol Surv 56:159, 2001.
13. Chervenak FA, Skupski DW, Romero R, et al: How accurate is fetal biometry in the assessment of fetal age? Am J Obstet Gynecol 178:678, 1998.
14. Mongelli M, Wilcox M, Gardosi J: Estimating the date of confinement: ultrasonographic biometery versus certain menstrual dates. Am J Obstet Gynecol 174:278, 1996.
15. Savitz DA. Terry JW Jr, Dole N, et al: Comparison of pregnancy dating by last menstrual period, ultrasound scanning, and their combination. Am J Obstet Gynecol 187:1660, 2002.
16. Rahim RR, Cuckle HS, Sehmi IK, et al: Compromise ultrasound dating policy in maternal serum screening for Down syndrome. Prenat Diagn 22:1181, 2002.
17. Ewigman BG, Crane JP, Frigoletto FD, et al: Effect of prenatal ultrasound screening on perinatal outcome. N Engl J Med 329: 821, 1993.
18. Bergsjo P, Villar J: Scientific basis for the content of routine antenatal care. II. Power to eliminate or alleviate adverse newborn outcomes; some special conditions and examinations. Acta Obstet Gynecol Scand 76:15, 1997.
19. Pearce JM, Campbell S: A comparison of symphysis-fundal height and ultrasound as screening tests for light-for-gestational age infants. Br J Obstet Gynaecol 94:100, 1987.
20. Hepburn M, Rosenberg K: An audit of the detection and management of small-for-gestational age babies. Br J Obstet Gynaecol 93:212, 1986.
21. Bais JM, Eskes M, Pel M, et al: Effectiveness of detection of intrauterine growth retardation by abdominal palpation as screening test in a low risk population: an observational study. Eur J Obstet Gynecol Reprod Biol 116:164, 2004.
22. Harding K, Evans S, Newnham J: Screening for the small fetus: a study of the relative efficacies of ultrasound biometry and symphysiofundal height. Aust N Z J Obstet Gynaecol 35:160, 1995.
23. Jahn A, Razum O, Berle P: Routine screening for intrauterine growth retardation in Germany: low sensitivity and questionable benefit for diagnosed cases. Acta Obstet Gynecol Scand 77:643, 1998.
24. Bricker L, Neilson JP: Routine ultrasound in late pregnancy (after 24 weeks gestation). Cochrane Database Syst Rev 2:CD001451, 2000.
25. Brenner WE, Edelman DA, Hendricks CH: A standard of fetal growth for the United States of America. Am J Obstet Gynecol 126:555, 1976.
26. Hadlock FP, Harrist RB, Martinez-Poyer J: In utero analysis of fetal growth: a sonographic weight standard. Radiology 181:129, 1991.
27. Doubilet PM, Benson CB, Nadel AS, et al: Improved birth weight table for neonates developed from gestations dated by early ultrasonography. J Ultrasound Med 16:241, 1997.
28. Gardosi J, Chang A, Kalyan B, et al: Customised antenatal growth charts. Lancet 339:283, 1992.

29. Clausson B, Gardosi J, Francis A, et al: Perinatal outcome in SGA births defined by customised versus population-based birthweight standards. Br J Obstet Gynecol 108:830, 2001.
30. Campbell S, Thoms A: Ultrasound measurement of fetal head to abdomen circumference ratio in the assessment of growth retardation. Br J Obstet Gynaecol 84:165, 1977.
31. David C, Gabrielli S, Pilu G, et al: The head-to-abdomen circumference ratio: a reappraisal. Ultrasound Obstet Gynecol 5:256, 1995.
32. Williams MC, O'Brien WF: A comparison of birth weight and weight/length ratio for gestation as correlates of perinatal morbidity. J Perinatol 17:346, 1997.
33. Smith-Bindman R, Chu PW, Ecker JL, et al: US evaluation of fetal growth: prediction of neonatal outcomes. Radiology 223:153, 2002.
34. Nyberg DA, Abuhamad A, Ville Y: Ultrasound assessment of abnormal fetal growth. Semin Perinatol 23:3, 2004.
35. Hadlock F: Evaluation of fetal weight estimation procedures. *In* Deter R, Harist R, Birnholz J, et al (eds): Quantitative Obstetrical Ultrasonography. New York, Weley, 1986, p 113.
36. Sherman DJ, Arieli S, Tovbin J, et al: A comparison of clinical and ultrasound estimation of fetal weight. Obstet Gynecol 91:212, 1998.
37. Baum JD, Gussman D, Wirth JC 3rd: Clinical and patient estimation of fetal weight vs. ultrasound estimation. J Reprod Med 47:194, 2002.
38. Robson SC, Gallivan S, Walkinshaw SA, et al: Ultrasonic estimation of fetal weight: use of targeted formulas in small for gestational age fetuses. Obstet Gynecol 82:359, 1993.
39. Combs CA, Rosenn B, Miodovnik M, et al: Sonographic EFW and macrosomia: is there an optimum formula to predict diabetic fetal macrosomia? J Matern Fetal Med 9:55, 2000.
40. Jouannic JM, Grange G, Goffinet F, et al: Validity of sonographic formulas for estimating fetal weight below 1,250g: a series of 119 cases. Fetal Diagn Ther 16:254, 2001.
41. Lee W, Deter RL, Ebersole JD, et al: Birth Weight Prediction by three-dimensional ultrasonography: fractional limb volume. J Ultrasound Med 20:1283, 2001.
42. Gonen R, Spiegel D, Abend M: Is macrosomia predictable, and are shoulder dystocia and birth trauma preventable? Obstet Gynecol 88:526, 1996.
43. Warren WB, Timor-Tritsch I, Peisner DB, et al: Dating the early pregnancy by sequential appearance of embryonic structures. Am J Obstet Gynecol 161:747, 1989.
44. Blaas HG, Eik-Nes SH, Kiserud T, et al: Early development of the abdominal wall, stomach and heart from 7 to 12 weeks of gestation: a longitudinal ultrasound study. Ultrasound Obstet Gynecol 6:240, 1995.
45. Rosati P, Guariglia L: Transvaginal sonographic assessment of the fetal urinary tract in early pregnancy. Ultrasound Obstet Gynecol 7:95, 1996.
46. Laboda LA, Estroff JA, Benacerraf BR: First trimester bradycardia. A sign of impending fetal loss. J Ultrasound Med 8:561, 1989.
47. Haak MC, Twisk JW, Van Vugt JM: How successful is fetal echocardiographic examination in the first trimester of pregnancy? Ultrasound Obstet Gynecol 20:9, 2002.
48. Tongsong T, Srisomboon J, Wanapirak C, et al: Pregnancy outcome of threatened abortion with demonstrable fetal cardiac activity: a cohort study. J Obstet Gynaecol 21:331, 1995.
49. Smith KE, Buyalos RP: The profound impact of patient age on pregnancy outcome after early detection of fetal cardiac activity. Fertil Steril 65:35, 1996.
50. Maso G, D'Ottavio G, De Seta F, et al: First-trimester intrauterine hematoma and outcome of pregnancy. Obstet Gynecol 105:339, 2005.
51. Tongsong T, Wanapirak C, Srisomboon J, et al: Transvaginal ultrasound in threatened abortions with empty gestational sacs. Int J Gynaecol Obstet 46:297, 1994.
52. Pennell RG, Needleman L, Pajak T, et al: Prospective comparison of vaginal and abdominal sonography in normal early pregnancy. J Ultrasound Med 10:63, 1991.
53. Stampone C, Nicotra M, Muttinelli C, et al: Transvaginal sonography of the yolk sac in normal and abnormal pregnancy. J Clin Ultrasound 24:3, 1996.
54. Rowling SE, Coleman BG, Langer JE, et al: First-trimester US parameters of failed pregnancy. Radiology 203:211, 1997.
55. Nicolaides KH: Nuchal translucency and other first-trimester sonographic markers of chromosomal abnormalities. Am J Obstet Gynecol 191:45, 2004.
56. Taipale P, Ammala M, Alonen R, et al: Two-stage ultrasonography in screening for fetal anomalies at 13–14 weeks and 18–22 weeks. Acta Obstet Gynecol Scan 83:1141, 2004.
57. VanDorsten JP, Hulsey TC, Newman RB, et al: Fetal anomaly detection by second-trimester ultrasonography in a tertiary center. Am J Obstet Gynecol 178:742, 1998.
58. American Institute of Ultrasound in Medicine: AIUM Practice Guideline for the performance of an antepartum obstetric ultrasound examination. J Ultrasound Med 22:1116, 2003.
59. Levitsky DB, Mack LA, Nyberg DA, et al: Fetal aqueductal stenosis diagnosed sonographically: how grave is the prognosis? AJR Am J Roentgenol 164:725, 1995.
60. Pilu G, Falco P, Gabrielli S, et al: The clinical significance of fetal isolated cerebral borderline ventriculomegaly: report of 31 cases and review of the literature. Ultrasound Obstet Gynecol 14:320, 1999.
61. Ghidini A, Strobelt N, Locatelli A, et al: Isolated fetal choroid plexus cysts: role of ultrasonography in establishment of the risk of trisomy 18. Am J Obstet Gynecol 182:972, 2000.
62. Blaas HG, Eriksson AG, Salvesen KA, et al: Brains and faces in holoprosencephaly: pre- and postnatal description of 30 cases. Ultrasound Obstet Gynecol 19:24, 2002.
63. Ulm B, Ulm MR, Deutinger J, et al: Dandy-Walker malformation diagnosed before 21 weeks of gestation: Associated malformations and chromosomal abnormalities. Ultrasound Obstet Gynecol 10:167, 1997.
64. Bernard JP, Moscoso G, Renier D, et al: Cystic malformations of the posterior fossa. Prenat Diagn 21:1064, 2001.
65. Boddaert N, Klein O, Ferguson N, et al: Intellectual prognosis of the Dandy-Walker malformation in children: the importance of vermian lobulation. Neuroradiology 45:320, 2003.
66. Bannister CM, Russell SA, Rimmer S, et al: Fetal arachnoid cysts: their site, progress, prognosis and differential diagnosis. Eur J Pediatr Surg 9(Suppl 1):27, 1999.
67. Chatzipapas IK, Whitlow BJ, Economides DL: The "Mickey Mouse" sign and the diagnosis of anencephaly in early pregnancy. Ultrasound Obstet Gynecol 13:196, 1999.
68. Bannister CM, Russell SA, Rimmer S, et al: Can prognostic indicators be identified in a fetus with an encephalocele? Eur J Pediatr Surg 10(Suppl 1):20, 2000.
69. Nicolaides KH, Campbell S, Gabbe SG, et al: Ultrasound screening for spina bifida: cranial and cerebellar signs. Lancet 2:72, 1986.
70. Van den Hof MC, Nicolaides KH, Campbell J, et al: Evaluation of the lemon and banana signs in one hundred thirty fetuses with open spina bifida. Am J Obstet Gynecol 162:322, 1990.
71. Revillon Y, Jan D, Plattner V, et al: Congenital cystic adenomatoid malformation of the lung: prenatal management and prognosis. J Pediatr Surg 28:1009, 1993.
72. Roggin KK, Breuer CK, Carr SR, et al: The unpredictable character of congenital cystic lung lesions. J Pediatr Surg 35:801, 2000.
73. Lopoo JB, Goldstein RB, Lipshutz GS, et al: Fetal pulmonary sequestration: a favorable congenital lung lesion. Obstet Gynecol 94: 567, 1999.
74. DeVore GR: Influence of prenatal diagnosis on congenital heart defects. Ann N Y Acad Sci 847:46, 1998.
75. Abuhamed A: A Practical Guide to Fetal Echocardiography. Philadelphia, Lipincott-Raven, 1997, p 1.
76. Wimalasundera RC, Gardiner HM: Congenital heart disease and aneuploidy. Prenat Diagn 30:1116, 2004.
77. Barisic I, Clementi M, Hausler M, et al: Evaluation of prenatal ultrasound diagnosis of fetal abdominal wall defects by 19 European registries. Ultrasound Obstet Gynecol 18:309, 2001.
78. Hwang PJ, Kousseff BG: Omphalocele and gastroschisis: an 18-year review study. Genet Med 6:232, 2004.
79. Corteville JE, Gray DL, Crane JP: Congenital hydronephrosis: correlation of fetal ultrasonographic findings with infant outcome. Am J Obstet Gynecol 165:384, 1991.
80. Stocks A, Richards D, Frentzen B, et al: Correlation of prenatal renal pelvic anteroposterior diameter with outcome in infancy. J Urol 155:1050, 1996.
81. Campbell J, Henderson A, Campbell S: The fetal femur/foot length ratio: a new parameter to assess dysplastic limb reduction. Obstet Gynecol 72:181, 1988.

82. Kurjak A, Zalud I, Jurkovic D, et al: Ultrasound diagnosis and evaluation of fetal tumors. J Perinat Med 17:173, 1989.
83. Perrelli L, D'Urzo C, Manzoni C, et al: Sacrococcygeal teratoma. Outcome and management. An analysis of 17 cases. J Perinat Med 30:179, 2002.
84. Santolaya J, Alley D, Jaffe R, et al: Antenatal classification of hydrops fetalis. Obstet Gynecol 79:256, 1992.
85. Hernandez-Andrade E, Scheier M, Dezerega V, et al: Fetal middle cerebral artery peak systolic velocity in the investigation of non-immune hydrops. Ultrasound Obstet Gynecol 23:442, 2004.
86. Descamps P, Jourdain O, Paillet C, et al: Etiology, prognosis and management of nuchal cystic hygroma: 25 new cases and literature review. Eur J Obstet Gynecol Reprod Biol 71:3, 1997.
87. Campbell S, Allan L, Griffin D, et al: Early diagnosis of fetal structural abnormalities. Prog Clin Biol Res 163B:187, 1985.
88. Chitty LS, Hunt GH, Moore J, et al: Effectiveness of routine ultrasonography in detecting fetal structural abnormalities in a low risk population. BMJ 303:1165, 1991.
89. Grandjean H, Larroque D, Levi S, et al: The performance of routine ultrasonographic screening of pregnancies in the Eurofetus Study. Am J Obstet Gynecol 181:446, 1999.
90. Filly RA: Obstetrical sonography: the best way to terrify a pregnant woman. J Ultrasound Med 19:1, 2000.
91. Vintzileos AM, Campbell WA, Rodis JF, et al: The use of second-trimester genetic sonogram in guiding clinical management of patients at increased risk for fetal trisomy 21. Obstet Gynecol 87:948, 1996.
92. Application for Practice Accreditation, AIUM Ultrasound Practice Accreditation Commission. Laurel, MD, American Institute of Ultrasound in Medicine.
93. Saari-Kemppainen A, Karjalainen O, Ylostalo P, et al: Fetal anomalies in a controlled one-stage ultrasound screening trial. A report from the Helsinki Ultrasound Trial. J Perinat Med 22:279, 1994.
94. American Institute of Ultrasound in Medicine Official Statement: Clinical safety. Approved March 26, 1997. Laurel MD, American Institute of Ultrasound in Medicine.
95. DeVore GR: The Routine Antenatal Diagnostic Imaging with Ultrasound Study: another perspective. Obstet Gynecol 84:622, 1994.
96. Chervenak FA, McCullough LB: Ethical dimensions of ultrasound screening for fetal anomalies. Ann N Y Acad Sci 847:185, 1998.

Fetal Therapy

MARK I. EVANS, YUVAL YARON, JAN DEPREST, ALAN W. FLAKE,
CHARLES KLEINMAN, AND MICHAEL R. HARRISON

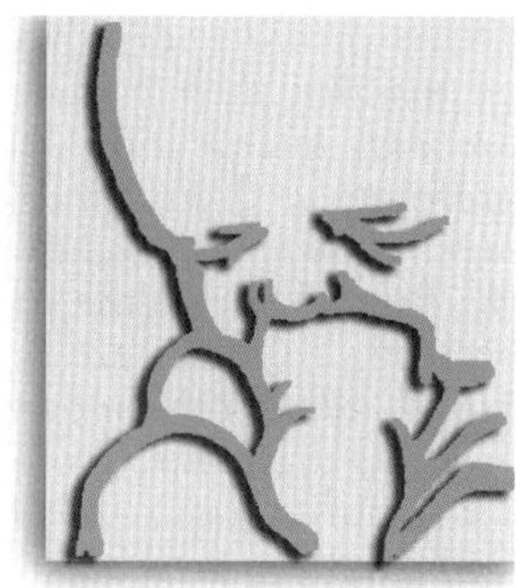

CHAPTER 10

KEY ABBREVIATIONS

Arterioarterial	AA
Arteriovenous	AV
Bone marrow transplantation	BMT
Congenital adrenal hyperplasia	CAH
Congenital cystic adenomatoid malformation	CCAM
Congenital diaphragmatic hernia	CDH
Central nervous system	CNS
Fetoscopic endoluminal tracheal occlusion	FETO
Graft-versus-host disease	GVHD
Hematopoietic stem cell	HSC
Human leukocyte antigen	HLA
Intermittent absent or reversed end-diastolic flow	iA/REDF
Intrauterine fetal death	IUFD
Intrauterine growth restriction	IUGR
Left-sided CDH	LCDH
Lower urinary tract obstruction	LUTO
Lung-to-head ratio	LHR
Methyl tetrahydrofolate reductase	MTHFR
Monochorionic	MC
Neural tube defect	NTD
Polymerase chain reaction	PCR
Preterm labor	PTL
Preterm premature rupture of the membranes	PPROM
Severe combined immunodeficiency syndrome	SCID
Termination of pregnancy	TOP
Thyroid-stimulating immunoglobulin	TSI
Tracheal occlusion	TO
Twin reversed arterial perfusion	TRAP
Twin-to-twin transfusion syndrome	TTTS
Venovenous	VV

INTRODUCTION

Traditionally, one of the major complaints by opponents of prenatal diagnosis was that the only treatment option following the diagnosis of an anomaly was termination of the pregnancy (TOP). Despite the fallacy of such an argument, it has been accepted by too many physicians and the public. In reality, there has been a nearly 40-year history of trying to treat birth defects in utero. Particularly over the last 2 decades, fetal therapy has evolved into four major areas: open surgical approaches, "closed" endoscopic surgical approaches, pharmacologic therapy, and stem cell/gene therapy. Progress in the field has been characterized by dramatic successes but also by frustration at technical challenges. Concurrently, targets change as ancillary therapies alter the risk/reward equations[1] for performing fetal surgery.

If a disorder can be treated safely and adequately postnatally, then in general, there is no justification for prenatal intervention. However, for many conditions, profound and irreparable damage occurs before birth, making fetal intervention the best or sometimes only way to ameliorate the pathology. Some procedures have been rare. Others are more common, but the expectation is that with improvements and increasing use of prenatal diagnosis, more women will chose to consider the opportunities to treat fetuses before birth.[2] It cannot be overemphasized, however, that opportunities for treatment depend on accurate, early diagnosis.

PERCUTANEOUS SURGICAL THERAPY

Obstructive Uropathies

Lower urinary tract obstructions (LUTOs) are heterogeneous and affect 1:5,000 to 8,000 newborn male infants. Posterior urethral valves or urethral atresias are the most common disorders, but stenosis of the urethral meatus, anterior urethral valves, ectopic insertion of a ureter, and tumors of the bladder have been observed. Massive distention of the bladder, followed by compensatory hypertrophy and hyperplasia of the smooth muscle, can be seen within the bladder wall. Compliance and elasticity decrease; poor postnatal function generally requires surgical reconstruction.[3] Elevated intravesicular pressures prevent urine inflow from the ureters; distortion of the ureterovesicle angles contributes further to reflux hydronephrosis. Progressive pyelectasis and calyectasis compress the delicate renal parenchyma within the encasing serosal capsule, leading to functional abnormalities within the medullary and, eventually, the cortical regions. Focal compressive hypoxia likely contributes to the progressive fibrosis. Perturbations in tubular function result in urinary hypertonicity. These obstructive processes eventually lead to type IV cystic dysplasia and renal insufficiency.[4–7]

Progressive oligo/anhydramnios can also lead to compressive abdominal deformations as seen in Potter sequence, which include extremity contractures and facial dysmorphology. Absence of normal amniotic fluid volume also interferes with pulmonary growth and development. Constant compressive pressure on the fetal thorax restricts expansion of the chest through normal physiologic "breathing movements." In fact, babies born with LUTO generally die from pulmonary complications because they do not live long enough to develop clinical renal failure.

The prenatal sonographic diagnosis of LUTO includes dilated and thickened walls of the bladder, hydronephrosis, and oligohydramnios. Urethral strictures or atresia, urethral agenesis, megalourethra, ureteral reflux, and cloacal anomalies may show a very similar appearance on ultrasound. The typical "keyhole sign" of proximal urethral dilation is secondary to urethral obstruction present in the posterior urethral valve or atresia. However, the precise pathophysiology can only be determined after birth.[7]

The prenatal evaluation and management of fetuses with the sonographic findings of LUTO are complex.[4–6] Other congenital anomalies, such as cardiac and neural tube defects, must be excluded before intervention can be considered. Karyotyping is needed to confirm a normal male chromosomal status; most are in fact normal. Affected female fetuses almost always have more complex syndromes of cloacal malformations and, hence, would not benefit from in utero shunt therapy. Given oligo/anhydramnios, which makes amniocentesis difficult, we commonly obtain karyotypes by transabdominal chorionic villus sampling.

Evaluation of underlying renal status in the fetus has become the key element pre-operatively. Over the past 15 years, we have developed a multicomponent approach for the analysis of fetal urine that evaluates proximal tubular and possible glomerular status using sodium, chloride, osmolality, calcium, beta-2 microglobulin, albumin, and total protein concentrations. Serial assessments are optimally performed at 48- to 72-hour intervals.[5,6] Using such an approach, one can directly correlate the degree of impaired renal function and damage with the extent of urinary hypertonicity and proteinuria. With these data, our ability to counsel patients about the renal status of their fetus and the long-term prognosis has improved dramatically.

Vesicoamniotic catheter shunts bypass the urethral obstruction, diverting urine into amniotic space. This allows drainage of the upper urinary tract and thus prevents pulmonary hypoplasia and physical deformations (Fig. 10-1). Fetuses with isolated LUTO, a normal male karyotype, and progressively improving urinary profile who meet threshold parameters have undergone successful intervention through percutaneous vesicoamniotic shunt therapy.

Experience has been widely varied and is related both to the etiology of obstruction as well as to the extent of prenatal evaluation before shunt placement. Freedman et al.[7] confirmed that infants with "prune belly" syndrome who have complete urethral obstructions have very good renal outcomes following vesicoamniotic shunt therapy. Although significant improvement in survival and renal function has been seen in infants with posterior urethral valves treated by shunting, many still show mild to moderate renal insufficiency at birth. Several of these infants have progressed to renal failure, dialysis, and transplantation. Infants with the worst prognosis are those with urethral atresia.

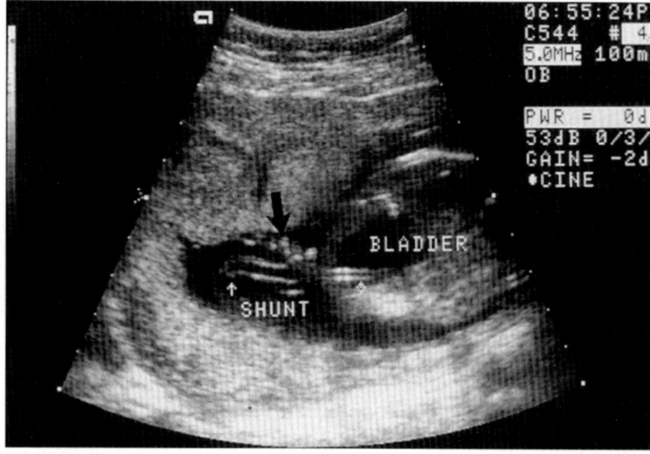

Figure 10-1. Bladder shunt. Catheter can be seen transversing bladder into amniotic cavity.

More recent data suggest that patients having bladder shunts have a 90-percent survival rate, but long-term renal function remains problematic. Just under half had "normal renal function," and about a quarter had mild impairments. Follow-up pediatric urologic/renal function assessment is critical. The Paris group found that about 25 percent of children had serious, long-term renal impairments, and about 15 percent developed end stage renal disease requiring transplant.[4] Therefore, parents must weigh the benefits of survival versus serious risks of poor postnatal renal function.

Other Shunts

Cephalic

Shunting was first attempted in the late 1970s for obstructive hydrocephalus,[5] but results were nearly uniformly disastrous. In retrospect, most subjects were very poor candidates for intervention. Many had multisystem disorders, aneuploidy, or such hopeless anomalies as holoprosencephaly.

Accordingly, ventriculoamniotic shunts have been abandoned since the early 1980s. With a better understanding of the poor natural history of the anomaly, and better, more accurate diagnostic techniques, we have recently speculated that there may be limited applications for prenatal neurologic shunting in cases of early onset, isolated, progressive obstructive hydrocephaly.

Thoracic

Percutaneously placed shunts have also been used to treat thoracic abnormalities.[6,7] The macrocystic form of congenital cystic adenomatous malformation can present with a very large intrathoracic mass and a single dominant macrocyst. This may cause cardiac and mediastinal shift and concomitant hemodynamic changes, as well as pulmonary compression and lung hypoplasia. Effects of dominant cysts can be ameliorated using pleuroamniotic shunts to drain these structures, reducing their volume and diminishing their space-occupying effects within the thoracic cavity.

Isolated pleural effusions can cause hemodynamic changes and lead to generalized hydrops as well as pulmonary compression that interferes with normal lung development. Small, unilateral effusions generally do not warrant intervention but must be followed closely because they have the potential for rapid progression and development of generalized hydrops.[8]

As with all fetal interventions, prenatal evaluation before intervention is critical for appropriate case selection. Seemingly isolated effusions may be the first sign of a cardiac malformation, aneuploidy, anemia, or infectious process. Thoracoamniotic shunting is effective only in carefully evaluated cases in which the risk of pulmonary hypoplasia from large effusions early in gestation is present, or in which exists early signs of progressive hydrops (unilateral or bilateral effusion, skin or scalp edema, ascites, pericardial effusion). Fetal anemia, per se, is not an indication for thoracoamniotic effusion shunting. Hydropic changes usually resolve with timely fetal transfusion therapy. However, when the fetus develops significant ascites, the prognosis diminishes considerably even with successful shunt intervention.[8] However, several cases with suddenly progressive pleural effusions and onset of generalized hydrops (skin/scalp edema, pericardial effusion, and moderate ascites) have been treated with complete resolution of all hydropic complications. Infants were normal after birth.

FETOSCOPY

Instruments

Fetoscopes are supplied by the same manufacturers who have developed hysteroscopic and laparoscopic counterparts. There is no indication that one particular brand performs better than another. Each scope strives for a combination of minimal diameter, appropriate length and maximal resolution. In Europe, considerable investment has been made by the European Commission to support instrument development by a partner of the Eurofoetus research consortium (Karl Storz Endoskope). As a result, a wide and still expanding range of 20 to 30 cm fetoscopes with diameters of 1.0 to 2.3 mm, sheaths, and specially designed instruments are now available.[9] There are two general types of endoscopes. First, semiflexible 0-degree fiberoptic scopes come in any length desired and have diameters of 1.0, 1.2, or 2.0 mm. These choices, in turn, determine the resolution and light transmission. A direct relationship exists between diameter and working length because light is lost with passage through the lens system. Larger diameter rod lens scopes are derived from hysteroscopic instruments but might be useful for diagnostic purposes. Image quality is better given their larger diameter. As technology evolves, more fibers can be packed in a given diameter. That fiber-endoscopes can be curved allows the scope to be directed toward an anteriorly located placenta or toward specific fetal structures like the urinary tract or trachea.[10] Rod lens telescopes with angles of inclination up to 30 degrees are available. To be functional, scopes are used within a sheath, allowing instrument insertion and irrigation. Investing in good-quality video-endoscopic hardware is essential, including a high-quality light fountain, video camera, and monitor. We also use a "twin video system," which mixes sonographic and endoscopic images and is projected onto a screen. Appropriate energy sources are needed for coagulating. For vessel or interstitial laser coagulation this could be a Nd:YAG (minimal power requirements 60 to 100 W) or diode laser (30 to 60 W). Monopolar and bipolar energy are readily available in all operation rooms. There are also proponents of the use of radiofrequency for intrafetal vessel ablation. A special generator is required if this approach is selected.

Twin-To-Twin Transfusion Syndrome

Background

Monochorionic (MC) twins by definition share a single placenta. In nearly all cases, vascular anastomoses connect the circulation of both babies. Intertwin transfusion is a constant, but balanced, phenomenon in the majority of MC twins, but if a specific pattern of anastomoses is present, twin-to-twin transfusion syndrome (TTTS) may occur. The exact incidence of TTTS remains to be determined, but an estimate of 10 to 15 percent is usually cited. In TTTS, a chronic imbalance in net flow occurs from one fetus (the donor) to the other (the recipient). Typically this occurs between 16 and 26 weeks of gestation. Hypovolemia, oliguria, and oligohydramnios develop in the donor, resulting in the "stuck twin" phenomenon. Hypervolemia, polyuria and hydramnios evolve in the recipient, which may develop circulatory overload and hydrops. TTTS is a *sonographic* diagnosis limited to twins believed to be MC. In Europe, the following additional stringent criteria were adopted: polyuric hydramnios in the recipient (defined as deepest vertical pocket of greater than 6 cm before 16 weeks; greater than 8 cm between 16 and 20 weeks; greater than 10 cm above 20 weeks) *combined* with oligohydramnios in the donor's sac (deepest vertical pocket <2 cm) secondary to oliguria. In the United States, a cutoff of 8 cm is used for the latter gestational age group.[11] Growth restriction may coincide, but is not part of the diagnostic criteria. The condition does not encompass the acute intertwin transfusion in MC twins that occurs only around birth or at the time of intrauterine fetal death (IUFD).

Pathophysiology

The pathophysiology of this condition is a subject in itself, and for discussion, we refer the reader elsewhere.[9] Briefly, vascular anastomoses provide the anatomic basis, and additional hemodynamic and hormonal factors contribute in variable degrees to precise clinical manifestation. The different manifestations are usually described by the sonographic staging system introduced by Quintero[12] (see box, "Twin-to-Twin Transfusion Syndrome") Staging implies that TTTS is progressive in character, but this is not obligatory. IUFD (stage V) may occur in a stage I patient without passing through hydrops (stage IV). Even if TTTS does not necessarily proceed through each stage, the staging system is useful in emphasizing the importance of strict criteria and thorough assessment. Doppler investigation is an integral part of evaluating the pregnancy suspected to have TTTS. Doppler may detect congestive heart failure in the recipient (negative or reversed a wave in the ductus venosus, pulsatile flow in the umbilical vein, tricuspid regurgitation) and signs of hypovolemia or increased vascular resistance in the donor (absent or reversed flow in the umbilical artery).[13]

Twin-to-Twin Transfusion Syndrome

Stage 1	Polyhydramnios/oligohydramnios with donor bladder visible.
Stage 2	Donor bladder not visible.
Stage 3	Presence of either absent or reverse end diastolic velocity of the umbilical artery, reverse flow in the ductus venosus, or pulsatile umbilical venous flow in either twin.
Stage 4	Hydrops in either twin.
Stage 5	Demise of one or both twins.

Classification of Quintero (11)

Vascular anastomoses are traditionally classified as arterioarterial (AA), venovenous (VV) or arteriovenous (AV) (Fig. 10-2).[14] AA and VV anastomoses are typically superficial, bidirectional anastomoses on the surface of the chorionic plate. AV anastomoses are usually referred to as deep anastomoses and, in reality, are no more than a shared cotyledon, receiving arterial supply from one twin and draining on the venous side to the other twin or both twins. All of these anastomoses are identifiable at the chorionic surface; in fact, this feature is a prerequisite for laser coagulation. However, recent work has shown that placental angioarchitecture may be more complex. Anastomoses invisible at the surface exist and might explain some failures of surgery. No imaging modalities can demonstrate their presence, and ablative therapy is not possible.[12,15]

Net chronic fetofetal transfusion triggers a series of fetal events, beginning with discrepant urine production. In the recipient, these include systemic hypertension, and in some cases, hypertrophic outflow tract obstruction. In the donor, increased placental vascular resistance in utero[16] and reduced arterial compliance in infancy are observed. The discordant long-term vascular programming in genetically identical TTTS survivors can be prevented with timely intrauterine therapy,[17] thus implicating deranged fetoplacental vascular function in utero.[18] As mentioned earlier, intrauterine growth restriction (IUGR) may be associated with TTTS and may influence clinical manifestation, management and eventual outcome. However, TTTS per se may contribute to poor growth. After successful generation of distinct chorionic circulations by laser or selective feticide, catch up growth can be observed in the previously growth restricted donor.[19] Also absent end-diastolic flow in the umbilical artery has been shown to disappear acutely following cord occlusion of the recipient, showing that it was not a manifestation of increased down-stream placental resistance.

Conservative Treatment

Untreated, TTTS has a very poor outcome. Hydramnios may lead to fetal demise or extreme preterm delivery. IUFD may result from cardiac failure in the recipient or poor perfusion in the donor; postmortem fetofetal hemorrhage of one twin may lead to death or cerebral sequelae in the survivor.[20,21] Therefore, therapy is essential. There are three treatment options applicable to *all* fetuses: serial amnioreduction, septostomy, and fetoscopic laser coagulation of vascular anastomoses. (TOC and selective feticide are not discussed here.)

The purpose of intentional puncturing of the intertwin septum ("septostomy") is normalizing the amniotic fluid of the donor. Actually, there is no evidence in support of septostomy as a primary, therapeutic technique, nor a good pathophysiologic mechanism through which it might work. In a recent randomized trial, survival proved no better than with drainage, although the need for

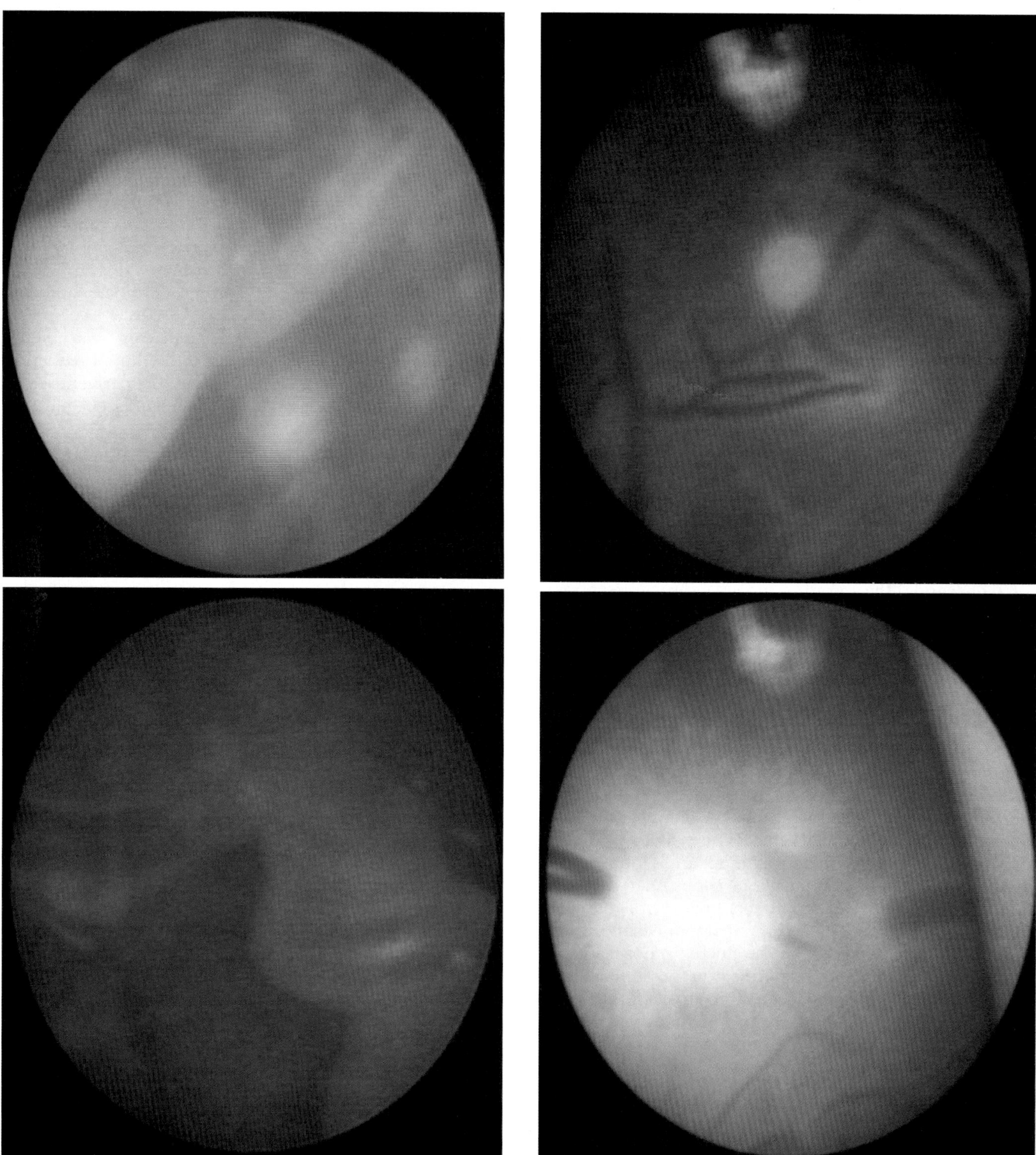

Figure 10-2. Fetoscopic vascular anastomoses. Communicating vessels (*left*) create hemodynamic imbalance, laser is used to ablate anastomosis between fetal circulation.

repeat drainage was decreased.[17,22] *Serial amnioreduction* reduces hydramnios and, hence, intrauterine pressure, thus alleviating symptoms and prolonging pregnancy. This may also temporarily improve fetal hemodynamics by reducing the amniotic fluid pressure and thereby enhancing uteroplacental perfusion.[23,24] Amnioreduction is easy and straightforward, and has a complication rate (including preterm premature rupture of the membranes [PPROM], abruption) of about 1 to 4 percent per intervention.[25] Amniodrainage leaves the angioarchitecture unchanged; thus, the procedure needs to be repeated. In the event of a single IUFD, the survivor remains at risk for fetofetal hemorrhage and its consequences. Although some still believe amniodrainage has a place in the earlier stages of TTTS, it clearly performs poorly in stage III and IV.[26] The overall perinatal survival rate according to Skupski was 61 percent (double survival: 50 percent, single survival rate: 20 percent).[27]

Laser Therapy

Whereas the procedures described earlier are palliative, fetoscopic laser coagulation of the vascular anastomoses seeks to address the underlying cause through a single intervention. Treatment inherently involves drainage of excessive amniotic fluid as well. First described by De Lia,[27a,27b] the strategy is ablating all anastomosing vessels, that might connect both fetuses, using either Nd:YAG, KTP or diode laser and 400 to 600 µm fibers in a nontouch technique. The procedure is performed percutaneously under local or regional anaesthesia. An endoscopic cannula is inserted into the amniotic cavity of the recipient fetus under ultrasound guidance at an angle perpendicular to the presumed vascular equator. The position of the fetuses, umbilical cord insertions, and placenta are mapped by ultrasound. Initial landmarks include both umbilical cord insertions and intertwin membrane. One visualizes the entire vascular equator and coagulates all visible anastomoses using a nontouch technique. Sections of approximately 1 to 2 cm are coagulated with pulses of 3 to 4 seconds, the duration judged by tissue response. Arteries are distinguishable from veins because they have a darker color and pass over the veins. Occasionally, it may be physically impossible to determine whether vessels anastomose or not. In these instances, vessels are still coagulated. When the placenta is anterior, operative conditions are more difficult. Special instruments have been proposed, including curved sheaths, flexible endoscopes, and a double insertion technique.[28] Most centers hospitalize patients for 1 or 2 postoperative days. Ultrasound is performed to document fetal viability and record changes in the phenotypic features of TTTS, that is amniotic fluid volume, bladder filling, and Doppler flow parameters. The donor typically develops relative hypervolemia, accounting for (transient) hydropic signs in 25 percent,[29] Similarly, 27 percent of donors demonstrate absent or reversed a wave in the ductus venosus. When absent end-diastolic flow was present in the donor before laser treatment, reappearance of positive end-diastolic flow was observed in 53 percent.[30] Discordant umbilical venous blood flow between donor and recipient may disappear as well.

There are three important complications in the postoperative period. Postoperative IUFD occurs in 18 percent of cases within 48 hours, usually involving the donor. The cause is unclear and not predictable. PPROM is another significant complication, accounting for high morbidity and mortality if the membranes rupture before viability. Intra-amniotic injection of platelets and clotting factors may be successful for treating early postoperative PPROM.[31] We perform Doppler investigations daily in the first 2 postoperative days and at least weekly thereafter in the first month. We measure of middle cerebral artery peak systolic velocity to detect anemia/polycythaemia in survivors.[20] Treatment may include intrauterine transfusion/exchange transfusion, repeat laser therapy, or cord occlusion (see later).

Results of Fetoscopic Laser Coagulation

In uncontrolled series, the overall fetal survival has been consistently between 55 and 68 percent, with a risk for neurologic morbidity in survivors of 2 percent to 11 percent. More than 80 percent of pregnancies have at least one survivor. Hecher et al.[32] demonstrated a learning curve, arguing against scattering the experience over too many centers. Comparative data are limited to the controlled series by Hecher and the Eurofoetus randomized controlled trial.[33] The latter compared serial amnioreduction with laser coagulation as a primary therapy. Laser yielded better survival and better neurologic outcome Survival of at least one twin was 76 percent versus 51 percent, median gestational age at delivery was higher (33.3 versus 29.0 weeks) Infants in the amnioreduction group had a higher incidence of cystic periventricular leukomalacia (14-percent versus 6-percent laser), particularly in recipients.

The staging system does not dictate therapeutic strategy; however, outcomes are related to the stage at the time of treatment.[21,34] When only amniotic fluid changes (stage I and II) are present, outcomes are better than in cases with circulatory compromise (stage III and IV). This applies to serial amnioreduction as well as laser treatment. Other factors play an equally important role. TTTS may trigger cervical changes, increasing the risk of PPROM and preterm labor (PTL). This change does not necessarily disappear after laser therapy.[35,36] It is unclear what cervical changes mean with respect to therapeutic strategy.

Longer term follow-up studies of patients treated by laser invariably show better outcomes than in drainage patients. In donors, renal function was shown to be normal. Recipient survivors have up to a 7-percent risk for pulmonary valve stenosis.[37] Neurologic outcomes improve with increasing experience.[38]

In conclusion, laser coagulation is the first-line treatment option for TTTS. Still, results remain far from optimal. Future trials will need to elucidate the role of so-called step-up therapies, in which one first offers either expectant management or amniodrainage in earlier stages of the disease, perhaps in the presence of only AA anastomoses. Interventions should not be practiced outside of such trials, because any previous procedure may hamper a subsequent laser procedure or cause inadvertent septostomy and, hence, lead to an iatrogenic monoamniotic pregnancy.

Cord Occlusion

Background: Elective, Prophylactic, and Rescue Feticide

Selective feticide necessitating cord occlusion can be considered in several circumstances not involving MC twin or higher order multiple pregnancies. These include:

1. Severe discordant structural or chromosomal abnormalities,
2. Severe discordant growth with high risk of IUFD,

3. Twin reversed arterial perfusion sequence (TRAP), and
4. Severe TTTS with associated discordant anomaly or in which inspection of the chorionic plate was precluded by position of the fetus and placenta.

In TRAP sequence, artery-to-artery anastomoses result in the donor pumping blood to its acardiac twin; polyhydramnios may occur and endanger the normal fetus. There is thus no ethical dilemma when the pregnancy as a whole is threatened in TRAP. The same holds for severe TTTS with associated anomalies, or with impending IUFD. Selective feticide is needed to rescue the healthy twin. However, discordant chromosomal, or much more common, discordant structural anomalies may also exist. Although these do not necessarily pose an immediate or even remote risk for IUFD of the anomalous fetus, the predictable poor quality of life for the abnormal twin may not be acceptable to the parents. Instead of termination of the entire pregnancy, selective feticide may be a more valuable option. Often such dilemms arise early in pregnancy, at which time it is impossible to predict reliably the natural history of the condition. An argument may thus be raised whether, analogous to feticide in dichorionic twins, early intervention is better. A representative situation is TRAP in which early parameters predict impeding heart failure, polyhydramnios or IUFD. It is tempting to treat such cases *prophylactically,* realizing this may constitute unnecessary treatment and complications.

INDICATIONS

DISCORDANT ANOMALIES

In monozygotic twins, the anomaly rate is 2 to 3 times higher than for dizygtic twins.[39] In more than 80 percent of cases, only one fetus is affected.[40] Although uncommon, even discordance for human aneuploidies (trisomy 13, trisomy 21, monosomy X) has been reported. This is referred to as heterokaryotypic monozygotism.[41] The diagnosis of heterokaryotic MC twins can be made only by amniocentesis of both amniotic sacs.[42] There are three management options for discordant structural and chromosomal anomalies: conservative management, selective feticide, or TOP. Given parents who do not accept the live birth of the affected twin with nonlethal anomalies, selective feticide may be an alternative to TOP of the entire pregnancy. Risk-benefit analysis needs to be considered because the healthy twin may be lost from feticide-related complications. Later, the argument will be made for late intervention to minimize the consequences of such complications. For anomalies with a high risk of in utero demise, this need not apply. Irrespective, one wants to avoid spontaneous IUFD with its associated risks.

SELECTIVE INTRAUTERINE GROWTH RESTRICTION

Selective IUGR (sIUGR) is usually defined as fetal growth below the 10th percentile for gestational age, together with an intertwin weight discordance of greater than 25 percent. The latter, calculated as ([larger twin-smaller twin]/larger twin), complicates 7 percent of MC

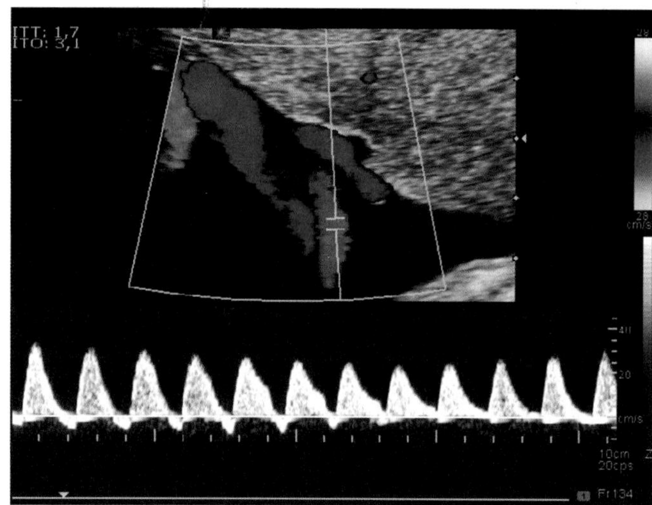

Figure 10-3. Color flow Doppler demonstrating intermittent absent and reversed end-diastolic flow.

twins.[43] Feticide is a theoretical option when IUFD before viability is imminent. Defining the latter is difficult, however, because Doppler studies may not be so conclusive as in non-MC pregnancies. In up to 50 percent, a pattern of intermittent absent or reversed end-diastolic flow (iA/REDF) in the umbilical artery may be present.[44,45] iA/REDF is unique to MC twins, and characterized by presence or absent and/or reversed end-diastolic flow in the umbilical artery, alternating over seconds or minutes with positive diastolic flow (Fig. 10-3). This reflects retrograde transmission of an arterioarterial waveform in the umbilical artery through intertwin placental arterioarterial anastomoses. In its absence, conventional surveillance methods and decision making can be used, as in other cases of growth restriction. In its presence, active management before viability might include selective feticide or laser coagulation of chorionic plate vessels to generate two distinct chorionic circulations. In the presence of iA/REDF, sudden IUFD in the small twin occurs in up to 25 percent of cases and neurologic damage of the appropriately grown twin may develop in up to 30 percent of the cases.[46,47]

The mere presence of iA/REDF and the associated large-diameter AA-anastomosis has two implications. Despite severe sIUGR, the smaller twin will not necessarily show signs of deterioration, being "rescued" by the intertwin transfusion. Furthermore, hemodynamic imbalances over the large anastomoses may already have caused damage to both twins, before more critical growth problems, thus prompting intervention. The clinical management of all of these cases constitutes at present a dilemma. In theory, laser coagulation of placental anastomoses, including the AA anastomoses, is a potential therapeutic option, disconnecting the two fetal circulations and protecting fetuses from each other. Coagulation also makes Doppler investigation a more reliable tool for subsequent monitoring of fetal well-being. In a small and heterogeneous series, Quintero et al.[48] compared coagulation cases with 17 cases managed expectantly. There were no significant differences in survival or neurologic morbidity.[49] Operative conditions in the absence of polyhdramnios are not comparable but theoretically can be overcome by amnioinfusion; however, vessels may be too large for coagulation. Therefore selective feticide would be an option. None of these options will, however, solve the problem of damage incurred before the procedure.

Twin Reversed Arterial Perfusion

This sequence complicates about 1 percent of MC twins. Through AA anastomoses, deoxygenated blood flows from an umbilical artery of the pump twin in reversed direction into the umbilical artery of the (recipient) perfused twin. This puts the (anatomically normal) pump twin at risk for high-output cardiac failure.[50] Reported survival rates range widely, from 14[51] to 90 percent.[52] Prediction of outcome, has not been established, but acardiac/pump weight ratio,[53] may be indicative. An increased ratio reflects rapid increase in the acardiac mass[54] and small differences in the umbilical artery Doppler values.[55,56]

Twin-to-Twin Transfusion Syndrome

Laser can salvage fetuses at all stages of this disease. Thus, there are few firm grounds to perform feticide in advanced disease, despite claims to the contrary as sometimes proposed.[57] Feticide may occasionally be performed when there are other fetal complications or when laser coagulation is technically impossible. At best, feticide yields by definition a 50-percent survival rate. Taking into account the well-defined complication rates and neurologic morbidity, overall survival will probably be 40 percent. Feticide also leads to the difficult decision of selecting a target among these two structurally normal fetuses. When one chooses the donor, the problem is accessing the anhydramniotic sac. Even when Doppler studies are abnormal, however, these can normalize after successful laser coagulation. Recipients appear to be at higher risk of neurologic[58] and cardiac sequelae,[59] but again their circulatory problems can normalize.

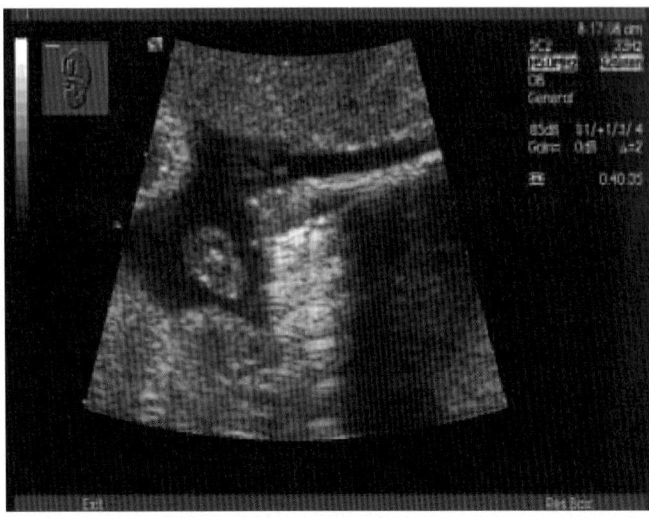

Figure 10-4. Fetoscopic bubbles reflecting heat generated by laser occludes blood flow of umbilical cord.

Techniques

In MC twins, selective feticide cannot be performed by injection of potassium chloride into the target fetus. The cotwin would be exposed to a substantial risk of cotwin death or brain injury due to agonal intertwin transfusion. Neither are cord embolization techniques an option.[60] Other minimally invasive techniques proposed to arrest and isolate the target twin's circulation[60] have considerably higher risks for fetal loss compared with the injection of potassium chloride. Bipolar coagulation is probably the most universally applicable technique, even later in gestation.[61] The site of port insertion is chosen according to the position of the placenta, the amniotic sac of the target fetus, and its umbilical cord. Preferentially, the other sac is avoided, eventually by using amnioinfusion to expand the target sac. Bipolar coagulation can use either 3.0- or 2.4-mm forceps, according to the cord diameter. The target fetus is medicated, certainly at later gestational age. Under ultrasound guidance, a portion of the umbilical cord is grasped while avoiding direct contact with the placenta, fetus, or membranes. Usually coagulation is effective at 25 Watts, as demonstrated by the appearance of turbulence and steam bubbles (Fig. 10-4). Limiting energy avoids tissue carbonization and cord perforation. Doppler studies can confirm arrest of flow, but we nonetheless coagulate three sections. In monoamniotic twins, we transect the umbilical cord to avoid cord entanglement. Patients are cared for as after laser coagulation, including Doppler interrogation of the middle cerebral artery velocities to detect fetal anemia.

Other approaches include laser to coagulate the umbilical cord, but this might fail later in the second trimester. One may use monopolar radiofrequency or laser energy for interstitial ablation of fetal vessels, for example, at the level of the cord insertion or aorta. As far as we know, reproducible results with the latter techniques have been described only in TRAP, in which low flow exists in target vessels.

Results

Bipolar umbilical cord coagulation has been shown to be an effective method, with survival rates of about 80 percent.[37,40,62] The largest experience that includes long-term follow-up is our series of 80 consecutive cord occlusions (seven triplets).[63] Survival was 83 percent, with no difference between twins and triplets. We observed one iatrogenic cord perforation.[64] Half of the in utero losses occurred in the immediate postoperative period. This is potentially related to incomplete occlusion, given its more likely occurrence after laser coagulation. Since we became aware of this problem, we screen postoperatively for fetal anemia, which can be treated by transfusion.[66] Other losses are thought mainly to be due to cord complications, raising the argument against intertwin septostomy. PPROM is the most common complication. It is obviously associated with a high risk for preterm delivery, and coincides with most perinatal deaths and cases with neurologic impairment after the age of 1 year (7 percent) There was a clear benefit of operator experience. Following 40 procedures, there is a dramatic decrease in PPROM and increase in intact survival. Results are equally good irrespective of the indications. One series reported lower survival rate in TRAP sequence, but our experience has been similar to that involving other indications.[66,67]

It is not possible to determine which method of feticide is optimal and when is the ideal time point in MC pregnancies. Because situations differ, the surgeon should ideally be familiar with several techniques in order to tailor therapy to the individual requirements of each case. These results also support the argument for selective feticide as late in gestation as possible in order to avoid the risks of early iPPROM and its consequences. Of course, this may or may not be an option in all countries.

Congenital Diaphragmatic Hernia

Background

Congenital diaphragmatic hernia (CDH) is usually a sporadic anomaly occurring 1/2–5,000 live births. In just over half the cases, the condition is an isolated anomaly; CDH fetuses with associated anomalies invariably have a poor prognosis. Despite optimal care, many neonates still die because of the consequences of pulmonary hypoplasia and pulmonary hypertension. A recent review of a British based regional case registry confirmed the overall mortality of 30 percent in antenatal diagnosed and live-born cases of isolated CDH.[68] Once diagnosed, patients should thus be referred in utero to specialized tertiary centers for prenatal evaluation, establishment of diagnosis and derivation of prognosis, determination of time for delivery, and preparation for neonatal resuscitation and delayed repair.[69]

Pivotal to defining options is ability to demonstrate *lethal* pulmonary hypoplasia in the previable period. Several imaging techniques quantifying lung development are being evaluated.[70] This can be done for left-sided CDH (LCDH) on the basis of presence of herniation of the left liver lobe into the thorax[71] and derivation of the lung-to-head ratio (LHR) during midgestation.[72] The best powered validation study involved 184 fetuses with isolated LCDH assessed between 22 and 28 weeks, and expectantly managed until both after 30 weeks.[73] When the liver is down, LHR does not reliably predict outcome. However, fetuses with liver up have an overall 50-percent chance to survive. With LHR, less than 1.6, survival is 66 percent; above LHR 1.6, survival is 83 percent.[14] LHR equal to 1.0 is useful demarcation, with only 11 percent of fetuses with liver up surviving till discharge.

In Utero Therapy

Any prenatal intervention that can reverse lung hypoplasia should theoretically improve prognosis. Tracheal occlusion (TO) prevents egress of tracheal fluid, in turn, leading to increased of lung tissue stretch. The reader is referred elsewhere for discussion of the experimental basis for TO.[74] Clinical experience with external tracheal clipping, initially through hysterotomy and later through fetoscopy, led to the conclusion that an endoluminal occlusion method might better prevent local complications.[74,75] In the late 1990s, we described fetoscopic endoluminal tracheal occlusion (FETO) in lambs, using a balloon[76] that could accommodate for increasing tracheal diameters as the fetus grows, without inducing tracheal damage.[77] Quintero first demonstrated clinical feasibility of a percutaneous approach, and we reported the first survivors in 2004.[78,79] Very soon thereafter, a randomized controlled trial comparing fetal endoscopic TO with standard postnatal care demonstrated no benefit from prenatal intervention (survival 73 percent in TO group versus 77 percent in postnatal management group).[80] The TO group had a modest improvement in pulmonary compliance with a lower alveolar-arterial oxygen difference.[81] This important trial confirms at closer reading that fetuses with isolated CDH who have a LHR between 1.0 and 1.4 have an 80-percent likelihood of survival, and are thus unlikely to benefit from fetal surgery. Overall, the number of fetuses potentially benefiting from prenatal intervention (LHR < 1.0) was low, and whether they would have benefited from prenatal TO could not be determined.

In the current European FETO program, selection criteria are (1) singleton pregnancy with severe CDH in an anatomically and chromosomally normal fetus (2) who presents with herniation of the liver into the thorax and also have an LHR of less than 1.0. (3) TO is then performed at 26 to 28 weeks, (4) Prenatal removal of the balloon is scheduled at 34 weeks. Interventions are done under local or regional anaesthesia with fetal analgesia for immobilization. A 10 French cannula, a 1.2-mm fetoscope within a 3.0 mm sheath (Karl Storz), and a detachable balloon occlusion system are used (Fig. 10-5). In 24 consecutive cases of LCDH, mean gestational age at delivery was 34 weeks (80 percent = 32 weeks). Preterm prelabor rupture of the membrane occurred in 15 percent before 28 weeks and in 30 percent before 32 weeks, suggesting iatrogenic cause (iPPROM). Early neonatal survival was 75 percent, and survival until hospital discharge was 50 percent. By contrast, in untreated controls, more than 90 percent of neonates succumbed to pulmonary hypoplasia. Surgical repair of the diaphragmatic hernia was needed in more than 90 percent requiring a patch.[82] An important predictor of outcome is LHR before FETO.[83] Among 28 fetuses undergoing FETO, the survival rate was 57 percent. Survival increased from 17 percent for LHR 0.4 to 0.5 to 62 percent for LHR 0.6 to 0.7 and 78 percent for LHR 0.8 to 0.9.

In summary, use of TO to treat CDH has a limited role but can be selectively effective.

Open Surgical Approaches

For a limited number of indications, open fetal surgery has been performed since the mid-1980s.[2] Appropriate concerns for maternal risk, rigorous selection criteria, and somewhat frustrating results have limited its use. There has been continuing innovation and development of instruments and techniques, motivated by the goal of safer open fetal surgery for both fetus and mother.

Congenital Diaphragmatic Hernia

The fetal approach to CDH has undergone continuous evolution since the first attempted CDH repair in 1986

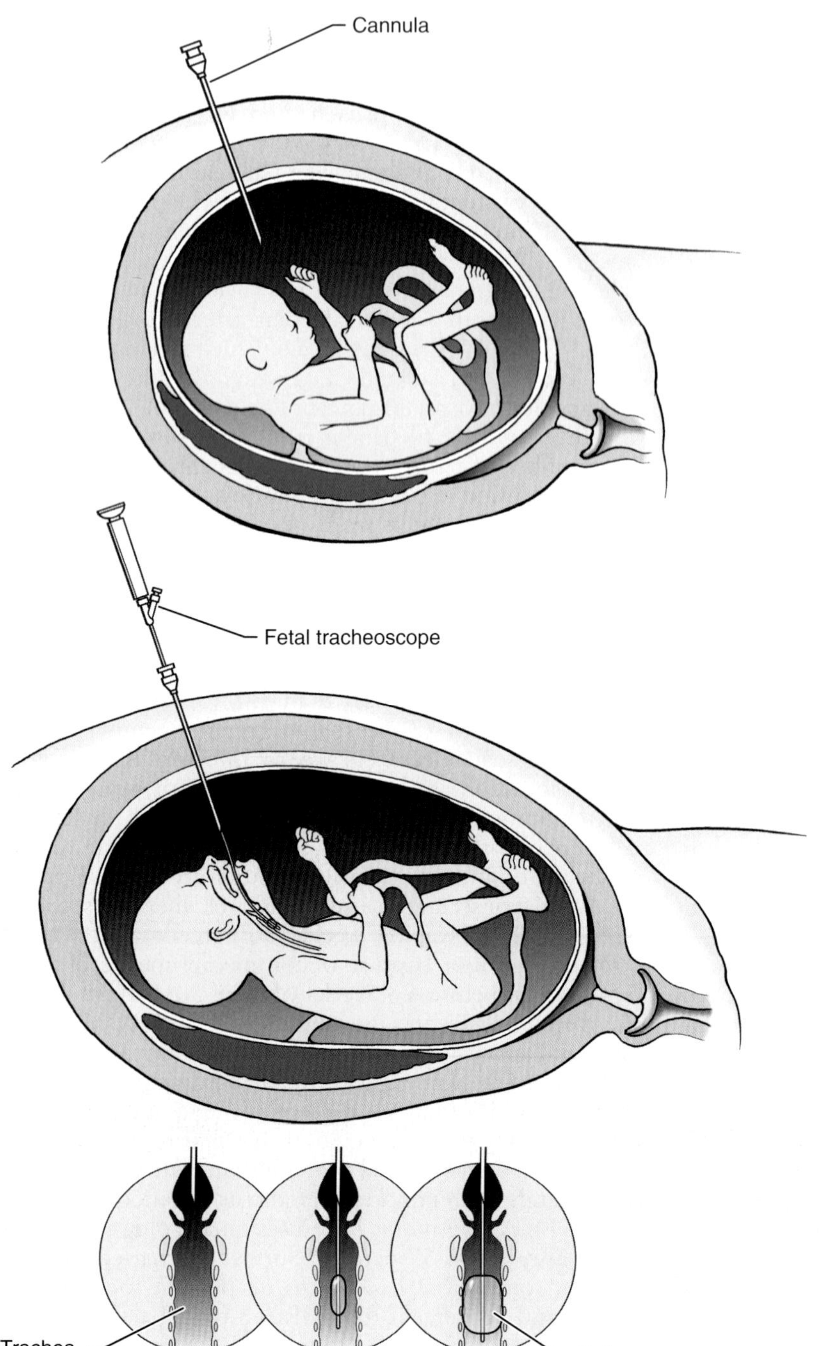

Figure 10-5. Balloon congenital diaphragmatic hernia. Trocar is inserted through fetal mouth and balloon expanded to completely occlude trachea.

and our first success in 1989.[84–86] However, definitive repair of CDH by reduction of viscera from the chest, diaphragmatic patch placement, and abdominal procedures (to reduce intraabdominal pressure) showed unacceptable mortality. With advances in neonatal care, open fetal repair proved no better than postnatal repair.[87,88] Definitive repair was abandoned and in utero tracheal occlusion took its place (Fig. 10-6).[89–96]

Already discussed in the context of fetoscopic approaches, TO increases lung size by accumulation of pulmonary secretions, which reduce the herniated viscera from the chest and decreases the risk for lung hypoplasia. However, the technique of achieving reliable, complete and reversible tracheal occlusion has evolved. Initially, this could only be accomplished by open fetal surgery and fetal neck dissection (taking care to avoid the recurrent laryngeal nerves) and placement of occlusive hemoclips. Next, fetoscopic techniques were developed to accomplish neck dissection and place a tracheal clip (the Fetendo clip procedure).[97–99] Finally, a simpler technique was developed in which a fetoscope passed through a single port was advanced into the fetal trachea (fetal bronchoscopy); a detachable silicone balloon was then inflated to occlude the trachea. It is this approach that was discussed earlier.

Overall, open surgery was used progressively less for CDH. Increasing sophistication of the surgical approach has been coupled with concomitant improvements in neonatal care using extracorporeal membrane oxygenation. This has made it difficult to determine the relative benefits of each approach without a prospective, randomized comparison that takes into account confounding variables. For this reason, a randomized trial of surgery for CDH versus optimal postnatal care was funded by National Institute for Child and Human Development.[93] The principal component of the trial was that patients in the postnatal care (control) arm would receive the same neonatal care by the same center as the surgical arm. It was originally expected that patients having surgery would show a survival rate of about 70 percent, compared with the best data on controls of 35 percent. The surgically treated patients achieved expected survival. However, the trial was stopped prematurely, because controls at the same tertiary specialty centers as the surgical group showed similar survival. This illustrates well the problem of the so-called moving target, that is, change in cost-benefits ratio as neonatal survival and surgical therapy concurrently improve. Irrespective, our use of technology must adapt to changing conditions.[100]

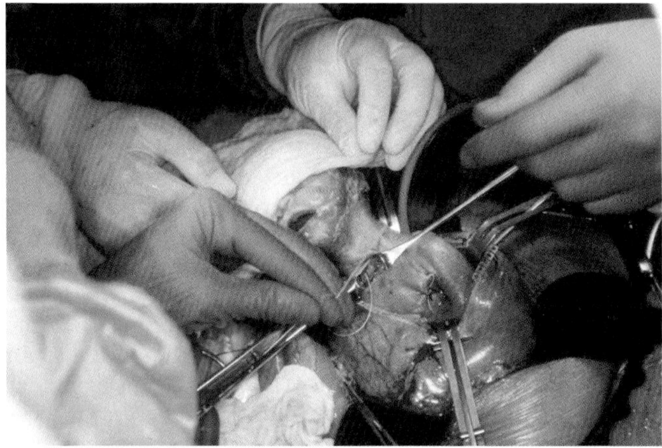

Figure 10-6. Open congenital diaphragmatic hernia repair by tracheal ligation. Fetus is excavated to extend balloon which is removed at delivery by EXIT procedure.

Congenital Cystic Adenomatoid Malformation

Congenital cystic adenomatoid malformation (CCAM) is a space-occupying congenital cystic lesion of the lung that may grow and induce hydrops by causing mediastinal shift and compromise venous return to the heart. When fetuses with CCAM develop hydrops, the fetal mortality rate approaches 100 percent (Fig. 10-7).[97–99] Fetal resection of CCAM reverses hydrops and has improved survival dramatically.[101–103] The fetal operation is performed by exposure through the maternal hysterotomy of fetal arm and chest wall on the side of the lesion. A large muscle-sparing thoracotomy is performed through the midthorax of the fetus, and the lobe containing the CCAM is isolated. The attachments of the lobe to adjacent lung tissue are bluntly divided and the lobar hilum divided by use of a TIA stapler or a bulk ligature. During the remainder of the pregnancy, the remaining normal lung shows compensatory growth to fill the space previously occupied by the mass.

Sacrococcygeal Teratoma

Fetal sacrococcygeal teratoma arises from the presacral space and may grow to massive proportions. In some fetuses, high-output failure is induced from tumor

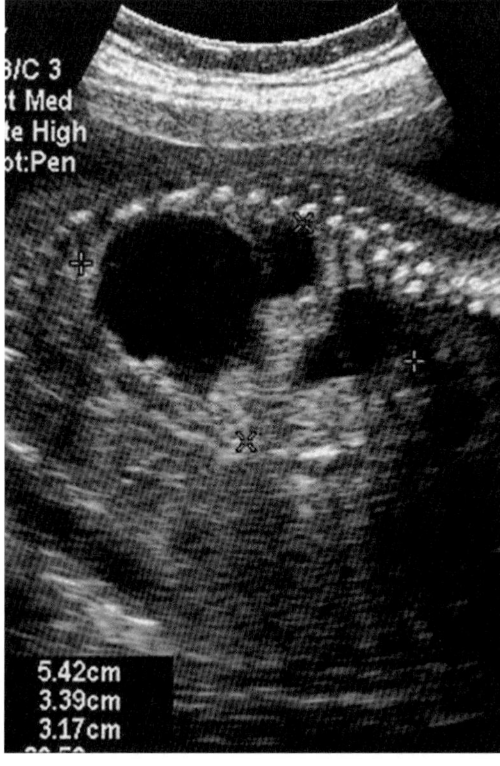

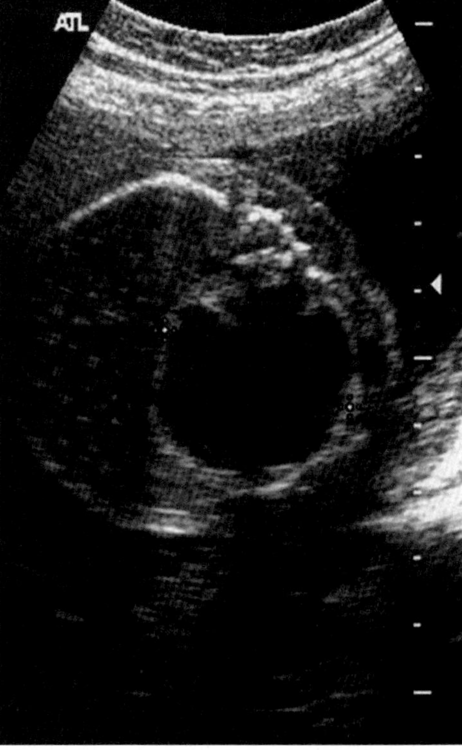

Figure 10-7. Microcystic congenital cystic adenomatoid malformation on ultrasound before surgery. Large cystic areas are common.

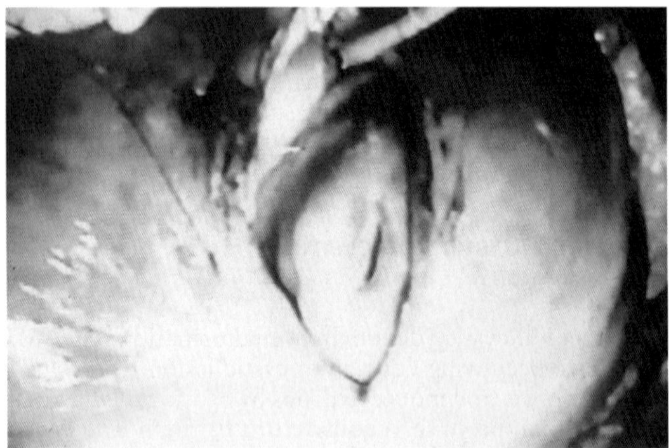

Figure 10-8. The EXIT procedure. Under heavy tocolytic anesthesia, tracheal clips are removed prior to delivery.

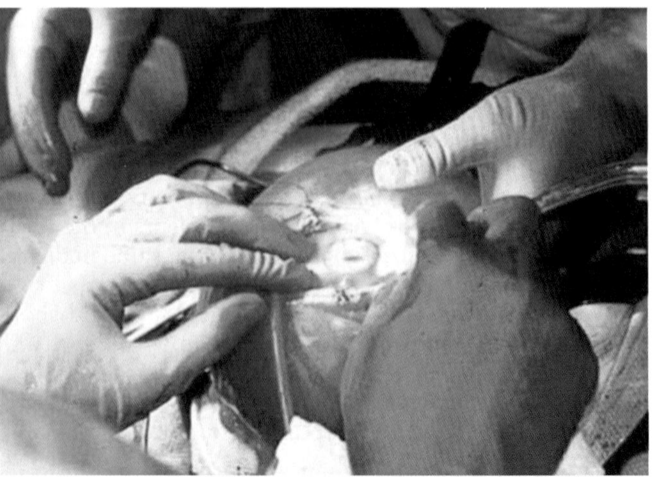

Figure 10-9. Myelomeningocele surgery.

vascular "steal." Fetal sacrococcygeal teratoma with high output physiology and associated placentomegaly or hydrops uniformly results in fetal demise.[100,101] The pathophysiologic rationale involves ligation of the vascular connections to the tumor, removal of the vascular "steal," and reversal of the high output physiology. The entire fetal procedure can be performed in less than 15 minutes with minimal blood loss. Because of the increase in afterload following ligation of the low resistance tumor circuit, the fetal hemodynamic status must be monitored by fetal echocardiography during and in the immediate period following ligation.

The EXIT Procedure

The EXIT procedure is a modified cesarean delivery that may be applied to deliver fetuses following fetal surgical procedures such as tracheal ligation, or to use for fetuses expected to have difficult airway problems owing to massive cervical teratomas or cystic hygromas.[102,103] The key component of the EXIT procedure is maintenance of uteroplacental perfusion until the fetal airway is secured and ventilation is established. This is in direct contrast to cesarean delivery, in which uterine contraction for hemostasis is encouraged. Instead, in the EXIT procedure, uterine relaxation is maintained by deep general anesthesia (Fig. 10-8). Fetal manipulations are then performed with maternal support through the placenta. Clips can be removed, chest masses removed, bronchoscopy performed, and stable airway access established in otherwise very difficult circumstances with this approach. Once the fetus is ready for transport to the nursery or adjacent operating suite, the cord is clamped and cut, and the cesarean delivery completed.

Meningomyelocele

Babies with myelingomyloceles have impaired lower motor function, loss of bowel control, and loss of bladder control. Many develop obstructive hydrocephalus and require ventriculoperitoneal shunting.[104] Experience from the 1970s and 1980s showed that babies with meningomyelocele delivered atraumatically by cesarean section had a relatively better level of motor function for their given level of anatomic defect than babies delivered through the vaginal canal.[105] Such data suggested that compression and trauma to the cord in the delivery process can exert permanent long-term sequelae to motor function. Therefore, it followed that trauma to the spinal cord in utero, either from continuous contact with the uterine wall or from toxic effects of the amniotic fluid, could be detrimental to the spinal cord function. Furthermore, investigators questioned the traditional dogma that the pathogenesis of meningomyelocele was strictly due to an abnormally developed spinal cord that did not engender the proper development of the bony spinal column. Possibly the primary defect was in the bony spinal column, exposing a once presumptively undamaged spinal cord. The cord might then be damaged only secondarily by toxic effects of amniotic fluid or trauma from the uterine environment. Thus, a rationale exists to cover and protect the spinal cord in utero.[106]

Three groups have done most of the work in this area and have attempted to repair meningomyeloceles in utero, both as an open surgical procedure and endoscopically, with the stated attempt to reduce long-term morbidity and mortality.[107–109] There is much controversy surrounding the data.[33] To date, the principal benefit seems to be only secondary, that is, a significant reduction in the number of babies requiring ventriculoperitoneal shunting for obstructive hydrocephalus (Fig. 10-9).[110,111] Major functional improvement has not been demonstrated. A randomized, prospective trial comparing fetal with postnatal neurosurgical closure begun in 2003 will still require several years to be completed. A major milestone of this trial has been the agreement among the participating centers not to perform any procedures outside the trial, and other centers around the country have agreed not to start programs until the trial is completed.

MEDICAL THERAPIES

Neural Tube Defects

Neural tube defects (NTDs) result from abnormal closure of the neural tube, which normally occurs between the third and fourth week of gestational age. The etiology includes both genetic and environmental factors. Socioeconomic status, geographic area, occupational exposure and maternal use of antiepileptic drugs have been associated with variations in the incidence.[112] Smithells et al. first showed that vitamin supplementation containing 0.36 mg folate could reduce the frequency of NTD recurrence by sevenfold.[113–115] In 1991, a randomized double-blinded trial demonstrated that preconceptual folate reduces the risk of recurrence in high-risk patients.[116] Subsequently, it was shown that preparations containing folate and other vitamins also reduce the occurrence of first time NTDs.[117] NTD recurrence prevention is now very well established. Current guidelines call for consumption of 4.0-mg/day folic acid by women with a prior child affected with a NTD, for at least 1 month before conception through the first 3 months of pregnancy. A total of 0.4 mg/day folic acid is recommended for women planning a pregnancy, to began preconceptually.

Since January, 1998, the U.S. Food and Drug Administration has mandated supplementation of breads and grains with folic acid. NTDs birth prevalence during the years 1990 to 1999 was evaluated by assessing birth certificate reports before and after mandatory fortification decreased by 19 percent.[115] Evans et al. have shown a nearly 30-percent drop in high maternal serum alpha-fetoprotein values in the United States comparing 2,000 values versus values (1997) before the introduction of folic acid supplementation.[118]

Folate plays a central part in embryonic and fetal development because of its role in nucleic acid synthesis is mandatory for cell division that takes place during embryogeneiss. Folate deficiency can occur either because of low dietary folate intake or because of increased metabolic requirement. The latter theoretically involves specific genetic perturbations such as the polymorphism of the thermolabile enzyme methylterahydrofolate reductase (MTHFR). Actually, evidence regarding the role of MTHFR in NTD is unsupported, except in certain populations, suggesting that these variants are not large contributors to the etiology of NTDs.[117,119] Candidate genes other than MTHFR may be responsible for an increased risk to NTDs.[120] Methionine synthase polymorphisms is associated with an increased risk for NTDs that is not influenced by maternal preconception folic acid intake at doses of 0.4 mg/day.[121] Other candidate genes include the mitochondrial membrane transporter gene *UCP2*.[122] Initial studies suggesting that zinc deficiency plays a role in the etiology of NTDs[123,124] were not confirmed.[126,127] Because methionine deficiency may be involved in NTDs, administration of methionine may be beneficial in NTD risk reduction.[127] In conclusion, preconceptional folic acid intake, either as a sole vitamin or as part of multivitamin supplementation, reduces the risk of recurrence and first time NTDs. The role of other dietary supplements remains unclear.

Adrenal Disorders

Congenital Adrenal Hyperplasia

Congenital adrenal hyperplasia (CAH) is actually a collection of autosomal recessive metabolic disorders, characterized by enzymatic defects in the steroidogenetic pathway.[128] Compensatory increase in adrenocorticotrophic hormone secretion leads to overproduction of steroid precursors in the adrenal cortex, resulting in adrenal hyperplasia. Excess precursors may be converted to androgens that may result in virilization of female fetuses. The phenotype is determined by the severity of the cortisol deficiency and the nature of the steroid precursors that accumulate proximal to the enzymatic block. The most common abnormality, which is responsible for greater than 90 percent of patients with CAH, is caused by a deficiency of the 21-hydroxylase enzyme. Less common causes for CAH include deficiencies in 11β-hydroxylase and 17α-hydroxylase. Reduced 21-hydroxylase activity results in accumulation of 17-hydroxyprogesterone as a result of impaired conversion to 11-deoxycorticosterone. Excess 17-hydroxyprogesterone is then converted through androstenedione to androgens, levels of which can increase by as much as several hundred fold. Excess androgens virilize the undifferentiated female external genitalia, ranging from mild clitoral hypertrophy to complete formation of a phallus and scrotum. In contrast, genital development in male fetuses is normal, although excess androgens cause postnatal virilization in both genders and may manifest in precocious puberty.[129] A severe enzyme deficiency or even a complete block of enzymatic activity produces the classic form of CAH. Two thirds to three fourths of cases have salt loss, which may be life threatening.

For 2 decades, it has been known that the fetal adrenal gland can be pharmacologically suppressed by maternal replacement doses of dexamethasone.[130] Suppression can prevent masculinization of affected female fetuses in couples who are carriers of classic CAH. Evans et al. were first to administer dexamethasone to a carrier mother beginning at 10 weeks of gestation in an attempt to prevent masculinization.[131] Differentiation of the external genitalia begins at about 7 weeks of gestation. Chorionic villus sampling has traditionally been the earliest approach for determining gender, although earlier detection should now be possible by molecular testing for Y-sequences in maternal blood. Pharmacologic therapy can be initiated before diagnosis, but therapy is continued only if the fetus is an affected female. Detailed inclusion criteria for treatment have been issued by the European Society for Pediatric Endocrinology and Wilkins Pediatric Endocrine Society[131]; hundreds of fetuses have been treated successfully with prevention or amelioration of masculinization.[129,133,135]

Hyperthyroidism

Neonatal hyperthyroidism is rare, with an incidence of 1:4,000 to 1:40,000/live births.[131] Fetal thyrotoxic goiter is usually secondary to maternal autoimmune disease, most commonly Graves' disease or Hashimoto's thyroiditis. As many as 12 percent of infants of mothers with a known history of Graves' disease are affected with neonatal thyrotoxicosis. This can occur even if the mother is euthyroid.[134] The underlying mechanism is transplacental passage of maternal IgG antibodies. These antibodies, known as thyroid-stimulating antibody or thyroid-stimulating immunoglobulin, are predominantly directed against the thyroid-stimulating hormone receptor. Often fetal goiter is diagnosed on ultrasound in pregnancies in which the mother has elevated thyroid-stimulating antibodies. In some cases, fetal goiters are incidentally detected on routine ultrasonography. In still others, detection follows scan for polyhydramnios. Untreated fetal hyperthyroidism may be associated with a mortality rate of 12 to 25 percent owing to high-output cardiac failure.[135]

Hypothyroidism

Congenital hypothyroidism is relatively rare, affecting about 1:3,000 to 1:4,000 infants.[136] About 85 percent of the cases are the result of thyroid dysgenesis, a heterogeneous group of developmental defects characterized by inadequate thyroid tissue. Congenital hypothyroidism is only rarely associated with errors of thyroid hormone synthesis, thryroid-stimulating hormone insensitivity, or absence of the pituitary gland. Fetal hypothyroidism may not necessarily manifest in a goiter before birth because maternal thyroid hormones may cross the placenta. Congenital hypothyroidism presenting with a goiter is observed in only about 10 to 15 percent of cases.[137]

Fetal goiterous hypothyroidism also follows maternal exposure to thyrostatic agents like propylthiouracil and radioactive I^{131} used to treat maternal hyperthyroidism.[138] Maternal ingestion of amiodarone or lithium may also cause hypothyroidism in the fetus. Fetal hypothyroidism may also follow transplacental passage of maternal blocking antibodies (known as TBIAb or TBII). Rarely, defects in fetal thyroid hormone biosynthesis may exist.[138]

An enlarged fetal goiter may cause esophageal obstruction and polyhydramnios, leading to preterm delivery or premature rupture of membranes. A goiter may even lead to high-output fetal heart failure.[142] A large fetal goiter can also cause extension of the fetal neck, leading to dystocia. Fetal hypothyroidism itself may be devastating, and without treatment, postnatal growth delay and severe mental retardation ensue. Even with immediate diagnosis and treatment at birth, children with congenital hypothyroidism demonstrate lower scores on long-term perceptual-motor, visuospatial, and language tests.[135]

INBORN ERRORS OF METABOLISM

Fetal treatment has been attempted for many inborn errors of metabolism, including methylmalonic academia, multiple carboxylase deficiency, Smith-Lemli-Opitz syndrome, and galactosemia,

Methylmalonic academia is an especially good example of a rare disorder in which pharmacologic alteration of the fetal environment can be demonstrated. However, postnatal significance is questionable. Extensive discussions of these disorders can be found in Evans et al.[140]

In Utero Cardiac Therapy

The ability to diagnose structural or functional heart disease prenatally has predictably led to a growth of interest in the potential for prenatal therapy. As in all fetal therapy (surgical or medical), it is necessary to identify fetal conditions that, if left untreated, will result in fetal death or a compromised condition that will render the neonate into a condition that will result in a lower likelihood of cure or functional survival than would be the case if the fetus were to undergo the proposed therapy. It is essential, of course, to consider the potential risks to both the mother and fetus, whose states of well-being are inextricably interwoven. The subject of fetal echocardiography and treatment has filled entire textbooks, so this section need only provide a brief overview.

Fetal antiarrhythmic therapy has evolved into a more invasive direction over the past decades, including injection of medication directly into the amniotic fluid, intramuscular administration of medication directly to the fetus, and direct, repetitive, administration of intravenous medication through the fetal umbilical vein.[139,142–144]

Direct instrumentation of the fetal heart was initially attempted in an effort to institute transcatheter pacing of a moribund fetus with congenital complete heart block and hydrops fetalis.[147] Subsequently there were reports of attempted catheter treatment of congenital cardiac malformations, with varied success. Several centers have investigated techniques for the institution of surface cooling and rewarming, and for the provision of cardiopulmonary bypass in fetal animal models.[146,147]

FETAL ANTIARRHYTHMIC THERAPY

The Fetus with Tachycardia

The administration of antiarrhythmic therapy to the pregnant mothers of fetuses with sustained supraventricular tachycardia represented the first examples of successful prenatal cardiac therapy. Multiple publications described treatment protocols for this arrhythmia. Characteristics of fetuses needing treatment include hydrops fetalis in the face of sustained arrhythmia, and a gestational age too early to preclude safe delivery and postnatal treatment. In such cases, therapy is best initiated with medications that have a relatively broad therapeutic margin and a low risk of proarrhythmia (unwanted precipitation or exacerbation of arrhythmia) for fetus or mother.[148,149]

The Fetus with Bradycardia

The most important sustained bradyarrhythmia is congenital complete heart block. Fetuses with this condition may develop hydrops fetalis and often have associated congenital heart disease. Clinical heart failure with congenital heart block, with or without congenital heart disease, represents an absolute indication for electrical pacemaker therapy in the neonate.[151] Hydrops fetalis in the presence of complete heart block in utero is a dire finding. The association of hydrops fetalis, complete heart block, and complex congenital heart disease is almost invariably fatal, with or without fetal therapy.[150]

The initial report of the application of electrical pacemaker therapy for fetal congenital heart block involved a fetus presenting with congenital heart block in the absence of congenital heart disease.[152] Presenting with several bradycardia and hydrops fetalis, this fetus had a heart block presumably arising on the basis of immune complex–mediated damage to fetal conduction tissue and myocardium. In desperation, the treating physicians placed a pacing catheter within the fetal heart through percutaneous puncture of the maternal abdomen, uterus, and fetal thorax and ventricular wall. Fetal ventricular capture was demonstrated, albeit without clinical improvement in the fetus. Subsequent attempts to use similar techniques had similarly discouraging outcomes.

MEDICAL TREATMENT OF CONGESTIVE HEART FAILURE IN THE FETUS

There are many anecdotal reports of administration of digoxin to pregnant women whose fetuses have evidence of impaired cardiac pump function. These have included cases in which structural heart disease (e.g., aortic stenosis) was associated with ventricular dysfunction and hydrops fetalis and in which initiation of digoxin therapy was temporally associated with improved ventricular shortening, resolution of hydrops fetalis, and postnatal salvage of the child.[153,154] In addition, there is a close temporal association between initiation of maternally administered digoxin and both improved ventricular shortening as well as resolving of hydrops fetalis in fetuses presumed to have viral myocarditis due to adenovirus, parvovirus, and coxsackievirus. In these cases, fetomaternal infection has been confirmed by viral studies (polymerase chain reaction) of maternal and fetal blood and amniotic fluid. In two fetuses that showed initial improvement but eventually underwent neonatal demise, adenoviral genome was detected by polymerase chain reaction in the infant's myocardial tissue. We have also recently demonstrated improved myocardial shortening and improved right ventricular dP/dT (calculated from the tricuspid regurgitant flow waveform) in two fetuses who had progressively dilating right ventricles,[155] progressive tricuspid regurgitation, and abnormal inferior vena caval flow waveforms in the face of large hemangiomas with significant arteriovenous shunting. The findings of cardiomegaly, tricuspid regurgitation, and abnormal venous Doppler studies in the vena cavae were similar to those described by Tulzer and colleagues in justification of the invasive pulmonary balloon valvuloplasties of two fetuses with pulmonary stenosis/atresia.[156] Digoxin has been used empirically to treat fetuses with severe dilated cardiomyopathy and marked cardiomegaly, bilateral atrioventricular valve regurgitation, and abnormal venous pulsatility. In all fetuses, a remarkable improvement occurred in biventricular shortening with partial amelioration of atrioventricular valve regurgitation and improved biventricular dP/dT.

Digoxin has been used for more than 200 years but is still administered largely on an empiric basis. Although its popularity waxes and wanes, recent studies have suggested some justified inclusion in the therapeutic arsenal. It is, however, unclear whether the salutary effects are related to Na^{+}/K^{+} ATPase inhibition and enhanced calcium availability to the myofilaments, or whether alterations of catecholamine concentration or effect alter the neuroendocrine manifestations of congestive heart failure. Irrespective, the underlying rationale for its use remains obvious efficacy ("it works"). On the other hand, it is also possible that some ostensible improvement in the days following digoxin administration coincide with spontaneous recoverey from the underlying pathology that caused circulatory failure. The conclusion was, therefore, that digoxin administration was serendipitous to clinical improvement. However, in a case in which a fetus had electron transfer, deficiency was present the underlying nature of the cardiomyopathy would not logically have been expected to improve.[155]

INTERVENTIONAL CARDIAC CATHETERIZATION OF THE HUMAN FETUS

Aortic Balloon Valvuloplasty

Motivated by a dismal postnatal outcome for fetuses diagnosed with critical aortic stenosis prenatally, the group from Guy's Hospital in London embarked upon an innovative program for percutaneous cardiac catheterization and aortic balloon valvuloplasty of fetuses with this condition. Although the initial experience was unsuccessful, the feasibility of a percutaneous approach was demonstrated. The maternal abdomen, uterus, fetal chest, and left ventricle were transversed with subsequent wire entry into the ascending aorta; angioplasty balloon catheter was passed, and subsequently retrieved.[157] This group reported percutaneous procedures with one surviving infant.[158] These initial reports suggested that balloon valvuloplasty was feasible but that the prognosis for the fetus was dependent on ability to relieve aortic stenosis and to prevent or reverse damage to the left ventricular myocardium. Despite survival of a single patient, this group declared a moratorium on such procedures until a clearer appreciation of hemodynamics and improvement in catheter technology was in place.[159] Indeed, follow-up studies from that same center a few years later documented improved survival in neonates who had not undergone fetal intervention. This undermined the rationale for introduction of fetal intervention as an alternative approach to an otherwise hopeless condition.[160]

PRENATAL HEMATOPOIETIC STEM CELL TRANSPLANTATION

Engraftment and clonal proliferation of a relatively small number of normal hematopoietic stem cells (HSCs) can sustain normal hematopoiesis for a lifetime. This observation provides a compelling rationale for bone marrow transplantation (BMT) and is now supported by thousands of long-term survivors of BMT who otherwise would have succumbed to lethal hematologic disease.[161–163] Realization of the full potential of BMT, however, continues to be limited by a critical shortage of immunologically compatible donor cells, the inability to control the recipient or donor immune response, and the requirement for recipient myeloablation to achieve engraftment. Human leukocyte antigen (HLA) mismatch is highly deleterious; the greater the mismatch, the higher the graft failure, and the greater the risk for graft-versus-host disease (GVHD) and delayed immunologic reconstitution. Current methods of myeloablation have high morbidity and mortality birth in children and adults. In combination, these problems remain daunting for many patients who might benefit from BMT. A theoretically attractive alternative is in utero transplantation of HSC.[165] This approach is potentially applicable to any congenital hematopoietic disease that can be diagnosed prenatally and can be cured or improved by engraftment of normal HSCs.

Rationale for In Utero Transplantation

The rationale for in utero transplantation is to take advantage of the window of opportunity created by normal hematopoietic and immunologic ontogeny. Before population of the bone marrow and before thymic processing of self-antigen, the fetus theoretically should be receptive to engraftment of foreign HSC without rejection and without the need for myeloablation. In the human fetus, the ideal window would appear to be before 14 weeks' gestation, before release of differentiated T lymphocytes into the circulation, and while the bone marrow is just beginning to develop sites for hematopoiesis.[165] The window may extend later beyond in immunodeficiency states, particularly when T-cell development is abnormal. During this time, presentation of foreign antigen by thymic dendritic cells theoretically should result in clonal deletion of reactive T-cells during the negative selection phase of thymic processing. The diagnosis of a large number of congenital hematologic diseases is possible during the first trimester. Technical advances in fetal intervention also make transplantation feasible by 12 to 14 weeks' gestation. The ontologic window of opportunity thus falls well within diagnostic and technical constraints, making application of this approach a realistic possibility.

Prenatal HSC transplantation could theoretically obviate many of the current limitations of postnatal BMT. There would be no requirement for HLA matching, thus resulting in expansion of the donor pool. Transplanted cells would not be rejected, and space would be readily available in the bone marrow, thus eliminating the need for toxic immunosuppressive and myeloablative drugs. The mother's uterus might prove to be the ideal sterile isolation chamber, eliminating the necessity for the 2 to 4 months isolation required after postnatal BMT and before immunologic reconstitution. Finally, prenatal transplantation and correction would preclude postnatal clinical manifestations of the disease, avoiding the recurrent infections, multiple transfusions, growth delay, and other complications that often compromise postnatal treatment.

Source of Donor Cells

Identifying the best source of donor cells may ultimately prove to be the most critical factor for the success of engraftment. The most obvious advantage of using fetal hematopoietic stem cells is the minimal number of mature T cells in fetal liver-derived populations before 14 weeks' gestation. This alleviates any concern about GVHD and avoids the necessity of T-cell depletion processes, which can negatively impact potential engraftment.[165,166] The disadvantage of using fetal or embryonic tissue relate not only to limited availability and quality control, but also to some perceived ethical problems regarding use of fetal tissue. At present, these issues remain prohibitive in the United States, limiting investigation and use of potentially efficacious donor sources.

Diseases Amenable to Prenatal Treatment

Generally speaking, any disease is a target if it can be diagnosed early in gestation, improved by BMT, and treated postnatal by BMT. Some diseases, however, are far more likely to benefit from prenatal transplantation than others. The list can be stratified into three general categories: hemoglobinopathies, immunodeficiency disorders, and inborn errors of metabolism. Each has unique considerations, and in fact each disease may respond differently (Table 10-1). Issues that need to be considered include availability of engraftment sites within the bone marrow at time of transplantation and capacity of a needed enzyme to cross the blood-brain barrier at a given gestational age. Of particular relevance for a prenatal approach in which experimental levels of engraftment have been relatively low is the observation that in many of the target diseases, engrafted normal cells would be predicted to have a significant survival advantage over diseased cells. This would have the salutary clinical effect of amplifying the specific lineage; a survival advantage would exist. In addition, even with minimal levels of engraftment, specific tolerance for donor antigen should be induced, allowing additional cells from the same donor to be given to the tolerant recipient after birth.[167,168]

Hemoglobinopathies

The sickle cell anemias and thalassemia syndromes make up the largest patient groups potentially treatable by prenatal stem cell transplantation.[165,169–171] Both groups can be diagnosed within the first trimester. Both have been cured by postnatal BMT, although BMT is not recommended routinely because of its prohibitive morbidity and mortality and the relative success of modern medical management. In both diseases, the success of BMT is indirectly related to the morbidity of the disease. That is, the younger the patient, the fewer transfusions received; therefore, the less organ compromise from iron overload, the better the results. In both disorders, there is a survival advantage for normal erythrocytes, resulting in amplification of normal bone marrow engraftment in the peripheral red cell compartment. Thus, patients with relatively low levels of mixed chimerism after postnatal BMT have demonstrated high levels of normal hemoglobin peripherally with partial or complete ameliora-

Table 10-1. Potential Candidates for in Utero Stem Cell Fetal Therapy

Hematopoietic Disorders	
Disorders affecting lymphocytes	
SCID (sex linked)	
SCID (adenosine deaminase deficiency)	
Ommen syndrome	
Agammaglobinemia	
Bare lymphocyte syndrome	
Disorders affecting granulocytes	
Chronic granulomatous disease	
Infantile agranulocytosis	
Neutrophil membrane GP-180	
Lazy leukocyte syndrome	
Disorders affecting erythrocytes	
Sickle cell disease	
α-Thalassemia	
β-Thalassemia	
Hereditary spherocytosis	
Fanconi's anemia	
Mannosidosis	
α-Mannosidosis	
β-Thalassemia	
Mucolipodoses	
Gaucher's disease	
Metachromatic leukocystrophy	
Krabbe's disease	
Niemann-Pick disease	
β-Glucoronidase deficiency	
Fabry's disease	
Adrenal leukodystrophy	
Mucopolysaccharidoses (MPS)	
MPS I	(Hurler's Disease)
MPS II	(Hunter's Disease)
MPS IIIB	(Sanfilippo B)
MPS IV	(Morquio)
MPS VI	(Maroteaux-Lamy)

SCID, Severe Combined Immunodeficiency Syndrome.

tion of their disease.[166,167] Experimentally, this has been shown to be true after in utero transplantation as well, with relatively high levels of circulating donor derived erythrocytes despite low levels of mixed chimerism in the bone marrow.[172] In combination with the observation that engraftment can be enhanced after birth using non-myeloablative approaches in the tolerant recipient,[170,171] this approach makes it likely that hemoglobinopathies will be successfully treated by in utero transplantation in the future.

Immunodeficiency Diseases

Immunodeficiency diseases represent an extremely heterogeneous group of diseases that differ in their likelihood of cure by their capacity to develop hematopoietic chimerism.[173,174] Once again, those diseases in which a survival advantage exists for normal cells would be most likely to benefit from even low levels of donor cell engraftment. The best example is severe combined immunodeficiency syndrome (SCID). Several different molecular causes of SCID have been identified, with approximately two thirds of cases due to X-linked recessive inheritance (X-SCID). The genetic basis of X-SCID is[175] a mutation of the gene encoding the common-γ chain, (-γc), a common component of several members of the cytokine receptor superfamily. Children affected with X-SCID have a block in thymic T-cell development and diminished T-cell response. Although present in normal or even increased numbers, B cells are dysfunctional, secondary either to a lack of helper T-cell function or to an intrinsic defect in B-cell maturation. Clinical experience with HLA-matched sibling bone marrow, fetal liver, or thymus transplantation generally has been successful without myeloablative therapy, suggesting that the lymphoid progeny of relatively few engrafted normal HSC have a selective growth advantage in vivo over genetically defective cells.[176]

The competitive advantage of normal cell populations in X-SCID is best supported by demonstrating skewed X-inactivation in female carriers.[177] Only T cells containing the normal X chromosome were found to be present in the circulation of carriers. Adenosine deaminase deficiency or other mutations in cytokine receptor signaling pathways (e.g., Jak 3 or ZAP-70) that result in SCID should also be favorable candidate diseases for in utero HSC transplantation. Ideally, results of in utero treatment for SCID should be compared with early postnatal transplantation protocols to determine whether there is an advantage favoring utero therapy. Such trials may not be possible owing to the rarity of these diseases and the perception that postnatal therapy is adequate.[178]

Unfortunately, other diseases such as chronic granulomatous disease would not be expected to provide a competitive advantage for donor cells. Nevertheless, even partial engraftment and expression of a normal cell phenotype might mitigate against the clinical manifestations of the disease and, hence, enhance donor-specific tolerance for later transplantation. If higher levels of engraftment are needed, further HSC transplants from the same donor could be performed after birth without fear of rejection.

Flake et al.[179] reported successful treatment of a fetus with X-linked SCIDS in a family in which a previously affected child died at 7 months of age. Diagnosis by chorionic villus sampling at 12 weeks showed another affected male infant. For this couple, abortion was not an option. After informed consent, paternal bone marrow was harvested, T cells depleted, and enriched stem cell populations injected intraperitoneally into the fetus beginning about 16 weeks of gestation. Subsequent injections were performed at 17 and 18 weeks. The child presently shows chimerism: all his T cells are of paternal origin, whereas the majority of B cells are his. The child has normal developmental milestones and has had no serious infections through 10 years of age.[180] Additional cases reported by Porta et al.[181] and Westgren et al.[178] showed similarly favorable results.

Inborn Errors of Metabolism

An even more heterogeneous group of diseases—inborn errors of metabolism—can be caused by a deficiency of a specific lysosomal hydrolase, which results in the accumulation of substrates such as mucopolysaccharide, glycogen, and sphingolipid.[181] Depending on the specific enzyme abnormality and the compounds that accumulate, certain patterns of tissue damage and organ failure occur. These include central nervous system (CNS) deterioration, growth failure, dysostosis multiplex and joint abnormalities, hepatosplenomegaly, myocardial or cardiac disease, upper airway obstruction, pulmonary infiltration, corneal clouding, and hearing loss. Potential efficacy of prenatal HSC transplantation for the treatment of these diseases must be considered on an individual disease basis. The purpose of BMT in these diseases is to provide HSC-derived mononuclear cells that can repopulate various organs, including the liver (Kupffer cells), skin (Langerhans' cells), lung (alveolar macrophages), spleen (macrophages), lymph nodes, tonsils, and the brain (microglia).[183] Disorders that have been corrected by postnatal BMT—Gaucher's disease or Maroteaux-Lamy syndrome (minimal CNS involvement)—are reasonable candidates for prenatal treatment. In many cases, postnatal BMT has corrected the peripheral manifestations of the disease and arrested the neurologic deterioration; however, postnatal BMT has not reversed neurologic injury in disorders such as metachromatic leukodystrophy and Hurler's disease.[184,185] In these cases, the neurologic injury must have begun before birth. Postnatal maturation of the blood-brain barrier presumably restricts access to the CNS of transplanted cells or the deficient enzyme. Thus, a compelling rationale exists for prenatal therapy of these diseases. The primary question is whether donor HSC-derived microglial elements would populate the CNS, providing the necessary metabolic correction inside the blood-brain barrier. Based on experimental results with in utero HSC transplantation alone for these disorders, it seems likely that a combination of in utero HSC transplantation and CNS-directed cellular or gene therapy will be needed to correct CNS manifestations of these diseases.[186]

To summarize, the only definitively successful HSC transplants to date have been for SCIDS. All others have either failed to engraft or showed GVHD. Despite only limited evidence of clinical efficacy, however, interest in the field continues to gain momentum. Concomitant advances in prenatal screening, molecular diagnosis and knowledge of the genome make it likely that opportunities to apply this approach will increase.

CONCLUSION

Increasing numbers of congenital and genetic abnormalities are amenable to in utero treatment is possible. In some cases, treatment is relatively routine. Advances in therapies have progressed at different paces for different disorders, but there is great hope and enthusiasm that progress will continue to expand the number of disorders for which therapy can be effective.[187]

KEY POINTS

- Accurate, early diagnosis is a pivotal prerequisite for fetal surgery, especially excluding fetuses with aneuploidy or multiple malformations.
- Intervention through fetal surgery is appropriate only if a given disorder can not be treated safety and adequately after birth.
- LUTOs can be treated by *percutaneous* placement of a vesicoamniotic catheter, which drains the obstructed urinary tract into the amniotic space; fetal surgery for LUTO is applicable only after serial analysis of fetal urine verifies adequate fetal renal status.
- Theoretical advantages of using a fetoscope of small diameter must be balanced against better visualization and instrument flexibility provided by larger diameter instruments.
- In TTTS, MC twins undergo vascular anastomoses, the donor twin shows *hypovolemic* and oligohydramnios (so-called stuck twin) and the recipient the converse. Laser coagulation of anastomoses on the chorionic place is superior to amnioreduction and septostomy.
- Cord occlusion by coagulation becomes applicable if the alternative is loss of the entire pregnancy, as would occur in some TTTS and in TRAP.
- Surgical removal of CCAM or sacrococcygeal teratoma is an accepted indication for open fetal surgery.
- The EXIT procedure is a modified cesarean delivery in which uterine relaxation is maintained under general *anesthesia* in order to allow persisting uteroplacental perfusion while delivery of fetuses having prior tracheal ligation or in whom airway problems can be anticipated can be treated.
- Administration of dexamethasone to the mother can prevent external genital masculinization in a female fetus affected with CAH, usually due to 21-hydroxylase deficiency.
- In utero stem cell transplantation (engraftment) should occur before 14 weeks' gestation in order to facilitate acceptance of HLA mismatched T cells that are still undifferentiated antigenically.

REFERENCES

1. Evans MI, Bui TH (eds): The Genome Revolution and Obstetrics and Gynecology. Balliere's Best Practice and Research in Clinical Obstetrics and Gynecology. Harcourt Brace Publishing Co., London, 16: 2002.
2. Harrison MR, Evans MI, Adzick NS, Holzgrove W: The Unborn Patient. Philadelphia, W.B. Saunders, 2000.
3. Johnson MP, Flake AW, Quintero RA, Evans MI: Shunt Procedures. *In* Evans MI, Johnson MP, Moghissi KS (eds): Invasive Outpatient Procedures in Reproductive Medicine. New York, Raven Press, 1997.

4. Muller F, Dreux S, Audibert F, et al: Fetal serum ss2-microglobulin and cystatin C in the prediction of post-natal renal function in bilateral hypoplasia and hyperechogenic enlarged kidneys. Prenatal Diag 24:327, 2004.
5. Drugan A, Krause B, Canady A, et al: The natural history of prenatally diagnosed ventriculomegaly. JAMA 261:1785, 1989.
6. Ahmad FK, Sherman SJ, Hagglund KH, et al: Isolated unilateral pleural effusion: The role of sonographic surveillance and in utero therapy. Fetal Diagn Ther 11:383, 1996.
7. Nicolaides KH, Azar GB: Thoracoamniotic shunting. Fetal Diagn Ther 5:153, 1990.
8. Lewi L, Dennes WJB, Fisk NM, Deprest J: Twin to twin transfusion syndrome. *In* Van Vught J, Schulman L (eds): Fetal Medicine. New York, M Dekker Publishers, 2006, p 447.
9. Deprest J, Ville Y, Barki G, et al: Endoscopy in fetal medicine. The Eurofoetus Group. Deprest J (ed): Karl Storz In, Tuttlingen, Germany, Endopress, 2004, p 1.
10. Jani J, Keller RL, Benachi A, et al: Prenatal prediction of survival in isolated left-sided diaphragmatic hernia. Ultrasound Obstet Gynecol 27:18, 2006.
11. Quintero RA, Morales WJ, Allen MH, et al: Staging of twin-twin transfusion syndrome. J Perinatol 19(8 Pt 1):550, 1999.
12. Zikulnig L, Hecher K, Bregenzer T, et al: Prognostic factors in severe twin-twin transfusion syndrome treated by endoscopic laser surgery. Ultrasound Obstet Gynecol 14:380, 1999.
13. Moise KJ, Dorman K, Lamvu G, et al: A randomized trial of amnioreduction versus septostomy in the treatment of twin-twin transfusion syndrome. Am J Obstet Gynecol 193:701, 2005.
14. Wee LY, Taylor M, Watkins N, et al: Characterisation of deep arterio-venous anastomoses within monochorionic placentae by vascular casting. Placenta 26:19, 2005.
15. Lewi L, Jani J, Cannie M, et al: Intertwin anastomoses in monochorionic placentas after fetoscopic laser coagulation for severe twin-to-twin transfusion syndrome: is there more than meets the eye? Am J Obstet Gynecol 194:790, 2006.
16. Robyr R, Lewi L, Salomon L, et al: Prevalence and management of late fetal complications following successful selective laser coagulation of chorionic plate anastomoses in twin-to-twin transfusion syndrome. Am J Obstet Gynecol 194:796, 2005.
17. Taylor MJ, Govender L, Jolly M, et al: Validation of the Quintero staging system for twin-twin transfusion syndrome. Obstet Gynecol 100:1257, 2002.
18. Gardiner HM, Taylor MJ, Karatza A, et al: Twin-twin transfusion syndrome: the influence of intrauterine laser photocoagulation on arterial distensibility in childhood. Circulation 107:1906, 2003.
19. Sutcliffe AG, Sebire NJ, Pigott AJ, et al: Outcome for children born after in utero laser ablation therapy for severe twin-to-twin transfusion syndrome. BJOG 108:1246, 2001.
20. Bajoria R, Wee LY, Anwar S, Ward S: Outcome of twin pregnancies complicated by single intrauterine death in relation to vascular anatomy of the monochorionic placenta. Hum Reprod 14:2124, 1999.
21. Nicolini U, Poblete: Single intrauterine death in monochorionic twins pregnancies. Ultrasound Obstet Gynecol 14:297, 1999.
22. Johnson JR, Rossi KQ, O'Shaughnessy RW: Amnioreduction versus septostomy in twin-twin transfusion syndrome. Am J Obstet Gynecol 185:1044, 2001.
23. Fisk NM, Vaughan J, Talbert D: Impaired fetal blood gas status in polyhydramnios and its relation to raised amniotic pressure. Fetal Diagn Ther 9:7, 1994.
24. Bower SJ, Flack NJ, Sepulveda W, et al: Uterine artery blood flow response to correction of amniotic fluid volume. Am J Obstet Gynecol 173:502, 1995.
25. Mari G, Roberts A, Detti L, et al: Perinatal morbidity and mortality rates in severe twin-twin transfusion syndrome: results of the International Amnioreduction Registry. Am J Obstet Gynecol 185:708, 2001.
26. Quintero RA, Dickinson JE, Morales WJ, et al: Stage-based treatment of twin-twin transfusion syndrome. Am J Obstet Gynecol 188:1333, 2003.
27. Skupski DW, Gurushanthaiah K, Chasen S: The effect of treatment of twin-twin transfusion syndrome on the diagnosis-to-delivery interval. Twin Res 5:1, 2002.
27a. De Lia JE, Cruikshank DP, Keve WR Jr: Fetoscopic neodymium: YAG laser occlusion of placental vessels in severe twin-twin transfusion syndrome. Obstet Gynecol 75:1046, 1990.
27b. De Lia JE, Kuhlmann RS, Harstad TW, Cruikshank DP: Fetoscopic laser ablation of placental vessles in severe previable twin-twin transfusion syndrome. Am J Obstet Gynecol 172:1202, 1995.
28. Deprest J, Barki G, Lewi L, et al: Fetoscopic instrumentation and techniques. *In* Van Vught J, Shulman L (eds): Fetal Medicine. New York, M Dekker Publishers, 2006, p 473.
29. Gratacos E, Van Schoubroeck D, Carreras E, et al: Transient hydropic signs in the donor fetus after fetoscopic laser coagulation in severe twin-twin transfusion syndrome: incidence and clinical relevance. Ultrasound Obstet Gynecol 19:449, 2002.
30. Zikulnig L, Hecher K, Bregenzer T, et al: Prognostic factors in severe twin-twin transfusion syndrome treated by endoscopic laser surgery. Ultrasound Obstet Gynecol 14:380, 1999.
31. Lewi L, Van Schoubroeck D, Van Ranst M, et al: Successful patching of iatrogenic rupture of the fetal membranes. Placenta 25:352, 2004.
32. Hecher K, Diehl W, Zikulnig L, et al: Endoscopic laser coagulation of placental anastomoses in 200 pregnancies with severe mid-trimester twin-to-twin transfusion syndrome. Eur J Obstet Gynecol Reprod Biol 92:135, 2000.
33. Robyr R, Salomon LJ, Yamamoto M, et al: Prevalence and management of late fetal complications following successful selective laser coagulation of chorionic plate anastomoses in twin to twin transfusion syndrome. Am J Obstet Gynecol 194:796, 2006.
34. Senat MV, Deprest J, Boulvain M, et al: Endoscopic laser surgery versus serial amnioreduction for severe twin-to-twin transfusion syndrome. N Engl J Med 351:136, 2004.
35. De Lia JE, Carr MH: Pregnancy loss after successful laser surgery for previable twin-twin transfusion syndrome. Am J Obstet Gynecol 187:517; author reply 518, 2002.
36. Robyr R, Boulvain M, Ortqvist L, et al: OC119: Prognostic factors for preterm delivery in twin-to-twin transfusion syndrome (TTTS) treated by laser coagulation. Ultrasound in Obstetrics and Gynecology 24:249, 2004.
37. Ville Y, Hecher K, Bui TH: Eurofetus update 2006 (unpublished)
38. Banek CS, Hecher K, Hackeloer BJ, Bartmann P: Long-term neurodevelopmental outcome after intrauterine laser treatment for severe twin-twin transfusion syndrome. Am J Obstet Gynecol 188:876, 2003.
39. Baldwin VJ: Anomalous development in twins. In Pathology of Multiple Pregnancies. New York, Springer-Verlag, 1994, p 169.
40. Bryan E, Little J, Burn J: Congenital anomalies in twins. Baillieres Clin Obstet Gynecol 1:697, 1987.
41. Lewi L, Van Schoubroeck D, Gloning K-P, et al: Selective feticide by cord occlusion in four sets of heterokarytypic monochorionic twins. J Soc Gynecol Investig 10(Suppl):97A, 2003.
42. Nieuwint A, Van Zalen-Sprock R, Hummel P, et al: 'Identical' twins with normal karyotypes. Prenat Diagn 19:72, 1999.
43. Sebire NJ, Snijders RJ, Hughes K, et al: The hidden mortality of monochorionic twin pregnancies. Br J Obstet Gynaecol 104:1203, 1997.
44. Nakai Y, Ishoko O, Nishio J, et al: Cyclic changes in the umbilical arterial flow in monochorionic diamniotic twin pregnancy. Eur J Obstet Gynecol Reprod Biol 101:135, 2002.
45. Gratacós E, Lewi L, Carreras E, et al: Incidence and characteristics of umbilical intermittent absent and/or reversed diastolic flow in complicated and uncomplicated monochorionic twin pregnancy. Ultrasound Obstet Gynecol 23:456, 2004.
46. Gratacós E, Lewi L, Carreras E, et al: Incidence and characteristics of umbilical intermittent absent and/or reversed diastolic flow in complicated and uncomplicated monochorionic twin pregnancy. Ultrasound Obstet Gynecol 23:456, 2004.
47. Quintero RA, Bornick PW, Morales WJ, et al: Selective photocoagulation of the communicating vessels in the treatment of monochorionic twins with selective growth retardation. Am J Obstet Gynecol 185:689, 2001.
48. Quintero RA, Bornick PW, Morales WJ, et al: Selective photocoagulation of the communicating vessels in the treatment of

monochorionic twins with selective growth retardation. Am J Obstet Gynecol 185:689, 2001.
49. Myers SA, Bennett TL: Selective photocoagulation of monochorionic twin pregnancy. Letter. Am J Obstet Gynecol 187:1, 2002.
50. Gilliam DL, Hendricks CH: Holoacardius: review of literature and case report. Obstet Gynecol 2:647, 1953.
51. Sogaard K, Skibsted L, Brocks V: Acardiac twins: pathophysiology, diagnosis, outcome and treatment. Six cases and review of the literature. Fetal Diagn Ther 14:53, 1999.
52. Sullivan AE, Varner MW, Ball RH, et al: The management of acardiac twins: a conservative approach. Am J Obstet Gynecol 189:1310, 2003.
53. Moore TR, Gale S, Benirschke K: Perinatal outcome of forty-nine pregnancies complicated by acardiac twinning. Am J Obstet Gynecol 163:907, 1990.
54. Brassard M, Fouron JC, Leduc L, et al: Prognostic markers in twin pregnancies with an acardiac fetus. Obstet Gynecol 94:409, 1999.
55. Sherer DM, Armstrong B, Shah YG, et al: Prenatal sonographic diagnosis, Doppler velocimetric umbilical cord studies, and subsequent management of an acardiac twin pregnancy. Obstet Gynecol 74:472, 1989.
56. Dashe JS, Fernandez CO, Twickler DM: Utility of Doppler velocimetry in predicting outcome in twin reversed-arterial perfusion sequence. Am J Obstet Gynecol 185:135, 2001.
57. Taylor MJ, Shalev E, Tanawattanacharoen S, et al: Ultrasound-guided umbilical cord occlusion using bipolar diathermy for Stage III/IV twin-twin transfusion syndrome. Prenat Diagn 22:70, 2002.
58. Senat MV, Deprest J, Boulvain M, et al: Endoscopic laser surgery versus serial amnioreduction for severe twin-to-twin transfusion syndrome. N Engl J Med 8:136–144, 2004.
59. Zosmer N, Bajoria R, Weiner E, et al: Clinical and echocardiographic features of in utero cardiac dysfunction in the recipient twin in twin-twin transfusion syndrome. Br Heart J 72:74, 1994.
60. Challis D, Gratacós E, Deprest J: Selective termination in monochorionic twins. J Perinat Med 27:327, 1999.
61. Ville Y: Selective feticide in monochorionic pregnancies: toys for the boys or standard of care? Ultrasound Obstet Gynecol 22:448, 2003.
62. Robyr R, Boulvain M, Lewi L, et al: Cervical length as a prognostic factor for preterm delivery in twin to twin transfusion syndrome treated by fetoscopic laser coagulation of chorionic plate anastomoses. Ultrasound Obstet Gynecol 25:37, 2005.
63. Lewi L, Jani J, Cannie M, et al: Intertwin anastomoses in monochorionic placentas after fetoscopic laser coagulation for twin to twin transfusion syndrome: is there more than meets the eye? Am J Obstet Gynecol 194:790, 2006.
64. Nicolini U, Poblete A, Boschetto C, et al: Complicated monochorionic twin pregnancies: experience with bipolar cord coagulation. Am J Obstet Gynecol 185:703, 2000.
65. Robyr R, Quarello E, Ville Y: Management of fetofetal transfusion syndrome. Prenat Diagn 25:786, 2005.
66. Quintero RA, Chmait RH, Murakoshi T, et al: Surgical management of twin reversed arterial perfusion sequence. Am J Obstet Gynecol 194:982, 2006.
67. Quintero RA, Munoz H, Hasbun J, et al: Fetal endoscopic surgery in a case of twin pregnancy complicated by reversed arterial perfusion sequence (TRAP sequence). Rev Chil Obstet Gynecol 60:112, 1995.
68. Stege G, Fenton A, Jaffray B: Nihilism in the 1990s. The true mortality of CDH. Pediatrics 112:532, 2003.
69. Chiu PP, Sauer C, Mihailovic A, et al: The price of success in the management of congenital diagphragmatic hernia: is improved survival accompanied by an increase in long term morbidity. J Pediatr Surg 41:888, 2006.
70. Deprest J, Jani J, Cannie M, et al: Progress in intra-uterine assessment of the fetal lung and prediction of neonatal function. Ultrasound Obstet Gynaecol 25:108, 2005.
71. Albanese CT, Lopoo DV, Paek BW, et al: Fetal liver position and perinatal outcome for congential diaphragmatic hernia. Prenat Diagn 18:1138, 1998.
72. Metkus AP, Filly RA, Stringer MD, et al: Sonographic predictors of survival in fetal diaphragmatic hernia. J Pediatr Surg 31:148, 1996.
73. Nelson S, Cameron A, Deprest J: Fetoscopic surgery for in utero management of Congenital Diaphragmatic Hernia. Fet Mat Med Rev 17:69, 2006.
74. Flake A, Crombleholme T, Johnson M, et al: Treatment of severe congenital diaphragmatic hernia by fetal tracheal occlusion: clinical experience with fifteen cases. Am J Obstet Gynecol 183:1059, 2000.
75. Harrison MR, Sydorak RM, Farrell JA, et al: Fetoscopic temporary tracheal occlusion for congenital diaphragmatic hernia: prelude to a randomized controlled trial. J Pediatr Surg 38:1012, 2003.
76. Deprest JA, Evrard VA, Van Ballaer PP, et al: Tracheoscopic endoluminal plugging using an inflatable device in the fetal lamb model. Eur J Obstet Gynaecol Reprod Biol 81:165, 1998.
77. Deprest J, Evrard V, Verbeken E, et al: Tracheal side effects of endoscopic balloon tracheal occlusion in the fetal lamb model. Eur J Obstet Gynecol Reprod Biol 92:119, 2000.
78. Quintero RA, Morales WJ, Bornick PW, et al: Minimally invasive intraluminal tracheal occlusion in a human fetus with left congenital diaphragmatic hernia at 27 weeks gestation via direct fetal laryngoscopy. Prenat Neonat Med 5:134, 2000.
79. Deprest J, Gratacos E, Nicolaides KH on behalf of the FETO task group: Fetoscopic tracheal occlusion (FETO) for severe congenital diaphragmatic hernia: evolution of a technique. Ultrasound Obstet Gynaecol 24:121, 2004.
80. Harrison MR, Keller RL, Hawgood SB, et al: A randomized trial of fetal endoscopic tracheal occlusion for severe fetal congential diaphragmatic hernia. N Engl J Med 349:1916, 2005.
81. Keller RL, Hawgood S, Neuhaus JM, et al: Infant pulmonary function in a randomized trial of fetal tracheal occlusion for severe congenital diaphragmatic hernia. Pediatr Res 56:818, 2004.
82. Jani J, Gratacos E, Greenough A, et al and the FETO task group: Percutaneous fetal endoscopic tracheal occlusion (FETO) for severe left sided congenital diaphragmatic hernia. Clin Obstet Gynecol N Am 48:910, 2005.
83. Jani J, Nicolaides KH, Gratacos E, et al and the FETO task group: Fetal lung-to-head ratio in the prediction of survival in severe left-sided diaphragmatic hernia treated by fetal endoscopic tracheal occlusion (FETO). Am J Obstet Gynecol 195:1646, 2006.
84. Adzick N, Harrison M, Flake A, et al: Automatic uterine stapling devices in fetal surgery: Experience in a primate model. Surgical Forum XXXVI:479, 1985.
85. Jennings RW, Adzick NS, Longaker MT, et al: New techniques in fetal surgery. J Pediatr Surg 27:1329, 1992.
86. Jennings RW, Adzick NS, Longaker MT, et al: Radiotelemetric fetal monitoring during and after open fetal operation. Surg Gynecol Obstet 176:59, 1993.
87. Harrison MR, Longaker MT, Adzick NS, et al: Successful repair in utero of a fetal diaphragmatic hernia after removal of herniated viscera from the left thorax. N Engl J Med 322:1582, 1990.
88. Harrison MR, Adzick NS, Flake AW, et al: Correction of congenital diaphragmatic hernia in utero: VI. Hard-learned lessons. J Pediatr Surg 28:1141; discussion 1417, 1993.
89. Harrison MR, Keller RL, Hawgood SB, et al: A randomized trial of et al endoscopic tracheal occlusion for severe fetal congenital diaphragmatic hernia. N Engl J Med 349:1916, 2003.
90. Harrison MR, Sydorak RM, Farrell JA, et al: Fetoscopic temporary tracheal occlusion for congenital diagphragmatic hernia: prelude to a randomized, controlled trial. J Pediatr Surg 38:1012, 2003.
91. Heerema AE, Rabban JT, Sydorak RM, et al: Lung pathology in patients with congenital diaphragmatic hernia treated with fetal surgical intervention, including tracheal occlusion. Pediatr Dev Pathol 6:536, 2003.
92. Sydorak RM, Harrison MR: Congenital diaphragmatic hernia: Advances in prenatal therapy. Clin Perinatol 30:465, 2003.
93. Danzer E, Sydora RM, Harrison MR, Albanese CT: Minimal access fetal surgery. Eur J Obstet Gynecol Reprod Biol 108:3, 2003.

94. Evans MI, Harrison MR, Flake AW, Johnson MP: Fetal therapy. Best Pract Res Clin Obstet Gynaecol 16:671, 2002.
95. Paek BW, Coakley FV, Lu Y, et al: Congenital diaphragmatic hernia: prenatal evaluation with mr lung volumetry—preliminary experience. Radiology 220:63, 2001.
96. Wenstrom KD: Fetal surgery for congenital diaphragmatic hernia. N Engl J Med 349:1887, 2003.
97. Adzick NS, Kitano Y: Fetal surgery for lung lesions, congenital diaphragmatic hernia, and saccrococcygeal teratoma. Semin Pediatr Surg 12:154, 2003.
98. Adzick NS, Harrison MR, Crombleholme TM, et al: Fetal lung: Management and outcome. Am J Obstet Gynecol 179:884, 1998.
99. Crombleholme TM, Coleman BG, Howell LJ, et al: elevated cystic adenomatoid malformation volume (CVR) outcome in prenatal diagnosis of cystic adenomatoid malformation of the lung. J Pediatr Surg 37:331, 2002.
100. Hotterman AX, Filiatrault D, Lallier M, et al: The natural history of sacrococcygeal teratomas diagnosed through routine obstetric sonogram: A single institution experience. J Pediatr Surg 37:331, 2002.
101. Paek B, Vaezy S, Fujimoto V, et al: Tissue ablation using high-intensity focused ultrasound. potential for fetal treatment. Am J Obstet Gynecol 189:702, 2003.
102. Liechty KW, Crombleholme TM, Flake AW, et al: Intrapartum Airway Management for giant neck masses. The EXIT (ex utero Intrapartum Treatorus procedure. Am J Obstet Gynecol 177:870, 1997.
103. Hedrick HL: Ex utero intrapartum therapy. Semin Perinatol 12:190, 2003.
104. Adzick NS, Walsh DS: Meningomyelocele: Prenatal diagnosis, pathophysiology & management. Semin Pediatr Surg 12:168, 2003.
105. Lemire RJ: Neural tube defects. JAMA 259:558, 1988.
106. Meuli M, Meuli-Simmen C, Hutchins GM, et al: In utero surgery rescues neurological function at birth in sheep with spina bifida. Nature Med 1:342, 1995.
107. Bruner JP, Tulipan N, Paschall RL, et al: Fetal surgery for myelomeningocele and the incidence of shunt-dependent hydrocephalus. JAMA 282:1819, 1999.
108. Sutton LN, Adzick NS, Bilaniuk LT, et al: Improvement in hindbrain. JAMA 282:312, 1999.
109. Tulipan N, Hermanz-Schulman M, Bruner JP: Reduced hirdbrain hermination after intrauterine myelomingocele repair. A report of four cases. Pediatr Neurosurg 29:274, 1998.
110. Bruner JP, Tulipan N, Paschall RL, et al: Intrauterine repair of myelomingocele, "hirdbrain hermination", and the incidence of shunt dependent hydrocephalus. JAMA 282:1819, 1999.
111. Johnson MP, Adzick WS, Rintoul N, et al: Fetal myelomeningocele repair: Short term outcomes. Am J Obstet Gynecol 189:482, 2003.
112. Lemire RJ: Neural tube defects. JAMA 259:558, 1988.
113. Frey L, Hauser WA: Epidemiology of neural tube defects. Epilepsia 44(Suppl 3):4, 2003.
114. Smithells RW, Sheppard S, Schorah CJ, et al: Possible prevention of neural tube defects by preconceptual vitamin supplementation. Lancet 1:399, 1980.
115. Honein MA, Paulozzi LJ, Mathews TJ, et al: Impact of folic acid fortification of the US food supply on the occurrence of neural tube defects. JAMA 285:2981, 2001.
116. MRC Vitamin Study Research Group: Prevention of neural tube defects: results of the MRC vitamin study. Lancet 338:132, 1991.
117. Finnell RH, Shaw GM, Lammer EJ, Volcik KA: Does prenatal screening for 5,10-methylenetetrahydrofolate reductase (MTHFR) mutations in high-risk neural tube defect pregnancies make sense? Genet Test 6:47, 2002.
118. Evans MI, Llurba E, Landsberger EJ, et al: Impact of folic acid supplementation in the United States: markedly diminished high maternal serum AFPs. Obstet Gynecol 103:474, 2004.
119. Parle-McDermott A, Mills JL, Kirke PN, et al: Analysis of MTHFR 1298AC and 677 CT polymorphisms as risk factor neural tube defects. J Hum Genet 48:190, 2003.
120. Rampersaud E, Melvin EC, Siegel D, et al: Updated investigations of the role of methylenetetrahydrofolate reductase in human neural tube defects. Clin Genet 63:210, 2003.
121. Zhu H, Wicker NJ, Shaw GM, et al: Homocysteine remethylation enzyme polymorphisms and increased risks for neural tube defects. Mol Genet Metab 78:216, 2003.
122. Opitz JM: RSH-SLO ("Smith-Lemli-Opitz") syndrome: historical, genetic, and development considerations. Am J Med Genet 50:344, 1994.
123. Sever LE: Zinc deficiency in man. Lancet I:887, 1973.
124. McMichael AJ, Dreosti IE, Gibson GT: A prospective study of serial maternal serum zinc levels and pregnancy outcome. Early Hum Dev 7:59, 1982.
125. Stoll C, Dott B, Alembik Y, Koehl C. Maternal trace elements, vitamin B_{12}, vitamin A, folic acid, and fetal malformations. Rep Toxicol 13:53, 1999.
126. Hambidge M, Hackshaw A, Wald N: Neural tube defects and serum zinc. Br J Obstet Gynecol 100:746, 1993.
127. Shoob HD, Sargent RG, Thompson SJ, et al: Dietary methionine is involved in the etiology of neural defect-affected pregnancies in humans. J Nutr 131:2653, 2001.
128. MacLaughton DT, Donahoe PK: Sex determination and differentiation. N Engl J Med 350:367, 2004.
129. Clayton PE, Miller WL, Oberfield SE, et al; ESPE/ LWPES CAH Working Group: Consensus statement on 21-hydroxylase deficiency from the European Society for Paediatric Endocrinology and the Lawson Wilkins Pediatric Endocrine Society. Horm Res; 58:188, 2002.
130. Evans MI, Chrousos GP, Mann DL, et al: Pharmacologic suppression of the fetal adrenal gland in utero: attempted prevention of abnormal external genital masculinization in suspected congenital adrenal hyperplasia. JAMA 253:1015, 1985.
131. Forrest M, David M: Prenatal treatment of congenital adrenal hyperplasia due to 21-hydroxylase deficiency. 7th International Congress of Endocrinology, Abstract y11, Quebec, Canada, 1984.
132. New MI, Carlson A, Obeid J, et al: Prenatal diagnosis for congenital adrenal hyperplasia in 532 pregnancies. Clin Endocrinol Metab 86:5651, 2001.
133. Fisher DA, Klein AH: Thyroid development and disorders of thyroid function in the newborn. N Engl J Med 304:702, 1981.
136. Bruinse HW, Vermeulen-Meiners C, Wit JM: Fetal treatment for thyrotoxicosis in non-thyrotoxic pregnant women. Fetal Ther 3:152, 1988.
135. Rovet J, Ehrlich R, Sorbara D: Intellectual outcome in children with fetal hypothyroidism. J Pediatr 110:700, 1987.
136. Fisher DA: Neonatal thyroid disease of women with autoimmune thyroid disease. Thyroid Today 9:1, 1986.
137. Volumenie JL, Polak M, Guibourdenche J, et al: Management of fetal thyroid goitres: a report of 11 cases in a single perinatal unit. Prenat Diagn 20:799, 2000.
138. Morine M, Takeda T, Minekawa R, et al: Antenatal diagnosis and treatment of a case of fetal goitrous hypothyroidism associated with high-output cardiac failure. Ultrasound Obstet Gynecol 19:506, 2002.
139. Kleinman CS, Copel JA, Nehgme RA: The fetus with cardiac arrhythmia. *In* Harrison MR, Evans MI, Adzick NS, Holzgreve W (eds): The Unborn Patient: The Art and Science of Fetal Therapy. Philadelphia, WB Saunders, 2001, p 417.
140. Evans MI, Johnson MP, Yaron Y, Drugan A (eds): Prenatal Diagnosis: Genetics, Reproductive Risks, Testing, and Managment. New York, McGraw Hill Publishing Co., 2006.
141. Kleinman CS, Donnerstein RL, DeVore GR, et al: Fetal echocardiography for evaluation of in utero congestive heart failure: A technique for study of nonimmune fetal hydrops. N Engl J Med 306:568, 1982.
142. Weiner CP, Thompson MIB: Direct treatment of fetal supraventricular tachycardia after failed transplacental therapy. Am J Obstet Gynecol 158:570, 1988.
143. Hansmann M, Gembruch U, Bald RK, et al: Fetal tachyarrhythmias: Transplacental and direct treatment of the fetus. A report of 60 cases. Ultrasound Obstet Gynecol 1:162, 1991.
144. Younis JS, Granat M: Insufficient transplacental digoxin transfer in severe hydrops fetalis. Am J Obstet Gynecol 157:1268, 1987.
145. Simpson PC, Trudinger BJ, Walker A, Baird PJ: The intrauterine treatment of fetal cardiac failure in a twin pregnancy with an

acardiac, acephalic monster. Am J Obstet Gynecol 147:842, 1983.

146. Slate RK, Stevens MB, Verrier ED, et al: Intrauterine repair of pulmonary stenosis in fetal sheep. Surg Forum 36:246, 1985.
147. Turley K, Vlahakes GI, Harrison MR, et al: Intrauterine cardiothoracic surgery: The fetal lamb model. Ann Thorac Surg 34:422, 1982.
148. Morganroth J: Risk factors for the development of proarrhythmic events. Am J Cardiol 59:32E, 1987.
149. Wellens JHH, Durrer D: Effect of digitalis on atrioventriciular conduction and circus movement tachycardia in patients with the Wolff-Parkinson-White syndrome. Circulation 47:1229, 1973.
150. Michaelsson M, Engle MA: Congenital complete heart block: An international study of the natural history. Cardiovascular Clin 4:85, 1972.
151. Anandakumar C, Biswas A, Chew SS, et al: Direct fetal therapy for hydrops secdondary to congenital atrioventricular heart block. Obstet Gynecol 87:835, 1996.
152. Carpenter RJ, Strasburger JF, Garson A Jr, et al: Fetal ventricular pacing for hydrops secondary to complete atrioventricular block. J Am Coll Cardiol 8:1434, 1986.
153. Bitar FF, Byrum CJ, Kveselis DA, et al: In utero management of hydrops fetalis caused by critical aortic stenosis. Am J Perinatol 14:389, 1997.
154. Schmider A, Henrich W, Dahnert I, Dudenhausen JW: Prenatal therapy of non-immunologic hydrops fetalis caused by severe aortic stenosis. Ultrasound Obstet Gynecol 16:275, 2000.
155. Kleinman CS, Donnerstein RL: Ultrasonic assessment of cardiac function in the intact human fetus. J Am Coll Cardiol 5(Suppl 1):84S-94S, 1985.
156. Yagel S, Weissman A, Rotstein Z, et al: Congenital heart defects: Natural course and in utero development. Circulation 96:550, 1997.
157. Maxwell D, Allan L, Tynan MJ: Balloon dilatation of the aortic valve in the fetus. A report of two cases. Br Heart J 65:256, 1991.
158. Allan LD, Maxwell DJ, Carminati, Tynan MJ: Survival after fetal aortic balloon valvoplasty. Ultrasound Obstet Gynecol. 5:90, 1995.
159. Kohl T, Szabo X, Suda K, et al: Fetoscopic and open transumbilical fetal cardiac catheterization in sheep. Potential approaches for human fetal cardiac intervention. Circulation 95:1048, 1997.
160. Simpson JM, Sharland GK: Natural history and outcome of aortic stenosis diagnosed prenatally. Heart 77:205, 1997.
161. Lucarelli G, Clift RA, Galimberti M, et al: Bone marrow transplantation in adult thalassemic patients. Blood 93:1164, 1999.
162. Walters MC, Patience M, Leisenring W, et al: Bone marrow transplantation for sickle cell disease. N Engl J Med 335:369, 1996.
163. Walters MC, Storb R, Patience M, et al: Impact of bone marrow transplantation for symptomatic sickle cell disease: an interim report. Multicenter investigation of bone marrow transplantation for sickle cell disease. Blood 95:1918, 2000.
164. Flake AW, Zanjani ED: In utero hematopoietic stem cell transplantation: Ontogenicopportunities ad biologic barriers. Blood 94:2179, 1999.
165. Flake AW, Zanjani ED: In utero hematopoietic stem cell transplantation. A status report. JAMA 278:932, 1997.
166. Touraine JL, Raudrant D, Laplace S: Transplantation of hematopoietic cells from the fetal liver to treat patients with congenital disease postnatally or prenatally. Transplant Proc 29:712, 1997.
167. Hayashi S, Peranteau WH, Shaaban AF, Flake AW: Complete allogeneic hematopoietic chimerism achieved by a combined strategy of in utero hematopoietic stem cell transplantation and postnatal donor lymphocyte infusion. Blood 100:804, 2002.
168. Peranteau WF, Hayashi S, Hsieh M, et al: High level allogeneic chimerism achieved by prenatal tolerance induction and postnatal non-myeloablative bone marrow transplantation. Blood 100:2225, 2002.
169. Hayward A, Ambruso D, Battaglia F, et al: Microchimerism and tolerance following intrauterine transplantation and transfusion for alpha-thalassemia-1. Fetal Diagn Ther 13:8, 1998.
170. Westgren M, Ringden O, Eik Nes S, et al: Lack of evidence of permanent enfragment after in utero fetal stem cell transplantiation in congenital hemoglobinopathies. Transplantation 61:1176, 1996.
171. Touraine JL, Raudrant D, Royo C, et al: In utero transplantation of hematopoietic stem cells in humans. Transplant Proc 23:1706, 1991.
172. Hayashi S, Abdulmalik O, Peranteau WH, et al: Mixed chimerism following in utero hematopoietic stem cell transplantation in murine models of hemoglobinopathy. Exp Hematol 31:176, 2003.
173. Flake AW: Stem cell and genetic therapies for the fetus. Semin Pediatr Surg 12:202, 2003.
174. Shields LE, Lindton BIM, Andrews RG, Westgren M: Fetal hematopoietic stem cell transplantation: a challenge for the twenty-first century. J Hematother Stem Cell Res 11:617, 2002.
175. Noguchi M, Yi H, Rosenblatt HM, et al: Interleukin-2 receptor gamma chain mutation results in X-linked severe combined immunodeficiency in humans. Cell 73:17, 1993
176. Slavin S, Naparstek E, Ziegler M, Lewin A: Clinical application of intrauterine bone marrow transplantation for treatment of genetic diseases-feasibility studies. Bone Marrow Transplant 9:189, 1992.
177. Buckley RH, Schiff SE, Schiff RI, et al: Hematopoietic stem-cell transplantation for the treatment of severe combined immunodeficiency. N Engl J Med 340:508, 1999.
178. Westgren M, Ringden O, Bartmann P, et al: Prenatal T-cell reconstitution after in utero transplantation with fetal liver cells in a patient with X-linked severe combined immunodeficiency. Am J Obstet Gynecol 187:475, 2002.
179. Flake AW, Roncarolo MG, Puck JM, et al: Treatment of x-linked severe combined immunodeficiency by in utero transplantation of paternal bone marrow. N Engl J Med 335:1806, 1996.
180. Flake AW, Zanjani ED: Treatment of severe combined immunodeficiency syndrome. N Engl J Med 341:291, 1999.
181. Pirovano S, Notarangelo LD, Malacarne F, et al: Reconstitution of T-cell compartment after in utero stem cell transplantation: analysis of T-cell repertoire and thymic output. Haematologica 89:450, 2004.
182. Moses S: Pathophysiology and dietary treatment of the glycogen storage diseases. J Pediatr Gastro Nutrit 11:155, 1990.
183. Kaye E: Therapeutic approaches to lysosomal storage diseases. Curr Opin Pediatr 7:650, 1995.
184. Imaizumi M, Gushi K, Kurobane I, et al: Long-term effects of bone marrow transplantation for inborn errors of metabolism: a study of four patients with lysosomal storage diseases. Acta Paediatr Japon 36:30, 1994.
185. Krivit W, Lockman L, Watkins P, et al: The future for treatment by bone marrow transplantation for adrenoleukodystrophy, metachromatic leukodystrophy, globoid cell leukodystrophy and Hurler syndrome. J Inherit Metabol Dis 18:398, 1995.
186. Westlake V, Jolly R, Jones B, et al: Hematopoietic cell transplantation in fetal lambs with ceroid-lipofuscinosis. Am J Med Genet 57:365, 1995.
187. Tulipan N, Hermanz-Schulman M, Bruner JP: Reduced hirdbrain hernination after intrauterine myelomingocele repair. A report of four cases. Pediatr Neurosurg 29:274, 1998.

Antepartum Fetal Evaluation

MAURICE L. DRUZIN, JAMES F. SMITH JR., STEVEN G. GABBE, AND KATHRYN L. REED

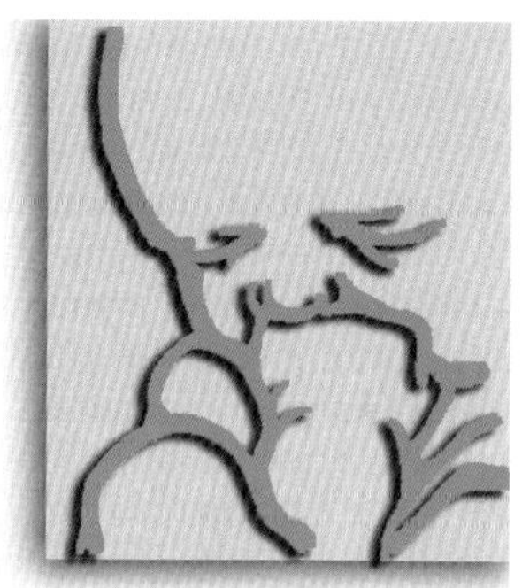

CHAPTER 11

KEY ABBREVIATIONS

American College of Obstetricians and Gynecologists	ACOG
Amniotic fluid index	AFI
Biophysical profile	BPP
Central nervous system	CNS
Contraction stress test	CST
Fetal breathing movement	FBM
Foam stability index	FSI
Intrauterine growth restriction	IUGR
Lecithin/sphingomyelin ratio	L/S
National Center for Health Statistics	NCHS
Nonstress test	NST
Oxytocin challenge test	OCT
Perinatal mortality rate	PMR
Phosphatidylglycerol	PG
Rapid eye movement	REM
Respiratory distress syndrome	RDS
Surfactant albumin ratio	SAR
Systolic/diastolic ratio	S/D
Vibroacoustic stimulation	VAS
World Health Organization	WHO

Not too long ago, the first aim of obstetric care was to prevent maternal death due to tuberculosis, syphilis, difficult deliveries, and hemorrhage. When this battle was won, at least in developed countries, and when perinatal mortality had dropped spectacularly, more time and interest could be focused on the fetus.[1]

Although antepartum fetal deaths are infrequent, they occur 10 times more frequently than sudden infant death. In 2002, there were approximately 26,000 stillbirths in the United States.[2] Antepartum fetal deaths now account for about 50 percent of all perinatal mortality in the United States.[3] The obstetrician must be concerned not only with prevention of this mortality but with the detection of fetal compromise and the timely delivery of such infants in an effort to maximize their future potential.[4] This chapter reviews the definition and causes of perinatal mortality, the techniques available for assessing fetal condition, how one may evaluate their diagnostic accuracy, and the clinical application of these techniques to obstetric practice.

THE ETIOLOGY OF PERINATAL MORTALITY

The perinatal mortality rate (PMR) has been defined by the National Center for Health Statistics (NCHS) as the number of late fetal deaths (fetal deaths of 28 weeks' gestation or more) plus early neonatal deaths (deaths of infants 0 to 6 days of age) per 1,000 live births plus fetal deaths.[5] A live birth is the complete expulsion or extraction of a product of conception from its mother, irrespective of the duration of the pregnancy, that, after separation, breathes or shows any evidence of life, such as beating of the heart, pulsation of the umbilical cord, or definite movement of voluntary muscles, whether or not the umbilical cord has been cut or the placenta is attached; each product of such a birth is considered live born. According to the NCHS, the neonatal mortality rate is defined as the number of neonatal deaths (deaths of infants 0 to 27 days of age) per 1,000 live births; the postneonatal mortality rate, the number of postneonatal deaths (the number of infants 28 to 365 days of age) per 1,000 live births; and the infant mortality rate, the number of infant deaths (deaths of infants under 1 year of age) per 1,000 live births. The definition of PMR provided by the World Health Organization (WHO) is somewhat different, including the number of fetuses and live births weighing at least 500 g or, when birth weight is unavailable, the corresponding gestational age (22 weeks) or body length (25 cm crown-heel) dying before day 7 of life per 1,000 such fetuses and infants.[6] The American College of Obstetricians and Gynecologists (ACOG) has recommended that only deaths of fetuses and infants weighing 500 g or more at delivery be used to compare data among states in the United States.[7] For international comparisons, only deaths of fetuses and infants weighing 1,000 g or more at delivery should be included,[7] bearing in mind that in developing countries, antepartum fetal deaths and preterm deliveries are likely to be significantly underreported.[2]

Since 1965, the PMR in the United States has fallen steadily. Using the NCHS definition, the PMR reported in 1997 was 7.3 per 1,000.[3] The neonatal mortality rate was 3.8 per 1,000, with fetal deaths at 3.5 per 1,000. The PMR for blacks, 13.2 per 1,000, was more than twice that of whites, 6.3 per 1,000. The significantly greater PMR in blacks results from higher rates of *both* neonatal and fetal deaths.

Although the majority of fetal deaths occur before 32 weeks' gestation, in planning a strategy for antepartum fetal monitoring, one must examine the risk of fetal death in the population of women who are still pregnant at that point in pregnancy.[8,9] When this approach is taken, one finds that fetuses at 40 to 41 weeks are at a threefold greater risk and those at 42 or more weeks are at a 12-fold greater risk for intrauterine death than fetuses at 28 to 31 weeks. The risks are even higher in multiple gestations, as pregnancy progresses. For twin gestations, the optimal time for delivery to prevent late gestation perinatal deaths is by 39 weeks, and for triplets, 36 weeks.[10]

The overall pattern of perinatal deaths in the United States has changed considerably during the past 40 years. Data collected between 1959 and 1966 by the Collaborative Perinatal Project revealed that 30 percent of perinatal deaths could be attributed to complications of the cord and placenta.[11] Other major causes of perinatal loss were maternal and fetal infections (17 percent), prematurity (10 percent), congenital anomalies (8 percent), and erythroblastosis fetalis (4 percent). In this series, 21 percent of the deaths were of unknown causes. In 1982, the major cause of early neonatal death was attributed to conditions originating in the perinatal period, such as infections, intraventricular hemorrhage, hydrops, meconium aspiration, and maternal complications such as diabetes mellitus and hypertension.[4] Congenital anomalies were the second leading cause of early neonatal death, accounting for 23 percent of such losses, whereas intrauterine hypoxia and birth asphyxia were responsible for 5 percent. In 2002, there were approximately 26,000 stillbirths, for a rate of 6.4 per 1000 total births. There were 28,000 infant deaths (7.0 per 1000 live births), and 19,000 (4.7 per 1000 live births) neonatal deaths.[6,12]

The stillbirth rate has shown a decline in the last 50 years but not to the same extent as the decline in infant deaths. The infant mortality rate has fallen progressively from 47.0 per 1,000 in 1940 to 26.0 per 1,000 in 1960, 12.6 per 1,000 in 1980, 9.2 per 1,000 in 1990, 7.2 per 1,000 in 1997, to 7.0 per 1000 in 2002.[6,13] Although the infant mortality rate includes all deaths of infants younger than 1 year of age, 50 percent of all infant deaths occur in the first week of life, and 50 percent of these losses result during the first day of life.[7] Clearly, perinatal events play an important role in infant mortality.[14] In 1994, the leading cause of infant mortality reported by the NCHS was "perinatal conditions not separately listed," including maternal complications such as hypertension and substance abuse, multiple pregnancy, placenta previa and abruption, breech delivery, prolonged pregnancy and macrosomia, congenital pneumonia and viral infections, meconium aspiration, and Rh isoimmunization. This diverse category accounted for 25.4 percent of infant mortality, whereas congenital anomalies and sudden infant death syndrome were responsible for 20.3 and 14.8 percent, respectively. Short gestation and low birth weight contributed 12.3 percent and respiratory distress syndrome (RDS) 6.7 percent. Only 2.1 percent of infant mortality was attributed to intrauterine hypoxia-birth asphyxia. Birth defects have been the single most important contributor to infant mortality for the past 20 years.[14] In 1995, malformations were responsible for 22 percent of all infant deaths, with one third caused by cardiac abnormalities and respiratory, central nervous system (CNS), and chromosomal defects each contributing approximately 15 percent.[15]

Fetal deaths may be divided into those that occur during the antepartum period and those that occur during labor, intrapartum stillbirths. From 70 to almost 90 percent of fetal deaths occurred before the onset of labor.[16] Manning et al.[17] point out that antepartum deaths may be divided into four broad categories: (1) chronic asphyxia of diverse origin; (2) congenital malformations; (3) superimposed complications of pregnancy, such as Rh isoimmunization, placental abruption, and fetal infection; and (4) deaths of unexplained cause. If it is to succeed, a program of antenatal surveillance must identify malformed fetuses (see Chapter 9) and recognize those at risk for asphyxia.

Recent data describing the specific etiologies of fetal deaths in the United States are not available. Fretts and colleagues[18,19] have analyzed the causes of deaths in fetuses weighing more than 500 g in 94,346 births at the Royal Victoria Hospital in Montreal from 1961 to 1993. The population studied was predominantly white and included patients from all socioeconomic groups. Approximately 95 percent made four or more prenatal visits. The autopsy rate in this series was greater than 95 percent. Overall, the fetal death rate declined by 70 percent, from 11.5 per 1,000 in the 1960s to 3.2 per 1,000 during 1990 to 1993.[19] The decline in the fetal death rate may be attributed to the prevention of Rh sensitization, antepartum fetal surveillance, improved detection of intrauterine growth restriction (IUGR) and fetal anomalies with ultrasound, and improved care of maternal diabetes mellitus and preeclampsia. Fetal deaths attributable to intrapartum asphyxia and Rh isoimmunization fell dramatically, from 13.1 to 1.2 per 1,000 for intrapartum asphyxia and 4.3 to 0.7 per 1,000 for Rh disease.[18] Deaths caused by lethal anomalies declined by 50 percent, 10.8 to 5.4 per 1,000, because early terminations of pregnancy were performed for anencephaly. Studies have documented an inverse association between fetal deaths for anomalies after 20 weeks and elective terminations before 20 weeks, suggesting that antenatal diagnosis of anomalies may influence the stillbirth rate.[20,21] Whereas fetal mortality resulting from IUGR fell 60 percent, 17.9 to 7.0 per 1,000 births, the growth-restricted fetus still had a more than 10-fold greater risk for fetal death than an appropriately grown fetus (see Chapter 29).

Fretts et al. noted that most of these deaths occurred between 28 and 36 weeks' gestation and that the diagnosis of IUGR was rarely identified before death. In addition to IUGR, leading causes of fetal death after 28 weeks' gestation included abruption and unexplained antepartum losses. Despite a marked fall in unexplained fetal deaths, 38.1 to 13.6 per 1,000, these losses were still responsible for more than 25 percent of all stillbirths. Fetal-maternal hemorrhage may occur in 10 to 15 percent of cases of unexplained fetal deaths. Fetal deaths caused by infection, most often associated with premature rupture of the membranes before 28 weeks' gestation, did not decline over the 30 years of the study, and accounted for about 19 percent of fetal deaths. Fretts et al.[19] also noted that, after controlling for risk factors such as multiple gestation, hypertension, diabetes mellitus, placenta previa and abruption, previous abortion, and prior fetal death, women 35 years of age or older had a nearly twofold greater risk for fetal death than women younger than 30 years. Data from Denmark have confirmed the J-shaped curve relationship between maternal age and fetal deaths, with the highest rates in teenagers and women older than 35 years of age.[22,23]

Schauer et al.[24] summarized data from seven studies evaluating the causes of fetal death after 20 weeks. The largest group was unexplained, mostly asphyxial intrauterine deaths, 9 to 50 percent; major anomalies, 7 to 21 percent; antepartum hemorrhage with or without verified abruption (as in the Fretts et al. data the single largest known cause of fetal death), 12 to 17 percent; IUGR, 7 to 15 percent; hypertension, 1.9 to 15.7 percent; isoimmunization, 2.3 to 7.7 percent; diabetes mellitus, less than 1 to 4.8 percent; and infection, 2.1 to 6.1 percent. In a prospective study of 107 late fetal deaths, all of which had a full autopsy, Schauer et al.[24] observed a similar distribution of causes: asphyxia, 66 percent; multiple anomalies, 6 percent; chromosomal disorders, 6 percent; infection, 3 percent, and unknown, 19 percent. The chromosomal abnormalities included trisomy 21, trisomy 18, and 45,XO.

In summary, based on available data, approximately 30 percent of antepartum fetal deaths may be attributed to asphyxia (IUGR, prolonged gestation), 30 percent to maternal complications (placental abruption, hypertension, preeclampsia, and diabetes mellitus), 15 percent to congenital malformations and chromosomal abnormalities, and 5 percent to infection. At least 20 percent of stillbirths have no obvious fetal, placental, maternal, or obstetric etiology, and this percentage increases with advancing gestational age. That is, late gestation stillbirths are more likely to have no identifiable etiology.[6]

Can these antepartum fetal deaths be prevented? Grant and Elbourne[9] have noted that "antepartum late fetal death is the component of perinatal mortality that has shown greatest resistance to change over recent years. In part, this reflects its relative unpredictability; in part, it reflects the relatively long period of time over which it can occur." Obstetric and pediatric assessors reviewed the circumstances surrounding each case of perinatal death in the Mersey region of England to identify any avoidable factors contributing to the death.[25] There were 309 perinatal deaths in this population, consisting of 157 stillbirths and 152 deaths in the first week of life. Of the 309 perinatal deaths, 182 (58.9 percent) were considered to have had avoidable factors. Most avoidable factors were found to be obstetric rather than pediatric or maternal and social. A high proportion (73.8 percent) of normal-birth-weight infants with no fetal abnormalities and no maternal complications had avoidable factors. The failure to respond appropriately to abnormalities during pregnancy and labor, including results from the monitoring of fetal growth or intrapartum fetal well-being, significant maternal weight loss, or reported reductions in fetal movement, constituted the largest groups of avoidable factors. Kirkup and Welch[26] confirmed these results in an analysis of avoidable factors contributing to fetal death in nonmalformed infants weighing 2,500 g or more. Patients at highest risk for fetal death included women of a parity of three or more and those who had no prenatal care before 20 weeks. The Mersey Region Working Party on Perinatal Mortality concluded that, in light of increasing public awareness about obstetric management and, in some instances, an antipathy toward modern procedures, the failure to act on abnormalities discovered during monitoring would assume greater importance.[25] These workers found that in no case was the induction of labor as a result of such monitoring considered an avoidable factor. In an interesting application of a sensitivity analysis of antepartum testing late in pregnancy in the older population, Fretts et al. found that although testing was associated with the most significant decrease in stillbirth, it was associated with a higher risk of induction of labor and cesarean delivery.[27] However, for the multiparous women of advanced age, with an odds ratio of fetal death of 3.3 compared with the younger patient, approximately 14 additional cesarean deliveries for failed inductions would be done to prevent a single stillbirth, a number many would consider acceptable.

A large clinical experience has demonstrated that antepartum fetal assessment can have a significant impact on the frequency and causes of antenatal fetal deaths. Schneider and colleagues[28] reviewed a decade of experience with antepartum fetal heart rate monitoring from 1974 through 1983. The contraction stress test (CST) was used primarily during the first 2 years of the study, followed by the nonstress test (NST). Overall, the PMR was found to be 22.4 per 1,000 in the nontested population and 11.8 per 1,000 in the tested high-risk population, a highly significant difference. The stillbirth rate in the nontested population, 11.1 per 1,000, was twice that of patients who were followed with antepartum surveillance. When corrected for congenital anomalies, the stillbirth rate in the tested high-risk population was only 2.2 per 1,000. Of 18 stillbirths within 7 days of testing, the majority were because of congenital anomalies and placental abruption.

In a carefully performed study, Stubblefield and Berek[29] reviewed the causes of perinatal death in term and postterm births. The most frequent cause of death of a term or postterm infant was extrinsic perinatal hypoxia, and the second most common cause was a lethal malformation. Overall, extrinsic perinatal hypoxia accounted for 56.1 percent of the deaths of term infants and 71.4 percent of the deaths of postterm infants. Major malformations were implicated in 26.3 percent of the deaths of term infants. Twenty-nine of the 32 antenatal deaths occurred between 37 and 42 weeks' gestation. The authors concluded that two thirds of the antenatal deaths were associated with chronic processes such as placental infarction that might have been detected had routine antepartum fetal surveillance been used. In obstetric populations in which high-risk patients are monitored, the majority of stillbirths now occur in what had previously been considered normal pregnancies.

APPLICATION OF ANTEPARTUM FETAL TESTING

Before using antepartum fetal testing, the obstetrician must ask several important questions[30]:

1. Does the test provide information not already known by the patient's clinical status?
2. Can the information be helpful in managing the patient?
3. Should an abnormality be detected, is there a treatment available for the problem?
4. Could an abnormal test result lead to increased risk for the mother or fetus?
5. Will the test ultimately decrease perinatal morbidity and mortality?

Unfortunately, few of the tests commonly employed today in clinical practice have been subjected to prospective and randomized evaluations that can answer these questions.[31–34] In most cases, when the test has been applied and good perinatal outcomes were observed, the test has gained further acceptance and has been used more widely. In such cases, one cannot be sure whether it is actually the information provided by the test that has led to the improved outcomes or whether it is the total program of care that has made the difference. When prospective randomized investigations are conducted, large numbers of patients must be studied, because many adverse outcomes such as intrauterine death are uncommon even in high-risk populations.[32] Although several controlled trials have failed to demonstrate improved outcomes with nonstress testing, the study populations ranged from only 300 to 530 subjects.[35–38]

The information one might predict from an antepartum fetal test is listed in the box "Aspects of Fetal Condition that Might be Predicted by Antepartum Testing." Although one would want to detect IUGR or discover the presence of a significant congenital malformation, the most valuable information provided by antepartum fetal assessment may be that the fetus is well and requires no intervention. In this way, the pregnancy may be safely prolonged and the fetus allowed to gain further maturity.[34] The second box lists those aspects of obstetric management that might be influenced by antepartum testing. Certainly, one would not want to begin a program of testing unless one were prepared to use the information.

Aspects of Fetal Condition That Might be Predicted by Antepartum Testing

- Perinatal death
- Intrauterine growth restriction (IUGR)
- Nonreassuring fetal status, intrapartum
- Neonatal asphyxia
- Postnatal motor and intellectual impairment
- Premature delivery
- Congenital abnormalities
- Need for specific therapy

Adapted from Chard T, Klopper A (eds): Introduction. *In* Placental Function Tests. New York, Springer-Verlag, 1982, p 1.

Obstetric Management That Might be Influenced by Antepartum Testing

- Preterm delivery
- Route of delivery
- Bed rest
- Observation
- Drug therapy
- Operative intervention in labor
- Neonatal intensive care
- Termination of pregnancy for a congenital anomaly

Adapted from Chard T, Klopper A (eds): Introduction. *In* Placental Function Tests. New York, Springer-Verlag, 1982, p 1.

Using the information has invariably meant prompt intervention by delivery that may not be indicated and could lead to potentially avoidable complications of prematurity. A more current approach is to use the term *intervention* to describe other types of procedures short of premature delivery. This strategy would include using combinations of antepartum tests in an organized sequence to evaluate the fetus further; administration of antenatal steroids; bed rest; prolonged oxygen therapy; and correction of maternal metabolic, cardiopulmonary, or other medical disorders. *Intervention* may also refer to fetal therapy such as intrauterine transfusion for anemia, removal of fluid from body cavities, diagnostic procedures, and direct administration of medication to the fetus.

Testing can be initiated at early gestational ages, 25 to 26 weeks, to identify the fetus at risk. Maternal and fetal interventions can then be considered. Obviously, safe prolongation of intrauterine life is the primary goal, and better understanding of the pathophysiology of the premature fetus and the use of combinations of tests will allow this to be accomplished. In the event of impending in utero death or severe compromise, premature delivery, although the last resort, is a reasonable option, given the remarkable survival statistics being reported in modern neonatal intensive care units (see Chapters 20 and 26). The use of postnatal surfactant and improved mechanical ventilators are only some of the advances leading to survival and intact neurologic survival statistics that would have been incomprehensible in previous decades.[39–41]

In selecting the population of patients for antepartum fetal evaluation, one would certainly include those pregnancies known to be at high risk of uteroplacental

Indications for Antepartum Fetal Monitoring

1. Patients at high risk of uteroplacental insufficiency
   - Prolonged pregnancy
   - Diabetes mellitus
   - Hypertension
   - Previous stillbirth
   - Suspected IUGR
   - Advanced maternal age
   - Multiple gestation with discordant growth
   - Antiphospholipid syndrome
2. When other tests suggest fetal compromise
   - Suspected IUGR
   - Decreased fetal movement
   - Oligohydramnios
3. Routine antepartum surveillance

IUGR, intrauterine growth restriction.

insufficiency (see the box "Indications for Antepartum Fetal Monitoring").[34]

The question of routine antepartum fetal surveillance must be carefully examined. Antepartum fetal testing can more accurately predict fetal outcome than antenatal risk assessment using an established scoring system.[42] Patients judged to be at high risk based on known medical factors but whose fetuses demonstrated normal antepartum fetal evaluation had a lower PMR than did patients considered at low risk, whose fetuses had abnormal antepartum testing results. Routine antepartum fetal evaluation would be necessary to detect most infants dying in utero as the result of hypoxia and asphyxia.[29] It would seem reasonable, therefore, to consider extending some form of antepartum fetal surveillance to all obstetric patients. As described later, assessment of fetal activity by the mother may be an ideal technique for this purpose.

STATISTICAL ASSESSMENT OF ANTEPARTUM TESTING

To determine the clinical application of antepartum diagnostic testing, the predictive value of the tests must be considered.[43,44] This information can most easily be presented in a 2 × 2 matrix. Table 11-1 presents this matrix using the CST and intrauterine fetal death as examples. The sensitivity of the test is the probability that the test will be positive or abnormal when the disease is present. The specificity of the test is the probability that the test result will be negative when the disease is not present. Note that the sensitivity and specificity refer not to the actual numbers of patients with a positive or abnormal result but to the proportion or probability of these test results. The predictive value of an abnormal test would be that fraction of patients with an abnormal test result who have the abnormal condition, and the predictive value of a normal test would be the fraction of patients with a normal test result who are normal (Table 11-1).

Antepartum fetal tests may be used to screen a large obstetric population to detect fetal disease. In this setting, a test of high sensitivity is preferable, because one would not want to miss patients whose fetuses might be compromised. One would be willing to overdiagnose the

Table 11-1. Two-by-Two Matrix of Possible Results for the Contraction Stress Test

	PERINATAL OUTCOME	
TEST RESULT	NORMAL (NORMAL NEWBORN)	ABNORMAL (INTRAUTERINE FETAL DEATH)
Normal (negative CST)	A True-negative	B False-negative
Abnormal (positive CST)	C False-positive	D True-positive

Sensitivity = D/(D + B).
Specificity = A/(A + C).
Predictive value of a positive test = D/(C + D).
Predictive value of a negative test = A/(A + B).

Table 11-2. Fifty Percent Prevalence

	PERINATAL OUTCOME	
TEST RESULT	NORMAL	ABNORMAL
Normal	490 True negative	125 False negative
Abnormal	10 False positive	375 True positive

Sensitivity = 75%.
Specificity = 98%.
Predictive value of a positive test = 97.4% (375 of 385).
Predictive value of a negative test = 79.6% (490 of 615).

problem, that is, accept some false-positive diagnoses. In further evaluating the patient whose fetus may be at risk and when attempting to confirm the presence of disease, one would want a test of high specificity. One would not want to intervene unnecessarily and deliver a fetus that was doing well. In this setting, multiple tests may be helpful. When multiple test results are normal, they tend to exclude disease. When all are abnormal, however, they tend to support the diagnosis of fetal disease.

The prevalence of the abnormal condition has great impact on the predictive value of antepartum fetal tests. Table 11-2 presents data for a population of 1,000 patients in whom the prevalence of the disease is 50 percent. The sensitivity of the test being evaluated is 75 percent, and its specificity is 98 percent. These figures are similar to those observed for several antepartum tests now in use. In this setting, an abnormal test result is likely to be associated with a true fetal abnormality. The predictive value of a positive test is 97.4 percent. However, when the prevalence of the disease falls to 2 percent, as it may be for intrauterine fetal deaths, even tests with a high sensitivity and specificity are associated with many false predictions (Table 11-3). In this circumstance, an abnormal test is more likely to indicate a false-positive diagnosis (n = 20) than it is a true-positive diagnosis (n = 15).

In interpreting the results of studies of antepartum testing, the obstetrician must consider the application of that test to his or her own population. If the study has been done in a population of patients at great risk, it is more likely that an abnormal test will be associated with

Table 11-3. Two Percent Prevalence

	PERINATAL OUTCOME	
TEST RESULT	**NORMAL**	**ABNORMAL**
Normal	960 True-negative	5 False-negative
Abnormal	20 False-positive	15 True-positive

Sensitivity = 75%.
Specificity = 98%.
Predictive value of a positive test = 42.8% (15 of 35).
Predictive value of a negative test = 99.4% (960 of 965).

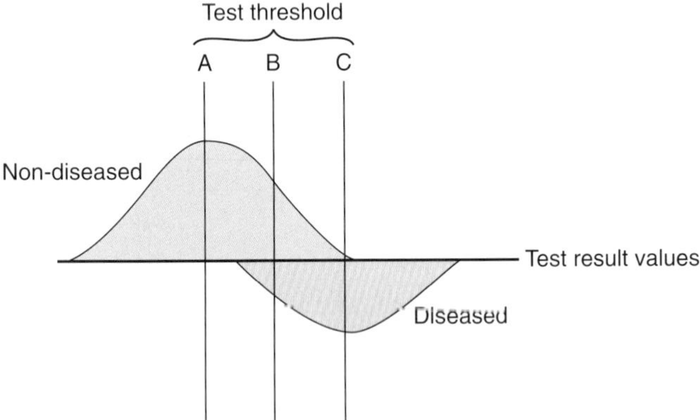

Figure 11-1. Hypothetical distribution of test results in a normal and diseased population, demonstrating the differences in test sensitivity and specificity with a change in test threshold. Making it more difficult for the fetus to pass the test by raising the test threshold (A) will increase the sensitivity, but decrease the specificity, of the test. On the other hand, making the test easier to pass by decreasing the test threshold (C) will increase the specificity of the test, but decrease the sensitivity. (Adapted from Carpenter M, Coustan D: Criteria for screening tests for gestational diabetes. Am J Obstet Gynecol 144:768, 1982.)

an abnormal fetus. If the obstetrician is practicing in a community with patients who are, in general, at low risk, however, an abnormal test result would more likely be associated with a false-positive diagnosis.

For most antepartum diagnostic tests, a cut-off point used to define an abnormal result must be arbitrarily established.[45] The cut-off point is selected to maximize the separation between the normal and diseased populations (Fig. 11-1). Changing the cut-off will have a great impact on the predictive value of the test. For example, suppose that 10 accelerations in 10 minutes were required for a fetus to have a reactive NST (threshold A). The fetus who fulfilled this rigid definition would almost certainly be in good condition. However, many fetuses who failed to achieve 10 accelerations in 10 minutes would also be in good condition, but would be judged to be abnormal by this cut-off. In this instance, the test would have many abnormal results. It would be highly sensitive and capture all of the abnormal fetuses, but it would have a low specificity. If the number of accelerations required to pass a NST were lowered to 1 in 10 minutes, it would decrease the sensitivity of the test (threshold C). That is, one might miss a truly sick fetus. At the same time, however, one would improve the specificity of the test or its ability to predict that percentage of the patients who are normal. Using the criterion of two accelerations of the fetal heart rate in 20 minutes for a reactive NST (threshold B), one hopes to have a test with both high sensitivity and high specificity.

BIOPHYSICAL TECHNIQUES OF FETAL EVALUATION

Fetal State

When interpreting tests that monitor fetal biophysical characteristics, one must appreciate that, during the third trimester, the normal fetus may exhibit marked changes in its neurologic state.[46,47] Four fetal states have been identified. The near-term fetus spends approximately 25 percent of its time in a quiet sleep state (state 1F) and 60 to 70 percent in an active sleep state (state 2F). Active sleep is associated with rapid eye movement (REM). In fetal lambs, electrocortical activity during REM sleep is characterized by low-voltage, high-frequency waves. The fetus exhibits regular breathing movements and intermittent abrupt movements of its head, limbs, and trunk. The fetal heart rate in active sleep (state 2F) exhibits increased variability and frequent accelerations with movement. During quiet, or non-REM, sleep, the fetal heart rate slows and heart rate variability is reduced. The fetus may make infrequent breathing movements and startled movements. Electrocortical activity recordings at this time reveal high-voltage, low-frequency waves. Near term, periods of quiet sleep may last 20 minutes, and those of active sleep approximately 40 minutes.[47] The mechanisms that control these periods of rest and activity in the fetus are not well established. External factors such as the mother's activity, her ingestion of drugs, and her nutrition may play a role.

When evaluating fetal condition using the NST or the biophysical profile (BPP), one must ask whether a fetus that is not making breathing movements or shows no accelerations of its baseline heart rate is in a quiet sleep state or is neurologically compromised. In such circumstances, prolonging the period of evaluation usually allows a change in fetal state, and more normal parameters of fetal well-being appear.

Maternal Assessment of Fetal Activity

Maternal assessment of fetal activity is a simple yet valuable method for monitoring fetal condition. Most patients can understand and follow protocols for counting fetal activity, and this method is obviously inexpensive. Therefore, maternal assessment of fetal activity may be ideal for routine antepartum fetal surveillance.

Studies performed using real-time ultrasonography have demonstrated that during the third trimester, the human fetus spends 10 percent of its time making gross fetal body movements and that 30 such movements are made each hour.[48] Periods of active fetal body movement last approximately 40 minutes, whereas quiet periods last about 20 minutes. Patrick et al.[48] noted that the longest period without fetal movements in a normal fetus was approximately 75 minutes. The mother is able to appreciate about 70 to 80 percent of gross fetal movements. The fetus does make fine body movements such as limb flexion and extension, hand grasping, and sucking, which probably reflect more coordinated CNS function. However, the mother is generally unable to perceive these fine movements. Fetal movement appears to peak between 9:00 p.m. and 1:00 a.m., a time when maternal glucose levels are falling.[47,48] In a study in which maternal glucose levels were carefully controlled with an artificial pancreas, Holden et al.[49] found that hypoglycemia was associated with increased fetal movement. Fetal activity does not increase after meals or after maternal glucose administration.[50,51]

Maternal evaluation of fetal activity may reduce fetal deaths caused by asphyxia. Using a sheep model, Natale et al.[52] demonstrated that fetal activity is extremely sensitive to a decrease in fetal oxygenation. A small fall in fetal Po_2 was associated with a cessation of limb movements in the fetal lamb.

Several methods have been used to monitor fetal activity in clinical practice. In general, the presence of fetal movements is a reassuring sign of fetal health. However, the absence of fetal activity requires further assessment before one can conclude that fetal compromise exists. Sadovsky et al.[53] recommended that mothers count fetal activity for 30 to 60 minutes each day, two or three times daily. If the mother has fewer than three movements in 1 hour, or if she appreciates no movements for 12 hours, the movement alarm signal, further evaluation of fetal condition must be made. Rayburn et al.[54] suggested that patients count fetal activity at least 60 minutes each day. Fewer than three movements an hour for 2 consecutive days may be a sign of fetal compromise. Pearson and Weaver[55] advocated the use of the Cardiff Count-to-Ten chart. They found that only 2.5 percent of 1,654 daily movement counts recorded by 61 women who subsequently delivered healthy infants fell below 10 movements per 12 hours. Therefore, they accepted 10 movements as the minimum amount of fetal activity the patient should perceive in a 12-hour period. The patient is asked to start counting the movements in the morning and to record the time of day at which the 10th movement has been perceived. Should the patient not have 10 movements during 12 hours, or should it take longer each day to reach 10 movements, the patient is told to contact her obstetrician. Sadovsky et al.[56] found that, of those techniques currently used in clinical management, the movement alarm signal and the technique of Pearson and Weaver are the most valuable.

Whatever technique is used must be carefully explained to the patient. Although most women are reassured by keeping a fetal activity chart and maternal-fetal attachment may be enhanced, some patients do become more anxious.[57,58] Women who were concerned about monitoring fetal movement complained that they were not given adequate information about variations in fetal activity patterns and maternal perception of movement.

Although there will be a wide but normal range in fetal activity, with fetal movement counting, each mother and her fetus serve as their own control.[9] Fetal and placental factors that influence maternal assessment of fetal activity include placental location, the length of fetal movements, the amniotic fluid volume, and fetal anomalies.[59] If the placenta is anterior, maternal perception of fetal movements may be decreased. Movements lasting 20 to 60 seconds are most likely to be felt by the mother.[60] Hydramnios reduces the mother's appreciation of fetal activity. Hydramnios may be associated with a fetal anomaly and should be further evaluated using ultrasonography. Rayburn and Barr[60] reported that 26 percent of fetuses with major malformations show decreased fetal activity compared with only 4 percent of normal fetuses. Anomalies of the CNS are most commonly associated with decreased activity.

Approximately 80 percent of all mothers are able to comply with a program of counting fetal activity.[9,62] Maternal factors that influence the evaluation of fetal movement include maternal activity, obesity, and medications. Mothers appear to appreciate fetal movements best when resting in the left lateral recumbent position. Therefore, patients should be told to lie down when counting fetal movement, an additional benefit of this approach to fetal evaluation. Obesity decreases maternal appreciation of fetal activity. Maternal medications such as narcotics or barbiturates may depress fetal movement.

Several large clinical studies have demonstrated the efficacy of maternal assessment of fetal activity in preventing unexplained fetal deaths. In a prospective randomized study, Neldam[62,63] asked one group of 1,562 pregnant patients at 32 weeks' gestation to count fetal activity three times each week for 2 hours after their main meals. Fewer than three fetal movements each hour was regarded as a sign of potential fetal compromise and was further evaluated with an ultrasound examination and an NST. In the monitored group of patients, only one stillbirth occurred. Ten stillbirths were noted in a control population of 1,549 women. Overall, 4 percent of patients in the monitored group reported their baby was not moving adequately, a low figure, but one similar to that observed in other studies. Of these 60 patients, almost 25 percent were found to have a fetus in distress based on further antepartum testing. Neldam[63] attributed the prevention of 14 fetal deaths to the use of maternal assessment of fetal activity.

Rayburn[64] found that in the 5 percent of his patients who reported decreased fetal activity the incidence of stillbirths was 60 times higher, the risk of fetal distress in labor 2 to 3 times higher, the incidence of low Apgar scores at delivery 10 times greater, and the incidence of severe growth restriction 10 times higher. Rayburn also observed that the normal fetus does *not* decrease activity in the week before delivery.

Using the Cardiff Count-to-Ten chart, Liston et al.[65] noted that 11 of 150 high-risk patients (7.3 percent) reported fewer than 10 movements in a 12-hour period. Two of these patients suffered perinatal deaths, and 33 percent experienced fetal distress in labor. Overall, 60 percent of patients who reported decreased fetal activity did exhibit evidence of fetal compromise. The number of false alarms was manageable.

Two prospective studies have yielded conflicting results regarding the efficacy of fetal movement counting as a technique for preventing fetal deaths. Grant and coworkers[66] recruited 68,000 European women who were randomly allocated within 33 pairs of clusters to either routine fetal movement counting using the Cardiff Count-to-Ten method or to standard care. Women counted for an average of almost 3 hours per day, and about 7 percent of the charts showed at least one alarm. Of concern, the rate of compliance for reporting decreased fetal movement was only 46 percent. Furthermore, compliance for charting movements and reporting alarms was lower among women who had a late fetal death. The antepartum death rates for nonmalformed singleton fetuses were equal in both experimental groups. However, in none of the 17 cases in which reduced movements were recognized and the fetus was still alive when the patient arrived at the hospital was an emergency delivery attempted. Why? Grant et al.[66] believe that intervention was not undertaken because of false reassurance from follow-up testing, especially heart rate monitoring, and because of errors in clinical judgment. One might conclude that this large prospective study failed to demonstrate a reduction in the antepartum fetal death rate as a result of fetal movement counting. However, what it seems to prove most clearly is that patient compliance is an essential part of this program, as is appropriate evaluation of the patient who presents with decreased fetal activity.

In contrast, an investigation by Moore and Piacquadio[67] demonstrated an impressive reduction in fetal deaths resulting from a formal program of fetal movement counting. Patients used the Count-to-Ten approach but were told to monitor fetal activity in the evening, a time of increased fetal movement. Most women observed 10 movements in an average of 21 minutes, and compliance was greater than 90 percent. Patients who did not perceive 10 movements in 2 hours, a level of fetal activity slightly more than 5 SD below the mean, were told to report immediately for further evaluation. During a 7-month control period, a fetal mortality rate of 8.7 per 1,000 was observed in 2,519 patients, and 11 of 247 women who came to the hospital with a complaint of decreased fetal movement had already suffered an intrauterine death. During the study period, the fetal death rate fell to 2.1 per 1,000, and only 1 of 290 patients with decreased fetal movement presented after fetal death had occurred. The number of antepartum tests required to assess patients with decreased fetal activity rose 13 percent during the study period. This investigation has been expanded to include almost 6,000 patients, and a fetal death rate of 3.6 per 1,000, less than half that found in the control period, has been achieved.[68]

Froen has recently advanced an reanalysis of the study by Grant, as well as review of current literature on maternal perception of fetal movement, and suggests a benefit to this form of antepartum testing.[69] However, for fetal movement counting to reduce the rate of stillbirth, diligence from the patient, to accurately and timely report diminished fetal movements, and providers, to determinatively and comprehensively assess fetal condition, must be emphasized.

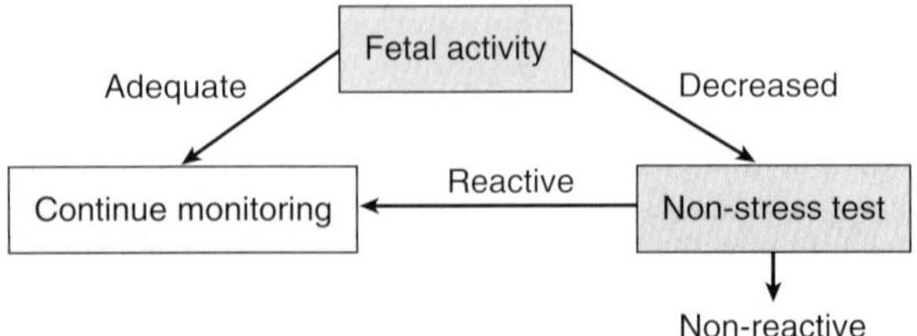

Figure 11-2. Maternal assessment of fetal activity is a valuable screening test for fetal condition. Should the mother report decreased fetal activity, an NST is performed. In this situation, most NSTs are reactive. NST, nonstress test.

In conclusion, there is a clearly established relationship between decreased fetal activity and fetal death. Therefore, it would seem prudent to request that *all* pregnant patients, regardless of their risk status, monitor fetal activity starting at 28 weeks' gestation (Fig. 11-2). The Count-to-Ten approach developed by Moore and Piacquadio[68] seems ideal.

Contraction Stress Test

The CST, also known as the oxytocin challenge test (OCT), was the first biophysical technique widely applied for antepartum fetal surveillance. It was well known that uterine contractions produced a reduction in blood flow to the intervillous space. Analyses of intrapartum fetal heart rate monitoring had demonstrated that a fetus with inadequate placental respiratory reserve would demonstrate late decelerations in response to hypoxia (see Chapter 15). The CST extended these observations to the antepartum period. The response of the fetus at risk for uteroplacental insufficiency to uterine contractions formed the basis for this test.

Performing the Contraction Stress Test

The CST may be conducted in the labor and delivery suite or in an adjacent area, although the likelihood of fetal distress requiring immediate delivery in response to uterine contractions or hyperstimulation is extremely small. The CST should be performed by staff familiar with the principles and technique of such testing. In many institutions, an antenatal diagnostic unit has been developed for this purpose. The patient is placed in the semi-Fowler's position at a 30- to 45-degree angle with a slight left tilt to avoid the supine hypotensive syndrome. The fetal heart rate is recorded using a Doppler ultrasound transducer, and uterine contractions are monitored with the tocodynamometer. Maternal blood pressure is determined every 5 to 10 minutes to detect maternal hypotension.[70] Baseline fetal heart rate and uterine tone are first recorded for a period of approximately 10 to 20 minutes. In some cases, adequate uterine activity occurs spontaneously, and additional uterine stimulation is not necessary. An adequate CST requires uterine contractions of moderate intensity lasting approximately 40 to 60 seconds with a frequency of three in 10 minutes. These criteria were selected to approximate the stress experienced by the fetus during the first stage of labor. If uterine activity is absent or inadequate, nipple stimulation is used to initiate contractions or intravenous oxytocin is begun. Oxytocin is administered by an infusion pump at 0.5 mU/min. The infusion rate is doubled every 20 minutes until adequate uterine contractions have been achieved.[34] One does not usually need to exceed 10 mU/min to produce adequate uterine activity. After the CST has been completed, the patient should be observed until uterine activity has returned to its baseline level. With nipple stimulation, the test may take approximately 30 minutes. If oxytocin is needed, 90 minutes may be required to perform the CST.

Contraindications to the test include those patients at high risk for premature labor, such as patients with premature rupture of the membranes, multiple gestation, and cervical incompetence, although the CST has not been associated with an increased incidence of premature labor.[71] The CST should also be avoided in conditions in which uterine contractions may be dangerous, such as placenta previa and a previous classic cesarean section or uterine surgery.

Interpreting the Contraction Stress Test

Most clinicians use the definitions proposed by Freeman to interpret the CST[71,72] (Table 11-4). In an attempt to decrease the frequency of suspicious tests that would require further evaluation, Martin and Schifrin[73] developed the "10-minute window" concept. A positive test would be any 10-minute segment of the tracing that includes three contractions, all showing late decelerations. A negative test is one in which no positive window is seen and there is at least one negative window, three uterine contractions in 10 minutes with no late decelerations (Figs. 11-3 and 11-4). The CST would be read as negative and not suspicious if an occasional late deceleration were seen, but a negative window was also present. They used the term *equivocal* rather than *suspicious* for a CST with an occasional late deceleration but no negative window. Equivocal implies that one is unable to make a determination of fetal condition based on the available information. A CST with both a positive and negative window would be interpreted as positive.

Variable decelerations that occur during the CST may indicate cord compression often associated with oligohydramnios. In such cases, ultrasonography should be performed to assess amniotic fluid volume. However, even if the amniotic fluid volume is demonstrated to be adequate, cord compression patterns need careful follow-up, because cord accidents with subsequent fetal death may occur in the presence of normal amounts of amniotic fluid on sonography. What appears to be a normal volume of amniotic fluid may contain meconium, which has a specific gravity different from clear amniotic fluid and therefore does not allow the cord to float freely. In cases of early placental insufficiency, the amount of

Table 11-4. Interpretation of the Contraction Stress Test

INTERPRETATION	DESCRIPTION	INCIDENCE (%)
Negative	No late decelerations appearing anywhere on the tracing with adequate uterine contractions (three in 10 minutes)	80
Positive	Late decelerations that are consistent and persistent, present with the majority (>50 percent) of contractions without excessive uterine activity; if persistent late decelerations seen before the frequency of contractions is adequate, test interpreted as positive	3–5
Suspicious	Inconsistent late decelerations	5
Hyperstimulation	Uterine contractions closer than every 2 minutes or lasting >90 seconds, or five uterine contractions in 10 minutes; if no late decelerations seen, test interpreted as negative	5
Unsatisfactory	Quality of the tracing inadequate for interpretation or adequate uterine activity cannot be achieved	5

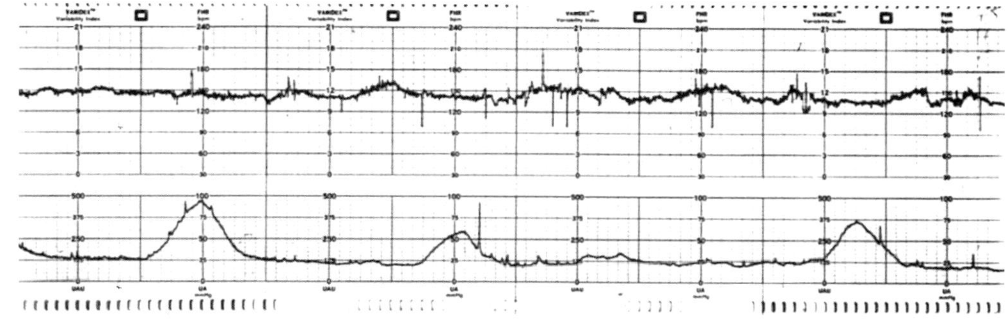

Figure 11-3. A reactive and negative CST. With this result, the CST would ordinarily be repeated in 1 week. CST, contraction stress test.

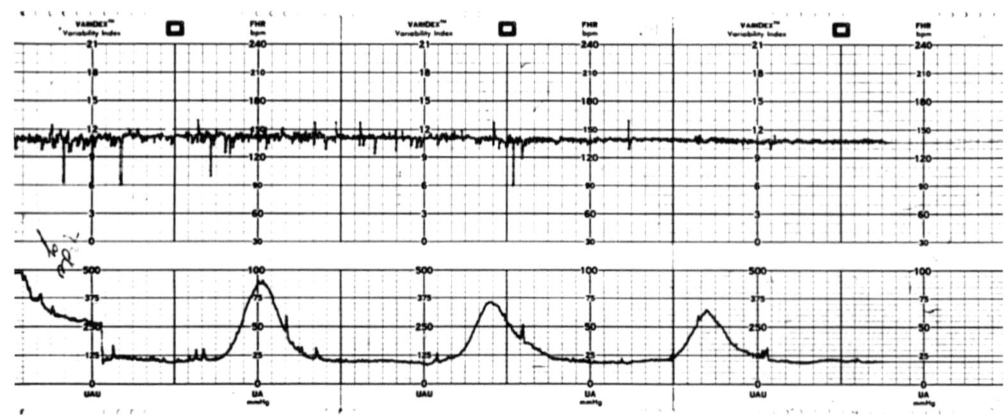

Figure 11-4. A nonreactive and negative CST. After this result, the test would ordinarily be repeated in 24 hours.

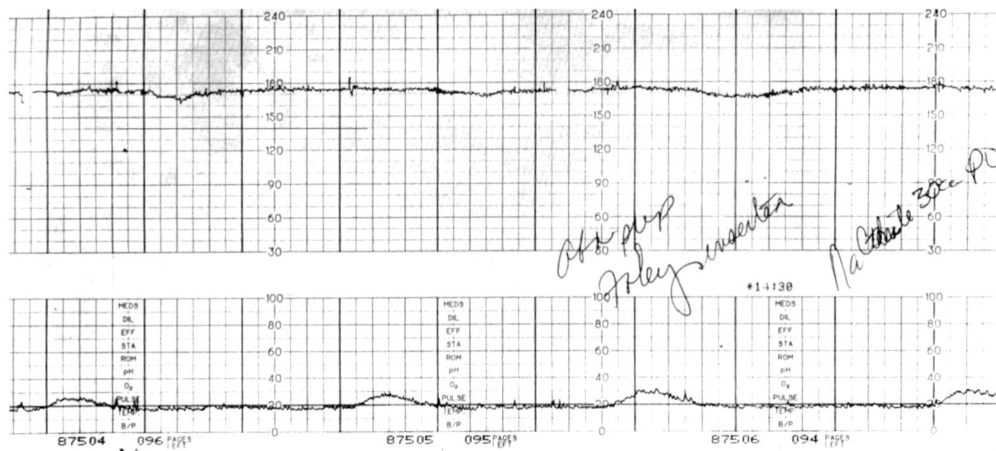

Figure 11-5. A nonreactive and positive CST with fetal tachycardia. At 34 weeks, a poorly compliant patient with type 1 diabetes mellitus reported decreased fetal activity. The NST revealed a fetal tachycardia of 170 bpm and was nonreactive. The CST was positive, and a BPP score was 2. The patient's cervix was unfavorable for induction. The patient underwent a low transverse cesarean delivery of a 2,200-g male infant with Apgar scores of 1 and 3. The umbilical arterial pH was 7.21. BPP, biophysical profile; CST, contraction stress test; NST, nonstress test.

Wharton's jelly in the umbilical cord may be diminished before the clinical appearance of oligohydramnios. The loss of the protective Wharton's jelly may make the umbilical vessels vulnerable to compression and lead to diminished blood flow.

A negative CST has been consistently associated with good fetal outcome. Therefore, a negative result permits the obstetrician to prolong a high-risk pregnancy safely. Nageotte et al.[74] reported only one preventable fetal death in 1,337 high-risk patients within 7 days after a negative CST. In a series of 679 pregnancies complicated by a prolonged gestation, Freeman et al.[75] observed no perinatal deaths when the CST was used as the primary method of surveillance. Of 337 women with a previous intrauterine fetal death, none had a stillbirth during a pregnancy in which they were followed with CSTs.[76] Druzin et al.[77] reported no antepartum deaths in a series of 819 patients tested at 280 days or more gestation, using both the NST and nipple stimulation CST. There were no differences in perinatal outcome in the group with a reactive NST, irrespective of the CST result. Similarly, Gabbe et al.[78] and Lagrew et al.[79] have reported only one fetal death within 1 week of a negative CST in 811 pregnancies complicated by type 1 diabetes mellitus. Other studies have shown the incidence of perinatal death within 1 week of a negative CST to be less than 1 per 1,000.[80–82] Many of these deaths, however, can be attributed to cord accidents, malformations, placental abruption, and acute deterioration of glucose control in patients with diabetes. Thus, the CST, like most methods of antepartum fetal surveillance, cannot predict acute fetal compromise. If the CST is negative, a repeat study is usually scheduled in 1 week. Changes in the patient's clinical condition may warrant more frequent studies.

A positive CST has been associated with an increased incidence of intrauterine death, late decelerations in labor, low 5-minute Apgar scores, IUGR, and meconium-stained amniotic fluid (Fig. 11-5).[82] In a prospective and blinded study, Ray et al.[83] observed three fetal deaths in 15 patients with positive CSTs. The incidence of low Apgar scores in this group was 53 percent. Overall, the likelihood of perinatal death after a positive CST has ranged from 7 to 15 percent. On the other hand, there has been a significant incidence of false-positive CSTs that, depending on the end point used, will average approximately 30 percent.[84] The positive CST is more likely to be associated with fetal compromise if the baseline heart rate lacks accelerations or "reactivity" and the latency period between the onset of the uterine contractions and the onset of the late deceleration is less than 45 seconds.[85,86]

There is no doubt that the high incidence of false-positive CSTs is one of the greatest limitations of this test, because such results could lead to unnecessary premature intervention. False-positive CSTs may be attributable to misinterpretation of the tracing; supine hypotension, which decreases uterine perfusion; uterine hyperstimulation, which is not appreciated using the tocodynamometer; or an improvement in fetal condition after the CST has been performed. The high false-positive rate also indicates that a patient with a positive CST need not necessarily require an elective cesarean delivery. If a trial of labor is to be undertaken after a positive CST, the cervix should be favorable for induction so that direct fetal heart rate monitoring and careful assessment of uterine contractility with an intrauterine pressure catheter can be performed. False-positive results are not increased when the CST is used early in the third trimester.[84] A negative or positive CST obtained between 28 and 33 weeks' gestation appears to have the same diagnostic significance as it would later in gestation. Merrill et al.[87] reported prolongation of pregnancy for up to 13 days in the presence of a nonreactive NST and a positive CST test if the BPP score was 6 or greater. This approach should be used only in the premature fetus and when careful follow-up with daily assessment, using the NST, CST, and BPP can be reliably performed.

A suspicious or equivocal CST should be repeated in 24 hours. Most of these tests will become negative. Bruce et al.[88] did observe that 5 of 67 patients (7.5 percent) with an initially suspicious CST exhibited positive tests on further evaluation. In 36 patients, the CST became negative, whereas in 26 patients it remained suspicious. Like the suspicious CST, a test that is unsatisfactory or shows hyperstimulation should be repeated in 24 hours.

In follow-up studies of children who demonstrated a positive CST, few have exhibited abnormalities in neurologic and psychological development.[89–91] An important determinant in the long-term outcome for these children would be the early recognition of nonreassuring fetal heart rate patterns and the prevention of intrapartum compromise.

The Nipple Stimulation Contraction Stress Test

Many centers use nipple stimulation to produce the uterine contractions needed for the CST. With nipple stimulation, the CST can generally be completed in less time, and an intravenous infusion is not required. Therefore, this approach would appear to be an ideal first step in performing a CST.

Several methods have been used to induce adequate uterine activity.[34,92,93] The patient may first apply a warm moist towel to each breast for 5 minutes. If uterine activity is not adequate, the patient is asked to massage one nipple for 10 minutes. Using this protocol, Oki et al.[92] achieved adequate uterine contractions in 30 minutes or less in 87.5 percent of 657 patients tested. The incidence of negative tests (72 percent) and positive tests (2 percent) was not different from that seen with the oxytocin-induced CST. Huddleston et al.[94] reported great success using intermittent nipple stimulation. The patient gently strokes the nipple of one breast with the palmar surface of her fingers through her clothes for 2 minutes and then stops for 5 minutes. This cycle is repeated only as necessary to achieve adequate uterine activity. In a series of 193 patients and 345 CSTs, 97 percent of the tests required only three cycles of stimulation. The average time for a CST performed in this way was 45 minutes, and 67.5 percent of the patients completed their tests in 40 minutes or less. The nipple stimulation CST was negative in 80.3 percent of patients and positive in 2.6 percent of patients. All of the patients in the Huddleston et al.[94] series were able to achieve adequate uterine contractions with nipple stimulation, and none required an oxytocin infusion. Intermittent rather than continuous nipple stimulation is important in avoiding hyperstimulation. Defined as contractions lasting more than 90 seconds or five or more contractions in 10 minutes, hyperstimulation has been reported in approximately 2 percent of tests when intermittent nipple stimulation is employed.[95,96]

The Nonstress Test

In 1969, Hammacher[97] noted that "the fetus can be regarded as safe, especially if reflex movements are accompanied by an obvious increase in the amplitude of oscillations in the basal fetal heart rate." This observation that accelerations of the fetal heart rate in response to fetal activity, uterine contractions, or stimulation reflect fetal well-being has formed the basis for the NST, the most widely applied technique for antepartum fetal evaluation.

In late gestation, the healthy fetus exhibits an average of 34 accelerations above the baseline fetal heart rate each hour.[98] These accelerations, which average 20 to 25 bpm in amplitude and approximately 40 seconds in duration, require intact neurologic coupling between the fetal CNS and the fetal heart.[98] Fetal hypoxia disrupts this pathway. At term, fetal accelerations are associated with fetal movement more than 85 percent of the time, and more than 90 percent of gross movements are accompanied by accelerations. Fetal heart rate accelerations may be absent during periods of quiet fetal sleep. Studies by Patrick et al.[98] demonstrated that the longest time between successive accelerations in the healthy term fetus is approximately 40 minutes. However, the fetus may fail to exhibit heart rate accelerations for up to 80 minutes and still be normal.

Although an absence of fetal heart rate accelerations is most often attributable to a quiet fetal sleep state, CNS depressants such as narcotics and phenobarbital, as well as the β-blocker propranolol, can reduce heart rate reactivity.[99,100] Chronic smoking is known to decrease fetal oxygenation through an increase in fetal carboxyhemoglobin and a decrease in uterine blood flow. Fetal heart rate accelerations are also decreased in smokers.[101]

The NST is usually performed in an outpatient setting. In most cases, only 10 to 15 minutes are required to complete the test. It has virtually no contraindications, and few equivocal test results are observed. The patient may be seated in a reclining chair, with care being taken to ensure that she is tilted to the left to avoid the supine hypotensive syndrome.[34,102] The patient's blood pressure should be recorded before the test is begun and then repeated at 5- to 10-minute intervals. Fetal heart rate is monitored using the Doppler ultrasound transducer, and the tocodynamometer is applied to detect uterine contractions or fetal movement. Fetal activity may be recorded by the patient using an event marker or noted by the staff performing the test. The most widely applied definition of a reactive test requires that at least two accelerations of the fetal heart rate of 15 bpm amplitude and 15 seconds' duration be observed in 20 minutes of monitoring (Fig. 11-6).[102] Because almost all accelerations are accompanied by fetal movement, fetal movement need not be recorded with the accelerations for the test to be considered reactive. However, fetal movements do provide another index of fetal well-being.

If the criteria for reactivity are not met, the test is considered nonreactive (Fig. 11-7). The most common cause for a nonreactive test is a period of fetal inactivity or quiet sleep. Therefore, the test may be extended for an additional 20 minutes with the expectation that fetal state will change and reactivity will appear. Keegan et al.[103] noted that approximately 80 percent of tests that were nonreactive in the morning became reactive when repeated later the same day. In an effort to change fetal state, some clinicians have manually stimulated the fetus or attempted to increase fetal glucose levels by giving the mother orange juice. There is no evidence that such efforts will increase fetal activity.[104–107] If the test has been extended for 40 minutes, and reactivity has not been seen, a BPP or CST should be performed. Of those fetuses that exhibit a nonreactive NST, approximately 25 percent will have a positive CST on further evaluation.[102,108,109] Reactivity that occurs during preparations for the CST has proved to be a reliable index of fetal well-being.

Overall, on initial testing, 85 percent of NSTs are reactive and 15 percent are nonreactive (Fig. 11-8).[102] Fewer than 1 percent of NSTs prove unsatisfactory because of inadequately recorded fetal heart rate data. On rare occasions, a sinusoidal heart rate pattern may be observed, as described in Chapter 15. This undulating heart rate pattern with virtually absent variability has been associated with fetal anemia, fetal asphyxia, congenital malformations, and medications such as narcotics. In one of the earliest reports on the use of the NST, Rochard et al.[110] described a sinusoidal pattern in 20 of 50 pregnancies complicated by Rh isoimmunization. One half of these pregnancies ended in a perinatal death, and 40 percent of the surviving infants required prolonged hospitalization. Only 10 percent of the babies with a sinusoidal pattern had an uncomplicated course.

The NST is most predictive when normal or reactive. Overall, a reactive NST has been associated with a peri-

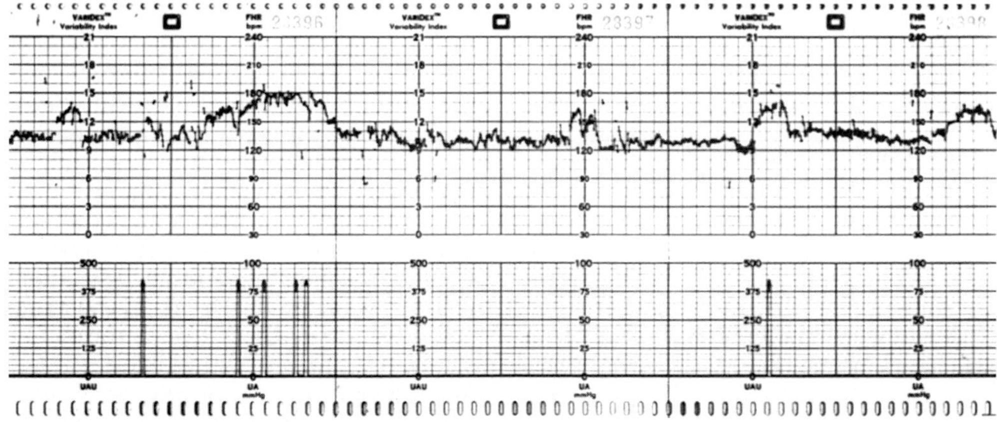

Figure 11-6. A reactive NST. Accelerations of the fetal heart that are greater than 15 bpm and last longer than 15 seconds can be identified. When the patient appreciates a fetal movement, she presses an event marker on the monitor, creating the arrows on the lower portion of the tracing. NST, nonstress test.

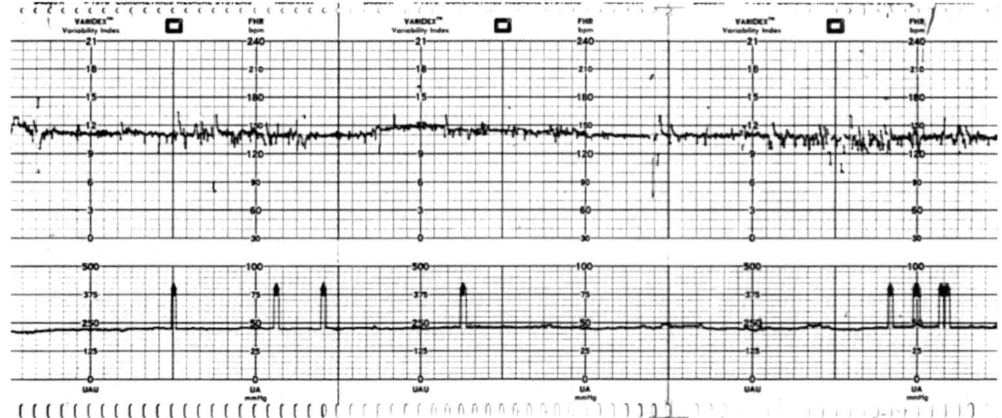

Figure 11-7. A nonreactive NST. No accelerations of the fetal heart rate are observed. The patient has perceived fetal activity as indicated by the arrows in the lower portion of the tracing. NST, nonstress test.

natal mortality of approximately 5 per 1,000.[102,111] At least one half of the deaths of babies dying within 1 week of a reactive test may be attributed to placental abruption or cord accidents. The PMR associated with a nonreactive NST, 30 to 40 per 1,000, is significantly higher, for this group includes those fetuses who are truly asphyxiated. On the other hand, when considering perinatal asphyxia and death as end points, a nonreactive NST has a considerable false-positive rate. Most fetuses exhibiting a nonreactive NST are not compromised but simply fail to exhibit heart rate reactivity during the 40-minute period of testing. Malformed fetuses also exhibit a significantly higher incidence of nonreactive NSTs.[112] Overall, the false-positive rate associated with the nonreactive NST is approximately 75 to 90 percent.[102]

The likelihood of a nonreactive test is substantially increased early in the third trimester.[113] Between 24 and 28 weeks' gestation, approximately 50 percent of NSTs are nonreactive.[114] Fifteen percent of NSTs remain nonreactive between 28 and 32 weeks.[115,116] After 32 weeks, the incidences of reactive and nonreactive tests are comparable to those seen at term. In summary, when accelerations of the baseline heart rate are seen during monitoring in the late second and early third trimesters, the NST has been associated with fetal well-being.

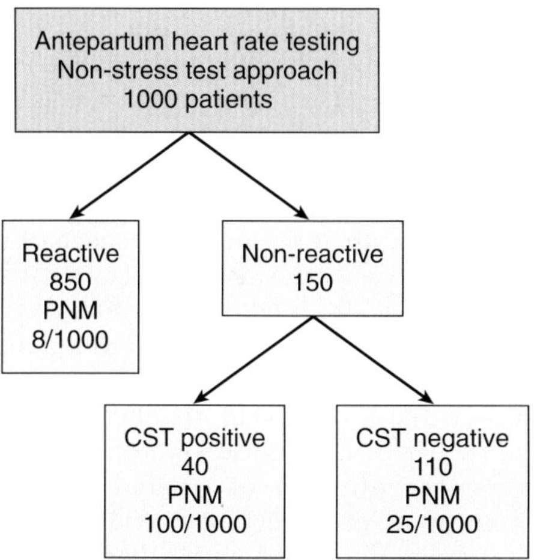

Figure 11-8. Results of nonstress testing (NST) in 1,000 high-risk patients. In general, 85 percent of the NSTs are reactive and 15 percent nonreactive. Of those patients with a nonreactive NST, approximately 25 percent will have a positive contraction stress test (CST) on further evaluation. The highest perinatal mortality (PNM) will be observed in patients with a nonreactive NST and positive CST. Patients with a nonreactive NST and negative CST will have a perinatal mortality rate higher than that found in patients whose NST is initially reactive. (PNM rates based on data from Evertson et al.[99])

Before 27 weeks' gestation, the normal fetal heart rate response to fetal movement may in fact be a bradycardia.[117] However, in some settings such as IUGR associated with antiphospholipid syndrome, bradycardia at a gestational age of 26 to 28 weeks may be a predictor of fetal compromise and impending fetal death. Druzin et al.[118] reported three cases in which antenatal steroid administration and elective premature delivery led to good perinatal outcome. In these challenging cases, the entire clinical situation needs to be evaluated, and a full discussion with the patient, including neonatal consultation, should be initiated before intervention and delivery of the very preterm fetus exhibiting fetal heart rate decelerations.

When nonreactive, the NST is extended in an attempt to separate the fetus in a period of prolonged quiet sleep from those who are hypoxemic or asphyxiated.[119–121] In three studies, approximately 3 percent of fetuses tested remained nonreactive after 80 to 90 minutes of evaluation. Brown and Patrick[119] noted that all NSTs that were to become reactive did so by 80 minutes or remained nonreactive for up to 120 minutes. Two stillbirths and one neonatal death occurred in seven cases with prolonged absence of reactivity. The mean arterial cord pH at delivery in this group was 6.95! In 27 pregnancies in which the fetus failed to exhibit accelerations during 80 minutes of monitoring, Leveno et al.[120] reported 11 perinatal deaths. In this study, IUGR was documented in 74 percent of cases, oligohydramnios in 81 percent, fetal acidosis in 41 percent, meconium staining of the amniotic fluid in 30 percent, and placental infarction in 93 percent. Therefore, if the NST is extended and a persistent absence of reactivity is observed, the fetus is likely to be severely compromised.

Vibroacoustic stimulation (VAS) may be used to change fetal state from quiet to active sleep and shorten the length of the NST (Fig. 11-9). Most studies have employed an electronic artificial larynx that generates sound pressure

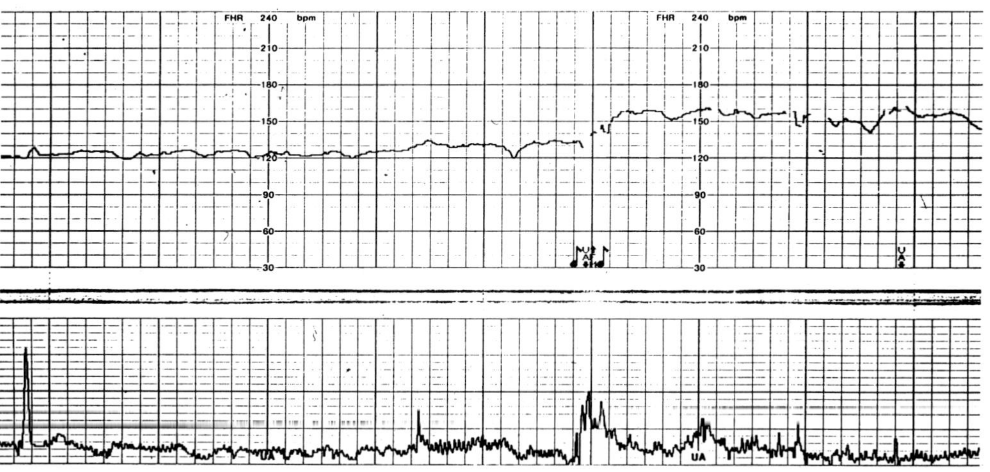

Figure 11-9. Reactive NST after VAS. The stimulus was applied in panel 54042, at the point marked by the musical notes. A sustained fetal heart rate acceleration was produced. NST, nonstress test; VAS, vibroacoustic stimulation.

levels measured at 1 m in air of 82 dB with a frequency of 80 Hz and a harmonic of 20 to 9,000 Hz.[122] Whether it is the acoustic or vibratory component of this stimulus that alters fetal state is unclear. Gagnon et al.[123] reported that a low-frequency vibratory stimulus applied at term changed fetal state within 3 minutes and was associated with an immediate and sustained increase in long-term fetal heart rate variability, heart rate accelerations, and gross fetal body movements. VAS may produce a significant increase in the mean duration of heart rate accelerations, the mean amplitude of accelerations, and the total time spent in accelerations.[124] Using VAS, the incidence of nonreactive NSTs was reduced from 12.6 to 6.1 percent in a retrospective study and from 14 to 9 percent in a prospective investigation.[125,126] A reactive NST after VAS stimulation appears to be as reliable an index of fetal well-being as spontaneous reactivity. However, those fetuses that remain nonreactive even after VAS may be at increased risk for poor perinatal outcome.[127] Intrapartum fetal distress, growth restriction, and low Apgar scores were increased in fetuses that were nonreactive after acoustic stimulation.[128] Auditory brain stem response appears to be functional in the fetus at 26 to 28 weeks' gestation.[127] VAS significantly increases the incidence of reactive NSTs after 26 weeks' gestation, and reduces the testing time, making this a potentially useful adjunct to antepartum fetal testing.[129,130]

In most centers that use VAS, the baseline fetal heart rate is first observed for 5 minutes.[122] If the pattern is nonreactive, a stimulus of 3 seconds or less is applied near the fetal head. If the NST remains nonreactive, the stimulus is repeated at 1-minute intervals up to three times. If there continues to be no response to VAS, further evaluation should be carried out with a BPP or CST. In summary, VAS may be helpful in shortening the time required to perform an NST and may be especially useful in centers where large numbers of NSTs are done.

Could the sound generated by an electronic artificial larynx damage the fetal ear? Using intrauterine microphones, Smith and colleagues[131] documented baseline intrauterine sound levels of up to 88 dB during labor. Transabdominal stimulation with an electronic artificial larynx increased these levels minimally, up to 91 to 111 dB. Sound vibrations and intensity are attenuated by amniotic fluid.[132] Therefore, a 90-dB sound pressure produced by VAS in air results in exposure of the fetal ear to the equivalent of 40 dB, the level of normal conversation at about 3 feet. Arulkumaran et al.[132] concluded that intrauterine sound levels from VAS were not hazardous to the fetal ear. Two studies have confirmed the safety of VAS use during pregnancy with no long-term evidence of hearing loss in children followed in the neonatal period and up to 4 years of age.[133,134]

Significant fetal heart rate bradycardias have been observed in 1 to 2 percent of all NSTs.[135–140] Druzin et al.[135] defined such bradycardias as a fetal heart rate of 90 bpm or a fall in the fetal heart rate of 40 bpm below the baseline for 1 minute or longer (Fig. 11-10). This definition has been most widely applied. In a review of 121 cases, bradycardia was associated with increased perinatal morbidity and mortality, particularly antepartum fetal death, cord compression, IUGR, and fetal malformations.[141] Although about one half of the NSTs associated with bradycardia were reactive, the incidence of a nonreassuring fetal heart rate pattern in labor leading to emergency delivery in this group was identical to that of patients exhibiting nonreactive NSTs. Clinical management decisions should be based on the finding of bradycardia, *not* on the presence or absence of reactivity. Bradycardia has a higher positive predictive value for fetal compromise (fetal death or fetal intolerance of labor) than does the nonreactive NST. In this setting, antepartum fetal death is most likely due to a cord accident.[135,139,140]

If a bradycardia is observed, an ultrasound examination should be performed to assess amniotic fluid volume and to detect the presence of anomalies such as renal agenesis. Expectant management in the setting of a bradycardia has been associated with a PMR of 25 percent. Therefore, several reports have recommended that delivery be undertaken if the fetus is mature. When the fetus is premature, one might elect to administer corticosteroids to accelerate fetal lung maturation before delivery. Continuous fetal heart rate monitoring is necessary if expectant management is followed.

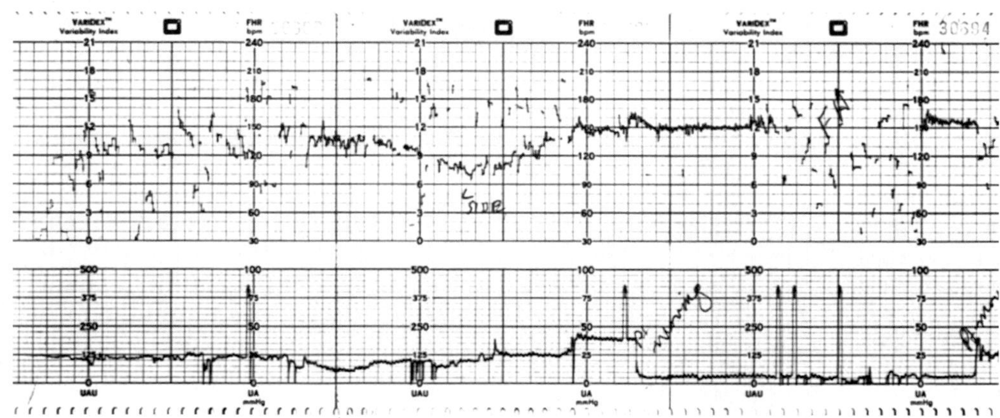

Figure 11-10. An NST in this primigravid patient of 43 weeks' gestation reveals a spontaneous bradycardia (panel 30692). The fetal heart rate has fallen from a baseline of 150 to 100 bpm. Upon induction of labor, the patient required cesarean delivery for fetal distress associated with severe variable decelerations. The amniotic fluid was decreased in amount and was meconium stained. NST, nonstress test.

In most cases, mild variable decelerations are not associated with poor perinatal outcome. Meis et al.[142] reported that variable decelerations of 20 bpm or more below the baseline heart rate but lasting less than 10 seconds were noted in 50.7 percent of patients having an NST. Whereas these decelerations were more often associated with a nuchal cord, they were not predictive of IUGR or a nonreassuring fetal heart rate pattern, or more severe variable decelerations during labor. Phelan[122] has added, however, that when mild variable decelerations are observed, even if the NST is reactive, an ultrasound examination should be performed to rule out oligohydramnios. A low amniotic fluid index and mild variable decelerations increase the likelihood of a cord accident.

In selected high-risk pregnancies, the false-negative rate associated with a weekly NST may be unacceptably high.[143,144] Boehm et al.[145] reported a reduction in the fetal death rate in their high-risk population from 6.1 to 1.9 per 1,000 when the frequency of the NST was increased from once to twice weekly. Barrett et al.[143] have emphasized that in pregnancies complicated by IUGR and diabetes mellitus, twice-weekly testing should be used. In reviewing the literature, they noted that the fetal death rate within 1 week after a nonreactive NST was significantly increased in both diabetes mellitus (14 per 1,000) and IUGR (20 per 1,000). Miyazaki and Miyazaki,[146] reported an 8 percent false-negative rate in 125 prolonged gestations evaluated with the NST. In the prolonged pregnancy and IUGR, oligohydramnios may occur, leading to cord compression and fetal demise. The assessment of amniotic fluid volume has clearly proved important in such cases. Barss and co-workers[147] reviewed the incidence of stillbirths within 1 week of a reactive test in patients with a prolonged gestation. For the general high-risk population, a false-negative rate of 2.7 per 1,000 was reported. Although the incidence in pregnancies complicated by a prolonged gestation was not higher (2.8 per 1,000), Barss et al.[147] noted that even this low rate can be considered excessively high in view of the fact that these fetuses are otherwise normal and mature. In summary, it appears that the frequency of the NST should be increased to *twice* weekly in pregnancies complicated by diabetes mellitus, prolonged gestation, and IUGR.[145]

Which antepartum heart rate test is best? The NST has proved to be an ideal screening test and remains the primary method for antepartum fetal evaluation at most centers. It can be quickly performed in an outpatient setting and is easily interpreted. In contrast, the CST is usually performed near the labor and delivery suite, may require an intravenous infusion of oxytocin, and may be more difficult to interpret. In initial studies, a reactive NST appeared to be as predictive of good outcome as a negative CST. Nevertheless, as more data have been gathered, it appears that the ability of the CST to stress the fetus and evaluate its response to intermittent interruptions in intervillous blood flow provides an earlier warning of fetal compromise. Murata et al.[148] found that, in the dying fetal rhesus monkey, the fetal pH at which late decelerations appear is significantly higher (7.32) than the pH at which fetal heart rate accelerations disappear (7.22). In a large collaborative project in which 1,542 patients were evaluated primarily with the NST and 4,626 with the CST, Freeman et al.[149] observed that the corrected perinatal mortality associated with a reactive NST, 3.2 per 1,000, was significantly higher than that observed with a negative CST, 1.4 per 1,000. Whereas both fetal death rates are extremely low for a high-risk population, that associated with the CST is clearly better.

The healthy fetus should exhibit a reactive baseline heart rate with no late decelerations when a CST is performed. However, as the fetus deteriorates, one will first observe late decelerations, and finally, the most ominous fetal heart rate pattern, the nonreactive NST and positive CST[80,86,150] (Fig. 11-5). When a nonreactive NST is followed by a positive CST, the incidence of perinatal mortality has been approximately 10 percent, a nonreassuring fetal heart rate pattern has occurred in most laboring patients, and IUGR has been reported in 25 percent of cases. The unusual combination of a reactive NST and a positive CST has been associated with a higher incidence of IUGR and late decelerations in labor than that seen with a negative CST.[151] The likelihood of fetal death is increased in patients demonstrating a nonreactive NST followed by a negative CST.[81,152,153] Consequently, repeating the NST in 24 hours appears the prudent course in such cases (Fig. 11-11).

Finally, arguments about the "best test" are counterproductive. Each test has its strengths and weaknesses, and a thorough understanding of the nature of the antepartum test, taking into consideration its advantages and disadvantages, is essential. The type of test and its application should be "condition" or diagnosis specific in

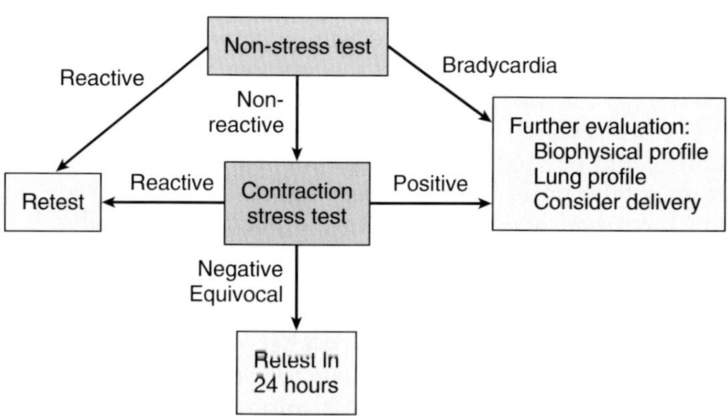

Figure 11-11. A branched testing scheme using the NST, CST, and BPP. Delivery is considered when the NST is nonreactive and the CST is positive. Delivery is also considered when a bradycardia is observed during the NST. The fetal BPP may be used to decrease the incidence of unnecessary premature intervention. BPP, biophysical profile; CST, contraction stress test; NST, nonstress test.

which a similar basic screening approach is used, adding different types of evaluation and increased frequency of testing as appropriate for the clinical situation.

Fetal Biophysical Profile

The use of real-time ultrasonography to assess antepartum fetal condition has enabled the obstetrician to perform an in utero physical examination and evaluate dynamic functions reflecting the integrity of the fetal CNS.[154] As emphasized by Manning et al.,[155] "fetal biophysical scoring rests on the principle that the more complete the examination of the fetus, its activities, and its environment, the more accurate may be the differentiation of fetal health from disease states."

Fetal breathing movements were the first biophysical parameter to be assessed using real-time ultrasonography. It is thought that the fetus exercises its breathing muscles in utero in preparation for postdelivery respiratory function. With real-time ultrasonography, fetal breathing movement (FBM) is evidenced by downward movement of the diaphragm and abdominal contents, and by an inward collapsing of the chest. Fetal breathing movements become regular at 20 to 21 weeks and are controlled by centers on the ventral surface of the fourth ventricle of the fetus.[156] They are observed approximately 30 percent of the time, are seen more often during REM sleep, and, when present, demonstrate intact neurologic control. Although the absence of FBMs may reflect fetal asphyxia, this finding may also indicate that the fetus is in a period of quiet sleep.[46,47]

Several factors other than fetal state and hypoxia can influence the presence of FBM. As maternal glucose levels rise, FBM becomes more frequent, and during periods of maternal hypoglycemia, FBM decreases. Maternal smoking reduces FBM, probably as a result of fetal hypoxemia.[157] Narcotics that depress the fetal CNS also decrease FBM.

Platt and colleagues[158] were among the first to examine the ability of FBM to predict perinatal outcome. Using real-time ultrasonography, they judged FBM to be present if at least one episode of FBM of at least 60 seconds' duration was observed within any 30-minute period of observation. Of 136 fetuses studied, 116 (85 percent) exhibited FBM. The incidence of fetal distress was significantly higher in fetuses without FBM, 60 percent (12 of 20), as was the incidence of low Apgar scores at 5 minutes, 50 percent (10 of 20). The comparable figures for fetuses demonstrating FBM were 3 percent (4 of 116) for a nonreassuring fetal heart rate pattern and 4 percent (5 of 116) for low Apgar scores.

Further research demonstrated that the evaluation of FBM could be used to distinguish the truly positive CST from a false-positive CST. Those fetuses that displayed FBM but had a positive CST were unlikely to exhibit fetal distress in labor. However, when a fetus failed to show FBM and demonstrated late decelerations during the CST, the likelihood of fetal compromise was great. A pattern emerged from these studies that as long as one antepartum biophysical test was normal, the likelihood that the fetus would have a normal outcome was high.[159,160] As the number of abnormal tests increased, however, the likelihood that fetal asphyxia was present increased as well.

Using these principles, Manning et al.[161] developed the concept of the fetal BPP score. These workers elected to combine the NST with four parameters that could be assessed using real-time ultrasonography: FBM, fetal movement, fetal tone, and amniotic fluid volume. FBM, fetal movement, and fetal tone are mediated by complex neurologic pathways and should reflect the function of the fetal CNS at the time of the examination. On the other hand, amniotic fluid volume should provide information about the presence of chronic fetal asphyxia. Finally, the ultrasound examination performed for the BPP has the added advantage of detecting previously unrecognized major fetal anomalies.

Vintzileos et al.[156] stressed that those fetal biophysical activities that are present earliest in fetal development are the last to disappear with fetal hypoxia. The fetal tone center in the cortex begins to function at 7.5 to 8.5 weeks. Therefore, fetal tone would be the last fetal parameter to be lost with worsening fetal condition. The fetal movement center in the cortex-nuclei is functional at 9 weeks and would be more sensitive than fetal tone. As noted earlier, FBM becomes regular at 20 to 21 weeks. Finally, fetal heart rate control, residing within the posterior hypothalamus and medulla, becomes functional at the end of the second trimester and early in the third trimester. An alteration in fetal heart rate would theoretically be the earliest sign of fetal compromise.

A BPP score was developed that is similar to the Apgar score used to assess the condition of the newborn.[161] The presence of a normal parameter, such as a reactive NST, was awarded 2 points, whereas the absence of that parameter was scored as 0. The highest score a fetus can receive is 10, and the lowest score is 0. The BPP may be used as early as 26 to 28 weeks' gestation. The time required for the fetus to achieve a satisfactory BPP score is closely related to fetal state, with an average of only 5 minutes if the fetus is in a 2F state but over 25 minutes if it is in a 1F state.[162] Twice-weekly testing is recommended in pregnancies complicated by IUGR, diabetes mellitus, prolonged gestation, and hypertension with proteinuria. The criteria proposed by Manning et al.,[161] and the clinical actions recommended in response to these scores, are presented in Tables 11-5 and 11-6. Regardless of a low score on the BPP, Manning et al. have emphasized that vaginal delivery is attempted if other obstetric factors are favorable.

In a prospective blinded study of 216 high-risk patients, Manning and colleagues[161] found no perinatal deaths when all five variables described earlier were normal, but a PMR of 60 percent in fetuses with a score of zero. Fetal deaths were increased 14-fold with the absence of fetal movement, and the PMR was increased 18-fold if FBM was absent. Any single test was associated with a significant false-positive rate ranging from 50 to 79 percent. However, combining abnormal variables significantly decreased the false-positive rate to as low as 20 percent. The false-negative rate, that is, the incidence of babies who were compromised but who had normal testing, was low, ranging from a PMR of 6.9 per 1,000 for infants with normal amniotic fluid volume to 12.8 per 1,000 for fetuses demonstrating a reactive NST. These

Table 11-5. Technique of Biophysical Profile Scoring

BIOPHYSICAL VARIABLE	NORMAL (SCORE = 2)	ABNORMAL (SCORE = 0)
Fetal breathing movements	At least one episode of >30 seconds' duration in 30 minutes' observation	Absent or no episode of ≥30 seconds' duration in 30 minutes
Gross body movement	At least three discrete body/limb movements in 30 minutes (episodes of active continuous movement considered a single movement)	Up to two episodes of body/limb movements in 30 minutes
Fetal tone	At least one episode of active extension with return to flexion of fetal limb(s) or trunk, opening and closing of hand considered normal tone	Either slow extension with return to partial flexion or movement of limb in full extension or absent fetal movement
Reactive fetal heart rate	At least two episodes of acceleration of ≥15 bpm and 15 seconds/duration associated with fetal movement in 30 minutes	Fewer than two accelerations or acceleration <15 bpm in 30 minutes
Qualitative anmiotic fluid volume	At least one pocket of amniotic fluid measuring 2 cm in two perpendicular planes	Either no amniotic fluid pockets or a pocket <2 cm in two perpendicular planes

Adapted from Manning FA: Biophysical profile scoring. *In* Nijhuis J (ed): Fetal Behaviour. New York, Oxford University Press, 1992, p 241.

Table 11-6. Management Based on Biophysical Profile

SCORE	INTERPRETATION	MANAGEMENT
10	Normal infant; low risk of chronic aphyxia	Repeat testing at weekly intervals; repeat twice weekly in diabetic patients and patients at 41 weeks' gestation
8	Normal infant; low risk of chronic aphyxia	Repeat testing at weekly intervals; repeat testing twice weekly in diabetics and patients at 41 weeks' gestation; oligohydramnios is an indication for delivery
6	Suspect chronic asphyxia	If 36 weeks' gestation and conditions are favorable, deliver; if at >36 weeks and L/S <2.0, repeat test in 4–6 hours; deliver if oligohydramnios is present
4	Suspect chronic asphyxia	If 36 weeks' gestation, deliver; if <32 weeks' gestation, repeat score
0–2	Strongly suspect chronic asphyxia	Extend testing time to 120 minutes; if persistent score ≤4, deliver, regardless of gestational age

Adapted from Manning FA, Harman CR, Morrison I, et al: Fetal assessment based on fetal biophysical profile scoring. Am J Obstet Gynecol 162:703, 1990; and Manning FA: Biophysical profile scoring. *In* Nijhuis J (ed): Fetal Behaviour. New York, Oxford University Press, 1992, p 241.

investigators found that, in most cases, the ultrasound-derived BPP parameters and NST could be completed within a relatively short time, each requiring approximately 10 minutes.

Manning et al.[153] have presented their experience with 26,780 high-risk pregnancies followed with the BPP. In Manning et al.'s protocol, a routine NST is not performed if all of the ultrasound parameters are found to be normal for a score of 8.[164] An NST is performed when one ultrasound finding is abnormal. The corrected PMR in this series was 1.9 per 1,000, with less than 1 fetal death per 1,000 patients within 1 week of a normal profile. Of all patients tested, almost 97 percent had a score of 8, which means that only 3 percent required further evaluation for scores of 6 or less. In a study of 525 patients with scores of 6 or less, poor perinatal outcome was most often associated with either a nonreactive NST and absent fetal tone or a nonreactive NST and absent FBM.[165] A significant inverse linear relationship was observed between the last BPP score and both perinatal morbidity and mortality (Figs. 11-12 and 11-13).[163] The false-positive rate, depending on the end point used, ranges from 75 percent for a score of 6 to less than 20 percent for a score of 0. Manning[166] has summarized the data reported in eight investigations using the BPP for fetal evaluation. Overall, 23,780 patients and 54,337 tests were reviewed. The corrected PMR, excluding lethal anomalies, was 0.77 per 1,000.

The BPP correlates well with fetal acid-base status. Vintzileos et al.[167] studied 124 patients undergoing cesarean birth *before* the onset of labor. Deliveries were undertaken for severe preeclampsia, elective repeat cesarean section, growth restriction, breech presentation, placenta previa, and fetal macrosomia. Acidosis was defined as an umbilical cord arterial pH less than 7.20. The earliest manifestations of fetal acidosis were a nonreactive NST and loss of FBM. With scores of 8 or more, the mean arterial pH was 7.28, and only two of 102 fetuses were acidotic. Nine fetuses with scores of 4 or less had a mean pH of 6.99, and all were acidotic.

Recent studies have demonstrated that antenatal corticosteroid administration may have an effect on the BPP, decreasing the profile score. Because corticosteroids are used in cases of anticipated premature delivery (24 to 34 weeks), any false-positive results on biophysical testing may lead to inappropriate intervention and delivery. Kelly et al. reported that BPP scores were decreased in more than one third of the fetuses tested at 28 to 34

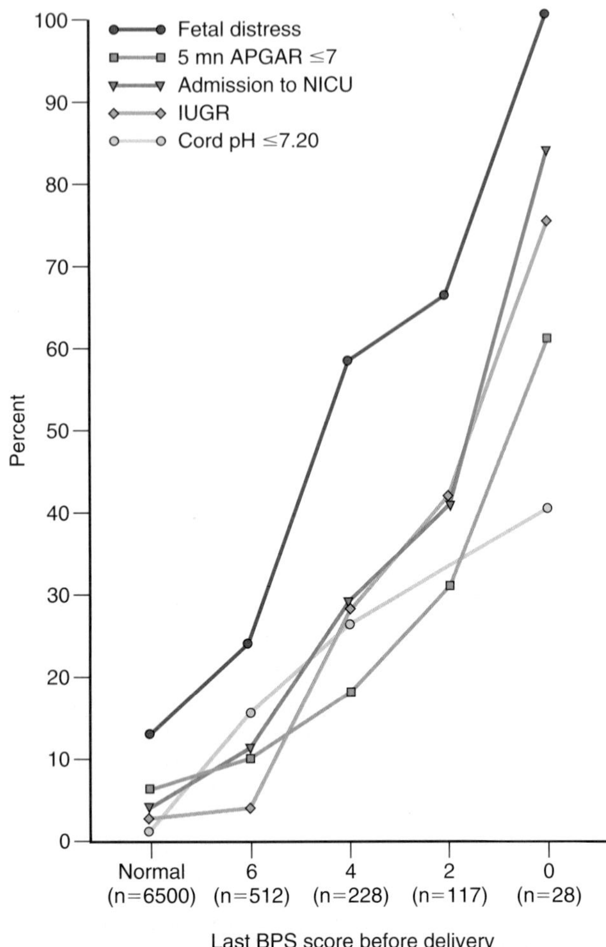

Figure 11-12. The relationship between five indices of perinatal morbidity and last biophysical profile score before delivery. A significant inverse linear correlation is observed for each variable. (From Manning FA, Harman CR, Morrison I, et al: Fetal assessment based on fetal biophysical profile scoring. Am J Obstet Gynecol 162:703, 1990, with permission.)

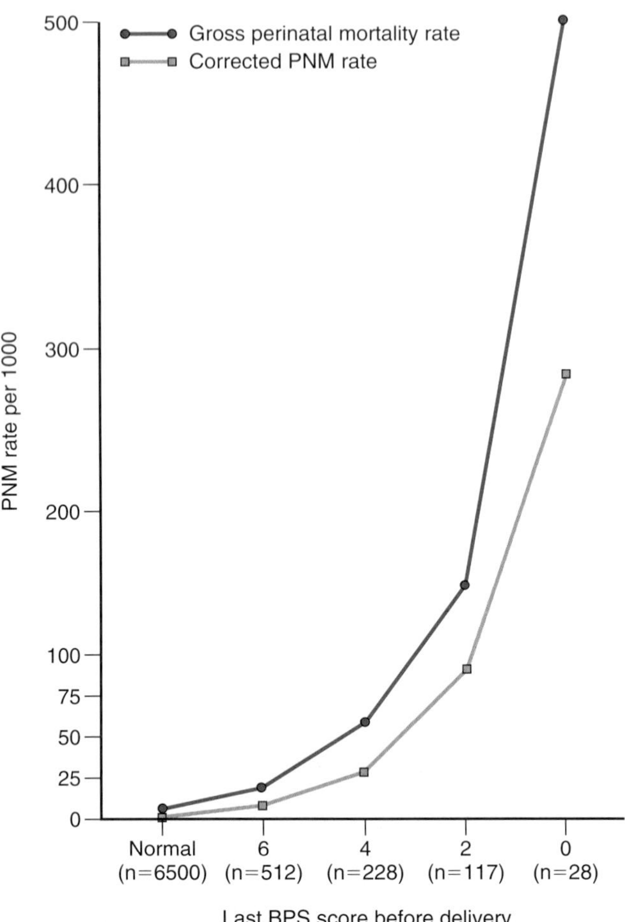

Figure 11-13. The relationship between perinatal mortality, both total and corrected for major anomalies, and the last BPP score before delivery. A highly significant inverse and exponential relationship is observed. BPP, biophysical profile. (From Manning FA, Harman CR, Morrison I, et al: Fetal assessment based on fetal biophysical profile scoring. Am J Obstet Gynecol 162:703, 1990, with permission.)

weeks' gestation. This effect was seen within 48 hours of corticosteroid administration. Neonatal outcome was not affected. Repeat BPPs within 24 to 48 hours were normal in cases in which the BPP score had decreased by 4 points. The most commonly affected variables were FBM and the NST.[168] Similarly Deren et al.[169] and Rotmensch et al.[170] reported transient suppression of FBM, fetal body movements, and heart rate reactivity following corticosteroid administration at less than 34 weeks' gestation. These parameters returned to normal by 48 to 96 hours after corticosteroid treatment. This effect must be considered at institutions where daily BPPs are used to evaluate the fetus in cases of preterm labor or preterm premature rupture of the membranes.

There has been some controversy concerning the utility of the BPP in predicting chorioamnionitis in pregnancies complicated by preterm labor or preterm premature rupture of the membranes. Sherer et al.[171] reported that the absence of FBM is associated with histologic evidence of fetal inflammation and intrauterine infection in patients with preterm labor and intact membranes before 32 weeks' gestation. However, they recommend that this finding not be used to guide clinical management because of the low positive predictive value of absent FBM. Lewis et al.[172] performed a randomized trial of daily NSTs versus BPP in the management of preterm premature rupture of the membranes. They concluded that neither daily NSTs nor BPPs had high sensitivity in predicting infectious complications in these patients. Daily BPPs increased cost without apparent benefit.

Manning et al. have described the correlation between biophysical scoring and the incidence of cerebral palsy in Manitoba. In patients referred for a BPP, there was an inverse, exponential, and highly significant relationship between last BPP score and the incidence of cerebral palsy. Scores of 6 or less had a sensitivity of 49 percent. The more abnormal the last BPP, the greater the risk of cerebral palsy. Gestational age, birth weight, or assumed timing of the injury were not related to the incidence of cerebral palsy. The incidence of cerebral palsy ranged from 0.7 per 1,000 live births, for a normal BPP score; to 13.1 per 1,000 live births, for a score of 6; and 333 per 1,000 live births, for a score of 0.[173]

Is an NST needed if all ultrasound parameters of the BPP are normal? Prospective and blinded studies by Platt et al.[174] and Manning et al.[175] using both the BPP and NST have demonstrated that each of these tests is a valuable predictor of normal outcome. In the experience of Manning et al., an NST was needed in less than 5 percent of tests. As emphasized by Eden et al.,[176] however, the NST allows the detection of fetal heart rate decelerations. In the presence of reduced amniotic fluid, these decelerations may be associated with a cord accident. Eden et al. reported that when spontaneous fetal heart rate decelerations lasting at least 30 seconds with a decrease of at least 15 bpm are seen in the presence of normal amniotic fluid, there is an increased likelihood of late decelerations in labor and cesarean delivery for fetal distress.

Several drawbacks of the BPP should be considered. Unlike the NST and CST, an ultrasound machine is required, and unless the BPP is videotaped, it cannot be reviewed. If the fetus is in a quiet sleep state, the BPP can require a long period of observation. The present scoring system does not consider the impact of hydramnios. In a pregnancy complicated by diabetes mellitus, the presence of excessive amniotic fluid is of great concern.

The false-positive (false-abnormal) rate of a particular test has always been of concern because of the possibility of unnecessary intervention (usually delivery) and subsequent iatrogenic complications. The BPP was developed in part to address the issue of the high false-abnormal rate of the CST and the NST. There has been little attention paid to the possible false-positive rate of the abnormal or equivocal BPP. This is particularly relevant because the BPP is most commonly used as the final backup test in the NST and CST sequence of testing and is critically important when dealing with the premature fetus. As noted earlier, the false-positive rate of a score of 0 is less than 20 percent, but for a score of 6, it is up to 75 percent. Inglis et al.[177] used VAS to define fetal condition with BPP scores of 6 or less in 81 patients at 28 to 42 weeks. Obstetric and neonatal outcomes of 41 patients whose score improved to normal after VAS were compared with those of 238 patients who had normal scores without VAS. The obstetric and neonatal outcomes were not significantly different between the two groups. VAS improved the BPP in about 80 percent of cases. Use of VAS for an equivocal BPP did not increase the false-negative rate and may reduce the likelihood of unnecessary obstetric intervention.[177]

Doppler Ultrasound

With the introduction of Doppler ultrasound, noninvasive assessment of the fetal, maternal, and placental circulations became possible. Evaluation of blood flow in the fetus and placenta had previously entailed such invasive procedures as injection of radioactive microspheres or direct application of transducers, with the potential of jeopardy to the fetus and mother. Investigators could now examine the association of changes in umbilical blood flow with fetal morbidity in the ongoing human pregnancy.

The Doppler principle is based on changes in the frequency of sound (or light) produced by a changing relationship between two objects. The frequency of sound produced by an object moving away from an observer is perceived as lower than the same frequency of sound produced by an object moving toward the observer.[178] A common example of this is the sound of a train horn as it moves toward, then past and away from the listener. Ultrasound waves beamed with a particular frequency will return to a receiver at a lower frequency when the target is moving away from the transducer, and at a higher frequency when the target is moving toward the transducer. The speed and direction of moving red blood cells have been investigated using this information, and converting it into waveforms interpretable by the human eye and ear. By convention, information received from objects moving away from the transducer is recorded below a zero line, and information received from objects moving toward the transducer is recorded above a zero line (Figs. 11-14 and 11-15). The frequency of the reflected sound is proportional to the velocity of the moving red blood cells. Information about blood flow velocity provides an indirect assessment of changes in blood flow. Calculation of flow velocity is derived from the equation

$$f_d = 2\, f_0 \frac{V_{\cos}\theta}{c},$$

where f_d is the change in ultrasound frequency or Doppler shift, f_0 is the transmitted frequency of the ultrasound beam, V is the velocity of the red blood cells, θ is the angle between the beam and the direction of movement of the reflector or red blood cells, and c is the velocity of sound in the medium (Fig. 11-16). The speed of sound in tissues is 1,540 m/sec. The number 2 in the equation accounts for the time spent from the transmission of the sound signal at its origin to its return. Volume flow may be calculated by multiplying the mean velocity by the cross-sectional area of the vessel. Velocities are measured in meters per second.

The combination of real-time ultrasound imaging with pulsed wave Doppler allows the identification of a spe-

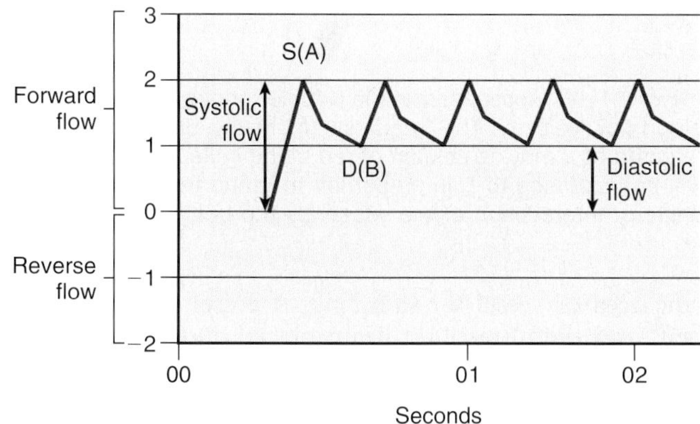

Figure 11-14. Diagram of a normal umbilical artery flow velocity waveform. Note the forward flow during both systole and diastole, the latter indicating low resistance in the placental bed. (Adapted from Warsof SL, Levy DL: Doppler blood flow and fetal growth retardation. *In* Gross TL, Sokol RJ [ed]: Intrauterine Growth Retardation, A Practical Approach. Chicago, Year Book, 1989, p 158.)

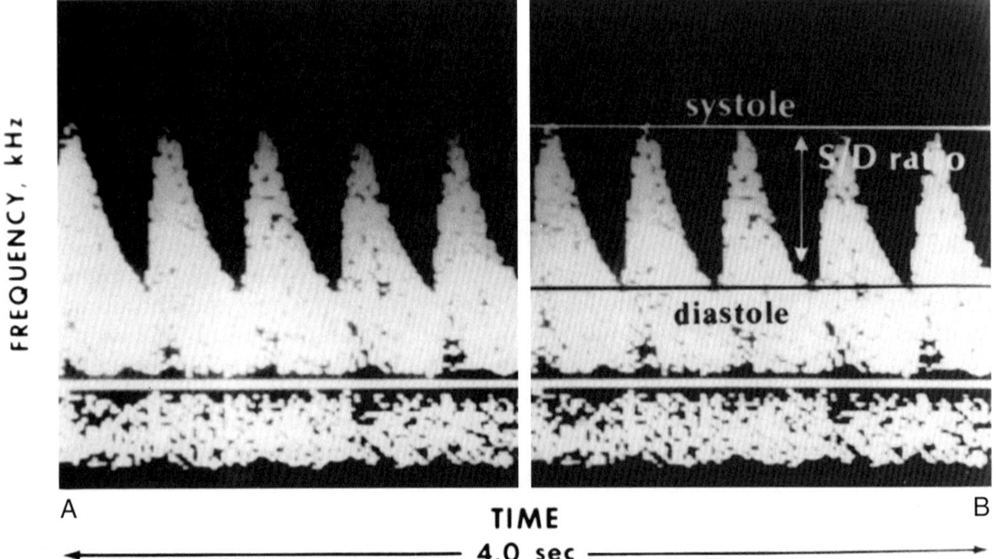

Figure 11-15. Doppler flow velocity waveforms of the normal umbilical artery. Note that umbilical arterial flow velocities are recorded above the baseline, whereas nonpulsatile umbilical vein flow in the opposite direction is found below the baseline (a). Measurement of the S/D ratio is also illustrated (b). S/D, systolic/diastolic. (From Bruner JP, Gabbe SG, Levy DW, et al: Doppler ultrasonography of the umbilical cord in normal pregnancy. J South Med Assoc 86:52, 1993, with permission.)

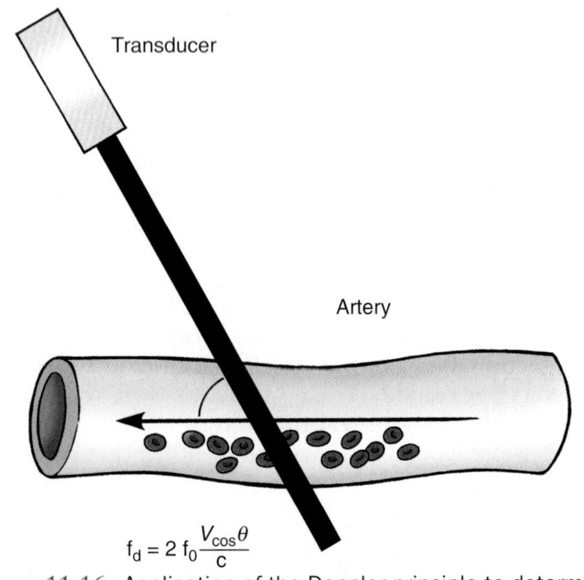

Figure 11-16. Application of the Doppler principle to determine blood flow velocity. The frequency (f_0) of the ultrasound beam directed at a moving column of red blood cells with velocity (V) will be increased to f_d in proportion to V and the cosine of the angle of intersection of the vessel by the beam (θ).

cific area or vessel for sampling. A vessel can be identified, and the ultrasound beam placed across that vessel using range gating. Ideally, the angle between the beam and the insonated vessel should less than 30 degrees. As the angle increases, large errors may be made in estimating flow velocity. Determinations of the volume of blood flow require accurate measurements of the diameter of the vessel studied in order to calculate its cross-sectional area. A small error in the measurement of the diameter can produce substantial errors in the determination of the volume of blood flow, because the radius is squared to calculate the area of the blood vessel. If blood flow is expressed in milliliters per kilogram per minute, fetal weight must be accurately estimated. Usually, a minimum of three to five waveforms is used to obtain measurements. In umbilical vessels, multiple sites are sampled.

Given the difficulty of estimating the angle between the Doppler ultrasound beam and the direction of blood flow in a particular vessel, a variety of angle-independent indices have been developed to characterize flow velocity waveforms produced. Indices rely on systolic, diastolic, and mean velocities. Systolic velocities are peak velocities that result from cardiac contraction. Diastolic velocities result from an interaction between peak flows, vessel compliance, heart rate, and the vascular impedance of the sites perfused. These indices do not measure the volume of blood flow. A commonly used index is the systolic (S)/diastolic (D) velocity ratio, the S/D ratio (Figs. 11-14 and 11-15). The pulsatility index is calculated as the systolic minus diastolic values divided by the mean of the velocity waveform (S-D/mean). An additional ratio, the resistance index, or Pourcelot ratio, is expressed as S-D/S. The latter two ratios are useful when the diastolic flow is absent or reversed. Higher indices occur with relatively lower diastolic velocities that are thought to be the result of increased resistance or vascular impedance.[179–181]

Variations in umbilical artery blood flow occur during episodes of fetal breathing (Fig. 11-17).[182] Changes in abdominal and thoracic pressure that occur with fetal breathing produce changes in preload, stroke volume, and afterload. Variations in fetal heart rate may shorten or lengthen diastole, with changes in stroke volume and less or more time for diastolic run-off, resulting in subsequent changes in both systolic and diastolic velocities. Sites closer to the fetal abdomen have relatively higher diastolic velocities, and sites closer to the placenta have relatively lower diastolic velocities.[183] For these reasons, it is recommended that umbilical velocity studies be per-

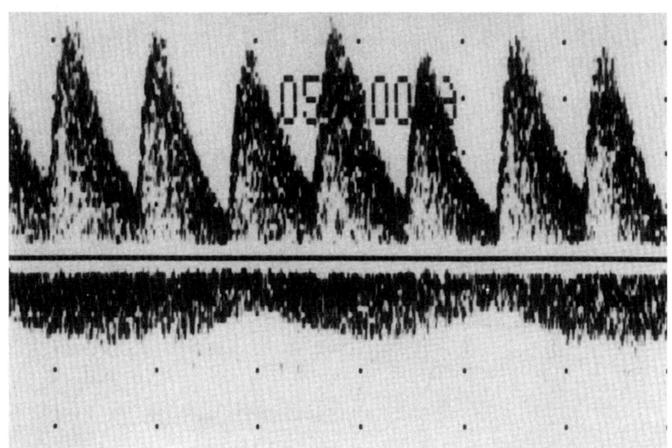

Figure 11-17. Umbilical arterial and venous Doppler flow velocity waveforms during an episode of fetal breathing. Venous velocities vary with every two to three arterial waveforms.

formed in midportions of the umbilical cord while fetuses are relatively quiet.

Values of normal umbilical artery flow velocity waveforms during pregnancy have been reported by many investigators (Fig. 11-18).[184,185] Before 15 weeks' gestation, diastolic flow is not consistently identified in the umbilical artery.[186] As the normal pregnancy progresses, there is proportionately more blood flow during diastole, and indices decrease. The normal decrease in umbilical artery velocity indices is consistent with a decrease in placental resistance with advancing gestational age.[187]

The main application of umbilical artery Doppler flow velocity measurements has been in the pregnancy at risk for or demonstrating IUGR (see Chapter 29).[188] IUGR is seen more often in fetuses with umbilical artery velocity indices that are elevated for their gestational age.[189] In some cases, end-diastolic flow is absent or reversed (Figs. 11-19 and 11-20).

The association of umbilical artery flow velocity waveform indices with alterations in placental blood flow

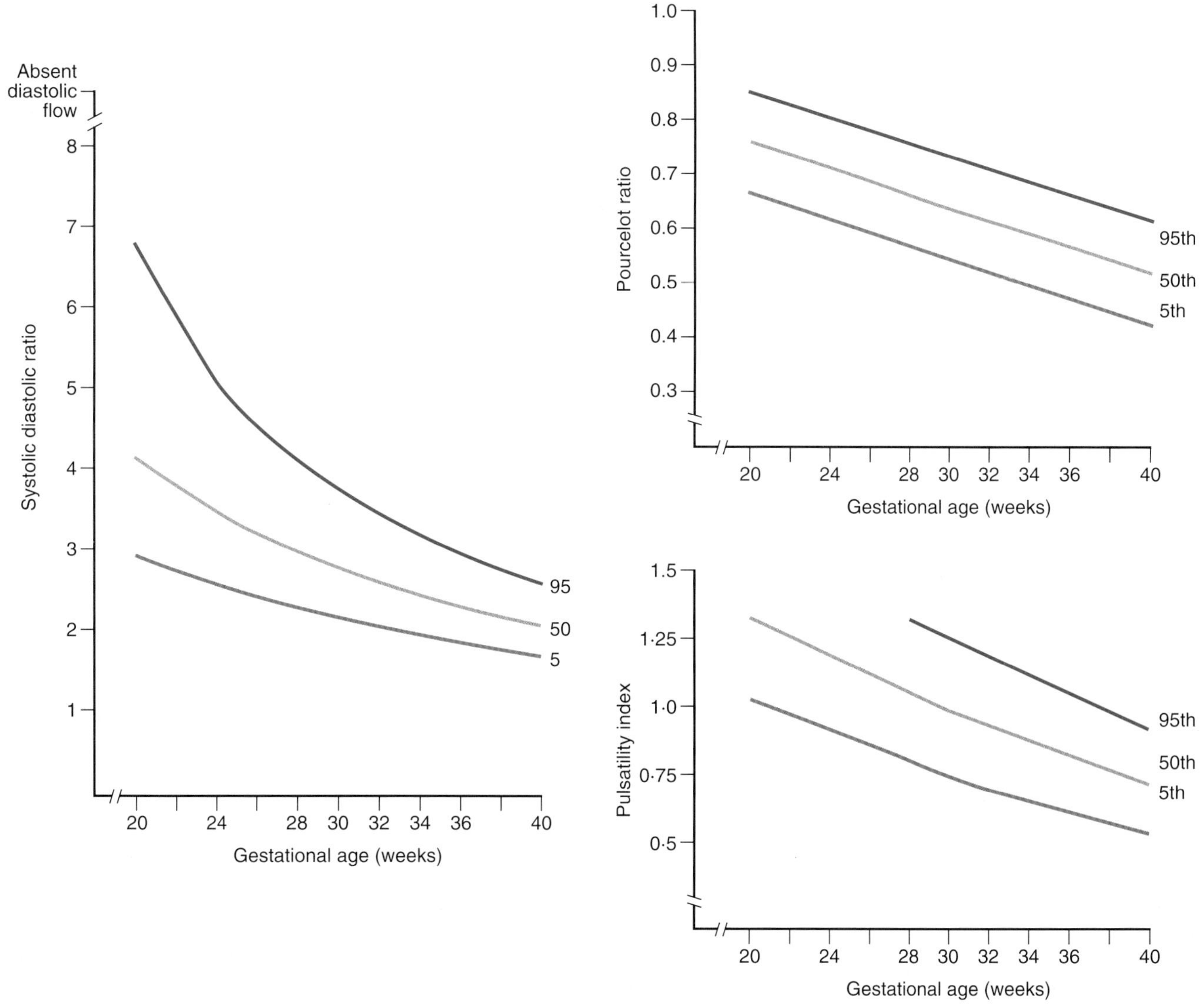

Figure 11-18. Normal ranges for the various indices used to quantify the flow velocity waveform patterns of the umbilical artery during pregnancy. (Modified from Thompson RS, Trudinger BJ, Cook CM, et al: Umbilical artery velocity waveforms: normal reference values for A/B ratio and Pourcelot ratio. Br J Obstet Gynaecol 95:589, 1988.)

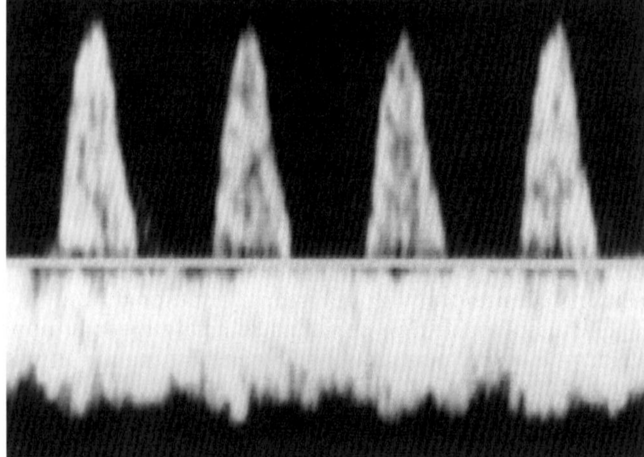

Figure 11-19. Umbilical arterial waveforms with absent end-diastolic velocities. In this case, venous velocities also demonstrate variation with the arterial waveforms.

was examined by Trudinger et al. in a sheep model.[190] The umbilical placental circulation was embolized with microspheres each day for 9 days in late gestation. The umbilical artery S/D ratio increased at 4 days, as did vascular resistance in the placental bed. The volume of umbilical blood flow did not fall significantly until the end of the study period. Using a similar experimental model, Morrow and Ritchie[191] reported a progressive increase in the S/D ratio leading to absent and then reversed diastolic flow. Hypoxia did not alter the S/D ratio, an observation also reported by Copel et al.[192] using a sheep model in which umbilical blood flow and S/D ratio were measured shortly after placental embolization. Copel et al. reported normal umbilical artery S/D ratios in the presence of fetal acidosis. Therefore, the umbilical artery S/D ratio more likely reflects placental vascular resistance than acute fetal hypoxemia. In an ovine model, Galan et al. have convincingly shown that fetal sheep with IUGR exist in a fetoplacental circulatory state characterized by high resistance and hypertension, and this is associated with abnormal umbilical artery indices.[193]

The most extreme abnormalities in umbilical artery waveforms are those in which the velocities are absent or reversed.[194,195] Absence of end-diastolic velocities is associated with an increase in perinatal morbidity and mortality. Reverse flow is even more predictive of poor perinatal outcome than absent diastolic flow. In addition to an association with IUGR, markedly abnormal Doppler studies have been reported in fetuses with congenital malformations, including chromosomal abnormalities. Farine et al.[195] summarized information from 31 studies with a total of 904 fetuses demonstrating absent or reversed end-diastolic velocities. They found a perinatal mortality of 36 percent. Eighty percent of the fetuses were below the 10th percentile in weight for gestational age. Abnormal karyotypes were found in 6 percent and malformations in 11 percent. The average duration from diagnosis to delivery ranged from 0 to 49 days, averaging 6 to 8 days. Absence or reversal of end-diastolic flow velocities in the umbilical artery, although not an indication for immediate delivery, is considered an indication for immediate and intensive ongoing fetal surveillance. Delivery is usually based on the results of fetal heart rate monitoring or the BPP, with consideration of maternal condition and gestational age.[194]

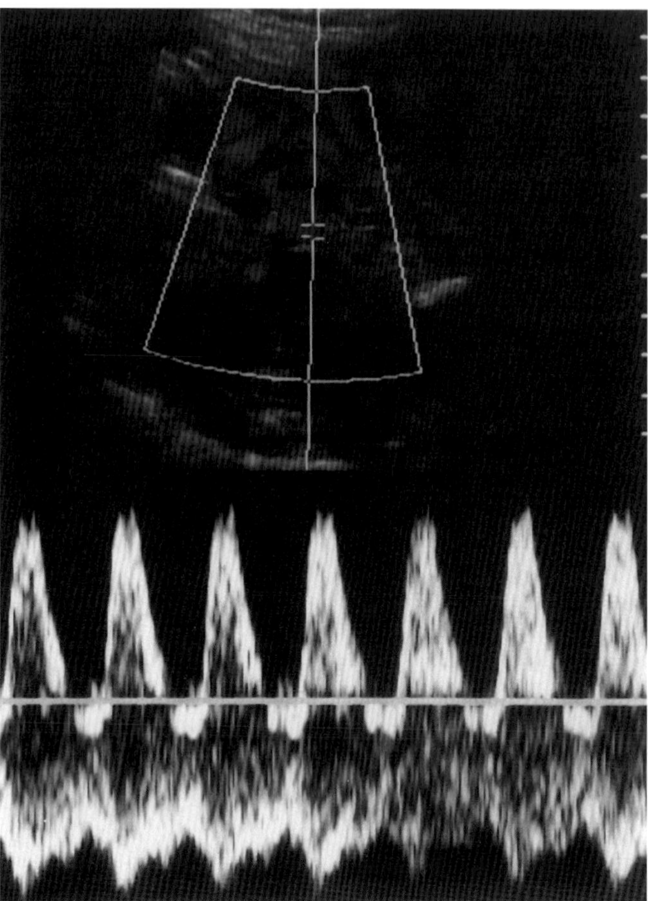

Figure 11-20. Umbilical arterial waveforms with reverse flow at end-diastole. Umbilical venous velocities have marked pulsations.

Most Doppler ultrasound studies of the fetus have focused on the umbilical arterial circulation. Examination of the fetal venous circulation has allowed some refinement in our understanding of the normal fetal circulation as well as fetal well-being. Most commonly, the fetal umbilical venous blood flow is monophasic (see Fig. 11-15). Fetuses with abnormal arterial velocities, or with abnormal cardiac function, may develop "pulsations" in the venous velocity waveform (see Fig. 11-19).[196] These pulsations occur during late diastole, and can be distinguished from breathing changes produced during fetal breathing episodes by their regularity, persistence, and association with the fetal heart rate. Umbilical venous pulsations can be produced in fetal lambs by volume-loading the venous circulation, and are associated with increases in central venous pressure.[197] Serial studies of human fetuses with absent end-diastolic velocities in the umbilical artery showed that the development of umbilical venous pulsations was associated with a shorter time between diagnosis and delivery with the deliveries performed for abnormal fetal heart rate patterns.[198] Fetuses with abnormally high umbilical artery velocity indices have a higher perinatal morbidity and mortality if abnormal venous velocities also develop.[199] Umbilical

Table 11-7. Doppler Changes During Antenatal Fetal Evaluation in Fetuses with Intrauterine Growth Restriction

VESSEL	CHANGE INDICATING FETAL COMPROMISE	PATHOPHYSIOLOGIC MECHANISM
Early Changes		
1. Umbilical Artery	Reduced, absence or reversed end-diastolic flow	Feto-placental circulatory resistance and hypertension
2. Middle Cerebral Artery	Decreased S/D or pulsatility index	Dilation of cerebral vessels ("brain sparing")
Late Changes		
3. Umbilical vein or ductus venosus	Pulsatility in umbilical vein or abnormal S/a Wave or reverse a-wave flow	Increased central venous pressure or diminished cardiac compliance
4. Pulmonary Artery	Decreased peak systolic velocity	Systemic hypertension and increased afterload
5. Aorta	Decreased peak systolic velocity	Systemic hypertension and increased afterload

Adapted from Ferrazzi E, Bozzo M, Rigano S, et al: Temporal sequence of abnormal Doppler changes in the peripheral and central circulatory systems of the severely growth-restricted fetus. Ultrasound Obstet Gynecol 19:140, 2002.

venous pulsations have been demonstrated in fetuses with late decelerations, during the deceleration itself.[200] These findings suggest that fetuses with abnormal umbilical arterial velocities may develop higher central venous pressures and umbilical venous pulsations as their condition deteriorates. Furthermore, fetuses with abnormal cardiac function or cardiac failure may demonstrate umbilical venous velocity pulsations even when umbilical arterial velocities are normal. Studies using Doppler assessment of peripheral and central fetal circulation in cases of IUGR has been performed, in an attempt to assess temporal and sequential relationships in Doppler changes as well as correlation with fetal heart rate patterns and BPP scores (see Chapter 29). In a prospective study by Ferrazzi et al.,[201] 26 women with growth restricted fetuses were followed, and five vessels were interrogated. These included the umbilical artery, middle cerebral artery, ductus venosus, pulmonary artery, and aorta. They found that serial changes in the velocimetry of these vessels followed a pattern that may be useful in identifying fetuses at risk for perinatal death. Early changes included absent end diastolic velocities of the umbilical artery, and persistent decreased indices of the middle cerebral artery, suggesting persistent dilation and "brain sparing." Subsequently, late changes occurred including reversed diastolic flow in the umbilical artery, abnormal ductus venosus waveforms and decreased aortic and pulmonary artery peak systolic velocities (Table 11-7). These circulatory patterns were identified before changes in fetal heart rate patterns, and generate interest as potential markers for worsening fetal status before changes in fetal heart rate patterns. Interestingly, however, 60 percent of the IUGR fetuses demonstrated abnormal fetal heart rate tracings in the absence of late changes in circulatory velocimetry. Furthermore, in a study of fetuses with IUGR by Baschat et al.,[202] concordance for compromise of the Doppler assessment and BPP occurred in only 44.5 percent of cases, and no consistent relationship between Doppler assessment and BPP results could be determined. Fetal deterioration appears to be independently reflected in the two modalities, and further research will be required to elucidate appropriate testing strategies utilizing the combination for fetuses affected with IUGR.

Although randomized trials are difficult to construct and complete, Williams et al.[203] compared NSTs with umbilical artery Doppler assessments for surveillance of pregnancies complicated by prolonged gestation, decreased fetal movement, diabetes mellitus, hypertension, and IUGR. Those patients randomized to Doppler assessments demonstrated a significant reduction in the cesarean delivery rate for fetal distress (4.6 percent versus 8.7 percent). The reduction was most pronounced in the subgroups of hypertension and suspected IUGR. Alternatively, in a decision-analysis model, Obido et al.[204] compared BPP scoring and Doppler assessment in monitoring fetus with IUGR. They concluded that a model using BPP only would be best to minimize neonatal death or disability. The assessment of the fetal condition by NST, CST, or assessment of the fetal biophysical state by BPP is currently the cornerstone of management planning for high-risk fetal conditions.

The effectiveness of umbilical artery Doppler studies as an antepartum fetal surveillance technique has been summarized in an editorial by Divon and Ferber, in which the results of several meta-analyses were reviewed.[194] A meta-analysis by Giles and Bisit of six published, peer-reviewed, randomized controlled, clinical trials showed a reduction in perinatal mortality in the 2,102 fetuses studied with Doppler compared with the 2,133 fetuses not evaluated with this technique.[205] An analysis of 12 published and unpublished randomized controlled clinical trials in 7,474 high-risk patients revealed fewer antenatal admissions, inductions of labor, cesarean deliveries for fetal distress, and perinatal mortality in high-risk pregnancies monitored with Doppler velocimetry.[206] A recent report by Neilson and Alfirevic confirmed these findings.[207] Divon and Ferber conclude that Doppler ultrasound is useful in high-risk pregnancies and will decrease perinatal mortality without increasing maternal or neonatal morbidity. Studies of low-risk pregnancies have not shown a benefit from the use of Doppler ultrasound.[208,209] Although the use of Doppler ultrasound in current obstetric practice is evolving, certain recommendations regarding its use have been made.[208] These include providing the availability of Doppler ultrasound for the assessment of fetoplacental circulation in high-risk pregnancies with suspected placental insufficiency, increasing fetal surveillance when reduced, absent, or reversed umbilical artery end diastolic velocities are encountered, and assessing fetal well-being when umbilical venous pulsations are encountered.[208]

THE ASSESSMENT OF FETAL PULMONARY MATURATION

This section reviews those techniques that enable the obstetrician to predict accurately the risks of RDS for the infant requiring premature delivery and to avoid the unnecessary complications of iatrogenic prematurity. It is the risk of iatrogenic prematurity for the neonate that is balanced against the risk of continued antepartum assessment of the potentially compromised fetus that determines ultimate management strategies. As such, incorporation of the discussion of assessment of fetal pulmonary maturity with that of antepartum assessment is critical.

RDS is caused by a deficiency of pulmonary surfactant, an antiatelectasis factor that is able to maintain a low stable surface tension at the air-water interface within alveoli. Surfactant decreases the pressure needed to distend the lung and prevents alveolar collapse (see Chapter 20). The type II alveolar cell is the major site of surfactant synthesis. Surfactant is packaged in lamellar bodies, discharged into the alveoli, and carried into the amniotic cavity with pulmonary fluid.

Phospholipids account for more than 80 percent of the surface active material within the lung, and more than 50 percent of this phospholipid is dipalmitoyl lecithin. The latter is a derivative of glycerol phosphate and contains two fatty acids as well as the nitrogenous base choline. Other phospholipids contained in the surfactant complex include phosphatidylglycerol (PG), phosphatidylinositol, phosphatidylserine, phosphatidylethanolamine, sphingomyelin, and lysolecithin. PG is the second most abundant lipid in surfactant and significantly improves its properties.

An accurate assessment of gestational age and fetal maturity is essential before an elective induction of labor or cesarean delivery or before the delivery of a patient whose fetus may not have matured normally such as a growth-restricted fetus or the fetus of a poorly controlled diabetic mother. Many of the techniques used in clinical practice in the past not only failed to predict gestational age but provided little information about fetal pulmonary maturation.[210]

Before the now-common practice of using ultrasound to establish gestational age and amniotic fluid studies to assess fetal pulmonary maturation, iatrogenic prematurity was an important clinical problem. In 1975, Goldenberg and Nelson[211] concluded that untimely or unwarranted intervention was responsible for 15 percent of their cases of RDS. In a similar study published in 1976, Hack et al.[212] observed that 12 percent of all infants with RDS in their neonatal intensive care unit were born after elective deliveries. None of these infants had had documentation of pulmonary maturation before delivery. Almost 30 years later, and despite widely publicized guidelines for assuming fetal lung maturation by the ACOG, iatrogenic causes of RDS in "term" neonates remains a potentially preventable problem. In a review of 35,031 deliveries occurring at 37 0/7 to 40 6/7 weeks, Wax et al.[213] found 18 infants with RDS requiring mechanical ventilation. Of the 16 infants born between 37 0/7 weeks and 38 6/7 weeks, six had been electively delivered without documented lung maturity. The importance of assessing pulmonary maturity and balancing the risks of neonatal respiratory distress is underscored.

Several changes in clinical practice appear to have decreased the incidence of RDS caused by iatrogenic prematurity. Patients who have had a single previous low transverse cesarean delivery may attempt a vaginal birth. In such cases, because the onset of spontaneous labor is awaited, documentation of fetal pulmonary maturation before elective intervention is not required. Most important, ultrasound documentation of gestational age in the first trimester or early in the second trimester has proven extremely reliable in timing elective inductions or cesarean deliveries (see Chapter 9). Many patients are currently requesting a repeat cesarean delivery after having a previous cesarean, to avoid the risks associated with uterine scar disruption in labor. In assessing the effect of cesarean delivery on respiratory distress in the neonate, Gerten et al.[214] found that cesarean delivery was an independent risk for RDS, with an odds ratio of 2.3. Labor prior to cesarean reduced the odds ratio to 1.9, but did not eliminate the increased risk of respiratory distress. This highlights the importance of assuring lung maturation before elective cesarean delivery.

Assessment of Fetal Pulmonary Maturity

Available methods for evaluating fetal pulmonary maturity can be divided into three categories: (1) quantitation of pulmonary surfactant, such as the lecithin/sphingomyelin (L/S) ratio; (2) measurement of surfactant function including the shake test; and (3) evaluation of amniotic fluid turbidity.[215,216] The first category has become the most common and reliable in current practice.

With the exception of amniotic fluid specimens obtained from the vaginal pool, the evaluation of fetal pulmonary maturation requires that a sample of amniotic fluid be obtained by amniocentesis. In the past, third-trimester amniocentesis was associated with significant fetal and maternal risks. Fetal complications have included fetal bleeding from laceration of the placenta or umbilical cord, fetomaternal bleeding, premature labor and premature rupture of the membranes, placental abruption, and fetal injury. Maternal complications, although rare, have included hemorrhage, in some cases from perforation of the uterine vessels, abdominal wall hematomas, Rh sensitization, and infection.

Ultrasound guidance for third-trimester amniocentesis has significantly decreased the risks of the procedure. In a review of seven studies that included 4,115 third-trimester amniocenteses, the frequency of complications was 3 percent for rupture of the membranes within 24 hours, 7 percent for a bloody tap, 4.4 percent for failed amniocentesis, 3.3 percent for labor within 24 hours, 1 percent for fetal trauma, and 0.05 percent for fetal death.[217] More recently, a review of amniocentesis for assessment of fetal lung maturity in 913 patients was completed by Stark et al.[218] They found that 15 procedures (1.6%) were unsuccessful, and complications requiring same-day delivery were present in only 6 patients (0.7%). Complications included fetal heart rate abnormalities, placental bleeding, abruption, and uterine rupture. Only one of six complications was associated with a single-needle pass and withdrawal of clear fluid.

Before the routine use of ultrasound guidance, failure to retrieve fluid from third trimester amniocentesis occurred in up to 11 percent of procedures, and bloody amniotic fluid was found in up to 15 percent.[219] Currently, only 1 to 2 percent of procedures fail to yield fluid, and bloody fluid is encountered in only 6 to 7 percent.[218] A bloody tap warrants careful observation[220] but does not necessarily mean immediate delivery. Only two of 62 bloody amniocenteses in the analysis of Stark were associated with the need for immediate delivery. At term, the fetal blood volume is relatively small, and fetal bleeding may have important clinical consequences. When a bloody tap occurs, the patient should be evaluated with continuous electronic fetal heart rate monitoring. An Apt test or Kleihauer-Betke test may confirm that the blood is of maternal origin, and the fetus has demonstrated no evidence of compromise. Should a nonreassuring fetal heart rate pattern be observed, consideration for cesarean delivery is prudent. When fetal blood is recovered and fetal maturity is ascertained, delivery may be considered even in the absence of fetal compromise by heart rate testing. For those fetuses demonstrating lack of pulmonary maturity, careful fetal assessment following a bloody tap is warranted, and treatment with corticosteroids followed by delivery thereafter may be beneficial.[221]

QUANTITATION OF PULMONARY SURFACTANT

LECITHIN/SPHINGOMYELIN RATIO

The L/S ratio was the first reliable assay for the assessment of fetal pulmonary maturity.[222,223] The amniotic fluid concentration of lecithin increases markedly at approximately 35 weeks' gestation, whereas sphingomyelin levels remain stable or decrease. Rather than determine the concentration of lecithin that could be altered by variations in amniotic fluid volume, Gluck and coworkers used sphingomyelin as an internal standard and compared the amount of lecithin with that of sphingomyelin. Amniotic fluid sphingomyelin exceeds lecithin until 31 to 32 weeks, when the L/S ratio reaches 1. Lecithin then rises rapidly, and an L/S ratio of 2.0 is observed at approximately 35 weeks. Wide variation in the L/S ratio at each gestational age has been noted. Nevertheless, a ratio of 2.0 or greater has repeatedly been associated with pulmonary maturity. In more than 2,100 cases, a mature L/S ratio predicted the absence of RDS in 98 percent of neonates.[224] With a ratio of 1.5 to 1.9, approximately 50 percent of infants will develop RDS. Below 1.5, the risk of subsequent RDS increases to 73 percent. Thus, the L/S ratio, like most indices of fetal pulmonary maturation, rarely errs when predicting fetal pulmonary maturity but is frequently incorrect when predicting subsequent RDS.[225] Many neonates with an immature L/S ratio do not develop RDS.

Several important variables must be considered in interpreting the predictive accuracy of the L/S ratio. A prolonged interval between the determination of an immature L/S ratio and delivery will necessarily increase the number of falsely immature results. It is probably best to discard amniotic fluid samples heavily contaminated by blood or meconium, because the effects of these compounds on the determination of the L/S ratio are unpredictable.[226,227] Blood has been reported both to increase and decrease the ratio, and meconium can produce falsely mature results. The presence of PG in a bloody or meconium-stained amniotic fluid sample remains a reliable indicator of pulmonary maturity.[228] PG is not normally found in blood, and meconium generally does not interfere with the identification of PG.[229,230] Finally, it is essential that the obstetrician know the analytic technique used and the predictive value of a mature L/S ratio in his or her laboratory.

Many perinatal processes alter the final interpretation of the L/S ratio. Surfactant deficiency, immaturity, and intrapartum complications are the prime factors in determining the pathogenesis of RDS.[231] Birth asphyxia may lead to RDS in many infants despite an L/S ratio greater than 2.0. In earlier studies, infants with severe Rh disease and infants of diabetic mothers were reported to have developed RDS despite mature L/S ratios. More recent data indicate that the L/S ratio is reliable in both high-risk conditions.[232,233] Kjos and colleagues[233] found no cases of RDS caused by surfactant deficiency in a study of women with pregestational and gestational diabetes.

PG, which does not appear until 35 weeks' gestation and increases rapidly between 37 to 40 weeks, is a marker of completed pulmonary maturation.[234] Most infants who lack PG but who have a mature L/S ratio fail to develop RDS. However, PG may provide further insurance against the onset of RDS despite intrapartum complications.

SLIDE AGGLUTINATION TEST FOR PHOSPHATIDYLGLYCEROL

A rapid immunologic semiquantitative agglutination test (Amniostat-FLM) can be used to determine the presence of PG.[235] This assay can detect PG at a concentration greater than 0.5 µg/ml of amniotic fluid. The test takes 20 to 30 minutes to perform and requires only 1.5 ml of amniotic fluid. Besides being highly sensitive, several studies have found a positive Amniostat-FLM to correlate well with the presence of PG by thin-layer chromatography and the absence of subsequent RDS. In a study evaluating samples from the vaginal pool and those obtained by amniocentesis, the overall concordance for the Amniostat-FLM and thin-layer chromatography results was 89 percent.[235] No cases of RDS were observed when the Amniostat-FLM assay demonstrated PG. This technique can be applied to samples contaminated by blood and meconium, but it is not commonly used in current practice.

FLUORESCENCE POLARIZATION

TDX TEST (SURFACTANT ALBUMIN RATIO)

The TDx analyzer, an automated fluorescence polarimeter, has been used to assess surfactant content in amniotic fluid.[236–239] The test requires 1 ml of amniotic fluid and can be run in less than 1 hour. The surfactant albumin ratio (SAR) is determined with amniotic fluid albumin used as an internal reference. A value of 70 was considered mature with the original assay, whereas with the newer FLM-II test, 55 is the mature cut-off.[215] A mature value reliably predicts the absence of RDS requiring intubation in infants of diabetic mothers.[240] The TDx test correlates well with the L/S ratio and has few falsely mature results, making it an excellent screening test.[221,241] The TDx assay proved to be reliable in predicting fetal lung maturity in vaginal pool specimens in patients with preterm premature rupture of the membranes at 30 to 36 weeks.[242] Approximately 50 percent of infants with an immature TDx result develop RDS. The test has gained wide popularity because of its ease, low cost, and reproducibility, and is commonly available in practice.

MEASUREMENT OF SURFACTANT FUNCTION

FOAM STABILITY INDEX

The test is based on the manual foam stability index (FSI), and is a variation of the shake test.[243] The kit currently available contains test wells with a predispensed volume of ethanol. The addition of 0.5-ml amniotic fluid to each test well in the kit produces final ethanol volumes of 44 to 50 percent. A control well contains sufficient surfactant in 50-percent ethanol to produce an example of the stable foam end point. The amniotic fluid/ethanol mixture is first shaken, and the FSI value is read as the highest value well in which a ring of stable foam persists.[244]

This test appears to be a reliable predictor of fetal lung maturity.[245] Subsequent RDS is very unlikely with an FSI value of 47 or higher. The methodology is simple, and the test can be performed at any time of day by persons who have had only minimal instruction. The assay appears to be extremely sensitive, with a high proportion of immature results being associated with RDS, as well as moderately specific, with a high proportion of mature results predicting the absence of RDS. Contamination of the amniotic fluid specimen by blood or meconium invalidates the FSI results. The FSI can function well as a screening test, but has lost popularity in current practice to other more reliable and convenient tests.

EVALUATION OF AMNIOTIC FLUID TURBIDITY

VISUAL INSPECTION

During the first and second trimesters, amniotic fluid is yellow and clear. It becomes colorless in the third trimester. By 33 to 34 weeks' gestation, cloudiness and flocculation are noted, and, as term approaches, vernix appears. Amniotic fluid with obvious vernix or fluid so turbid it does not permit the reading of newsprint through it will usually have a mature L/S ratio.[246]

LAMELLAR BODY COUNTS

Lamellar bodies are the storage form of surfactant released by fetal type II pneumocytes into the amniotic fluid. Because they have the same size as platelets, the amniotic fluid concentration of lamellar bodies may be determined using a commercial cell counter.[247–250] The test requires less than 1 ml of amniotic fluid and takes only 15 minutes to perform. A lamellar body count greater than 30,000 to 55,000/μl is highly predictive of pulmonary maturity, whereas a count below 10,000/μl suggests a significant risk for RDS. Lewis et al. have recently reported that a lamellar body count of less than 8,000 predicted an immature L/S and PG assay in all cases, whereas a value greater than 32,000 predicted a mature L/S or PG assay in 99 percent of cases.[251] The cutoff used to predict fetal pulmonary status depends on the type of cell counter used and the speed of centrifugation of the amniotic fluid specimen. Neither meconium nor lysed blood has a significant effect on the lamellar body count. The ease and relatively low cost of this test has contributed to its popularity, although poor concordance among various instruments for the assay of lamellar body counts has been noted.[252]

Determination of Fetal Pulmonary Maturation in Clinical Practice

A large number of techniques are now available to assess fetal pulmonary maturation.[215] Several rapid screening tests, including the TDx test and lamellar body count, appear to be highly reliable when mature. In an uncomplicated pregnancy, when a screening test such as the TDx demonstrates fetal pulmonary maturation, one can safely proceed with delivery.[239,251] The more complicated, expensive, and timely L/S ratio may be reserved for those borderline TDx or lamellar body count results in the clinical circumstance of a fetus that may benefit from delivery if maturity is ultimately confirmed with advanced testing. This sequential approach is also extremely cost effective.[215,216,253,254] When the screening test is immature, the L/S ratio and PG assessment should be considered.

As data has been assimilated in recent years related to lung maturity assessment and its role in high-risk pregnancy management, new important paradigms are emerging. Traditionally, lung maturity tests have been interpreted in categorical fashion, usually as either "positive" indicating lung maturity and a low risk of RDS, or "negative" indicating the absence of maturity and a higher risk of RDS. However, the presence of RDS in neonates is associated with both gestational age and lung maturity assessments. As further information has been gathered, it is now possible to stratify risk of RDS based on both gestational age and lung maturity assessment. This represents a more appropriate use of the lung maturity tests. For instance, the risk of RDS given an FLM result of 30 to 40 mg/g is about 50 percent at 28 weeks, about 25 percent at 32 weeks, and only about 10 percent at 36 weeks.[255] In assessing the risk of RDS complicating subsequent delivery,[256–259] results from fetal lung maturity testing are most appropriately correlated with the gestational age at the time of fluid retrieval.

A PRACTICAL APPROACH TO TESTING

How can one most efficiently use all the techniques available for antepartum fetal surveillance? Obstetricians should take a "diagnosis-specific" or "condition-specific" approach to testing.[260] That is, they must consider the pathophysiology of the disease process that will be evaluated and then select the best method or methods of testing for that problem. For example, in the pregnancy complicated by significant Rh isoimmunization, one might want to use serial evaluations of fetal hemoglobin. In a pregnancy complicated by diabetes mellitus, careful monitoring of maternal glucose levels should accompany antepartum heart rate testing. In contrast, in a pregnancy complicated by suspected growth restriction, one would want to make serial evaluations of amniotic fluid volume with ultrasound to detect oligohydramnios.

In a prolonged pregnancy, one would use a parallel testing scheme. In this situation, the obstetrician is not concerned with fetal maturity, but rather with fetal well-being. Several tests are performed at the same time, such as antepartum fetal heart rate testing and the BPP. It is acceptable in this high-risk situation to intervene when a single test is abnormal. One is willing to accept a false-positive test result to avoid the intrauterine death of a mature and otherwise healthy fetus. In a study of prolonged gestations in Canada between 1980 and 1995, Sue-A-Quan et al. reported a decline in the stillbirth rate for deliveries at 41 or more weeks' gestation that they attributed to an increased rate of labor induction.[261] Patients may have been induced electively or selectively for abnormal tests of fetal well-being.

In most other high-risk pregnancies, such as those complicated by diabetes mellitus or hypertension, it is preferable to allow the fetus to remain in utero as long as possible. In these situations, a branched testing scheme is used. To decrease the likelihood of unnecessary premature intervention, the obstetrician uses a series of tests and, under most circumstances, would only deliver a premature infant when all parameters suggest fetal compromise. In this situation, one must consider the likelihood of neonatal RDS as predicted by the evaluation of amniotic fluid indices and review these risks with colleagues in neonatology.

Maternal assessment of fetal activity would appear to be an ideal first-line screening test for both high-risk and low-risk patients. The use of this approach may decrease the number of unexpected intrauterine deaths in so-called normal pregnancies. Although a negative CST has been associated with fewer intrauterine deaths than a reactive NST, the NST appears to have significant advantages in screening high-risk patients. It can be easily and rapidly performed in an outpatient setting. Most clinicians use the BPP or CST to assess fetal condition in patients exhibiting a persistently nonreactive NST. This sequential approach may be particularly valuable in avoiding unnecessary premature intervention.

MODIFIED BIOPHYSICAL PROFILE

Figure 11-21 presents a practical testing scheme that has been used successfully by several centers.[122,154,262,263] The NST, an indicator of present fetal condition, may be combined with the amniotic fluid index (AFI) (see Chapters 9 and 31), a marker of long-term status, in a modified BPP. In this setting, an AFI greater than 5 cm is usually considered normal, although different criteria have been applied.[264] VAS may be used to shorten the time required to achieve a reactive NST. Although most patients are evaluated weekly, patients with diabetes mellitus, IUGR, or a prolonged gestation are tested twice weekly. If the NST is nonreactive despite VAS or extended monitoring, or if the AFI is abnormal, either a full BPP or CST is performed. Using this approach, Clark et al.[262] found no unexpected antepartum fetal deaths in a series of 2,628 high-risk pregnancies. VAS shortened the mean testing time to 10 minutes. Only 2 percent of all NSTs were nonreactive. However, 17 percent of these were followed by a positive CST or BPP score of 4 or less. Clark et al. have extended their experience with this technique to include an additional 3,005 tests. One fetus died 2 days after a reactive NST because of a cord accident. Therefore, only one fetal death has been observed in almost 9,000 tests after a reactive NST and normal AFI, indicating a high detection rate with the use of the modified BPP. In a series of 6,543 fetuses, Vintzileos et al.[265] reported no fetal deaths attributable to hypoxia within 1 week of a reactive NST and an ultrasound study demonstrating normal amniotic

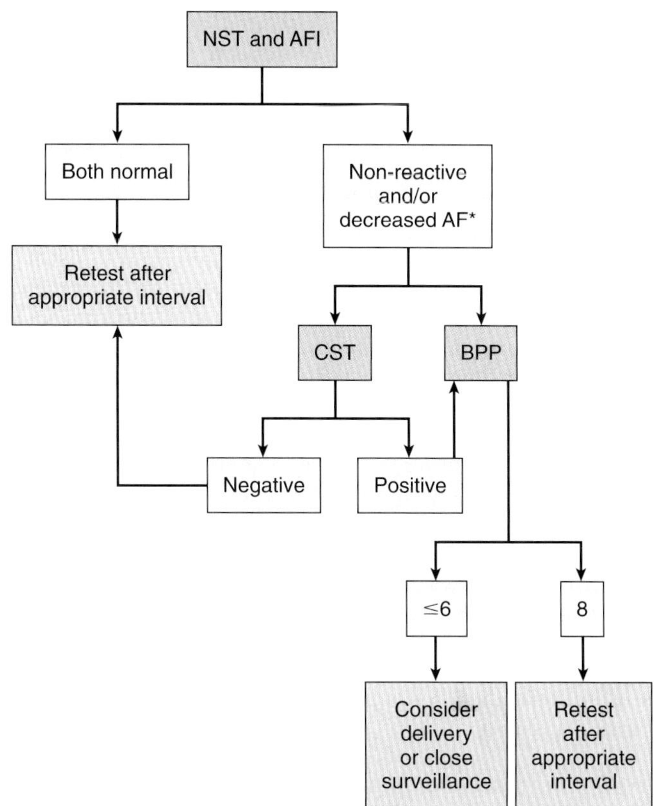

Figure 11-21. Flow chart for antepartum fetal surveillance in which the NST and AFI are used as the primary methods for fetal evaluation. A nonreactive NST and decreased AF are further evaluated using either the CST or the BPP. Further details regarding the use of the BPP are provided in Table 11-6. *If the fetus is mature and amniotic fluid volume is reduced, delivery should be considered before further testing is undertaken. AFI, amniotic fluid index; BPP, biophysical profile; CST, contraction stress test; NST, nonstress test. (Adapted from Finberg HJ, Kurtz AB, Johnson RL, et al: The biophysical profile: a literature review and reassessment of its usefulness in the evaluation of fetal well-being. J Ultrasound Med 9:583, 1990.)

fluid. Nageotte et al.[266] demonstrated that the modified BPP was as good a predictor of adverse fetal outcome as a negative CST. Furthermore, the CST as a backup test was associated with a higher rate of intervention for an abnormal test than the use of a complete BPP as a backup test. Miller et al. described 56,617 antepartum tests in 15,482 women identified as high risk.[267] Six indications (prolonged pregnancy, diabetes mellitus, decreased fetal movement, suspected IUGR, hypertension, and a history of previous stillbirth) accounted for more than 90 percent of patients tested. The modified BPP including the NST and AFI was used primarily with the full BPP as a backup test. Sixty percent of those delivered for an abnormal test had no evidence of fetal compromise. However, false-positive tests led to preterm deliveries in only 1.5 percent of those tested before 37 weeks. The false-negative rate was similar to that of the CST and complete BPP, 0.8 per 1,000 women tested. Overall, the modified BPP had a false-positive rate comparable to the NST but higher than the CST and full BPP. The low false-negative rate and ease of performance of the modified BPP make it an excellent approach for the evaluation of large numbers of high-risk patients. As such, although potentially still a useful test, the CST is becoming less frequently used in current practice.[268,269]

STRATEGIES TO REDUCE ANTEPARTUM FETAL DEATHS

What strategies can be used to reduce antepartum fetal deaths?[270] (See the box "Strategies to Reduce Antepartum Fetal Deaths.") First, it is important to determine the cause of a fetal death so that the patient and her partner can be counseled, the risk of recurrence described, and a plan of care for subsequent pregnancies developed. The obstetrician should write a detailed note describing the stillborn fetus, amniotic fluid, umbilical cord, placenta, and membranes. If the infant is malformed, growth restricted, or hydropic, chromosomal studies should be obtained. An autopsy should be requested.[270,271] Incerpi et al.[272] observed that an autopsy and evaluation of the placenta were the most valuable tests in determining the cause of fetal death, and following a protocol for assessment of fetal death, they were able to determine a cause in 72 percent of stillbirths. Postmortem magnetic resonance imaging is being used more frequently in antenatal diagnosis, and its use in the case of fetal death has been investigated and compared with autopsy.[273] Tests for syphilis, and the acquired and inherited thrombophilias including antiphospholipid antibodies, and the lupus anticoagulant, deficiencies in protein C, protein S, and antithrombin 3, and DNA mutation analysis for factor V, factor II and the methyltetrahydrofolate reductase gene, should be done. If the patient has not been screened for diabetes mellitus during gestation, a fasting glucose test should be ordered. Because significant fetal-maternal hemorrhage has been observed in approximately 5 percent of all fetal deaths, a Kleihauer-Betke test should be obtained.

To prevent antepartum deaths, routine fetal movement counting should be considered in all pregnancies, starting at 28 weeks' gestation. The modified Count-to-Ten method developed by Moore and Piacquadio is a simple and valuable technique.[67] To reduce fetal deaths resulting from fetal malformations, second-trimester serum analyte screening should be offered and routine ultrasound performed at 18 to 20 weeks (see Chapters 6 and 9). Additionally, first-trimester screening may be beneficial for aneuploidy screening and offers advantages of earlier detection. To detect IUGR, careful serial measurements of fundal height should be performed with an ultrasound examination at 30 to 32 weeks in high-risk patients including those with vascular disease and in patients with lagging uterine growth (see Chapter 29). Finally, to reduce fetal deaths caused by placental abruption, patients who are hypertensive should be followed closely and managed with antihypertensive medication, and those known to be abusing cocaine should be counseled and enrolled in treatment programs.

Strategies to Reduce Antepartum Fetal Deaths

- Determination of the cause of fetal death
- Antepartum fetal evaluation in all pregnancies with routine fetal movement counting
- Surveillance for fetal malformations in all pregnancies with a triple screen and routine ultrasound at 18–20 weeks
- Surveillance for detection of IUGR with fundal height measurements and ultrasound at 30–32 weeks in high-risk patients and patients with lagging growth
- Programs to identify and treat cocaine abuse in pregnancy

IUGR, intrauterine growth restriction.
From Gabbe SG: Prevention of antepartum fetal deaths. OB/GYN Clinical Alert, April 1998, p 94, with permission.

Key Points

- The prevalence of an abnormal condition (i.e., fetal death) has great impact on the predictive value of antepartum fetal tests.
- Intrauterine fetal deaths occur in the United States approximately 10 times more frequently than sudden infant death.
- The near-term fetus spends approximately 25 percent of its time in a quiet sleep state (state 1F) and 60 to 70 percent in an active sleep state (state 2F).
- Approximately 5 percent of women monitoring fetal movement report decreased fetal activity.
- The observation that accelerations of the fetal heart rate in response to fetal activity, uterine contractions, or stimulation reflect fetal well-being is the basis for the NST.
- The frequency of the NST should be increased to twice weekly in pregnancies complicated by diabetes mellitus, prolonged gestation, and IUGR.
- Use of VAS for a nonreactive NST or equivocal BPP does not increase the false-negative rate and

may reduce the likelihood of unnecessary obstetric intervention.

❑ Reversed end-diastolic flow in the umbilical artery flow velocity waveform has been associated with an increased PMR.

❑ Most amniotic fluid tests of fetal pulmonary maturation accurately predict maturity, but improved accuracy in predicting subsequent RDS is noted when the indices are correlated with gestational age.

❑ The NST, an indicator of present fetal condition, and the AFI, a marker of long-term fetal status, have been combined in the modified BPP.

REFERENCES

1. Eskes TKAB: Introduction. *In* Nijhuis J (ed): Fetal Behaviour. New York, Oxford University Press, 1992, p xv.
2. Fretts RC: Etiology and prevention of stillbirth. Am J Obstet Gyncecol 193:1923, 2005.
3. Centers for Disease Control and Prevention, NCHS, National Vital Statistics System: Vital statistics of the United States, vol. II, mortality, Part A; Infant mortality rates, fetal mortality rates, and perinatal mortality rates, according to race: United States, selected years 1950–1998. Public Health Service, Washington, DC, U.S. Govt. Printing Office.
4. Chard T, Klopper A (eds): Introduction. *In* Placental Function Tests. New York, Springer-Verlag, 1982, p 1.
5. Friede A, Rochat R: Maternal mortality and perinatal mortality: definitions, data, and epidemiology. *In* Sachs B (ed): Obstetric Epidemiology. Littleton, MA, PSG Publishing Company, 1985, p 35.
6. World Health Organization. The OBSQUID Project: Quality development in perinatal care, final report. Publ Eur Surv, 1995.
7. American College of Obstetricians and Gynecologists: Perinatal and infant mortality statistics. Committee Opinion 167, December 1995.
8. Cotzias CS, Paterson-Browm S, Fisk NM: Prospective risk of unexplained stillbirth in singleton pregnancies at term: population based analysis. BMJ 319:287, 1999.
9. Grant A, Elbourne D: Fetal movement counting to assess fetal well-being. *In* Chalmers I, Enkin M, Keirse MJNC (eds): Effective Care in Pregnancy and Childbirth. Oxford, Oxford University Press, 1989, p 440.
10. Kahn B, Lumey LH, Zybert PA, et al: Prospective risk of fetal death in singleton, twin, and triplet gestations: implications for practice Obstet Gynecol 102:685, 2003.
11. Naeye RL: Causes of perinatal mortality in the United States Collaborative Perinatal Project. JAMA 238:228, 1977.
12. Martin JA, Hamilton BE, Sutton PD, et al: Births: final data for 2002. Natl Vital Stat Rep 52:1, 2003.
13. Guyer B, Strobino DM, Ventura SJ, Singh GK: Annual summary of vital statistics 1994. Pediatrics 96:1029, 1995.
14. March of Dimes Perinatal Profiles: Health Indicators, 1990–1997. New York, The March of Dimes Perinatal Data Center and Planning and Community Services Divison, 2000.
15. Morbidity and Mortality Weekly Report: Trends in infant mortality attributable to birth defects—United States, 1980–1995. Boston, Massachusetts Medical Society, 2000.
16. Lammer EJ, Brown LE, Anderka MT, Guyer B: Classification and analysis of fetal deaths in Massachusetts. JAMA 261:1757, 1989.
17. Manning FA, Lange IR, Morrison I, Harman CR: Determination of fetal health: methods for antepartum and intrapartum fetal assessment. *In* Leventhal J (ed): Current Problems in Obstetrics and Gynecology. Chicago, Year Book Medical Publishers, 1983.
18. Fretts RC, Boyd ME, Usher RH, Usher H: The changing pattern of fetal death, 1961–1988. Obstet Gynecol 79:35, 1992.
19. Fretts RC, Schmittdiel J, McLean FH, et al: Increased maternal age and the risk of fetal death. N Engl J Med 333:953, 1995.
20. Liu S, Joseph KS, Kramer MS, et al: Relationship of prenatal diagnosis and pregnancy termination to overall infant mortality in Canada. JAMA 287:1561, 2002.
21. Forrester MB, Merz RD: Inclusion of early fetal deaths in a birth defects surveillance system. Teratology 64:S20, 2001.
22. Andersen AMN, Wohlfahrt J, Christens P, et al: Maternal age and fetal loss: population based register linkage study. BMJ 320:1708, 2000.
23. Stein Z, Susser M: The risks of having children in later life. BMJ 320:1681, 2000.
24. Schauer GM, Kalousek DK, Magee JF: Genetic causes of stillbirth. Semin Perinatol 16:341, 1992.
25. Mersey Region Working Party on Perinatal Mortality: Perinatal health. Lancet 1:491, 1982.
26. Kirkup B, Welch G: "Normal but dead": perinatal mortality in the non-malformed babies of birthweight 2–5 kg and over in the Northern Region in 1983. Br J Obstet Gynaecol 97:381, 1990.
27. Fretts RC, Elkin EB, Myers ER, Heffner LJ: Should older women have anteparatum testing to preven unexplained stillbirth? Obstet Gynecol 104:56, 2004.
28. Schneider EP, Hutson JM, Petrie RH: An assessment of the first decade's experience with antepartum fetal heart rate testing. Am J Perinatol 5:134, 1988.
29. Stubblefield P, Berek J: Perinatal mortality in term and postterm births. Obstet Gynecol 56:676, 1980.
30. Duenhoelter J, Whalley P, MacDonald P: An analysis of the utility of plasma immunoreactive estrogen measurements in determining delivery time of gravidas with a fetus considered at high risk. Am J Obstet Gynecol 125:889, 1976.
31. Mohide P, Keirse MJNC: Biophysical assessment of fetal well-being. *In* Chalmers I, Enkin M, Keirse MJNC (eds): Effective Care in Pregnancy and Childbirth. Oxford, Oxford University Press, 1989, p 477.
32. Thornton JG, Lilford RJ: Do we need randomised trials of antenatal tests of fetal wellbeing? Br J Obstet Gynaecol 100:197, 1993.
33. Divon MY, Ferber A: Evidence-based antepartum fetal testing. *In* Prenatal and Neonatal Medicine. New York, The Parthenon Publishing Group, 2000.
34. American College of Obstetricians and Gynecologists: Antepartum fetal surveillance. Practice Bulletin 9, October 1999.
35. Flynn AM, Kelly J, Mansfield H, et al: A randomized controlled trial of non-stress antepartum cardiotocography. Br J Obstet Gynaecol 89:427, 1982.
36. Brown VA, Sawers RS, Parsons RJ, et al: The value of antenatal cardiotocography in the management of high-risk pregnancy: a randomized controlled trial. Br J Obstet Gynaecol 89:716, 1982.
37. Lumley J, Lester A, Anderson I, et al: A randomized trial of weekly cardiotocography in high-risk obstetric patients. Br J Obstet Gynaecol 90:1018, 1983.
38. Kidd LC, Patel NB, Smith R: Non-stress antenatal cardiotocography: a prospective randomized clinical trial. Br J Obstet Gynaecol 92:1156, 1985.
39. Ferrera TB, Hoekstra RF, Couser RJ, et al: Survival and follow-up of infants born at 23–26 weeks gestational age: effects of surfactant therapy. J Pediatr 124:119, 1994.
40. Allen M, Donohue P, Dushman A: The limit of viability: neonatal outcome of infants born at 22–25 weeks gestation. N Engl J Med 329:1597, 1993.
41. Schwartz RM, Luby AM, Scanlon JW, Kellog RJ: Effect of surfactant on morbidity, mortality and resource use in newborn infants weighing 500–1500 grams. N Engl J Med 330:1476, 1994.
42. Schifrin B, Foye G, Amato J, et al: Routine fetal heart rate monitoring in the antepartum period. Obstet Gynecol 54:21, 1979.
43. Stempel L: Eenie, meenie, minie, mo . . . what do the data really show? Obstet Gynecol 144:745, 1982.
44. Peipert JF, Sweeney PJ: Diagnostic testing in obstetrics and gynecology: a clinician's guide. Obstet Gynecol 82:619, 1993.

45. Carpenter M, Coustan D: Criteria for screening tests for gestational diabetes. Am J Obstet Gynecol 144:768, 1982.
46. Manning FA: Assessment of fetal condition and risk: analysis of single and combined biophysical variable monitoring. Semin Perinatol 9:168, 1985.
47. Van Woerden EE, VanGeijn HP: Heart-rate patterns and fetal movements. *In* Nijhuis J (ed): Fetal Behaviour. New York, Oxford University Press, 1992, p 41.
48. Patrick J, Campbell K, Carmichael L, et al: Patterns of gross fetal body movements over 24-hour observation intervals during the last 10 weeks of pregnancy. Am J Obstet Gynecol 142:363, 1982.
49. Holden K, Jovanovic L, Druzin M, Peterson C: Increased fetal activity with low maternal blood glucose levels in pregnancies complicated by diabetes. Am J Perinatol 1:161, 1984.
50. Phelan JP, Kester R, Labudovich ML: Nonstress test and maternal glucose determinations. Obstet Gynecol 67:4, 1982.
51. Druzin ML, Foodim J: Effect of maternal glucose ingestion compared with maternal water ingestion on the nonstress test. Obstet Gynecol 67:4, 1982.
52. Natale R, Clewlow F, Dawes G: Measurement of fetal forelimb movements in the lamb in utero. Am J Obstet Gynecol 140:545, 1981.
53. Sadovsky E, Yaffe H, Polishuk W: Fetal movement monitoring in normal and pathologic pregnancy. Int J Gynaecol Obstet 12:75, 1974.
54. Rayburn W, Zuspan F, Motley M, Donaldson M: An alternative to antepartum fetal heart rate testing. Am J Obstet Gynecol 138:223, 1980.
55. Pearson J, Weaver J: Fetal activity and fetal well being: an evaluation. BMJ 1:1305, 1976.
56. Sadovsky E, Ohel G, Havazeleth H, et al: The definition and the significance of decreased fetal movements. Acta Obstet Gynecol Scand 62:409, 1983.
57. Draper J, Field S, Thomas H: Women's views on keeping fetal movement charts. Br J Obstet Gynaecol 93:334, 1986.
58. Mikhail MS, Freda MC, Merkatz RB, et al: The effect of fetal movement counting on maternal attachment to fetus. Am J Obstet Gynecol 165:988, 1991.
59. Sorokin Y, Kierker L: Fetal movement. Clin Obstet Gynecol 25:719, 1982.
60. Johnson TRB, Jordan ET, Paine LL: Doppler recordings of fetal movement: II. Comparison with maternal perception. Obstet Gynecol 76:42, 1990.
61. Rayburn W, Barr M: Activity patterns in malformed fetuses. Am J Obstet Gynecol 142:1045, 1982.
62. Neldam S: Fetal movements as an indicator of fetal well being. Lancet 1:1222, 1980.
63. Neldam S: Fetal movements as an indicator of fetal well being. Dan Med Bull 30:274, 1983.
64. Rayburn W: Antepartum fetal assessment. Clin Perinatol 9:231, 1982.
65. Liston R, Cohen A, Mennuti M, Gabbe S: Antepartum fetal evaluation by maternal perception of fetal movement. Obstet Gynecol 60:424, 1982.
66. Grant A, Valentin L, Elbourne D, Alexander S: Routine formal fetal movement counting and risk of antepartum late death in normally formed singletons. Lancet 2:345, 1989.
67. Moore TR, Piacquadio K: A prospective evaluation of fetal movement screening to reduce the incidence of antepartum fetal death. Am J Obstet Gynecol 160:1075, 1989.
68. Moore TR, Piacquadio K: Study results vary in count-to-10 method of fetal movement screening. Am J Obstet Gynecol 163:264, 1990.
69. Froen JF: A kick from within-fetal movement counting and the concelled progress in antenatal care. J Perinatal Med 32:13–24, 2004.
70. Collea J, Holls W: The contraction stress test. Clin Obstet Gynecol 25:707, 1982.
71. Braly P, Freeman R, Garite T, et al: Incidence of premature delivery following the oxytocin challenge test. Am J Obstet Gynecol 141:5, 1981.
72. Freeman R: The use of the oxytocin challenge test for antepartum clinical evaluation of uteroplacental respiratory function. Am J Obstet Gynecol 121:481, 1975.
73. Martin C, Schifrin B: Prenatal fetal monitoring. *In* Aladjem S, Brown A (eds): Perinatal Intensive Care. St. Louis, CV Mosby, 1977, p 155.
74. Nageotte MP, Towers CV, Asrat T, et al: The value of a negative antepartum test: contraction stress test and modified biophysical profile. Obstet Gynecol 84:231, 1994.
75. Freeman R, Garite T, Modanlou H, et al: Postdate pregnancy: utilization of contraction stress testing for primary fetal surveillance. Am J Obstet Gynecol 140:128, 1981.
76. Freeman RK, Dorchester W, Anderson G, Garite TJ: The significance of a previous stillbirth. Am J Obstet Gynecol 151:7, 1985.
77. Druzin ML, Karver ML, Wagner W, et al: Prospective evaluation of the contraction stress test and non stress tests in the management of postterm pregnancy. Surg Gynecol Obstet 174:507, 1992.
78. Gabbe SG, Mestman JH, Freeman RK, et al: Management and outcome of diabetes mellitus, classes B-R. Am J Obstet Gynecol 129:723, 1977.
79. Lagrew DC, Pircon RA, Towers CV, et al: Antepartum fetal surveillance in patients with diabetes: when to start? Am J Obstet Gynecol 168:1820, 1993.
80. Evertson L, Gauthier R, Collea J: Fetal demise following negative contraction stress tests. Obstet Gynecol 51:671, 1978.
81. Grundy H, Freeman RK, Lederman S, Dorchester W: Nonreactive contraction stress test: clinical significance. Obstet Gynecol 64:337, 1984.
82. Freeman R, Anderson G, Dorchester W: A prospective multi-institutional study of antepartum fetal heart rate monitoring. I. Risk of perinatal mortality and morbidity according to antepartum fetal heart rate test results. Am J Obstet Gynecol 143:771, 1982.
83. Ray M, Freeman R, Pine S, et al: Clinical experience with the oxytocin challenge test. Am J Obstet Gynecol 114:1, 1972.
84. Gabbe S, Freeman R, Goebelsmann U: Evaluation of the contraction stress test before 33 weeks' gestation. Obstet Gynecol 52:649, 1978.
85. Bissonnette J, Johnson K, Toomey C: The role of a trial of labor with a positive contraction stress test. Am J Obstet Gynecol 135:292, 1979.
86. Braly P, Freeman R: The significance of fetal heart rate reactivity with a positive oxytocin challenge test. Obstet Gynecol 50:689, 1977.
87. Merrill PM, Porto M, Lovett SM, et al: Evaluation of the nonreactive positive contraction stress test prior to 32 weeks: the role of the biophysical profile. Am J Perinatol 12:229, 1995.
88. Bruce S, Petrie R, Yeh S-Y: The suspicious contraction stress test. Obstet Gynecol 51:415, 1978.
89. Scanlon J, Suzuki K, Shea E, Tronick E: A prospective study of the oxytocin challenge test and newborn neurobehavioral outcome. Obstet Gynecol 54:6, 1979.
90. Crane J, Anderson B, Marshall R, Harvey P: Subsequent physical and mental development in infants with positive contraction stress tests. J Reprod Med 26:113, 1981.
91. Beischer N, Drew J, Ashton P, et al: Quality of survival of infants with critical fetal reserve detected by antenatal cardiotocography. Am J Obstet Gynecol 146:662, 1983.
92. Oki EY, Keegan KA, Freeman RD, Dorchester W: The breast-stimulated contraction stress test. J Reprod Med 32:919, 1987.
93. Keegan KA, Helm DA, Porto M, et al: A prospective evaluation of nipple stimulation techniques for contraction stress testing. Am J Obstet Gynecol 157:121, 1987.
94. Huddleston J, Sutliff G, Robinson D: Contraction stress test by intermittent nipple stimulation. Obstet Gynecol 63:669, 1984.
95. Curtis P, Evens S, Resnick J, et al: Patterns of uterine contractions and prolonged uterine activity using three methods of breast stimulation for contraction stress tests. Obstet Gynecol 73:631, 1989.
96. Devoe LD, Morrison J, Martin J, et al: A prospective comparative study of the extended nonstress test and the nipple stimulation contraction stress test. Am J Obstet Gynecol 157:531, 1987.
97. Hammacher K: The clinical significance of cardiotocography. *In* Huntingford P, Huter K, Saling E (eds): Perinatal Medicine. 1st European Congress, Berlin. San Diego, Academic, 1969, p 80.

98. Patrick J, Carmichael L, Chess L, Staples C: Accelerations of the human fetal heart rate at 38 to 40 weeks' gestational age. Am J Obstet Gynecol 148:35, 1984.
99. Margulis E, Binder D, Cohen A: The effect of propranolol on the nonstress test. Am J Obstet Gynecol 148:340, 1984.
100. Keegan K, Paul R, Broussard P, et al: Antepartum fetal heart rate testing. III. The effect of phenobarbital on the nonstress test. Am J Obstet Gynecol 133:579, 1979.
101. Phelan J: Diminished fetal reactivity with smoking. Am J Obstet Gynecol 136:230, 1980.
102. Lavery J: Nonstress fetal heart rate testing. Clin Obstet Gynecol 25:689, 1982.
103. Keegan K, Paul R, Broussard P, et al: Antepartum fetal heart rate testing. V. The nonstress test: an outpatient approach. Am J Obstet Gynecol 136:81, 1980.
104. Druzin M, Gratacos J, Paul R, et al: Antepartum fetal heart rate testing. XII. The effect of manual manipulation of the fetus on the nonstress test. Am J Obstet Gynecol 151:61, 1985.
105. Eglinton G, Paul R, Broussard P, et al: Antepartum fetal heart rate testing. XI. Stimulation with orange juice. Am J Obstet Gynecol 150:97, 1984.
106. Tan KH, Sabapathy A: Maternal glucose administration for facilitating tests of fetal wellbeing. Cochrane Database Syst Rev 4: CD003397, 2001.
107. Tan KH, Sabathy A: Fetal Manipulation for facilitating tests of fetal wellbeing. Cochrane Database syst Rev 4:CD003396, 2001.
108. Keegan K, Paul R: Antepartum fetal heart rate testing. IV. The nonstress test as a primary approach. Am J Obstet Gynecol 136:75, 1980.
109. Evertson L, Gauthier R, Schifrin B, et al: Antepartum fetal heart rate testing. I. Evolution of the nonstress test. Am J Obstet Gynecol 133:29, 1979.
110. Rochard F, Schifrin B, Goupil F, et al: Nonstressed fetal heart rate monitoring in the antepartum period. Am J Obstet Gynecol 126:699, 1976.
111. Phelan J: The nonstress test: a review of 3,000 tests. Am J Obstet Gynecol 139:7, 1981.
112. Phillips W, Towell M: Abnormal fetal heart rate associated with congenital abnormalities. Br J Obstet Gynaecol 87:270, 1980.
113. Natale R, Nasello C, Turliuk R: The relationship between movements and accelerations in fetal heart rate at twenty-four to thirty-two weeks' gestation. Am J Obstet Gynecol 148:591, 1984.
114. Bishop E: Fetal acceleration test. Am J Obstet Gynecol 141:905, 1981.
115. Lavin J, Miodovnik M, Barden T: Relationship of nonstress test reactivity and gestational age. Obstet Gynecol 63:338, 1984.
116. Druzin ML, Fox A, Kogut E, et al: The relationship of the nonstress test to gestational age. Am J Obstet Gynecol 153:386, 1985.
117. Aladjem S, Vuolo K, Pazos R, et al: Antepartum fetal testing: evaluation and redefinition of criteria for clinical interpretation. Semin Perinatol 5:145, 1981.
118. Druzin ML, Lockshin M, Edersheim T, et al: Second trimester fetal monitoring and preterm delivery in pregnancies with systematic lupus erythematosus and/or circulating anticoagulant. Am J Obstet Gynecol 157:1503, 1987.
119. Brown R, Patrick J: The nonstress test: how long is enough? Am J Obstet Gynecol 141:646, 1981.
120. Leveno K, Williams M, DePalma R, et al: Perinatal outcome in the absence of antepartum fetal heart rate acceleration. Obstet Gynecol 61:347, 1983.
121. DeVoe L, McKenzie J, Searle N, et al: Clinical sequelae of the extended nonstress test. Am J Obstet Gynecol 151:1074, 1985.
122. Phelan JP: Antepartum fetal assessment: new techniques. Semin Perinatol 12:57, 1988.
123. Gagnon R, Foreman J, Hunse C, et al: Effects of low-frequency vibration on human germ fetuses. Am J Obstet Gynecol 161:1479, 1989.
124. Gagnon R, Hunse C, Foreman J: Human fetal behavioral states after vibratory stimulation. Am J Obstet Gynecol 161:1470, 1989.
125. Smith CV, Phelan JP, Paul RH, et al: Fetal acoustic stimulation testing: a retrospective experience with the fetal acoustic stimulation test. Am J Obstet Gynecol 153:567, 1985.
126. Smith CV, Phelan JP, Platt LD, et al: Fetal acoustic stimulation testing. II. A randomized clinical comparison with the nonstress test. Am J Obstet Gynecol 155:131, 1986.
127. Kuhlman KA, Depp R: Acoustic stimulation testing. Obstet Gynecol Clin North Am 15:303, 1988.
128. Trudinger BJ, Boylan P: Antepartum fetal heart rate monitoring: value of sound stimulation. Obstet Gynecol 55:265, 1980.
129. Druzin ML, Edersheim TG, Hutson JM, et al: The effect of vibroacoustic stimulation on the nonstress test at gestational ages of thirty-two weeks or less. Am J Obstet Gynecol 1661:1476, 1989.
130. Tan KH, Smyth R: Fetal vibroacoustic stimulation for facilitation of tests of fetal wellbeing. Cochrane Database Syst Rev 1: CD002963, 2001.
131. Smith CV, Satt B, Phelan JP, et al: Intrauterine sound levels: intrapartum assessment with an intrauterine microphone. Am J Perinatol 7:312, 1990.
132. Arulkumaran S, Talbert D, Hsu TS, et al: In-utero sound levels when vibroacoustic stimulation is applied to the maternal abdomen: an assessment of the possibility of cochlea damage in the fetus. Br J Obstet Gynaecol 99:43, 1992.
133. Arulkumaran S, Mircog B, Skurr BA, et al: No evidence of hearing loss due to fetal acoustic stimulation test. Obstet Gynecol 78:2, 1991.
134. Ohel G, Horowitz E, Linder N, et al: Neonatal auditory acuity following in utero vibratory acoustic stimulation. Am J Obstet Gynecol 157:440, 1987.
135. Druzin M, Gratacos J, Keegan K, et al: Antepartum fetal heart rate testing. VII. The significance of fetal bradycardia. Am J Obstet Gynecol 139:194, 1981.
136. Druzin ML: Antepartum Fetal Assessment. Cambridge, MA, Blackwell Scientific Publications, 1992, p 13.
137. Phelan J, Lewis P: Fetal heart rate decelerations during a nonstress test. Obstet Gynecol 57:288, 1981.
138. Pazos R, Vuolo K, Aladjem S, et al: Association of spontaneous fetal heart rate decelerations during antepartum nonstress testing and intrauterine growth retardation. Am J Obstet Gynecol 144:574, 1982.
139. Dashow E, Read J: Significant fetal bradycardia during antepartum heart rate testing. Am J Obstet Gynecol 148:187, 1984.
140. Bourgeois F, Thiagarajah S, Harbert G: The significance of fetal heart rate decelerations during nonstress testing. Am J Obstet Gynecol 150:215, 1984.
141. Druzin ML: Fetal bradycardia during antepartum testing, further observations. J Reprod Med 34:47, 1989.
142. Meis P, Ureda J, Swain M, et al: Variable decelerations during non-stress tests are not a sign of fetal compromise? Am J Obstet Gynecol 154:586, 1994.
143. Barrett J, Salyer S, Boehm F: The nonstress test: an evaluation of 1,000 patients. Am J Obstet Gynecol 141:153, 1981.
144. Miller JM Jr, Horger EO III: Antepartum heart rate testing in diabetic pregnancy. J Reprod Med 30:515, 1985.
145. Boehm FH, Salyer S, Shah DM, et al: Improved outcome of twice weekly nonstress testing. Obstet Gynecol 67:566, 1986.
146. Miyazaki F, Miyazaki B: False reactive nonstress tests in postterm pregnancies. Am J Obstet Gynecol 140:269, 1981.
147. Barss V, Frigoletto F, Diamond F: Stillbirth after nonstress testing. Obstet Gynecol 65:541, 1985.
148. Murata Y, Martin C, Ikenoue T, et al: Fetal heart rate accelerations and late decelerations during the course of intrauterine death in chronically catheterized rhesus monkeys. Am J Obstet Gynecol 144:218, 1982.
149. Freeman R, Anderson G, Dorchester W: A prospective multi-institutional study of antepartum fetal heart rate monitoring. II. Contraction stress test versus nonstress test for primary surveillance. Am J Obstet Gynecol 143:778, 1982.
150. Slomka C, Phelan J: Pregnancy outcome in the patient with a nonreactive nonstress test and a positive contraction stress test. Am J Obstet Gynecol 139:11, 1981.
151. Devoe L: Clinical features of the reactive positive contraction stress test. Obstet Gynecol 63:523, 1984.
152. Druzin M, Gratacos J, Paul R: Antepartum fetal heart rate testing. VI. Predictive reliability of "normal" tests in the prevention of antepartum death. Am J Obstet Gynecol 137:746, 1980.

153. Kadar N: Perinatal mortality related to nonstress and contraction stress tests. Am J Obstet Gynecol 142:931, 1982.
154. Finberg HJ, Kurtz AB, Johnson RL, et al: The biophysical profile: a literature review and reassessment of its usefulness in the evaluation of fetal well-being. J Ultrasound Med 9:583, 1990.
155. Manning FA, Morrison I, Lange IR, et al: Fetal assessment based on fetal biophysical profile scoring: experience in 12,620 referred high-risk pregnancies. Am J Obstet Gynecol 151:343, 1985.
156. Vintzileos A, Campbell W, Ingardia C, Nochimson D: The fetal biophysical profile and its predictive value. Obstet Gynecol 62:271, 1983.
157. Gennser G, Marsal K, Brantmark B: Maternal smoking and fetal breathing movements. Am J Obstet Gynecol 123:861, 1975.
158. Platt L, Manning F, Lemay M, Sipos L: Human fetal breathing: relationship to fetal condition. Am J Obstet Gynecol 132:514, 1978.
159. Manning F, Platt L, Sipos L, Keegan K: Fetal breathing movements and the nonstress test in high-risk pregnancies. Am J Obstet Gynecol 135:511, 1979.
160. Schifrin B, Guntes V, Gergely R, et al: The role of real-time scanning in antenatal fetal surveillance. Am J Obstet Gynecol 140:525, 1981.
161. Manning F, Platt L, Sipos L: Antepartum fetal evaluation: development of a fetal biophysical profile. Am J Obstet Gynecol 136:787, 1980.
162. Pillai M, James D: The importance of behavioral state in biophysical assessment of the term human fetus. Br J Obstet Gynaecol 97:1130, 1990.
163. Manning FA, Harman CR, Morrison I, et al: Fetal assessment based on fetal biophysical profile scoring. Am J Obstet Gynecol 162:703, 1990.
164. Manning FA, Morrison I, Lange IR, et al: Fetal biophysical profile scoring: selective use of the nonstress test. Am J Obstet Gynecol 156:709, 1987.
165. Manning FA, Morrison I, Harman CR, et al: The abnormal fetal biophysical profile score. V. Predictive accuracy according to score composition. Am J Obstet Gynecol 162:918, 1990.
166. Manning FA: Biophysical profile scoring. *In* Nijhuis J (ed): Fetal Behaviour. New York, Oxford University Press, 1992, p 241.
167. Vintzileos AM, Gaffney SE, Salinger LM, et al: The relationship between fetal biophysical profile and cord pH in patients undergoing cesarean section before the onset of labor. Obstet Gynecol 70:196, 1987.
168. Kelly MK, Schneider EP, Petrikovsky BM, Lesser ML: Effect of antenatal steroid administration on the fetal biophysical profile. J Clin Ultrasound 28:224, 2000.
169. Deren O, Karaer C, Önderoglu L, et al: The effect of steroids on the biophysical profile of the healthy preterm fetus and its relationship with time. Am J Obstet Gynecol 185:S108, 2000.
170. Rotmensch S, Liberati M, Celentano C, et al: The effect of betamethasone on fetal biophysical activities and Doppler velocimetry of umbilical and middle cerebral arteries. Acta Obstet Gynecol Scand 78:768, 1999.
171. Sherer DM, Spong CY, Salafia CM: Fetal breathing movements within 24 hours of delivery in prematurity are related to histologic and clinical evidence of amnionitis. Am J Perinatol 14:337, 1997.
172. Lewis DF, Adair CD, Weeks JW, et al: A randomized clinical trial of daily nonstress testing versus biophysical profile in the management of preterm premature rupture of the membranes. Am J Obstet Gynecol 181:1495, 1999.
173. Manning FA: Fetal biophysical profile. Obstet Gynecol Clin North Am 26:557, 1999.
174. Platt L, Eglinton G, Sipos L, et al: Further experience with the fetal biophysical profile. Obstet Gynecol 61:480, 1983.
175. Manning F, Lange I, Morrison I, et al: Fetal biophysical profile score and the nonstress test: a comparative trial. Obstet Gynecol 64:326, 1984.
176. Eden RD, Seifert LS, Kodack LD, et al: A modified biophysical profile for antenatal fetal surveillance. Obstet Gynecol 71:365, 1988.
177. Inglis SR, Druzin ML, Wagner WE, Kogut E: The use of vibroacoustic stimulation during the abnormal or equivocal biophysical profile. Obstet Gynecol 82:371, 1993.
178. Hatle L, Angelsen B: Doppler Ultrasound in Cardiology. Philadelphia, Lea & Febiger, 1985, p 1.
179. Warsof SL, Levy DL: Doppler blood flow and fetal growth retardation. *In* Gross TL, Sokol RJ (ed): Intrauterine Growth Retardation, A Practical Approach. Chicago, Year Book, 1989, p 158.
180. Bruner JP, Gabbe SG, Levy DW, et al: Doppler ultrasonography of the umbilical cord in normal pregnancy. J South Med Assoc 86:52, 1993.
181. Morrow RJ, Hill AA, Adamson SL: Experimental models used to investigate the diagnostic potential of Doppler ultrasound in the umbilical circulation. *In* Copel JA, Reed KL (eds): Doppler Ultrasound in Obstetrics and Gynecology. New York, Raven Press, 1995, p 5.
182. Indik JH, Reed KL: Variation and correlation in human fetal umbilical velocities with fetal breathing: evidence of the cardiac-placental connection. Am J Obstet Gynecol 163:1792, 1990.
183. Sonesson SE, Fouron JC, Drblik SP, et al: Reference values for Doppler velocimetric indices from the fetal and placental ends of the umbilical artery during normal pregnancy. J Clin Ultrasound 21:317, 1993.
184. Thompson RS, Trudinger BJ, Cook CM, et al: Umbilical artery velocity waveforms: normal reference values for A/B ratio and Pourcelot ratio. Br J Obstet Gynaecol 95:589, 1988.
185. Hendricks SK, Sorensen TK, Wang KY, et al: Doppler umbilical artery waveform indices—normal values from fourteen to forty-two weeks. Am J Obstet Gynecol 161:761, 1989.
186. Rizzo G, Arduini D, Romanini C: First trimester fetal and uterine Doppler. *In* Copel JA, Reed KL (eds): Doppler Ultrasound in Obstetrics and Gynecology. New York, Raven Press, 1995, p 105.
187. Itskovitz J: Maternal-fetal hemodynamics. *In* Maulik D, McNellis D (eds): Reproductive and Perinatal Medicine (VIII) Doppler Ultrasound Measurement of Maternal-Fetal Hemodynamics. Ithaca, NY, Perinatology Press, 1987, p 13.
188. McCowan LME, Harding JE, Stewart AW: Umbilical artery Doppler studies in small for gestational age babies reflect disease severity. Br J Obstet Gynaecol 107:916, 2000.
189. Pollock RN, Divon MY: Intrauterine growth retardation: diagnosis. *In* Copel JA, Reed KL (eds): Doppler Ultrasound in Obstetrics and Gynecology. New York, Raven Press, 1995, p 171.
190. Trudinger BJ, Stevens D, Connelly A, et al: Umbilical artery flow velocity waveforms and placental resistance: the effects of embolization of the umbilical circulation. Am J Obstet Gynecol 157:1443, 1987.
191. Morrow R, Ritchie K: Doppler ultrasound fetal velocimetry and its role in obstetrics. Clin Perinatol 16:771, 1989.
192. Copel JA, Schlafer D, Wentworth R, et al: Does the umbilical artery systolic/diastolic ratio reflect flow or acidosis? Am J Obstet Gynecol 163:751, 1990.
193. Galan HL, Anthony RV, Rigano S, et al: Fetal hypertension and abnormal Doppler velocimetry in an oving model of intrueterine growth restriction. Am J Obstet Gynecol 192:272, 2005.
194. Divon MY, Ferber A: Evidence-based antepartum fetal testing. Perinatal Neonatal Med 5:3, 2000.
195. Farine D, Kelly EN, Ryan G, et al: Absent and reversed umbilical artery end-diastolic velocity. *In* Copel JA, Reed KL (eds): Doppler Ultrasound in Obstetrics and Gynecology. New York, Raven Press, 1995, p 187.
196. Indik JH, Chen V, Reed KL: Association of umbilical venous with inferior vena cava blood flow velocities. Obstet Gynecol 77:551, 1991.
197. Reed KL, Chaffin D, Anderson CF: Umbilical venous Doppler velocity pulsations and inferior vena cava pressure elevations in fetal lambs. Obstet Gynecol 87:617, 1996.
198. Arduini D, Rizzo G, Romanini C: The development of abnormal heart rate patterns after absent end-diastolic velocity in umbilical artery: analysis of risk factors. Am J Obstet Gynecol 168:50, 1993.
199. Hecher K, Campbell S, Doyle P, et al: Assessment of fetal compromise by Doppler investigation of the fetal circulation. Circulation 91:129, 1995.
200. Damron DP, Chaffin DG, Anderson CF, Reed KL: Umbilical artery velocity ratios and venous pulsations in fetuses with late decelerations. Obstet Gynecol 84:1038, 1994.

201. Ferrazzi E, Bozzo M, Rigano S, et al: Temporal sequence of abnormal Doppler changes in the peripheral and central circulatory systems of the severely growth-restricted fetus. Ultrasound Obstet Gynecol 19:140, 2002.
202. Baschat AA, Galan HL, Bhide A, et al: Doppler and biophysical assessment in growth restricted fetuses: distribution of test results. Ultrasound Obstet Gynecol 27:41, 2006.
203. Williams KP, Farquharson DF, Bebbington M, et al: Screening for fetal well-being in a high-risk pregnant population comparing the nonstress test with umbilical artery Doppler velocimetry: A randomized controlled clinical trial. Am J Obstet Gynecol 188:1366, 2003.
204. Obido AO, Quinones JN, Lawrence-Cleary K, et al: What antepartum test should guide the timing of delivery of the preterm growth restricted fetus? A decision-analysis. Am J Obstet Gynecol 191:1477, 2004.
205. Giles WB, Bisits A: Clinical use of Doppler in pregnancy: information from six randomized trials. Fetal Diagn Ther 8:247, 1993.
206. Alfirevic Z, Neilson JP: Doppler ultrasonography in high-risk pregnancies: systematic review with meta-analysis. Am J Obstet Gynecol 172:1379, 1995.
207. Neilson JP, Alfirevic Z: Doppler ultrasound in high-risk pregnancies (Cochrane Review). *In* The Cochrane Library, Issue 4. Oxford, Update Software, 1999.
208. Gagnon, R, Van den Hof M: Diagnostic Imagin Committee, Executive and Council of the Society of Obstetricians and Gynaecologists of Canada. The use of fetal Doppler in obstetrics. J Obstet Gynecol Can 25:601, 2003.
209. Goffinet F, Paris-Llado J, Nisand I, Breart G: Umbilical artery Doppler velocimetry in unselected and low risk pregnancies: a review of randomized controlled trials. Br J Obstet Gynaecol 104:425, 1997.
210. Strassner H, Nochimson D: Determination of fetal maturity. Clin Perinatol 9:297, 1982.
211. Goldenberg R, Nelson K: Iatrogenic respiratory distress syndrome. Am J Obstet Gynecol 123:617, 1975.
212. Hack M, Fanaroff A, Klaus M, et al: Neonatal respiratory distress following elective delivery: a preventable disease? Am J Obstet Gynecol 126:43, 1976.
213. Wax JR, Herson V, Carignan E, et al: Contribution of elective delivery to severe respiratory distress at term. Am J Perinatol 19:81, 2002.
214. Gerten KA, Coonrod DV, Bay RC, Chambliss LR: Cesarean delivery and respiratory distress syndrome: does labor make a difference? Am J Obstet Gynecol 193:1061, 2005.
215. Assessment of Fetal Lung Maturity, ACOG Educational Bulletin, Number 230, 1996.
216. Dunn LR: The clinical use of fetal lung maturity testing. Resident Reporter 3:32, 1998.
217. Newton ER, Cetrulo CL, Kosa DJ: Biparietal diameter as a predictor of fetal lung maturity. J Reprod Med 28:480, 1983.
218. Stark CM, Smith RS, Lagrandeur RM, et al: Need for urgent delivery after third-trimester amniocentesis. Obstet Gynecol 95:48, 2000.
219. Sabbagha R, Salvino C: Report on third trimester amniocentesis at Prentice Women's Hospital of Northwestern University Medical School, Chicago, Illinois. *In* Antenatal diagnosis. NIH Consensus Statement. National Institutes of Health, Bethesda, Maryland, 1979, p 61.
220. Golde S, Platt L: The use of ultrasound in the diagnosis of fetal lung maturity. Clin Obstet Gynecol 27:391, 1984.
221. Liu KZ, Shaw RA, Dembinski TC, et al: Comparison of infrared spectroscopic and fluorescence depolarization assays for fetal lung maturity. Am J Obstet Gynecol 183:181, 2000.
222. Gluck L, Kulovich M, Borer R, et al: The interpretation and significance of the lecithin/sphingomyelin ratio in amniotic fluid. Am J Obstet Gynecol 120:142, 1974.
223. Kulovich M, Hallman M, Gluck L: The lung profile. Am J Obstet Gynecol 135:57, 1979.
224. Harvey D, Parkinson C, Campbell S: Risk of respiratory distress syndrome. Lancet 1:42, 1975.
225. Creasy G, Simon N: Sensitivity and specificity of the L/S ratio in relation to gestational age. Am J Perinatol 1:302, 1984.
226. Buhi W, Spellacy W: Effects of blood or meconium on the determination of the amniotic fluid lecithin/sphingomyelin ratio. Am J Obstet Gynecol 121:321, 1975.
227. Tabsh K, Brinkman C, Bashore R: Effect of meconium contamination on amniotic fluid lecithin:sphingomyelin ratio. Obstet Gynecol 58:605, 1981.
228. Stedman C, Crawford S, Staten E, et al: Management of preterm premature rupture of membranes: assessing amniotic fluid in the vagina for phosphatidylglycerol. Am J Obstet Gynecol 140:34, 1981.
229. Strassner H, Golde S, Mosley G, et al: Effect of blood in amniotic fluid on the detection of phosphatidylglycerol. Am J Obstet Gynecol 138:697, 1980.
230. Hill L, Ellefson R: Variable interference of meconium in the determination of phosphatidylglycerol. Am J Obstet Gynecol 147:339, 1983.
231. Thibeault D, Hobel C: The interrelationship of the foam stability test, immaturity, and intrapartum complications in the respiratory distress syndrome. Am J Obstet Gynecol 118:56, 1974.
232. Horenstein J, Golde SH, Platt LD: Lung profiles in the isoimmunized pregnancy. Am J Obstet Gynecol 153:443, 1985.
233. Kjos SL, Walther FJ, Montoro M, et al: Prevalence and etiology of respiratory distress in infants of diabetic mothers: predictive value of fetal lung maturation tests. Am J Obstet Gynecol 163:898, 1990.
234. Kulovich M, Gluck L: The lung profile. II. Complicated pregnancy. Am J Obstet Gynecol 135:64, 1979.
235. Towers CV, Garite TJ: Evaluation of the new Amniostat-FLM test for the detection of phosphatidylglycerol in contaminated fluids. Am J Obstet Gynecol 160:298, 1989.
236. Steinfeld JD, Samuels P, Bulley MA, et al: The utility of the TDx test in the assessment of fetal lung maturity. Obstet Gynecol 79:460, 1992.
237. Bayer-Zwirello LA, Jertson J, Rosenbaum J, et al: Amniotic fluid surfactant-albumin ratio as a screening test for fetal lung maturity: two years of clinical experience. J Perinatol XIII:354, 1993.
238. Apple FS, Bilodeau L, Preese LM, Benson P: Clinical implementation of a rapid, automated assay for assessing fetal lung maturity. J Reprod Med 39:883, 1994.
239. Bonebrake RG, Towers CV, Rumney PJ, Peimbold P: Is fluorescence polarization reliable and cost efficient in a fetal lung maturity cascade? Am J Obstet Gynecol 177:835, 1997.
240. Livingston EG, Herbert WNP, Hage ML, et al: Use of the TDx-FLM assay in evaluating fetal lung maturity in an insulin-dependent diabetic population. Obstet Gynecol 86:826, 1995.
241. Kesselman EJ, Figueroa R, Garry D, Maulik D: The usefulness of the TDx/TDxFLx fetal lung maturity II assay in the initial evaluation of fetal lung maturity. Am J Obstet Gynecol 188:1220, 2003.
242. Edwards RK, Duff P, Ross KC: Amniotic fluid indices of fetal pulmonary maturity with preterm premature rupture of membranes. Obstet Gynecol 96:102, 2000.
243. Sher G, Statland B, Freer D, Hisley J: Performance of the amniotic fluid foam stability-50 percent test. A bedside procedure for the prenatal detection of hyaline membrane disease. Am J Obstet Gynecol 134:705, 1979.
244. Sher G, Statland B: Assessment of fetal pulmonary maturity by the Lumadex Foam Stability Index Test. Obstet Gynecol 61:444, 1983.
245. Lockitch G, Wittmann BK, Snow BE, et al: Prediction of fetal lung maturity by use of the Lumadex-FSI test. Clin Chem 32:361, 1986.
246. Strong TH Jr, Hayes AS, Sawyer AT, et al: Amniotic fluid turbidity: a useful adjunct for assessing fetal pulmonary maturity status. Int J Gynecol Obstet 38:97, 1992.
247. Ashwood ER, Palmer SE, Taylor JS, Pingree SS: Lamellar body counts for rapid fetal lung maturity testing. Obstet Gynecol 81:619, 1993.
248. Fakhoury G, Daikoku NH, Benser J, Dubin NH: Lamellar body concentrations and the prediction of fetal pulmonary maturity. Am J Obstet Gynecol 170:72, 1994.
249. Greenspoon JS, Rosen DJD, Roll K, Dubin SB: Evaluation of lamellar body number density as the initial assessment in a fetal lung maturity test cascade. J Reprod Med 40:260, 1995.

250. Dalence CR, Bowie LJ, Dohnal JC, et al: Amniotic fluid lamellar body count: a rapid and reliable fetal lung maturity test. Obstet Gynecol 86:235, 1995.
251. Lewis PS, Lauria MR, Dzieczkowski J, et al: Amniotic fluid lamellar body count: cost-effective screening for fetal lung maturity. Obstet Gynecol 93:387, 1999.
252. Szallasi A, Gronowski AM, Eby CS: Lamellar body count in amniotic fluid: a comparative study of four different heatologic analyzers. Clin Chem 49:994, 2003.
253. Garite TJ, Freeman RK, Nageotte MP: Fetal maturity cascade: a rapid and cost-effective method for fetal lung maturity testing. Obstet Gynecol 67:619, 1986.
254. Herbert WNP, Chapman JF: Clinical and economic considerations associated with testing for fetal lung maturity. Am J Obstet Gynecol 155:820, 1986.
255. McElrath TF, Colon I, Hecht J, Tanasijevic MJ, Norwitz ER: Neonatal respiratory distress syndrome as a function of gestational age and an assay for surfactant-to-albumin ration. Obstet Gynecol 103:463, 2004.
256. Karcher R, Sykes E, Batton D, et al: Gestational age–specific predicted risk of neonatal respiratory distress syndrome using lamellar body count and surfactant-to-albumin ratio in amniotic fluid. Am J Obstet Gynecol 193:1680, 2005.
257. Parvin CA, Kaplan LA, Chapman JF, et al: Predicting respiratory distress syndrome using gestational age and fetal lung maturity by fluorescent polarization. Am J Obstet Gynecol 192:199, 2005.
258. Pinette MG, Blackstone J, Wax JR, Cartin A: Fetal lung maturity indices—a plea for gestational age–specific interpretation: a case report and discussion. Am J Obstet Gynecol 187:1721, 2002.
259. Stubblefield PG: Using the TDx-FLM assay and gestational age together for more accurate prediction of risk for neonatal respiratory distress syndrome. Am J Obstet Gynecol 187:1429, 2002.
260. Kontopoulos EV, Vintzileos AM: Condition-specific antepartum fetal testing. Am J Obst Gynecol 191:1546, 2004.
261. Sue-A-Quan AK, Hannah ME, Cohen MM, et al: Effect of labour induction on rates of stillbirth and cesarean section in post-term pregnancies. Can Med Assoc J 160:1145, 1999.
262. Clark SL, Sabey P, Jolley K: Nonstress testing with acoustic stimulation and amniotic fluid volume assessment: 5973 tests without unexpected fetal death. Am J Obstet Gynecol 160:694, 1989.
263. Mills MS, James KD, Slade S: Two-tier approach to biophysical assessment of the fetus. Am J Obstet Gynecol 163:12, 1990.
264. Magann EF, Isler CM, Chauhan SP, Martin JN: Amniotic fluid volume estimation and the biophysical profile: a confusion of criteria. Obstet Gynecol 96:640, 2000.
265. Vintzileos AM, Campbell WA, Nochimson DJ, et al: The use and misuse of the fetal biophysical profile. Am J Obstet Gynecol 156:527, 1987.
266. Nageotte MP, Towers CV, Asrat T, Freeman RK: Perinatal outcome with the modified biophysical profile. Am J Obstet Gynecol 170:1672, 1994.
267. Miller DA, Rabello YA, Paul RH: The modified biophysical profile: antepartum testing in the 1990s. Am J Obstet Gynecol 174:812, 1996.
268. Huddleston EF: Continued utility of the contractions stress test? Clin Obstet Gynecol 45:1005–14, 2002.
269. Chaffin DG: Death knell for the contraction stress test? Am J Obstet Gynecol 172:1329, 1995.
270. Bove KE: Autopsy Committee of the College of American Pathologists: Practice Guidelines for Autopsy Pathology. Arch Pathol Lab Med 121:368, 1997.
271. Doyle LW: Effects of perinatal necropsy on counselling. Lancet 355:2093, 2000.
272. Incerpi MH, Miller DA, Samadi R, et al: Stillbirth evaluation: what tests are needed? Am J Obstet Gynecol 178:1121, 1998.
273. Woodward PJ, Sohaey R, Harris DP, et al: Postmortem fetal MR imaging: comparison with findings at autopsy. Am J Roentgenol 168:41, 1997.

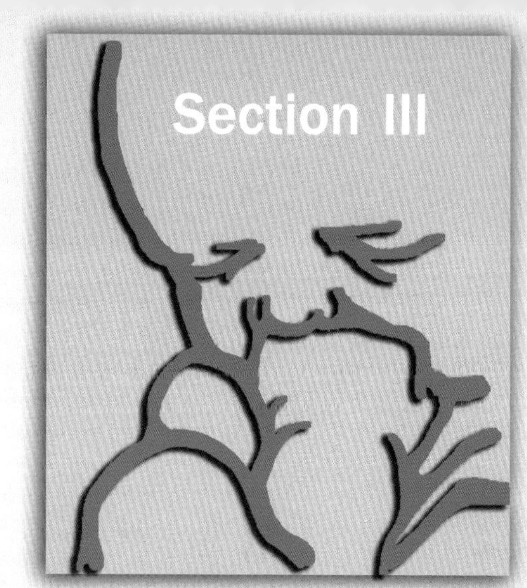

Intrapartum Care

Normal Labor and Delivery

SARAH KILPATRICK AND ETOI GARRISON

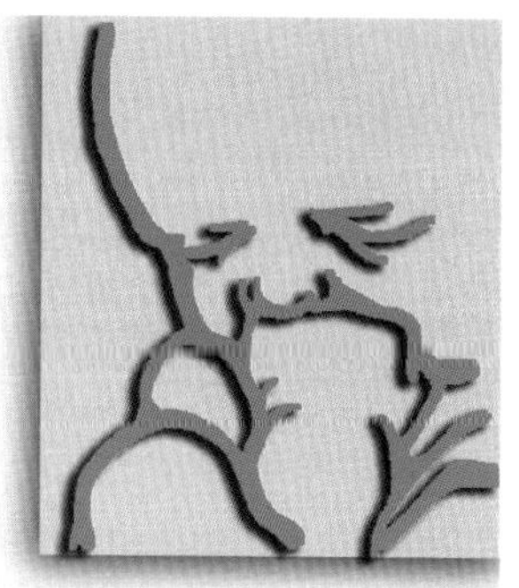

CHAPTER 12

KEY ABBREVIATIONS

American College of Obstetricians and Gynecologists	ACOG
Cephalopelvic disproportion	CPD
Left occiput anterior	LOA
Occiput anterior	OA
Occiput posterior	OP
Occiput transverse	OT
Prostaglandins	PG
Randomized controlled trial	RCT
Right occiput anterior	ROA

LABOR: DEFINITION AND PHYSIOLOGY

Labor is defined as the process by which the fetus is expelled from the uterus. More specifically, labor requires regular, effective contractions that lead to dilation and effacement of the cervix. This chapter describes the physiology and normal characteristics of term labor and delivery.

The physiology of labor initiation has not been completely elucidated but the putative mechanisms have been recently reviewed by Liao et al.[1] Labor initiation is species specific, and the mechanisms in human labor are unique. The four phases of labor from quiescence to involution are outlined in Figure 12-1.[2] The first phase is quiescence and represents that time in utero before labor begins when uterine activity is suppressed by the action of progesterone, prostacyclin, relaxin, nitric oxide, parathyroid hormone–related peptide, and possibly other hormones. During the activation phase, estrogen begins to facilitate expression of myometrial receptors for prostaglandins (PG) and oxytocin, which results in ion channel activation and increased gap junctions. This increase in the gap junctions between myometrial cells facilitates effective contractions.[3] In essence, the activation phase readies the uterus for the subsequent stimulation phase, when uterotonics, particularly PG and oxytocin, stimulate regular contractions. In the human, this process at term may be protracted, occurring over days to weeks. The final phase, uterine involution, occurs after delivery and is mediated primarily by oxytocin. The first three phases of labor require endocrine, paracrine, and autocrine interaction between the fetus, membranes, placenta, and mother.

The fetus has a central role in the initiation of term labor in nonhuman mammals; in humans, the fetal role is not completely understood (Fig. 12-2).[2–5] In sheep, term labor is initiated through activation of the fetal hypothalamic-pituitary-adrenal axis, with a resultant increase in fetal adrenocorticotrophic hormone and cortisol.[4,5] Fetal cortisol increases production of estradiol and decreases production of progesterone by a shift in placental metabolism of cortisol dependent on placental 17α-hydroxylase. The change in the progesterone/estradiol ratio stimulates placental production of oxytocin and PG, particularly $PGF_{2\alpha}$.[4] If this increase in fetal adrenocorticotrophic hormone and cortisol is blocked, parturition is delayed.[5] In contrast, humans lack placental 17α-hydroxylase and there is no increase in fetal cortisol near term. Rather, in humans, uterine activation may be potentiated in part by increased fetal adrenal production of dehydroepiandrostenidione, which is converted in the placenta to estradiol and estriol. Placental estriol stimulates an increase in maternal (likely decidual) $PGF_{2\alpha}$, PG receptors, oxytocin receptors, and gap junctions. In humans, there is no documented decrease in progesterone near term and a fall in progesterone is not necessary for labor initiation. However, recent research suggests the possibility of a "functional progesterone withdrawal" in humans: Labor is accompanied by a decrease in the con-

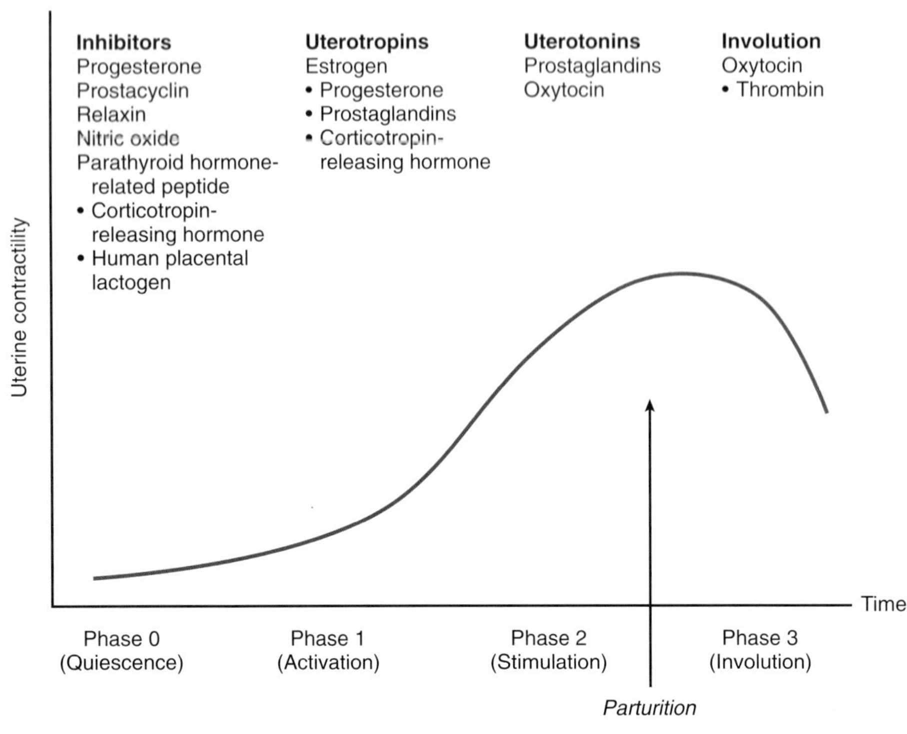

Figure 12-1. Regulation of uterine activity during pregnancy and labor. (Adapted from Challis JRG, Gibb W: Control of parturition. Prenat Neonat Med 1:283, 1996.)

centration of progesterone receptors, as well as a change in the ratio of progesterone receptor isoforms A and B in both the myometrium[6,7] and membranes.[8] More research is needed to elucidate the precise mechanism through which the human parturition cascade is activated. Fetal maturation may play an important role, as well as maternal cues that impact circadian cycling. There are distinct diurnal patterns of contractions and delivery in most species, and in humans, the majority of contractions occur at night.[2,9]

Oxytocin is used commonly for labor induction and augmentation; a full understanding of the mechanism of oxytocin action is helpful. Oxytocin is a peptide hormone synthesized in the hypothalamus and released from the posterior pituitary in a pulsatile fashion. At term, oxytocin is a potent endogenous uterotonic agent that is capable of stimulating uterine contractions at intravenous infusion rates of 1 to 2 mIU/min.[10] Oxytocin is inactivated largely in the liver and kidney, and during pregnancy, it is degraded primarily by placental oxytocinase. Its biologic half life is approximately 3 to 4 minutes but appears to be shorter when higher doses are infused. Concentrations of oxytocin in the maternal circulation do not change significantly during pregnancy or before the onset of labor, but they do rise late in the second stage of labor.[10,11] Studies of fetal pituitary oxytocin production and the umbilical arteriovenous differences in plasma oxytocin strongly suggest that the fetus secretes oxytocin that reaches the maternal side of the placenta.[10,12] The calculated rate of active oxytocin secretion from the fetus increases from a baseline of 1 mIU/min before labor to around 3 mIU/min after spontaneous labor.

Significant regional differences in myometrial oxytocin receptor distribution have been reported, with large numbers of fundal receptors and fewer receptors in the lower uterine segment and cervix.[13] Myometrial oxytocin receptors increase on average by 100- to 200-fold during pregnancy, reaching a maximum during early labor.[10,11,14,15] This rise in receptor concentration is paralleled by an increase in uterine sensitivity to circulating oxytocin. Specific high-affinity oxytocin receptors have also been isolated from human amnion and decidua parietalis but not decidua vera.[10,13] It has been suggested that oxytocin plays a dual role in parturition. First, through its receptor, oxytocin directly stimulates uterine contractions. Second, oxytocin may act indirectly by stimulating the amnion and decidua to produce PG.[13,16,17] Indeed, even when uterine contractions are adequate, induction of labor at term is successful only when oxytocin infusion is associated with an increase in PGF production.[13]

Oxytocin binding to its receptor activates phospholipase C. In turn, phospholipase C increases intracellular calcium both by stimulating the release of intracellular calcium and by promoting the influx of extra cellular calcium. Oxytocin stimulation of phospholipase C can be blocked by increased levels of cyclic adenosine monophosphate. Increased calcium levels stimulate the calmodulin-mediated activation of myosin light-chain kinase. Oxytocin may also stimulate uterine contractions via a calcium independent pathway by inhibiting myosin phosphatase which in turn increases myosin phosphorylation. These pathways ($PGF_{2\alpha}$ and intracellular calcium) have been the target of multiple tocolytic agents: indomethacin, calcium channel blockers, beta mimetics (through stimulation of cyclic adenosine monophosphate) and magnesium.

MECHANICS OF LABOR

Labor and delivery are not passive processes in which uterine contractions push a rigid object through a fixed

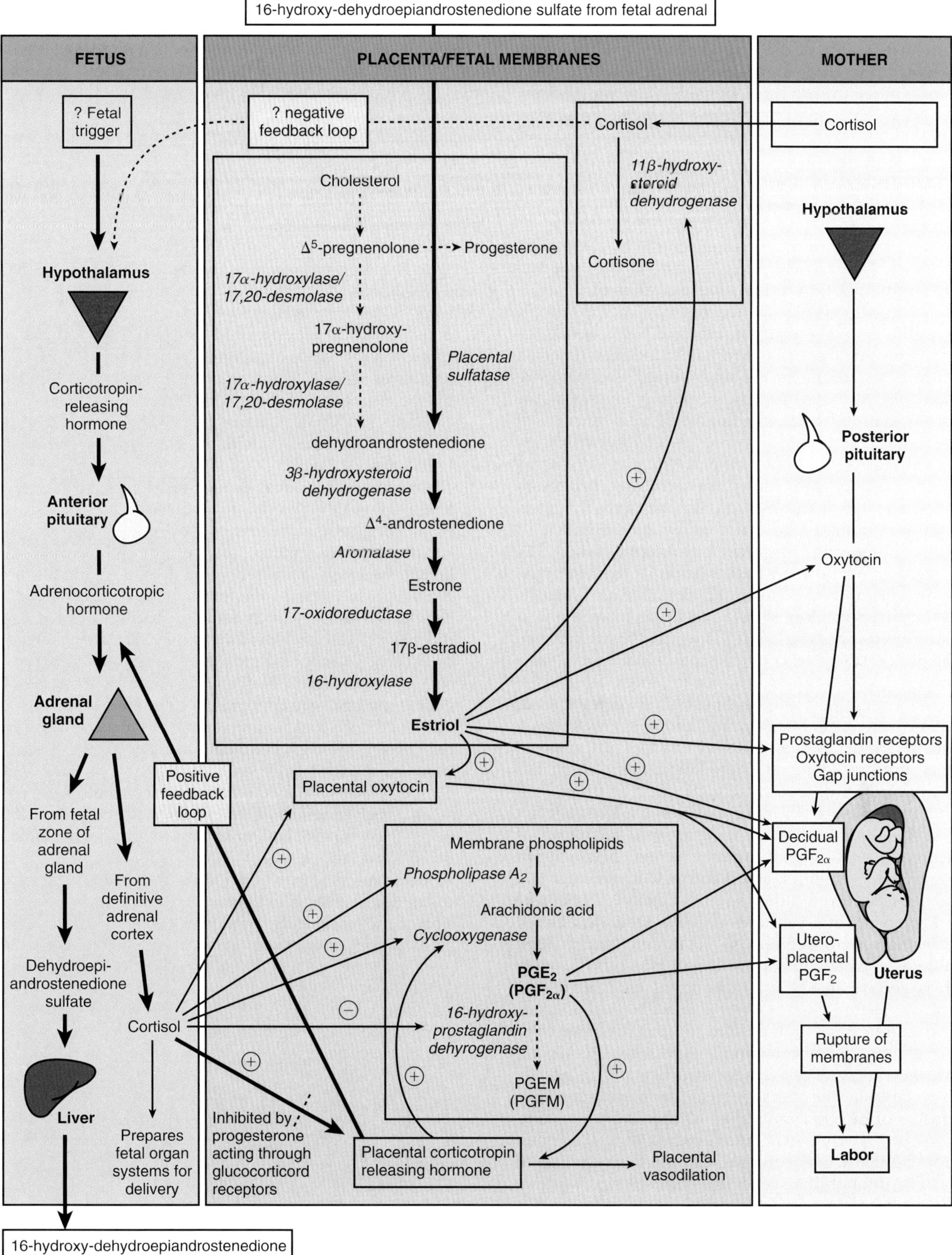

Figure 12-2. Proposed "parturition cascade" for labor induction at term. The spontaneous induction of labor at term in the human is regulated by a series of paracrine/autocrine hormones acting in an integrated parturition cascade responsible for promoting uterine contractions. PGE_2, prostaglandin E_2; PGEM, 13, 14-dihydro 15 keto PGE_2; $PGF_{2\alpha}$, prostaglandin $F_{2\alpha}$; PGFM, 13, 14-dihydro-15keto-$PGF_{2\alpha}$. (Modified from Norwitz ER, Robinson JN, Repke JT: The initiation of parturition: a comparative analysis across the species. Curr Prob Obstet Gynecol Fertil 22:41, 1999.)

aperture. The ability of the fetus to successfully negotiate the pelvis during labor and delivery is dependent on the complex interaction of three variables: uterine activity, the fetus, and the maternal pelvis (Powers, Passenger, Passage).

Uterine Activity (Powers)

The powers refer to the forces generated by the uterine musculature. Uterine activity is characterized by the frequency, amplitude (intensity), and duration of contractions. Assessment of uterine activity may include simple observation, manual palpation, external objective assessment techniques (such as external tocodynamometry), and direct measurement via an internal uterine pressure catheter. External tocodynamometry measures the change in shape of the abdominal wall as a function of uterine contractions and, as such, is qualitative rather than quantitative. Although it permits graphic display of uterine activity and allows for accurate correlation of fetal heart rate patterns with uterine activity, external tocodynamometry does not allow measurement of contraction intensity or basal intrauterine tone. The most precise method for determination of uterine activity is the direct measurement of intrauterine pressure. However, this procedure should not be performed unless indicated given the small but finite associated risks of uterine perforation, placental disruption and intrauterine infection.

Despite technologic improvements, the definition of "adequate" uterine activity during labor remains unclear. Classically, three to five contractions per 10 minutes has been used to define adequate labor; this pattern has been observed in approximately 95 percent of women in spontaneous labor. In labor, patients usually contract every 2 to 5 minutes, with contractions becoming as frequent as every 2 to 3 minutes in late active labor and during the second stage. Abnormal uterine activity can also be observed either spontaneously or resulting from iatrogenic interventions. Tachysystole is defined as more than 5 contractions in 10 minutes for at least 20 minutes. Hyperstimulation is defined as tachysytole which is accompanied by an abnormal fetal heart rate pattern.[18]

Various units have been devised to objectively measure uterine activity, the most common of which is the *Montevideo unit,* a measure of average frequency and amplitude above basal tone (the average strength of contractions in millimeters of mercury multiplied by the number of contractions per 10 minutes). Two hundred to 250 Montevideo units define adequate labor in the active phase of labor.[19,20] Although it is generally believed that optimal uterine contractions are associated with an increased likelihood of vaginal delivery, there are limited data to support this assumption. If uterine contractions are "adequate" to effect vaginal delivery, one of two things will happen: either the cervix will efface and dilate, and the fetal head will descend, or there will be worsening caput succedaneum (scalp edema) and molding of the fetal head (overlapping of the skull bones) without cervical effacement and dilatation. The latter situation suggests the presence of cephalopelvic disproportion (CPD), which can be either absolute (in which a given fetus is simply too large to negotiate a given pelvis) or relative (in which delivery of a given fetus through a given pelvis would be possible under optimal conditions but is precluded by malposition or abnormal attitude of the fetal head).

The Fetus (Passenger)

The passenger, of course, is the fetus. There are several fetal variables that influence the course of labor and delivery. These are summarized below.

1. Fetal *size* can be estimated clinically by abdominal palpation or with ultrasound, but both are subject to a large degree of error. Fetal macrosomia (defined by the American College of Obstetricians and Gynecologists [ACOG] as actual birth weight greater than 4,500 g[21]) is associated with an increased likelihood of failed trial of labor.[22]
2. *Lie* refers to the longitudinal axis of the fetus relative to the longitudinal axis of the uterus. Fetal lie can be either longitudinal, transverse, or oblique (Fig. 12-3). In a singleton pregnancy, only fetuses in a longitudinal lie can be safely delivered vaginally.
3. *Presentation* refers to the fetal part that directly overlies the pelvic inlet. In a fetus presenting in the longitudinal lie, the presentation can be cephalic (vertex) or breech. Compound presentation refers to the presence of more than one fetal part overlying the pelvic inlet. Funic presentation refers to presentation of the umbilical cord and is rare at term. In a cephalic fetus, the presentation is classified according to the leading bony landmark of the skull, which can be either the occiput (vertex), the chin (mentum), or the brow (Fig. 12-4). *Malpresentation,* referring to any presentation other than vertex, is seen in approximately 5 percent of all term labors.
4. *Attitude* refers to the position of the head with regard to the fetal spine (the degree of flexion and/or extension of the fetal head). Flexion of the head is important to facilitate *engagement* of the head in the maternal

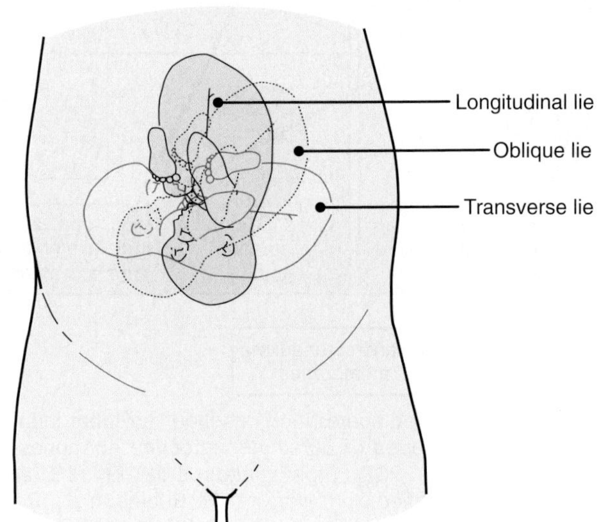

Figure 12-3. Examples of different fetal lie.

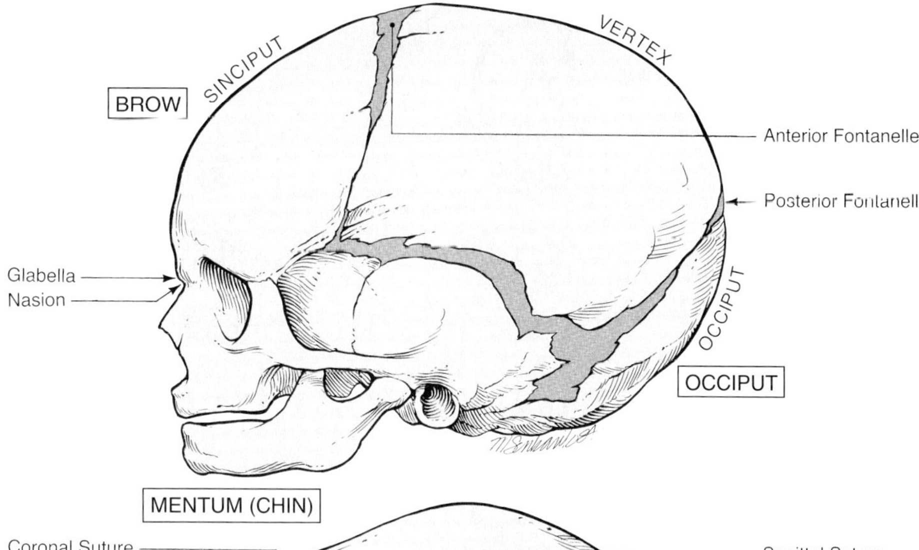

Figure 12-4. Landmarks of fetal skull for determination of fetal position.

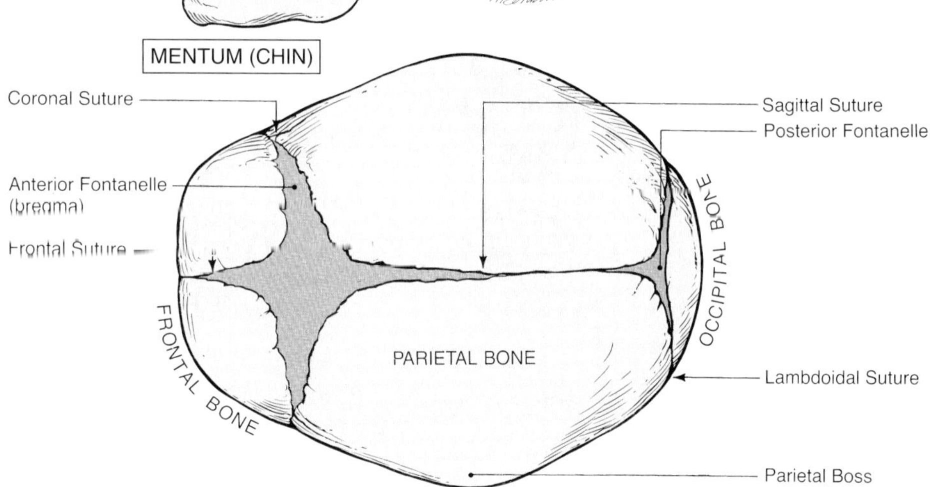

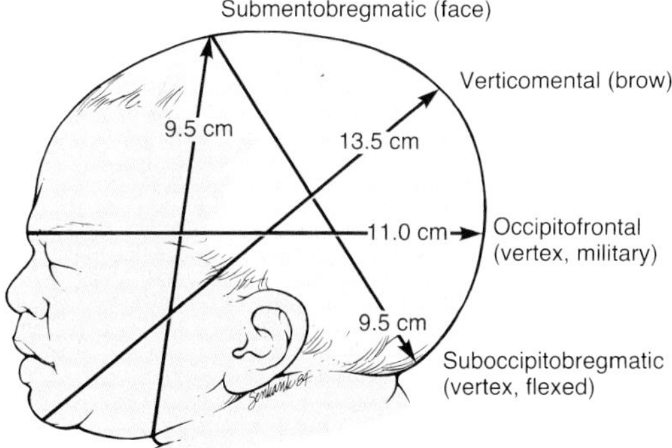

Figure 12-5. Presenting diameters of the average term fetal skull.

pelvis. When the fetal chin is optimally flexed onto the chest, the suboccipitobregmatic diameter (9.5 cm) presents at the pelvic inlet (Fig. 12-5). This is the smallest possible presenting diameter in the cephalic presentation. As the head deflexes (extends), the diameter presenting to the pelvic inlet progressively increases even before the malpresentations of brow and face are encountered (see Fig. 12-5), and may contribute to failure to progress in labor. The architecture of the pelvic floor along with increased uterine activity may correct deflexion in the early stages of labor.

5. *Position* of the fetus refers to the relationship of the fetal presenting part to the maternal pelvis, and it can be assessed most accurately on vaginal examination. For cephalic presentations, the fetal occiput is the reference. If the occiput is directly anterior, the position is occiput anterior (OA). If the occiput is turned toward the mother's right side, the position is right occiput anterior (ROA). In the breech presentation, the sacrum is the reference (right sacrum anterior). The various positions of a cephalic presentation are illustrated in Figure 12-6. In a vertex presentation, position can be determined by palpation of the fetal sutures. The sagittal suture is the easiest to palpate. Palpation of the distinctive lamdoid sutures should identify the position of the fetal occiput. The frontal suture can also be used to determine the position of the front of the vertex. Most commonly, the fetal head enters the pelvis in a transverse position and, then as a normal part of labor, rotates to an OA position. Most fetuses deliver in the OA, LOA, or ROA position. In the past, less than 10 percent of presentations were occiput posterior (OP) at delivery.[23] However epidural analgesia is associated with an increased risk of OP presentation (observed in 12.9 percent of women with epidural analgesia).[24] Asynclitism occurs when the sagittal suture is not directly central relative to the maternal pelvis. If the fetal head is turned such that more parietal bone is present posteriorly, the sagittal suture is more anterior and this is referred to as posterior asynclitism. Anterior asynclitism occurs when there is more parietal bone presenting anteri-

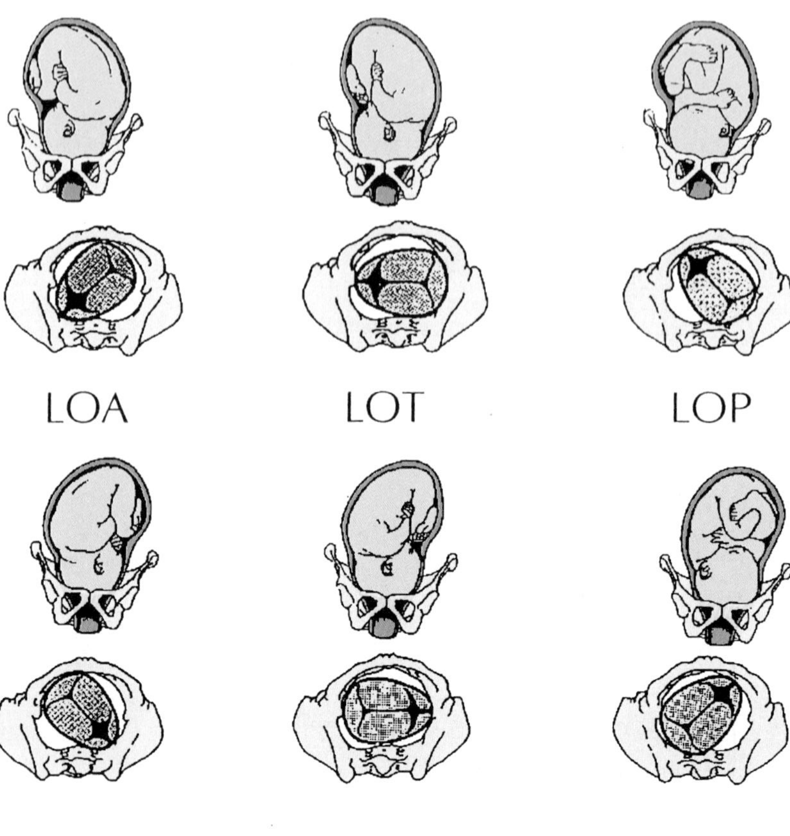

Figure 12-6. Fetal presentations and positions in labor. LOA, left occiput anterior; LOP, left occiput posterior; LOT, left occiput transverse; ROA, right occiput anterior; ROT, right occiput transverse; ROP, right occiput posterior. (Adapted from Norwitz ER, Robinson J, Repke JT: The initiation and management of labor. *In* Seifer DB, Samuels P, Kniss DA [eds]: The Physiologic Basis of Gynecology and Obstetrics. Philadelphia, Lippincott Williams & Wilkins, 2001.)

orly. The occiput transverse (OT) and OP positions are less common at delivery and more difficult to deliver. *Malposition* refers to any position in labor that is not ROA, OA, or LOA.

6. *Station* is a measure of descent of the bony presenting part of the fetus through the birth canal (Fig. 12-7). The current standard classification (–5 to +5) is based on a quantitative measure in centimeters of the distance of the leading bony edge from the ischial spines. The midpoint (0 station) is defined as the plane of the maternal ischial spines. The ischial spines can be palpated on vaginal examination at approximately 8 o'clock and 4 o'clock. For the right-handed person, they are most easily felt on the maternal right.

An abnormality in any of the above-mentioned fetal variables may affect both the course of and the likelihood of vaginal delivery. Failure to progress in labor should prompt a careful reevaluation of the above-mentioned fetal parameters to exclude absolute or relative CPD.

The Maternal Pelvis (Passage)

The passage consists of the bony pelvis (composed of the sacrum, ilium, ischium, and pubis) and the resistance provided by the soft tissues. The bony pelvis is divided into the false (greater) and true (lesser) pelvis by the pelvic brim, which is demarcated by the sacral promontory, the anterior ala of the sacrum, the arcuate line of the ilium, the pectineal line of the pubis, and the pubic crest culmi-

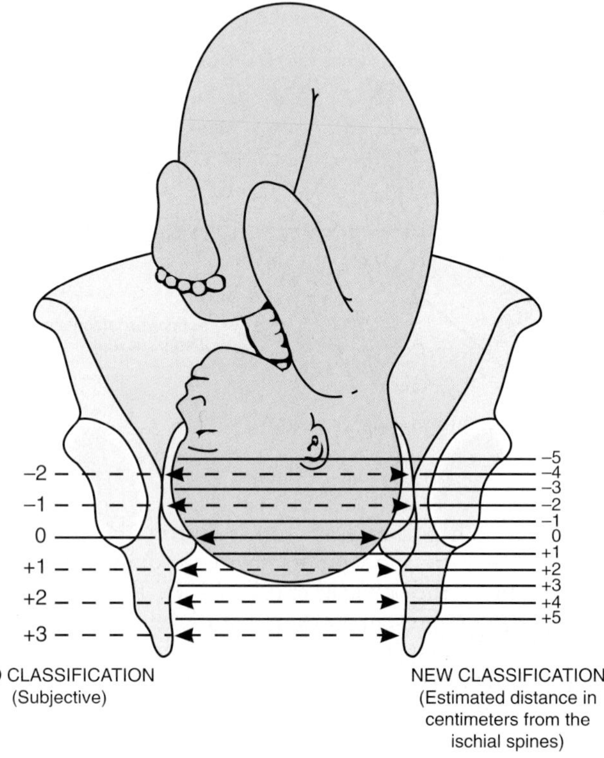

Figure 12-7. The relationship of the leading edge of the presenting part of the fetus to the plane of the maternal ischial spines determines the station. Station +1/+3 (old classification) or +2/+5 (new classification) is illustrated.

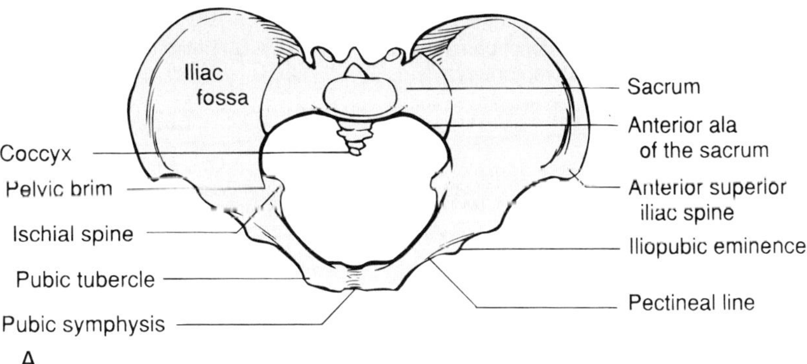

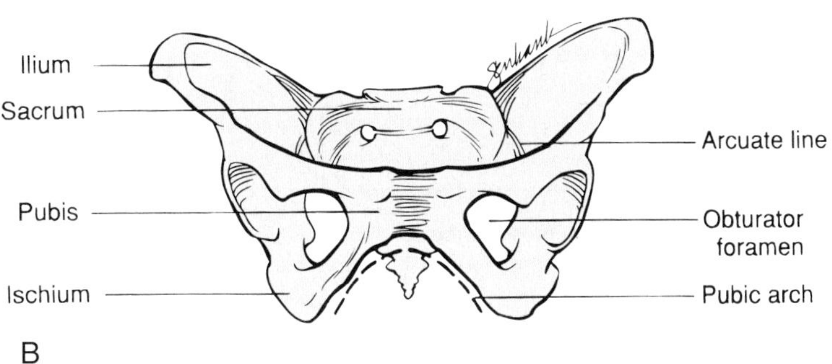

Figure 12-8. Superior (*A*) and anterior (*B*) view of the female pelvis. (From Repke JT: Intrapartum Obstetrics. New York, Churchill Livingstone, 1996, p 68, with permission.)

nating in the symphysis (Fig. 12-8). Measurements of the various parameters of the bony female pelvis have been made with great precision, directly in cadavers and using radiographic imaging in living women. Such measurements have divided the true pelvis into a series of planes that must be negotiated by the fetus during passage through the birth canal, which can be broadly classified into the pelvic inlet, midpelvis and pelvic outlet. X-ray pelvimetry has defined average and critical limit values for the various parameters of the bony pelvis (Table 12-1).[25] Critical limit values are measurements that are associated with a significant probability of CPD.[26] Computed tomography also has the potential for highly reproducible measurements of the bony pelvis.[27] However, both computed tomography and X-ray pelvimetry are rarely used, having been replaced in large part by a clinical trial of the pelvis (labor).

Clinical pelvimetry is currently the only method of assessing the shape and dimensions of the bony pelvis in labor. A useful protocol for clinical pelvimetry is detailed in Figure 12-9 and involves the assessment of the pelvic inlet, midpelvis, and pelvic outlet. The inlet of the true pelvis is largest in its transverse diameter (usually >12.0 cm). The *diagonal conjugate* (the distance from the sacral promontory to the inferior margin of the symphysis pubis as assessed on vaginal examination) is a clinical representation of the anteroposterior diameter of the pelvic inlet. The *true conjugate* (or *obstetric conjugate*) of the pelvic inlet is the distance from the sacral promontory to the superior aspect of the symphysis pubis. This measurement cannot be made clinically but can be estimated by subtracting 1.5 to 2.0 cm from the diagonal conjugate. This is the smallest diameter of the inlet, and it usually measures approximately 10 to 11 cm. The limiting factor in the midpelvis is the interspinous diameter (the measurement between the ischial spines), which is usually the smallest diameter of the pelvis but should be greater than 10 cm. The pelvic outlet is rarely of clinical significance. The anteroposterior diameter from the coccyx to the symphysis pubis is approximately 13 cm in most cases, and the transverse diameter between the ischial tuberosities is approximately 8 cm.

Table 12-1. Average and Critical Limit Values for Pelvic Measurements by X-ray Pelvimetry

DIAMETER	AVERAGE VALUE	CRITICAL LIMIT*
Pelvic inlet		
Anteroposterior (cm)	12.5	10.0
Transverse (cm)	13.0	12.0
Sum (cm)	25.5	22.0
Area (cm^2)	145.0	123.0
Pelvic midcavity		
Anteroposterior (cm)	11.5	10.0
Transverse (cm)	10.5	9.5
Sum (cm)	22.0	19.5
Area (cm^2)	125.0	106.0

*The critical limit values cited imply a high likelihood of cephalopelvic disproportion.

Adapted from O'Brien WF, Cefalo RC: Labor and delivery. *In* Gabbe SG, Niebyl JR, Simpson JL (eds): Obstetrics: Normal and Problem Pregnancies, 3rd ed. New York, Churchill Livingstone, 1996, p 377.

The shape of the female bony pelvis can be classified into four broad categories: gynecoid, anthropoid, android, and platypelloid (Fig. 12-10). This classification, based on the radiographic studies of Caldwell and Moloy, separates those with favorable characteristics (gynecoid, anthropoid) from those that are less favorable

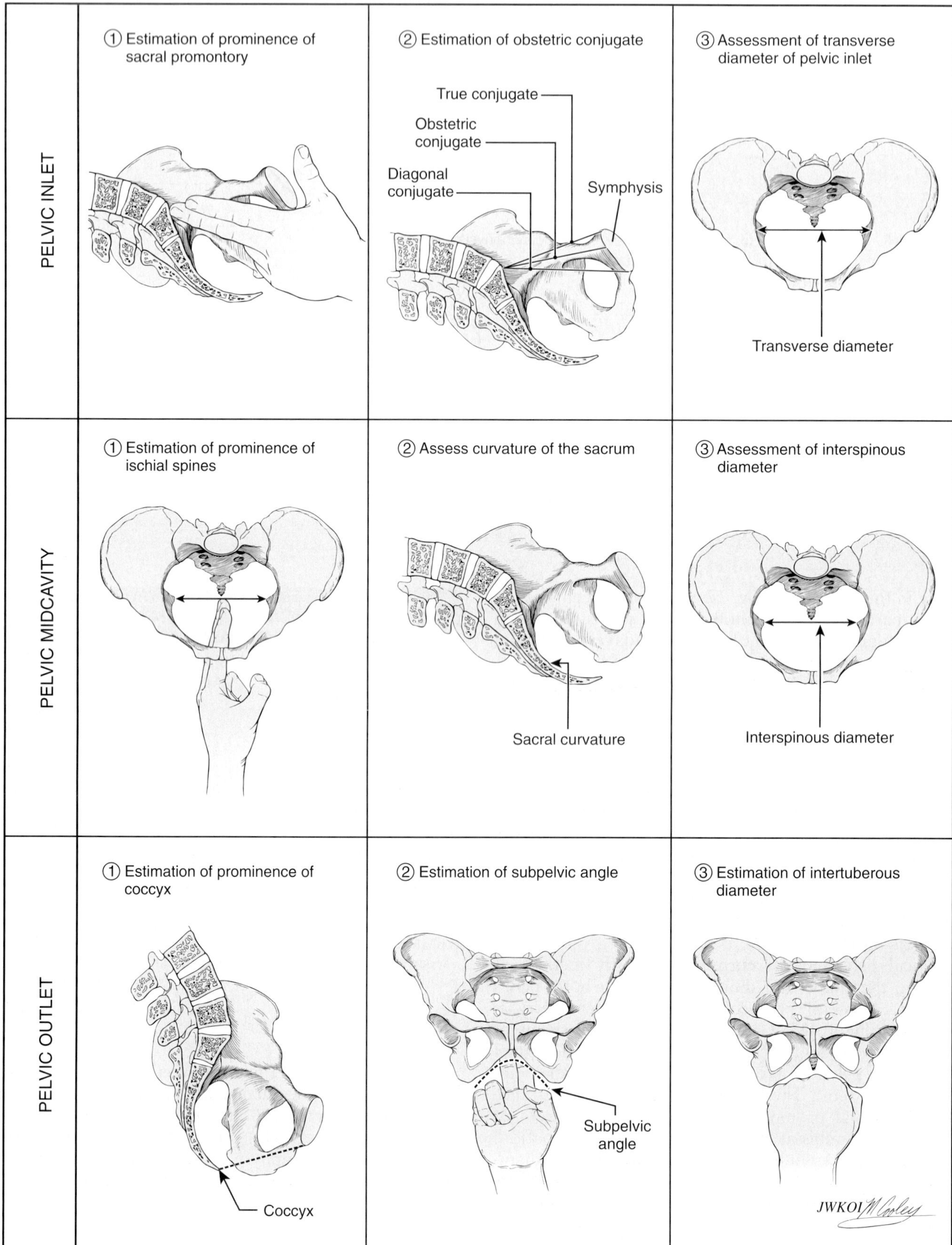

Figure 12-9. A protocol for clinical pelvimetry.

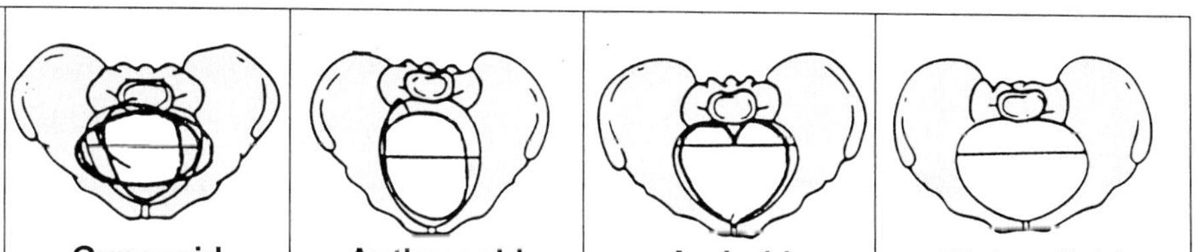

		Gynecoid	Anthropoid	Android	Platypelloid
Pelvic inlet 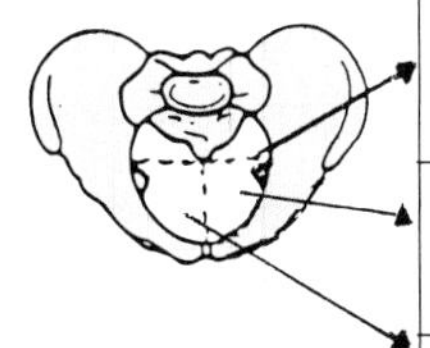	Widest transverse diameter of inlet	12 cm	< 12 cm	12 cm	12 cm
	Anteroposterior diameter of inlet	11 cm	> 12 cm	11 cm	10 cm
	Forepelvis	Wide	Divergent	Narrow	Straight
Pelvic midcavity 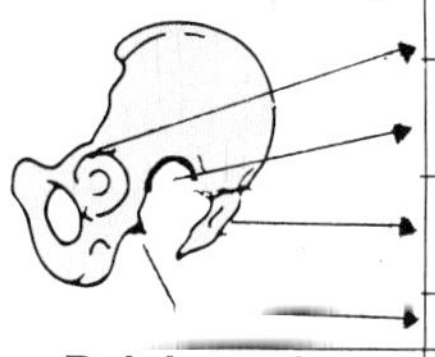	Side walls	Straight	Narrow	Convergent	Wide
	Sacrosciatic notch	Medium	Backward	Narrow	Forward
	Inclination of sacrum	Medium	Wide	Forward (lower third)	Narrow
	Ischial spines	Not prominent	Not prominent	Not prominent	Not prominent
Pelvic outlet 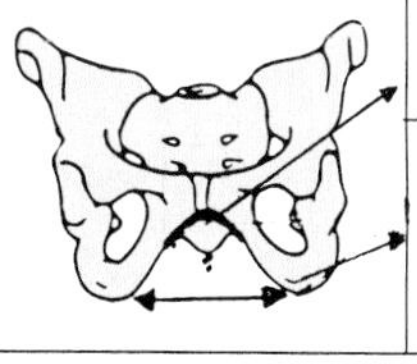	Subpubic arch	Wide	Medium	Narrow	Wide
	Transverse diameter of outlet	10 cm	10 cm	< 10 cm	10 cm

Figure 12-10. Characteristics of the four types of female bony pelvis. (Modified from Callahan TL, Caughey AB, Heffner LJ [eds]: Blueprints in Obstetrics & Gynecology. Malden, MA, Blackwell Science, 1998, p 45.)

for vaginal delivery (android, platypelloid).[28] In reality, however, many women fall into intermediate classes, and the distinctions become arbitrary. The gynecoid pelvis is the classic female shape with an oval-shaped inlet, diverging midpelvic sidewalls, and far-spaced ischial spines. The anthropoid pelvis has an exaggerated oval shape to the inlet, with the largest diameter being anteroposterior, and with limited anterior capacity to the pelvis. Such pelves are more often associated with delivery in the occiput posterior position. The android pelvis is male in pattern, with a heart-shaped inlet, prominent sacral promontory and ischial spines, shallow sacrum, and converging midpelvic sidewalls theoretically increasing the risk of CPD. The platypelloid pelvis is a broad, flat pelvis with an exaggerated oval-shaped inlet, but with the largest diameter being the transverse diameter theoretically predisposing to transverse arrest. Although the assessment of fetal size along with pelvic shape and capacity is still of clinical utility, it is a very inexact science. An adequate trial of labor is the only definitive method to determine whether a given fetus will be able to safely negotiate a given pelvis.

Pelvic soft tissues may provide resistance in both the first and second stages of labor. In the first stage, resistance is offered primarily by the cervix; whereas in the second stage, it is by the muscles of the pelvic floor. It has been proposed that rapid labors result from low pelvic resistance rather than from high myometrial activity.[29] When cervical ripening is used before augmentation of labor, subsequent intrauterine pressures are lower compared with augmentation alone.[30] However, this hypothesis has not received wide acceptance. In the second stage of labor, the resistance of the pelvic musculature is believed to play an important role in the rotation and movement of the presenting part through the pelvis.

CARDINAL MOVEMENTS IN LABOR

The mechanisms of labor, also known as the cardinal movements, refer to the changes in position of fetal head during its passage through the birth canal. Because of the asymmetry of the shape of both the fetal head and the maternal bony pelvis, such rotations are required for the fetus to successfully negotiate the birth canal. Although labor and birth is a continuous process, seven discrete cardinal movements of the fetus are described: engagement, descent, flexion, internal rotation, extension, external rotation or restitution, and expulsion (Fig. 12-11).

Engagement

Engagement refers to passage of the widest diameter of the presenting part to a level below the plane of the pelvic inlet (Fig. 12-12). In the cephalic presentation with a well-

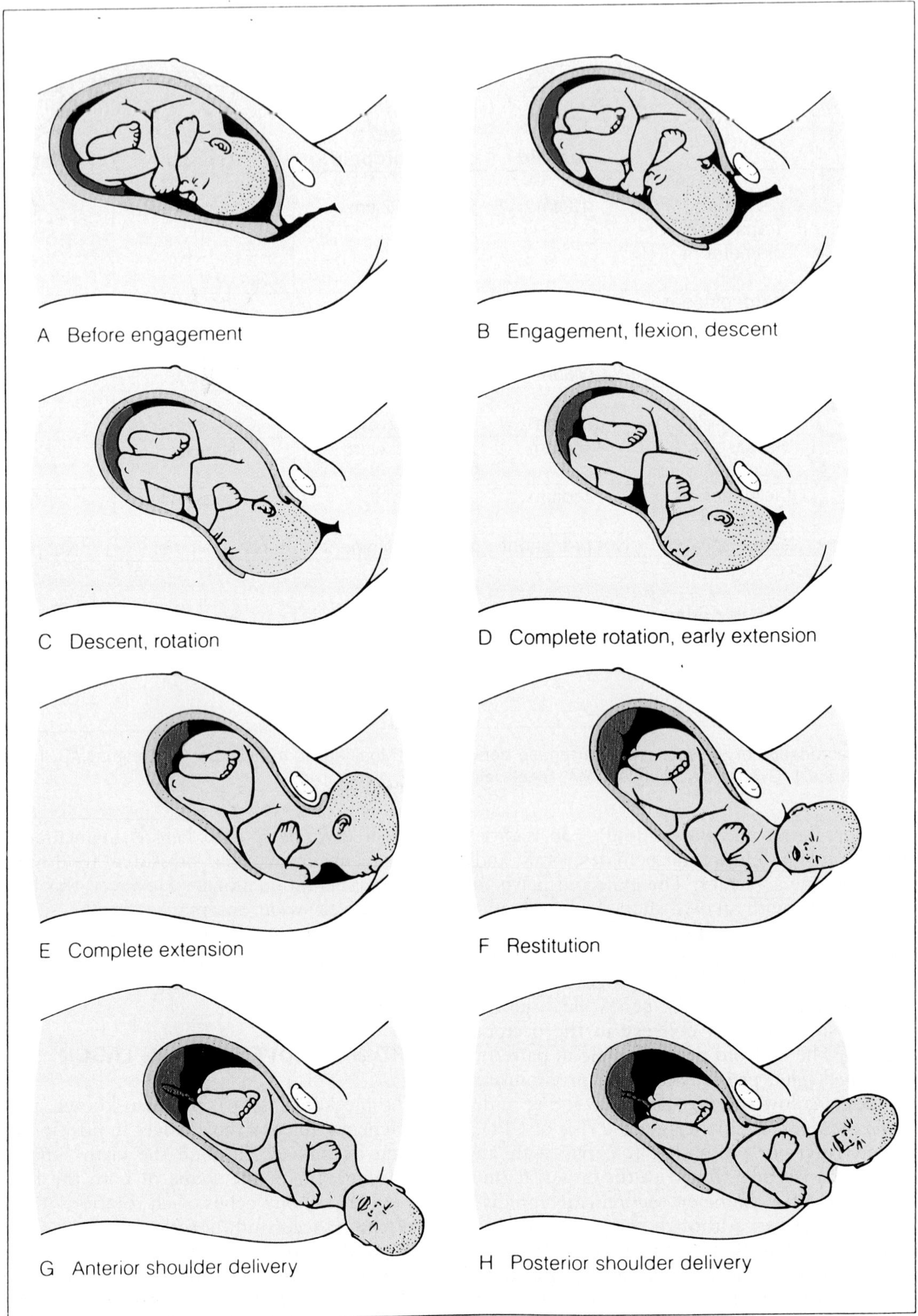

Figure 12-11. Cardinal movements of labor.

flexed head, the largest transverse diameter of the fetal head is the biparietal diameter (9.5 cm). In the breech, the widest diameter is the bitrochanteric diameter. Clinically, engagement can be confirmed by palpation of the presenting part both abdominally and vaginally. With a cephalic presentation, engagement is achieved when the presenting part is at 0 station (at the level of the maternal ischial spines) on vaginal examination. Engagement is considered an important clinical prognostic sign because it demonstrates that, at least at the level of the pelvic

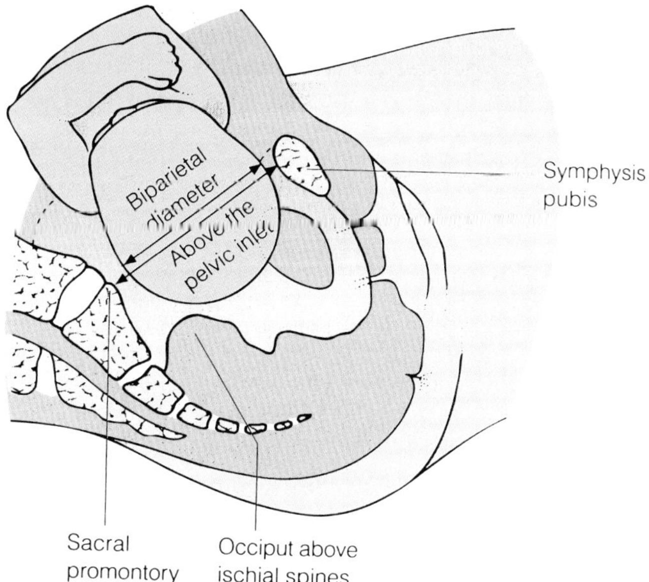

Figure 12-12. Engagement of the fetal head.

inlet, the maternal bony pelvis is sufficiently large to allow descent of the fetal head. In nulliparas, engagement of the fetal head usually occurs by 36 weeks' gestation. In multiparas, however, engagement can occur later in gestation or even during the course of labor.

Descent

Descent refers to the downward passage of the presenting part through the pelvis. Descent of the fetus is not continuous; the greatest rates of descent occur during the deceleration phase of the first stage of labor and during the second stage of labor.

Flexion

Flexion of the fetal head occurs passively as the head descends owing to the shape of the bony pelvis and the resistance offered by the soft tissues of the pelvic floor. Although flexion of the fetal head onto the chest is present to some degree in most fetuses before labor, complete flexion usually occurs only during the course of labor. The result of complete flexion is to present the smallest diameter of the fetal head (the suboccipitobregmatic diameter) for optimal passage through the pelvis.

Internal Rotation

Internal rotation refers to rotation of the presenting part from its original position as it enters the pelvic inlet (usually OT) to the anteroposterior position as it passes through the pelvis. As with flexion, internal rotation is a passive movement resulting from the shape of the pelvis and the pelvic floor musculature. The pelvic floor musculature, including the coccygeus and ileococcygeus muscles, forms a V-shaped hammock that diverges anteriorly. As the head descends, the occiput of the fetus rotates towards the symphysis pubis (or, less commonly, towards the hollow of the sacrum), thereby allowing the widest portion of the fetus to negotiate the pelvis at its widest dimension. Owing to the angle of inclination between the maternal lumbar spine and pelvic inlet, the fetal head engages in an asynclitic fashion (i.e., with one parietal eminence lower than the other). With uterine contractions, the leading parietal eminence descends and is first to engage the pelvic floor. As the uterus relaxes, the pelvic floor musculature causes the fetal head to rotate until it is no longer asynclitic.

Extension

Extension occurs once the fetus has descended to the level of the introitus. This descent brings the base of the occiput into contact with the inferior margin at the symphysis pubis. At this point, the birth canal curves upward. The fetal head is delivered by extension and rotates around the symphysis pubis. The forces responsible for this motion are the downward force exerted on the fetus by the uterine contractions along with the upward forces exerted by the muscles of the pelvic floor.

External Rotation

External rotation, also known as restitution, refers to the return of the fetal head to the correct anatomic position in relation to the fetal torso. This can occur to either side depending on the orientation of the fetus. This is again a passive movement resulting from a release of the forces exerted on the fetal head by the maternal bony pelvis and its musculature and mediated by the basal tone of the fetal musculature.

Expulsion

Expulsion refers to delivery of the rest of the fetus. After delivery of the head and external rotation, further descent brings the anterior shoulder to the level of the symphysis pubis. The anterior shoulder is delivered in much the same manner as the head, with rotation of the shoulder under the symphysis pubis. After the shoulder, the rest of the body is usually delivered without difficulty.

NORMAL PROGRESS OF LABOR

Progress of labor is measured with multiple variables. With the onset of regular contractions, the fetus descends in the pelvis as the cervix both effaces and dilates. The clinician must assess not only cervical effacement and dilation but fetal station and position with each vaginal examination to judge labor progress. This assessment depends on skilled digital palpation of the fetal presenting part and maternal cervix. Cervical effacement refers to the length of the remaining cervix and can be reported in length or as a percentage. If percentage is used, then

0 percent effacement refers to at least a 2 cm long, or a very thick cervix, and 100-percent effacement refers to no length remaining or a very thin cervix. Most clinicians use percentage to follow cervical effacement during labor. Generally, ≥80 percent effacement is required for the diagnosis of active labor. Dilation, perhaps the easiest assessment to master, ranges from closed or 0 cm dilation to complete or 10 cm dilated. For most people, a cervical dilation that accommodates a single index finger is equal to 1 cm and 2 index fingers dilation is equal to 3 cm. If no cervix can be palpated around the presenting part, then the cervix is 10 cm or completely dilated. The assessment of station (see earlier) is important to document progress, but it is also critical when determining if an operative vaginal delivery is feasible. Fetal head position is another aspect that must be assessed; ideally, head position should be determined before significant caput has developed, obscuring the sutures. Like station, knowledge of the fetal position is critical before performing an operative vaginal delivery.

Labor has two categorizations: phases and stages. Phases are divided into latent and active. The latent phase of labor is defined as the period between the onset of labor and the point when labor becomes active. The onset of labor is difficult to identify objectively. Usually, it is defined by the initiation of regular painful contractions. Patients are frequently at home at this time, therefore, the identification of latent labor depends on patient memory. The beginning of active labor is a retrospective diagnosis because the definition of the active phase of labor is when the slope of cervical dilation accelerates. In general, active labor requires ≥80 percent effacement and ≥4 cm dilation of the cervix. In addition, there are three stages of labor. The first stage is from labor onset until full dilation. The second stage is from full dilation until delivery of the baby, and the third stage is from the delivery of the baby until the delivery of the placenta.

The work of Dr. Emanuel Friedman in the 1950s and 1960s was seminal to the current knowledge of labor progress in nulliparous and multiparous women. He analyzed labor progress in 500 nulliparous and multiparous women, and reported normative data that are still useful today.[31,32] Of note, Friedman's second-stage lengths are somewhat artificial because most nulliparous women in that era had a forceps delivery once the duration of the second stage reached 2 hours. More recent data evaluating women in spontaneous labor without augmentation or operative delivery from multiple countries are amazingly similar in the means, suggesting that these normative data are reliable and useful (Table 12-2).[33–36] Of interest, epidural use appears to add about 2 hours to the first stage and about 20 minutes to the second stage in both multiparous and nulliparous women.[36] Friedman's data popularized the use of the labor graph, first depicting only cervical dilation and then modified to include descent and dilation.[37] Rates of 1.5 cm and 1.2 cm dilation per hour in the active phase for multiparous and nulliparous women, respectively, represent the 5th percentile for rates of dilation[32] and have led to the general concept that in active labor, dilation of at least 1 cm per hour should occur (Table 12-3). The exact time when an individual patient enters the active phase becomes obvious only retrospectively.

Table 12-2. Summary of Means and 95th Percentiles for Duration of First- and Second-Stage Labor

PARAMETER	MEAN	95TH PERCENTILE
Nulliparas		
Latent Labor	7.3–8.6 h	17–21 h
1st Stage	7.7–13.3 h	16.6–19.4 h
1st Stage epidural	10.2 h	19 h
2nd Stage	53–57 m	122–147 m
2nd Stage epidural	79 m	185 m
Multiparas		
Latent Labor	4.1–5.3 h	12–14
First Stage	5.7–7.5 h	12.5–13.7 h
First Stage epidural	7.4 h	14.9 h
Second Stage F2	17–19 m	57–61 m
Second Stage epidural	45 m	131 m

Friedman,[31,32] 1955–56, Albers,[33] 1996, Kilpatrick,[36] 1989, Schulman,[39] 1964

Table 12-3. Median Duration of Time Elapsed in Hours* for Each Centimeter of Dilation During Labor

CERVICAL DILATION (CM)	BEFORE PERIOD	AFTER PERIOD	*P* VALUE
3–4	2.03	2.30	.36
4–5	1.29	2.17	<.01
5–6	0.66	0.67	.84
6–7	0.62	0.54	.32
7–8	0.44	0.51	.25
8–9	0.41	0.52	.05
9–10	0.44	0.50	.27

*An interval-censored regression model with a log normal distribution was fitted to adjust for maternal age, prepregnancy BMI, and gravidity.

From Vahratian A, Zhang J, Hasling J, et al: The effect of early epidural versus early intravenous analgesia use on labor progression: a natural experiment. Am J Obstet Gynecol 191:259, 2004.

Limits of lengths of first and second stages incorporating the effect of epidural use are helpful in identifying those women who may benefit from interventions (see Table 12-2).[33,35] Second-stage durations of 1 hour for multiparous women without an epidural, 2 hours for multiparous women with an epidural and nulliparous women without an epidural, and 3 hours for nulliparous women with an epidural identify clinical outliers. Although there is no indication that these limits should be used arbitrarily to justify ending the second stage, they identify a subset of women who require further evaluation.

A more practical approach to following labor progress was introduced by Schulman and Ledger, when they published a modified labor graph that evaluated labor progress focused on latent and active phase only, and this is the graph most commonly used today (Fig. 12-13).[39] When evaluating labor progress, it is extremely important to understand that progress in latent phase is slower and less predictable both in multiparas and nulliparas. Mean latent phase lengths and 95th percentile limits for multipara and nullipara are shown in Table 12-2. Factors affecting the duration of labor include parity, maternal

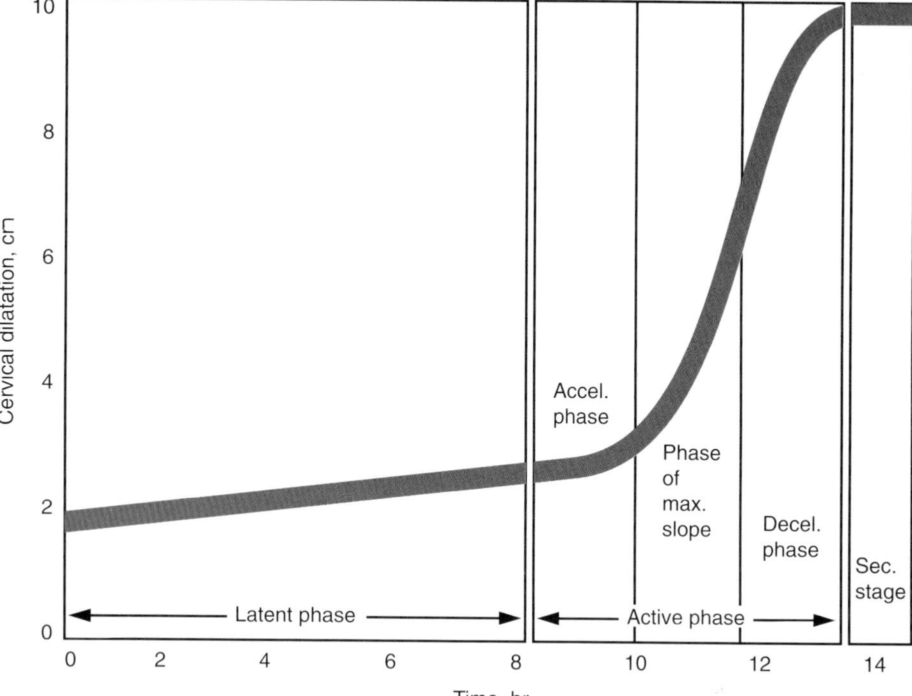

Figure 12-13. Modern labor graph. Characteristics of the average cervical dilatation curve for nulliparous labor. (Adapted from Friedman EA: Labor: Clinical Evaluation and Management, 2nd ed. Norwalk, CT, Appleton-Century-Crofts, 1978.)

body mass index, fetal position, and fetal size. Longer labors are associated with increased maternal body mass index[40] and fetal position other than OA.[41]

Mean lengths of the third stage of labor are not affected by parity. In a case series of nearly 13,000 singleton vaginal deliveries greater than 20 weeks' gestation, the median third stage duration was 6 minutes and exceeded 30 minutes in a mere 3 percent of women.[42] A threshold of 30 minutes was associated with a significantly increased risk of a greater than 500-ml blood loss, a drop in postdelivery hematocrit by greater than or equal to 10 percent, or a need for dilation and curettage.[42] This suggests that manual removal and or extraction of the placenta is indicated after 30 minutes. Factors significantly associated with a prolonged second stage included preterm delivery, ≥3 previous abortions, induced labor, chorioamnionitis, and parity ≥5.

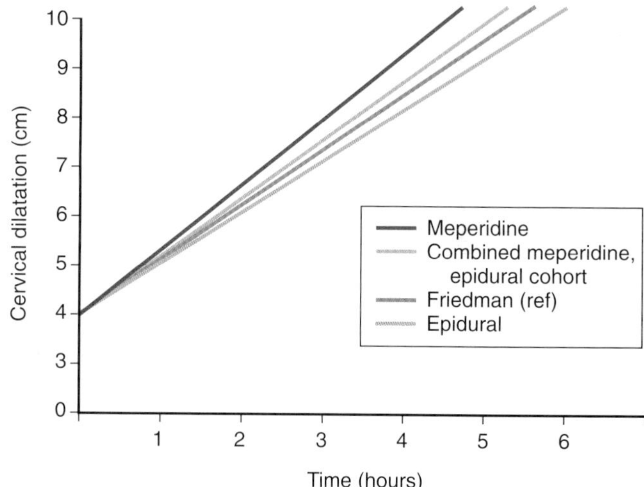

Figure 12-14. Comparison of the rates of cervical dilation during the active phase of labor originally reported by Friedman and now reported for the women who received patient-controlled intravenous meperidine, patient-controlled epidural analgesia, and the combined cohort. (From Alexander JM, Sharma SK, McIntire DD, Leveno KJ: Epidural analgesia lengthens the Friedman active phase of labor. Obstet Gynecol 100:46, 2002.)

Maternal Activity, Positions, and Labor Support

Various interventions have been suggested to encourage normal labor progress, including maternal ambulation during active labor (Fig. 12-14). However, a well-designed randomized trial of over 1,000 women in active labor comparing ambulation with usual care found no differences in the duration of the first stage, need for oxytocin, use of analgesia, or route of delivery.[43] In contrast, other interventions such as the presence of a labor doula may be effective. In a recent meta-analysis of 11 trials, continuous doula support compared with no support was associated with a significant reduction in use of analgesia, oxytocin, and operative or cesarean delivery.[44] In addition, continuous doula support was associated with significantly shorter length of labor.

Active Management of Labor

Dystocia is the second most common indication for cesarean delivery, following previous cesarean delivery. In the late 1980s, in an effort to reduce the rapidly rising cesarean delivery rate, active management of labor was popularized in the United States based on findings in Ireland, where the routine use of active management was associated with very low rates of cesarean delivery.[45] Protocols for active management included admission only when labor was established (painful contractions and spontaneous rupture of membranes, 100-percent effacement, or passage of blood stained mucus); artificial rupture of membranes on diagnosis of labor; aggressive oxytocin augmentation for labor progress of less than 1 cm/h with high-dose oxytocin (6 mIU/min initial dose, increased by 6 mIU/min every 15 minutes to a maximum of 40 mIU/min); and patient education.[45] Observational data suggested that this management protocol was associated with rates of cesarean delivery of 5.5 percent and delivery within 12 hours in 98 percent of women.[45] Only 41 percent of the nulliparas actually required oxytocin augmentation. Multiple nonrandomized studies were subsequently published attempting to duplicate these results in the United States and Canada.[46–48] Two of these reported a significant reduction in cesarean delivery when compared with historical controls.[46,48] However, in two of three randomized controlled trials (RCTs), there was no significant decrease in the rate of cesarean delivery with active compared with routine management of labor.[49,50] In the third RCT, the overall cesarean delivery rate was not significantly different; however, when controlled for confounding variables, cesarean delivery was significantly lower in the actively managed group.[51] In all randomized trials, labor duration was significantly decreased by a range of 1.7 to 2.7 hours, and neonatal morbidity was not different between groups. This reduction in labor duration has significant cost and bed management implications, especially for busy labor and delivery units. Perhaps the most important factor in active management is delaying admission until active labor has been established.

Second Stage of Labor

Abnormal progress in fetal descent is the dystocia of the second stage. The diagnostic parameters are outlined in Table 12-2. For practical purposes the 95th percentiles for length of second stage is 1 hour for multiparas without epidural analgesia, 2 hours for multiparas with epidural analgesia or nulliparas without epidural analgesia, and 3 hours for nulliparas with epidural analgesia.[32] Other models include prospectively determined second-stage partograms in which the median second-stage lengths are similar to those outlined in Table 12-2.[52] Women with a prolonged second stage by these criteria should be evaluated for potential interventions. As with active labor, poor progress may be related to inadequate contractions; initiating oxytocin in the second stage may be effective if contraction frequency is diminished. If malposition is diagnosed, rotation to OA (either manually or by forceps) may be indicated in the second stage. If neither uterine forces nor fetal position are abnormal, the default diagnosis is fetal pelvic disproportion. No excess neonatal morbidity has been reported in association with a prolonged second stage in the absence of nonreassuring fetal heart rate tracings. Therefore, if steady progress is observed, there is no need for arbitrary time cut-offs.[53–57] In contrast, maternal morbidity, including perineal trauma, postpartum hemorrhage, and chorioamnionitis, is significantly higher in women with a second stage lasting longer than 2 hours.[57] However, it is important to note that performing an instrument-assisted vaginal delivery is unlikely to reduce perineal trauma and morbidity. If the fetal heart rate tracing is reassuring, continuing the second stage beyond 3 hours is reasonable. After 4 hours, the likelihood of vaginal delivery declines while maternal morbidity increases. The incidence of a vaginal delivery, including operative delivery, in women with a second stage length of less than 2 hours, 2 to 4 hours, and longer than 4 hours is 99 percent, 91 percent, and 66 percent, respectively.[57]

There are multiple factors that influence the duration of the second stage including epidural analgesia, nulliparity, older maternal age, longer active phase, larger birth weight, and excess maternal weight gain.[58,59] Modifiable factors that have been evaluated in the management of the second stage include maternal position, decreasing epidural analgesia (see Chapter 16), and delayed pushing. Two of three RCTs of decreased second stage epidural analgesia found no difference in outcome or second-stage length.[60,61] One reported a decrease in second-stage length and operative delivery in the group that was randomized to reduced levels of epidural analgesia.[60] Epidural analgesia is clearly associated with an increased rate of operative delivery rate and associated perineal injury.[62,63] Delayed pushing has also been studied in nulliparas with epidural analgesia to determine if this strategy reduces the need for operative delivery, but little benefit has been demonstrated.[63–66] Only one trial reported a significant decrease in operative deliveries and that was limited to midpelvic deliveries.[64] Conversely, the risk of delayed pushing appears to be negligible. Finally, the effect of maternal position has been evaluated.[67,68] Randomization to squatting using a birth cushion was associated with a significant reduction in operative deliveries and a significantly shorter second stage in nulliparas compared with delivery in the lithotomy position.[67] In a second trial randomizing women to either a routine delivery position or any upright position (squatting, kneeling, sitting, or standing per patient choice), no difference in operative deliveries was noted between groups but a significant increase in the percent of women with an intact perineum was noted in the upright group.[68] Therefore, allowing women to choose alternate positions during the second stage may be beneficial, especially in nulliparas.

SPONTANEOUS VAGINAL DELIVERY

Preparation for delivery should take into account the patient's parity, the progression of labor, fetal presentation, and any labor complications. In women in whom fetal manipulation is anticipated (shoulder dystocia risk factors or multiple gestation), transfer to a larger and better equipped delivery room, removal of the foot of the bed, and delivery in the lithotomy position may be appropriate. If no complications are anticipated, delivery can be accomplished with the mother in her preferred position. Common positions include the lateral (Sims) position or the partial sitting position.

The goals of clinical assistance at spontaneous delivery are the reduction of maternal trauma, prevention of fetal injury, and initial support of the newborn, if required. When the fetal head crowns and delivery is imminent, gentle pressure should be used to maintain flexion of the fetal head and to control delivery, potentially protecting against perineal injury. Once the fetal head is delivered, external rotation (restitution) is allowed; if shoulder dystocia is anticipated, it is appropriate to proceed directly with gentle downward traction of the fetal head before restitution occurs. During restitution, nuchal umbilical cords should be identified and reduced; in rare cases in which simple reduction is not possible, the cord can be doubly clamped and transected. Although suction of the fetal oropharynx is appropriate, there is no evidence that additional DeLee suction reduces the risk of meconium aspiration syndrome in the presence of meconium.[69] The anterior shoulder should then be delivered by gentle downward traction in concert with maternal expulsive efforts. The posterior shoulder is then delivered by upward traction. These movements should be performed with the minimal force possible to avoid perineal injury and traction injuries to the brachial plexus. The timing of cord clamping should be dictated by convenience and is usually performed immediately after delivery. Although transfer of blood from the placenta to the fetus can continue for up to 3 minutes after birth, the volume of transfusion that results from delayed cord clamping is not clinically significant in most cases. After delivery, the infant should be held securely or placed on the mother's abdomen and wiped dry, while any mucus remaining in the airway is suctioned.

DELIVERY OF THE PLACENTA AND FETAL MEMBRANES

The third stage of labor can be managed either passively or actively. Passive management is characterized by patiently waiting for the classic signs of placental separation: (1) lengthening of the umbilical cord, and (2) a gush of blood from the vagina signifying separation of the placenta from the uterine wall. In addition, two techniques of controlled cord traction are commonly used to facilitate separation and delivery of the placenta: the *Brandt-Andrews maneuver* (in which an abdominal hand secures the uterine fundus to prevent uterine inversion while the other hand exerts sustained downward traction on the umbilical cord) or the *Créde maneuver* (in which the cord is fixed with the lower hand while the uterine fundus is secured and sustained upward traction is applied using the abdominal hand). Care should be taken to avoid avulsion of the cord. Active management with uterotonic agents such as oxytocin administered at delivery hasten delivery of the placenta and may reduce the incidence of postpartum hemorrhage and total blood loss.[70] Conversely, other studies have shown no benefit to active management in the second stage.[71]

After delivery, the placenta, umbilical cord, and fetal membranes should be examined. Placental weight (excluding membranes and cord) varies with fetal weight, with a ratio of approximately 1:6. Abnormally large placentae are associated with such conditions as hydrops fetalis and congenital syphilis. Inspection and palpation of the placenta should include the fetal and maternal surfaces and may reveal areas of fibrosis, infarction, or calcification. Although each of these conditions may be seen in the normal term placenta, extensive lesions should prompt histologic examination. Adherent clots on the maternal placental surface may indicate recent placental abruption; however, their absence does not exclude the diagnosis. A missing placental cotyledon or a membrane defect (suggesting a missing succenturiate lobe) suggests retention of a portion of placenta and should prompt further clinical evaluation. There is no need for routine manual exploration of the uterus after delivery unless there is suspicion of retained products of conception or a postpartum hemorrhage.

The site of insertion of the umbilical cord into the placenta should be noted. Abnormal insertions include marginal insertion (in which the cord inserts into the edge of the placenta) and membranous insertion (in which the vessels of the umbilical cord course through the membranes before attachment to the placental disk). The cord itself should be inspected for length, the correct number of umbilical vessels (normally two arteries and one vein), true knots, hematomas, and strictures. The average cord length is 50 to 60 cm. A single umbilical artery discovered on pathologic examination is associated with other fetal structural anomalies in 27 percent of cases.[72,73] Therefore, this finding should be relayed to the attending neonatologist or pediatrician.

EPISIOTOMY, PERINEAL INJURY, AND PERINEAL REPAIR

Following delivery of the placenta, the cervix, vagina, and perineum should be carefully examined for evidence of injury. If a laceration is seen, its length and position should be noted and repair initiated. Adequate analgesia (either regional or local) is essential for repair (see Chapter 16). Special attention should be paid to repair of the perineal body, the external anal sphincter, and the rectal mucosa. Failure to recognize and repair rectal injury can lead to serious long-term morbidity, most notably fecal incontinence.

Perineal injuries, either spontaneous or with episiotomy, are the most common complications of spontaneous or operative vaginal deliveries. A first-degree tear is defined as a superficial tear confined to the epithelial layer. Second-degree tears extend into the perineal body but not into the external anal sphincter. Third-degree tears involve superficial or deep injury to the external anal sphincter, whereas a fourth-degree tear extends completely through the rectal mucosa. Significant morbidity is associated with third- and fourth-degree tears, including risk of flatus and stool incontinence, rectal vaginal fistula, infection, and pain. Primary approximation of perineal laceration affords the best opportunity for functional repair, especially if there is evidence of rectal sphincter injury. The external anal sphincter should be repaired by direct apposition or overlapping the cut ends and securing them using interrupted sutures.

Episiotomy is an incision into the perineal body made during the second stage of labor to facilitate delivery. It

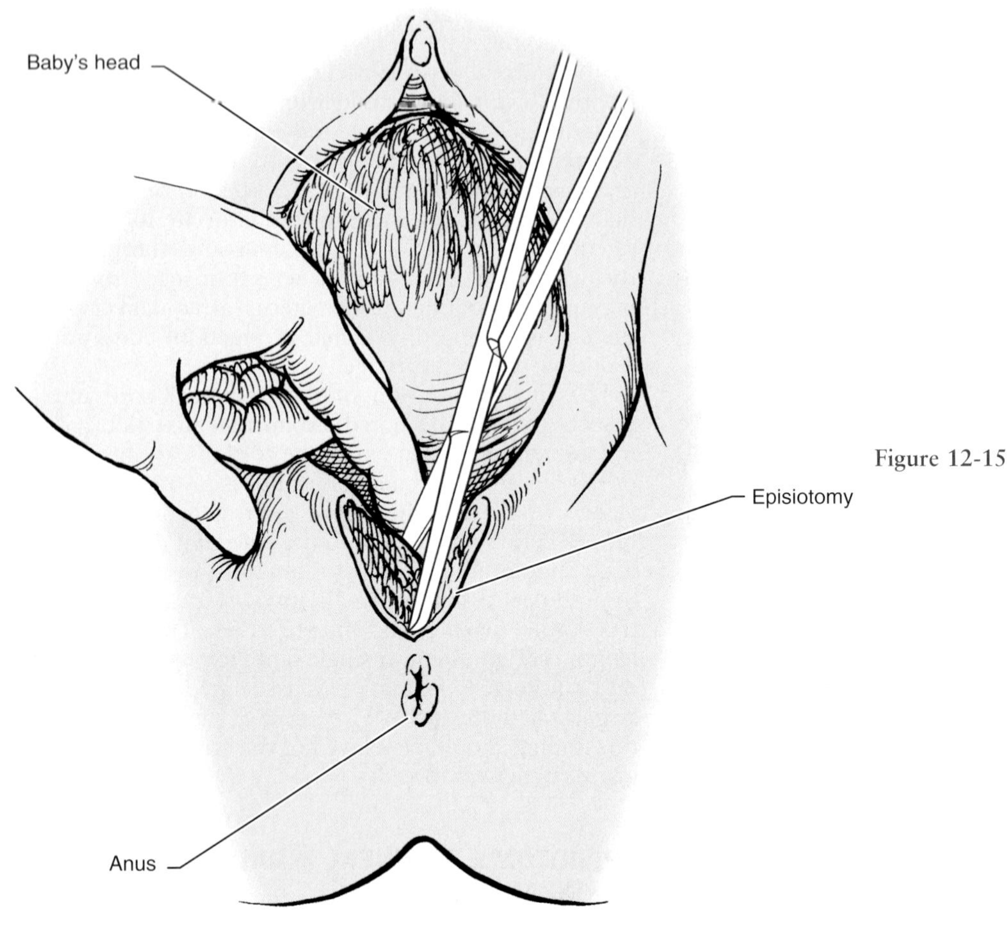

Figure 12-15. Cutting a midline episiotomy.

is by definition a second-degree tear. Episiotomy can be classified into two broad categories: median and mediolateral. Median (midline) episiotomy refers to a vertical midline incision from the posterior forchette toward the rectum, and is preferred in the United States (Fig. 12-15). After adequate analgesia, either local or regional, has been achieved, straight Mayo scissors are generally used to perform the episiotomy. Care should be taken to displace the perineum from the fetal head. The size of the incision depends on the length of the perineum but is generally approximately one half of the length of the perineum, and should be extended vertically up the vaginal mucosa for a distance of 2 to 3 cm. Every effort should be made to avoid direct injury to the anal sphincter. Complications of median episiotomy include increased blood loss, especially if the incision is made too early, fetal injury, and localized pain. With a mediolateral episiotomy, the incision is made at a 45-degree angle from the inferior portion of the hymeneal ring (Fig. 12-16). The length of the incision is less critical than with median episiotomy, but longer incisions require lengthier repair. The side to which the episiotomy is performed is usually dictated by the dominant hand of the practitioner. Because such incisions appear to be moderately protective against severe perineal trauma, they are the procedure of choice for women with inflammatory bowel disease because of the critical need to prevent rectal injury. Although it is often said that mediolateral episiotomy causes more pain in the postpartum period than medial episiotomy, only one poorly designed trial has directly compared midline and mediolateral episiotomy.[74] This study received a poor-quality rating in a recent analysis owing to inadequate randomization, lack of allocation concealment, and failure to mask outcome assessors as potential sources of bias.[75] Although no differences were found in postpartum pain or dyspareunia, initiation of sexual intercourse occurred earlier in women with midline episiotomy. Chronic complications such as unsatisfactory cosmetic results and inclusions within the scar may be more common with mediolateral episiotomies and blood loss is greater.

Historically, it was believed that episiotomy improved outcome by reducing pressure on the fetal head, protecting the maternal perineum from extensive tearing, and subsequent pelvic relaxation. However, consistent data since the late 1980s confirm that midline episiotomy actually increases the risk of third- and fourth-degree tears. Therefore, there should be no role for routine episiotomy in modern obstetrics.[76,77] Midline episiotomy is associated with a significant increase of third- and fourth-degree lacerations in spontaneous vaginal delivery in nulliparous women both with spontaneous and operative vaginal

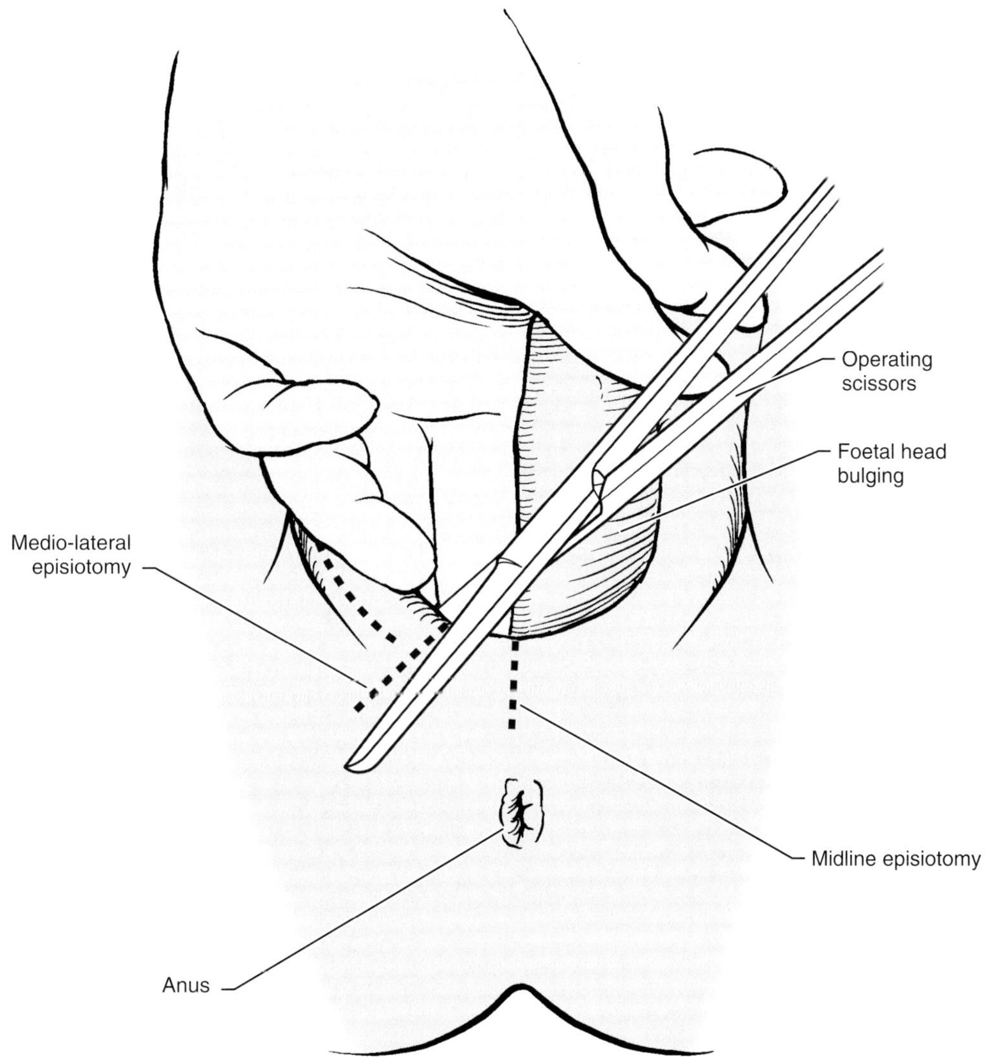

Figure 12-16. Cutting a medio-lateral episiotomy.

delivery.[77–83] Based on these data and ACOG recommendations,[84] rates of midline episiotomy have decreased, although episiotomies are performed in 10 to 17 percent of deliveries, suggesting that elective episiotomy continues to be performed.[85,86] Decreasing episiotomy rates from 87 percent in 1976 to 10 percent in 1994 were associated with a parallel decrease in the rates of third- or fourth-degree lacerations (9 to 4 percent) and an increase in the incidence of an intact perineum (10 to 26 percent).[85] Randomized trials comparing routine to indicated use of episiotomy report a 23-percent reduction in perineal lacerations requiring repair (11 to 35 percent).[86] Although there is no role for routine episiotomy, indicated episiotomy should be performed in select situations and providers should receive training in the skill.[87] Indications for episiotomy include the need to expedite delivery in the setting of fetal heart rate abnormalities or for relief of shoulder dystocia.

KEY POINTS

- Labor is a clinical diagnosis that includes regular painful uterine contractions and progressive cervical effacement and dilatation.
- The fetus likely plays a key role in determining the onset of labor, although the precise mechanism by which this occurs is not clear.
- The ability of the fetus to successfully negotiate the pelvis during labor and delivery is dependent on the complex interaction of three variables: uterine force, the fetus, and the maternal pelvis.
- Routine median episiotomy is associated with a significant increase in the incidence of severe perineal trauma and should be avoided.

REFERENCES

1. Liao JB, Buhimschi CS, Norwitz ER: Normal labor: mechanism and duration. Obstet Gynecol Clin N Am 32:145, 2005.
2. Challis JRG, Gibb W: Control of parturition. Prenat Neonat Med 1:283, 1996.
3. Garfield RE, Blennerhassett MG, Miller SM: Control of myometrial contractility: Role and regulation of gap junctions. Oxf Rev Reprod Biol 10:436, 1988.
4. Liggins GC: Initiation of labour. Biol Neonate 55:366, 1989.
5. Nathanielsz PW: Comparative studies on the initiation of labor. Eur J Obstet Gynecol Reprod Biol 78:127, 1998.
6. Pieber D, Allport VC, Hills F, et al: Interactions between progesterone receptor isoforms in myometrial cells in human labour. Mol Hum Reprod 7:875, 2001.
7. Mesiano S, Chan EC, Fitter JT, et al: Progesterone withdrawal and estrogen activation in human parturition are coordinated by progesterone receptor A expression in the myometrium. J Clin Endocrinol Metab 87:2924, 2002.
8. Oh SY, Kim CJ, Park I, et al: Progesterone receptor isoform (A/B) ratio of human fetal membranes increases during term parturition. Am J Obstet Gynecol 193:1156, 2005.
9. Honnebier M, Nathanielsz P: Primate parturition and the role of the maternal circadian system. Eur J Obstet Gynecol Reprod Biol 55:193, 1994.
10. Zeeman GG, Khan-Dawood FS, Dawood MY: Oxytocin and its receptor in pregnancy and parturition: current concepts and clinical implications. Obstet Gynecol 89:873, 1997.
11. Fuchs AR, Fuchs F: Endocrinology of human parturition: a review. Br J Obstet Gynaecol 91:948, 1984.
12. Dawood MY, Wang CF, Gupta R, et al: Fetal contribution to oxytocin in human labor. Obstet Gynecol 52:205, 1978.
13. Fuchs AR: The role of oxytocin in parturition. *In* Huszar G (ed): The Physiology and Biochemistry of the Uterus in Pregnancy and Labour. Boca Raton, FL, CRC Press, 1986, p 163.
14. Fuchs AR, Fuchs F, Husslein P, et al: Oxytocin receptors and human parturition: a dual role for oxytocin in the initiation of labor. Science 215:1396, 1982.
15. Fuchs AR, Fuchs F, Husslein P, et al: Oxytocin receptors in the human uterus during pregnancy and parturition. Am J Obstet Gynecol 150:734, 1984.
16. Husslein P, Fuchs A-R, Fuchs F: Oxytocin and the initiation of human parturition. II Stimulation of prostaglandin production in human deciduas by oxytocin. Am J Obstet Gynecol 141:694, 1981.
17. Fuchs A-R, Husslein P, Fuchs F: Oxytocin and the initiation of human parturition. II. Stimulation of prostaglandin production in human decidua by oxytocin. Am J Obstet Gynecol 141:694, 1981.
18. Howarth, GR, Botha, DJ: Amniotomy plus intravenous oxytocin for induction of labour. The Cochrane Database of Systematic Reviews 2005:1.
19. Caldeyro-Barcia R, Sica-Blanco Y, Poseiro JJ, et al: A quantitative study of the action of synthetic oxytocin on the pregnant human uterus. J Pharmacol Exp Ther 121:18, 1957.
20. Miller FC: Uterine activity, labor management, and perinatal outcome. Semin Perinatol 2:181, 1978.
21. American College of Obstetricians and Gynecologists: Fetal macrosomia, ACOG Practice Bulletin No. 22. Washington, DC, American College of Obstetricians and Gynecologists, 2000.
22. Spellacy WN, Miller S, Winegar A, Peterson PQ: Macrosomia-maternal characteristics and infant complications. Obstet Gynecol 66:158, 1985.
23. Friedman EA, Kroll B: Computer analysis of labor progression II. Distribution of data and limits of normal. J Reprod Med 6:20, 1971.
24. Lieberman E, Davidson K, Lee-Parritz A, Shearer E: Changes in fetal position during labor and their association with epidural analgesia. Obstet Gynecol 105:974, 2005.
25. O'Brien WF, Cefalo RC: Evaluation of x-ray pelvimetry and abnormal labor. Clin Obstet Gynecol 25:157, 1982.
26. Joyce DN, Giva-Osagie F, Stevenson GW: Role of pelvimetry in active management of labor. Br Med J 4:505, 1975.
27. Morris CW, Heggie JC, Acton CM: Computed tomography pelvimetry: accuracy and radiation dose compared with conventional pelvimetry. Australas Radiol 37:186, 1993.
28. Caldwell WE, Moloy HC: Anatomical variations in the female pelvis and their effect in labor with a suggested classification. Am J Obstet Gynecol 26:479, 1933.
29. Crawford JW: Computor monitoring of fetal heart rate and uterine pressure. Am J Obstet Gynecol 21:342, 1975.
30. Lamont RF, Neave S, Baker AC, et al: Intrauterine pressures in labours induced by amniotomy and oxytocin or vaginal prostaglandin gel compared with normal labour. Br J Obstet Gynaecol 98:441, 1991.
31. Friedman EA: Primigravid labor. Obstet Gynecol 6:567, 1955.
32. Friedman EZ: Labor in multiparas. Obstet Gynecol 9:691, 1956.
33. Albers LL, Schiff M, Gorwoda JG: The length of active labor in normal pregnancies. Obstet Gynecol 87:355, 1996.
34. Bergsjo P, Halle C: Duration of the second stage of labor. Acta Obstet Gynecol Scand 59:193, 1980.
35. Duignan NM: Characteristics of normal labour in different racial groups. Br J Obstet Gynecol 82:593, 1975.
36. Kilpatrick SJ, Laros RK: Characteristics of normal labor. Obstet Gynecol 74:85, 1989.
37. Friedman E, Sachtleben M: Station of the fetal presenting part. I. Pattern of descent. Am J Obstet Gynecol 93:522, 1965.
38. Schifrin BS, Cohen WR: Labor's dysfunctional lexicon. Obstet Gynecol 74:121, 1989.
39. Schulman H, Ledger W: Practical applications of the graphic portrayal of labor. Obstet Gynecol 23:442, 1964.
40. Vahratian A, Zhang J, Troendle JF, et al: Maternal prepregnancy overweight and obesity and the pattern of labor progression in term nulliparous women. Obstet Gynecol 104:943, 2004.
41. Sheiner E, Levy A, Feinstein U, et al: Risk factors and outcome of failure to progress during the first stage of labor: a population-based study. Acta Obstet Gynecol Scand 81:222, 2002.
42. Combs CA, Laros R: Prolonged third stage of labor: Morbidity and risk factors. Obstet Gynecol 77:863, 1991.
43. Bloom SL, McIntire DD, Kelly MA, et al: Lack of effect of walking on labor and delivery. N Engl J Med 339:76, 1998.
44. Scott KD, Berkowitz G, Klaus M: A comparison of intermittent and continuous support during labor: A meta-analysis. Am J Obstet Gynecol 180:1054, 1999.
45. O'Driscoll K, Foley M, MacDonald D: Active management of labor as an alternative to cesarean section for dystocia. Obstet Gynecol 63:485, 1984.
46. Akoury H, Brodie G, Caddick R, et al: Active management of labor and operative delivery in nulliparous women. Am J Obstet Gynecol 158:255, 1988.
47. Akoury HA, MacDonald FJ, Brodie G, et al: Oxytocin augmentation of labor and perinatal outcomes in nulliparas. Obstet Gynecol 78:227, 1991.
48. Boylan P, Frankowski R, Rountree R, et al: Effect of active management of labor on the incidence of cesarean section for dystocia in nulliparas. Am J Perinatol 375:389, 1991.
49. Frigoletto FD, Lieberman E, Lang JM, et al: A clinical trial of active management of labor. N Engl J Med 333:745, 1995.
50. Rogers R, Gilson GJ, Miller AC, et al: Active management of labor: Does it make a difference? Am J Obstet Gynecol 177:599, 1997.
51. Lopez-Zeno J, Peaceman A, Adashek J, Socol ML: A controlled trial of a program for the active management of labor. N Engl J Med 326:450, 1992.
52. Sizer AR, Evans J, Bailey SM, Wiener J: A second-stage partogram. Obstet Gynecol 96:678, 2000.
53. Cohen W: Influence of the duration of second stage labor on perinatal outcome and puerperal morbidity. Obstet Gynecol 49:266, 1977.
54. Derham R, Crowhurst J, Crowther C: The second stage of labour: durational dilemmas. Aust NZ J Obstet Gynaecol 31:31, 1991.
55. Menticoglou SM, Manning F, Harman C, Morrison I: Perinatal outcome in relation to second-stage duration. Am J Obstet Gynecol 173:906, 1995.
56. Moon JM, Smith CV, Rayburn WF: Perinatal outcome after a prolonged second stage of labor. J Reprod Med 35:229, 1990.

57. Myles TD, Santolaya J: Maternal and neonatal outcomes in patients with a prolonged second stage of labor. Obstet Gynecol 102:52, 2003.
58. Kadar N, Cruddas M, Campbell S: Estimating the probability of spontaneous delivery conditional on time spent in the second stage. Br J Obstet Gynecol 93:568. 1986.
59. Piper JM, Bolling DR, Newton ER: The second stage of labor: Factors influencing duration. Am J Obstet Gynecol 165:976, 1991.
60. Chestnut DH, Bates JN, Choi WW: Continuous infusion epidural stage of labour. Obstet Gynecol 69:323, 1987.
61. Chestnut DH, Laszowski LJ, Pollack KL, et al: Continuous epidural infusion of 0.0625 percent Bupivacaine—0.0002 percent Fentanyl during the second stage of labor. Anesthesiology 72:613, 1990.
62. Chestnut DH, Vanderwalker GE, Owen CI, et al: The influence of continuous epidural bupivacaine analgesia on the second stage of labor and method of delivery in nulliparous women. Anesthesiology 66:774, 1987.
63. Manyonda I, Shaw D, Drife J: The effect of delayed pushing in the second stage of labor with continuous lumbar epidural analgesia. Acta Obstet Gynecol Scand 69:291, 1990.
64. Fraser W, Marcoux S, Krauss I, et al: Multicenter, randomized, controlled trial of delayed pushing for nulliparous women in the second stage of labor with continuous epidural analgesia. Am J Obstet Gynecol 182:1165, 2000.
65. Hansen S, Clark S, Foster J: Active pushing versus passive fetal descent in the second stage of labor: a randomized controlled trial. Obstet Gynecol 99:29, 2002.
66. Plunkett BA, Lin A, Wong CA, et al: Management of the second stage of labor in nulliparas with continuous epidural analgesia. Obstet Gynecol 102:109, 2003.
67. Ardosi J, Hutson N, B-Lynch C: Randomised, controlled trial of squatting in the second stage of labour. Lancet 7:74, 1989.
68. Gardosi J, Sylvester S, B-Lynch C: Alternative positions in the second stage of labour: a randomized controlled trial. Br J Obstet Gynecol 96:1290, 1989.
69. Vain NE, Szyld EG, Prudent LM, et al: Oropharyngeal and nasopharyngeal suctioning of meconium-stained neonates before delivery of their shoulders: multicentre, randomised controlled trial. Lancet 364:597, 2004.
70. Rogers J, Wood J, McCandlish R, et al: Active versus expectant management of third stage of labour: the Hinchingbrooke randomised controlled trial. Lancet 351:693, 1998.
71. Jackson KW, Albert JR, Schemmer GK, et al: A randomized controlled trial comparing oxytocin administration before and after placental delivery in the prevention of postpartum hemorrhage. Am J Obstet Gynecol 185:873, 2001.
72. Prucka S, Clemens M, Craven C, McPherson E: Single umbilical artery: what does it mean for the fetus? A case-control analysis of pathologically ascertained cases. Genet Med 6:54, 2004.
73. Thummala MR, Raju TN, Langenberg P: Isolated single umbilical artery anomaly and the risk for congenital malformations: a meta-analysis. J Pediatr Surgery 33:580, 1998.
74. Coates PM, Chan KK, Wilkins M, et al: A comparison between midline and mediolateral episiotomies. Br J Obstet Gynaecol 87:408, 1980.
75. Hartmann K, Viswanathan M, Palmieri R, et al: Outcomes of routine episiotomy: a systematic review. JAMA 293:2141, 2005.
76. Thorp JM, Bowes W: Episiotomy: can its routine use be defended? Am J Obstet Gynecol 160:1027, 1989.
77. Shiono P, Klebanoff M, Carey C: Midline episiotomies: more harm than good. Obstet Gynecol 75:765, 1990.
78. Angioli R, Gomez-Marin O, Cantuaria G, O'Sullivan M: Severe perineal lacerations during vaginal delivery: The University of Miami experience. Am J Obstet Gynecol 182:1083, 2000.
79. Bansal R, Tan W, Ecker J, et al: Is there a benefit to episiotomy at spontaneous vaginal delivery? A natural experiment. Am J Obstet Gynecol 175:897, 1996.
80. Robinson JN, Norwitz ER, Cohen AP, et al: Epidural analgesia and the occurrence of third and fourth degree obstetric laceration in nulliparas. Obstet Gynecol 94:259, 1999.
81. Helwig JT, Thorp JM Jr, Bowes WA Jr: Does midline episiotomy increase the risk of third- and fourth-degree lacerations in operative vaginal deliveries? Obstet Gynecol 82:276,1993.
82. Ecker J, Tan W, Bansal R, et al: Is there a benefit to episiotomy at operative vaginal delivery? Observations over ten years in a stable population. Am J Obstet Gynecol;176:411–4, 1997.
83. Robinson J, Norwitz E, Cohen A, et al: Episiotomy, operative vaginal delivery, and significant perineal trauma in nulliparous women. Am J Obstet Gynecol 181:1180, 1999.
84. Gilstrap LC, Oh W: Guidelines for Perinatal Care, 5th ed. Washington, DC, American College of Obstetrics and Gynecologists. American Academy of Pediatrics, 2002.
85. Bansal R, Tan W, Ecker J, et al: Is there a benefit to episiotomy at spontaneous vaginal delivery? A natural experiment. Am J Obstet Gynecol 175:897, 1996.
86. Clemons JL, Towers GD, McClure GB, O'Boyle AL: Decreased anal sphincter lacerations associated with restrictive episiotomy use. Am J Obstet Gynecol 192:1620, 2005.
87. Eason E, Labrecque M, Wells G, Feldman P: Preventing perinaeal trauma during childbirth: a systematic review. Obstet Gynecol 95:464, 2000.

Abnormal Labor and Induction of Labor

LEAH R. BATTISTA AND DEBORAH A. WING

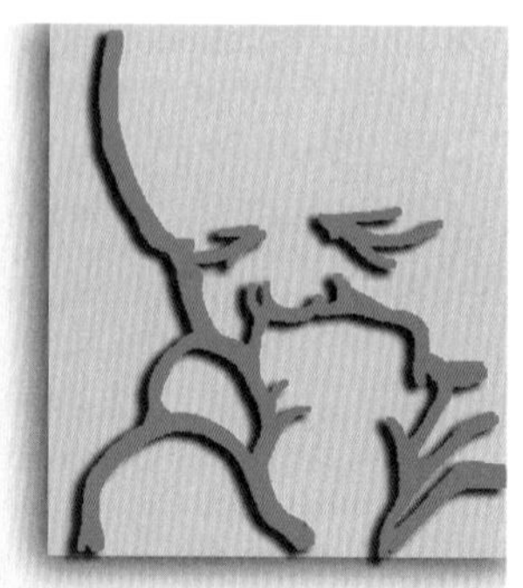

CHAPTER 13

KEY ABBREVIATIONS

American College of Obstetricians and Gynecologists	ACOG
Active management of risk in pregnancy at term	AMOR-IPAT
Cephalopelvic disproportion	CPD
Confidence interval	CI
Electronic fetal monitoring	EFM
Extra-amniotic saline infusion	EASI
Food and Drug Administration	FDA
Group B streptococcus	GBS
Intrauterine pressure catheter	IUPC
Occiput posterior	OP
Odds ratio	OR
Premature rupture of membranes	PROM
Prostaglandin	PG
Prostaglandin E_1 (misoprostol)	PGE_1
Prostaglandin E_2 (dinoprostone)	PGE_2
Relative risk	RR

INTRODUCTION

Labor is the physiologic process by which a fetus is expelled from the uterus to the outside world. A switch from contractures (long-lasting, low-frequency activity) to contractions (frequent, high-intensity, high-frequency activity) occurs before progressive cervical effacement and dilatation of the cervix and regular uterine contractions.[1] The timing of the switch varies from patient to patient. The exact trigger for the onset of labor is unknown, but there is considerable evidence to suggest that the fetus provides the stimulus through complex neuronal-hormonal signaling.[2–4]

The mean duration of a human singleton pregnancy is 280 days or 40 weeks from the first day of the last menstrual period. *Term* is defined as the period from 36 completed ($37^{0/7}$) to 42 weeks of gestation. *Preterm* labor refers to the onset of labor before 36 completed weeks of gestation. Prolonged or *postterm pregnancy* refers to gestation continuing beyond 42 completed weeks.

DIAGNOSIS

Labor is a clinical diagnosis defined as uterine contractions resulting in progressive cervical effacement and dilatation, often accompanied by a bloody discharge referred to as bloody show, which results in birth of the baby. The diagnosis of bona fide labor is often elusive. There are wide variations in the clinical spectrum of normal labor as well as many opinions of the definitions for normal and abnormal labor progress. In order to gain an understanding of abnormal labor progress and induction of labor, a fundamental understanding of normal spontaneous labor is needed.

PHYSIOLOGY OF NORMAL LABOR AT TERM

Most guidelines for normal human labor progress are derived from Friedman's clinical observations of women in labor.[5,6] Friedman characterized a sigmoid pattern for labor when graphing cervical dilatation against time (Fig. 13-1).[7] He divided labor into three functional divisions: the *preparatory division, dilatational division,* and *pelvic division.* The preparatory division is better known as the *latent phase,* during which little cervical dilatation occurs but considerable changes are taking place in the con-

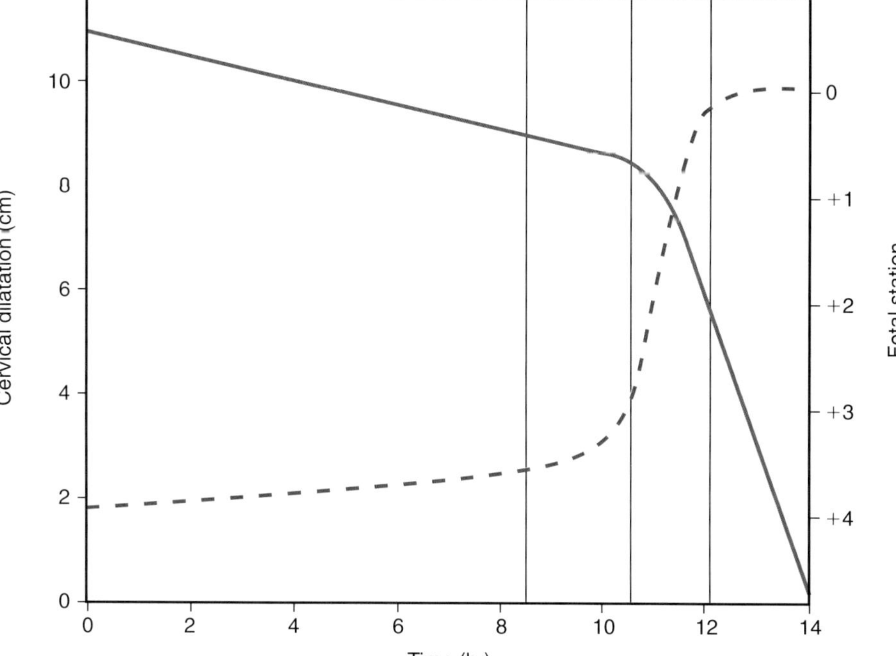

Figure 13-1. Characteristics of the average cervical dilatation curve for nulliparous labor. (Adapted from Friedman EA: Labor: Clinical Evaluation and Management, 2nd ed. Norwalk, CT, Appleton-Century-Crofts, 1978.)

nective tissue components of the cervix. The dilatation division or *active phase* is the time period when dilatation proceeds at its most rapid rate to complete cervical dilatation. These two phases together make up the *first stage of labor*. The *pelvic division* or *second stage of labor* refers to the time of full cervical dilatation to the delivery of the infant.

Latent Phase

The onset of latent labor as defined by Friedman is the point at which regular uterine contractions are perceived.[8] Friedman found the mean duration of latent labor was 6.4 hours for nulliparas and 4.8 for multiparas. The 95th percentiles for maximum length in latent labor was 20 hours for nulliparous women and 14 hours for multiparous women.[7] These are considered the upper limits for time spent in latent labor (Table 13-1).[6,9,10]

Disorders of the Latent Phase

Latent phase arrest implies that labor has not truly begun. Prolonged latent phase refers to a latent phase lasting longer than 20 hours for nulliparas women and 14 hours or longer for multiparas women.[11] Because the duration of latent labor is highly variable, expectant management is most appropriate. Some women can spend days in latent labor; provided there is no indication for delivery, awaiting active labor is appropriate. If expeditious delivery is indicated, then augmentation of labor may be initiated with a pharmacologic agent such as oxytocin. Another option is to administer "therapeutic rest" especially if contractions are painful, with an analgesic agent such as morphine. A recommended dosing regimen is a single administration of 15 to 20 mg of morphine subcutaneously or intramuscularly. Often this will help abate or alleviate painful contractions and allow the patient to rest comfortably until active labor begins. The onset of regular contractions is often unpredictable after amniotomy and, therefore, is not recommended in nulliparas with prolonged latent phase. Early amniotomy may increase the risk of prolonged membrane rupture and its associated infectious morbidity.

Table 13-1. Progression of Spontaneous Labor At Term

PARAMETER	MEDIAN MEAN OR	5TH CENTILE
Nulliparas		
Total duration	10.1 h	25.8 h
Stages		
First	9.7 h	24.7 h
Second	33.0 min	117.5 min
Third	5.0 min	30 min
Latent phase (duration)	6.4 h	20.6 h
Maximal dilation (rate)	3.0 cm/h	1.2 cm/h
Descent (rate)	3.3 cm/h	1.0 cm/h
Multiparas		
Total duration	6.2 h	19.5 h
Stages		
First	8.0 h	18.8 h
Second	8.5 min	46.5 min
Third	5.0 min	30 min
Latent phase (duration)	4.8 h	13.6 h
Maximal dilation (rate)	5.7 cm/h	1.5 cm/h
Descent (rate)	6.6 cm/h	2.1 cm/h

Data from Friedman EA: Primigravid Labor: A graphicostatistical analysis. Obstet Gynecol 6:567, 1955; Friedman EA: Labor in Multiparas: A graphicostatistical analysis. Obstet Gynecol 8:691, 1956; Cohen W, Friedman EA (eds): Management of Labor. Baltimore, University Park Press, 1983.

Active Phase

Active labor demarcates a rapid change in cervical dilatation. The active phase begins once cervical dilatation progresses at a minimum rate of 1.2 cm/h for nulliparous women and 1.5 cm/h for multiparous women. This change to active phase usually occurs when the cervix is dilated between 3 to 5 cm, but the most accurate diagnosis is retrospective. In the presence of regular uterine contractions accompanied by cervical dilatation of 3 to 4 cm, the threshold for active labor has likely been reached. Friedman observed that the mean duration of active phase labor in nulliparas women was 4.9 hours, with a standard deviation of 3.4 hours.[6] There was a large variation in his results, with the maximum duration of active phase reported to be 11.7 hours. Rates of cervical dilatation varied as much from 1.2 to 6.8 cm/h.

Disorders of the Active Phase

Active-phase disorders may be divided into *protraction* (primary dysfunctional labor) and *arrest* (secondary arrest) disorders.[8] Protraction is defined as a slow rate of cervical change less than 1.2 cm/h for the nullipara and less than 1.5 cm/h for the multipara. These rates represent less than the 5th percentile for most gravidas (Fig. 13-2).[5,6,12] Rates of cervical change may be protracted by the use of epidural anesthesia.[13,14] In one investigation including 199 nulliparous women all entering labor spontaneously, labor progress was compared in women receiving epidural analgesia with those receiving intravenous meperidine.[15] The mean cervical dilatation on admission and at the time of initiation of analgesia was the same in each group (3 to 4 cm). Women receiving epidural analgesia required more oxytocin for longer intervals and had longer first and second stages of labor. The total admission to delivery interval was prolonged by approximately 2 hours. These data suggest that patients receiving epidural analgesia may require modification of the guidelines for labor progress in the first stage. Similar modifications have been established for the second stage of labor with epidural use.[16]

The most common cause of a protraction disorder is inadequate uterine activity. External tocodynamometry is used to evaluate the duration of and time interval between contractions but cannot be used to evaluate the strength of uterine contractions. The external monitor is held against the abdominal wall and records a relative measurement of uterine contraction intensity reflecting its movement with uterine shape change. Precise measurements of uterine activity must be obtained with an *intrauterine pressure catheter* (IUPC). After amniotomy, an IUPC can be placed into the uterus to measure the pressure generated during a uterine contraction. An IUPC is frequently used when inadequate uterine activity is suspected owing to a protraction or arrest disorder. It can also be used to monitor and titrate oxytocin augmentation of labor to desired uterine effect. The lower limit of contraction pressure required to dilate the cervix is observed to be 15 mm Hg over baseline.[17] Normal spontaneous contractions often exert pressures up to 60 mm Hg.[18]

Once inadequate uterine activity is diagnosed with an IUPC, oxytocin is usually administered. Typically, the dose is increased until there is normal progression of labor, resulting in strong contractions occurring at 2- to 3-minute intervals lasting 60 to 90 seconds, with a peak intrauterine pressure of 50 to 60 mm Hg and a resting

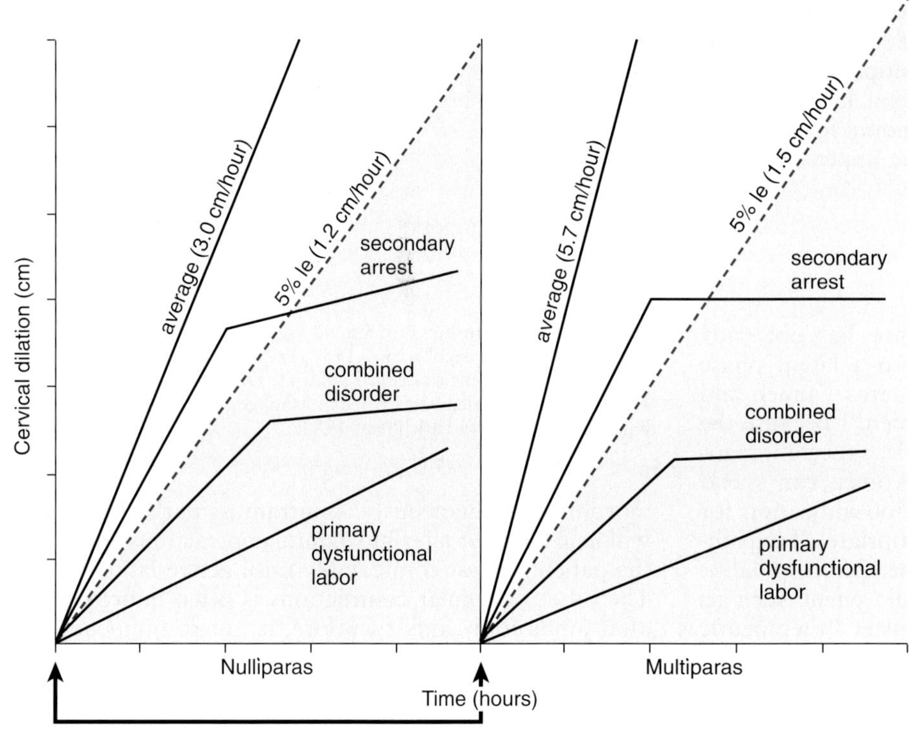

Figure 13-2. Disorders of the first stage of labor. Combined disorder implies an arrest in a gravida previously exhibiting primary dysfunctional labor.

tone of 10 to 15 mm Hg, or in uterine activity equal to 150 to 350 Montevideo units.[15] Montevideo units are calculated by subtracting the baseline uterine pressure from the peak contraction pressure of each contraction in a 10-minute window and adding the pressures generated by each contraction.[19]

Another common cause of protraction disorders is abnormal positioning of the fetal presenting part. Some examples of malpresentation are an extended (rather than flexed) fetal head, brow presentation, and occiput posterior (OP) position. When persistent OP position is present, labor is reported to be prolonged an average 1 hour in multiparous women and 2 hours in nulliparous women.[20] In one series, sonography showed OP position in 35 percent of women in early active labor,[21] indicating that this may contribute to prolongation of labor in many women. In another recent investigation, the prevalence of persistent OP position at the time of vaginal delivery regardless of parity was 5.5 percent, 7.2 percent in nulliparas and 4.0 percent in multiparas.[22] The OP position was found to be associated with longer first and second stages, and a lower rate of vaginal delivery (26 percent for nulliparas and 57 percent for multiparas) when compared with the occiput anterior (OA) position. Most fetuses in the OP position undergo spontaneous anterior rotation during the course of labor, and expectant management is generally indicated. However, approximately 5 percent remain in persistent OP position or transverse arrest, which often requires either an operative vaginal delivery or cesarean delivery.

Cephalopelvic disproportion (CPD) refers to the disproportion between the size of the fetus relative to the mother and can be the cause of a protraction or arrest disorder. This is a diagnosis of exclusion, often made at the time a protracted labor course is observed. Most frequently, malposition of the fetal presenting part is the culprit rather than true CPD. Unfortunately there is no way to accurately predict CPD. It is estimated that thousands of unnecessary cesarean deliveries would need to be performed in low-risk pregnancies to prevent one diagnosis of true CPD.[23,24]

Secondary arrest is defined as cessation of previously normal active phase cervical dilatation for a period of 2 hours or more.[25,26] Evaluation of this disorder includes an assessment of uterine activity with an IUPC, performance of clinical pelvimetry, and evaluation of fetal presentation, position, station, and estimated fetal weight. Amniotomy and oxytocin therapy can be initiated if uterine activity is found to be inadequate. The majority of gravidas respond to this intervention, and resume progression of cervical dilatation and achieve vaginal delivery.[27] Rouse et al.[28] found that at least 4 hours of oxytocin augmentation can be administered before secondary arrest of labor is diagnosed without incurring additional maternal or fetal compromise.

COMBINED DISORDER

A combined disorder of active phase dilatation is defined as arrest of dilatation occurring when a patient has previously exhibited a primary protracted labor. This pattern is associated with less favorable outcomes with regard to vaginal delivery when compared with patients with secondary arrest alone.[25] If diagnosed, an evaluation of uterine activity is necessary, as is an assessment of pelvic capacity, fetal position, station, and estimated fetal weight.

An alternative classification system for disorders of the active phase of labor is based on the electromechanical state of the uterus regarding uterine tone.[19,29] *Hypotonic dysfunction* reflects an inefficient generation and propagation of action potentials through the myometrium or lack of contractile response of myometrial cells to the contractile signal. Hypotonic uterine contractions are infrequent, of low amplitude, and accompanied by low or normal baseline intrauterine pressures. Maternal discomfort is minimal. Oxytocin augmentation is usually applied in this clinical situation if active labor has already begun.

Hypertonic dysfunction is primarily a condition of primiparas and usually occurs in early labor. It is characterized by the presence of regular uterine contractions that fail to effect cervical effacement and dilatation. Frequent contractions of low amplitude are often associated with an elevated basal intrauterine pressure. Maternal discomfort is usually significant. Therapeutic rest can be initiated in this clinical situation if the patient is in latent labor or expectant management can be applied. When diagnosed, the most likely scenario is that the patient will soon enter active labor. If the patient is in active labor and found to have hypertonic dysfunction, amniotomy can be performed with or without concomitant oxytocin administration.

Second Stage

The second stage of labor begins when the cervix becomes fully dilated (first stage) and ends with the delivery of the infant. Although fetal descent begins before the cervix becomes fully dilated, the majority of fetal descent occurs once full cervical dilatation is achieved. Also when the cervix becomes fully dilated, maternal expulsion efforts may begin.

DISORDERS OF THE SECOND STAGE

Protraction of descent is defined as descent of the presenting part during the second stage of labor occurring at less than 1 cm/h in nulliparas women and less than 2 cm/h in multiparas women.[30] *Arrest (failure) of descent* refers to no progress in descent. Both diagnoses require prompt evaluation of uterine activity, maternal expulsive efforts, fetal heart rate status, fetal position, clinical pelvimetry, and a reevaluation of estimated fetal weight. Decisions then may be made regarding interventions, such as increasing or initiating oxytocin infusion to improve maternal expulsion efforts, or proceeding with operative vaginal or cesarean delivery. Management of the second stage of labor can be difficult, and decisions regarding intervention must be individualized.

The median duration of the second stage is 50 minutes for nulliparas and 20 minutes for multiparas, but this is highly variable, and these estimations do not account for anesthesia.[31] The upper limit for the duration of the second stage of labor was previously defined to be 2 hours.[32,33] However, the use of regional anesthesia increases the mean duration of the second stage by 20 to 30 minutes.[31,34] Other factors influence the length of the second stage as well such as parity, maternal size, birth weight, occiput posterior position, and fetal station at complete dilatation.[35] Many authors have studied the perinatal effects of a prolonged second stage and found no increase in infant morbidity or mortality with a second stage lasting longer than 2 hours,[36,37] although the rate of vaginal delivery precipitously decreases after 3 hours in the second stage. These data led to amendment of the American College of Obstetricians and Gynecologists (ACOG) guidelines for the definition of prolonged second stage provided the fetal heart rate tracing is normal and there is some degree of labor progress. These guidelines are as follows: For nulliparous women, the diagnosis for a prolonged second stage should be considered when the second stage exceeds 3 hours if regional anesthesia has been administered or 2 hours if no regional anesthesia is used. In multiparous women, the diagnosis can be made when the second stage exceeds 2 hours with regional anesthesia or 1 hour without.[16] Although perinatal outcomes are not compromised with a prolonged second stage of labor, there is evidence that maternal morbidities such as perineal trauma, chorioamnionitis, instrumental delivery, and postpartum hemorrhage, increase with prolonged second stages lasting greater than 2 hours.[38] Effective management of the second stage should be individualized.

Third Stage

The third stage of labor refers to the time period from delivery of the infant to the expulsion of the placenta. Separation of the placenta is the consequence of continued uterine contractions. Signs of placental separation include a gush of blood, lengthening of the umbilical cord, and change in shape of the uterine fundus from discoid to globular with elevation of the fundal height. The interval between delivery of the infant and delivery of the placenta and fetal membranes is usually less than 10 minutes and is complete within 15 minutes in 95 percent of deliveries.[39] The most important risk associated with a prolonged third stage is hemorrhage; this risk increases proportionally with increased duration.[40] Because of the associated increased incidence of hemorrhage after 30 minutes, most practitioners diagnose retained placenta after this time interval has elapsed. Interventions to expedite placental delivery are usually undertaken at this time.[41]

Management of the third stage of labor may be expectant or active. Expectant management refers to the delivery of the placenta without cord clamping, cord traction, or the administration of uterotonic agents such as oxytocin. Active management consists of early cord clamping, controlled cord traction, and administration of a uterotonic agent. Oxytocin is the usual uterotonic agent given, but others have been used, such as misoprostol or other prostaglandin compounds. Comparing active to expectant management of the third stage, there appears to be a reduced risk of postpartum hemorrhage and prolongation when active management is used.[42] There is some debate regarding the timing of oxytocin administration when the active management of the third stage is practiced: after the placenta has delivered versus after the anterior shoulder of the fetus has delivered. A randomized controlled trial including 1,486 women comparing the effects of oxytocin administration upon delivery of the anterior shoulder to administration after delivery of the placenta showed no significant differences in blood loss or retained placenta between the groups.[43]

Retained placenta can usually be treated with measures such as manual removal. This procedure can be performed under regional anesthesia or conscious sedation. If attempt at manual removal is not successful, a sharp curettage can be performed under sonographic guidance. Prophylactic broad-spectrum antimicrobial agents are often administered when manual removal of the placenta is performed, although there is little evidence to support (or refute) their use.[44]

Precipitous Labor

Precipitous labor refers to delivery of the infant in less than 3 hours.[45] This occurs in approximately 2 percent of all deliveries in the United States.[46] Precipitous labor and delivery alone is not usually associated with significant maternal and infant morbidity and mortality. Short labors can be associated with placental abruption, uterine tachysystole, and recent maternal cocaine use—all of which are major contributors to poor outcomes for mothers and infants.[47] Other investigators have looked at intrapartum risk factors associated with permanent brachial plexus injury and found that a precipitous second stage is the most common labor abnormality associated with shoulder dystocia, although the rates of permanent injury did not increase.[48]

INDUCTION AND AUGMENTATION OF LABOR

Induction of labor is one of the most commonly performed obstetric procedures in the United States.[49] Induction of labor refers to the iatrogenic stimulation of uterine contractions before the onset of spontaneous labor to accomplish vaginal delivery. Augmentation of labor refers to increasing the frequency and improving the intensity of existing uterine contractions in a patient who is in labor and not progressing adequately, in order to accomplish vaginal delivery.

Indications and Contraindications

Generally, induction of labor should be undertaken when the benefits of expeditious delivery to either mother or fetus outweigh the risk of continuing the pregnancy.[50] There are many accepted medical and obstetric indications for labor induction and several relative indications for labor induction (Table 13-2). Contraindications are those that preclude vaginal delivery among others (Table 13-3).

Careful examination of the maternal and fetal condition is required before undertaking labor induction (Table 13-4). Indications and contraindications for induction should be reviewed as well as the alternatives. Risks and benefits of labor induction should be discussed with the patient, including the risk of cesarean delivery (to be discussed later). Confirmation of gestational age is critical, and evaluation of fetal lung maturity status should be performed if indicated (Table 13-5).[51] Fetal weight should be estimated and clinical pelvimetry performed. Fetal presentation and position should be confirmed. A cervical examination should be performed and documented as well. In addition, labor induction should be performed at a location where personnel are available who are familiar with the process and its potential complications. Uterine activity and electronic fetal monitoring (EFM) are recommended for any gravida receiving uterotonic drugs.

Table 13-2. Indications for Induction of Labor

ACCEPTED ABSOLUTE INDICATIONS	RELATIVE INDICATIONS
Hypertensive disorders	**Hypertensive disorders**
• Preeclampsia/eclampsia	• Chronic hypertension
Maternal medical conditions	**Maternal medical conditions**
• Diabetes mellitus	• Systemic lupus erythematosus
• Renal disease	• Gestational diabetes
• Chronic pulmonary disease	• Hypercoagulable disorders
	• Cholestasis of pregnancy
Prelabor rupture of membranes	**Polyhydramnios**
Chorioamnionitis	**Fetal anomalies requiring specialized neonatal care**
Fetal compromise	**Logistic factors**
• Fetal growth restriction	• Risk of rapid labor
• Isoimmunization	• Distance from hospital
• Nonreassuring antepartum fetal testing	• Psychosocial indications
• Oligohydramnios	• Advanced cervical dilation
Fetal demise	**Previous stillbirth**
Prolonged pregnancy (>42 weeks)	**Postterm pregnancy (>41 weeks)**

Table 13-3. Contraindications to Labor Induction

ACCEPTED ABSOLUTE CONTRAINDICATIONS	RELATIVE CONTRAINDICATIONS
Prior classic uterine incision or transfundal uterine surgery	
Active genital herpes infection	Cervical carcinoma
Placenta or vasa previa	
Umbilical cord prolapse	Funic presentation
Transverse or oblique fetal lie	Malpresentation (breech)
Absolute cephalopelvic disproportion (as in women with pelvic deformities)	

Elective Induction of Labor

Elective induction of labor refers to the initiation of labor for convenience in an individual with a term pregnancy who is free of medical or obstetric indications. The rate of elective induction in the United States has increased dramatically from 9.5 percent to 19.4 percent from 1989 to 1998.[52] Factors associated with higher induction rates are white race, higher education, and early initiation of prenatal care. Although elective induction is not recommended or encouraged, it may be appropriate in specific instances such as a history of very short labors or for patients who live a great distance from the hospital. Also a patient who has experienced a prior stillbirth at or near term may require labor induction to ease anxiety and fears about the loss of a subsequent pregnancy. In addition, there are certain maternal medical conditions that require multispecialty participation in which the benefit of a planned delivery to have experienced personnel readily available is most appropriate. Examples of such cases are pregnancies with maternal cardiac disease that may require invasive monitoring during labor or those complicated by chronic renal disease in which considerations for hemodialysis may dictate a scheduled birth.

The major risks of elective induction of labor at term are increased rates of cesarean delivery, especially in nulliparas, and iatrogenic prematurity. The risk of cesarean delivery following elective induction, especially for the nullipara with an unfavorable cervix, is clearly established in the literature. Macer et al.[53] conducted a retrospective review of more than 500 women who either underwent elective induction of labor or spontaneous labor at term. They found no statistical significant differences in cesarean delivery or instrumented delivery between the groups when all subjects regardless of cervical condition or parity status were included. When

Table 13-4. Evaluation before Induction of Labor

PARAMETER	CRITERIA
Maternal	Confirm indication for induction
	Review contraindications to labor and/or vaginal delivery
	Perform clinical pelvimetry to assess pelvic shape and adequacy of bony pelvis
	Assess cervical condition (assign Bishop score)
	Review risks, benefits and alternatives of induction of labor with patient
Fetal/neonatal	Confirm gestational age
	Assess need to document fetal lung maturity status
	Estimate fetal weight (either by clinical or ultrasound examination)
	Determine fetal presentation and lie
	Confirm fetal well-being

Table 13-5. Criteria for Confirmation of Gestational Age and Fetal Pulmonary Maturity

	PARAMETERS
Clinical criteria	1. ≥39 weeks' gestation have elapsed since the first day of the last menstrual period in a women with a regular menstrual cycle. 2. Fetal heart tones have been documented for ≥20 weeks' gestation by nonelectronic fetoscope or for ≥30 weeks by Doppler ultrasound.
Laboratory determination	1. ≥36 weeks' gestation have elapsed since a positive serum human chorionic gonadotropin pregnancy test. 2. Ultrasound estimation of gestational age is considered accurate if it is based on crown-rump measurements obtained at 6 to 11 weeks' gestation or it is based on biparietal diameter measurements obtained before 20 weeks' gestation.
Fetal pulmonary maturity	According to the Guidelines for Perinatal care,[51] term gestation can be confirmed if two or more of the above-mentioned obstetric clinical or laboratory criteria are present. If term gestation cannot be confirmed, amniotic fluid analyses can be used to provide evidence of fetal lung maturity. A variety of tests are available. The parameters for evidence of fetal pulmonary maturity are listed below: 1. Lecithin/sphingomyelin (L/S) ratio >2.1 2. Presence of phosphatidylglycerol (PG) 3. TDxFLM assay ≥70 mg surfactant per 1 g albumin present 4. Presence of saturated phosphatidylcholine (SPC) ≥ 500 ng/mL in nondiabetic patients (≥1000 ng/mL for pregestational diabetic patients)

Data from the American Academy of Pediatrics and American College of Obstetricians and Gynecologists: Guidelines for Perinatal Care, 5th ed. American College of Obstetricians and Gynecologists, Kearneysville, WV, 2002.

stratifying by parity, they found that the rate of cesarean delivery did not differ among elective induction and spontaneous labor groups regardless of initial cervical status in multiparous subjects. For nulliparous women with an unfavorable cervix (Bishop score = 6) undergoing induction, however, the cesarean delivery rate was 50 percent compared with 22 percent in the spontaneous labor group (relative risk [RR] 2.48 95-percent confidence interval [CI] 1.27 to 4.87). The nulliparous women with a favorable cervix undergoing elective induction had similar cesarean delivery rates as nulliparous women in spontaneous labor. However, this finding should be treated with caution given the small sample size and retrospective study design.

To demonstrate the risk of cesarean delivery in nulliparous women undergoing elective induction of labor in a major metropolitan setting, Seyb et al. followed a cohort of 1,561 nulliparous women with term, uncomplicated singleton pregnancies. The women were divided into three groups: those who underwent spontaneous labor, elective induction, and medically indicated induction. They found a 7.8-percent rate of cesarean delivery in the spontaneous labor group and nearly an 18-percent rate in both the elective induction group and the medically indicated induction group.[54] The women who underwent induction of labor were also at increased risk for other complications such as chorioamnionitis. The mean time spent on labor and delivery was almost twice as long, and the postpartum stays were prolonged if labor induction was undertaken. The total cost associated with hospitalization for elective induction was 17.4 percent higher than for spontaneous labor, including costs for labor and delivery, pharmacy, and postpartum care.

These findings were confirmed by an investigation undertaken by Maslow and Sweeney[55] of 263 women with singleton term gestations who underwent elective induction compared with 872 women who had spontaneous onset of labor. They found a threefold and twofold higher risk of cesarean delivery for the nulliparous patients and the multiparous patients in the elective induction group respectively. Rates for cesarean delivery for nulliparous and multiparous subjects with induced labor were 17.5 percent and 6.9 percent compared with 6 percent and 3.1 percent in the spontaneous labor group. They also found that there was a higher cost and more hospital care required for the elective induction group compared with the spontaneous labor group. These data reinforce the finding that labor induction remains a significant predictor of cesarean delivery for both nulliparous and multiparous women and contributes to rising health care costs.

The largest trial to date examining outcomes after elective labor induction in nulliparous women was performed in Flanders, Belgium by Cammu et al.[56] These investigators performed a matched cohort study that included 7,683 nulliparas undergoing elective labor induction and 7,683 nulliparas in spontaneous labor. Women were recruited from all 80 labor wards in Flanders, and each had a term singleton pregnancy, a fetus in a cephalic presentation, and with a birth weight between 3,000 and 4,000 g. Each woman with induced labor and the corresponding woman with spontaneous labor came from the same ward and had babies of the same sex. Cesarean delivery was significantly more common in the elective induction group occurring in 9.9 percent of patients compared with 6.5 percent of the spontaneous labor group (RR 1.52 95-percent CI 1.37 to 1.70). Most of these cesarean deliveries were a result of a higher incidence of first-stage disorders. In addition, babies who were born after induced labor were transferred more often to the neonatal ward.

Kaufman et al.[57] studied the economic consequences of elective induction of labor at term. Using decision analysis, these researchers examined a hypothetical cohort of 100,000. Pregnant patients for whom an initial decision was made to either induce labor at 39 weeks' or to follow the patient expectantly through the remainder of pregnancy. All patients in this model underwent elective induction at 42 weeks' gestation. Clinical outcomes of patients undergoing expectant management were evaluated. Using baseline estimates, the investigators concluded that elective induction would result in more than 12,000 excess cesarean deliveries and impose an annual cost to the medical system of nearly $100 million. A policy of induction at any gestational age, regardless of parity or cervical ripeness, required economic expenditures by the medical system. Although never cost saving, inductions were less expensive at later gestational ages, for multiparous patients, and for those women with a favorable cervix. The inductions most costly to the health care system were those performed in nulliparas with unfavorable cervices at 39 weeks. When nulliparous women with favorable cervices undergo labor induction, the estimated cost is approximately halved, but is still considerably higher than allowing spontaneous labor.

One approach called the Active Management of Risk in Pregnancy at Term (AMOR-IPAT) with promise for reducing the risk of cesarean delivery following induction of labor has been described.[58] Using a retrospective cohort design, delivery outcomes of 100 women with a tailored approach to prenatal care and individualization of risk of cesarean delivery were compared with 300 nonexposed women. Consideration was given to the most common indications for nonelective cesarean delivery: cephalopelvic disproportion and uteroplacental insufficiency. A hypothetical ceiling for gestational age at delivery, always less than or equal to 41 weeks' and more than or equal to 38 weeks', was set for each subject. Cervical ripening was used for all women with Bishop scores of less than 5. Despite an increase in the labor induction rate in the women participating in AMOR-IPAT (63 versus 26 percent, $p < 0.001$), there was a significant reduction in cesarean deliveries in the exposed group (4 versus 17 percent, $p < 0.001$). Prospective trials are underway to verify these results, which were obtained in a university-based, primarily indigent patient population. These results may reflect selection bias of the prospectively followed cohort or an example of the Hawthorne effect. Some studies suggest that in the context of the prolonged pregnancy, routine labor induction may result in fewer cesarean deliveries compared with expectant management.[59,60] A recent meta-analysis included 16 studies that compared induction and expectant management for uncomplicated, singleton pregnancies of at least 41 weeks' gestation.[61] Compared with women allocated to expectant management, those who underwent labor induction had lower cesarean delivery rates (20 versus 22 percent, odds ratio [OR] 0.88, 95-percent CI 0.78 to 0.99). There were no statistically significant differences in perinatal mortality rates, neonatal intensive care admission rates, meconium aspiration, or abnormal APGAR scores. Therefore, after 41 weeks' gestation, elective labor induction appears to be justified.

Cervical Ripening

The condition of the cervix influences the success of inducing labor. For this reason, a cervical examination is essential before labor induction is initiated. In 1964, Bishop developed a scoring system to evaluate multiparous women for elective induction at term.[62] The scoring system is based on properties of the cervix that may be assessed clinically at the time of pelvic examination such as dilatation, effacement, consistency, and position as well as the station of the fetal presenting part (Table 13-6).[62,63]

Although Bishop originally used this scoring system to prevent iatrogenic prematurity in an era before the widespread use of sonography, it is now widely used to predict the success of labor induction. The higher the Bishop score, the more "ripe" or "favorable" the cervix is for labor induction. A low Bishop score, usually considered less than or equal to 5, is "unripened" or "unfavorable" and will benefit from cervical ripening. For example, the likelihood of a vaginal delivery after labor induction is similar to that after spontaneous onset of labor if the Bishop score is greater than or equal to 8 in multiparous patients.[62] A low Bishop score is particularly predictive of failure in nulliparous women who undergo induction of labor at term. The high risk of cesarean delivery associated with failure of induction in nulliparous women at term with low Bishop scores is well established in the literature.[64,65] Seminal data from Singapore from the 1980s revealed a 45-percent likelihood of cesarean delivery for failed induction for nulliparous women with an unfavorable cervix (Bishop score less than 6) in an era when oxytocin was used for both cervical ripening and labor induction.

Recently, the rates of cesarean delivery were compared in 4,635 nulliparas women in spontaneous labor with 2,647 nulliparas women who underwent induction of labor.[66] Cesarean delivery was performed in 11.5 percent

Table 13-6. Modified Bishop Score

SCORE PARAMETER	0	1	2	3
Dilatation (cm)	Closed	1–2	3–4	5 or more
Effacement (%)	0–30	40–50	60–70	80 or more
Length (cm)*	*>4*	*2–4*	*1–2*	*1–2*
Station	−3	−2	−1 or 0	+1 or +2
Consistency	Firm	Medium	Soft	
Cervical Position	Posterior	Midposition	Anterior	

Bishop EH: Pelvic scoring for elective induction. Obstet Gynecol 24:266, 1964.

*Modification by Calder AA, Brennand JE: Labor and normal delivery: Induction of labor. Curr Opin Obstet Gynecol 3:764, 1991. This modification replaces percent effacement as one of the parameters of the Bishop score.

Table 13-7. Methods of Cervical Ripening

PHARMACOLOGIC METHODS	MECHANICAL METHODS
Oxytocin	Membrane stripping
Prostaglandins	Amniotomy
E_2 (dinoprostone, Prepidil gel and Cervidil time-released vaginal insert)	
E_1 (misoprostol, Cytotec)	
Estrogen	Mechanical dilators
	Laminaria tents
	Dilapan
	Lamicel
Relaxin	Transcervical balloon catheters
	With extra-amniotic saline infusion
	With concomitant oxytocin administration
Hyaluronic acid	
Progesterone receptor antagonists	

of the spontaneous labor group and 23.7 percent of the labor induction group. The most important variable in predicting the risk of cesarean delivery was a Bishop score at the initiation of labor induction with a 31.5 percent cesarean section rate among patients with a Bishop score less than 5 versus 18.1 percent for patients with a Bishop = 5.

Cervical ripening methods fall into two main categories: pharmacologic and mechanical (Table 13-7). Examples of pharmacologic methods include administration of oxytocin, prostaglandins, estrogens, relaxin, hyaluronic acid, and progesterone receptor antagonists. Mechanical methods include membrane stripping, amniotomy, and balloon dilators, among others.

Pharmacologic Methods

Oxytocin

Oxytocin is a polypeptide hormone produced in the hypothalamus and secreted from the posterior lobe of the pituitary gland in a pulsatile fashion. It is identical to its synthetic analog, which is among the most potent uterotonic agents known. Synthetic oxytocin is an effective means of labor induction.[67] Exogenous oxytocin administration produces periodic uterine contractions first demonstrable at approximately 20 weeks' gestation, with increasing responsiveness with advancing gestational age primarily due to an increase in myometrial oxytocin binding sites.[68] There is little change in myometrial sensitivity to oxytocin from 34 weeks to term; however, once spontaneous labor begins, the uterine sensitivity to oxytocin increases rapidly.[69] This physiologic mechanism makes oxytocin more effective in augmenting labor than in inducing labor, and even less successful as a cervical ripening agent.

Oxytocin is most often given intravenously. It cannot be given orally because the polypeptide is degraded to small, inactive forms by gastrointestinal enzymes. The plasma half life is short, estimated at 3 to 6 minutes,[70] and steady-state concentrations are reached within 30 to 40 minutes of initiation or dose change.[71] Synthetic oxytocin is generally diluted by placing 10 units in 1,000 mL of an isotonic solution, such as normal saline, yielding an oxytocin concentration of 10 mU/mL. It is given by infusion pump to allow continuous, precise control of the dose administered.

Although oxytocin is an effective means of labor induction in women with a favorable cervix as noted earlier, it is less effective as a cervical ripening agent. Many randomized controlled trials comparing oxytocin with various prostaglandin (PG) formulations and other methods of cervical ripening confirm this observation. Lyndrup et al.[72] compared the efficacy of labor induction with vaginal PGE_2 with continuous oxytocin infusion in 91 women with an unfavorable cervix (Bishop score = 6). They found PGE_2 more efficacious for labor induction in 12 to 24 hours, with fewer women undelivered at 24 hours. However, by allowing the inductions to proceed for 48 hours, they found no difference in vaginal delivery rates after 48 hours between the two groups. In a larger study involving 200 women with an unfavorable cervix undergoing labor induction, vaginally applied prostaglandin E_2 was compared with continuous oxytocin infusion.[73] These investigators found a shorter time interval to active labor, a significantly greater change in Bishop score, fewer failed inductions, and fewer multiple-day inductions with PGE_2 compared with oxytocin. No difference in the rate of cesarean delivery was found between the groups overall.

In a Cochrane review of 110 trials including more than 11,000 women comparing oxytocin with any vaginal prostaglandin formulation for labor induction, oxytocin alone was associated with an increase in unsuccessful vaginal delivery within 24 hours (52 versus 28 percent, RR 1.85, 95-percent CI 1.41 to 2.43). There was no difference in the rate of cesarean delivery between groups. When intracervical prostaglandins were compared with oxytocin alone for labor induction, oxytocin alone was associated with an increase in unsuccessful vaginal delivery within 24 hours (51 versus 35 percent, RR 1.49, 95-percent CI 1.12 to 1.99) and an increase in cesarean delivery (19 versus 13 percent, RR 1.42, 95-percent CI 1.11 to 1.82).[67]

In the setting of premature rupture of membranes (PROM) at term (defined as rupture of membranes before the onset of labor), labor induction is recommended if spontaneous labor does not ensue within a reasonable amount of time because as the time between rupture of membranes and the onset of labor increases, so may the risk of maternal and fetal infection.[74–77] A series of systematic reviews examined the outcomes of pregnancies with PROM at or near term.[74,76,77] One trial accounts for most of the patients included in the analysis.[78] Hannah et al. studied 5,041 women with PROM at term. Subjects were randomly assigned to receive intravenous oxytocin, vaginal prostaglandin E_2 gel, or expectant management for up to 4 days, with labor induced with either intravenous oxytocin or vaginal prostaglandin E_2 gel. Those randomized to the expectant management group were induced if complications such as chorioamnionitis developed. The rates of neonatal infection and cesarean delivery were not statistically different between the groups. Rates of clinical chorioamnionitis were less in the group receiving intravenous oxytocin. When oxytocin alone was compared with vaginal prostaglandins in 14 trials for labor induction after PROM by Cochrane reviewers, both medications were found to be equally efficacious.[65] Thus, both can be used in this clinical setting. Because the majority of women with PROM enter labor spontaneously, a policy of expectant management for up to 24 hours is not unreasonable.[79] However, active management of PROM does not increase the risk of cesarean delivery and significantly shortens the time until delivery. Therefore, patients should be offered a choice between active and expectant management, although more prefer active management.[78]

The optimal regimen for oxytocin administration is debatable, although success rates for varying protocols are similar. Protocols differ as to the initial dose, incremental time period, and steady state dose (Table 13-8).[50] A maximum oxytocin dose has not been established, but most protocols do not exceed 42 mU/min.

Low-Dose Oxytocin Dosing

Low-dose protocols mimic endogenous maternal physiology and are associated with lower rates of uterine hyperstimulation.[80] Low-dose oxytocin is initiated at 0.5 to 1 mU and increased by 1 mU per minute at 40- to 60-minute intervals. Slightly higher doses beginning at 1 to 2 mU/min increased by 1 to 2 mU/min, with shorter incremental time intervals of 15 to 30 minutes have also been recommended.[80] Pulsatile oxytocin administration, which truly mimics endogenous oxytocin release from the posterior pituitary, at 8- to 10-minute intervals, is considered a variant of low-dose oxytocin administration. It has the advantage of reducing total oxytocin requirements by 20 to 50 percent.[81–83]

High-Dose Oxytocin Dosing

High-dose oxytocin regimens are often employed in active management of labor protocols. These regimens are largely used for labor augmentation, rather than for labor induction. Examples of these protocols start with an initial oxytocin dose of 6 mU/min increased by 6 mU/min at 20 minute intervals[81] or start at 4 mU/min with 4 mU/min incremental increases.[84] A prospective study involving nearly 5,000 women at Parkland Hospital comparing low-dose with high-dose oxytocin regimens for labor induction and augmentation was undertaken.[85] The high-dose protocol allowed for reduction of the dosage to 3 mU/min in the presence of uterine hyperstimulation. The results indicated that subjects given the high-dose regimen had a significantly shorter mean admission to delivery time, fewer failed inductions, fewer forceps deliveries, fewer cesarean deliveries for failure to progress, less chorioamnionitis, and less neonatal sepsis than subjects given the low-dose regimen. Notably, these subjects had a higher rate of cesarean delivery performed for "fetal distress," but no difference in neonatal outcomes was observed. Merrill and Zlatnik[86] conducted a randomized, double-masked trial including 1,307 patients, comparing high-dose (4.5 mU/min initially increased by 4.5 mU/min every 30 minutes) with low-dose (1.5 mU/min initially, increased by 1.5 mU/min every 30 minutes) oxytocin for augmentation and induction of labor. Oxytocin solutions were prepared by a central pharmacy and infusion volumes were identical to ensure double masking. In the group receiving high-dose oxytocin, labor was significantly shortened when used for induction (8.5 versus 10.5 hours, $P < 0.001$), and augmentation (4.4 versus 5.1 hours, $P = 0.3$). There was no significant difference in rates of cesarean delivery between the two regimens (15 versus 11.3 percent, $P = 0.17$). There were, however, more decreases or discontinuations of oxytocin in the high-dose group both for uterine hyperstimulation and fetal heart rate abnormalities. Discontinuation of oxytocin did not appear to have an adverse impact on the rate of cesarean delivery or lengthening of labor. Neonatal outcomes were observed to be similar in both groups.

In contemporary obstetric practice, based on the above-mentioned evidence, oxytocin is most often used to augment labor in patients with inadequate uterine activity or to induce labor in a patient with a favorable cervical status. One of many dosing regimens may be used depending on the standard practice in the community or the preference of the individual practitioner. Satin et al.[85] studied the differences in outcomes when oxytocin was used to augment as opposed to induce labor. These investigators prospectively studied 2,788 consecutive women with singleton pregnancies. Indications for oxytocin stimulation were divided into augmentation (n = 1,676) and induction (n = 1,112). The low-dose regimen consisted of a starting dose of 1 mU/min with incremental increases of 1 mU/min at 20-minute intervals until 8 mU/min, then 2 mU/min increases up to a maximum of 20-mU/min, and was used first for 5 months in 1,251 pregnancies.

Table 13-8. Labor Stimulation with Oxytocin: Examples of Low- and High-Dose Oxytocin Dosing Regimens

REGIMEN	STARTING DOSE (mU/MIN)	INCREMENTAL INCREASE (mU/MIN)	DOSAGE INTERVAL (MIN)
Low-Dose	0.5–1.0	1	30–40
	1–2	2	15
High-Dose	~6	~6	15
	6	6*, 3, 1	15

*The incremental increase is reduced to 3 mU/min in the presence of hyperstimulation and reduced to 1 mU/min with recurrent hyperstimulation.
American College of Obstetricians and Gynecologists. Induction of Labor. ACOG Practice Bulletin No. 10. Washington, DC. ©ACOG, 1999.

The high-dose regimen consisted of a starting dose of 6 mU/min with increases of 6 mU/min at 20-minute intervals up to a maximum dose of 42 mU/min, and was used for the subsequent 5 months in 1,537 pregnancies. Labor augmentation was more than 3 hours shorter in the high-dose group compared with that of the low-dose group. High-dose augmentation resulted in fewer cesarean deliveries for labor dystocia and fewer failed inductions when compared with the low-dose regimen, although cesarean deliveries for fetal distress were performed more frequently. When making decisions regarding which oxytocin regimen to use, the risks and benefits need to be carefully considered depending on the ultimate outcome desired.

Oxytocin Dosing Intervals

Varying dosing intervals have also been studied[87,88] and, in contemporary practice, vary from 15 to 40 minutes. One comparison of the efficacy and outcomes with differing oxytocin dosing intervals[89] included 1,801 consecutive pregnancies receiving high-dose oxytocin (starting dose of 6 mU/min with incremental increases of 6 mU/min) at 20- and 40-minute intervals. In this study, 949 women received oxytocin at 20-minute intervals (n = 603 labor augmentations and n = 346 labor inductions) and 852 women received oxytocin at 40-minute dosing intervals (n = 564 labor augmentations and n = 288 labor inductions). The rates of cesarean delivery for dystocia or fetal distress were not statistically different between groups; however, the 20-minute regimen for augmentation was associated with a significant reduction in cesarean delivery for dystocia (8 versus 12 percent, P = .05). The incidence of uterine hyperstimulation was greater with the 20-minute regimen for induction compared with the 40-minute regimen (40 versus 31 percent; P = .02) but did not result in an increased rate of cesarean delivery for nonreassuring fetal status. Neonatal outcomes were unaffected by the dosing interval.

Prostaglandins

Administration of PG results in dissolution of collagen bundles and an increase in submucosal water content of the cervix.[90] These changes in cervical connective tissue at term are similar to those observed in early labor. PGs are endogenous compounds found in the myometrium, deciduas, and fetal membranes during pregnancy. The chemical precursor is arachidonic acid. PG formulations have been used since they were first synthesized in the laboratory in 1968. Prostaglandin analogs were originally given by intravenous and oral routes. Later, local administration of prostaglandins in the vagina or the endocervix became the route of choice because of fewer side effects and acceptable clinical response.[91,92] Side effects of all PG formulations and routes may include fever, chills, vomiting, and diarrhea.[91]

The efficacy of locally applied PG (vaginal or intracervical) for cervical ripening and labor induction as compared with oxytocin (alone or in combination with amniotomy) has been demonstrated in a Cochrane review involving more than 10,000 women. Overall, induction with PG was associated with an increase in successful vaginal delivery within 24 hours, a reduction in the rate of cesarean delivery, a lower likelihood that the cervix would remain unchanged (or unfavorable) at 24 to 48 hours, and a reduction in the use of epidural analgesia.[93]

The optimal route, frequency, and dose of prostaglandins of all types and formulations for cervical ripening and labor induction have not been determined. Also, prostaglandin formulations of any kind should be avoided in women with a prior uterine scar such as a prior cesarean delivery or myomectomy because their use appears to increase the risk for uterine rupture.[94,95]

Prostaglandin E_2

One of the first randomized controlled trials using intravaginal PG was conducted in 1979 by Liggins et al.[96] Eighty-four term women with singleton pregnancies were randomly assigned to three groups receiving placebo, 0.2 mg or 0.4 mg PGE_2 compound. Labor was established in 48 hours in 9.3 percent of placebo women, 65.4 percent of women receiving 0.2 mg PGE_2 and 85.7 percent of women receiving 0.4 mg PGE_2. Rayburn[97] summarized the experience with more than 3,313 pregnancies representing 59 prospective clinical trials in which either intracervical or intravaginal PGE_2 was used for cervical ripening before the induction of labor. He concluded that local administration of PGE_2 is effective in enhancing cervical effacement and dilatation, reducing the failed induction rate, shortening the induction to delivery interval, and reducing oxytocin use and cesarean delivery for failure to progress. These findings were confirmed in a meta-analysis of 44 controlled trials performed worldwide using various PG compounds and dosing regimens.[92] Because there appears to be no difference in clinical outcomes when comparing intravaginal or intracervical PGE_2 preparations, and for ease of administration and patient satisfaction, vaginal administration is recommended.[98] A sustained-release vaginal pessary for PGE_2 has been developed. Its use eliminates the need for repeated dosing. Although data are limited, when comparing the efficacy of the intravaginally applied PGE_2 to the sustained-release suppository, there appears to be no difference in rates of vaginal delivery, fetal heart rate abnormalities, or uterine hyperstimulation.[99,100]

Currently, there are two PGE_2 preparations approved by the United States Food and Drug Administration (FDA) for cervical ripening. There is a variety of other PGE_2 compounds such as suppositories available in the United States and tablets available in Europe, although these latter formulations are not approved for use by the FDA for cervical ripening. Many clinicians and pharmacists may prepare their own formulations of PGE_2 gel by thawing and resuspending 20 mg PGE_2 suppositories in small amounts of methylcellulose gel. The resulting gel preparation is then frozen in plastic syringes in various doses ranging from 1 to 6 mg.

Prepidil (Upjohn Pharmaceuticals, Kalamazoo, Michigan) contains 0.5 mg of dinoprostone in 2.5 mL of gel for intracervical administration. The dose can be repeated in 6 to 12 hours if there is inadequate cervical change and minimal uterine activity following the first dose. The manufacturer recommends that the maximum cumulative dose of dinoprostone not exceed 1.5 mg (three doses) within a 24-hour period. Oxytocin should not be initiated until 6 to12 hours after the last dose because of the potential for uterine hyperstimulation with concurrent oxytocin and prostaglandin administration.

Cervidil (Forest Pharmaceuticals, St. Louis, Missouri) is a vaginal insert containing 10 mg of dinoprostone in a timed-release formulation. The vaginal insert administers the medication at 0.3 mg/h and may be left in place for up to 12 hours. An advantage of the vaginal insert over the gel formulation is that the insert may be removed with the onset of active labor, rupture of membranes, or with the development of uterine hyperstimulation. This abnormality of uterine contractions is more often defined as six or more contractions in 10 minutes for a total of 20 minutes with concurrent fetal heart rate tracing abnormalities.[101] Per the manufacturer's recommendations, oxytocin may be initiated 30 to 60 minutes after removal of the insert.

These two preparations are relatively expensive, costing approximately $168 for a single application of dinoprostone gel and $210 for each dinoprostone vaginal insert.[102] These agents also require refrigerated storage and become unstable at room temperature.

Prostaglandin E_1

Misoprostol (Cytotec, Searle Pharmaceuticals, Chicago, Illinois) is a synthetic prostaglandin E_1 analog available as 100 mcg and 200 mcg tablets. The current FDA approved use for misoprostol is for the treatment and prevention of peptic ulcer disease related to chronic nonsteroidal anti-inflammatory use. Administration of misoprostol for preinduction cervical ripening is considered a safe and effective "off-label" use by the ACOG.[103] Misoprostol is inexpensive, with a cost of approximately $1.20 per 100-mcg tablet.[102] It is also stable at room temperature. Misoprostol can be administered both orally or placed vaginally with few systemic side effects. Although not scored, the tablets are usually divided to provide 25- or 50-mcg doses.

Multiple studies suggest that misoprostol tablets placed vaginally are either superior to or equivalent in efficacy compared with intracervical PGE_2 gel.[104–108] More recently a meta-analysis of 70 trials revealed the following points regarding the use of misoprostol compared with other methods of cervical ripening and labor induction.[109] Misoprostol improved cervical ripening compared with placebo and was associated with a reduced failure to achieve vaginal delivery within 24 hours (RR 0.36, 95-percent CI 0.19 to 0.68). There was a trend toward fewer cesarean deliveries that did not reach statistical significance. Compared with other vaginal prostaglandins for labor induction, vaginal misoprostol was more effective in achieving vaginal delivery within 24 hours (RR 0.80, 95-percent CI 0.73 to 0.87). Compared with vaginal or intracervical PGE_2, oxytocin augmentation was also less common with misoprostol (RR 0.65, 95-percent CI 0.57 to 0.73). However, uterine hyperstimulation with fetal heart rate changes (RR 2.04, 95-percent CI 1.49 to 2.80) and meconium-stained amniotic fluid (RR 1.42, 95-percent CI 1.11–1.81) was more common. Most studies suggested that restricting the dose of misoprostol to 25 mcg every 4 hours significantly reduced the risk of uterine hyperstimulation with and without fetal heart rate changes and meconium passage. Most important, regardless of misoprostol dose, there were no significant differences in immediate neonatal outcomes.

Although ACOG, based on its review of the existing evidence, recommends 25 mcg dosing every 3 to 6 hours with vaginally applied misoprostol, the optimal dose and timing interval is not known.[110] Oxytocin may be initiated, if necessary, 4 hours after the final misoprostol dose. A meta-analysis comparing 25-mcg with 50-mcg dosing reported that 50-mcg dosing resulted in a higher rate of vaginal delivery within 24 hours with higher rates of uterine hyperstimulation and meconium passage but without compromising in neonatal outcomes.[111] A statistically significant difference in fetal acidosis defined as a umbilical arterial pH of less than 7.16 was found in infants born to mothers given 50 mcg of intravaginally applied misoprostol every 3 hours compared with those born to mothers given 25 mcg every 3 hours.[112,113] In their Committee Opinions on the use of misoprostol for labor induction, the ACOG concludes that safety using the higher 50-mcg dosing could not be adequately evaluated and suggests the higher dose could be used only in select circumstances.[103,114]

Oral administration of misoprostol for cervical ripening has also been studied.[115–122] Oral administration has the promise for offering more patient comfort, satisfaction, and convenience of administration. Most of these studies compared lower oral doses of misoprostol such as 50 mcg given every 3 to 6 hours and compared them to similar vaginal misoprostol dosing regimens such as 25 to 50 mcg given every 3 to 6 hours. This oral regimen of dosing appears to be less effective than vaginal administration for achieving vaginal delivery, requires more oxytocin use, and results in longer inductions.[123] When higher doses of oral misoprostol such as 100 mcg are compared with 25 mcg administered vaginally, oral misoprostol was more effective, with fewer women failing to achieve vaginal delivery after 24 hours.[124] However, 100-mcg oral dosing was associated with higher rates of uterine hyperstimulation. Some investigators have described titrating oral misoprostol to its desired effect of achieving regular and painful uterine contractions.[122,125] This method appears to achieve vaginal delivery rates similar to vaginally administered misoprostol with less uterine hyperstimulation. The consequence of this approach is prolongation of induction times by 3 to 4 hours. More data are needed to shed light on the optimal dosing and safety of oral misoprostol for cervical ripening and labor induction.

Other novel approaches include buccal and sublingual misoprostol administration. The theory is that avoiding first-pass hepatic circulation from oral administration will lead to bioavailability similar to that achieved with vaginal administration. This hypothesis has been substantiated by pharmacokinetic studies that have shown that the buccal and sublingual routes of administration are associated with rapid onset of action and greater bioavailability than other routes.[126] In a randomized controlled trial including 250 women admitted for labor induction, 50 mcg of sublingual misoprostol was compared to 100 mg of orally administered misoprostol given every 4 hours to a maximum of five doses. Sublingual misoprostol appeared to have the same efficacy as orally administered misoprostol to achieve vaginal delivery within 24 hours with no increase in uterine hyperstimulation.[127] However, the 100-mcg oral dose has higher rates of hyperstimulation than 25 mcg administered vaginally. A randomized controlled trial including 152 women received either 200 mcg of buccal misoprostol every 6 hours or 50 mcg of misoprostol administered vaginally every 6 hours.[128] There was no statistically significant difference in time interval to vaginal delivery, the rate of vaginal delivery, or the rate of uterine hyperstimulation between the two groups. However, given the concerns of more uterine hyperstimulation with oral routes of administration compared with vaginal administration, more data are needed to clarify the efficacy and safety of oral, buccal, and sublingual misoprostol use. Optimal dosing regimens are yet to be defined, and additional concern exists because of the greater bioavailability associated with these routes of administration when compared with vaginal use.

Progesterone Receptor Antagonists (Mifepristone)

RU-486 (mifepristone) is a competitive steroid receptor antagonist. It is a more selective progesterone antagonist and has been used for early pregnancy termination. Because of its antiprogestational action, it has been studied as a potential alternative for cervical ripening and labor induction in term pregnancies.[129–133] These studies comparing mifepristone with placebo demonstrate mifepristone is more effective than placebo for cervical ripening. There are no studies to date comparing mifepristone to other agents such as prostaglandins used for cervical ripening and labor induction.[134] At this time, access to this medication limits widespread research and use.

Other Methods

Estrogen

Seminal parturition studies in sheep showed that there is a prelabor rise in estrogen associated with a decrease in progesterone.[135,136] These changes stimulate prostaglandin production and may help initiate labor. Through this mechanism, estrogen has been suggested and studied as a cervical ripening agent and labor induction agent.[137–140] This approach has limited widespread clinical applicability, because there is no discussion of rates of vaginal delivery achieved within 24 hours or cervical status change after 12 to 24 hours. Of note, the investigators reported that when comparing estrogen with placebo, there were no differences in the rate of cesarean deliveries or in uterine hyperstimulation between groups. At this time, estrogen is not currently used in common practice as an induction agent, and there is insufficient evidence to draw any conclusions regarding its efficacy.[141]

Relaxin

Relaxin is a protein hormone thought to have a promoting effect on cervical ripening through connective tissue remodeling. The main source of human relaxin is the corpus luteum of pregnancy. Its use was thought to have advantages over other agents that promoted uterine activity by potentially decreasing the risk of uterine hyperstimulation. Most research on induction of labor with relaxin has used porcine or bovine preparations and demonstrated improved efficacy over a placebo for cervical ripening.[142–144] With the advent of DNA technology, human recombinant relaxin has become available for evaluation. Two studies totaling 113 women who received human recombinant relaxin for induction of labor compared with placebo showed no effect on cervical ripening or labor induction.[145,146] The place of relaxin as an induction or cervical priming agent is unclear, and further trials are needed to determine its effect and place in current clinical practice.[147]

Hyaluronic Acid

The cervix is a fibrous organ composed principally of hyaluronic acid, collagen, and proteoglycan. Hyaluronic acid increases as pregnancy progresses, peaks after the onset of labor, and decreases rapidly after birth of the infant.[148] The increase in the level of hyaluronic acid is associated with an increase in tissue water content of the cervix, which is one of the mechanisms involved in cervical ripening. In the past, investigators postulated that cervical injection of hyaluronic acid would lead to cervical ripening. Although there is a theoretical physiologic mechanism for hyaluronic acid as a cervical ripening agent, there are no published studies using this agent for this indication. No data are available to assess its use for cervical ripening or labor induction.[149]

Mechanical Methods

Mechanical methods of cervical ripening have been available and used for centuries. They were among the first methods used for labor induction. Advantages to a mechanical approach are that they are often less costly, result in less hyperstimulation, are easy to store, and may result in fewer side effects for mother and fetus.[150] Disadvantages include the risk of infection, disruption of a low-lying placenta, and some maternal discomfort on manipulation of the cervix.

Membrane Stripping

Stripping or sweeping of the fetal membranes refers to digital separation of the chorioamniotic membrane from the wall of the cervix and lower uterine segment. This procedure was first reported for induction of labor at term in 1810 by Hamilton in England.[151] For membrane stripping, the fetal vertex should be well applied to the cervix, and the cervix should be dilated sufficiently to allow introduction of the examiner's finger. This process of membrane stripping is presumed to cause the release of endogenous prostaglandins from the adjacent membranes and decidua, as well as from the cervix.[152,153] Many investigations have been conducted using routine membrane stripping at 38 or 39 weeks to either prevent prolonged pregnancies or decrease the frequency of more formal inductions occurring after 41 weeks.[154–161] A meta-analysis including 19 trials demonstrated that routine membrane stripping at term will reduce the interval to spontaneous labor by 3 days, decrease the frequency of pregnancies continuing beyond 41 and 42 weeks, and lower the frequency of formal induction.[162,163] There was no difference in the maternal or neonatal infection rate, or the rates of membrane rupture or cesarean delivery. Complications that can result from membrane stripping include rupture of membranes, hemorrhage from disruption of an occult placenta previa, and the development of chorioamnionitis. There does not appear to be a contraindication to membrane stripping in Group B streptococcus (GBS)–colonized women. In accordance with Centers for Disease Control and Prevention guidelines, antibiotic prophylaxis should be administered to any GBS-colonized woman once labor ensues or membrane rupture occurs.[164]

Amniotomy

Amniotomy, artificial rupture of membranes, is a technique involving the perforation of the chorioamniotic membranes. It is an effective method of labor induction performed in multiparous women with favorable cervices.[165] Before amniotomy is performed, confirmation is essential that the fetal vertex, and not the umbilical cord or other fetal part, is presenting and is well applied to the cervix. These precautions are taken to prevent umbilical cord prolapse, which often necessitates emergent cesarean delivery. The amniotomy procedure usually involves a toothed clamp such as an Allis clamp, or more commonly, a plastic hook that is applied to the membranes and manipulated so as to hitch or scratch the membranes. The fetal heart rate status before and after the procedure should be monitored, and the character and color of the amniotic fluid should be recorded. Combined use of amniotomy and intravenous oxytocin is more effective than amniotomy alone, with fewer women undelivered vaginally after 24 hours.[166] This conclusion is demonstrated by a multicenter study including 925 women in labor.[165] Patients were randomized once they reached cervical dilatation of 3 cm to receive early amniotomy along with conventional labor management (which included oxytocin use) or conservative labor management without oxytocin use. The early amniotomy group had fewer protracted labor disorders, and the median length of time from randomization to full cervical dilatation was 136 minutes shorter. Additionally, less oxytocin was required in the early amniotomy group. The cesarean delivery rate was similar between the groups. In another study including 196 women with favorable cervices randomized to receive either amniotomy alone or amniotomy followed by oxytocin infusion, women who received oxytocin infusion with amniotomy had a shorter induction-to-delivery interval of 6 hours (95-percent CI 5.0 to 6.5 hours) compared with 9 hours (95-percent CI 7.0 to 10.0 hours) in the group receiving amniotomy alone.[168] Two studies[169,170] that, in combination, included 160 women found more postpartum hemorrhage in the amniotomy and intravenous oxytocin group with 11 (13.75 percent) cases compared with 2 (2.5 percent) cases in the vaginal prostaglandin group.

Mechanical Dilators

Mechanical dilators placed in the lower uterine segment release endogenous prostaglandins from the fetal membranes and maternal decidua. In addition, the osmotic properties of hygroscopic dilators promote cervical ripening. These hygroscopic dilators absorb endocervical and local tissue fluids that cause swelling and allow for controlled dilatation by mechanical pressure. One such synthetic osmotic dilator, Dilapan (JCEC Company, Kendell Park, New Jersey) is currently unavailable for clinical use in the United States. Another device known as Lamicel (Merocel Corporation, Mystic, Connecticut) is commercially available.

Laminaria

Natural osmotic dilators are derived from the seaweed *Laminaria japonicum*. The dried seaweed has the ability to double in size from its initial size of 2 mm to 6 mm. Maximal dilatation occurs after 6 to 12 hours following application. Laminaria have been found to be at least as effective in promoting cervical dilatation as PGE_2 gel.[171] A significant disadvantage of the use of laminaria for cervical ripening is patient discomfort both at the time of insertion and with progressive cervical dilatation. With other equally effective agents available, there is no obvious benefit to support their routine use. In specific clinical circumstances in which prostaglandins should be avoided or are unavailable because of supply or cost, laminaria can be used both safely and effectively.

Transcervical Balloon Catheters

A deflated Foley catheter, usually a 16 French 30 mL balloon, can be passed through an undilated cervix into the extra-amniotic space and then inflated. The balloon is then retracted to rest against the internal os. Some clinicians remove the top of the catheter before insertion although there is no data to suggest that this is necessary. To add more traction, pressure may be applied by attaching a weight such as a liter of intravenous fluid to the end of the catheter and suspending it with the force of gravity or by taping the catheter under tension to the patient's inner thigh. The benefit of traction has not been proven, and may confer no added clinical benefit. This technique appears to be as effective for preinduction cervical ripening as prostaglandin E_2 gel and intravaginal misoprostol in most studies.[172–174] Transcervical Foley catheter placement is a superior method of preinduction cervical ripening when compared with intravenous oxytocin and has been associated with a lower rate of cesarean delivery in one investigation.[150] Some studies show more rapid cervical ripening, a shortened induction to delivery interval, and reduced frequency of patients undelivered in 24 hours when combining a transcervical balloon catheter with a pharmacologic method of cervical ripening such as a prostaglandin,[175] whereas others do not.[174] No increased risk of preterm delivery in subsequent pregnancies following the placement of balloon catheters in the lower uterine segment was found by Sciscione et al.[176] in 126 women.

Trials using the transcervical Foley catheter with simultaneous oxytocin infusion compared with vaginally administered misoprostol have been described.[173–175] In all of these studies, researchers used extra-amniotic saline infusion (discussed later), along with the transcervical Foley catheter. The largest trial by Buccellato et al. included 250 women undergoing labor induction with an unfavorable cervix who were randomly assigned to receive either a transcervical Foley catheter with concomitant oxytocin infusion or vaginally administered misoprostol 50 µg every 4 hours for a maximum of three doses. There were no significant differences in the rate of cesarean delivery, rate of uterine hyperstimulation, or time intervals to vaginal delivery, indicating that both methods of labor induction appear to be equally effective. Mullin et al. studied 200 women undergoing labor induction with an unfavorable cervix. Subjects were randomized to receive a transcervical Foley catheter with extra-amniotic saline infusion with concomitant oxytocin infusion or vaginally administered misoprostol 25 µg every 4 hours for a maximum of six doses. They found that subjects receiving misoprostol had a longer average interval from labor induction to delivery of 1,323 minutes compared with 970 minutes for subjects receiving the transcervical Foley catheter. There were no differences in cesarean births between the two groups. These data indicate that the transcervical Foley catheter with simultaneous oxytocin infusion may be just as efficacious as the usual dosing regimen for vaginally administered misoprostol for preinduction cervical ripening, and may, in fact, result in shorter induction to delivery time intervals.

The use of the Atad double-balloon device has also been described in a limited group of studies.[180–182] One investigation included 95 women with Bishop scores no more than 4 and randomly assigned them to vaginally administered PGE_2, Atad balloon dilator technique, or continuous oxytocin for labor induction. They found a significant mean change in Bishop score after 12 hours in the PGE_2 group and Atad balloon dilator group of 5 compared with 2.5 in the oxytocin group. In addition they found a higher rate of failed induction in the oxytocin group (58 percent) compared with 20 percent in the PGE_2 and 5.7 percent in the Atad balloon dilator groups. Vaginal delivery rates in the oxytocin group were 26.7 percent compared with 77 percent and 70 percent in the Atad balloon dilator and PGE_2 groups, respectively.

Extra-Amniotic Saline Infusion

Infusion of isotonic fluid into the extraovular space has been employed as an adjunct to transcervical balloon catheter placement in the lower uterine segment. The hypothesis for this approach is that this disruption of the fetal-maternal interface will result in added release of endogenous prostaglandins and other parturition-related hormones to facilitate the onset of spontaneous uterine activity. Most commonly, isotonic saline is used; hence, the name extra-amniotic saline infusion (EASI) and is infused continuously at rates of 20 to 40 ml/h. The use of EASI with a transcervical Foley balloon catheter appears to be effective for cervical ripening when compared with intravaginal prostaglandins,[177,183] although EASI does not appear to improve induction outcomes over those observed with the use of Foley catheter alone.[184] A Cochrane review comparing EASI to any prostaglandin for cervical ripening showed that EASI infusion was significantly less likely to result in vaginal delivery within 24 hours (43 versus 58 percent RR 1.33, 95-percent CI 1.02 to 1.75), had a higher risk of cesarean delivery (31 versus 22 percent, RR 1.48, 95-percent CI 1.14 to 1.90), and did not reduce the risk of hyperstimulation.[150] From these data, there is little support for the use of EASI as an adjunct to transcervical balloon catheter placement.

Prediction of Labor Induction Success

Because of the risk of cesarean delivery and the rising costs of health care associated with labor induction, some researchers have tried to identify, with varying success, biochemical and biophysical assays to predict the probability of vaginal delivery following labor induction.[185–192] These measures include digital evaluation of the cervix, ultrasonographic cervical length measurements, and use of fetal fibronectin before labor induction. Fetal fibronectin is available for the prediction of preterm birth within 2 weeks and has been studied for its ability to predict successful induction of labor. Garite et al.[193] investigated 160 patients undergoing labor induction at term. A vaginal swab immunoassay for fetal fibronectin was performed in all patients before the induction. Patients with a positive result ($n = 108$) had a lower rate of cesarean delivery (15 versus 27 percent, $p = 0.05$) and shorter intervals to delivery. Although there was a trend toward a decrease in cesarean deliveries for nulliparous women with a positive fetal fibronectin who underwent inductions with a Bishop score of 5 and shorter time intervals to vaginal delivery, this difference was not statistically significant.

Reis et al.[194] prospectively studied 134 patients who were undergoing labor induction at term. A clinical history was first taken regarding prior vaginal delivery. All participants underwent a digital cervical examination, sonographic measurement of cervical length, and fetal fibronectin assay before the start of labor induction. The performance of each test in predicting vaginal delivery within 24 hours of labor induction was evaluated. Only obstetric history and digital examination (Bishop score) were found to predict accurately vaginal delivery within 24 hours and were independently associated with labor duration. Fetal fibronectin and ultrasound measurements both failed to predict the outcome of the induced labor. The investigators did not stratify their data based on parity, and conclusions could not be made regarding the role of these tools in nulliparous patients.

Bailit et al.[195] used a decision analysis to determine if the vaginal delivery rate is increased in nulliparous women undergoing elective labor induction following fetal fibronectin testing. In this model, three management strategies were evaluated presuming fetal fibronectin testing was performed in select groups at 39 weeks of pregnancy: (1) No elective induction of labor for any candidate until 41 weeks' gestation (spontaneous labor), (2) induction only of those patients with a positive fetal fibronectin result at 39 weeks, and (3) elective induction for every woman at no less than 39 weeks' gestation without performance of a fetal fibronectin test. The investigators based estimates and assumptions for their statistical model on previous published clinical studies regarding rates of cesarean delivery for women in spontaneous labor, rates of cesarean delivery after an induction for a prolonged pregnancy, distribution of fetal fibronectin results at 39 weeks' gestation, and percentage of pregnancies beyond 41 weeks. Investigators found that the spontaneous labor strategy had the highest rate of vaginal delivery (90 percent) and the elective induction strategy had the lowest rate (79 percent). When fetal fibronectin test results were used to screen candidates for elective induction, the rate of vaginal delivery was higher than the induction strategy but lower than the spontaneous labor strategy (83 percent). These investigators concluded that the best approach to improve vaginal delivery rates was to avoid elective induction in nulliparous women. Fetal fibronectin may, however, improve chances of vaginal delivery over nonselective induction. Larger trials are needed to further clarify the role of fetal fibronectin in predicting the success of labor induction in the nulliparous patient and the cost effectiveness of this approach.

MANAGEMENT OF ABNORMAL LABOR AND DELIVERY

Oxytocin Augmentation

When the first stage of labor is protracted or an arrest disorder is diagnosed, an evaluation of uterine activity, clinical pelvimetry, and fetal position, station, and estimated weight should be performed. If uterine activity is found to be suboptimal, the most common remedy is oxytocin augmentation, because once labor is initiated, the uterus becomes more sensitive to oxytocin stimulation. Various oxytocin dosing regimens have been described in the obstetric literature. Local protocols for oxytocin administration should specify the dose of oxytocin being delivered (milliunits per minute) as opposed to the volume of fluid being infused (milliliters per minute), initial doses, incremental increases with periodicity, and maximum dose.

Side Effects

Uterine Overactivity

The most frequently encountered complication of oxytocin or prostaglandin administration is uterine overactivity. The most commonly used terms to describe this activity are hyperstimulation, tachysystole, and hypertonus. There are no uniform definitions for these terms. The ACOG offers the following definitions[16]:

Hyperstimulation can be defined as a persistent pattern of more than five contractions in 10 minutes, uterine contractions lasting at least 2 minutes, or contractions of normal duration occurring within 1 minute of each other, with or without fetal heart rate changes.

Tachysystole can be defined as hyperstimulation without fetal heat rate changes.

Hyperstimulation syndrome has been used to describe hyperstimulation or tachysystole associated with fetal heart rate abnormalities.

Other authorities use alternative terminology.[109,196] The term "uterine hyperstimulation without fetal heart rate changes" has been used to describe the uterine tachysystole (more than 5 contractions per 10 minutes for at least 20 minutes). Uterine hypersystole/hypertonus (a contraction lasting at least 2 minutes) and the term "uterine hyperstimulation with fetal heart rate changes" have been used to denote uterine hyperstimulation syndrome (tachysystole or hypersystole with fetal heart rate changes such as persistent decelerations, tachycardia, or decreased short-term variability). These differences are semantic but can be a source of confusion if the reader is unaware of the discrepancies.

One of the advantages of oxytocin administration is that if uterine hyperstimulation is encountered, the infusion can quickly be stopped. This usually results in the resolution of such uterine overactivity. In addition, placing the woman in the left lateral position, administering oxygen, and increasing intravenous fluids may be of benefit. If fetal heart rate tracing abnormalities persist and uterine hyperstimulation is ongoing, the use of a tocolytic, such as terbutaline, may be considered. Oxytocin may then be reinitiated if appropriate once uterine tone has returned to baseline and fetal status is reassuring.

Water Intoxication

Oxytocin is structurally and functionally related to vasopressin, or antidiuretic hormone. It binds to vasopressin and oxytocin receptors in the kidney and the brain. Oxytocin can have an antidiuretic effect at high doses and can, in extreme situations, result in water intoxication. Severe symptomatic hyponatremia can result if oxytocin is administered at high concentrations (e.g., 40 mU/min) in large quantities of hypotonic solutions (more than 3 liters) for prolonged periods of time.[197] Symptoms of severe acute hyponatremia include headache, anorexia, nausea, vomiting, abdominal pain, lethargy, drowsiness, unconsciousness, grand mal seizures, and potentially irreversible neurologic injury. Fortunately, this side effect is extremely rare even with high dose oxytocin regimens.

If water intoxication occurs, oxytocin and any hypotonic solutions should be stopped. Correction of hyponatremia must be performed carefully and consists of restricting water intake and careful administration of hypertonic saline. Correction of hyponatremia must occur slowly and cautiously because overly rapid correction can be deleterious.

Hypotension

Historically, bolus injections of oxytocin were thought to cause hypotension.[198] Current practice for labor management is administration by infusion pump or slow drip. Mean arterial blood pressure and peripheral vascular resistance have been noted to decrease 30 percent and 50 percent, respectively, after oxytocin bolus injection of 5 to 10 units. This caused increases of 30 percent in heart rate, 25 percent in stroke volume, and 50 percent in cardiac output when compared with patients receiving slow dilute infusions. Fewer cardiovascular side effects are observed when oxytocin is given as a slow intravenous infusion or intramuscularly, as may be needed for third-stage labor management. However, a more recent report by Davies et al.[199] revealed that a 10-IU bolus of oxytocin given in the third stage of labor was not associated with adverse hemodynamic responses compared with oxytocin given as an infusion. Although multiple boluses during labor are not recommended, consideration may be given to its use in the third stage of labor as a single bolus.

Uterine Rupture

Uterine rupture is rare and in most instances occurs in women with prior uterine surgery such as cesarean delivery or myomectomy. Other risk factors for uterine rupture are grand multiparity; marked uterine overdistention either with a macrosomic fetus, multiple gestation, or polyhydramnios; and fetal malpresentation. Although there is no association between maximum dose of oxtyocin and risk of uterine rupture,[200] it is likely that some cases of uterine rupture can be avoided by using the lowest dose of oxytocin possible that produces regular contractions and cervical change. Data regarding the safety of oxytocin for induction of labor in the setting of a prior cesarean birth are largely retrospective in nature and lack of reporting on some important confounding variables. However most studies suggest that the use of oxytocin for labor induction or augmentation in not associated with a significant increase in the risk of uterine rupture in women with a prior cesarean delivery.[201–203] Furthernore, there does not appear to be a difference in a population-based, retrospective cohort study of more than 20,000 women with a single prior cesarean delivery the uterine rupture rates (per 1,000) were 5.2 for women in spontaneous labor, 7.7 for women induced without prostaglandins, and 24.5 for women induced with prostaglandins.[95] Therefore, prostaglandins are not recommended for cervical ripening or induction in women with a prior uterine scar.[204] Use of intrauterine pressure catheters does not appear to be helpful in diagnosis of uterine rupture, because the ruptures usually evolve gradually in labor and are often heralded by abnormal fetal heart rate patterns.[205,206] There is no evidence that amnioinfusion increases the risk of uterine rupture; however, studies to date have been small and retrospective.[207]

Key Points

- The ability of the fetus to successfully negotiate the pelvis during labor and delivery is dependent on the complex interaction of three variables: the powers, the passenger, and the passage. Abnormalities in labor progress can arise with any of these three factors.
- When induction of labor is attempted against an unfavorable cervix, the likelihood of a successful outcome is reduced. The choice of which method to use to promote cervical maturation and to induce labor should be individualized. A single technique is rarely effective, and a combination of maneuvers may be required.
- Membrane sweeping is effective in reducing the interval to spontaneous onset of labor and the overall duration of pregnancy when performed at term. It is not associated with increased maternal or neonatal infection but can cause maternal discomfort and vaginal bleeding.
- In women with intact membranes, amniotomy should be performed where feasible before or concomitant with administration of intravenous oxytocin.
- The two major potential complications of elective induction of labor are iatrogenic prematurity and increased cesarean delivery resulting from failed induction.
- Recent studies have demonstrated that routine induction of labor at 41 weeks' gestation is not associated with an increased risk of cesarean delivery regardless of parity, state of the cervix, or method of induction. This indicates that some target populations may be appropriate for elective induction without incurring the added risks of cesarean delivery.
- Induction of labor with intravenous oxytocin, intravaginal prostaglandin compounds, and expectant management (with defined time limits) are all reasonable options for women and their infants in the face of PROM at term, because they result in similar rates of neonatal infection and cesarean delivery.
- There are a variety of different dosing protocols and dosing intervals for the administration of oxytocin for labor induction and augmentation. In general, higher doses are associated with shorter times to delivery but more uterine hyperstimulation than are lower doses. Lower doses of oxytocin do not increase operative delivery rates or prolong delivery intervals.
- Complications of oxytocin administration include water intoxication, uterine hyperstimulation, and uterine rupture. These complications are most commonly seen with high-dose, prolonged infusions.
- The condition of the cervix at the start of labor induction is critical to the success of the induction attempt. There are both pharmacologic and mechanical methods of cervical ripening available.

REFERENCES

1. Nathanielsz PW, Giussani DA, Wu WX: Stimulation of the switch in myometrial activity from contractures to contractions in the pregnant sheep and nonhuman primate. Equine Vet J Suppl 24:83, 1997.
2. Liggins GC, Fairclough RJ, Grieves SA, et al: The mechanism of initiation of parturition in the ewe. Recent Prog Horm Res 29:111, 1973.
3. Liggins GC, Kennedy PC, Holm LW: Failure of initiation of parturition after electrocoagulation of the pituitary of the fetal lamb. Am J Obstet Gynecol 182:473, 2000.
4. McDonald TJ, Nathanielsz PW: Bilateral destruction of the fetal paraventricular nuclei prolongs gestation in sheep. Am J Obstet Gynecol 165:764, 1991.
5. Friedman E: The graphic analysis of labor. Am J Obstet Gynecol 68:1568, 1954.
6. Friedman EA: Primigravid labor; a graphicostatistical analysis. Obstet Gynecol 6:567, 1955.
7. Friedman EA: Labor: Clinical Evaluation & Management, 2nd ed. New York, Appleton-Century-Crofts, 1978.
8. Friedman EA: An objective approach to the diagnosis and management of abnormal labor. Bull N Y Acad Med 48:842, 1972.
9. Friedman EA: Labor in multiparas; a graphicostatistical analysis. Obstet Gynecol 8:691, 1956.
10. Cohen W, Friedman EA: Management of Labor. Baltimore, University Park Press, 1983.
11. Friedman EA, Sachtleben MR: Dysfunctional labor. I. Prolonged latent phase in the nullipara. Obstet Gynecol 17:135, 1961.
12. Friedman EA: The functional divisions of labor. Am J Obstet Gynecol 109:274, 1971.
13. Thorp JA, Hu DH, Albin RM, et al: The effect of intrapartum epidural analgesia on nulliparous labor: a randomized, controlled, prospective trial. Am J Obstet Gynecol 169:851, 1993.
14. Newton ER, Schroeder BC, Knape KG, Bennett BL: Epidural analgesia and uterine function. Obstet Gynecol 85:749, 1995.
15. Alexander JM, Lucas MJ, Ramin SM, et al: The course of labor with and without epidural analgesia. Am J Obstet Gynecol 178:516, 1998.
16. ACOG Practice Bulletin Number 49, December 2003: Dystocia and augmentation of labor Obstet Gynecol 102:1445, 2003.
17. Caldeyro-barcia R, Alvarez H, Reynolds SRM: A better understanding of uterine contractility through simultaneous recording with an internal and seven channel external method. Surg Gynecol Obstet 91:641, 1950.
18. Hendricks CH, Quilligan EJ, Tyler CW, Tucker GJ: Pressure relationships between the intervillous space and the amniotic fluid in human term pregnancy. Am J Obstet Gynecol 77:1028, 1959.
19. Caldeyro-Barcia R, Poseiro JJ: Physiology of the uterine contraction. Clin Obstet Gynaecol 3:386, 1960.
20. Phillips RD, Freeman M: The management of the persistent occiput posterior position. A review of 552 consecutive cases. Obstet Gyneco; 43:171, 1974.
21. Akmal S, Kametas N, Tsoi E, et al: Ultrasonographic occiput position in early labour in the prediction of caesarean section. Br J Obstet Gynaecol 111:532, 2004.
22. Ponkey SE, Cohen AP, Heffner LJ, Lieberman E: Persistent fetal occiput posterior position: obstetric outcomes. Obstet Gynecol 101:915, 2003.
23. Rouse DJ, Owen J, Goldenberg RL, Cliver SP: The effectiveness and costs of elective cesarean delivery for fetal macrosomia diagnosed by ultrasound. JAMA 276:1480, 1996.
24. Rouse DJ, Owen J: Prophylactic cesarean delivery for fetal macrosomia diagnosed by means of ultrasonography—A Faustian bargain? Am J Obstet Gynecol 181:332, 1999.
25. Friedman EA, Sachtleben MR: Dysfunctional labor. III. Secondary arrest of dilatation in the nullipara. Obstet Gynecol 19:576, 1962.
26. Friedman EA, Sachtleben MR: Dysfunctional labor VI. Abnormal progress in the multipara. Obstet Gynecol 22:478, 1963.
27. Friedman EA, Sachtleben MR: Dysfunctional labor, V. Therapeutic trial of oxytocin in secondary arrest. Obstet Gynecol 21:13, 1963.
28. Rouse DJ, Owen J, Hauth JC: Active-phase labor arrest: oxytocin augmentation for at least 4 hours. Obstet Gynecol 93:323, 1999.
29. Jacoate TN, Baker K, Martin RB: Inefficient uterine activity. Surg Gynecol Obstet 95:257, 1952.
30. Friedman EA, Sachtleben MR: Station of the fetal presenting part. V. Protracted descent patterns. Obstet Gynecol 36:558, 1970.
31. Kilpatrick SJ, Laros RK Jr: Characteristics of normal labor. Obstet Gynecol 74:85, 1989.
32. Hellman LM, Prystowsky H: The duration of the second stage of labor. Am J Obstet Gynecol 63:1223, 1952.
33. Hamilton G: Classical observations and suggestions in obstetrics. Edinburgh Med J 7:313, 1861.
34. Zhang J, Yancey MK, Klebanoff MA, et al: Does epidural analgesia prolong labor and increase risk of cesarean delivery? A natural experiment. Am J Obstet Gynecol 185:128, 2001.
35. Piper JM, Bolling DR, Newton ER: The second stage of labor: factors influencing duration. Am J Obstet Gynecol 165:976, 1991.
36. Cohen WR: Influence of the duration of second stage labor on perinatal outcome and puerperal morbidity. Obstet Gynecol 49:266, 1977.
37. Menticoglou SM, Manning F, Harman C, Morrison I: Perinatal outcome in relation to second-stage duration. Am J Obstet Gynecol 173(3 Pt 1):906, 1995.
38. Myles TD, Santolaya J: Maternal and neonatal outcomes in patients with a prolonged second stage of labor. Obstet Gynecol 102:52, 2003.
39. Dombrowski MP, Bottoms SF, Saleh AA, et al: Third stage of labor. analysis of duration and clinical practice. Am J Obstet Gynecol 172:1279, 1995.
40. Hibbard BM: Obstetrics in general practice. The third stage of labour. Br Med J 5396:1485, 1964.
41. Combs CA, Laros RK Jr: Prolonged third stage of labor: morbidity and risk factors. Obstet Gynecol 77:863, 1991.
42. Prendiville WJ, Elbourne D, McDonald S: Active versus expectant management in the third stage of labour. Cochrane Database Syst Rev 2:CD000007, 2000.
43. Jackson KW Jr, Allbert JR, Schemmer GK, et al: A randomized controlled trial comparing oxytocin administration before and after placental delivery in the prevention of postpartum hemorrhage. Am J Obstet Gynecol 185:873, 2001.
44. American College of Obstetricians and Gynecologists: Prophylactic antibiotics in labor and delivery. Obstet Gynecol 102:875, 2003.
45. Hughes EC: Obstetric-Gynecologic Terminology. Philadelphia: Davis, 1972.
46. Ventura SJ, Martin JA, Curtin SC, et al: Births: final data for 1998. Natl Vital Stat Rep 48:1, 2000.
47. Mahon TR, Chazotte C, Cohen WR: Short labor: characteristics and outcome. Obstet Gynecol 84:47, 1994.
48. Poggi SH, Stallings SP, Ghidini A, et al: Intrapartum risk factors for permanent brachial plexus injury. Am J Obstet Gynecol 189:725, 2003.
49. Martin JA, Hamilton BE, Sutton PD, et al: Births: final data for 2002. Natl Vital Stat Rep 52:1, 2003.
50. American College of Obsetricians and Gynecologists: Induction of Labor (1999). ACOG Practice bulletin #10. Washington, DC.
51. American Academy of Pediatrics and American College of Obstetricians and Gynecologists: Guidelines for Perintal Care, 5th ed. American College of Obstetricians and Gynecologists, Kearneysville, WV, 2002.
52. Zhang J, Yancey MK, Henderson CE: U.S. national trends in labor induction, 1989–1998. J Reprod Med 47:120, 2002.
53. Macer JA, Macer CL, Chan LS: Elective induction versus spontaneous labor: a retrospective study of complications and outcome. Am J Obstet Gynecol 166:1690, 1992.
54. Seyb ST, Berka RJ, Socol ML, Dooley SL: Risk of cesarean delivery with elective induction of labor at term in nulliparous women. Obstet Gynecol 94:600, 1999.
55. Maslow AS, Sweeny AL: Elective induction of labor as a risk factor for cesarean delivery among low-risk women at term. Obstet Gynecol 95:917, 2000.
56. Cammu H, Martens G, Ruyssinck G, Amy JJ: Outcome after elective labor induction in nulliparous women: a matched cohort study. Am J Obstet Gynecol 186:240, 2002.

57. Kaufman KE, Bailit JL, Grobman W: Elective induction: an analysis of economic and health consequences. Am J Obstet Gynecol 187:858, 2002.
58. Nicholson JM, Kellar LC, Cronholm PF, Macones GA: Active management of risk in pregnancy at term in an urban population: an association between a higher induction of labor rate and a lower cesarean delivery rate. Am J Obstet Gynecol 191:1516, 2004.
59. Hannah ME, Hannah WJ, Hellmann J, et al: Induction of labor as compared with serial antenatal monitoring in post-term pregnancy. A randomized controlled trial. The Canadian Multicenter Post-term Pregnancy Trial Group. N Engl J Med 326:1587, 1992.
60. McNellis D, Medearis AL, Fowler S, et al: A clinical trial of labor versus expectant managment in postterm pregnancy. Am J Obstet Gynecol 170:716, 1994.
61. Sanchez-Ramos L, Olivier F, Delke I, Kaunitz AM: Labor induction versus expectant management for postterm pregnancies: a systematic review with meta-analysis. Obstet Gynecol 101:1312, 2003.
62. Bishop EH: Pelvic scoring for elective induction. Obstet Gynecol 24:266, 1964.
63. Calder AA, Brennand JE: Labor and normal delivery: Induction of labor. Curr Opin Obstet Gynecol 3:764, 1991.
64. Arulkumaran S, Gibb DM, TambyRaja RL, et al: Failed induction of labour. Aust N Z J Obstet Gynaecol 25:190, 1985.
65. Xenakis EM, Piper JM, Conway DL, Langer O: Induction of labor in the nineties: conquering the unfavorable cervix. Obstet Gynecol 90:235, 1997.
66. Johnson DP, Davis NR, Brown AJ: Risk of cesarean delivery after induction at term in nulliparous women with an unfavorable cervix. Am J Obstet Gynecol 188:1565, 2003.
67. Kelly AJ, Tan B: Intravenous oxytocin alone for cervical ripening and induction of labour. Cochrane Database Syst Rev 3: CD003246, 2001.
68. Fuchs AR, Fuchs F, Husslein P, Soloff MS: Oxytocin receptors in the human uterus during pregnancy and parturition. Am J Obstet Gynecol 150:734, 1984.
69. Caldeyro-barcia R, Sereno JA: The response of human uterus to oxytocin throughout pregnancy. London, Pergamon Press, 1959.
70. Ryden G, Sjoholm I: The metabolism of oxytocin in pregnant and non-pregnant women. Acta Obstet Gynecol Scand Suppl 9(Suppl):37, 1971.
71. Seitchik J, Amico J, Robinson AG, Castillo M: Oxytocin augmentation of dysfunctional labor. IV. Oxytocin pharmacokinetics. Am J Obstet Gynecol 150:225, 1984.
72. Lyndrup J, Legarth J, Dahl C, et al: Induction of labour: the effect of vaginal prostaglandin or i.v. oxytocin—a matter of time only? Eur J Obstet Gynecol Reprod Biol 37:111, 1990.
73. Pollnow DM, Broekhuizen FF: Randomized, double-blind trial of prostaglandin E2 intravaginal gel versus low-dose oxytocin for cervical ripening before induction of labor. Am J Obstet Gynecol 174:1910, 1996.
74. Tan BP, Hannah ME: Oxytocin for prelabour rupture of membranes at or near term. Cochrane Database Syst Rev 2:CD000157, 2000.
75. Hannah ME, Huh C, Hewson SA, Hannah WJ: Postterm pregnancy: putting the merits of a policy of induction of labor into perspective. Birth 23:13, 1996.
76. Tan BP, Hannah ME: Prostaglandins versus oxytocin for prelabour rupture of membranes at or near term. Cochrane Database Syst Rev 2:CD000158, 2000.
77. Tan BP, Hannah ME: Prostaglandins for prelabour rupture of membranes at or near term. Cochrane Database Syst Rev 2: CD000178, 2000.
78. Hannah ME, Ohlsson A, Farine D, et al: Induction of labor compared with expectant management for prelabor rupture of the membranes at term. TERMPROM Study Group. N Engl J Med 334:1005, 1996.
79. Duff, P: Premature rupture of the membranes at term. N Engl J Med 334:1053, 1996.
80. Blakemore KJ, Qin NG, Petrie RH, Paine LL: A prospective comparison of hourly and quarter-hourly oxytocin dose increase intervals for the induction of labor at term. Obstet Gynecol 75:757, 1990.
81. O'Driscoll K, Foley M, MacDonald D: Active management of labor as an alternative to cesarean section for dystocia. Obstet Gynecol 63:485, 1984.
82. Willcourt RJ, Pager D, Wendel J, Hale RW: Induction of labor with pulsatile oxytocin by a computer-controlled pump. Am J Obstet Gynecol 170:603, 1994.
83. Odem RR, Work BA Jr, Dawood MY: Pulsatile oxytocin for induction of labor: a randomized prospective controlled study. J Perinat Med 16:31, 1988.
84. Xenakis EM, Langer O, Piper JM, et al: Low-dose versus high-dose oxytocin augmentation of labor–a randomized trial. Am J Obstet Gynecol 173:1874, 1995.
85. Satin AJ, Leveno KJ, Sherman ML, et al: High- versus low-dose oxytocin for labor stimulation. Obstet Gynecol 80:111, 1992.
86. Merrill DC, Zlatnik FJ: Randomized, double-masked comparison of oxytocin dosage in induction and augmentation of labor. Obstet Gynecol 94:455, 1999.
87. Orhue AA: A randomised trial of 45 minutes and 15 minutes incremental oxytocin infusion regimes for the induction of labour in women of high parity. Br J Obstet Gynaecol 100:126, 1993.
88. Orhue AA: A randomized trial of 30-min and 15-min oxytocin infusion regimen for induction of labor at term in women of low parity. Int J Gynaecol Obstet 40:219, 1993.
89. Satin AJ, Leveno KJ, Sherman ML, McIntire D: High-dose oxytocin: 20- versus 40-minute dosage interval. Obstet Gynecol 83:234, 1994.
90. Rayburn WF, Lightfoot SA, Newland JR, et al: A model for investigating microscopic changes induced by prostaglandin E2 in the term cervix. J Mat Fet Invest 4:137, 1994.
91. Prins RP, Neilson DR Jr, Bolton RN, et al: Preinduction cervical ripening with sequential use of prostaglandin E_2 gel. Am J Obstet Gynecol 154:1275, 1986.
92. Keirse MJ: Prostaglandins in preinduction cervical ripening. Meta-analysis of worldwide clinical experience. J Reprod Med 38(1 Suppl):89, 1993.
93. Kelly AJ, Kavanagh J, Thomas J: Vaginal prostaglandin (PGE2 and PGF2a) for induction of labour at term. Cochrane Database Syst Rev 2:CD003101, 2001.
94. Wing DA, Lovett K, Paul RH: Disruption of prior uterine incision following misoprostol for labor induction in women with previous cesarean delivery. Obstet Gynecol 91:828, 1998.
95. Lydon-Rochelle M, Holt VL, Easterling TR, Martin DP: Risk of uterine rupture during labor among women with a prior cesarean delivery. N Engl J Med 345:3, 2001.
96. Liggins GC: Controlled trial of induction of labor by vaginal suppositories containing prostaglandin E_2. Prostaglandins 18:167, 1979.
97. Rayburn WF: Prostaglandin E_2 gel for cervical ripening and induction of labor: a critical analysis. Am J Obstet Gynecol 160:529, 1989.
98. Kelly AJ, Kavanagh J, Thomas J: Vaginal prostaglandin (PGE2 and PGF2a) for induction of labour at term. Cochrane Database Syst Rev 4:CD003101, 2003.
99. Perryman D, Yeast JD, Holst V: Cervical ripening: a randomized study comparing prostaglandin E_2 gel to prostaglandin E_2 suppositories. Obstet Gynecol 79:670, 1992.
100. Smith CV, Rayburn WF, Connor RE, et al: Double-blind comparison of intravaginal prostaglandin E_2 gel and "chip" for preinduction cervical ripening. Am J Obstet Gynecol 163:845, 1990.
101. Rayburn WF, Wapner RJ, Barss VA, et al: An intravaginal controlled-release prostaglandin E_2 pessary for cervical ripening and initiation of labor at term. Obstet Gynecol 79:374, 1992.
102. Red book: pharmacy's fundamental reference.(2004) Montvale, NJ: Thomson PDR.
103. ACOG Committee Opinion: Number 283, May 2003. New U.S. Food and Drug Administration labeling on Cytotec (misoprostol) use and pregnancy. Obstet Gynecol 101:1049, 2003.
104. Chuck FJ, Huffaker BJ: Labor induction with intravaginal misoprostol versus intracervical prostaglandin E_2 gel (Prepidil gel): randomized comparison. Am J Obstet Gynecol 173:1137, 1995.

105. Varaklis K, Gumina R, Stubblefield PG: Randomized controlled trial of vaginal misoprostol and intracervical prostaglandin E_2 gel for induction of labor at term. Obstet Gynecol 86:541, 1995.
106. Wing DA, Rahall A, Jones MM, et al: Misoprostol: an effective agent for cervical ripening and labor induction. Am J Obstet Gynecol 172:1811, 1995.
107. Wing DA, Jones MM, Rahall A, et al: A comparison of misoprostol and prostaglandin E_2 gel for preinduction cervical ripening and labor induction. Am J Obstet Gynecol 172:1804, 1995.
108. Sanchez-Ramos L, Peterson DE, Delke I, et al: Labor induction with prostaglandin E_1 misoprostol compared with dinoprostone vaginal insert: a randomized trial. Obstet Gynecol 91:401 1998.
109. Hofmeyr GJ, Gulmezoglu AM: Vaginal misoprostol for cervical ripening and induction of labour. Cochrane Database Syst Rev 1: CD000941, 2003.
110. Induction of Labor with Misoprostol. ACOG Committee Opinion #228 November, 1999.
111. Sanchez-Ramos L, Kaunitz AM, Wears RL, et al: Misoprostol for cervical ripening and labor induction: a meta-analysis. Obstet Gynecol 89:633, 1997.
112. Farah LA, Sanchez-Ramos L, Rosa C, et al: Randomized trial of two doses of the prostaglandin E_1 analog misoprostol for labor induction. Am J Obstet Gynecol 177:364, 1997.
113. Sanchez-Ramos L, Kaunitz AM, Delke I: Labor induction with 25 microg versus 50 microg intravaginal misoprostol: a systematic review. Obstet Gynecol 99:145, 2002.
114. Response to Searl's drug warning on misoprostol. ACOG committee opinion #243, 2000.
115. Wing DA, Ham D, Paul RH: A comparison of orally administered misoprostol with vaginally administered misoprostol for cervical ripening and labor induction. Am J Obstet Gynecol 180:1155,1999.
116. Ngai SW, To WK, Lao T, Ho PC: Cervical priming with oral misoprostol in pre-labor rupture of membranes at term. Obstet Gynecol 87:923, 1996.
117. Windrim R, Bennett K, Mundle W, Young DC: Oral administration of misoprostol for labor induction: a randomized controlled trial. Obstet Gynecol 89:392, 1997.
118. Toppozada MK, Anwar MY, Hassan HA, el-Gazaerly WS: Oral or vaginal misoprostol for induction of labor. Int J Gynaecol Obstet 56:135, 1997.
119. Bennett KA, Butt K, Crane JM, et al: A masked randomized comparison of oral and vaginal administration of misoprostol for labor induction. Obstet Gynecol 92:481, 1998.
120. Adair CD, Weeks JW, Barrilleaux S, et al: Oral or vaginal misoprostol administration for induction of labor: a randomized, double-blind trial. Obstet Gynecol 92:810, 1998.
121. le Roux PA, Olarogun JO, Penny J, Anthony J: Oral and vaginal misoprostol compared with dinoprostone for induction of labor: a randomized controlled trial. Obstet Gynecol 99:201, 2002.
122. Hofmeyr GJ, Alfirevic Z, Matonhodze B, et al: Titrated oral misoprostol solution for induction of labour: a multi-centre, randomised trial. Br J Obstet Gynaecol 108:952, 2001.
123. Alfirevic Z: Oral misoprostol for induction of labour. Cochrane Database Syst Rev 2:CD001338, 2001.
124. Wing DA, Park MR, Paul RH: A randomized comparison of oral and intravaginal misoprostol for labor induction. Obstet Gynecol 95:905, 2000.
125. Dallenbach P, Boulvain M, Viardot C, Irion O: Oral misoprostol or vaginal dinoprostone for labor induction: a randomized controlled trial. Am J Obstet Gynecol 188:162, 2003.
126. Tang OS, Schweer H, Seyberth HW, et al: Pharmacokinetics of different routes of administration of misoprostol. Hum Reprod 17:332, 2002.
127. Shetty A, Mackie L, Danielian P, et al: Sublingual compared with oral misoprostol in term labour induction: a randomised controlled trial. Br J Obstet Gynaecol 109:645, 2002.
128. Carlan SJ, Blust D, O'Brien WF: Buccal versus intravaginal misoprostol administration for cervical ripening. Am J Obstet Gynecol 186:229, 2002.
129. Frydman R, Lelaidier C, Baton-Saint-Mleux C, et al: Labor induction in women at term with mifepristone (RU 486): a double-blind, randomized, placebo-controlled study. Obstet Gynecol 80:972, 1992.
130. Giacalone PL, Targosz V, Laffargue F, et al: Cervical ripening with mifepristone before labor induction: a randomized study. Obstet Gynecol 92:487, 1998.
131. Wing DA, Fassett MJ, Mishell DR: Mifepristone for preinduction cervical ripening beyond 41 weeks' gestation: a randomized controlled trial. Obstet Gynecol 96:543, 2000.
132. Stenlund PM, Ekman G, Aedo AR, Bygdeman M: Induction of labor with mifepristone—a randomized, double-blind study versus placebo. Acta Obstet Gynecol Scand 78:793, 1999.
133. Elliott CL, Brennand JE, Calder AA: The effects of mifepristone on cervical ripening and labor induction in primigravidae. Obstet Gynecol 92:804, 1998.
134. Neilson JP: Mifepristone for induction of labour. Cochrane Database Syst Rev 4:CD002865, 2000.
135. Klopper AI, Dennis KJ: Effect of oestrogens on myometrial contractions. Br Med J 5313:1157, 1962.
136. Pinto RM, Rabow W, Vtta RA: Uterine cervix ripening in term pregnancy due to the action of estradiol-17-beta. A histological and histochemical study. Am J Obstet Gynecol 92:319, 1965.
137. Magann EF, Perry KG Jr, Dockery JR Jr, et al: Cervical ripening before medical induction of labor: a comparison of prostaglandin E_2, estradiol, and oxytocin. Am J Obstet Gynecol 172:1702, 1995.
138. Peedicayil A, Jasper P, Balasubramaniam N, Jairaj P: A randomized controlled trial of extra-amniotic ethinyloestradiol in ripening the cervix at term. Br J Obstet Gynaecol 96:973, 1989.
139. Quinn MA, Murphy AJ, Kuhn RJ, et al: A double blind trial of extra-amniotic oestriol and prostaglandin F_2 alpha gels in cervical ripening. Br J Obstet Gynaecol 88:644, 1981.
140. Tromans PM, Beazley J, Shenouda PI: Comparative study of oestradiol and prostaglandin E_2 vaginal gel for ripening the unfavourable cervix before induction of labour. Br Med J (Clin Res Ed) 282:679, 1981.
141. Thomas J, Kelly AJ, Kavanagh J: Oestrogens alone or with amniotomy for cervical ripening or induction of labour. Cochrane Database Syst Rev 4:CD003393, 2001.
142. MacLennan AH, Green RC, Bryant-Greenwood GD, et al: Ripening of the human cervix and induction of labour with purified porcine relaxin. Lancet 1:220, 1980.
143. MacLennan AH, Green RC, Grant P, Nicolson R: Ripening of the human cervix and induction of labor with intracervical purified porcine relaxin. Obstet Gynecol 68:598, 1986.
144. Evans MI, Dougan MB, Moawad AH, et al: Ripening of the human cervix with porcine ovarian relaxin. Am J Obstet Gynecol 147:410, 1983.
145. Brennand JE, Calder AA, Leitch CR, et al: Recombinant human relaxin as a cervical ripening agent. Br J Obstet Gynaecol 104:775, 1997.
146. Bell RJ, Permezel M, MacLennan A, et al: A randomized, double-blind, placebo-controlled trial of the safety of vaginal recombinant human relaxin for cervical ripening. Obstet Gynecol 82:328, 1993.
147. Kelly AJ, Kavanagh J, Thomas J: Relaxin for cervical ripening and induction of labour. Cochrane Database Syst Rev 2: CD0031032001.
148. Kobayashi H, Sun GW, Tanaka Y, et al: Serum hyaluronic acid levels during pregnancy and labor. Obstet Gynecol 93:480, 1999.
149. Kavanagh J, Kelly AJ, Thomas J: Hyaluronidase for cervical priming and induction of labour. Cochrane Database Syst Rev 2:CD003097, 2001.
150. Boulvain M, Kelly A, Lohse C, et al: Mechanical methods for induction of labour. Cochrane Database Syst Rev 4:CD001233, 2001.
151. Kerr JM: Historical Review of British Obstetrics and Gynaecology, 1800–1950. London, E & S Livingston, 1954.
152. McColgin SW, Bennett WA, Roach H, et al: Parturitional factors associated with membrane stripping. Am J Obstet Gynecol 169:71, 1993.
153. Mitchell MD, Flint AP, Bibby J, et al: Rapid increases in plasma prostaglandin concentrations after vaginal examination and amniotomy. Br Med J 2:1183, 1977.
154. Berghella V, Rogers RA, Lescale K: Stripping of membranes as a safe method to reduce prolonged pregnancies. Obstet Gynecol 87:927, 1996.

155. Cammu H, Haitsma V: Sweeping of the membranes at 39 weeks in nulliparous women: a randomised controlled trial. Br J Obstet Gynaecol 105:41, 1998.
156. Wiriyasirivaj B, Vutyavanich T, Ruangsri RA: A randomized controlled trial of membrane stripping at term to promote labor. Obstet Gynecol 87:767, 1996.
157. Crane J, Bennett K, Young D, et al: The effectiveness of sweeping membranes at term: a randomized trial. Obstet Gynecol 89:586, 1997.
158. McColgin SW, Hampton HL, McCaul JF, et al: Stripping membranes at term: can it safely reduce the incidence of post-term pregnancies? Obstet Gynecol 76:678, 1990.
159. McColgin SW, Patrissi GA, Morrison JC: Stripping the fetal membranes at term. Is the procedure safe and efficacious? J Reprod Med 35:811, 1990.
160. Allott HA, Palmer CR: Sweeping the membranes: a valid procedure in stimulating the onset of labour? Br J Obstet Gynaecol 100:898, 1993.
161. Boulvain M, Fraser WD, Marcoux S, et al: Does sweeping of the membranes reduce the need for formal induction of labour? A randomised controlled trial. Br J Obstet Gynaecol 105:34, 1998.
162. Boulvain M, Irion O, Marcoux S, Fraser W: Sweeping of the membranes to prevent post-term pregnancy and to induce labour: a systematic review. Br J Obstet Gynaecol 106:481, 1999.
163. Boulvain M, Stan C, Irion O: Membrane sweeping for induction of labour. Cochrane Database Syst Rev 2:CD000451, 2001.
164. Schrag S, Gorwitz R, Fultz-Butts K, Schuchat A: (2005) Prevention of perinatal group B streptococcal disease: Revised guidelines from CDC. MMWR 51[RR11]:1, 2002.
165. Booth JH, Kurdyak VB: Elective induction of labour: a controlled study. Can Med Assoc J 103:245, 1970.
166. Howarth GR, Botha DJ: Amniotomy plus intravenous oxytocin for induction of labour. Cochrane Database Syst Rev 3: CD003250, 2001.
167. Fraser WD, Marcoux S, Moutquin JM, Christen A: Effect of early amniotomy on the risk of dystocia in nulliparous women. The Canadian Early Amniotomy Study Group. N Engl J Med 328:1145, 1993.
168. Moldin PG, Sundell G: Induction of labour: a randomised clinical trial of amniotomy versus amniotomy with oxytocin infusion. Br J Obstet Gynaecol 103:306, 1996.
169. Kennedy JH, Stewart P, Barlow DH: Induction of labour: a comparison of a single prostaglandin E_2 vaginal tablet with amniotomy and intravenous oxytocin. Br J Obstet Gynaecol 89:704, 1982.
170. Orhue AA: Induction of labour at term in primigravidae with low Bishop's score: a comparison of three methods. Eur J Obstet Gynecol Reprod Biol 58:119, 1995.
171. Sanchez-Ramos L, Kaunitz AM, Connor PM: Hygroscopic cervical dilators and prostaglandin E_2 gel for preinduction cervical ripening. A randomized, prospective comparison. J Reprod Med 37:355, 1992.
172. St Onge RD, Connors GT: Preinduction cervical ripening: a comparison of intracervical prostaglandin E_2 gel versus the Foley catheter. Am J Obstet Gynecol 172:687, 1995.
173. Sciscione AC, Nguyen L, Manley J, et al: A randomized comparison of transcervical Foley catheter to intravaginal misoprostol for preinduction cervical ripening. Obstet Gynecol 97:603, 2001.
174. Chung JH, Huang WH, Rumney PJ, et al: A prospective randomized controlled trial that compared misoprostol, Foley catheter, and combination misoprostol-Foley catheter for labor induction. Am J Obstet Gynecol 189:1031, 2003.
175. Perry KG Jr, Larmon JE, May WL, et al: Cervical ripening: a randomized comparison between intravaginal misoprostol and an intracervical balloon catheter combined with intravaginal dinoprostone. Am J Obstet Gynecol 178:1333, 1998.
176. Sciscione A, Larkin M, O'Shea A, et al: Preinduction cervical ripening with the Foley catheter and the risk of subsequent preterm birth. Am J Obstet Gynecol 190:751, 2004.
177. Vengalil SR, Guinn DA, Olabi NF, et al: A randomized trial of misoprostol and extra-amniotic saline infusion for cervical ripening and labor induction. Obstet Gynecol 91:774, 1998.
178. Buccellato CA, Stika CS, Frederiksen MCL: A randomized trial of misoprostol versus extra-amniotic sodium chloride infusion with oxytocin for induction of labor. Am J Obstet Gynecol 182:1039, 2000.
179. Mullin PM, House M, Paul RH, Wing DA: A comparison of vaginally administered misoprostol with extra-amniotic saline solution infusion for cervical ripening and labor induction. Am J Obstet Gynecol 187:847, 2002.
180. Atad J, Bornstein J, Calderon I, et al: Nonpharmaceutical ripening of the unfavorable cervix and induction of labor by a novel double balloon device. Obstet Gynecol 77:146, 1991.
181. Atad J, Hallak M, Auslender R, et al: A randomized comparison of prostaglandin E_2, oxytocin, and the double-balloon device in inducing labor. Obstet Gynecol 87:223, 1996.
182. Atad J, Hallak M, Ben-David Y, et al: Ripening and dilatation of the unfavourable cervix for induction of labour by a double balloon device: experience with 250 cases. Br J Obstet Gynaecol 104:29, 1997.
183. Lyndrup J, Nickelsen C, Weber T, et al: Induction of labour by balloon catheter with extra-amniotic saline infusion (BCEAS): a randomised comparison with PGE2 vaginal pessaries. Eur J Obstet Gynecol Reprod Biol 53:189, 1994.
184. Guinn DA, Davies JK, Jones RO, et al: Labor induction in women with an unfavorable Bishop score: randomized controlled trial of intrauterine Foley catheter with concurrent oxytocin infusion versus Foley catheter with extra-amniotic saline infusion with concurrent oxytocin infusion. Am J Obstet Gynecol 191:225, 2004.
185. Ahner R, Egarter C, Kiss H, et al: Fetal fibronectin as a selection criterion for induction of term labor. Am J Obstet Gynecol 173:1513, 1995.
186. Lockwood CJ, Moscarelli RD, Wein R, et al: Low concentrations of vaginal fetal fibronectin as a predictor of deliveries occurring after 41 weeks. Am J Obstet Gynecol 171:1, 1994.
187. Pandis GK, Papageorghiou AT, Ramanathan VG, et al: Preinduction sonographic measurement of cervical length in the prediction of successful induction of labor. Ultrasound Obstet Gynecol 18:623, 2001.
188. Chandra S, Crane JM, Hutchens D, Young DC: Transvaginal ultrasound and digital examination in predicting successful labor induction. Obstet Gynecol 98:2, 2001.
189. Blanch G, Olah KS, Walkinshaw S: The presence of fetal fibronectin in the cervicovaginal secretions of women at term—its role in the assessment of women before labor induction and in the investigation of the physiologic mechanisms of labor. Am J Obstet Gynecol 174:262, 1996.
190. Kiss H, Ahner R, Hohlagschwandtner M, et al: Fetal fibronectin as a predictor of term labor: a literature review. Acta Obstet Gynecol Scand 79:3, 2000.
191. Tam WH, Tai SM, Rogers MS: Prediction of cervical response to prostaglandin E2 using fetal fibronectin. Acta Obstet Gynecol Scand 78:861, 1999.
192. Ojutiku D, Jones G, Bewley S: Quantitative foetal fibronectin as a predictor of successful induction of labour in post-date pregnancies. Eur J Obstet Gynecol Reprod Biol 101:143, 2002.
193. Garite TJ, Casal D, Garcia-Alonso A, et al: Fetal fibronectin: a new tool for the prediction of successful induction of labor. Am J Obstet Gynecol 175:1516, 1996.
194. Reis FM, Gervasi MT, Florio P, et al: Prediction of successful induction of labor at term: role of clinical history, digital examination, ultrasound assessment of the cervix, and fetal fibronectin assay. Am J Obstet Gynecol 189:1361, 2003.
195. Bailit JL, Downs SM, Thorp JM: Reducing the caesarean delivery risk in elective inductions of labour: a decision analysis. Paediatr Perinat Epidemiol 16:96, 2002.
196. Curtis P, Evens S, Resnick J: Uterine hyperstimulation. The need for standard terminology. J Reprod Med 32:91, 1987.
197. Whalley PJ, Pritchard JA: Oxytocin and water intoxication. JAMA 186:601, 1963.
198. Weis FR Jr, Markello R, Mo B, Bochiechio P: Cardiovascular effects of oxytocin. Obstet Gynecol 46:211, 1975.
199. Davies GA, Tessier JL, Woodman MC, et al: Maternal hemodynamics after oxytocin bolus compared with infusion in the third stage of labor: a randomized controlled trial. Obstet Gynecol 105:294, 2005.

200. Goetzl L, Shipp TD, Cohen A, et al: Oxytocin dose and the risk of uterine rupture in trial of labor after cesarean. Obstet Gynecol 97:381, 2001.
201. Sanchez-Ramos L, Gaudier FL, Kaunitz AM: Cervical ripening and labor induction after previous cesarean delivery. Obstet Gynecol 43:513, 2000.
202. Zelop CM, Shipp TD, Repke JT, et al: Uterine rupture during induced or augmented labor in gravid women with one prior cesarean delivery. Am J Obstet Gynecol 181:882, 1999.
203. Locatelli A, Regalia AL, Ghidini A, et al: Risks of induction of labour in women with a uterine scar from previous low transverse cesarean section. Br J Obstet Gynaecol 111:1394, 2004.
204. Induction of labor for vaginal birth after cesarean delivery. ACOG Committee Opinion No. 271. American College of Obstetricians and Gynecologists. Obstet Gynecol 99:679, 2002.
205. Rodriguez MH, Masaki DI, Phelan JP, Diaz FG: Uterine rupture: are intrauterine pressure catheters useful in the diagnosis? Am J Obstet Gynecol 161:666, 1989.
206. Devoe LD, Croom CS, Youssef AA, Murray C: The prediction of "controlled" uterine rupture by use of the intrauterine pressure catheters. Obstet Gynecol 80:626, 1992.
207. Ouzounian JG, Miller DA, Paul RH: Amnioinfusion in women with previous cesarean births: a preliminary report. Am J Obstet Gynecol 174:783, 1996.

Operative Vaginal Delivery

PETER E. NIELSEN, HENRY L. GALAN, SARAH KILPATRICK, AND ETOI GARRISON

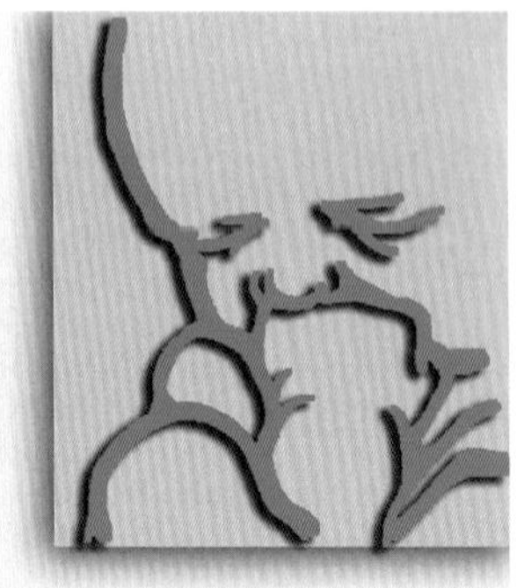

CHAPTER 14

KEY ABBREVIATIONS

American College of Obstetricians and Gynecologists	ACOG
Biparietal diameter	BPD
Confidence interval	CI
Food and Drug Administration	FDA
Intracranial hemorrhage	ICH
Intelligence quotient	IQ
Left occiput anterior	LOA
Left occiput posterior	LOP
Maternal fetal	MF
Neonatal intensive care unit	NICU
Occiput anterior	OA
Occiput posterior	OP
Occiput transverse	OT
Odds ratio	OR
Relative risk	RR
Right occiput anterior	ROA

INTRODUCTION

Obstetric forceps are the one instrument that makes the practice of obstetric care unique to obstetricians. The proper use of these instruments has afforded safe and timely vaginal delivery to those whose abnormal labor course and/or urgent need for delivery required their use. Following the introduction of forceps by Chamberlin during the 1600s, much discussion about the proper use and timing of forceps application ensued. Following Smellie's retirement from practice in 1760, forceps began to be used very frequently, resulting in an increase in both maternal and neonatal injury owing to the application techniques used at the time. In his 1788 text entitled "An Introduction to the Practice of Midwifery," Thomas Denman stated that ". . . the head of the child shall have rested for 6 hours as low as the perineum before the forceps are applied though the pains should have ceased during that time".[1] Denman's Law then became widely accepted as the standard of this time. However, after the news of Princess Charlotte's death following the birth of a stillborn Prince on November 6, 1817, a review of Denman's Law ensued with much public discussion regarding the timely use of forceps. Princess Charlotte's labor had been managed by one of Denman's students and son-in-law, Sir Richard Croft, whose second-stage labor management during this delivery came into question. Croft had permitted the second stage to last 24 hours, including 6 hours on the perineum, as Denman's Law had advised. However, the Princess delivered a 9 pound stillborn male heir, and within 24 hours of delivery the Princess herself died of a massive postpartum hemorrhage. Disturbed with depression and despair at the blame for the death of both the Princess and the heir to the British throne, Croft shot himself three months later. During a lecture delivered at the Royal College of Obstetricians and Gynaecologists on September 28, 1951, Sir Eardley Holland named his lecture on these events "A Triple Obstetric Tragedy" in which he described a mother, baby and accoucheur all dead, victims of a mistaken system.[2] In a subsequent text in 1817, Denman wrote: "Care is also to be taken that we do not, through an aversion to the use of instruments, too long delay that assistance we have the power of affording them".[3] The debate regarding the use of these instruments continued into the 20th century, with prophylactic forceps delivery advocated by DeLee in 1920.[4] This clinical management strategy resulted in forceps delivery rates in excess of 65 percent by 1950.

With these lessons in mind, a review of operative vaginal delivery in modern obstetric practice is extremely important and timely. Rates of cesarean delivery have risen in both the United States and the United Kingdom,[5,6] reaching a rate of approximately 25 percent of all deliveries in the United States, whereas rates of forceps delivery have declined from 17.7 percent in 1980 to 4 percent in 2000[5] in the United States, and from 8.6 percent in 1989 to 6.2 percent in 1993 in the United Kingdom.[7] Conversely, the rate of vacuum-assisted vaginal delivery more than doubled in the United States between 1980 and 2000 to 8.4 percent.[4] Most residency training programs in the United States still expect proficiency in outlet and low forceps (less than or greater than 45-degree rotation), whereas less than 40 percent expect proficiency in midforceps delivery.[8] However, to make education and teaching of these procedures even more challenging, new resident work hour restrictions have resulted in a decline in resident experience with both primary cesarean delivery and vacuum-assisted vaginal delivery, despite increased institutional volumes of these procedures. In a study by Blanchard,[9] the decrease in experience with these procedures has been dramatic, noting a 54-percent decline in experience with primary cesarean delivery and a 56-percent decline in vacuum-assisted vaginal delivery. Because both forceps and vacuum extractors are acceptable and safe instruments for operative vaginal delivery, operator experience is the determining factor in which instrument should be used in a specific clinical situation.[10] Declining use and resident experience may make it difficult to provide the level of operator experience required for proficiency of this obstetric art. However, because most women prefer a vaginal delivery, focused experience with the use of these instruments during residency training is crucial to ensure safe, timely, and effective vaginal delivery because women are more likely to achieve a spontaneous vaginal delivery in a subsequent pregnancy after forceps delivery than after cesarean delivery (78 versus 31 percent).[11–14] The challenge, therefore, is to ensure that women who experience second-stage labor abnormalities are afforded options for safe and timely delivery.

OPERATIVE VAGINAL DELIVERY

Classification, Prerequisites and Indications

The use of a well-defined and consistent classification system for operative vaginal deliveries makes comparison of maternal and neonatal outcomes among spontaneous delivery, cesarean delivery, and operative vaginal delivery as well as instruction in these techniques easier. It is intuitive that not all operative vaginal deliveries are the same with respect to degree of difficulty or maternal and fetal risk. Therefore, classification systems have been developed and modified over time. In 1949, Titus created a classification system that permitted general practitioners to perform operative vaginal delivery without consultation from a specialist.[15] This system divided the pelvis into thirds from the spines to the inlet and, in the opposite direction, in thirds to the outlet. Dennen proposed an alternative classification system in 1952 that was based on the four major obstetric planes of the pelvis with the following definitions: high forceps as the biparietal diameter (BPD) in the plane of the inlet, but above the ischial spines, midforceps as the BPD just at or below the ischial spines and the sacral hollow not filled, low-midforceps as the BPD below the ischial spines, the leading bony part within a fingerbreadth of the perineum between contractions and the hollow of the sacrum filled, and outlet as the BPD below the level of the ischial spines, the sagittal suture in the anteroposterior diameter and the head visible at the perineum during a contraction.[15]

In 1965, the American College of Obstetricians and Gynecologists (ACOG) created a classification system that defined midforceps extremely broadly (from the ischial spines to the pelvic floor and any rotation). This category clearly included many forceps operations that ranged from delivery of a straightforward anteroposterior position of the fetal vertex to complex rotations.[16] The broad category for these operations lead many practicing clinicians to question whether the classification should be narrowed to reflect the clinically significant differences between deliveries such as these. Therefore, in 1988, ACOG revised the classification of forceps operations to address two significant shortcomings of the previous system, that midforceps was too widely defined and outlet forceps too narrowly defined.[17] This system was validated in 1991 by Hagadorn-Freathy,[18] demonstrating that 25 percent of deliveries in this study that would have been previously classified as midforceps (but were reclassified into the low-forceps [>45-degree] rotation and midforceps categories) were associated with 41 percent of episiotomy extensions and 50 percent of the lacerations in the cohort. Clearly the outcomes of these operations confounded the relatively low-risk group of low-forceps operations with up to 45-degree rotation (which would also have been classified as midforceps by the previous system). In short, these investigators validated the 1988 ACOG classification scheme by demonstrating that the higher station and more complex deliveries carried a greater risk of maternal and fetal injury compared with those that were more straightforward. This differentiation was lost in the 1965 classification scheme owing to the broad definition of low forceps. It is extremely important to appropriately classify operative vaginal delivery based on this system, including accurate determination of fetal station and position.

With respect to operative vaginal delivery of the vertex, station is defined as the relationship of the estimated distance, in centimeters, between the leading bony portion of the fetal head and the level of the maternal ischial spines, and position refers to the relationship of the occiput to a denominating location on the maternal pelvis. Operative vaginal delivery with a fetus in the left occiput anterior (LOA) position, with the leading bony portion of the

Table 14-1. Prerequisites for Forceps or Vacuum Extractor Application

Engaged fetal vertex
Ruptured membranes
Fully dilated cervix
Position is precisely known
Assessment of maternal pelvis reveals adequacy for the estimated fetal weight
Adequate maternal analgesia is available
Bladder drained
Knowledgeable operator
Willingness to abandon the procedure, if necessary
Informed consent has been obtained
Necessary support personnel and equipment are present

vertex 3 cm below the ischial spines (+3 station) would be classified as a low forceps, less than 45-degree rotation delivery. It is also important to note that this classification system applies to both forceps and vacuum extraction instruments, and that the precise position and station must be known before the placement of either instrument.

In addition to precise evaluation of the position and station, several other extremely important data are necessary before performing operative vaginal delivery. The prerequisites for application of either forceps or vacuum extractor are listed in Table 14-1. When these prerequisites have been met, the following indications are appropriate for consideration of either forceps delivery or vacuum extraction:

- Prolonged second stage
  - Nulliparous women: lack of continuing progress for 3 hours with regional analgesia or 2 hours without regional analgesia
  - Multiparous women: lack of continuing progress for 2 hours with regional analgesia or 1 hour without regional analgesia
- Suspicion of immediate or potential fetal compromise
- Nonreassuring fetal heart rate tracing
- Shortening of the second stage of labor for maternal benefit (i.e., maternal exhaustion, maternal cardiopulmonary or cerebrovascular disease)

OPERATIVE VAGINAL DELIVERY INSTRUMENTS

Forceps Instruments

Invention and modification have led to a description and use of more than 700 varieties of forceps instruments. Most of them are of historic interest only, but many common features remain among those still in use. Forceps are paired instruments, except when used at cesarean delivery and are broadly categorized according to their intended use: "classic" forceps, rotational forceps, and specialized forceps designed to assist vaginal breech deliveries. Each forceps type consists of two halves joined by a lock, which may be sliding or fixed. The key structures of forceps include the blade, shank, lock, finger guards, and handle (Fig. 14-1). The toe refers to the tip of the blade and the heel to the end of the blade that is attached to the shank at the posterior lip of the fenestration (if present). The cephalic curve is defined by the radius of the two blades when in opposition and the pelvic curve by the upward (or reverse as in the case of Kielland and Piper forceps) curve of the blades from the shank. The handles transmit the applied force, the screw or lock represent the fulcrum, and the blades transmit the load (Fig. 14-2).[19,20]

The pelvic curve permits ease of application along the maternal pelvic axis (see Fig. 14-2). Forceps have two functions, traction and rotation, both of which can only be accomplished by some degree of compression on the fetal head. The cephalic curvature of the blade is designed to aid in the even distribution of force about the fetal parietal bone and fetal malar eminence. Blades may be solid (Tucker-McLane), fenestrated (Simpson), or pseudofenestrated (Luikart-Simpson). The pseudofenestration modification can be applied to the design of any type of forceps and is known as the Luikart modification. In general, use of solid or pseudofenestrated blades results in less risk of maternal soft tissue injury, especially during rotation, but fenestrated blades provide improved traction in comparison to solid blades.

"Classic" Forceps

Classic forceps instruments are typically used when rotation of the vertex is not required for delivery. However, they may be used for rotations such as the Scanzoni-Smellie maneuver. All classic forceps have a cephalic curve, a pelvic curve, and an English lock, in which the articulation is fixed in a slot into which the shank of the opposite blade fits. The type of classic forceps instrument is determined by its shank, whether overlapping or parallel. Examples of classic forceps with parallel shanks include Simpson, DeLee, Irving, and Hawks-Dennen forceps. Classic forceps with overlapping shanks include Elliott and Tucker-McLane. Because these instruments have a more rounded cephalic curve than the Simpson forceps, they are often used for assisting delivery of the unmolded head, such as that commonly encountered in the multiparous patient. In addition, because the Tucker-McLane forceps have a shorter, solid blade and overlapping shanks, they are more often used for rotations than other classic instruments.

Rotational Forceps

Forceps instruments used for rotation are characterized as having a cephalic curve amenable to application to the molded vertex, and either only a slight pelvic curve or none at all. The absence of a pelvic curve in these instruments facilitates rotation of the vertex without moving the handles of the instrument through a wide arch, as is necessary when using one of the classic instruments to accomplish rotation. Forceps that may be used for rotation include some of the classic instruments (e.g., Tucker-McLane) and those with minimal pelvic curvature (e.g., Kielland and Leff). In 1916, Christian Kielland of Norway described the rationale for the introduction of his new forceps:

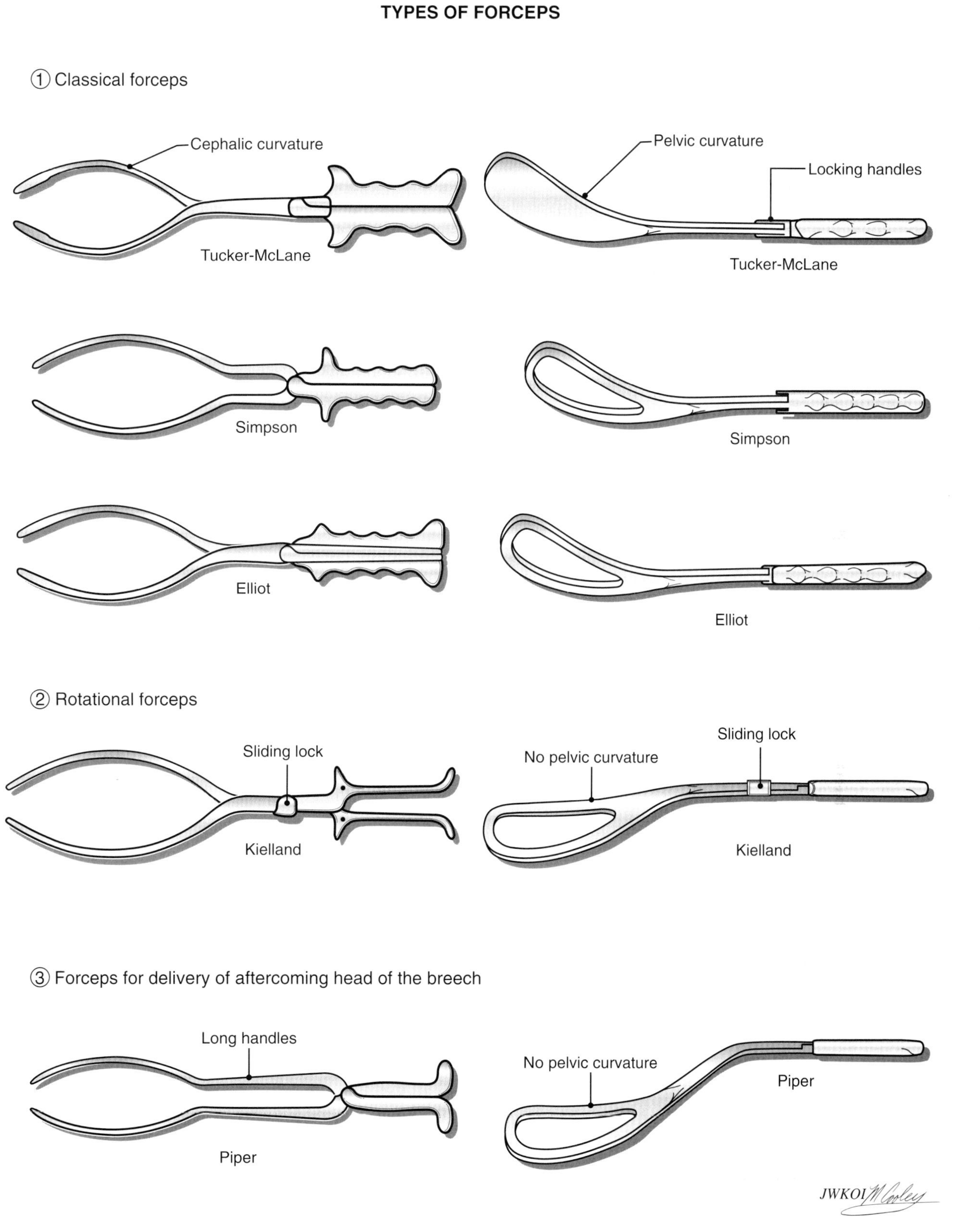

TYPES OF FORCEPS

① Classical forceps

Cephalic curvature

Tucker-McLane

Pelvic curvature

Locking handles

Tucker-McLane

Simpson

Simpson

Elliot

Elliot

② Rotational forceps

Sliding lock

Kielland

No pelvic curvature

Sliding lock

Kielland

③ Forceps for delivery of aftercoming head of the breech

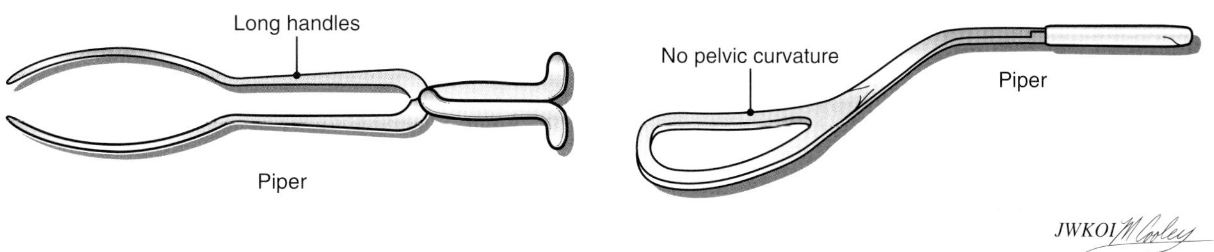

JWKO1/M Cooley

Figure 14-1. Classification of forceps.

When the head is high it has to be pulled through a greater length of the birth canal, which is incompletely prepared. The child's head is in such a position that it cannot be grasped by the blades of the forceps in the way which is possible when the head is low and completely rotated. The forceps do not hold the head in the biparietal diameter, but over the occipital and frontal areas which cannot withstand much pressure. These factors are responsible for the difficulties which occur in such a delivery, but they do not entirely explain the amount of force required nor the resistance which is encountered. In the search for an explanation of the chief cause for the remarkable amount

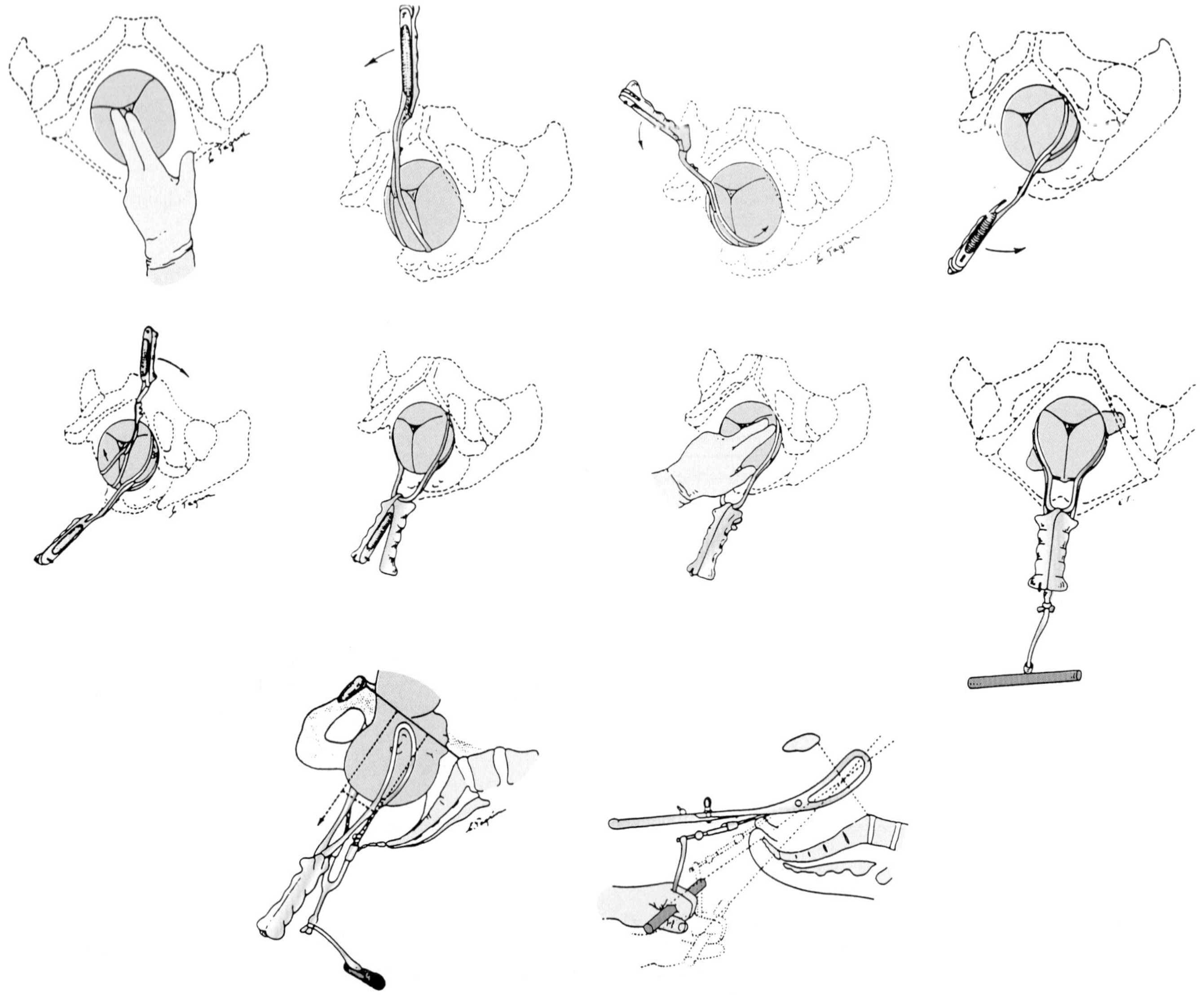

Figure 14-2. Stepwise approach to application of obstetric forceps.

of force, which had to be used, it was thought that traction might be in the wrong direction, because the blade of the ordinary forceps is curved to correspond with the birth canal. This type of forceps cannot be depressed sufficiently low against the perineum without the risk of damaging it or losing the good position on the fetal head when an attempt is made to exert traction in the pelvic axis.[21]

Following their introduction, Kielland forceps have become a frequently used instrument for rotation of the vertex (see Fig. 14-1). These forceps have a slightly backward pelvic curve with overlapping shanks and a sliding lock. The advantages of the Kielland forceps compared with the classic instruments for rotation include:

- A straight design that places the handle and shanks in the same plane as the long axis of the fetal head, permitting the toe to travel through a very small arch during rotation.
- The distance between the heel and the intersecting point of the shanks is long, which accommodates heads of various shapes and sizes associated with unusual molding.
- A slight degree of axis traction is produced by the reverse pelvic curve.
- The sliding lock permits placement of the handles at any level on the shank to accommodate the asynclitic head and subsequent correction of asynclitism.

In 1955, another forceps used for rotation of the vertex was introduced by Leff.[22] These forceps have a locking shank with short, straight and narrow blades and a smaller cephalic curve than the Kielland forceps. In a series of 104 consecutive rotational forceps deliveries (>90 degrees) using Leff forceps compared with 163 nonrotational forceps deliveries with traditional instruments, Feldman demonstrated a lower episiotomy (66 versus 82 percent) and perineal laceration rate (16 versus 23 percent) with the Leff forceps compared with the nonrotational forceps group, attributed to a 40 percent spontaneous vaginal delivery rate after Leff forceps rotation.[23] In addition, there was no difference in the low incidence of fetal bruising between the groups (3 percent in each). They concluded that Leff forceps were also a safe option for rotation of the persistent occipitoposterior fetal position.

Other Specialized Instruments

Forceps to assist with delivery of the aftercoming head during vaginal breech delivery (Piper forceps) have a cephalic curve, a reverse pelvic curve, long parallel shanks and an English lock (see Fig. 14-1). This design provides easy application to the aftercoming head, stabilizing and protecting the fetal head and neck during delivery. The long shanks permit the body of the breech to rest against it during delivery of the head.

Vacuum Extraction Devices

The Swedish obstetrician, Tage Malmstrom was credited with the introduction of the first successful vacuum cup into the field of modern obstetrics in 1953. It consisted of a metal cup, suction tubing, and a traction chain.[24,25] Vacuum devices are classified by the material used to make the cup: either stainless steel or plastic (silicone). Plastic ("soft") cups are used much more commonly in the United States than the stainless steel cups owing to the lower rates of scalp trauma associated with these devices.[26] These devices consist of the cup, which is connected to a handle grip and tubing that connects them both to a vacuum source (Fig. 14-3). The vacuum generated through this tubing attaches the fetal scalp to the cup and allows traction on the vertex. The vacuum force can be generated either from wall suction or by a hand-held device with a pumping mechanism.

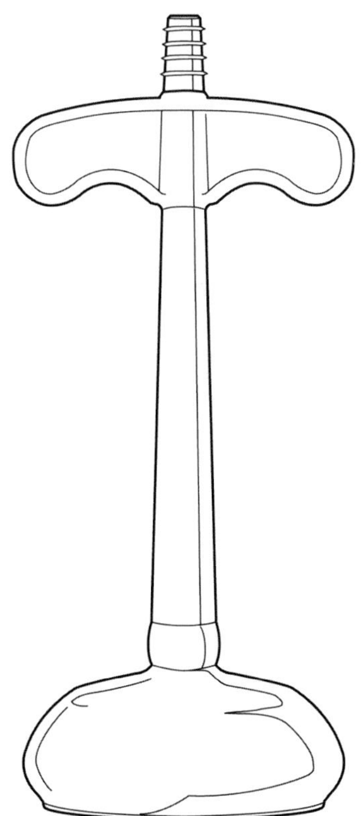

Figure 14-3. "M" style mushroom vacuum extractor cup with a centrally located stem and handle.

Stainless Steel Devices

The Malmstrom device is the most commonly used instrument for vacuum extraction in the world.[27] This device consists of a mushroom-shaped stainless steel cup, two vacuum hoses, a traction chain and attached metallic disk, a traction handle, and a vacuum source. The cup is available in 40-, 50-, and 60-mm diameter sizes and is designed such that the diameter of the opening is smaller than the internal diameter of the cup. Therefore, when vacuum is established, the fetal scalp fills the internal dimension of the cup and an artificial caput succedaneum is formed (the "chignon"). This allows for appropriate traction force to be applied to the vertex without a "pop off" or detachment.

Soft Cup Devices

These devices may be classified into three groups by the shape of the cup: funnel shaped, bell shaped and mushroom shaped (Figs. 14-4 and 14-5). The Kobayashi style funnel-shaped Silastic cup is the prototype and the largest cup available (65 mm). It was designed to fit over the fetal occiput without requiring formation of a chignon. This feature results in a lower rate of scalp trauma and more rapid time to effect delivery compared with the stainless steel devices but with a slightly higher failure rate owing to "pop off."[26,28] Bell-shaped cups are available from a number of vendors and include the following brands: Mityvac (Prism Enterprises, San Antonio, Texas), Kiwi (Clinical Innovations, Murray, Utah) and CMI (Utah Medical, Midvale, Utah). When compared with the funnel-shaped Silastic cups, these devices are easier to place owing to their smaller size and fail less often owing to loss of suction.[29] The mushroom-shaped cups are a hybrid of the stainless steel and plastic devices. Examples of these devices include the M-cup (Mityvac, Prism Enterprises, San Antonio, Texas), the Flex Cup (CMI, Utah Medical, Midvale, Utah) and the Omni-cup (Kiwi, Clinical Innovations, Murray, Utah). The maneuverability of these devices is superior to either the funnel-shaped or bell-shaped devices owing to their smaller size and increased flexibility of the traction stem relative to the cup. However, they (like other vacuum devices) are still limited in their use for either occiput posterior (OP) or occiput transverse (OT) positions owing to an inability to achieve the proper median flexing application. Recent advances to the Kiwi product have resulted in a style of cup in which the stem is completely collapsible against the cup (see Fig. 14-4), thus allowing placement of the vacuum on the point of flexion of the head that is asynclitic or in the OP position.

OPERATIVE VAGINAL DELIVERY TECHNIQUES

Classical Forceps: Application for Occiput Anterior and Occiput Posterior Positions

Forcep blades are labeled left and right based on the maternal side into which they are placed. For example,

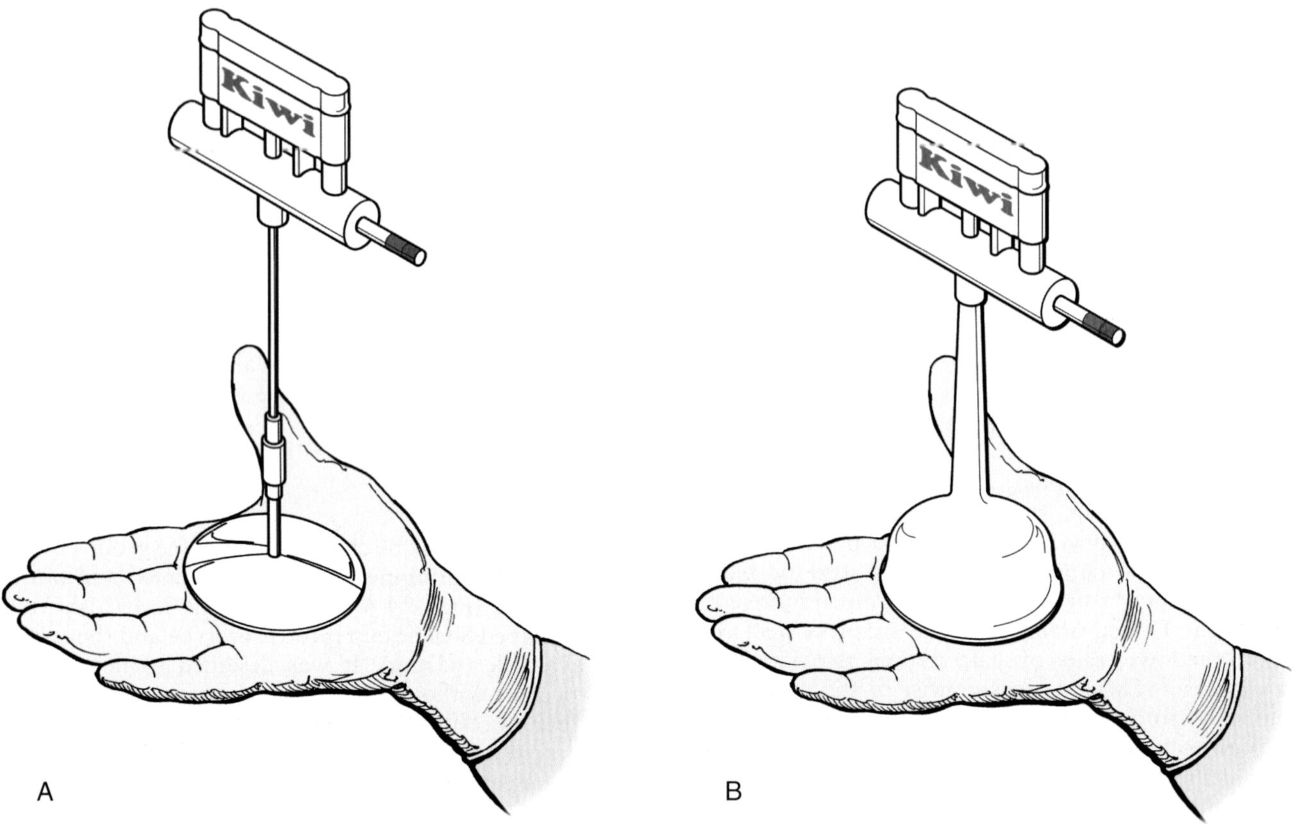

Figure 14-4. Depicted are two kiwi vacuum devices demonstrating the hand-held pump and pressure gauge device. Unlike the cup in *B*, the stem on the cup in *A*, OmniCup is flexible and can be laid flat against the cup. (From Vacca A: Handbook of Vacuum Delivery in Obstetric Practice. Albion, Australia, Vacca Research Pty. Ltd., 2003.)

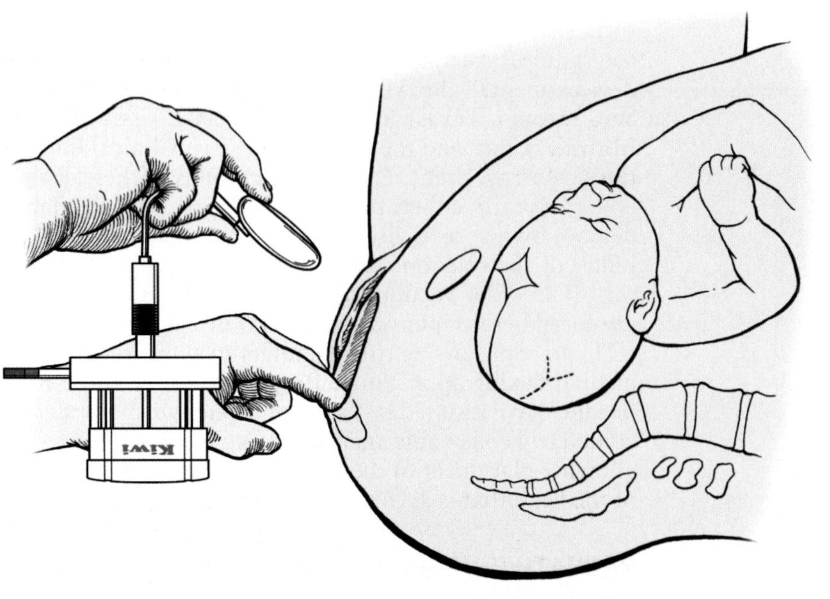

Figure 14-5. Placement of the OmniCup with flexible stem at the point of flexion of a fetal head in the occiput posterior position, which is otherwise difficult to accomplish with the traditional vacuum devices. (From Vacca A: Handbook of Vacuum Delivery in Obstetric Practice. Albion, Australia, Vacca Research Pty, Ltd., 2003.)

the left blade refers to the maternal left side and its handle is held in the operator's left hand for placement (see Fig. 14-2).[30] The posterior blade is conventionally placed first because it provides a splint for the fetal head to prevent rotation from the occiput anterior (OA) position to a more OP position when the second blade is applied. Therefore, when the fetus is OA or LOA, the left blade is placed first. The operator holds the handle of the left blade in his or her left hand, with the toe of the blade directed towards the floor. With the plane of the shank perpendicular to the floor, the cephalic curve of the blade is to be applied to the curve of the fetal head.

To protect the vaginal sidewalls, the fingers of the right hand are placed within the left vagina with the palm of the hand facing the fetal skull. The cephalic curve of the blade should lie evenly against the fetal skull as the toe of the blade is placed at approximately 6 o'clock. The operator's right thumb guides the heel of the blade and the right index finger guides the toe of the blade gently over the left parietal bone. The handle of the blade should be held lightly with the left thumb and index finger. As the blade is inserted into the pelvis, its shank and handle are to be rotated counterclockwise toward the right maternal thigh and then inward toward the maternal midline. This movement will guide the toe of the blade over the left parietal bone and onto the left malar eminence. The force applied by the left thumb and index finger on the handle should be minimal as the blade enters the maternal pelvis. If there is any resistance to blade entry into the maternal pelvis, the blade should be removed and the application technique re-evaluated. Once the blade has been applied, an assistant may hold it in place. To place the right blade, this process is repeated with opposite hands doing the maneuvers described earlier.

When the fetus is in a right occiput anterior (ROA) position, the right fetal parietal bone is located in the posterior maternal pelvis so the posterior blade will be the right blade, and this is placed first. Once both blades are in place, if the handles do not lock easily, the application is incorrect. The blades should have a bimalar, biparietal placement when applied properly (Fig. 14-6). Once the handles are locked, proper blade location must be confirmed. Identification of the posterior fontanel, sagittal suture, lamdoid sutures, and blade fenestrations, if present, enable the operator to confirm proper forceps blade placement before their use. The three criteria needed to confirm proper forceps application are (1) the posterior fontanel should be one finger breath above the plane of the shanks and midway between the blades or the lamdoid sutures (or anterior fontanelle for the OP fetus) should be equidistant from the upper edge of each blade; (2) the sagittal suture should be perpendicular to the plane of the shanks; and (3) if using fenestrated blades, the fenestrations should be barely palpable.[30] The operator should not be able to place more than one fingertip between the fenestration and the fetal head.

The direction of traction on the fetal head is determined by the station of the BPD. For example, higher fetal stations require a steeper angle of traction below the horizontal. The shape of the maternal pelvis may be visualized as the terminal end of the letter "J." As the fetal head descends within the pelvis, the axis of traction follows a curved line upward from the floor. The axis of traction rises above the horizontal as the fetal head crowns and extends just as the head does in a spontaneous vaginal delivery. With the axis traction principle, force is directed in two vectors—downward and out. One hand holds the shanks and exerts downward traction while the operator's other hand holds the handles and exerts traction outward. An alternative method may be employed by the use of an axis traction instrument. This attachment may be joined to the handle to facilitate traction below the handles in the line of the pelvic axis (see Fig. 14-1). Forceps traction should begin with the uterine contraction and coincide with maternal pushing efforts until the contraction ends. Fetal heart tones should be monitored. Descent should occur with each pull, and if no descent occurs after two to three pulls, the operative delivery should be halted and measures should be taken to proceed with cesarean delivery. Switching to a vacuum should be done very cautiously.

Forceps may also be appropriate for OP, left occiput posterior (LOP), or right occiput posterior (ROP) positions if the station of the bony part of the head is truly at least +2 station. Infants in persistent OP presentation present a unique challenge. With a deflexed or extended head, a wider diameter presents through the pelvic outlet. This requires more force for descent of the fetal head. Proper assessment of fetal station can be made complex by extension and molding of the fetal head.[30] With fetal molding, the widest diameter of the fetal head may be at a much higher station than the leading bony part, thus making traction within the proper pelvic axis difficult to ascertain. There is a tendency to overestimate station in OP presentations, so the operator must be confident in their station assessment.

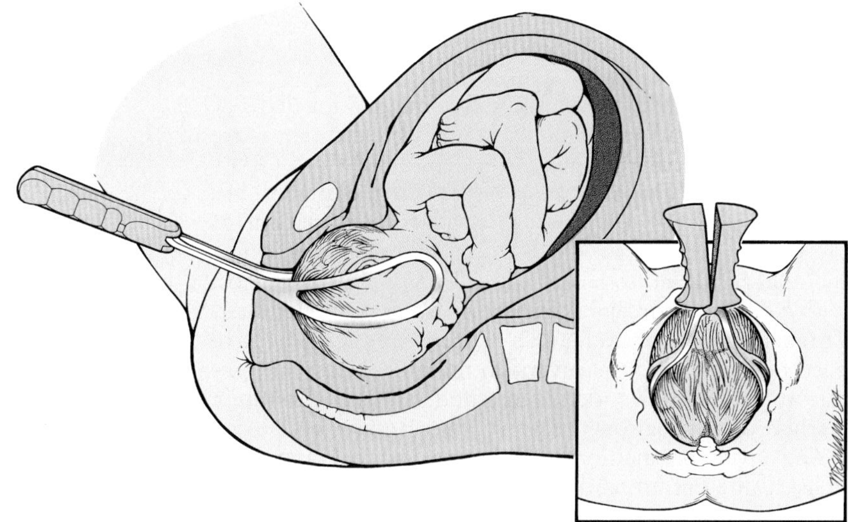

Figure 14-6. Proper application of obstetric forceps. (From O'Brien WF, Cefalo RC: Labor and delivery. *In* Gabbe SG, Niebyl JR, Simpson JL [eds]: Obstetrics: Normal and Problem Pregnancies, 3rd ed. New York, Churchill Livingstone, 1996, p 377, with permission.)

Rotational Forceps: Application for Occiput Transverse Positions

Rotation must be accomplished from the OT position before delivery of the fetal head. This may happen spontaneously, with manual assistance, or with use of forceps, when appropriate. The reader is referred to *Dennen's Forceps Deliveries* for more extensive review of forceps rotation techniques.[30] Forcep rotations should be attempted only with an experienced operator.

CLASSIC FORCEPS

For LOT presentations, the posterior left blade should be applied first. The toe of the blade is placed at 6 o'clock, and the cephalic curve is applied to the fetal head. The handle is lowered to facilitate blade entry into the posterior pelvis and rests below the horizontal, the degree of which will be determined by fetal station. The anterior right blade is labeled the wandering blade. The right blade is inserted with the right hand posteriorly at approximately 7 o'clock. Upward pressure on the blade is exerted with the fingers of the left hand as the right hand moves the handle in a clockwise arc across the left thigh toward the floor. The toe of the blade "wanders" from posterior to anterior, around the frontal bone, to rest anterior to the right ear. Elevation of the handle of the right blade permits movement of the blade further into the pelvis beyond the symphysis and articulation at the handles. The proper attitude of flexion is created by moving the handles toward the pelvic midline. Rotation of the fetal head is accomplished by counterclockwise rotation of the handles in a wide arc across the left thigh toward 12 o'clock. With classic forceps a wide rotational arc at the handles produces the desired smaller arc of rotation at the toe of the blades. Once the OA position is reached, the blades may be readjusted before the generation of traction. This same procedure may be employed for the right OT presentation with classic forceps. In this instance, however, the right blade is posterior and should be applied first.

KEILLAND FORCEPS

Keilland's forceps were originally designed for delivery of the fetal head in deep transverse arrest.[21] They are now also used for rotation of the fetal head from OP or OT positions. The advantage of Keilland's forceps lies in the reverse pelvic curve, which permits placement of the blades in the direct OT position without elevation of the fetal head and loss of station. Unlike classic forceps, with Keilland's forceps the anterior blade is applied first. Three methods of Keilland's forceps application have been described: (1) the inversion method ("classic application"), (2) the wandering method, and (3) the direct method of application.[30]

The inversion method may be used in OT and LOP or ROP presentations. In left OT presentation, the right anterior blade is gently guided below the symphysis with assistance from the operator's left hand. With this application, the cephalic curve is facing up and beyond the symphysis, the handle is dropped below the horizontal, and the blade is rotated 180 degrees toward the midline until the cephalic curve rests on the parietal bone and malar eminence. If resistance is met with the inversion technique, the wandering technique may be used.

The wandering method for Keilland's forceps is similar to that used for classic forceps. The wandering method requires initial placement of the anterior blade onto the posterior parietal bone, with the cephalic curve directly applied to the fetus. The blade is then gently advanced around the face and frontal bone until it rests above the anterior fetal ear.

The direct method of application is preferred when the head is at low fetal station near the pelvic outlet. If the anterior ear is palpable beyond the symphysis, the forceps may be directly applied, often with less difficulty than the other two methods. With the cephalic curve facing the fetus, the blade is applied by lowering the handle toward the floor. The toe is then gently advanced with guidance from the operator's opposite hand. The posterior blade is then inserted at 6 o'clock, with the cephalic curve facing the fetal skull. The operator's free hand is inserted into posterior pelvis palm side up, and the blade is gently guided into position over the posterior ear. The sliding lock will permit closure of the blades and correction of asynclitism. Unlike rotation with classic forceps, the reverse pelvic curve of Keilland's forceps permits rotation directly on the axis of the shanks.[30] The shanks and handles are rotated around the midline point of application and should be held during rotation in a plane perpendicular to the plane of the fetal BPD. After successful rotation, proper forceps placement should be confirmed before traction. Alternatively, Keilland's forceps could be removed, and classic forceps placed before traction.

Forceps Rotation: Application for the Occiput Posterior Position

The fetal head may be rotated from OP to OA by use of the Scanzoni-Smellie technique using classic forceps.[31] The posterior blade should be applied first and then appropriate placement of forceps confirmed. Minimal elevation of the fetal head upward within the pelvis will facilitate rotation. Movement of the handles in a wide arc toward the fetal back will enable rotation from the LOP position to OA. After rotation of the handles in a wide arc, the toe of the blades will be upside down with respect to the fetal malar eminence. They must then be removed and replaced properly before traction on the fetal head. Rotation from OP may also be accomplished with Keilland's forceps. After successful rotation, traction can be applied for delivery of the fetal head.

Vacuum Extraction

As with forceps, successful use of the vacuum extractor is determined by (1) proper application on the fetal head and (2) traction within the pelvic axis.[32,33] The leading point of the fetal head is the ideal position for vacuum cup placement. It is labeled the flexion point or pivot point and is located on the sagittal suture 2 to 3 cm below the posterior fontanel for the OA presentation and 2 to 3 cm above the posterior fontanel for the OP presentation.[32,34] Placement of the vacuum cup over the pivot point maintains the attitude of flexion for a well-flexed head and creates flexion in a deflexed head if traction is applied correctly. Incorrect placement on an asynclitic head results in unequal distribution of force and increase the risk of neonatal intracranial injury and scalp lacerations.[33,35] Therefore, knowledge of exact fetal position is important for efficacious vacuum placement. The force generated by vacuum suction is substantial, with recommended pressures ranging from 550 to 600 mm Hg (11.6 psi).[36] After initial placement of the cup, correct application must be confirmed, including determining that there is no vaginal tissue caught underneath the vacuum cup, before the vacuum pressure is raised to the desired level. Just as with forceps, traction should begin with each contraction and coincide with maternal pushing efforts. Routine traction between contractions should be avoided. In the absence of maternal pushing, traction alone increases the force required for fetal descent and increases the risk of cup detachment.[33] Twisting or rocking of the vacuum cup to facilitate descent of the fetal head is not recommended because there is an increased risk of scalp laceration and intracranial hemorrhage (ICH).[33,37]

With correct application, however, traction in the pelvic axis often results in flexion and autorotation, depending on fetal station and the vacuum cup selected.[32,35]

Detachment of the vacuum cup during traction should be viewed as an indication for re-evaluation of the site of application, direction of axis traction, and fetal maternal pelvic dimensions. The rapid decompression resulting from cup detachment for the soft and rigid vacuum cups has been associated with scalp injury, and it should not be viewed as a safety mechanism that is without potential for fetal risk.[35,38] There are limited data to provide evidence-based support for the maximum duration of safe vacuum application, maximum number of pulls required before delivery of the fetal head, and the maximum number of popoffs or cup detachments before abandonment of the procedure.[33,35,39–41] There is a general consensus, however, that descent of the fetal head should occur with each pull, and if no descent occurs after three pulls, then the operative attempt should be stopped. Most authorities have recommended that the maximum number of cup detachments be limited to two or three and the duration of vacuum application prior to abandonment of the procedure a maximum of 20 to 30 minutes.[41–43] A randomized controlled trial (RCT) compared maintenance of suction of 600 mm Hg throughout the operative delivery to reduction of suction to 100 mm Hg between contractions and found no differences in duration of operative delivery or in neonatal outcome.[44] Finally, vacuum cup selection may play a role in the likelihood of successful vaginal delivery. The soft cup instruments used in modern practice are associated with less scalp trauma but have a higher failure rate than rigid metal vacuum cups.[42] A meta-analysis of nine RCTs of soft versus rigid vacuum extractor cups determined that the average failure rates were 16 and 9 percent for the soft and metal cups, respectively. The detachment rates were 22 and 10 percent for the soft and metal cups, respectively. Higher failure rates with the soft cup may be secondary to difficulties associated with proper placement and traction, particularly if the fetus is deflexed, malpositioned, or at higher station.[31,32,42]

RISKS AND BENEFITS OF OPERATIVE VAGINAL DELIVERY

Benefits of Operative Vaginal Delivery

Most women desire a vaginal delivery.[14] As such, the safe and effective application of instrumental delivery during the second stage of labor is crucial. In addition, acknowledging the benefits of operative vaginal delivery and the maternal views following these interventions is an important component to enhance counseling. In a cohort study of 393 women who had either a "difficult" operative vaginal delivery performed in the operating suite or a cesarean delivery for an arrest disorder in the second stage of labor, an equal proportion of patients in both groups desired future pregnancy (51 versus 54 percent) when asked before hospital discharge. However, women who had an operative vaginal delivery were much more likely to desire a subsequent vaginal delivery compared with women delivered by cesarean section when asked immediately postpartum (79 versus 39 percent)[11] and when asked again 3 years later (87 percent versus 33 percent).[12] In addition, of those patients who achieved pregnancy within 3 years of the index delivery in this cohort, substantially more women who had an operative vaginal delivery achieved subsequent vaginal delivery compared with those who had a prior cesarean delivery (78 versus 31 percent).[12] Johanson followed patients 5 years after a randomized trial comparing forceps with vacuum extraction and demonstrated that more than 75 percent achieved a spontaneous vaginal delivery with a larger fetus in their second pregnancy.[45]

Because women report fear of childbirth as a common reason for avoiding future pregnancies,[12] patients who had an operative delivery were asked about their views on this procedure including preparation for this type of delivery. Most women felt that their birth plan or antenatal classes had not properly prepared them for the possibility of an operative delivery in the second stage of labor.[13] In addition, most had difficulty understanding the need for the intervention despite a review of the indications by the medical staff before discharge. These patients desired more focused antenatal information on operative delivery and a postdelivery debriefing by their delivering physician or midwife focusing on the reasons for the intervention and their future pregnancy and delivery implications.[13]

Maternal Risks

The focus of recent attention regarding operative vaginal delivery has been the risk of perineal trauma and subsequent pelvic floor dysfunction. The principle risks appear to be those of urinary and fecal incontinence. However, the difficulty in establishing the precise risks of this dysfunction in patients who have had an operative vaginal delivery compared with those who have not is confounded by many factors including the indication for the operative delivery, number of deliveries, maternal weight, neonatal birth weight and head circumference, perineal body length, episiotomy, and the effects of maternal aging.[46] We will examine three aspects of maternal risk associated with operative vaginal delivery: significant perineal trauma (third- and fourth-degree laceration), urinary incontinence, and fecal incontinence.

Perineal Trauma

Significant perineal trauma is generally defined as a third-degree laceration, involving the anal sphincter, or fourth degree laceration, involving the rectal mucosa. Estimated frequencies of these injuries vary based on multiple maternal factors including parity, birth weight, type of delivery, and use of episiotomy. In a large, population-based retrospective study of more than 2 million vaginal deliveries, the frequency of severe perineal injury was noted to be 11.5 percent in nulliparous patients, 13.8 percent in patients with a successful vaginal birth after cesarean delivery, and 1.8 percent in multiparous patients.[47] Increased risks of anal sphincter injuries were found to be associated with primiparity, macrosomia, shoulder dystocia, maternal diabetes mellitus, prolonged pregnancy, nonreassuring fetal heart rate patterns, and operative vaginal delivery. In contrast to other studies demonstrating a much larger risk of severe perineal injury due to forceps and vacuum delivery (seven- to eightfold), the study by Handa and colleagues observed an odds ratio (OR) of only 1.4 for forceps delivery and 2.3 for vacuum delivery, suggesting that operative vaginal delivery may be associated with a much lower risk of third- and fourth-degree lacerations than was previously thought.[48,49] In addition, Handa found that episiotomy was associated with a 10-percent decrease in anal sphincter laceration. Other studies have also observed that episiotomy associated with forceps use either did not increase the risk of third- or fourth-degree lacerations[49] or reduced their risk.[50] However, other investigations have noted an increased risk of severe perineal injury with episiotomy use.[51] Finally, in a retrospective review of more than 2,000 consecutive deliveries, reduction in episiotomy use was found to be associated with an increased rate of vaginal lacerations, a decreased rate of fourth-degree lacerations and no change in the rate of third-degree lacerations over a ten year period from one institution.[52] Whether more liberal use of episiotomy affects the rate of severe perineal lacerations remains to be evaluated in a prospective randomized trial.

Urinary Incontinence

Stress urinary incontinence is defined as the involuntary leakage of urine during effort or exertion and occurs at least once weekly in one third of adult women.[53] Both pregnancy and the interval time following pregnancy predispose women to urinary incontinence. Viktrup and colleagues observed that 32 percent of nulliparous women developed urinary incontinence during pregnancy and 7 percent after delivery. One year following delivery, only 3 percent reported incontinence; however, 5 years later, 19 percent of women asymptomatic following delivery had incontinence.[54,55] The Norwegian EPINCONT study, with an 80-percent response rate to a survey of more than 11,000 nulliparous patients, observed a 24-percent prevalence of urinary incontinence and increased urinary incontinence symptoms with increasing age, body mass index (BMI), and number of years since their delivery.[56] In addition, incontinence was significantly associated with birth weight greater than 4,000 g and fetal head circumference greater than 38 cm. Having at least one vacuum or forceps delivery in this cohort did not affect the risk of developing urinary incontinence. In a prospective study of the short- and long-term effects of forceps delivery compared with spontaneous vaginal delivery, which included both patient survey and clinical examination data, Meyer observed a similar incidence of urinary incontinence at both 9 weeks (32 versus 21 percent) and 10 months (20 versus 15 percent).[57] In addition, bladder neck behavior, urethral sphincter function, and intravaginal pressures were similar between the groups. The only difference noted was an increased incidence of a weak pelvic floor in the forceps group (20 versus 6 percent) at the 10 month examination. In a 5-year follow-up study of patients randomized to either forceps or vacuum delivery, Johanson observed no difference in the incidence of urinary dysfunction between these groups.[58] However, Arya in a prospective observational study using patient survey data reported that urinary incontinence after forceps delivery was more likely to persist at 1 year compared with spontaneous vaginal delivery or vacuum delivery (11 versus 3 percent).[59] The only prospective randomized trial to assess urinary incontinence symptoms after planned elective cesarean delivery compared with planned vaginal delivery is the Term Breech Trial.[60] At 3 months postpartum, women randomized to cesarean delivery reported less urinary incontinence compared with those in the planned vaginal delivery group (4.5 versus 7.3 percent; relative risk 0.62, 95-percent confidence interval [CI] 0.41 to 0.93). Finally, in a long-term (34-year) follow-up study of patients following either forceps, spontaneous vaginal delivery, or an elective cesarean delivery without labor, urinary incontinence was found more frequently in those women who had a spontaneous vaginal delivery compared with those who had a forceps delivery (19 versus 7 percent). In addition, the total number of vaginal deliveries was the only risk factor attributed to urinary incontinence in this cohort (OR 19.5; 95-percent CI, 4.01 to 34.8; P = 0.001).[61] The precise association between mode of vaginal delivery (spontaneous, forceps, or vacuum) and urinary incontinence remains unclear at this time in light of the many other factors that appear to contribute to this condition. However, there appears to be little if any effect of forceps delivery on the subsequent development of urinary incontinence. Therefore, it is reasonable to counsel patients that the use of forceps or vacuum for an appropriate obstetric indication likely has no increased long-term affect on urinary incontinence compared with spontaneous vaginal delivery.

Fecal Incontinence

Overall rates of anal sphincter injury noted at the time of vaginal delivery in nulliparous patients are reported to be between 7 to 11.5 percent.[47,62,63] Operative vaginal delivery has been associated with an increased risk of perineal injury, specifically third- and fourth-degree lacerations.[47–49] However, what is not clear is the precise incidence of occult anal sphincter injury in patients delivering vaginally and the resulting affect on fecal incontinence. In the largest prospective study evaluating the prevalence of anal sphincter injury after forceps delivery in nulliparous women using endoanal ultrasound, de Parades examined 93 patients 6 weeks after delivery and found a 13-percent prevalence of anal sphincter injury.[64] These findings are in contrast to other studies that have evaluated fewer patients each, but found a higher prevalence of anal sphincter injury shortly following forceps delivery[64–72] (Table 14-2).

The difficulty with many of these studies noted in Table 14-2 is the extremely low number of patients that return for the endoanal ultrasound following delivery. For example, even though Sultan recruited patients from a previous RCT of forceps and vacuum delivery, only 44 of the original 313 patients (14 percent) were assessed.[71] Because not all patients were evaluated, it is possible that significant selection bias occurred and that the actual prevalence of anal sphincter injury was lower because those patients most symptomatic would be likeliest to return for endoanal ultrasound. Indeed, in the largest randomized trial to date evaluating anal sphincter function following forceps or vacuum extraction, Fitzpatrick was able to follow up on all 61 patients randomized to forceps delivery and demonstrated a much lower rate of anal sphincter injury than previously reported (56 percent). Even though more patients who delivered by forceps compared with vacuum delivery in this study described altered fecal continence (59 versus 33 percent), there were no differences seen in endoanal ultrasound defects or in anal manometry results. In addition, there were no differences in symptom scores between the groups and the degree of disturbance to continence was low in both groups, with the most common symptom being occasional flatal incontinence.[72]

However, de Parades found lower rates of anal sphincter injury (13 percent) and complaints of altered fecal continence (30 percent) following forceps delivery. Most symptomatic patients complained of persistence of incontinence of flatus (17/28), as noted in the study by Fitzpatrick. In addition, a significant increase in the daily number of stools was associated with anal sphincter defects visible on endoanal ultrasound, but the development of altered fecal continence symptoms was not.[64]

Even though it appears that immediate complaints of altered fecal continence and evidence of anal sphincter injury may be as high as 60 percent immediately following operative vaginal delivery, data from long-term follow-up does not bear this figure out. For example, Johanson followed patients 5 years after randomization to either forceps or vacuum delivery and found no significant difference in complaints of altered fecal continence between the groups (15 versus 26 percent).[58] In addition, most patients in the forceps and vacuum groups who noted altered fecal continence had occasional incontinence of flatus or diarrhea as their only symptom (70 and 68 percent, respectively). In addition, 34-year follow-up data on 42 patients delivered by forceps compared with 41 patients delivered by spontaneous vaginal delivery demonstrated a higher rate of anal sphincter injury on ultrasonography in the forceps group (44 versus 22 percent), but no difference in the rate of altered fecal continence (14 versus 10 percent).[61] These data suggest that forceps delivery is a risk for sphincter injury but not for long-term fecal incontinence. In fact, logistic regression revealed that the largest neonatal birth weight, and not forceps delivery, was the contributing risk for significant fecal incontinence in this study.[61] Therefore, based on these data, the anal sphincter injury rate in women who deliver by forceps may be higher; however, long-term rates of fecal incontinence appear to be no different than in women who deliver spontaneously. These findings could reflect the body's ability to heal and compensate for anal sphincter injury over time and may also be the basis for questioning the importance and validity of early outcome assessments of anal incontinence.

Table 14-2. Prevalence of Anal Sphincter Injury Following Forceps Delivery

STUDY	FORCEPS DELIVERIES (N)	IAS INJURY (N)	EAS INJURY (N)	IAS AND EAS INJURY (N)	TOTAL ANAL INJURY (%) SPHINCTER
Sultan[65]	10	2	1	5	80
Sultan[66]	26	7	3	11	81
Rieger[70]	4	0	0	0	0
Sultan[71]	19	MD	MD	MD	79
Varma[67]	6	0	5	0	83
Abramowitz[68]	35	MD	MD	MD	63
Belmonte-Montes[69]	17	0	11	2	76
Fitzpatrick[72]	61	0	34	0	56
De Parades[64]	93	0	11	1	13

EAS, external anal sphincter; IAS, internal anal sphincter; MD, missing data.

Fetal Risks

The focus of possible fetal injury associated with operative vaginal delivery includes craniofacial/intracranial injury and neurologic/cognitive effects. The risks of fetal injury are generally instrument specific, with vacuum deliveries accounting for statistically significantly higher rates of cephalohematoma, and subgaleal and retinal hemorrhages, and forceps deliveries accounting for a nonsignificantly higher rate of scalp/facial injuries.[73] In addition, the sequential use of vacuum and forceps requires particular attention because use in this manner is associated with a maternal and neonatal risk, which is greater than the sum of the individual risks of these instruments.[63]

CRANIOFACIAL AND INTRACRANIAL INJURY

CEPHALOHEMATOMA AND SUBGALEAL HEMORRHAGE

Rates of subperiosteal cephalohematoma in vacuum-assisted vaginal deliveries are higher than rates for either forceps or spontaneous vaginal delivery (112/1,000, 63/1,000 and 17/1,000, respectively).[74,75] However, the most clinically significant and potentially life-threatening injury in this category is a subgaleal hemorrhage (see Chapter 20). This "false cephalohematoma" was first described by Naegele in 1819 to differentiate it from a true subperiosteal cephalohematoma.[76] Subgaleal hemorrhage occurs when blood collects in the loose areolar tissue in the space between the galea aponeurotica and the periosteum. If the veins that connect the dural sinus and the scalp rupture in this layer due to shear forces, the potential space within this loosely applied connective tissue in the subgaleal space may expand with blood well beyond the limits of the suture lines (unlike a subperiosteal cephalohematoma, which is limited to blood and fluid collections within the margins of the suture lines). This space has the potential volume of several hundred milliliters of blood, which may produce profound neonatal hypovolemia, leading to hypoxia, disseminated intravascular coagulation (DIC), end-organ injury and death.[77] Older literature cites several causes of subgaleal hemorrhage with the source as follows: vacuum extraction, 48 percent; spontaneous vaginal delivery, 28 percent, forceps, 14 percent, and cesarean delivery, 9 percent.[76] Although this is older literature reporting in an era when a "low-forceps" delivery was broadly defined by the 1965 ACOG Classification scheme, it is most important to note that these potentially life-threatening bleeds can also occur with spontaneous vaginal deliveries. More recent data suggests that subgaleal hemorrhage occurs nearly exclusively with the vacuum device.[78–80] In an older, 1979 literature review, Plauche et al.[81] report a range for the rate of subgaleal hemorrhage of 0.32 to 9.7 percent, and these occurred primarily with metal cups. More recent data suggests an incidence of subgaleal bleeding of 26–45/1,000.[82] Benaron et al.[83] reported an incidence of 1/200 with soft silicone vacuum cups.

Subgaleal hemorrhage has an estimated incidence of approximately 4 per 10,000 spontaneous vaginal deliveries.[76] In a 30-month prospective study, Boo[84] evaluated more than 64,000 neonates and found that the incidence per live birth was much higher for vacuum extraction than other modes of delivery (41 per 1,000 versus 1 per 1,000). Both the type of cup and the duration of its use are predictors of scalp injury. Soft cups are more likely to be associated with a decreased incidence of scalp injuries but may not be less likely to result in a subgaleal hemorrhage.[4] In one study, vacuum application duration of more than 10 minutes was the best predictor of scalp injury.[85] In May 1998, the Food and Drug Administration (FDA) issued a public health advisory regarding the use of vacuum-assisted delivery devices. The advisory cited a fivefold increase in the rate of deaths and serious morbidity during the previous 4 years compared with the past 11 years and recommended use of these devices only when a specific obstetric indication is present. Other recommendations included the following:

- Persons who use vacuum devices for assisted delivery are versed in their use, and that they are aware of the indications, contraindications, and precautions as supported in the accepted literature and current device labeling.
- The recommended use for all these products is to apply steady traction in the line of the birth canal. Rocking movements or applying torque to the device may be dangerous. Because the instructions may be different for each device type or style, it is important to use the instructions provided by the manufacturer of the particular product being used.
- Alert those who will be responsible for the infant's care that a vacuum assisted delivery device has been used, so that they can monitor the infant for signs of complications.
- Educate the neonatal care staff about the complications of vacuum-assisted delivery devices that have been reported to the FDA and in the literature. They should watch for the signs of these complications in any infant in whom a vacuum-assisted delivery device was used.
- Report reactions associated with the use of vacuum-assisted delivery devices to the FDA.[37]

Despite the fact that many recommend allowing no more than three pop-offs before successful delivery, there is no clear evidence that three applications are safe because if the cup slips during traction without descent of the vertex, neonatal scalp injury may still occur.[85] For example, Benaron[83] demonstrated that the risk of injury and bleeding is increased in nulliparous patients and in those with severe dystocia, malposition, and forceful, prolonged vacuum extractor use. Therefore, caution must be taken with the use of vacuum extractor devices to avoid prolonged (>30 minutes) or forceful use.

INTRACRANIAL HEMORRHAGE

Rates of clinically significant ICH for vacuum, forceps and cesarean delivery during labor are similar (1/860, 1/664 and 1/907 respectively) but are higher than for cesarean delivery without labor (1/2,750) or spontaneous vaginal delivery (1/1,900).[87] Because cesarean delivery following abnormal labor was associated with the same rate of ICH as forceps and vacuum in this study, it is likely that the common risk factor for any increased risk of ICH is abnormal labor and not the type of operative vaginal delivery performed. In fact, because the prevalence of clinically silent subdural hemorrhages is approximately 6 percent following uncomplicated spontaneous vaginal delivery, the presence of this hemorrhage in an otherwise asymptomatic neonate does not necessarily indicate excessive birth trauma and again reflects the natural history of labor and delivery.[88] In these neonates with silent subdural hemorrhages, all resolved within 4 weeks of delivery.

Neurologic and Cognitive Effects

Vacuum-assisted vaginal deliveries increase the risk of neonatal retinal hemorrhages by approximately twofold compared with forceps deliveries.[73] Despite this finding, data on the long-term consequences of these hemorrhages does not demonstrate any significant effect. Johanson followed a cohort of children 5 years following an RCT of forceps versus vacuum extraction and found a 13-percent rate of visual problems in the group. However, there was no difference between those delivered by forceps compared with those delivered by vacuum extraction (12.8 versus 12.5 percent).[58] Seidman was also unable to detect any increased risk of vision abnormalities in a cohort of 1,747 individuals delivered by vacuum extraction compared with more than 47,000 individuals delivered by spontaneous vaginal delivery and examined at age 17 years by the Israeli Defense Forces draft board.[89] There also does not appear to be any long-term effect of operative vaginal delivery on cognitive development. Seidman demonstrated that mean intelligence scores at age 17 years were no different between those delivered by forceps or vacuum extraction compared were spontaneous vaginal delivery. However, the mean intelligence scores for those delivered by cesarean delivery were significantly lower than those of the spontaneous delivery group.[89] Similarly, in a 1993 report from patients within the Kaiser system in Oakland CA, Wesley was unable to detect a difference in cognitive development by measuring intelligence quotient (IQ) in 1,192 children delivered by forceps compared with 1,499 who delivered spontaneously and were examined at age 5 years. Furthermore, of the 1,192 forceps deliveries, there were 114 midforceps, and no differences in IQ were seen at age 5 compared with 1,500 controls.[90] Finally, there also appears to be no association between forceps delivery and epilepsy in adulthood. Murphy and colleagues evaluated a cohort of more than 21,000 individuals and found forceps delivery was not associated with an increased risk of epilepsy or anticonvulsant therapy when compared with other methods of delivery.[91]

Most studies focusing on long-term neurodevelopmental outcomes have focused on IQ from 3 to 7 years after birth. These reports can be divided into older literature (using the 1965 ACOG classification scheme) and recent literature (using the 1988 classification scheme). The older studies reveal mixed results regarding IQ in childhood. Studies by Friedman in 1977 and Richardson in 1983 both showed a significant reduction in IQ associated with spontaneous vaginal delivery and midforceps deliveries for both black and white subgroups at ages 3 to 4 years. In 1983, Friedman conducted a follow-up study of children at age 7 years and found a significant reduction in IQ between spontaneous vaginal delivery and midforceps deliveries. Conversely, Broman used the same database as Friedman, which was the Collaborative Perinatal Project involving over 12,000 deliveries, but he stratified the data by socioeconomic status, race, and gender and found no differences in IQ at 3 to 4 years of age.

Dierker[91a] followed 110 infants for 5 years delivered by midforceps and matched with infants born by cesarean delivery for the same indications and found no differences in IQ or neurologic abnormalities. Interestingly, in a 1984 Scandinavian study by Nilsen,[91b] a significant increase in the IQ of male children delivered by Kielland's rotational forceps was observed, a finding not seen in the girls in this study.

Complex Operative Vaginal Delivery Procedures

Rotations Greater than 45 Degrees

The correct application and delivery technique using forceps is critical to the safe performance of this procedure. The outcomes of forceps delivery are often directly compared to and contrasted with those of spontaneous vaginal delivery. When these comparisons are made, forceps deliveries are associated with a higher rate of maternal injury than spontaneous vaginal delivery. However, the comparison of these two modes of delivery is not appropriate because forceps applications require an indication for use that confounds the clinical outcome when compared with spontaneous vaginal delivery. A more appropriate comparison to forceps delivery (or operative vaginal delivery in general) is cesarean delivery for second-stage arrest disorder. Unfortunately, there are no prospective, randomized trials directly comparing these two modes of delivery. However, numerous retrospective studies comparing midcavity and rotational forceps delivery with cesarean delivery demonstrate no increased risk of fetal/neonatal adverse outcomes including Apgar score, umbilical cord blood gas values, birth trauma, and neonatal intensive care unit (NICU) admission.[92–95] Specifically, the rates of neonatal morbidity associated with Kielland forceps rotation are similar to cesarean delivery including rates of cephalohematoma (9 to 17 percent), facial bruising (13 to 18 percent), facial nerve injury (1 to 5 percent) and brachial plexus injury (<1 percent).[96–98] Interestingly, rates of maternal morbidity (intraoperative and postoperative complications, blood loss and length of stay) have been found to be higher in patients delivered by cesarean delivery compared with those delivered by midcavity forceps delivery.[92,93]

The outcomes of rotational forceps deliveries have also been evaluated and compared with nonrotational forceps delivery. Healy evaluated 552 Kielland's forceps rotations, 95 Scanzoni-Smellie maneuvers with classic instruments, and 160 manual rotations followed by delivery with a classic instrument and found no difference in neonatal outcomes between the groups.[99] Krivac et al.[100] compared 55 Kielland's forceps rotations with 213 nonrotational forceps deliveries. Fifteen of the rotations were greater than 90 degrees, and 40 were less than 90 degrees, but greater than 45 degrees. They found that the Kielland forceps rotation group had both a longer labor and longer second stage than the nonrotational group and a higher rate of 1-minute Apgar scores less than 6 and meconium at delivery. However, the nonrotational forceps group had a greater incidence of postpartum hemorrhage (14 versus 7 percent) and a higher rate of third- and fourth-degree lacerations (24 versus 14 percent). No other differences in maternal or neonatal morbidity were noted including no difference in rates of nerve compromise (<1 percent), facial bruising (7 percent), shoulder dystocia (1 percent), or NICU admissions. Hankins et al.[101] performed a retrospective case-controlled study comparing 113 forceps deliveries greater than 90 degrees compared with 167 forceps deliveries less than 45 degrees. No differences in major fetal injury were demonstrated between these two groups. Major fetal injury was defined as skull fracture, subdural hematoma and brachial plexus or facial nerve injury, and fetal acidemia (pH <7.0). Finally, Feldman compared 104 rotational forceps deliveries using Leff forceps for persistent OP position with 163 nonrotational forceps deliveries and found lower rates of episiotomy (66 versus 82 percent) and perineal lacerations (16 percent versus 23 percent) in the forceps rotation group and no differences in the rates of neonatal morbidity between the groups.[102] These data suggest that when properly applied and used, forceps deliveries requiring greater than 45 degree rotation may be safely accomplished without increased risk of maternal or neonatal morbidity and, therefore, should remain a management option for women with second-stage labor abnormalities.

Midpelvic Cavity Delivery

Like rotational forceps deliveries, delivery of the fetus from a 0 or +1 station (midpelvic or midforceps) requires a specific set of skills and precautions. In 1988, ACOG reported on required conditions for a midforceps delivery that included the following: (1) an experienced person performing or supervising the procedure, (2) adequate anesthesia, (3) assessment of maternal-fetal size, and (4) willingness to abandon the attempt at delivery. This information should be taken together with the prerequisites set forth by Richardson et al.[103]: the midforceps procedure (1) must rationally be needed as an alternative method of delivery to cesarean delivery, (2) must be associated with demonstrably less maternal morbidity than cesarean section, and (3) should not result in fetal harm. Several studies that compare cesarean delivery to midforceps procedures show that midforceps delivery is not associated with more adverse neonatal outcomes including cord blood gases, Apgar scores, NICU admissions, and birth trauma.[92,93,104] In 1997, Revah et al.[104] reported their findings of a retrospective chart review of 401 cesarean deliveries over a 7-year period in which a trial of operative delivery (forceps or vacuum) was conducted in 75 cases. There were no differences between cesarean delivery with a trial of operative delivery versus without an operative delivery attempt for any maternal or fetal outcome. Although the outcomes of these studies are reassuring, because of the technical skills required, it is most reasonable to abide by the guidance set forth in the ACOG practice bulletin published in 2000, which states "Unless the preoperative assessment is highly suggestive of successful outcome, trial of operative vaginal delivery is best avoided."[82] In short, following the ACOG statement and the above-stated prerequisites provides the skilled practitioner with guidelines and support for attempting a safe midpelvic cavity delivery.

Sequential Use of Vacuum and Forceps

The sequential use of these instruments appears to increase the likelihood of adverse maternal and neonatal outcomes more than the sum of the relative risks of each instrument.[63,75] Compared with spontaneous vaginal delivery, deliveries by sequential use of vacuum and forceps are associated with significantly higher rates of ICH (RR 3.9; 95-percent CI, 1.5 to 10.1), brachial plexus injury (RR 3.2; 95-percent CI, 1.6 to 6.4), facial nerve injury (RR 3.0; 95-percent CI, 4.7 to 37.7), neonatal seizures (RR 13.7; 95-percent CI, 2.1 to 88.0), requirement for mechanical ventilation of the neonate (RR 4.8, 95-percent CI, 2.1 to 11.0), severe perineal lacerations (RR 6.2, 95 percent CI, 6.4 to 20.1) and postpartum hemorrhage (RR 1.6, 95-percent CI, 1.3 to 2.0).[63] Therefore, care should be taken to avoid the sequential use of these instruments to reduce maternal and neonatal morbidity.

Vacuum Delivery and the Preterm Fetus

There is no quality data for firm recommendations regarding a gestational age limit below which the vacuum extractor should not be used. There are two studies reporting the use of soft cups without adverse outcomes in preterm fetuses. However, these studies were small and lacked power to demonstrate significance. There are no RCTs comparing forceps versus vacuums or comparing different vacuum types to pass judgment on a gestational age cut-off. ACOG reports that most experts in operative vaginal delivery limit the vacuum procedure to fetuses greater than 34 weeks' gestation.[82] This is a reasonable cut-off, given that the premature head is likely at greater risk for compression-decompression injuries simply due to the pliability of the preterm skull and the more fragile soft tissues of the scalp.

COUNSELING: FORCEPS, VACUUM, OR CESAREAN DELIVERY

The increasing use of vacuum extraction over forceps has resulted in numerous publications comparing efficacy and morbidity between methods. Table 14-3 provides a summary of the disadvantages associated with both methods. In a Cochrane meta-analysis including 10 RCTs of vacuum and forceps use, vacuum extraction had a greater failure rate than that of forceps.[105]

Table 14-3. Comparative Morbidities Associated with Forceps Delivery and Vacuum Extraction

FORCEPS	VACUUM EXTRACTION
Greater third- and fourth-degree and vaginal lacerations	Higher failure rate than forceps
Greater maternal discomfort postpartum	Increased risk of neonatal injury:
Greater duration of training needed	Minor: cephalohematoma, retinal homorrhage
Increased risk of neonatal facial nerve injury	Major: subarachnoid hemorrhage, subgaleal homorrhage
	Less need for maternal anesthesia

Adapted from Johanson RB, Menon BK: Vacuum extraction versus forceps for assisted vaginal delivery. Cochrane Database Syst Rev (2): CD000224, 2000.

Vacuum extraction was associated with less maternal trauma, including third- and fourth-degree extensions, and vaginal lacerations, than forceps use.[105] Less maternal regional and general anesthesia was used for vacuum extractions. There were no differences in significant neonatal injury between the two groups. Despite small sample sizes, vacuum extraction was associated with an increased risk of cephalohematoma and retinal hemorrhage when compared with forceps use. Cephalohematoma formation with vacuum extraction was reported to have a mean incidence of 6 percent, with no difference between soft or rigid vacuum cups, and is considered to be a finding of little significance.[35,105]

Unless a patient is willing to undergo cesarean delivery before the onset of advanced labor, there does not appear to be any advantage to avoiding operative vaginal delivery in an attempt to reduce the long-term risks of incontinence. The effects of both forceps and vacuum delivery on the risk of developing urinary incontinence appear to be the same as that of spontaneous vaginal delivery with between 5 to 20 percent of women developing long-term persistent urinary incontinence regardless of vaginal delivery method. In addition, despite evidence that the anal sphincter injury rate in women who deliver by forceps is higher, it is not clear that the long-term rates of fecal incontinence in these women is any different than those who deliver spontaneously. Approximately 10 to 30 percent of women develop some degree of altered fecal continence following vaginal delivery, with cesarean delivery before the onset of labor as the only reliable means of reducing this risk.

The greatest risk for urinary incontinence appears to be the total number of vaginal deliveries, and the greatest risk for subsequent development of fecal incontinence appears to be related to the effect of the largest neonate delivered vaginally, irrespective of mode of delivery. Regarding fetal risks, vacuum deliveries appear to increase the incidence of cephalohematoma, and subgaleal and retinal hemorrhages compared with forceps or spontaneous vaginal deliveries. Forceps deliveries increase the risk of facial bruising and transient facial nerve palsies compared with vacuum or spontaneous vaginal deliveries. However, there is no evidence that these immediate neonatal morbidities result in any long-term visual, neurologic, or cognitive developmental abnormalities. Finally, patients delivered by cesarean delivery in the second stage have a higher risk of intraoperative and postoperative complications, higher rates of blood loss, and longer hospital stays than those delivered by operative vaginal delivery.

Patients should also be informed that substantially more women who have an operative vaginal delivery achieve subsequent vaginal delivery in the next pregnancy compared with those who have a cesarean delivery (78 versus 31 percent). Therefore, it is reasonable to counsel patients that the options for second-stage assisted delivery include both forceps and vacuum when appropriate, because the proper application of these instruments and execution of these deliveries can avoid the maternal morbidity associated with cesarean delivery and increase the likelihood of a subsequent vaginal delivery for the next pregnancy without additional long-term maternal or neonatal risk.

In a Cochrane review of 10 randomized studies comparing the use of forceps to vacuum extraction for assisted vaginal delivery, vacuum devices were found more likely to fail than forceps.[74] However, vacuum use was also more likely to result in vaginal delivery, probably because failed vacuum extraction led to the use of forceps and subsequent vaginal delivery due to a lower forceps failure rate. A lower failure rate is not the only reason to consider forceps. Forceps may be the only acceptable instrument to effect an operative vaginal delivery in some circumstances. Some examples of these clinical situations include delivery of the head at assisted breech delivery, assisted delivery of a preterm infant younger than 34 weeks' gestation, delivery with a face presentation, suspected coagulopathy or thrombocytopenia in the fetus, and instrumental delivery for maternal medical conditions that preclude pushing.[14] Because the specific clinical situation and operator experience are the key factors that contribute to the choice of instrument, it is critical that students of obstetrics be thoroughly familiar with the use of both instruments.

RESIDENCY TRAINING AND OPERATIVE VAGINAL DELIVERY

The overall incidence of operative vaginal delivery has remained stable over the past 15 years. Interestingly, over this same time span, vacuum extraction procedures have overtaken forceps procedures as the instrument of choice (Fig. 14-7).

A 1992 report of a survey conducted by Ramin et al. of U.S. residency training programs reported that most programs use the 1988 classification scheme and that 86 percent taught midforceps.[106] It should be noted that even though a large percentage of programs teach the complex forceps procedures, the number of such procedures to reach proficiency has not been elucidated. In short, the overall decline in forceps procedures performed, the complexity of midpelvic cavity deliveries, and the shift from complex rotational deliveries to vacuum extraction and cesarean deliveries by younger faculty as shown by Tan et al. and Jain et al.[97,107] may make the midforceps pro-

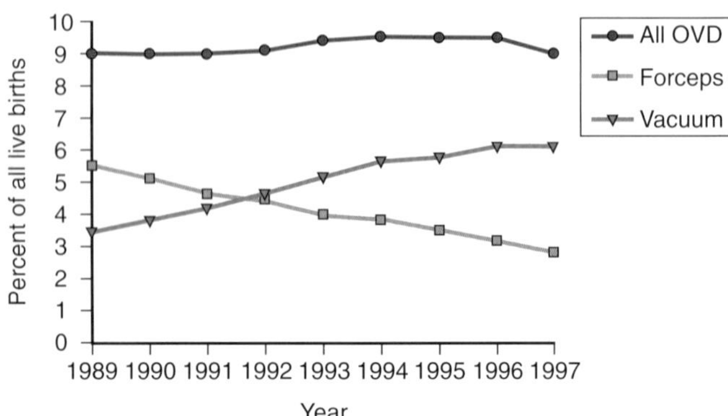

Figure 14-7. The overall incidence of operative vaginal delivery has remained stable over the last 15 years. Interestingly, over this same time span, vacuum extraction procedures have overtaken forceps procedures as the instrument of choice. (Modified from Miksovsky P, Watson WJ: Obstetric vacuum extraction: state of the art in the new millennium. Obstet Gynecol Surv 56:736, 2001.)

Table 14-4. Modes of Delivery and Birth Outcomes Before and After Initiation of Dedicated Obstetrics Staff Located on Labor and Delivery

	BEFORE	AFTER	*p*
Births	3,481	4,338	0.0001
Cesarean section	888 (26%)	1,183 (27%)	NS
Operative vaginal delivery	394 (11%)	461 (11%)	NS
Forceps	172 (5%)	337 (8%)	0.00001
Vacuum	222 (6%)	124 (3%)	0.00001
3rd or 4th degree lacerations	126 (4%)	134 (3%)	NS
Birth injury	8 (0.2%)	13 (0.3%)	NS
AS <7 at 5 minutes	67 (2%)	104 (2%)	NS

cedure obsolete in the near future.[106] In response to these types of concerns, Kim et al.[108] conducted a unique study to determine whether the rates of vacuum extraction and forceps procedures could be reversed without an increase in morbidity in a residency program. This retrospective study compared outcomes 2 years before and 2 years after an obstetrics faculty member was dedicated to the labor floor from Monday through Thursday, 7 a.m. to 5 p.m. Table 14-4 depicts how such a dedicated instructor can increase the number of forceps relative to vacuum extractions without increasing third- or fourth-degree lacerations or adverse neonatal outcomes.

Although the early 1990 report by Ramin et al.[106] provided encouraging information regarding the use of the 1988 classification scheme, a more recent study by Carollo et al.[109] is unsettling. In this 2004 study, Carollo conducted a survey of several teaching hospitals in the Denver area asking the following important questions: (1) How do you define fetal station? (2) How do you think a majority of your colleagues define fetal station? (3) How do you think the ACOG defines the classification of fetal station? and (4) How important do you think these distinctions are? What makes this study additionally unique is that these questions were asked of both attendings and residents in obstetrics and gynecology as well as nurses. Approximately 35 percent of attending physicians still defined station by dividing the pelvis into thirds rather than centimeters, as set forth in the old 1965 ACOG classification scheme. In addition, nearly 15 percent used the BPD rather than the presenting part as the landmark on the fetus to define station. These percentage numbers were higher for nurses and residents. The percent of correctly used techniques for defining station was highest at the university teaching hospital. These data suggest that, although we do fairly well at teaching proper technique for determining station, we are poor at disseminating the information into practice. Operative vaginal deliveries will be more difficult and dangerous if misunderstandings in defining fetal station persist.

Key Points

- Obstetric forceps are the one instrument that makes the practice of obstetric care unique to obstetricians. The proper use of these instruments has afforded safe and timely vaginal delivery to those whose abnormal labor course and urgent need for delivery require their use.
- Rates of cesarean delivery have risen in the United States, reaching a rate of approximately 25 percent of all deliveries in the United States, whereas rates of forceps deliveries have declined from 17.7 percent in 1980 to 4 percent in 2000.
- Resident work hour restrictions have resulted in a decline in resident experience with both primary cesarean delivery and vacuum-assisted vaginal delivery.
- Treat the vacuum extractor with the same respect as the forceps. The prerequisites for application of forceps or vacuum extractor are identical.
- When using vacuum extraction, descent of the fetal head should occur with each pull. If no descent occurs after three pulls, then the operative attempt should be stopped.
- There appears to be little if any effect of forceps delivery on the subsequent development of urinary incontinence.
- The rate of anal sphincter injury in women who deliver by forceps may be higher; however, long-term rates of fetal incontinence appear to be no different than in women who deliver spontaneously.
- The risks of fetal injury associated with operative vaginal delivery are generally instrument specific, with vacuum deliveries accounting for higher rates of cephalohematoma, and subgaleal and retinal hemorrhages, and forceps deliveries accounting for a nonsignificantly higher rate of scalp and facial injuries.

❑ Numerous retrospective studies comparing midcavity and rotation forceps delivery with cesarean delivery demonstrate no increased risk of fetal or neonatal adverse outcomes including Apgar score, umbilical cord blood gas values, trauma, and neonatal intensive care unit admission.

❑ When properly applied and used, forceps deliveries requiring greater than 45 degrees may be safely accomplished without increased risk of maternal or neonatal morbidity and therefore should remain a management option for women with second-stage labor abnormalities.

❑ The sequential use of vacuum extraction and forceps increases the likelihood of adverse maternal and neonatal outcomes more than the sum of the relative risks of each instrument.

REFERENCES

1. Denman T: An Introduction to the Practice of Midwifery, ed 1. London, 1788.
2. Holland E: The Princess Charlotte of Wales: A triple obstetric tragedy. J Obstet Gynaecol Br Emp 58:905, 1951.
3. Denman T: Aphorisms on the Application and use of the Forceps, ed 6, London, 1817.
4. DeLee JB: The prophylactic forceps operation. Am J Obstet Gynecol 1:34, 1920.
5. Kozak LJ, Weeks JD: US trends in obstetric procedures. 1990–2000. Birth 29:157, 2002.
6. Thomas J, Paranjoth S: National sentinel caesarean section audit report. London: Royal College of Obstetricians and Gynaecologists Clinical Effectiveness Support Unit, 2001.
7. Meniru GI: An analysis of recent trends in vacuum extraction and forceps delivery. Br J Obstet Gynaecol 103:168, 1996.
8. Hankins GD, Uckan E, Rowe TF, Collier S: Forceps and vacuum delivery: expectations of residency and fellowship training program directors. Am J Perinatol 16:23, 1999.
9. Blanchard MH, Amini SB, Frank TM: Impact of work hour restrictions on resident case experience in an obstetrics and gynecology residency program. Am J Obstet Gynecol 191:1746, 2004.
10. American College of Obstetricians and Gynecologists Practice Bulletin Number 17. Operative Vaginal Delivery. June 2000.
11. Murphy DJ, Liebling RE: Cohort study of maternal views on future mode of delivery following operative delivery in the second stage of labor. Am J Obstet Gynecol 188:542, 2003.
12. Bahl R, Strachan B, Murphy DJ: Outcome of subsequent pregnancy three years after previous operative delivery in the second stage of labour: cohort study. BMJ 328:311, 2004.
13. Murphy DJ, Pope C, Frost J, Liebling RE: Women's views on the impact of operative delivery in the second stage of labour—qualitative study. BMJ 327:1132, 2003.
14. Patel RR, Murphy DJ: Forceps delivery in modern practice. BMJ 328:1302, 2004.
15. Dennen EH: A classification of forceps operations according to station of head in pelvis. Am J Obstet Gynecol 63:272, 1952.
16. American College of Obstetricians and Gynecologists: Manual of Standards of Obstetric-Gynecologic Practice: American College of Obstetricians and Gynecologists, 2nd ed. Washington, DC, ACOG, 1965.
17. American College of Obstetricians and Gynecologists, Committee on Obstetrics, Maternal and Fetal Medicine: Obstetric Forceps. Technical Bulletin No. 59, February 1988.
18. Hagadorn-Freathy AS, Yeomans ER, Hankins GDV: Validation of the 1988 ACOG Forceps Classification System. Obstet Gynecol 77:356, 1991.
19. Laube DW: Forceps delivery. Clin Obstet Gynecol 29:286, 1986.
20. Laufe LE: Obstetric Forceps. New York, Harper and Row. Hoeber Medical Division. 1968.
21. Kielland C: The application of forceps to the unrotated head. A description of a new type of forceps and a new method of insertion. Translated from the original article in Monafs schrift fur Geburshilfe und Gynakologie 43:48, 1916.
22. Lett M: An obstetric forceps for rotation of the fetal head. Am J Obstet Gynecol 70:208, 1955.
23. Feldman DM, Borgida AF, Sauer F, Rodis JF: Rotational versus nonrotational forceps: Maternal and neonatal outcomes. Am J Obstet Gynecol 181:1185, 1999.
24. Malmstrom T: Vacuum extractor: An obstetrical instrument. Gothenburg, Sweden, Northern Association of Obstetrics and Gynecologists, 1954, p 1.
25. Malmstrom T: The vacuum extractor: an obstetrical instrument. Acta Obstet Gynecol Scand 36:5, 1957.
26. Kuit JA, Eppinga HG, Wallenburg HC, Hiukeshoven FJ: A randomized comparison of vacuum extraction delivery with a rigid and a pliable cup. Obstet Gynecol 82:280, 1993.
27. Hillier CEM, Johanson RB: Worldwide survey of assisted vaginal delivery. Int J Gynecol Obstet 47:109, 1994.
28. Hammarstrom M, Csemiczky G, Belfrage P: Comparison between the conventional Malmstrom extractor and a new extractor with Silastic cup. Acta Obstet Gynecol Scand 65:791, 1986.
29. Dell DL, Sightler SE, Plauche WC: Soft cup vacuum extraction: a comparison of outlet delivery. Obstet Gynecol 66:624, 1985.
30. Hale RW (ed): Dennen's Forceps Deliveries, 4th ed. Washington, D.C., American College of Obstetrics and Gynecology, 2001.
31. Scanzoni FW: Lehrbuch der Geburtshulfe, 3rd ed. Vienna, Seidel, 1853, p 838.
32. Bird GC: The importance of flexion in vacuum extractor delivery. Br J Obstet Gynecol 83:194, 1976.
33. Mikovsky P, Watson WJ: Obstetric Vacuum extraction: State of the art in the new millenium. Obstet Gynecol Surv 56:736, 2001.
34. Lucas MJ: The role of vacuum in modern obstetrics. Clin Obstet Gynecol 37:794, 1994.
35. Vacca A: Vacuum assisted delivery. Best Pract Res Clin Obstet Gynecol 16:17, 2002.
36. Vacca A: Handbook of Vacuum Extraction in Obstetrical Practice. London, Edward Arnold, 1992.
37. Center for Devices and Radiological Health. FDA Public Health advisory: Need for caution when using vacuum assisted delivery devices. Rockville, MD: Food and Drug Administration. Accessed December 5, 2006. Available from: http://www.fda.gov/cdrh/feta1598.html
38. Plauche WC: Fetal cranial injuries related to delivery with the Malmstrom vacuum extractor. Obstet Gynecol 53:750, 1979.
39. O'Grady JP, Pope CS, Patel SS: Vacuum extraction in modern obstetric practice: a review and critique. Curr Opin Obstet Gynecol 12:475, 2000.
40. Bird GC: The use of the vacuum extractor. Clin Obstet Gynecol 25:167, 1982.
41. Bofill JA, Rust OA, Schorr SJ, et al: A randomized prospective trial of obstetric forceps versus the m-cup vacuum extractor. Am J Obstet Gynecol 175:1325, 1996.
42. Johanson R, Menon V: Soft vs. rigid vacuum extractor cups for assisted vaginal delivery. Cochrane Database Syst Rev (2): CD000446, 2000.
43. Operative vaginal delivery. Guideline 26. Royal College of Obstetricians and Gynecologists, 2005. Accessed December 5, 2006. Available from: http://www.rcog.org.uk/resources/Public/pdf/operative_vaginal_delivery.pdf.
44. Bofill JA, Rust OA, Schorr SJ, et al: A randomized trial of two vacuum extraction techniques. Obstet Gynecol 89:758, 1997.
45. Johanson RB, Heycock E, Carter J, et al: Maternal and child health after assisted vaginal delivery: Five-year follow up of a randomized controlled study comparing forceps and ventouse. Br J Obstet Gynaecol 106:544, 1999.
46. Handa VL, Harris TA, Ostergard DR: Protecting the pelvic floor: obstetric management to prevent incontinence and pelvic organ prolapse. Obstet Gynecol 88:470, 1996.
47. Handa VL, Danielsen BH, Gilbert WM: Obstetric anal sphincter lacerations. Obstet Gynecol 98:225, 2001.

48. Angioli R, Gomez-Marin O, Cantuaria G, O'Sullivan MJ: Severe perineal lacerations during vaginal delivery: The University of Miami experience. Am J Obstet Gynecol 182:1083, 2000.
49. Robinson JN, Norwitz ER, Cohen AP, et al: Episiotomy, operative vaginal delivery, and significant perineal trauma in nulliparous women. Am J Obstet Gynecol 181:1180, 1999.
50. Bodner-Alder B, Bodner K, Kimberger O, et al: Management of the perineum during forceps delivery: Association of episiotomy with the frequency and severity of perineal trauma in women undergoing forceps delivery. J Reprod Med 48:239, 2003.
51. Christianson LM, Bovbjerg VE, McDavitt EC, Hullfish KL: Risk factors for perineal injury during delivery. Am J Obstet Gynecol 189:255, 2003.
52. Ecker JL, Tan WM, Bansal RK, et al: Is there a benefit to episiotomy at operative vaginal delivery? Observations over ten years in a stable population. Am J Obstet Gynecol 176:411, 1997.
53. Nygaard IE, Heit M: Stress urinary incontinence. Obstet Gynecol 104:607, 2004.
54. Viktrup L, Lose G, Rolff M, Barfoed K: The symptom of stress incontinence caused by pregnancy or delivery in primiparas. Obstet Gynecol 79:945, 1992.
55. Viktrup L, Lose G: The risk of stress incontinence 5 years after first delivery. Am J Obstet Gynecol 185:82, 2001.
56. Rortveit G, Daltveit AK, Hannestad YS, Hunskaar S: Vaginal delivery parameters and urinary incontinence: The Norwegian EPINCONT study. Am J Obstet Gynecol 189:1268, 2003.
57. Meyer S, Hohlfeld P, Achtare C, et al: Birth trauma: short and long term effects of forceps delivery compared with spontaneous delivery on various pelvic floor parameters. Br J Obstet Gynaecol 107:1360. 2000.
58. Johanson RB, Heycock E, Carter J, et al: Maternal and child health after assisted vaginal delivery: five-year follow up of a randomized controlled study comparing forceps and ventouse. Br J Obstet Gynaecol 106:544, 1999.
59. Arya LA, Jackson ND, Myers DL, Verma A: Risk of new-onset urinary incontinence after forceps and vacuum delivery in primiparous women. Am J Obstet Gynecol 185:1318, 2001.
60. Hannah ME, Hannah WJ, Hodnett ED, et al: Outcomes at 3 months after planned cesarean versus planned vaginal delivery for breech presentation at term: the International Randomized Term Breech Trial. JAMA 287:1822, 2002.
61. Bollard RC, Gardiner A, Duthie GS: Anal sphincter injury, fetal and urinary incontinence: A 34-year follow-up after forceps delivery. Dis Colon Rectum 46:1083, 2003.
62. Richter HE, Brumfield CG, Cliver SP, et al: Risk factors associated with anal sphincter tear: A comparison of primiparous patients, vaginal births after cesarean deliveries and patients with previous vaginal delivery. Am J Obstet Gynecol 187:1194, 2002.
63. Gardella G, Taylor M, Benedetti T, et al: The effect of sequential use of vacuum and forceps for assisted vaginal delivery on neonatal and maternal outcomes. Am J Obstet Gynecol 185:896, 2001.
64. deParades V, Etienney I, Thabut D, et al: Anal sphincter injury after forceps delivery: Myth or reality? Dis Colon Rectum 47:24, 2004.
65. Sultan AH, Kamm MA, Hudson CN, et al: Anal-sphincter disruption during vaginal delivery. N Engl J Med 329:1905, 1993.
66. Sultan AH, Kamm MA, Bartram CI, Hudson CN: Anal sphincter trauma during instrumental delivery. Int J Gynecol Obstet 43:263, 1993.
67. Varma A, Gunn J, Gardiner A, et al: Obstetric anal sphincter injury: prospective evaluation of incidence. Dis Colon Rectum 42:1537, 1999.
68. Abramowitz L, Sobhani I, Ganansia R, et al: Are sphincter defects the cause of anal incontinence after vaginal delivery? Results of a prospective study. Dis Colon Rectum 43:590, 2000.
69. Belmontes-Montes C, Hagerman G, Vega-Yepez PA, et al: Anal sphincter injury after vaginal delivery in primiparous females. Dis Colon Rectum 44:1244, 2001.
70. Rieger N, Schloithe A, Saccone G, Wattchow D: A prospective study of anal sphincter injury due to childbirth. Scand J Gastroenterol 33:950, 1998.
71. Sultan AH, Johanson RB, Carter JE: Occult anal sphincter trauma following randomized forceps and vacuum delivery. Int J Gynecol Obstet 61:113, 1998.
72. Fitzpatrick M, Behan M, O'Connell PR, O'Herlihy C: Randomised clinical trial to assess anal sphincter function following forceps or vacuum assisted vaginal delivery. BJOG 110:424, 2003.
73. Johanson RB, Menon V: Vacuum extraction versus forceps for assisted vaginal delivery. [revised 23 Nov 2001] *In* The Cochrane Pregnancy and Childbirth Database. The Cochrane Collaboration; Issue 1, Oxford, Update Software; 2002.
74. Johnson JH, Figueroa R, Garry D, et al: Immediate maternal and neonatal effects of forceps and vacuum-assisted deliveries. Obstet Gynecol 103:513, 2004.
75. Demissie K, Rhoads GG, Smulian JC, et al: Operative vaginal delivery and neonatal and infant adverse outcomes: population based retrospective analysis. BMJ 329:24, 2004.
76. Plauche WC: Subgaleal haematoma: a complication of instrumental delivery. JAMA 244:1597, 1980.
77. Eliachar E, Bret AJ, Bardiaux M, et al: Hematome souscutane cranien du nouveau-ne. Arch Fr Pediatr 20:1105, 1963.
78. Govaert P, Defoort P, Wigglesworth JS: Cranial haemorrhage in the term newborn infant. Clin Dev Med 129:1, 1993.
79. Ngan HY, Miu P, Ko L, Ma HK: Long-term neurological sequelae following vacuum extractor delivery. Aust N Z J Obstetr Gynaecol 30:111, 1990.
80. Chadwick LM, Pemberton PJ, Kurinczuk JJ: Neonatal subgaleal haematoma: associated risk factors, complications and outcome. J Paediatr Child Health 32:228, 1996.
81. Plauche WC: Fetal cranial injuries related to delivery with the Malmstrom vacuum extractor. Obstet Gynecol 53:750, 1979.
82. ACOG Practice Bulletin, No 17, June 2000; or ACOG Compendium of Selected Publications, 2005, p 640.
83. Benaron DA: Subgaleal hematoma causing hypovolemic shock during delivery after failed vacuum extraction: case report. J Perinatol 12:228, 1993.
84. Boo N: Subaponeurotic haemorrhage in Malaysian neonates. Singapore Med J 31:207, 1990.
85. Teng FY, Sayer JW: Vacuum extraction: Does duration predict scalp injury? Obstet Gynecol 89:281, 1997.
86. Uchil D, Arulkumaran S: Neonatal subgaleal hemorrhage and its relationship to delivery by vacuum extraction. Obstet Gynecol Surv 58:687, 2003.
87. Towner D, Castro MA, Eby-Wilkens E, Gilbert WM: Effect of mode of delivery in nulliparous women on neonatal intracranial injury. N Engl J Med 341:1709, 1999.
88. Whitby EH, Griffiths PD, Rutter S, et al: Frequency and natural history of subdural haemorrhages in babies and relation to obstetric factors. Lancet 363:846, 2004.
89. Seidman DS, Laor A, Gale R, et al: Long-term effects of vacuum and forceps deliveries. Lancet 337:15835, 1991.
90. Wesley BD, van den Berg BJ, Reece EA: The effect of forceps delivery on cognitive development. Am J Obstet Gynecol 169:1091, 1993.
91. Murphy DJ, Libby G, Chien P, et al: Cohort study of forceps delivery and the risk of epilepsy in adulthood. Am J Obstet Gynecol 191:392, 2004.
91a. Dierker LJ Jr, Rosen MG, Thompson K, Lynn P: Midforceps deliveries: long-term outcome of infants. Am J Obstet Gynecol 154:764, 1986.
91b. Nilsen ST: Boys born by forceps and vacuum extraction examined at 18 years of age. Acta Obstet Gynecol Scand 63:549, 1984.
92. Bashore RA, Phillips WH Jr, Brickman CR 3rd: A comparison of the morbidity of midforceps and cesarean delivery. Am J Obstet Gynecol 162:1428, 1990.
93. Traub AI, Morrow RJ, Ritchie JW, et al: A continuing use for Kielland's forceps? Br J Obstet Gynaecol 91:894, 1984.
94. Murphy DJ, Liebling RE, Verity L, et al: Early maternal and neonatal morbidity associated with operative delivery in the second stage of labour: A cohort study. Lancet 358:1203, 2001.
95. Hinton L, Ong S, Danielian PJ: Kiellands forceps delivery—quantification of neonatal and maternal morbidity. Int J Gynecol Obstet 74:289, 2001.

96. Rubin L, Coopland AT: Kielland's forceps. Can Med Assoc J 103:505, 1970.
97. Tan KH, Sim R, Yam KL: Kielland's forceps delivery: Is it a dying art? Singapore Med J 33:380, 1992.
98. Hankins GDV, Rowe TF: Operative vaginal delivery—Year 2000. Am J Obstet Gynecol 175:275, 1996.
99. Healy DL, Quinn MA, Pepperell RJ: Rotational delivery of the fetus; Kielland's forceps and two other methods compared Br J Obstet Gynaecol 89:501, 1982.
100. Krivac TC, Drewes P, Horowitz GM, et al: Kielland vs. non rotational forceps for the second stage of labor. J Reprod Med 44:511, 1999.
101. Hankins GDV, Leicht T, Van Hook J, Uckan EM: The role of forceps rotation in maternal and neonatal injury. Am J Obstet Gynecol 180:231, 1999.
102. Feldman DM, Borgida AF, Sauer F, Rodis JF: Rotational versus nonrotational forceps: Maternal and neonatal outcomes. Am J Obstet Gynecol 181:1185, 1999.
103. Richardson DA, Evans MI, Cibils LA: Midforceps delivery: a critical review. Am J Obstet Gynecol 145:621, 1983.
104. Revah A, Ezra Y, Farine D, Ritchie K: Failed trail of vacuum or forceps-maternal and fetal outcome. Am J Obstet Gynecol 176:200, 1997.
105. Johanson R, Menon V: Vacuum extraction vs. forceps delivery. Cochrane Pregnancy and Childbirth Group Cochrane Database of Systematic Reviews 2, 2005.
106. Ramin SM, Little BB, Gilstrap LC 3rd: Survey of forceps delivery in North American in 1990. Obstet Gynecol 81:307, 1993.
107. Jain V, Guleria K, Gopalan S, Narang A: Mode of delivery in deep transverse arrest. Int J Gynecol Obstet 43:129, 1993.
108. Kim M, Simpson W, Moore T: Teaching forceps: the impact of proactive faculty. Am J Obstet Gynecol 184:S185, 2001.
109. Carollo TC, Reuter JM, Galan HL, Jones RO: Defining fetal station. Am J Obstet Gynecol 191:1793, 2004.

Intrapartum Fetal Evaluation

THOMAS J. GARITE

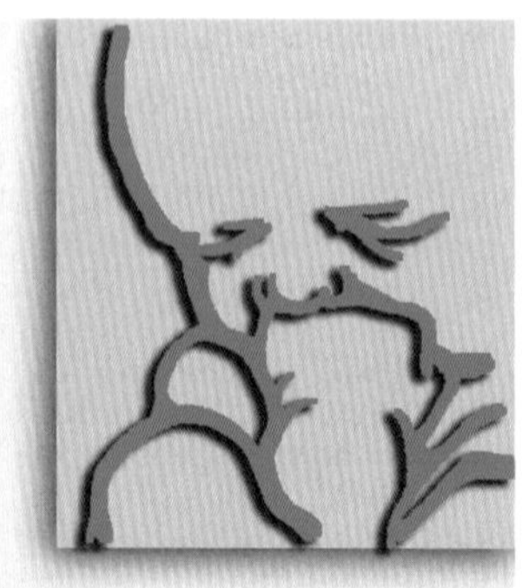

CHAPTER 15

KEY ABBREVIATIONS

American College of Obstetricians and Gynecologists	ACOG
Beats per minute	bpm
Cardiotocography	CTG
Central nervous system	CNS
Electrocardiogram	ECG
Electronic fetal monitoring	EFM
Fetal heart rate	FHR
Human immunodeficiency virus	HIV
Magnesium sulfate	$MgSO_4$
Nonreassuring fetal status	NRFS
National Institute of Child Health and Human Development	NICHD
Premature rupture of the membranes	PROM

The question being asked by the clinician evaluating the fetus in labor is simple: How well oxygenated is the fetus? If hypoxia is severe enough and lasts long enough, fetal tissue and organ damage will result, which may result in long-term injuries or death. Hypoxia severe enough to cause tissue damage virtually always occurs only in the face of a significant metabolic acidosis, and the term asphyxia is used in this situation (Fig. 15-1). To clarify the terminology used in these situations, a glossary is provided at the end of the chapter.

Although there are other less frequent causes of fetal injury or death in labor (e.g., infection, hemorrhage), hypoxia is by far the most common etiology and the one for which medical and surgical interventions have the potential for preventing injury and death. Before intensive intrapartum fetal heart rate (FHR) monitoring, relatively uniform intrapartum fetal death rates of 3 to 4 per 1,000 were reported.[1] Thus, on an obstetric service of 200 to 300 monthly deliveries, 1 intrapartum death would occur each month; but now such events are extremely rare in monitored fetuses. Fetal hypoxia that is severe and associated with metabolic acidosis, but not sufficient to result in death, may alternatively cause asphyxial injury to the fetus and newborn. The fetal central nervous system (CNS) is the organ system most vulnerable to long-term injury. However, the fetus destined to have permanent neurologic damage virtually always has multiorgan dysfunction in the newborn period. Usually, complications such as seizures, respiratory distress, pulmonary hypertension with persistent fetal circulation, renal failure, bowel dysfunction, and pulmonary hemorrhage are seen in the baby who will ultimately have permanent neurologic injury.[2] Babies who recover from these complications and survive may be normal or may develop cerebral palsy.

Cerebral palsy is defined as a movement disorder, usually spastic in nature, that is present at birth, is nonprogressive, and often, but not always, associated with varying degrees of mental retardation.[3] Seizures are often seen in children with cerebral palsy. However, mental retardation or seizures, in the absence of spasticity, are rarely the result of peripartum asphyxia. It is still unclear whether other neurologic dysfunction in children, such as learning and behavioral disorders, can be the result of perinatal asphyxia. Cerebral palsy will develop in 0.5 percent of all births and is prevalent in about 0.1 percent of all school-age children.[3,4] Prematurity remains the leading cause of cerebral palsy. It is estimated that peripartum events contribute to no more than 25 percent of the overall rate of this disease.[5]

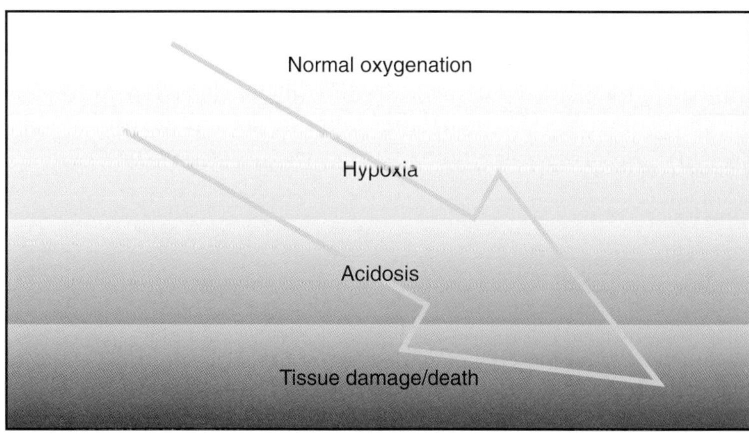

Figure 15-1. The purpose of FHR monitoring is to detect fetal hypoxia and metabolic acidosis. Many fetuses develop hypoxia intermittently but never progress to metabolic acidosis. The ideal is to avoid intervention for hypoxia, but to intervene in the presence of early metabolic acidosis before it can result in tissue damage or fetal death.

Thus, the goal of intrapartum monitoring is to detect hypoxia in labor and allow the clinician to implement nonoperative interventions such as positioning and oxygen (O_2) administration to correct or ameliorate the oxygen deficiency. If this is unsuccessful, the monitor should help the clinician to determine the severity and duration of the hypoxia and whether there is a metabolic acidosis. And finally, if there is sufficient hypoxia and metabolic acidosis present, the monitor should give adequate warning and time to permit the clinician to deliver the baby expeditiously, whether by operative vaginal means or cesarean delivery, thereby preventing damage or death from occurring. Unfortunately, the fetus is inaccessible, and until recently, we have had crude and limited tools available to determine all of the above-mentioned information necessary to make correct and timely decisions to accomplish these goals.

HISTORY OF FETAL MONITORING

Because of the inaccessible location of the fetus, evaluating fetal well-being, or more specifically, fetal oxygen status, has been an ongoing and difficult challenge. In the 1600s, Kilian first proposed that the FHR might be used to diagnose fetal distress and to indicate when the clinician should intervene on behalf of the fetus. The sound of the fetal heart had first been detected by Marsac of France in the 1600s and described in a poem by his colleague, Phillipe LeGaust. This observation went unnoticed until 1818, when Mayor, and subsequently Kergaradec, described the fetal heart sounds by placing an ear on the maternal abdomen. Kergaradec suggested that auscultation of the fetal heart could be used to determine fetal viability and fetal lie. In 1893, VonWinckel described the criteria for fetal distress that were to remain essentially unchanged until the arrival of electronic FHR monitoring. These included tachycardia (FHR > 160 beats per minute [bpm]), bradycardia (FHR < 100 bpm), irregular heart rate, passage of meconium, and gross alteration of fetal movement.[1]

These criteria went unquestioned until 1968, when Benson et al.[6] published the results of the Collaborative Project. These authors reviewed the benefits of auscultation in more than 24,000 deliveries and concluded that "there was no reliable indicator of fetal distress in terms of fetal heart rate save in extreme degree." Thus, it became apparent that other, more sophisticated means of intrapartum fetal evaluation were required. In 1906, Cremer described the use of the fetal electrocardiogram (ECG) using abdominal and intravaginal electrical leads.[7] Several investigators made attempts using ECG waveforms to detect fetal hypoxia but ultimately concluded that there were no consistent fetal ECG changes with fetal distress.[8] The subsequent history of electronic FHR monitoring (EFM) is a story of technological development and empiric observations of alterations in FHR associated with various causes of fetal hypoxia and acidosis.

In 1958, Edward Hon, called the father of EFM in the United States, reported on the instantaneous recording of the fetal ECG from the maternal abdomen.[9] He and his colleagues painstakingly measured R-R intervals from a continuous ECG tracing and mathematically converted these to rate, in beats per minute, and then hand recorded each interval on graph paper. From these efforts, Hon, Caldeyro-Barcia in Uruguay, and Hammacher in Germany began to describe various FHR patterns associated with fetal distress.[10–12] Despite attempts by these and subsequent leaders in the field, universal standards for monitoring and terminology were never established. For example, Europeans tend to refer to electronic FHR monitoring (EFM in the United States) as cardiotocography (CTG) and run their tracings at a paper speed of 1 cm/min as compared with 3 cm/min in this country. The first commercially available electronic fetal monitor was produced in the late 1960s, and by the mid-1970s, EFM was in use in most labor and delivery units in the United States. Today, most women giving birth in the United States have electronic FHR monitoring during labor.

INSTRUMENTATION FOR ELECTRONIC FETAL HEART RATE MONITORING

Many technologic advances have been made since the first monitors were produced. External FHR monitoring using electrocardiography did not function well in labor, and phonocardiography was subject to fetal and maternal movement and other external noise. Doppler became the dominant modality for external monitoring. Initially, this modality was difficult to use because the complex Doppler signal made it difficult to determine which point within that signal the computer should use to measure the interval from beat to beat to convert to rate (Fig. 15-2). Logic, or computer processing formulas, were used to get apparently good continuous signals, but this process introduced artifact, and the apparent variability and other aspects of the FHR were often inaccurate. Ultimately, better Doppler devices coupled with autocorrelation formulas for processing the signal have resulted in excellent external FHR signals that can be relied upon clinically. External monitoring is necessary at all times when the membranes are intact and cannot or should not be ruptured (Fig. 15-3). In addition, certain clinical situations make it unwise to puncture the skin with a fetal electrode for fear of vertical transmission of infection to the fetus. Such conditions include maternal infection with human immunodeficiency virus (HIV), hepatitis C, and herpes simplex.

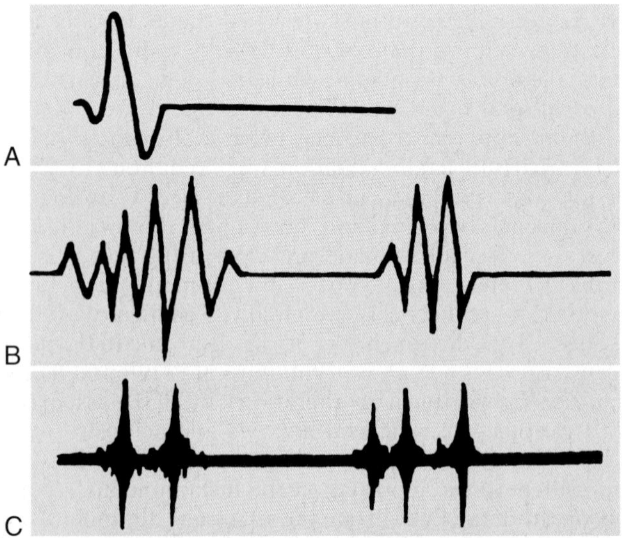

Figure 15-2. These complexes represent the types of signals that the FHR may be required to count. *A,* ECG; *B,* Doppler; *C,* phonocardiogram. Note the complexity of the Doppler signal. To consistently count the same place in the signal complex and avoid artifactually increasing variability, complex signal processing formulas are required.

It is often necessary to apply an internal electrode to obtain a high-quality, accurate, continuous FHR tracing. This is especially true in patients who are obese, those with a premature fetus, or when the mother or fetus is moving too much to obtain an adequate signal. The original internal electrode was made from a modified skin clip that required a special instrument to place it on the fetal scalp. In the mid-1970s, an easier-to-insert and less traumatic spiral electrode was introduced (Fig. 15-4). This electrode is applied to the fetal scalp manually without additional instruments and without the requirement for a speculum to visualize the scalp. The electrical circuit for this electrode includes the spiral electrode for one pole and a small metal bar at the base of the plastic, which, bathed in vaginal secretions, completes the circuit through the mother's body. The spiral electrode has remained in use without substantial change since its introduction. The FHR tracing results from the signal processor, which counts every R-R interval of the ECG from the scalp electrode, converts this interval to rate, and displays every interval (in rate as beats per minute) on the top channel of the two-channel fetal monitor recording paper. The signal is amplified by an automatic gain amplifier, which increases the amplitude (gain) until an adequate signal is available to count (Fig. 15-5). It must be remembered that when the fetus is dead, the amplifier may increase the gain of the small maternal ECG transmitted through the dead fetus, and this may be easily misinterpreted as a fetal bradycardia (Fig. 15-6).

It is clear that the term electronic fetal monitoring, unlike the European version cardiotocography, undervalues the lower channel of the fetal monitor tracing, which provides information about the uterine contractions in labor. Contractions can also be monitored externally or internally. The external monitoring device, or tocodynamometer, is basically a ring-style pressure transducer attached to the maternal abdomen via a belt that main-

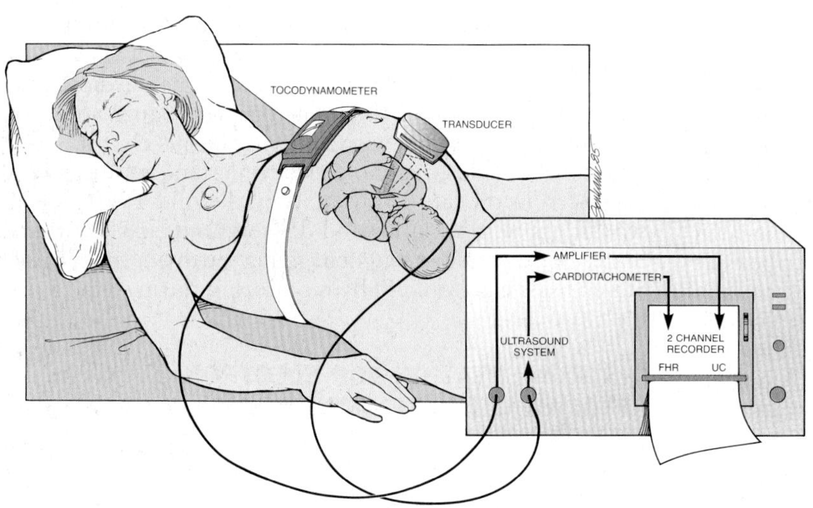

Figure 15-3. Instrumentation for external monitoring. Contractions are detected by the pressure-sensitive tocodynamometer, amplified, and then recorded. Fetal heart rate is monitored using the Doppler ultrasound transducer, which both emits and receives the reflected ultrasound signal that is then counted and recorded.

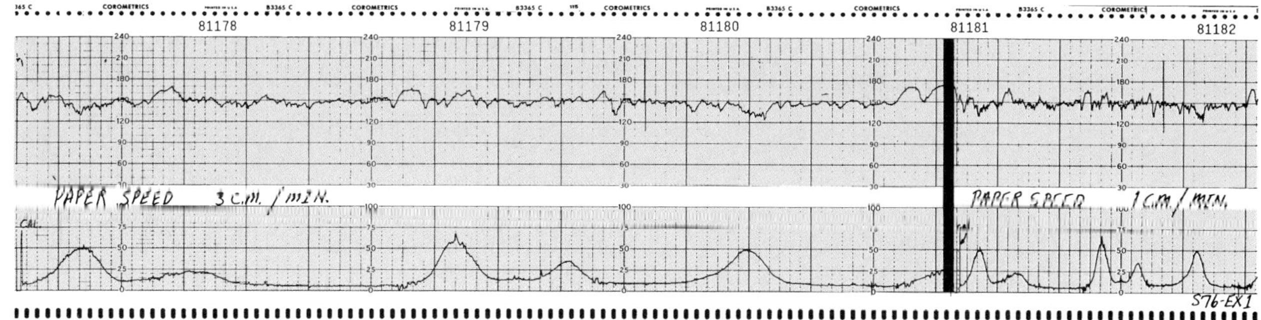

Figure 15-4. Internal fetal heart rate data gathered at the standard recording speed of 3 cm/min for the first portion. The same data are being recorded at a speed of 1 cm/min in the last segment. Normal long-term and short-term variabilities are present. Note that the uterine activity channel has been calibrated so that the intrauterine pressure readings can be measured correctly.

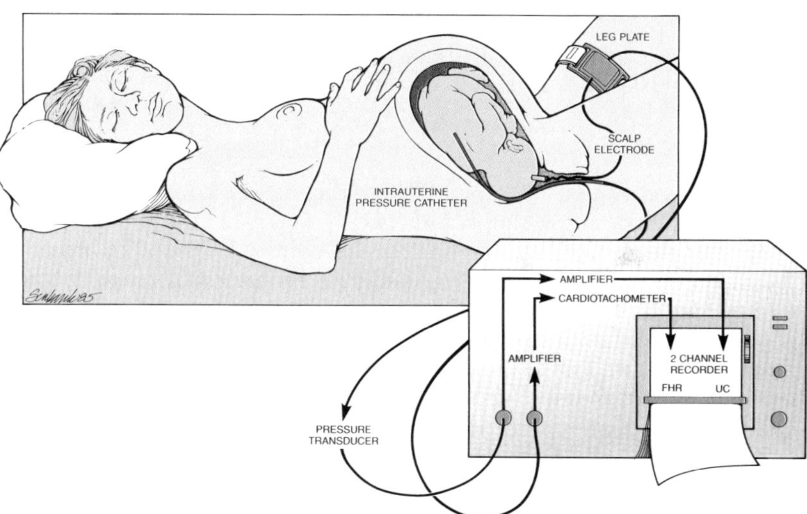

Figure 15-5. Techniques used for direct monitoring of fetal heart rate and uterine contractions. Uterine contractions are assessed with an intrauterine pressure catheter connected to a pressure transducer. This signal is then amplified and recorded. The fetal electrocardiogram is obtained by direct application of the scalp electrode, which is then attached to a leg plate on the mother's thigh. The signal is transmitted to the monitor, where it is amplified, counted by the cardiotachometer, and then recorded.

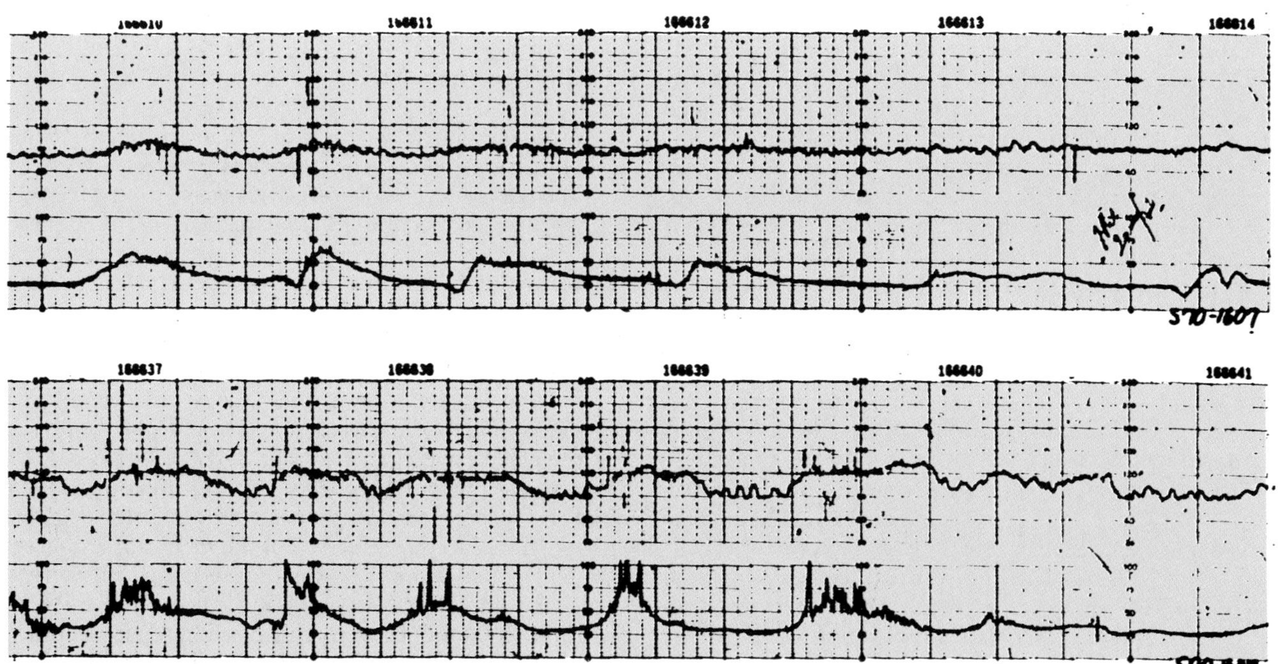

Figure 15-6. This is a tracing from an internal electrode demonstrating an apparent bradycardia with a rate of about 90 bpm. In actuality, this tracing is from a dead fetus, and the automatic gain amplifier increases the amplitude of the maternal ECG signal, allowing the monitor to count and display the maternal heart rate.

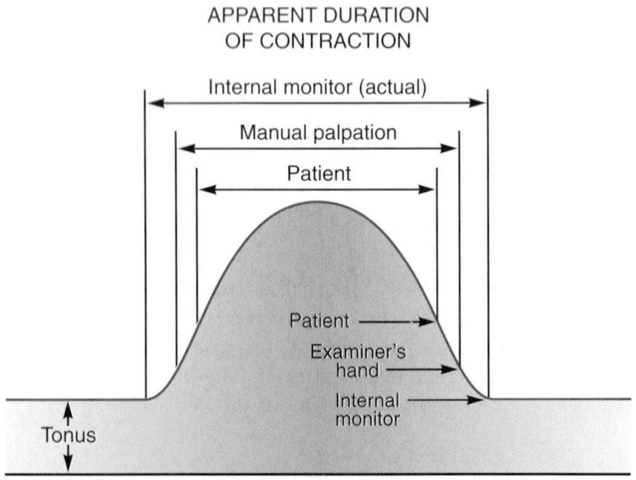

Figure 15-7. The sensitivity of the device used to monitor a uterine contraction can affect not only the apparent strength of the contraction but also the apparent duration of the contraction.

tains tight continuous contact. When the uterus contracts, the change in its shape and rigidity depresses the plunger of the sensor, which changes the voltage of the electrical current. The change in voltage is proportional to the strength of the uterine contractions. The tocodynamometer depicts the frequency of the contractions accurately, but the strength of the contractions only relatively, becaise it cannot measure actual intrauterine pressure. In addition, the apparent duration of the contraction varies with the sensitivity of the monitor, which is negatively affected by variables such as maternal obesity and premature gestational age (Fig. 15-7). The advantage of the external monitor is that it can be used when membranes are intact and it is noninvasive. Its disadvantages, in addition to its inherently limited accuracy, is that it is more uncomfortable for the mother and limits her mobility. Contractions can be more accurately monitored through an intrauterine pressure catheter. The catheters require that the membranes be ruptured and are inserted transcervically beyond and above the fetal presenting part to rest within the uterine cavity. The original pressure catheters were open water-filled systems attached to a pressure transducer adjacent to the fetal monitor. These systems, while accurate, required frequent adjustments and flushing. Newer catheters have closed systems with the strain gauges in the tips or with sensors that relay the signal to a strain gauge at the base of the catheter. Although they are more expensive, they are easier to use and require less nursing attention. Once the catheter is electronically calibrated, the contractions are accurately recorded in terms of frequency, duration, and intensity on the lower channel of the two-channel recording paper or television monitor. This channel is conveniently calibrated at 0 to 100 mm Hg on its vertical scale, from which contraction amplitude can be read. These catheters also are often made with a second port through which saline can be infused for amnioinfusion (see later).

The goal of monitoring is to maintain adequate, high-quality, continuous FHR and contraction tracings while maintaining maximum maternal comfort and avoiding the risk of trauma or infection to the fetus and mother. External devices minimize risk but often give less accurate information and are more uncomfortable for the mother. In general, when the FHR is reassuring and there is an adequate tracing and when the progress of labor is adequate, the external devices are fine. When a better quality FHR tracing is required or it becomes important to accurately assess uterine contraction duration and intensity, then internal devices may be necessary.

THE PHYSIOLOGIC BASIS OF FETAL HEART RATE MONITORING

The basis of FHR monitoring is, in a real sense, fetal brain monitoring. The fetal brain is constantly responding to stimuli, both peripheral and central, with signals to the fetal heart that alter the heart rate on a moment-to-moment basis. Such stimuli to which the brain responds include chemoreceptors, baroreceptors, and direct effects of metabolic changes within the brain itself. The benefit for the brain to modulate the FHR is derived from its goal of maintaining optimal perfusion to the brain without compromising blood flow to other organs any more than is necessary. It should be intuitively obvious, therefore, that the use of FHR to monitor fetal oxygenation is inherently crude and nonspecific, because many stimuli other than oxygen will either cause the brain to alter the fetal heart rate or may have a direct effect on the fetal heart itself. This really explains the most important basic premise of EFM: when the FHR is normal in appearance, one can be assured with high reliability that the fetus is well oxygenated, but when the FHR is not entirely normal, it may be the result of hypoxia or of other variables that may also affect the fetal heart rate. In the past when the FHR became abnormal and the clinician decided intervention was necessary because of concern over fetal hypoxia, the term fetal distress was used. More often than not, however, such intervention results in the delivery of a well-oxygenated, nonacidotic, vigorous newborn. Thus, more recently, on the basis of recommendations of the American College of Obstetricians and Gynecologists (ACOG), the terminology was changed to reflect the inherent inaccuracy of the abnormal FHR. The term fetal distress has been abandoned in favor of the more intellectually honest term nonreassuring fetal status (NRFS).[13]

Fetal oxygenation is determined by many factors. The placenta functions as the fetal lung. Oxygen transfer across the placenta, as in the lung or any membrane, is proportional to the difference between partial pressures of oxygen between the mother and the fetus, the blood flow to the placenta, a coefficient of diffusion for the gas, and the surface area of the placenta. Transfer is inversely proportional to the thickness of the membrane (placenta). Under normal circumstances during labor, the only variable that alters fetal oxygenation is the temporary interruption in blood flow to the placenta that occurs as a result of the compression of the spiral arteries by the wall of the uterus at the peak of the contraction. The duration that the spiral arteries is compressed thus depends on the duration and strength of the contraction (Fig. 15-8).

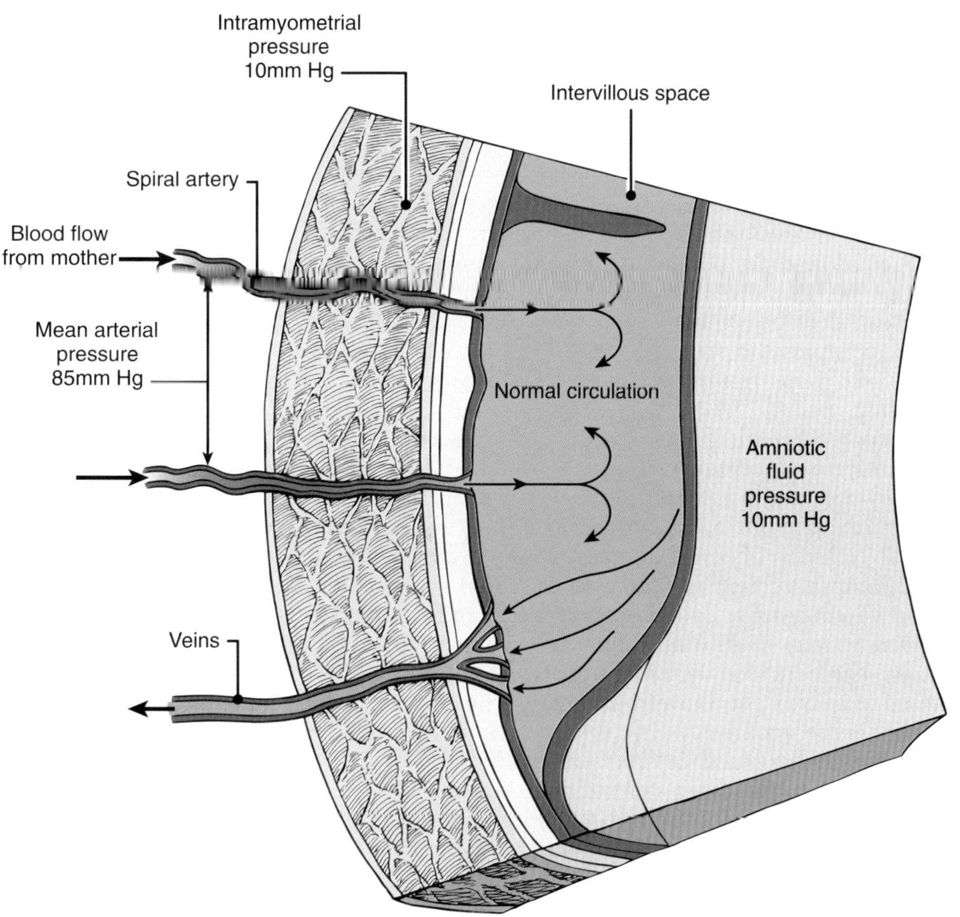

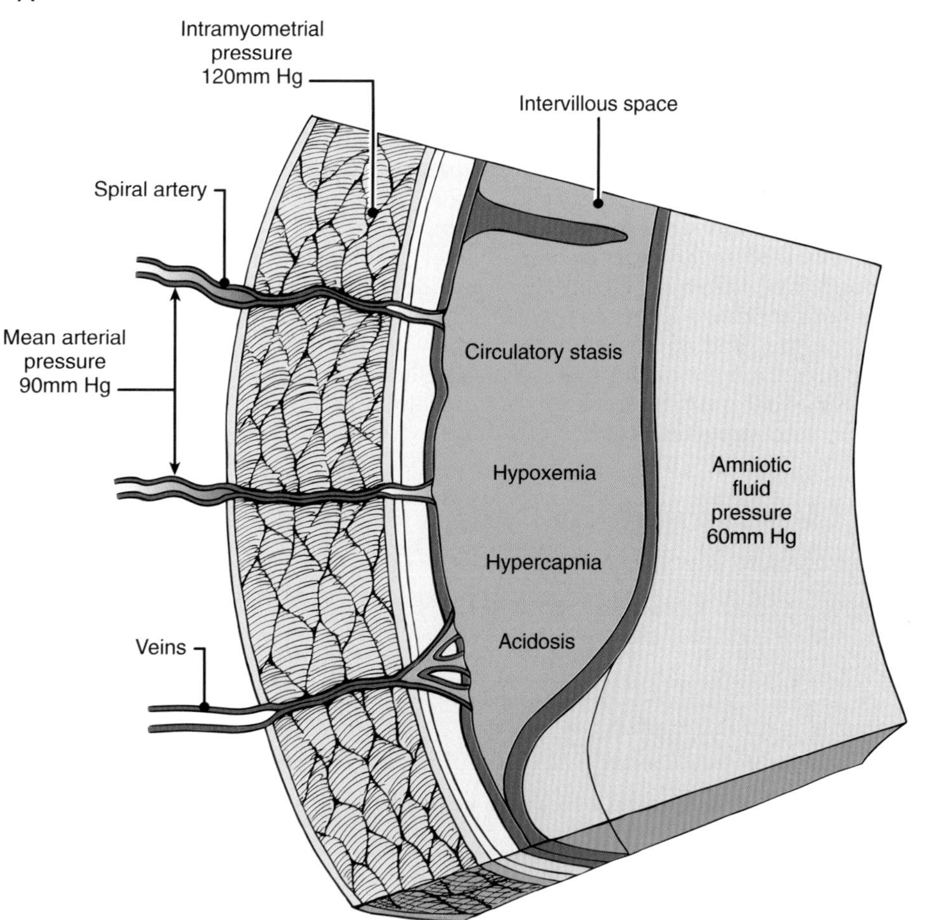

Figure 15-8. In the resting state between contractions *A,* the intraluminal pressure within the spiral arteries exceeds the intramyometrial pressure. Thus uteroplacental blood flow is sustained. However, at the peak of a uterine contraction *B,* the myometrial presure can exceed the arterial pressure and uterine blood flow will be transiently interrupted, temporarily halting oxygen delivery to the placenta.

Under normal circumstances, the fetus tolerates these periods of stasis well without a significant change in its oxygen content. Contractions that are unusually long or unusually strong may, however, result in transient periods of fetal hypoxemia.

Other variables that have the potential for altering fetal oxygenation most commonly include those that affect uterine perfusion. A laboring woman in the supine position can develop supine hypotension as a result of vena caval compression from the uterus. Maternal hypotension with redistribution of blood flow away from the placenta occurs frequently with regional anesthesia. Maternal hemorrhage associated with placenta previa or abruptio placentae may have similar effects. There are several microvascular diseases that can impair fetal oxygenation from poor perfusion within the uteroplacental vascular bed. Examples include hypertension, preeclampsia/eclampsia, collagen vascular disease, diabetic vasculopathy, and prolonged pregnancy. Abruptio placentae may compromise fetal oxygenation in several ways. These include maternal hypotension, as previously noted, a decrease in the surface area of the placenta, and uterine hyperactivity.

Although the placenta functions as the fetal lung, the umbilical cord functions as its trachea, leading oxygen to the baby and carbon dioxide (CO_2) away. Alteration in umbilical cord blood flow is a very common occurrence during labor, either from direct compression or from stretch. Direct compression may occur when the cord becomes impinged between any part of the fetal body and the uterine wall, either with contractions or with fetal movement. This is especially common when there is oligohydramnios, because there is less amniotic fluid to provide a cushion for the cord.[14] Alternatively, cord stretch may occur as the fetus descends into the pelvis. Typically, this is seen just before complete dilation, when descent of the vertex normally occurs. There are three potent stimuli that produce spasm of the umbilical vessels and are intended to allow cessation of fetal umbilical cord blood flow following birth. These include a lower ambient temperature, a higher oxygen tension as the baby begins breathing, and the stretch of the umbilical cord as the baby falls from the birth canal.[15] Thus, it should not be surprising that transient cessation of cord blood flow will occur with stretching of the cord during descent if the cord is looped around the baby's neck and descent of the vertex occurs.

It becomes important, therefore, to understand the physiologic mechanisms that control the FHR. This is so not only because the FHR may be used to determine the severity of the hypoxia and whether a metabolic acidosis is ensuing, but also because the FHR pattern can elucidate the mechanism of the reduction in fetal oxygenation. Thus, by knowing the cause of any hypoxia, the treatment, when possible, can be more specifically directed at the cause. Finally, an understanding of the mechanism and progression of the FHR pattern can often also provide an opportunity to predict how fetal oxygenation will progress over time.

The FHR has many characteristics that we are able to use to accomplish this interpretation. These include the *baseline rate*; the *variability* of the FHR from beat to beat; transient alterations below the baseline, termed *decelerations*; and transient alterations above the baseline, termed *accelerations*. Rate and variability are generally included as *characteristics of the baseline* FHR, and decelerations and accelerations as *periodic changes*.*

Tachycardia

The baseline FHR is typically between 120 and 160 bpm. In very early gestation (15 to 20 weeks), the FHR is significantly higher than in the term fetus. The decline in FHR represents a maturation of fetal vagal tone with progressing gestation.[18] If atropine or other vagolytic drugs are administered, the FHR regresses to the higher baseline of 160 bpm. Thus, the baseline heart rate is largely a function of vagal activity. Many factors have the potential to alter the fetal baseline. Rates above 160 bpm are called *tachycardia*. Tachycardia may have great clinical significance. The two most common causes of tachycardia are maternal fever and drugs that directly raise the fetal heart rate. Maternal fever raises the core temperature of the fetus, which is always about 1°F higher than the maternal temperature. With maternal fever, virtually all fetuses have tachycardia (Fig. 15-9). The FHR rises approximately 10 bpm for each 1°F increase in maternal temperature. Because at term with chorioamnionitis only 1 to 2 percent of fetuses are septic, the tachycardia is

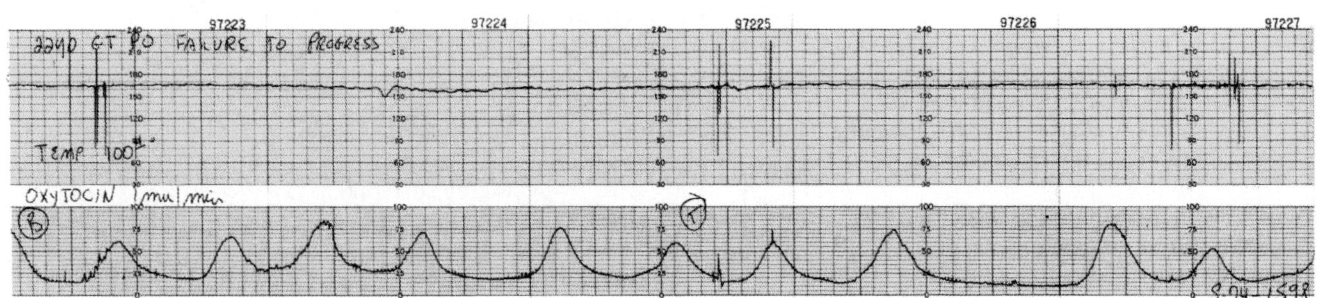

Figure 15-9. A tachycardia with a fetal heart rate of 170 bpm seen in association with a maternal fever of 100.4°F.

*The terminology used in this chapter is fairly standard and is consistent with the most recent ACOG Technical Bulletin (Number 207 July, 1995)[16]; however, a recent publication from the National Institute of Child Health and Human Development Research Planning Workshop has some notable differences, and these are discussed.[17]

unlikely to indicate fetal sepsis but rather is probably caused by an increase in fetal metabolic rate associated with the elevated temperature. Drugs that elevate the FHR fall into one of two categories: vagolytic and β-sympathomimetic. Commonly used drugs that are vagolytic include scopalomine, atropine and phenothiazines, and hydroxyzine. These drugs, however, rarely raise the FHR above 160 bpm. β-Sympathomimetics include terbutaline and ritodrine, used for preterm labor, and terbutaline and epinephrine, used for bronchospasm. Other less common causes of fetal tachycardia include fetal hyperthyroidism, fetal anemia, fetal heart failure, and fetal tachyarrhythmias. As fetal hypoxia becomes progressively worse and persists over time, fetal tachycardia often develops. However, when contractions are present, tachycardia is not the first physiologic response to hypoxia and, in the absence of decelerations, in the laboring patient, is rarely if ever caused by hypoxia.[19]

Bradycardia

An FHR less than 120 bpm is termed a *bradycardia*. One must distinguish between a baseline FHR less than 120 bpm and a deceleration from a previous normal baseline. Not only is a deceleration that is prolonged difficult to distinguish from a baseline change, but there is also some disagreement over terminology. This is an important issue, because a baseline bradycardia is usually innocuous (Fig. 15-10), whereas a prolonged deceleration to less than 120 bpm lasting more than 60 to 90 seconds may often indicate significant fetal hypoxia (Fig. 15-11). True fetal bradycardias are due to several possible causes. In the range of 90 to 120 bpm, a bradycardia may often be a normal variant, and these fetuses are usually bradycardic after birth but are otherwise well oxygenated and normal. As with tachycardia and fever, maternal hypothermia may cause fetal bradycardia. This is commonly seen with patients on magnesium sulfate ($MgSO_4$) who are vasodilated, and it has also been described with maternal hypoglycemia and hypothermia.[20,21] A number of drugs may also result in fetal bradycardia. A fetal baseline heart rate in the range of 80 bpm or less, especially with reduced variability, may be caused by a complete heart block. Complete heart block may result from antibodies associated with maternal lupus erythematosus, may be seen with congenital cardiac anomalies, or is idiopathic.[22] Although a heart block is not associated with hypoxia, it makes the FHR essentially useless in monitoring fetal oxygenation, because the fetal brain is no longer communicating with the ventricle of the heart that is being monitored. Finally, when a patient is admitted with a baseline bradycardia, one should also consider the possibility of maternal heart rate being recorded with a dead fetus (whether internal or external monitor) (Fig. 15-6). Real-time ultrasound is used to verify that the bradycardia is fetal in origin.

Variability

The fetal cardiotachometer is unique among adult monitors in that it records the interval-to-interval difference in rate for every heart beat. Thus, differences in heart rate from beat to beat are recorded as variability reflected visually as a line that fluctuates above and below the baseline.

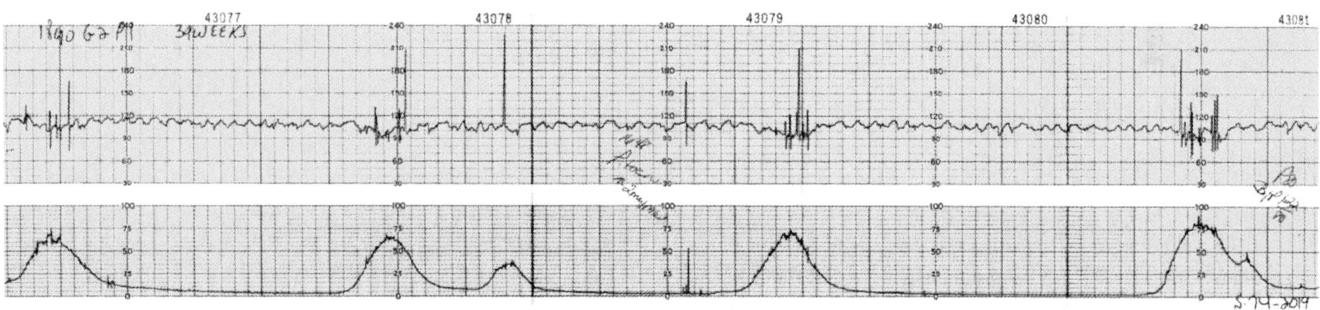

Figure 15-10. A bradycardia with a fetal heart rate of 110 bpm. This patient is in premature labor at 34 weeks' gestation and is being treated with magnesium sulfate. The fetal bradycardia is probably because of maternal hypothermia, which can be seen with vasodilation caused by the magnesium sulfate.

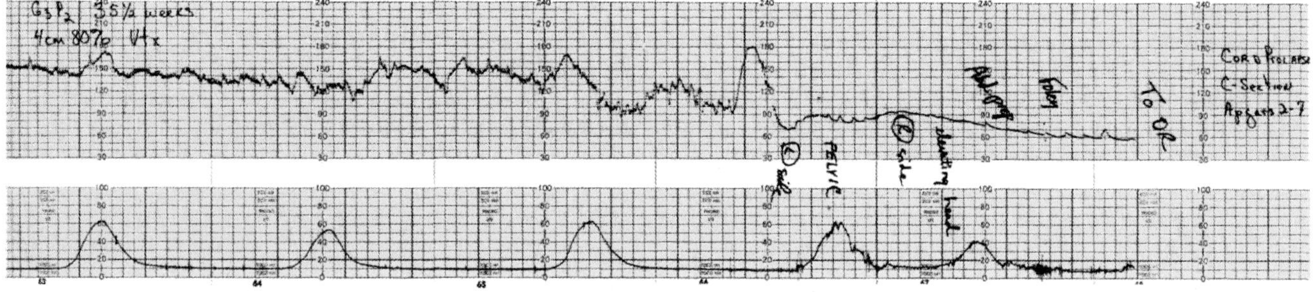

Figure 15-11. The prolonged deceleration to 60 bpm, in this case due to umbilical cord prolapse, should be distinguished from a fetal bradycardia, which is defined as the baseline heart rate.

This variability is a reflection of neuromodulation of the FHR by an intact and active CNS and also reflects normal cardiac responsiveness. Generally, the variability of the FHR is described as having two components: *short-term* and *long-term variability*. Short-term variability is the beat-to-beat irregularity in the FHR and is caused by the difference in rates between successive beats of the FHR. It is caused by the push-pull effect of sympathetic and parasympathetic nerve input, but the vagus nerve has the dominant role in affecting variability. Long-term variability is the waviness of the FHR tracing, and is generally seen in three to five cycles per minute. Previous texts spent considerable effort in distinguishing between the significance of short- and long-term variability, but in general, they are reduced or increased together, and there is no clear evidence that distinguishing between the two is helpful clinically. The National Institute of Child Health and Human Development (NICHD) Research Planning Workshop also concluded that no distinction should be made between short- and long-term variability.[17]

This characteristic of the fetal baseline, if interpreted correctly, can be one of the most useful single parameters in determining the severity of fetal hypoxia. The simplest way to describe the causes of alterations, especially reductions, in FHR variability is to say that this parameter reflects the activity of the fetal brain. When the fetus is alert and active, the FHR variability is normal or increased. When the fetus is obtunded, owing to whatever cause, the variability is reduced. Because severe hypoxia, especially when it reaches the level of metabolic acidosis, always depresses the CNS, normal variability reliably indicates the absence of severe hypoxia and acidosis (Fig. 15-12*A*). Unfortunately, the converse is not true, because there are many factors that cause the CNS to be depressed

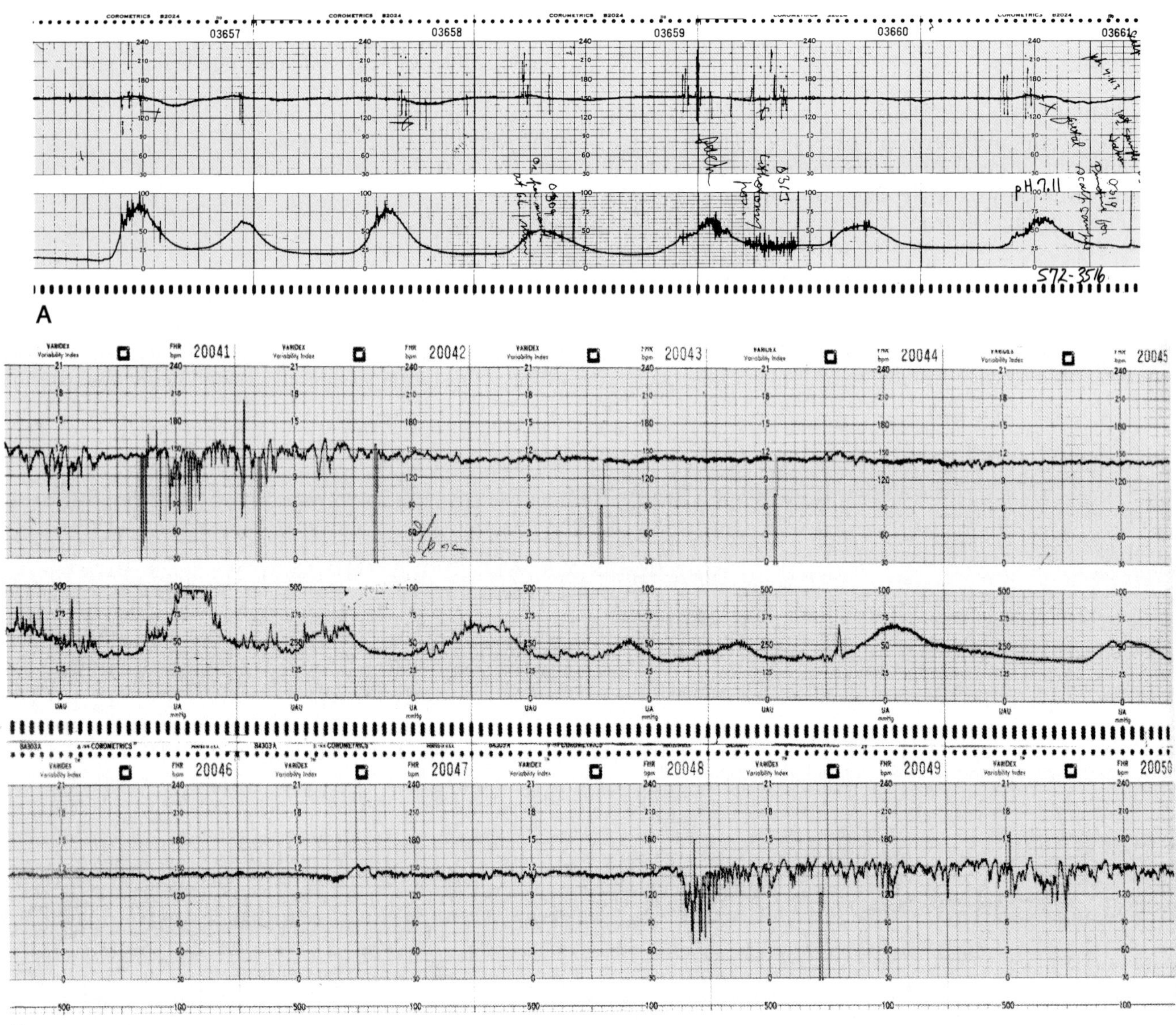

Figure 15-12. *A,* The markedly decreased variability seen in this case is in association with persistent late decelerations. A scalp pH of 7.11 confirms that the loss of variability is because of CNS depression caused by acidosis. *B,* The abrupt decrease in variability seen here, in contrast to *A*, is not seen in association with any decelerations that might suggest hypoxia. Thus, the decreased variability must be because of another reason, and in this case, given the equally abrupt return to normal variability in *B,* is probably caused by a fetal sleep cycle.

(see box, Potential Causes of Decreased Variability of the Fetal Heart Rate); thus, reduced variability is a very nonspecific finding and must be interpreted in the context of other indicators of hypoxia, and other causes of reduced variability must be considered (Fig. 15-12*B*). In general, anything that is associated with depressed or reduced brain function will diminish variability. These include fetal sleep cycles; drugs, especially CNS depressants; fetal anomalies, especially of the CNS; and previous insults that have damaged the fetal brain. FHR variability is also affected by gestational age, and very immature fetuses of less than 26 weeks' gestation often have reduced variability from an immature CNS, although this situation varies from fetus to fetus. In addition, as heart rate increases with fetal tachycardia, variability is often reduced from the rate alone, as sympathetic dominance overrides the natural influence of the vagus.

Increased FHR variability, original referred to as a salutatory FHR pattern, in nonlaboring animals has been shown to be associated with very early or minimal hypoxia.[23] This is a rare pattern and difficult to interpret. In labor, late, variable, or prolonged decelerations virtually always present with early hypoxia, and increased variability is not consistent with an acidotic fetus; so this finding can be interpreted in context with the entire FHR pattern.

Another problem with variability besides its nonspecificity, is that the interpretation of variability is quite subjective. Variability is usually described quantitatively, as normal, increased, reduced, or absent. The National Institute of Child Health and Human Development (NICHD) Research Planning Workshop suggested that FHR variability be defined as follows:

Absent: amplitude undetectable
Minimal: amplitude > undetectable and ≤5 bpm
Moderate: amplitude 6 to 25 bpm
Marked: >25 bpm.[17]

Experts given tracings to interpret often disagree on the quantification of variability even using just these four categories. Trying to categorize variability any further is fraught with even more potential for disagreement and does not appear to have predictive value.

Potential Causes of Decreased Variability of the Fetal Heart Rate

Depression due to hypoxia and acidosis
Fetal anomalies, especially of the CNS
Fetal sepsis
Tumors of the CNS
Fetal heart block
Tachycardia
Extreme prematurity
Previous neurologic insult
Fetal sleep cycles
Drugs/medications
- Narcotics
- Barbiturates
- Tranquilizers
- Phenothiazines
- Parasympatholytics
- General anesthetics

CNS, central nervous system.

PERIODIC CHANGES

Variability, tachycardia, and bradycardia are characteristic alterations of the baseline heart rate. Periodic changes of the FHR include decelerations and accelerations. These are transient changes in the fetal heart rate of relatively brief duration, with return to the original baseline FHR. In labor, these changes usually occur in response to uterine contractions but may also occur with fetal movement.

Decelerations

There are four principal types of decelerations: *early*, *late*, *variable*, and *prolonged*. These are named for their timing, relationship to contractions, duration, and shape, but they are important distinctions more because they describe the cause of the decelerations.

EARLY DECELERATIONS

Early decelerations are shallow, symmetric, uniform decelerations with onset and return that are gradual, resulting in a U-shaped deceleration (Fig. 15-13). They begin early in the contraction, have their nadir coincident with the peak of the contraction, and return to the baseline by the time the contraction is over. Early decelerations are not associated with accelerations that precede or follow the deceleration. These decelerations rarely descend more than 30 to 40 bpm below the baseline rate. They are thought to be caused by compression of the fetal head by the uterine cervix as it overrides the anterior fontanel of

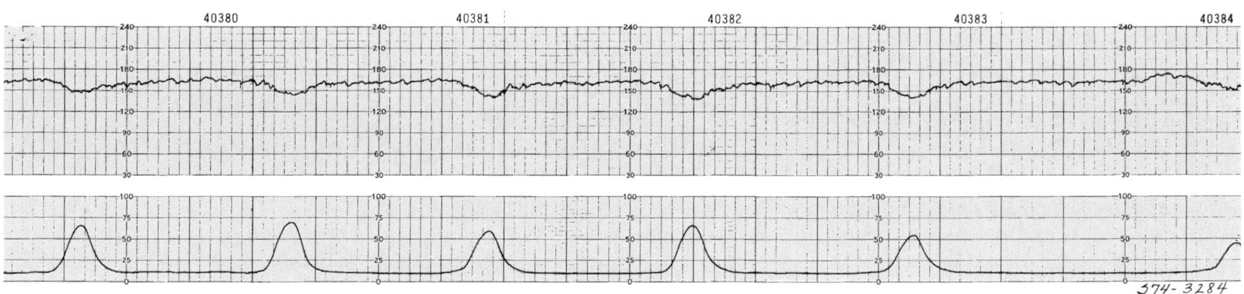

Figure 15-13. Early decelerations.

the cranium.[24] This results in altered cerebral blood flow, precipitating a vagal reflex with the resultant slowing of the FHR. More nonspecific head compression can result in decelerations that are indistinguishable from variable decelerations. Because of the similar cause, these latter decelerations have often been called early decelerations but are by definition not so. Because the cervix creates the pressure, these decelerations are usually seen between 4 and 6 cm of dilation (E.H. Hon, personal communication). They do not indicate fetal hypoxia and are only significant in that they may be easily confused with late decelerations because of their similar shape and depth. They are the most infrequent of decelerations, occurring in about 5 to 10 percent of all fetuses in labor.

Late Decelerations

Late decelerations are similar in appearance to early decelerations. They, too, are of gradual onset and return, U-shaped, and generally descend below the baseline no more than 30 to 40 bpm, although there are exceptions. However, in contrast to early decelerations, late decelerations are delayed in timing relative to the contraction. They begin usually about 30 seconds after the onset of the contraction or even at or after its peak. Their nadir is after the peak of the contraction. FHR variability may be unchanged or even increased during the decelerations. These decelerations are not associated with accelerations immediately preceding or following their onset and return (Fig. 15-14).

The physiology of late decelerations is quite complex, but an understanding of the physiology pays dividends in terms of interpreting and managing these important FHR changes. Late decelerations are generally said to be caused by uteroplacental insufficiency. This implies that uteroplacental perfusion is temporarily interrupted during the peak of strong contractions. The fetus that normally will not become hypoxic with this temporary halt in blood flow may do so if there is insufficient perfusion or oxygen exchange at other times. Whereas this may be a correct idealized description, in reality any compromise of delivery, exchange, or uptake in fetal oxygen, other than by umbilical cord compression, can result in a late deceleration if the insult is sufficient. Physiologically, oxygen sensors within the fetal brain detect a relative drop in fetal oxygen tension in association with the uterine contraction. This change initially results in an increase in sympathetic neuronal response, causing an elevation in fetal blood pressure that, when detected by baroreceptors, produces a protective slowing in the FHR in response to the increase in peripheral vascular resistance. This has been referred to as the reflex type of late deceleration. This complex double reflex is probably the reason the deceleration is delayed.[25] During this type of reflex, the depth of the deceleration is proportional to the severity of the hypoxia and the deceleration moves closer to the contraction as the hypoxia becomes more severe. However, there is also a second type of late deceleration, caused by myocardial depression. As the hypoxia continues and becomes more severe, late decelerations are no longer vagally mediated and are seen even with interruption of the vagus nerve; thus, they are directly myocardial in origin. These decelerations are *not* proportional in their depth to the severity of the hypoxia, and actually may become more shallow as the hypoxia becomes severe. Because of this latter type of deceleration, it is generally agreed that the depth of the late deceleration cannot be used to judge the severity of the hypoxia. Because of the mechanisms causing these changes, *late decelerations always indicate fetal hypoxia.* Only the severity of the hypoxia and the overall duration of the late decelerations will determine whether a metabolic acidosis will occur, and this is highly unpredictable. One reason this may be so is found in recent data suggesting that the oxygen threshold that triggers the brain to slow the fetal heart in this characteristic way may be more related to the relative drop from baseline oxygenation rather than an absolute number.[26] Thus, the fetus accustomed to higher than average oxygen saturation may have a drop in oxygen at or only slightly below the normal range; a level deep enough to signal a late deceleration but not low enough to require anaerobic metabolism. Another important point in understanding the results of hypoxia associated with late decelerations is that the placenta's capacity for exchanging oxygen is substantially less than its capacity for exchanging carbon dioxide. In situations in which there are persistent late decelerations and the fetus becomes sufficiently hypoxic to develop a metabolic acidosis, there may be no reten-

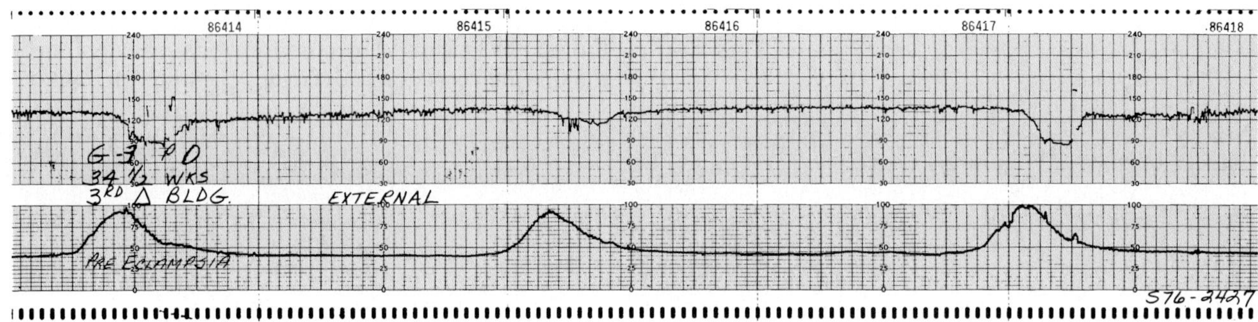

Figure 15-14. A case complicated by third-trimester bleeding in which the external heart rate and uterine activity data are collected. Note the presence of persistent late decelerations with only three contractions in 20 minutes as well as the apparent loss of variability of the fetal heart rate. The rise in baseline tone of the uterine activity channel cannot be evaluated with the external system.

tion of carbon dioxide. This is analogous to the adult with lung disease but no airway disease in whom hypoxia is often seen without difficulty in eliminating CO_2. Thus, the metabolic acidosis is usually not mixed with a respiratory acidosis. The only common exception to this is with abruptio placentae, in which CO_2 retention is seen with late decelerations.[27]

Causes of late decelerations include any factor that can alter delivery, exchange, or uptake of oxygen at the fetal-maternal interface within the placenta. Most commonly, late decelerations are observed in patients without inherent pathology. Excessive uterine contractions, usually seen with oxytocin, are the single most common cause of late decelerations. In these situations, the duration of interruption of uterine blood flow is prolonged and the hypoxia is more than the normal fetus can endure, and late decelerations are expressed. Conduction anesthesia (spinal or epidural) can cause either systemic or local hypoperfusion/hypotension, and thus the level of contractions required to interrupt uterine blood flow is lower, and again the duration of interruption of uterine blood flow is prolonged (Fig. 15-15). The most common pathologic conditions of the placenta associated with late decelerations are those characterized by either microvascular disease in the placenta or local vasospasm compromising blood flow and thus exchange. Common causes include postmaturity, maternal hypertension (chronic hypertension or preeclampsia), collagen vascular diseases, and diabetes mellitus in its more advanced stages. Besides altering perfusion, abruptio placentae is an example of altered placental exchange caused by a combination of reduced placental surface area and increased contractions that typically result in late decelerations when the separation is sufficient to cause fetal hypoxia. Severe maternal anemia or maternal hypoxemia may compromise oxygen delivery and result in late decelerations. Conversely, chronic fetal anemia may diminish fetal oxygen uptake and be associated with late decelerations.

Variable Decelerations

The most common type of decelerations seen in the laboring patient is variable decelerations. Variable decelerations are, in general, synonymous with umbilical cord compression, and anything that results in the interruption of blood flow within the umbilical cord will result in a variable deceleration. The variable deceleration is the most difficult pattern to describe verbally, but the easiest to recognize visually. First and foremost, the term variable is by far the best single word to describe this type of deceleration. They are variable in all ways: size, shape, depth, duration, and timing relative to the contraction. The onset is usually abrupt and sharp. The return is similarly abrupt in most situations. The depth and duration are proportional to the severity and duration of interruption of cord blood flow. Variable decelerations are usually seen with accelerations immediately preceding the onset of the deceleration and immediately following the return to baseline. The NICHD Research Planning Workshop proposed that the duration of a variable deceleration should be limited to 2 minutes, and that beyond 2 minutes, it should be called a prolonged deceleration.[17] However, most definitions in the past have not put a limit on duration but rely more on the appearance of the deceleration. More than 50 years ago, Barcroft first described the variable deceleration when he ligated the umbilical cord of a fetal goat (Fig. 15-16).[28] In 1975, Lee externalized the human umbilical cord at cesarean section before delivery and demonstrated that the reflex involved in the complex pattern of the variable deceleration is one that is caused primarily by changes in systemic blood pressure in the fetus and is mediated through baroreceptors (Fig. 15-17).[29] When the umbilical cord is gradually compressed, the thinner walled umbilical vein collapses first and blood flow returning to the fetus is interrupted. This results in decreased cardiac return, fetal hypotension, and a baroreceptor reflex that leads the brain to accelerate the heart rate in order to maintain cardiac output. This increase in

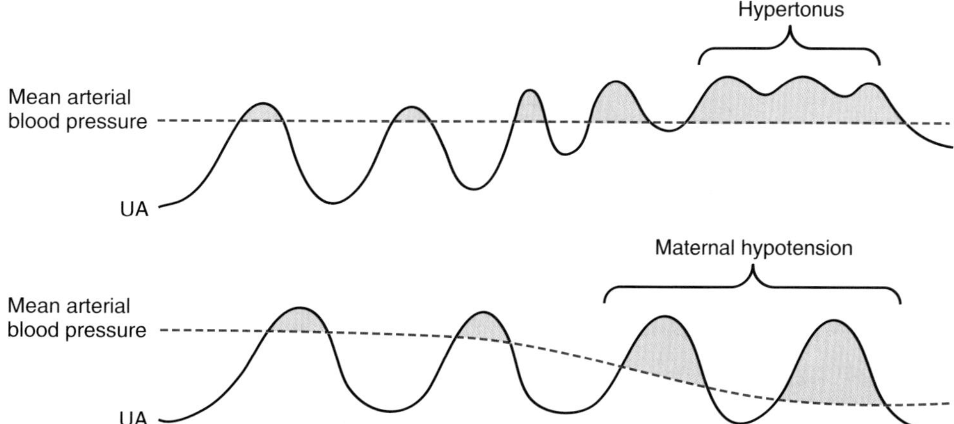

Figure 15-15. The two most common causes of late decelerations in labor are excessive uterine contractions (usually caused by oxytocin) and maternal hypotension. Both result in decrease in uteroplacental perfusion, hypertonus by interrupting the transmyometrial perfusion for a prolonged period, and hypotension by dropping the perfusion pressure, thus increasing the amount of time perfusion is interrupted even with a normal contraction. UA, uterine artery.

heart rate is the acceleration that precedes the variable deceleration. With continuing compression, the umbilical artery is compressed, and the fetus detects an increase in systemic vascular resistance as the previously low-resistance placental bed, to which 50 percent of fetal cardiac output normally flows, is occluded. The baroreceptors detect the increase in resistance, and the heart slows as a protective mechanism. As the cord vessels gradually open, the arteries open first and the heart rate returns to baseline; but if the flow in the vein is still blocked, an acceleration of the same mechanism of the one that preceded the deceleration occurs. Although this model is idealized, one might surmise that the orderly occlusion of vein, vein and artery, vein does not always occur. This is probably the reason that with variable decelerations, any combination of deceleration with acceleration preceding, preceding and following, following only, neither, or even acceleration alone may be seen with cord compression, as in Figure 15-18.

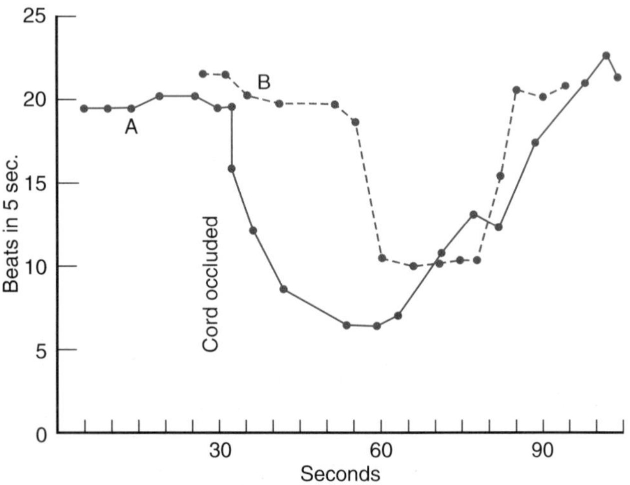

Figure 15-16. This is the original description of a variable deceleration in a fetal goat by Barcroft. The *solid line A* represents the fetal heart rate with temporary umbilical cord occlusion and the *dotted line B* is the fetal heart rate with temporary cord occlusion after the vagal nerve has been severed.

In reality, although we refer to umbilical cord compression as the single mechanism for interruption of cord blood flow, there are probably several different mechanisms that may have the same end result. Compression may be the mechanism that occurs when the cord is impinged between a fetal body part and the uterine wall during contractions or with fetal movement. As previously mentioned, cord stretch may be the reason the flow is compromised with nuchal cords and seen as the baby descends through the pelvis. If cold saline is infused too rapidly with amnioinfusion, the FHR may slow, presumably caused by cord spasm, the natural fetal reflex to cold stimulus. Whatever the mechanism, it is most important to realize that variable decelerations are initially caused by a reflex in response to changes in pressure and not hypoxia. Thus, variable decelerations (even deep and prolonged) can be seen in fetuses with no change in oxygen saturation (Fig. 15-19).

Variable decelerations are seen in the vast majority of all labors, and most often, these decelerations occur without fetal hypoxemia. It is apparent that additional criteria are needed to separate those benign variable

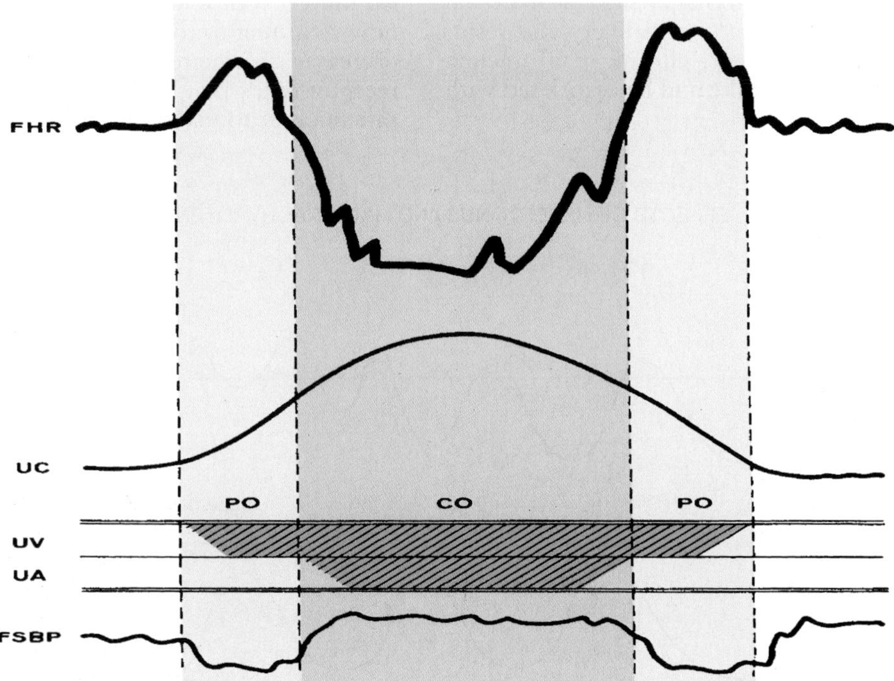

Figure 15-17. This figure represents fetal heart rate (FHR) and fetal systemic blood pressure (FSBP) occurring during compression of the umbilical vein (UV) and umbilical artery (UA). UC is the uterine contraction. Note the acceleration of the FHR as the FSBP is decreased, marking a baroreceptor response to decreased cardiac return, and the deceleration of the FHR when the FSBP is increased, the baroreceptor response to increased peripheral resistance. CO, complete occlusion; PO, partial occlusion.

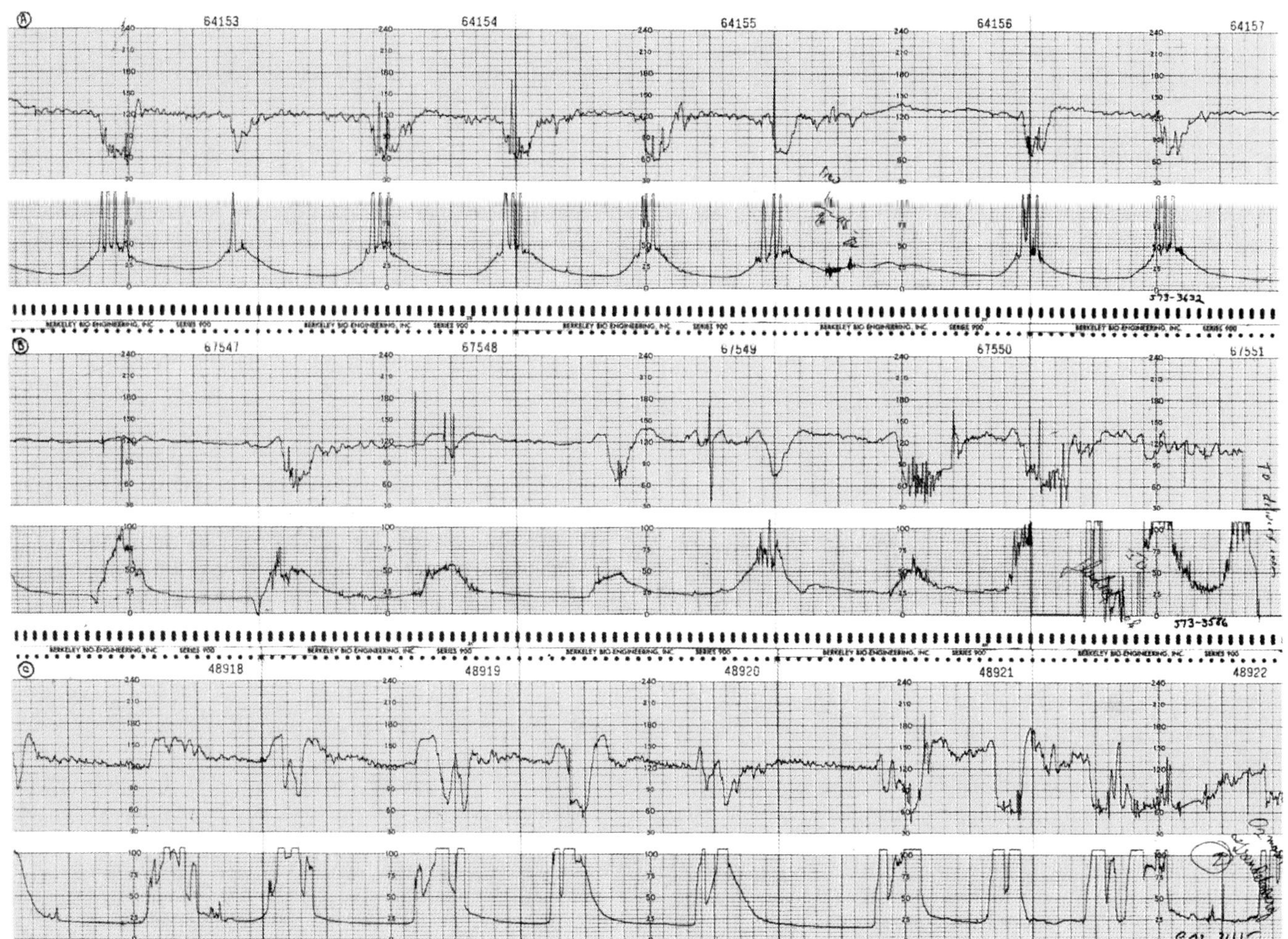

Figure 15-18. These are typical variable decelerations. Note that such decelerations are often recognized by the accelerations that precede and follow the decelerations.

decelerations not likely to be associated with hypoxia from those that are. Kubli et al.[30] described a category of mild, moderate, and severe variable decelerations based on depth and duration (see box, Classifications of the Severity of Variable Decelerations). Although there is indeed a correlation between the severity of these decelerations and the likelihood of hypoxia, one can see from Figure 15-19 that it is difficult to pick a specific depth and duration that always predicts oxygen compromise. Therefore, in addition, characteristics of the fetal baseline are also used, including the development of tachycardia and loss of variability (Fig. 15-20). When cord compression occurs with each contraction and is sustained for a prolonged period of time, there will be a change from the usual abrupt return to baseline to a slow or delayed return to baseline (Fig. 15-21). This is also often called a late component, although a combined pattern of late and variable decelerations (Fig. 15-22) should be distinguished from progressive, severe variable decelerations that result in slow return to baseline, as the etiologies and thus the potential treatments will differ. This particular discriminator of variable decelerations can be one of the most confusing aspects in all of fetal monitoring. Because a slow return to baseline can represent fetal hypoxia from either progressive cord compression or from a coincident late deceleration, the question is, Does this finding always represent hypoxia? Many times this sign appears without significant cord compression preceding its onset; therefore, it is unlikely that a substantial oxygen deficit has developed. Thus, many times these are benign findings and may represent more slow release of the cord or some other unexplained phenomenon. Finally, in extreme situations in which there is profound fetal hypoxia and acidosis, the variable decelerations will appear smoother and rounded or "blunted" rather than having the usual abrupt changes seen with the more common benign decel-

Classifications of the Severity of Variable Decelerations

Mild
- Deceleration of a duration of <30 seconds, regardless of depth
- Decelerations not below 80 bpm, regardless of duration

Moderate
- Deceleration with a level <80 bpm

Severe
- Deceleration to a level <70 bpm for >60 seconds

Data from Kubli et al.[30]

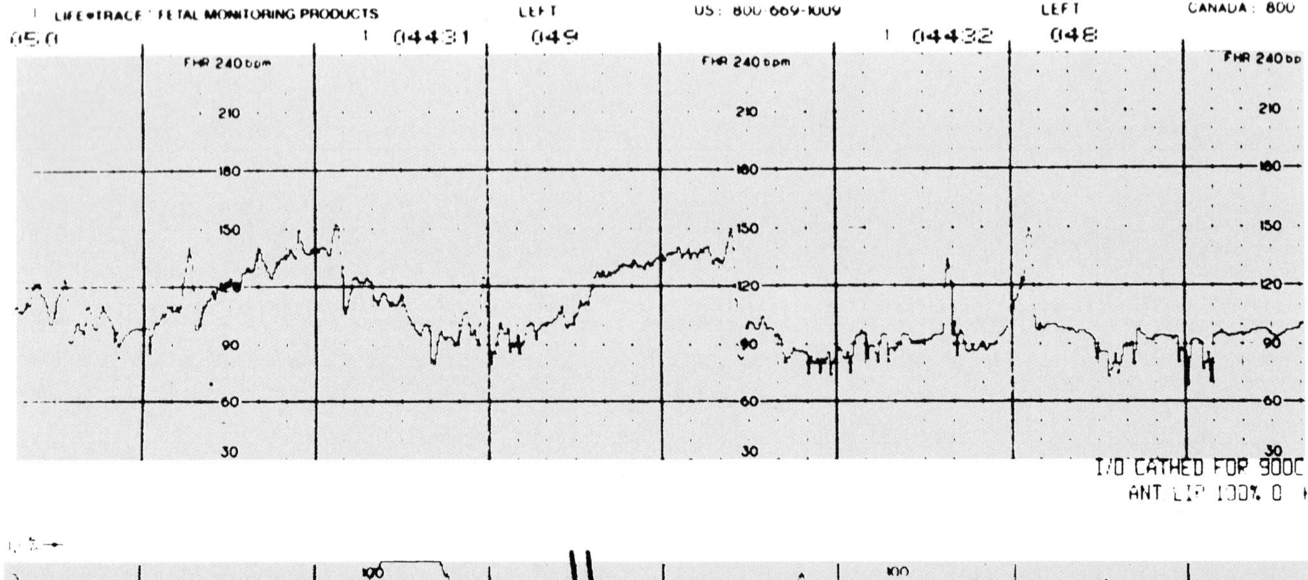

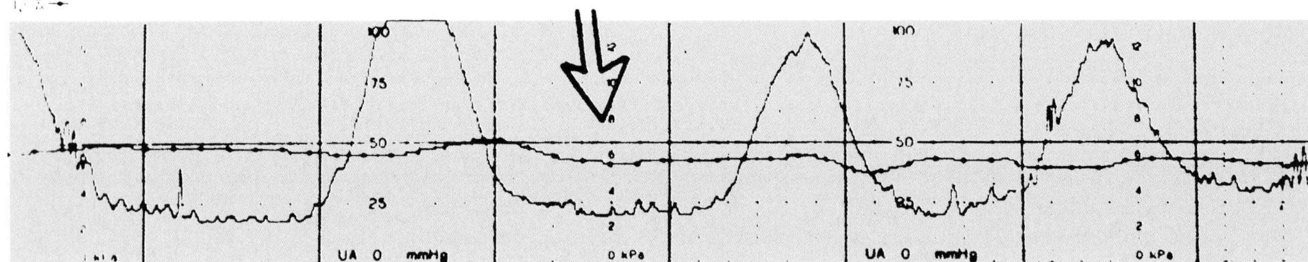

Figure 15-19. Superimposed on the contraction monitor tracing is a continuous tracing using a newly approved fetal pulse oximeter. The tracing shows an fetal oxygen saturation value ranging from 50 to 40 percent (normal = 35 to 60 percent). Note the consistently normal saturation values despite the prolonged FHR decelerations to 80 bpm.

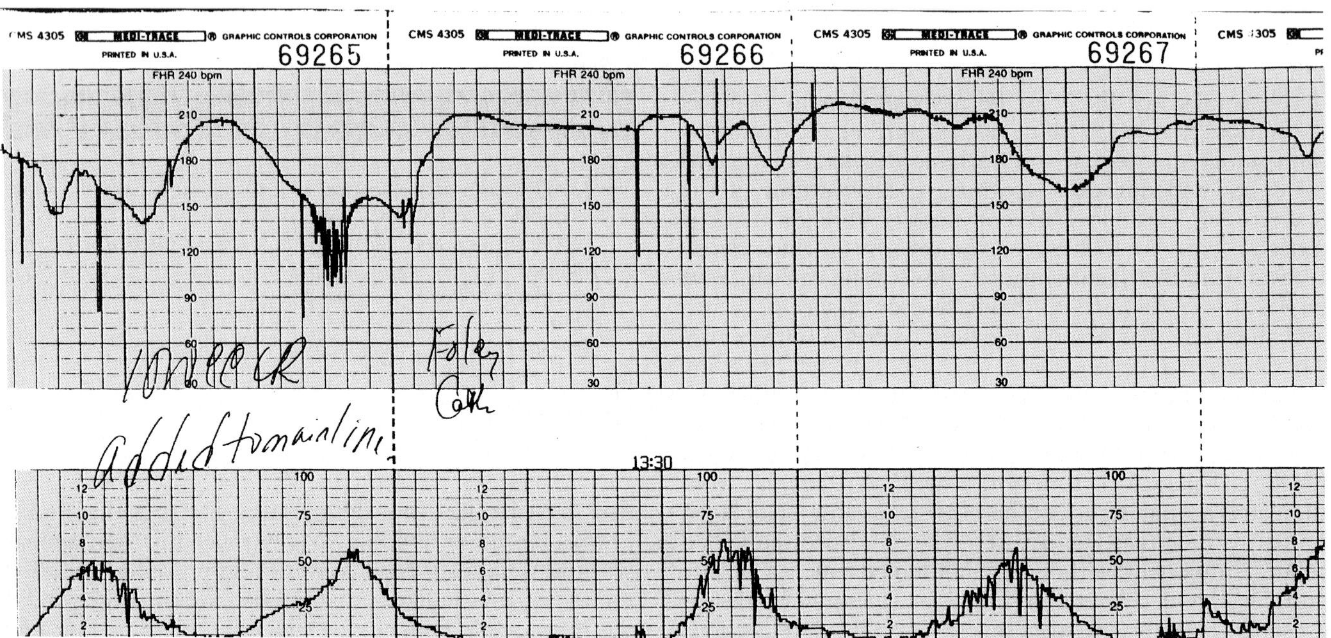

Figure 15-20. The association of loss of variability and tachycardia in association with these variable decelerations make this a nonreassuring FHR pattern.

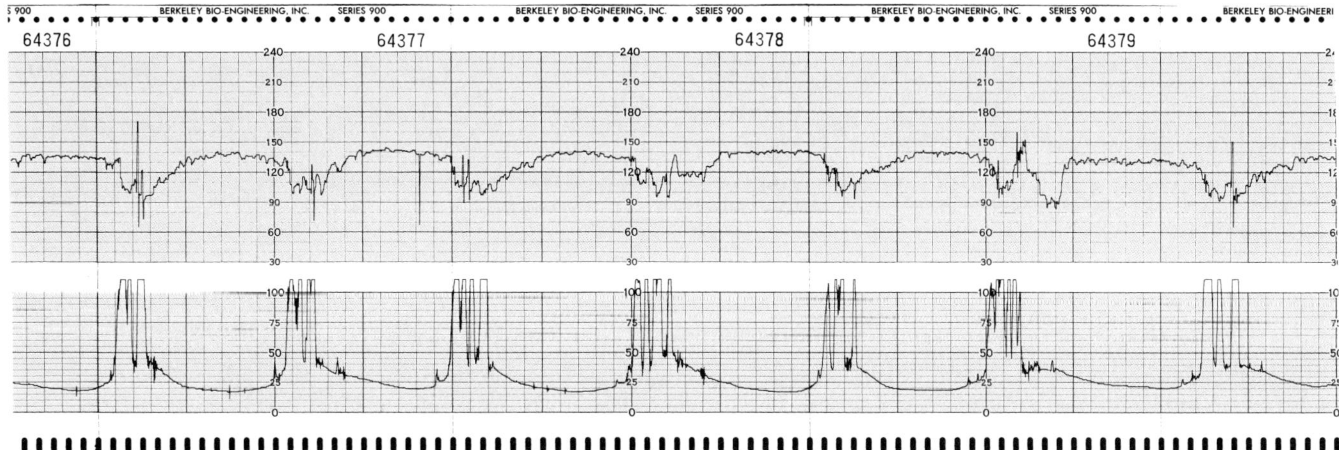

Figure 15-21. These variable decelerations, although mild in depth and duration, are associated with a slow, rather than abrupt, return to baseline. This may be a sign of developing hypoxia as a result of repetitive umbilical cord compression with inadequate opportunity to reoxygenate between events. Generally, this finding makes the variable decelerations nonreassuring.

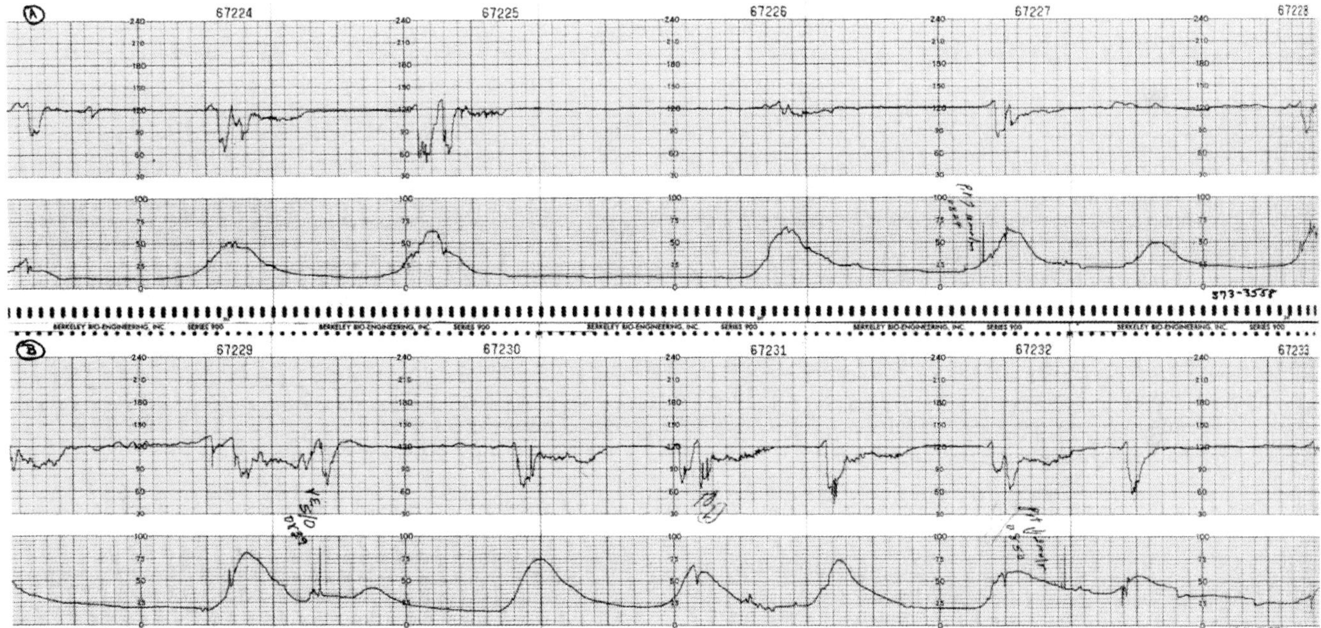

Figure 15-22. Here are repetitive variable decelerations with a slow return to baseline. However, the minimal depth and duration of the variable decelerations and the fact that one can see an independent late deceleration with the third contraction would suggest that this pattern is actually a combined one of mild variable and persistent late decelerations.

erations. Such cases are virtually always seen in association with absent FHR variability and they can also be followed by a blunted acceleration following the return to baseline described by Goodlin and Lowe as overshoot (Fig. 15-23).[31] This is a rare situation and is seen only when all criteria are met including absent variability, blunted variable decelerations, no acceleration preceding the variable deceleration, and no other spontaneous accelerations of the FHR.

There are four categories of causes of cord compression patterns that are useful to consider from a management standpoint. Variable decelerations appearing early in labor are often caused by oligohydramnios. Other variable decelerations often first appear when the patient reaches 8 to 9 cm of dilation, the time in labor when the curve for descent of the presenting part becomes steep. This is probably most often because of nuchal cords, wherein the cord becomes stretched with descent of the fetal head, and as previously described, cord stretch is a profound stimulus for vasospasm in the cord vessels.[15] Unusual types of abnormal umbilical cords, such as short cords, true knots, velamentous cord insertion, cord looped around the extremities, occult cord prolapse, and velamentous insertion of the cord will produce unpredictable onsets in the timing of the appearance of variable decelerations. And finally, the rarest form of cord compression, and one that usually requires rapid delivery by cesarean section, is true umbilical cord prolapse.

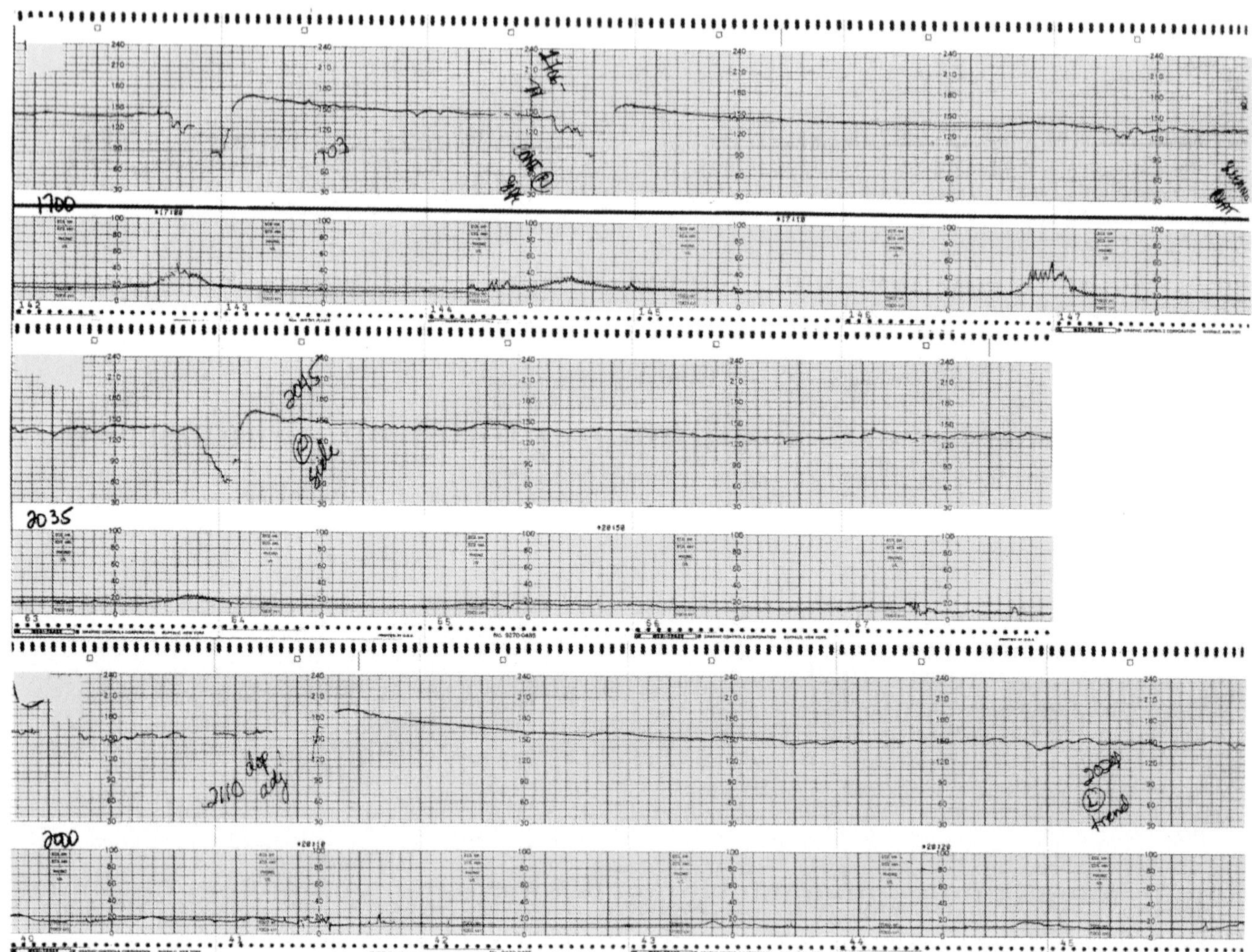

Figure 15-23. The accelerations following these variable decelerations, without any acceleration preceding, in association with absent variability fulfill the criteria to describe the accelerations as "overshoot." Such a finding can be an ominous finding and is often associated with marked metabolic acidosis.

Because the umbilical cord is most analogous to the adult trachea, interruption in cord flow results in both retention of CO_2 and cessation of O_2 delivery. When this becomes progressive, the intermittent compression often first leads to a progressive increase in fetal CO_2, which results in a respiratory acidosis. If the cord compression continues and also is sufficiently severe to cause insufficient delivery of oxygen, then a metabolic acidosis can also develop. Thus, in a fetal acidosis resulting from cord compression, the acidosis can be respiratory or combined respiratory and metabolic but should not be metabolic alone.

Prolonged Decelerations

Prolonged decelerations are isolated decelerations lasting 90 to 120 seconds or more. The NICHD Research Planning Workshop proposed that prolonged decelerations be defined as those lasting 2 to 10 minutes, and that beyond 10 minutes, it is a baseline change.[17] Although this proposal is meant to create uniform definitions, it belies the pathophysiology of the deceleration, because the sudden drop in FHR is the result of some adverse afferent stimulus and if sustained will result in a prolonged decrease in FHR. Thus, this is not really a baseline change, because the FHR will return to or near its original baseline when the stimulus is removed. Unlike the other three decelerations, in which the type of deceleration defines the pathophysiologic mechanism, prolonged decelerations may be caused by virtually any of the mechanisms previously described, but usually are of a more profound and sustained nature. Prolonged umbilical cord compression, profound placental insufficiency, or possibly even sustained head compression may lead to prolonged decelerations.

The presence of and severity of hypoxia are thought to correlate with the following variables with a prolonged deceleration: the depth and duration of the deceleration, how abruptly it returns to baseline, how much variability is lost during the deceleration, and whether there is a rebound tachycardia and loss of variability following the deceleration (Fig. 15-24). Examples of the more profound stimuli that may result in this type of deceleration include

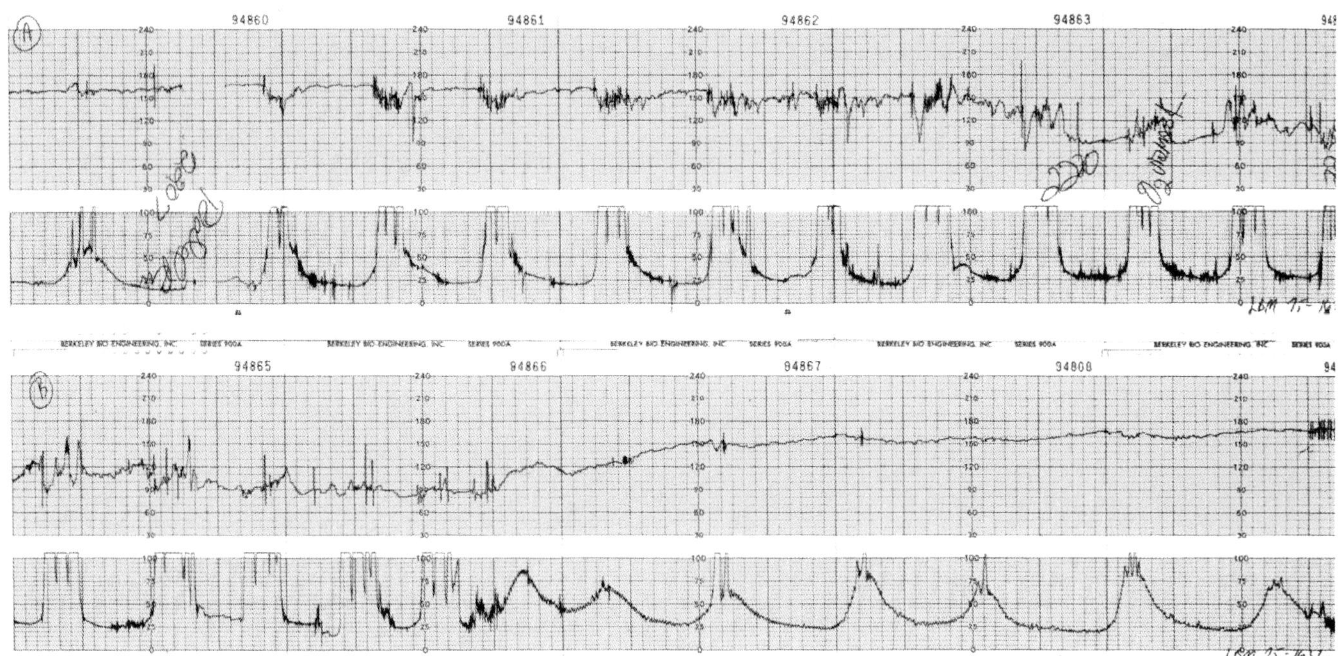

Figure 15-24. Often following a prolonged deceleration, as with the one shown in this figure, there is a temporary period of tachycardia and loss of variability. Such a response would suggest that this was a significant hypoxic event. The etiology of this deceleration is not clear but may have been because of excessive uterine contractions compounded by maternal pushing.

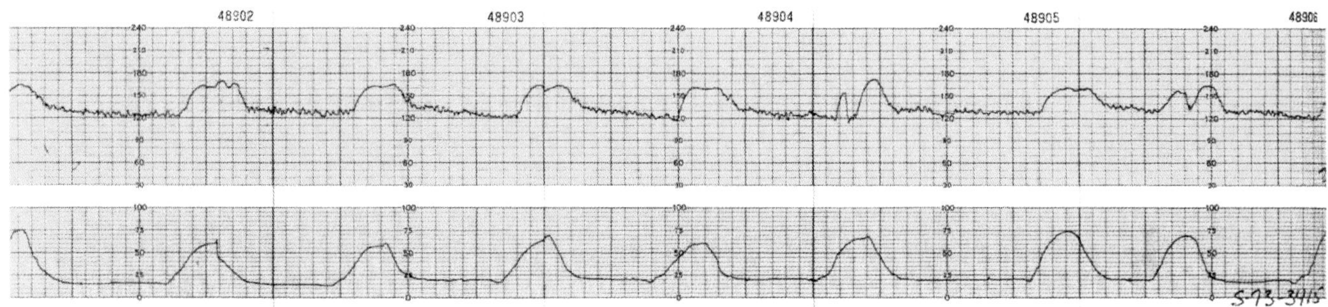

Figure 15-25. These are accelerations of the fetal heart. They are usually seen with fetal movement, and are often coincident with uterine contractions as well, as in this patient.

a prolapsed umbilical cord or other forms of prolonged cord compression, prolonged uterine hyperstimulation, hypotension following conduction anesthesia, severe degrees of abruptio placentae, paracervical anesthesia, an eclamptic seizure, and rapid descent through the birth canal. Occasionally, less severe stimuli such as examination of the fetal head, Valsalva's maneuvers, or application of a scalp electrode may cause milder forms of prolonged decelerations.

Accelerations

Accelerations are periodic changes of the FHR above the baseline (Fig. 15-25). They are not classified by type. Except for those accelerations previously described that are associated with variable decelerations, virtually all accelerations are a physiologic response to fetal movement.[32] Accelerations are usually short in duration, lasting no more than 30 to 90 seconds, but in an unusually active fetus, they can be sustained as long as 30 minutes or more. Again, the NICHD Research Planning Workshop disagrees somewhat on this definition. They propose that accelerations of more than 10 minutes be defined as a change in baseline.[17] However, sustained accelerations (Fig. 15-26) are associated with an actively moving fetus, and when the fetus becomes quiet, the FHR will return to baseline. It is important that these accelerations not be confused with a baseline change, because sustained accelerations, which are consistent with a well-oxygenated, vigorous fetus, can be confused visually with fetal tachycardia, and the return of the FHR to the original baseline can be confused with decelerations.

The presence of accelerations has virtually the same meaning as normal FHR variability, but the absence of accelerations means only that the baby is not moving. Because accelerations can be quantified in beats per minute above the baseline and duration, their pres-

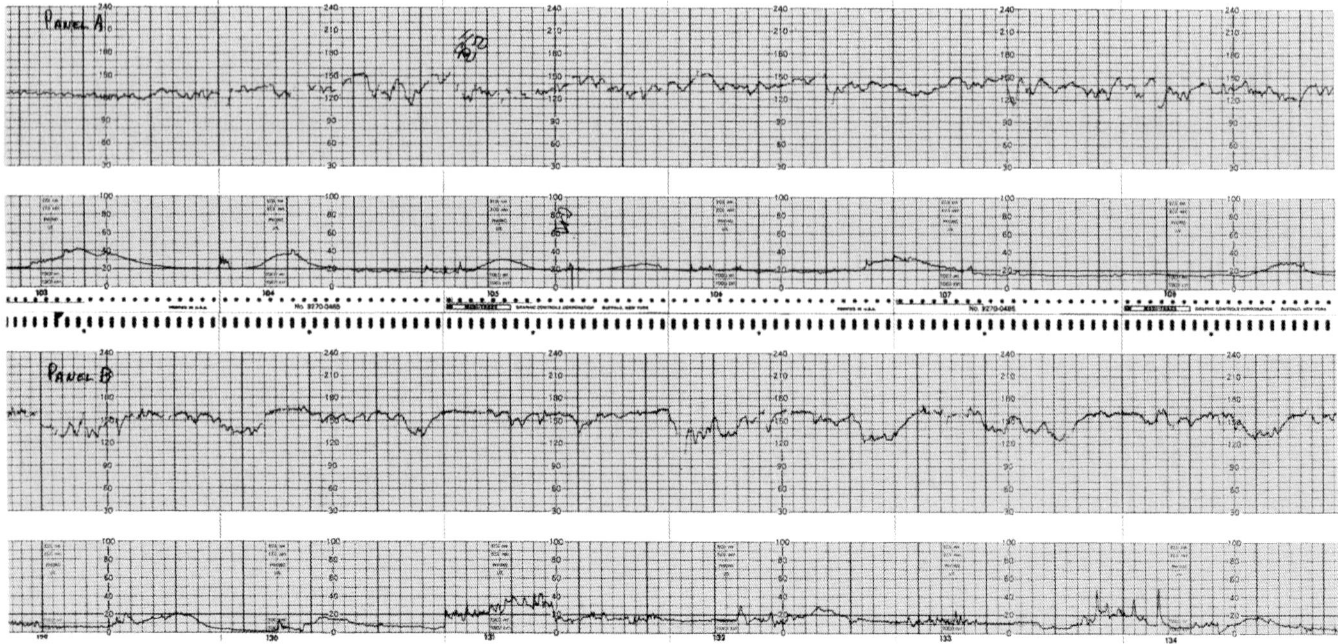

Figure 15-26. This figure shows prolonged and repetitive accelerations, especially on the lower panel. Accelerations that are sustained or confluent can be easily confused with a tachycardia and the return to baseline can be confused with decelerations.

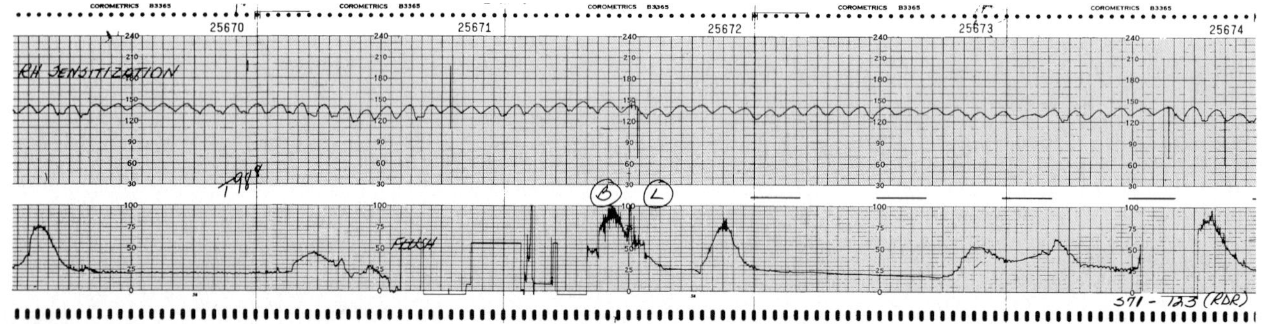

Figure 15-27. The sinusoidal heart rate pattern with its even undulations is demonstrated. Internal monitoring shows the absence of beat-to-beat variability characteristic of true sinusoidal patterns.

ence is less subjective than quantifying FHR variability. The 15 bpm above the baseline lasting for more than 15 seconds definition of an acceleration, first described with the nonstress test, is the definition usually used for defining accelerations in labor. Earlier in gestation, accelerations are less frequent and of lower amplitude. Fetuses of younger than 32 weeks have been defined as having accelerations if they exceed 10 bpm for more than 10 seconds.[17] Clark et al.[33] made the observation that in fetuses having otherwise nonreassuring FHR patterns, the presence of accelerations, using this definition, virtually always ruled out a pH less than 7.20 on scalp sampling. Subsequently, these authors and others have confirmed that the presence of spontaneous accelerations or accelerations induced by stimulation of the fetal scalp or acoustic stimulation with a vibroacoustic stimulator has the same reliability.[34,35] If there is no acceleration in the face of an otherwise nonreassuring FHR, most studies have shown that about 50 percent of these fetuses have an acidotic pH value on scalp sampling. However, the absence of accelerations in a fetus without a nonreassuring deceleration pattern rarely indicates fetal acidosis.

Sinusoidal Patterns

This pattern was originally described by Kubli et al. in 1972[36] and Shenker in 1973,[37] and is rare but significant. This pattern is strongly associated with fetal hypoxia, most often seen in the presence of severe fetal anemia. Using strict criteria for this pattern, defined by Modanlou et al.,[38] there will be a high correlation with significant fetal acidosis or severe anemia. These criteria for identifying a sinusoidal FHR include (1) a stable baseline FHR of 120 to 160 bpm with regular sine wavelike oscillations, (2) an amplitude of 5 to 15 bpm, (3) a frequency of 2 to 5 cycles/min, (4) fixed or absent short-term variability, (5) oscillation of the sine wave above and below the baseline, and (6) absence of accelerations (Fig. 15-27). The pathophysiology of the sinusoidal pattern

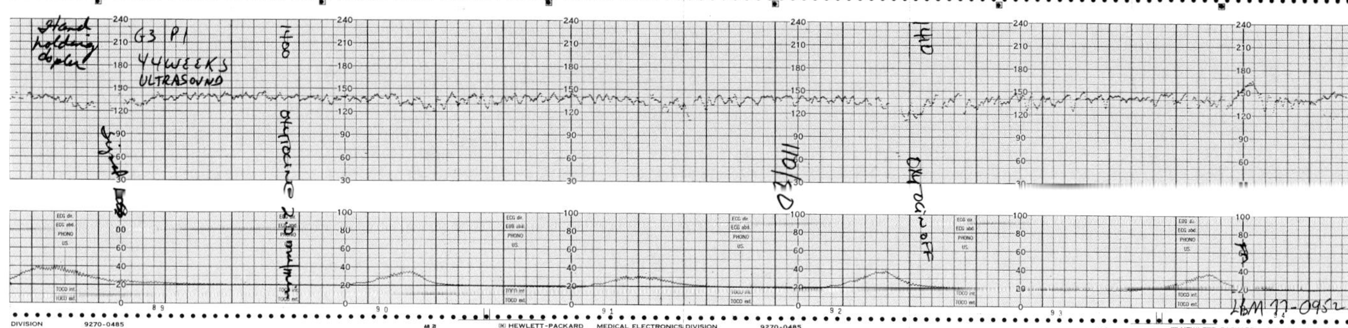

Figure 15-28. More common than sinusoidal tracings are those that are actually normal or "pseudosinusoidal" but can easily be confused with a sinusoidal pattern. There are often small accelerations or above-average variability that mimics the sine wave-like pattern. It is important to use the strict criteria defined in the text before interpreting a pattern as sinusoidal.

has been elucidated by Murata et al.,[39] who correlated the pattern with levels of fetal arginine vasopressin and subsequently reproduced the pattern with vagotomy and injection of arginine vasopressin. Arginine vasopressin is elevated with hemorrhage or acidosis, and it appears that in such situations with a severely compromised fetus and little vagal activity, the hormone directly affects the fetal heart and this FHR pattern results. The sinusoidal pattern has also been described after injection of certain narcotics such as butorphanol (Stadol)[40] or meperidine (Demerol).[41]

Unfortunately, there are relatively commonly seen FHR patterns that mimic sinusoidal patterns (pseudosinusoidal) that are associated with well-oxygenated and nonanemic fetuses.[38] These patterns can easily be confused with sinusoidal FHR patterns (Fig. 15-28); therefore, it is important to strictly apply all of the above six criteria before calling a pattern sinusoidal.

Evolution of Fetal Heart Rate Patterns

One of the sources of greatest confusion regarding FHR pattern interpretation and management is that the patterns have very poor specificity in terms of predicting fetal hypoxia and acidosis, newborn depression, or need for resuscitation. When patterns are normal or reassuring, there is almost always normal oxygenation and the baby is born vigorous, with normal pH and Apgar scores. However, when the pattern is nonreassuring, the baby is more often normal than depressed or acidotic.

In addition to the inherent problem we have in trying to use EFM, a nonspecific modality, to determine fetal oxygenation, there is another reason why many studies have demonstrated such poor correlation with adverse perinatal outcome. Investigators have tried to correlate specific FHR findings in isolation without taking into account the expected evolution of the FHR patterns.[19,30] For example, if one attempts to correlate FHR variability with acidosis or depression, normal variability will correlate well with a normal pH and normal Apgar scores, but reduced or absent variability will correlate poorly with acidosis or depression. This is partly because of the multiple causes of reduced variability. However, in the fetus with persistent late decelerations who then loses FHR variability, the correlation with acidosis and depression should improve substantially because there was evidence that *hypoxia led to the acidosis*. This is a critical concept in understanding FHR monitoring. Murata and coworkers demonstrated in the fetal monkey, whose oxygenation was progressively reduced, that late decelerations consistently *preceded* the loss of variability and accelerations.[42] Decelerations are the indicators of hypoxia. If hypoxia is the cause of the reduced variability, then those decelerations indicative of hypoxia should *precede* the development of tachycardia, loss of variability, or disappearance of accelerations (Fig. 15-29). Furthermore, the duration and appearance of the decelerations should be of sufficient magnitude to suggest that CNS depression could have resulted.

Therefore, the fetus who develops one of the latter variables (e.g., loss of accelerations) in the absence of decelerations is not likely to have hypoxia, and another cause should be considered (e.g., drugs, sleep cycle). It must be remembered that when the fetus demonstrates one of these baseline changes or absence of accelerations on admission, it is not possible to know whether evidence of hypoxia preceded these changes. In addition, this approach does not apply antepartum, when the nonstress test is used. Contractions are not present, and there will not be an opportunity to assess for the presence or absence of decelerations in response to contractions.

MANAGEMENT OF NONREASSURING FETAL HEART RATE PATTERNS

Traditionally, an FHR pattern that suggested fetal hypoxia would be called fetal distress if it was sufficiently concerning to warrant immediate operative intervention. But, as previously mentioned, in most cases, when a cesarean or forceps delivery was done for fetal distress, the fetus was delivered without evidence of significant hypoxia or acidosis. This has led to the recommendation from ACOG to use the term nonreassuring fetal status to indicate a more accurate description of the indication for such intervention.[13] This is also descriptive of the approach to the management of the fetus with concerning FHR patterns. That is, when the FHR pattern is suggestive of hypoxia, and therefore nonreassuring, other means of reassurance should be used when possible.

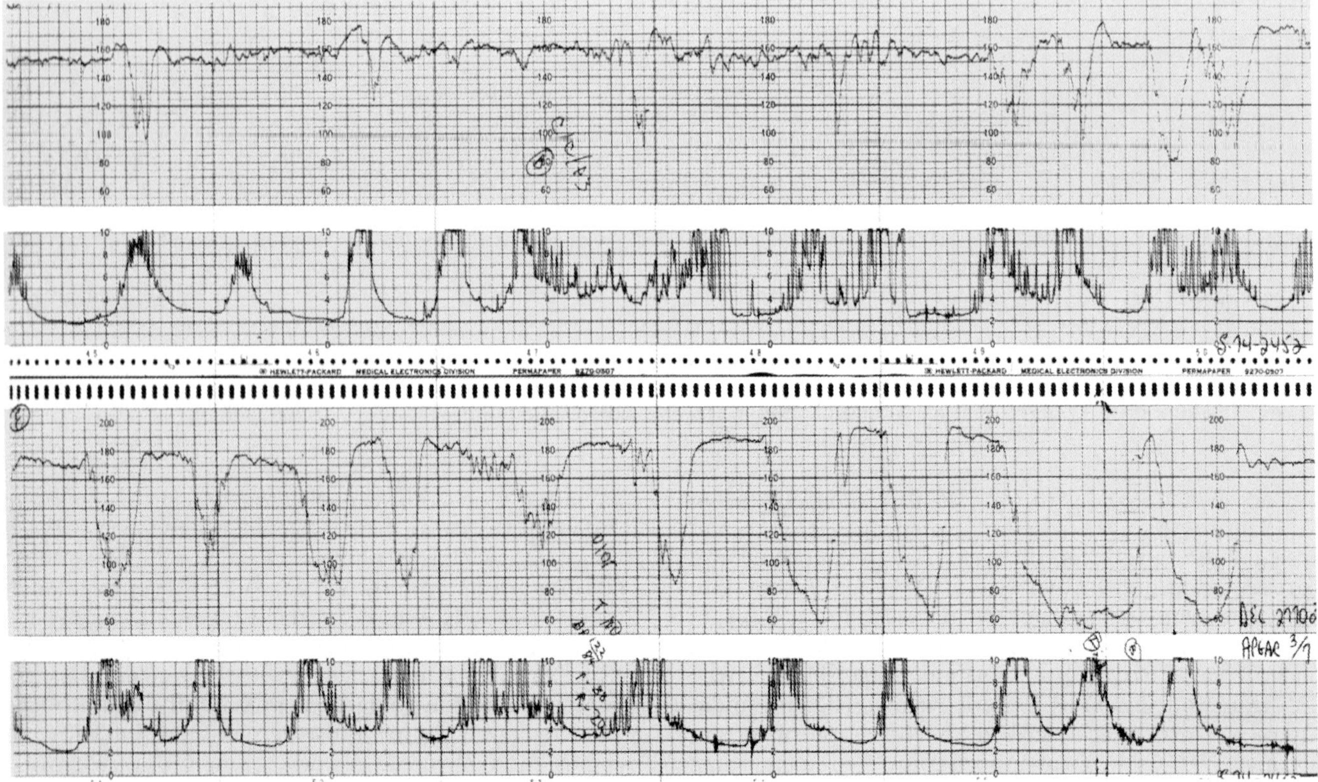

Figure 15-29. Loss of variability and tachycardia should be interpreted as indicative of hypoxia and developing acidosis only when they are associated with decelerations that suggest progressive hypoxia, as with these variable decelerations, which are becoming deeper and more prolonged.

Interventions for Nonreassuring Fetal Status

The ideal intervention for fetal hypoxia is a cause-specific, noninvasive one that permanently reverses the problem. Although it is not always possible, this should certainly be the goal. Obviously, the first step in achieving this goal is to recognize the cause of the abnormal FHR pattern. A thorough knowledge of the pathophysiology of FHR changes coupled with a careful clinical patient evaluation and a knowledge of common causes of specific FHR changes will maximize the opportunity for this goal to succeed. In addition to cause-specific types of interventions, virtually all cases of hypoxia should theoretically also benefit by more generic interventions that have the potential to maximize oxygen delivery and placental exchange.

NONSURGICAL INTERVENTIONS

OXYGEN ADMINISTRATION

One of the most obvious ways to maximize oxygen delivery to the fetus is to give additional oxygen to the mother. Although there is no incontrovertible evidence that oxygen administration to the mother does improve oxygenation in the fetus,[43] some recent evidence suggests the hypoxic fetus will become less so with maternal oxygen through a face mask.[44] Therefore, when the fetal heart rate has decelerations suggestive of hypoxia, oxygen administration to the mother is indicated. However, the practice of administering oxygen for patterns such as isolated loss of variability or loss of accelerations without decelerations or for mild variable decelerations does not make physiologic sense and may have some negative effects by increasing patient discomfort and unnecessarily frightening the mother in labor.

LATERAL POSITIONING

Ideally, all patients should labor in the lateral recumbent position, at least from the standpoint of maximizing uterine perfusion. The reasons for this are, at least theoretically, twofold: (1) in being inactive and recumbent, the body is required to deliver the least amount of blood flow to other muscles; and (2) in the lateral position, there is no compression by the uterus on the vena cava or aorta, thus maximizing cardiac return and cardiac output.

HYDRATION

Most patients in labor are either restricted or prohibited from taking oral fluids for fear of requiring an urgent operative delivery in the presence of a full stomach. If not fluid restricted, individuals involved in sustained exercise, and possibly by inference in active labor, do not voluntarily ingest adequate amounts of fluid because of a phenomenon called autodehydration.[45] In addition, recent evidence would suggest that the usual amount of intravenous fluid of 125 ml/h is a gross underestimate of the replacement required in labor.[46] Thus, by increasing fluid administration, there is the potential to maximize intravascular volume and thus uterine perfusion.

Oxytocin

In a patient with a nonreassuring pattern, the more time there is between contractions, the more time to maximally perfuse the placenta and deliver oxygen. In patients receiving oxytocin, there is potential to improve oxygenation by decreasing or discontinuing oxytocin. Often, however, this becomes a difficult situation, because many patients will stop progressing in labor in terms of continued dilation or descent if the oxytocin is discontinued. It is often necessary to restart the oxytocin, and this may be appropriate, especially if there are accelerations or other means to document the absence of acidosis. Written documentation explaining the necessity and appropriateness of continuing oxytocin in this situation is especially important. The situation with patients who develop persistently nonreassuring patterns, especially with loss of accelerations or absence of other reassurance, and who require discontinuation of oxytocin, but then fail to progress because adequate contractions cannot be sustained, is often referred to as fetal intolerance to labor.

Tocolytics

There are numerous references in the obstetric literature describing the use of tocolytics to maximize oxygen delivery, by essentially the same mechanism described in the previous paragraph on discontinuing oxytocin.[46–50] Tocolytics are appropriate in at least two situations: (1) When patients are having spontaneous excessive contractions, leading to nonreassuring FHR patterns, especially prolonged decelerations (Fig. 15-30) (different tocolytics have been described, but the most commonly used one, and perhaps the one that provides the most rapid response, is subcutaneous terbutaline, 0.25 mg); and (2) intrauterine resuscitation after the decision is made to perform an operative delivery while waiting for preparations to be made. Subcutaneous terbutaline has been demonstrated to improve Apgar scores and cord pH values without apparent complications, such as postpartum hemorrhage.[51]

Amnioinfusion

In situations in which variable decelerations appear to be caused by oligohydramnios, reestablishing intrauterine fluid volume through a process called amnioinfusion has been demonstrated in numerous randomized studies to ameliorate the variable decelerations, improve Apgar scores and cord pH values, and even reduce the need for cesarean delivery for NRFS.[52–54] Reference to this idea can be found as far back as 1925[55] but was rediscovered and proposed by Miyazaki and Taylor in 1983.[56] Intrauterine pressure catheters are now made with a port that allows the simultaneous administration of saline to accomplish this goal. Thus, in the patient with variable decelerations that suggest progression to more nonreasurring types, and when the cause is likely to be caused by oligohydramnios, the implementation of amnioinfusion is warranted. What has not yet been established is whether in some situations amnioinfusion should be started prophylactically when there is an unusually high risk for the development of variable decelerations from oligohydramnios, such as preterm premature rupture of membranes (PROM).

Theoretically, using amnioinfusion before the onset of the decelerations in certain fetuses, such as very premature ones or those with intrauterine growth restriction who will progress to acidosis and depression much more rapidly with cord compression, will prevent the rapid evolution of hypoxia and acidosis. No studies are available as of yet to compare therapeutic as opposed to prophylactic amnioinfusion. Amnioinfusion also has been proposed, in several prospective randomized trials, to be used to avoid the fetal/neonatal pulmonary problems in the presence of meconium.[57] The evidence for efficacy in this setting is good. However, clear evidence that this modality avoids the meconium aspiration syndrome is lacking, because this complication is relatively infrequent. Some of these problems will be avoided with good oropharyngeal suctioning on the perineum and neonatal suctioning below the vocal cords when necessary. The theory behind this use of amnioinfusion is that (1) it dilutes the meconium by increasing fluid volume, and (2) by avoiding fetal gasping, which can occur with significant hypoxic episodes (i.e., sustained cord compression), the likelihood of meconium aspiration before delivery is reduced. Surveys of university hospitals suggest that amnioinfusion is used for both variable decelerations and meconium in the vast majority.[58]

Meconium

The presence of meconium is an extremely confusing issue when evaluating the fetus in labor. The quandary arises from the fact that although a hypoxic insult eliciting a significant vagal response from the fetus often results in the passage of meconium from the fetal gut, passage of meconium can also occur in the absence of any

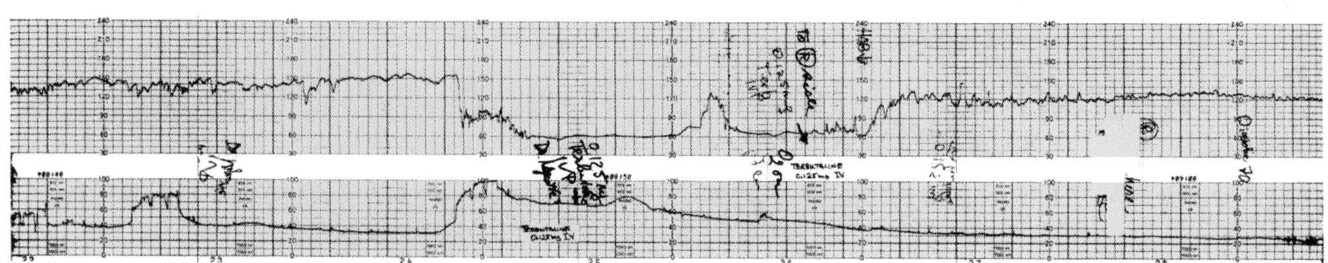

Figure 15-30. This prolonged deceleration in a patient with a spontaneous prolonged contraction is treated with subcutaneous terbutaline with apparent resolution of both the contraction and the deceleration.

significant or sustained hypoxia. Meconium is not only a potential sign of fetal hypoxia but is also a potential toxin if the fetus aspirates this particulate matter with a gasping breath in utero or when it takes its first breaths following birth. The thickness of the meconium is also a reflection of the amount of amniotic fluid, and thick meconium virtually always reflects some degree of oligohydramnios. Thus, there may be a vicious circle in such a situation. Oligohydramnios often leads to cord compression; the vagal response to cord compression may also lead to further passage of meconium, but also when it is sustained or prolonged, it may lead to fetal gasping, increasing the likelihood that meconium aspiration can occur before birth. Furthermore, because oligohydramnios may be an indicator of failing placental function, meconium may also indicate that the fetus is at risk for placental insufficiency. In general, meconium should alert the clinician to the potential for oligohydramnios, umbilical cord compression, placental insufficiency, and meconium aspiration. Fortunately, a reassuring FHR tracing is generally reliable, and patients with meconium can be managed expectantly. But in the presence of meconium, especially thick meconium, the risk factors associated with meconium should be entered in the equation when managing relatively nonreassuring patterns, as should all clinical variables.

Alternatives for Evaluating the Fetus with a Nonreassuring Fetal Heart Rate Pattern

In the fetus with a persistently nonreassuring FHR pattern, in whom nonsurgical efforts at reversing or improving the pattern fail, the next step is to attempt to find out whether the hypoxia has progressed to metabolic acidosis.

Fetal Scalp pH

Determination of fetal scalp pH is historically the oldest and most well-tested method for determining if the fetus is acidotic. Technically, a plastic cone is inserted transvaginally against the fetal vertex. The cervix needs to be at least 4 to 5 cm dilated and the vertex at a −1 station or below to accomplish this. Mineral oil or another lubricant is applied to the scalp so blood will bead, and then using a lancet, the scalp is pricked and blood is then collected in a long capillary tube (Fig. 15-31). The tube will hold about 100 µl of blood, and about 30 µl is needed to perform a pH test alone and 70 µl to determine Pco_2 as well. To determine if an acidosis is metabolic or respiratory, the Pco_2 is needed. This is an important distinction, Because the question being asked is whether there has been sufficient hypoxia to lead to metabolic acidosis. Respiratory acidosis is far less concerning, but without determining Pco_2, this cannot be sorted out. Unfortunately, it is difficult to obtain enough blood for both pH and Pco_2 in most instances. Pco_2 determination is especially important when doing scalp pH for variable decelerations, because most acidosis is respiratory in this situation. A scalp pH less than 7.20 is consistent with fetal acidosis and a pH of 7.20 to 7.25 is borderline and should be repeated immediately. A reassuring value over 7.25 must be repeated every 20 to 30 minutes as long as the pattern persists and the fetus is not acidotic. In practice, because this technique is cumbersome, fraught with technical inaccuracy, uncomfortable for the patient, and with the requirement of performing repeated samples, it is used very infrequently.[59] Even in large teaching services

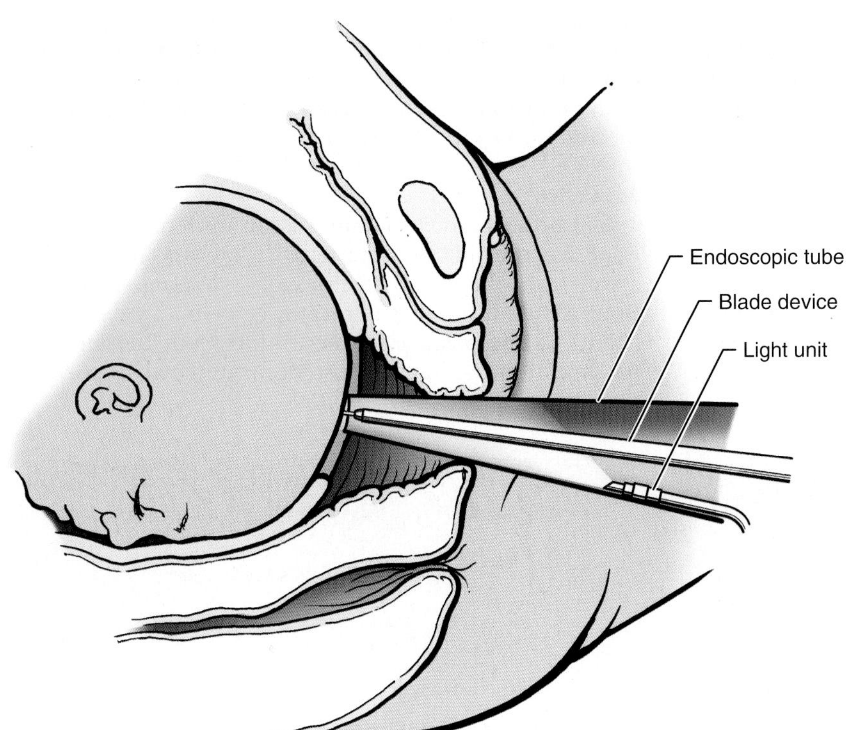

Figure 15-31. Technique of fetal scalp blood sampling.

accustomed to using this technique, its abandonment, coupled with an appreciation of the utility of accelerations for predicting the presence or absence of acidosis, does not appreciably increase the need for operative intervention.[60]

Accelerations

In the fetus with a nonreassuring pattern, spontaneous accelerations have the same significance as those elicited by scalp or acoustic stimulation. Thus, any acceleration—either spontaneous or induced—indicates the absence of acidosis. It should be emphasized that the absence of accelerations as well as the absence of decelerations or other patterns suggesting hypoxia should not elicit concern. The fetus is often not moving in labor, and from a pathophysiologic perspective, without evidence of hypoxia, the fetus cannot develop a metabolic acidosis. Thus, the application of the interpretation of accelerations should generally be restricted to the fetus with an otherwise nonreassuring FHR pattern, when the question is being asked: Hypoxia is present. Is the fetus now developing a metabolic acidosis?

Fetal Pulse Oximetry

One important recent development in obstetrics is the introduction of fetal pulse oximetry. Because FHR monitoring is specifically intended to monitor fetal oxygenation and because this modality is so nonspecific, it stands to reason that what we should be using ideally is a device that directly monitors fetal oxygenation or pH, or both.

Fetal pulse oximetry was approved by the Food and Drug Administration for use in fetuses with nonreassuring FHR patterns in May 2000. The approval was made on the basis of the previously mentioned data and the results of a large multicenter trial of more than 1,000 patients comparing FHR monitoring alone versus FHR monitoring backed up by pulse oximetry in fetuses already having nonreassuring FHR patterns.[61] Whereas the trial did not demonstrate an overall reduction in cesarean delivery, there was a reduction in cesarean delivery for NRFS and an improved specificity and sensitivity of operative intervention for the fetus with depression, acidosis, and in need of resuscitation. Most importantly, in following the fetus with a nonreassuring FHR tracing but a reassuring oxygen saturation value (>30 percent), there was no increase in babies with adverse outcomes.

Therefore, fetal pulse oximetry may prove to be a potentially valuable alternative to fetal scalp pH monitoring in patients with nonreassuring FHR patterns and may allow continued monitoring and avoid intervention of fetuses with apparently nonreassuring FHR patterns but with normal oxygenation. Because at this time there is such limited clinical experience in this country with pulse oximetry and few confirmatory studies of its value in practice are available, it is difficult to determine how it will impact practice; however, its potential is quite promising. The ACOG has taken the position that it cannot currently recommend the use of fetal pulse oximetry until further studies are available to confirm its efficacy and safety. It remains to be seen whether this modality will ultimately find its place in clinical practice.

Fetal Electrocardiogram for Intrapartum Monitoring

Another recent addition to the technology of evaluating fetal oxygenation in labor is computerized interpretation of the fetal ECG complex. This modality has become used commonly in parts of Europe and has recently been approved for use in the United States. Assessment of changes in the ST interval and T wave height gives information on the metabolic energy balance in the myocardium. An increase in T wave amplitude occurs with hypoxia. This is due to the surge of epinephrine, activating beta-receptors, which stimulates cyclic AMP production, the phosphorylase enzyme, and glycogenolysis. This causes potassium ions to be set free and an increase of the T wave amplitude.[63,64] Lactate is also produced, contributing to the development of metabolic acidosis. The rate of increase in T wave amplitude depends on the amount of glycogen used to maintain myocardial energy balance. The ratio between the height of the T wave and the QRS amplitude provides the T/QRS ratio, which serves as a reflection of changes in T wave height. A normal fetus under perfect conditions of signal quality will have a T/QRS less than 0.25. An increase can occur over a shorter or longer period (episodic or baseline rise). Initial hypoxia can also cause a downsloping ST segment (biphasic ST). A biphasic ST is also seen if the fetal heart has a reduced capacity to respond because it has been exposed to previous stress and has limited reserve as in infections, malformations, or in premature fetuses. A biphasic ST is graded 1 to 3 according to the degree of sloping. A significant increase in T/QRS or more than two consecutive biphasic ECG complexes in combination with a nonreassuring heart rate tracing indicates fetal distress and calls for intervention.[65] A multicenter randomized controlled trial in Europe comparing FHR monitoring alone with FHR monitoring and fetal ECG ST analysis demonstrated a significant and substantial lowering of the rate of metabolic acidosis and a minimal, but statistically significant reduction in cesarean delivery with the use of this technology.[66] Again, as with fetal pulse oximetry, it is too early to assess whether this will have a significant impact on the practice of intrapartum fetal assessment in the United States.

Operative Intervention for Nonreassuring Fetal Status

When the fetus is determined to have a persistently nonreassuring FHR pattern and back-up methods (scalp pH, accelerations, pulse oximetry) cannot provide reassurance that the fetus is not acidotic, operative intervention is indicated to expeditiously deliver the baby to avoid further deterioration. Several questions arise when the decision has been made for intervention for NRFS. What is the best choice, operative vaginal delivery or cesarean section? How much time do we have to perform the delivery? What anesthetic should be used? What is the prognosis of the baby? And, finally, are there situations where the baby is already damaged or otherwise not likely to benefit from this intervention?

Choosing operative vaginal delivery or cesarean section is not difficult if the patient is in early labor. For the patient near or at complete dilation, this becomes a question of judgment. Which route is more likely to create the more rapid delivery while at the same time result in the least complications for mother and baby? When the clinician is unsure whether an attempt at operative vaginal delivery will succeed, the question is even more difficult. This decision will depend not only on the variables that predict success for an operative vaginal delivery (e.g., station, clinical pelvimetry, size of the baby, skill of the clinician) but also on the severity of the FHR pattern and whether there is time to find out whether an operative delivery will succeed. The time for intervention also is a question of judgment. Except for the situation of a prolonged deceleration to less than 70 bpm with loss of variability that will not recover and requires the most rapid intervention safely possible, most other situations require judgment and integration of the entire clinical picture of mother and baby.

The question of how much time is available to perform an operative intervention in the face of a nonreassuring FHR pattern is a complex one, muddied not only by the unpredictability of the nonreassuring pattern but also by the medicolegal pressures that have arisen as a result of EFM. The ACOG recommends that "all hospitals have the capability of performing a cesarean delivery within 30 minutes of the decision to operate,"[67] but that "not all indications for a cesarean delivery will require a 30-minute response time." The examples given that mandate an expeditious delivery include hemorrhage from placenta previa, abruptio placentae, prolapse of the umbilical cord, and ruptured uterus. In some situations (e.g., sustained prolonged deceleration to <70 bpm with loss of variability), 30 minutes may be too long to avoid damage; in others, this may be too restrictive and may result in suboptimal anesthetic choices and compromised preoperative preparation. Thus, a judgment made on the basis of the severity of the FHR pattern and the overall clinical status of mother and baby must be integrated into this difficult decision.

MANAGEMENT OF NONREASSURING FHR PATTERNS—A PROPOSED PROTOCOL

The following algorithm for management of nonreassuring patterns is proposed.

1. When the pattern suggests the beginning development of hypoxia or is already nonreassuring:
   a. When possible, identify the cause of the problem (e.g., hypotension from an epidural).
   b. Correct the cause (e.g., fluids and ephedrine to correct the hypotension).
   c. Give measures to maximize placental oxygen delivery and exchange: oxygen by face mask, lateral positioning, hydration, consider decreasing or discontinuing oxytocin.
2. If the pattern becomes or remains nonreassuring and the above measures have been completed:
   a. Attempt to provide other measures of reassurance to rule out metabolic acidosis.
      - Accelerations-spontaneous or elicited
      - Scalp pH
      - Fetal pulse oximetry, Fetal ECG/ST Segment analysis
   b. If reassurance using one of the above methods can be provided, and the pattern persists, continuous or intermittent (every 30 minutes) evidence of absence of acidosis must be ascertained.
   c. If reassurance of the absence of acidosis cannot be provided, deliver expeditiously by the safest and most reasonable means (operative vaginal or cesarean section).

Patterns that qualify as nonreassuring and cannot be corrected and therefore warrant evidence of the absence of metabolic acidosis include:

1. Persistent late decelerations (>50 percent of contractions).
2. Nonreassuring variable decelerations.
   a. Progressively severe.
   b. With developing tachycardia and loss of variability.
   c. With developing slow return to baseline.
3. Sinusoidal tracing.
4. Recurrent prolonged decelerations.
5. The confusing pattern.
   a. The patient presents with a pattern of absent variability but without explanatory decelerations.
   b. An unusual pattern that does not fit into one of the categories defined above but does not have elements of a reassuring pattern.

Several of the above-mentioned presentations and others warrant additional discussion. Prolonged decelerations that will not return to baseline are a potentially ominous situation. Causes of these patterns include virtually any substantial insult that can cause severe hypoxia, especially when the FHR goes below 80 bpm. Examples include abruptio placentae, ruptured uterus, cord prolapse or sustained cord compression, profound hypotension, maternal seizure or respiratory arrest, and rapid descent and impending delivery of the fetus.

Generally, the following approach to these sustained prolonged decelerations should be taken. First, be patient. Often these patterns are noticed on the central monitor, and caregivers unnecessarily run to the room and frighten the patient and family. Because the vast majority of these decelerations spontaneously resolve in 1 to 3 minutes, such action is usually unwarranted. If the deceleration does not resolve, the patient should be examined to rule out cord prolapse or sudden descent. If these are not present, determine if there is an apparent cause that can be specifically corrected. If the cause cannot be found, the general explanation by process of elimination is sustained cord compression, and repositioning the patient, oxygen administration, and discontinuing oxytocin is all that can be provided. Should none of these measures work, operative delivery is required unless spontaneous delivery is imminent. How long one should wait for the corrective measures or spontaneous recovery to occur is somewhat variable. This will be determined by the depth of the deceleration, the loss of variability during the deceleration, whether evidence of hypoxia preceded the deceleration, and whether the heart rate is intermittently returning toward baseline or is just staying down. Evidence to recommend a precise amount of time wherein intervention must occur is difficult to integrate, because the vast majority of time, we are dealing with relative hypoxia rather than complete anoxia. Complete anoxia in real life probably occurs only with severe degrees of uterine rupture and complete abruption. Even with cord prolapse, the vast majority of time there is some cord blood flow. Windle[68] performed the classic experiment using complete anoxia in fetal monkeys. Monkeys allowed to breathe in 6 minutes or less showed no clinical or pathologic ill effects. Asphyxiation for 7 to 12 minutes resulted in transient motor and behavioral changes, with some scarring in certain specific brain areas in some animals. Those who are anoxic for 12 to 17 minutes, if death did not occur, had the most severe neurologic and clinical effects. Therefore, in the worst case of all, if delivery occurs in less than 12 minutes from the onset of the deceleration, damage will be unlikely, unless there was some hypoxia before the deceleration.

The most difficult pattern to manage is in the fetus with recurrent prolonged decelerations that do recover (Fig. 15-32). Generally, these can be managed using the same algorithm for nonreassuring patterns as described earlier. However, even if one can provide reassurance that acidosis does not exist following any of the decelerations, there is a concern that this pattern portends a deceleration that will recur and will not recover, and one will be placed in the situation described in the previous paragraph. Therefore, there will be occasions when the recurrent prolonged decelerations are concerning enough that operative intervention is warranted even if there is no concern about acidosis at the present moment. One must integrate the frequency, severity, and duration of the deceleration; the fetal response in terms of tachycardia and loss of variability; and how much time is expected before spontaneous delivery will occur to make this difficult decision. Therefore, for example, in the nulliparous patient at 4 cm, having decelerations lasting 4 minutes to 70 bpm every 10 minutes, operative delivery may be warranted. Whereas in the multipara at 8 cm making normal progress with similar or less frequent decelerations, it may be justified to manage these expectantly, but with all preparations made for immediate delivery should one of the decelerations not recover.

Auscultation as an Alternative

Almost all randomized controlled trials have demonstrated that intermittent auscultation is as effective as EFM in detecting fetal hypoxia in labor. There are some limitations to this statement, however. Virtually all of these trials compared EFM to intermittent auscultation with one-on-one nursing, in which the auscultation was performed every 15 minutes in the first stage and every 5 minutes in the second stage, and the auscultation was performed for a period of 60 seconds through and following an entire uterine contraction. This is a situation that is difficult to duplicate in everyday practice because of lower nurse/patient ratios and because emergencies with

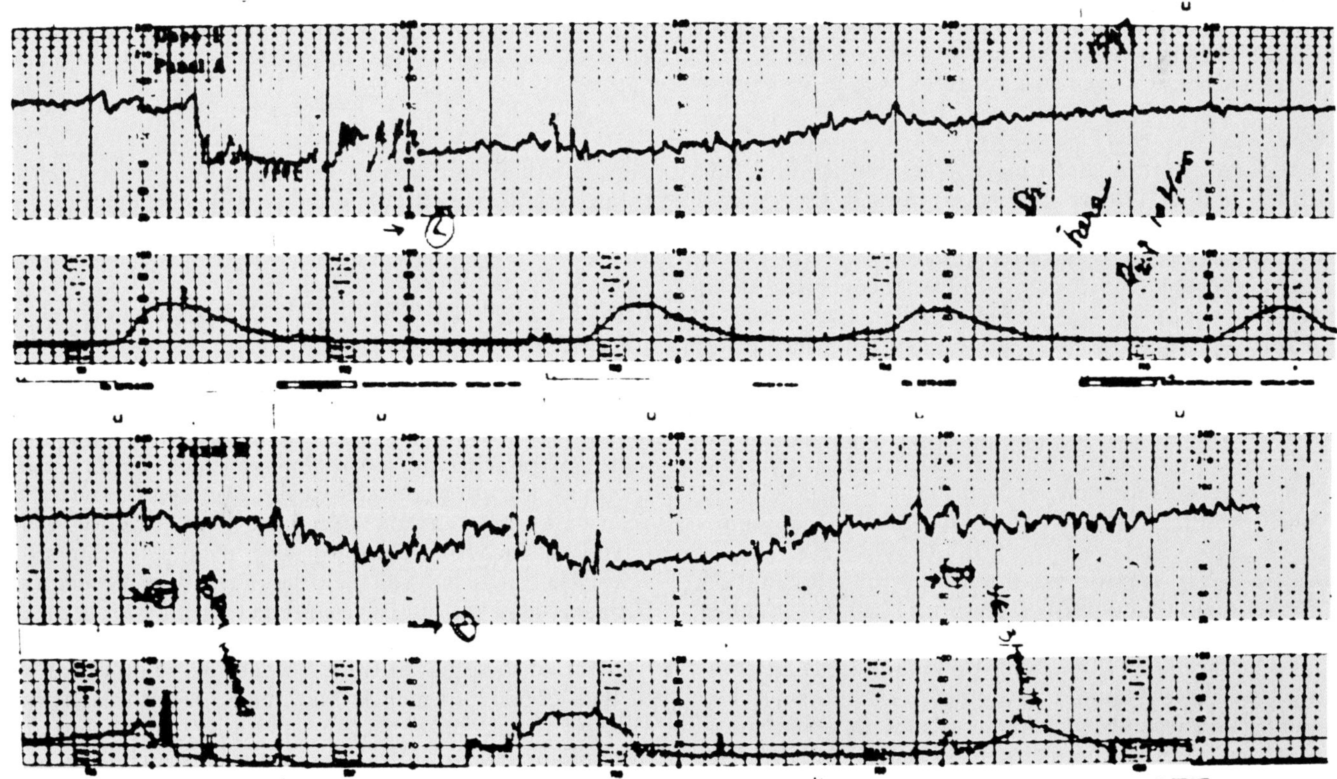

Figure 15-32. Recurrent unexplained prolonged decelerations.

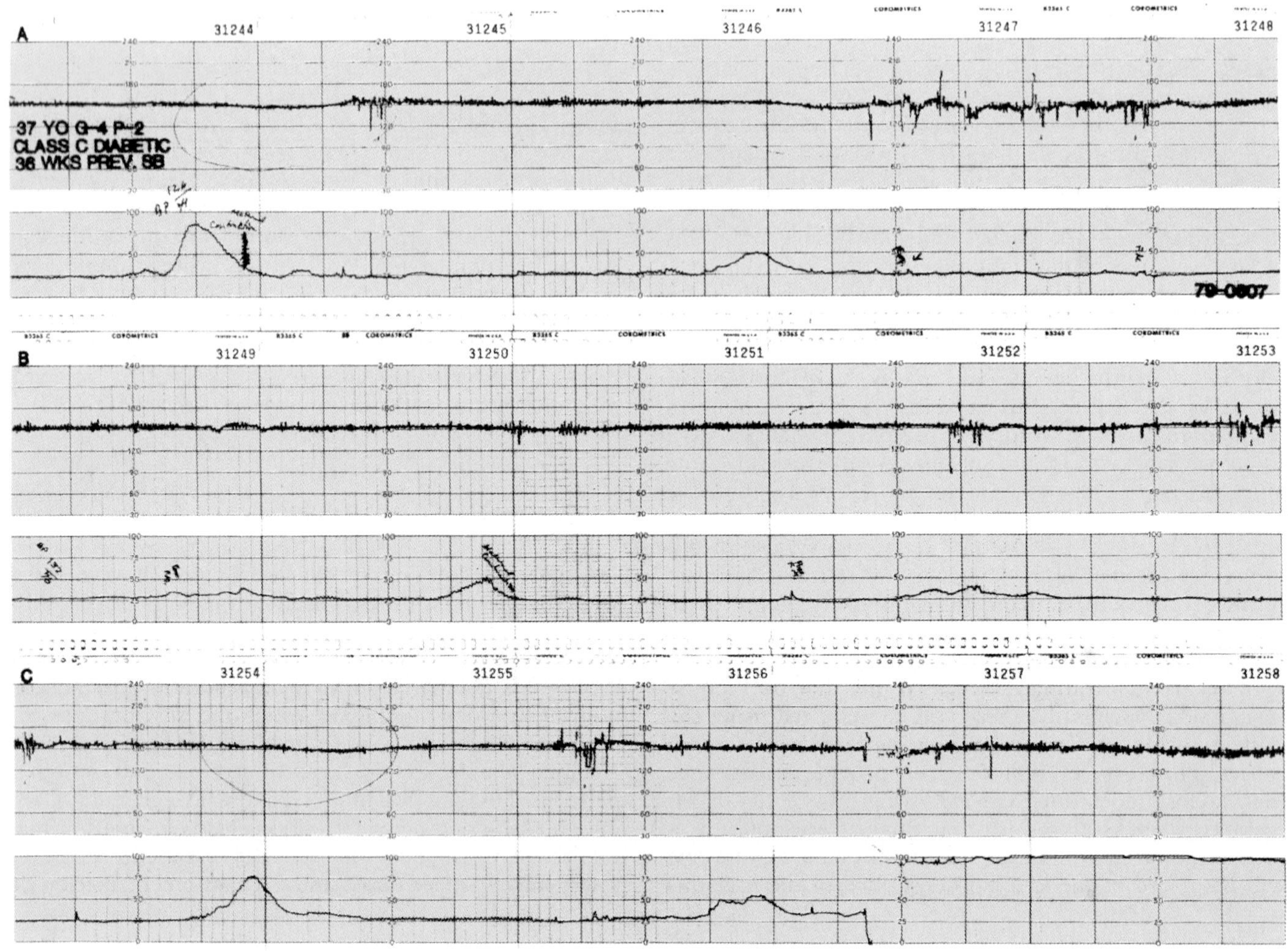

Figure 15-33. These persistent late decelerations associated with absent variability are difficult to recognize even with an internal electrode. This is a nonreassuring FHR pattern, which is often ominous. It is unlikely that such decelerations, associated with a normal baseline rate, would be recognized with intermittent auscultation.

other patients often take a nurse away from the bedside for long periods of time. Second, in most of the studies, fetuses who entered labor may have been monitored electronically before randomization, and often very-high-risk patients were excluded from study. Ingemarsson et al. have shown that 50 percent of patients who develop nonreassuring FHR patterns in labor have a nonreassuring FHR pattern on admission.[69] And finally, in virtually all of the studies comparing EFM with auscultation, when the auscultated FHR was abnormal, the patient was then monitored electronically. Furthermore, there are nonreassuring FHR tracings that are indicative of hypoxia and acidosis that are not likely to be detected with auscultation (Fig. 15-33).

Therefore, it is reasonable to conclude that auscultation is an acceptable option for monitoring the fetus in labor when certain conditions are in place. The fetus should have a reassuring FHR on admission monitored electronically. The patient should have one-on-one nursing. The standards for frequency from the ACOG for auscultation are at least every 30 minutes in the first stage and every 15 minutes in the second stage for the low-risk patient and every 15 minutes in the first stage and every 5 minutes in the second stage for the high-risk patient.[16] Fetuses with abnormal FHR patterns on auscultation should have electronic monitoring to define the pattern and monitor for progression to worsening or nonreassuring patterns.

ASSESSMENT OF FETAL CONDITION AT BIRTH

The Apgar score was originally introduced as a tool to be used in guiding the need for neonatal resuscitation. Subsequently, this means of fetal assessment became used routinely for all births. However, the Apgar score has been expected to predict far more than was originally intended. Such expectations have included evaluating acid-base status at birth (i.e., the presence or absence of perinatal asphxia) and even predicting long-term prognosis. Unfortunately, the Apgar score is a nonspecific measure of these parameters, because many other causes of fetal depression may mimic that seen with asphyxia, such as drugs, anomalies, prematurity, suctioning for meconium, and so forth. In situations in which FHR patterns have been concerning and other back-up methods for evaluating fetal oxygenation or fetal acid-base status have been used, or in cases in which the baby is unex-

Table 15-1. Normal Blood Gas Values of Umbilical Artery and Vein

	MEAN VALUE	NORMAL RANGE*
Artery		
pH	7.27	7.15 to 7.38
Pco_2	50	35 to 70
Bicarbonate	23	17 to 28
Base excess	−3.6	−2.0 to −9.0
Vein		
pH	7.34	7.20 to 7.41
Pco_2	40	33 to 50
Bicarbonate	21	15 to 26
Base excess	−2.6	−1.0 to −8.0

*Values are ±2 SD and represent a composite of multiple studies.
Data derived from Thorp and Rushing.[69]

pectedly depressed, it is important to specifically evaluate these parameters at birth, using umbilical cord blood gases. To accomplish this, a doubly clamped 10- to 30-cm section of umbilical cord is taken after the orginal cord clamping and separation of the baby from the cord. Using heparinized syringes, samples of umbilical artery and vein are separately obtained. These samples are evaluated for respiratory gases.[70] Normal ranges for umbilical cord gases are shown in Table 15-1. Cord blood Po_2 or O_2 saturation is not useful, because many normal newborns are initially hypoxemic until normal extrauterine respiration is established. Although cord pH, especially arterial pH, is the essential value, Pco_2 is also very important, because if the pH is low, the Pco_2 is used to determine whether the acidosis is respiratory or metabolic. Respiratory acidosis is not predictive of newborn or long-term injury and should correlate with little or no need for resuscitation. In addition, the cord gases should be used to correlate interpretation of the FHR patterns, as previously described in the sections on their pathophysiology and to determine the appropriateness of operative intervention or lack of it. These gases can help the pediatrician in determining the etiology of immediate complications and the need for more intense observation of the baby. In addition, these values are often useful if the baby develops any long-term neurologic injury in determining whether any such injury may have been related to peripartum asphyxia. Studies have shown that if such asphyxia is present, in order for it to result in long-term injury it must have been severe (metabolic acidosis with a pH < 7.0 to 7.05) and be associated with multiple organ dysfunction in the newborn period.[2]

RISKS AND BENEFITS OF ELECTRONIC FETAL MONITORING

EFM was introduced with the hope that this modality would reduce or eliminate the devastating consequences of asphyxia. Enthusiasm for this new technology established the role of continuous FHR monitoring in labor before studies demonstrated its accuracy. Initial retrospective studies evaluated more that 135,000 patients and showed more than a threefold improvement in the intrapartum fetal death rate for patients monitored electronically.[1] However, the majority of subsequent prospective, randomized, controlled trials have failed to demonstrate an improvement in the intrapartum fetal death rate using EFM.[71–77] In these studies, however, electronic FHR monitoring was compared with frequent intermittent auscultation with one-on-one nursing, a standard that is difficult to maintain. Many patients with abnormal FHR patterns on admission were not randomized, and virtually always, patients with an abnormal FHR on auscultation were ultimately monitored electronically. A more recent randomized controlled trial of EFM versus intermittent auscultation did demonstrate a significant improvement in perinatal mortality in the electronically monitored group.[78] The past three decades have not shown a change in the 2 per 1,000 incidence of cerebral palsy, suggesting that the widespread use of EFM has not affected this problem. However, these data are somewhat difficult to analyze because of other changes occurring simultaneously. There has been a dramatic improvement in the survival of very-low-birthweight premature babies during this time period, and prematurity accounts for the majority of cerebral palsy. Second, term babies with asphyxia have had an increase in survival during this time period, thus allowing for a potential increase in surviving children with brain damage. Any of these factors may obscure an effect that FHR monitoring may have had in reducing the incidence of cerebral palsy. EFM has other potential benefits. These include an ability to understand the mechanism of developing hypoxia and treat it more specifically. It provides the ability to accurately monitor uterine contractions so we can better understand progress or lack of progress in labor, as well as monitor the effects of oxytocin-stimulated contractions on fetal oxygenation. The monitor is ultimately, like all other monitors in intensive care situations, a labor-saving device allowing nurses to perform other tasks simultaneously.

EFM has several disadvantages, however. During the period in which FHR monitoring has risen in popularity, there was a parallel increase in the cesarean section rate. Certainly, this was not all caused by EFM, because there were many other changes in obstetric practice during this time period. In virtually all of the randomized controlled trials, EFM resulted in an increase in the cesarean section rate over intermittent auscultation without a concomitant improvement in outcome. There is also, however, a desire to deliver babies before significant hypoxia has any potential to damage the baby, and the nonspecific changes in FHR only fuel this concern, setting up the current environment of excessive intervention. In reality, metabolic acidosis occurs in only about 2 percent of all labors, and even allowing for a reasonable amount of latitude in early intervention, cesarean section rates should not exceed 4 to 5 percent for this indication. Unfortunately, rates of 10 percent for NRFS are common. Thus, the need for better, more specific modalities to allow us to evaluate hypoxia and acidosis in the fetus with a nonreassuring FHR pattern are needed. Fetal pulse oximetry appears to have great potential, but its effect on cesarean section rates in real practice remains to be seen.

The second major problem associated with EFM is the fear of a lawsuit should the child be compromised in any way. The monitor has created an expectation of perfect outcome. The interpretation of abnormal FHR tracings is highly subjective and variable, and experts often give diametrically opposed interpretations of the same tracing. The modality itself is nonspecific, and babies with anomalies or preexisting brain damage will often have abnormal FHR tracings easily confused with ongoing hypoxia. Finally, a jury cannot help but be sympathetic to a family and baby with disfiguring and debilitating cerebral palsy, and large financial awards seem to be the only way at present to compensate these unfortunate victims. However, these outcomes are not consistent with what we know about asphyxia. More than 75 percent of brain-damaged children have causes that are *not* related to perinatal asphyxia. Many cases of asphyxia occur *before* labor or early in labor before the patient arrives in the hospital. Very few of these cases are truly preventable. Again, a modality such as fetal pulse oximetry would seem to have the potential to clarify whether an abnormal FHR pattern is truly hypoxic in origin and eliminate any subjectivity in interpretation. One can only hope that once these pressures are removed from the labor and delivery suite, the opportunity to do what is best for the fetus and mother will be enhanced and this will be the only motivating force.

SUMMARY

EFM has become the standard means for evaluating fetal oxygenation in labor. Because of fetal inaccessibility and the lack of alternatives to more specifically evaluate fetal oxygenation, this modality has been the only alternative. FHR monitoring is reliable when it tells us the fetus is well oxygenated, but it is more often unreliable when it suggests the fetus is "in distress." The recent change in terminology describing the abnormal FHR pattern as nonreassuring is a more accurate and honest depiction of the limitations of EFM in this situation. Despite or even because of these limitations, it is imperative that the clinician understand as much as possible about the underlying physiologic explanations of normal and abnormal FHR patterns, because this allows the only reasonable opportunity to appropriately evaluate and manage these changes. The goal of FHR monitoring should be to carefully and thoroughly monitor all patients in active labor; avoid unnecessary operative and nonoperative intervention for benign and innocuous FHR patterns; correct nonreassuring FHR patterns with noninvasive, etiology-specific therapies when possible; or if this is not possible, use appropriate means such as scalp pH, accelerations, or fetal pulse oximetry to rule out acidosis; and finally, if acidosis cannot be ruled out, operatively intervene in an expeditious manner appropriate for the entire clinical situation.

Acknowledgment

A special acknowledgment and thank you is expressed to Dr. Isis Amer-Whalin from the Department of Obstetrics and Gynecology at the Karolinska University Hospital in Stockholm, Sweden for her contribution to the section on fetal EKG for intrapartum monitoring.

KEY POINTS

- The goals of intrapartum fetal evaluation by EFM and available back-up methods are to detect fetal hypoxia, reverse the hypoxia with nonsurgical means, or if unsuccessful, determine if the hypoxia has progressed to metabolic acidosis, and if so, deliver the baby expeditiously to avoid the hypoxia and acidosis from resulting in any damage to the baby.

- EFM is an inherently suboptimal method of determining fetal hypoxia and acidosis, because many factors besides these variables may alter the FHR and mimic changes caused by hypoxia and acidosis. When the FHR is normal, its reliability in predicting the absence of fetal compromise is high, but when the FHR is abnormal, its reliability in predicting the presence of asphyxia is poor.

- The term fetal distress should be abandoned in favor of nonreassuring fetal status, because when the fetal monitor suggests that there may be a problem, in most circumstances, we can only say that we are no longer reassured with a high degree of certainty that the fetus is well oxygenated.

- Late decelerations are always indicative of relative fetal hypoxia, and are caused by inadequate oxygen delivery, exchange, or uptake that is aggravated by the additional hypoperfusion of the placenta caused by contractions. Variable decelerations are caused by a decrease in umbilical cord flow resulting from cord compression or cord stretch. Prolonged decelerations may be caused by any mechanism that decreases fetal oxygenation.

- In labor, loss of variability, loss of accelerations, and tachycardia should be interpreted only as indicative of fetal compromise in the presence of nonreassuring decelerations (late, nonreassuring variable or prolonged decelerations), as signs of hypoxia should always precede signs of neurologic depression secondary to hypoxia.

- In the presence of oligohydramnios and variable decelerations, or with meconium, intrapartum amnioinfusion has been shown to decrease rates of cesarean delivery for NRFS and may decrease neonatal respiratory complications caused by meconium aspiration.

- In the presence of an otherwise nonreassuring FHR pattern, the presence of accelerations of the FHR, either spontaneous or elicited by scalp stimulation or vibroacoustic stimulation, indicate the absence of fetal acidosis. Their absence is associated with a 50 percent chance of fetal acidosis, but only in the setting of a nonreassuring FHR.

- Umbilical cord blood gases should be obtained and documented in situations in which there is a nonreassuring or confusing FHR pattern during labor, there is neonatal depression following birth, with premature babies, and when suctioning for meconium is performed. These values will help clarify the reasons for abnormal FHR patterns or for neonatal depression.

❑ Fetal pulse oximetry was approved in May 2000 by the Food and Drug Administration for use in term (≥ 36 weeks) patients with nonreassuring FHR patterns. This technology may improve our ability to more accurately interpret nonreassuring FHR patterns and may have the potential to decrease cesarean deliveries for NRFS.

❑ Although there is correlation between a nonreassuring FHR pattern and neonatal depression, the FHR is a poor predictor of long-term neurologic sequelae. Furthermore, fetuses with previous neurologic insults may have significantly abnormal FHR patterns, even when they are well oxygenated in labor.

Glossary

Acidemia increased hydrogen ion concentration in blood.

Acidosis increased hydrogen ion concentration in tissue.

Asphyxia hypoxia with metabolic acidosis.

Base deficit buffer base content lower than normal (this is calculated from a normogram using pH and Pco_2).

Base excess buffer base content higher than normal.

Hypoxemia decreased oxygen concentration in blood.

Hypoxia decreased oxygen concentration in tissue.

pH the negative log of hydrogen ion concentration ($7.0 = 1 \times 10^{-7}$).

REFERENCES

1. Freeman RK, Garite TJ, Nageotte MP (eds): Clinical management of fetal distress. *In* Fetal Heart Rate Monitoring, 2nd ed. Baltimore, Williams & Wilkins, 1991.
2. American College of Obstetricians and Gynecologists: Fetal and Neonatal Neurologic Injury. Technical Bulletin No. 163, January 1992.
3. Eastman NJ, Kohl SG, Maisel JE, et al: The obstetrical background of 753 cases of cerebral palsy. Obstet Gynecol Surv 17:459, 1962.
4. Nelson KB, Ellenberg JH: Epidemiology of cerebral palsy. *In* Schoenberg BS (ed): Advances in Neurology, Vol. 19. New York, Raven Press, 1979.
5. Wegman M: Annual summary of vital statistics. Pediatrics 70:835, 1982.
6. Benson RC, Shubeck F, Deutschberger J, et al: Fetal heart rate as a predictor of fetal distress: a report from the Collaborative Project. Obstet Gynecol 32:529, 1968.
7. Cremer M: Munch. Med Wochensem 58:811, 1906.
8. Hon EH, Hess OW: The clinical value of fetal electrocardiography. Am J Obstet Gynecol 79:1012, 1960.
9. Hon EH: The electronic evaluation of the fetal heart rate. Am J Obstet Gynecol 75:1215, 1958.
10. Hon EH: Observations on "pathologic" fetal bradycardia. Am J Obstet Gynecol 77:1084, 1959.
11. Caldeyro-Barcia R, Mendez-Bauer C, Poseiro JJ, et al: Control of human fetal heart rate during labor. *In* Cassels D (ed): The Heart and Circulation in the Newborn Infant. New York, Grune & Stratton, 1966.
12. Kaser O, Friedberg V, Oberk K (eds): Gynakologie v Gerburtshilfe BD II. Stutgart, Georg Thieme Verlag, 1967.
13. American College of Obstetricians and Gynecologists: Fetal Distress and Birth Asphyxia. Washington, DC, American College of Obstetricians and Gynecologists, ACOG Committee Opinion 137.
14. Vintzileos M, Campbell WA, Nochimson DJ, Weinbaum PJ: Degree of oligohydramnios and pregnancy outcome in patients with PROM. Obstet Gynecol 66:162, 1985.
15. Roach MR: The umbilical vessels. *In* Goodwin JM, Godden DO, Chance GW (eds): Perinatal Medicine. Baltimore, Williams & Wilkins, 1976, p 136.
16. American College of Obstetricians and Gynecologists: Fetal Heart Rate Patterns: Monitoring, Interpretation and Management. Technical Bulletin No. 207, July 1995.
17. Electronic Fetal Heart Rate Monitoring: Research Guidelines For Interpretation, National Institute of Child Health and Human Development Research Planning Workshop. Am J Obstet Gynecol 177:1385, 1997.
18. Schifferli P, Caldeyro-Barcia R: Effects of atropine and beta adrenergic drugs on the heart rate of the human fetus. *In* Boreus L (ed): Fetal Pharmacology. New York, Raven Press, 1973, p 259.

19. Bisonette JM: Relationship between continuous fetal heart rate patterns and Apgar score in the newborn. Br J Obstet Gynaecol 82:24, 1975.
20. Langer O, Cohen WR: Persistent fetal bradycardia during maternal hypoglycemia. Am J Obstet Gynecol 149:688, 1984.
21. Parsons MT, Owens CA, Spellacy WN: Thermic effects of tocolytic agents: decreased temperature with magnesium sulfate. Obstet Gynecol 69:88, 1987.
22. Gembruch U, Hansmann M, Redel DA, et al: Fetal complete heart block: antenatal diagnosis, significance and management. Eur J Obstet Gynecol Reprod Biol 31:9, 1989.
23. Druzen M, Ikenoue T, Murata Y, et al: A possible mechanism for the increase in FHR variability following hypoxemia. Presented at the 26th Annual Meeting of the Society for Gynecological Investigation, San Diego, California, March 23, 1979.
24. Paul WM, Quilligan EJ, MacLachlan T: Cardiovascular phenomenon associated with fetal head compression. Am J Obstet Gynecol 90:824, 1964.
25. Martin CB Jr, de Haan J, van der Wildt B, et al: Mechanisms of late deceleration in the fetal heart rate. A study with autonomic blocking agents in fetal lambs. Eur J Obstet Gynecol Reprod Biol 9:361, 1979.
26. Garite TJ: The relationship between late decelerations and fetal oxygen saturation. (Work in progress.)
27. Francis J, Garite T: The association between abruptio placentae and abnormal FHR patterns. (Submitted for publication.)
28. Barcroft J: Researches on Prenatal Life. Oxford, Blackwell Scientific Publications, 1946.
29. Lee ST, Hon EH: Fetal hemodynamic response to umbilical cord compression. Obstet Gynecol 22:554, 1963.
30. Kubli FW, Hon EH, Khazin AE, et al: Observations on heart rate and pH in the human fetus during labor. Am J Obstet Gynecol 104:1190, 1969.
31. Goodlin RC, Lowe EW: A functional umbilical cord occlusion heart rate pattern. The significance of overshoot. Obstet Gynecol 42:22, 1974.
32. Navot D, Yaffe H, Sadovsky E: The ratio of fetal heart rate accelerations to fetal movements according to gestational age. Am J Obstet Gynecol 149:92, 1984.
33. Clark S, Gimovsky M, Miller FC: Fetal heart rate response to scalp blood sampling. Am J Obstet Gynecol 144:706, 1982.
34. Clark S, Gimovsky M, Miller F: The scalp stimulation test: a clinical alternative to fetal scalp blood sampling. Am J Obstet Gynecol 148:274, 1984.
35. Smith C, Hguyen H, Phelan J, Paul R: Intrapartum assessment of fetal well-being: A comparison of fetal acoustic stimulation with acid base determinations. Am J Obstet Gynecol 155:776, 1986.
36. Kubli F, Ruttgers H, Haller U, et al: Die antepartale fetale Herzfrequenz. II. Verhalten von Grundfrequenz, Fluktuation und Dezerationo bei antepartalem Fruchttod, Z. Gerburtshilfe Perinatol 176:309, 1972.
37. Shenker L: Clinical experience with fetal heart rate monitoring of 1000 patients in labor. Am J Obstet Gynecol 115:1111, 1973.
38. Modanlou H, Freeman RK: Sinusoidal fetal heart rate pattern: its definition and clinical significance. Am J Obstet Gynecol 142:1033, 1982.
39. Murata Y, Miyake Y, Yamamoto T, et al: Experimentally produced sinusoidal fetal heart rate pattern in the chronically instrumented fetal lamb. Am J Obstet Gynecol 153:693, 1985.
40. Angel J, Knuppel R, Lake M: Sinusoidal fetal heart rate patterns associated with intravenous butorphanol administration. Am J Obstet Gynecol 149:465, 1984.
41. Epstein H, Waxman A, Gleicher N, et al: Meperidine induced sinusoidal fetal heart rate pattern and reversal with naloxone. Obstet Gynecol 59:225, 1982.
42. Murata Y, Martin CB, Ikenoue T, et al: Fetal heart rate accelerations and late decelerations during the course of intrauterine death in chronically catheterized rhesus monkeys. Am J Obstet Gynecol 144:218, 1982.
43. Dildy G, Clark S, Loucks C: Intrapartum fetal pulse oximetry: the effects of maternal hyperoxia on fetal oxygen saturation mark. Am J Obstet Gynecol 171:1120, 1994.
44. Haydon ML, Gorenberg DM, Garite TJ, et al: The effect of maternal oxygen administration during labor on fetal pulse oximetry: a pilot study. Presented at the 26th Annual Meeting of the Society for Maternal Fetal Medicine. Miami, FL Jan 29–Feb. 4, 2006.
45. Noakes TD: Fluid replacement during exercise. Exerc Sport Sci Rev 21:297, 1993.
46. Garite TJ, Weeks J, Peters-Phair K, et al: A randomized controlled trial of the effect of increased intravenous hydration on the course of labor in nulliparas. Am J Obstet Gynecol 813:1049, 2000.
47. Lipshitz J: Use of B2 sympathomimetic drug as a temporizing measure in the treatment of acute fetal distress. Am J Obstet Gynecol 129:31, 1977.
48. Tejani N, Verma UL, Chatterjee S, et al: Terbutaline in the management of acute intrapartum fetal acidosis. J Reprod Med 28:857, 1983.
49. Arias F: Intrauterine resuscitation with terbutaline: a method for the management of acute intrapartum fetal distress. Am J Obstet Gynecol 131:39, 1977.
50. Patriarcho MS, Viechnicki BN, Hutchinson TA: A study on intrauterine fetal resuscitation with terbutaline. Am J Obstet Gynecol 157:383, 1987.
51. Burke MS, Porreco RP, Day D, et al: Intrauterine resuscitation with tocolysis: an alternate month clinical trail. J Perinatol 10:296, 1989.
52. Miyazaki F, Nevarez F: Saline amnioinfusion for relief of repetitive variable decelerations: a prospective randomized study. Am J Obstet Gynecol 153:301, 1985.
53. Nageotte MP, Freeman RK, Garite TJ, et al: Prophylactic intrapartum amnioinfusion in patients with preterm premature rupture of membranes. Am J Obstet Gynecol 153:557, 1985.
54. Owen J, Henson BV, Hauth JC: A prospective randomized study of saline solution amnioinfusion. Am J Obstet Gynecol 162:1146, 1990.
55. Delee JB, Pollack C: Intrauterine injection of saline to replace the amniotic fluid. Obstet Gynecol 1925.
56. Miyazaki F, Taylor N: Saline amnioinfusion for relief of variable or prolonged decelerations. Am J Obstet Gynecol 14:670, 1983.
57. Pierce J, Gaudier FL, Sanchez-Ramos L: Intrapartum amnioinfusion for meconium-stained fluid: meta-analysis of prospective clinical trials. Obstet Gynecol 95:1051, 2000.
58. Wenstrom K, Andrews WW, Maher JE: Amnioinfusion survey: prevalence, protocols and complications. Obstet Gynecol 86:572, 1995.
59. Clark SL, Paul RH: Intrapartum fetal surveillance: the role of fetal scalp blood sampling. Am J Obstet Gynecol 153:717, 1985.
60. Goodwin TM, Milner-Masterson C, Paul R: Elimination of fetal scalp blood sampling on a large clinical service. Obstet Gynecol 83:971, 1994.
61. Garite TJ, Dildy GA, McNamara H, et al: A multicenter controlled trial of fetal pulse oximetry in the intrapartum management of non-reassuring fetal heart rate patterns. Am J Obstet Gynecol 183:1049, 2000.
62. Fetal Pulse Oximtery. ACOG Committeee Opinion No. 258, Sept. 2001.
63. Rosen KG, Kjellmer I: Changes in the fetal heart rate and ECG during hypoxia. Acta Physiol Scand 93:59, 1975.
64. Greene KR, Dawes GS, Lilja H, Rosen KG: Changes in the ST waveform of the fetal lamb electrocardiogram with hypoxemia. Am J Obstet Gynecol 144:950, 1982.
65. Lilja H, Greene KR, Karlsson K, Rosen KG: ST waveform changes of the fetal electrocardiogram during labour—a clinical study. Br J Obstet Gynaecol; 92:611, 1985.
66. Amer-Wahlin I, Hellsten C, Noren H, et al: Cardiotocography only versus cardiotocography plus ST analysis of fetal electrocardiogram for intrapartum fetal monitoring: a Swedish randomised controlled trial. Lancet 358:534, 2001.
67. Guidelines for Perinatal Care: American Academy of Pediatrics and American College of Obstetricians and Gynecologists, 4th ed. Washington, DC, ACOG, 1997, p 112.
68. Windle WF: Neuropathology of certain forms of mental retardation. Science 140:1186, 1963.
69. Ingemarsson I, Arulkumaran S, Ingemarsson E, et al: Admission test: a screening test for fetal distress in labor. Obstet Gynecol 68:800, 1986.

70. Thorp JA, Rushing RS: Umbilical cord blood gas analysis. Obstet Gynecol Clin North Am 26:695, 1999.
71. Haverkamp AD, Thompson HE, McFee JG, et al: The evaluation of continuous fetal heart rate monitoring in high risk pregnancy. Am J Obstet Gynecol 125:310, 1976.
72. Haverkamp AD, Orleans M, Langendoerfer S, et al: A controlled trial of the differential effects of intrapartum fetal monitoring. Am J Obstet Gynecol 134:399, 1979
73. Renou P, Chang A, Anderson I, et al: Controlled trial of fetal intensive care. Am J Obstet Gynecol 126:470, 1976.
74. Kelso IM, Parsons RJ, Lawrence GF, et al: An assessment of continuous fetal heart rate monitoring in labor: a randomized trial. Am J Obstet Gynecol 131:526, 1978.
75. Wood C, Renou P, Oates J, et al: A controlled trial of fetal heart rate monitoring in a low-risk population. Am J Obstet Gynecol 141:527, 1981.
76. McDonald D, Grant A, Sheridan-Pereira M, et al: The Dublin randomized control trial of intrapartum fetal heart rate monitoring. Am J Obstet Gynecol 152:524, 1985.
77. Leveno KJ, Cunningham FG, Nelson S, et al: A prospective comparison of selective and universal electronic fetal monitoring in 34,995 pregnancies. N Engl J Med 315:615, 1986
78. Vintzileos AM, Antsaklis A, Varvarigos I, et al: A randomized trial of intrapartum electronic fetal heart rate monitoring versus intermittent auscultation. Obstet Gynecol 81:899, 1993.

Obstetric Anesthesia

JOY L. HAWKINS, LAURA GOETZL, AND DAVID H. CHESTNUT

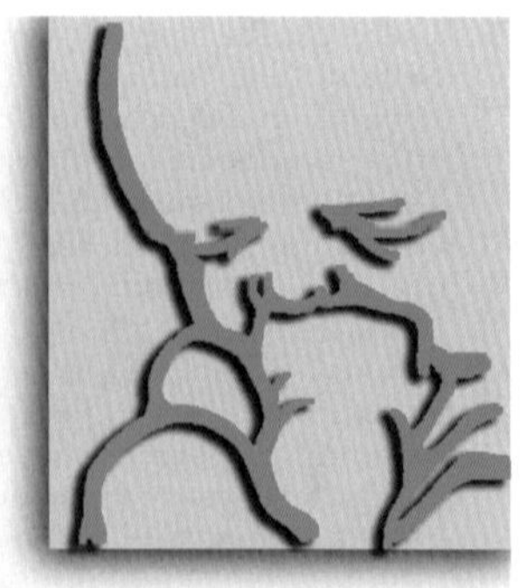

CHAPTER 16

KEY ABBREVIATIONS

American Society of Anesthesiologists	ASA
Confidence interval	CI
Central nervous system	CNS
Combined spinal-epidural	CSE
Effective dose	ED
Induction-to-delivery interval	I-D
Occiput anterior	OA
Occiput posterior	OP
Odds ratio	OR
Patient-controlled analgesia	PCA
Patient-controlled epidural analgesia	PCEA
Patient-controlled intravenous analgesia	PCIA
Postdural puncture headache	PDPH
Relative risk	RR
Uterine incision-to-delivery interval	U-D

Obstetric anesthesia encompasses all techniques used by anesthesiologists and obstetricians to alleviate the pain associated with labor and delivery: general anesthesia, regional anesthesia, local anesthesia, and analgesia. Relief from pain during labor and delivery is an essential part of good obstetric care. Unique clinical considerations guide anesthesia provision for obstetric patients; physiologic changes of pregnancy and increases in certain complications must be considered. This chapter reviews the various methods that can be used for obstetric analgesia and anesthesia, as well as their indications and complications.

PERSONNEL

Anesthesiologists, working either independently or supervising a team of residents or certified nurse anesthetists provide anesthesia for 98 percent of obstetric procedures in larger hospitals in the United States.[1] Nurse anesthetists, independent of anesthesiologists, rarely provide anesthesia for obstetric cases in larger hospitals but provide anesthesia for 34 percent of obstetric procedures in hospitals with fewer than 500 births per year.[1] Almost all hospitals with more than 300 beds have an anesthesiologist on the medical staff, whereas only 16 percent of hospitals with fewer than 50 beds have an anesthesiologist available.[2] In this situation, most states require that nurse anesthetists be supervised by the operating surgeon or obstetrician, who will ultimately be responsible for treatment and the outcome of any adverse events. Recognizing that this represents less than optimal care, The American Society of Anesthesiologists partnered with the American College of Obstetricians and Gynecologists to issue the Joint Statement on the Optimal Goals for Anesthesia Care in Obstetrics,[3] recommending that a qualified anesthesiologist assume responsibility for anesthetics in every hospital providing obstetric care. The statement notes: "There are many obstetric units where obstetricians or obstetrician-supervised nurse anesthetists administer anesthetics. The administration of general or regional anesthesia requires both medical judgment and technical skills. Thus, a physician with privileges in anesthesiology should be readily available."[3]

PAIN PATHWAYS

Pain during the first stage of labor results from a combination of uterine contractions and cervical dilation. Painful sensations travel from the uterus through visceral afferent (sympathetic) nerves that enter the spinal cord through the posterior segments of thoracic spinal nerves 10, 11, and 12 (Fig. 16-1). During the second stage of

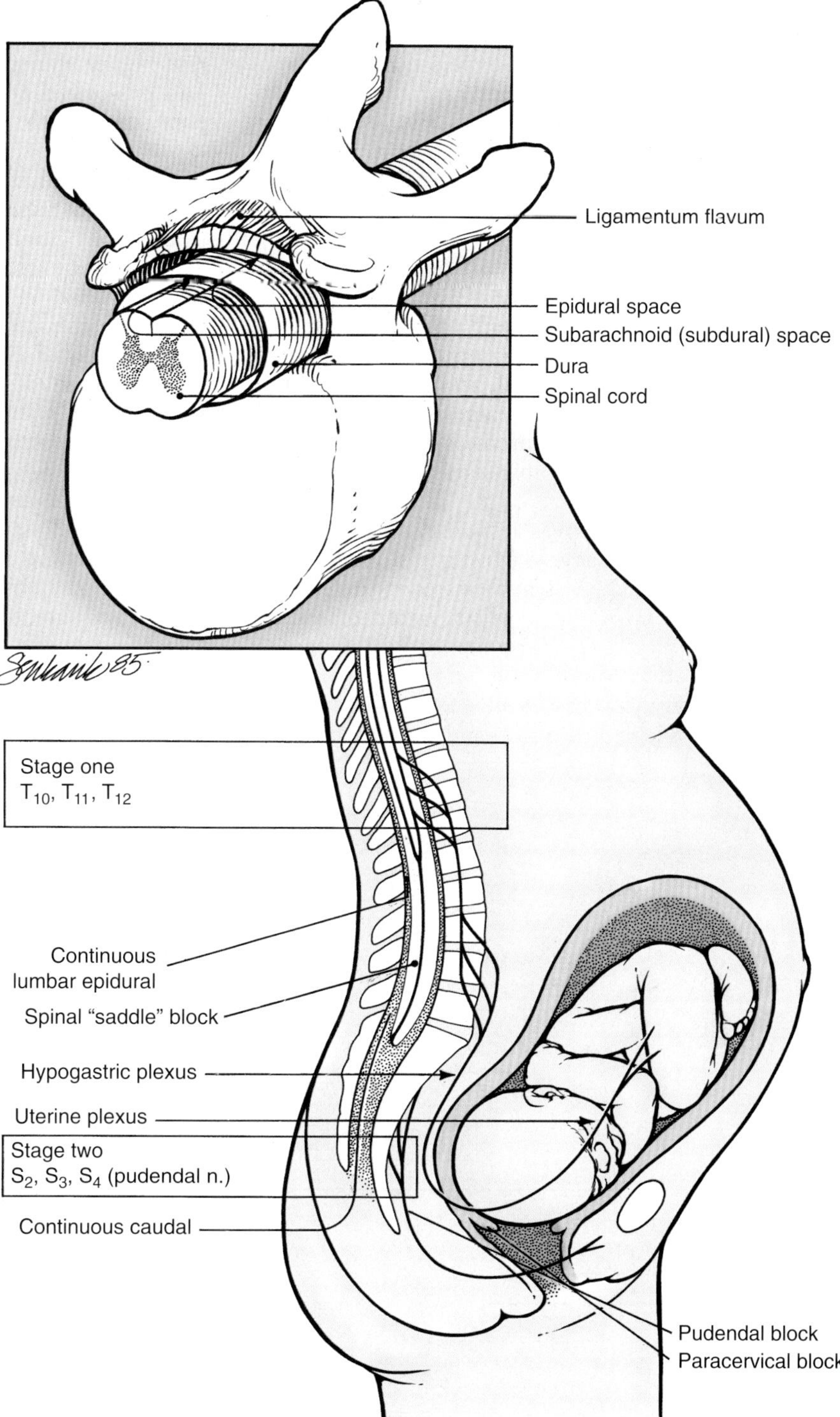

Figure 16-1. Pain pathways of labor and delivery and nerves blocked by various anesthetic techniques.

labor, additional painful stimuli are added as the fetal head distends the pelvic floor, vagina, and perineum. The sensory fibers of sacral nerves 2, 3, and 4 (i.e., the pudendal nerve) transmit painful impulses from the perineum to the spinal cord during second stage and any perineal repair (see Fig. 16-1). During cesarean delivery, although the incision is usually around thoracic spinal nerve 12 dermatome, anesthesia is required to a level of thoracic spinal nerve 4 to completely block peritoneal discomfort, especially during uterine exteriorization. Pain after cesarean delivery is due to both incisional pain and uterine involution.

EFFECTS OF PAIN AND STRESS

The process of labor involves significant pain and stress for the majority of women. Using the McGill Pain

Questionnaire, which measures intensity and quality of pain, Melzack and colleagues[4] provided a sophisticated and in-depth report on the labor experience of 87 nulliparous and 54 parous patients. Pain rating index scores were assigned to each parturient's description of labor pain and compared with those of nonobstetric patients. It is enlightening to consider that 59 percent of nulliparous and 43 percent of parous patients described their labor pain in terms more severe than did those suffering from cancer pain. In contrast, only 24 percent of parous patients and 9 percent of nulliparous patients described the pain as relatively minor. Although those with childbirth training reported less pain than those without such training, the differences were small, and training did not affect patients' use of epidural analgesia (81 versus 82 percent). The most substantial predictors of pain intensity were ultimately socioeconomic status and prior menstrual difficulties.

The maternal and fetal stress response to the pain of labor has been difficult to assess. Most investigators have described and quantified stress in terms of the release of adrenocorticotropic hormone, cortisol, catecholamines, and β-endorphins (Fig. 16-2). Early labor is accompanied by sustained elevations in plasma adrenocorticotropic hormone and cortisol levels,[5,6] followed by increases in epinephrine, norepinephrine, and β-endorphins throughout labor.[7,8] Stress may not be a beneficial response because β-adrenergic agents have uterine relaxant effects and higher epinephrine levels are associated with anxiety and prolonged labor.[9] Furthermore, animal studies indicate that both epinephrine and norepinephrine can decrease uterine blood flow in the absence of maternal heart rate and blood pressure changes, contributing to occult fetal asphyxia.[10] Maternal psychological stress (induced by bright lights or toe clamp) can detrimentally affect uterine blood flow and fetal acid-base status as demonstrated in baboons and monkeys.[11] In pregnant sheep, catecholamines increase and uterine blood flow decreases after electrically induced painful stimuli and after nonpainful stimuli (such as loud noises) induce fear and anxiety, as evidenced by struggling[12] (Fig. 16-3).

Although some of the physiologic stress of labor is unavoidable, analgesia and anesthesia may reduce additional increments in the stress response that are secondary to pain. Postpartum women suffer objective deficits in cognitive and memory function when compared with nonpregnant women.[13] Intrapartum analgesia does not exacerbate, but rather *lessens* the cognitive defect compared with unmedicated parturients. Presumably, cognitive function is adversely affected by the stress of labor, which is mitigated by judicious use of analgesics. Epidural analgesia prevents increases in both cortisol

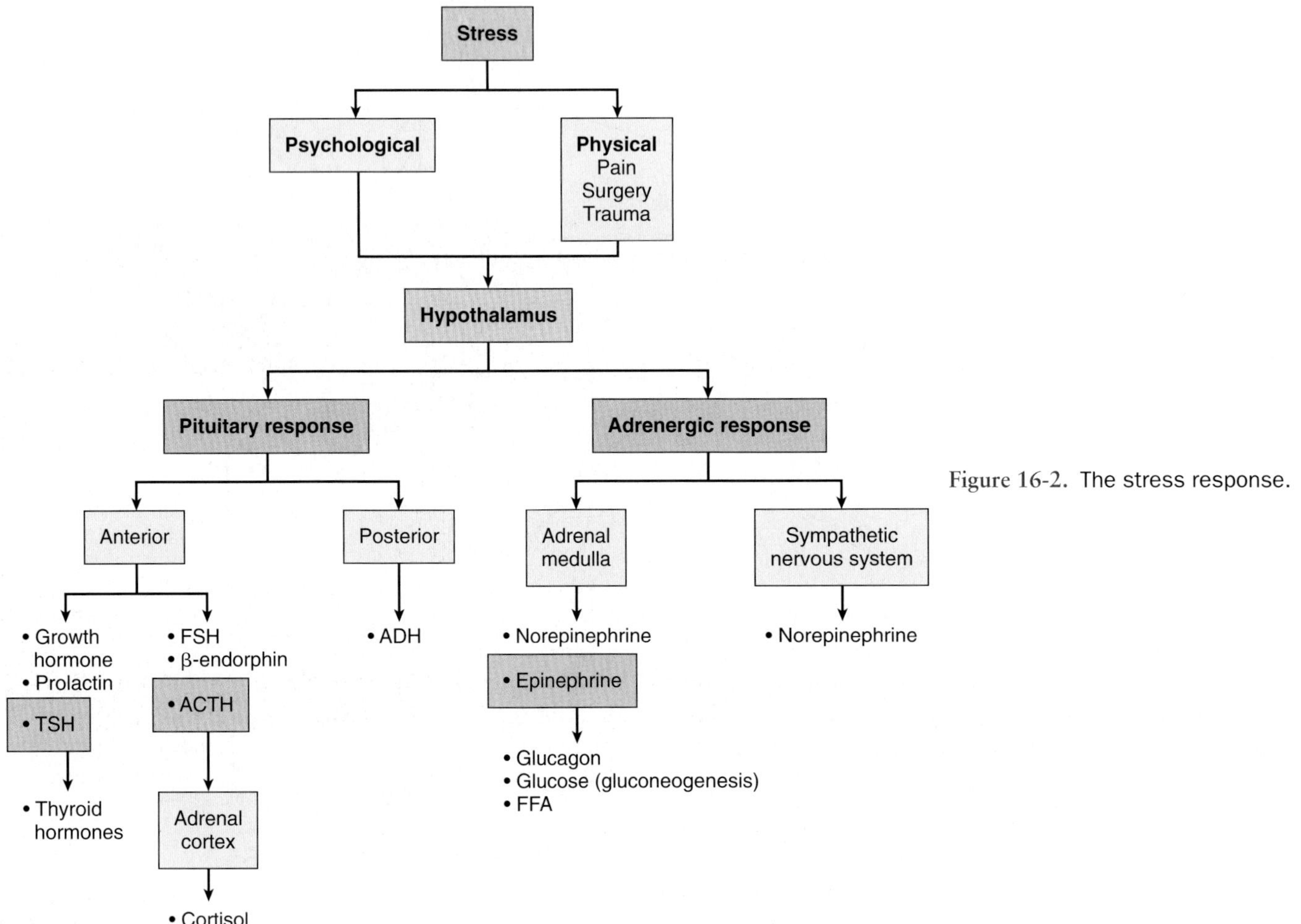

Figure 16-2. The stress response.

and 11-hydroxycorticosteroid levels during labor,[14] but systemically administered opioids do not.[15] Epidural analgesia also attenuates elevations of epinephrine, norepinephrine,[7] and endorphin levels.[16] Presumably, regional anesthesia blocks afferent stimuli to the hypothalamus and, thus, inhibits the body's response to stress[17] (Fig. 16-4).

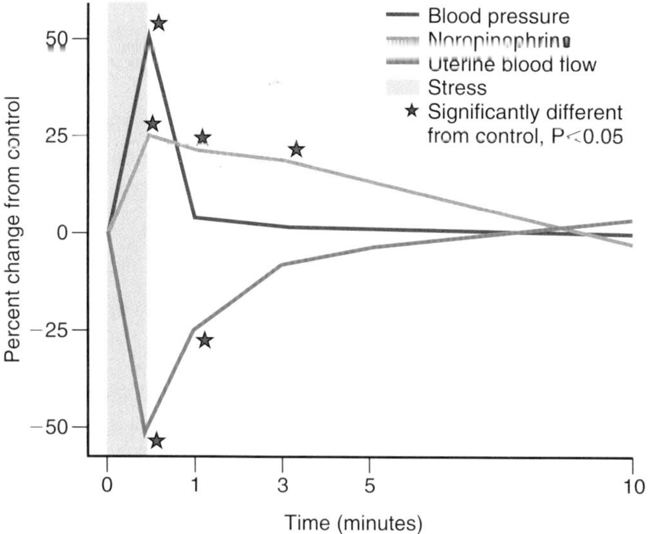

Figure 16-3. Effects of electrically induced stress (30 to 60 seconds) on maternal mean arterial blood pressure, plasma norepinephrine levels, and uterine blood flow. (Modified from Shnider SM, Wright RG, Levinson G, et al: Uterine blood flow and plasma norepinephrine changes during maternal stress in the pregnant ewe. Anesthesiology 50:526, 1979.)

There is convincing evidence that anesthesia, sedation, or both effectively decrease the physiologic effects of pain and stress in monkey and baboon fetuses.[11,18] Assuming any hypotension is rapidly treated and perfusion is preserved by uterine displacement, fetal acid-base status (as measured by base excess) of human infants whose mothers receive epidural anesthesia during the first stage of labor is altered less than infants of mothers who receive systemic opioid analgesia.[19]

ANALGESIA FOR LABOR

Table 16-1 presents the frequency with which the various forms of analgesia are used during labor. The data are from a large survey of hospitals in the United States, stratified by the size of their delivery service.[1]

Psychoprophylaxis

Psychoprophylaxis is any nonpharmacologic method of minimizing the perception of painful uterine contractions. Relaxation, concentration on breathing, gentle massage, and partner or doula participation contribute to effectiveness. One of the method's most valuable contributions is that it is often taught in prepared childbirth classes, where parents tour the labor and delivery suite and learn

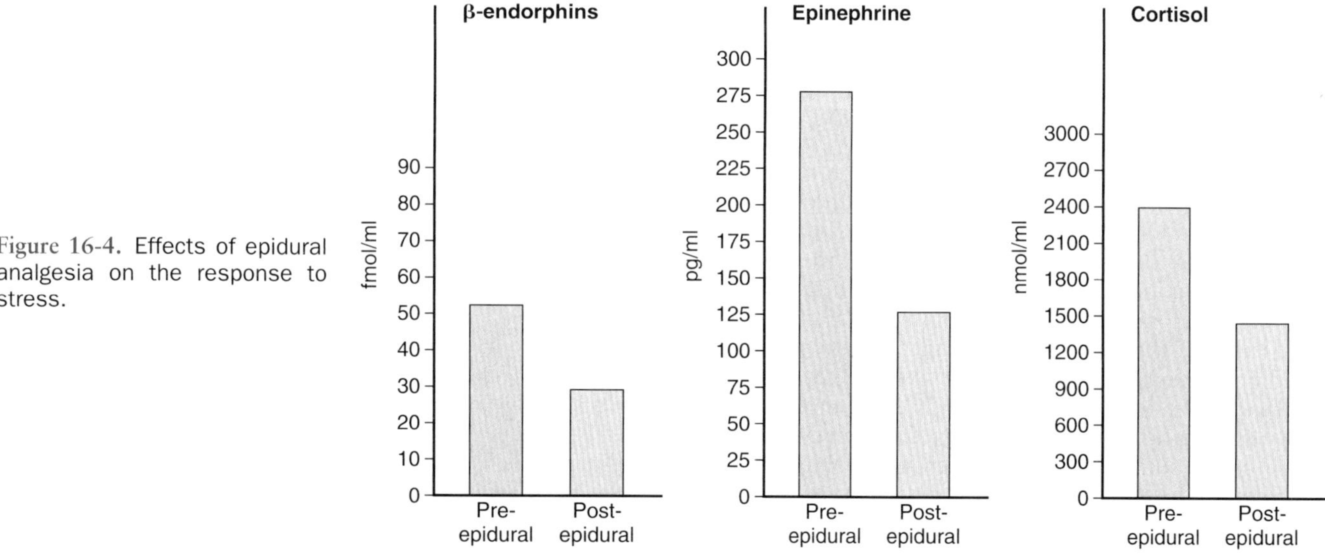

Figure 16-4. Effects of epidural analgesia on the response to stress.

Table 16-1. Analgesic Procedures Used for Labor Pain Relief in 2001 According to Size of Delivery Service

HOSPITAL SIZE (BIRTHS/YEAR)	NO ANESTHESIA (%)	NARCOTICS BARBITURATES TRANQUILIZERS (%)	PARACERVICAL BLOCK (%)	SPINAL OR EPIDURAL BLOCK (%)
<500	12	37	3	57
500–1,499	10	42	3	59
>1,500	6	34	2	77

Adapted from Bucklin BA, Hawkins JL, Anderson JR, Ullrich FA: Obstetric anesthesia workforce survey. Anesthesiology 103:645, 2005.

about the normal processes of labor and delivery, in many instances mitigating their fear of the unknown.

Although psychoprophylactic techniques can be empowering, the majority of women will still ultimately blend them with pharmacologic methods.[1] A disadvantage to the teachings of some philosophies of psychoprophylaxis is the belief that use of drug-induced pain relief represents failure or will harm the child. Because the majority of first-time mothers choose epidural analgesia (even 57 percent of those strongly wishing to avoid it), these teachings are counterproductive and can heighten fear and anxiety during labor.[20]

Nonpharmacologic techniques for labor analgesia may be used alone, or in conjunction with parenteral or regional techniques.[21] A systematic review of acupuncture concluded the evidence for efficacy is promising but that there is a paucity of data.[22] From the three randomized clinical trials they reviewed, the authors suggest that acupuncture alleviates labor pain and reduces use of both epidural analgesia and parenteral opioids. Acupuncture may be helpful for patients who feel strongly about avoiding epidural analgesia in labor, although arranging to have a qualified and credentialed provider available at the time of delivery may be challenging. A randomized controlled trial of laboring in water found no advantage in labor outcome or in reducing the need for analgesia, but the request for epidural analgesia was delayed by about 30 minutes.[23] The American Academy of Pediatrics Committee on Fetus and Newborn has expressed concerns about *delivering* in water because of the lack of trials demonstrating safety and the rare but reported unusual complications such as infection or asphyxia.[24] They state that "... underwater birth should be considered an experimental procedure that should not be performed except within the context of an appropriately designed RCT after informed parental consent." Intracutaneous sterile water injections are simple to perform and have good evidence for efficacy, perhaps by a similar gating mechanism as acupuncture.[25] An intradermal injection of 0.1 ml of sterile water at four sites in the lower back significantly lowers visual analog pain scores during labor.[26] A number of studies have examined transcutaneous electrical nerve stimulation during labor. Patients tend to rate the device as helpful, despite the fact it does not decrease pain scores or the use of additional analgesics. As one study noted, transcutaneous electrical nerve stimulation units appear not to change the degree of pain, but somehow may have made the pain less disturbing.[27] Although the efficacy of these techniques is largely unproven because of a lack of randomized clinical trials, there are no serious safety concerns with any of these techniques, which is attractive to patients and their caregivers. Women expect to have choices and a degree of control during their childbirth, and their caregivers should provide analgesic options for them to choose from, including nonpharmacologic methods.

Systemic Opioid Analgesia

Opioids (also known as narcotics) are drugs possessing morphine-like pharmacologic activity. Morphine and codeine are natural alkaloids derived from opium. Opioids such as hydromorphone (Dilaudid) and heroin are semisynthetic compounds made by a simple alteration of the morphine molecule. Meperidine (Demerol) and fentanyl are synthetic compounds resembling morphine. Opioids can be given in intermittent doses by intramuscular or intravenous routes at the patient's request, or through patient-controlled administration. All opioids provide sedation and a sense of euphoria, but their analgesic effect in labor is limited and their primary mechanism of action is sedation.[28] Opioids can also produce nausea and respiratory depression in the mother, the degree of which is usually comparable for equipotent analgesic doses. Also, all opioids freely cross the placenta to the newborn, decreasing beat-to-beat variability, and can increase the likelihood of significant respiratory depression in the newborn at birth, with subsequent need for treatment.[29,30] A meta-analysis that aggregates the results of several randomized trials reveals that opioid treatment is associated with an increased risk of Apgar scores less than 7 at 5 minutes (odds ratio [OR] 2.6; 95 percent confidence interval [CI] 1.2–5.6) and increased need for neonatal naloxone (OR 4.17; 95 percent CI 1.3–14.3) although the overall incidence of both was low.[31]

If left untreated, hypoventilation from neonatal depression can result in hypoxia, hypercapnia, and acidosis, which, in turn, may lead to neonatal injury. If properly cared for, infants with opioid-induced depression will suffer no ill effects. Proper care includes ventilation, oxygenation, gentle stimulation, and the judicious use of the opioid antagonist naloxone. Positive-pressure ventilation is the single most effective measure and can be provided through facemask or intubation. Naloxone is a useful drug that should be available whenever opioids are used. However, it is an adjunct to ventilation, not a substitute for it. Opioids also may produce neurobehavioral changes in the newborn. Agents such as meperidine have active metabolites that persist in the newborn for as long as 2 to 4 days.[32] Although there has been some concern that neurobehavioral effects may persist and be influential in later life, persistent effects have not been demonstrated.[33] The trend in modern obstetric care is to use short-acting medications that are quickly cleared from the newborn and do not have active metabolites.

An important and significant disadvantage of opioid analgesia is the prolonged effect of these agents on maternal gastric emptying. When parenteral or epidural opioids are used, gastric emptying is prolonged, and if general anesthesia becomes necessary, the risk of aspiration is increased.[34,35] The opioids in common use today are meperidine, nalbuphine, butorphanol, and fentanyl. Morphine fell out of favor in the 1960s to 1970s because of a single study reporting increased respiratory depression in the newborn compared with meperidine, but no recent study has compared their relative safety for the newborn in the setting of modern practice.[36]

Patient-Controlled Analgesia

The infusion pump is programmed to give a predetermined dose of drug upon patient demand. The physician will program the pump to include a lockout interval to limit the total dose administered per hour. Advantages of this method include the sense of autonomy, which patients appreciate, and elimination of delays in treatment while the patient's nurse obtains and administers the dose. In general, patient-controlled analgesia (PCA) results in a decreased total dose of opioid during labor.[37,38] Fentanyl and meperidine are the opioids most commonly employed with this technique.

MEPERIDINE (DEMEROL)

Meperidine is a synthetic opioid. Meperidine 100 mg is roughly equianalgesic to morphine 10 mg, but has been reported to have a somewhat less depressive effect on respiration.[36] Usually, 25 to 50 mg are administered intravenously; it may also be used intramuscularly or in a patient-controlled analgesia (PCA) pump delivering 15 mg of meperidine every 10 minutes as needed until delivery.[39] The analgesic action of meperidine begins after approximately 10 to 20 minutes and persists for 2 to 3 hours after intramuscular administration. Plasma concentrations of meperidine are higher after deltoid injection than after gluteus muscle injection,[40] suggesting that the deltoid muscle may be the preferred intramuscular site during labor. Intravenously, the onset of analgesia begins almost immediately and lasts approximately 1.5 to 2 hours. Side effects may include tachycardia, nausea and vomiting, and a delay in gastric emptying.

Normeperidine is an active metabolite of meperidine, potentiating meperidine's depressant effects in the newborn. Normeperidine concentrations increase slowly, and therefore, it exerts its effect on the newborn during the second hour after administration.[29] Multiple doses of meperidine result in greater accumulation of both meperidine and normeperidine in fetal tissues[41,42]; thus, administration of large doses of meperidine in the first stage of labor (rather than during the second stage of labor) leads to high doses accumulated in the fetus. A randomized controlled study using intravenous PCA meperidine for labor analgesia found 3.4 percent of infants required naloxone at delivery (versus 0.8 percent with epidural analgesia).[43] Normeperidine accumulation in the fetus can result in prolonged neonatal sedation and neurobehavioral changes.[44,45] These neurobehavioral changes are evident into day 2 and day 3 of life.[46,47] In contrast, fentanyl also crosses the placenta but has no active metabolites and has not been associated with neonatal depression, so its administration can continue into the second stage of labor.[48]

NALBUPHINE (NUBAIN)

Nalbuphine is a synthetic agonist-antagonist opioid, meaning it has opioid blocking properties as well as analgesic properties. Its analgesic potency is similar to that of morphine when compared on a milligram-per-milligram basis, and usual doses are 5 to 10 mg intravenously every 3 hours. A reported advantage of nalbuphine is its ceiling effect for respiratory depression,[49] that is, respiratory depression from multiple doses appears to plateau. One limitation of nalbuphine is that its antagonist activity may also limit the analgesia it can produce, and it may interfere with spinal and epidural opioids given as part of a neuraxial technique. Nalbuphine causes less maternal nausea and vomiting than meperidine, but it tends to produce more maternal sedation, dizziness, and dysphoria, as well as the risk of opioid withdrawal in susceptible patients.[50]

BUTORPHANOL (STADOL)

Butorphanol is also a synthetic agonist-antagonist opioid analgesic drug. The dosage of 1 to 2 mg is administered intravenously and compares favorably with 40 to 80 mg of meperidine or 5 to 10 mg morphine.[51] Nausea and vomiting appear to occur less often with butorphanol than with other opioids.[51] Like nalbuphine, the major advantage is a ceiling effect for respiratory depression, and the side effects of the two drugs are similar.[52] Rarely, a pseudosinusoidal fetal heart rate pattern may occur after administration, but this is not unique to butorphanol.

FENTANYL

Fentanyl is a fast-onset, short-acting synthetic opioid with no active metabolites. In a randomized comparison with meperidine, fentanyl 50 to 100 µg every hour provided equivalent analgesia, with fewer neonatal effects and less maternal sedation and nausea.[48] The main drawback of fentanyl is its short duration of action requiring frequent redosing or the use of a patient-controlled intravenous infusion pump.[38,53] A sample PCA setting for fentanyl is a 50 µg incremental dose with a 10-minute lockout and no basal rate.[38]

Sedatives

Sedatives do not possess analgesic qualities and are most often used early in labor to relieve anxiety or to aid in sleep. All sedatives and hypnotics cross the placenta freely, and except for the benzodiazepines, they have no known antagonists. Those most frequently used are barbiturates, phenothiazines, and benzodiazepines.

BARBITURATES

Because barbiturates and other sedatives are not analgesic, patients may be less able to cope with pain than if they had received no pharmacologic assistance at all; that is, normal coping mechanisms may be blunted.[54] Although barbiturates can depress both cardiovascular and respiratory functions in mother and newborn, low doses have little effect. Effects that do occur may persist for a prolonged time. For example, attention span can be depressed for as long as 2 to 4 days. Thus, these drugs should rarely be used during labor.

PHENOTHIAZINES

Promethazine (Phenergan) is perhaps the most widely used phenothiazine. When given in small doses in combination with an opioid, these drugs do not seem to produce additional neonatal depression.[55] However, like the barbiturates, these agents rapidly cross the placenta and, in large doses, can depress the fetus for a significant period and therapeutic antagonists are not available. Promethazine is a weak antiemetic agent and causes significant sedation in the mother and occasional extrapyramidal symptoms. Sedation is rarely desirable during the childbirth experience. Promethazine may actually impair the analgesic efficacy of opioids. In a randomized double blind trial, women received placebo, metoclopramide, or promethazine as an antiemetic with meperidine analgesia.[56] Analgesia after placebo or metoclopramide was significantly better than that after promethazine as measured by pain scores and need for supplemental analgesics. Metoclopramide 10 mg has also been shown to improve PCA analgesia during second-trimester termination of pregnancy.[57,58] In two randomized double-blind studies, the group receiving metoclopramide (versus saline) used 54 percent and 66 percent less intravenous morphine.

By using opioids with less potential to cause nausea and vomiting such as fentanyl, routine use of promethazine should be unnecessary. To prevent polypharmacy, antiemetic treatment should only be used in symptomatic patients. If used, promethazine should be given intravenously as intramuscular injection is very painful. Ondansetron (Zofran) is a potent antiemetic with few side effects and should be used instead of promethazine whenever possible. Metoclopramide may be used as a prophylactic antiemetic with little sedation and possible potentiation of analgesia.

BENZODIAZEPINES

All of the benzodiazepines are associated with significant maternal amnesia; therefore, their use should be avoided during labor and especially delivery.[59] Indications for benzodiazepine treatment include management of severe anxiety disorders and treatment of seizures due to eclampsia or local anesthetic toxicity. Diazepam was the first widely used benzodiazepine. A major disadvantage of diazepam is that it disrupts thermoregulation in newborns, which renders them less able to maintain body temperature.[60] Presumably this can occur with any of the benzodiazepines. As with many drugs, beat-to-beat variability of the fetal heart rate can be reduced even with a single intravenous dose, although these changes do not reflect alterations in the acid-base status of the newborn. Unlike diazepam, midazolam is water soluble, and it is shorter acting than diazepam.[61] There are no data on its use in labor, and there are conflicting data regarding its effects on the fetus/neonate when used as an induction agent for cesarean delivery.[62,63] Flumazenil, a specific benzodiazepine antagonist, can reliably reverse benzodiazepine-induced sedation and ventilatory depression.[64]

PLACENTAL TRANSFER

Essentially, all analgesic and anesthetic agents except highly ionized muscle relaxants cross the placenta freely (see box, "Factors Influencing Placental Transfer from Mother to Fetus").[65,66] The limited transfer of muscle relaxants such as succinylcholine enables anesthesiologists to use general anesthesia for cesarean delivery without causing fetal paralysis.

Because the placenta has the properties of a lipid membrane, most drugs and all anesthetic agents cross by simple diffusion. Thus, the amount of drug that crosses the placenta increases as concentrations in the maternal circulation and total area of the placenta increase. Diffusion is also affected by the properties of the drug itself, including molecular weight, spatial configuration, degree of ionization, lipid solubility, and protein binding. For example, bupivacaine is highly protein bound, a characteristic that some believe explains why fetal blood concentrations are so much lower than with other local anesthetics. On the other hand, bupivacaine is also highly lipid soluble. The more lipid soluble a drug is, the more freely it passes through a lipid membrane. Furthermore, once in the fetal system, lipid solubility enables the drug to be taken up by fetal tissues rapidly, that is, redistribution, which again contributes to the lower blood concentration of the agent.

The degree of ionization of a drug is also important. Most drugs exist in both an ionized and nonionized state, with the nonionized form more freely crossing lipid membranes. The degree of ionization is influenced by the pH; this may become relevant in situations in which there is a significant pH gradient between mother (normal pH 7.40) and an acidotic infant (pH < 7.2). For example, local anesthetics are more ionized at a lower pH, so the nonionized portion of the drug in the maternal circulation (normal pH) crosses to the acidotic fetus, becomes ionized, and thus remains in the fetus, potentially leading to higher local anesthetic concentrations in the fetus/newborn (Fig. 16-5).[67] Whether this has relevant adverse clinical effects on the fetus is unknown.

Factors Influencing Placental Transfer form Mother to Fetus

- Drug
  - Molecular weight
  - Lipid solubility
  - Ionization, pH of blood
  - Spatial configuration
- Maternal
  - Uptake into bloodstream
  - Distribution via circulation
  - Uterine blood flow
    - Amount
    - Distribution (myometrium versus placenta)
- Placental
  - Circulation: intermittent spurting arterioles
  - Lipid membrane: Fick's law of simple diffusion
- Fetal
  - Circulation: ductus venosus, foramen ovale, ductus arteriosus

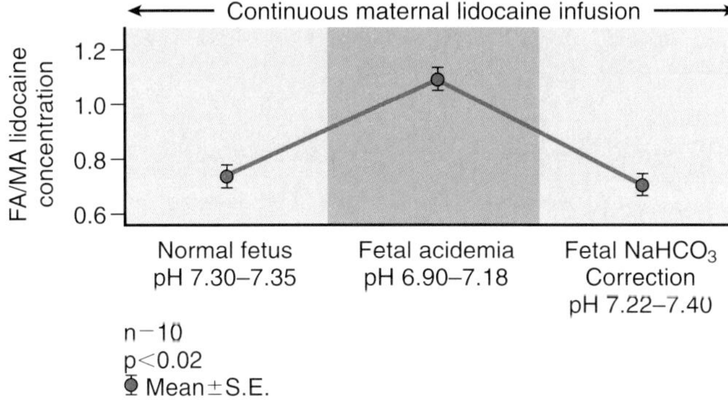

Figure 16-5. Fetal-maternal arterial (FA/MA) lidocaine ratios were significantly higher ($p < 0.02$) during fetal acidemia than during control or when pH was corrected with bicarbonate ($N = 10$; mean ± SE). (From Biehl D, Shnider SM, Levinson G, Callender K: Placental transfer of lidocaine: effects of fetal acidosis. Anesthesiology 48:409, 1978, with permission.)

Regional Analgesic/Anesthetic Techniques

Regional analgesic/anesthetic techniques use local anesthetics to provide sensory as well as various degrees of motor blockade over a specific region of the body. In obstetrics, regional techniques include major blocks, such as lumbar epidural and spinal, and minor blocks such as paracervical, pudendal, and local infiltration (see Fig. 16-1).

Lumbar Epidural Analgesia/Anesthesia

Epidural blockade is a major regional anesthetic used to provide *analgesia* during labor, or surgical *anesthesia* for vaginal or cesarean delivery. Epidural analgesia offers the most effective form of pain relief[68] and is used by the majority of women in the United States.[1] In most obstetric patients, the primary indication for epidural analgesia is the patient's desire for pain relief. Medical indications for epidural analgesia during labor may include anticipated difficulty in intubation, a history of malignant hyperthermia, selected forms of cardiovascular and respiratory disease, and prevention or treatment of autonomic hyperreflexia in parturients with a high spinal cord lesion. Epidural block is placed using a large-bore needle (16-, 17-, or 18-gauge) to locate the epidural space. Next, a catheter is inserted through the needle, and the needle is removed over the catheter. After aspirating the catheter, a test dose of local anesthetic with a "marker" such as epinephrine may be given first to be certain the catheter has not been unintentionally placed in the subarachnoid (spinal) space or in a blood vessel. Intravascular placement will lead to maternal tachycardia due to the epinephrine, and rapid onset of sensory and motor block will occur if the local anesthetic is placed in the spinal fluid. Once intravascular and intrathecal placement have been ruled out, local anesthetic is injected through the catheter, which remains taped in place to the mother's back to enable subsequent injections throughout labor (see Figs. 16-1 and 16-6). Thus, it is often called continuous epidural analgesia.

Two forms of epidural analgesia are used for labor: lumbar and caudal. The catheter is placed through a lumbar interspace in lumbar analgesia and through the sacral hiatus in caudal analgesia (see Fig. 16-1). Because of the large volume of local anesthetic used, adverse effects on muscle tone in the legs and pelvic floor, and the highly variable anatomy of the sacral hiatus in adults, the caudal approach has fallen out of favor for labor analgesia. A rare but serious complication of caudal anesthesia is accidental injection of local anesthetic into the fetal head, leading to newborn apnea, bradycardia, and convulsions.[69]

Most anesthesiologists now prefer the lumbar approach and use a technique described as segmental epidural analgesia (Fig. 16-7). Low concentrations of local anesthetic (0.25 percent bupivacaine) are injected at L2-L5, affecting the small easily blocked sympathetic nerves that mediate early labor pain, but sparing the sensation of pressure and motor function of the perineum and lower extremities. The patient should be able to move about in bed and perceive the impact of the presenting part on the perineum. Patients vary in their responses to local anesthetics, and infusions may need to be adjusted to a lower rate or concentration if the patient develops excessive motor block. If perineal anesthesia is needed for delivery, a larger volume of local anesthetic can be administered at that time through the catheter (see Fig. 16-7). Alternatively, for perineal anesthesia, the obstetrician can perform a pudendal block or local infiltration of the perineum.

A variant of the epidural technique involves passing a small-gauge pencil-point spinal needle through the epidural needle before catheter placement. This combined spinal-epidural (CSE) or coaxial technique provides more rapid onset of analgesia using a very small dose of opioid or a local anesthetic and opioid combination.[70] Because the dose of drug used in the subarachnoid space is much smaller than that used for epidural analgesia, the risks of local anesthetic toxicity or high spinal block are avoided. Side effects are usually mild and easily treated, and include pruritus and nausea. Pruritus occurs in as many as 80 percent of women after intrathecal opioid administration, although only about 10 percent request treatment. Small doses of nalbuphine or naloxone are effective therapies for pruritus, or less commonly, propofol, ondansetron, or diphenhydramine may be used. The risk of postdural puncture headache following CSE is no different than that with epidural analgesia alone, approximately 1.5 percent.[71]

Nonreassuring fetal heart rate changes occur in equivalent numbers of patients receiving spinal or epidural analgesia in labor: 21.5 percent of patients receiving intrathecal sufentanil and 23.4 percent of patients receiving epidural bupivacaine.[72] Although the incidence of hypotension is also similar between the two techniques, the etiology of fetal bradycardia after spinal analgesia may relate to uterine hypertonus rather than hypotension. Rapid onset of spinal analgesia decreases maternal catecholamines, specifically epinephrine, which may have been causing uterine relaxation through its beta-

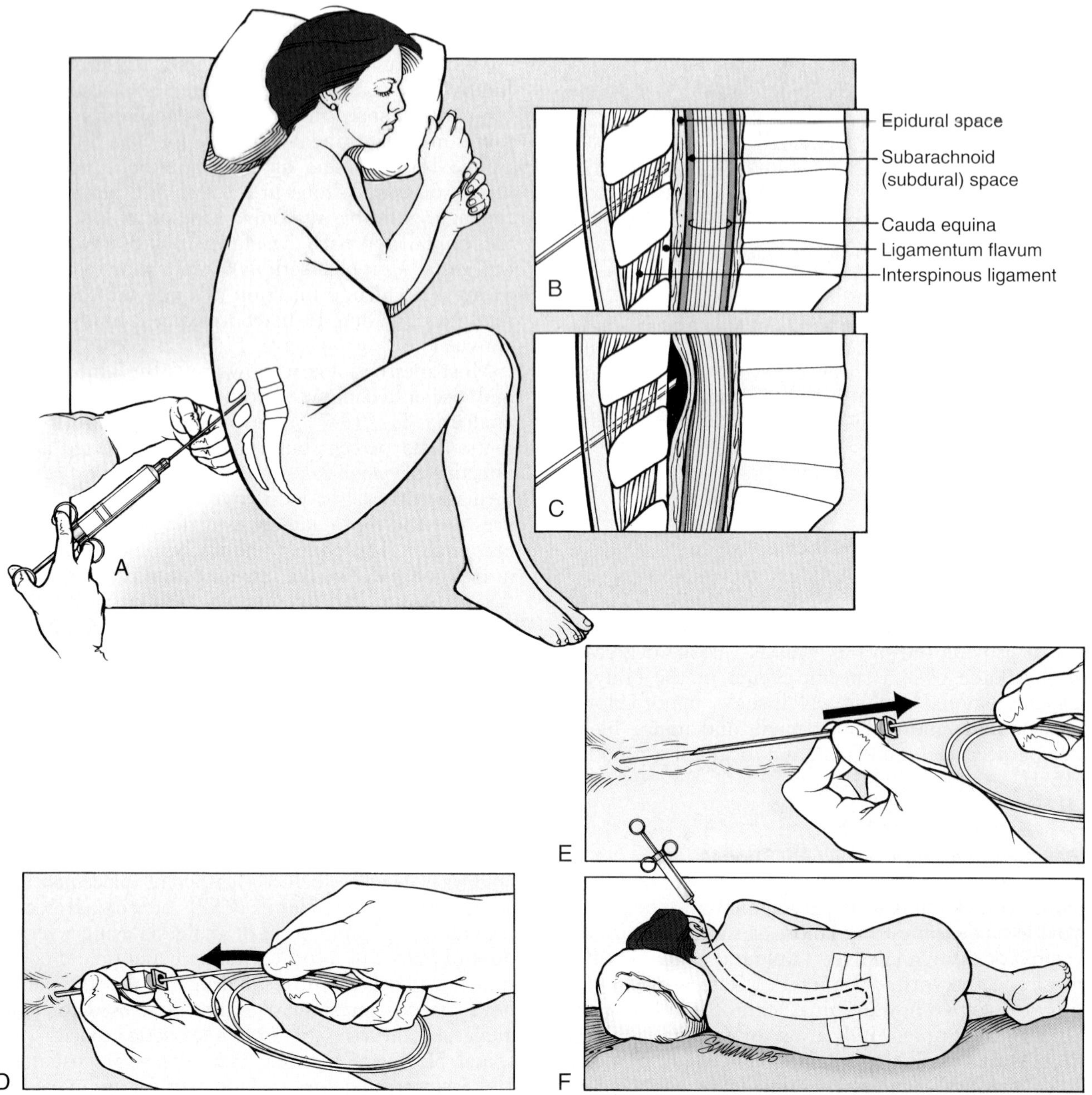

Figure 16-6. Technique of lumbar epidural puncture by the midline approach. *A,* This side view shows left hand held against patient's back, with thumb and index finger grasping hub. Attempts to inject solution while point of needle is in the interspinous ligament meet resistance. *B,* Point of needle is in the ligamentum flavum, which offers marked resistance and makes it almost impossible to inject solution. *C,* Entrance of the needle's point into epidural space is discerned by sudden lack of resistance to injection of saline. Force of injected solution pushes dura-arachnoid away from point of needle. *D,* Catheter is introduced through needle. Note that hub of needle is pulled caudad toward the patient, increasing the angle between the shaft of the needle and the epidural space. Also note technique of holding the tubing: It is wound around the right hand. *E,* Needle is withdrawn over tubing and held steady with the right hand. *F,* Catheter is immobilized with adhesive tape. Note the large loop made by the catheter to decrease risk of kinking at the point where the tube exits from the skin. (From Bonica JJ: Obstetric Analgesia and Anesthesia. Amsterdam, World Federation of Societies of Anesthesiologists, 1980, with permission.)

agonist activity. Fortunately these nonreassuring fetal heart rate changes do not seem to affect labor outcome. In a review of 2,380 deliveries in a community hospital, there was no increase in emergency cesarean delivery in the 1,240 patients who received regional analgesia for labor (98 percent of which were CSE) versus the 1,140 patients who received systemic or no medication.[73] A systematic review of randomized comparisons of intrathecal opioid analgesia versus epidural or parenteral opioids in labor found the use of intrathecal opioids significantly increased the risk of fetal bradycardia (OR 1.8; 95-percent confidence interval, 1.0 to 3.1).[74] However, the risk of cesarean delivery for fetal heart rate abnormalities was similar in the two groups (6.0 versus 7.8 percent). Fetal heart rate should be monitored during and after the administration of either epidural or

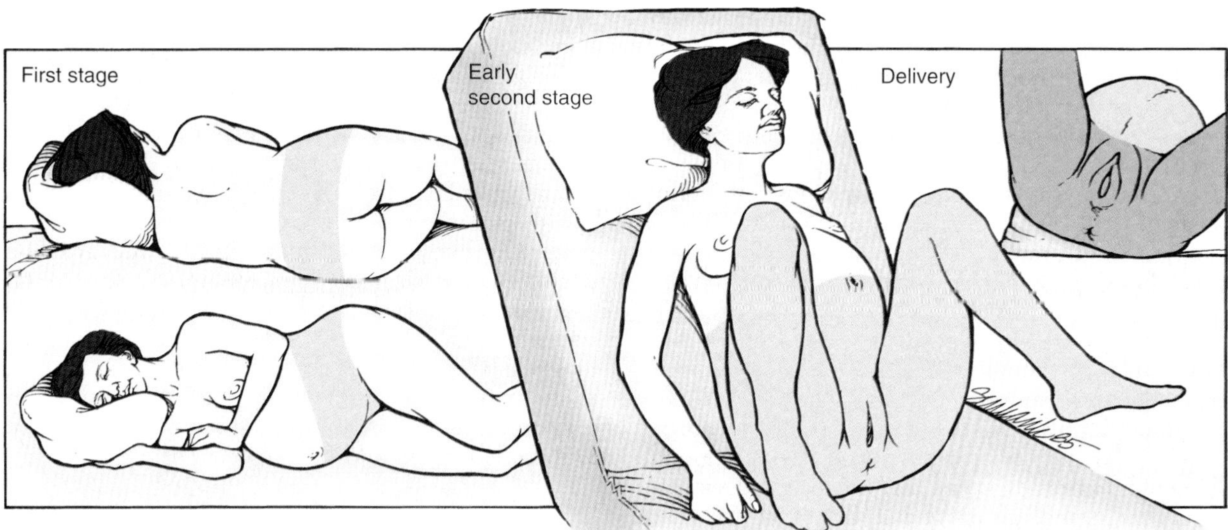

Figure 16-7. Segmental epidural analgesia for labor and delivery. A single catheter is introduced into the epidural space and advanced so that its tip is at L2. Initially, small volumes of low concentrations of local anesthetic are used to produce segmental analgesia. For the second stage, the analgesia is extended to the sacral segments by injecting a larger amount of the same concentration of local anesthetic, with the patient in the semirecumbent position. After internal rotation, a higher concentration of local anesthetic is injected to produce motor block of the sacral segments and thus achieve perineal relaxation and anesthesia. The wedge under the right buttock causes the uterus to displace to the left. (From Bonica JJ: Obstetric Analgesia and Anesthesia. Amsterdam, World Federation of Societies of Anesthesiologists, 1980, with permission.)

intrathecal medications to allow for timely intrauterine resuscitation.

Some practitioners have used an opioid only or opioid plus local anesthetic technique to allow parturients to ambulate during labor (the "walking epidural") because there is little or no interference with motor function.[70] One randomized study found that use of intrathecal opioids increased speed of cervical dilatation and decreased length of labor when compared with conventional epidural analgesia.[75] Another randomized trial compared early (<4 cm dilatation) administration of intrathecal opioids to parenteral opioids, both followed by epidural analgesia. The use of intrathecal opioids improved pain control in early labor without increasing the risk of cesarean delivery.[76] This option, which avoids maternal sedation and decreases nausea and vomiting, is likely to become increasingly popular.

Side effects of epidural or combined spinal-epidural analgesia include hypotension, local anesthetic toxicity, allergic reaction, high or total spinal anesthesia, neurologic injury, and spinal headache. In addition, epidural analgesia use increases the rate of intrapartum fever and possibly operative vaginal delivery. The effect of epidural analgesia on labor progression, fetal position, and risk of cesarean delivery is controversial and is discussed in detail below. Because epidural anesthesia is associated with side effects and complications, some of which are dangerous, those who administer it must be thoroughly familiar not only with the technical aspects of its administration but also with the signs and symptoms of complications and their treatment. Specifically, the American Society of Anesthesiologists and American College of Obstetricians and Gynecologists have stated: "Persons administering or supervising obstetric anesthesia should be qualified to manage the infrequent but occasionally life-threatening complications of major regional anesthesia such as respiratory and cardiovascular failure, convulsions due to toxic levels of local anesthetic, or vomiting and aspiration. Mastering and retaining the skills and knowledge necessary to manage these complications require adequate training and frequent application."[3]

HYPOTENSION

Hypotension is defined variably but most often as a systolic blood pressure less than 100 mm Hg or a 20-percent decrease from baseline. It occurs after approximately 10 to 30 percent of spinal or epidural blocks given during labor.[43,77] Hypotension occurs primarily as a result of the effects of local anesthetic agents on sympathetic fibers, which normally maintain blood vessel tone. Vasodilation results in decreased venous return of blood to the right side of the heart, with subsequent decreased cardiac output and hypotension. A secondary mechanism may be decreased maternal endogenous catecholamines following pain relief. Hypotension threatens the fetus by decreasing uterine blood flow. However, when recognized promptly and treated effectively, few, if any, untoward effects accrue to either mother or fetus (Table 16-2).[77,78] Special care should be taken to avoid or promptly treat hypotension, especially in situations in which acute or chronic fetal compromise is suspected.

Treatment of hypotension begins with prophylaxis, which includes (1) intravenous access for volume expansion and administration of pressors and (2) left uterine displacement to maintain cardiac preload. Isotonic crystalloid infusion may mitigate against the effects of vasodilation. Rapid boluses should not contain dextrose because of the association with subsequent neonatal hypoglycemia.[79] Proper treatment of hypotension depends on immediate diagnosis. Therefore, the individual administering the anesthesia must be present and attentive. Once diagnosed, hypotension is corrected by increasing the rate of intravenous fluid infusion and exaggerating left uterine displacement. If these simple measures do not suffice, a vasopressor is indicated.

The vasopressor of choice is evolving from ephedrine, given in 5- to 10-mg doses to phenylephrine, in 50- to 100-μg increments. Ephedrine is a mixed α- and β-agonist, and was thought to be less likely to compromise uteroplacental perfusion than the pure α-agonists.[80] Recent clinical studies have suggested that phenylephrine may be given safely to treat hypotension during regional anesthesia for cesarean delivery, and the drug indeed may lead to higher umbilical artery pH values in the fetus and less maternal nausea and vomiting.[81,82] Of concern, ephedrine is associated with fetal tachycardia.[83] When compared with phenylephrine for treatment of hypotension following regional analgesia in a randomized trial, ephedrine was associated with higher degrees of fetal acidosis.[82] The beta-agonist action of ephedrine may increase fetal oxygen requirements, leading to hypoxia in cases of uteroplacental insufficiency.[84] Phenylephrine corrects maternal hypotension, apparently without causing clinically significant uterine artery vasoconstriction or decreased placental perfusion even in extremely high doses.[85] Rather than causing abnormal increases in systemic vascular resistance, these doses may simply return vascular tone to normal after spinal anesthesia. It is also possible that constricting peripheral arteries may preferentially shunt blood to the uterine arteries. The parturient has decreased sensitivity to all vasopressors, and that may also protect the fetus from excessive vasoconstriction. Adrenergic agents such as methoxamine and phenylephrine cause reflex bradycardia that may be useful when a parturient is excessively tachycardic in association with hypotension, or if tachycardia associated with ephedrine would be detrimental.

Table 16-2. Epidural Analgesia: Hypotension Versus No Hypotension*

	HYPOTENSION† (N = 5)	NO HYPOTENSION (N = 20)
Umbilical artery		
pH	7.269	7.311
BE (mEq/L)	1.4	1.3
Po_2 (mm Hg)	23.6	23.2
Sao_2 (%)	48.2	50.2
Umbilical vein		
pH	7.344	7.366
BE (mEq/L)	1.8	1.5
Po_2 (mm Hg)	41	33.7
Svo_2 (%)	84.6	72

BE, base excess.

*Values are means; they indicate that properly treated hypotension need not result in a compromised fetus.

†Hypotension was severe enough to be treated with the vasopressor ephedrine.

Modified from James FM III, Crawford JS, Hopkinson R, et al: A comparison of general anesthesia and lumbar epidural analgesia for elective cesarean section. Anesth Analg 56:228, 1977.

Local Anesthetic Toxicity

The incidence of systemic local anesthetic toxicity (high blood concentrations of local anesthetic) after lumbar epidural analgesia is 0.01 percent.[86] However, convulsions due to local anesthetic toxicity were the most common damaging events during regional anesthesia in obstetric patients in the American Society of Anesthesiologists (ASA) Closed Claims Project database, with 85 percent associated with epidural anesthesia. In 75 percent of these cases, neurologic injury or death to the mother, newborn, or both occurred.[87] Maternal mortality data also show that local anesthetic toxicity is the most common cause of death resulting from regional anesthesia during cesarean delivery.[88] Most often, toxicity occurs when the local anesthetic is injected into a vessel rather than into the epidural space or when too much is administered even though injected properly. These reactions can also occur during placement of pudendal or paracervical blocks. All local anesthetics have maximal recommended doses, and these should not be exceeded. For example, the maximum recommended dose of lidocaine is 4 mg/kg when used without epinephrine and 7 mg/kg when used with epinephrine. Epinephrine delays and decreases the uptake of local anesthetic into the blood stream. Package inserts for all local anesthetics contain appropriate dosing information (Table 16-3).

Local anesthetic reactions have two components, central nervous system (CNS) and cardiovascular. Usually, the CNS component precedes the cardiovascular component. Prodromal symptoms of the CNS reaction include

Table 16-3. Maximal Recommended Doses of Common Local Anesthetics

	WITH EPINEPHRINE*		WITHOUT EPINEPHRINE	
LOCAL ANESTHETIC	MG/KG	DOSE (MG/70 KG)	MG/KG	TOTAL (MG/70 KG)
Bupivacaine	2.5	175	3.0	1,225
Chloroprocaine	11.0	800	14.0	1,000
Etidocaine	4.0	300	5.5	1,400
Lidocaine	4.0	300	7.0	1,500
Mepivacaine	5.0	400	—	—
Tetracaine	1.5	100	—	—

*All epinephrine concentrations 1:200,000.

Table 16-4. Blood Gas Determinations During and After Local Anesthetic–Induced Convulsions

			BLOOD-GAS VALUES				
CONVULSION	TIME	OXYGEN	pH	P_{CO_2} (mm Hg)	P_{O_2} (mm Hg)	HCO_3 (mEq/L)	BASE EXCESS (mEq/L)
Patient 1							
1st	19:50:00	10*	—	—	—	—	—
2nd	9:50:30		7.27	48	48	21.5	−14.2
3rd	9:51:00			—	—	—	—
4th	9:53:00		7.09	59	33	17.1	−10.2
Cessation	9:54:00		—	—	—	—	
	9:55:30	6†	7.01	71	210	17.2	−11.2
	10:22:00	Room air	7.25	48	99	20.5	−5.2
			7.56	25	106	22.5	−10.2
Patient 2							
1st	19:47:00	—	—	—	—	—	—
2nd	9:47:30		6.99	76	87	17.4	−10.2
3rd	9:48:00		—	—	—	—	—
Cessation	9:50:00		—	—	—	—	—
	10:02:00	10*	7.16	54	140	18.5	−6.9

*Bag and mask with oral Guedel airway and artificial respiration.
†Nasal prongs.
Modified from Moore DC, Crawford RD, Scurlock JE: Severe hypoxia and acidosis following local anesthetic-induced convulsions. Anesthesiology 53:259, 1980.

excitation, bizarre behavior, ringing in the ears, and disorientation. These symptoms may culminate in convulsions, which are usually brief. After the convulsions, depression follows, manifested by the postictal state. The cardiovascular component of the local anesthetic reaction usually begins with hypertension and tachycardia but is soon followed by hypotension, arrhythmias, and in some instances, cardiac arrest. Thus, the cardiovascular component also has excitant and depressant characteristics. One frequently sees the CNS component without the more serious cardiovascular component. Bupivacaine may represent an exception to this principle.[89,90] Resuscitation of patients who receive an intravascular injection of bupivacaine is extremely challenging, likely owing to the prolonged blocking effect on sodium channels.[91] Laboratory evidence supports bupivacaine's increased cardiotoxicity over equianalgesic doses of other amide local anesthetics such as ropivacaine and lidocaine.[92–94] The manufacturers of bupivacaine have recommended that the 0.75-percent concentration not be used in obstetric patients or for paracervical block.[95] However, use of a more dilute concentration does not guarantee safety; bupivacaine and all local anesthetics should be administered by slow, incremental injection.[96] Local anesthetic toxicity has also decreased, with greater emphasis on use of a test dose, typically containing 15 µg of epinephrine to exclude unintentional intravenous or subarachnoid catheter placement.[97,98] Others have questioned the lack of specificity of test doses during labor and the potential harm to the fetus or hypertensive mother.[99] Intravascular injection of 15 µg epinephrine produces maternal tachycardia, which may be difficult to differentiate from that seen during a contraction. Nonreassuring fetal heart tones due to decreased uterine blood flow may also occur after intravascular epinephrine.

Treatment of a local anesthetic reaction depends on recognizing the signs and symptoms. Prodromal symptoms should trigger the immediate cessation of the injection of local anesthetic. If convulsions have already occurred, treatment is aimed at maintaining proper oxygenation and preventing the patient from harming herself. Convulsions use considerable amounts of oxygen, which results in hypoxia and acidosis (Table 16-4).[100] Should the convulsions continue for more than a brief period, small intravenous doses of thiopental (25 to 50 mg) or a benzodiazepine (2 to 5 mg midazolam) are useful. The depressant effects of these agents add to the depressant phase of the local anesthetic reaction; therefore, appropriate equipment and personnel must be available to maintain oxygenation, a patent airway, and cardiovascular support. Rarely, succinylcholine is needed for paralysis to prevent the muscular activity and to facilitate ventilation and perhaps intubation. In cases of complete cardiac collapse, delivery of the infant may facilitate maternal resuscitation. The American Heart Association has stated: "Several authors now recommend that the decision to perform a peri-mortem cesarean section should be made rapidly, with delivery effected within 4 to 5 minutes of the arrest."[101]

Allergy to Local Anesthetics

There are two classes of local anesthetics: amides and esters. A true allergic reaction to an amide-type local anesthetic (e.g., lidocaine, bupivacaine, ropivacaine) is extremely rare. Allergic reactions to the esters (2-chloroprocaine, procaine, tetracaine) are also uncommon but can occur. They are often associated with a reaction to para amino benzoic acid (PABA) in skin creams or suntan lotions. When a patient reports that she is "allergic" to local anesthetics, she is frequently referring to a normal reaction to the epinephrine that is occasionally added to local anesthetics, particularly by dentists. Epinephrine can cause increased heart rate, pounding in the ears, and nausea, symptoms that may be interpreted as an allergy. Therefore, it is important to document the specific agents and clinical symptoms with any history of allergy. If a specific local anesthetic can be identified, choosing one from the other class should be safe, or meperidine can be used as an alternative to local anesthetics in the subarachnoid space.[102]

HIGH SPINAL OR "TOTAL SPINAL" ANESTHESIA

This complication occurs when the level of anesthesia rises dangerously high, resulting in paralysis of the respiratory muscles, including the diaphragm (C3-C5). The incidence of total spinal anesthesia after epidural anesthesia is less than 0.03 percent and after spinal anesthesia is 0.2 percent.[86,103] Total spinal anesthesia can result from a miscalculated dose of drug, unintentional subarachnoid injection during an epidural block, or improper positioning of a patient after spinal block with hyperbaric local anesthetic solutions. The accessory muscles of respiration are paralyzed earlier, and their paralysis may result in apprehension and anxiety and a feeling of dyspnea. The patient usually can breathe adequately as long as the diaphragm is not paralyzed, but treatment must be individualized. Dyspnea, real or imagined, should always be considered an effect of paralysis until proved otherwise. Cardiovascular effects, including hypotension and even cardiovascular collapse, may accompany total spinal anesthesia.

Treatment of total spinal anesthesia includes rapidly assessing the true level of anesthesia. Therefore, individuals who administer major regional anesthesia should be thoroughly familiar with dermatome charts (Fig. 16-8) and should also be able to recognize what a certain sensory level of anesthesia means with regard to innervation of other organs or systems. For example, a T4 sensory level may represent total sympathetic nervous system blockade. Numbness and weakness of the fingers and hands indicates that the level of anesthesia has reached the cervical level (C6 to C8), which is dangerously close to the innervation of the diaphragm. If the diaphragm is not paralyzed, the patient is breathing adequately, and cardiovascular stability is maintained, administration of oxygen and reassurance may suffice. If the patient remains

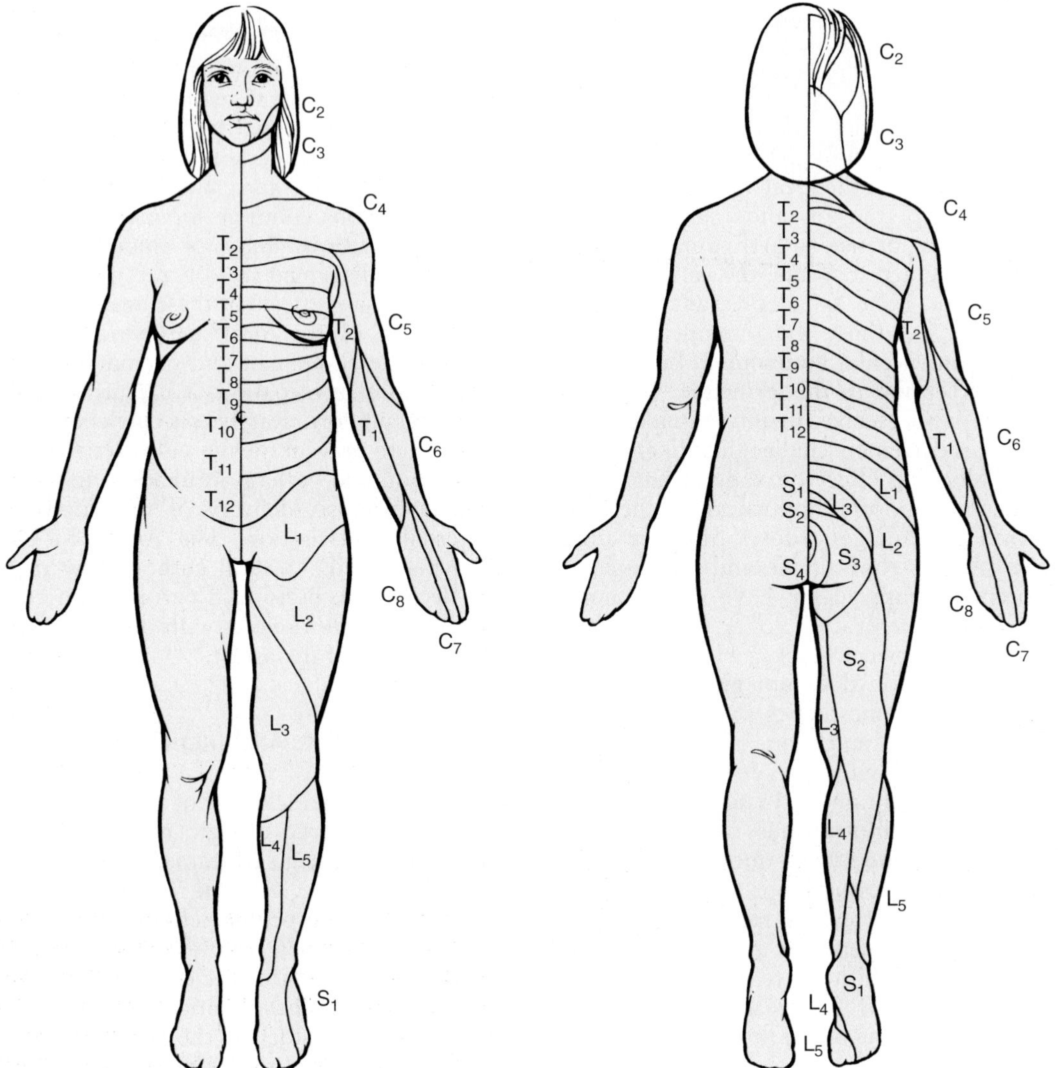

Figure 16-8. Dermatome chart. (Adapted from Haymaker L, Woodhall B: Peripheral Nerve Injuries. Philadelphia, WB Saunders Company, 1945.)

anxious or if the level of anesthesia seems to be involving the diaphragm, then assisted ventilation is indicated and endotracheal intubation will be necessary to protect the airway. Induction of general anesthesia will facilitate the process. Cardiovascular support is provided as necessary. With prompt and adequate treatment, serious sequelae should be extremely rare.

Paralysis and Nerve Injury

Paralysis after either epidural or spinal anesthesia is extremely rare; even minor injuries such as foot-drop and segmental loss of sensation are uncommon. Nerve injury occurs in 0.06 percent of spinal anesthetics and 0.02 percent of epidural anesthetics.[86] With commercially prepared drugs, ampules, and disposable needles, infection and caustic injury rarely occur. In the past, there were case reports of neurologic deficit after use of 2-chloroprocaine, primarily after unintentional subarachnoid (i.e., spinal) injection of large volumes of the drug.[104] The consensus is that 2-chloroprocaine itself is not neurotoxic, but that the combination of low pH of the local anesthetic solution with the sodium bisulfite preservative found in earlier formulations may produce neurologic dysfunction.[105] The current formulation does not contain preservatives, and is even being investigated as a possible short-acting spinal anesthetic agent.[106]

When nerve damage follows regional analgesia during obstetric or surgical procedures, the anesthetic technique must be suspected, although causation is rare.[107] Other potential etiologies include incorrectly positioned stirrups, difficult forceps applications, or abnormal fetal presentations.[108] During abdominal procedures, overzealous or prolonged application of pressure with retractors on sensitive nerve tissues may also result in injury. Fortunately, most neurologic deficits after labor and delivery are minor and transient[109]; however, consultation with a neurologist or neurosurgeon should be considered.

One of the more dramatic and correctable forms of nerve damage follows compression of the spinal cord by a hematoma that has formed during the administration of spinal or epidural anesthesia, presumably from accidental puncture of an epidural vessel. If the condition is diagnosed early, usually with the aid of a neurologist or neurosurgeon, the hematoma can be removed by laminectomy and the problem resolved without permanent damage. Fortunately, this is a rare complication. Nonetheless, spinal and epidural blocks are contraindicated if the patient has a coagulopathy, if the patient is pharmacologically anticoagulated, or if the platelet count is less than 75,000 μl. Hemolysis, elevated liver enzymes and low platelets (HELLP) syndrome may be a particularly strong risk factor because of multifactorial sources for coagulation defects.[110] Any significant motor or sensory deficit after regional anesthesia should be investigated immediately and thoroughly.

Spinal Headache

Spinal headache may follow uncomplicated spinal anesthesia, but it is far more common when, during the process of administering an epidural block, the dura is punctured and spinal fluid leaks out (i.e., "wet tap"). The incidence of this complication varies between 1 and 3 percent, and its occurrence depends an the experience of the person performing the epidural block.[111] Once a wet tap occurs, a spinal headache results in as many as 70 percent of patients. The incidence is much less following spinal anesthesia, because smaller atraumatic (pencil-point) needles are used. Characteristically, a spinal headache is more severe in the upright position and is relieved by the supine position. A differential diagnosis should include migraine, pneumocephalus from the loss of resistance to air technique, infection, cortical vein thrombosis, preeclampsia, and intracerebral or subarachnoid hemorrhage. A spinal headache is thought to be caused by loss of cerebrospinal fluid, which allows the brain to settle and thus meninges and vessels to stretch. Hydration, bedrest, abdominal binders, and the prone position have all been advocated as prophylactic measures after known dural puncture. However, most anesthesiologists now agree that these actions are of little value.[111]

When a patient develops a postdural puncture headache (PDPH), she should be counseled about the cause and potential treatment options, which range from conservative to aggressive. If the headache is mild and interferes minimally with activity, treatment may be initiated with oral analgesics and caffeine or theophylline, which are cerebral vasoconstrictors that may provide symptomatic relief.[112] If simple measures prove ineffective, an epidural blood patch should be considered. Approximately 20 ml of the patient's own blood is placed aseptically into the epidural space; providing a tamponade effect that may result in immediate relief. It may also coagulate over the hole and prevent further cerebrospinal fluid leakage.[113] Patients can be released within 1 to 2 hours.[114] Patients should be instructed to avoid coughing or straining for the first several days after insertion of the blood patch. The epidural blood patch has been found to be remarkably effective and nearly complication free, despite the fact that it is an iatrogenic epidural hematoma.[115–117] Prophylactic epidural blood patches inserted through the epidural catheter immediately after delivery are not effective in preventing headaches.[118] A preventive measure that may be effective is passing the epidural catheter through the dural hole at the time of wet tap to provide continuous spinal anesthesia, with removal of the catheter 24 hours after delivery.[119] Injecting preservative-free saline through the catheter before removing the spinal catheter may also decrease the incidence of headache, although these data are preliminary.[120]

Back Pain

Back pain is a common peripartum complaint, and a common concern for women considering regional anesthesia for their delivery. An antepartum survey of pregnant patients, before their delivery or any use of regional anesthesia, found that 69 percent of patients reported back pain, 58 percent reported sleep disturbances due to back pain, 57 percent said it impaired activities of daily living, and 30 percent had stopped at least one daily activity because of pain.[121] Only 32 percent informed their obstetric providers they had back pain, and only 25 percent of those providers recommended treatment. Despite concerns that using regional anesthesia contributes to back pain, postpartum surveys indicate that the incidence of back pain after childbirth is the same whether women had regional analgesia for their delivery or not; approximately 40 to 50 percent at 2 and 6 months postpartum.[122,123]

Breast-Feeding Issues

Some patients and providers are concerned that regional analgesia may hinder the newborn's ability to breastfeed effectively.[124] Observational studies showing an association between difficult breast-feeding and anesthetic use during labor do not account for obstetric events such as prolonged labor or operative delivery, factors that can cause difficulty with early breast-feeding. Local anesthetic agents, opioids, and barbiturates are distributed to the fetus and could theoretically reduce the newborn's ability to breast-feed.[125,126] There are no randomized trials comparing breastfeeding outcomes in patients who received epidural analgesia or no medication. However, two prospective cohort studies have found no difference in the number of women successfully breastfeeding at 1, 4, and 6 weeks after delivery, whether or not they used epidural analgesia during labor.[127,128] Not surprisingly, women treated with epidural analgesia for postoperative pain control after cesarean delivery are more successful at breast-feeding than those treated with systemic opioids.[129] Infants of women treated with intravenous PCA after cesarean delivery were less alert and had more neonatal neurobehavioral depression after meperidine than after morphine, probably due to meperidine's active metabolites.[44] Other factors contributing to successful breast-feeding include lactation consultation services, maternal motivation, and support from obstetricians and pediatricians.

Effects on Labor and Method of Delivery

Significant controversy surrounds how to appropriately counsel patients regarding the effect of regional analgesia on their labor course, incidence of malposition, need for instrument-assisted vaginal delivery, and risk of cesarean delivery.

Study Design

Multiple prospective randomized studies of epidural analgesia have been performed both in nulliparous populations and in mixed populations. However, the poor quality of analgesia provided by systemic opioids typically leads to high rates of crossover of control patients into the epidural analgesia arm. Neither intent-to-treat analysis nor actual-use analysis are entirely satisfactory in this situation. Studies with the lowest crossover rates have accomplished their goal through the use of substantial doses of parenteral opioids, resulting in higher than expected rates of neonatal resuscitation in the opioid groups.[39,43] Nonrandomized studies provide interesting observational data; however, careful analysis of potential confounders is critical, because patients who self-select epidural analgesia are clearly different from patients who avoid it. Furthermore, with declining rates of operative vaginal delivery and increasing rates of cesarean delivery, up-to-date studies are needed to examine these outcomes. Of concern, randomized studies are often conducted in academic centers where operative delivery rates in low-risk patients may be significantly lower than in community hospitals. Finally, regional analgesia techniques vary and modifications in technique occur continuously. More modern techniques use lower concentrations of local anesthetic and titrate the dose to the specific needs of the patient, potentially lowering the risk of operative delivery. Despite these limitations, the published literature offers considerable insight regarding the effects of regional analgesia on the progress of labor and method of delivery.

Progress Of Labor

Randomized studies support the conclusion that epidural analgesia results in a modest prolongation of both the first and second stages of labor; not surprisingly, these effects are most pronounced in nulliparous patients. Similarly, epidural analgesia is associated with a significant increase in the use of oxytocin for labor augmentation; the relative risk (RR) of oxytocin treatment after initiation of epidural analgesia varies considerably depending on obstetric practice such as rates of induction and active management of labor. Despite aggressive use of oxytocin, it appears that an effect on the length of active labor persists. A meta-analysis evaluated data from 2,703 nulliparous patients randomized to epidural analgesia or parenteral opioids in five trials from a single institution (1993–2000).[130] Of note, 22 percent of patients were not compliant with their assigned method of analgesia; statistically, this would tend to bias results toward the null hypothesis and reduce the magnitude of the effect of epidural analgesia. Additionally, the concentration of bupivacaine given through epidural infusion decreased from 0.125 percent to 0.0625 percent over the 7-year inclusion period. Using an intent-to-treat analysis, the average duration of labor from initiation of analgesia to complete cervical dilation was approximately 36 minutes longer in patients randomized to receive epidural analgesia, despite a significantly increased rate of oxytocin use in the epidural analgesia group. The average second stage of labor was 13 minutes longer in nulliparas with epidural analgesia ($p < 0.001$). More important, these studies incorporated either discontinuing or decreasing the rate of epidural infusion in the second stage and a significantly higher rate of operative vaginal deliveries in the epidural groups that likely shortened the average duration of the second stage. In a subanalysis including only protocol-compliant women ($n = 2,116$), the effects of epidural analgesia were more pronounced: a 90-minute prolongation in the average duration of the first stage of labor and a 38-percent increase in the duration of the second stage (17 minutes). A recent multicenter randomized trial of patient-controlled epidural analgesia (PCEA) versus patient-controlled intravenous opioids (PCIA) also found a 23-minute prolongation in the duration of the second stage, despite a relatively high crossover rate and a practice of allowing the fetal head to descend to the perineum before encouraging maternal expulsive efforts.[131]

Both the timing and technique of regional analgesia have the potential to affect the length of labor. Vahratian et al.[132] analyzed nulliparous labor curves from Tripler Army Medical Center in the year before (n = 223) and after (n = 278) regional analgesia became widely available in that hospital. The rate of epidural analgesia use rose precipitously from 2 to 92 percent in nulliparas admitted at or before 4-cm cervical dilation. Introduction of epidural analgesia was associated with an increase in the median duration of the first stage of labor by 48 minutes. After multivariate analysis was performed to adjust for the upward trends in maternal age and body mass index (BMI), the majority of this delay was attributed to slower cervical change between 4 and 5 cm dilation. Alexander et al.[133] also reported slower cervical change over time in women randomized to receive epidural analgesia, but this study was designed to detect overall changes in linear rates of cervical change rather than more complicated patterns. Patients randomized to PCEA versus intermittent bolus epidural analgesia had a similar duration of the first stage but a longer average second stage of labor (70 versus 54 minutes, $p < 0.05$).[134] This 16-minute increase in second-stage duration may have been secondary to increased sensory or motor block in PCEA patients who received higher total doses of bupivacaine (45.2 mg versus 33.4 mg, $p < 0.001$). Pain scores were significantly lower in the PCEA group at full cervical dilatation, but there was no difference in motor block as measured by Bromage scale.

Wong et al.[76] randomized patients requesting pain medication at a cervical dilation of <4 cm to receive 25 mcg intrathecal fentanyl or parenteral hydromorphone. Both groups of patients were eventually treated with PCEA (0.0625 percent bupivacaine with 2 ug/ml of fentanyl); roughly 60 percent of patients in each group were dilated 4 or more cm at the time epidural infusion was initiated, and there was no difference in the duration of epidural analgesia between the two groups. As expected, patients randomized to intrathecal opioids in early labor had less emesis and better pain control compared with patients in the parenteral opioids group. Of greater interest was the significantly shorter interval between initiation of analgesia and complete cervical dilation in the intrathecal opioid group (90 minutes median difference, $p < 0.001$). Although it is tempting to conclude that intrathecal opioids speed early labor, these results may have been partly due to the higher proportion of patients in the parenteral opioid group with a cervical dilation of ≤1.5 cm (42 versus 31 percent, $p = 0.007$) at randomization. Regardless, it is reassuring that intrathecal fentanyl was not associated with slower cervical dilation or prolonged labor in this study. Therefore, early intrathecal opioids followed by continuous epidural infusion in active labor may be a good option for women desiring regional analgesia, offering superior pain control until active labor has been achieved.

Fetal Position at Delivery

One possible mechanism by which epidural analgesia could increase the length of the second stage is by increasing the incidence of fetal malposition: occiput posterior (OP) or occiput transverse. Few randomized studies have specifically addressed this issue in nulliparous patients. Two randomized studies with crossover rates of 20 to 30 percent (underestimating the possible effect of epidural analgesia) reported an increased relative risk of malpresentation of 1.1 to 1.3, but in both cases, the 95-percent confidence interval crossed unity.[135,136] One small randomized trial with a low rate of crossover reported a relative risk of 4.2 (1.0;18.5) for OP position.[137] In contrast, Yancey et al.[138] noted a steady rate of OP position (6.0 versus 5.7 percent) before and after the introduction of widely available epidural analgesia. More recently, Lieberman et al. followed a prospective cohort of 1,562 nulliparous women with serial ultrasound examinations to assess fetal position: at enrollment, at request for epidural analgesia or 4 hours after admission, at greater than 8-cm cervical dilation, and at delivery.[139] Women requesting epidural analgesia were not more likely to have a fetus in OP position at enrollment (23.4 verusus 26 percent, $p = 0.9$) and OP position was not associated with increased complaints of "back labor." Epidural analgesia was associated with an increased likelihood of OP position at delivery (RR 4.0, 95-percent CI 1.4 to 11.1) after controlling for other risk factors. Of interest, 69 percent of infants born in the OP position were not OP at enrollment. This suggests two potential mechanisms, failure to convert away from OP position as well as de novo conversion. Surprisingly, malposition was not associated with an increased risk of operative vaginal delivery in this study (17.5 percent OA (occiput anterior), 17.9 percent OP, 12.7 percent occiput transverse, $p = 0.4$), which may be due to decreasing obstetric comfort with difficult operative vaginal deliveries and increasing reliance on cesarean delivery.

Operative Vaginal Delivery Rate and Perineal Injury

Any analysis of the relationship between regional analgesia and instrument-assisted vaginal delivery is complicated by the strong influence of obstetric practice and the obstetrician's attitude towards operative vaginal delivery. Despite restricting this discussion to studies prohibiting elective procedures, indications vary widely and include: nonreassuring fetal status, inadequate maternal effort, and prolonged second stage. Meta-analyses of randomized controlled trials consistently confirm that epidural analgesia is associated with a significant increased risk (RR of 1.9 to 2.1) of nonelective instrument-assisted vaginal delivery.[130,140] This increased risk may be due to the association between epidural analgesia and OP position, longer second stage, and less effective expulsive efforts. Therefore, obstetricians may be more likely to perform elective instrument-assisted delivery in patients with effective anesthesia. However, compiled data suggest that instrument-assisted vaginal delivery, especially forceps delivery, is associated with a significantly increased risk of third- or fourth-degree perineal laceration in both nulliparous and multiparous patients,[141] which, in turn, places affected women at increased risk of fecal incontinence.[142] The association between epidural analgesia and increased rates of instrument-assisted delivery, combined with the increased risk of perineal injury associated with instrument-assisted deliveries, provides an explanation for studies demonstrating an increased risk of perineal injury in women with epidural analgesia.[143]

Potential strategies for decreasing the risk of instrument-assisted delivery include reduced density of epidural analgesia during the second stage, delayed pushing, and avoiding arbitrary definitions of a prolonged second stage, provided that consistent progress is observed. However, the evidence for these strategies is conflicting. One study examining delayed pushing reported no decrease in instrumental delivery, but rates of operative delivery and episiotomy were unacceptably high (50 percent and 70 percent), clearly demonstrating the inclusion of elective operative procedures.[144] All women in this study were evaluated for endosonographic evidence of external anal sphincter damage, and forceps delivery was associated with a 55 percent rate of injury. Others have reported a decrease in forceps delivery with delayed pushing, although the statistical significance was borderline ($p = 0.06$).[145] Multiple studies have suggested that the risk of anal sphincter injury is increased after median episiotomy; therefore, if operative vaginal delivery must be performed, routine episiotomy should be avoided.[146,147]

Cesarean Delivery Rate

Several well-designed randomized studies suggest that, in settings with baseline low rates of cesarean delivery, epidural analgesia does not increase the risk of cesarean delivery.[39,43] Similarly, Zhang et al.[148] compared rates of cesarean delivery in more than 1,000 nulliparous patients before and after on-demand labor epidural analgesia became available in their hospital. Despite an increase from less than 1 percent to 84 percent in labor epidural analgesia use, the rate of cesarean delivery did not increase (14.4 versus 12.2 percent). However, given the evidence that epidural analgesia may slow labor and increase the risk of malposition, it is appropriate to remain concerned regarding the possible effects of epidural analgesia in practices with higher rates of cesarean delivery. In the aforementioned studies, the rate of primary cesarean delivery ranged from 7 to 14.4 percent, far below the national cesarean rate of 17.9 percent in nulliparas during the same time period.[149] This discrepancy may be due, in part, to the significantly younger age distribution and higher rates of rapid delivery described in many of the randomized trials. In low-risk patients, provider practice patterns significantly influence cesarean delivery rates.[150] Therefore, in a given population, the risk of cesarean delivery may vary depending on epidural analgesia technique, patient population, obstetric management, protocols for oxytocin augmentation, obstetric and patient attitudes toward cesarean delivery, provider comfort with instrument-assisted vaginal delivery, and other risk factors.

The debate regarding the ideal timing of epidural analgesia will likely fade with the increasing popularity of combined spinal-epidural techniques. In the randomized study described earlier, Wong et al. convincingly demonstrated that the pain of latent labor is more effectively managed with pure intrathecal opioids followed by CSE compared with parenteral opioids followed by epidural analgesia after 4-cm cervical dilation, without an increased rate of cesarean delivery in the early CSE group (17.8 percent vs. 20.7 percent, $p = 0.31$).[75] In settings in which CSE is unavailable, the timing of traditional epidural analgesia administration remains controversial. Chestnut et al.[151,152] reported no increased risk of cesarean delivery with early versus late epidural analgesia, in nulliparous women in spontaneous labor and also in women undergoing oxytocin induction of labor. However, when analyzed by intent to treat, the absolute difference in cervical dilation at randomization was slight (4 cm versus 5 cm), significantly decreasing the power of the studies to detect a difference in cesarean delivery rates. In contrast, Thorp et al.[137] suggested that epidural analgesia's detrimental effect on labor progression occurs largely before 5 cm cervical dilation. This finding is consistent with the report by Vahratian et al., described earlier, that epidural analgesia's detrimental effect on labor progression occurs largely between 4 and 5 cm of dilation. Therefore, it remains possible that early administration of epidural local anesthetic solutions could significantly slow labor and contribute to an increased risk of cesarean delivery. One study also suggested that patients randomized to PCEA are exposed to higher total local anesthesia doses and are more likely to deliver by cesarean than patients receiving standard intermittent bolus epidural analgesia (16.3 percent versus 6.7 percent, $p < 0.05$).[134] Management of epidural analgesia and timing of administration should be individualized to the patient's needs and level of pain. Attention should be focused on minimizing local anesthetic concentrations while still providing adequate pain control and on avoiding routine administration of epidural analgesia in latent labor.

Fever

Epidural analgesia during labor is associated with an increase in maternal temperature, but the risk of fever is strongly dependent on the duration of exposure.[153] Therefore, the majority of the risk is confined to nulliparous patients. In a well-designed study with a low crossover rate (6 percent), Sharma et al. reported a 33 percent rate of intrapartum fever greater than 37.5°C in nulliparous patients randomized to epidural analgesia, compared with 7 percent in those receiving parenteral opioids.[130] This more than fourfold increased risk of fever occurred despite relatively minor prolongations in the mean duration of labor (50 minutes). Multiparous women deliver shortly after the onset of active labor, resulting in a short duration of exposure to epidural analgesia, and are not at significantly increased risk for fever (3 versus 2 percent).[154] Similarly, Yancey et al.[155] described an 18-fold increase in the rate of intrapartum fever in nulliparous patients (from 0.6 percent to 11 percent) in a single year following the introduction of an epidural analgesia service in their hospital.

The etiology of this febrile response is not well understood; possible mechanisms include noninfectious inflammatory activation, changes in thermoregulation, and acquired intrapartum infection. Intrapartum fever after epidural analgesia is associated with increased serum levels of inflammatory cytokines in the mother and fetus.[156] In addition, one study suggested that placental inflammation is more common with epidural analgesia (61 versus

36 percent), but this study was limited by the high rate of chorioamnionitis that was documented on pathologic examination, even in the absence of maternal fever (36 percent).[157] Although infants of women randomized to epidural analgesia have a 1.5-fold increase (95-percent CI 1.1 to 2.0) in neonatal sepsis evaluations, no increased risk of documented sepsis has been reported.[154,158] Despite the lack of infectious morbidity, intrapartum exposure to hyperthermia may not be benign for the neonate. Animal study indicates that the presence of hyperthermia during an ischemic event increases susceptibility to hypoxic-ischemic insult.[159] Impey et al.[160] reported a 10-fold higher risk of neonatal encephalopathy in term infants exposed to intrapartum fever, defined as an oral temperature greater than 37.5°C (OR 10.8, 95-percent CI 4.0 to 29.3). The absolute risk of encephalopathy in neonates born to febrile mothers was 2.1 percent. Finally, although the absolute risk is low, maternal temperature greater than 38°C is associated with 9.3-fold increased risk of cerebral palsy in term infants (95-percent CI 2.7 to 31).[161] Acetaminophen, the standard therapy used to ameliorate hyperthermia, is not effective in preventing fever secondary to epidural analgesia.[162]

Paracervical Block

Paracervical block analgesia is a simple and effective procedure when performed properly (see Table 16-1). Commonly, 5 to 6 ml of a dilute solution of local anesthetic without epinephrine (e.g., 1 percent lidocaine or 1 or 2 percent 2-chloroprocaine) is injected into the mucosa of the cervix at the 3- and 9-o'clock positions (Fig. 16-9). The duration of analgesia depends on the local anesthetic used. This technique has fallen out of favor owing to its association with the fetal bradycardia that follows in 2 to 70 percent of applications. Occurring within 2 to 10 minutes and persisting from 3 to 30 minutes, these bradycardias are usually benign. However cases of fetal acidosis and death have been reported.[163] A significant fall in pH and a rise in base deficit occur only in those fetuses with bradycardia persisting more than 10 minutes.[164] Paracervical block should be used cautiously at all times and should not be used at all in mothers with fetuses in either acute or chronic distress.

There is no consensus regarding the mechanism of post-paracervical block bradycardia. High fetal blood concentrations of local anesthetic could occur if local anesthetic injected close to the uterine artery passed to the fetus. This theory is consistent with the finding that infants who suffer bradycardia frequently have higher local anesthetic concentrations than their mothers.[163] Alternatively, bradycardia may result from uterine artery vasoconstriction secondary to a direct effect of the local anesthetic on the uterine artery (Fig. 16-10).[165,166] The fetal electrocardiogram (ECG) pattern during one of these episodes suggests hypoxia, a finding that supports the uterine artery vasoconstriction theory.[164] Furthermore, the high concentrations of local anesthetic required to produce vasoconstriction during the administration of a paracervical block can be achieved close to the uterine artery (see Fig. 16-10). A third theory is based on the possibility that local anesthetic injected directly into the uterine musculature increases uterine tone.

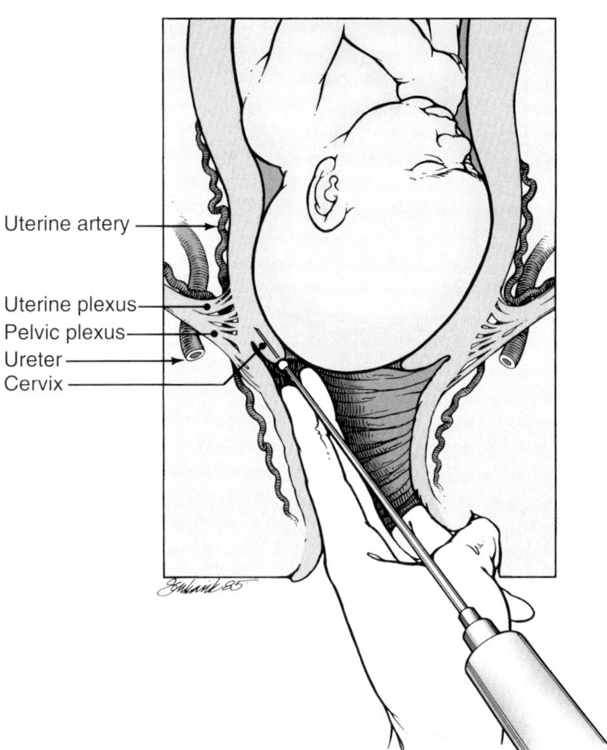

Figure 16-9. Technique of paracervical block. Schematic coronal section (enlarged) of lower portion of cervix and upper portion of vagina shows relation of needle to paracervical region. (Modified from Bonica JJ: Principles and Practice of Obstetric Analgesia and Anesthesia. Philadelphia, FA Davis, 1967, p 234.)

Sterile Water Injection

A novel way to provide relief of severe lower back pain during the first stage of labor involves subcutaneous or intracutaneous injection of sterile water at four points on the lower back.[26,167] In a randomized controlled trial, the median reductions in the visual analog pain scores were 4 to 5 compared with 1 in the placebo group.

ANESTHESIA FOR VAGINAL DELIVERY

The goal of pain relief for vaginal delivery is to match the patient's wishes with the requirements of the delivery without subjecting either mother or fetus to unnecessary risk.

Local Anesthesia

In the form of perineal infiltration, local anesthesia is widely used and very safe. Spontaneous vaginal delivery, episiotomy, and perhaps outlet vacuum deliveries can be accomplished with this simple technique. Local anesthetic toxicity may occur if large amounts of local anesthetic are

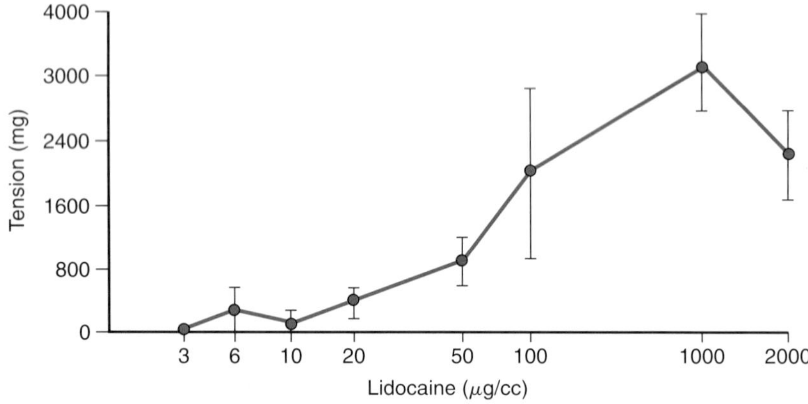

Figure 16-10. Dose-response curve of the pregnant human uterine artery to lidocaine hydrochloride (mean ± SEM; *N* = 9). (From Gibbs CP, Noel SC: Response of arterial segments from gravid human uterus to multiple concentrations of lignocaine. Br J Anaesth 45:409, 1977, with permission.)

Table 16-5. Lidocaine Concentrations at Delivery in Maternal Plasma and Umbilical Cord Vein After Perineal Infiltration

	CONCENTRATION (NG/mL)	
SAMPLE (N = 15)	MEAN ± SD	RANGE
Maternal plasma		
Peak concentration	648 ± 666	60–2,400
At delivery	548 ± 468	33–1,474
Umbilical cord vein	420 ± 406	45–1,380
Fetal/maternal ratio*	1.32 ± 1.46	0.05–4.66

SD, standard deviation.

*Ratio of level in cord vein to level in maternal vein at delivery (mean of individual ratios, not ratio of means).

From Philipson EH, Kuhnert BR, Syracuse CD: Maternal, fetal, and neonatal lidocaine levels following local perineal infiltration. Am J Obstet Gynecol 149:403, 1984, with permission.

used or if an inadvertent intravascular injection occurs. Usually, 5 to 15 ml of 1-percent lidocaine suffices. There is rapid and significant transfer of lidocaine to the fetus after perineal infiltration.[168] In 5 of 15 infants, the concentration of lidocaine at delivery was greater in the umbilical vein than in the mother (Table 16-5).

Pudendal Nerve Block

Pudendal nerve block is a minor regional block that also is reasonably effective and very safe. The obstetrician, using an Iowa trumpet and a 20-gauge needle, injects 5 to 10 ml of local anesthetic just below the ischial spine. Because the hemorrhoidal nerve may be aberrant in 50 percent of patients,[169] some physicians prefer to inject a portion of the local anesthetic somewhat posterior to the spine (Fig. 16-11). Although a transperineal approach to the ischial spine is possible, most prefer the transvaginal approach. One-percent lidocaine or 2-percent 2-chloroprocaine can be used.

Pudendal block is generally satisfactory for all spontaneous vaginal deliveries and episiotomies, and for some outlet or low operative vaginal deliveries, but it may not be sufficient for deliveries requiring additional manipulation. The potential for local anesthetic toxicity is higher with pudendal block compared with perineal infiltration because of large vessels proximal to the injection site (see Fig. 16-11). Therefore, aspiration before injection is particularly important. When perineal and labial infiltration are required in addition to pudendal block, it is critically important to closely monitor the total amount of local anesthetic given.

Monitored Anesthesia Care Analgesia

For urgent or unanticipated instrumental deliveries, an anesthesiologist or nurse anesthetist may administer inhalation or intravenous analgesia while still maintaining protective laryngeal and cough reflexes. The obstetrician should add local infiltration or a pudendal block. The combined effects are additive and satisfactory for most operative vaginal deliveries, shoulder dystocias, and head entrapments. The anesthesiologist frequently questions the patient to determine the level of anesthesia and to ensure that deeper planes of anesthesia are avoided. Such precautions are important because if the patient becomes unconscious, all of the hazards associated with general anesthesia are possible, including inadequate airway, hypoxia, and aspiration. Because continual assessment of the patient's state of consciousness is required and is sometimes difficult, only anesthesiologists or nurse anesthetists should administer inhalation analgesia. Furthermore, in the United States, this technique requires the use of the anesthesia machine, misuse of which can prove disastrous. Most frequently, the anesthesiologist uses 50-percent nitrous oxide or, for intravenous analgesia, ketamine, 0.25 to 0.5 mg/kg. This latter agent may be particularly effective in the labor room when an anesthesia machine is not available, or for the patient who cannot or will not tolerate an anesthetic face mask. Inhalation or intravenous analgesia renders some patients amnesic of the event, a characteristic that may be undesirable.

Spinal (Subarachnoid) Block

A saddle block is a spinal block in which the level of anesthesia is limited to little more than the perineum. Spinal anesthesia is reasonably easy to perform and usually

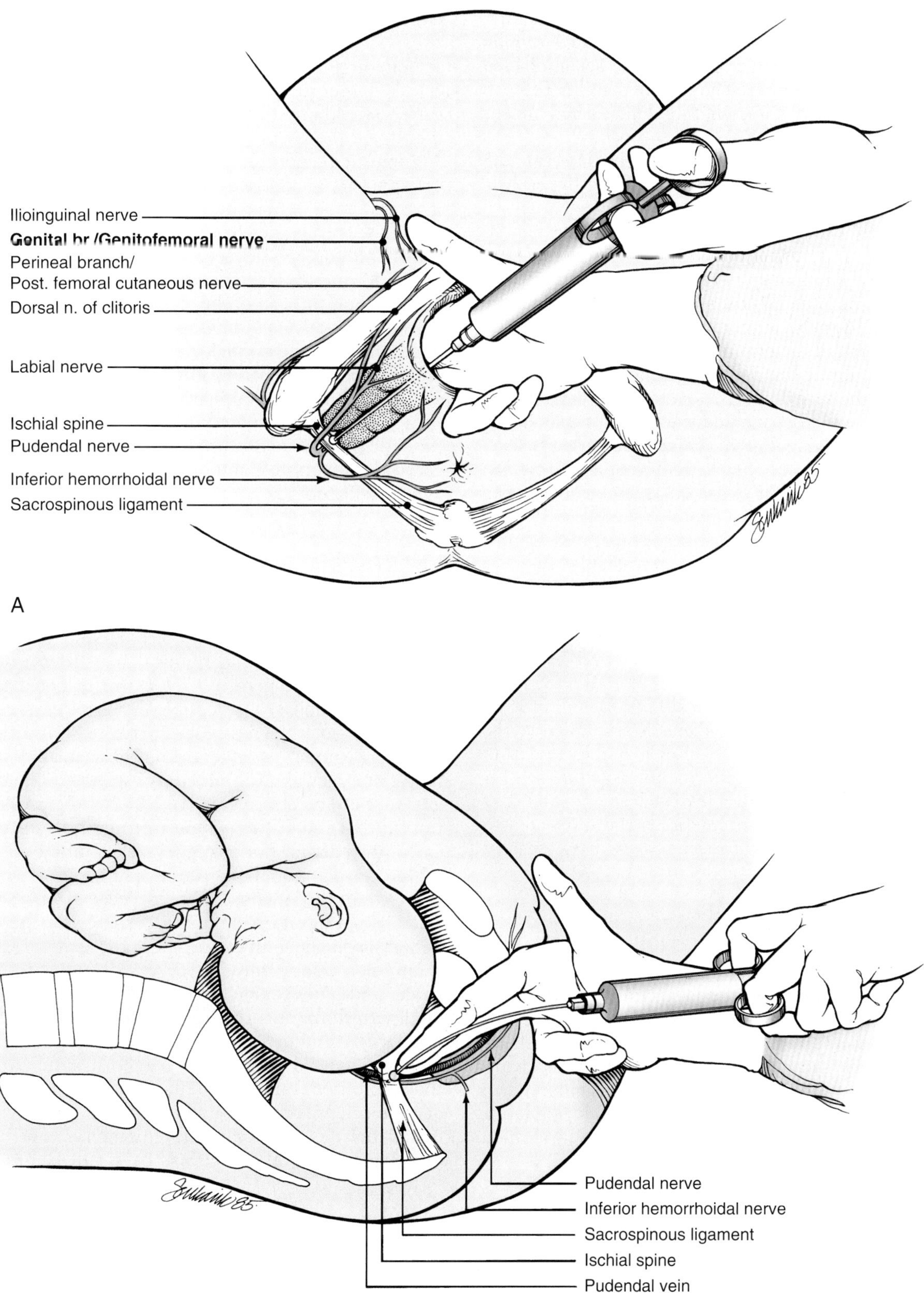

Figure 16-11. *A* and *B*, Anatomy of the pudendal nerve and techniques of pudendal block.

provides total pain relief in the blocked area. Therefore, spontaneous delivery, forceps delivery, perineal repairs and more complicated deliveries can all be accomplished without pain for the mother. The patient's ability to push may be compromised somewhat by diminished motor strength as well as significant sensory block.

Usually spinal anesthesia is achieved by injecting 25 to 50 mg hyperbaric lidocaine or 5 to 7.5 mg hyperbaric bupivacaine into the subarachnoid space through a 24- to 27-gauge spinal needle. It is preferable to use a pencil-point needle of the smallest possible gauge, because these needles reduce the risk of spinal headache. Fentanyl 10 to 25 μg may also be added to the spinal anesthetic. Because the solution is hyperbaric relative to cerebrospinal fluid, the most important determinant of anesthesia level is gravity. For example, the sitting position causes the level to fall toward the sacral nerve roots for a perineal block. Less controllable factors include the Valsalva maneuver, coughing, and straining, any of which will cause the level to rise. Injecting the local anesthetic during a contraction may result in higher than expected levels of anesthesia and should be avoided.

Persons other than anesthesiologists sometimes administer spinal anesthesia, which is technically easy to perform. In such situations, it is important to remember that all hazards associated with major blocks are possible, including hypotension and "total spinal." The person who administers spinal anesthesia must never leave the patient unattended without ensuring that another competent individual will assume responsibility for monitoring the blood pressure and level of anesthesia. Usually, the level of the spinal block will be complete and fixed within 5 to 10 minutes, but it may continue to creep upward for 20 minutes or longer. Left uterine displacement should be maintained after the local anesthetic has been injected to maintain venous return and prevent excess hypotension.

Single-Dose Caudal and Lumbar Epidural Anesthesia

Single-dose epidural anesthesia techniques are used much less frequently than in the past. The relative difficulty, slow onset, and large amounts of local anesthetic required to block sacral nerves are significant disadvantages compared with spinal anesthesia. Usually, when these techniques are used they are instituted during labor as continuous techniques and maintained or intensified for the delivery.

General Anesthesia

General anesthesia is rarely indicated for vaginal delivery. Whether given for a brief or a prolonged period of time, general anesthesia engenders considerable risk and, therefore, should not be used without strong indication. An unanticipated breech presentation, shoulder dystocia, internal version, and extraction of a second twin or uterine inversion may represent rare indications for general anesthesia. General anesthesia may rarely be indicated for a difficult forceps delivery in a patient in whom major regional anesthesia is contraindicated. When general anesthesia is indicated, the technique specific for cesarean delivery is used, including administration by experienced and competent personnel, rapid-sequence induction, and endotracheal intubation. For breech delivery or delivery of a second twin, administration of a high concentration of a volatile halogenated agent (e.g., isoflurane, desflurane, or sevoflurane) is used to effect uterine and perhaps cervical relaxation. Equipotent doses of any of these three agents will provide equivalent uterine relaxation.[170]

ANESTHESIA FOR CESAREAN DELIVERY

In the United States, general anesthesia is used for about 10 percent of cesarean births (depending on size of hospital), and spinal and epidural anesthetics are used for approximately 90 percent (Table 16-6).[1] Local anesthesia for cesarean delivery is possible but is only rarely used.[171] Although general anesthesia carries excess risk for the mother, regional or general anesthesia results in similar fetal outcomes as ascertained by Apgar scores and blood gas measurements (Table 16-7).[170,172] Neurobehavioral testing that quantifies responses to certain stimuli in the early postpartum hours suggests that infants of mothers who receive regional anesthesia achieve somewhat higher scores than those whose mothers receive general anesthesia.[173,174] In addition, infants do somewhat better when ketamine is the induction agent for general anesthesia than when thiopental is used.[175] Lidocaine, 2-chloroprocaine, and bupivacaine for regional anesthesia are associated with similar neurobehavior scores.[176] When the Food and Drug Administration appointed a committee to study neurobehavioral changes in newborns after anesthesia, the committee concluded that, although anesthetic agents can alter neurobehavioral performance, there was no evidence that they affect later development.[33] The usefulness of neurobehavioral testing has been called into question

Table 16-6. Anesthetic Procedures Used for Cesarean Delivery in 2001 According to Size of Delivery Service

HOSPITAL SIZE (BIRTHS/YEAR)	EPIDURAL BLOCK (%)		SPINAL BLOCK (%)		GENERAL ANESTHESIA (%)	
	ELECTIVE	EMERGENT	ELECTIVE	EMERGENT	ELECTIVE	EMERGENT
<500	14	14	80	59	3	25
500–1,499	17	21	75	48	5	30
>1,500	22	36	67	45	3	15

Adapted from Bucklin BA, Hawkins JL, Anderson JR, Ullrich FA: Obsetric anesthesia workforce survey. Anesthesiology 103:645, 2005.

Table 16-7. Elective Cesarean Section—Blood Gas and Apgar Scores

	GENERAL ANESTHESIA* (N = 20)	EPIDURAL ANESTHESIA* (N = 15)	SPINAL ANESTHESIA† (N = 15)
Umbilical vein			
pH	–7.38	–7.359	–7.34
Po_2 (mm Hg)	35	36	37
Pco_2 (mm Hg)	38	42	48
Apgar < 6			
1	–1	–0	–0
5	–0	–0	–0
Umbilical artery			
pH	–7.32	–7.28	–7.28
Po_2 (mm Hg)	22	18	18
Pco_2 (mm Hg)	47	55	63
BE (mEq^hL)	–1.80	–1.60	–1.40

BE, base excess.

*Data from James FM III, Crawford JS, Hopkinson R, et al: A comparison of general anesthesia and lumbar epidural analgesia for elective cesarean section. Anesth Analg 56:228, 1977.

†Data from Datta S, Brown WU: Acid-base status in diabetic mothers and their infants following general or spinal anesthesia for cesarean section. Anesthesiology 47:272, 1977.

Advantages and Disadvantages of General Anesthesia for Cesarean Delivery

Advantages
- Patient does not have to be awake during a major operation.
- General anesthesia provides total pain relief.
- Operating conditions are optimal.
- The mother can be given 100% oxygen if needed.

Disadvantages
- Patients will not be awake during childbirth, although there is a small risk of undesirable awareness.
- There is a slight risk of fetal depression.
- Intubation causes hypertension and tachycardia, which may be particularly dangerous in severely preeclamptic patients.
- Intubation can be difficult or impossible.
- Aspiration of stomach contents is possible.

because of poor inter-rater reliability.[177,178] Neurobehavioral considerations do not weigh heavily in the choice of anesthesia or anesthetic agent; the choice can be based on the preferences of the mother, the obstetrician, and the anesthesiologist, as well as on the demands of the particular clinical situation.

General Anesthesia

Balanced general anesthesia, referring to a combination of various agents including barbiturates, inhalation agents, opioids, and muscle relaxants as opposed to high concentrations of potent inhalation agents alone, is preferred for obstetric applications (see box, "Advantages and Disadvantages of General Anesthesia for Cesarean Delivery").

Failure to intubate and aspiration continue to be major causes of anesthesia-related maternal mortality, and as a result, many anesthesiologists now prefer regional anesthesia over general anesthesia.[88,179–181] Data from both the ASA Closed Claims study[87] and the Centers for Disease Control and Prevention[88,181] indicate that maternal mortality rates are as much as seven times higher during general anesthesia as during regional anesthesia, although the absolute risk is very low. Case fatality rates are 16.8 maternal deaths per million general anesthetics and 2.5 per million regional anesthetics. To understand how these complications arise, the obstetrician should be aware of the sequence of events during general anesthesia.

Premedication

Premedication using sedative or opioid agents is usually omitted because these agents cross the placenta and can depress the fetus. Sedation should be unnecessary if the procedure is explained well.

Antacids

Use of a clear antacid is considered routine for all parturients prior to surgery. Additional aspiration prophylaxis using an H_2-receptor blocking agent and metoclopramide may be given to parturients with risk factors such as morbid obesity, diabetes mellitus, a difficult airway, or those who have previously received opioids. As soon as it is known that the patient requires cesarean delivery, be it with regional or general anesthesia, 30 ml of a clear, nonparticulate antacid, such as 0.3 M sodium citrate,[182] Bicitra,[183] or Alka Seltzer, 2 tablets in 30 ml water,[184] is administered to decrease gastric acidity and ameliorate the consequences of aspiration, should it occur. The chalky white particulate antacids are avoided because they can produce lung damage (Fig. 16-12).[185]

Left Uterine Displacement

As during labor, the uterus may compress the inferior vena cava and the aorta during cesarean delivery; aor-

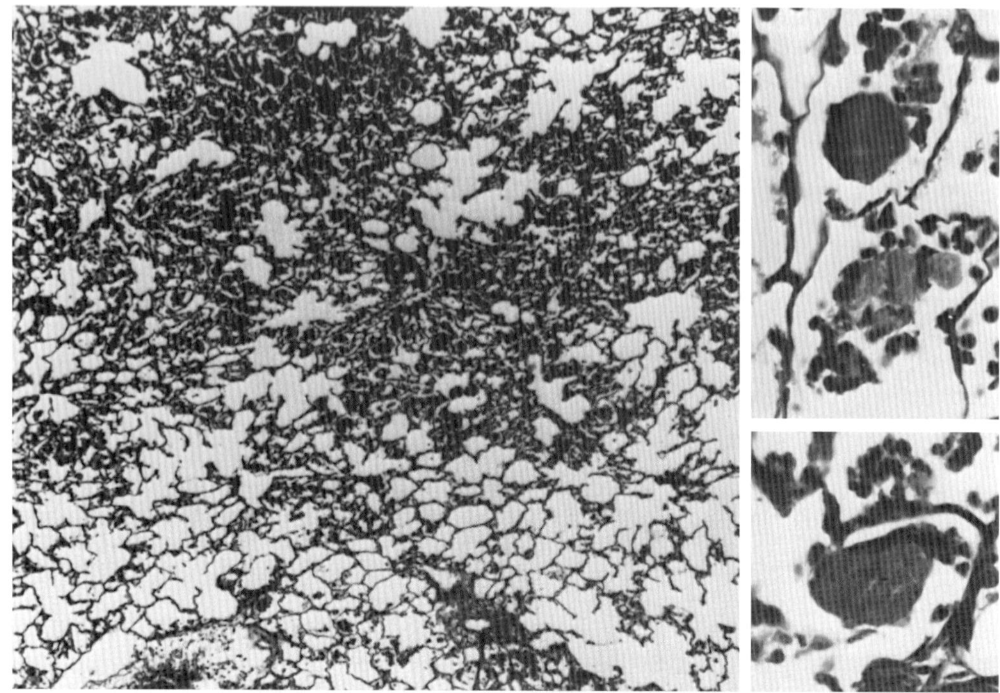

Figure 16-12. Lung after aspiration of particulate antacid. Note marked extensive inflammatory reaction. The alveoli are filled with polymorphonuclear leukocytes and macrophages in approximately equal numbers. Insets at right show large and small intra-alveolar particles surrounded by inflammatory cells (48 hours). Later, the reaction changed to an intra-alveolar cellular collection of clusters of large macrophages with abundant granular cytoplasm, in some of which were small amphophilic particles similar to those seen in the insets. No fibrosis or other inflammatory reaction was seen (28 days). (From Gibbs CP, Schwartz DJ, Wynne JW, et al: Antacid pulmonary aspiration in the dog. Anesthesiology 51:380, 1979, with permission.)

tocaval compression is detrimental to both mother and fetus. The duration of anesthesia has little effect on neonatal acid-base status when left uterine displacement is practiced; however, when patients remain supine, Apgar scores decrease as time of anesthesia increases.[186,187]

Preoxygenation

Preoxygenation is especially important in pregnant patients who have decreased functional residual capacity and are more likely than nonpregnant patients to rapidly become hypoxemic if untoward events accompanied by apnea occur.[188] Before starting induction, 100-percent oxygen should be administered through a face mask for 2 to 3 minutes. In situations of dire emergency, four vital capacity breaths of 100 percent oxygen through a tight circle system will provide similar benefit.[189]

Induction

The anesthesiologist rapidly administers thiopental (a short-acting barbiturate) to render the patient unconscious. An appropriate dose has little effect on the fetus.[172,190,191] Other induction agents that may be used are propofol,[192] etomidate,[193] and ketamine,[194] all of which are rapidly redistributed in the mother and fetus. Women who receive ketamine for induction require less analgesic medications in the first 24 hours after their cesarean delivery compared with those who have thiopental.[195] Its antagonism of NMDA receptors may prevent central hypersensitization, providing preemptive analgesia.

Although obstetricians are often concerned about the induction-to-delivery interval (I-D) during general anesthesia, uterine incision-to-delivery interval (U-D) is more predictive of neonatal status.[187,196] With a prolonged I-D interval, there is fetal uptake of the inhaled anesthetic and depressed Apgar scores (i.e., sleepy babies), but fetal acid-base status is normal and effective ventilation is all that is needed. Prolonged U-D intervals greater than 3 minutes lead to depressed Apgar scores with regional or general anesthesia, and they are associated with elevated fetal umbilical artery norepinephrine concentrations and associated fetal acidosis.[196]

Muscle Relaxants

Immediately after administration of thiopental or ketamine, the anesthesiologist gives a muscle relaxant to facilitate intubation. Succinylcholine, a rapid-onset, short-acting muscle relaxant, remains the agent of choice in most patients.

Cricoid Pressure

In rapid-sequence induction, as the induction agent begins to take effect and the patient approaches unconsciousness, an assistant applies pressure to the cricoid cartilage, just below the thyroid cartilage, and does not release the pressure until an endotracheal tube is placed, its position verified by end-tidal carbon dioxide measurement, and the cuff on the tube inflated.[197] Pressure on the cricoid closes off the esophagus and is extremely important in preventing aspiration should regurgitation or vomiting occur. It is a simple, safe, effective maneuver that should not be omitted.

Intubation

Usually, intubation proceeds smoothly. However, in approximately 1:238 obstetric patients, it is difficult, delayed, or impossible. The incidence of failed intubation in obstetric patients is about seven times more common than in patients in the general operating room (i.e., 1:230 to 280 in obstetric patients versus 1:2,230 in surgical patients).[198,199] When the delay is prolonged or the intubation impossible, the critical factors include delivering oxygen to the now unconscious and paralyzed patient and preventing aspiration.[200] Delay in intubation is associated with escalating aspiration risk. Therefore, it is particularly important during a difficult intubation that the person applying cricoid pressure not release that pressure until told to do so by the anesthesiologist.

The patient at risk for a difficult or impossible intubation can often be identified before surgery. Examination of the airway is a critical part of the preanesthetic evaluation. The anesthesiologist will assess (1) the ability to visualize oropharyngeal structures (Mallampati classification[201]); (2) range of motion of the neck; (3) presence of a receding mandible, which indicates the depth of the submandibular space; and (4) whether protruding maxillary incisors are present.[202] Obstetricians should be alert to the presence of obesity, severe edema, anatomic abnormalities of the face or neck or spine, including trauma or surgery, abnormal dentition, difficulty opening the mouth, extremely short stature, short neck or arthritis of the neck, or goiter. When the obstetrician recognizes airway abnormalities, patients should be referred for an early preoperative evaluation by the anesthesiologist.

Proper Tube Placement

Before the operation begins, the anesthesiologist must ensure that the endotracheal tube is properly positioned within the trachea. End-tidal carbon dioxide analysis is the preferred method to confirm that the tube is within the trachea.[203] Of course, the anesthesiologist will also confirm that breath sounds are bilateral and equal. The operation should not proceed until the airway is secure, because the patient cannot be allowed to awaken after the abdomen is opened.

When intubation cannot be accomplished and cesarean delivery is not urgent, the decision to delay the operation and allow the mother to awaken is easy. However, if the operation is being done because of rapidly worsening fetal condition or maternal hemorrhage, allowing the mother to awaken may further jeopardize the fetus or mother. Continued fetal heart rate monitoring during induction of anesthesia may help guide anesthetic and obstetric management in situations of failed intubation. Rarely, in situations of dire fetal compromise, the anesthesiologist and obstetrician may jointly decide to proceed with cesarean delivery while the anesthesiologist provides oxygenation, ventilation, and anesthesia by face mask ventilation or laryngeal mask airway,[204] with an additional person maintaining continuous cricoid pressure. In these emergency situations, it may be necessary to have additional trained personnel to provide assistance. After delivery, the obstetrician may need to obtain temporary hemostasis and then halt surgery while the anesthesiologist secures the airway by fiberoptics or other methods.

An algorithm for management of failed intubation in the obstetric patient is shown in Figure 16-13. Nursing

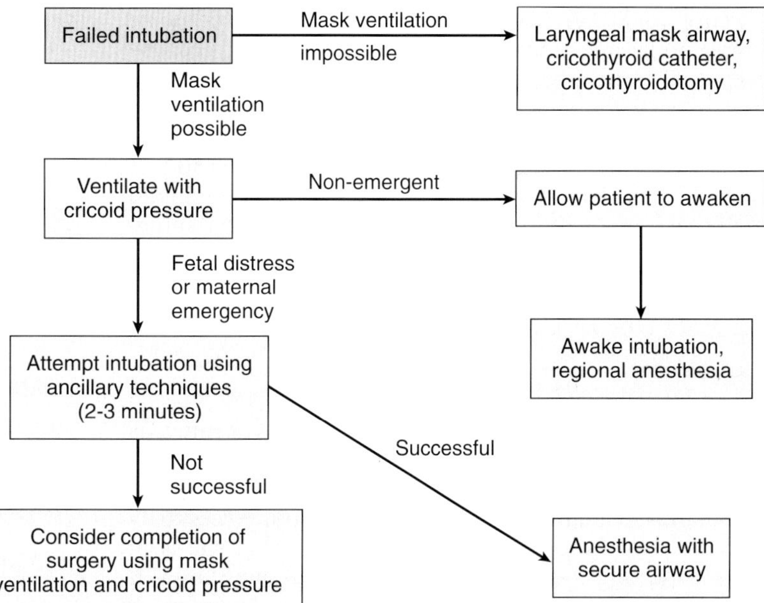

Figure 16-13. An algorithm for the management of failed intubation in the obstetric patient.

staff should also be familiar with the difficult airway algorithm in case they are called upon to assist during an airway emergency. Equipment to manage the difficult airway must be immediately available in the labor and delivery suite.[205,206]

Nitrous Oxide and Oxygen

Once the endotracheal tube is in place, a 50:50 mixture of nitrous oxide and oxygen, which is safe for both mother and fetus, is added to provide analgesia and amnesia.[207]

Volatile Halogenated Agent

Usually, in addition to the nitrous oxide, an analgesic quantity (low concentration) of a volatile halogenated agent (e.g., isoflurane, sevoflurane, or desflurane) is added to provide maternal amnesia and additional analgesia. These agents, in low concentrations, are not harmful to mother or fetus. Uterine relaxation does not result from low concentrations of these agents and bleeding should not be increased secondary to its addition.[170,172,208,209] Proceeding without a potent inhalation agent results in an unacceptably high incidence of maternal awareness and recall. Even with the use of one of these agents, maternal awareness and recall occasionally occur.[210] Therefore, it is important that all operating room personnel use discretion in conversation and conduct themselves as if the patient were awake.

Postdelivery

The concentration of nitrous oxide can usually be increased after delivery. In addition, the volatile halogenated agent is continued at a low concentration, and pain relief is supplemented with an opioid such as fentanyl or morphine. Other intravenous agents such as benzodiazepines may also be added to ensure maternal amnesia. Twenty to 80 U/L oxytocin are infused intravenously. Large bolus injections of oxytocin are avoided because they can cause a drop in systemic vascular resistance, hypotension, and tachycardia.[211] Maternal deaths have been reported following intravenous bolus oxytocin in the setting of hypovolemia or pulmonary hypertension.[212] Recent work has shown the effective dose (ED) ED90 for bolus oxytocin during cesarean delivery under spinal anesthesia to be 0.35 IU and the ED100 to be 1.0 IU.[213] Larger bolus doses should be unnecessary.

Extubation

Because the patient can aspirate while awakening as well as during induction, extubation is not done until the patient is awake and can respond appropriately to commands. Coughing and bucking do not necessarily indicate that the patient is awake, merely that she is in the second stage—the excitement stage—of anesthesia. It is during this period of anesthesia that laryngospasm is most likely to occur should any foreign body, including the endotracheal tube or bits of stomach contents, stimulate the larynx. The patient must therefore be awake and conscious, not merely active, before extubation.

Aspiration

Aspiration is a serious and often fatal complication of general anesthesia and, therefore, deserves specific attention. In most instances, it can be prevented. When it cannot, the consequences depend in part on the volume and nature of the aspirate. The conventional wisdom is that patients are at risk when their stomach contents are greater than 25 ml and when the pH of those contents is less than 2.5.[214] Pregnant patients are at higher risk for aspiration.[215] The enlarged uterus increases intraabdominal pressure and thus intragastric pressure. The gastroesophageal sphincter is distorted by the enlarged uterus, making it less competent, and possibly explaining the high incidence of heartburn that occurs during pregnancy. Increased progesterone levels affect smooth muscle, delaying gastric emptying and relaxing the gastroesophageal sphincter. Gastrin, the hormone that increases both acidity and volume of gastric contents, is increased during pregnancy, and motilin, a hormone that speeds gastric emptying, is decreased during pregnancy. Labor itself delays gastric emptying, primarily when patients have received opioids.[216] Many patients undergo cesarean delivery after a prolonged labor, during which they may have received several doses of opioids.[42]

The severity of lung damage, and rates of morbidity after aspiration vary and depend on the type of material aspirated. Less acidic aspirates (pH > 2.5) fill the alveoli decreasing $Pa{O_2}$ without a significant destructive or inflammatory effect. Aspirates with a pH of less than 2.5 cause hemorrhage, inflammatory exudates, and edema resulting in lower $Pa{O_2}$. Aspiration of partially digested food produces the most severe physiologic and histologic alterations. $Pa{O_2}$ decreases more than with any other type of aspiration, and lung damage is considerably more destructive[217] (Table 16-8).

Although acidic stomach contents can be neutralized safely and effectively with clear antacids or an H_2-receptor antagonist,[182–184,218,219] antacids cannot ameliorate the risks of aspiration after food intake. Aspiration

Table 16-8. Arterial Blood Gas Tensions and pH of Dogs 30 Minutes After Aspiration of 2 CC^{h}KG of Various Materials

ASPIRATE		RESPONSE		
COMPOSITION	pH	$P{O_2}$ (mm Hg)	$PC{O_2}$ (mm Hg)	pH
Saline	5.9	61	34	7.37
HCl	1.8	41	45	7.29
Food particles	5.9	34	51	7.19
Food particles	1.8	23	56	7.13

From Gibbs CP, Modell JH: Management of aspiration pneumonitis. *In* Miller RD (ed): Anesthesia, 3rd ed. New York, Churchill Livingstone, 1990, p 1293, with permission.

of partially digested food causes significant hypoxia and lung damage, even at a pH level as high as 5.9.[217] To decrease aspiration risk in cases of unplanned cesarean delivery, oral intake during labor should be limited to modest amounts of clear liquids or ice chips.[205]

Regional Anesthesia

If the fetal status permits and there are no maternal contraindications, regional anesthesia is preferred for cesarean delivery (see box, "Advantages and Disadvantages of Regional Anesthesia"). Contraindications to regional anesthesia include significant hemorrhage, infection at the site of needle insertion, coagulopathy, increased intracranial pressure caused by a mass lesion, patient refusal, and perhaps some forms of heart disease. Ongoing hemorrhage is a firm contraindication to regional anesthesia because the sympathetic blockade overrides compensatory vasoconstriction, potentially precipitating cardiovascular decompensation.

In the setting of maternal heart disease, the choice of anesthesia depends on the specific lesion. Epidural analgesia is the anesthetic technique of choice for patients with mitral valvular disease. In patients with aortic stenosis, pulmonary hypertension, or a right-to-left shunt who are unable to tolerate a decrease in systemic vascular resistance or a decrease in venous return of blood to the right side of the heart, regional analgesia or anesthesia should be used with caution and single-dose spinal or epidural anesthesia is contraindicated.[220] Rather, there should be slow, careful induction of continuous spinal or epidural anesthesia performed by an anesthesiologist with experience in the use of regional anesthesia in high-risk obstetric patients. Although there have been reports of successful administration of epidural anesthesia to patients with aortic stenosis[221] and Eisenmenger's syndrome,[222] the administration of general anesthesia remains most common. Intrathecal or epidural *opioid* analgesia does not decrease systemic vascular resistance and has emerged as an attractive choice of analgesia during labor in these complex patients,[223–225] but because neuraxial opioids provide inadequate anesthesia, they are not appropriate if cesarean delivery is required. However, even if general anesthesia is used, neuraxial opioids can provide postoperative analgesia.

The use of regional anesthesia in patients with fetal compromise depends on the severity of fetal condition and the presence of preexisting epidural anesthesia. If the situation is severe and acute, it is usually prudent not to delay delivery to perform a regional technique de novo. Furthermore, if hypotension occurs, the risk to the already compromised fetus is compounded. Ongoing acute fetal deterioration is usually an indication for general anesthesia. However, one should not indiscriminately perform rapid sequence induction.[226] A history and/or suspicion of difficult intubation should prompt performance of either awake intubation or regional anesthesia, despite the presence of fetal compromise because of the risk of maternal death from unsuccessful intubation. Lesser degrees of fetal compromise may permit regional anesthesia.[227,228] For example, if an epidural catheter has been placed earlier, a partial level of anesthesia already exists, and there is hemodynamic stability, extension of epidural anesthesia may be appropriate for cesarean delivery. The anesthesiologist may give additional local anesthetic while the urethral catheter is inserted and the abdomen is prepared and draped. Often, there will be satisfactory anesthesia when the surgeon is ready to make the skin incision. If not, the ongoing fetal heart rate pattern will dictate whether a delay is acceptable. When partial but inadequate epidural anesthesia results, one may consider supplemental local infiltration of local anesthetic, but most often general anesthesia will be indicated.

In cases in which the fetal heart rate tracing is not critical, de novo spinal or epidural anesthesia may be performed for cesarean delivery. In cases in which extension of existing epidural anesthesia is unsuccessful, spinal anesthesia should be placed with caution as the risk of high spinal anesthesia is increased.[103]

In healthy patients, the choice between epidural, spinal, and CSE anesthesia primarily rests with the anesthesiologist. With the recent availability of small-gauge spinal needles with pencil-point tip design, the risk of headache is no different after spinal or epidural anesthesia.[72] Most consider spinal block to be easier and quicker to perform, and most believe that the resulting anesthesia will be more solid and complete.[229] Perhaps the most significant advantage of spinal anesthesia is that it requires considerably less local anesthetic, and therefore, the potential for local anesthetic toxicity is less. Either technique is satisfactory, however, and should provide safe, effective anesthesia for mother, newborn, and obstetrician.

Advantages and Disadvantages of Regional Anesthesia

Advantages
- The patient is awake and can participate in the birth of her child.
- There is little risk of drug depression or aspiration and no intubation difficulties.
- Newborns generally have good neurobehavioral scores.
- The father is more likely to be allowed in the operating room.
- Postoperative pain control using neuraxial opioids may be superior to intravenous PCA.

Disadvantages
- Patients may prefer not to be awake during major surgery.
- An inadequate block may result.
- Hypotension, perhaps the most common complication of regional anesthesia, occurs during 25 to 75 percent of spinal or epidural anesthetics.
- Total spinal anesthesia may occur.
- Local anesthetic toxicity may occur.
- Although extremely rare, permanent neurologic sequelae may occur.
- There are several contraindications.

Local Anesthesia

Although rarely indicated, it is possible to use local anesthesia to perform a cesarean delivery.[171] The obstetrician must be thoroughly familiar with the recommended maximal dosages of the anesthetic used because large amounts may be necessary (see Table 16-3). The obstetrician should give a dilute solution of local anesthetic (e.g., 0.5-percent lidocaine or 1.0-percent 2-chloroprocaine) to allow for administration of a sufficiently large volume. It may be necessary to dilute a stock solution of 1-percent lidocaine or 2-percent 2-chloroprocaine to provide the recommended dilute solution. The patient must be familiar with the procedure and willing to cooperate. When the technique is used successfully, the operation must be performed skillfully and with minimal tissue trauma. Such requirements are often difficult to meet during an emergency cesarean section, particularly one for severe fetal distress or massive hemorrhage. When a major operation proceeds with local anesthesia, the initial stages of the operation may be accomplished easily, but later, the need may arise to progress more rapidly or to use maneuvers that require more tugging and pulling than anticipated. For example, the fetal head may be impacted in the pelvis, or a uterine vein may be lacerated. In these situations, the obstetrician must proceed with extreme haste, and a patient under local anesthesia may not be able to tolerate the manipulation. With an anesthesiologist in attendance, general anesthesia can be instituted immediately and the situation resolved. Therefore, the obstetrician must seriously consider all consequences before beginning an emergency cesarean delivery without an anesthesiologist in attendance.

Rarely, local anesthesia is requested by a patient in whom a regional block is technically impossible or contraindicated so that the patient can be awake for the delivery of the infant. In these cases, general anesthesia can be initiated after the patient sees her baby to complete the cesarean procedure.

Postoperative Pain Management

If spinal or epidural anesthesia is used for cesarean delivery, excellent postoperative analgesia can be obtained by addition of opioids to the local anesthetic solution.[230] The more lipid-soluble opioids such as fentanyl or sufentanil provide fast onset of analgesia with minimal side effects but have a short duration of 2 to 4 hours. They are often used in combination with a local anesthetic in a continuous or patient-controlled epidural infusion to improve the quality of the block. In contrast, morphine is hydrophilic, which gives it a prolonged duration of up to 24 hours, and it can be given as a single dose at the time of cesarean delivery. Unfortunately, its water solubility gives it a long onset time and higher incidence of side effects. The most common side effects of spinal and epidural opioids are itching and nausea. Respiratory depression is a rare but serious complication.[230,231] Several studies have shown that spinal or epidural opioids provide superior pain relief when compared with parenteral (intramuscular or intravenous PCA) opioids with a trend toward earlier hospital discharge and lower cost.[232]

If general anesthesia was used or neuraxial opioids provide inadequate pain control, an intravenous PCA can be used. Morphine, hydromorphone (Dilaudid), and fentanyl have all been used successfully. When nursing parturients were randomized to PCA morphine or meperidine after cesarean delivery, neurobehavioral scores were higher in the morphine group, and those infants were more alert and oriented to animate human cues.[45] A hospital quality improvement study of pain management after cesarean delivery allocated women to regimens using morphine or meperidine by intramuscular or intravenous PCA administration. Morphine was superior to meperidine for pain control and breast-feeding success, and women used less morphine when administered by PCA than when given intramuscularly.[233]

When intravenous PCA is used, the pump settings include an incremental dose, usually 1 to 2 mg morphine, 0.2 to 0.4 mg hydromorphone, or 10 to 25 μg fentanyl; a lockout interval of 6 to 10 minutes, and possibly a basal or continuous infusion rate. Usually basal rates are unnecessary for pain control and only increase maternal sedation and side effects. Using PCA provides better patient satisfaction by allowing her to control her pain medication.

The addition of nonsteroidal anti-inflammatory agents significantly improves pain scores with neuraxial morphine and reduces use of PCA opioids.[234,235] Intravenous ketorolac, rectal indomethacin, or oral ibuprofen can be used depending on the patient's ability to tolerate oral intake. Contraindications for nonsteroidal use include renal dysfunction or low urine output, use of gentamicin or similar drugs with renal toxicity, coagulopathy and uterine atony. Although the package insert for ketorolac states that it is contraindicated for use in breast-feeding mothers, the American Academy of Pediatrics approves its use while women are breast-feeding.

Key Points

- Analgesia during labor can reduce or prevent potentially adverse stress responses to the pain of labor.
- Parenteral opioids for labor analgesia work primarily by sedation and, except at high doses, result in minimal reduction of maternal pain. Side effects include maternal nausea and respiratory depression in both the mother and newborn. The routine use of promethazine (Phenergan) in conjunction with opioids should be avoided.
- Placental transfer of a drug between mother and fetus is governed by the characteristics of the drug (including its size, lipid solubility, and ionization), maternal blood levels and uterine blood flow, placental circulation, and the fetal circulation.
- Continuous regional analgesia is the most effective form of intrapartum pain relief currently available, and has the flexibility to provide additional anesthesia for spontaneous or instrumental delivery, cesarean delivery, and postoperative pain control.

❑ Spinal opioids provide excellent analgesia during much of the first stage of labor, whereas decreasing or avoiding the risks of local anesthetic toxicity, high spinal anesthesia, and motor block. Most patients need additional analgesia later in labor and during the second stage.

❑ Side effects and complications of regional anesthesia include hypotension, local anesthetic toxicity, total spinal anesthesia, neurologic injury, and spinal headache. Personnel providing anesthesia must be available and competent to treat these problems.

❑ Epidural analgesia prolongs labor and increases the rate of instrument-assisted vaginal deliveries. The preponderance of contemporary evidence suggests that epidural analgesia does not increase the cesarean delivery rate. Maternal-fetal factors and obstetric management are the most important determinants of the cesarean delivery rate.

❑ Epidural analgesia is associated with an increased rate of maternal fever during labor. This increases the rate of neonatal sepsis evaluation but not the rate of documented neonatal sepsis. Other neonatal implications are unclear.

❑ General anesthesia is used for less than 5 percent of elective and roughly 25 percent of emergent cesarean deliveries. Although safe for the newborn, general anesthesia can be associated with failed intubation and aspiration, the leading causes of anesthesia-related maternal mortality.

❑ Aspiration of gastric contents is most detrimental when food particles are present or the pH is less than 2.5; therefore, patients should be encouraged not to eat during labor, and acid-neutralizing medications should be used before operative deliveries.

❑ The use of regional anesthesia is not absolutely contraindicated in cases of nonreassuring fetal testing; the method of anesthesia should be chosen based on the degree of fetal compromise and maternal safety.

REFERENCES

1. Bucklin BA, Hawkins JL, Anderson JR, Ullrich FA: Obstetric anesthesia workforce survey. Anesthesiology 103:645, 2005.
2. Orkin FK: The geographic distribution of anesthesiologists during rapid growth in their supply [abstract]. Anesthesiology 81:A1295, 1994.
3. Joint Statement on the Optimal Goals for Anesthesia Care in Obstetrics: American Society of Anesthesiologists/American College of Obstetricians and Gynecologists, Park Ridge, IL, 2001.
4. Melzack R: The myth of painless childbirth. Pain 19:321, 1984.
5. Burns JK: Relation between blood levels of cortisol and duration of human labour. J Physiol (Lond) 254:12P, 1976.
6. Tuimala RJ, Kauppila JI, Haapalahti J: Response of pituitary-adrenal axis on partial stress. Obstet Gynecol 46:275, 1975.
7. Falconer AD, Powles AB: Plasma noradrenaline levels during labour: influence of elective lumbar epidural blockade. Anaesthesia 37:416, 1982.
8. Goland RS, Wardlaw SI, Stark RI, Frantz AG: Human plasma beta-endorphin during pregnancy, labor, and delivery. J Clin Endocrinol Metab 52:74, 1981.
9. Lederman RP, Lederman E, Work BA Jr, et al: The relationship of maternal anxiety, plasma catecholamines, and plasma cortisol to progress in labor. Am J Obstet Gynecol 132:495, 1978.
10. Rosenfeld CR, Barton MD, Meschia G: Effects of epinephrine on distribution of blood flow in the pregnant ewe. Am J Obstet Gynecol 124:156, 1976.
11. Morishima HO, Yeh M-N, James LS: Reduced uterine blood flow and fetal hypoxemia with acute maternal stress: experimental observation in the pregnant baboon. Am J Obstet Gynecol 134:270, 1979.
12. Shnider SM, Wright RG, Levinson G, et al: Uterine blood flow and plasma norepinephrine changes during maternal stress in the pregnant ewe. Anesthesiology 50:524, 1979.
13. Eidelman AI, Hoffmann NW, Kaitz M: Cognitive deficits in women after childbirth. Obstet Gynecol 81:764, 1993.
14. Maltau JM, Eielsen OV, Stokke KT: Effect of the stress during labor on the concentration of cortisol and estriol in maternal plasma. Am J Obstet Gynecol 134:681, 1979.
15. Thornton CA, Carrie LES, Sayers I, et al: A comparison of the effect of extradural and parenteral analgesia on maternal plasma cortisol concentrations during labour and the puerperium. Br J Obstet Gynaecol 83:631, 1976.
16. Abboud TK, Sarkis F, Hung TT, et al: Effects of epidural anesthesia during labor on maternal plasma beta-endorphin levels. Anesthesiology 59:1, 1983.
17. Abboud TK, Artal R, Henriksen EH, et al: Effects of spinal anesthesia on maternal circulating catecholamines. Am J Obstet Gynecol 142:252, 1982.
18. Myers R, Myers SE: Use of sedative, analgesic, and anesthetic drugs during labor and delivery: bane or boon? Am J Obstet Gynecol 133:83, 1979.
19. Reynolds F, Sharma SK, Seed PT: Analgesia in labour and fetal acid-base balance: a meta-analysis comparing epidural with systemic opioid analgesia. Br J Obstet Gynaecol 109:1344, 2002.
20. Goldberg AB, Cohen A, Lieberman E: Nulliparas' preferences for epidural analgesia: their effects on actual use in labor. Birth 26:139, 1999.
21. Eappen S, Robbins D: Nonpharmacological means of pain relief for labor and delivery. International Anesthesiology Clinics 40:103, 2002.
22. Lee H, Ernst E: Acupuncture for labor pain management: a systematic review. Am J Obstet Gynecol 191:1573, 2004.
23. Cluett ER, Pickering RM, Getliffe K, St. George Saunders NJ: Randomised controlled trial of labouring in water compared with standard of augmentation for management of dystocia in first stage of labour. BMJ 328:314, 2004.
24. Committee on Fetus and Newborn of the American Academy of Pediatrics: Underwater births. Pediatrics 115:1413, 2005.
25. Huntley AL, Coon JT, Ernst E: Complementary and alternative medicine for labor pain: a systematic review. Am J Obstet Gynecol 191:36, 2004.
26. Ader L, Hansson B, Wallin G: Parturition pain treated by intracutaneous injections of sterile water. Pain 41:133, 1990.
27. Harrison RF, Woods T, Shore M, et al: Pain relief in labour using transcutaneous electrical nerve stimulation (TENS). Br J Obstet Gynaecol 93:739, 1989.
28. Olofsson C, Ekblom A, Ekman-Ordeberg G, et al: Lack of analgesic effect systemically administered morphine or pethidine on labour pain. Br J Obstet Gynaecol 103:968, 1996.
29. Kuhnert BR, Kuhnert PM, Tu AL, Lin DCK: Meperidine and normeperidine levels following meperidine administration during labor. II. Fetus and neonate. Am J Obstet Gynecol 133:909, 1979.
30. Pittman KA, Smyth RD, Losada M, et al: Human perinatal distribution of butorphanol. Am J Obstet Gynecol 138:797, 1980.
31. Halpern SH, Leighton BL, Ohlsson A, et al: Effect of epidural vs parenteral opioid analgesia on the progress of labor: a meta-analysis. JAMA 280:2105, 1998.
32. Corke BC: Neurobehavioural responses of the newborn: the effect of different forms of maternal analgesia. Anaesthesia 32:539, 1977.

33. Kolata GB: Scientists attack report that obstetrical medications endanger children. Science 204:391, 1979.
34. Wright PMC, Allen RW, Moore J, et al: Gastric emptying during lumbar extradural analgesia in labour: effect of fentanyl supplementation. Br J Anaesth 68:248, 1992.
35. O'Sullivan GM, Sutton AJ, Thompson SA, et al: Noninvasive measurement of gastric emptying in obstetric patients. Anesth Analg 66:505, 1987.
36. Way WL, Costley EC, Way EL: Respiratory sensitivity of the newborn infant to meperidine and morphine. Clin Pharmacol Ther 6:454, 1965.
37. Rayburn W, Leuschen MP, Earl R, et al: Intravenous meperidine during labor: a randomized comparison between nursing- and patient-controlled administration. Obstet Gynecol 174:702, 1989.
38. Campbell DC: Parenteral opioids for labor analgesia. Clin Obstet Gynecol 46:616, 2003.
39. Sharma SK, Alexander JM, Messick G, et al: A randomized trial of epidural analgesia versus intravenous meperidine analgesia during labor in nulliparous women. Anesthesiology 96:546, 2002.
40. Lazebnik N, Kuhnert BR, Carr PC, et al: Intravenous, deltoid, or gluteus administration of meperidine during labor? Am J Obstet Gynecol 160:1184, 1989.
41. Kuhnert BR, Philipson EH, Kuhnert PM, Syracuse CD: Disposition of meperidine and normeperidine following multiple doses during labor. I. Mother. Am J Obstet Gynecol 151:406, 1985.
42. Kuhnert BR, Kuhnert PM, Philipson EH, Syracuse CD: Disposition of meperidine and normeperidine following multiple doses during labor. II Fetus and neonate. Am J Obstet Gynecol 151:410, 1985.
43. Sharma SK, Sidawi JE, Ramin SM, et al: A randomized trial of epidural versus patient-controlled meperidine analgesia during labor. Anesthesiology 87:487, 1997.
44. Wittels B, Scott DT, Sinatra RS: Exogenous opioids in human breast milk and acute neonatal neurobehavior: a preliminary study. Anesthesiology 73:864, 1990.
45. Wittels B, Glosten B, Faure EA, et al: Postcesarean analgesia with both epidural morphine and intravenous patient-controlled analgesia: neurobehavioral outcomes among nursing neonates. Anesth Analg 85:600, 1997.
46. Hodgkinson R, Bhatt M, Wang CH: Double-blind comparison of the neurobehaviour of neonates following the administration of different doses of meperidine to the mother. Can Anaesth Soc J 25:405, 1978.
47. Kuhnert BR, Linn PL, Kennard MJ, Kuhnert PM: Effects of low doses of meperidine on neonatal behavior. Anesth Analg 64:335, 1985.
48. Rayburn WF, Smith CV, Parriot JE, Wood RE: Randomized comparison of meperidine and fentanyl during labor. Obstet Gynecol 74:604, 1989.
49. Romagnoli A, Keats AS: Ceiling effect for respiratory depression by nalbuphine. Clin Pharmacol Ther 27:478, 1980.
50. Wilson CM, McClean E, Moore J, Dundee JW: A double-blind comparison of intramuscular pethidine and nalbuphine in labour. Anaesthesia 41:1207, 1986.
51. Maduska AL, Hajghassemali M: A double-blind comparison of butorphanol and meperidine in labour: maternal pain relief and effect on the newborn. Can Anaesth Soc J 25:398, 1978.
52. Kallos T, Caruso FS: Respiratory effects of butorphanol and pethidine. Anaesthesia 34:633, 1979.
53. Rosaeg OP, Kitts JB, Koren G, et al: Maternal and fetal effects of intravenous patient-controlled fentanyl analgesia during labour in a thrombocytopenic parturient. Can J Anaesth 39:277, 1992.
54. Dundee JW: Alterations in response to somatic pain associated with anaesthesia. II. The effect of thiopentone and pentobarbitone. Br J Anaesth 32:407, 1960.
55. McQuitty FM: Relief of pain in labour. A controlled double-blind trial comparing pethidine and various phenothiazine derivatives. J Obstet Gynaecol Br Cmnwlth 74:925, 1967.
56. Vella L, Francis D, Houlton P, Reynolds F: Comparison of the antiemetics metoclopramide and promethazine in labour. BMJ 290:1173, 1985.
57. Rosenblatt WH, Cioffi AM, Sinatra R, Silverman DG: Metoclopramide-enhanced analgesia for prostaglandin-induced termination of pregnancy. Anesth Analg 75:760, 1992.
58. Rosenblatt WH, Cioffi AM, Sinatra R, et al: Metoclopramide: an analgesic adjunct to patient-controlled analgesia. Anesth Analg 73:553, 1991.
59. Camann W, Cohen MB, Ostheimer GW: Is midazolam desirable for sedation in parturients? Anesthesiology 65:441, 1986.
60. Owen JR, Irani SF, Blair AW: Effect of diazepam administered to mothers during labour on temperature regulation of neonate. Arch Dis Child 47:107, 1972.
61. Wilson CM, Dundee JW, Moore J, et al: A comparison of the early pharmacokinetics of midazolam in pregnant and nonpregnant women. Anaesthesia 42:1057, 1987.
62. Ravlo O, Carl P, Crawford ME, et al: A randomized comparison between midazolam and thiopental for elective cesarean section anesthesia. II. Neonates. Anesth Analg 68:234, 1989.
63. Bland BAR, Lawes EG, Duncan PW, et al: Comparison of midazolam and thiopental for rapid sequence anesthetic induction for elective cesarean section. Anesth Analg 66:1165, 1987.
64. Gross JB, Weller RS, Conard P: Flumazenil antagonism of midazolam-induced ventilatory depression. Anesthesiology 75:179, 1991.
65. Dilts PV: Placental transfer. Clin Obstet Gynecol 24:555, 1981.
66. Santos AC, Finster M: Perinatal pharmacology. *In* Hughes SC, Levinson G, Rosen MA (eds): Anesthesia for Obstetrics, 4th ed. Baltimore, Lippincott Williams & Wilkins, 2002, p 61.
67. Biehl D, Shnider SM, Levinson G, Callender K: Placental transfer of lidocaine: effects of fetal acidosis. Anesthesiology 48:409, 1978.
68. American College of Obstetricians and Gynecologists: Obstetric analgesia and anesthesia. ACOG Practice Bulletin 32. Washington, D.C., 2002.
69. Sinclair JC, Fox HA, Lentz JF, et al: Intoxication of the fetus by a local anesthetic. N Engl J Med 273:1173, 1965.
70. Eisenach JC: Combined spinal-epidural analgesia in obstetrics. Anesthesiology 91:299, 1999.
71. Norris MC, Fogel ST, Conway-Long C: Combined spinal-epidural versus epidural labor analgesia. Anesthesiology 95:913, 2001.
72. Nielsen PE, Erickson JR, Abouleish EI, et al: Fetal heart rate changes after intrathecal sufentanil or epidural bupivacaine for labor analgesia: incidence and clinical significance. Anesth Analg 83:742, 1996.
73. Albright GA, Forster RM: Does combined spinal-epidural analgesia with subarachnoid sufentanil increase the incidence of emergency cesarean delivery? Reg Anesth 22:400, 1997.
74. Mardirosoff C, Dumont L, Boulvain M, Tramer MR: Fetal bradycardia due to intrathecal opioids for labor analgesia: a systematic review. Br J Obstet Gynaecol 109:274, 2002.
75. Tsen LC, Thue B, Datta S, Segal S: Is combined spinal-epidural analgesia associated with more rapid cervical dilation in nulliparous patients when compared with conventional epidural analgesia? Anesthesiology 91:920, 1999.
76. Wong CA, Scavone BM, Peaceman AM, et al: The risk of cesarean delivery with neuraxial analgesia given early versus late in labor. N Engl J Med 352:655, 2005.
77. Cohen SE, Cherry CM, Holbrook RH, et al: Intrathecal sufentanil for labor analgesia—sensory changes, side effects, and fetal heart rate changes. Anesth Analg 77:1155, 1993.
78. Brizgys RV, Dailey PA, Shnider SM, et al: The incidence and neonatal effects of maternal hypotension during epidural anesthesia for cesarean section. Anesthesiology 67:782, 1987.
79. Kenepp NB, Sheley WC, Kumar S, et al: Effects on newborn of hydration with glucose in patients undergoing caesarean section with regional anesthesia. Lancet 1:645, 1980.
80. Ralston DH, Shnider SM, deLorimier AA: Effects of equipotent ephedrine, metaraminol, mephentermine, and methoxamine on uterine blood flow in the pregnant ewe. Anesthesiology 40:354, 1974.
81. Lee A, Ngan Kee WD, Gin T: A quantitative systematic review of randomized controlled trials of ephedrine versus phenylephrine for the management of hypotension during spinal anesthesia for cesarean section. Anesth Analg 94:920, 2002.
82. Cooper DW, Carpenter M, Mowbray P, et al: Fetal and maternal effects of phenylephrine and ephedrine during spinal anesthesia for cesarean delivery. Anesthesiology 97:1582, 2002.

83. Wright RG, Shnider SM, Levinson G, et al: The effect of maternal administration of ephedrine on fetal heart rate and variability. Obstet Gynecol 57:734, 1981.
84. Riley ET: Spinal anesthesia for caesarean delivery: keep the pressure up and don't spare the vasoconstrictors (editorial). Br J Anaesth 92:459, 2004.
85. Ngan Kee WD, Khaw KS, Ng FF: Comparison of phenylephrine infusion regimens for maintaining maternal blood pressure during spinal anaesthesia for caesarean section. Br J Anaesth 92:469, 2004.
86. Auroy Y, Narchi P, Messiah A, et al: Serious complications related to regional anesthesia. Anesthesiology 87:479, 1997.
87. Ross BK: ASA closed claims in obstetric: lessons learned. Anesthesiology Clin N Am 21:183, 2003.
88. Hawkins JL, Koonin LM, Palmer SK, et al: Anesthesia-related deaths during obstetric delivery in the United States, 1979–1990. Anesthesiology 86:277, 1997.
89. Albright GA: Cardiac arrest following regional anesthesia with etidocaine or bupivacaine. Anesthesiology 51:285, 1979.
90. Santos AC, DeArmas PI: Systemic toxicity of levobupivacaine, bupivacaine, and ropivacaine during continuous intravenous infusion to nonpregnant and pregnant ewes. Anesthesiology 95:1256, 2001.
91. Clarkson CW, Hondeghem LM: Mechanism for bupivacaine depression of cardiac conduction: fast block of sodium channels during the action potential with slow recovery from block during diastole. Anesthesiology 62:396, 1985.
92. Morrison SG, Dominguez JJ, Frascarolo P, Reiz S: A comparison of the electrocardiographic cardiotoxic effects of racemic bupivacaine, levobupivacaine, and ropivacaine in anesthetized swine. Anesth Analg 90:1308, 2000.
93. Groban L, Deal DD, Vernon JC, et al: Cardiac resuscitation after incremental overdosage with lidocaine, bupivacaine, levobupivacaine, and ropivacaine in anesthetized dogs. Anesth Analg 92:37, 2001.
94. Ohmura S, Masayuki K, Ohta T, et al: Systemic toxicity and resuscitation in bupivacaine-, levobupivacaine-, or ropivacaine-infused rats. Anesth Analg 93:743, 2001.
95. Abbott Laboratories: Letter to doctors: urgent new recommendations about bupivacaine. Breon Laboratories, Westboro, MA, Astra Pharmaceutical Products, Inc, 1984.
96. Writer WDR, Davies JM, Strunin L: Trial by media: the bupivacaine story. Can Anaesth Soc J 31:1, 1984.
97. Moore DC, Batra MS: The components of an effective test dose prior to epidural block. Anesthesiology 55:693, 1981.
98. Abraham RA, Harris AP, Maxwell LG, Kaplow S: The efficacy of 1.5 percent lidocaine with 7.5 percent dextrose and epinephrine as an epidural test dose for obstetrics. Anesthesiology 64:116, 1986.
99. Leighton BL, Norris MC, Sosis M, et al: Limitations of epinephrine as a marker of intravascular injection in laboring women. Anesthesiology 66:688, 1987.
100. Weinberg GL: Current concepts in resuscitation of patients with local anesthetic cardiac toxicity. Reg Anesth Pain Med 27:568, 2002.
101. American Heart Association guidelines for cardiopulmonary resuscitation and emergency cardiovascular care. Circulation 112:1, 2005.
102. Camann W, Bader A: Spinal anesthesia with meperidine as the sole agent. Int J Obstet Anesth 1:156, 1992.
103. Dadarkar P, Philip J, Weidner C, et al: Spinal anesthesia for cesarean section following inadequate labor epidural analgesia: a retrospective audit. Int J Obstet Anesth 13:239, 2004.
104. Moore DC, Spierdijk J, Van Kleef JD, et al: Chloroprocaine neurotoxicity: four additional cases. Anesth Analg 61:155, 1982.
105. Gissen AJ, Datta S, Lambert D: The chloroprocaine controversy, II. Is chloroprocaine neurotoxic? Reg Anesth 9:135, 1984.
106. Drasner K: Chloroprocaine spinal anesthesia: back to the future? Anesth Analg 100:549, 2005.
107. Wong CA: Neurologic deficits and labor analgesia. Reg Anesth Pain Med 29:341, 2004.
108. Martin JT: Lithotomy positions. *In* Martin JT, Warner MA (eds): Positioning in Anesthesia and Surgery. Philadelphia, WB Saunders Company, 1997, p 47.
109. Ong BY, Cohen MM, Esmail A, et al: Paresthesias and motor dysfunction after labor and delivery. Anesth Analg 66:18, 1987.
110. Moen V, Dahlgren N, Irestedt L: Severe neurological complications after central neuraxial blockades in Sweden 1990–1999. Anesthesiology 101:950, 2004.
111. Turnbull DK, Shepherd DB: Post-dural puncture headache: pathogenesis, prevention and treatment. Br J Anaesth 91:718, 2003.
112. Camann WR, Murray RS, Mushlin PS, et al: Effects of oral caffeine on postdural puncture headache. Anesth Analg 70:181, 1990.
113. Kroin JS, Nagalla SKS, Buvanendran A, et al: The mechanisms of intracranial pressure modulation by epidural blood and other injectates in a postdural puncture rat model. Anesth Analg 95:423, 2002.
114. Ravindran RS: Epidural autologous blood patch on an outpatient basis. Anesth Analg 63:962, 1984.
115. Abouleish E, de la Vega S, Blendinger I, Tio TO: Long-term follow-up of epidural blood patch. Anesth Analg 54:459, 1975.
116. Hebl JR, Horlocker TT, Chantigian RC, Schroeder DR: Epidural anesthesia and analgesia are not impaired after dural puncture with or without epidural blood patch. Anesth Analg 89:390, 1999.
117. Woodward WM, Levy DM, Dixon AM: Exacerbation of postdural puncture headache after epidural blood patch. Can J Anaesth 41:628, 1994.
118. Scavone BM, Wong CA, Sullivan JT, et al: Efficacy of a prophylactic epidural blood patch in preventing post dural puncture headache in parturients after inadvertent dural puncture. Anesthesiology 101:1422, 2004.
119. Ayad S, Demian Y, Narouze SN, Tetzlaff JE: Subarachnoid catheter placement after wet tap for analgesia in labor: influence on the risk of headache in obstetric patients. Reg Anesth Pain Med 28:512, 2003.
120. Kuczkowski KM, Benumof JL: Decrease in the incidence of postdural puncture headache: maintaining CSF volume. Acta Anaesthesiol Scand 47:98, 2003.
121. Wang SM, Dezinno P, Maranets I, et al: Low back pain during pregnancy: prevalence, risk factors, and outcomes. Obstet Gynecol 104:65, 2004.
122. Howell CJ, Dean T, Lucking L, et al: Randomised study of long term outcome after epidural versus non-epidural analgesia during labour. BMJ 325:357, 2002.
123. Loughnan BA, Carli F, Romney J, et al: Epidural analgesia and backache: a randomized controlled comparison with intramuscular meperidine for analgesia during labour. Br J Anaesth 89:466, 2002.
124. Walker M: Do labor medications affect breastfeeding? J Hum Lact 13:131, 1997.
125. Rajan L: The impact of obstetric procedures and analgesia/anaesthesia during labour and delivery on breastfeeding. Midwifery 10:87, 1994.
126. Ransjo-Arvidson AB, Matthiesen AS, Lilja G, et al: Maternal analgesia during labor disturbs newborn behavior: effects on breastfeeding, temperature and crying. Birth 28:5, 2001.
127. Halpern S, MacDonell J, Levine NT, Wilson D: Does epidural analgesia influence breast-feeding outcomes six weeks postpartum? Birth 26:83, 1999.
128. Albani A, Addamo P, Rehghi A, et al: The effect on breastfeeding rate of regional anesthesia technique for cesarean and vaginal childbirth. Minerva Anestesiol 65:625, 1999.
129. Hirose M, Hara Y, Hosokawa T, Tanaka Y: The effect of postoperative analgesia with continuous epidural bupivacaine after cesarean section on the amount of breast feeding and infant weight gain. Anesth Analg 82:1166, 1996.
130. Sharma SK, McIntire DD, Wiley J, Leveno KJ: Labor analgesia and cesarean delivery; an individual patient meta-analysis of nulliparous women. Anesthesiology 100:142, 2004.
131. Halpern SH, Muir H, Breen TW, et al: A multicenter randomized controlled trial comparing patient-controlled epidural with intravenous analgesia for pain relief in labor. Anesth Analg 99:1532, 2004.
132. Vahratian A, Zhang J, Hasling J, et al: The effect of early epidural versus early intravenous analgesia use on labor progression: a natural experiment. Am J Obstet Gynecol 191:259, 2004.

133. Alexander JM, Sharma SK, McIntire DD, Leveno KJ: Epidural analgesia lengthens the Friedman active phase of labor. Obstet Gynecol 100:46, 2002.
134. Halonen P, Sarvela J, Saisto T, et al: Patient-controlled epidural technique improves analgesia for labor but increases cesarean delivery rate compared with the intermittent bolus technique. Acta Anaesth Scand 48:732, 2004.
135. Bofill JA, Vincent RD, Ross EL, et al: Nulliparous active labor, epidural analgesia, and cesarean delivery for dystocia. Am J Obstet Gynecol 177:1465, 1997.
136. Howell CJ, Kidd C, Roberts W, et al: A randomized controlled trial of epidural compared with non-epidural analgesia in labor. Br J Obstet Gynaecol 108:27, 2001.
137. Thorp JA, Hu DH, Albin RM, et al: The effect of intrapartum epidural analgesia on nulliparous labor: a randomized, controlled, prospective trial. Am J Obstet Gynecol 169:851, 1993.
138. Yancey MK. Zhang J, Schweitzer DL, et al: Epidural analgesia and fetal head malposition at vaginal delivery. Obstet Gynecol 97:608, 2001.
139. Lieberman E, Davidson K, Lee-Parritz A, Shearer E: Changes in fetal position during labor and their association with epidural analgesia. Obstet Gynecol 105:974, 2005.
140. Leighton BL, Halpern SH: The effects of epidural analgesia on labor, maternal, and neonatal outcomes: a systematic review. Am J Obstet Gynecol 186:S69, 2002.
141. Christianson LM, Bovbjerg VE, McDavitt EC, Hullfish KL: Risk factors for perineal injury during delivery. Am J Obstet Gynecol 189:255, 2003.
142. Hall W, McCracken K, Osterweil P, Guise JM: Frequency and predictors for postpartum fecal incontinence. Am J Obstet Gynecol 188:1205, 2003.
143. Robinson JN, Norwitz ER, Cohen AP, et al: Epidural analgesia and third- or fourth-degree lacerations in nulliparas. Obstet Gynecol 94:259, 1999.
144. Fitzpatrick M, Harkin R: A randomized clinical trial comparing the effects of delayed versus immediate pushing with epidural analgesia on mode of delivery and faecal continence. Br J Obstet Gynaecol 109:1359, 2002.
145. Maresh M, Choong KH, Beard RW: Delayed pushing with lumbar epidural analgesia in labour. Br J Obstet Gynaecol 90:623, 1983.
146. Yancey MK, Herpolsheimer A, Jordan GD, et al: Maternal and neonatal effects of outlet forceps delivery compared with spontaneous vaginal delivery in term pregnancies. Obstet Gynecol 78:646, 1991.
147. Eason E, Labrecque M, Marcoux S, Mondor M: Anal incontinence after childbirth. CMAJ 166:326, 2002.
148. Zhang J, Yancey MK, Klebanoff MA, et al: Does epidural analgesia prolong labor and increase risk of cesarean delivery? A natural experiment. Am J Obstet Gynecol 185:128, 2001.
149. American College of Obstetricians and Gynecologists: Task Force on Cesarean Delivery Rates, 2000.
150. Fischer A, LaCoursiere DY, Barnard P, et al: Differences between hospitals in cesarean rates for term primigravidas with cephalic presentation. Obstet Gynecol 105:816, 2005.
151. Chestnut DH, McGrath JM, Vincent RD, et al: Does early administration of epidural analgesia affect obstetric outcome in nulliparous women who are in spontaneous labor? Anesthesiology 80:1201, 1994.
152. Chestnut DH, Vincent RD Jr, McGrath JM, et al: Does early administration of epidural analgesia affect obstetric outcome in nulliparous women who are receiving intravenous oxytocin? Anesthesiology 80:1193, 1994.
153. Fusi L, Steer PJ, Maresh MJ, Beard RW: Maternal pyrexia associated with the use of epidural analgesia in labour. Lancet 1:1250, 1989.
154. Philip J, Alexander JM, Sharma SK, et al: Epidural analgesia during labor and maternal fever. Anesthesiology 90:1271, 1999.
155. Yancy MK, Zhang J, Schwarz J, et al: Labor epidural analgesia and intrapartum maternal hyperthermia. Obstet Gynecol 98:763, 2001.
156. Goetzl L, Evans T, Rivers J, et al: Elevated maternal and fetal serum interleukin-6 levels are associated with epidural fever. Am J Obstet Gynecol 187:834, 2002.
157. Dashe JS, Rogers BB, McIntire DD, Leveno KJ: Epidural analgesia and intrapartum fever: placental findings. Obstet Gynecol 93:341, 1999.
158. Lieberman E, Lang JM, Frigoletto F, et al: Epidural analgesia, intrapartum fever, and neonatal sepsis evaluation. Pediatrics 99:415, 1997.
159. Tomimatsu T, Fukuda H, Kanagawa T, et al: Effects of hyperthermia on hypoxic-ischemic brain damage in the immature rat: its influence on caspase-3-like protease. Am J Obstet Gynecol 188:768, 2003.
160. Impey L, Greenwood C, MacQuillan K, et al: Fever in labour and neonatal encephalopathy: a prospective cohort study. Br J Obstet Gynecol 108:594, 2001.
161. Wu YW, Escobar GJ, Grether JK, et al: Chorioamnionitis and cerebral palsy in term and near term infants. JAMA 290:2677, 2003.
162. Goetzl L, Rivers J, Wali A, et al: Prophylactic acetaminophen does not prevent epidural fever in nulliparous women: a double-blind placebo-controlled trial. Am J Perinatology 24:471, 2004.
163. Shnider SM, Asling JH, Holl JW, Margolis AJ: Paracervical block anesthesia in obstetrics. I. Fetal complications and neonatal morbidity. Am J Obstet Gynecol 107:619, 1970.
164. Freeman RK, Gutierrez NA, Ray ML, et al: Fetal cardiac response to paracervical block anesthesia. Part I. Am J Obstet Gynecol 113:583, 1972.
165. Gibbs CP, Noel SC: Response of arterial segments from gravid human uterus to multiple concentrations of lignocaine. Br J Anaesth 45:409, 1977.
166. Greiss FC Jr, Still JG, Anderson SG: Effects of local anesthetic agents on the uterine vasculatures and myometrium. Am J Obstet Gynecol 124:889, 1976.
167. Martensson L, Wallin G: Labour pain treated with cutaneous injections of sterile water: a randomised controlled trial. Br J Obstet Gynaecol 106:633, 1999.
168. Philipson EH, Kuhnert BR, Syracuse CD: Maternal, fetal, and neonatal lidocaine levels following local perineal infiltration. Am J Obstet Gynecol 149:403, 1984.
169. Klink EW: Perineal nerve block: an anatomic and clinical study in the female. Obstet Gynecol 1:137, 1953.
170. Gambling DR, Sharma SK, White PF, et al: Use of sevoflurane during elective cesarean birth: a comparison with isoflurane and spinal anesthesia. Anesth Analg 81:90, 1995.
171. Cooper MG, Feeney EM, Joseph M, McGuinness JJ: Local anaesthetic infiltration for caesarean section. Anaesth Intensive Care 17:198, 1989.
172. Kuczkowski KM, Reisner LS, Lin D: Anesthesia for cesarean section. *In* Chestnut DH (ed): Obstetric Anesthesia: Principles and Practice, 3rd ed. Philadelphia, Elsevier Mosby, 2004, p 421.
173. Scanlon JW, Brown WU Jr, Weiss JB, Alper MH: Neurobehavioral responses of newborn infants after maternal epidural anesthesia. Anesthesiology 40:121, 1974.
174. Brockhurst NJ, Littleford JA, Halpern SH: The neurologic and adaptive capacity score. Anesthesiology 92:237, 2000.
175. Hodgkinson R, Bhatt M, Kim SS, et al: Neonatal neurobehavioral tests following cesarean section under general and spinal anesthesia. Am J Obstet Gynecol 132:670, 1978.
176. Abboud TK, Khoo SS, Miller F, et al: Maternal, fetal, and neonatal responses after epidural anesthesia with bupivacaine, 2-chloroprocaine, or lidocaine. Anesth Analg 61:638, 1982.
177. Halpern SH, Littleford JA, Brockhurst NJ, et al: The neurologic and adaptive capacity score is not a reliable method of newborn evaluation. Anesthesiology 94:958, 2001.
178. Camann W, Brazelton TB: Use and abuse of neonatal neurobehavioral testing. Anesthesiology 92:3, 2000.
179. Cooper GM, McClure JH: Maternal deaths from anaesthesia. An extract from *Why Mothers Die 2000–2002,* the confidential enquiries into maternal deaths in the United Kingdom. Br J Anaesth 94:417, 2005.
180. Morgan M: Anaesthetic contribution to maternal mortality. Br J Anaesth 59:842, 1987.
181. Hawkins JL, Chang J, Callaghan W, et al: Anesthesia-related maternal mortality in the United States, 1991–1996. An update. Anesthesiology 97:A1046, 2002.
182. Gibbs CP, Spohr L, Schmidt D: The effectiveness of sodium citrate as an antacid. Anesthesiology 57:44, 1982.
183. Gibbs CP, Banner TC: Effectiveness of Bicitra as a preoperative antacid. Anesthesiology 61:97, 1984.
184. Chen CT, Toung TJ, Cameron JL: Alka-Seltzer® for prophylactic use in prevention of acid aspiration pneumonia. Anesthesiology 57:A103, 1982.

185. Gibbs CP, Schwartz DJ, Wynne JW, et al: Antacid pulmonary aspiration in the dog. Anesthesiology 51:380, 1979.
186. Crawford JA, Burton M, Davies P: Time and lateral tilt at caesarean section. Br J Anaesth 44:477, 1972.
187. Datta S, Ostheimer GW, Weiss JB, et al: Neonatal effect of prolonged anesthetic induction for cesarean section. Obstet Gynecol 58:331, 1981.
188. Archer GW, Marx GF: Arterial oxygen tension during apnoea in parturient women. Br J Anaesth 46:358, 1974.
189. Norris MC, Dewan DM: Preoxygenation for cesarean section: a comparison of two techniques. Anesthesiology 62:827, 1985.
190. Morgan DJ, Blackman GL, Paull JD, Wolf LJ: Pharmacokinetics and plasma binding of thiopental. II. Studies at cesarean section. Anesthesiology 54:474, 1981.
191. Holdcroft A, Morgan M: Intravenous induction agents for caesarean section [editorial]. Anaesthesia 44:719, 1989.
192. Gin T. Propofol during pregnancy. Acta Anaesthesiol Sin 32:127, 1994.
193. Gregory MA, Davidson DG: Plasma etomidate levels in mother and fetus. Anaesthesia 46:716, 1991.
194. Bernstein K, Gisselsson L, Jacobsson T, Ohrlander S: Influence of two different anaesthetic agents on the newborn and the correlation between foetal oxygenation and induction-delivery time in elective caesarean section. Acta Anaesthesiol Scand 29:157, 1985.
195. Kee WDN, Khaw KS, Ma ML, et al: Postoperative analgesic requirement after cesarean section: a comparison of anesthetic induction with ketamine or thiopental. Anesth Analg 85:1294, 1997.
196. Bader AM, Datta S, Arthur GR, et al: Maternal and fetal catecholamines and uterine incision-to-delivery interval during elective cesarean. Obstet Gynecol 75:600, 1990.
197. Sellick BA: Cricoid pressure to control regurgitation of stomach contents during induction of anesthesia. Lancet 2:404, 1961.
198. Samsoon GLT, Young JRB: Difficult tracheal intubation: a retrospective study. Anaesthesia 42:487, 1987.
199. Barnardo PD, Jenkins JG: Failed tracheal intubation in obstetrics: a 6-year review in a UK region. Anaesthesia 55:690, 2000.
200. Rahman K, Jenkins JG: Failed tracheal intubation in obstetrics: no more frequent but still managed badly. Anaesthesia 60:168, 2005.
201. Mallampati SR, Gatt SP, Gugino LD, et al: A clinical sign to predict difficult tracheal intubation: a prospective study. Can Anaesth Soc J 32:429, 1985.
202. Rocke DA, Murray WB, Rout CC, et al: Relative risk analysis of factors associated with difficult intubation in obstetric anesthesia. Anesthesiology 77:67, 1992.
203. American Society of Anesthesiologists: Standards for Basic Anesthetic Monitoring. Park Ridge, IL, American Society of Anesthesiologists, 2004.
204. Awan R, Nolan JP, Cook TM: Use of a ProSeal™ laryngeal mask airway for airway maintenance during emergency caesarean section after failed tracheal intubation. Br J Anaesth 92:144, 2004.
205. American Society of Anesthesiologists Task Force on Obstetrical Anesthesia: Practice guidelines for obstetrical anesthesia. Anesthesiology 106, 2007 (in press).
206. American Society of Anesthesiologists Task Force on Difficult Airway Management: Practice guidelines for management of the difficult airway: an updated report. Anesthesiology 98:1269, 2003.
207. Marx GF, Joshi CW, Orkin LR: Placental transmission of nitrous oxide. Anesthesiology 32:429, 1970.
208. Kan K, Shigihara A, Tase C, et al: Comparison of sevoflurane and other volatile anesthetics for cesarean section. J Anesth 9:363, 1995.
209. Warren TM, Datta S, Ostheimer GW, et al: Comparison of the maternal and neonatal effects of halothane, enflurane, and isoflurane for cesarean delivery. Anesth Analg 62:516, 1983.
210. Chin KJ, Yeo SW: Bispectral index values at sevoflurane concentrations of 1 percent and 1.5 percent in lower segment cesarean delivery. Anesth Analg 98:1140, 2004.
211. Pinder AJ, Dresner M, Calow C, et al: Haemodynamic changes caused by oxytocin during caesarean section under spinal anaesthesia. Int J Obstet Anesth 11:156, 2002.
212. Thomas TA, Cooper GM: Maternal deaths from anaesthesia. An extract from *Why Mothers Die 1997–1999*, the confidential enquiries into maternal deaths in the United Kingdom. Br J Anaesth 89:499, 2002.
213. Carvalho JCA, Balki M, Kingdom J, Windrim R: Oxytocin requirements at elective cesarean delivery: a dose-finding study. Obstet Gynecol 104:1005, 2004.
214. Roberts RB, Shirley MA: Reducing the risk of acid aspiration during cesarean section. Anesth Analg 53:859, 1974.
215. O'Sullivan GM, Guyton TS: Aspiration: risk, prophylaxis, and treatment. *In* Chestnut DH (ed): Obstetric Anesthesia, ed 3, Philadelphia, Elsevier Mosby, 2004, p 523.
216. O'Sullivan GM, Bullingham RE: Noninvasive assessment by radiotelemetry of antacid effect during labor. Anesth Analg 64:95, 1985.
217. Schwartz DJ, Wynne JW, Gibbs CP, et al: The pulmonary consequences of aspiration of gastric contents at pH values greater than 2.5. Am Rev Respir Dis 121:119, 1980.
218. Eyler SW, Cullen BF, Murphy ME, Welch WD: Antacid aspiration in rabbits: a comparison of Mylanta and Bicitra. Anesth Analg 61:288, 1982.
219. Hodgkinson R, Glassenberg R, Joyce TH, et al: Comparison of cimetidine (Tagamet®) with antacid for safety and effectiveness in reducing gastric acidity before elective cesarean section. Anesthesiology 59:86, 1983.
220. Ray P, Murphy GJ, Shutt LE: Recognition and management of maternal cardiac disease in pregnancy. Br J Anaesth 93:428, 2004.
221. Easterling TR, Chadwick HS, Otto CM, Benedetti TJ: Aortic stenosis in pregnancy. Obstet Gynecol 72:113, 1988.
222. Bonnin M, Mercier FJ, Sitbon O, et al: Severe pulmonary hypertension during pregnancy. Anesthesiology 102:1133, 2005.
223. Ahmad S, Hawes D, Dooley S, et al: Intrathecal morphine in a parturient with a single ventricle. Anesthesiology 54:515, 1981.
224. Abboud TK, Raya J, Noveihed R, Daniel J: Intrathecal morphine for relief of labor pain in a parturient with severe pulmonary hypertension. Anesthesiology 59:477, 1983.
225. Pollack KL, Chest DH, Wenstrom KD: Anesthetic management of a parturient with Eisenmenger's syndrome. Anesth Analg 70:212, 1990.
226. ACOG Committee on Obstetric Practice: Committee Opinion #197: Inappropriate use of the terms fetal distress and birth asphyxia. Washington, DC, American College of Obstetricians and Gynecologists, 1998.
227. Marx GF, Luykx WM, Cohen S: Fetal-neonatal status following caesarean section for fetal distress. Br J Anaesth 56:1009, 1984.
228. Chestnut DH: Anesthesia for fetal distress. *In* Chestnut DH (ed): Obstetric Anesthesia: Principles and Practice, ed 3, Philadelphia, Elsevier Mosby, 2004, p 447.
229. Riley ET, Cohen SE, Macario A, et al: Spinal versus epidural anesthesia for cesarean section: a comparison of time efficiency, costs, charges, and complications. Anesth Analg 80:709, 1995.
230. Abouleish E, Rawal N, Rashad MN: The addition of 0.2 mg subarachnoid morphine to hyperbaric bupivacaine for cesarean delivery: a prospective study of 856 cases. Reg Anesth 16:137, 1991.
231. Ferouz, F, Norris MC, Leighton BL: Risk of respiratory arrest after intrathecal sufentanil. Anesth Analg 85:1088, 1997.
232. Cohen SE, Subak LL, Brose WG, et al: Analgesia after cesarean delivery: patient evaluations and costs of five opioid techniques. Reg Anesth 16:141, 1991.
233. Yost NP, Bloom SL, Sibley MK, et al: A hospital-sponsored quality improvement study of pain management after cesarean delivery. Am J Obstet Gynecol 190:1341, 2004.
234. Lowder JL, Shackelford DP, Holbert D, Beste TM: A randomized, controlled trial to compare ketorolac tromethamine versus placebo after cesarean section to reduce pain and narcotic usage. Am J Obstet Gynecol 189:1559, 2003.
235. Angle PJ, Halpern SH, Leighton BL, et al: A randomized controlled trial examining the effect of naproxen on analgesia during the second day after cesarean delivery. Anesth Analg 95:741, 2002.

Malpresentations

SUSAN M. LANNI AND JOHN W. SEEDS

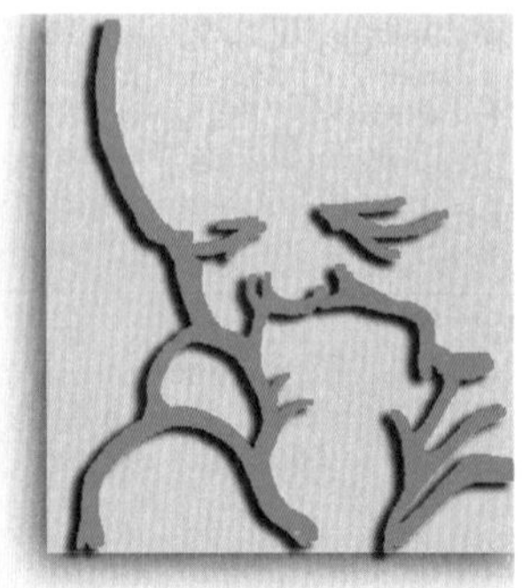

CHAPTER 17

KEY ABBREVIATIONS

Anteroposterior	AP
Cerebral palsy	CP
Computerized tomography	CT
Confidence interval	CI
External cephalic version	ECV
Magnetic resonance imaging	MRI
Odds ratio	OR
Perinatal mortality rate	PMR
Periventricular leukomalacia	PVL
Preterm premature rupture of the membranes	PPROM
Relative risk	RR

Near term or during labor, the fetus normally assumes a vertical orientation or lie and a cephalic presentation, with the fetal vertex flexed on the neck (Fig. 17-1). In about 5 percent of cases, however, deviation occurs from this normal lie, presentation, or flexion attitude; such deviation constitutes a fetal malpresentation. The word "malpresentation" suggests the possibility of adverse consequences, and malpresentation is typically associated with increased risk to both the mother and the fetus. Malpresentation once led to a variety of maneuvers intended to facilitate vaginal delivery, and early in the 20th century, such interventions included destructive operations leading, predictably, to fetal death. Later, manual or instrumental attempts to convert the malpresenting fetus to a more favorable orientation were devised. Internal podalic version, followed by a complete breech extraction was once advocated as a solution to many malpresentation situations. However, internal podalic version along with most manipulative efforts to achieve vaginal delivery were associated with a high fetal or maternal morbidity or mortality rate and have been largely abandoned. In contemporary practice, cesarean delivery has become the recommended alternative to manipulative vaginal techniques when normal progress toward vaginal delivery is not observed.

This chapter examines malpresentations, possible etiologies, and the mechanics of labor and vaginal delivery unique to each situation.

CLINICAL CIRCUMSTANCES ASSOCIATED WITH MALPRESENTATION

Generally, factors associated with malpresentation include (1) diminished vertical polarity of the uterine cavity, (2) increased or decreased fetal mobility, (3) obstructed pelvic inlet, and (4) fetal malformation. The association of great parity with malpresentation is presumably related to laxity of maternal abdominal muscular support and, therefore, loss of the normal vertical orientation of the uterine cavity. Placentation either high in the fundus or low in the pelvis (Fig. 17-2) is another factor that diminishes the likelihood of a fetus assuming a longitudinal axis. Uterine myomata, intrauterine synechiae, and müllerian duct abnormalities such as septate uterus or uterus didelphys are likewise associated with a higher than expected rate of malpresentation. Because both prematurity and hydramnios permit increased fetal mobility, there is a greater probability of a noncephalic presentation if labor or rupture of membranes occurs. Furthermore, preterm birth involves a fetus that is small relative to the maternal pelvis and may result in morbidity often secondary to prematurity. Pelvic engagement

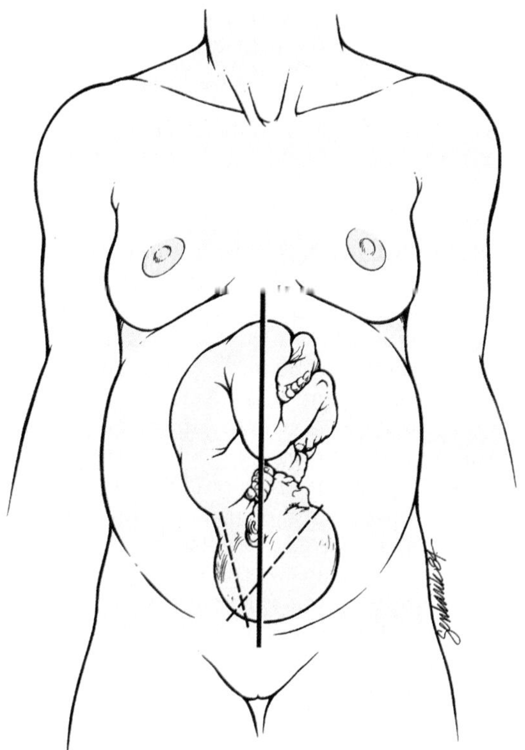

Figure 17-1. Frontal view of a fetus in a longitudinal lie with fetal vertex flexed on the neck.

and descent with labor or rupture of membranes can occur despite malpresentation. In contrast, conditions such as aneuploidies, myotonic dystrophy, joint contractures from various etiologies, arthrogryposis or oligohydramnios, and fetal neurologic dysfunction that result in decreased fetal muscle tone, strength, or activity are also associated with an increased incidence of fetal malpresentation. Finally, the cephalopelvic disproportion associated with severe fetal hydrocephalus or with a contracted maternal pelvis is frequently implicated as an etiology of malpresentation because normal engagement of the fetal head is prevented.

ABNORMAL AXIAL LIE

The fetal "lie" indicates the orientation of the fetal spine relative to the spine of the mother. The normal fetal lie is longitudinal and by itself does not indicate whether the presentation is cephalic or breech. If the fetal spine or long axis crosses that of the mother, the fetus may be said to occupy a transverse or oblique lie (Fig. 17-3), which may cause either an arm, foot, or a shoulder to be the presenting part (Fig. 17-4). The lie may be termed unstable if the fetal membranes are intact and there is great fetal mobility resulting in frequent changes of lie or presentation.[1]

Abnormal fetal lie is diagnosed in approximately 1 in 300 cases, or 0.33 percent of pregnancies at term.[2–8] Prematurity is often a factor, with abnormal lie reported to occur in about 2 percent of pregnancies at 32 weeks, or six times the rate found at term.[9] Persistence of a trans-

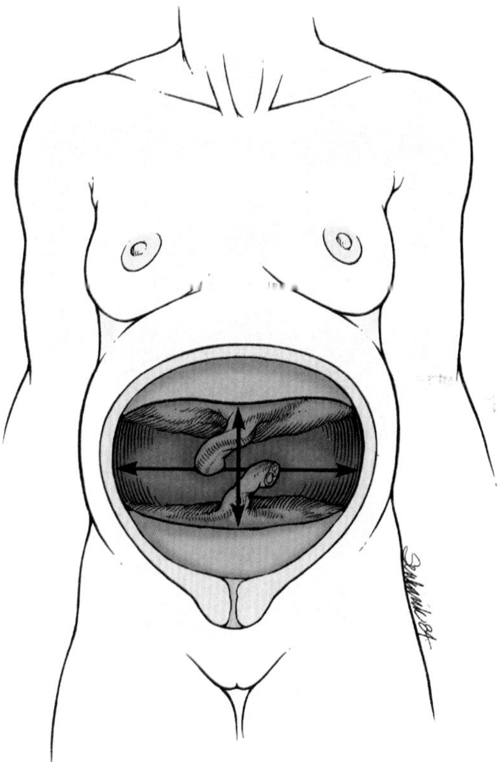

Figure 17-2. Either the high fundal or low implantation of the placenta illustrated here would normally be in the vertical orientation of the intrauterine cavity and increase the probability of a malpresentation.

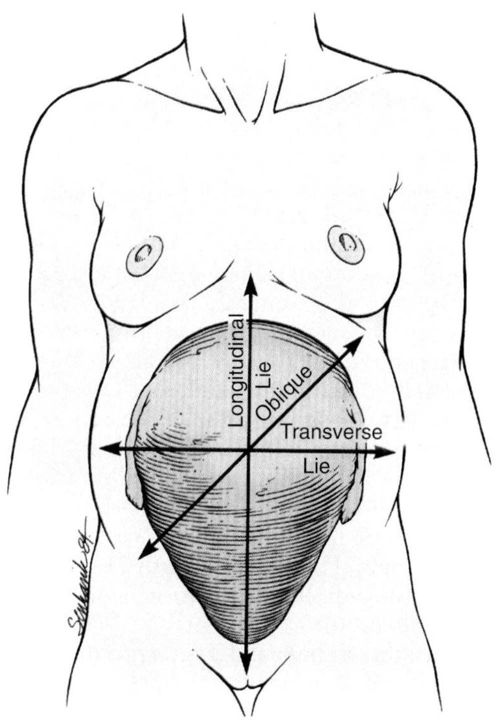

Figure 17-3. A fetus may occupy a longitudinal, oblique, or transverse axis, as illustrated by these vectors. The lie does not indicate whether the vertex or the breech is closest to the cervix.

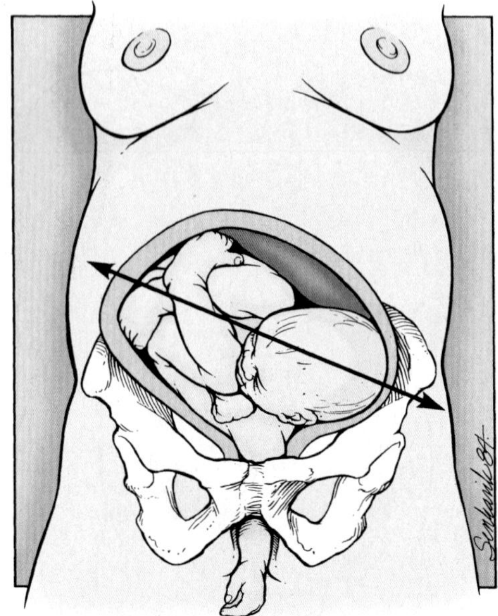

Figure 17-4. This fetus lies in an oblique axis with an arm prolapsing.

verse, oblique, or unstable lie beyond 37 weeks requires a systematic clinical assessment and a plan for management, because rupture of membranes without a fetal part filling the inlet of the pelvis imposes a high risk of cord prolapse, fetal compromise, and maternal morbidity if neglected.

Great parity, prematurity, contraction or deformity of the maternal pelvis, and abnormal placentation are the most commonly reported clinical factors associated with abnormal lie,[2,5,9] although Cockburn and Drake found many cases that manifested none of these factors.[3] In fact, any condition that alters the normal vertical polarity of the intrauterine cavity will predispose to abnormal lie.

Diagnosis of the abnormal lie may be made by palpation or vaginal examination and verified by ultrasound. Routine use of Leopold's maneuvers may assist detection, but Thorp et al.[10] found the sensitivity of Leopold's maneuvers for the detection of malpresentation to be only 28 percent and the positive predictive value only 24 percent compared with immediate ultrasound verification. Others have observed prenatal detection in as few as 41 percent of cases before labor.[3] A fetal loss rate of 9.2 percent with an early diagnosis versus a loss rate of 27.5 percent with a delayed diagnosis indicates that early diagnosis improves fetal outcome.[3]

Reported perinatal mortality for unstable or transverse lie (corrected for lethal malformations and extreme prematurity) varies from 3.9 percent[11] to 24 percent,[1] with maternal mortality as high as 10 percent. Maternal deaths are usually related to infection after premature rupture of membranes, hemorrhage secondary to abnormal placentation, complications of operative intervention for cephalopelvic disproportion, or traumatic delivery.[7,9] Fetal loss of phenotypically and chromosomally normal gestations at ages considered to be viable is primarily associated with neglect, prolapsed cord, or traumatic delivery.[9] Cord prolapse occurs 20 times as often with abnormal axial lie as it does with a cephalic presentation.

MANAGEMENT OF A SINGLETON GESTATION

The normally grown singleton infant at term cannot undergo a safe vaginal delivery from an abnormal axial lie,[4,7] and a search for a potentially dangerous or compromising etiology of the malpresentation is indicated. A transverse/oblique or unstable lie late in the third trimester necessitates ultrasound examination to exclude a major fetal malformation and abnormal placentation. Fortunately, most cases of fetal anomalies or abnormal placentation are diagnosed long before the third trimester. Elective hospitalization may permit observation and early recognition of cord prolapse, and provides proximity to immediate care.[6,11] Phelan et al.[12] reported 29 patients with transverse lie diagnosed at or beyond 37 weeks' gestation and managed expectantly. Eighty-three percent (24 of 29) spontaneously converted to breech (9 of 24) or vertex (15 of 24) before labor; however, the overall cesarean delivery rate was 45 percent, and there were two cases of cord prolapse, one uterine rupture, and one neonatal death. Such outcomes suggest that active intervention at or beyond 37 weeks or after confirmation of fetal lung maturity may be of benefit. External cephalic version with subsequent induction of labor, if successful, might diminish the risk of adverse outcome.

In cases of an abnormal lie, the risk of fetal death varies with the obstetric intervention. Fetal mortality should approach zero for cesarean birth but has been reported as high as 10 percent in older reports compared with 25 to 90 percent when internal podalic version and breech extraction are performed.[3,4,7–9,13] A mortality rate of 6 percent was reported for successful external version and vertex vaginal delivery in papers published more than 40 years ago.[8,9] External cephalic version followed by induction of labor after 37 weeks in the case of abnormal lie is a reasonable alternative to both expectant management and elective cesarean delivery. External cephalic version has been found to be safe, with close monitoring, and is effective in the majority of cases.[3,14,15] Using such a protocol, Edwards and Nicholson[6] reported 86 of 96 cases delivered vaginally, with fetal compromise detected in only four and no fetal losses.

If external version is unsuccessful or unavailable, if spontaneous rupture of membranes occurs, or if active labor has begun with an abnormal lie, cesarean delivery is the treatment of choice for the potentially viable infant.[1,3,14] There is no place for internal podalic version and breech extraction in the management of transverse or oblique lie or unstable presentation in singleton pregnancies because of the unacceptably high rate of fetal and maternal complications.[2]

A persistent abnormal axial lie, particularly if accompanied by ruptured membranes, also alters the choice of uterine incision at cesarean delivery. Although a low transverse cervical incision has many surgical advantages, up to 25 percent of transverse incisions require vertical extension for delivery of an infant from an abnormal lie to allow access to and atraumatic delivery of the vertex entrapped in the muscular fundus.[3,14] Furthermore, the lower uterine segment is often poorly developed. Deciding on a cesarean delivery to minimize birth trauma, then choosing a transverse uterine incision, which can potentially make fetal extraction more difficult, is not logical. Therefore, when managing a transverse or oblique lie with ruptured membranes or a poorly developed lower segment, a vertical incision is more prudent. Intraoperative cephalic version may allow the use of a low transverse incision, as reported by Pelosi et al., but ruptured membranes or oligohydramnios makes this difficult.[14]

DEFLECTION ATTITUDES

"Attitude" refers to the position of the fetal head in relation to the neck. The normal attitude of the fetal vertex during labor is one of full flexion on the neck, with the fetal chin against the upper chest. Deflexed attitudes include various degrees of deflection or even extension of the fetal head on the neck (Fig. 17-5). Spontaneous conversion to a more normal flexed attitude or further extension of an intermediate deflection to a fully extended position commonly occurs as labor progresses owing to resistance exerted by the bony pelvis and soft tissues. Although safe vaginal delivery is possible in many cases, experience indicates that cesarean delivery is the only appropriate alternative when arrest of progress is observed.

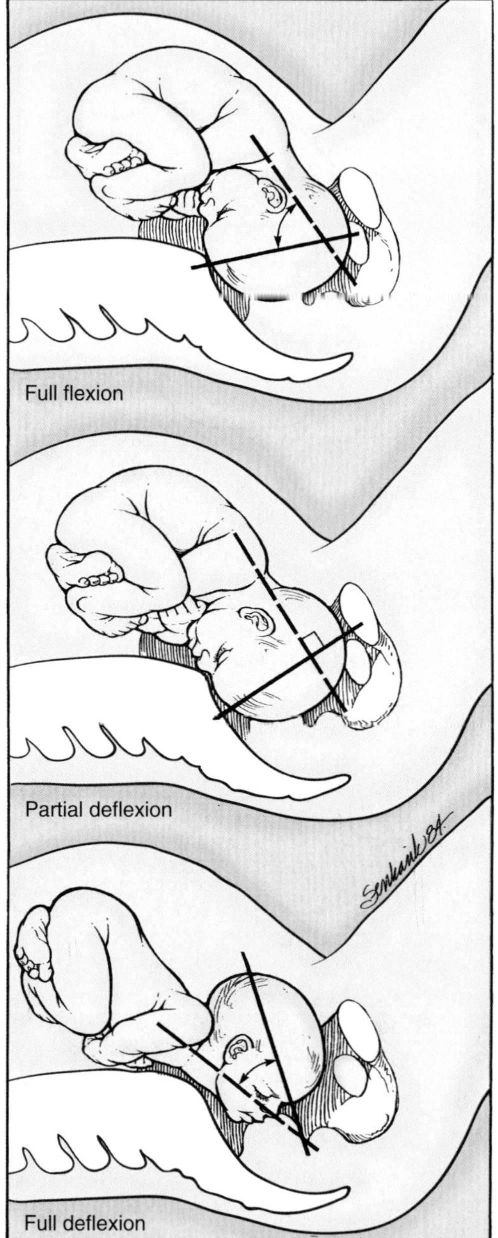

Figure 17-5. The normal "attitude" *(top view)* shows the fetal vertex flexed on the neck. Partial deflexion *(middle view)* shows the fetal vertex intermediate between flexion and extension. Full deflexion *(lower view)* shows the fetal vertex completely extended, with the face presenting.

FACE PRESENTATION

A face presentation is characterized by a longitudinal lie and full extension of the fetal head on the neck, with the occiput against the upper back (Fig. 17-6). The fetal chin (mentum) is chosen as the point of designation during vaginal examination. For example, a fetus presenting by the face whose chin is in the right posterior quadrant of the maternal pelvis would be called a *right mentum posterior* (Fig. 17-7). The reported incidence of face presentation ranges from 0.14 to 0.54 percent, averaging about 0.2 percent, or 1 in 500 live births overall.[8,16–21] Reported perinatal mortality, corrected for nonviable malformations and extreme prematurity, varies from 0.6 percent to 5 percent, averaging about 2 to 3 percent.[22,23]

All clinical factors known to increase the general rate of malpresentation (see the box, "Etiologic Factors in Malpresentation") have been implicated in face presentation, but Browne and Carney emphasized that many infants with a face presentation are malformed.[24] Anencephaly, for instance, is found in about one third of cases of face presentation.[5,25,26] Fetal goiter as well as tumors of the soft tissues of the neck may also cause deflexion of the head. Frequently observed maternal factors include a contracted pelvis or cephalopelvic disproportion in 10 to 40 percent of cases.[17,20,23] In a review of face presentation, Duff found that one of these etiologic factors was found in up to 90 percent of cases.[18]

Early recognition of the face presentation is important, and the diagnosis can be suspected anytime abdominal palpation finds the fetal cephalic prominence on the same side of the maternal abdomen as the fetal back (Fig. 17-8); however, face presentation is more often discovered by vaginal examination. In practice, fewer than 1 in 20 infants with face presentation is diagnosed by abdominal examination.[22] In fact, only half of these infants are found to have a face presentation by any means before the second stage of labor,[20,22,26,27] and half of the remaining cases are undiagnosed until delivery.[20,23] Perinatal mortality may be higher, however, with late diagnosis.[17]

Mechanism of Labor

Knowledge of the early mechanism of labor for face presentation is incomplete. Many infants with a face

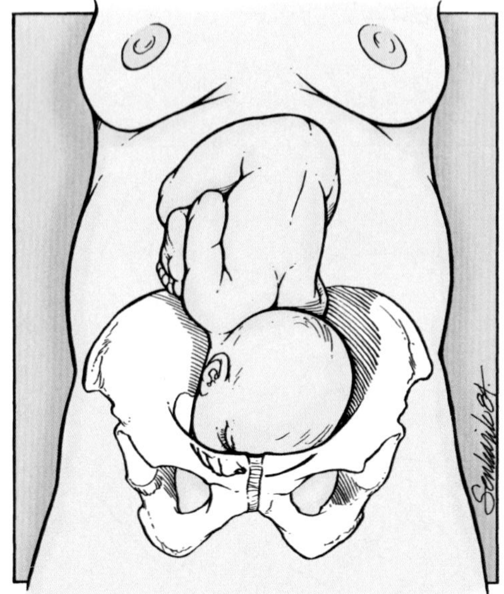

Figure 17-6. This fetus with the vertex completely extended on the neck enters the maternal pelvis in a face presentation. The cephalic prominence would be palpable on the same side of the maternal abdomen as the fetal spine.

presentation probably begin labor in the less extended brow position. With descent into the pelvis, the forces of labor press the fetus against maternal tissues; either flexion or full extension of the head on the spine then often occurs. The labor of a face presentation must include engagement, descent, internal rotation generally

Etiologic Factors in Malpresentation
Maternal
Great parity
Pelvic tumors
Pelvic contracture
Uterine malformation
Fetal
Prematurity
Multiple gestation
Hydramnios
Macrosomia
Hydrocephaly
Trisomies
Anencephaly
Myotonic dystrophy
Placenta previa

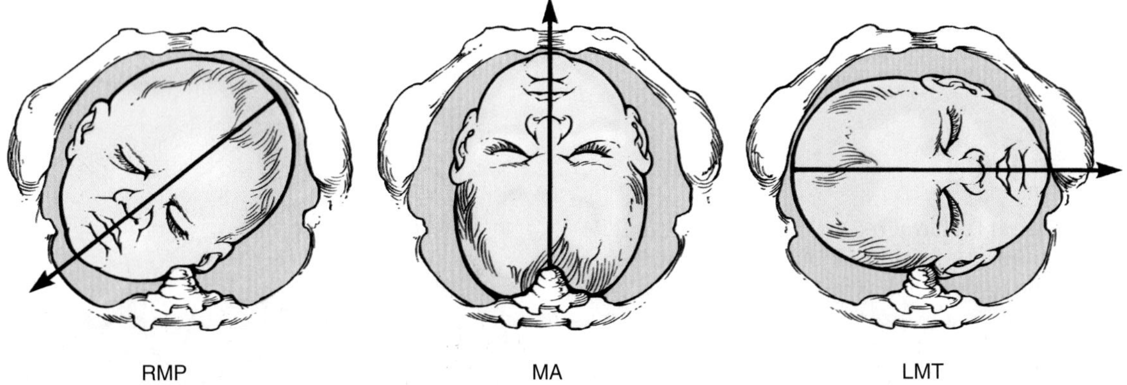

Figure 17-7. The point of designation from digital examination in the case of a face presentation is the fetal chin relative to the maternal pelvis. *Left,* Right mentum posterior (RMP). *Middle,* Mentum anterior (MA). *Right,* Left mentum transverse (LMT).

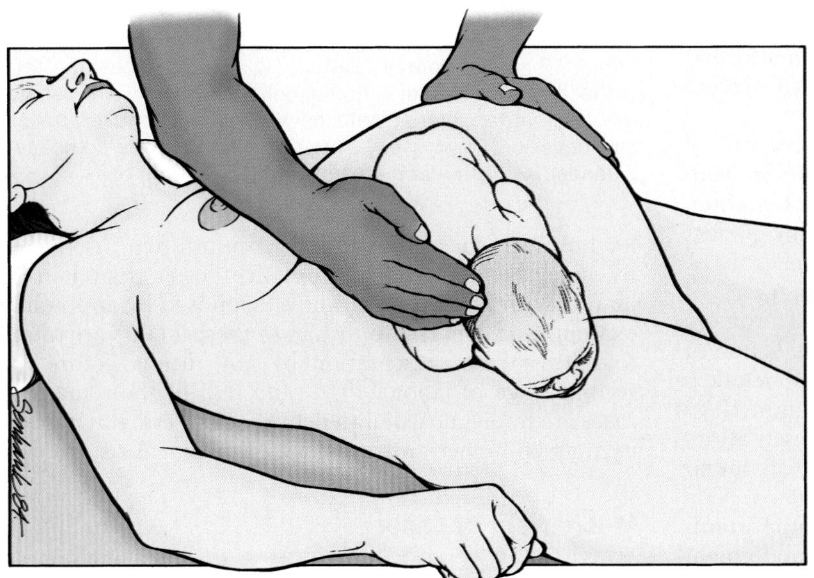

Figure 17-8. Palpation of the maternal abdomen in the case of a face presentation should find the fetal cephalic prominence on the side away from the fetal small parts instead of on the same side as in the case of a normally flexed fetal head.

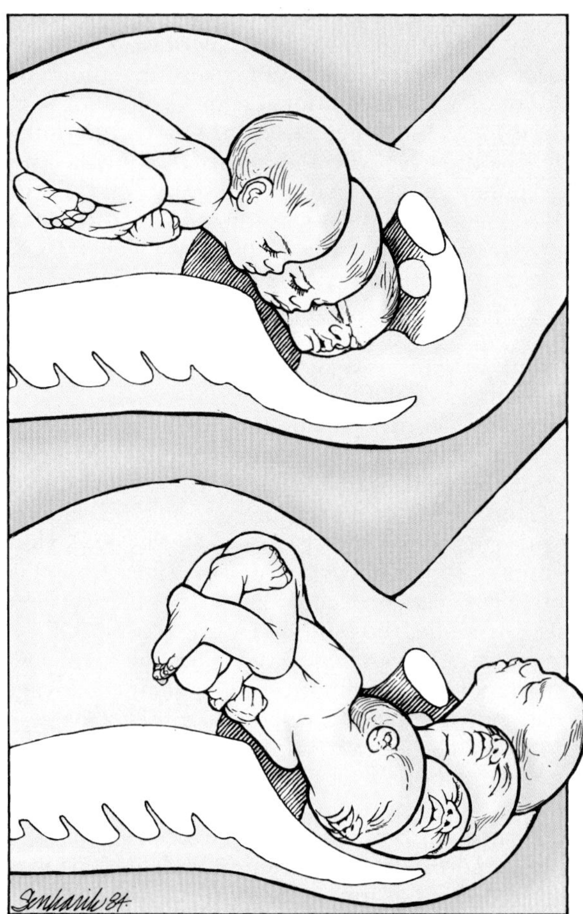

Figure 17-9. Engagement, descent, and internal rotation remain cardinal elements of vaginal delivery in the case of a face presentation, but successful vaginal delivery of a term-size fetus presenting a face generally requires delivery by flexion under the symphysis from a mentum anterior position, as illustrated here.

to a mentum anterior position, and delivery by flexion as the chin passes under the symphysis (Fig. 17-9). However, flexion of the occiput may not always occur. Borrell and Fernstrom[28] have proposed that delivery in the fully extended attitude may be common.

The prognosis for labor with a face presentation depends on the orientation of the fetal chin. At diagnosis, 60 to 80 percent of infants with a face presentation are mentum anterior,[5,20,22,29] 10 to 12 percent are mentum transverse,[5,22,29] and 20 to 25 percent are mentum posterior.[5,20,22,29] Almost all average-sized infants presenting mentum anterior with adequate pelvic dimensions will achieve spontaneous or easily assisted vaginal delivery.[5,22,30,31] Furthermore, most mentum transverse infants will rotate to the mentum anterior position and deliver vaginally, and even 25 to 33 percent of mentum posterior infants will rotate and deliver vaginally in the mentum anterior position.[5,16,20] In a review of 51 cases of persistent face presentation, Schwartz et al.[29] found that the mean birth weight of those infants in mentum posterior who did rotate and deliver vaginally was 3,425 g, compared with 3,792 g for those infants who did not rotate and deliver vaginally. Persistence of mentum posterior with an infant of normal size, however, makes safe vaginal delivery less likely. Overall, 70 to 80 percent of infants with face presentation can be delivered vaginally, either spontaneously or by low forceps, whereas 12 to 30 percent require cesarean delivery.[5,20,22,23] Manual attempts to convert the face to a flexed attitude or to rotate a posterior position to a more favorable mentum anterior are rarely successful and increase both maternal and fetal risks.[16,22,26,32] In 1965, Campbell[22] reported fetal losses of up to 60 percent with internal podalic version and breech extraction for face presentation. Maternal deaths from uterine rupture and trauma after version with extraction have also been documented. Thus, contemporary management through spontaneous delivery or cesarean delivery are the preferred routes for maternal and fetal safety.[16,22,26]

Prolonged labor is a common feature of face presentation and has been associated with an increased number of intrapartum deaths.[5,8,17] Therefore, prompt attention to an arrested labor pattern is recommended. In the case of an average or small fetus, adequate pelvis, and hypotonic labor, oxytocin may be considered. No absolute contraindication to oxytocin augmentation of hypotonic labor in face presentations exists, but an arrest of progress despite adequate labor should call for cesarean delivery.[8]

Worsening of the fetal condition in labor is common. Salzmann et al.[26] observed a 10-fold increase in fetal compromise with face presentation. Several other observers have also found that abnormal fetal heart rate patterns occur more often with face presentation.[16,18] Continuous intrapartum electronic fetal heart rate monitoring of a fetus with face presentation is considered mandatory, but extreme care must be exercised in the placement of an electrode, because ocular or cosmetic damage is possible. If external Doppler heart rate monitoring is inadequate and an internal electrode is considered necessary, placement of the electrode on the fetal chin is often recommended. Cesarean delivery is warranted if a nonreassuring heart rate pattern is identified, even if sufficient progress in labor is occurring.

Safe vaginal delivery may be accomplished in many cases of face presentation, and a trial of labor with careful monitoring of fetal condition and labor progress is not contraindicated unless macrosomia or a small maternal pelvis is identified. However, cesarean delivery has been reported in as many as 60 percent of cases of face presentation.[18,27] If cesarean delivery is warranted, care should be taken to flex the head gently both to accomplish elevation of the head through the hysterotomy incision as well as to avoid potential nerve damage to the neonate. Forced flexion may also result in damage, especially with fetal goiter, or neck tumors.

Laryngeal and tracheal edema resulting from pressures of the birth process might require immediate nasotracheal intubation.[33] Nuchal tumors or simple goiters, fetal anomalies that might have caused the malpresentation, require expert neonatal management.

BROW PRESENTATION

A fetus in a brow presentation occupies a longitudinal axis, with a partially deflexed cephalic attitude, midway between full flexion and full extension (Fig. 17-10).[24] The frontal bones are the point of designation. If the anterior fontanel is on the mother's left side, with the sagittal suture in the transverse pelvic axis, the fetus would be in a left frontum transverse position (Fig. 17-11). The reported incidence of brow presentation varies widely, from 1 in 670 to 1 in 3,433, averaging about 1 in 1,500 deliveries.[34,35] Brow presentation is detected more often in early labor before flexion occurs to a normal attitude. Less frequently, further extension results in a face presentation.

Perinatal mortality corrected for lethal anomalies and very low birth weight varies from 1 to 8 percent.[36] In a study of 88,988 deliveries, corrected perinatal mortality rates for brow presentations depended on the mode of delivery, and a loss rate of 16 percent, the highest in this study, was associated with manipulative vaginal birth.[37]

In general, factors that delay engagement are associated with persistent brow presentation. Cephalopelvic disproportion, prematurity, and great parity are often found and have been implicated in more than 60 percent of cases of persistent brow presentation.[5,35,38,39]

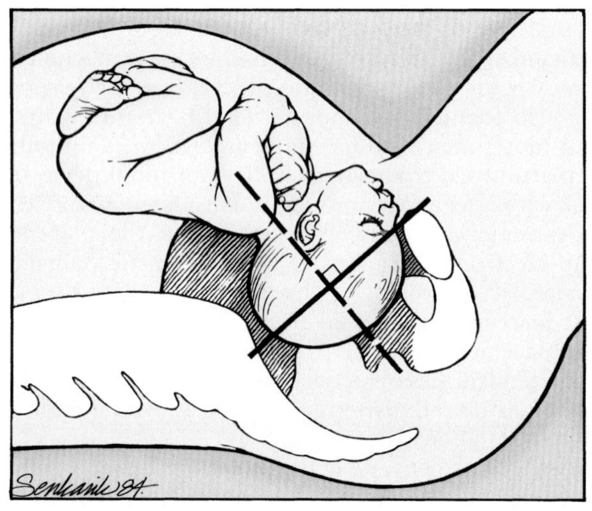

Figure 17-10. This fetus is a brow presentation in a frontum anterior position. The head is in an intermediate deflexion attitude.

Detection of a brow presentation by abdominal palpation is unusual in practice. More often, a brow presentation is detected on vaginal examination. As in the case of a face presentation, diagnosis in labor is more likely. Fewer than 50 percent of brow presentations are detected before the second stage of labor, with most of the remainder undiagnosed until delivery.[34,37–39] Frontum anterior is reportedly the most common position at diagnosis, occurring about twice as often as either transverse or posterior positions. Although the initial position at diagnosis may be of limited prognostic value, Skalley and Kramer[39] reported the cesarean delivery rate to be higher with frontum transverse or frontum posterior than with frontum anterior.

A persistent brow presentation requires engagement and descent of the largest (mento-occipital) diameter or profile of the fetal head.[40] This process is possible only with a large pelvis or a small infant, or both. However, brow presentations convert spontaneously by flexion or further extension to either a vertex or a face presentation and are then managed accordingly.[34,35] The earlier the diagnosis is made, the more likely conversion will occur spontaneously. Fewer than half of fetuses with persistent brow presentations undergo spontaneous vaginal delivery, but in most cases, a trial of labor is not contraindicated.[5,36]

Prolonged labors have been observed in 33 to 50 percent of brow presentations,[5,20,35,38,39] and secondary arrest is not uncommon.[34] Forced conversion of the brow to a more favorable position with forceps is contraindicated,[34,35,38] as are attempts at manual conversion. One unexpected cause of persistent brow presentation may be an open fetal mouth pressed against the vaginal wall, splinting the head and preventing either flexion or extension[28,35] (Fig. 17-12).

In most brow presentations, as with face presentations, minimal manipulation yields the best results if the fetal heart rate pattern remains reassuring.[35,41] Expectant management may be justified only with a large pelvis, a small fetus, and adequate progress, according to one large study.[37] If a brow presentation persists with a large baby, successful vaginal delivery is unlikely, and cesarean delivery may be most prudent.[20]

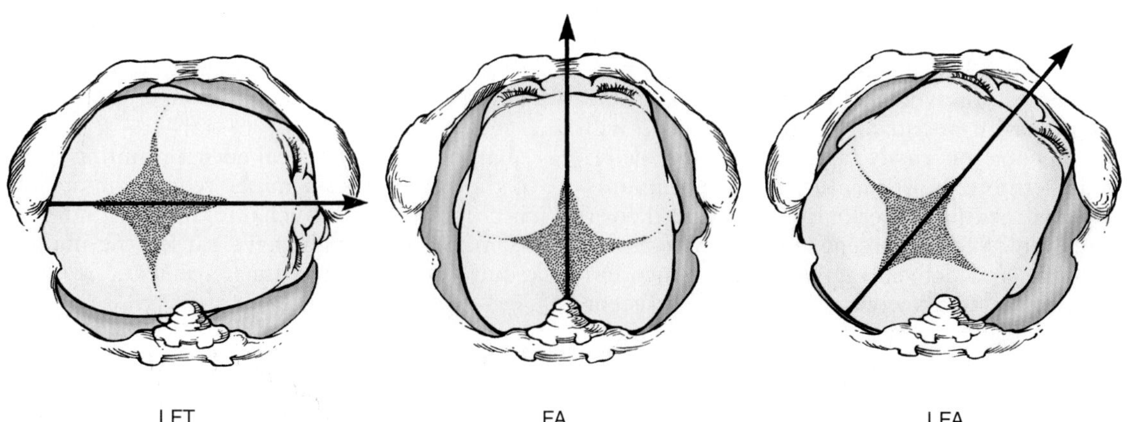

Figure 17-11. In brow presentation, the anterior fontanel (frontum) relative to the maternal pelvis is the point of designation. *Left,* Fetus in left frontum transverse (LFT). *Middle,* Frontum anterior (FA). *Right,* Left frontum anterior (LFA).

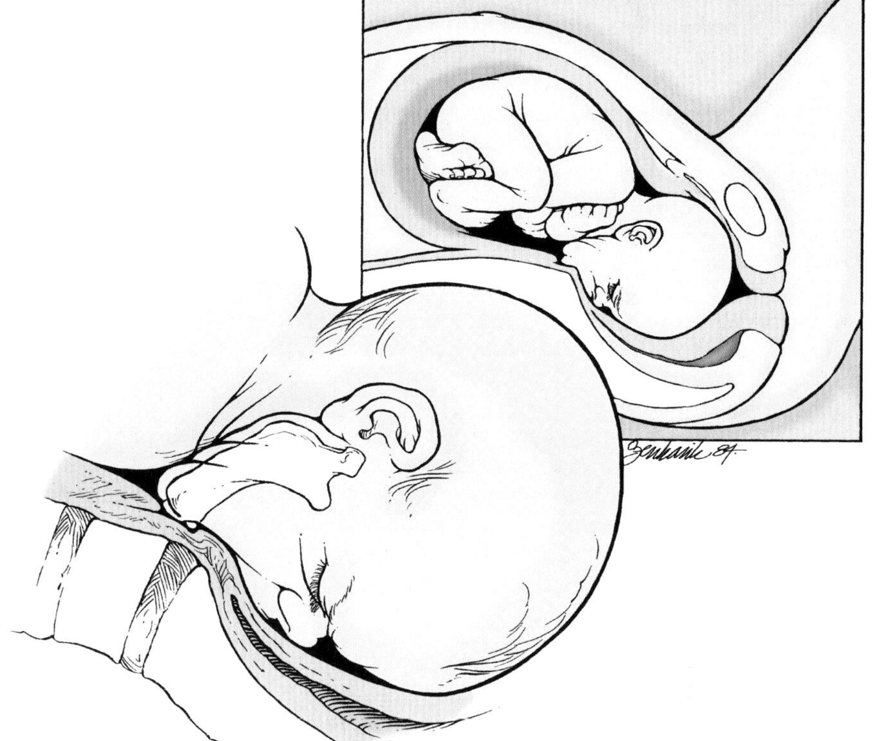

Figure 17-12. The open fetal mouth against the vaginal sidewall may brace the head in the intermediate deflexion attitude as shown here.

Radiographic or computed tomographic (CT) pelvimetry might be helpful. Despite this, one report states that although 91 percent of cases with adequate pelvimetry converted to a vertex or a face and delivered vaginally, 20 percent with some form of pelvic contracture did also.[5] Therefore, regardless of pelvic dimensions, consideration of a trial of labor with careful monitoring of maternal and fetal condition may be appropriate. As in the case of a face presentation, oxytocin may be used cautiously to correct hypotonia, but prompt resumption of progress toward delivery should follow.

COMPOUND PRESENTATION

Whenever an extremity is found prolapsed beside the main presenting fetal part, the situation is referred to as a compound presentation[42] (Fig. 17-13). The reported incidence ranges from 1 in 377 to 1 in 1213 deliveries.[5,42–45] The combination of an upper extremity and the vertex is the most common.

This diagnosis should be suspected with any arrest of labor in the active phase or failure to engage during active labor.[44] Diagnosis is made by vaginal examination by discovery of an irregular mobile tissue mass adjacent to the larger presenting part. Recognition late in labor is common, and as many as 50 percent of persisting compound presentations are not detected until the second stage.[42] Delay in diagnosis may not be detrimental because it is likely that only the persistent cases require intervention.

Although maternal age, race, parity, and pelvic size have been associated with compound presentation, prematurity is the most consistent clinical finding.[5,42–44] The very small premature fetus is at great risk of persistent compound presentation. In late pregnancy, external cephalic version of a fetus in breech position increases the risk of a compound presentation.[46]

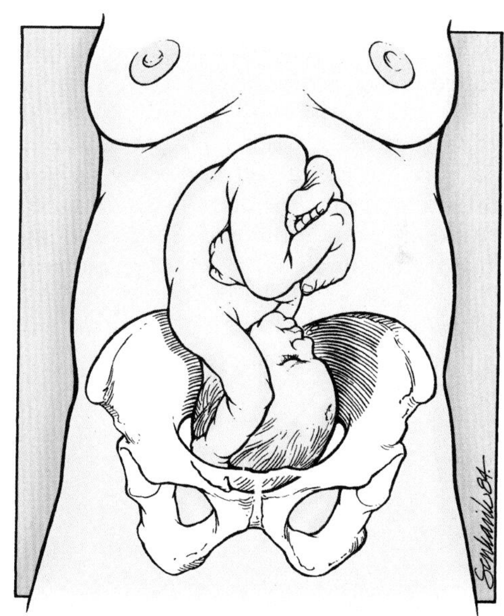

Figure 17-13. The compound presentation of an upper extremity and the vertex illustrated here most often spontaneously resolves with further labor and descent.

Older, uncontrolled studies report elevated perinatal mortality with a compound presentation, with an overall rate of 93 per 1000.[5] Higher loss rates of 17 to 19 percent have been reported when the foot prolapses.[43] As with other malpresentations, fetal risk is directly related to the method of management. A fetal mortality rate of 4.8 percent has been noted if no intervention is required compared with 14.4 percent with intervention other than cesarean delivery. A 30-percent fetal mortality rate has been observed with internal podalic version and breech extraction.[43] These figures may demonstrate selection bias because it is possible that difficult cases were chosen for manipulative intervention. When intervention is necessary, cesarean delivery appears to be the only safe choice.

Fetal risk in compound presentation is specifically associated with birth trauma and cord prolapse. Cord prolapse occurs in 11 to 20 percent of cases, and it is the most frequent single complication of this malpresentation.[5,43,44] Cord prolapse probably occurs because the compound extremity splints the larger presenting part, resulting in an irregular fetal aggregate that incompletely fills the pelvic inlet. In addition to the hypoxic risk of cord prolapse, common fetal morbidity includes neurologic and musculoskeletal damage to the involved extremity. Maternal risks include soft tissue damage and obstetric laceration.

Despite these dangers, labor is not necessarily contraindicated with a compound presentation; however, the prolapsed extremity should not be manipulated.[42–44,47] The accompanying extremity may retract as the major presenting part descends. Seventy-five percent of vertex/upper extremity combinations deliver spontaneously.[5] Occult or undetected cord prolapse is possible, and therefore, continuous electronic fetal heart rate monitoring is recommended.

The primary indications for surgical intervention are cord prolapse, nonreassuring fetal heart rate patterns, and arrest of labor.[5] Cesarean delivery is the only appropriate clinical intervention, because both version extraction and repositioning the prolapsed extremity are associated with adverse outcome and are to be avoided.[42–44] Two to 25 percent of compound presentations require abdominal delivery.[42,44] Protraction of the second stage of labor and dysfunctional labor patterns have been noted to occur more frequently with persistent compound presentation.[42] As in other malpresentations, spontaneous resolution occurs more often and surgical intervention is less frequently necessary in those cases diagnosed early in labor. Small or premature fetuses are more likely to have persistent compound presentations but are also more likely to have a successful vaginal delivery. Persistent compound presentation with parts other than the vertex and hand in combination in a term-sized infant has a poor prognosis for safe vaginal delivery, and cesarean delivery is usually necessary. However, a simple compound presentation (e.g., hand) may be allowed to labor if progressing normally with reassuring fetal status.

BREECH PRESENTATION

The infant presenting as a breech occupies a longitudinal axis with the cephalic pole in the uterine fundus. This presentation occurs in 3 to 4 percent of labors overall, although it is found in 7 percent of pregnancies at 32 weeks and in 25 percent of pregnancies of less than 28 weeks' duration.[48] The three types of breech are noted in Table 17-1. The infant in the frank breech position is flexed at the hips with extended knees. The complete breech is flexed at both joints, and the footling breech has one or both hips partially or fully extended (Fig. 17-14).

The diagnosis of breech presentation may be made by abdominal palpation or vaginal examination and

Table 17-1. Breech Categories

TYPE	OVERALL PERCENT OF BREECHES	RISK (%) PROLAPSE	PREMATURE
Frank breech	48–73[31,46,48,54,93]	0.5[50]	38[48]
Complete	4.6–11.5[31,48,54,93]	4–6[50]	12[48]
Footling	12–38[31,48,54]	15–18[50]	50[48]

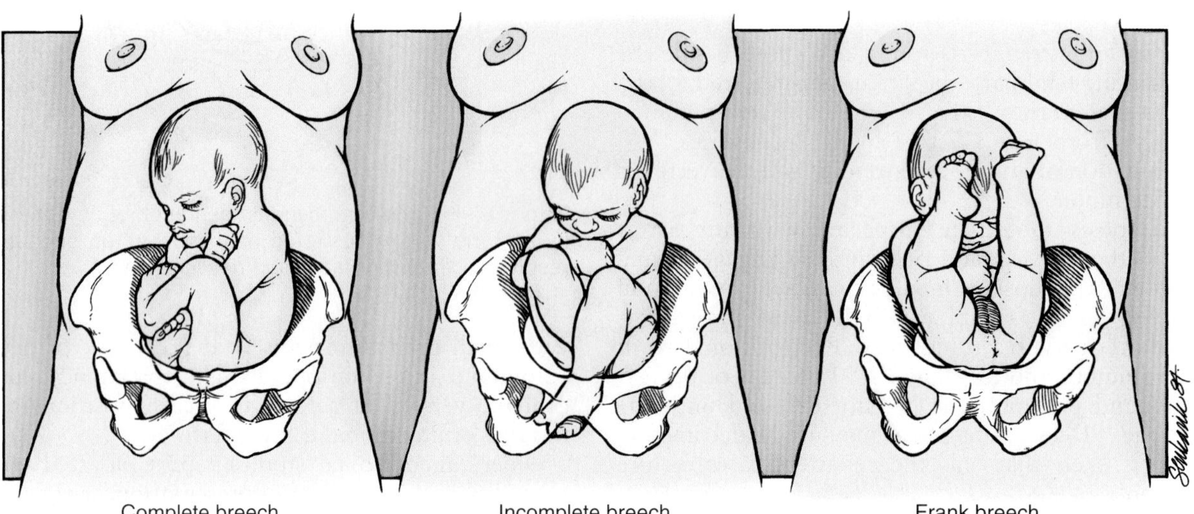

Complete breech Incomplete breech Frank breech

Figure 17-14. The complete breech is flexed at the hips and flexed at the knees. The incomplete breech shows incomplete deflexion of one or both knees or hips. The frank breech is flexed at the hips and extended at the knees.

confirmed by ultrasound. Prematurity, fetal malformation, müllerian anomalies, and polar placentation are commonly observed causative factors. High rates of breech presentation are noted in certain fetal genetic disorders, including trisomies 13, 18, and 21; Potter's syndrome; and myotonic dystrophy.[49] Thus, conditions that alter fetal muscular tone and mobility such as increased and decreased amniotic fluid, for example, also increase the frequency of breech presentation.

Mechanism and Conduct of Labor and Vaginal Delivery

The two most important elements for the safe conduct of vaginal breech delivery are continuous electronic fetal heart rate monitoring and noninterference until spontaneous delivery of the breech to the umbilicus has occurred. Early in labor, the capability for immediate cesarean delivery should be established. Anesthesia should be available, the operating room readied, and appropriate informed consent obtained (discussed later). Two obstetricians should be in attendance as well as a pediatric team. Appropriate training and experience with vaginal breech delivery are fundamental to success. The instrument table should be prepared in the customary manner, with the addition of Piper forceps and extra towels. There is no contraindication to epidural analgesia in labor; many even view epidural anesthesia as an asset in the control and conduct of the second stage.

The infant presenting in the frank breech position usually enters the pelvic inlet in one of the diagonal pelvic diameters (Fig. 17-15). Engagement has occurred when the bitrochanteric diameter of the fetus has progressed beyond the plane of the pelvic inlet, although by vaginal examination, the presenting part may be palpated only at -2 to -4 station (out of 5). As the breech descends and encounters the levator ani muscular sling, internal rotation usually occurs to bring the bitrochanteric diameter into the anteroposterior (AP) axis of the pelvis. The point of designation in a breech labor is the fetal sacrum and, therefore, when the bitrochanteric diameter is in the AP axis of the pelvis, the fetal sacrum will lie in the transverse pelvic diameter (Fig. 17-16).

If normal descent occurs, the breech will present at the outlet and begin to emerge, first as a sacrum transverse, then rotating to sacrum anterior. Crowning occurs when the bitrochanteric diameter passes under the pubic

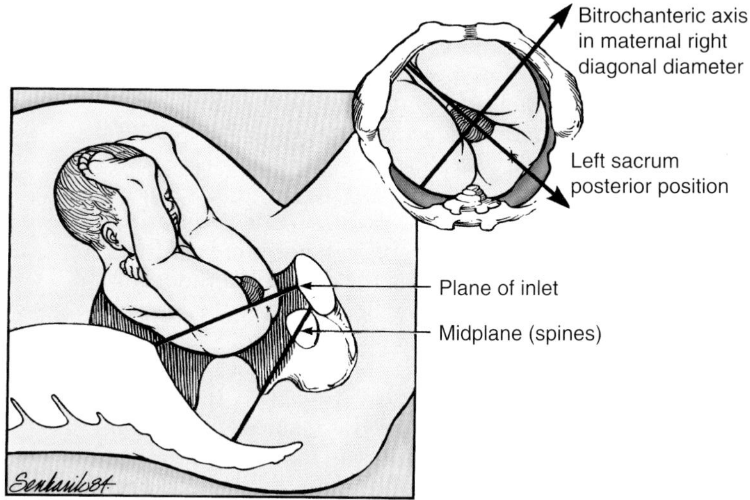

Figure 17-15. The breech typically enters the inlet with the bitrochanteric diameter aligned with one of the diagonal diameters, with the sacrum as the point of designation in the other diagonal diameter. This is a case of left sacrum posterior (LSP).

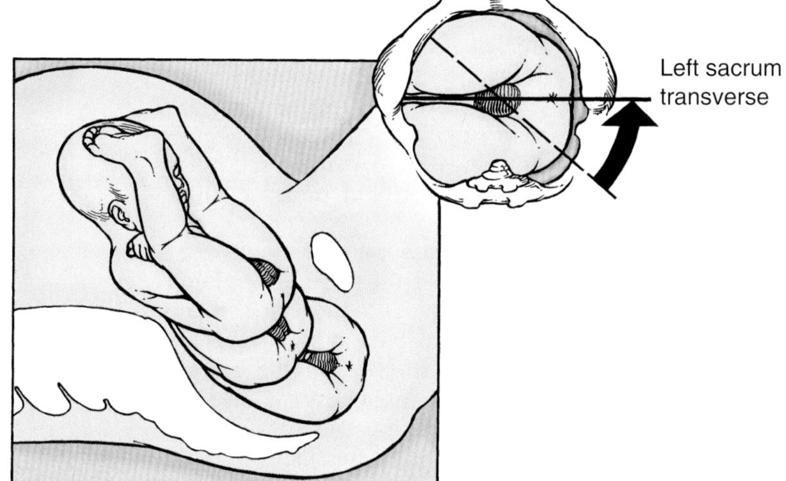

Figure 17-16. With labor and descent, the bitrochanteric diameter generally rotates toward the anteroposterior axis and the sacrum toward the transverse.

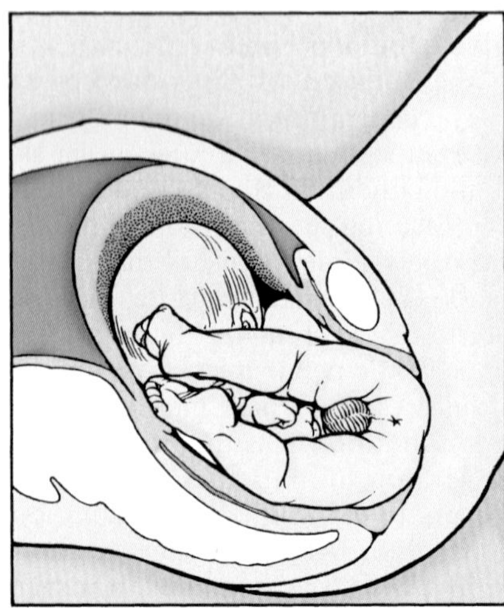

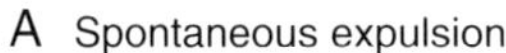

A Spontaneous expulsion

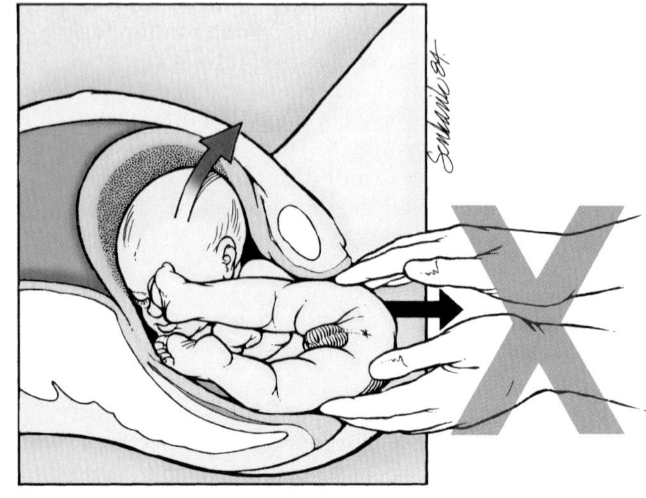

B Undesired deflexion

Figure 17-17. The fetus emerges spontaneously *(A),* whereas uterine contractions maintain cephalic flexion. Premature aggressive traction *(B)* encourages deflexion of the fetal vertex and increases the risk of head entrapment or nuchal arm entrapment.

symphysis. An episiotomy may facilitate delivery but should be delayed until crowning begins. As the infant emerges, rotation begins, usually toward a sacrum anterior position. This direction of rotation may reflect the greater capacity of the hollow of the posterior pelvis to accept the fetal chest and small parts. It is important to emphasize that operator intervention is not yet needed or helpful other than possibly to perform the episiotomy and encourage maternal expulsive efforts.

Premature or aggressive assistance may adversely affect the delivery in at least two ways. First, complete cervical dilatation must be sustained for sufficient duration to retard retraction of the cervix and entrapment of the after-coming fetal head. Rushing the delivery of the trunk may result in cervical retraction. Second, the safe descent and delivery of the breech infant must be the result of uterine and maternal expulsive forces only, in order to maintain neck flexion. Any traction by the provider in an effort to speed delivery would encourage deflexion of the neck and result in the presentation of the larger occipitofrontal fetal cranial profile to the pelvic inlet (Fig. 17-17). Such an event could be catastrophic. Rushed delivery also increases the risk of a nuchal arm, with one or both arms trapped behind the head above the pelvic inlet. Entrapment of a nuchal arm makes safe vaginal delivery much more difficult, because it dramatically increases the aggregate size of delivering fetal parts that must pass through the birth canal. Safe breech delivery of an average-sized infant, therefore, depends predominantly on maternal expulsive forces, and patience, not traction, from the provider.

As the frank breech emerges further, the fetal thighs are typically flexed firmly against the fetal abdomen, often splinting and protecting the umbilicus and cord. The Pinard maneuver may be needed to facilitate delivery of the legs in a frank breech presentation. After the umbilicus has been reached, pressure is applied to the medial aspect of the knee, which causes flexion and subsequent delivery of the lower leg. Simultaneous to this, the fetal pelvis is rotated away from that side (Fig. 17-18). This results in external rotation of the thigh at the hip, flexion

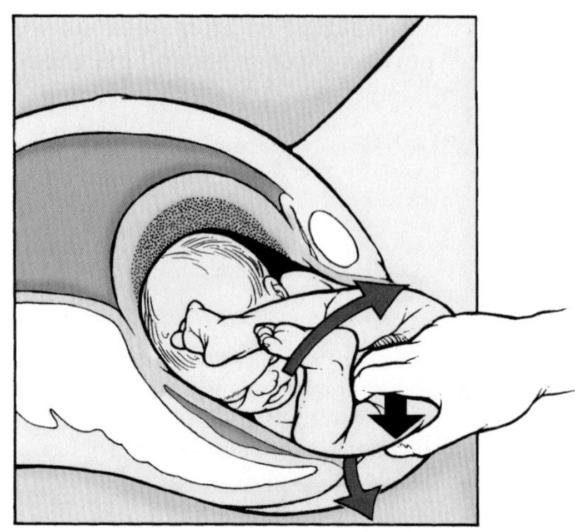

A

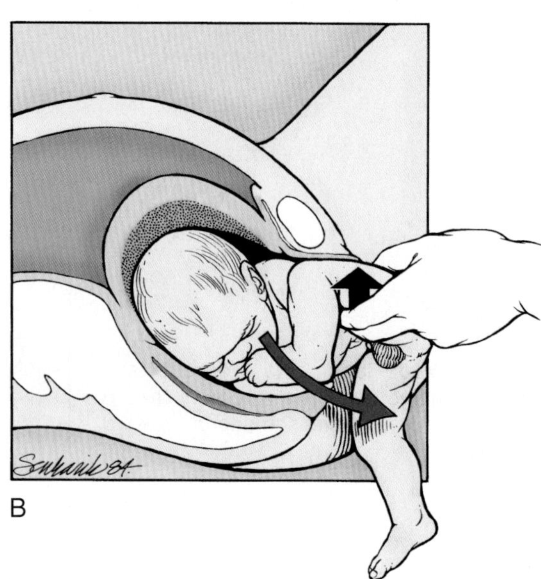

B

Figure 17-18. After spontaneous expulsion to the umbilicus, external rotation of each thigh *(A)* combined with opposite rotation of the fetal pelvis results in flexion of the knee and delivery of each leg *(B).*

of the knee, and delivery of one leg at a time. The dual movement of counterclockwise rotation of the fetal pelvis as the operator externally rotates the right thigh, and clockwise rotation of the fetal pelvis as the operator externally rotates the fetal left thigh is most effective in facilitating delivery. The fetal trunk is then wrapped with a towel to provide secure support of the body while further descent results from expulsive forces from the mother. The operator primarily facilitates the delivery of the fetus by guiding the body through the introitus. The operator is not applying outward traction on the fetus that might result in deflexion of the fetal head or nuchal arm.

When the scapulae appear at the outlet, the operator may slip a hand over the fetal shoulder from the back (Fig. 17-19), follow the humerus, and with movement from medial to lateral, sweep first one and then the other arm across the chest and out over the perineum. Gentle rotation of the fetal trunk counterclockwise assists delivery of the right arm, and clockwise rotation assists delivery of the left arm (turning the body "into" the arm). This accomplishes delivery of the arms by drawing them across the fetal chest in a fashion similar to that used for delivery of the legs (Fig. 17-20). Once both arms have been delivered, if the vertex has remained flexed on the neck, the chin and face will appear at the outlet, and the airway may be cleared and suctioned (Fig. 17-21).

With further maternal expulsive forces alone, spontaneous controlled delivery of the fetal head often occurs. If not, delivery may be accomplished with a simple manual effort to maximize flexion of the vertex using pressure on the fetal maxilla (not mandible), the Mauriceau-Smellie-Veit maneuver, along with suprapubic pressure (Credé's maneuver) and gentle downward traction (Fig. 17-22). Although maxillary pressure facilitates flexion, the main force effecting delivery remains the mother.

Alternatively, the operator may apply Piper forceps to the after-coming head. The application requires *very slight* elevation of the fetal trunk by the assistant, while the operator kneels and applies the Piper forceps directly to the fetal head in the pelvis. The position of the operator for applying the forceps is depicted in Figure 17-23, which also demonstrates how *excessive* elevation by the assistant may potentially cause harm to the neonate. Hyperextension of the fetal neck from excessive eleva-

A

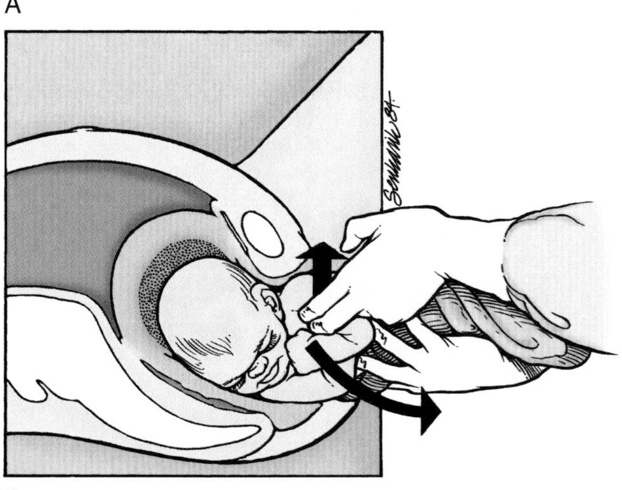

B

Figure 17-19. When the scapulae appear under the symphysis, the operator reaches over the left shoulder, sweeps the arm across the chest *(A)*, and delivers the arm *(B)*.

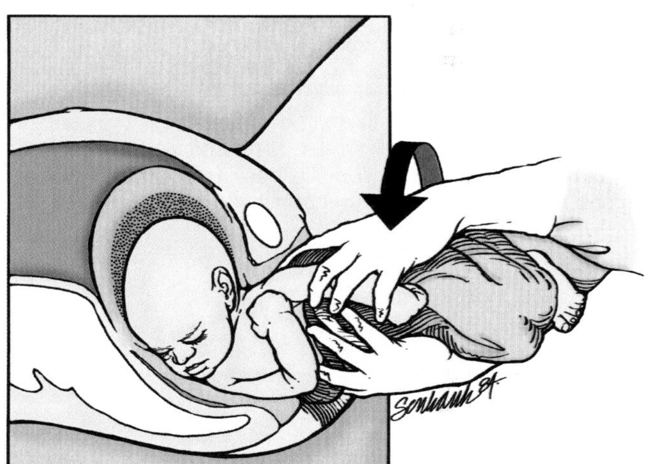

Figure 17-20. Gentle rotation of the shoulder girdle facilitates delivery of the right arm.

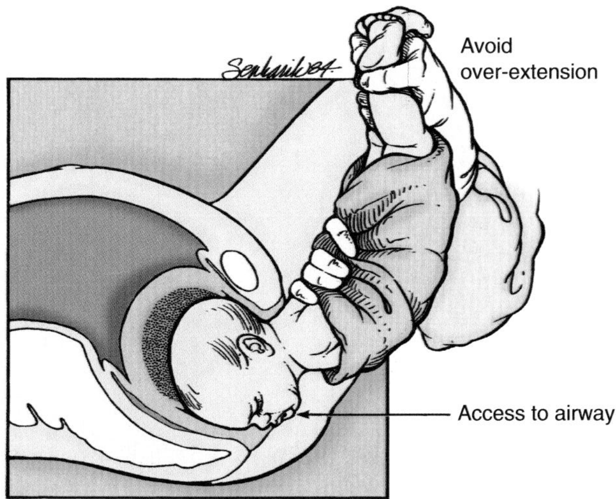

Figure 17-21. Following delivery of the arms, the fetus is wrapped in a towel for control and slightly elevated. The fetal face and airway may be visible over the perineum. Excessive elevation of the trunk is avoided.

tion of the fetal trunk, shown in Figure 17-23, should be avoided.

Piper forceps are characterized by absence of pelvic curvature. This modification allows *direct* application to the fetal head and avoids conflict with the fetal body that would occur with the application of standard instruments from below. The forceps are inserted into the vagina from beneath the fetus. The blade to be placed on the maternal left is held by the handle in the operator's left hand and the blade inserted with the operator's right hand in the vagina along the left maternal sidewall and placed against the right fetal parietal bone. The handle of the right blade is then held in the operator's right hand and inserted by the left hand along the right maternal sidewall and placed against the left fetal parietal bone. Gentle downward traction on the forceps with the fetal trunk supported on the forceps shanks results in controlled delivery of the vertex (Fig. 17-24). Forceps application controls the fetal head and prevents extension of the head on the neck. Routine use of Piper forceps to the after-coming head may be advisable both to ensure control of the delivery and to maintain optimal operator proficiency in anticipation of deliveries that may require their use.

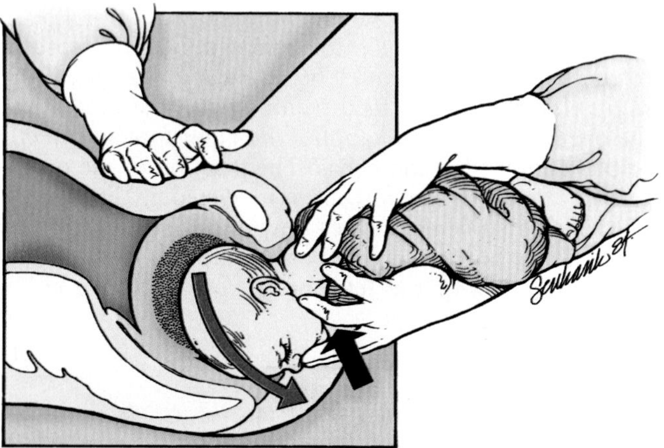

Figure 17-22. Cephalic flexion is maintained by pressure *(heavy arrow)* on the fetal maxilla (not mandible!). Often, delivery of the head is easily accomplished with continued expulsive forces from above and gentle downward traction.

Arrest of spontaneous progress in labor with adequate uterine contractions necessitates consideration of cesarean delivery. Any evidence of fetal compromise or sustained cord compression on the basis of continuous electronic fetal monitoring also requires consideration of cesarean delivery. Vaginal interventions directed at facilitating delivery of the breech that is complicated by an arrest of spontaneous progress are discouraged, because fetal and maternal morbidity and mortality are both greatly increased. However, if labor is deemed to be hypotonic by internally monitored uterine pressures, oxytocin is not contraindicated.[50–52]

Mechanisms of descent and delivery of the incomplete and the complete breech are not unlike those used for the frank breech described earlier; at least one leg may not require attention. The risk of cord prolapse or entangle-

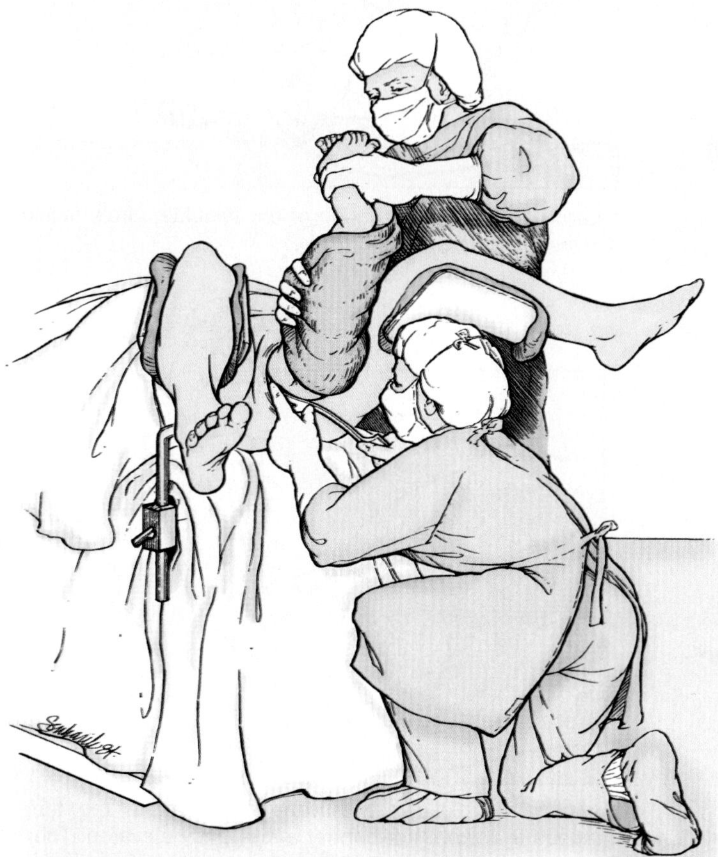

Figure 17-23. Demonstration of INCORRECT assistance during the application of Piper forceps; the assistant hyperextends the fetal neck. Positioning as such increases the risk for neurologic injury.

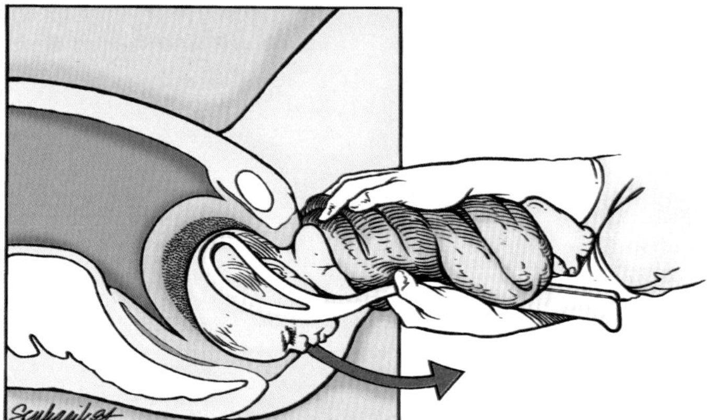

Figure 17-24. The fetus may be laid on the forceps and delivered with gentle downward traction, as illustrated here.

ment is greater, and hence, the possibility of emergency cesarean delivery is increased. Furthermore, incomplete and complete breeches may not be as effective as cervical dilators as either the vertex or the larger aggregate profile of the thighs and buttocks of the frank breech. Thus, the risk of entrapment of the after-coming head is increased, and as a result, primary cesarean delivery is often advocated for nonfrank breech presentations. However, the randomized trial of Gimovsky et al.[53] found the vaginal delivery of the non-frank breech to be reasonably safe as well.

Management of the Term Breech

Debate remains over the proper management of the term breech. Much of what we know is derived from relatively few studies of varied methodologies, patient populations, and multiple retrospective cohort analyses, which are subject to bias. These reports indicate that the perinatal mortality rate for the vaginally delivered breech appears to be greater than for its cephalic counterpart; to what degree and why being cornerstones of the debate. The reported perinatal mortality rate associated with breech presentation has varied from 9 to 25 percent in older series,[54,55] which is three to five times that of the cephalic fetus at term.[56–58] But the excess deaths associated with breech presentation are largely due to lethal anomalies and complications of prematurity, both of which are found more frequently among breech infants. Excluding anomalies and extreme prematurity, the corrected perinatal mortality reported by some investigators approaches zero regardless of the method of delivery, whereas others find that even with exclusion of these factors, the term breech infant has been found to be at higher risk for birth trauma and asphyxia.[59–62] To date, only three randomized trials have been reported.[50,53,62] Therefore, conclusions regarding safety of breech delivery from a fetal standpoint vary. A summary of some of the reported complications is listed in Table 17-2. Overall, consideration of a potential breech vaginal delivery often involves bias, and yet must be mutually agreed upon by the patient and the physician. A cooperative, compliant patient makes the most appropriate candidate for breech vaginal delivery. Complete informed consent is essential.

Table 17-2. Incidence of Complications Seen with Breech Presentation

Complication	Incidence
Intrapartum fetal death	Increased 16 fold[65,66]
Perinatal mortality	1.3%[62]
Intrapartum asphyxia	Increased 3.8 fold[73,77]
Cord prolapse	Increased 5 to 20 fold[48,50,55] 1.3%[62]
Birth trauma	Increased 13 fold[48] 1.4%[62]
Dystocia, difficulty delivering head	4.6[62] to 8.8%[48]
Spinal cord injuries with extended head	21%[30,113]
Major anomalies	6–18%[55,73,77]
Prematurity	16–33%[31,54,60,64,68,96,97]
Hyperextension of head	5%[112]
Fetal heart rate abnormalities	15.2%[62]

Route of Delivery for the Term Frank or Complete Breech

The cesarean delivery rate for breech presentation began to approach 90 percent in some centers in the mid-1970s without a consequent proportionate drop in perinatal mortality.[63–65] Maternal mortality is clearly higher with cesarean delivery, ranging from 0.2 to 0.43 percent.[50,66] Maternal morbidity is also higher with abdominal delivery. Some institutions reported a 50-percent incidence of postcesarean maternal morbidity compared with as little as 5 percent with vaginal delivery.[50,67] In an attempt to balance both maternal and fetal risks, plans were proposed to select appropriate candidates for a trial of labor.

In 1965, Zatuchni and Andros retrospectively analyzed 182 breech births, of which 25 infants had poor outcomes.[68] Therefore, these investigators devised a score based on six clinical variables at the time of admission (Table 17-3) that identified those patients destined to manifest difficulties in labor for whom prompt and appropriate interventions could be made. The score used parity, gestational age, estimated weight, prior successful breech vaginal delivery, dilation and station to ascertain likelihood of successful vaginal delivery. However, the parturient herself could increase the score by presenting

Table 17-3. Zatuchni-Andros System

Factor	0	1	2
Parity	Nullipara	Multipara	Multipara
Gestational age	39	38	37
Estimated fetal weight	8 lb	7–8 lb	7 lb
Previous breech	No	One	Two
Dilatation	2	3	4 or more
Station	−3 or >	−2	−1 or less

From Zatuchni GI, Andros GJ: Prognostic index for vaginal delivery in breech presentation at term. Am J Obstet Gynecol 93:237, 1965, with permission.

later in labor; other factors that affect the score are less modifiable. At least three subsequent prospective studies applied the Zatuchni-Andros system and found it to be both sensitive and accurate in selecting candidates for successful vaginal delivery.[69–71] A Zatuchni-Andros score of less than 4 in these studies accurately predicted poor outcomes in patients with infants presenting as a breech. Furthermore, in applying the scoring system, only 21 to 27 percent of patients failed to qualify for a trial of labor.[69,70] Previous breech delivery, one of the items scored in the Zatuchni-Andros system, has a significant odds ratio (OR) for recurrence of breech (4.32, 95-percent confidence interval [CI], 4.08 to 4.59) after one breech delivery, and up to 28.1 (95 percent CI, 12.2 to 64.8) after three. This study did not, however, control for recurrent causes of breech presentation such as uterine malformations and abnormal placentation.[72]

Because most reports of breech delivery are of level II to III evidence, their validity and, most importantly, universal applicability may be questioned. Many data were gathered before electronic fetal heart rate monitoring became commonplace. Until 2000, only one randomized trial (level I evidence) had examined term frank breech and method of delivery.[50] Improved perinatal survival had been reported for abdominally delivered breeches, and there is some evidence, although inconsistent, that the method of delivery may also impact on the quality of survival.[55,60,62,73–75] Functional neurologic defects were found by 2 years of age in 24 percent of breech infants born vaginally but only in 2.5 percent of those breech weight- and age-matched infants born by cesarean delivery.[76] However, in comparing 175 breech infants having a 94-percent cesarean delivery rate with 595 historical controls having a 22-percent rate of abdominal delivery, Green et al.[77] found no significant differences in outcome. Neurologic outcomes were reviewed for 239 of 348 infants delivered from breech position.[78] Examinations performed at 3 to 10 years of age showed no statistically significant neurologic differences between neonates delivered by vaginal breech versus matched vertex controls. Thus, these authors concluded that breech outcomes relate to degree of prematurity, maternal pregnancy complications, and fetal malformations, as well as birth trauma or asphyxia.

Pelvimetry is frequently employed when deciding to allow trial of labor in a breech presenting fetus. Clinical pelvimetry is an acceptable technique and can be used to determine the dimensions of the midpelvis and the outlet, and the inlet by way of surrogate measurement (the obstetric conjugate). The reader is referred to the Intrapartum Care section, in Chapter 12 on normal labor and delivery for discussion and demonstration of clinical pelvimetry. Radiographic pelvimetry has been included in the management of the breech presentation with little objective validation. Regardless, it is expected to predict successful vaginal delivery when adequate pelvic dimensions are present. There are at least four techniques for pelvimetry that are presently in common usage worldwide, including conventional plain film radiography using up to three films, CT with up to three views (lateral, AP, and axial slice), magnetic resonance imaging (MRI), and digital fluorography, not presently used in the United States. MRI is the only technique not associated with radiation exposure, and CT pelvimetry using a single lateral view results in the lowest exposure dose.[79] Air gap technique with conventional radiography will lower the radiation dosage. Current trends show a move toward the lower dose CT techniques of up to three images.[80]

Management of the Breech

Trial of labor may be considered if
- Estimated fetal weight (EFW) = 2,000 to 3,800 g
- Frank breech
- Adequate pelvis
- Flexed fetal head
- Fetal monitoring
- Zatuchni-Andros score ≥4
- Ripid cesarean possible
- Good progress maintained in labor
- Experience and training available
- Informed consent possible

Cesarean delivery may be prudent if
- EFW <1,500 or >4,000 g
- Footling presentation
- Small pelvis
- Hyperextended fetal head
- Zatuchni-Andros score <4
- Absence of expertise
- Nonreassuring fetal heart rate pattern
- Arrest of progress

The clinician must possess the necessary training and experience to offer a patient with a persistent breech presentation a trial of labor. Furthermore, the relationship between the patient and the clinician should be well established and the discussions of risks and benefits must be objective and nondirective with accurate documentation of the discussion. If any of these factors are lacking, cesarean delivery becomes the safer choice. However, even if a clinician has made the choice that he or she will never prospectively offer a patient with breech presentation a trial of labor, the burden of responsibility to know and understand the mechanism and management of a breech delivery is not relieved. No one active in obstetrics will avoid the occasional emergency breech delivery. Regular review of principles, and practice with simulations using a mannequin and model pelvis with an experienced colleague, can increase the skills and improve the performance of anyone facing such an emergency.

Factors that impact the decision to deliver a breech vaginally or by cesarean section are listed in the box, "Management of the Breech." The obvious implication of the dramatically diminished experience in training programs with vaginal breech delivery is that inexperience itself will constitute an indication for cesarean delivery. Certainly, in no case should a woman with an infant presenting as a breech be allowed to labor unless (1) anesthesia coverage is immediately available, (2) cesarean delivery can be undertaken promptly, (3) continuous fetal heart rate monitoring is used, and (4) the delivery is attended by a pediatrician and two obstetricians, of whom at least one is experienced with vaginal breech birth.

THE TERM BREECH TRIAL

One of the most influential publications of the last decade was the multicenter prospective study called the Term Breech Trial. The impetus for this investigation was a series of retrospective studies that demonstrated increased morbidity and mortality of neonates after vaginal breech delivery including neonatal intensive care unit admission, hyperbilirubinemia, bone fracture, intracranial hemorrhage, neonatal depression,[67] convulsions, and death.[81] Other studies, however, found that emergent cesarean delivery was also associated with poor neonatal outcomes. Irion et al.[82] reported similarly poor neonatal outcomes from cesarean deliveries of 705 singleton breeches, and concluded that as a result of the increased *maternal* morbidity associated with cesarean birth, delivery of the breech by cesarean section was not firmly indicated. This opinion was supported by Brown et al.[52] in their prospective case series, noting that the corrected perinatal mortality rate did not differ for neonates weighing ≥ 1,500 g.

In October 2000, the first results from the Term Breech Trial were published.[62] Overall, 2,088 patients from 121 centers in 26 countries with varied national perinatal mortality statistics, according to the World Health Organization, were enrolled in the study, with random assignment of 1041 to the planned cesarean delivery group, and 1,042 to the planned vaginal delivery group. The data were analyzed by the intention to treat method, and 941/1,041 (90.4 percent) and 591/1,042 (56.7 percent) delivered by their intended route of delivery, cesarean section and vaginal birth, respectively. Intrapartum events, including cord prolapse and fetal heart rate abnormalities, occurred at rates similar to prior studies. Maternal and fetal/neonatal short-term (immediate, 6 weeks, and 3 months) and long-term (2-year) outcome data were presented in this and subsequent reports. For both countries with low and high perinatal mortality rates (PMR), the occurrence of perinatal mortality, or serious neonatal morbidity (defined within the report) was significantly lower in the planned cesarean delivery group than the planned vaginal delivery group (relative risk [RR] = 0.33 [0.19–0.56], $p < 0.0001$). In countries with an already low PMR, there was a proportionately greater risk reduction in PMR in the planned cesarean delivery. The effects of operator experience and prolonged labor did not affect the direction of the risk reduction and marginally affected the amplitude. No differences existed in maternal mortality or serious maternal morbidity between the groups.[62]

The effects on the correlation between labor and delivery factors were assessed in a separate regression analysis, using only delivery mode in one regression, and only labor factors including all other variables, such as fetal monitoring, length of labor, and medications in the other. Mode of delivery and birth weight were both significantly associated with adverse fetal outcome, without a significant degree of interaction of these variables. Essentially, smaller infants (<2,800 g) were at greatest risk (OR 2.13[1.2–3.8] $p = 0.01$). Birth weights greater than 3,500 g showed a trend toward more adverse outcomes, but the trend did not reach significance. The analysis of the labor data shows a "dose response relationship between the progression of labour and the risk of adverse perinatal outcome," such that a prelabor cesarean delivery is associated with the lowest rates of adverse outcome compared with vaginal breech delivery.[83] Maternal outcomes at 3 months showed a reduced rate (RR = 0.62, 0.41 to 0.93) of urinary incontinence in the planned cesarean delivery group,[84] but 2 years after delivery, no differences in urinary incontinence or breastfeeding, medical, sexual, social, pain, or reproductive issues, as outlined in the text, existed.[85] Neonatal outcomes at 2 years showed no difference in mortality rates or neurodevelopmental delay between the planned cesarean section and planned vaginal delivery groups.[86] Thus, the term breech trial can be summarized as follows: If a trial of labor is attempted and is successful, babies born by planned vaginal delivery have a small but significant risk of dying or sustaining a debilitating insult in the short term. If they survive, there is no difference in the mortality rate or in the presence of developmental delay when compared with those children born by planned cesarean delivery.

The worldwide repercussions of the Term Breech Trial are still being realized. Eighty of the collaborating centers in 23 of 26 countries responded to a follow-up questionnaire regarding change in practice patterns after the results of the Term Breech Trial were published. A plurality stated that practice had changed (92.5 percent). Eighty five percent of respondents reported that an analysis of relative costs would not affect the continued implementation of a policy of planned cesarean delivery for the breech at term.[87]

A Dutch study examining the effects on delivery statistics and outcomes following the Term Breech Trial showed an increase in the cesarean delivery rate for the term breech from 50 to 80 percent, which was associated with a concomitant reduction in perinatal mortality from 0.35 to 0.18 percent.[88]

The total cesarean delivery rate in the United States in 2004 was 29.1 percent of all deliveries.[89] In 1978, the rate of cesarean deliveries in the United States was 24.4 percent of deliveries, with a drastic variation in rates in the intervening years. The 1981 National Institutes of Health Consensus Report found that 12 percent of cesarean deliveries in 1978 were performed for breech presentation and that this indication contributed 10 to 15 percent to the overall rise in the rate of cesarean births. At least a portion of the increase in cesarean delivery rates is a response to the perceived risk of morbidity and mortality associated with the breech presentation.[62–64,77] In the United States, the cesarean delivery rate for breech presentation increased from 11.6 to 79.1 percent between 1970 and 1985.[77,90] Comparing the U.S. cesarean delivery rates from 1998 and 2002, before and after the Term Breech Trial's publication, one notes a marked increase in the rates for cesarean section: 21.2 percent of all live births in 1998, compared to 26.1 percent in 2002, and 29.1 percent in 2004. Both rates of primary and repeat cesarean deliveries increased. This may be in part because of the staggering number of multiple births and their related degree of prematurity, the relative reduction in vaginal birth after cesarean section,[89] and the self-fulfilling prophecy of lack of experience owing to increasing trends toward cesarean delivery for breech, leaving a void of experienced operators to perform breech vaginal deliveries (see Chapter 19). The rates for cesarean delivery for breech presentation showed an increase over this period from 84.2 percent in 1998 compared with 86.9 percent in 2002. Although not as large a percentage increase as compared with the Netherlands, this constitutes a significant trend.[91,92] The implications for future pregnancies has not been studied but may be implied by the trend toward decreasing attempts at vaginal birth after cesarean section: maternal morbidity and mortality rates are significantly increased with each subsequent cesarean birth.

Even though greater risks appear to face the breech infant, there remain many who believe that complete abandonment of vaginal delivery for the breech is not yet justified.[93,94] The Term Breech Trial also has its detractors, who state inclusion of fetuses with estimated weights up to 4 kg and less than 2,500 g, and procedural aberrations in labor assessment and adequacy (length of time permitted for first and second stage of labor, liberal use of induction and augmentation of labor), as well as worldwide differences in standards of obstetric care and its providers make the trial's results suspect and not generalizable. No study is perfect in its methodology or results; the Term Breech Trial certainly adds to the body of literature on breech vaginal delivery but may not be the final answer to the question of the safety of vaginal breech delivery.

Special Clinical Circumstances and Risks—Preterm Breech, Hyperextended Head, Footling Breech

The various categories of breech presentation clearly demonstrate dissimilar risks, and management plans might vary among these situations.[66,95] The premature breech, the breech with a hyperextended head, and the footling breech are categories that have high rates of fetal morbidity or mortality. Complications associated with incomplete dilatation and cephalic entrapment may be more frequent. For these three breech situations, in general, cesarean delivery appears to optimize fetal outcome and, therefore, is recommended.

Low birth weight (<2,500 g) is a confounding factor in about one third of all breech presentations.[54,60,64,68,96,97] Whereas the benefit of cesarean delivery for the breech infant weighing 1,500 to 2,500 g remains controversial,[11,35,52,55,97–103] some studies showed improved survival with abdominal delivery in the 1,000- to 1,500-g weight group.[60,100] A recent multicenter study of long-term outcomes of vaginally delivered infants at 26 to 31 weeks' gestation found no differences in rates of death or developmental disability within 2 years of follow-up.[104] Traumatic morbidity is reportedly decreased in both weight groups by the use of cesarean delivery, including a lower rate of both intra- and periventricular hemorrhage.[103] Although some advocate a trial of labor in the frank breech infant weighing over 1,500 g, others recommend labor only when the infant exceeds 2,000 g.[35,64,96,105] There are proportionately fewer frank breech presentations in the low-birth-weight group.[31,60] In fact, most infants weighing less than 1,500 g and presenting as a breech are footling breeches.[105] Although most deaths in the very-low-birth-weight breech group are due to prematurity or lethal anomalies,[97,99,105,106] cesarean delivery has been shown by some to decrease corrected perinatal mortality in this weight group compared with that in similar-sized vertex presentations.[60,107] Other authors suggest that improved survival in these studies relates to improved neonatal care of the premature infant when compared with the outcomes of historical controls.[108] When vaginal delivery of the preterm breech is chosen or is unavoidable, however, conduction anesthesia and the use of forceps for the delivery of the after-coming head appear to decrease fetal morbidity and mortality.[97,109,110]

Preterm premature rupture of the fetal membranes (PPROM) is associated with prematurity and chorioamnionitis, both of which have been found to be independent risk factors for the development of cerebral palsy (CP). PPROM is associated with a high rate of malpresentations because of prematurity and decreased amniotic fluid. Knowing the association of chorioamnionitis with periventricular leukomalacia (PVL), a lesion found to precede development of CP in the premature neonate, Baud et al.[111] correlated the mode of delivery with PVL, and subsequent CP in breech preterm deliveries. The authors found that in the presence of chorioamnionitis, delivery by elective cesarean section was associated with a dramatic decrease in the incidence of PVL.

Hyperextension of the fetal head has been consistently associated with a high (21-percent) risk of spinal cord injury if the breech is delivered vaginally.[30,112,113] In such cases, it is important to differentiate simple deflexion of the head from clear hyperextension, given that Ballas et al.[114] have shown that simple deflexion carries no excess risk. The issue of simple deflexion of the fetal vertex as opposed to hyperextension is similar to the relationships between the occipitofrontal cranial plane and the axis of the fetal cervical spine illustrated in Figure 17-5. Often, as labor progresses, spontaneous flexion will occur in response to fundal forces.

Finally, the footling breech carries a prohibitively high (16- to 19-percent) risk of cord prolapse during labor. In many cases, cord prolapse is manifest only late in labor, after commitment to vaginal delivery may have been made.[60,99] Cord prolapse necessitates prompt cesarean delivery. Furthermore, the footling breech is a poor cervical dilator, and cephalic entrapment becomes more likely.

Breech Second Twin

Approximately one third of all twin gestations present as vertex/breech (i.e., first twin is a vertex, and the second is a breech; see also Chapter 28, Multiple Gestations).[115] The management alternatives in the case of the vertex/breech twin pregnancy in labor include cesarean delivery, vaginal delivery of the first twin and attempted external cephalic version of the second twin, or internal podalic version and extraction of the second twin. Blickstein et al.[115] compared the obstetric outcomes of 39 cases of vertex/breech twins with the outcomes of 48 vertex/vertex twins. Although the breech second twin had a higher incidence of low birth weight and a longer hospital stay, the authors found no basis for elective cesarean delivery in this clinical circumstance. The outcomes of another study of 136 pairs of vertex/nonvertex twins weighing more than 1,500 g allows us to conclude that breech extraction of the second twin appears to be a safe alternative to cesarean delivery.[116] Laros and Dattel[117] studied 206 twin pairs and likewise found no clear advantage to arbitrary cesarean delivery because of a specific presentation. When comparing outcomes of 390 vaginally delivered second twins (207 delivered vertex; 183 delivered breech), with 95 percent of the breech deliveries being total breech extractions, it is noted that no significant differences existed between the vertex and breech infants, even when stratified by birth weight.[118] These outcomes assume the skills and experience required to perform a successful breech extraction. Any clinician uncomfortable with the prospective delivery of a singleton breech, however, would be unwise to consider a breech extraction of a second twin.

Vaginal delivery followed by external version is a viable alternative, using ultrasound in the delivery room to directly visualize the fetus. Often there is a transient decrease in uterine activity after the delivery of the first infant, which can be used to advantage in the performance of a cephalic version. Description of experience with 30 malpositioned second twins (12 transverse and 18 breech) shows that version after birth of the first twin was successful in 11 of the 12 transverse infants and in 16 of the 18 breech infants.[119] These twins were all older than 35 weeks' gestation, with intact membranes of the second twin after delivery of the first, no evidence of anomalies, and normal amniotic fluid volume.

If internal podalic version/extraction of the second twin is to be performed, it can be facilitated by ultrasonic guidance. A hand is inserted into the uterus, both fetal feet are identified and grasped with membranes intact, and traction is applied to bring the feet into the pelvis and out the introitus, with maternal expulsive efforts remaining the major force in effecting descent of the fetus. Membranes are left intact until both feet are at the introitus.[120] Once membranes are ruptured, the delivery is subsequently managed as a footling breech delivery. If the operator has difficulty identifying the fetal feet, intrapartum ultrasound may be of assistance.

During breech extraction, and perhaps more often with a breech extraction of a smaller twin, the fetal head can become entrapped in the cervix. In such cases, the operator's entire hand is placed in the uterus, the fetal head is cradled, and as the hand is withdrawn, the head is protected.[121] This splinting technique has also been used for the safe extraction of the breech head at the time of cesarean delivery. Head entrapment may also occur because of increased uterine tone, or contractions. In this case, a uterine relaxing agent may be employed, with nitroglycerin (50 to 200 μg intravenously) being one of the fastest acting, safest agents in appropriately selected patients. Terbutaline, ritodrine, or inhalational anesthesia may also be used.

A small, prospective trial in the near-term gestation (>35 weeks) found no difference in neonatal morbidity between vaginal delivery and cesarean birth of vertex/nonvertex twins. However, increased maternal morbidity with cesarean delivery was found.[120] Again, safe vaginal delivery of the breech second twin by podalic version and extraction requires specific skills and experience.

External Cephalic Version

External cephalic version (ECV) is a third alternative to vaginal delivery or cesarean delivery for the breech fetus.[15,54,56,122–125] Many have found that ECV significantly reduces the incidence of breech presentation in labor and is associated with few complications such as cord compression or placental abruption.[15,125] Reported success with ECV varies from 60 to 75 percent, with a similar percentage of these remaining vertex at the time of labor.[15,126–129] Although many infants in breech presentation before 34 weeks will convert spontaneously to a cephalic presentation, few will do so afterward.[125] Repetitive external version applied weekly after 34 weeks in one report was successful in converting more than two thirds of cases and reducing their breech presentation rate by 50 percent.[125] In another randomized trial of ECV in low-risk pregnancies between 37 and 39 weeks, success was achieved in 68 percent of 25 cases in the version group, whereas only four of the 23 controls converted to a vertex spontaneously before labor.[122] All of those in whom external version was successful presented in labor as a vertex.[122] In another prospective, controlled study of ECV performed weekly between 33 weeks and term, 48 percent of the study group were vertex in labor compared with only 26 percent of controls. Another experience with 112 patients demonstrated a 49-percent success rate with ECV. The cesarean delivery rate was 17 percent among those patients with successful ECV compared with 78 percent among those patients with an unsuccessful version attempt.[130]

A review of English language reports on outcomes of pregnancies after ECV concluded that it was a safe and effective intervention.[15] The overall success rate among investigators in the United States was 65 percent, with an average cesarean delivery rate of 37 percent among those undergoing an attempted version compared with 83 percent among controls. Successful version was reported more often in parous than nulliparous women and more often between 37 and 39 weeks than after 40 weeks. Fetal complications include abruption, a nonreassuring fetal heart rate pattern, rupture of membranes, cord prolapse, spontaneous conversion back to breech, and fetomaternal hemorrhage. Maternal complications include a high rate of cesarean delivery (up to 64 percent in one study; two- to fourfold risk in another), primarily for dystocia, despite successful conversion.[131,132]

Gentle constant pressure applied in a relaxed patient with frequent fetal heart rate assessments are elements of success stressed by all investigators.[54,56,122] Methodology varies, although the "forward roll" is more widely supported than the "back flip" (Fig. 17-25).[122] The mechanical goal is to squeeze the fetal vertex gently out of the fundal area to the transverse and finally into the lower segment of the uterus.

Tocolysis, regional anesthesia, and ultrasound during the procedure may also be helpful. Use of a number of tocolytics have been reported; however, considerable experience has been reported using intravenous ritodrine. Because of maternal side effects, however, this agent has fallen out of favor in this country. Other agents used are hexoprenaline, salbutamol, nitroglycerin,[133] and terbutaline. A randomized trial of 103 nulliparous patients found success rates with subcutaneous terbutaline were 52 percent compared with 27 percent in the control group. No adverse maternal effects resulting from the drug were found.[134] A randomized trial of 58 patients at 37 to 41 weeks' gestation with breech presentation found no benefit from β-mimetic tocolysis, with success rates of approximately two thirds in each group.[127] Factors associated with failure of version included obesity, deep pelvic engagement of the breech, oligohydramnios, and posterior positioning of the fetal back.[128] The use of epidural anesthesia for external cephalic version has also been controversial. Many believe that operators might apply excessive pressure to the maternal abdomen when epidural anesthesia is employed, which might make fetal compromise more likely, indicated by fetal heart rate decelerations and possibly related to placental abruption. However, a randomized trial of 69 women using epidural anesthesia demonstrated a better than twofold increase in success of the procedure when epidural was employed.[135]

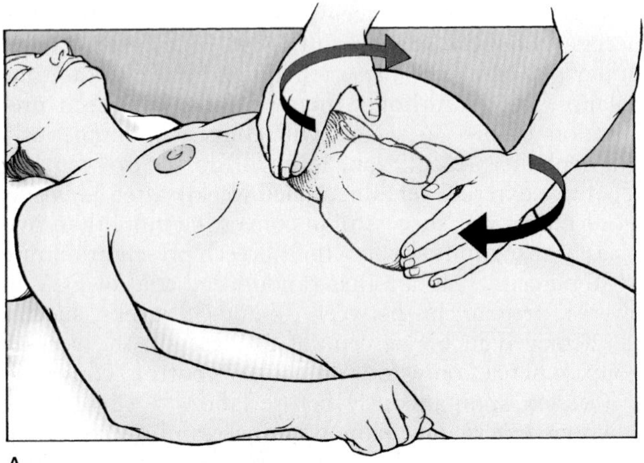

A

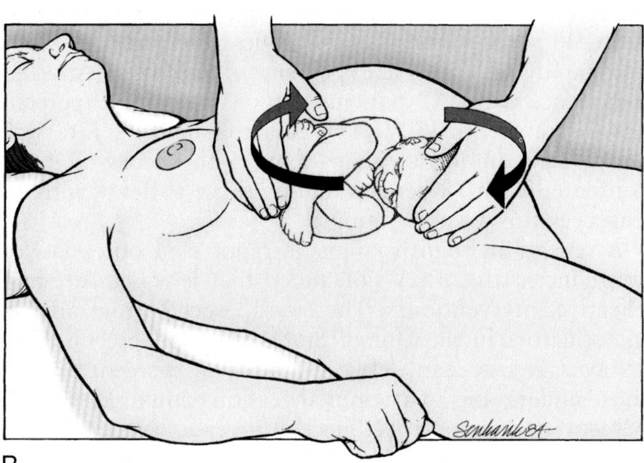

B

Figure 17-25. External cephalic version is accomplished by gently "squeezing" the fetus out of one area of the uterus and into another (*A*). Here, the "forward roll," often the most popular, is illustrated (*B*).

A Cochrane database study of the effects of tocolysis, regional anesthesia, vibroacoustic stimulation and transabdominal amnioinfusion for ECV was performed and reported in 2004. Tocolysis reduced the failure rate of ECV (RR = 0.74, 95-percent CI, 0.64 to 0.87). The reduction of noncephalic presentations at birth did not reach significance, but the cesarean delivery rate was reduced (RR = 0.85, 95-percent CI, 0.72 to 0.99). Regional anesthesia also showed a reduced rate of cesarean sections and noncephalic presentations at birth in two out of five trials included. No other interventions improved success rates of ECV.[136] Performing the version before term does not appear to significantly impact the likelihood of noncephalic presentations at term, (RR = 1.02, 95-percent CI, 0.89 to 1.17); cesarean delivery (RR = 1.10, 95-percent CI, 0.78 to 1.54); low Apgar scores (RR = 0.81, 95-percent CI, 0.44 to 1.49); or perinatal mortality (RR = 1.19, 95-percent CI, 0.46 to 3.05).[137] Fetomaternal transfusion has been reported to occur in up to 6 percent of patients undergoing external version,[138] and thus, Rh-negative unsensitized women should receive Rh-immune globulin. Quantitation of fetomaternal hemorrhage with the Kleihauer-Betke or flow cytometry test will determine the number of ampules of Rh immune globulin to be administered.

In the case of the gravida with a previous cesarean delivery, ECV has also been controversial. Studies of limited sample size have concluded that ECV is safe for mother and fetus, and results in increased vaginal delivery rates. Success rates of up to 82 percent in patients with a previous cesarean delivery have been reported.[139] Use of intravenous ritodrine tocolysis in 11 patients with history of previous low cervical transverse cesarean section resulted in no uterine dehiscences found clinically or at the time of cesarean delivery.[140]

Of interest are the recent trials employing moxibustion of accupoint BL 67 (Zhiyin; beside the outer corner of the 5th toenail) to resolve breech presentation, with and without acupuncture or percutaneous low-frequency electrical stimulation, also applied to the same accupoint. Moxibustion is a traditional Chinese method that uses the application of heat generated by the combustion of herbs to provide stimulation to accupoints. The particular herb used, *Artemisia vulgaris* (mugwort), is purported to work by stimulating fetal movements. Of 130 patients in the treatment group of one study, only one required cephalic version, whereas 24 of 130 in the controls group required this procedure. Seventy-five percent of the treatment group, and 62 percent of the control group were cephalic at birth.[141] When acupuncture is used in conjunction with moxibustion, rates of spontaneous conversion approach 54 percent compared with the observed group (37 percent, $p = 0.01$).[142] Another study noted significantly higher spontaneous and moxibustion-induced correction rates of breech presentation: 74 versus 92.5 percent, respectively.[143] This study enrolled patients on average 4 weeks earlier than the prior study. No fetal heart rate abnormalities have been noted with the use of acupuncture and moxibustion in combination.[144] The role for traditional Chinese medicine in modern obstetrics, while promising, remains to be further elucidated.

SHOULDER DYSTOCIA

Shoulder dystocia is diagnosed when, after delivery of the fetal head, further expulsion of the infant is prevented by impaction of the fetal shoulders within the maternal pelvis. Specific efforts are necessary to facilitate delivery (Fig. 17-26).

Although a difficult shoulder dystocia occurs infrequently, one does not soon forget the experience. Often, but not always, at the end of a difficult labor, the fetal head may be delivered spontaneously or by forceps, but the neck then retracts. The fetal head appears to be drawn back with the chin close to the maternal perineum or thigh, creating difficulty suctioning the infant's mouth. As maternal expulsive efforts are encouraged, the fetal head becomes plethoric, and the danger to the infant is apparent if delivery cannot be promptly accomplished.

Shoulder dystocia has been reported in 0.15 to 1.7 percent of all vaginal deliveries.[145,146] All investigators have documented increased perinatal morbidity and mortality with shoulder dystocia.[145,146] Mortality varies from 21 to 290 in 1,000 when shoulder girdle impaction occurs, and neonatal morbidity has been reported to be immediately obvious in 20 percent of infants.[145] In reviewing 131 macrosomic infants, Boyd et al.[147] found that only half of all cases of brachial palsy occurring in macrosomic infants also carried a diagnosis of shoulder dystocia. Obviously, brachial palsy was noted in half of these cases without a clinical diagnosis of shoulder dystocia. Severe asphyxia was observed in 143 of 1,000 births with shoulder dystocia compared with 14 of 1,000 overall.[147] Fetal morbidity is not always immediately apparent. McCall[148] found 28 percent of infants born with shoulder dystocia demonstrated some neuropsychiatric dysfunction at 5- to 10-year follow-up. Fewer than one half of these children had immediate morbidity. The neonatal morbidity of greatest concern is brachial plexus injury, resulting from trauma to cervical nerve root 5 and 6. Fortunately, most cases are transient, with full recovery observed in 90 to 95 percent of infants.[149]

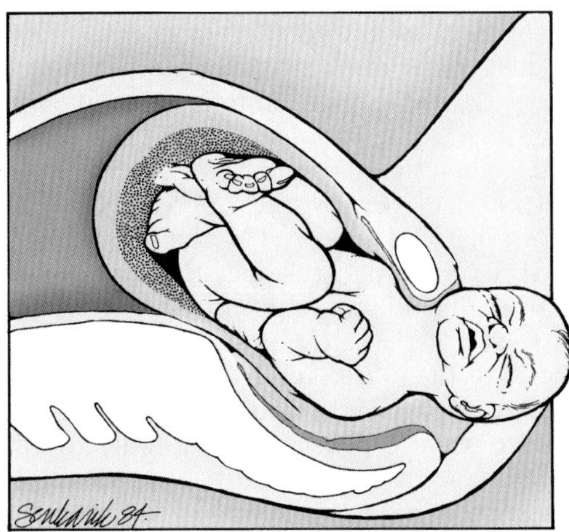

Figure 17-26. When delivery of the fetal head is not followed by delivery of the shoulders, the anterior shoulder has often become caught behind the symphysis, as illustrated here. The head may retract toward the perineum. Desperate traction on the fetal head is not likely to facilitate delivery and may lead to trauma.

Although shoulder dystocia has traditionally been strongly associated with macrosomia, up to one half of cases of shoulder dystocia occur in neonates weighing less than 4,000 g.[150,151] However, Acker et al.[151] found that the relative probability of shoulder dystocia in the 7 percent of infants weighing more than 4,000 g was 11 times greater than the average, and in the 2 percent of infants weighing more than 4,500 g it was 22 times greater. With macrosomia or continued fetal growth beyond term, the trunk and particularly the chest grow larger relative to the head. Chest circumference exceeds the head circumference in 80 percent of cases.[150] Arms also contribute to the greater dimensions of the upper body. Macrosomia shows the strongest correlation with shoulder dystocia of any clinical factor and occurs more often with gestational diabetes and twice as often in prolonged pregnancies. Other clinical factors associated with shoulder dystocia appear to be related to macrosomia as well and include maternal obesity,[147,152] previous birth of an infant weighing more than 4,000 g,[147,150,152,153] diabetes mellitus,[152,153] prolonged second stage of labor,[151–153] prolonged deceleration phase (8 to 10 cm), instrumental midpelvic delivery,[154] and previous shoulder dystocia,[153] which has been found to have a recurrence risk of almost 14 percent. Increased maternal age and excess maternal weight gain have been found by some but not all investigators[147,152–154] to increase the risk of macrosomia and shoulder dystocia.[153] Father's birth weight and adult size during young adulthood have also been found to correlate with fetal weight in addition to the traditional determinants.[156]

Macrosomia has been variously defined as a birth weight greater than either 4,000 g or 4,500 g.[145,147,157,159,160] Male predominance is routinely observed, and the condition is associated with the clinical features described earlier. The two most common complications observed with macrosomia are postpartum hemorrhage and shoulder dystocia.[152] Golditch and Kirkman[158] observed shoulder dystocia in 3 percent of deliveries of infants weighing between 4,100 and 4,500 g and in 8.2 percent of those weighing more than 4,500 g. Benedetti and Gabbe[145] reported that fetal injury occurred in 47 percent of infants weighing more than 4,000 g who were delivered from the midpelvis and had shoulder dystocia.

Clinical efforts to detect macrosomia prenatally could be helpful in anticipating problems with delivery of the shoulders. Such efforts, however, have been disappointing.[160] Numerous sonographic markers have been assessed to determine their usefulness in predicting macrosomia. These include the estimation of fetal weight using a variety of fetal dimensions and the comparison of chest to head circumference. Most recently, the fetal abdominal diameter–biparietal diameter difference was evaluated retrospectively both in diabetic and in nondiabetic women.[161] A difference of greater than or equal to 2.6 cm was found to predict shoulder dystocia with sensitivity and specificity of 100 and 46 percent, respectively, with positive and negative predictive values of 30 and 100 percent, respectively. Furthermore, a fetal abdominal circumference of 35 cm or greater has been found to identify more then 90 percent of macrosomic infants.[162] Both of these studies are retrospective and limited by difficulty measuring the fetal abdominal outline at advanced gestational age caused by acoustic shadowing. Parks and Ziel[152] found that of 110 macrosomic infants, the diagnosis was made prenatally in only 20 percent. The clinical estimate of birth weight was more than 3 lb in error in 6 percent of cases. Numerous efforts in the literature repeatedly demonstrate the shortcomings of both clinical and ultrasonographic estimations of fetal weight, and have concluded that the best estimation is a combination of the two.

There is a growing trend to consider cesarean delivery of any infant with an estimated weight more than 4,500 g or of any infant of a diabetic mother with an estimated weight more than 4,000 g[151,154,160] to avoid birth trauma, particularly brachial plexus injury. Any consideration of elective abdominal delivery on the basis of estimated fetal weight alone, however, must consider the technical error of the method. If 90 percent confidence is desired that the actual fetal weight is at least 4,000 g, the sonographic estimate by most current methods must exceed 4,600 g. This is a result of the expected methodologic error of ±10 percent (±1 standard deviation). Furthermore, the fetal vertex is often too deeply engaged in the pelvis to allow accurate measurement of head circumference. Estimated fetal weight should be only one of several factors considered in the management of the laboring patient. In the obese diabetic patient with an estimated fetal weight more than 4,500 g and showing poor progress in labor, cesarean delivery may be the most prudent course. However, in most other cases, the risks of cesarean delivery to the mother, the accuracy of prediction of macrosomia, and the alternative of a carefully monitored trial of labor should be discussed. Gross et al.[163] carefully reviewed the clinical characteristics of 394 mothers delivering infants weighing more than 4,000 g and concluded that although birth weight, prolonged deceleration phase, and length of second stage were all individually predictive, no prospective model adequately discriminated the infant destined to sustain trauma from shoulder dystocia from the infant not so destined. Taking this one step further, identifying macrosomic fetuses for the ultimate prevention of neurologic injury has been the subject of studies that report a significant increase in annual cost for routine cesarean deliveries for macrosomia in the nondiabetic population but improved ratios of cost per brachial plexus injury prevented per year in the diabetic population. Ultrasound detection and elective cesarean delivery of the macrosomic infant of the nondiabetic mother has been predicted to result in $4.9 million of expenditure to prevent one permanent neurologic injury, whereas one maternal death would result from cesarean delivery for every 3.2 neonatal nerve injuries prevented.[164] Elective cesarean delivery for fetuses of diabetic mothers (both gestational and pregestational) has also been controversial. Langer et al.[165] found that 76 percent of shoulder dystocias could be prevented if a policy of elective cesarean delivery was instituted at an estimated weight of 4,250 g, whereas Acker et al.[151] found that using a fetal weight threshold of 4,000 g, 55 percent could be prevented in the diabetic poplation. Although many clinicians perform an elective cesarean delivery in a patient with diabetes mellitus and an estimated fetal weight of 4,000 to 4,500 g,[165,166] Keller expressed concern about the inaccuracy of ultrasound estimation of fetal weight in the gestational diabetic population, with 50 percent of shoulder dystocias occurring in fetuses who weighed less than 4,000 g.[167]

Whereas in the past, it was believed that brachial plexus injury resulted primarily from operator-induced excess traction in the setting of shoulder dystocia, evidence now exists that such injuries may result from endogenous forces during the second stage of labor. Shoulder dystocia itself places the brachial plexus on stretch. Maternal endogenous forces may actually exceed clinician applied exogenous forces as well.[167a,167b]

The occurrence of brachial plexus injury in the absence of shoulder dystocia has been described and attributed to in utero forces, such as the posterior shoulder impacting on the sacral promontory (although anterior injuries have been described as well),[168] malpresentations,[169] and dysfunctional labor, mostly precipitate labor.[151,170] Interestingly, in neonates with brachial plexus injury without shoulder dystocia, there was a trend toward lower birth weight, more clavicular fractures, and longer persistence of the condition than their counterparts in the shoulder dystocia-present group.[168,170a]

The most effective preventive measure is to be familiar with the normal mechanism of labor and to be constantly prepared to deal with shoulder dystocia.[171] Normally, after the delivery of the head, external rotation (restitution) occurs, returning the head to its natural perpendicular relationship to the shoulder girdle. The fetal sagittal suture is usually oblique to the AP diameter of the outlet, and the shoulders occupy the opposite oblique diameter of the inlet (Fig. 17-27). As the shoulders descend in response to maternal pushing, the anterior shoulder emerges from its oblique axis under one of the pubic rami. However, if the anterior shoulder descends in the AP diameter of the outlet and the fetus is relatively large for the outlet, impaction behind the symphysis can occur, and further descent is blocked.[146] Shoulder dystocia also occurs with an extremely rapid delivery of the head, as can occur with vacuum extraction or forceps or precipitous labor.

Successful treatment follows anticipation and preparation.[171] Anticipation involves the prenatal suspicion of macrosomia by clinical and sonographic means. One must be aware of the clinical features that have been cited and consider a pregnancy at high risk for macrosomia and, therefore, for shoulder dystocia.

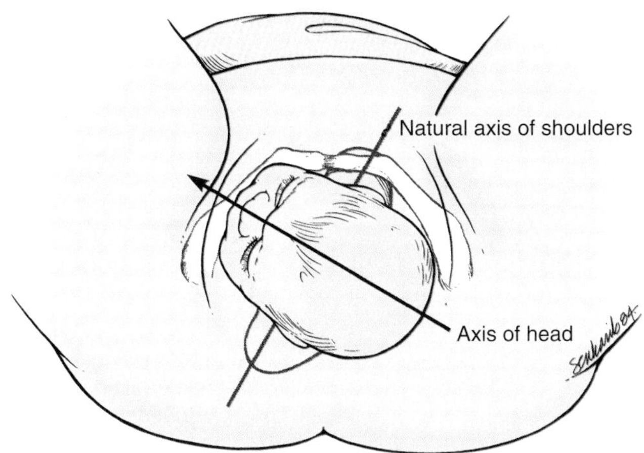

Figure 17-27. After delivery of the head, "restitution" results in the long axis of the head reassuming its normal orientation to the shoulders as seen here.

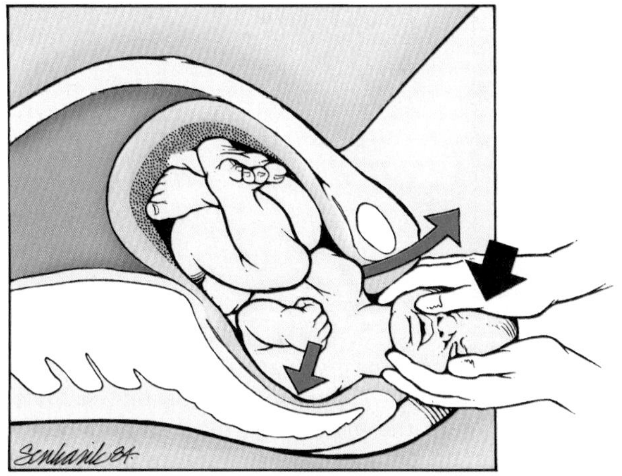

Figure 17-28. Gentle, symmetric pressure on the head will move the posterior shoulder into the hollow of the sacrum and encourage delivery of the anterior shoulder. Care should be taken not to "pry" the anterior shoulder out asymmetrically, because this might lead to trauma to the anterior brachial plexus.

Such deliveries are best managed in a delivery room. Deliveries in bed increase the difficulty of reducing a shoulder dystocia because the bedding precludes fullest use of the posterior pelvis and outlet. Strong consideration for cesarean delivery is recommended when a prolonged second stage occurs in association with macrosomia.

Once a vaginal delivery has begun, the obstetrician must resist the temptation to rotate the head forcibly to a transverse axis. Maternal expulsive efforts should be used rather than traction. Gentle manual pressure on the fetal head inferiorly and posteriorly will push the posterior shoulder into the hollow of the sacrum, increasing the room for the anterior shoulder to pass under the pubis (Fig. 17-28). This pressure is not outward traction and must be symmetric. If the head is pressed asymmetrically, as if to "pry" the anterior shoulder out, brachial plexus injury is more likely.

If delivery is not accomplished, a deliberate, planned sequence of efforts should then be initiated.[171] One must not pull desperately on the fetal head. Fundal expulsive efforts, including maternal pushing and any fundal pressure, should be temporarily stopped. Aggressive fundal pressure before disimpaction or rotation of the shoulders will not facilitate delivery and may work against rotation and disimpaction.

The McRoberts maneuver[172] is a simple, logical, and usually successful measure to promote delivery of the shoulders. The McRoberts maneuver involves hyperflexion of maternal legs on the maternal abdomen that results in flattening of the lumbar spine and ventral rotation of the maternal pelvis and symphysis (Fig. 17-29). This maneuver may increase the useful size of the posterior outlet, resulting in easier disimpaction of the anterior shoulder. Gonik et al.[173] showed that the McRoberts maneuver significantly reduces shoulder extraction forces, brachial plexus stretching, and likelihood of clavicular fracture. In a retrospective review of shoulder dystocia, Gherman et al. found that the McRoberts maneuver was the only step required in 42 percent of 236 cases.[174] When shoulder dystocia occurs because of failure of the bisacromial diameter to engage, the Walcher position, which entails dropping the maternal legs down toward the floor with concurrent suprapubic pressure in a dorsal-caudal direction, has been advocated. Only then, while constant suprapubic pressure is being maintained, should the parturient be placed in the McRoberts position; this may allow for the disimpaction of the fetal shoulder from the symphysis by increasing the AP diameter of the inlet before increasing the outlet.[175] Additionally, the "all fours," or Gaskin maneuver, which differs from the knee-chest position, may relieve the dystocia.[176] Use of this maneuver is reasonable only in the setting of a mobile parturient with no significant motor blockade from regional anesthetic, and a stable and wide surface on which to assume this position in order to avoid the potential for injury during transition to this position.

If the shoulders remain undelivered, often only moderate suprapubic pressure is required to disimpact the anterior shoulder and allow delivery (Fig. 17-30). If this is not effective, the operator's hand may be passed behind the occiput into the vagina, and the anterior shoulder may be pushed forward to the oblique, after which, with maternal efforts and gentle posterior pressure, delivery should occur (Fig. 17-31).[171] Alternatively, the posterior shoulder may be rotated forward, through a 180-degree arc, and passed under the pubic ramus as in turning a screw (Wood's screw maneuver). As the posterior shoulder rotates anteriorly, delivery will often occur.[177]

Many authorities have advocated delivery of the posterior arm and shoulder should the above-mentioned methods fail. The operator's hand is passed into the vagina, following the posterior arm of the fetus to the elbow. The arm is flexed and swept out over the chest and the perineum (Fig. 17-32). In some cases, delivery will now occur without further manipulation. In others, rotation of the trunk, bringing the freed posterior arm anteriorly, is required.[150,171] These maneuvers are highly likely to fracture the clavicle (up to 25 percent), humerus (up to 15 percent), or both, or they may result in transient or permanent nerve injury in up to approximately 9 percent of cases.[177] Overall, similar rates of bone fracture were noted when any type of manipulation was performed to accomplish delivery of an impacted fetal

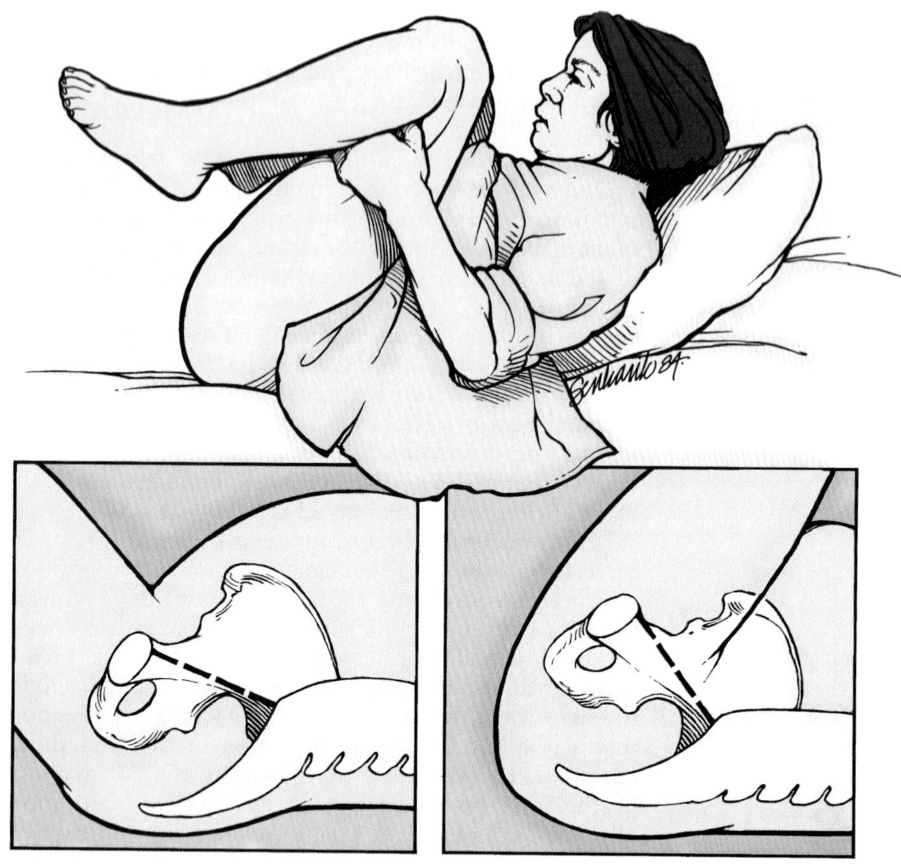

Figure 17-29. The least invasive maneuver to disimpact the shoulders is the McRoberts maneuver. Sharp ventral flexion of the maternal hips results in ventral rotation of the maternal pelvis and an increase in the useful size of the outlet.

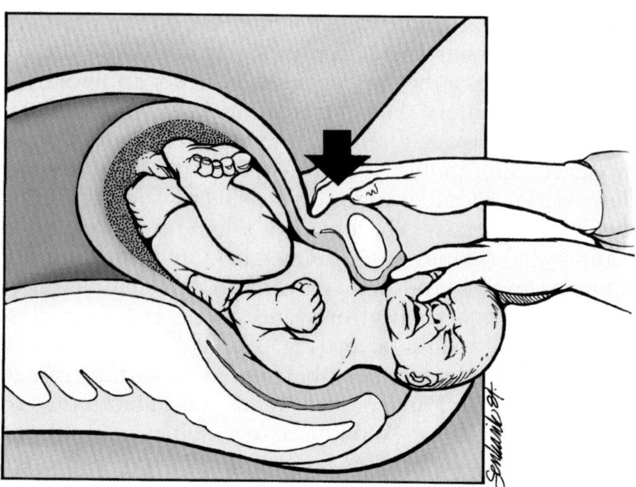

Figure 17-30. Moderate suprapubic pressure will often disimpact the anterior shoulder.

shoulder.[178] Deliberate fracture of the clavicle is possible and will facilitate delivery by diminishing the rigidity and size of the shoulder girdle. It is best if the pressure is exerted in a direction away from the lung to avoid puncture. Sharp instrumental transection of the clavicle is not recommended, because lung puncture is common with such a method, and infection of the bone through the open wound is a serious possible complication.

Maneuvers to prevent shoulder dystocia have been evaluated in two separate studies: one compared McRoberts position and suprapubic pressure to no intervention,[178a] while the other examined the use of lithotomy vs. McRoberts position.[178b] In the first study, head to body delivery times did not differ significantly. The "prophylactic" group had greater numbers of subjects who required cesarean delivery, and, when these were included in the analysis, results strongly favored use of prophylactic measures for reducing incidence of shoulder dystocia (RR = 0.33, 95-percent CI, 0.12 to 0.86). A greater number of patients required additional maneuvers to relieve the shoulder dystocia in the control group. Additionally, no differences were noted in NICU admissions or birth injuries. This study does not support routine use of these maneuvers in cases of suspected shoulder dystocia. The study by Poggi et al.[178b] compared the traditional lithotomy postion to McRoberts position, and additionally evaluated the forces required to release the shoulder with force sensing gloves. The study concluded that peak forces and force rates did not differ between groups. The head to body delivery time was longer by 4 seconds in the prophylactic group, which was statistically significant. There were similar numbers of actual shoulder dystocias (one per group) encountered in each arm. In summary, it is unclear whether the use of prophylactic measures in patients at risk for shoulder dystocia are of benefit.

Two techniques rarely used in the United States for the management of shoulder dystocia include vaginal replacement of the fetal head with cesarean delivery (Zavanelli maneuver) and subcutaneous symphysiotomy. Sandberg reviewed the Zavanelli maneuver for both the vertex- and breech-presenting undeliverable

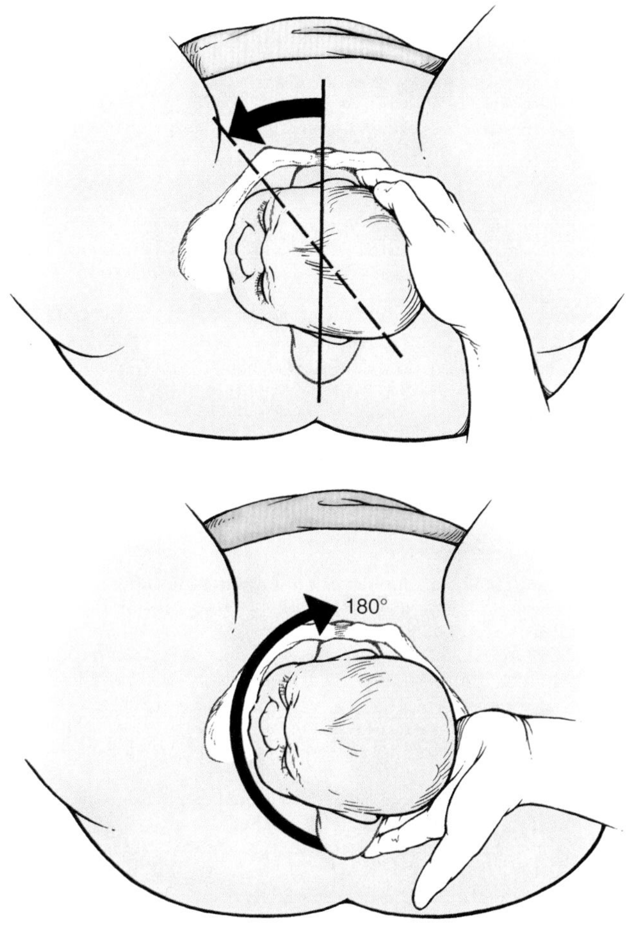

Figure 17-31. Rotation of the anterior shoulder forward through a small arc or the posterior shoulder forward through a larger one will often lead to descent and delivery of the shoulders. Forward rotation is preferred, because it tends to compress and diminish the size of the shoulder girdle, whereas backward rotation would open the shoulder girdle and increase the size.

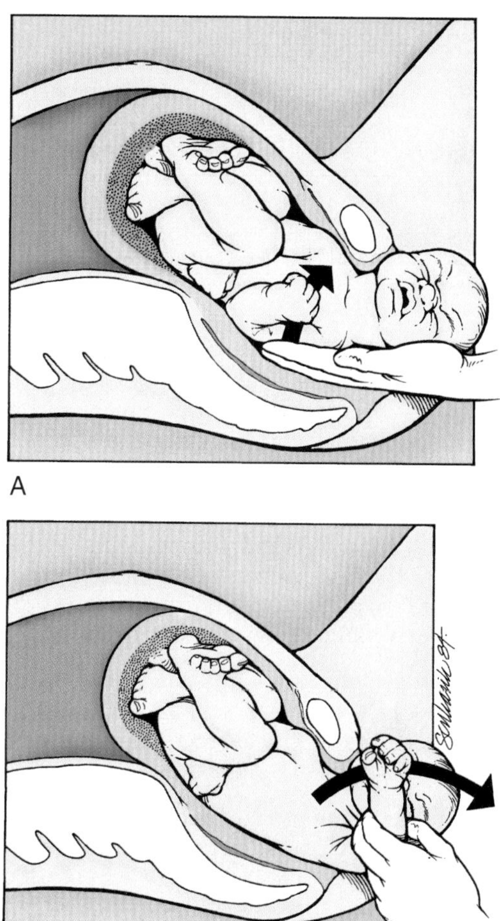

Figure 17-32. The operator here inserts a hand (*A*) and sweeps the posterior arm across the chest and over the perineum (*B*). Care should be taken to distribute the pressure evenly across the humerus to avoid unnecessary fracture.

fetuses. Cephalic replacement was successful in 84 of 92 vertex-presenting fetuses, and in 11 of 11 breech-presenting, podalic replacement was successful. Maternal risks included soft tissue trauma and sepsis, but the fetal risks were described as "minimal," with no fetal injuries attributed to the maneuver; this may be misleading because of the presence of a multitude of etiologies for permanent injury or death, likely from attempts at disimpaction, prolonged delivery time, and hypoxia.[179] O'Leary and Cuva[180] described 35 cases, 31 of which were considered successful and one of which needed a hysterotomy incision to allow manual disimpaction of the fetal shoulders and facilitate vaginal delivery when the fetal head could not be replaced into the vagina from below.

Subcutaneous symphysiotomy has been practiced in remote areas of the world for many years as an expedient alternative to cesarean delivery with very good results.[181] In a case series of three symphysiotomies, the procedure was used as a last resort and was associated with the death of all three neonates because of hypoxic complications. The procedure was concluded to be safe and effective as long as attention is paid to the three main points in the procedure: lateral support of the legs, partial sharp dissection of the symphysis, and displacement of the urethra to the side with an indwelling urinary catheter.[182] However, neither cephalic replacement nor symphysiotomy has been widely or often used in obstetric practice in the United States. Attempted implementation of either method by the inexperienced practitioner before the trial of more conventional remedies may increase risk to the child, the mother, and the clinician.

In summary, shoulder dystocia is not precisely predictable but may be anticipated in the case of a variety of predisposing clinical conditions. Shoulder dystocia will, in most cases, respond to any or all of several prudent interventions. The specific method used to disimpact the shoulder is probably not as critical as the practice of a careful, methodical approach to the problem and the avoidance of desperate, potentially traumatic or asymmetric traction. The maneuvers used should be carefully described in the delivery note. There may not be any complication of labor and delivery when forethought is more important to a successful outcome than shoulder dystocia.

Key Points

- The "fetal lie" indicates the orientation of the fetal spine relative to that of the mother. Normal fetal lie is longitudinal and by itself does not connote whether the presentation is cephalic or breech.
- Cord prolapse occurs 20 times as often with an abnormal axial lie as it does with a cephalic presentation.
- Fetal malformations are observed in more than half of infants with a face presentation.
- Fetal malpresentation requires timely diagnostic exclusion of major fetal or uterine malformations and/or abnormal placentation.
- With few exceptions, a closely monitored labor and vaginal delivery is a safe possibility with most malpresentations. However, cesarean delivery is the only acceptable alternative if normal progress toward spontaneous vaginal delivery is not observed.
- External cephalic version of the infant in breech presentation near term is a safe and often successful management option. Use of tocolytics and epidural anesthesia may improve success.
- Appropriate training and experience is a prerequisite to the safe vaginal delivery of selected infants in breech presentation.
- Simple compound presentation may be permitted a trial of labor as long as labor progresses normally with reassuring fetal status. Compression or reduction of the fetal part may result in damage, however.
- Shoulder dystocia cannot be precisely predicted or prevented but is often associated with macrosomia, maternal obesity, gestational diabetes, and a prolonged pregnancy.
- The clinician must be prepared to deal with shoulder dystocia at every vaginal delivery with a deliberate, controlled sequence of interventions.

REFERENCES

1. Yates MJ: Transverse fetal lie in labour. J Obstet Gynaecol Br Commonw 71:237, 1964.
2. MacGregor WG: Aetiology and treatment of the oblique, transverse and unstable lie of the foetus with particular reference to antenatal care. J Obstet Gynaecol Br Commonw 71:237, 1964.
3. Cockburn KG, Drake RF: Transverse and oblique lie of the foetus. Aust N Z J Obstet Gynaecol 8:211, 1968.
4. Sandhu SK: Transverse lie. J Indian Med Assoc 68:205, 1977.
5. Cruikshank DP, White CA: Obstetric malpresentations-twenty years' experience. Am J Obstet Gynecol 116:1097, 1973.
6. Edwards RI, Nicholson HO: The management of the unstable lie in late pregnancy. J Obstet Gynaecol Br Commonw 76:713, 1969.
7. Flowers CE: Shoulder presentation. Am J Obstet Gynecol 96:145, 1966.
8. Johnson CE: Abnormal fetal presentations. Lancet 84:317, 1964.
9. Johnson CE: Transverse presentation of the fetus. JAMA 187:642, 1964.
10. Thorp JM, Jenkins TJ, Watson W: Utility of Leopold maneuvers in screening for malpresentation. Obstet Gynecol 78:394, 1991.
11. Hourihane MJ: Etiology and management of oblique lie. Obstet Gynecol 32:512, 1968.
12. Phelan JP, Boucher M, Mueller E, et al: The nonlaboring transverse lie. J Reprod Med 31:184, 1986.
13. Cackins LA, Pearce EWJ: Transverse presentation. Obstet Gynecol 9:123, 1957.
14. Pelosi MA, Apuzzio J, Fricchione D, et al: The intraabdominal version technique for delivery of transverse lie by low segment cesarean section. Am J Obstet Gynecol 136:1009, 1979.
15. Zhang J, Bowes WA, Fortney JA: Efficacy of external cephalic version: a review. Obstet Gynecol 82:306, 1993.
16. Benedetti TJ, Lowensohn RI, Trluscott AM: Face presentation at term. Obstet Gynecol 55:199, 1980.
17. Copeland GN, Nicks FI, Christakos AC: Face and brow presentations. N C Med J 29:507, 1968.
18. Duff P: Diagnosis and management of face presentation. Obstet Gynecol 57:105, 1981.
19. Groenig DC: Face presentation. Obstet Gynecol 2:495, 1953.
20. Magid R, Gillespie CF: Face and brow presentation. Obstet Gynecol 9:450, 1957.
21. Prevedourakis CN: Face presentation. Am J Obstet Gynecol 94:1092, 1966.
22. Campbell JM: Face presentation. Aust N Z J Obstet Gynaecol 5:231, 1965.
23. Dede JA, Friedman EA: Face presentation. Am J Obstet Gynecol 87:515, 1963.
24. Browne ADH, Carney D: Management of malpresentations in obstetrics. Br Med J 5393:1295, 1964.
25. Gomez HE, Dennen EH: Face presentation. Obstet Gynecol 8:103, 1956.
26. Salzmann B, Soled M, Gilmour T: Face presentation. Obstet Gynecol 16:106, 1960.
27. Cucco UP: Face presentation. Am J Obstet Gynecol 94:1085, 1966.
28. Borrell U, Fernstrom A: Face I: the mechanism of labor. Radiol Clin North Am 5:73, 1966.
29. Schwartz A, Dgani R, Lancet M, et al: Face presentation. Aust N Z J Obstet Gynaecol 26:172, 1986.
30. Abroms IF, Bresnan MJ, Zuckerman JE, et al: Cervical cord injuries secondary to hyperextension of the head in breech presentations. Obstet Gynecol 41:369, 1973.
31. Adams CM: Review of breech presentation. S D J Med 32:15, 1979.
32. Gold S: The conduct and management of face presentations. J Int Coll Surg 43:253, 1965.
33. Lansford A, Arias D, Smith BE: Respiratory obstruction associated with face presentation. Am J Dis Child 116:318, 1968.
34. Meltzer RM, Sachtleban MR, Friedman EA: Brow presentation. Am J Obstet Gynecol 100:255, 1968.
35. Kovacs SG: Brow presentation. Med J Aust 2:820, 1970.
36. Levy DL: Persistent brow presentation—a new approach to management. South Med J 69:191, 1976.
37. Ingolfsson A: Brow presentations. Acta Obstet Gynecol Scand 48:486, 1969.
38. Bednoff SL, Thomas BE: Brow presentation. N Y J Med 67:803, 1967.
39. Skalley TW, Kramer TF: Brow presentation. Obstet Gynecol 15:616, 1960.
40. Moore EJT, Dennen EH: Management of persistent brow presentation. Obstet Gynecol 6:186, 1955.
41. Jennings PN: Brow presentation with vaginal delivery. Aust N Z J Obstet Gynaecol 8:219, 1968.
42. Breen JL, Wiesmeien E: Compound presentation—a survey of 131 patients. Obstet Gynecol 32:419, 1968.
43. Goplerud J, Eastman NJ: Compound presentation. Obstet Gynecol 1:59, 1953.
44. Weissberg SM, O'Leary JA: Compound presentation of the fetus. Obstet Gynecol 41:60, 1973.

45. Dignam WJ: Difficulties in delivery, including shoulder dystocia and malpresentations of the fetus. Clin Obstet Gynecol 19:577, 1976.
46. Ang LT: Compound presentation following external version. Aust N Z J Obstet Gynaecol 19:213, 1978.
47. Douglas HGK, Savage PE: An unusual case of compound presentation. J Obstet Gynaecol Br Commonw 77:1036, 1970.
48. Collea JV: Current management of breech presentation. Clin Obstet Gynecol 23:525, 1980.
49. Braun FHT, Jones KL, Smith DW: Breech presentation as an indicator of fetal abnormality. J Pediatr 86:419, 1975.
50. Collea JV, Chein C, Quilligan EJ: The randomized management of term frank breech presentation—a study of 208 cases. Am J Obstet Gynecol 137:235, 1980.
51. Flanagan TA, Mulchahey KM, Korenbrot CC, et al: Management of term breech presentation. Am J Obstet Gynecol 156:1492, 1987.
52. Brown L, Karrison T, Cibils L: Mode of delivery and perinatal results in breech presentation. Am J Obstet Gynecol 171:28, 1994.
53. Gimovsky ML, Wallace RL, Schifrin BS, et al: Randomized management of the non-frank breech presentation at term—a preliminary report. Am J Obstet Gynecol 146:34, 1983.
54. Fall O, Nilsson BA: External cephalic version in breech presentation under tocolysis. Obstet Gynecol 53:712, 1979.
55. Kubli F: Risk of vaginal breech delivery. Contrib Gynecol Obstet 3:80, 1977.
56. Hibbard LT, Schumann WR: Prophylactic external cephalic version in an obstetric practice. Am J Obstet Gynecol 116:511, 1973.
57. Kauppila O, Gronroos M, Aro P, et al: Management of low birth weight breech delivery—should cesarean section be routine? Obstet Gynecol 57:289, 1981.
58. Rovinsky JJ, Miller JA, Kaplan S: Management of breech presentation at term. Am J Obstet Gynecol 115:497, 1973.
59. de la Fuente P, Escalante JM, Hernandez-Garcia JM: Perinatal mortality in breech presentations. Contrib Gynecol Obstet 3:108, 1977.
60. Goldenberg RL, Nelson KG: The premature breech. Am J Obstet Gynecol 127:240, 1977.
61. NIH consensus development statement on cesarean childbirth. Obstet Gynecol 57:537, 1981.
62. Hannah ME, Hannah WJ, Hewson SA, et al: Planned caesarean section versus planned vaginal birth for breech presentation at term: a randomised multicentre trial. Term Breech Trial Collaborative Group. Lancet 356:1375, 2000.
63. Mansani FE, Cerutti M: The risk in breech delivery. Contrib Gynecol Obstet 3:86, 1977.
64. Seitchik J: Discussion of "breech delivery-evaluation of the method of delivery on perinatal results and maternal morbidity" by Bowes et al. Am J Obstet Gynecol 135:970, 1979.
65. Wolter DF: Patterns of management with breech presentation. Am J Obstet Gynecol 125:733, 1976.
66. Bowes WA, Taylor ES, O'Brien M, et al: Breech delivery—evaluation of the method of delivery on perinatal results and maternal morbidity. Am J Obstet Gynecol 135:965, 1979.
67. Diro M, Puangsricharem A, Royer L, et al: Singleton term breech deliveries in nulliparous and multiparous women: a 5 year experience at the University of Miami/Jackson Memorial Hospital. Am J Obstet Gynecol 181:247, 1999.
68. Zatuchni GI, Andros GJ: Prognostic index for vaginal delivery in breech presentation at term. Am J Obstet Gynecol 93:237, 1965.
69. Bird CC, McElin TW: A six year prospective study of term breech deliveries utilizing the Zatuchni-Andros prognostic scoring index. Am J Obstet Gynecol 121:551, 1975.
70. Mark C, Roberts PHR: Breech scoring index. Am J Obstet Gynecol 101:572, 1968.
71. Zatuchni GI, Andros GJ: Prognostic index for vaginal delivery in breech presentation at term. Am J Obstet Gynecol 98:854, 1967.
72. Albrechtsten S, Rasmussen S, Dalaker K, Irgens L: Reproductive career after breech presentation: subsequent pregnancy rates, interpregnancy interval and recurrence. Obstet Gynecol 92:345, 1998.
73. Brenner WE, Bruce RD, Hendricks CH: The characteristics and perils of breech presentation. Am J Obstet Gynecol 118:700, 1974.
74. Lyons ER, Papsin FR: Cesarean section in the management of breech presentation. Am J Obstet Gynecol 130:558, 1978.
75. Spanio P, Elia F, DeBonis F, et al: Fetal-neonatal mortality and morbidity in cesarean deliveries. Contrib Gynecol Obstet 3:130, 1977.
76. Westgren M, Ingemarsson I, Svenningsen NW: Long-term follow up of preterm infants in breech presentation delivered by cesarean section. Dan Med Bull 26:141, 1979.
77. Green JE, McLean F, Smitt LP, et al: Has an increased cesarean section rate for term breech delivery reduced the incidence of birth asphyxia, trauma, and death? Am J Obstet Gynecol 142:643, 1982.
78. Faber-Nijholt R, Huisjes JH, Touwen CL, et al: Neurological follow up of 281 children born in breech presentation-a controlled study. BMJ 286:9, 1983.
79. Badr I, Thomas SM, Cotterill AD, et al: X-ray pelvimetry—which is the best technique? Clin Radiol 52:136, 1997.
80. Thomas SM, Bees NR, Adam EJ: Trends in the use of pelvimetry techniques. Clin Radiol 53:293, 1998.
81. Roman J, Bakos O, Cnattingius S: Pregnancy outcomes by mode of delivery among term breech births: Swedish experience 1987–1993. Obstet Gynecol 92:945, 1998.
82. Irion O, Almagbaly PH, Morabia A: Planned vaginal delivery versus elective cesarean section: a study of 705 singleton term breech presentations. Br J Obstet Gynaecol 105:710, 1998.
83. Su M, McLeod L, Ross S, et al: Term Breech Trial Collaborative Group: Factors associated with adverse perinatal outcome in the Term Breech Trial. Am J Obstet Gynecol 189:740, 2003.
84. Hannah ME, Hannah WJ, Hodnett ED, et al: Term Breech Trial 3-Month Follow-up Collaborative Group: Outcomes at 3 months after planned cesarean vs planned vaginal delivery for breech presentation at term: the international randomized Term Breech Trial. JAMA 287:1822, 2002.
85. Hannah ME, Whyte H, Hannah WJ, et al: Term Breech Trial Collaborative Group: Maternal outcomes at 2 years after planned cesarean section versus planned vaginal birth for breech presentation at term: the international randomized Term Breech Trial. Am J Obstet Gynecol 191:917, 2004.
86. Whyte H, Hannah ME, Saigal S, et al: Term Breech Trial Collaborative Group: Outcomes of children at 2 years after planned cesarean birth versus planned vaginal birth for breech presentation at term: the International Randomized Term Breech Trial. Am J Obstet Gynecol 191:864, 2004.
87. Hogle KL, Hewson S, Gafini A, et al: Impact of the international term breech trial on clinical practice and concerns: a survey of center collaborators. J Obstet Gynaecol Can 25:14, 2003.
88. Rietberg CC, Elferick-Stinkens PM, Visser GH: The effect of the Term Breech trial on medical intervention behaviours and neonatal outcome in the Netherlands: an analysis of 35,453 term breech infants. BJOG 112:205, 2005.
89. Martin JA, Hamilton BE, Menacker F, et al: Preliminary births for 2004: Infant and maternal health. Health E-stats. Hyattsville, MD, National Center for Health Statistics. Released November 15, 2005.
90. Croughan-Minihane MS, Petitt DB, Gordis L, Golditch I: Morbidity among breech infants according to method of delivery. Obstet Gynecol 75:821, 1990.
91. Martin JA, Hamilton BE, Sutton PD, et al: National Vital Statistics Reports, Vol 52, No 10, Centers for Disease Control and Prevention, National Center for Health Statistics, National Vital Statistics System December 17, 2003.
92. Ventura SJ, Martin JA, Curtin SC, et al: National Vital Statistics Reports, Vol 48, No 3, Centers for Disease Control and Prevention, National Center for Health Statistics, National Vital Statistics System, March 28, 2000.
93. Graves WK: Breech delivery in twenty years of practice. Am J Obstet Gynecol 137:229, 1980.
94. Niswander KR: Discussion of "The randomized management of term frank breech presentation—vaginal delivery versus cesarean section" by Collea et al. Am J Obstet Gynecol 131:193, 1978.
95. Lewis BV, Sene Viratne HR: Vaginal breech delivery or cesarean section. Am J Obstet Gynecol 134:615, 1979.

96. De Crespigny LJC, Pepperell RJ: Perinatal mortality and morbidity in breech presentation. Obstet Gynecol 53:141, 1979.
97. Cruikshank DP, Pitkin RM: Delivery of the premature breech. Obstet Gynecol 50:367, 1977.
98. Cruikshank DP: Premature breech [letter to the editor]. Am J Obstet Gynecol 130:500, 1978.
99. Woods JR: Effects of low birth weight breech delivery on neonatal mortality. Obstet Gynecol 53:735, 1979.
100. Ulstein M: Breech delivery. Ann Chir Gynaecol Fenn 69:70, 1980.
101. Weissman A, Blazer S, Zimmer EZ, et al: Low birthweight breech infant: short term and long term outcome by method of delivery. Am J Perinatol 5:289, 1988.
102. Anderson G, Strong C: The premature breech: caesarean section or trial of labour? J Med Ethics 14:18, 1988.
103. Tejani N, Verma U, Shiffman R, et al: Effect of route of delivery on periventricular/intraventricular hemorrhage in the low birthweight fetus with a breech presentation. J Reprod Med 32:911, 1987.
104. Wolf H, Schaap HP, Brunise HW, et al: Vaginal delivery compared with cesarean section in early preterm breech delivery: a comparison of long term outcome. Br J Obstet Gynaecol 106:486, 1999.
105. Karp LE, Doney JR, McCarthy T, et al: The premature breech-trial of labor or cesarean section? Obstet Gynecol 53:88, 1979.
106. Mann LI, Gallant JM: Modern management of the breech delivery. Am J Obstet Gynecol 134:611, 1979.
107. Duenhoelter JH, Wells CE, Reisch JS, et al: A paired controlled study of vaginal and abdominal delivery of the low birth weight breech fetus. Obstet Gynecol 54:310, 1979.
108. Cox C, Kendall AC, Hommers M: Changed prognosis of breech-presenting low birthweight infants. Br J Obstet Gynaecol 89:881, 1982.
109. Milner RDG: Neonatal mortality of breech deliveries with and without forceps to the aftercoming head. Br J Obstet Gynaecol 82:783, 1975.
110. Milner RDG: Neonatal mortality of breech deliveries with and without forceps to the aftercoming head. Contrib Gynecol Obstet 3:113, 1977.
111. Baud O, Ville Y, Zupan V, et al: Are neonatal brain lesions due to infection related to mode of delivery? Br J Obstet Gynaecol 105:121, 1998.
112. Caterini H, Langer A, Sama JC, et al: Fetal risk in hyperextension of the fetal head in breech presentation. Am J Obstet Gynecol 123:632, 1975.
113. Daw E: Hyperextension of the head in breech presentation. Am J Obstet Gynecol 119:564, 1974.
114. Ballas S, Toaff R, Jaffa AJ: Deflexion of the fetal head in breech presentation. Obstet Gynecol 52:653, 1978.
115. Blickstein I, Schwartz-Shoham Z, Lancet M: Vaginal delivery of the second twin in breech presentation. Obstet Gynecol 69:774, 1987.
116. Gocke SE, Nageotte MP, Garite T, et al: Management of the nonvertex second twin: primary cesarean section, external version, or primary breech extraction. Am J Obstet Gynecol 161:111, 1989.
117. Laros RK, Dattel BJ: Management of twin pregnancy: the vaginal route is still safe. Am J Obstet Gynecol 158:1330, 1988.
118. Fishman A, Grubb DK, Kovacs BW: Vaginal delivery of the nonvertex second twin. Am J Obstet Gynecol 168:861, 1993.
119. Tchabo JG, Tomai T: Selected intrapartum external cephalic version of the second twin. Obstet Gynecol 79:421, 1992.
120. Rabinovici J, Reichman B, Serr DM, et al: Internal podalic version with unruptured membranes for the second twin in transverse lie. Obstet Gynecol 71:428, 1988.
121. Druzin ML: Atraumatic delivery in cases of malpresentation of the very low birthweight fetus at cesarean section: the splint technique. Am J Obstet Gynecol 154:941, 1986.
122. Van Dorsten JP, Schifrin BS, Wallace RL: Randomized control trial of external cephalic version with tocolysis in late pregnancy. Am J Obstet Gynecol 141:417, 1981.
123. Hanley BJ: Editorial—fallacy of external version. Obstet Gynecol 4:124, 1954.
124. Thornhill PE: Changes in fetal polarity near term spontaneous and external version. Am J Obstet Gynecol 93:306, 1965.
125. Ylikorkala O, Hartikainen-Sorri A: Value of external version in fetal malpresentation in combination with use of ultrasound. Acta Obstet Gynecol Scand 56:63, 1977.
126. Stine LE, Phalen JP, Wallace R, et al: Update on external cephalic version performed at term. Obstet Gynecol 65:642, 1985.
127. Robertson AW, Kopelman JN, Read JA, et al: External cephalic version at term: is a tocolytic necessary? Obstet Gynecol 70:896, 1987.
128. Fortunato SJ, Mercer LJ, Guzick DS: External cephalic version with tocolysis: factors associated with success. Obstet Gynecol 72:59, 1988.
129. Marchick R: Antepartum external cephalic version with tocolysis: a study of term singleton breech presentations. Am J Obstet Gynecol 158:1339, 1988.
130. Hanss JW: The efficacy of external cephalic version and its impact on the breech experience. Am J Obstet Gynecol 162:1459, 1990.
131. Shupski DW, Harrison-Restelli C, Dupont RB: External cephalic version: an approach with few complications. Gynecol Obstet Invest 56:83, 2003.
132. Vezina Y, Bujold E, Varin J, et al: Cesarean delivery after successful external cephalic version of breech presentation at term: a comparative study. Am J Obstet Gynecol 190:763, 2004.
133. Belfort MA: Intravenous nitroglycerine as a tocolytic for intrapartum external cephalic version. S Afr Med J 83:656, 1993.
134. Fernandez CO, Bloom SL, Smulian JC, et al: A randomized placebo controlled evaluation of terbutaline for external cephalic version. Obstet Gynecol 90:775, 1997.
135. Schorr SJ, Speights SE, Ross EL, et al: A randomized trial of epidural anesthesia to improve external cephal version success. Am J Obstet Gynecol 177:1133, 1997.
136. Hofmeyr GJ, Gyte G: Interventions to help external cephalic version for breech presentation at term. The Cochrane Database of Systematic Reviews 2004, Issue 1.
137. Hofmeyr GJ: External cephalic version for breech presentation before term. The Cochrane Database of Systematic Reviews 1996, Issue 1.
138. Marcus RG, Crewe-Brown H, Krawitz S, et al: Fetomaternal hemorrhage following successful and unsuccessful attempts at external cephalic version. Br J Obstet Gynaecol 82:578, 1975.
139. Flamm BL, Fried MW, Lonky NM, Giles SW: External cephalic version after previous cesarean section. Am J Obstet Gynecol 165:370, 1991.
140. Schachter M, Kogan S, Blickstein I: External cephalic version after previous cesarean section-a clinical dilemma. Int J Gynecol Obstet 45:17, 1994.
141. Cardini F, Weixin H: Moxibustion for the correction of breech presentation: a randomized controlled trial. JAMA 280:1580, 1998.
142. Neri I, Airola G, Contu G, et al: Accupuncture plus moxibustion to resolve breech presentation: a randomized controlled study. J Matern Fetal Neonatal Med 15:247, 2004.
143. Kanakura Y, Kometani K, Nagata T, et al: Moxibustion treatment of breech presentation. Am J Chin Med 29:37, 2001.
144. Neri I, Fazzio M, Menghini S, et al: Non-stress test changes during acupuncture plus moxibustion on BL 67 point in breech presentations. J Soc Gynecol Investig 9:158, 2002.
145. Benedetti TJ, Gabbe SG: Shoulder dystocia—a complication of fetal macrosomia and prolonged second stage of labor with midpelvic delivery. Obstet Gynecol 52:526, 1978.
146. Swartz DP: Shoulder girdle dystocia in vertex delivery-clinical study and review. Obstet Gynecol 15:194, 1960.
147. Boyd ME, Usher RH, McLean FH: Fetal macrosomia—prediction, risks, and proposed management. Obstet Gynecol 61:715, 1983.
148. McCall JO: Shoulder dystocia—a study of after effects. Am J Obstet Gynecol 83:1486, 1962.
149. Sandmire HF, DeMott RK: The Green Bay cesarean section study IV. The physician factor as a determinant of cesarean birth rates for the large fetus. Am J Obstet Gynecol 174:1557, 1996.

150. Seigworth GR: Shoulder dystocia—review of 5 years' experience. Obstet Gynecol 28:764, 1966.
151. Acker DB, Sachs BP, Friedman EA: Risk factors for Erb-Duchenne palsy. Obstet Gynecol 66:764, 1985.
152. Parks DG, Ziel HK: Macrosomia—a proposed indication for primary cesarean section. Obstet Gynecol 52:407, 1978.
153. Lewis DF, Edwards MS, Asrat T, et al: Can shoulder dystocia be predicted? J Reprod Med 43:654, 1998.
154. Acker DB, Gregory KD, Sachs BP, et al: Risk factors for Erb-Duchenne palsy. Obstet Gynecol 71:389, 1988.
155. Lewis DF, Raymond RC, Perkins MB, et al: Recurrence rate of shoulder dystocia. Am J Obstet 172:1369, 1995.
156. Klebanoff MA, Mednick BR, Schulsinger C, et al: Father's effect on infant birthweight. Am J Obstet Gynecol 178:1022, 1998.
157. Modanlou HD, Dorchester WL, Thorosian A, et al: Macrosomia—maternal, fetal, and neonatal implications. Obstet Gynecol 55:420, 1980.
158. Golditch IM, Kirkman K: The large fetus—management and outcome. Obstet Gynecol 52:26, 1978.
159. Modanlou HD, Komatsu G, Dorchester W, et al: Large for gestational age neonates: anthropometric reasons for shoulder dystocia. Obstet Gynecol 60:417, 1982.
160. Chauhan SP, Grobman WA, Gherman RA, et al: Suspicion and treatment of the macrosomic fetus: a review. Am J Obstet Gynecol 193:332, 2005.
161. Cohen B, Penning S, Major C, et al: Sonographic prediction of shoulder dystocia in infants of diabetic mothers. Obstet Gynecol 88:10, 1996.
162. Jazayeri A, Heffron JA, Phillips R, Spellacy WN: Macrosomia prediction using ultrasound fetal abdominal circumference of 35 centimeters or more. Obstet Gynecol 93:523, 1999.
163. Gross TL, Sokol RJ, Williams T, et al: Shoulder dystocia: a fetal—physician risk. Am J Obstet Gynecol 156:1408, 1987.
164. Rouse DJ, Owen J, Goldenberg RL, Cliver SP: The effectiveness and costs of elective cesarean delivery for fetal macrosomia diagnosed by ultrasound. JAMA 276:1480, 1996.
165. Langer O, Berkus MD, Huff RW, Samueloff A: Shoulder dystocia: should the fetus weighing >4000g be delivered by cesarean section? Am J Obstet Gynecol 165:831, 1991.
166. ACOG practice bulletin clinical management guidelines for obstetrician-gynecologists. Obstet Gynecol 100:1045, 2002.
167. Keller JD, Lopez-Zano JA, Dooley SL, Socol ML: Shoulder dystocia and birth trauma in gestational diabetes: a five year experience. Am J Obstet Gynecol 165:928, 1991.
167a. Gonik B, Walker A, Grimm M: Mathematical modeling of forces associated with shoulder dystocia: the use of a mathematic dynamic model. Am J Obstet Gynecol 182:689, 2000.
167b. Gonik B, Zhang N, Grimm M: Prediction of brachial plexus stretching during shoulder dystocia using a computer simulation model. Am J Obstet Gynecol 189:1168, 2003.
168. Gherman RB, Ouzounian JG, Miller DA, et al: Spontaneous vaginal delivery: a risk for Erb's palsy? Am J Obstet Gynecol 178:423, 1998.
169. Gilbert WM, Nesbitt TS, Danielsen B: Associated factors in 1611 cases of brachial plexus injury. Obstet Gynecol 93:536, 1999.
170. Sandmire HF, DeMott RK: Erb's palsy: concepts and causation. Obstet Gynecol 95:940, 2000.
170a. Gurewitsch ED, Johnson E, Hamzehzadeh S, Allen RH: Risk factors for brachial plexus injury with and without shoulder dystocia. Am J Obstet Gynecol 194:486, 2006.
171. Gherman RB: Shoulder dystocia: prevention and management. Obstet Gynecol Clin North Am 32:297, 2005.
172. Gonik B, Stringer CA, Held B: An alternate maneuver for management of shoulder dystocia. Am J Obstet Gynecol 145:882, 1983.
173. Gonik B, Allen R, Sorab J: Objective evaluation of the shoulder dystocia phenomenon: effect of maternal pelvic orientation on force reduction. Obstet Gynecol 74:44, 1989.
174. Gherman RB, Goodwin TM, Souter I, et al: The McRobert's maneuver for the alleviation of shoulder dystocia: how successful is it? Am J Obstet Gynecol 176:656, 1997.
175. Pecorari D: A guest editorial from abroad: meditations on a nightmare of modern midwifery: shoulder dystocia. Obstet Gynecol Surv 54:353, 1999.
176. Brunner JP, Drummond SB, Meenan AL, Gaskin IM: All fours maneuver for reducing shoulder dystocia during labor. J Reprod Med 43:439, 1998.
177. Gross SJ, Shime J, Farine D: Shoulder dystocia: predictors and outcome. Am J Obstet Gynecol 156:334, 1987.
178. Gherman RB, Ouzounian JG, Goodwin TM: Obstetric maneuvers for shoulder dystocia and associated fetal morbidity. Am J Obstet Gynecol 178:1126, 1998.
178a. Beall MH, Spong CY, Ross MG: A randomized controlled trial of prophylactic maneuvers to reduce head-to-body delivery time in patients at risk for shoulder dystocia. Obstet Gynecol 102:31, 2003.
178b. Poggi SH, Allen RH, Patel CR, et al: Randomized trial of McRoberts versus lithotomy positioning to decrease the force that is applied to the fetus during delivery. Am J Obstet Gynecol 191:874, 2004.
179. Sandberg EC: The Zavanelli maneuver: 12 years of recorded experience. Obstet Gynecol 93:312, 1999.
180. O'Leary JA, Cuva A: Abdominal rescue after failed cephalic replacement. Obstet Gynecol 80:514, 1992.
181. Hartfield VJ: Symphysiotomy for shoulder dystocia [letter]. Am J Obstet Gynecol 155:228, 1986.
182. Goodwin TM, Banks E, Millar LK, Phelan JP: Catastrophic shoulder dystocia and emergency symphysiotomy. Am J Obstet Gynecol 177:463, 1997.

Antepartum and Postpartum Hemorrhage

KARRIE E. FRANCOIS AND MICHAEL R. FOLEY

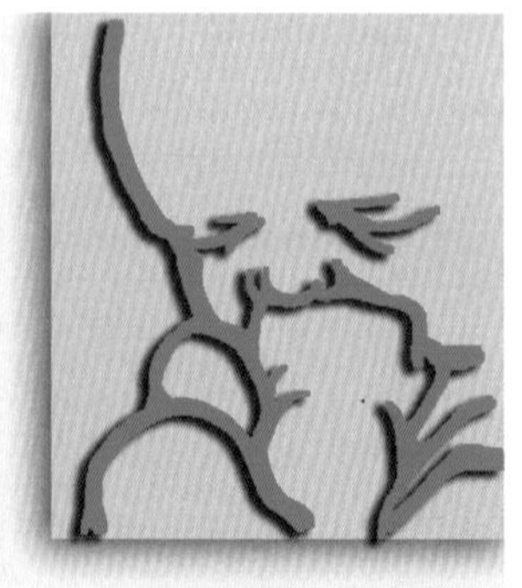

CHAPTER 18

KEY ABBREVIATIONS

Disseminated intravascular coagulation	DIC
Fresh frozen plasma	FFP
Packed red blood cells	prbc

INTRODUCTION

Antepartum and postpartum hemorrhage remain one of the leading causes of obstetric morbidity and mortality throughout the world. Between 17 and 25 percent of all pregnancy-related deaths can be directly attributed to hemorrhage.[1,2] Because of this significant contribution to maternal mortality, it is critical for the obstetrician to have a thorough understanding of the hemodynamic changes that accompany pregnancy and the maternal adaptations that occur with excessive blood loss.

PREGNANCY-RELATED HEMODYNAMIC CHANGES

Pregnancy is associated with four significant hemodynamic changes (see Chapter 3). The first of these is plasma volume expansion. The average singleton pregnancy has a 40- to 50-percent increase in plasma volume, which occurs by the 30th week of gestation. This increase in plasma volume is accompanied by an increase in red blood cell mass. With appropriate substrate availability, red blood cell mass can be expected to increase 20 to 30 percent by the end of pregnancy.[3] Maternal cardiac output rises with normal pregnancy owing to both increased stroke volume and heart rate. Consensus exists that the average rise in cardiac output is 30 to 50 percent above nonpregnant levels, with the peak occurring in the early third trimester.[4] Systemic vascular resistance falls in parallel with this rise in cardiac output and blood volume expansion.[5] Finally, fibrinogen and the majority of procoagulant blood factors (I, VII, VIII, IX, and X) increase during pregnancy.[6] These four physiologic changes are protective of maternal hemodynamic status and, in doing so, allow for further physiologic adaptations that accompany obstetric hemorrhage.

PHYSIOLOGIC ADAPTATION TO HEMORRHAGE

During pregnancy and the puerperium, a defined sequence of physiologic adaptations occur with hemorrhage (Fig. 18-1). When 10 percent of the circulatory blood volume is lost, vasoconstriction occurs in both the arterial and venous compartments in order to maintain blood pressure and preserve blood flow to essential organs. As blood loss reaches 20 percent or more of the total blood volume, increases in systemic vascular resistance can no longer compensate for the lost intravascular volume and blood pressure decreases. Cardiac output falls in parallel due to a loss in preload, resulting in poor end-organ perfusion. If the intravascular volume is not appropriately replaced, cardiogenic shock will ensue (Fig. 18-1).

In severe preeclampsia, these physiologic adaptations are altered. Unlike most pregnant patients, the protective mechanism of blood volume expansion is diminished with severe preeclampsia. It is estimated that plasma volume expansion is 9 percent lower in preeclamptic patients.[7] In addition, because of the significant vasoconstriction that accompanies preeclampsia, blood loss in these patients may be underestimated because blood pressure may be maintained in the normotensive range despite significant hemorrhage. Finally, in preeclampsia, oliguria may not be as reliable an indicator of poor end-organ perfusion secondary to hemorrhage because reduced urine output is often a manifestation of the severity of the hypertensive disorder.

CLASSIFICATION OF HEMORRHAGE

A standard classification for acute blood loss is illustrated in Table 18-1. Understanding the physiologic responses that accompany varying degrees of volume deficit can assist the clinician when caring for patients experiencing hemorrhage. Determination of the hemorrhage class reflects the volume deficit, which may not be the same as volume loss. The average 60-kg pregnant woman maintains a blood volume of 6,000 ml by 30 weeks' gestation.

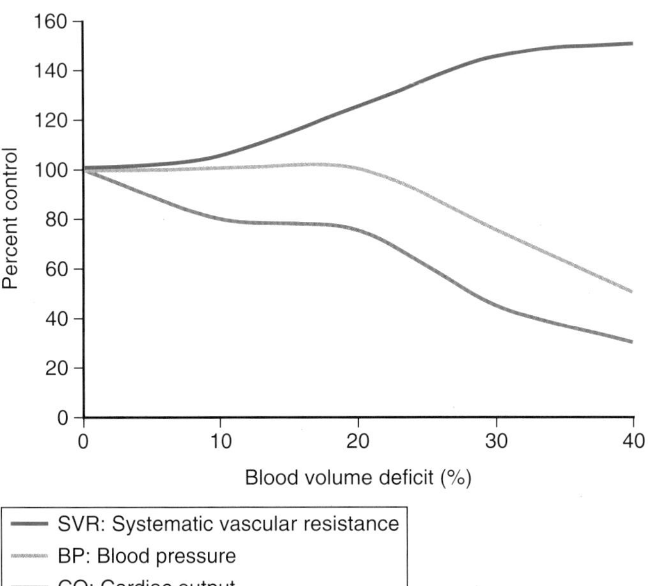

Figure 18-1. Relationships among systemic vascular resistance, blood pressure, and cardiac output in the face of progressive blood volume deficit.

Class 1 hemorrhage corresponds to a 900-ml blood loss. This blood loss typically correlates to a 15-percent volume deficit. Women with this amount of volume deficit rarely exhibit physiologic changes owing to the hemodynamic adaptations that accompany pregnancy.

Class 2 hemorrhage is characterized by 1,200- to 1,500-ml blood loss or a 20- to 25-percent volume deficit. Early physical changes that occur during this hemorrhage class include tachycardia and tachypnea. Although tachycardia is usually recognized as a compensatory mechanism to increase cardiac output, the significance of tachypnea is unclear and often unappreciated clinically. Tachypnea can represent a sign of impending clinical decompensation.

Narrowing of the pulse pressure is another sign of class 2 hemorrhage. The pulse pressure represents the difference between the systolic and diastolic blood pressures. Pulse pressure is a good reflection of stroke volume and β-1 stimulation. Similarly diastolic blood pressure is a reflection of systemic vasoconstriction. Therefore, the systolic blood pressure represents the interrelationship between these entities. With a class 2 volume deficit, the sympathoadrenal system is activated, resulting in a diversion of blood away from nonvital organs (skin, muscle, kidney) and a redistribution of the circulation to vital body organs, the brain, and heart. The end result is increased vasoconstriction, increased diastolic blood pressure, maintenance of systolic blood pressure, and a narrowing of the pulse pressure. With greater narrowing of the pulse pressure, more compensatory vasoconstriction is occurring to accommodate for a loss in stroke volume. A final physiologic response of class 2 hemorrhage is orthostatic hypotension. Although blood pressure comparisons can be made in the supine, sitting, and standing positions to document this response, a practical approach is to assess the time needed to refill a blanched hypothenar area on the patient's hand. Typically, a patient with normal volume status can reperfuse this area within 1 to 2 seconds after pressure is applied. A patient with class 2 hemorrhage and orthostatic hypotension will have significant reperfusion delay.

Class 3 hemorrhage is defined as a blood loss of 1,800 to 2,100 ml and corresponds to a volume deficit of 30 to 35 percent. Within this hemorrhage class, the physiologic

Table 18-1. Classification of Hemorrhage*

HEMORRHAGE CLASS	ACUTE BLOOD LOSS	% LOST	PHYSIOLOGIC RESPONSE
1	900 ml	15	Asymptomatic
2	1,200–1,500 ml	20–25	Tachycardia and tachypnea Narrowed pulse pressure Orthostatic hypotension Delayed hypothenar refilling
3	1,800–2,100 ml	30–35	Worsening tachycardia and tachypnea Hypotension Cool extremities
4	>2,400 ml	40	Shock Oliguria/Anuria

*Total blood volume = 6,000 ml.

responses noted in class 2 hemorrhage are exaggerated. Patients demonstrate significant tachycardia (120 to 160 beats/minute), tachypnea (30 to 50 breaths/minute), overt hypotension, and cool extremities.

Class 4 hemorrhage is characterized by more than a 2,400-ml blood loss. This amount of blood loss exceeds 40 percent of the patient's total blood volume. The clinical manifestations of this volume deficit include absent distal pulses, cardiogenic shock, and oliguria/anuria. When a large hemorrhage occurs, renal blood flow is reduced and redirected from the outer renal cortex to the juxtamedullary region. In this region, increased water and sodium absorption occur, resulting in less urine volume, lower urinary sodium concentration, and increased urine osmolarity. A urine sodium concentration less than 10 to 20 mEq/L or a urine/serum osmolar ratio greater than 2 indicates significantly reduced renal perfusion in the face of hemorrhage.

ANTEPARTUM HEMORRHAGE

Placental Abruption

Definition and Pathogenesis

Placental abruption, or abruptio placenta, refers to the premature separation of a normally implanted placenta from the uterus. Typically, defective maternal vessels in the deciduas basalis rupture and cause the separation. On rare occasions, the separation may be caused by a disruption of the fetal-placental vessels.[8] The damaged vessels cause bleeding, which results in a decidual hematoma that can lead to placental separation, destruction of placental tissue, and a loss of maternal-fetal surface area for nutrient and gas exchange.[9]

Incidence

Placental abruption complicates 1 in 75 to 1 in 226 deliveries.[9–12] The range in incidence likely reflects variable criteria for diagnosis as well as an increased recognition in recent years of milder forms of abruption. Approximately one third of all antepartum bleeding can be attributed to placental abruption.[8]

Clinical Manifestations

The clinical manifestations of placental abruption include vaginal bleeding or occult uterine bleeding, abdominal pain, uterine contractions or hypertonus, uterine tenderness, nonreassuring fetal heart rate patterns or fetal death, and disseminated intravascular coagulation (DIC).[9,14–16] Approximately 80 percent of placental abruptions occur before the onset of labor.[13] The diagnosis is confirmed with certainty by the macroscopic inspection of a placenta with adherent retroplacental clot and depression/disruption of the underlying placental tissue.

Placental abruption can be broadly classified into three grades that correlate with the following clinical and laboratory findings:

Grade 1: A mild abruption characterized by slight vaginal bleeding and minimal uterine irritability. Maternal blood pressure and fibrinogen levels are unaffected, and the fetal heart rate pattern is normal. Approximately 40 percent of placental abruptions are grade 1.

Grade 2: A partial abruption with mild to moderate vaginal bleeding and significant uterine irritability or contractions. Maternal blood pressure is maintained, but the pulse is often elevated and postural blood volume deficits may be present. The fibrinogen level may be decreased, and the fetal heart rate often shows signs of fetal compromise. Grade 2 abruptions account for 45 percent of all placental abruptions.

Grade 3: A large or complete abruption characterized by moderate to severe vaginal bleeding or occult uterine bleeding with painful, tetanic uterine contractions. Maternal hypotension and coagulopathy are frequently present along with fetal death. Approximately 15 percent of placental abruptions are recognized as grade 3.

Risk Factors

Although the exact etiology of placental abruption is unclear, a variety of risk factors have been identified (Table 18-2).

Increasing Parity and/or Maternal Age

Several studies have noted a higher incidence of placental abruption with increasing parity.[15,17,18] Among primigravid women, the frequency of placental abruption is less than 1 percent; however, 2.5 percent of grand multiparas experience placental abruption.[19] Theories suggest that damaged endometrium, impaired decidualization, and aberrant vasculature may have a causal role with increasing parity and/or age.[8]

Maternal age is often cited as an associated risk factor for placental abruption. Although a 15-year population-based study in Norway was able to demonstrate a strong relationship between maternal age and placental abruption for all levels of parity, others studies suggest that

Table 18-2. Placental Abruption Risk Factors
Increasing parity and/or maternal age
Cigarette smoking
Cocaine abuse
Trauma
Maternal hypertension
Preterm premature rupture of membranes
Multiple gestation
Polyhydramnios with rapid uterine decompression
Inherited or acquired thrombophilia
Uterine malformations or fibroids
Placental anomalies
Previous abruption

there is no increased risk for placental abruption among older women when parity and hypertensive disease are excluded.[17,18,20]

Cigarette Smoking

Cigarette smoking is associated with a significantly increased incidence of placental abruption and fetal death.[18,21–23] There appears to be a dose-response relationship with the number of cigarettes smoked and the risk of placental abruption, as well as perinatal mortality.[24,25] When compared with nonsmokers, smokers have a 40-percent increased risk of fetal death from abruption with each pack of cigarettes smoked.[26] The proposed causation of this increased risk is decidual ischemia and necrosis.[19]

Cocaine Abuse

Cocaine abuse in the third trimester has been associated with as high as a 10-percent placental abruption rate.[27,28] The pathogenesis appears to be related to cocaine-induced vasospasm and resulting decidual ischemia, reflex vasodilation, and vascular disruption within the placental bed.[8]

Trauma

Blunt or penetrating trauma to the gravid abdomen has been associated with placental abruption. After a minor trauma, the risk of placental abruption is between 1 and 5 percent, whereas the risk may be as high as 50 percent after severe injury.[29] The two most common causes of maternal trauma are motor vehicle accidents and domestic abuse. With motor vehicle accidents, uterine stretch, direct penetration, and placental shearing from acceleration-deceleration forces are the primary causes of trauma-related placental abruption.

Maternal Hypertension

Maternal hypertension is the most consistently identified risk factor for placental abruption.[30] This relationship has been noted with both chronic and pregnancy-related hypertension. Compared with normotensive women, hypertensive women have a fivefold increased risk of placental abruption. This relationship is most strongly associated with grade 3 abruption, in which 40 to 50 percent of cases have underlying hypertensive disease.[30,31] Maternal vascular disease is hypothesized as the common etiology for hypertension and placental abruption.

Preterm Premature Rupture of Membranes

Placental abruption occurs in 2 to 5 percent of pregnancies with preterm premature rupture of membranes.[32–34] This risk may be increased with intrauterine infection and oligohydramnios.[33] Nonreassuring fetal heart rate patterns accompany nearly half of pregnancies with preterm premature rupture of membranes and placental abruption.[34]

It is unclear whether placental abruption is the cause or consequence of preterm premature rupture of membranes.[8] Hemorrhage and associated thrombin generation may stimulate cytokine and protease production, resulting in membrane rupture. Alternatively, the cytokine/protease cascade that follows ruptured membranes may cause damage to the decidual vasculature, predisposing the placenta to an abruption.

Rapid Uterine Decompression Associated with Multiple Gestation and Polyhydramnios

Rapid decompression of an overdistended uterus can cause placental abruption. This may occur in the setting of multiple gestation or with polyhydramnios. Compared with singletons, twins have been reported to have nearly a threefold increased risk of placental abruption.[35] Although the exact timing of placental abruption in multiple gestations is difficult to ascertain, it has been attributed to rapid decompression of the uterus after the delivery of the first twin. Likewise, rapid loss of amniotic fluid in pregnancies complicated by polyhydramnios has been implicated in placental abruption. This can occur with spontaneous rupture of membranes or may follow therapeutic amniocentesis.

Inherited Thrombophilia

Recent evidence has implicated the presence of inherited or acquired thrombophilias as a significant factor in the etiology of placental abruption.[36–41] The thrombophilias most commonly cited include factor V Leiden mutation, prothrombin G20210A mutation, thermolabile methylene tetrahydrofolate reductase mutation (C677T) with associated hyperhomocysteinemia, type 1 plasminogen activator inhibitor, protein C deficiency, protein S deficiency, antithrombin III deficiency, hypofibrogenemia or dysfibrinogenemia, and antiphospholipid antibody syndrome.[42] There appears to be a dose-response increase in the risk of placental abruption with increasing numbers or combinations of thrombophilias.[43]

Uterine and Placental Factors

Placental implantation over a uterine malformation (e.g., septum) or fibroid, as well as placental abnormalities (e.g., circumvallate placenta), can be associated with placental abruption.

Prior Abruption

A previous abruption is associated with a risk of recurrence between 5 to 17 percent.[14,15,30] After two consecutive abruptions, the recurrence risk rises to 25 percent. In the largest series of grade 3 placental abruptions with resultant fetal death, the recurrence rate of another grade 3 placental abruption and subsequent fetal demise was 11 percent.

Diagnosis

The diagnosis of placental abruption is primarily clinical, with supportive evidence from sonographic, laboratory, and pathologic studies. Any vaginal bleeding in the third trimester of pregnancy should prompt an investigation to determine its etiology. Although vaginal bleeding is the hallmark sign of placental abruption, 10 to 20 percent of affected women may have an occult or concealed hemorrhage.

Sonography

Although early studies evaluating the use of ultrasound for the diagnosis of placental abruption identified less than 2 percent of cases, recent advances in imaging and its interpretation have improved detection rates. Early hemorrhage is typically hyperechoic or isoechoic, whereas resolving hematomas are hypoechoic within 1 week and sonolucent within 2 weeks of the abruption.[44] Acute hemorrhage has been misinterpreted as a thickened placenta or fibroid.

Ultrasound can identify three predominant locations for placental abruption. These are subchorionic (between the placenta and the membranes), retroplacental (between the placenta and the myometrium), and preplacental (between the placenta and the amniotic fluid). Figure 18-2 illustrates the classification of hematomas in and

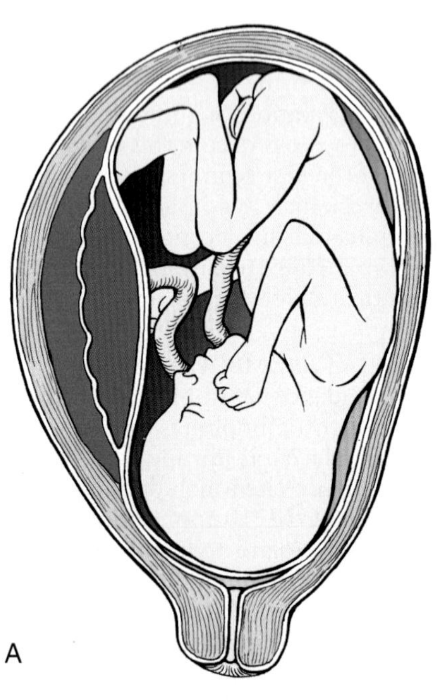

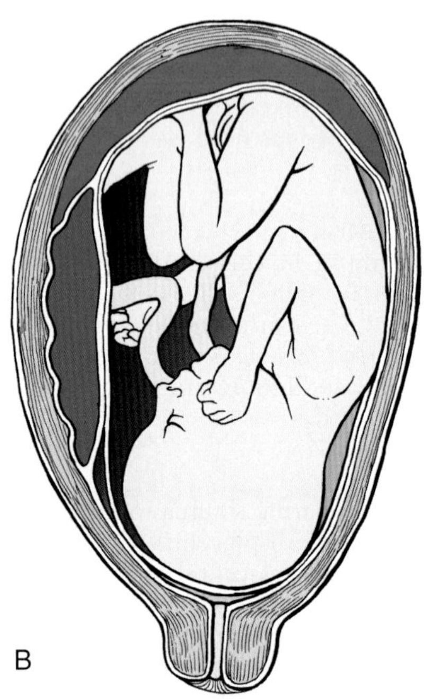

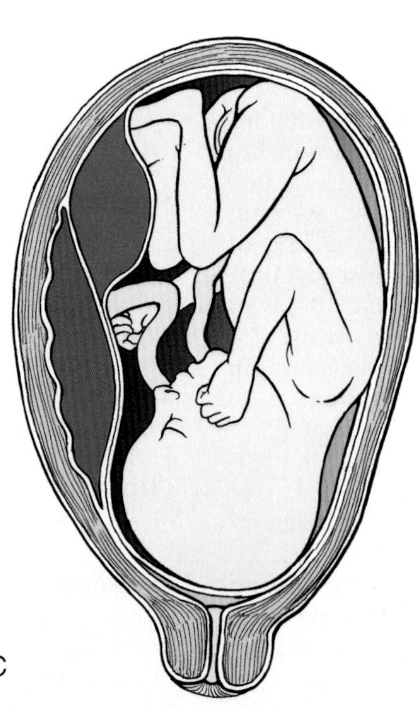

Figure 18-2. Drawings demonstrating the classification system of placental abruption. *A,* Retroplacental abruption: The bright red area represents a blood collection behind the placenta (dark red). *B,* Subchorionic abruption: The bright red area represents subchorionic bleeding, which is observed to dissect along the chorion. *C,* Preplacental abruption: The bright red area represents a blood collection anterior to the placenta within the amnion and chorion (subamniotic). (From Trop I, Levine D: Hemorrhage during pregnancy: Sonography and MR imaging. AJR Am J Roentgenol 176:607, 2001. Copyright 2001 American Roentgen Ray Society.)

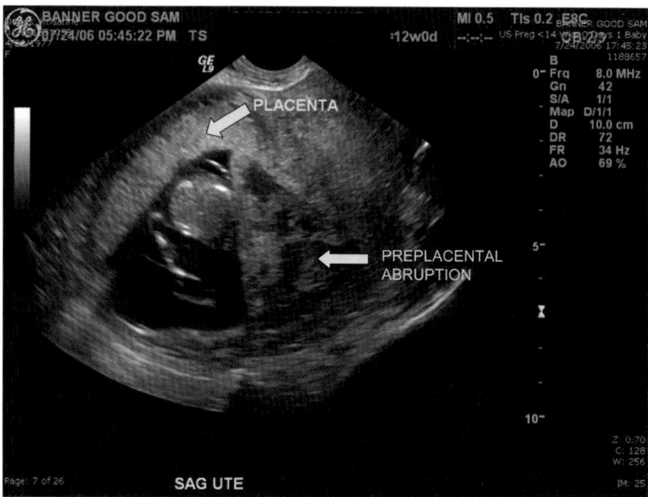

Figure 18-3. Ultrasonic image of a preplacental abruption. (Courtesy of WH Clewell.)

around the placenta. Figure 18-3 demonstrates an ultrasonic representation of a preplacental abruption.

The location and extent of the placental abruption identified on ultrasound examination is of clinical significance. Retroplacental hematomas are associated with a worse prognosis for fetal survival than subchorionic hemorrhage. The size of the hemorrhage is also predictive of fetal survival. Large retroplacental hemorrhages (>60 ml) are associated with a 50 percent or greater fetal mortality, whereas similar sized subchorionic hemorrhages are associated with a 10 percent mortality risk.[45]

Laboratory Findings

Few laboratory studies can assist in the diagnosis of placental abruption. Hypofibrinogenemia and evidence of DIC are supportive of the diagnosis; however, clinical correlation is necessary. As noted earlier, most abruptions are not accompanied by coagulopathy.

Pathologic Studies

Macroscopic inspection of the placenta demonstrates adherent clot and depression of the placental surface. Fresh or acute placental abruptions may not have any identifiable evidence on pathologic examination.

Management

Nearly half of all placental abruptions will result in delivery at less than 37 weeks' gestation.[20] Gestational age at the time of presentation is an important prognostic factor. In patients presenting at less than 20 weeks, 82 percent can be expected to have a term delivery despite evidence of placental abruption. However, if the presentation occurs after 20 weeks' gestation, only 27 percent will deliver at term.

Once the diagnosis of placental abruption has been made, precautions should be taken to anticipate the possible life-threatening consequences for both mother and fetus. These precautions include baseline laboratory assessment (hemoglobin, hematocrit, platelet count, type and screen, fibrinogen, and coagulation studies), appropriate intravenous access (large-bore catheter), availability of blood products, continuous fetal heart rate and contraction monitoring, and communication with operating room and neonatal personnel.

The timing and mode of delivery are dependent on the severity of the maternal-fetal condition, the gestational age, and the cervical examination. In the case of a grade 1 abruption that is remote from term, hospitalization with expectant management may be warranted.[46] A trial of tocolysis for documented preterm labor and administration of antenatal corticosteroid therapy can be considered if maternal-fetal status is stable. Reported series of expectant management in preterm gestations with placental abruption have shown a significant prolongation of the pregnancy (>1 week) in more than 50 percent of patients without adverse maternal or fetal outcomes.[47,48] In a large series of preterm patients who presented with placental abruption and received tocolysis, approximately one third delivered within 48 hours of admission, one third delivered within 7 days, and one third delivered greater than 1 week from initial presentation. There were no cases of intrauterine demise in women presenting with a live fetus.[49] Although these results are encouraging, the clinician must always keep in mind that placental abruption can result in both maternal and fetal morbidity. Any attempt to arrest preterm labor in a known or suspected placental abruption must be weighed against the likelihood of neonatal survival and morbidity, the severity of the abruption, and the safety of the mother.

Women presenting at or near term with a placental abruption should undergo delivery. Induction or augmentation of labor is not contraindicated in the setting of an abruption; however, close surveillance for any evidence of maternal or fetal compromise is advised. Continuous fetal heart rate monitoring is recommended because 60 percent of fetuses may exhibit nonreassuring intrapartum heart rate patterns. Intrauterine pressure catheters and fetal scalp electrodes can assist the clinician during the intrapartum course. Intrauterine pressure catheter monitoring can demonstrate elevated uterine resting tone. This may be associated with deficits in uterine blood flow and fetal oxygenation. Maternal hemodynamic and clotting parameters must be followed closely in order to detect signs of evolving coagulopathy. Although vaginal delivery is generally preferable, operative delivery is often necessary owing to fetal and maternal decompensation.

The management of women with severe coagulopathy and fetal demise requires a thorough knowledge of the natural history of severe placental abruption. Nearly 4 decades ago, Pritchard and Brekken noted several clinically important and relevant observations concerning the natural course of placental abruption.[50] These include the following: (1) approximately 40 percent of patients with grade 3 placental abruption will demonstrate signs of DIC; (2) within 8 hours of initial symptoms in such women, hypofibrinogenemia will be present; (3) severe hypofibrinogenemia will not recover without blood product replacement; and (4) the time course for recovery from hypofibrinogenemia is roughly 10 mg/dl per hour after delivery of the fetus and placenta.

When managing patients with severe or grade 3 placental abruptions with intrauterine fetal demise, maintenance of maternal volume status and replacement of blood products is essential. Although operative delivery may appear to lead to the most rapid resolution of the problem, it may pose significant risk to the patient. Unless the coagulopathy is corrected, surgery can result in uncontrollable bleeding and increased need for hysterectomy. The uterus does not need to be evacuated before coagulation status can be restored. Blood product replacement and delayed delivery until hematologic parameters have improved are generally associated with good maternal outcomes.

When operative delivery is necessary, a Couvelaire uterus characterized by extravasation of blood into the myometrium may be found in 8 percent of patients. This finding may be associated with significant uterine atony. Administration of uterotonic therapy usually improves the condition. Hysterectomy should be reserved for cases of atony and hemorrhage unresponsive to conventional uterotonic therapies.

Neonatal Outcome

Placental abruption has been uniformly associated with increased perinatal mortality (20 to 30 percent), preterm delivery, and intrauterine growth restriction.[11,51,52] When compared with normal controls, women with placental abruption have a ninefold increased risk of intrauterine fetal demise, a fourfold increased risk of preterm delivery, and a twofold increased risk of intrauterine growth restriction.[53] A case-control study has also shown a greater risk for adverse long-term neurobehavioral outcomes in infants delivered after placental abruption.[54] Neonates at risk for an abnormal outcome had a higher incidence of abnormal fetal heart rate tracings (45 percent) and emergency cesarean delivery (53 percent) when compared with controls (10 percent and 10 percent, respectively). Finally, an increased incidence of sudden infant death syndrome has been noted in newborns following placental abruptions.[55]

Placenta Previa

Definition and Pathogenesis

Placenta previa is defined as the presence of placental tissue over or adjacent to the cervical os. Traditionally three variations of placenta previa are recognized: complete, partial, and marginal. Although complete placenta previa referred to the total coverage of the cervical os by placental tissue, the differences between partial (placental edge at the cervical os) and marginal (placental edge near the cervical os) are often subtle and vary by the timing and method of diagnosis. In more recent years, ultrasound technology and precision have advanced allowing for more accurate assessments of the placental location in relation to the cervical os. With this in mind, contemporary classification of placenta previa consists of two variations: *placenta previa,* in which the cervical os is covered by placental tissue, and *marginal placenta previa,* in which the placenta lies within 2 to 3 cm of the cervical os but does not cover it.[56]

Incidence

The overall reported incidence of placenta previa at delivery is 4/1,000 deliveries.[57] In the second trimester, placenta previa may be found in 4 to 6 percent of pregnancies.[58–60] The term placental migration has been used to explain this "resolution" of placenta previa that is noted near term. Two theories have been suggested to account for this phenomenon. The first hypothesis proposes that as the pregnancy advances the stationary lower placental edge relocates away from the cervical os with the development of the lower uterine segment. Indeed the lower uterine segment has been noted to increase from 0.5 cm at 20 weeks to more than 5 cm at term.[61] The second hypothesis suggests that trophotropism, or the growth of trophoblastic tissue away from the cervical os toward the fundus, results in resolution of the placenta previa.[62]

Clinical Manifestations

Placenta previa typically presents as painless vaginal bleeding in the second or third trimester. Some patients present with uterine contractions that precede a bleeding episode.[58,63] The bleeding is believed to occur from disruption of placental blood vessels in association with the development and thinning out of the lower uterine segment.

Risk Factors

Several risk factors for placenta previa have been noted (Table 18-3). Additionally, some reports have documented a higher association of fetal malpresentation, preterm premature rupture of membranes, and intrauterine growth restriction with placenta previa.[58,64–66]

Increasing Parity and Maternal Age

Studies have reported more cases of placenta previa with increasing parity. Grand multiparas have been reported to have a 5-percent risk for placenta previa as compared with a 0.2-percent among nulliparous women.[61] Maternal age also seems to influence the occurrence of placenta

Table 18-3. Placenta Previa Risk Factors
Increasing parity
Increasing maternal age
Cigarette smoking
Residence in higher altitude
Multiple gestations
Previous placenta previa
Prior curettage
Prior cesarean delivery

previa formation. Women older than 35 years of age have more than a fourfold increased risk of placenta previa, and women older than 40 years of age have a ninefold greater risk.[67,68]

Cigarette Smoking and Residence at Higher Elevation

Cigarette smoking has been associated with as high as a threefold increased risk of previa formation.[69] Likewise, residence at higher elevations may contribute to previa development.[58] The need for increased placental surface area secondary to decreased uteroplacental oxygenation may contribute to these associations.

Multiple Gestations

Controversy exists regarding an increased risk of placenta previa with multiple gestations. Although some studies have shown a higher incidence of placenta previa among twins, others have not documented a significantly increased risk.[35,70,71]

Previous Placenta Previa

Having had a previous placenta previa increases the risk for the development of another previa in a subsequent pregnancy. This association has been reported to be as high as an eightfold relative risk.[72] The exact etiology for this increased risk is unclear but may be attributed to a genetic predisposition for the phenomenon.

Prior Curettage and Prior Cesarean Delivery

Prior uterine surgery has been associated with placenta previa formation. Although a history of curettage has a slightly elevated previa risk (1.3 relative risk), prior cesarean delivery is a significant risk factor.[73] In the pregnancy following a cesarean delivery, the risk of placenta previa has been reported to be between 1 and 4 percent.[74–78] There is a linear increase in placenta previa risk with the number of prior cesarean deliveries. In patients with four or more cesarean deliveries, the risk of placenta previa approaches 10 percent.[75] Endometrial scarring is thought to be the etiologic factor for this increased risk.

Diagnosis

The timing of the diagnosis of placenta previa has undergone significant change in the last 2 decades. Painless third-trimester bleeding was a common presentation for placenta previa in the past, whereas most cases of placenta previa are now detected antenatally with ultrasound before the onset of significant bleeding.

Sonography

Transabdominal and transvaginal ultrasound provide the best means for diagnosing placenta previa. Although transabdominal ultrasound can detect at least 95 percent of placenta previa cases, transvaginal ultrasound has a reported diagnostic accuracy approaching 100 percent.[79,80] Typically, a combined approach can be used in which transabdominal ultrasound is employed as the initial diagnostic modality and transvaginal ultrasound is reserved for uncertain cases. Of note, good images can be obtained using transvaginal ultrasound without the probe contacting the cervix (Fig. 18-4). Also, translabial ultrasound can be used to assist in the diagnosis if reservation exists regarding the use of a transvaginal probe.[81]

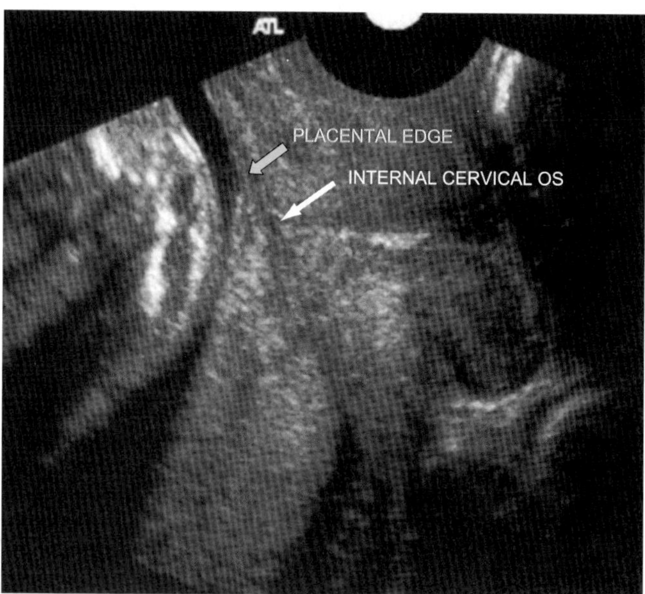

Figure 18-4. Transvaginal ultrasound. Diagnosis of placenta previa. The arrow identifies the caudal edge of the placenta covering the internal cervical os. (From Gillen-Goldstein J, Lockwood CJ: Abruptio placentae. *www.uptodate.com*.)

If placenta previa is diagnosed before 24 weeks' gestation, repeat sonography should be obtained between 28 and 32 weeks' gestation. More than 90 percent of the cases of placenta previa diagnosed in the midtrimester resolve by term.[82] The potential for resolution of the placenta previa is dependent on whether the previa is complete versus marginal. Complete placenta previa diagnosed in the second trimester will persist into the third trimester in 26 percent of cases, whereas marginal placenta previa will persist in only 2.5 percent of cases.[83]

Management

General management principles for patients with placenta previa in the third trimester include serial sonography to assess placental location and fetal growth, avoidance of cervical examinations and coitus, activity restrictions, counseling regarding labor symptoms and vaginal bleeding, dietary/nutrient supplementation to avoid maternal anemia, and early medical attention if any vaginal bleeding occurs.[84]

Outpatient Management

Asymptomatic patients with placenta previa or patients with a history of a small bleed that has resolved for greater than 7 days are potential candidates for outpatient management. Several studies have documented the safety, efficacy, and cost savings of outpatient versus inpatient management in such cases.[60,85,86] Candidates for outpatient management must be highly compliant, live within 15 minutes from the hospital, have 24-hour emergency transportation to the hospital, and verbalize a thorough understanding of the risks associated with placenta previa and outpatient management.

Expectant Management of Preterm Patients

Patients with placenta previa who present preterm with vaginal bleeding require hospitalization and immediate evaluation to assess maternal-fetal stability. Studies have demonstrated that immediate delivery can be delayed and a significant prolongation (>2 weeks) of pregnancy can occur even in patients with initial bleeding episodes greater than 500 ml.[58]

In order to optimize maternal-fetal outcome, patients should initially be managed in a labor and delivery unit with continuous fetal heart rate and contraction monitoring. Large-bore intravenous access and baseline laboratory studies (hemoglobin, hematocrit, platelet count, blood type and screen, and coagulation studies) should be obtained. If the patient is less than 34 weeks' gestation, administration of antenatal corticosteroids should be undertaken as well as an assessment of the facility's emergency resources for both the mother and the neonate. In some cases, maternal transport and consultation with a maternal-fetal medicine specialist and a neonatologist may be warranted. Finally, tocolysis can be employed if the vaginal bleeding is preceded by or associated with uterine contractions. Magnesium sulfate is generally considered superior to β-mimetic therapy, given its reduced potential for hemodynamic-related side effects[87] (see Chapter 26).

Once stabilized, patients can be maintained on hospitalized bed rest and expectantly managed. Although some authorities have recommended prophylactic transfusions to keep the maternal hematocrit greater than 30 percent, alternative options to increase endogenous red blood cell formation should be considered,[88] including oral iron, vitamin C, and folate supplementation, intravenous iron sucrose administration, and recombinant erythropoietin alpha administration. The use of facility-based blood conservation programs can assist the clinician in conservative options for blood product replacement. Lastly, consideration of autologous blood donation may be appropriate for stable patients who are candidates for this service.[89,90]

Although maternal hemorrhage is of utmost concern, fetal blood can also be lost during the process of placental separation. Rh-immune globulin should be given to all Rh-negative, unsensitized women with third-trimester bleeding from placenta previa. A Kleihauer-Betke preparation of maternal blood should be performed. This test detects the occasional patient with a fetomaternal hemorrhage of greater than 30 ml who requires additional doses of RhoGAM. Thirty-five percent of infants whose mothers have received antepartum transfusion will also be anemic and need a transfusion when delivered.[58]

Delivery

Cesarean delivery is indicated for all patients with sonographic evidence of placenta previa. In patients with a marginal placenta previa in which the placental edge is clearly 2 to 3 cm from the cervical os, vaginal delivery may be considered; however, precautions should be made for the possibility of an emergent cesarean delivery with labor.

When performing cesarean delivery for placenta previa, the surgeon should be aware of the potential for rapid blood loss during the delivery process. Patients should have 2 to 4 units of packed red blood cells available at the time of delivery. In addition, before incising the lower uterine segment, the surgeon should assess the vascularity of this region. Although a low transverse incision is not contraindicated in patients with placenta previa, performing a vertical uterine incision may be preferable in selected cases. This is particularly true with an anterior placenta previa. Ideally, the placenta should not be disrupted when entering the uterus. If the placenta is disrupted, expedited delivery is essential. Once the fetus has been removed from the uterus, the cord blood should be "milked" to the fetus in order to avoid immediate neonatal hypovolemia and anemia. Given the potential for placenta accreta, the physician should allow the placenta to spontaneously deliver. If it does not separate easily, precautions should be taken for dealing with a placenta accreta (see later). Once the placenta separates, bleeding is controlled by the contraction of uterine myometrial fibers around the spiral arterioles. Because the lower uterine segment often contracts poorly, significant bleeding can occur from the placental implantation site. Aggressive uterotonic therapy and surgical intervention should be undertaken to rapidly control the bleeding.

Associated Conditions

Placenta Accreta

Definition and Pathogenesis

Placenta accreta represents the abnormal attachment of the placenta to the uterine lining due to an absence of the deciduas basalis and an incomplete development of the fibrinoid layer. Variations of placenta accreta include placenta increta and placenta percreta, in which the placenta extends to and through the uterine myometrium, respectively (Fig. 18-5).

Incidence and Risk Factors

The overall incidence of placenta accreta or one of its variations is 1 in 533 deliveries.[91] The two most significant risk factors for placenta accreta are placenta previa and prior cesarean delivery. The risk of placenta accreta in patients with placenta previa and an unscarred uterus is approximately 3 percent.[75] This risk dramatically increases with one or more cesarean deliveries (Table 18-4). Placenta previa with a history of one prior cesarean delivery is associated with nearly a 11-percent risk of placenta accreta. This risk rises to 67 percent when placenta previa occurs with a history of four or more cesarean deliveries.[75]

Other risk factors that have been reported include increasing parity and maternal age, prior uterine surgery, and endometrial defects.[92]

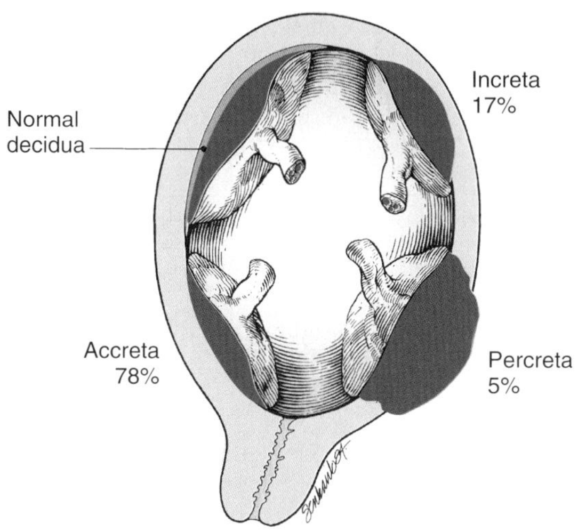

Figure 18-5. Uteroplacental relationships found in abnormal placentation.

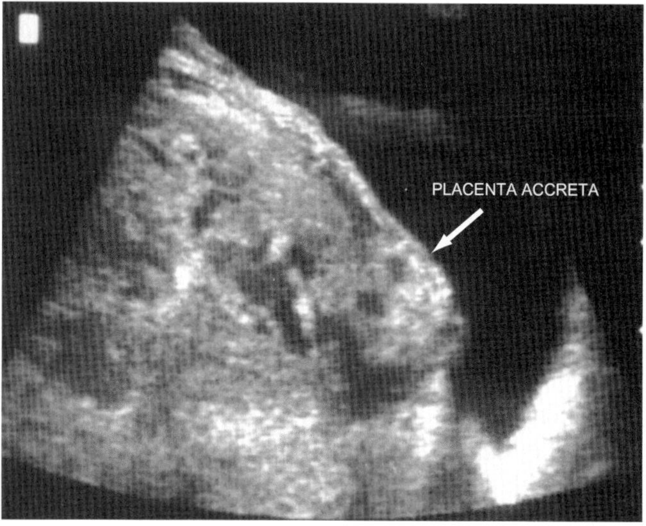

Figure 18-6. Ultrasonic image of focal placenta accreta. Arrow identifies an area at the uterine placental interface that demonstrates a loss of the normal hypoechoic zone, thinning and disruption of the uterine serosa-bladder interface and a focal exophytic mass within the placenta.

Table 18-4. Risk of Placenta Accreta with Placenta Previa and Prior Cesarean Delivery

NUMBER OF CESAREAN DELIVERIES	PLACENTA ACCRETA RISK (%)
0	3
1	11
2	40
3	61
≥4	67

From Silver RM, Landon MB, Rouse DJ, et al: Maternal morbidity associated with multiple repeat cesarean deliveries. Obstet Gynecol 107:1226, 2006.

Clinical Manifestations

The clinical manifestations are similar to those of placenta previa.

Diagnosis

In the past, placenta accreta was usually diagnosed intrapartum by the difficult or incomplete removal of the placenta and associated postpartum hemorrhage. Today with advanced radiographic technology, the diagnosis can be made antenatally.

Ultrasound is the best radiographic modality for the diagnosis of placenta accreta. Findings that are suggestive of placenta accreta include a loss of the normal hypoechoic retroplacental-myometrial zone, thinning and disruption of the uterine serosa-bladder interface, focal exophytic masses within the placenta, and numerous intraplacental vascular lacunae (Fig. 18-6).[93,94] The diagnostic sensitivity and specificity approaches 85 to 90 percent with experienced sonographers.[93] Color and power Doppler ultrasound have also proven to be useful in diagnosing placenta accreta.[95,96] Magnetic resonance imaging can be used in conjunction with sonography to assess a placenta at risk for abnormal invasion. Magnetic resonance imaging is useful in cases with equivocal ultrasound findings or with a posterior placental location.[97,98] Unexplained elevations in maternal serum alpha-fetoprotein have been associated with placenta accreta.[99,100]

Management

Because placenta accreta poses a risk for massive postpartum hemorrhage, at least two thirds of the patients require cesarean hysterectomy.[58,101,102] Ideally a multidisciplinary team approach should be assembled for these cases. Preoperative assessments by blood conservation teams, anesthesiologists, advanced pelvic surgeons, and urologists (especially for a suspected placenta percreta) are recommended. The delivery should occur at a facility that is prepared to manage significant obstetric hemorrhage. Adequate intravenous access with two large-bore catheters and ample blood product availability are mandatory. When performing the surgery, it is recommended that the uterus be incised above the placental attachment site and the placenta left in situ after clamping the cord because disruption of the implantation site may result in rapid blood loss. Adjuvant use of aortic and/or internal iliac artery balloon occlusion catheters and post-surgical embolization may be considered.[103–106]

When future fertility is desired, a variety of uterine conservation techniques can be considered. These techniques include delayed manual removal of the placenta, packing of the lower uterine segment, curettage, oversewing of the placental implantation site, uterine artery embolization, and administration of methotrexate.[102,106–112]

Vasa Previa

Definition and Pathogenesis

Vasa previa is defined as the velamentous insertion of fetal vessels over the cervical os. Typically, the fetal vessels lack protection from Wharton's jelly and are prone to rupture. When the vessels rupture, the fetus is at high risk for exsanguination. The overall perinatal mortality for vasa previa is between 58 and 73 percent.[113,114]

Incidence and Risk Factors

The incidence of vasa previa has been reported as 1/2,000 to 5,000 deliveries.[115] Reported risk factors for vasa previa include bilobed, succenturiate-lobed, and low-lying placentas; pregnancies resulting from in vitro fertilization; multiple gestations; and history of second-trimester placenta previa.[116–119]

Clinical Manifestations

Vasa previa usually presents after rupture of membranes with the acute onset of vaginal bleeding from a lacerated fetal vessel. If immediate intervention is not provided, fetal bradycardia and subsequent death occur.

Diagnosis

In the past, vasa previa was usually detected by palpation of the fetal vessels within the membranes during labor or with the acute onset of vaginal bleeding and subsequent fetal bradycardia or death after membrane rupture. With the use of sonography and Doppler imaging, vasa previa is being detected more frequently antenatally.[116,119–123] Transabdominal, transvaginal, and translabial approaches have been used. The diagnosis is confirmed when umbilical arterial waveforms are documented at the same rate as the fetal heart rate (Figs. 18-7*A* and *B*).

Management

When diagnosed antenatally, vasa previa should be managed similarly to placenta previa. Some authorities have recommended hospitalization in the third trimester with the administration of antenatal corticosteroids, serial antepartum testing, and cesarean delivery at approximately 36 weeks' gestation.[124] If an intrapartum diagnosis of vasa previa is made, expeditious delivery is needed. Immediate neonatal blood transfusion is often required.

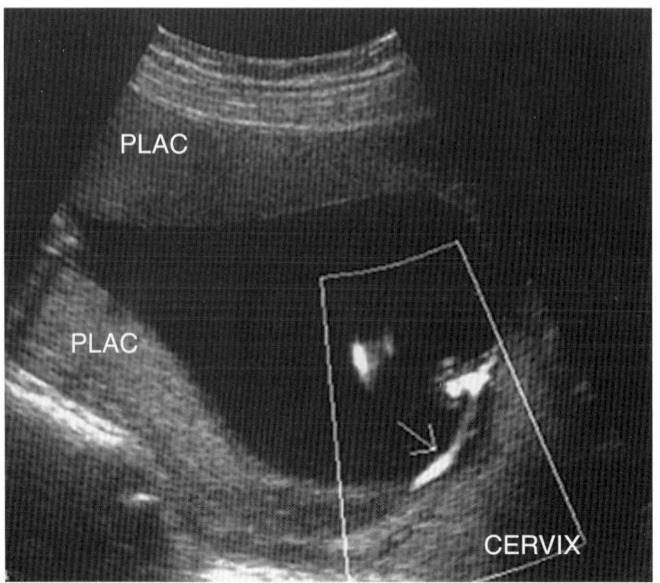

A

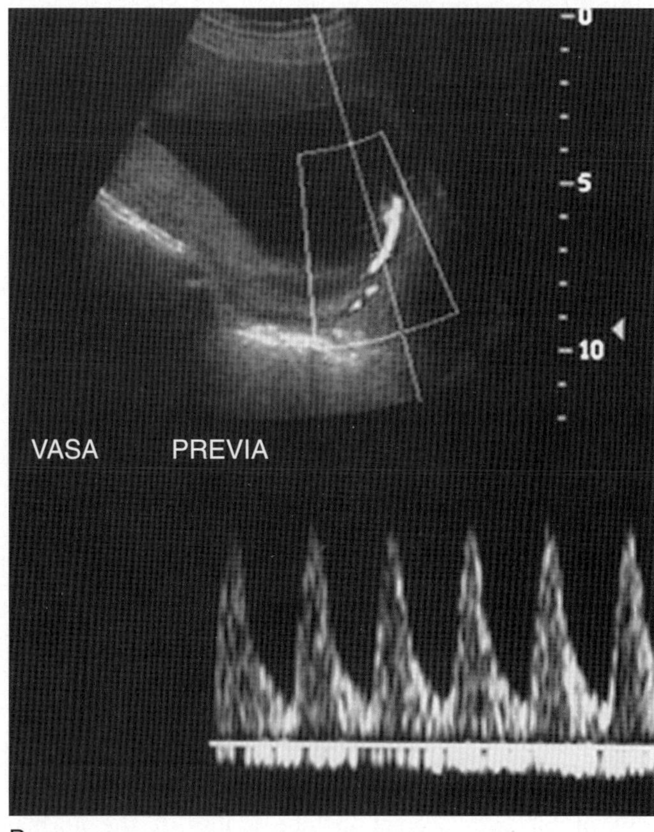

B

Figure 18-7. *A,* The arrow indicates a vasa previa overlying the cervix. *B,* An ultrasonic/Doppler image demonstrating vasa previa. (Note the diagnosis of vasa previa is confirmed when the arterial waveforms of the vessels crossing the internal cervical os are consistent with the fetal heart rate.) (From Gillen-Goldstein J, Lockwood CJ: Abruptio placentae. *www.uptodate.com*.)

POSTPARTUM HEMORRHAGE

Normal Blood Loss and Postpartum Hemorrhage

Normal delivery-related blood loss depends upon the type of delivery. The average blood loss for a vaginal delivery, cesarean delivery, and cesarean hysterectomy is 500 ml, 1,000 ml, and 1,500 ml, respectively.[125] These values are often underestimated and unappreciated clinically owing to the significant blood volume expansion that accompanies normal pregnancy.

Postpartum hemorrhage has been variably defined in the literature. Definitions have included subjective assessments greater than the standard norms, a 10-percent decline in hematocrit, and the need for a blood transfusion. Because of these varied definitions, the exact incidence of postpartum hemorrhage is difficult to ascertain; however, estimates suggest that postpartum hemorrhage complicates 4 to 6 percent of all deliveries.[126,127]

Postpartum Hemorrhage Etiologies

The etiologies of postpartum hemorrhage can be categorized as early, those occurring within 24 hours of delivery, and late, those occurring from 24 hours until 6 weeks postdelivery. Table 18-5 lists the most common causes of early and late postpartum hemorrhage. Because the obstetrician is typically faced with early postpartum hemorrhage more often than the late variety, the remainder of this discussion focuses on its causes and management (Fig. 18-8).

UTERINE ATONY

DEFINITION AND PATHOGENESIS

Uterine atony, or the inability of the uterine myometrium to contract effectively, is the most common cause of early postpartum hemorrhage. At term, blood flow through the placental site averages 600 ml/min. After placental delivery, the uterus controls bleeding by contracting its myometrial fibers in a "tourniquet" fashion around the spiral arterioles. If inadequate uterine contraction occurs, rapid blood loss will ensue.

Table 18-5. Etiologies of Postpartum Hemorrhage

Early	Uterine atony
	Lower genital tract lacerations (perineal, vaginal, cervical, periclitoral, labial, periurethral, rectum)
	Upper genital tract lacerations (broad ligament)
	Lower urinary tract lacerations (bladder, urethra)
	Retained products of conception (placenta, membranes)
	Invasive placentation (placenta accreta, placenta increta, placenta percreta)
	Uterine rupture
	Uterine inversion
	Coagulopathy (hereditary, acquired)
Late	Infection
	Retained products of conception
	Placental site subinvolution
	Coagulopathy

INCIDENCE AND RISK FACTORS

Uterine atony complicates 1 in 20 deliveries.[128] Risk factors for uterine atony include uterine overdistention (multiple gestation, polyhydramnios, fetal macrosomia), prolonged oxytocin use, rapid or prolonged labor, grand multiparity, chorioamnionitis, placenta previa, and use of uterine-relaxing agents (tocolytic therapy, halogenated anesthetics, nitroglycerin).

CLINICAL MANIFESTATIONS AND DIAGNOSIS

Uterine atony is diagnosed clinically by rapid uterine bleeding associated with a lack of myometrial tone and an absence of other etiologies for postpartum hemorrhage. Typically, bimanual palpation of the uterus confirms the diagnosis.

PREVENTION AND MANAGEMENT

By recognizing high-risk factors for uterine atony and quickly initiating a treatment cascade, the clinician can decrease blood loss. Two preventive methods that have been suggested to reduce postpartum hemorrhage from uterine atony are active management of the third stage of labor and spontaneous delivery of the placenta after cesarean delivery. A recent Cochrane review compared

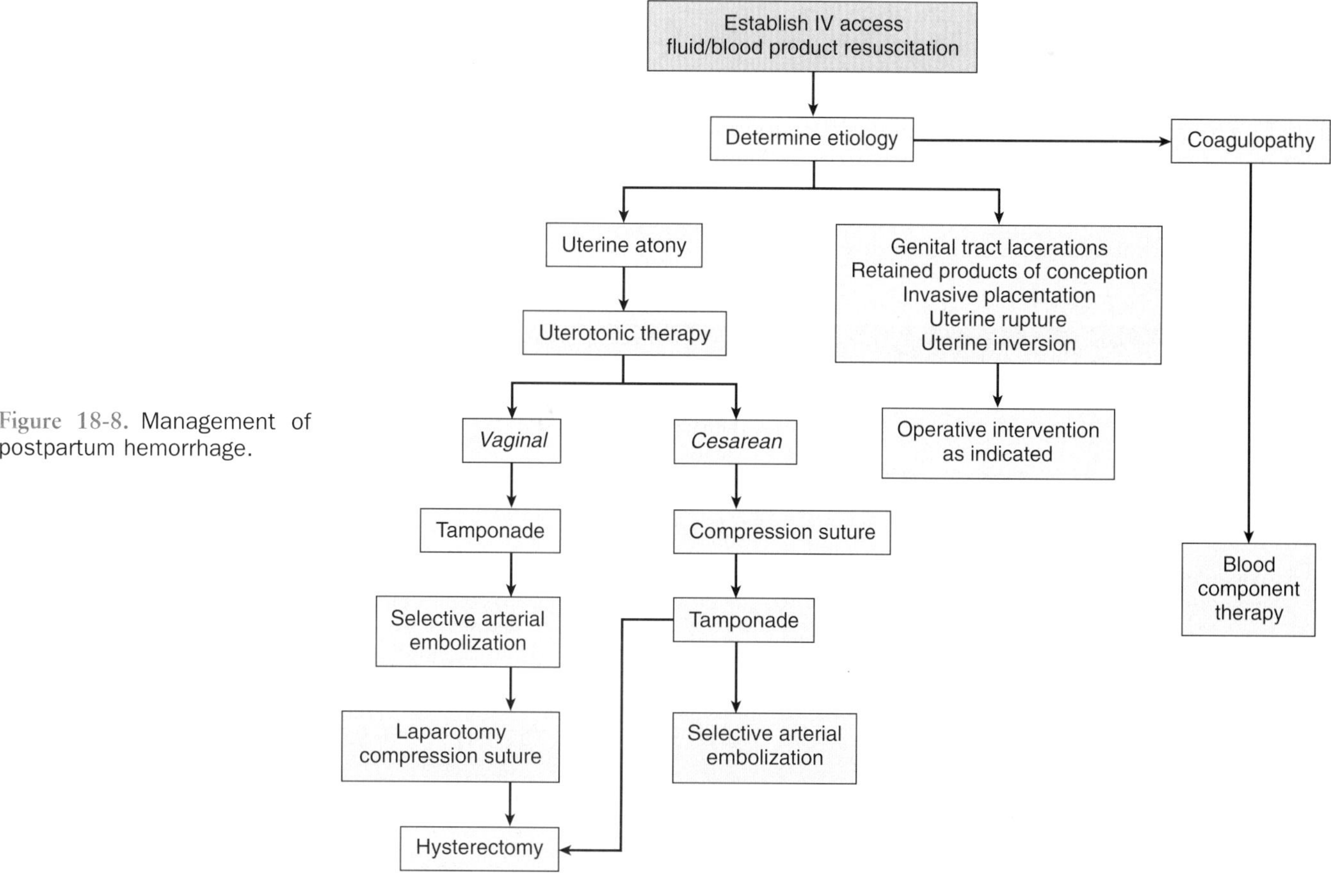

Figure 18-8. Management of postpartum hemorrhage.

the effect of prophylactic oxytocin administration in the third stage of labor versus no uterotonic therapy.[129] Treated patients had significant reductions in mean blood loss, postpartum hemorrhage, and the need for additional uterotonic therapies. Controversy exists regarding the timing of oxytocin administration. Although some studies suggest that giving oxytocin before delivery of the placenta results in less blood loss and fewer postpartum transfusions, other trials have found no significant differences in these outcomes.[130,131] Spontaneous delivery of the placenta during cesarean delivery is also associated with reduced blood loss. In one controlled study, spontaneous delivery reduced blood loss by 30 percent and postpartum endometritis by sevenfold when compared with manual removal.[132]

If preventive measures are unsuccessful, medical treatment for uterine atony should be initiated. This treatment includes bimanual uterine massage and uterotonic therapy.

Bimanual Uterine Massage

Figure 18-9 demonstrates the proper technique for bimanual uterine massage. In order to provide effective massage, the uterus should be compressed between the external fundally placed hand and the internal intravaginal hand. Care must be taken to avoid aggressive massage that can injure the large vessels of the broad ligament.

Uterotonic Therapy

Uterotonic medications represent the mainstay of drug therapy for postpartum hemorrhage secondary to uterine atony. Table 18-6 lists available uterotonic agents with their dosages, side effects, and contraindications. Oxytocin (Pitocin) is usually given as a first-line agent. Intravenous therapy is the preferred route of administration, but intramuscular and intrauterine dosing is possible. Initial treatment starts with 10 to 20 units of oxytocin in 1,000 ml of crystalloid solution. Higher doses (80 units in 1,000 ml) have proven safe and efficacious, with a 20-percent reduction in the need for additional uterotonic therapy when compared with standard dosing.[133]

When oxytocin fails to produce adequate uterine tone, second-line therapy must be initiated. Currently, a variety of other uterotonic agents are available for use. The choice of a second-line agent depends upon its side effect profile as well as its contraindications. Methylergonovine (Methergine) is an effective uterotonic agent but has limited usefulness owing to its potential for worsening hypertension in patients with a preexisting hypertensive disease. Prostaglandins are highly effective uterotonic agents. Both natural and synthetic prostaglandin formulations are available. Intramuscular and intrauterine administration of 15-methyl prostaglandin $F_{2\alpha}$ (Hemabate) can be used for control of atony. Recurrent doses (250 µg) can be administered every 15 minutes, if needed, to a maximum of eight doses (2 mg). Asthma is

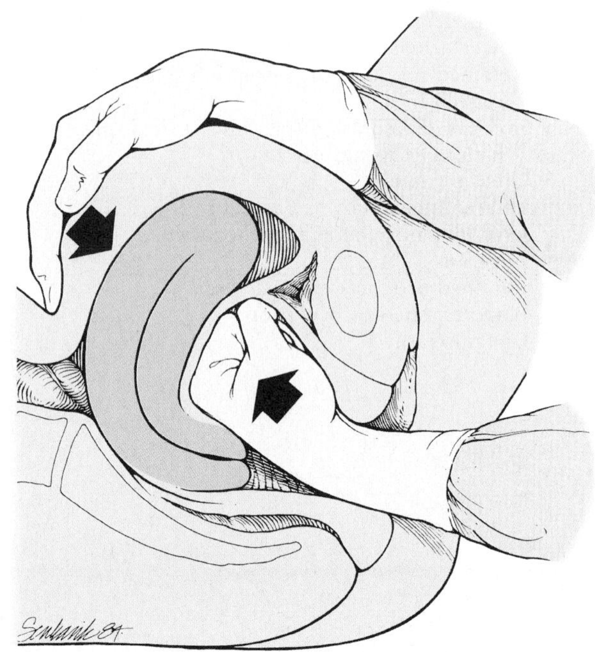

Figure 18-9. Bimanual uterine massage.

Table 18-6. Uterotonic Therapy

AGENT	DOSE	ROUTE	DOSING FREQUENCY	SIDE EFFECTS	CONTRAINDICATIONS
Oxytocin (Pitocin)	10–80 units in 1,000 ml of crystalloid solution	First line: IV Second line: IM or IU	Continuous	Nausea, emesis, water intoxication	None
Methylergonovine (Methergine)	0.2 mg	First line: IM Second line: IU or PO	Every 2–4 h	Hypertension, hypotension, nausea, emesis	Hypertension, preeclampsia
15-Methyl Prostaglandin $F_{2\alpha}$ (Hemabate)	0.25 mg	First line: IM Second line: IU	Every 15–90 min (8-dose maximum)	Nausea, emesis, diarrhea, flushing, chills	Active cardiac, pulmonary, renal or hepatic disease
Prostaglandin E_2 (Dinoprostone)	20 mg	PR	Every 2 h	Nausea, emesis, diarrhea, fever, chills, headache	Hypotension
Misoprostol (Cytotec)	600–1000 mcg	First line: PR Second line: PO	Single dose	Tachycardia, fever	None

IM, intramuscular; IU, intrauterine; IV, intravenous; PR, per rectum; PO, per oral.

a strong contraindication to its use because it has bronchoconstrictive properties. Prostaglandin E_2 (Prostin) is a naturally occurring oxytocic that can dramatically improve uterine tone; however, it has an unfavorable side effect profile that includes fever/chills, nausea/vomiting, diarrhea, and headaches. Finally, misoprostol (Cytotec), a synthetic prostaglandin E_1 analogue, has promise both for the prevention and treatment of postpartum hemorrhage.[134–139] Unlike the other prostaglandin formulations, misoprostol is extremely cost effective and has no significant contraindications to its use. Unfavorable side effects include tachycardia and fever.

When atony is due to tocolytic therapy, that is, those medications that impair calcium entry into the cell (magnesium sulfate, nifedipine), calcium gluconate should be considered as an adjuvant therapy. Given as an intravenous push, one ampule (1 g) of calcium gluconate can effectively improve uterine tone and resolve bleeding due to atony.

If pharmacologic methods fail to control atony-related hemorrhage, alternative measures must be undertaken. These include uterine tamponade, selective arterial embolization, and surgical intervention.

Uterine Tamponade

Uterine packing is a safe, simple, and effective way to control postpartum hemorrhage by providing tamponade to the bleeding uterine surface.[140–142] Although packing techniques vary, a few basic principles should be followed. The pack should be made of a long, continuous gauze (e.g., Kerlex) rather than multiple small sponges. Placement of the gauze within a sterile plastic bag or glove can ease removal of the pack. When packing the uterus, placement should begin at the fundus and progress downward in a side-to-side fashion to avoid dead space for blood accumulation.[128] Transurethral Foley catheter placement and prophylactic antibiotic use should be considered to prevent urinary retention and infection, respectively. Finally, prolonged packing should be avoided (not more than 12 to 24 hours), and close attention to the patient's vital signs and hemoglobin/hematocrit should be paid while the pack is in place in order to minimize unrecognized ongoing bleeding.

Recently, a tamponade-balloon has been developed as an alternative to packing (SAS Bakri Tamponade Balloon, Cook OB/GYN Products, Fig. 18-10). This catheter balloon is inserted into the uterus and inflated with 500 ml of saline. The balloon provides a tamponade to the uterine surface, while the catheter allows drainage of blood from the uterine cavity.[143,144]

Selective Arterial Embolization

Selective arterial embolization is an increasingly common therapeutic option for patients with postpartum hemorrhage that are hemodynamically stable.

The technique involves pelvic angiography to visualize the bleeding vessels and placement of Gelfoam (gelatin) pledgets into the vessels for occlusion. A cumulative success rate of 97 percent has been reported.[128]

Selective arterial embolization has several advantages over surgical intervention. First, it allows for selective occlusion of bleeding vessels. This can be extremely valuable in circumstances of aberrant pelvic vasculature, for example, uterine arteriovenous malformations. Second, the uterus and potential future fertility are preserved. Cases series have reported successful pregnancies after pelvic embolization.[145–147] Finally, the procedure has minimal morbidity, enables the physician to forego or

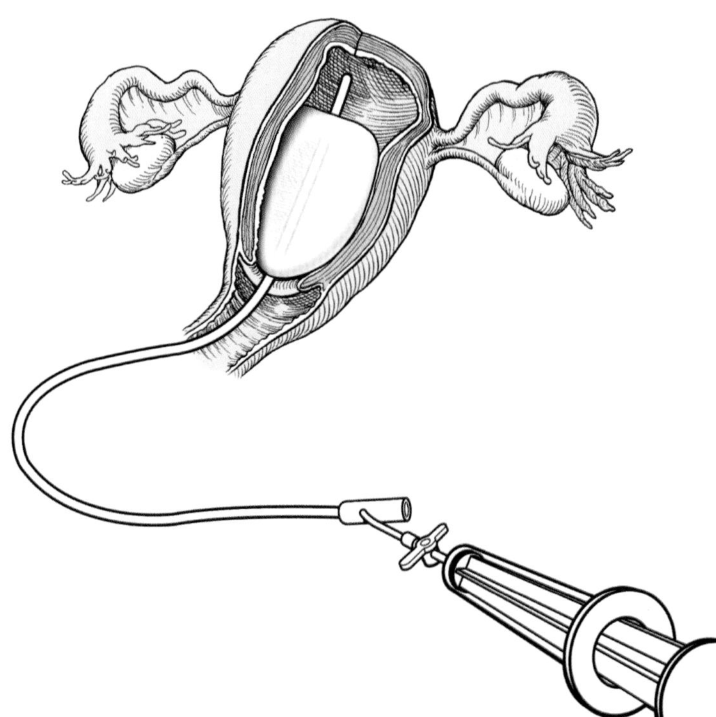

Figure 18-10. The SOS Bakri Tamponade Balloon. (Courtesy of Cook OB/GYN Products.)

delay surgical intervention, and can be performed in coagulopathic patients, allowing more time for blood and clotting factor replacement.[148] Procedure-related complications occur in less than 10-percent of cases. Reported complications include postembolization fever, infection, ischemic pain, and tissue necrosis.[148] A relative disadvantage of the procedure is its limited availability. Timely coordination of services between the obstetric team and interventional radiology is necessary to provide this treatment option.

Surgical Intervention

When uterine atony is unresponsive to conservative management, surgical intervention through laparotomy is necessary. Possible interventions include arterial ligation, various uterine suturing techniques, and hysterectomy.

The goal of arterial ligation is to decrease uterine perfusion and subsequent bleeding. Success rates have varied from 40 to 95 percent in the literature depending on which vessels are ligated.[149] Arterial ligation may be performed on the ascending uterine arteries, the utero-ovarian arteries, the infundibulopelvic ligament vessels, and the hypogastric arteries. Because hypogastric arterial ligation can be technically challenging and time-consuming, it is not advised as a first-line technique unless the surgeon is extremely skilled in performing the procedure. Instead, a stepwise progression of uterine vessel ligation is recommended.

Nearly 40 years ago, O'Leary described a technique of bilateral uterine artery ligation for control of postpartum hemorrhage.[150] Today, it is still considered the best initial ligation technique given its ease in performance and the accessibility of the uterine artery. To perform the procedure, the ascending uterine artery should be located at the border of the upper and lower uterine segment. Absorbable suture is passed through the uterine myometrium at the level of the lower uterine segment and laterally around the uterine vessels through the broad ligament. The suture is then tied to compress the vessels against the uterine wall (Fig. 18-11). Because the suture is placed fairly high in the lower uterine segment, the ureter is not in jeopardy and the bladder does not need to be mobilized. Unilateral artery ligation will control hemorrhage in 10 to 15 percent of cases, whereas bilateral ligation will control an additional 75 percent.[151]

If bleeding persists, the utero-ovarian and infundibulopelvic vessels should be ligated. The utero-ovarian arteries can be ligated similarly to what has been described for the ascending uterine vessels. If this measure is unsuccessful, interruption of the infundibulopelvic vessels can be undertaken. Although the ovarian blood supply may be decreased with an infundibulopelvic vessel ligation, successful pregnancy has been reported.[152]

In addition to arterial ligation, uterine suturing techniques have been described for atony control. These include placement of a B-Lynch compression suture and multiple square sutures.[153,154] To place a B-Lynch compression suture, the patient should lie in the dorsal lithotomy position so that an assessment of vaginal bleeding can occur. A large absorbable suture is anchored within the uterine myometrium both anteriorly and posteriorly. It is passed in a continuous fashion around the external surface of the uterus and tied firmly so that adequate uterine compression occurs. Figure 18-12 demonstrates proper placement of this suture. Several case reports have documented successful resolution of uterine atony with the B-Lynch compression suture.[153,155–157]

A recent report demonstrated efficacy of multiple square sutures within the uterine wall to control hemorrhage.[154] This technique involves the use of a large absorbable suture on a blunt straight needle. The needle is passed from the anterior to the posterior aspects of the uterus and back in the opposite directions to form a square. The suture is tied firmly to provide compression to the bleeding surfaces. Like the B-Lynch compression suture, this technique has proved successful for the treatment of uterine atony.

The final surgical intervention for refractory bleeding due to atony is hysterectomy (see Chapter 19). Hysterectomy provides definitive therapy. Because blood loss may be massive, it may be prudent to perform a supracervical hysterectomy. This consideration is especially important when the patient is hemodynamically unstable.

Genital Tract Lacerations

Definition and Pathogenesis

Genital tract lacerations may occur with both vaginal and cesarean deliveries. These lacerations involve the

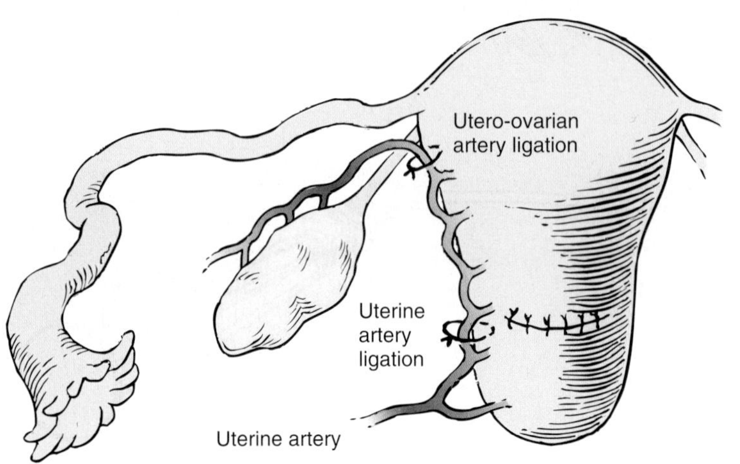

Figure 18-11. Uterine artery ligation.

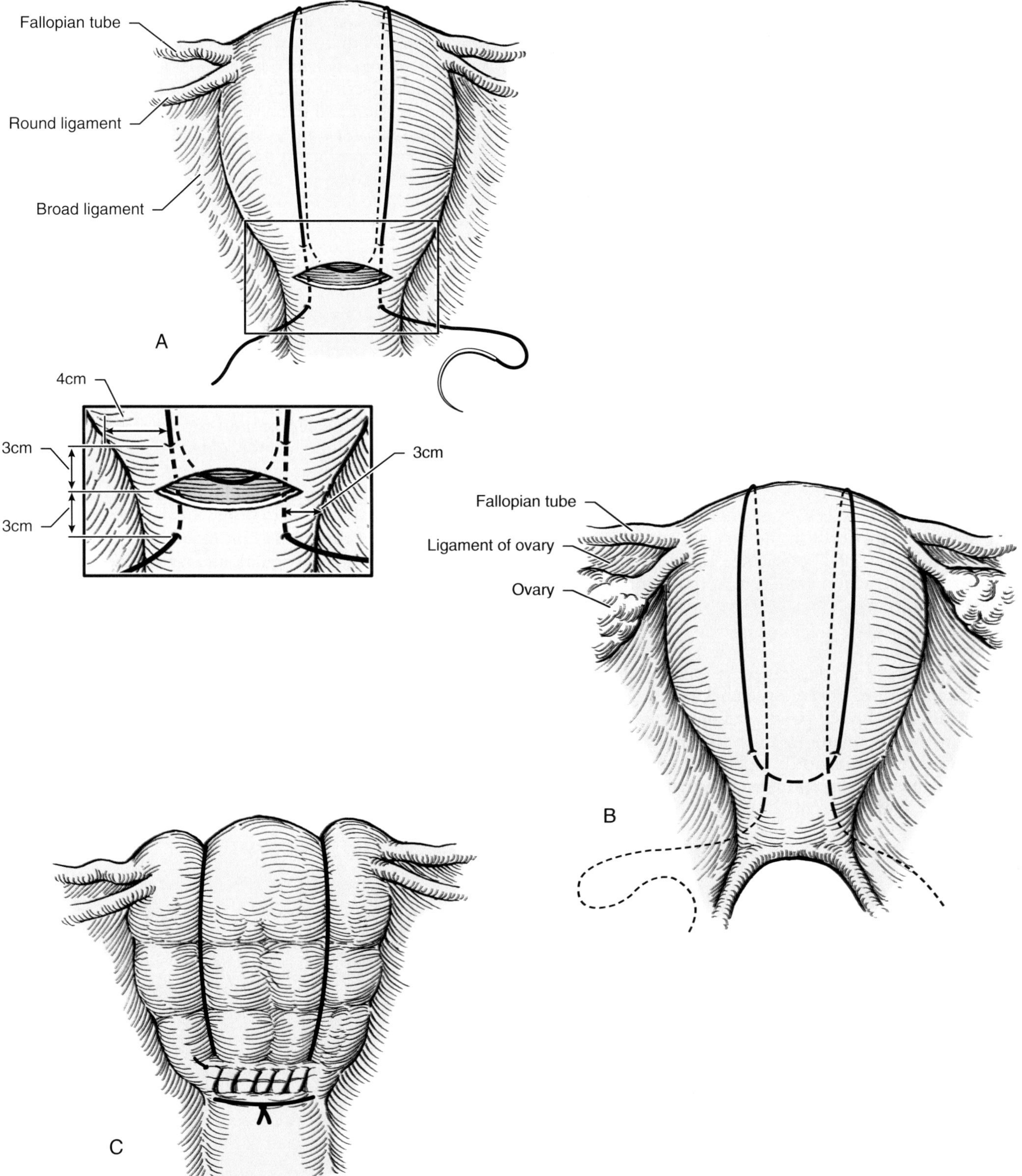

Figure 18-12. B-Lynch compression suture. (From B-Lynch C, Coker A, Lawal AH, et al: The B-Lynch surgical technique for control of massive postpartum haemorrhage: an alternative to hysterectomy? Five cases reported. Br J Obstet Gynaecol 104:275, 1997.)

maternal soft tissue structures and can be associated with large hematomas and rapid blood loss if unrecognized. The most common lower genital tract lacerations are perineal, vulvar, vaginal, and cervical. Upper genital tract lacerations are typically associated with broad ligament and retroperitoneal hematomas.

Incidence and Risk Factors

Although it is difficult to ascertain their exact incidence, genital tract lacerations are the second leading cause of postpartum hemorrhage. Risk factors include operative vaginal delivery, fetal malpresentation, fetal macrosomia, episiotomy, precipitous delivery, prior cerclage placement, Duhrssen's incisions, and shoulder dystocia.

Clinical Manifestations and Diagnosis

A genitourinary tract laceration should be suspected if bleeding persists after delivery despite adequate uterine tone. Occasionally, the bleeding may be masked owing to its location, that is, the broad ligament. In these circumstances, large amounts of blood loss may occur in an unrecognized hematoma. Pain and hemodynamic instability may be the primary presenting symptoms.

For diagnosis, it is best to evaluate the lower genital tract starting superiorly at the cervix and progressing inferiorly to the vagina, perineum, and vulva. Adequate exposure and retraction are essential to diagnosing many of these lacerations.

Management

Once a genital tract laceration is diagnosed, management depends upon its severity and location.

Lacerations of the cervix and vaginal fornices are often difficult to repair owing to their location. In these circumstances, relocation to an operating room for better pain relief, pelvic relaxation, and visualization are recommended. If the laceration is adjacent to the urethra or bowel, the use of additional instrumentation (e.g., transurethral catheter) can protect uninjured organs and allow for more efficient repair.

Careful inspection of the cervix and vagina will often indicate the source of the bleeding. Figures 18-13 through 18-15 illustrate second-, third-, and fourth-degree lacerations of the perineum and techniques for their repair. Adequate exposure for the repair of such lacerations is critical and, if needed, assistance should be summoned to aid in retraction.

In cervical laceration, it is important to secure the base of the laceration, which is often a major source of bleeding. However, this area is frequently the most difficult to suture. Valuable time can be lost trying to expose the angle of such a laceration. A helpful technique to use in these cases, especially when help is limited or slow in responding, is to start to suture the laceration at its proximal end, using the suture for traction to expose the more distal portion of the cervix until the apex is in view (Fig. 18-16). The technique has the added advantage of arresting significant bleeding from the edges of laceration.

On occasion, a blood vessel laceration may lead to the formation of a pelvic hematoma in the lower or upper genital tract. The three most common locations for a pelvic hematoma are vulvar, vaginal, and retroperitoneal.

Vulvar Hematoma

Vulvar hematomas usually result from lacerated vessels in the superficial fascia of the anterior and/or posterior pelvic triangle. Blood loss is tamponaded by Colle's fascia, the urogenital diaphragm, and anal fascia (Fig. 18-17). Because of these fascial boundaries, the mass will extend to the skin and a visible hematoma results (Fig. 18-18).

Surgical drainage is the primary treatment for a vulvar hematoma. A wide linear incision through the

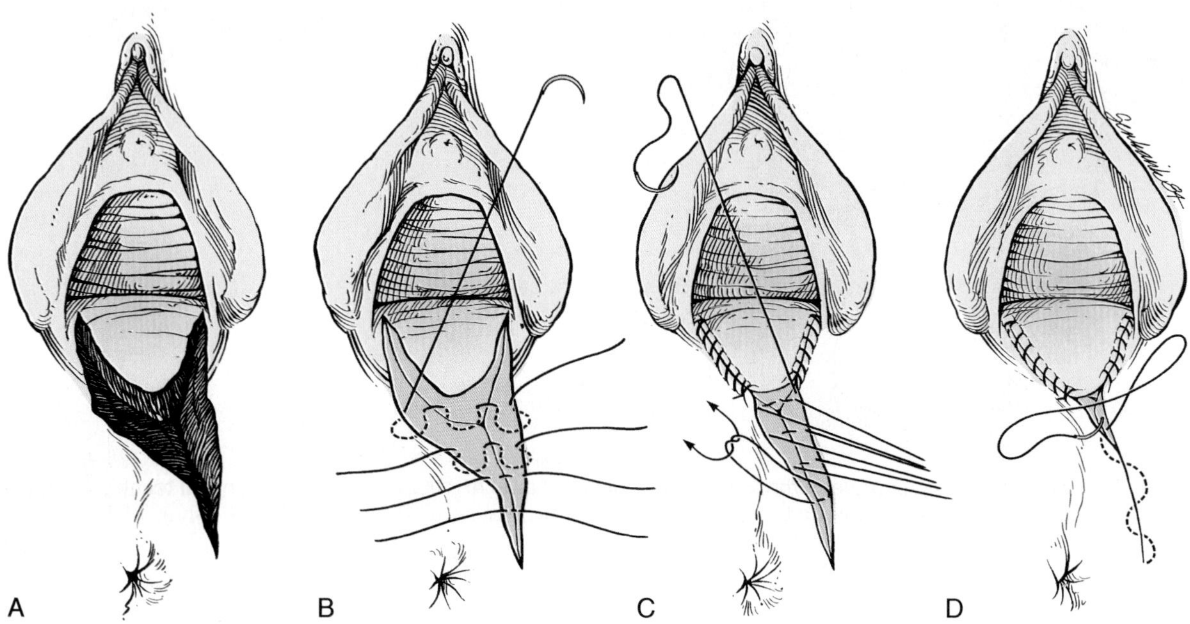

Figure 18-13. Repair of a second-degree laceration. A first-degree laceration involves the fourchet, the perineal skin, and the vaginal mucous membrane. A second-degree laceration also includes the muscles of the perineal body. The rectal sphincter remains intact.

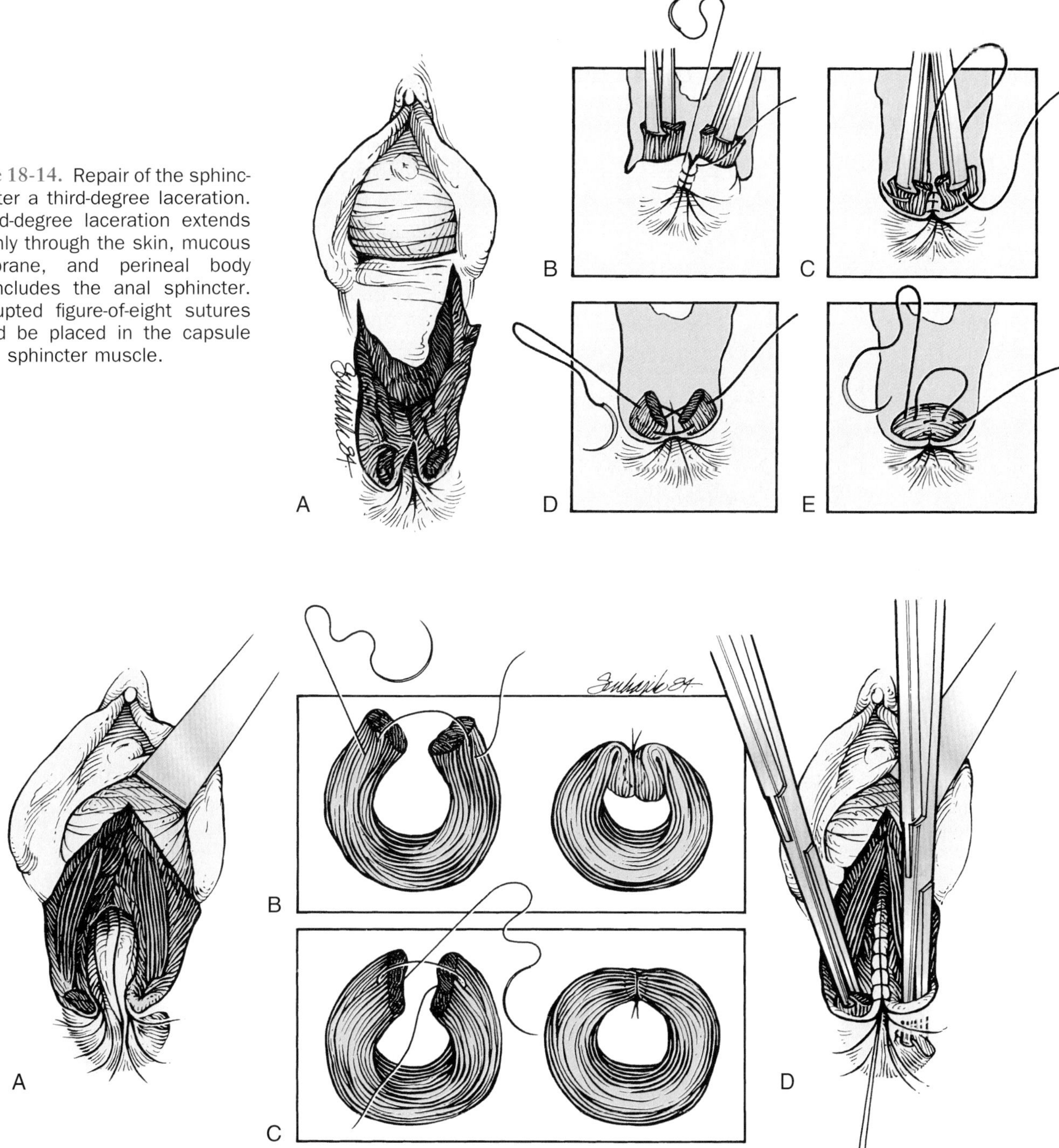

Figure 18-14. Repair of the sphincter after a third-degree laceration. A third-degree laceration extends not only through the skin, mucous membrane, and perineal body but includes the anal sphincter. Interrupted figure-of-eight sutures should be placed in the capsule of the sphincter muscle.

Figure 18-15. Repair of a fourth-degree laceration. This laceration extends through the rectal mucosa. *A,* The extent of this laceration is shown, with a segment of the rectum exposed. *B,* Approximation of the rectal submucosa. This is the most commonly recommended method for repair. *C,* Alternative method of approximating the rectal mucosa in which the knots are actually buried inside the rectal lumen. *D,* After closure of the rectal submucosa, an additional layer of running sutures may be placed. The rectal sphincter is then repaired.

skin is recommended. Typically, the bleeding is due to multiple small vessels; hence, vessel ligation is not possible. Once the hematoma is evacuated, the dead space should be closed in layers with absorbable suture and a sterile pressure dressing applied. A transurethral Foley catheter should be placed until significant tissue edema subsides.

Vaginal Hematoma

Vaginal hematomas result from delivery-related soft tissue damage. These hematomas accumulate above the pelvic diaphragm (Fig. 18-19). It is unusual for large amounts of blood to collect in this region, and protrusion of the hematoma into the vaginal-rectal area is common.

Like vulvar hematomas, vaginal hematomas are due to multiple small vessel lacerations and require surgical drainage. Unlike vulvar hematomas, the incision of a vaginal hematoma does not require closing; rather a vaginal pack should be placed to tamponade the raw edges. If bleeding persists, selective arterial embolization may be considered.

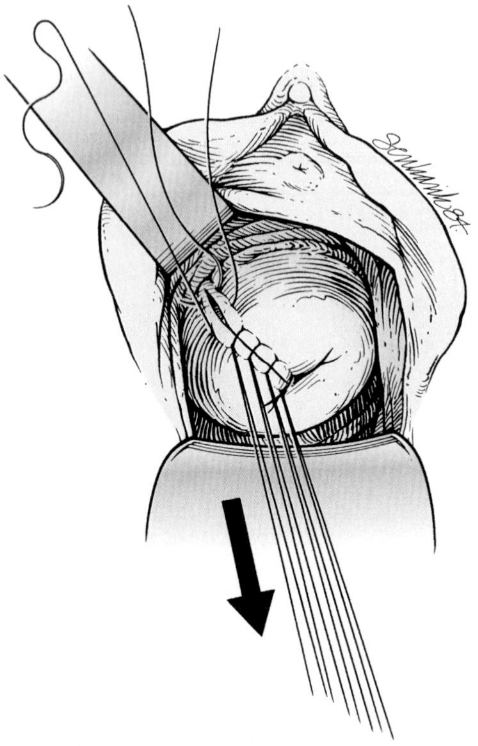

Figure 18-16. Repair of a cervical laceration, which begins at the proximal part of the laceration, using traction on the previous sutures to aid in exposing the distal portion of the defect.

Retroperitoneal Hematoma

Although they are infrequent, retroperitoneal hematomas are the most serious and life threatening. The early symptoms of a retroperitoneal hematoma are often subtle, with the hematoma being unrecognized until the patient is hemodynamically unstable from massive hemorrhage. These hematomas usually occur after a vessel laceration from the hypogastric arterial tree (Fig. 18-20). Such lacerations may result from inadequate hemostasis of the uterine arteries at the time of cesarean delivery or after rupture of a low transverse cesarean scar during a trial of labor. Treatment of a retroperitoneal hematoma typically involves surgical exploration, hematoma evacuation, and arterial ligation. In some situations, selective arterial embolization may be necessary as an adjunctive treatment.

Retained Products of Conception

Definition and Pathogenesis

Retained products of conception, namely placental tissue and amniotic membranes, can inhibit the uterus from adequate contraction and result in hemorrhage.

Incidence and Risk Factors

Retained products of conception complicate 1 in 100 to 1 in 200 deliveries.[158] Risk factors include midtrimester delivery, chorioamnionitis, and accessory placental lobes.

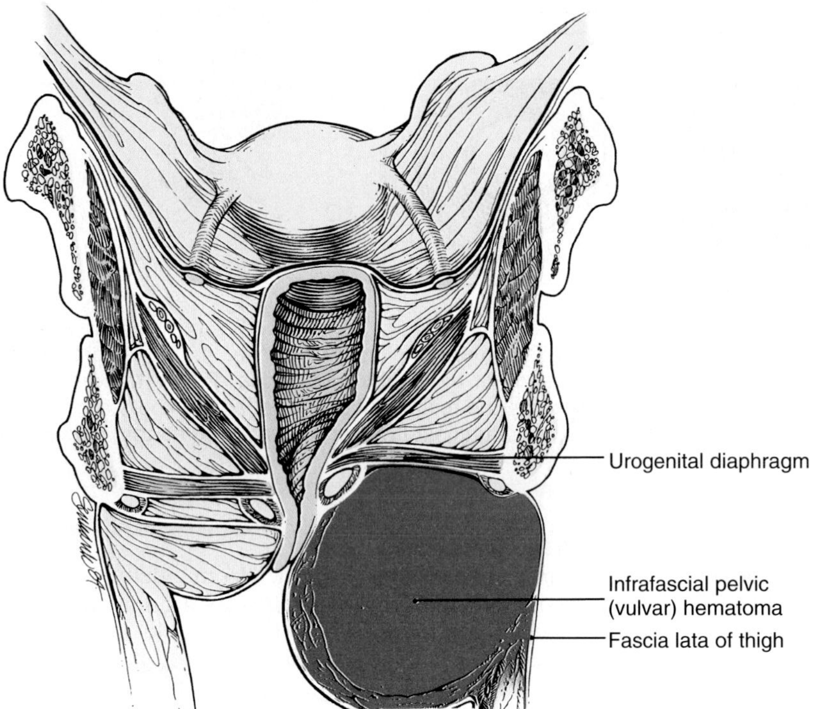

Figure 18-17. Vulvar hematoma fascial boundaries.

Clinical Manifestations and Diagnosis

Uterine bleeding, often associated with atony, may be due to retained products of conception. To assess the uterus for retained products of conception, the uterine cavity needs to be explored. Manual exploration is not only diagnostic but therapeutic as well (Fig. 18-21). By wrapping the examination hand with moist gauze, removal of retained placental fragments and amniotic membranes can be facilitated. If manual access to the uterine cavity is difficult or limited owing to maternal body habitus or inadequate pain relief, transabdominal or transvaginal ultrasound may be used to determine if retained placental fragments are present.

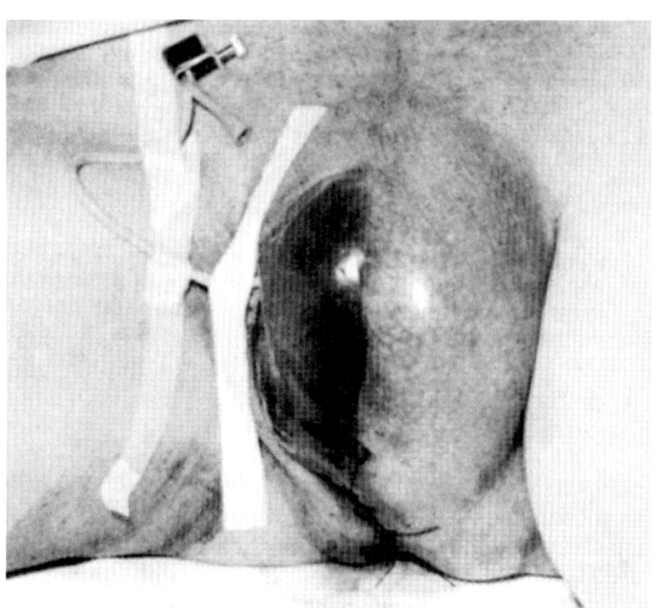

Figure 18-18. Large vulvar hematoma.

Management

Once a diagnosis of retained products of conception is made, removal must be undertaken. Therapeutic options include manual extraction, as noted previously, or uterine curettage. Although uterine curettage may be performed in a delivery room, excessive bleeding mandates that an operating room be used for the procedure. A large Banjo curette should be employed with gentle traction in order to avoid uterine perforation. Transabdominal ultrasound guidance is helpful in determining that the evacuation of tissue is complete.

Umbilical vein injection with normal saline and oxytocin has proved effective in reducing the need for manual extraction of a retained placenta; however, further studies are needed before universal endorsement of this technique.[159]

Uterine Rupture

Definition and Pathogenesis

Uterine rupture refers to the complete nonsurgical disruption of all uterine layers (endometrium, myometrium, and serosa).[160] The severity of hemorrhage and maternal-fetal morbidity depends upon the extent of the rupture. A large rupture may be associated with massive hemorrhage and extrusion of the fetus and placenta into the maternal abdomen, whereas a small rupture may have minimal bleeding and insignificant maternal-fetal consequences. The terms "uterine dehiscence" and "incomplete uterine rupture" are often used to describe the latter type of disruption (see Chapter 19).

Incidence and Risk Factors

The overall incidence of uterine rupture is 1 in 2,000 deliveries; however, this number varies depending on the presence of a prior uterine scar. A prior low transverse uterine incision is associated with 0.2- to 1.5-percent risk

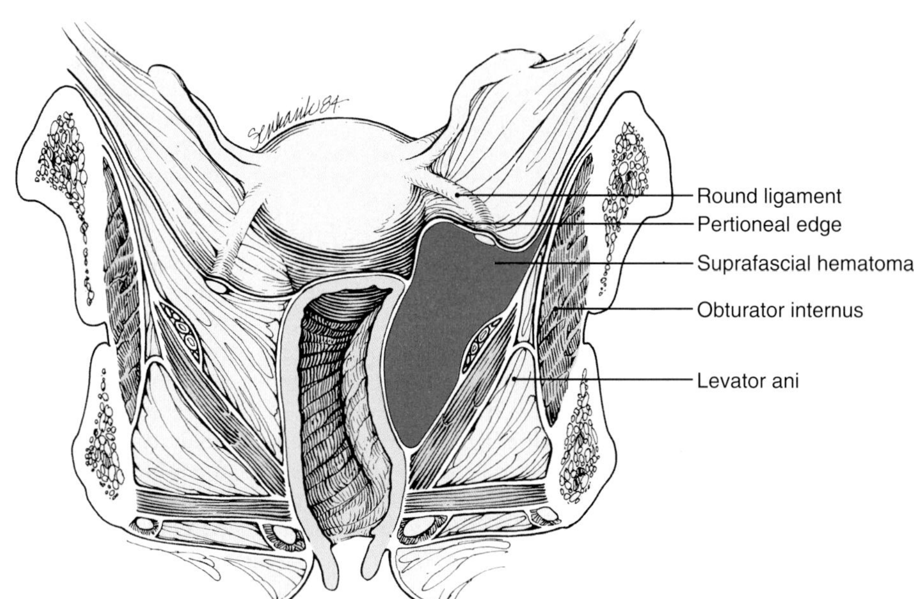

Figure 18-19. Vaginal hematoma.

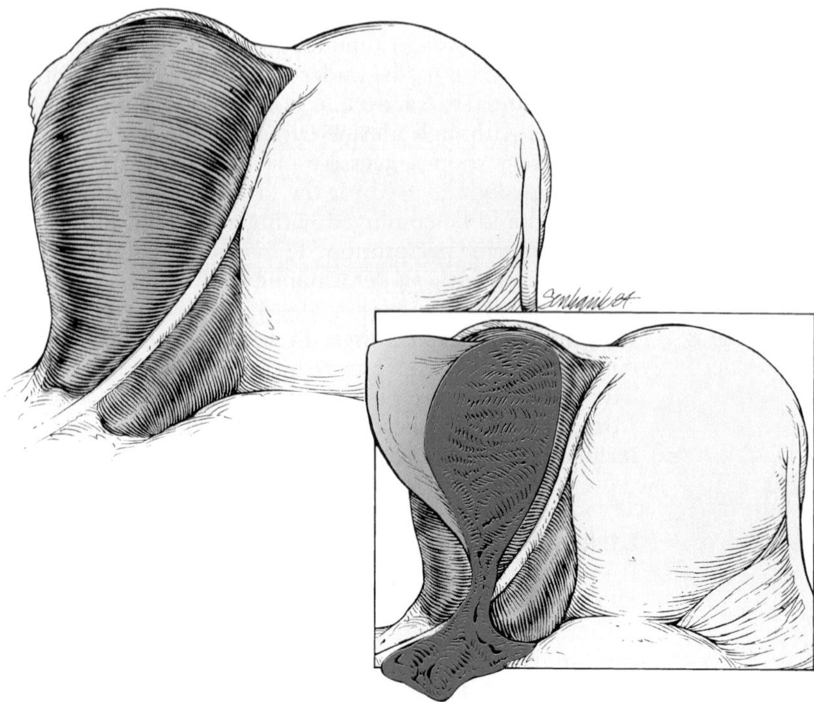

Figure 18-20. Retroperitoneal hematoma.

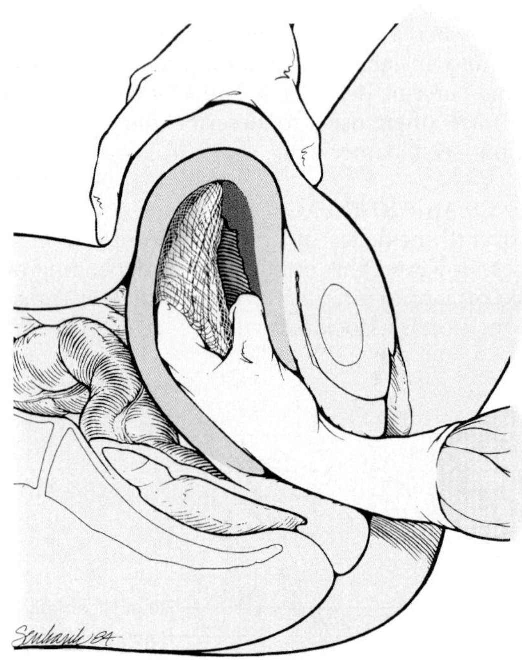

Figure 18-21. Manual uterine exploration.

of uterine rupture, whereas a classical or T-shaped incision and low vertical incision are associated with a 4- to 9-percent and a 1- to 7-percent risk, respectively.[161]

Multiple risk factors for uterine rupture have been documented. The most significant risk factor is a trial of labor after a prior cesarean delivery.[162] Induction of labor and multiple prior cesarean deliveries have been reported to increase the risk.[163,164] Other risk factors include maternal age, multiparity, fetal malpresentation, obstructed labor, multiple gestation, prior hysterotomy/myomectomy, uterine manipulation (e.g., internal podalic version), mid- to high-operative vaginal delivery, trauma, interdelivery interval less than 18 months, postpartum fever after prior cesarean delivery, and one-layer closure of a prior uterine incision.[165–172]

Clinical Manifestations and Diagnosis

Uterine rupture is associated with both fetal and maternal clinical manifestations. A nonreassuring fetal heart rate pattern is the most common fetal finding, including variable and late decelerations, followed by bradycardia.[173] In some circumstances, a loss of fetal station in labor may occur. The maternal presentation with uterine rupture includes constant abdominal pain, uterine tenderness, a change in uterine shape, cessation of contractions, hematuria (if extension into the bladder has occurred), and signs of hemodynamic instability.[160]

Uterine rupture is suspected clinically but confirmed surgically. Laparotomy will demonstrate complete disruption of the uterine wall, with bleeding and partial or complete extravasation of the fetus into the maternal abdomen.

Management

Once the fetus and placenta are delivered, the site of rupture should be assessed to determine if it can be repaired. If feasible, the rupture can be repaired in multiple layers with absorbable suture. Hysterectomy should be reserved for cases in which the defect is large and difficult to close or when the mother is hemodynamically unstable.

Maternal and Neonatal Outcomes

Although maternal mortality is uncommon with a uterine rupture, significant morbidity can occur. A large review of the literature concerning uterine ruptures related to trial of labor after prior cesarean delivery found increased risks of blood transfusion, hysterectomy, and genitourinary injury.[174] With regard to perinatal outcome, increased rates of low 5-minute Apgar scores (<5), umbilical artery pH less than 7.0, admission to the neonatal intensive care unit, hypoxic-ischemic encephalopathy, and neonatal death have been documented.[175–177]

Uterine Inversion

Definition and Pathogenesis

Uterine inversion refers to the collapse of the fundus into the uterine cavity. Uterine inversion may be incomplete, complete, or prolapsed. Incomplete uterine inversion represents a partial extrusion of the fundus into the uterine cavity. With complete uterine inversion, the internal lining of the fundus crosses through the cervical os, forming a rounded mass in the vagina with no palpable fundus abdominally. Prolapsed uterine inversion refers to the entire uterus prolapsing through the cervix with the fundus passing out of the vaginal introitus.

The two most commonly proposed etiologies for uterine inversion include excessive umbilical cord traction with a fundally attached placenta and fundal pressure in the setting of a relaxed uterus.[178]

Incidence and Risk Factors

Uterine inversion is a rare event, complicating approximately 1 in 2,500 deliveries.[179] Proposed risk factors for uterine inversion include uterine overdistention, fetal macrosomia, prolonged labor, uterine malformations, invasive placentation, short umbilical cord, tocolysis, oxytocin use, primiparity, and manual extraction of the placenta.[158] Uterine inversion is more commonly found in women with collagen disorders such as Ehlers Danlos syndrome.

Clinical Manifestations and Diagnosis

Uterine inversion should be suspected with the sudden onset of brisk vaginal bleeding in association with an absent palpable fundus abdominally and maternal hemodynamic instability. It may occur before or after placental detachment. The diagnosis is made clinically with bimanual examination, during which the uterine fundus is palpated in the lower uterine segment or within the vagina. Sonography can be used to confirm the diagnosis if the clinical examination is unclear.[180]

Management

Once diagnosed, uterine inversion requires rapid intervention to restore maternal hemodynamic stability and to control hemorrhage. Maternal fluid resuscitation through a large-bore intravenous catheter is recommended. The uterus must be replaced to its proper orientation to resolve the hemorrhage. This is best accomplished in an operating room with the assistance of an anesthesiologist. The uterus and cervix should initially be relaxed with a tocolytic agent (e.g. magnesium sulfate, β-mimetic), nitroglycerin, or a halogenated anesthetic.[181–183] Once relaxed, gentle manual pressure is applied to the uterine fundus in order to return it to its proper abdominal location (Fig. 18-22). Uterotonic therapy should then be given to assist with uterine contraction and prevent recurrence of the inversion.[184]

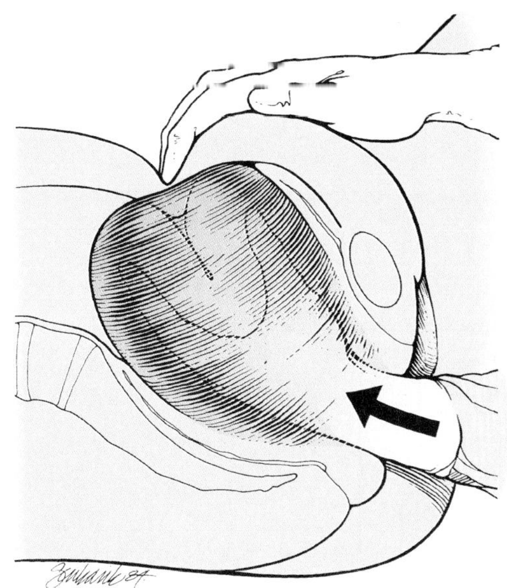

Figure 18-22. Manual replacement of uterine inversion.

If manual repositioning is unsuccessful, other options include hydrostatic pressure and surgical correction. To provide hydrostatic pressure, a silicone cup (i.e., vacuum extraction cup) is placed into the vagina and warmed saline is infused in order to create increased intravaginal pressure and resultant correction of the inversion.[185,186] Surgical options include the Huntington and Haultain procedures. The Huntington procedure involves a laparotomy with serial clamping and upward traction of the round ligaments to restore the uterus to its proper position.[187] If this technique fails, the Haultain procedure, which uses a vertical incision within the inversion and manual repositioning of the fundus, can be attempted.[188] As with the manual technique, uterotonic therapy should be administered immediately after uterine replacement.

Coagulopathy

Definition and Pathogenesis

Coagulopathy represents an imbalance between the clotting and fibrinolytic systems. This imbalance may be hereditary or acquired in origin. Hereditary coagulopathies are relatively rare and have variable etiologies. Given their rarity, the reader is referred to Chapter 41 for further discussion.

Although acquired coagulopathy can be due to iatrogenic causes such as the administration of anticoagulants, it is usually the result of DIC. Figure 18-23 demonstrates the pathophysiology of DIC and its association with hemorrhage.

Incidence and Risk Factors

The overall incidence of DIC in the obstetric population has not been reported; however, several risk factors

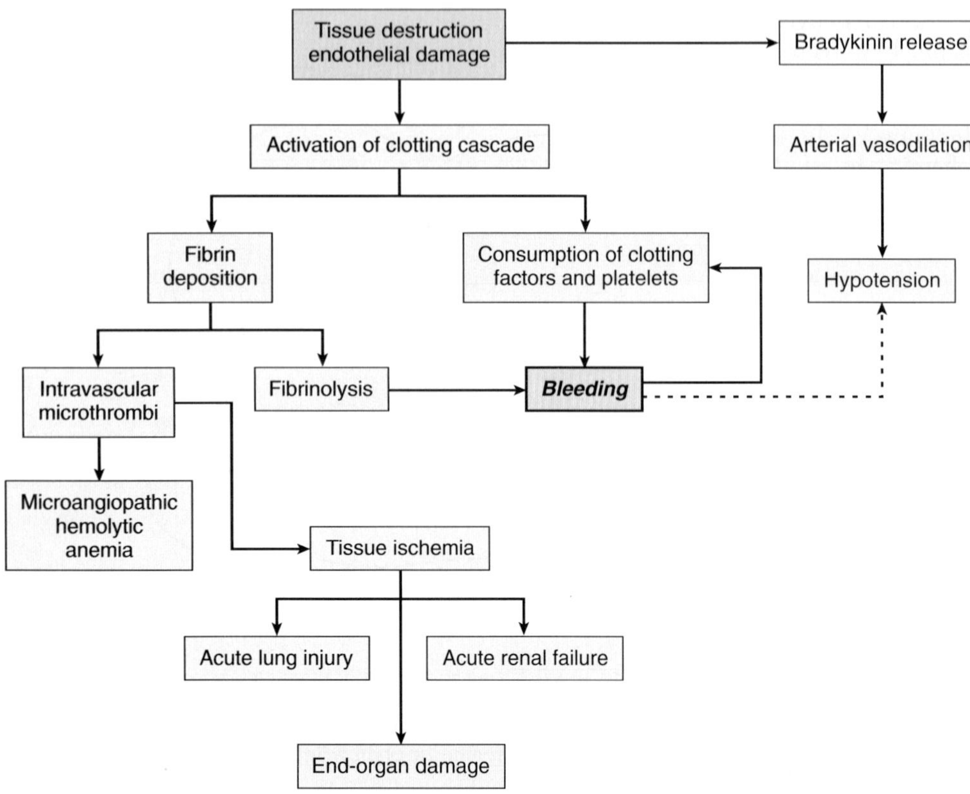

Figure 18-23. Pathophysiology and clinical manifestations of disseminated intravascular coagulation.

have been documented. These include massive antepartum or postpartum hemorrhage, sepsis, severe preeclampsia, amniotic fluid embolism, tissue necrosis (e.g., retained intrauterine fetal demise and trauma), placental abruption, saline abortion, and acute fatty liver of pregnancy.

Clinical Manifestations and Diagnosis

The primary clinical manifestations of DIC include bleeding, hypotension out of proportion to blood loss, microangiopathic hemolytic anemia, acute lung injury, acute renal failure, and ischemic end-organ tissue damage (e.g., liver/gastrointestinal tract dysfunction, central nervous system dysfunction, etc.).

The diagnosis of DIC is primarily clinical, with the recognition of hemorrhage and impaired clot formation. Laboratory studies that are helpful to confirm the diagnosis include thrombocytopenia, hemolytic changes on the peripheral blood smear, decreased fibrinogen, elevated fibrin degradation products, and prolonged prothrombin time and activated partial thromboplastin time. If rapid laboratory assessment is not possible, drawing 5 ml of maternal blood into an empty red top tube and observing for clot formation provides the clinician a rough estimate of the degree of existing coagulopathy. If a clot is not visible within 6 minutes or forms and lyses within 30 minutes, the fibrinogen level is likely less than 150 mg/dl.

Management

The most important factor in the successful treatment of DIC is identifying and correcting the underlying etiology. For most obstetric causes, delivery of the fetus initiates resolution of the coagulopathy. In addition, rapid replacement of blood products and clotting factors should occur simultaneously. The patient should have two large-bore intravenous catheters for fluid and blood component therapy. Laboratory studies should be drawn serially every 2 to 4 hours until resolution of the DIC is evident. The obstetrician should attempt to achieve a platelet count greater than 50,000/μl and a fibrinogen level greater than 100 mg/dl.

Adjuvant therapies to consider in DIC management include vitamin K administration and recombinant activated factor VIIa.

Vitamin K

Factors II, VII, IX, and X are vitamin K–dependent clotting factors. In DIC, these clotting factors are consumed. Administration of vitamin K (5 to 10 mg) by the subcutaneous, intramuscular, or intravenous routes can assist with endogenous replenishment of these procoagulants.

Recombinant Activated Factor VIIa

Factor VII is a precursor for the extrinsic clotting cascade. When massive procoagulant factor consumption occurs, factor replacement is necessary. Human recombinant factor VIIa has been used successfully in cases of DIC attributed to postpartum hemorrhage.[189–191] The dosage of this intravenous therapy is 60 to 100 μg/kg. An important advantage of this therapy is its rapid bioavailability and reversal of DIC (10 minutes); however, the disadvantages include its short half life (2 hours) and cost. Recombinant activated factor VIIa should be considered in cases of refractory DIC or when blood component replacement is delayed.

Blood Component Therapy

All obstetricians will encounter antepartum and postpartum hemorrhage. In most instances, fluid resuscitation and blood component therapy is life saving. Therefore, every physician should have a thorough understanding of appropriate volume and transfusion therapy, alternative treatment options, and their risks.

Volume Resuscitation

Initial management of a hemorrhaging patient requires appropriate volume resuscitation. Two large-bore intravenous catheters are recommended. Warmed crystalloid solution in a 3:1 ratio to the estimated blood loss should be rapidly infused. If the hemorrhage is easily controlled, this may be the only volume resuscitation needed. The patient should have serial assessments of her vital signs and hematologic profiles to confirm hemodynamic stability.

Colloid Solutions

Colloid solutions contain larger particles, called colloids, which are less permeable across vascular membranes. These solutions provide a greater increase in colloid oncotic pressure and plasma volume; however, they are more expensive than crystalloids and may be associated with anaphylactoid reactions. Examples of colloid solutions include albumin, hetastarch, and dextran.

Blood Component Therapy

Whole Blood

Whole blood contains red cells, clotting factors, and platelets. Whole blood is rarely used in modern obstetrics because of its many disadvantages, including a short storage life (24 hours), large volume (500 ml per unit), and potential for hypercalemia.

Packed Red Blood Cells

Packed red blood cells (prbc) are the most appropriate therapy for patients requiring red blood cell replacement for hemorrhage. They are the only blood product to provide oxygen-carrying capacity. Each prbc unit contains approximately 300 ml of volume: 250 ml red blood cells and 50 ml of plasma. In a 70-kg patient, one unit of prbc will raise the hemoglobin by 1 g/dl and the hematocrit by 3 percent. Transfusion of prbc should be considered in any gravida with a hemoglobin less than 8 g/dl or with active hemorrhage and DIC.

Platelet Concentrates

Platelets are separated from whole blood and stored in plasma. Because one unit of platelets provides an increase of only approximately 7,500/mm^3, platelet concentrates of 6 to 10 units need to be transfused. Platelet concentrates can be derived from multiple donors or single donors. The single donor concentrates are preferred because they expose the patient to fewer potential antigenic and immunologic risks. Transfusion of a single donor platelet concentrate will increase the circulating platelet count by 30,000 to 60,000/mm^3. Because sensitization can occur, it is important for platelets to be ABO and Rh specific. Transfusion of platelets should be considered when the platelet count is less than 20,000/mm^3 after a vaginal delivery, less than 50,000/mm^3 after a cesarean delivery, or if there is evidence of DIC.

Fresh Frozen Plasma

Fresh frozen plasma (FFP) is plasma that is extracted from whole blood. FFP primarily contains fibrinogen, antithrombin III, and clotting factors V, XI, XII. Transfusing FFP not only assists with coagulation but provides the patient with volume resuscitation because each unit contains approximately 250 ml. Typically, fibrinogen levels are used to monitor a patient's response to FFP. Each unit of FFP should raise the fibrinogen level by 5 to 10 mg/dl. FFP does not need to be ABO or Rh compatible. FFP should be considered for hemorrhaging patients with evidence of DIC, coagulopathic liver disease, or warfarin reversal.

Cryoprecipitate

Cryoprecipitate is the precipitate that results from thawed FFP. It is rich in fibrinogen, factor VIII, von Willebrand's factor, and factor XIII. Like FFP, cryoprecipitate can be measured clinically by the fibrinogen response, which should increase by 5 to 10 mg/dl per unit. Unlike FFP, each unit of cryoprecipitate provides minimal volume (40 ml), so it is an ineffective agent for volume resuscitation. Cryoprecipitate is indicated for patients with DIC and concerns of volume overload, hypofibrinogenemia, factor VIII deficiency, and von Willebrand's disease.

Table 18-7 contains a summary of the available blood component therapies.

Table 18-7. Blood Component Therapy

COMPONENT	CONTENTS	VOLUME	ANTICIPATED EFFECT (PER UNIT)
Packed red blood cells	rbc, wbc, plasma	300 ml	Increase in hemoglobin by 1 g/dl
Platelets*†	platelets, rbc, wbc, plasma	50 ml	Increase in platelet count by 7,500/mm^3
Fresh frozen plasma	fibrinogen, antithrombin III, clotting factors, plasma	250 ml	Increase in fibrinogen by 5–10 mg/dl
Cryoprecipitate	fibrinogen, factor VIII, vWF, factor XIII	40 ml	Increase in fibrinogen by 5–10 mg/dl

*Given as a pooled concentrate or 6–10 units.
†A "single-donor platelet concentrate" contains a variable volume and increases the circulating platelet count between 30,000 and 60,000/mm^3.
rbc, red blood cells; vWF, von Willebrand factor; wbc, white blood cells.

Transfusion Risks and Reactions

Metabolic Abnormalities and Hypothermia

When prbc are stored, leakage of potassium and ammonia can occur into the plasma. This may result in hyperkalemia and high ammonia concentrations in patients requiring massive transfusion. In addition, because most prbc units are stored with a calcium-chelating agent, hypocalcemia may occur. Serial assessments of metabolic profiles and ionized calcium levels can assist the clinician in managing these changes.

In addition to metabolic abnormalities, hypothermia may complicate the clinical course of massive transfusion and result in cardiac arrhythmias. Hypothermia can be prevented by warming prbc units before transfusion and by providing alternative heating devices to the patient (e.g., "bear-hugger" anesthesia warmer).

Immunologic Reactions

Transfusions introduce interactions between inherited or acquired antibodies and the foreign antigens of the transfused blood products.[192] The most common immunologic reactions are febrile nonhemolytic transfusion reactions and urticarial reactions. Transfusion of leukoreduced blood products has been proposed to decrease the frequency of these reactions. Retrospective cohort studies have demonstrated a mild improvement in the occurrence of adverse reactions with universal leukoreduction.[193–195] Rare immunologic complications include acute or delayed hemolytic transfusion reactions, anaphylaxis, posttransfusion purpura, and graft-versus-host disease.

Infection Risks

All blood products have the potential to transmit viral and bacterial infections. Although transmission rates have substantially decreased in the past decade, they are still a potential risk that must be disclosed when a transfusion is needed. Table 18-8 lists current transfusion-related infection risks.

Acute Lung Injury

Acute lung injury complicates 1 in 2,000 transfusions.[196] This complication is characterized by acute respiratory distress, hypoxemia, hypotension, fever, and pulmonary edema.[197] Symptoms can be mild or severe, and resolution is usually complete within 96 hours. A pulmonary agglutinin reaction is thought to be responsible for the acute lung injury.[192] Treatment consists of supportive care with oxygen administration and diuresis.

Table 18-8. Transfusion-Related Infection Risks

INFECTION	TRANSMISSION RISK
HIV-1, HIV-2	1 in 1,900,000
Hepatitis B	1 in 140,000
Hepatitis C	1 in 1,000,000
HTLV I and II	1 in 650,000
Bacterial Contamination	
• Red cells	1 in 600,000
• Platelet	1 in 12,000

HIV, human immunodeficiency virus; HTLV, human t-cell lymphotropic virus.

Autologous Transfusion

Autologous transfusion refers to the collection and reinfusion of the patient's own prbc. Although it is unreasonable to have all pregnant individuals consider autologous donation, patients at high risk for transfusion (e.g., placenta previa or accreta) may be good candidates. Guidelines for autologous donation are as follows: minimum predonation hemoglobin of 11 g/dl, first donation within 6 weeks of anticipated delivery due to prbc storage life of 42 days, weekly interval between donations, and no donation within 2 weeks of anticipated delivery.[198]

Autologous transfusion should be used selectively. Autologous donation is significantly more expensive than homologous transfusion, and risks of bacterial contamination and subsequent homologous transfusion are not completely eliminated.

Alternative Management Approaches

Acute Normovolemic Hemodilution

Acute normovolemic hemodilution refers to a blood conservation technique in which blood is removed from a patient immediately before surgery, the patient is given crystalloid or colloid solution to maintain normovolemia during surgery, and then the blood is reinfused to the patient after surgery. The goal is for more dilute blood loss at the time of surgery. Acute normvolemic hemodilution can be considered for patients with good initial hemoglobin concentrations who are expected to have a blood loss of at least 1,000 ml during surgery (e.g., patients with suspected placenta accreta).

Autotransfusion

Autotransfusion is the collection of blood from the operative field, filtering the blood, and then reinfusing the red cells back to the patient. The most widely known device for autotransfusion is the Cell Saver. Although autotransfusion is often used in trauma cases, it has had limited application in obstetrics due to theoretical concerns regarding the risk of infection and amniotic fluid embolism. Several small studies have documented the safety and effectiveness of autotransfusion in the obstetrical setting.[199–202] Autotransfusion has many advantages over homologous transfusion. Not only does it eliminate the risk of infectious disease transmission, isoimmunization, and immunologic transfusion reactions, but it can rapidly provide the patient with red cells (1 unit in a 3-minute interval).

Alternative Oxygen Carriers

Because some patients refuse to accept blood products (e.g., Jehovah's Witness patients) or are unable to be transfused owing to a lack of compatible blood, new oxygen carriers are being developed and have promise as alternatives to transfusion therapy.[203] The two primary products are hemoglobin-based oxygen carriers and perfluorocarbons. Hemoglobin-based oxygen carriers use hemoglobin from animals, outdated human blood, or recombinant technology. The hemoglobin is separated from the red cell stroma and undergoes multiple filtration and polymerization processes before use. Perfluorocarbons are inert compounds that can dissolve gases, including oxygen. Both products have high oxygen-carrying capacities and have been used in phase III trials for elective surgery and in patients with hemorrhagic shock.

KEY POINTS

- Hemorrhage is a major cause of obstetric morbidity and mortality throughout the world.
- Understanding the hemodynamic changes of pregnancy and the physiologic responses that occur with hemorrhage assist in appropriate management.
- Placental abruption is diagnosed primarily by clinical findings and confirmed by laboratory, sonographic, and pathologic studies.
- Placenta previa remote from term can be expectantly managed.
- Placenta previa in association with a prior cesarean delivery is a major risk factor for placenta accreta.
- Placenta accreta is best managed with a multidisciplinary team approach.
- Postpartum hemorrhage affects 4 to 6 percent of all deliveries.
- Management of uterine atony should follow a rapidly initiated sequenced protocol.
- DIC mandates treatment of the initiating event and rapid replacement of consumed blood products.
- Although the risks of transfusion therapy are low, alternative measures for blood replacement should be considered if clinically appropriate.

REFERENCES

1. Chang J, Elam-Evans L, Berg CJ, et al: Pregnancy-related mortality surveillance-United States, 1991–1999. MMWR 52:1, 2003.
2. World Health Organization, Regional Office for Africa. *http://www.afro.who.int/press/2003* Accessed August 2004.
3. Pritchard J: Changes in blood volume during pregnancy and delivery. Anesthesiology 26:393, 1965.
4. van Oppen A, Stigter R, Bruinse H: Cardiac output in normal pregnancy: a critical review. Obstet Gynecol 87:310, 1996.
5. Clark S, Cotton D, Lee W, et al: Central hemodynamic assessment of normal term pregnancy. Am J Obstet Gynecol 161:1439, 1989.
6. Lochitch G: Clinical biochemistry of pregnancy. Crit Rev Clin Lab Sci 34:67, 1997.
7. Bletka M, Hlavaty V, Trnkova M, et al: Volume of whole blood and absolute amount of serum proteins in the early stage of late toxemia in pregnancy. Am J Obstet Gynecol 106:10, 1970.
8. Gillen-Goldstein J, Lockwood CJ: Abruptio placentae. *www.uptodate.com* Accessed September 2006.
9. Clark SL: Placenta previa and abruptio placentae. *In* Creasy RK, Resnik R (eds): Maternal-Fetal Medicine: Principles and Practice, 5th ed, Philadelphia, WB Saunders Company, 2004, p 713.
10. Knab DR: Abruptio placentae: An assessment of the time and method of delivery. Obstet Gynecol 52:625, 1978.
11. Karegard M, Gennser G: Incidence and recurrence rate of abruption placentae in Sweden. Obstet Gynecol 67:523, 1986.
12. Abdella TN, Sibai BM, Hays JM, et al: Relationship of hypertensive disease to abruption placentae. Obstet Gynecol 63:365, 1984.
13. Hurd WW, Miodovnik M, Hertzberg V, et al: Selective management of abruption placentae: A prospective study. Obstet Gynecol 61:467, 1983.
14. Pritchard J: Obstetric hemorrhage. *In* Pritchard J, MacDonald (eds): Williams Obstetrics. New York, Appleton-Century-Crofts, 1980. p 485.
15. Hibbard BM, Jeffcoate TN: Abruptio placentae. Obstet Gynecol 27:155, 1966.
16. Sher G: Pathogenesis and management of uterine inertia complicating abruption placentae with consumption coagulopathy. Am J Obstet Gynecol 129:164, 1977.
17. Ananth CV, Wilcox AJ, Savitz DA, et al: Effect of maternal age and parity on the risk of uteroplacental bleeding disorders in pregnancy. Obstet Gynecol 88:511, 1996.
18. Kramer MS, Usher RH, Pollack R, et al: Etiologic determinants of abruptio placentae. Obstet Gynecol 89:221, 1997.
19. Clark SL: Placenta previa and abruptio placentae. *In* Creasy RK, Resnik R (eds): Maternal-Fetal Medicine: Principles and Practice, 5th ed. Philadelphia, WB Saunders Company, 2004, p 714.
20. Rasmussen S, Irgens L, Bergsojo P, et al: The occurrence of placental abruption in Norway 1967–1991. Acta Obstet Gynecol Scand 75:222, 1996.
21. Ananth CV, Savitz DA, Bowes WA Jr, et al: Influence of hypertensive disorders and cigarette smoking on placental abruption and uterine bleeding during pregnancy. Br J Obstet Gynaecol 04:572, 1997.
22. Ananth CV, Smulian JC, Vintzileos AM: Incidence of placental abruption in relation to cigarette smoking and hypertensive disorders during pregnancy: A meta-analysis of observational studies. Obstet Gynecol 93:622, 1999.
23. Castles A, Adams EK, Melvin CL, et al: Effects of smoking during pregnancy. Five meta-analyses. Am J Prev Med 16:208, 1999.
24. Ananth CV, Smulian JC, Demissie K, et al: Placental abruption among singleton and twin births in the United States: Risk factor profiles. Am J Epidemiol 153:177, 2001.
25. Kyrklund-Blomberg NB, Genner G, Cnattingius S: Placental abruption and perinatal death. Paediatr Perinat Epidemiol 15:290, 2001.
26. Raymond EG, Mills JL: Placental abruption: Maternal risk factors and associated fetal conditions. Acta Obstet Gynaecol Scand 72:633, 1993.
27. Hoskins IA, Friedman DM, Frieden FJ, et al: Relationship between antepartum cocaine abuse, abnormal umbilical artery Doppler velocimetry, and placental abruption. Obstet Gynecol 78:279, 1991.
28. Hulse GK, Milne E, English DR, et al: Assessing the relationship between maternal cocaine use and abruptio placentae. Addiction 92:1547, 1997.
29. Harris CM: Trauma and pregnancy. In Foley MR, Strong TH Jr, Garite TJ (eds): Obstetric Intensive Care Manual, 2nd ed. New York, McGraw-Hill, 2004, p 239.
30. Pritchard J, Mason R, Corley M, et al: The genesis of severe placental abruption. Am J Obstet Gynecol 108:22, 1970.
31. Naeye R, Harkness WL, Utts J: Abruptio placentae and perinatal death: A prospective study. Am J Obstet Gynecol 128:740, 1977.
32. Vintzileos AM, Campbell WA, Nochimson DJ, et al: Preterm premature rupture of membranes: A risk factor for the development of abruptio placentae. Am J Obstet Gynecol 156:1235, 1987.
33. Ananth CV, Oyelese Y, Srinivas N, et al: Preterm premature rupture of membranes, intrauterine infection, and oligohydramnios: Risk factors for placental abruption. Obstet Gynecol 104:71, 2004.
34. Major CA, deVeciana M, Lewis DF, et al: Preterm premature rupture of membranes and abruptio placentae: Is there an asso-

ciation between these pregnancy complications? Am J Obstet Gynecol 172:672, 1995.
35. Spellacy WN, Handler A, Ferre CD: A case-control study of 1253 twin pregnancies from 1982–1987 perinatal data base. Obstet Gynecol 75:168, 1990.
36. Kupferminc MJ, Eldor A, Steinmen N, et al: Increased frequency of genetic thrombophilia in women with complications of pregnancy. N Engl J Med 340:9, 1999.
37. Vollset SE, Refsum H, Irgens LM, et al: Plasma total homocysteine, pregnancy complications, and adverse pregnancy outcomes: The Hordaland Homocysteine study. Am Clin Nutr 71:962, 2000.
38. Lockwood CJ: Heritable coagulopathies in pregnancy. Obstet Gynecol Surv 54:754, 1999.
39. Prochazka M, Happach C, Marsal K, et al: Factor Vleiden in pregnancies complicated by placental abruption. Br J Obstet Gynecol 110:462, 2003.
40. Facchinetti F, Marozio L, Grandone E, et al: Thrombophilic mutations are a main risk factor for placental abruption. Haematologica 88:785, 2003.
41. Nurk E, Tell GS, Refsum H, et al: Associations between maternal methylenetetrahydrofolate reductase polymorphisms and adverse outcomes of pregnancy: The Hordaland Homocysteine study. Am J Med 117:26, 2004.
42. Ness PM, Budzynski AZ, Olexa SA, et al: Congenital hypofibrinogenemia and recurrent placental abruption. Obstet Gynecol 61:519, 1983.
43. Roque H, Paidas MJ, Funal EF, et al: Maternal thrombophilias are not associated with early pregnancy loss. Thromb Haemost 91:290, 2004.
44. Nyberg DA, Cyr DR, Mack LA, et al: Sonographic spectrum of placental abruption. Am J Roentgenol 148:161, 1987.
45. Nyberg DA, Mack LA, Benedetti TJ, et al: Placental abruption and placental hemorrhage: Correlation of sonographic findings with fetal outcome. Radiology 358:357, 1987.
46. Sholl JS: Abruptio placentae: Clinical management in nonacute cases. Am J Obstet Gynecol 156:40, 1987.
47. Bond A, Edersheim T, Curry L, et al: Expectant management of abruptio placentae before 35 weeks gestation. Am J Perinatol 6:121, 1989.
48. Combs C, Nyberg D, Mack L, et al: Expectant management after sonographic diagnosis of placental abruption. Am J Perinatol 9:170, 1992.
49. Saller DJ: Tocolysis in the management of third trimester bleeding. J Perinatol 10:125, 1990.
50. Pritchard JA, Brekken AL: Clinical and laboratory studies on severe abruption placenta. Am J Obstet Gynecol 108:22, 1967.
51. Lowe TW, Cunningham FG: Placental abruption. Clin Obstet Gynecol 33:406, 1990.
52. Saftlas A, Olsen D, Atrash H, et al: National trends in the incidence of abruptio placenta. Obstet Gynecol 78:1081, 1991.
53. Ananth CV, Berkowitz GS, Savitz DA, et al: Placental abruption and adverse perinatal outcomes. JAMA 282:1646, 1999.
54. Spinillo A, Fazzi E, Stronati E, et al: Severity of abruptio placenta and neurodevelopmental outcome in low birth weight infants. Early Hum Dev 35:44, 1993.
55. Li DK, Wi S: Maternal placental abnormality and the risk of sudden infant death syndrome. Am J Epidemiol 149:608, 1999.
56. Clark SL: Placenta previa and abruptio placentae: In Creasy RK, Resnik R (eds): Maternal-Fetal Medicine: Principles and Practice, 5th ed. Philadelphia, WB Saunders Company, 2004, p 707.
57. Faiz AS, Anath CV: Etiology and risk factors for placenta previa: An overview and metaanalysis of observational studies. J Matern Fetal Neonatal Med 13:175, 2003.
58. Cotton DB, Read JA, Paul RH, et al: The conservative aggressive management of placenta previa. Am J Obstet Gynecol 137:687, 1980.
59. Rosati P, Guariglia L: Clinical significance of placenta previa at early routing transvaginal scan. J Ultrasound Med 19:581, 2000.
60. Mouer JR: Placenta previa: Antepartum conservative management, inpatient versus outpatient. Am J Obstet Gynecol 170:1683, 1994.
61. Lavery JP: Placenta previa. Clin Obstet Gynecol 33:414, 1990.
62. Strassmann P: Placenta praevia. Arch Gynecol 67:112, 1902.
63. Silver R, Depp R, Sabbagha RE, et al: Placenta previa: Aggressive expectant management. Am J Obstet Gynecol 150:15, 1984.
64. Sheiner E, Shoham-Vardi I, Hallak M, et al: Placenta previa: Obstetric risk factors and pregnancy outcome. J Matern Fetal Med 10:414, 2001.
65. Varma TR: Fetal growth and placental function in patients with placenta praevia. J Obstet Gynaecol Br Commonw 80:311, 1973.
66. Newton ER, Barss V, Cetrulo CL: The epidemiology and clinical history of asymptomatic midtrimester placenta previa. Am J Obstet Gynecol 148:743, 1984.
67. Iyasu S, Saftlas AK, Rowley DL, et al: The epidemiology of placenta previa in the United States, 1979 through 1987. Am J Obstet Gynecol 168:1424, 1993.
68. Ananth CV, Wilcox AJ, Savitz DA, et al: Effect of maternal age and parity on the risk of uteroplacental bleeding disorders in pregnancy. Obstet Gynecol 88:511, 1996.
69. Chelmow D, Andrew DE, Baker ER: Maternal cigarette smoking and placenta previa. Obstet Gynecol 87:703, 1996.
70. Strong TH, Brar HS: Placenta previa in twin gestations. J Reprod Med 34:415, 1989.
71. Francois K, Johnson J, Harris C: Is placenta previa more common in multiple gestations? Am J Obstet Gynecol 188:1226, 2003.
72. Monica G, Lilja C: Placenta previa, maternal smoking, and recurrence risk. Acta Obstet Gynaecol Scand 74:341, 1995.
73. Taylor VM, Kramer MD, Vaughan TL, et al: Placenta previa and prior cesarean delivery: How strong is the association? Obstet Gynecol 84:55, 1994.
74. Brenner W, Edelman D, Hendricks C: Characteristics of patients with placenta previa and results of "expectant management." Am J Obstet Gynecol 132:180, 1978.
75. Silver RM, Landon MB, Rouse DJ, et al: Maternal morbidity associated with multiple repeat cesarean deliveries. Obstet Gynecol 107:1226, 2006.
76. Nielsen TF, Hagberg H, Ljungblad U: Placenta previa and antepartum hemorrhage after previous cesarean section. Gynecol Obstet Invest 27:88, 1989.
77. Singh P, Rodrigues C, Gupta PA: Placenta previa and previous cesarean section. Acta Obstet Gynecol Scand 60:367, 1981.
78. Chattopadhyay S, Kharif H, Sherbeeni J: Placenta previa and accreta after previous cesarean section. Eur J Obstet Gynecol Reprod Biol 52:151, 1993.
79. Bowie JD, Rochester D, Cadkin AV, et al: Accuracy of placental localization by ultrasound. Radiology 128:177, 1978.
80. Timor-Tritsch IE, Monteagudo A: Diagnosis of placenta previa by transvaginal sonography. Ann Med 25:279, 1993.
81. Dawson WB, Dumas MD, Romano WM, et al: Translabial ultrasonography and placenta previa: Does measurement of the os-placenta distance predict outcome? J Ultrasound Med 15:441, 1996.
82. Farine D, Peisner DB, Timor-Trisch IE: Placenta previa—Is the traditional diagnostic approach satisfactory? J Clin Ultrasound 18:328, 1990.
83. Zelop C, Bromley B, Frigoletto FJ, et al: Second trimester sonographically diagnosed placenta previa: Prediction of persistent previa at birth. Int J Gynaecol Obstet 44:207, 1994.
84. Russo-Stieglitz K, Lockwood CJ: Placenta previa and vasa previa. *www.uptodate.com* Accessed March 2006.
85. Wing DA, Paul RH, Millar LK: Management of the symptomatic placenta previa: A randomized, controlled trial of inpatient versus outpatient expectant management. Am J Obstet Gynecol 75:806, 996.
86. D'Angelo LJ, Irwin LF: Conservative management of placenta previa: A cost-benefit analysis. Am J Obstet Gynecol 148:320, 1984.
87. Watson P, Cefalo R: Magnesium sulfate tocolysis in selected patients with symptomatic placenta previa. Am J Perinatol 1990;7:251.
88. Mabie WC: Placenta previa. Clin Perinatol 19:425, 1992.
89. Dinsmoor MJ, Hogg BB: Autologous blood donation with placenta previa: Is it feasible? Am J Perinatol 12:382, 1995.
90. Toedt ME: Feasilibity of autologous blood donation in patients with placenta previa. J Fam Pract 48:219, 1999.
91. Resnik R: Diagnosis and management of placenta accreta. *www.uptodate.com* Accessed June 2006.

92. Miller DA, Chollet JA, Goodwin TM: Clinical risk factors for placenta previa-placenta accreta. Am J Obstet Gynecol 177:210, 1997
93. Finberg H, Williams J: Placenta accreta: Prospective sonographic diagnosis in patients with placenta previa and prior cesarean section. J Ultrasound Med 11:333, 1992.
94. Comstock CH, Love JJ, Bronsteen RA, et al: Sonographic detection of placenta accreta in the second and third trimesters of pregnancy. Am J Obstet Gynecol 190:1135, 2004.
95. Levine D, Hulka CA, Ludmir J, et al: Placenta accreta: Evaluation with color Doppler US, power Doppler US, and MR imaging. Radiology 205:773, 1997.
96. Chou MM, Ho ES, Lee YH: Prenatal diagnosis of placenta previa accreta by transabdominal color Doppler ultrasound. Ultrasound Obstet Gynecol 15:28, 2000.
97. Maldjian C, Adam R, Pelosi M, et al: MRI appearance of placenta percreta and placenta accreta. Magn Reson Imaging 17:965, 1999.
98. Kirkinen P, Helin-Martikainen HL, Vanninen R, et al: Placenta accreta: Imaging by gray-scale and contrast-enhanced color Doppler sonography and magnetic resonance imaging. J Clin Ultrasound 26:90, 1998.
99. Kupferminc MJ, Tamura RK, Wigton TR, et al: Placenta accreta is associated with elevated maternal serum alpha-fetoprotein. Obstet Gynecol 82:266, 1993.
100. Hung TH, Shau WY, Hsieh CC, et al: Risk factors for placenta accreta. Obstet Gynecol 93:545, 1999.
101. Read J, Cotton D, Miller F: Placenta accreta: Changing clinical aspects and outcome. Obstet Gynecol 56:31, 1980.
102. Druzin ML: Packing of lower uterine segment for control of post-cesarean bleeding in instances of placenta previa. Surg Gynecol Obstet 169:543, 1980.
103. Dubois J, Garel L, Grignon A, et al: Placenta percreta: Balloon occlusion and embolization of the internal iliac arteries to reduce Intraoperative blood loss. Am J Obstet Gynecol 176:723, 1997.
104. Paull JD, Smith J, Williams L, et al: Balloon occlusion of the abdominal aorta during caesarean hysterectomy for placenta percreta. Anaesth Intensive Care 23:731, 1995.
105. Kidney DD, Nguyen AM, Ahdoot D, et al: Prophylactic perioperative hypogastric artery balloon occlusion in abnormal placentation. Am J Roentgenol 176:1521, 2001.
106. Hong TM, Tseng HS, Lee RC, et al: Uterine artery embolization: An effective treatment for intractable obstetric hemorrhage. Clin Radiol 59:96, 2004.
107. Cho J, Kim S, Cha K, et al: Interrupted circular suture: Bleeding control during cesarean delivery in placenta previa accreta. Obstet Gynecol 78:876, 1991.
108. Kayem G, Davy C, Goffinet F, et al: Conservative versus extirpative management in cases of placenta accreta. Obstet Gynecol 104:531, 2004.
109. Arulkumaran S, Ng CS, Ingemarsson I, et al: Medical treatment of placenta accreta with methotrexate. Acta Obstet Gynecol Scand 65:285, 1986.
110. Rziel A, Golan A, Ariely S, et al: Repeated ultrasonography and intramuscular methotrexate in conservative management of residual adherent placenta. J Clin Ultrasound 20:288, 1992.
111. Legros RS, Price FV, Hill LM, et al: Nonsurgical management of placenta percreta: A case report. Obstet Gynecol 83:847, 1994.
112. Mussalli GM, Shah J, Berck DJ, et al: Placenta accreta and methotrexate therapy: Three case reports. J Perinatol 20:331, 2000.
113. Rucker MP, Tureman GR: Vasa previa. Virginia Med Monthly 72:202, 1952.
114. Torrey WE: Vasa previa. Am J Obstet Gynecol 63:146, 1952.
115. Quek SP, Tan KL: Vasa previa. Aust N Z J Obstet Gynaecol 12:206, 1972.
116. Lee W, Lee VL, Kirk JS, et al: Vasa previa: Prenatal diagnosis, natural evolution, and clinical outcome. Obstet Gynecol 95:572, 2000.
117. Oyelese KO, Turner M, Lees C, et al: Vasa previa: An avoidable obstetric tragedy. Obstet Gynecol Survey 54:138. 1999.
118. Francois K, Mayer S, Harris, C, et al: Association of vasa previa with a history of second-trimester placenta previa. J Reprod Med 48:771, 2003.
119. Catanzarite V, Maida C, Thomas W, et al: Prenatal sonographic detection of vasa previa: Ultrasound findings and obstetric outcome in ten cases. Ultrasound Obstet Gynecol 18:109, 2001.
120. Gianopoulos J, Carver T, Tomich PG, et al: Diagnosis of vasa previa with ultrasonography. Obstet Gynecol 69:488, 1987.
121. Nelson LH, Melone PJ, King M: Diagnosis of vasa previa with transvaginal and color flow Doppler ultrasound. Obstet Gynecol 76:506, 1990.
122. Meyer WJ, Blumenthal L, Cadkin A, et al: Vasa previa: Prenatal diagnosis with transvaginal color Doppler flow imaging. Am J Obstet Gynecol 169:1627, 1993.
123. Hertzberg BS, Kliewer MA: Vasa previa: Prenatal diagnosis by transperineal sonography with Doppler evaluation. J Clin Ultrasound 26:405, 1998.
124. Oyelese Y, Catanzarite V, Perfumo F, et al: Vasa previa: The impact of prenatal diagnosis on outcomes. Obstet Gynecol 103:937, 2004.
125. Pritchard JA, Baldwin RM, Dickey JC, et al: Blood volume changes in pregnancy and the puerperium. II. Red blood cell loss and changes in apparent blood volume during and following vaginal delivery, cesarean section, and cesarean section plus total hysterectomy. Am J Obstet Gynecol 84;1271, 1962.
126. Combs CA, Murphy EL, Laros RK Jr: Factors associated with postpartum hemorrhage with vaginal birth. Obstet Gynecol 77:69, 1991.
127. Combs CA, Murphy EL, Laros RK Jr: Factors associated with hemorrhage in cesarean deliveries. Obstet Gynecol 77:77, 1991.
128. Dildy GA: Postpartum hemorrhage: New management options. Clin Obstet Gynecol 45:330, 2002.
129. Elbourne DR, Prendiville WJ, Carroli G, et al: Prophylactic use of oxytocin in the third stage of labour. Cochrane Database Syst Rev 4:CD001808, 2001.
130. Prendiville W, Harding J, Elbourne D, et al: The Briston third stage trial: Active vs. physiological management of the third stage of labor. BMJ 297:1295, 1988.
131. Jackson KW Jr, Allbert JR, Schemmer GK, et al: A randomized controlled trial comparing oxytocin administration before and after placental delivery in prevention of postpartum hemorrhage. Am J Obstet Gynecol 185:873, 2001.
132. McCurdy CM, Magann EF, McCurdy CJ, et al: The effect of placental management at cesarean delivery on operative blood loss. Am J Obstet Gynecol 167:1363, 1993.
133. Munn MB, Owen J, Vincent R, et al: Comparison of two oxytocin regimens to prevent uterine atony at cesarean delivery: A randomized controlled trial. Obstet Gynecol 98:386, 2001.
134. El-Rafaey H, O'Brien P, Morafa W, et al: Use of oral misoprostol in the prevention of postpartum haemorrhage. Br J Obstet Gynecol 104:336, 1997.
135. El-Rafaey H, Nooh R, O'Brien P, et al: The misoprostol third stage of labour study: A randomized controlled comparison between orally administered misoprostol and standard management. Br J Obstet Gynecol 107:1104, 2000.
136. Gulmezoglu AM, Villar J, Ngoc NT, et al: WHO multicenter randomized trial of misoprostol in the management of the third stage of labor. Lancet 358:689, 2001.
137. Gulmezoglu AM: Prostaglandins for prevention of postpartum hemorrhage. Cochrane Database Syst Rev CD000494, 2000.
138. O'Brien P, El-Rafaey H, Gordan A, et al: Rectally administered misoprostol for the treatment of postpartum hemorrhage unresponsive to oxytocin and ergometrine: A descriptive study. Obstet Gynecol 92:212, 1998.
139. Lokugamage AU, Sullivan KR, Niculescu I, et al: A randomized study comparing rectally administered misoprostol versus Syntometrine combined with an oxytocin infusion for the cessation of primary postpartum hemorrhage. Acta Obstet Gynecol Scand 80:835, 2001.
140. Maier RC: Control of postpartum hemorrhage with uterine packing. Am J Obstet Gynecol 169:317, 1993.
141. Hester JD: Postpartum hemorrhage and reevaluation of uterine packing. Obstet Gynecol 45:501, 1975.
142. Hsu S, Rodgers B, Lele A, et al: Use of packing in obstetric hemorrhage of uterine origin. J Reprod Med 48:69, 2003.
143. Bakri YN, Amri A, Abdul Jabber F: Tamponade-balloon for obstetrical bleeding. Int J Gynecol Obstet 74:139, 2001.

144. Condous GS, Arulkumaran S, Symonds I, et al: The "tamponade test" in the management of massive postpartum hemorrhage. Obstet Gynecol 101:767, 2003.
145. Salomon LJ, deTayrac R, Castaigne-Meary V, et al: Fertility and pregnancy outcome following pelvic arterial embolization for severe post-partum haemorrhage. A cohort study. Hum Reprod 18:849, 2003.
146. Ornan D, White R, Pollack J, et al: Pelvic embolization for intractable postpartum hemorrhage: Long-term follow-up and implications for fertility. Obstet Gynecol 102:904, 2003.
147. Wang H, Garmel S: Successful term pregnancy after bilateral uterine artery embolization for postpartum hemorrhage. Obstet Gynecol 102:603, 2003.
148. Jacobs AJ: Treatment of postpartum hemorrhage. *www.uptodate.com* Accessed August 2006.
149. Mousa HA, Walkinshaw S: Major postpartum haemorrhage. Curr Opin Obstet Gynecol 13:595, 2001.
150. O'Leary JL, O'Leary JA: Uterine artery ligation in the control of intractable postpartum hemorrhage. Am J Obstet Gynecol 94:920, 1966.
151. Adrabbo F, Salah J: Stepwise uterine devascularization: A novel technique for management of uncontrollable postpartum hemorrhage with preservation of the uterus. Am J Obstet Gynecol 171:694, 1984.
152. Mengert W, Burchell R, Blumstein R, et al: Pregnancy after bilateral ligation of internal iliac and ovarian arteries. Obstet Gynecol 34:664, 1969.
153. B-Lynch C, Coker A, Lawal AH, et al: The B-Lynch surgical technique for control of massive postpartum haemorrhage: an alternative to hysterectomy? Five cases reported. Br J Obstet Gynaecol 104:275, 1997.
154. Cho JH, Jun HS, Lee CN: Hemostatic suturing technique for uterine bleeding during cesarean delivery. Obstet Gynecol 96:129, 2000.
155. Gerfguson JE, Bourgeois FJ, Underwood PB: B-Lynch suture for postpartum hemorrhage. Obstet Gynecol 95:1020, 2000.
156. Dacus JV, Busowski MT, Busowski JD, et al: Surgical treatment of uterine atony employing the B-Lynch technique. J Matern Fet Med 9:194, 2000.
157. Vansgaard K: B-Lynch suture in uterine atony. Ugeskr Laeger 162:3468, 2000.
158. Silverman F: Management of the third stage of labor. *www.uptodate.com* Accessed July 2006.
159. Carroli G, Bergel E: Umbilical vein injection for management of retained placenta, Cochrane Database Syst Rev 4:CD001337, 2001.
160. Welischar J, Quirk JG: Vaginal birth after cesarean delivery. *www.uptodate.com* Accessed August 2006.
161. Vaginal birth after previous cesarean delivery. ACOG practice bulletin #54. Obstet Gynecol 104:203, 2004.
162. Guise JM, McDonagh MS, Osterweil P, et al: Systematic review of the incidence and consequences of uterine rupture in women with previous cesarean section. BJM 329:19, 2004.
163. Lydon-Rochelle M, Holt VL, Easterling TR, et al: Risk of uterine rupture during labor among women with a prior cesarean delivery. N Engl J Med 345:3, 2001.
164. Caughey AB, Shipp TD, Repke JT, et al: Rate of uterine rupture during a trial of laboring women with one or two prior cesarean deliveries. Am J Obstet Gynecol 181:872, 1999.
165. Shipp TD, Zelop C, Repke JT, et al: The association of maternal age and symptomatic uterine rupture during a trial of labor after prior cesarean delivery. Obstet Gynecol 99:585, 2002.
166. Fuchs K, Peretz BA, Marcovici R, et al: The "grand multipara"—is it a problem? A review of 5785 cases. Int J Gynaecol Obstet 23;321, 1985.
167. Hamiliton EF, Bujold E, McNamara H, et al: Dystocia among women with symptomatic uterine rupture. Am J Obstet Gynecol 184:620, 2001.
168. Shipp TD, Zelop C, Repke JT, et al: Interdelivery interval and risk of symptomatic uterine rupture. Obstet Gynecol 97:175, 2001.
169. Esposito MA, Menihan CA, Malee MP: Association of interpregnancy interval with scar failure in labor: A case-control study. Am J Obstet Gynecol 183:1180, 2000.
170. Shipp TD, Zelop C, Cohen A, et al: Post-cesarean delivery fever and uterine rupture in a subsequent trial of labor. Obstet Gynecol 101:136, 2003.
171. Bujold E, Bujold C, Hamiliton EF, et al: The impact of a single-layer or double-layer closure on uterine rupture. Am J Obstet Gynecol 186:1326, 2002.
172. Durnwald C, Mercer B: Uterine rupture, perioperative and perinatal morbidity after single-layer and double-layer closure at cesarean delivery. Am J Obstet Gynecol 189:925, 2003.
173. Ridgeway JJ, Weyrich DL, Benedetti TJ: Fetal heart rate changes associated with uterine rupture. Obstet Gynecol 103:506, 2004.
174. Chauhan SP, Martin JN Jr, Henrichs CE, et al: Maternal and perinatal complications with uterine rupture in 142,075 patients who attempted vaginal birth after cesarean delivery: A review of the literature. Am J Obstet Gynecol 189:408, 2003.
175. Leung AS, Leung EK, Paul RH: Uterine rupture after previous cesarean delivery: Maternal and fetal consequences. Am J Obstet Gynecol 169:945, 1993.
176. Bujold E, Gauthier B: Neonatal morbidity associated with uterine rupture: What are the risk factors? Am J Obstet Gynecol 186:311, 2002.
177. Landon MB, Hauth JC, Leveno KJ, et al: Maternal and perinatal outcomes associated with a trial of labor after prior cesarean delivery. N Engl J Med 351:2581, 2004.
178. Lipitz S, Frenkel Y: Puerperal inversion of the uterus. Eur J Obstet Gynecol Reprod Biol 27:271, 1988.
179. Brar HS, Greenspoon JS, Platt LD, et al: Acute puerperal uterine inversion: new approaches to management. J Reprod Med 34:173, 1989.
180. Hseih TT, Lee JD: Sonographic findings in acute puerperal uterine inversion. J Clin Ultrasound 19:306, 1991.
181. Grossman RA: Magnesium sulfate for uterine inversion. J Reprod Med 26:261, 1981.
182. Catanzarite VA, Moffitt KD, Baker ML, et al: New approaches to the management of acute uterine inversion. Obstet Gynecol 68:78, 1986.
183. Altabef KM, Spencer JT, Zinberg S: Intravenous nitroglycerin for uterine relaxation of an inverted uterus. Am J Obstet Gynecol 166:1237, 1992.
184. Johnson AB: A new concept in the replacement of the inverted uterus and a report of nine cases. Am J Obstet Gynecol 57:557, 1949.
185. Momani AW, Hassan A: Treatment of puerperal uterine inversion by the hydrostatic method; reports of five cases. Eur J Obstet Gynecol Reprod Biol 32:281, 1989.
186. Ogueh O, Ayida G: Acute uterine inversion: A new technique of hydrostatic pressure replacement. Br J Obstet Gynaecol 104:951, 1997.
187. Huntington JL: Acute uterine inversion of the uterus. Boston Med Surg J 15:376, 1921.
188. Haultain FWN: The treatment of chronic uterine inversion by abdominal hysterotomy with a successful case. Br Med J 2:974, 1901.
189. Bouwmeester FW, Jonkhoff AR, Verheijen RH, et al: Successful treatment of life-threatening postpartum hemorrhage with recombinant activated factor VII. Obstet Gynecol 101:1172, 2003.
190. Moscardo F, Perez F, de la Rubia J, et al: Successful treatment of severe intra-abdominal bleeding associated with disseminated intravascular coagulation using recombinant activated factor VII. Br J Haematol 114:174, 2001.
191. Segal S, Shemesh IY, Blumental R, et al: The use of recombinant factor VIIa in severe postpartum hemorrhage. Acta Obstet Gynecol Scand 83:771, 2004.
192. Silvergleid AJ: Immunologic blood transfusion reactions. *www.uptodate.com* Accessed May 2006.
193. Yazer MH, Podlosky L, Clarke G, et al: The effect of prestorage WBC reduction on rates of febrile nonhemolytic transfusion reactions to platelet concentrates and RBC. Transfusion 44:10, 2004.
194. Paglino JC, Pomper GJ, Fisch GS, et al: Reduction in febrile but not allergic reactions to rbcs and platelets after conversion to universal prestorage leukoreduction. Transfusion 44:16, 2004.
195. King KE, Shirey RS, Thoman SK, et al: Universal leukoreduction decreases the incidence of febrile nonhemolytic transfusion reactions to RBCS. Transfusion 44:25, 2004.

196. Silliman CC, Paterson AJ, Dickey WO, et al: The association of biologically active lipids with the development of transfusion-related acute lung injury: A retrospective study. Transfusion 37:719, 1997.
197. Popovsky MA, Chaplin HC Jr, Moore SB: Transfusion-related acute lung injury: A neglected, serious complication of hemotherapy. Transfusion 32:589, 1992.
198. Martin SR, Strong TH Jr: Transfusion of blood components and derivatives in the obstetric intensive care patient. *In* Foley MR, Strong TH Jr, Garite TJ (eds): Obstetric Intensive Care Manual, 2nd ed. New York, McGraw-Hill, 2004, p 19.
199. Zichella L, Gramolini R: Autotransfusion during cesarean section. Am J Obstet Gynecol 162:295, 1990.
200. Merril BS, Mitts DL, Rogers W, et al: Autotransfusion: Intraoperative use in ruptured ectopic pregnancy. J Reprod Med 24:14, 1980.
201. Jongen VHWM: Autotransfusion and ectopic pregnancy: An experience from Tanzania. Trop Doct 27:78, 1997.
202. Rebarber A, Lonser R, Jackson S, et al: The safety of intraoperative autologous blood collection and autotransfusion during cesarean section. Am J Obstet Gynecol 179:715, 1998.
203. Fridey JL: Oxygen carriers as alternatives to red cell transfusion. *www.uptodate.com* Accessed June 2006.

Cesarean Delivery

Mark B. Landon

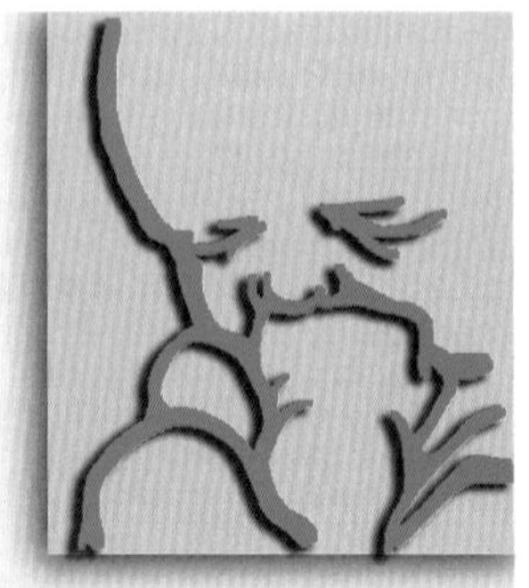

CHAPTER 19

KEY ABBREVIATIONS

American College of Obstetricians and Gynecologists	ACOG
Cephalopelvic disproportion	CPD
Computerized tomography	CT
Deep venous thrombosis	DVT
Fetal heart rate	FHR
Hypoxic-ischemic encephalopathy	HIE
Maternal-Fetal Medicine Units Network	MFMU
National Institute of Child Health and Human Development	NICHD
National Institutes of Health	NIH
Odds ratio	OR
Pulmonary embolus	PE
Relative risk	RR
Trial of labor	TOL
Vaginal birth after cesarean delivery	VBAC

DEFINITION

Cesarean section has classically been defined as delivery of a fetus through a surgically created incision in the anterior uterine wall. Because cesarean and section both refer to an incision, some prefer the terms cesarean delivery or cesarean birth to describe the procedure. This chapter reviews the history of cesarean delivery, trends in cesarean section rates, and indications, techniques, and complications of this procedure.

HISTORY OF CESAREAN DELIVERY

Cesarean delivery has been described since ancient times, and there is evidence from both early Western and non-Western societies of this surgical procedure being performed. The evolution of the term "cesarean" has been debated over time. Although this term was originally believed to have been derived from the birth of Julius Caesar, it is unlikely that his mother, Aurelia, would have survived the operation. Her knowledge of her son's invasion of Europe many years later indicates that she survived childbirth. In Caesar's time, surgical delivery was reserved for cases when the mother was dead or dying. Roman law under Caesar specified surgical removal of the fetus before burial of deceased pregnant women. Religious edicts required separate burial for the infant and mother. Thus, the term cesarean more likely refers to being cut open as the Latin verb "caedare" means to cut. Cesarean operation was the preferred term before the 1598 publication of Guillimeau, who introduced the term "section."[1]

Although sporadic reports of heroic life saving efforts through cesarean childbirth existed for hundreds of years, it was not until the later part of the 19th century that the operation began to be established as part of obstetric practice. This coincided with the gradual transition of childbirth as primarily a midwife attended event, often in rural settings, to an urban hospital experience. The wide emergence of hospitals laid the foundation for establishing obstetrics as a hospital-based specialty. As new methods for anesthesia emerged, cesarean delivery for obstructed labor gained popularity over destructive procedures such as craniotomy accompanying difficult vaginal births. Despite the dangers that still existed with cesarean delivery, the operation was viewed as preferable to a difficult high forceps delivery, which was associated with fetal injury and deep pelvic lacerations. Whereas refinements in anesthesia techniques allowed the operation to be performed, mortality rates remained very high, with sepsis and peritonitis as leading causes of postoperative deaths. Primitive surgical techniques and lack of antisepsis clearly contributed to such outcomes. Surgeons attempted to complete the operation without closing the uterus, fearing that the suture material itself would promote infection, and that the uterus would best heal by intention. As a result, women were placed at risk for both hemorrhage and infection.

In 1876, Eduardo Porro advocated hysterectomy with cesarean delivery in order to control bleeding and to prevent postoperative infection.[2] Shortly thereafter, surgeons gained experience with internal suturing because silver wire stitches were developed by the gynecologist J. Marion Sims. Sims had perfected the use of these sutures in the treatment of vesicovaginal fistulas resulting from obstructed labors.

Because gynecologic surgeons performed more cesarean deliveries and the outcomes improved, great attention was placed on technique including the site of uterine incision. Between 1880 and 1925, surgeons began employing transverse incisions of the uterus. It was noted that such incisions reduced the rate of infection and the risk for rupture with subsequent pregnancies.[3] However, owing to the risk of peritonitis, extraperitoneal cesarean was advocated by Frank (1907) and Latzko (1909) and was popularized by Beck (1919) in the United States.[4–6]

The introduction of penicillin in 1940 also dramatically reduced the risks of infection associated with childbirth. As antibiotic therapy emerged, the need for extraperitoneal dissection and incision diminished. The low cervical incision introduced by Munro Kerr (1926) became further established as the technique of choice.[7] As technology including improved anesthesia developed and the medical management of pregnancy and childbirth accelerated, cesarean delivery became more commonplace in obstetrics. Obstetricians over time have evaluated the risk and benefits of this procedure, and a liberalized approach to using cesarean childbirth has emerged in the United States over the past 35 years. In 1970, the cesarean delivery rate was approximately 5 percent. By 2004, it had reached 29.1 percent, the highest rate ever recorded in the United States.[8]

TRENDS IN CESAREAN DELIVERY RATES

The cesarean delivery rate describes the proportion of women undergoing cesarean delivery of all women giving birth during a specific time period. The cesarean delivery rate may be further subdivided into the primary cesarean (first-time operation) and repeat cesarean delivery rate, both as a proportion of the entire obstetric population. Cesarean delivery rates have risen in the United States in a dramatic fashion from less than 5 percent in the 1960s to nearly 30 percent by 2004. Over the past 35 years, an increase in international cesarean delivery rates has also been documented, yet for most European nations, the overall rate remains significantly lower than in the United States.[9]

Given the discrepancy in cesarean delivery rates between the United States and other countries without a perceivable benefit in neonatal outcomes, health policy groups have critically evaluated this issue including its cause and possible solutions. Twenty-five years ago, the National Institutes of Health (NIH) established a task force on cesarean childbirth and sponsored a consensus development conference on this subject.[10] It was recognized that almost all of the increase in cesarean section rates was due to increased repeat operations, and primary cesarean deliveries for dystocia and fetal distress (Table 19-1).

Table 19-1. Factors Responsible for Increased Cesarean Delivery Rates

Obstetric Factors

- Increased primary cesarean delivery rate
  - Failed induction/increased utilization of induction of labor
  - Decreased utilization of operative vaginal delivery
  - Increased macrosomia/elective cesarean delivery for macrosomia
  - Decline in vaginal breech delivery
- Increased repeat cesarean delivery rate
  - Decreased utilization of VBAC

Maternal Factors

- Increased proportion of women > age 35
- Increased nulliparous women
- Increased elective primary cesarean deliveries

Physician Factors

- Malpractice litigation concerns

With expanding indications for cesarean delivery, and little enthusiasm for vaginal birth after cesarean (VBAC) before 1980, it was obvious that prior cesarean delivery had emerged as a major indication. Dystocia was also being diagnosed more frequently through the 1970s and 1980s, along with a parallel decline in operative vaginal delivery rates.[11] Not surprisingly, the increased cesarean delivery rates in the United States compared with European countries can be explained almost entirely by cephalopelivc disproportion and repeat cesarean delivery as the dominant indications for the operation.[12]

Fear of litigation is also recognized as liberalizing the indications for cesarean section particularly with respect to labor management and the diagnosis of fetal distress or nonreassuring fetal heart rate (FHR) patterns. Despite knowledge that intrapartum electronic FHR monitoring has not been shown to reduce the risk of metabolic acidosis, birth asphyxia, or cerebral palsy compared with intermittent auscultation, its widespread use has been cited as a factor in increasing the diagnosis of fetal distress and thus cesarean delivery.[13,14] The NIH task force recommended that both dystocia and elective repeat cesarean deliveries clearly required further study and institution of strategies to reduce their contribution to the overall rise in cesarean delivery. This recommendation was appealing in that these two categories contributed greatly to the rise in cesarean section, and they represent indications that would likely be amenable to a reduction since physician practice patterns clearly influence these categories of cesarean delivery.

Cesarean delivery accounts for more than one million major operations performed annually in the United States.[1] It is the most common major surgical procedure undertaken today. Following efforts championed by institutions and payors to reduce the cesarean section rate, between 1988 and 1996, the overall cesarean delivery rate in the United States fell from 24.7 percent to a nadir of 20.7 percent. This decline can be largely attributed to the increased practice of trial of labor (TOL) after prior cesarean birth.[15] However, over the past decade, cesarean rates have steadily climbed and exceed those of the late 1980s. This rise is reflected by an increase in the primary cesarean rate and a steep drop in the rate of vaginal births after previous cesarean deliveries. VBAC rates plummeted from a peak of 28.3 percent in 1996 to 9.2 percent in 2004[8] (Fig. 19-1).

The rise in cesarean section rates has prompted increased interest in the indications, complications, and techniques involved with this procedure. Despite clear documentation of the prevalence of cesarean section, there is remarkably little prospectively gathered information concerning a variety of issues related to abdominal delivery. The overwhelming economic burden of cesarean birth on health care delivery continues to focus efforts on strategies aimed at reducing cesarean delivery rates. Because cesarean section carries with it a risk for uncommon complications such as maternal mortality and more often observed infectious complications extending the mother's length of stay in the hospital, cesarean section data continue to be employed as an indicator to reflect overall quality of care for obstetric services. The appropriate use of a TOL in women with a prior cesarean section has also been a focus for providers and payors of obstetric care.

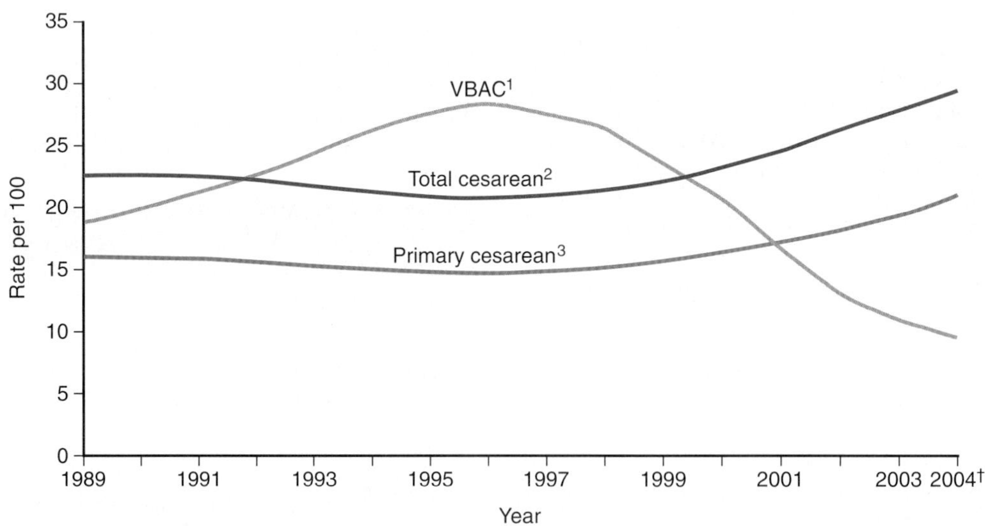

†Preliminary data
¹Number of vaginal births after previous cesarean per 100 live births: to women with a previous cesarean delivery
²Percentage of all live births by cesarean delivery.
³Number of primary cesarean deliveries per 100 live births: to women who have not had a previous cesarean.
Note: Due to changes in data collection from implementation of the 2003 revision of the U.S. Standard Certificate of Live Birth, there may be small discontinuities in values of primary cesarean delivery and VBAC in 2000 and 2004; see "Technical Notes."

Figure 19-1. Total and primary cesarean rate and vaginal birth after previous cesarean (VBAC): United States, 1989 to 2004. (From Martin JA, Hamilton BE, Menachker F, et al: Preliminary births for 2004. Health E-Stats. National Center for Health Statistics. [*www.cdc.gov/nchs/products/pubs/pubd/hestats/prelimbirths/prelimbirths04.htm*])

MONITORING CESAREAN DELIVERY RATES

It is not possible to determine an optimal cesarean delivery rate because an "ideal" rate must be a function of multiple clinical factors that vary in each population and are influenced by the level of obstetric care provided. Further complicating this issue is the absence of complete and accurate data that focus on both maternal and infant outcomes. Thus, although cesarean delivery rates can be considered a measure of a specific health care process (mode of delivery), these rates are not outcome measures because they do not indicate whether cesarean or vaginal birth results in optimal perinatal outcomes. In spite of these limitations, the observation of wide variation in cesarean delivery rates according to geographic region and more importantly among physicians within the same institutions with similar patient populations provide at least indirect evidence that excess use of cesarean delivery is a significant quality of care issue to be considered.

Both the *Health People 2000* report and the recent *Healthy People 2010* document suggest an overall target cesarean delivery rate of 15 percent.[16,17] Trends in cesarean delivery rates in the United States would strongly indicate that this challenge will not be met. Among the reasons for this fact are (1) continued increase in primary cesarean deliveries for dystocia, failed induction, and abnormal presentation; (2) an increase in the proportion of women with obesity, diabetes mellitus, and multiple gestation, which predispose to cesarean delivery; (3) increased practice of elective cesarean delivery in order to preserve pelvic floor function; and (4) limited use of TOL after cesarean delivery owing to both safety and medicolegal concerns (see Table 19-1).

In spite of little consensus regarding the best mode of delivery for many complicated pregnancies, third-party payors and institutions continue to rely on expert opinion concerning optimal cesarean delivery rates without the benefit of risk stratification. It follows that institutions involved in tertiary obstetric care thus managing a large number of preterm deliveries and maternal complications of pregnancy should have higher cesarean rates than primary care facilities.[18] Several models have been developed to provide risk-adjusted cesarean delivery rates.[19] Use of hospital billing information consisting of International Classification of Diseases codes is a common methodology; however, important information such as parity and other demographics are lacking with this approach. In contrast, Leiberman and colleagues employed a case-mix system, which stratified women according to parity, prior cesarean delivery, presentation, gestational age, and the presence of medical conditions precluding a TOL.[20] In their study, the crude cesarean delivery rate was higher for hospital-based practice physicians (24.4 percent) than for community-based practitioners (21.5 percent). However, the proportion of women falling into categories conferring a high risk of cesarean delivery was twice as high for the hospital-based practice. Standardizing the case mix resulted in an overall cesarean rate of 20.1 percent for the hospital-based physicians.

In 2000, the American College of Obstetricians and Gynecologists (ACOG) developed a simple formula to help institutions and physicians assess their risk-adjusted cesarean delivery rates.[21] Two populations were targeted that included (1) nulliparous women with a singleton vertex gestation at 37 weeks or greater without other complications and; (2) women with one prior low-transverse cesarean delivery, delivering a single vertex fetus at 37 weeks or greater without other complications. For "first-time cesareans," the benchmark rate set by ACOG for 2010 is 15.5 percent, which represents the 25th percentile of state rankings (national rate was 17.9 percent in 1996). For "repeat cesareans," the benchmark rate for vaginal delivery after a prior cesarean is 37 percent, a figure which represents the 75th percentile of state rankings (1996 national VBAC rate was 30.3 percent). The use of these simple case-mix adjusted rates should make comparative evaluation of cesarean delivery rates more meaningful. As data becomes more unified and methodologically sound, the quality of obstetric care can be better assessed.

Using raw and risk-adjusted data, institutions have sought to reduce cesarean birth rates through quality improvement initiatives.[22] Myers and Gleicher successfully reduced overall cesarean rates from 17.5 percent to 11.9 percent after developing guidelines in concert with a comprehensive data collection process and intensive feedback to physicians.[23] Outliers were identified and subjected to "one-on-one" reviews of their individual practices. Other successful programs aimed at lowering cesarean rates have also relied on the combination of providing quality data and counseling to physicians who become invested in changing their practice pattern.[21] The 2000 ACOG report on evaluation of cesarean delivery concludes with two major observations:

1. Improved residency or post-residency training in operative (forceps or vacuum-assisted) vaginal delivery is recommended to foster better understanding of the use of these techniques and the normal progression of labor. Surveys show operative vaginal delivery is less than 15 percent among ACOG Fellows and residents in the United States yet safe use of these techniques may help reduce the cesarean delivery rate (see Chapter 14).
2. Certain management practices may affect cesarean delivery rates, so institutions and physicians should consider some changes if their cesarean delivery rates are believed to be too high. The continuous presence of nurses or other trained individuals who provide comfort and support to women in labor may lead to lower rates. In addition, 24-hour dedicated in-house obstetric coverage by hospitals and practice groups may help reduce cesarean delivery rates.

INDICATIONS FOR CESAREAN DELIVERY

Maternal indications for cesarean delivery are relatively few and can be considered as medical or mechanical in nature (Table 19-2). Although somewhat debatable, certain maternal cardiac conditions such as unstable ischemic coronary artery disease and a dilated aortic root

Table 19-2. Indications for Cesarean Delivery

Maternal
- Specific cardiac disease (Marfan's syndrome, unstable coronary artery disease)
- Specific respiratory disease (Guillian-Barré syndrome)
- Conditions associated with increased intracranial pressure
- Mechanical obstruction of the lower uterine segment (tumors, fibroids)
- Mechanical vulvar obstruction (condylomata)

Fetal
- Nonreassuring fetal status
- Breech or transverse lie
- Maternal herpes
- Congenital anomalies

Maternal-fetal
- Cephalopelvic disproportion
- Placental abruption
- Placenta previa
- Elective cesarean delivery

with Marfan's syndrome have been considered indications for cesarean section. These diagnoses may pose a risk for deterioration of maternal condition with the stress of labor. Serious respiratory disease requiring assisted ventilation and conditions resulting in altered mental status might also mandate cesarean delivery. Central nervous system abnormalities in which increased intracranial pressure would be undesirable such as accompanies the second stage of labor have also led some to recommend cesarean section.

Alterations in the capacity of the maternal pelvis can be indications for cesarean delivery. Mechanical vaginal obstruction due to pelvic masses such as lower segment myomata or ovarian neoplasm are examples. Finally, women with massive condylomata may require cesarean section as well.

Elective Cesarean Delivery

Elective cesarean delivery also known as "cesarean section on demand" has emerged as a widely debated topic in obstetrics over the past several years. Feldman and Freiman first proposed elective cesarean delivery in order to prevent fetal morbidity and mortality associated with intrapartum events.[24] In their 1985 publication, the fetal benefits of elective cesarean were weighed against the increased risk of maternal mortality with cesarean section. The increasing safety of cesarean delivery over the next 20 years and emergence of improved data concerning benefits and risks has rekindled interest in this subject. In 2000, Harer[25] endorsed elective cesarean delivery, citing better infant outcomes compared with vaginal birth as well as lower rates of pelvic floor injury. Several years later, ACOG eventually acknowledged that in certain cases, elective cesarean delivery might be performed provided the physician believed that the procedure would promote the overall health and welfare of the woman and her fetus.[26]

Two principal benefits of elective cesarean are a reduction in perinatal mortality and morbidity, as well as a

Table 19-3. Risks and Benefits of Elective Cesarean Delivery

Potential Benefits
- Reduction in perinatal morbidity and mortality
  - Elimination of intrapartum events associated with perinatal asphyxia
  - Reduction in traumatic birth injuries
  - Reduction in stillbirth beyond 30 weeks' gestation
- Possible protective effect against pelvic floor dysfunction

Potential Risks
- Increased short-term morbidity
  - Increased endometritis, transfusion, venous thrombosis rates
  - Increased length of stay and longer recovery time
- Increased long term morbidity
  - Increased risk for placenta accreta, hysterectomy with subsequent cesarean deliveries

protective effect against pelvic floor dysfunction (Table 19-3). Perinatal mortality is several times lower with a planned cesarean delivery compared with labor and vaginal birth.[27] Additionally, hypoxic ischemic encephalopathy of the newborn related to intrapartum events including abruption, cord prolapse, and progressive asphyxia may occur in approximately 1 in 3,000 to 5,000 births.[28] Many of these cases presumably would be prevented by elective cesarean delivery, as would unexplained stillbirths occurring beyond 39 weeks' gestation. Traumatic birth injuries including intracranial hemorrhage, fractures, and brachial plexus injury are reduced with cesarean delivery as well.[29]

Increased maternal risks attributed to vaginal delivery include urinary and fetal incontinence, pelvic prolapse, and sexual dysfunction. The precise contribution of vaginal delivery versus pregnancy and labor to these complications has been difficult to ascertain. In a survey of 2,000 women, Wilson and colleagues reported a prevalence of incontinence of 24.5 percent following vaginal delivery compared with 5.2 percent after cesarean section.[30] In primiparous women, cesarean delivery significantly reduced the risk for incontinence (relative risk [RR] = 0.2) compared with vaginal birth. However, these authors noted that in women with more than three cesarean deliveries, no difference was noted when compared with rates in women delivered vaginally. In a Norwegian study of 15,000 women, Rortveit reported a 10.1 percent rate of incontinence in nulliparous women, 15.9 percent in those having cesarean section, and 21 percent in the vaginal delivery group.[31] These authors concluded that pregnancy itself can cause pelvic floor damage and that cesarean delivery may not be completely protective. MacLennan's survey of 3,000 women also supports an increased risk of prolapse with all methods of delivery. These authors concluded that pregnancy, more than mode of delivery, appeared to contribute to long-term pelvic floor damage.[32] Nonetheless, Minkoff and Chervenak[33] assert that a policy of prophylactic cesarean delivery might reduce the risk of significant urinary incontinence from 10 percent to 5 percent.

The maternal risks of elective cesarean delivery have been considered marginal compared with those of vaginal delivery. Rates of maternal mortality (excluding non-elective cesarean deliveries) are comparable to vaginal delivery. Sachs and colleagues reported a cesarean mortality rate of 22.3/100,000 compared with 10.9/100,000 for vaginal delivery; however, the rates were comparable excluding medical complications.[34] A British survey reported one death in 78,000 cesareans, which was lower than the rate for vaginal births.[35] In contrast, a population based seven year study (1992 to 1998) revealed cesarean section to be associated with a fourfold increased risk of maternal death, when controlling for various pregnancy complications.[36]

Cesarean delivery does increase maternal morbidity.[36] The rate of endometritis (3.0 percent) versus vaginal birth (0.4 percent) is increased, yet one study indicates comparable rates of postpartum hemorrhage, transfusion, and deep venous thrombosis.[37] Other reports confirm increased risks for these morbidities with cesarean section including major complication rates as high as 4.5 percent.[38] Cesarean delivery also presents a risk for future placental abnormalities including placenta previa and placenta accreta. These risks increase with the increasing number of cesarean deliveries performed for each woman and are substantial with more than three operations.[39] Thus, the decision to undergo elective cesarean delivery must include thoughtful consideration of future childbearing plans.

Fetal Indications

Fetal indications are primarily recognized distress with the potential for long-term consequences of metabolic acidosis. Somewhere between 1 and 3 percent of women undergo cesarean section for a nonreassuring FHR pattern. The diagnosis of fetal distress has been cited as the third leading cause for the rise in cesarean birth over the past several decades.[40] It is noteworthy that no apparent reduction in the frequency of cerebral palsy has accompanied this rise and has led to challenge the benefit of continuous electronic fetal monitoring and associated increases in the cesarean delivery rate.[41] Haverkamp and colleagues[42] first noted that cesarean delivery is more often performed for labor abnormalities in women who undergo continuous fetal monitoring compared with controls. This finding is of particular interest considering a more recent randomized trial involving the use of continuous fetal pulse oximetry during labor.[43] Whereas, women monitored with this device demonstrated a 50-percent reduction in the number of cesarean deliveries for nonreassuring fetal status compared with continuous FHR monitoring, the overall cesarean delivery rates between study groups was not different. The women monitored with fetal pulse oximetry had an increased rate of cesarean delivery for dystocia.

Other fetal indications for cesarean delivery include risk of transmission of infection or potential for fetal trauma. Examples of these categories would include active maternal herpes infection and breech delivery in which head entrapment is a possibility. By the mid 1990s, the cesarean delivery rate for breech presentation had reached nearly 85 percent in the United States, and following current recommendations from ACOG, it will likely rise further.[44] Excessive fetal size or suspected macrosomia has been increasingly designated as an indication for cesarean delivery, yet little data exist to support this approach in the nondiabetic woman.[45] Certain birth defects such as hydrocephalus with macrocrania and neural tube defects have traditionally undergone cesarean delivery, yet insufficient data exist to make this an absolute indication. Similarly, little data exist to suggest a benefit for cesarean delivery with fetal abdominal wall defects, such as omphalocele and gastroschisis.[46] Exceptions to this approach might include cases of extraabdominal liver involvement with omphalocele.

Maternal-Fetal Indications

The majority of cesarean deliveries are performed for conditions that might pose a threat to both mother and fetus if vaginal delivery occurred. Placenta previa and placental abruption with the potential for hemorrhage are clear examples. Dystocia presents a risk for both direct fetal and maternal trauma. It may also compromise fetal oxygentation and metabolic status. Cephalopelvic disproportion (CPD) is a diagnosis that is generally made on a relative basis after a trial of sufficient labor often with oxytocin augmentation. The criteria for CPD remains subjective, and at present, norms for progress during labor have been challenged.[47] Although failure to make sufficient progress in the active phase of labor has been attributed to deficiencies in uterine activity, the failure to progress may also be the potential of varying physician approaches to the management of labor itself. The proper length of time for an adequate TOL oxytocin stimulation in protraction disorders is undefined, with most practitioners allowing "a few hours." Because it has been shown that oxytocin has not been employed at all in many cesarean deliveries performed for dystocia, it can be concluded that inadequate trials of oxytocin stimulation may be a significant factor in the performance of some unnecessary cesarean deliveries.[48]

Blumenthal and colleagues[49] found a large difference between the incidence of dystocia in public and private patients, and concluded that the difference probably resulted from differences in criteria used for the two groups. However, they were unable to determine whether the difference resulted from excessive intervention in the private group or from less than optimal intervention in the public groups. Haynes de Regt[50] and colleagues similarly demonstrated an overall cesarean section rate of 17.1 percent in nonprivate versus 21.4 percent in private patients. In this study, private patients giving birth to their first child were significantly more likely than clinic patients to undergo cesarean delivery if dystocia, malpresentation, or fetal distress were diagnosed. Unfortunately, this large retrospective study could not provide detailed information concerning criteria used to diagnose both dystocia and suspected fetal compromise.

Understanding that physician characteristics may affect cesarean delivery rates, Berkowitz and colleagues[51] analyzed 6,327 deliveries performed by 48 different practitioners between 1983 and 1985. Although no significant differences were found according to gender or practice setting of the physicians, older, more experienced physicians performed significantly fewer cesarean sections for dystocia and a higher percentage of forceps deliveries for breech extractions. This finding is of great interest inasmuch as Frigoletto and coworkers[52] noted that between 30 and 40 percent of primary cesarean deliveries at both Brigham and Women's Hospital and Northwestern University are performed during the second stage of labor in contrast to less than 5 percent at the National Maternity Hospital in Dublin. These findings may provide insight into potential strategies to further reduce cesarean deliveries performed for dystocia.

TECHNIQUE OF CESAREAN SECTION

Site Preparation

Preparation of the skin is performed in order to reduce the risk of wound infection by decreasing the amount of skin flora and contaminants at the incision site. Incision site preparation is accomplished in the operating room through application of a surgical scrub, which generally includes an antimicrobial agent. Before applying a scrub solution, hair is removed from the operative site. Removal with a razor may actually increase the risk of infection by breaks in the skin allowing entry of bacteria. For this reason, some advocate clipping of the hair before surgery.[53] In either case, only enough hair should be removed to allow good approximation of skin edges. Cesarean delivery wounds are considered to be clean contaminated. In both this type of wound and clean incisions, the type of surgical scrub or duration has not been associated with any change in the frequency of wound infections.[54] Some surgeons employ a scrub for several minutes, whereas others apply a single swab of bactericidal solution, which takes less than 1 minute. The rate of wound infection following cesarean delivery is approximately 5 percent and is not influenced by preparation technique.[55]

Administration of Prophylactic Antibiotics

Prophylactic antibiotics are of clear benefit in reducing the frequency of postcesarean endomyometritis and wound infection. This is particularly true for cases of prolonged labor and ruptured membranes. The comprehensive Cochrane Review demonstrates a benefit to antibiotic prophylaxis in both elective (non-laboring) and nonelective (laboring) cesarean delivery.[56] The preferred agents for prophylaxis are cefazolin or cefotetan. A randomized trial of 377 women undergoing cesarean delivery revealed no significant difference in outcome between those given cefazolin versus cefotetan.[57] Single-dose therapy given following cord clamping is as effective as multidose therapy.[58,59] There is no apparent advantage to more broad-spectrum antibiotic prophylaxis. Penicillin allergic patients may receive a single dose of 500 mg of metronidazole. For women with clinical chorioamnionitis, treatment with combination antibiotic therapy supplants the need for prophylaxis. This therapy should be instituted promptly (before delivery) and continued until the patient exhibits a clinical response.

Incision Type

The surgeon has a choice of a vertical or transverse skin incision, with the transverse Pfannenstiel being the most common incision type (Fig. 19-2). Factors that influence the type of incision include the urgency of the delivery, prior incision type, and the potential need to explore the upper abdomen for nonobstetric pathology. Although some prefer a vertical incision in emergent situations, a Pfannenstiel actually adds relatively little extra operative time, particularly in a nonobese individual. The skin incision used in the previous procedure is usually repeated in most cesarean deliveries. There is a continued debate as to the surgical merits of a transverse skin incision. Although these incisions are more cosmetic and less painful, it is unclear whether the risk for subsequent herniation and other postoperative complications are influenced by incision type. The author prefers a Pfannenstiel incision in most cases in which a transverse incision is to be made. Occasionally, a transverse incision of the rectus sheath and muscles (Maylard incision) is necessary for proper exposure and room to deliver the fetus. In these cases, only the medial half of the muscle is incised to avoid lacerating the deep epigastric vessels. Complete transection of the rectus muscles is the Cherney incision, which requires identification of the epigastric vessels and ligation bilaterally.

When a transverse skin incision is employed, it is made approximately 3 cm above the symphysis in the midline

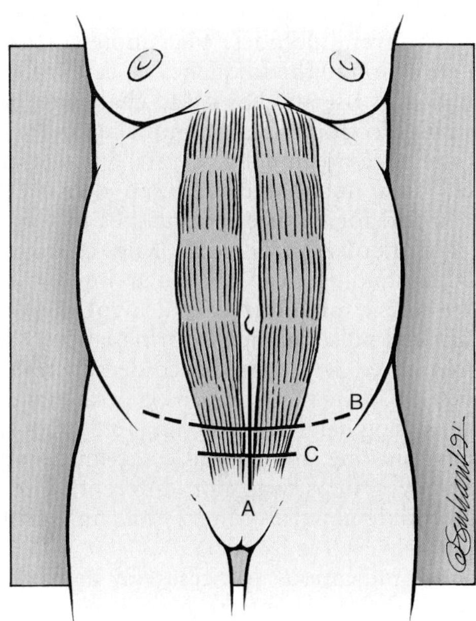

Figure 19-2. The obstetrician most commonly uses one of three abdominal incisions: (*A*) midline, (*B*) Maylard, or (*C*) Pfannenstiel. *Hatched lines* indicate possible extension. (Modified from Baker C, Shingleton HM: Incisions. Clin Obstet Gynecol 31:701, 1988.)

and extended laterally in a slightly curvilinear manner. In obese individuals, the incision preferably should not be made in the underside of the panniculus. The length of the incision should be based on the estimated fetal size and can be enlarged after deeper dissection. The subcutaneous tissue can then be bluntly pushed away to identify the underlying fascia. In repeat operations, sharp dissection of the subcutaneous adipose tissue is generally required. The fascia is incised and dissected in a curvilinear manner bilaterally. It should be tented with the surgeon's forceps to separate it from the underlying muscle and to identify perforating vessels, which require ligation or coagulation. Curvilinear extension is essential because direct transverse extension often leads to inadvertent muscle incisions and bleeding. Once the fascial incision is completed, the fascia is then grasped in the midline bilaterally and is separated from the underlying rectus muscles superiorly and inferiorly by blunt and sharp dissection from the median raphe. The rectus muscles are generally separated in the midline to reveal the posterior rectus sheath and peritoneum, which are incised sharply. The peritoneum is tented and palpated for underlying bowel and then entered with a scalpel or scissors. The point of entry should be as superior as possible to avoid bladder injury, particularly in repeat operations in which the bladder may be adherent superiorly.

Uterine Incision and Development of the Bladder Flap

A low transverse uterine incision is employed in more than 90 percent of cases (Fig. 19-3). It is preferred because it does not compromise the upper uterine segment and it is easier to perform and repair. It is also associated with less blood loss. This incision type provides for the option of subsequent TOL because the rate of subsequent rupture is lower than with incisions incorporating the upper uterine segment.

A vertical uterine incision is either low or classic and should have clear indications. A vertical uterine incision is performed if the lower uterine segment is poorly developed or if the fetus is in a backdown transverse lie. A vertical incision is recommended for a preterm breech delivery as well (Table 19-4). This approach is advised unless the lower segment is extremely well developed. A vertical incision is performed in most cases of a complete anterior placenta previa or if there are leiomyomata obstructing the lower segment. Other indications include certain fetal abnormalities such as massive hydrocephalus or a very large sacrococcygeal teratoma.

The classic uterine incision includes the upper uterine segment. The decision to use this incision depends on the need to extend a vertical cut, as in cases of anterior pla-

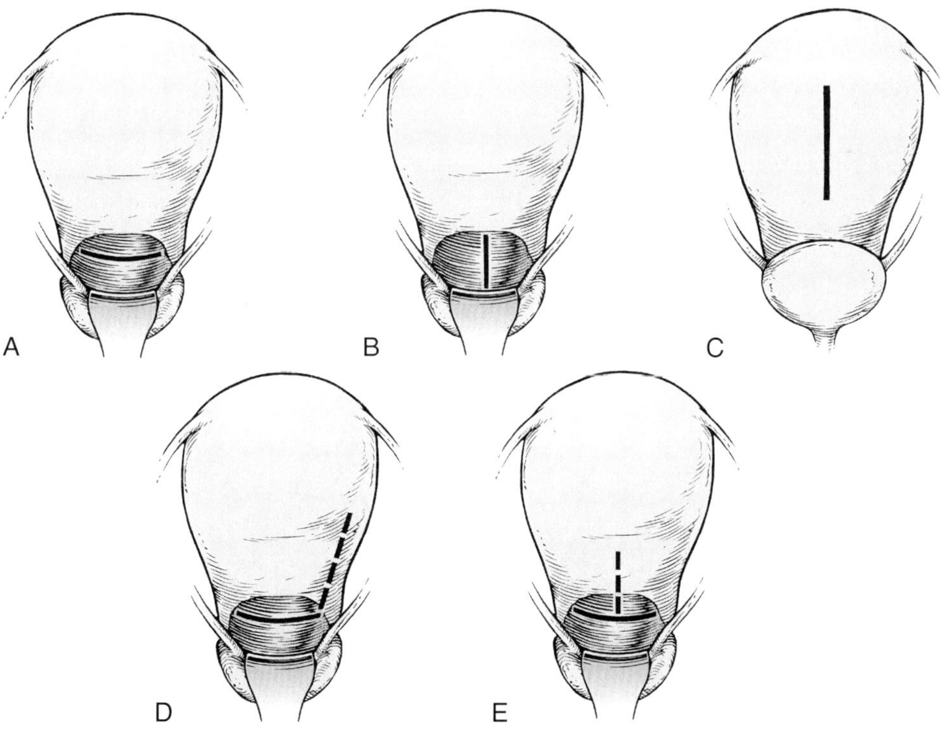

Figure 19-3. Uterine incisions for cesarean delivery. *A,* Low transverse incision. The bladder is retracted downward, and the incision is made in the lower uterine segment, curving gently upward. If the lower segment is poorly developed, the incision can also curve sharply upward at each end to avoid extending into the ascending branches of the uterine arteries. *B,* Low vertical incision. The incision is made vertically in the lower uterine segment after reflecting the bladder, avoiding extension into the bladder below. If more room is needed, the incision can be extended upward into the upper uterine segment. *C,* Classic incision. The incision is entirely within the upper uterine segment and can be at the level shown or in the fundus. *D,* J incision. If more room is needed when an initial transverse incision has been made, either end of the incision can be extended upward into the upper uterine segment and parallel to the ascending branch of the uterine artery. *E,* T incision. More room can be obtained in a transverse incision by an upward midline extension into the upper uterine segment.

centa previa or certain birth defects as described earlier. The disadvantages of a classic incision are its tendency for greater adhesion formation and a greater risk of uterine rupture with subsequent pregnancy.

Following full entry into the peritoneal cavity, the surgeons should palpate the uterus for fetal presentation and alignment, and then place a bladder retractor to expose the lower uterine segment. The uterus is often dextrorotated, and its position must be appreciated to plan the incision site. Creation of a bladder flap versus a direct uterine incision above the bladder fold has been compared in a randomized trial of 102 women. Bladder flap development was associated with a longer incision to delivery interval and total operating time, and a greater fall in maternal hemoglobin.[60] Consideration to not developing a bladder flap may be reasonable, given these findings. When developing the bladder flap, the vesicouterine serosa is picked up with smooth forceps and is incised in the midline with Metzenbaum scissors. The incision is carried out laterally in a curvilinear manner. The vesicouterine fold is then tented with forceps or a pair of hemostats, which allows direct visualization as the bladder flap is bluntly created using the index and middle fingers of the surgeon's hand. Sharp dissection may be necessary, particular in repeat operations. The surgeon then bluntly sweeps out laterally on each side to allow just enough room for insertion of the bladder blade. A Richardson retractor is then inserted laterally, and continuous suction is made available for preparation of the uterine incision.

Table 19-4. Potential Indications for Vertical Uterine Incision

Underdeveloped lower uterine segment
Breech or transverse lie with undeveloped lower uterine segment
Inability to develop bladder flap with repeat cesarean delivery
Lower segment anterior myoma
Anterior placenta previa

In cases of a low transverse incision, the incision is begun at least 2 cm above the bladder margin. Suction is applied. However, tamponade with sponges superiorly and inferiorly is performed if considerable bleeding is encountered. This technique allows better visualization and minimizes the chance of fetal laceration. The incision is extended laterally and superiorly at the angles by either sharp dissection or blunt spreading using the index fingers. The latter method is best suited for well-developed lower segments, although the choice is made by the operator based on experience with the goal being to avoid lateral extension into the uterine vessels and broad ligament. Two randomized trials have compared sharp versus blunt extension of the uterine incision. Sharp extension appears to be associated with increased blood loss and carries with it the potential risk of cutting the umbilical cord or direct fetal injury.[61,62]

The low vertical incision depends on the downward displacement of the bladder in order to confine the incision to the true lower segment (Fig. 19-4). The incision is begun as inferiorly as possible and extended cephalad with the bandage scissors. If the thick myometrium of the upper segment is incised, the incision becomes a classic one, and should be described as such in the dictated operative report.

Extraction of the Fetus

Once an adequate uterine incision has been completed, the fetal head is extracted by elevation and flexion using the operator's hand as a fulcrum. If the head is not easily delivered, the uterine incision may be extended. Adequate exposure by the assistant is critical to prevent lateral extension into the broad ligament. Rarely, a T-

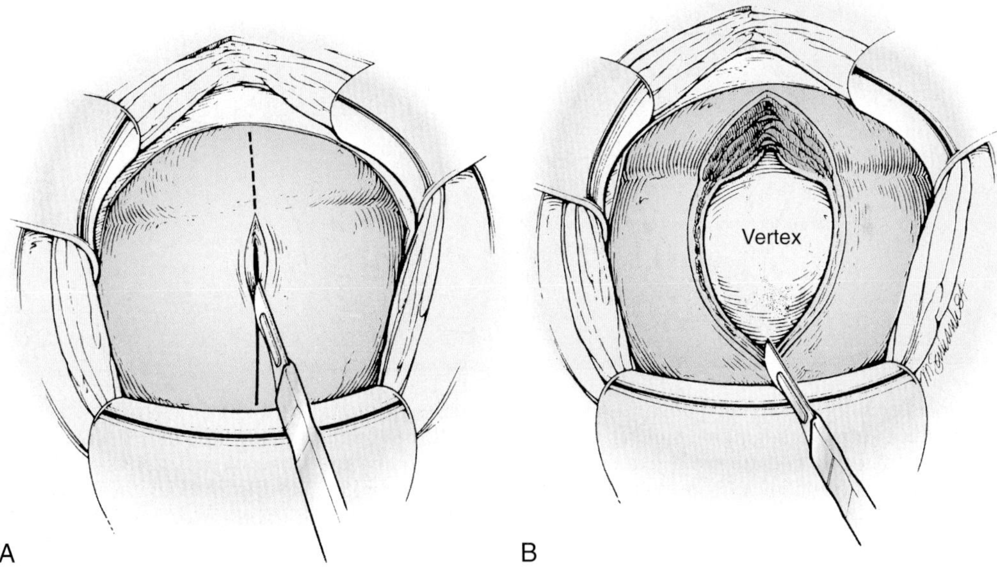

Figure 19-4. Low vertical incision. *A,* Ideally, a vertical incision is contained entirely in the lower uterine segment. *B,* Extension into the upper uterine segment, either inadvertently or by choice, is common.

incision will be made to facilitate delivery. Most such cases involve an attempt at delivery of a preterm malpresentation through a poorly developed lower uterine segment.[63] In cases in which the vertex is wedged in the maternal pelvis, an assistant may need to vaginally displace the presenting part upward. Vacuum extraction or short Simpson forceps may also be applied to the fetal vertex, although this is rarely necessary if the abovementioned steps are taken. Following nasal and oropharynx suction, fundal pressure is applied to extract the fetal body. The cord is clamped and cut, and the infant is passed from the field.

Placental Extraction and Uterine Repair

Following delivery of the infant, prophylactic antibiotics are administered along with intravenous oxytocin as a drip (20 units/L). Removal of the placenta may be accomplished by either manual extraction or spontaneous expulsion with gentle cord traction. Several randomized trials have demonstrated greater blood loss and a higher rate of endometritis with manual extraction method.[64–66]

The uterine repair may be greatly facilitated by lifting the fundus and delivering the uterus through the abdominal incision. This facilitates better visualization of the extent of the incision to be repaired as well as the adnexae. The disadvantage of elevation of the uterus is that it may increase patient discomfort or lead to nausea or vomiting. There is no apparent increased risk for either blood loss or infection with exteriorization of the uterus.[65] Bleeding along the incision line is temporarily controlled by using Ring clamps because they are less traumatic than other instruments. The uterus is then manually curetted with a moistened sponge, and all obvious placental fragments or membranes are teased away from the uterine wall. If the patient has not labored and the cervix is not dilated, the cervix may be opened from above by the surgeon's index finger. This is less traumatic than using an instrument. The surgeon's gloves are then changed prior to uterine closure.

The uterine incision should be well inspected before closure. The lateral aspects of the incision may encroach upon the ascending branch of the uterine artery, making palpation of its pulse a requirement before suturing. Any inferior extensions of the incision should be visualized and repaired separately before closure. The lower uterine incision may be closed as either a single layer of running locking sutures or a second imbricating (non-locking) running layer may be employed as well (Fig. 19-5). There is controversy as to whether an increased risk for subsequent uterine rupture accompanies the single layer closure technique.[67–69] The locking of the primary layer of closure facilitates hemostatsis and may not be necessary if the incision is fairly hemostatic before closure. Number 1 or 0 chromic gut or a synthetic suture of similar gauge is employed. The single layer closure method has gained great popularity in recent years because it significantly decreases operating time with less extra hemostatic suturing required and no difference in the rate of infection.[70]

A vertical uterine incision generally requires a two-layer closure technique. This may be accomplished by first running a locking continuous layer (Fig. 19-6). For cases in which there is wide separation, this author prefers a second interrupted layer in which each side is sutured twice before securing the knot. Myometrium is gathered laterally with this method as the needle is placed parallel to the uterus while incorporating the myometrium. The serosa is not pierced with the needle. The assistant then pinches each segment for the surgeon tying the knot. This technique is somewhat more time consuming than a second continuous layer, however, it is often more hemostatic and leads to better tissue approximation.

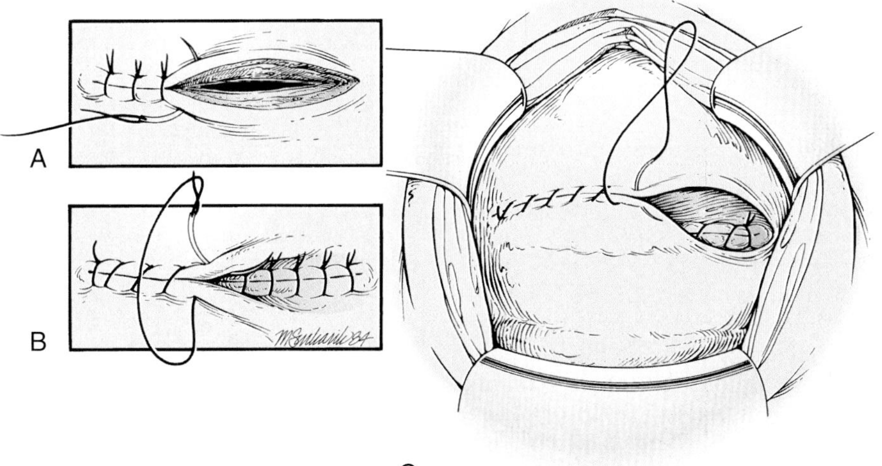

Figure 19-5. Closure of low transverse incision. *A,* The first layer can be either interrupted or continuous. A continuous locking suture is less desirable, despite its reputed hemostatic abilities, because it may interfere with incision vasculature and, hence, with healing and scar formation. *B,* A second inverted layer created by using a continuous Lembert's or Cushing's stitch is customary but is really needed only when apposition is unsatisfactory after application of the first layer. Inclusion of too much tissue produces a bulky mass that may delay involution and interfere with healing. *C,* The bladder peritoneum is reattached to the uterine peritoneum with fine suture.

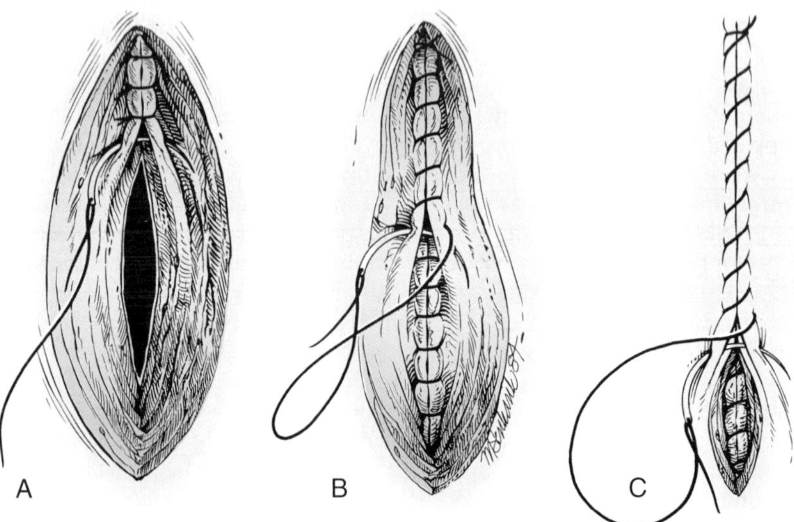

Figure 19-6. Repair of a classic incision. Three-layer closure of a classic incision, including inversion of the serosal layer to discourage adhesion formation. The knot at the superior end of the incision of the second layer can be buried by medial to lateral placement of the suture from within the depth of the incision and subsequent lateral to medial reentry on the opposing side with resultant knot placement within the incision.

The vesicouterine serosa may be approximated with a 2-0 or 3-0 suture. However, most surgeons today omit this step before reperitonealization occurs spontaneously over several days. Additionally, allowing for spontaneous reperitonealization may be associated with less postoperative discomfort and more prompt return of bowel function.[71,72]

The uterine incision is inspected for hemostasis before returning it to the peritoneal cavity. Individual bleeding points are cauterized or ligated with as little suture placement as possible. The adnexae are inspected, and tubal ligation is performed, if so desired. Following return of the uterus, the pelvis may be irrigated with warm saline. Sponge and needle counts are then performed before abdominal closure.

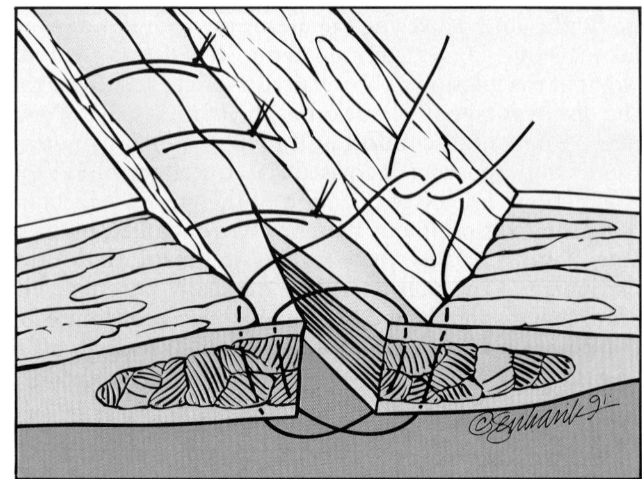

Figure 19-7. Modification of far-near, near-far Smead-Jones suture. Suture passes deeply through lateral side of anterior rectus fascia and adjacent fat, crosses the midline of the incision to pick up the medial edge of the rectus fascia, then catches the near side of the opposite rectus sheath, and, finally, returns to the far margin of the opposite rectus sheath and subcutaneous fat. (Modified from American College of Obstetricians and Gynecologists: Prolog. In Gynecologic Oncology and Surgery. Washington, DC, ACOG, 1991, p 187.)

Abdominal Closure

The parietal peritoneum is not reapproximated because spontaneous closure will occur within days. The rectus fascia is closed with either a continuous nonlocking or interrupted technique. A suture with good tensile strength and relatively delayed absorption is preferred. Synthetic braided or monofilament sutures are best to use. In closing the fascia, placement of sutures should be at a minimum 1.5 cm from the margin of the incision. In most cases of wound disruption, the suture remains intact but has cut through the fascia as a result of placement too close to the cut margin. Patients at risk for wound disruption may benefit from either the Smead Jones technique or interrupted figure-of-eight suturing, both employing delayed absorption suture material such as monofilament polyglycolic acid. Sutures are placed at 1-cm intervals. In most instances, a running continuous monofilament propylene suture will suffice for a transverse incision. The Smead Jones closure technique is preferred for vertical incisions in high-risk cases (Fig. 19-7). A suture with either far-near, near-far placement that passes through the lateral side of the anterior rectus fascia and adjacent subcutaneous adipose tissue and then crosses the midline of the incision to pick up the medial edge of the rectus fascia, then catches the near side of the opposite rectus sheath before returning to the far margin of the opposite rectus sheath and subcutaneous fat accomplishes this technique.

The subcutaneous tissue is closed if it will facilitate skin closure or the fat thickness exceeds 2 cm. It appears that closure of the subcutaneous tissue decreases the risk of wound disruption by 34 percent in women with excessive subcutaneous fat.[73] Subcutaneous drainage through a separate stab site is employed in obese individuals if the incision is not perfectly hemostatic, although its benefit for routine use over subcutaneous closure alone has not been established. The skin is closed with either a staple device or a subcuticular closure for transverse incisions.

Evidence-Based Recommendations for Cesarean Delivery Techniques

The aim of proper technique at cesarean delivery should be to minimize complications and morbidity associated with the procedure. Berghella and colleagues[74] have provided evidence-based guidance for surgical decisions regarding technique employed at cesarean delivery. Based upon their review, the following summarizes evidence-based *good quality recommendations*:

- Prophylactic antibiotic administration for all cesarean deliveries (either ampicillin or first generation cephalosporin for one dose)
- Use of blunt uterine incision expansion
- Spontaneous placental removal
- Nonclosure of both visceral and parietal peritoneum
- Suture closure or drainage of the subcutaneous tissue when the thickness is greater than 2 cm.

COMPLICATIONS OF CESAREAN DELIVERY

Intraoperative Complications

Women undergoing cesarean delivery are at risk for several intraoperative complications including hemorrhage and injury to adjacent organs. Injury to the bowel, bladder, and ureters is uncommon; however, the obstetrician must be familiar with management of these problems. The key element is to recognize and define the extent of these injuries and to promptly institute repair. Consultation with a urologist, general surgeon, or gynecologic oncologist may be necessary depending on the skill level of the obstetrician and the complexity of the injury encountered.

Uterine Lacerations

Lacerations of the uterine incision most commonly involve extension of a low transverse incision following arrest of descent in the second stage or with delivery of a large fetus. Most lacerations are myometrial extensions and can be closed with a running locking suture independently or in conjunction with closure of the primary uterine incision. High lateral extensions may require unilateral ascending uterine artery branch ligation. In cases that extend laterally and inferiorly, care must be taken to avoid ureteral injury. On occasion, if the extension involves bleeding into the broad ligament, opening this space and identifying the ureters before suture placement may be helpful. On rare occasions, retrograde ureteral stent placement may be necessary. Opening the dome of the bladder is the preferred technique for retrograde stent placement.

Bladder Injury

Minor injury to the bladder from vigorous retraction and bruising with resultant hematuria is common. More significant injury such as a bladder dome laceration is infrequent but can occur on entering the peritoneum, particularly with multiple repeat operations. Bladder injury is also encountered with development of the bladder flap in cases in which scarring increases adherence to the lower anterior uterine wall. Sharp dissection is preferred to "take the bladder" down; however, cystotomy may not be avoided in such cases. If the bladder is very adherent and tacked high, it may be advisable to proceed with a vertical uterine incision to avoid bladder disruption.

Bladder dome lacerations are generally repaired with a double-layer closure technique employing 2-0 or 3-0 chromic suture. The mucosa is avoided with closure, although this is not imperative. If there is any question regarding possible trigone or ureteral injury before repair, intravenous indigo carmine is administered, and the ureteral orifices are visualized for dye spillage. Retrograde filling of the bladder with sterile milk may be useful following closure to ensure its integrity. Continuous Foley drainage should be accomplished for several days following repair of a bladder injury.

Ureteral Injury

Ureteral injury has been reported to occur in 1 in 1,000 cesarean deliveries.[75] The frequency of injury increases with cesarean hysterectomy. Most injuries follow attempts to control bleeding from lateral extensions into the broad ligament. As described previously, opening the broad ligament before suture placement may reduce the risk for this complication. If the integrity of the ureter is in doubt, the dome of the bladder may be opened and intravenous indigo carmine administered. The ureteral orifices are visualized for dye spillage, signifying ureteral patency. If ureteral injury is recognized postoperatively, cystoscopy with stent placement or nephrostomy with radiologic imaging may define the extent of injury and help in planning appropriate management.

Gastrointestinal Tract Injury

Bowel injury during cesarean section is rare. Most cases involve incidental enterotomy on entering the abdomen for a repeat laparotomy. Careful incision of the peritoneum with tenting, exposing a clear space, significantly reduces the risk of bowel injury. Defects in the bowel serosa are closed with interrupted suture of fine silk using an atraumatic needle. If the lumen of the small bowel is lacerated, closure is accomplished in two layers. A 3-0 absorbable suture is preferred for mucosa followed by interrupted silk suture for the serosa.

Large defects of the small bowel or colonic injuries generally require consultation with a general surgeon or gynecologic oncologist. Small defects may be closed primarily; however, large defects with fecal contamination may require a temporary colostomy. Broad spectrum antibiotic coverage is recommended for such cases, which must include administration of an aminoglycoside in addition to metronidazole or clindamycin.

Uterine Atony

A more complete review of the management of uterine atony is found in Chapter 18. Uterine atony can be controlled in most cases by a combination of uterine massage and uterotonic agents. Intravenous oxytocin in dosages up to 40 units/L running wide open is attempted initially. If this fails to result in uterine contraction, either methergine, 0.2 mg administered intramuscularly or 0.25 mg of 15-methylprostaglandin F2 α (Hemabate) is administered intramuscularly or directly into the myometrium. Several successive doses of Hemabate every 10 to 15 minutes may be tried (up to 1.0 mg) if necessary. However, most individuals respond to one or two doses so that surgical treatment should be planned accordingly. The initial surgical approach is bilateral ascending uterine artery branch ligation, especially if future fertility is desired. If this fails, hypogastric artery ligation or hysterectomy is generally undertaken (Fig. 19-8). Hypogastric artery ligation is effective in less than 50 percent of cases.[76]

Placenta Accreta

Placenta accreta has increased in frequency with rising cesarean delivery rates, and in some series of cesarean hysterectomy, placenta accreta is the most common indication.[77] The risk for placenta accreta increases with each repeat cesarean delivery and is substantially increased by the presence of placenta previa (see Chapter 18).[78,79]

Focal placenta accreta may be managed by oversewing the implantation site with figure-of-eight absorbable sutures. However, hemostasis must be ensured. If the lower segment continues to bleed, it should be packed tightly to reduce blood loss while proceeding with hysterectomy. In cases of total placenta previa with clinically apparent placenta accreta, it may be advisable to leave the placenta attached while proceeding with hysterectomy. This approach may lower blood loss considerably. Most cases of placenta accreta with previa require complete hysterectomy because of placental attachment to the relatively hypocontractile lower uterine segment.

Maternal Mortality

Maternal morbidity and mortality are increased in cesarean delivery compared with vaginal birth, even when controlling for conditions that might predispose to cesarean section. Given the infrequent nature of maternal death arising from cesarean delivery, it is not

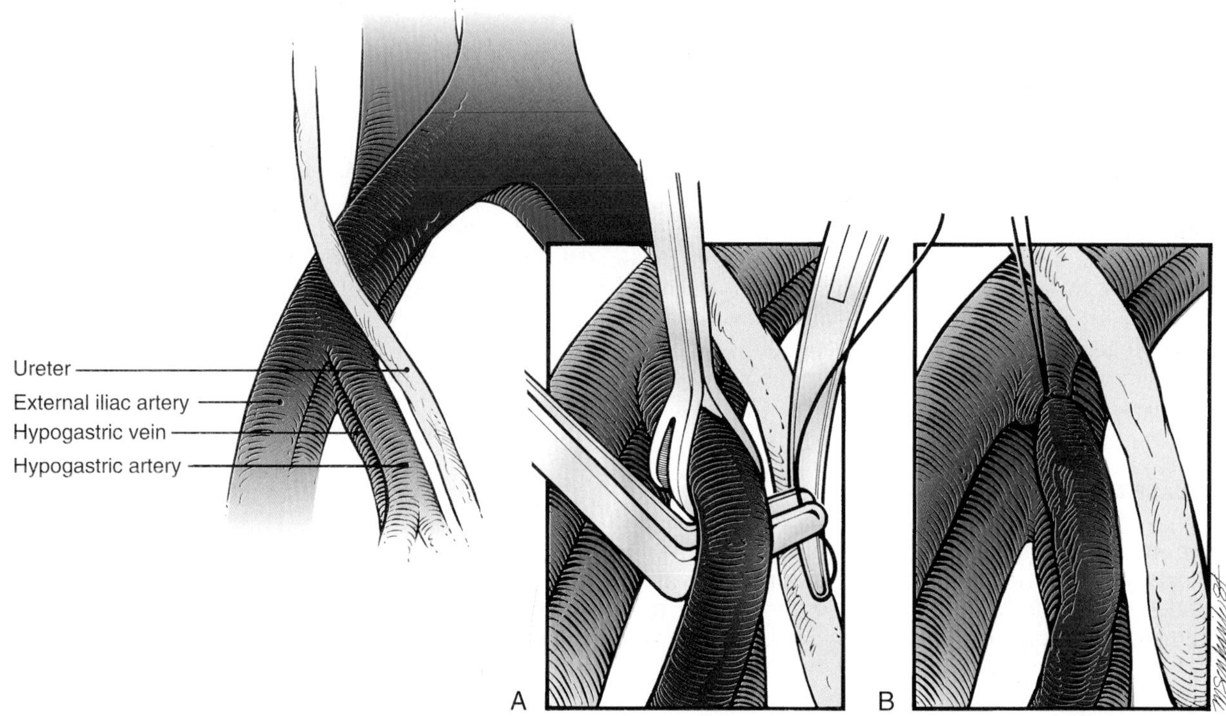

Figure 19-8. Hypogastric artery ligation. Approach to the hypogastric artery through the peritoneum, parallel and just lateral to the ovarian vessels, exposing the interior surface of the posterior layer of the broad ligament. The ureter will be found attached to the medial leaf of the broad ligament. The bifurcation of the common iliac artery into its external and internal (hypogastric) branches is exposed by blunt dissection of the loose overlying areolar tissues. Identification of these structures is essential. *A* and *B,* To avoid traumatizing the underlying hypogastric vein, the hypogastric artery is elevated by means of a Babcock clamp before passing an angled clamp to catch a free tie. (Adapted from Breen J, Cregori CA, Kindierski JA: Hemorrhage in Gynecologic Surgery. Hagerstown, MD, Harper & Row, 1981, p 438.)

surprising that the attributable death rate has ranged from 6/100,000 to 22/100,000. In a study of 250,000 deliveries, Lilford and colleagues[80] reported the RR for maternal death from cesarean delivery compared with vaginal birth to be approximately seven fold more likely when preexisting medical conditions were excluded. In contrast, Lydon-Rochelle noted similar rates of maternal death among women delivered by cesarean section versus vaginal birth when adjusting for maternal age and the presence of severe preeclampsia.[81]

The principle causes of morbidity related to cesarean section are infectious and thromboembolic disease. Anesthesia-related morbidity and mortality has been substantially reduced through the expanded use of regional anesthesia and the employment of awake intubation for patients requiring general anesthesia who may have a difficult airway for standard intubation.

Maternal Postoperative Morbidity

Endomyometritis

Postcesarean endomyometritis remains the most common complication of cesarean delivery despite its reduced frequency as a result of the use of prophylactic antibiotic regimens. In the past, primary cesarean section with labor was associated with an average rate of endometritis of 30 to 40 percent without administration of prophylaxis.[82] Recent data would suggest the risk for this complication is considerably lower. In a prospective observational study of 17,341 women delivered by primary cesarean section, Goepfert and coworkers reported endometritis in 1,496 (8.6 percent) cases.[83] Labor, prolonged rupture of membranes, and lower socioeconomic status appear to be the factors that most influence the rate of this complication.[83] Before the institution of protocols using broad-spectrum antibiotic coverage to cover anaerobic bacteria, severe complications such as a pelvic abscess necessitating hysterectomy or superimposed septic thrombophlebitis although rare, were encountered in a few percent of refractory cases. The general perception is that the frequency of these severe complications has been reduced. In Goepfert's series, pelvic abscess developed in 0.47 percent of cases following the diagnosis of chorioamnionitis compared with only 0.1 percent if fever was not observed during labor.[83]

The majority of cases of endomyometritis arise from ascending infection from cervicovaginal flora. Infections past the deepest part of the uterine incision may extend to the uterine musculature and, if not adequately treated, may produce peritonitis, abscess, and septic phlebitis. The diagnosis of endomyometritis often rests on clinical risk factors in a febrile postoperative patient. The presence of chorioamnionitis, prolonged labor, and ruptured membranes should especially prompt early treatment in suspected cases. The utility of endometrial cultures is limited owing to contamination with vaginal flora and the fact that therapy is rarely guided by these results. Treatment is primarily based on clinical findings including uterine tenderness, leukocytosis, and fever.

Parenteral antibiotics employing a regimen directed against possible anaerobic infection are the preferred therapeutic agents. Clindamycin and an aminoglycoside such as gentamicin is commonly employed or a single agent penicillin based regimen using β-lactamase inhibition to allow for anaerobic coverage.

For women who fail to respond to antibiotic therapy over 2 to 3 days, an alternative source for the fever such as a wound infection, deep abscess, hematoma, or septic pelvic thrombophlebitis should be considered. On occasion, mastitis may produce significant temperature elevations (Figs. 19-9 and 19-10).

Wound Infection

Wound infection complicates approximately 1 to 5 percent of cesarean deliveries.[82] Most cesarean section wounds are considered "clean contaminated" owing to the interface with the lower reproductive tract. Emergent cesarean deliveries or those associated with chorioamnionitis are considered "contaminated" and have higher wound infection rates.

The diagnosis of wound infection is usually straightforward in patients who present with tenderness, erythema, or discharge. Early wound infection (first 2 postoperative days) is often a result of streptococcal infection, whereas later wound infection is generally caused by overgrowth of staphylococcus or a mixed aerobic/anaerobic infection. Extreme wound discoloration or anesthesia of the surrounding tissue should prompt consideration of necrotizing fasciitis, particularly if the patient is very ill with a marked leukocytosis. Necrotizing fasciitis has been

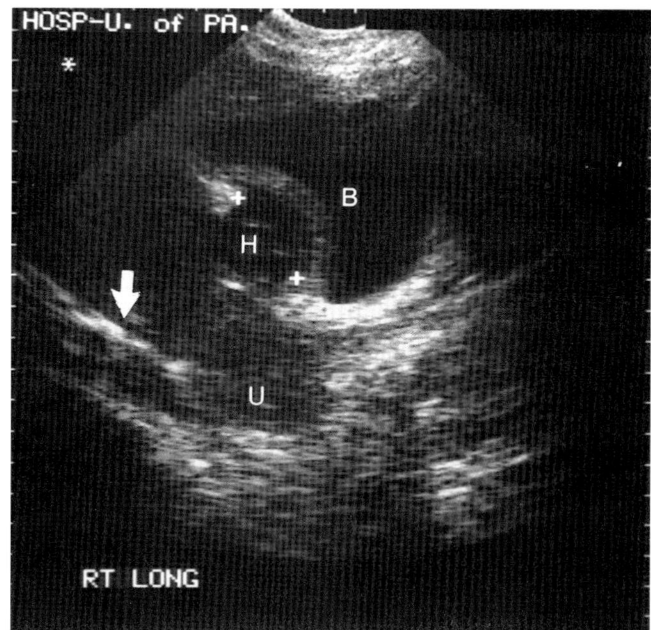

Figure 19-9. Ultrasound of infected bladder flap hematoma marked by cursors (+). The patient presented approximately 1 week after cesarean delivery with fever. She responded to antibiotics. Note that the full bladder (B) enhances visualization of the hematoma (H). The arrow designates the endometrial cavity of the uterus (U).

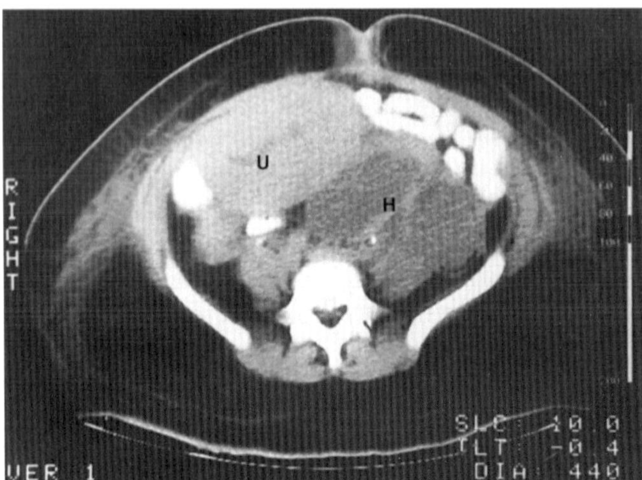

Figure 19-10. Computed tomography scan of pelvis 6 days after a cesarean section showing left-sided broad ligament hematoma (H). The uterus (U) is displaced to the right. The patient responded to antibiotics. (Courtesy of Dr. Michael Blumenfeld, Department of Obstetrics and Gynecology, Ohio State University, Columbus, OH.)

reported to develop in 1 in 2,500 of women undergoing primary cesarean delivery.[83]

Wound discharge should be sent for culture before instituting therapy. The infected portion of the wound should be opened, inspected, irrigated, and debribed as necessary. In most cases, this alone will suffice for therapy, and the wound is left to close by secondary intention. If extensive infection, discoloration, gangrene, or bullae are encountered, the wound should be inspected and debribed under general anesthesia. Examination of histologic specimens may aid in the diagnosis of necrotizing infection. In such cases, all nonviable tissue should be removed, and consultation with an experienced surgeon is recommended. Antibiotic coverage, which is rarely necessary for simple wound infections, should be instituted promptly for advanced serious wound disruptions.

Thromboembolic Disease

Deep venous thrombosis is not uncommonly encountered during pregnancy secondary to higher levels of clotting factors and venous stasis (see Chapter 41). The puerperal period is a risk along with cesarean delivery contributing further to the likelihood of thrombosis. Other risk factors are immobility, obesity, advanced age, and parity. In a 2-year analysis of data from the Maternal-Fetal Medicine Unit (MFMU) Network Cesarean Registry (1999 to 2000), Hauth and colleagues[81] reported deep venous thrombosis occurring in 67 (0.17 percent) of 39,285 women undergoing cesarean birth. Untreated deep venous thrombosis can progress to life-threatening pulmonary embolism in up to 25 percent of cases. Prompt treatment with anticoagulation reduces this risk substantially. In Hauth's report, pulmonary embolism developed in 48 women (0.12 percent).[84]

Deep venous thrombosis (DVT) is suggested by the presence of unilateral leg pain and swelling. A significant difference in the calf or thigh diameter may be present; however, error with this measurement is possible. The presence of Homan's sign (pain with foot dorsiflexion) is often observed if the calf is involved. Many cases of DVT present as pulmonary embolus (PE), particularly in the postoperative patient. Tachypnea, dyspnea, tachycardia, and pleuritic pain are the classic symptoms, with cough and specific pulmonary auscultatory findings less common.

If DVT is suggested, Doppler studies may be useful for proximal disease but are less sensitive for calf thrombosis. Impedance plethysmography is also helpful in detecting proximal disease. However, it is of limited value in the diagnosis of pelvic thrombosis. If DVT is highly suspected and the above studies are inconclusive, a venogram should be obtained. The work-up for suspected PE includes first an arterial blood gas and chest film, followed by ventilation/perfusion study or spiral computerized tomography (CT) study. Oxygen should be administered and heparin begun if a clinical PE appears likely. An indeterminate perfusion scan requires pulmonary angiography to establish or rule out the diagnosis of PE.

Septic Pelvic Thrombophlebitis

It is likely that less than 1 percent of women with endomyometritis will develop septic pelvic thrombophlebitis; however, accurate figures for the frequency of this condition in current practice are lacking. Septic pelvic thrombophlebitis is most often a diagnosis of exclusion established in refractory cases of women being treated for endomyometritis. A pelvic CT scan may aid in the diagnosis, although the sensitivity and specificity of this technique are clearly difficult to establish. In practice, a febrile patient who has undergone cesarean delivery and fails to respond to appropriate broad coverage antibiotic therapy for suspected uterine infection is begun on full-dose heparin therapy, which is continued for several days following a clinical response. Long-term anticoagulation is not prescribed. Patients with septic pelvic phlebitis may present with spiking nocturnal fever and chills. However, these findings may be absent, and a persistent febrile state may be all that is present. In cases in which there is no response to anticoagulation therapy, imaging studies including pelvic CT are indicated to rule out an abscess or hematoma. Refractory cases may require laparotomy and hysterectomy (Fig. 19-11).

VAGINAL BIRTH AFTER CESAREAN DELIVERY

Trends in Vaginal Birth After Cesarean Delivery-Trial of Labor

In 1980, Bottoms and colleagues concluded that primary emphasis should be placed on reducing cesarean section for dystocia and repeat operations because these two indications had increased the rate of cesarean section far beyond any other indications.[85] The modest decline in cesarean delivery observed from 1988 to 1996

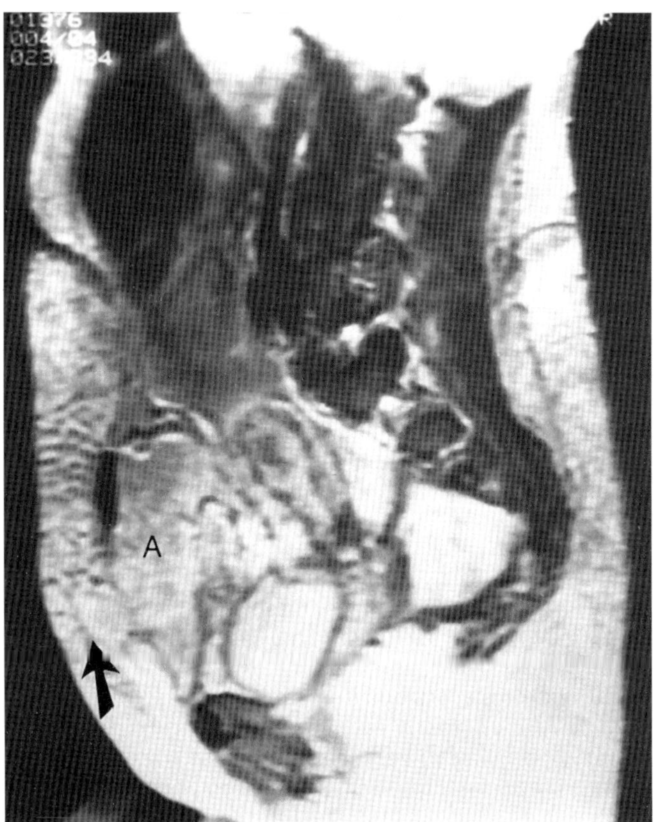

Figure 19-11. Magnetic resonance imaging (MRI) scan of abdominal wall abscess. This patient presented 1 week after a cesarean delivery with fever and an abdominal mass. The differential diagnosis included an intraperitoneal infection with extension or a wound abscess. This MRI shows a wound abscess (A) above fascia that extended to the abdominal wall (*arrow*). The abscess responded to drainage and antibiotics.

was largely due to an increased TOL rate in women with a prior cesarean section. However, at the present time, only 9.2 percent of women with a prior cesarean delivery undergo a TOL in the United States. It has been established that approximately two thirds of women with a prior cesarean delivery are actually candidates for a TOL.[86] Thus, the majority of repeat operations are elective and are often influenced by physician discretion.[87] A comparison of TOL rates between the United States and several European nations reveals significant underutilization of TOL in this country.[88] Given this information and the fact that 8 to 10 percent of the obstetric population has had a previous cesarean delivery, more widespread use of TOL continues to have the potential to decrease the overall cesarean section rate by approximately 5 percent.[89]

The evolution in management of the woman with a prior cesarean delivery can be traced through several ACOG documents and key studies over the past 15 years. In 1988, ACOG published "Guidelines for Vaginal Delivery After a Previous Cesarean Birth," recommending VBAC-TOL as it became clear that this procedure was safe and did not appear to be associated with excess perinatal morbidity compared with elective cesarean delivery.[90] They recommended that each hospital develop its own protocol for the management of VBAC patients and that a women with one prior low transverse cesarean section should be counseled and encouraged to attempt labor in the absence of a contraindication such as a prior classic incision. This recommendation was supported by several large case series attesting to the safety and effectiveness of TOL.[91–95] With this information, VBAC rates reached a peak of 28.3 percent. Some third-party payors and managed care organizations began to mandate a TOL for women with a prior cesarean delivery. Physicians, feeling institutional pressure to lower cesarean section rates, began to offer a TOL liberally and likely included less-than-optimal candidates. With the rise in VBAC experience, a number of reports appeared in the literature suggesting a possible increase in uterine rupture and its maternal and fetal consequences.[96–99] Sachs and colleagues[100] reported a tripling of the incidence of uterine rupture in Massachusetts from 1985 to1995. Further descriptions of uterine rupture with hysterectomy and adverse perinatal outcomes including fetal death and neonatal brain injury set the stage for the precipitous decline in VBAC during the last decade.[101–104]

In 1999, ACOG issued a practice bulletin that acknowledged the apparent statistically small but significant risks of uterine rupture with poor outcomes for both women and their infants. It was also recognized that such adverse events during a TOL may lead to malpractice suits.[105] These developments have led to a more conservative approach to TOL, even by ardent supporters of VBAC, and have illustrated the need to reevaluate VBAC recommendations.[106] Nonetheless, this practice bulletin and its updated 2004 version consistently conclude that most women with one previous cesarean delivery with a low-transverse incision are candidates for VBAC and should be counseled about VBAC and offered a TOL.[106] ACOG has acknowledged that insufficient data existed to provide counseling for patients presenting with a prior low vertical incision, multiple gestation, breech presentation, or an estimated fetal weight greater than 4,000 g.

Candidates for Trial of Labor

Most women who have had a low transverse uterine incision with a prior cesarean delivery and have no contraindications to vaginal birth can be considered candidates for a TOL. The following are selection criteria suggested by ACOG[106] for identifying candidates for VBAC:

- One previous low-transverse cesarean delivery
- Clinically adequate pelvis
- No other uterine scars or previous rupture
- Physicians immediately available throughout active labor capable of monitoring labor and performing an emergency cesarean delivery

Additionally, several retrospective studies indicate that it may be reasonable to offer a TOL to women in other clinical situations. These would include more than one previous cesarean delivery, macrosomia, gestation beyond 40 weeks, previous low-vertical incision, unknown uterine scar type, and twin gestation.[106]

A TOL is contraindicated in women at high risk for uterine rupture. A TOL should not be attempted in the following circumstances:

- Previous classical or T-shaped incision, or extensive transfundal uterine surgery
- Previous uterine rupture
- Medical or obstetric complications that preclude vaginal delivery
- Inability to perform an emergency cesarean delivery because of unavailable surgeon, or anesthesia, insufficient staff or resources at the hospital.

Success Rates for Trial of Labor

The overall success rate for VBAC appears to be in the 70–80 percent range according to published reports.[107–109] At the peak of VBAC experience with high TOL rates, success was observed in only 60 percent of cases.[110] More selective criteria resulting in TOL rates in the 30-percent range have yielded a higher number of vaginal births, 70 to 75 percent.[111,112] Predictors of successful TOL are well described. The prior indication for cesarean delivery clearly impacts the likelihood of successful VBAC. A history of prior vaginal birth or a nonrecurring condition such as a breech or fetal distress is associated with the highest success rates for VBAC[113] (Table 19-5). Although many authors have attempted to predict the success of VBAC based on present and prior labor characteristics, such scoring systems are at best only moderately successful.[114] Understanding that there is no reliable method to predict success of a TOL for an individual woman, a number of factors that have been studied are summarized in the following sections.

In the largest such study of 5,003 women with an overall VBAC success rate of 74 percent, Flamm and Geiger[114] identified five significant variables which were incorporated into a weighted scoring system. These factors included age younger than 40, prior indication, and cervical dilation 4 cm or more at admission. Rates of successful vaginal birth ranged from 49 percent in patients scoring 0 to 2 to 95 percent in patients scoring 8 to 10. However, only 234 (4.7 percent) of women had a score of 0 to 2. Beyond this score, the majority of women had a successful VBAC. The utility of this scoring system is thus limited by the requirement for implementation at the time of admission rather than providing an assessment of the likelihood of success prior to the decision to undergo a TOL.

Table 19-5. Success Rates for Trial of Labor (TOL)

	VBAC SUCCESS (%)
Prior Indication	
CPD/FTP	63.5
NRFWB	72.6
Malpresentation	83.8
Prior Vaginal Delivery	
Yes	86.6
No	60.9
Labor Type	
Induction	67.4
Augmented	73.9
Spontaneous	80.6

CPD, cephalopelvic disproportion; FTP, failure to progress; NRFWB, nonreassuring fetal well-being.

Adapted from Landon MB, Leindecker S, Spong CY, et al: Factors affecting the success of trial of labor following prior cesarean delivery. Am J Obstet Gynecol 193:1016, 2005.

Maternal Demographics

Race, age, body mass index, and insurance status have all been demonstrated to impact the success of TOL.[111] In a multicenter study of 14,529 term pregnancies undergoing TOL, white women had a 78-percent success rate compared with 70 percent in nonwhite women.[111] Obese women are more likely to fail a TOL, as are women older than age 40.[111] Conflicting data exists with regard to payor status.[111,115]

Prior Indication for Cesarean Delivery

Success rates for women whose first cesarean delivery was performed for a nonrecurring indication (breech, nonreassuring fetal well-being) are similar to vaginal delivery rates for nulliparous women.[113] Prior cesarean delivery for a breech presentation is associated with the highest reported success rate of 89 percent.[111,113] In contrast, prior operative delivery for cephalopelvic disproportion/failure to progress is associated with success rates ranging from 50 to 67 percent.[116,117] Whereas Ollendorf and colleagues could not demonstrate a relationship between prior maximal cervical dilation reached and subsequent VBAC success, Hoskins and Gomez reported that if dystocia was diagnosed between 5 and 9 cm in a prior labor, 67 to 73 percent of VBAC attempts are successful compared to only 13 percent if prior cesarean delivery was performed during the second stage of labor.[118]

Prior Vaginal Delivery

Prior vaginal delivery including prior successful VBAC can be considered the greatest predictor for successful TOL.[111] In one series, prior vaginal delivery had an 87-percent success rate compared with a 61-percent success in women without a prior vaginal delivery. Caughey and colleagues reported that for patients with a prior VBAC, the success rate is 93 percent compared with 85 percent in women with a vaginal delivery before their cesarean birth but who had not had a successful VBAC.[119]

Birth Weight

Increased birth weight is associated with a lower likelihood of a successful VBAC.[112] Birth weight greater than 4,000 g in particular is associated with a significantly higher risk of failed VBAC.[112] However, 60 to 70 percent of women who attempt VBAC with a macrosomic fetus are successful.[120]

Table 19-6. Success Rates for Trial of Labor (TOL) with Two Prior Cesarean Deliveries

AUTHOR	N	SUCCESS RATE (%)
Miller[126]	2,936	75.3
Caughey[125]	134	62.0
Macones[128]	1,082	74.6
Landon[127]	876	67.0

Table 19-7. Risk of Uterine Rupture with Trial of Labor (TOL)

PRIOR INCISION TYPE	RUPTURE RATE (%)
Low Transverse	0.5–1.0
Low Vertical	0.8–1.1
Classic or T	4–9

Labor Status and Cervical Examinations

Both labor status and cervical examination upon admission influence the success of a TOL.[121] Flamm and colleagues reported an 86-percent success rate in women presenting with cervical dilation greater than 4 cm.[111] A VBAC success rate of 67 percent has been reported if the cervical examination is less than 4 cm on admission.[114]

Not surprisingly, women who undergo induction of labor are at higher risk for repeat cesarean delivery compared with those who enter spontaneous labor.[111,122] This risk is approximately 1.5 to 2.0 fold higher. In a study of 429 women undergoing induction with a prior cesarean delivery, Grinstead and Grobman[123] reported an overall 78-percent success rate. These authors noted several factors in addition to past obstetric history, including indication for induction and the need for cervical ripening as determinants of VBAC success.[123]

Previous Incision Type

Previous incision type cannot be ascertained in certain patients, which may challenge the obstetrician. It appears that women with an unknown scar have VBAC success rates similar to those of women with documented prior low transverse incisions.[111] Similarly, women with previous low vertical incisions do not appear to have lower VBAC success rates.[124]

Multiple Prior Cesarean Deliveries

Women with more than one prior cesarean delivery have been demonstrated to consistently have a lower likelihood of achieving VBAC[125–127] (Table 19-6). Caughey and colleagues reported a 75-percent success rate for women with one prior cesarean delivery compared with 62 percent in women with two prior operations.[125] In contrast, a larger multicenter study of 13,617 women undergoing a TOL revealed a 75.5-percent success rate for women with two prior cesarean deliveries, which was not statistically different than the 75-percent success rate in women with one prior operation.[128]

RISKS OF VAGINAL BIRTH AFTER CESAREAN-TRIAL OF LABOR

Uterine Rupture

The principal risk of VBAC-TOL is uterine rupture. This complication is directly attributable to attempted VBAC, because symptomatic rupture is rarely observed in elective repeat operations.[129,130] It is important to differentiate between uterine rupture and uterine scar dehiscence. This distinction is clinically relevant because dehiscence most often represents an occult scar separation observed at laparotomy in women with a prior cesarean section. The serosa of the uterus is intact, and hemorrhage with its potential for fetal and maternal sequelae are absent. In contrast, uterine rupture is a through-and-through disruption of all uterine layers, with consequences of hemorrhage, fetal distress, stillbirth and significant maternal morbidity, and the potential for mortality. Terminology, definitions, and ascertainment for uterine rupture vary significantly in the existing VBAC literature.[131] A review of 10 observational studies providing the best evidence on the occurrence of symptomatic rupture with TOL revealed rupture rates ranging form 0/1,000 in a small study to 7.8/1,000 in the largest study, with a pooled rate of 3.8 percent per 1,000 trials of labor.[131,132] The recent large multicenter prospective observational MFMU Network Study reported a 0.69 percent incidence with 124 symptomatic ruptures occurring in 17,898 women undergoing a TOL.[133]

The rate of uterine rupture depends on both the type and location of the previous uterine incision (Table 19-7). Uterine rupture rates are highest with a previous classical or T-shaped incision with a range reported between 4 and 9 percent.[134] The risk for rupture with a previous low vertical incision has been difficult to estimate owing to imprecision with the diagnosis and the uncommon utilization of this incision type. Naif and colleagues reported a 1.1-percent risk for rupture in174 women with a prior low vertical scar undergoing TOL, whereas Shipp reported a 0.8-percent (3/377) risk of rupture with a prior low vertical incision.[134,135] On the basis of these two studies, the authors concluded that women with a prior low vertical uterine incision are not at increased risk for rupture compared with women with prior low transverse incisions.

Women with an unknown type of scar do not appear to be at increased risk for uterine rupture. Among 3,206 women with an unknown scar in the MFMU Network report, uterine rupture occurred in 0.5 percent of the trials of labor.[133]

The most serious sequelas of uterine rupture include perinatal death, hypoxic-ischemic encephalopathy, and hysterectomy. It is unclear from published studies how often uterine rupture results in perinatal death.[130] Citing six deaths in 74 uterine ruptures among 11 studies, Guise and colleagues[132] calculated 0.14 additional perinatal deaths per 1000 trials of labor. This figure is remark-

Table 19-8. Risk of Perinatal Death Related to Uterine Rupture

AUTHOR	NO. RUPTURES	PERINATAL DEATHS/ TRIALS OF LABOR
Guise (pooled data)[132]	74	0.14/1,000
Landon[133]	123	0.11/1,000
Chauhaun (pooled date)[136]	880	0.4/1,000

Table 19-9. Perinatal Outcomes after Uterine Rupture in Term Pregnancies

OUTCOME	TERM PREGNANCIES WITH UTERINE RUPTURE (N = 114)
Intrapartum stillbirth	0
Hypoxic-ischemic encephalopathy	7 (6.2)
Neonatal death	2 (1.8)
Admission to the neonatal intensive care unit	46 (40.4)
5-Minute Apgar score ≤5	16 (14.0)
Umbilical artery blood pH ≤7.0	23 (33.3)

Adapted from Landon MB, Hauth JC, Leveno KJ, et al for the National Institute of Child Health and Human Development Maternal-Fetal Medicine Units Network: Maternal and perinatal outcomes associated with a trial of labor after prior cesarean section. N Engl J Med 351:2581, 2004.

ably similar to the National Institute of Child Health and Human Development (NICHD) MFMU Network study, in which there were two neonatal deaths among 124 ruptures, for an overall rate of rupture related perinatal death of 0.11 per 1,000 TOLs.[133] An all-inclusive review of 880 maternal uterine ruptures in studies of varying quality during a 20-year period showed 40 perinatal deaths in 91,039 trials of labor, for a rate of 0.4 per 1,000[136] (Table 19-8).

Perinatal hypoxic brain injury is recognized as an underreported adverse outcome related to uterine rupture. Perinatal asphyxia has been poorly defined in VBAC studies, and variables such as cord blood gas levels and Apgar scores are reported in only a fraction of cases.[136] Landon and colleagues[131] found a significant increase in the rate of hypoxic-ischemic encephalopathy (HIE) related to uterine rupture among the offspring of women who underwent a TOL at term, as compared with the children of women who underwent an elective repeat cesarean delivery (0.46 per 1,000 trials of labor versus no cases, respectively). In 114 cases of uterine rupture at term, seven (6.2 percent) infants sustained HIE, and two of these infants died in the neonatal period (Table 19-9).

Maternal hysterectomy may be a complication of uterine rupture, if the defect cannot be repaired or is associated with uncontrollable hemorrhage. In five studies reporting on hysterectomies related to rupture, seven cases occurred in 60 symptomatic ruptures (13 percent; range 4 to 27 percent), indicating that 3.4 per 10,000 women electing a TOL sustain a rupture that necessitates hysterectomy.[131] The NICHD MFMU Network study included 5/124 (4 percent) cases requiring hysterectomy in which the uterus could not be repaired following rupture.[133]

Risk Factors for Uterine Rupture

Rates of uterine rupture vary significantly depending on a variety of associated risk factors. In addition to the type of uterine scar, characteristics of the obstetric history including number of prior cesarean deliveries, prior vaginal delivery, interdelivery interval, and uterine closure technique have been reported to affect the risk of uterine rupture. Similarly, factors related to labor management, including induction and the use of oxytocin augmentation, have been studied.

Number of Prior Cesarean Deliveries

In a large single center study of more than 1,000 women with multiple prior cesarean deliveries undergoing a TOL, Miller and colleagues[126] reported uterine rupture in 1.7 percent of women with two or more previous cesarean deliveries compared with a frequency of 0.6 percent in those with one prior operation (odds ratio 3.06; 95 percent confidence interval 1.95 to 4.79). Interestingly, the risk for uterine rupture was not increased further for women with three prior cesarean deliveries. Caughey and colleagues[125] conducted a smaller study of 134 women with two prior cesarean deliveries and controlled for labor characteristics as well as obstetric history. These authors reported a rate of uterine rupture of 3.7 percent among these 134 women compared to 0.8 percent in the 3,757 women with one previous scar (odds ratio 4.5, 95-percent confidence interval 1.18 to 11.5). The risk was 4.8 times greater for these women after multivariate analysis. This information led to the ACOG recommendation that a TOL for women with two prior cesarean deliveries be limited to those with a history of a prior vaginal delivery.[106] Recently, Macones and colleagues[128] reported a rate of uterine rupture of 20/1082 (1.8 percent) in women with two prior cesarean deliveries compared with 113/12,535 (0.9 percent) in women with one prior operation (adjusted odds ratio 2.3, 95 percent confidence interval 1.37 to 3.85).[128] In contrast, Landon's analysis from the MFMU Network Cesarean Registry found no significant difference in rupture rates in women with one prior cesarean; 115/16,916 (0.7 percent) versus multiple prior cesareans; 9/975 (0.9 percent).[127] It thus appears that if multiple prior cesarean section is associated with an increased risk for uterine rupture, the magnitude of any additional risk is fairly small (Table 19-10).

Prior Vaginal Delivery

Prior vaginal delivery appears to be protective against uterine rupture following TOL. In a study of 3,783 women undergoing a TOL, Zelop and colleagues[137] noted the rate of uterine rupture among women with a prior vaginal birth was 0.2 percent (2/1021) compared with 1.1 percent (30/2,762) among women with no prior vaginal

Table 19-10. Risk of Uterine Rupture Following Multiple Prior Cesarean Deliveries

		RUPTURE RATE		
AUTHOR	N	SINGLE PRIOR	MULTIPLE PRIOR	RR (CI)
Miller[126]	3,728	0.6%	1.7%	3.1 (1.9–4.8)
Caughey[125]	134	0.8%	3.7%	4.5 (1.2–11.5)
Macones[128]	1,082	0.9%	1.8%	2.3 (1.4–3.9)
Landon[127]	975	0.7%	0.9%	1.4 (0.7–2.7)

CI, confidence interval; N, number of women with multiple prior cesarean sections attempting vaginal birth after cesarean; RR, relative risk.

deliveries. After controlling for demographic differences and labor characteristics, women having one or more vaginal deliveries had a rate of uterine rupture that was one fifth that of women without prior vaginal birth (odds ratio [OR] 0.2, 95 percent confidence interval 0.04 to 0.8). A similar protective effect of prior vaginal birth has been reported in two large multicenter studies.[127,138] There is currently no information as to whether a history of successful VBAC is also protective against uterine rupture.

Uterine Closure Technique

Over the past 15 years, the single-layer closure technique has gained popularity because it has appeared to be associated with shorter operating time and comparable short-term complications compared with the traditional two-layer technique. A retrospective review of 292 women undergoing a TOL found similar rates of scar separation and uterine rupture for women with one- and two-layer closures.[67] In a randomized trial, Chapman and colleagues[68] compared the incidence of uterine rupture in 145 women who received either one- or two-layer closure at their primary cesarean delivery. Following TOL, no cases of uterine rupture were found in either group; however, the study is underpowered to detect a potential difference. A large observational cohort study identified an approximate four fold increased rate of rupture following single closure technique when compared to previous double layer closure.[69] This study included detailed review of operative reports in which the rate of rupture was 15/489 (3.1 percent) with single-layer closure versus 8/1,491 (0.5 percent) with a previous double-layer closure.

Interpregnancy Interval

Three studies have addressed whether a short interpregnancy interval may be associated with an increased risk for uterine rupture with a TOL.[139–141] Shipp and colleagues reported an incidence of rupture of 2.3 percent (7/311) in women with an interdelivery interval less than 18 months compared with 1.1 percent (22/2,098) with a longer interdelivery interval.[139] After controlling for demographic characteristics and oxytocin use, women with a shorter interpregnancy interval were 3 times more likely to experience uterine rupture. In a study of 1,185 women undergoing a TOL, Huang and colleagues[140] found no increased risk for uterine rupture with an interdelivery interval of less than 18 months. Using a multivariate approach, Bujold et al.[141] have reported an interdelivery interval of less than 24 months to be associated with an almost threefold increased risk for uterine rupture. In this study, the rate of rupture was 2.8 percent in women with a short interval versus 0.9 percent in women with greater than 2 years since the prior cesarean birth.

Table 19-11. Risk of Uterine Rupture Following Labor Induction

AUTHOR	LYDON-ROCHELLE[142]	LANDON[133]
All inductions	24/2,326 (1.0)	48/4,708 (1.0)
Spontaneous	56/10,789 (0.5)	24/6,685 (0.4)
Prostaglandins	9/366 (2.5)	0/227 (0.0)
Prostaglandin + Oxytocin	—	13/926 (1.4)

Induction of Labor

Induction of labor may be associated with an increased risk of uterine rupture.[133,138,142] In a population-based retrospective cohort analysis, Lydon-Rochelle and colleagues[142] reported a rate of uterine rupture of 24/2,326 (1.0 percent) for women undergoing induction compared with 56/10,789 (0.5 percent) in women with the spontaneous onset of labor. In the prospective MFMU Network cohort analysis, Landon and coworkers noted the risk for uterine rupture to be nearly threefold elevated (OR 2.86, 95-percent CI, 1.75 to 4.67) with induction 48/4,708 (1.0 percent) versus spontaneous labor 24/6,685 (0.4 percent).[133] In controlling for various potential confounders, Zelop and colleagues[137] compared the risk of uterine rupture in women undergoing labor induction with oxytocin versus spontaneous labor. Induction of labor with oxytocin was found to be associated with a 4.6-fold increased risk of uterine rupture (rupture rate of 2.0 percent versus 0.7 percent). Despite these analyses, it remains unclear whether induction causes uterine rupture or whether an associated risk factor is present (Table 19-11). There is also conflicting data concerning whether various induction methods increase the risk for uterine rupture.[143] Lydon-Rochelle's[142] study suggested an increased risk for uterine rupture with the use of prostaglandins for labor induction. Uterine rupture was noted in 15/1,960 (0.8 percent) of women induced without prostaglandins compared with 9/366 (2.5 percent) for those induced with prostaglandin. Unfortunately, these authors could not determine which specific prostaglandin agent was used.

Neither Landon nor Macones confirmed the findings of Lydon-Rochelle of an increased risk of rupture associated with the use of prostaglandin agents alone for induction.[133,138] Macones did report an increased risk for rupture in women undergoing induction only if they received both prostaglandins *and* oxytocin.[138] The methodology in this study did allow the authors to distinguish between induction methods. This was also not possible in Lydon-Rochelle's report, which relied on procedure codes for the use of prostaglandins that did not exclude the concomitant use of oxytocin. Interestingly, in the MFMU Network Study, there were no cases of uterine rupture when prostaglandin alone was used for induction, including 52 cases in which misoprostol was used.[133] The safety of this medication, which is popular for cervical ripening and labor induction (see Chapter 13), has been challenged for women attempting VBAC. Plaut[144] reported a uterine rupture rate of 5.6 percent (5/89) in women receiving misoprostol for labor induction. However, as in other series, it is unclear whether these women received oxytocin as well. The timing (delay) of uterine rupture in relation to misoprostol administration also calls into question cause and effect. Following several case reports of uterine rupture with misoprostol use, Wing and colleagues[145] conducted a randomized trial of intravaginal misoprostol versus oxytocin in women attempting VBAC. Seventeen women received misoprostol and 21 oxytocin. The study was stopped prematurely because two emergency cesarean deliveries were performed with uterine disruption in patients receiving misoprostol. Despite several studies that have not demonstrated an increased risk for uterine rupture with prostaglandins and the lack of studies or meta-analyses of sufficient size to detect a statistically increased risk for rupture with misoprostol, ACOG has issued a Committee Opinion discouraging the use of prostaglandins for cervical ripening or induction in women attempting VBAC-TOL.[146]

Labor Augmentation

Excessive use of oxytocin may be associated with uterine rupture, and careful labor augmentation should be practiced in women attempting TOL. A meta-analysis concluded that oxytocin use does not appear to influence the risk of a dehiscence or uterine rupture.[93] In a case-control study, Leung and colleagues[103] reported an OR of 2.7 for uterine rupture in women receiving oxytocin augmentation. Dysfunctional labor including arrest disorders actually increased the risk sevenfold and, thus, may be the primary factor responsible for rupture. In contrast to Leung's data, Zelop[137] found that labor augmentation with oxytocin did not significantly increase the risk for rupture. In another study, the rate of uterine rupture with oxytocin augmentation was 52/6,009 (0.9 percent) compared with 24/6,685 (0.4 percent) without oxytocin use.[133] In summary, oxytocin use may marginally increase the risk for uterine rupture in women undergoing a TOL. Therefore, judicious use of labor stimulation should be employed in these patients.

Other Risks Associated with Vaginal Birth After Cesarean-Trial of Labor

In the absence of randomized controlled trials, there are limited data to inform women and health care providers about adverse outcomes associated with a TOL. Meta-analysis of these data have been criticized owing to lack of comparability between women undergoing a TOL and those having an elective repeat cesarean delivery.[130]

It has generally been accepted that vaginal delivery is associated with lower morbidity and mortality rates than is cesarean delivery. In contrast to Mozurkevich's meta-analysis of 15 studies, Landon and colleagues found an increased risk for both postpartum endometritis and the need for blood transfusion in women undergoing a TOL compared with elective repeat cesarean delivery without labor[130,133] (Table 19-12). However, the exclusion of women who presented in early labor who subsequently underwent repeat operation may have lowered the risk of complications in the elective repeat cesarean group. Nonetheless, most of the excess adverse events accompanying a TOL are attributable to the failure group who require a repeat cesarean operation[133,147] (Table 19-13).

An increased risk for maternal mortality accompanying all cases of cesarean delivery has been extrapolated to women undergoing an elective repeat operation versus a planned TOL, although the data to support this suggestion are limited. The infrequency of maternal death, confounding variables such as maternal disease, and the classification of an elective or nonelective procedure, complicate comparisons of mortality. Maternal death attributable to uterine rupture is exceedingly rare.[101] The MFMU Cesarean Registry study found that maternal deaths were not significantly more common with elective

Table 19-12. Comparison of Maternal Complications in a Trial of Labor (TOL) versus Elective Repeat Cesarean Delivery

COMPLICATION	TRIAL OF LABOR (N = 17,898)	ELECTIVE REPEAT CESAREAN DELIVERY (N = 15,801)	ODDS RATIO (98% CI)
Uterine rupture	124 (0.7)	0	—
Hysterectomy	41 (0.2)	47 (0.3)	0.77 (0.51–1.17)
Thromboembolic disease	7 (0.04)	10 (0.1)	0.62 (0.24–1.62)
Transfusion	304 (1.7)	158 (1.0)	1.71 (1.41–2.08)
Endometritis	517 (2.9)	285 (1.8)	1.62 (1.40–1.87)
Maternal death	3 (0.02)	7 (0.04)	0.38 (1.10–1.46)
One or more of the above	978 (5.5)	563 (3.6)	1.56 (1.41–1.74)

Adapted from Landon MB, Hauth JC, Leveno KJ, et al for the National Institute of Child Health and Human Development Maternal-Fetal Medicine Units Network: Maternal and perinatal outcomes associated with a trial of labor after prior cesarean section. N Engl J Med 351:2581, 2004.

Table 19-13. Maternal Complications According to the Outcome of a Trial of Labor (TOL)

COMPLICATION	FAILED VAGINAL DELIVERY (N = 4,759)	SUCCESSFUL VAGINAL DELIVERY (N = 13,139)	ODDS RATIO (95% CI)	P VALUE
Uterine rupture	110 (2.3)	14 (0.1)	22.18 (12.70–38.72)	<0.001
Uterine dehiscence	100 (2.1)	19 (0.1)	14.82 (9.06–24.23)	<0.001
Hysterectomy	22 (0.5)	19 (0.1)	3.21 (1.73–5.93)	<0.001
Thromboembolic disease*	4 (0.1)	3 (0.02)	3.69 (0.83–16.51)	0.09
Transfusion	152 (3.2)	152 (1.2)	2.82 (2.25–3.54)	<0.001
Endometritis	365 (7.7)	152 (1.2)	7.10 (5.86–8.60)	<0.001
Maternal death	2 (0.04)	1 (0.01)	5.52 (0.50–60.92)	0.17
Other maternal adverse events†	63 (1.3)	1 (0.01)	176.24 (24.44–1,271.05)	<0.001
One or more of the above	669 (14.1)	309 (2.4)	6.81 (5.93–7.83)	<0.001

CI, confidence interval.

*Thromboembolic disease includes deep venous thrombosis or pulmonary embolism.

†Other adverse events include broad ligament hematoma, cystotomy, bowel injury, and ureteral injury.

Adapted from Landon MB, Hauth JC, Leveno KJ, et al for the National Institute of Child Health and Human Development Maternal-Fetal Medicine Units Network: Maternal and perinatal outcomes associated with a trial of labor after prior cesarean section. N Engl J Med 351:2581, 2004.

repeat cesarean delivery. However, the study was not powered to detect a difference between this group and women attempting VBAC.[133]

Management of Vaginal Birth After Cesarean-Trial of Labor

Because uterine rupture may be a catastrophic event, ACOG recommends that VBAC should only be attempted in institutions equipped to respond to emergencies, with physicians immediately available to provide emergency care.[98] Thus, both in house obstetric and obstetric anesthesia coverage are necessary to comply with this recommendation.

The management of labor in women undergoing a TOL is primarily based upon opinion. Women attempting VBAC should be encouraged to contact their health care provider promptly when labor or ruptured membranes occurs. Continuous electronic fetal monitoring is prudent, although the need for intrauterine pressure catheter monitoring is controversial. Studies that have examined FHR patterns before uterine rupture consistently report that nonreassuring signs, particularly significant variable decelerations or bradycardia, are the most common finding accompanying uterine rupture.[148,149] Leung analyzed FHR and contraction patterns in association with 78 cases of uterine rupture.[103] Prolonged decelerations (FHR less than 90 bpm exceeding 1 minute without return to baseline) occurred in 55 of 78 cases (71 percent) of uterine rupture. Prolonged deceleration was also noted in 36/36 (100 percent) of cases in which the fetus was extruded from the uterus.

Despite the presence of adequate personnel to conduct an emergency cesarean delivery, prompt intervention does not always prevent fetal neurologic injury or death.[132,150] It appears that a nonreassuring FHR pattern occurring before uterine rupture identified cases in which the amount of time necessary to deliver an intact fetus is limited (Fig. 19-12). In Leung's study, significant neonatal morbidity occurred when 18 minutes or longer elapsed between the onset of FHR deceleration and delivery.[103] In cases in which prolonged deceleration was preceded by severe variable or late decelerations, fetal injury was noted as early as 10 minutes from the onset of a prolonged deceleration. In contrast to Leung's findings, Bujold and Gauthier[151] reported that less than 18 minutes elapsed between prolonged decelerations and delivery in two of three neonates diagnosed with HIE in 23 cases of uterine rupture.

TOL is not a contraindication to the use of epidural analgesia and does not appear to affect success rates.[111] Epidural analgesia also does not mask the signs and symptoms of uterine rupture. The role of oxytocin augmentation in uterine rupture has been discussed previously. Most studies, again, do not support a marked increased risk for associated uterine rupture.[152] In a case-control study, Goetzl and colleagues[152] reported no association between uterine rupture and oxytocin-dosing intervals, total dose used, and the mean duration of oxytocin administration.

The conduct of vaginal delivery itself is not altered by a history of prior cesarean birth. Most individuals do not routinely explore the uterus in order to detect asymptomatic scar dehiscences because these generally heal well. However, excessive vaginal bleeding or maternal hypotension should be promptly evaluated including assessment for possible uterine rupture. Of 124 cases of uterine rupture accompanying 17,898 trials of labor, 14 (11 percent) were identified following vaginal delivery.[133]

Counseling for Vaginal Birth After Cesarean-Trial of Labor

A pregnant women with a previous cesarean delivery is at risk for both maternal and perinatal complications whether undergoing TOL or choosing an elective repeat

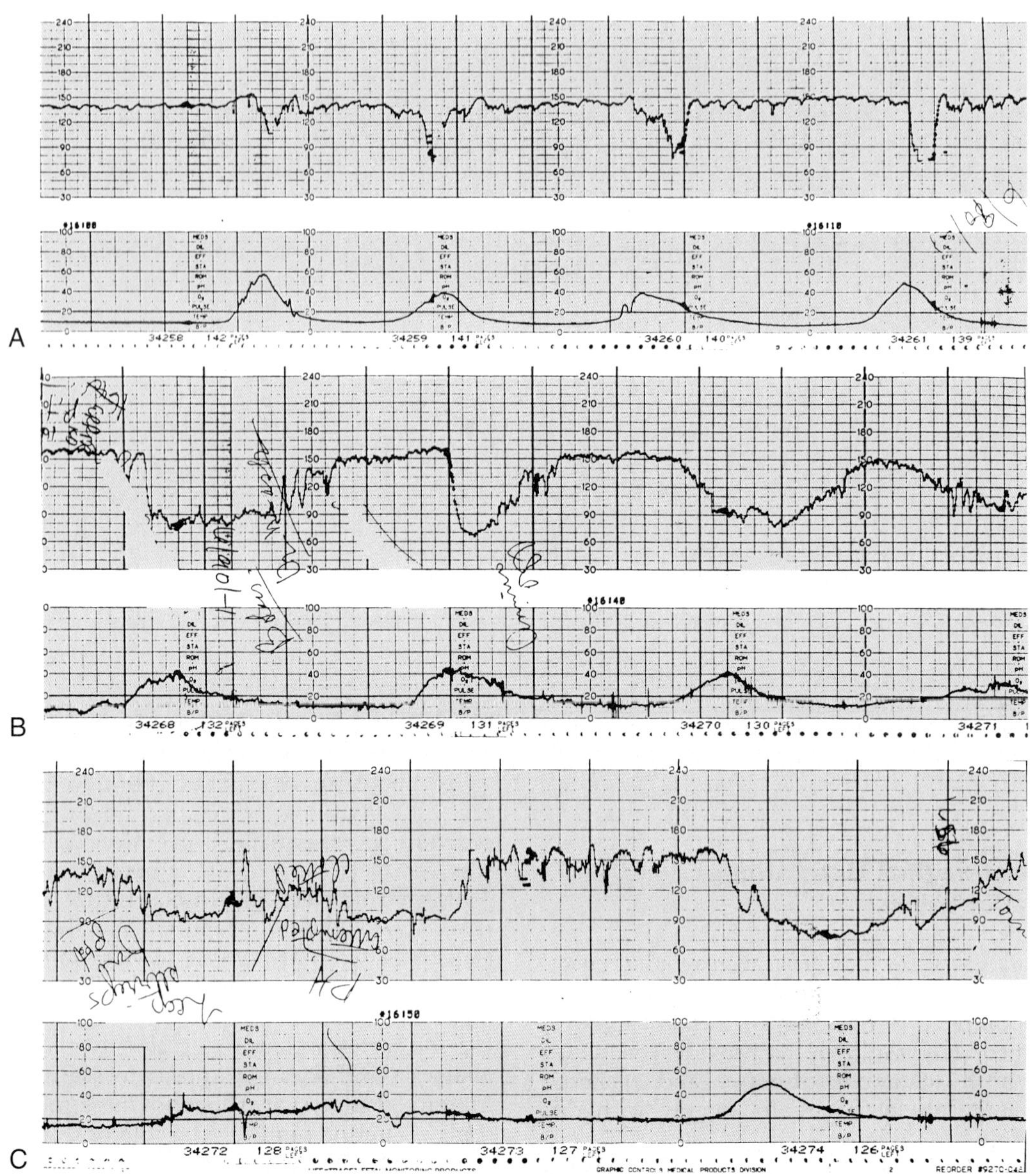

Figure 19-12. *A*, The patient is a 37-year-old gravida 7 para 3 Ab3 woman at 41 weeks' gestation who presented for induction of labor. She had had two prior vaginal deliveries but her last baby was born at 33 weeks by low transverse cesarean section for nonimmune hydrops caused by a cardiac malformation. The patient's induction was begun with prostaglandin gel. Her cervix changed from fingertip dilated, 50-percent effaced, to 1-cm dilated, 70-percent effaced with a cephalic presentation at –2 station. Oxytocin was then begun at 1 milliunit/min. The patient progressed well, and epidural anesthesia was administered at 4 to 5 cm dilation, 90 percent effaced, and 0 station. The patient was at 6 cm dilation with a tracing demonstrating normal heart rate variability and variable decelerations. *B*, 30 minutes after the above tracing was recorded, the fetal heart rate pattern changed to severe variable decelerations. *C*, The tracing then demonstrated prolonged decelerations at 90 bpm. The patient was taken to the operating room for an emergency cesarean delivery. Uterine rupture had occurred along the site of the previous uterine incision. A female fetus weighting 3,200 g with Apgar scores of 7 and 8 was delivered. The umbilical arterial pH was 7.17 and the venous pH 7.22. The uterine incision had not extended and was easily closed. The baby did well.

operation. Complications of both procedures should be discussed and an attempt should be made to include an individualized risk assessment for both uterine rupture and the likelihood of successful VBAC (Table 19-14). For example, a woman who might require induction of labor may be at a slight increased risk for uterine rupture and is also less likely to achieve vaginal delivery. Future childbearing and the risks of multiple cesarean deliveries including the risks of placenta previa and placenta accreta should be considered as well (Table 19-15).

It is essential to make every effort to make every effort possible to obtain records of the prior cesarean delivery in order to ascertain previous uterine incision type. This is particularly relevant to cases of prior preterm breech delivery in which a vertical uterine incision or a low transverse incision in an undeveloped lower uterine segment might preclude a TOL. If previous uterine incision type is unknown, the implications of this missing information should be discussed as well.

Following complete informed consent detailing the risks and benefits for the individual woman, the delivery plan should be formulated by both the patient and physician. It is inappropriate to mandate VBAC-TOL because many women desire an elective repeat operation after thorough counseling. However, VBAC-TOL should continue to remain an option for most women with a prior cesarean delivery, particularly when one considers the magnitude of risks accompanying TOL. The attributable risk for a serious adverse perinatal outcome (perinatal death or HIE) at term appears to be approximately 1 in 2,000 trials of labor.[133] Combining an independent risk for hysterectomy attributable to uterine rupture at term with the risk for newborn HIE indicates the chance of one of these adverse events occurring to be approximately 1 in 1,250 cases.

The decision to elect a TOL may also increase the risk for perinatal death and HIE unrelated to uterine rupture. For women awaiting spontaneous labor beyond 39 weeks, there is a small possibility of unexplained stillbirth that might be avoidable with a scheduled repeat operation. A risk for fetal hypoxia and its sequelas may also accompany labor events unrelated to the uterine scar. In the MFMU Network Study, five cases of non-rupture-related HIE occurred in term infants in the TOL group compared with none in the elective repeat cesarean population.[133]

Table 19-14. Risks Associated with Trial of Labor (TOL)

Uterine rupture and related morbidity	
Uterine rupture	(0.5–1.0/100 TOL)
Perinatal death and/or encephalopathy	(0.5/1000 TOL)
Hysterectomy	(0.3/1000 TOL)
Increased maternal morbidity with failed TOL	
Transfusion	
Endometritis	
Length of stay	
Potential risk for perinatal asphyxia with labor (cord prolapse, abruption)	
Potential risk for antepartum stillbirth beyond 39 weeks' gestation	

Table 19-15. Risks Associated with Elective Repeat Cesarean Delivery

- Increased maternal morbidity compared with successful trial of labor
- Increased length of stay and recovery
- Increased risks for abnormal placentation and hemorrhage with successive cesarean operations

CESAREAN HYSTERECTOMY

Cesarean hysterectomy refers to the removal of the uterus at the time of a planned or unplanned cesarean delivery. The reported incidence of cesarean hysterectomy is 5 to 8 per 1,000 cesarean deliveries.[78,153,154] Postpartum hysterectomy encompasses both cesarean hysterectomy as well as removal of the uterus following vaginal delivery. In most cases of hysterectomy following vaginal birth, the indication for the procedure is uterine atony with uncontrolled hemorrhage that has failed to respond to conservative measures (see Chapter 18). In contrast, placenta accreta is the most common indication for post-cesarean hysterectomy (Table 19-16). In a series of 186 cesarean hysterectomies, 37 percent were performed for placenta accreta, whereas 35 percent had atony as the primary indication. Of the 71 placenta accreta cases, 58 (81 percent) accompanied a repeat cesarean delivery.[154] There appears to be a trend of increasing cesarean hysterectomy as a result of an increased frequency of prior cesarean birth, itself a risk factor for placenta accreta. Nearly 25 percent of women with placenta previa and prior cesarean delivery develop placenta accreta, which in most cases, requires a hysterectomy to control bleeding.[78] With two or more prior cesarean deliveries and an existing placenta previa, the risk for cesarean hysterectomy ranges from 30 to 50 percent.[79,153] Although placenta accreta itself poses a risk for peripartum hysterectomy, its association with prior uterine scarring (such as a cesarean delivery incision) is responsible for the approximately 50- to 100-fold increased risk for hysterectomy following cesarean section compared with vaginal delivery. A history of prior cesarean section is now present in

Table 19-16. Indications for Cesarean Hysterectomy

	CLARK ET AL[153] (1978–82)		STANCO[78] (1985–90)		ZELOP[155]* (1983–91)		SHELLHAAS[154] (1999–2001)	
	NO.	PERCENT	NO.	PERCENT	NO.	PERCENT	NO.	PERCENT
Placenta accreta	21	30	55	45	75	64	69	37
Placenta percreta	—	—	6	5	—	—	—	
Uterine atony	30	43	25	20	25	21	65	35
Bleeding	—	—	19	16	—	—	—	
Uterine rupture	9	13	14	11	10	9	10	5
Fibroids with bleeding	3	4	3	2	2	2	9	5
Uterine infection	—	—	1	1	3	3	—	
Scar extension/other	7	10	—	—	2	2	2	10

*Abnormal placentation.

†82 (67%) had at least one prior cesarean delivery.

57 to 67 percent of women undergoing a peripartum hysterectomy.

Most cesarean hysterectomies are emergent procedures performed to control hemorrhage when conservative measures have failed. Occasionally, cesarean hysterectomy is planned for the treatment of cervical cancer or large myomata. The most common indications for emergency cesarean hysterectomy are placenta accreta, uterine atony, and uterine rupture. In Shellhaas' series from the MFMU Network, these accounted for over 75 percent of the procedures.[154]

Before the introduction of effective oxytocics such as prostaglandin $F_{2\alpha}$, uterine atony was the most common indication for cesarean hysterectomy. Improved oxytocics coupled with a rising rate of cesarean delivery, which again has increased the frequency of abnormal placentation that has resulted in placenta accreta becoming the most common indication for cesarean hysterectomy. In two reports from Los Angeles County–University of Southern California Medical Center over an 18-year period, placenta accreta accounted for 30 percent of peripartum hysterectomies initially and later was associated with 45 percent of procedures.[79,153] The frequency of atony associated with peripartum hysterectomy fell from 43 to 20 percent from 1978 to 1990.[79,153]

In the above-mentioned series, uterine rupture was responsible for 11 to 13 percent of peripartum hysterectomies. In most cases of symptomatic rupture, the uterus can be preserved if so desired. The decision to proceed with hysterectomy ultimately depends on the ability to satisfactorily repair the uterus with hemostasis as well as the patients' wishes for future childbearing. Small dehiscences discovered at cesarean delivery or following successful VBAC are generally not indications for cesarean hysterectomy.

Technique and Complications

A peripartum hysterectomy including cesarean hysterectomy may be subtotal (supracervical) or total depending upon the clinical circumstances. In most planned procedures, a total hysterectomy is performed, whereas a subtotal hysterectomy may be preferable in cases in which emergency surgery is necessary for life-threatening hemorrhage and dissection of the cervix is difficult. Subtotal hysterectomy is a faster procedure and has been suggested in unstable patients, yet a comparison of this procedure with total hysterectomy was not associated with less blood loss, operative time, or morbidity.[38] However, selection bias is probable in that women with significant bleeding from atony or placenta accreta are more likely to undergo subtotal hysterectomy.[155]

Subtotal hysterectomy is more likely to be performed in cases of atony. In one series of 30 cases of peripartum hysterectomy for atony, a subtotal procedure was accomplished in 77 percent of patients.[153] Subtotal hysterectomy is less often performed in cases of placenta previa/accreta because lower uterine segment bleeding with these conditions often requires a total hysterectomy to control hemorrhage. In Shellhaas' series of 186 procedures, 66 percent were total hysterectomies.[154]

The operative technique for cesarean hysterectomy consists of the same general surgical considerations for the procedure performed in the nonpregnant individual. Specific considerations include adequate inferior displacement of the bladder if possible before the hysterectomy because taking the bladder down may be difficult following uterine incision and delivery of the infant. Additionally, care must be taken to avoid bladder and ureteral injury, which appears to be relatively common with peripartum hysterectomy. Cystotomy has been reported to occur in up to 5 to 9 percent of cases, although many of these represent intentional procedures.[156] Ureteral injury is observed in 1 in 200 operations.[157] The ureter is particularly vulnerable to injury if broad ligament bleeding occurs and lateral clamping is necessary to control this. If ureteral injury is suspected, the dome of the bladder may be incised and retrograde stenting of the uterus is performed. Intravenous infection of indigo carmine may also be useful in identifying a ureteral injury or detecting a suspected ligature.

The sequence of maneuvers for hysterectomy is not different from the procedure in the nonpregnant state. As mentioned previously, efforts to displace the bladder inferiorly before delivery are advised. Following delivery and removal of the placenta, the uterine incision is frequently reapproximated or attention is given to securing hemostasis by ligating the uteroovarian anastamosis bilaterally. The bladder should be inspected and mobilized by blunt and sharp dissection. In most cases, the ovaries are left, although the adnexa in the pregnant state are vulnerable to hematoma formation, which has necessitated salpingoophorectomy in as many as 17 percent of emergent procedures.[155] The avascular portion of the broad ligaments are incised and the uterine vessels are identified, clamped, and suture ligated (see Figs. 19-13 and 19-14). Clamps are placed tightly along the lateral aspect of the uterus to prevent injury to the ureter and hematoma formation. At this point, the decision is often made whether to proceed with subtotal versus total hysterectomy. In most instances, a total procedure is performed unless the patient is unstable and bleeding can be adequately controlled by the subtotal approach. If the cervix is amputated, it is closed with figure-of-eight sutures, and reperitonealization may or may not be performed (Fig. 19-15). If total hysterectomy is to be accomplished, after further consideration, the cervical stump is elevated with traction and is separated from the cardinal and uterosacral ligaments by clamping and ligature (Fig. 19-16). The vagina is then entered anteriorly or at the lateral angle above a curved clamp. An effort should be made to be certain the cervix is completely removed, although in cases following labor, this may be difficult. Similarly, excess portions of the superior vagina should not be excised. In order to minimize these complications, some surgeons prefer to insert a finger through an incision in the lower uterine segment in order to identify the cervicovaginal junction before excision of the cervix (Fig. 19-17). The vaginal cuff is supported by approximation to the cardinal and uterosacral ligament pedicles (Figs. 19-18 and 19-19). The cuff may be left open or closed in an interrupted or running locking continuous suture (Fig. 19-20). If significant bleeding is a concern, the cuff

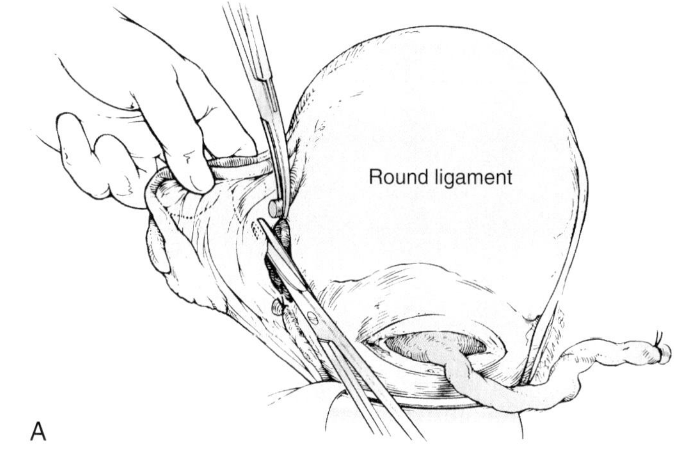

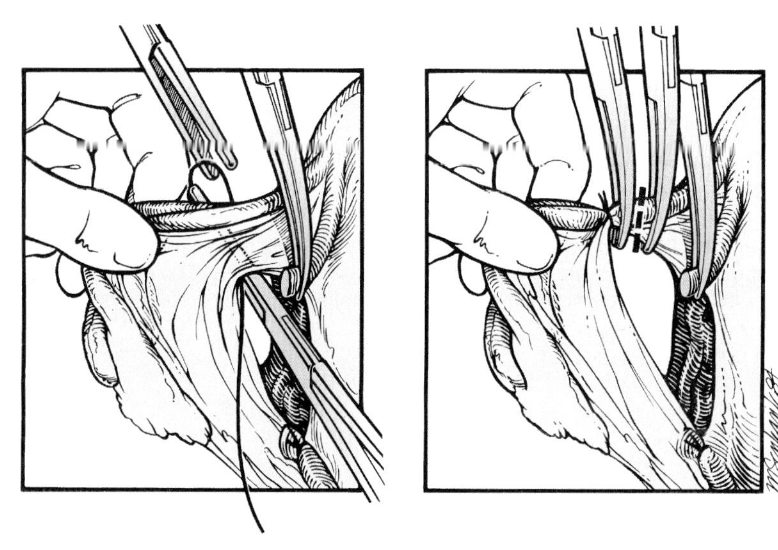

Figure 19-13. Cesarean hysterectomy. *A,* After extending the bladder flap, each round ligament is cut and ligated. The posterior leaf of the broad ligament can be opened for a short distance, taking care to incise only the surface layer. The avascular space beneath the utero-ovarian ligament may be opened by blunt finger dissection to isolate the adnexal pedicle. *B,* A free tie is passed through the avascular space and firmly tied. The advantage of this tie is to secure the vessels within the pedicle before it is cut (*right*). The adnexal pedicle is doubly clamped and cut. In addition, a transfixing suture will then be placed around the pedicle.

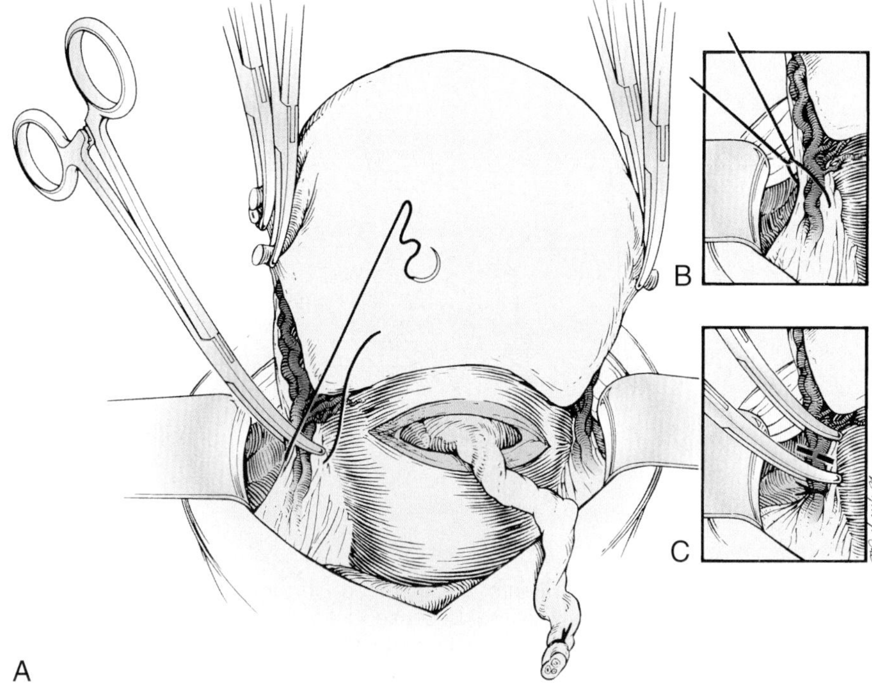

Figure 19-14. *A,* The ascending branches of the uterine artery are clamped, cut, and a suture is placed just below the tip of the clamp and immediately next to the uterine wall. *B,* After removing the clamp, the suture is tied, thus securing the vessel before they are cut. *C,* The pedicle is regrasped just above the tie and then doubly ligated.

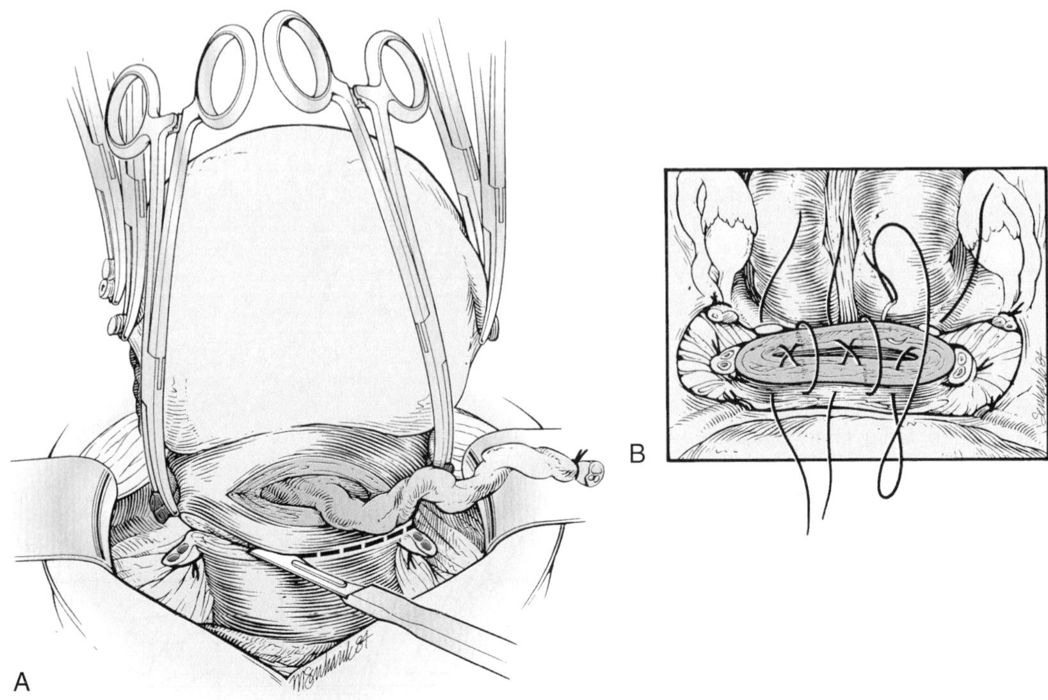

Figure 19-15. Subtotal hysterectomy. *A,* The cervix is incised just below the level of the ligated pedicles of the uterine arteries, amputating the uterine corpus from its cervical stump. *B,* The cervical stump may be closed with several interrupted figure-of-eight sutures; reperitonealization is then accomplished as in a total hysterectomy.

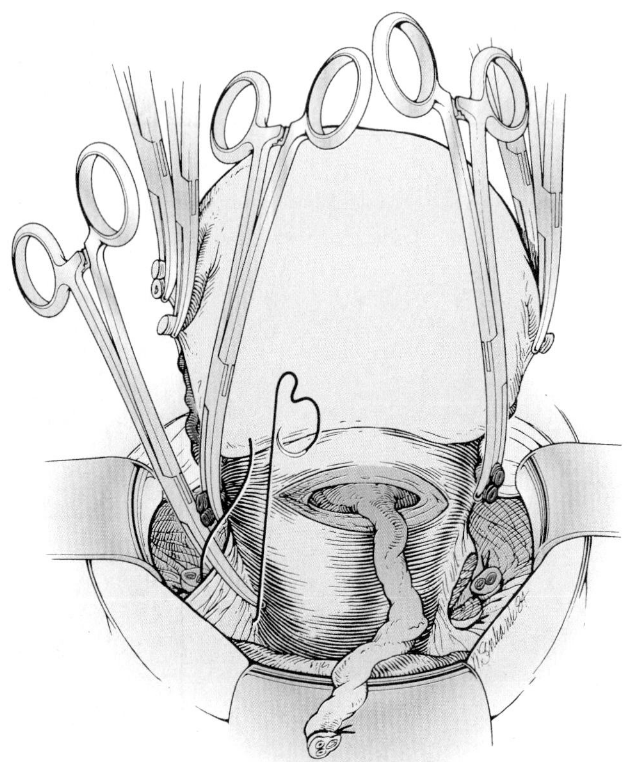

Figure 19-16. The cardinal ligaments are clamped at their point of insertion, cut, and singly ligated. Because these structures are hypertrophied, several bites may be necessary. Some physicians clamp, cut, and ligate the uterosacral ligaments separately.

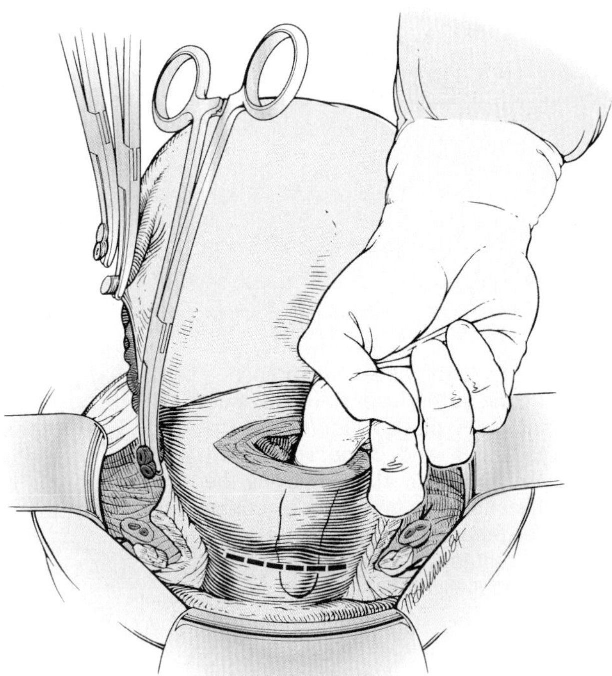

Figure 19-17. Because the cervix is elongated, it may be useful to insert an index finger through the cervical canal to demarcate the vaginal incision and to ensure complete removal of the cervix and avoid unnecessary removal of vaginal length.

is better left open for dependent drainage or placement of a drain. Reperitonealization has become less favored and has been replaced by many with fixation of the ovarian pedicles to the round ligaments, so as to reduce the chance of adhesion to the vaginal cuff (Fig. 19-21).

The principal complications of cesarean hysterectomy are urologic injury, as discussed erarlier, and hemorrhage. The average blood loss varies, with an excess of 500 ml to 1,000 ml beyond a routine cesarean delivery. The frequency of transfusion has been reported to be 75 percent[154] (Table 19-17). In many cases, the indication for hysterectomy is hemorrhage itself with a large preexisting blood loss before commencing the hysterectomy. Febrile morbidity is common, particularly with an unplanned cesarean hysterectomy, with infection rates of 25 to 30 percent observed, despite prophylactic antibiotic administration.[79,155] With the friability of pelvic tissues, as well as the indications for hysterectomy often resulting in coagulopathy, postsurgical bleeding is observed with increased frequency following peripartum hysterectomy.

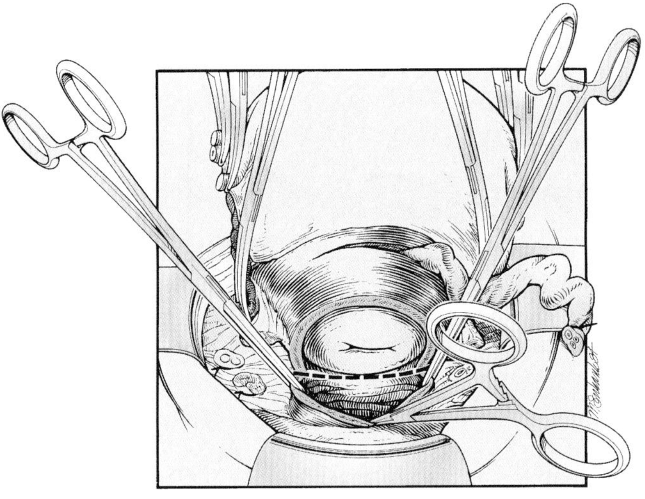

Figure 19-18. The vagina is circumferentially incised at its cervical attachment and grasped with four clamps.

Reexploration has been reported in 2 to 4 percent of cases.[79,155]

TUBAL STERILIZATION

Surgical approach to tubal sterilization is influenced by whether the procedure is being performed on a postpartum or on an interval basis. Advantages to the postpartum approach include the use of one anesthesia for labor, delivery, and sterilization, and only one hospitalization.[158] Tubal ligations after vaginal delivery are performed through a minilaparotomy incision at the level of the uterine fundus, usually subumbilically. The same surgical techniques are applied if tubal ligation is performed at the time of cesarean section. Interval sterilizations are performed by laparoscopy or minilaparotomy.

The choice of surgical approach influences the choice of methods of tubal occlusion. For example, most procedures performed through a minilaparotomy use some type of partial salpingectomy technique as the method of tubal occlusion. Most laparoscopic sterilizations use either coagulation, application of silicone rubber bands, or application of clips as the method of tubal occlusion.[159] The long-term failure rate is approximately 1 percent overall.

Modified Pomeroy

The method of tubal occlusion used by Pomeroy was described in 1930,[160] and it is the most popular means of postpartum tubal ligation because of its simplicity. The Pomeroy technique as originally described included grasping the fallopian tube at its midportion, creating a small knuckle, and then ligating the loop of tube with a double strand of catgut suture. It is critical that the fallopian tube be conclusively identified. Visualizing the fimbriated portion of the tube and identifying the round ligament as a separate structure can accomplish this.

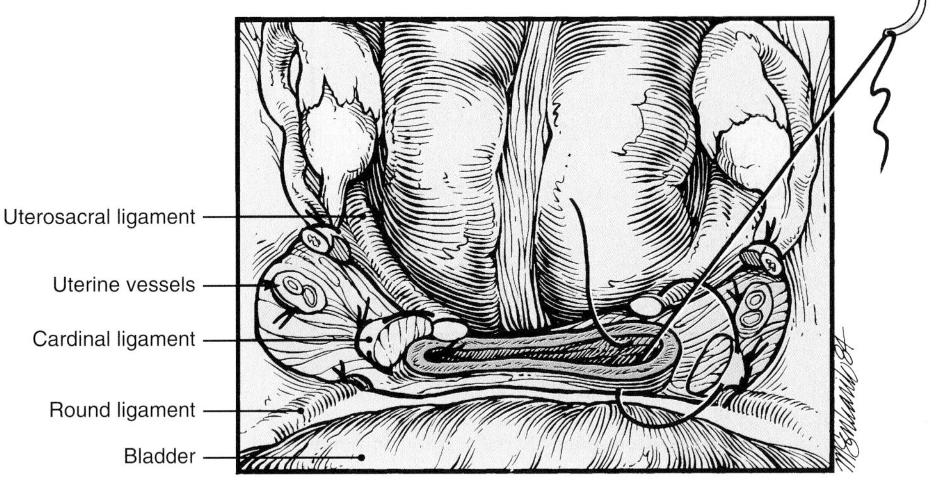

Figure 19-19. The angles of the vaginal cuff are closed with sutures to include the cardinal and uterosacral ligaments, thus providing fascial support to the vaginal vault. A simple loop suture is commonly used at this location to reduce the likelihood of breakage during the state of postoperative edema.

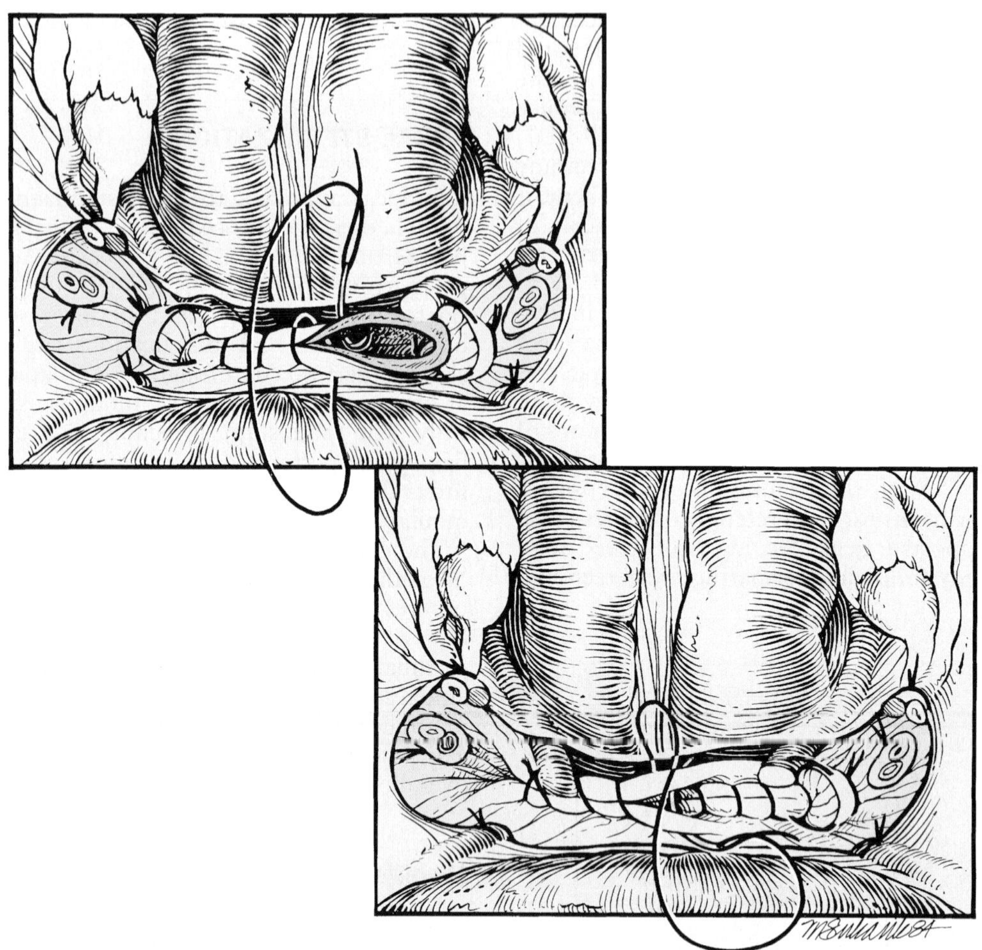

Figure 19-20. There are a number of methods of closing the vaginal cuff. Illustrated is a two-layer closure. The first layer closes the vagina, and the second layer closes the endopelvic fascia. Many operators prefer to leave the cuff "open" by using one continuous suture that circles the cuff, approximating the cut edge to its surrounding fascia.

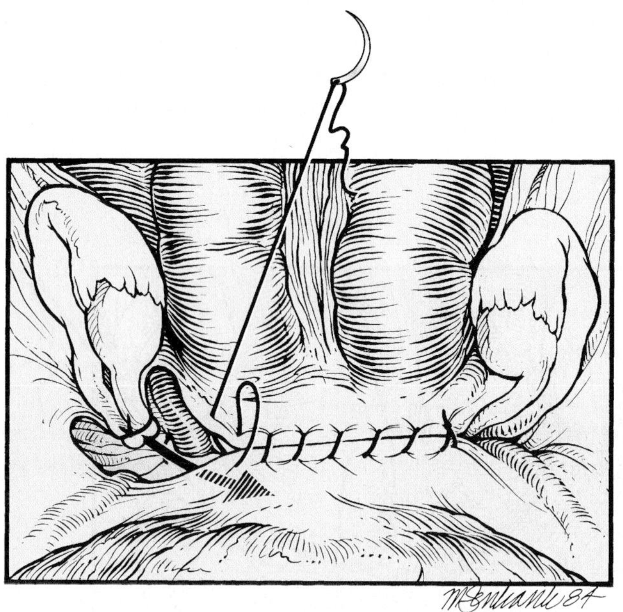

Figure 19-21. The bladder flap is closed with a continuous suture that inverts the pedicles of the round ligaments and adnexae. Note that these structures have not been attached to the vaginal cuff.

Absorbable sutures are used so that the tubal ends will separate quickly after surgery, leaving a gap between the proximal and distal ends. In performing the procedure, care should be taken to make the loop of fallopian tube sufficient in size to ensure that complete transection of the tubal lumen will occur. After the loop of fallopian tube is ligated, the mesosalpinx of the ligated loop should be perforated using scissors, and the knuckle of the tube is transected (Fig. 19-22). It is important not to resect the fallopian tube so close to the suture that the remaining portion of the fallopian tube slips out of the ligature and causes delayed bleeding.

The Irving Procedure

Irving first reported his sterilization technique in 1924, with a modification in 1950.[161] In the modified procedure, a window is created in the mesosalpinx, and the fallopian tube is doubly ligated with No. 1 chromic catgut. The fallopian tube is then transected approximately 4 cm from the uterotubal portion; the two free ends of the ligation stitch on the proximal tubal segment are held long. The proximal portion of the fallopian tube is dis-

Table 19-17. Cesarean Hysterectomy Morbidity and Mortality

	CLARK ET AL (1978–82)		STANCO ET AL (1985–90)		ZELOP ET AL (1983–91)		SHELLHAAS ET AL (1999–2001)	
	NO.	PERCENT	NO.	PERCENT	NO.	PERCENT	NO.	PERCENT
Procedures	70		123		117		186	
Subtotal	38	54%	65	53%	25	21%	63	34%
Operative time (mean)	3.1 h		NA		3.0 h		2.8 h	
Blood loss (mean)	3,575 mi		3,000 ml		3,000 ml*		—	
Hemorrhage					102	87		
Transfused patients	67	96	102	83	102	87		80%
Reexplored	—	—	—	—	3	1	7	3.8%
Infect Morbidity	—	—	—	—	58	50		
Febrile	35	50	NA		39	33	21	11%
UTI			NA		7	6	6	3.2%
Wound infection	8	12	11	9	4	6	2	1.1%
Urologic injury	3	4	4	3	10	9		
Cystotomy		0	12†		9	8	18	9.7%
Ureteral	3	4	—		3	3	0	
Maternal Death	1‡	1	0		0		3	1.6%

UTI, urinary tract infection.
*Median value 50% >3,000 ml and 50% <3,000 ml.
†Intentional cystotomies for ureteral stent passage.
‡Cardiac arrest secondary to amniotic fluid embolus.
Data from Clark et al,[153] Stanco et al,[78] Zelop et al,[155] and Shellhaas et al.[154]

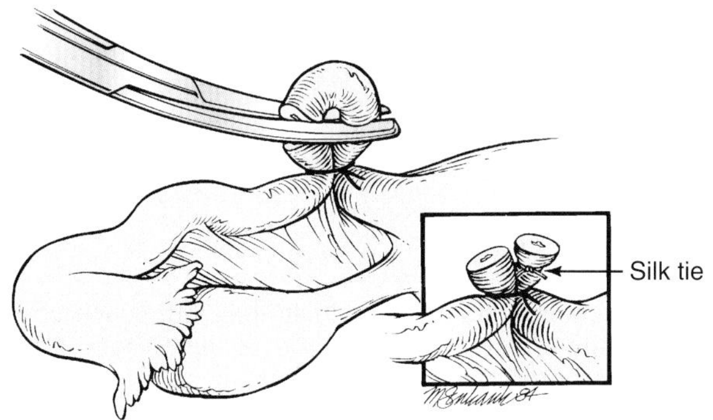

Figure 19-22. Pomeroy sterilization. A knuckle of tube is ligated with absorbable suture, and a small segment is being excised. Note that the ligation is performed at a site that will favor reanastomosis, should that become desirable. Some surgeons place an extra tie of nonabsorbable suture around the proximal stump as added protection against recanalization.

sected free from the mesosalpinx and then buried into an incision in the myometrium of the posterior uterine wall, near the uterotubal junction. This is accomplished by first creating a tunnel approximately 2 cm in length with a mosquito clamp in the uterine wall. The two free ends of the ligation stitch on the proximal tubal segment are then brought deep into the myometrial tunnel, and brought out through the uterine serosa. Traction is then placed on the sutures to draw the proximal tubal stump into the myometrial tunnel; tying the free sutures fixes the tube in that location. No treatment of the distal tubal stump is necessary, but some choose to bury the segment in the mesosalpinx (Fig. 19-23). Although this technique is slightly more complicated than the others, it has the lowest failure rate.[162]

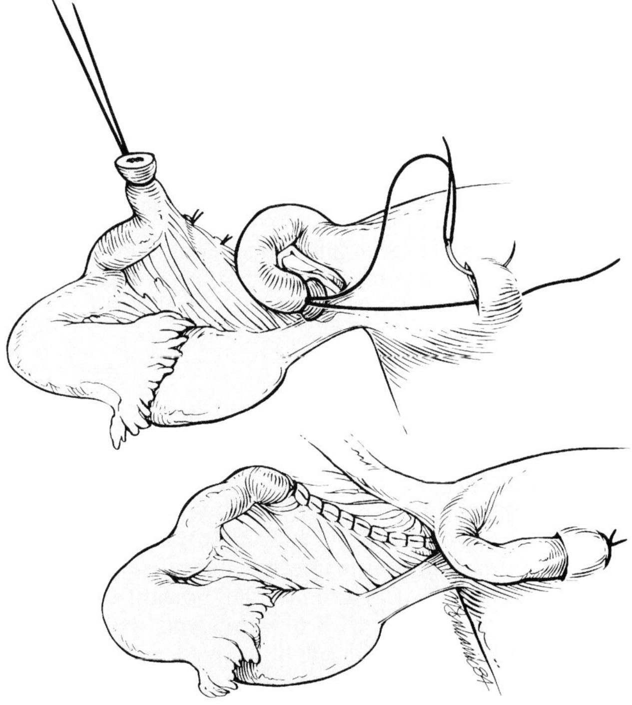

Figure 19-23. Irving sterilization. The tube is transected 3 to 4 cm from its insertion, and a short tunnel is created by means of a sharp-nosed hemostat in either the anterior or posterior uterine wall. The cut end of the tube can then be buried in the tunnel and, if necessary, further secured by an interrupted suture at the opening of the tunnel. The distal cut end is buried between the leaves of the broad ligament.

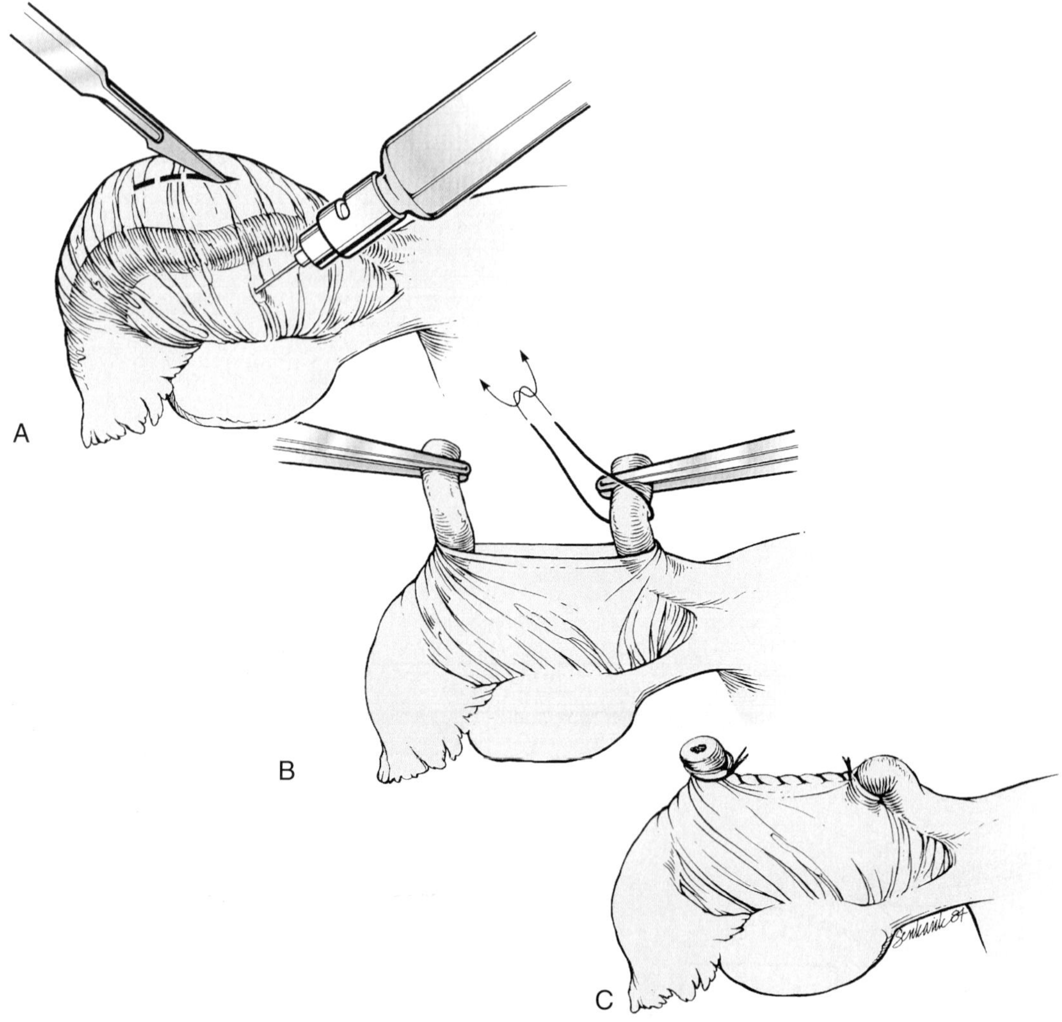

Figure 19-24. Uchida sterilization. The leaves of the broad ligament and peritubal peritoneum are infiltrated with saline so that the tube can be easily isolated from these structures (*A*), divided (*B*), and ligated (*C*). The broad ligament is then closed, burying the proximal stump between the leaves and including the distal stump in the line of closure.

The Uchida Procedure

In this sterilization procedure,[163] the muscular portion of the fallopian tube is separated from its serosal cover and grasped approximately 6 to 7 cm from the uterotubal junction. Saline solution is injected subserosally, and the serosa is then incised. The muscular portion of the fallopian tube is grasped with a clamp and divided. The serosa over the proximal tubal segment is bluntly dissected toward the uterus, exposing approximately 5 cm of the proximal tubal segment. The tube is then ligated with chromic suture near the uterotubal junction, and approximately 5 cm of the tube is resected. The shortened proximal tubal stump is allowed to retract into the mesosalpinx. The serosa around the opening in the mesosalpinx is sutured in a purse-string with a fine absorbable stitch; when the suture is tied the mesosalpinx is gathered around the distal tubal segment (Fig. 19-24). Some surgeons choose to excise only 1 cm of fallopian tube rather than the recommended 5 cm in case the patient wishes to have a tubal reanastomosis in the future.

KEY POINTS

- In 1970, the cesarean delivery rate was approximately 5 percent. By 2004, it had reached 29.1 percent, the highest rate ever recorded in the United States. VBAC rates have plummeted from a peak of 28.3 percent in 1996 to 9.2 percent in 2004.
- A *Healthy People 2010* document suggests an overall target cesarean delivery rate of 15 percent. Factors that will make this rate difficult to achieve include (1) continued increase in primary cesarean deliveries for dystocia, failed induction, and abnormal presentation; (2) an increase in the proportion of women with obesity, diabetes mellitus, and multiple gestation; (3) increased use of elective cesarean delivery to preserve pelvic floor function; and (4) limited use of TOL after cesarean delivery due to both safety and medicolegal concerns.

❑ The rate of wound infection following cesarean delivery is approximately 5 percent and is not influenced by preparation technique.

❑ A vertical uterine incision is performed for cesarean delivery if the lower uterine segment is poorly developed or if the fetus is in a backdown transverse lie. A vertical incision is recommended for a preterm breech delivery.

❑ Prophylactic antibiotics are of clear benefit in reducing the frequency of postcesarean endomyometritis and wound infection.

❑ Two randomized trials have compared sharp versus blunt extension of the uterine incision. Sharp extension appears to be associated with increased blood loss as well as the potential risk of cutting the umbilical cord or direct fetal injury.

❑ Several randomized trials have demonstrated greater blood loss and a higher rate of endometritis with manual extraction of the placenta at cesarean delivery. Thus, spontaneous expulsion of the placenta with gentle cord traction is preferred.

❑ When closing the abdomen after a cesarean delivery, the subcutaneous tissue is closed if its thickness exceeds 2 cm. This approach reduces the risk of wound disruption by 34 percent in women with excessive subcutaneous fat.

❑ The risk of uterine rupture in a TOL depends greatly on the previous uterine incision, ranging from 0.5 to 1.0 percent with a prior low transverse cesarean delivery to 4 to 9 percent with a prior classic or T-incision.

❑ Oxytocin use may marginally increase the risk for uterine rupture in women undergoing a TOL. Therefore, judicious stimulation of labor should be used in these patients.

❑ A nonreassuring FHR pattern, particularly significant variable decelerations or bradycardia, is the most common finding accompanying uterine rupture.

REFERENCES

1. Sewell JE: Cesarean Section—A Brief History. Washington DC, American College of Obstetricians and Gynecologists, 1993.
2. Porro E: Della Amputazione Utero-ovarica. Milan, 1876.
3. Eastman NJ: The role of Frontier America in the development of cesarean section. Am J Obstet Gynecol 24:919, 1932.
4. Frank F: Suprasymphysial delivery and its relation to other operations in the presence of contracted pelvis. Arch Gynaekol 81:46, 1907.
5. Latzko W: Ueber den extraperitonealen Kaiserschnitt. Zentralbl Gynaekol 33:275, 1989.
6. Beck AC: Obeservations in a series of cesarean sections done at the Long Island College Hospital during the past six years. Am J Obstet Gynecol 79:197, 1919.
7. Kerr JMM: The technique of cesarean section with special reference to the lower uterine segment incision. Am J Obstet Gynecol 12:729, 1926.
8. Martin JA, Hamilton BE, Menachker F, et al: Preliminary births for 2004. Health E-Stats. National Center for Health Statistics. *www.cdc.gov/nchs/products/pubs/pubd/hestats/prelim*births/prelimbirths04.htm. Accessed June 1, 2005.
9. Notzon FC: International differences in the use of obstetric interventions. JAMA 264:3286, 1990.
10. Cesarean Childbirth: Report of a Consensus Development Conference Sponsored by the National Institute of Child Health and Human Development. DHHS Publ No 82-2067. Washington, DC, U.S. Government Printing Office, October 1981.
11. American College of Obstetricians and Gynecologists: ACOG Executive Summary: Evaluation of Cesarean Delivery. Washington, DC, ACOG, 2000.
12. Notzon FC, Placek PJ, Taffel SM: Comparison of national cesarean section rates. N Engl J Med 316:386, 1987.
13. Freeman R: Intrapartum fetal monitoring—a disappointing story. N Engl J Med 322:624, 1990.
14. Shy KK, Luthy DA, Bennett FC, et al: Effects of electronic fetal heart monitoring, as compared with periodic auscultation on the neurologic development of premature infants. N Engl J Med 322:588, 1990.
15. Taffel SM, Placek PJ, Moien M, Kosary CL: 1989 US cesarean section rate steadies—VBAC rises to nearly one in five. Birth 18:73, 1991.
16. Public Health Service. Healthy People 2000: National Health Promotion and Disease Prevention Objectives: Full Report with Commentary. Washington, D.C.: Government Printing Office, 1990:378. (DHHS publication no. (PHS) 91-50212.
17. Public Health Service. Healthy People 2010: With Understanding and Improving Health and Objectives for Improving Health, 2nd ed. Washington, D.C.: Government Printing Office, November 1:45, 2000.
18. Socol ML, Garcia PM, Peaceman AD, Dooley SL: Reducing cesarean births at a primarily private university hospital. Am J Obstet Gynecol 168:1748, 1993.
19. Bailit JL, Dooley SL, Peaceman AN: Risk adjustment for interhospital comparison of primary cesarean rates. Obstet Gynecol 93:1025, 1999.
20. Lieberman E, Ernst EK, Rooks JP, et al: Results of the national study of vaginal birth after cesarean section. Obstet Gynecol 104:933, 2004.
21. Lomas J: Opinion leaders versus audit feedback to implement practice guidelines: delivery after previous cesarean section. JAMA 265:2202, 1991.
22. Main EK: Reducing cesarean birth rates with data driven quality improvement activities. Pediatrics 103(Supp E):374, 1999.
23. Myers SA, Gleicher N: A successful program to lower cesarean section rates. N Engl J Med 319:1511, 1988,
24. Feldman GB, Frieman JA: Prophylactic cesarean section at term? N Engl J Med 312:1264, 1985.
25. Harer WB: Informed consent for delivery. ACOG Clin Rev 5:13, 2000.
26. American College of Obstetricians and Gynecologists: ACOG Committee Opinion. Surgery and patient choice: the ethics of decision making. Obstet Gynecol 287:2684, 2003.
27. Smith GC, Pell JP, Cameron AD, et al: Risk of perinatal death associated with labor after previous cesarean delivery in uncomplicated term pregnancies. JAMA 287:2684, 2002.
28. Badawi N, Kurinczuk JJ, Keogh JM, et al: Intrapartum risk factors for newborn encephalopathy: the Western Australian case-control study. BMJ 317:1554, 1998.
29. Towner D, Castro MA, Eby-Wilkens E, et al: Effect of mode of delivery in nulliparous women on neonatal intracranial injury. N Engl J Med 341:1709, 1999.
30. Wilson PD, Herbison RM, Herbison GP: Obstetric practice and the prevalence of urinary incontinence three months after delivery. Br J Obstet Gynaecol 103:154, 1996.
31. Rortviet G, Daltveit AK, Hannestad YS, Hunskaar S: Urinary incontinence after vaginal delivery or cesarean section. N Engl J Med 348:900, 2003.
32. Mac Lennan AH, Taylor AW, Wilson DH, Wilson D: the prevalence of pelvic floor disorders and their relationship to gender, age, parity, and mode of delivery. Br J Obstet Gynaecol 107:1460, 2000.

33. Minkoff H, Chervenak FA: Elective primary cesarean delivery. N Engl J Med 248:946, 2003.
34. Sachs BP, Yeh J, Acher D, et al: Cesarean section-related maternal mortality in Massachusetts, 1954–1985. Obstet Gynecol 71:385, 1988.
35. Lucas DN, Yentis SM, Kinsella SM, et al: Urgency of cesarean section: A new classification. JR Soc Med 93:346, 2000.
36. Burrows LJ, Meyn LA, Weber AM: Maternal morbidity associated with vaginal versus cesarean delivery. Obstet Gynecol 103:907, 2004.
37. Harper MA, Byington RP, Espeland MA, et al: Pregnancy related death and healthcare services. Am J Obstet Gynecol 102:273, 2003.
38. VanHorn MA, Van Dongen PW, Mulder J: Maternal consequences of cesarean section. A retrospective study of intraoperative and postoperative maternal complications of cesarean section during a 10-year period. Eur J Obstet Gynecol 74:1, 1997.
39. Jackson N, Paterson-Brown S: Physical sequelae of cesarean section. Best Practice and Research 15:49, 2001.
40. Placek PJ, Taffel SM, Keppel KG: Maternal and infant characteristics associated with cesarean section delivery. Department of Health and Human Services. Publ No PHS 84–1232. Hyattsville, MD, National Center of Health Statistics, December 1983.
41. Freeman R, Nelson KB: Intrapartum asphyxia and cerebral palsy. Pediatrics 82:240, 1988.
42. Haverkamp AD, Orleans M, Langendoerfet S, et al: A controlled trial of the differential effects of intrapartum fetal monitoring. Am J Obstet Gynecol 134:399, 1979.
43. Garite T, Dildy GA, McNamara H, et al: A multicenter controlled trial of fetal pulse oximetry in the intrapartum management of nonreassuring fetal heart rate patterns. Am J Obstet Gynecol 183:1049, 2000.
44. American College of Obstetricians and Gynecologists (ACOG): Mode of term singleton breech delivery, ACOG Committee Opinion 265. Washington, DC, ACOG 2001.
45. Rouse DJ, Owen J: Prophylactic cesarean delivery for fetal macrosomia diagnosed by means of ultrasonography—A Faustian bargain? Am J Obstet Gynecol 181:33, 1999.
46. How HY, Harris BJ, Pietrantoni M, et al: Is vaginal delivery preferable to elective cesarean delivery in fetuses with a known vertical wall defect? Am J Obstet Gynecol 182:1527, 2000.
47. Rouse DJ, Owen J, Hauth JC: Active-phase labor arrest: Oxytocin augmentation for at least 4 hours. Obstet Gynecol 93:323, 1999.
48. Alexander J, for the NICHD MFMU Network. MFMU Cesarean Registry: A Comparison of Maternal and Neonatal outcomes when primary cesarean delivery is performed in the second stage versus the first stage of labor. Am J Obstet Gynecol Abstract #178, 187:S109, 2003.
49. Blumenthal NJ, Harris RS, O'Conner MC, et al: Changes cesarean section rates experience at a Sydney obstetric teaching hospital. Aust NZ J Obstet Gynaecol 24:246, 1984.
50. Haynes de Regt RH, Minkoff HL, Feldman J, et al: Relation of private or clinic care to the cesarean birth rate. N Engl J Med 315:619, 1986.
51. Berkowitz GS, Fiarman GS, Mijicca MA, et al: Effect of physician characteristics on the cesarean birth rate. Am J Obstet Gynecol 161:146, 1989.
52. Frigoletto FD, Lieberman E, Lang JM, et al: A clinical trial of active management of labor. N Engl J Med 338:745, 1995.
53. Alexander JW, Fischer JE, Bovajian M, et al: The influence of hair removal methods on wound infections. Arch Surg 118:347, 1983.
54. Alexander JW, Aerni S, Plettner JP: Development of a safe and effective one minute preoperative skin preparation. Arch Surg 120:1357, 1985.
55. Gibbs RS, Sweet RL, Duff WP: Maternal and fetal infectious disorders. *In* Creasy RK, Resnik R (eds): Maternal-Fetal Medicine Principles and Practice. Philadelphia, WB Saunders, 2004, p 752.
56. Smaill F, Hofmeyr GJ: Antiobiotic prophylaxis for cesarean section. Cochrane Database Syst Rev 2005;1.
57. Carlson C, Duff P: Antibiotic prophylaxis for cesarean delivery: is an extended-spectrum agent necessary? Obstet Gynecol 76:343, 1990.
58. Hopkins L, Smaill F: Antibiotic prophylaxis regimens and drugs for cesarean section (Cochrane Review). In: the Cochrane Library, Issue 2, 2003. Oxford: Update Software.
59. Faro S, Martens MG, Hammill HA, et al: Antibiotic prophylaxis: Is there a difference? Am J Obstet Gynecol 162:900, 1990.
60. Hohlagschwandtner M, Ruecklinger E, Husslein P, Joura EA: Is the formation of a bladder flap at cesarean necessary? A randomized trial. Obstet Gynecol 98:1089, 2001.
61. Rodriguez A, Porter KB, O'Brien WF: Blunt versus sharp expansion of the uterine incision in low-segment transverse cesarean section. Am J Obstet Gynecol 171:1022, 1994.
62. Magann EG, Chauhan SP, Bufkin L, et al: Intraoperative haemorrhage by blunt versus sharp expansion of the uterine incision at cesarean delivery: a randomized clinical trial. Br J Obstet Gynaecol 109:448, 2002.
63. Boyle J, Gabbe SG: T and J vertical extensions in low transverse cesarean births. Obstet Gynecol 87:238, 1996.
64. McCurdy CM, Magann EF, McCurdy CJ, et al: The effect of placenta management at cesarean delivery on operative blood loss. Am J Obstet Gynecol 167:1363, 1992.
65. Magann EF, Dodson MK, Albert JR, et al: Blood loss at time of cesarean section by method of placental removal and exteriorization versus in situ repair of the uterine incision. Surg Gynecol Obstet 177:389, 1993.
66. Atkinson MW, Owen J, Wren A, Hauth JC: The effect of manual removal of the placenta on post-cesarean endometritis. Obstet Gynecol 87:99, 1996.
67. Tucker JM, Hauth JC, Hodgkins P, et al: Trial of labor after a one- or two-layer closure of a low transverse uterine incision. Obstet Gynecol 168:545, 1993.
68. Chapman SJ, Owen J, Hauth JC: One-versus two-layer closure of a low transverse cesarean: the next pregnancy. Obstet Gynecol 89:16, 1997.
69. Bujold E, Bujold C, Hamilton EF, et al: The impact of a single-layer or double-layer closure on uterine rupture. Am J Obstet Gynecol 186:1326, 2002.
70. Hauth JC, Owne J, Davis RO: Transverse uterine incision closure: one versus two layers. Am J Obstet Gynecol 167:1108, 1992.
71. Pietrantoni M, Parsons MT, O'Brien WF, et al: Peritoneal closure or non-closure at cesarean. Obstet Gynecol 77:293, 1991.
72. Hull DB, Varner MW: A randomized study of closure of the peritoneum at cesarean delivery. Obstet Gynecol 77:818, 1991.
73. Chelmow D, Rodriguez EF, Sabatini MM: Suture closure of subcutaneous fat and wound disruption after cesarean delivery: a meta-analysis. Obstet Gynecol 103:974, 2004.
74. Berghella V, Baxter JK, Chauhan SP: Evidence-based surgery for cesarean delivery. Am J Obstet Gynecol 193:107, 2005.
75. Eisenkop SM, Richman R, Platt LD, et al: Urinary tract injury during cesarean section. Obstet Gynecol 60:591, 1982.
76. Clark SL, Phelan YP, Yeh SY, et al: Hypogastric artery ligation for the control of obstetric hemorrhage. Obstet Gynecol 66:35, 1985.
77. Bakshi S, Meyer BA: Inductions for and outcomes of emergency peripartum hysterectomy: a fiver-year review. J Reprod Med 44:733, 2000.
78. Stanco LM, Schrimmer DB, Paul RH, Mischell DR Jr: Emergency peripartum hysterectomy and associated risk factors. Am J Obstet Gynecol 168:879, 1993.
79. Silver RM, Landon MB, Rouse DJ, et al: Maternal morbidity associated with multiple repeat cesarean deliveries. Obstet Gynecol 107:1226, 2006.
80. Lilford RJ, Van Coeverden SC, De Groot HA, et al: The relative risks of cesarean section (intrapartum and elective) and vaginal delivery: A detailed analysis to exclude the effects of medical disorders and other acute pre-existing physiological disturbance. Br J Obstet Gynaecol 97:883, 1990.
81. Lydon-Rochelle M, Holt V, Easterling TR, et al: Cesarean delivery and postpartum mortality among primiparas in Washington State, 1987–1986. Obstet Gynecol 97:169:2001.
82. Smaill F, Hofmeyr GJ: Antibiotic prophylaxis for cesarean section (Cochrane Review). In: the Cochrane Library, Issue 2, 2003. Oxford: Update Software.
83. Goepfert A: The MFMU Cesarean Registry: Infectious Morbidity Following Primary Cesarean Section. SMFM Abstract #410. Am J Obstet Gynecol 185:S192, 2001.

84. Hauth J, for the NICHD MFMU Network. MFMU Cesarean Registry: Thromboembolism—Occurrence and risk factors in 39,285 cesarean births. SMFM Abstract #207. Am J Obstet Gynecol 189: S120, 2003.
85. Bottoms SF, Rosen MG, Sokol RJ: The increase in the cesarean birth. N Engl J Med 302:559, 1980.
86. Flamm BL: Vaginal birth after cesarean section: controversies old and new. Clin Obstet Gynecol 28:735, 1985.
87. Goldman G, Pineault R, Pitvin L, et al: Factors influencing the practice of vaginal birth after cesarean section. Am Public Health 83:1104, 1993.
88. Shiono PH, Fielden JR, McNellis D, et al: Recent trends in cesarean birth and trial of labor rates in the United States. JAMA 257:494, 1987.
89. American College of Obstetricians and Gynecologists: Vaginal Delivery After Previous Cesarean Birth. Practice Patterns, No. 1. Washington, DC, ACOG, 1995.
90. American College of Obstetricians and Gynecologists: Guidelines for Vaginal Delivery After a Previous Cesarean Birth. Committee Opinion NO 143 [replaces No. 64, October 1988]. Washington, DC, ACOG, 1994.
91. Flamm BL, Newman LA, Thomas SJ, et al: Vaginal birth after cesarean delivery: results of a 5-year multicenter collaborative study. Obstet Gynecol 76:750, 1990.
92. Flamm B, Goings J, Yunbao L, Wolde-Tsadik G: Elective repeat cesarean section delivery versus trial of labor: a prospective multicenter study. Obstet Gynecol 83:927, 1994.
93. Rosen MG, Dickinson JC,Westhoff CL: Vaginal birth after cesarean: A meta-analysis of morbidity and mortality. Obstet Gynecol 77:465, 1991.
94. Paul RH, Phelan JP, Yeh S: Trial of labor in the patient with a prior cesarean birth. Am J Obstet Gynecol 151:297, 1985.
95. Martin JN Jr, Harris BA Jr, Huddleston JF, et al: Vaginal delivery following previous cesarean birth. Am J Obstet Gynecol 146:255, 1983.
96. Beall M, Eglinton GS, Clark SL, et al: Vaginal delivery after cesarean section in women with unknown types of uterine scars. J Reprod Med 29:31, 1984.
97. Pruett K, Kirshon B, Cotton D: Unknown uterine scar in trial of labor. Am J Obstet Gynecol 159:807, 1988.
98. Scott J: Mandatory trial of labor after cesarean delivery: an alternative viewpoint. Obstet Gynecol 77:811, 1991.
99. Pitkin RM: Once a cesarean? Obstet Gynecol 77:939, 1991.
100. Sachs BP, Kobelin C, Castro MA, Frigoletto F: The risks of lowering the cesarean-delivery rate. N Engl J Med 340:54, 1990.
101. Farmer RM, Kirschbaum T, Potter D, et al: Uterine rupture during a trial of labor after previous cesarean section. Am J Obstet Gynecol 165:996, 1991.
102. Boucher M, Tahilramaney MP, Eglinton GS, et al: Maternal morbidity as related to trial of labor after previous cesarean delivery: a quantitative analysis. J Reprod Med 29:12, 1984.
103. Leung AS, Farmer RM, Leung EK, et al: Risk factors associated with uterine rupture during trial of labor after cesarean delivery: a case controlled study. Am J Obstet Gynecol 168:1358, 1993.
104. Arulkumaran S, Chua S, Ratnam SS: Symptoms and signs with scar rupture—value of uterine activity measurements. Aust N Z J Obstet Gynaecol 32:208, 1992.
105. Vaginal birth after previous cesarean delivery: clinical management guidelines for obstetricians-gynecologists. ACOG practice bulletin no. 5. Washington D.C.: American College of Obstetricians and Gynecologists, July 1999.
106. Vaginal birth after previous cesarean delivery: clinical management guidelines for obstetrician-gynecologists. ACOG Practice Bulletin No. 54. Washington D.C. American College of Obstetricians and Gynecologists, July 2004.
107. Whiteside DC, Mahan SC, Cook JC: Factors associated with successful vaginal delivery after cesarean section. J Reprod Med 28:785, 1983.
108. Silver RK, Gibbs RS: Prediction of vaginal delivery in patients with a previous cesarean section who require oxytocin. Am J Obstet Gynecol 156:57, 1987.
109. Flamm BL: Vaginal birth after cesarean section. *In* Flamm BL, Quilligan EJ (eds): Cesarean section: guidelines for appropriate utilization. New York: Springer-Verlag, 1995, p 51.
110. Gregory KD, Korst LM, Cane P, et al: Vaginal birth after cesarean and uterine rupture rates in California. Obstet Gynecol 93:985, 1999.
111. Landon MB, Leindecker S, Spong CY for the National Institute of Child Health and Human Development Maternal-Fetal Medicine Units Network: The MFMU Cesarean Registry: Factors affecting the success and trial of labor following prior cesarean delivery. Am J Obstet Gynecol 193:1016, 2005.
112. Elkousky MA, Samuel M, Stevens E, et al: The effect of birthweight on vaginal birth after cesarean delivery success rates. Am J Obstet Gynecol 188:824, 2003.
113. Coughlan C, Kearney R, Turner MJ: What are the implications for the next delivery in primigravidae who have an elective cesarean section for breech presentation? Br J Obstet Gynaecol 109:624, 2002.
114. Flamm BL, Geiger AM: Vaginal birth after cesarean delivery: an admission scoring system. Obstet Gynecol 90:907, 1997.
115. Abitol MM, Castillo I, Taylor UB, et al: Vaginal birth after cesarean section: the patient's point of view. Am Fam Physician 47:129, 1993.
116. Ollendorff DA, Goldberg JM, Minoque JP, Socol ML: Vaginal birth after cesarean section for arrest of labor: is success determined by maximum cervical dilatation during the prior labor? Am J Obstet Gynecol 159:636, 1988.
117. Jongen VHWM, Halfwerk MGC, Brouwer WK: Vaginal delivery after previous cesarean section for failure of second stage of labour. Br J Obstet Gynecol 195:1079, 1998.
118. Hoskins IA, Gomez JL: Correlation between maximum cervical dilation at cesarean delivery and subsequent vaginal birth after cesarean delivery. Obstet Gynecol 89:591, 1997.
119. Caughey AB, Shipp TD, Repke JT, et al: Trial of labor after cesarean delivery: The effects of previous vaginal delivery. Am J Obstet Gynecol 179:938, 1998.
120. Flamm BL, Goings JR: Vaginal birth after cesarean section: is suspected fetal macrosomia a contraindication? Obstet Gynecol 74:694, 1989.
121. Weinstein D, Benshushan A, Tanos V, et al: Predictive score for vaginal birth after cesarean section. Am J Obstet Gynecol 174:192, 1996.
122. Shipp TD, Zelop CM, Repke JT, et al: Labor after previous cesarean: influence of prior indication and parity. Obstet Gynecol 95:913, 2000.
123. Grinstead J, Grobman WA: Induction of labor after one prior cesarean: predictors of vaginal delivery. Obstet Gynecol 103:534, 2004.
124. Rosen MG, Dicknson JC: Vaginal birth after cesarean: a meta-analysis of indicators for success. Obstet Gynecol 76:865, 1990.
125. Caughey AB, Shipp TD, Repke JT, et al: Rate of uterine rupture during a trial of labor in women with one or two prior cesarean deliveries. Am J Obstet Gynecol 181:872, 1999.
126. Miller DA, Diaz FG, Paul RH: Vaginal birth after cesarean: a 10 year experience. Obstet Gynecol 84:255, 1994.
127. Landon MB, Spong CY, Thom E for the National Institute of Child Health and Human Development Maternal-Fetal Medicine Units Network. Risk of uterine rupture with a trial of labor in women with multiple and single prior cesarean delivery. Obstet Gynecol 108:12, 2006.
128. Macones GA, Cahill A, Para E, et al: Obstetric outcomes in women with two prior cesarean deliveries: Is vaginal birth after cesarean delivery a viable option? Am J Obstet Gynecol 1223, 2005.
129. Kieser KE, Baskett TF: A 10-year population-based study of uterine rupture. Obstet Gynecol 100:749, 2002.
130. Mozurkewich EL, Hutton EK: Elective repeat cesarean delivery versus trial of labor: a meta-analysis of the literature from 1989 to 1999. Am J Obstet Gynecol 183:1187, 2000.
131. Vaginal Birth After Cesarean (VBAC). Rockville, Md.: Agency for Health Care Research and Quality. March 2003. (AHRQ publication no. 03-E018.)
132. Guise JM, McDonagh MS, Osterweil P, et al: Systematic review of the incidence and consequences of uterine rupture in women with previous cesarean section. BMJ 329:19, 2004.
133. Landon MB, Hauth JC, Leveno KJ, et al for the National Institute of Child Health and Human Development Maternal-Fetal Medicine Units Network: Maternal and perinatal outcomes associated

with a trial of labor after prior cesarean delivery. N Engl J Med 351:2581, 2004.
134. Naif RW 3rd, Ray MA, Chauhan SP, et al: Trial of labor after cesarean delivery with a lower-segment, vertical uterine incision: is it safe? Am J Obstet Gynecol 172:1666, 1995.
135. Shipp TD, Zelop CM, Repke TJ, et al: Intrapartum uterine rupture and dehiscence in patients with prior lower uterine segment vertical and transverse incisions. Obstet Gynecol 94:735, 1999.
136. Chauhan SP, Martin JN Jr, Henrichs CE, et al: Maternal and perinatal complications with uterine rupture in 142,075 patients who attempted vaginal birth after cesarean delivery: a review of the literature. Am J Obstet Gynecol 189:408, 2003.
137. Zelop CM, Shipp TD, Repke JT, et al: Uterine rupture during induced or augmented labor in gravid women with one prior cesarean delivery. Am J Obstet Gynecol 181:882, 1999.
138. Macones G, Peipert J, Nelson D, et al: Maternal complications with vaginal birth after cesarean delivery: a multicenter study. Am J Obstet Gynecol 193:1656, 2005.
139. Shipp TD, Zelop CM, Repke JT, et al: Interdelivery interval and risk of symptomatic uterine rupture. Obstet Gyencol 97:175, 2001.
140. Huang WH, Nakashima DK, Rummey PJ, et al: Interdelivery interval and the success of vaginal birth after cesarean delivery. Obstet Gynecol 99:41, 2002.
141. Bujold E, Mehta SH, Bujold C, Gauthier RJ: Interdelivery interval and uterine rupture. Am J Obstet Gynecol 187:199, 2002.
142. Lydon-Rochelle M, Holt V, Easterling TR, Martin DP: Risk of uterine rupture during labor among women with a prior cesarean delivery. N Engl J Med 345:36, 3001.
143. Stone JL, Lockwood CJ, Berkowitz G, et al: Use of cervical prostaglandin E_2 gel in patients with previous cesarean section. Am J Perinatol 11:309, 1994.
144. Plaut MM, Schwartz ML, Lubarsky SL: Uterine rupture ssociated with the use of misoprostol in the gravid patient with a previous cesarean section. Am J Obstet Gynecol 180:1535, 1999.
145. Wing DA, Lovett K, Paul RH: Disruption of prior uterine incision following misoprostol for labor induction in women with previous cesarean delivery. Obstet Gynecol 91:828, 1998.
146. ACOG Practice Bulletin: Induction of Labor. No 10, 1999.
147. McMahon MJ, Luther ER, Bowes WA, Olshan AF: Comparison of a trial of labor with an elective second cesarean section. N Engl J Med 335:689, 1996.
148. Jones R, Nagashima A, Hartnett-Goodman M, Goodlin R: Rupture of low transverse cesarean scars during trial of labor. Obstet Gynecol 77:815, 1991.
149. Rodriguez M, Masaki D, Phelan J, Diaz F: Uterine rupture: are intrauterine pressure catheters useful in the diagnosis? Am J Obstet Gynecol 161:666, 1989.
150. Clark SL, Scott JR, Porter TF, et al: Is vaginal birth after cesarean less expensive than repeat cesarean delivery? Am J Obstet Gynecol 182:599, 2000.
151. Bujold E, Gauthier RJ: Should we allow a trial of labor after a previous cesarean for dystocia in the second stage of labor? Obstet Gynecol 99:520, 2002.
152. Goetzel L, Shipp TD, Cohen A, et al: Oxytocin dose and the risk of uterine rupture in trial of labor after cesarean. Obstet Gynecol 97:381, 2001.
153. Clark SL, Yeh S-Y, Phelan JP, et al: Emergency hysterectomy for obstetric hemorrhage. Obstet Gynecol 64:376, 1984.
154. Shellhaas C for the NICHD MFMU Network. The MFMU Cesarean Registry: Hysterectomy—Its indications, morbidities, and mortalities. Abstract No. 155. Am J Obstet Gynecol 185: S123, 2002.
155. Zelop CM, Harlow BL, Frigoletto FD Jr, et al: Emergency peripartum hysterectomy. Am J Obstet Gynecol 168:1443, 1993.
156. Eisenkep SM, Richman R, Platt LD, et al: Urinary tract injury during cesarean section. Obstet Gynecol 60:591, 1982.
157. Mickal A, Begneaud WP, Hawes TP Jr: Pitfalls and complications of cesarean section hysterectomy. Clin Obstet Gynecol 12:660, 1969.
158. Viscomi CM, Rathmell JP: Labor epidural catheter reactivation or spinal anesthesia for delayed postpartum tubal ligation: a cost comparison. J Clin Anesth 7:380, 1995.
159. Peterson HB, Xia Z, Hughes JM, et al: The risk of pregnancy after tubal sterilization: findings from the U.S. Collaborative Review of Sterilization. Am J Obstet Gynecol 174:1161, 1996.
160. Bishop E, Nelms WF: A simple method of tubal sterilization. N Y State J Med 30:214, 1930.
161. Irving FC: Tubal sterilization. Am J Obstet Gynecol 60:1101, 1950.
162. Lopez-Zeno JA, Muallem NS, Anderson JB: The Irving sterilization technique: a report of a failure. Int J Fertil 35:23, 1990.
163. Uchida H: Uchida tubal sterilization. Am J Obstet Gynecol 121:153, 1975.

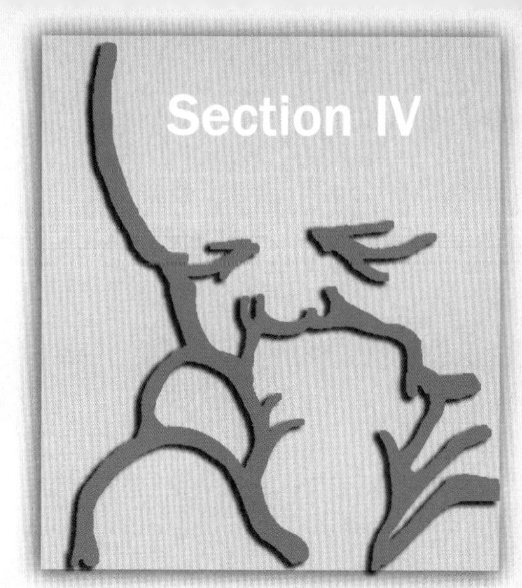

Postpartum Care

The Neonate

ADAM A. ROSENBERG

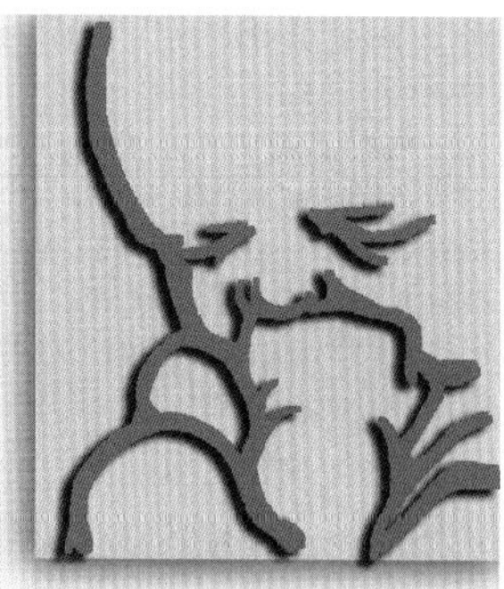

CHAPTER 20

KEY ABBREVIATIONS

Appropriate for gestational age	AGA
Central nervous system	CNS
Chronic lung disease	CLD
Computed tomography	CT
Cyclic adenosine monophosphate	cAMP
Dipalmitoylphosphatidylcholine	DPPC
Docohexanoic acid	DHA
Functional residual capacity	FRC
Glucose-6-phosphate dehydrogenase	G6PD
Group B streptococcus	GBS
Hyaline membrane disease	HMD
Human immunodeficiency virus	HIV
Idiopathic thrombocytopenic purpura	ITP
Inferior vena cava	IVC
Intrauterine growth restriction	IUGR
Large for gestational age	LGA
Magnetic resonance imaging	MRI
Meconium aspiration syndrome	MAS
Necrotizing enterocolitis	NEC
Periventricular/intraventricular hemorrhage	PVH/IVH
Periventricular leukomalacia	PVL
Persistent pulmonary hypertension of the newborn	PPHN
Pulmonary vascular resistance	PVR
Rapid eye movement sleep	REM
Respiratory distress syndrome	RDS
Small for gestational age	SGA
Surfactant protein	SP
Thyroid-releasing hormone	TRH
Thyroid-stimulating hormone	TSH
Uridine diphosphoglucuronosyl transferase	UDPGT

The first 4 weeks of an infant's life, the neonatal period, are marked by the highest mortality rate in all of childhood. The greatest risk occurs during the first several days after birth. Critical to survival during this period is the infant's ability to adapt successfully to extrauterine life. During the early hours after birth, the newborn must assume responsibility for thermoregulation, metabolic homeostasis, and respiratory gas exchange, as well as undergo the conversion from fetal to postnatal circulatory pathways. This chapter reviews the physiology of a successful transition as well as the implications of circumstances that disrupt this process. Implicit in these considerations is the understanding that the newborn reflects the sum total of its genetic and environmental past as well as any minor or major insults to which it was subjected during gestation and parturition. The period of neonatal adaptation is then most meaningfully viewed as continuous with fetal life.

CARDIOPULMONARY TRANSITION

Pulmonary Development

Lung development and maturation require a carefully regulated interaction of anatomic, physiologic, and biochemical processes. The outcome of these events provides an organ with adequate surface area, sufficient vascularization, and the metabolic capability to sustain oxygenation and ventilation during the neonatal period. Five stages of morphologic lung development have been identified in the human fetus[1]:

1. Embryonic period—3 to 7 weeks postconception
2. Pseudoglandular period—5th to 17th weeks
3. Canalicular period—16th to 26th weeks
4. Saccular period—24th to 38th weeks
5. Alveolar period—36 weeks to 2 years after birth

The lung arises as a ventral diverticulum from the foregut during the fourth week of gestation. During the ensuing weeks, branching of the diverticulum occurs, leading to a tree of narrow tubes with thick epithelial walls composed of columnar-type cells. Experimental studies demonstrate that this patterning of the developing lung is regulated by interactions with surrounding mesenchyme.[2] Molecular mechanisms involved in these early phases of lung development include expression of transcription factors that are important for specification of the foregut endoderm, endogenous secretion of polypeptides that are important for pattern formation, growth and differentiation factors critical to cell development, and involvement of exogenous agents such as retinoic acid.[3–5] By 16 weeks, the conducting portion of the tracheobronchial tree up to and including terminal bronchioles has been established. The vasculature derived from the pulmonary circulation develops concurrently with the conducting airways, and by 16 weeks preacinar blood vessels are formed.[6,7] The canalicular stage is characterized by differentiation of the airways, with widening of the airways and thinning of epithelium. In addition, primitive respiratory bronchioles begin to form, marking the start of the gas-exchanging portion of the lung. Vascular proliferation continues, along with a relative decrease in mesenchyme, bringing the vessels closer to the airway epithelium. The saccular stage is marked by the development of the gas-exchanging portion of the tracheobronchial tree (acinus) composed of respiratory bronchioles, alveolar ducts, terminal saccules, and finally, alveoli. During this stage, the pulmonary vessels continue to proliferate with the airways and surround the developing air sacs. The final phase of prenatal lung development (alveolar) is marked by the formation of thin secondary alveolar septae and the remodeling of the capillary bed. Several million alveoli will form before birth, which emphasizes the importance of the last few weeks of pregnancy to pulmonary adaptation. Postnatal lung growth is characterized by generation of alveoli. At birth, there are approximately 50 million airspaces, and by 8 years of age, there are 300 million.[1]

The critical determinants of extrauterine survival are the formation of the thin air-blood barrier and production of surfactant. By the time of birth, the epithelial lining of the gas-exchanging surface is thin and continuous with two alveolar cell types (types I and II). Type I cells contain few subcellular organelles, whereas type II cells contain abundant mitochondria, endoplasmic reticulum, Golgi apparatus, and osmiophilic lamellar bodies known to contain surfactant. The synthesis and metabolism of surfactant is presented in Figure 20-1. Surfactant lipids are processed in the Golgi apparatus to multivesicular bodies that associate with surfactant protein B and C. This complex is stored in membrane enclosed structures called lamellar bodies. Surfactant is secreted by exocytosis as lamellar bodies unravel into tubular myelin. The other surfactant proteins (A and D) are secreted independently of the lamellar bodies. Tubular myelin is a loose lattice of phospholipids and surfactant-specific proteins. The surface active component of surfactant then adsorbs at the alveolar interface between air and water in a monolayer.[8] With repetitive expansion and compression of the surface monolayer, material is extruded that is either cleared by alveolar macrophages through endocytic pathways or taken up by the type II cell for recycling back into lamellar bodies.[9]

Because of the development of high surface forces along the respiratory epithelium when breathing begins, the availability of surfactants in terminal airspaces is critical to postnatal lung function. Just as surface tension acts to reduce the size of a bubble in water, so, too, it acts to reduce lung inflation, promoting atelectasis. This is described by the LaPlace relationship, which states that the pressure, P, within a sphere is directly proportional to surface tension, T, and inversely proportional to the radius of curvature, r (Fig. 20-2). Surfactant has the physical property of variable surface tension dependent on the degree of surface area compression. In other words, as the radius of the alveolus decreases, surfactant serves to reduce surface tension, preventing collapse of the alveolus. If this property is extrapolated to the lung, smaller alveoli will remain stable because of lower surface tension than other larger alveoli. This feature is emphasized in Figure 20-3, which compares pressure-volume curves from surfactant-deficient and surfactant-treated preterm rabbits. Surfactant deficiency is characterized by high opening pressure, low maximal lung volume, and lack of deflation stability at low pressures.[10]

Saturated phosphatidylcholine (the surface tension-reducing component of surfactant) is found in lung tissue of the human fetus earlier in gestation than in other species (Fig. 20-4).[11] Tissue stores of surfactant are considerable at term. Surfactant is released from storage pools into fetal lung fluid at a basal rate during late gestation. Secretion is stimulated by labor and the initiation of air breathing.[12]

Natural surfactant contains 80 percent phospholipids, 10 percent neutral lipids, and 10 percent protein (Fig. 20-5).[10,13] Approximately half of the protein is

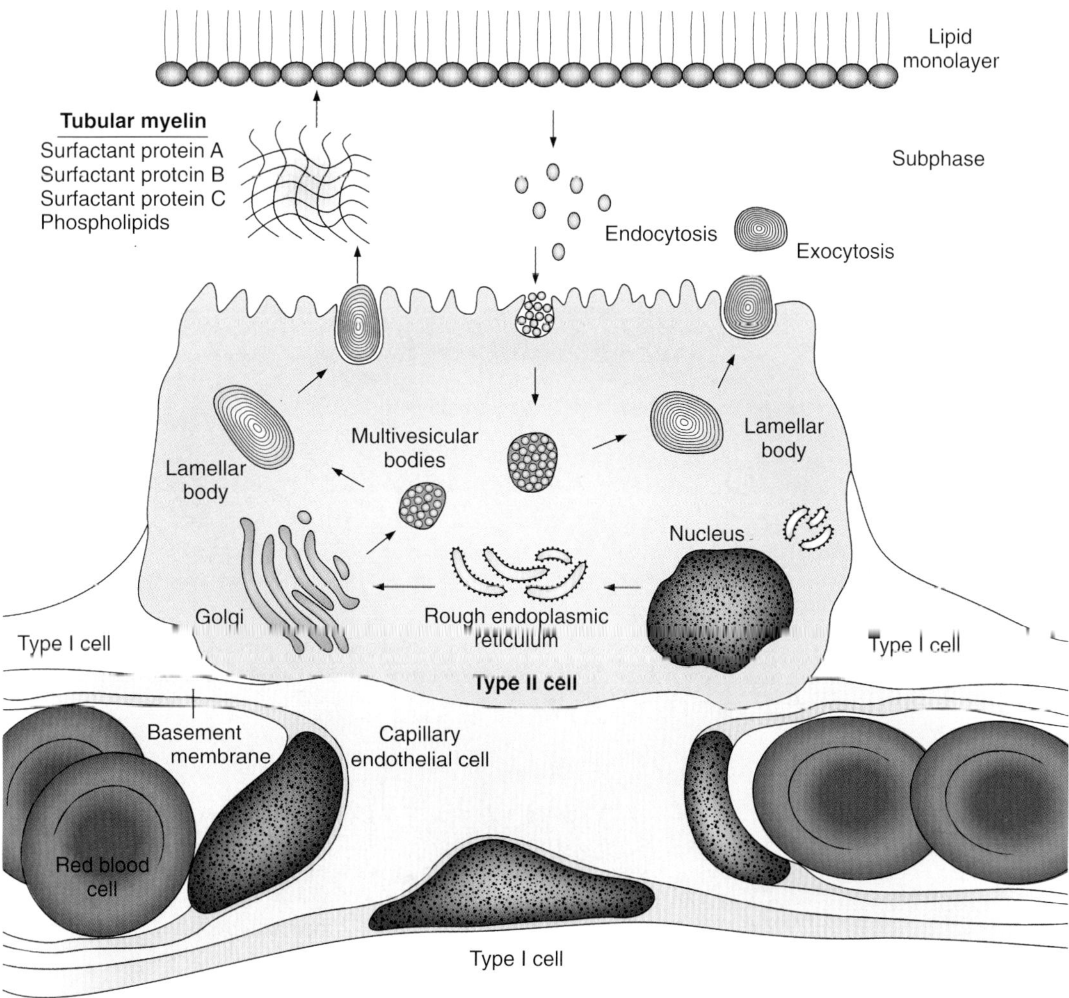

Figure 20-1. Metabolism of surfactant. Surfactant phospholipids are synthesized in the endoplasmic reticulum, transported through the Golgi apparatus to multivesicular bodies, and finally packaged in lamellar bodies. After lamellar body exocytosis, phospholipids are organized into tubular myelin before aligning in a monolayer at the air-fluid interface in the alveolus. Surfactant phospholipids and proteins are taken up by type II cells and either catabolized or reused. Surfactant proteins are synthesized in polyribosomes, modified in endoplasmic reticulum, Golgi apparatus, and multivesicular bodies. (Adapted from Whitsett JA, Pryhuber GS, Rice WR, et al: Acute respiratory disorders. *In* Avery GB, Fletcher MA, MacDonald MG [eds]: Neonatology: Pathophysiology and Management of the Newborn, 5th ed. Philadelphia, Lippincott Williams & Wilkins, 1999, p 485, with permission.)

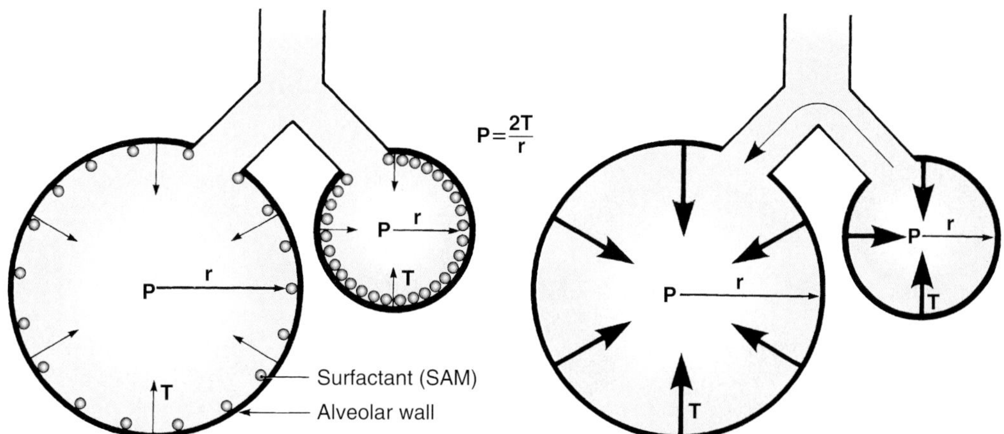

Figure 20-2. LaPlace's law. The pressure, P, within a sphere is directly proportional to surface tension, T, and inversely proportional to the radius of curvature, r. In the normal lung, as alveolar size decreases, surface tension is reduced because of the presence of surfactant. This serves to decrease the collapsing pressure that needs to be opposed and maintains equal pressures in the small and large interconnected alveoli. (Adapted from Netter FH: The Ciba Collection of Medical Illustrations. The Respiratory System, Vol 7. Summit, NJ, Ciba-Geigy, 1979, with permission.)

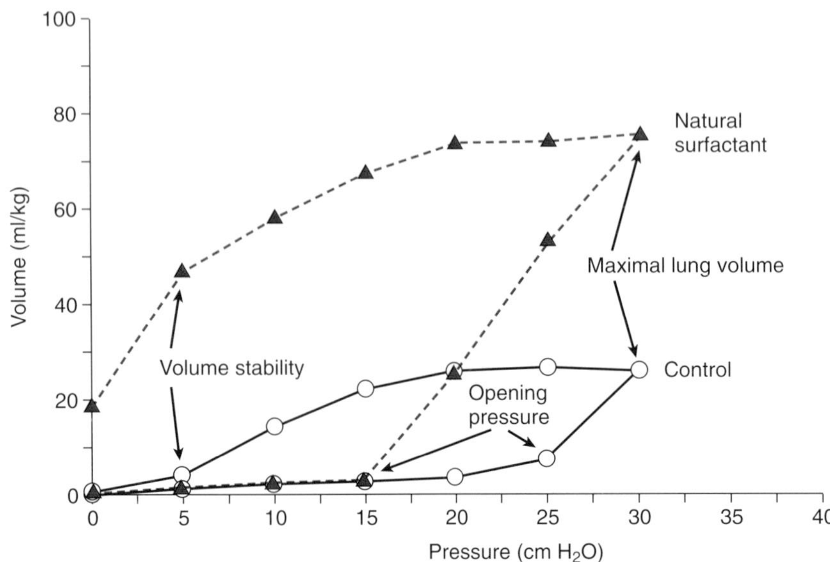

Figure 20-3. Pressure-volume relationships for the inflation and deflation of surfactant-deficient and surfactant-treated preterm rabbit lungs. Surfactant deficiency is indicated by high opening pressure, low maximal volume at a distending pressure of 30 cm of water, and the lack of deflation stability at low pressures on deflation. (Adapted from Jobe AH: Lung development and maturation. *In* Fanaroff AA, Martin RJ [eds]: Neonatal-Perinatal Medicine: Diseases of the Fetus and Infant, 7th ed. St. Louis, Mosby Inc, 2002, p 973, with permission.)

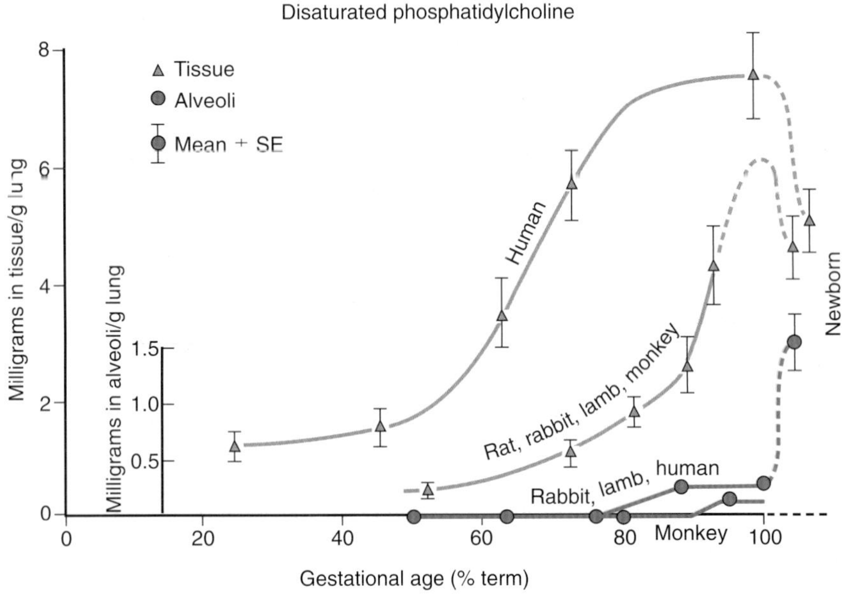

Figure 20-4. Accumulation of saturated phosphatidylcholine during gestation. Gestational age is plotted as percentage of term. (Adapted from Clements JA, Tooley WH: Kinetics of surface-active material in the fetal lung. *In* Hodson WA [ed]: Development of the Lung. New York, Marcel Dekker, 1977, with permission.)

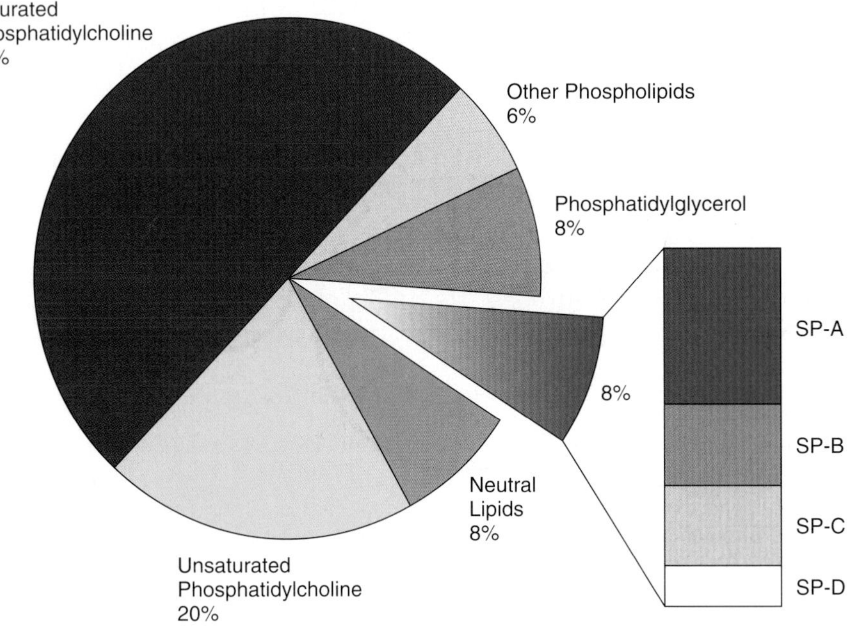

Figure 20-5. Composition of pulmonary surfactant. SP, surfactant protein. (Adapted from Jobe AH: Lung development and maturation. *In* Fanaroff AA, Martin RJ [eds]: Neonatal-Perinatal Medicine: Diseases of the Fetus and Infant, 7th ed. St Louis, Mosby Inc, 2002, p 973, with permission.)

specific for surfactant. The principal classes of phospholipids are saturated phosphatidylcholine compounds, 45 percent (more than 80 percent of which are dipalmitoylphosphatidylcholine [DPPC]); 25 percent unsaturated phosphatidylcholine compounds; and 10 percent phosphatidylglycerol, phosphatidylinositol, and phosphatidylethanolamine. Four unique surfactant-associated proteins have been identified.[13] All are synthesized and secreted by type II alveolar cells. DPPC is the molecule critical to the surface tension–lowering property of surfactant at the air-liquid interface in the alveolus. Surfactant protein (SP)–A functions cooperatively with the other surfactant proteins and lipids to enhance the biophysical activity of surfactant, but its most important role is in innate host defense of the lung.[13] SP-B and SP-C are lipophilic proteins that facilitate the adsorption and spreading of lipid to form the surfactant monolayer. SP-B deficiencies are associated with neonatal pulmonary complications and death.[14] SP-D plays a role in the regulation of surfactant lipid homeostasis, inflammatory responses, and host defense mechanisms.[13]

Several hormones and growth factors contribute to the regulation of pulmonary phospholipid metabolism and lung maturation: glucocorticoids, thyroid hormone, thyrotropin-releasing hormone, retinoic acid, cyclic adenosine monophosphate (cAMP), epidermal growth factor, and others. Glucocorticoids are the most important of the stimulating factors. They augment the synthesis of all surfactant components and accelerate morphologic development.[15,16]

Pregnant women with anticipated preterm delivery have received corticosteroid treatment since 1972.[17] Numerous controlled trials have since been done and have been cumulatively evaluated using meta-analysis.[18] Based on such analysis, a significant reduction of about 50 percent in the incidence of respiratory distress syndrome (RDS) is seen in infants born to mothers who received antenatal corticosteroids. In secondary analysis, a 70-percent reduction in RDS was seen among babies born between 24 hours and 7 days after corticosteroid administration. In addition, evidence suggests a reduction in mortality and RDS even with treatment started less than 24 hours before delivery. Although most babies in the trials were between 30 and 34 weeks' gestation, clear reduction in RDS was evident when the population of babies less than 31 weeks was examined. Gender and race do not influence the protective effect of corticosteroids. In the population of patients with preterm premature rupture of the membranes, antenatal corticosteroids also reduce the frequency of RDS.

Corticosteroids also accelerate maturation of other organs in the developing fetus, including cardiovascular, gastrointestinal, and central nervous system (CNS). Corticosteroid therapy reduces the chances of both periventricular-intraventricular hemorrhage (PVH/IVH) and necrotizing enterocolitis (NEC).[18,19] The significant reductions in serious neonatal morbidity are also reflected in a reduction in the risk of early neonatal mortality. The short-term beneficial effects of antenatal corticosteroids are enhanced by reassuring reports about long-term outcome. The children of mothers treated with antenatal corticosteroids show no lag in intellectual or motor development, no increase in learning disabilities or behavioral disturbances, and no effect on growth compared with untreated infants.[20,21]

Since the advent of antenatal steroids for the prevention of RDS, other maternal and neonatal therapies have been introduced that decrease mortality and morbidity. Surfactant replacement therapy to treat specifically the surfactant deficiency that is the cause of RDS has been shown to decrease mortality and the severity of RDS.[22–25] The effects of antenatal corticosteroids and postnatal surfactant appear to be additive in terms of decreasing the severity of and mortality caused by RDS.[26] Thyroid-releasing hormone (TRH) has also been used as an agent to accelerate lung maturation. TRH crosses the placenta and elicits a striking fetal thyroid-stimulating hormone (TSH) response.[27] Animal studies have demonstrated improvement in fetal pulmonary maturation after maternal administration of TRH.[28] The collective results of human clinical trials, however, suggest that a combination of prenatal glucocorticoids and postnatal surfactant replacement is not enhanced by the administration of TRH.[29]

The First Breaths

A critical step in the transition from intrauterine to extrauterine life is the conversion of the lung from a dormant fluid-filled organ to one capable of gas exchange. This requires aeration of the lungs, establishment of an adequate pulmonary circulation, ventilation of the aerated parenchyma, and diffusion of oxygen and carbon dioxide through the alveolar-capillary membranes. This process has its origins in utero as fetal breathing.

Fetal Breathing

Fetal breathing has been demonstrated in a large number of mammalian species.[30] Fetal breathing has been most extensively studied in fetal sheep and to a lesser degree in humans. Fetal breathing in third-trimester fetal sheep occurs primarily during periods of low-voltage electrocortical activity (rapid-eye-movement [REM] sleep).[31,32] The predominant respiratory pattern is one of rapid, irregular movements varying in amplitude at a rate of 60 to 120 per minute. Isolated deep inspiratory efforts can occur at one to three times per minute unassociated with any particular stage of sleep. During high-voltage electrocortical activity (quiet sleep), only occasional breaths occur after tonic muscular discharges associated with body movements. The onset of breathing in the fetal sheep has been noted as early as 40 days of gestation. By days 90 through 115, breathing is almost continuous, with rare apneic pauses of less than 2 minutes' duration. From day 115 to term, breathing is episodic, as described earlier. Human fetal breathing is similar to that observed in fetal sheep.[33] Respiratory activity is initially detectable at 11 weeks. The most prevalent pattern is rapid, small-amplitude movements (60 to 90 per minute) present 60 to 80 percent of the time. Less commonly, irregular low-amplitude movements interspersed with slower larger amplitude movements are seen.

Initially, fetal breathing was thought to depend on behavioral influences. However, subsequent work has shown responses to chemical stimuli and other agents. Acute hypercapnea stimulates breathing in both human and sheep fetuses.[34,35] Hypoxia abolishes fetal breathing,[35] whereas an increase in oxygen tension to levels above 200 mm Hg induces continuous fetal breathing.[36] Hyperglycemia after bolus injections of glucose to the mother or after ingestion of a meal increases fetal breathing in humans.[37,38] Of the pulmonary reflexes, the inflation reflex (decreasing frequency of breathing) is active in fetal life.[39] Peripheral and central chemoreflexes as well as vagal afferent reflexes can be demonstrated in the fetus, but their role in spontaneous fetal breathing appears minimal.[40]

Breathing is intermittent in the fetus and becomes continuous after birth. The mechanism responsible for this transition is unknown. In the fetal lamb, the REM sleep dependence of breathing can be overcome in a number of ways. The most profound continuous intrauterine breathing is caused by prolonged infusion of large doses of prostaglandin synthesis inhibitors,[41] suggesting that prostaglandins may be involved in the transition to continuous postnatal respiration. Other factors surrounding birth, including blood gas changes and various sensory stimuli, are also postulated to be involved.[10,12] Another factor possibly involved is the "release" from a placental inhibitory factor that is removed after cord occlusion.[43]

The role of fetal breathing in the continuum from fetal to neonatal life is still not completely understood. Fetal respiratory activity is probably essential to the development of chest wall muscles (including diaphragm) and serves as a regulator of lung fluid volume and thus lung growth.[40]

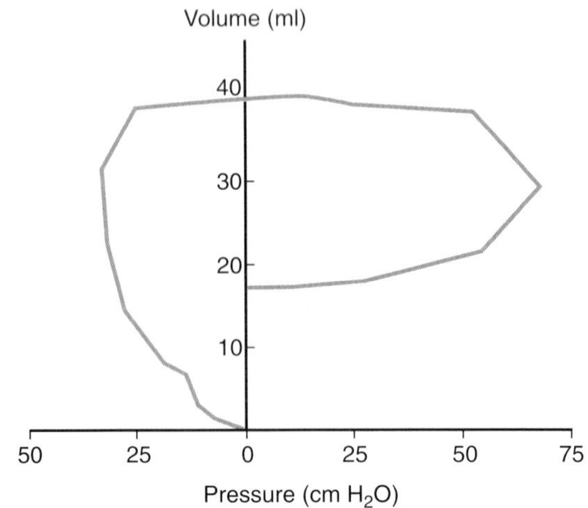

Figure 20-6. Pressure-volume loop of the first breath. Air enters the lung as soon as intrathoracic pressure falls and expiratory pressure greatly exceeds inspiratory pressure. (Modified from Milner AD, Vyas H: Lung expansion at birth. J Pediatr 101:879, 1982, with permission.)

Mechanics of the First Breath

With its first breaths, the neonate must overcome several forces resisting lung expansion: (1) viscosity of fetal lung fluid, (2) resistance provided by lung tissue itself, and (3) the forces of surface tension at the air-liquid interface.[44] Viscosity of fetal lung fluid is a major factor as the neonate attempts to displace fluid present in the large airways. As the passage of air moves toward small airways and alveoli, surface tension becomes more important. Resistance to expansion by the lung tissue itself is less significant. The process begins as the infant passes through the birth canal. The intrathoracic pressure caused by vaginal squeeze is up to 200 cm H_2O.[45,46] With delivery of the head, approximately 5 to 28 ml of tracheal fluid is expressed. Subsequent delivery of the thorax causes an elastic recoil of the chest. With this recoil, a small passive inspiration (no more than 2 ml) occurs.[45] This is accompanied by glossopharyngeal forcing of some air into the proximal airways (frog breathing)[47] and the introduction of some blood into pulmonary capillaries.[48,49] This pulmonary vascular pressure may have a role in producing initial continuous surfaces throughout the small airways of the lung into which surfactant can deploy.[49]

The initial breath is characteristically a short inspiration, followed by a more prolonged expiration (Fig. 20-6).[45,50,51] The initial breath begins with no air volume and no transpulmonary pressure gradient. Considerable negative intrathoracic pressure during inspiration is provided by diaphragmatic contraction and chest wall expansion. An opening pressure of about 25 cm H_2O usually is necessary to overcome surface tension in the smaller airways and alveoli before air begins to enter. The volume of this first breath varies between 30 and 67 ml and correlates with intrathoracic pressure. The expiratory phase is prolonged, because the infant's expiration is opposed by intermittent closure at the pharyngolaryngeal level[47] with the generation of large positive intrathoracic pressure. This pressure serves to aid both in maintenance of a functional residual capacity (FRC) and with fluid removal from the air sacs. The residual volume after this first breath ranges between 4 and 30 ml, averaging 16 to 20 ml. There are really no major systematic differences among the first three breaths, demonstrating similar pressure patterns of decreasing magnitude. The FRC rapidly increases with the first several breaths and then more gradually. By 30 minutes of age, most infants attain a normal FRC with uniform lung expansion.[52] The presence of functional surfactant is instrumental in the accumulation of an FRC.[12]

In utero, alveoli are open and stable at nearly neonatal lung volume because they are filled with fetal lung liquid, probably produced by ultrafiltration of pulmonary capillary blood as well as by secretion by alveolar cells.[53] Transepithelial chloride secretion appears to be a major factor responsible for the production of luminal liquid in the fetal lung.[54,55] Normal expansion and aeration of the neonatal lung is dependent on removal of fetal lung liquid. Liquid is removed by a combination of mechanical drainage and absorption across the lung epithelium.[56] This process begins before a normal term birth because of decreased fluid secretion and increased absorption. Once labor is initiated, there is a reversal of liquid flow across the lung epithelium.[57] Active transcellular sodium absorption drives liquid from the lumen to interstitial space, where it is drained through the pulmonary circulation and lymphatics.[56,58–60] In normal circumstances, the process is complete within 2 hours of birth. Cesarean-delivered infants without benefit of labor and premature infants have delayed lung fluid clearance. In both groups, the prenatal decrease in lung water does not occur.[56,61] In addition, in the premature neonate, fluid clearance is diminished by increased alveolar surface tension, increased left atrial pressure, and hypoproteinemia.[62]

Circulatory Transition

The circulation in the fetus (Fig. 20-7) has been studied in a variety of species using several techniques (see Chapter 2).[63,64]

Umbilical venous blood, returning from the placenta, has a Po_2 of about 30 to 35 mm Hg. Because of the left shift of the oxyhemoglobin disassociation curve caused by fetal hemoglobin, this corresponds to a saturation of 80 to 90 percent. About 60 percent of this blood passes through the liver (mainly to the middle and left lobes). This blood ultimately enters the inferior vena cava (IVC) through the hepatic veins. The remainder (40 percent midgestation; 20 percent at term) bypasses the hepatic circulation through the ductus venosus, which empties directly into the IVC.[65,66] Because of streaming in the IVC, the more oxygenated blood from the ductus venosus and left hepatic vein, as it enters the heart, is deflected by the crista dividens through the foramen ovale to the left atrium. The remainder of left atrial blood is the small amount of venous return from the pulmonary circulation. The remainder of return from the IVC, less oxygenated blood from the lower body, renal, mesenteric, and right hepatic veins, streams across the tricuspid valve to the right ventricle. Almost all the return from the superior vena cava (SVC) and the coronary sinus passes through the tricuspid valve to the right ventricle, with only 2 to 3 percent crossing the foramen ovale. In the near-term fetus, the combined ventricular output is about 450 ml/kg/min. Two thirds of the cardiac output is from the right ventricle, and one third is from the left ventricle. The blood in the left ventricle has a Po_2 of 25 to 28 mm Hg (saturation of 60 percent) and is distributed to the coronary circulation, brain, head, and upper extremities, with the remainder (10 percent of combined output) passing into the descending aorta. The major portion of the right ven-

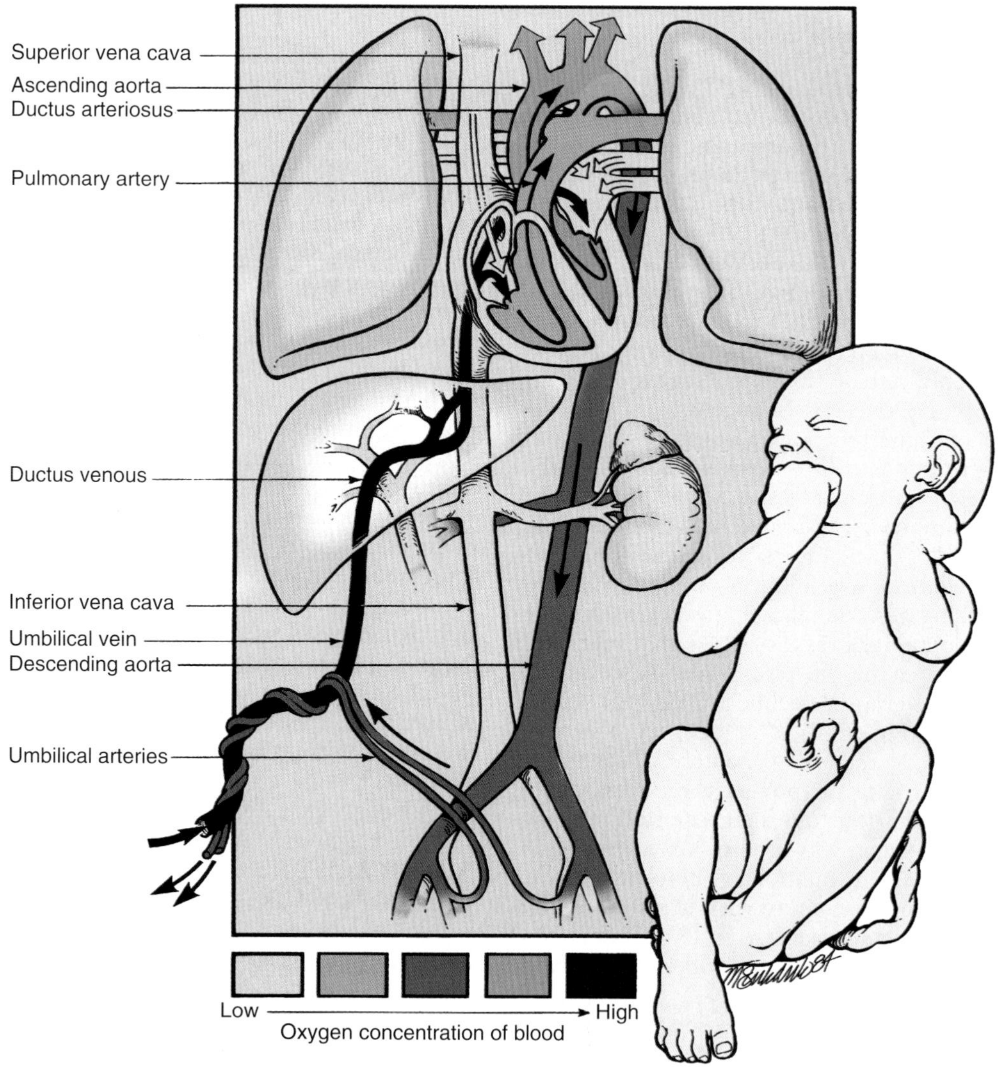

Figure 20-7. The fetal circulation.

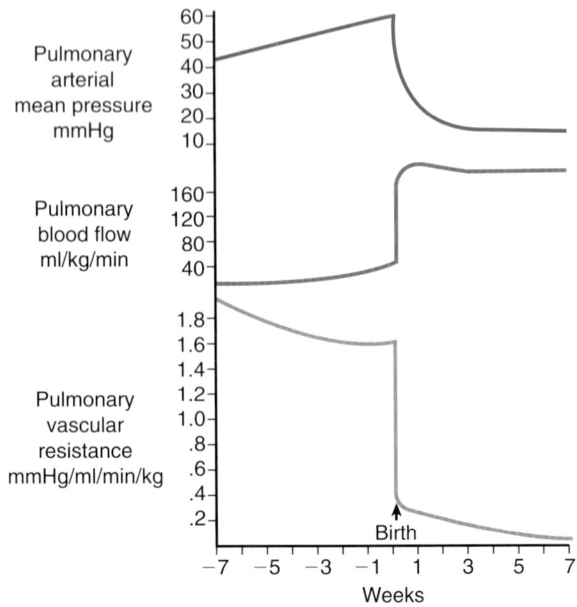

Figure 20-8. Representative changes in pulmonary hemodynamics during transition from the late-term fetal circulation to the neonatal circulation. (Adapted from Rudolph AM: Fetal circulation and cardiovascular adjustments after birth. *In* Rudolph CD, Rudolph AM, Hostetter MK, et al [eds]: Rudolph's Pediatrics, 21st ed. New York, McGraw-Hill, 2003, p 1749, with permission.)

tricular output (60 percent of combined output) is carried by the ductus arteriosus to the descending aorta, with only 7 percent of combined output going to the lungs. Thus, 70 percent of combined output passes through the descending aorta, with a Po_2 of 20 to 23 mm Hg (saturation of 55 percent) to supply the abdominal viscera and lower extremities. Forty-five percent of combined output goes through the umbilical arteries to the placenta. This arrangement provides blood of a higher Po_2 to the critical coronary and cerebral circulations and serves to divert venous blood to where oxygenation occurs.

The diversion of right ventricular output away from the lungs through the ductus arteriosus is caused by the very high pulmonary vascular resistance (PVR) in the fetus. This high pulmonary pressure results from chronic exposure to a low Po_2, causing vasoconstriction and an increase in the medial muscle layer in pulmonary arteries.[63] With advancing gestational age, an increase in the number of small pulmonary vessels occurs that increases the cross-sectional area of the pulmonary vasculature. This contributes to the gradual decline in PVR that begins during later gestation (Fig. 20-8). With delivery, a variety of factors interact to decrease PVR acutely. Mechanical expansion of the lungs with a hypoxic gas mixture causes a decrease in PVR and a fourfold increase in pulmonary blood flow.[67] When oxygen was used to ventilate in this study, a further increase in pulmonary blood flow was seen, caused by an increase in oxygen tension of the blood. Central to the acute decrease in PVR associated with birth is increased production of endothelium-derived relaxing factor or nitric oxide.[68,69]

With the increase in pulmonary flow, left atrial return increases with a rise in left atrial pressure (Table 20-1).

Table 20-1. Pressures in the Perinatal Circulation

	FETAL (MM HG)	NEONATAL (MM HG)
Right atrium	4	5
Right ventricle	65/10	40/5
Pulmonary artery	65/40	40/25
Left atrium	3	7
Left ventricle	60/7	70/10
Aorta	60/40	70/45

Modified from Nelson NM: Respiration and circulation after birth, In Smith CA, Nelson NM (eds): The Physiology of the Newborn Infant, 4th ed. Springfield, IL, Charles C Thomas, 1976, p 117.

In addition, with the removal of the placenta, IVC return to the right atrium is diminished. The foramen ovale is a flap valve, and when left atrial pressure increases over that on the right side, the opening is functionally closed. It is still possible to demonstrate patency with insignificant right-to-left shunts in the first 12 hours of life in a human neonate, but in a 7- to 12-day newborn, such a shunt is rarely seen, although anatomic closure is not complete for a longer time.

With occlusion of the umbilical cord, the large run-off of blood to the placenta is interrupted, causing an increase in systemic pressure. This, coupled with the decrease in right-sided pressures, serves to reverse the shunt through the ductus arteriosus to a predominantly left-to-right shunt. By 15 hours of age, shunting in either direction is physiologically insignificant.[70] Although functionally closed by 4 days of age,[71] the ductus is not irreversibly and anatomically occluded for 1 month. The role of an increased oxygen environment in ductal closure is well established.[72] Prostaglandin metabolism has also been shown to play an important role in ductal patency in utero and in closure after birth.[72] Ductal closure appears to occur in two phases: constriction and anatomic occlusion. Initially, the muscular wall constricts, followed by permanent closure achieved by endothelial destruction, subintimal proliferation, and connective tissue formation.[72] The ductus venosus is functionally occluded shortly after the umbilical circulation is interrupted.

Shortly after birth in the neonatal lamb, resting cardiac output is about 350 ml/kg/min.[63] This represents an increase in left ventricular output from about 150 (fetal) to 350 (postnatal) ml/kg/min, whereas right ventricular output increases from 300 (fetal) to 350 (postnatal) ml/kg/min. The most dramatic increase in individual organ blood flow is that to the lungs (30 to 350 ml/kg/min). Myocardial, renal, and gastrointestinal blood flows also increase, whereas adrenal, cerebral, and carcass flows decrease.[73]

ABNORMALITIES OF CARDIOPULMONARY TRANSITION

Birth Asphyxia

Even normal infants may experience some limitation of oxygenation (asphyxia) during the birth process. A variety of circumstances can exaggerate this problem, resulting in a depressed infant, including (1) acute interruption of umbilical blood flow, as occurs during cord compression; (2) premature placental separation; (3) maternal hypotension or hypoxia; (4) any of the above-mentioned problems superimposed on chronic uteroplacental insufficiency; and (5) failure to execute a proper resuscitation.[74] Other contributing factors include anesthetics and analgesics used in the mother, mode and difficulty of delivery, maternal health, and prematurity.

The neonatal response to asphyxia follows a predictable pattern demonstrable in a number of species. Dawes[75] investigated the responses of the newborn rhesus monkey (Fig. 20-9). After delivery, the umbilical cord was tied and the monkey's head was placed in a saline-filled plastic bag. Within about 30 seconds, a short series of respiratory efforts began. These were interrupted by a convulsion or a series of clonic movements accompanied by an abrupt fall in heart rate. The animal then lay inert with no muscle tone. Skin color became progressively cyanotic and then blotchy because of vasoconstriction in an effort to maintain systemic blood pressure. This initial period of apnea lasted about 30 to 60 seconds. The monkey then began to gasp at a rate of three to six per minute. The gasping lasted for about 8 minutes, becoming weaker terminally. The time from onset of asphyxia to last gasp could be related to postnatal age and maturity at birth; the more immature the animal, the longer the time. Secondary or terminal apnea followed and, if resuscitation was not quickly initiated, death ensued. As the animal progressed through the phase of gasping and then on to terminal apnea, heart rate and blood pressure continued to fall, indicating hypoxic depression of myocardial function. As the heart failed, blood flow to critical organs decreased, resulting in organ injury.

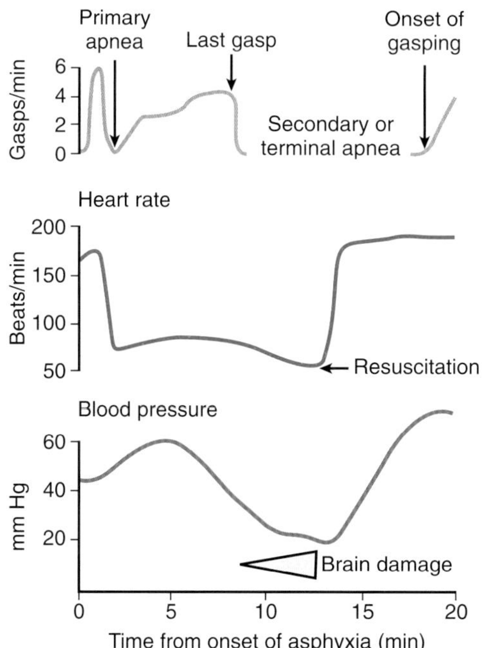

Figure 20-9. Schematic depiction of changes in rhesus monkeys during asphyxia and on resuscitation by positive-pressure ventilation. (Adapted from Dawes GS: Foetal and Neonatal Physiology. Chicago, Year Book, 1968, with permission.)

The response to resuscitation has also been described in great detail and is qualitatively similar in all species, including humans.[76,77] During the first period of apnea, almost any physical or chemical stimulus causes the animal to breathe. If gasping has already ceased, the first sign of recovery with initiation of positive-pressure ventilation is an increase in heart rate. The blood pressure then rises, rapidly if the last gasp has only just passed, but more slowly if the duration of asphyxia has been longer. The skin then becomes pink, and gasping ensues. Rhythmic spontaneous respiratory efforts become established after a further interval. For each 1 minute past the last gasp, 2 minutes of positive-pressure breathing is required before gasping begins and 4 minutes to reach rhythmic breathing. Not until some time later do the spinal and corneal reflexes return. Muscle tone gradually improves over the course of several hours.

Delivery Room Management of the Newborn

A number of situations during pregnancy, labor, and delivery place the infant at increased risk for asphyxia: (1) maternal diseases, such as diabetes and hypertension, third-trimester bleeding, and prolonged rupture of membranes; (2) fetal conditions, such as prematurity, multiple births, growth restriction, fetal anomalies, and rhesus isoimmunization; and (3) conditions related to labor and delivery, including fetal distress, meconium staining, breech presentation, and administration of anesthetics and analgesics.

When an asphyxiated infant is expected, a resuscitation team should be in the delivery room. The team should have at least two persons, one to manage the airway and one to monitor heart rate and provide whatever assistance is needed. The necessary equipment for an adequate resuscitation is listed in Table 20-2. The equipment should be checked regularly and should be in a continuous state of readiness.

Steps in the resuscitation process[78,79] are as follows (Fig. 20-10):

1. Dry the infant well and place under the radiant heat source on the back or side with the neck slightly extended. Do not allow the infant to become hyperthermic.
2. Gently suction the oropharynx and then the nose.
3. Assess the infant's condition (Table 20-3). The best criteria to assess are the infant's respiratory effort (apneic, gasping, regular) and heart rate (more or less than 100). A depressed heart rate indicative of hypoxic myocardial depression is the single most reliable indicator of the need for resuscitation.[77,80]
4. Generally, infants who are breathing with heart rates over 100 bpm require no further intervention. If the infant is breathing with an adequate heart rate, but is cyanotic, provide supplemental oxygen. Infants with heart rates less than 100 bpm with apnea or irregular respiratory efforts should be vigorously stimulated by rubbing the baby's back with a towel while blowing oxygen over the face.

Table 20-2. Equipment for Neonatal Resuscitation

CLINICAL NEEDS	EQUIPMENT
Thermoregulation	Radiant heat source with platform, mattress covered with warm sterile blankets, servo control heating, temperature probe
Airway management	*Suction:* bulb suction, meconium aspirator, wall vacuum suction with sterile catheters *Ventilation:* manual infant resuscitation bag connected to a pressure manometer capable of delivering 100% oxygen, appropriate masks for term and preterm infants, oral airways, stethoscope, gloves *Intubation:* neonatal laryngoscope with #0 and #1 blades; extra bulbs and batteries; endotracheal tubes 2.5, 3.0 and 3.5 mm OD with stylet; scissors, adhesive tape, end tidal CO_2 detection device
Gastric decompression	Nasogastric tube, 8 Fr with 20-ml syringe
Administration of drugs/volume	Sterile umbilical catheterization tray, umbilical catherters (3.5 and 5 Fr), volume expanders (normal saline), drug box with appropriate neonatal vials and dilutions (see Table 20-5), sterile syringes and needles
Transport	Warmed transport isolette with an oxygen source

5. If the baby fails to respond rapidly to tactile stimulation, proceed to bag and face mask ventilation with 100% oxygen, using a soft mask that seals well around the mouth and nose. Choice of ventilation bags includes a flow-inflating bag (500 to 750 ml) with a pressure gauge and flow control valve or a self-inflating bag (240 to 750 ml) with an oxygen reservoir and pressure release valve (Fig. 20-11). A T-piece resuscitation device may also be used. For the initial inflations, pressures of 30 to 40 cm H_2O may be necessary to overcome surface active forces in the lungs. Adequacy of ventilation is assessed by observing expansion of the infant's chest with bagging and a gradual improvement in color, perfusion, and heart rate. After the first few breaths, attempts should be made to lower the peak pressure to 15 to 20 cm H_2O. Rate of bagging should not exceed 40 to 60 bpm.
6. Most neonates can be effectively resuscitated with a bag and face mask. If the infant does not initially respond to bag and mask ventilation, try to reposition the head (slight extension), reapply the mask to achieve a good seal, consider suctioning the mouth and oropharynx, and try ventilating with the mouth open. It may be necessary to increase the pressure used. However, if there is no favorable response in 30 to 40 seconds, one can proceed to intubation:
   a. The head should be stable, with the nose in the sniffing position (pointing straight upward).

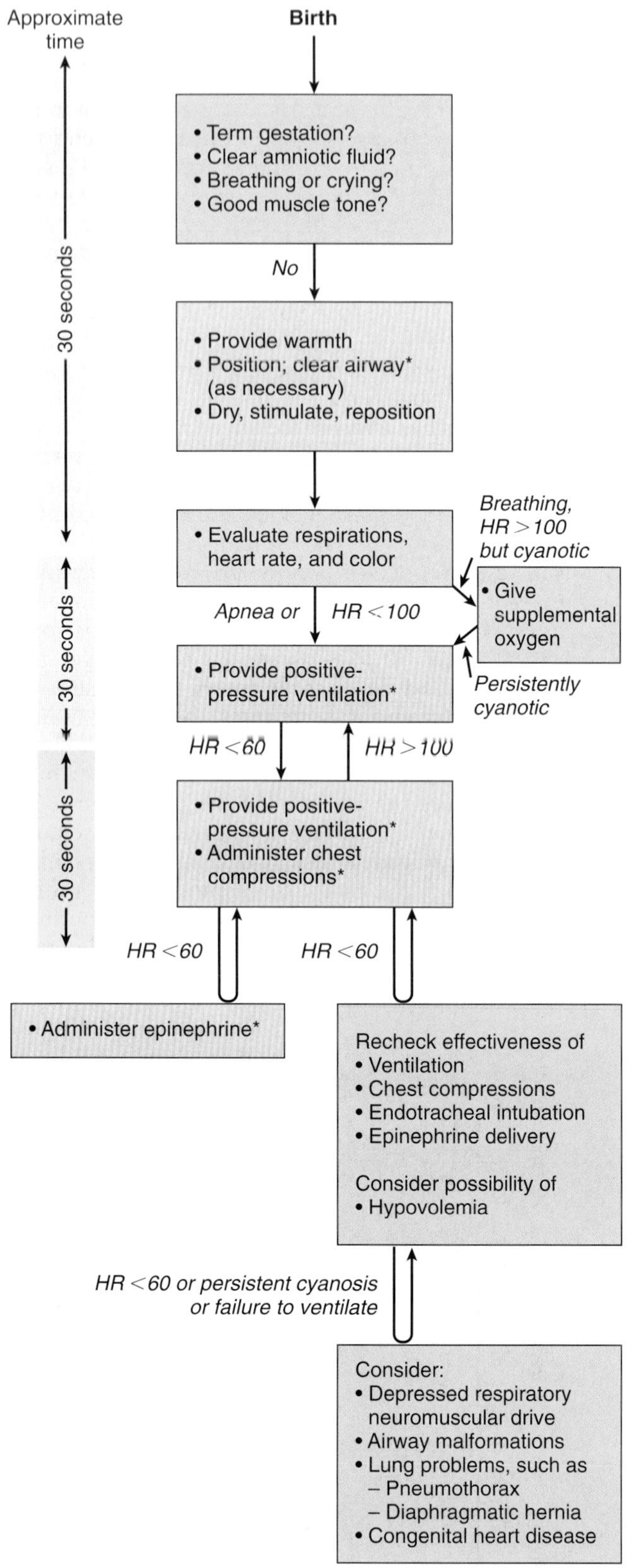

Figure 20-10. Delivery room management of the newborn. (Reproduced with permission from American Heart Association, American Academy of Pediatrics: Neonatal Resuscitation Textbook, 2006.)

b. Insert the laryngoscope blade, and sweep the tongue to the left.
c. Advance the blade to the base of the tongue, and identify the epiglottis.
d. Pick up the proper size endotracheal tube (2.5 mm OD for infants <1,000 g, 3.0 mm for infants 1,000 to 2,000 g, and 3.5 mm for larger infants) with the right hand.
e. Slide the laryngoscope anterior to the epiglottis, and gently lift along the angle of the handle of the laryngoscope (Fig. 20-12).
f. Identify the vocal cords.
g. Insert the tube in the right side of the mouth, and visualize the tube passing through the vocal cords. The tube should be located 7 cm at the lip for a 1,000 g infant, 8 cm for a 2,000-g infant, and 9 cm for a 3,000-g infant.
h. Ventilate as described earlier.
i. Failure to respond to intubation and ventilation can result from mechanical causes or severe asphyxia.

Table 20-3 The Apgar Scoring System

SIGN	0	1	2
Heart rate	Absent	<100 bpm	>100 bpm
Respiratory effort	Apneic	Weak, irregular, gasping	Regular
Reflex irritability*	No response	Some response	Facial grimace, sneeze, cough
Muscle tone	Flaccid	Some flexion	Good flexion of arms and legs
Color	Blue, pale	Body pink, hands and feet blue	Pink

*Elicited by suctioning the oropharynx and nose.
Modified from Apgar V: A proposal for a new method of evaluation of the newborn infant. Anesth Analg 32:260, 1953.

j. The mechanical causes listed in Table 20-4 should be quickly ruled out. Check to be sure the endotracheal tube passes through the vocal cords. A CO_2 detector placed between the endotracheal tube and the bag can be very helpful as a rapid confirmation of tube position in the airway. Occlusion of the tube should be suspected when there is resistance to bagging and no chest wall movement. If the endotracheal tube is in place and not occluded, and the equipment is functioning, a trial of bagging with higher pressures is indicated. The other causes listed in Table 20-4 are rare compared with equipment failure or tube problems. A pneumothorax is characterized by asymmetric breath sounds not corrected by repositioning the tube above the carina. Pleural effusions usually occur with fetal hydrops, whereas a diaphragmatic hernia should be ruled out in the setting of asymmetric breath sounds and a scaphoid abdomen. Pulmonary hypoplasia should be considered if the pregnancy has been complicated by oligohydramnios. It is very unusual for a neonatal resuscitation to require either cardiac massage or drugs. Almost all newborns respond to ventilation with 100 percent oxygen.

7. If mechanical causes are ruled out, external cardiac massage should be performed for persistent heart rate at less than 60 bpm after intubation and positive pressure ventilation for 30 seconds. Compression of ⅓ the anteroposterior diameter of the chest should be performed, interposed with ventilation at a 3:1 ratio (90 compressions, 30 breaths per minute).
8. If drugs are needed for a persistent heart rate less than 60 bpm after ventilation and chest compressions (Table 20-5), the drug of choice is 0.1 to 0.3 ml/kg of 1:10,000 epinephrine through the endotracheal tube or preferably an umbilical venous line. Sodium bicarbonate 1 to 2 mEq/kg of the neonatal dilution (0.5 mEq/ml) can be used in prolonged resuscitation efforts in which response to other measures is poor or with a documented metabolic acidosis. If volume loss is suspected (e.g., documented blood loss with clini-

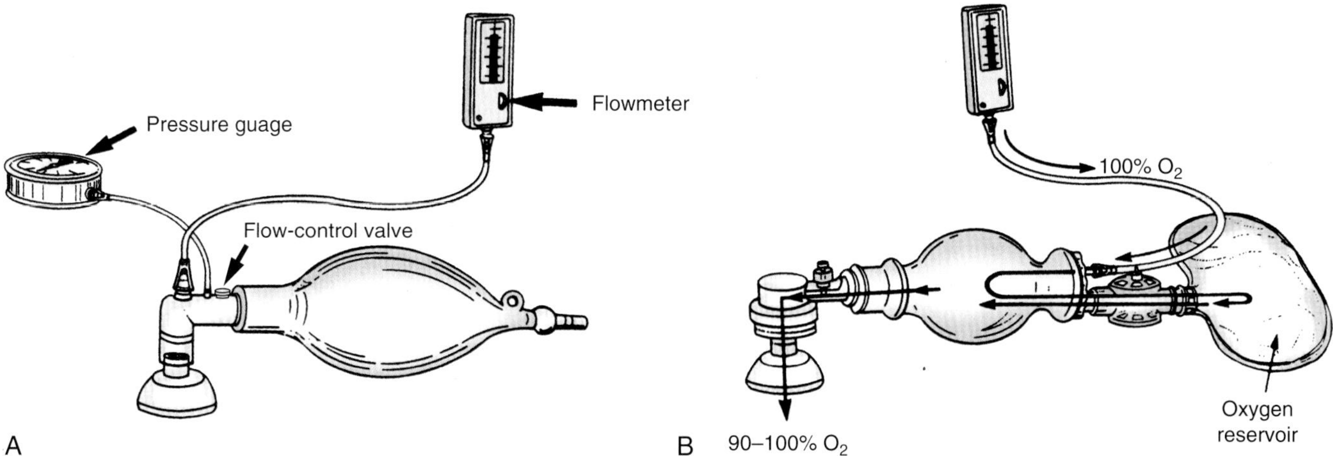

Figure 20-11. Bags used for neonatal resuscitation. Panel *A*, A flow-inflating bag with a pressure manometer and flow control valve. *B*, A self-inflating bag with an oxygen reservoir to maintain 90 to 100 percent oxygen. (From the American Heart Association and American Academy of Pediatrics: Neonatal Resuscitation Textbook, 2000, with permission.)

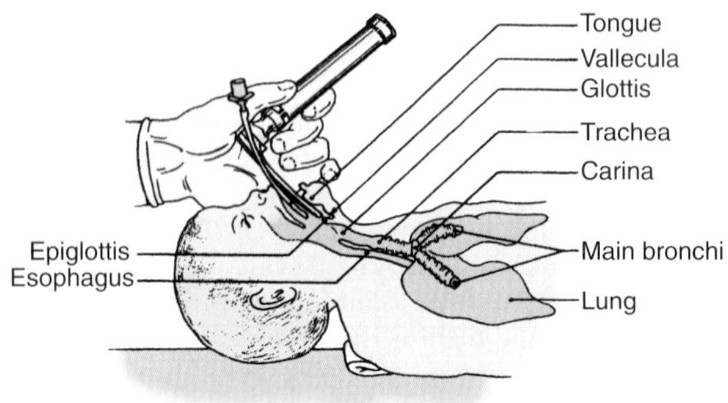

Figure 20-12. Anatomy of laryngoscopy for endotracheal intubation. (From the American Heart Association and American Academy of Pediatrics: Neonatal Resucitation Textbook, 2000, with permission.)

Table 20-4. Mechanical Causes of Failed Resuscitation

CATEGORY	EXAMPLES
Equipment failure	Malfunctioning bag, oxygen not connected or running
Endotracheal tube malposition	Esophagus, right mainstem bronchus
Occluded endotracheal tube	
Insufficient inflation pressure to expand lungs	
Space-occupying lesions in the thorax	Pneumothorax, pleural effusions, diaphragmatic hernia
Pulmonary hypoplasia	Extreme prematurity, oligohydramnios

Table 20-5. Neonatal Drug Doses

DRUG	DOSE	ROUTE	HOW SUPPLIED
Epinephrine	0.1–0.3 ml/kg	IV or ET	1:10,000 dilution
Sodium bicarbonate*	1–2 mEq/kg	IV	0.5 mEq/ml (4.2% solution)
Volume†	10 ml/kg	IV	Normal saline, whole blood
Naloxone‡	0.1 mg/kg	IV, ET, IM, SC	1 mg/ml

*For correction of metabolic acidosis only after adequate ventilation has been achieved; give slowly over several minutes.

†Infuse slowly over 5 to 10 minutes.

‡After proceeding with proper airway management and other resuscitative techniques IV, intravenous, ET, endotracheal, IM, intramuscular, SC, subcutaneous.

Modified from American Heart Association and American Academy of Pediatrics: Neonatal Resuscitation Textbook. American Heart Association and American Academy of Pediatrics, 2000.

cal evidence of hypovolemia), 10 ml/kg of a volume expander (normal saline) should be administered through an umbilical venous line. The appropriateness of continued resuscitative efforts should always be reevaluated in an infant who fails to respond to all of the above-mentioned efforts. Today, resuscitative efforts are made even in "apparent stillbirths," that is, infants whose 1-minute Apgar scores are 0 to 1. However, efforts should not be sustained in the face of little or no improvement over a reasonable period of time (i.e., 10 to 15 minutes).[81]

A few special circumstances merit discussion at this point. Infants in whom respiratory depression secondary to narcotic administration is suspected may be given naloxone (Narcan). However, this should not be done until the airway has been managed and the infant resuscitated in the usual fashion. In addition, naloxone should not be given to the infant of an addicted mother, because it will precipitate withdrawal. A second special group are preterm infants. Minimizing heat loss improves survival, so prewarmed towels should be available, and the environmental temperature of the delivery suite should be raised. In the extremely-low-birth-weight infant (<1,000 g), proceed quickly to intubation. Volume expanders and sodium bicarbonate should be infused slowly to avoid rapid swings in blood pressure.

Finally, there is the issue of meconium-stained amniotic fluid. Meconium aspiration syndrome (MAS) is a form of aspiration pneumonia that occurs most often in term or postterm infants who have passed meconium in utero (10 to 15 percent of all deliveries[82]). Overall, 4 to 6 percent of children born through meconium-stained fluid are diagnosed with MAS, and an additional 4 to 9 percent are diagnosed with other respiratory disorders.[82] Delivery room management of meconium in the amniotic fluid has been based on the notion that aspiration takes place with the initiation of extrauterine respiration and that the pathologic condition is related to the aspirated contents. This resulted in the practice of oropharyngeal suction on the perineum after delivery of the head followed by airway visualization and suction by the resuscitator after delivery.[83] Both of these assumptions are likely not entirely true. Meconium is found below the vocal cords in 35 percent of births from meconium-stained fluid.[84] In utero aspiration has been induced in animal models[84,85] and confirmed in autopsies of human stillbirths.[84,86] In addition, the combined suction approach to prevention of MAS has not been uniformly successful in decreasing the incidence of MAS.[84,87,88] Further concern was raised by the experience that routine suctioning of the neonatal airway itself was associated with respiratory morbidity.[89,90] These data have been confirmed by a large multicenter, prospective, randomized controlled trial assessing selective intubation of apparently vigorous meconium-stained infants.[91] Compared with expectant management, intubation and tracheal suction did not result in a decreased incidence of MAS or other respiratory disorders. Finally, the role of suction on the perineum before delivery of the shoulders has now been shown not to prevent MAS.[92]

In terms of the role of meconium in the genesis of MAS, 35 percent of infants born with meconium in the amniotic fluid have meconium in the lungs. Up to 55 percent have abnormal chest radiographs, yet respiratory distress develops in only 5 to 10 percent of these infants.[84] Severe MAS is associated with persistent pulmonary hypertension of the newborn and is likely the result of a long-standing intrauterine process with meconium only a marker of intrauterine hypoxia.[93]

Current clinical and experimental data support that MAS is the result of intrauterine asphyxia. The best method of prevention is to identify the fetus at risk (prolonged pregnancy, oligohydramnios). Intrapartum management should emphasize treatments that enhance uteroplacental perfusion. Aminoinfusion in cases with oligohydramnios may reduce cord compression, gasping, and intrapartum aspiration.[94] The management of the infant's airway remains controversial, although postnatal prevention of MAS will often not be possible. In light of the above-mentioned information, the current approach to the meconium stained infant is as follows:

1. The obstetrician carefully suctions the oropharynx and nasopharynx after delivery of the baby.
2. If the baby is active and breathing and requires no resuscitation, the airway need not be inspected, thus avoiding the risk of inducing vagal bradycardia.
3. Any infant in need of resuscitation should have the airway inspected and suctioned before instituting positive-pressure ventilation.
4. Suction the stomach when airway management is complete and vital signs are stable.

One additional point to mention about neonatal resuscitation is that a fair amount of data now exist to support resuscitation with room air in lieu of 100 percent oxygen.[95] Concerns have been raised about the potential harmful effects of 100 percent oxygen, in particular the generation of oxygen free radicals.[96] With that in mind, air may be a more appropriate gas than 100 percent oxygen. Current recommendations regarding the use of 100 percent oxygen have not changed,[78] but new recommendations may evolve over the next several years. It is acceptable to begin resuscitations with less than 100% oxygen and assess the infant's response.

Sequelae of Birth Asphyxia

The incidence of birth asphyxia is about 1 percent in term and near-term infants, with an increased incidence in infants of lower gestational age.[97] In a study involving more than 38,000 deliveries, MacDonald et al.[97] reported an incidence of 0.4 percent in infants older than 38 weeks and 62.3 percent in those younger than 27 weeks. The acute sequelae that need to be managed in the neonatal period are listed in Table 20-6. It is evident that widespread organ injury occurs. Management focuses on supportive care and treatment of specific abnormalities. This includes careful fluid management, blood pressure support, intravenous glucose, and treatment of seizures. Phenobarbital (40 mg/kg) 1 to 6 hours after the event given as neuroprotective therapy is associated with an improved neurologic outcome.[98] The roles of hypothermia (selective head cooling or whole body hypothermia), oxygen free radical scavengers, excitatory amino acid antagonists, and calcium channel blockers in minimizing cerebral injury after asphyxia are still investigational.[99–102]

If the infant survives, the major long-term concern is permanent CNS damage. The challenge is identifying criteria that can provide information about the risk of future problems for a given infant. A variety of markers have been examined to identify birth asphyxia and risk for adverse neurologic outcome.[84,103–109] Meconium in the amniotic fluid considered in isolation does not increase the risk of unfavorable outcome.[84] Marked fetal bradycardia is associated with some increase in risk, but use of electronic fetal monitoring and cesarean delivery have not altered the incidence of cerebral palsy over the last several decades.[103–106] Low Apgar scores at 1 and 5 minutes are not very predictive of outcome, but infants with low scores that persist at 15 and 20 minutes after birth have a 50-percent chance of manifesting cerebral palsy if they survive.[107] Cord pH is predictive of adverse outcome only after the pH is less than 7.00.[108] The best predictor of outcome is the severity of the neonatal neurologic syndrome.[109] Infants with mild encephalopathy survive and are normal on follow-up examination. Moderate encephalopathy carries a 25 to 50 percent risk of severe handicap or death, whereas the severe syndrome carries a greater than 75-percent risk of death or disability. Diagnostic aids including electroencephalograms, evoked potentials, computed tomography (CT) and magnetic resonance imaging (MRI) scans, and Doppler flow studies can also aid in predicting outcome.[109,110] It is also important to keep in mind that the circulatory response to hypoxia is to redistribute blood flow to provide adequate oxygen delivery to critical organs (e.g., brain, heart) at the expense of other organs. Thus, it is hard to imagine an insult severe enough to damage the brain without evidence of other organ dysfunction.

The long-term neurologic sequelae of intrapartum asphyxia are cerebral palsy with or without associated cognitive deficits and epilepsy.[103,111,112] Although cerebral palsy can be related to intrapartum events, the large majority of cases are of unknown cause.[112,113] Furthermore, cognitive deficits and epilepsy, unless associated with cerebral palsy, cannot be related to asphyxia or to other intrapartum events.[111,112] To attribute cerebral

Table 20-6. The Acute Sequelae of Asphyxia

SYSTEM	MANIFESTATIONS
Central nervous system	Cerebral edema, seizures, hemorrhage and hypoxic-ischemic encephalopathy
Cardiac	Papillary muscle necrosis—transient tricuspid insufficiency, cardiogenic shock
Pulmonary	Aspiration syndromes (meconium, clear fluid), acquired surfactant deficiency, persistent pulmonary hypertension, pulmonary hemorrhage
Renal	Acute tubular necrosis with anuria or oliguria
Adrenal	Hemorrhage with adrenal insufficiency
Hepatic	Enzyme elevations, liver failure
Gastrointestinal	Necrotizing enterocolitis, feeding intolerance
Metabolic	Hypoglycemia, hypocalcemia
Hematologic	Coagulation disorders, thrombocytopenia

Table 20-7. Relationship of Intrapartum Events and Cerebral Palsy

Essential Criteria:

Evidence of a metabolic acidosis in fetal umbilical cord arterial blood obtained at delivery (pH < 7.00 and base deficit ≥12 mmol/L)
Early onset of severe or moderate neonatal encephalopathy in infants born at 34 or more weeks' gestation
Cerebral palsy of the spastic quadriplegic or dyskinetic type
Exclusion of other identifiable etiologies such as trauma, coagulation disorders, infectious conditions, or genetic disorders

Criteria that Suggest Intrapartum Timing but are not Specific to Asphyxial Insults:

A sentinel hypoxic event occurring immediately before or during labor
A sudden sustained fetal bradycardia or the absence of fetal heart rate variability in the presence of persistent late or variable decelerations, usually after a hypoxic sentinel event when the pattern was previously normal
Apgar scores of 0–3 beyond 5 minutes
Onset of multisystem involvement within 72 hours of birth
Early imaging study showing evidence of acute nonfocal cerebral abnormality

Adapted from American College of Obstetricians and Gynecologists, American Academy of Pediatrics: Neonatal encephalopathy and cerebral palsy: defining pathogenesis and pathophysiology. Washington DC, ACOG, 2003.

Table 20-8. Birth Injuries

CLASSIFICATION	EXAMPLE
Soft tissue injuries*	Lacerations, abrasions, fat necrosis
Extracranial bleeding	Cephalohematoma*, subgaleal bleed
Intracranial hemorrhage	Subarachnoid, subdural, epidural, cerebral, cerebellar
Nerve injuries	Facial nerve*, cervical nerve roots (brachial plexus palsies*, phrenic n., Horner's syndrome), recurrent laryngeal n. (vocal cord paralysis)
Fractures	Clavicle*, facial bones, humerus, femur, skull, nasal bones
Dislocations	Extremities, nasal septum
Eye injuries	Subconjunctiva* and retinal hemorrhages, orbital fracture, corneal laceration, breaks in Desçemet's membrane with corneal opacification
Torticollis†	
Spinal cord injuries	
Visceral rupture	Liver, spleen
Scalp laceration*	Fetal scalp electrode, scalpel
Scalp abcess	Fetal scalp electrode

*More common occurrences.
†Secondary to hemorrhage into the sternocleidomastoid muscle.

palsy to peripartum asphyxia, there must be an absence of other demonstrable causes, substantial or prolonged intrapartum asphyxia (fetal heart rate abnormalities, fetal acidosis), and clinical evidence during the first days of life of neurologic dysfunction in the infant (Table 20-7).[114]

BIRTH INJURIES

Birth injuries are defined as those sustained during labor and delivery. Factors predisposing to birth injury include macrosomia, cephalopelvic disproportion, shoulder dystocia, prolonged or difficult labor, precipitous delivery, abnormal presentations (including breech), and use of forceps (especially midforceps).[115] Injuries range from minor (requiring no therapy) to life threatening (Table 20-8).

Soft tissue injuries are most common. Most are related to dystocia and to the use of forceps. Accidental lacerations of the scalp, buttocks, and thighs may be inflicted with the scalpel during cesarean delivery. Cumulatively, these injuries are of a minor nature and respond well to therapy. Hyperbilirubinemia, particularly in the premature infant, is the major neonatal complication related to soft tissue damage.

A cephalohematoma occurs in 0.2 to 2.5 percent of live births.[116] Caused by rupture of blood vessels that traverse from the skull to the periosteum, the bleeding is subperiosteal and therefore limited by suture lines, with the most common site of bleeding being over the parietal bones. Associations include prolonged or difficult labor and mechanical trauma from operative vaginal delivery with a greater incidence seen with vacuum delivery from forceps. Linear skull fractures beneath the hematoma have been reported in 5.4 percent of cases[116] but are of no major consequence except in the unlikely event that a leptomeningeal cyst develops. Most cephalhematomas are reabsorbed in 2 weeks to 3 months. Subgaleal bleeds, which are not limited by suture lines, can occur in association with vacuum extraction (especially with multiple applications) and difficult forceps deliveries, and can result in life-threatening anemia, hypotension, or consumptive coagulopathy. Depressed skull fractures are also seen in neonates, but most do not require surgical elevations.

Intracranial hemorrhages related to trauma include epidural, subdural, subarachnoid, and intraparenchymal bleeds.[117] With improvements in obstetric care, subdural hemorrhages fortunately are now rare. Three major varieties of subdural bleeds have been described: (1) posterior fossa hematomas due to tentorial laceration with rupture of the straight sinus, vein of Galen, or transverse sinus or due to occipital osteodiastasis (a separation between the squamous and lateral portions of the occipital bone); (2) falx laceration, with rupture of the inferior sagittal sinus; and (3) rupture of the superficial cerebral veins. The clinical symptoms are related to the location of bleeding. With tentorial laceration, bleeding is infratentorial, causing brain stem signs and a rapid progression to death. Falx tears cause bilateral cerebral signs (e.g., seizures and focal weakness) until blood extends infratentorially to the brain stem. Subdural hemorrhage over the cerebral convexities can cause several clinical states, ranging from an asymptomatic newborn to one with seizures and focal neurologic findings. Infants with lacerations of the tentorium and falx have a poor outlook. In contrast, the prognosis for rupture of the superficial cerebral veins is much better, with the majority of survivors being normal. Primary subarachnoid hemorrhage is the most common variety of neonatal intracranial hemorrhage.[117] Clinically, these infants are often asymptomatic, although they may present with a characteristic seizure pattern. The seizures begin on day 2 of life, and the infants are "well" between convulsions. In general, the prognosis for subarachnoid bleeds is good.

Trauma to peripheral nerves produces another major group of birth injuries. Brachial plexus injuries are caused by stretching of the cervical roots during delivery, usually when shoulder dystocia is present. Upper arm palsy (Erb-Duchenne), the most common brachial plexus injury, is caused by injury to the fifth and sixth cervical nerves; lower arm paralysis (Klumpke) results from damage to the eighth cervical and first thoracic nerves. Damage to all four nerve roots produces paralysis of the entire arm. Outcome for these injuries is variable, with some infants left with significant residual.[118,119] Horner's syndrome due to damage to sympathetic outflow through nerve root T1 may accompany Klumpke's palsy, and approximately 5 percent of patients with Erb's palsy have an associated phrenic nerve paresis. Facial palsy is another fairly common injury caused either by pressure from the sacral promontory or fetal shoulder as the infant passes through the birth canal or by forceps. Most of these palsies resolve, although in some infants, paralysis is persistent.

The majority of bone fractures resulting from birth trauma involve the clavicle and result from shoulder dystocia or breech extractions that require vigorous manipulations. Clinically, many of these fractures are asymptomatic, and when present, symptoms are mild. Prognosis for clavicular as well as limb fractures is uniformly good. The most commonly fractured long bone is the humerus.

Spinal cord injuries are a relatively infrequent but often severe form of birth injury. Accurate incidence is difficult to assess, because symptoms mimic other neonatal diseases and autopsies often do not include a careful examination of the spine. Depressed tone, hyporeflexia, and respiratory failure are clues to this diagnosis. Excessive longitudinal traction and head rotation during forceps delivery predispose to spinal injury, and hyperextension of the head in a footling breech is particularly dangerous. Outcomes include death or stillbirth caused by high cervical or brain stem lesions, long-term survival of infants with paralysis from birth, and minimal neurologic symptoms or spasticity.

NEONATAL THERMAL REGULATION

Physiology

The human newborn is a homeotherm possessing the ability to maintain a stable core body temperature over a range of environmental temperatures. The range of environmental temperatures over which the neonate can operate is narrower than that of an adult as a result of the infant's inability to dissipate heat effectively in warm environments and, more critically, to maintain temperature in response to cold.

Heat Production

The heat production within the body is a by-product of metabolic processes and must equal heat losses through the skin and lungs. In the adult, heat production in response to cold can come from voluntary muscle activity, involuntary muscle activity (shivering), and nonshivering chemical thermogenesis. Although some increases in activity and shivering have been observed, nonshivering thermogenesis is the most important means of increased heat production in the cold-stressed newborn.[120,121] Nonshivering thermogenesis can be defined as an increase in total heat production without detectable (visible or electrical) muscle activity. From both animal[122] and human[123] observations, it has been inferred that the site of this increased heat production is brown fat. This fat is located between the scapulae; around the muscles and blood vessels of the neck, axillae, and mediastinum; between the esophagus and trachea; and around the kidneys and adrenal glands. Brown fat differs both morphologically and metabolically from white fat. Brown fat cells contain more mitochondria and fat vacuoles, and have a richer blood and sympathetic nerve supply. The initiation of nonshivering thermogenesis at birth depends on cooling, which results in increased sympathetic activity with release of norepinephrine from nerve endings that terminate in brown adipocytes. This results in an increase in lipase activity with hydrolysis of triglycerides and phospholipids forming fatty acids and glycerol. These can be oxidized with release of heat.[124,125]

Heat Loss

Heat loss to the environment is dependent on both an internal temperature gradient (from within the body to the surface) and an external gradient (from the surface to the environment). The infant can change the internal gradient by altering vasomotor tone and, to a lesser extent, by postural changes that decrease the amount of exposed surface area. The external gradient is dependent on purely physical variables. Heat transfer from the surface to the environment involves four routes: radiation, convection, conduction, and evaporation. Radiant heat loss, heat transfer from a warmer to a cooler object that is not in contact, depends on the temperature gradient between the objects. Heat loss by convection to the surrounding gaseous environment depends on air speed and temperature. Conduction or heat loss to a contacting cooler object is minimal in most circumstances. Heat loss by evaporation is cooling secondary to water loss at the rate of 0.6 cal/g water evaporated and is affected by relative humidity, air speed, exposed surface area, and skin permeability. In infants in excessively warm environments, under overhead radiant heat sources, or in very immature infants with thin, permeable skin, evaporative losses increase considerably.

Compared with an adult, the newborn is compromised in the ability to conserve as well as dissipate heat. Conservation of heat is impaired because of a large surface area/body weight ratio and less tissue insulation because of less subcutaneous fat.[126] With a cold stress, heat is conserved chiefly by vasoconstriction in both mature and immature neonates. When the environment is too warm, heat loss is augmented by vasodilation of skin vessels and an increase in evaporative heat loss by sweating. Sweating is present in term infants when rectal temperatures rise above 37.2°C.[127] With sweating, evaporative heat losses can increase two- to fourfold in term babies, but this is not enough to prevent a rise in core temperature. Table 20-9 summarizes the neonate's efforts to maintain a stable core temperature in the face of cold or heat stress.

Table 20-9. Neonatal Response to Thermal Stress

STRESSOR	RESPONSE	TERM	PRETERM
Cold	Vasoconstriction	++	++
	↓ Exposed surface area (posture change)	±	±
	↑ Oxygen consumption	++	+
	↑ Motor activity, shivering	+	−
Heat	Vasodilation	++	++
	Sweating	+	−

++, Maximum response; +, intermediate; ±, may have a role; −, no response.

Neutral Thermal Environment

Although most available information confirms that the human neonate is a homeotherm, the range of temperatures over which core body temperature remains stable is narrower than in an adult and decreases with decreasing gestational age. Therefore, it is advantageous to maintain an infant in a neutral thermal environment (Fig. 20-13). A neutral thermal environment makes minimal demands on the neonate's energy reserves, core body temperature being regulated by changes in skin blood flow and posture. Body temperature remains normal, whereas oxygen consumption and heat production are minimal and match heat loss.[120,128] With a drop in environmental temperature out of the thermoneutral range, the infant increases oxygen consumption and thus heat production to keep up with heat losses and maintain a stable core temperature. Core temperature is maintained until heat loss exceeds the infant's ability to increase heat production further. When the infant is placed in an environment warmer than neutral thermal zone, hyperthermia rapidly occurs because of the neonate's inability to dissipate heat and an increase in oxygen consumption that ensues as the infant's body temperature rises. The neutral thermal environment for a given infant depends on size, gestational age, and postnatal age.[129] The optimal thermal environment for naked babies and cot-nursed (dressed and bundled) babies has been defined (Fig. 20-14).[128,130] It is important to note that the environmental temperatures shown in Figure 20-14 are operative temperatures for an infant in an incubator. The operative temperature

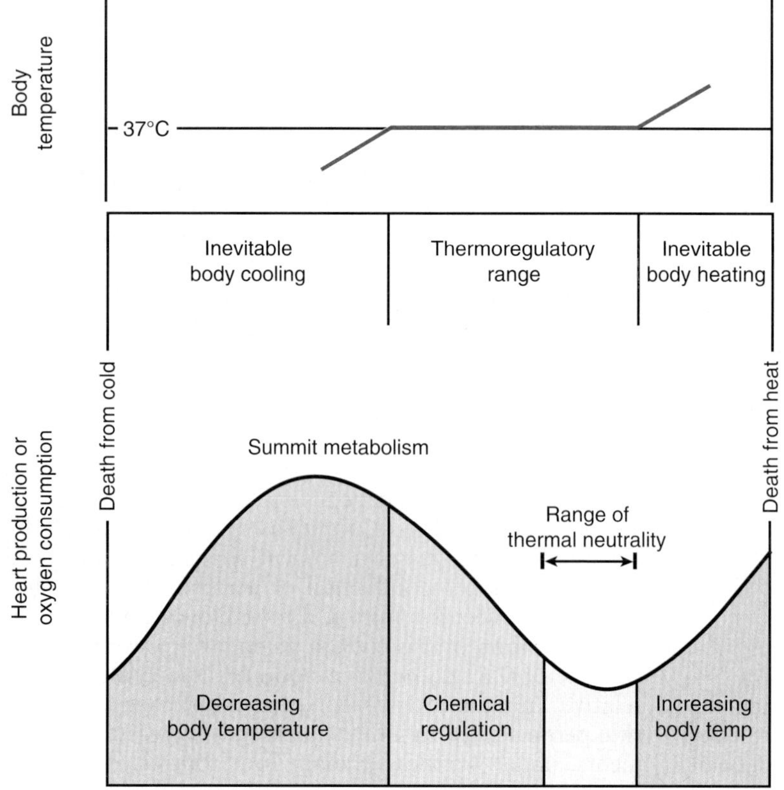

Figure 20-13. Effect of environmental temperature on oxygen consumption and body temperature. (Adapted from Klaus MH, Fanaroff AA: The physical environment. *In* Klaus MH, Fanaroff AA [eds]: Care of the High-Risk Neonate, 5th ed. Philadelphia, WB Saunders Company, 2001, p 130, with permission.)

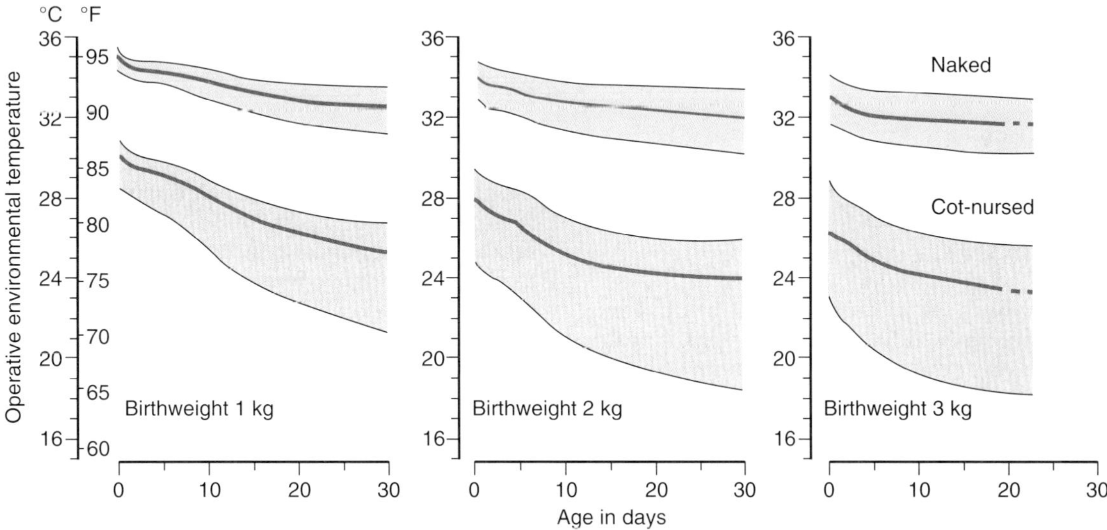

Figure 20-14. Range of environmental temperatures to maintain naked or cot-nursed 1-kg, 2-kg, and 3-kg infants in a neutral thermal environment. (From Klaus MH, Fanaroff AA: The physical environment. *In* Klaus MH, Fanaroff AA [eds]: Care of the High Risk Neonate, 5th ed. Philadelphia, WB Saunders Company, 2001, p 130, with permission.)

can differ from the measured environmental temperature because of changes in relative humidity and temperature of the incubator walls. Incubator wall temperature will vary as a function of room temperature. In general, maintaining the abdominal skin temperature at 36.5°C minimizes oxygen consumption.[131]

CLINICAL APPLICATIONS

Delivery Room

In utero, fetal thermoregulation is the responsibility of the placenta and is dependent on maternal core temperature, with fetal temperature 0.5°C higher than maternal temperature.[124,132] At birth, the infant's core temperature drops rapidly from 37.8°C because of evaporation from its wet body and radiant and convective losses to the cold air and walls of the room. Even with an increase in oxygen consumption to the maximum capability of the newborn (15 ml/kg/min), the infant can produce only 0.075 cal/kg/min and will rapidly lose heat. Measures taken to reduce heat loss after birth depend on the clinical situation. For the well term infant, drying the skin and wrapping the baby with warm blankets is sufficient. When it is necessary to leave an infant exposed for close observation or resuscitation, the infant should be dried and placed under a radiant heat source. Room temperature can be elevated as an added precaution for the low-birth-weight infant.

Nursery

Babies are cared for in the newborn nursery wrapped in blankets in bassinets (cot-nursed), in isolettes, or under a radiant heat source. Healthy full-term infants (weighing >2.5 kg) need only be clothed and placed in a bassinet under a blanket. A nursery temperature of 25°C should be adequate (Fig. 20-14). Infants weighing 2 to 2.5 kg who are either slightly premature or growth restricted should be allowed 12 to 24 hours to stabilize in an isolette and then advanced to a bassinet. Lower birth weight babies (<2 kg) will require care in either isolettes or under radiant heat sources. Adequate thermal protection of the low-birth-weight infant is essential. This is especially important for the very-low-birth-weight infant (<1.5 kg), who often does not behave like a mature homeotherm. These neonates can react to a small change in environmental temperature with a change in body temperature rather than a change in oxygen consumption. In addition, warmer environments have also been shown to hasten growth of the premature infant.[133]

The isolette, which heats by convection, is the most commonly used heating device for the low-birth-weight nude infant. The major source of heat loss while in a neutral thermal environment is radiant to the walls of the isolette. The magnitude of this loss is predictable if room temperature is known. These losses can be minimized using double-walled isolettes in which the inner wall temperature is very close to the air temperature within the isolette. An isolette permits adequate observation of the infant and is suitable for caring for the most sick low-birth-weight or full-sized infants. Once clinical status has been stabilized, the child can be dressed, which will afford increased thermal stability.

Radiant warmers can also be used to ensure thermal stability of both low-birth-weight and full-sized infants. Radiant warmers are used most effectively for short-term warming during initial resuscitation and stabilization as well as for performing procedures. They provide easy access to the infant while ensuring thermal stability. The main heat losses are convection, which can be significant because of variable air speed in a room, and evaporation. Evaporative heat loss resulting in significant fluid losses is a major concern for the very-low-birth-weight premature cared for under a radiant warmer. Placing a plastic shield over the infant or covering the skin with a semipermeable membrane can minimize these fluid losses.[134,135]

The most economical means of thermal support for the low-birth-weight infant is skin-to-skin contact with a parent. This "kangaroo" care has been shown to reduce serious illness and enhance lactation while providing adequate thermal support.[136–139]

NEONATAL NUTRITION AND GASTROENTEROLOGY

At birth, the newborn infant must assume various functions performed during fetal life by the placenta. Cardiopulmonary transition and thermoregulation have already been discussed. The final critical task for the newborn is the assimilation of calories, water, and electrolytes.

Nutritional Requirements

The required caloric, water, and electrolyte intake of the newborn depends on body stores and normal rate of energy expenditure. Body composition varies considerably with gestational age (Fig. 20-15).[140–142] The average 1-kg neonate consists of 85 percent water, 10 percent protein, and 3 percent fat as compared with 74 percent water, 12 percent protein, and 11 percent fat at term. Carbohydrate stores in the term infant are eight times higher. Rates of energy expenditure differ as well. Although basal metabolic rate is lower in premature than in term infants, the premature infant frequently has increased metabolic demand secondary to cold stress and work of breathing. The small-for-gestational-age (SGA) infant provides another special consideration, possessing a higher basal metabolic rate per kilogram than a normally grown infant.[143]

Water and Electrolyte

Maintenance water requirements are dependent on metabolic rate (evaporative losses to dissipate the heat of oxidation) and the necessary water to excrete the renal solute load. Other pertinent factors, especially for the premature infant, include environmental variation in insensible water losses and diminished ability to concentrate urine.[144] An individual infant's water requirement can be determined by measuring urine and stool losses and estimating insensible losses through skin and mucosa. It is normal during the first 3 to 4 postnatal days for an infant to experience a weight loss of up to 10 percent as the physiologic contraction of extracellular body fluid takes place. Maintenance electrolyte requirements are 2 to 3 mEq/kg/day for sodium, chloride, and bicarbonate and 1 to 2 mEq/kg/day for potassium. During periods of rapid growth, requirements will be higher.

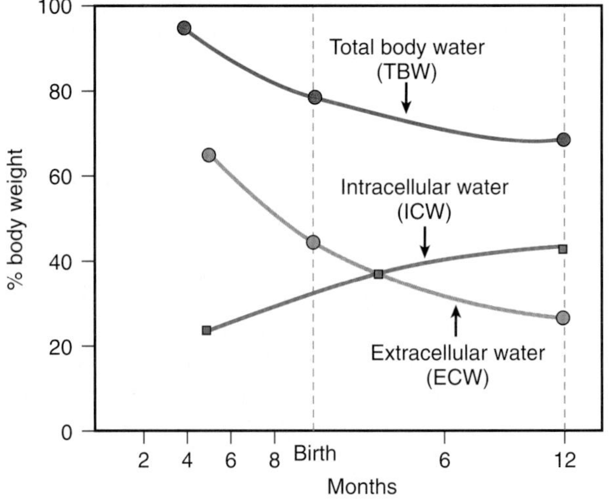

Figure 20-15 Changes in body water during gestation and infancy. (Adapted from Friis-Hansen B: Water distribution in the foetus and newborn infant. Acta Paediatr Scand Suppl 305:7, 1983, with permission.)

Calories

Caloric needs are primarily dependent on oxygen consumption. The character of the feeding also affects caloric needs by altering specific dynamic action and fecal losses. The average caloric requirement for a normal full-term infant is estimated to be about 100 to 110 kcal/kg/day. The needs of the low-birth-weight infant are more variable, but usually 105 to 130 kcal/kg/day is adequate.[145] Standard infant formulas and breast milk provide approximately 20 kcal/oz. Therefore, volumes of 150 to 180 ml/kg/day will provide the necessary caloric intake of 100 to 120 kcal/kg/day for the average term or preterm infant beyond 32 to 34 weeks' gestation. Infants weighing less than 1,500 g should be fed with either formulas designed specifically for the premature or fortified breast milk. The goal for the growing premature is growth at a rate comparable to intrauterine growth during the third trimester. The nutritional needs of the full-term and premature infant are shown in Table 20-10.

Protein

Both the quantity and quality of protein intake are important for adequate growth, particularly for the premature infant.[145,146] Suggested intakes range from 2.25 to 4.0 g/kg/day (~3.5 g/kg/day for the premature infant). The "gold standard" for amino acid content is that which provides a plasma amniogram as close as possible to that seen with human milk.[146]

Fat and Carbohydrate

Before birth, glucose is the major energy source for the human fetus. After birth, 40 to 50 percent of the calories oxidized are fat.[147] Besides its role as an energy source, fat is an important component of cellular membranes, a carrier of fat-soluble vitamins, and a source of essential fatty acids. The brain and retina contain large quantities of long chain ω-3 and ω-6 polyunsaturated fatty acids, particularly docohexanoic acid (DHA) and arachadonic acid (AA). The precursor of DHA and AA is

Table 20-10. Nutritional Needs of the Full-Term and Premature Infant

	PREMATURE		
	<1 KG	<1–2.5 KG	FULL-TERM
		per kg/day	
Protein (g)	4	3.5	2
Na (mEq)	3.5	3	3
Cl (mEq)	3.1	2.5	2.3
K (mEq)	2.5	2.5	2.4
Ca (mg)	210	185	130
P (mg)	140	123	70
Mg (mg)	10	8.5	5
Fe (mg)	2–4	1–2	2
Biotin (μg)	1–1.4	1–2	1–2
Pantothenic acid (mg)	5–9	1–1.4	1–1.4
Choline (mg)	5–9	5–9	5–9
		per day	
Fluoride (mg)	0.1 (?)	0.1 (?)	0.1 (?)
Cu (mg)	0.17	0.1–0.5	0.5–1
Zn (mg)	1.5	1.5–3	3–5
Mn (mg)	0.01–0.02	0.02–0.04	0.3–1
Cr (μg)	2–4	2–6	10–40
I (μg)	5	5–10	10–15
Se (μg)	1.5–2.5	1.5–7.5	10–60
Mo (μg)	2–3	2–7.5	30–80
Vitamin A (IU)	1000	1000	1000
Vitamin D (IU)	400	400	400
Vitamin E (IU)	5–25	5–25	4
Vitamin K (μg)	5	5	5
Vitamin C (mg)	60	60	35
Vitamin B_1 (mg)	0.2	0.2	0.2
Vitamin B_2 (mg)	0.4	5	5
Vitamin B_6 (mg)	0.2	0.2	0.2
Vitamin B_{12} (μg)	0.15	0.15	0.15
Niacin (mg)	5	5	5
Folic acid (μg)	50	50	50

Reproduced with permission from Pereira GR: Nutritional assessment. *In* Polin RA, Fox WW, Abman SH (eds): Fetal and Neonatal Physiology. Philadelphia, WB Saunders Company, 2004, p 291.

alpha linolenic acid. It is unlikely that synthesis of DHA from alpha linolenic acid can meet the need for optimal brain DHA accumulation.[148] Human infants born at term accumulate DHA during the third trimester by maternal transfer across the placenta.[149] Transfer continues after birth through breast milk. Since 2002, infant formulas have been supplemented with DHA and AA. Published studies as yet have not demonstrated a consistent benefit from supplementation on either visual function or neurodevelopmental outcome.[150,151] Fat is also not completely absorbed; more so in the premature than in the term infant.[147] For that reason, preterm formulas provide a portion of the fat energy as medium-chain triglycerides.

Intestinal disaccharidases develop early in fetal life, with lactase reaching mature levels at term.[152] Both term and preterm infants can digest lactose, the major sugar in human milk and standard infant formulas. Although lactase levels are lower in preterm infants and can lead to feeding intolerance, early initiation of enteral feeds can lead to a rapid increase in lactase.[153] Carbohydrate represents 40 to 50 percent of total calories in most formulas as well as human milk. These levels are more than adequate to maintain normal blood glucose levels and prevent ketosis.

Vitamins and Minerals

Published requirements are available for all major minerals and vitamins for term and preterm infants.[145,154] Information on trace minerals[145,154] is available as well.

Infant Feeding

For the well term or slightly preterm infant, institution of oral feeds within the first 2 to 4 hours of life is reasonable practice. For infants who are SGA or large for gestational age (LGA), feeds within the first hour or two of life may be indicated to avoid hypoglycemia. Premature infants (<31 weeks' gestation) who are unable to nipple feed present a more complex set of circumstances. In addition to an inability to suck and swallow efficiently, such infants face a number of problems: (1) relatively high caloric demand; (2) small stomach capacity; (3) incompetent esophageal-cardiac sphincter, leading to gastroesophageal reflux; (4) poor gag reflex, creating a tendency for aspiration; (5) decreased digestive capability (especially for fat); and (6) slow gastric emptying and intestinal motility. These infants can initially be supported adequately with parenteral nutrition, followed by institution of nasogastric tube feedings when their cardiopulmonary status is stable.

Although a wide range of infant formulas satisfy the nutritional needs of most neonates, breast milk remains the standard on which formulas are based. The distribution of calories in human milk is 7 percent protein, 55 percent fat, and 38 percent carbohydrate. The whey/casein ratio is 70:30, enhancing ease of protein digestion and gastric emptying, while fat digestion is augmented by the presence of a breast milk lipase. In addition to easy digestibility, the amino acid make-up is well suited for the newborn. Despite the low levels of several vitamins and minerals, bioavailability is high. Besides the nutritional features, breast milk's immunochemical and cellular components provide protection against infection.[155]

The growth demands of the low-birth-weight infant exceed the contents of human milk for protein, calcium, phosphorus, sodium, zinc, copper, and possibly other nutrients.[156] These shortcomings can be addressed through the addition of human milk fortifiers to mother's preterm breast milk.[156] Advantages of breast milk for the premature include its anti-infective properties, possible protection against NEC, and its role in enhancing neurodevelopmental outcome.[157–160]

Few contraindications to breast-feeding exist. Infants with galactosemia should not ingest lactose-containing milk. Infants with other inborn errors such as phenylketonuria may ingest some human milk, with close monitoring of the amount. The presence of environmental pollutants has been documented in breast milk, but to date no serious side effects have been reported. Most drugs do not contraindicate breast-feeding, but there are a few exceptions (see Chapter 8). Transmission of some viral infections via breast milk is a concern as well. Mothers who are hepatitis B surface antigen (HB_sAg) or human immunodeficiency virus (HIV) positive should not breast-feed. The nursery staff must be aware of problems associated with breast-feeding and use lactation consultants to deal with poor infant latching, sore nipples, poor milk supply, and excessive hyperbilirubinemia. The obstetrician and pediatrician should serve as a source of knowledge and, most importantly, support. Table 20-11 illustrates what a mother can expect as she breast-feeds her infant.

Neonatal Hypoglycemia

Glucose is a major fetal fuel transported by facilitated diffusion across the placenta. After birth, before an appropriate supply of exogenous calories is provided, the newborn must maintain blood glucose through endogenous sources. This homeostasis depends on an adequate supply of gluconeogenic substrates (amino acids, lactate, glycerol), functionally intact hepatic glycogenolytic and gluconeogenic enzyme systems, and a normal endocrine counterregulatory hormone system (glucagon, catecholamines, growth hormone, cortisol) integrating and modulating these processes. Hepatic glycogen stores are almost entirely depleted within the first 12 hours after birth in the healthy term neonate and more rapidly in the preterm or stressed infant if there is no other glucose source. Fat and protein stores are then used for energy, while glucose levels are maintained by hepatic gluconeogenesis.

In utero, fetal blood glucose concentration is 15 mg/dl lower than maternal levels. In the healthy unstressed neonate, glucose falls over the first 1 to 2 hours after birth, stabilizes at a minimum of about 40 mg/dl, and then rises to 50 to 80 mg/dl by 3 hours of life.[161] Hypoglycemia can be defined as blood glucose levels less than 45 mg/dl. Infants at risk for hypoglycemia and in whom glucose should be monitored include preterm infants, SGA infants, hyperinsulinemic (LGA) infants, and infants with perinatal stress or asphyxia. As in term babies, blood sugar drops after birth in preterm babies, but the latter are less able to mount a counterregulatory response.[162] In addition, the presence of respiratory distress, hypothermia, and other factors can increase glucose demand, exacerbating hypoglycemia. SGA infants are at risk for hypoglycemia resulting from decreased glycogen stores as well as impaired gluconeogenesis and ketogenesis.[163] Onset of hypoglycemia in SGA and preterm infants usually occurs at 2 to 6 hours of life. Hyperinsulinemia occurs in the infant of a diabetic mother as well as other rare conditions, including Beckwith-Weidemann syndrome and congenital hyperinsulinism.[161] Onset of hypoglycemia in these infants can be in the first 30 to 60 minutes after birth. In the case of perinatal asphyxia, hypoglycemia is the result of excessive glucose demand.[164] Infants with recurrent hypoglycemia over 3 to 4 days should be evaluated for endocrine (hyperinsulinism, decreased counterregulatory hormones) and inborn errors of metabolism disorders (Table 20-12).

Symptoms of hypoglycemia include jitteriness, seizures, cyanosis, respiratory distress, apathy, hypotonia, and eye rolling.[161] However, many infants, particularly premature infants, are asymptomatic. Because of the risk of subsequent brain injury,[165] hypoglycemia, when present, should be aggressively treated. However, the single best treatment is prevention by identifying infants at risk, including premature, SGA, LGA, and any stressed infant. These newborns should have blood glucose screened with a bedside glucose meter. All values less than or equal to 45 mg/dl should be confirmed with a laboratory or rapid glucose analyzer measurement of whole blood glucose. Treatment is provided by early institution of feeds or an intravenous glucose bolus (2 ml/kg of $D_{10}W$ solution) followed by a glucose infusion at a rate of 6 mg/kg/min.

Congenital Gastrointestinal Surgical Conditions

Several congenital surgical conditions of the gastrointestinal tract interfere with a normal transition. Many of these conditions can be diagnosed with antenatal ultrasound, allowing transfer of the mother to a perinatal center for delivery.

Gastrointestinal Tract Obstruction

Tracheoesophageal fistula and esophageal atresia are characterized by a blind esophageal pouch and a fistulous connection between either the proximal or distal esophagus and the airway.[166] Eighty-five percent of infants with these conditions have the fistula between the distal esophagus and the airway. Polyhydramnios is common because of the high level of gastrointestinal obstruction. Infants present in the first hours of life with copious secretions, choking, cyanosis, and respiratory distress. Diagnosis can be confirmed with chest radiography after careful placement of a nasogastric tube to the point where resistance is met. The tube will be seen in the blind esophageal pouch. If a tracheoesophageal fistula is present to the distal esophagus, gas will be present in the abdomen.

Infants with high intestinal obstruction present early in life with either bilious or nonbilious vomiting.[167] A history of polyhydramnios is common, and the amniotic fluid, if bile stained, can easily be confused with thin meconium staining. In duodenal atresia, vomitus may or may not contain bile, whereas malrotation with midgut volvulus and high jejunal atresia are characterized by bilious vomiting. Malrotation and midgut volvulus involve torsion of the intestine around the superior mesenteric artery, causing occlusion of the vascular supply to most of the small intestine. If not treated promptly, the infant can lose most of the small bowel due to ischemic injury. Therefore, bilious vomiting in the neonate demands immediate attention and evaluation. Diagnosis of high intestinal obstruction can be confirmed with radiographs. Duodenal atresia is characterized by a "double-bubble sign" (stomach and dilated duodenum). Diagnosis of midgut

Table 20-11. Guidelines for Successful Breast Feeding

	FIRST 8 HOURS	8–24 HOURS	DAY 2	DAY 3	DAY 4	DAY 5	DAY 6 ONWARD
Milk Supply	You may be able to express a few drops of milk.		Milk *should* come in between the 2nd and 4th day.			Milk should be in. Breasts may be firm and/or leak milk.	Breasts should feel softer after nursing.
Baby's Activity	Baby is usually wide awake in the first hour of life. Put baby to breast within ½ hour of birth.	Wake up your baby. Babies may not wake up on their own to feed.	Baby should be more cooperative and less sleepy.	Look for early feeding cues such as rooting, lip smacking, and hands to face.			Baby should appear satisfied after feedings.
Feeding Rountine	Baby may go into a deep sleep 2–4 hours after birth.	Feed your baby every 1 to 4 hours, as often as wanted, a minimum of 8–12 times each day.	Use chart on back side of page to write *down* time and length of each feeding.			May go *one* longer interval (up to 5 hours) between feeds in a 24-hour period.	
Breast-Feeding	Baby will wake up and be alert and responsive for several more hours after initial deep sleep.	As long as Mom is comfortable, nurse at both breasts as long as baby is actively sucking.	Try to nurse both sides each feeding, aiming for 10 minutes each side. Expect some nipple tenderness.	Consider hand expressing or pumping a few drops of milk to soften the nipple if the breast is too firm for the baby to latch on.	Nurse a minimum of 10–30 minutes each side every feeding for the first few weeks of life. Once your milk supply is well established, allow your baby to finish the first breast before offering the second.		Mom's nipple tenderness is improving or is gone.
Baby's Urine Output		Baby must have a minimum of 1 wet diaper in first 24 hours.	Baby must have at least one wet diaper every 8–11 hours.	You should see an increase in wet diapers to 4–6 times in 24 hours.	Baby's urine should be light yellow or clear.	Baby should have 6–8 wet diapers each day of colorless or light yellow urine.	
Baby's Stools		Baby should have a black-green stool (meconium stool).	Baby may have a second very dark (meconium) stool.	Baby's stools should be changing color from black-green to yellow.		Baby should have 3–4 yellow, soft stools a day.	The number of stools may decrease gradually after 4–6 weeks of life.

Courtesy of Beth Gabrielski, RN: The Children's Hospital, Denver, 1999 with permission.

Table 20-12. Etiologies of Neonatal Hypoglycemia

I. Transient neonatal hypoglycemia
  A. Preterm and IUGR infants
  B. Transient hyperinsulinism (IDM)
  C. Perinatal stress (hypoxia, RDS)
II. Persistent neonatal hypoglycemia
  A. Hyperinsulinism
    1. potassium-ATP channel
    2. glucokinase hyperinsulinism
    3. glutamate dehydrogenase hyperinsulinism
    4. Beckwith-Wiedemann syndrome
  B. Counterregulatory hormone deficiency (hypopituitarism)
  C. Inborn errors of metabolism
    1. Glycogenolysis disorders
    2. Gluconeogenesis disorders
    3. Fatty acid oxidation disorders

ATP, adenosine triphosphate; IDM, infant of a diabetic mother; IUGR, intrauterine growth restriction; RDS, respiratory distress syndrome.

volvulus can be confirmed with an upper gastrointestinal tract series, looking for contrast not to pass the ligament of Treitz. Approximately 30 percent of cases of duodenal atresia are associated with Down syndrome.[167]

Low intestinal obstruction presents with increasing intolerance of feeds (spitting progressing to vomiting), abdominal distention, and decreased or absent stool.[167] Differential diagnosis of lower intestinal obstruction includes imperforate anus, Hirschsprung disease, meconium plug syndrome, small left colon, colonic and ileal atresia, and meconium ileus. Plain x-ray study of the abdomen shows gaseous distention, with air through a considerable portion of the bowel and air-fluid levels. Diagnosis of meconium ileus, meconium plug, and small left colon syndrome can be made by appearance on contrast enema. Rectal biopsy searching for absence of ganglion cells confirms the diagnosis of Hirschsprung disease. Infants with meconium ileus and meconium plug should be screened for cystic fibrosis.

Abdominal Wall Defects

Omphaloceles[168] are formed by incomplete closure of the anterior abdominal wall after return of the midgut to the abdominal cavity. The size of the defect is variable, but usually the omphalocele sac contains some intestine, stomach, liver, and spleen. The abdominal cavity is small and underdeveloped. The umbilical cord can be seen to insert onto the center of the omphalocele sac. There is a high incidence of associated anomalies, including cardiac, other gastrointestinal anomalies, and chromosomal syndromes (trisomy 13). Delivery room treatment involves covering the defect with sterile warm saline to prevent fluid loss and nasogastric tube decompression.[169]

Gastroschisis[168] is a defect in the anterior abdominal wall lateral to the umbilicus with no covering sac, with the herniated viscera usually limited to intestine. Furthermore, the intestine has been exposed to amniotic fluid and has a thickened, beefy red appearance. The herniation is thought to occur as a rupture through an ischemic portion of the abdominal wall. Other than intestinal atresia, associated anomalies are uncommon. Delivery room management is as described for omphalocele.

Diaphragmatic Hernia

In diaphragmatic hernia,[170] herniation of abdominal organs into the hemithorax (usually left) occurs because of a posterolateral defect in the diaphragm. Infants usually present in the delivery room with respiratory distress, cyanosis, decreased breath sounds on the side of the hernia, and shift of the mediastinum to the side opposite the hernia. The rapidity and severity of presentation with respiratory distress is dependent on the degree of associated pulmonary hypoplasia. The ipsilateral and to some extent contralateral lung are compressed in utero because of the hernia. Delivery room treatment is to intubate, to ventilate, and to decompress the gastrointestinal tract with a nasogastric tube. A chest radiograph confirms the diagnosis. The mortality due to diaphragmatic hernia is 25 to 40 percent, with survival dependent upon the degree of lung hypoplasia and the presence of associated congenital heart disease.[171] See Chapter 10 for a discussion of fetal surgical approaches to diaphragmatic hernia aimed at minimizing lung hypoplasia.[172,173]

Necrotizing Enterocolitis

NEC is the most common acquired gastrointestinal emergency in the neonatal intensive care unit. This disorder predominantly affects premature infants, with higher incidences present with decreasing gestational age, although it is seen in term infants with polycythemia, congenital heart disease, and birth asyphyxia.[174,175] The pathogenesis is multifactorial, with intestinal ischemia, infection, provision of enteral feedings, and gut maturity playing roles to varying degrees in individual patients.[174] Tocolysis with indomethacin presumably related to changes in intestinal circulation has been associated with an increased incidence of NEC and isolated intestinal perforation, whereas antenatal betamethasone may decrease the incidence.[18,176,177]

Clinically, there is a varied spectrum of disease, from a mild gastrointestinal disturbance to a rapid fulminant course characterized by intestinal gangrene, perforation, sepsis, and shock. The hallmark symptoms are abdominal distention, ileus, delayed gastric emptying, and bloody stools. The radiographic findings are bowel wall edema, pneumatosis intestinalis, biliary free air, and free peritoneal air. Associated symptoms include apnea, bradycardia, hypotension, and temperature instability.

Neonatal Jaundice

The most common problem encountered in a term nursery population is jaundice. Neonatal hyperbilirubinemia occurs when the normal pathways of bilirubin

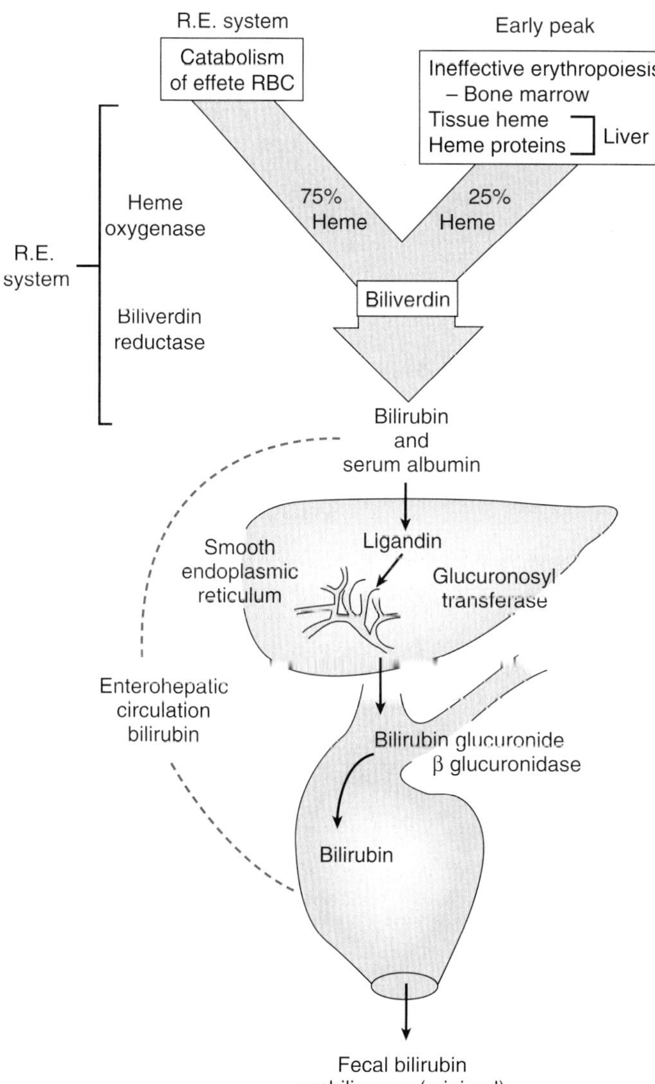

Figure 20-16. Neonatal bile pigment metabolism. (Adapted from Maisels MJ: Jaundice. *In* Avery GB, Fletcher MA, MacDonald MG [eds]: Neonatology: Pathophysiology and Management of the Newborn, 5th ed. Philadelphia, Lippincott Williams & Wilkins, 1999, p 765, with permission.)

metabolism and excretion are altered. Figure 20-16 demonstrates the metabolism of bilirubin. The normal destruction of circulating red cells accounts for about 75 percent of the newborn's daily bilirubin production. The remaining sources include ineffective erythropoiesis and tissue heme proteins. Heme is converted to bilirubin in the reticuloendothelial system. Unconjugated bilirubin is lipid soluble and transported in the plasma reversibly bound to albumin. Bilirubin enters the liver cells by dissociation from albumin in the hepatic sinusoids. Once in the hepatocyte, bilirubin is conjugated with glucuronic acid in a reaction catalyzed by uridine diphosphoglucuronosyl transferase (UDPGT). The water-soluble conjugated bilirubin is sufficiently polar to be excreted into bile or filtered through the kidney. After conjugation, bilirubin is excreted rapidly into the bile canaliculi and into the small intestine. The enzyme β-glucuronidase is present in small bowel and hydrolyzes some of the conjugated

Table 20-13. Risk Factors for Significant Hyperbilirubinemia

Jaundice observed at less than 24 hours
Blood group incompatability with positive direct Coombs' test
Other hemolytic disease (G6PD deficiency)
Gestational age 35–36 weeks
Previous sibling needing phototherapy
Cephalohematoma, subgaleal blood collection, bruising
Exclusive breast feeding, especially if nursing not going well
East Asian race

G6PD, glucose-6-phosphate dehydrogenase.
Adapted from American Academy of Pediatrics Subcommittee on Hyperbilirubinemia: Management of hyperbilirubinemia in the newborn infant 35 or more weeks gestation. Pediatrics 114:297, 2004.

bilirubin. This unconjugated bilirubin can be reabsorbed into the circulation, adding to the total unconjugated bilirubin load (enterohepatic circulation). Major predisposing factors of neonatal jaundice are (1) increased bilirubin load because of increased red cell volume with decreased cell survival, increased ineffective erythropoiesis, and the enterohepatic circulation; and (2) decreased hepatic uptake, conjugation, and excretion of bilirubin. These factors result in the presence of clinically apparent jaundice in approximately two thirds of newborns during the first week of life.[178] This transient jaundice has been called physiologic jaundice. Infants whose bilirubin levels are above the 95th percentile for age in hours and infants in high-risk groups to develop hyperbilirubinemia require close follow-up (Fig. 20-17 and Table 20-13).[179]

Pathologic jaundice during the early neonatal period is indirect hyperbilirubinemia usually caused by overproduction of bilirubin. The leading cause in this group of patients is hemolytic disease, of which fetomaternal blood group incompatibilities (ABO, Rh and other minor antibodies) are the most common (see Chapter 30). Other causes of hemolysis include genetic disorders such as hereditary spherocytosis and nonspherocytic hemolytic anemias, such as glucose-6-phosphate dehydrogenase (G6PD) deficiency. Other etiologies of bilirubin overproduction include extravasated blood (bruising, hemorrhage), polycythemia, and exaggerated enterohepatic circulation of bilirubin because of mechanical gastrointestinal obstruction or reduced peristalsis from inadequate oral intake. Disease states involving decreased bilirubin clearance must be considered in the patients in whom no cause of overproduction can be identified. Causes of indirect hyperbilirubinemia in this category include familial deficiency of UDPGT (Crigler-Najjar syndrome), Gilbert's syndrome, breast milk jaundice, and hypothyroidism. Mixed or direct hyperbilirubinemia are rare during the first week of life.

A strong association exists between breast-feeding and neonatal hyperbilirubinemia. The syndrome of breast milk jaundice is characterized by full-term infants who have jaundice that persists into the second and third weeks of life with maximal bilirubin levels of 10 to 30 mg/dl. If breast-feeding is continued, the levels persist for 4 to 10 days and then decline to normal by 3 to 12 weeks.

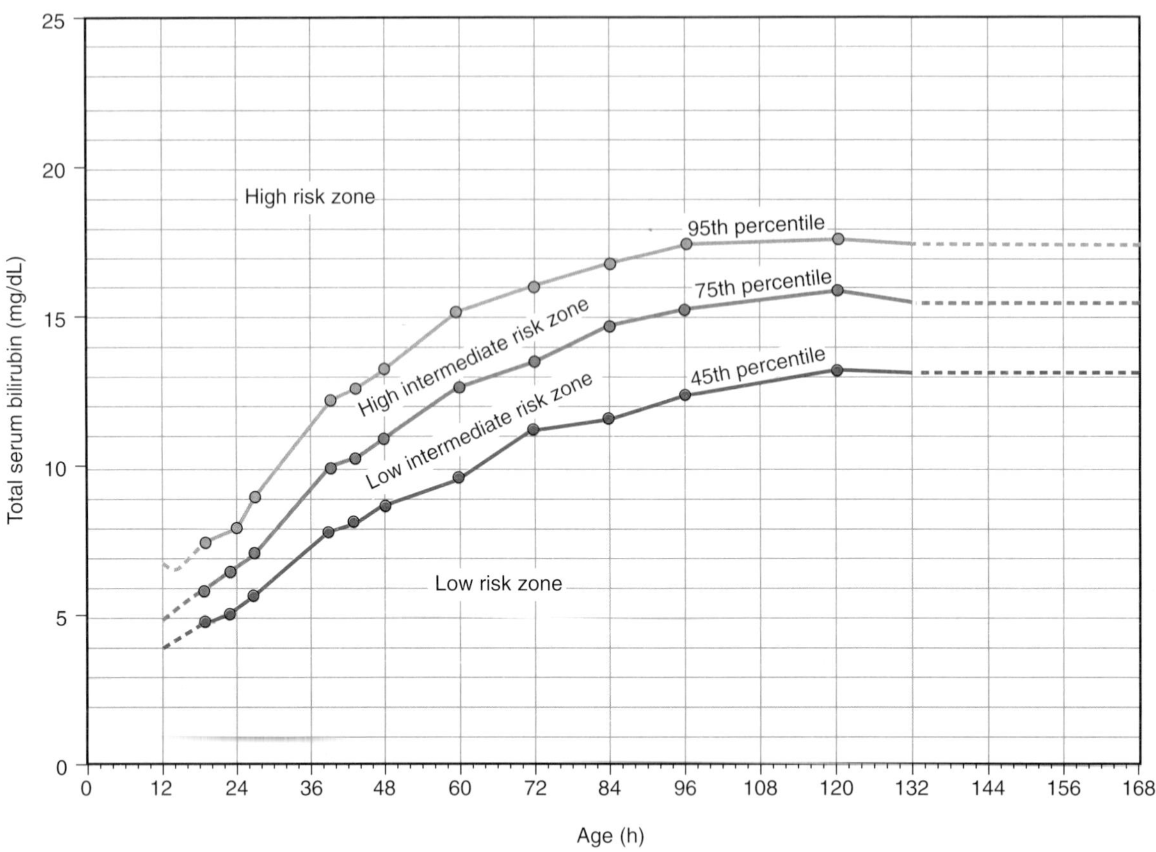

Figure 20-17. Risk of developing significant hyperbilirubinemia in term and near-term infants based on hour-specific bilirubin determinations. (From Bhutani VK, Johnson L, Sivieri EM: Predictive ability of a predischarge hour-specific serum bilirubin for subsequent significant hyperbilirubinemia in healthy term and near-term newborns. Pediatrics 103:6, 1999. Copyright 1999 American Academy of Pediatrics, with permission.)

Interruption of breast-feeding is associated with a prompt decline in 48 hours.[180] In addition to this syndrome, breast-fed infants as a whole have higher bilirubin levels over the first 3 to 5 days of life than their formula-fed counterparts (Fig. 20-18).[181] Rather than interrupting breast-feeding, this early jaundice is responsive to increased frequency of breast-feeding. Suggested mechanisms for breast-feeding–associated jaundice include decreased early caloric intake, inhibitors of bilirubin conjugation in breast milk, and increased intestinal reabsorption of bilirubin.[182] In some patients, there is considerable overlap in these described syndromes.

The overriding concern with neonatal hyperbilirubinemia is the development of bilirubin toxicity causing the pathologic entity of kernicterus, the staining of certain areas of the brain (basal ganglia, hippocampus, geniculate bodies, various brain stem nuclei, and cerebellum) by bilirubin. Neuronal necrosis is the dominant histopathologic feature at 7 to 10 days of life. The early symptoms of bilirubin encephalopathy consist of lethargy, hypotonia and poor feeding progressing to high-pitched cry, hypertonicity, and opisthotonos. Survivors usually suffer sequelae, including athetoid cerebral palsy, high-frequency hearing loss, paralysis of upward gaze, and dental dysplasia.[183] The risk of bilirubin encephalopathy in a given infant is not well defined. The only group that one can speak of with any certainty is those infants with Rh isoimmunization in whom a level of 20 mg/dl has been associated with an increased risk of kernicterus.[184] This observation has been extended to the management of other neonates with hemolytic disease, although no definitive data exist regarding these infants. The risk is probably small for term infants without hemolytic disease even at levels higher than 20 mg/dl.[185–187] Recent descriptions of bilirubin encephalopathy in breast-fed infants with dehydration and hyperbilirubinemia in whom an adequate supply of breast milk has not been established mandates close follow-up of all breast-feeding mothers.[188] The true risk for nonhemolytic hyperbilirubinemia to produce brain damage in the preterm in the current era of liberal use of phototherapy that prevents marked elevation of severe bilirubin in these infants is unknown. However, most currently available data would suggest this risk is low.[189]

NEONATAL HEMATOLOGY

Anemia

Early hematopoietic cells originate in the yolk sac. By 8 weeks' gestation, erythropoiesis is taking place in the liver, which remains the primary site of erythroid production through the early fetal period. By 6 months of gestation, the bone marrow becomes the principal site of red cell development.[190] Normal hemoglobin levels at

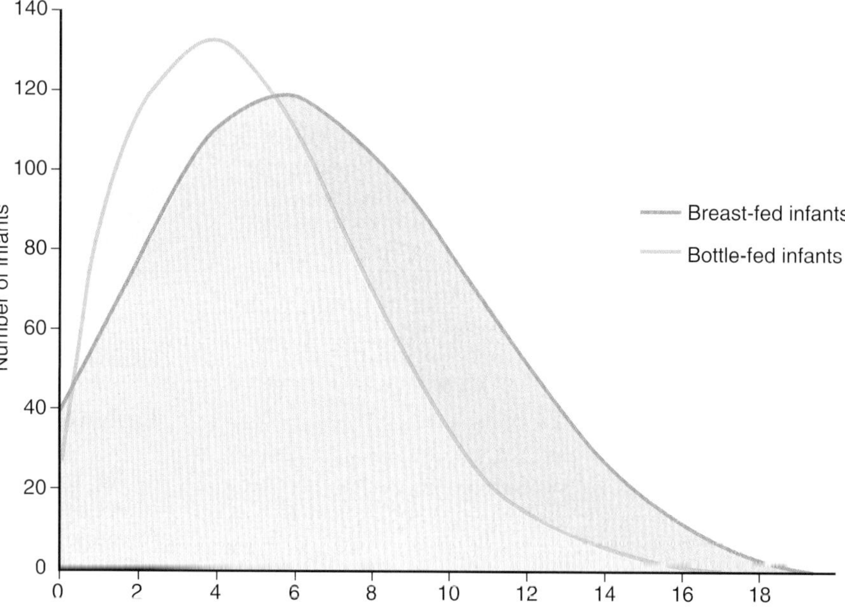

Figure 20-18. Distribution of maximum serum bilirubin concentrations in white infants who weigh more than 2,500g. (Adapted from Maisels MJ, Gifford KL: Normal serum bilirubin levels in the newborn and the effect of breast-feeding. Pediatrics 78:837, 1986, with permission.)

term range from 13.7 to 20.1 g/dl.[191] In the very preterm infant, values as low as 12 g/dl are acceptable.[192] Anemia at birth or appearing in the first few weeks of life is the result of blood loss, hemolysis, or underproduction of erythrocytes.[193] Blood loss resulting in anemia can occur prenatally, at the time of delivery, or postnatally. In utero blood loss can be the result of fetomaternal bleeding, twin-to-twin transfusion, or blood loss resulting from trauma (maternal trauma, amniocentesis, external cephalic version). The diagnosis of fetomaternal hemorrhage large enough to cause anemia can be made using the Kleihauer-Betke technique of acid elution to identify fetal cells in the maternal circulation. Blood loss at delivery can be caused by umbilical cord rupture, incision of the placenta during cesarean delivery, placenta previa, or abruptio placentae. Internal hemorrhage can occur in the newborn, often related to a difficult delivery. Sites include intracranial, cephalhematomas, subgaleal space, retroperitoneal, liver capsule, and ruptured spleen. When blood loss has been chronic (e.g., fetomaternal), infants will be pale at birth but well compensated and without signs of volume loss. The initial hematocrit will be low. Acute bleeding will present with signs of hypovolemia (tachycardia, poor perfusion, hypotension). The initial hematocrit can be normal or decreased, but after several hours of equilibration, it will be decreased. Anemia caused by hemolysis from blood group incompatibilities is common in the newborn period. Less common causes of hemolysis include erythrocyte membrane abnormalities, enzyme deficiencies, and disorders of hemoglobin synthesis. Impaired erythrocyte production is a rare cause of neonatal anemia.

Polycythemia

Elevated hematocrits occur in 1.5 to 4 percent of live births.[194] Although 50 percent of polycythemic infants are appropriate for gestational age (AGA), the proportion of polycythemic infants is greater in the SGA and LGA populations.[194] Causes of polycythemia include twin-to-twin transfusion, maternal-to-fetal transfusion, intrapartum transfusion from the placenta associated with fetal distress, chronic intrauterine hypoxia (SGA infants, LGA infants of diabetic mothers), delayed cord clamping, and chromosomal abnormalities.[195] The consequence of polycythemia is hyperviscosity, resulting in impaired perfusion of capillary beds. Therefore, clinical symptoms can be related to any organ system (Table 20-14). Because viscosity measurements are not routinely performed at most institutions, hyperviscosity is inferred from hematocrit because the major factor influencing viscosity in the newborn is red cell mass. Cord blood hematocrit greater than or equal to 57 percent[196] and capillary hematocrit of at least 70 percent are indicative of polycythemia. Confirmation of the diagnosis is a peripheral venous hematocrit of at least 64 percent.[196] Reduction of venous hematocrit to less than 60 percent may improve acute symptoms, but it has not been shown to improve long-term neurologic outcome.[197–199]

Table 20-14. Organ-Related Symptoms of Hyperviscosity

Central nervous system	Irritability, jitteriness, seizures, lethargy
Cardiopulmonary	Respiratory distress caused by congestive heart failure or persistent pulmonary hypertension
Gastrointestinal	Vomiting, heme-positive stools, abdominal distention, necrotizing enterocolitis
Renal	Decreased urine output, renal vein thrombosis
Metabolic	Hypoglycemia
Hematologic	Hyperbilirubinemia, thrombocytopenia

Table 20-15. Differential Diagnosis of Neonatal Thrombocytopenia

DIAGNOSIS	COMMENTS
Immune	Passively acquired antibody (e.g., idiopathic thrombocytopenic purpura, systemic lupus erythematosus, drug induced)
	Alloimmune sensitization to HPA-1a antigen
Infections	Bacterial; congenital viral infections (e.g., cytomegalovirus, rubella)
Syndromes	Absent radii; Fanconi's anemia
Giant hemangioma	
Thrombosis	
High-risk infant with respiratory distress syndrome, pulmonary hypertension, and so forth	Disseminated intravascular coagulation
	Isolated thrombocytopenia

HPA-1a, human platelet antigen-1a.

Thrombocytopenia

Neonatal thrombocytopenia can be isolated or occur associated with deficiency of clotting factors. A differential diagnosis is presented in Table 20-15. The immune thrombocytopenias have implications for perinatal care. In idiopathic thrombocytopenic purpura (ITP), maternal antiplatelet antibodies that cross the placenta lead to destruction of fetal platelets. However, only 10 to 15 percent of infants born to mothers with ITP have platelet counts less than 100,000 and even in infants with severe thrombocytopenia, serious bleeding is rare.[200–203] Alloimmune thrombocytopenia occurs when an antigen is present on fetal platelets but is not present on maternal platelets. On exposure to fetal platelets, the mother develops antiplatelet antibodies that cross the placenta causing destruction of fetal platelets. In the largest series of cases of suspected alloimmune thrombocytopenia, the majority were caused by HPA-1a alloantibodies.[204] Because the maternal platelet count is normal, the diagnosis is suspected on the basis of a history of a previously affected pregnancy. Intracranial hemorrhage is common with this condition (10 to 20 percent) and can occur in the antenatal or intrapartum periods.[205,206] Percutaneous umbilical blood sampling (PUBS) can be performed to measure fetal platelet count. Antenatal treatment options include fetal platelet transfusions treatment with corticosteroids and administration of weekly intravenous immunoglobulin infusions to the mother.[205–207]

Vitamin K Deficiency Bleeding of the Newborn

Vitamin K1 oxide (1 mg) should be given intramuscularly to all newborns to prevent hemorrhagic disease caused by a deficiency in vitamin K–dependent clotting factors (II, VII, IX, X).[208] Babies born to mothers who are on anticonvulsant medication are particularly at risk of having vitamin K deficiency. Bleeding occurs in 0.25 to 1.4 percent of newborns who do not receive vitamin K prophylaxis, generally in the first 5 days to 2 weeks but as late as 12 weeks. Oral vitamin K has been shown to be effective in raising vitamin K levels but is not as effective in preventing late hemorrhagic disease of the newborn. Late hemorrhagic disease of the newborn most commonly occurs in breast-fed infants whose courses have been complicated by diarrhea.

PERINATAL INFECTION

Early-Onset Bacterial Infection

The unique predisposition of the neonate to bacterial infection is related to defects in both innate and acquired immune responses.[209]

The incidence of bacterial infection in infants younger than 5 days of age is 4 to 5/1000 live births. Rupture of membranes for more than 12 to 18 hours increases the risk of infection with the rate of infection 1 in 100 births after 24 hours. The presence of chorioamnionitis further increases the risk to 1 in 10.[210–213] Maternal fever from other etiologies (e.g., epidural anesthesia) does not increase the risk of neonatal infection and merits only close observation of the newborn. Irrespective of membrane rupture, infection rates are higher in preterm infants. Maternal colonization with group B streptococcus (GBS) carries a 1 in 100 risk to the newborn of early onset sepsis. The majority of early-onset bacterial infection presents on day 1 of life, with respiratory distress the most common presenting symptom. These infections are most often caused by GBS and gram-negative enteric pathogens. The algorithm for prevention of early-onset GBS infections is presented in Figure 20-19, with the approach to the newborn shown in Figure 20-20.[214] Other etiologies of infection in the newborn are covered in Chapter 49.

RESPIRATORY DISTRESS

The establishment of respiratory function at birth is dependent on expansion and maintenance of air sacs, clearance of lung fluid, and provision of adequate pulmonary perfusion. In many premature and other high-risk infants, developmental deficiencies or unfavorable perinatal events hamper a smooth respiratory transition. Furthermore, a neonate has a limited number of ways to respond symptomatically to a variety of pathophysiologic insults. The presentation of respiratory distress is among the most common symptom complexes seen in the newborn and may be secondary to both noncardiopulmonary and cardiopulmonary etiologies (Table 20-16). The symptom complex includes an elevation of the respiratory rate to greater than 60 bpm with or without cyanosis, nasal flaring, intercostal and sternal retractions, and expiratory grunting. The retractions are the result of the neonate's efforts to expand a lung with poor compliance using a very compliant chest wall. The expiratory grunt is caused by closure of the glottis during expira-

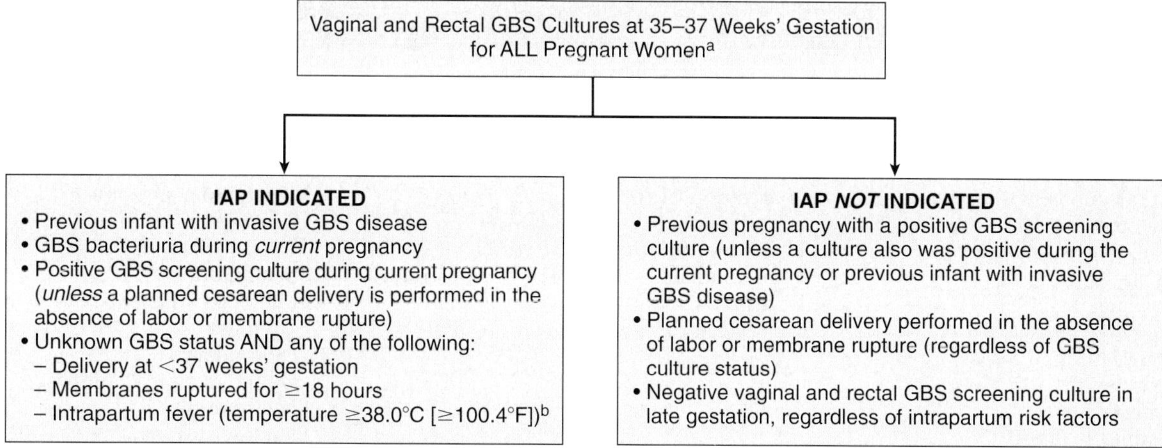

Vaginal and Rectal GBS Cultures at 35–37 Weeks' Gestation for ALL Pregnant Women[a]
IAP INDICATED
• Previous infant with invasive GBS disease
• GBS bacteriuria during *current* pregnancy
• Positive GBS screening culture during current pregnancy (*unless* a planned cesarean delivery is performed in the absence of labor or membrane rupture)
• Unknown GBS status AND any of the following:
– Delivery at <37 weeks' gestation
– Membranes ruptured for ≥18 hours
– Intrapartum fever (temperature ≥38.0°C [≥100.4°F])[b]
IAP *NOT* INDICATED
• Previous pregnancy with a positive GBS screening culture (unless a culture also was positive during the current pregnancy or previous infant with invasive GBS disease)
• Planned cesarean delivery performed in the absence of labor or membrane rupture (regardless of GBS culture status)
• Negative vaginal and rectal GBS screening culture in late gestation, regardless of intrapartum risk factors
[a] Exceptions: women with GBS bacteriuria during the current pregnancy or women with a previous infant with invasive GBS disease.
[b] If chorioamnionitis is suspected, broad-spectrum antimicrobial therapy that includes an agent known to be active against GBS should replace GBS IAP.
GBS = group B streptococcus, IAP = intrapartum antimicrobial prophylaxis

Figure 20-19. Indications for intrapartum antimicrobial prophylaxis to prevent early onset GBS disease using a universal prenatal culture screening strategy at 35 to 37 weeks' gestation for all pregnant women. (Reproduced with permission from the American Academy of Pediatrics: RedBook 2003 Report of the Committee on Infectious Disease, 2003.)

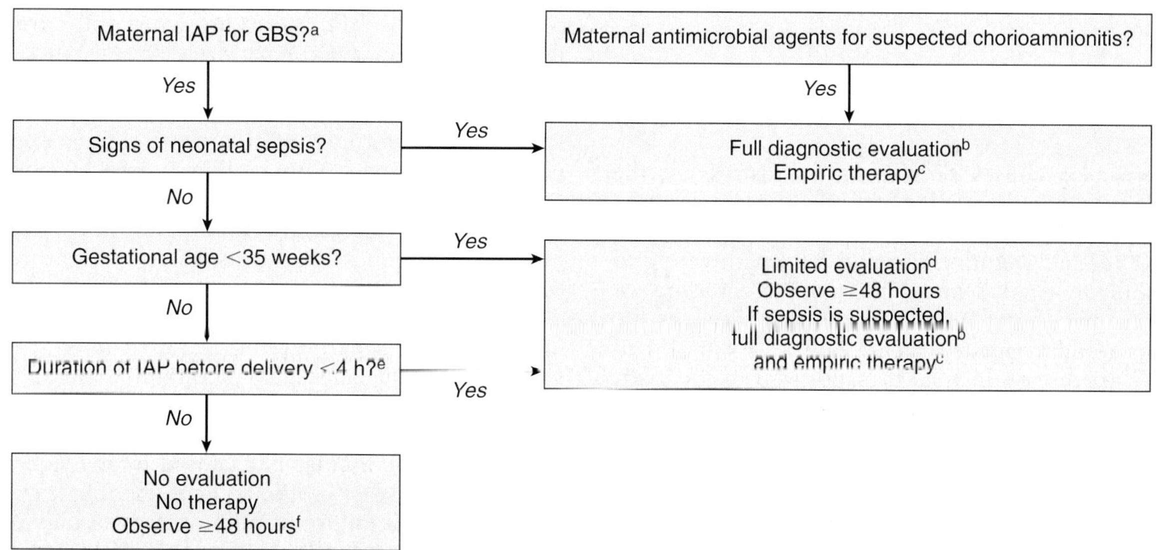

Maternal IAP for GBS?[a]
Maternal antimicrobial agents for suspected chorioamnionitis?
Yes
Yes
Signs of neonatal sepsis?
Yes
Full diagnostic evaluation[b]
Empiric therapy[c]
No
Gestational age <35 weeks?
Yes
Limited evaluation[d]
Observe ≥48 hours
If sepsis is suspected, full diagnostic evaluation[b] and empiric therapy[c]
No
Duration of IAP before delivery <4 h?[e]
Yes
No
No evaluation
No therapy
Observe ≥48 hours[f]
[a] If no maternal IAP for GBS was administered despite an indication being present, data are insufficient on which to recommend a single management strategy.
[b] Includes complete blood cell (CBC) count with differential, blood culture, and chest radiograph if respiratory abnormalities are present. When signs of sepsis are present, a lumbar puncture, if feasible, should be performed.
[c] Duration of therapy varies depending on results of blood culture, cerebrospinal fluid findings (if obtained), and the clinical course of the infant. If laboratory results and clinical course do not indicate bacterial infection, duration may be as short as 48 hours.
[d] CBC including (WBC) count with differential and blood culture.
[e] Applies only to penicillin, ampicillin, or cefazolin and assumes recommended dosing regimens.
[f] A healthy-appearing infant who was ≥38 weeks' gestation at delivery and whose mother received ≥4 hours of IAP before delivery may be discharged home after 24 hours if other discharge criteria have been met and a person able to comply fully with instructions for home observation will be present. If any one of these conditions is not met, the infant should be observed in the hospital for at least 48 hours and until criteria for discharge are achieved.

Figure 20-20. Empiric management of a neonate born to a mother who received intrapartum antimicrobial prophylaxis (IAP) for prevention of early onset GBS disease or chorioamnionitis. (Reproduced with permission from the American Academy of Pediatrics: RedBook 2003 Report of the Committee on Infectious Disease, 2003.)

Table 20-16. Respiratory Distress in the Newborn

NONCARDIOPULMONARY	CARDIOVASCULAR	PULMONARY
Hypo- or hyperthermia	Left-sided outflow obstruction	Upper airway obstruction
Hypoglycemia	Hypoplastic left heart	Choanal atresia
Metabolic acidosis	Aortic stenosis	Vocal cord paralysis
Drug intoxications; withdrawal	Coarctation of the aorta	Meconium aspiration
Polycythemia	Cyanotic lesions	Clear fluid aspiration
Central nervous system insult	Transposition of the great vessels	Transient tachypnea
Asphyxia	Total anomalous pulmonary venous return	Pneumonia
Hemorrhage	Tricuspid atresia	Pulmonary hypoplasia
Neuromuscular disease	Right-sided outflow obstruction	Primary
Werdnig-Hoffman disease		Secondary
Myopathies		Hyaline membrane disease
Phrenic nerve injury		Pneumothorax
Skeletal abnormalities		Pleural effusions
Asphyxiating thoracic dystrophy		Mass lesions
		Lobar emphysema
		Cystic adenomatoid malformation

tion in an effort to increase expiratory pressure to help maintain functional residual capacity. The evaluation of such an infant requires use of history, physical examination, and laboratory data to arrive at a diagnosis. It is important to consider causes other than those related to the heart and lungs, because one's natural tendency is to focus immediately on the more common cardiopulmonary etiologies.

Cardiovascular Causes

Cardiovascular causes of respiratory distress in the neonatal period can be divided into two major groups—those with structural heart disease and those with persistent right-to-left shunting through fetal pathways and a structurally normal heart. The two presentations of serious structural heart disease in the first week of life are cyanosis and congestive heart failure. Examples of cyanotic heart disease include transposition of the great vessels, tricuspid atresia, certain types of truncus arteriosus, total anomalous pulmonary venous return, and right-sided outflow obstruction including tetralogy of Fallot and pulmonary stenosis or atresia. Although cyanosis is the central feature in these disorders, tachypnea develops in many infants because of increased pulmonary blood flow or secondary to metabolic acidosis from hypoxia. Infants with congestive heart failure generally have some form of left-sided outflow obstruction (e.g., hypoplastic left heart syndrome, coarctation of the aorta). Left-to-right shunt lesions such as ventricular septal defect do not present with increased pulmonary blood flow and congestive heart failure until pulmonary vascular resistance is low enough to permit a significant shunt (usually 3 to 4 weeks of age at sea level). Infants with left-sided outflow obstruction generally do well the first day or so until the source of systemic flow, the ductus arteriosus, narrows. With ductal narrowing, dyspnea, tachypnea, and tachycardia develop, followed by rapid progression to congestive heart failure and metabolic acidosis. On examination, these infants have pulse abnormalities. With hypoplastic left heart syndrome and critical aortic stenosis, pulses are profoundly diminished in all extremities, whereas infants with coarctation of the aorta and interrupted aortic arch have differential pulses when the arms and legs are compared.

The syndrome of persistent pulmonary hypertension of the newborn (PPHN) occurs when the normal postnatal decrease in pulmonary vascular resistance does not occur, maintaining right-to-left shunting across the patent ductus arteriosus and foramen ovale.[215] Most infants with PPHN are full term or postmature and have experienced perinatal asphyxia. Other clinical associations include hypothermia, MAS, hyaline membrane disease (HMD), polycythemia, neonatal sepsis, chronic intrauterine hypoxia, pulmonary hypoplasia, and premature closure of the ductus arteriosus in utero.

On the basis of developmental considerations, these infants can be separated into three groups[216]: (1) acute vasoconstriction caused by perinatal hypoxia, (2) prenatal increase in pulmonary vascular smooth muscle development, and (3) decreased cross-sectional area of the pulmonary vascular bed caused by inadequate vessel number. In the first group, an acute perinatal event leads to hypoxia and failure of pulmonary vascular resistance to drop. In the second, abnormal muscularization of the pulmonary resistance vessels results in PPHN after birth. The third circumstance includes infants with pulmonary hypoplasia (e.g., diaphragmatic hernia). Clinically, the syndrome is characterized by cyanosis, often unresponsive to increases in FiO_2, respiratory distress, an onset at less than 24 hours, evidence of right ventricular overload, systemic hypotension, acidosis, and no evidence of structural heart disease. There have been considerable advances in treatment for this condition using high frequency ventilation, inhaled nitric oxide, and in refractory cases, extracorporeal membrane oxygenation.[217,218] Nitric oxide is identical or similar to endogenously produced endothelium-derived relaxing factor and is used as a selective pulmonary vasodilator in infants with PPHN.[219]

Pulmonary Causes

Of the causes of respiratory distress related to the airways and pulmonary parenchyma listed in Table 20-16, the differential diagnosis in a term infant includes transient tachypnea, aspiration syndromes, congenital pneumonia, and spontaneous pneumothorax. The syndrome of transient tachypnea (wet lung or type II RDS) presents as respiratory distress in nonasphyxiated term infants or slightly preterm infants. The clinical features include various combinations of cyanosis, grunting, nasal flaring, retracting, and tachypnea during the first hours after birth. The chest radiograph is the key to the diagnosis, with prominent perihilar streaking and fluid in the interlobar fissures. The symptoms generally subside in 12 to 24 hours, although they can persist longer. The preferred explanation for the clinical features is delayed reabsorption of fetal lung fluid.[220] Transient tachypnea is seen more commonly in infants delivered by elective cesarean section or in the slightly preterm infant (see Mechanics of the First Breath, earlier).

At delivery, the neonate may aspirate clear amniotic fluid or fluid mixed with blood. Whether infants can aspirate a sufficient volume of clear fluid to cause symptoms is controversial. However, there are a group of infants whose clinical course is more prolonged (4 to 7 days) and severe than that of infants with transient tachypnea. These infants have a radiologic picture similar to transient tachypnea often associated with more marked hyperexpansion. Occasionally, the infiltrates are impressive, with evidence of far more fluid than is seen with transient tachypnea.

MAS occurs in full-term or postmature infants. The perinatal course is often marked by fetal distress and low Apgar scores. These infants exhibit tachypnea, retractions, cyanosis, overdistended and barrel-shaped chest, and coarse breath sounds. Chest radiography reveals coarse, irregular pulmonary densities with areas of diminished aeration or consolidation. There is a high incidence of air leaks, and many of the infants exhibit persistent pulmonary hypertension.[84,93]

The lungs represent the most common primary site of infection in the neonate. Both bacterial and viral infections can be acquired before, during, or after birth. The most common route of infection, particularly for bacteria, is ascending from the genital tract before or during labor. Infants with congenital pneumonia present with symptoms from very early in life, including tachypnea, retractions, grunting, nasal flaring, and cyanosis. The chest radiograph pattern is often indistinguishable from other causes of respiratory distress, particularly HMD.[221]

Spontaneous pneumothorax occurs in 1 percent of all deliveries, but a much lower percent result in symptoms.[222] The risk is increased by manipulations such as positive-pressure ventilation. Respiratory distress is usually present from shortly after birth, and breath sounds may be diminished on the affected side. The majority of these problems resolve spontaneously without specific therapy.

Despite improved understanding and recent advances, HMD remains the most common etiology for respiratory distress in the neonatal period. It was the initial reports of Avery and Mead[223] demonstrating a high surface tension in extracts of lungs from infants dying of RDS that led to the present understanding of the role of surfactant in the pathogenesis of HMD. The deficiency of surfactant in the premature infant increases alveolar surface tension and, according to LaPlace's law (Fig. 20-2), increases the pressure necessary to maintain patent alveoli. The end result is poor lung compliance, progressive atelectasis, loss of FRC, alterations in ventilation-perfusion mismatch, and uneven distribution of ventilation.[224,225] HMD is further complicated by the weak respiratory muscles and compliant chest wall of the premature infant. Hypoxemia and respiratory and metabolic acidemia contribute to increased pulmonary vascular resistance, right-to-left ductal shunting, and worsening ventilation-perfusion mismatch that exacerbate hypoxemia. Hypoxemia and hypoperfusion result in alveolar epithelial damage, with increased capillary permeability and leakage of plasma into alveolar spaces. Leakage of protein into airspaces serves to inhibit surfactant function, exacerbating the disease process.[224,225] The materials in plasma and cellular debris combine to form the characteristic hyaline membrane seen pathologically. The recovery phase is characterized by regeneration of alveolar cells, including type II cells, with an increase in surfactant activity.

Clinically, neonates with HMD demonstrate tachypnea, nasal flaring, subcostal and intercostal retractions, cyanosis, and expiratory grunting. As the infant begins to tire with progressive disease, apneic episodes occur. If some intervention is not undertaken at this point, death ensues. The radiologic appearance of the lungs is what would be expected in an extensive atelectatic process. The infiltrate is diffuse, with a ground-glass appearance. Major airways are air filled and contrast with the atelectatic alveoli, creating the appearance of air bronchograms, whereas the diaphragms are elevated because of profound hypoexpansion. Acute complications of HMD include infection, air leaks, and persistent patency of the ductus arteriosus.

Of more concern than acute complications are the long-term sequelae suffered by infants with HMD. The major long-term consequences are chronic lung disease (CLD) requiring prolonged ventilator and oxygen therapy and significant neurologic impairment. In 1967, Northway et al.[226] first described the syndrome of bronchopulmonary dysplasia in infants surviving severe HMD requiring mechanical ventilation. Today, many infants who develop CLD are extremely-low-birth-weight infants who require prolonged ventilation for apnea and poor respiratory effort who initially did not have severe HMD.[227] The incidence is especially high in infants born at less than 800 g. The severity is variable, ranging from very mild pulmonary insufficiency to severe disease with prolonged mechanical ventilation, frequent readmissions for respiratory exacerbations after nursery discharge, and a higher incidence of neurodevelopmental sequelae compared with very-low-birth-weight controls.[228] Although pulmonary function improves over time and most children do well, long-term pulmonary sequelae are evident.[229,230] Factors involved in the etiology of CLD are gestational age, elevated inspired oxygen concentration, ventilator volutrauma, severity of underlying disease, inflammation, and infection.[231]

Table 20-17. Cumulative Results of Placebo-Controlled Surfactant Trials*

	MODIFIED NATURAL† (%)		SYNTHETIC‡ (%)	
	SURFACTANT	CONTROL	SURFACTANT	CONTROL
Mortality	15	24	11	18
Patent ductus arteriosus	46	43	44	48
Severe ICH	19	19	7	8
Chronic lung disease	37	37	11	11

*Higher incidences of intracranial hemorrhage (ICH) and chronic lung disease in modified natural surfactant studies reflects the lower gestational age on average in both groups in these studies compared to the artificial surfactant studies.
†Studies with Survanta, Curosurf, and Infasurf; 2,000 patients.
‡Studies with Exosurf; 4,400 patients.

Treatment for HMD involves supplemental oxygen, early use of nasal continuous positive airway pressure (CPAP) to maintain FRC, mechanical ventilation, and surfactant replacement therapy.[23,25,232,233] Modified natural surfactant, which is extracted by alveolar lavage or from lung tissue (usually bovine) and then modified by selective addition or removal of components, and true artificial surfactant, which is a mixture of synthetic compounds that may or may not be components of natural surfactant, have been used extensively. These agents (administered intratracheally) have shown efficacy in decreasing the severity of acute HMD and the frequency of air leak complications. Efficacy has been demonstrated when used in the delivery room to "prevent" or when used as a rescue treatment for established HMD. Although surfactant replacement therapy has decreased mortality and acute pulmonary morbidity, this therapy has not affected the frequency of other complications of prematurity (Table 20-17). Of note is that, despite resulting in lower ventilator settings and Fio_2 concentration over the first several days of life, the incidence of CLD has not been changed. However, the severity of long-term pulmonary complications is less. Long-term neurodevelopment follow-ups show rates of handicap similar to placebo-treated infants.[234]

NEONATAL NEUROLOGY

Intraventricular Hemorrhage and Periventricular Leukomalacia

Periventricular/intraventricular hemorrhage (PVH/IVH) and periventricular leukomalacia (PVL) are the most common neurologic complications of prematurity. The overall incidence of PVH/IVH is 20 to 30 percent in infants weighing less than 1,500 g or at <31 weeks' gestation with severe bleeds (grades 3 and 4) at 10 percent.[235,236] The highest incidence is seen in babies of the lowest gestational age and birth weight; nearly 50 and 25 percent, respectively, for all IVH and severe bleeds for babies born at less than 700 g.[235,236] Bleeds are graded according to severity as indicated in Table 20-18.[237] Diagnosis is confirmed with real-time ultrasound. PVL is reported in about 2 to 4 percent of infants younger than 32 weeks' gestation,[235] but the cystic PVL reported likely underestimates the full spectrum of PVL (see later).

Table 20-18. Classification of Intraventricular Hemorrhage

GRADE	DEFINITION
I	Subependymal hemorrhage
II	Intraventricular hemorrhage without ventricular dilatation
III	Intraventricular hemorrhage with ventricular dilatation
IV	Intraventricular hemorrhage with associated parenchymal hemorrhage

Adapted from Papile LA, Burstein J, Burstein R, Koffler H: Incidence and evolution of subependymal and intraventricular hemorrhage: a study of infants with birth weights less than 1500 gm. J Pediatr 92:529, 1978.

Bleeding originates in the subependymal germinal matrix located ventrolateral to the lateral ventricles in the caudothalamic groove. The germinal matrix is made up of a rete or meshwork of thin-walled vessels in the process of remodeling into a capillary network and a mass of undifferentiated cells that are destined to become cortical neurons, astrocytes, and oligodendroglia. Rupture of a germinal matrix hemorrhage into the ventricular system leads to intraventricular hemorrhage. A proposed pathogenesis derived from a review of available information is presented in Figure 20-21. The critical predisposing event is likely an ischemia-reperfusion injury to the capillaries in the germinal matrix. Physiologic data from beagle puppies have shown that the germinal matrix is a low blood flow region prone to ischemia.[238] Furthermore, IVH is most reliably produced in these puppies by a sequence of hemorrhagic hypotension followed by hypertension.[239] The amount of bleeding is then influenced by a variety of factors that affect the pressure gradient across the injured capillary wall. Likewise, for babies who manifest parenchymal bleeding (grade 4) and PVL, the inciting event is likely ischemia with reperfusion injury. The periventricular white matter is a border zone for cerebral blood flow in the preterm infant and is vulnerable to ischemic injury. Although cystic PVL (multifocal areas of necrosis with cyst formation in deep periventricular white matter) has been well characterized by ultrasound, the expanded use of MRI scans in preterm infants has identified infants (especially among those of lower gestational age) with diffuse white matter injury.[240,241] These infants have diffuse exces-

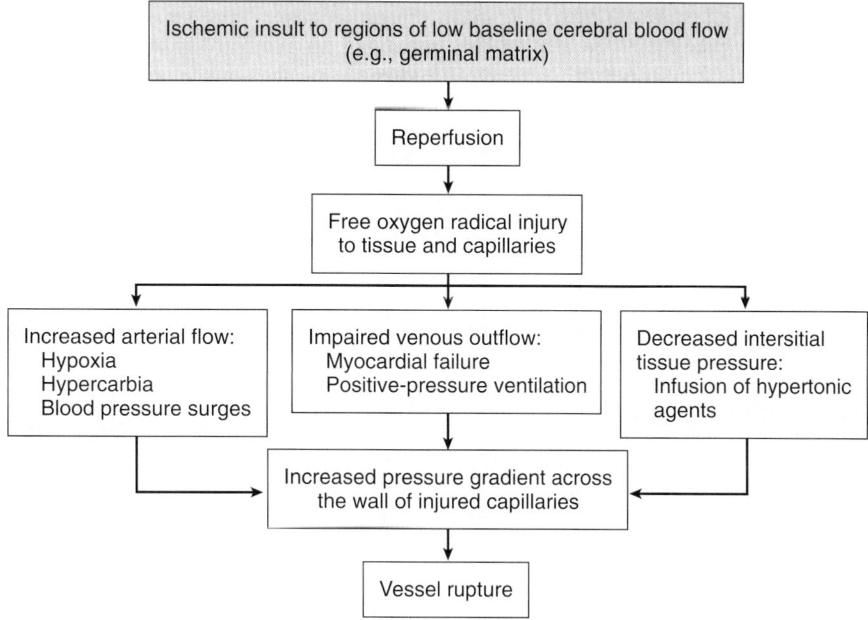

Figure 20-21. Pathogenesis of periventricular/intraventricular hemorrhage in the preterm infant

sive high signal intensities on T2-weighted MRI[242] often accompanied by ventricular dilation at term. These findings are far more common in the preterm population than cystic PVL,[242] and certainly represent part of the spectrum of PVL. The other important clinical correlate of PVL is maternal chorioamnionitis and neonatal infection.[243,244] Data from a variety of studies suggest that infection and ischemia are additive in the pathogenesis of PVL with the critical injury to preoligodendrocytes caused by reactive oxygen and nitrogen species.[245–248]

The neurodevelopmental outcome of infants with IVH is related to the severity of the original bleed, development of posthemorrhagic hydrocephalus, and the degree of associated parenchymal injury. Infants with grade I or II IVH have neurodevelopmental outcomes similar to those of preterm infants without IVH, although reports of outcome in school-aged children do show that survivors of mild IVH display a variety of subtle neurologic and cognitive abnormalities, including motor incoordination, hyperactivity, attention and learning deficits, and visual motor difficulties.[249,250] On the other hand, infants with progressive ventricular dilatation (grade III) or periventricular hemorrhagic infarction (grade IV) are at high risk for major neurodevelopmental handicap as well as less severe neurologic and cognitive disabilities.[251,252] The presence of severe PVL carries a guarded prognosis with a high risk of cerebral palsy and associated cognitive deficit.[253,254]

Although the incidence and severity of intracranial hemorrhage have progressively decreased as a result of advances in both obstetric and neonatal care, the therapeutic focus continues to be on strategies to prevent this complication of prematurity. Both antenatal and postnatal approaches have been developed. For the most part, postnatal pharmacologic strategies have not had a major effect in decreasing the incidence and severity of IVH. Because IVH and PVL are likely perinatal events, antenatal prevention holds the most promise. Both vitamin K and phenobarbital have been administered in this way.[255] Antenatal phenobarbital resulted in a decrease in both frequency and severity of IVH. The proposed mechanism of action is thought to be scavenging of oxygen free radicals, although phenobarbital does decrease both brain blood flow and cerebral metabolic rate. However, two large randomized prospective studies failed to confirm the positive effects of phenobarbital shown in previous smaller studies.[256,257] One reason for the discrepancy is likely due to the widespread use of antenatal corticosteroids in the more recent studies. Antenatal corticosteroids, although not used specifically to decrease the incidence of IVH and PVL, do appear to decrease the frequency of these complications and likely represent the most important antenatal strategy to prevent intracranial hemorrhage.[18,19] Phenobarbital may still have a role in the mother who has not been "prepared" with betamethasone and is delivering at under 28 weeks' gestation.

Seizures

Newborns rarely have well-organized tonic-clonic seizures because of incomplete cortical organization and a preponderance of inhibitory synapses. Newborn seizures can be classified into four subtypes.[258] The first is the subtle seizure characterized by ocular phenomena, oral-buccal-lingual movements, peculiar limb movements (e.g., bicycling movements), autonomic alterations, and apnea. Clonic seizures are characterized by rhythmic (one to three jerks per second) movements that can be focal or multifocal. The third seizure type is focal or generalized tonic seizures marked by extensor posturing. The fourth seizure type is myoclonic activity that is distin-

Table 20-19. Differential Diagnosis of Neonatal Seizures

DIAGNOSIS	COMMENTS
Hypoxic-ischemic encephalopathy	Most common etiology (60%, onset first 24 hours)
Intracranial hemorrhage	≤15% of cases; PVH/IVH, subdural or subarachnoid bleeds, stroke
Infection	12% of cases
Hypoglycemia	SGA, IDM
Hypocalcemia, hypomagnesemia	Low-birth-weight infant, IDM
Hyponatremia	Rare, seen with syndrome of inappropriate secretion of antidiuretic hormone (SIADH)
Disorders of amino and organic acid metabolism, hyperammonemia	Associated acidosis, altered level of consciousness
Pyridoxine dependency	Seizures refractory to routine therapy; cessation of seizures after administration of pyridoxine
Developmental defects	Other anomalies, chromosomal syndromes
Drug withdrawal	
Benign familial neonatal seizures	
No cause found	10% of cases

IDM, infant of diabetic mother; PVH/IVH, periventricular/intraventricular hemorrhage; SGA, small for gestational age.

guished from clonic seizures by the more rapid speed of the myoclonic jerk and the predilection for flexor muscle groups. The differential diagnosis of neonatal seizures is presented in Table 20-19. The most frequent cause of neonatal seizures is hypoxic ischemic encephalopathy, with the second leading cause being intracranial hemorrhage. The prognosis for neonatal seizures depends on the cause. Difficult-to-control seizure activity caused by hypoxic ischemic encephalopathy and hypoglycemic seizures in particular have a high incidence of long-term sequelae.

CLASSIFICATION OF NEWBORNS BY GROWTH AND GESTATIONAL AGE

In assessing the risk for mortality or morbidity in a given neonate, evaluation of birth weight and gestational age together provide the clearest picture. This requires an accurate assessment of the infant's gestational age. When large populations are considered, maternal dates remain the single best determinant of gestational age. Early obstetric ultrasound is also a very useful adjunct in determining pregnancy dating. However, in the individual neonate, especially when dates are uncertain, a reliable postnatal assessment of gestational age is necessary. A scoring system appraising gestational age on the basis of physical and neurologic criteria was developed by Dubowitz et al.[259] and later simplified and updated by Ballard et al.[260,261] (Fig. 20-22). The Ballard examination is less accurate before 28 weeks' gestation,[262] but additional features can be examined to aid in the determination of an accurate gestational age. The anterior vascular capsule of the lens reveals complete coverage of the lens by vessels at 27 to 28 weeks. Foot length (from the heel to the tip of the largest toe) is 4.5 cm at 25 weeks and increases by 0.25 cm/wk. Infants can then be classified, using growth parameters and gestational age, by means of intrauterine growth curves such as those developed by Lubchenco et al.[263] (Fig. 20-23). Infants born between 37 and 42 weeks are classified as term; less than 37 weeks, preterm; and greater than 42 weeks, postterm. In each grouping, infants are then identified according to growth as AGA if birth weight falls between the 10th to 90th percentile, SGA if birth weight is below the 10th percentile, and LGA if birth weight is above the 90th percentile. Knowledge of a baby's birth weight in relation to gestational age is helpful in anticipating neonatal problems.

There are numerous causes of growth restriction (see Chapter 29). Those operative early in pregnancy such as chromosomal aberrations, congenital viral infections, and some drug exposures induce symmetric restriction of weight, length, and head circumference. In most cases, the phenomenon occurs later in gestation and leads to more selective restriction of birth weight alone. Such factors include hypertension or other maternal vascular disease and multiple gestation.[264] Neonatal problems besides chromosomal abnormalities and congenital viral infections common in SGA infants include birth asphyxia, hypoglycemia, polycythemia, and hypothermia. In addition, congenital malformations are seen more frequently among undergrown infants.[265]

The most common identifiable conditions leading to excessive infant birth weight are maternal diabetes and maternal obesity. Other conditions associated with macrosomia are erythroblastosis fetalis, other causes of fetal hydrops, and Beckwith-Wiedemann syndrome. LGA infants are at risk for hypoglycemia, polycythemia, congenital anomalies, cardiomyopathy, hyperbilirubinemia, and birth trauma.

NURSERY CARE

Nurseries are classified on the basis of level of care provided (Table 20-20). Level I nurseries care for infants presumed healthy, with an emphasis on screening and surveillance. Level II nurseries can care for infants more than 32 weeks' gestation, who weigh at least 1,500 g, and who require special attention, but will probably not need subspeciality services. Level III nurseries care for all newborn infants who are critically ill regardless of the level of support required.[266] A perinatal center encompasses both high-risk obstetric services and level III nursery services.

Care of the normal newborn involves observation of transition from intrauterine to extrauterine life, establishing breast- or bottle-feeds, noting normal patterns of stooling and urination, and surveillance for neonatal problems. Signs suggestive of illness include temperature instability, change in activity, refusal to feed, pallor, cyanosis, jaundice, tachypnea and respiratory distress, delayed (beyond 24 hours) passage of first stool or

Neuromuscular Maturity

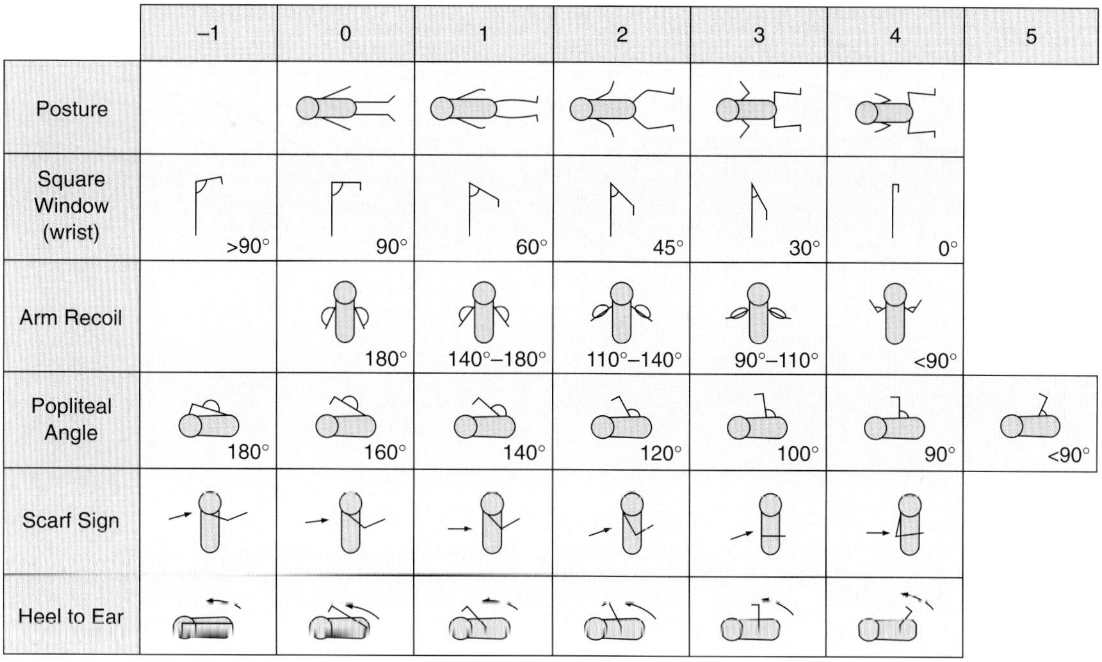

	−1	0	1	2	3	4	5
Posture							
Square Window (wrist)	>90°	90°	60°	45°	30°	0°	
Arm Recoil		180°	140°–180°	110°–140°	90°–110°	<90°	
Popliteal Angle	180°	160°	140°	120°	100°	90°	<90°
Scarf Sign							
Heel to Ear							

Physical Maturity

Skin	sticky friable transparent	gelatinous red, translucent	smooth pink, visible veins	superficial peeling &/or rash, few veins	cracking pale areas rare veins	parchment deep cracking no vessels	leathery cracked wrinkled
Lanugo	none	sparse	abundant	thinning	bald areas	mostly bald	
Plantar Surface	heel-toe 40–50 mm: −1 < 40 mm: −2	> 50 mm no crease	faint red marks	anterior transverse crease only	creases ant. 2/3	creases over entire sole	
Breast	imperceptible	barely perceptible	flat areola no bud	stippled areola 1–2 mm bud	raised areola 3–4 mm bud	full areola 5–10 mm bud	
Eye/Ear	lids fused loosely: −1 tightly: −2	lids open pinna flat stays folded	sl. curved pinna; soft; slow recoil	well-curved pinna; soft but ready recoil	formed & firm instant recoil	thick cartilage ear stiff	
Genitals male	scrotum flat, smooth	scrotum empty faint rugae	testes in upper canal rare rugae	testes descending few rugae	testes down good rugae	testes pendulous deep rugae	
Genitals female	clitoris prominent labia flat	prominent clitoris small labia minora	prominent clitoris enlarging minora	majora & minora equally prominent	majora large minora small	majora cover clitoris & minora	

Maturity Rating

score	weeks
−10	20
-5	22
0	24
5	26
10	28
15	30
20	32
25	34
30	36
35	38
40	40
45	42
50	44

Figure 20-22. Assessment of gestational age. (From Ballard JL, Khoury JC, Wedig K, et al: New Ballard Score, expanded to include extremely premature infants. J Pediatr 119:417, 1991, with permission.)

void, and bilious vomiting. In addition, the following laboratory screens should be performed: (1) blood type and direct and indirect Coombs' test on infants born to mothers with type O or Rh-negative blood; (2) glucose screen in infants at risk for hypoglycemia; (3) hematocrit in infants with signs and symptoms of anemia or polycythemia; and (4) mandated screening for inborn errors of metabolism, such as PKU and galactosemia, sickle cell disease, hypothyroidism, cystic fibrosis, and congenital adrenal hyperplasia. In addition to the state-sponsored screen, many centers are offering expanded newborn screening by tandem mass spectroscopy that

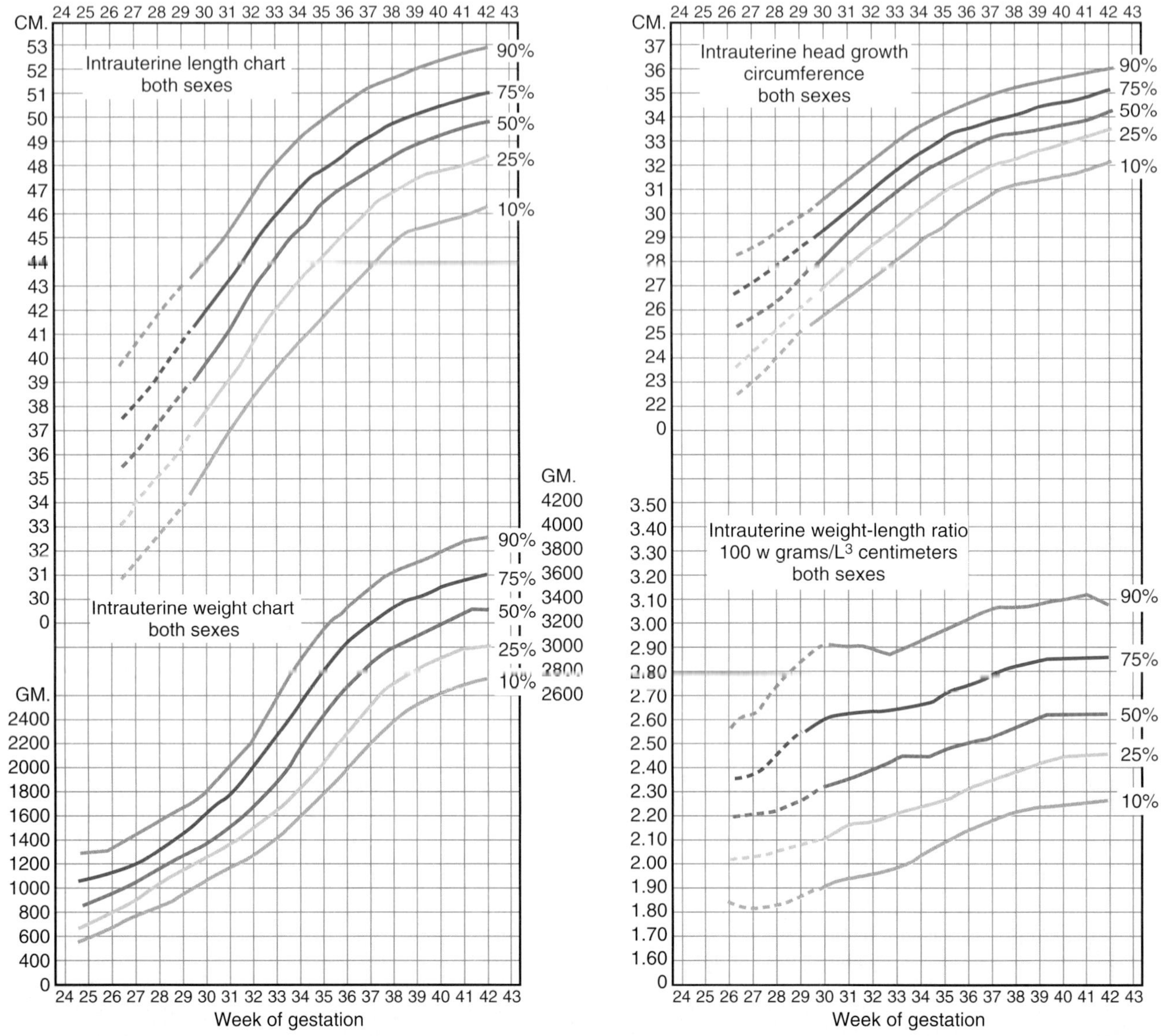

Figure 20-23. Intrauterine growth curves for weight, length, and head circumference for singleton births in Colorado. (From Lubchenco LO, Hansman C, Boyd E: Intrauterine growth in length and head circumference as estimated from live births at gestational ages from 26 to 42 weeks. Pediatrics 37:403, 1966, with permission.)

looks for a variety of other inborn metabolic errors.[267] All newborns should also have an initial hearing screen performed before discharge.[268] Finally, babies routinely receive 1 mg intramuscular of vitamin K to prevent vitamin K–deficient hemorrhagic disease of the newborn and either 1 percent silver nitrate or erythromycin ointment to prevent gonococcal ophthalmia neonatorum. Hepatitis B vaccine and hepatitis B immunoglobulin are administered to infants born to HB_sAg-positive mothers. All infants should be vaccinated against hepatitis B, but the first dose can wait until 1 to 2 months if the mother is HBsAg negative. Infants should be positioned supine or lying on the right side with the dependent arm forward for sleep to minimize the risk of sudden infant death syndrome.[269]

It is now common on most services for mothers and babies to be discharged within 24 to 36 hours of delivery. Criteria for early discharge are presented in Table 20-21.[270,271] Discharge at 24 to 36 hours appears safe and appropriate for most infants without contraindications, provided a follow-up at 48 to 72 hours after discharge is ensured.[271]

Circumcision is an elective procedure to be performed only in healthy, stable infants. The procedure probably has medical benefits, including prevention of phimosis, paraphimosis, and balanoposthitis, as well as a decreased incidence of cancer of the penis, cervical cancer (in partners of circumcised men), sexually transmitted diseases (including HIV), and urinary tract infection in male infants.[272] Most parents, however, make the decision regarding circumcision for nonmedical reasons. The risks of the procedure include local infection, bleeding, removal of too much skin, and urethral injury. The combined incidence of these complications is less than 1 percent. Local anesthesia (dorsal penile nerve block or circumferential ring block) with 1 percent lidocaine without epinephrine is safe and effective, and should always be used.[272] Techniques that allow visualization of the glans

Table 20-20. Levels of Nursery Care

Level 1: A nursery with personnel and equipment to perform neonatal resuscitation, evaluate and provide newborn care for healthy infants, stabilize and provide care for infants born at 35–37 weeks' gestation who remain physiologically stable, and stabilize ill or less than 35 weeks' gestation infants before transport to a higher level facility.
Level 2: A facility able to provide care to infants born at more than 32 weeks' gestation weighing more than 1500 g who have physiologic immaturity; who are moderately ill with problems expected to resolve quickly, and who do not need urgent subspecialty care. Can provide convalescent care for infants after intensive care. A level 2A does not do mechanical ventilation or nasal continuous positive airway pressure, whereas a 2B can do short-term (less than 24 hours) of ventilation.
Level 3: Provide care for the sickest and most complex infants
3A: Care for infants beyond 28 weeks and 1000 g in need of conventional mechanical ventilation.
3B: Can provide care for infants less than 28 weeks and 1000 g, high-frequency ventilation, inhaled nitric oxide, on-site subspecialists, advanced imaging, on-site or nearby pediatric surgeons and anesthesiologists.
3C: Can provide ECMO and repair of complex congenital heart disease.

ECMO, extracorporeal membrane oxygenation.
Adapted from American Academy of Pediatrics Committee on Fetus and Newborn: Levels of neonatal care. Pediatrics 114:1341, 2004.

Table 20-21. Infant Criteria for Early Discharge

1. Uncomplicated antepartum, intrapartum and postpartum course.
2. Vaginal delivery with 5 minute Apgar ≥7.
3. Term singleton (38–42 weeks) who is appropriately grown.
4. Normal vital signs stable for at least 12 hours before discharge; axillary temperature of 36.1 to 37.2°C; heart rate 100–160 bpm; respiratory rate 40–60 breaths/min.
5. The infant has urinated and passed a stool.
6. Completion of two successful feeds; if breast feeding observation by an experienced caregiver of at least one feed.
7. Normal physical examination.
8. No bleeding from circumcision site for 2 hours.
9. No jaundice in the first 24 hours.
10. Completion of hearing screen, newborn metabolic screen and blood type and Coombs' test (type O and Rh-negative mothers).
11. Maternal labs available and reviewed.
12. Hepatitis B vaccine given or outpatient arrangements made.
13. Infant teaching completed; home safety and social supports evaluated.
14. Forty-eight hour follow-up visit scheduled.
15. Infants born to group B streptococcus positive mothers with inadequate antenatal chemoprophylaxis or born to mothers with >12 hours ruptured membranes are observed for 48 hours.

throughout the procedure (Plastibell and Gomco clamp) are preferred to a "blind" technique (Mogen clamp) because of occasional amputation of the glans with the latter. Circumcision is contraindicated in infants with genital abnormalities. Appropriate laboratory evaluation should be performed before the procedure in infants with a family history of bleeding disorders.

Care of the Parents

Klaus and Kennell[273] outline these steps in maternal-infant attachment: (1) planning the pregnancy; (2) confirming the pregnancy; (3) accepting the pregnancy; (4) noting fetal movement; (5) accepting the fetus as an individual; (6) going through labor; (7) giving birth; (8) hearing and seeing the baby; (9) touching, smelling, and holding the baby; (10) caretaking; and (11) accepting the infant as a separate individual. Numerous influences can affect this process. A mother's and father's actions and responses are derived from their own genetic endowment, their own interfamily relationships, cultural practices, past experiences with this or previous pregnancies, and, most importantly, how they were raised by their parents.[273] Also critical is the in-hospital experience surrounding the birth-how doctors and nurses act, separation from the baby, and hospital practices.

The 60- to 90-minute period after delivery is a very important time. The infant is alert, active, and able to follow with his or her eyes,[274] allowing meaningful interaction to transpire between infant and parents. The infant's array of sensory and motor abilities evokes responses from the mother and initiates communication that may be helpful for attachment and induction of reciprocal actions. Whether a critical time period for these initial interactions exists is not clear, but improved mothering behavior does seem to occur with increased contact over the first 3 postpartum days.[275] The practical implications of this information are that labor and delivery should pose as little anxiety as possible for the mother, and parents and baby should have time together immediately after delivery if the baby's medical condition permits.

Mothers with high-risk pregnancies are at increased risk for subsequent parenting problems. It is important for both obstetrician and pediatrician alike to be involved prenatally, allowing time to prepare the family for anticipated aspects of the baby's care as well as providing reassurance that the odds are heavily in favor of a live baby who will ultimately be healthy. If before birth one can anticipate a need for neonatal intensive care (known congenital anomaly, refractory premature labor), maternal transport to a center with a unit that can care for the baby should be planned. In this way, a mother can be with her baby during its most critical care. Before delivery, it is also very helpful to allow the parents to tour the unit their baby will occupy.

The single basic principle in dealing with parents of a sick infant is to provide essential information clearly and accurately to both parents, preferably when they are together. With improved survival rates, especially in premature infants, most babies, despite early problems, will do well. Therefore, it is reasonable in most circumstances to be positive about the outcome. There is also no reason to emphasize problems that might occur in the future or to deal with individual worries of the physician. Questions, if asked, need to be answered honestly, but the list of parents' worries does not need to be voluntarily increased.

Before the parents' initial visit to the unit, a physician or nurse should describe what the baby and the equipment look like. When they arrive in the nursery, this can again be reviewed in detail. If a baby must be moved to another hospital, the mother should be given time to see and to touch her infant before the transfer. The father should be encouraged to meet the baby at the receiving hospital so he can become comfortable with the intensive care unit. He can serve as a link between baby and mother with information and photographs.

As a baby's course proceeds, the nursery staff can help the parents become comfortable with their infant. This can include participation in caretaking as well as skin-to-skin contact with the infant (Kangaroo care).[276] Individualized developmentally based care has also shown some benefit for high-risk infants.[277] It is also important for the staff to discuss among themselves any problems that parents may be having as well as to keep a record of visits and phone calls. This approach will allow early intervention to deal with potential problems.

The birth of an infant with a congenital malformation provides another situation in which staff support is essential. Parents' reactions to the birth of a malformed infant follow a predictable course. For most, there is initial shock and denial, a period of sadness and anger, gradual adaptation, and finally an increased satisfaction with and the ability to care for the baby. The parents must be allowed to pass through these stages and, in effect, to mourn the loss of the anticipated normal child.[278]

The death of an infant or a stillborn is a highly stressful family event. This fact has been emphasized by Cullberg,[279] who found that psychiatric disorders developed in 19 of 56 mothers studied 1 to 2 years after the deaths of their neonates. One of the major predispositions was a breakdown of communication between parents. The health care staff need to encourage the parents to talk with each other, discuss their feelings, and display emotion. The staff should talk with the parents at the time of death and then several months later to review the findings of the autopsy, answer questions, and see how the family is doing.

OUTCOME OF NEONATAL INTENSIVE CARE AND THRESHOLD OF VIABILITY

More sophisticated neonatal care has resulted in improved survival of very-low-birth-weight (<1,500 g) infants, in particular those less than 1,000 g (Fig. 20-24). Current survival rates are 90 percent or greater for infants greater than 1,000 g and 28 weeks' gestation, 85 percent at 800 to 1,000 g and 26 to 27 weeks' gestation, and nearly 70 to 75 percent for infants 700 to 800 g and 25 weeks' gestation, with a considerable drop in survival below 700 g and 25 weeks.[235,280] It is important to note that survival in terms of best obstetric estimate is greater at very low gestational ages than survival in terms of postnatal assessment of gestational age. The numbers in terms of best obstetric estimate based on data at the institution of birth should be referred to for antenatal counseling. This improved survival comes with a price, because a variety of morbidities are seen in these infants. Major neurologic morbidities seen in very-low-birth-weight infants include cerebral palsy (spastic diplegia, quadriplegia, hemiplegia, or paresis), cognitive delay, and hydrocephalus. Lesser disabilities include learning and behavior difficulties that can cause problems when school age is attained. The rate of severe neurologic disability is fairly constant at 10 percent of all very-low-birth-weight survivors from 1,000 to 1,500 g. The number increases from 10 to 25 percent in infants of extremely low birth weight (<1,000 g) and is particularly troubling for infants born at less than 25 weeks' gestation.[281–285] In these infants, approximately half of the survivors have moderate or severe neurosensory disability.[283] In addition to the modest increase in severe disability, these infants have an increased rate of lesser disabilities including subnormal mental performance, behavior problems and the need for special education in school (Fig. 20-25).[285,286] Risk factors for neurologic morbidity include seizures, major intracranial hemorrhage or PVL, severe intrauterine growth restriction (IUGR), need for mechanical ventilation, CLD, poor early head growth, retinopathy of prematurity and low socioeconomic class.[251–254,287–289]

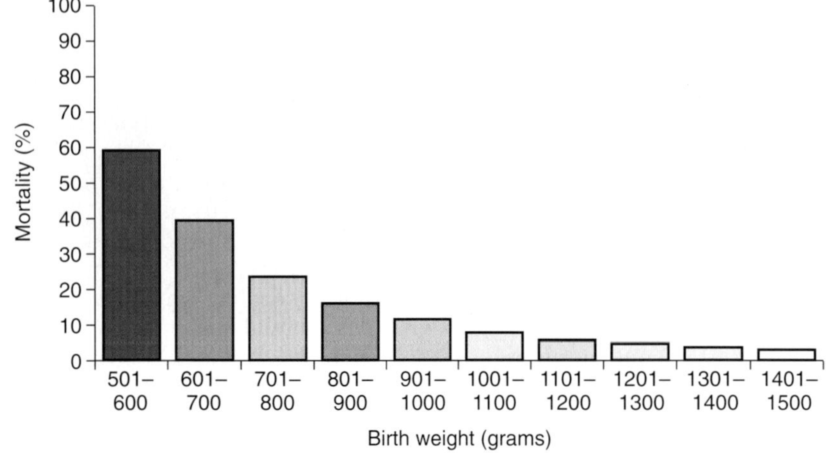

Figure 20-24. Survival by birth weight. (Reproduced with permission from the Vermont Oxford Network 2003 Report, published 2004.)

There are other morbidities that need to be considered as well. Because the number of survivors weighing less than 1,000 g has increased, a reemergence of retinopathy of prematurity has been seen. This disorder, caused by retinal vascular proliferation leading to hemorrhage, scarring, retinal detachment, and blindness, originally was thought to be caused solely by inappropriate exposure to high concentrations of oxygen. It is now thought that the origin is multifactorial, with extreme prematurity a critical factor.[290] Incidence of acute proliferative retinopathy by birth weight is less than 10 percent in infants weighing more than 1,250 g, 20 percent in those 1,000 to 1,250 g, 50 to 60 percent in those 750 to 1,000 g, and 70 percent in those less than 750 g.[235,291] Severe retinopathy is evident in 5 percent of the infants 1,000 to 1,250 g, in 10 percent of infants 750 to 1,000 g, and 25 to 40 percent of infants less than 750 g. Of the infants with severe retinopathy, 10 percent (4 percent of the total population) will go on to have severe visual problems. The other major neurosensory morbidity is hearing loss, which occurs in 2 percent of neonatal intensive care unit survivors.[292] Other sequelae of neonatal intensive care include CLD, growth failure, short gut, and need for postdischarge rehospitalization.

The information presented earlier on outcome is relevant to discussions about obstetric and neonatal intervention at the threshold of viability. If one considers the end point of survival without major disability, this occurs in 0 percent at 22 weeks, less than 10 percent at 23 weeks, approximately 20 to 25 percent at 24 weeks and approximately 45 to 50 percent at 25 weeks.[283,293] With this information in mind, most neonatologists believe that care is clearly beneficial beyond 25 completed weeks, whereas less than half believe that way at 24 to 24 6/7 weeks and virtually none at less than 24 completed weeks.[294] Having said that, more than half would intervene on behalf of an infant beyond 23 weeks' gestation. These discussions need to be modified depending on circumstances. For instance, morbidity and mortality would increase in the face of overt infection or severe IUGR.[295] A reasonable approach would seem to be to encourage interventions on behalf of the fetus or newborn beyond 25 completed weeks' gestation and not intervene at less than 23 to 24 weeks' gestation. The range between 23 and 25 weeks should be evaluated on a case-by-case basis.

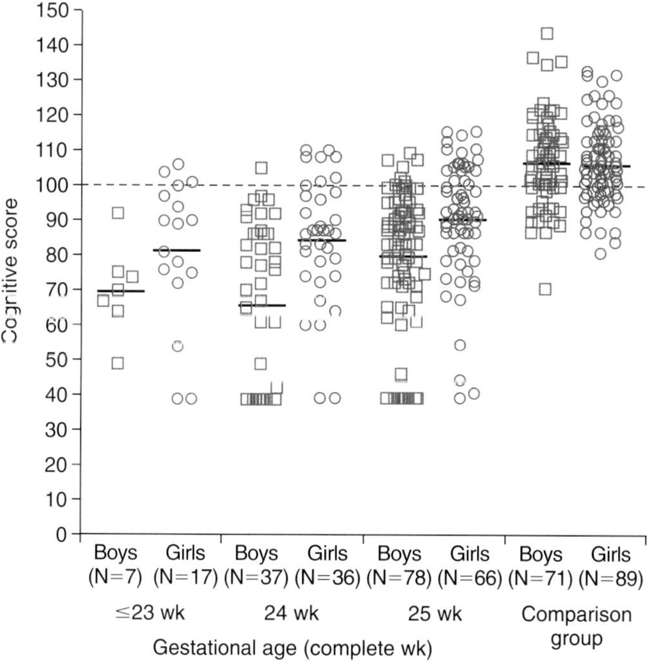

Figure 20-25. Cognitive scores for 241 extremely preterm children and 160 age-matched classmates who were full term at birth, according to sex and completed weeks of gestation at birth. The scores are the Kaufman Assessment Battery for Children scores for the Mental Processing Composite or developmental scores according to the Griffiths Scales of Mental Development and NEPSY. *Bars* indicate mean scores. *Dashed line* is the mean of a standardized population. (Reproduced with permission from Marlow N, Wolke D, Bracewell MA, et al: Neurologic and developmental disability at six years of age after extremely preterm birth. N Engl J Med 352:9, 2005)

Key Points

- Surfactant maintains lung expansion on expiration by lowering surface tension at the air-liquid interface in the alveolus.
- Respiratory distress syndrome in premature infants is in part caused by a deficiency of surfactant and can be treated with surfactant replacement therapy.
- Antenatal corticosteroids accelerate fetal lung maturation and decrease neonatal mortality and respiratory distress syndrome in preterm infants. In addition, corticosteroids are associated with a decrease in intracranial hemorrhage and NEC.
- Transition from intrauterine to extrauterine life requires removal of fluid from the lungs, switching from a fetal to neonatal circulation, and establishment of a normal neonatal lung volume.
- The most important step in neonatal resuscitation is to achieve adequate expansion of the lungs.
- MAS likely is the result of intrauterine asphyxia with mortality related to associated persistent pulmonary hypertension.
- The best predictor of neurologic sequelae of birth asphyxia is the presence of hypoxic ischemic encephalopathy in the neonatal period. The neurologic sequelae of birth asphyxia is cerebral palsy. However, the large majority of cerebral palsy is of unknown origin or etiologies other than perinatal asphyxia.
- The major neurologic complications seen in premature infants are PVH/IVH and PVL.
- Hypoglycemia is a predictable and preventable complication in the newborn.
- Survival, in particular for infants weighing less than 1,000 g, has increased with improved methods of neonatal intensive care, including provision of exogenous surfactant.

REFERENCES

1. Wert SE: Normal and abnormal structural development of the lung. *In* Polin RA, Fox WW, Abman SH (eds): Fetal and Neonatal Physiology, 3rd ed. Philadelphia, WB Saunders Company, 2004, p 783.
2. Shannon JM, Deterding RR: Epithelial-mesnechymal interactions in lung development. *In* MacDonald JA (ed): Lung Growth and Development. New York, Marcel Dekker, 1997 p 81.
3. Perl A-KT, Whitsett JA: Molecular mechanisms controlling lung morphogenesis. Clin Genet 56:14, 1999.
4. Kaplan F: Molecular determinants of fetal lung organogenesis. Mol Genet Metabol 71:321, 2000.
5. Cardoso WV: Molecular regulation of lung development. Annu Rev Physiol 63:471, 2001.
6. Morrell NW, et al: Development of the pulmonary vasculature. *In* Gaultier C, Bourbon JR, Post M, et al (eds): Lung Development. New York, Oxford University Press, 2000 p 152.
7. Hall SM, Hislop AA, Haworth SG: Origin, differentiation, and maturation of human pulmonary veins. Am J Respir Cell Mol Biol 26:333, 2002.
8. Wright JR, Clements JA: Metabolism and turnover of lung surfactant. Am Rev Respir Dis 136:426, 1987.
9. Rider ED, Ikegami M, Jobe AH: Localization of alveolar surfactant clearance in rabbit lung cells. Am J Physiol 283:L201, 1992.
10. Jobe AH: Lung development and maturation. *In* Fanaroff AA, Martin RJ (eds): Neonatal-Perinatal Medicine: Diseases of the Fetus and Infant, 7th ed. St. Louis, Mosby Inc, 2002, p 973.
11. Clements JA, Tooley WH: Kinetics of surface-active material in the fetal lung. *In* Hodson WA (ed): Development of the Lung. New York, Marcel Dekker, 1977.
12. Jobe AH: The role of surfactant in neonatal adaptation. Semin Perinatol 12:113, 1988.
13. Whitsett JA: Composition of pulmonary surfactant lipids and proteins. In Polin RA, Fox WW, Abman SH (eds): Fetal and Neonatal Physiology, 3rd ed. Philadelphia, WB Saunders Company, 2004, p 1005.
14. Cole FS, Hamvas A, Nogee LM: Genetic disorders of neonatal respiratory function. Pediatr Res 50:157, 2001
15. Ballard PL: Hormonal regulation of pulmonary surfactant. Endocr Rev 10:165, 1989.
16. Gross I, Ballard PL: Hormonal therapy for prevention of respiratory distress syndrome. *In* Polin RA, Fox WW, Abman SH (eds): Fetal and Neonatal Physiology, 3rd ed. Philadelphia, WB Saunders Company, 2004, p 1069.
17. Liggins GC, Howie RN: A controlled trial of antepartum glucocorticoid treatment for prevention of the respiratory distress syndrome in premature infants. Pediatrics 50:515, 1972.
18. Crowley PA: Antenatal corticosteroid therapy: a meta-analysis of the randomized trials, 1972–1994. Am J Obstet Gynecol 173:322, 1995.
19. Leviton A, Kuban KC, Pagano M, et al: Antenatal corticosteroids appear to reduce the risk of postnatal germinal matrix hemorrhage in intubated low birth weight newborns. Pediatrics 91:1083, 1993.
20. Schmand B, Neuvel J, Smolders-de-Haas H, et al: Psychological development of children who were treated antenatally with corticosteroids to prevent respiratory distress syndrome. Pediatrics 86:58, 1990.
21. Smolders-de-Haas H, Neuvel J, Schmand B, et al: Physical development and medical history of children who were treated antenatally with corticosteroids to prevent respiratory distress syndrome: a 10- to 12-year follow-up. Pediatrics 86:65, 1990.
22. Halliday HL: Overview of clinical trials comparing natural and synthetic surfactants. Biol Neonate 67(Suppl 1):32, 1995.
23. Jobe AH: Pulmonary surfactant therapy. N Engl J Med 328:861, 1993.
24. Pramanik AK, Holtzman RB, Merritt TA: Surfactant replacement therapy for pulmonary diseases. Pediatr Clin North Am 40:913, 1993.
25. Merritt TA, Soll RF, Hallman M: Overview of exogenous surfactant replacement therapy. J Intensive Care Med 8:205, 1993.
26. Jobe AH, Mitchell BR, Gunkel JH: Beneficial effects of the combined use of prenatal corticosteroids and postnatal surfactant on preterm infants. Am J Obstet Gynecol 168:508, 1993.
27. Thorpe-Beeston JG, Nicolaides KH, Snijders RJM, et al: Fetal thyroid stimulating hormone response to maternal administration of thyrotropin-releasing hormone. Am J Obstet Gynecol 164:1244, 1991.
28. Rooney SA, Marino PA, Gobran LJ, et al: Thyrotropin-releasing hormone increases the amount of surfactant in lung lavage from fetal rabbits. Pediatr Res 13:623, 1979.
29. Gross I, Moya FR: Is there a role for antenatal TRH in the prevention of neonatal respiratory disorders? Semin Perinatol 25:406, 2001.
30. Jansen AH, Chernick V: Development of respiratory control. Physiol Rev 63:437, 1983.
31. Dawes GS, Fox HE, Leduc BM, et al: Respiratory movements and rapid eye movement sleep in the foetal lamb. J Physiol (Lond) 220:119, 1972.
32. Rigatto H, Moore M, Cates D, et al: Fetal breathing and behavior measured through a double-wall Plexiglas window in sheep. J Appl Physiol 61:160, 1986.
33. Kaplan M: Fetal breathing movements, an update for the pediatrician. Am J Dis Child 137:177, 1983.
34. Connors G, Hunse C, Carmichael L, et al: The role of carbon dioxide in the generation of human fetal breathing movements. Am J Obstet Gynecol 158:322, 1988.
35. Boddy K, Dawes GS, Fisher R, et al: Foetal respiratory movements, electrocortical and cardiovascular responses to hypoxaemia and hypercapnia in sheep. J Physiol (Lond) 243:599, 1974.
36. Baier RJ, Hasan SU, Cates DB, et al: Effects of various concentrations of O_2 and umbilical cord occlusion on fetal breathing and behavior. J Appl Physiol 68:1597, 1990.
37. Goodman JDS: The effect of intravenous glucose on human fetal breathing measured by Doppler ultrasound. Br J Obstet Gynaecol 87:1080, 1980.
38. Patrick J, Campbell K, Carmichael L, et al: Patterns of human fetal breathing during the last 10 weeks of pregnancy. Obstet Gynecol 56:24, 1980.
39. Maloney JE, Adamson TM, Brodecky V, et al: Modification of respiratory center output in the unanesthetized fetal sheep "in utero." J Appl Physiol 39:552, 1975.
40. Jansen AH, Chernick V: Fetal breathing and development of control of breathing. J Appl Physiol 70:1431, 1991.
41. Kitterman JA, Liggins GC, Clements JA, Tooley WH: Stimulation of breathing movements in fetal sheep by inhibitors of prostaglandin synthesis. J Dev Physiol 1:453, 1979.
42. James LS, Weisbrot IM, Prince CE, et al: The acid-base status of human infants in relation to birth asphyxia and the onset of respiration. J Pediatr 52:379, 1958.
43. Alvaro RE, de Almeida V, Al-Alaiyan S, et al: A placental factor inhibits breathing induced by umbilical occlusion in fetal sheep. J Dev Physiol 19:23, 1993.
44. Agostoni E, Taglietti A, Agostoni AF, Setnikar I: Mechanical aspects of the first breath. J Appl Physiol 13:344, 1958.
45. Milner AD, Vyas H: Lung expansion at birth. J Pediatr 101:879, 1982.
46. Karlberg P, Adams FH, Geubelle F, Wallgren G: Alteration of the infant's thorax during vaginal delivery. Acta Obstet Gynaecol Scand 41:223, 1962.
47. Bosma J, Lind J: Upper respiratory mechanisms of newborn infants. Acta Paediatr Scand (Suppl 135):132, 1962.
48. Jäykkä S: Capillary erection and lung expansion. Acta Paediatr Scand 46(Suppl 112):9, 1957.
49. Talbert DG: Role of pulmonary vascular pressure in the first breath: engineering reassessment of Jaykka's experimental findings. Acta Paediatr Scand 81:737, 1992.
50. Karlberg P, Cherry RB, Escardó FE, Koch G: Respiratory studies in newborn infants. II. Pulmonary ventilation and mechanics of breathing in the first minutes of life, including the onset of respiration. Acta Paediatr Scand 51:121, 1962.
51. Karlberg P: The adaptive changes in the immediate postnatal period, with particular reference to respiration. J Pediatr 56:585, 1960.
52. Klaus M, Tooley WH, Weaver KH, Clements JA: Lung volume in the newborn infant. Pediatrics 30:111, 1962.
53. Oliver RE, Strang LB: Ion fluxes across the pulmonary epithelium and the secretion of lung liquid in the foetal lamb. J Physiol (Lond) 241:327, 1974.

54. Carlton DP, Cummings JJ, Chapman DL, et al: Ion transport regulation of lung liquid secretion in foetal lambs. J Dev Physiol 17:99, 1992.
55. Carlton DP, Cummings JJ, Poulain FR, et al: Increased pulmonary vascular filtration pressure does not alter lung liquid secretion in fetal sheep. J Appl Physiol 72:650, 1992.
56. Barker PM, Southern KW: Regulation of liquid secretion and absorption by the fetal and neonatal lung. *In* Polin RA, Fox WW, Abman SH (eds): Fetal and Neonatal Physiology, 3rd ed. Philadelphia, WB Saunders Company, 2004, p 822.
57. Brown MJ, Olver RE, Ramsden CA, et al: Effects of adrenaline and of spontaneous labor on the secretion and absorption of lung liquid in the fetal lamb. J Physiol (Lond) 344:137, 1983
58. Bland RD, Hansen TN, Haberkern CM, et al: Lung fluid balance in lambs before and after birth. J Appl Physiol 53:992, 1982.
59. Raj JU, Bland RD: Lung luminal liquid clearance in newborn lambs. Effect of pulmonary microvascular pressure elevation. Am Rev Respir Dis 134:305, 1986.
60. Jain L: Alveolar fluid clearance in developing lungs and its role in neonatal transition. Clin Perinatol 26:585, 1999.
61. Bland RD, Bressack MA, McMillan DD: Labor decreases the lung water content of newborn rabbits. Am J Obstet Gynecol 135:364, 1979.
62. Bland RD, Carlton DP, Scheerer RG, et al: Lung fluid balance in lambs before and after premature birth. J Clin Invest 84:568, 1989.
63. Rudolph AM: Fetal circulation and cardiovascular adjustments after birth. *In* Rudolph CD, Rudolph AM, Hostetter MK, et al (eds): Rudolph's Pediatrics, 21st ed. New York, McGraw-Hill, 2003, p 1749.
64. Adamson SL, Myatt L, Byrne BMP: Regulation of umbilical flow. *In* Polin RA, Fox WW, Abman SH (eds): Fetal and Neonatal Physiology, 3rd ed. Philadelphia, WB Saunders Company, 2004, p 748.
65. Bellotti M, Pennati G, DeGasperi C, et al: Role of ductus venosus in distribution of umbilical blood flow in human fetuses during second half of pregnancy. Am J Physiol Heart Circ Physiol 279: H1256, 2000.
66. Kiserud T: The ductus venosus. Semin Perinatol 25:11, 2001.
67. Teitel DF, Iwamato HS, Rudolph AM: Changes in the pulmonary circulation during birth-related events. Pediatr Res 27:372, 1990.
68. Kinsella JP, McQueston JA, Rosenberg AA, Abman SH: Hemodynamic effects of exogenous nitric oxide in ovine transitional pulmonary circulation. Am J Physiol 263:H875, 1992.
69. Abman SH, Chatfield BA, Hall SL, McMurtry IF: Role of endothelium-derived relaxing factor during transitional pulmonary circulation at birth. Am J Physiol 259:H1921, 1990.
70. Moss AJ, Emmanoulides G, Duffie ER Jr: Closure of the ductus arteriosus in the newborn infant. Pediatrics 32:25, 1963.
71. Gentile R, Stevenson G, Dooley T, et al: Pulse Doppler echocardiographic determination of time of ductal closure in normal newborn infants. J Pediatr 98:443, 1981.
72. Clyman RI: Mechanisms regulating closure of the ductus arteriosus. *In* Polin RA, Fox WW, Abman SH (eds): Fetal and Neonatal Physiology 3rd ed. Philadelphia, WB Saunders Company, 2004, p 743.
73. Behrman RE, Lees MH: Organ blood flows of the fetal, newborn and adult rhesus monkey. Biol Neonate 18:330, 1971.
74. Phibbs RH: Delivery room management. *In* Avery GB, Fletcher MA, MacDonald MG (eds): Neonatology: Pathophysiology and Management of the Newborn, 5th ed. Philadelphia, Lippincott Williams & Wilkins, 1999, p 279.
75. Dawes GS: Foetal and Neonatal Physiology. Chicago, Year Book, 1968.
76. Cross KW: Resuscitation of the asphyxiated infant. Br Med Bull 22:73, 1966.
77. Gupta JM, Tizard JPM: The sequence of events in neonatal apnea. Lancet 2:55, 1967.
78. American Heart Association and American Academy of Pediatrics: Neonatal Resuscitation Textbook. American Academy of Pediatrics and American Heart Association, 2006.
79. Niermeyer S: Resuscitation of the newborn infant. *In* Thureen PJ, Deacon J, Hernandez JA, et al (eds): Assessment and Care of the Well Newborn. St Louis, Elsevier, 2005, p 43.
80. Apgar V: A proposal for a new method of evaluation of the newborn infant. Anesth Analg 32:260, 1953.
81. Jain L, Ferre C, Vidyasagar D: Cardiopulmonary resuscitation of apparently stillborn infants: survival and long-term outcome. J Pediatr 118:778, 1991.
82. Wiswell TE, Fuloria M: Management of meconium-stained amniotic fluid. Clin Perinatol 26:659, 1999.
83. Carson BS, Losey RW, Bowes WA, Simmons MA: Combined obstetric and pediatric approach to prevent meconium aspiration syndrome. Am J Obstet Gynecol 126:712, 1976.
84. Katz VL, Bowes WA: Meconium aspiration syndrome: reflections on a murky subject. Am J Obstet Gynecol 166:171, 1992.
85. Block MF, Kallenberger DA, Kern JD, Nepveux RD: In utero meconium aspiration by the baboon fetus. Obstet Gynecol 57:37, 1981.
86. Brown BL, Gleicher N: Intrauterine meconium aspiration. Obstet Gynecol 57:26, 1981.
87. Falciglia HS: Failure to prevent meconium aspiration syndrome. Obstet Gynecol 71:349, 1988.
88. Falciglia HS, Henderschott C, Potter P, Helmchen R: Does DeLee suction at the perineum prevent meconium aspiration syndrome? Am J Obstet Gynecol 167:1243, 1992
89. Linder N, Aranda JV, Tsur M, et al: Need for endotracheal intubation and suction in meconium-stained neonates. J Pediatr 112:613, 1988.
90. Yoder BA: Meconium-stained amniotic fluid and respiratory complications: impact of selective tracheal suction. Obstet Gynecol 83:77, 1994.
91. Wiswell TE, Gannon CM, Jacob J, et al: Delivery room management of the apparently vigorous meconium-stained neonate: Results of the multicenter international collaborative trial. Pediatrics 105:1, 2000.
92. Vain NE, Szyld EG, Wiswell TE, et al: Oropharyngeal and nasopharyngeal suctioning of meconium-stained neonates before delivery of their shoulders: multicentre, randomized controlled trial. Lancet 364:597, 2004.
93. Murphy JD, Vawter GF, Reid LM: Pulmonary vascular disease in fatal meconium aspiration. J Pediatr 104:758, 1984.
94. Pierce J, Gaudier FL, Sanchez-Ramos L: Intrapartum amnioinfusion for meconium-stained fluid: meta-analysis of prospective clinical trials. Obstet Gynecol 95:1051, 2000.
95. Davis PG, Tan A, O'Donnel CPF, et al: Resuscitation of newborn infants with 100% oxygen or air: a systematic review and meta-analysis. Lancet 364:1329, 2004.
96. Saugstad OD: Is oxygen more toxic than currently believed? Pediatrics 108:1203, 2001.
97. MacDonald HM, Mulligan JC, Allen AC, Taylor PM: Neonatal asphyxia. I. Relationship of obstetric and neonatal complications to neonatal mortality in 38,405 consecutive deliveries. J Pediatr 96:898, 1980.
98. Hall RT, Hall FK, Daily DK: High dose phenobarbital therapy in term newborn infants with severe perinatal asphyxia: a randomized prospective study with three-year follow-up. J Pediatr 132:345, 1998.
99. Shankaran S: The postnatal management of the asphyxiated term infant. Clin Perinatol 29:675, 2002
100. Vannucci RC, Perlman JM: Interventions for perinatal hypoxic-ischemic encephalopathy. Pediatrics 100:1004, 1997.
101. Gluckman PD, Wyall JS, Azzopardi D, et al: Selective head cooling with mild systemic hypothermia after neonatal encephalopathy: multicentre randomized trial. Lancet 365:663, 2005.
102. Jacobs S, Hunt R, Tarnow-Mordi W, et al: Cooling for newborns with hypoxic-ischemic encephalopathy. Cochrane Database Sys Rev 4:CD003311, 2003.
103. Nelson KB, Emery ES III: Birth asphyxia and the neonatal brain: what do we know and when do we know it? Clin Perinatol 20:327, 1993.
104. Scheller JM, Nelson KB: Does cesarean delivery prevent cerebral palsy or other neurologic problems of childhood? Obstet Gynecol 83:624, 1994.
105. Grant A, Joy M-T, O'Brien N, et al: Cerebral palsy among children born during the Dublin randomised trial of intrapartum monitoring. Lancet 2:1233, 1989.
106. Nelson KB, Dambrosia JM, Ting TY, et al: Uncertain value of electronic fetal monitoring in predicting cerebral palsy. N Engl J Med 334:613, 1996.

107. Nelson KB, Ellenberg JH: Obstetric complications as risk factors for cerebral palsy or seizure disorders. JAMA 251:1843, 1984.
108. Goldaber KB, Gilstrap LC, Leveno KJ, et al: Pathologic fetal acidemia. Obstet Gynecol 78:1103, 1991.
109. Allan WC: The clinical spectrum and prediction of outcome in hypoxic-ischemic encephalopathy. Neoreviews 3:e108, 2002.
110. Huppi PS: Advances in postnatal neuroimaging: relevance to pathogenesis and treatment of brain injury. Clin Perinatol 29:827, 2002.
111. Freeman JM, Nelson KB: Intrapartum asphyxia and cerebral palsy. Pediatrics 82:240, 1988.
112. Freeman JM (ed): Prenatal and Perinatal Factors Associated with Brain Disorders, Publication No. 85-1149. Bethesda, MD, NIH, 1985.
113. Nelson KB, Ellenberg JH: Antecedents of cerebral palsy: multivariate analysis of risk. N Engl J Med 315:81, 1986.
114. American College of Obstetricians and Gynecologists: American Academy of Pediatrics: Neonatal encephalopathy and cerebral palsy: defining pathogenesis and pathophysiology. Washington, DC, ACOG, 2003
115. Rosenberg AA: Traumatic birth injury. Neoreviews 4:e273, 2003
116. Zelson C, Lee SJ, Pearl M: The incidence of skull fractures underlying cephalohematomas in newborn infants. J Pediatr 85:371, 1974.
117. Volpe JJ (ed): Intracranial hemorrhage: subdural, primary subarachnoid, intracerebellar, intraventricular (term infant) and miscellaneous. *In* Neurology of the Newborn, 4th ed. Philadelphia, WB Saunders Company, 2001, p 397.
118. Noetzel MJ, Park TS, Robinson S, et al: Prospective study of recovery following neonatal brachial plexus injury. J Child Neurol 16:488, 2001.
119. van Ouwerkerk WJR, Vander Sluijis JA, Nollet F, et al: Management of obstetric brachial plexus lesions: state of the art and future developments. Child Nerv Syst 16:630, 2000.
120. Sahni R, Schulze K: Temperature control in newborn infants. *In* Polin RA, Fox WW, Abman SH (eds): Fetal and Neonatal Physiology, 3rd ed. Philadelphia, WB Saunders Company, 2004, p 548.
121. Adamsons K Jr, Gandy GM, James LS: The influence of thermal factors upon oxygen consumption of the newborn human infant. J Pediatr 66:495, 1965.
122. Dawkins MJR, Hull D: Brown adipose tissue and the response of new-born rabbits to cold. J Physiol (Lond) 172:216, 1964.
123. Aherne W, Hull D: The site of heat production in the newborn infant. Proc R Soc Med 57:1172, 1962.
124. Power GG, Blood AB, Hunter CJ: Perinatal thermal physiology. *In* Polin RA, Fox WW, Abman SH (eds): Fetal and Neonatal Physiology, 3rd ed. Philadelphia, WB Saunders Company, 2004, p 541.
125. Gunn TR, Ball KT, Power GG, Gluckman PD: Factors influencing the initiation of nonshivering thermogenesis. Am J Obstet Gynecol 164:210, 1991.
126. Hey EN, Katz G, O'Connell B: The total thermal insulation of the new-born baby. J Physiol (Lond) 207:683, 1970.
127. Hey EN, Katz G: Evaporative water loss in the newborn baby. J Physiol (Lond) 200:605, 1969.
128. Hey EN, Katz G: The optimum thermal environment for naked babies. Arch Dis Child 45:328, 1970.
129. Scopes JW: Metabolic rate and temperature control in the human body. Br Med Bull 22:88, 1966.
130. Hey EN, O'Connell B: Oxygen consumption and heat balance in the cot-nursed baby. Arch Dis Child 45:335, 1970.
131. Silverman WA, Sinclair JC, Agate FJ Jr: The oxygen cost of minor changes in heat balance of small newborn infants. Acta Paediatr Scand 55:294, 1966.
132. Adamsons K Jr, Towell ME: Thermal homeostasis in the fetus and newborn. Anesthesiology 26:531, 1965.
133. Glass L, Silverman WA, Sinclair JC: Effect of the thermal environment on cold resistance and growth of small infants after the first week of life. Pediatrics 41:1033, 1968.
134. Mancini AJ, Sookdeo-Drost S, Madison KC, et al: Semipermeable dressings improve epidermal barrier function in premature infants. Pediatr Res 36:306, 1994.
135. Vobra S, Roberts RS, Zhang B, et al: Heat loss prevention (HELP) in the delivery room: a randomized, controlled trial of polyethylene occlusive skin wrapping in very preterm infants. J Pediatr 145:750, 2004.
136. Sloan NL, Camacho LWL, Rojas EP, et al: Kangaroo mother method: randomized controlled trial of an alternative method of care for stabilized low-birth weight infants. Lancet 344:782, 1994.
137. Bauer K, Uhrig C, Sperling P, et al: Body temperatures and oxygen consumption during skin-to-skin (kangaroo) care in stable preterm infants weighing less than 1500 grams. J Pediatr 130:240, 1997.
138. Bauer J, Sontheimer G, Fischer C, et al: Metabolic rate and energy balance in very low birth weight infants during kangaroo holding by their mothers and fathers. J Pediatr 129:608, 1996.
139. Bier JB, Ferguson AE, Morales Y, et al: Comparison of skin to skin contact with standard contact in low birth weight infants who are breast fed. Arch Pediatr Adolesc Med 150:1265, 1996.
140. Ziegler EE, O'Donnell AM, Nelson SE, Fomon SJ: Body composition of the reference fetus. Growth 40:329, 1976.
141. Friis-Hansen B: Water distribution in the foetus and newborn infant. Acta Paediatr Scand Suppl 305:7, 1983.
142. Lorenz JM: Fetal and neonatal body water compartment volumes with reference to growth and development. *In* Polin RA, Fox WW, Abman SH (eds): Fetal and Neonatal Physiology, 3rd ed. Philadelphia, WB Saunders Company, 2004, p 1351.
143. Sinclair JC, Silverman WA: Intrauterine growth in active tissue mass of the human fetus, with particular reference to the undergrown baby. Pediatrics 38:48, 1966.
144. Bell EF, Oh W: Fluid and electrolyte management. *In* Avery GB, Fletcher MA, MacDonald MG (eds): Neonatology: Pathophysiology and Management of the Newborn, 5th ed. Philadelphia, Lippincott Williams & Wilkins, 1999, p 345.
145. Committee on Nutrition, American Academy of Pediatrics: Nutritional needs of preterm infants. *In* Kleinman RE (ed): Pediatric Nutrition Handbook, 5th ed. Elk Grove Village, IL, American Academy of Pediatrics, 2004, p 23.
146. Heird WC, Kashyap S: Protein and amino acid metabolism and requirements. *In* Polin RA, Fox WW, Abman SH (eds): Fetal and Neonatal Physiology, 3rd ed. Philadelphia, WB Saunders Company, 2440, p 527.
147. Putet G: Lipids as an energy source for the premature and full-term neonate. *In* Polin RA, Fox WW, Abman SH (eds): Fetal and Neonatal Physiology, 3rd ed. Philadelphia, WB Saunders Company, 2004, p 415.
148. Su HM, Huang MC, Saad NM, et al: Fetal baboons convert 18: 3n-3 to 22: 6n-3 in vivo. A stable isotope tracer study. J Lip Res 42:581, 2001.
149. Dutta-Roy AK: Transport mechanisms for long-chain polyunsaturated fatty acids in the human placenta. Am J Clin Nut 71:315S, 2000.
150. Forsyth JS, Carlton SE: Long chain polyunsaturated fatty acids in infant nutrition: effects on infant development. Curr Opin Clin Nutr Metab Care 4:1, 2001.
151. Un S, Carlson SE: Long chain fatty acids in the developing retina and brain. *In* Polin RA, Fox WW, Abman SH (eds): Fetal and Neonatal Physiology, 3rd ed. Philadelphia, WB Saunders Company, 2004, p 429.
152. Auricchio S, Rubino A, Murset G: Intestinal glycosidase activities in the human embryo, fetus, and newborn. Pediatrics 35:944, 1965.
153. Shulman RJ, Schanler RJ Lau C, et al: Early feeding, feeding tolerance, and lactase activity in preterm infants. J Pediatr 133:645, 1998.
154. Pereira G: Nutritional assessment. *In* Polin RA, Fox WW, Abman SH (eds): Fetal and Neonatal Physiology, 3rd ed. Philadelphia, WB Saunders Company, 2004, p 291.
155. Heinig MJ: Host defense benefits of breast feeding for the infant: effect of breast-feeding duration and exclusivity. Pediatr Clin North Am 48:105, 2001.
156. Schanler RJ, Hurst NM, Lau C: The use of human milk and breastfeeding in premature infants. Clin Perinatol 26:379, 1999.
157. Lucas A, Cole TJ: Breast milk and necrotizing enterocolitis. Lancet 336:1519, 1990.
158. Lucas A, Morley R, Cole TJ, et al: Breast milk and subsequent intelligence quotient in children born preterm. Lancet 339:261, 1992.

159. Lucas A, Morley R, Cole TJ, Gore SM: A randomised multicenter study of human milk versus formula and later development in preterm infants. Arch Dis Child 70:F141, 1994.
160. Morley R, Lucas A: Nutrition and cognitive development. Br Med Bull 53:123, 1997.
161. McGowan J: Neonatal hypoglycemia. NeoReviews 20:e6, 1999.
162. Hawdon JM, Ward Platt MP, Aynsley-Green A: Patterns of metabolic adaptation for preterm and term infants in the first neonatal week. Arch Dis Child 67:357, 1992.
163. Hawdon JM, Ward Platt MP: Metabolic adaptation in small for gestational age infants. Arch Dis Child 68:262, 1993.
164. Hawdon JM, Ward Platt MP, Aynsley-Green A: Prevention and management of neonatal hypoglycemia. Arch Dis Child 70:F60, 1994.
165. Vannucci RC, Vannucci S: Hypoglycemic brain injury. Semin Neonatol 6:147, 2001.
166. Reyes HM, Meller JL, Loeff D: Management of esophageal atresia and tracheoesophageal fistula. Clin Perinatol 16:79, 1989.
167. Kays DW: Surgical conditions of the neonatal intestinal tract. Clin Perinatol 23:353, 1996.
168. Meller JL, Reyes HN, Loeff DS: Gastroschisis and omphalocoele. Clin Perinatol 16:113, 1989.
169. Chahine AA, Ricketts RR: Resuscitation of the surgical neonate. Clin Perinatol 26:693, 1999.
170. Van Meurs K, Short BL: Congenital diaphragmatic hernia: the neonatologists perspective. NeoReviews 20:e79, 1999.
171. Cohen MS, Rychik J, Bush DM: Influence of congenital heart disease on survival in children with congenital diaphragmatic hernia. J Pediatr 141:25, 2002.
172. Benachi A, Chailley-Heu B, Delezoide A-L, et al: Lung growth and maturation after tracheal occlusion in diaphragmatic hernia. Am J Respir Crit Care Med 157:921, 1998.
173. Harrison MR, Keller RL, Hawgood SB, et al: A randomized trial of fetal endoscopic tracheal occlusion for severe congenital diaphragmatic hernia. N Engl J Med 349:1916, 2003.
174. Caplan MS, Jilling T: The pathophysiology of necrotizing enterocolitis. Neoreviews 2:e103, 2001.
175. Dimmit RA, Moss RL: Clinical management of necrotizing enterocolitis. Neoreviews 2:e110, 2001.
176. Norton ME, Merrill J, Cooper BAB, et al: Neonatal complications after the administration of indomethacin for preterm labor. N Engl J Med 329:1602, 1993.
177. Major CA, Lewis DF, Harding JA, et al: Tocolysis with indomethacin increases the incidence of necrotizing enterocolitis in the low-birth-weight neonate. Am J Obstet Gynecol 170:102, 1994.
178. Cashore WJ: Bilirubin metabolism and toxicity in the newborn. *In* Polin RA, Fox WW, Abman SH (eds): Fetal and Neonatal Physiology, 3rd ed. Philadelphia, WB Saunders Company, 2004, p 1199.
179. American Academy of Pediatrics Subcommittee on Hyperbilirubinemia: Management of hyperbilirubinemia in the newborn infant 35 or more weeks of gestation. Pediatrics 114:297, 2004.
180. Auerbach KG, Gartner LM: Breast feeding and human milk: their association with jaundice in the neonate. Clin Perinatol 14:89, 1987.
181. Maisels MJ, Gifford KL: Normal serum bilirubin levels in the newborn and the effect of breast-feeding. Pediatrics 78:837, 1986.
182. Gourley GR: Breast feeding, diet, and neonatal hyperbilirubinemia. NeoReviews 1:e25, 2000.
183. Perlstein MA: The late clinical syndrome of posticteric encephalopathy. Pediatr Clin North Am 7:665, 1960.
184. Hsia DY, Allen FH Jr, Gellis SS, Diamond LK: Erythroblastosis fetalis. VIII. Studies of serum bilirubin in relation to kernicterus. N Engl J Med 247:668, 1952.
185. Newman TB, Maisels MJ: Does hyperbilirubinemia damage the brain of healthy full-term infants? Clin Perinatol 17:331, 1990.
186. Johnson L, Bhutani VK: Guidelines for management of the jaundiced term and near-term infant. Clin Perinatol 25:555, 1998.
187. Newman TB, Maisels MJ: Evaluation and treatment of jaundice in the term newborn: a kinder, gentler approach. Pediatrics 89:809, 1992.
188. Davidson L, Thilo L: How to make kernicterus a never event. Neoreviews 4:e308, 2003.
189. Watchko JF, Oski FA: Kernicterus in preterm newborns: past, present, and future. Pediatrics 90:707, 1992.
190. Yoder MC: Embryonic hematopoiesis. *In* Christensen RD (ed): Hematologic Problems of the Neonate. Philadelphia, WB Saunders Company, 2000, p 3.
191. Christensen RD: Expected hematologic values for term and preterm neonates. *In* Christensen RD (ed): Hematologic Problems of the Neonate. Philadelphia, WB Saunders Company, 2000, p 117.
192. Forestier F, Daffos F, Catherine N, et al: Developmental hematopoesis in normal human fetal blood. Blood 77:2360, 1991.
193. Widness JA: Pathophysiology, diagnosis, and prevention of neonatal anemia. Neoreviews 1:e61, 2000.
194. Werner EJ: Neonatal polycythemia and hyperviscosity. Clin Perinatol 22:693, 1995.
195. Black VD, Lubchenco LO: Neonatal polycythemia and hyperviscosity. Pediatr Clin North Am 29:1137, 1982.
196. Ramamurthy RS, Berlanga M: Postnatal alteration in hematocrit and viscosity in normal and polycythemic infants. J Pediatr 110:929, 1987.
197. Black VD, Camp BW, Lubchenco LO, et al: Neonatal hyperviscosity association with lower achievement and IQ scores at school age. Pediatrics 83:662, 1989.
198. Schimmel MS, Bromiker R, Soll RF: Neonatal polycythemia: is partial exchange transfusion justified? Clin Perinatol 31:545, 2004.
199. Bada HS, Korones SB, Pourcyrous M, et al: Asymptomatic syndrome of polycythemia hyperviscosity: effect of partial exchange transfusion. J Pediatr 120:579, 1992.
200. Burrows R, Kelton J: Fetal thrombocytopenia and its relation to maternal thrombocytopenia. N Engl J Med 329:1463, 1993.
201. McCrae KR, Samuels P, Schreiber AD, et al: Pregnancy-associated thrombocytopenia: pathogenesis and management. Blood 80:2697, 1992.
202. Sainio S, Jousti L, Jarvenpaa AL, et al: Idiopathic thrombocytopenic purpura in pregnancy. Acta Obstet Gynecol Scand 77:272, 1998.
203. Cook RL, Miller RC, Katz VL, et al: Immune thrombocytopenic purpura in the pregnancy: a reappraisal of management. Obstet Gynecol 78:578, 1991.
204. Mueller-Eckhardt C, Kiefel V, Grubert A, et al: 348 cases of suspected neonatal alloimmune thrombocytopenia. Lancet 1:363, 1989.
205. Johnson JM, Ryan G, Al-Muse A, et al: Prenatal diagnosis and management of neonatal alloimmune thrombocytopenia. Semin Perinatol 21:45, 1997.
206. Bussel JB, Zabusky MR, Berkowitz RL, et al: Fetal alloimmune thrombocytopenia. N Engl J Med 337:22, 1997.
207. Bussel JB: Alloimmune thrombocytopenia in the fetus and newborn. Semin Thromb Hemost 27:245, 2001.
208. American Academy of Pediatrics Committee on the Fetus and Newborn: Controversies concerning vitamin K and the newborn. Pediatrics 112:191, 2003.
209. Lapine TR, Hill HR: Host defense mechanisms against bacteria. In Polin RA, Fox WW, Abman SH (eds): Fetal and Neonatal Physiology, 3rd ed. Philadelphia, WB Saunders Company, 2004, p 1475.
210. Gibbs RS, Schrag S, Schuchat A: Perinatal infections due to group B streptococci. Obstet Gynecol 104:1062, 2004.
211. Stoll BJ: The global impact of neonatal infection. Clin Perinatol 24:1, 1997.
212. St. Geme JW Jr, Murray DL, Carter J, et al: Perinatal bacterial infection after prolonged rupture of amniotic membranes: an analysis of risk and management. J Pediatr 104:608, 1984.
213. Belady PH, Farkouh LJ, Gibbs RS: Intra-amniotic infection and premature rupture of the membranes. Clin Perinatol 25:123, 1998.
214. Schrag S, Gorwitz R, Fultz-Butts K, et al: Prevention of perinatal group B streptococcal disease. Revised guidelines from CDC. MMWR 51(RR11):1, 2002.
215. Walsh-Sukys MC: Persistent pulmonary hypertension of the newborn: the black box revisited. Clin Perinatol 20:127, 1993.
216. Rudolph AM: High pulmonary vascular resistance after birth. 1. Pathophysiologic considerations and etiologic classification. Clin Pediatr 19:585, 1980.

217. Kinsella JP, Abman SH: Inhaled nitric oxide: current and future uses in neonates. Semin Perinatol 24:387, 2000.
218. Schumacher RE, Baumgart S: Extracorporeal membrane oxygenation 2001: the odessey continues. Clin Perinatol 28;629, 2001.
219. Kinsella JP, Shaul PW: Physiology of nitric oxide in the developing lung. *In* Polin RA, Fox WW, Abman SH (eds): Fetal and Neonatal Physiology. Philadelphia, WB Saunders Company, 2004, p 733.
220. Avery ME, Gatewood OB, Brumley G: Transient tachypnea of the newborn. Am J Dis Child 111:380, 1966.
221. Ablow RC, Driscoll SG, Effman EL, et al: A comparison of early-onset group B streptococcal neonatal infection and the respiratory-distress syndrome of the newborn. N Engl J Med 294:65, 1976.
222. Whitsett JA, Pryhuber GS, Rice WR, et al: Acute respiratory disorders. *In* Avery GB, Fletcher MA, MacDonald MG (eds): Neonatology: Pathophysiology and Management of the Newborn, 5th ed. Philadelphia, Lippincott Williams & Wilkins, 1999, p 485.
223. Avery ME, Mead J: Surface properties in relation to atelectasis and hyaline membrane disease. Am J Dis Child 97:517, 1959.
224. Cotton RB: Pathophysiology of hyaline membrane disease (excluding surfactant). *In* Polin RA, Fox WW, Abman SH (eds): Fetal and Neonatal Physiology, 3rd ed. Philadelphia, WB Saunders Company, 2004, p 926.
225. Jobe AH, Ikegami M: Pathophysiology of respiratory distress syndrome and surfactant metabolism. *In* Polin RA, Fox WW, Abman SH (eds): Fetal and Neonatal Physiology, 3rd ed. Philadelphia, WB Saunders Company, 2004, p 1055.
226. Northway WH Jr, Rosan RC, Porter DY: Pulmonary disease following respiratory therapy of hyaline membrane disease. N Engl J Med 276:357, 1967.
227. Farrell PA, Fiascone JM: Bronchopulmonary dysplasia in the 1990's: a review for the pediatrician. Curr Probl Pediatr 27:129, 1997.
228. Bregman J, Farrell EE: Neurodevelopmental outcome in infants with bronchopulmonary dysplasia. Clin Perinatol 19:673, 1992.
229. Jacob SV, Coates AL, Lands LC, et al: Long-term pulmonary sequelae of severe bronchopulmonary dysplasia. J Pediatr 133:193, 1998.
230. Northway WH Jr, Moss RB, Carlisle KB, et al: Late pulmonary sequelae of bronchopulmonary dysplasia. N Engl J Med 323:1793, 1990.
231. Jobe AH, Bancalari E: Bronchopulmonary dysplasia. Am J Respir Crit Care Med 163:1723, 2001.
232. Kattwinkel J: Surfactant. Evolving issues. Clin Perinatol 25:17, 1998.
233. Narendran V, Donovan EF, Hoath SB, et al: Early bubble CPAP and outcomes in ELBW preterm infants. J Perinatol 23:195, 2003.
234. Survanta: Multidose Study Group: Two-year follow-up of infants treated for neonatal respiratory distress syndrome with bovine surfactant. J Pediatr 124:962, 1994.
235. Vermont Oxford Neonatal Network: Vermont Oxford Network Annual VLBW Database Summary 2003, Burlington, Vermont Oxford Network, 2004.
236. Hamrick SEG, Miller SP, Leonard C, et al: Trends in severe brain injury and neurodevelopmental outcome in premature newborns: the rate of cystic periventricular leukomalacia. J Pediatr 145:593, 2004.
237. Papile L-A, Burstein J, Burstein R, Koffler H: Incidence and evolution of subependymal and intraventricular hemorrhage: a study of infants with birth weight less than 1500gm. J Pediatr 92:529, 1978.
238. Pasternak JF, Groothuis DR, Fischer JM, Fischer DP: Regional cerebral blood flow in the newborn beagle pup: the germinal matrix is a "low-flow" structure. Pediatr Res 16:499, 1982.
239. Goddard J, Lewis RM, Armstrong DL, Zeller RS: Moderate, rapidly induced hypertension as a cause of intraventricular hemorrhage in the newborn beagle model. J Pediatr 96:1057, 1980.
240. Counsell SJ, Allsop JM, Harrison MC, et al: Diffusion-weighted imaging of the brain in preterm infants with focal and diffuse white matter abnormality. Pediatrics 112:1, 2003.
241. Volpe JJ: Cerebral white matter injury of the premature infant—more common than you think. Pediatrics 112:176, 2003.
242. Maalouf EF, Duggan PJ, Counsell S, et al: Comparison of findings on cranial ultrasound and magnetic resonance imaging in preterm infants. Pediatrics 107:719, 2001.
243. Perlman JM, Risser R, Broyles S: Bilateral cystic periventricular leukomalacia in the premature infant: associated risk factors. Pediatrics 97:822, 1996.
244. Dammann D, Leviton A: Maternal intrauterine infection, cytokines and brain damage in the preterm newborn. Pediatr Res 42:1, 1997.
245. Back SA, Luo NL, Borenstein NS, et al: Late oligodendrocyte progenitors coincide with the developmental window of vulnerability for human perinatal white matter injury. J Neurosci 21:1302, 2001.
246. Haynes RL, Folkerth RD, Keefe R et al: Nitrosative and oxidative injury to premyelinating oligodendrocytes in periventricular leukomalacia. J Neuropath Exp Neurol 62:441, 2003.
247. Back SA, Gan X, Li Y: Maturation dependent vulnerability of oligodendrocytes to oxidative stress—induced death caused by glutathione depletion. J Neurosci 18:6241, 1998.
248. Eklind S, Mallard C, Leverin A-L, et al: Bacterial endotoxin sensitizes the immature brain to hypoxic—ischaemic injury. Eur J Neurosci 13:1101, 2001.
249. Ford LM, Steichen J, Steichen Asch PA, et al: Neurologic status and intracranial hemorrhage in very-low-birth-weight preterm infants: outcome at 1 and 5 years. Am J Dis Child 143:1186, 1989.
250. Lowe J, Papille LA: Neurodevelopmental performance of very-low-birth-weight infants with mild periventricular, intraventricular hemorrhage. Outcome at 5 to 6 years of age. Am J Dis Child 144:1242, 1990.
251. Guzzetta F, Shackelford GD, Volpe S, et al: Periventricular echodensities in the premature newborn: critical determinant of neurologic outcome. Pediatrics 78:995, 1986.
252. Shankaran S, Koepke T, Woldt E, et al: Outcome after posthemorrhagic ventriculomegaly in comparison with mild hemorrhage without ventriculomegaly. J Pediatr 114:109, 1989.
253. deVries LS, van Haastert IC, Rademaker KJ, et al: Ultrasound abnormalities preceding cerebral palsy in high risk preterm infants. J Pediatr 144:815, 2004.
254. Perlman JM: White matter injury in the preterm infant: an important determination of abnormal neurodevelopmental outcome. Early Hum Dev 53:99, 1998.
255. Rosenberg AA, Galan HC: Fetal drug therapy. Pediatr Clin North Am 44:113, 1997.
256. Thorp JA, Ferrette-Smith D, Gaston LA, et al: The effect of combined antenatal vitamin K and phenobarbital therapy for preventing intracranial hemorrhage in newborns less than 34 weeks gestation. Obstet Gynecol 86:1, 1995.
257. Shankaran S, Papile L-A, Wright LL, et al: The effect of antenatal phenobarbital therapy on neonatal intracranial hemorrhage in preterm infants. N Engl J Med 337:466, 1997.
258. Scher MS: Seizures in the newborn infant. Diagnosis, treatment, and outcome. Clin Perinatol 24:735,1997.
259. Dubowitz LMS, Dubowitz V, Goldberg C: Clinical assessment of gestational age in the newborn infant. J Pediatr 77:1, 1970.
260. Ballard JL, Kazmaier K, Driver M: A simplified assessment of gestational age. Pediatr Res 11:374, 1977.
261. Ballard JL, Khoury JC, Wedig K, et al: New Ballard Score, expanded to include extremely premature infants. J Pediatr 119:417, 1991.
262. Donovan EF, Tyson JE, Ehrenkranz RA, et al: Inaccuracy of Ballard scores before 28 weeks' gestation. J Pediatr 135:147, 1999.
263. Lubchenco LO, Hansman C, Boyd E: Intrauterine growth in length and head circumference as estimated from live births at gestational ages from 26 to 42 weeks. Pediatrics 37:403, 1966.
264. Lin C-C, Santoloya-Forgas J: Current concepts of fetal growth restriction: Part I. Causes, classification, and pathophysiology. Obstet Gynecol 92:1044, 1998.
265. Khoury MJ, Erickson JD, Cordero JF, McCarthy BJ: Congenital malformations and intrauterine growth retardation: a population study. Pediatrics 82:83, 1988.
266. American Academy of Pediatrics Committee on Fetus and Newborn: Levels of neonatal care. Pediatrics 114:1341, 2004.
267. Schulze A, Lindner M, Kohmuller D, et al: Expanded newborn screening for inborn errors of metabolism by electrospray ioniza-

tion—tandem mass spectroscopy: results, outcome and implications. Pediatrics 111:1399, 2003.
268. Thompson DC, McPhillips H, Davis RL, et al: Universal newborn hearing screening. Summary of evidence. JAMA 286:2000, 2001.
269. American Academy of Pediatrics Task Force on Infant Positioning and SIDS: Positioning and sudden infant death syndrome (SIDS): update. Pediatrics 98:1216, 1996.
270. Conrad PD, Wilkening RB, Rosenberg AA: Safety of newborn discharge in less than 36 hours in an indigent population. Am J Dis Child 143:98, 1989.
271. American Academy of Pediatrics, American College of Obstetricians and Gynecologists: Guidelines for Perinatal Care, 5th ed. Elk Grove Village, IL, American Academy of Pediatrics, 2002.
272. American Academy of Pediatrics Task Force on Circumcision: Circumcision policy statement. Pediatrics 103:686, 1999.
273. Klaus MH, Kennel JH: Care of the parents. *In* Klaus MH, Fanaroff AA (eds): Care of the High-Risk Neonate, 5th ed. Philadelphia, WB Saunders Company, 2001, p 195.
274. Brazelton TB, Scholl ML, Robey JS: Visual responses in the newborn. Pediatrics 37:284, 1966.
275. Klaus MH, Jerauld R, Kreger NC: Maternal attachment: importance of the first post-partum days. N Engl J Med 286:460, 1972.
276. Whitelaw A: Kangaroo baby care: just a nice experience or an important advance for preterm infants? Pediatrics 85:604, 1990.
277. Als H, Lawhon G, Duffy FH: Individual developmental care for the very low birth weight preterm infant. Medical and neurofunctional effects. JAMA 272:853, 1994.
278. Solnit AJ, Stark MH: Mourning and the birth of a defective child. Psychoanal Study Child 16:523, 1961.
279. Cullberg J: Mental reactions of women to perinatal death. *In* Morris N (ed): Psychosomatic Medicines in Obstetrics and Gynecology. New York, S Karger, 1972, p 326.
280. Horbar JD, Badger GJ, Carpenter JH, et al: Trends in mortality and morbidity for very low birth weight infants, 1991–1999. Pediatrics 110:143, 2002.
281. Hack M, Fanaroff AA: Outcomes of children of extremely low birthweight and gestational age in the 1990's. Early Hum Dev 53:193, 1999.
282. Wood NS, Marlow N, Costeloe K, et al: Neurologic and developmental disability after extremely preterm birth. N Engl J Med 343:378, 2000.
283. Marlow N, Wolke D, Bracewell MA, et al: Neurologic and developmental disability at six years of age after extremely preterm birth. N Engl J Med 352:9, 2005.
284. Saigal S, den Ouden L, Wolke D, et al: School age outcomes in children who were extremely low birth weight from four international population-based cohorts. Pediatrics 112:943, 2003.
285. Anderson P, Doyle LW: Neurobehavioral outcomes of school age children born extremely low birth weight or very preterm in the 1990's. JAMA 289:3264, 2003.
286. Hack M, Taylor G, Klein N, et al: School-age outcomes in children with birth weights under 750g. N Engl J Med 331:753, 1994.
287. Schmidt B, Asztalos EV, Roberts RS, et al: Impact of bronchopulmonary dysplasia, brain injury, and severe retinopathy on the outcome of extremely low-birth-weight infants at 18 months. JAMA 289:1124, 2003.
288. Hack M, Breslau N, Weissman B, et al: Effect of very low birth weight and subnormal head size on cognitive abilities at school age. N Engl J Med 325:231, 1991.
289. Kok JH, Den Ouden AL, Verloove-Vanhornick SP, et al: Outcome of very preterm small for gestational age infants: the first nine years of life. Br J Obstet Gynaecol 105:162, 1998.
290. Lucey JF, Dangman B: A reexamination of the role of oxygen in retrolental fibroplasia. Pediatrics 73:82, 1984.
291. Valentine PH, Jackson JC, Kalina RE, Woodrum DE: Increased survival of low birth weight infants: impact on the incidence of retinopathy of prematurity. Pediatrics 84:442, 1989.
292. Kramer SJ, Vertes DR, Condom M: Auditory brainstem responses and clinical followup of high risk infants. Pediatrics 83:385, 1989.
293. Levene M: Is intensive care for very immature babies justified? Acta Paediatr 93:149, 2004.
294. Peerzada JM, Richardson DM, Burns JP: Delivery room decision-making at the threshold of viability. J Pediatr 145:492, 2004.
295. Lucey JF, Rowan CA, Shiono P, et al: Fetal infants: the fate of 4172 infants with birth weights of 401–500 grams—the Vermont Oxford experience (1996–2000). Pediatrics 113:1559, 2004.

Postpartum Care

Vern L. Katz

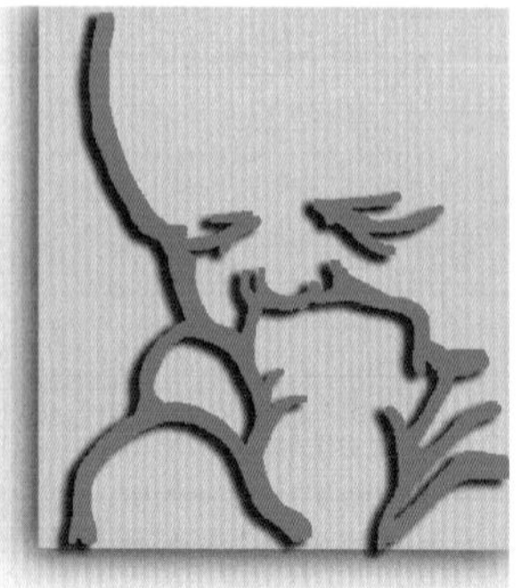

CHAPTER 21

Key Abbreviations

Depot medroxyprogesterone acetate	DMPA
Edinburgh Postnatal Depression Scale	EPDS
Food and Drug Administration	FDA
Follicle-stimulating hormone	FSH
Intrauterine device	IUD
Postpartum thyroiditis	PPT

The postpartum time period, also called the puerperium, lasts from delivery of the placenta until 6 to 12 weeks after delivery. Most of the physiologic changes in pregnancy will have returned to prepregnancy physiology by 6 weeks. However, many of the cardiovascular changes and psychological changes may persist for many more months. This chapter examines the physiologic adjustments of the postpartum period, the return of the female genital tract to its prepregnancy state (involution), the major puerperal disease states, and the natural course of lactation.

The postpartum period is associated with as much tradition and superstition as any other rite of passage in life, because the health of a new infant is so important to the survival of any family or clan. In order to support the successful recovery of the mother, and the healthy transition through the neonatal period, customs, taboos, and rituals have developed in most cultures. Indeed, many of the current medical recommendations about puerperium have developed from adaptations of socially acceptable traditions, rather than science. For example, the 6-week postpartum check approximates the end of the 40 days of rest and sexual separation required in traditional societies.

Cultures throughout the world have specific postpartum traditions that include both restrictions on activity and prescribed activities, different foods for the newly delivered mother, as well as particular and unique taboos regarding postpartum care (Table 21-1). For example, bathing is a taboo in some cultures. Because women often cherish these rituals, it is essential for physicians, midwives, and nurses to be sensitive to these customs even though a woman's place of delivery may be far from her native country.

This chapter examines the normal physiologic changes of the puerperium and the transitions to prepregnancy physiology. With respect to these changes, we evaluate the principles and practices of postpartum care, the role of the provider being to help the patient through the transition. As is true of most physiologic changes, disease may occur when the change is exaggerated or insufficient.

POSTPARTUM INVOLUTION

The Uterus

The crude weight of the pregnant uterus at term (excluding the fetus, placenta, membranes, and amniotic fluid) is approximately 1,000 g, approximately 10- to 20-fold heavier than the nonpregnant uterus.[2] The specific time course of uterine involution has not been fully elucidated, but within 2 weeks after birth, the uterus has usually returned to the pelvis, and by 6 weeks, it is usually normal size, as estimated by palpation. The gross

Table 21-1. Examples of Postpartum Rituals

- In the rural Philippines, the mother, who works up until she goes into labor, is prohibited from working after delivery, and she is given a new name. The maternal grandmother visits daily and does the housework and cooking for 8 weeks. The mother is bathed by the grandmother daily. When the umbilical cord falls off the infant, a feast is prepared. The cord is blessed at the feast. The new father is prohibited from building stone walls and from driving nails for 6 months. For 2 months, the relatives tend the fields.
- Postpartum taboos related to *hot and cold* are found worldwide.
  - In Asian, African, and Latin American cultures, heat and cold must be maintained in balance to promote health and prevent disease. Because blood, which is "hot," is lost during delivery, the parturient must replenish her "heat" by staying bundled and drinking warm liquids.
  - Several traditional Middle Eastern areas see the bones as open after delivery, and exposure to cold creates a vulnerability to disease. Bathing is often taboo for traditional women; sponge baths may be substituted.
  - In parts of rural India, the new mother returns to her mother's house for 16 weeks. She is given a hot bath every day. Cold baths are taboo, because cold water is associated with disease.
  - Many cultures have rituals regarding treatment of the placenta. It may be dried and turned to powder for its "medical" powers. The umbilical cord was hung in a nearby tree by some eastern Native American tribes. In Eastern European tradition, it was buried under certain corners of the house, to ensure prosperity.

anatomic and histologic characteristics of the involutional process are based on the study of autopsy, hysterectomy, and endometrial biopsy specimens.[2–4] The decrease in the size of the uterus and cervix during the puerperium has been demonstrated with serial magnetic resonance imaging as illustrated in Figure 21-1.[5] The findings are consistent with those of serial sonography and computed tomography.[4–6]

Immediately after delivery, rapidly decreasing endometrial surface area facilitates placental shearing at the decidual layer. The average diameter of the placenta is 18 cm; in the immediate postpartum uterus, the average diameter of the site of placental attachment measures 9 cm. In the first 3 days after delivery the placental site is infiltrated with granulocytes and mononuclear cells, a reaction that extends into the endometrium and superficial myometrium. By the 7th day, there is evidence of the regeneration of endometrial glands, often appearing atypical, with irregular chromatin patterns, misshapen and enlarged nuclei, pleomorphism, and increased cytoplasm. By the end of the first week, there is also evidence of the regeneration of endometrial stroma, with mitotic figures noted in gland epithelium; by postpartum day 16, the endometrium is fully restored.

Decidual necrosis begins on the first day, and by the 7th day, a well-demarcated zone can be seen between necrotic and viable tissue. An area of viable decidua remains between the necrotic slough and the deeper endomyometrium. Sharman[3] described how the non-necrotic decidual cells participate in the reconstruction of the endometrium, a likely role, given their original role as endometrial connective tissue cells. By the 6th week, decidual cells are rare. The immediate inflammatory cell infiltrate of polymorphonuclear leukocytes and lymphocytes persists for about 10 days, presumably serving as an antibacterial barrier. The leukocyte response diminishes rapidly after the 10th day, and plasma cells are seen for the first time. The plasma cell and lymphocyte response may last as long as several months. In fact, endometrial stromal infiltrates of plasma cells and lymphocytes are the sign (and may be the only sign) of a recent pregnancy.

Hemostasis immediately after birth is accomplished by arterial smooth muscle contraction and compression of vessels by the involuting uterine muscle. Vessels in the placental site are characterized during the first 8 days by thrombosis, hyalinization, and endophlebitis in the veins, and by hyalinization and obliterative fibrinoid endarteritis in the arteries. The mechanism for hyalinization of arterial walls, which is not completely understood, may be related to the previous trophoblastic infiltration of arterial walls that occurs early in pregnancy. Many of the thrombosed and hyalinized veins are extruded with the slough of the necrotic placental site, but hyalinized arteries remain for extended periods as stigmata of the placental site. Restoration of the endometrium in areas other than the placental site occurs rapidly, with the process being completed by day 16 after delivery. The gland epithelium does not undergo the reactivity or the pseudoneoplastic appearance noted in placental site glands.[5]

The postpartum uterine discharge or lochia begins as a flow of blood lasting several hours, rapidly diminishing to a reddish brown discharge through the 3rd or 4th day postpartum. This is followed by a transition to a mucopurulent, somewhat malodorous discharge, called lochia serosa, requiring the change of several perineal pads per day. The median duration of lochia serosa is 22 to 27 days.[6,7] However, 10 to 15 percent of women will have lochia serosa at the time of the 6-week postpartum examination. In the majority of patients, the lochia serosa is followed by a yellow-white discharge, called lochia alba. Breast-feeding or the use of oral contraceptive agents does not affect the duration of lochia. Frequently, there is a sudden but transient increase in uterine bleeding between 7 and 14 days postpartum. This corresponds to the slough of the eschar over the site of placental attachment. Myometrial vessels of greater than 5 mm in diameter are present for up to 2 weeks postpartum, which accounts for the dramatic bleeding that can occur with this phenomenon.[6] Although it can be profuse, this bleeding episode is usually self-limited, requiring nothing more than reassurance of the patient. If it does not subside within 1 or 2 hours, the patient should be evaluated for possible retained placental tissue.

Ultrasound may be helpful in the management of abnormal postpartum bleeding. The empty uterus with a clear midline echo can often be distinguished from the uterine cavity expanded by clot (sonolucent) or retained tissue (echo dense). Serial ultrasound examinations of postpartum patients showed that in 20 to 30 percent, there was some retained blood or tissue within 24 hours

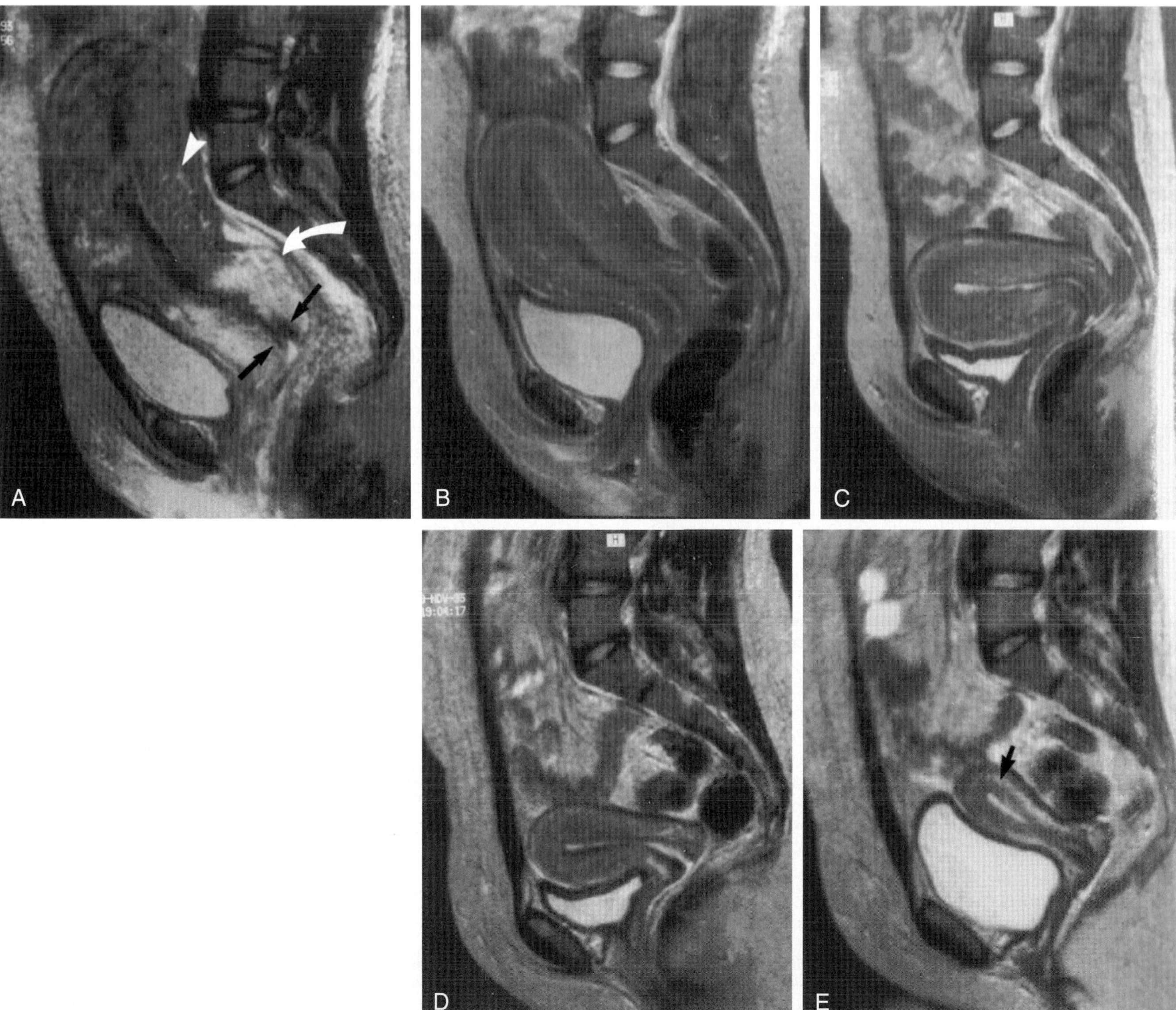

Figure 21-1. Sagittal T2-weighted fast-spin echo magnetic resonance images (3/500/100) obtained serially after uncomplicated vaginal delivery. *A,* Initial image obtained less than 30 hours after delivery. Uterus and cervix are large and thick walled. The uterine cervix is clearly distinguished from the uterine corpus by the high-signal-intensity outer cervical stroma (OCS) *(white arrow).* The low-signal-intensity inner cervical stroma (ICS) is apparent *(black arrows).* The myometrium has heterogeneous signal intensity, and prominent myometrial vessels are seen *(arrowhead).* The myometrial vessels remained prominent on images obtained 1 week *(B)* and 2 weeks *(C)* after delivery. At 1 week, the uterus and cervix have diminished substantially in size, the OCS has diminished in signal intensity, and the ICS is more clearly defined. The low signal intensity in the endometrial canal in *A* and *B* likely represents blood products. At 2 weeks *(C),* 6 weeks *(D),* and 6 months *(E),* the uterus has progressively deceased in size. At 2 weeks, the endometrium has returned to a normal high signal intensity. By 6 months, the junctional zone has been restored (*arrow* in *E*); however, it is broadened, measuring approximately 7 mm. (From Willms AB, Brown ED, Kettritz UI, et al: Anatomic changes in the pelvis after uncomplicated vaginal delivery: evaluation with serial MR imaging. Radiology 195:91, 1995, with permission.)

after delivery. By the 4th postpartum day, only about 8 percent of patients showed endometrial cavity separation, a portion of which eventually had abnormal postpartum bleeding because of retained placental tissue.[8] In cases of abnormal postpartum bleeding, ultrasound examination may be a useful adjunct in detecting patients who have retained tissue or clot and, therefore, who will benefit from uterine evacuation and curettage. Those who have an empty uterine cavity will respond to therapy with oxytocin or methylergonovine.[9]

The Cervix

During pregnancy, the cervical epithelium increases in thickness, and the cervical glands show both hyperplasia and hypertrophy. Within the stroma, a distinct decidual reaction occurs. These changes are accompanied by a substantial increase in the vascularity of the cervix.[10] Colposcopic examination performed after delivery has demonstrated ulceration, laceration, and ecchymosis of the cervix.[11] Regression of the cervical epithelium begins within the first 4 days after delivery, and by the end of the first week, edema and hemorrhage within the cervix are minimal. Vascular hypertrophy and hyperplasia persist throughout the first week postpartum. By 6 weeks' postpartum, most of the antepartum changes have resolved, although round cell infiltration and some edema may persist for several months.[12]

The Fallopian Tube

The epithelium of the fallopian tube during pregnancy is characterized by a predominance of nonciliated cells, a phenomenon that is maintained by the balance between the high levels of progesterone and estrogen.[13] After delivery, in the absence of progesterone and estrogen, there is further extrusion of nuclei from nonciliated cells and diminution in height of both ciliated and nonciliated cells. Andrews[13] demonstrated that the number and height of ciliated cells can be increased in the puerperium by treatment with estrogen.

Fallopian tubes removed between postpartum days 5 and 15 demonstrate inflammatory changes of acute salpingitis in 38 percent of cases, but no bacteria are found. The specific cause of the inflammatory change is unknown.[13] Furthermore, there is no correlation between the presence of histologic inflammation in the fallopian tubes and puerperal fever or other clinical signs of salpingitis.

Ovarian Function

It has long been recognized that women who breast-feed their infants are amenorrheic for long periods of time, often until the infant is weaned. Several studies, using a variety of methods to indicate ovulation, have demonstrated that ovulation occurs as early as 27 days after delivery, with the mean time being approximately 70 to 75 days in nonlactating women.[14,15] Among those women who are breast-feeding their infants, the mean time to ovulation is about 6 months.

Menstruation resumes by 12 weeks' postpartum in 70 percent of women who are not lactating, and the mean time to the first menstruation is 7 to 9 weeks. In one study of lactating women, it was 36 months before 70 percent began to menstruate. The duration of anovulation depends on the frequency of breast-feeding, the duration of each feed, and the proportion of supplementary feeds.[16] The risk of ovulation within the first 6 months' postpartum in a woman exclusively breast-feeding is 1 to 5 percent.

The hormonal basis for puerperal ovulation suppression in lactating women appears to be the persistence of elevated serum prolactin levels.[17] Prolactin levels fall to the normal range by the 3rd week postpartum in nonlactating women, but remain elevated into the 6th week postpartum in lactating patients. Estrogen levels fall immediately after delivery in both lactating and nonlactating women, and remain depressed in lactating patients. In those who are not lactating, estrogen levels begin to rise 2 weeks after delivery and are significantly higher than in lactating women by postpartum day 17. Follicle-stimulating hormone (FSH) levels are identical in breast-feeding and non-breast-feeding women, suggesting that the ovary does not respond to FSH stimulation in the presence of increased prolactin levels.

Weight Loss

One of the most welcomed changes for the majority of women who have recently given birth is the loss of the weight that was accumulated during pregnancy. The immediate loss of 10 to 13 lb is attributed to the delivery of the infant, placenta, and amniotic fluid and to blood loss.[18] However, most women will not manifest that loss until 1 to 2 weeks after delivery owing to fluid retention immediately after delivery. Women may be reassured about the temporary dependent edema secondary to this fluid retention. For most women, weight loss postpartum does not tend to compensate for weight gain during gestation. By 6 weeks postpartum, only 28 percent of women will have returned to their prepregnant weight.[19] The remainder of any weight loss occurs from 6 weeks postpartum until 6 months after delivery, with the majority of weight loss concentrated in the first 3 months. Women with excess weight gain in pregnancy (>35 lb) are likely to have a net gain of 11 lb.[19] Breast-feeding has relatively little effect on postpartum weight loss.[20] With a program of diet and exercise, weight loss of approximately 0.5 kg/wk between 4 and 14 weeks' postpartum in breast-feeding overweight women did not affect the growth weight of their infants.[21] Similarly, aerobic exercise had no adverse effect on lactation.[22] In a longitudinal study of pregnancy weight gain, 540 women were followed for 5 to 10 years (mean 8.5) after their index pregnancy. Women who returned to pre-pregnancy weight by 6 months after delivery were much more likely to have gained less weight at the 5- to 10-year follow-up compared with women who retained their pregnancy weight gains. In this cohort, breastfeeding and aerobic exercise were associated with a significantly lower weight gain over time.[23]

Thyroid Function

Thyroid size and function throughout pregnancy and the puerperium have been quantitated with ultrasonography and thyroid hormone levels.[24] Thyroid volume increases approximately 30 percent during pregnancy and regresses to normal size gradually over a 12-week period. Thyroxine and triiodothyronine, which are both elevated throughout pregnancy, return to normal within 4 weeks postpartum. For women taking thyroid medications, it is appropriate to check thyroid levels at 6 weeks postpartum to adjust dosing. It is now recognized that the postpartum period is associated with an increased risk for the development of a transient autoimmune thyroiditis that may in some cases evolve into permanent hypothyroidism.[25] The relationship of subclinical thyroid dysfunction and postpartum depression is controversial.[26–29] Postpartum thyroiditis (PPT) an autoimmune disease that may present with hyperthyroid or hypothyroid symptoms occurs in 2 to 17 percent of women, with a mean incidence about 10 percent. Women with type I diabetes have up to a 25-percent risk of PPT. Women with gestational diabetes and type II diabetes also have a slightly increased risk. Only that subset of women who develop symptoms should be treated. Puerperal hypothyroidism often presents with symptoms that include mild dysphoria; consequently, thyroid function studies are suggested in the evaluation of patients with suspected postpartum depression that occurs 2 to 3 months after delivery. Hyperthyroid symptoms are best treated with beta blockers, and hypothyroid symptoms with thyroid supplementation. Both are acceptable with breast-feeding. Methimazole and propylthiouracil are also safe with lactation. From 5 to 30 percent of women with PPT eventually develop hypothyroidism. If a woman becomes symptomatic and is treated, it is reasonable to stop medications after 1 year and re-evaluate thyroid status before the patient considers becoming pregnant again.[26–29]

Cardiovascular System and Coagulation

Blood volume increases throughout pregnancy to levels in the third trimester about 35 percent above nonpregnant values.[30] The greatest proportion of this increase consists of an expansion in plasma volume that begins in the first trimester and amounts to an additional 1,200 ml of plasma, representing a 50 percent increase by the third trimester. Red blood cell volume increases by about 250 ml.

Immediately after delivery, plasma volume is diminished by approximately 1,000 ml secondary to blood loss. By the third postpartum day, the plasma volume is replenished by a shift of extracellular fluid into the vascular space.[31] In contrast, the total blood volume declines by 16 percent of the predelivery value, suggesting a relative and transient anemia.[32] By 8 weeks postpartum, the red cell mass has rebounded and the hematocrit is normal in the majority of women.[33] As total blood volume normalizes, venous tone also returns to baseline. In a prospective evaluation of 42 women, at 4 and 42 days postpartum, Macklon and Greer[34] demonstrated significant reduction in deep vein vessel size and a concomitant increase in venous flow velocity in the lower extremities.

Pulse rate increases throughout pregnancy, as does stroke volume and cardiac output. Immediately after delivery, these remain elevated or rise even higher for 30 to 60 minutes. Following delivery, there is a transient rise of approximately 5 percent in both diastolic and systolic blood pressures throughout the first 4 days postpartum.[35] Data are scant regarding the rate at which cardiac hemodynamics return to prepregnancy levels. Early studies suggested cardiac output had returned to normal when measurements were made 8 to 10 weeks postpartum.[36] Clapp and Capeless[37] performed longitudinal evaluations of cardiac function at bimonthly intervals in 30 healthy women using M-mode ultrasound before pregnancy; during gestation; and at 12, 24, and 52 weeks postpartum. Cardiac output and left ventricular volume peaked at 24 weeks' gestation. There was a slow return to prepregnancy values over the year of study. However, even 1 year after delivery, there was a significantly higher cardiac output in both nulliparous and multiparous women than prepregnancy values. The authors suggested that this "cardiac remodeling" from pregnancy may last for an extended time in healthy women. Anecdotally, elite athletes have tried to take advantage of this physiologic boost to cardiac function, by planning pregnancies a year before major sporting events.

Pregnancy is known to be a time of significantly increased coagulability that persists into the postpartum period.[38,39] The greatest level of coagulability is observed immediately postpartum through 48 hours. Fibrinogen concentrations gradually diminish over the first 2 weeks postpartum. Compared with antepartum values, there is a rapid decrease in platelets in some patients and no change or an increase in others. Within 2 weeks after delivery, the platelet count rises, possibly as a marker of increased bone marrow output as red cell mass is replaced. Fibrinolytic activity increases in the first 1 to 4 days after delivery and returned to normal in 1 week, as measured by levels of plasminogen activation inhibitor 1. D-dimer levels are increased over pregnancy levels and are a poor marker of thrombus formation. Protein-S levels and activated protein-C resistance are decreased for up to 6 weeks or longer. In general, tests for thrombophilia and hemostasis should be delayed, if possible, for 10 to 12 weeks. The changes in the coagulation system, together with vessel trauma and immobility account for the increased risk of thromboembolism noted in the puerperium, especially when an operative delivery has occurred.

The Urinary Tract and Renal Function

It is generally accepted that the urinary tract becomes dilated during pregnancy, especially the renal pelves and the ureters above the pelvic brim. These findings, demonstrated 70 years ago by Baird,[40] affect the collecting system of the right kidney more than that of the left and are caused by compression of the ureters by the adjacent vasculature and enlarged uterus, combined with the effects of progesterone. Ultrasound studies of the urinary tract also document the enlargement of the collecting system throughout pregnancy.[41] A study of serial ultrasound examinations of the urinary tract in 20 women throughout pregnancy included a single postpartum examination 6 weeks after delivery.[42] The overall trend was that of dilatation of the collecting system throughout pregnancy, estimated by measurements of the separation of the pelvis-calyceal echo complex, from a mean of 5.0 mm (first trimester) to 10 mm (third trimester) in the right kidney and from 3.0 to 4.0 mm in the left collecting system. Measurements in all but two patients had returned to prepregancy status at the time of the 6-week postpartum examination. Cietak and Newton[43] performed serial nephrosonography on 24 patients throughout pregnancy and the puerperium. At 12 weeks postpartum, more than half of the patients demonstrated persistence of urinary stasis, described as a slight separation of the renal pelvis. This finding is evidence of hyperdistensibility and suggests that pregnancy has a permanent effect on the size of the upper renal tract. The intravenous urography studies performed by Dure-Smith[44] also suggest that subtle anatomic changes take place in the ureters that persist long after the pregnancy has ended. Ureteral tone above the pelvic brim, which in pregnancy is higher than normal, returns to nonpregnant levels immediately after cesarean delivery.[45]

Studies in which water cystometry and uroflowmetry were performed within 48 hours of delivery and again 4 weeks postpartum demonstrated a slight but significant decrease in bladder capacity (from 395.5 to 331 ml) and volume at first void (from 277 to 224 ml) in the study interval. Nevertheless, all the urodynamic values studied were within normal limits on both occasions. The results were not affected by the weight of the infant or by an episiotomy. However, prolonged labor and the use of epidural anesthesia appeared to diminish postpartum bladder function transiently.[46]

The most detailed study of renal function in normal pregnancy is that of Sims and Krantz,[47] who studied 12 patients with serial renal function tests throughout pregnancy and for up to 1 year after delivery. Glomerular filtration, which increased by 50 percent early in pregnancy and remained elevated until delivery, returned to normal nonpregnant levels by postpartum week 8. Endogenous creatinine clearance, similarly elevated throughout pregnancy, also returned to normal by the eighth postpartum week. Renal plasma flow increased by 25 percent early in pregnancy, gradually diminished in the third trimester (even when measured in the lateral recumbent position), and continued to decrease to below-normal values in the postpartum period for up to 24 weeks.[48] Normal values were finally established by 50 to 60 weeks after delivery. The reason for the prolonged postpartum depression of renal plasma flow is not clear. Because of the variable changes in renal clearance, mothers who are taking medications in which doses have been changed (due to the physiologic adaptations of pregnancy) will need to have their medication levels rechecked. This may be done at 4 to 6 weeks postpartum.

Other Changes

Hair growth is altered in pregnancy and postpartum. After delivery, there is a more rapid hair turnover for up to 3 months. As a greater percentage of hair begins to undergo the growth phase, more hair falls out with combing and brushing. The loss is in a diffuse, not balding, pattern. This transient phenomenon is called *telogen effluvium,* and the patient may be reassured that her hair growth will return to normal within a few months and that the excess hair in the comb or brush will regrow.[49]

Several investigators have reported on bone mineral changes with lactation and the associated amenorrhea. After delivery, there is a generalized decrease in bone mineralization that is temporary and resolves by 12 to 18 months postpartum in most women.[50] Bone loss appears to be greater in the femoral neck than in other areas of the skeleton.[51,52] Calcium supplementation does not seem to ameliorate the bone loss because it is not a problem of inadequate calcium stores, nor does exercise prevent it.[53] For almost all women, the bone loss is self limited and reversible.

Management of the Puerperium

For most parturients, the immediate puerperium is spent in the hospital or birthing center. The ideal duration of hospitalization for patients with uncomplicated vaginal births has been controversial and culturally determined. During World War II, early discharge with nurse follow-up was initiated to support the "war bride" baby boom.[54] In the 1950s, the lying-in period after delivery was 8 to 14 days.[55] At present, most women stay in the hospital 24 to 48 hours after a vaginal birth. For patients with an uncomplicated postoperative course following cesarean delivery, the postpartum stay is 2 to 4 days. The optimal time is dependent on a patient's needs and home support. Approximately 3 percent of women who have vaginal deliveries and 9 percent of women who have cesarean deliveries have at least one childbirth-related complication requiring longer hospitalization after delivery or readmission to the hospital.[56] Studies that have evaluated the safety and outcomes of early discharge (48 hours) have relied on nurse or midwife home visits. Unfortunately, in most areas of the United States insurance does not cover this service.

In a recent study, 1,249 randomly selected patients were questioned 8 weeks following delivery about health problems that occurred during the puerperium.[57] Eighty-five percent reported at least one problem during their hospitalization, and 76 percent noted at least one problem that persisted for 8 weeks. A wide range of problems were reported by the patients, including a painful perineum, difficulties with breast-feeding, urinary infections, urinary and fecal incontinence, and headache. Three percent of the patients had been rehospitalized, most commonly for abnormal bleeding or infection. This study draws attention to a substantial amount of symptomatic morbidity that occurs during the puerperium. Although longer hospitalization may not improve perineal pain or incontinence, open lines of communication with patients between discharge and the 6-week visit affect patient self-care and promote a more positive patient experience. In particular, lactation consultation may help to improve effective breast feeding and consideration should be given to postponing discharge in primparas until this service can be performed.

If a patient has adequate support at home (i.e., help with housekeeping and meal preparation), there is little value in an extended hospital stay, provided the mother is adequately educated about infant care and feeding and in the identification of danger signs in either the infant or herself. Except for an increased incidence of rehospitalization of some neonates for hyperbilirubinemia, there are few disadvantages to postpartum hospitalization of less than 48 hours for many patients.[58–61] For mothers who do not have adequate support at home and who are insecure about infant care and feeding, extending the hospital stay will provide time for mothers to gain adequate education and some measure of self-confidence, but this extra time may not be covered by insurance.[62] Written and video presentations are also efficient means of patient education. Home nursing visits can be helpful in providing support, education, and advice to mothers in selected situations. Written materials or handouts are particularly necessary because memory is temporarily affected by the sleep deprivation that is the rule in the first few days after delivery. Before discharge, women should be offered any vaccines that may be necessary to protect immunity. Rubella, varicella, hepatitis B, and influenza are the four most common vaccines given. All are safe with breastfeeding.[63]

The time from delivery until complete physiologic involution and psychological adjustment has been called "the fourth trimester."[64] Patients should understand that lochia will persist for 3 to 8 weeks, and that on days 7 to 14, there is often an episode of heavy vaginal bleeding, which occurs when the placental eschar sloughs. Tampons are permissible if they are comfortable upon insertion and are changed frequently, and if there are no perineal, vaginal, or cervical lacerations, which preclude insertion of a tampon until healing has occurred. Physical activity, including walking up and down stairs, lifting moderately heavy objects, riding in or driving a car, and performing muscle-toning exercises, can be resumed without delay if the delivery has been uncomplicated. Instructions regarding exercise are patient specific. Studies have found that exercise postpartum does not affect lactation and may decrease anxiety levels.[65,66] As such, exercise may have benefits beyond the mother's desire to "get back into shape." The most troublesome complaint is lethargy and fatigue. Consequently, every task or activity should be a brief one in the first few days of the puerperium. Mothers whose lethargy persists beyond several weeks must be evaluated, especially for thyroid dysfunction and postpartum depression.

Sexual activity may be resumed when the perineum is comfortable and when bleeding has diminished. The desire and willingness to resume sexual activity in the puerperium varies greatly among women, depending on the site and state of healing of perineal or vaginal incisions and lacerations, the amount of vaginal atrophy secondary to breast-feeding, and the return of libido.[67] Although the median time to resuming intercourse after delivery is 6 to 7 weeks, approximately one half of women who do so have dyspareunia. In a substantial number, dyspareunia lasts for a year or more.[68,69] Signorello et al.[70] noted a 2.5-fold increased risk of dyspareunia at 6 months following operative vaginal delivery compared with other subsets of postpartum women. For all women, breastfeeding at 6 months is associated with a more than fourfold increase in dyspareunia. Similarly, a recent large review of studies examining postpartum sexuality noted the greatest incidence of sexual dysfunction to be associated with operative vaginal delivery.[71] In contrast, 25 percent of all women reported a heightened sexual pleasure at 6 months after delivery. Postpartum dyspareunia is not always related to vulvar trauma and occurs in some women who have a cesarean delivery. It is also observed in women who use oral contraceptives and do not breastfeed, suggesting that lack of estrogen effect on the vagina is not the major cause of postpartum dyspareunia. In a study of 50 parturients, Ryding[72] found that 20 percent had little desire for sexual activity 3 months after delivery, and an additional 21 percent had complete loss of desire or aversion to sexual activity. This variation in attitude, desire, and willingness must be acknowledged when counseling women about the resumption of sexual activity. Women who breastfeed tend to begin intercourse later than average, and women who deliver by cesarean section tend to begin sooner.[73] Clinicians commonly advise pregnant women on the use of vaginal lubricants for sexual activity in the first few months postpartum, because of the decreased natural lubrication with lower estrogen levels. This may be included in the written handouts given to patients when they go home. Astro-glide gel (Biofilm Inc., Vista, CA) is one of the more commonly recommended lubricants, along with other, water-soluble lubricants. If patients are using barrier contraception, they should be advised against the use of petroleum-based lubricants such as Vaseline (Unilever, London, UK). If dyspareunia persists, a small amount of estrogen cream applied daily to the vagina may be helpful in breastfeeding women with atrophic changes.

Many patients return to work situations outside the home after their pregnancies. Frequently, the physician must complete insurance or employer forms to establish maternity leave for patients. Six weeks is regarded as the normal period of "disability" following delivery,[74] although some mothers return to work sooner. As mentioned earlier, the 6 weeks is derived from tradition. In China, 30 days is common and in Western Europe, many months and even up to a year of maternity leave is offered.

Health Maintenance

A follow-up examination is frequently scheduled for 6 weeks after delivery. Several studies have shown that a routine postpartum visit to the physician at 1 or 2 weeks after delivery or a home visit by a nurse midwife does not reduce maternal or infant morbidity.[75,76] Nevertheless, for some patients, an appointment approximately 2 weeks postpartum or a home visit by a visiting nurse or nurse midwife is more productive in detecting problems and providing support for a mother. Late puerperal infections, postpartum depression, and problems with infant care and feeding often occur before the 6-week postpartum visit. As mentioned later, open-ended questions should be asked to detect problems. At the 6-week visit questions regarding depression, energy, sexuality, contraception, and future pregnancies should be addressed. A copy of the Edinburgh Postpartum Depression Scale (EPDS) is in Table 21-2. It may be used as a fast, reliable, and user-friendly tool to screen for depression. A Pap smear is usually done at this time. It is helpful to solicit questions about the delivery, because women may be hesitant to ask them spontaneously, especially regarding sexuality and incontinence. If there are health issues that need addressing, such as glucose screens, thyroid levels, or other tests, they may be performed or scheduled at this visit.

Women with chronic medical diseases, such as collagen vascular disease, autoimmune disorders, and neuro-

Table 21-2. Edinburgh Postnatal Depression Scale (EPDS)

In the past 7 days:

1. **I have been able to laugh and see the funny side of things:**
   As much as I always could
   Not quite so much now
   Definitely not so much now
   Not at all
2. **I have looked forward with enjoyment to things:**
   As much as I ever did
   Rather less than I used to
   Definitely less than I used to
   Hardly at all
3. **I have blamed myself unnecessarily when things went wrong:**
   Yes, most of the time
   Yes, some of the time
   Not very often
   No, never
4. **I have been anxious or worried for no good reason:**
   No, not at all
   Hardly ever
   Yes, sometimes
   Yes, very often
5. **I have felt scared or panicky for no very good reason:**
   Yes, quite a lot
   Yes, sometimes
   No, not much
   No, not at all
6. **Things have been getting on top of me:**
   Yes, most of the time I haven't been able to cope at all
   Yes, sometimes I haven't been coping as well as usual
   No, most of the time I have coped quite well
   No, I have been coping as well as ever
7. **I have been so unhappy that I have had difficulty sleeping:**
   Yes, most of the time
   Yes, sometimes
   Not very often
   No, not at all
8. **I have felt sad or miserable:**
   Yes, most of the time
   Yes, quite often
   Not very often
   No, not at all
9. **I have been so unhappy that I have been crying:**
   Yes, most of the time
   Yes, quite often
   Only occasionally
   No, never
10. **The thought of harming myself has occurred to me:**
    Yes, quite often
    Sometimes
    Hardly ever
    Never

Response categories are scored 0, 1, 2, and 3 according to increased severity of the symptom. Items in bold type are reverse scored (3, 2, 1, 0). The total score is calculated by adding together the scores for each of the 10 items.

From Cox JL, Holden JM, Sagovsky R: Detection of postnatal depression. Development of the 10-item Edinburgh Postnatal Depression Scale. Br J Psychiatry 150:782, 1987, with permission.

logic conditions, should be seen at close intervals. Many patients with these disorders may experience "flares" of their symptoms after delivery. Ideally, these visits should be scheduled in advance with the patient's primary care or subspecialty physician. Prophylactic therapy is not recommended for women with systemic lupus or multiple sclerosis. However, warning patients to be attuned to signs and symptoms that reflect a flare of their illness allows for early and more effective interventions.

Perineal Care

Many women who give birth have spontaneous lacerations of the perineum or vagina or less commonly, episiotomies. In the United States, episiotomies are more often performed as midline than as mediolateral incisions. Provided that the incision or the laceration does not extend beyond the transverse perineal muscle, that there is no hematoma or extensive ecchymosis, and that a satisfactory repair has been accomplished, there is little need for perineal care beyond routine cleansing with a bath or shower. Analgesia can be accomplished in most patients with nonsteroidal anti-inflammatory drugs such as ibuprofen. These drugs have been shown to be superior to acetaminophen or propoxyphene for episiotomy pain and uterine cramping.[77] Furthermore, because of a low milk/maternal plasma drug concentration ratio, a short half life, and transformation into glucuronide metabolites, ibuprofen is safe for nursing mothers.

A patient who has had a mediolateral episiotomy, third- or fourth-degree perineal laceration, periurethral lacerations, or extensive perineal bruising may experience considerable perineal pain.[78] Occasionally, the pain and periurethral swelling prevent the patient from voiding, making urethral catheterization necessary. When a patient complains of inordinate perineal pain, the first and most important step is to reexamine the perineum, vagina, and rectum to detect and drain a hematoma or to identify a perineal infection. Perineal pain may be the first symptom of the rare but potentially fatal complications of angioedema, necrotizing fasciitis, or perineal cellulitis.[79–81]

In cases of moderate perineal pain, sitz baths will provide additional pain relief. Although hot sitz baths have long been customary therapy for perineal pain, Droegemueller[82] outlined the rationale for using cold or "iced" sitz baths. This therapy is similar to that for the treatment of athletic injuries, for which considerable success has been achieved with cold therapy. Cold provides immediate pain relief as a result of decreased excitability of free nerve endings and decreased nerve conduction. Further pain relief comes from local vasoconstriction, which reduces edema, inhibits hematoma formation, and decreases muscle irritability and spasm. Patients who have alternated using hot and cold sitz baths usually prefer the cold. The technique for administering a cold sitz bath is first to have the patient sit in a tub of water at room temperature to which ice cubes are then added. This avoids the sensation of sudden immersion in ice water. The patient remains in the ice water for 20 to 30 minutes. Patients with perineal incisions or lacerations should be advised to postpone sexual intercourse until there is no perineal discomfort. Tampons may be inserted whenever the patient is comfortable doing so. However, to avoid any risk of toxic shock syndrome, the use of tampons should be confined to the daytime to prevent leaving a tampon in the vagina for prolonged periods.

Frequently, what appears to be severe perineal pain is, in fact, the pain of prolapsed hemorrhoids. Witch hazel compresses, suppositories containing corticosteroids, or local anesthetic sprays or emollients may be helpful. Occasionally, a thrombus occurs in a prolapsed hemorrhoid. It is a simple task to remove the thrombus through a small scalpel incision using local anesthesia by an obstetrician trained in this procedure or a general surgeon. Dramatic relief of pain usually follows this procedure.

Urinary and anal incontinence are a significant problem in women following delivery.[83] Approximately one third of women at 8 weeks and 15 percent of women at 12 weeks have urinary incontinence. A strong predictor for incontinence after delivery is a history of prior urinary incontinence or new-onset incontinence during the index pregnancy. In addition to urinary incontinence, approximately 5 percent of women have anal incontinence 3 months after vaginal birth, with the majority experiencing flatal rather than fecal incontinence.[84,85] Forceps, but not vacuum, assisted vaginal delivery is associated with an twofold increased risk of fecal incontinence in primparas.[86] Similarly, anal sphincter disruption in nulliparas is associated with a 2.3-fold increase in anal incontinence five years after delivery.[87] Nulliparous women with sphincter disruption or operative vaginal delivery should be screened specifically for symptoms at follow-up visits.

Perineal exercises were developed by Kegel in 1948 and involve voluntary contraction of the pelvic floor. A recent meta-analysis reviewed the effectiveness of perineal exercise in treating incontinence. Harvey's review[85] found that only when the exercises are performed with a vaginal biofeedback device was there improvement in the incidence of urinary incontinence. If symptoms of either urinary or flatal incontinence persist for more than 6 months, studies should be undertaken to define the specific neuromuscular or anatomic abnormality so that the appropriate pharmacologic, biophysical, or surgical treatment can begin. Women should be counseled regarding this plan at their postpartum visit so that they can return if symptoms persist.

Delayed Postpartum Hemorrhage and Postpartum Anemia

The causes and management of immediate postpartum hemorrhage are discussed in Chapter 18. Delayed postpartum uterine bleeding of sufficient quantity to require medical attention occurs in 1 to 2 percent of patients. One of the most common causes of postpartum hemorrhage that occurs 2 to 5 days after delivery is von Willebrand's disease. Von Willebrand's factor increases in pregnancy, and thus excessive bleeding usually does not occur in the first 48 hours after birth. Women presenting in this time frame should be screened for this condition. Uterine atony and postpartum hemorrhage are responsible for approximately eight maternal deaths each year in the United States.[88] The bleeding occurs most frequently between days 8 and 14 of the puerperium.[89] Significant bleeding may require treatment with utertonic agents or curettage. When suction evacuation and curettage are performed, retained gestational products, usually in small amounts, will be found in about 40 percent of cases.[90,91] Whether small placental remnants are the cause is not known. In the management of patients with heavy delayed bleeding, ultrasound examination usually determines if there is a significant amount of retained material, although it is sometimes difficult to distinguish between blood clot and retained placental fragments. Suction evacuation of the uterus is successful in arresting the bleeding in almost all cases whether or not there is histologic confirmation of retained gestational products. If curettage is required at this time, especially if a sharp curette is used, a course of antibiotics begun before surgery is advisable for its possible benefit in reducing the formation of uterine synechiae. The curettage should be performed with care, because the postpartum uterine wall is soft and easier to perforate. In those rare instances in which delayed postpartum hemorrhage does not respond to the use of oxytocic agents and curettage, selective arterial embolization may be effective in controlling the bleeding.[92] Women with postpartum hemorrhage, and subsequent anemia, often have excessive fatigue in the postpartum period. Some investigators have advocated the use of recombinant erythropoietin as an alternative to transfusion for symptomatic women with anemia.[93,94]

Postpartum Infection

Although the standard definition of postpartum febrile morbidity is a temperature of 38.0°C (100.4°F) or higher on any two of the first 10 days after delivery, exclusive of the first 24 hours, most clinicians do not wait two full days to begin evaluation and treatment of patients who develop a fever in the puerperium.[95] The most common cause of postpartum fever is endometritis, which occurs after vaginal delivery in approximately 2 percent of patients and after cesarean delivery in about 10 to 15 percent. The differential diagnosis includes urinary tract infection, lower genital tract infection, wound infections, pulmonary infections, thrombophlebitis, and mastitis. The diagnosis and management of postpartum infection are discussed in detail in Chapter 49. Although almost all antibiotics are safe with lactation, antibiotics in the quinolone group and metronidazole should be avoided. Sulfa-based antibiotics cross poorly into breast milk but should be avoided with ill, premature, or jaundiced neonates. If there is no good alternative, these agents may be used and breast milk discarded for 24 hours after the last dose. Single-dose fluconazole is considered safe with lactation, but continued dosing (5 to 7 days) has not been well studied[96] (see Chapter 8).

Maternal-Infant Attachment

Klaus et al.[97] were among the first investigators to study maternal-infant attachment and to bring attention to the importance of the first few hours of maternal-infant association. Their studies as well as those of others have contributed substantially to major changes in hospital policies dealing with patients in labor and delivery and during the postpartum confinement. It is now recognized that there should be opportunities for parents to be with their newborns particularly from the first few moments after birth and as frequently as possible during the first days thereafter. Skin-to-skin contact is recommended. These associations are usually characterized by fondling, kissing, cuddling, and gazing at the infant, which are manifestations of maternal commitment and protectiveness toward her infant. Separation of mother and infant in the first hours after birth has been shown to diminish or delay the development of these characteristic mothering behaviors,[98] a problem that is intensified when medical, obstetric, or newborn complications require intensive care for either the mother or her newborn infant.

Robson and Powell[99] summarized the literature on early maternal attachment and emphasized how difficult it is to accomplish good research studies about this phenomenon. Although it is generally agreed that early association of the mother and infant is beneficial and should not be interfered with unnecessarily, there are still doubts about the long-term implications, if any, of a lack of early maternal-infant association. In their monograph summarizing their investigations about parent-infant attachment, Klaus and Kennel[100] warn against drawing far-reaching conclusions. Although favoring the theory of a "sensitive period" soon after birth, during which close parent-infant interaction facilitates subsequent attachment and beneficial parenting behavior, these investigators concur that humans are highly adaptable and state that "there are many fail-safe routes to attachment." This appears to be the prevailing view among experts at this time.

The modern hospital maternity ward should enhance and encourage parent-infant attachment by such policies as flexible visiting hours for the father, encouragement of the infant rooming with the mother, and strongly supportive attitudes about breast-feeding. These policies also allow the nursing staff to observe parenting behavior and to identify inept, inexperienced, or inappropriate behavior toward the infant. Some situations may call for more intensive follow-up by visiting nurses, home health visitors, or social workers to provide further support for the family during the posthospital convalescence. The role of postpartum home visits in enhancing parenting behavior is controversial. Gray et al.[101] found this approach beneficial. Siegel et al.[102] studied the effect of early and prolonged mother-infant contact in the hospital and a postpartum visitation program on attachment and parenting behavior. They found that early and prolonged maternal-infant contact in the hospital had a significant effect on enhancing subsequent parenting behavior, but the postpartum home visitations had no impact.

The development of the qualities associated with good parenting depends on many factors. Certainly, it does not depend solely on what transpires in the few hours surrounding the birth experience. There is evidence that specific identification of an infant with its mother's voice begins in utero during the third trimester.[103] Furthermore, the parents' own experiences as children, as well as their intellectual and emotional attitudes about children, must play a large role in their own parenting behavior. Areskog et al.[104] showed that women who expressed fear of childbirth during the antenatal period had more complications and more pain in labor, and also had more difficulties in attachment to their infants. Consequently, the peripartum period provides opportunities to enhance parenting behavior and to identify families for which follow-up after birth may be necessary to ensure the most favorable child development. For example, adolescents, particularly primiparous adolescents, are a particularly high-risk group. Rates of domestic abuse are especially high in adolescent mothers.

In summary, the postpartum ward should be an environment that provides parents ample opportunity to interact with their newborn infants. Personnel, including nurses, nurses' aides, and physicians caring for mothers and infants should be alert to signs of abnormal parenting (e.g., refusal of the mother to care for the infant, the use of negative or abusive names in describing or referring to the infant, inordinate delay in naming the infant, or obsessive and unrealistic concerns about the infant's health). These or other signs that maternal-infant attachment is delayed or endangered are as deserving of frequent follow-up during the postpartum period as are any of the traditional medical or obstetric complications.

LACTATION AND BREAST-FEEDING

Lactation and breast-feeding are reviewed in detail in Chapter 22. One of the important objectives of the puerperium is to enhance the maternal-infant interaction as regards nutrition of the infant. After several decades during which interest in breast-feeding languished in Western cultures, there has been renewed interest, enthusiasm, and acknowledgment for what is clearly the most reasonable means of feeding most all newborn infants (Fig. 21-2). In the United States, the proportion of mothers who breast-fed their infants has steadily increased over the past 2 decades.[105] Although the increase in breast-feeding is seen in all demographic groups, it is greatest in upper income and more highly educated groups. The increase in the popularity of breast-feeding is due in part to an increasing awareness of the advantages. Nevertheless, additional knowledge about breast-feeding may be gained during prenatal care from well-informed, enthusiastic, and supportive physicians and nurses, by reading from one of several lay books on breast-feeding, and by participating in classes on prepared childbirth. A variety of hospital practices, including the use of audiovisual aids, telephone hotlines, and in-service training for personnel, have been shown to increase the incidence of successful breast-feeding.[106]

The prenatal physical examination may identify problems that will affect breast-feeding. These include inverted nipples, which can be corrected in part by wearing breast shields, or *Candida* vaginal infections, which should be treated to avoid thrush in the infant, and painful *Candida* infection of the nipples. There are very few contraindications to breast-feeding. Reduction mammoplasty with autotransplantation of the nipple simply makes breast-

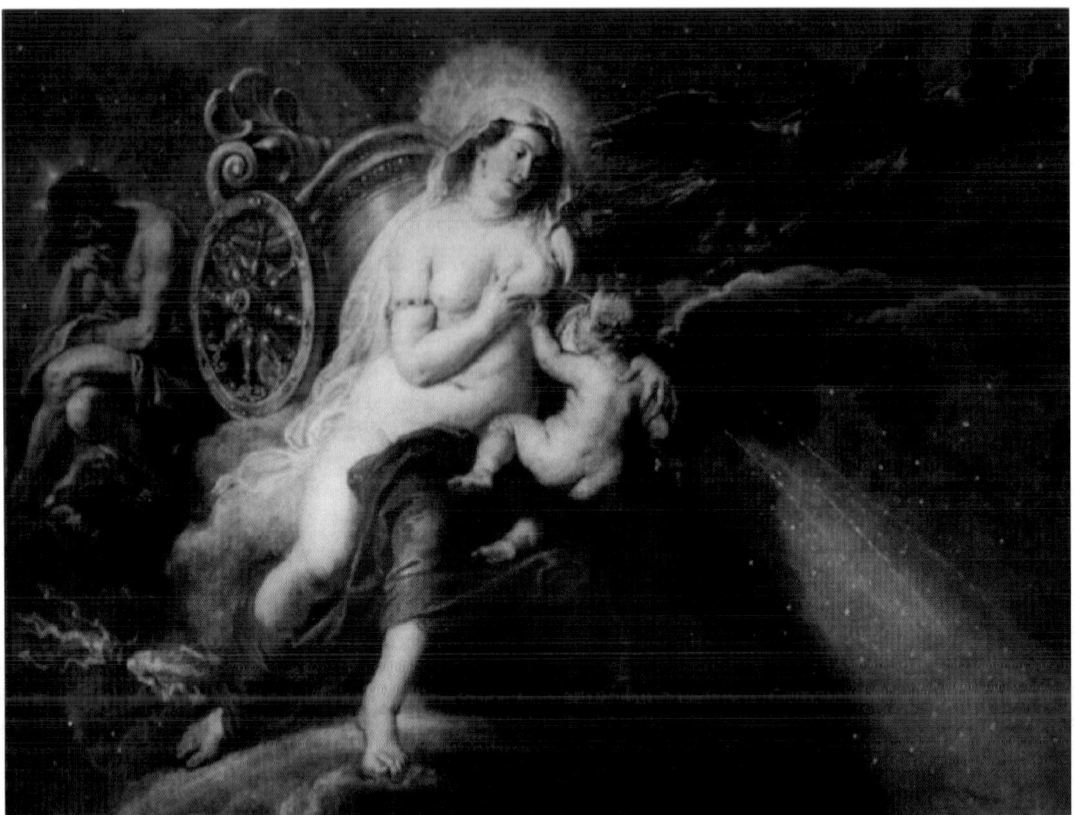

Figure 21-2. Lactation has long been considered sacred and divine. The term galaxy, is derived from the Greek word Galaxos—for breast milk from the Greek mythologic explanation for the Milky Way. The Greek god, Zeus, had his mortal son, Hercules, brought to nurse at the breast of the sleeping Hera, since breast-feeding from a goddess would convey immortality. Hera awoke and, not recognizing the strange infant, pushed him away. Her breast milk spilled out into the sky and formed the *Galaxia Kuklos,* Greek for *path of breast milk.* In Latin, this was translated *Via Lactea,* or *roadway of breast milk,* or as we know it, in English, Milky Way. (From Birth of the Milky Way by Peter Rubens, Prado Museum, Madrid, Spain.)

feeding impossible. Puerperal infections, including acute mastitis, can be managed successfully while the mother continues to breast-feed. There is the possibility of transmitting certain viral infections in the breast milk, including cytomegalovirus, herpes simplex, hepatitis B virus, and human immunodeficiency virus. Most medications taken by the mother enter the breast milk to a small degree. Because of the short duration for which most medications are prescribed, however, and the minimal amounts of drug that reach the breast milk (usually in concentrations similar to or less than in maternal plasma), it is usually safe to recommend that the infant continue nursing. If there is any doubt about the effect of a specific drug taken by a mother and whether she should continue breast-feeding, one should consult a recent reference about the effects of drugs in the nursing infant (see Chapter 8).

Complications of Breast-Feeding

The most common complication of breast-feeding is puerperal mastitis. This condition, which is characterized by fever, myalgias, and an area of pain and redness in either breast, usually has its onset before the end of the 2nd postpartum week, but there is also an increase in its incidence in the 5th and 6th weeks postpartum. Niebyl et al.[107] reported 20 women in whom puerperal mastitis developed. The women were treated with penicillin V, ampicillin, or dicloxacillin and allowed to continue breast-feeding their infants. No abscess developed. This experience is similar to that of others,[108] who have found that breast-feeding need not be discontinued in women with mastitis. In fact, the combination of a penicillinase-resistant penicillin and continued breast-feeding promptly result in resolution of the infection in 96 percent of cases. In 3 to 4 percent of cases, the mastitis may progress to abscess formation, which requires drainage. In addition, fungal or yeast mastitis is common. This usually presents with redness in both breasts and very tender nipples. The symptom of bilateral nipple tenderness may help to differentiate bacterial from fungal mastitis. Significant mastitis is best treated with systematic antifungals such as fluconazole. Mild cases respond to topical antifungals or gentian violet. The infant may continue to breast-feed during this time.

Lactation Suppression

For those patients who for personal or medical reasons will not breast-feed, breast support, ice packs, and analgesic medications are helpful in ameliorating the symptoms of breast engorgement. The new mother should avoid suckling or other means of milk expression, and the natural inhibition of prolactin secretion will result in breast involution. In 30 to 50 percent of patients, this process will be associated with breast engorgement and pain that may last for most of the first postpartum week.[109]

Bromocriptine is not approved by the Food and Drug Administration (FDA) for lactation suppression. This ergot derivative is a dopamine receptor agonist with prolonged action that inhibits the release of prolactin. Twenty-three percent of patients have side effects, including symptomatic hypotension, nausea, and vomiting, and 18 to 40 percent have rebound breast secretion, congestion, or engorgement following the termination of therapy. Furthermore, there have been reports of puerperal stroke, seizures, and myocardial infarctions in association with the use of bromocriptine prescribed for lactation suppression.[110–113] Although these events are rare and a causal relationship with bromocriptine has not been established, the manufacturers' prescription recommendations include instructions to avoid the use of this medication in patients with hypertensive complications of pregnancy and to monitor blood pressure periodically during the time the patient is using the drug. Consequently, it can be questioned whether it is prudent to use a medication for 2 weeks that has this incidence of side effects, possibly life-threatening complications, and the requirement for blood pressure monitoring during therapy. Puerperal breast engorgement, although painful, in most instances resolves within the first postpartum week.

PREGNANCY PREVENTION AND BIRTH CONTROL

The immediate postpartum period is a convenient time for a discussion of family planning with patients; however, ideally these conversations should begin during prenatal care. The period of anovulation infertility lasts from 5 weeks in nonlactating women to 8 weeks or more in women who breast-feed their infants without supplementation.[10] With exclusive breast-feeding, the pregnancy rate during lactational amenorrhea is 1 percent at 1 year postpartum.[114] However exclusive breastfeeding for this period of time is uncommon in the United States, and women are unlikely to know the actual duration they will breast-feed at hospital discharge. Even for women who leave the hospital breast-feeding exclusively, the majority will stop breast-feeding or begin supplementation at 6 weeks postpartum, especially if they return to work. Robson et al.[115] found that most women have resumed intercourse by 3 months, and for some, resumption of an active sexual life begins much earlier. Consequently, it is important that a decision be made about pregnancy prevention before the patient leaves the hospital, although it is usually the last thing on a new mother's mind. Part of the discussion about contraception should include recommendations about pregnancy intervals. Siblings may have less health problems and the incidence of adverse outcomes is less if the spacing between births is 18 to 36 months.[116]

A patient should be made aware of the various options of pregnancy prevention and birth control in terms that she and her partner can understand. This may be done by individual instruction from nurses, physicians, or midwives or by a variety of films or videotapes. One study found that written material, plus a discussion, given at the time of hospitalization, is most helpful to mothers.[116] The decision about family planning methods depends on the patient's motivation, number of children, state of health, whether she is breast-feeding, and on the religious background of the couple. It cannot be assumed that because a woman has used a method of contraception effectively before the current pregnancy that she will need no counseling thereafter. Debrovner and Winikoff[117] found that more than one half of patients change contraceptive techniques between pregnancies.

Natural Methods

The natural family planning methods, which depend on predicting the time of ovulation by use of basal body temperature or assessment of cervical mucus, cannot be used until regular menstrual cycles have resumed.[118] In the first weeks or months following birth, provided there is little or no supplemental feeding for the infant, breast-feeding will provide 98 percent contraceptive protection for up to 6 months. At 6 months, or if menses return, or if breast-feeding ceases to be full or nearly full before the 6th month, the risk of pregnancy increases.[119] Once regular menses have resumed, natural family planning methods, which depend on detection of the periovulation period using changes in cervical mucus or basal body temperature or both, can be employed. However, it is important to note that a woman will have ovulated once before the resumption of normal menses as a warning flag. In women with regular cycles, for whom periods of abstinence are acceptable to her and to her partner, natural family planning techniques are associated with pregnancy rates very close to those for barrier methods of contraception (with spermicides).[120]

Barrier Methods

Barrier methods of contraception and vaginal spermicides were long used in Europe and England before they were manufactured in this country beginning in the 1920s.[121] The failure rate for the diaphragm varies from 2.4 to 19.6 per 100 woman-years. Because this method of contraception requires substantial motivation, instruction, and experience, it is more effective in older women who are familiar with the technique. Vessey and Wiggins[122] found a failure rate of 2.4 per 100 woman-years among diaphragm users who were older than 25 years of age and who had a minimum of 5 months' experience using it. The proper size of the diaphragm should be determined at the 6-week postpartum visit, even in patients who previously used this form of contraception. In women who are breast-feeding, anovulation leads to vaginal dryness and tightness, which may make the proper fitting of a diaphragm more difficult. The diaphragm should be used with one of the spermicidal lubricants, all of which contain nonoxynol-9.

The use of condoms alone or in combination with spermicides is often advised for women who wish to postpone a decision about sterilization or oral contraceptive therapy until the postpartum visit. Pregnancy rates for the condom are reported to be from 1.6 to 21 per 100 woman-years, depending on the age and motivation of the population studied.[123]

Hormonal Contraceptive Medications

The combined estrogen-progestin preparations have proved to be the most effective method of contraception, with pregnancy rates reported as less than 0.5 per 100 woman-years. Most compounds include 35 μg or less of estrogen and varying amounts of progestins. Compounds containing the progestational components desogestrel, gestodene, or norgestimate appear to be less androgenic and have less impact on carbohydrate and lipid metabolism than compounds containing levonorgestrel or norethindrone.[124] Cardiovascular complications, including hypertension, venous thrombosis, stroke, and myocardial infarction, have been substantially reduced with the reduction in estrogen content. The cardiovascular complications are found predominantly in women who smoke or have a family history of thromboembolic disease.[125] In nonsmoking women, the risk-benefit ratio is clearly in favor of using oral contraceptive agents. This is particularly true when the additional benefits of these agents are considered, which include lowered risks of benign breast disease, ovarian and endometrial cancer, iron deficiency anemia, toxic shock syndrome, pelvic inflammatory disease, and ectopic pregnancy.[126]

In patients who are not breast-feeding, combined hormonal contraceptive agents, oral or transdermal, can be taken as early as 2 to 3 weeks after delivery. The effect of oral contraceptive agents on lactation is controversial. Controlled studies of the combined-type oral contraceptive agents with doses of ethinyl estradiol or mestranol of 50 μg or more demonstrated a suppressive effect on lactation. The common contraceptives with 35 μg or less of estrogen still have some suppressive effects. Progestin-only medications (e.g., norethindrone 0.35 mg every day) do not diminish lactation performance and may, in fact, increase the quality and duration of lactation.[127] There is no evidence that progestin-only contraceptive agents taken before the onset of lactation affect lactation success. A recent study by Halderman and Nelson found that initiation of progestin-only contraception at the time of hospital discharge did not affect lactation patterns, incidence of supplementation, or discontinuation of breast-feeding.[128] Depot medroxyprogesterone acetate (DMPA) 150 mg intramuscularly every 3 months, which has a contraceptive efficiency exceeding 99 percent, is used by many women following delivery.[129] The most troublesome side effect is unpredictable spotting and bleeding. Long-term DMPA use has been associated with reversible reduction in bone density and unfavorable changes in lipid metabolism. The major advantages of this form of contraception are the ease of administration and patient convenience. Progestin-only oral contraceptives should be avoided in Hispanic women with gestational diabetes who are breast-feeding, because of an increased risk for the subsequent development of type II diabetes.[130]

Diaz et al.[131] studied the effect of a low-dose combination oral contraceptive containing 0.03 mg ethinyl estradiol and 0.15 mg levonorgestrel. The medication was begun after all women had been nursing for 1 month. Among those women taking the oral contraceptive medications, there was a small but significant decrease in lactation performance and in the weight gain of their infants compared with controls. In women whose motivation to breast-feed is marginal, the slight inhibition of lactation induced by oral contraceptive agents may be sufficient to discourage them from continuing to nurse their infants, and so progestin-only preparations may be offered to these women. Combined hormonal vaginal rings have not been well studied. Use at 2 to 3 weeks after delivery may be problematic in some women due to perineal and vaginal healing. However, in the nonlactating mother, use at 2 to 3 weeks is reasonable if there is no discomfort.

Levonorgestrel subdermal implants were approved by the FDA for contraceptive use in the United States in 1990.[132] Implants inserted 4 weeks after delivery have no effect on lactation or growth of an infant who is nursing, even though small amounts of levonorgestrel are excreted in the milk. Although the usual time of insertion is 4 to 6 weeks following delivery, the implants can be inserted in the immediate puerperium in women who are breast-feeding. Irregular uterine bleeding, expense, and the occasional difficulty in removing the implants are the major drawbacks to the use of this form of contraception. Despite the proven contraceptive effectiveness of levonorgestrel implants, there has been a decline in the perceived desirability of this method of birth control in recent years.[133] The contraceptive patch has not been well studied in the post partum period for its effects on lactation. Many clinicians assume that it will have a lesser effect than oral contraceptives but that it will still have some effect; therefore, it may be reasonable to initiate its use after lactation has been established.[134]

Intrauterine Devices

The copper-containing and the progesterone-releasing device (IUD) is highly effective in preventing pregnancy at rates that are comparable to tubal ligation (<1 pregnancies per 100 woman-years), yet with the added benefit of reversibility.[135] Excellent candidates for an IUD include: women who desire an interpregnancy interval of more than 2 to 3 years, women who desire long-term contraception but prefer to avoid sterilization, breast-feeding women, women with side effects from hormonal contraception, and women with prior birth control failures. The IUD is an ideal form of birth control in breast-feeding mothers owing to its lack of effect on milk production. Furthermore, in a multicenter study, Cole et al.[136] observed that breast-feeding did not increase the risk of expulsion or other complications regardless of the time of insertion of the device. Significant complications of the

IUD are infrequent and include uterine perforation (<0.7 percent), expulsion (5 to 10 percent) and discontinuation secondary to side effects (4 to 14 percent).[137] Multiple studies now suggest no increased risk of pelvic inflammatory disease in women with an IUD after the initial insertion.[138] Although the overall risk of ectopic pregnancy is lower in women using the IUD when compared with women using no contraception, the chances that a pregnancy will be ectopic is 7 to 10 times higher in the IUD user. Therefore, all women receiving an IUD should be counseled to present immediately to their physician if they suspect pregnancy, so that the location of the pregnancy can be determined without delay.

Increased vaginal bleeding is noted in some women using copper-containing IUDs, but vaginal bleeding is decreased in women using progesterone-containing IUDs. Therefore, a woman's menstrual history is helpful in determining which type of IUD is ideal for her situation and decreasing copper IUD removal secondary to vaginal bleeding or dysmenorrhea.[139] Similarly, women who will be uncomfortable with amenorrhea should not be counseled for a progesterone-containing IUD. Contraindications to IUD insertion include postpartum endometritis, uterine anomalies, incomplete uterine involution, and for IUDs containing copper, Wilson's disease or a known allergy to copper. Syncope as a result of the vagal response at the time of IUD insertion is uncommon with IUD insertion at 6 weeks, given that the cervix remains slightly dilated.[140] Mishell and Roy[141] demonstrated no increase in perforation 4 to 8 weeks after delivery using a withdrawal method for insertion which appears to reduce the risk of this complication. Insertion of the IUD immediately following delivery is an alternate strategy. Surprisingly, this practice is associated with fewer perforations than are insertions between 1 and 8 weeks. Not surprising, however, is the finding of a higher expulsion rate (10 to 21 percent).[142]

The biologic action of IUDs is a matter of concern to those who might object to this method if its principal action is prevention of implantation of the blastocyst. The investigations of Alvarez et al.[143] convincingly support the concept that the principal mode of action of IUDs is by a method other than destruction of live embryos. Both the World Health Organization and the American College of Obstetricians and Gynecologists have reviewed the evidence and concluded that the IUD is not an abortifacient.[144]

Sterilization

Tubal sterilization is the most frequently used method of contraception in the United States.[145] The puerperium is a convenient time for tubal ligation procedures to be performed in women who desire sterilization. The procedure can be performed at the time of a cesarean delivery or within the first 24 to 48 hours after delivery. In some hospitals, the operation is performed immediately after delivery in uncomplicated patients, especially when epidural anesthesia was given for labor analgesia. With the use of small paraumbilical incision, the procedure seldom prolongs the patient's hospitalization.

The 10-year failure rate of postpartum partial salpingectomy is 0.75 percent.[146] There are several modifications of this procedure: the Pomeroy, Parkland, Uchida, and Irving (see Chapter 23).[147,148] Because of the relaxed abdominal wall and the easy accessibility of the fallopian tubes, the minilaparotomy has the advantages of convenience and speed without the possible risks of visceral injury that might occur with the trocar of the laparoscope. More important than the type of procedure is the discussion with the mother about the timing of the procedure. Puerperal sterilization compared with interval sterilization is associated with increased incidence of guilt and regret.[149] Postponing tubal ligation procedures until 6 to 8 weeks after delivery is less convenient but does provide time to ensure that the infant is healthy and to review all the implications of the decision. Importantly, interval tubal ligation may not be covered by Medicaid in some states. Laparoscopic tubal ligation can be accomplished as an outpatient procedure, with a minimum of morbidity.

The risks of tubal ligation procedures, whether performed in the puerperium or as an interval procedure, include the short-term problems of anesthetic accidents, hemorrhage, injury of the viscera, and infection. These complications are infrequent, and deaths from the procedure occur in two to 12 per 100,000 procedures. Long-term complications are less well defined and more controversial. About 10 to 15 percent of patients have irregular menses and increased menstrual pain after tubal sterilization. This so-called post-tubal syndrome is sufficiently severe in some cases to require hysterectomy. Well-controlled prospective studies, however, have failed to provide convincing evidence that these symptoms occur more commonly after tubal sterilization than in control patients of the same age and previous menstrual history.[150,161]

There has also been concern about poststerilization depression.[152] Because depression is common in women of childbearing age and is even more common in the puerperium, it is unlikely that sterilization procedures are independent risk factors for depression. It is obvious, however, that the loss of fertility associated with a sterilization procedure will have important conscious and subconscious implications for many women. Therefore, it is not surprising that some patients manifest transient grief reactions in response to tubal ligation. The loss of libido that may occur in such situations may be frightening to some women and equally disturbing to their partners. Reassurance that such reactions are temporary and are not necessarily symptoms of a seriously disturbed psyche is an important means of support during this crisis. Both partners must be aware of the dynamics of this situation to avoid a sense of estrangement.

Obstetricians must remember that vasectomy is often a more advisable and desirable alternative for a couple considering sterilization.[153,154] It can be performed as an outpatient procedure under local anesthesia with insignificant loss of time from work or family. Furthermore, almost all the failures (about three to four per 1,000 procedures) can be detected by a postoperative semen analysis. This is a decided advantage over the tubal ligation, in which failures are discovered only when a pregnancy occurs.

Furthermore, vasectomy is less expensive and overall is associated with fewer complications. In addition, women whose husbands undergo vasectomy are less likely to have hysterectomies than are women who have had tubal sterilization.[155] Studies of long-term health effects of vasectomy found no evidence of an increased risk of atherosclerotic heart disease or other chronic illnesses.[153,156]

Tubal ligation can be reversed but is expensive and often not covered by insurance. A patient should not undergo sterilization if she is contemplating reversal. Success as measured by the occurrence of pregnancy following tubal reanastamosis varies from 40 to 85 percent, depending on the type of tubal ligation performed and on the length of functioning tube that remains. Success rates for vas reanastamosis vary from 37 to 90 percent, with higher success rates being associated with shorter intervals from the time of vas ligation.

Hysterectomy has been advocated as a means of sterilization that has the advantage of protecting the patient from future uterine or cervical cancer. However, the morbidity of cesarean or puerperal hysterectomy operations is sufficiently great to preclude their consideration for elective sterilization.[157]

POSTPARTUM PSYCHOLOGICAL REACTIONS

The psychological reactions experienced following childbirth include the common, relatively mild, physiologic, and transient "maternity blues" (50 to 70 percent of women), true depression occurring in 8 to 20 percent of women, and frank puerperal psychosis occurring in 0.14 to 0.26 percent. These problems are discussed in Chapter 50. In patients with underlying depression, a previous history of postpartum depression or in those who report symptoms that develop during the immediate postpartum period, it is essential that a postpartum visit be scheduled sooner than the traditional 6 weeks. Other risk factors for postpartum depression include a family history of depression, a mother with postpartum depression, a poor social situation, and prolonged separation from her infant. The moderately depressed mother often experiences such guilt and embarrassment secondary to her sense of failure in her mothering role that she will be unable to call her physician or admit the symptoms of her depression. Consequently, ample time must be set aside to explore in depth even the slightest symptoms or sign of depression. Home visits in this situation may be appropriate to assess the patient. When a patient calls with a seemingly innocuous question, she should be asked two or three open-ended questions about her general status. These questions allow the patient to open up if there is an underlying depression that she is too guilty or afraid to express initially; for example:

1. How do you feel things are going?
2. How are things with the baby?
3. Are you feeling like you expected?

Because nursing staff often triage phone calls for physicians and midwives, it is important that such personnel be instructed to be alert to this protocol. Additionally, we recommend that both parents be warned before hospital discharge that if the maternity blues seem to be lasting longer than 2 weeks, or become "too tough" to handle, then either partner should call. An easy screening depression scale, the EPDS, is shown (see Table 21-2). Puerperal thyroid disease will often present with symptoms that include mild dysphoria; consequently, thyroid function studies are suggested in the evaluation of patients with suspected postpartum depression that occurs 2 to 3 months after delivery.

MANAGING PERINATAL GRIEVING

For the most part, perinatal events are happy ones and are occasions for rejoicing. When a patient and her family experience a loss associated with a pregnancy, special attention must be given to the grieving patient and her family.

The most obvious cases of perinatal loss are those in which a fetal or neonatal death has occurred. Other more subtle losses can be associated with a significant amount of grieving, such as the birth of a critically ill or malformed infant, an unexpected hysterectomy performed for intractable postpartum hemorrhage, or even a planned postpartum sterilization procedure. Grief occurs with any significant loss whether it is the actual death of an infant or the loss of an idealized child in the case of the birth of a handicapped infant.[158]

Mourning is as old as the human race, but the clinical signs and symptoms of grief and their psychological ramifications as they relate to loss suffered by women during their pregnancies have been given special consideration in recent years. In studying the relatives of servicemen who died in World War II, Lindemann[159] recognized five manifestations of normal grieving. These include somatic symptoms of sleeplessness, fatigue, digestive symptoms, and sighing respirations; preoccupation with the image of the deceased; feelings of guilt; feelings of hostility and anger toward others; and disruption of the normal pattern of daily life. He also described the characteristics of what is now recognized as pathologic grief, which may occur if acute mourning is suppressed or interrupted. Some of the manifestations of this so-called morbid grief reaction are overactivity without a sense of loss; appearance or exacerbations of psychosomatic illness; alterations in relationships with friends and relatives; furious hostility toward specific persons; lasting loss of patterns of social interaction; activities detrimental to personal, social, and economic existence; and agitated depression.

Kennel et al.[160] studied the reaction of 20 mothers to the loss of their newborn infants. Characteristic signs and symptoms of mourning occurred in all the patients, even in situations in which the infant was nonviable. Similar grief reactions occurred in most of the parents of 101 critically ill infants who survived after referral to a regional neonatal intensive care unit,[161] showing that separation from a seriously ill newborn is sufficient to provoke typical grief reaction.

It is important that the characteristics of the grieving patient be recognized and understood by health professionals caring for such patients; otherwise, substantial misunderstanding and mismanagement of the patient will occur. For example, if the patient's reaction of anger and hostility is not anticipated, a nurse or physician may take personally statements or actions by the patient or her family and avoid the patient at the very time she needs the most consolation and support. Because of their own discomfort with the implications of death, physicians, nurses, and others on the postpartum unit often find it uncomfortable to deal with patients whose fetus or infant has died. As a consequence, there is a reluctance to discuss the death with the patient and a tendency to rely on the use of sedatives or tranquilizers to deal with the patient's symptoms of grief.[162–164] What is actually beneficial at such a time is a sympathetic listener and an opportunity to express and discuss feelings of guilt, anger, and hopelessness, and the other symptoms of mourning.

It is not surprising that postpartum depression is more common and more severe in families that have suffered a perinatal loss. In one study, the prolonged grief response occurred more often in those women who became pregnant within 5 months of the death of the infant.[165] This finding suggests that in counseling women after the loss of an infant, one should avoid the traditional advice of encouraging the family to embark soon on another pregnancy as a "replacement" for the infant who died. Just how long the normal grief reaction lasts is not known, and surely it varies with different families. Lockwood and Lewis[166] studied 26 patients who had suffered a stillbirth; they followed several patients for as long as 2 years. Their data suggest that grief in this situation is usually resolved within 18 months, invariably with a resurgence of symptoms at the first anniversary of the loss.

Somatic symptoms of grief, such as anorexia, weakness, and fatigue, are now well recognized; other psychological manifestations are also reported. Spontaneous abortion and infertility increase among couples who attempt to conceive after the loss of an infant.[167] Physical changes that occur with grieving may account for this increase in poor reproductive success. Schleifer et al.[168] found significant suppression of lymphocyte stimulation in the spouses of women with advanced breast carcinoma. Although the most intense suppression was noted within the month after bereavement, a modified response was noted for as long as 14 months.

The regionalization of perinatal health care has resulted in a large proportion of the perinatal deaths occurring in tertiary centers. In some of these centers, teams of physicians, nurses, social workers, and pastoral counselors have evolved to aid specifically in the management of families suffering a perinatal loss.[169–172] Although this approach ensures an enlightened, understanding, and consistent approach to bereaved families, it suggests that the support of a grieving patient is a highly complex endeavor, to be accomplished only by a few specially trained individuals who care for postpartum patients. Enlightened and compassionate counseling of parents who have suffered a perinatal loss may be accomplished by any of the mother's health care professionals by using the guidelines listed in Table 21-3.[172] Clearly, management of grief is not solely a postpartum responsibility.

Table 21-3. Guidelines for Managing Perinatal Loss

Keep parents informed; be honest and forthright.
Recognize and facilitate anticipatory grieving.
Inform parents about the grieving process.
Encourage support person to remain with the mother throughout labor.
Encourage the mother to make as many choices about her care as possible.
Support parents in seeing, touching, or holding the infant.
Describe the infant in detail, especially for couples who choose not to see the infant.
Allow photographs of the infant.
Prepare the couple for hospital paperwork, such as autopsy requests.
Discuss funeral or memorial services.
Assist the couple in how to inform siblings, relatives, and friends.
Discuss subsequent pregnancy.
Liberal use of follow-up home or office visits.

Modified from Kowalski K: Managing perinatal loss. Clin Obstet Gynecol 23:1113, 1980.

This is particularly true when a prenatal diagnosis is made of fetal death or fetal abnormality. A continuum of support is essential as the patient moves from the prenatal setting, to labor and delivery, to the postpartum ward, and finally to her home. Relaxation of many of the traditional hospital routines may be necessary to provide the type of support these families need. For example, allowing a loved one to remain past visiting hours, providing a couple a private setting to be with their deceased infant, or allowing unusually early discharge with provisions for frequent phone calls and follow-up visits often facilitates the resolution of grief.

It is also important to realize that the fathers of infants who die have somewhat different grief responses than do the mothers. In a study of 28 fathers who had lost infants, Mandell et al.[173] found their grief characterized by the necessity to keep busy with increased work, feelings of diminished self-worth, self-blame, and limited ability to ask for help. Stoic responses are typical of men and may obstruct the normal resolution of grief.

Postpartum Posttraumatic Stress

Posttraumatic stress disorder may occur after any physical or psychological trauma. It may lead to behavioral sequelae including flashbacks, avoidance, and inability to function. Emergency operative deliveries, both vaginal and abdominal, and severe unexpected pain have been reported to have produced posttraumatic stress. The reaction may lead to fear of a subsequent delivery that may become incapacitating, as well as generalized symptoms of this disorder. Whenever an emergency procedure is indicated, debriefing afterward, both early and a few weeks later, may help to decrease the incidence of this problem. Women with adverse outcomes frequently experience transference of their previous experience as the next delivery approaches.[174–177]

KEY POINTS

- By 6 weeks postpartum, only 28 percent of women have returned to their prepregnant weight.
- Approximately 50 percent of parturients experience diminished sexual desire during the 3 months following delivery.
- Postpartum uterine bleeding of sufficient quantity to require medical attention occurs in 1 to 2 percent of parturients. In patients requiring curettage, 40 percent will be found to have retained placental tissue.
- *Candida* infection is a common cause of persistent nipple soreness in women who are breast-feeding.
- Most women with puerperal mastitis can be adequately treated with dicloxacillin or a first generation cephalosporin while they continue to breast-feed their infants.
- Breast-feeding results in 98-percent contraceptive protection for up to 6 months following delivery, provided there is little or no supplemental feeding of the infant.
- Progestin-only contraceptive medication does not diminish lactation performance.
- Postpartum, major depression occurs in 8 to 20 percent of parturients, if possible, risk factors should be used to identify patients for increased screening and surveillance.
- Puerperal hypothyroidism often presents with symptoms that include mild dysphoria; consequently, thyroid function studies are suggested in the evaluation of patients with suspected postpartum depression that occurs 2 to 3 months after delivery.

REFERENCES

1. Williams JS: Regeneration of the uterine mucosa after delivery, with special reference to the placental site. Am J Obstet Gynecol 122:664, 1981.
2. Hytten FE, Cheyne GA: The size and composition of the human pregnant uterus. J Obstet Gynaecol Br Commonw 76:400, 1969.
3. Sharman A: Postpartum regeneration of the human endometrium. J Anat 87:1, 1953.
4. Anderson WR, Davis J: Placental site involution. Am J Obstet Gynecol 102:23, 1968.
5. Willms AB, Brown ED, Kettritz UI, et al: Anatomic changes in the pelvis after uncomplicated vaginal delivery: evaluation with serial MR imaging. Radiology 195:91, 1995.
6. Oppenheimer LS, Sheriff EA, Goodman JDS, et al: The duration of lochia. Br J Obstet Gynaecol 93:754, 1986.
7. Visness CM, Kennedy KI, Ramos R: The duration and character of postpartum bleeding among breast-feeding women. Obstet Gynecol 89:159, 1997.
8. Lipinski JK, Adam AH: Ultrasonic prediction of complications following normal vaginal delivery. J Clin Ultrasound 9:17, 1981.
9. Chang YL, Madrozo B, Drukker BH: Ultrasonic evaluation of the postpartum uterus in management of postpartum bleeding. Obstet Gynecol 58:227, 1981.
10. Glass M, Rosenthal AH: Cervical changes in pregnancy, labor and puerperium. Am J Obstet Gynecol 60:353, 1950.
11. Coppleson M, Reid BL: A colposcopic study of the cervix during pregnancy and the puerperium. J Obstet Gynaecol Br Commonw 73:575, 1966.
12. McLaren HC: The involution of the cervix. Br Med J 1:347, 1952.
13. Andrews MC: Epithelial changes in the puerperal fallopian tube. Am J Obstet Gynecol 62:28, 1951.
14. Cronin TJ: Influence of lactation upon ovulation. Lancet 2:422, 1968.
15. Perex A, Uela P, Masnick GS, et al: First ovulation after childbirth: the effect of breast feeding. Am J Obstet Gynecol 114:1041, 1972.
16. Gray RH, Campbell ON, Apelo R, et al: Risk of ovulation during lactation. Lancet 335:25, 1990.
17. Bonnar J, Franklin M, Nott PN, et al: Effect of breast-feeding on pituitary-ovarian function after childbirth. Br Med J 4:82, 1975.
18. Crowell DT: Weight change in the postpartum period: a review of the literature. J Nurse Midwifery 40:418, 1995.
19. Scholl TO, Hediger ML, Schall JI, et al: Gestational weight gain, pregnancy outcome, and postpartum weight retention. Obstet Gynecol 86:423, 1995.
20. Schauberger CW, Rooney BL, Brimer LM: Factors that influence weight loss in the puerperium. Obstet Gynecol 79:424, 1992.
21. Lovelady CA, Garner KE, Thoreno KL, et al: The effect of weight loss in overweight, lactating women on the growth of their infants. N Engl J Med 342:449, 2000.
22. Dewey KG, Lovelady CA, Nommsen-Rivers LA, et al: A randomized study of the effects of aerobic exercise by lactating women on breast-milk volume and composition. N Engl J Med 330:449, 1994.
23. Rooney BL, Schauberger CW: Excess pregnancy weight gain and long-term obesity: one decade later. Obstet Gynecol 100:245, 2002.
24. Rasmusen NG, Hornnes PJ, Hegedus L: Ultrasonographically determined thyroid size in pregnancy and postpartum: the goitrogenic effect of pregnancy. Am J Obstet Gynecol 160:1216, 1989.
25. Jausson R, Dahlberg PA, Winsa B, et al: The postpartum period constitutes an important risk for the development of clinical Graves disease in young women. Acta Endocrinol 116:321, 1987.
26. Kent GN, Stuckey BGA, Allen JR, et al: Post partum thryoid dysfunction: clinical assessment and relationship to psychiatric affective morbidity. Clin Endocrinol 51:429, 1999.
27. Pedersen CA, Stern RA, Pate J, et al: Thyroid and adrenal measures during late pregnancy and the puerperium in women who have been major depressed or who become dysmorphic postpartum. J Affect Disord 29:201, 1993.
28. Terry AJ, Hague WM: Postpartum thyroiditis. Semin Perinatol 22:497, 1998.
29. Stagnaro-Green A: Postpartum thyroiditis. Best Prac Res Clin Endocrinol Metab 18:303, 2004.
30. Walters WAW, Limm VL: Blood volume and haemodynamics in pregnancy. Clin Obstet Gynaecol 2:301, 1975.
31. Lindesman R, Miller MM: Blood volume changes during the immediate postpartum period. Obstet Gynecol 21:40, 1963.
32. Ueland K: Maternal cardiovascular dynamics. VIII. Intrapartum blood volume changes. Am J Obstet Gynecol 126:671, 1976.
33. Paintin DB: The size of the total red cell volume in pregnancy. J Obstet Gynaecol Br Commonw 69:719, 1962.
34. Macklon NS, Greer IA: The deep venous system in the puerperium: an ultrasound study. Br J Obstet Gynaecol 104:198, 1997.
35. Walters WAW, MacGregor WG, Hills M: Cardiac output at rest during pregnancy and the puerperium. Clin Sci 30:1, 1966.
36. Walters BNJ, Thompson ME, Lea E, DeSwiet M: Blood pressure in the puerperium. Clin Sci 71:589, 1986.
37. Clapp JF III, Capeless E: Cardiovascular function before, during, and after the first and subsequent pregnancies. Am J Cardiol 80:1469, 1997.
38. Ygge J: Changes in blood coagulation and fibrinolysis during the puerperium. Am J Obstet Gynecol 104:2, 1969.

39. Hellgren M: Hemostasis during normal pregnancy and puerperium. Semin Thromb Hemost 29:125, 2003.
40. Baird D: The upper urinary tract in pregnancy and puerperium, with special reference to pyelitis of pregnancy. J Obstet Gynaecol Br Emp 42:733, 1935.
41. Peake SL, Roxburgh HB, Langlois SL: Ultrasonic assessment of hydronephrosis of pregnancy. Radiology 146:167, 1983.
42. Fried AM, Woodring JH, Thompson DJ: Hydronephrosis of pregnancy: a prospective sequential study of the course of dilatation. J Ultrasound Med 2:255, 1983.
43. Cietak KA, Newton JR: Serial qualitative maternal nephrosonography in pregnancy. Br J Radiol 58:399, 1985.
44. Dure-Smith P: Pregnancy dilatation of the urinary tract. Radiology 96:545, 1970.
45. Rubi RA, Sala NC: Ureteral function in pregnant women. III. Effect of different positions and of fetal delivery upon ureteral tonus. Am J Obstet Gynecol 101:230, 1968.
46. Kerr-Wilson RHJ, Thompson SW, Orr JW Jr, et al: Effect of labor on the postpartum bladder. Obstet Gynecol 64:115, 1984.
47. Sims EAH, Krantz KE: Serial studies of renal function during pregnancy and the puerperium in normal women. J Clin Invest 37:1764, 1958.
48. DeAlvarez RR: Renal glomerulotubular mechanisms during normal pregnancy. Am J Obstet Gynecol 75:931, 1958.
49. Burke KE: Hair loss: What causes it and what can be done about it. Hair Loss 85:52, 1989.
50. Polatti F, Capuzzo E, Viazzo F, et al: Bone mineral changes during and after lactation. Obstet Gynecol 94:52, 1999.
51. Holmberg-Marttila D, Sievanen H: Prevalence of bone mineral changes during postpartum amenorrhea and after resumption of menstruation. Am J Obstet Gynecol 180:537, 1999.
52. Lasky MA, Prentice A: Bone mineral changes during and after lactation. Obstet Gynecol 94:608, 1999.
53. Little KD, Clapp JF III: Self-selected recreational exercise has no impact on early postpartum lactation-induced bone loss. Med Sci Sports Exerc 30:831, 1998.
54. Temkin E: Driving through: Postpartum care during World War II. Am J Public Health 89:587, 1999.
55. Brown S, Small R, Faber B, et al: Early postnatal discharge from hospital for healthy mothers and term infants. The Cochrane Library 4:1, 2004.
56. Hebert PR, Reed G, Entman SS, et al: Serious maternal morbidity after childbirth: prolonged hospital stays and readmissions. Obstet Gynecol 94:942, 1999.
57. Glazener CMA, Abdalla M, Stroud P, et al: Postnatal maternal morbidity: extent, causes, prevention and treatment. Br J Obstet Gynaecol 102:282, 1995.
58. Liu LL, Clemens CJ, Shay DK, et al: The safety of early newborn discharge: the Washington state experience. JAMA 278:293, 1997.
59. Mandl KD, Brennan TA, Wise PH, et al: Maternal and infant health: effects of moderate reductions in postpartum length of stay. Arch Pediatr Adolesc Med 151:915, 1997.
60. Britton JR, Britton HL, Gronwaldt V: Early perinatal hospital discharge and parenting during infancy. Pediatrics 104:1070, 1999.
61. Brumfield CG: Early postpartum discharge. Clin Obstet Gynecol 41:611, 1998.
62. Moran CF, Holt VL, Martin DP: What do women want to know after childbirth? Birth 24:27, 1997.
63. Bohlke K, Galil K, Jackson L, et al: Postpartum varicella vaccination: Is the vaccine virus excreted in breast milk? Obstet Gynecol 102:970, 2003.
64. Jennings B, Edmundson M: The postpartum periods: after confinement: the fourth trimester. Clin Obstet Gynecol 23:1093, 1980.
65. Koltyn KF, Schultes SS: Psychological effects of an aerobic exercise session and a rest session following pregnancy. J Sports Med Phys Fitness 37:287, 1997.
66. Sampselle CM, Seng J, Yeo S, et al: Physical activity and postpartum well-being. J Obstet Gynecol Neonatal Nurs 28:41, 1999.
67. Reamy K, White SE: Sexuality in pregnancy and the puerperium: a review. Obstet Gynecol Surv 40:1, 1985.
68. Glazener CMA: Sexual function after childbirth: women's experiences, persistent morbidity and lack of professional recognition. Br J Obstet Gynaecol 104:330, 1997.
69. Goetsch MF: Postpartum dysparunia. An unexplored problem. J Reprod Med 44:963, 1999.
70. Signorello L, Harlow B, Chekos A, et al: Postpartum sexual functioning and its relationship to perineal trauma: A retrospective cohort study of primiparous women. Am J Obstet Gynecol 184:881, 2001.
71. Hicks TL, Forester-Goodall S, Quattrone EM, et al: Postpartum sexual functioning and method of delivery: Summary of the evidence. Am College Nurse-Midwives 49:430, 2004.
72. Ryding E-L: Sexuality during and after pregnancy. Acta Obstet Gynecol Scand 63:679, 1984.
73. Byrd JE, Shibley-Hyde J, DeLamater J, et al: Sexuality during pregnancy and the year postpartum. J Family Practice 47:305, 1998.
74. American College of Obstetricians and Gynecologists: Pregnancy, Work, and Disability. Technical Bulletin No. 58. Washington, DC, ACOG, 1980.
75. Gagnon AJ, Edgar L, Kramer MS, et al: A randomized trial of a program of early postpartum discharge with nurse visitation. Am J Obstet Gynecol 176:205, 1997.
76. Gunn J, Lumley S, Chondros P, Young D: Does an early postnatal check-up improve maternal health: results from a randomized trial in Australian general practice. Br J Obstet Gynaecol 105:991, 1998.
77. Windle ML, Booker LA, Rayburn WF: Postpartum pain after vaginal delivery: a review of comparative analgesic trials. J Reprod Med 34:891, 1989.
78. Macarthur AJ, Macarthur C: Incidence, severity and determinants of perineal pain after vaginal delivery: A prospective cohort study. Am J Obstet Gynecol 191:1199, 2004.
79. Shy KK, Eschenbach DA: Fatal perineal cellulitis from episiotomy site. Obstet Gynecol 54:929, 1979.
80. Stiller RJ, Kaplan BM, Andreoli JW Jr: Hereditary angioedema and pregnancy. Obstet Gynecol 64:133, 1984.
81. Ewing TL, Smale LE, Eliot FA: Maternal deaths associated with postpartum vulvar edema. Am J Obstet Gynecol 134:173, 1979.
82. Droegemueller W: Cold sitz baths for relief of postpartum perineal pain. Clin Obstet Gynecol 23:1039, 1980.
83. Connolly AM, Thorp JM Jr: Childbirth-related perineal trauma: clinical significance and prevention. Clin Obstet Gynecol 42:820, 1999.
84. Chaliha C, Kalia V, Stanton S, et al: Antenatal prediction of postpartum fecal incontinence. Obstet Gynecol 94:689, 1999.
85. Harvey MA: Pelvic floor exercises during and after pregnancy: A systematic review of their role in preventing pelvic floor dysfunction. J Obstet Gynecol Can 25:487, 2003.
86. MacArthur C, Glazener C, Lancashire R, et al: Faecal incontinence and mode of first and subsequent delivery: a six-year longitudinal study. Br J Obstet Gynaecol 112:1075, 2005.
87. Pollack J, Nordenstam J, Brismar S, et al: Anal incontinence after vaginal delivery: a five-year prospective cohort study. Obstet Gynecol 104:1397, 2004.
88. Chichakli LO, Atrash HK, Mackay AP, et al: Pregnancy-related mortality in the United States due to hemorrhage: 1979–1992. Obstet Gynecol 94:721, 1999.
89. King PA, Duthie SJ, Dip V, et al: Secondary postpartum hemorrhage. Aust N Z J Obstet Gynaecol 29:394, 1989.
90. Boyd BK, Katz VL, Hansen WF: Delayed postpartum hemorrhage: A retrospective analysis. J Maternal-Fetal Med 4:19, 1995.
91. Hoveyda F, MacKenzie IZ: Secondary postpartum haemorrhage: Incidence, morbidity and current management. Br J Obstet Gynaecol 108:927–30, 2001.
92. Pelage J-P, Phillippe S, Repiquet D, et al: Secondary postpartum hemorrhage: treatment with selective arterial embolization. Radiology 212:385, 1999.
93. Kotto-Kome AC, Calhoun DA, Montenegro R, et al: Effect of administering recombinant erythropoietin to women with postpartum anemia: a meta-analysis. J Perinatol 24:11, 2004.
94. Breymann C, Richter C, Huttner C, et al: Effectiveness of recombinant erythropoietin and iron sucrose vs iron therapy only, in patients with postpartum anaemia and blunted erythropoiesis. Eur J Clin Invest 30:154, 2000.
95. Charles J, Charles D: Postpartum infection. *In* Charles D (ed): Obstetric and Perinatal Infections. St Louis, Mosby Year Book, 1993, p 60.

96. Hale E, Keltz-Pomeranz M: Dermatologic agents during pregnancy and lactation: an update and clinical review. Int J Dermatol 41:197, 2002.
97. Klaus MH, Jerauld R, Kreger NC, et al: Maternal attachment: importance of the first postpartum days. N Engl J Med 286:460, 1972.
98. McClellan MS, Cabianca WC: Effects of early mother-infant contact following cesarean birth. Obstet Gynecol 56:52, 1980.
99. Robson KM, Powell E: Early maternal attachment. *In* Brickington IF, Kumar R (eds): Motherhood and Mental Illness. San Diego, Academic Press, 1982, p 155.
100. Klaus M, Kennel J: Parent-Infant Bonding. St Louis, CV Mosby, 1982.
101. Gray J, Butler C, Dean J, et al: Prediction and prevention of child abuse and neglect. Child Abuse Neglect 1:45, 1977.
102. Siegel E, Cauman KE, Schaefer ES, et al: Hospital and home support during infancy: impact on maternal attachment, child abuse and neglect and health care utilization. Pediatrics 66:183, 1980.
103. DeCasper AJ, Fifer W: Of human bonding: newborns prefer their mother's voices. Science 208:1174, 1980.
104. Areskog B, Uddenberg N, Kjessler B: Experience of delivery in women with and without antenatal fear of childbirth. Gynecol Obstet Invest 16:1, 1983.
105. Healthy People, Progress Review, May 5, 1999, DHHS, Public Health Service.
106. Winikoff B, Myers D, Laukaran VH, Stone R: Overcoming obstacles to breast-feeding in a large municipal hospital: applications of lessons learned. Pediatrics 80:423, 1987.
107. Niebyl JR, Spence MR, Parmley TH: Sporadic (nonepidemic) puerperal mastitis. J Reprod Med 20:97, 1978.
108. Thomsen AC, Espersen T, Maigaard S: Course and treatment of milk statis, noninfectious inflammation of the breast, and infectious mastitis in nursing women. Am J Obstet Gynecol 149:492, 1984.
109. Spitz AM, Lee NC, Peterson HB: Treatment for lactation suppression: little progress in one hundred years. Am J Obstet Gynecol 179:1485, 1998.
110. Willis J (ed): Postpartum hypertension, seizures, and strokes reported with bromocriptine. FDA Drug Bull 14:3, 1984.
111. Katz M, Kroll I, Pak I, et al: Puerperal hypertension, stroke, and seizures after suppression of lactation with bromocriptine. Obstet Gynecol 66:822, 1985.
112. Iffy L, TenHove W, Frisoli G: Acute myocardial infarction in the puerperium in patients receiving bromocriptine. Am J Obstet Gynecol 155:371, 1986.
113. Ruch A, Duhring J: Postpartum myocardial infarction in a patient receiving bromocriptine. Obstet Gynecol 74:448, 1989.
114. Kazi A, Kennedy KI, Visness CM, Kahn T: Effectiveness of the lactational amenorrhea method in Pakistan. Fertil Steril 64:717, 1995.
115. Robson KM, Brant H, Kumar R: Maternal sexuality during first pregnancy after childbirth. Br J Obstet Gynaecol 88:882, 1981.
116. Klebanoff MA: The interval between pregnancies and the outcome of subsequent births. N Engl J Med 340:643, 1999.
117. Debrovner CH, Winikoff B: Trends in postpartum contraceptive choice. Obstet Gynecol 63:65, 1984.
118. Flynn AM: Natural methods of family planning. Clin Obstet Gynaecol 11:661, 1984.
119. Rojnik B, Kosmelj K, Andolsek-Jeras L: Initiation of contraception postpartum. Contraception 51:75, 1995.
120. Sanford JB, Thurnau PB, Lemaire JC: Physicians' knowledge and practices regarding natural family planning. Obstet Gynecol 94:672, 1999.
121. Wortman J: The diaphragm and other intravaginal barriers—a review. Popul Rep H:58, 1979.
122. Vessey M, Wiggins P: Use-effectiveness of the diaphragm in a selected family planning clinic population in the United Kingdom. Contraception 9:15, 1974.
123. Mills A: Barrier contraception. Clin Obstet Gynaecol 11:641, 1984.
124. Speroff L, DeCherney A: Evaluation of a new generation of oral contraceptives. Obstet Gynecol 81:1034, 1993.
125. Kay CR: The Royal College of General Practitioners' oral contraceptive study: some recent observations. Clin Obstet Gynaecol 11:759, 1984.
126. Baird DT, Glasier AF: Hormonal contraception. N Engl J Med 328:1543, 1993.
127. Koetsawang S: The effects of contraceptive methods on the quality and quantity of breast milk. Int J Gynaecol Obstet 25 (Suppl):115, 1987.
128. Halderman LD, Nelson AL: Impact of early postpartum administration of progestin-only hormonal contraceptives compared with nonhormonal contraceptives on short-term breast-feeding patterns. Am J Obstet Gynecol 186:1250, 2002.
129. Kaunitz AM: Long-acting injectable contraception with depot medroxyprogesterone acetate. Am J Obstet Gynecol 170:1543, 1994.
130. Kjos SL, Peters RK, Xiang A, et al: Contraception and the risk of type 2 diabetes mellitus in Latina women with prior gestational diabetes mellitus. JAMA 280:533, 1998.
131. Diaz S, Peralta G, Juez C, et al: Fertility regulation in nursing women: III. Short-term influence of low-dose combined contraceptive upon lactation and infant growth. Contraception 27:1, 1983.
132. Sivin I, Campodonica I, Kiriwat O, et al: The performance of levonoregestrel rod and Norplant contraceptive implants: a 5 year randomized study. Hum Reprod 13:3371, 1998.
133. Berenson AB, Wiemann CM, McCombs SL, Soma-Garcia A: The rise and fall of levonogestrel implants: 1992–1996. Obstet Gynecol 92:790, 1998.
134. Sonnenberg FA, Burkman RT, Speroff L, et al: Cost-effectiveness and contraceptive effectiveness of the transdermal contraceptive patch. Am J Obstet Gyn 192:1, 2005.
135. Federal Drug Administration Guide to Contraception, 2003.
136. Cole LP, McCann MF, Higgins JE, et al: Effects of breast feeding on IUD performance. Am J Public Health 73:384, 1983.
137. Espy E, Ogburn T: Perpetuating negative attitudes about the intrauterine device: textbooks lag behind the evidence. Contraception 65:389, 2002.
138. Farley TMM, Rosenberg MJ, Rowe PJ, et al: Intrauterine devices and pelvic inflammatory disease: an international perspective. Lancet 339:785, 1992.
139. Stanback J, Grimes D: Can intrauterine device removals for bleeding or pain be predicted at a one-month follow-up visit? A multivariate analysis. Contraception 58:357, 1998.
140. Farmer M, Webb A: Intrauterine device insertion–related complications: can they be predicted? J Fam Plan Repro Health Care 29:227, 2003.
141. Mishell DR Jr, Roy S: Copper intrauterine contraceptive device event rate following insertion 4 to 8 weeks postpartum. Am J Obstet Gynecol 143:29, 1982.
142. Grimes D, Schulz K, vanVliet H, et al: Immediate post-partum insertion of intrauterine devices: a Cochrane review. Hum Reprod 17:549, 2002.
143. Alvarez T, Brache V, Fernandez E, et al: New insights on the mode of action of intrauterine contraceptive devices in women. Fertil Steril 49:768, 1988.
144. Rivera R, Yacobson I, Grimes D: The mechanism of action of hormonal contraceptives and intrauterine contraceptive devices. Am J Obstet Gynecol 181:1263, 1999.
145. Peterson LS: Contraceptive use in the United States: 1982–1990. Advanced Data from Vital Health Statistics. No. 260 Hyattsville, MD: National Center for Health Statistics, 1995 (DHHS publication no. PHS 95-1250).
146. Peterson HB, Xia Z, Hughes JM, et al: The risk of pregnancy after tubal sterilization: findings from The U.S. Collaborative Review of Sterilization. Am Obstet Gynecol 174:1161, 1996.
147. Cunningham FG, MacDonald PC, Leveno KJ, et al: Williams Obstetrics, 19th ed. Norwalk, CT, Appleton & Lange, 1993.
148. Irving FC: A new method of insuring sterility following cesarean section. Am J Obstet Gynecol 8:335, 1924.
149. Hillis SD, Marchbanks PA, Taylor LR, Peterson HB: Poststerilization regret: findings from the United States Collaborative Review of Sterilization. Obstet Gynecol 93:889, 1999.
150. Vessy M, Huggins G, Lawless M, et al: Tubal sterilization: findings in a large prospective study. Br J Obstet Gynaecol 90:203, 1983.

151. Bhiwandiwala PP, Mumford SD, Feldblum PJ: Menstrual pattern changes following laparoscopic sterilization with different occlusion techniques: a review of 10,004 cases. Am J Obstet Gynecol 145:684, 1983.
152. Bledin KD, Brice B: Psychological conditions in pregnancy and the puerperium and their relevance to postpartum sterilization: a review. Bull WHO 61:533, 1983.
153. Peterson HB, Huber DH, Belker AM: Vasectomy: an appraisal for the obstetrician-gynecologist. Obstet Gynecol 76:568, 1990.
154. Hendrix NW, Chauhan SP, Morrison JC: Sterilization and its consequences. Obstet Gynecol Surv 54:766, 1999.
155. Hillis SD, Marchbanks PA, Taylor LR, Peterson HB: Higher hysterectomy risk for sterilized than nonsterilized women: findings from the U.S. Collaborative Review of Sterilization Working Group. Obstet Gynecol 91:241, 1998.
156. Walker MW, Jick H, Hunter JR: Vasectomy and non-fatal myocardial infarction. Lancet 1:13, 1981.
157. Haynes DM, Martin BJ: Cesarean hysterectomy: a twenty-five year review. Am J Obstet Gynecol 46:215, 1975.
158. Drotar D, Baskiewicz A, Irvin N, et al: The adaptation of parents to the birth of an infant with a congenital malformation: a hypothetical model. Pediatrics 56:710, 1975.
159. Lindemann E: Symptomatology and management of acute grief. Am J Psychol 101:141, 1944.
160. Kennel JH, Slyter H, Claus MKH: The mourning response of parents to the death of a newborn. N Engl J Med 83:344, 1970.
161. Benfield DG, Leib SA, Reuter J: Grief response of parents after referral of the critically ill newborn to a regional center. N Engl J Med 294:975, 1976.
162. Giles PFH: reactions of women to perinatal death. Aust N Z J Obstet Gynaecol 10:207, 1970.
163. Zahourek R, Jensen J: Grieving and the loss of the newborn. Am J Nurs 73:836, 1973.
164. Seitz PM, Warrick LH: Perinatal death: the grieving mother. Am J Nurs 74:2028, 1974.
165. Rowe J, Clyman R, Green C, et al: Follow-up of families who experience perinatal death. Pediatrics 62:166, 1978.
166. Lockwood S, Lewis IC: Management of grieving after stillbirth. Med J Aust 2:308, 1980.
167. Mandell F, Wolf LC: Sudden infant death syndrome and subsequent pregnancy. Pediatrics 56:774, 1975.
168. Schleifer SJ, Keller SE, Camerimo M, et al: Suppression of lymphocyte stimulation following bereavement. JAMA 250:374, 1983.
169. Lake M, Knuppel R, Murphy J, et al: The role of a grief support team following stillbirths. Am J Obstet Gynecol 61:497, 1983.
170. Furlong R, Hobbins J: Grief in the perinatal period. Obstet Gynecol 61:497, 1983.
171. Condon JT: Management of established pathological grief reaction after stillbirth. Am J Psychiatry 143:987, 1986.
172. Kowalski K: Managing perinatal loss. Clin Obstet Gynecol 23:1113, 1980.
173. Mandell F, McAnulty E, Race RM: Observations of paternal response to sudden unanticipated infant deaths. Pediatrics 65:221, 1980.
174. Saisto T, Ylikorkala O, Halmesmaki E: Factors associated with fear of delivery in second pregnancies. Obstet Gynecol 94:679, 1999.
175. Fisher J, Astbury J, Smith A: Adverse psychological impact of operative obstetric interventions: a prospective longitudinal study. Aust N Z J Psychiatry 31:728, 1997.
176. Reynolds JL: Post-traumatic stress disorder after childbirth: the phenomenon of traumatic birth. Can Med Assoc J 156:831, 1997.
177. Ryding EL, Wijma K, Wijma B: Predisposing psychological factors for posttraumatic stress reactions after emergency cesarean section. Acta Obstet Gynecol Scand 77:351, 1998.

Breast-Feeding

Edward R. Newton

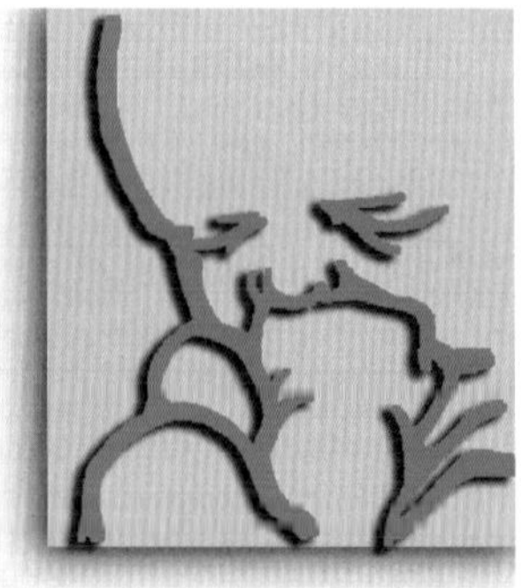

CHAPTER 22

Key Abbreviations

confidence interval	CI
Human immunodeficiency virus	HIV
Immunoglobulin A	IgA
Potassium chloride	KOH
Luteinizing hormone	LH
Messenger RNA	mRNA
Odds ratio	OR
Purified protein derivative	PPD
Secretory immunoglobulin A	sIgA
United Nations Children's Fund	UNICEF
World Health Organization	WHO

Breast-feeding and breast milk are the global standard for infant feeding in undeveloped and developed countries. This statement is supported by the World Health Organization, the U.S. Surgeon General, the American Academy of Pediatrics, the American College of Obstetricians and Gynecologists, the American Academy of Family Practice, and the Academy of Breastfeeding Medicine. The American Academy of Pediatrics has recently published an endorsement for breast-feeding at least through the first year of life and as an exclusive method for the first 6 months.[1,2] Unfortunately, the majority of American infants are not given this opportunity.[3–5] Figures 22-1 and 22-2 describes the incidence of breast-feeding in the United States.[3,4] These data are the result of serial mail surveys sent to postpartum women. The response rate is consistently about 50 percent, and minority women are underrepresented. The data for minority women are derived by major statistical manipulation. The latest survey (conducted in 2002)[4] reports that 70.1 percent of women initiate breast-feeding in the hospital and only 46.1 percent of those are still breast-feeding at 6 months. Approximately 20 percent of American infants meet the standard of breast-feeding 1 year or more.

Specific populations are at greater risk for the failure to initiate and continue breast-feeding. Lower socioeconomic classes, those who lack of education, and teenagers initiate breast-feeding at about one half to two thirds the rate of middle and upper class, mature high school graduates (Tables 22-1 and 22-2).[3–5] Fortunately, since 1989, more women at greatest risk for feeding their infants artificial breast milk are initiating breast-feeding in the hospital.[3] Perceived breast milk insufficiency, sore nipples and breasts, the lack of family and professional support, and the decision to return to work are the most often cited reasons for early weaning. Cultural attitudes underlie many of these risk factors for failure to breast-feed successfully.

Dysfunctional cultural and familial attitudes are outside the direct control of medicine and may directly affect the care delivered by physicians. The normal function of the breasts, specifically to produce breast milk, is muted by two cultural attitudes. One cultural attitude is the association of breasts with sexual attraction. The media is replete with examples that show beautiful, well-formed breasts as a sexual ideal. A corollary of this attitude is that breast-feeding will cause the breasts to sag and lose their sex appeal. The other opposing cultural attitude is that breast-feeding restricts self-fulfillment; mothers who stay at home to breast-feed and care for their babies are considered poor examples of the modern, independent professional woman. These attitudes are exacerbated by a lack of knowledge about breast-feeding and lactation. The normal function of the breasts is excluded from the curriculum of primary and secondary schools

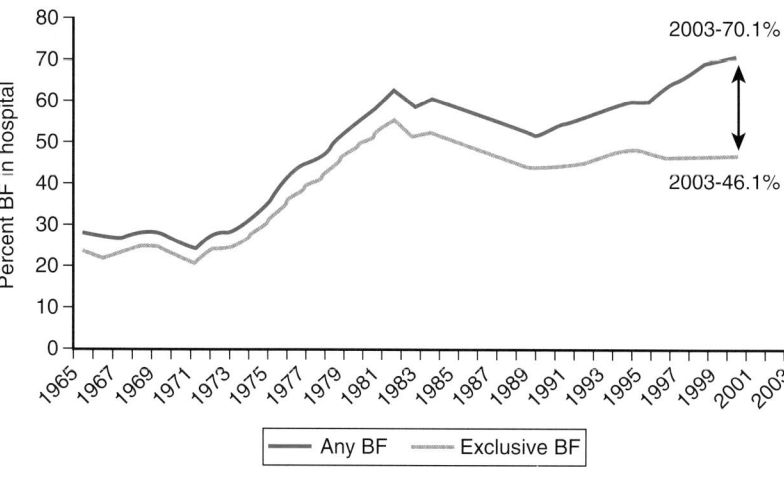

Figure 22-1. Incidence of breast-feeding in the hospital. (Data from American Academy of Pediatrics, Work Group on Breastfeeding: Breastfeeding and the use of human milk. Pediatrics 100:1035, 1997.)

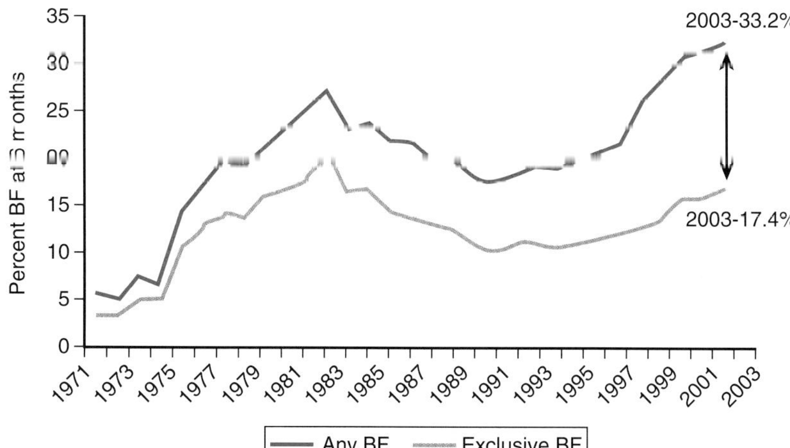

Figure 22-2. Incidence of breast-feeding at 6 months. (Data from American Academy of Pediatrics, Work Group on Breastfeeding: Breastfeeding and the use of human milk. Pediatrics 100:1035, 1997.)

Table 22-1. Predictors of Breastfeeding Initiation: PRAMS 1993–1998

HELPFUL FACTORS	ADJUSTED OR (95% CI)
Year of birth	1.08 (1.04–1.12)
Married	1.47 (1.33–1.63)
Parity >/= 1	1.48 (1.33–1.65)
Non-WIC participant	1.22 (1.10–1.35)
No prenatal discussion of nutrition	1.24 (1.09–1.42)
Normal birth weight	1.23 (1.14–1.34)
OBSTACLES	**ADJUSTED OR (95% CI)**
Black race	0.59 (0.53–0.65)
Maternal age <20	0.66 (0.57–0.77)
Maternal age 20–29	0.79 (0.77–0.86)
Maternal education: < high school	0.41 (0.36–0.46)
Maternal education: high school only	0.50 (0.46–0.54)
No prenatal discussion of breastfeeding	0.68 (0.60–0.76)
Cesarean delivery	0.71 (0.64–0.78)

CI, confidence interval; OR, odds ratio; WIC, The Special Supplemental Nutrition Program for Women, Infants, and Children.
Adapted from Newton ER: The epidemiology of breastfeeding. Clin Obstet Gynecol 47:613, 2004; Ahluwalia I, Morrow B, Hsia J, et al: Who is breastfeeding? Recent trends from the Pregnancy Risk Assessment and Monitoring System. J Pediatr 142:486, 2003.

Table 22-2. Predictors of Breast-Feeding Continuation More Than 10 Weeks: PRAMS 1993–1998

HELPFUL FACTORS	ADJUSTED OR (95% CI)
Married	1.43 (1.26–1.63)
Non-WIC participant	1.20 (1.05–1.36)
Normal birth weight	1.37 (1.23–1.53)
OBSTACLES	**ADJUSTED OR (95% CI)**
Maternal age <20	0.50 (0.41–0.61)
Maternal age 20–29	0.72 (0.65–0.79)
Maternal education: < high school	0.64 (0.54–0.76)
Maternal education: high school only	0.68 (0.61–0.75)
Parity >/= 1	0.72 (0.64–0.82)
Parity >/= 2	0.79 (0.70–0.89)
Cesarean delivery	0.82 (0.72–0.93)

CI, confidence interval; OR, odds ratio; WIC, The Special Supplemental Nutrition Program for Women, Infants, and Children.
Adapted from Newton ER: The epidemiology of breastfeeding. Clin Obstet Gynecol 47:613, 2004; Ahluwalia I, Morrow B, Hsia J, et al: Who is breastfeeding? Recent trends from the Pregnancy Risk Assessment and Monitoring System. J Pediatr 142:486, 2003.

on the basis of the connection between breasts and sex. After completion of their education, few women experience any examples of successful breast-feeding. Only 25 percent of grandmothers initiated breast-feeding (from 1965 to 1975), and few of the new mothers have breast-fed more than a few weeks. The lack of exposure to successful, experienced breast-feeding mothers seriously compromises the chances of success for the women who attempt to breast-feed.

Physicians are products of the same culture of the women they help. Unfortunately, many have the same cultural biases as their patients and the same lack of primary and secondary education regarding the normal physiology of breast-feeding. The curricula of medical school and residency training programs compound the lack of education. Most physicians reflecting on their own education on breast-feeding will identify neither a structured curriculum nor practical experiences with successfully breast-feeding mother-infant dyads. At most, he or she has experienced only one or two lectures regarding breast-feeding, often focused on breast anatomy or the endocrinology of lactation. In fact, the most commonly cited resource for physicians is another nonmedical individual or their breast-feeding spouse. On obstetric rotations, medical students and obstetrics residents rarely see normal breast-feeding dyads longer than 1 to 3 days postpartum. On pediatric rotations, learners often see the baby only in the nursery and rarely see the normal mother breast-feed as an inpatient or at newborn visits. Although pediatric residents observe and support the mother who pumps or nurses her growing preterm infant, the exposure is not normal and often is negative. As a result, there are serious gaps in physician knowledge as they attempt to serve the over 2 million newborns and mothers per year who attempt to breast-feed. A national survey of physician knowledge revealed that 20 to 40 percent of physicians (obstetricians, pediatricians, and family practitioners) did not know that breast-feeding is the "gold standard" for infant feeding, and similar percentages have serious and sometimes dangerous gaps in their knowledge in the management of breast-feeding problems.[6] A 1999 survey of fellows of the American Academy of Pediatricians revealed that only 65 percent recommended exclusive breast-feeding during the first month of life, and more than half agreed with or had a neutral opinion about the statement that breast-feeding and formula-feeding are equally acceptable methods for feeding infants.[7]

The purpose of this chapter is to begin the educational process through which obstetricians will adopt the lactating mother as their patient. In order to support the breast-feeding mother, the obstetrician must be convinced of the biologic superiority of breast-feeding and human breast milk over artificial breast milk (formula). This chapter reviews the morbidity and mortality associated with infant feeding using artificial breast milk and discusses the limitations of the current research. Subsequently, this chapter addresses breast anatomy and physiology of lactation in a framework pertinent to breast-feeding management. This chapter describes the vast differences between breast milk and artificial breast milk, a difference directly related to unique needs of the human infant. Specific issues related to the obstetrician (or other health care provider) are addressed and include the role of the obstetrician in preconceptional counseling, prenatal care, delivery room management, and postpartum care for the breast-feeding mother.

MORBIDITY AND MORTALITY ASSOCIATED WITH ARTIFICIAL BREAST MILK

Epidemiologic research shows that human milk and breast-feeding of infants provide significant advantages to general health, growth, and development. In contrast, infant feeding with artificial breastmilk, or "formula," is associated with higher incidences of acute and chronic diseases than in infants who are fed human milk through breast-feeding. The studies of predominantly middle class populations in developed countries show that infant feeding with artificial breast milk is associated with higher incidences and greater severity of diarrhea,[8–10] lower respiratory infection,[11–13] otitis media,[14–16] bacteremia,[17–21] bacterial meningitis,[17–21] urinary tract infection,[22,23] and necrotizing enterocolitis[24,25] than similar populations who were breast-fed. Numerous studies show higher incidences of sudden infant death syndrome,[26,27] type 1 and 2 diabetes mellitus,[28–30] adolescent-adult obesity,[31–34] Crohn's disease,[35,36] ulcerative colitis,[35,36] childhood cancers,[37] allergic diseases,[38–41] asthma among infants[42–46] and systemic infection in preterm infants fed artificial breast milk.[47] In high-risk populations such as preterm infants and infants with phenylketonuria, as well as healthy middle class populations of infants, breast-feeding has been associated with enhancement of cognitive development and intelligence quotients.[48–54] Using a sample representative of the United States population, Chen et al.[55] examined the role of breast-feeding on post neonatal mortality (28 days to 1 year). Not breast-feeding was associated with a 21-percent increase in postneonatal mortality. Infection and trauma were the predominant causes of the excess mortality. This translates to 720 postneonatal deaths that might have been prevented if exclusive breast-feeding had been used.[55]

One major challenge of breast-feeding research is the inability to assign research subjects to breast-feeding or feeding artificial breast milk: self-selection bias. In most studies, the demographic differences between women who breast-feed and those who do not can be adjusted statistically. Recently, newer population research designs reduce the self-selection bias. Cluster-randomized trials of breast-feeding promotion modeled on the WHO/UNICEF Baby-Friendly Hospital initiative have been used in two separate populations.[56–58] In these studies, maternity clinics and hospitals are assigned randomly to receive intensive educational programs to increase breast-feeding rates. The outcomes of interest are breast-feeding rates and short-term neonatal morbidities (infections, atopic dermatitis, etc.). In both studies, exclusive breast-feeding rates at 3 months were improved significantly ($P < 0.001$). The rates were 43.4 percent versus 6.4 percent in Belarus[56,57] and 79 percent versus 48 percent in India.[58] The intervention communities were associated with a 30- to 50-percent lower prevalence of gastrointestinal infections and atopic dermatitis, and better infant growth.[56–58]

An increase in acute medical diseases leads to higher costs of medical care for those families who choose to feed their infant artificial breast milk.[59–62] Among Medicaid populations in Colorado, California, and health maintenance organizations in Arizona,[47] the medical cost of artificial breast milk feeding amounts to $300 to $500 dollars per year per infant. Among patients who belonged to a large health maintenance organization in Tucson, Arizona, the excess yearly medical costs of 1,000 never-breast-fed infants versus 1,000 infants who were exclusively breast-fed for at least 3 months was $331,041[60,62] (Table 22-3).

The nonmedical costs of artificial breast milk, or "formula," feeding is considerably higher than breast-feeding. The direct cost of artificial breast milk feeding includes the cost of the artificial formula (900 ml/day), bottles, and supplies. In January, 2006 in eastern North Carolina the average retail cost of 900 ml of prepared formula was about $6.00 daily ($2190 yearly); of concentrate, about $4.25 daily ($1,550 yearly); and of powdered formula, about $3.25 daily ($1,190 yearly). A major indirect cost of artificial breast milk feeding is the environmental impact of large dairy herds to supply the milk substrate.

Breast-feeding provides the right amount of a superior product at precisely the right time and at the right temperature. The nonmedical costs of breast-feeding include the cost of increased maternal calorie and protein needs ($1 to $2 daily), nursing bras and breast pads, and an increased number of diapers in the first 2 to 3 months. If an electric breast pump is used when the woman returns to work, the cost of breast-feeding increases $2 to $4 per day.

Breast-feeding accrues multiple benefits to the mother that are not shared by women who feed their infants artificial breast milk.[63,64] Breast-feeding through increased release of oxytocin results in faster uterine involution and less postpartum blood loss[65]; the incidence of postpartum anemia may be reduced. Breast-feeding is associated with 1 to 3 kg (more in African-American women) less retained postpartum weight.[66] Decreased retained postpartum weight may reduce or delay the onset of chronic disease in older women, obesity,[34] type 2 diabetes mellitus,[29] and hypertension.[63,64,67] A recent study[68] showed breast-feeding was inversely associated with large vessel (carotid) atherosclerosis at 65-year follow-up versus individuals fed artificial breast milk (adjusted odds ratio [OR] [95-percent confidence interval (CI)]; 0.54 [0.29–0.92]) after controlling for age, gender, socioeconomic variables, smoking, drinking, blood pressure, adiposity, cholesterol, insulin resistance, and C reactive protein. Research demonstrates that exclusive breast-feeding delays ovulation with increased child spacing,[69] improved bone mineralization postpartum with reduction in hip fractures in the postmenopausal period,[70–72] and a reduced risk of ovarian cancer[63,64] and premenopausal breast cancer.[63,73–75]

Table 22-4 depicts the major long-term risks associated with exclusive artificial breast-milk infant feeding after the first week postpartum.

Table 22-3. Excess Medical Cost Among 1,000 Never Breast-Fed Vs 1,000 Exclusive (>3 Months) Breast-Fed Infants

	EXCESS SERVICES PER YEAR/1,000 NEVER BREAST-FED	TOTAL EXCESS COST
Office visits	1,693	$111,315
Follow-up visits	340	$22,355
Medications*	609	$7,669
Chest radiography	51	$1,836
Days of hospitalization†	212	$187,866
Total excess cost per year		$331,031

*Lower respiratory infection, otitis media.
†Lower respiratory infection, gastroenteritis.
Adapted from Ball TM, Wright AL: Health care costs of formula-feeding in the first year of life. Pediatrics 103:870, 1999.

Table 22-4. Long-Term Risks of Exclusive Use of Artificial Breast Milk: Results of Meta-Analyses

AUTHOR (YEAR)	OUTCOME	ADJUSTED ODDS RATIO (95TH CI)
McVea (2000)[27]	Sudden infant death	2.11 (1.66–2.68)
Sadauskaie (2004)[28]	Type 1 diabetes	1.85 (1.23–2.78)
Stuebe (2005)[29]	Adult type 2 diabetes	Increased 14% (7%–21%)
Arenz (2004)[32]	Childhood obesity	1.28 (1.18–1.41)
Owen (2005)[34]	Adult obesity	1.15 (1.13–1.15)
Klement (2004)[35]	Crohn's disease	2.22 (1.27–3.85)
Klement (2004)[35]	Ulcerative colitis	1.79 (1.23–2.63)
Gdalevich (2001)[41]	Atopic dermatitis	1.47 (1.14–1.92)
Anderson (1999)[53]	Intelligence quotient (IQ)	Minus 3.16 points (2.35–3.95)
Martin (2005)[37]	Childhood cancer	Increased 9%–41%
Martin (2005)[73]	Premenopausal breast cancer	1.14 (1.02–1.27)

CI, confidence interval.

LIMITATIONS OF BREAST-FEEDING RESEARCH

In the past, there have been major flaws in the designs and conclusions of epidemiologic research regarding the benefits or lack of benefits of breast-feeding. In the last 10 years, the quality has improved, but several cautions are warranted. A major confounder is the difference in the demographic characteristics between women who breast-feed and women who use artificial breast milk (see Tables 22-1 and 22–2). Many outcomes, such as infections and chronic diseases, are also more prevalent in lower socio-economic groups. When comparing outcomes between breast-feeding and artificial breast milk feeding, the effect of demographic differences should be analyzed and controlled in the analysis. In addition, cultural support and demographic differences of women who breast-feed their infants have changed. In the 1950s and 1960s cultural pressures pushed better educated, wealthier middle class women away from breast-feeding; the incidence of initiation of breast-feeding reached its nadir in the early 1970s. This change is important when considering recall data used in studies evaluating differences in chronic diseases in the older adult, especially breast cancer.

Much of the older epidemiologic research has relied on self-report and recall data, usually long after the event has occurred. Memory is not perfect, and biases are often introduced, such as combining events into convenient ages or socially acceptable times of weaning. One major area of recall bias is the definition of partial breast-feeding. An example of the confounding nature of this bias is a serial survey of nurses.[75] The study showed no significant benefit of breast-feeding in the reduction of premenopausal breast cancer, which was touted by the authors as evidence of no relationship between infant feeding and breast cancer. Because this was a population of nurses, in which a significant number were working at the time they were feeding their infant, a variable that was not measured, the definition of breast-feeding may reflect intent more than the actual degree of breast-feeding.

After statistical control for demographic variables, an unavoidable self-selection bias remains. Intrinsic personality characteristics may be determinants of feeding choice; a random allocation of feeding method is not possible. There is also evidence that women who breast-feed exhibit more nurturing behavior than women who feed their infants artificial breast milk.[76]

When analyzing any article involving breast-feeding, it is important to understand the author's definition of breast-feeding. Exclusive breast-feeding is considered when the infant does not receive any additional food or nutriment other than breast milk. Partial breast-feeding needs to be defined by the proportion of feeds that are breast milk or artificial breast milk. If an infant consumes 700 ml of artificial breast milk per day, then the proportion of breast milk consumed is small regardless of the frequency of breast-feeding episodes. Control for the "dose" effect is important in physiologic as well as epidemiologic studies. The content and character of breast milk are affected by the frequency of feeds, the duration of the feed, when in the feed the breast milk is collected, the method of breast milk collection, and the time of day of the collection.

One common design mistake is the failure to understand the effect of duration of breast-feeding. Breast-feeding has immediate and long-term benefits. The immediate benefits accrue only when a significant proportion of the infant's diet is breast milk. For example, the protection against gastroenteritis is afforded by the presence of antigen-specific immunoglobulin A (IgA) in breast milk. This protection is present only when the infant is breast-feeding. On the other hand, breast milk modulates the infant's immune system and improves response to infection well after breast-feeding has ceased. Although it appears that there is a dose-dependent relationship between the duration of exclusive breast-feeding and many long-term benefits, the effective dose (duration of exclusive breast-feeding) varies by benefit and is unknown. Most studies have arbitrarily determined the "effective" dose and challenge the benefits of breast-feeding based on that "effective" dose. For example, Agre[77] concluded that exclusive breast-feeding for 3 months had no bearing on the frequency of infection in the first year of life. However, his outcome variable, frequency of infection in the first 12 months, did not stratify the outcome by when the infant was actually breast-feeding. An episode of gastroenteritis at 10 months was counted as a breast-feeding "failure" even though the infant breast-fed only 6 months.

In summary, good breast-feeding research must demonstrate appropriate definitions of breast-feeding, control for the "dose" effect, control for demographic differences between breast-feeding and non-breast-feeding populations, and appropriate linkage between behavior and outcomes.

BREAST ANATOMY AND DEVELOPMENT

The size and shape of the breast vary greatly by stage of development, physiologic state, and phenotype. The breast is located in the superficial fascia between the second rib and sixth intercostal cartilage in the midclavicular line. There is usually a projection of the central disk into each axilla, the *tail of Spence.* The mature breast weighs about 200 g in the nonpregnant state; during pregnancy, 500 g; and during lactation, 600 to 800 g. As long as glandular tissue and the nipple are present, the size or shape of the breast has little to do with the functional success of the breast. The adequacy of glandular tissue for breast-feeding is ascertained by inquiring whether a woman's breasts have enlarged during pregnancy. If there is failure of the breast to enlarge as the result of pregnancy, especially if associated with minimal breast tissue on examination, the clinician should be wary of primary failure of lactation.

The nipple, or *papilla mammae,* is a conical elevation in the middle of the areola, or *areola mammae.* The areola is a circular pigmented area that darkens during pregnancy. The contrast with the fairer skin of the body provides a visual cue for the newborn who is attempting to latch-on. The areola contains multiple small elevations, *Montgomery's tubercles,* which enlarge during pregnancy and lactation. Montgomery's tubercles contain multiple ductular openings of sebaceous and sweat glands. These glands secrete lubricating and anti-infective substances (IgA) that protect the nipples and areola during nursing. These substances are washed away when the breasts and nipples are washed with soap or alcohol-containing compounds, leaving the nipple prone to cracking and infection.

Unlike the dermis of the body of the breast, which includes fat, the areola and nipple contain smooth muscle and collagenous and elastic tissue. With light touch or anticipation, these muscles contract and the nipple erects to form a teat. The contraction pulls the lactiferous sinuses into the nipple-areola complex, which allows the infant to milk the breast milk from these reservoirs.

The tip of the nipple contains the openings (0.4 to 0.7 mm in diameter) of 15 to 20 milk ducts (2 to 4 mm in diameter). Each of the milk ducts empties one tubuloalveolar gland, which is embedded in the fat of the body of the breast. A sphincter mechanism at the opening of the duct limits the ejection of milk from the breast. The competency of this mechanism is variable. About 20 percent of women do not demonstrate milk ejection from the contralateral breast when milk ejection is stimulated. If milk leakage is demonstrated from the contralateral breast during nursing, there is supporting evidence of an intact let-down reflex and is highly suggestive of milk transfer to the infant.

Five to 10 mm from their exit, the milk ducts widen (5 to 8 mm) into the lactiferous sinuses (Fig. 22-3). When these sinuses are pulled into the teat during nursing, the infant's tongue, facial muscles, and mouth squeeze the milk from the sinuses into the infant's oropharnyx.[78,79] The tubuloalveolar glands (15 to 20) form lobi, which are arranged in a radial fashion from the central nipple-areola complex. The lobi and lactiferous ducts extend into the tail of Spence. Ten to 40 lactiferous ducts connect to each lactiferous sinus, each forming a lobulus. Each lobulus arborizes into 10 to 100 alveoli for tubulosaccular secretory units. The alveoli are the critical units of the production and ejection of milk. A sac of alveolar cells is surrounded by a basket of myoepithelial cells. The alveolar cells are stimulated by prolactin to produce milk. The myoepithelial cells are stimulated by oxytocin to contract and eject the recently produced milk into the lactiferous ducts, lactiferous sinuses, and beyond.

The radial projection of lactiferous ducts prompts important considerations relative to breast surgery on women who are breast-feeding or who will breast-feed. Surgical skin incisions parallel to the circumareolar line, especially at the circumareolar line, have better cosmetic healing and are often chosen by surgeons. However, if the incision is taken deep into the parenchyma, the lactiferous ducts may be compromised; a superficial, parallel skin incision and a deep radial incision are preferred. In women who intend to breast-feed, a circumareolar incision is to be avoided. The incision compromises breast-feeding in three ways: occlusion of lactiferous ducts, restriction of the formation of a teat during nursing, and injury to the lateral cutaneous branch of the fourth intercostal nerve.

Surgical disruption of the lateral cutaneous branch of the fourth intercostal nerve can have devastating effects on the success of breast-feeding.[80,81] This nerve is critical to the production and ejection of breast milk (see The Physiology of Lactation, below). Furthermore, the nerves provide organ-specific control of regional blood flow, and a tremendous increase in mammary blood flow occurs during a nursing episode.[82] Disruption of this autonomic control may severely compromise lactation performance. The rate of breast-feeding failure is two to three times higher when a circumareolar incision is performed.[80] The obstetrician needs to be alert to old surgical incisions when a pregnant patient expresses a desire to breast-feed or when a breast biopsy is anticipated in a reproductive-aged woman.

As mammals, humans have the potential to develop mammary tissue, glandular or nipple tissue, anywhere along the milk line *(galactic band)*. The milk line extends from the axilla and inner upper arm to its current position, down the abdomen along the midclavicular line to the upper lateral mons and upper inner thigh. When accessory glands occur, this is termed hypermastia. This may involve accessory glandular tissue, supernumerary nipples, or both. Two to 6 percent of women have hypermastia, and the response to pregnancy and lactation is variable. The most common site for accessory breast tissue is the axilla. These women may present at 2 to 5 days postpartum (galactogenesis) with painful enlargements in the axilla. Ice and symptomatic therapy for 24 to 48 hours are sufficient. Supernumerary nipples *(polythelia)* are associated with renal abnormalities (11 percent).

THE PHYSIOLOGY OF LACTATION

The physiology of lactation has three major components: stages of lactogenesis, endocrinology of lactogenesis, and nursing behavior/milk transfer.

Stages of Lactogenesis

Full alveolar development and maturation of the breast must await the hormones of pregnancy (progesterone, prolactin, and human placental lactogen) for completion of the developmental process. By midpregnancy, the gland is competent to secrete milk (colostrum), although full function is not attained until the tissues are released from the inhibition of high levels of circulating progesterone. This is termed *lactogenesis stage 1*. Lactogenesis stage 2 occurs as the progesterone levels fall after delivery of the placenta, during the first 2 to 4 days after birth. Stage 2 includes dramatic increases in mammary blood flow, and oxygen and glucose uptake by the breast. At 2 to 3 days postpartum, the secretion of milk is copious and "the milk comes in." This is the most common time for engorgement if the breasts are not drained by efficient, frequent nursing. Until lactogenesis stage 2 is developed, the breasts secrete colostrum. Colostrum is very different than mature milk in volume and constituents.[83,84] Colostrum has more protein, especially secretory immunoglobulins, lactose, and lower fat content than mature

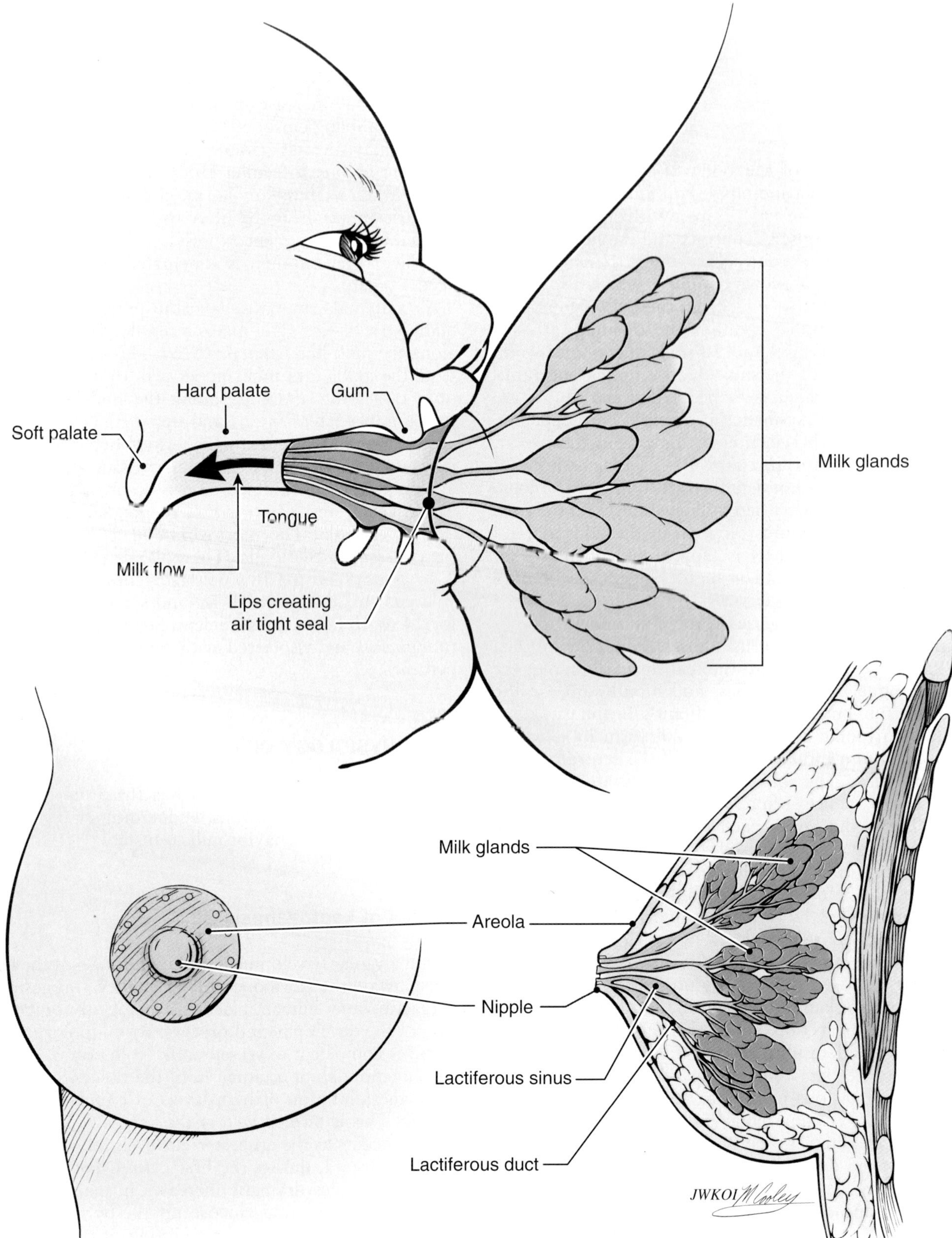

Figure 22-3. Anatomy of the breast.

milk. Prolactin and glucocorticoids play important promoter roles in this stage of development.

After lactogenesis stage 2 (4 to 6 days postpartum), lactation enters an indefinite period of milk production formerly called galactopoiesis, now termed lactogenesis stage 3. The duration of this stage is dependent on the continued production of breast milk and the efficient transfer of the breast milk to the infant. Prolactin appears to be the single most important galactopoietic hormone because selective inhibition of prolactin secretion by bromocriptine disrupts lactogenesis. Oxytocin appears to be the major galactokinetic hormone. Stimulation of the nipple and areola or behavioral cues cause a reflex contraction of the myoepithelial cells that surround the alveoli and ejection of milk from the breast.

The final stage of development is involution and cessation of breast-feeding. As the frequency of breast-feeding is reduced to less than six episodes in 24 hours and milk volume decreases to less than 400 ml/24 h, prolactin levels fall and a cyclic pattern ends in the total cessation of milk production. After 24 to 48 hours of no transfer of breast milk to the infant, intraductal pressure[85] and lactation inhibitory factor[86] appear to initiate apoptosis of the secretory epithelial cells and proteolytic degradation of the basement membrane. Lactation inhibitory factor is a protein secreted in the milk, whose increasing concentration in the absence of drainage appears to decrease milk production by the alveolar cells.[85–88] It counterbalances pressures such as the increased frequency of nursing to increase milk supply and allows for the day-to-day adjustment in infant demands.

The Endocrinology of Lactogenesis

Prolactin is the major hormone promoting milk production. Prolactin induces the synthesis of messenger RNAs (mRNAs) for the production of enzymes and milk proteins by binding to membrane receptors of the mammary epithelial cells. Thyroid hormones selectively enhance the secretion of lactalbumin. Cortisol, insulin, parathyroid hormone and growth hormone are supportive metabolic hormones in the production of carbohydrates and lipids in the milk. Ovarian hormones are not required for the maintenance of established milk production and are suppressed by high levels of prolactin.

The alveolar cell is the principal site for the production of milk. Neville[84,89] describes five pathways for milk synthesis and secretion in the mammary alveolus, including four major transcellular pathways and one paracellular pathway. They are (1) exocytosis (merocrine secretion) of milk protein and lactose in Golgi-derived secretory vesicles, (2) milk fat secretion through milk fat globules (apocrine secretion), (3) secretion of ions and water across the apical membrane, (4) pinocytosis-exocytosis of immunoglobulins, and (5) paracellular pathway for plasma components and leukocytes. During lactation as opposed to during pregnancy, very few of the constituents of breast milk are transferred directly from maternal blood. The junctions between cells, called *tight junctions,* are closed. As weaning occurs, the tight junctions are released, and sodium and other minerals easily cross to the milk, changing the taste of the milk.

The substrates for milk production are primarily absorbed from the maternal gut or produced in elemental form by the maternal liver. Glucose is the major substrate for milk production. Glucose serves as the main source of energy for other reactions and is a critical source of carbon. The synthesis of fat from carbohydrates plays a predominant role in fat production in human milk. Proteins are built from free amino acids derived from the plasma.

A sizable proportion of breast milk is produced during the nursing episode. In order to supply the substrates for milk production, there is a 20- to 40-percent increase in blood flow to the mammary glands as well as increased blood flow to the gastrointestinal tract and liver. Cardiac output is increased by 10 to 20 percent during a nursing episode.[82] The vasodilation of the regional vascular beds is under the control of the autonomic nervous system. Oxytocin may play a critical role in directing the regional distribution of maternal cardiac output through an autonomic, parasympathetic action.

Given that milk is produced during the nursing episode, variation in content during a feed is expected. During a feeding episode, the lipid content of milk rises by more than two- to threefold (1 to 5 percent), with a corresponding 5-percent fall in lactose concentration.[90] The protein content remains relatively constant. At the extreme, there can be a 30- to 40-percent difference in the volume obtained from each breast.[90–92] Likewise, there are intraindividual variations in lipid and lactose concentrations.

The rising lipid content during a feed has practical implications in breast-feeding management. If a woman limits her feeds to less than 4 minutes but nurses more frequently, the calorie density of the milk is lower and the infant's hunger may not be satiated. The infant wishes to feed sooner, and the frequency of nursing accelerates. This stimulates more milk production and creates a scenario of a hungry infant despite apparent good volume and milk transfer.[93] Lengthening the nursing episode or using one breast for each nursing episode often solves the problem.

The volume and concentration of constituents also vary during the day.[91,92] Volume per feed increases by 10 to 15 percent in the late afternoon and evening. Nitrogen content peaks in the late afternoon and falls to a nadir at 5 a.m. Fat concentrations peak in the early morning and reach a nadir at 9 p.m. Lactose levels stay relatively stable throughout the day. The variation in milk volume and content in working women who nurse only when at home has not been studied. Presumably, the variation in volume and content is preserved if the woman pumps during the day.

Does diet affect the volume and constitution of breast milk? For the average American woman with the range of diets from teenagers to mature, health-conscious adults, the answer is "no." There is no convincing evidence that the macronutrients in breast milk, protein, fats, and carbohydrates vary across the usual range of American diets. Volume may vary in the extremes. In developing countries where there is widespread starvation and daily calorie intake is less than 1,600 kcal during prepregnancy and pregnancy, milk volume and calorie density are minimally decreased (5 to 10 percent) in underweight breast-feeding mothers, if at all.[94] In a controlled experiment,[95] well-nourished European women reduced their calorie intake by 33 percent for 1 week. Milk volume was not reduced when the diet was maintained at greater than 1,500 kcal/day. If the daily energy intake was less than 1,500 kcal/day, milk volume was reduced 15 percent. Moderate dieting and weight loss postpartum (4.5 lb/month) are not associated with changes in milk volume,[84] nor does aerobic exercise have any adverse effect.[96,97]

In the first year of life, the infant undergoes tremendous growth; infants double their birth weight in 180 days. Infants fed artificial breast milk lose up to 5 percent of their birth weight during the first week of life, whereas breast milk–fed infants lose about 7 percent of their birth weight. A maximum weight loss of 10 percent of birth weight is tolerated in the first week of life in breast-fed infants. If this threshold is exceeded, the breast-feeding dyad needs immediate intervention by a trained health care provider. Although supplementation with donor breast milk or artificial breast milk may be a necessary part of the intervention, the key focus of intervention is establishing good breast milk transfer by ensuring adequate production, correct nursing behavior, and adequate frequency. Once stage 3 of lactogenesis occurs, "the milk has come in"; the term breast-fed infant will gain about 0.75 to 1 oz/day with adequate milk transfer. By 14 days, the breast-fed infant should have returned to its birth weight.

Food intake and energy needs are not constant. The infant's need for energy and fluids varies by day or week with growth spurts, greater activity, fighting illness, or greater fluid losses, as in hot weather. Mammals have developed an extremely efficient mechanism to adjust milk supply within 24 to 48 hours depending on demand through oxytocin and the let-down reflex, and prolactin production. The prolactin and oxytocin travel to their target cells—prolactin to the alveolar epithelium in the breast, and oxytocin to the myoepithelial cells that shroud the alveolar epithelium. The pituitary's prolactin and luteinizing hormone (LH) response to nursing frequency is depicted in Figure 22-4. In lactating women, baseline prolactin levels are 200 ng/ml at delivery, 75 ng/ml between 10 and 90 days postpartum, 50 ng/ml between 90 and 180 days postpartum, and 35 ng/ml after 180 days postpartum. Maternal serum prolactin levels rise by 80 to 150 percent of baseline levels within seconds of nipple stimulation. As long as nursing frequency is maintained at greater than eight episodes a day for 10 to 20 minutes with each episode, the serum prolactin levels will suppress the LH surges and ovarian function.[89,98]

Serum oxytocin levels also rise with nipple stimulation. However, the oxytocin response is much more affected by operant conditioning, and its response may precede the rise in prolactin levels. The maternal cerebrum is influenced by exposure to nursing cues as well as to the influences of nipple stimulation. The cerebrum either stimulates or inhibits the hypothalamus to increase or decrease the production of prolactin inhibitory factor (dopamine) and, subsequently, the release of oxytocin from the posterior pituitary. Cerebral influences have a lesser effect on the release of prolactin. Positive sights, sounds, or smells related to nursing often stimulate the production of oxytocin, which, in turn, causes the myoepithelial cells to contract and milk to leak from the breasts. This observation is a good clinical clue indicating an uninhibited let-down reflex.

In a classic series of experiments, Newton and Egli[99] demonstrated the power of noxious influences to inhibit

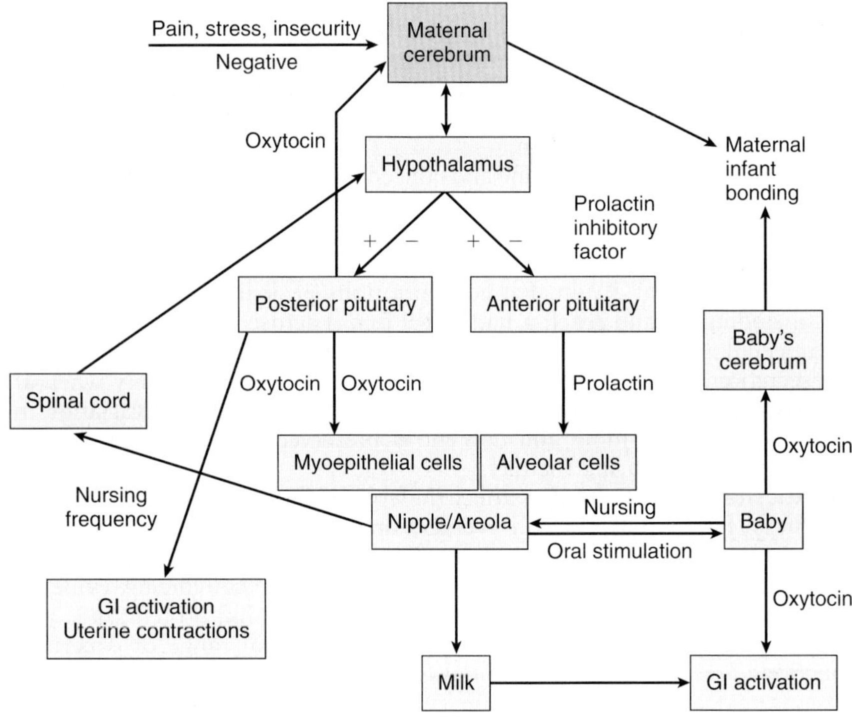

Figure 22-4. Oxytocin and the let-down reflex. The major reflex includes feedback stimulation from the nipple/areola to the hypothalamus to increase/decrease the release of oxytocin from the posterior pituitary and prolactin inhibitor factor (PIF-dopamine). The PIF affects the release of prolactin. Prolactin increases milk production. Oxytocin causes milk ejection. The release of both hormones is affected by positive or negative influences from the upper central nervous system. Oxytocin has three different target sites, the gastrointestinal tract (GI), uterus (contractions), and the upper central nervous system (mother-infant bonding). Oral stimulation in the infant initiates oxytocin release to improve GI activities and maternal-infant bonding. (From Rolland R, DeJong FH, Schellekens LA, et al: The role of prolactin in the restoration of ovarian function during the early postpartum period in the human: a study during inhibition of lactation by bromergocryptine. Clin Endocrinol 4:23, 1975, with permission.)

the release of oxytocin and to reduce milk transfer to the infant. The baseline milk production per feed was measured in controlled situations, about 160 g per feed. During a consecutive feed, a noxious event (i.e., saline injection) was administered during the feed. The amount of milk produced was cut in half, 80 to 100 g. Subsequently, the milk production was measured in a trial in which a noxious event was administered and intranasal oxytocin was given concomitantly. The milk production was restored to almost 90 percent of baseline production, 130 to 140 g. A wide variety of noxious events were able to elicit the same decrease in milk production. The noxious events included placing the mother's feet in ice water, applying electric shocks to her toes, having her trace shapes while looking only through a mirror, or requiring her to proofread a document in a timed fashion. These observations have important implications concerning the management of breast-feeding. Pain, anxiety, and insecurity may be hidden reasons for breast-feeding failure through the inhibitions of the let-down reflex. In contrast, the playing of a soothing motivational/educational audio tape to women who were pumping milk for their premature infants has improved milk yields.[100] These observations have been confirmed by measuring the inhibition of oxytocin release by psychological stress.[101,102] The positive and negative influences of the cerebrum are further highlighted by the observation[102–104] that 75 percent of women who had a positive attitude during pregnancy were likely to be successful at breast-feeding. In contrast, 75 percent of women who had a negative attitude during pregnancy had an unsuccessful breast-feeding experience. This observation has been confirmed more recently.[105] When the mother's attitude was very good or good and family was present, the exclusive breast-feeding rate was 20 percent at 6 months. If the mother's attitude was fair, the breast-feeding rate at 6 months was 5 percent.

Oxytocin has additional target cells in the mother. The effect of oxytocin on uterine activity is well known. Uterine involution is enhanced with breast-feeding. Animal and human research suggests that oxytocin is a neurohormone. Oxytocin is associated with an antifight/flight response in the autonomic nervous system, and so the mother tolerates stress better, and maternal-infant bonding is improved. In addition, gastrointestinal mobility and absorption are enhanced.[106,107]

In addition to the antistress effect, surges in oxytocin levels are associated with the release of gastrointestinal hormones and increased gastrointestinal motility.[106] In the mother, these actions enhance the absorption of substrates necessary for lactogenesis. In infants, there is a growing body of knowledge that indicates similar associations with oxytocin surges. Skin-to-skin contact and the oral stimulation of nursing stimulate a para-sympathetic, antifight/flight response in the infant. Kangaroo care of premature newborns (skin-to-skin contact) is associated with a physiologically stable state, improved stress responses, and improved weight gain.[106–108] Oxytocin appears to mediate this response.[108,109] Breast-feeding is associated with far more skin-to-skin contact and maternal behaviors than bottle-feeding.

Although the central nervous system locus for imprinting is unknown, imprinting immediately after birth is an important predictor of breast-feeding success. The survival of lambs depends on nursing within an hour after birth. If the lamb has not nursed during the critical period, maternal-infant bonding becomes dysfunctional and the lamb fails to thrive. In humans, the consequences are not nearly as drastic. Several trials with random assignment of subjects to early nursing (delivery room) or late nursing (2 hours after birth) demonstrated a 50- to 100-percent increase in the number of mothers who were breast-feeding at 2 to 4 months postpartum after nursing was begun in the delivery room.[110] One of the keys to obstetric management is to have the mother nurse her newborn in the delivery room.

Milk Transfer

Milk transfer to the infant is a key physiologic principle in lactation.[111] The initial step of this process is good latch-on. With light tactile stimulation of the cheek and lateral angle of the mouth, the infant reflexively turns its head and opens its mouth, as in a yawn (Fig. 22-5). The nipple is tilted slightly downward using a "C-hold," or *palmar grasp*. In this hand position, the fingers support the breast from underneath and the thumb lightly grasps the upper surface 1 to 2 cm above the areola-breast line. The infant is brought firmly to the breast by the supporting arms while being careful to not push the back of the baby's head. The nipple and areola are drawn into the mouth as far as the areola-breast line (Figs. 22-6 and 22-7). The posterior areola may be less visible than the anterior areola, and the lower lip of the infant is often curled out. The infant's lower gum lightly fixes the teat over the lactiferous sinuses. A slight negative pressure

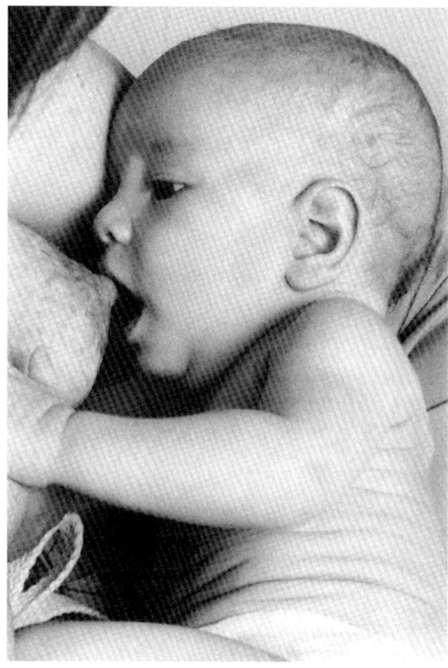

Figure 22-5. The latch-on reflex.

exerted by the oropharynx and mouth holds the length of the teat and breast in place and reduces the "work" to refill the lactiferous sinuses after they are drained. The milk is extracted, not by negative pressure, but by a peristaltic action from the tip of the tongue to the base. There is no stroking, friction, or in-and-out motion of the teat; it is more of an undulating action. The buccal mucosa and tongue mold around the teat, leaving no space.

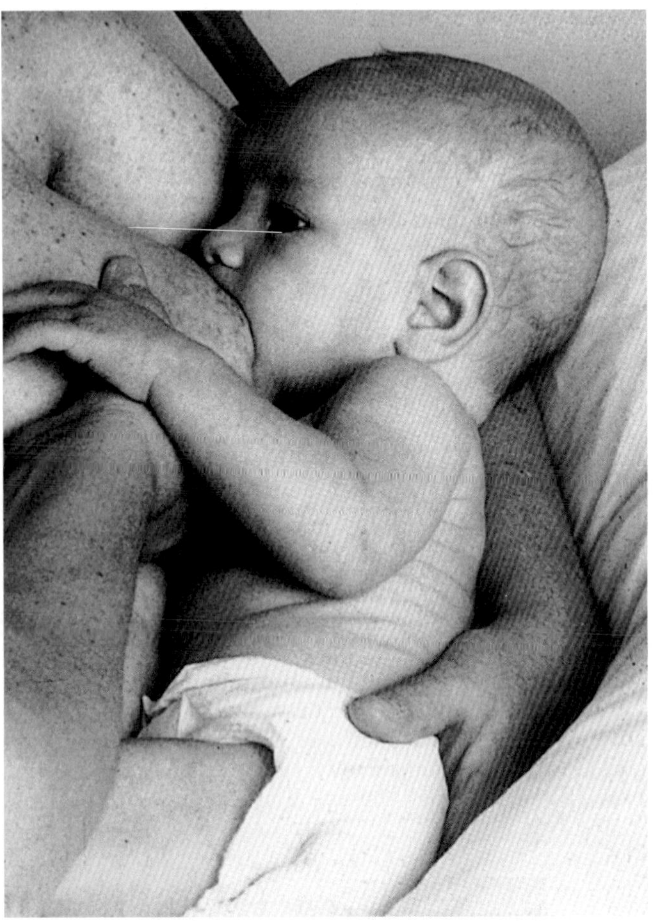

Figure 22-6. Appropriate latch-on.

The peristaltic movement of the infant's tongue is most frequent in the first 3 minutes of a nursing episode; the mean latency from latch-on to milk ejection is 2.2 minutes. After milk flow is established, the frequency of sucking falls to a much slower rate.[78,79,98,112] The change in cadence is recognizable as "suck-suck-swallow-breath." Audible swallowing of milk is a good sign of milk transfer. At the start of a feed, the infant obtains 0.10 to 0.20 ml per suck. As the infant learns how to suck and matures, he or she becomes more efficient at obtaining more milk in a shorter period of time. Eighty to 90 percent of the milk is obtained in the first 5 minutes the infant nurses on each breast, but the fat-rich and calorie-dense hind milk is obtained in the remainder of the time sucking at each breast, usually less than 20 minutes total.[18,98,113,114] A bottle-feeding infant sucks steadily in a linear fashion, receiving about 80 percent of the artificial breast milk in the first 10 minutes.

Sucking on a bottle is mechanically very different than nursing on the human teat (Fig. 22-8). The relatively inflexible artificial nipple resists the milking motion of the infant's tongue and mouth. The diameter of the artificial nipple expands during a suck, whereas the human teat collapses during the milk flow. The infant who is sucking on a bottle learns to generate strong negative pressures (>100 mm Hg) in order to suck the milk out of the bottle. Because rapid flow from the bottle can gag the infant, he or she quickly learns to use the tongue to regulate the flow. When the infant who has learned to bottle-feed is put to the breast, the stopper function of the tongue may abrade the tip of the nipple and force the nipple out of the infant's mouth. The efficiency of milk transfer falls drastically, and the hungry infant becomes frustrated and angry. A similar rejection may occur at 4 to 8 weeks when the exclusively breast-feeding infant is given a bottle in preparation for the mother's return to work.

Milk transfer is made more efficient by proper positioning of the infant to the breast. Proper positioning places

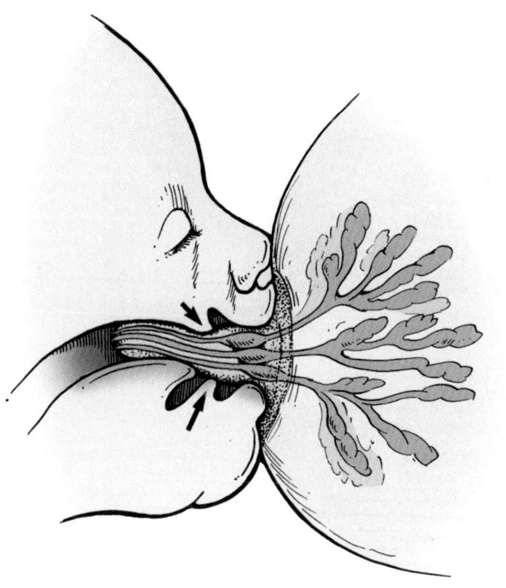

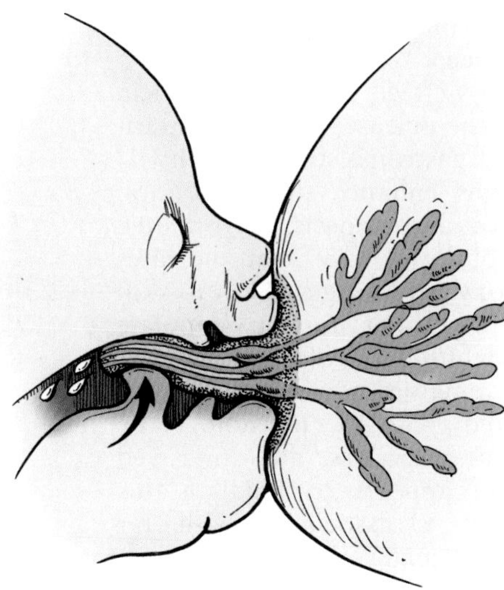

Figure 22-7. The mechanics of nursing.

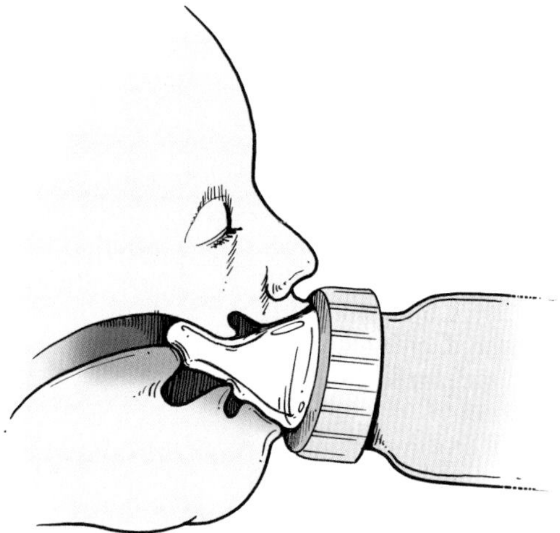

Figure 22-8. The mechanics of bottle feeding.

the infant and mother chest-to-chest. The infant's ear, shoulder, and hip are in line. The three most common maternal positions are cross arm chest-to-chest, side-lying, or the football hold (Figs. 22-6, 22-9, and 22-10). Each has its own advantages. Rotating positions of nursing allows improved drainage of different lobules, an observation important in the management of a "plugged" duct. Maternal comfort and convenience are the major reasons for changing nursing positions; the football hold position and the side-lying position are more comfortable if there is an abdominal incision.

Baseline prolactin levels appear to be the major determinant of the hormonal state during lactation, a state of high-prolactin, low-estrogen, and low-progesterone levels. As the frequency of nursing decreases below eight in 24 hours, the baseline prolactin levels drop to a level below which ovulation is suppressed (35 to 50 ng/ml), LH levels then rise, and menstrual cycling is initiated.[89,98,113,115] The intensity (adjusted OR) of factors that initiate the onset of menses are the duration of sucking episodes less than 7 minutes (OR 2.4), night feeds less than four per 24 hours (OR 2.3), maternal age 15 to 24 years (OR 2.1), maternal age 25 to 34 years (OR 1.7), and day feeds less than seven per 24 hours (OR 1.6).[116] Serum prolactin levels in women who feed their infants artificial breast milk exclusively drop to prepregnant levels (8 to 14 ng/ml) within days. The total number of nursing episodes per day (more than eight per 24 hours) and night nursings are critical to the successful management of breast-feeding.

One of the major determinants of nursing frequency is the introduction of substitute nutriment sources for the infant, artificial breast milk or solids. Breast milk has the nutritional content to satisfy the growth needs of the infant for at least 6 months postpartum. In the first 6 months, feeding with artificial breast milk affects the physiology of successful lactation in three ways. Substitution with artificial breast milk reduces proportionally the nutriment requirements from breast milk, increases the gastric emptying time (slower digestion than breast milk) with a subsequent decrease in the frequency of nursing episodes, and reduces the efficiency of nursing by the use of an opposing sucking technique on the artificial nipple.

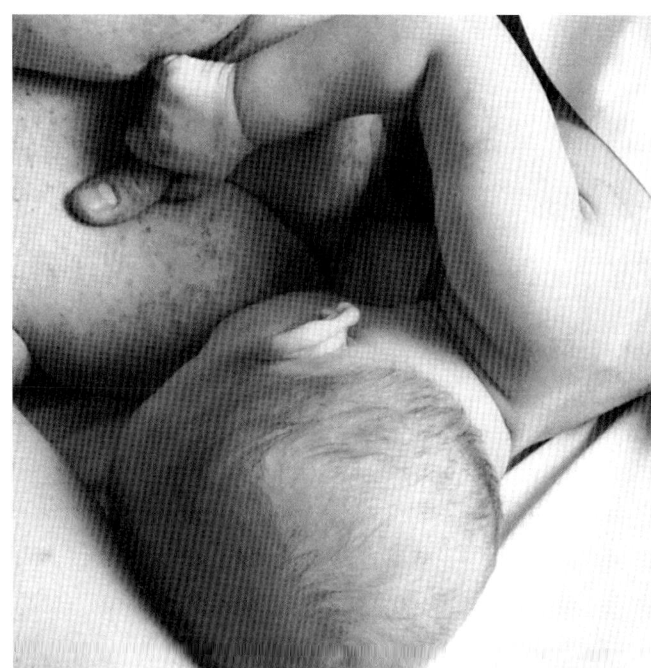

Figure 22-9. Side-lying nursing.

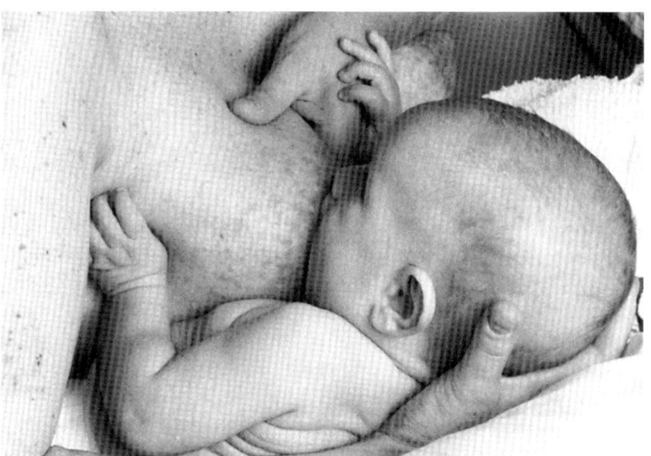

Figure 22-10. The football hold.

As depicted in Figure 22-4, prolactin falls, and menses resume.

Solid foods (e.g., eggs, cereals, pureed food) have a similar effect on the hormonal milieu of the lactating woman. One of the errors in Western child care is the early, forced introduction of solids. In most cases, the infant's gut is filled with slowly digesting food with less nutritional quality than either artificial breast milk or breast milk. The long-term result may be childhood and adolescent obesity. The most logical time to start solid food substitution is when the infant has reached the neurologic maturity to grasp and bring food to its mouth from his or her mother's plate. The required neurologic maturity to perform this behavior usually occurs at about 6 months. As the infant matures, his or her ability to feed improves and the proportion of the diet supplied by solid food gradually increases.

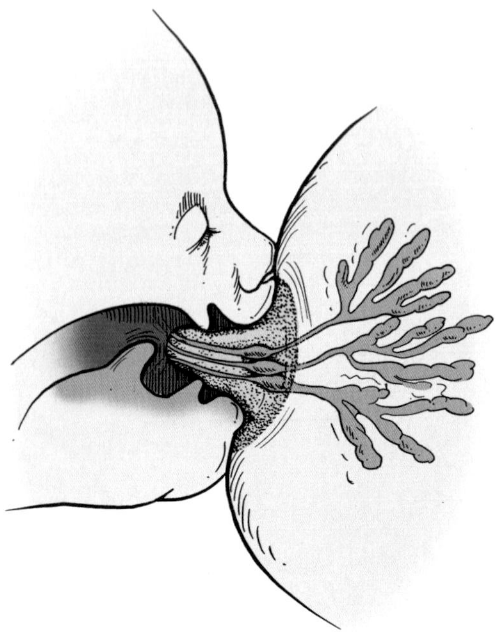

Figure 22-11. Breast-feeding and engorgement. The firm swollen breast parenchyma pushes the newborn's face away, and she is unable to pull the teat into her mouth. Her tongue abrades the tip of the nipple.

The failure to develop good milk transfer is the major cause of lactational failure and breast pain, especially in the neonatal period. Inhibition of the let-down reflex and failure to empty the breasts completely leads to ductal distention and parenchymal swelling (engorgement). Engorgement compromises the mechanics of nursing (Fig. 22-11), and alveolar distention reduces secretion of milk by the alveolar cells. Without adequate transfer of milk to the infant, lactation is doomed to fail. Distention of the alveoli by retained milk causes a rapid (6 to 12 hours) decrease in milk secretion and enzyme activity by the alveolar epithelium. The decreased production of milk is explained by pressure inhibition and by an inhibitor that is secreted in breast milk.[85–88] Distention of the alveoli inhibits secretion directly rather than indirectly by a decrease in nutriment or hormonal access.

BREAST MILK: THE GOLD STANDARD

One of the most common misperceptions by physicians and the lay public is that modern formulas for artificial breast milk are equivalent to breast milk. Human breast milk is uniquely suited to our biologic needs and remains the best source of nutrition for the human infant. Human breast-milk has a composition very different than that of bovine milk or soybean plants from which artificial breast milk is produced.[117]

In contrast with most other animals, the human secretory immune system is not completely functional at birth. Although the passive transplacental transfer of maternal IgG starts at 20 weeks, fetal levels do not approach maternal levels until term. By 3 months of age, the infant must rely on its own secretory response. The newborn's IgM and IgA responses are näive and incomplete. For example, in the presence of active antigen-positive cytomegalovirus infection at birth, 20 percent of infants are IgM negative. A newborn's cellular response is likewise immature; functional impairment is evident for months after birth. Breast milk provides necessary support for the developing immune system.[118,119] The powerful anti-infective qualities of breast milk are measured by decreased infant mortality in developing countries, where exclusive breast-feeding is the norm. In first-world countries, the anti-infective benefits of exclusive breast-feeding are measured by decreased mortality[55] and fewer hospitalizations.[60]

The composition of mature human milk is very different from artificial breast milk or "formula." Most artificial breast milk products use bovine milk as a substrate. Minerals, vitamins, protein, carbohydrates, and fats are added to pasteurized bovine milk for perceived nutritional needs as well as marketing needs in order to make a product that will successfully compete with human breast milk. Human breast milk appears "thinner" than bovine milk. Artificial breast milk manufacturers add constituents to make artificial breast milk appear rich and creamy. Fats such as palm or coconut oil are useful in producing a thick, creamy appearance.

Extensive research has described the unique composition of human milk. The infant formula industry has produced even greater volumes of data concerning their attempts to exactly reproduce human milk. The complete review of the composition of human milk is well beyond the scope of this chapter.[120] In 1980, the U.S. Congress passed the Infant Formula Act (with revisions in 1985) as the result of severe health consequences when artificial breast milk failed to include key vitamins and minerals in new formula compositions. This law now requires that all formulas for artificial breast milk contain minimum amounts of essential nutriments, vitamins, and minerals. Although life-threatening omissions are unlikely, current formulas for artificial breast milk have major differences in the total quantities and qualities of proteins, carbohydrates, and fats when compared with human milk.[117,121,122]

The nutritional differences between artificial breast milk and human milk are reflected in differences in the growth patterns of infants who are exclusively breast-fed for 4 to 6 months and infants who are fed artificial breast milk.[123] In general, breast-fed infants have faster linear and head growth, whereas artificial breast milk–fed infants tend to have greater weight gain and fat deposition. The greater deposition in fat may relate in part to the earlier introduction of solid foods in the infant fed artificial breast milk, a factor that has not been adequately controlled in current studies. Regardless of the cause, greater fat deposition in infants fed artificial breast milk has important adverse effects on the child and the future health of the society. Infant feeding using artificial breast milk is associated with a higher incidence of adolescent obesity, which predicts significant increases in adult morbidity such as obesity, type 2 diabetes mellitus, coronary heart disease, and hypertension[67,68,124] (see Table 22-4).

At birth, the fetus enters an unsterile world with an immature immune system. Full development of the immune system may take up to 6 years. Breast milk has a wide array of anti-infective properties that will support the developing immune system.[118,119,125] The major mechanisms for the protective properties of breast milk include active leukocytes, antibodies, antibacterial products, and competitive inhibition.[125] Active leukocytes[126] are completely eliminated by pasteurization or freezing. Breast milk contains 4,000 cells/mm^3: 90 percent macrophages, 5 percent T-cell lymphocytes, 3 percent B-cell lymphocytes, and 2 percent plasma cells/neutrophils. The concentration of these cells is higher in the first week of breast-feeding. Later, the concentration decreases, but the change in the absolute number is not dramatic.

A critical event in host resistance is the recognition of pathogenic agents in the environment and the production of an antigen-specific response. Breast-feeding provides a unique system to help the infant fight infection with antigen-specific responses. The infant is at risk for infection by the same organism that is likely to infect the mother. Through breast milk, the neonate takes advantage of maternal recognition of these infectious agents. This important mechanism is depicted in Figure 22-12 and reviewed by Slade and Schwartz.[127] An antigen or infectious agent (virus, bacteria, fungus, and protozoa) stimulates the activity of leukocytes in the gastrointestinal or respiratory tract of the mother. Lymphocytes, which are encoded with the antigen signature, travel to the nearest lymph node and stimulate lymphoblasts to develop cytotoxic T cells, helper T cells, and plasma cells programmed to destroy the initiating antigen through phagocytosis or complement/immunoglobulins produced by the B cells. The response is amplified by the migration of committed helper lymphocytes to other sites of white blood cell production, the spleen and bone marrow, where they stimulate the production of antigen-specific committed white blood cells. Some of the committed, antigen-specific helper lymphocytes travel to the mucosa of the breast in the lactating mother. They may migrate into the breast milk (macrophages) or may produce immunoglobulin (lymphocytes or plasma cells). Both are uniquely programmed to fight the specific infectious agent challenging the mother.

Immunoglobulins are a unique component of breast milk but are absent in artificial breast milk.[118,119,125–127] Immunoglobulins constitute a sizable portion of the protein content of early milk (colostrum) for the first 2 to 4 days. In serum, the concentration of monomeric IgA is one fifth the concentration of IgG. In breast milk, the ratio is reversed. During the first day of lactation, the concentrations of immunoglobulins are IgA, 600 mg/dl; IgM, 125 mg/dl; and IgG, 80 mg/dl. By day 4, the concentration, but not absolute amount, has fallen to a steady level; IgA, 80 mg/dl; IgM, 30 mg/dl; and IgG, 16 mg/dl. Other immunoglobulin classes are found in small amounts, but their function is not well understood. In contrast to monomeric serum IgA, the secretory immunoglobulin A (sIgA) in breast milk is dimeric or polymeric. Polymerization improves transport across the mucous membrane into

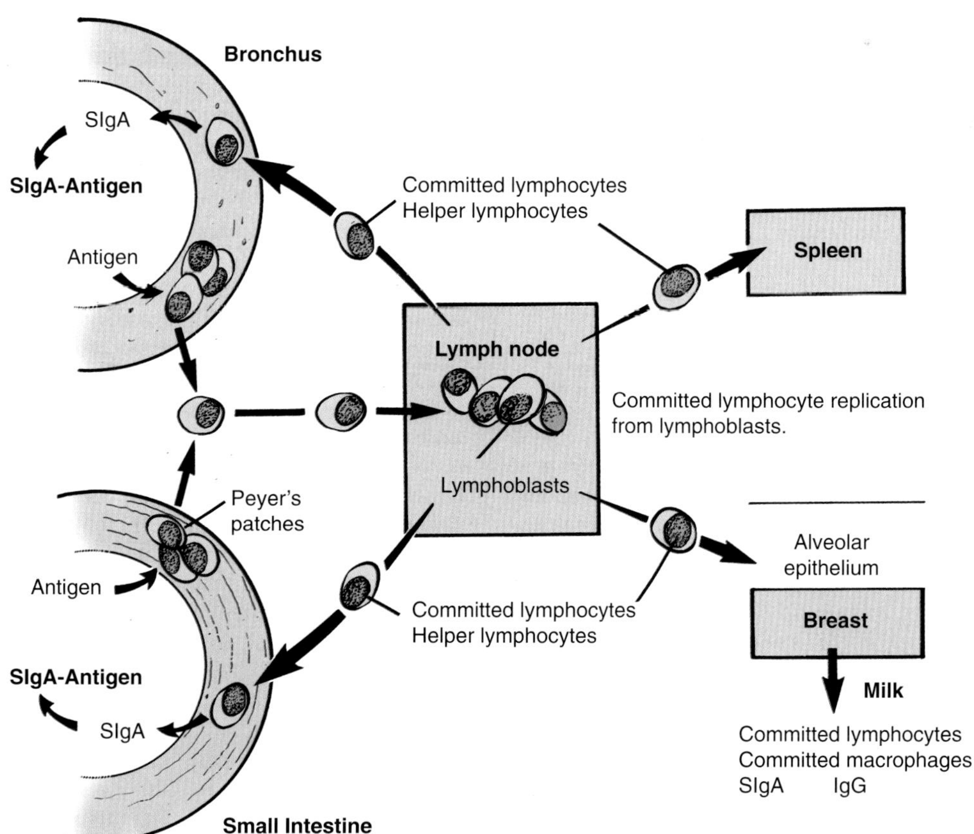

Figure 22-12. The immunology of the breast.

the breast milk. The sIgA is produced locally by plasma cells. Plasma cells, which produce sIgA, constitute 50 to 80 percent of the leukocytes in the breast submucosa.

The immunoglobulins in breast milk appear to be fully functional. sIgA does not activate complement or promote opsonic complement subfragments. As a consequence, sIgA is not bactericidal. It appears that sIgA blocks the mucosal receptors (adhesins) on the infectious agent. The virulence of pathogens is related to their ability to use adhesins capable of interacting with complementary epithelial cell–surface receptors. When the antigen-specific sIgA attaches, the pathogen is effectively neutralized.

Certain vitamins and minerals are essential for the growth of pathogenic bacteria. A major mechanism by which breast milk protects the infant is the competition for "essential" nutriments of pathogenic bacteria. Iron and vitamin B_{12} are two essential nutriments for pathogenic bacteria that have been studied relative to breast milk. Breast milk contains lactoferrin, an iron-binding glycoprotein, in large quantities (5.5 mg/ml in the colostrum to 1.5 mg/ml in mature milk) and is absent in artificial breast milk. The free iron form of lactoferrin competes with siderophilic bacteria for ferric iron, and thus disrupts the proliferation of these organisms.[128] The binding of iron to lactoferrin also enhances iron absorption; less iron is required in breast milk in order to satisfy the iron needs of the infant. The antibacterial role of lactoferrin is more complex than simple competition for ferric iron.[129] Lactoferrin causes a release of lipopolysaccharide molecules from the bacterial cell wall. This process appears to sensitize the cell wall to attack by lysozyme. Lactoferrin and lysozyme work together to destroy the pathogenic organisms.[130–133]

In summary, breast milk is uniquely composed to satisfy the biologic needs of the human infant. In particular, the uniquely human need for brain development and immune system support are provided by breast milk and not by artificial breast milk. Many of the documented benefits of breast-feeding are directly related to the unique composition of breast milk and the failure of artificial breast milk to replicate human milk.

THE ROLE OF THE OBSTETRICIAN AND GYNECOLOGIST

The gynecologist plays a primary role in the initiation of breast-feeding.[134] Fifty percent of women choose the method they will use to feed their infant before their pregnancy. The gynecologist needs to start promotion before the first pregnancy. As the reproductive-aged woman seeks initially family planning advice and contraception, there is high likelihood that she will become pregnant in the next 2 to 5 years. The breast examination is a regular part of the family planning visit, performed to screen for breast cancer despite its rare occurrence at the ages of usual pregnancies, which is younger than 35 years of age. This visit is a good opportunity to reassure the woman of her normal breast anatomy and build her self-efficacy for lactation success through vocal and visible support of breast-feeding.

The obstetrician/gynecologist amplifies support for breast-feeding by community advocacy, office environment, and personal choices. The office environment needs to be "breast-feeding friendly." Visible, active support of breast-feeding includes the presence of breast-feeding mothers, patient educational programs on breast-feeding, a quiet area for nursing mothers, the absence of material supplied by formula companies, and visible support for office personnel who choose to breast-feed. The physician, especially the young female obstetrician/gynecologist, is an important role model for patients. Women will ask the female gynecologist whether and how long she breast-fed her children. Her answers will have a powerful influence.

The support of the obstetrician begins at the first prenatal visit and continues through the mother's total breast-feeding experience. At the first prenatal visit, the method of infant feeding is identified, her choice to breast-feed is verbally reinforced, gaps in her knowledge are identified, and an educational plan is recommended. The educational plan may include reference reading, specific classes on breast-feeding, identification of a "breast-feeding–friendly pediatrician," and introduction to community resources, such as support groups (La Leche League International). At the initial physical examination, the breasts are examined for anatomic abnormalities that might influence the success of breast-feeding, such as hypoplasia, nipple inversion, and surgical scars.

At the 36-week visit, the obstetrician readdresses the mother's choice and knowledge regarding breast-feeding. Simple concepts of breast-feeding physiology are reinforced: early feeds, frequent feeds (>10 per day), reinforcing environment, and no supplementation unless directed by a pediatrician. The obstetrician reinforces the appropriate way to latch the baby to the breast and ensures that the increase in her breast size reflects the hormonal readiness for breast-feeding. The patient is warned of hospital policies and attitudes that interfere with breast-feeding success. The 36-week visit is a good time to address the appropriateness of medications and breast-feeding.

At delivery and during the postpartum hospitalization, the obstetrician is the champion for the application of breast-feeding physiology; early to the breast (<1 hour) after birth, frequent feeds (>10 per day), appropriate nursing behavior (latch-on), continuous mother-infant contact (rooming-in), and no infant supplementation unless directed by the infant's physician. As an advocate for breast-feeding, the obstetrician must be willing to confront administrative and nursing protocols that are designed for control and efficiency rather than optimal care for the breast-feeding dyad.

National and international health organizations have long recognized the barriers that modern medical care and hospitals raise against successful breast-feeding. In 1989, WHO initiated the Baby Friendly Hospital initiative. The 10 steps by which a hospital might be designated "baby friendly" are outlined in Table 22-5. The United States is the only developed country not to fully endorse the initiative, primarily as a result of the influence on Congress by the powerful formula company lobby. As of the year 2006, less than 70 of the more than 2,000 hospitals worldwide that have been designated baby

Table 22-5. Ten Steps to Successful Breast-Feeding

1. Have a written policy to support breast-feeding.
2. Train all health care providers.
3. Inform all pregnant women about the benefits of management of breast-feeding.
4. Initiate breast-feeding within 1 hour after birth.
5. Show mothers how to breast-feed and maintain lactation even if they are separated from their infants.
6. Give newborn infants no food or drink other than breast milk, unless medically indicated.
7. Allow mothers and infants to remain together 24 hours a day, that is, rooming in.
8. Encourage breastfeeding on demand.
9. Give no artificial teats or pacifiers.
10. Foster the establishment of breastfeeding support groups and refer mothers to them on discharge from the hospital or clinic.

Adapted from WHO/UNICEF: Protesting, promoting, and supporting breastfeeding: The special role of maternity services, a joint WHO/UNICEF statement, Geneva, 1989, World Health Organization.

friendly are in the United States. The biggest challenge to hospitals in the United States in becoming baby friendly is the forbearance of artificial breast milk donations and direct in-hospital marketing by the artificial breast milk companies. The obstetrician has a role in supporting the baby-friendly initiative.

After postpartum discharge, the obstetrician is primarily focused on maternal concerns about breast-feeding: maternal diet, breast symptoms and signs, hormonal function postpartum, contraception, and maternal medications. The obstetrician is also a breast-feeding advocate when the mother is referred to other specialists. A secondary but equally important focus is the growth and development of the infant. Traditionally, the obstetrician sees the mother at 4 to 6 weeks postpartum, but often the obstetrician and the mother communicate before that visit. By inquiring about the growth and feeding of her infant, the obstetrician provides an important reinforcement of the mother's decision to breast-feed and an important screen for the pediatrician regarding the growth and feeding of the infant. The obstetrician can identify critical or developing problems regarding infant growth and feeding for the pediatrician. The obstetrician must know the indicators of adequate infant growth and clinical indicators that milk is being produced and transferred. When the obstetrician remains a verbal participant in the mother's breast-feeding experience at the 4- to 6-week postpartum visit, the likelihood that the mother will continue to breast-feed at 16 weeks is almost doubled.[135] During the interpregnancy interval, the obstetrician/gynecologist identifies the challenges, myths, and obstacles in the last pregnancy and helps correct them for the subsequent lactational period.

SUCCESSFUL MANAGEMENT OF BREAST-FEEDING

The successful management of breast-feeding requires the active cooperation of the mother, her support group, the obstetric care provider, and infant care provider. In our current culture, a lactation consultant often becomes an active participant in the care of the breast-feeding dyad. There are numerous reliable reference texts for additional information. They include *Breastfeeding: a Guide For The Medical Profession*,[136] *The Breastfeeding Answer Book*,[137] *The Womanly Art of Breastfeeding*,[138] *Drugs In Pregnancy and Lactation*,[139] *Medication and Mother's Milk*,[140] and *Breastfeeding Handbook for Physicians*.[141]

ANATOMIC ABNORMALITIES OF THE BREAST

The relationship between breast anatomy and lactation should be addressed during the well-woman or family planning visits in women who anticipate future pregnancy. During pregnancy, infant feeding becomes a major focus, and the woman needs this issue addressed, because often there are hidden questions and concerns regarding her adequacy to breast-feed. The breast examination at the first prenatal visit is an excellent opportunity to address infant feeding concerns and myths relative to her breast anatomy. Self-doubt concerning the size or shape of the breasts should be addressed, and the patient should be reassured that less than 5 percent of lactational failures are caused by faulty anatomy.

Congenital abnormalities of the breasts (excluding inverted nipples) are rare; these abnormalities are present in less than 1 in 1,000 women. The most significant defect is glandular hypoplasia. These women have no development or abnormal development of one or both breasts during sexual maturation. Women with no development of the breasts often have normally shaped and sized nipples and areolas, and they may have sought consultation from a plastic surgeon. One manifestation of abnormal development is referred to as the *tubular breast*. The nipple and areola, which are often normal in size, shape, and appearance, are attached to a tube of fibrous cords. Whatever the shape or size of the breasts in a nonpregnant woman, the final evaluation of adequate glandular tissue must await the expected growth during pregnancy. The size of the average breast will grow from 200 g to 600 g during pregnancy; most women will easily recognize this growth. A routine screening question at the 36-week prenatal visit should be, "Have your breasts grown during pregnancy?" If the response is negative in a woman with unusually small or abnormally shaped breasts, lactational failure is a possibility, and prenatal consultation with a lactation expert is recommended. Unilateral abnormalities are usually not a problem except for increased asymmetry, because the normal breast can usually produce more than enough milk for the infant. The texture of the breast and tethering of the nipple are also assessed. An inelastic breast gives the impression that the skin is fixed to dense underlying tissue, whereas the elastic breast allows elevation of the skin and subcutaneous tissue from the parenchyma. Lack of elasticity may complicate nursing because of increased rigidity with engorgement. Massage of the periareolar tissue four times a day for 10 minutes is recommended. Engorgement should be assiduously avoided in the postpartum period by early, frequent nursing.

Congenital tethering of the nipple to underlying fascia is diagnosed by squeezing the outer edge of the areola (Fig. 22-13); normally, the nipple will protrude. Severe tethering is manifested by an inverted nipple. The most severe forms of tethering occur in less than 1 percent of women. Although successful breast-feeding is possible in these severe cases, prenatal consultation and close follow-up are very important to identify and treat poor milk transfers. Flat or inverted nipples are much less likely to preclude successful breast-feeding. Three prenatal methods of treating tethered nipples have been described: nipple pulling, Hoffman's exercises, and nipple cups (shells). A controlled trial failed to demonstrate efficacy[142] of either shells or Hoffman's exercises and recommended that these should be abandoned.

In the early neonatal period, a breast pump may be of help in women with flat or inverted nipples. The breast is gently pumped at low settings until the teat is drawn out. The infant is immediately offered that breast. The same procedure is performed on the other side. Usually, this is only required for a few days. If it is required for more than a few days, a relatively cheap alternative can be created from a 10- or 20-ml plastic syringe, the sizes depending on the size of the nipple.[143] The end of the syringe where the needle attaches is removed and the plunger is reversed. The nipple is placed in the smooth, plunger end of the syringe and gentle traction is applied until the nipple everts. Although pumping and syringe suction are practical solutions, no controlled trials have supported their efficacy.

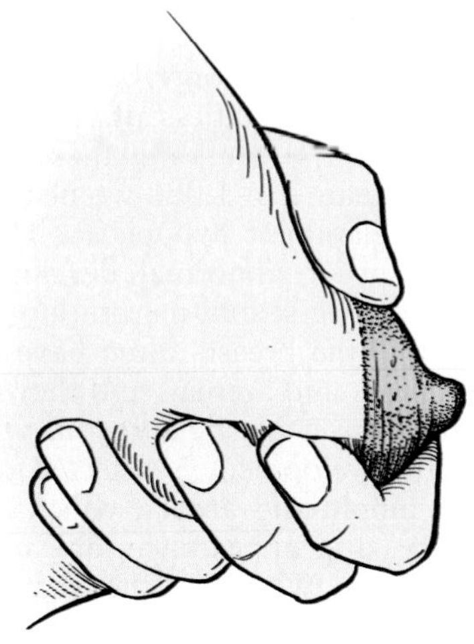

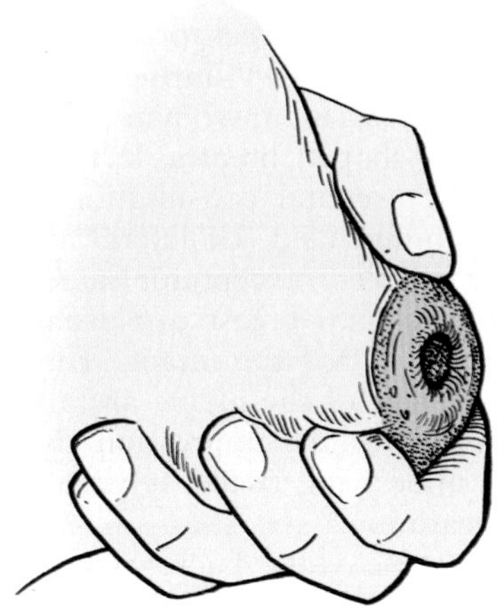

Figure 22-13. Assessment of nipple tethering.

Modern clothing (especially protective brassieres) prevents friction that toughens the skin and helps protect the nipple from cracking during early lactation. In the second half of pregnancy, nipple skin may be toughened by wearing a nursing brassiere with the flaps open. However, washing with harsh soaps; buffing the nipple with a towel; and using alcohol, benzoin, or other drying agents are not helpful and may increase the incidence of cracking. Normally, the breast is washed with clean water and should be left to air dry. A cautiously used sunlamp or hair dryer may facilitate drying. Trials involving application of breast cream or expression of colostrum have not shown a reduction in nipple trauma or sensitivity, when compared with those with untreated nipples.

Previous breast surgery may have significant adverse effects on breast-feeding success. The major issues are loss of sensation in the nipple or areola by nerve injury or compromise of the lactiferous ducts. Women who have had breast surgery, breast biopsy, chest surgery, or augmentation have a threefold higher incidence of unsuccessful breast-feeding.[80] Circumareolar skin incisions, which are used for cosmetic considerations in breast biopsies or breast augmentation, may compromise both the nerve and ducts. Breast augmentation has significant potential to disrupt breast-feeding.[144] In a carefully studied, prospective series, 27 of 42 (64 percent) of women who exclusively breast-fed after preconceptional breast augmentation had insufficient lactation, and the infant growth rate was less than 20 g/day. Circumareolar incision was the dominant predictor. One half of women with a submammary or axillary incision had insufficient lactation, whereas all 11 women after a circumareolar incision for breast augmentation had lactation failure. Loss of nipple sensation occurs in one third to one half of patients after circumareolar incision. If the woman has had a silicone implant, she can be reassured that there is no evidence that breast-feeding places her infant at risk. The concentration of silicone in artificial formula or cow's milk is 5 to 10 times higher than in breast milk from women who have silicone implants.[145] Large epidemiologic studies of infants who have nursed from breasts with silicone implants have not shown excess adverse events.[146]

Reduction mammoplasty is always associated with lactation insufficiency if exclusive breast-feeding is relied on for infant nutrition. If the reduction involves the removal of greater than 500 g per breast or the procedure uses the free nipple graft technique, the production of a nominal amount of breast milk is rare. If the nipple and areola are relocated on a pedicle of vascular tissue and ducts, partial breast-feeding is a possibility. In any case of reconstructive surgery on the breast (e.g., augmentation or reduction), the breast-feeding dyad is considered at high risk for lactation failure. This observation was recently confirmed by a controlled study.[147] The control and mammoplasty groups reported any breast-feeding at 1 month at a rate of 94 percent and 58 percent, respectively. Similarly, the rate of exclusive breast-feeding at 1 month was 70 percent and 21 percent in the respective groups. Prenatal referral to an expert on lactation is appropriate.

LABOR AND DELIVERY MANAGEMENT

Approximately 15 percent of women who state they wish to breast-feed at the onset of term labor are discharged either completely feeding their infant artificial breast milk or giving the majority of the infant's feeds as artificial breast milk. A combination of obstetric management, hospital policies, and pediatric management contribute to this attrition. Obstetric interventions are often critical for the health of the mother or infant, but they may affect the success of lactation.[148] Few, if any, interventions directly inhibit the physiology of lactation. Most obstetric interventions reduce the success of lactation by indirect interference with physiology. Induction of labor is not associated with lactation failure, but a long, tiring induction and labor will reduce the likelihood that the mother will get appropriate amounts of infant contact in the delivery room and in the first 24 hours after birth. Cesarean delivery reduces the incidence of breast-feeding by 10 to 20 percent in the first week after birth.[149] After most cesarean deliveries[149] and difficult vaginal deliveries,[150] the infant is not put to the breast immediately after birth, nor will the mother breast-feed her infant more than eight times in the first 24 hours. Well-meaning nurses become concerned for the baby's nutrition, and artificial breast milk is given to the infant until the mother "recovers." Labor analgesia (i.e., meperidine and promethazine) has long been associated with poor breast-feeding success. Intrapartum narcotics appear to adversely affect the infant's ability to nurse effectively.[111,151–153] Epidural anesthesia with local anesthetic agents seems to be better for breast-feeding than parenteral narcotics. Epidural anesthesia with local anesthetics does not appear to have a major effect. The impact of epidural or intrathecal narcotics on sucking behavior and lactation success has been shown to decrease breast-feeding success in a double-blind study with random assignment of subjects.[153] The presence of a doula, or a labor companion other than family, appears to be an effective method to reduce the need for epidural anesthesia and operative deliveries.[154,155] An added benefit is earlier initiation and longer duration of breast-feeding.[155] Postsurgical pain control is best achieved with morphine rather than meperidine, which adversely affects neonatal behavior. Obstetric and pediatric protocols can be very effective in separating mother and baby. Several prominent examples include magnesium sulfate therapy for preeclampsia, a positive maternal group B streptococcus culture, maternal fever work-up, and diabetes mellitus/hypoglycemia protocols. All of these medical interventions produce major barriers to delivery room nursing and an inadequate frequency of nursing in the first 24 to 48 hours.

The peripartum period is critical for achieving successful lactation. The obstetrician must apply the five basic principles of lactation physiology: early imprinting, frequent nursing, good latch-on, a confident and comfortable mother, and no supplementation unless medically indicated. Nursing should be initiated within 30 minutes after birth, preferably in the delivery room. Contraindications include (1) a heavily medicated mother; (2) an infant with a 5-minute Apgar score result less than 6; or (3) a premature infant at less than 36 weeks' gestation.

The instructor should pay special attention to the mother's position during the first feeding; she should be in a relaxed, comfortable position. With skin-to-skin contact, the infant is presented to the breast with its ventral surface to the mother's ventral surface. A dry neonate, skin-to-skin contact, and supplemental radiant heating will prevent neonatal cold stress. Routine eye treatment should be delayed, because it may disrupt the important family bonding process.

In the recovery room and on the ward, the best place for the neonate is with the mother. This maximizes mother-infant bonding and allows "on-demand" feeding every 1 to 2 hours. Rooming-in allows the mother to participate in the care of her baby and gives her an opportunity to ask questions. The mother should be encouraged to sleep when the neonate sleeps. Because the hospital runs on an adult diurnal pattern, the patient should be discharged early in order to get her rest.

The frequency of early feeding is proportional to milk production and weight gain in neonates.[156] Therefore, supplementation with glucose or formula should be discouraged. Supplementation decreases milk production through a reduction in nursing frequency by satiation of the neonate and slower digestion of formula. Supplementation also undermines the mother's confidence about her lactational adequacy.[111,158] When obstetricians give information at the first prenatal visit about breast-feeding that was developed by makers of artificial breast milk, the duration of breast-feeding is significantly reduced when compared to packet information on breast-feeding developed by "breast-feeding–friendly" obstetricians and pediatricians. A randomized assignment to give or not to give free formula samples at the time of discharge demonstrated a significantly reduced incidence of breast-feeding at 1 month and an increased likelihood of solid food introduction by the mothers given the formula samples.[157–159] This was most significant in high-risk groups: those less educated, primiparas, and those reporting illness since leaving the hospital.

Other factors influencing the success of lactation are improper positioning and nursing technique, which can lead to increased nipple trauma and incomplete emptying. In the early postpartum period, nursing technique should be evaluated in three areas: presentation and latching-on, maternal-infant positioning, and breaking of the suction. The infant should not have to turn its head to nurse. A ventral surface-to-ventral surface presentation is necessary. When latching-on to the nipple, the neonate should take as much of the areola as possible into its mouth. This is facilitated by gently stimulating the baby's cheek to elicit a yawn-like opening of its mouth and rapid placement of the breast into it. A supporting hand on the breast helps; the C-hold involves four fingers cupping and supporting the weight of the breast, which is especially important in the weak or premature neonate, whose lower jaw may be depressed by the weight of the breast. The thumb rests above and 1 to 2 cm away from the areolar edge and points the nipple downward. Retraction by the thumb will pull the areola away from the mouth and cause an incorrect placement. Any position that is comfortable and convenient, while allowing the appropriate mouth-areola attachment, should be encouraged; the sitting position is the most common. In patients who have had a cesarean delivery in whom pressure on the abdomen is uncomfortable, a side-lying or football hold may be better. A rotation of positions is recommended to reduce focal pressure on the nipple and to ensure complete emptying. Removal of the nursing infant can be a problem; suction by the neonate can injure the nipple if it is not broken before disengagement. A finger inserted between the baby's lips and the breast will break the suction.

The single most difficult management issue is the control of routines and hospital attitudes detrimental to lactation. Policies that worked against the physiology of lactation included formula distribution and supplementation without a medical indication, constant questioning of the mother about breast-feeding, preprinted orders for lactation suppression medication, pediatric clearance before the first feeding, limited maternal access to the infant, and little educational material for new mothers or staff.

When providers are not well informed or are apathetic about lactation, success of lactation is unlikely. This theme underscores the role of the physician in educating patients, nursing staff, and support personnel about the physiology and benefits of lactation.

MATERNAL NUTRITION

The efficiency of conversion of maternal foodstuff to milk is about 80 to 90 percent. If the average milk volume per day is 900 ml, and milk has an average energy content of 75 kcal/dl, the mother must consume an extra 794 kcal/day, unless stored energy is used. During pregnancy, most women store an extra 2 to 5 kg (19,000 to 48,000 kcal) in tissue, mainly as fat, in physiologic preparation for lactation.[160] These calories and nutrients supplement the maternal diet during lactation. As a result, the required dietary increases are easily attainable in healthy mothers and infants.

In lactation, most vitamins and minerals should be increased 20 to 30 percent over nonpregnant requirements. Folic acid should be doubled. Calcium, phosphorus, and magnesium should be increased by 40 to 50 percent, especially in the teenager who is lactating. In practical terms, these needs can be supplied by the following additions to the diet: 2 cups of milk, 2 oz of meat or peanut butter, a slice of enriched or whole wheat bread, a citrus fruit, a salad, and an extra helping (one half to three quarters of a cup) of a dark green or yellow vegetables. The appropriate intake of vitamins can be ensured by continuing prenatal vitamins with 1 mg of folic acid through the lactation. The mother should drink at least 1 extra liter of fluid per day to make up for the fluid loss through milk.

Vegetarianism has become increasingly more common, and if this is the case, dietary deficiencies may include B vitamins (especially B_{12}), total protein, and the full complement of essential amino acids. The recommendation should be to take a good dietary history with the focus on protein, iron, calcium, and vitamins D and B; supplement with soy flour, molasses, or nuts; use complementary vegetable protein combinations; and avoid excess phytate and bran.

Many women are concerned about losing weight postpartum.[160,161] If 700 to 1,200 kcal are used daily to nourish an infant, a mother could lose weight by not increasing her caloric intake, but a thoughtful selection of food groups and the elimination of "empty calories" are necessary. A reduction of total calories (<25 kcal/kg) and total protein (<0.6 g/kg) may reduce the daily milk volume by 20 to 30 percent but not the milk quality, unless the mother is more than 10 percent below her ideal body weight. Because dieting mobilizes fat stores that may contain environmental toxins, women with high exposure to such toxins should not lose weight during lactation.

BREAST AND NIPPLE PAIN

Breast or nipple pain is one of the most frequent complaints of lactating mothers.[161] The frequency is related to failure in the initial management of lactation: late first feed, decreased frequency of feedings, poor nipple grasp, or poor positioning. The differential diagnosis of breast pain includes problems with latching-on, engorgement, nipple trauma, mastitis, and occasionally, the let-down reflex.

Symptoms and the infant's personality help make the differential diagnosis. In some cases, the nipple and breast pain starts with latching-on and diminishes with let-down. Women describe the let-down reflex as painful; this occurs after the first minute of sucking and usually lasts only a minute or two as the ductal swelling is relieved by nursing. Classically, the anxious, vigorous infant, who sucks strongly against empty ducts until the let-down occurs, is associated with this pain pattern. Contact pain suggests nipple trauma and may persist as long as the nipple is manipulated. The nipple-confused infant who chews on the nipple and abrades the tip with his tongue is associated with this pattern. Engorgement causes a dull, generalized discomfort in the whole breast, worse just before a feed and relieved by it. Localized, unilateral, and continuous pain in the breast may be caused by mastitis.[162]

A physical examination and observation of nursing technique can confirm the impression left by a good history. Through observation of a nursing episode, an infant's personality and nursing technique can be assessed. The whole of the nipple and much of the areola should be included in the infant's mouth. An examination of the nipple may reveal a fissure or blood blister. Bilateral breast firmness and tenderness may indicate engorgement. Engorgement may be peripheral, periareolar, or both. Mastitis is characterized by fever, malaise, localized erythema, heat, tenderness, and induration (see later).

Infection may be a cofactor associated with the pain of nipple injury. When the microbiology of the nipple/milk of 61 lactating women with nipple pain was compared with that of 64 lactating women without nipple pain and 31 nonlactating women, *Candida albicans* (19 percent) and *Staphylococcus aureus* (30 percent) were more common in women with pain and nipple fissures than in controls (3 to 5 percent).[163] Antibiotics may be effective in the treatment of nipple pain and trauma.[164]

The management of breast pain consists of general as well as specific steps. Prevention is a key component. Appropriate nursing technique and positioning will prevent, or significantly decrease, the incidence of nipple trauma, engorgement, and mastitis. Rotation of nursing position reduces the suction pressure on the same part of the nipple, as well as ensuring complete emptying of all lobules of the breast. Frequent nursing reduces engorgement and milk stasis. The use of soaps, alcohol, and other drying agents on the nipples tends to increase nipple trauma and pain. The nipples should be air dried for a few minutes after each feed, and clean water is sufficient to cleanse the breast, if necessary. Some experts recommend that fresh breast milk be applied to the nipples and allowed to dry after each feed.

Stimulating a let-down and manual expression of milk is useful in the management of many breast problems. The flow of milk can be improved by placing the mother in a quiet, relaxed environment. The breast is massaged in a spiral fashion, starting at the top and moving toward the areola; the fingers are moved in a circular fashion from one spot to another, much like a breast examination. After the massage, the breast is stroked from the top of the breast to the nipple with a light stroke and shaken, while the woman leans forward. Once milk starts to flow, manual expression is begun.

Manual expression is performed by holding the thumb and first two fingers on either side of the areola, in a half circle, but the breast should not be cupped. The hand pushes the breast straight into the chest wall, as the thumb and fingers are rolled forward. Large, pendulous breasts may need lifting before this. The maneuver is repeated in all four quadrants of the areola to drain as many reservoirs as possible. The procedure is repeated rhythmically and gently, because squeezing, sliding, or pulling may injure the breast. The sequence of massage, stroke, shake, and express is useful in providing milk immediately for the vigorous infant, in allowing an improved latch-on by reducing periareolar engorgement, and in reducing high suction pressures on a traumatized nipple. The let-down produced by manual expression is never as complete as a normally elicited one. An effective let-down can by elicited by initiating nursing on the side without nipple trauma or mastitis. This will effectively reduce breast pain.

In the first 5 days after birth, about 35 percent of the nipples of breast-feeding mothers show damage, and 69 percent of mothers have nipple pain.[163–165] The management of painful, tender, or injured nipples includes prefeeding manual expression, correction of latching-on, rotation of positions, and initiation of nursing on the less painful side first, with the affected side exposed to air. Drying is facilitated by the cautious application of dry heat (e.g., with hair dryer on low setting) for 20 minutes four times per day. Aspirin or codeine (15 to 30 mg) given 30 minutes before nursing may be helpful in severe cases. Engorgement can be avoided, but if it occurs, feeding frequency should be maintained or increased by pumping. A wide variety of preparations have been applied to traumatized nipples, including lanolin, A & D ointment, white petrolatum, antibiotics, vitamin E oil, and used tea bags, but few of these methods have been evaluated scientifically. Soap and alcohol have been shown to injure nipples. Nipple shields should be used only as a last resort because of a 20- to 60-percent reduction in milk consumption. Thin latex shields may be better than the traditional red rubber ones, although milk flow is still reduced by 22 percent.[166]

Engorgement of the breast occurs when there is inadequate drainage of milk.[167] Swollen, firm, and tender breasts are caused by distention of the ducts and increased extravascular fluid. Aside from the discomfort, engorgement leads to dysfunctional nursing behavior and nipple trauma. The firm breast tissue pushes the infant's face away from the nipple. The widened base of the nipple disrupts the attachment, and the infant's thrusting tongue abrades the tip. This leads to further engorgement, decreased milk production, and in some cases, early termination of breast-feeding.

The best treatment is prevention, but when this has not occurred, management is centered on symptomatic support and relief of distention. Proper elevation of the breasts is important. The mother should wear a firm-fitting nursing brassiere, with neither thin straps nor plastic lining. A warm shower or bath, with prefeed manual expression, is effective. Frequent suckling (every 1 to 2 hours) is the most effective mechanism to relieve engorgement; postfeed electric pumping from each breast may be helpful. In selected cases, intranasal oxytocin may be given just before each feed if let-down seems to be inhibited.

MASTITIS AND BREAST ABSCESS

Mastitis is an infectious process of the breast characterized by high fever (39° to 40°C), localized erythema, tenderness, induration, and palpable heat over the area. Often, these signs are associated with nausea, vomiting, malaise, and other flulike symptoms. Mastitis occurs most frequently in the first 2 to 4 weeks postpartum and at times of marked reduction in nursing frequency. Risk factors include maternal fatigue, poor nursing technique, nipple trauma, and epidemic *S. aureus*. The most common organisms associated with mastitis are *S. aureus*, *S. epidermidis*, streptococci and, occasionally, gram-negative rods. The incidence of sporadic mastitis is 2 to 10 percent in lactating and less than 1 percent in nonlactating mothers.[168,169]

Until recently, the management of mastitis has been directed by retrospective clinical reviews of experience. In most cases, this consisted of bed rest, continued lactation, and antibiotics, with an 80- to 90-percent cure rate, a 10-percent abscess rate, a 10-percent recurrence rate, and a 50-percent cessation of breast-feeding. Starting in 1982, Thomsen et al.[170] published important articles concerning pathophysiology, diagnosis, and treatment of mastitis. He observed that the diagnosis and prognosis of inflammatory symptoms of the breast could be established by counts of leukocytes and bacteria in breast milk. This is obtained after careful washing of the mother's hands and breasts with a mild soap. The milk is manually expressed, and the first 3 ml discarded. A microscopic analysis is performed on an unspun specimen. When the leukocyte count was greater than 10^6 leukocytes/ml and the bacterial count less than 10^3 bacteria/ml, the diagnosis was noninfectious inflammation of the breast. With no treatment, the inflammatory symptoms lasted 7 days; 50 percent developed mastitis, and only 21 percent returned to normal lactation. When the breast was emptied frequently by continued lactation, the symptoms lasted 3 days, and 96 percent returned to normal lactation.

If the breast milk showed greater than 10^6 leukocytes/ml and greater than 10^3 bacteria/ml, the diagnosis was mastitis. Delay in therapy resulted in abscess formation in 11 percent, and only 15 percent returned to normal lactation. Frequent emptying of the infected breast by continued nursing eliminated abscess formation, but only 51 percent returned to normal lactation. Additional antibiotic therapy increased the return to normal lactation in 97 percent with resolution of symptoms in 2.1 days.

In summary, the management of mastitis includes the following: (1) breast support; (2) fluids; (3) assessment of nursing technique; (4) nursing initiated on the uninfected side first to establish let-down; (5) the infected side emptied by nursing with each feed (occasionally, a breast pump helps to ensure complete drainage); and (6) dicloxacillin, 250 mg every 6 hours for 7 days. Erythromycin may be used in patients allergic to penicillin. It is important to continue antibiotics for a full 7 days, because abscess formation is more likely with shorter courses. Hand washing before each feed and by nursing staff reduces nosocomial infection rates. Rooming-in does not reduce the acquisition of hospital strains of *S. aureus* or infection rates. During epidemics, early discharge may reduce infection rates.

Breast abscess occurs in about 10 percent of women who are treated for mastitis. The signs include a high fever (39° to 40°C), and a localized area of erythema, tenderness, and induration. In the center, a fluctuant area may be difficult to palpate. The patient feels ill. Abscesses usually occur in the upper outer quadrants and *S. aureus* is usually cultured from the abscess cavity.

The management of breast abscess is similar to that for mastitis, except that (1) drainage of the abscess is indicated and (2) breast-feeding should be limited to the uninvolved side during the initial therapy. The infected breast should be mechanically pumped every 2 hours and with every let-down. Serial percutaneous needle aspiration under ultrasound guidance[171] is the best and standard method to drain the abscess. Occasionally, surgical drainage is required. The skin incision should be made over the fluctuant area in a manner parallel to and as far as possible from the areolar edge. Although the skin incision follows skin lines, the deeper extension should be made bluntly in a radial direction. Sharp dissection perpendicular to the lactational ducts increases blood loss, the risk of a fistula, and the risk of ductal occlusion. Once the abscess cavity is entered, all loculations are bluntly reduced and the cavity is irrigated with saline. American surgeons pack the wound open for drainage and secondary closure. British surgeons advocate removal of the abscess wall and primary closure. In either case, wide closure sutures should be avoided, because they may compromise the ducts. Patients have a protracted recovery of 18 to 32 days and recurrent abscess formation in 9 to 15 percent of cases. Breast-feeding from the involved side may be resumed if skin erythema and underlying cellulitis have resolved, which may occur in 4 to 7 days.

C. albicans infection is considered a common cause of breast pain.[163] Candida infection of the breast is a commonly diagnosed by clinical presentation. Women describe severe pain when the infant nurses. She will describe the pain as "like a red hot poker being driven through my chest." Often she has received antibiotics recently, has diabetes, or the infant has evidence of oral thrush or diaper rash *(C. albicans)*. A potassium hydroxide (KOH) smear can confirm the diagnosis. A drop of midstream milk is combined with a drop of 10-percent KOH and examined under high-power light microscopy. A typical pattern of hyphae and spores will be visualized. The initial treatment is to massage nystatin cream or miconazole oral gel into both nipples after each feed and in the infant's mouth three times a day for 2 weeks. Recurrent or persistent candida mastitis can be treated by swabbing the infant's mouth with gentian violet liquid (0.5 percent) and immediately latching the baby to the breast, twice a day for 3 days. The major disadvantage of this therapy is the permanent staining associated with gentian violet. An alternative therapy in severe cases is oral fluconazole, 200-mg loading dose followed by 100 mg/day for 14 days.

MILK TRANSFER AND INFANT GROWTH

When is an exclusive diet of breast milk insufficient to supply the nutritional needs of the growing infant? Women who wean in the first 8 weeks most often say that insufficient milk is the reason for quitting, and well-meaning family members often ask, "When are you going to start feeding your child real food?"

Correct answers are not readily available. Many nondietary factors affect the growth of infants, including high birth order, younger maternal age, low maternal weight, poor maternal nutrition during pregnancy, birth interval, birth weight less than 2.4 kg, multiple gestation, infection, death of either parent, and divorce or separation.

In addition, there are inconsistencies in the standard reference charts for growth or nutritional needs. Most growth charts are based on formula-fed infants, who often receive solid food supplementation earlier and in greater proportion than comparable breast-fed infants. Reference charts with sufficiently large numbers of exclusively breast-fed infants from developed countries are lacking. Because milk volume is a quantitative measure of nutrition, variations in volume and concentrations of constituents caused by individual variation and different methods of collection compound the interpretation.

Despite the latter concerns, it is apparent that a healthy and successfully breast-feeding mother can supply enough nutrition through breast milk alone for 6 months. The clinical markers for adequate breast milk transfer include an alert, healthy-appearing infant with good muscle tone, good skin turgor, six wet diapers per day, eight or more nursing episodes per day, three or four loose stools per day, consistent evidence of a let-down with operant conditioning, and consistent weight gain.

The term "failure to thrive" has been used loosely to include all infants who show any degree of growth failure. For the breast-feeding mother, it may just be a matter of comparing the growth of her infant to growth charts compiled from formula-fed infants. The loosely applied term can seriously undermine the mother's confidence, and ill-advised supplementation further compromises milk volume and may mask other important underlying causes. The infant should be evaluated for failure to thrive or slowed growth if (1) it continues to lose weight after 7 days of life (after "the milk has come in," the infant should gain 0.75–1 oz/day); (2) does not regain birth weight by 2 weeks; or (3) gains weight at a rate below the 10th percentile beyond the first months of age. If the infant is premature, ill, or small for gestational age, weight, height, and skin-fold thickness can be used to define adequate growth. The cause of failure to thrive is often complex and is beyond the scope of this chapter.

JAUNDICE IN THE NEWBORN

Ten to fifteen percent of breast-fed neonates have jaundice defined by a peak serum bilirubin greater than 12 mg/dl in term infants.[172] Pediatric concerns include hemolysis, liver disease, or infection as underlying causes, and kernicterus as a consequence. Unconjugated serum bilirubin greater than 20 mg/dl is considered the critical level for the development of kernicterus in term infants. When the serum bilirubin is greater than 5 mg/dl in the first 24 hours, a serious disease process such as hemolysis may be present, and intervention is appropriate.

The focus on breast-feeding as related to neonatal jaundice results from the characterization of two syndromes: breast-feeding jaundice syndrome and breast milk jaundice syndrome.[172] In the early 1960s, 5 to 10 percent of lactating women were found to have a steroid metabolite of progesterone, 5β-pregnane-3(α), 20(β)-diol, in their icterogenic milk, but the compound was not found in the milk of women whose infants were normal (breast milk jaundice syndrome). This metabolite is associated with an inhibition of glucosyl transferase in the liver, differences in the metabolism of long-chain unsaturated fatty acids, and increased resorption of bile acids in jaundiced infants.

In breast milk jaundice syndrome, the neonates are healthy and active. The hyperbilirubinemia develops after the fourth day of life and may last several months, with a gradual fall in level. When breast-feeding is stopped for 24 to 48 hours, there is a 30- to 50-percent decline in bilirubin levels. With resumption of nursing, serum levels will rise slightly (1 to 2 mg/dl), plateau, and then start to fall slowly, regardless of feeding method. After excluding other causes of jaundice, and with careful monitoring of serum bilirubin, breast-feeding can continue.

Unfortunately, the focus on rare breast milk jaundice cases, the concern about kernicterus, and the increased bilirubin in many breast-fed neonates between 2 and 7 days old led to routine supplementation of infants with water, glucose, and formula, even when bilirubin concentrations were in the moderate range of 8 to 12 mg/dl. These interventions have led to the breast-feeding jaundice syndrome, or starvation jaundice. The cause of the elevated bilirubin—reduced feeding frequency or low milk transfer—is often unrecognized. It has been clearly demonstrated that feeding frequency greater than eight feedings per 24 hours is associated with lower bilirubin levels. Likewise, water supplementation studied in a controlled fashion does not decrease the peak serum bilirubin. Management consists of prevention by improvement in the quality and frequency of nursing. Rooming-in and night feedings should be encouraged.

GALACTOGOGUES: DRUGS TO IMPROVE MILK PRODUCTION

Obstetricians may interface with the breast-feeding dyad when there is a question of adequate milk production and transfer by the mother. The mother and the pediatrician will ask for a galactogogue to be prescribed by the obstetrician.

Numerous agents have been shown to increase prolactin production, and galactorrhea is a clinical issue for women on phenothiazine or metoclopramide. It is reasonable that these drugs might be used when milk supply seems insufficient.[173] The most understandable clinical scenarios include premature delivery requiring mechanical pumping, glandular hypoplasia, reduction mammoplasty, and relactation (nursing an adoptive child). The most common clinical presentation is perceived poor milk supply or inhibited milk let-down (oxytocin inhibition). Clinical trials with random assignment of subjects have demonstrated the effectiveness of metoclopramide, sulpiride, and nasal oxytocin for increasing milk production. In one randomized study of mothers of premature infants, metoclopramide did not improve breast milk volume or duration of breast feeding.[174]

Metoclopramide (Reglan) is used to promote gastrointestinal tone; however, a secondary effect is to increase prolactin levels. Most studies demonstrate a multiple fold increase in basal prolactin levels and a 60- to 100-percent increase in milk volume. The effects of metoclopramide are very dose dependent; the usual dose is 10 to 15 mg three times a day. The side effects, including gastric cramping, diarrhea, and depression, may limit its use. The incidence of depression increases with long-term use; treatment should be tapered over time and limited to less than 4 weeks. There appears to be little effect on the infant. The dose that the infants received is much less than the amount used therapeutically to treat esophageal reflux, regardless of the time postpartum.

Sulpiride is a selective dopamine antagonist used in Europe as an antidepressant and antipsychotic. Smaller doses (50mg twice daily) do not produce neuroleptic effects in the mother, but prolactin and milk production are increased significantly. Clinical studies suggest an increase in milk production (20 to 50 percent) less than that seen with metoclopramide. In a placebo-controlled study with random assignment of 130 subjects, sulpiride 50mg twice daily for the first 7 days postpartum increased the total milk yield from 916 ± 66ml in the control group to 1211 ± 65ml in the sulpiride-treated group. The transfer of sulpiride to the breast milk was minimal, and no adverse effects were seen in the infants. Sulpiride is not available in the United States.

Intranasal oxytocin substitutes for endogenous oxytocin to contract the myoepithelial cells and cause milk let-down. In theory, its use is to overcome an inhibited let-down reflex. Oxytocin is destroyed by gastrointestinal enzymes and is not given orally. Until recently, oxytocin intranasal spray was available commercially, but it has been taken off the market. A pharmacist can prepare an intranasal spray with a concentration of 2 IU per drop. The let-down dose is a spray (3 drops) to each nostril; the total let-down dose is approximately 12 IU. This is taken within 2 or 3 minutes of each nursing episode. The suggested duration of therapy is unclear. Underlying causes for an inhibited let-down reflex need to be identified and controlled.

There have been few clinical trials using oxytocin alone to improve milk production. In a double-blind group sequential trial, intranasal oxytocin alone was used to enhance milk production in women during the first 5 days after delivery of a premature infant. The cumulative volume of breast milk obtained between the second and fifth days was 3.5 times greater in primiparas given intranasal oxytocin than in primiparas given placebo. Because of oxytocin's complementary mechanism to prolactin-stimulating medications, they are often used in combination.

Although metoclopramide, sulpiride, and oxytocin appear to be effective and relatively safe for the mother and infant, they are only secondary support interventions. The primary focus should be to enhance prolactin and oxytocin through the natural mechanisms, such as appropriate and frequent stimulation of the nipple and areola. Galactagogues should only be used for a short duration (2 to 4 weeks) and in conjunction with hands-on counseling by an individual with the time, energy, and knowledge to enhance the "natural" production of breast milk.

MATERNAL DISEASE

In the vast majority of cases of lactating mothers with intercurrent disease, there is no medical reason to stop breast-feeding.[175] However, appropriate management requires individualizing the care of the nursing dyad in order to preserve the supply-and-demand relationship of lactation. For example, a hospitalized nursing mother should have her nursing baby with her in the hospital for on-demand feedings. This situation may stretch the flexibility of hospital administrators and nursing services, but the problem can be overcome by education.

The first principle is to maintain lactation. An acute hospitalization for a surgical procedure is a common complication. If breast milk was the neonate's only source of nutrition, an acute reduction in nursing may lead to breast engorgement, confusing postoperative fever, and mastitis. The infant should be put to the breast just before premedication, and the breasts should be emptied in the recovery room. The most effective way is to have the mother nurse. Although some anesthetic may be present in the milk, most are compatible with lactation.[176] If there is legitimate concern or if the mother cannot communicate (on a ventilator), the breasts should be pumped mechanically and subsequently emptied every 2 to 3 hours by nursing or pumping.

The second principle is to adjust for the special nutritional requirements of nursing mothers. This principle is especially pertinent when intake is restricted postoperatively and when the maternal diet must be manipulated. In the postoperative period, the surgeon must account for the calories and fluid required for lactation. Until oral intake is established, a lactating mother needs an additional 500 to 1,000ml of fluid per day. Early return to a balanced diet is essential to offset the additional energy and protein requirements of lactation and wound healing.

The third principle is to ensure that the maternal disease will not harm the infant. This is most pertinent with infectious disease, but it is equally important in cases in which a mother's judgment is in question, such as severe mental illness, substance abuse, or a history of physical abuse. The benefits of breast-feeding in the latter situations must be carefully evaluated, using the resources of the patient, her family, and social services.

Infection is the most common area where breast-feeding is questioned. In general, the necessary exposure of the infant to the mother in day-to-day care is such that breast-feeding does not add to the risk. This recommendation assumes that appropriate therapy is being given to both mother and infant. Isolation of infected areas should still be practiced, such as a mask in the case of respiratory infection and lesion isolation in herpes. The three acute infections in which breast-feeding is contraindicated are herpes simplex lesions of the breast, untreated active (not just purified protein derivative [PPD]–positive) tuberculosis, and human immunodeficiency viral (HIV) disease.

The fourth principle is to evaluate adequately the need and type of medication used for therapy (see Chapter 8). The drug management of chronic hypertension illustrates this principle. First, the need for medication must be scrutinized. There is considerable controversy in the literature as to whether or not to treat patients with mild chronic hypertension (diastolic blood pressure 90 to 100mmHg). The desire of a mother with mild hypertension to breast-feed may change the risk-benefit ratio so that antihypertensive drug therapy should be delayed until after lactation. Second, the medication should be evaluated for its effect on milk production. In the first 3 to 4 months of therapy, diuretics reduce intravascular volume and, subsequently, milk volume. On the other hand, if a patient has been on low doses of thiazide diuretics for more than

6 months, the effect on milk volume is minimal, as long as adequate oral intake is maintained. Third, the medication should be evaluated for its secretion in breast milk and its possible effects on the infant. Thiazide diuretics, ethacrynic acid, and furosemide also cross into breast milk in small amounts. These agents have the potential to displace bilirubin, and their use during lactation is of concern when the infant is less than 1 month old or is jaundiced. In general, most other antihypertensive drugs are compatible with breast-feeding. Although new drugs come onto the market frequently, it is wise to use drugs that have had a long history of clinical use.

DRUGS IN BREAST MILK

Most medications taken by the mother appear in the milk (see Chapter 8), but the calculated dose consumed by the nursing infant ranges from 0.001 to 5 percent of the standard therapeutic doses and are tolerated by infants without toxicity.[176] Two good references are *Drugs in Pregnancy and Lactation*[139] and *Medications in Mother's Milk*.[140] Very few drugs are absolutely contraindicated. These include anticancer agents, radioactive materials, chloramphenicol, phenylbutazone, and atropine.

The following guidelines are helpful:

1. Evaluate the therapeutic benefit of medication. Diuretics given for ankle swelling provide very different benefits from those given for congestive heart failure. Are drugs really necessary, and are there safer alternatives?
2. Choose drugs most widely tested and with the lowest milk/plasma ratio.
3. Choose drugs with the lowest oral bioavailability.
4. Select the least toxic drug with the shortest half life.
5. Avoid long-acting forms. Usually, these drugs are detoxified by the liver or bound to protein.
6. Schedule doses so that the least amount gets into the milk. The rate of maternal absorption and the peak maternal serum concentration are helpful in scheduling dosage. Usually, it is best for the mother to take the medication immediately after a feeding.
7. Monitor the infant during the course of therapy. Many pharmacologic agents for maternal use are also used for infants. This implies the availability of knowledge about therapeutic doses and the signs and symptoms of toxicity.
8. Contact the infant's caregivers to assure them of the safety of the drug in lactation.

BREAST MASSES DURING LACTATION

Breast cancer is the most common cancer of the female reproductive organs. Although the risk of breast cancer increases tremendously after the age of 40, 1 to 3 percent of all breast cancers occur during pregnancy and lactation. Breast cancer diagnosed during lactation may have its origin before or during pregnancy. As a result of this assumption and small numbers of pregnant or lactating women, most studies have lumped the populations together. Recently, researchers in Japan have analyzed breast cancer in age-matched control women (n = 192), women who were pregnant at diagnosis (n = 72), and women who were lactating at diagnosis (n = 120).[177] The prognosis for breast cancer that is diagnosed during pregnancy or lactation is poorer than for breast cancer diagnosed at other times. The 10-year survival for age-matched controls without lymph node metastasis was 93 percent; for women who were diagnosed during pregnancy or lactation, the survival rate was 85 percent. When the lymph nodes are involved, the 10-year survival rate was 62 percent and 37 percent in controls and women who were diagnosed during pregnancy or lactation, respectively. The difference in survival is partially explained by a longer duration of symptoms before diagnosis (6.3 versus 5.4 months), tumor size on palpation (4.6 versus 3.0 cm), and tumor size on cut surface (4.3 versus 2.6 cm), in lactating women versus control women, respectively. The delay in diagnosis and the greater size at diagnosis in lactating women reflects the reluctance of the obstetric care provider and the lactating woman to aggressively sample a breast mass.

The lactating woman is most likely to recognize a breast mass through her daily manipulations of her breasts. In her framework of reference, she usually considers this mass a "plugged duct." She should be encouraged to report a plugged duct that persists more than 2 weeks despite efforts to initiate drainage of that lobule. Her provider faces an expanded differential diagnosis. Fibromas and fibroadenomas are more common in young women. These solid tumors are rubbery, nodular, and mobile, and they may grow rapidly with the hormonal stimulation of pregnancy. The most common diagnosis is a dilated milk duct, a completely benign diagnosis.

A needle aspiration of the mass is the mainstay of diagnosis. Percutaneous fine-needle aspiration is performed in the same manner as in nonpregnant women. The use of local anesthetic is optional; infiltration of the area around a small lesion may increase the likelihood of a nondiagnostic aspiration. The area over the mass is swabbed with iodine or alcohol and, using sterile techniques, the lesion is fixed between the thumb and fingers of the nondominant hand. Using a 22-gauge needle attached to a 20-ml syringe, the center of the lesion is probed. Initial aspiration usually reveals the nature of the lesion. If milk or greenish fluid (fibrocystic disease) is found and the lesion disappears, no further diagnostic procedures need to be performed. If the tumor is solid or fails to disappear completely after aspiration, the needle is passed several times through the lesion under strong negative pressure. The aspirated tissue fluid is air-dried on a slide and sent for cytologic evaluation. The pathology requisition should note the age and lactating status. Fine-needle aspiration biopsy appears to have the same accuracy in pregnancy and lactation as in the nonpregnant, nonlactating woman. Gupta et al.[178] performed 214 fine-needle aspirations during pregnancy and lactation. Eight (13.7 percent) were cancer, and the sensitivity, specificity, and positive predictive value was 100, 81, and 61 percent, respectively.

Ultrasound is an expensive but accurate method of determining the cystic nature of a breast mass in lactating women. Mammography is more difficult to interpret during lactation. Young breasts are generally more dense, and the massive increase in functioning glands may obscure small cancers. However, the accuracy is still good if the films are interpreted by experienced radiologists. In general, mammography is a secondary diagnostic modality.

A core biopsy using ultrasound or radiographic guidance is a reasonable option to avoid a surgical procedure. If a surgical biopsy is required, the surgeon usually needs guidance regarding the management of lactation. Most breast biopsies can be performed under local anesthesia. If the mother nurses just before the procedure, she will empty the breast, which makes the surgery easier, and will allow 3 to 4 hours until the next feed. Local anesthetics are not absorbed orally and pose no risk to the infant. The mother should be allowed to nurse on demand. Most anesthetics used for general anesthesia enter the breast milk in small amounts (1 to 3 percent) of the maternal dose, and minimal behavioral effects in infants have been observed. In most cases, the mother can nurse within 4 hours of the anesthetic. The mother's breasts should be pumped 3 to 4 hours after the last feed regardless of the anesthetic status. She will begin to feel the discomfort of engorgement, and the fever of engorgement may confuse the postoperative picture as early as 8 or 10 hours. The failure to empty the breasts within 12 hours will begin to adversely affect milk supply.

Surgical biopsy usually has little effect on breast-feeding performance unless the procedure is done in the periareolar area or the nerves supplying the nipple are compromised. Circumareolar incisions are to be avoided, if possible. Milk fistulas are an uncommon risk (5 percent) of central biopsy. The fistulas are usually self-limited and will spontaneously heal over several weeks. Prohibiting breast-feeding does not change the likelihood of ultimate healing.

BACK-TO-WORK ISSUES

In 1984, approximately 26 percent of new mothers had full-time employment, and an additional 15 percent had part-time employment.[179,180] At 5 or 6 months postpartum, 12.3 percent of full-time employees were breast-feeding, as were 29 percent of part-time employees or unemployed mothers. Two thirds of the working mothers were supplementing their infants' diets with formula. In 1992, approximately 34 percent of new mothers had full-time employment, and an additional 15 percent had part-time employment. Full-time employees were breast-feeding at one half (13 percent) the rate of breast-feeding among part-time employees (26 percent) or the unemployed (27 percent).[181]

The separation of mother and infant adversely affects the psychology and physiology of lactation through a decrease in the frequency of nursing, breast engorgement, and unsatisfied needs of the baby. The anxiety and fatigue associated with the combination of employment and lactation inhibits the let-down reflex, weakens maternal host defenses, and disrupts family dynamics. The infant must adapt to another caregiver, a new sucking technique, and unfamiliar infectious agents found in day-care settings. Therefore, it is not surprising that formula feeding is viewed as an improvement in mothers' lives, but it does create feelings of inadequacy and guilt in some women.

Breast-feeding during employment is both possible and fulfilling.[179,180] Preparation, milk storage, and choice of child care are the cornerstones to easy adaptation to employment. Preparation involves preemployment change in lifestyle to accommodate the increased stresses. Lactation should be well established with frequent nursing (10 to 14 times per day) and no supplementation before return to work. Return to full-time work before 4 months has a greater negative impact than return to work after 4 months.[179,180] Part-time work lessens the impact. About 2 weeks before her return to work, the mother should change her nursing schedule at home. During the workday, she should express or pump her breasts two or three times, while increasing her nursing with short, frequent feeds before and after work times. The infant is fed bottles of stored breast milk by a different person in a different place to allow it to adapt more easily.

During the 2 weeks before employment, the day-care arrangements should be carefully selected and observed. In addition to references, several questions are pertinent to the selection of the day-care setting. Is the sitter a mother herself, and does the sitter have experience with nursing babies? Is the mother welcome to use the child-care site for a midday nursing? Does the day-care center provide in-arm feeding, or does it use high chairs and propped bottle-feedings? Is the time and activity of the center highly structured and rigid, or is it flexible to mother or infant needs and requests? Does the staff treat the parents and children with respect? Many of these questions can be answered by an extended (1 to 2 hours) observation of the center and its children.

Fatigue is the number one enemy of the working mother. Emotional and physical support of the mother is critical. Some helpful suggestions include (1) bringing the infant's bed into the parents' room, or the construction of a temporary extension to the parents' bed; (2) use of labor-saving devices, division of domestic chores, and the elimination of less important household chores to reduce the workload; and (3) taking naps and frequent rest periods to conserve energy.

Continued stimulation of the breast during working hours is important. Pumping not only improves milk supply but also supplies human milk for the infant. Manual expression and mechanical pumping should be performed more frequently (two to three times) in the first 6 months postpartum. After 6 months, the frequency can be reduced and eliminated as the infant is supplemented by fluids or solids during the day.

The collection of breast milk has become simple with the wide variety of mechanical pumps available in the market. Mechanical pumps that employ a bulb syringe produce the least amount of milk and have the highest rate of bacterial contamination. Cyclic electric pumps produce the most milk with the least amount of nipple trauma. Water-driven pumps are both cheap and relatively effective. The most efficient pumps are not as effective as the efficiently nursing baby in increasing milk volume and raising prolactin levels.[182]

The concern about bacterial growth in expressed and stored milk has been alleviated by recent studies showing that bacterial contamination does not increase significantly for up to 6 hours after expression, when the milk is stored at room temperature, nor were there differences in bacterial counts between specimens stored at room temperature and those stored under refrigeration for 10 hours.[183] Freshly refrigerated milk should be used within 2 days. Four to 6 oz of human milk can be frozen in partially filled resealable (Ziploc) plastic bags. When human milk is frozen, it should be cooled briefly before transfer to the freezer. The milk will keep for 2 to 4 weeks in the refrigerator freezer and up to 6 months in a freezer set at 0°F. The individual packets of milk should be stored with the newest packet on the bottom of the stack. The next used packet (the oldest) is thawed quickly in warm tap water just prior to use. Frozen milk should not be thawed in the microwave, because the heating is uneven and severe oral burns have been reported. After it is thawed, it should be used within 6 to 8 hours.

WEANING

The American Academy of Pediatrics recommends exclusive breast-feeding for the first 6 months of life and continuation at least through the first 12 months of life. This recommendation in 1997 initiated a firestorm of controversy regarding "the excessive duration of breast-feeding." Breast-feeding is both a biologic process and a culturized activity. In the United States, breast-feeding has been culturized to no breast-feeding or breast-feeding for less than 6 months. From a broader biologic and historical perspective, the United States experience reflects cultural bias, not biologic reality. In remarkable reviews, Dettwyler[184,185] makes a very cogent argument for the "natural" age of weaning in the human to be 3 to 4 years. She has several arguments. Traditional and prehistoric societies wean between the third and fourth year. Based on weaning when the infant weight is four times its birth weight, similar to other primates, weaning should occur between 2 and 3 years. If weaning corresponds to attainment of one third the adult weight, then weaning would occur between 3 and 4 years. If humans behaved like chimpanzees or gorillas and weaned at six times the gestational period, humans would wean at 4.5 years. The dental, neurologic, and immunologic systems are still developing until 6 years of age; breast-feeding and breast milk provide unique support for these systems up to 4 to 6 years. Developmentally, the infant is able to place solid food in its mouth at 6 months, but this intake, if left to the infant's own skills, would not reach a significant proportion of the nutritional requirements until 18 to 24 months. The ability to drink from a cup occurs close to the second year. As the infant supplements an increasing proportion of its nutritional needs with solid or liquid food, the mother will begin to ovulate. Subsequent pregnancy is increasingly more likely. Breast-feeding, through its suppression of gonadal function, maintains a birth interval of 3 to 4 years. Clearly, breast-feeding into the third or fourth year is a cultural exception in the United States, but prolonged breast-feeding does not constitute abnormal or deviant behavior as expressed by many "modern" Americans. As we learn more about the benefits of long-term lactation, our culture may return to more reasonable expectations for duration of breast-feeding.

KEY POINTS

- WHO, the U.S. Surgeon General, the American Academy of Pediatrics, the American Academy of Family Practice, the American College of Obstetricians and Gynecologists, and the Academy of Breastfeeding Medicine endorse breast-feeding as the gold standard for infant feeding.

- Breast-feeding accrues many health benefits for the infant, including protection against infection, less allergy, better growth, better neurodevelopment, and lower rates of chronic disease such as type 1 diabetes mellitus and childhood cancer.

- Breast-feeding accrues more health benefits for the mother, including faster postpartum involution of the uterus, improved postpartum weight loss, less premenopausal breast cancer, better mother-infant bonding, and less economic burden.

- Artificial breast milk lacks key components including defenses against infection; hormones and enzymes to aid digestion; polyunsaturated fatty acids, which are necessary for optimal brain growth; and adequate composition for efficient digestion.

- Contact with the breast within one half hour after birth increases the duration of breast feeding. A frequency of nursing greater than eight per 24 hours, night nursing, and a duration of nursing longer than 15 minutes are needed to maintain adequate prolactin levels and milk supply.

- Prolactin is the major promoter of milk synthesis. Oxytocin is the major initiator of milk ejection. The release of prolactin and oxytocin results from the stimulation of the sensory nerves supplying the areola and nipple.

- Oxytocin released from the posterior pituitary can be operantly conditioned and is influenced negatively by pain, stress, or loss of self-esteem.

- The nursing actions on a human teat versus on an artificial teat are very different. Poor lactation is the major cause of nipple injury and poor milk transfer. Perceived or real lack of milk transfer is the major reason why lactation fails.

- Milk production is reduced by an autocrine pathway through a protein that inhibits milk production by the alveolar cells, and by distention and pressure against the alveolar cells.

REFERENCES

1. American Academy of Pediatrics, Work Group on Breastfeeding: Breastfeeding and the use of human milk. Pediatrics 100:1035, 1997.
2. American College of Obstetricians and Gynecologists: Breastfeeding: Maternal and Infant Aspect Educational Bulletin, 258, July 2000.
3. Newton ER: The epidemiology of breastfeeding. Clin Obstet Gynecol 47:613, 2004.
4. Ryan A, Wenjun Z, Acosta A: Breastfeeding continues to increase in the new millennium. J Pediatr 110:1103, 2002.
5. Ahluwalia I, Morrow B, Hsia J, et al: Who is breastfeeding? Recent trends from the Pregnancy Risk Assessment and Monitoring System. J Pediatr 142:486, 2003.
6. Freed G, Clark S, Sorenson J, et al: National assessment of physicians' breast-feeding knowledge, attitudes, training and experience. JAMA 273:472, 1995.
7. Schanler RJ, O'Connor KG, Lawrence RA: Pediatricians' practices and attitudes regarding breastfeeding promotion. Pediatrics 103: E35, 1999.
8. Beaudry M, Dufour R, Marcoux S: Relation between infant feeding and infections during the first six months of life. J Pediatr 126:191, 1995.
9. Tellez A, Winiechka-Krusnell J, Paniagua M, Linder E: Antibodies in mother's milk protect children against giardiasis. Scandinavian J Infect Dis 5:322, 2003.
10. Golding J, Emmett PM, Rogers IS: Gastroenteritis, diarrhea and breastfeeding. Early Hum Dev 49 Suppl:S83, 1997.
11. Frank AL, Taber LH, Glezen WP, et al: Breast-feeding and respiratory virus infection. Pediatrics 70:239, 1982.
12. Wright AI, Holberg CJ, Martinez FD, et al: Breast feeding and lower respiratory tract illness in the first year of life. BMJ 299:945, 1989.
13. Nafstad P, Jaakkola JJ, Hagen JA, et al: Breastfeeding, maternal smoking and lower respiratory tract infections. Eur Respir J 9:2623, 1996.
14. Duncan B, Ey J, Holberg CJ, et al: Exclusive breast-feeding for at least 4 months protects against otitis media. Pediatrics 91:867, 1993.
15. Owen MJ, Baldwin CD, Swank PR, et al: Relation of infant feeding practices, cigarette smoke exposure, and group child care to the onset and duration of otitis media with effusion in the first two years of life. J Pediatr 123:702, 1993.
16. Paradise JL, Rockette HE, Colborn DK, et al: Otitis media in 2253 Pittsburgh-area infants: prevalence and risk factors during the first two years of life. Pediatrics 99:318, 1997.
17. Cochi SL, Fleming DW, Hightower AW, et al: Primary invasive *Haemophilus influenzae* type b disease; a population-based assessment of risk factors. J Pediatr 108:887, 1986.
18. Duffy LC, Faden H, Wasielewski R, et al: Exclusive breastfeeding protects against bacterial colonization and day care exposure to otitis media. Pediatrics 100:E7, 1997.
19. Takala AK, Eskola J, Palmgren J, et al: Risk factors of invasive *Haemophilus influenzae* type b disease among children in Finland. J Pediatr 115:694, 1989.
20. Istre GR, Conner JS, Broome CV, et al: Risk factors for primary invasive *Haemophilus influenzae* disease: increased risk from day care attendance and school-aged household members. J Pediatr 106:190, 1985.
21. Silfverdal SA, Bodin L, Hugosson S, et al: Protective effect of breastfeeding on invasive *Haemophilus influenzae* infection: a case-control study in Swedish preschool children. Int J Epidemiol 26:443, 1997.
22. Pisacane A, Graziano L, Mazzarella G, et al: Breast-feeding and urinary tract infection. J Pediatr 120:87, 1992.
23. Marild S, Hansson S, Jodal U, et al: Protective effect of breastfeeding against urinary tract infection. Acta Paediatr 93:164, 2004.
24. Lucas A, Cole TJ: Breast milk and neonatal necrotizing enterocolitis. Lancet 336:1519, 1990.
25. Covert RF, Barman N, Domanico RS, et al: Prior enteral nutrition with human milk protects against intestinal perforation in infants who develop necrotizing enterocolitis. Pediatr Res 37:305A, 1995.
26. Alm B, Wennergren G, Norvenious SG, et al: Breast feeding and the sudden infant death syndrome in Scandinavia, 1992–95. Arch Dis Child 86:400, 2002.
27. McVea KL, Turner PD, Peppler DK: The role of breastfeeding in sudden infant death syndrome. J Hum Lact 16:13, 2000.
28. Sadauskaite-Kuehne V, Ludvigsson J, Padaiga Z, et al: Longer breastfeeding is an independent protective factor against development of type 1 diabetes mellitus in childhood. Diabetes Metab Rev 20:150, 2004.
29. Stuebe AM, Rich-Edwards JW, Willett WC, et al: Duration of lactation and incidence of type 2 diabetes. JAMA 294:2601, 2005.
30. Pettitt DJ, Forman MR, Hanson RL, et al: Diabetes and Arthritis Epidemiology Section, Breastfeeding and incidence on non-insulin-dependent diabetes mellitus in Pima Indians. Lancet 350:166, 1997.
31. Knip M, Akerblom HK: Early nutrition and later diabetes risk. Adv Exp Med Biol 569:142, 2005.
32. Arenz R: Breast-feeding and childhood obsesity—a systematic review. Intern J Obes Rel Metab Disord 28:1247, 2004.
33. Martorell R, Stein AD, Schroeder DG: Early nutrition and later adiposity. J Nutr 131:874S, 2004.
34. Owen CG, Martin RM, Whincup PH, et al: Effect of infant feeding on the risk of obesity across the life course: a quantitative review of published evidence. Pediatrics 115:1367, 2005.
35. Klement E, Cohen RV, Boxman J, et al: Breastfeeding and risk of inflammatory bowel disease: a systematic review with meta-analysis. Am J Clin Nutr 80:1342, 2004.
36. Corrao G, Tragnone A, Caprilli R, et al: Risk of inflammatory bowel disease attributable to smoking, oral contraception and breastfeeding in Italy: a nationwide case-control study. Cooperative Investigators of the Italian Group for the Study of the colon and the Rectum. Int J Epidemiol 27:397, 1998.
37. Martin RM, Gunnell D, Owen CG, Smith GD: Breast-feeding and childhood cancer: A systematic review with metaanalysis. Int J Cancer 117:1020, 2005.
38. Saarinen VM, Kajosaari M: Breast feeding as prophylaxis against atopic disease: prospective follow-up until 17 years old. Lancet 346:1065, 1995.
39. Scariati PD, Grummer-Strawn LM, Fein SB: A longitudinal analysis of infant morbidity and the extent of breastfeeding in the United States. Pediatrics 99:5, 1997.
40. Van Odijk J, Kull I, Borres MP, et al: Breastfeeding and allergic disease: a multidisciplinary review of the literature (1966–2001) on the mode of early feeding in infancy and its impact on later atopic manifestations. Allergy 58:833, 2003.
41. Gdalevick M, Mimouni D, David M, Mimouni M: Breast-feeding and the onset of atopic dermatitis in childhood: a systematic review and meta-analysis of prospective studies. J Am Acad Dermatol 45:520, 2001.
42. Oddy WH, de Klerk NH, Sly PD, Holt PG: The effects of respiratory infections, atopy, and breastfeeding on childhood asthma. Eur Respir J 19:899, 2002.
43. Oddy WH: A review of the effects of breastfeeding on respiratory infections, atopy, and childhood asthma. J Asthma 41:605, 2004.
44. Friedman NJ: The role of breast-feeding in the development of allergies and asthma. J Allergy Clin Immunol 115:1238, 2005.
45. Oddy WH, Sly PD, de Klerk NH, Landau LI, et al: Breast feeding and respiratory morbidity in infancy: a birth cohort study. Arch Dis Child 88:224, 2004.
46. Futrakul S, Deerojanawong J, Prapphal N: Risk factors of bronchial hyperresponsiveness in children with wheezing-associated respiratory infection. Pediatr Pulmonol 40:81, 2005.
47. Hylander MA, Strobino DM, Dhanireddy R: Human milk feedings and infection among very low weight infants. Pediatrics 102: E38, 1998.
48. Lucas A, Morley R, Cole TJ: Randomized trial of early diet in preterm babies and later intelligence quotient. BMJ 317:1481, 1998.
49. Riva E, Agostoni C, Biasucci G, et al: Early breastfeeding is linked to higher intelligence quotient scores in dietary treated phenylketonuric children. Acta Paediatr 85:56, 1996.
50. Horwood LJ, Darlow BA, Mogridge N: Breast milk feeding and cognitive ability at 7–9 years. Arch Dis Child 84:F23, 2001.

51. Gustafsson PA, Duchen K, Birberg U, Karlsson T: Breastfeeding, very long polyunsaturated fatty acids (PUFA) and IQ at 6 1/2 years of age. Acta Paediatr 93:1280, 2004.
52. Gomez-Sanchiz M, Canete R, Rodero I, et al: Influence of breast-feeding on mental and psychomotor development. Clin Pediatr 42:35, 2003.
53. Anderson JW, Johnstone BM, Remley DT: Breast-feeding and cognitive development: a meta-analysis. Am J Clin Nutr 70:525, 1999.
54. Slykerman RF, Thompson JM, Becroft DM, Robinson E, et al: Breastfeeding and intelligence of preschool children. Acta Paediatr 94:832, 2005.
55. Chen A, Rogan WJ: Breastfeeding and the risk of postneonatal death in the United States. Pediatrics. 113:e435, 2004.
56. Kramer MS, Chalmers B, Hodnett ED, et al: Promotion of Breast-feeding Intervention Trial (PROBIT): a randomized trial in the Republic of Belarus. JAMA 285:413, 2001.
57. Kramer MS, Chalmers B, Hodnett ED, et al: Promotion of Breast-feeding Intervention Trial (PROBIT): a randomized trial in the Republic of Belarus. JAMA 285:413, 2001.
58. Bhandari N, Bahl R, Mazumdar S, et al: Effect of community-based promotion of exclusive breastfeeding on diarrheal illness and growth: a cluster randomized controlled trial. Lancet 361(9367):1418, 2003.
59. Wright AL, Bauer M, Naylor A, et al: Increasing breastfeeding rates to reduce infant illness at the community level. Pediatrics 101:837, 1998.
60. Ball TM, Wright AL: Health care costs of formula-feeding in the first year of life. Pediatrics 103:870, 1999.
61. Ball TM, Bennett DM: The economic impact of breastfeeding. Pediatr Clin N Am 48:253, 2001.
62. Madden JM, Soumerai SB, Lieu TA, et al: Effects on breastfeeding of changes in maternity length-of-stay policy in a large health maintenance organization. Pediatrics 111:519, 2003.
63. Labbok MH: Health sequelae of breastfeeding for the mother. Clin Perinatol 26:491, 1999.
64. Schack-Nielsen L, Larnkjaer A, Michaelsen KF: Long term effects of breastfeeding on the infant and mother. Adv Exp Med Biol 569:16, 2005.
65. Chua S, Arulkumaran S, Lim I, et al: Influence of breastfeeding and nipple stimulation on postpartum uterine activity. Br J Obstet Gynaecol 101:804, 1994.
66. Dewey KG, Heinig MJ, Nommsen LA: Maternal weight-loss patterns during prolonged lactation. Am J Clin Nutr 58:162, 1993.
67. Lee SY, Kim MT, Jee SH, Yang HP: Does long-term lactation protect premenopausal women against hypertension risk? A Korean women's cohort study. Prev Med 41:433, 2005.
68. Martin RM, Ebrahim S, Griffin M, et al: Breastfeeding and atherosclerosis: intima-media and plaques at 65-year follow-up of the Boyd-Orr cohort. Atheroscler Thromb Vasc Biol 25:1482, 2005.
69. Short RV, Lewis PR, Renfree MB, et al: Contraceptive effects of extended lactational amenorrhea; beyond the Bellagio consensus. Lancet 337:715, 1991.
70. Melton LJ, Bryant SC, Wahner HW, et al: Influence of breast-feeding and other reproductive factors on bone mass later in life. Osteoporos Int 3:76, 1993.
71. Kalkwarf HJ: Lactation and maternal bone health. Adv Exp Med Biol 554:101, 2004.
72. Huo D, Lauderdale DS, Li L: Influence of reproductive factors on hip fracture risk in Chinese women. Osteoporos Int 14:694, 2003.
73. Martin RM, Middleton N, Gunnell D, et al: Breast-feeding and cancer: the Boyd Orr cohort and a systematic review with meta-analysis. J Natl Cancer Inst 97:1446, 2005.
74. Collaborative Group on Hormonal Factors in Breast Cancer: Breast cancer and breastfeeding: collaborative reanalysis of individual data from 47 epidemiological studies in 30 countries, including 50302 women with breast cancer and 96973 women with the disease. Lancet 360:187, 2002.
75. Michels KB, Willett WC, Rosner BA, et al: Prospective assessment of breastfeeding and breast cancer incidence among 89,887 women. Lancet 347:431, 1996.
76. Crow RA, Fawcett JN, Wright P: Maternal behavior during breast- and bottle-feeding. J Behav Med 3:259, 1980.
77. Agre F: The relationship of mode of infant feeding and location of care to frequency of infection. Am J Dis Child 139:809, 1985.
78. Woolridge MW: The anatomy of infant sucking. Midwifery 2:164, 1986.
79. Weber F, Woolridge MW, Baum JD: An ultrasonographic study of the organization of sucking and swallowing by newborn infants. Dev Med Child Neural 28:19, 1986.
80. Neifert M, DeMarzo S, Seacat J, et al: The influence of breast surgery, breast appearance, and pregnancy-induced breast changes on lactation sufficiency as measured by infant weight gain. Birth 17:31, 1990.
81. Neifert MR: Clinical aspects of lactation: promoting breastfeeding success. Clin Perinatol 26:281, 1999.
82. Katz M, Creasy RK: Mammary blood flow regulation in the nursing rabbit. Am J Obstet Gynecol 150:497, 1984.
83. Saint L, Smith M, Hartmann PE: The yield and nutrient content of colostrum and milk of women from giving birth to 1 month post-partum. Br J Nutr 52:87, 1984.
84. Neville MC: Determinants of milk volume and composition. *In* Jensen RG (ed): Handbook for Milk Composition. San Diego, Academic Press, 1995, p 87.
85. Peaker M: The effect of raised intramammary pressure on mammary function in the goat in relation to the cessation of lactation. J Physiol (Lond) 310:415, 1980.
86. Wilde CJ, Addey CVP, Boddy LM, et al: Autocrine regulation of milk secretion by a protein in milk. Biochem J 305:51, 1995.
87. Lund LR, Romer J, Thomasset N, et al: Two distinct phases of apoptosis in mammary gland involution: proteinase-independent and -dependent pathways. Development 122:181, 1996
88. Prentice A, Addey CP, Wilde CJ: Evidence for local feedback control of human milk secretion. Biochem Soc Trans 16:122, 1989.
89. Neville MC: Physiology of lactation. Clin Perinatol 26:251, 1999.
90. Hall B: Changing composition of human milk and early development of an appetite control. Lancet 1:779, 1975.
91. Neville MC, Keller R, Seacat J, et al: Studies in human lactation: milk volumes in lactating women during the onset of lactation and full lactation. Am J Clin Nutr 48:1375, 1988.
92. Neville MC, Keller RP, Seacat J, et al: Studies on human lactation. 1. Within-feed and between-breast variation in selected components of human milk. Am J Clin Nutr 40:635, 1984.
93. Woolridge MW, Fisher C: Colic, "overfeeding" symptoms of lactose malabsorption in the breast-fed baby a possible artifact of feed management. Lancet 2:382, 1988.
94. Rasmussen KM: Maternal nutritional status and lactational performance. Clin Nutr 7:147, 1988.
95. Strode MA, Dewey KG, Lonnerdal B: Effects of short-term caloric restriction on lactational performance of well-nourished women. Acta Paediatr Scand 75:222, 1986.
96. Dewey KG, Lovelady CA, Nommsen-Rivers LA, et al: A randomized study of the effects of aerobic exercise by lactating women on breast-milk volume and composition. N Engl J Med 330:449, 1994.
97. Lovelady CA: The impact of energy restriction and exercise in lactating women. Adv Exp Med Biol 554:115, 2004.
98. Hartmann PE, Cregan MD, Ramsay DT, et al: Physiology of lactation in preterm mothers: Initiation and maintenance. Pediatr Ann 32:351, 2003.
99. Newton M, Egli GE: The effect of intranasal administration of oxytocin on the let-down of milk in lactating women. Am J Obstet Gynecol 76:103, 1958.
100. Feher SDK, Berger LR, Johnson JD, et al: Increasing breast milk production for premature infants with a relaxation/imagery audiotape. Pediatrics 83:57, 1989.
101. Ueda T, Yokoyama Y, Irahara M, et al: Influence of psychological stress on suckling-induced pulsatile oxytocin release. Obstet Gynecol 84:259, 1994.
102. Dewey KG: Maternal and fetal stress are associated with impaired lactogenesis in humans. J Nutr 131:3012S, 2001.
103. Losch M, Dungy CI, Russell D, et al: Impact of attitudes on maternal decisions regarding infant feeding. J Pediatr 126:507, 1996.
104. Newton N, Newton M: Relationship of ability to breast-feed and maternal attitudes toward breast-feeding. Pediatrics 5:869, 1950.

105. Cernadas JM, Nocess G, Barrena L, et al: Maternal and prenatal factors influence duration of exclusive breastfeeding. J Hum Lact 19:136, 2003.
106. Uvnas-Moberg K: Oxytocin linked antistress effects—the relaxation and growth response. Acta Physiol Scand Suppl 640:38, 1997.
107. Carter CS, Altemus M: Integrative functions of lactational hormones in social behavior and stress management. Ann N Y Acad Sci 807:164, 1997.
108. Kennel JH, Klaus MH: Bonding: recent observations that alter perinatal care. Pediatr Rev 19:4, 1998.
109. Mikiel-Kostyra K, Mazur J, Boltruszko I: Effect of early skin-to-skin contact after delivery on duration of breastfeeding: a prospective cohort study. Acta Paediatr 91:1301, 2002.
110. Lindenberg CS, Artola RC, Jimenez V: The effect of early post-partum mother-infant contact and breastfeeding promotion on the incidence and continuation of breastfeeding. Int J Nurs Stud 27:179, 1990.
111. Neifert M: Breastmilk Transfer: positioning, latch-on, and screening for problems in milk transfer. Clin Obstet Gynecol 47:656, 2004.
112. Woolridge MW, How TV, Drewett RF, et al: The continuous measurement of milk intake at a feed in breast-babies. Early Hum Dev 6:365, 1982.
113. Howie PW, McNeilly AS, McArdle T, et al: The relationship between suckling-induced prolactin response and lactogenesis. J Clin Endocrinol Metab 50:670, 1980.
114. Lucas A, Lucas PI, Baum JD: Differences in the pattern of milk intake between breast and bottle fed infants. Early Hum Dev 5:195, 1981.
115. Anderson AN, Schioler V: Influence of breast-feeding pattern on the pituitary-ovarian axis of a woman in an industrialized country. Am J Obstet Gynecol 143:673, 1982.
116. Jones RE: A hazards model analysis of breastfeeding variables and maternal age on return to menses postpartum in rural Indonesian women. Hum Biol 60:853, 1988.
117. Newton ER: Breastmilk: The gold standard. Clin Obstet Gynecol 47:632, 2004.
118. Goldman AS, Chheda S, Kenney SE, et al: Immunologic protection of the premature newborn by human milk. Semin Perinatol 19:495, 1994.
119. Garofalo RP, Goldman AS: Expression of functional immunomodulatory and anti-inflammatory factors in human milk. Clin Perinatol 26:361, 1999.
120. International code of marketing of breastmilk substitutes, Geneva, World Health Organization, 1981.
121. Kunz C, Rodriquez-Palmero M, Koletzko B, et al: Nutritional and biochemical properties of human milk, part I: general aspects, proteins, and carbohydrates. Clin Perinatol 26:307, 1999.
122. Rodriquez-Palmero M, Koletzko B, Kunz C, et al: Nutritional and biochemical properties of human milk, part II: lipids, micronutrients, and bioactive factors. Clin Perinatol 26:335, 1999.
123. Dewey KG: Growth characteristics of breast-fed compared to formula-fed infants. Biol Neonate 74:94, 1998.
124. Ravelli AC, van der Meulen JH, Osmond C, et al: Infant feeding and adult glucose tolerance, lipid profile, blood pressure, and obesity. Arch Dis Child 82:248, 2000.
125. Hanson LA: Human milk and host defence: immediate and long-term effects. Acta Paediatr Suppl 88:42, 1999.
126. Xanthou M: Human milk cells. Acta Paediatr 86:1288, 1997.
127. Slade HB, Schwartz SA: Mucosal immunity: the immunology of breast milk. J Allergy Clin Immunol 80:346, 1987.
128. Ellison RT, Giehl TJ: Killing of gram-negative bacteria by lactoferrin and lysozyme. J Clin Invest 88:1080, 1991.
129. Iyer S, Lonnerdal B: Lactoferrin, lactoferrin receptors and iron metabolism. Eur J Clin Nutr 47:232, 1993.
130. Dai D, Walker WA: Protective nutrients and bacterial colonization in the immature human gut. Adv Pediatr 46:353, 1999.
131. Newburg DS, Ruiz-Palacious GM, Morrow AL: Human milk glycans protect infants against enteric pathogens. Annu Rev Nutr 25:37, 2005.
132. Schwiertz A, Gruhl B, Lobnitz M, et al: Development of the intestinal bacterial composition in hospitalized preterm infants in comparison with breast-fed, full-term infants. Pediatr Res 54:393, 2003.
133. Morrow AL, Ruiz-Palacious GM, Altaye M, et al: Human milk oligosaccharides are associated with protection against diarrhea in breast-fed infants. J Pediatr 145:297, 2004.
134. Nichols-Johnson V: Promoting breastfeeding as an obstetrician/gynecologist. Clin Obstet Gynecol 47:624, 2004.
135. Mansbach IK, Palti H, Pevsner B, et al: Advice from the obstetrician and other sources: do they affect women's breast feeding practices? A study among different Jewish groups in Jerusalem. Soc Sci Med 19:157, 1984.
136. Lawrence RA: Breastfeeding, A Guide for the Medical Profession, 6th ed. St. Louis, Mosby, 2005.
137. Mohrbacher N, Stock J: The Breastfeeding Answer Book, revised ed. Schaumburg, IL, La Leche League International, 2003.
138. The Womanly Art of Breastfeeding, 6th revised ed. Schaumburg, IL, La Leche League Internal, 2002.
139. Briggs GG, Freeman RK, Yaffe SJ: Drugs in Pregnancy and Lactation, 7th ed. Baltimore, Williams & Wilkins, 2005.
140. Hale TW: Medications and Mothers' Milk, 11th ed. Amarillo, TX, Pharmsoft Medical Publishers, 2004.
141. American Academy of Pediatrics and The American College of Obstetricians and Gynecologists: Breastfeeding Handbook for Physicians. Washington, DC, 2006.
142. Alexander JM, Grant AM, Campbell MJ: Randomized controlled trial of breast shells and Hoffman's exercises for inverted and non-protractile nipples. BMJ 304:1030, 1990.
143. Kesaree N, Banapurmath CR, Banapurmath S, et al: Treatment of inverted nipples using a disposable syringe. J Hum Lact 9:27, 1993.
144. Hurst NM: Lactation after augmentation mammoplasty. Obstet Gynecol 87:30, 1996.
145. Semple JL, Lugowski SJ, Baines CJ, et al: Breast milk contamination and silicone implants: preliminary results using silicon as a proxy measurement for silicone. Plast Reconstr Surg 102:528, 1998.
146. Kjoller K, McLaughlin JK, Friis S, et al: Health outcomes in offspring of mothers with breast implants. Pediatrics 102:1112, 1998.
147. Souto GC, Giugliani ER, Giugliani C, et al: The impact of breast reduction surgery on breastfeeding performance. J Hum Lact 19:43–9, 2003.
148. Dewey KG, Nommsen-Rivers LA, Heinig MJ, et al: Risk factors for suboptimal infant breastfeeding behavior, delayed onset of lactation, and excess neonatal weight loss. Pediatrics 112:6079, 2003.
149. Evans KC, Evans RG, Royal R, et al: Effect of caesarean section on breast milk transfer to the normal term newborn over the first week of life. Arch Dis Child Fetal Neonatal Ed 88:F380, 2003.
150. Patel RR, Liebling RE, Murphy DJ: Effect of operative delivery in the second stage of labor on breastfeeding success. Birth 30:255, 2003.
151. Righard L, Alade MO: Effect of delivery room routines on success of first breast-feed. Lancet 336:1105, 1990.
152. Diek MJ, Evans ML, Arthurs JB: Predicting early breastfeeding attrition. J Hum Lact 18:21, 2002.
153. Beilin Y, Bodian CA, Weiser J, et al: Effect of labor epidural anesthesia with or without fentanyl on infant breastfeeding: a prospective, randomized, double-blind study. Anesthesiology 103:1211, 2005.
154. Zhang J, Bernasko JW, Leybovich E, et al: Continuous labor support from labor attendant for primiparous women: a meta-analysis. Obstet Gynecol 88:739, 1996.
155. Hofmeyr CJ, Nikodem VC, Wolman WL, et al: Companionship to modify the clinical birth environment: effects of progress and perceptions of labour, and breastfeeding. Br J Obstet Gynaecol 98:756, 1991.
156. Egli GE, Egli NS, Newton M: The influence of the number of breast-feedings on milk production. Pediatrics 27:314, 1961.
157. Howard C, Howard F, Lawrence R, et al: Office prenatal formula advertising and its effect on breast-feeding patterns. Obstet Gynecol 95:296, 2000.

158. Howard FM, Howard CR, Weitzman ML: The physician a advertiser: the unintentional discouragement of breast-feeding. Obstet Gynecol 95:296, 2000.
159. Bergcuim Y, Daugherty C, Kramer MS: Do infant formula samples shorten the duration of breastfeeding? Lancet 1:1148, 1983.
160. Sadurskis A, Kabir N, Wager J, et al: Encrgy metabolism, body composition, and milk production in healthy Swedish women during lactation. Am J Clin Nutr 28:44, 1988.
161. Brewer MM, Bates MR, Vannoy LP: Postpartum changes in maternal weight and body fat depots in lactating vs nonlactating women. Am J Clin Nutr 49:259, 1989.
162. Mass S: Breast Pain: Engorgement, nipple pain and mastitis. Clin Obstet Gynecol. 47:676, 2004.
163. Amir L, Garland SM, Dennerstein L, et al: *Candida albicans:* is it associated with nipple pain in lactating women? Gynecol Obstet Invest 41:30, 1996.
164. Livingston V, Stringer LJ: The treatment of Staphylococcus infected sore nipples: A randomized comparative study. J Hum Lact 15:241, 1999.
165. Cable B, Stewart M, Davis J: Nipple wound care: a new approach to an old problem. J Hum Lact 13:313, 1997
166. Woolridge MW, Baum JD, Drewett RF: Effect of traditional and of a new nipple shield on sucking patterns and milk flow. Early Hum Dev 4:357, 1980.
167. Hill PD, Humenick SS: The occurrence of breast engorgement. J Hum Lact 10:79, 1994.
168. Foxman B, D'Arcy H, Gillespie B, et al: Lactation mastitis: Occurrence and medical management among 946 breastfeeding women in the United States. Am J Epidemiol 155:103, 2002.
169. Kinlay Jr, O'Connell DL, Kinlay S: Incidence of mastitis in breastfeeding women during the six months after delivery: a prospective cohort study. Med J Aust 169:310, 1998.
170. Thomsen AC, Espersen T, Maignard S: Course and treatment of milk stasis, non-infectious inflammation of the breast, and infectious mastitis in nursing women. Am J Obstet Gynecol 149:492, 1984.
171. O'Hara RJ, Dexter SPL, Fox JN: Conservative management of infective mastitis and breast abscesses after ultrasonographic assessment. Br J Surg 83:1413, 1996.
172. Gartner LM, Herschel M: Jaundice and breastfeeding. Pediatr Clin North Am 48:389, 2001.
173. Emery MM: Galacatogogues: drugs to induce lactation. J Hum Lact 12:55, 1996.
174. Hansen WF, McAndrew S, Harris K, et al: Metoclopramide effect on breastfeeding the preterm infant: A randomized trial. Obstet Gynecol 105:383, 2005.
175. Howard CR, Howard F: Management of breastfeeding when the mother is ill. Clin Obstet Gynecol 47:683, 2004.
176. Hale T: Maternal Medications during breastfeeding. Clin Obstet Gynecol 47:696, 2004.
177. Ishida T, Yoke T, Kasumi F, et al: Clinicopathologic characteristics and prognosis of breast cancer patients associated with pregnancy and lactation: analysis of case-control study in Japan. Jpn J Cancer Res 83:1143, 1992.
178. Gupta RK, McHutchison AG, Dowle CS, et al: Fine-needle aspiration cytodiagnosis of breast masses in pregnant and lactating women and its impact on management. Diagn Cytopathol 9:156, 1993.
179. Meek JY: Breastfeeding in the workplace. Pediatr Clin North Am 48:461, 2001.
180. Neilsen J: Return to work: practical management of breastfeeding. Clin Obstet Gynecol 47:724, 2004.
181. Fein SB, Roe B: The effect of work status on initiation and duration of breast-feeding. Am J Public Health 88:1042, 1998.
182. Zinaman MJ, Hughes V, Queenan JT, et al: Acute prolactin and oxytocin responses and milk yield to infant suckling and artificial methods of expression in lactating women. Pediatrics 89:437, 1992.
183. Hamosh M, Ellis LA, Pollock DR, et al: Breast-feeding and the working mother: effect of time and temperature of short-term storage on proteolysis lipolysis, and bacterial growth in milk. Pediatrics 97:492, 1996.
184. Dettwyler KA: A time to wean: the hominid blueprint for the natural age of weaning in modern human populations. *In* Stuart-MacAdam P, Dettwyler KA (eds): Breastfeeding: Biocultural Perspectives. New York, Aldine de Gruyter, 1995, p 39.
185. Dettwyler K: When to wean: biological versus cultural perspectives. Clin Obstet Gynecol 47:712, 2004.

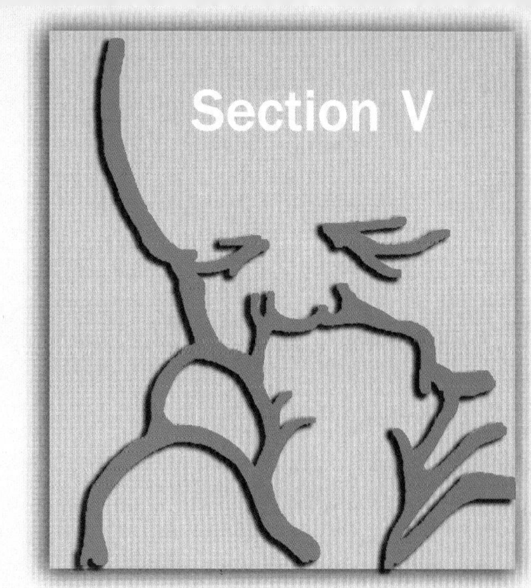

Complicated Pregnancy

Surgical Procedures in Pregnancy

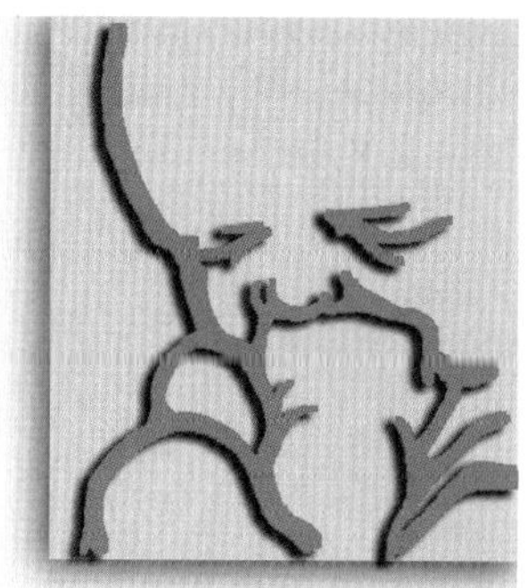

Erika J. Lu and Myriam J. Curet

CHAPTER 23

KEY ABBREVIATIONS

Cardiopulmonary resuscitation	CPR
Computed tomography	CT
Magnetic resonance imaging	MRI

One of the greatest challenges to both the obstetrician and surgeon is the care of the pregnant patient. Physiologic changes during pregnancy alter classic complaints, presentations, and treatments. In addition, outcomes of disease management affect two patients, both the mother and fetus. Abdominal emergencies in pregnant patients are notoriously difficult to diagnose, and management of cases that are straightforward in the nonpregnant woman become complicated in the pregnant state.

This chapter reviews the physiologic changes that affect the diagnosis and management of the acute abdomen in pregnancy. Common surgical conditions are reviewed. Particular discussion is dedicated to the use of minimally invasive surgery in pregnancy, because operative laparoscopy has become increasingly common in pregnant women over the past decade. Last, we review the principles of managing a pregnant trauma patient.

PHYSIOLOGIC CHANGES IN PREGNANCY

Physiologic changes unique to pregnancy alter the patterns of evaluation for the gravid surgery patient. Changes in cardiac, respiratory, renal, and gastrointestinal physiology are important concepts to keep in mind when evaluating the pregnant patient (Table 23-1).

DIAGNOSTIC IMAGING

The selection of diagnostic imaging studies in the pregnant patient is frequently a source of anxiety for the patient, obstetrician, and surgeon. The use of diagnostic radiology is often curtailed because of the concern for fetal injury. Fortunately, most radiologic studies are benign and expose the fetus to relatively low doses of radiation, typically less than 1 rad. Conventional X-ray examinations expose the fetus to less than 0.2 rad. Computed tomography (CT) exposes the fetus to higher doses of radiation, as outlined in Table 23-2.[1]

Current literature suggests that diagnostic imaging that exposes the fetus to less than 5 rad does not cause birth defects, intrauterine growth restriction, or spontaneous abortion, even during the first trimester. Although there is concern about teratogenicity of exposure from 5 to 10 rad, serious risk to the fetus is known to occur only above 10 rad.[2] Direct fetal irradiation of greater than 10 rad is associated with microcephaly, intrauterine growth restriction, developmental delay, and even fetal death. Lead shielding of the abdomen should be used whenever possible to reduce the dose of radiation to the fetus.

In certain situations, diagnostic radiology is an unavoidable part of evaluation of the pregnant surgical patient, and the benefits of such procedures should be weighed against an accurate assessment of the risk.

The following guidelines from The American College of Obstetricians and Gynecologists outline the use of radiographic exams during pregnancy[3]:

- Pregnant patients should be counseled that exposure from a single radiographic procedure does not result in harmful effects to the fetus. Specifically, exposure of less than 5 rad is not associated with an increased risk of fetal anomalies or spontaneous abortion.
- Concern about potential adverse effects of high-dose ionizing radiation should not prevent medically indicated diagnostic imaging.

Table 23-1. Physiologic Changes During Pregnancy

Blood Volume	↑ by 30–50%	Significant blood loss may occur (up to 2 liters) before hemodynamic alterations are appreciated. By this time, the patient may already be volume depleted
Hematocrit	30–50% normal	
SVR	↓ in BP	↓ in SBP by 5–10 mm Hg ↓ in DBP by 10–20 mm Hg
Heart rate	↑ by 10–15 bpm	
Clotting factors	↑ in Factors II, VII, VIII, IX, X, fibrinogen	4–6 fold increased risk of thromboembolism, particularly during periods of venous stasis, an in surgery. DVT prophylaxis in the form of SCDs should always be used
WBC	10,000 to 14,000 normal	Physiologic leukocytosis during pregnancy makes it more difficult to evaluate infectious abdominal processes, particularly late in the 3rd trimester, when the WBC is even higher.
Platelets	Low to normal	
FRC	Decreased FRC	The mother has lower threshold for hypoxemia, and atelectasis is more common postoperatively
Minute Ventilation	Increased minute ventilation, with $P_{CO_2} \approx 30$ mm Hg	Physiology maternal hyperventilation causes a compensatory metabolic acidosis with a decrease in maternal HCO_3. The mother therefore has less buffering capacity for metabolic acidosis
Progesterone-mediated smooth muscle relaxation	Decreased LES tone and GERD	Increased risk of aspiration with general anesthesia
	Decreased bowel peristalsis	Increased period of postoperative ileus; increased postoperative nausea and vomiting
	Abdominal wall laxity	More difficult to appreciate peritoneal signs in the acute abdomen, such as rebound and guarding
	Gallbladder stasis	Increased incidence of cholecystitis
	Hydroureter and urinary stasis	Increased risk of pyelonephritis, which must be ruled out when evaluating for acute abdomen

DBP, diastolic blood pressure; DVT, deep vein thrombosis; FRC, functional residual capacity; GERD, gastroesophageal reflux; LES, lower esophageal sphincter; SBP; systolic blood pressure; SCD, sequential compression device; SVR, systemic vascular resistance; WBC, white blood count.

Table 23-2. Approximate Fetal Doses from Common Diagnostic Procedures

PROCEDURE	FETAL EXPOSURE (RAD)
Chest radiograph (2 views)	0.00002–0.00007
Abdominal radiograph (1 view)	0.1–0.4
Computed tomography (CT) of the chest	0.6–0.96
Computed tomography (CT) of the abdomen	0.8–4.9
Computed tomography (CT) of the pelvis	2.5–7.9

Data from Lowe SA: Diagnostic radiography in pregnancy: risks and reality. Aust N Z J Obstet Gynecol 44:191, 2004.

- During pregnancy, nonionizing imaging procedures such as ultrasound and magnetic resonance imaging (MRI) should be considered whenever possible.

COMMON GENERAL SURGERY PROBLEMS IN PREGNANCY

Appendicitis

Appendicitis is the most common nongynecologic cause of the acute surgical abdomen during pregnancy, occurring in as many as 1 in 1,500 pregnancies.[4] Unfortunately, it is also the most frequently delayed surgical intervention because of its challenging diagnosis and a general reluctance to operate unnecessarily on a pregnant patient. Diagnostic delay and subsequent appendiceal perforation is the cause of preterm labor and fetal loss in as many as 36 percent of cases.[4–6] Early diagnosis and surgical intervention prevent fetal loss, with only a 1- to 5-percent fetal loss rate in unperforated cases.[7] Some authors have reported that delay of more than 24 hours in surgical intervention results in perforation in two thirds of the patients.[8] This is of greatest concern late in pregnancy, when the incidence of perforative appendicitis is highest and fetal viability is most likely. During the third trimester, appendiceal perforation is twice as common compared with the first and second trimesters (69 versus 31 percent).[9]

Maternal mortality from appendicitis is now very uncommon and usually associated with significant surgical delay. Over the past 30 years, the incidence of mortality has dropped dramatically to nearly zero because of prompt surgical intervention and improved antibiotic coverage.[6]

When appendicitis is suspected, the decision to operate should be based on clinical grounds, just as in the nonpregnant patient. Larger series report no pathology found at 20 to 35 percent of laparotomies, with greater accuracy of diagnosis during the first trimester.[6]

Clinical Presentation

The diagnosis of appendicitis during pregnancy is difficult because the hallmarks of appendicitis such as anorexia, nausea, vomiting, and leukocytosis are already present in the normal obstetric population. The most reliable symptom in pregnant patients with appendicitis is right lower quadrant pain.[10] Classic teaching maintains that this pain moves from the right lower quadrant in first trimester presentations toward the right upper quadrant in third-trimester presentations. This migration was first described in by Baer in 1932, who demonstrated cephalad displacement of the appendix by the expanding uterus using barium radiographs.[11] However, modern clinical experience does not confirm this assertion, with recent studies demonstrating that the most frequent location of pain remains in the right lower quadrant, regardless of trimester.[10]

Rebound tenderness and guarding are not particularly reliable symptoms to aid in the diagnosis of appendicitis in the gravid patient because of the laxity of abdominal musculature in the latter half of pregnancy.[12] Furthermore, fever is not present in the majority of pregnant patients with appendicitis, with up to 70 percent of patients having temperatures of less than 99.6°F.[13]

Laboratory Data

There are several pitfalls associated with the interpretation of laboratory data in the pregnant patient. Evaluation of the white blood cell count may not be helpful owing to the physiologic leukocytosis present in normal pregnancy, particularly during the third trimester. Although elevated neutrophil counts traditionally suggest infectious etiologies, one study found that only 59 percent of patients with proven appendicitis had a left shift.[13] The same authors suggest that urinalysis can also be confusing, with 20 percent of women with appendicitis having abnormal results. This can lead to the incorrect diagnosis of urinary tract infection[13] and further delay surgical therapy. Recent series have questioned the utility of using laboratory tests to confirm or reject the diagnosis of appendicitis at all.[10]

Imaging

Ultrasound is the initial imaging modality of choice in the pregnant patient. It has a sensitivity of 86 percent in the nonpregnant patient, with similar accuracy in the first and second trimesters of pregnancy.[12] During the third trimester, ultrasound examination is technically difficult and may be nondiagnostic. In these cases, helical CT should be considered. It exposes the fetus to only 0.3 rads[6] and can be completed in 15 minutes. In a recent study of seven patients with suspected appendicitis, helical CT correctly identified the two cases of pathologically proven appendicitis and allowed surgery to be avoided in the remaining five cases.[14]

Management

When preparing the pregnant patient for surgery, timely consultation between surgical, obstetric, and neonatal services should take place. External fetal monitoring should be considered intraoperatively if the gestational age is in the range of fetal viability (>24 weeks' gestation). In open laparotomy, a sterile plastic bag may be wrapped around the fetal heart rate monitor and displaced from the skin incision. In laparoscopic surgery, intraoperative fetal monitoring should be considered even at previable gestational ages so that if fetal heart rate abnormalities develop, pneumoperitoneum can be desufflated in an attempt to correct the problem. With laparoscopy, transvaginal ultrasound should be used because with transabdominal ultrasound monitoring, the signal is lost during abdominal insufflation.[15]

Various incisions have been described for open appendectomy in the pregnant patient. The most popular is a muscle-splitting incision over the point of maximal tenderness, which is of particular significance in the second and third trimesters, when the appendix may be significantly displaced by the gravid uterus. Paramedian and midline vertical incisions should be used if there is significant doubt as to the diagnosis in order to gain easier access to the adnexa. Uterine manipulation is avoided to decrease the risk of uterine irritability and preterm labor.

Laparoscopic appendectomy is an option for women up to 28 weeks' of gestation, before the size of the gravid uterus prevents visualization of the operative field.[16] Special precautions unique to laparoscopic surgery are detailed in subsequent sections.

In cases in which perforation has occurred, a critical part of therapy is the use of copious irrigation and broad-spectrum antibiotics with anaerobic coverage. The use of intraperitoneal drains has been advocated in these cases.[6]

Preterm contractions are common after appendectomy, occurring in approximately 80 percent of patients. However, preterm labor with cervical change and subsequent preterm delivery is relatively uncommon, occurring in 5 to 14 percent of patients.[10] Although tocolytic agents have not been shown to be helpful in preventing preterm delivery, they are frequently used in clinical practice.

Symptomatic Cholelithiasis

Symptomatic cholelithiasis is the second most common nongynecologic condition requiring surgery during pregnancy, occurring in 1 of 1,600 pregnancies.[9] The overall incidence of biliary tract disease during pregnancy ranges from 0.05 to 0.3 percent.[17,18] Many studies have shown that multiparity and abnormal gallbladder motility during pregnancy increase the risk of developing gallstones.[19,20]

When managing a gravid patient with biliary tract disease, the clinician must consider differences in outcome between conservative management and definitive surgical therapy. Although there is consensus that surgical intervention is necessary in complicated gallstone disease, the management of symptomatic cholelithiasis remains controversial with regard to medical versus surgical management.

Patients with obstructive jaundice, acute cholecystitis failing medical management, gallstone pancreatitis, or suspected peritonitis[17,19,21] should be treated surgically. Gallstone pancreatitis is particularly morbid and is associated with a significant maternal mortality rate of 15 to 60 percent and a fetal mortality rate near 60 percent.[18] Timely surgical intervention, typically during the same hospitalization after a period of bowel rest, is warranted.

Clinical Presentation

Pregnant patients with symptomatic cholelithiasis present with the same symptoms as nonpregnant patients, including nausea, vomiting, and the acute onset of stabbing right upper quadrant or midabdominal pain. Murphy's sign, with tenderness on deep inspiration under the right costal margin, is less common in the pregnant patient.

Laboratory Studies

Laboratory studies of serum transaminases and direct bilirubin can be elevated in biliary tract disease. Alkaline phosphatase is elevated during normal pregnancy and is therefore less helpful in diagnosis. Leukocytosis is also a part of normal pregnancy and not helpful in differentiating between biliary colic and acute cholecystitis.

Imaging

Ultrasound is the diagnostic modality of choice in pregnancy because of its noninvasiveness, speed and accuracy. It has a sensitivity of 95 percent for detecting gallstones and usually produces good views of the gallbladder, even without fasting.[22]

Medical Management

Traditional treatment of symptomatic cholelithiasis and acute cholecystitis during pregnancy has been conservative, particularly during the third trimester. This involves the use of supportive intravenous hydration, bowel rest with nasogastric suction and no oral intake, and narcotics. Antibiotics are indicated for signs of cholecystitis or infection. Surgery was usually reserved for refractory cases failing medical management after several days, or for patients with recurrent bouts of biliary colic. Recent studies have challenged this approach in favor of more aggressive early surgical intervention.

Surgical Management

Since the late 1980s, several authors have argued that early surgical management of biliary colic resulted in better pregnancy outcomes than in medically managed patients.[23–25] A recent study suggests that pregnant patients with symptomatic cholelithiasis have a high rate of symptomatic relapse during pregnancy, with more severe disease during relapse, including choledocholithiasis and gallstone pancreatitis.[25]

The safest time to operate on the pregnant patient is during the second trimester, when the risks of teratogenesis, miscarriage, and preterm delivery are lowest. The risk of teratogenesis is usually limited to the first trimester, and the incidence of spontaneous miscarriage dramatically decreases during the second trimester. During the third trimester, the gravid uterus obscures the operative field, making laparoscopy difficult. Patients presenting with simple biliary colic during the first or third trimesters should be managed medically and offered elective cholecystectomy in the second trimester or immediately postpartum. Any patient whose clinical condition deteriorates despite medical therapy should undergo cholecystectomy or cholecystostomy regardless of the trimester.[26]

Uncomplicated open cholecystectomy is associated with rare maternal mortality, 5 percent fetal death, and 7 percent preterm labor.[27] Percutaneous cholecystostomy can be an effective management option that avoids the use of general anesthesia but is infrequently performed.

Laparoscopic biliary tract surgery has emerged as a safe modality for cholecystectomy during pregnancy. Since it was first performed in a pregnant patient in 1991, numerous studies have shown that it reduces postoperative pain and recovery time, results in less fetal exposure to narcotics, and decreases the risk of incisional hernias compared to open cholecystectomy.[15,16] It is more likely to be technically feasible later in pregnancy than laparoscopic appendectomy because the uterus does not completely obscure the operative field, even during the third trimester. In general, 28 weeks' of gestation appears to be the limit for successful completion of laparoscopic surgery, although reports of surgery in later gestational ages have been published. Cholangiography should be performed selectively with a single film and use of lead shielding to protect the fetus from radiation exposure.[28] Conversion to open cholecystectomy should always be performed if intraoperative conditions make continued laparoscopic surgery unsafe.[29]

LAPAROSCOPY IN PREGNANCY

Laparoscopic surgery has revolutionized the field of general surgery over the past 15 years. Numerous authors have shown that the advantages of minimally invasive surgery, including decreased pain, shorter hospitalization, and quicker return to normal activity, apply to the pregnant population.[16,27,30] Historically, most surgeons considered pregnancy to be a contraindication to laparoscopy. However, recent literature has shown that minimally invasive surgery can be performed safely during pregnancy with acceptable maternal and fetal morbidity.[15–19,21,25,28,31] The second trimester is by far the best time to perform laparoscopic surgery, with a fetal loss rate of only 5.6 percent compared with 12 percent in

Table 23-3. Reported Cases of Laparoscopic Biliary Tract Surgeries During Pregnancy Trimester

SOURCE	NO. OF PATIENTS	1ST NO. PATIENTS	2ND NO. PATIENTS	3RD NO. PATIENTS	PTD (%)	MEAN GESTATIONAL AGE OF PTD	NO. OF FETAL DEATHS
Rollins et al[57]	31	3	19	9	6 (20%)	33.8 weeks	1
Afflect et al[58]	42	3	28	11	5 (11.9%)	35.5 weeks	0
Muench et al[59]	16	9	6	1	0	...	0
Sungler et al[60]	9	0	8	1	0	...	0
Cosenza et al[32]	12	...	...	...	0	...	0
Daradkeh et al[61]	16	2	10	4	0	...	0
Graham et al[62]	6	2	4	0	0	...	0
Glasgow et al[63]	14	3	11	0	1	35 weeks	0
Gouldman et al[21]	8	1	7	0	0	...	0
Lu et al[25]	6	0	6	0	0	...	0
Comitalo et al[64]	4	0	4	0	1	37 weeks	0
Soper et al[31]	5	0	5	0	0	...	0
Morrell et al[65]	5	0	5	0	2	33 weeks	0
Lanzafame et al[19]	5	0	3	2	0	...	0

PTD, preterm delivery.

the first trimester. Furthermore, the rate of premature labor is 0 percent in the second trimester compared with 40 percent during the third trimester.[17] There are more than 50 reports in the English literature documenting the use of laparoscopic cholecystectomy during pregnancy. The largest series are documented in Table 23-3. One hundred and seventy-one cases of laparoscopic biliary surgery are discussed, with only one fetal loss. This compares favorably with a 3 percent rate of fetal loss in open cholecystectomy for uncomplicated biliary tract disease.[32] In one study by Amos et al.,[33] there were four fetal losses among seven patients who underwent laparoscopic cholecystectomy. Although this series addresses the risks of laparoscopy, it should be noted that the pregnancies that resulted in fetal death involved long operative times and complicated biliary tract disease such as gallstone pancreatitis, which is inherently associated with a fetal loss rate of up to 60 percent.[18,25]

In addition to the safety of laparoscopy in pregnancy, there are the added benefits of decreased preterm delivery secondary to decreased uterine manipulation and less fetal depression secondary to reduced narcotic use.[15,30] This has popularized operative laparoscopy for various indications during pregnancy, including appendicitis and cholecystitis.

The proven benefits of laparoscopic surgery during pregnancy must be weighed against the risks. In addition to its technical difficulty due to the gravid uterus, the surgeon must consider the unknown risks of fetal acidosis caused by carbon dioxide absorption, decreased uterine blood flow resulting from increased intraabdominal pressure, and fetal hypotension from decreased maternal cardiac output.

The concern for fetal hypotension with pneumoperitoneum is theoretical, but is not believed to be of clinical significance given the presence of increased intraabdominal pressure in other states such as the maternal Valsalva's maneuver, coughing, and straining.[31] Although there are no reports of deleterious effects of pneumoperitoneum gas on the human fetus, animal studies have raised concern for fetal acidosis.

The following practice guidelines are based on the SAGES Guidelines of Laparoscopic Surgery During Pregnancy.[34] They should be followed when performing minimally invasive surgery in the pregnant patient to reduce adverse effects on the mother or fetus.

1. Obstetric consultation should be obtained to aid in perioperative management.
2. When possible, surgery should be deferred until the second trimester, when the risk to the fetus is lowest.
3. Aspiration precautions should be taken, because the pregnant woman has a decreased lower esophageal sphincter pressure and delayed gastric emptying.
4. The patient should be placed in left lateral decubitus position with minimal reverse. Trendelenburg to decrease uterine compression of the inferior vena cava.
5. Antiembolic stockings should be used to prevent deep venous thrombosis, especially given the increased levels of clotting factors and fibrinogen creating a procoagulable state during pregnancy.
6. Use an open Hasson technique for entering the abdominal cavity. Although several authors have successfully used the Veress needle, puncture of the uterus has been reported. There is a higher risk of abdominal visceral injury with increasing gestational age, making the Veress needle contraindicated.
7. Maintain carbon dioxide pneumoperitoneum at 12 to 15 mm Hg, keeping intraabdominal pressure at the minimum level to achieve adequate visualization.
8. Maternal end tidal carbon dioxide should be continuously monitored and maintained at 25 to 30 mm Hg to minimize maternal and thereby fetal acidosis. Prompt adjustments to the minute ventilation are critical.
9. If the fetus is of viable gestational age, continuous fetal monitoring should be employed. Transvaginal ultrasound is often needed because transabdominal ultrasound is made difficult by the presence of pneumoperitoneum. If there is evidence of fetal distress, pneumoperitoneum should be released immediately. If the fetus is not of viable gestational age, then pre-

operative and postoperative fetal heart tones should be documented.
10. Lead shielding of the fetus should be used whenever cholangiography is used. Fluoroscopy should be limited.
11. Minimize operative time. Several studies have shown an increase in $Paco_2$ with increased operative time.

TRAUMA IN PREGNANCY

Trauma is the leading cause of maternal death secondary to nonobstetric etiologies.[35] Major trauma affects as many as 8 percent of pregnant women.[36] Therefore, experience with evaluating and managing the pregnant trauma victim is important to both the surgeon and obstetrician.

Blunt Trauma

Blunt trauma during pregnancy is most commonly the result of motor vehicle collisions, falls, and violence. Of particular clinical significance are motor vehicle collisions, which are the leading cause of death in girls and women age 6 to 29 years, according to the National Highway and Traffic Safety Administration.[37] Physical abuse in pregnancy occurs in as many as 10 percent of pregnant women, frequently resulting in blunt abdominal trauma.[38]

Motor vehicle collisions account for the great majority of blunt trauma in pregnancy. Maternal death is the major cause of fetal death following a motor vehicle collision.[39] In 1971, Crosby et al.[39] demonstrated a reduction in maternal death rate from 33 to 5 percent with the use of two-point restraints A more recent study demonstrated that the proper use of seatbelts, along with crash severity, is the number one predictor of maternal and fetal outcome.[40] Ejection from the vehicle and associated head trauma are correlated with poor fetal outcome. Although there is no large-scale data on the safety of airbag use in pregnancy, the National Highway and Traffic Safety Administration does not consider pregnancy as an indicator for deactivation of airbags. In general, it is believed that airbags, in combination with the proper positioning of a three-point restraint across the maternal pelvis, provide the greatest protection to the mother and unborn child.

Mechanisms of Maternal Injury

Two physiologic changes unique to the pregnant patient change the mechanism of injury compared with that in the nonpregnant patient. First, the transmission of force in the gravid abdomen is different than in the nonpregnant patient owing to the relative cephalad displacement of abdominal contents. Bowel injury tends to be seen with less frequency.[41]

Second, increased vascularity during pregnancy makes splenic and retroperitoneal injury more common. It has been shown that 25 percent of pregnant women suffering from severe blunt trauma have hemodynamically significant splenic or hepatic injuries.[42]

Mechanisms of Fetal Injury

Clinically evident placental abruption occurs in up to 40 percent of severe blunt abdominal trauma and in 3 percent of minor traumas with direct uterine force.[43] It is caused by the shearing force placed on the placental-uterine interface. Abruption compromises fetal oxygenation, and the patient must be monitored closely for signs of fetal distress, which may necessitate delivery.

Uterine rupture is a rare but serious complication of severe blunt abdominal trauma. It is estimated to occur in less than 1 percent of all pregnant trauma victims[44] but must be quickly assessed given its grave consequences. Fetal death almost always occurs, and the rate of maternal death can be as high as 10 percent.[45] Before 12 weeks' gestation, the small size of the uterus allows it to be protected by its pelvic location, making it less prone to injury. As the pregnancy continues, the propensity for uterine rupture increases as it becomes more of an abdominal organ. By the third trimester, increased pelvic blood flow raises the likelihood of serious hemorrhage with uterine injury. Rupture is usually related to severe direct abdominal impact.

Direct fetal injuries are another rare occurrence in trauma, which is seen in approximately 1 percent of cases with severe abdominal or pelvic force.[46] It usually occurs late in pregnancy in patients with other significant injuries. Fetal skull and brain injuries tend to occur with maternal pelvic fractures late in the third trimester, when the fetal head is already engaged in the maternal pelvis.[47] In high-speed motor vehicle accidents, fetal brain injuries can also occur as a result of deceleration force.

Penetrating Trauma

The most common causes of penetrating trauma in the pregnant patient are gunshot and stab wounds. Other mechanisms are rare and not discussed here. The gravid trauma victim is unique in the pattern of injury sustained. The upper abdomen is the most common site of stab wounds in the pregnant patient. In late pregnancy, small bowel injury becomes more common in upper abdominal stabbings secondary to the cephalad displacement of the bowel loops by the gravid uterus.[42] These injuries should be managed operatively, as discussed later.

The maternal death rate in penetrating trauma is two-thirds lower than in nongravid patients secondary to the protective effects of the uterus on other abdominal organs. One study demonstrates a reduction in mortality in abdominal gunshot wounds from 12.5 to 3.9 percent.[46] Conversely, the fetal death rate is significant—as high as 71 percent with gunshot wounds[48] and 42 percent with abdominal stab wounds.[49]

Principles of Trauma Management in Pregnancy

Primary Survey and Initial Resuscitation

With few exceptions, priorities of initial resuscitation are similar to those in nonpregnant patients. Initial attempts at stabilization should be directed towards establishment of the airway, maintenance of oxygenation, and fluid resuscitation for the mother. Most situations that cause maternal instability are also harmful to the fetus. During resuscitation, several obstetric issues should be considered.

When establishing an airway, guidelines for intubation and mechanical ventilation are similar to those in the nonpregnant patient. However, pregnant women should be managed as high-risk for aspiration, because they are more prone to pulmonary aspiration of gastric contents.

Volume resuscitation is complicated by several factors in the gravid patient. First, aortocaval compression causes compromise of maternal perfusion and decreases cardiac output by 25 percent.[50] Therefore, left lateral displacement of the uterus should be performed in any patient at greater than 24 weeks' gestation. This can be accomplished by tilting the entire backboard, or if backboard tilt is contraindicated, manual lateral displacement of the uterus. Second, with expansion of the blood volume by 40 to 50 percent during pregnancy, it can be difficult to interpret maternal blood loss. Clinically significant blood loss of up to 2 liters, or 30 percent of the total blood volume, may not be readily apparent. The clinician must be wary of a falsely reassuring hemodynamic state masking ongoing hemorrhage. Third, the acute use of inotropes or vasopressors may be needed to sustain maternal blood flow. This reduces uteroplacental blood flow, but maternal considerations should take precedence.

Diagnosis of the acute abdomen is difficult in the gravid patient. Chronic stretching of the peritoneum during pregnancy diminishes the typical signs of peritoneal irritation.[35] Therefore, direct peritoneal lavage with open insertion of a peritoneal catheter is advocated by several authorities as the preferred technique of evaluation in pregnancy.[51] This has not been shown to adversely affect the outcome of pregnancy.

Surgery for Penetrating Trauma

Surgeons have had a traditionally low threshold for surgical exploration of the pregnant patient with penetrating abdominal injury. All posterior and upper abdominal wounds should be explored, as well as gunshot wounds in the uterine area. With maternal or fetal compromise, surgery should be considered.

Some data suggest that anterior abdominal entry wounds below the level of the uterine fundus may be managed conservatively.[52] Diagnostic peritoneal lavage, fistulogram, and ultrasound may aid in management of the stable lower abdominal penetrating injury.

If exploratory laparotomy is undertaken, a thorough inspection of the uterus should always be performed to rule out injury. Delivery of the fetus is rarely indicated unless there is direct perforating uterine injury, nonreassuring fetal status, fetal death, or the gravid uterus is preventing adequate exposure for repair of maternal injuries.[36] In cases of direct uterine injury, management should involve consideration of gestational age, injuries present, and the maternal and fetal prognosis if the baby is undelivered. In cases of fetal death, labor induction postoperatively may be a better option to uterine evacuation during laparotomy in an unstable patient.[35]

Secondary Survey. Fetal Evaluation

Fetal evaluation should be a part of the secondary survey in the pregnant trauma patient. As previously discussed, placental abruption is one of the most common causes of fetal compromise in the gravid trauma patient. Ultrasonography has not been found to reliably detect placental abruption.[53] Cardiotocography is the preferred method of stratifying risk in these cases. One study demonstrated that the presence of more than one contraction every 10 minutes was associated with a 20 percent risk of placental abruption. If cardiotocography fails to reveal frequent contractions, the fetal heart rate is reassuring, and there is no other clinical evidence of placental abruption, such as vaginal bleeding, fetal heart rate and contraction monitoring should still be continued for a minimum of 4 to 6 hours. Even with reassuring fetal heart rate monitoring, a small risk of abruption persists up to several days after the trauma.[54]

During secondary evaluation of the fetus, the clinician should test the mother for evidence of a fetomaternal hemorrhage. Ten to 30 percent of pregnant trauma patients have some level of fetomaternal hemorrhage.[45] For all unsensitized Rh-negative mothers, anti-D immunoglobulin should be considered. The Kleihauer-Betke test is recommended for Rh negative patients in order to quantify the fetomaternal hemorrhage and calculate the correct dose of anti-D immunoglobulin.

CARDIAC ARREST IN THE PREGNANT PATIENT

Cardiopulmonary resuscitation (CPR) is not particularly effective in increasing cardiac output or organ perfusion. This, coupled with the effect of aortocaval compression on venous return, makes CPR in the gravid patient relatively inefficient. In animal data in which partial occlusion of the inferior vena cava was used to mimic aortocaval compression in pregnancy, there was a dramatic decrease in the effectiveness of chest compressions.[55] This was reflected in an increase in catecholamine need, an increase in metabolic acidosis, and the need for CPR 10 times longer to recover from bupivicaine-induced cardiac arrest. Therefore, left lateral tilt is recommended to reduce the effects of aortocaval compression in patients at greater than 24 weeks' of gestation. However, the use of lateral tilt decreases the total compressive force generated by CPR by virtue of vector physics, further reducing the efficacy of chest compressions.

Because of the relative inefficiency of CPR, some authors advocate the use of early open cardiac massage to increase organ perfusion. However, prospective data are lacking to support its true efficacy, and its use should be guided on a case by case basis.

Perimortem cesarean delivery has been advocated for both maternal and fetal indications. Bedside cesarean delivery should always be considered to aid in maternal resuscitation if chest compressions are unsuccessful within 5 minutes. This improves outcome in cases in which aortocaval compression hinders the efficacy of CPR. Cesarean delivery should also be undertaken if the fetus is viable and maternal cardiopulmonary arrest appears untreatable. In a retrospective review of 269 cases of perimortem cesarean section, Katz et al.[56] demonstrated that all babies delivered within 5 minutes of maternal death appeared to be neurologically intact. Overall, fetal survival ranged from 50 to 70 percent, with outcome diminishing as time from maternal arrest to delivery increased. In patients with longer periods of maternal arrest, such as those transported to the hospital in arrest, cesarean delivery is still an option but the rate of intact neonatal survival diminishes.

CONCLUSION

Management of surgical diseases occurring during pregnancy can be a challenge for obstetricians and surgeons. When evaluating the gravid surgical patient, it is important to keep in mind the unique physiologic changes during pregnancy that affect management. With symptoms such as nausea and vomiting common especially in early pregnancy, and with limitations on the use of radiography, acute illnesses such as appendicitis may be difficult to diagnose. When caring for a pregnant patient, it is preferable to operate in the second trimester if possible, as with uncomplicated biliary tract disease. When considering surgical approaches, laparoscopy offers significant advantages, with good maternal and fetal outcomes, when guidelines for safety are followed. Management of the pregnant trauma patient should always be directed toward stabilization of the mother first, with evaluation of the fetus in the secondary survey.

KEY POINTS

- Use of nonionizing imaging procedures such as ultrasound and MRI should be considered whenever possible to minimize fetal irradiation.
- The diagnosis of acute abdomen is difficult in the gravid patient for numerous reasons.
- Operative delay in a pregnant patient with appendicitis increases risk of perforation and significantly increases the rate of preterm labor and fetal loss.
- Pregnant patients with complicated gallstone disease, particularly gallstone pancreatitis, should be treated surgically.
- The second trimester is the safest time to operate on the pregnant patient.
- Pregnant women with uncomplicated gallstone disease should be managed medically during the first and third trimesters, then offered elective laparoscopic cholecystectomy in the second trimester or in the postpartum period.
- Laparoscopic surgery can be performed safely during pregnancy.
- The SAGES guidelines for laparoscopic surgery during pregnancy should be followed in all pregnant patients undergoing laparoscopic surgery.
- Expansion of maternal blood volume during pregnancy may mask signs of maternal hemorrhage, and clinically significant blood loss can occur before hemodynamic changes are evident.
- Management of the pregnant trauma patient should always be directed toward stabilization of the mother first, with evaluation of the fetus during the secondary survey.

REFERENCES

1. Lowe SA: Diagnostic radiography in pregnancy: risks and reality. Aust N Z J Obstet Gynaecol 44:191, 2004.
2. Schwartz HM, Reichling BA: Hazards of radiation exposure for pregnant women. JAMA 239:1908, 1978.
3. American College of Obstetricians and Gynecologists: Guidelines for diagnostic imaging during pregnancy. Committee Opinion. www.acog.org, American College of Obstetricians and Gynecologists, 1995.
4. Babaknia A, Parsa H: Appendicitis during pregnancy. Obstet Gynecol 50:40, 1977.
5. Horowitz MD, Gomez GA, Santiesteban R: Acute appendicitis in pregnancy. Arch Surg 120:1362, 1995.
6. Sharp HT: The acute abdomen during pregnancy. Clin Obstet Gynecol 45:405, 2002.
7. Firstenberg MS, Malangoni MA: Gastrointestinal surgery during pregnancy. Gastroenterol Clin North Am 27:73, 1998.
8. Tamir IL, Bongard FS, Klein SR: Acute appendicitis in the pregnant patient. Am J Surg 160:571, 1990.
9. Weingold AB: Appendicitis in pregnancy. Clin Obstet Gynecol 26:801, 1983.
10. Mourad J, Elliot JP, Erickson L: Appendicitis in pregnancy: New information that contradicts long-held clinical beliefs. Am J Obstet Gynecol 182:1027, 2000.
11. Baer JL, Reirs RA, Arens RA: Appendicitis in pregnancy with changes in position and axis of the normal appendix in pregnancy. JAMA 52:1359, 1932.
12. Martin C, Varner MW: Physiologic changes in pregnancy: surgical implications. Clin Obstet Gynecol 37:241, 1994.
13. Masters K, Levine BA, Gaskill HV: Diagnosing appendicitis during pregnancy. Am J Surg 148:768, 1984.
14. Castro MA, Shipp TD, Castro EE: The use of helical computed tomography in pregnancy for the diagnosis of acute appendicitis. Am J Obstet Gynecol 184:184, 2001.
15. Hart RO, Tamadon A, Fitzgibbons RJ, Fkeming A: Open laparoscopic cholecystectomy in pregnancy. Surg Laparosc Endosc 3:13, 1993.
16. Curet MJ, Allen D, Josloff RK, et al: Laparoscopy during pregnancy. Arch Surg 131:546, 1996
17. McKellar DP, Anderson CT, Boynton CJ, Peoples JB: Cholecystectomy during pregnancy without fetal loss. Surg Gynecol Obstetr 174:465, 1992.
18. Printen KJ, Ott RA: Cholecystectomy during pregnancy. Am J Surg 44:432, 1978.

19. Lanzafame RJ: Laparoscopic cholecystectomy. Surgery 118:627, 1995.
20. Scott LD: Gallstone disease and pancreatitis in pregnancy. Gastroenterol Clin North Am 21:803, 1992.
21. Gouldman JW, Sticca RP, Rippon MB, McAlhany JC: Laparoscopic cholecystectomy in pregnancy. Am Surg 64:93, 1998.
22. Stauffer RA, Adams A, Wygal J: Gallbladder disease in pregnancy. Am J Obstetr Gynecol 6:661, 1982.
23. Dixon NP, Faddis DM, Silberman H: Aggressive surgical management of cholecystitis during pregnancy. Am J Surg;154:292, 1987.
24. Lee S, Bradley JP, Mele MM: Cholelithiasis in pregnancy: surgical versus medical management. Obstet Gynecol 95:S70, 2000.
25. Lu EJ, Curet MJ, El-Sayed YY, Kirkwood KS: Medical versus surgical management of biliary tract disease in pregnancy. Am J Surg 188:755, 2004.
26. Weber RA, Smith RW, Wright RC: Percutatneous cholecystostomy during pregnancy: a new treatment for acute cholecystitis in pregnancy? Contemporary Surgical Resident 1:21, 1993.
27. Curet MJ: Special problems in laporoscopic surgery. Surg Clin North Am 80:1095, 2000.
28. Chandra M, Shipro SJ, Gordon LA: Laparoscopic cholecystectomy in the first trimester of pregnancy. Surg Laparosc Endosc 4:68, 1994.
29. Barone JE, Bears S, Chen S, et al: Outcome study of cholecystectomy during pregnancy. Am J Surg 177:232, 1999.
30. Bisharah M, Tulandi T: Laparoscopic surgery in pregnancy. Clin Obstet Gynecol 46:92, 2003.
31. Soper NJ, Hunter J, Petrie RH: Laparoscopic cholecystectomy during pregnancy. Surg Endosc 6:115, 1992.
32. Cosenza CA, Saffari B, Jabbour N, et al: Surgical management of biliary gallstone disease during pregnancy. Am J Surg 178:545, 1999.
33. Amos JD, Schorr SJ, Norman PF, et al: Laparoscopic surgery during pregnancy. Am J Surg 171:435, 1996.
34. Society of American Gastrointestinal Endoscopic Surgeons (SAGES): Guidelines for laparoscopic surgery during pregnancy. Surg Endosc 12:189, 1998.
35. Moise KJ, Belfort MA: Damage control for the pregnant patient. Surg Clin North Am 77:835, 1997.
36. Lavery JP, Staten-McCormick M: Management of moderate to severe trauma in pregnancy. Obstet Gynecol Clin North Am 22:69, 1995.
37. Administration NHTSA. Motor vehicle crashes as a leading cause of death in US, 2002. www.nra.nhtsa.dot.gov/pdf/nra-30Incsa/rph/2005/809843.pdf
38. Van Hook JW, Hankins GDV: Trauma and envenomation. *In* Clark SL, Cotton DB, Hankins GDV, Phelan JP (eds): Critical Care Obstetrics, 3rd ed. Oxford, Blackwell Scientific, 1997, p 597.
39. Crosby WM, Costiloe JP: Safety of lap-belt restraint for pregnant victims of automobile collisions. N Engl J Med 284:632, 1971.
40. Pearlman MD, Klinich KD, Schneider LW: A comprehensive program to improve safety for pregnant women and fetuses in motor vehicle crashes: a preliminary report. Am J Obstet Gynecol 182:1554, 2000.
41. Pearlman MD, Tintinalli JE, Lorenz RP: A prospective controlled study of outcome after trauma during pregnancy. Am J Obstet Gynecol 162:1502, 1990.
42. Kuhlmann RS, Cruikshank DP: Maternal trauma during pregnancy. Clin Obstet Gynecol 37:274, 1994.
43. Lane PL: Traumatic fetal deaths. J Emerg Med 7:433, 1989.
44. Pearlman MD: Trauma and pregnancy. *In* Hankins GDV, Clark SL, Cunningham FG (eds): Operative Obstetrics. Norwalk, Appleton & Lange, 1999, p 651.
45. Pearlman MD, Tintinalli JE: Evaluation and treatment of the gravida and fetus following trauma during pregnancy. Obstet Gynecol Clin North Am 18:371, 1991.
46. Van Hook JW: Trauma in pregnancy. Clin Obstet Gynecol 45:414, 2002.
47. Hartl R, Ko K: In utero skull fracture: case report. J Trauma 41:549, 1996.
48. Sandy EA, Koerner M: Self-inflicted gunshot wound to the pregnant abdomen: report of a case and review of the literature. Am J Perinatol 6:30, 1989.
49. Sakala EP, Kort DD: Management of stab wounds to the pregnant uterus: A case report and review of the literature. Obstet Gynecol Surv 43:319, 1988.
50. Lees M, Scott D, Carr MG: Circulatory effects of recumbent postural changes in late pregnancy. Clin Sci 32:453, 1967.
51. Brundage SI, Davies JK, Jurkovich GJ: Trauma to the pregnant patient. *In* Grenvik A, Ayers SM, Holbrook PR (eds): Critical Care, 4th ed. Philadephia, WB Saunders, 2000, p 383.
52. Awwad JT, Azar GB: High-velocity penetrating wounds of the gravid uterus: review of 16 years of civil war. Obstet Gynecol 83:259, 1994.
53. Dalmus MA, Sibai BM: Blunt abdominal trauma: are there predictive factors for abruptio placentae or maternal-fetal distress? Am J Obstet Gynecol 169:1054, 1993.
54. Higgins SD, Garite TJ: Late abruptio placenta in trauma patients: implications for monitoring. Obstet Gynecol 63:10S, 1984.
55. Kasten GW, Martin ST: Resuscitation from bupivicaine-induced cardiovasccular toxicity during partial inferior vena cava occlusion. Anesth Analg 65:341, 1986.
56. Katz VL, Dotter DJ, Droegemueller W: Perimortem cesarean delivery. Obstet Gynecol 68:571, 1986.
57. Rollins MD, Chan JK, Price RR: Laparoscopy for appendicitis and cholelithiasis during pregnancy. Surg Endosc 18:237, 2004.
58. Affleck DG, Handrahan DL, Egger MJ, Price RR: The laparoscopic management of appendicitis and cholelithiasis during pregnancy. Am J Surg 178:523, 1999.
59. Muench J, Akbrink M, Seragini F, et al: Delay in treatment of biliary disease during pregnancy increases morbidity and can be avoided with safe laparoscopic cholecystectomy. Am Surg 67:539, 2001.
60. Sungler P, Heinerman PM, Steiner H, et al: Laparoscopic cholecystectomy and interventional endoscopy for gallstone complications during pregnancy. Surg Endosc 14:267, 2000.
61. Daradkeh S, Sumrein I, Zaiden K, Abu-Khalaf M: Management of gallbladder stones during pregnancy: conservative treatment or laparoscopic cholecystectomy? Hepatogastroenterology 46:3074, 1999.
62. Graham G, Baxi L, Tharakan T: Laparoscopic cholecystectomy during pregnancy: a case series and review of the literature. Obstet Gynecol Surv 53:566, 1998.
63. Glasgow RE, Visser BC, Harris HW, et al: Changing management of gallstone disease during pregnancy. Surg Endosc 12:241, 1998.
64. Comitalo JB, Lynch D: Laparoscopic cholecystectomy in the pregnant patient. Surg Laparosc Endosc 4:268, 1994.
65. Morrell DG, Mullins JR, Harrison PB: Laparoscopic cholecystectomy during pregnancy in symptomatic patients. Surgery 112:856, 1992.

Pregnancy Loss

JOE LEIGH SIMPSON AND ERIC R. M. JAUNIAUX

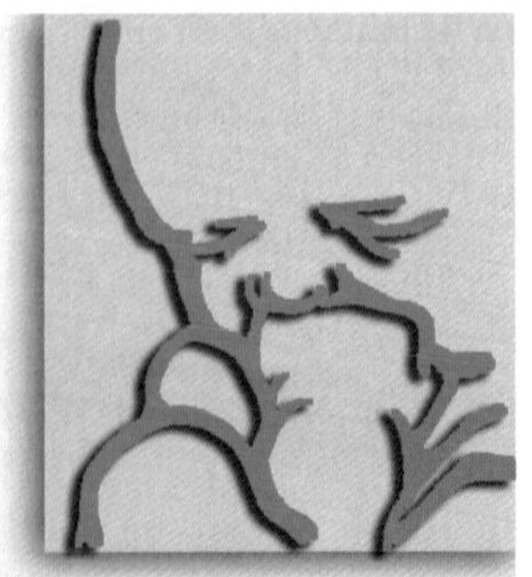

CHAPTER 24

KEY ABBREVIATIONS

American College of Obstetricians and Gynecologists	ACOG
Anticardiolipin	aCL
Antiphospholipid antibodies	aPL
Assisted reproductive technologies	ART
β-human chorionic gonadotropin	β-hCG
Clusters of differentiation	CD
Confidence interval	CI
Fluorescence in situ hybridization	FISH
Human chorionic gonadotropin	hCG
Human leukocyte antigen	HLA
Immunoglobulin A	IgA
Immunoglobulin G	IgG
Interleukin	IL
Interferon	INF
Lupus anticoagulant	LAC
Luteinizing hormone	LH
Luteal phase defect	LPD
National Institute of Child Health and Human Development	NICHD
Oxygen	O_2
Preimplantation genetic diagnosis	PGD
Rhesus (D antigen)	Rh(D)
Royal College of Obstetricians and Gynaecologists	RCOG
Standard deviation	SD
T-helper	Th
Three-dimensional	3D
Thyroid receptor β	TRβ
Thyroid-stimulating hormone	TSH

Not all conceptions result in a live-born infant, and overall human reproduction is described as being extremely inefficient compared with that of other mammals species. It has been estimated that approximately 50 to 70 percent of spontaneous conceptions are lost before completion of the first trimester, most of them during the first month after the last menstrual period. They are often ignored as conceptions, particularly if they occur around the time of an expected menstrual period. Of clinically recognized pregnancies, 10 to 15 percent are lost. Among married women in the United States, 4 percent have experienced two fetal losses, and 3 percent have experienced three or more.[1] It is accepted that a subset of women manifest repetitive spontaneous miscarriages, as opposed to randomly having repeated untoward events. This chapter considers the causes of fetal wastage, and the management of couples experiencing repetitive losses.

FREQUENCY AND TIMING OF PREGNANCY LOSSES

Pregnancy loss occurs throughout gestation, beginning before implantation. Not surprisingly, losses are more frequent among morphologically abnormal than among morphologically normal embryos. Within 10 to 14 days after implantation, β-human chorionic gonadotropin (β-hCG) assays can detect preclinical pregnancies. This is still before when pregnancy is recognized clinically, usually 5 to 6 weeks after the last menstrual period. About two thirds of implanted pregnancies that miscarry are lost before clinical recognition, based on cohort studies in which daily urinary hCG assays were performed beginning around the expected time of implantation (day 20 of gestation).[2] Of pregnancies detected in this fashion, 31 percent (61 of 198) were lost; the preclinical loss rate was 22 percent (43 of 198), and the clinically recognized loss rate was 12 percent (19 of 155). Data later in gestation were gathered by Mills and colleagues[3,4] in a National Institute of Child Health and Human Development (NICHD) collaborative study, in which serum β-hCG assays were performed 28 to 35 days after the previous menses. The total fetal loss rate (preclinical and clinical) for pregnancies was 16 percent for these pregnancies. Mean gestational age was 4 to 5 weeks or approximately 10 days later than those ascertained by Wilcox et al.[2] Spandorfer et al.[5] found a loss rate of 11.6 percent (233/2014) when in vitro fertilization pregnancies were assessed at 7-week ultrasound. The mean age of the sample was 35 to 36 years, older than in the study by Simpson et al.[4] but several weeks later in gestation.

Clinically recognized first-trimester fetal loss rates are 10 to 12 percent, which are well documented in both retrospective and prospective cohort studies.[6] Higher loss rates have reported, but these probably reflect unwitting inclusion of surreptitious illicit abortions, a common occurrence where legal termination is proscribed. As is discussed in this chapter, loss rates reflect many factors. However, two associations are worth emphasizing here at the onset. First, maternal age greatly increases risk, a 40-year-old woman carrying twice the risk of a 20-year-old woman. Second, prior pregnancy history is pivotal. Loss rates are lowest (6 percent) among nulliparous women who have never experienced a loss,[7] rising to 25 to 30 percent after three or more miscarriages. Recurrence risk data are invariably derived from studying women whose losses were usually not recognized until 9 to 12 weeks' gestation. However, the same counseling figures are appropriate for couples whose pregnancies are ascertained in the fifth week of gestation.[8]

Loss rates may be lower when conception occurs on days other than the date of ovulation or the day prior (optimal interval). In the Wilcox et al.[9] cohort of 189 pregnancies, 141 lasted beyond 6 weeks. Among the implantations leading to a clinical pregnancy, 84 percent originated on days 8, 9, or 10 after ovulation. No pregnancies occurred when implantation took place beyond day 12. The loss rate was 13 percent if implantation occurred by day 9, increasing to 26 percent, 52 percent, and 82 percent on the next 3 days, respectively. Gray et al. reported that in couples with prior abortions, loss rates are 7 percent when conception occurred on the day of ovulation or 1 day earlier, but 23 percent when conception occurred on other (non-optimal) days of the cycle.[10]

Fetal demise occurs *before* clinical signs are manifested, as evidenced by only 2 to 3 percent of viable pregnancies being lost after 8 weeks' gestation.[4,11-13] Given the well-accepted clinical loss rate of 10 to 12 percent, it can be deducted that fetal viability ceases weeks before maternal symptoms appear. Thus, most fetuses aborting clinically at 9 to 12 weeks must have died weeks previously. Thus, almost all losses are "missed abortions," that is, retained in utero for an interval before clinical recognition; thus, the term is archaic.

If the fetus is alive at 8 to 9 weeks, 2 to 3 percent are lost thereafter. Most losses occur in the next 2 months. Loss rates are perhaps 1 percent in women confirmed by ultrasound to have viable pregnancies at 16 weeks, and even lower after 20 weeks.[14] Loss rates have been estimated to be 0.54 percent at age 20, increasing to 0.6 to 0.9 percent by ages 34 to 38 years, and 2.1 percent by age 43 years.[15]

ETIOLOGY OF PRECLINICAL LOSSES

Decades ago, Hertig and Rock[16-18] examined the fallopian tubes, uterine cavities, and endometria of women undergoing elective hysterectomy. These women were of proved fertility, with a mean age of 33.6 years. Coital times were recorded before hysterectomy. Eight preimplantation embryos (<6 days from conception) were recovered (Fig. 24-1A). Four of these eight embryos were morphologically abnormal. The four abnormal embryos presumably would not have implanted or, if implanted, would not have survived long thereafter. Nine of 26 implanted embryos (6 to 14 embryonic days) were morphologically abnormal (Fig. 24-1B). The validity of these conclusions was confirmed in the modern era, when aneuploidy was detected in embryos by fluorescence in situ hybridization (FISH).

The frequency of losses among human preimplantation embryos is very high,[19,20] as witnessed in assisted reproductive technology (ART). Pregnancy rates (positive pregnancy test) are 25 to 35 percent per embryo, and these rates are naturally lower with morphologically abnormal embryos. Of morphologically normal embryos, at least 25 percent show chromosomal abnormalities (aneuploidy or polyploidy),[21] based on studies using FISH with chromosome-specific probes for 7 to 9 chromosomes.[21] The 25-percent aneuploidy rate in morphologically normal embryos is also consistent with 6-percent aneuploidy in sperm from ostensibly normal men[22,23] and in 20 percent of oocytes.[24,25] Prevalence of abnormalities is higher in many studies using FISH on polar bodies or oocytes.[23] Aneuploidy rates in embryos rise strikingly as maternal age increases, being 40 to 45 percent in women older than the age of 40 years. Blastocyst transfer is popular in ART, and some have claimed this selects against genetically abnormal embryos. However, this is not true to a clinically meaningful extent.

Chromosomal abnormalities are even more frequent in morphologically abnormal embryos. Studies in the 1980s initially used metaphase analysis, finding chromosomal abnormalities in 78 percent of fragmented embryos, compared with 12.5 percent in morphologically normal embryos.[19] Using FISH with chromosome-specific probes, abnormality rates of 50 to 75 percent are observed, even though not all chromosomes were tested.[21]

Overall, many embryos are morphologically abnormal. Chromosomal abnormalities would be expected to be the most frequent explanation for morphologically abnormal embryos, as initially recovered by Hertig et al.[16–18]

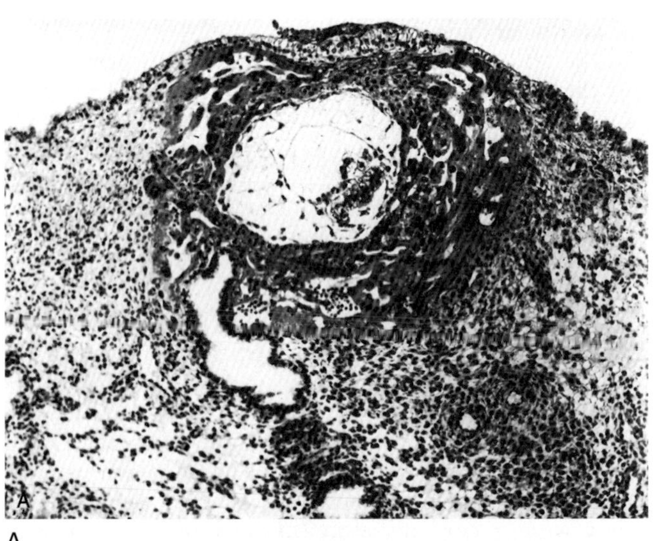

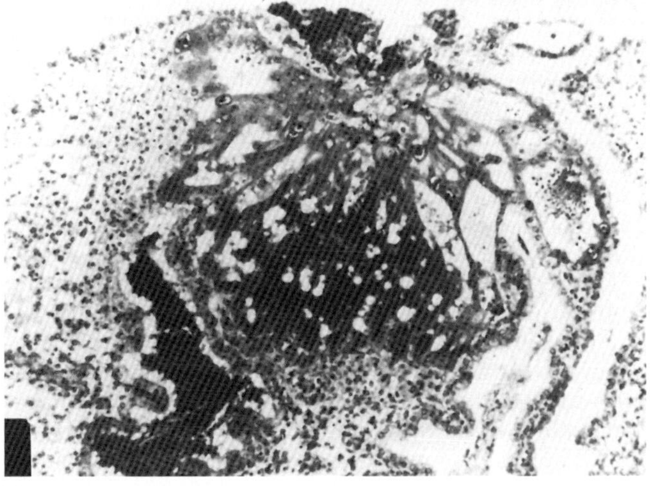

Figure 24-1. Cross section of endometrium containing an abnormal 14-day-old embryo *(A)* compared with a normal 11-day-old embryo. *B,* In the abnormal embryo, no embryonic disk is present and only syncytiotrophoblasts are identifiable. (From Hertig A, Rock J: A series of potentially abortive ova recovered from fertile women prior to the first missed menstrual period. Am J Obstet Gynecol 58:968, 1949, with permission.)

PLACENTAL ANATOMIC CHARACTERISTICS OF SUCCESSFUL AND UNSUCCESSFUL PREGNANCIES

As judged by adult tissue criteria, the human fetus develops in a low oxygen (O_2) environment (see Chapter 1). The human gestational sac is designed to minimize the flux of O_2 from maternal blood to the fetal circulation. In particular, the extravillous trophoblast that migrates inside the uterine tissue to anchor the pregnancy creates a cellular shell with plugs inside the tip of the uteroplacental arteries This additional barrier keeps most of the maternal circulation outside the placenta and thus reduces the chemical activity of free oxygen radicals inside the placenta during most of the first trimester of the human pregnancy.[26] In normal pregnancies, the onset of the maternal circulation is a progressive phenomenon, starting around 9 weeks at the periphery and gradually extending toward the center of the placenta.[27] This process correlates closely with the pattern of trophoblast invasion across the placental bed (Fig. 24-2).

In about two thirds of early pregnancy failures, there is anatomic evidence of defective placentation, which is mainly characterized by a thinner and fragmented trophoblast shell and reduced cytotrophoblast invasion of the lumen at the tips of the spiral arteries.[28] This is associated with premature onset of the maternal circulation throughout the placenta in most cases of miscarriages.[26,29,30] These defects are similar in euploid and most aneuploid miscar-

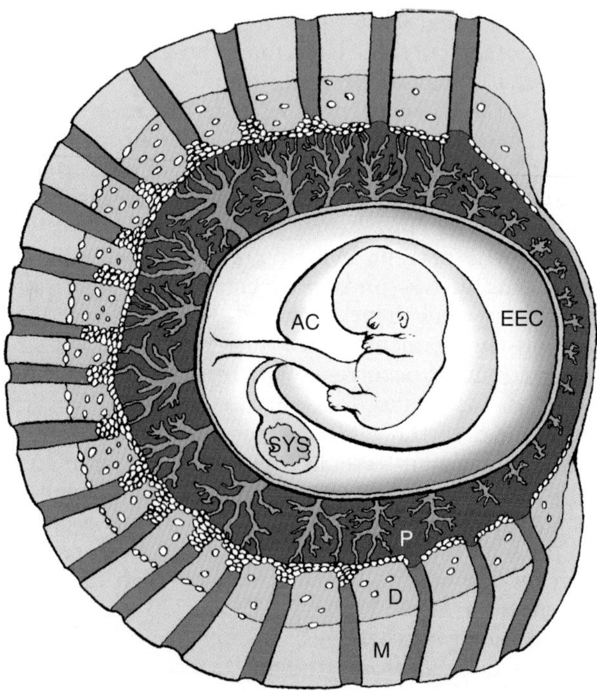

Figure 24-2. A gestational sac at the end of the second month (8 to 9 weeks) showing the myometrium (M), the decidua (D), the placenta (P), the exo-coelomic cavity (ECC), the amniotic cavity (AC) and the secondary yolk sac (SYS). (From Jauniaux E, Cindrova-Davies T, Johns T, et al: Distribution and transfer pathways of antioxidant molecules inside the first trimester human gestational sac. J Clin Endocrinol Metab 89:1452, 2004.)

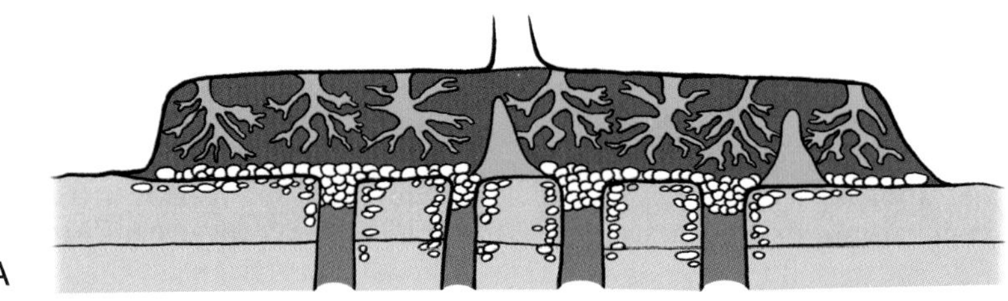

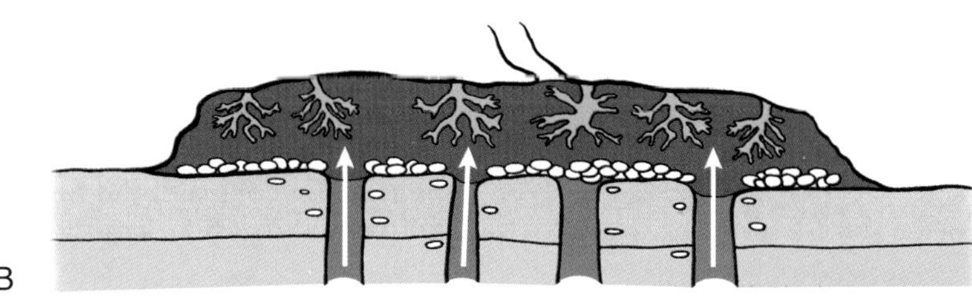

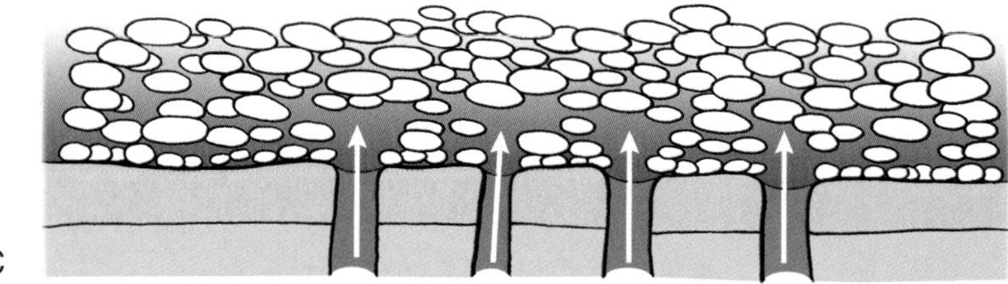

Figure 24-3. Placentation in a normal ongoing pregnancy *(A)*, in an early pregnancy failure *(B)*, and in a complete hydatidiform mole *(C)*. Note in *A*, the continuous trophoblastic shell, the plugs in the lumens of the spiral arteries, and the interstitial migration of the extravillous trophoblast through the decidua down to the superficial layer of the myometrium; in *B*, the discontinuous trophoblastic shell, the absence of plugs and the reduced migration of extravillous trophoblastic cells; in *C*, the absence of trophoblastic plugs and interstitial migration. (From Jauniaux E, Burton GJ: Pathophysiology of histological changes in early pregnancy loss. Placenta 26:114, 2005.)

riages but are more pronounced in hydatidiform moles (Fig. 24-3). In vivo ultrasound data and histopathologic data indicate that in most early pregnancy loss the onset of the intervillous circulation is premature and widespread owing to incomplete transformation and plugging of the uteroplacental arteries.[30] In about 80 percent of the cases of missed miscarriage, the onset of the maternal placental circulation is both precocious and generalized throughout the placenta. This finding is independent of the karyotype of the conceptus.[31] This leads to higher O_2 concentrations during early pregnancy, widespread trophoblastic oxidative damage, and placental degeneration. Although in vitro studies have demonstrated the ability of damaged syncytium to regenerate from the underlying cytotrophoblast, it is likely that in the face of extensive damage, this ability will be overwhelmed, leading to complete pregnancy failure.[32]

CHROMOSOMAL ABNORMALITIES ARE THE MOST FREQUENT CAUSE OF CLINICALLY RECOGNIZED LOSS

Chromosomal abnormalities are the major cause of clinically recognized pregnancy loss. At least 50 percent of clinically recognized pregnancy losses result from a chromosomal abnormality,[33–35] and the frequency is probably higher. If one analyzes chorionic villi after ultrasound diagnosis of fetal demise, rather than relying on later recovery of spontaneously expelled products, the frequency of chromosomal abnormalities is 75 to 90 percent.[36,37] Maternal age is increased in these cases. Comparative genome hybridization (microarray analysis) detects abnormalities in abortuses not evident by karyotype.[14]

Among second-trimester losses, one observes chromosomal abnormalities more similar to those seen in live-born infants: trisomies 13, 18, and 21 as well as monosomy X and sex chromosomal polysomies. This also holds among third-trimester losses (stillborn infants), in which the frequency of chromosomal abnormalities is approximately 5 percent.[38] This frequency is less than that observed in earlier abortuses but much higher than that found among live-born infants (0.6 percent).

Table 24-1. Chromosomal Completion in Spontaneous Abortions; Recognized Clinically in the First Trimester*

COMPLETION	FREQUENCY	PERCENT
Normal 46,XX or 46,XY		54.1
Triploidy		7.7
69,XXX	2.7	
69,XYX	0.2	
69,XXY	4.0	
Other	0.8	
Tetraploidy		2.6
92,XXX	1.5	
92,XXYY	0.55	
Not Stated	0.55	
Monosomy X		18.6
Structural abnormalities		1.5
Sex chromosomal polysomy		0.2
47,XXX	0.05	
47,XXY	0.15	
Autosomal monosomy (G)		0.1
Autosomal trisomy for chromosomes		22.3
1	0	
2	1.11	
3	0.25	
4	0.64	
5	0.04	
6	0.14	
7	0.89	
8	0.79	
9	0.72	
10	0.36	
11	0.04	
12	0.18	
13	1.07	
14	0.82	
15	1.68	
16	7.27	
17	0.18	
18	1.15	
19	0.01	
20	0.61	
21	2.11	
22	2.26	
Double trisomy		0.7
Mosaic trisomy		1.3
Other abnormalities or not specified		0.9
		100.0

*Pooled data from several series, as referenced elsewhere by Simpson and Bombard.[35]

Autosomal Trisomy

Autosomal trisomies comprise the largest (approximately 50 percent) single class of chromosomal complements in cytogenetically abnormal spontaneous abortions. Frequencies of various trisomies are listed in Table 24-1. Trisomy for every chromosome has been observed, including chromosome 1.[39,40] The most common trisomy is trisomy 16. Most trisomies show a maternal age effect, but the effect varies markedly among chromosomes. The maternal age effect is especially impressive for double trisomies.

Attempts have been made to correlate placental morphologic abnormalities with specific trisomies, but these relationships are imprecise. The comparison of ultrasound findings and placental histology indicates that villous changes following in utero fetal demise could explain the low predictive value of placental histology itself in identifying an aneuploidy or another nonchromosomal etiology. By contrast, the histologic features of complete and partial hydatidiform molar gestations are so distinctive that most molar miscarriages are correctly diagnosed by histologic examination alone.

Trisomies incompatible with life predictably show slower growth than trisomies compatible with life (e.g., trisomies 13, 18, 21). The mean crown-rump length in abortuses shown to be trisomic for 13, 18, and 21 is 20.65 mm compared with only 10.66 mm for trisomies that virtually never survive to term (e.g., trisomy 10 or 16).[41] Either the former survive longer or the latter show greater intrauterine growth restriction, or both. Abortuses from the former group tend to show anomalies consistent with those found in full-term live-born trisomic infants.[41,42] The malformations present have been said to be more severe than those observed in induced abortuses following prenatal diagnosis.

Aneuploidy usually results from errors at meiosis I, specifically maternal meiosis I. In trisomy 13 and trisomy 21, 90 percent of these maternal cases arise at meiosis I; almost all trisomy 16 cases arise in maternal meiosis I.[43] A notable exception is trisomy 18, in which two thirds of the 90 percent of maternal meiotic cases arise at meiosis II.[44,45]

Errors of maternal meiosis I are associated with advanced maternal age and, in turn, with decreased or absent meiotic recombination.[44–46] The hypothesis invoked to explain this relationship is the product-line hypothesis, which states that oocytes ovulated earlier in life are characterized by more genetic recombination and, hence, less likelihood for nondisjunction.[47] However, recent work indicates that the situation is more complex, the location and type of recombination being pivotal and influenced by maternal age.[48]

Errors in *paternal* meiosis account for 10 percent of acrocentric (13, 14, 15, 21, and 22) trisomies.[49] In trisomy 21, paternal meiotic errors are equally likely to arise in meiosis I or II,[50] a circumstance that contrasts with the situation in maternal meiotic errors. Among nonacrocentric chromosomes, paternal contribution is uncommon. A surprising exception involves trisomy 2.

Polyploidy

In polyploidy, there are more than two haploid chromosomal complements. Nonmosaic triploidy (3n = 69) and tetraploidy (4n = 92) is common in abortuses. This phenomenon is presumably distinct from the diploid/triploid mosaicism that is found in some 30 percent of blastocysts.[51] Triploid abortuses are usually 69,XXY or 69,XXX, resulting from dispermy.[52,53] An association exists between diandric (paternally inherited) triploidy and hydatidiform mole, a "partial mole" said to exist if molar tissue and fetal parts coexist. The more common "complete" (classic) hydatidiform mole is 46,XX, of androgenetic origin and is made exclusively of villous tissue.[53] Pathologic findings in diandric triploid and tetraploid placentas include a disproportionately large gestational sac, focal (partial) hydropic degeneration of placental villi, and trophoblast hyperplasia.[54] Placental hydropic changes are progressive and thus may be difficult to identify in early pregnancy. By contrast, placental villi often undergo hydropic degeneration after fetal demise. This can happen in all types of miscarriage; thus, histologic and cytogenetic investigations are essential to differentiate between true and pseudomole, because a true mole can be associated with persistent trophoblastic disease. Fetal malformations associated with triploid miscarriage include neural tube defects and omphaloceles, anomalies reminiscent of those observed in triploid conceptuses surviving to term. Facial dysmorphia and limb abnormalities have also been reported.

Tetraploidy is uncommon, rarely progressing beyond 2 to 3 weeks of embryonic life. This chromosomal abnormality can also be associated with persistent trophoblastic disease and thus needs to be identified in order to offer the woman an hCG follow-up.

Monosomy X

Monosomy X is the single most common chromosomal abnormality among spontaneous abortions, accounting for 15 to 20 percent of abnormal specimens. Monosomy X embryos usually consist of only an umbilical cord stump. Later in gestation, anomalies characteristic of the Turner syndrome may be seen, such as cystic hygromas and generalized edema (Fig. 24-4). Unlike live-born 45,X individuals, 45,X abortuses show germ cells; however, germ cells rarely develop beyond the primordial germ cell stage. The pathogenesis of 45,X germ cell failure thus involves not so much failure of germ cell development as more rapid attrition in 45,X compared with 46,XX embryos.[55,56] Incidentally, this observation makes plausible the rare but well-documented pregnancies occurring in 45,X individuals.[57]

Monosomy X usually (80 percent) occurs as a result of paternal sex chromosome loss.[58] This observation is consistent with the lack of a maternal age effect in 45,X or possibly even an inverse age effect.

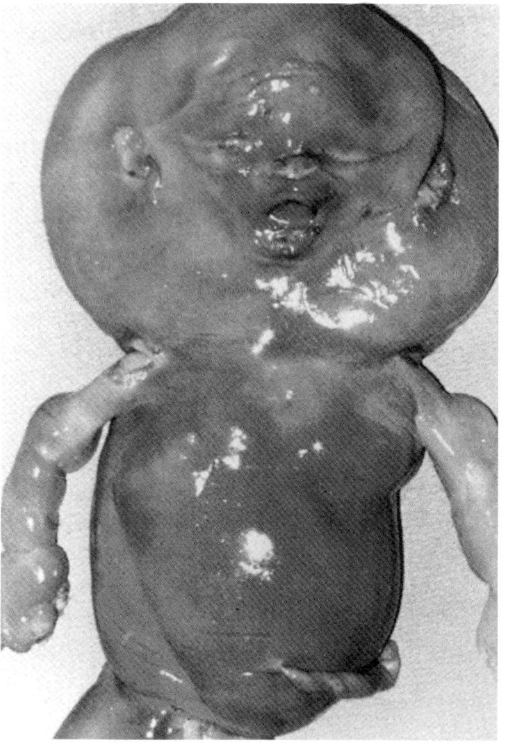

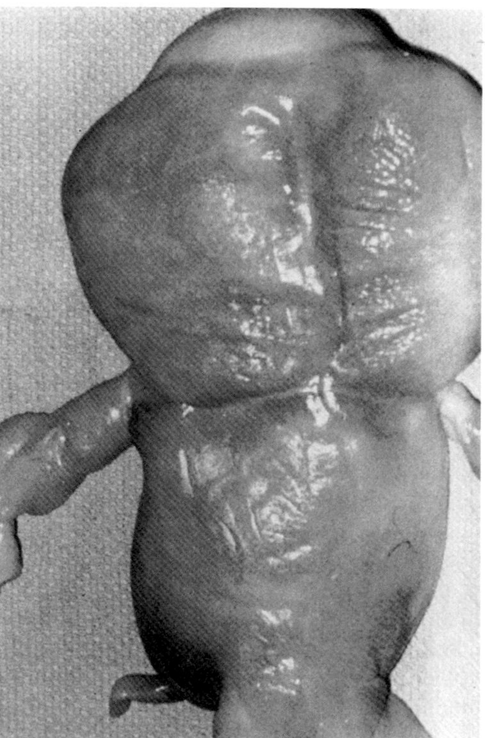

Figure 24-4. Photograph of a 45,X abortus. (From Simpson JL, Bombard AT: Chromosomal abnormalities in spontaneous abortion: frequency, pathology and genetic counseling. *In* Edmonds K, Bennett MJ [eds]: Spontaneous Abortion. London, Blackwell, 1987, p 51, with permission.)

Structural Chromosomal Rearrangement

Structural chromosomal rearrangements account for 1.5 percent of all abortuses (see Table 24-1). Rearrangements (e.g., translocation) may either arise de novo during gametogenesis or be inherited from a parent carrying a "balanced" translocation or inversion. Phenotypic consequences depend on the specific duplicated or deficient chromosomal segments. Although not a common cause of sporadic losses, inherited translocations are an important cause of *repeated* fetal wastage.

Sex Chromosomal Polysomy (X or Y)

The complements 47,XXY and 47,XYY each occur in about 1 per 800 live-born male births; 47,XXX occurs in 1 per 800 female births. X or Y polysomies are only slightly more common in abortuses than in liveborns.

MENDELIAN AND POLYGENIC/ MULTIFACTORIAL ETIOLOGY

The 30 to 50 percent of first-trimester abortuses that show no chromosomal abnormalities could still have undergone fetal demise as a result of other genetic etiologics. Neither mendelian nor polygenic/multifactorial disorders show chromosomal abnormalities, and yet these etiologies are more common explanations of congenital anomalies than chromosomal abnormalities. It would be very naïve to assume mendelian and polygenic/multifactorial factors do not play pivotal roles in embryonic mortality. Baek[59] enumerated more than 30 plausible candidate genes. Especially consistent with mendelian or polygenic etiologies are abortuses who demonstrate structural anomalies and no chromosomal abnormalities. However, lack of cytogenetic data on the dissected specimens makes it nearly impossible to determine the precise role of noncytogenetic mechanisms in early embryonic maldevelopment. Philipp and Kalousek[60] correlated cytogenetic status of missed abortuses with morphologic abnormalities at embryoscopy. Embryos with chromosomal abnormalities usually showed one or more external anomalies, but some euploid embryos also showed anatomic anomalies.

In addition to recognized mendelian etiology, novel nonmendelian forms of inheritance probably play a greater role in embryonic loss than in live-born abnormalities. Normal chromosomal complement does not necessarily exclude numeric perturbations. Mosaicism may be restricted to the placenta, the embryo per se being normal. This phenomenon is termed "confined placental mosaicism." Losses caused by this mechanism may already be reflected in extant data because most studies have involved analysis only of villous material. Related to confined placental mosaicism is uniparental disomy, a phenomenon in which both homologues for a given chromosome are derived from a single parent. This probably occurs as result of expulsion of a chromosome from a trisomic zygote ("trisomic rescue"). The karyotype would appear normal (46,XX or 46,XY), but genes on the involved chromosome would lack contribution of one parent or the other. For example, uniparental disomy for chromosome 21 has been detected in an embryonic abortus.[61]

Another unusual mechanism that could be responsible for spontaneous abortions is skewed X-inactivation. In one study of 48 women having two prior losses without explanation, seven (14.6 percent) had highly skewed X-inactivation, defined as 90 percent of their X chromosomes originating from one specific parent versus the expected of 50 percent; only one of the 67 controls (1.5 percent) showed skewed X-inactivation.[62] All male offspring of a woman with skewed X-inactivation might be aborted. A pedigree consistent with this hypothesis has been reported.[63] This could be explained by X-linked lethality, or by the uniparental disomy of a zygote benefiting from trisomic rescue; the fewer surviving cells at the time of X-inactivation would increase the likelihood of skewing.

RECURRENCE RISKS AND COUNSELING

Faced with a couple having experienced a spontaneous abortion, the obstetrician has several immediate obligations: (1) inform the couple concerning the overall frequency of fetal wastage (10 to 12 percent of clinically recognized pregnancies, and many more unrecognized) and its likely etiology (genetic and especially cytogenetic), (2) provide applicable recurrence risks, and (3) determine the necessity for a formal clinical evaluation. The responsibility to inform patients can be fulfilled by summarizing the salient facts cited in this chapter, emphasizing common etiologies responsible for fetal losses that we shall cover. Explicitly worth citing is the positive correlation between loss rates and both maternal age and prior losses. The maternal age effect is not solely the result of increased trisomic abortions but presumably reflects endometrial factors as well.

Recurrence Risks

Loss rates are definitely increased among women who have experienced previous losses but not nearly to the extent once thought (Table 24-2). For decades, obstetricians believed in the concept of "habitual abortion." After three losses, the risk of subsequent losses was thought to rise sharply. Such beliefs were based on calculations made in 1938 by Malpas,[64] who concluded that following three abortions the likelihood of a subsequent one was 80 to 90 percent. Thus, occurrence of three consecutive spontaneous abortions was said for decades to confer on a woman the designation of "habitual aborter." These risk figures not only proved incorrect but were and unfortunately still seem subconsciously to be used as "controls" for clinical studies evaluating various treatment plans. This practice led to unwarranted acceptance of certain interventions, the most unfortunate of which was diethylstilbestrol treatment.

In 1964, Warburton and Fraser[65] showed that the likelihood of recurrent abortion rose only to 25 to 30

Table 24-2. Approximate Recurrence Risk Figures Useful for Counseling Women with Repeated Spontaneous Abortions*

	PRIOR ABORTIONS	RISK (%)
Women with live-born infants	0	5–10
	1	20–25
	2	25
	3	30
	4	30
Women without live-born infant	3	30–40

*Recurrence risks are slightly higher for older women.
Regan L: A prospective study on spontaneous abortion. *In* Beard RW, Sharp F (eds): Early Pregnancy Loss: Mechanisms and Treatment, London, Springer-Verlag 1988, p 22; Warburton D, Fraser FC: Spontaneous abortion risks in man: data from reproductive histories collected in a medical genetic unit. Am J Hum Genet 16:1, 1964; Poland BJ, Miller JR, Jones DC, et al: Reproductive counseling in patients who have had a spontaneous abortion. Am J Obstet Gynecol 127:685, 1977.

percent, irrespective of whether a woman had previously experienced one, two, three, or even four spontaneous abortions. This concept has been confirmed in many subsequent studies, with the additional observation that if no previous live-born infants have occurred, the loss rate is somewhat higher.[66] The lowest risks (5 percent) are observed in nulliparous women with no prior losses.[7] Women who smoke cigarettes or drink alcohol moderately are at slightly higher risk.[67] Recurrence risks are slightly higher if the abortus is cytogenetically normal than cytogenetically abnormal.[68]

Taking all of the above-mentioned factors into account, the prognosis is reasonably good even with no therapy, the predicted success rate being 70 percent. Indeed, Vlaanderen and Treffers[69] reported successful pregnancies in each of 21 women having unexplained prior repetitive losses but subjected to no intervention. Other groups reached similar conclusions.[70,71] Therefore, to be judged efficacious, therapeutic regimens must achieve successes greater than 70 percent.

When Is Formal Evaluation Necessary?

A couple experiencing even one loss should be counseled and provided recurrence risk rates. However, not every couple needs formal assessment and a battery of tests. Infertile couples who are in their fourth decade may choose to be evaluated formally after only two losses. After three losses, traditionally all couples should be offered formal evaluation. There is no scientific basis for waiting until 3 losses, although this is the benchmark for the Royal College of Obstetricians and Gynaecologists (RCOG). The American College of Obstetricians and Gynecologists (ACOG) defines recurrent loss as either two or three "consecutive" losses, the number is perhaps more defensible, but the "consecutive" is very arguable. Once a couple enters evaluation, they should undergo all tests employed by a given practitioner. There is no rationale for performing certain studies after two losses yet deferring others until three losses have occurred.

Any couple having a stillborn or anomalous live born infant should undergo cytogenetic studies unless the stillborn was known to have a normal chromosome complement. Parental chromosomal (conventional metaphase) rearrangements (i.e., translocations or inversions) should be excluded. If chromosomal studies on the stillborn were unsuccessful, common trisomies can still be ruled out by performing FISH on stored deparaffined tissue.

ETIOLOGY AND CLINICAL EVALUATION OF REPETITIVE ABORTIONS

Translocations

Structural chromosomal abnormalities are accepted as one explanation for repetitive abortions. The most common structural rearrangement encountered is a translocation, which is found in about 5 percent of couples experiencing repeated losses.[72,73] Individuals with balanced translocations are phenotypically normal, but their offspring (abortuses or abnormal live-born infants) may show chromosomal duplications or deficiencies as a result of normal meiotic segregation. Among couples with repetitive abortions, about 60 percent of translocations are reciprocal and 40 percent robertsonian. Women are about twice as likely as men to show a balanced translocation.[74]

The clinical consequences of a balanced translocation are illustrated in Figure 24-2. If a child has Down syndrome as a result of a centric fusion (robertsonian) translocation, the rearrangement will prove to have originated de novo in 50 to 75 percent of cases. That is, a balanced translocation will not exist in either parent. The likelihood of Down syndrome recurring in subsequent offspring is minimal. On the other hand, the risk is significant in the 25 to 50 percent of families in which individuals have Down syndrome as the result of a balanced parental translocation (e.g., parental complement 45,XX,-14,-21,+t[14q;21q]). The theoretical risk of having a child with Down syndrome is 33 percent, but empirical risks are considerably less. The risk is only 2 percent if the father carries the translocation and 10 percent if the mother carries the translocation.[75,76] If robertsonian (centric-fusion) translocations involve other chromosomes, empirical risks are lower. In t(13q;14q), the risk for live-born trisomy 13 is 1 percent or less.

Reciprocal translocations do not involve centromeric fusion, but represent interchanges between two or more chromosomes. Empirical data for specific translocations are usually not available, but useful generalizations can be made on the basis of pooled data derived from many different translocations. Again, theoretical risks for abnormal offspring (unbalanced reciprocal translocations) are far greater than empirical risks. Overall, the risk is 12 percent for offspring of either female heterozygotes or male heterozygotes.[75,76] Thus, detecting a chromosomal rearrangement profoundly affects subsequent pregnancy management. Antenatal cytogenetic studies should be offered. The frequency of unbalanced fetuses is lower if parental balanced translocations are ascertained through repetitive abortions (3 percent) than through anomalous live-born infants (nearly 20 percent).[75] Presumably more unbalanced products are lethal.

Preimplantation genetic diagnosis (PGD) has provided relevant information. When a balanced translocation is detected in a couple experiencing recurrent abortions, prognosis for a live-born infant is little different than if a translocation had not been detected.[77] However, certain couples show repeated abortions. When studied by PGD, lethal products are observed in up to 90 to100 percent of cases.[78] Thus, PGD is used to identify and transfer the few balanced embryos, increasing the statistical likelihood of conception.[79]

Rarely, a translocation precludes normal live-born infants. This occurs when a translocation involves homologous chromosomes (e.g., t[13q13q] or t[21q21q]). If the father carries such a structural rearrangement, artificial insemination may be appropriate. If the mother carries the rearrangement, donor oocytes or donor embryos and ART should be considered.

Inversions

An uncommon parental chromosomal rearrangement responsible for repetitive pregnancy losses is an inversion. In inversions, the order of genes is reversed. Analogous to translocations, individuals heterozygous for an inversion should be normal if their genes are merely rearranged. However, individuals with inversions suffer untoward reproductive consequences as a result of normal meiotic phenomena. Crossing-over involving the inverted segment yields unbalanced gametes (see Simpson and Elias for more details).[80] Pericentric inversions are present in perhaps 0.1 percent of women and 0.1 percent of men experiencing repeated spontaneous abortions. Paracentric inversions are even rarer.

Overall, women with a *pericentric* inversion have a 7-percent risk of abnormal live-born infantss; men carry a 5-percent risk. Pericentric inversions ascertained through phenotypically normal probands are less likely to result in abnormal live-born infants.

Inversions involving only a small portion of the total chromosomal length paradoxically may be less significant clinically because large duplications or deficiencies arise following crossing-over, and these are usually lethal. By contrast, inversions involving only 30 to 60 percent of the total chromosomal length are relatively more likely to be characterized by duplications or deficiencies compatible with survival.[81]

Data are limited on recurrence risks involving *paracentric* inversions. Theoretically, there should be less risk for unbalanced products than with pericentric inversions because paracentric recombinants should nearly all be lethal. On the other hand, abortions and abnormal live-born infants have been observed within the same kindred, and the risk for unbalanced viable offspring has been tabulated at 4 percent.[82] Antenatal cytogenetic studies should be offered.

Recurrent Aneuploidy

Already discussed as the most common overall cause for sporadic abortions, numeric chromosomal abnormalities (aneuploidy) may be responsible for both recurrent as well as sporadic losses. This reasoning is based on observations that the complements of successive abortuses in a given family are more likely to be either recurrently normal or recurrently abnormal (Table 24-3). If the complement of the first abortus is abnormal, the likelihood is increased the complement of the second abortus will also be abnormal.[83] The recurrence usually involves trisomy.

These data suggest that certain couples are predisposed toward chromosomally abnormal conceptions. Although corrections for maternal age account for some of the ostensible nonrandom distribution, the risks seem clearly increased compared with normal women of comparable age. If couples are predisposed to recurrent aneuploidy, they might logically be at increased risk not only for aneuploid abortuses but also for aneuploid live-born infants. The trisomic autosome in a subsequent pregnancy might not always confer lethality, but rather might be compatible with life (e.g., trisomy 21). Indeed, the risk of live-born trisomy 21 following an aneuploid abortus is about 1 percent.[84] Further in support of recurrent aneuploidy is that a tendency for trisomic preimplantation embryos to recur in successive ART cycles. Both Rubio et al.[85] and Munné et al.[86] found increased aneuploid embryos in couples with repeated abortions, compared with couples undergoing PGD for mendelian indications. In the former study, the difference was 71 percent versus

Table 24-3. Recurrent Aneuploidy: The Relationship Between Karyotypes of Successive Abortuses

COMPLEMENT OF FIRST ABORTUS	COMPLEMENT OF SECOND ABORTUS					
	NORMAL	TRISOMY	MONOSOMY	TRIPLOIDY	TETRAPLOID	DE NOVO REARRANGEMENT
Normal	142	18	5	7	3	2
Trisomy	31	30	1	4	3	1
Monosomy X	7	5	3	3	0	0
Triploidy	7	4	1	4	0	0
Tetraploidy	3	1	0	2	0	0
De novo rearrangement	1	3	0	0	0	0

Warburton D, Kline J, Stein Z, et al: Does the karyotype of a spontaneous abortion predict the karyotype of a subsequent abortion? Evidence from 273 women with two karyotyped spontaneous abortions. Am J Hum Genet 41:465, 1987.

21 percent to 45 percent in women of mean age 36 years. In the latter, findings were 37 percent versus 21 percent in women younger than age 35 years. In these same women, trisomic clinical abortions have been observed. Transferring euploid embryos clearly decreases the frequency of abortions.

If recurrent aneuploidy is a genuine phenomenon, the frequency of chromosomal abnormalities in recurrent abortuses (i.e., in which the same women has had a previous abortus) should be approximately the same as in first-time abortuses. Some authors indeed observed this frequency, indicating that recurrent aneuploidy is likely to be a common cause of recurrent abortion. Treatment for nongenetic causes should then generally be eschewed. Others have found lower frequencies in recurrent abortuses and, hence, concluded that sporadic cases were mostly genetic but recurrent cases mostly nongenetic. If validated, the latter conclusion would have important implications. The actual data are mixed for diagnosis, therapy, and prognosis.

Among 420 abortuses that were obtained from women with repeated losses, Stephenson et al.[87] found 54 percent chromosomal abnormalities, of which 31 percent of the original sample were trisomic. Among unselected pooled data 48 percent of abortuses were abnormal of which 27 percent of the original sample were trisomic. Stern et al.[88] found a 57-percent frequency of chromosomal abnormalities among repetitively aborting women and an identical frequency among sporadically aborting women. Other studies have found higher order abortuses more likely to be cytogenetically normal. With abortuses of 4 or higher the rate of chromosomal abnormalities decreases.[89] This suggests that higher order abortuses are relatively more likely to be due to "maternal" factors. It is logical that this could be true for consecutive losses of four or more, but more arguable with two or three losses.

No information concerning fetal chromosomal status may be available in couples having repetitive abortions. Sometimes, one can obtain paraffin-blocked products of conception and perform FISH for chromosomes most likely to be trisomic (13, 14, 16, 18, 21, 22). If no information exists, it is unclear whether antenatal diagnostic tests are appropriate. Risks for abnormal offspring are probably increased; however, the small but finite risk of amniocentesis or chorionic villus sampling is especially troublesome to couples who have had difficulty achieving pregnancy. Noninvasive approaches (see Chapter 7) may be the preferable initial option.

Luteal Phase Defects

Implantation in an inhospitable endometrium is a plausible explanation for spontaneous abortion. The hormone usually hypothesized to be deficient is progesterone, the deficiency of which might fail to prepare the estrogen-primed endometrium for implantation. Luteal phase defects (LPDs) is the term used to describe the endometrium manifesting an inadequate progesterone effect. Progesterone secreted by the corpus luteum is necessary to support the endometrium until the trophoblast produces sufficient progesterone to maintain pregnancy, an event occurring around 7 gestational (menstrual) weeks or 5 weeks after conception. Plausible pathogenic mechanisms underlying LPD include decreased gonadotropin-releasing hormone, decreased follicle-stimulating hormone, inadequate luteinizing hormone (LH), inadequate ovarian steroidogenesis, or endometrial receptor defects. Once almost universally accepted as a very common cause for fetal wastage, LPD now is considered an uncommon cause.

A major difficulty is lack of standard diagnostic criteria in LPD. LPD was originally defined on the basis of an endometrial biopsy lagging at least 2 days behind the actual postovulation date. This dating was determined by counting backward from the next menstrual period, assuming 14 days from the date of ovulation to menses. This method remains the standard. However, even the original report of Noyes et al.[90] showed a mean error of 1.81 days in dating, suggesting that an endometrial biopsy should be designated "out-of-phase" only if it lags 3 or more days behind the actual postovulation date. Interobserver variation is considerable. Endometrial biopsies (n = 62) read by five different pathologists resulted in differences in interpretation that would have altered management in approximately one third of patients.[91] Reading coded endometrial biopsy slides a second time, the same pathologist agreed with his or her initial diagnosis in only 25 percent of samples.[92] Histology identical to that observed with luteal phase "defects" is found often in fertile women. When regularly menstruating fertile women with no history of abortions were biopsied in serial cycles, the frequency of LPD was 51.4 percent in any single cycle and 26.7 percent in sequential cycles.[93] Other diagnostic criteria have been proposed, such as integrated serum progesterone (three values).[94] However, hormone levels seem to be no more specific than endometrial biopsy. Indeed, in patients with two or more spontaneous abortions, a low serum progesterone level in the luteal phase is only 71 percent predictive of an LPD as defined on the basis of an abnormal endometrial biopsy.[95] In an attempt to characterize gonadotropin and progesterone secretion in LPD, it has been suggested that the diagnosis is best made on the basis of a single assay of three pooled blood samples[96,97]; a level of 10 ng/ml of less connotes LPD.[98] Highly relevant is the NICHD collaborative Reproductive Medicine study showing that out-of-phase biopsies distinguished poorly between fertile and infertile women. This authoritative group recommended against endometrial biopsy in the evaluation of infertility.[99]

In addition to the lack of set criteria for diagnosis, there are still no randomized studies showing LPD to be a genuine entity. Some studies[100] have been cited as evidence of efficacy, but their experimental designs are not optimal[101] because concurrent control groups were not recruited. A recent meta-analysis showed no beneficial effect of progesterone treatment.[102]

Relevant also are observations suggesting a relationship between fetal loss and either oligomenorrhea[103] or clinically evident polycystic ovarian syndrome.[104] These observations could be consistent with studies cited earlier showing pregnancy loss is lowest when conceptions occur in midcycle.[10] The pathogenesis could be endometrial dyssynchrony mediated through perturbations of LH. Regan et al.[105] reported increased pregnancy loss in 20 women with elevated LH; however, treatment to lower LH failed to decrease the pregnancy loss rate.[106] Several studies have failed to show an elevated LH.[107–109]

In summary, LPD is a questionable entity. If it does exist, whether progesterone or progestational agents can be used to treat LPD successfully is also controversial.

Thyroid Abnormalities

Decreased conception rates and increased fetal losses are associated with overt hypothyroidism or hyperthyroidism. Subclinical thyroid dysfunction has generally not been considered an explanation for repeated losses,[110] but the situation is complex. Bussen and Steck[111] studied 22 women with a history of habitual abortion and similar numbers of nulligravid and multigravid controls. Thyroid antibodies were increased in the former. Stagnaro-Green et al.[112] and Glinoer et al.[113] concluded that antithyroid antibodies and mild thyroid disease were associated with spontaneous abortions, whereas Singh et al.[114] thought that thyroid antibodies were a useful marker for clinical losses in the ART population. Pratt et al.[115] reported increased antithyroid antibodies in euthyroid women experiencing first-trimester losses, but the same group[116] also concluded that the ostensible association was secondary to nonspecific organ antibodies. Rushworth et al.[117] followed women in a repetitive abortion clinic who had antibodies against thyroglobulin or thyroid microsomal factors. The overall prevalence of antibodies in 164 women was 19 percent. However, subsequent outcomes were not significantly different whether thyroid antibody-positive or -negative. Overall, thyroid antibodies in asymptomatic women would still not seem to be a major cause of early pregnancy loss. Neither the RCOG nor ACOG recommend ordering thyroid antibody tests in otherwise healthy women.

Elevations of maternal thyroid hormone are, however, clearly deleterious. This effect was shown by analysis of a family from the Azores in which a gene conferring resistance to thyroid hormone was segregating.[118] In this family, this autosomal dominant disorder was caused by a point mutation in the thyroid receptor β (TRβ) gene (Arg243Gln). Those with the receptor mutation must secrete large amounts of thyroid-stimulating hormone (TSH) to compensate. In pregnancy, the fetus is exposed to high levels of maternal TSH because it crosses the placenta. Pregnancy loss rates were compared among individuals who did and did not have the mutation. Loss rates were 22.8 percent in offspring of mothers who had the Arg243Gln mutation, 2.0 percent in normal mothers whose male partner was affected, and 4.4 percent in couples in which neither partner had the mutation.

Diabetes Mellitus

Women whose diabetes mellitus is poorly controlled are at increased risk for fetal loss. Mills et al.[3] showed in a NICHD collaborative study that women whose glycosylated hemoglobin level was greater than 4 standard deviations (SD) above the mean showed higher pregnancy loss rates than women with lower glycosylated hemoglobin levels. This finding has also been found in retrospective studies.[119] Poorly controlled diabetes mellitus should be considered one cause for early pregnancy loss, but well-controlled or subclinical diabetes is probably not a cause of early miscarriage. Neither the RCOG nor ACOG recommend testing for occult diabetes mellitus.

Intrauterine Adhesions (Synechiae)

Intrauterine adhesions could interfere with implantation or early embryonic development. Adhesions may follow overzealous uterine curettage during the postpartum period, intrauterine surgery (e.g., myomectomy), or endometritis. Curettage is the usual explanation, with adhesions most likely to develop if curettage is performed 3 or 4 weeks after delivery. Individuals with uterine synechiae usually manifest hypomenorrhea or amenorrhea, but perhaps 15 to 30 percent show repeated abortions. If adhesions are detected in a woman experiencing repetitive losses, lysis under direct hyperoscopic visualization should be performed. Postoperatively, an intrauterine device or inflated Foley catheter may be inserted in the uterus to discourage reapposition of healing uterine surfaces. Estrogen administration should also be initiated. Approximately 50 percent of patients conceive after surgery, but the frequency of abortions remains high.

Incomplete Müllerian Fusion

Second Trimester

Müllerian fusion defects are an accepted cause of second-trimester losses and pregnancy complications. Low birth weight, breech presentation, and uterine bleeding are other abnormalities associated with müllerian fusion defects compared with women having hysterosalpingogram-proven normal uteri.[120] However, most reports lack any type of controls.[121–126] A few studies claim that the poorer outcomes are associated with septate uteri[123] or T-shaped uteri,[122] but others discern few differences among various anomalies.[127]

When patients presented after a first-trimester pregnancy loss and showed a divided uterine cavity, losses were associated with a uterine septum but not bicornuate uterus.[128] In 509 women with recurrent losses studied by three-dimensional (3D) ultrasound, Salim et al.[129] found greater uterine distortion in those recounting histories of losses. However, the major problem in attributing cause and effect for second-trimester complications and uterine anomalies is that uterine anomalies are so frequent that adverse outcomes could be coincidental. For example, in the Salim et al. study, 23.8 percent of women with recurrent miscarriage had some uterine anomalies on 3D ultrasound.[129] Unsuspected bicornuate uteri were found in 1.2 percent of 167 women undergoing laparoscopic sterilization; 3.6 percent had a severely septate uterus, whereas 15.3 percent had fundal anomalies.[130] Other authors have found müllerian defects in 3.2 percent (22 of 679) of fertile women; 20 of the 22 defects were septate.[131]

Treatment has traditionally involved surgical correction, such as metroplasty. Ludmir et al.[132] wondered if aggressive nonsurgical treatment may be just as efficacious. A total of 101 women with an uncorrected malformation were tracked longitudinally. After first being followed with no surgery and with no defined nonsurgical regimen, women with anomalies underwent a conservative but aggressive protocol consisting of decreased physical and tocolysis. Fetal survival rates in both bicornuate and septate groups were, however, not significantly different before (52 and 53 percent, respectively) or after (58 and 65 percent, respectively) the protocol.

First Trimester

First-trimester abortions might also be caused by müllerian fusion defects. Septate uteri might raise the risk of poor implantation on a poorly vascularized and inhospitable surface. Abortions occurring after ultrasonographic confirmation of a viable pregnancy at 8 or 9 weeks may properly be attributed to uterine fusion defects; however, losses lacking confirmation of fetal viability are more likely to represent missed abortions in which fetal demise occurred before 8 weeks. Women experiencing second-trimester abortions can be assumed to benefit from uterine reconstruction, but reconstructive surgery is not necessarily advisable if losses are restricted to the first trimester.

Leiomyomas

Although leiomyomas are frequent, relatively few women develop symptoms requiring medical or surgical therapy. That leiomyomas cause first- or second-trimester pregnancy wastage per se, rather than obstetric complications like prematurity, is thus plausible but probably uncommon. Analogous to uterine anomalies, the coexistence of two common phenomenon, uterine leiomyomas and reproductive losses, need not necessarily imply a causal relationship.

Location of leiomyomas is probably more important than size, submucous leiomyomas being most likely to cause abortion. Postulated mechanisms leading to pregnancy loss include (1) thinning of the endometrium over the surface of a submucous leiomyoma, predisposing to implantation in a poorly decidualized site; (2) rapid growth caused by the hormonal milieu of pregnancy, compromising the blood supply of the leiomyoma and resulting in necrosis ("red degeneration") that, in turn, leads to uterine contractions and eventually fetal expulsion; and (3) encroachment of leiomyomas on the space required by the developing fetus, leading to premature delivery through mechanisms presumably analogous to those operative in incomplete müllerian fusion. Relative lack of space can also lead to fetal deformations (i.e., positional abnormalities arising in a genetically normal fetus).

Hartmann et al.[133] has conducted a study correlating ultrasonographically detected leiomyomas with pregnancy outcome in a cohort of North Carolina women. Of 1,313 women ascertained early in pregnancy, the 131 with leiomyomas had an increased prior spontaneous abortion rate (odds ratio 2.17). A pitfall is that uterine contractions could mimic fibroids and reflect increased uterine activity that itself was the primary or secondary explanation for the loss.

Surgical procedures to reduce leiomyomata may occasionally be warranted in women experiencing repetitive second-trimester abortions. More often, however, leiomyomata have no etiologic relationship to pregnancy loss. Surgery should be reserved for women whose abortuses were both phenotypically and karyotypically normal and in which viability until at least 9 to 10 weeks was documented.

Incompetent Internal Cervical Os

A functionally intact cervix and lower uterine cavity are prerequisites for a successful pregnancy. Characterized by painless dilation and effacement, cervical incompetence usually occurs during the middle second or early third trimester. This condition is usually considered to have followed traumatic events like cervical amputation, cervical lacerations, forceful cervical dilatation, or conization. However, etiology may be genetic, for example perturbation of a pivotal connective tissue gene (e.g., collagen, fibrillin). Surgical techniques to correct cervical incompetence are discussed in Chapter 25.

Infections

Infections are accepted causes of late fetal wastage and logically could be responsible for early fetal loss as well. Microorganisms and conditions reported to be associated with spontaneous abortion include variola, vaccinia, *Salmonella typhi, Vibrio fetus,* malaria, cytomegalovirus, *Brucella, Toxoplasma, Mycoplasma hominis, Chlamydia trachomatis,* and *Ureaplasma urealyticum.* Transplacental infection doubtless occurs with each of these microorganisms, and sporadic losses could logically be caused by any. However, confirmation of this relationship has not been forthcoming. In fact, polymerase chain reaction analysis of villi from 54 chromosomally normal abortuses showed no amplification for *Urealyticum, M. hominis, cytomegalovirus,* and adeno-associated virus; there was 1 sample positive for *Chlamydia trachomatis* and 8 for human papillomavirus (HPV).[134] Other studies have generally not found differences in outcome between women treated and not treated with antibiotics. Unanswered also is whether the infectious agents were causative in the fetal losses or merely arose secondarily after demise caused by a noninfectious etiology. Confounding variables (e.g., maternal age, prior pregnancy history) are rarely taken into account. Overall, an association between a common microorganism and pregnancy loss could easily reflect chance findings.

Of the potential organisms, *Ureaplasma* and *Chlamydia* are not only the most commonly implicated in *repetitive* abortion but also fulfill prerequisites necessary for a causal relationship. Both organisms can exist in an asymptomatic state, and neither is necessarily so severe as to cause infertility. In an older but still informative study, 46 women with histories of three or more consecutive losses of unknown etiology were followed by Stray-Pedersen et al.[135] *Ureaplasma* was recovered significantly more often among women with repetitive abortions (28 percent) than among controls (7 percent). Infected women and their husbands (n = 43) were then treated with doxycycline, with subsequent cultures confirming eradication of *Ureaplasma*. Nineteen of the 43 women became pregnant; of the 19, three experienced another spontaneous abortion and 16 had normal full-term infants. Among 18 women with untreated *Ureaplasma*, only five full-term pregnancies occurred.

Because of the presence of antibodies to chlamydia in the sera of women who experienced repeated losses, an association has been sought on the basis of high titers.[136,137] However, other data have not confirmed this,[138,139] and an immunohistochemical study found no difference in the frequency of cytomegalovirus antigen in karyotypically normal and abnormal abortuses.[140] Paukku et al.[141] found no differences in the frequencies of IgG-IgA antibodies to *C. trachomatis* in 70 Finnish women with multiple losses.

Toxoplasma antibodies have been observed in Mexican and in Egyptian women having repetitive losses,[142,143] but whether frequencies are higher in those general populations is unclear. In general, toxoplasmosis is not considered a significant cause of pregnancy loss.[144]

A key question is whether infectious agents *cause* fetal losses or merely arise following fetal demise due to other etiologies. Cohort surveillance for infections beginning in early pregnancy is necessary in order to determine the etiologic role of infections in pregnancy loss. Using a NICHD cohort study, Simpson et al.[145] analyzed data collected on clinical infections in 818 women followed from early in the first trimester. No clinical evidence was found that infection occurred more often in the 112 subjects experiencing pregnancy loss compared with the 706 having successful pregnancies. This observation held both for the 2-week interval in which a given loss was recognized clinically as well as in the prior 2-week interval. These data suggest that the attributable risk of infection in first-trimester spontaneous abortion is low.

Given this uncertainty, what evaluation and management is recommended? Culturing the endometrium for *U. urealyticum* or performing DNA-based tests seems reasonable but is expensive. Vibramycin therapy is so innocuous that empiric treatment with doxycycline (100 mg orally twice a day for 10 days for both husband and nonpregnant wife) can be recommended empirically. This same regimen can be used to treat chlamydia.

Antifetal Antibodies

Perturbations of the immune system can be responsible for fetal wastage. However, the nature of the immunologic process responsible for maintaining pregnancy is complex.

Antifetal antibodies are predictably deleterious. These antibodies are directed against the fetus on the basis of genetic dissimilarities. Fetal loss is well documented in Rh-negative (D-negative) women having anti-D antibodies. More apropos for early pregnancy loss is the presence of anti-P antibodies. Most individuals are genotype Pp or PP, but one may be homozygous for p (pp). If a woman of genotype pp has a Pp or PP mate, resulting offspring may or must be Pp. If the mother develops anti-P antibodies, Pp fetuses will be rejected (aborted) early in gestation. Plasmapheresis may be efficacious.[146,147]

Cytokines

Cytokines could be primarily involved, or they could be mediators of other phenomena. Hill and colleagues[148] proposed that perturbations of cytokines cause repetitive abortions in women through T-helper cell abnormalities. The rationale is based on T-helper 1 (Th1) cytokines being deleterious, whereas Th2 cytokines are not. Th1 cytokines include tumor necrosis factor, interleukin (IL)–2, and interferon (IFN)–γ. Th2 cytokines include IL-4, IL-5, IL-6, and IL-10, all of which are secreted by activated T cells expressing the CD4 phenotype. Natural killer cells expressing CD56 also produce salutary cytokines. In women with recurrent loss, immune cell responsiveness becomes activated to produce increased IFN-γ and tumor necrosis factor.[149] Supporting the hypothesis that Th1 cytokines are deleterious, down-regulation of Th1 cytokines in certain mammalian species improves pregnancy outcome.[150,151] Progesterone therapy is said by some to mitigate against the deleterious effects.

Acquired Thrombophilias

An association between second-trimester pregnancy loss and certain autoimmune diseases is generally accepted.[152,153] Antibodies found in women with pregnancy loss encompass nonspecific antinuclear antibodies as well as antibodies against such cellular components as phospholipids, histones, and double- or single-stranded DNA. Acquired aPL antibodies, in turn, represent a broad category that encompasses lupus anticoagulant (LAC) antibodies and anticardiolipin antibodies (aCL). Diagnosis requires two positive tests, taken at least 6 weeks apart, for lupus anticoagulant or IgG or IgM aCL antibodies, in moderate or higher titers. Most investigators[154] agree that mid-trimester fetal death is increased in women with LAC or aCL, perhaps dramatically so. Controversy centers on the role of these antibodies in first-trimester losses.

Initially descriptive studies seemed to show increased aCL antibodies in women with first-trimester pregnancy losses. However, frequencies of various antiphospholipid antibodies (LAC, aPL, aCL) were later shown to be similar in women who experience and who do not experience first-trimester abortions.[155–158] Furthermore, an unavoidable pitfall in assessing the role these antibodies play in first-trimester losses is the selection bias of studying couples only after they have presented with spontaneous abortions. That antibodies did not arise until *after* the pregnancy loss cannot be excluded. To address this pitfall, Simpson et al.[159] analyzed sera obtained prospectively from women within 21 days of conception. A total of 93 women who later experienced pregnancy loss were matched 2:1 with 190 controls who subsequently had a normal live-born offspring.[159] No association was observed between pregnancy loss and presence of either aPL or aCL.

Although neither aPL nor aCL would seem to contribute substantively to first-trimester pregnancy loss in the general population, the issue is not completely resolved. Some believe that more specific assays are needed, such as antiphosphatidylethanolamine.[160] Another pitfall is that marked variation in aPL antibodies occurs during pregnancy.[161] Power calculations are also inadequate to exclude an effect limited to selected subsets, such as the 3 to 4 percent of women with three or more repetitive losses; however, one third of women in the cohort study of Simpson et al.[159] experienced at least one prior loss, and in that group, the frequency of aPL and aCL was not increased compared with those of women without prior losses.[162]

In conclusion, a relationship between first-trimester loss and aPL and aCL seems unlikely to be applicable to more than a small subset of cases. Given this, treatment regimens may be offered with aspirin and heparin.[163,164] Treating these patients with intravenous immunoglobulin or with steroids is not recommended.[165]

Inherited Thrombophilias

Given that any relationship between fetal loss and aPLs or aCLs must involve placental thrombosis, maternal hypercoagulable states could also be associated with increased fetal losses. Inherited hypercoagulable associations include factor V Leiden (1691G→A), prothrombin (Factor II, 20210G→A) and homozygosity for the 677C→T polymorphism in the methylenetetrahydrofolate reductase gene.

Studying sera from women previously experiencing repetitive losses, Rai and coworkers[166] found an association between activated protein C resistance and second-trimester losses. The prevalence of factor V Leiden was 7.1 percent in women with abortions[167] versus 4 to 5 percent in the general population; no association was observed between factor V Leiden and aPLs or aCLs. Women with histories of repetitive abortions who had factor V Leiden and then became pregnant had a lower likelihood (4/11 or 30 percent) of delivering a live birth than women who lacked factor V Leiden (77/177 or 60 percent).[168] This group also found thromboelastographic abnormalities to be more common in women with repetitive abortions than in controls,[169] offering a way to identify high-risk women. In a later contribution,[170] they showed that acquired activated protein C resistance but not congenital (factor V Leiden) activated protein C resistance was more common in aborters. To evaluate acquired activated protein C resistance, they studied 904 women with three or more consecutive losses less than 12 weeks and 207 women with at least one loss after 12 weeks. *Acquired* activated protein C resistance Leiden mutation was more common in both groups (8.8 percent early losses, 8.7 percent late losses) than in 150 controls (3.3 percent). By contrast, factor V Leiden, the congenital form of acquired activated protein C resistance, was similar among all three groups (3.3 percent of 1,808 women with recurrent early loss, 3.9 percent of 414 women with late loss, and 4.0 percent of 300 controls). In Brazilian women, Souza and coworkers[171] found factor V Leiden in four of 56 (7.1 percent) women who aborted compared with 6 of 384 controls (1.6 percent). Factor II G20210A (prothrombin) was found in 2 of the 56 (3.6 percent) versus 1 percent of controls.

Not all authors agree that a relationship is established.[172,173] Pauer and colleagues,[174] and Balasch et al.[175] failed to find a relationship between early losses and factor V Leiden. Deficiencies of antithrombin, protein C, or protein S were not found by Kutteh and coworkers[176] to be any more frequent in 50 women with three or more losses than in 50 controls. Coumans et al.[177] assessed 52 women with two or more losses before 12 weeks' gestation for markers, and found no relationship with any of these same hemostatic markers. An increased frequency of hyperhomocystinemia was observed in women with repeated losses (six of 35 patients tested or 17.1 percent) compared with controls (4.5 percent). Such a relationship was also shown by Grandone et al.[178] and Ridker and colleagues.[179]

Overall, hypercoagulable states, or at least factor V Leiden and prothrombin 20120G→A, seem plausible causes of repetitive losses. However, most women with these conditions are normal, and ordering tests seems arguable if losses have occurred only in the first trimester, or no maternal signs of hypercoagulabity exist. In these circumstances, our treatment should be safe (e.g., aspirin). If losses occur in the second trimester, cause and effect seem more likely.

Alloimmune Disease (Shared Parental Antigens)

In contrast to Rh(D) isoimmunization, it may be paradoxically beneficial for mother and father and, hence, mother and fetus to be genetically dissimilar. If fetal rejection indeed occurs as result of diminished fetal-maternal immunologic interaction (alloimmune factors), immunotherapy might be beneficial on the grounds of generating blocking antibodies directed at the few loci differing between father and mother and, hence, mother and fetus. Indeed, the first prospective randomized trial produced impressive results.[180] Virtually all subsequent studies have been far less so. A 1994 multicenter effort pooling results of immunotherapy by injection of paternal leukocytes reported a scant 11 percent increase in the pregnancy rate in the immunized group.[181] Meta-analysis by Fraser et al.[182] found the odds ratio to be only 1.3 in favor of a beneficial effect. In 1999, Ober et al.[183] reported a definitive NICHD collaborative effort involving six U.S. and Canadian centers. Women with three or more spontaneous abortions of unknown cause were randomized into one arm (n = 91) subjected to immunization with paternal mononuclear cells; control women in the other arm were given saline (n = 92). Pregnancy beyond 28 weeks occurred in 46 percent (31 of 68) of the immunized group versus 65 percent (41 of 63) in the nonimmunized group. These findings were the opposite of expectation if immunotherapy were salutary.

Overall, the attributable role of human leukocyte antigen (HLA) sharing in pregnancy losses in the general population must be low, if not negligible, and immunotherapy is not indicated.[163] In the United States, the Food and Drug Administration requires clinicians performing immunotherapy to hold an Investigational New Drug application.[184] Although HLA sharing per se is not worth testing, several different HLA-G alleles single nucleotide polymorphisms have been claimed to be associated with increased pregnancy loss.[185,186]

Drugs, Chemicals, and Noxious Agents

Various exogenous agents have been implicated in fetal losses. Of course, the problem is that every pregnant woman is exposed to low doses of ubiquitous agents. Rarely are data adequate to determine the true role of these exogenous factors in early pregnancy losses.

Outcomes following exposures to exogenous agents are usually derived on the basis of case-control studies (see Chapter 8). In such studies, women who aborted claimed exposure to the agent in question more often than controls. However, case-control studies have certain inherent biases. The primary bias is recall, control women having less incentive to recall antecedent events than subjects experiencing an abnormal outcome. Employers also naturally attempt to limit exposure of women in the reproductive age group; thus, exposures to potentially dangerous chemicals are usually unwitting and, hence, poorly documented. Pregnant women are also exposed to many agents concurrently, making it nearly impossible to attribute adverse effects to a single agent. Given these caveats, physicians should be cautious about attributing pregnancy loss to exogenous agents. On the other hand, common sense dictates that exposure to potentially noxious agents be minimized.

X-Irradiation

Irradiation and antineoplastic agents in high doses are acknowledged abortifacients. Of course, therapeutic x-rays or chemotherapeutic drugs are administered during pregnancy only to seriously ill women whose pregnancies often must be terminated for maternal indications. On the other hand, pelvic x-ray exposure of up to perhaps 10 rad places a woman at little to no increased risk. The exposure is usually to doses that are far less (1 to 2 rad). Still, it is prudent for pregnant hospital workers to avoid handling chemotherapeutic agents and to minimize potential exposures during diagnostic x-ray procedures.

Cigarette Smoking

Smoking during pregnancy is accepted as being associated with spontaneous abortion,[187] but in most studies, it is difficult to exclude confounding variables. Increased abortion rates are seen in smokers, independent of maternal age and independent of alcohol consumption.[188] The relationship between pregnancy loss and tobacco use is best evaluated using urinary cotinine levels. Four hundred women with spontaneous abortions were compared with 570 who experienced ongoing pregnancies.[188] Women with urinary cotinine had increased risk of abortion, but the odds ratio reached only 1.8 (95-percent confidence interval [CI], 1.3 to 2.6). Smoking 10 or more cigarettes per day for at least 10 years and during pregnancy is associated with increased chromosomal instability in amniocytes.[189,190] Chromosomal region 11q23, known to be involved in leukemogenesis, seems especially sensitive to genotoxic compounds contained in tobacco. Within this context, the direct damage to placental tissue could explain the higher rate of miscarriage in heavy smokers.

Caffeine

In data gathered in cohort fashion, Mills et al.[149] showed that the odds ratio for association between pregnancy loss and caffeine (coffee and other dietary forms) was only 1.15 (95-percent CI, 0.89 to 1.49).[149] Women exposed to higher levels may have a greater risk as shown by the finding of Klebanoff et al.[191] of an association between pregnancy losses and caffeine ingestion greater than 300 mg daily (1.9-fold increase). A confounding problem with caffeine studies is difficulty in taking into account the effects of nausea, which is more common in successful pregnancies. However, in general, reassurance can be given concerning moderate caffeine exposure and pregnancy loss.

Alcohol

Alcohol consumption should be avoided during pregnancy for reasons independent of pregnancy loss (see Chapters 5 and 8). However, alcohol may increase pregnancy loss only slightly. In one study,[187] 616 women suffering spontaneous abortions were compared with 632 women delivering at 28 gestational weeks or more. Among women whose pregnancies ended in spontaneous abortion, 17 percent drank at least twice per week; only 8.1 percent of controls drank similar quantities of alcohol. Some authors also found a slightly increased risk for abortion in women who drank in the first trimester,[192] whereas others[193] found alcohol consumption to be nearly identical in women who did and did not experience an abortion; 13 percent of women who aborted and 11 percent of control women drank on average three to four drinks per week; other investigations have reached a similar conclusion.[188,194] Armstrong et al.[190] found the odds ratio to be 1.82 with 20 drinks or more per week.

Overall, alcohol shows only a small effect, potentially explained entirely by confounders. Abstinance is unlikely to prevent pregnancy loss. Thus, women should not attribute a loss to alcohol exposure during early gestation. Evaluation for other causes is still in order.

CONTRACEPTIVE AGENTS

Conception with an intrauterine device in place increases the risk of fetal loss, and can rarely result in second trimester sepsis characterized by a flulike syndrome. If the device is removed before pregnancy, there is no increased risk of spontaneous abortion.

Oral contraceptives use before or during pregnancy is not associated with fetal loss, nor is spermicide exposure before or after conception.

ENVIRONMENTAL CHEMICALS

Limiting exposure to potential toxins in the workplace is prudent for pregnant women. The difficulty lies in defining the precise effect of lower exposures and attributing a specific risk. False alarms concerning potential toxins are frequent. Among the many chemical agents variously claimed to be associated with fetal losses, consensus seems to be evolving around only a few.[195] These include anesthetic gases, arsenic, aniline dyes, benzene, solvents, ethylene oxide, formaldehyde, pesticides, and certain divalent cations (lead, mercury, cadmium). Workers in rubber industries, battery factories, and chemical production plants are among those at potential risk. This topic is discussed in Chapter 8.

Trauma

Women commonly attribute pregnancy losses to trauma, such as a fall or blow to the abdomen. Actually, fetuses are well protected from external trauma by intervening maternal structures and amniotic fluid. The temptation to attribute a loss to minor traumatic events should be avoided. A nested case-control study of 392 cases and 807 controls showed no relationship between physical violence and abortions.[196]

Psychological Factors

That impaired psychological well-being predisposes to early fetal losses has been claimed but never proved. Certainly, neurotic or mentally ill women experience losses as do normal women. Whether the frequency of losses is higher in the former is less certain because potential confounding variables have not been taken into account, and genetic factors not considered.

Investigations cited as proving a benefit of psychological well-being are those of Stray-Pedersen et al.[197] Pregnant women who previously experienced repetitive abortions received increased attention but no specific medical therapy ("tender loving care"). These women (n = 16) were more likely (85 percent) to complete their pregnancy than women (n = 42) not offered such close attention (36 percent). One pitfall was that only women living "close" to the university were eligible to be placed in the increased-attention group. Women living farther away served as "controls"; however, these women may have differed from the experimental group in other ways as well.

Several other studies have also reported a beneficial effect of psychological well-being.[70,71,198] Again, pitfalls exist in study design, and the biologic explanation for this effect remains obscure.

Severe Maternal Illness

Many debilitating maternal diseases are associated with increased early abortion. Pathogenesis is not necessarily independent of mechanisms discussed previously, specifically endocrinologic or immunologic. Symptomatic maternal diseases established as causes of fetal wastage include Wilson's disease, maternal phenylketonuria, cyanotic heart disease, hemoglobinopathies, and inflammatory bowel disease. Any life-threatening disease would be expected to be associated with an increased pregnancy loss, and indeed one would expect this teleologically. Overall, relatively few fetal losses will be the result of severe maternal disease. This applies even more for repetitive losses.

RECOMMENDED EVALUATION FOR RECURRENT PREGNANCY LOSSES

1. Couples experiencing only one first-trimester abortion should receive pertinent information, but not necessarily be evaluated formally. Mention the relatively high (10 to 15 percent) pregnancy loss rate in the general population and the beneficial effects of abortion in eliminating abnormal conceptuses. Provide relevant recurrence risks, usually 20 to 25 percent subsequent loss in the presence of a prior live-born infant and somewhat higher in the absence of a prior live-born infant. Risks are higher for older women. If a specific medical illness exists, treatment is obviously necessary. It is recommended that lysis of intrauterine adhesions be performed. Otherwise, no further evaluation need be undertaken, even if uterine anomalies or leiomyomas are present.
2. Investigation may or may not be necessary after two spontaneous abortions, depending on the patient's age and personal desires. After three spontaneous abortions, evaluation is usually indicated. One should then (a) obtain a detailed family history, (b) perform a complete physical examination, (c) discuss recurrence risks, and (d) order the selected tests cited later. Occurrence of an anomalous stillborn or live-born infant warrants genetic evaluation irrespective of the number of pregnancy losses.

3. Parental chromosomal studies should be undertaken on all couples having repetitive losses. Antenatal chromosomal studies should be offered if a balanced chromosomal rearrangement is detected in either parent or if autosomal trisomy occurred in any previous abortus.
4. Although it is impractical to karyotype all abortuses, cytogenetic information on abortuses may be useful. Detection of a trisomic abortus suggests recurrent aneuploidy, justifying prenatal cytogenetic studies in future pregnancies. Performing prenatal cytogenetic studies solely on the basis of repeated losses is more arguable, but not unreasonable among women aged 30 to 34 years.
5. LPD as a discrete entity seems arguable. Timed endometrial biopsies are not reliable, nor is measuring progesterone levels. If performed, progesterone levels should be determined late in the luteal phase in two or more cycles. Progesterone therapy has been proposed, but its efficacy is unproved.
6. Other endocrine causes for repeated fetal losses include poorly controlled diabetes mellitus, overt thyroid dysfunction, and elevated maternal TSH levels. Subclinical diabetes or thyroid disease should not be considered causes.
7. To determine the role of infectious agents, the endometrium may be cultured for *U. urealyticum*. Alternatively, a couple could be treated empirically with vibramycin or doxycycline. Of other infections agents, only *C. trachomatis* seems of equal plausibility. These two agents are more likely to cause sporadic than repetitive losses.
8. If an abortion occurs after 8 to 10 weeks' gestation, a uterine anomaly or submucous leiomyoma should be considered. The uterine cavity should be explored by hysteroscopy or hysterosalpingography. As noted in item #1, intrauterine adhesions should be lysed. If a müllerian fusion defect (septate or bicornuate uterus) is detected in a woman experiencing one or more second-trimester spontaneous abortions, surgical correction may be warranted. A large submucous leiomyoma may also justify myomectomy or reduction. However, the same statements do not necessarily apply following first-trimester losses. Cervical incompetence should be managed by cervical cerclage during the next pregnancy.
9. To exclude autoimmune disease involving aPL antibodies, assessment should include aPL and aCL. Women with antibodies who experience midtrimester losses may benefit from treatment with heparin and aspirin, but the same does not necessarily hold when these antibodies are detected in asymptomatic women having first-trimester pregnancy losses. This recommendation also holds for women undergoing ART.
10. Determining parental HLA types is not recommended. Immunotherapy by inoculation of the mother with her husband's leukocytes is unequivocally ineffective.
11. One should discourage exposure to cigarettes and alcohol, yet not necessarily ascribe cause and effect in an individual case. Similar counsel should apply for exposures to other potential toxins.

Key Points

- Approximately 22 percent of all pregnancies detected on the basis of urinary hCG assays are lost, usually before clinical recognition. The loss of preimplanation embryos is even higher, 25 to 50 percent of morphologically normal and 50 to 75 percent of morphologically abnormal embryos.

- Fetal demise occurs before clinical signs are manifested, as evidenced by only 2 to 3 percent of viable pregnancies being lost after 8 weeks' gestation. Thus, most fetuses aborting clinically at 9 to 12 weeks must have died weeks previously. Almost all losses are thus "missed abortions," that is, retained in utero for an interval before clinical recognition; thus, the term missed abortion is archaic.

- If the pregnancy is ultrasonographically viable at 8 to 9 weeks, 2 to 3 percent are lost thereafter. Most losses occur in the next 2 months. Loss rates are perhaps 1 percent in women confirmed by ultrasound to have viable pregnancies at 16 weeks, and even lower after 20 weeks.

- The clinical loss rate is 10 to 12 percent. Loss rates are age dependent, a 40-year-old women having twice the loss rate of a 20-year-old women. Most of these pregnancies are lost before 8 weeks' gestation.

- Pregnancy losses may be recurrent, although increasing after one loss. The recurrence risk generally reaches no more than 30 percent after three or four losses.

- By far the most common causes of pregnancy losses are chromosomal abnormalities. At least 50 percent if not 80 to 90 percent of clinically recognized pregnancy losses show a chromosomal abnormality. The types of chromosomal abnormalities in abortuses differ from those found in live-born infants, but autosomal trisomy still accounts for 50 percent of abnormalities. A balanced translocation is present in about 5 percent of couples having repeated spontaneous abortions.

- Many nongenetic causes of repetitive abortions have been proposed, but not all are proved. It is reasonable to evaluate couples for these conditions, but efficacy of treatment remains uncertain.

- Uterine anomalies are accepted causes of *second-trimester* losses, and couples experiencing such losses may benefit from metroplasty or hysteroscopic resection of a uterine septum. Uterine anomalies are not common causes of first-trimester losses.

- Drugs, toxins, and physical agents are associated with spontaneous abortion, but usually not in repetitive pregnancies. Avoiding potential toxins is desirable, but one should not assume that such exposures explain repetitive losses. Smoking during pregnancy is accepted as associated with spontaneous abortions, but it is difficult to exclude confounding variables.

- LAC antibodies, aPL, and aCL, are associated with second-trimester losses, but their role in first-trimester losses is arguable. Immunotherapy for couples sharing HLA antigens or otherwise showing blunted maternal response to paternal antigens (alloimmune disease) is not recommended. Determining parental HLA types in the absence of other immunologic evaluations is not recommended.

- Despite a history of recurrent abortions, prognosis is reasonably good even without therapy. The success rate is 30 to 40 percent even with repeated losses and no prior live-born infants. An efficacious therapeutic regimen should show success greater than 70 percent in a randomized control trial.

REFERENCES

1. U.S. Department of Health and Human Services: Reproductive impairments among married couples., U.S. Vital and Health Statistics Series 23, No. 11, Hyattsville, MD, 1982, p.5.
2. Wilcox AJ, Weinberg CR, O'Connor JF, et al: Incidence of early loss of pregnancy. N Engl J Med 319:189, 1988.
3. Mills JL, Simpson JL, Driscoll SG, et al: Incidence of spontaneous abortion among normal women and insulin-dependent diabetic women whose pregnancies were identified within 21 days of conception. N Engl J Med 319:1617, 1988.
4. Simpson JL, Mills JL, Holmes LB, et al: Low fetal loss rates after ultrasound-proved viability in early pregnancy. JAMA 258:2555, 1987.
5. Spandorfer SD, Davis OK, Barmat LI, et al: Relationship between maternal age and aneuploidy in *in vitro* fertilization pregnancy loss. Fertil Steril 81:1265, 2004.
6. Simpson JL, Carson SA: Causes of fetal loss. *In* Gray R, Leridon L, Spira F (eds): Symposium on Biological and Demographic Determinants of Human Reproduction. Oxford, Oxford University Press, 1993, p 287.
7. Regan L: A prospective study on spontaneous abortion. *In* Beard RW, Sharp F (eds): Early Pregnancy Loss: Mechanisms and Treatment. London, Springer-Verlag, 1988, p 22.
8. Simpson JL, Gray RH, Queenan JT, et al: Risk of recurrent spontaneous abortion for pregnancies discovered in the fifth week of gestation. Lancet 344:964, 1994.
9. Wilcox AJ, Baird DD, Weinberg CR: Time of implantation of the conceptus and loss of pregnancy. N Engl J Med 340:1796, 1999.
10. Gray RH, Simpson JL, Kambic RT, et al: Timing of conception and the risk of spontaneous abortion among pregnancies occurring during the use of natural family planning. Am J Obstet Gynecol 172:1567, 1995.
11. Wilson RD, Kendrick V, Wittmann BK, et al: Risk of spontaneous abortion in ultrasonically normal pregnancies. Lancet 2:920, 1984.
12. Gilmore DH, McNay MB: Spontaneous fetal loss rate in early pregnancy. Lancet 1:107, 1985.
13. Hoesli IM, Walter-Gobel I, Tercanli S, et al: Spontaneous fetal loss rates in a non-selected population. Am J Med Genet 100:106, 2001.
14. Ellett K, Buxton EJ, Luesley DM: The effect of ethnic origin on the rate of spontaneous late mid-trimester abortion. Ethn Dis 2:84, 1992.
15. Wyatt PR, Owolabi T, Meier C, et al: Age-specific risk of fetal loss observed in a second trimester serum screening population. Am J Obstet Gynecol 192:240, 2005.
16. Hertig AT, Rock J, Adams EC: Description of human ova within the first 17 days of development. Am J Anat 98:435, 1956.
17. Hertig AT, Rock J, Adams EC, et al: Thirty-four fertilized human ova, good, bad and indifferent, recovered from 210 women of known fertility. Pediatrics 25:202, 1959.
18. Hertig AT, Rock J: Searching for early fertilized human ova. Gynecol Invest 4:121, 1973.
19. Plachot M, Junca AM, Mandelbaum J, et al: Chromosome investigations in early life. II. Human preimplantation embryos. Hum Reprod 2:29, 1987.
20. Munné S, Grifo J, Cohen J, et al: Chromosome abnormalities in human arrested preimplantation embryos: A multiple-probe FISH study. Am J Hum Genet 55:150, 1994.
21. Munné S, Alikani M, Tomkin G, et al: Embryo morphology, developmental rates, and maternal age are correlated with chromosome abnormalities. Fertil Steril 64:382, 1995.
22. Egozcue J, Blanco J, Vidal F: Chromosome studies in human sperm nuclei using fluorescence in-situ hybridization (FISH). Hum Reprod Update 3:441, 1997.
23. Pellestor F, Anahory T, Hamamah S: The chromosomal analysis of human oocytes. An overview of established procedures. Hum Reprod Update 11:15, 2005.
24. Plachot M: Genetics in human oocytes. *In* Boutaleb Y, Gzouli A (ed): New Concepts in Reproduction. Lanes, England, Parthenon Pub Group, 1992, p 367.
25. Martin R: Chromosomal abnormalities in human sperm. Adv Exp Med Biol 518:181, 2003.
26. Jauniaux E, Gulbis B, Burton GJ: The human first trimester gestational sac limits rather than facilitates oxygen transfer to the foetus—a review. Placenta 24(Suppl A):S86, 2003.
27. Jauniaux E, Hempstock J, Greenwold N, et al: Trophoblastic oxidative stress in relation to temporal and regional differences in maternal placental blood flow in normal and abnormal early pregnancies. Am J Pathol 162:115, 2003.
28. Hustin J, Jauniaux E, Schaaps JP: Histological study of the materno-embryonic interface in spontaneous abortion. Placenta 11:477, 1990.
29. Jauniaux E, Zaidi J, Jurkovic D, et al: Comparison of colour Doppler features and pathological findings in complicated early pregnancy. Hum Reprod 9:2432, 1994.
30. Jauniaux E, Greenwold N, Hempstock J, et al: Comparison of ultrasonographic and Doppler mapping of the intervillous circulation in normal and abnormal early pregnancies. Fertil Steril 79:100, 2003.
31. Greenwold N, Jauniaux E, Gulbis B, et al: Relationship among maternal serum endocrinology, placental karyotype, and intervillous circulation in early pregnancy failure. Fertil Steril 79:1373, 2003.
32. Hempstock J, Jauniaux E, Greenwold N, et al: The contribution of placental oxidative stress to early pregnancy failure. Hum Pathol 34:1265, 2003.
33. Boué J, Boué A, Lazar P: Retrospective and prospective epidemiological studies of 1500 karyotyped spontaneous human abortions. Teratology 12:11, 1975.
34. Hassold TJ: A cytogenetic study of repeated spontaneous abortions. Am J Hum Genet 32:723, 1980.
35. Simpson JL, Bombard AT: Chromosomal abnormalities in spontaneous abortion: frequency, pathology and genetic counseling. *In* Edmonds K (ed): Spontaneous Abortion. London, Blackwell, 1987, p 51.
36. Sorokin Y, Johnson MP, Uhlmann WR, et al: Postmortem chorionic villus sampling: correlation of cytogenetic and ultrasound findings. Am J Med Genet 39:314, 1991.
37. Strom CM, Ginsberg N, Applebaum M, et al: Analyses of 95 first-trimester spontaneous abortions by chorionic villus sampling and karyotype. J Assist Reprod Genet 9:458, 1992.
38. Kuleshov NP: Chromosome anomalies of infants dying during the perinatal period and premature newborn. Hum Genet 31:151, 1976.
39. Simpson JL: Genetics of spontaneous abortions. *In* Carp H (ed): Recurrent Pregnancy Loss. Taylor and Francis Medical Books, UK, 2006, In Press.
40. Banzai M, Sato S, Matsuda H, et al: Trisomy 1 in a case of a missed abortion. J Hum Genet 49:396, 2004.
41. Warburton D, Byrne J, Canik N: Chromosome Anomalies and Prenatal Development: An Atlas. New York, Oxford University Press, 1991.
42. Kalousek DK: Pathology of abortion: chromosomal and genetic correlations. *In* Kraus FT, Damjanov IK (eds): Pathology of Reproductive Failure. Baltimore, Williams & Wilkins, 1991, p 228.

43. Hassold T, Merrill M, Adkins K, et al: Recombination and maternal age-dependent nondisjunction: molecular studies of trisomy 16. Am J Hum Genet 57:867, 1995.
44. Fisher JM, Harvey JF, Morton NE, et al: Trisomy 18: studies of the parent and cell division of origin and the effect of aberrant recombination on nondisjunction. Am J Hum Genet 56:669, 1995.
45. Bugge M, Collins A, Petersen MB, et al: Non-disjunction of chromosome 18. Hum Mol Genet 7:661, 1998.
46. Hassold TJ: Nondisjunction in the human male. Curr Top Dev Biol 37:383, 1998.
47. Henderson SA, Edwards RG: Chiasma frequency and maternal age in mammals. Nature 217:22, 1968.
48. Lamb NE, Yu K, Shaffer J, et al: Association between maternal age and meiotic recombination for trisomy 21. Am J Hum Genet 76:91, 2005.
49. Hassold T, Abruzzo M, Adkins K, et al: Human aneuploidy: incidence, origin, and etiology. Environ Mol Mutagen 28:167, 1996.
50. Savage AR, Petersen MB, Pettay D, et al: Elucidating the mechanisms of paternal non-disjunction of chromosome 21 in humans. Hum Mol Genet 7:1221, 1998.
51. Clouston HJ, Herbert M, Fenwick J, et al: Cytogenetic analysis of human blastocysts. Prenat Diagn 22:1143, 2002.
52. Jacobs PA, Angell RR, Buchanan IM, et al: The origin of human triploids. Ann Hum Genet 42:49, 1978.
53. Beatty RA: The origin of human triploidy: An integration of qualitative and quantitative evidence. Ann Hum Genet 41:299, 1978.
54. Jauniaux E, Burton GJ: Pathophysiology of histological changes in early pregnancy loss. Placenta 26:114, 2005.
55. Singh RP, Carr DH: The anatomy and histology of XO human embryos and fetuses. Anat Rec 155:369, 1966.
56. Jirasek JE: Principles of reproductive embryology. *In* Simpson JL (ed): Disorders of Sex Differentiation: Etiology and Clinical Delineation. San Diego, Academic Press, 1976, p 51.
57. Simpson JL: Pregnancies in women with chromosomal abnormalities. *In* Schulman JD, Simpson JL (eds): Genetic Diseases in Pregnancy. New York, Academic Press, 1981, p 439.
58. Chandley AC: The origin of chromosomal aberrations in man and their potential for survival and reproduction in the adult human population. Ann Genet 24:5, 1981.
59. Baek KH: Aberrant gene expression associated with recurrent pregnancy loss. Mol Hum Reprod 10:291, 2004.
60. Philipp T, Kalousek DK: Generalized abnormal embryonic development in missed abortion: embryoscopic and cytogenetic findings. Am J Med Genet 111:43, 2002.
61. Henderson DJ, Sherman LS, Loughna SC, et al: Early embryonic failure associated with uniparental disomy for human chromosome 21. Hum Mol Genet 3:1373, 1994.
62. Lanasa MC, Hogge WA, Kubik C, et al: Highly skewed X-chromosome inactivation is associated with idiopathic recurrent spontaneous abortion. Am J Hum Genet 65:252, 1999.
63. Pegoraro E, Whitaker J, Mowery-Rushton P, et al: Familial skewed X inactivation: a molecular trait associated with high spontaneous-abortion rate maps to Xq28. Am J Hum Genet 61:160, 1997.
64. Malpas P: A study of abortion sequences. J Obstet Gynaecol Br Emp 45:932, 1938.
65. Warburton D, Fraser FC: Spontaneous abortion risks in man: data from reproductive histories collected in a medical genetic unit. Am J Hum Genet 16:1, 1964.
66. Poland BJ, Miller JR, Jones DC, et al: Reproductive counseling in patients who have had a spontancous abortion. Am J Obstet Gynecol 127:685, 1977.
67. Kline J, Stein ZA, Susser M, et al: Smoking: a risk factor for spontaneous abortion. N Engl J Med 297:793, 1977.
68. Boué J, Boué A: Chromosomal analysis of two consecutive abortuses in each of 43 women. Humangenetik 19:275, 1973.
69. Vlaanderen W, Treffers PE: Prognosis of subsequent pregnancies after recurrent spontaneous abortion in first trimester. Br Med J 295:92, 1987.
70. Liddell HS, Pattison NS, Zanderigo A: Recurrent miscarriage—outcome after supportive care in early pregnancy. Aust N Z J Obstet Gynaecol 31:320, 1991.
71. Houwert-de Jong MH, Termijtelen A, Eskes TK, et al: The natural course of habitual abortion. Eur J Obstet Gynecol Reprod Biol 33:221, 1989.
72. Simpson JL, Meyers CM, Martin AO, et al: Translocations are infrequent among couples having repeated spontaneous abortions but no other abnormal pregnancies. Fertil Steril 51: 811, 1989.
73. De Braekeleer M, Dao TN: Cytogenetic studies in couples experiencing repeated pregnancy losses. Hum Reprod 5:519, 1990.
74. Simpson JL, Elias S, Martin AO: Parental chromosomal rearrangements associated with repetitive spontaneous abortions. Fertil Steril 36:584, 1981.
75. Boué A, Gallano P: A collaborative study of the segregation of inherited chromosome structural rearrangements in 1,356 prenatal diagnoses. Prenat Diagn 4:45, 1984.
76. Daniel A, Hook EB, Wulf G: Risks of unbalanced progeny at amniocentesis to carriers of chromosome rearrangements: data from United States and Canadian laboratories. Am J Med Genet 33:14, 1989.
77. Carp H, Feldman B, Oelsner G, et al: Parental karyotype and subsequent live births in recurrent miscarriage. Fertil Steril 81:1296, 2004.
78. Mackie OC, Scriven PN: Meiotic outcomes in reciprocal translocation carriers ascertained in 3-day human embryos. Eur J Hum Genet 10:801, 2002.
79. Verlinsky Y, Tur-Kaspa I, Cieslak J, et al: Preimplantation testing for chromosomal disorders improves reproductive outcome of poor-prognosis patients. Reprod Biomed Online 11:219, 2005.
80. Simpson JL, Elias S: Genetics in Obstetrics and Gynecology, 3rd ed. Philadelphia, WB Saunders, 2003.
81. Sutherland GR, Gardiner AJ, Carter RF: Familial pericentric inversion of chromosome 19, inv (19) (p13q13) with a note on genetic counseling of pericentric inversion carriers. Clin Genet 10:54, 1976.
82. Pettenati MJ, Rao PN, Phelan MC, et al: Paracentric inversions in humans: a review of 446 paracentric inversions with presentation of 120 new cases. Am J Med Genet 55:171, 1995.
83. Warburton D, Kline J, Stein Z, et al: Does the karyotype of a spontaneous abortion predict the karyotype of a subsequent abortion? Evidence from 273 women with two karyotyped spontaneous abortions. Am J Hum Genet 41:465, 1987.
84. Alberman ED: The abortus as a predictor of future trisomy 21. *In* Cruz DI, Gerald PS (eds): Trisomy 21 (Down syndrome), Baltimore, Raven, 1981, p 69.
85. Rubio C, Simon C, Vidal F, et al: Chromosomal abnormalities and embryo development in recurrent miscarriage couples. Hum Reprod 18:182, 2003.
86. Munné S, Sandalinas M, Magli C, et al: Increased rate of aneuploid embryos in young women with previous aneuploid conceptions. Prenat Diagn 24:638, 2004.
87. Stephenson MD, Awartani KA, Robinson WP: Cytogenetic analysis of miscarriages from couples with recurrent miscarriage: a case-control study. Hum Reprod 17:446, 2002.
88. Stern C, Chamley L, Hale L, et al: Antibodies to beta$_2$ glycoprotein I are associated with in vitro fertilization implantation failure as well as recurrent miscarriage: results of a prevalence study. Fertil Steril 70:938, 1998.
89. Ogasawara M, Kajiura S, Katano K, et al: Are serum progesterone levels predictive of recurrent miscarriage in future pregnancies? Fertil Steril 68:806, 1997.
90. Noyes RW, Hertig AT, Rock J: Dating the endometrial biopsy. Fertil Steril 1:3, 1950.
91. Scott RT, Snyder RR, Strickland DM, et al: The effect of interobserver variation in dating endometrial histology on the diagnosis of luteal phase defects. Fertil Steril 50:888, 1988.
92. Li TC, Dockery P, Rogers AW, et al: How precise is histologic dating of endometrium using the standard dating criteria? Fertil Steril 51:759, 1989.
93. Davis OK, Berkeley AS, Naus GJ, et al: The incidence of luteal phase defect in normal, fertile women, determined by serial endometrial biopsies. Fertil Steril 51:582, 1989.
94. Jordan J, Craig K, Clifton DK, et al: Luteal phase defect: the sensitivity and specificity of diagnostic methods in common clinical use. Fertil Steril 62:54, 1994.

95. Daya S, Ward S, Burrows E: Progesterone profiles in luteal phase defect cycles and outcome of progesterone treatment in patients with recurrent spontaneous abortion. Am J Obstet Gynecol 158: 225, 1988.
96. Soules MR, Clifton DK, Cohen NL, et al: Luteal phase deficiency: abnormal gonadotropin and progesterone secretion patterns. J Clin Endocrinol Metab 69:813, 1989.
97. Soules MR, McLachlan RI, Ek M, et al: Luteal phase deficiency: characterization of reproductive hormones over the menstrual cycle. J Clin Endocrinol Metab 69:804, 1989.
98. Soules MR, Wiebe RH, Aksel S, et al: The diagnosis and therapy of luteal phase deficiency. Fertil Steril 28:1033, 1977.
99. Coutifaris C, Myers ER, Guzick DS, et al: NICHD National Cooperative Reproductive Medicine Network. Histological dating of timed endometrial biopsy tissue is not related to fertility status. Fertil Steril 82:1264, 2004.
100. Phung TT, Byrd JR, McDonough PG: Etiologies and subsequent reproductive performance of 100 couples with recurrent abortion. Fertil Steril 32:389, 1979.
101. Simpson JL: Fetal wastage. *In* Gabbe SG, Niebyl JR, Simpson JL (eds): Obstetrics: Normal and Problem Pregnancies. New York, Churchill Livingstone, 1996, p 729.
102. Karamardian LM, Grimes DA: Luteal phase deficiency: effect of treatment on pregnancy rates. Am J Obstet Gynecol 167:1391, 1992.
103. Quenby SM, Farquharson RG: Predicting recurring miscarriage: what is important? Obstet Gynecol 82:132, 1993.
104. Sagle M, Bishop K, Ridley N, et al: Recurrent early miscarriage and polycystic ovaries. BMJ 297:1027, 1988.
105. Regan L, Owen EJ, Jacobs HS: Hypersecretion of luteinising hormone, infertility, and miscarriage. Lancet 336:1141, 1990.
106. Clifford K, Rai R, Watson H, et al: Does suppressing luteinising hormone secretion reduce the miscarriage rate? Results of a randomised controlled trial. BMJ 312:1508, 1996.
107. Carp HJ, Hass Y, Dolicky M, et al: The effect of serum follicular phase luteinizing hormone concentrations in habitual abortion: correlation with results of paternal leukocyte immunization. Hum Reprod 10:1702, 1995.
108. Bussen S, Sutterlin M, Steck T: Endocrine abnormalities during the follicular phase in women with recurrent spontaneous abortion. Hum Reprod 14:18, 1999.
109. Tulppala M, Stenman UH, Cacciatore B, et al: Polycystic ovaries and levels of gonadotrophins and androgens in recurrent miscarriage: prospective study in 50 women. Br J Obstet Gynaecol 100:348, 1993.
110. Montoro M, Collea JV, Frasier SD, et al: Successful outcome of pregnancy in women with hypothyroidism. Ann Intern Med 94:31, 1981.
111. Bussen S, Steck T: Thyroid autoantibodies in euthyroid nonpregnant women with recurrent spontaneous abortions. Hum Reprod 10:2938, 1995.
112. Stagnaro-Green A, Roman SH, Cobin RH, et al: Detection of at-risk pregnancy by means of highly sensitive assays for thyroid autoantibodies. JAMA 264:1422, 1990.
113. Glinoer D, Soto MF, Bourdoux P, et al: Pregnancy in patients with mild thyroid abnormalities: maternal and neonatal repercussions. J Clin Endocrinol Metab 73:421, 1991.
114. Singh J, Hunt P, Eggo MC, et al: Thyroid-stimulating hormone rapidly stimulates inositol polyphosphate formation in FRTL-5 thyrocytes without activating phosphoinositidase C. Biochem J 316:175, 1996.
115. Pratt DE, Kaberlein G, Dudkiewicz A, et al: The association of antithyroid antibodies in euthyroid nonpregnant women with recurrent first trimester abortions in the next pregnancy. Fertil Steril 60:1001, 1993.
116. Pratt D, Novotny M, Kaberlein G, et al: Antithyroid antibodies and the association with non-organ-specific antibodies in recurrent pregnancy loss. Am J Obstet Gynecol 168:837, 1993.
117. Rushworth FH, Backos M, Rai R, et al: Prospective pregnancy outcome in untreated recurrent miscarries with thyroid autoantibodies. Hum Reprod 15:1637, 2000.
118. Anselmo J, Cao D, Karrison T, et al: Fetal loss associated with excess thyroid hormone exposure. JAMA 292:691, 2004.
119. Miodovnik M, Mimouni F, Tsang RC, et al: Glycemic control and spontaneous abortion in insulin-dependent diabetic women. Obstet Gynecol 68:366, 1986.
120. Ben Rafael Z, Seidman DS, Recabi K, et al: Uterine anomalies. A retrospective, matched-control study. J Reprod Med 36:723, 1991.
121. Michalas SP: Outcome of pregnancy in women with uterine malformation: evaluation of 62 cases. Int J Gynaecol Obstet 35:215, 1991.
122. Makino T, Sakai A, Sugi T, et al: Current comprehensive therapy of habitual abortion. Ann N Y Acad Sci 626:597, 1991.
123. Moutos DM, Damewood MD, Schlaff WD, et al: A comparison of the reproductive outcome between women with a unicornuate uterus and women with a didelphic uterus. Fertil Steril 58:88, 1992.
124. Golan A, Langer R, Neuman M, et al: Obstetric outcome in women with congenital uterine malformations. J Reprod Med 37:233, 1992.
125. Candiani GB, Fedele L, Parazzini F, et al: Reproductive prognosis after abdominal metroplasty in bicornuate or septate uterus: a life table analysis. Br J Obstet Gynaecol 97:613, 1990.
126. Makino T: Management of uterine congenital malformations: evaluation of outcome. *In* Hedon B, Springer J, Mores P (eds): Proceedings of the 15th World Congress on Fertility and Sterility. Montpellier, France 17-22 September, 1995. New York, Parthenon, 1995, p 135.
127. Stein AL, March CM: Pregnancy outcome in women with mullerian duct anomalies. J Reprod Med 35:411, 1990.
128. Proctor JA, Haney AF: Recurrent first trimester pregnancy loss is associated with uterine septum but not with bicornuate uterus. Fertil Steril 80:1212, 2003.
129. Salim R, Regan L, Woelfer B, et al: A comparative study of the morphology of congenital uterine anomalies in women with and without a history of recurrent first trimester miscarriage. Hum Reprod 18:162, 2003.
130. Stampe SS: Estimated prevalence of mullerian anomalies. Acta Obstet Gynecol Scand 67:441, 1988.
131. Simon C, Martinez L, Pardo F, et al: Mullerian defects in women with normal reproductive outcome. Fertil Steril 56:1192, 1991.
132. Ludmir J, Samuels P, Brooks S, et al: Pregnancy outcome of patients with uncorrected uterine anomalies managed in a high-risk obstetric setting. Obstet Gynecol 75:906, 1990.
133. Hartmann KE, Herring AH: Predictors of the presence of uterine fibroids in the first trimester of pregnancy: A prospective cohort study. J Soc Gynecol Investig 11[Abstract 789], 340A, 2004.
134. Matovina M, Husnjak K, Milutin N, et al: Possible role of bacterial and viral infections in miscarriages. Fertil Steril 81:662, 2004.
135. Stray-Pedersen B, Eng J, Reikvam TM: Uterine T-mycoplasma colonization in reproductive failure. Am J Obstet Gynecol 130:307, 1978.
136. Quinn PA, Petric M, Barkin M, et al: Prevalence of antibody to *Chlamydia trachomatis* in spontaneous abortion and infertility. Am J Obstet Gynecol 156:291, 1987.
137. Witkin SS, Ledger WJ: Antibodies to Chlamydia trachomatis in sera of women with recurrent spontaneous abortions. Am J Obstet Gynecol 167:135, 1992.
138. Rae R, Smith IW, Liston WA, et al: Chlamydial serologic studies and recurrent spontaneous abortion. Am J Obstet Gynecol 170: 782, 1994.
139. Olliaro P, Regazzetti A, Gorini G, et al: Chlamydia trachomatis infection in "sine causa" recurrent abortion. Boll Ist Sieroter Milan 70:467, 1991.
140. van Lijnschoten G, Stals F, Evers JL, et al: The presence of cytomegalovirus antigens in karyotyped abortions. *In* van Lijnschoten G (ed): Morphology and Karyotype in Early Abortions, Amsterdam, 1993, p 79.
141. Paukku M, Tulppala M, Puolakkainen M, et al: Lack of association between serum antibodies to *Chlamydia trachomatis* and a history of recurrent pregnancy loss. Fertil Steril 72:427, 1999.
142. Zavala-Velazquez J, Guzman-Marin E, Barrera-Perez M, et al: [Toxoplasmosis and abortion in patients at the O'Horan Hospital of Merida, Yucatan]. Salud Publica Mex 31:664, 1989.
143. el Ridi AM, Nada SM, Aly AS, et al: Toxoplasmosis and pregnancy: an analytical study in Zagazig, Egypt. J Egypt Soc Parasitol 21:81, 1991.
144. Sahwi SY, Zaki MS, Haiba NY, et al: Toxoplasmosis as a cause of repeated abortion. J Obstet Gynaecol 21:145, 1995.

145. Simpson JL, Mills JL, Kim H, et al: Infectious processes: an infrequent cause of first trimester spontaneous abortions. Hum Reprod 11:668, 1996.
146. Rock JA, Shirey RS, Braine HG, et al: Plasmapheresis for the treatment of repeated early pregnancy wastage associated with anti-P. Obstet Gynecol 66:57S, 1985.
147. Strowitzki T, Wiedemann R, Heim MU, et al: [Pregnancy with an extremely rare P blood group with anti-PP1Pk]. Geburtshilfe Frauenheilkd 51:710, 1991.
148. Hill JA, Polgar K, Anderson DJ: T-helper 1-type immunity to trophoblast in women with recurrent spontaneous abortion. JAMA 273:1933, 1995.
149. Mills JL, Holmes LB, Aarons JH, et al: Moderate caffeine use and the risk of spontaneous abortion and intrauterine growth retardation. JAMA 269:593, 1993.
150. Raghupathy R: Th1-type immunity is incompatible with successful pregnancy. Immunol Today 18:478, 1997.
151. Wegmann TG, Lin H, Guilbert L, et al: Bidirectional cytokine interactions in the maternal-fetal relationship: is successful pregnancy a TH2 phenomenon? Immunol Today 14:353, 1993.
152. Cowchock S: Autoantibodies and pregnancy wastage. Am J Reprod Immunol 26:38, 1991.
153. Branch DW, Ward K: Antibodies and pregnancy wastage. Semin Reprod Endocrinol 1:168, 1989.
154. Scott JR, Rote NS, Branch DW: Immunologic aspects of recurrent abortion and fetal death. Obstet Gynecol 70:645, 1987.
155. Petri M, Golbus M, Anderson R, et al: Antinuclear antibody, lupus anticoagulant, and anticardiolipin antibody in women with idiopathic habitual abortion. A controlled, prospective study of forty-four women. Arthritis Rheum 30:601, 1987.
156. Carp HJ, Menashe Y, Frenkel Y, et al: Lupus anticoagulant. Significance in habitual first-trimester abortion. J Reprod Med 38:549, 1993.
157. Mishell DR, Jr: Recurrent abortion. J Reprod Med 38:250, 1993.
158. Eroglu GE, Scopelitis E: Antinuclear and antiphospholipid antibodies in healthy women with recurrent spontaneous abortion. Am J Reprod Immunol 31:1, 1994.
159. Simpson JL, Carson SA, Chesney C, et al: Lack of association between antiphospholipid antibodies and first-trimester spontaneous abortion: prospective study of pregnancies detected within 21 days of conception. Fertil Steril 69:814, 1998.
160. Sugi T, Katsunuma J, Izumi S, et al: Prevalence and heterogeneity of antiphosphatidylethanolamine antibodies in patients with recurrent early pregnancy losses. Fertil Steril 71:1060, 1999.
161. Topping J, Quenby S, Farquharson R, et al: Marked variation in antiphospholipid antibodies during pregnancy: relationships to pregnancy outcome. Hum Reprod 14:224, 1999.
162. Simpson JL, Carson SA, Chesney C, et al: Lack of association between antiphospholipid antibodies and first-trimester spontaneous abortion: prospective study of pregnancies detected within 21 days of conception. Fertil Steril 69:814, 1998.
163. Royal College of Obstetricians and Gynecologists Guidelines: The investigation and treatment of couples with recurrent miscarriages. London, Royal College of Obstetricians and Gynecologists, 17, 2003.
164. ACOG Practice Bulletin 24: Management of recurrent early pregnancy loss. Washington, DC, American College of Obstetricians and Gynecologists, 2001.
165. ASM Practice Committee: Intravenous immunoglobulin (IVIG) and recurrent spontaneous pregnancy loss. Fertil Steril 86:[suppl 4] 226, 2006.
166. Rai R, Regan L, Hadley E, et al: Second-trimester pregnancy loss is associated with activated C resistance. Br J Haematol 92:489, 1996.
167. Rai R, Chilcott IT, Backos M, et al: Prevalence of factor V Leiden genotype amongst 785 consecutive women with recurrent miscarriage. Hum Reprod 14:O-130, 1999.
168. Rai R, Backos M, Chilcott IT: Prospective outcome of untreated pregnancies amongst women with the factor V Leiden genotype and recurrent miscarriages. Hum Reprod 14:O-037, 1999.
169. Rai R, Chilcott IT, Tuddenham EG, et al: Computerized thromboelastographic parameters amongst women with recurrent miscarriage-evidence for a pro-thrombotic state. Hum Reprod 14: O-132, 1999.
170. Rai R, Shlebak A, Cohen H, et al: Factor V Leiden and acquired activated protein C resistance among 1000 women with recurrent miscarriage. Hum Reprod 16:961, 2001.
171. Souza SS, Ferriani RA, Pontes AG, et al: Factor V leiden and factor II G20210A mutations in patients with recurrent abortion. Hum Reprod 14:2448, 1999.
172. Preston FE, Rosendaal FR, Walker ID, et al: Increased fetal loss in women with heritable thrombophilia. Lancet 348:913, 1996.
173. Dizon-Townson DS, Kinney S, Branch DW, et al: The factor V Leiden mutation is not a common cause of recurrent miscarriage. J Reprod Immunol 34:217, 1997.
174. Pauer HU, Neesen J, Hinney B: Factor V Leiden and its relevance in patients with recurrent abortions. Am J Obstet Gynecol 178:629, 1998.
175. Balasch J, Reverter JC, Fabregues F, et al: First-trimester repeated abortion is not associated with activated protein C resistance. Hum Reprod 12:1094, 1997.
176. Kutteh WH, Park VM, Deitcher SR: Hypercoagulable state mutation analysis in white patients with early first-trimester recurrent pregnancy loss. Fertil Steril 71:1048, 1999.
177. Coumans AB, Huijgens PC, Jakobs C, et al: Haemostatic and metabolic abnormalities in women with unexplained recurrent abortion. Hum Reprod 14:211, 1999.
178. Grandone E, Margaglione M, Colaizzo D, et al: Factor V Leiden is associated with repeated and recurrent unexplained fetal losses. Thromb Haemost 77:822, 1997.
179. Ridker PM, Miletich JP, Buring JE, et al: Factor V Leiden mutation as a risk factor for recurrent pregnancy loss. Ann Intern Med 128:1000, 1998.
180. Mowbray JF, Gibbings C, Liddell H, et al: Controlled trial of treatment of recurrent spontaneous abortion by immunisation with paternal cells. Lancet 1:941, 1985.
181. Recurrent Miscarriage Immunotherapy Trials Group: World-wide collaborative observational study and meta-analysis on allogenic leukocyte immunotherapy for recurrent spontaneous abortion. Am J Reprod Immunol 32:55, 1985.
182. Fraser EJ, Grimes DA, Schulz KF: Immunization as therapy for recurrent spontaneous abortion: a review and meta-analysis. Obstet Gynecol 82:854, 1993.
183. Ober C, Karrison T, Odem RR, et al: Mononuclear-cell immunisation in prevention of recurrent miscarriages: a randomised trial. Lancet 354:365, 1999.
184. CBER Letter. Lymphocyte Immune Therapy (LIT) [http: and *www.fda.gov/cber/ltr/lit013002.htm]*. Microbiology relevant to recurrent miscarriage. Clin Obstet Gynaecol 37:722, 1994.
185. Aldrich CL, Stephenson MD, Karrison T, et al: HLA-G genotypes and pregnancy outcome in couples with unexplained recurrent miscarriage. Mol Hum Reprod 7:1167, 2001.
186. Ober C, Aldrich CL, Chervoneva I, et al: Variation in the HLA-G promoter region influences miscarriage rates. Am J Hum Genet 72:1425, 2003.
187. Kline J, Shrout P, Stein Z, et al: Drinking during pregnancy and spontaneous abortion. Lancet 2:176, 1980.
188. Ness RB, Grisso JA, Hirschinger N, et al: Cocaine and tobacco use and the risk of spontaneous abortion. N Engl J Med 340:333, 1999.
189. de la Chica RA, Ribas I, Giraldo J, et al: Chromosomal instability in amniocytes from fetuses of mothers who smoke. JAMA 293:1212, 2005.
190. Armstrong BG, McDonald AD, Sloan M: Cigarette, alcohol, and coffee consumption and spontaneous abortion. Am J Public Health 82:85, 1992.
191. Klebanoff MA, Levine RJ, DerSimonian R, et al: Maternal serum paraxanthine, a caffeine metabolite, and the risk of spontaneous abortion. N Engl J Med 341:1639, 1999.
192. Harlap S, Shiono PH: Alcohol, smoking, and incidence of spontaneous abortions in the first and second trimester. Lancet 2:173, 1980.
193. Halmesmaki E, Valimaki M, Roine R, et al: Maternal and paternal alcohol consumption and miscarriage. Br J Obstet Gynaecol 96:188, 1989.
194. Parazzini F, Bocciolone L, La Vecchia C, et al: Maternal and paternal moderate daily alcohol consumption and unexplained miscarriages. Br J Obstet Gynaecol 97:618, 1990.

195. Savitz DA, Sonnenfeld NL, Olshan AF: Review of epidemiologic studies of paternal occupational exposure and spontaneous abortion. Am J Ind Med 25:361, 1994.
196. Nelson DB, Grisso JA, Joffe MM, et al: Violence does not influence early pregnancy loss. Fertil Steril 80:1205, 2003.
197. Stray-Pedersen B, Stray-Pedersen S: Recurrent abortion: the role of psychotherapy. *In* Beard RW, Sharp F (eds): Early Pregnancy Loss: Mechanism and Treatment. London, Royal College of Obstetricians and Gynecologists, 1988, p 433.
198. Clifford K, Rai R, Regan L: Future pregnancy outcome in unexplained recurrent first trimester miscarriage. Hum Reprod 12:387, 1997.
199. Hertig AT, Rock J: A series of potentially abortive ova recovered from fertile women prior to the first missed menstrual period. Am J Obstet Gynecol 58:968, 1949.
200. Gropp A: Chromosomal animal model of human disease. Fetal trisomy and development failure. *In* Berry L, Poswillo DE (eds), Teratology, Berlin, Springer-Verlag, 1975, p 17.

Cervical Incompetence

JACK LUDMIR AND JOHN OWEN

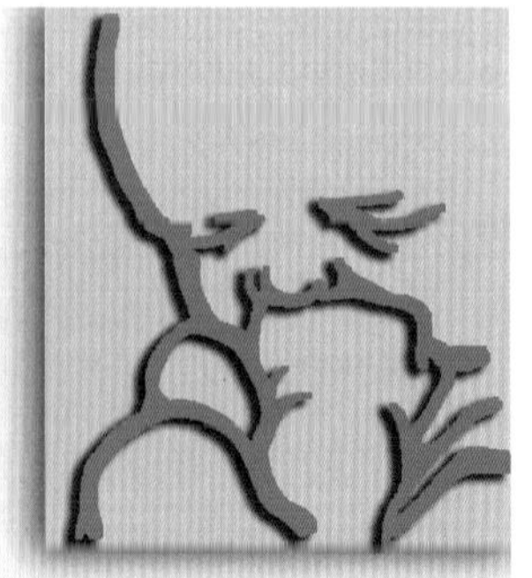

CHAPTER 25

KEY ABBREVIATIONS

Confidence interval	CI
Diethylstilbestrol	DES
Lactate dehydrogenase	LDH
Loop electrosurgical excision procedure	LEEP
Maternal-Fetal Medicine	MFM
National Institutes of Child Health and Human Development	NICHD

Since the initial description in 1658 of the cervix being "so slack that it cannot keep in the seed" by Cole and Culpepper,[1] few subjects in obstetrics have generated as much controversy as the term "cervical incompetence," or as more recently referred "cervical insufficiency." The competent or "sufficient" human uterine cervix is a complex organ that undergoes extensive changes throughout gestation and parturition. It is a key structure responsible for keeping the fetus inside the uterus until the end of gestation, and for undergoing significant changes that allows the delivery of the baby during labor. The cervix is primarily fibrous connective tissue composed of an extracellular matrix consisting of collagen types I and II, elastin and proteoglycans, and a cellular portion consisting of smooth muscle and blood vessels. A complex remodeling process of the cervix occurs during gestation involving timed biochemical cascades, interactions between the extracellular and cellular compartments, and cervical stromal infiltration by inflammatory cells.[2] Any disarray in this timed interactions could result in early cervical change, cervical insufficiency, and preterm delivery.

The incidence of cervical insufficiency in the general obstetric population is reported to vary between approximately 1 : 100 and 1 : 2000.[3–5] Wide variation is likely due to real biologic differences among study populations, the criteria used to establish the diagnosis, and reporting bias between general practitioners and referral centers.

THE DIAGNOSIS OF CERVICAL INCOMPETENCE

Cervical insufficiency is primarily a clinical diagnosis, characterized by recurrent painless dilation and spontaneous midtrimester birth, usually of a living fetus. The diagnosis is usually retrospective and made only after poor obstetric outcomes have occurred (or rarely, are in evolution). Because there are few proven objective criteria, and lack of a specific histologic diagnosis other than a rare, gross cervical malformation, a careful history and review of the past obstetric records are crucial to making an accurate diagnosis. Unfortunately, in many instances, the records are incomplete or unavailable, and many women cannot provide a reliable history. Even with excellent records and a complete history, clinicians might disagree on the diagnosis in all but the most classic cases. Confounding factors in the history, medical records, or current physical assessment might be used to either support or refute the diagnosis, based on their perceived importance. The physician managing a patient who experiences a spontaneous midtrimester birth is in the optimal position to assess whether the typical clinical criteria for cervical incompetence were present. Possibly a more specific diagnosis of cervical incompetence can be made by witnessing "incompetence in evolution," a possible indication for emergent cerclage that will be covered later. Because cervical incompetence is generally a retrospective diagnosis and depends on a history of untoward outcomes, clinicians have sought criteria that might lead

Table 25-1. Diagnostic Criteria for Cervical Incompetence

Historical Factors:
- History of painless cervical dilatation with preterm (midtrimester) delivery

Index Gestation:
- Painless cervical shortening and dilatation detected by serial digital evaluations.
- Short cervix detected by sonography in women with a clinical history.

to a prospective and more objective diagnosis. In women considered to be "at risk" for cervical incompetence, based on an atypical history or because of other identified "risk factors," serial examinations may be performed to detect progressive shortening and dilation, leading to a presumptive diagnosis of incompetence, which may be amenable to therapeutic intervention (Table 25-1).

THE SPONTANEOUS PRETERM BIRTH SYNDROME

Because spontaneous preterm birth is not a discrete, well-characterized disease process, it is best characterized as a *syndrome* comprising several anatomic and related functional components.[6] These include the uterus and its myometrial contractile function (e.g., preterm labor), decidual activation and loss of chorioamnionic integrity (e.g., preterm rupture of membranes), and finally, diminished cervical competence, either from a primary anatomic defect or from early pathologic cervical ripening (e.g., cervical incompetence). In a particular pregnancy, a single anatomic feature may appear to predominate, even though it is more likely that most cases of spontaneous preterm birth result from the interaction of multiple stimuli and pathways which culminate in the overt clinical syndrome. Nevertheless, the relative importance of these components varies not only among different women but also in successive pregnancies for a particular patient.

Because the underlying processes (i.e., infection, inflammation, and so on) and their interactions with the anatomic components of the syndrome remain poorly characterized, the specific series of events leading to spontaneous preterm birth cannot be accurately determined, either during pregnancy, when the syndrome is recognized and managed, or by a careful retrospective analysis of the past obstetric events. Thus, finding effective preventive management strategies has been generally unsuccessful and only empirically based.

CERVICAL COMPETENCE AS A BIOLOGIC CONTINUUM

As early as 1962 Danforth and Buckingham[7] suggested that cervical incompetency was not an all or none phenomenon. Rather, it comprised degrees of incompetency, and combinations of factors could cause "cervical failure." This concept never gained wide acceptance in spite of the obvious heterogeneity observed in clinical practice. Cervical incompetence was generally viewed as dichotomous, possibly because available treatment strategies were similarly devised. These classic investigations demonstrated that the normal cervix is comprised predominantly of connective tissue, unlike the uterine corpus. This fibrous band is the chief mechanical barrier against the loss of the enlarging products of conception. The cervix and mucous glands also play an important immunologic role in preventing organisms from ascending into the normally sterile intrauterine environment.

In a subsequent report, these investigators analyzed cervical biopsies taken from postpartum women and compared them with hysterectomy specimens from nonpregnant patients.[8] Pregnancy was associated with increased water content, a marked decline in collagen and glycoprotein, and increased glycosaminoglycans. The cellular and biochemical changes suggested that cervical dilation in pregnancy is a dynamic process, and this might explain why a woman could have a pregnancy outcome consistent with cervical incompetence in one pregnancy but, then without treatment, have a subsequent term birth. Presumably, the factors inciting the pathologic cervical changes might vary among pregnancies. Women with a more muscular cervix might have an unusual susceptibility or lower threshold for the effects of the factors that precipitated the clinical syndrome of preterm birth.

These earlier observations were enlarged by Leppert and colleagues,[9] who reported an absence of elastic fibers in the cervix of women with clinically well-characterized cervical incompetence on the basis of their reproductive history. Conversely, cervical biopsy specimens from women with normal pregnancies showed normal amounts and orientation of these elastic fibers. Rechberger and colleagues[10] also compared cervical biopsy specimens among nonpregnant controls, women in the midtrimester with clinically defined cervical incompetence and normal postpartum gravidas. Compared with normal postpartum patients, they found increased collagen extractability and collagenolytic activity in women with cervical incompetence, suggesting a high collagen turnover characterized by higher proportions of newly synthesized collagen with lower mechanical strength. It is unknown whether these microstructural and biochemical phenomena were congenital, acquired from previous trauma, or the result of other pregnancy-associated pathology. Collectively, these biochemical and ultrastructural findings support the variable, and often unpredictable, clinical course of women with a history of cervical incompetence.[11]

Although the traditional paradigm has depicted the cervix as either competent or incompetent, recent evidence, including clinical data[12–15] and interpretative reviews[16–18] suggest that, as with most other biologic processes, cervical competence is rarely an all or none phenomenon and more likely functions along a continuum of reproductive performance. Although some women have tangible anatomic evidence of poor cervical integrity, most women with a clinical diagnosis of cervical incompetence have ostensibly normal cervical anatomy. In a proposed model of cervical competence as a continuum, a poor obstetric history results from a process of premature cervical ripening, induced by a myriad of underlying factors, including infection, inflammation, local or systemic hormonal effects, or even genetic predisposition. If and when cervical integrity is compromised, other processes may be stimulated, appearing clinically as other components of the spontaneous preterm birth syndrome (i.e., premature membrane rupture, or preterm labor). A decision as to whether diminished cervical competence arises through primary endogenous mechanical deficiencies or exogenous factors, would define the optimal therapy. Thus, a more rational concept of cervical incompetence is to view the cervix as an interdependent participant in the multifactorial model of the spontaneous preterm birth syndrome.

TESTS FOR CERVICAL INCOMPETENCE

Because the diagnosis of cervical incompetence has been determined primarily from past reproductive performance and physical examination findings, the obvious limitations associated with the clinical diagnosis have prompted the search for sensitive and specific tests that could be applied in a prospective manner to women deemed at risk for cervical incompetence, thus obviating the need for recurrent pregnancy loss. Such a test might provide a timely diagnosis and the potential for optimal therapeutic intervention.

Most of the earlier reported tests for cervical incompetence were based on the functional anatomy of the interval os in the nonpregnant state and are of historical interest. Attempts at objective assessments include passage of a #8 Hegar dilator into the nonpregnant cervical canal without resistance[19] and traction forces required to dislodge a Foley catheter whose balloon was placed above the internal os and filled with 2 to 3 mm of water.[20] Subjectively effortless passage of the dilator or removal of the Foley balloon with less than 600 g of force would confirm an objective diagnosis.

In 1988 Kiwi and colleagues[21] estimated the elastic properties of the nonpregnant cervix in two cohorts of women: 247 women with a poor obstetric history and 42 controls. Although women in the poor obstetric history group had significantly lower elastance values than the controls, there was significant overlap between the two groups. They reported no subsequent pregnancy outcomes, proposed no clinically useful cutoff for their evaluation, and could only suggest that such objective evaluation might ultimately prove to be clinically useful to accurately select patients for cerclage.

In 1993, Zlatnick and Burmeister[22] reported their experience with a cervical compliance score derived from the results of three other tests: hysterosalpingography, passage of a #8 Hegar dilator, and intrauterine balloon traction performed in 138 nonpregnant women. Their histories included prior delivery less than 34 weeks following clinically diagnosed preterm labor or preterm membrane rupture, with or without antecedent bleeding. A small portion of their cohort had a questionable history of cervical incompetence. Scores could range from 0 to 5, and women with low scores of 2 or less were more likely to have been delivered at 27 to 34 weeks as compared with women with higher scores, who were more likely to have been delivered in the midtrimester at 14 to 26 weeks ($P < .01$). In subsequent pregnancies, cerclage was recommended in all women with a high score of greater than 2, and most underwent surgery. Surprisingly, in spite of surgical intervention, more women with high scores delivered at 14 to 29 weeks' gestation ($P = .07$) casting doubt on the clinical utility of this scoring system.

All such attempts at providing an objective diagnosis of cervical incompetence failed because the tests were not evaluated with regard to standard characteristics (i.e., sensitivity, specificity) against some reference standard for the diagnosis. Moreover, none of these tests could reasonably predict pregnancy-associated conditions that would lead to premature ripening and cervical dilation. Finally, because there is no universally applicable standard for the diagnosis of incompetence, and because the results of such tests were never evaluated and linked to a proved effective treatment, their clinical utility was, at best, theoretical. Since no test for cervical incompetence in the nonpregnant patient has been validated, none of these tests are in common use today. Clinical assessment of the cervix is performed in the index pregnancy when the diagnosis of cervical insufficiency is suspected.

CAN SONOGRAPHIC EVALUATION OF THE CERVIX DIAGNOSE INCOMPETENCE?

Over the past 2 decades numerous investigators have suggested that cervical incompetence can be diagnosed by midtrimester sonographic evaluation of the cervix. Various sonographic findings including cervical length, funneling at the internal os, and dynamic response to provocative maneuvers (e.g., fundal pressure) have been used to select women for treatment, generally cerclage (Fig. 25-1). In these earlier reports, the sonographic evaluations were not blinded, leading to uncontrolled interventions and difficulty determining their value. A representative sample of numerous reports linking the findings from cervical sonography to a diagnosis of cervical incompetence is depicted in Table 25-2. Note that the diagnostic criteria are disparate and, in some cases, not described in a quantitative or reproducible manner.

More recently large, blinded observational studies using reproducible methods have been published.[13,23–26] These investigators reported the relationship between midtrimester cervical sonographic findings and preterm birth. The National Institutes of Child Health and Human Development (NICHD) Maternal-Fetal Medicine (MFM) Units Network[13] completed a study of 2,915 unselected women with a singleton pregnancy who underwent a blinded cervical sonographic evaluation at 24 weeks' gestation. The relative risk of spontaneous preterm birth increased inversely proportionally to cervical length. In spite of this highly significant relationship, as a test for predicting spontaneous preterm birth of less than 35 weeks, a cervical length cutoff of less than 26 mm (the population 10th percentile) had low sensitivity (37 percent), and poor positive predictive value (18 percent).

In a subsequent study, the NICHD MFM Units Network[26] examined the utility of cervical ultrasound as

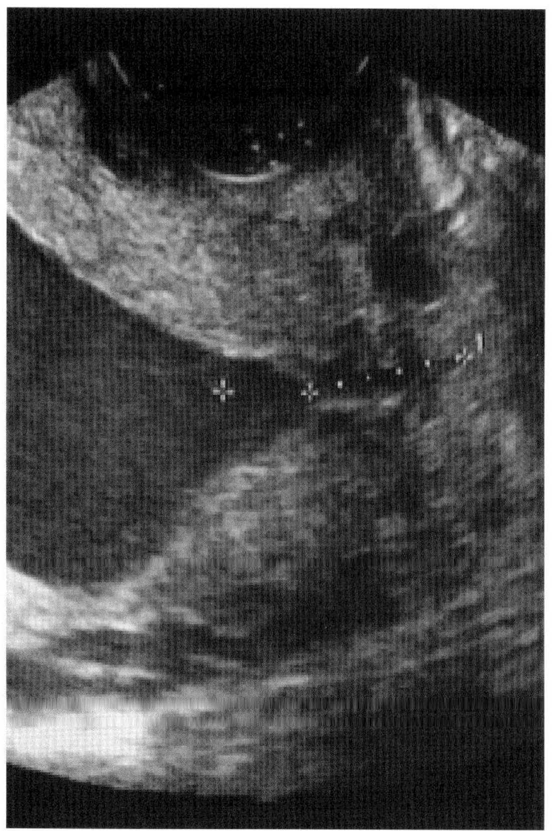

Figure 25-1. Short cervix (dotted line) by transvaginal sonogram at 22 weeks' gestation.

a predictor of spontaneous preterm birth of less than 35 weeks in high-risk women, defined as at least one prior spontaneous preterm birth of less than 32 weeks. Women believed to have cervical incompetence (based on a clinical history) were not eligible. Beginning at 16 to 18 weeks of gestation, 183 gravidas underwent serial, biweekly sonographic evaluations until the 23rd week of gestation. The study design permitted analysis of the shortest observed cervical length over time, which also included any fundal pressure-induced (or spontaneously occurring) cervical length shortening. As in the previous study,[13] there was a highly significant inverse relationship between cervical length and spontaneous preterm birth. However, in this high-risk population, at a cervical length cutoff of less than 25 mm, the sensitivity increased to 69 percent and the positive predictive value to 55 percent. A secondary analysis of the data suggested that these high-risk women with shortened cervical length may have a clinically significant *component* of diminished cervical competence, because there was a preponderance of midtrimester births of less than 27 weeks in this group.[27]

These reports[13,26] support the concept that cervical length, as a surrogate function for cervical competence, operates along a continuum of reproductive performance and provides prospective confirmation of an earlier published retrospective analysis.[12] Nevertheless, in spite of the consistent relationship between shortened cervical length and spontaneous preterm birth, the actual identification of an appropriate cervical length action cutoff and confirmation of the potential contribution of related cervical sonographic findings (e.g., funneling at the internal os), remains problematic. Clearly, cervical sonography performs poorly as a screening test in low-

Table 25-2. Published Reports of the Sonographic Diagnosis of Cervical Incompetence

AUTHOR, YEAR	POPULATION	N	GA	COMMENT	CRITERIA FOR CERVICAL INCOMPETENCE
Varma, '86 (114)	At risk	115	10–32 weeks	40 received cerclage	Not explicitly stated. Cervical canal width >8 mm implied
Michaels, '86 (115)	At risk	107	N/S	32 received cerclage for sonographic CI	Membrane prolapse >6 mm and "short cervix"
Ayers, '88 (15)	Prior MT loss	88	N/S	70 received cerclage	CL <40 mm (–2 standard deviations from the mean)
Fox, '96 (116)	At risk	19	14–28 weeks	Used sonography to avoid cerclage in women with classic history; 12 of 19 underwent cerclage	>1 cm decrease in CL and/or funneling
Guzman, '97 (117)	At risk	10	N/S	Examined natural history of fundal pressure response	CL <10 mm or cervix dilated on physical exam
Guzman, '97 (118)	At risk	89	MT	Transfundal pressure and other provocative maneuvers	Progressive cervical changes to CL <26 mm
Wong, '97 (119)	High risk	41	17–33	16 had prophylactic cerclage. Postural test evaluated as a provocative maneuver	33% decrease in CL
Guzman, '98 (120)	At risk	57	MT	Retrospective cohort study. Elective vs. ultrasound indicated	CL <20 mm with or without fundal pressure
MacDonald, '01 (121)	High risk	106	<24 wk	Serial scans	CL <10 mm with or without fundal pressure

CI, cervical incompetence; CL, cervical length; GA, gestational age; MT, midtrimester; N/S, not stated.

risk women,[12,13] but it appears to have significant clinical utility in high-risk women, defined as a prior early spontaneous preterm birth.[24–26] Whether cervical ultrasound has similar predictive values in other populations of at risk women (e.g., diethylstilbestrol [DES], prior cervical surgery, multiple induced abortions, and so on) remains speculative, because it has not been well studied. Although some investigators have included women with these risk factors in their study populations composed primarily of women with previous spontaneous preterm birth, the results could not be subcategorized because of small sample sizes.[28] However, in a recent series of 64 women with various uterine anomalies, the authors observed an overall preterm delivery rate of less than 35 weeks of 11 percent and a significant relationship between cervical length of less than 25 mm and preterm birth,[29] with summary predictive values similar to other high-risk populations.[26]

Use of cervical ultrasound in twin gestations has also been reported.[31,32] However, the test characteristics, especially sensitivity and positive predictive value (<40 percent), appear to be generally lower than for women with a prior early spontaneous preterm birth. A recent systematic review[30] summarized the predictive value of vaginal sonography for preterm birth in 46 published series of both asymptomatic and symptomatic gravidas carrying singleton or twin gestations.

RISK FACTORS FOR CERVICAL INCOMPETENCE

Based largely on the epidemiologic associations between the clinical diagnosis of cervical incompetence and antecedent historic factors, numerous "risk factors" for cervical incompetence have been recognized. These include prior cervical surgery (i.e., trachelectomy, cone biopsy), in utero DES exposure, prior induced or spontaneous first- and second-trimester abortions, uterine anomalies, multiple gestations or prior spontaneous preterm births that did not meet typical criteria for cervical incompetence. Because DES usage was effectively curtailed in the early 1970s, this congenital risk factor should soon be of only historic interest.

Cervical damage from surgery is diminishing as indications for cone biopsy and more radical surgical procedures are diminishing. More common is the patient who has undergone a loop electrosurgical excision procedure (LEEP), usually for cervical dysplasia. These procedures are plausibly a risk factor for cervical incompetence. Regrettably, it has not been feasible to simultaneously control for the epidemiologic risk factors that are associated with both preterm birth and dysplasia. In 1995, Ferenczy[33] reported 574 women who had undergone LEEP and examined the reproductive performance of 55 women who conceived after the surgery. Their goal had been to obtain a nominal 7-mm thick specimen and cited a maximum excisional depth of 1.5 cm. In this series, there were no spontaneous preterm births before 37 weeks observed. Data from a similar series of 52 women revealed an incidence of spontaneous preterm birth of less than 10 percent and no midtrimester losses that might suggest a clinical diagnosis of cervical incompetence.[34] A more recent and much larger retrospective cohort study by Sadler et al.[35] examined 652 women treated with laser conization, laser ablation, or LEEP, and compared these with a cohort of 426 untreated patients. The overall adjusted rates of preterm birth before 37 weeks' gestation were similar; however, the group with the highest tertile of cone height (≥1.7 cm) did have more than a threefold increased risk of preterm chorioamnion rupture compared with untreated women. Even considering the effect on preterm membrane rupture, the overall effect on preterm birth was not statistically significant, as the 95-percent confidence interval (CI) included 1.0.

Published data on cone biopsy is similarly reassuring. Weber[36] reported an incidence of preterm birth of only 7 percent in 577 pregnancies of women with a prior cone biopsy. Leiman[37] concluded that the risk of preterm birth was greater only when the maximum cone height was greater than 2 cm or the volume removed was greater than 4 cc. Raio and colleagues[38] performed a matched cohort study of 64 women who had undergone prior laser conization and observed no difference in the incidence of preterm birth compared with their controls (9.4 percent versus 4.7 percent), and statistically similar gestational ages at delivery and birth weights. However, in a secondary analysis, a laser cone height greater than 10 mm was a significant independent risk factor for preterm birth. Other earlier reports have also suggested that larger cone biopsies increased the risk of preterm birth. Nevertheless, the distribution of preterm births in these populations did not confirm a disproportionate incidence of midtrimester loss consistent with cervical incompetence.

Kuoppala and Saarikoski[39] retrospectively reviewed 62 women who had undergone cone biopsy and an equal number of matched control patients. The pregnancy outcomes of 22 who underwent elective cerclage were similar to those managed without cerclage, with fetal salvage rates of 97 percent and 100 percent, respectively. On the basis of their findings and review of seven other published reports, they concluded that prophylactic cerclage was not routinely indicated. Of note, in the largest published randomized trial of cerclage[39] (summarized later), women with one or more cone biopsies or cervical amputations had an overall preterm birth rate of 35 percent. However, in this population, there was no benefit from prophylactic cerclage placement.

In summary, most women with prior LEEP or cone biopsy do not appear to have a clinically significant rate of second-trimester loss or preterm birth. However, women in whom a large cone specimen was removed or destroyed (including cervical amputations), or who have undergone multiple prior procedures, probably have an increased risk of spontaneous preterm birth. Whether prophylactic cerclage would be an effective preventive strategy in these at-risk women remains speculative. The available clinical trial data does not suggest a benefit from prophylactic cerclage, and so these women may be followed clinically for evidence of premature cervical changes. Women with a history of prior cervical surgery and spontaneous midtrimester loss, suggesting a clinical diagnosis of incompetence, should be considered for prophylactic cerclage in future pregnancies.

USE OF CERCLAGE FOR RISK FACTORS

Because of epidemiologic associations, clinicians have tried to expand the role of cerclage to include women with "risk factors." To date there have been four randomized clinical trials that included women with various risk factors for spontaneous preterm birth and whose managing physicians did not believe they required a prophylactic cerclage for a typical history of cervical incompetence. Three of these trials[40–42] were relatively small series and included women based on a scoring system[40]: twin gestation[41] and recurrent spontaneous preterm birth.[42] None of these trials showed a benefit to cerclage but generally confirmed a higher rate of hospitalizations and medical interventions in the surgical intervention groups.

The largest randomized trial of cerclage was conducted by the Royal College of Obstetricians and Gynecologists between 1981 and 1988.[43] A total of 1,292 women were enrolled in 12 countries because of uncertainty on the part of their managing physicians as to whether a prophylactic cerclage was indicated. As anticipated, these patients comprised a heterogeneous group with at least six distinct risk-factor subgroups identified on the basis of their dominant history or physical examination findings. Although women assigned to cerclage had a statistically significant lower rate of preterm birth less than 33 weeks (13 percent versus 17 percent; P = .03), the investigators estimated that approximately 25 cerclage procedures would be required to prevent one such birth. Moreover, women assigned to cerclage received more tocolytic medications and spent more time in the hospital. Puerperal fever was significantly more common in the cerclage group. Of interest is the finding in a secondary analysis that only the subgroup of women with multiple pregnancies affected, defined as at least three prior spontaneous preterm births including midtrimester losses, appeared to benefit from cerclage (15 percent versus 32 percent; P = .02). This secondary analysis confirmed the importance of assessing clinical history in considering the diagnosis and treatment of cervical incompetence.

CERCLAGE FOR CERVICAL SONOGRAPHIC INDICATIONS

Under the presumption that shortened cervical length (with or without funneling at the internal os) is diagnostic of cervical incompetence, several investigators have studied the effect of sonographically indicated cerclage on reproductive performance. Several investigators published retrospective analyses of uncontrolled use of cerclage in various "at-risk" populations with conflicting results, suggesting that cerclage was either effective[44,45] or ineffective.[46–49] In addition to the inherent biases present in these study designs and differences among study populations, small sample size, variable sonographic criteria, type of cerclage, inclusion of ancillary clinical findings, and definition of pregnancy outcome led to an inconclusive analysis.

Currently, four randomized trials of cerclage for sonographic indications have been published (Table 25-3). Althuisius and her colleagues in the Netherlands,[50,51] performed a two-tiered randomized clinical trial of high-risk patients, the majority of whom were believed to have cervical incompetence based on their obstetric history. In the first tier, eligible patients were randomly assigned to receive either prophylactic cerclage or to begin sonographic surveillance. Thirty-five of the patients assigned to the cervical ultrasound group were found to have a shortened cervical length less than 25 mm and underwent a second randomization to either cerclage or no cerclage. Both cerclage and no cerclage groups were instructed to use modified home rest. Of the 19 assigned to cerclage, there were no preterm births before 34 weeks versus a 44 percent preterm birth rate in the no cerclage-home rest group (P = .002). None of the women who maintained a cervical length of at least 25 mm experienced a preterm birth. Interestingly, the women who received cerclage for shortened cervical length had outcomes almost identical to women who received the earlier prophylactic cerclage. Rust and colleagues[52] enrolled 138 women who had various risk factors for preterm birth (including 12 percent with multiple gestations) and randomly assigned

Table 25-3. Randomized Trials of Cerclage for Sonographically Suspected Cervical Incompetence in Singleton Gestations

AUTHOR, YEAR	POPULATION	N	SELECTION CRITERIA	GA	PRIMARY OUTCOME CRITERION	CERCLAGE	NO CERCLAGE	BENEFIT
Althuisius, 2001 (51)	High-risk history consistent with CI	35	CL <25 mm	<27 weeks	Preterm birth <34 weeks	0%	44%	Yes
Rust, 2001 (52)	Unselected, but many had risk factors	113	CL <25 mm or >25% funneling	16–24 weeks	Preterm birth <34 weeks	35%	36%	No
To, 2004 (53)	Unselected, low risk	253	CL 15 mm	22–24 weeks	Preterm birth <33 weeks	22%	26%	No
Berghella, 2004 (54)	Unselected, but most had risk factors	61	CL <25 mm or >25% funneling	14–23 weeks	Preterm birth <35 weeks	45%	47%	No

CI, cervical incompetence; CL, cervical length; GA, gestational age.

them to receive a McDonald cerclage or no cerclage after their cervical length shortened to less than 25 mm or they developed funneling less than 25 percent. Preterm birth before 34 weeks was observed in 35 percent of the cerclage group versus 36 percent of the control group.

In a multinational trial comprising 12 hospitals in six countries, To and colleagues[53] screened 47,123 unselected women at 22 to 24 weeks' gestation with vaginal ultrasound to identify 470 with a shortened cervical length of 15 mm or less. Of these 470, 253 participated in a randomized trial whose primary outcome was the intergroup rates of delivery before 33 weeks' gestation. Women assigned to the cerclage group (N = 127) underwent a Shirodkar procedure. They had a similar rate of preterm birth as the control population (N = 126), 22 percent versus 26 percent; p = .44. The authors did not specifically comment on the proportion of women in the control group who were delivered in the midtrimester after a presentation consistent with clinically defined cervical incompetence; however, they observed four stillbirths attributed to birth at 23 to 24 weeks and five neonatal deaths in deliveries at 23 to 26 weeks. In the cerclage group, the respective counts were three and four.

Berghella and colleagues[54] screened women with various risk factors for spontaneous preterm birth (prior preterm birth, curettages, cone biopsy, DES exposure) with vaginal scans every 2 weeks from 14 to 23 weeks' gestation and randomly assigned 61 with a cervical length less than 25 mm or funneling less than 25 percent to a McDonald cerclage or to a no-cerclage control group. Preterm birth before 35 weeks was observed in 45 percent of the cerclage group and 47 percent of the control group.

Of the four published randomized trials, the findings of Rust and colleagues[52] and Berghella[54] seem most applicable to obstetric practice in the United States, and these reports did not support the use of cerclage for sonographic findings commonly cited as "abnormal" in women with various types of risk factors. The multinational trial by To et al. confirmed that shortened cervical length less than 15 mm identified a very high-risk group; however, approximately 1,000 women in a general obstetric population would have to be screened to find one with this risk factor. None of these demonstrated an appreciable benefit from ultrasound-indicated cerclage.

The trial by Althuisius and colleagues[50,51] focused on women whom they believed had a clinical diagnosis of cervical incompetence and who would have likely been candidates for prophylactic cerclage in the United States. Nevertheless, their study does suggest a potential role for cervical ultrasound in women with a clinical diagnosis of cervical incompetence, if the intent is to *avoid* cerclage when the cervical length is maintained at greater than 25 mm. This has also been the conclusion of other investigators.[55] In a similar report, Fejgin and colleagues[56] presented a case series of 35 women in whom cerclage had been placed in prior pregnancies for questionable indications. Collectively, these women had been managed through 58 pregnancies with cerclage. These investigators followed the cohort through an additional 52 pregnancies managed with clinical examinations and sonography up to 28 weeks' gestation without elective, prophylactic cerclage. Compared with the pregnancies managed with elective cerclage, fewer perinatal losses were observed in the group managed with serial examinations (0 percent versus 16 percent in the elective cerclage group; P = .01).

A recently published meta-analysis[57] of the four randomized trials[51–54] described earlier, analyzed patient-level data to determine if certain subgroups of women with midtrimester cervical shortening might benefit from cerclage defined as a reduction in the relative risk of preterm birth before 35 weeks. They observed a marginal benefit from cerclage in women with singleton gestations and particularly those who had experienced a prior spontaneous preterm birth (relative risk 0.61, 95-percent CI 0.4 to 0.9). Paradoxically, they demonstrated a significant *detriment* in women with multiple gestations (relative risk 2.15, 95-percent CI 1.15 to 4.01), although this has not been confirmed in other series.[48,49] Large, multicenter randomized trials in high-risk women defined as one or more prior early spontaneous preterm births, but who lack a clinical history of cervical incompetence, are needed to further define the potential utility of cervical ultrasound screening to select patients for interventions such as cerclage and are currently in progress.[58]

PATIENT SELECTION FOR CERCLAGE

Most of what is known about the management of the incompetent cervix is based on case series that reported surgical correction of the presumed underlying mechanical defect in the cervical stroma. The contemporary mainstay of treatment has been a surgical approach using one of the classic cerclage procedures, although both medical treatments and other mechanical supportive therapies have been used. Like many aspects of clinical medicine, current therapeutic standards are often based more on expert opinion and results of studies using uncontrolled interventions than the findings of randomized clinical trials.[58a] This is particularly true for cervical incompetence in which, to date, there have been no published placebo-controlled randomized trials of cerclage in women with a typical clinical history.

Branch in 1986[59] and Cousins in 1980[60] collectively tabulated over 25 case series of cerclage efficacy published between 1959 and 1981. Branch[59] estimated a pre-cerclage survival range of 10 to 32 percent versus a perinatal survival range of 75 to 83 percent in the same cohorts of women managed with Shirodkar cerclage. Similarly, case series that used McDonald cerclage reported a cohort perinatal survival range of 7 to 50 percent before and 63–89 percent after cerclage. Cousins[60] estimated a "mean" survival before Shirodkar of 22 percent versus 82 percent post therapy and 27 percent and 74 percent, respectively, for investigators who used the McDonald technique. In total, more than 2,000 patients have been reported in these historic cohort comparisons. Interpretation of these series, as noted by Cousins,[60] is limited by the fact that (1) diagnostic criteria were not consistent or always reported; (2) definitions of treatment success were inconsistent (but generally recorded as perinatal survival, as opposed to a gestational age-based end point); (3) treatment approaches were not always detailed and might involve multiple combinations of surgery, medication, bed rest, and other uncontrolled therapies; and (4) cases were not subcategorized according to etiology (i.e., anatomic defects versus a presumed functional cause). Nevertheless, based on compelling but potentially biased efficacy data, the surgical management of women with clinically defined cervical incompetence has become standard practice, and it is unlikely that a well-designed intervention trial for classic cervical incompetence will ever be performed if it includes a placebo or no-treatment group. Although interpretation of efficacy based on historic control groups is always problematic, collectively these reports demonstrate that even women with typical histories may have successful pregnancies without cerclage and that cerclage as a treatment is not universally effective. Both of these observations support the multiple etiologies and interactive pathways characteristic of the spontaneous preterm birth syndrome.

Because of its unproven efficacy in randomized clinical trials, and the attendant surgical risks, the recommendation for prophylactic cerclage should be limited to women with recurrent spontaneous preterm birth syndrome, when a careful history and physical examination suggest a dominant cervical component. Unless the physical examination confirms a significant cervical anatomic defect, consistent with disruption of its circumferential integrity, the clinician should assess the history for other components of the preterm birth syndrome: cervical incompetence remains a diagnosis of exclusion.

Women with cervical incompetence often have some premonitory symptoms such as increased pelvic pressure, vaginal discharge, and urinary frequency. These symptoms, although neither specific for cervical incompetence nor uncommon in a normal pregnancy, should not be immediately dismissed, particularly in women with risk factors for spontaneous preterm birth. Thus, the history of rapid, relatively painless labor should perhaps better characterize the diagnosis of cervical incompetence.

Although a history of preterm labor is generally considered to exclude the diagnosis of incompetence, patients may develop some clinically evident uterine activity once their cervix has spontaneously dilated (Ferguson's reflex) but generally have a rapid progress in labor.

Similarly, a history of midtrimester spontaneous membrane rupture alone can neither confirm nor refute the diagnosis of cervical incompetence, since spontaneous membrane rupture may occur after some pathologic cervical ripening and dilation has exposed the membranes to the genital tract flora. After spontaneous membrane rupture occurs, chorioamnionitis, vaginal bleeding (placental abruption), or labor may ensue, and these events may obscure the underlying etiology. However, if midtrimester membrane rupture occurs in the setting of a closed cervix on physical examination, or if it is followed by a typical course of either spontaneous or induced labor, causes other than cervical incompetence should be emphasized. Conversely, if physical examination after membrane rupture shows marked cervical softening, effacement, and dilation with no antecedent history of painful contractions, the diagnosis of cervical incompetence is supported, particularly if followed by a rapid and relatively painless labor.

A legitimate clinical question arises over the optimal management of a patient who has experienced one spontaneous midtrimester birth, and causes other than cervical incompetence have been excluded by history and physical examination. The observation of a second similar midtrimester birth increases the specificity of the diagnosis and also the likelihood that prophylactic cerclage would be an effective treatment in the next pregnancy. Clearly, if the index midtrimester birth was associated with an identifiable anatomic defect, interval repair or prophylactic cerclage should be encouraged in the next pregnancy. However, in contemporary obstetric practice, such anatomic defects are increasingly uncommon. Although controlled clinical data are lacking, it seems reasonable to follow a patient with this history, using serial clinical evaluations in the second trimester instead of empirically recommending cerclage. Currently, the use of cervical ultrasound to select patients for cerclage is considered investigational,[58] although in selected cases, with worrisome symptoms or pelvic findings, it may be useful.[45]

INCOMPETENCE IN EVOLUTION

Although the efficacy of cerclage for the treatment of a clinically defined history of cervical incompetence remains unproven in controlled studies, women who present with incompetence in evolution, generally defined as a midtrimester cervical dilation of at least 2 cm and no other predisposing cause (labor, infection, bleeding, ruptured membranes), are often considered for an emergent cerclage. Similar to case series proposing the presumed benefit of prophylactic cerclage, reports describing the outcome of women who present with cervical incompetence in evolution generally have not always included a contemporary control group managed with bed rest or other therapy.

Aarts and colleagues[61] reviewed eight series published between 1980 and 1992 comprising 249 patients who received an emergent midtrimester cerclage and estimated a mean neonatal survival rate of 64 percent (reported range 22 to 100 percent). Novy and colleagues[45] published 35 cases of incompetence in evolution (cervical dilation 2 to 5 cm); the two cohorts included 19 women who received emergent cerclage, and 16 who were managed with bed rest. Neonatal survival was 80 percent in the cerclage cohort versus 75 percent in the bed rest group.

In a prospective, although uncontrolled evaluation of cerclage versus bed rest (cerclage was utilized at the discretion of the attending physician), Olatunbosun and colleagues[62] studied women presenting with more advanced cervical dilation greater than 4 cm. The cerclage group comprised 22 women versus 15 in the bed-rest group. Although neonatal survival was not significantly different (17/22 with cerclage versus 9/15 with bed rest, $p = .3$) gestational age at birth was a mean 4 weeks older in the cerclage group (33 versus 29 weeks, $p = .001$). Rates of chorioamnionitis were similar between the two groups.

Although these reports are not of sufficient scientific quality on which to base firm management recommendations, collectively they demonstrate several important concepts. The earlier the gestational age at presentation and the more advanced the cervical dilation, the greater the risk of poor neonatal outcome. The finding of membrane prolapse into the vagina is also a significant risk factor for poor outcome.[63]

Recently, Althuisius and colleagues[64] published a randomized clinical trial of emergency cerclage plus bed rest versus bed rest alone in 23 women who presented with cervical dilation and membranes prolapsing to or beyond the external os before 27 weeks' gestation. Both singleton and twin gestations were eligible; however, no information on the amount of cervical dilation was reported, and so it is not known whether the groups were comparable in this important aspect. They observed a longer mean interval from presentation to delivery (54 days versus 20 days; $p = .046$) in the cerclage group. Neonatal survival was 9/16 with cerclage and 4/14 in the bed rest group. Although the survival differences were not statistically significant, there was significantly lower neonatal composite morbidity (which included death) in the cerclage and bed rest group (10/16 versus 14/14 in the bed rest alone group; $p = .02$).

Other reports show that women who present with cervical incompetence in evolution have an appreciable (nominal 50 percent) incidence of bacterial colonization of their amniotic fluid or other markers of subclinical chorioamnionitis[65–67] or proteomic markers of inflammation or bleeding.[68] Women with abnormal amniotic fluid markers have a much shorter presentation-to-delivery interval, regardless of whether they receive a cerclage or are managed expectantly with bed rest.

Mays and colleagues[66] performed amniocentesis in 18 women who presented with this syndrome and analyzed the amniotic fluid for glucose, lactate dehydrogenase (LDH), Gram's stain, and culture; abnormal results suggested subclinical infection. Of 11 women who underwent cerclage with no evidence of subclinical infection, the neonatal survival was 100 percent, and the mean latent phase duration from presentation to delivery was 93 days. Of the 7 women with abnormal biochemistries in whom cerclage was withheld, no neonatal survivors were observed, and the mean latent phase was 4 days. Recognizing that at least a portion of the 7 women who declined amniocentesis, but who received emergent cerclage, also had subclinical infection, it was predictable that the mean latent phase in this cohort was intermediate (17 days) as compared with the groups with amniotic fluid analyses. These investigators suggested that amniocentesis could aid in selecting candidates for emergent therapeutic cerclage.

In summary, the optimal management of women who present with cervical incompetence in evolution remains indefinite. Although emergent cerclage may benefit some, patient selection remains largely empiric. Although not standard care, the evaluation of amniotic fluid makers of infection and inflammation appears to have important prognostic value, although it is still unclear whether and to what extent the results should direct patient management.

CERCLAGE TECHNIQUE

Prophylactic Cerclage

In 1950, Lash and Lash described repair of the cervix in the nonpregnant state involving partial excision of the cervix to remove the area of presumed weakness.[69] Unfortunately, this technique had a high incidence of subsequent infertility. In 1955, Shirodkar reported successful management of cervical incompetence with the use of a submucosal band.[70] Initially, he used catgut as suture material, and later he used Mersilene placed at the level of the internal cervical os. The procedure required anterior displacement of the bladder in an attempt to place the suture as high as possible at the level of cervical internal os. This type of procedure resulted in a greater number of patients being delivered by cesarean delivery because of the difficulty in removing the suture buried under the cervical surface and may require leaving the suture in place postpartum. Several years later, McDonald described a suture technique in the form of a purse string, not requiring cervical dissection, which was easily placed during pregnancy.[71] This technique involves taking four or five bites as high as possible in the cervix, trying to avoid injury to the bladder or the rectum, with placement of a knot anteriorly to facilitate removal (Fig. 25-2). Several types of suture material have been used.[72] We have been successful in using a Mersilene tape. However, the use of thinner suture material, such as Prolene or other synthetic nonabsorbable sutures like Ethibond, is advocated by others, with the argument that the width of the Mersilene tape places the patient at greater risk for infection.[72,73] Currently, there is no evidence that placing two sutures results in better outcomes than placing one.[74–76] Preoperative patient preparations, including the use of prophylactic antibiotics or tocolytics, have not been proven to be of benefit. We perform a culture for group B streptococcus and give preoperative penicillin to the patient with a positive culture. Prophylactic cerclage placement is performed after the first trimester, to avoid the risk of spontaneous loss most likely attributable to chromosomal abnormalities.[74,75] The choice of anesthesia for cerclage varies.[77] Chen et al.[78] did not show a difference in outcome between general versus regional anesthesia. In our experience, a short-acting regional anesthetic is sufficient. We advise patients to remain on bed rest for the first 48 hours after cerclage and to avoid intercourse until their follow-up postoperative visit. Decisions regarding physical activity and intercourse are individualized, and based on the status of the cervix as determined by outpatient digital evaluation or sonographic findings (Fig. 25-3).[79] The suture is usually removed electively at 37 weeks. However, recent data suggests that removing the cerclage at the time of labor does not result in greater morbidity for the mother.[80]

In patients with a hypoplastic cervix, such as those exposed to DES in utero, history of a large cervical conization, or a prior history of failed vaginal cerclage, an abdominal cerclage has been recommended.[81] This procedure is usually done between 11 and 13 weeks, and requires a laparotomy. A bladder flap is created, and a Mersilene tape is placed at the level of the junction

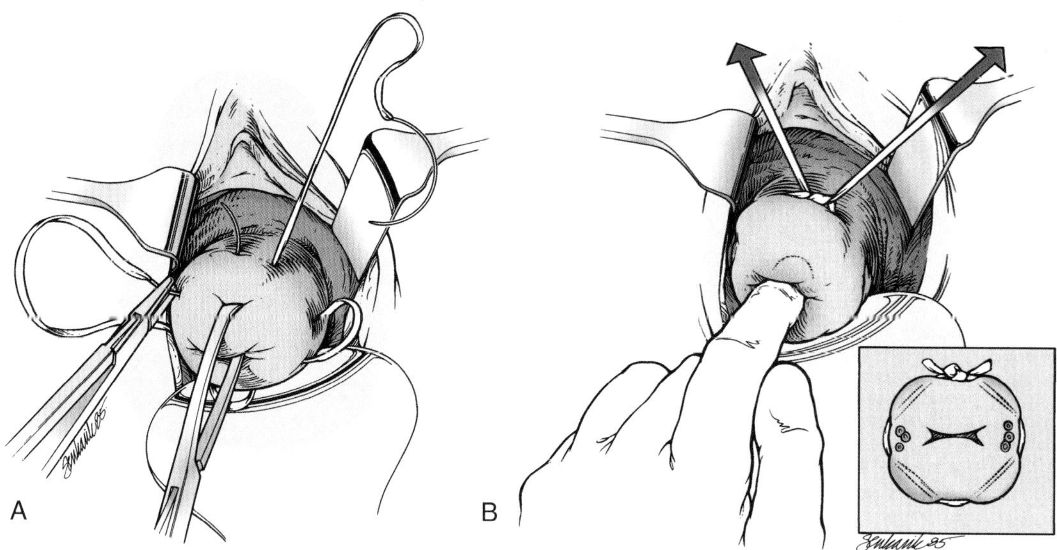

Figure 25-2. Placement of sutures for McDonald cerclage. *A,* We use a double-headed Mersilene band with four bites in the cervix, avoiding the vessels. *B,* The suture is placed high up in the cervix, close to the cervicovaginal junction, approximately at the level of the internal os.

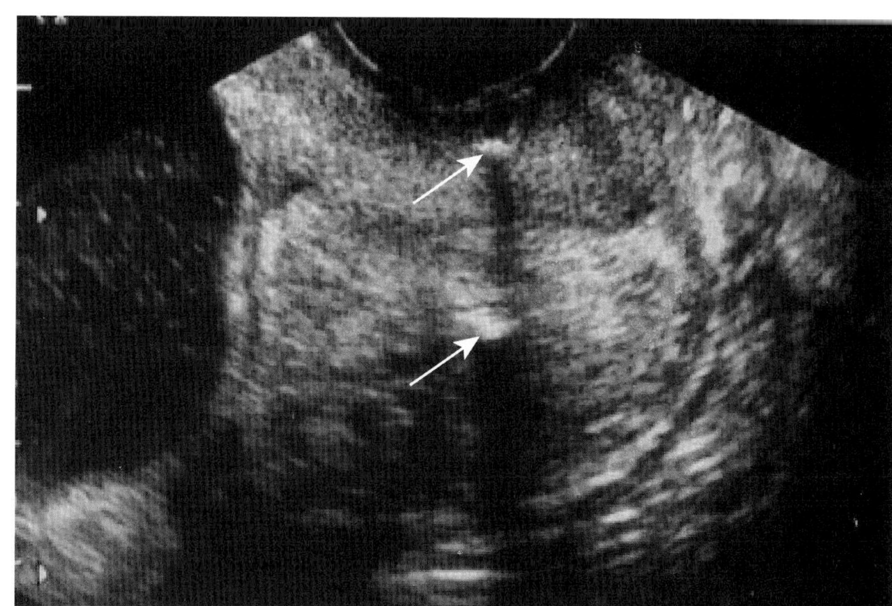

Figure 25-3. Transvaginal sonogram of the cervix after cerclage placement. The internal os is closed, and there is no funneling. Echogenic spots in the cervix correspond to cerclage (arrows).

between the lower uterine segment and the cervix, lateral to the uterus and medial to the uterine vessels (Fig. 25-4). Greater morbidity including injury to the uterine vessels requires expertise with this procedure. In our experience with more than 60 cases, we have found it helpful to have an assistant provide fundal traction, whereas the surgeon grasps the uterine vessels and retracts them laterally, exposing an avascular space between the artery and the cervix. A right angle clamp is passed anteriorly to posterior through this avascular space, tenting and incising the posterior leaf of the broad ligament and grasping a Mersilene tape that is brought back through the space. The same procedure is repeated on the opposite side, and the tape is tied anteriorly (Figs. 25-5 to 25-8). Novy et al.[82] have reported extensive experience with this procedure, with low morbidity and favorable outcome.

Cesarean delivery is necessary, and the suture is left in place if future fertility is desired. In cases of pregnancy complications requiring midtrimester delivery, we have either performed a posterior colpotomy, cutting the tape and allowing for vaginal delivery, or performed laparotomy and hysterotomy, leaving the suture intact. In most of the reported series of abdominal cerclage including ours, this surgical procedure was performed during gestation.[82] However, recently Groom and colleagues[83] described this procedure as an interval cerclage in the nonpregnant state with subsequent good pregnancy outcome. Advantages of an interval procedure include avoidance of laparotomy in pregnancy and less bleeding morbidity. Disadvantages include inability to become pregnant and the difficulties of pregnancy management if the gestation results in a first trimester miscarriage. Currently, there are no studies

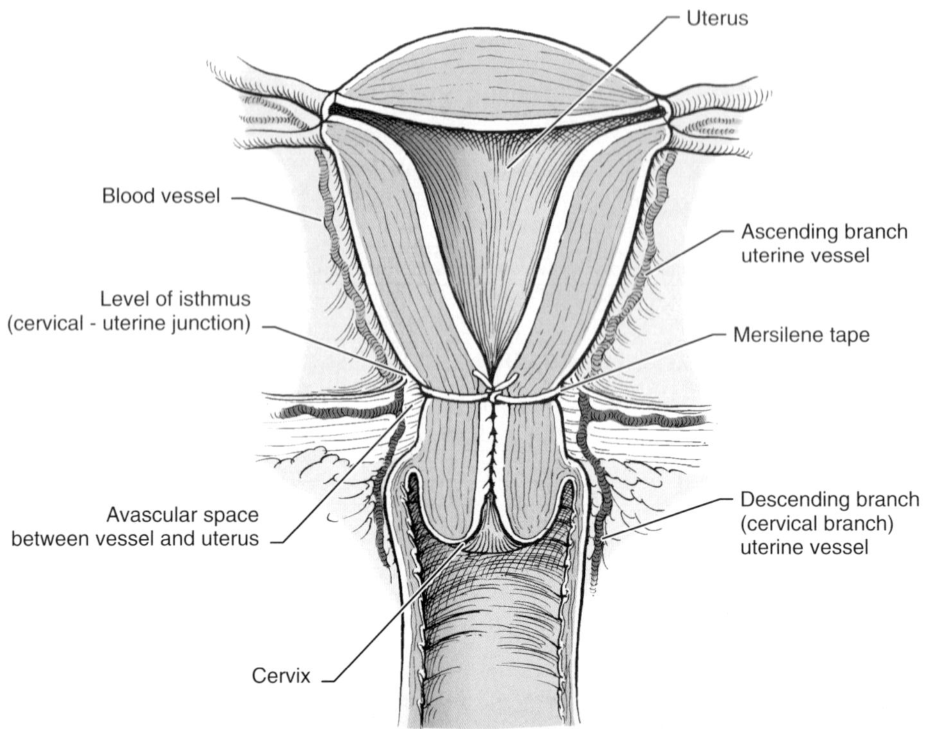

Figure 25-4. Abdominal cerclage. Surgical placement of circumferential mersilene tape around uterine isthmus and median to uterine vessels. Knot is tied anteriorly.

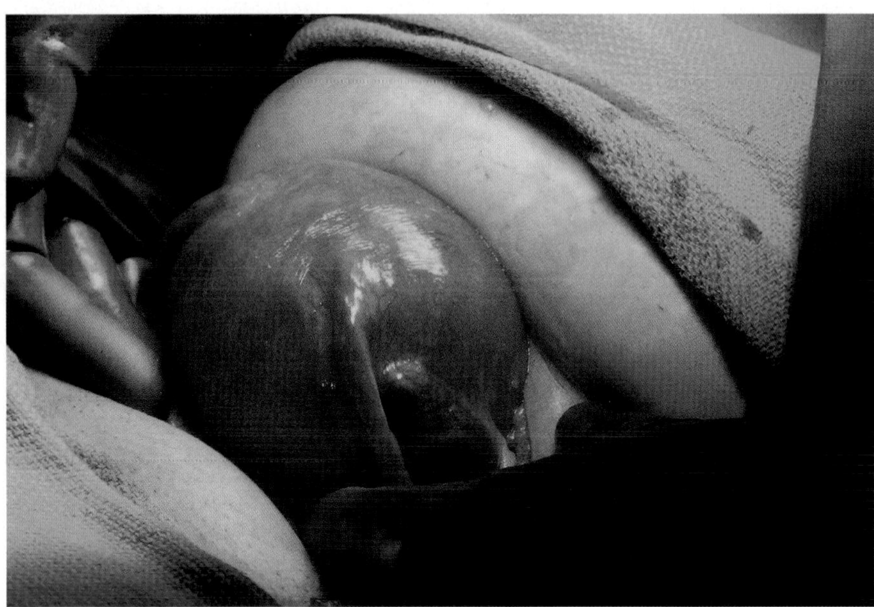

Figure 25-5. Abdominal cerclage at 12 weeks' gestation. Uterus is exteriorized.

comparing interval versus abdominal cerclage during gestation that enable us to make specific recommendations about timing of the procedure.

To avoid an abdominal procedure in selected patients, we have described the placement of a transvaginal cerclage in cases of a hypoplastic cervix, or when the cervix is flush against the vaginal wall.[84] Under ultrasound guidance, the supravaginal portion of the cervix is dissected away from the bladder and a suture is placed either in a purse-string fashion, or in cross fashion from 12 to 6 o'clock and 3 to 9 o'clock (Fig. 25-9). We have performed this procedure in 22 patients, avoiding an abdominal procedure, with successful pregnancy outcome. Fifty percent of patients had a cesarean delivery, and the rest delivered vaginally after the suture was cut through a small posterior colpotomy incision. In the last few years, a laparoscopic abdominal approach to the cervix has been described using the same principles as an abdominal cerclage.[85,86] The procedure has been described primarily in the nonpregnant state with subsequent good pregnancy outcome. Recently, Cho and colleagues[87] performed laparoscopic abdominal cerclage during pregnancy in 20

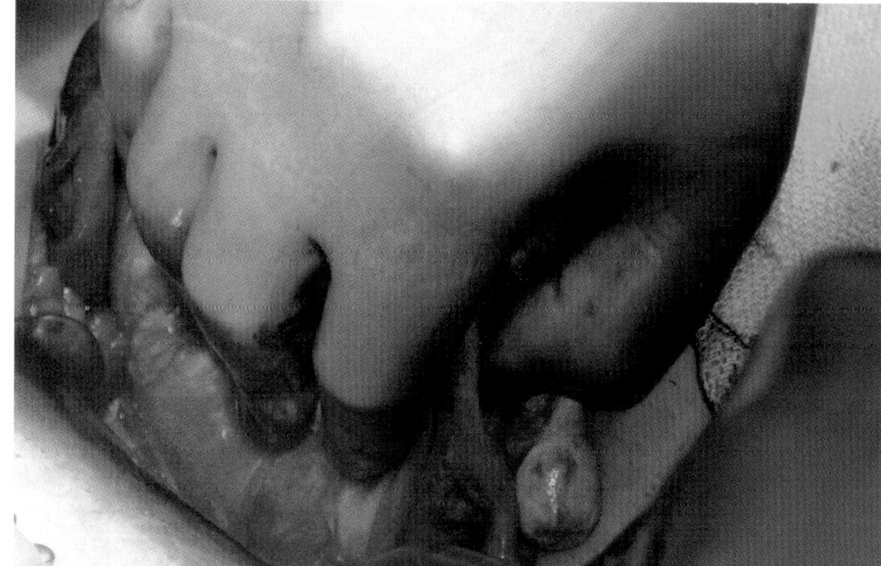

Figure 25-6. Abdominal cerclage. Bladder flap has been created and surgeon identifies and palpates uterine vessel.

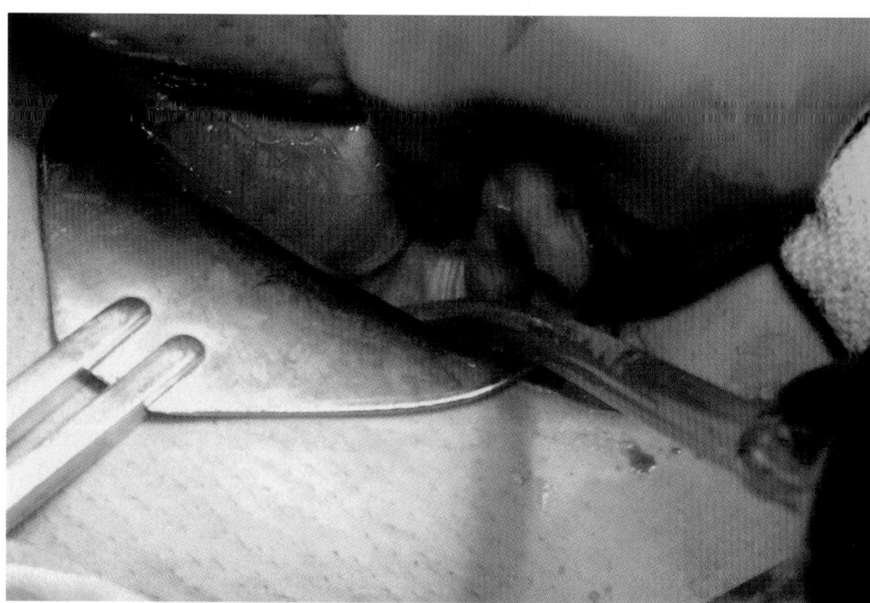

Figure 25-7. Abdominal cerclage. Surgeon retracts uterine vessel laterally to create an avascular space between uterus and vessel, before passing right angle clamp with Mersilene tape through this space.

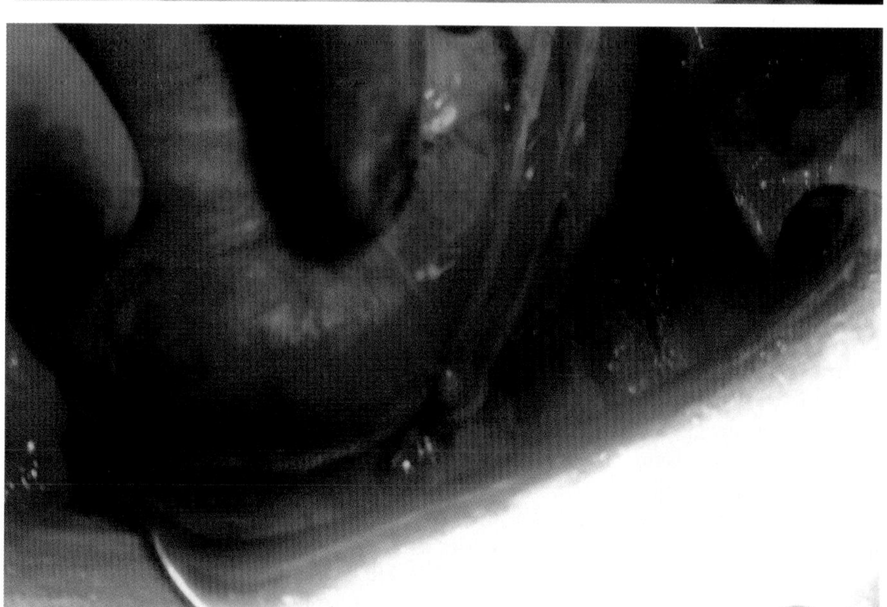

Figure 25-8. Abdominal cerclage. Mersilene tape has been placed circumferencially around uterine isthmus and tied anteriorly. Notice ballooning of the lower uterine segment above suture.

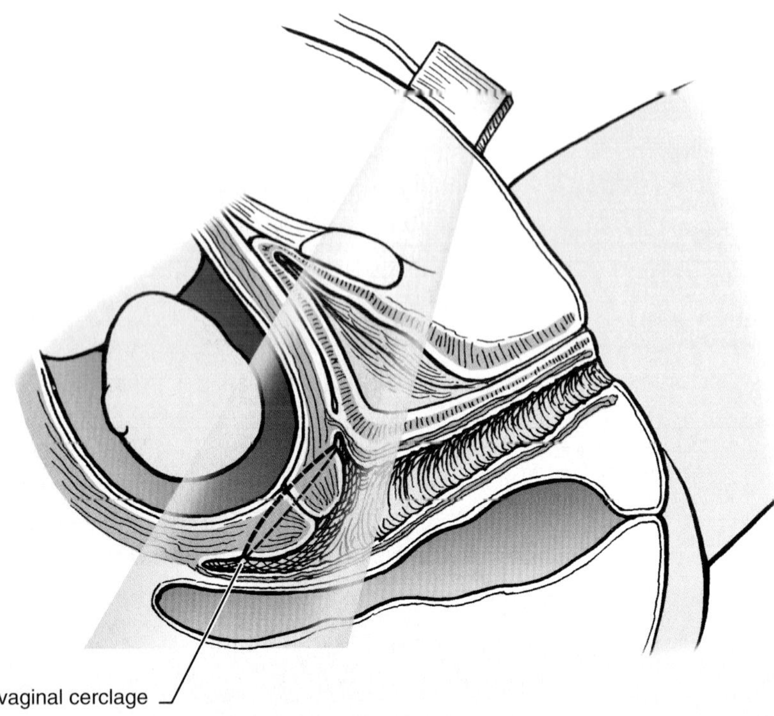

Figure 25-9. Transvaginal cerclage under ultrasound guidance. (Modified from Ludmir J, Jackson GM, Samuels P: Transvaginal cerclage under ultrasound guidance in cases of severe cervical hypoplasia. Obstet Gynecol 75:1067, 1991.)

patients with minimal morbidity, and successful outcome in 19 of them. There is a need for randomized trials evaluating this new technique in the nonpregnant and pregnant state, compared with a vaginal approach to determine the best approach to patients with a history of failed cerclage.

Therapeutic and Emergent Cerclage

Patients demonstrating cervical change either by digital evaluation or transvaginal sonography may benefit from a therapeutic cerclage.[88–91] However, the gestational age limit for cerclage placement is ill defined. Although some clinicians offer this therapeutic modality up to 28 weeks,[92] we do not advocate the use of therapeutic cerclage beyond 24 weeks' gestation, because of fetal viability concerns and the potential to cause a preterm delivery while placing the cerclage. Some of these patients have been managed successfully with strict bed rest.[93] If the decision is made to place a cerclage, we treat preoperatively with antibiotics and nonsteroidal anti-inflammatory agents, such as indomethacin. The patient is placed on strict bed rest for the first 72 hours and is advised to refrain from intercourse and strenuous physical activity for the remainder of the pregnancy. We follow these patients with frequent sonographic assessment of the cervix and recommend strict bed rest if the membranes are prolapsing to the level of the suture.[94] Prophylactic tocolytics are not used after the procedure.

In situations in which the cervix has dilated enough to allow visualization of the membranes or the membranes have prolapsed into the vagina, placing an emergent cerclage constitutes a heroic maneuver.[92,95–98] These patients are at high risk of having a subclinical infection and subsequent poor outcome, as described previously.[95,99] To rule out infection, some clinicians advocate amniocentesis before cerclage placement.[100] Several techniques have been described to reduce the prolapsing membranes, including the following: placing the patient in Trendelenburg position; the use of a pediatric Foley catheter to tease the membranes into the endocervical canal, and instilling 1 L of saline into the bladder with upper displacement of the lower uterine segment (Fig. 25-10).[97–101] The efficacy of antibiotics or tocolytics has not been properly studied, but most series advocate their use. Although clinicians have been reluctant to offer cerclage in patients with protruding membranes, some reports have suggested salvage rate in excess of 70 percent despite advanced cervical dilatation.[102–104]

Risks of Cerclage

Cervical lacerations at the time of delivery are one of the most common complications from a cerclage, occurring in 1 to 13 percent of patients.[74] Three percent of patients require cesarean delivery because of the inability of the cervix to dilate secondary to cervical scarring and dystocia.[74] Although the risk of infection is minimal with a prophylactic cerclage, the risk increases significantly in cases of advanced dilatation with exposure of membranes to the birth canal.[99] However, this infectious morbidity may be the result of subclinical chorioamnionitis. Cervical cerclage displacement occurs in a small number of patients. We have not performed revision of the cerclage during the index pregnancy, although small series have reported successful surgical treatment of a failed cerclage.[76] When the clinician is faced with premature rupture of membranes distant from term in a patient

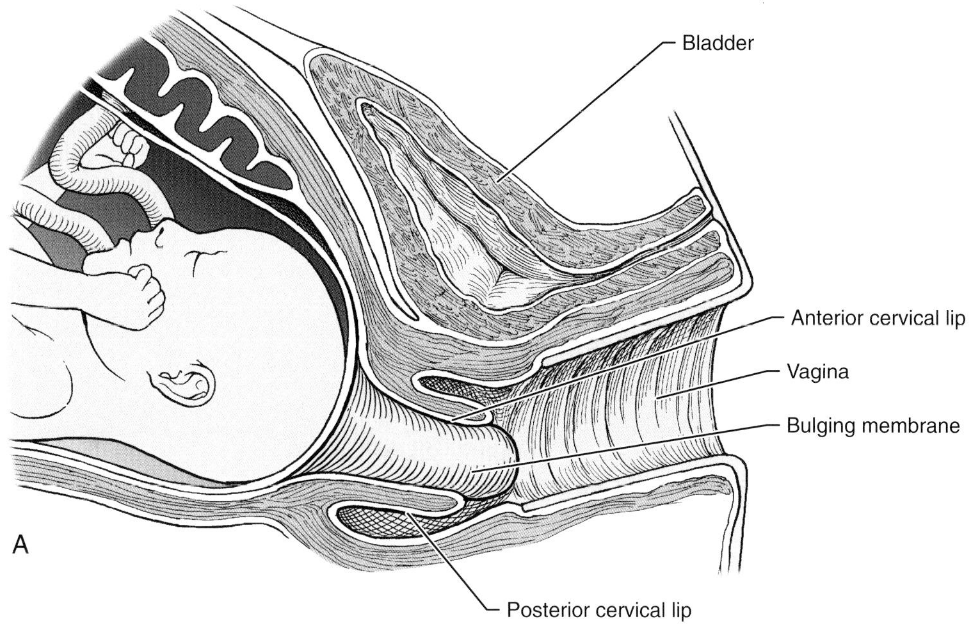

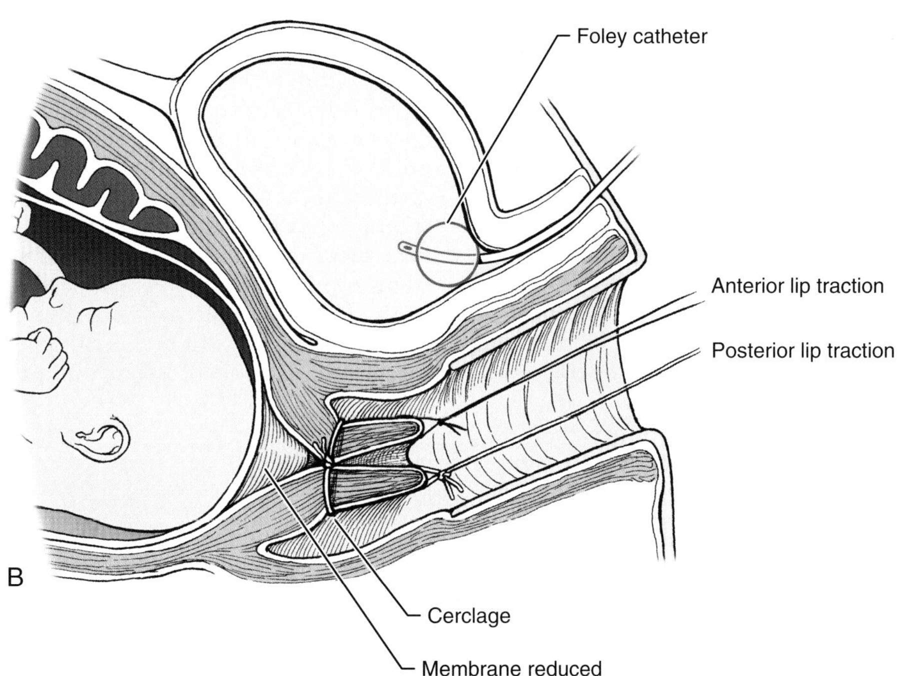

Figure 25-10. Emergent cerclage for bulging membranes at 23 weeks. *A*, Cervix dilated 3 cm with membranes protruding through the external cervical os into the vagina. *B*, Patient placed in Trendelenburg position, and bladder filled with saline. Stay silk sutures placed on anterior and posterior lip for traction while reducing membranes. McDonald cerclage placed distal to reduced membranes.

with cerclage, the decision to remove or leave the suture is controversial. Our own data suggests that with suture retention, there is an increased period of latency, at the expense of an increased risk for neonatal sepsis and mortality.[105] These data have been challenged by reports from Jenkins and colleages[106] suggesting an increased latency period (244 versus 119 hours) without an increase in neonatal morbidity, in cases of retained cerclage, and by McElrath et al.,[107] who did not find differences in latency or neonatal outcome in patients when the suture was left in situ after rupture of the membranes. Decisions to remove the suture at the time of ruptured membranes should be individualized until more information becomes available. Finally, even though cerclage placement is considered a benign procedure, a maternal death secondary to sepsis in a patient with retained cerclage has been reported.[108] Because of associated risks, and questionable effectiveness, the liberal use of this surgical procedure is discouraged and the decision should be carefully balanced against potential harm, in particular for patients in whom the indications for cerclage are not clear.

Alternative Treatments to Cervical Cerclage

Nonsurgical interventions have been advocated for patients with presumed cervical incompetence. The rationale for the recommendation for bed rest alone, or in conjunction with cerclage, relies in the theoretical concept of putting less pressure on the cervix while in the recumbent position. The validity of this concept has not been scientifically proven and to date there are no proper studies evaluating this intervention alone versus cerclage, in a randomized prospective fashion. The efficacy of pharmacologic agents such as indomethacin, progesterone, antibiotics, and others remains to be elucidated. Recently the MFM Units Network reported their results, comparing weekly injections of 17α-hydroxyprogesterone caproate for the prevention of preterm birth in women with history of prior spontaneous preterm delivery. Patients receiving the progestational agent had a 33 percent reduction in preterm birth compared with those receiving placebo.[109] At this time, it is unclear how this information may be applied to patients with a clinical history of cervical insufficiency, and further investigation is necessary.

Since the description by Vitsky in 1961 of the use of a vaginal pessary instead of cerclage for patients with cervical incompetence,[110] several studies mainly in Europe suggest the same outcome for patients managed with this noninvasive modality compared with a surgical intervention.[111] Recently Arabin et al.[112] studied the use of a vaginal pessary in patients with a sonographically detected short cervix (Fig. 25-11). Patients managed with a pessary gained 99 days compared to 67 days for patients managed with bed rest alone ($p = 0.02$). We have reported our initial experience[113] using the same type of vaginal pessary studied by Arabin in patients with sonographic cervical shortening and a prior history of preterm delivery. When compared with bed rest alone, patients with pessaries gained significantly greater gestational age (10.0 ± 41 weeks versus 5.1 ± 3.6 weeks $p = 0.03$). Further prospective, randomized trials comparing pessary, cerclage, and bed rest are necessary before conclusions regarding the efficacy of any of these interventions can be established.

SUMMARY

Cervical incompetence is rarely a distinct and well-defined clinical entity but only one piece of a larger and more complex spontaneous preterm birth syndrome. The original paradigm of obstetric and gynecologic trauma as a common antecedent of cervical incompetence has been replaced by the recognition of functional, as opposed to anatomic, deficits as the more prevalent basis. Cervical competence functions along a continuum, influenced by both endogenous and exogenous factors that interact through various pathways with other recognized components of the preterm birth syndrome: uterine contractions and decidual/membrane activation. Thus, the convenient term, *cervical incompetence,* may actually represent an oversimplified, incomplete version of the broader, though poorly understood, pathophysiologic process. Consequently, the continued use of traditional therapies, unsubstantiated by results of clinical trials, must be questioned. Effective, evidence-based management guidelines will stem from a more complete understanding of the preterm birth syndrome. This will improve patient selection and permit specifically tailored treatment regimens, confirmed by the results of well-designed intervention trials.

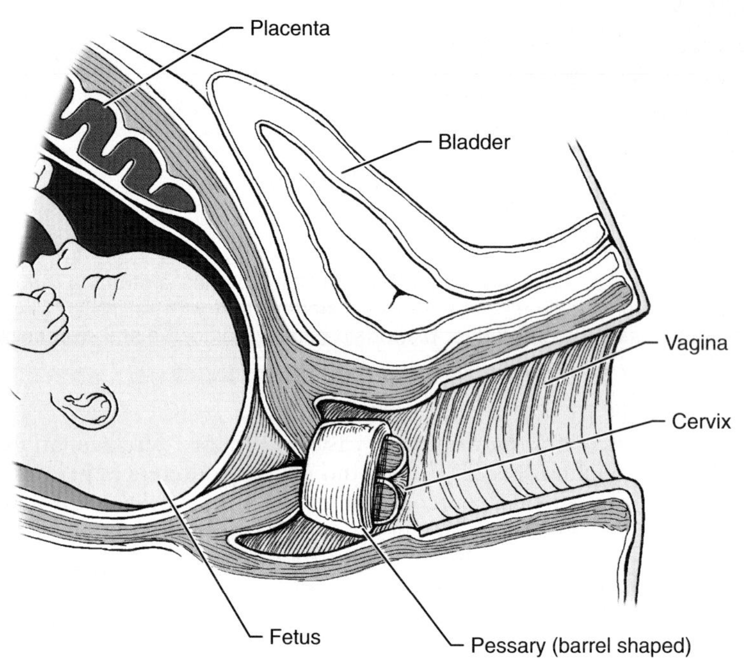

Figure 25-11. Vaginal pessary (Arabin type) placed at 22 weeks in patient with cervical length of 2.2 cm, funneling, and prior history of preterm delivery at 26 weeks.

Cervical incompetence remains a clinical diagnosis, because a clinically useful, objective test coupled with an effective therapy, has not been identified. At present, cervical ultrasound represents a powerful research instrument that can be used to screen selected high-risk populations, identify patients who may have a treatable *component* of cervical insufficiency, and recommend effective interventions. Surgical intervention in the form of prophylactic cerclage, sonographically indicated cerclage, emergent cerclage, and abdominal/laparoscopic cerclage may be reasonable in carefully selected patients. Alternative treatments such as bed rest and a vaginal pessary require further investigation.

KEY POINTS

- Cervical incompetence or insufficiency is primarily a clinical diagnosis characterized by recurrent painless dilatation and spontaneous midtrimester loss.
- Cervical incompetence is rarely a distinct and well-defined clinical entity, but only one component of the larger and more complex spontaneous preterm birth syndrome.
- Current evidence suggests that cervical competence functions along a continuum, influenced by both endogenous and exogenous factors, such as uterine contractions and decidual/membrane actuation.
- There is no objective diagnostic test for cervical incompetence.
- Cervical ultrasound performs poorly as a screening test in low-risk women, but it may be helpful in selected high-risk populations who may have a treatable component of cervical insufficiency.
- Prophylactic cerclage for patients with clinical history of cervical insufficiency remains a reasonable approach.
- Serial ultrasound evaluations of the cervix in patients at risk for cervical insufficiency may be an acceptable alternative approach to prophylactic cerclage.
- The benefit of cerclage for a sonographically defined short cervix in various high-risk populations remains unproven.
- Ultrasound-indicated cerclage for women at risk for preterm delivery not attributable to cervical insufficiency, does not improve outcome.
- Emergent cerclage may be beneficial in reducing preterm birth in a subgroup of patients without markers of infection.
- There is a need for randomized studies to evaluate alternative treatments for cervical insufficiency such as bed rest, pharmacologic therapy, and vaginal pessary.

REFERENCES

1. Anonymous. In Culpepper N, Cole A, Rowland W (eds): The Practice of Physick. London, George Strawbridge, 1678, p 502.
2. Ludmir J, Sehdev HM: Anatomy and physiology of the cervix. Clin Obstet Gynecol 43:433, 2000.
3. Barter RH, Dusbabek JA, Riva HL, Parks JL: Surgical closure of the incompetent cervix during pregnancy Am J Obstet Gyneccol 75:511, 1958.
4. Jennings CL: Temporary submucosal cerclage for cervical incompetence: Report of forty-eight cases. Am J Obstet Gynecol 113:1097, 1972.
5. Kuhn R, Pepperell R: Cervical ligation: a review of 242 pregnancies. Aust N Z J Obstet Gynaecol 17:79–83, 1977.
6. Romero R, Mazor M, Munoz H, et al: The preterm labor syndrome. Ann N Y Acad Sci 734:414, 1994.
7. Danforth DN, Buckingham JC: Cervical incompetence: A re-evaluation. Postgrad Med 32:345, 1962.
8. Danforth DN, Veis A, Breen M, et al: The effect of pregnancy and labor on the human cervix: Changes in collagen, glycoproteins and gycosaminoglycans. Am J Obstet Gynecol 120:641, 1974.
9. Leppert PC, Yu SY, Keller S, et al: Decreased elastic fibers and desmosine content in incompetent cervix. Am J Obstet Gynecol 157:1134, 1987.
10. Rechberger T, Uldbjerg N, Oxlund H: Connective tissue changes in the cervix during normal pregnancy and pregnancy complicated by cervical incompetence. Obstet Gynecol 71:563, 1988.
11. Dunn LJ, Dana P. Subsequent obstetrical performance of patients meeting the historical criteria for cervical incompetence. Bull Sloan Hosp Women 7:43, 1962.
12. Iams JD, Johnson FF, Sonek J, et al: Cervical competence as a continuum: a study of ultrasonography cervical length and obstetric performance. Am J Obstet Gynecol 172:1097, 1995.
13. Iams JD, Goldenberg RL, Meis PJ, et al: The length of the cervix and the risk of spontaneous premature delivery. N Engl J Med 334:567,1996.
14. Buckingham JC, Buethe RA, Danforth DN: Collagen-muscle ratio in clinically normal and clinically incompetent cervixes. Am J Obstet Gynecol 91:232, 1965.
15. Ayers JWR, DeGrood RM, Compton AA, et al: Sonographic evaluation of cervical length in pregnancy: diagnosis and management of preterm cervical effacement in patients at risk for premature delivery. Obstet Gynecol 71:939, 1988.
16. Craigo SD: Cervical incompetence and preterm delivery [editorial]. N Engl J Med 334:595, 1996.
17. Olah KS, Gee H: The prevention of preterm delivery—can we afford to continue to ignore the cervix? Br J Obstet Gynaecol 99:278, 1992.
18. Romero R, Gomez R, Sepulveda W: The uterine cervix, ultrasound and prematurity [editor comments]. Ultrasound Obstet Gynecol 2:385, 1992.
19. Toaff R, Toaff ME: Diagnosis of impending late abortion. Obstet Gynecol 43:756, 1974.
20. Bergman P, Svenerund A: Traction test for demonstrating incompetence of internal os of the cervix. Int J Fertil 2:163, 1957.
21. Kiwi R, Neuman MR, Merkatz IR, et al: Determination of the elastic properties of the cervix. Obstet Gynecol 71:568, 1988.
22. Zlatnik KFJ, Burmeister LF: Interval evaluation of the cervix for predicting pregnancy outcome and diagnosing cervical incompetence. J Repro Med 38:365, 1993.
23. Tongsong T, Kamprapanth P, Srisomboon J, et al: Single transvaginal sonographic measurement of cervical length early in the third trimester as a predictor of preterm delivery. Obstet Gynecol 86:184, 1995.
24. Berghella V, Tolosa JE, Kuhlman K, et al: Cervical ultrasonography compared with manual examination as a predictor of preterm delivery. Am J Obstet Gynecol 177:723, 1997.
25. Andrews WW, Copper R, Hauth JC, et al: Mid-trimester cervical ultrasound findings predict recurrent early preterm birth. Obstet Gynecol 95:222, 2000.
26. Owen J, Yost N, Berghella V, et al: Mid-trimester endovaginal sonography in women at high risk for spontaneous preterm birth. JAMA 286:1340, 2001.

27. Owen J, Yost N, Berghella V, et al: Can shortened mid-trimester cervical length predict very early spontaneous preterm birth? Am J Obstet Gynecol 191:298, 2004.
28. Berghella V, Tolosa JE, Kuhlman K, et al: Cervical ultrasonography compared with manual examination as a predictor of preterm delivery. Am J Obstet Gynecol 177:723, 1997.
29. Airoldi J, Berghella V, Sehdev H, Ludmir J: Transvaginal Ultrasonography of the cervix to predict preterm birth in women with uterine anomalies. Obstet Gynecol 106:553, 2005.
30. Honest H, Bachman LM, Coomarasamy A, et al: Accuracy of cervical transvaginal sonography in predicting preterm birth; a systematic review. Ultrasound Obstet Gynecol 22:305, 2003.
31. McMahon KS, Neerhof MC, Haney EI, et al: Prematurity in multiple gestations: identification of patients who are at low risk. Am J Obstet Gynecol 186:1137, 2002.
32. Imseis HM, Albert TA, Iams JD: Identifying twin gestations at low risk for preterm birth with a transvaginal ultrasonographic cervical measurement at 24 to 26 weeks' gestation. Am J Obstet Gynecol 177:1149, 1997.
33. Ferenczy A, Choukroun D, Falcone T, Franco E: The effect of cervical loop electrosurgical excision on subsequent pregnancy outcome: North American experience. Am J Obstet Gynecol 172:1246, 1995.
34. Althuisius SM, Shornagel GA, Dekker GA, van Geijn HP, Hummel P: Loop electrosurgical excision procedure of the cervix and time of delivery in subsequent pregnancy. Int J Gynecol Obstet 72:31, 2001.
35. Sadler L, Saftkas A, Wang W, et al: Treatment for cervical intraepithelial neoplasis and risk of preterm delivery. JAMA 29:2100, 2004.
36. Weber T, Obel E: Pregnancy complications following conization of the uterine cervix. Acta Obstet Gynecol Scand 58:259, 1979.
37. Leiman G, Harrison NA, Rubin A: Pregnancy following conization of the cervix: complications related to cone size. Am J Obstet Gynecol 136:14, 1980.
38. Raio L, Ghezzi F, Di Naro E, et al: Duration of pregnancy after carbon dioxide laser conization of the cervix: influence of cone height. Obstet Gynecol 90:978, 1997.
39. Kuoppala T, Saarikoski S: Pregnancy and delivery after cone biopsy of the cervix. Arch Gynecol 237:149, 1986.
40. Lazar P, Gueguen S, Dreyfus J, et al: Multicentred controlled trial of cervical cerclage in women at moderate risk of preterm delivery. Br J Obstet Gynaecol 91:731, 1984.
41. Dor J, Shalev J, Mashiach S, et al: Elective cervical suture of twin pregnancies diagnosed ultrasonically in the first trimester following induced ovulation. Gynecol Obstet Invest 13:55, 1982.
42. Rush RW, Isaacs S, McPherson K, et al: A randomized controlled trial of cervical cercalge in women at high risk for preterm delivery. Br J Obstet Gynaecol 91:724, 1984.
43. MacNaughton MC, Chalmers IG, Dubowitz V, et al: Final report of the Medical Research Council/Royal College of Obstetrics and Gynaecology multicentre randomized trial of cervical cerclage. Br J Obstet Gynaecol 100:516, 1993.
44. Heath VCF, Souka AP, Erasmus I, et al: Cervical length at 23 weeks of gestation: The value of Shirodkar suture for the short cervix. Ultrasound Obstet Gynecol 12:318, 1998.
45. Novy MJ, Gupta A, Wothe DD, et al: Cervical cerclage in the second trimester of pregnancy: A historical cohort study. Am J Obstet Gynecol 184:1447, 2001.
46. Berghella V, Daly SF, Tolosa JE, et al: Prediction of preterm delivery with transvaginal ultrasonography of the cervix in patients with high-risk pregnancies: Does cerclage prevent prematurity? Am J Obstet Gynecol 181:809, 1999.
47. Hassan SS, Romero R, Maymon E, et al: Does cervical cerclage prevent preterm delivery in patients with a short cervix? Am J Obstet Gynecol 184:1325, 2001.
48. Newman RB, Krombach SR, Myers MC, McGee DL: Effect of cerclage on obstetrical outcome in twin gestations with a shortened cervical length. Am J Obstet Gynecol 186:634, 2002.
49. Roman AS, Rebarber A, Pereria L, et al: The efficacy of sonographically indicated cerclage in multiple gestations. J Ultrasound Med 24:763, 2005.
50. Althuisius SM, Dekker GA, van Geijn HP, et al: Cervical Incompetence Prevention Randomized Cerclage Trial (CIPRACT): Study design and preliminary results. Am J Obstet Gynecol 183:823, 2000.
51. Althuisius SM, Dekker GA, Hummel P, et al: Final results of the cervical incompetence prevention randomized cerclage trial (CIPRACT): therapeutic cerclage with bed rest versus bed rest alone. Am J Obstet Gynecol 185:1106, 2001.
52. Rust OA, Atlas RO, Reed J, et al: Revisiting the short cervix detected by transvaginal ultrasound in the second trimester: why cerclage may not help. Am J Obstet Gynecol 185:1098, 2001.
53. To MS, Alfirevic Z, Heath VCF, et al: on behalf of the Fetal Medicine Foundation Second Trimester Screening Group: Cervical cerclage for prevention of preterm delivery in women with short cervix: randomized controlled trial. Lancet 363:1849, 2004.
54. Berghella V, Odibo AO, Tolosa JE: Cerclage for prevention of preterm birth in women with a short cervix found on transvaginal ultrasound: A randomized trial. Am J Obstet Gynecol 191:1311, 2004.
55. Berghella V, Haas S, Chervoneva I, Hyslop T: Patients with prior second-trimester loss: prophylactic cerclage or serial transvaginal sonograms. Am J Obstet Gynecol 187:747, 2002.
56. Fejgin MD, Gabai B, Golberger S, et al: Once a cerclage, not always a cerclage. J Reprod Med 39:880, 1994.
57. Berghella V, Odibo AO, To MS, et al: Cerclage for short cervix on ultrasonography, meta-analysis of trials using individual patient-level data. Obstet Gynecol 106:181, 2005.
58. Owen J, Iams JD, Hauth JC: Vaginal sonography and cervical incompetence. Am J Obstet Gynecol 188:586, 2003.
58a. Romero R, Espinoza J, Erez O, Hassam S: The role of cervical cerclage in obstetric practice: Can the patient who could benefit from this procedure be identified? Am J Obstet Gynecol 194:1, 2006.
59. Branch DW: Operations for cervical incompetence. Clin Obstet Gynecol 29:240,1986.
60. Cousins JM: Cervical incompetence: 1980. A time for reappraisal. Clin Obstet Gynecol 23:467, 1980.
61. Aarts JM, Jozien T, Brons J, Bruinse HW: Emergency cerclage: A review. Obstet Gynecol Survey 50:459, 1995.
62. Olatunbosun OA, Al-Nuaim L, Turnell RW: Emergency cerclage compared with bedrest for advanced cervical dilatation in pregnancy. Int Surg 80:170, 1995.
63. Kokia E, Dor J, Blankenstein J, et al: A simple scoring system for treatment of cervical incompetence diagnosed during the second trimester. Gynceol Obstet Invest 31:12, 1991.
64. Althuisius SM, Dekker GA, Hummel P, van Geijn HP: Cervical incompetence prevention randomized cerclage trial: Emergency cerclage with bedrest versus bedrest alone. Am J Obstet Gynecol 189:907, 2003.
65. Romero R, Gonzalez R, Sepulveda W, et al: Infection and Labor VIII. Microbial invasion of the amniotic cavity in patients with suspected cervical incompetence: Prevalence and clinical significance. Am J Obstet Gynecol 167:1086, 1992.
66. Mays JK, Figuerioa R, Shah J, et al: Amniocentesis for selection before rescue cerclage. Obstet Gynecol 95:652, 2000.
67. Treadwell MC, Bronsteen RA, Bottoms SF: Prognostic factors and complication rates for cervical cerclage: A review of 482 cases. Am J Obstet Gynecol 165:555, 1991.
68. Weiner CP, Lee KY, Buhimschi CS, et al: Proteomic biomarkers that predict the clinical success of rescue cerclage. Am J Obstet Gynecol 192:710, 2005.
69. Lash AF, Lash SR: Habitual abortion: the incompetent internal os of the cervix. Am J Obstet Gynecol 59:68, 1950.
70. Shirodkar VN: A new method of operative treatment for habitual abortions in the second trimester of pregnancy. Antiseptic 52:299, 1955.
71. McDonald IA: Suture of the cervix for inevitable miscarriage. J Obstet Gynecol Br Empire 64:346, 1957.
72. Abdelhak YE, Sheen JJ, Kuczynski E, et al: Comparison of delayed absorbable suture v. non-absorbable suture for the treatment of incompetent cervix. J Perinatal Med 27:250, 1999.
73. Aarnoudse JG, Huisjes HJ: Complications of cerclage. Acta Obstet Gynecol Scand 58:225, 1979.
74. Harger JH: Comparison of success and morbidity in cervical cerclage procedures. Obstet Gynecol 53:534, 1980.
75. McDonald IA: Incompetence of the cervix. Aust N Z J Obstet Gynaecol 18:34, 1978.
76. Schulman H, Farmakides G: Surgical approach to failed cervical cerclage: a report of three cases. J Reprod Med 30:626, 1985.

77. Steinberg ES, Santos AC: Surgical anesthesia during pregnancy. Int Anesthesiol Clin 28:58, 1980.
78. Chen L, Ludmir J, Miller FL, et al: Is regional better than general anesthesia for cervical cerclage? Nine years experience. Anesth Analg 70:Sl, 1990.
79. Ludmir J, Cohen BF, Wong GP, et al: Managing the patient with cerclage: Bedrest versus amulation based on sonographic findings. Presented at the 17th Annual Meeting of the Society of Perinatal Obstetricians, Anaheim, CA 1997.
80. Abdelhak YE, Aronov R, Roque H, Young BK: Management of cervical cerclage at term: remove the suture in labor? J Perinat Med 28:453, 2000.
81. Novy MJ: Transabdominal cervicoisthmic cerclage for the management of repetitive abortion and premature delivery. Am J Obstet Gynecol 143:44, 1982.
82. Novy MJ: Transabdominal cervicoisthmic cerclage: a reappraisal 25 years after its introduction. Am J Obstet Gynecol 164:163, 1991.
83. Groom KN, Jones BA, Edmonds DK, Bennett PR: Preconception Transabdominal cervicoisthmic cerclage. Am J Obstet Gynecol, 191:230, 2004.
84. Ludmir J, Jackson GM, Samuels P: Transvaginal cerclage under ultrasound guidance in cases of severe cervical hypoplasia. Obstet Gynecol 78:1087, 1991.
85. Scarantino SE, Reilly JG, Moretti ML, Pillari VT: Laparoscopic removal of a transabdominal cervical cerclage. Am J Obstet Gynecol 182:1086, 2000.
86. Gallot D, Savary D, Laurichesse H, et al: Experience with three cases of laparoscopic transabdominal cervioisthmic cerclage and two subsequent pregnancies. Br J Obstet Gynaecol 110:696, 2003.
87. Cho CH, Kim TH, Kwon SH, et al: Laparoscopic transabdominal cervicoisthmid cerclage during pregnancy. J Am Gynecol Laparosc 10:363, 2003.
88. Harger JH: Cervical cerclage: patient selection, morbidity, and success rates. Clin Perinatol 10:321, 1983.
89. Cardosi RJ, Chez RA: Comparison of elective and empiric cerclage and the role of emergency cerclage. J Matern Fetal Med 7:230, 1998.
90. Ludmir J, Landon MB, Gabbe SG, et al: Management of the diethylstilbestrol-exposed pregnant patient: a prospective study. Am J Obstet Gynecol 157:665, 1987.
91. Guzman ER, Forster JK, Vintzileos AM, et al: Pregnancy outcomes in women treated with elective versus ultrasound-indicated cervical cerclage. Ultrasound Obstet Gynecol 12:323, 1998.
92. Benifla JL, Goffinet F, Darai E, et al: Emergency cervical cercalge after 20 weeks' gestation: a retrospective study of 16 years' practice in 34 cases. Fetal Diagn Ther 12:274, 1997.
93. Berghella V, Daly SF, Tolosa JE, et al: Prediction of preterm delivery with transvaginal ultrasonography of the cervix in patients with high-risk pregnancies: does cerclage prevent prematurity? Am J Obstet Gynecol 181:809, 1999.
94. Althuisius SM, Dekker GA, van Geijin HP, et al: The effect of McDonald Cerclage on cervical length as assessed by transvaginal ultrasonography. Am J Obstet Gynecol 180:366, 1999.
95. Minakami H, Matsubara S, Izumi A, et al: Emergency cervical cercalge: relation between its success, perioperative serum level of C-reactive protein and WBC count, and degree of cervical dilatation. Gynecol Obstet Invest 47:157, 1999.
96. Aarts JM, Brons JT, Bruinse HW, et al: Emergency cerclage: a review. Obstet Gynecol Surv 50:459, 1995.
97. Caruso A, Trivellini C, DeCarolis S, et al. Emergency cerclage in the presence of protruding membranes: is pregnancy outcome predictable? Acta Obstet Gynaecol Scand 79:265, 2000.
98. Barth WH Jr., Yeomans ER, Hankins GDV, et al: Emergent cerclage. Surg Gynaecol Scand 58:225, 1979.
99. Charles D, Edwards WR: Infectious complications of cerclage. Am J Obstet Gynecol 141:1065, 1981.
100. Mays JK, Figuerioa R, Shah J, et al: Amniocentesis for selection before rescue cerclage. Obstet Gynecol 95:652, 2000.
101. Scheerer LJ, Lam F, Bartololucci L, et al: A new technique for reduction of prolapsed fetal membranes for emergency cervical cerclage. Obstet Gynecol 74:408, 1989.
102. Kurup M, Goldkrand JW: Cervical incompetence: elective, emergent, or urgent cerclage. Am J Obstet Gynecol 181:240, 1999.
103. Wu MY, Yang YS, Huang SC, et al: Emergent and elective cerclage for cervical incompetence. Int J Gynaecol Obstet 54:23, 1996.
104. Lipitz S, Libshsitz A, Oelsner G, et al: Outcome of second-trimester, emergency cervical cerclage in patients with no history of cervical incompetence. Am J Perinatol 13:419, 1996.
105. Ludmir J, Bader T, Chen L, et al: Poor perinatal outcome associated with retained cerclage in patients with premature rupture of membranes. Obstet Gynecol 84:823, 1994.
106. Jenkins TM, Bergehlla V, Shlossman PA, et al: Timing of cerclage removal after preterm premature rupture of membranes: Maternal and neonatal outcomes. Am J Obstet Gynecol 183:847, 2000.
107. McElrath TF, Norwitz ER, Lieberman ES, Heffner LJ: Management of cervical cerclage and preterm premature rupture of the membranes: Should the stitch be removed? Am J Obstet Gynecol 183:840, 2000.
108. Dunn LE, Robinson JC, Steer CM: Maternal death following suture of incompetent cervix during pregnancy. Am J Obstet Gynecol 78:335, 1959.
109. Meis PJ, Klebanoff M, Thom E, Dombrowski MP, et al: Prevention of recurrent preterm delivery 17 alpha hydroxyprogesterone caproate. N Engl J Med 348:2379, 2003.
110. Vitsky M: Simple treatment of the incompetent cervical os. Am J Obstet Gynecol 81:1194, 1961.
111. Forster F, Dunng R, Schwartz G: Therapy of cervix insufficiency—cerclage or support pessary? Sentrablbl Gynaekol 108:230, 1986.
112. Arabin B, Halbesma JR, Vork F, et al: Is treatment with vaginal pessaries an option in patients with a sonographically detected short cervix? J Perinat Med 31:122, 2003.
113. Ludmir J, Mantione JR, Debbs RH, Sehdev HM: Is pessary a valid treatment for cervical change during the late midtrimester? J Soc Gynecol Investig 9(Suppl):11, 2002.
114. Varma TR, Patel RH, Pillai U: Ultrasonic assessment of cervix in "at risk" patient. Acta Obstet Gynaecol Scand 65:146, 1986.
115. Michaels WH, Montgomery C, Karo J, et al: Ultrasound differentiation of the competent from the incompetent cervix: prevention of preterm delivery. Am J Obstet Gynecol 151:537, 1986.
116. Fox R, James M, Tuohy J, Wardle P: Transvaginal ultrasound in the management of women with suspected cervical incompetence. Br J Obstet Gynaecol 103:921, 1996.
117. Guzman ER, Vintzileos AM, McLean DA, et al: The natural history of a positive response to transfundal pressure in women at risk for cervical incompetence. Am J Obstet Gynecol 176:634, 1997.
118. Guzman ER, Pisatowski DM, Vintzileos AM, et al: A comparison of ultrasonographically detected cervical changes in response to transfundal pressure, coughing, and standing in predicting cervical incompetence. Am J Obstet Gynecol 177:660, 1997.
119. Wong G, Levine D, Ludmir J: Maternal postural challenge as a functional test for cervical incompetence. J Ultra Med 16:169, 1997.
120. Guzman ER, Mellon R, Vintzileos AM, et al: Relationship between endocervical canal length between 15–24 weeks gestation and obstetric history. J Maternal Fetal Med 7:269, 1998.
121. MacDonald R, Smith P, Vyas S: Cervical incompetence: the use of transvaginal sonography to provide an objective diagnosis. Ultra Obstet Gynecol 18:211, 2001.

Preterm Birth

JAY D. IAMS AND ROBERTO ROMERO

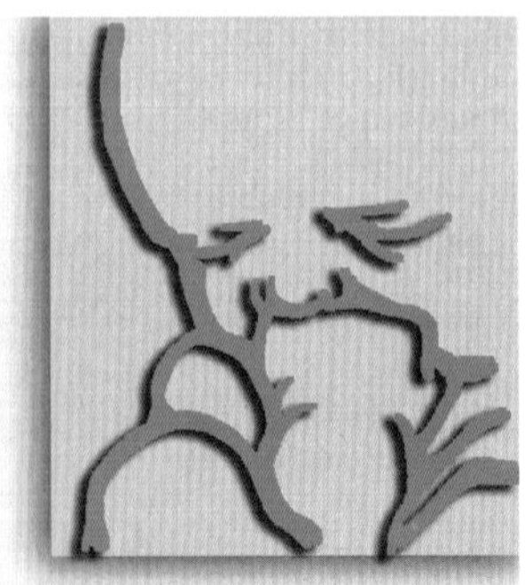

CHAPTER 26

KEY ABBREVIATIONS

Adrenocorticotrophic hormone	ACTH
Assisted reproductive techniques	ART
Bacterial vaginosis	BV
Bronchopulmonary dysplasia	BPD
Confidence interval	CI
Corticotropin-releasing hormone	CRH
Cyclic adenosine monophosphate	cAMP
Cyclooxygenase	COX
Estrogen receptor	ER
Extremely low birth weight	ELBW
Fetal inflammatory response syndrome	FIRS
Gelatinase-B	MMP-9
Group B streptococcus	GBS
In vitro fertilization	IVF
Inducible form of nitric oxide synthase	iNOS
Interstitial collagenase	MMP-1
Intravenous	IV
Intraventricular hemorrhage	IVH
Low birth weight	LBW
Myosin light-chain kinase	MLCK
National Institute of Child Health and Human Development	NICHD
Necrotizing enterocolitis	NEC
Neutrophil collagenase	MMP-8
Nonsteroidal anti-inflammatory drugs	NSAIDs
Odds ratio	OR
Patent ductus arteriosus	PDA
Prelabor rupture of membranes	PROM
Progesterone receptor	PR
Relative risk	RR
Respiratory distress syndrome	RDS
Thyrotropin-releasing hormone	TRH
Tumor necrosis factor-α	TNF-α
U.S. Food and Drug Administration	FDA
Very low birth weight	VLBW
White blood cell	WBC

INTRODUCTION

Birth before term (37 to 41 weeks' gestation) is associated with death and disability in infants and children. Perinatal mortality and morbidity occur most commonly in infants born before 37 weeks' and especially before 32 weeks' gestation. Prematurity-related disorders cause more than 70 percent of fetal and neonatal deaths in the United States annually.[1] In 2002, nearly 40 percent of neonatal deaths (between birth and one month of age) and about 25 percent of infant deaths (from birth to 1 year of age) occurred in infants who were preterm and low birth weight (LBW).[1] Infants born preterm are more likely to develop visual and hearing impairment, chronic lung disease, cerebral palsy, and delayed development in childhood. Although advances in neonatal care have led to increased survival and reduced short- and long-term morbidity for preterm infants, the percentage of births before 37 weeks' has risen steadily to one of every eight babies born in 2003.

DEFINITIONS

A *preterm birth* is defined as one that occurs before the completion of 37 menstrual weeks of gestation, regardless of birth weight. *LBW* is defined by the size of the infant at birth, regardless of gestational age. Gestational age and birth weight are related by the terms *small for gestational age* (birth weight less than the 10th percentile for gestational age), *appropriate for gestational age* (birth weight between the 10th and 90th percentiles), and *large for gestational age* (birth weight above the 90th percentile). A *preterm* or *premature* infant is one born before 37 weeks of gestation (259 days from the first day of the mother's last normal menstrual period, or 245 days after conception). An LBW infant is one whose birth weight is less than 2,500 g, a *very low birth weight* (VLBW) infant is one whose birth weight is less than 1,500 g, and an *extremely low birth weight* (ELBW) infant is one whose birth weight is less than 1,000 g.

FREQUENCY OF PRETERM AND LOW BIRTH WEIGHT DELIVERY

The frequency of preterm birth increased from 10.6 to 12.5 percent of live births in the United States between 1990 and 2004.[2,3]

Preterm births after 32 weeks account for most of the increase. Births before 32 weeks increased slightly from 1.91 to 1.96 percent between 1992 and 2003 but rose again to 2.0 percent in 2004. See bar graphs in Figure 26-1.

The most recent rates of preterm and LBW for 2003 and 2004 according to the race and Hispanic origin of the mother are shown in Table 26-1.

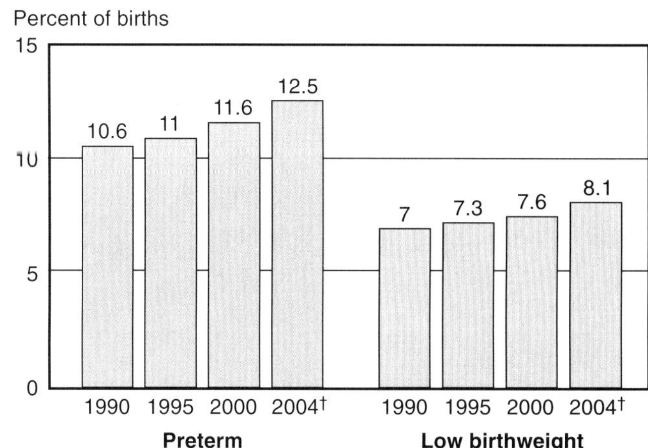

Figure 26-1. Percentage of infants born preterm and born low birth weight: United States, 1990, 1995, 2000, and 2004. (From Martin JA, Hamilton BE, Menacker F, et al: Preliminary births for 2004: Infant and maternal health. Health E-stats. Released November 15, 2005.)

Table 26-1. Percentage of Live Births Preterm and very Preterm and Percentage of Live Births Low and very Low Birth Weight, by Race and Hispanic Origin of Mother: United States, Final 2003 and Preliminary 2004.[2]

	PRETERM				LOW BIRTH WEIGHT			
	TOTAL		VERY PRETERM		TOTAL		VERY LOW BIRTH WEIGHT	
RACE AND HISPANIC ORIGIN OF MOTHER	2004	2003	2004	2003	2004	2003	2004	2003
All races and origins	12.5	12.3	2.00	1.97	8.1	7.9	1.47	1.45
Non-Hispanic white	11.5	11.3	1.63	1.60	7.2	7.0	1.20	1.18
Non-Hispanic black	17.9	17.8	4.04	3.99	13.7	13.6	3.14	3.12
American Indian total	13.7	13.5	2.17	2.17	7.5	7.4	1.28	1.30
Asian or Pacific Islander total	10.6	10.5	1.49	1.43	7.9	7.8	1.14	1.09
Hispanic	12.0	11.9	1.76	1.73	6.8	6.7	1.19	1.16

From Martin JA, Hamilton BE, Menacker F, et al: Preliminary births for 2004: Infant and Maternal health. 11-15-2005. Hyattsville, Maryland, National Center for Health Statistics. Health E-stats.

The rise in preterm births has been attributed to increased use of assisted reproductive technologies (ART)[4] and increased willingness to choose delivery when medical or obstetric complications threaten the health of the mother or fetus after 32 to 34 weeks' gestation.[5]

The perinatal mortality rate has declined over this time as the preterm birth rate has risen.[6,7]

The proportion of LBW infants who are preterm versus term varies widely between developed and underdeveloped nations. In underdeveloped countries, most LBW infants are born after 37 weeks, their LBW the result of poor intrauterine nutrition and chronic maternal illness and/or malnutrition. In developed nations, most LBW infants are preterm, although there are wide variations within the United States according to race, parity, fetal gender, and environmental factors such as maternal cigarette smoking and altitude. The rates of preterm birth across the United States in 2003 are shown in Figure 26-2.

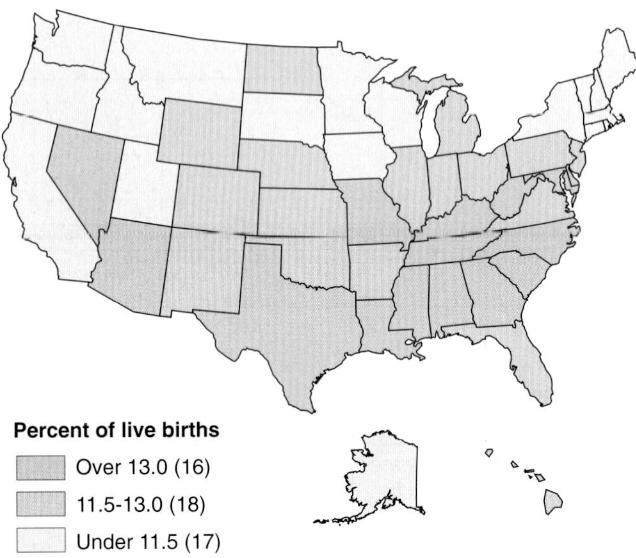

Figure 26-2. The rates of preterm birth across the United States in 2003. (Copyright March of Dimes, 2005; with permission.)

PERINATAL MORTALITY AND MORBIDITY

Perinatal mortality is reported based on available data and is most broadly defined as the sum of stillbirths after 20 weeks' gestation plus neonatal deaths through 28 days of life per 1,000 total births (live births + stillbirths). A recent report from the National Center for Health Statistics chose to define the *perinatal mortality rate* as the number of *late* fetal deaths (after 28 weeks) plus infant deaths within 7 days of birth per 1,000 total births after 28 weeks.[6] Using this definition, the perinatal mortality rate declined steadily from 32.5 in 1950, to 9.1 in 1990, and 6.9 in 2001.

The perinatal mortality rate is twice as high for infants born to black than to white mothers. In a study that defined perinatal mortality to include all stillbirths after 22 weeks plus neonatal deaths through 28 days of life,[5] perinatal mortality rates were nearly double in black women compared with whites. Perinatal mortality rates declined between 1989 and 2000 for both black and white women (Table 26-2), whereas preterm birth rates between 1989 and 2000 rose from 8.4 percent to 10.4 percent among whites, and decreased from 19.0 percent to 17.4 percent in blacks.

Regardless of definition, the leading cause of perinatal mortality is preterm birth. Perinatal mortality increases markedly as gestational age and birth weight decline. In 2001, 41 percent of all infants born before 28 weeks of gestation died within 1 year, compared with 5 percent of infants born at 28 to 31 weeks, 1 percent of infants born at 32 to 35 weeks and 0.3 percent of infants born at term.[8]

The infant mortality rate is the number of deaths of live-born infants before 1 year of age per 1,000 live births. The two leading causes of all infant deaths are congenital anomalies and complications of prematurity. In 2003, conditions related to preterm birth caused 20.3 percent of deaths from birth to 1 year, whereas 20.0 percent were related to congenital anomalies.[9]

The threshold for survival fell steadily after the introduction of neonatal intensive care but has plateaued recently.[10] In 1970, most hospitals did not expect infants born before 28 weeks or with birth weight below 1,000 g

Table 26-2. Changes in Crude Perinatal Mortality Rates Among White and Black Women: United States, 1989 and 2000

	WHITE WOMEN			BLACK WOMEN		
	PERIOD OF BIRTH			PERIOD OF BIRTH		
PERINATAL MORTALITY RATE*	1989	2000	RR (95% CI)	1989	2000	RR (95% CI)
Overall perinatal mortality rate	7.8	5.4	0.70 (0.69–0.71)	14.8	10.8	0.73 (0.70–0.75)
Among all preterm births	50.6	36.2	0.71 (0.69–0.73)	54.1	47.4	0.87 (0.84–0.91)
Ruptured membranes	60.8	42.6	0.69 (0.63–0.74)	74.9	70.9	0.94 (0.85–1.05)
Medically indicated	64.7	44.4	0.67 (0.64–0.70)	63.0	51.4	0.81 (0.75–0.87)
Spontaneous	41.6	29.3	0.70 (0.67–0.73)	47.2	41.1	0.87 (0.82–0.91)

*per 1000 births.
CI, confidence interval; RR, relative risk.
Relative risk (95% confidence interval) denotes changes in perinatal mortality rates between 1989 and 2000.
From Ananth CVP, Joseph KSM, Oyelese YM, et al: Trends in preterm birth and perinatal mortality among singletons: United States, 1989 Through 2000. Obstet Gynecol 105:1084, 2005.

to survive. Major advances in care since then include regionalized care for high-risk mothers and preterm LBW infants, antenatal administration of corticosteroids, neonatal administration of exogenous pulmonary surfactant, and improved ventilator technology. These changes in perinatal care have produced survival rates that now exceed 90 percent for infants born at 28 weeks' gestation or 1,000 g birth weight.[11]

In a study of live-born singleton infants delivered at Canadian tertiary perinatal centers between 1991 and 1996, 56.1 percent born at 24 weeks (n = 406) and 68 percent born at 25 weeks' (n = 454) survived to discharge from the hospital.[12] Figure 26-3 shows survival and mortality rates for 8,523 infants born in 1997 to 1998 at a single U.S. center.[13] After 23 to 25 weeks, the majority of infants in this center survived to hospital discharge.

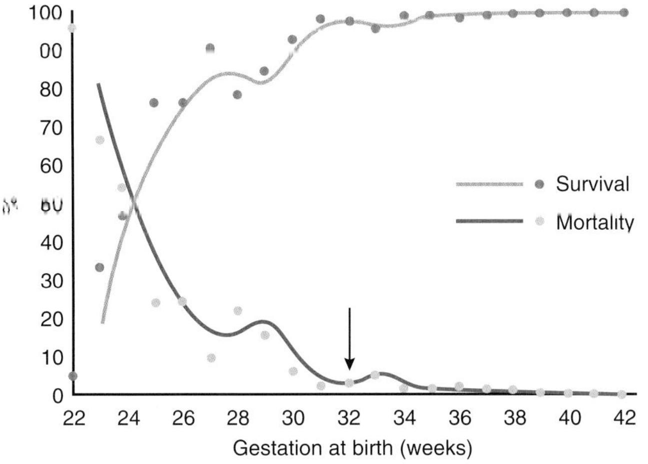

Figure 26-3. Perinatal mortality and gestational age. (Modified from Mercer BMM: Preterm premature rupture of the membranes. Obstet Gynecol 101:178, 2003.)

Data from the Vermont, Oxford and National Institute of Child Health and Human Development (NICHD) Neonatal Research Networks suggest that improvements in survival and morbidity for infants born between 23 and 25 weeks' have reached a limit. Between 1996 and 2000, survival rates for babies born into the tertiary nurseries of the NICHD Neonatal Research Network improved from 20 to 30 percent at 23 weeks, 58 to 60 percent at 24 weeks, and 75 to 80 percent at 25 weeks.[14] In the Vermont Oxford data, mortality and morbidity among infants weighing 501 to 1500 g declined steadily between 1991 and 1995 but did not improve further between 1995 and 1999.[10] In 2002, the American Academy of Pediatrics[15] and the American College of Obstetricians and Gynecologists[16] issued joint statements on perinatal care at the limit of viability that base recommendations for care and communication with the patients and families on the data reported by Lemons et al.[11] (Fig. 26-4).

Survival among infants with birthweights less than 500 g is rare but has attracted attention because of successes among infants previously thought to be nonviable. Of 4,172 live-born infants who weighed between 401 and 500 g at birth, 48 percent died in the delivery room.[17] The mean gestational age of infants in this study was 23.3 weeks; among the 17 percent who survived to hospital discharge, the mean gestational age was 25.3 weeks. Survivors had substantial morbidity.

Further precision in estimating neonatal mortality rates can be made by considering birth weight and maternal race/ethnicity as well as gestational age.[18] A review that accounted for these factors[18] found that the risk of neonatal mortality does not exceed 50 percent for babies of any ethnicity or race until the gestational age at birth is less than 24 weeks and birth weight is below 500 g. The analysis also confirmed higher rates of preterm and LBW

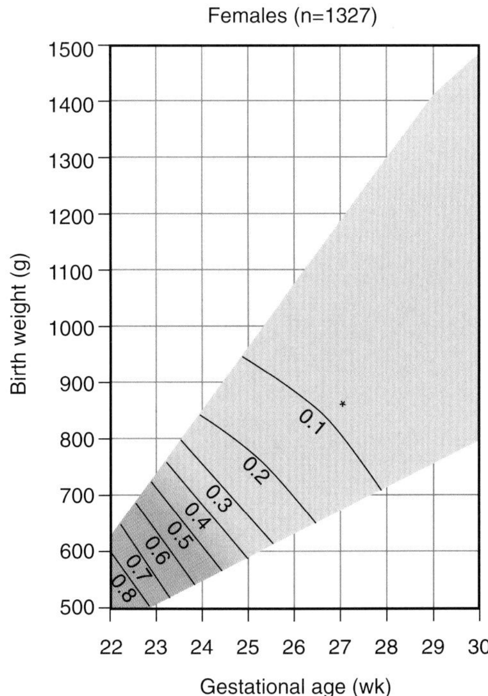

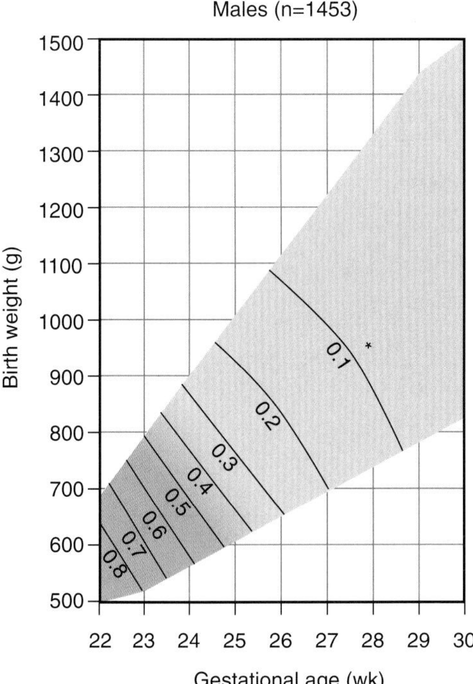

Figure 26-4. Low birth weight mortality charts for male and female infants. *, Numbers in graphs refer to mortality rate before hospital discharge for infants born alive between 22 and 30 weeks of gestation. (From Lemons JA, Bauer CR, Oh W, et al: Very low birth weight outcomes of the National Institute of Child Health and Human Development Neonatal Research Network, January 1995 through December 1996. Pediatrics 107:E1, 2001.)

delivery and lower rates of neonatal mortality for black preterm LBW infants as seen in previous studies.

Other factors that affect mortality rates for preterm and very LBW infants include advantages for infants who are female (odds ratio [OR] 0.42, 95-percent confidence interval [CI] 0.29 to 0.61), small for gestational age (OR 0.58, 95-percent CI 0.38 to 0.88), and who have antenatal treatment with corticosteroids (OR 0.52, 95-percent CI 0.36 to 0.76) or neonatal treatment with surfactant.[12,19,20] Intrauterine infection adversely influences survival and morbidity,[20] as does an expectation by the health care team that the infant will not survive.[21,22] Mortality rates also vary among neonatal intensive care units, despite similar care practices and patient demographics.[23] Thus, local statistics are preferred when counseling patients.

Perinatal Morbidity

Preterm infants are at risk for specific diseases related to the immaturity of various organ systems and the cause and circumstances of preterm birth.[24] Common complications in premature infants include respiratory distress syndrome (RDS), intraventricular hemorrhage (IVH), bronchopulmonary dysplasia (BPD), patent ductus arteriosus (PDA), necrotizing enterocolitis (NEC), sepsis, apnea, and retinopathy of prematurity. Typical rates for the most common neonatal morbidities are shown in Figure 26-5, from the dataset cited previously of 8,523 infants born in 1997 to 1998.[13]

The frequency of major morbidity rises as gestational age decreases, especially below 30 weeks. There is wide geographic variation in the frequency of neonatal morbidities especially for very LBW infants.[23] Reports of survival and morbidity also vary according to the denominator employed. Obstetric datasets include all living fetuses at entry to the obstetric suite,[25] whereas neonatal datasets exclude intrapartum and delivery room deaths and thus report rates based on newborns admitted to the nursery.[11,12] Rates of survival and morbidity at the same gestational age or birth weight are thus somewhat higher in neonatal datasets.

Long-Term Outcomes

Major neonatal morbidities related to preterm birth that carry lifetime consequences include chronic lung disease, grades III and IV IVH (associated with cerebral palsy), NEC, and vision and hearing impairment. Follow-up studies of infants born preterm and LBW infants reveal increased rates of cerebral palsy, neurosensory impairment, reduced cognition and motor performance, academic difficulties, and attention deficit disorders.[23,25–27] The incidence of long-term morbidity in survivors is especially increased for those born before 26 weeks. In a study from the United Kingdom, 78 percent of 308 survivors born before 25 weeks were followed and compared with classmates of normal birth weight. Almost all had some disability at age six: 22 percent had severe neurocognitive disabilities (cerebral palsy, intelligence quotient >3 standard deviatons below the mean, blind, or deaf), 24 percent had moderate disability, 34 percent had mild disability, and 20 percent had no neurocognitive disability.[28]

Health care workers regularly overestimate the likelihood and severity of neurologic morbidity in infants born preterm (Figs. 26-6 and 26-7).

Similarly, self-esteem among prematurely born adolescents is higher than expected. A report of self-described quality of life among 132 adolescents who weighed less

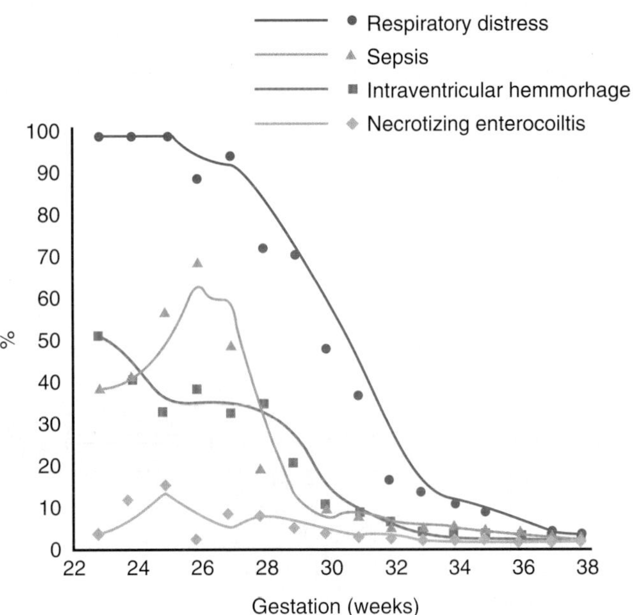

Figure 26-5. Survival and mortality rates for 8,523 infants born in 1997 to 1998 at a single U.S. center. (From Mercer BMM: Preterm Premature rupture of the membranes. Obstet Gynecol 101:178, 2003.)

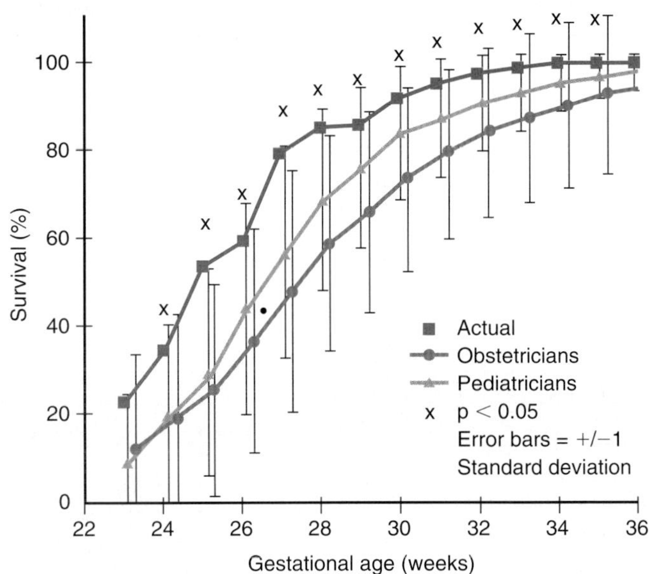

Figure 26-6. Estimated versus actual survival rates. (From Morse SB, Haywood JL, Goldenberg RL, et al: Estimation of neonatal outcome and perinatal therapy use. Pediatrics 105:1046, 2000.)

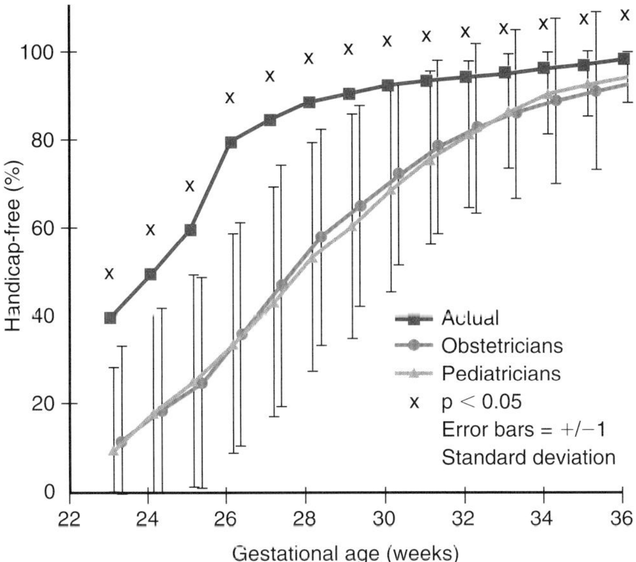

Figure 26-7. Estimated versus actual rates of handicap-free survival. (From Morse SB, Haywood JL, Goldenberg RL, et al: Estimation of neonatal outcome and perinatal therapy use. Pediatrics 105:1046, 2000.)

than 1 kg at birth found that although 24 percent had significant sensory deficits, they did not differ from controls of normal birth weight in their self-perception of global self-worth, scholastic or job competence, or social acceptance.[29]

EPIDEMIOLOGY OF PRETERM BIRTH

Numerous maternal and fetal diagnoses precede preterm birth: Preterm labor, preterm ruptured membranes, preeclampsia, abruptio placenta, multiple gestation, placenta previa, fetal growth retardation, excessive or inadequate amniotic fluid volume, fetal anomalies, amnionitis, incompetent cervix, and maternal medical problems such as diabetes, asthma, drug abuse, and pyelonephritis have been linked to preterm delivery. Maternal characteristics reported more frequently in women who deliver preterm include black ethnicity, low socioeconomic status, poor nutrition, periodontal disease, low prepregnancy weight (body mass index <19.6), absent or inadequate prenatal care, age younger than 18 years or older than 35 years, strenuous work, high level of personal stress, anemia, cigarette smoking, genitourinary colonization or infection, cervical injury or abnormality, uterine anomaly or fibroids, excessive uterine contractility, premature cervical dilation of more than 1 cm or effacement greater than 80 percent, and most strongly, a history of preterm birth.

These clinical disorders and risk factors have been usefully organized into two broad categories, *spontaneous* and *indicated,* based on the presence or absence of factors that place the mother or fetus at risk.[30–32]

Indicated preterm deliveries account for about 25 percent of preterm births in the United States, and follow medical or obstetric conditions that create undue risk for the mother (e.g., maternal sepsis or hypoxia), the fetus (e.g., poorly controlled maternal diabetes or intrauterine growth restriction), or both (e.g., maternal hypertension, placenta previa, or abruption) should the pregnancy continue. The most common diagnoses that precede an indicated preterm birth are preeclampsia (40 percent), fetal distress (25 percent), intrauterine growth restriction (10 percent), placental abruption (7 percent), and fetal demise (7 percent).[32] Illicit drug use in pregnancy, especially cocaine ingestion, has been associated with indicated preterm birth.[33] Maternal asthma has been linked to preterm birth in the past, but a recent prospective study found no relationship between the severity of asthma and the risk of preterm birth or LBW delivery.[34] Preterm and LBW were found to be related to the use of systemic, but not inhaled corticosteroids, in women with asthma in this study.[35]

Spontaneous preterm births follow preterm labor, preterm ruptured membranes, or related diagnoses such as incompetent cervix or amnionitis, when labor begins in the absence of overt maternal or fetal illness. Risk factors associated with spontaneous preterm birth include genital tract infection, nonwhite race, multiple gestation, bleeding in the second trimester, low prepregnancy weight, and a history of previous preterm birth.[36,37] Approximately 75 percent of preterm births are spontaneous.[30–32]

Epidemiologic studies of spontaneous preterm birth reveal two patterns of preterm birth characterized by the gestational age at delivery and the likelihood of recurrent preterm birth in subsequent pregnancies.[38] Births before 32 weeks' are often associated with infection, are more often followed by long-term morbidity for the infant, and are associated with a greater likelihood of recurrent preterm delivery in subsequent pregnancies. Births after 32 weeks are often associated with increased uterine contraction frequency, increased uterine volume due to hydramnios or multiple gestation; are less likely to be complicated by infection or followed by long-term morbidity; and carry a somewhat lower risk of recurrence.

CLINICAL RISK FACTORS FOR PRETERM BIRTH

Obstetric History

A history of preterm birth confers an approximately twofold increase in the risk of early delivery in subsequent pregnancies. The risk of a subsequent preterm birth rises as the number of prior preterm births increases, and it declines with each birth that is not preterm. The recurrence risk in the third pregnancy for women whose first birth was preterm and whose second birth was at term is substantially less than the risk for women with two successive preterm deliveries (Table 26-3).

Recurrent preterm birth is associated with genitourinary infection, maternal ethnicity, and the gestational age of a prior preterm birth—the earlier the birth, the greater the likelihood of recurrence.[37] Black women have rates of recurrent preterm birth that are higher than other racial and ethnic groups.[39]

There is conflicting evidence as to whether or not a history of a prior elective termination of pregnancy

Table 26-3. Risk of Preterm Delivery by Obstetrical History

		% PTB IN NEXT PREGNANCY		
FIRST BIRTH	SECOND BIRTH	N	PERCENT	RR
Term		25,817	4.4	1.0
Preterm		1,860	17.2	3.9
Term	Term	24,689	2.6	.6
Preterm	Term	1,540	5.7	1.3
Term	Preterm	1,128	11.1	2.5
Preterm	Preterm	320	28.4	6.5

PTB, preterm birth; RR, relative risk.

From Bakketeig LS, Hoffman HJ: Epidemiology of preterm birth: Results from a longitudinal study of births in Norway. *In* Elder MG, Hendricks CH (eds): Preterm Labor. London: Butterworths, 1981.

increases the risk of preterm birth. A recent study reported that an elective abortion increased the risk for subsequent preterm birth between 22 and 32 weeks of gestation (OR 1.5, 95-percent CI 1.1 to 2.0). Women with more than one elective termination had a higher risk, especially for preterm births before 28 weeks' gestation.[40]

Infection

Systemic and genital tract infections are significantly associated with preterm birth.[41] In women in spontaneous preterm labor and intact membranes, lower genital tract flora are commonly found in the amniotic fluid, placenta, and membranes. The flora include *Ureaplasma urealyticum, Mycoplasma hominis, Fusobacterium species, Gardnerella vaginalis,* peptostreptococci, and bacteroides species.[42,43] *Trichomonas vaginalis* has also been linked to preterm birth but the OR is modest (1.3, 95-percent CI 1.1 to 1.4).[44]

Clinical and histologic evidence of infection are more common as the gestational age at delivery decreases, especially before 30 to 32 weeks. Positive cultures of fetal membranes[45] and amniotic fluid[46] have been reported in 20 to 60 percent of women with preterm labor before 34 weeks' gestation. The frequency of positive cultures increases as gestational age decreases, from 20 to 30 percent after 30 weeks to 60 percent at 23 to 24 weeks' gestation. Evidence of infection is less common after 34 weeks.

Bacterial vaginosis (BV) is a condition in which the ecosystem of the vagina is altered so that gram-negative anaerobic bacteria (e.g., *Gardnerella vaginalis,* Bacteroides, Prevotella, Mobiluncus, and Mycoplasma species) largely replace the normally predominant lactobacilli. BV is associated with a twofold increased risk of spontaneous preterm birth.[47] The association between BV and preterm birth is stronger when BV is detected early in pregnancy.[48] Despite the association of BV with preterm birth, antibiotic treatment has not consistently produced a decline in preterm birth,[49–51] suggesting the mechanism of the relationship is more complex than originally thought.[52]

Infections outside the genital tract have also been related to preterm birth, most commonly to urinary tract and intra-abdominal infections, for example, pyelonephritis and appendicitis.[53] The presumed mechanism of disease is inflammation of the nearby reproductive organs, but infections at remote sites, especially if they are chronic, have also been associated with increased risk of spontaneous preterm birth. Recent literature links maternal periodontal infection and inflammation to preterm birth.[54–56] This association remains significant after adjusting for confounding variables. It is possible that the effect of periodontal disease is mediated through cytokines produced during the local inflammatory process, or by entry of periodontal organisms through the maternal circulation into the placenta. Interestingly, periodontitis is similar to BV as a condition characterized by altered host flora.

Maternal Ethnic Background

Preterm delivery occurs in black women at nearly twice the rate observed in women from other ethnic groups. In 2003, 17.8 percent of births to non-Hispanic black women occurred before 37 completed weeks' gestation, compared with 11.9 percent for Hispanic women and 11.3 percent of non-Hispanic white women.[7] The reasons for this disparity are not clear. Although the rate of preterm birth declines with advancing education among blacks, it remains higher than the rate among nonblack women at all educational levels.[57] Most but not all studies find lower rates of preterm delivery among black women born outside the United States than the 16 to 18 percent rate reported for American black women.[58–60]

Sociodemographic factors do not explain the higher rate of preterm birth in American-born black women. Several studies report consistently higher rates of preterm and LBW infants in black versus white women despite controlling for social disadvantage.[61]

BV has been studied as a potential explanation for the higher rate of preterm birth in blacks. A large observational study of vaginal flora in pregnancy found organisms associated with BV more often in black women, even when differences in health behaviors were controlled. Coital frequency and number of partners did not differ by race.[62] However, subsequent studies have not found a decline in preterm birth rates when BV was identified and successfully treated in either black or white women.[49]

Variations in host response to microbial colonization that might occur due to genetic polymorphisms that influence the inflammatory response, have been proposed as contributors to the increased rate of preterm birth in blacks.[63–67]

Environmental factors such as stress and maternal smoking may affect the risk of preterm birth by altering the inflammatory response.[68–71] It is likely that a combination of genetic and environmental factors may account for some fraction of the disparity in the frequency of preterm birth among ethnic groups. Genetic factors that control the immune response, as well as environmental factors such as chronic stress (even cultural racism), may play a role and are being investigated.[72]

The paradigm of variable response to inflammatory stimuli has been most studied for infection-driven preterm birth, but it may also apply to other risk factors.

Bleeding

Vaginal bleeding in pregnancy is a risk factor for preterm birth due to placenta previa, placental abruption, and when the origin is unclear.[31,38,73,74] Unexplained vaginal bleeding has been more strongly associated with subsequent preterm birth when it is persistent and when it occurs in white women.[75] An increase in maternal serum alpha-fetoprotein in the absence of structural fetal anomalies is a marker of fetomaternal bleeding that has also been associated with an increased incidence of preterm birth,[75,76] suggesting that occult placental hemorrhage may lead to eventual preterm delivery. The magnitude of the risk for preterm birth attributable to bleeding may be related not only to the amount and gestational age at which bleeding occurs during pregnancy, but also to the cause or causes of bleeding.

Uterine Factors

Cervical Length

When measured by transvaginal ultrasonography, cervical length is inversely and continuously related to the risk of preterm birth in both singleton[77,78] and multifetal pregnancies.[79,80] Between 18 and 32 weeks of gestation, the risk of spontaneous premature birth increases as the cervical length decreases.[77,78,81] Cervical length measurements before 16 weeks are not related to preterm birth risk, owing to increased variability of cervical length measurements as the cervix and lower segment are difficult to distinguish before 16 to 20 weeks.[82] After 16 weeks, the relationship between cervical length and preterm birth risk is evident throughout the range of cervical length: The risk rises as the length declines even for values above the median (35 mm at 24 to 28 weeks) (Fig. 26-8).

Sonographic cervical length provides an indirect assessment of cervical competence or sufficiency. Women whose cervical length at 22 to 24 weeks' gestation was at or below the 10th percentile (25 mm by endovaginal ultrasound) had a 6.5-fold increased risk (95-percent CI, 4.5 to 9.3) of preterm birth before 35 weeks' and a 7.7-fold increased risk (95-percent CI 4.5 to 13.4) of preterm birth before 32 weeks' gestation when compared with women whose cervical length measurement was greater than the 75th percentile.[79] Cervical length is strongly related to a history of spontaneous preterm birth and to the risk of recurrent preterm birth. For women with a prior preterm birth, the likelihood of recurrent preterm birth before 35 weeks declines from 31 percent when the cervical length at 24 weeks is 25 mm or less, to 16 percent when the cervical length was 26 to 35 mm, and to just 8 percent when the cervical length was 36 mm or more (35 mm = the 50th percentile). In contrast, among women whose only prior birth or births were at term, the rate of birth less than 35 weeks was 8 percent when the cervix was 25 mm or less, 4 percent when it was 26 to 35 mm, and 2 percent when it was 36 mm or more.[83] This relationship persists when other factors such as maternal ethnicity and genitourinary tract infection are controlled. The explanation for the linkage between cervical length and preterm

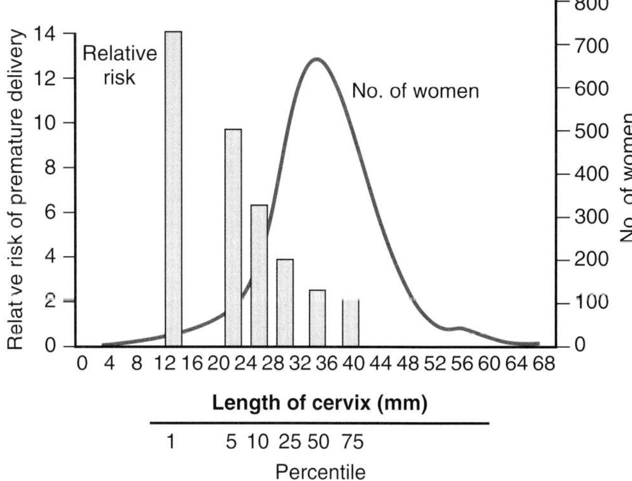

Figure 26-8. Distribution of subjects by percentile of cervical length measured by transvaginal sonography at 24 weeks *(solid line)* and relative risk of spontaneous preterm birth before 35 weeks according to percentiles of cervical length *(bars)*. Relative risk of spontaneous preterm delivery for women at the 1st, 5th, 10th, 25th, 50th, and 75th percentiles are compared with the risks among women with cervical lengths higher than the 75th percentile. (From Iams JD, Goldenberg RL, Meis PJ, et al: The length of the cervix and the risk of spontaneous premature delivery. N Engl J Med 334:567, 1996.)

birth risk is not fully elucidated, but it is likely that the normal biologic variation in size or length of the cervix is modulated by exogenous factors such as uterine volume, contractions, and genital tract infection.[84]

Congenital Abnormalities

Congenital structural abnormalities of the uterus, known as müllerian fusion defects, may affect the cervix, the uterine corpus, or both. The risk of preterm births in women with uterine malformations is 25 to 50 percent depending on the specific malformation.[85] Abnormal cervical development may cause reduced cervical sufficiency (see Chapter 25). Implantation of the placenta on a uterine septum may lead to preterm birth by means of placental separation and hemorrhage. A T-shaped uterus in women exposed in utero to diethylstilbestrol has also been associated with an increased risk of preterm labor and birth.[86]

Multiple Gestation

There is a strong association between multifetal gestation and risk of preterm birth. Rates of preterm, very preterm, LBW, and VLBW births according to fetal number are shown in Table 26-4.

The risk of early birth rises with the number of fetuses, suggesting uterine overdistention and fetal signaling as potential pathways to early initiation of labor. Nevertheless, almost 50 percent of women with twins deliver after 37 weeks, suggesting that uterine stretch or distention

Table 26-4. Preterm and Low Birth Weight Births by Number of Fetuses

BIRTHS	TWIN	TRIPLET	QUADRUPLETS	QUINTUPLETS
<32 wk	12%	36%	60%	78%
<37 wk	58%	92%	97%	91%
Mean GA	35 wk	32 wk	30 wk	28 wk
<1.5 kg	10%	34%	61%	84%
<2.5 kg	55%	94%	99%	94%

GA, gestational age.

From Centers for Disease Control and Prevention: Use of assisted reproductive technology. MMWR 51:97–101, 2002.

Table 26-5. Perinatal Outcomes in Singletons After IVF Meta-Analysis of 15 Studies

Data from 12,283 IVF and 1,900,000 spontaneous births

■ Perinatal mortality ↑ in IVF	(OR 2.2, CI 1.6, 3.0)
■ Preterm birth ↑ in IVF	(OR 2.0, CI 1.7, 2.2)
■ Low birth weight ↑ in IVF	(OR 1.8, CI 1.4, 2.2)
■ Very low birth weight ↑ in IVF	(OR 2.7, CI 2.3, 3.1)
■ SGA ↑ in IVF	(OR 1.6, CI 1.3, 2.0)

IVF, in vitro fertilization; OR, odds ratio; SGA, small for gestational age.

Data from Jackson RA, Gibson KA, et al: Perinatal outcomes in singletons following in vitro fertilization: A meta-analysis. Obstet Gynecol 103:551, 2004.

Table 26-6. Perinatal Outcomes in Singletons After IVF, SART, ASRM, and CDC Study 1996–2000

ART Singletons in 2000 had:

↑ Low birth weight—RR 1.62, CI 1.49 to 1.75
↑ Very low birth weight—RR 1.79, CI 1.45 to 2.12
↑ Preterm birth—RR 1.41, CI 1.32 to 1.51
↑ Preterm (1.74) and term (1.39) low birth weight/IUGR

ART, assisted reproductive techniques; ASRM, American Society for Reproductive Medicine; CDC, Centers for Disease Control and Prevention; CI, 95% confidence interval; IUGR, intrauterine growth restriction; IVF, in vitro fertilization; RR, risk ratio; SART, Society for Assisted Reproductive Technology.

Data from Schieve LA, Ferre C, Peterson HB, et al: Perinatal outcome among singleton infants conceived through assisted reproductive technology in the United States. Obstet Gynecol 103:1144, 2004, and ACOG Committee Opinion #324: Perinatal risks associated with assisted reproductive technology. Obstet Gynecol 106:1143, 2005.

is variably accommodated according to other maternal characteristics including cervical length,[80] physical activity, uterine tone, and the presence or absence of other risk factors.

In addition to spontaneous preterm labor, multiple gestations are more commonly complicated by medical and obstetric disorders that lead to preterm delivery. Discordant fetal growth, fetal anomalies, hypertension, abruptio placenta, and fetal compromise are more common in multiple gestation, and increase with the number of fetuses.[87]

Infants born of multifetal gestation contribute disproportionately to perinatal mortality and morbidity. Newman and Luke[89] estimated the contribution of multiple gestation to perinatal mortality and morbidity, and found that multiple gestations, while accounting for 2.9 percent of all births, were associated with 13 percent of perinatal deaths, 16 percent of neonatal deaths, 10 percent of fetal deaths, and 15 percent of cases of cerebral palsy.

As the incidence of multiple gestation has increased owing to ART,[89] the proportion of preterm births caused by multiple gestation has also increased.[90] Of 31,582 births after ART in the United States in 2000, 45.6 percent were singletons, 44.5 percent were twins, 9.3 percent were triplets, and 0.6 percent were higher order (more than three fetuses).[91] In Europe, 26.3 percent of ART pregnancies result in a multifetal gestation owing to the European practice of limiting the number of embryos placed in the uterus after in vitro fertilization. Increased attention in the United States to the issue of higher order multiples has led to a plateau in the previously rising rate of such pregnancies.[92]

Assisted Reproductive Technologies

Preterm and LBW deliveries occur more commonly in pregnancies conceived after ovulation induction and ART including in vitro fertilization (IVF) and gamete and zygote intrafallopian transfer, frozen embryo transfer, and donor embryo transfer.[93] The increased rate of preterm birth after ART is due not only to the increased occurrence of multiple gestations but to an increased rate of preterm births in singleton pregnancies as well. Although rates of LBW, VLBW, and preterm birth decreased for singleton ART pregnancies between 1996 and 2000, they were still significantly higher than spontaneously conceived singleton gestations, with a relative risk of 1.41 (95-percent CI 1.32 to 1.51).[94] A meta-analysis of 15 studies that compared 12,283 IVF pregnancies with 1.9 million spontaneously conceived singleton births found approximately twofold increased rates of perinatal mortality, preterm birth, LBW and VLBW and small for gestational age for infants born after IVF[95] (Tables 26-5 and 26-6). A twofold increased risk has been reported by others[96,97] and Helmerhorst et al. found a threefold increased risk of births before 32 weeks in a review of 27 studies (RR 3.27, 95-percent CI 2.03 to 5.28). Rates of preterm birth among multiple gestations do not appear to be increased for ART relative to spontaneously conceived twins and triplets, so the explanation for the increased rates for ART singletons is not clear. Microbial colonization of the upper genital tract,[98] increased stress among infertility patients, side effects of superovulation,[99] and increased rates of birth defects[100] have been proposed.

Lifestyle-Related Risks for Preterm Birth

Maternal stress, maternal cigarette smoking, sexual practices, and the nature, duration, and intensity of work have been suggested to contribute to risk for preterm birth. Smoking has been consistently related to preterm as well as LBW deliveries, particularly to preterm ruptured membranes.[101,102] A possible relationship between sexual activity and preterm birth is based on observations of increased contraction frequency following coitus[103] and to sexual activity as an opportunity to acquire genital tract infections that could influence preterm birth risk, but data to establish an increased risk are lacking. The duration and intensity of work were reported to be risk factors for preterm birth in 1984,[104] but more recent data show only a modest relationship between physically demanding work and preterm birth.[105,106]

PATHOPHYSIOLOGY*

Term and preterm parturition share anatomic, physiologic, and biochemical features that are considered part of the common pathway of parturition. This pathway includes (1) increased uterine contractility, (2) cervical ripening, and (3) membrane/decidual activation. However, although spontaneous labor at term results from physiologic activation of the common pathway of parturition, preterm labor/delivery is the result of a pathologic activation of this pathway. The insult responsible for activation may lead to asynchronous recruitment of each pathway. Asynchrony is recognized clinically as (1) cervical insufficiency when the process affects predominantly the cervix; (2) preterm uterine contractions when the process affects the myometrium; or (3) preterm premature rupture of membranes if the insult targets the chorioamniotic membranes. Synchronous activation in the preterm gestation would be labeled as preterm labor with intact membranes. Whether at or before term, parturition culminates in a common pathway composed of cervical changes, persistent uterine contractions, and activation of the decidua and membranes. The fundamental difference is that labor at term is a normal physiologic activation of the common pathway, whereas preterm parturition is the result, entirely or in part, of pathologic processes that activate one or more of the components of the common pathway.

Although labor is of short duration (hours or days at the most), parturition is a longer process that includes a preparatory phase of the key organs involved in the common pathway. Thus, cervical changes occur over weeks, there is increased myometrial contractility before the onset of labor, and the appearance of fetal fibronectin in the cervicovaginal mucous can be considered to reflect extracellular matrix degradation, indicating activation of the decidua and membranes.

Normal parturition at term is currently understood as beginning several weeks before actual labor during which cervical ripening occurs as evidenced by changes in cervical consistency and effacement. A fetal maturity-based signal for labor originates in the fetal hypothalamus and leads to increased secretion of corticotropin-releasing hormone, which, in turn, stimulates adrenocorticotrophic hormone and cortisol production by the fetal adrenals,[107–109] which ultimately leads to activation of the common pathway of parturition.[110,111] The fetus may contribute to the onset of preterm labor in the context of the fetal inflammatory response syndrome (see later).[112,113]

Spontaneous preterm birth may best be understood as a syndrome, in which the clinical presentations of preterm labor, preterm ruptured membranes, and preterm cervical effacement and dilation without labor occur as the result of multiple etiologies that can occur alone or in combination. Some act to initiate preterm parturition acutely, for example, an acute post-traumatic placental abruption, but most follow a more subacute or indolent path over several weeks. It is helpful to remember that the normal process of parturition proceeds for several weeks before clinically evident labor begins.[114] Thus, pathological stimuli of parturition may act in concert with the normal physiologic preparation for labor, especially after 32 weeks of pregnancy. Before 30 to 32 weeks, a greater degree of pathologic stimulus may be required to initiate labor.

A fetal contribution to the genesis of preterm labor is also suggested by comparison of birth weights of infants born preterm to fetal weights at the same gestational ages for infants ultimately born at term.[115,116] Similar data from Gardosi et al.[117] (Fig. 26-9) show a skewed distribution of birth weights at 32 weeks' gestation.

Cervical Changes (Ripening)

The remarkable task of the cervix is to facilitate conception, retain the conceptus throughout pregnancy, dilate to allow safe delivery, and to repeat this process in subsequent pregnancies. These functions depend on regulation of the extracellular matrix, which is composed of collagen, elastin, and fibronectin. Collagen is

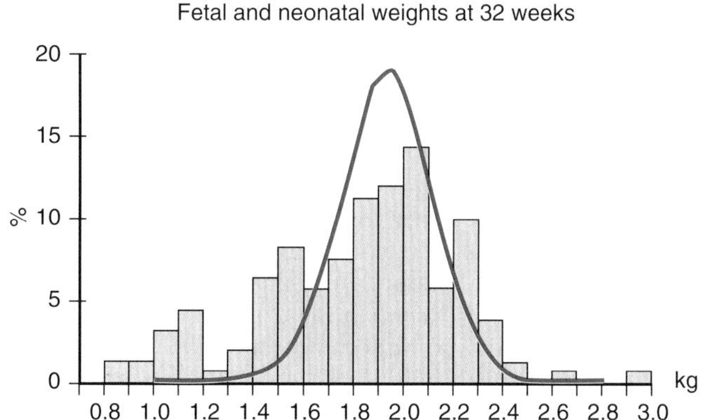

Figure 26-9. Impairment of growth in fetuses destined to deliver preterm (*blue bars*) compared to in utero weights of fetuses at same gestational age born at term (*red line*). (From Gardosi JO: Prematurity and fetal growth restriction. Early Hum Dev 81:43, 2005.)

*This section is based substantially on a chapter by Romero et al. (Romero R, Espinoza J, Mazor M, Chaiworapongsa T: The preterm parturition syndrome. *In* Critchley H, Bennett P, Thornton S (eds): Preterm Birth. London, RCOG Press, 2004, pp 28–60) with the permission of the publisher.

the principal determinant of the tensile strength of the cervix. Cervical ripening occurs as the consequence of decreased total collagen content, increased collagen solubility, and increased collagenolytic activity by collagenase and leucocyte elastase. Extracellular matrix turnover in the cervix is high, and thus, the mechanical properties of the cervix can change rapidly.[118] Changes in extracellular matrix during cervical ripening include an influx of inflammatory cells (macrophages, neutrophils, mast cells, eosinophils, and so on) into the cervical stroma in a process similar to an inflammatory response. These cells produce cytokines and prostaglandins that affect extracellular matrix metabolism.[119–123] Prostaglandins effect cervical ripening physiologically and have been widely used as pharmacological agents to ripen the cervix for induction of labor. Cervical ripening is influenced by estrogen, which induces ripening by stimulating collagen degradation, and by progesterone, which blocks these estrogenic effects. Furthermore, administration of progesterone receptor antagonist can induce cervical ripening,[124] and administration of progesterone has been reported to reverse ripening.[125] Another mediator implicated in the mechanisms of cervical ripening is nitric oxide (NO),[126] which can act as an inflammatory mediator.[127–129] Animal and human studies have found that the inducible form of nitric oxide synthase (iNOS) and NO production in the cervix increase during labor,[130] that administration of L-nitro-arginine methylester (a nonspecific inhibitor of iNOS) blocks cervical ripening,[130] and that direct application of sodium nitroprusside, a NO donor, to the cervix can induce cervical ripening.[131–135]

Cervical changes normally precede the onset of labor, are gradual, and develop over several weeks.[136] Preterm birth is often preceded by cervical ripening over a period of weeks in the second and third trimesters, evidenced in clinical examination by softening and thinning of the cervix[137] and in ultrasound examination of the cervix by cervical "funneling" and shortening of the length of the endocervical canal.[77,78]

Increased Uterine Contractility

Labor is characterized by a change in uterine contractility from episodic uncoordinated myometrial contractures that last several minutes and produce little increase in intrauterine pressure to more coordinated contractions of short duration that produce marked increases in intrauterine pressure that ultimately effect delivery.[138,139] The change from the contracture to the contraction pattern typically begins at night, suggesting neural control.[140,141] The transition from contractures to contractions may progress to normal labor[142] or may occur dyssynchronously as the result of inflammation, for example, with maternal infection or abdominal surgery.[143–145] Fasting may also induce the switch in humans.[146,147] Oxytocin is produced by the decidua and the paraventricular nuclei of the hypothalamus, indicating both an endocrine and paracrine role.[148–156] Plasma concentrations of oxytocin mirror uterine contractility,[140] suggesting that oxytocin may mediate the circadian rhythm in uterine contractility.

Cellular communication is another feature of labor, promulgated by formation of gap junctions that develop in the myometrium before labor and disappear after delivery.[157–161] Gap junction formation and the expression of the gap junction protein connexin 43 in human myometrium is similar in term and preterm labor.[162–166] These findings suggest that the appearance of gap junctions and increased expression of connexin 43 may be part of the underlying molecular and cellular events responsible for the switch from contractures to contractions before the onset of parturition. Estrogen, progesterone and prostaglandins have been implicated in the regulation of gap junction formation, as well as in influencing the expression of connexin 43.[167–169] Lye et al.[164,170,171] have proposed that changes in a set of distinct proteins called "contraction-associated proteins" is characteristic of this stage of parturition.

Decidual Membrane Activation

The maternal decidua and adjacent fetal membranes undergo anatomic and biochemical changes over the final weeks of gestation that ultimately result in spontaneous rupture of membranes. Premature activation of this mechanism leads to preterm prelabor rupture of membranes (PROM), the clinical antecedent for up to 40 percent of all preterm deliveries. Although rupture of membranes normally occurs during the first stage of labor, histologic studies of prematurely ruptured membranes show decreased amounts of collagen types I, III, and V and an increased expression of tenascin (expressed during tissue remodelling and wound healing) and disruption of the normal wavy collagen pattern,[172] suggesting that preterm rupture is a process that precedes the onset of labor.

Structural extracellular matrix proteins such as collagens have been implicated in the tensile strength of the membranes, whereas the viscoelastic properties were attributed to elastin.[173,174] Dissolution of extracellular cements (i.e., fibronectins) is thought to be responsible for the process that allows the membranes to separate from the decidua after the birth of the infant.[175–179] Degradation of the extracellular matrix, assessed by the detection of oncofetal fibronectin, is part of the common pathway of parturition. The presence of fetal fibronectin in cervicovaginal secretions between 22 and 37 weeks is evidence of disruption of the decidual-chorionic interface and is associated with an increased risk of preterm birth.

The precise mechanism of membrane-decidual activation is uncertain, but matrix-degrading enzymes and apoptosis (programmed cell death) have been proposed. Increased levels of matrix metalloproteinase 1 (MMP-1) (interstitial collagenase),[180] MMP-8 (neutrophil collagenase),[181] MMP-9 (gelatinase-B) and neutrophil elastase[182] has been documented in the amniotic fluid of women with preterm PROM.[183] Regulation of tissue inhibitors of MMPs (TIMPs) may also participate.[184]

Apoptosis may also play a role in the mechanism of membrane rupture,[185,186] through increased expression of proapoptotic genes and decreased expression of antiapoptotic genes.[187] MMP-9 may induce apoptosis in amnion.[188–190]

Fetal Participation in the Onset of Labor

A fetal signal contributes to the onset of labor in animals and humans. Destruction of the paraventricular nucleus of the fetal hypothalamus results in prolongation of pregnancy in sheep.[191,192] The human counterpart to this animal experiment is anencephaly, which is also characterized by prolonged pregnancy when women with polyhydramnios are excluded.[193] The current paradigm is that once maturity has been reached, the fetal brain, specifically the hypothalamus, increases corticotrophin-releasing hormone (CRH) secretion, which, in turn, stimulates adrenocorticotrophic hormone (ACTH) and cortisol production by the fetal adrenals.[107–109] This increase in cortisol in sheep and dehydroepiandrosterone sulfate in primates eventually leads to activation of the common pathway of parturition.[110,111] A role for the human fetus in the onset of preterm labor has been proposed in the context of the fetal inflammatory response syndrome.[112,113]

The Preterm Parturition Syndrome

Obstetric taxonomy is largely based on clinical presentation, not the mechanism of disease. Premature labor may occur as the common clinical presentation of infection, vascular insult, uterine overdistension, abnormal allogeneic recognition, stress, or other pathologic processes. Often more than one of these factors is operative in the same patient. Thus, preterm labor is a syndrome for which there is no single diagnostic test or treatment. Obstetric syndromes[194] share the following features:

- Multiple etiologies
- Chronicity
- Fetal involvement
- Clinical manifestations that are adaptive
- Variable susceptibility due to gene-environment interactions.

Each of these features are true of preterm birth. There are clearly *multiple etiologies* for preterm labor, as listed earlier. Pathways to preterm labor are demonstrated to be *chronic,* as seen in the time interval between observation of a short cervix or increased concentrations of fetal fibronectin in vaginal fluid in the midtrimester of pregnancy and subsequent preterm labor or delivery.[47,195–197] *Fetal involvement* has been demonstrated in women with microbial invasion of the amniotic cavity, in which fetal bacteremia and cytokine production have been detected in 30 percent of women with preterm PROM and a positive amniotic fluid culture for microorganisms.[198] Similarly, neonates born after spontaneous preterm labor or preterm PROM are more likely to be small for gestational age, suggesting chronically compromised fetal supply.[115,116,199–203] Preterm labor may be seen as an *adaptive* mechanism of host defense against infection that allows the mother to eliminate an infected tissue and the fetus to exit from a hostile environment.[112,204] If the clinical manifestations are adaptive, it is not surprising that treatments aimed at the common terminal pathway of parturition, such as tocolysis or cerclage, and not at the fundamental mechanism of disease-inducing activation of the pathway (myometrial contractility, cervical dilatation and effacement), would not be effective. There is increasing evidence of gene-environment interaction in the steps leading to preterm labor, complicated by the presence, and even perhaps the conflicting interests, of two genomes (maternal and fetal). This is most evident in studies of the relationship between maternal genital tract colonization and preterm birth. Finally, there may be additional mechanisms not yet identified.

Pathologic processes implicated in the preterm parturition syndrome include intrauterine infection, uterine ischemia, uterine overdistention, abnormal allograft reaction, allergy-induced, cervical insufficiency, and endocrine disorders (Fig. 26-10).

Intrauterine Infection

Systemic maternal infections such as pyelonephritis and pneumonia are frequently associated with the onset of premature labor in humans.[205–217] Intrauterine infection is a frequent and important mechanism of disease leading to preterm delivery.[43,218–220] Intrauterine infection or systemic administration of microbial products to pregnant animals can result in preterm labor and delivery,[221–230] and there is substantial evidence that subclinical intrauterine infections are associated with preterm labor and delivery.[231] Moreover, fetal infection and inflammation have been implicated in the genesis of fetal or neonatal injury leading to cerebral palsy and chronic lung disease. Microbiologic and histopathologic studies suggest that infection-related inflammation may account for 25 to 40 percent of cases of preterm delivery.[232]

Frequency of Intrauterine Infection in Spontaneous Preterm Birth

The prevalence of positive amniotic fluid cultures for microorganisms in women with preterm labor and intact membranes is approximately 13 percent.[233] The earlier the gestational age at preterm birth, the more likely that microbial invasion of the amniotic cavity is present.[46] In preterm PROM, the prevalence of positive amniotic fluid cultures for microorganisms is approximately 32 percent.[233] Among women presenting with a dilated cervix in the midtrimester, the prevalence of positive amniotic fluid cultures is 51 percent.[234] Microbial invasion of the amniotic cavity occurs in 12 percent of twin gestations presenting with preterm labor and delivering a preterm neonate.[235,236] The most common microorganisms found in the amniotic cavity are *genital Mycoplasmas* and *U. urealyticum.*

Intrauterine Infection as a Chronic Process

Evidence in support of chronicity of intrauterine inflammation/infection is derived from studies of the microbiologic state of the amniotic fluid, as well as the concentration of inflammatory mediators at the

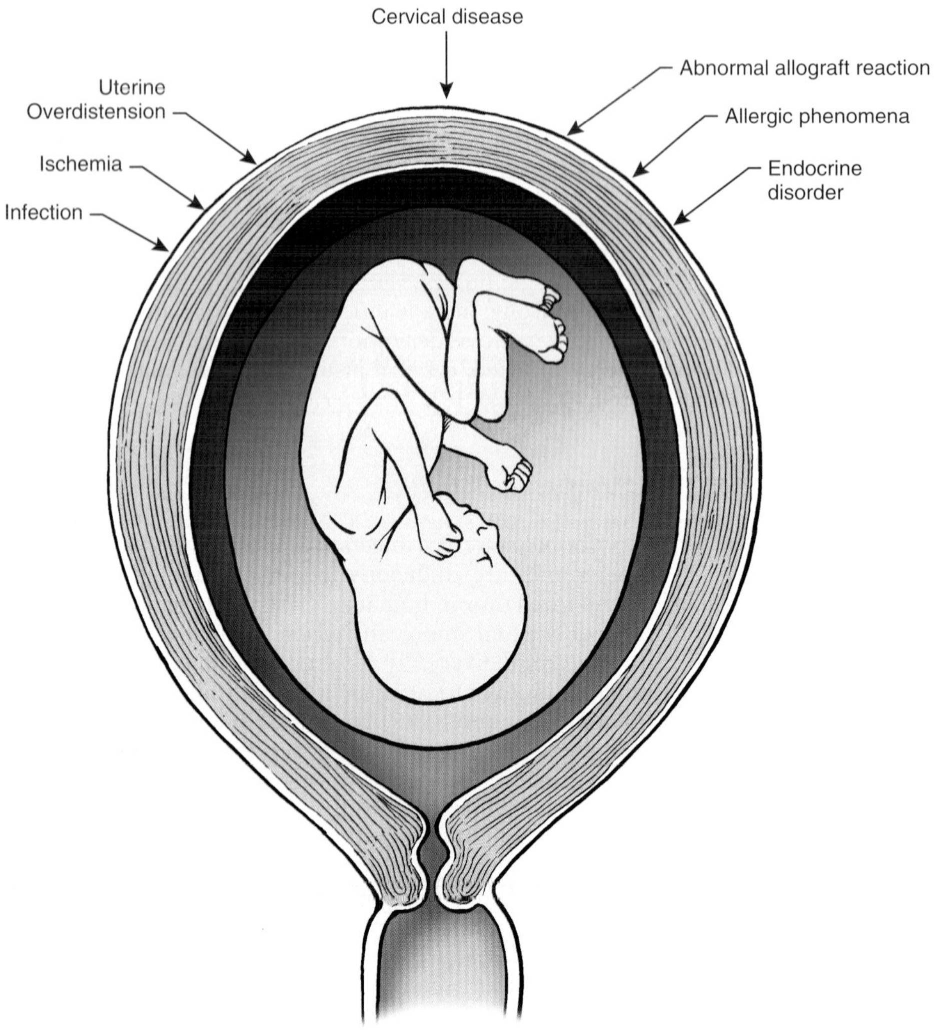

Figure 26-10. Pathological processes implicated in the preterm parturition syndrome include intrauterine infection, uterine ischemia, uterine overdistension, abnormal allograft reaction, allergy-induced, cervical insufficiency and endocrine disorders. (From Romero R, Espinoza J, Mazor M, Chaiworapongsa T: The preterm parturition syndrome. *In* Critchley H, Bennett P, Thornton S [eds]: Preterm Birth. London, RCOG Press, 2004, pp 28–60.)

time of genetic amniocentesis. Genital mycoplasmas including *M. hominis* and *U. urealyticum* have been recovered from amniotic fluid samples obtained at second-trimester genetic amniocentesis,[237–239] with subsequent preterm delivery and histologic chorioamnionitis, especially in those with *U. urealyticum.*[240] Increased levels of inflammatory markers such as interleukin 6 (IL-6),[240–242] MMP-8,[243] tumor necrosis factor-α (TNF-α),[244] and angiogenin[244a] have been found in second-trimester amniotic fluid samples obtained from women who subsequently delivered preterm. These observations suggest that microbial invasion of the amniotic cavity in the midtrimester of pregnancy can lead to pregnancy loss or preterm delivery weeks later. The most advanced stage of ascending intrauterine infection is fetal infection. Fetal bacteremia has been detected in blood obtained by cordocentesis in 33 percent of fetuses with positive amniotic fluid culture and 4 percent of those with negative amniotic fluid culture.[198]

Molecular mediators that trigger parturition (cytokines and other inflammatory mediators) are similar to those that protect the host against infection. The onset of preterm labor in response to intrauterine infection is thus very likely a host defense mechanism with survival value for mother and, after viability, for the fetus as well.

Infection, Preterm Labor, and Neonatal Outcomes

The scenario postulated from the preceding evidence is that microorganisms that reside in or ascend to reach the decidua may, depending on host defense and environmental influences, stimulate a local inflammatory reaction as well as the production of proinflammatory cytokines, chemokines, and inflammatory mediators (platelet activating factor, prostaglandins, leucotrienes, reactive oxygen species, NO, and so on). This inflammatory process, which is initially extra-amniotic, may produce cervical effacement, further inflammation of the choriodecidual interface, uterine contractions, may progress to the amniotic fluid and, ultimately, the fetus as well. Microorganisms are known to cross intact membranes into the amniotic cavity, where inflammatory mediators are produced by resident macrophages and other host cells within the amniotic cavity.[245–248] Finally, microorganisms that gain access to the fetus may elicit a systemic inflammatory response, the fetal inflammatory response syndrome (FIRS), characterized by increased concentrations of IL-6[204] and other cytokines,[249–251] as well as cellular evidence of neutrophil and monocyte activation.[252] FIRS is a subclinical condition originally described in fetuses of mothers presenting with preterm labor and intact membranes and preterm PROM.[204] IL-6 is a major mediator of the host response to infection and tissue damage, and is capable of eliciting biochemical, physiologic, and immunologic changes in the host, including stimulation of the production of C-reactive protein by liver cells, activation of T and natural killer cells, and so on. Fetuses with FIRS have a higher rate of neonatal complications and are frequently born to mothers with subclinical microbial invasion of the amniotic cavity.[191] Evidence of multisystemic involvement in cases of FIRS includes increased concentrations of fetal plasma MMP-9,[250] neutrophilia, a higher number of circulating nucleated red blood cells, and higher plasma concentrations of G-CSF.[249] The histologic hallmark of FIRS is inflammation in the umbilical cord (funisitis) or chorionic vasculitis.[253] The systemic fetal inflammatory response may result in multiple organ dysfunction,[254] septic shock, and death in the absence of timely delivery. Newborns with funisitis are at increased risk for neonatal sepsis[255] as well as long-term handicap, including BPD[256] and cerebral palsy.[257,258]

When the inflammatory process does not involve the chorioamniotic membranes and decidua, systemic fetal inflammation and injury may occur in the absence of labor with eventual delivery at term. An example of this is fetal alloimmunization in which there is an elevation of fetal plasma concentrations of interleukin 6, but not preterm labor.

Gene-Environment Interactions

Gene-environment interactions underlie many complex disorders such as atherosclerosis and cancer. A gene-environment interaction is said to be present when the risk of a disease (occurrence or severity) among individuals exposed (to both genotype and an environmental factor) is greater or lower than that which is predicted from the presence of either the genotype or the environmental exposure alone.[259,260] The inflammatory response to the presence of microorganisms is modulated by interactions between the host genotype and environment that determine the likelihood and course of some infectious diseases. An example of such an interaction has been reported for BV, an allele for TNF-α and preterm delivery. Maternal BV is a consistently reported risk factor for spontaneous preterm delivery,[47,195–197] yet treatment of BV does not reliably prevent preterm birth in women with BV.[49–51,66,261–271] One potential explanation has come from a study of preterm birth rates in women according to their carriage of BV and whether or not they had allele 2 of TNF-α known to be associated with spontaneous preterm birth.[66] Both BV (OR 3.3; 95-percent CI 1.8 to 5.9) and TNF-α allele 2 (OR 2.7; 95-percent CI 1.7 to 4.5) were associated with increased risk for preterm delivery, but the risk of spontaneous preterm birth was substantially increased (OR 6; 95-percent CI 1.9 to 21.0) in women with both BV and the TNF-α allele 2, suggesting that a gene-environmental interaction predisposes to preterm birth. It is reasonable to assume that other gene-environment interactions, such as intrauterine infection, microbial invasion of the fetus, membrane integrity, uterine contractile response, and the likelihood of perinatal injury, may influence other aspects of preterm parturition.

Uteroplacental Ischemia/ Decidual Hemorrhage

After inflammation, the most common abnormalities seen in placental pathology specimens from spontaneous preterm births are vascular lesions of the maternal and fetal circulations.[273] Maternal lesions include failure of physiologic transformation of the spiral arteries, atherosis, and thrombosis. Fetal abnormalities include decreased number of villous arterioles and fetal arterial thrombosis.

One proposed mechanism linking vascular lesions and preterm labor/delivery is uteroplacental ischemia, evidenced in primate models[274] and in studies that found failure of physiologic transformation in the myometrial segment of the spiral arteries, a phenomenon typical of pre-eclampsia and intrauterine growth restriction, in women with preterm labor and intact membranes and preterm PROM as well.[275,276] Abnormal uterine artery Doppler velocimetry indicating increased impedance to flow in the uterine circulation has been reported in women with apparently idiopathic preterm labor.[277–279] Finally, the frequency of small-for-gestational-age infants is increased in women delivering after preterm labor with intact membranes and preterm PROM.[115,116,199–203]

The mechanisms responsible for preterm parturition in cases of ischemia have not been determined, but uterine ischemia has been postulated to lead to increased production of uterine renin[280,281] from the fetal membranes.[282] Angiotensin II can induce myometrial contractility directly[283] or through the release of prostaglandins.[284]

Uteroplacental ischemia may also lead to decidual necrosis and hemorrhage, and activation of parturition through production of thrombin, which stimulates myometrial contractility in a dose-dependent manner.[285,286] Thrombin also stimulates production of MMP-1,[287] urokinase-type plasminogen activator (uPA), and tissue-type plasminogen activator (tPA) by endometrial stromal cells in culture.[288] MMP-1 can digest collagen directly, whereas urokinase-type plasminogen activator and tissue-type plasminogen activator catalyse the transformation of plasminogen into plasmin, which, in turn, can degrade type III collagen and fibronectin,[289] important components of the extracellular matrix in the chorioamniotic membranes.[290] Thrombin/antithrombin complexes, a marker of in vivo generation of thrombin, are increased in plasma[291] and amniotic fluid[292] of women with preterm labor and preterm PROM. Decidua is a rich source of tissue factor, the primary initiator of coagulation and of thrombin activation.[292] These observations are consistent with clinical associations among vaginal bleeding, retroplacental hematomas, and preterm delivery.[294–298]

Uterine ischemia should not be equated with fetal hypoxemia. Studies of fetal cord blood do not support fetal hypoxemia as a cause of preterm parturition.[299,300]

Uterine Overdistention

The mechanisms responsible for the increased frequency of preterm birth in multiple gestations and other disorders associated with uterine overdistension are unknown.[301–305] Central questions are how the uterus senses stretch, and how these mechanical forces induce biochemical changes that lead to parturition. Increased expression of oxytocin receptor,[306] connexin 43,[166] and the *c-fos* mRNA have been consistently demonstrated in the rat myometrium near term.[307–311] Progesterone blocks stretch-induced gene expression in the myometrium.[171] Mitogen-activated protein kinases have been proposed to mediate stretch-induced *c-fos* mRNA expression in myometrial smooth muscle cells.[307–311] Stretch can have effects on the chorioamniotic membranes.[312–326] For example, in vitro studies have demonstrated an increase in the production of collagenase, IL-8,[122,318] and prostaglandin E_2 (PGE_2),[317] as well as the cytokine pre–B-cell colony-enhancing factor.[321] These observations provide a possible link between the mechanical forces operating in an overdistended uterus and rupture of membranes.

Abnormal Allograft Reaction

The fetoplacental unit has been considered nature's most successful semiallograft. Abnormal recognition and adaptation to fetal antigens has been proposed as a mechanism of recurrent pregnancy loss, intrauterine growth restriction, and pre-eclampsia.[327–329] Chronic villitis, a lesion indicative of placental rejection, has been found in the placentas of some women who deliver after spontaneous preterm labor.[330]

Allergy-Induced Preterm Labor

Case reports indicate that preterm labor has occurred after exposure to an allergen that generates an allergic-like mechanism (type I hypersensitivity reaction) and that a subgroup of patients with preterm labor have eosinophils as the predominant cells in amniotic fluid,[331–333] suggesting a form of uterine allergy. There is substantial evidence to support this hypothesis. Mast cells present in the uterus produce histamine and prostaglandins, both of which can induce myometrial contractility.[334,335] Premature labor and delivery can be induced by exposure to an allergen in sensitized animals, and can be prevented by treatment with a histamine H_1 receptor antagonist.[336]

Cervical Insufficiency

Although cervical insufficiency (formerly called cervical incompetence) is traditionally considered a cause of midtrimester delivery, accumulating evidence suggests that it also is a contributing factor to spontaneous preterm births before 32 weeks' gestation.[337] The understanding of cervical function has changed from a categorical concept of cervical "incompetence" versus "competence" to one in which cervical function is described by a bell curve.[78,338] The risk of spontaneous preterm birth increases as cervical length decreases, with the greatest risk for spontaneous preterm birth in women whose cervical length lies below the 5th to 10th percentile (see Fig. 26-8). Cervical insufficiency may be the result of a congenital disorder (e.g., hypoplastic cervix or diethylstilboestrol exposure in utero), surgical trauma (e.g., conization resulting in substantial loss of connective tissue) or traumatic damage to the structural integrity of the cervix (e.g., repeated cervical dilatation associated with termination of pregnancy).[339] Some cases presenting with the clinical characteristics of cervical insufficiency may be due to infection, estimated to include as many as 50 percent of women presenting with acute cervical insufficiency.[234] The optimal means to diagnose cervical insufficiency, the role of cervical length determination during pregnancy in the prediction of preterm birth, and of cerclage in its prevention are discussed in Chapter 25.

Endocrine Disorders

Estrogen and progesterone play a central role in the endocrinology of pregnancy.[340] Progesterone is thought to maintain myometrial quiescence, down-regulate gap junction formation, and inhibit cervical ripening.[341–343] Estrogens have been implicated in increasing myometrial contractility and excitability, as well as in the induction of cervical ripening prior to the onset of labor.[342,343] In many species, a fall in maternal serum progesterone concentration occurs before spontaneous parturition, but the mechanism for this progesterone withdrawal depends primarily on whether the placenta or the corpus luteum is the major source of progesterone.[344,345]

A fall in serum progesterone levels has not been demonstrated before parturition in humans. Nevertheless, inhibition of progesterone action could result in parturition.[340,341,346,347] Alternative mechanisms posited to explain a suspension of progesterone action without a serum progesterone withdrawal include binding of progesterone to a high-affinity protein and, thus, reduced functional active form[348,349]; increased cortisol concentration that competes with progesterone for binding to the glucocorticoid receptors, resulting in functional progesterone withdrawal[350]; and conversion of progesterone to an inactive form within the target cell before interacting with its receptor.[351,352] None of these hypotheses are proven.[353] Recent research has focused on alterations in the number and function of estrogen-progesterone receptors and progesterone binding.[354–356]

The human progesterone receptor (PR) exists as two major subtypes, PR-A and PR-B. Another isoform, PR-C, has recently been described, but its function is not well understood. The human estrogen receptor (ER) also exists as two major subtypes, ERα and ERβ. A functional progesterone withdrawal has been proposed in which expression of PR-A in myometrium suppresses progesterone responsiveness and that functional progesterone withdrawal occurs by increased expression of the ERα.[357] An alternative mechanism of functional progesterone withdrawal has been proposed wherein activation of nuclear factor κ B in amnion represses progesterone function.[358–362] Regardless of the mechanism, there is a consensus that a localized functional progesterone withdrawal occurs in intrauterine tissues during human parturition. Changes in the ratio of estrogen and progesterone receptors can activate the three components of the common pathway of parturition.

However, the pathologic mechanisms responsible for suspension of progesterone action in preterm parturition remain to be elucidated. In the case of infection, IL-1 and TNF-α can induce activation of nuclear factor κ B and this, in turn, may influence progesterone function.[358]

Summary of the Preterm Parturition Syndrome

Preterm parturition is a syndrome caused by multiple etiologies with several clinical presentations including uterine contractility (preterm labor), preterm cervical ripening without significant clinical contractility (cervical insufficiency or advanced cervical dilation and effacement), or rupture of the amniotic sac (preterm PROM). The clinical presentation varies with the type and timing of the insult or stimulus to the components of the common pathway of parturition, the presence or absence of environmental cofactors, and individual variations in host response by both mother and fetus. This conceptual framework has implications for the understanding of the mechanisms responsible for the initiation of preterm parturition, as well as the diagnosis, treatment, and prevention of preterm birth.

CLINICAL CARE FOR WOMEN IN PRETERM LABOR

Clinical evaluation of preterm parturition begins with assessment of potential causes of labor, looking first for conditions that threaten the health of mother and fetus. Acute maternal conditions, for example, pyelonephritis, pneumonia, asthma, peritonitis, trauma, and hypertension, or obstetric conditions including preeclampsia, placental abruption, placenta previa, and chorioamnionitis may mandate delivery. Fetal compromise may be acute, manifested by an abnormal fetal heart rate tracing, or chronic, indicated by fetal growth restriction or oligohydramnios, and may require delivery depending on the severity and potential for *in utero* versus *ex utero* treatment. Fetal growth restriction is more common in infants delivered after preterm labor or preterm PROM, even in apparently otherwise uncomplicated pregnancies.[115,116]

Conditions that suggest specific therapy such as preterm ruptured membranes or cervical insufficiency should then be sought and treated accordingly.

The next concerns are the accuracy of preterm labor diagnosis and the balance of risks and benefits that accompany continued pregnancy versus allowing delivery. Several issues arise:

- What is the gestational age, and what is the level of confidence about the accuracy of the gestational age?
- What, in the absence of advanced labor (cervical effacement >80 percent with dilation >2 cm) and a clear cause of preterm labor, is the accuracy of the diagnosis of preterm labor?
- Are confirmatory diagnostic tests such as cervical sonography, fetal fibronectin, or amniocentesis for infection necessary?
- What is the anticipated neonatal morbidity and mortality at this gestational age in this clinical setting?
- Should labor be stopped?
- Is transfer to a more appropriate hospital required?
- Should fetal lung maturity be tested?
- What interventions can be applied that will reduce the risks of perinatal morbidity and mortality?
- Should drugs to arrest labor (tocolytics), glucocorticoids, and/or antibiotics be given?

DIAGNOSIS OF PRETERM LABOR

Given the pathways for preterm parturition described earlier, clinical recognition of preterm labor requires attention to the biochemical as well as the biophysical features of the onset of labor. Pathologic uterine contractility rarely occurs in isolation; cervical ripening and decidual membrane activation are almost always in progress as well, most often before uterine contractions are clinically evident. Therefore, preterm labor must be considered whenever a pregnant woman reports recurrent abdominal or pelvic symptoms that persist for more than an hour in the second half or pregnancy. Symptoms of preterm labor such as pelvic pressure, increased vaginal discharge, backache, and menstrual-like cramps occur frequently in normal pregnancy, and suggest preterm labor more by persistence than severity. Contractions may be painful or painless, depending on the resistance offered by the cervix. Contractions against a closed, uneffaced cervix are likely to be painful, but persistence of recurrent pressure or tightening may be the only symptoms when cervical effacement precedes the onset of contractions.[363]

The traditional criteria to diagnose preterm labor are persistent uterine contractions accompanied by dilation and effacement of the cervix as determined by digital examination. These criteria assume a crisp transition from "preterm parturition" to "preterm labor" that is increasingly understood as being more gradual than previously thought. The symptoms and signs of preterm labor are thus initially imprecise and become more accurate only when preterm labor is well established. Optimal criteria for initiation of treatment are not clear. Contraction frequency of six or more per hour, cervical dilation of 3 cm, effacement of 80 percent, ruptured membranes and bleeding are symptoms of preterm labor most often associated with preterm delivery.[364,365] When lower thresholds for contraction frequency and cervical change are used, "false-positive" diagnosis (defined in randomized controlled trials as delivery at term after treatment with placebo only[366,367]) occurs in nearly 40 percent of women, but sensitivity does not rise.[368] Difficulty in accurate diagnosis is the product of the high prevalence of the symptoms and signs of early preterm labor in normal pregnancy,[103] the gradual onset of preterm labor discussed earlier, and the imprecision of digital examination of the cervix below 3 cm dilation and 80 percent effacement.[369] The practice of initiating tocolytic drugs for contraction frequency without additional diagnostic criteria results in unnecessary treatment of women who do not actually have preterm labor.

Diagnostic Tests for Preterm Labor

Women with symptoms whose cervical dilation is less than 2 cm and whose effacement is less than 80 percent present a diagnostic challenge. Diagnostic accuracy may be improved in these patients by testing other features of parturition, such as cervical ripening, assessed by transvaginal sonographic measurement of cervical length; and decidual activation, tested by an assay for fetal fibronectin in cervicovaginal fluid.[370–372] Both tests aid diagnosis primarily by reducing false-positive diagnosis. Transabdominal sonography has poor reproducibility for cervical measurement and should not be used clinically without confirmation by a transvaginal ultrasound.[373,374] A cervical length of 30 mm or more by endovaginal sonography indicates that preterm labor is unlikely in symptomatic women if the examination is properly performed (Fig. 26-11).[370]

Similarly, a negative fibronectin test in women with symptoms before 34 weeks' gestation with cervical dilation less than 3 cm can also reduce the rate of false-positive diagnosis if the result is returned promptly and the clinician is willing to act on a negative test result by not initiating treatment.[375] When both tests were performed in a study of 206 women with possible preterm labor, the fetal fibronectin test improved the performance of sonographic cervical length only when the sonographic cervical length was less than 30 mm (Table 26-7; also see box entitled "Clinical Evaluation of Patients with Possible Preterm Labor").[376]

Amniocentesis for Women with Preterm Labor

The goal of care for women with preterm labor is to reduce perinatal morbidity and mortality, most of which is caused by immaturity of the respiratory, gastrointestinal, coagulation, and central nervous systems of the preterm infant. Fetal pulmonary immaturity is the most frequent cause of serious newborn illness, and the fetal pulmonary system is the only organ system whose function is directly testable before delivery. If the quality of obstetric dating is good and intrauterine fetal well-being is not compromised, the likelihood of neonatal RDS may

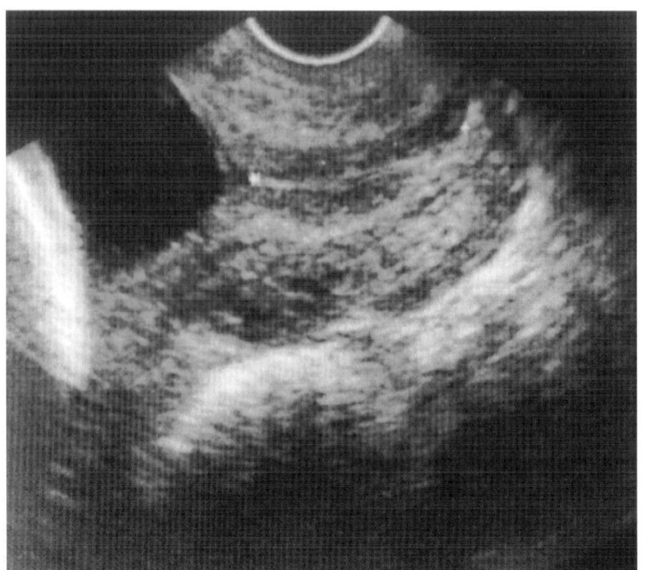

A

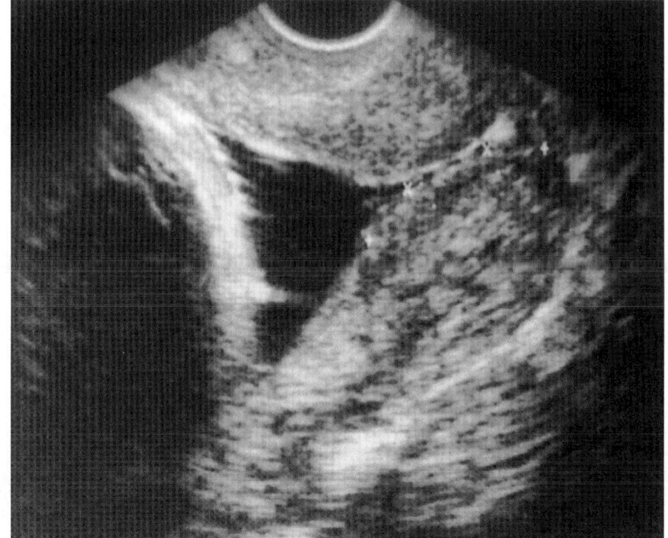

B

Figure 26-11. *A,* Transvaginal ultrasound image of the cervix at 28 weeks in a normal pregnancy. Calipers (+) are placed at the notches marking the internal and external os where the anterior and posterior walls of the cervical canal touch. *B,* Transvaginal ultrasound image of the cervix at 28 weeks in a patient with preterm labor. The (X) calipers mark the length of the cervical canal that is used for clinical evaluation. The (+) calipers are placed at the outer edges of the cervix; this length is not useful clinically because of wide variation among patients.

Table 26-7. Frequency of Spontaneous Preterm Delivery According to Cervical Length (Cutoff 30 mm) and Vaginal Fibronectin Results in Women with Symptoms of Preterm Labor

CERVICAL LENGTH <30 MM	FETAL FIBRONECTIN +	DELIVERY WITHIN 48 HOURS	DELIVERY WITHIN 7 DAYS	DELIVERY ≤32 WKS	DELIVERY ≤35 WKS
No	No	2.2% (2/93)	2.2% (2/93)	0% (0/47)	1.1% (1/93)
No	Yes	0% (0/14)	7.1% (1/14)	0% (0/5)	21.4% (3/14)
Yes	No	7.1% (5/70)	11.4% (8/70)	6.5% (2/31)	17.1% (12/70)
Yes	Yes	26.3% (10/38)	44.7% (17/38)	38.9% (7/18)	47.4% (18/38)
Prevalence of the outcome		7.9% (17/215)	13.0% (28/215)	8.9% (9/101)	15.8% (34/215)

From Gomez R, Romero R, Medina L, et al: Cervicovaginal fibronectin improves the prediction of preterm delivery based on sonographic cervical length in patients with preterm uterine contractions and intact membranes. Am J Obstet Gynecol 192:350, 2005.

Clinical Evaluation of Patients with Possible Preterm Labor

1. **Patient presents with signs/symptoms of preterm labor:**
   Persistent contractions (painful or painless)
   Intermittent abdominal cramping, pelvic pressure, or backache
   Increase or change in vaginal discharge
   Vaginal spotting or bleeding
2. **General physical examination:**
   Sitting pulse and blood pressure
   Temperature
   External fetal heart rate and contraction monitor
3. **Sterile speculum examination**
   pH
   Fern
   Pooled fluid
   Fibronectin swab (posterior fornix or external cervical os, avoiding areas with bleeding)
   Cultures for chlamydia (cervix), and *Neisseria gonorrhea* (cervix), and group B streptococcus (outer third of vagina and perineum)
4. **Transabdominal ultrasound examination**
   Placental location
   Amniotic fluid volume
   Estimated fetal weight and presentation
   Fetal well being
5. **Cervical examination** (after ruptured membranes excluded)
   a. **Cervix ≥3 cm dilation /80% effaced**
   Preterm labor diagnosis confirmed. Evaluate for tocolysis
   b. **Cervix 2 to 3 cm dilation / < 80% effaced**
   Preterm labor likely but not established. Monitor contraction frequency and repeat digital examination in 30–60 minutes. Diagnose preterm labor if cervical change. If not, send fibronectin or obtain transvaginal cervical ultrasound. Evaluate for tocolysis if any cervical change, cervical length <20 mm or positive fibronectin.
   c. **Cervix <2 cm dilation and <80% effaced**
   Preterm labor diagnosis uncertain. Monitor contraction frequency, send fibronectin and/or obtain cervical sonography, and repeat digital examination in 1 to 2 hours. Evaluate for tocolysis if there is a 1-cm change in cervical dilation, effacement >80%, cervical length <20 mm or positive fibronectin
6. **Use of Cervical Ultrasound**
   Cervical length <20 mm *and* contraction criteria met = preterm labor
   Cervical length 20–30 mm *and* contraction criteria met = probable preterm labor
   Cervical length >30 mm = preterm labor *very unlikely* regardless of contraction frequency

be estimated from the gestational age (see Figs. 26-3, 26-4, and 26-5).

Amniotic fluid studies may be useful in women with possible preterm labor in the following circumstances:

1. Fetal pulmonary maturity testing
   a. When dates are uncertain (e.g., late prenatal care, fetal size larger than expected for dates, suggesting a more advanced gestation, maternal glucose intolerance, or size less than expected suggesting fetal growth restriction)
   b. When a chronic hostile intrauterine environment may be present, for example, maternal hypertension, poor fetal growth, decreased amniotic fluid volume, substance abuse
2. Testing for infection/inflammation
   a. For glucose (amniotic fluid glucose levels less than 20 mg/dl suggest intra-amniotic infection), Gram's stain for white blood cells (WBC) and bacteria, and culture and when maternal fever or leukocytosis is present, or tocolysis is ineffective
3. Determining fetal karyotype
   a. The presence of polyhydramnios or a fetal anomaly suggests that preterm labor may have occurred due to uterine distention or placental insufficiency associated with fetal aneuploidy. Fluorescence in situ hybridization studies for the most common aneuploid conditions can be available within 48 hours.

GOALS OF TREATMENT FOR WOMEN IN PRETERM LABOR

Treatment with drugs to arrest labor after contractions and cervical change are well established or membranes have ruptured does not prolong pregnancy sufficiently to allow further intrauterine growth and maturation, but their use can often delay preterm birth long enough to permit three interventions that have been shown to reduce neonatal morbidity and mortality:

1. Antenatal transfer of the mother and fetus to the most appropriate hospital.
2. Antibiotics in labor to prevent neonatal infection with the group B streptococcus (GBS).
3. Antenatal administration of glucocorticoids to the mother to reduce neonatal morbidity and mortality due to respiratory distress, intraventricular hemorrhage, and other causes.

Maternal Transfer

Many states have adopted systems of regionalized perinatal care in recognition of the advantages of concentrating care for preterm infants, especially those born before 32 weeks. Hospitals and birth centers caring for normal mothers and infants are designated as Level I. Larger hospitals that care for the majority of maternal and infant complications are designated as Level II centers; these hospitals have neonatal intensive care units staffed and equipped to care for most infants with birth weights greater than 1,500 g. Level III centers typically provide care for the sickest and smallest infants, and for maternal complications requiring intensive care. This approach has been associated with improved outcomes for preterm infants.[377,378]

Antibiotics

Women with preterm labor should be treated with antibiotics to prevent neonatal GBS infection (see Chapter 49). Because preterm infants have a greater risk of neonatal GBS infection than infants born at term, intrapartum prophylaxis with penicillin or ampicillin is recommended.[39] This policy has successfully reduced the incidence of neonatal GBS infection to such a degree that most GBS infections now occur in full-term infants. There is also evidence that infants born to women with preterm PROM have reduced perinatal morbidity when antepartum antibiotic prophylaxis has been administered for 3 to 7 days.[380,381]

Antibiotic therapy to prolong pregnancy in women with preterm labor and intact membranes is not effective for that purpose. This use has been studied extensively with disappointing results.[382–386] The failure of antibiotics to improve clinical outcome in this setting may be attributed to treatment of women whose preterm labor did not result from infection, and to the timing of treatment relative to the infectious process. Rather than an acute infection due to the recent ascent of vaginal organisms into the uterus, the pathologic sequence in which infection-driven preterm labor occurs is often much more indolent.[52,387] Antimicrobial therapy of women in preterm labor should be limited to GBS prophylaxis, women with preterm PROM, or treatment of a specific pathogen.

Antenatal Corticosteroids

Glucocorticoids act generally in the developing fetus to promote maturation over growth.[388] In the lung, corticosteroids promote surfactant synthesis, increase lung compliance, reduce vascular permeability, and generate an enhanced response to postnatal surfactant treatment. Glucocorticoids have similar maturational effects on other organs including the brain, kidneys, and gut.[389]

Studies by Liggins of mechanisms of parturition in sheep led to the discovery of the beneficial effect of antenatal glucocorticoids on the maturation and performance of the lung in prematurely born infants.[390] Subsequent studies have shown conclusively that antepartum administration of the glucocorticoids betamethasone or dexamethasone to the mother reduces the risk of death, RDS, intraventricular hemorrhage, NEC, and PDA in the preterm neonate.[391] Guidelines for appropriate clinical use of antenatal glucocorticoids have evolved from initial skepticism and selective use, through a period of broad and repeated treatment following the first NICHD panel report in 1994,[392] to the current practice of a single course of treatment recommended by the NICHD Consensus Panel in 2000.[393] Betamethasone and dexamethasone, the only drugs found beneficial for this purpose, are potent glucocorticoids with limited if any mineralocorticoid effect. A course of treatment consists of two doses of 12 mg of betamethasone (the combination of 6 mg each of betamethasone acetate and betamethasone phosphate) administered intramuscularly twice, 24 hours apart, or four doses of 6 mg of dexamethasone given intramuscularly every 12 hours. Other corticosteroids (prednisolone, prednisone) and routes of administration (oral) are not suitable alternates because of reduced placental transfer, lack of demonstrated benefit, and in the case of oral dexamethasone, increased risk of adverse effects when compared with the intramuscular route.[394]

Fetal Effects

Randomized placebo-controlled trials and meta-analyses confirm the beneficial effects of antenatal corticosteroids. Infants born to treated women were significantly less likely to experience RDS (OR 0.53), IVH (OR 0.38), and neonatal death (OR 0.60).[391] The beneficial effects on IVH are independent of the effects on respiratory function. Other morbidities of preterm birth are also reduced by antenatal glucocorticoids, including NEC, PDA, and BPD. Betamethasone and dexamethasone are apparently equally effective in reducing perinatal morbidity, but one study of infants born between 24 and 31 weeks' gestation noted that the rate of periventricular leukomalacia was 4.4 percent among 361 infants who were treated antenatally with betamethasone, 11.0 percent among 165 infants who received dexamethasone, and 8.4 percent among 357 infants who were not treated with antenatal glucocorticoids.[395]

Other Fetal Effects of Glucocorticoids

Transient reduction in fetal breathing and body movements sufficient to affect the interpretation of the biophysical profile have been described with both drugs but are more common after betamethasone, typically lasting 48 to 72 hours after the second dose.[393–395] Transient suppression of neonatal cortisol levels has been reported, but neonatal response to ACTH stimulation was unimpaired.[399–401]

Maternal Effects

Antenatal glucocorticoids produce a transient rise in maternal platelet and WBC count lasting 72 hours; WBC counts in excess of 20,000 are rarely due to steroids. Maternal glucose tolerance is challenged as well and often requires insulin therapy to maintain euglycemia in women with previously well-controlled gestational or pregestational diabetes. Maternal blood pressure is unaffected by antenatal steroid treatment; neither betamethasone nor dexamethasone has significant mineralocorticoid effect. Women treated with multiple courses of steroids during pregnancy had a blunted response to ACTH stimulation later in pregnancy or the puerperium.[402]

Duration of Benefit

The duration of the beneficial fetal effects after a single course of glucocorticoids is not clear. The issue is difficult to study because the interval between treatment and delivery in clinical trials is variable, and because some effects may be transient whereas others are permanent. Neonatal benefit has been most easily observed when the interval between the first dose and delivery exceeds 48 hours, but some benefit is evident after an incomplete course. One large multicenter trial[403] found evidence of benefit for as long as 18 days after the initial course of treatment. Other meta-analyses report reduced morbidity for weeks after a single course of antenatal steroids when compared with untreated infants.

RISKS OF ANTENATAL CORTICOSTEROID TREATMENT

The recommendation of the 1994 NICHD Consensus Conference[404] to increase the use of antenatal steroids, coupled with uncertainty about the duration of neonatal protection from a single course of treatment and difficulty in predicting imminent preterm delivery, resulted in increased treatment of mothers at risk. Although more women received treatment, many did not deliver within 7 days but remained at risk and were treated weekly until delivery or 34 weeks' gestation. The safety and benefit of one course of steroids has never been questioned. Long-term follow-up studies of infants in the original cohorts of infants treated with a single course of antenatal steroids have displayed no differences in physical characteristics or mental function when compared with gestational age–matched controls.[405] The increasing use of repeated courses prompted animal and human studies that have raised concerns about the effects of prolonged exposure to steroids on fetal growth and neurologic function. The animal studies may be summarized as showing reduced fetal growth and adverse brain and neurologic development in several species.[406–411]

Human studies also found reduced growth in fetuses exposed to multiple courses of antenatal steroids. An Australian study found a twofold increase in birth weights below the 10th percentile and significantly reduced head circumference in infants exposed to more than three antenatal courses of steroids.[412] Others have also found reduced head circumference.[413] The NICHD reconvened the Consensus Panel in 2000 to review available information about repeated courses of steroids. The panel reemphasized the benefit and safety of a single course of antenatal corticosteroids (given either as two doses of 12 mg intramuscularly [IM], 24 hours apart or four doses of dexamethasone every 12 hours) for women between 24 and 34 weeks of pregnancy who are deemed to be at risk of preterm delivery within 7 days. The NICHD Panel found data that suggested neonatal benefit after repeat versus single courses of steroids, but in the absence of appropriate clinical studies, recommended that "repeat courses of corticosteroids . . . should not be used routinely . . . (but) should be reserved for patients enrolled in randomized controlled trials."

Results of three prospective randomized clinical trials of repeat antenatal corticosteroids in 551 women were reviewed by the Cochrane Database.[414] One trial compared weekly betamethasone to rescue treatment from enrollment through 34 weeks. Notably, more than 75 percent of women in the weekly treatment group received corticosteroids within a week of preterm birth, compared with only 37 percent of women assigned to receive rescue steroids ($p = 0.001$), indicating the difficulty in predicting imminent preterm delivery.[415] The NICHD MFMU Network Study[416] randomized 495 women, of whom 492 (591 infants) were available for analysis, and 252 received repetitive steroids. There were no differences in the adverse outcomes for infants who were exposed to multiple courses versus placebo (7.7 percent versus 9.2 percent, $P = 0.67$). Trends toward improvement were seen in the repeat steroids group including reduced use of surfactant (12.5 percent versus 18.4 percent, $P = 0.02$), reduced need for mechanical ventilation (15.5 percent versus 23.5 percent $P = 0.005$), and less treatment for hypotension (5.7 percent versus 11.2 percent, $P = 0.02$). Among infants delivered before 32 weeks, morbidity was less common in the repeat steroids group (21.3 versus 38.5 percent, $P = 0.083$). However, repeated courses were associated with insignificant trends toward reduced infant weight (2,194 versus 2,289 g, $P = .09$) and length (44.2 versus 44.7 cm, $P = .09$). Infants exposed to four or more courses had a significant decrease in birth weight (2,396 versus 2,561 g, $P = 0.01$).[416] The current consensus based on these data is to limit antenatal steroids to a single course given when significant risk of preterm birth is first recognized after 24 weeks' gestation.

Other Antenatal Treatments to Reduce Fetal Morbidity

RESPIRATORY DISTRESS

The occurrence of RDS among infants born to women treated with steroid therapy has led to investigation of alternative treatment approaches to further enhance pulmonary maturation. Neonatal treatment with surfactant is an effective adjunctive therapy that adds independently and synergistically to the benefit of corticosteroids in reducing RDS-related morbidity. More than 4,600 women have been enrolled into 13 trials of maternal treatment with antenatal thyrotropin-releasing hormone (TRH) to reduce neonatal lung disease. There were no benefits compared with corticosteroids alone for any neonatal outcome. Prenatal treatment with TRH actually increased risk of adverse outcomes for infants in some trials.[417]

NEUROLOGIC MORBIDITY

Antenatal maternal treatment with phenobarbital, vitamin K, and magnesium sulfate has been studied to reduce or prevent neonatal neurologic morbidity. Phenobarbital was not effective in reducing intraventricular hemorrhage when given alone[418] or in combination with vitamin K.[419] Antenatal maternal treatment with magnesium has been inconsistently associated with reduced rates of intraventricular hemorrhage, cerebral palsy and perinatal mortality in premature infants.[420–425] A randomized placebo-controlled trial of antenatal magnesium conducted in 1,062 women delivered before 30 weeks' gestation found significantly lower rates of gross motor dysfunction and nonsignificant trends of reduced mortality and cerebral palsy in surviving infants in the treated group at 2 years of age.[426] There were no significant adverse effects noted in infants exposed to antenatal magnesium sulfate. A similar American trial is ongoing.

Tocolysis

Efficacy

The efficacy of tocolytic drugs has been addressed through studies that compare one tocolytic drug with another, or less commonly, to a placebo in their ability to prolong pregnancy for 48 hours (the time sufficient to attain the benefit of antenatal corticosteroids), or 1 week (the time considered sufficient to gain significant additional in utero fetal maturation). No studies have shown that any tocolytic can reduce the rate of preterm birth. Most are too small to allow firm conclusions so that reviews or meta-analyses, wherein several studies of similar design are combined, are the best available means to judge efficacy. The Cochrane Collaboration *(www.cochrane.org/index0.htm)* regularly produces meta-analyses of obstetric interventions including tocolytic drugs. Recent Cochrane meta-analyses of tocolytic agents indicate that calcium channel blockers[427] and oxytocin antagonists[428] can delay delivery by 2 to 7 days with the most favorable ratio of benefit to risk, that β-mimetic drugs delay delivery by 48 hours but carry greater side effects,[429] that there is insufficient evidence regarding COX inhibitors[430] and that magnesium sulfate is ineffective.[431]

Meta-analyses of studies of individual tocolytic drugs typically report limited prolongation of pregnancy but no decrease in preterm birth and rarely offer information about whether prolongation of pregnancy was accompanied by improved infant outcomes. Delayed delivery for 48 hours to allow antenatal transport and corticosteroids to reduce neonatal morbidity and mortality are thus the main rationale for use of these drugs.

Choosing a Tocolytic Agent

Pharmacology

A brief review of myometrial activity and the sites of action of the various tocolytic agents is appropriate. The key process in actin-myosin interaction, and thus contraction, is myosin light-chain phosphorylation. This reaction is controlled by myosin light-chain kinase (MLCK). The activity of tocolytic agents can be explained by their effect on the factors regulating the activity of this enzyme, notably calcium and cyclic adenosine monophosphate (cAMP). Calcium is essential for the activation of MLCK and binds to the kinase as calmodulin-calcium complex. Intracellular calcium levels are regulated by two general mechanisms: (1) influx across the cell membrane and (2) release from intracellular storage sites. Entry of calcium into cells occurs by at least two mechanisms. Depolarization leads to calcium influx through specific calcium channels that are voltage dependent. This is the site of action of the calcium channel blockers. Calcium can also enter through voltage-independent mechanisms, most notably the calcium-magnesium-ATPase system. Magnesium ions may interact here and also may compete with calcium for the voltage-dependent channels. Calcium is stored within cells in the sarcoplasmic reticulum and in mitochondria. Progesterone and cyclic AMP (cAMP) promote calcium storage at these sites, while prostaglandin $F_{2\alpha}$ ($PGF_{2\alpha}$) and oxytocin stimulate its release MLCK is also regulated by cAMP, which directly inhibits MLCK function through phosphorylation. Levels of cAMP are increased by the action of adenylate cyclase, which, in turn, is stimulated by β-mimetic agents. Therefore, β-mimetic tocolytics act through adenylate cyclase to increase cAMP, which inhibits MLCK activity both by direct phosphorylation and by reducing intracellular free calcium (by inhibiting calcium release from storage vesicles). β-Mimetics also interact with surface receptors on the trophoblast, leading to increased cAMP, which in this tissue, increases production of progesterone.[425] For the myometrium to contract in a coordinated and effective manner (i.e., labor, whether term or preterm), individual smooth muscle cells must be functionally interconnected and able to communicate with adjacent cells. The key element of intercellular coordination of effective labor contractions is the gap junction. Estrogens and progesterone regulate formation of gap junctions and the concentration of oxytocin receptors.[432]

Contraindications to Tocolysis

Common maternal contraindications to tocolysis include hypertension, bleeding, and cardiac disease. Preterm labor accompanied by maternal hypertension places both mother and fetus at risk of acute hypertensive crises, and may occur in response to fetal stress or distress, uterine ischemia, or occult placental abruption. Although vaginal spotting may occur in women with preterm labor because of cervical effacement or dilation, any bleeding beyond light spotting is rarely due to labor alone. Placenta previa and abruption must be considered, because both may be accompanied by uterine contractions. In general, both diagnoses contraindicate tocolytic treatment. However, in rare instances, prophylactic use of tocolysis in women with these dangerous diagnoses may be considered to achieve time for corticosteroids in the setting of extreme prematurity when the bleeding is believed to occur in response to contractions. Such treatment is fraught with difficulty, because even low doses of some tocolytic agents can be hazardous in a patient with bleeding. β-Mimetic agents and calcium channel blockers may hamper maternal cardiovascular response to hypotension, and prostaglandin inhibitors are known to impair maternal platelet function. Cardiac disease is a contraindication because of the risks of tocolytic drug treatment in these patients. Fetal contraindications to tocolysis include gestational age of greater than 37 weeks, fetal demise or lethal anomaly, chorioamnionitis, and evidence of acute or chronic fetal compromise.

Tocolytic drugs may be safely used when standard protocols are followed. The choice of tocolytic requires consideration of the efficacy, risks, and side effects for each patient.

Calcium Channel Blockers

Calcium channel blockers marketed for treatment of hypertension, angina, and arrhythmias are increasingly being used without U.S. Food and Drug Administration (FDA) approval as tocolytic drugs. The pharmacologic effect is believed to occur through inhibition of the voltage-dependent channels of calcium entry into smooth muscle cells, resulting in a direct decrease in intracellular calcium as well as decreased release of calcium from intracellular storage sites. Nifedipine is the agent most studied as a tocolytic agent; it more selectively inhibits uterine contractions compared with other calcium blockers such as verapamil. Calcium channel blockers are rapidly absorbed after oral administration. Pharmacokinetics in pregnancy are similar to those used in the nonpregnant state. After oral administration, nifedipine appears in plasma within a few minutes, reaches peak concentrations at 15 to 90 minutes, and has a half life of 81 minutes.[433] Placental transfer occurs within 2 to 3 hours after oral nifedipine. The duration of action of a single dose is up to 6 hours. There are no placebo-controlled trials of calcium channel blockers as tocolytics. The Cochrane Collaboration meta-analyses support calcium channel blockers as short-term tocolytics compared with other available agents because of relatively greater contraction suppression and fewer side effects than other agents in 12 reported trials.[427] Rates of birth within 7 days of treatment (RR 0.76, 95 percent CI 0.60 to 0.97) and before 34 weeks' gestation (RR 0.83, 95-percent CI 0.69 to 0.99) were significantly reduced with calcium channel blockers, as were the rates of neonatal morbidities including RDS (RR 0.63, 95 percent CI 0.46 to 0.88), NEC (RR 0.21, 95-percent CI 0.05 to 0.96), IVH (RR 0.59, 95-percent CI 0.36 to 0.98), and jaundice (RR 0.73, 95-percent CI 0.57 to 0.93) when compared with treatment with other tocolytics. Fewer women treated with calcium channel blockers ceased treatment owing to adverse drug reactions (RR 0.14, 95-percent CI 0.05 to 0.36).

Maternal Effects Nifedipine has fewer side effects when compared with β-mimetics[427,434] and magnesium sulfate.[435] Hypotension occurs frequently with nifedipine, but other side effects are more frequent with magnesium and β-mimetics. Nicardipine displayed similar advantages when compared in a randomized trial with magnesium.[436] Pretreatment with fluids may reduce the incidence of maternal side effects related to hypotension such as headache (20 percent), flushing (8 percent), dizziness, and nausea (6 percent). Most effects are mild, but serious complications have been reported, including a documented myocardial infarction 45 minutes after the second dose of nifedipine given to a young healthy woman.[437] Simultaneous or sequential use of calcium channel blockers with β-mimetics is not recommended, nor is concurrent administration of magnesium, owing to reports of skeletal muscle blockade when nifedipine was given with magnesium sulfate.[438,439]

Fetal Effects Initial animal studies raised questions of fetal hypotension, but a study of women treated for preterm labor revealed no changes in fetal middle cerebral artery, renal artery, ductus arteriosus, umbilical artery, or maternal vessels.[440]

Treatment Protocol When used as a tocolytic, nifedipine is commonly given as a 10- to 20-mg initial dose, repeated every 3 to 6 hours until contractions are rare, followed by long-acting formulations of 30 or 60 mg every 8 to 12 hours for 48 hours until antenatal steroids have been administered. The long acting preparations reduce side effects.

Summary of Treatment with Calcium Channel Blockers

Nifedipine has been used increasingly as a tocolytic because of its low incidence of significant maternal and fetal side effects and ease of administration. Nifedipine should not be combined with magnesium or β-mimetics, and should be avoided in the presence of intrauterine infection, maternal hypertension, and cardiac disease. Use should follow published dosage schedules, and the cautions noted should be kept in mind.

MAGNESIUM SULFATE

Intravenous magnesium sulfate has been used to inhibit preterm labor since the 1970s.[441] Magnesium apparently acts by competition with calcium either at the motor end plate, reducing excitation, or at the cell membrane, reducing calcium influx into the cell at depolarization. Evidence to support magnesium sulfate as an effective tocolytic is weak,[431,442,443] but it remains a common choice because clinicians are familiar with its use as treatment for preeclampsia, and its presumed safety relative to β-mimetics. The Cochrane Library reviewers found no significant advantage in the rates of delivery within 48 hours or before 34 or 37 weeks in studies of women treated with magnesium.[431]

Maternal Effects Magnesium has a low rate of serious maternal side effects, but flushing, nausea, vomiting, headache, generalized muscle weakness, diplopia, and shortness of breath occur frequently. Chest pain and pulmonary edema have been reported with a frequency similar to that of β-mimetics.[444]

Neonatal Effects Magnesium crosses the placenta and achieves serum levels comparable to maternal levels, but serious short-term neonatal complications are uncommon. Lethargy, hypotonia, and respiratory depression may occur. Prolonged treatment for more than 7 days has been associated with neonatal bone abnormalities.[445] One small trial suggested that magnesium sulfate may have adverse effects on neonatal and infant morbidity and mortality,[423] but these observations were not confirmed by larger studies that enrolled more than 10 times as many subjects.[426,446]

Treatment Protocol Magnesium sulfate must be given parenterally to achieve serum levels greater than the normal range. Therapeutic dosage regimens are similar to those used for intravenous seizure prophylaxis of preeclampsia. A loading dose of 4 to 6 g is given over 30 minutes, followed by an infusion of 1 to 4 g per hour.[444] Serum magnesium levels do not appear to be related to therapeutic effect.[447] Mean serum magnesium levels in patients with successful tocolysis were similar to those in patients in whom tocolysis failed.

If renal function is normal, magnesium is excreted rapidly in the urine. In patients with evidence of renal impairment, for example, oliguria or serum creatinine levels greater than 0.9 mg/dl, magnesium should be administered cautiously, followed with frequent vital signs, deep tendon reflexes and serum levels, and doses adjusted accordingly. Magnesium sulfate should not be used in patients with myasthenia gravis because the magnesium ion competes with calcium.

A clinical protocol for magnesium sulfate as a tocolytic is shown here:

1. Administer loading dose of 4 to 6 g magnesium sulfate in 10- to 20-percent solution over 30 minutes (60 ml of 10 percent magnesium sulfate in 1 L D5 0.9 normal saline).
2. Maintenance dose of 2 g/h (40 g of magnesium sulfate added to 1 L D5 0.9 normal saline or Ringer's lactate at 50 ml/h).
3. Increase magnesium sulfate by 1 g/h until the patient has fewer than one contraction per 10 minutes or a maximum dose of 4 g/h is reached.
4. Limit intravenous (IV) fluid to 125 ml/h. Follow fluid status closely; an indwelling urinary catheter is recommended.
5. Maintenance of magnesium sulfate tocolysis for 12 hours after contractions have stopped or decreased to less than 1 per 10 to 15 minutes is common but unsupported by data. Therapy may be stopped without tapering the dose.
6. Recurrent or persistent contractions require reevaluation to look for an underlying cause of the preterm labor such as amnionitis or occult abruption. Amniocentesis should be considered. The accuracy of the original diagnosis of preterm labor should be reconsidered with cervical sonography or fibronectin.
7. Patients treated with magnesium sulfate should be assessed with the following examinations:
   a. Deep tendon reflexes and vital signs including respiratory rate should be recorded hourly
   b. Intake and output every 2 to 4 hours
   c. Magnesium levels if any clinical concern about side effects or if infusion equals or exceeds 4 g/h
8. Calcium gluconate should be readily available to reverse the respiratory effects of magnesium.

Summary of Treatment with Magnesium Sulfate Magnesium sulfate is a familiar agent, but tocolytic efficacy is poor. Magnesium may be a useful choice when the diagnosis of preterm labor is early and uncertain, and in patients in whom other agents are contraindicated, for example, in patients with insulin-dependent diabetes.

Cyclooxygenase Inhibitors

Prostaglandins are mediators of the final pathways of uterine muscle contraction. Prostaglandins cause an increase in free intracellular calcium levels in myometrial cells and increased activation of MLCK, resulting in uterine contractions. Myometrial gap junction formation, an important step in synchronized uterine activity, is enhanced by prostaglandins. Prostaglandins given to pregnant women can ripen the cervix or induce labor, depending on the dosage and route of administration. Prostaglandin synthase, also known as cyclooxygenase (COX), converts arachidonic acid to prostaglandin G_2. Prostaglandin synthesis is increased when the COX-2 form of this enzyme is induced by cytokines, bacterial products such as phospholipases and endotoxins, and corticosteroids, and reduced by inhibition of COX by nonsteroidal anti-inflammatory drugs (NSAIDs). The NSAID agents vary in their activity, potency and side effect profile. Indomethacin is the NSAID most often used as a tocolytic. Indomethacin crosses the placenta. Unlike aspirin, indomethacin binds reversibly to COX, so that inhibition lasts only until the drug is excreted. Umbilical artery serum concentrations equal maternal levels within 6 hours of oral administration. The half life in the mother is 4 to 5 hours, and in a full-term infant is 15 hours, but is significantly longer in preterm infants. The Cochrane Review concluded that indomethacin administration was associated with a significant reduction in births before the 37th week, increased gestational age and increased birth weight, but found inadequate data to assess fetal safety.[430]

Maternal Effects Prostaglandin inhibition has multiple side effects because of the abundance of prostaglandin-mediated physiologic functions. Nevertheless, serious maternal side effects are uncommon when the agent is used in a brief course of tocolysis. As with any NSAID, gastrointestinal side effects such as nausea, heartburn, and vomiting are common but usually mild. Less common but more serious complications include gastrointestinal bleeding, prolonged bleeding time,[441] thrombocytopenia, and asthma in aspirin-sensitive patients. Prolonged treatment with NSAIDs can lead to renal injury, especially when other nephrotoxic drugs are used. Hypertensive women may rarely experience acute increased blood pressure after indomethacin treatment. The antipyretic effect of an NSAID may obscure a clinically significant fever. Maternal contraindications to indomethacin tocolysis include renal or hepatic disease, active peptic ulcer disease, poorly controlled hypertension, asthma, and coagulation disorders.

Fetal and Neonatal Effects In contrast to the generally favorable maternal side effect profile, the potential for fetal and neonatal complications of COX inhibitors such as indomethacin tocolysis is worrisome. In actual practice, serious complications have been rare, but there is risk of injury to the fetus if treatment protocols are not followed carefully. Three principal side effects raise concern: (1) constriction of the ductus arteriosus, (2) oligohydramnios, and (3) neonatal pulmonary hypertension. The ductal constriction occurs because formation of prostacyclin and PGE_2, which maintain ductal vasodilation, is inhibited by indomethacin.[449] Doppler evidence of ductal constriction was found in seven of 14 fetuses of women treated with indomethacin between 27 and 31 weeks of pregnancy but resolved within 24 hours after the medication was discontinued.[450] The likelihood of ductal constriction increased from 5 to 10 percent[442] before 32 weeks to 50 percent after 48 hours of treatment at 32 to 35 weeks. Ductal constriction is usually transient and responds to discontinuation of the drug, but persistent ductal constriction and irreversible right heart failure have been reported.[451] A review of fetal echocardiographs obtained from 61 women treated with indomethacin for preterm labor found evidence of ductal constriction in 50 percent of fetuses.[452] Constriction was detected at an average of 30.9 ± 2.3 weeks after an average of 5.1 ± 6.0 days of indomethacin therapy, and reversed in all fetuses after cessation of medication.

Oligohydramnios associated with indomethacin tocolysis is due to reduced fetal urine production, which is caused by indomethacin-induced reduction of normal prostaglandin inhibition of anti-diuretic hormone and by direct effects on fetal renal blood flow. These effects are dose related and reversible, but neonatal renal insufficiency and death after several weeks of antenatal maternal treatment has been reported.[453]

Primary pulmonary hypertension in the neonate is a potentially fatal illness that has also been associated with prolonged (>48 hours) indomethacin therapy.[454,455] Primary neonatal pulmonary hypertension has not been reported with 24 to 48 hours of therapy, but the incidence may be as high as 5 to 10 percent with long-term therapy.[456]

Other complications, including NEC, small bowel perforation, PDA, jaundice, and IVH, have been observed when indomethacin administration was outside of standardized protocols that did not limit the duration of treatment or employed the drug after 32 weeks.[457] No association with IVH was noted in studies in which standard protocols were used.[458,459] A review of outcomes of 1,621 fetuses treated in utero with indomethacin found no significant differences compared with 1,387 infants not exposed.[illegible]

Sulindac is an NSAID that has less placental transfer than indomethacin, but tocolytic efficacy has not been studied in large numbers.[460] Because of the effect on fetal urine production and amniotic fluid volume, indomethacin may be an appropriate tocolytic when preterm labor is associated with polyhydramnios. Indomethacin has been used to treat preterm labor in women with polyhydramnios,[461] and for polyhydramnios without labor.[462] Uterine activity and pain associated with degenerating uterine fibroids in pregnancy also respond well to indomethacin.

Treatment Protocol Indomethacin is well absorbed orally. The usual regimen is a 50 mg oral loading dose followed by 25 to 50 mg by mouth every 6 hours. Therapy is limited to 2 to 3 days because of concern about side effects described earlier.

Protocol for Indomethacin Tocolysis.

1. Limit use to preterm labor before 32 weeks' gestation in women with normal amniotic fluid volume and normal renal function.
2. Loading dose is 50 milligrams by mouth.
3. Give 25 milligrams orally every 6 hours for 48 hours.
4. Check amniotic fluid volume prior to initiation and at 48 to 72 hours. If amniotic fluid is significantly reduced, the drug should be discontinued.
5. Use the drug for no longer than 48 to 72 consecutive hours. Treatment beyond 48 hours requires extraordinary circumstances. Ductal flow should be evaluated with Doppler echocardiography.
6. Discontinue therapy promptly if delivery seems imminent.
7. Fetal contraindications to use of indomethacin include growth restriction, renal anomalies, chorioamnionitis, oligohydramnios, ductal dependent cardiac defects, and twin-twin transfusion syndrome.

Summary of Treatment with Indomethacin Indomethacin is an effective tocolytic agent that is generally well tolerated by the mother. Concern about fetal side effects has appropriately limited use of indomethacin to brief courses of therapy in patients with preterm labor before 32 weeks.

β-Mimetic Tocolytics

β-sympathomimetic drugs including terbutaline, ritodrine, and others have been widely used as tocolytics for many years. Structurally related to epinephrine and norepinephrine, these agents act to relax smooth muscle, for example, in the bronchial tree, blood vessels, and myometrium, through stimulation of the β-receptors. β-receptors are divided into β1- and β2-subtypes. The β1-receptors are largely responsible for the cardiac effects, whereas β2-receptors mediate smooth muscle relaxation, hepatic glycogen production, and islet cell release of insulin. Variable ratios of β2- to β-receptors occur in body tissues. For example, the heart is primarily stimulated by β1-agonists, but 14 percent of its β-receptors are β2. Stimulation of β-receptors in the heart, vascular system and liver accounts for the side effects of these drugs. The most commonly used β-mimetic in the United States is terbutaline (marketed as a drug for asthma), but others including albuterol, fenoterol, hexoprenaline, metaproterenol, nylidrin, orciprenaline, and salbutamol are used in other countries. Ritodrine was approved by the FDA as a parenteral tocolytic in 1980, but it did not achieve wide use because of frequent maternal side effects. Ritodrine is no longer marketed in the United States. Terbutaline has a rapid effect when given subcutaneously (3 to 5 minutes). Published protocols often employ subcutaneous administration, with a usual dose of 0.25 mg (250 μg) every 4 hours.[463] A single subcutaneous dose of terbutaline to arrest contractions during the initial evaluation of preterm contractions may aid in the diagnosis of preterm labor. In one study,[464] women whose contractions persisted or recurred after a single dose were more likely to have true preterm labor; those whose contractions ceased were probably not in labor. The Cochrane Database reported an analysis of 1,332 women enrolled into 11 randomized placebo-controlled trials of β-mimetic drugs found that treated subjects were less likely to deliver within 48 hours (RR 0.63, 95-percent CI 0.53 to 0.75) but not within 7 days.[429] Although a 48-hour delay in delivery allows sufficient time for in utero transfer and treatment with steroids, perinatal and neonatal death, and perinatal morbidity were not reduced in this analysis. Side effects requiring change or cessation of treatment were frequent. Previous reviews have found similar results.[465]

Side Effects and Complications of β-Mimetic Tocolysis

Maternal side effects of the β-mimetic drugs are common and diverse owing to the abundance of β-receptors in the body. Maternal tachycardia, chest discomfort, palpitation, tremor, headache, nasal congestion, nausea and vomiting, hyperkalemia and hyperglycemia are significantly more common in women treated with β-mimetics.[429] Most are mild and of limited duration, but serious maternal cardiopulmonary and metabolic complications have been reported.

Cardiopulmonary Complications of β-Mimetics. The β-mimetic agents produce a mild (5- to 10-mm Hg) fall in diastolic blood pressure, and the extensive peripheral vasodilatation makes it difficult for the patient to mount a normal response to hypovolemia. Signs of excessive blood loss, for example, maternal and fetal tachycardia, are masked by β-mimetics, so their use may be dangerous in women with antepartum hemorrhage.[466] The most important steps to prevent cardiac complications are (1) excluding patients with prior cardiac disease and (2) limiting infusion rates so that maternal pulse does not exceed 130 beats per minute. Symptomatic cardiac arrhythmias and myocardial ischemia have occurred during β-agonist tocolytic therapy; myocardial infarction leading to death has been reported.[466] The placental arteriovenous shunt diminishes aortic diastolic blood pressure, and the tachycardia created by β-stimulation shortens diastole, thus reducing myocardial perfusion. Tocolysis should be discontinued and oxygen administered whenever a patient develops chest pain during tocolytic therapy. Premature ventricular contraction, premature nodal contractions, and atrial fibrillation noted in association with β-mimetic therapy[466] usually respond to discontinuation of the drug and oxygen administration. Baseline or routine electrocardiograms before or during treatment are not helpful.[467] Nonetheless, an electrocardiogram is indicated if there is no response to oxygen and cessation of β-mimetic therapy. Pulmonary edema has been reported with all tocolytics, most commonly after β-mimetic therapy. Restricting the duration of treatment to less than 24 hours, careful attention to fluid status, and detection of complicating conditions such as intrauterine infection may reduce this risk.

Metabolic Complications. β-mimetic agents induce transient hyperglycemia and hypokalemia during treatment. Measurement of glucose and potassium before initiating therapy and on occasion during the first 24 hours of treatment is appropriate to identify significant hyperglycemia (>180 mg/dl) or hypokalemia (<2.5 mEq/L). These metabolic changes are mild and transient, but prolonged treatment beyond 24 hours may induce significant alterations in maternal blood sugar, insulin levels, and energy expenditure.[468] The risk of abnormal glucose metabolism is further increased by simultaneous treatment with corticosteroids,[469] a common combination for threatened preterm labor. Other agents should be chosen for women with pregestational diabetes, and usually for those with gestational diabetes as well. β-mimetic treatment in these women requires frequent monitoring and insulin infusion to maintain euglycemia.

Neonatal Effects. Neonatal hypoglycemia, hypocalcemia, and ileus may follow treatment with β-mimetics, and can be clinically significant if the maternal infusion is not discontinued 2 hours or more before delivery.[470] Of concern, a study in rats found "biochemical alterations and structural damage in the immature brain" in rat pups exposed in utero at a neurodevelopmental gestational age comparable to clinical use of tocolytics in humans, and declared terbutaline to be a "developmental neurotoxicant."[471] Long-term data in humans are lacking.

Long-term or maintenance use of β-mimetic drugs has been championed by clinicians who advocate detection and suppression of contractions to prevent preterm labor. Protocols for continuous subcutaneous infusion of terbutaline have been reported to have fewer side effects than oral administration[472,473] but have had no effect on rates of preterm birth or perinatal morbidity in randomized placebo-controlled trials.[474–476] Subcutaneous infusion of terbutaline has been the subject of an FDA advisory: "*Published studies on the safety of this use (subcutaneous infusion) are seriously limited by methodologic inadequacies. In the absence of data establishing the effectiveness and safety of the drug/device (for subcutaneous infusion) the FDA is alerting practitioners . . . and others that continuous administration of subcutaneous terbutaline sulfate has not been demonstrated to be effective and is potentially dangerous.*"[477] No placebo-controlled trials demonstrating effectiveness have been reported since the FDA advisory was issued.

Given their potential for clinically significant side effects and the availability of alternate choices, the β-sympathomimetic agents should not be used in women with known or suspected heart disease, severe preeclampsia or eclampsia, pregestational gestational diabetes requiring insulin, or hyperthyroidism. These drugs are contraindicated when suspected preterm labor is complicated by maternal fever, fetal tachycardia, leukocytosis, or other signs of possible chorioamnionitis.

Summary of Treatment with β-Mimetic Tocolysis

β-Mimetic drugs were once the most commonly used tocolytics but are being replaced by agents with better safety and side effect profiles. Terbutaline has relatively few serious side effects when used as a single subcutaneous injection of 0.25 mg to facilitate maternal transfer or to initiate tocolysis, while another agent with a slower onset of action is being given. Long-term oral or subcutaneous treatment has not been shown in controlled trials to reduce prematurity or neonatal morbidity.

Other Tocolytic Agents

The oxytocin antagonist atosiban was investigated in a randomized, placebo-controlled trial in which 501 subjects with acute preterm labor were randomized to receive either IV and subcutaneous atosiban or IV and subcutaneous placebo.[156] Subjects with persistent contractions and progressive cervical change after 1 hour of initial treatment in either the placebo or atosiban arms were treated with an open label "rescue" tocolytic agent of the clinician's choice. For women enrolled after 28 weeks' gestation, those who received atosiban were more likely to remain undelivered without an alternate tocolytic at 24 hours (73 percent versus 58 percent, OR 1.93, 95-percent CI 1.30 to 2.86), at 48 hours (67 percent versus 56 percent, OR 1.62, 95-percent CI 1.62 to 2.37) and at 7 days (62 percent vs. 49 percent, OR 1.70, 95-percent CI 1.17 to 2.46). There were no advantages over placebo for subjects enrolled between 20 and 28 weeks. Maternal side effects of atosiban were few except for injection site inflammation. Although the differences in pregnancy prolongation were significant, the FDA did not approve atosiban because of an unexpected finding of more perinatal deaths among infants born to women enrolled into the atosiban arm before 26 weeks. This was due to an imbalance in the number of very early gestations enrolled in the atosiban arm versus the placebo arm of the study. As in other placebo-controlled tocolytic trials, the rate of "successful" treatment in the placebo group was 50 percent or more. A companion trial compared subcutaneous infusions of atosiban to placebo.[478] The interval from the start of maintenance infusion therapy to the first recurrence of preterm labor was longer for the atosiban group, but there were no differences in the rate of preterm birth before 28, 32, or 37 weeks' gestation. An international study group compared the efficacy and side effect profile of atosiban with ritodrine.[479] Efficacy to delay delivery for 48 hours (about 85 percent for both drugs) and 7 days (about 75 percent for both drugs) was similar, but cardiovascular side effects were much less common for atosiban (4 percent) than for ritodrine (84 percent).

The NO donor glyceryl trinitrate has been studied in a trial in which 245 women with acute preterm labor were randomly assigned to receive either transdermal glyceryl trinitrate or standard ritodrine tocolysis.[480] The rate of prolongation to 37 weeks was 74 percent in both treatment arms. Headache occurred in 30 percent of the patients who received glyceryl trinitate. In a recent report, treatment of preterm labor with transdermal nitroglycerin before 28 weeks was associated with a significant decrease in neonatal morbidity in a randomized placebo-controlled trial.[480a]

Management of Persistent Contractions Despite 12–24 Hours of Tocolysis

1. Is the patient infected? Repeat clinical examination, white blood cell counts, and fetal assessment. Consider amniocentesis for glucose, Gram's stain, and culture.
2. Is the fetus compromised? Review the fetal heart tracings and do a biophysical assessment.
3. Is there evidence of abruption? Is there a suspicion of uterine anomaly with implantation of the placenta on the septum? Repeat hemoglobin, hematocrit, and fibrinogen, and abdominal sonography for placental implantation site.
4. Is the diagnosis of preterm labor correct? Is the cervix changing? Do a transvaginal cervical ultrasound to measure cervical length and look for funneling or separation of the membranes from the lower segment. Send a fibronectin swab.
5. If infection, fetal compromise, and abruption can be excluded, stop parenteral tocolysis for 24 hours and observe. Most patients will stop contraction spontaneously.

Clinical Use of Tocolytic Drugs

Tocolytic therapy is employed in several clinical circumstances. In a patient who presents in active labor with advanced cervical effacement, the diagnosis is not in question and the goal is prompt treatment to allow maternal transfer and time for steroids and GBS prophylaxis. In this setting, initial treatment with subcutaneous terbutaline or oral nifedipine may be the best choice to stop contractions promptly. Treatment for preterm labor may be continued until contractions have stopped, or occur less frequently than four times per hour without additional cervical change. When labor has been difficult to stop in a patient with complete cervical effacement, acute treatment may be continued until a full course of steroid therapy is completed (48 hours).

Persistent Contractions

If contractions persist despite therapy, the wisdom of tocolytic treatment should be reevaluated. The cervix should be reexamined; if cervical dilation has progressed beyond 4 cm, tocolytic therapy in most cases should be discontinued. Fetal well-being and the possibility of placental abruption or intra-amniotic infection should be considered. If these concerns can be excluded, the accuracy of the original diagnosis is in doubt, remembering that significant effacement, softness, and development of the lower uterine segment are the features of the digital examination that most reliably indicate preterm labor. If a fibronectin swab was collected before therapy was begun, it should be sent for analysis. A positive result is not confirmatory, but a negative fibronectin, if collected before performance of a digital examination, provides evidence that the patient's contractions are benign.[371] Alternately, a transvaginal cervical ultrasound examination may be performed. A length of 30 mm or more essentially excludes the diagnosis.[370]

Serum levels are not clinically helpful to adjust the dose of tocolytics. A change to a second agent, or combination therapy with multiple agents, may slow contractions but may result in increased side effects. Sustained treatment with multiple tocolytics increases the risk of significant side effects and should be avoided.[481,482] Combined use of β-mimetics or magnesium sulfate with calcium channel blockers should also be avoided (see box entitled "Management of Persistent Contractions Despite 12 to 24 Hours of Tocolysis").

Care After Acute Treatment for Preterm Labor

Maintenance Tocolytic Treatment

Continued suppression of contractions after acute tocolysis does not reduce the rate of preterm birth.[483–487] Meta-analyses of these data also find no evidence of prolongation of pregnancy or decline in the frequency of preterm birth.[488,489]

Posthospitalization surveillance with outpatient monitoring of uterine contractions did not improve the rate of delivery before 37 weeks, birth weight, or gestational age at delivery in any of three randomized trials[490–492] or in a meta-analysis of these.[442] A multicenter randomized trial in which uterine activity was monitored but the data were ignored in one group also found no improvement in preterm birth rate when contraction data were used.[493]

The duration of hospitalization for an episode of preterm labor varies according to several factors including the dilation, effacement, and sonographic length of the cervix, ease of tocolysis, gestational age, obstetric history, distance from hospital, and the availability of home care and family support. Associated risk factors that may complicate or increase the risk of recurrent preterm labor, such as a positive genital culture for chlamydia or gonorrhea, urinary tract infection, and anemia should be addressed before discharge from hospital care. Social issues such as homelessness, availability of child care, or protection from an abusive partner are important determinants of a patient's ability to comply with medical care, and these issues must be considered before the patient is discharged from the hospital.

CONDUCT OF LABOR AND DELIVERY FOR THE PRETERM INFANT

Intrapartum care for women in labor before term is often complicated by conditions such as hypertension, amnionitis, abruption, oligohydramnios, or fetal growth restriction that increase the chance of intrapartum fetal compromise. When labor is induced preterm for maternal or fetal indications, the lower uterine segment and cervix may not be well prepared for labor, leading to a prolonged latent phase.

Intrapartum Assessment of the Preterm Fetus

Careful fetal surveillance has been associated with significantly improved outcome for preterm infants.[494,495] Ominous heart rate tracings have the same associations with fetal acidosis as they do later in gestation. Mean fetal heart rate falls continuously, from 160 bpm at 22 weeks gestation, to 140 bpm at term due to a gradual increase in parasympathetic tone. Fetal heart rate patterns should be interpreted in the preterm fetus as they are at term.

Labor and Delivery

The course of labor in preterm gestation may be shorter than that of term pregnancy. The active phase and the second stage may be particularly brief. Care should be taken to ensure that the fetus does not have a precipitous delivery without control of the fetal head. There is no benefit for prophylactic forceps to "protect" the fetal head.[496] The neonatal care team should be alerted to the circumstances of a preterm birth well in advance of the delivery so that appropriate personnel and equipment are available.

Cesarean Delivery

Routine cesarean delivery of all preterm or VLBW infants is not justified.[497–499] Trends favoring cesarean section disappear after adjustment for confounding factors.[499] A review of studies of neonatal and maternal morbidities after vaginal versus cesarean delivery for infants born between 24 and 36 weeks[500] found increased maternal morbidity without clear benefit for the infant. Neonatal intracranial hemorrhage occurs as often before and after labor as it does during labor and delivery.

For infants in breech presentation, there are intuitive reasons for cesarean birth, particularly to avoid trapping of the after-coming head and other manipulations that could lead to trauma or hypoxia. Older retrospective studies that suggested a benefit for cesarean delivery led to the current custom of cesarean delivery for preterm breech fetuses, but support for this practice remains weak.[501] It is illogical to perform a cesarean to avoid a traumatic vaginal delivery only to encounter a difficult cesarean birth because of an inadequate abdominal or uterine incision. The operation should be conducted to ensure an atraumatic delivery through as generous an incision as necessary. In a study of delivery mode for "high-risk" VLBW infants (e.g., preeclampsia, vaginal bleeding, abnormal heart rate tracing) versus "low-risk" VLBW infants (e.g., preterm labor, incompetent cervix), cesarean section was of no value in the low-risk group, but was associated with significantly improved survival rates in the high-risk group.[502] Considering the above-mentioned factors, optimal delivery of the VLBW fetus may at times appropriately lead to a decision to perform a cesarean without labor.

PREVENTION OF PRETERM BIRTH

Care of preterm birth may be described according to the public health model as *tertiary* (treatment initiated after the parturitional process has begun to limit perinatal morbidity and mortality), *secondary* (identification and treatment for individuals with increased risk), or *primary* (prevention and reduction of risk in the population). Previous sections of this chapter have described tertiary care for preterm birth. Tests to predict preterm birth have been vigorously sought but there is no test with ideal sensitivity or predictive value.

Clinical Predictors

Among the clinical risk factors for preterm birth described earlier in the chapter, several confer substantial increased risk, including multiple gestation (RR five to sixfold), a history of preterm birth (RR two to fourfold), and vaginal bleeding after the first trimester (RR threefold). However, these factors are present only in a minority of women who ultimately deliver preterm and thus have low sensitivity. More prevalent risk factors such as low prepregnancy weight, genitourinary colonization or infection, and black ethnicity have lower relative risks of 1.5- to 2-fold. Clinical risk scoring systems have been devised but have a sensitivity of only about 25 percent,[36,38] and derive much of their sensitivity from a history of prior preterm delivery. More than 50 percent of women who deliver preterm have no apparent clinical risk factors.

Biophysical Predictors

Uterine Contractions

Detection of uterine contractions through maternal self perception[36] and electronic tocodynamometry[503,504] has been studied to predict risk of preterm delivery. Although an increased frequency of self-reported[37] and electronically detected[504] contractions has been significantly associated with preterm delivery, contraction frequency does not perform well to predict preterm birth because contractions occur so commonly in normal pregnancy. The result is very low sensitivity and positive predictive value (Table 26-8).

Table 26-8. Prediction at 22 to 24 and 27 to 28 Weeks of Spontaneous Preterm Birth

TEST	SENSITIVITY %	SPECIFICITY %	PVP %	PVN %
At 22 to 24 weeks				
UC ≥ 4/h	6.7	92.3	25.0	84.7
Bishop ≥ 4	32.0	91.4	42.1	87.4
CL ≤ 25 mm	40.8	89.5	42.6	88.8
fFN ≥ 50 ng/ml	18.0	95.3	42.9	85.6
At 27 to 28 weeks				
UC ≥ 4/h	28.1	88.7	23.1	91.1
Bishop ≥ 4	46.4	77.9	18.8	92.9
CL ≤ 25 mm	53.6	82.2	25.0	94.1
fFN ≥ 50 ng/ml	21.4	94.5	30.0	91.6

Bishop, Bishop score; CL, cervical length by endovaginal ultrasound; fFN, cervicovaginal fetal fibronectin; PVN, predictive value of a negative result; PVP, predictive value of a positive result; UC, uterine contractions per hour by ambulatory tocodynamometry.

From Iams JD, Newman RB, Thom EA, et al: Frequency of uterine contractions and the risk of spontaneous preterm delivery. N Engl J Med 346:250, 2002.

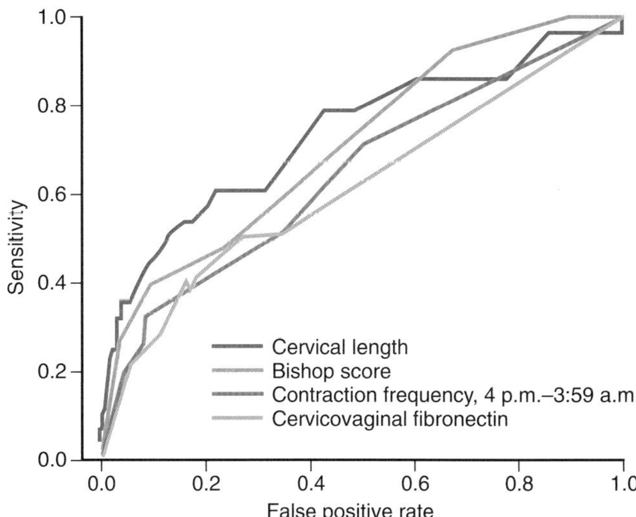

Figure 26-12. Receiver-operating-characteristic curves for cervical length, Bishop score, frequency of contractions between 4 p.m. and 3:59 a.m., and Presence or Absence of Fetal Fibronectin in Cervicovaginal Secretions at 27 to 28 Weeks in the Prediction of Spontaneous Preterm Delivery (Less Than 35 Weeks). (From Iams JD, Newman RB, Thom EA, et al: Frequency of uterine contractions and the risk of spontaneous preterm delivery. N Engl J Med 346:25, 2002.)

Cervical Examination

Cervical dilation, effacement, consistency, position, and station of the presenting part as determined by manual examination have been related to an increased risk of preterm birth[36,78,137] but also suffer from low sensitivity and positive predictive values (Fig. 26-12).[78] Cervical length measured with transvaginal ultrasound has also been related to an increased risk of preterm birth as cervical length decreases. The relative risk of preterm birth before 35 weeks is increased six- to eightfold in women whose cervical length is less than the 10th percentile (25 mm) when compared with women with a cervical length above the 75th percentile (40 mm) at 20 to 24 weeks. The reported sensitivity is somewhat better than other tests, but positive predictive value is low, and the equipment required is not universally available.[78,81,504]

Biochemical Predictors

Cervicovaginal secretions contain biochemical markers that have been tested as screening tests for preterm birth, including fetal fibronectin,[38,505] IL-6 and IL-8,[506,507] TNF-α, and matrix metalloproteinases. Fetal fibronectin, a glycoprotein of fetal origin that normally resides at the decidual-chorionic interface, has been studied extensively and is marketed in the United States as a diagnostic test for preterm labor. Fibronectin is present in cervicovaginal secretions in 3 to 4 percent of pregnant women between 21 and 37 weeks.[176,505] A positive test in asymptomatic women at 24 weeks has a sensitivity for spontaneous preterm birth before 35 weeks of 20 percent to 30 percent.[504,505] The sensitivity of fibronectin for early preterm births before 28 weeks was 63 percent in one study.[505] Fibronectin is a better screening test for risk of delivery within 2 weeks of sampling than for delivery before a specific gestational week of pregnancy.[508]

Altered levels of serum biomarkers including alpha-fetoprotein, alkaline phosphatase, granulocyte-macrophage colony–stimulating factor, defensins, and CRH have been linked to increased risk of preterm birth but are not sensitive when used alone.[509,510] Increased sensitivity has been reported when serum markers are used in combination with other markers such as fetal fibronectin and cervical length.[509]

BV has been studied as a marker because of consistent reports linking BV to increased risk. The sensitivity of tests for BV to identify women at risk is low because the strength of the association is modest and BV is highly prevalent some populations.[511]

Vogel et al.[512] summarized biomarkers for preterm birth in Table 26-9.

Interventions to Prevent Preterm Birth

Interventions have been based on identifying and correcting each potential cause or risk factor for preterm birth, with the expectation that the rate of preterm birth would decline in accordance with the contribution of that factor to the prematurity rate. Trials have addressed early identification of preterm labor through patient education, detection and pharmacologic suppression of uterine contractions[513]; antimicrobial therapy of vaginal microorganisms[50,51,514,515]; cerclage sutures to bolster the cervix[516]; reduction of maternal stress[517,518]; improved nutrition[519] and access to prenatal care[520]; and reduced physical activity.[521–523] Some trials enrolled women with the risk factor in question without regard to obstetric history (e.g., antibiotics for women with a positive culture for a genital

Table 26-9. Selected Biomarkers to Predict Preterm Birth in Asymptomatic Women

BIOMARKER	NUMBER OF SUBJECTS	COMPARTMENT	GA AT SAMPLING	END POINT	LR+	SENSITIVITY%	FP%	REFERENCE*
Multiple (≥2 out of 5)	177	S/P, C, V + C	24	<32	24	59	2	(58) Goldenberg et al. AJOG 2001
U. urealyticum	254	Amniotic fluid	<17	<37	10	88	9	(9) Gerber et al. J Infect Dis 2003
Relaxin	176	S/P	<24	<34	6.8	27	4	(64) Vogel et al. AJOG 2001
Cervical length	Meta analysis	Cervix	<24	<34	6.3	—	—	(29) Honest et al. Ultrasound Obstet Gynecol 2003
Alk phos	1868	S/P	<20	<37	4.6	14	3	(69) Meyer et al. AJOG 1995
CRH	860	S/P	<30	<37	3.0	39	13	(40) McLean et al. AJOG 1999
G-CSF	388	S/P	24	<32	3.3	49	15	(16) Goldenberg et al. AJOG 2000
Interleukin-6	250	V + C	24	<32	3.3	20	6	(15) Goepfert et al. AJOG 2001
Interleukin-6	580	Amniotic fluid	<20 ?	<34	2.8	14	5	(14) Wenstrom et al. AJOG 1996
FFN	Meta analysis	V + C	>20	<37	2.9	—	—	(22) Honest et al. BMJ 2002
AFP	254	S/P	24	<35	2.6	35	13	(58) Goldenberg et al. AJOG 2001
Chlamydia	380	U	24	<37	2.5	16	6	(10) Andrews et al. AJOG 2000
Ferritin	100	S/P	34	<37	2.2	75	33	(70) Goel et al. Acta Obstet Gynecol Scand 2003
Ferritin	364	V + C	<25	<37	1.4	35	25	(71) Ramsey et al. AJOG 2002
C-RP	484	S/P	<21	<37	1.8	26	15	(75) Hvilsom et al. Acta Obstet Gynecol Scand 2002
BV	Meta analysis	V + C	<24	<37	1.6	—	—	(8) Honest et al. BMJ 2004

Modified from Vogel I, Thorsen P, Curry A, et al: Biomarkers for the prediction of preterm delivery. Acta Obstet Gynecol Scand 84:516, 2005.

AFP, alpha-fetoprotein; Alk phos, alkaline phosphatase; BV, bacterial vaginosis; C, cervical secretions; C-RP, C-reactive protein; CRH, corticotropin-releasing hormone; FFN, fetal fibronectin; FP, false-positive rate; GA, gestational age; G-CSF, granulocyte colony–stimulating factor; LR, likelihood ratio; S/P, serum or plasma; V, vaginal secretions, U, urine.

*Ref Column Refers to Citations in the Paper by Vogel et al 2005.

microorganism), whereas others were limited to women with a prior preterm delivery (e.g., the European cerclage trials or the recent progesterone supplementation studies).[524,525] Successful elimination of single risk factors has been accomplished but has not produced a decrease in preterm birth. Because preterm birth is increasingly understood to be a syndrome with diverse causal pathways, these efforts summarized in Table 26-10 are now understood to have been simplistic.

Social Support and Improved Access to Prenatal Care

Improved access to care and social support has had some success,[526,527] but other trials have found no benefit.[517,518]

Activity Modification

Bed rest is prescribed for as many as 20 percent of pregnancies in the United States,[521] with little evidence of benefit. One study of a prematurity prevention program suggested that activity restriction may have contributed to a reduction in preterm births,[522] but a Cochrane Review of the effectiveness of bed rest to prevent singleton preterm birth found no evidence of reduced preterm birth.[523] Adverse effects of bed rest include venous thrombosis, muscle atrophy, osteoporosis, cardiovascular deconditioning, and psychological and economic impact on the mother and family.[529–531]

Early Detection of Preterm Labor

Early diagnosis of preterm labor has been studied in the belief that tocolytic drugs would be more effective if given before significant cervical change occurs. An initial

Table 26-10. Summary of Studies of Interventions to Prevent Preterm Birth in Asymptomatic Women

RISK FACTOR	INTERVENTION	STUDY	OUTCOME	REFERENCE
Nutritional Deficiencies				
Calcium	Calcium	RCT in 190	↓ PTB	Villar & Repke AJOG 1990
	Calcium	RCT in 456	↓ PTB	Crowther Aust NZ J Obstet Gynecol 1999
	Calcium	RCT in 4589	No Δ in PTB	Levine NEJM 1997
Vitamins	Vitamin C	RCT in 200	↑ in PTB	Steyn J Obstet Gynaecol 2003
	Vitamin C	Meta-analysis of 766 in RCTs	No Δ in PTB, but ?↑ in PTB	Rumbold & Crowther Cochrane Database 2006
	Vitamin E	Meta-analysis of 566 in RCTs	No Δ in PTB	Rumbold & Crowther Cochrane Database 2006
	Vitamins C + E	RCT in 2410 with risk of preeclampsia	No Δ in PTB ↑ in LBW	Poston et al Lancet 2006
	Vitamins C + E	RCT in 1877 in nulliparas	No Δ in PTB	Rumbold et al NEJM 2006
	Multivitamins	RCT peri-conception MV in 5502	No Δ in PTB	Czeizel Arch Gynecol Obstet 1994
Social Support				
	Nurse visits	RCT	↓ PTB in teens <17 yrs old	Olds et al Pediatrics 1986
	Social support	RCT in 2235 women with increased risk	No Δ in PTB or LBW	Villar et al NEJM 1992
	Nurse visits	RCT in 1139 with social risk	No Δ in PTB or LBW	Kitzman et al JAMA 1997
	Teen prenatal clinics	RCT in 651 teens	↓ PTB	Quinlivan & Evans BJOG 2004
	Social support	Meta-analysis	No Δ in PTB or LBW	Hodnett & Fredericks Cochrane Database 2005
Bed Rest				
	Bed rest for women with twins or risk of PTB	Meta-analyses	No Δ in PTB or LBW	Goldenberg Obstet Gynecol Sosa Cochrane Database 2006
Risk Scoring and Education				
	Frequent visits and education for high risk women	RCT of 2395 women at 5 sites	No Δ in PTB or LBW	March of Dimes Collaborative AJOG 1993
Maintenance Tocolysis				
After treatment of preterm labor	Oral tocolysis subcutaneous pump	Meta-analyses of small RCT's	No Δ in PTB or LBW	Macones Obstet Gynecol 1995 Sanchez-Ramos Clin Perinatol 2003 Berkman AJOG 2003 Dodd Cochrane Database 2006 Nanda Cochrane Database 2006
Uterine Contraction Monitoring				
	Monitoring contractions to detect recurrent preterm labor	3 RCT's in women treated for PTL	No Δ in PTB or LBW	Iams et al Am J Perinatol 1990 Nagey et al Obstet Gynecol 1993
		Meta-analysis		Brown et al AJOG 1999 Berkman et al AJOG 2003
	Monitoring contractions to detect early PTL	RCT in 2422 at risk of PTB	No Δ in PTB or LBW	Dyson et al NEJM 1998
		Review		ACOG Practice Bulletin 31, Obstet Gynecol 2001
Cervical Cerclage				
	Cervical cerclage	RCT in women with a prior PTB	Mixed but mostly negative results	MacNaughton BJOG 1993 To et al Lancet 2004
		Reviews and meta-analyses		Owen et al AJOG 2003 Drakeley et al Cochrane Database 2006 Berghella Obstet Gynecol 2005
		Observational study	? benefit if no cervical inflammation*	Sakai et al AJOG 2006*
Progesterone supplementation				
	Progesterone	RCT in 142 women with risk	↓ PTB	da Fonseca AJOG 2003
	17 α OH progesterone caproate	RCT in 459 women with a prior PTB	↓ PTB	Meis et al NEJM 2003
		Meta-analyses	↓ PTB	Dodd Acta Obstet Gynecol Scand 2005 Sanchez Ramos Obstet Gynecol 2005 Mackenzie AJOG 2006

LBW, low birth weight; PTB, preterm birth; RCT, randomized controlled trial.

promising report was not confirmed in larger studies.[533,534] This approach was expanded using outpatient electronic monitoring of uterine contractions accompanied by daily nursing contact, but large randomized controlled trials in women at risk found no effect on the rate of preterm birth or neonatal outcomes.[493,535] The largest such trial[513] randomized more than 2,400 women and found no effect of close monitoring of symptoms or contractions on rates of preterm birth or eligibility for tocolysis.

Antibiotics to Prevent Preterm Birth

A trial of antibiotic prophylaxis for urinary tract infection unexpectedly reported a lower rate of LBW in women who received tetracycline compared with placebo.[536] This report has been followed by a mixed literature of success and failure as shown in Table 26-11.

Antibiotic treatment has been reported to reduce the risk of recurrent preterm delivery in women with BV who also have a prior preterm birth,[263,269] but metronidazole treatment had no effect on the rate of preterm birth in a placebo-controlled trial of 1,900 women with asymptomatic BV.[49] Analysis by obstetric history of preterm birth, race, gestational age at initiation of treatment, eradication of BV, and prepregnancy weight did not reveal any subgroup in which treatment improved perinatal outcome. Placebo-controlled trials of clindamycin administered orally (n = 485)[538] or vaginally (n = 409)[539] to women with BV reported reductions in preterm birth, especially if treatment was administered early in pregnancy, but two other trials of vaginal clindamycin found no benefit. One found no difference in preterm birth rates despite successful elimination of BV in treated women (n = 601),[540] and the other[541] found an increased rate of preterm birth less than 34 weeks in women who were fully compliant with clindamycin treatment compared with placebo (9 percent versus 1.4 percent). Reviews of randomized trials of antibiotic treatment of BV to reduce preterm birth have found no benefit in low risk women with BV, and inconsistent evidence of possible benefit in women with a prior preterm birth.[50,51,268]

These studies led to investigation of preconceptional antibiotics for women with a history of preterm birth. There was no benefit for women treated with metronidazole and azithromycin between pregnancies in a recently reported trial[387] in which there was a possibility that antibiotics might actually have increased the likelihood of preterm birth. This unexpected effect was also seen in a trial of metronidazole for women with *T. vaginalis*.[515] Although they are preliminary, the data from these two studies argue for restraint in clinical use of antibiotics given solely to reduce preterm birth. The relationship between genital tract microorganisms and preterm birth is more complex than a simple infection.[52,67]

Reports of increased risk of preterm birth in women with periodontal disease[54–56,542,542a] have led to studies of screening and treatment of periodontal disease in pregnant women to reduce preterm birth.[543] One study

Table 26-11. Studies of Antibiotics to Prevent Preterm Birth

AUTHOR	YEAR	ENTRY CRITERIA	ANTIBIOTICS	OUTCOME
Elder	1971	Bacteriuria	Oral tetracycline	↓ LBW
Romero	1989	Bacteriuria	Meta-analysis	↓ LBW
Smaill	2001	Bacteriuria	Meta-analysis	↓ LBW
Eschenbach	1991	*Ureaplasma urealyticum*	Oral erythromycin	no effect
Klebanoff	1995	Group B strep	Oral erythromycin	no effect
Hauth	1995	Prior PTD or weight <50 kg	Oral metronidazole and erythromycin	No effect if BV–, ↓ PTD if BV+
Joesoef	1995	BV	Vaginal clindamycin	No effect
McDonald	1997	BV	Oral metronidazole	none if no Hx PTD, benefit if Hx PTD
Gichangi	1997	Poor Ob Hx* (African pop)	Cefetamet-pivoxil	↓ LBW
Vermeulen	1999	Prior preterm birth	Vaginal 2% clindamycin vs placebo at 26 & 32 weeks	No benefit; >PTD & infections in compliant Clindamycin received
Carey	2000	BV	Oral metronidazole	No effect in Asx women or Hx PTD
Klebanoff	2001	Trichomonas	Oral metronidazole	↑ PTD
Rosenstein	2000	BV	Vaginal clindamycin	No difference in PTD
Kurkinen-Raty	2001	BV at 12 weeks'	Vaginal 2% clindamycin	No difference in PTD
Kekki	2001	BV at 10–17 weeks'	Vaginal 2% clindamycin vs. placebo at 10 to 17 weeks'	No difference in PTD
Ugwumadu	2003	BV	Oral clindamycin	↓ PTD
Lamont	2003	BV	Vaginal clindamycin	↓ PTD, no Δ LBW
Andrews	2003	Positive fibronectin	Oral MTZ + Erythromycin	no effect
Kiss	2004	Gram's stain for BV, Trichomonas, yeast	Medication as detected	↓ PTD
Shennan	2006	Clinical risk of PTB and possible fFN 24–27 wks	Metronidazole	Study stopped due to 2 X increase in births <37 wk in metronidazole group

BV, bacterial vaginosis; Hx, history of; LBW, low birth weight; MTZ, metronidazole; PTD, preterm delivery.

enrolled 366 women who were randomized at 21 to 25 weeks to receive routine dental care plus placebo medication, intensive physical treatment of periodontal plaque plus metronidazole (250 mg TID for 1 week), or intense periodontal cleaning plus placebo medication. Rates of preterm birth before 35 weeks' were 4.9 percent, 3.3 percent, and 0.8 percent, respectively. A larger randomized trial of intensive periodontal care during pregnancy versus postpartum found similar rates of preterm birth in both groups.[543a] The role of periodontal care to reduce preterm birth is thus uncertain.[544]

Prophylactic Cerclage for Women with Risk of Preterm Birth

Recognition that some early preterm births may be due to variant clinical presentations of cervical insufficiency led to consideration of cervical cerclage treatment for women with such a history. A randomized trial of cerclage for women with prior preterm birth found fewer preterm births before 33 weeks in women with multiple prior early births, but no effect on the overall prematurity rate.[544a] The introduction of cervical sonography spawned additional trials in women with a prior preterm birth and ultrasound evidence of cervical effacement,[545,546] and in women with ultrasound findings alone.[547,548] These studies have been usefully reanalyzed by the original authors using the original data.[516] When data from women with singleton pregnancies enrolled into these four trials were combined, the risk of birth before 35 weeks' was significantly reduced with cerclage treatment for women with a prior preterm birth and a short cervix in the current pregnancy (RR 0.63, 95-percent CI 0.48 to 0.85), but there was no advantage of cerclage treatment for women with a short cervix who did not have a prior preterm birth (RR 0.84, 95-percent CI 0.60 to 1.17). The authors recommended that these data be confirmed by a larger prospective trial. Notably, analysis of outcomes in the 49 women with twin gestations in these trials showed an *increased* rate of preterm birth in women treated with cerclage (RR 2.15, 95-percent CI 1.15 to 4.01).

Prophylactic Medications

Tocolytic agents have been studied as prophylaxis but without evident benefit.[549,550] Progesterone supplementation, administered as either weekly intramuscular injections of 250 mg of 17α-hydroxyprogesterone caproate[525] or daily progesterone vaginal suppositories,[524] has been revisited as a method to prevent preterm birth in two recent randomized trials that enrolled women with a previous preterm birth. The risk of recurrent preterm birth was reduced in both studies by about one third.[524,525] When these studies were included in meta-analyses with earlier trials of supplemental progesterone, the risk of recurrent preterm birth was reduced by 40 to 55%.[551,552] Unlike strategies targeted at a specific risk factor such as infection, supplemental progesterone was effective in reducing preterm birth in women chosen only because of a prior preterm birth. This suggests three possibilities: (1) that it is effective in inhibiting a pathway shared by diverse causes of preterm birth, (2) that it has diverse effects that act on several different pathways, or (3) that it is very effective against one highly prevalent pathway or cause.

Although progesterone supplementation is promising, there are several questions about its use that remain incompletely answered:

1. How does it work? The original rationale for progesterone prophylaxis was as a uterine relaxant, but other studies indicate effects on the inflammatory response[553] and gap junction formation.[554]
2. Is it safe? There is little evidence in human studies of teratogenic risk,[555] but theoretical concern remains that it may blunt a fetal signal for labor generated by an in utero risk. Physical and developmental examinations at age 4 of children born to mothers enrolled in the NICHD study[525] of prophylactic 17 OH-P did not differ between those exposed in utero to placebo or 17 OH-P.[555a]
3. Who should receive it? Data showing benefit is available only for women with a prior preterm birth between 18 and 36 weeks. There is evidence that progesterone offers greatest benefit for women with a prior preterm birth before 34 weeks' gestation.[556] There are as yet no studies of 17 OH-P in women with risk factors such as a multiple gestation, short cervix, positive fibronectin, a history of cervical insufficiency or cerclage, or preterm labor in the current pregnancy. The American College of Obstetricians and Gynecologists Committee on Obstetric Practice issued an opinion[394] recommending that use of supplemental progesterone in either formulation be limited to women with a prior preterm birth until further studies are conducted to evaluate the use of progesterone in women with other risk factors for preterm delivery. Treatment with 17 OH-P did not reduce the rate of preterm birth in a placebo controlled trial conducted in 655 women with twins.[556a] Studies in other risk groups are ongoing.

SUMMARY

Preterm birth is a syndrome, the final result of several pathways that often overlap to initiate parturition. Obstetric interventions to reduce infant morbidity such as antenatal glucocorticoids and antibiotics are effective tertiary therapies but can never be wholly effective in eliminating the morbidity and mortality due to prematurity. Recent advances in detection of pregnancies at risk have not yet led to reduction in preterm birth, but recent studies of progesterone prophylaxis hold promise.

Key Points

- More than 70 percent of fetal, neonatal, and infant morbidity and mortality occurs in infants born preterm.
- The rate of preterm birth has increased to one in eight births in 2005 owing primarily to the rising number of multifetal gestations associated with infertility treatment.

- Major risk factors for preterm birth are a history of previous preterm delivery, multifetal gestation, bleeding after the first trimester of pregnancy, and a low maternal body mass index, but most women who deliver preterm have no apparent risk factors. Every pregnancy is potentially at risk.
- Spontaneous preterm birth is a syndrome in which the parturitional process may be initiated by one or more pathways culminating in cervical ripening, decidual activation, uterine contractions, and ruptured membranes.
- The most common clinical disorders that result in preterm birth are preterm labor and preterm ruptured membranes.
- Accurate early diagnosis of preterm labor is a major problem. Up to 50 percent of patients diagnosed with preterm labor do not actually have preterm labor, yet as many as 20 percent of symptomatic patients diagnosed as not being in labor will deliver prematurely.
- Three interventions have been shown to reduce perinatal morbidity and mortality:
  - Transfer of the mother and fetus to an appropriate hospital.
  - Administration of antibiotics to prevent neonatal GBS infection.
  - Administration of corticosteroids to reduce neonatal RDS and intraventricular hemorrhage.
- Although the mechanism of action is unclear, the risk of recurrent preterm birth may be reduced in women with a prior preterm birth by administration of prophylactic supplemental progesterone, given as 17-α hydroxyprogesterone caproate.

REFERENCES

1. Anderson RL, Smith BL: Deaths: Leading Causes for 2002. Hyattsville, MD, National Center for Health Statistics, 2005, p 53.
2. Martin JA, Hamilton BE, Menacker F, et al: Preliminary Births for 2004: Infant and Maternal Health. Hyattsville, Maryland, National Center for Health Statistics. Health E-stats. 11–15-2005.
3. Martin JA, Hamilton BE, Sutton PD, et al: Births: Final Data for 2003. Hyattsville, Maryland, National Center for Health Statistics, 2005, p 54.
4. Wright VC, Chang J, Jeng G, Macaluso M: Assisted reproductive technology surveillance, United States, 2003. MMWR 55:2, 2006.
5. Ananth CVP, Joseph KSM, Oyelese YM, et al: Trends in preterm birth and perinatal mortality among singletons: United States, 1989 Through 2000. Obstet Gynecol 105:1084, 2005.
6. Health, United States, 2004 with Chartbook on Trends in the Health of Americans. Hyattsville, Maryland, National Center for Health Statistics, 2004.
7. Hamilton BE, Martin JA, Sutton PD: Births: Preliminary Data for 2003. Hyattsville, Maryland, National Vital Statistics Reports, 2004.
8. Martin JA, Hamilton BE, Sutton PD, et al: Births: Final Data for 2002. Hyattsville, Maryland: National Center for Health Statistics, 2003.
9. Hoyert DL, Heron M, Murphy SL, Kung HC: Deaths: Final Data for 2003. Health E-Stats, 2006.
10. Horbar JD, Badger GJ, Carpenter JH, et al: Trends in mortality and morbidity for very low birth weight infants, 1991–1999. Pediatrics 110:143, 2002.
11. Lemons JA, Bauer CR, Oh W, et al: Very low birth weight outcomes of the National Institute of Child Health and Human Development Neonatal Research Network, January 1995 Through December 1996. Pediatrics 107:e1, 2001.
12. Effer SBA, Moutquin J-M, Farine D, et al: Neonatal survival rates in 860 singleton live births at 24 and 25 weeks gestational age. A Canadian multicentre study. Br J Obstet Gynaecol 109:740, 2002.
13. Mercer BMM: Preterm premature rupture of the membranes. [Editorial]. Obstetr Gynecol 101:178, 2003.
14. Fanaroff AA, Hack M, Walsh MC: The NICHD neonatal research network: changes in practice and outcomes during the first 15 years. Semin Perinatol 27:281, 2003.
15. MacDonald H: Perinatal care at the threshold of viability. Pediatrics 110:1024, 2002.
16. Clinical Management Guidelines for Obstetrician-Gynecologists. Number 38, September 2002 (Replaces Committee Opinion Number 163, November 1995): Perinatal care at the threshold of viability. Obstet Gynecol 100:617, 2002.
17. Lucey JF, Rowan CA, Shiono P, et al: Fetal infants: The fate of 4172 infants with birth weights of 401 to 500 grams—The Vermont Oxford Network Experience (1996–2000). Pediatrics 113:1559, 2004.
18. Alexander GR, Kogan M, Bader D, et al: US birth weight/gestational age-specific neonatal mortality: 1995–1997 rates for whites, hispanics, and blacks. Pediatrics 111:e61, 2003.
19. Tyson J, Younes N, Verter J, et al: Viability, morbidity, and resource use among newborns of 501- to 800-g birth weight. JAMA 276:1645, 1996.
20. Barton L, Hodgman J, Pavlova Z: Causes of death in the extremely low birth weight infant. Pediatrics 102:446, 1999.
21. Bottoms SF, Paul RH, Iams JD, et al: Obstetric determinants of neonatal survival of extremely low birth weight infants. Am J Obstet Gynecol 176:960, 1997.
22. Shankaran S, Fanaroff A, Wright L, et al: Risk factors for early death among extremely low-birth-weight infants. Am J Obstet Gynecol 186:796, 2002.
23. Vohr BR, Wright LL, Dusick AM, et al: Center differences and outcomes of extremely low birth weight infants. Pediatrics 113:781, 2004.
24. Villar J, Abalos E, Carroli G, et al: Heterogeneity of perinatal outcomes in the preterm delivery syndrome. Obstet Gynecol 104:78, 2004.
25. Wood NS, Marlow N, Costeloe K, et al: Neurologic and developmental disability after extremely preterm birth. EPICure Study Group. N Engl J Med 343:378, 2000.
26. Hack M, Flannery DJ, Schluchter M, et al: Outcomes in young adulthood for very-low-birth-weight infants. N Engl J Med 346:149, 2002.
27. Bhutta AT, Cleves MA, Casey PH, et al: Cognitive and behavioral outcomes of school-aged children who were born preterm: a meta-analysis. JAMA 288:728, 2002.
28. Marlow N, Wolke D, Bracewell MA, Samara M: The EPICure Study Group: Neurologic and developmental disability at six years of age after extremely preterm birth. N Engl J Med 352:9, 2005.
29. Saigal S, Lambert M, Russ C, Hoult L: Self-esteem of adolescents who were born prematurely. Pediatrics 109:429, 2002.
30. Meis P, Ernest J, Moore M, et al: Regional program for prevention of premature birth in northwestern North Carolina. Am J Obstet Gynecol 157:550, 1987.
31. Meis P, Michielutte R, Peters T, et al: Factors associated with preterm birth in Cardiff, Wales. Am J Obstet Gynecol 173:597, 1995.
32. Meis P, Goldenberg R, Mercer B, et al: The preterm prediction study: Risk factors for indicated preterm births. Am J Obstet Gynecol 178:562, 1998.

33. Shiono P, Klebanoff M, Nugent R, et al: The impact of cocaine and marijuana use on low birth weight and preterm birth: A multicenter study. Am J Obstet Gynecol 172:19, 1995.
34. Dombrowski MP, Schatz M, Wise R, et al: Asthma during pregnancy. Obstet Gynecol 103:5, 2004.
35. Schatz M, Dombrowski M, Wise R, et al: The relationship of asthma medication use to perinatal outcomes. J Allergy Clin Immunol 113:1040, 2004.
36. Mercer BM, Goldenberg RL, Das A, et al: The Preterm Prediction Study: A clinical risk assessment system. Am J Obstet Gynecol 174:1885, 1996.
37. Mercer B, Goldenberg R, Moawad A, et al: The Preterm Prediction Study: Effect of gestational age and cause of preterm birth on subsequent obstetric outcome. Am J Obstet Gynecol 181:1216, 1999.
38. Goldenberg RL, Iams JD, Mercer BM, et al: The preterm prediction study: the value of new vs standard risk factors in predicting early and all spontaneous preterm births. NICHD MFMU Network. Am J Public Health 88:233, 1998.
39. Adams MMP, Elam-Evans LDP, Wilson HGP, Gilbertz DAM: Rates of and factors associated with recurrence of preterm delivery. JAMA 283:1591, 2000.
40. Moreau C, Kaminski M, Ancel PY, et al: Previous induced abortions and the risk of very preterm delivery: results of the EPIPAGE study. Br J Obstet Gynaecol 112:430, 2005.
41. Goldenberg RL, Hauth JC, Andrews WW: Intrauterine infection and preterm delivery. N Engl J Med 342:1500, 2000.
42. Krohn M, Hillier S, Nugent R, et al: The genital flora of women with intra-amniotic infection. J Infect Dis 171:1475–80, 1995.
43. Goncalves LF, Chaiworapongsa T, Romero R: Intrauterine infection and prematurity. Ment Retard Dev Disabil Res Rev 8:3, 2002.
44. Cotch MF, Pastorek JGI, Nugent RPP, et al: *Trichomonas vaginalis* associated with low birth weight and preterm delivery. Sex Transm Dis 24:353, 1997.
45. Hillier SL, Martius J, Krohn M, et al: A case-control study of chorioamnionic infection and histologic chorioamnionitis in prematurity. N Engl J Med 319:972, 1988.
46. Watts DH, Krohn MA, Hillier SL, Eschenbach DA: The association of occult amniotic fluid infection with gestational age and neonatal outcome among women in preterm labor. Obstet Gynecol 79:351, 1992.
47. Hillier SL, Nugent RP, Eschenbach DA, et al: Association between bacterial vaginosis and preterm delivery of a low-birth-weight infant. N Engl J Med 333:1737, 1995.
48. Riduan J, Hillier S, Utomo B, et al: Bacterial vaginosis and prematurity in Indonesia: Association in early and late pregnancy. Am J Obstet Gynecol 169:175, 1993.
49. Carey JC, Klebanoff MA, Hauth JC, et al: Metronidazole to prevent preterm delivery in pregnant women with asymptomatic bacterial vaginosis. National Institute of Child Health and Human Development Network of Maternal-Fetal Medicine Units. N Engl J Med 342:534, 2000.
50. Guise JM, Mahon SM, Aickin M, et al: Screening for bacterial vaginosis in pregnancy. Am J Prev Med 20:62, 2001.
51. Okun N, Gronau KA, Hannah ME: Antibiotics for bacterial vaginosis or *Trichomonas vaginalis* in pregnancy: a systematic review. Obstet Gynecol 105:857, 2005.
52. Espinoza J, Erez O, Romero R: Preconceptional antibiotic treatment to prevent preterm birth in women with a previous preterm delivery. Am J Obstet Gynecol 194:630, 2006.
53. Romero R, Oyarzun E, Mazor M, et al: Meta-analysis of the relationship between asymptomatic bacteriuria and preterm delivery/low birth weight. Obstet Gynecol 73:576, 1989.
54. Offenbacher S, Lieff S, Boggess K, et al: Maternal periodontitis and prematurity. Part I: Obstetric outcome of prematurity and growth restriction. Ann Periodontol 6:164, 2001.
55. Jeffcoat MK, Geurs NC, Reddy MS, et al: Periodontal infection and preterm birth: Results of a prospective study. J Am Dent Assoc 132:875, 2001.
56. Goepfert AR, Jeffcoat MK, Andrews WW, et al: Periodontal disease and upper genital tract inflammation in early spontaneous preterm birth. Obstet Gynecol 104:777, 2004.
57. Kogan MD, Alexander GR: Social and behavioral factors in preterm birth. Prenat Neonat Med 3:29, 1998.
58. Cabral H, Fried LE, Levenson S, et al: Foreign-born and US-born black women: differences in health behaviors and birth outcomes. Am J Public Health 80:70, 1990.
59. Martin JA, Hamilton BE, Ventura SJ, et al: Births: Final data for 2000. Hyattsville, Maryland, National vital statistics reports; National Center for Health Statistics, 2002, p 1.
60. Feresu SA, Harlow SD, Welch K, Gillespie BW: Incidence of and socio-demographic risk factors for stillbirth, preterm birth and low birthweight among Zimbabwean women. Paediatr Perinat Epidemiol 18:154, 2004.
61. Goldenberg R, Cliver S, Mulvihill X, et al: Medical, psychosocial, and behavioral risk factors do not explain the increased risk for low birth weight among black women. Am J Obstet Gynecol 175:1317, 1996.
62. Goldenberg R, Klebanoff M, Nugent R, et al: For the Vaginal Infections in Pregnancy Study Group: Bacterial colonization of the vagina in four ethnic groups. Am J Obstet Gynecol 174:1618, 1996.
63. Genç MR, Gerber S, Nesin M, Witkin SS: Polymorphism in the interleukin-1 gene complex and spontaneous preterm delivery. Am J Obstet Gynecol 187:157, 2002.
64. Simhan H, Krohn M, Roberts J, et al: Interleukin-6 promoter -174 polymorphism and spontaneous preterm birth. Am J Obstet Gynecol 189:915, 2003.
65. Moore S, Ide M, Randhawa M, et al: An investigation into the association among preterm birth, cytokine gene polymorphisms and periodontal disease. Br J Obstet Gynaecol 111:125, 2004.
66. Macones GA, Parry S, Elkousy M, et al: A polymorphism in the promoter region of TNF and bacterial vaginosis: preliminary evidence of gene-environment interaction in the etiology of spontaneous preterm birth. Am J Obstet Gynecol 190:1504, 2004.
67. Romero RM, Chaiworapongsa TM, Kuivaniemi HM, Tromp GP: Bacterial vaginosis, the inflammatory response and the risk of preterm birth: A role for genetic epidemiology in the prevention of preterm birth. Am J Obstet Gynecol 190:1509, 2004.
68. Kiecolt-Glaser JK, McGuire L, Robles TF, Glaser R: Psychoneuroimmunology: Psychological influences on immune function and health. J Consult Clin Psychol 70:537, 2002.
69. Glaser R, Kiecolt-Glaser J: Stress-induced immune dysfunction: implications for health. Nat Rev Immunol 5:243, 2005.
70. Ruiz RJR, Fullerton JC, Dudley DJM: The interrelationship of maternal stress, endocrine factors and inflammation on gestational length. Obstet Gynecol Surv 58:415, 2003.
71. Annells MF, Hart PH, Mullighan CG, et al: Interleukins-1, -4, -6, -10, tumor necrosis factor, transforming growth factor-β, FAS, and mannose-binding protein C gene polymorphisms in Australian women: Risk of preterm birth. Am J Obstet Gynecol 191:2056, 2004.
72. Hogue CR, Bremner JD: Stress model for research into preterm delivery among black women. Am J Obstet Gynecol 192:s47, 2005.
73. Ekwo EE, Gosselink CA, Moawad A: Unfavorable outcome in penultimate pregnancy and premature rupture of membranes in successive pregnancy. Obstet Gynecol 80:166, 1992.
74. Yang J, Hartmann KE, Savitz DA, et al: Vaginal bleeding during pregnancy and preterm birth. Am J Epidemiol 160:118, 2004.
75. Burton BK: Elevated maternal serum alpha-fetoprotein:Interpretation and follow-up. Clin Obstet Gynecol 31:293, 1988.
76. Chandra S, Scott H, Dodds L, et al: Unexplained elevated maternal serum α-fetoprotein and/or human chorionic gonadotropin and the risk of adverse outcomes. Am J Obstet Gynecol 189:771, 2003.
77. Andersen HF, Nugent CE, Wanty SD, et al: Prediction of risk for preterm delivery by ultrasonographic measurement of cervical length. Am J Obstet Gynecol 163:859, 1990.
78. Iams JD, Goldenberg RL, Meis PJ, et al: The length of the cervix and the risk of spontaneous premature delivery. N Engl J Med 334:567, 1996.
79. Goldenberg RL, Iams JD, Miodovnik M, et al: National Institute of Child Health and Human Development Maternal-Fetal Medicine Units Network: The preterm prediction study: risk factors in twin gestations. Am J Obstet Gynecol 175:1047, 1996.

80. Imseis H, Albert T, Iams JD: Identifying twin gestations at low risk for preterm birth with a transvaginal ultrasonographic cervical measurement at 24 to 26 weeks' gestation. Am J Obstet Gynecol 177:1148, 1997.
81. Taipale P, Hiilesmaa V: Sonographic measurement of uterine cervix at 18–22 weeks' gestation and the risk of preterm delivery. Obstet Gynecol 92:902, 1998.
82. Berghella V, Talucci M, Desai A: Does transvaginal sonographic measurement of cervical length before 14 weeks predict preterm delivery in high-risk pregnancies? Ultrasound Obstet Gynecol 21:140, 2003.
83. Iams J, Goldenberg R, Mercer B, et al: The Preterm Prediction Study: Recurrence risk of spontaneous preterm birth. Am J Obstet Gynecol 178:1035, 1998.
84. Heath V, Southall T, Souka A, et al: Cervical length at 23 weeks of gestation: prediction of spontaneous preterm delivery. Ultrasound Obstet Gynecol 12:312, 1998.
85. Raga F, Bauset C, Remohi J, et al: Reproductive impact of congenital Mullerian anomalies. Hum Reprod 12:2277, 1997.
86. Kaufman RH, Adam ERVI, Hatch EE, et al: Continued follow-up of pregnancy outcomes in diethylstilbestrol-exposed offspring. Obstet Gynecol 96:483, 2000.
87. Gardner MO, Goldenberg RL, Cliver SP, et al: The origin and outcome of preterm twin pregnancies. Obstet Gynecol 85:553, 1995.
88. Newman R, Luke B: Multifetal Pregnancy. Philadelphia, Lippincott Williams & Wilkins, 2001, p 244.
89. Wilcox L, Kiely J, Melvin C, Martin M: Assisted reproductive technologies: estimates of their contribution to multiple births and newborn hospital days in the United States. Fertil Steril 65:361, 1996.
90. Martin JA, Hamilton BE, Ventura SJ, et al: Births: Final data for 2001. Hyattsville, Maryland: National Center for Health Statistics, 2002, p 1.
91. Green NS: Risks of birth defects and other adverse outcomes associated with assisted reproductive technology. Pediatrics 114:256, 2004.
92. Jain T, Missmer SA, Hornstein MD: Trends in embryo-transfer practice and in outcomes of the use of assisted reproductive technology in the United States. N Engl J Med 350:1639, 2004.
93. ACOG Committee Opinion 324: Perinatal risks associated with assisted reproductive technology. Obstet Gynecol 106:1143, 2005.
94. Schieve LA, Ferre C, Peterson HB, et al: Perinatal outcome among singleton infants conceived through assisted reproductive technology in the United States. Obstet Gynecol 103:1144, 2004.
95. Jackson RA, Gibson KA, Wu YW, Croughan MS: Perinatal outcomes in singletons following in vitro fertilization: a meta-analysis. Obstet Gynecol 103:551, 2004.
96. McGovern PG, Llorens AJ, Skurnick JH, et al: Increased risk of preterm birth in singleton pregnancies resulting from in vitro fertilization-embryo transfer or gamete intrafallopian transfer: A meta-analysis. Fertil Steril 82:1514, 2004.
97. Helmerhorst FM, Perquin DA, Donker D, Keirse MJ: Perinatal outcome of singletons and twins after assisted conception: a systematic review of controlled studies. BMJ 328:261, 2004.
98. Romero R, Espinoza J, Mazor M: Can endometrial infection/inflammation explain implantation failure, spontaneous abortion, and preterm birth after in vitro fertilization? Fertil Steril 82:799, 2004.
99. Weiss G, Goldsmith LT, Sachdev R, et al: Elevated first-trimester serum relaxin concentrations in pregnant women following ovarian stimulation predict prematurity risk and preterm delivery. Obstet Gynecol 82:821, 1993.
100. Hansen M, Kurinczuk JJ, Bower C, Webb S: The risk of major birth defects after intracytoplasmic sperm injection and in vitro fertilization. N Engl J Med 346:725, 2002.
101. Kyrklund-Blomberg NB, Cnattingius S: Preterm birth and maternal smoking: Risks related to gestational age and onset of delivery. Am J Obstet Gynecol 179:1051, 1998.
102. Savitz DA, Dole N, Terry JWJ, et al: Smoking and pregnancy outcome among African-American and white women in central North Carolina. Epidemiology 12:636, 2001.
103. Moore TR, Iams JD, Creasy RK, et al: Diurnal and gestational patterns of uterine activity in normal human pregnancy. The Uterine Activity in Pregnancy Working Group. Obstet Gynecol 83:517, 1994.
104. Mamelle N, Laumon B, Lazar P: Prematurity and occupational activity during pregnancy. Am J Epidemiol 119:309, 1984.
105. Mozurkewich EL, Luke B, Avni M, Wolf FM. Working conditions and adverse pregnancy outcome: a meta-analysis. Obstet Gynecol 95:623, 2000.
106. Newman RB, Goldenberg RL, Moawad AH, et al: Occupational fatigue and preterm premature rupture of membranes. Am J Obstet Gynecol 184:438, 2001.
107. Kendall JZ, Challis JR, Hart IC, et al: Steroid and prostaglandin concentrations in the plasma of pregnant ewes during infusion of adrenocorticotrophin or dexamethasone to intact or hypophysectomized foetuses. J Endocrinol 75:59, 1977.
108. Liggins G, Holm LW, Kennedy PC: Prolonged pregnancy following surgical lesions of the foetal lamb pituitary. J Reprod Fertil 12:419, 1966.
109. Mecenas CA, Giussani DA, Owiny JR, et al: Production of premature delivery in pregnant rhesus monkeys by androstenedione infusion. Nat Med 2:443, 1996.
110. Rees LH, Jack PM, Thomas AL, Nathanielsz PW: Role of foetal adrenocorticotrophin during parturition in sheep. Nature 253:274, 1975.
111. Liggins GC: Premature parturition after infusion of corticotrophin or cortisol into foetal lambs. J Endocrinol 42:323, 1968.
112. Romero R, Gomez R, Ghezzi F, et al: A fetal systemic inflammatory response is followed by the spontaneous onset of preterm parturition. Am J Obstet Gynecol 179:186, 1998.
113. Nathanielsz PW, Jenkins SL, Tame JD, et al: Local paracrine effects of estradiol are central to parturition in the rhesus monkey. Nat Med 4:456, 1998.
114. Casey ML, MacDonald PC: The endocrinology of human parturition. Ann NY Acad Sci 828:273, 1997.
115. Zeitlin J, Ancel PY, Saurel-Cubizolles MJ, Papiernik E: The relationship between intrauterine growth restriction and preterm delivery: an empirical approach using data from a European case-control study. Br J Obstet Gynaecol 107:750, 2000.
116. Bukowski R, Gahn D, Denning J, Saade G: Impairment of growth in fetuses destined to deliver preterm. Am J Obstet Gynecol 185:463, 2001.
117. Gardosi JO: Prematurity and fetal growth restriction. Early Hum Dev 81:43, 2005.
118. Uldbjerg N, Ekman G, Malmstrom A: Ripening of the human uterine cervix related to changes in collagen, glycosaminoglycans and collagenolytic activity. Am J Obstet Gynecol 147:662, 1982.
119. Ito A, Hiro D, Sakyo K, Mori Y: The role of leukocyte factors on uterine cervical ripening and dilation. Biol Reprod 37:511, 1987.
120. Ito A, Hiro D, Ojima Y, Mori Y: Spontaneous production of interleukin-1-like factors from pregnant rabbit uterine cervix. Am J Obstet Gynecol 159:261, 1988.
121. Ito A, Leppert PC, Mori Y: Human recombinant interleukin-1 alpha increases elastase-like enzyme in human uterine cervical fibroblasts. Gynecol Obstet Invest 30:239, 1990.
122. Maradny EE, Kanayama N, Halim A, et al: Stretching of fetal membranes increases the concentration of interleukin-8 and collagenase activity. Am J Obstet Gynecol 174:843, 1996.
123. Osmers RG, Blaser J, Kuhn W, Tschesche H: Interleukin-8 synthesis and the onset of labor. Obstet Gynecol 86:223, 1995.
124. Chwalisz K, Shi Shao O, Neff G, Egler J: The effect of antigestagen ZK 98, 199 on the uterine cervix. Acta Endocrinologica 283:113, 1987.
125. Stys S, Clewell W, Meschia G: Changes in cervical compliance at parturition independent of uterine activity. Am J Obstet Gynecol 130:414, 1978.
126. Chwalisz K, Garfield RE: Role of nitric oxide in the uterus and cervix: implications for the management of labor. J Perinat Med 26:448, 1998.
127. Chwalisz K, Buhimschi I, Garfield RE: The role of nitric oxide in obstetrics. Prenat Neonat Med 4:292, 1996.
128. Evans CH, Stefanovic-Racic M, Lancaster J: Nitric oxide and its role in orthopaedic disease. Clin Orthop 312:275, 1995.

129. Romero R: Clinical application of nitric oxide donors and blockers. Hum Reprod 13:248, 1998.
130. Buhimschi I, Ali M, Jain V, et al: Differential regulation of nitric oxide in the rat uterus and cervix during pregnancy and labour. Hum Reprod 11:1755, 1996.
131. Ekerhovd E, Weijdegard B, Brannstrom M, et al: Nitric oxide induced cervical ripening in the human: Involvement of cyclic guanosine monophosphate, prostaglandin F(2 alpha), and prostaglandin E(2). Am J Obstet Gynecol 186:745, 2002.
132. Facchinetti F, Piccinini F, Volpe A: Chemical ripening of the cervix with intracervical application of sodium nitroprusside: a randomized controlled trial. Hum Reprod 15:2224, 2000.
133. Ledingham MA, Thomson AJ, Young A, et al: Changes in the expression of nitric oxide synthase in the human uterine cervix during pregnancy and parturition. Mol Hum Reprod 6:1041, 2000.
134. Thomson AJ, Lunan CB, Cameron AD, et al: Nitric oxide donors induce ripening of the human uterine cervix: a randomised controlled trial. Br J Obstet Gynaecol 104:1054, 1997.
135. Tschugguel W, Schneeberger C, Lass H, et al: Human cervical ripening is associated with an increase in cervical inducible nitric oxide synthase expression. Biol Reprod 60:1367, 1999.
136. Bishop EH: Pelvic scoring for elective induction. Obstet Gynecol 24:266, 1964.
137. Copper RL, Goldenberg RL, Davis RO, et al: Warning symptoms, uterine contractions, and cervical examination findings in women at risk of preterm delivery. Am J Obstet Gynecol 162:748, 1990.
138. Nathanielsz P, Honnebier M: Myometrial function. *In* Drife J, Calder A (eds): Prostaglandins and the Uterus. London, Springer-Verlag, 1992, p 161.
139. Hsu HW, Figueroa JP, Honnebier MB, et al: Power spectrum analysis of myometrial electromyogram and intrauterine pressure changes in the pregnant rhesus monkey in late gestation. Am J Obstet Gynecol 161:467, 1989.
140. Honnebier MB, Jenkins SL, Wentworth RA, et al: Temporal structuring of delivery in the absence of a photoperiod: preparturient myometrial activity of the rhesus monkey is related to maternal body temperature and depends on the maternal circadian system. Biol Reprod 45:617, 1991.
141. Katz M, Newman RB, Gill PJ: Assessment of uterine activity in ambulatory patients at high risk of preterm labor and delivery. Am J Obstet Gynecol 154:44, 1986.
142. Taylor NF, Martin MC, Nathanielsz PW, Seron-Ferre M: The fetus determines circadian oscillation of myometrial electromyographic activity in the pregnant rhesus monkey. Am J Obstet Gynecol 146:557, 1983.
143. Binienda Z, Rosen ED, Kelleman A, et al: Maintaining fetal normoglycemia prevents the increase in myometrial activity and uterine 13,14-dihydro-15-keto-prostaglandin F2 alpha production during food withdrawal in late pregnancy in the ewe. Endocrinology 127:3047, 1990.
144. Nathanielsz P, Poore E, Brodie A, et al: Update on molecular events of myometrial activity during pregnancy. *In* Nathanielsz P, Parer J (eds): Research in Perinatal Medicine. Ithaca, NY, Perinatology, 1987, p 111.
145. Romero R, Avila C, Sepulveda W, et al: The role of systemic and intrauterine infection in preterm labor. *In* Fuchs A, Fuchs F, Stubblefield P (eds): Preterm Birth: Causes, Prevention, and Management. New York, McGraw-Hill, 1993, p 97.
146. Maymon E, Mazor M, Romero R, et al: The Yom Kippur effect on human parturition. Am J Obstet Gynecol 176:S115, 1997.
147. Kaplan M, Eidelman AI, Aboulafia Y: Fasting and the precipitation of labor. The Yom Kippur effect. JAMA 250:1317, 1983.
148. Effectiveness and safety of the oxytocin antagonist atosiban versus beta-adrenergic agonists in the treatment of preterm labour. The Worldwide Atosiban versus Beta-agonists Study Group. Br J Obstet Gynaecol 108:133, 2001.
149. Blanks AM, Thornton S: The role of oxytocin in parturition. Br J Obstet Gynaecol 110(Suppl)20:46, 2003.
150. Chibbar R, Miller FD, Mitchell BF: Synthesis of oxytocin in amnion, chorion, and decidua may influence the timing of human parturition. J Clin Invest 91:185, 1993.
151. Coomarasamy A, Knox EM, Gee H, Khan KS: Oxytocin antagonists for tocolysis in preterm labour—a systematic review. Med Sci Monit 8:RA268, 2002.
152. European Atosiban Study Group: The oxytocin antagonist atosiban versus the beta-agonist terbutaline in the treatment of preterm labor. A randomized, double-blind, controlled study. Acta Obstet Gynecol Scand 80:413, 2001.
153. French/Australian Atosiban Investigators Group: Treatment of preterm labor with the oxytocin antagonist atosiban: a double-blind, randomized, controlled comparison with salbutamol. Eur J Obstet Gynecol Reprod Biol 98:177, 2001.
154. Miller FD, Chibbar R, Mitchell BF: Synthesis of oxytocin in amnion, chorion and decidua: a potential paracrine role for oxytocin in the onset of human parturition. Regul Pept 45:247, 1993.
155. Moutquin JM, Sherman D, Cohen H, et al: Double-blind, randomized, controlled trial of atosiban and ritodrine in the treatment of preterm labor: a multicenter effectiveness and safety study. Am J Obstet Gynecol 182:1191, 2000.
156. Romero R, Sibai BM, Sanchez Ramos L, et al: An oxytocin receptor antagonist (atosiban) in the treatment of preterm labor: a randomized, double-blind, placebo-controlled trial with tocolytic rescue. Am J Obstet Gynecol 182:1173, 2000.
157. Cole WC, Garfield RE, Kirkaldy JSL: Gap junctions and direct intercellular communication between rat uterine smooth muscle cells. Am J Physiol 249:C20, 1985.
158. Garfield RE, Sims S, Daniel EE: Gap junctions: their presence and necessity in myometrium during parturition. Science 198:958, 1977.
159. Garfield RE, Sims SM, Kannan MS, Daniel EE: Possible role of gap junctions in activation of myometrium during parturition. Am J Physiol 235:C168, 1978.
160. Garfield RE, Hayashi RH: Appearance of gap junctions in the myometrium of women during labor. Am J Obstet Gynecol 140:254, 1981.
161. Garfield RE, Puri CP, Csapo AI: Endocrine, structural, and functional changes in the uterus during premature labor. Am J Obstet Gynecol 142:21, 1982.
162. Balducci J, Risek B, Gilula NB, et al: Gap junction formation in human myometrium: a key to preterm labor? Am J Obstet Gynecol 168:1609, 1993.
163. Chow L, Lye SJ: Expression of the gap junction protein connexin-43 is increased in the human myometrium toward term and with the onset of labor. Am J Obstet Gynecol 170:788, 1994.
164. Lefebvre DL, Piersanti M, Bai XH, et al: Myometrial transcriptional regulation of the gap junction gene, connexin-43. Reprod Fertil Dev 7:603, 1995.
165. Orsino A, Taylor CV, Lye SJ: Connexin-26 and connexin-43 are differentially expressed and regulated in the rat myometrium throughout late pregnancy and with the onset of labor. Endocrinology 137:1545, 1996.
166. Ou CW, Orsino A, Lye SJ: Expression of connexin-43 and connexin-26 in the rat myometrium during pregnancy and labor is differentially regulated by mechanical and hormonal signals. Endocrinology 138:5398, 1997.
167. Cook JL, Zaragoza DB, Sung DH, Olson DM: Expression of myometrial activation and stimulation genes in a mouse model of preterm labor: myometrial activation, stimulation, and preterm labor. Endocrinology 141:1718, 2000.
168. Lye SJ, Nicholson BJ, Mascarenhas M, et al: Increased expression of connexin-43 in the rat myometrium during labor is associated with an increase in the plasma estrogen:progesterone ratio. Endocrinology 132:2380, 1993.
169. Petrocelli T, Lye SJ: Regulation of transcripts encoding the myometrial gap junction protein, connexin-43, by estrogen and progesterone. Endocrinology 133:284, 1993.
170. Lye SJ: The initiation and inhibition of labour: towards a molecular understanding. Semin Reprod Endocrinol 12:284, 1994.
171. Lye SJ, Mitchell J, Nashman N, et al: Role of mechanical signals in the onset of term and preterm labor. Front Horm Res 27:165, 2001.
172. Skinner SJ, Liggins GC: Glycosaminoglycans and collagen in human amnion from pregnancies with and without premature rupture of the membranes. J Dev Physiol 3:111, 1981.

173. Hieber AD, Corcino D, Motosue J, et al: Detection of elastin in the human fetal membranes: proposed molecular basis for elasticity. Placenta 18:301, 1997.
174. Bryant-Greenwood GD: The extracellular matrix of the human fetal membranes: structure and function. Placenta 19:1, 1998.
175. Iams JD, Casal D, McGregor JA, et al: Fetal fibronectin improves the accuracy of diagnosis of preterm labor. Am J Obstet Gynecol 173:141, 1995.
176. Lockwood CJ, Senyei AE, Dische MR, et al: Fetal fibronectin in cervical and vaginal secretions as a predictor of preterm delivery. N Engl J Med 325:669, 1991.
177. Nageotte MP, Casal D, Senyei AE: Fetal fibronectin in patients at increased risk for premature birth. Am J Obstet Gynecol 170:20, 1994.
178. Oshiro B, Edwin S, Silver R: Human fibronectin and human tenascin production in human amnion cells. J Soc Gynecol Invest 3:351A. 1996.
179. Feinberg RF, Kliman HJ, Lockwood CJ: Is oncofetal fibronectin a trophoblast glue for human implantation? Am J Pathol 138:537, 1991.
180. Maymon E, Romero R, Pacora P, et al: Evidence for the participation of interstitial collagenase (matrix metalloproteinase 1) in preterm premature rupture of membranes. Am J Obstet Gynecol 183:914, 2000.
181. Maymon E, Romero R, Pacora P, et al: Human neutrophil collagenase (matrix metalloproteinase 8) in parturition, premature rupture of the membranes, and intrauterine infection. Am J Obstet Gynecol 183:94, 2000.
182. Helmig BR, Romero R, Espinoza J, et al: Neutrophil elastase and secretory leukocyte protease inhibitor in prelabor rupture of membranes, parturition and intra-amniotic infection. J Matern Fetal Neonatal Med 12:237, 2002.
183. Vadillo-Ortega F, Hernandez A, Gonzalez-Avila G, et al: Increased matrix metalloproteinase activity and reduced tissue inhibitor of metalloproteinases-1 levels in amniotic fluids from pregnancies complicated by premature rupture of membranes. Am J Obstet Gynecol 174:1371, 1996.
184. Maymon E, Romero R, Pacora P, et al: A role for the 72 kDa gelatinase (MMP-2) and its inhibitor (TIMP-2) in human parturition, premature rupture of membranes and intraamniotic infection. J Perinat Med 29:308, 2001.
185. Lei H, Furth EE, Kalluri R, et al: A program of cell death and extracellular matrix degradation is activated in the amnion before the onset of labor. J Clin Invest 98:1971, 1996.
186. Fortunato SJ, Menon R, Bryant C, Lombardi SJ: Programmed cell death (apoptosis) as a possible pathway to metalloproteinase activation and fetal membrane degradation in premature rupture of membranes. Am J Obstet Gynecol 182:1468, 2000.
187. Fortunato SJ, Menon R, Lombardi SJ: Support for an infection-induced apoptotic pathway in human fetal membranes. Am J Obstet Gynecol 184:1392, 2001.
188. Lei H, Kalluri R, Furth EE, et al: Rat amnion type IV collagen composition and metabolism: implications for membrane breakdown. Biol Reprod 60:176, 1999.
189. McLaren J, Taylor DJ, Bell SC: Increased incidence of apoptosis in non-labour-affected cytotrophoblast cells in term fetal membranes overlying the cervix. Hum Reprod 14:2895, 1999.
190. McLaren J, Taylor DJ, Bell SC: Increased concentration of pro-matrix metalloproteinase 9 in term fetal membranes overlying the cervix before labor: implications for membrane remodeling and rupture. Am J Obstet Gynecol 182:409, 2000.
191. McDonald TJ, Nathanielsz PW: Bilateral destruction of the fetal paraventricular nuclei prolongs gestation in sheep. Am J Obstet Gynecol 165:764, 1991.
192. Gluckman PD, Mallard C, Boshier DP: The effect of hypothalamic lesions on the length of gestation in fetal sheep. Am J Obstet Gynecol 165:1464, 1991.
193. Honnebier WJ, Swaab DF: The influence of anencephaly upon intrauterine growth of fetus and placenta and upon gestation length. J Obstet Gynaecol Br Commonw 80:577, 1973.
194. Romero R: The child is the father of the man. Prenat Neonat Med 1:8, 1996.
195. Eschenbach DA, Gravett MG, Chen KC, et al: Bacterial vaginosis during pregnancy. An association with prematurity and postpartum complications. Scand J Urol Nephrol Suppl 86:213, 1984.
196. Flynn CA, Helwig AL, Meurer LN: Bacterial vaginosis in pregnancy and the risk of prematurity: a meta-analysis. J Fam Pract 48:885, 1999.
197. Meis PJ, Goldenberg RL, Mercer B, et al: The preterm prediction study: significance of vaginal infections. National Institute of Child Health and Human Development Maternal-Fetal Medicine Units Network. Am J Obstet Gynecol 173:1231, 1995.
198. Carroll SG, Papaioannou S, Ntumazah IL, et al: Lower genital tract swabs in the prediction of intrauterine infection in preterm prelabour rupture of the membranes. Br J Obstet Gynaecol 103:54, 1996.
199. MacGregor SN, Sabbagha RE, Tamura RK, et al: Differing fetal growth patterns in pregnancies complicated by preterm labor. Obstet Gynecol 72:834, 1988.
200. Ott WJ: Intrauterine growth retardation and preterm delivery. Am J Obstet Gynecol 168:1710, 1993.
201. Tamura RK, Sabbagha RE, Depp R, et al: Diminished growth in fetuses born preterm after spontaneous labor or rupture of membranes. Am J Obstet Gynecol 148:1105, 1984.
202. Weiner CP, Sabbagha RE, Vaisrub N, Depp R: A hypothetical model suggesting suboptimal intrauterine growth in infants delivered preterm. Obstet Gynecol 65:323, 1985.
203. Williams MC, O'Brien WF, Nelson RN, Spellacy WN: Histologic chorioamnionitis is associated with fetal growth restriction in term and preterm infants. Am J Obstet Gynecol 183:1094, 2000.
204. Gomez R, Romero R, Ghezzi F, et al: The fetal inflammatory response syndrome. Am J Obstet Gynecol 179:194, 1998.
205. Benedetti TJ, Valle R, Ledger WJ: Antepartum pneumonia in pregnancy. Am J Obstet Gynecol 144:413, 1982.
206. Cunningham FG, Morris GB, Mickal A: Acute pyelonephritis of pregnancy: A clinical review. Obstet Gynecol 42:112, 1973.
207. Fan YD, Pastorek JG, Miller JM Jr, Mulvey J: Acute pyelonephritis in pregnancy. Am J Perinatol 4:324–26, 1987.
208. Finland M, Dublin TD: Pneumococcic pneumonia complicating pregnancy and the puerperium. JAMA 112:1027, 1939.
209. Gilles HM, Lawson JB, Sibelas M, et al: Malaria, anaemia and pregnancy. Ann Trop Med Parasitol 63:245, 1969.
210. Herd N, Jordan T: An investigtion of malaria during pregnancy in Zimbabwe. Afr J Med 27:62, 1981.
211. Hibbard L, Thrupp L, Summeril S, et al: Treatment of pyelonephritis in pregnancy. Am J Obstet Gynecol 98:609, 1967.
212. Kass E: Maternal urinary tract infection. NY State J Med 1:2822, 1962.
213. Madinger NE, Greenspoon JS, Ellrodt AG: Pneumonia during pregnancy: has modern technology improved maternal and fetal outcome? Am J Obstet Gynecol 161:657, 1989.
214. McLane CM: Pyelitis of pregnancy: a five-year study. Am J Obstet Gynecol 38:117, 1939.
215. Oxhorn H: The changing aspects of pneumonia complicating pregnancy. Am J Obstet Gynecol 70:1057, 1955.
216. Stevenson CS, Glasko AJ, Gillespie EC: Treatment of typhoid in pregnancy with chloramphenicol (chloromycetin). JAMA 146:1190, 1951.
217. Wing ES, Troppoli DV: The intrauterine transmission of typhoid. JAMA 95:405, 1930.
218. Minkoff H: Prematurity: infection as an etiologic factor. Obstet Gynecol 62:137, 1983.
219. Romero R, Mazor M, Wu Y, et al: Infection in the pathogenesis of preterm labor. Semin Perinatol 12:262, 1988.
220. Romero R, Sirtori M, Oyarzun E, et al: Infection and labor. V. Prevalence, microbiology, and clinical significance of intraamniotic infection in women with preterm labor and intact membranes. Am J Obstet Gynecol 161:817, 1989.
221. Bang B: The etiology of epizootic abortion. J Comp Anthol Ther 10:125, 1987.
222. Fidel PL Jr, Romero R, Wolf N, et al: Systemic and local cytokine profiles in endotoxin-induced preterm parturition in mice. Am J Obstet Gynecol 170:1467, 1994.
223. Kullander S: Fever and parturition. An experimental study in rabbits. Acta Obstet Gynecol Scand Suppl 66:77, 1977.
224. McDuffie RS Jr, Sherman MP, Gibbs RS: Amniotic fluid tumor necrosis factor-alpha and interleukin-1 in a rabbit model of bacterially induced preterm pregnancy loss. Am J Obstet Gynecol 67:1583, 1992.

225. McKay DG, Wong TC: The effect of bacterial endotoxin on the placenta of the rat. Am J Pathol 42:357, 1963.
226. Rieder RF, Thomas L: Studies on the mechanisms involved in the production of abortion by endotoxin. J Immunol 84:189, 1960.
227. Romero R, Munoz H, Gomez R, et al: Antibiotic therapy reduces the rate of infection-induced preterm delivery and perinatal mortality. Am J Obstet Gynecol 170:390, 1994.
228. Skarnes RC, Harper MJ: Relationship between endotoxin-induced abortion and the synthesis of prostaglandin F. Prostaglandins 1:191, 1972.
229. Takeda Y, Tsuchiya I: Studies on the pathological changes caused by the injection of the Shwartzman filtrate and the endotoxin into pregnant rabbits. Jap J Exper Med 21:9, 1953.
230. Zahl PA, Bjerknes C: Induction of decidua-placental hemorrhage in mice by the endotoxins of certain gram-negative bacteria. Proc Soc Exper Biol Med 54:329, 1943.
231. Gomez R, Ghezzi F, Romero R, et al: Premature labor and intra-amniotic infection. Clinical aspects and role of the cytokines in diagnosis and pathophysiology. Clin Perinatol 22:281, 1995.
232. Romero R, Salafia CM, Athanassiadis AP, et al: The relationship between acute inflammatory lesions of the preterm placenta and amniotic fluid microbiology. Am J Obstet Gynecol 166:1382, 1992.
233. Romero R, Espinoza J, Chaiworapongsa T, Kalache K: Infection and prematurity and the role of preventive strategies. Semin Neonatol 7:259, 2002.
234. Romero R, Gonzalez R, Sepulveda W, et al: Infection and labor. VIII. Microbial invasion of the amniotic cavity in patients with suspected cervical incompetence: prevalence and clinical significance. Am J Obstet Gynecol 167:1086, 1992.
235. Romero R, Shamma F, Avila C, et al: Infection and labor. VI. Prevalence, microbiology, and clinical significance of intraamniotic infection in twin gestations with preterm labor. Am J Obstet Gynecol 163:757, 1990.
236. Romero R, Nores J, Mazor M, et al: Microbial invasion of the amniotic cavity during term labor. Prevalence and clinical significance. J Reprod Med 38:543, 1993.
237. Cassell GH, Davis RO, Waites KB, et al: Isolation of *Mycoplasma hominis* and *Ureaplasma urealyticum* from amniotic fluid at 16–20 weeks of gestation: potential effect on outcome of pregnancy. Sex Transm Dis 10:294, 1983.
238. Gray DJ, Robinson HB, Malone J, Thomson RB Jr: Adverse outcome in pregnancy following amniotic fluid isolation of Ureaplasma urealyticum. Prenat Diagn 12:111, 1992.
239. Horowitz S, Mazor M, Romero R, et al: Infection of the amniotic cavity with *Ureaplasma urealyticum* in the midtrimester of pregnancy. J Reprod Med 40:375, 1995.
240. Romero R, Munoz H, Gomez R, et al: Two thirds of spontaneous abortion/fetal deaths after genetic amniocentesis are the result of a pre-existing sub-clinical inflammatory process of the amniotic cavity. Am J Obstet Gynecol 172:261, 1995.
241. Wenstrom KD, Andrews WW, Tamura T, et al: Elevated amniotic fluid interleukin-6 levels at genetic amniocentesis predict subsequent pregnancy loss. Am J Obstet Gynecol 175:830, 1996.
242. Wenstrom KD, Andrews WW, Hauth JC, et al: Elevated second-trimester amniotic fluid interleukin-6 levels predict preterm delivery. Am J Obstet Gynecol 178:546, 1998.
243. Yoon BH, Oh SY, Romero R, et al: An elevated amniotic fluid matrix metalloproteinase-8 level at the time of mid-trimester genetic amniocentesis is a risk factor for spontaneous preterm delivery. Am J Obstet Gynecol 185:1162, 2001.
244. Ghidini A, Eglinton GS, Spong CY, et al: Elevated mid-trimester amniotic fluid tumor necrosis alpha levels: a predictor of preterm delivery. Am J Obstet Gynecol 174:307, 1996.
244a. Spong CY, Ghidini A, Sherer DM, et al: Angiogenin: a marker for preterm delivery in midtrimester amniotic fluid. Am J Obstet Gynecol 176:415, 1997.
245. Romero R, Avila C, Santhanam U, Sehgal PB: Amniotic fluid interleukin 6 in preterm labor. Association with infection. J Clin Invest 85:1392, 1990.
246. Romero R, Sepulveda W, Kenney JS, et al: Interleukin 6 determination in the detection of microbial invasion of the amniotic cavity. Ciba Found Symp 167:205, 1992.
247. Romero R, Yoon BH, Kenney JS, et al: Amniotic fluid interleukin-6 determinations are of diagnostic and prognostic value in preterm labor. Am J Reprod Immunol 30:167, 1993.
248. Yoon BH, Romero R, Kim CJ, et al: Amniotic fluid interleukin-6: a sensitive test for antenatal diagnosis of acute inflammatory lesions of preterm placenta and prediction of perinatal morbidity. Am J Obstet Gynecol 172:960, 1995.
249. Berry SM, Gomez R, Athayde N, et al: The role of granulocyte colony stimulating factor in the neutrophilia observed in the fetal inflammatory response syndrome. Am J Obstet Gynecol 178: S202, 1998.
250. Romero R, Athayde N, Gomez R, et al: The fetal inflammatory response syndrome is characterized by the outpouring of a potent extracellular matrix degrading enzyme into the fetal circulation. Am J Obstet Gynecol 178:S3, 1998.
251. Romero R, Maymon E, Pacora P, et al: Further observations on the fetal inflammatory response syndrome: a potential homeostatic role for the soluble receptors of tumor necrosis factor alpha. Am J Obstet Gynecol 183:1070, 2000.
252. Berry SM, Romero R, Gomez R, et al: Premature parturition is characterized by in utero activation of the fetal immune system. Am J Obstet Gynecol 173:1315, 1995.
253. Pacora P, Chaiworapongsa T, Maymon E, et al: Funisitis and chorionic vasculitis: the histological counterpart of the fetal inflammatory response syndrome. J Matern Fetal Med 11:18, 2002.
254. Romero R, Gomez R, Ghezzi F, et al: A novel form of fetal cardiac dysfunction in preterm premature rupture of membranes. Am J Obstet Gynecol 180:S27, 1999.
255. Yoon BH, Romero R, Park JS, et al: The relationship among inflammatory lesions of the umbilical cord (funisitis), umbilical cord plasma interleukin 6 concentration, amniotic fluid infection, and neonatal sepsis. Am J Obstet Gynecol 183:1124, 2000.
256. Yoon BH, Romero R, Kim KS, et al: A systemic fetal inflammatory response and the development of bronchopulmonary dysplasia. Am J Obstet Gynecol 181:773, 1999.
257. Yoon BH, Romero R, Yang SH, et al: Interleukin-6 concentrations in umbilical cord plasma are elevated in neonates with white matter lesions associated with periventricular leukomalacia. Am J Obstet Gynecol 174:1433, 1996.
258. Yoon BH, Romero R, Park JS, et al: Fetal exposure to an intra-amniotic inflammation and the development of cerebral palsy at the age of three years. Am J Obstet Gynecol 182:675, 2000.
259. Clayton D, McKeigue PM: Epidemiological methods for studying genes and environmental factors in complex diseases. Lancet 358:1356, 2001.
260. Tiret L: Gene-environment interaction: a central concept in multifactorial diseases. Proc Nutr Soc 61:457, 2002.
261. US Preventive Services Task Force: Screening for bacterial vaginosis in pregnancy. Recommendations and rationale. Am J Prev Med 20:59, 2001.
262. Centers for Disease Control and Prevention: Sexually transmitted diseases treatment guidelines 2002. MMWR 51:1, 2002.
263. Hauth JC, Goldenberg RL, Andrews WW, et al: Reduced incidence of preterm delivery with metronidazole and erythromycin in women with bacterial vaginosis. N Engl J Med 333:1732, 1995.
264. Klebanoff MA, Guise JM, Carey JC: Treatment recommendations for bacterial vaginosis in pregnant women. Clin Infect Dis 36:1630–31, 2003.
265. Koumans EH, Markowitz LE, Hogan V: Indications for therapy and treatment recommendations for bacterial vaginosis in non-pregnant and pregnant women: a synthesis of data. Clin Infect Dis 35:S152, 2002.
266. Lamont RF: Infection in the prediction and antibiotics in the prevention of spontaneous preterm labour and preterm birth. Br J Obstet Gynaecol 110 Suppl 20:71, 2003.
267. Leitich H, Brunbauer M, Bodner-Adler B, et al: Antibiotic treatment of bacterial vaginosis in pregnancy: a meta-analysis. Am J Obstet Gynecol 188:752, 2003.
268. McDonald H, Brocklehurst P, Parsons J: Antibiotics for treating bacterial vaginosis in pregnancy. Cochrane Database Syst Rev 1: CD000262, 2005.
269. McDonald HM, O'Loughlin JA, Vigneswaran R, et al: Impact of metronidazole therapy on preterm birth in women with bacterial

vaginosis flora *(Gardnerella vaginalis)*: a randomised, placebo controlled trial. Br J Obstet Gynaecol 104:1391, 1997.
270. McGregor JA, French JI, Parker R, et al: Prevention of premature birth by screening and treatment for common genital tract infections: results of a prospective controlled evaluation. Am J Obstet Gynecol 173:157, 1995.
271. Morales WJ, Schorr S, Albritton J: Effect of metronidazole in patients with preterm birth in preceding pregnancy and bacterial vaginosis: a placebo-controlled, double-blind study. Am J Obstet Gynecol 171:345–47, 1994.
272. Roberts AK, Monzon-Bordonaba F, Van Deerlin PG, et al: Association of polymorphism within the promoter of the tumor necrosis factor alpha gene with increased risk of preterm premature rupture of the fetal membranes. Am J Obstet Gynecol 180:1297, 1999.
273. Romero R, Sepulveda W, Baumann P, et al: The preterm labor syndrome: Biochemical, cytologic, immunologic, pathologic, microbiologic, and clinical evidence that preterm labor is a heterogeneous disease. Am J Obstet Gynecol 168:288, 1993.
274. Combs CA, Katz MA, Kitzmiller JL, Brescia RJ: Experimental preeclampsia produced by chronic constriction of the lower aorta: validation with longitudinal blood pressure measurements in conscious rhesus monkeys. Am J Obstet Gynecol 169:215, 1993.
275. Kim YM, Chaiworapongsa T, Gomez R, et al: Failure of physiologic transformation of the spiral arteries in the placental bed in preterm premature rupture of membranes. Am J Obstet Gynecol 187:1137, 2002.
276. Kim YM, Bujold E, Chaiworapongsa T, et al: Failure of physiologic transformation of the spiral arteries in patients with preterm labor and intact membranes. Am J Obstet Gynecol 189:1063, 2003.
277. Brar HS, Medearis AL, DeVore GR, Platt LD: Maternal and fetal blood flow velocity waveforms in patients with preterm labor: prediction of successful tocolysis. Am J Obstet Gynecol 159:947, 1988.
278. Brar HS, Medearis AL, De Vore GR, Platt LD: Maternal and fetal blood flow velocity waveforms in patients with preterm labor: relationship to outcome. Am J Obstet Gynecol 161:1519, 1989.
279. Strigini FA, Lencioni G, De Luca G, et al: Uterine artery velocimetry and spontaneous preterm delivery. Obstet Gynecol 85:374, 1995.
280. Woods LL, Brooks VL: Role of the renin-angiotensin system in hypertension during reduced uteroplacental perfusion pressure. Am J Physiol 257:R204, 1989.
281. Katz M, Shapiro WB, Porush JG, et al: Uterine and renal renin release after ligation of the uterine arteries in the pregnant rabbit. Am J Obstet Gynecol 136:676, 1980.
282. Poisner AM: The human placental renin-angiotensin system. Front Neuroendocrinol 19:232, 1998.
283. Lalanne C, Mironneau C, Mironneau J, Savineau JP: Contractions of rat uterine smooth muscle induced by acetylcholine and angiotensin II in Ca2+-free medium. Br J Pharmacol 81:317, 1984.
284. Campos GA, Guerra FA, Israel EJ: Angiotensin II induced release of prostaglandins from rat uterus. Arch Biol Med Exp (Santiago) 16:43, 1983.
285. Elovitz MA, Saunders T, Ascher-Landsberg J, Phillippe M: Effects of thrombin on myometrial contractions in vitro and in vivo. Am J Obstet Gynecol 183:7994, 2000.
286. Elovitz MA, Baron J, Phillippe M: The role of thrombin in preterm parturition. Am J Obstet Gynecol 185:1059, 2001.
287. Rosen T, Schatz F, Kuczynski E, et al: Thrombin-enhanced matrix metalloproteinase-1 expression: a mechanism linking placental abruption with premature rupture of the membranes. J Matern Fetal Neonatal Med 11:11, 2002.
288. Lockwood CJ, Krikun G, Aigner S, Schatz F: Effects of thrombin on steroid-modulated cultured endometrial stromal cell fibrinolytic potential. J Clin Endocrinol Metab 81:107, 1996.
289. Lijnen HR: Matrix metalloproteinases and cellular fibrinolytic activity. Biochemistry (Mosc) 67:92, 2002.
290. Aplin JD, Campbell S, Allen TD: The extracellular matrix of human amniotic epithelium: ultrastructure, composition and deposition. J Cell Sci 79:119, 1985.
291. Chaiworapongsa T, Espinoza J, Yoshimatsu J, et al: Activation of coagulation system in preterm labor and preterm premature rupture of membranes. J Matern Fetal Neonatal Med 11:368, 2002.
292. Gomez R, Athayde N, Pacora P, et al: Increased thrombin in intrauterine inflammation. Am J Obstet Gynecol 178:S62, 1998.
293. Lockwood CJ, Krikun G, Papp C, et al: The role of progestationally regulated stromal cell tissue factor and type-1 plasminogen activator inhibitor (PAI-1) in endometrial hemostasis and menstruation. Ann N Y Acad Sci 734:57, 1994.
294. Funderburk SJ, Guthrie D, Meldrum D: Outcome of pregnancies complicated by early vaginal bleeding. Br J Obstet Gynaecol 87:100, 1980.
295. Ghezzi F, Ghidini A, Romero R, et al: Doppler velocimetry of the fetal middle cerebral artery in patients with preterm labor and intact membranes. J Ultrasound Med 14:361, 1995.
296. Nagy S, Bush M, Stone J, et al: Clinical significance of subchorionic and retroplacental hematomas detected in the first trimester of pregnancy. Obstet Gynecol 102:94, 2003.
297. Signore CC, Sood AK, Richards DS: Second-trimester vaginal bleeding: correlation of ultrasonographic findings with perinatal outcome. Am J Obstet Gynecol 178:336, 1998.
298. Williams MA, Mittendorf R, Lieberman E, Monson RR: Adverse infant outcomes associated with first-trimester vaginal bleeding. Obstet Gynecol 78:14, 1991.
299. Gomez R, Romero R, Ghezzi F, et al: Are fetal hypoxia and acidemia causes of preterm labor and delivery? Am J Obstet Gynecol 176:S115, 1997.
300. Carroll SG, Papaioannou S, Nicolaides KH: Assessment of fetal activity and amniotic fluid volume in the prediction of intrauterine infection in preterm prelabor amniorrhexis. Am J Obstet Gynecol 172:1427, 1995.
301. Besinger R, Carlson N: The physiology of preterm labor. *In* Keith L, Papiernik E, Keith D, Luke B (eds): Multiple Pregnancy: Epidemiology, Gestation and Perinatal Outcome. London, Parthenon Publishing, 1995, p 415.
302. Hill LM, Breckle R, Thomas ML, Fries JK: Polyhydramnios: ultrasonically detected prevalence and neonatal outcome. Obstet Gynecol 69:21, 1987.
303. Ludmir J, Samuels P, Brooks S, Mennuti MT: Pregnancy outcome of patients with uncorrected uterine anomalies managed in a high-risk obstetric setting. Obstet Gynecol 75:906, 1990.
304. Phelan JP, Park YW, Ahn MO, Rutherford SE: Polyhydramnios and perinatal outcome. J Perinatol 10:347, 1990.
305. Weiner CP, Heilskov J, Pelzer G, et al: Normal values for human umbilical venous and amniotic fluid pressures and their alteration by fetal disease. Am J Obstet Gynecol 161:714, 1989.
306. Ou CW, Chen ZQ, Qi S, Lye SJ: Increased expression of the rat myometrial oxytocin receptor messenger ribonucleic acid during labor requires both mechanical and hormonal signals. Biol Reprod 59:1055, 1998.
307. Mitchell JA, Lye SJ: Regulation of connexin43 expression by c-fos and c-jun in myometrial cells. Cell Commun Adhes 8:299, 2001.
308. Mitchell JA, Lye SJ: Differential expression of activator protein-1 transcription factors in pregnant rat myometrium. Biol Reprod 67:240, 2002.
309. Oldenhof AD, Shynlova OP, Liu M, et al: Mitogen-activated protein kinases mediate stretch-induced c-fos mRNA expression in myometrial smooth muscle cells. Am J Physiol Cell Physiol 283:C1530, 2002.
310. Piersanti M, Lye SJ: Increase in messenger ribonucleic acid encoding the myometrial gap junction protein, connexin-43, requires protein synthesis and is associated with increased expression of the activator protein-1, c-fos. Endocrinology 136:3571, 1995.
311. Shynlova OP, Oldenhof AD, Liu M, et al: Regulation of c-fos expression by static stretch in rat myometrial smooth muscle cells. Am J Obstet Gynecol 186:1358, 2002.
312. Barclay CG, Brennand JE, Kelly RW, Calder AA: Interleukin-8 production by the human cervix. Am J Obstet Gynecol 169:625, 1993.
313. Calder AA: Prostaglandins and biological control of cervical function. Aust N Z J Obstet Gynaecol 34:347, 1994.

314. Chwalisz K, Benson M, Scholz P, et al: Cervical ripening with the cytokines interleukin 8, interleukin 1 beta and tumour necrosis factor alpha in guinea-pigs. Hum Reprod 9:2173, 1994.

315. Denison FC, Calder AA, Kelly RW: The action of prostaglandin E_2 on the human cervix: stimulation of interleukin 8 and inhibition of secretory leukocyte protease inhibitor. Am J Obstet Gynecol 180:614, 1999.

316. el Maradny E, Kanayama N, Halim A, et al: Interleukin-8 induces cervical ripening in rabbits. Am J Obstet Gynecol 171:77, 1994.

317. Kanayama N, Fukamizu H: Mechanical stretching increases prostaglandin E_2 in cultured human amnion cells. Gynecol Obstet Invest 28:123, 1989.

318. Maehara K, Kanayama N, Maradny EE, et al: Mechanical stretching induces interleukin-8 gene expression in fetal membranes: a possible role for the initiation of human parturition. Eur J Obstet Gynecol Reprod Biol 70:191, 1996.

319. Mazor M, Hershkovitz R, Ghezzi F, et al: Intraamniotic infection in patients with preterm labor and twin pregnancies. Acta Obstet Gynecol Scand 75:624, 1996.

320. Millar LK, Stollberg J, DeBuque L, Bryant-Greenwood G: Fetal membrane distention: determination of the intrauterine surface area and distention of the fetal membranes preterm and at term. Am J Obstet Gynecol 182:128, 2000.

321. Nemeth E, Tashima LS, Yu Z, Bryant-Greenwood GD: Fetal membrane distention: I. Differentially expressed genes regulated by acute distention in amniotic epithelial (WISH) cells. Am J Obstet Gynecol 182:50, 2000.

322. Nemeth E, Millar LK, Bryant-Greenwood G: Fetal membrane distention: II. Differentially expressed genes regulated by acute distention in vitro. Am J Obstet Gynecol 182:60, 2000.

323. Rajabi M, Solomon S, Poole AR: Hormonal regulation of interstitial collagenase in the uterine cervix of the pregnant guinea pig. Endocrinology 128:863, 1991.

324. Sennstrom MK, Brauner A, Lu Y, et al: Interleukin-8 is a mediator of the final cervical ripening in humans. Eur J Obstet Gynecol Reprod Biol 74:89, 1997.

325. Stjernholm YM, Sahlin L, Eriksson HA, et al: Cervical ripening after treatment with prostaglandin E_2 or antiprogestin (RU486). Possible mechanisms in relation to gonadal steroids. Eur J Obstet Gynecol Reprod Biol 84:83, 1999.

326. Yoon BH, Park KH, Koo JN, et al: Intra-amniotic infection of twin pregnancies with preterm labor. Am J Obstet Gynecol 176:535, 1997.

327. McLean JM: Early embryo loss. Lancet 1:1033, 1987.

328. Aksel S: Immunologic aspects of reproductive diseases. JAMA 268:2930–34, 1992.

329. Kilpatrick DC: Immune mechanisms and pre-eclampsia. Lancet 2:1460, 1987.

330. Benirschke K, Kaufmann P: Villitis of unknown etiology. *In* Benirschke K, Kaufmann P (eds): Pathology of the Human Placenta. New York, Springer-Verlag, 1995, p 596.

331. Romero R, Mazor M, Avila C, et al: Uterine "allergy": A novel mechanism for preterm labor. Am J Obstet Gynecol 164:375, 1991.

332. Holgate ST: The epidemic of allergy and asthma. Nature 402: B2, 1999.

333. Corry DB, Kheradmand F: Induction and regulation of the IgE response. Nature 402:B18, 1999.

334. Padilla L, Reinicke K, Montesino H, et al: Histamine content and mast cell distribution in mouse uterus: the effect of sexual hormones, gestation and labor. Cell Mol Biol 36:93, 1990.

335. Rudolph MI, Bardisa L, Cruz MA, Reinicke K: Mast cell mediators evoke contractility and potentiate each other in mouse uterine horns. Gen Pharmacol;23:833, 1992.

336. Bytautiene E, Romero R, Vedernikov Y, et al: Induction of premature labor and delivery by allergic reaction and prevention by histamine H1 receptor antagonist. Am J Obstet Gynecol 191:1356, 2004.

337. Iams JD, Johnson FF, Sonek J, et al: Cervical competence as a continuum: a study of ultrasonographic cervical length and obstetric performance. Am J Obstet Gynecol 172:1097, 1995.

338. Harger JH: Cerclage and cervical insufficiency: an evidence-based analysis. Obstet Gynecol 100:1313, 2002.

339. Romero R, Mazor M, Gomez R: Cervix incompetence and premature labor. Fetus 3:1, 1993.

340. Mesiano S: Roles of estrogen and progesterone in human parturition. Front Horm Res 27:86, 2001.

341. Chwalisz K: The use of progesterone antagonists for cervical ripening and as an adjunct to labour and delivery. Hum Reprod 9(Suppl 1):131, 1994.

342. Gorodeski IG, Geier A, Lunenfeld B, et al: Progesterone (P) receptor dynamics in estrogen primed normal human cervix following P injection. Fertil Steril 47:108, 1987.

343. Stjernholm Y, Sahlin L, Akerberg S, et al: Cervical ripening in humans: potential roles of estrogen, progesterone, and insulin-like growth factor-I. Am J Obstet Gynecol 174:1065, 1996.

344. Bernal AL: Overview of current research in parturition. Exp Physiol 86:213, 2001.

345. Young IR: The comparative physiology of parturition in mammals. *In* Smith R (ed): The Enodocrinology of Parturition. Basel, Reinhardt Druck, 2001, p 10.

346. Bygdeman M, Swahn ML, Gemzell-Danielsson K, Gottlieb C: The use of progesterone antagonists in combination with prostaglandin for termination of pregnancy. Hum Reprod 9(Suppl 1):121, 1994.

347. Puri CP, Patil RK, Elger WA, Pongubala JM: Effects of progesterone antagonist ZK 98 299 on early pregnancy and foetal outcome in bonnet monkeys. Contraception 41:197, 1990.

348. McGarrigle HH, Lachelin GC: Increasing saliva (free) oestriol to progesterone ratio in late pregnancy: a role for oestriol in initiating spontaneous labour in man? Br Med J 289:457, 1984.

349. Westphal U, Stroupe SD, Cheng SL: Progesterone binding to serum proteins. Ann N Y Acad Sci 286:10, 1977.

350. Karalis K, Goodwin G, Majzoub JA: Cortisol blockade of progesterone: a possible molecular mechanism involved in the initiation of human labor. Nat Med 2:556, 1996.

351. Milewich L, Gant NF, Schwarz BE, et al: Initiation of human parturition. VIII. Metabolism of progesterone by fetal membranes of early and late human gestation. Obstet Gynecol 50:45, 1977.

352. Mitchell BF, Wong S: Changes in 17 beta,20 alpha-hydroxysteroid dehydrogenase activity supporting an increase in the estrogen/progesterone ratio of human fetal membranes at parturition. Am J Obstet Gynecol 168:1377, 1993.

353. Pieber D, Allport VC, Hills F, et al: Interactions between progesterone receptor isoforms in myometrial cells in human labour. Mol Hum Reprod 7:875, 2001.

354. Rezapour M, Backstrom T, Lindblom B, Ulmsten U: Sex steroid receptors and human parturition. Obstet Gynecol 89:918, 1997.

355. How H, Huang ZH, Zuo J, et al: Myometrial estradiol and progesterone receptor changes in preterm and term pregnancies. Obstet Gynecol 86:936, 1995.

356. Henderson D, Wilson T: Reduced binding of progesterone receptor to its nuclear response element after human labor onset. Am J Obstet Gynecol 185:579, 2001.

357. Mesiano S, Chan EC, Fitter JT, et al: Progesterone withdrawal and estrogen activation in human parturition are coordinated by progesterone receptor A expression in the myometrium. J Clin Endocrinol Metab 87:2924, 2002.

358. Allport VC, Pieber D, Slater DM, et al: Human labour is associated with nuclear factor-kappaB activity which mediates cyclo-oxygenase-2 expression and is involved with the 'functional progesterone withdrawal.' Mol Hum Reprod 7:581, 2001.

359. Belt AR, Baldassare JJ, Molnar M, et al: The nuclear transcription factor NF-kappaB mediates interleukin-1beta-induced expression of cyclooxygenase-2 in human myometrial cells. Am J Obstet Gynecol 181:359, 1999.

360. Bennett P, Allport V, Loudon J, Elliott C: Prostaglandins, the fetal membranes and the cervix. Front Horm Res 27:147, 2001.

361. Kalkhoven E, Wissink S, Van der Saag PT, van der BB: Negative interaction between the RelA(p65) subunit of NF-kappaB and the progesterone receptor. J Biol Chem 271:6217, 1996.

362. Pieber D, Allport VC, Bennett PR: Progesterone receptor isoform A inhibits isoform B-mediated transactivation in human amnion. Eur J Pharmacol 427:7, 2001.

363. Olah K, Gee H: The prevention of preterm delivery—can we afford to continue to ignore the cervix? Br J Obstet Gynecol 99:278,1992.
364. Hueston WJ: Preterm contractions in community settings: II. Predicting preterm birth in women with preterm contractions. Obstet Gynecol 92:43, 1998.
365. Macones GA, Segel SY, Stamilio DM, Morgan MA: Prediction of delivery among women with early preterm labor by means of clinical characteristics alone. Am J Obstet Gynecol 181:1414, 1999.
366. King JF, Grant A, Keirse MJNC: Beta-mimetics in preterm labour: An overview of the randomized controlled trials. Br J Obstet Gynaecol 95:211, 1988.
367. Merkatz IR, Peter JB, Barden TP: Ritodrine hydrochloride: A betamimetic agent for use in preterm labor. Obstet Gynecol 56:7, 1980.
368. Peaceman A, Andrews W, Thorp J, et al: Fetal fibronectin as a predictor of preterm birth in patients with symptoms: A multicenter trial. Am J Obstet Gynecol 177:13, 1997.
369. Jackson GM, Ludmir J, Bader TJ: The accuracy of digital examination and ultrasound in the evaluation of cervical length. Obstet Gynecol 79:214–18, 1992.
370. Leitich H, Brumbauer M, Kaider A, et al: Cervical length and dilation of the internal os detected by vaginal ultrasonography as markers for preterm delivery: A systematic review. Am J Obstet Gynecol 181:1465, 1999.
371. Leitich H, Egarter C, Kaider A, et al: Cervicovaginal fetal fibronectin as a marker for preterm delivery: A meta-analysis. Am J Obstet Gynecol 180:1169, 1999.
372. Management of preterm labor. ACOG Practice Bulletin No. 43. American College of Obstetricians and Gynecologists. Obstet Gynecol 101:1039, 2003.
373. Anderson HF: Transvaginal and transabdominal ultrasonography of the uterine cervix during pregnancy. J Clin Ultrasound 19:77, 1991.
374. Mason GC, Maresh MJA: Alterations in bladder volume and the ultrasound appearance of the cervix. Br J Obstet Gynaecol 97:457–58, 1990.
375. Chien PF, Khan KS, Ogston S, Owen P: The diagnostic accuracy of cervico-vaginal fetal fibronectin in predicting preterm delivery: an overview. Br J Obstet Gynaecol 104:436, 1997.
376. Gomez R, Romero R, Medina L, et al: Cervicovaginal fibronectin improves the prediction of preterm delivery based on sonographic cervical length in patients with preterm uterine contractions and intact membranes. Am J Obstet Gynecol 192:350, 2005.
377. Yeast J, Poskin M, Stockbauer J, Shaffer S: Changing patterns in regionalization of perinatal care and the impact on neonatal mortality. Am J Obstet Gynecol 178:131, 1998.
378. Towers CV, Bonebrake R, Padilla G, Rumney P: The effect of transport on the rate of severe intraventricular hemorrhage in very low birth weight infants. Obstet Gynecol 95:291, 2000.
379. Schrag S, Gorwitz R, Fultz-Butts K, Schuchat A: Prevention of perinatal group B streptococcal disease. Revised guidelines from CDC. MMWR 51:1, 2002.
380. Mercer B, Miodovnik M, Thurnau G, et al: Antibiotic therapy for reduction of infant morbidity after preterm premature rupture of the membranes. A randomized controlled trial. National Institute of Child Health and Human Development Maternal-Fetal Medicine Units Network. JAMA 278:989, 1997.
381. Kenyon S, Taylor D, Tarnow-Mordi W: Broad-spectrum antibiotics for preterm, prelabour rupture of fetal membranes: the ORACLE I randomised trial. Lancet 357:979, 2001.
382. Newton ER, Dinsmoor MJ, Gibbs RS: A randomized, blinded, placebo-controlled trial of antibiotics in idiopathic preterm labor. Obstet Gynecol 74:562, 1989.
383. Newton E, Shields L, Ridgway LI, et al: Combination antibiotics and indomethacin in idiopathic preterm labor: a randomized double-blind clinical trial. Am J Obstet Gynecol 165:1753, 1991.
384. Romero R, Sibai B, Caritis S, et al: Antibiotic treatment of preterm labor with intact membranes: a multicenter, randomized, double-blinded, placebo-controlled trial. Am J Obstet Gynecol 169:764, 1993.
385. Norman K, Pattinson R, de Souza I, et al: Ampicillin and metronidazole treatment in preterm labour: a multicentre, randomised controlled trial. Br J Obstet Gynaecol 101:404, 1994.
386. Gordon M, Samuels P, Shubert P, et al: A randomized, prospective study of adjunctive ceftizoxime in preterm labor. Am J Obstet Gynecol 172:1546, 1995.
387. Andrews WW, Goldenberg RL, Hauth JC, et al: Interconceptional antibiotics to prevent spontaneous preterm birth: A randomized trial. Am J Obstet Gynecol 194:617, 2006.
388. Loeb J: Corticosteroids and growth. N Engl J Med 295:547, 1976.
389. Ballard PL, Ballard RA: Scientific basis and therapeutic regimens for use of antenatal glucocorticoids. Am J Obstet Gynecol 173:254, 1995.
390. Liggins GC, Howie RN: A controlled trial of antepartum glucocorticoid treatment for prevention of the respiratory distress syndrome in premature infants. Pediatrics 50:515, 1972.
391. Crowley P: Prophylactic corticosteroids for preterm birth. Cochrane Database Syst Rev CD000065, 1996.
392. National Institutes of Health Consensus Development Conference Statement: Effect of corticosteroids for fetal maturation on perinatal outcomes. Am J Obstet Gynecol 173:246, 1995.
393. Antenatal corticosteroids revisited: repeat courses—National Institutes of Health Consensus Development Conference Statement, August 17–18, 2000. Obstet Gynecol 98:144, 2001.
394. Use of progesterone to reduce preterm birth. ACOG Committee Opinion No. 291. American College of Obstetricians and Gynecologists. Obstet Gynecol 102:1115, 2003.
395. Baud O, Foix-L'Helias L, Kaminski M, et al: Antenatal glucocorticoid treatment and cystic periventricular leukomalacia in very premature infants. N Engl J Med 341:1190, 1999.
396. Mulder EJ, Derks JB, Visser GH: Antenatal corticosteroid therapy and fetal behaviour: a randomised study of the effects of betamethasone and dexamethasone. Br J Obstet Gynaecol 104:1239, 1997.
397. Senat MV, Minoui S, Multon O, et al: Effect of dexamethasone and betamethasone on fetal heart rate variability in preterm labour: a randomised study. Br J Obstet Gynaecol 105:749, 1998.
398. Rotmensch S, Liberati M, Vishne TH, et al: The effect of betamethasone and dexamethasone on fetal heart rate patterns and biophysical activities. A prospective randomized trial. Acta Obstet Gynecol Scand 78:493, 1999.
399. Teramo DA, Hallman M, Raivo KO, et al: Neonatal effects and serum cortisol levels after multiple courses of maternal corticosteroids. Obstet Gynecol 90:819, 1997.
400. Terrone DA, Smith LG, Jr, Wolf EJ, et al: Neonatal effects and serum cortisol levels after multiple courses of maternal corticosteroids. Obstet Gynecol 90:819, 1997.
401. Terrone DA, Rinehart BK, Rhodes PG, et al: Multiple courses of betamethasone to enhance fetal lung maturation do not suppress neonatal adrenal response. Am J Obstet Gynecol 180:1349, 1999.
402. McKenna DS, Wittber GM, Nagaraja HN, Samuels P: The effects of repeat doses of antenatal corticosteroids on maternal adrenal function. Am J Obstet Gynecol 183:669, 2000.
403. Gamsu HR, Mullinger BM, Donnai P, Dash CH: Antenatal administration of betamethasone to prevent respiratory distress syndrome in preterm infants: report of a UK multicentre trial. Br J Obstet Gynaecol 96:401, 1989.
404. Leviton LC, Goldenberg RL, Baker CS, et al: Methods to encourage the use of antenatal corticosteroid therapy for fetal maturation: a randomized controlled trial. JAMA 281:46, 1999.
405. Dessens AB, Haas HS, Koppe JG: Twenty-year follow-up of antenatal corticosteroid treatment. Pediatrics 105:E77, 2000.
406. Aghajafari F, Murphy K, Matthews S, et al: Repeated doses of antenatal corticosteroids in animals: a systematic review. Am J Obstet Gynecol 186:843, 2002.
407. Cotterrell M, Balazs R, Johnson AL: Effects of corticosteroids on the biochemical maturation of rat brain: postnatal cell formation. J Neurochem 19:2151, 1972.
408. Huang WL, Beazley LD, Quinlivan JA, et al: Effect of corticosteroids on brain growth in fetal sheep. Obstet Gynecol 94:213, 1999.

409. Jobe AH, Wada N, Berry LM, et al: Single and repetitive maternal glucocorticoid exposures reduce fetal growth in sheep. Am J Obstet Gynecol 178:880, 1998.
410. Quinlivan JA, Archer MA, Evans SF, et al: Fetal sciatic nerve growth is delayed following repeated maternal injections of corticosteroid in sheep. J Perinat Med 28:26, 2000.
411. Stewart JD, Gonzalez CL, Christensen HD, Rayburn WF: Impact of multiple antenatal doses of betamethasone on growth and development of mice offspring. Am J Obstet Gynecol 177:1138, 1997.
412. French NP, Hagan R, Evans SF, et al: Repeated antenatal corticosteroids: size at birth and subsequent development. Am J Obstet Gynecol 180:114, 1999.
413. Abbasi S, Hirsch D, Davis J, et al: Effect of single versus multiple courses of antenatal corticosteroids on maternal and neonatal outcome. Am J Obstet Gynecol 182:1243, 2000.
414. Crowther CA, Harding J: Repeat doses of prenatal corticosteroids for women at risk of preterm birth for preventing neonatal respiratory disease. Cochrane Database Syst Rev CD003935, 2003.
415. Mercer B, Egerman R, Beazley D, et al: Antenatal corticosteroids in women at risk for preterm birth: A randomized trial. Am J Obstet Gynecol 184:S6, 2001.
416. Wapner RJ, Sorokin Y, Thom EA, et al: Single versus weekly courses of antenatal corticosteroids: evaluation of safety and efficacy. Am J Obstet Gynecol 195:633, 2006.
417. Crowther CA, Alfirevic Z, Haslam RR: Thyrotropin-releasing hormone added to corticosteroids for women at risk of preterm birth for preventing neonatal respiratory disease. Cochrane Database Syst Rev CD000019, 2004.
418. Shankaran S, Papile LA, Wright LL, et al: The effect of antenatal phenobarbital therapy on neonatal intracranial hemorrhage in preterm infants. N Engl J Med 337:466, 1997.
419. Thorp JA, Ferrette-Smith D, Gaston LA, et al: Combined antenatal vitamin K and phenobarbital therapy for preventing intracranial hemorrhage in newborns less than 34 weeks' gestation. Obstet Gynecol 86:1, 1995.
420. Nelson KB, Grether J: Effect of $MgSO_4$ therapy on cerebral palsy rates in infants <1500 grams. J Pediatr 95:263, 1995.
421. Grether JK, Hoogstrate J, Selvin S, Nelson KB: Magnesium sulfate tocolysis and risk of neonatal death. Am J Obstet Gynecol 178:1, 1998.
422. Grether JK, Hoogstrate J, Walsh-Greene E, Nelson KB: Magnesium sulfate for tocolysis and risk of spastic cerebral palsy in premature children born to women without preeclampsia. Am J Obstet Gynecol 183:717, 2000.
423. Mittendorf R, Covert R, Boman J, et al: Is tocolytic magnesium sulphate associated with increased total paediatric mortality? Lancet 350:1517, 1997.
424. Paneth N, Jetton J, Pinto-Martin J, Susser M: Magnesium sulfate in labor and risk of neonatal brain lesions and cerebral palsy in low birth weight infants. The Neonatal Brain Hemorrhage Study Analysis Group. Pediatrics 99:E1, 1997.
425. Schendel DE, Berg CJ, Yeargin-Allsopp M, et al: Prenatal magnesium sulfate exposure and the risk for cerebral palsy or mental retardation among very low-birth-weight children aged 3 to 5 years. JAMA 276:1805, 1996.
426. Crowther CA, Hiller JE, Doyle LW, Haslam RR: Effect of magnesium sulfate given for neuroprotection before preterm birth: a randomized controlled trial. JAMA 290:2669, 2003.
427. King JF, Flenady VJ, Papatsonis DN, et al: Calcium channel blockers for inhibiting preterm labour. Cochrane Database Syst Rev CD002255, 2003.
428. Papatsonis D, Flenady V, Cole S, Liley H: Oxytocin receptor antagonists for inhibiting preterm labour. Cochrane Database Syst Rev CD004452, 2005.
429. Anotayanonth S, Subhedar NV, Garner P, et al: Betamimetics for inhibiting preterm labour. Cochrane Database Syst Rev CD004352, 2004.
430. King J, Flenady V, Cole S, Thornton S: Cyclo-oxygenase (COX) inhibitors for treating preterm labour. Cochrane Database Syst Rev CD001992, 2005.
431. Crowther CA, Hiller JE, Doyle LW: Magnesium sulphate for preventing preterm birth in threatened preterm labour. Cochrane Database Syst Rev CD001060, 2002.
432. Huszar G, Naftolin F: The myometrium and uterine cervix in normal and preterm labor. N Engl J Med 311:571, 1984.
433. Ferguson JE, Schutz T, Pershe R, et al: Nifedipine pharmacokinetics during preterm labor tocolysis. Am J Obstet Gynecol 161:1485, 1989.
434. Papatsonis DN, Van Geijn HP, Ader HJ, et al: Nifedipine and ritodrine in the management of preterm labor: a randomized multicenter trial. Obstet Gynecol 90:230, 1997.
435. Glock JL, Morales WJ: Efficacy and safety of nifedipine versus magnesium sulfate in the management of preterm labor: a randomized study. Am J Obstet Gynecol 169:960, 1993.
436. Larmon JE, Ross BS, May WL, et al: Oral nicardipine versus intravenous magnesium sulfate for the treatment of preterm labor. Am J Obstet Gynecol 181:1432, 1999.
437. Oei SG, Oei SK, Brolmann HA: Myocardial infarction during nifedipine therapy for preterm labor. N Engl J Med 340:154, 1999.
438. Snyder SW, Cardwell MS: Neuromuscular blockade with magnesium sulfate and nifedipine. Am J Obstet Gynecol 161:35, 1989.
439. Ben-Ami M, Giladi Y, Shalev E: The combination of magnesium sulphate and nifedipine: a cause of neuromuscular blockade. Br J Obstet Gynaecol 101:262, 1994.
440. Mari G, Kirshon B, Moise KJ Jr, et al: Doppler assessment of the fetal and uteroplacental circulation during nifedipine therapy for preterm labor. Am J Obstet Gynecol 161:1514, 1989.
441. Steer CM, Petrie RH: A comparison of magnesium sulfate and alcohol for the prevention of premature labor. Am J Obstet Gynecol 129:1, 1977.
442. Berkman N, Thorp JM Jr, Lohr KN, et al: Tocolytic treatment for the management of preterm labor: a review of the evidence. Am J Obstet Gynecol 188:1648, 2003.
443. Ramsey PS, Rouse DJ: Magnesium sulfate as a tocolytic agent. Semin Perinatol 25:236, 2001.
444. Elliott JP: Magnesium sulfate as a tocolytic agent. Am J Obstet Gynecol 147:277, 1983.
445. Holcomb WL Jr, Shackelford GD, Petrie RH: Magnesium tocolysis and neonatal bone abnormalities: a controlled study. Obstet Gynecol 78:611, 1991.
446. Rouse DJ, Hirtz DG, Thom E: Association between use of antenatal magnesium sulfate in preterm labor and adverse health outcomes in infants. Am J Obstet Gynecol 188:295, 2003.
447. Madden C, Owen J, Hauth JC: Magnesium tocolysis: serum levels versus success. Am J Obstet Gynecol 162:1177, 1990.
448. Lunt CC, Satin AJ, Barth WH Jr, Hankins GD: The effect of indomethacin tocolysis on maternal coagulation status. Obstet Gynecol 84:820, 1994.
449. Moise KJ Jr: Effect of advancing gestational age on the frequency of fetal ductal constriction in association with maternal indomethacin use. Am J Obstet Gynecol 168:1350, 1993.
450. Moise KJ Jr, Huhta JC, Sharif DS, et al: Indomethacin in the treatment of premature labor. Effects on the fetal ductus arteriosus. N Engl J Med 319:327, 1988.
451. Mohen D, Newnham JP, D'Orsogna L: Indomethacin for the treatment of polyhydramnios: a case of constriction of the ductus arteriosus. Aust N Z J Obstet Gynaecol 32:243, 1992.
452. Vermillion ST, Scardo JA, Lashus AG, Wiles HB: The effect of indomethacin tocolysis on fetal ductus arteriosus constriction with advancing gestational age. Am J Obstet Gynecol 177:256, 1997.
453. van der Heijden BJ, Carlus C, Narcy F, et al: Persistent anuria, neonatal death, and renal microcystic lesions after prenatal exposure to indomethacin. Am J Obstet Gynecol 171:617, 1994.
454. Manchester D, Margolis HS, Sheldon RE: Possible association between maternal indomethacin therapy and primary pulmonary hypertension of the newborn. Am J Obstet Gynecol 126:467, 1976.
455. Csaba IF, Sulyok E, Ertl T: Relationship of maternal treatment with indomethacin to persistence of fetal circulation syndrome. J Pediatr 92:484, 1978.
456. Besinger RE, Niebyl JR, Keyes WG, Johnson TR: Randomized comparative trial of indomethacin and ritodrine for the long-term treatment of preterm labor. Am J Obstet Gynecol 164:981, 1991.

457. Norton ME, Merrill J, Cooper BA, et al: Neonatal complications after the administration of indomethacin for preterm labor. N Engl J Med 329:1602, 1993.
458. Vermillion ST, Newman RB: Recent indomethacin tocolysis is not associated with neonatal complications in preterm infants. Am J Obstet Gynecol 181:1083, 1999.
459. Suarez RD, Grobman WA, Parilla BV: Indomethacin tocolysis and intraventricular hemorrhage. Obstet Gynecol 97:921, 2001.
459a. Loe SM, Sanchez-Ramos L, Kaunitz AM: Assessing the neonatal safety of indomethacin tocolysis: a systematic review with meta-analysis. Obstet Gynecol 106:173, 2005.
460. Carlan SJ, O'Brien WF, O'Leary TD, Mastrogiannis D: Randomized comparative trial of indomethacin and sulindac for the treatment of refractory preterm labor. Obstet Gynecol 79:223, 1992.
461. Mamopoulos M, Assimakopoulos E, Reece EA, et al: Maternal indomethacin therapy in the treatment of polyhydramnios. Am J Obstet Gynecol 162:1225, 1990.
462. Kirshon B, Mari G, Moise KJ Jr: Indomethacin therapy in the treatment of symptomatic polyhydramnios. Obstet Gynecol 75:202, 1990.
463. Stubblefield PG, Heyl PS: Treatment of premature labor with subcutaneous terbutaline. Obstet Gynecol 59:457, 1982.
464. Guinn DA, Goepfert AR, Owen J, et al: Management options in women with preterm uterine contractions: a randomized clinical trial. Am J Obstet Gynecol 177:814, 1997.
465. Gyetvai K, Hannah ME, Hodnett ED, Ohlsson A: Tocolytics for preterm labor: a systematic review. Obstet Gynecol 94:869, 1999.
466. Benedetti TJ: Maternal complications of parenteral beta-sympathomimetic therapy for premature labor. Am J Obstet Gynecol 145:1, 1983.
467. Hendricks SK, Keroes J, Katz M: Electrocardiographic changes associated with ritodrine-induced maternal tachycardia and hypokalemia. Am J Obstet Gynecol 154:921, 1986.
468. Smigaj D, Roman-Drago NM, Amini SB, et al: The effect of oral terbutaline on maternal glucose metabolism and energy expenditure in pregnancy. Am J Obstet Gynecol 178:1041, 1998.
469. Fisher JE, Smith RS, Lagrandeur R, Lorenz RP: Gestational diabetes mellitus in women receiving beta-adrenergics and corticosteroids for threatened preterm delivery. Obstet Gynecol 90:880, 1997.
470. Epstein MF, Nicholls E, Stubblefield PG: Neonatal hypoglycemia after beta-sympathomimetic tocolytic therapy. J Pediatr 94:449, 1979.
471. Rhodes MC, Seidler FJ, Abdel-Rahman A, et al: Terbutaline is a developmental neurotoxicant: effects on neuroproteins and morphology in cerebellum, hippocampus, and somatosensory cortex. J Pharmacol Exp Ther 308:529, 2004.
472. Lam F, Elliott J, Jones JS, et al: Clinical issues surrounding the use of terbutaline sulfate for preterm labor. Obstet Gynecol Surv 53:S85, 1998.
473. Perry KG Jr, Morrison JC, Rust OA, et al: Incidence of adverse cardiopulmonary effects with low-dose continuous terbutaline infusion. Am J Obstet Gynecol 173:1273, 1995.
474. Wenstrom KD, Weiner CP, Merrill D, Niebyl J: A placebo-controlled randomized trial of the terbutaline pump for prevention of preterm delivery. Am J Perinatol 14:87, 1997.
475. Guinn DA, Goepfert AR, Owen J, et al: Terbutaline pump maintenance therapy for prevention of preterm delivery: a double-blind trial. Am J Obstet Gynecol 179:874, 1998.
476. Macones GA, Berlin M, Berlin JA: Efficacy of oral beta-agonist maintenance therapy in preterm labor: a meta-analysis. Obstet Gynecol 85:313, 1995.
477. U.S. Food and Drug Administration (FDA): Warning on use of terbutaline sulfate for preterm labor. JAMA 279:9, 1998.
478. Valenzuela GJ, Sanchez-Ramos L, Romero R, et al: Maintenance treatment of preterm labor with the oxytocin antagonist atosiban. The Atosiban PTL-098 Study Group. Am J Obstet Gynecol 182:1184, 2000.
479. Moutquin JM, Sherman D, Cohen H, et al: Double-blind, randomized, controlled trial of atosiban and ritodrine in the treatment of preterm labor: a multicenter effectiveness and safety study. Am J Obstet Gynecol 182:1191, 2000.
480. Lees CC, Lojacono A, Thompson C, et al: Glyceryl trinitrate and ritodrine in tocolysis: an international multicenter randomized study. GTN Preterm Labour Investigation Group. Obstet Gynecol 94:403, 1999.
480a. Smith GN, Walker MC, Ohlsson A, et al for the Canadian Preterm Labour Nitroglycerin Trial Group: Randomized double-blind placebo-controlled trial of transdermal nitroglycerin for preterm labor. Am J Obstet Gynecol 196:37, 2007.
481. Ferguson JE, Hensleigh PA, Kredenster D: Adjunctive use of magnesium sulfate with ritodrine for preterm labor tocolysis. Am J Obstet Gynecol 148:166, 1984.
482. Hatjis CG, Swain M, Nelson LH, et al: Efficacy of combined administration of magnesium sulfate and ritodrine in the treatment of premature labor. Obstet Gynecol 69:317, 1987.
483. Carlan SJ, O'Brien WF, Jones MH, et al: Outpatient oral sulindac to prevent recurrence of preterm labor. Obstet Gynecol 85:769, 1995.
484. Creasy RK, Golbus MS, Laros RK Jr, et al: Oral ritodrine maintenance in the treatment of preterm labor. Am J Obstet Gynecol 137:212, 1980.
485. Holleboom CA, Merkus JM, van Elferen LW, Keirse MJ: Double-blind evaluation of ritodrine sustained release for oral maintenance of tocolysis after active preterm labour. Br J Obstet Gynaecol 103:702, 1996.
486. Lewis R, Mercer BM, Salama M, et al: Oral terbutaline after parenteral tocolysis: a randomized, double-blind, placebo-controlled trial. Am J Obstet Gynecol 175:834, 1996.
487. Rust OA, Bofill JA, Arriola RM, et al: The clinical efficacy of oral tocolytic therapy. Am J Obstet Gynecol 175:838, 1996.
488. Nanda K, Cook LA, Gallo MF, Grimes DA: Terbutaline pump maintenance therapy after threatened preterm labor for preventing preterm birth. Cochrane Database Syst Rev CD003933, 2002.
489. Sanchez-Ramos L, Huddleston JF: The therapeutic value of maintenance tocolysis: an overview of the evidence. Clin Perinatol 30:841, 2003.
490. Iams JD, Johnson FF, O'Shaughnessy RW: Ambulatory uterine activity monitoring in the post-hospital care of patients with preterm labor. Am J Perinatol 7:170, 1990.
491. Nagey DA, Bailey-Jones C, Herman AA: Randomized comparison of home uterine activity monitoring and routine care in patients discharged after treatment for preterm labor. Obstet Gynecol 82:319, 1993.
492. Brown HL, Britton KA, Brizendine EJ, et al: A randomized comparison of home uterine activity monitoring in the outpatient management of women treated for preterm labor. Am J Obstet Gynecol 180:798, 1999.
493. The Collaborative Home Uterine Monitoring Study (CHUMS) Group: A multicenter randomized controlled trial of home uterine monitoring: active versus sham device. Am J Obstet Gynecol 173:1120, 1995.
494. Luthy DA, Shy KK, van BG, Larson EB, et al: A randomized trial of electronic fetal monitoring in preterm labor. Obstet Gynecol 69:687, 1987.
495. Larson EB, van BG, Shy KK, Luthy DA, et al: Fetal monitoring and predictions by clinicians: observations during a randomized clinical trial in very low birth weight infants. Obstet Gynecol 74:584, 1989.
496. Barrett JM, Boehm FH, Vaughn WK: The effect of type of delivery on neonatal outcome in singleton infants of birth weight of 1,000 g or less. JAMA 250:625, 1983.
497. Hack M, Fanaroff AA: Outcomes of extremely-low-birth-weight infants between 1982 and 1988. N Engl J Med 321:1642, 1989.
498. Kitchen WH, Permezel MJ, Doyle LW, et al: Changing obstetric practice and 2-year outcome of the fetus of birth weight under 1000 g. Obstet Gynecol 79:268, 1992.
499. Malloy MH, Onstad L, Wright E: The effect of cesarean delivery on birth outcome in very low birth weight infants. National Institute of Child Health and Human Development Neonatal Research Network. Obstet Gynecol 77:498, 1991.
500. Grant A, Penn ZJ, Steer PJ: Elective or selective caesarean delivery of the small baby? A systematic review of the controlled trials. Br J Obstet Gynaecol 103:1197, 1996.
501. Wolf H, Schaap AH, Bruinse HW, et al: Vaginal delivery compared with caesarean section in early preterm breech delivery:

a comparison of long term outcome. Br J Obstet Gynaecol 106:486, 1999.

502. Dietl J, Arnold H, Mentzel H, Hirsch HA: Effect of cesarean section on outcome in high- and low-risk very preterm infants. Arch Gynecol Obstet 246:91, 1989.

503. Nageotte MP, Dorchester W, Porto M, et al: Quantitation of uterine activity in preceding preterm, term, and postterm labor. Am J Obstet Gynecol 158:1254, 1988.

504. Iams JD, Newman RB, Thom EA, et al: Frequency of uterine contractions and the risk of spontaneous preterm delivery. N Engl J Med 346:250, 2002.

505. Goldenberg RL, Mercer BM, Meis PJ, et al: The preterm prediction study: Fetal fibronectin testing and spontaneous preterm birth. Obstet Gynecol 87:643, 1996.

506. Goepfert A, Goldenberg RL, Andrews WW, et al: The Preterm Prediction Study: association between cervical interleukin 6 concentration and spontaneous preterm birth. National Institute of Child Health and Human Development Maternal-Fetal Medicine Units Network. Am J Obstet Gynecol 184:483, 2001.

507. Kurkinen-Raty M, Ruokonen A, Vuopala S, et al: Combination of cervical interleukin-6 and -8, phosphorylated insulin-like growth factor-binding protein-1 and transvaginal cervical ultrasonography in assessment of the risk of preterm birth. Br J Obstet Gynaecol 108:875, 2001.

508. Goldenberg RL, Mercer BM, Iams JD, et al: The preterm prediction study: Patterns of cervicovaginal fetal fibronectin as predictors of spontaneous preterm delivery. Am J Obstet Gynecol 177:8, 1997.

509. Goldenberg RL, Iams JD, Mercer BM, et al: The Preterm Prediction Study: toward a multiple-marker test for spontaneous preterm birth. Am J Obstet Gynecol 185:643, 2001.

510. Moawad AH, Goldenberg RL, Mercer B, et al: The Preterm Prediction Study: the value of serum alkaline phosphatase, alpha-fetoprotein, plasma corticotropin-releasing hormone, and other serum markers for the prediction of spontaneous preterm birth. Am J Obstet Gynecol 186:990, 2002.

511. Honest H, Bachmann LM, Knox EM, et al: The accuracy of various tests for bacterial vaginosis in predicting preterm birth: a systematic review. Br J Obstet Gynaecol 111:409, 2004.

512. Vogel I, Thorsen P, Curry A, et al: Biomarkers for the prediction of preterm delivery. Acta Obstet Gynecol Scand 84:516, 2005.

513. Dyson DC, Danbe KH, Bamber JA, et al: Monitoring women at risk for preterm labor. N Engl J Med 338:15, 1998.

514. Klebanoff MA, Regan JA, Rao VR, et al: Outcome of the Vaginal Infections and Prematurity Study: Results of a clinical trial of erythromycin among pregnant women colonized with group B streptococci. Am J Obstet Gynecol 172:1540, 1995.

515. Klebanoff MA, Carey JC, Hauth JC, et al: Failure of metronidazole to prevent preterm delivery among pregnant women with asymptomatic *Trichomonas vaginalis* infection. N Engl J Med 345:487, 2001.

516. Berghella V, Odibo A, To MS, et al: Cerclage for short cervix on ultrasonography; Meta-analysis of trials using individual patient data. Obstet Gynecol 106:181, 2005.

517. Villar J, Farnot U, Barros F, et al: A randomized trial of psychosocial support during high risk pregnancies Latin American Network for Perinatal and Reproductive Research. N Engl J Med 327:1266, 1992.

518. Klerman LV, Ramey SL, Goldenberg RL, et al: A randomized trial of augmented prenatal care for multiple-risk, Medicaid-eligible African American women. Am J Public Health 91:105, 2001.

519. Rumbold A, Crowther CA: Vitamin C supplementation in pregnancy. Cochrane Database Syst Rev CD004072, 2005.

520. Rogers MM, Peoples-Sheps MD, Suchindran C: Impact of a social support program on teenage prenatal care use and pregnancy outcomes. J Adolesc Health 19:132, 1996.

521. Goldenberg RL, Cliver SP, Bronstein J, et al: Bed rest in pregnancy. Obstet Gynecol 84:131, 1994.

522. Armson BA, Dodds L, Haliburton SC, et al: Impact of participation in the Halifax County preterm birth prevention project. J Obstet Gynaecol Can 25:209, 2003.

523. Sosa C, Althabe F, Belizan J, Bergel E: Bed rest in singleton pregnancies for preventing preterm birth. Cochrane Database Syst Rev CD003581, 2004.

524. da Fonseca EB, Bittar RE, Carvalho MH, et al: Prophylactic administration of progesterone by vaginal suppository to reduce the incidence of spontaneous preterm birth in women at increased risk: a randomized placebo-controlled double-blind study. Am J Obstet Gynecol 188:419, 2003.

525. Meis PJ, Klebanoff M, Thom E, et al: Prevention of recurrent preterm delivery by 17-alpha-hydroxyprogesterone caproate. N Eng J Med 348:2379, 2003.

526. Moore ML, Meis PJ, Ernest JM, et al: A randomized trial of nurse intervention to reduce preterm and low birth weight births. Obstet Gynecol 91:656, 1998.

527. Hobel CJ, Ross MG, Bemis RL, et al: The West Los Angeles Preterm Birth Prevention Project. I. Program impact on high-risk women. Am J Obstet Gynecol 170:54, 1994.

528. Spencer B, Thomas H, Morris J: A randomized controlled trial of the provision of a social support service during pregnancy: the South Manchester Family Worker Project. Br J Obstet Gynaecol 96:281, 1989.

529. Kovacevich GJ, Gaich SA, Lavin JP, et al: The prevalence of thromboembolic events among women with extended bed rest prescribed as part of the treatment for premature labor or preterm premature rupture of membranes. Am J Obstet Gynecol 182:1089, 2000.

530. Maloni JA, Brezinski-Tomasi JE, Johnson LA: Antepartum bed rest: effect upon the family. J Obstet Gynecol Neonatal Nurs 30:165, 2001.

531. Gupton A, Heaman M, Ashcroft T: Bed rest from the perspective of the high-risk pregnant woman. J Obstet Gynecol Neonatal Nurs 26:423, 1997.

532. Herron MA, Katz M, Creasy RK: Evaluation of a preterm birth prevention program: preliminary report. Obstet Gynecol 59:452, 1982.

533. Mueller-Heubach E, Reddick D, Barnett B, Bente R: Preterm birth prevention: evaluation of a prospective controlled randomized trial. Am J Obstet Gynecol 160:1172, 1989.

534. Collaborative Group on Preterm Birth Prevention: Multicenter randomized, controlled trial of a preterm birth prevention program. Am J Obstet Gynecol 169:352, 1993.

535. Hueston WJ, Knox MA, Eilers G, et al: The effectiveness of preterm-birth prevention educational programs for high-risk women: a meta-analysis. Obstet Gynecol 86:705, 1995.

536. Elder HA, Santamarina BA, Smith S, Kass EH: The natural history of asymptomatic bacteriuria during pregnancy: the effect of tetracycline on the clinical course and the outcome of pregnancy. Am J Obstet Gynecol 111:441, 1971.

537. Shennan A, Crawshaw S, Briley A, et al: A randomised controlled trial of metronidazole for the prevention of preterm birth in women positive for cervicovaginal fetal fibronectin: the PREMET Study. Br J Obstet Gynaecol 113:65, 2006.

538. Ugwumadu A, Manyonda I, Reid F, Hay P: Effect of early oral clindamycin on late miscarriage and preterm delivery in asymptomatic women with abnormal vaginal flora and bacterial vaginosis: a randomised controlled trial. Lancet 361: 983, 2003.

539. Lamont RF, Duncan SL, Mandal D, Bassett P: Intravaginal clindamycin to reduce preterm birth in women with abnormal genital tract flora. Obstet Gynecol 101:516, 2003.

540. Joesoef MR, Hillier SL, Wiknjosastro G, et al: Intravaginal clindamycin treatment for bacterial vaginosis: effects on preterm delivery and low birth weight. Am J Obstet Gynecol 173:1527, 1995.

541. Vermeulen GM, Bruinse HW: Prophylactic administration of clindamycin 2 percent vaginal cream to reduce the incidence of spontaneous preterm birth in women with an increased recurrence risk: A randomised placebo-controlled double-blind trial. Br J Obstet Gynaecol 106:652, 1999.

542. Boggess KAM, Moss K, Madianos PP, et al: Fetal immune response to oral pathogens and risk of preterm birth. Am J Obstet Gynecol 193:1121, 2005.

542a. Moore S, Ide M, Coward PY, et al: A prospective study to investigate the relationship between periodontal diseases and adverse pregnancy outcome. Br Dent J 197:251, 2004.

543. Jeffcoat MK, Hauth JC, Geurs NC, et al: Periodontal disease and preterm birth: results of a pilot intervention study. J Periodontol 74:1214, 2003.

543a. Michalowicz BS, Hodges JS, DiAngelis AJ, et al: Treatment of periodontal disease and the risk of preterm birth. N Engl J Med 355:1885, 2006.

544. Khader YS, Ta'ani Q: Periodontal diseases and the risk of preterm birth and low birth weight: a meta-analysis. J Periodontol 76:161, 2005.

544a. MacNaughton MC, Chalmers IG, Dubowitz V, et al: Final report of the Medical Research Council/Royal College of Obstetrics and Gynaecology multicentre randomised trial of cervical cerclage. Br J Obstet Gynaecol 100:516, 1993.

545. Althuisius SM, Dekker GA, Hummel P, et al: Final results of the cervical incompetence prevention randomized cerclage trial (CIPRACT): Therapeutic cerclage with bed rest versus bed rest alone. Am J Obstet Gynecol 185:1106, 2001.

546. Berghella V, Odibo AO, Tolosa JE: Cerclage for prevention of preterm birth in women with short cervix found on transvaginal ultrasound examination: a randomized trial. Am J Obstet Gynecol 191:1311, 2004.

547. Rust OA, Atlas RO, Reed J, et al: Revisiting the short cervix detected by transvaginal ultrasound in the second trimester: Why cerclage therapy may not help. Am J Obstet Gynecol 185:1098, 2001.

548. To MS, Alfirevic Z, Heath VCF, et al: Cervical cerclage for prevention of preterm delivery in women with short cervix: randomised controlled trial. Lancet 363:1849, 2004.

549. Berkman N, Thorp JM Jr, Lohr KN, et al: Tocolytic treatment for the management of preterm labor: a review of the evidence. Am J Obstet Gynecol 188:1648, 2003.

550. Sanchez-Ramos L, Kaunitz AM, Delke I: Progestational agents to prevent preterm birth: A meta-analysis of randomized controlled trials. Obstet Gynecol 105:273, 2005.

551. Dodd JM, Crowther CA, Cincotta R, et al: Progesterone supplementation for preventing preterm birth: a systematic review and meta-analysis. Acta Obstet Gynecol Scand 84:526, 2005.

552. Sanchez-Ramos L, Kaunitz AM, Delke I: Progestational agents to prevent preterm birth: A meta-analysis of randomized controlled trials. Obstet Gynecol 10:273, 2005.

553. Elovitz M, Wang Z: Medroxyprogesterone acetate, but not progesterone, protects against inflammation-induced parturition and intrauterine fetal demise. Am J Obstet Gynecol 190:693, 2004.

554. Garfield RE, Dannan MS, Daniel EE: Gap junction formation in myometrium: control by estrogens, progesterone, and prostaglandins. Am J Physiol 238:C81, 1980.

555. Meis PJM: For the Society for Maternal-Fetal Medicine: 17-Hydroxyprogesterone for the prevention of preterm delivery. Obstet Gynecol 105:1128, 2005.

555a. Northen A, NICHD MFMU Network: 4 year follow-up of children exposed to 17 Alpha hydroxyprogesterone caproate in utero. Am J Obstet Gynecol 195:S6, 2006.

556. Spong CY, Meis PJ, Thom EA, et al: Progesterone for prevention of recurrent preterm birth: impact of gestational age at previous delivery. Am J Obstet Gynecol 193:1127, 2005.

556a. Caritis S, Rouse D, NICHD MFMU Network: A randomized controlled trial of 17-hydroxyprogesterone caproate for the prevention of preterm birth in twins. Am J Obstet Gynecol 195:S2, 2006.

Premature Rupture of the Membranes

BRIAN M. MERCER

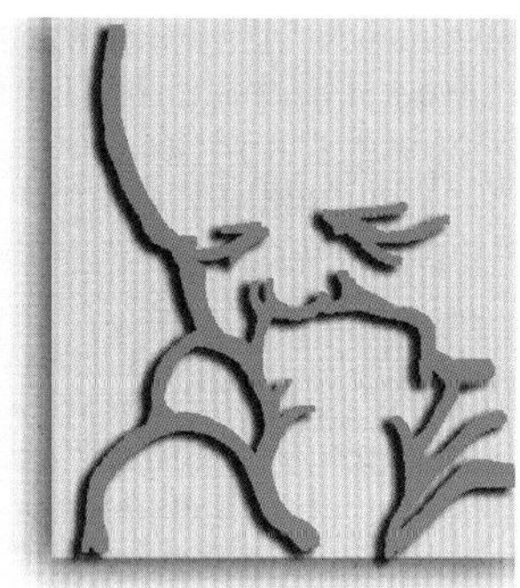

CHAPTER 27

KEY ABBREVIATIONS

By mouth	PO
Confidence interval	CI
Group B streptococcus	GBS
Herpes simplex virus	HSV
Human immunodeficiency virus	HIV
Intramuscular	IM
Intravenous	IV
Intraventricular hemorrhage	IVH
Lamellar body count	LB
Lecithin/sphingomyelin ratio	L/S
Maternal-Fetal Medicine Units	MFMU
Matrix metalloproteinases	MMP
National Institute of Child Health and Human Development	NICHD
Neonatal intensive care unit	NICU
Odds ratio	OR
Phosphatidylglycerol	PG
Premature rupture of the membranes	PROM
Respiratory distress syndrome	RDS
Surfactant/albumin 'ratio'	S/A
Tissue inhibitors of matrix metalloproteinases	TIMP
U.S. Food and Drug Administration	FDA

INTRODUCTION

Membrane rupture that occurs spontaneously before the onset of labor is described as premature rupture of membranes (PROM), regardless of gestational age at membrane rupture. PROM complicates approximately 8 to 10 percent of pregnancies. Preterm PROM, occurring before 37 weeks' of gestation, complicates 3 percent of pregnancies, is responsible for approximately one third of all preterm births,[1–4] and like preterm labor and incompetent cervix, it is considered a cause of "spontaneous preterm birth." Midtrimester PROM is PROM that occurs at or before 26 weeks' gestation, and the condition has been used in the past to indicate PROM occurring before the limit of potential neonatal survival (i.e., limit of viability).[5,6] As the limit of viability continues to decline, it is more relevant to differentiate preterm PROM into that which occurs before the limit of viability (i.e., previable PROM; currently before 23 weeks' gestation), preterm PROM remote from term (from the limit of viability to ~31 weeks' gestation), and preterm PROM near term (~32 to 36 weeks' gestation).

PROM at any gestational age is associated with brief latency from membrane rupture to delivery and also increased risks of perinatal infection and umbilical cord compression due to oligohydramnios. Because of this problem, term and preterm PROM are significant causes of perinatal morbidity and mortality. When PROM occurs at term, there is a low risk of severe neonatal complications with delivery of a noninfected and nonasphyxiated infant, and clinical management should be directed toward expeditious delivery with attention to risk factors for perinatal infection. Delivery at 32 to 36 weeks' gestation is generally associated with good infant outcomes, although complications can occur, particularly if the fetus is immature. Given the risks of continued pregnancy, delivery of the mature fetus is generally warranted. The immature fetus may benefit from measures to continue the pregnancy and accelerate fetal maturation. With immediate delivery after preterm PROM remote from term, there is a significant risk of perinatal morbidities and mortality that can be reduced thorough delay of delivery. In the absence of contraindications, management is directed toward continuing the pregnancy, with attention to potential risks of umbilical cord compression, intrauterine infection, and abruptio placentae. When PROM occurs before the limit of viability, neonatal death is inevitable with immediate delivery. Although conservative management can still lead to previable birth, some of these women benefit from extended latency, with delivery of a potentially viable infant. Regardless of the gestational age, the patient should be well informed regarding the potential maternal, fetal, and neonatal complications of PROM. These issues are discussed in detail in this chapter.

FETAL MEMBRANE ANATOMY AND PHYSIOLOGY

The fetal membranes are made up of a thin layer of amnion that lines the amniotic cavity, and a thicker outer layer of chorion that is directly apposed to maternal decidua. The amnion fuses to the chorion at near the end of the first trimester of pregnancy. These layers are subsequently connected by a collagen-rich connective tissue zone. Subsequently, the fetal membranes consist of single layer of cuboidal amnion epithelium with subjacent compact and spongy connective tissue layers, and a thicker chorion consisting of reticular and trophoblastic layers. Together, the amnion and chorion are stronger than either layer independently, although the amnion has greater tensile strength than the chorion. With advancing gestational age, changes in collagen content and type, and intercellular matrix, and cellular apoptosis result in structural weakening of the fetal membrane.[7–10] Membrane remodeling is more evident in the region of the internal cervical os in humans.[11–14] Membrane weakening appears to be stimulated by the presence of local matrix metalloproteinases (e.g., MMP-1, MMP-2, MMP-9), decreased levels of tissue inhibitors of matrix metalloproteinases (e.g., TIMP-1, TIMP-3) within the membranes, and increased poly[ADP-ribose]polymerase (PARP) cleavage.[12,15] With the onset of contractions, the amniochorionic membrane is subject to additional physical strain with increased intrauterine pressure that can lead to membrane rupture. Should the fetal membranes not rupture before active labor, advancing cervical dilatation decreases the work needed to cause membrane rupture over the internal cervical os, facilitating spontaneous membrane rupture in many cases.[7]

ETIOLOGY OF PREMATURE RUPTURE OF THE MEMBRANES

PROM occurring before term likely results from a variety of factors ultimately leading to accelerated membrane weakening through an increase in local cytokines and an imbalance in the interaction between MMPs and TIMPs,[16] increased collagenase and protease activity,[17] increased shear stress from uterine contractile activity, or from other factors that cause increased intrauterine pressure (e.g., polyhydramnios).[10,18] A number of clinical risk factors, including connective tissue disorders (e.g., Ehlers-Danlos syndrome), urogenital tract infection, abnormal genital tract colonization, chorioamnionitis, recent coitus, low socioeconomic status, uterine over-distention, second- and third-trimester bleeding, low body mass index (<19.8 kg/m^2), nutritional deficiencies of copper and ascorbic acid, antepartum bleeding in one or more trimesters, maternal cigarette smoking, cervical conization or cerclage, pulmonary disease in pregnancy, and preterm labor or symptomatic contractions in the current gestation have been linked to the occurrence of preterm PROM.[1–5,10,18–29] Each of these risk factors, individually or in concert, could lead to PROM through the mechanisms outlined earlier. However, the ultimate clinical cause of premature membrane rupture is often not apparent at delivery.

There is specific evidence linking preterm premature rupture of the membranes to infections involving the urogenital tract. Genital tract pathogens that have been associated with preterm PROM include *Neisseria gonorrhoeae, Chlamydia trachomatis, Trichomonas vaginalis*, and group B beta-hemolytic streptococci (GBS).[30–37] Although vaginal GBS colonization does not appear to be associated with PROM,[38,39] GBS bacteruria has been associated with preterm PROM and low birth weight infants.[40] A consistent association has been found between bacterial vaginosis and spontaneous preterm births, including those following preterm PROM.[41–43] It is not clear whether bacterial vaginosis is the inciting pathogen, facilitates ascent of other bacteria to the upper genital tract, or if it is a marker of maternal predisposition to abnormal genital track colonization. Bacterial invasion can facilitate membrane rupture through direct secretion of proteases, and also through stimulation of a host inflammatory response resulting in the elaboration of local cytokines, metalloproteases, and prostaglandins. Histologic studies of the membranes after preterm PROM often demonstrate significant bacterial contamination along the choriodecidual interface with minimal involvement of the amnion.[30] Women with preterm PROM have a high incidence of positive amniotic fluid cultures (25 to 35 percent) from amniocentesis specimens even when there is no clinical suspicion of infection.[44–52] Although some of these findings may reflect ascending infection subsequent to membrane rupture, it is probable that ascending colonization and infection is integral to the pathogenesis of preterm PROM in many cases.

Although the onset of vaginal fluid leakage is an acute event, there is evidence that the factors and events leading to membrane rupture are sometimes subacute or even chronic. Women with a prior preterm birth, especially one due to PROM, are at increased risk for recurrent preterm birth due to PROM. Preliminary studies have suggested an association between maternal genotype for inflammatory proteins and the risk of spontaneous preterm birth due to preterm labor or PROM.[53–57] Additionally, asymptomatic women with a short cervical length (<25 mm) at 22 to 24 weeks are at increased risk for PROM to occur weeks later.[39]

PREDICTION AND PREVENTION OF PRETERM PREMATURE RUPTURE OF THE MEMBRANES

Once preterm PROM occurs, delivery is often required or inevitable. Optimally, prediction and prevention of PROM would offer the best opportunity to prevent its complications. Prevention of preterm PROM requires an understanding of clinical markers for subsequent membrane rupture and interventions that could treat or ameliorate these underlying risk factors. Examples of specific risk factors whose treatment might reduce the risk of preterm PROM in certain individuals include cigarette smoking, urinary tract and sexually transmitted infections, and severe polyhydramnios. Alternatively, identification of women at high risk for PROM due to the presence of less specific risk factors might lead to development of more broad-based preventive strategies.

Prior preterm birth and especially preterm birth due to PROM has been associated with preterm PROM in a subsequent pregnancy.[58] The risk increases with decreasing gestational age of the index preterm birth. Those with a prior preterm birth near the limit of potential viability (23 to 27 weeks) have a 27.1-percent risk of subsequent preterm birth, and those with a prior history of preterm birth due to PROM have a 3.3-fold higher risk of preterm birth due to PROM (13.5 percent versus 4.1 percent, $p < 0.01$), and a 13.5-fold higher risk of preterm PROM before 28 weeks (1.8 versus 0.13 percent, $p < 0.01$) in a subsequent gestation. In a recent analysis from a prospective evaluation of preterm birth prediction, nulliparas and women with prior deliveries were evaluated separately because those without a prior birth lacked important historic information available to those with a prior term or preterm birth.[39] In that study, multivariable analysis revealed medical complications (including pulmonary disease in pregnancy), work during pregnancy, low maternal body mass index (<19.8 kg/m^2), and bacterial vaginosis to be significant markers for subsequent preterm birth in nulliparas, when assessed at 22 to 24 weeks' gestation (Table 27-1). Among women with prior deliveries, prior preterm birth due to preterm labor or PROM, and low maternal body mass index were the only statistically significant clinical markers for subsequent preterm PROM after controlling for other factors. A short cervical length (<25 mm) identified by transvaginal ultrasound was associated with an increased risk of subsequent PROM in both nulliparas and multiparas. Nulliparas with a positive cervicovaginal fetal fibronectin and a short cervix had a 16.7-percent risk of preterm birth due to preterm PROM. Among multiparas, women with a prior preterm birth due to PROM, a short cervix on ultrasound, and positive cervicovaginal fetal fibronectin screen had a 10.9-fold higher risk of PROM with delivery before 35 weeks' gestation (25 versus 2.3 percent) (Table 27-2). It must be noted, however, that such risk assessment systems identify only a small number of women who are at high risk and that the majority of preterm births due to PROM occur among "low-risk" women. Furthermore, although clinical and ancillary testing has increased our ability to identify women at increased risk, ancillary testing is expensive and inconvenient, and has not yet led to an effective intervention for the prevention of PROM. As such, routine ancillary testing cannot be recommended for this indication. Women determined to be at high-risk for preterm birth due to PROM based on clinical findings can be individually assessed for correctable risk factors, and encouraged to seek medical care should symptoms occur. There is current evidence to support progesterone treatment for women with a prior preterm birth due to PROM or preterm labor.[59,60] Such treatment has not yet received U.S. Food and Drug Administration (FDA) approval for this indication.

CLINICAL COURSE AFTER PREMATURE RUPTURE OF THE MEMBRANES

A hallmark of PROM is brief latency from membrane rupture to delivery. On average, latency increases with decreasing gestational age at membrane rupture. At term,

Table 27-1. Markers for Preterm PROM Before 37 Weeks*

	NULLIPARAS (N = 1,618)	MULTIPARAS (N = 1,711)
Medical complications	3.7 (1.5–9.0)	*
Work in pregnancy	3.0 (1.5–6.1)	*
Symptomatic contractions within 2 weeks	2.2 (1.2–7.5)	*
Bacterial vaginosis	2.1 (1.1–4.1)	*
Low body mass index (<19.8 kg/m^2)	2.0 (1.0–4.0)	1.8 (1.1–3.0)
Prior preterm birth due to PROM	*	3.1 (1.8–5.4)
Prior preterm birth due to preterm labor	*	1.8 (1.1–3.1)
Cervix ≤25 mm	3.7 (1.8–7.7)	2.5 (1.4–4.5)
Positive fetal fibronectin	*	2.1 (1.1–4.0)

PROM, Premature rupture of the membranes; not significant in final model.

Results of multivariable analyses for nulliparas and multiparas (presented as odds ratios with 95% confidence intervals).

*Adapted with permission from Mercer BM, Goldenberg RL, Meis PJ, et al and the NICHD-MFMU Network: The preterm prediction study: Prediction of preterm premature rupture of the membranes using clinical findings and ancillary testing. Am J Obstet Gynecol 183:738, 2000.

Table 27-2. Risk of Preterm Birth due to PROM before 37 and 35 Weeks Gestation Based on Parity, Cervical Length, Fetal Fibronectin, and Prior Obstetric History among Multiparas

	N	<37 WEEKS	<35 WEEKS
All multiparas	1,711	5.0	2.3
No risk factors present	1,351	3.2	0.8
Prior preterm birth due to PROM only	124	10.5	4.8
Prior preterm birth due to PROM and positive FFN	13	15.4	15.4
Prior preterm birth due to PROM and Short cervix	26	23.1	15.4
All 3 risk factors present	8	25.0	25.0

FFN, fetal fibronectin; Positive FFN, Cervicovaginal fetal fibronectin screen positive (>50 ng/ml) at 22–24 weeks' gestation; PROM, Premature rupture of the membranes; Short cervix, cervix length ≤25 mm on transvaginal ultrasound at 22–24 weeks gestation

Adapted with permission from Mercer BM, Goldenberg RL, Meis PJ, et al and the NICHD-MFMU Network: The preterm prediction study: Prediction of preterm premature rupture of the membranes using clinical findings and ancillary testing. Am J Obstet Gynecol 183:738, 2000.

one half of expectantly managed gravidas deliver within 5 hours and 95 percent deliver within 28 hours of membrane rupture.[61] Between 32 and 34 weeks, the mean interval between rupture and delivery is 4 days.[62] Of all women with PROM before 34 weeks, 93 percent deliver in less than 1 week. After excluding those admitted in labor or with amnionitis or nonreassuring fetal heart rate tracings, 50 to 60 percent of those conservatively managed will deliver within 1 week of membrane rupture.[29] When PROM occurs near the limit of viability, 30 to 40 percent remain pregnant for at least 1 week, and one in five conservatively managed women have a latency of 4 weeks or more.[5] A small proportion of women with membrane rupture can anticipate cessation of fluid leakage (2.6 to 13 percent), particularly those suffering membrane rupture subsequent to amniocentesis. Approximately 86 percent of those with leakage after amniocentesis will reseal.[6,27,63]

RISKS OF PREMATURE RUPTURE OF THE MEMBRANES

Maternal Risks

Infection of the amniotic cavity is the most common complication after preterm PROM. The risk of clinical chorioamnionitis increases with increasing duration of membrane rupture, and decreases with advancing gestational age at PROM.[64,65] Overall, 9 percent of gravidas with PROM at term develop chorioamnionitis.[66] This risk increases to 24 percent with membrane rupture longer than 24 hours. With PROM remote from term, chorioamnionitis occurs in 13 to 60 percent of pregnancies, and endometritis occurs in approximately 2 to 13 percent of cases.[67,68] Placental abruption may cause PROM or occur subsequent to membrane rupture, and affects 4 to 12 percent of these pregnancies.[21,69,70] Uncommon but serious complications of PROM managed conservatively near or before the limit of viability include retained placenta and hemorrhage requiring dilation and curettage (12 percent), maternal sepsis (0.8 percent), and maternal death (0.14 percent).[71]

Fetal and Neonatal Risks

Fetal complications after membrane rupture include infection and fetal distress due to umbilical cord compression or placental abruption. Umbilical cord compression due to oligohydramnios is a common finding after PROM.[72] Frank or occult umbilical cord prolapse can also occur, particularly with fetal malpresentation. Because of these factors, women with PROM have a higher risk of cesarean delivery for nonreassuring fetal heart rate patterns than those with isolated preterm labor (7.9 versus 1.5 percent). Fetal death occurs in 1 to 2 percent of cases of conservatively managed PROM.[25] Amnioinfusion may be of value to reduce umbilical cord compression secondary to oligohydramnios but is not recommend for routine use in the absence of fetal heart rate evidence of cord compression (see Chapter 15).

The frequency and severity of neonatal complications after PROM varies inversely with gestational age at membrane rupture and at delivery. Respiratory distress syndrome (RDS) is the most common serious acute morbidity after preterm PROM, Necrotizing enterocolitis, intraventricular hemorrhage (IVH), and sepsis are common with early preterm birth but relatively uncommon near term. Serious perinatal morbidity remote from term can lead to long-term sequelae such as chronic lung disease, visual or hearing difficulties, mental retardation, developmental and motor delay, cerebral palsy, or death. Although specific data are not available for those delivering after preterm PROM, general community-based survival and morbidity data reveal that long-term morbidities and death are uncommon with delivery after ~32 weeks' gestation.[73,74]

Neonatal sepsis is twofold more common after preterm birth due to PROM than after preterm labor with intact membranes. Neonatal infection can result from the same organisms present in the amniotic fluid, or from other organisms, and can present as acute congenital pneumonia, sepsis, meningitis, or late onset bacterial or fungal infections. Fortunately, most infants delivered in the setting of chorioamnionitis will not have a serious infection. There is accumulating evidence to suggest that fetal/neonatal infection and inflammation are associated with an increased risk of long-term neurologic complications. Cerebral palsy and cystic periventricular leukomalacia have been linked to amnionitis, which is more commonly seen after preterm PROM, and is more likely with increased latency.[75] Elevated amniotic fluid cytokines and fetal systemic inflammation have been associated with preterm PROM, periventricular leukomalacia, and cerebral palsy.[76–78] It has been postulated that infection- and inflammation-induced cytokines could have a direct neurotoxic effect that leads to these outcomes. Although there are no data to suggest that immediate delivery on admission with PROM will avert these sequelae, these findings highlight the importance of restricting conservative management after PROM to circumstances in which there is the potential to reduce neonatal morbidity through such measures (see later). Further study in this area is needed.

Pulmonary hypoplasia is a severe complication of PROM that occurs in the second trimester and carries a 70-percent mortality rate. Fetal lung development is particularly sensitive to membrane rupture in the second trimester.[79–84] Whether due to tracheobronchial collapse and fluid efflux with PROM or loss of intrinsic factors within the tracheobronchial fluid, pulmonary hypoplasia develops over weeks after membrane rupture owing to a lack of terminal bronchiole and alveolar development during the cannalicular phase of pulmonary development at 16 to 28 weeks' gestation.[85–88] Pulmonary hypoplasia is most accurately diagnosed pathologically based on radial alveolar counts and lung weights.[89,90] Clinical findings in the neonate such as a small chest circumference with severe respiratory distress and persistent pulmonary hypertension, and X-ray findings such as small well-aerated lungs with a bell-shaped chest and elevation of the diaphragm are also supportive of the diagnosis.[80,85]

Overall, pulmonary hypoplasia complicates up to 26.5 percent of cases in series of midtrimester PROM (mean 5.9 percent). The incidence of lethal pulmonary hypoplasia is inversely correlated with gestational age at rupture,[80,91] complicating nearly 50 percent of cases with membrane rupture before 19 weeks and prolonged latency.[83–85,92,93] Lethal pulmonary hypoplasia rarely occurs with PROM after 26 weeks of gestation (0 to 1.4 percent).[94] However, other pulmonary complications. such as pneumothorax and pneumomediastinum related to poor pulmonary compliance and high ventilatory pressures, can occur with lesser degrees of this condition.[80,94,95] Restriction deformities occur in approximately ~1.5 percent of infants delivered after conservative management after midtrimester PROM, but these deformities can complicate up to 27 percent of fetuses with prolonged oligohydramnios.[71,80,94–97]

DIAGNOSIS OF PREMATURE RUPTURE OF THE MEMBRANES

The diagnosis of PROM depends on history, physical examination, and laboratory information. More than 90 percent of cases can be confirmed based on the presence of a suspicious history or ultrasonographic findings, followed by documentation of fluid passing from the cervix or the presence of a nitrazine/ferning positive vaginal pool of fluid. In addition to providing confirmatory evidence of membrane rupture, sterile speculum examination can provide the opportunity to inspect for cervicitis, or umbilical cord or fetal prolapse; to assess cervical dilatation and effacement; and to obtain appropriate cultures (e.g., endocervical *Neisseria gonorrhoeae* and *Chlamydia trachomatis,* anovaginal *Streptococcus agalactiae*).

The diagnosis of membrane rupture is confirmed by the presence of the following findings:

- Visualization of a pool of fluid in the posterior vaginal fornix with evident clear fluid passing from the cervical canal.
- Vaginal pH of more than 6.0 to 6.5.
- Microscopic arborized crystals ("ferning") owing to the interaction of amniotic fluid proteins and salts, which is evident in vaginal secretions obtained by swabbing the posterior fornix with a sterile swab.

False-positive results may occur with blood or semen contamination, alkaline antiseptics, or bacterial vaginosis. Cervical mucus can yield a false-positive ferning pattern; however, the crystals appears as a more floral pattern. The fern test is unaffected by meconium, changes in vaginal pH, and blood/amniotic fluid ratios of up to 1:5. The fern pattern in samples heavily contaminated with blood is atypical and appears more "skeletonized."[98,99] Prolonged leakage with minimal residual fluid can lead to a "false-negative" inspection, or nitrazine or ferning test. Should initial testing be negative but a clinical suspicion of membrane rupture remain, the patient can be retested after prolonged recumbency or alternate measures can be considered. Cervicovaginal screening for fetal fibronectin or other markers such as prolactin or human chorionic gonadotrophin may be helpful in excluding the diagnosis. Alternatively, a positive test may reflect disruption of the decidua rather than membrane rupture. Other plausible causes of vaginal discharge (e.g., urinary incontinence, vaginitis, cervicitis, mucous "show" with cervical effacement and dilatation, semen, and vaginal douches) should be excluded if the diagnosis is unclear.

Ultrasound evaluation may prove useful if the diagnosis remains in doubt after speculum examination. Although oligohydramnios without evident fetal urinary tract malformations or fetal growth restriction may be suggestive of membrane rupture, ultrasound alone cannot diagnose or exclude membrane rupture with certainty. If the diagnosis is equivocal, the patient can be placed in a Trendelenburg position for a few hours and reexamined as outlined earlier. Alternatively, the diagnosis of membrane rupture can be made unequivocally with ultrasound guided dye amnioinfusion (1 ml indigo carmine + 9 ml sterile saline), followed by observation for passage of dye onto a perineal pad.

Some women presenting with a suspicious history for membrane rupture have negative speculum examination findings and a normal amniotic fluid volume on ultrasound, only to return subsequently with gross membrane rupture. Whether these women initially had a small amount of fluid transudation across a weakened membrane, or minimal leakage around a firmly applied presenting fetal part cannot generally be determined. Those with a suspicious history, but negative physical findings should be encouraged to return should they have persistent or recurrent symptoms.

MANAGEMENT OF PREMATURE RUPTURE OF THE MEMBRANES

General Considerations

Management of PROM is based primarily on an individual assessment of the estimated risk for fetal and neonatal complications should conservative management or expeditious delivery be pursued. The risks of maternal morbidity should also be considered, particularly when PROM occurs before the limit of potential viability (currently 23 weeks' gestation).

Initial Assessment and Care

At term, initial assessment is similar to that offered to woman presenting in labor with intact membranes. The diagnosis of membrane rupture is confirmed and the duration of membrane rupture assessed, to assist the pediatric caregivers with subsequent management decisions. The patient is assessed for fetal presentation, contractions, findings suggestive of intrauterine infection, and evidence of fetal well-being. GBS carriage is ascertained, if available, from a recent (i.e., performed within the past 5 weeks) anovaginal culture.

Although practice varies regarding the management of preterm PROM, there is general consensus regarding some issues. Gestational age should be established based on clinical history, and prior ultrasound assessment, where available (Fig. 27-1). If preterm PROM occurs, ultrasound should be performed to assess fetal growth, position, residual amniotic fluid volume, for gross fetal abnormalities that may cause polyhydramnios and PROM, and to assist in gestational age assignment if no prior ultrasound has been performed. Narrowing of the biparietal diameter (dolichocephaly) due to oligohydramnios can lead to underestimation of gestational age and fetal weight after PROM.[100] Tables using fetal head circumference can be used under this circumstance. The woman with preterm PROM should be evaluated clinically for evidence of advanced labor, chorioamnionitis, placental abruption, and fetal distress. Those with advanced labor, intrauterine infection, significant vaginal bleeding, or nonreassuring fetal testing are best delivered regardless of gestational age. If fetal malpresenta-

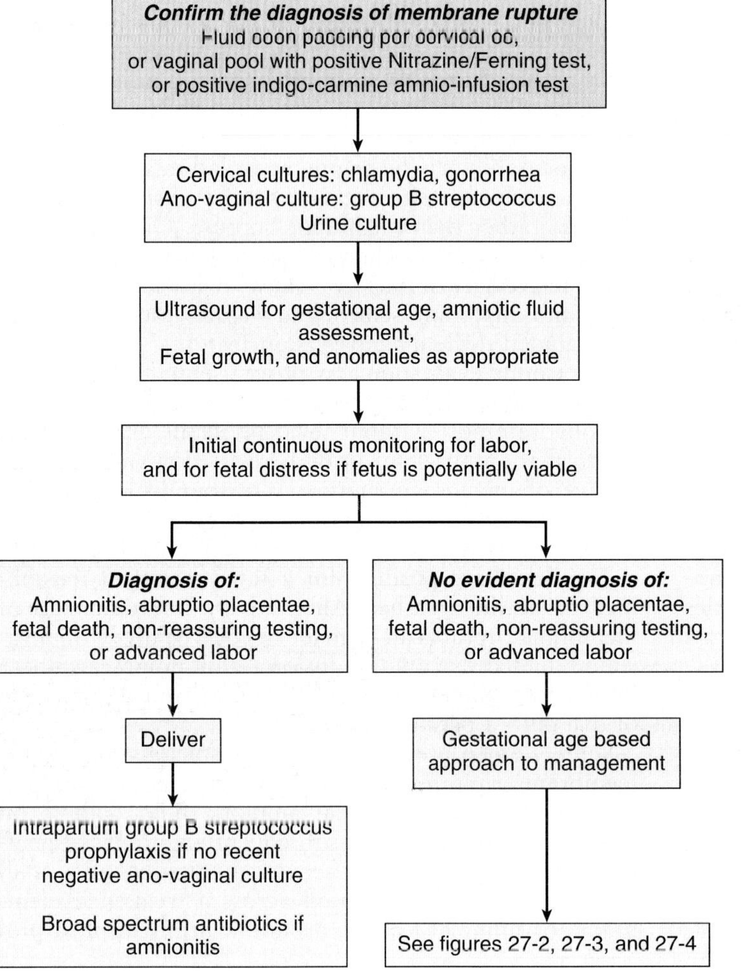

Figure 27-1. Initial assessment and management of women with preterm premature rupture of the membranes. (From Mercer BM: Preterm premature rupture of the membranes: diagnosis and management. Clin Perinatol 31:765, 2004.)

Corticosteroid Administration

Antenatal corticosteroid administration is one of the most effective obstetric interventions to reduce the risks of RDS, IVH, necrotizing enterocolitis, perinatal death, and long-term neurologic morbidity among women at high risk of delivering an immature preterm infant. Although it has been suggested that antenatal corticosteroids after preterm PROM may be ineffective because these women would deliver too quickly to accrue the potential benefits, and because PROM might accelerate fetal pulmonary maturation or be inappropriate because treatment might delay the diagnosis or increase the risk of perinatal infection, current evidence supports the administration of antenatal corticosteroids to the woman with PROM and suspected or documented fetal immaturity. The majority of women with preterm PROM will remain pregnant for at least 24 to 48 hours during conservative management. RDS remains the most common acute morbidity after preterm PROM, regardless of any potential maturational effect of PROM.[150] The most recent meta-analysis regarding antenatal corticosteroid administration after preterm PROM has confirmed steroid therapy to significantly reduce the risks of RDS (20 percent versus 35.4 percent), IVH (7.5 percent versus 15.9 percent), and necrotizing enterocolitis (0.8 percent versus 4.6 percent), without increasing the risks of maternal (9.2 percent versus 5.1 percent) or neonatal (7.0 percent versus 6.6 percent) infection.[151] The combined use of antibiotics and corticosteroids appears to confer greater benefit than either treatment alone for women with preterm PROM. In a randomized controlled trial of antenatal corticosteroids after antibiotic administration, Lewis et al.[152] found less frequent RDS (18.4 percent versus 43.6 percent, $p = 0.03$) with no evident increase in perinatal infections (3 percent versus 5 percent) after steroid administration. A second trial revealed no reduction in RDS with antenatal corticosteroids concurrent to antibiotic administration but did find a reduction in perinatal death among those remaining pregnant 24 hours or more (1.3 percent versus 8.3 percent, $p = 0.05$), and no increase in perinatal infectious morbidity with steroid treatment.[153] In a third trial of antibiotic treatments versus placebo in which all women received antenatal corticosteroids, the combination of neonatal mortality, sepsis, and respiratory morbidity was less common with antibiotics and steroids (29.3 percent vs. 48.6 percent, $p < 0.05$), a finding that was particularly evident for those with PROM before 27 weeks' gestation.[154]

Although there appears to be benefit to a single course of antenatal corticosteroids, either betamethasone (12 mg intramuscularly [IM], q24h × two doses) or dexamethasone (6 mg IM, q12h × four doses), after preterm PROM, data regarding the risks and benefits of repeated weekly courses is conflicting. Using multivariable regression analysis to control for gestational age and other factors in a retrospective analysis, Vermillion et al.[155] found repeated antenatal corticosteroid administration to be associated an increased risk of early neonatal sepsis among those receiving two or more courses of antenatal corticosteroids (15.3 percent) as compared with a single course (2 percent), or no courses (1.5 percent), $p < 0.001$; a finding that persisted after controlling for other characteristics (OR 2.9). Ghidini et al.[156] noted less IVH and amnionitis, and a trend toward less sepsis but no reduction in the risk of RDS with repeated antenatal corticosteroid doses. Alternatively, Abbassi et al.[157] observed a lower risk of RDS with more than one course of antenatal corticosteroids after PROM (34.9 percent versus 45.2 percent) without an apparent increase in the risk of neonatal sepsis (9.9 percent versus 6.2 percent). Given the potential risks and the absence of clear data supporting the benefit of repeated weekly antenatal corticosteroid administration, such treatment does not appear warranted. It remains to be determined if the patient treated with a single course of antenatal corticosteroids after PROM near the limit of viability could benefit from an additional single course at 30 to 32 weeks after extended latency, with the development of additional alveoli that were not present to benefit from initial therapy.

Antibiotic Administration

The goal of adjunctive antibiotic therapy during conservative management of preterm PROM remote from term is to treat or prevent ascending decidual infection in order to prolong pregnancy and offer the opportunity for reduced neonatal infectious and gestational age–dependent morbidity. Three meta-analyses summarize a large number of published reports of randomized, prospective clinical trials assessing the utility of adjunctive antibiotic therapy during expectant management of PROM.[29,158,159] One of these meta-analyses demonstrated that antibiotic treatment was associated with significant pregnancy prolongation, as well as reduced chorioamnionitis, postpartum endometritis, neonatal sepsis, pneumonia, and intraventricular hemorrhage, when compared with expectant management.[29] The other meta-analysis found a significant reduction in neonatal sepsis and IVH.[158] In the most recent meta-analysis, Kenyon found antibiotic administration to delay delivery and reduce major markers of neonatal morbidity but suggested that amoxicillin-clavulonic acid be avoided because of the increased risk of neonatal necrotizing enterocolitis.[159]

Two large multicenter clinical trials with different approaches to this issue have adequate power to evaluate the utility of adjunctive antibiotics after preterm PROM in reducing infant morbidity. The combination of these studies, as well as specific details from individual smaller trials, offers valuable insights regarding the potential role of adjunctive antibiotics in this setting. The National Institutes of Child Health and Human Development Maternal Fetal Medicine Units (NICHD-MFMU) Research Network elected to study women with preterm PROM from the limit of 24 to 32 weeks 0 days gestation to see if adjunctive antibiotic therapy would reduce the number of infants who were acutely ill after birth.[150,160] This trial used initial aggressive intravenous therapy (48 hours) with ampicillin (2 g IV q6h) and erythromycin (250 mg IV q6h), followed by limited duration oral therapy (5 days) with amoxicillin (250 mg by mouth [PO] q8h) and enteric-coated erythromycin-base (333 mg PO q8h) because these agents provide broad-spectrum antimicrobial coverage and have demonstrated safety when used in pregnancy. GBS carriers in both study arms were treated with ampicillin for 1 week and then again in labor, and were analyzed separately. This trial found that antibiotic treatment prolonged pregnancy, increasing twofold the likelihood that women would remain undelivered after 7 days of treatment. Treated women continued to be more likely to remain pregnant at up to 3 weeks after randomization, despite discontinuation of antibiotics at 7 days, suggesting that the therapy actually successfully treated subclinical infection rather than just suppressing it. Regarding infant morbidity, the NIH trial found that antibiotics improved neonatal health by reducing the number of babies with one or more major infant morbidity (composite morbidity: death, RDS, early sepsis, severe IVH, severe necrotizing enterocolitis) from 53 to 44 percent ($p < 0.05$). Additionally, aggressive antibiotic therapy was associated with significant reductions in individual gestational age–dependent morbidities including RDS (40.5 percent versus 48.7 percent), stage 3 to 4 necrotizing enterocolitis (2.3 percent versus 5.8 percent), patent ductus arteriosus (11.7 percent versus 20.2 percent), and chronic lung disease (bronchopulmonary dysplasia: 20.5 percent versus 13.0 percent), $p \leq 0.05$ for each. Regarding infectious morbidity, the antibiotic study group had a lower incidence of neonatal GBS sepsis (0 percent versus 1.5 percent, $p = 0.03$). Regarding individual infectious morbidities, amnionitis was reduced with study antibiotics (32.5 percent versus 23 percent, $p = 0.01$), and both neonatal sepsis (8.4 percent versus 15.6 percent, $p = 0.009$) and pneumonia (2.9 percent versus 7.0 percent, $p = 0.04$) were less frequent in the antibiotic group for those who were not GBS carriers. Because of these findings, limited duration aggressive antibiotic therapy is recommended during conservative management of preterm PROM remote from term. Although not specifically studied, recent shortages in antibiotic availability have led to the need for substitution of alternative antibiotic treatments. Oral ampicillin, erythromycin, and azithromycin are likely appropriate alternatives to the above-mentioned agents, as needed.

In a second large multicenter placebo controlled trial, Kenyon et al.[161] studied oral antibiotic therapy with erythromycin, amoxicillin-clavulonic acid, or both for up to 10 days after preterm PROM before 37 weeks. In summary, oral erythromycin therapy was associated with brief pregnancy prolongation (not significant at 7 days), reduced need for supplemental oxygen (31.1 percent versus 35.6 percent, $p = 0.02$), reduced positive blood cultures (5.7 percent versus 8.2 percent, $p = 0.02$), but no significant reduction in the primary outcome (a baby suffering one or more of the following: death, chronic lung disease, or major cerebral abnormality on ultrasonography, 12.7 percent versus 15.2 percent, $p = 0.08$). Oral amoxicillin-clavulonic acid prolonged pregnancy (43.3 percent versus 36.7 percent undelivered after 7 days, $p = 0.005$) and reduced the need for supplemental oxygen (30.1 percent versus 35.6 percent, $p = 0.05$), but was associated with an increased risk of necrotizing enterocolitis (1.9 percent vs. 0.5 percent, $p = 0.001$) without reducing other neonatal morbidity. The combination of oral amoxicillin-clavulonic acid and erythromycin yielded similar findings. Sub-analysis of women with preterm PROM remote from term was not presented but was reported to reveal the same pattern of findings as with amoxicillin-clavulonic acid alone. The authors concluded that oral erythromycin was effective in reducing infant complications but raised concern regarding the potential negative effects of oral amoxicillin-clavulonic acid. However, given the small differences in the actual incidences of morbidity in the study groups, many women would need to be treated with oral erythromycin to prevent one adverse outcome. Furthermore, the finding regarding increased necrotizing enterocolitis with oral amoxicillin-clavulonic acid is at odds with the NICHD-MFMU trial finding of reduced stage 3 to 4 necrotizing enterocolitis with aggressive antibiotic therapy in a higher risk population. Review of the literature does not reveal a consistent pattern regarding an increased risk of necrotizing enterocolitis with broad-spectrum antibiotic therapy during conservative management of PROM remote from term.

In summary, there appears to be a role for a 7-day course of parenteral and oral therapy with erythromycin and amoxicillin/ampicillin during conservative management of preterm PROM remote from term to prolong pregnancy, and to reduce infectious and gestational age–dependent neonatal morbidity. The combination of oral erythromycin and extended-spectrum ampicillin-clavulonic acid in a lower risk population near term does not appear to be beneficial and may be harmful. This latter regimen is not recommended. Several recent studies have attempted to determine whether brief duration antibiotic therapy is adequate after preterm PROM.[162,163] These studies are of inadequate size and power to demonstrate equivalent effectiveness against infant morbidity.

Tocolysis

There is some evidence from prospective studies that prophylactic tocolysis can prolong pregnancy briefly after preterm PROM,[164–168] particularly when beta-agonists are given before the onset of contractions. However, therapeutic tocolysis initiated only after the onset of contractions has not been shown to prolong latency in this setting. A report from the National Institutes of Health's Collaborative study on antenatal steroids suggested an association between tocolytic use after preterm PROM and subsequent neonatal RDS.[169] Although the biologic plausibility for this finding is not clear, subsequent small prospective studies have found neither an increase nor decrease in neonatal morbidity with tocolytic treatment. However, the available literature has not evaluated tocolytic therapy concurrent to antenatal corticosteroid and antibiotic administration. It is plausible that prophylactic tocolysis could result in initial uterine quiescence to allow antibiotic suppression of subclinical decidual infection, and allow additional time for initial corticosteroid effects on the fetus. This approach needs further study. In the mean time, tocolytic therapy after preterm PROM should not be considered an expected practice but may be appropriate in the pregnancy that is at high risk for neonatal complications after preterm birth or for transportation to a tertiary care institution.

Cerclage

Preterm PROM is a common complication after cervical cerclage, affecting about one in four pregnancies with a cerclage and about half of pregnancies requiring an emergent cerclage.[26,170,171] There are no prospective studies regarding the management of women with preterm PROM and a cervical cerclage in situ. Retrospective studies have found that the risk of adverse perinatal outcomes is not higher than after preterm PROM without a cerclage if the cerclage is removed on admission.[172,173] Studies comparing pregnancies in which the cerclage is retained or removed after preterm PROM have been small but have yielded consistent patterns.[174–176] Each has found insignificant trends toward increased maternal infectious morbidity, with only brief pregnancy prolongation, and one study found increased infant mortality and death due to sepsis when the cerclage was left in situ.[174] Although one study comparing differing practices at two institutions found significant pregnancy prolongation with cerclage retention, this finding could reflect population or practice differences at these institutions.[175] No controlled study has found cerclage retention to reduce the frequency or severity of infant morbidities after preterm PROM. Based on the available data suggesting potential risk with no evident fetal/neonatal benefit, early cerclage removal is recommended when PROM occurs, particularly if the history of incompetent cervix is not typical. The value of short-term cerclage retention while attempting to enhance fetal maturation with antenatal corticosteroids after early preterm PROM has not been determined.

Herpes Simplex Virus

Neonatal herpes simplex virus (HSV) infection most commonly results from direct maternal-fetal transmission during the delivery process, with infection rates of 34 to 80 percent after primary and 1 to 5 percent after secondary maternal infection.[177,178] When neonatal herpes infection occurs, the mortality rate is 50 to 60 percent, with up to 50 percent of survivors suffering serious sequelae.[179,180] Based on small case series of women with an active maternal genital herpes infection by Amstey (N = 9) and Nahmias (N = 26), both in 1971, the accepted belief has been that extended latency after membrane rupture (>4 to 6 hours) is associated with an increased risk of neonatal infection.[181–183] However, a recent case series published by Major and coworkers evaluated pregnancy outcomes of 29 gravidas managed expectantly with active *recurrent* HSV lesions and PROM before 32 weeks' gestation.[184] In this series, antenatal corticosteroids and antibiotics were not administered, nor were antiretroviral agents administered to all patients. Latency after membrane rupture ranged from 1 to 35 days, and cesarean delivery was performed if active lesions were present at the time of delivery. None of the 26 infants delivered under this regimen developed neonatal herpes infection (95-percent CI, 0 to 10.4 percent). These data are supportive of conservative management of PROM complicated by recurrent maternal HSV infection. Such treatment should be considered only at an early gestational age, when the likelihood of infant mortality and long-term morbidity with delivery is high. Prophylactic treatment with antiviral agents (e.g., acyclovir) to reduce viral shedding and the frequency of recurrences is appropriate under this circumstance.

Management of Previable Premature Rupture of the Membranes

The cause of previable PROM has implications for the anticipated pregnancy outcome and can be helpful in guiding counseling and management. Previable PROM subsequent to second-trimester amniocentesis, in most cases, is likely related to continued leakage of fluid through a small membrane defect without concurrent infection. Under this circumstance, there is a high likelihood that the membranes will reseal, and extended pregnancy can be anticipated. When previable PROM occurs subsequent to persistent second trimester bleeding, oligohydramnios, or an elevated maternal serum alpha-fetoprotein, membrane rupture likely reflects an abnormality of placentation and the prognosis for a favorable outcome is poor. Early in pregnancy, the line between a spontaneous miscarriage and PROM can be blurred. The patient with previable PROM and no other indication for immediate delivery should be counseled regarding the potential risks and benefits of expectant management. Counseling should include a realistic appraisal of fetal and neonatal outcomes, as well as the risks of maternal complications incurred with conservative management.

The majority of available data regarding these women are derived from retrospective studies conducted regarding maternal, fetal, and infant outcomes after midtrimester PROM at or before 26 weeks' gestation. In a review of women with midtrimester PROM, Schucker and Mercer found the maternal risks during conservative management of midtrimester PROM to include chorioamnionitis (39.3 percent), abruption (3.2 percent), retained placenta (11.9 percent), and endometritis (9.9 percent).[71] Maternal sepsis (0.8 percent) and death (0.14 percent) were rare but serious complications. Conservative management can also lead to less well-defined risks such as muscle wasting, bone demineralization, and deep venous thrombosis due to prolonged bed rest. Overall survival after conservatively managed midtrimester PROM occurs in 45 percent of cases, with stillbirth complicating 15 percent. Neonatal complications include pulmonary hypoplasia (5.9 percent), RDS (52 percent), IVH (24 percent), infection (15 percent), and necrotizing enterocolitis (6.4 percent), as well as long-term complications such as bronchopulmonary dysplasia (18 percent), retinopathy of prematurity (13 percent), hydrocephalus (12 percent), and contractures (1.5 percent). Despite the frequency of significant perinatal morbidities, 69 percent of survivors in the published literature are apparently neurologically intact at long-term follow-up. Although these studies provide helpful information, they are limited by the rarity of this condition, requiring data collection over extended periods of time, with evolving practice patterns and outcomes relating to a progressive decline in the limit of potential viability. Prediction of outcomes for the individual presenting with midtrimester PROM is extremely difficult, given our inability to predict those who will have extended latency and the ultimate gestational age at delivery in any given case.

There are no current data regarding outcomes after conservative management of PROM occurring before 23 weeks' gestation. Data available from eight studies regarding conservatively managed PROM before 23 weeks reveal uncommon infant survival (11.7 percent), and frequent stillbirth (28.1 percent) and chorioamnionitis (13.1 percent), with considerable variation in these studies.[95,96,185–190] Those with PROM between 16 and 19 weeks had similar rates of stillbirth (27.6 percent) and amnionitis (14.7 percent) but higher survival rates (17.9 percent).[95,185–188,191–193] This finding likely reflects significant underreporting of those presenting and delivering quickly before 20 weeks' gestation.

A potential management scheme for PROM before the limit of viability is presented in Figure 27-4. At present, there is no consensus regarding the advantages of inpatient versus outpatient management for the patient electing conservative management after previable PROM. The benefits of an initial period of inpatient observation may include strict bed and pelvic rest to enhance the opportunity for resealing, as well as early identification of infection and abruption. A number of novel treatments including amnioinfusion, and fibrin/platelet/cryoprecipitate or gel-foam sealing of the membranes have been preliminarily investigated.[194–196] The maternal risks and fetal benefits of these aggressive interventions have not been adequately demonstrated to suggest inclusion of such therapy be incorporated into routine clinical practice. Typically, women with previable PROM are readmitted to hospital for bed rest and observation for infection, abruption, labor, and nonreassuring fetal heart rate patterns once the pregnancy has reached the limit of viability. Administration of antenatal corticosteroids for fetal maturation is appropriate at this time.

During conservative management, serial ultrasound performed every 1 to 2 weeks can evaluate reaccumula-

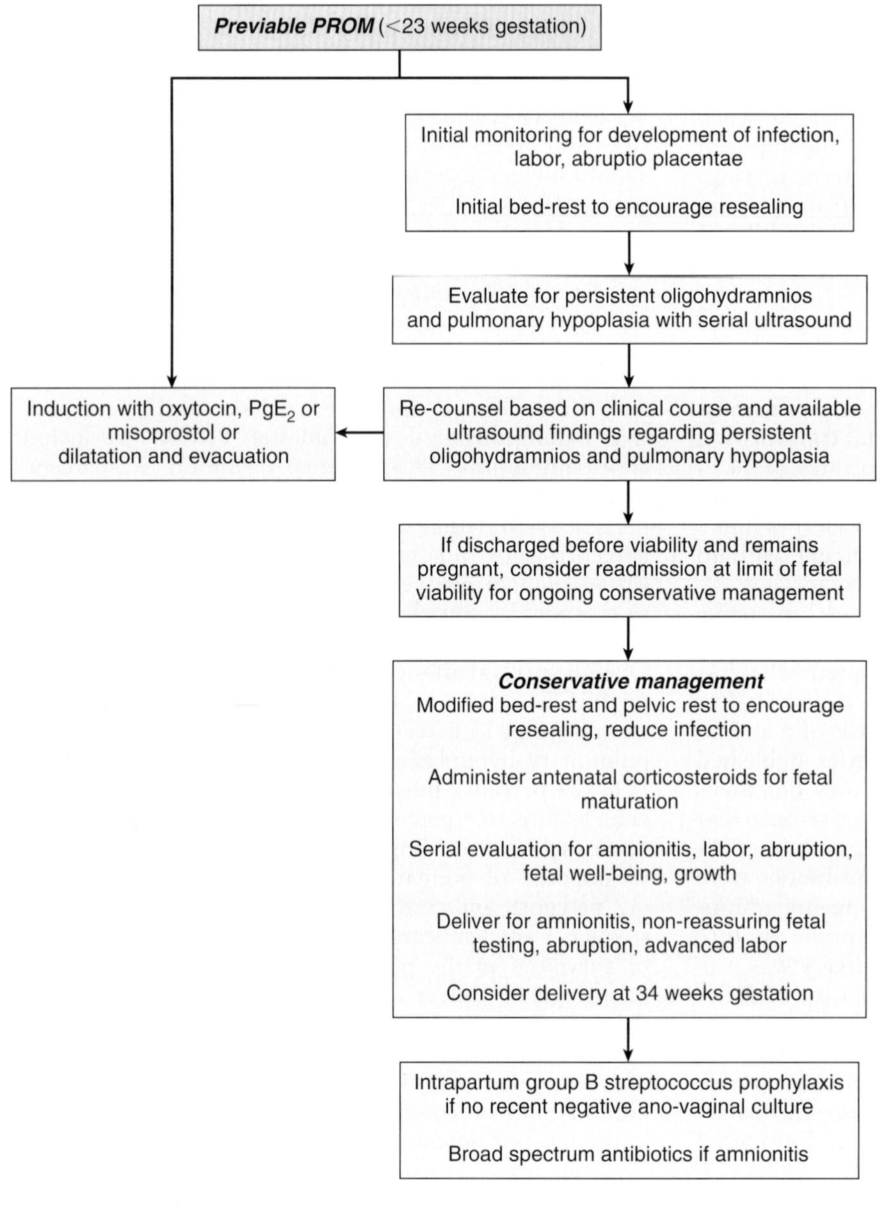

Figure 27-4. Management algorithm for preterm PROM before the limit of potential viability (currently 23 weeks' gestation). PgE_2, prostaglandin E_2. (From Mercer BM: Preterm premature rupture of the membranes: diagnosis and management. Clin Perinatol 31:765, 2004.)

tion of amniotic fluid and interval pulmonary growth. Although persistent severe oligohydramnios is the strongest marker for subsequent development of lethal pulmonary hypoplasia, serial fetal biometric evaluation (e.g., lung length, chest circumference), and ratios to adjust for overall fetal size (thoracic/abdominal circumference, thoracic circumference/femur length) can demonstrate a lack of fetal pulmonary growth over time and have a predictive value for neonatal mortality due to pulmonary hypoplasia.[85,93,197–200] However, these findings require weeks to become evident. Studies of pulmonary artery and ductus arteriosus waveform modulation with fetal breathing movements have shown some promise but can be technically difficult to perform.[93,197,201,202] Identification of lethal pulmonary hypoplasia before the limit of viability may offer the opportunity for the patient to reconsider the plan of conservative management.

Some women will not wish to incur the significant risk of adverse maternal and neonatal sequelae after previable PROM. Delivery can be accomplished by labor induction with high-dose oxytocin or with vaginal prostaglandin E_2, prostaglandin E_1 (misoprostol), or by dilatation and evacuation. The optimal approach depends on patient characteristics (e.g., gestational age, evident amnionitis, prior cesarean delivery), available facilities, and physician experience.

SUMMARY

The potential for significant perinatal morbidity and mortality exists when PROM occurs at term or preterm. Expeditious delivery of the patient with PROM at or near term can reduce the risk of perinatal infections without increasing the likelihood of operative delivery. Careful conservative management of PROM remote from term offers caregivers the potential to reduce infectious and gestational age–dependent morbidity. Early transfer to a facility capable of providing urgent obstetric and neonatal intensive care is important should adequate facilities not be available locally. Regardless of the management approach, infants delivering after preterm PROM and after PROM before the limit of potential viability are at high-risk for perinatal complications, many of which cannot be avoided with current technology and management algorithms.

KEY POINTS

- PROM complicates approximately 8 to 10 percent of pregnancies, is responsible for approximately one third of preterm births, and is a significant cause of gestational age-dependent and infectious perinatal morbidity and mortality.

- Latency from membrane rupture to delivery is typically brief, and decreases with increasing gestational age at membrane rupture.

- Chorioamnionitis is common after preterm PROM and increases in frequency with decreasing gestational age at membrane rupture.

- Women with a prior preterm birth due to PROM have a 3.3-fold higher risk of subsequent preterm birth due to PROM, and a 13.5-fold higher risk of preterm PROM before 28 weeks' gestation.

- Some potentially preventable causes of preterm PROM include urogenital tract infections, poor maternal nutrition with a low body mass index (<19.8 kg/m^2), and cigarette smoking.

- Vaginal fluid evaluated by L/S ratio, S/A ratio (TDx-FLM II assay), PG determination, and LB reliably predict the presence of fetal pulmonary maturity after preterm PROM.

- Conservative management of the pregnancy complicated by preterm PROM with documented fetal pulmonary maturity near term (32 to 36 weeks) prolongs latency only briefly but increases the risk of perinatal infection and does not improve neonatal outcomes.

- Antenatal corticosteroid administration and limited duration broad-spectrum antibiotic administration, given during conservative management of PROM remote from term, have been shown to reduce neonatal infectious and gestational age–dependent morbidity.

- Cervical cerclage retention after preterm PROM has not been shown to improve neonatal outcomes.

- Lethal pulmonary hypoplasia is common after PROM occurring before 20 weeks and can be predicted with serial ultrasound assessment of lung/chest growth.

REFERENCES

1. Meis PJ, Ernest JM, Moore ML: Causes of low birth weight births in public and private patients. Am J Obstet Gynecol 156:1165, 1987.
2. Tucker JM, Goldenberg RL, Davis RO, et al: Etiologies of preterm birth in an indigent population: is prevention a logical expectation? Obstet Gynecol 77:343, 1991.
3. Robertson PA, Sniderman SH, Laros RK Jr, et al: Neonatal morbidity according to gestational age and birth weight from five tertiary care centers in the United States, 1983 through 1986. Am J Obstet Gynecol 166:1629, 1992.
4. Ventura SJ, Martin JA, Taffel SM, et al: Advance report of final natality statistics, 1993. Monthly vital statistics report from the Centers for disease control and prevention 44:1, 1995.
5. Taylor J, Garite T: Premature rupture of the membranes before fetal viability. Obstet Gynecol 64:615, 1984.
6. Mercer BM: Management of premature rupture of membranes before 26 weeks' gestation. Obstet Gynecol Clin North Am 19:339, 1992.
7. Kitzmiller J: Preterm premature rupture of the membranes. *In* Fuchs F, Stubblefield PG (eds): Preterm Birth Causes, Prevention and Management. New York, Macmillan, 1984, p 298.
8. Lei H, Kalluri R, Furth EE, et al: Amnion type IV collagen composition and metabolism: implications for membrane breakdown. Biol Reprod 60:176, 1999.
9. Lei H, Furth EE, Kalluri R, et al: A program of cell death and extracellular matrix degradation is activated in the amnion before the onset of labor. J Clin Invest 98:1971, 1997.

10. Skinner SJM, Campos GA, Liggins GC: Collagen content of human amniotic membranes: Effect of gestation length and premature rupture. Obstet Gynecol 57:487, 1981.
11. Malak TM, Bell SC: Structural characteristic of term human fetal membranes: a novel zone of extreme morphological alteration within the rupture site. Br J Obstet Gynecol 101:375, 1994.
12. El Khwad M, Stetzer B, Moore RM, et al: Term human fetal membranes have a weak zone overlying the lower uterine pole and cervix before the onset of labor. Biol Reprod 72:720, 2005.
13. McLaren J, Taylor DJ, Bell, SC: Increased incidence of apoptosis in non-labor affected cytotrophoblast cells in term fetal membranes overlying the cervix. Hum Reprod 14:2:895, 1999.
14. McParland PC, Taylor DJ, Bell SC: Mapping of zones of altered morphology and choriodeciduaic connective tissue cellular phenotype in human fetal membranes (amnion and deciduas) overlying the lower uterine pole and cervix before labor at term. Am J Obstet Gynecol 189:1481, 2003.
15. McLaren J, Taylor DJ, Bell SC: Increased concentration of pro-matrix metalloproteinase 9 in term fetal membranes overlying the cervix before labor: implications for membrane remodeling and rupture. Am J Obstet Gynecol 182:409, 2000.
16. Athayde N, Edwin SS, Romero R, et al: A role for matrix metalloproteinase-9 in spontaneous rupture of the fetal membranes. Am J Obstet Gynecol 179:1248, 1998.
17. Parry S, Strauss JF: Premature rupture of the fetal membranes. N Engl J Med 338:663, 1998.
18. Lavery JP, Miller CE, Knight RD: The effect of labor on the rheologic response of chorioamniotic membranes. Obstet Gynecol 60:87, 1982.
19. Minkoff H, Grunebaum AN, Schwarz RH, et al: Risk factors for prematurity and premature rupture of membranes: A prospective study of the vaginal flora in pregnancy. Am J Obstet Gynecol 150:965, 1984.
20. Naeye R: Factors that predispose to premature rupture of the fetal membranes. Obstet Gynecol 60:93, 1982.
21. Meis PJ, Ernest JM, Moore ML: Causes of low birth-weight births in public and private patients. Am J Obstet Gynecol 156:1165, 1987.
22. Maradny EE, Kanayama N, Halim A, et al: Stretching of fetal membranes increases the concentration of interleukin-8 and collagenase activity. Am J Obstet Gynecol 174:843, 1996.
23. Ekwo EE, Gosselink CA, Moawad A: Unfavorable outcome in penultimate pregnancy and premature rupture of membranes in successive pregnancy. Obstet Gynecol 80:166, 1982.
24. Harger JH, Hsing AW, Tuomala RE, et al: Risk factors for preterm premature rupture of fetal membranes: A multicenter case-control study. Am J Obstet Gynecol 163:130, 1990.
25. Naeye RL, Peters EC: Causes and consequences of premature rupture of the fetal membranes. Lancet 1:192, 1980.
26. Charles D, Edwards WB: Infectious complications of cervical cerclage. Am J Obstet Gynecol 141:1065, 1981.
27. Gold RB, Goyer GL, Schwartz DB, et al: Conservative management of second trimester post-amniocentesis fluid leakage. Obstet Gynecol 74:745, 1989.
28. Hadley CB, Main DM, Gabbe SG: Risk factors for preterm premature rupture of the fetal membranes. Am J Perinatol 7:374, 1990.
29. Mercer B, Arheart K: Antimicrobial therapy in expectant management of preterm premature rupture of the membranes. Lancet 346:1271, 1995.
30. Romero R, Mazor M, Wu YK, et al: Infection in the pathogenesis of preterm labor. Semin Perinatol 12:262, 1988.
31. Heddleston L, McDuffie RS Jr, Gibbs RS: A rabbit model for ascending infection in pregnancy: intervention with indomethacin and delayed ampicillin-sulbactam therapy. Am J Obstet Gynecol 169:708, 1993.
32. McDonald HM, O'Loughlin JA, Jolley PT, et al: Changes in vaginal flora during pregnancy and association with preterm birth. J Infect Dis 170:724, 1994.
33. Regan JA, Chao S, James LS: Premature rupture of membranes, preterm delivery, and group B streptococcal colonization of mothers. Am J Obstet Gynecol 141:184, 1981.
34. Alger LS, Lovchik JC, Hebel JR, et al: The association of *Chlamydia trachomatis, Neisseria gonorrhoeae,* and group B streptococci with preterm rupture of the membranes and pregnancy outcome. Am J Obstet Gynecol 159:397, 1988.
35. Ekwo EE, Gosselink CA, Woolson R, Moawad A: Risks for premature rupture of amniotic membranes. Int J Epidemiol 22:495, 1993.
36. McGregor JA, French JI, Parker R, et al: Prevention of premature birth by screening and treatment for common genital tract infections: results of a prospective controlled evaluation. Am J Obstet Gynecol 173:157, 1995.
37. McGregor JA, Schoonmaker JN, Lunt BD, Lawellin DW: Antibiotic inhibition of bacterially induced fetal membrane weakening. Obstet Gynecol 76:124, 1990.
38. Romero R, Mazor M, Oyarzun E, et al: Is there an association between colonization with group B Streptococcus and prematurity? J Reprod Med 34:797, 1989.
39. Mercer BM, Goldenberg RL, Meis PJ, et al and the NICHD-MFMU Network: The preterm prediction study: Prediction of preterm premature rupture of the membranes using clinical findings and ancillary testing. Am J Obstet Gynecol 183:738, 2000.
40. Regan JA, Klebanoff MA, Nugent RP, et al: Colonization with group B streptococci in pregnancy and adverse outcome. VIP Study Group. Am J Obstet Gynecol 174:1354, 1996.
41. Romero R, Chaiworapongsa T, Kuivaniemi H, Tromp G. Bacterial vaginosis, the inflammatory response and the risk of preterm birth: a role for genetic epidemiology in the prevention of preterm birth. Am J Obstet Gynecol 190:1509, 2004.
42. American College of Obstetricians and Gynecologists: ACOG Practice Bulletin. Assessment of risk factors for preterm birth. Clinical management guidelines for obstetrician-gynecologists. Obstet Gynecol 98:709. 2001.
43. Hillier SL, Nugent RP, Eschenbach DA, et al: Association between bacterial vaginosis and preterm delivery of a low-birth-weight infant. The Vaginal Infections and Prematurity Study Group. N Engl J Med 333:1737, 1995.
44. Garite TJ, Freeman RK, Linzey EM, Braly P: The use of amniocentesis in patients with premature rupture of membranes. Obstet Gynecol 54:226, 1979.
45. Cotton DB, Gonik B, Bottoms SF: Conservative vs. aggressive management of preterm rupture of membranes. A randomized trial of amniocentesis. Am J Perinatol 1:322, 1984.
46. Fisk NM: A dipstick test for infection in preterm premature rupture of the membranes. J Perinat Med 15:565, 1987.
47. Romero R, Quintero R, Oyarzun E, et al: Intraamniotic infection and the onset of labor in preterm premature rupture of the membranes. Am J Obstet Gynecol 159:661, 1988.
48. Broekhuizen FF, Gilman M, Hamilton PR: Amniocentesis for gram stain and culture in preterm premature rupture of the membranes. Obstet Gynecol 66:316, 1985.
49. Dudley J, Malcolm G, Ellwood D: Amniocentesis in the management of preterm premature rupture of the membranes. Aust N Z J Obstet Gynaecol 31:331, 1991.
50. Gauthier DW, Meyer WJ: Comparison of gram stain, leukocyte esterase activity, and amniotic fluid glucose concentration in predicting amniotic fluid culture results in preterm premature rupture of membranes. Am J Obstet Gynecol 167:1092, 1992.
51. Mercer BM, Moretti ML, Prevost RR, Sibai BM: Erythromycin therapy in preterm premature rupture of the membranes: a prospective, randomized trial of 220 patients. Am J Obstet Gynecol 166:794, 1992.
52. Carroll SG, Papaioannou S, Davies ET, Nicolaides KH: Maternal assessment in the prediction of intrauterine infection in preterm prelabor amniorrhexis. Fetal Diagn Ther 10:290, 1995.
53. Millar LK, Boesche MH, Yamamoto SY, et al: A relaxin mediated pathway to preterm premature rupture of the fetal membranes that is independent of infection. Am J Obstet Gynecol 179:126, 1998.
54. Roberts AK, Monzon-Bordonaba F, Van Deerlin PG, et al: Association of polymorphism within the promoter of the tumor necrosis factor α gene with increased risk of preterm premature rupture of the fetal membranes. Am J Obstet Gynecol 180:1297, 1999.
55. Fujimoto T, Parry S, Urbanek M, et al: A single nucleotide polymorphism in the matrix metalloproteinase-1 (MMP-1) promoter influences amnion cell MMP-1 expression and risk for preterm premature rupture of the fetal membranes. J Biol Chem 277:6296, 2002.
56. Ferrand PE, Parry S, Sammel M, et al: A polymorphism in the matrix metalloproteinase-9 promoter is associated with increased

risk of preterm premature rupture of membranes in African Americans. Mol Hum Reprod 8:494, 2002.
57. Macones GA, Parry S, Elkousy M, et al: A polymorphism in the promoter region of TNF and bacterial vaginosis: preliminary evidence of gene-environment interaction in the etiology of spontaneous preterm birth. Am J Obstet Gynecol 190:1504, 2004.
58. Mercer BM, Goldenberg RL, Moawad AH, et al for the NICHD MFM Network: The preterm prediction study: Effect of gestational age and cause of preterm birth on subsequent obstetric outcome. Am J Obstet Gynecol 181:1216, 1999.
59. Meis PJ, Klebanoff M, Thom E, et al and the National Institute of Child Health and Human Development Maternal-Fetal Medicine Units Network: Prevention of recurrent preterm delivery by 17 alpha-hydroxyprogesterone caproate. N Engl J Med 348:2379, 2003.
60. da Fonseca EB, Bittar RE, Carvalho MH, Zugaib M: Prophylactic administration of progesterone by vaginal suppository to reduce the incidence of spontaneous preterm birth in women at increased risk: a randomized placebo-controlled double-blind study. Am J Obstet Gynecol 188:419, 2003.
61. Hannah ME, Ohlsson A, Farine D, et al: Induction of labor compared with expectant management for prelabor rupture of membranes at term. N Engl J Med 334:1005, 1996.
62. Dale PO, Tanbo T, Bendvold E, Moe N: Duration of the latency period in preterm premature rupture of the membranes. Eur J Obstet Gynecol Reprod Biol 30:257, 1989.
63. Johnson JWC, Egerman RS, Moorhead J: Cases with ruptured membranes that "reseal." Am J Obstet Gynecol 163:1024, 1990.
64. Hillier SL, Martius J, Krohn M, et al: A case-control study of chorioamnionic infection and histologic chorioamnionitis in prematurity. N Engl J Med 319:972, 1988.
65. Morales WJ: The effect of chorioamnionitis on the developmental outcome of preterm infants at one year. Obstet Gynecol 70:183, 1987.
66. Gunn GC, Mishell DR, Morton DG: Premature rupture of the fetal membranes: A review. Am J Obstet Gynecol 106:469, 1970.
67. Garite TJ, Freeman RK: Chorioamnionitis in the preterm gestation. Obstet Gynecol 59:539, 1982.
68. Simpson GF, Harbert GM Jr: Use of β-methasone in management of preterm gestation with premature rupture of membranes. Obstet Gynecol 66:168, 1985.
69. Gonen R, Hannah ME, Milligan JE: Does prolonged preterm premature rupture of the membranes predispose to abruptio placentae? Obstet Gynecol 74:347, 1989.
70. Vintzileos AM, Campbell WA, Nochimson DJ, Weinbaum PJ: Preterm premature rupture of the membranes: a risk factor for the development of abruptio placentae. Am J Obstet Gynecol 156:1235, 1987.
71. Schucker JL, Mercer BM: Midtrimester premature rupture of the membranes. Semin Perinatol 20:389, 1996.
72. Moberg LJ, Garite TJ, Freeman RK: Fetal heart rate patterns and fetal distress in patients with preterm premature rupture of membranes. Obstet Gynecol 64:60, 1984.
73. Mercer BM: Preterm premature rupture of the membranes. Obstet Gynecol 101:178, 2003.
74. Stevenson DK, Wright LL, Lemons JA, et al: Very low birth weight outcomes of the National Institute of Child Health and Human Development Neonatal Research Network, January 1993 through December 1994. Am J Obstet Gynecol 179:1632, 1998.
75. Wu YW, Colford JM Jr: Chorioamnionitis as a risk factor for cerebral palsy: A meta-analysis. JAMA 284:1417, 2000.
76. Yoon BH, Jun JK, Romero R, et al: Amniotic fluid inflammatory cytokines (interleukin-6, interleukin 1b, and tumor necrosis factor-α), neonatal brain white matter lesions, and cerebral palsy. Am J Obstet Gynecol 177:19, 1997.
77. Yoon BH, Romero R, Kim CJ, et al: High expression of tumor necrosis factor-alpha and interleukin-6 in periventricular leukomalacia. Am J Obstet Gynecol 177:406, 1997.
78. Yoon BH, Romero R, Yang SH, et al: Interleukin-6 concentrations in umbilical cord plasma are elevated in neonates with white matter lesions associated with periventricular leukomalacia. Am J Obstet Gynecol 174:1433, 1996.
79. Vergani P, Ghidini A, Locatelli A, et al: Risk factors for pulmonary hypoplasia in second-trimester premature rupture of membranes. Am J Obstet Gynecol 170:1359, 1994.
80. Rotschild A, Ling EW, Puterman ML, Farquharson D: Neonatal outcome after prolonged preterm rupture of the membranes. Am J Obstet Gynecol 162:46, 1990.
81. Hibbard JU, Hibbard MC, Ismail M, Arendt E: Pregnancy outcome after expectant management of premature rupture of the membranes in the second trimester. J Reprod Med 38:945, 1993.
82. Beydoun S, Yasin S: Premature rupture of the membranes before 28 weeks: Conservative management. Obstet Gynecol 155:471, 1986.
83. Moretti M, Sibai B: Maternal and perinatal outcome of expectant management of premature rupture of the membranes in midtrimester. Am J Obstet Gynecol 159:390, 1988.
84. Rib DM, Sherer DM, Woods JR: Maternal and neonatal outcome associated with prolonged premature rupture of membranes below 26 weeks' gestation. Am J Perinatol 10:369, 1993.
85. Lauria MR, Gonik B, Romero R: Pulmonary hypoplasia: pathogenesis, diagnosis, and antenatal prediction. Obstet Gynecol 86:466, 1995.
86. Nakayama DK, Glick PL, Harrison ML, et al: Experimental pulmonary hypoplasia due to Oligohydramnios and its reversal by relieving thoracic compression. J Pediatr Surg 18:347, 1983.
87. Adzick NS, Harrison MR, Glick PL, et al: Experimental pulmonary hypoplasia and Oligohydramnios: Relative contributions of lung fluid and fetal breathing movements. J Pediatr Surg 19:658, 1984.
88. Harding R, Hooper SB, Dickson KA: A mechanism leading to reduced lung expansion and lung hypoplasia in fetal sheep during Oligohydramnios. Am J Obstet Gynecol 163:1904, 1990.
89. Askenazi SS, Perlman M: Pulmonary hypoplasia; lung weight and radial alveolar count as criteria of diagnosis. Arch Dis Child 54:614, 1979.
90. Wigglesworth JS, Desai R: Use of DNA estimation for growth assessment in normal and hypoplastic fetal lungs. Arch Dis Child 56:601, 1981.
91. Carroll SG, Blott M, Nicolaides KH: Preterm prelabor amniorrhexis: Outcome of live births. Obstet Gynecol 86:18, 1995.
92. Moessinger AC, Collins MH, Blanc WA, et al: Oligohydramnios-induced lung hypoplasia: The influence of timing and duration in gestation. Pediatr Res 20:951, 1986.
93. Rizzo G, Capponi A, Angelini E, et al: Blood flow velocity waveforms from fetal peripheral pulmonary arteries in pregnancies with preterm premature rupture of the membranes: relationship with pulmonary hypoplasia. Ultrasound Obstet Gynecol 15:98, 2000.
94. Nimrod C, Varela-Gittings F, Machin G, et al: The effect of very prolonged membrane rupture on fetal development. Am J Obstet Gynecol 148:540, 1984.
95. Dowd J, Permezel M: Pregnancy outcome following preterm premature rupture of the membranes at less than 26 weeks' gestation. Aust N Z J Obstet Gynaecol 32:120, 1992.
96. Hadi HA, Hodson CA, Strickland D: Premature rupture of the membranes between 20 and 25 weeks' gestation: role of amniotic fluid volume in perinatal outcome. Am J Obstet Gynecol 170:1139, 1994.
97. Blott M, Greenough A: Neonatal outcome after prolonged rupture of the membranes starting in the second trimester. Arch Dis Child 63:1146, 1988.
98. Reece EA, Chervenak FA, Moya FR, Hobbins JC: Amniotic fluid arborization: Effect of blood, meconium, and pH alterations. Obstet Gynecol 64:248, 1984.
99. Rosemond RL, Lombardi SJ, Boehm FH: Ferning of amniotic fluid contaminated with blood. Obstet Gynecol 75:338, 1990.
100. Bottoms SF, Welch RA, Zador IE, Sokol RJ: Clinical interpretation of ultrasound measurements in preterm pregnancies with premature rupture of the membranes. Obstet Gynecol 69:358, 1987.
101. Schutte MF, Treffers PE, Kloosterman GJ, Soepatmi S: Management of premature rupture of membranes: The risk of vaginal examination to the infant. Am J Obstet Gynecol 146:395, 1983.
102. Lewis DF, Major CA, Towers CV, et al: Effects of digital vaginal examinations on latency period in preterm premature rupture of membranes. Obstet Gynecol 80:630, 1992.

103. Alexander JM, Mercer BM, Miodovnik M, et al: The impact of digital cervical examination on expectantly managed preterm rupture of membranes. Am J Obstet Gynecol 183:1003, 2000.
104. Brown CL, Ludwiczak MH, Blanco JD, Hirsch CE: Cervical dilation: Accuracy of visual and digital examinations. Obstet Gynecol 81:215, 1993.
105. Sbarra AJ, Blake G, Cetrulo CL, et al: The effect of cervical/vaginal secretions on measurements of lecithin/sphingomyelin ratio and optical density at 650 nm. Am J Obstet Gynecol 139:214, 1981.
106. Shaver DC, Spinnato JA, Whybrew D, et al: Comparison of phospholipids in vaginal and amniocentesis specimens of patients with premature rupture of membranes. Am J Obstet Gynecol 156:454, 1987.
107. Phillippe M, Acker D, Torday J, et al: The effects of vaginal contamination on two pulmonary phospholipid assays. J Reprod Med 27:283, 1982.
108. Lewis DF, Towers CV, Major CA, et al: Use of Amniostat-FLM in detecting the presence of phosphatidylglycerol in vaginal pool samples in preterm premature rupture of membranes. Am J Obstet Gynecol 169:573, 1993.
109. Estol PC, Poseiro JJ, Schwarcz R: Phosphatidylglycerol determination in the amniotic fluid from a PAD placed over the vulva: a method for diagnosis of fetal lung maturity in cases of premature ruptured membranes. J Perinat Med 20:65, 1992.
110. Russell JC, Cooper CM, Ketchum CH, et al: Multicenter evaluation of TDx test for assessing fetal lung maturity. Clin Chem 35:1005, 1989.
111. Edwards RK, Duff P, Ross KC: Amniotic fluid indices of fetal pulmonary maturity with preterm premature rupture of membranes. Obstet Gynecol 96:102, 2000.
112. Pastorek JG 2nd, Letellier RL, Gebbia K: Production of a phosphatidylglycerol-like substance by genital flora bacteria. Am J Obstet Gynecol 159:199, 1988.
113. Schumacher RE, Parisi VM, Steady HM, Tsao FH: Bacteria causing false positive test for phosphatidylglycerol in amniotic fluid. Am J Obstet Gynecol 151:1067, 1985.
114. Golde SH: Use of obstetric perineal pads in collection of amniotic fluid in patients with rupture of the membranes. Am J Obstet Gynecol 146:710, 1983.
115. Buhi WC, Spellacy WN: Effects of blood or meconium on the determination of the amniotic fluid lecithin/sphingomyelin ratio. Am J Obstet Gynecol 121:321, 1975.
116. Cotton DB, Spillman T, Bretaudiere JP: Effect of blood contamination on lecithin to sphingomyelin ratio in amniotic fluid by different detection methods. Clin Chim Acta 137:299, 1984.
117. Carlan SJ, Gearity D, O'Brien WF: The effect of maternal blood contamination on the TDx-FLM II assay. Am J Perinatol 14:491, 1997.
118. Ashwood ER, Palmer SE, Taylor JS, Pingree SS: Lamellar body counts for rapid fetal lung maturity testing. Obstet Gynecol 81:619, 1993.
119. Tabsh KM, Brinkman CR 3rd, Bashore R: Effect of meconium contamination on amniotic fluid lecithin: sphingomyelin ratio. Obstet Gynecol 58:605, 1981.
120. American College of Obstetricians and Gynecologists: ACOG Committee Opinion: number 279, December 2002. Prevention of early-onset group B streptococcal disease in newborns. Obstet Gynecol 100:1405, 2002.
121. American Academy of Pediatrics (Committee on Infectious Diseases and Committee on Fetus and Newborn of the American Academy of Pediatrics): Guidelines for the prevention of group B streptococcal (GBS) infection by chemoprophylaxis. Pediatrics 90:775, 1992.
122. Gibbs RS, Schrag S, Schuchat A: Perinatal infections due to group B streptococci. Obstet Gynecol 104:1062, 2004.
123. Mercer BM, Carr TL, Beazley DD, et al: Antibiotic use in pregnancy and drug-resistant infant sepsis. Am J Obstet Gynecol 181:816, 1999.
124. Stoll BJ, Hansen N, Fanaroff AA, et al: Changes in pathogens causing early-onset sepsis in very-low-birth-weight infants. N Engl J Med 347:240, 2002.
125. Towers CV, Carr MH, Padilla G, Asrat T: Potential consequences of widespread antepartal use of ampicillin. Am J Obstet Gynecol 179:879, 1998.
126. Duff P, Huff RW, Gibbs RS: Management of premature rupture of membranes and unfavorable cervix in term pregnancy. Obstet Gynecol 63:697, 1984.
127. Fayez JA, Hasan AA, Jonas HS, Miller GL: Management of premature rupture of the membranes. Obstet Gynecol 52:17, 1978.
128. Morales WJ, Lazar AJ: Expectant management of rupture of membranes at term. South Med J 79:955, 1986.
129. Van der Walt D, Venter PF: Management of term pregnancy with premature rupture of the membranes and unfavourable cervix. S Afr Med J 75:54, 1989.
130. Grant JM, Serle E, Mahmood T, et al: Management of prelabour rupture of the membranes in term primigravidae: report of a randomized prospective trial. Br J Obstet Gynaecol 99:557, 1992.
131. Ladfors L, Mattsson LA, Eriksson M, Fall O: A randomised trial of two expectant managements of prelabour rupture of the membranes at 34 to 42 weeks. Br J Obstet Gynaecol 103:755, 1996.
132. Shalev E, Peleg D, Eliyahu S, Nahum Z: Comparison of 12- and 72-hour expectant management of premature rupture of membranes in term pregnancies. Obstet Gynecol 85:1, 1995.
133. Tan BP, Hannah ME: Prostaglandins vs. oxytocin for prelabour rupture of membranes at term. The Cochrane Database of Systematic Reviews 2, 2005.
134. Strong TH Jr, Hetzler G, Sarno AP, Paul RH: Prophylactic intrapartum amnioinfusion: A randomized clinical trial. Am J Obstet Gynecol 162:1370, 1990.
135. Schrimmer DB, Macri CJ, Paul RH: Prophylactic amnioinfusion as a treatment for oligohydramnios in laboring patients: A prospective randomized trial. Am J Obstet Gynecol 165:972, 1991.
136. Naef RW 3rd, Allbert JR, Ross EL, et al: Premature rupture of membranes at 34 to 37 weeks' gestation: Aggressive vs. conservative management. Am J Obstet Gynecol 178:126, 1998.
137. Neerhof MG, Cravello C, Haney EI, Silver RK: Timing of labor induction after premature rupture of membranes between 32 and 36 weeks gestation. Am J Obstet Gynecol 180:349, 1999.
138. Cox SM, Leveno KJ: Intentional delivery vs. expectant management with preterm ruptured membranes at 30–34 weeks' gestation. Obstet Gynecol 86:875, 1995.
139. Mercer BM, Crocker L, Boe N, Sibai B: Induction vs. expectant management in PROM with mature amniotic fluid at 32–36 weeks: A randomized trial. Am J Obstet Gynecol 82:775, 1993.
140. Mercer BM in response to Repke JT, Berck DJ: Preterm premature rupture of membranes: a continuing dilemma. Am J Obstet Gynecol 170:1835, 1994.
141. Kovacevich GJ, Gaich SA, Lavin JP, et al: The prevalence of thromboembolic events among women with extended bed rest prescribed as part of the treatment for premature labor or preterm premature rupture of membranes. Am J Obstet Gynecol 182:1089, 2000.
142. Asrat T, Nageotte MP, Garite SE, Dorchester W: Gram stain results from amniocentesis in patients with preterm premature rupture of the membranes–comparison of maternal and fetal characteristics. Am J Obstet Gynecol 163:887, 1990.
143. Hanley ML, Vintzeleos AM: Biophysical testing in premature rupture of the membranes. Semin Perinatol 20:418, 1996.
144. Lewis DF, Adair CD, Weeks JW, et al: A randomized clinical trial of daily nonstress testing vs biophysical profile in the management of preterm premature rupture of membranes. Am J Obstet Gynecol 181:1495, 1999.
145. Romero R, Yoon BH, Mazor M, et al: A comparative study of the diagnostic performance of amniotic fluid glucose, white blood cell count, interleukin-6, and Gram stain in the detection of microbial invasion in patients with preterm premature rupture of membranes. Am J Obstet Gynecol 169:839, 1993.
146. Belady PH, Farhouh LJ, Gibbs RS: Intra-amniotic infection and premature rupture of the membranes. Clin Perinatol 24:43, 1997.
147. Sperling RS, Ramamurthy RS, Gibbs RS: A comparison of intrapartum vs. immediate postpartum treatment of intraamniotic infection. Obstet Gynecol 70:861, 1987.
148. Gibbs RS, Dinsmoor MJ, Newton ER, Ramamurthy RS: A randomized trial of intrapartum vs. immediate postpartum treatment of women with intra-amniotic infection. Obstet Gynecol 72:823, 1988.

149. Gilstrap LC 3rd, Leveno KJ, Cox SM, et al: Intrapartum treatment of acute chorioamnionitis: Impact on neonatal sepsis. Am J Obstet Gynecol 159:579, 1988.
150. Mercer B, Miodovnik M, Thurnau G, et al, and the NICHD-MFMU Network: Antibiotic therapy for reduction of infant morbidity after preterm premature rupture of the membranes: a randomized controlled trial. JAMA 278:989, 1997.
151. Harding JE, Pang J, Knight DB, Liggins GC: Do antenatal corticosteroids help in the setting of preterm rupture of membranes? Am J Obstet Gynecol 184:131, 2001.
152. Lewis DF, Brody K, Edwards MS, et al: Preterm premature ruptured membranes: A randomized trial of steroids after treatment with antibiotics. Obstet Gynecol 88:801, 1996.
153. Pattinson RC, Makin JD, Funk M, et al: The use of dexamethasone in women with preterm premature rupture of membranes—a multicentre, double-blind, placebo-controlled, randomised trial. Dexiprom Study Group. S Afr Med J 89:865, 1999.
154. Lovett SM, Weiss JD, Diogo MJ, et al: A prospective, double blind randomized, controlled clinical trial of ampicillin-sulbactam for preterm premature rupture of membranes in women receiving antenatal corticosteroid therapy. Am J Obstet Gynecol 176:1030, 1997.
155. Vermillion ST, Soper DE, Chasedunn-Roark J: Neonatal sepsis after betamethasone administration to patients with preterm premature rupture of membranes. Am J Obstet Gynecol 181:320, 1999.
156. Ghidini A, Salafia CM, Minior VK: Repeated courses of steroids in preterm membrane rupture do not increase the risk of histologic chorioamnionitis. Am J Perinatol 14:309, 1997.
157. Abbasi S, Hirsch D, Davis J, et al: Effect of single vs. multiple courses of antenatal corticosteroids on maternal and neonatal outcome. Am J Obstet Gynecol 182:1243, 2000.
158. Egarter C, Leitich H, Karas H, et al: Antibiotic treatment in premature rupture of membranes and neonatal morbidity: A meta-analysis. Am J Obstet Gynecol 174:589, 1996.
159. Kenyon S, Boulvain M, Neilson J: Antibiotics for preterm rupture of membranes. Cochrane Database Syst Rev CD001058, 2003.
160. Mercer BM, Goldenberg RL, Das AF, et al, and National Institute of Child Health and Human Development Maternal-Fetal Medicine Units Network: What we have learned regarding antibiotic therapy for the reduction of infant morbidity. Semin Perinatol 27:217, 2003.
161. Kenyon SL, Taylor DJ, Tarnow-Mordi W, and Oracle Collaborative Group: Broad spectrum antibiotics for preterm, prelabor rupture of fetal membranes: the ORACLE I Randomized trial. Lancet 357:979, 2001.
162. Lewis DF, Adair CD, Robichaux AG, et al: Antibiotic therapy in preterm premature rupture of membranes: Are seven days necessary? A preliminary, randomized clinical trial. Am J Obstet Gynecol 188:1413; discussion 1416, 2003.
163. Segel SY, Miles AM, Clothier B, et al: Duration of antibiotic therapy after preterm premature rupture of fetal membranes. Am J Obstet Gynecol 189:799, 2003.
164. Christensen KK, Ingemarsson I, Leideman T, et al: Effect of ritodrine on labor after premature rupture of the membranes. Obstet Gynecol 55:187, 1980.
165. Levy DL, Warsof SL: Oral Ritodrine and preterm premature rupture of membranes. Obstet Gynecol 66:621, 1985.
166. Weiner CP, Renk K, Klugman M: The therapeutic efficacy and cost-effectiveness of aggressive tocolysis for premature labor associated with premature rupture of the membranes. Am J Obstet Gynecol 159:216, 1988.
167. Garite TJ, Keegan KA, Freeman RK, Nageotte MP: A randomized trial of ritodrine tocolysis vs. expectant management in patients with premature rupture of membranes at 25 to 30 weeks of gestation. Am J Obstet Gynecol 157:388, 1987.
168. How HY, Cook CR, Cook VD, et al: Preterm premature rupture of membranes: aggressive tocolysis vs. expectant management. J Matern Fetal Med 7:8, 1998.
169. Curet LB, Rao AV, Zachman RD, et al: Association between ruptured membranes, tocolytic therapy, and respiratory distress syndrome. Am J Obstet Gynecol 148:263, 1984.
170. Treadwell MC, Bronsteen RA, Bottoms SF: Prognostic factors and complication rates for cervical cerclage: A review of 482 cases. Am J Obstet Gynecol 165:555, 1991.
171. Harger JH: Comparison of success and morbidity in cervical cerclage procedures. Obstet Gynecol 56:543, 1990.
172. Blickstein I, Katz Z, Lancet M, Molgilner BM: The outcome of pregnancies complicated by preterm rupture of the membranes with and without cerclage. Int J Gynaecol Obstet 28:237, 1989.
173. Yeast JD, Garite TR: The role of cervical cerclage in the management of preterm premature rupture of the membranes. Am J Obstet Gynecol 158:106, 1988.
174. Ludmir J, Bader T, Chen L, et al: Poor perinatal outcome associated with retained cerclage in patients with premature rupture of membranes. Obstet Gynecol 84:823, 1994.
175. Jenkins TM, Berghella V, Shlossman PA, et al: Timing of cerclage removal after preterm premature rupture of membranes: maternal and neonatal outcomes. Am J Obstet Gynecol 183:847, 2000.
176. McElrath TF, Norwitz ER, Lieberman ES, Heffner LJ: Perinatal outcome after preterm premature rupture of membranes with in situ cervical cerclage. Am J Obstet Gynecol 187:1147, 2002.
177. Brown ZA, Vontver LA, Benedetti J, et al: Effects on infants of a first episode of genital herpes during pregnancy. N Engl J Med 317:1246, 1987.
178. Chuang T: Neonatal herpes: Incidence, prevention and consequences. Am J Prev Med 4:47, 1988.
179. Visintine AM, Nahmias AJ, Josey WE: Genital herpes. Perinatal Care 2:32, 1978.
180. Stagno S, Whitley RJ: Herpes virus infections of pregnancy part II: Herpes simplex virus and Varicella zoster infections. N Engl J Med 313:1327, 1985.
181. Amstey MS: Management of pregnancy complicated by genital herpes virus infection. Obstet Gynecol 37:515, 1971.
182. Nahmias AJ, Josey WE, Naib ZM, et al. Perinatal risk associated with maternal genital herpes simplex virus infection. Am J Obstet Gynecol 110:825, 1971.
183. Gibbs RS, Amstey MS, Lezotte DC: Role of cesarean delivery in preventing neonatal herpes virus infection. JAMA 270:94, 1993.
184. Major CA, Kitzmiller JL: Perinatal survival with expectant management of midtrimester rupture of membranes. Am J Obstet Gynecol 163:838, 1990.
185. Morales WJ, Talley T: Premature rupture of membranes at <25 weeks: a management dilemma. Am J Obstet Gynecol 168:503, 1993.
186. Taylor J, Garite TJ: Premature rupture of membranes before fetal viability. Obstet Gynecol 64:615, 1984.
187. Moretti M, Sibai BM: Maternal and perinatal outcome of expectant management of premature rupture of membranes in the midtrimester. Am J Obstet Gynecol 159:390, 1988.
188. Farooqi A, Holmgren PA, Engberg S, Serenius F: Survival and 2-year outcome with expectant management of second-trimester rupture of membranes. Obstet Gynecol 92:895, 1998.
189. Beydoun SN, Yasin SY: Premature rupture of the membranes before 28 weeks: conservative management. Am J Obstet Gynecol 155:471, 1986.
190. Robson MS, Turner MJ, Stronge JM, O'Herlihy C: Is amniotic fluid quantitation of value in the diagnosis and conservative management of prelabour membrane rupture at term? Br J Obstet Gynaecol 97:324, 1990.
191. Bengtson JM, VanMarter LJ, Barss VA, et al: Pregnancy outcome after premature rupture of the membranes at or before 26 weeks' gestation. Obstet Gynecol 73:921, 1989.
192. Rib DM, Sherer DM, Woods JR Jr: Maternal and neonatal outcome associated with prolonged premature rupture of membranes below 26 weeks' gestation. Am J Perinatol 10:369, 1993.
193. Shumway JB, Al-Malt A, Amon E, et al: Impact of oligohydramnios on maternal and perinatal outcomes of spontaneous premature rupture of the membranes at 18–28 weeks. J Matern Fetal Med 8:20, 1999.
194. Sciscione AC, Manley JS, Pollock M, et al: Intracervical fibrin sealants: a potential treatment for early preterm premature rupture of the membranes. Am J Obstet Gynecol 184:368, 2001.
195. Quintero RA, Morales WJ, Bornick PW, et al: Surgical treatment of spontaneous rupture of membranes: the amniograft–first experience. Am J Obstet Gynecol 186:155, 2002.
196. O'Brien JM, Barton JR, Milligan DA: An aggressive interventional protocol for early midtrimester premature rupture of the membranes using gelatin sponge for cervical plugging. Am J Obstet Gynecol 187:1143, 2002.

197. Laudy JA, Tibboel D, Robben SG, et al: Prenatal prediction of pulmonary hypoplasia: clinical, biometric, and Doppler velocity correlates. Pediatrics 109:250, 2002.
198. Yoshimura S, Masuzaki H, Gotoh H, et al: Ultrasonographic prediction of lethal pulmonary hypoplasia: comparison of eight different ultrasonographic parameters. Am J Obstet Gynecol 175:477, 1996.
199. D'Alton M, Mercer B, Riddick E, Dudley D: Serial thoracic vs. abdominal circumference ratios for the prediction of pulmonary hypoplasia in premature rupture of the membranes remote from term. Am J Obstet Gynecol 166:658, 1992.
200. Vintzileos AM, Campbell WA, Rodis JF, et al: Comparison of six different ultrasonographic methods for predicting lethal fetal pulmonary hypoplasia. Am J Obstet Gynecol 161:606, 1989.
201. van Eyck J, van der Mooren K, Wladimiroff JW: Ductus arteriosus flow velocity modulation by fetal breathing movements as a measure of fetal lung development. Am J Obstet Gynecol 163:558, 1990.
202. Blott M, Greenough A, Nicolaides KH, Campbell S: The ultrasonographic assessment of the fetal thorax and fetal breathing movements in the prediction of pulmonary hypoplasia. Early Hum Dev 21:143, 1990.

Multiple Gestations

JANE CLEARY-GOLDMAN, USHA CHITKARA, AND RICHARD L. BERKOWITZ

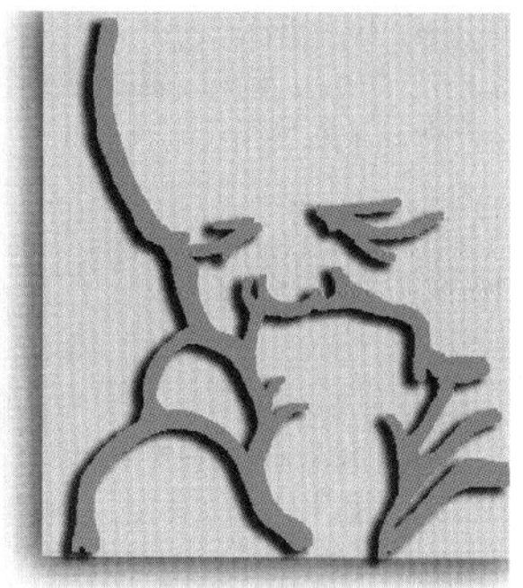

CHAPTER 28

KEY ABBREVIATIONS

Alpha-fetoprotein	AFP
Appropriate for gestational age	AGA
Arterioarterial	AA
Arteriovenous	AV
Assisted reproductive technology	ART
Beta-human chorionic gonadotropin	β-hCG
Biparietal diameter	BPD
Chorionic villus sampling	CVS
Crown-rump length	CRL
Dizygotic	DZ
Estimated fetal weight	EFW
Fetal fibronectin test	FFN
Head circumference	HC
Intrauterine fetal demise	IUFD
Intrauterine growth restriction	IUGR
In vitro fertilization	IVF
Monozygotic	MZ
Multiples of the median	MoM
Multifetal pregnancy reduction	MPR
Pregnancy-associated plasma protein-A	PAPP-A
Selective termination	ST
Small for gestational age	SGA
Systolic/diastolic	S/D
Twin-to-twin transfusion syndrome	TTTS
Twin reversed arterial perfusion	TRAP
Venovenous	VV

INTRODUCTION

The phenomenon of twinning has fascinated mankind throughout its recorded history. Twins have often been regarded as being inherently "different" from singletons, and societal responses to their birth have ranged from awe to fear. Researchers have been interested in exploiting their uniqueness in an attempt to separate the influences of genetic and environmental factors on both fetal and long-term development.[1] Obstetricians have long been aware that pregnancies complicated by twinning are by their very nature at higher risk than those of most singletons. Finally, parents and future siblings are often overjoyed or overwhelmed when they are told that twins are expected. They are virtually never neutral in their response.

Twins can be either monozygotic (MZ) or dizygotic (DZ). Zygosity refers to the genetic make-up of a pregnancy. In MZ twins, a single fertilized ovum splits into two distinct individuals after a variable number of divisions. Such twins are almost always genetically identical and, therefore of the same sex. On rare occasions, mutations can cause genetic discordance resulting in phenotypic and chromosomal dissimilarities between MZ twins. On the other hand, when two separate ova are fertilized, DZ twins result. These individuals are as genetically distinct as any other children born to the same couple. Sets of DZ twins may have the same or opposite gender. DZ half-siblings have been reported in which two ova were fertilized by different fathers, and it has been hypothesized that monovular dispermic fertilization may occur. These latter situations are very uncommon, however. In most cases, DZ twins are genetically dissimilar true siblings.

The frequency of MZ twins is fairly constant throughout the world at a rate of approximately 4 per 1,000 births. This rate does not seem to vary with maternal characteristics such as age or parity. DZ twinning, however, is associated with multiple ovulation, and its frequency varies between races and is affected by several identifiable factors including maternal age and parity.[1] In general, the frequency of DZ twins is low in Asians, intermediate in whites, and high in blacks. The Yorubas of western Nigeria have a frequency of 45 twins per 1,000 births, and about 90 percent are DZ.[2]

The different rates of DZ twinning may be due to racial or individual variations in pituitary gonadotropin production. Patients with fertility problems treated with clomiphene citrate or gonadotropins are well known to have a dose-dependent increase in multiple births when compared with patients who conceive without these agents.[3] Although DZ twins predominate in these patients, triplets and high-order multiples (pregnancies with greater than three fetuses) may also occur. The use of assisted reproductive technology (ART) such as in vitro fertilization (IVF) and embryo transfer has further increased the incidence of multiple pregnancies.[4] In the United States, since 1980, twin births have risen 65 percent and triplet and high-order multiple births have quadrupled.[5] In 2002, there were 31.1 twins per 1,000 live births and 184 triplets and high-order multiples per 100,000 live births.[5] This dramatic rise in multiple births is mainly attributed to the growing popularity of assisted conception as well as to the fact that many patients are delaying childbearing until they are of an older age. Nonetheless, although the twin birth rate continues to rise, the triplet and high-order multiple birth rate seems to have stabilized.[5] Refinements in assisted conception techniques and recommendations from the American Society for Reproductive Medicine limiting the number of embryos transferred during IVF cycles are probably affecting the incidence of triplets and high-order multiples.[5–7]

The cause of MZ twinning is unclear. Benirschke and Kim[8] state that it is an uncommon occurrence among other mammals. In two species of armadillo, however, polyembryony regularly follows implantation of a single blastocyst. Oxygen deprivation has been experimentally shown to enhance fission in fish embryos, and some teratogens have been associated with increased MZ twinning rates in laboratory animals. There is currently no satisfactory explanation for the fact that MZ twins occur in humans with such a constant frequency around the world. Although most multiples occurring after assisted conception result from implantation of multiple embryos, MZ twinning is also increased by ovulation induction and other ART methods.[9–13] Against a spontaneous rate of 0.4 percent in the general population, studies have reported that MZ twinning may be greater than 10 times higher in pregnancies conceived with fertility treatment.[10,13] One theory to explain these increased rates of MZ is that alterations in either the structure or physical properties of the zona pellucida surrounding the early embryo may be responsible for the increased tendency toward iatrogenic zygote splitting and resultant MZ twins. However, the exact etiology is unclear.[13]

PERINATAL MORBIDITY AND MORTALITY

Owing to advances in both maternal fetal medicine and neonatal care, a general decline in perinatal mortality has been reported over the past two decades from centers around the world for both singleton and multiple gestations. Nonetheless, complications secondary to prematurity, growth abnormalities, and monochorionicity continue to place the offspring of a multiple gestation at higher risk for perinatal morbidity and mortality than their singleton counterparts. Although perinatal mortality rates have decreased, the risk of prematurity in multifetal gestations has not changed significantly.[14] In 2002 in the United States, the mean age at delivery for twins was 35.3 weeks, 32.2 weeks for triplets, and 29.9 weeks for quadruplets as compared with 38.8 weeks for singletons.[5] Only 1.6 percent of singletons delivered before 32 weeks' gestation as compared with 11.9 percent of twins, 36.1 percent of triplets, and 59.9 percent of quadruplets. Although less than 1 percent of singletons deliver before 28 weeks' gestation, 5 percent of twins and 14 percent of triplets are born at that extremely early gestational age.[15,16] Offspring of multiple pregnancies weigh less than their singleton counterparts.[5] The mean birth weight for singletons is 3,332 g compared with 2,347 g for twins, 1,687 g for triplets, and 1,309 g for quadruplets.[5] Owing to the greater incidence of prematurity and low birth weight, the perinatal mortality rate for twins is greater than that of singletons. In a recent population database study that included more than 2.2 million Swedish births, the fetal and infant mortality rates for singletons was 4.1 and 5.0 per 1,000 births as compared with 12.0 and 16.0 per 1,000 births for twins.[17] In addition, same-sex twins had higher mortality rates than non–same-sex twins, suggesting that monochorionicity plays a role in the increased risk for perinatal mortality in multiple gestations. Recent National Vital Statistics data from the United States indicate that twins and triplets are approximately five and 12 times more likely to die by their first birthday than singletons.[18]

The literature on the perinatal outcome of triplets and high-order multiples is limited. Many studies report data that is not contemporary and thus does not reflect current improvements in neonatal care, including antenatal corticosteroid administration and surfactant therapy.[19] In addition, accurate knowledge regarding the outcome of high-order multiples remains limited because of the relatively small numbers in any reported series, especially for quadruplets and larger numbers. Many series present data on patients who were managed at several different centers and thus reflect the management of numerous physicians rather than one consistent perinatal and neonatal team.[16,20] Although perinatal outcomes have improved as a result of advances in neonatology, preterm delivery is still associated with significant morbidity and mortality. In pregnancies complicated by triplets and high-order multiples, premature delivery with its concomitant increase in perinatal morbidity and mortality is an important concern.[16,21] In a recent review of 100 triplet pregnancies that were managed at a single tertiary care center from 1992 to 1999, 42 percent delivered before 32 weeks' gestation and 14 percent delivered before 28 weeks.[16] The corrected perinatal mortality rate was 97/1,000 live births, which is a marked improvement when compared with earlier studies. One hundred percent of the infants born after 26 weeks' gestation survived, but neonatal morbidity was significant. Seventy-three percent of the 274 neonates were admitted to the neonatal intensive care unit. Respiratory distress syndrome complicated 21 percent of neonatal cases, chronic lung disease 4 percent, necrotizing enterocolitis 3 percent, and grade IV intraventricular hemorrhage less than 1 percent of cases. It is important to note that severe intraventricular hemorrhage, necrotizing enterocolitis, and retinopathy of prematurity was rarely diagnosed after 28 weeks' gestation, suggesting that long-term outcomes for the majority of triplet survivors should be favorable. In addition, triplet pregnancies with a monochorionic component are at increased risk for adverse outcomes compared to those that are trichorionic.[22]

The perinatal outcome data relating to quadruplets and greater is even more limited. Furthermore, these studies are often focused on those pregnancies that have reached viability, suggesting an artificially inflated view of the overall outcomes. Perinatal mortality rates ranging from 0 to 67 per 1,000 quadruplet births have been suggested in some series.[23,24] Recent data suggest that increasing maternal age may be associated with more favorable survival outcomes for the offspring of quadruplet and quintuplet pregnancies.[25] The precise reason for improved outcomes in these older patients is unclear.

Offspring of multiple pregnancies are also at increased risk for perinatal morbidity. Owing to prematurity and low birth weight, multiples comprise a disproportionate portion of neonatal intensive care admissions.[26] Neonates from multiple gestations are over-represented among preterm and low-birth-weight infants. Cerebral palsy also has been associated with multiple births.[27] Children from a multiple pregnancy have a four times higher risk of developing cerebral palsy compared with their singleton counterparts.[28] This risk is mostly related to the higher rates of prematurity.

Although the offspring of a multiple gestation may be born earlier than singletons, preterm twin and triplet neonates appear to have similar birth weight, morbidity, and mortality as gestational age-matched controls.[29–31] Garite et al.[32] reviewed neonatal records from 1997 to 2002 from a large prospectively recorded neonatal database. There were 12,302 twin, 2,155 triplet, and 36,931 singleton pregnancies included in the study. At all gestational ages until 29 weeks for triplets and 32 weeks for twins, average birth weights were similar for triplets, twins, and singletons. After 32 weeks, the differences between twin and singleton average birth weight were due to the weight of the smaller twin. At all weeks studied, the larger twins' mean weights were similar to that of singletons. Neonatal morbidities such as intraventricular hemorrhage, retinopathy of prematurity, and necrotizing enterocolitis were similar in the offspring of multiple gestations and singletons. Intrauterine growth restriction (IUGR) was associated with increased perinatal mortality at all gestational ages, whereas growth discordance alone was not. Prematurity and IUGR appear to contribute to the neonatal morbidity and mortality associated with multiple birth.

It is unclear if mode of conception has an impact on neonatal outcomes in patients carrying multiple fetuses. Several recent studies on assisted conception and perinatal outcomes have had conflicting results. Some have suggested that fertility treatment is associated with worse outcomes, whereas others have suggested that it improves outcomes, and still others have suggested that it has no effect.[33–35] Larger prospective studies taking into account confounding factors such as monochorionicity are needed before the influence of assisted conception on outcomes in multiples can be determined.

In addition, the increased incidence of multiple birth has an economic impact on society due to more frequent and longer maternal and neonatal hospital admissions.[36] For example, a review of 55 triplet pregnancies with 149 liveborn neonates delivered at a single tertiary care center from 1992 to 1996 found the mean charge for a triplet pregnancy was $190,000 (antepartum and neonatal care).[37] The majority of the increased costs were secondary to prolonged neonatal intensive care and were inversely proportional to gestational age at delivery. Other studies have looked at hospital expenditures in early childhood. These studies also found that multiple births were associated with increased inpatient costs, especially in the first year of life.[38]

DIAGNOSIS

Multiple gestations should be suspected whenever (1) the uterus seems to be larger than dates, (2) auscultation of more than one fetal heart is suspected, (3) the pregnancy has occurred following assisted conception, or (4) family history. Multiple gestations may also be diagnosed serendipitously at the time of ultrasound scanning, such as before a genetic amniocentesis or as a result of an elevated serum alpha-fetoprotein (AFP) level in mass-screening programs.

Separate gestational sacs with individual yolk sacs can be identified by ultrasound as early as 5 weeks from the first day of the last menstrual period.[39] However, approximately 15 percent of cases of multiple gestations may be missed between 5 and 6 weeks' gestation.[39] In general, the ultrasound diagnosis of multiple gestations within the first trimester is relatively straightforward. It is mandatory, however, to visualize separate fetuses. Retromembranous collections of blood or fluid or a prominent fetal yolk sac should not be confused with a twin gestation. Demonstration of the viability of each fetus at the time of the examination requires visualization of independent cardiac activity. Unfortunately, mistakes can be made regarding the number of fetuses present when scans are hastily interpreted. This is particularly true in the third trimester but may also occur in the first and second trimesters, especially when four or more fetuses are present.

It must be remembered that an ultrasound image, unlike a flat plate of the abdomen, does not provide a composite overview. The image displayed is only a tomographic slice through the area being studied. Therefore, it is possible to display two circular structures that may represent different fetal heads or, alternatively, the head and thorax of the same fetus in a tucked position. Misinterpretation in this setting has resulted in the incorrect diagnosis of twins when only one fetus was present. On the other hand, rapid and careless scanning may result in failure to detect a second fetus whose head is deeply engaged in the pelvis or pushed up under the mother's ribs. If a multiple gestation is suspected, the ultrasonologist must be compulsive in examining the entire uterine cavity. A scan should not be completed until the orientation of all the visualized fetal parts is understood.

An argument often used in support of universal ultrasound screening for all pregnant patients during the second trimester is that it would result in the early diagnosis of multiple pregnancies with almost 100 percent accuracy.[40] Persson and Kullander[41] reported the results of this type of screening program, which has been in effect at the Malmo General Hospital in Sweden since 1973. Originally, the program began with a single scan performed in the 30th week, but subsequently all patients were offered examinations at both 17 and 33 weeks. Between 1974 and 1982, 98 percent of 254 multiple gestations were detected by ultrasound screening. There were no false-positive diagnoses, but 2 percent of multiple gestations were missed on the first examination. These authors also reported a reduction in perinatal mortality from 107 per 1,000 to 34 per 1,000 when similar numbers of twins delivered between 1970 and 1974 were compared with those delivered from 1975 to 1982. Major morbidity (e.g., cerebral palsy, mental retardation, late motor development, and hearing defects) decreased from 9.6 to 3.6 percent, and the frequency of delivery before 38 weeks dropped from 34 to 15.8 percent. The marked improvement in these figures was obviously due to multiple factors, but early diagnosis was among them. Results of the Routine Antenatal Diagnostic Imaging with Ultrasound (RADIUS) study from the United States indicate a similar experience.[42] This study compared a group of low-risk pregnant patients who underwent routine ultrasound screening in the second and third trimesters of pregnancy with a control group who had an ultrasound examination only when medically indicated. The diagnosis of multiple gestations, when present, was made before 26 weeks" gestation in all patients who had the screening ultrasound examination. In contrast, 37 percent of multiple gestations were not identified in the control group until after 26 weeks' gestation, and in 13 percent, the diagnosis was not made until the delivery admission.

CHORIONICITY

Although zygosity refers to the genetic make-up of the twin pregnancy, chorionicity indicates the pregnancy's membrane composition (Fig. 28-1). Chorionicity is determined by the mechanism of fertilization and in MZ twins by the timing of embryo division. The vast majority of DZ twins have separate dichorionic diamniotic placentas, that is, each fetus has its own separate placenta and amniotic sac with a separate amnion and chorion. This is due to the fact that DZ twins result from the fertilization of two different ova by two separate sperm. Each blastocyst generates its own placenta. If implantation of these blastocysts is not proximal to each other, two separate placentas will result, each of which will have a chorion and an amnion. Should they implant side by side, intimate fusion of the placental disks occur, but these

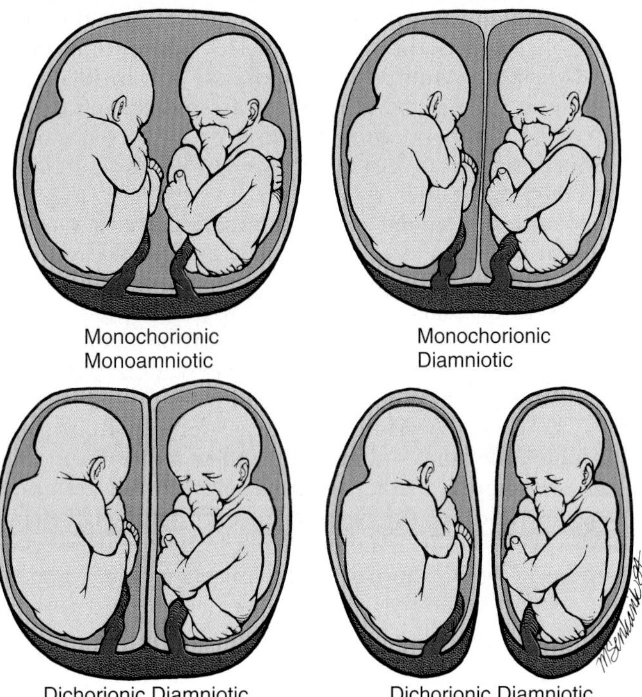

Figure 28-1. Placentation in twin pregnancies.

placentas are almost always diamniotic and dichorionic. Rare cases of DZ monochorionic twins conceived following ART have been reported.[43,44]

The type of placenta that develops in an MZ pregnancy is determined by the timing of cleavage of the fertilized ovum. If twinning is accomplished during the first 2 to 3 days, it precedes the setting aside of cells that eventually become the chorion. In that case, two chorions and two amnions are formed. After approximately 3 days, however, twinning cannot split the chorionic cavity, and from that time on a monochorionic placenta must result. If the split occurs between the third and eighth days, a diamniotic monochorionic placenta will develop. Between the 8th and 13th days, the amnion has already formed, and the placenta will therefore be monoamniotic and monochorionic. Embryonic cleavage between the 13th and 15th days will result in conjoined twins within a single amnion and chorion; beyond that point, the process of twinning cannot occur.

The frequency of placental types within a population is influenced by the rate of DZ twinning. In the United States, approximately 80 percent of spontaneously conceived twin placentas are dichorionic, and 20 percent are monochorionic. In Nigeria, where DZ twinning is much more common, the frequency of dichorionic placentas approaches 95 percent.[8] With triplets, quadruplets, and higher orders of multiple gestation, monochorionic and dichorionic placentations may coexist.

Because monochorionic placentas predominantly occur in MZ pregnancies, pathologic evaluation of placental membranes will establish zygosity in 20 percent of cases in the United States. In approximately 35 percent of cases, the twins will be of opposite sex and, therefore, most likely DZ. This leaves only 45 percent of cases (twins of like sex having dichorionic placentas) in whom further studies may be necessary in order to determine zygosity.[45,46]

Ultrasound Prediction of Amnionicity and Chorionicity

The determination of chorionicity is important in the management of multiple gestations because monochorionic twins are at increased risk for poor outcomes.[47] For example, the incidence of growth abnormalities is higher in monochorionic than in dichorionic twins, and the twin-to-twin transfusion syndrome (TTTS) occurs exclusively in monochorionic pregnancies. Antenatal knowledge of the type of placentation and chorionicity is not only helpful but, in some cases, is critical for determining optimal management. This is true when deciding whether IUGR in one fetus of a twin gestation is due to TTTS or uteroplacental insufficiency. When contemplating the selective termination of one abnormal twin, or when performing elective first trimester multifetal pregnancy reduction, precise knowledge of chorionicity is imperative. In these latter situations, if the gestation is monochorionic, a shared placental circulation could result in death or injury to a surviving fetus depending on the technique used for the termination procedure.

Chorionicity is most accurately determined in the first trimester. From 6 to 10 weeks, counting the number of gestational sacs and evaluating the thickness of the dividing membrane is the optimal method of determining chorionicity. Two separate gestational sacs, each containing a fetus and a thick dividing membrane, suggests a dichorionic diamniotic pregnancy, whereas one gestational sac with a thin dividing membrane and two fetuses suggests a monochorionic diamniotic pregnancy.[39] After 9 weeks, the dividing membranes become progressively thinner in monochorionic pregnancies, but in dichorionic pregnancies, they remain thick and easy to identify at the attachment to the placenta as a triangular projection which is also known as the lambda or twin peak sign.[48–50] At 11 to 14 weeks' gestation, sonographic examination of the base of the intertwin membrane for the presence or absence of the lambda sign provides reliable distinction between dichorionic and monochorionic pregnancies.[51] The number of yolk sacs can also be used as an indirect method of determining amnionicity.[52] Chorionicity and amnionicity diagnosed at early gestational ages should always be confirmed by a repeat ultrasound in 2 to 3 weeks as there have been cases of misdiagnosis.[53]

After the early second trimester (16 to 18 weeks), determination of chorionicity and amnionicity becomes less accurate, and different techniques are used. The sonographic prediction of chorionicity and amnionicity should be systematically approached by determining the number of placentas visualized and the sex of each fetus, and then by assessing the membranes that divide the sacs. The pregnancy is clearly dichorionic if two separate placental disks are seen. If the twins are different genders, the pregnancy is virtually always dichorionic. However, if the gender is unknown or the same for both fetuses, or if the placentas are adjacent or fused, chorionicity remains unknown.

When a single placenta is present and the twins are of the same sex, careful sonographic examination of the dividing membrane usually results in a correct diagnosis. Evaluation of three features in the intertwin membrane will provide an almost certain diagnosis about the chorionicity of a twin pregnancy. These are (1) thickness of the intertwin membrane, (2) number of layers visualized in the membrane, and (3) assessment of the junction of the membrane with the placental site for the "twin peak" sign. In dichorionic diamniotic pregnancies, the dividing membrane appears "thick"[54–56] and has a measured diameter of greater than or equal to 2 mm,[57] and either three or four layers can often be identified (Fig. 28-2).[58,59] With a monochorionic diamniotic pregnancy, only two layers of membranes are identified, and the membrane appears to be "thin and hairlike"[58] (Fig. 28-3). A floating monochorionic diamniotic membrane may fold back upon itself and give a false impression of having four layers. Inspection of the membranes near the placental insertion will reduce this artifact. It should be mentioned that significant magnification of the image is helpful in counting the number of layers.

Identifying the twin peak sign can also aid in the diagnosis of chorionicity.[48,49] The twin peak sign as a triangular projection of tissue with the same echogenicity as the placenta extending beyond the chorionic surface of the placenta. This tissue is insinuated between the layers of the intertwin membrane, wider at the chorionic surface, and tapering to a point at some distance inward from that

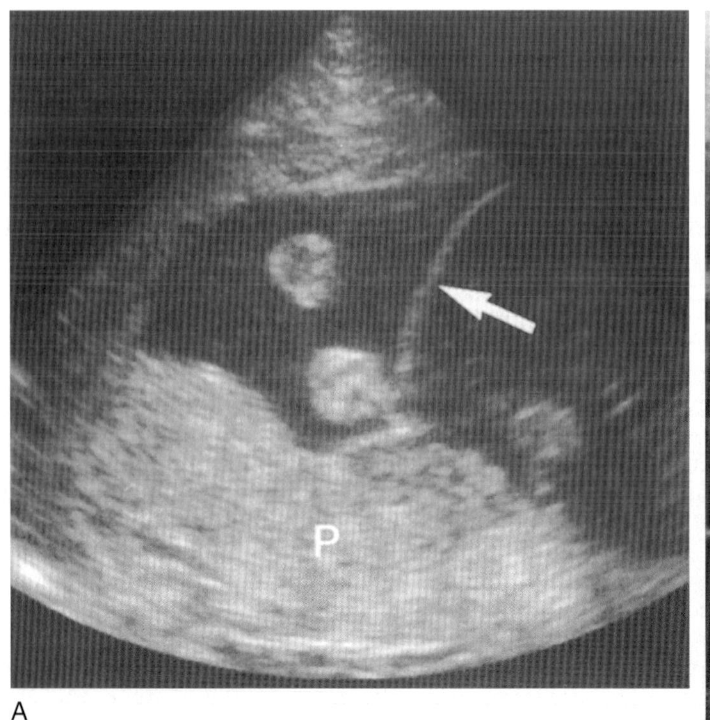

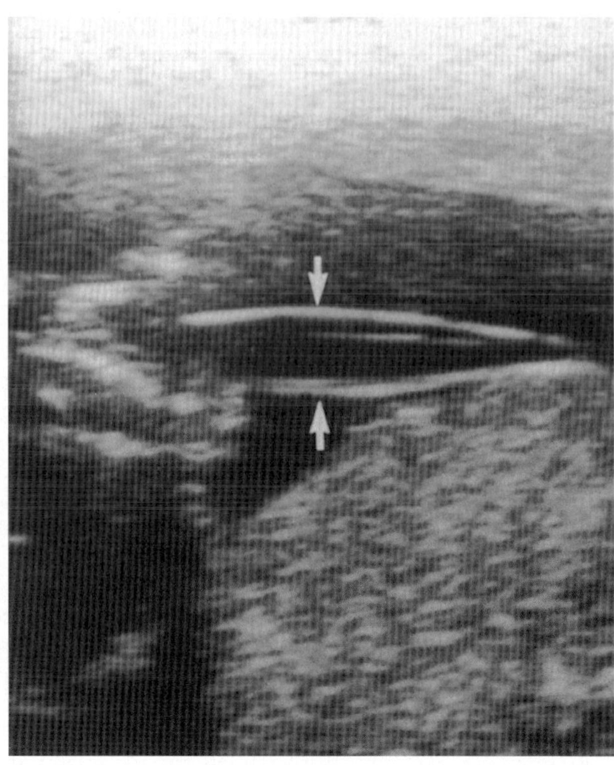

Figure 28-2. *A,* The dividing membrane (*arrow*) is thick, suggestive of a dichorionic diamniotic placentation. *B,* Visualization of four layers in the dividing membrane suggests dichorionic diamniotic placentation. P, placenta.

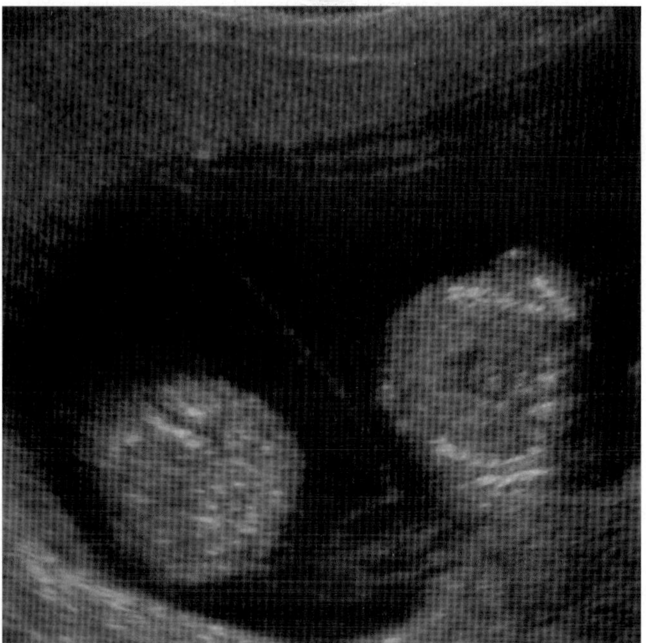

Figure 28-3. The dividing membrane is thin and hair-like, suggestive of monochorionic diamniotic placentation.

surface (Fig. 28-4). This finding is produced by extension of chorionic villi into the potential interchorionic space of the twin membrane. This space exists only in a dichorionic pregnancy and is produced by reflection of each chorion away from its placenta at the place where it encounters the chorion and placenta of the co-twin (Fig. 28-5*A*). The twin peak sign cannot occur in monochorionic placentation because the single continuous chorion does not extend into the potential interamniotic space of the monochorionic diamniotic twin membrane (Fig. 28-5*B*). In assessing the twin peak sign with ultrasonography, it is important that the zone of intersection of the membrane with the placenta be carefully scrutinized over as much length as can be detected. It should be mentioned that the absence of the twin peak sign alone does not guarantee that the pregnancy is monochorionic. Under these circumstances, evaluation of other features of the membrane previously described (i.e., thickness and number of layers) gives additional diagnostic clues regarding chorionicity and amnionicity.

In some pregnancies with monochorionic diamniotic placentation, the dividing membranes may not be sonographically visualized because they are very thin. In other cases, they may not be seen because severe oligohydramnios causes them to be closely apposed to the fetus in that sac. This results in a "stuck twin" appearance, in which the trapped fetus remains firmly held against the uterine wall despite changes in maternal position (Fig. 28-6). Diagnosis of this condition confirms the presence of a diamniotic gestation, which should be distinguished from a monoamniotic gestation where dividing membranes are absent. In the latter situation, free movement of both twins, and entanglement of their umbilical cords, can be demonstrated.[60]

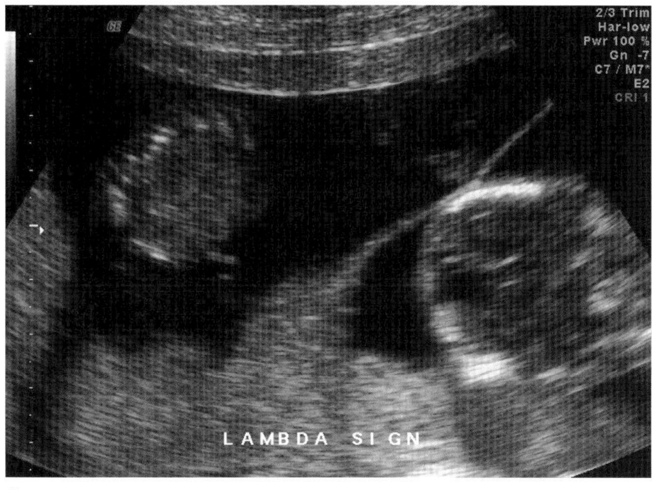

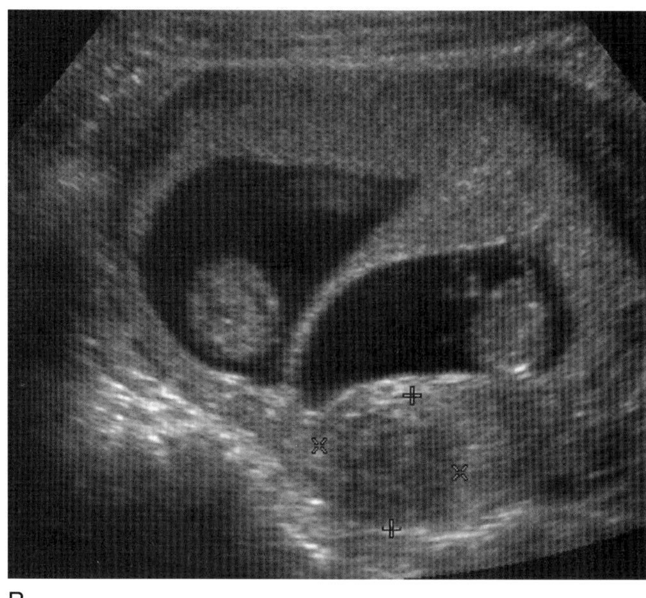

Figure 28-4. "Twin peak" sign appears as a triangular extension of placental tissue, wide at the placental surface and tapering to a point at its junction with the intertwin membrane.

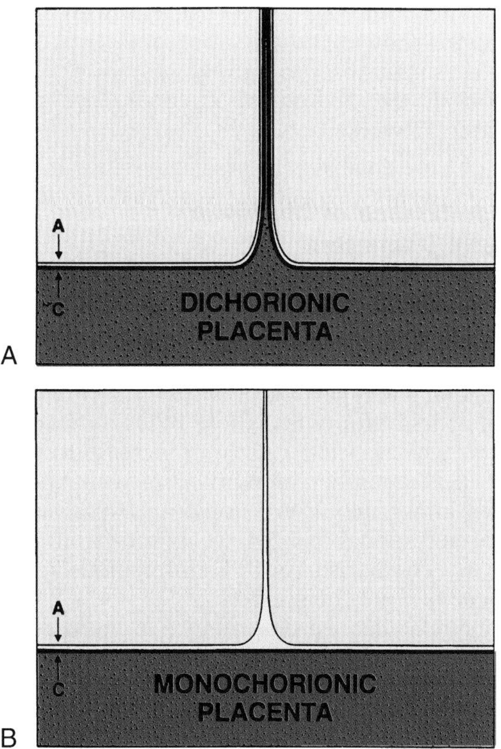

Figure 28-5. *A,* In a dichorionic pregnancy with fused placentas, both the amnions (A) and the chorions (C) reflect away from the placental surface at the point of origin of the septum. This creates a potential space in direct continuity with the chorionic villi and into which they can extend. *B,* In a monochorionic twin pregnancy, the septum is formed by reflection of the two amnions away from the placenta. There is a continuous single chorion, which provides an intact barrier, preventing extension of placental villi into the potential interamniotic space.

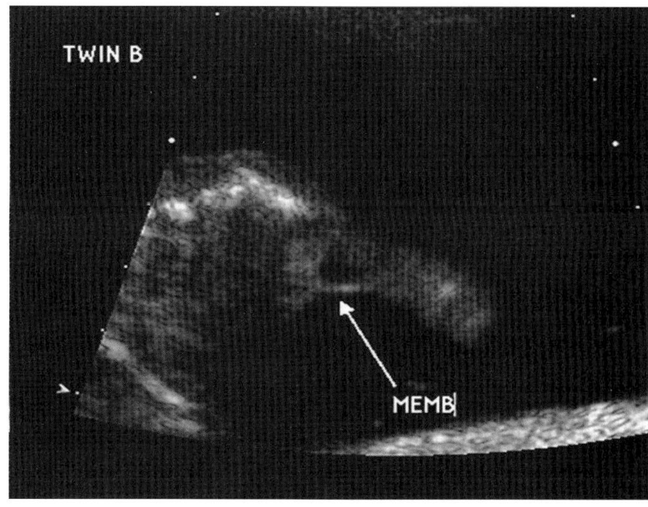

Figure 28-6. Twin gestation with severe oligohydramnios in sac of twin B. The separating membrane is closely apposed to this fetus and was only visualized with great difficulty.

FETAL GROWTH AND DEVELOPMENT

In multiple gestations, ultrasound is the most accurate method for assessing fetal growth. Normal twins grow at the same rate as singletons up to 30 to 32 weeks' gestation, after which they do not gain weight as rapidly as singletons of the same gestational age.[61] After 32 weeks, the combined weight gain of both twins is approximately equivalent to that gained by a singleton for the remaining portion of the pregnancy.[62] The restriction in each twin's somatic growth is thought to be related to "crowding" in utero. The implication of this concept is that at some point in the third trimester, the placenta can no longer keep pace with the nutrient requirements of both developing fetuses. This process occurs even earlier when more than two fetuses are present.

A study of specimens obtained by induced abortion performed between 8.5 and 21 weeks showed the relationship between body weight and length in twins to be the same as that for singletons.[63] This finding supports the concept that twins are not growth restricted during the first half of pregnancy. Fenner et al.[64] have provided insight into the other end of the gestational age spectrum by studying 146 twins admitted to their neonatal unit with gestational ages at birth ranging from 30 weeks to term. When data from those infants were plotted on Lubchenco's growth charts for singletons, the twins' birth weights dropped below the mean for singletons by 32 weeks but remained within the low-normal range until the 36th week, after which they fell progressively below the 10th percentile. Twin birth lengths and head circumferences, however, remained within the low-normal range for singletons throughout the entire pregnancy. The disparity between relatively normal head size and body length in association with somatic deprivation is compatible with the concept of asymmetric growth restriction. The latter is a mechanism whereby growth-restricted fetuses preferentially favor head growth at the expense of increases in body weight.[65] These studies suggest that alterations in twin growth occur primarily in the third trimester, worsen as gestational age progresses, and are usually asymmetric in nature.

In the large collaborative study conducted by Kohl and Casey,[66] birth weights differed between 500 and 999 g in 18 percent of the twin sets and were in excess of 1,000 g in 3 percent. Obviously these discrepancies in birth weight could be due, in part, to constitutional factors. Because DZ twins are genetically distinct individuals, it is not surprising that they could be programmed to have very different weights at birth. There are, however, several pathologic situations in which twins may be born with substantial weight differences. These include TTTS, the combination of an anomalous fetus with a normal co-twin, and IUGR, affecting only one twin because of local placental factors. IUGR, on the other hand, can affect both twins relatively equally, in which case they would both be small, but not discordant in size. Therefore, detection of differences in size in utero suggests that IUGR may be present but is not diagnostic of that condition. Conversely, the demonstration that twin fetuses have similar sizes does not rule out abnormal growth. Therefore, it is necessary to assess each twin individually if abnormal growth in utero is to be detected.

Are Singleton Nomograms Applicable to Twins?

The first question to be asked is whether ultrasound nomograms devised for singletons can be used to follow twins. Conflicting data exist in the published literature regarding this issue. Some investigators have found twins to have smaller biparietal diameters (BPDs) than those of singletons at all gestational ages,[67] whereas others have found mean BPD values corresponding to those of singletons until the third trimester but demonstrate progressive slowing in growth of the twin BPDs thereafter.[68–72] However, when 18 sets of concordant twins with verified menstrual dates were compared with values from singletons who were appropriate for gestational age (AGA) at birth, Crane et al.[73] found the two groups to have mean BPD values that were essentially identical throughout gestation. These authors conclude that normal twin BPD growth is similar to that of AGA singletons at all stages of gestation, and the conflicting results of earlier studies are due to the inclusion of discordant twins with IUGR in the study group. A similar conclusion was reached by Graham et al.,[74] who studied 104 twins with concordant growth, excellent gestational age assessment, and delivery after 36 weeks. They found almost identical results when BPD and femur length values were compared with those from a selected population of singletons. Other investigators[72,75] also found no significant difference in BPD between uncomplicated singleton and twin pregnancies, suggesting that charts derived from singleton pregnancies may be reliably used to estimate gestational age of twins.

Neonatal anthropometric data obtained from concordant twins suggests that although there is significant reduction of birth weights of twins in late pregnancy, head circumference and body lengths are generally similar to those of normal singletons at corresponding gestational age.[71,73] These findings are consistent with ultrasound observations showing twin femur length growth patterns similar to singletons throughout gestation,[70,74,76] but a reduction in the abdominal circumference growth in twins after 32 weeks.[70,71]

The Significance of Divergent Biparietal Diameters

Reports have suggested that as the difference between twin BPDs increases, the likelihood that the smaller fetus will be growth restricted increases.[77] Leveno et al.[78] reported that a comparison of twins with BPD differences of 4 mm or less with twins whose BPDs differed by 5 mm or greater was associated with an increase from 7 to 22 percent in the number of twin pairs with one growth-restricted infant. Houlton[79] noted an overall increase in small-for-gestational-age (SGA) infants from 40 to 71 percent in a comparison of BPD differentials below 6 mm with those of 6 mm or greater.

Crane et al.[73] defined discordance in utero as an intrapair difference in BPD of 5 mm or more and a fall in BPD below 2 standard deviations for gestational age on their normal twin curve. They suggested that head circumference (HC) be measured if BPD intrapair differences exceed 5 mm. Chitkara et al.[80] also found that BPD intrapair differentials of 5 mm or greater correlated with an increased incidence of significant birth weight differences. However, estimated fetal weight and abdominal circumference measurements were found to be better predictors of discordant size. Other investigators have corroborated these observations.[81]

This compilation of confusing and seemingly conflicting data can probably be summarized as follows. Significant differences in twin BPDs may indicate that one twin is growth restricted. However, the finding could be purely artifactual because of flattening of the head in association with malpresentation or in utero crowding. Measurements of several parameters, along with serial examinations, helps distinguish fetal growth abnormalities in most cases. Nevertheless, although major intrapair BPD differences may reflect IUGR in one fetus, it is not the only criterion that should be used to look for abnormal development in utero because it will not be present when both twins are growth restricted.

The Use of Multiple Parameters to Assess Intrauterine Growth Restriction and Growth Discordance in Multiple Gestations

How then should growth in utero be followed in multiple pregnancies? Serial ultrasound is the optimal method of assessing fetal growth in multiples. BPD alone, as an isolated variable, is a poor predictor of IUGR in twins. Neilson[82] retrospectively analyzed 66 twin pregnancies with good dates by plotting BPD values on a singleton nomogram. Only 56 percent of the 43 SGA neonates were found to have abnormal BPD growth, whereas 49 percent of the fetuses with abnormal BPD curves were found not to be growth restricted at delivery. A survey of multiple parameters on serial ultrasound examinations provides the most accurate assessment of the size of each individual fetus in twin gestations.[71,80,83,84] The highest accuracy for predicting either appropriate or restricted growth is obtained by estimating the fetal weight. Among individual parameters, abdominal circumference is the single most sensitive measurement in predicting both IUGR and growth discordance.[80,81,84,85] Studies suggest that an intrapair difference in abdominal circumference measurement of 2 cm or more can be effectively used as a screening test for discordant fetal growth and IUGR in the smaller twin.[81,84,85] On the other hand, individual measurements of BPD, HC, or femur length are relatively poor predictors for either IUGR or growth discordance.[80,84,85]

Probably the most important conclusions that can be drawn from these various studies are that it is technically feasible to measure multiple ultrasound parameters in twin pregnancies and that a consideration of as many variables as possible will maximize the effectiveness of an ultrasonic assessment of fetal size. The same general principles can be applied to the assessment of growth in triplets and high-order multiple gestations. Another point that should be stressed is that growth is a dynamic process and, therefore, patients with multiple gestations should be followed with serial scans. Because the predictive accuracy of any fetal measurement in utero is inversely proportional to the scan to delivery interval, we recommend that all patients with twins be scanned at least every 3 to 4 weeks after 20 weeks and more frequently if IUGR or growth discordance is suspected.

PRENATAL DIAGNOSIS

Prenatal diagnosis and genetic counseling are important in the management of patients with a multiple gestation because these pregnancies are at increased risk for chromosomal and structural anomalies. Likewise, because DZ twinning has been associated with advancing maternal age and because many patients who undergo assisted conception, which is associated with an increased risk for multiples, are of advancing maternal age, prenatal diagnosis has become a cornerstone in the management of patients pregnant with multiples.

Chromosomal Anomalies in Twins

Most known chromosomal anomalies have been reported in twins.[86] DZ twins are usually discordant for these anomalies and, surprisingly, MZ twins may be as well. In DZ pregnancies, the maternal age-related risk for chromosomal abnormalities for each twin is the same as in singleton pregnancies. Therefore, it has been suggested that the chance of at least one fetus being affected by a chromosomal defect is twice as high as in singleton pregnancies. In MZ twins, the risk for chromosomal abnormalities is the same as in singleton pregnancies, and in the vast majority of cases, both fetuses are affected. There are, however, occasional case reports of MZ twins discordant for abnormalities of autosomal or sex chromosomes, most commonly with one fetus having Turner's syndrome and the other having either a normal male or female phenotype.[87,88]

Genetic consultation should be offered to all patients of advanced maternal age with twins, triplets, and high-order multiples. In patients with singletons and monochorionic twins, advanced maternal age is currently defined as age greater than 35 years at expected date of delivery. In the literature, there is a range of maternal ages suggested for classifying patients with dichorionic twins as being advanced. Reports suggest that women with twins may be so labeled between the ages of 31 and 33 because their midtrimester risk of having one fetus with Down syndrome is similar to that of a 35-year-old woman with a singleton.[89–91] With high-order multiple gestations, this age is thought to be even younger. It is important to remember that in women who have pregnancies conceived with egg donation the age of the ovum donor should be used to determine the pregnancy's age related risk for aneuploidy.

SCREENING FOR ANEUPLOIDY

Second-Trimester Screening

In singletons, the second trimester quad test (combining second trimester serum AFP, beta human chorionic gonatotropin (β-hCG), unconjugated estriol, and inhibin-A with maternal age) detects greater than 75 percent of cases of Down syndrome with a 5 percent false-positive rate.[92] Second-trimester maternal serum screening for Down syndrome is more complex in patients with multiple gestations compared with those with singletons. On average, maternal serum biochemical markers are twice as high in twins as they are in singletons of the same gestational age.[93] In maternal serum screening programs for Down syndrome these serum markers can be measured in a woman with twins and then divided by the corresponding medians for normal twins. The process has been termed pseudo-risk estimation. Nonetheless, experience with maternal serum screening in twins during the second trimester has been limited and interpretation of the analyte data may be difficult. In cases discordant for anomalies, altered serum levels from the affected fetus will be brought closer to the mean by the unaffected twin. In addition, studies have suggested that when singletons are conceived following ART, there may be a small increased risk for false-positive serum screening results due to changes in fetoplacental endocrinologic metabolism.[94] Although this finding has not been confirmed in multiple gestations, larger studies are needed before the impact of ART on maternal serum analytes in twins can be determined. Owing to the fact that second-trimester maternal serum analytes are difficult to interpret in the setting of a twin pregnancy, many medical centers do not offer this screening modality routinely.

First-Trimester Screening

In the first-trimester, nuchal translucency ultrasound measurements combined with maternal age appears to be a promising method for aneuploidy screening in patients with multiple gestations. In singleton pregnancies, an enlarged nuchal translucency combined with maternal age has been shown to identify approximately 80 percent of fetuses with Down syndrome.[95] Because the nuchal translucency distribution does not differ significantly in singletons compared with twins, the Down syndrome detection rate in multiples using this modality is similar to that of singletons.[96] The prevalence of increased nuchal translucency appears to be higher in patients from monochoronic pregnancies than in those from dichorionic pregnancies, and it has been suggested that this may reflect an early manifestation of TTTS in some of these cases.[97] In contrast to other screening techniques, nuchal translucency can be performed in pregnancies complicated by triplets and high-order multiples with similar accuracy as in singletons.

In singletons, first-trimester combined screening—maternal age and nuchal translucency combined with maternal serum free β-hCG and pregnancy associated plasma protein-A (PAPP-A) has been shown to detect approximately 82 percent of cases of Down syndrome for a 5-percent false-positive rate.[98] In a recent prospective study, Spencer and Nicolaides[99] reported a 75-percent detection rate of Down syndrome for a 9-percent false-positive rate using nuchal translucency and first-trimester serum markers in 206 twin pregnancies. Of note, chorionicity is not thought to affect maternal serum biochemical markers in twin pregnancies.[100] The combination of nuchal translucency and biochemistry in twins may prove to give detection rates similar to singleton pregnancies. Nonetheless, this form of screening has been criticized because similar to second trimester serum screening, the analyte data is difficult to interpret. Larger prospective studies of first trimester combined screening in twins are needed before definitive conclusions and recommendations for practice can be made.

Screening for Neural Tube Defects in Multiple Gestations

In singletons, a second-trimester maternal serum AFP of greater than 2.5 multiples of the median (MoM) has been used to screen for neural tube defects. Different AFP cutoffs are needed for twin pregnancies owing to the fact that the maternal serum AFP level in a twin pregnancy is approximately double that of a singleton pregnancy. A cut-off of 4.5 MoM is often used for twins because it has a detection rate of 50 to 85 percent for a 5-percent false-positive rate.[101] If an abnormal serum AFP is found, ultrasound evaluation is required for further evaluation. It is important to note that similar to maternal serum screening for aneuploidy, maternal serum screening for neural tube defects in a twin pregnancy will always be limited by the fact that it is impossible to confirm which fetus is affected without performing an ultrasound examination. As a result, many centers do not offer this type of serum screening for twin pregnancies.

Screening for Anatomic Abnormalities

The fetuses of multiple gestations are at increased risk for anatomic abnormalities. As a result, it is important that careful evaluation of the anatomy of each fetus be obtained in these patients. No large-scale studies of ultrasound for fetal anatomy in multiple gestations have been performed. Nonetheless, small studies have attempted to determine the predictive value of ultrasound in the detection of fetal anomalies in multiple gestations, and it has been found to be effective in detecting anomalies in these pregnancies.[102]

PRENATAL DIAGNOSTIC TECHNIQUES IN MULTIPLE GESTATIONS

Amniocentesis

Midtrimester amniocentesis is an ultrasound-guided transabdominal invasive technique for withdrawing amniotic fluid for genetic analysis. In multiple gestations, it is suggested that fluid for genetic studies be obtained from each fetal sac.[103] If the pregnancy is DZ, the fetuses are genetically distinct individuals. If the pregnancy is MZ, there is the possibility of discordance for chromosomal abnormalities due to the phenomenon of postzygotic nondisjunction resulting in heterokaryotypic twins. Twins at risk for erythroblastosis fetalis should also have each sac tapped for Rh-determination if the father is a heterozygote, because one twin may be Rh-positive and the other Rh-negative.[104] It should be noted that twins in Rh-sensitized pregnancies have been successfully transfused in utero.[105]

Amniocentesis in a multiple pregnancy is often performed with an ultrasound-guided double needle technique. In a 1980, Elias et al.[106] reported that they were successful in obtaining fluid from both amniotic sacs in 19 of 20 pregnancies during the second trimester. These authors used ultrasound to identify the lie of each fetus and then introduced an amniocentesis needle into one

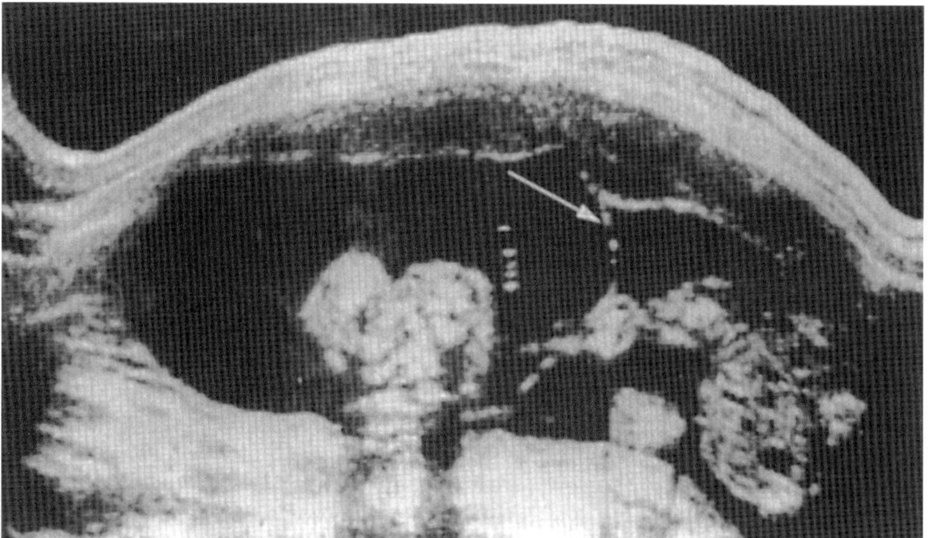

Figure 28-7. Sagittal scan with a single anterior placenta demonstrating a vertical membrane (*arrow*) separating the two sacs.

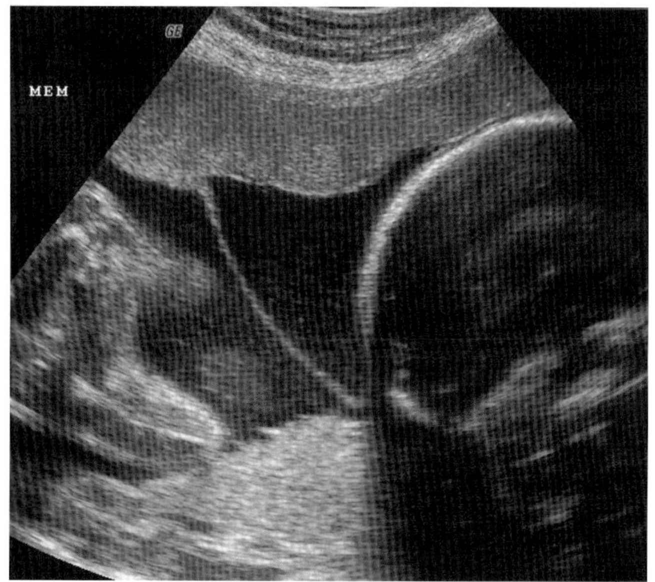

A

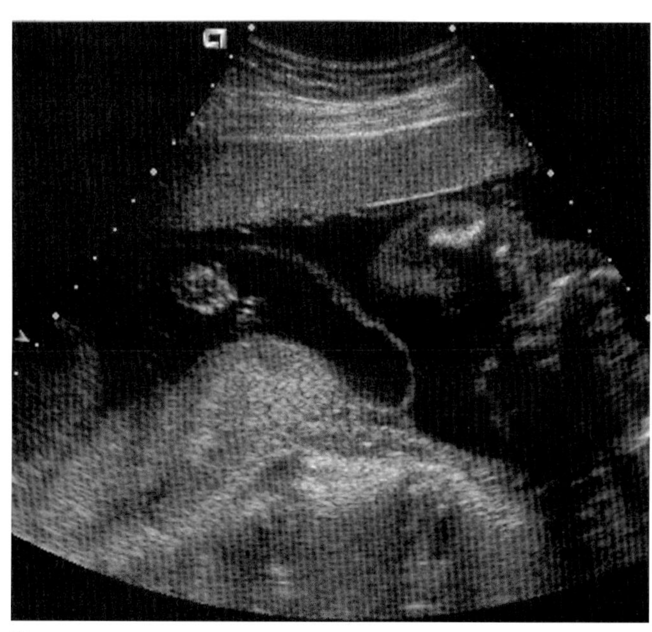

B

Figure 28-8. Individual anterior and posterior placentas with the membranes running horizontally between the two sacs.

sac using a standard insertion technique. After aspirating fluid, they introduced a blue dye, to serve as a marker, and then removed the needle. A different needle was then inserted and the aspiration of untinged fluid indicated that the second sac had been successfully entered.

Single uterine entry for genetic amniocentesis in twin pregnancies has been proposed.[107] After amniotic fluid is aspirated from the sac of one twin, the syringe is removed, the stylet replaced, and the needle advanced through the intertwin membrane under continuous ultrasound guidance into the sac of the second twin. When aspirating fluid from the second sac, discarding the first 1 ml is recommended in order to avoid possible contamination with amniotic fluid from the first sac. Although this method is technically feasible, we continue to recommend the technique using a separate needle insertions for each sac in order to eliminate any chance of contamination of fluid samples. Also, it is possible that the puncture site in the membrane separating the two sacs may inadvertently enlarge and lead to a cord accident later in pregnancy, as has been reported in cases of TTTS treated with septostomy.

When performing amniocentesis in a multiple pregnancy, several points should be noted:

1. The usual precautions applying to all cases of amniocentesis must be followed when multiple sacs are tapped. A thorough ultrasound examination should precede the amniocentesis, at which time the viability of all fetuses should be verified and their gestational ages and relative sizes assessed. The position of the placenta or placentas and dividing membranes should be noted (Figs. 28-7 and 28-8) and a search for gross fetal, uterine, and adnexal pathology performed. It is particularly important to note the position of one fetus relative to the other's, and to label the aspirated fluids appropriately. It is also important to place a drawing in the patient's chart so that at a later date, it is possible to correlate a particular fetus with its fluid speci-

men. This becomes critically important in the case of genetic studies if at a later date selective termination of one fetus is to be considered.

2. Direct ultrasonic visualization of the needle tip during its insertion allows for greater precision in guiding the needle to an optimal sampling site. It also reduces the potential for traumatizing the fetus.
3. Use of a marker dye is very helpful in performing amniocentesis on more than one sac, but methylene blue has been associated with fetal hemolysis when injected intraamniotically.[108] Furthermore, multiple ileal obstructions[109] or jejunal atresia[110,111] have been reported in twins whose sacs have been injected with 1-percent methylene blue at the time of a diagnostic tap in the second trimester. Therefore, it is recommended that either indigo carmine or Evan's blue be used rather than methylene blue. Whatever dye is used, it should not be red so as to avoid confusion in the event of a bloody tap.
4. When failure to see a separating membrane between the sacs suggests the possibility of a monoamniotic twin gestation, use of a marker dye alone may not definitively rule out this diagnosis, because aspiration of colored fluid on a second needle insertion may represent reentry into the first sac. Under these circumstances, a technique described by Tabsh[112] may be useful in differentiating a single monoamniotic sac from separate diamniotic sacs when the membrane is simply not being visualized. Leaving the needle in place after an initial sample of fluid is withdrawn, 0.1 ml of air drawn into the syringe through a micropore filter is mixed with 0.5 ml of marker dye and 5 ml of aspirated amniotic fluid. This mixture is then injected back into the sac under firm, gentle pressure in order to create microbubbles within the amniotic fluid. The microbubbles serve as ultrasonic contrast agents within the first sac and should demarcate it from a second sac if one is present. A site for needle insertion into the second sac can then be selected. Aspiration of colorless fluid confirms that a second sac has been entered, whereas fluid colored with dye indicates that the original sac has been reentered. If the microbubbles are seen around both fetuses, a diagnosis of monoamniotic twins can be confirmed.

Although second-trimester amniocentesis for genetic indications has become a well-accepted procedure, some studies have suggested a higher postprocedural fetal loss rate in twin pregnancies than in those with singletons.[113–115] These studies, however, did not address the question of whether the increased fetal wastage following amniocentesis is attributable to the procedure or to the twin gestation itself. In a case-controlled study, Ghidini et al.[116] concluded that second-trimester amniocentesis in twin pregnancies was not associated with excess pregnancy loss and that the likelihood of fetal loss secondary to this procedure is probably of the same order of magnitude as that in singletons. More recent studies have contradicted these authors' findings. In a retrospective study of 476 twins who underwent amniocentesis and 477 twins who did not, Yukobowich et al.[117] found statistically different loss rates (2.7 versus 0.6 percent). Toth-Pal et al.[118] compared pregnancy loss rates in 175 twin pregnancies that underwent amniocentesis to 300 controls. In the amniocentesis group, the loss rate was 3.87 versus 2.39 percent in the control group. Although these results were not statistically significant, the authors suggested that genetic amniocentesis in multiples slightly increases the loss rate.

Chorionic Villus Sampling

Chorionic villus sampling (CVS) is another procedure used for prenatal diagnosis of genetic disorders (see Chapter 7). Chorionic villi for chromosomal or DNA analysis can be obtained either by transcervical catheter or by transabdominal needle under ultrasound guidance. The advantage of this technique over amniocentesis is the earlier availability of results because the procedure is generally performed between 10.5 and 12 weeks' gestation. CVS is considered a safe alternative to amniocentesis in multiples.[103,119] The early diagnosis afforded by CVS is particularly important for patients who may be considering multifetal pregnancy reduction. The cytogenetic laboratory should be made aware when CVS is being performed on a multiple pregnancy because studies have suggested that as many as 4 percent of samples may show twin-to-twin contamination.[103] More recent studies have suggested that cross-contamination between placentas may be far less frequent.[120,121]

PROBLEMS SPECIFIC TO MULTIPLE GESTATIONS

Early Fetal Wastage

As a result of ultrasound studies performed during the first trimester, there is evidence to suggest that the incidence of multiple gestations is higher than is usually appreciated and that a significant amount of early wastage occurs in these pregnancies. This has led to the concept of the "vanishing twin." Landy et al.[122] reviewed nine series that have addressed this phenomenon. The series vary in regard to the populations studied, timing of the ultrasonography, and number of scans performed. Frequencies of twin "disappearance" in patients scanned before 14 weeks' gestation reportedly range from 13 to 78 percent. The higher rates were found in studies performed before 10 weeks' gestation.

One explanation for the disappearance of a gestational sac is resorption, which has been documented to occur in both human singleton pregnancies and lower animals. This phenomenon has been ultrasonically described in human multiple gestations between 7 and 12 weeks. The true incidence of resorption of one or more gestational sacs is unknown, but it can occur without adverse effects on a coexisting fetus. Another explanation for sac disappearance is the presence of a blighted ovum or anembryonic pregnancy. Robinson and Caines[123] define a blighted ovum as a gestational sac having a volume of 2.5 ml or more in which no fetus can be identified on ultrasound examination. It should be noted that the sac need not be totally anechoic, because disorganized echoes may be present in some cases. Several studies have reported that the only apparent complication of regression of a blighted ovum is slight vaginal bleeding. Regardless of whether vaginal bleeding accompanies regression of a blighted ovum, a coexisting normal pregnancy has a good prognosis for carrying to term. Furthermore, experience with patients undergoing elective first-trimester reduction of multifetal pregnancies suggests that the clinical course and outcome of these pregnancies is similar to that observed with the naturally occurring phenomenon of a blighted or "disappearing" co-twin.

Landy et al.[122] point out that pathologic evidence to confirm "disappearance" rates as high as 78 percent is lacking. Examination of the placenta and membranes after delivery of a singleton thought to be a surviving twin rarely shows evidence of the one that disappeared. It is also true that examination of the products of an abortion is usually not helpful in verifying the presence of a sac that has "vanished." The difficulty encountered in obtaining positive pathologic confirmation of the diagnosis, however, does not mean that it is incorrect. On the other hand, false diagnoses are certainly possible as a result of poor ultrasound studies. If equipment with inferior resolution is used, or if the types of artifacts described earlier are misread as being second sacs, the presence of multiple gestations may be overdiagnosed. Particular attention should be paid to the fact that pressure from the scanning transducer can create an hourglass appearance in a normal single sac that may be incorrectly interpreted as demonstrating two separate sacs.

Aside from first-trimester bleeding, there are no reported maternal complications associated with the early disappearance of a fetus.[122] The associated overall abortion rates in reported series range from 7 to 37 percent. However, in two studies, when a vanished sac was associated with vaginal bleeding during the first trimester, spontaneous abortions occurred in 26 percent[124] and 92 percent[125] of cases. In a retrospective review of the first trimester ultrasound data for 260 twin pregnancies in which one or both fetuses delivered at term, Dickey et al.[126] found that disparities in gestational sac diameter and crown-rump length (CRL) were good predictors of eventual outcome. When disparities of 3 mm or more were observed either between the twin gestational sac diameters (at <49 days' gestation) or between the twin CRL measurements (at <63 days' gestation), these were associated with an embryo loss rate of 50 percent or more. The incidence of these disparities was lower in pregnancies resulting from assisted reproductive technologies than spontaneous conceptions and was unrelated to differences in birth weight, length, or gender of the neonate.

Landy et al.[122] conclude that the phenomenon of the vanishing twin seems to truly exist. Although on the basis of current information it is impossible to determine the exact prevalence, their data suggest that a reasonable figure for its incidence may be as high as 21 percent.[127] These authors caution, however, that it is necessary to make "an accurate, faultless diagnosis" of multiple gestation in the first trimester before sharing this information with the mother because of its inevitable emotional impact.

Problems Related to Placentation

Patients with multiple gestations appear to be at increased risk for problems related to abnormal placentation. Benirschke and Kim[8] note that prolapse of the cord and rupture of a vasa previa with fetal exsanguination are more common in twins than in singletons. They attribute the latter to the fact that a velamentous cord insertion occurs in 7 percent of twin placentas as opposed to 1 percent in singletons. Robinson et al.[128] found that 7.1 percent of 72 pregnancies having a velamentous insertion of the cord had associated deformational defects of the neonate. This is defined as an alteration in shape or structure, or both, of a part of the fetus that has differentiated normally (e.g., clubfoot). These investigators speculate that competition for space between the developing fetus and the placenta due to mechanical factors that cause crowding in utero leads to fetal structural defects of a deformational nature and also alters the direction in which the placenta can grow. The latter situation secondarily causes velamentous insertion to occur when the bulk of the placental tissue is forced to grow laterally leaving the umbilical cord, which initially was located centrally, in an area that eventually becomes atrophic chorion laeve. The increased incidence of velamentous cord insertions in twin pregnancies may result from competition for space when two blastocysts happen to implant in close proximity. In support of this theory is the observation that velamentous insertions are more common in the most closely approximated twin placentas.

Twin-to-Twin Tranfusion Syndrome

TTTS is virtually always a complication of monochorionic pregnancies. It is characterized by an imbalance in the blood flow through communicating vessels across a shared placenta leading to underperfusion of the donor twin and overperfusion of the recipient. The donor twin often develops IUGR and oligohydramnios, whereas the recipient experiences volume overload and polyhydramnios that may lead to heart failure and hydrops. On echocardiography, the recipient may demonstrate decreased ventricular function, tricuspid regurgitation, and cardiomegaly.[129] These cardiac abnormalities can progress during pregnancy and persist into the neonatal period. To respond to the increased blood volume, the recipient also becomes hypertensive, and produces increasing amounts of atrial and natriuretic peptides.[130] Polyhydramnios can lead to uterine overdistention and increased uterine pressure, both of which may contribute to an increased risk for preterm labor and preterm premature rupture of membranes. Umbilical artery Doppler studies can vary. Absent end diastolic flow is more frequently found in the donor twin.[131,132] Studies of fetal blood sampling have suggested that the donor twin often has a significantly lower hematocrit than the recipient.[133]

Although all monochorionic twins share a portion of their vasculature, only about 15 percent will develop TTTS.[134] The syndrome can present at any gestational age. Earlier onset is often associated with poorer prognosis. The transfer of blood can occur in small increments

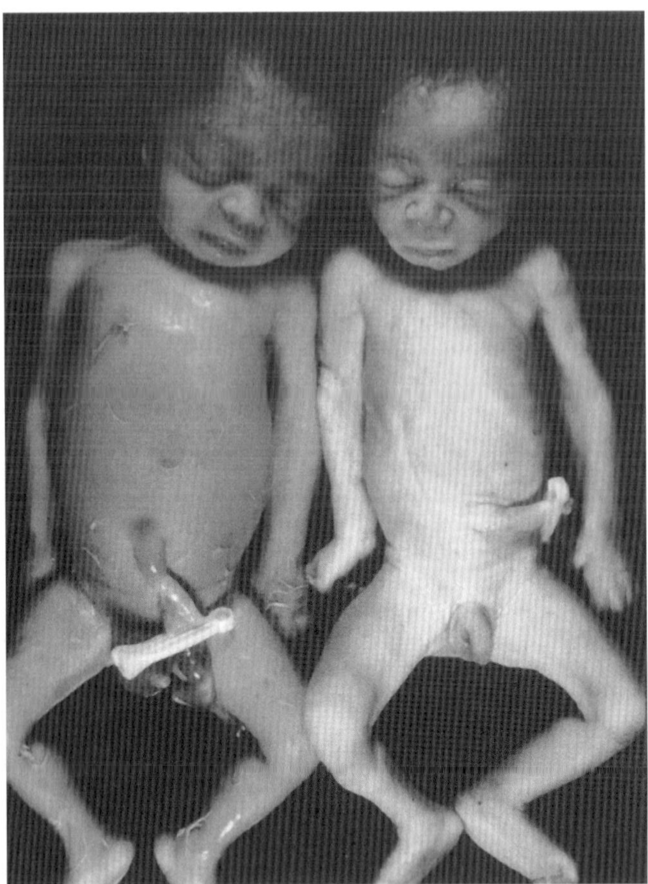

Figure 28-9. Stillborn male twins at 31 weeks' gestation, secondary to TTTS. The plethoric twin on the left weighed 1,670g and the anemic growth-restricted twin on the right weighed 1,300g.

chronically over the course of the pregnancy, or it can be acute. If untreated, the prognosis is poor with reported mortality rates for both twins ranging from 60 to 100 percent[135–137] (Figs. 28-9 and 28-10). If one fetus dies in utero, the surviving twin is at risk for multiorgan damage, including severe neurologic compromise. Even if both twins survive, the pathophysiology of TTTS can result in adverse neurologic sequelae to one or both.[138–147]

The following mechanism has been proposed to explain the etiology of TTTS.[148] In monochorionic placentas, there can be three types of vascular communications: arteriovenous (AV), arterioarterial (AA), and venovenous (VV). A cotyledon near the dividing membrane may receive arterial blood from one fetus and drain directly into the venous circulation of the other. AV shunts are usually deep in the placenta and are unidirectional. Superficial AA and VV connections are crucial for maintaining bidirectional flow. According to this theory, the absence of adequate superficial anastomoses, which maintain balanced blood flow, is the mechanism underlying TTTS.

The diagnosis of TTTS is made in utero with ultrasound. The four requirements, none of which is pathognomonic, include (1) the presence of a single placenta, (2) same-gender fetuses, (3) significant weight discordance, and (4) significant amniotic fluid discordance often with a "stuck twin." The most important element in diagnosing TTTS is disparity in the amniotic fluid volume (maximal vertical pocket less than 2cm for the donor twin, and maximal vertical pocket greater than 8cm for the recipient twin). The differential diagnosis of a "stuck twin" includes uteroplacental insufficiency, structural or chromosomal abnormality, abnormal cord insertion into the placenta, intrauterine infection with organisms such as cytomegalovirus, and growth discordance.

A staging system for TTTS was developed by Quintero et al.[149] in order to categorize disease severity and to standardize comparison of different treatment results. In stage 1, oligohydramnios is evident, but the donor twin's bladder is visible; in stage 2, the donor twin's bladder is no longer visible; in stage 3, the Doppler studies are abnormal (i.e., absent/reversed end-diastolic velocity in the umbilical artery, reversed flow in the ductus venosus, or pulsatile flow in the umbilical vein); stage 4 is complicated by hydrops; and in stage 5, one or both fetuses have died.

In addition to sonographically measuring biometry and amniotic fluid, several investigators have attempted to evaluate the role of Doppler velocimetry studies in making or confirming a diagnosis of TTTS. To date, these studies have provided conflicting results. Farmakides et al.[150] reported two cases in which umbilical artery waveforms of the twins were discordant and concluded that simultaneous observation of high- and low-resistance umbilical artery systolic/diastolic (S/D) ratios was highly suggestive of TTTS. On the other hand, in eight cases in which the diagnosis was documented or strongly suspected, Giles et al.[151] found no difference in interpair S/D ratios. Pretorius et al.[152] also reported eight cases of TTTS and found no consistent pattern of umbilical artery Doppler S/D ratios. The mortality rate was very high in that study, with five of eight pregnancies resulting in fetal or neonatal death of both twins. In all of these cases of perinatal loss, one or both of the twins had either absent or reversed diastolic flow. The authors concluded that, although evidence of greatly increased placental resistance (i.e., absent or reversed diastolic flow) is not helpful in identifying the donor from the recipient twin, it invariably predicts a poor outcome. Data from the Australian and New Zealand TTTS Registry[153] support the observations of Pretorius et al.[152] In their study of umbilical artery blood flow velocity waveforms, Ishimatsu and colleagues[154] were also unable to identify any distinctive findings in patients with TTTS. However, the presence of cardiomegaly in five recipient twins, with tricuspid regurgitation and a biphasic umbilical vein waveform in three others, led them to suggest that these findings may be more diagnostic than umbilical artery Doppler velocimetry and representative of the hemodynamic changes that occur in TTTS. It is interesting to note that AA anastomoses can be identified using Doppler ultrasound as early as the first trimester. As mentioned earlier, absence of these anastomoses has been found to be associated with an increased risk for TTTS.[134]

Expectant management is not recommended in TTTS because of the poor perinatal outcomes associated with the disorder.[155] Treatment depends on the gestational age at diagnosis. Patients with early-onset TTTS may opt for selective termination of one twin (usually the donor) or

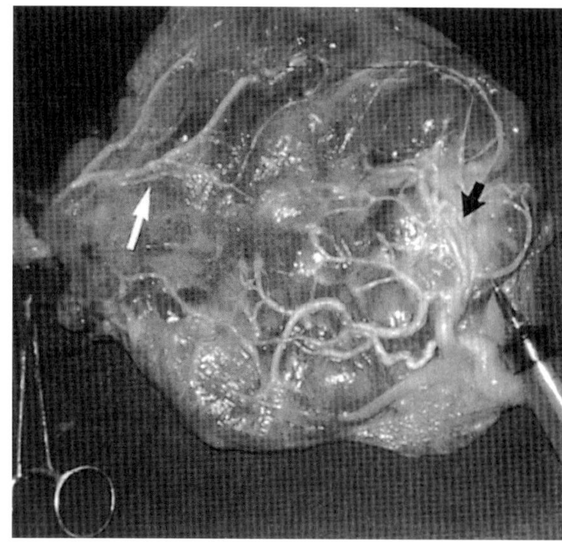
A

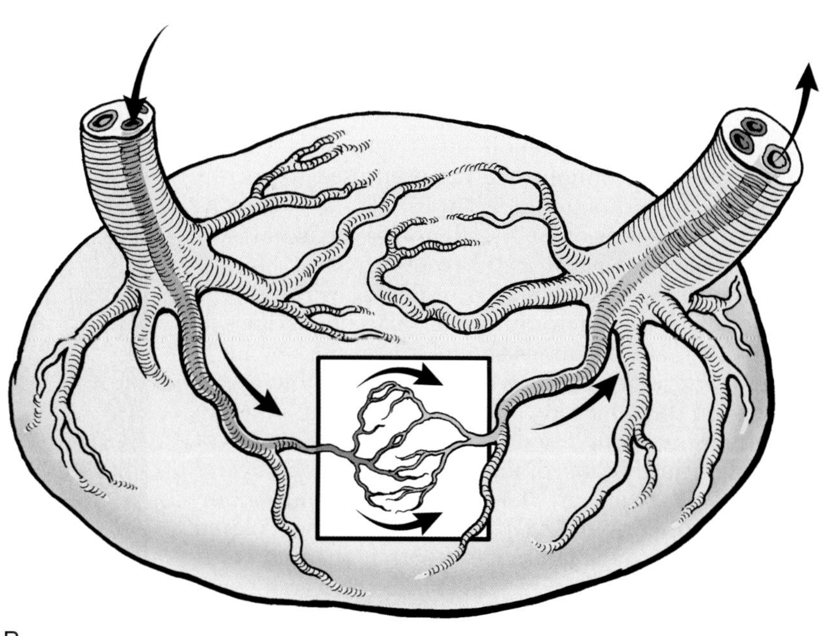
B

Figure 28-10. *A,* The placenta of a pregnancy complicated by TTTS. Milk has been injected into an artery on the "donor" side of the placenta (*black arrow*). It can be seen returning through the venous circulation on that side but is also evident in the venous circulation of the "recipient" (*white arrow*). *B,* The arteriovenous shunt shown in *A*.

termination of the entire pregnancy. If TTTS is diagnosed in the middle to late third trimester, treatment may be less aggressive depending on the disease severity and proximity to term.

In the midtrimester, aggressive management is recommended. Medical management with digoxin has been attempted.[156] Indomethacin is contraindicated due to reports of fetal demise following its use.[157] Current treatment for severe TTTS requires physical intervention. There are three main management options: (1) serial reduction amniocentesis, (2) amniotic septostomy, and (3) laser ablation of the anastomoses.

In serial reduction amniocentesis,[155,158] an 18-gauge spinal needle is placed into the polyhydramniotic sac under ultrasound guidance. If the patient can tolerate the procedure, amniotic fluid is withdrawn until the fluid level returns to normal. Amnioreduction is repeated as often as necessary to maintain a near-normal amniotic fluid volume. The mechanism by which this procedure restores the amniotic fluid balance is unknown. Removing excessive fluid from the sac with polyhydramnios may result in decreased pressure on the sac with oligohydramnios. This, in turn, may result in increased placental perfusion to the stuck twin with secondary improvement in its amniotic fluid volume. Studies have cited perinatal survival rates of 37 to 83 percent following serial amnioreductions.[131] The wide range in perinatal survival may be due to reporting bias, small sample sizes, and variation in the timing and amount of fluid removed.

Amniotic septostomy is another management option.[155,159] In this procedure, a 20-gauge spinal needle is inserted through the dividing membrane under ultrasound guidance. The amniotic fluid, then, sometimes equilibrates across the disrupted membrane. Similar to serial amnioreduction, the mechanism of action of this technique is unclear. It is possible that the defect in the membranes allows the donor to swallow a sufficient volume of fluid to augment its circulating blood volume, secondarily increasing its urine output. Unfortunately, studies regarding the effectiveness of this treatment modality have been conflicting. In one report of 12 cases, pregnancy was prolonged by 8 weeks with an 83-percent survival rate.[160] In another report of 14 patients (seven managed by serial amnioreduction and seven with amniotic septostomy) no differences in overall survival were noted. The septostomy patients, however, delivered significantly later.[161] In another report, all three of the treated pregnancies were lost within 5 days due to preterm premature rupture of membranes.[161] In a more recent study by Saade et al.[162] in which 32 patients were randomized to septostomy and 31 to amnioreduction, similar outcomes were noted between the groups. Both groups had a 65-percent survival.[162] Because septostomy can functionally create an iatrogenic monoamniotic pregnancy that has its own inherent complications and risks, the procedure has been criticized. Likewise, comparing amnioreduction to septostomy is challenging because both procedures use amnioreduction, and, alternatively, serial amnioreduction can be complicated by inadvertent septostomy.

Laser ablation of placental anastomoses is a third invasive treatment option that has been used to correct the underlying pathophysiology of TTTS and reduce its associated complications.[155,163] Reported perinatal survival rates have ranged from 53 to 69 percent.[131] In this procedure, a fetoscope is placed in the sac with polyhydramnios, and the anatomy of the placental vessels is evaluated. An arteriovenous shunt is diagnosed by identifying an artery that supplies a cotyledon without a vein returning on the same side of the dividing membrane. In that setting, a vein is usually seen on the other side of the dividing membrane draining the cotyledon toward the recipient twin. A 0.4-mm neodymium:yttrium-aluminum-garnet (Nd:YAG) laser fiber is then placed through a sleeve in the fetoscope to permit ablation of the communicating vessels (Fig. 28-11). Controversy exists about whether it is preferable to ablate all anastomoses (nonselective laser ablation) or just the AV anastomoses involved in the donor-to-recipient transfusion (selective laser ablation).[164] Reduction amniocentesis is simultaneously performed.

Senat et al.[163] recently published the results of the European prospective multicenter randomized controlled study of endoscopic laser (semiselective technique) versus serial amnioreduction for the treatment of severe TTTS between 15 and 26 weeks' gestation. As the result of an interim analysis demonstrating a significant benefit to the laser group, the study was stopped after 142 patients had been treated. Compared with the amnioreduction group, the laser group had a higher likelihood of survival of at least one twin to 28 days of life (76 percent versus 56 percent) and 6 months of age (76 percent versus 51 percent). The median gestational age at delivery was significantly older in the laser group than in the amnioreduction group (33.3 weeks versus 29.0 weeks). Thirty patients in the laser group (42 percent) and 48 in the amnioreduction group (69 percent) delivered before 32 weeks' gestation. Neonates from the laser group also had a lower incidence of periventricular leukomalacia and were more likely to be free of neurologic complications at 6 months of age (52 percent versus 31 percent). The authors concluded that endoscopic laser coagulation of anastomoses is a more effective first-line treatment than serial amnioreduction for severe TTTS diagnosed before 26 weeks' gestation.

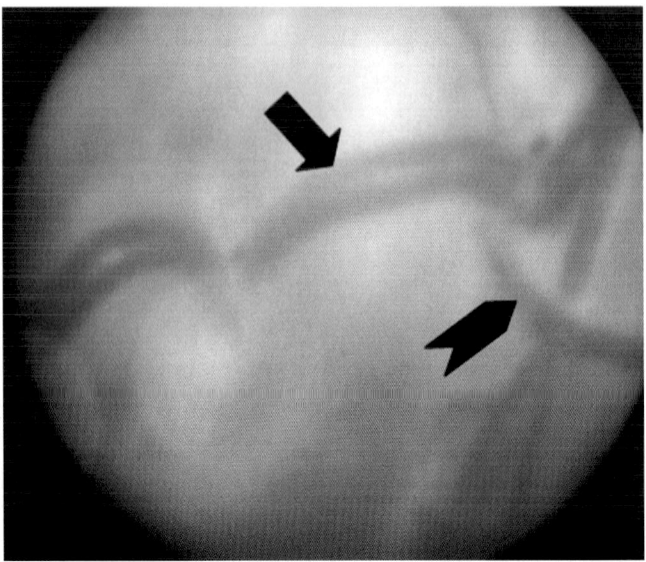

A

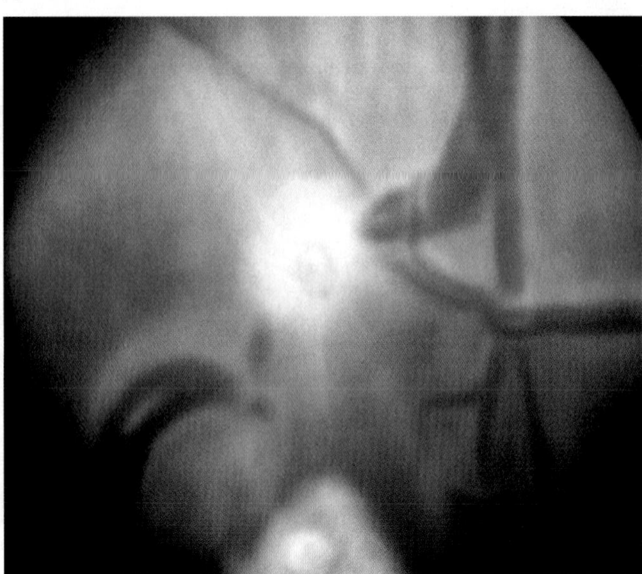

B

Figure 28-11. *A,* An artery from one twin going to a cotyledon, which is drained by a vein returning to the co-twin (*arrow*). The cotyledon is also perfused by a small artery from the co-twin (*arrowhead*) and drained by a large vein going also to the co-twin. In order to preserve this cotyledon for the co-twin, the arterial perfusion to the cotyledon from the other twin is interrupted by laser photocoagulating the other artery. *B,* The effect of photocoagulation. (Courtesy of Timothy M Crombleholme, MD, University of Cincinnati College of Medicine.)

While the findings in the study by Senat et al.[165] are important, many questions remain unanswered. The results reported by those authors should be replicated by others, and further studies are needed to determine the long-term cardiac, neurologic, and developmental outcomes in pediatric survivors of severe TTTS. As a result, no definitive recommendations regarding the treatment of this disorder can be made at the present time.

Growth Discordance

Growth discordance in utero is the difference in sonographic estimated fetal weights expressed as a percentage of the larger twin's estimated fetal weight. This can reflect a problem in multiple gestations and has been associated with an increased risk for adverse perinatal outcomes.[166] Abnormal growth discordance has been defined as ranging from 15 to 40 percent but is usually thought to be greater than 20 percent. Approximately 15 percent of twins are diagnosed with this condition.[166] Risk factors include monochorionicity, uteroplacental insufficiency, gestational hypertension, velamentous cord insertion, and antenatal bleeding.[167]

Growth discordance has different implications depending on chorionicity. In most cases, dichorionic diamniotic twins are distinct individuals with genetically different growth patterns, and it is not surprising that they may have divergent birth weights. Nonetheless, there are several pathologic conditions in which weight differences can occur in dichorionic pregnancies, including in utero crowding, unequal sharing of the placenta, and the combination of a normal fetus with one that is anomalous. Situations unique to monochorionic twinning, such as TTTS, can also result in significant growth discordance.

Although IUGR can complicate a pregnancy with growth discordance, the latter does not necessarily imply the former. However, growth discordance can be a marker for SGA/IUGR. Although some studies have demonstrated an increased risk for perinatal morbidity in growth discordant twins, others have not. In approximately two thirds of discordant twin pairs, the smaller twin has a birth weight of less than the 10th percentile.[168] In a study of more than 10,000 discordant twins, the neonatal mortality rates were 29 versus 11/1,000 live births when the smaller twin weighed less than the tenth percentile compared with those who were above it.[168] On the other hand, a recent study suggests that 20 percent growth discordance may result in an increased risk for some adverse outcomes but not for serious morbidity and mortality.[169] After adjusting for chorionicity, antenatal steroids, oligohydramnios, preeclampsia, and gestational age at delivery, discordant twins independent of SGA status were at increased risk for low or very low birth weight, admission to the neonatal intensive care unit (NICU), an oxygen requirement in the NICU, and hyperbilirubinemia. However, they did not seem to be at increased risk for serious neonatal morbidity and mortality.

Because the studies regarding growth discordance are conflicting with regard to increased risk for adverse perinatal outcomes, we follow these patients closely with serial growth scans and antenatal testing. In the absence of IUGR or nonreassuring fetal status, or both, pregnancies complicated by this problem without any other maternal or obstetric issues are delivered at term.

Monoamniotic Twins

Monoamniotic twinning is an uncommon form of twinning in which both twins occupy a single amniotic sac. It accounts for approximately 1 percent of all MZ twin pregnancies.[8] Historically, perinatal morbidity and mortality rates have been reported to be in excess of 50 percent.[170–173] This has been attributed to premature delivery, growth restriction, congenital anomalies, vascular anastomoses between twins, umbilical cord entanglement, and cord accidents. In addition, the incidence of discordant anatomic abnormalities is increased. More recent reviews of prenatally diagnosed cases suggest improved perinatal outcomes, with mortality rates ranging from 10 to 32 percent.[174–179] This decrease is likely due to prenatal diagnosis, the use of antenatal corticosteroids, intense fetal surveillance, and early elective delivery.

The prenatal diagnosis of monoamnionicity is established when an experienced sonographer cannot identify a dividing membrane separating like-gender twins that share a common placenta. The diagnosis can be confirmed after sonographic identification of entangled umbilical cords using color flow Doppler[180] (Fig. 28-12). Other techniques used to diagnose monoamnionicity have included the visualization of one yolk sac in a twin pregnancy at less than 10 weeks' gestation, and amniography with iopamidol or an indigo carmine air mixture.[52,112,181] Three-dimensional ultrasound has also been used to visualize monoamniotic fetuses lying in a single amniotic cavity.[182] If monoamnionicity is suspected early in pregnancy, a follow-up ultrasound examination is suggested to confirm the diagnosis.[53]

An alternative consideration in the differential diagnosis of monoamnionicity is the intrauterine rupture of a diamniotic twin membrane, which can mimic the sonographic appearance of true monoamniotic twins. However, because this has a perinatal mortality rate

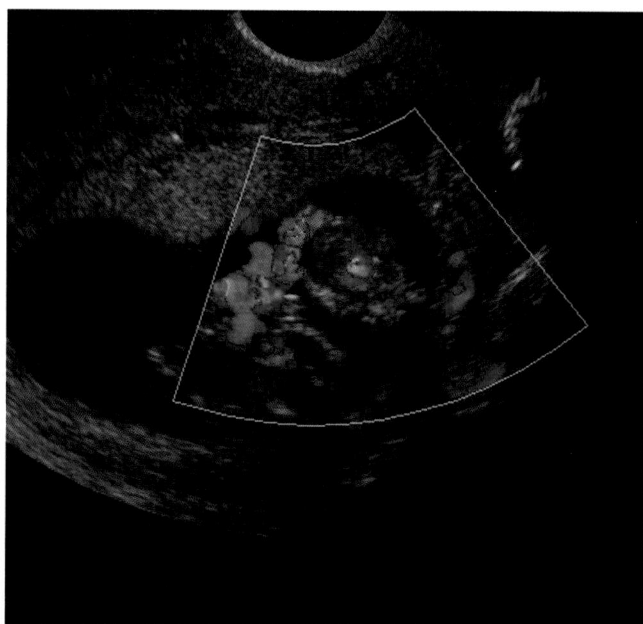

Figure 28-12. Doppler ultrasound of tangled umbilical cords in a monochorionic monoamniotic twin pregnancy.

similar to that of true monoamniotic gestations, distinguishing between these two conditions is not necessary.[183] When a previously identified dividing membrane can no longer be visualized, this clinical scenario should be suspected. Possible causes for intrauterine rupture include trauma during amniocentesis, infection, and developmental disturbances of the membranes.

Because umbilical cord accidents are the primary cause of fetal death, most management protocols emphasize intense fetal surveillance in an attempt to prevent that complication. This should be initiated as soon as possible after fetal viability has been achieved because intrauterine fetal demise (IUFD) has been documented to occur in monoamniotic twins throughout gestation.[101] Furthermore, this surveillance must be repeated frequently because fetal compromise and death can happen suddenly and without warning.

Many older reports on monoamniotic twins are not optimal for counseling patients because in most of those cases, the diagnosis of monoamnionicity was made postnatally. There have been several more recent series that are helpful. Rodis et al.[174] reviewed 13 cases of monoamnionicity at one tertiary care center over a 10-year period. All patients underwent serial ultrasound examinations and antenatal fetal surveillance two to seven times per week starting at 24 to 26 weeks' gestation. The average gestational age at diagnosis was 16.3 weeks' gestation. The mean gestational age at delivery was 32.9 weeks' gestation, with a mean birth weight of 1,669 g. All pregnancies exhibited cord entanglement at the time of delivery, with 62 percent having knotted cords (Fig. 28-13). Sixty-two percent of the pregnancies were delivered for abnormal fetal testing. All of these patients were delivered by cesarean section by 35 weeks' gestation, and there were no fetal deaths. Two neonates died during the perinatal period: one due to a congenital heart defect, and the other from asphyxia and sepsis. The latter did not receive antenatal testing more than twice a week. When compared with 77 sets of monoamniotic twins from the literature that had not been diagnosed prenatally, these patients had a 71-percent reduction in the relative risk of perinatal mortality.

A more recent study evaluated the impact of routine hospitalization for fetal monitoring on perinatal survival and neonatal morbidity in a multicenter retrospective cohort study of 96 monoamniotic twin gestations.[179] Forty-three patients were admitted electively for inpatient surveillance at a median gestational age of 26.5 weeks. The remainder were followed as outpatients and admitted only for routine obstetric indications. IUFD did not occur in any hospitalized patient, but the risk of IUFD in those women who were followed as outpatients was 14.8 percent (13/88). Statistically significant improvements in birth weight, gestational age at delivery, and neonatal morbidity were also noted for the women who were followed as inpatients. This study suggested that improved neonatal survival and decreased perinatal morbidity can be achieved in patients with monoamniotic twins who are admitted electively for inpatient fetal monitoring.

Maternal administration of the prostaglandin inhibitor sulindac is the only intervention that has been used in an attempt to reduce the incidence of cord accidents in monoamniotic twins. This medication results in decreased amniotic fluid volume, which theoretically stabilizes fetal lie and decreases cord compression.[185] Because of insufficient data regarding its safety and efficacy, this intervention is not commonly prescribed.

Although we acknowledge that the good outcomes obtained in the above-mentioned studies could be due to chance, we recommend intermittent daily fetal testing in hospital for all patients with monoamniotic twins starting at 24 to 26 weeks' gestation because of the risk for sudden IUFD from cord entanglement. Although cord accidents cannot be predicted, daily fetal heart rate monitoring may reveal an increasing frequency of variable decelerations. If these are identified, continuous monitoring is

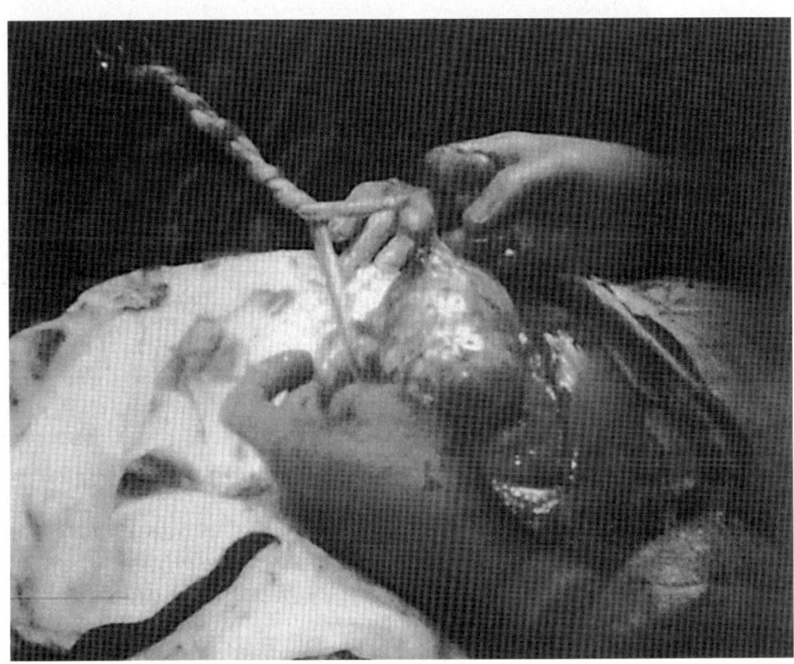

Figure 28-13. Entangled cords found during cesarean delivery in a case of monochorionic monoamniotic twins.

recommended, which may lead to an emergency delivery for nonreassuring fetal testing. Antenatal corticosteroids should be administered if delivery is anticipated between 24 and 34 weeks' gestation. Doppler studies of the umbilical arteries in monoamniotic twins that demonstrate a notch may also be suggestive of cord compression.[186]

In the absence of nonreassuring fetal testing, the timing of elective delivery is not well established.[187] Some authors have advocated delivery of all monoamniotic twin pregnancies as soon as fetal lung maturity has been demonstrated,[188] whereas others have recommended elective delivery at 32 weeks' gestation.[184] Still others suggest that it is unnecessary to deliver monoamniotic twins before term. In a retrospective evaluation of 24 sets of histologically confirmed monoamniotic twin pregnancies, Carr et al.[189] found no perinatal deaths after 30 weeks of gestation. They suggested that there is no advantage to elective premature delivery of these pregnancies. However, in their series, the diagnosis of monoamnioticity was made prenatally in 21 percent of the cases, and only 29 percent of the women were known to be carrying twins. Tessen and Zlatnik[190] reviewed 20 monoamniotic twin pregnancies. In this retrospective series, there were no perinatal deaths after 32 weeks of gestation, and the authors suggested that prophylactic premature delivery of these women might not be indicated. However, in a subsequent addendum to the original paper they reported a double fetal death at 35 weeks just after publication of their report.

Provided that the fetal status is reassuring, it is our practice to perform elective delivery following the administration of antenatal corticosteroid therapy at 34 weeks' gestation. Delivery at this time is associated with a low risk of neonatal morbidity when weighed against the uncertain risk of continuing the pregnancy. However, it may not be unreasonable to manage selected cases of monoamniotic twins expectantly beyond 34 weeks' gestation, with careful ongoing fetal surveillance.

The optimal mode of delivery of monoamniotic twins also remains controversial. Cesarean delivery has been recommended to eliminate the risk of intrapartum cord accidents, but vaginal delivery of these patients is not contraindicated. In one series, no fetal deaths and only one case of nonreassuring fetal testing requiring emergency cesarean delivery occurred during labor in 15 monoamniotic twin pregnancies delivered vaginally.[190] In another series of 24 cases, vaginal delivery was accomplished in 75 percent of individual neonates and in 48 percent of liveborn infants, although the antenatal diagnosis of monoamniotic twins was unknown in most cases and, therefore, could not have influenced management.[189] On the other hand, there are data suggesting potential difficulties with the vaginal delivery of monoamniotic twins. In one case, a nuchal cord affecting the first twin was cut to facilitate delivery, and following delivery of that twin's body, it was noted that the cut cord actually belonged to the second twin.[191,192] Given these issues and the high incidence of nonreassuring fetal testing, we deliver all monoamniotic twin pregnancies by cesarean section.

Twin Reversed Arterial Perfusion Sequence

Twin reversed arterial perfusion (TRAP) sequence, which is also known as acardia, is a malformation that occurs in monochorionic pregnancies with a frequency of approximately 1 per 30,000 deliveries.[8] These extremely malformed fetuses either have no heart at all (holoacardia) or only rudimentary cardiac tissue (pseudoacardia) in association with other multiple developmental abnormalities (Fig. 28-14). These patients always have monochorionic placentas and vascular anastomoses that sustain the life of the acardiac twin. Controversy exists regarding the etiology of this condition. Kaplan and Benirschke[193] believe that reversal of flow through the acardiac twin secondary to at least one artery-to-artery and one vein-to-vein connection in the placenta leads to the anomaly of TRAP. Retrograde fetal perfusion has been documented to occur by Doppler studies.[194,195] Other

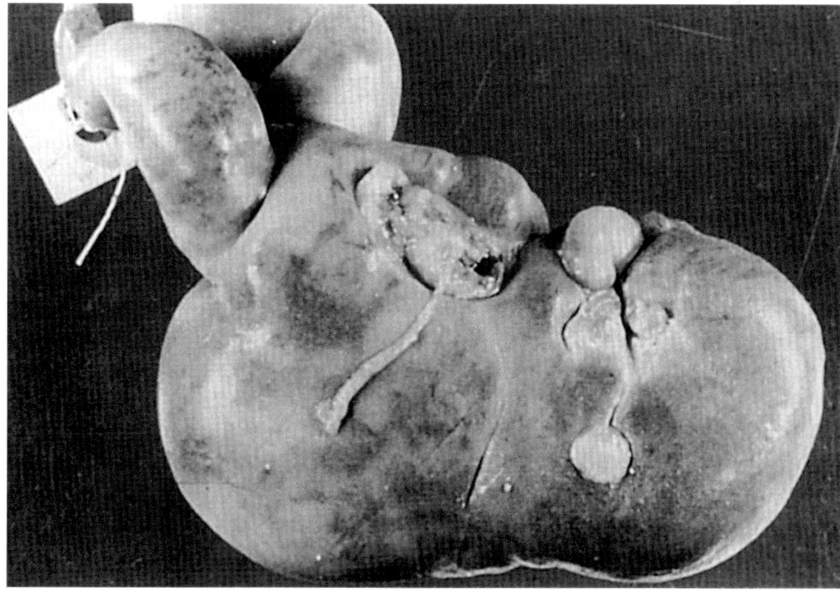

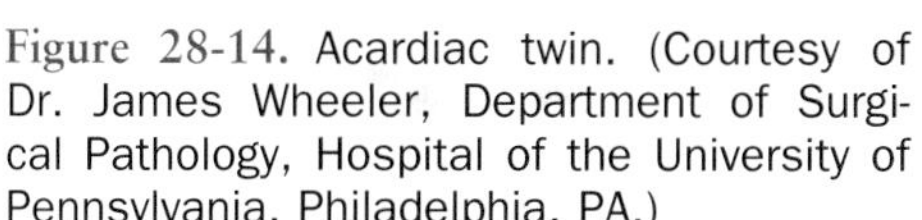

Figure 28-14. Acardiac twin. (Courtesy of Dr. James Wheeler, Department of Surgical Pathology, Hospital of the University of Pennsylvania, Philadelphia, PA.)

authors,[196] however, believe that acardia is a primary defect in cardiac development, and, although the placental vascular anastomoses are necessary for survival of the affected twin, these are not responsible for the abnormalities.

There is a high incidence of chromosomal abnormalities in these pregnancies. In 6 of the 12 acardiac cases reported by Van Allen et al.,[197] an abnormal karyotype was found in the perfused twin, whereas the karyotype of the pump twin was normal. The remaining six perfused twins were chromosomally normal.

Antenatal diagnosis by ultrasound of an acardiac fetus coexisting with a normal co-twin is fairly straightforward. The anomalous twin may appear to be an amorphous mass or may show a wide range of abnormalities that depend on which organ system has failed to develop. The lower extremities and body are typically more completely developed, whereas the most severe abnormalities involve the upper body. The heart is frequently absent or rudimentary, and a single umbilical artery is present in approximately half the cases. A retrograde pattern of fetal perfusion can be demonstrated to occur through the umbilical arteries by Doppler studies.

The pump twin, although structurally normal, is at increased risk for in utero cardiac failure, and mortality rates of 50 percent or higher have been reported.[198] When the size ratio of the acardiac to that of the pump twin is less than 25 percent, the mortality rate is diminished. However, the prognosis worsens when polyhydramnios, preterm labor, or cardiac decompensation of the pump twin are present.[198] Management of patients with pregnancies complicated by TRAP is controversial. Expectant management with serial ultrasound surveillance including fetal echocardiography is reasonable in the absence of poor prognostic features. If delivery is anticipated between 24 and 34 weeks' gestation, antenatal corticosteroid administration should be considered. Delivery may be indicated if signs of cardiac decompensation are noted. Maternal administration of digoxin and indomethacin have been reported as medical management of acardia, however, no series data are available.

Various techniques have been used to interrupt the vascular communication between the twins in an effort to improve outcome of the normal pump twin. These methods have included hysterotomy with physical removal of the acardiac twin, ultrasound-guided injection of thrombogenic materials into the umbilical circulation of the acardiac twin, ligation of the umbilical cord of the acardiac twin under fetoscopic guidance, and radiofrequency cord ablation.[199–204]

Conjoined Twins

Conjoined twins occur with a frequency of about 1 per 50,000 deliveries and are an extremely rare complication of monochorionic twinning.[131] The most famous conjoined twins were Chang and Eng Bunker, who were born in Siam in 1811. These xiphopagus twins (i.e., joined by a band of tissue extending from the umbilicus to the xiphoid cartilage) lived unseparated for 63 years. P.T. Barnum exhibited them extensively for a number of years. At the age of 31, they married two sisters who bore them a total of 26 children. They died within hours of each other.

The precise etiology of conjoined twinning is unknown, but the most widely accepted theory is that incomplete division of an MZ embryo occurs at approximately 13 to 15 days' postovulation. Most conjoined twins are female, with the ratio of women to men being reported as 2:1 or 3:1. Many of these infants are delivered prematurely and are stillborn. They are classified according to their site of union. The most common location is the chest (thoracopagus) (Fig. 28-15), followed by the anterior abdominal wall from the xiphoid to the umbilicus (xiphopagus), the buttocks (pygopagus), the ischium (ischiopagus), and the head (craniopagus).[131] Organs may be shared to varying degrees in different sets of twins. Major congenital anomalies of one or both twins are not uncommon. Polyhydramnios is said to be present in almost one half of the reported cases of conjoined twins.

Ultrasound is the most reliable way to establish this diagnosis in utero, and the diagnosis can be made as early as the first trimester of pregnancy by transvaginal ultrasound.[205,206] Color Doppler, fetal echocardiography, three-dimensional ultrasound, and magnetic resonance imaging can be effectively used to complement two-dimensional imaging, to confirm the diagnosis, as well as determine the extent of organ sharing and definitive classification of conjoined twinning.[207–209] If the diagnosis is

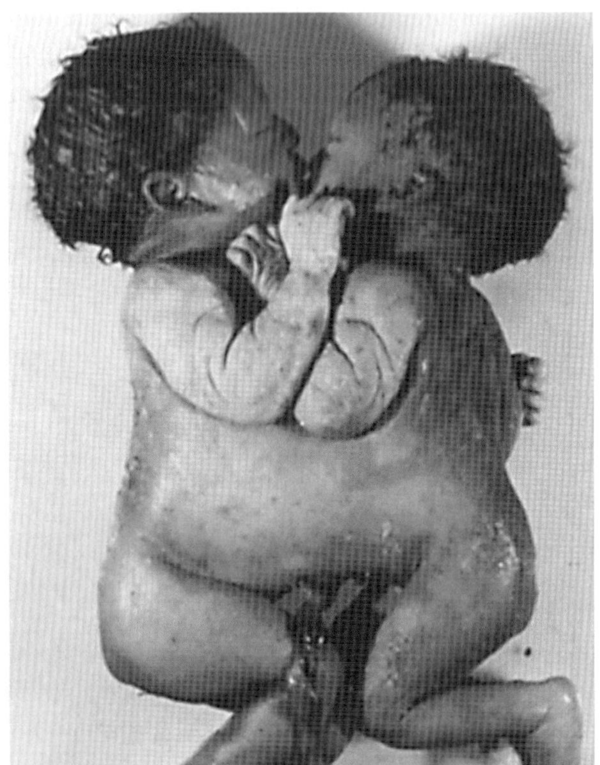

Figure 28-15. Conjoined twins attached at the chest or thoracopagus, the most common form of conjoined twins. They originate at the primitive streak stage of the embryonic plate (13 to 15 days). (Courtesy of Dr. James Wheeler, Department of Surgical Pathology, Hospital of the University of Pennsylvania, Philadelphia, PA.)

made early in the first trimester, a follow-up confirmatory ultrasound is suggested in approximately two weeks.[53]

Once the diagnosis of conjoined twins is made, management options should be discussed with the patient. If the diagnosis is confirmed before viability, pregnancy termination should be offered. If the patient desires expectant management, it is suggested that she be counseled that the prognosis for successful separation depends on the degree of organ and vascular sharing between the two fetuses, especially the heart. Prenatal evaluation includes transabdominal and transvaginal ultrasound, three-dimensional ultrasound, color Doppler, fetal echocardiography, and magnetic resonance imaging. Because structural abnormalities are often concomitant, a careful survey of the fetal anatomy is suggested. In order to optimize the postnatal management, patients with conjoined twins should be cared for by a multidisciplinary team in the antenatal period. This team should include maternal-fetal medicine specialists, neonatologists, pediatric anesthesiologists, pediatric surgeons, and appropriate pediatric subspecialists.[131]

Patients with conjoined twins should deliver at a tertiary-care facility where neonatal and pediatric specialists are available. Cesarean delivery near term is the preferred method of delivery to minimize maternal and fetal injury. If the twins are thought to have a poor chance of surviving and are small enough to pass through the birth canal without damaging the mother, vaginal delivery might be considered. Surgical separation of conjoined twins is beyond the scope of this chapter but has been discussed elsewhere.[210,211]

It is also interesting to note that although the long-term follow-up of conjoined twins who underwent surgical separation is limited, it seems favorable. Although survivors have required additional surgeries following the initial separation to correct urologic, orthopedic, and neurosurgical issues, the majority are achieving educational levels similar to their singleton peers.[212] There have even been case reports of separated conjoined twins having successful pregnancies themselves.[213]

Death of One Twin in Utero

IUFD of one twin occurs most commonly during the first trimester. This phenomenon is known as a "vanishing twin." Although it may be associated with vaginal spotting, the loss of one conceptus is often not clinically recognized, and the prognosis for the surviving twin is excellent.[122,127]

Single IUFD of one fetus in a multiple gestation in the second or third trimesters is much less common, complicating approximately 0.5 to 6.8 percent of twin pregnancies.[214–222] Monochorionic twins are at increased risk for single IUFD compared with dichorionic twins. It is estimated that there is a three- to fourfold increase in intrauterine death with monochorionic twins as compared with dichorionic twins.[221,223] In addition, a single fetal death is also more common among twins with a structural abnormality.[221] Demise of both fetuses in a twin pregnancy has been reported infrequently.[224] Studies have indicated single IUFD rates ranging from 4.3 to 17 percent in triplet pregnancies.[222,225,226] In high-order multiples, demise of a single fetus may be even more common.

The etiology of IUFD in a multiple pregnancy may be similar to that for singletons or be unique to the twinning process. Death in utero may be caused by genetic and anatomic anomalies, abruption, placental insufficiency, cord abnormalities such as a velamentous cord insertion, infection, and maternal diseases including diabetes and hypertension.[227] In monochorionic pregnancies, IUFD may result from complications of TTTS. In addition, monoamniotic twins are at increased risk of cord entanglement and subsequent IUFD. Similar to singletons, the etiology of IUFD often remains elusive.[228]

Single IUFD in a multiple gestation can adversely affect the surviving fetus or fetuses in two ways: (1) risk for multicystic encephalomalacia and multi-organ damage in monochorionic pregnancies and (2) preterm labor and delivery in both dichorionic and monochorionic twins.

Multicystic encephalomalacia results in cystic lesions within the cerebral white matter distributed in areas supplied by the anterior and middle cerebral arteries and is associated with profound neurologic handicap. The risk of this occurring following single IUFD in a monchorionic pregnancy may be greater than 20 percent for the surviving co-twin.[229–231]

Significant hypotension at the time of demise of the co-twin is thought to cause the neurologic injury in the surviving fetus. Blood from the survivor may rapidly "back-bleed" into the demised twin through placental anastomoses, which is a form of acute TTTS.[232,233] If the resulting hypotension is severe, the surviving twin is at risk for ischemic damage to vital organs.[227] Because the injury is coincident with the IUFD, rapid delivery of the co-twin following single IUFD in a monochorionic pregnancy is unlikely to improve the outcome.[234]

It is unclear how early in gestation the death of one fetus in a monochorionic pregnancy can cause adverse sequelae for the surviving co-twin. Neuropathologists have been unable to pinpoint the exact timing of insult. Of note, a case has recently been reported of an IUFD of one fetus at approximately 13 weeks in a monochorionic gestation that resulted in multicystic encephalomalacia in the co-twin.[235] Ultrasound and magnetic resonance imaging were performed in the second trimester demonstrating this injury (Figs. 28-16 and 28-17). The patient was counseled regarding the poor prognosis and opted for termination. Multicystic encephalomalacia was confirmed pathologically, although the exact timing could not be determined.

The determination of chorionicity is important for the counseling and management of patients with a single IUFD. Optimally, this has been established early in pregnancy. If, however, it has not been done before the IUFD, an attempt should be made to determine the chorionicity by ultrasound examination when the demise is discovered. Sonographic evaluation may not establish chorionicity with absolute certainty in some of these cases, and when the diagnosis is in doubt, DNA studies on amniocytes may be considered.[46]

The optimal treatment for IUFD in multiples is not well established owing to the paucity of reported cases. To

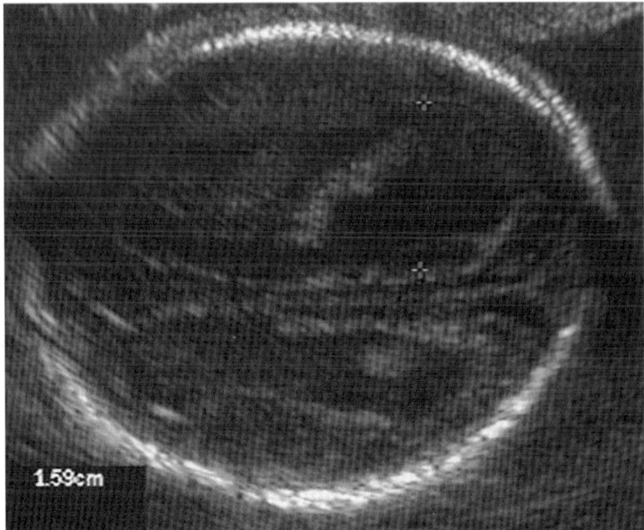

Figure 28-16. Ultrasound suggesting multicystic encephalomalacia in a surviving twin following early demise of its co-twin in a monochorionic pregnancy. (From Weiss JL, Cleary-Goldman J, Budorick N, et al: Multicystic encephalomalacia after first trimester intrauterine fetal death in monochorionic twins. Am J Obstet Gynecol 190:563, 2004, with permission.)

date, recommendations have been based on case reports, case series, and expert opinion. Referral to a tertiary-care perinatal unit is advised when one fetus in a multifetal gestation has died in utero. In some of these cases, labor will already have started, and in others, coexisting maternal illness or placental abruption may make it necessary to expeditiously deliver the surviving fetus or fetuses. Clinical management depends on the gestational age, fetal lung maturity, or detection of in utero compromise of the surviving fetus or fetuses. The goal is to optimize outcome for the survivor while avoiding prematurity and its potential adverse sequelae. Elective delivery is not recommended before 37 weeks' gestation unless antenatal surveillance is suggestive of fetal compromise. It should be emphasized, however, that close surveillance after the diagnosis of single IUFD in a monochorionic twin gestation cannot guarantee a good outcome for the surviving fetus.

Management protocols can be divided into (1) pregnancies complicated by IUFD after viability and (2) those in which this occurs before viability has been achieved. Patients with monochorionic placentation should be counseled about the risk for multicystic encephalomalacia if an IUFD of one twin occurs after viability has been reached. It is difficult to predict which surviving monochorionic twins will develop cerebral injury. The nonstress test and biophysical profile give insight into the physiologic status but may not reflect subtle central nervous system changes. Ultrasound examination of the fetal brain may be suggestive of multicystic encephalomalacia but cannot definitively rule it out. Antenatal magnetic resonance imaging of the fetal brain is investigational at this time but appears to be useful in detecting multicystic encephalomalacia in utero. As a consequence, we currently obtain fetal magnetic resonance imaging on all patients with monochorionic placentas approximately 2 weeks after the demise of one fetus has been detected. Although it is uncertain if normal magnetic resonance imaging definitively rules out brain abnormalities, it is a reassuring sign. A single course of antenatal corticosteroids is recommended if delivery is anticipated within 7 days and the gestational age is between 24 and 34 completed weeks. In monochorionic pregnancies, surviving offspring are monitored with weekly biophysical profiles and nonstress tests. Antenatal surveillance for dichorionic pregnancies complicated by IUFD is controversial. Weekly fetal testing may be considered because these patients have a history of unexplained stillbirth. If other abnormalities such as IUGR or oligohydramnios are evident, fetal testing is intensified.

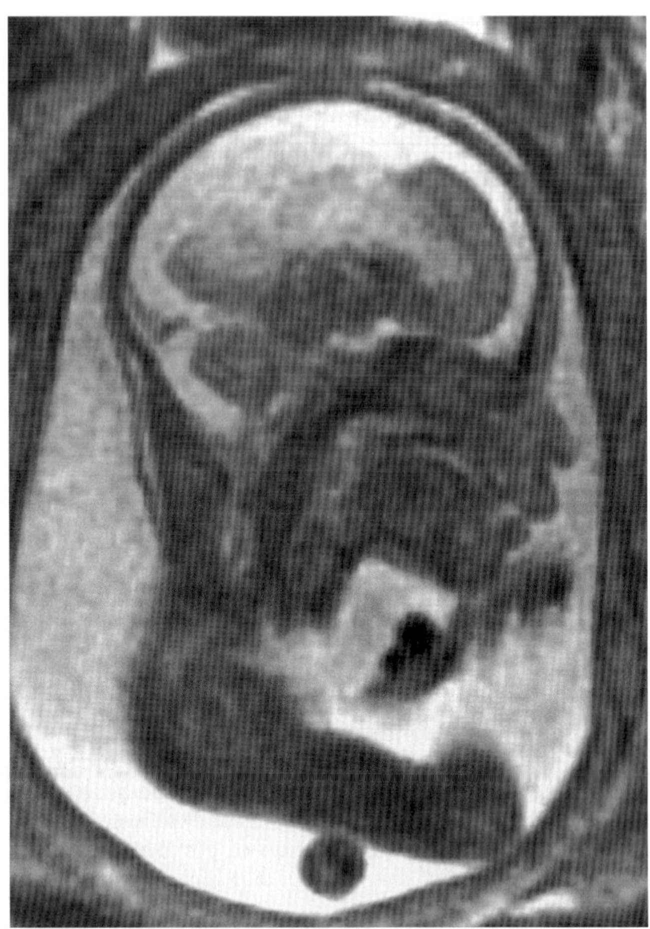

Figure 28-17. Magnetic resonance imaging suggesting multicystic encephalomalacia in a surviving twin following early demise of its co-twin in a monochorionic pregnancy. (From Weiss JL, Cleary-Goldman J, Budorick N, et al: Multicystic encephalomalacia after first trimester intrauterine fetal death in monochorionic twins. Am J Obstet Gynecol 190:563, 2004, with permission.)

In most cases, elective delivery is planned at approximately 37 weeks' gestation. If lung maturity is documented, delivery may be scheduled earlier. Nonreassuring fetal status should result in expedited delivery. Vaginal delivery is not contraindicated, and cesarean delivery is reserved for routine obstetric indications. At delivery, umbilical cord gas measurements should be performed. Autopsy should be offered for the stillborn fetus but may not be helpful if the demise has occurred several weeks earlier. Pathologic examination of the placenta is recommended. In addition, the pregnancy history should be communicated to the pediatricians caring for the neonate.

If IUFD occurs in a previable dichorionic pregnancy, the patient is managed expectantly until 37 weeks' gestation. Fetal surveillance should be considered once viability has been achieved. Monochorionic pregnancies complicated by IUFD before viability are more challenging. It is recommended that these patients be counseled regarding the risk of multiorgan injury including multicystic encephalomalacia. Ultrasound imaging and fetal magnetic resonance imaging can be helpful in making the diagnosis. Some patients may opt to terminate the entire pregnancy, whereas others will choose expectant management. Once the surviving co-twin reaches viability, these women should be managed according to the recommendations described earlier.

Besides fetal risks, there may be maternal risks associated with IUFD in a multiple pregnancy. For example, there is a theoretical possibility for maternal consumptive coagulopathy in twin pregnancies complicated by a single IUFD. It was originally estimated that there was a 25-percent incidence of maternal disseminated intravascular coagulation when a dead fetus was retained in a multiple gestation.[236] However, only a few cases of laboratory changes consistent with a subclinical coagulopathy have been reported under these circumstances, and the 25-percent incidence is certainly an overestimation.[132,237] In one series of 16 pregnancies complicated by IUFD of one twin, no cases of maternal disseminated intravascular coagulation were found.[220] In another series, transient fibrin-split products and hypofibrinogenemia were identified in 2 of 20 cases of single IUFD in twins, neither of which was clinically apparent or required medical therapy.[229] It is also reassuring to note that no cases of clinically significant coagulopathy have been reported in the extensive literature on selective termination (ST) and multifetal pregnancy reduction (MPR). When IUFD occurs in a multiple pregnancy, we recommend baseline maternal hematologic studies be obtained including a PT, PTT, fibrinogen level, and platelet count. If these values are within normal limits, further surveillance is not performed.

In addition, the IUFD of one twin can result in preterm delivery in both monochorionic and dichorionic pregnancies.[219,238,239] Carlson and Towers[219] reported that 76 percent of 17 twin pregnancies complicated by IUFD of one fetus delivered before 37 weeks. This is almost double the background incidence of reported preterm delivery in twins. Of note, mothers with a single IUFD do not appear to be at increased risk for infection due to a retained twin.[219] Cesarean delivery rates seem to be increased in these patients often because of nonreassuring fetal status of the living twin.[219] Finally, dystocia caused by the dead fetus may occasionally occur.

It is well known that the occurrence of IUFD in singleton pregnancies may cause feelings of loss, sadness, anxiety, and guilt. On the other hand, the psychological impact of this occurring in multiple pregnancies has not been well studied. In these women, bereavement may be underestimated because there is a shift in focus to the living offspring.[227,240] As a result, we suggest that patients with a multiple pregnancy complicated by IUFD of one fetus be offered psychological or bereavement counseling, or both.

Discordant Congenital Anomalies

There is general agreement that anomalies occur more frequently in twins than in singletons, but controversy exists regarding the degree of difference. A large series from Czechoslovakia[241] reported a rate of anomalies of 1.4 percent for singletons, 2.7 percent for twins, and 6.1 percent for triplets. Among cases of twins in which anomalies were detected, both twins were affected in 14.8 percent. There were no cases of triplets in which all three infants were affected. Hendricks[242] found the frequency of anomalies to be more than three times higher in twins than in singletons, whereas in Kohl and Casey's series,[illegible] the frequency was 1.5 to 2 times higher. Other studies cited by Benirschke and Kim[8] report smaller increases.

Nance[196] presents evidence to suggest that a group of birth defects involving midline structures, including symmelia, extrophy of the cloaca, and midline neural tube defects, may be associated in some way with the twinning process. Symmelia is a rare severe defect that results from fusion of the preaxial halves of the developing hindlimb buds, producing a single lower extremity with a knee that flexes in the opposite direction from normal. The incidence of this condition is 100 times higher in MZ births than in singletons. MZ twins have also been shown to have a higher frequency of neural tube defects than singletons,[243] and they are often discordant for the abnormality. Nance[196] suggests that the MZ twinning process, with its attendant opportunities for asymmetry, cytoplasmic deficiency, and competition in utero, may favor the discordant expression of midline neurologic defects in these twins. This author also cites evidence that 10 percent of all cases of extrophy of the cloaca occur in like-sex twins. In each of these instances, it is unclear whether the occurrence of a malformation somehow initiates the twinning process or whether a common factor predisposes to both events. Discordance is often, but not always, a feature of these midline defects in MZ twins.

The diagnosis of discordance for a major genetic disease or for an anatomic abnormality in the second trimester places the parents in an extremely difficult position. Management choices include (1) expectant management, (2) termination of the entire pregnancy, and (3) ST of the anomalous fetus. ST is different than MPR, which is discussed later in this chapter. The latter refers to reduction in the number of fetuses a woman is carrying in order to reduce her risk of preterm delivery. ST, on the other hand, refers to terminating a specific fetus that is known to be abnormal.

Several issues should be considered when counseling patients about the management of a multiple pregnancy complicated by a discordant anomaly. These include (1) severity of the anomaly, (2) chorionicity, (3) effect of the anomalous fetus on the remaining fetus or fetuses, and (4) the parents' ethical beliefs. It is important to counsel patients that conservative management can result in adverse outcomes for the healthy twin. Several studies have demonstrated that in a twin pregnancy discordant for major fetal anomalies, the normal fetus may be at increased risk for preterm delivery, low birth weight, and perinatal morbidity and mortality.[244–246]

Selective Termination of an Anomalous Fetus

Several techniques that have been successfully used to perform ST in the second trimester include cardiac puncture with exsanguination, removal of the affected twin at hysterotomy, cardiac puncture with intracardiac injection of calcium gluconate, air embolization through the umbilical vessels with fetoscopic guidance, and intracardiac injection of potassium chloride.[247–252] The latter approach has gained widespread acceptance for both ST and MPR procedures because of its proven safety and efficacy.[253]

Evans et al.[253] reported the outcome of 402 ST procedures from eight centers in four countries using ultrasound-guided intracardiac injection of potassium chloride. The overall results were excellent, with delivery of one or more viable infants in more than 90 percent of cases. There were no cases of disseminated intravascular coagulation or serious maternal complications. Similarly, Eddelman et al.[254] reported favorable outcomes in 200 ST cases performed in one institution on 164 twins, 32 triplets, and four quadruplets. The average gestational age at the time of the procedure was 19 2/7 weeks, with a range of 12 to 23 6/7 weeks. The indications for ST in that series included chromosomal abnormalities, structural anomalies, mendelian disorders, placental insufficiency, and cervical incompetence. The overall unintended pregnancy loss rate was 4 percent, but the losses were fivefold higher in triplets than in twins. The average gestational age at delivery was 36 1/7 weeks, and 84 percent delivered after 32 weeks' gestation.

In monochorionic twins, ST is more challenging. Complete ablation of the umbilical cord of the anomalous fetus is needed to avoid death or neurologic morbidity to the remaining normal fetus from a back bleed through the communicating vessels. Furthermore, in this situation, a lethal agent injected into the anomalous twin could enter the circulation of its normal sibling. Most reported attempts at ST in monochorionic pregnancies without occlusion of all vessels in the abnormal twin's cord have led to death of the second twin within a short time. Techniques used in an attempt to prevent this problem include surgical removal of the fetus by hysterotomy, cord ligation by fetoscopy, insertion of a helical metal coil or surgical silk suture soaked in ethanol to induce thrombosis, and radiofrequency cord ablation[131,255–261] (Fig. 28-18).

Immediate complications associated with ST procedures include selection of the wrong fetus, technical inability to accomplish the objective of the procedure, premature rupture of membranes, and infection with loss of the entire pregnancy. Before initiating the procedure, it is essential to correctly identify the abnormal fetus. When the indication for ST is an abnormal karyotype diagnosed by amniocentesis or chorionic villus sampling, a sonographically identifiable marker may or may not be present. If the gender of the twins is different, or the affected fetus has a gross morphologic anomaly such as hydrocephaly or an omphalocele, the abnormal twin can be easily identified by sonography. However, in the absence of such visible signs, one must rely on information provided from the original diagnostic procedure, which frequently has been performed elsewhere and several days or weeks before the patient presents for termination. In those cases if accurate localizing information is lacking, fetal blood sampling and rapid karyotype determination should be performed to identify the abnormal fetus before ST is attempted. Furthermore, in all cases, a sample of aspirated fetal blood or amniotic fluid should be obtained from the terminated twin at the time of the ST procedure to confirm that the correct fetus has been terminated. ST using intracardiac potassium chloride injection without concomitant cord occlusion is contraindicated if dichorionicity cannot be confirmed. To exclude monochorionicity, DNA zygosity studies may be useful.[46]

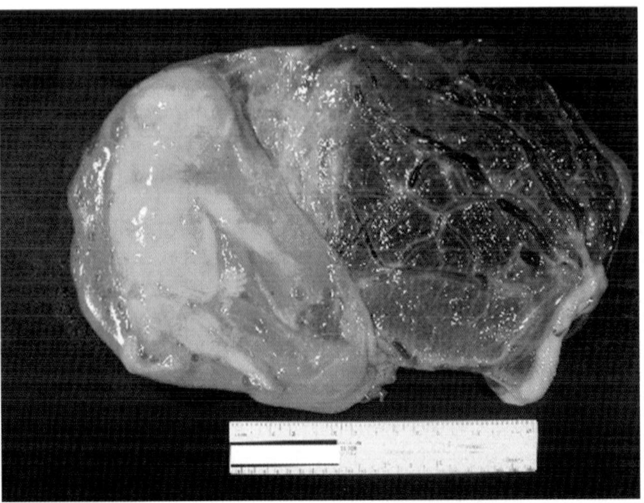

Figure 28-18. Placenta of a term delivery from a monochorionic twin pregnancy discordant for a fetal anomaly following early radiofrequency cord ablation. (From Shevell T, Malone FD, Weintraub J, et al: Radiofrequency ablation in a monochorionic twin discordant for fetal anomalies. Am J Obstet Gynecol 190:575, 2004, with permission.)

In summary, ST of an anomalous fetus in a multiple gestation is a medically acceptable option. It is important, however, to counsel the patient about the risks and benefits of the procedure versus expectant management. Furthermore, it is imperative to establish the chorionicity of the pregnancy and to be certain which fetus is abnormal before the procedure is performed.

First-Trimester Multifetal Pregnancy Reduction

The increasingly successful use of ovulation induction and ART has resulted in a growing number of multifetal pregnancies with three or more fetuses. Because the risk of preterm delivery is directly proportional to the number of fetuses being carried in the uterus, first-trimester reduction has been advocated as a method to reduce the risk of prematurity in these pregnancies. The original technique of transcervical aspiration of gestational sacs described by Dumez and Oury[262] has largely been abandoned. Currently, the method of choice consists of injecting a small dose of potassium chloride into the thorax of one or more of the fetuses, either transabdominally or transvaginally, under real-time sonographic guidance.[263] The latter approach is not used frequently because it is associated with more intrauterine infections and a higher loss rate than the former. In monochorionic pregnancies, the use of these techniques is contraindicated because vascular communications within the placenta can result in death or adverse long-term sequelae in the surviving fetus.

MPR is an outpatient procedure that results in the delivery of healthy infants close to term in the majority of cases.[264,265] It is usually performed between 11 and 13 weeks, and CVS can safely be performed on some or all of the fetuses before the procedure. Ultrasound is used to map the location of each fetus, and prophylactic antibiotics are often administered. Any fetus appearing to be anatomically abnormal, small for gestational age, or known to have a karyotypic abnormality is included amongst those that are reduced. Whenever possible, the fetus whose sac overlies the cervical os is not electively reduced, in order to minimize the risk of premature rupture of the membranes. Asystole is obtained by injecting an appropriate amount of potassium chloride into the thorax of one or more fetuses under direct sonographic observation. The patient is discharged after the operator is satisfied that no cardiac activity is evident in any of the fetuses that have undergone the procedure. Follow-up ultrasound examinations should be performed to confirm the success of the procedure and to monitor the growth of the remaining fetuses.

Evans et al.[264] published a series of 3,513 completed first-trimester MPR procedures from 11 centers in five countries. The overall rate of loss was 9.6 percent, but each of the participating centers showed significant improvement in this parameter as the operators developed more experience over time. The most recent collaborative overall rates of loss (1995 to 1998) were 4.5 percent for women starting with triplets, 7.3 percent for those with quadruplets, 11.4 percent for quintuplets, and 15.4 percent for sextuplets or higher. The rate of loss of those who reduced to twins was 6.0 percent, as compared with 18.4 percent for those who were left with triplets.

Stone and colleagues[265] reported the outcome of 1,000 consecutive patients undergoing MPR at a single institution. The overall unintended rate of pregnancy loss was 5.4 percent. The rate was 2.5 percent amongst those who reduced from twins to a singleton, and 12.9 percent for those who presented with 6 or more fetuses but was stable at 4.7 to 5.4 percent for women who started with either 3, 4, or 5 fetuses. The rates of loss were 16.7 percent, 5.5 percent, and 3.5 percent for those who reduced to triplets, twin and singletons respectively. Significantly, the mean gestational ages for surviving fetuses were 35.3 weeks and 33.5 weeks for twins and triplets, respectively, which is essentially identical to what would be expected if these women had initially conceived that number of fetuses.

While perinatal morbidity and mortality are clearly likely to improve when pregnancies with four or more fetuses are reduced to smaller numbers, the medical advantages of reducing triplets to twins remains unproven.[266] The significance of improving the mean gestational age at delivery by approximately 2 weeks when triplets are reduced to twins is probably marginal. Of greater importance, however, is the percentage of infants that deliver very prematurely. Women with triplets have approximately an 8-percent risk of delivering between 24 and 28 weeks, and a 25-percent risk of delivering between 24 and 32 weeks. In the series by Stone et al.,[265] these figures were 3.9 percent and 12.6 percent respectively for those who underwent MPR to twins. When larger series are accumulated, one would expect to see a reflection of these differences in both perinatal morbidity and mortality statistics. Several studies have suggested that patients undergoing reductions from triplets to twins have perinatal outcomes that are similar to unreduced twins, and better than those of expectantly managed triplets.[266,267] Nevertheless, much larger series are needed in order to meaningfully quantify the magnitude of improvement derived from reducing triplets to twins.

Following MPR to twins, women should be followed closely for all of the complications associated with multiple gestations. Because the majority of losses occur several weeks after the procedure, the period from 18 to 24 weeks should be one of heightened surveillance. It is also recommended that these patients not undergo second-trimester aneuploidy serum screening because maternal serum AFP levels have been shown to be significantly elevated as a result of the retained dead fetus(es).[268] Because the incidence of IUGR may be increased in the surviving fetuses following MPR procedures, serial sonographic growth assessment has been suggested.[269]

In a study of 100 women who had undergone MPR at one institution, Shreiner-Engel et al.[270] reported that in the vast majority of cases the primary rationale stated for undergoing the procedure was the couple's perception of the need to sacrifice the lives of some of their fetuses in order to maximize the potential benefits for those that remained. Almost all of the couples found the decision-making process and ensuing procedure to be extremely stressful and emotionally painful, but most were able to reconcile their grief reaction to the fetal loss or losses, bond normally to the remaining fetuses, and have few persistent negative feelings. Mild feelings of guilt and anger, and moderate sadness about the MPR persisted for many women. A small subset, however, continued to react to their reduction with considerable emotional distress, although not at the level of clinical significance.

Physically reducing the number of fetuses being carried is far from an ideal solution to the problems associated with multifetal pregnancies. It would certainly be better to avoid the problem altogether by effectively monitoring patients receiving ovulatory stimulants and minimizing the number of embryos transferred in IVF programs. It is recognized that even in the most skilled and conscientious hands the creation of multifetal pregnancies cannot be entirely eliminated in women receiving infertility therapy with existing technologies. Nevertheless, it should be possible to substantially reduce the number of cases of triplets currently being seen, and to virtually eliminate those with four or more fetuses. When, however, three or more fetuses have been conceived, the experience to date suggests that MPR is a relatively safe and effective option to consider for couples whose only choices in the past were either to accept a substantial risk of extreme prematurity or terminate the entire pregnancy.

MANAGEMENT OF MULTIPLE GESTATIONS

The Antepartum Period

PRETERM LABOR

Patients with a multiple gestation are at increased risk for preterm labor and delivery. Management strategies such as routine bed rest, prophylactic tocolytics, home uterine monitoring, and prophylactic cervical cerclage have not proven beneficial.[89]

Marivate and Norman[2] cite five studies that reported a reduction in perinatal mortality and prematurity rates and two others that found no difference in those variables when patients with twins who were routinely admitted to the hospital were compared with those treated as outpatients. Two prospective randomized trials published in 1984 and 1985 found no benefit from late elective hospital admission,[271,272] and in the latter study preterm delivery was more common among the hospitalized group.

Hawrylyshyn et al.[273] reported that in their series of 175 consecutive twin deliveries, bed rest after 30 weeks had no effect on perinatal mortality. Because 70 percent of the perinatal deaths in their study occurred before the 30th week, these workers concluded that elective hospitalization must include the period from 25 to 30 weeks in order to exert any significant impact on both the survival and the quality of survival of twins. In support of this concept, Chervenak et al.[274] found that 81 percent of the perinatal mortality in their series of 385 twin pregnancies occurred before the 29th week of gestation.

Two other studies that evaluated the role of early routine hospital admission for twin gestations came to similar conclusions. The first was a multicenter randomized study from Australia in which 11 hospitals participated.[275] Of 141 patients with twins in the study, 72 were assigned to outpatient care and 69 were hospitalized from 26 to 30 weeks' gestation. No differences between the groups could be demonstrated in the frequencies of major maternal complications, preterm delivery, or mean birth weights at delivery. Surprisingly, there was a trend toward greater frequency of preterm delivery and admission of neonates to the neonatal intensive care unit in the group admitted to the hospital. Leveno et al.[276] also observed no differences in pregnancy outcome between 134 patients with twin gestations that were hospitalized from 24 to 32 weeks as compared with 177 patients who were not routinely hospitalized.

Bed rest in the hospital is expensive and disrupts normal family life. Because there is no evidence to suggest that elective hospitalization is universally beneficial for patients with twins, we believe that these women should be hospitalized only for the same indications that would be used to admit those with singletons.

Prophylactic administration of tocolytic agents has been attempted with varying degrees of success. Marivate and Norman[2] cite one report in which pregnancy prolongation and increased birth weight were associated with this approach and three other series that found no improvement in those variables when prophylactic tocolysis was administered to patients with twins. Since an increased incidence of maternal cardiovascular complications has been reported in patients with multiple gestations who have been treated with β-agonists,[277] it seems prudent to restrict the use of those agents to women who are confirmed to be in preterm labor.

Results of studies using prophylactic cervical cerclage have been disappointing. A randomized trial of 128 patients with twins who were offered elective cerclage at 18 to 26 weeks did not demonstrate any benefit.[278] Likewise, prophylactic cerclage has not been shown to significantly improve perinatal outcomes in triplets.[279] Because this surgical procedure may be associated with adverse sequelae for both the mother and her fetuses, it is recommended that cerclage placement be restricted to women with either a strongly suggestive history or objectively documented cervical incompetence.

Ambulatory home monitoring of uterine contractions with a tocodynamometer used in an attempt to predict preterm labor has not been shown to be useful. A meta-analysis of 6 randomized trials was unable to demonstrate a significant benefit of home uterine activity monitoring to reduce the risk of preterm delivery in patients with twins.[280] Furthermore, a prospective trial of 2,422 patients, including 844 with twins, in which women were randomized to weekly nurse contact, daily nurse contact, or daily nurse contact in addition to home uterine activity monitoring, showed no difference in preterm delivery before 35 weeks' gestation.[281]

Houlton et al.[282] attempted to predict the onset of labor in a series of patients with twins by evaluating the effectiveness of a cervical assessment score derived by subtracting dilatation of the internal os in centimeters from the length of the cervix. These authors found a significant relationship between a low or serially decreasing score, and the onset of labor within the subsequent 14 days. Similar results were reported by Neilson et al.,[283] but O'Connor and colleagues found that routine cervical assessment and uterine activity measurements were not helpful in predicting preterm delivery.[284]

Premature cervical shortening and cervical funneling detected by transvaginal ultrasound examination have good predictive capabilities for the development of preterm labor and delivery in women with multiple gestations.[285–288] Studies suggest that a cervical length measurement of 35 mm at 24 to 26 weeks identifies women with twins who are at low risk for delivery before 34 weeks' gestation.[286] On the other hand, a cervical length of 25 mm or less with or without funneling at 24 weeks' gestation predicts a high risk for preterm labor and delivery.[285] A study by Goldenberg et al.[285] also found that a positive fetal fibronectin (FFN) test at 28 weeks is a significant predictor of spontaneous preterm labor before 32 weeks' gestation.

In the singleton population at high risk for preterm birth, weekly injections of 17 alpha-hydroxyprogesterone caproate have been shown to reduce the rate of preterm delivery.[289] It has been suggested that this treatment could reduce rates of preterm birth in patients with multiple gestations, and a Maternal-Fetal Medicine Network randomized trial did not show benefit of this hormone in twins.[289a]

Specialized Twin Clinics

The value of special twin clinics has been described.[290] In these clinics, where women known to be carrying twins are seen at regular intervals by the same medical team, several advantages accrue. Patients have the opportunity to develop rapport with a small group of caregivers. This results in an increased awareness of their special problems and may increase compliance with therapeutic directives. The patients can also talk with other women who are expecting twins, and they learn that their antenatal experiences are usually not unique. Furthermore, the medical personnel become more adept at detecting early signs of the special problems associated with twin pregnancies. Finally, and perhaps most importantly, the team of caregivers has the opportunity to develop antenatal management protocols that are maximally effective for this special group of patients.

Gestational Hypertension and Preeclampsia

Both gestational hypertension and preeclampsia are more common in women carrying a multiple gestation. In secondary analyses of prospective data from 684 twin pregnancies and 2,946 singletons from a multicenter trial of low-dose aspirin for the prevention of preeclampsia, rates of gestational hypertension and preeclampsia were twice as high in patients with twins.[291] In addition, women with twins whose pregnancies were complicated by gestational hypertension experienced higher rates of adverse perinatal outcomes such as preterm delivery and placental abruption. Rates of preeclampsia seem to be the same for both MZ and DZ twins.[292] Eclampsia also seems to be increased, although the etiology of these increased rates is unknown. In addition, when preeclampsia occurs in patients with a multiple gestation, it seems to occur earlier, is more severe, and is often atypical in presentation. Owing to the increased risk of preeclampsia, patients with multiple gestations require frequent monitoring for the early signs and symptoms of that disorder.

Other Maternal Complications

Patients with twins, triplets, and high-order multiple gestations are also at increased risk for other pregnancy complications such as threatened abortion, hyperemesis, anemia, urinary tract infections, musculoskeletal disorders, abnormal placentation, thromboembolism, preterm premature rupture of membranes, abruption, cesarean delivery, and postpartum hemorrhage.[16,89,93,293] Women with multiple pregnancies should receive extra iron supplementation. In addition, women with a multiple gestation may be prone to developing acute fatty liver of pregnancy.[294] This disease process is characterized by severe coagulopathy, hypoglycemia, hyperammonemia, and can cause maternal death. Whenever hepatic dysfunction is diagnosed in a patient with a multiple gestation, acute fatty liver should be considered in the differential diagnosis.

Antenatal Surveillance

Although it is prudent to follow fetal growth with serial ultrasound scans, routine antenatal testing in patients with an uncomplicated multiple gestation has not been demonstrated to improve outcomes.[89] Antenatal testing is suggested in all patients with multiple gestations complicated by IUGR, discordant growth, abnormal fluid volumes, TTTS, monoamnionicity, fetal anomalies, a single IUFD, and other medical/obstetric complications. For women with twins, options for antenatal testing include the nonstress test, the biophysical profile, and Doppler assessment.

Assessment of fetal well-being by simultaneous nonstress heart rate testing in twin pregnancies is both feasible and efficacious. DeVoe and Azor[295] followed 24 sets of twins who underwent 120 simultaneously recorded nonstress tests in the third trimester. Technical problems in obtaining readable tracings were encountered in only 15 percent of cases. Reactive nonstress tests were found to be associated with a good prognosis if delivery occurred within 1 week, whereas nonreactive nonstress tests were less specific but, in some cases, reflected nonreassuring fetal status in utero. These authors concluded that nonstress tests in twins, whether reactive or nonreactive, appear to be prognostically comparable to those previously reported in singleton third-trimester pregnancies. The study of Blake et al.[296] in 94 patients with multiple gestations confirmed that antepartum nonstress testing is a highly reliable and predictive test in the assessment of multiple gestations. As continuous monitoring of all fetuses in a triplet or high-order multiple gestations is challenging, a modified biophysical profile (8-point BPP without nonstress testing) is the most practical surveillance option for these patients. Nonstress testing may be used for fetuses with abnormal biophysical profile scores.[297]

When patients with a multiple gestation present for antenatal testing, and when they are being monitored in labor, each fetal heart rate tracing should be independently identified in order to know precisely which fetus is being monitored. Monitoring of triplets and high-order multiple gestations may require frequent sonographic identification of the appropriate fetus.

Routine Doppler studies have not been found to be helpful in the management of women with multiple gestations.[298,299] However, when IUGR or growth discordance is suspected in one or more fetuses, Doppler velocimetry is a useful adjunct in assessing and following these pregnancies. Furthermore, in cases of monochorionic twins with IUGR, discordant growth, or amniotic fluid volume abnormalities, Doppler studies of the ductus venosus may be helpful in identifying the possible overlapping pathologies of utero-placental insufficiency, and cardiac dysfunction.

Our protocol for the surveillance of patients with multiple gestations is as follows:

1. Ideally, an initial ultrasound is performed in the first trimester to determine the number of fetuses and the amnionicity/chorionicity in order to differentiate monochorionic and dichorionic gestations. Patients are also offered ultrasound for nuchal translucency at 10 3/7 to 13 6/7 weeks' gestation.
2. The second ultrasound evaluation is scheduled at 18 to 20 weeks' gestation. This includes standard biometry to confirm gestational age and the size of each fetus, assessment of amniotic fluid volume in each sac, and an anatomic survey of each fetus to rule out morphologic anomalies. If the patient did not have a first-trimester ultrasound, an attempt is made to determine chorionicity by examining fetal gender, the number of placentas, the thickness as well as number of layers in the membrane separating the sacs, and the presence or absence of the lambda or twin peak sign.
3. If the first two scans are normal and suggestive of dichorionic diamniotic twinning, subsequent scans for fetal growth are performed every 3 to 4 weeks thereafter as long as fetal growth and amniotic fluid volume in each sac remains normal.
4. If the initial scan is suggestive of monochorionic diamniotic placentation and, therefore, at potential risk for developing TTTS, subsequent scans are repeated every 2 to 3 weeks.
5. If there is evidence of IUGR, discordant fetal growth, or discordant fluid volumes, fetal surveillance is intensified and includes frequent nonstress testing, along with biophysical profile and Doppler velocimetry studies. Because absent end-diastolic or reversed diastolic flow can be a predictor of poor outcome or imminent death in utero, consideration should be given to delivering patients with these findings in one fetus if the other is mature enough for an elective delivery.
6. Daily nonstress testing starting at approximately 24 to 26 weeks' gestation is suggested for patients with monoamniotic twins because of their risk for sudden IUFD from cord entanglement. Although cord accidents cannot be predicted, daily fetal heart rate monitoring may reveal increasing frequency of variable decelerations. When variable decelerations are identified, continuous monitoring is recommended and may ultimately require delivery for nonreassuring fetal testing.

Fetal Lung Maturity

The clinical management of multiple gestations occasionally requires the assessment of fetal lung maturity. There is currently no consensus as to whether pulmonary maturation differs between singletons and multiples. In one study, it was found that after 31 weeks' gestation, twins exhibited higher TDx-FLM assay values compared with singletons.[300] The explanation for why twin gestations could have accelerated changes in their pulmonary maturity indices is not understood. Likewise, it is not known if these laboratory findings reflect relative differences in the risk of respiratory distress syndrome between singletons and multiples. If they do not, new parameters will be needed to avoid false-positive prediction of adequate lung maturity in twins.

If elective delivery is scheduled before 38 weeks' gestation, amniocentesis for fetal lung maturity determination may be considered. A recent study of fetal lung maturity in 58 diamniotic twins indicated that asynchronous pulmonary maturity may occur, regardless of fetal sex and size.[301] Twenty-five percent of twin pairs before 32 weeks' gestation had a significant disparity, usually due to the fact that one twin demonstrated greater lung maturity than expected for gestational age.[301] These data indicate that fetal lung maturity indices from one twin may not be predictive of its co-twin's status, particularly for pregnancies less than 32 weeks' gestation. Therefore, if technically feasible, it is suggested that the gestational sac of each twin be sampled when amniocentesis for lung maturity is required. For pregnancies with triplets and high-order multiple gestations, there are not enough data to make recommendations regarding amniocentesis for fetal lung maturity.

The Intrapartum Period

Mode of Delivery

A number of factors must be considered when determining the mode of delivery for patients with multiple gestations. These variables include the gestational age and estimated weights of the fetuses, their positions relative to each other, the availability of real-time ultrasound on the labor floor and in the delivery room, and the capability of monitoring each twin independently during the entire intrapartum period. Older series may not be applicable to current practice because our ability to monitor both twins closely during labor and delivery has increased considerably in recent years.

All combinations of intrapartum twin presentations can be classified into three groups: twin A vertex, twin B vertex; twin A vertex, twin B nonvertex; and twin A nonvertex, twin B either vertex or nonvertex. In a series of 362 twin deliveries presented by Chervenak et al.,[302] these presentations were found in 42.5, 38.4, and 19.1 percent of cases, respectively. In the series, 81.2 percent of the vertex-vertex twin gestations were delivered vaginally. These investigators believe that when both twins are in vertex presentation, a cesarean delivery should be considered only for the same indications applied to singletons. This recommendation holds true for any gestational age provided that both twins can be monitored during labor.

Cesarean delivery is the method of choice when the presenting twin is in a nonvertex position. External cephalic version of the presenting twin would be difficult, if not impossible, in these patients. Furthermore, if the second twin is in a vertex presentation and faces its sibling, the potential for locking exists. Khunda[303] states that the frequency of locking is approximately 1 per 1,000 twin deliveries, with an associated fetal mortality of 31 percent. This condition occurs most commonly in breech-vertex presentations, when the fetal chins overlie each other. It is usually not recognized until the body of the presenting twin is out of the vagina and the aftercoming head cannot be delivered. Eventually it becomes clear that entry of the first twin's head into the pelvis is being obstructed by that of the second twin. Sevitz and Merrell[304] described a case in which a vaginal delivery was accomplished and one twin survived after intravenous administration of a beta-mimetic agent to a woman whose twins had locked during delivery. The more devastating consequences of this disorder, however, have been aptly described by Nissen.[305] Finally, it is possible that the second twin could complicate the delivery of the first twin in more subtle ways, such as by deflexing its head.

The management of that subset of patients whose twins are in a vertex-breech or vertex-transverse lie is particularly controversial. Chervenak et al.[302] cite 11 references in which depressed Apgar scores and increased perinatal mortality rates associated with vaginal breech delivery of the second twin have led some investigators to recommend cesarean delivery whenever twin B is in a nonvertex lie. On the other hand, Acker et al.[306] compared 74 nonvertex first or second twins weighing more than 1,499 g delivered by cesarean section to 76 nonvertex second twins with similar birth weights delivered vaginally and found no perinatal deaths in either groups or statistically significant differences in low 5-minute Apgar scores.

Chervenak and colleagues[307] analyzed the intrapartum management of 93 vertex-breech and 42 vertex-transverse twin sets. Seventy-eight percent of the vertex-breech group and 53 percent of the vertex-transverse group were delivered vaginally. These authors state that their data do not definitively prove vaginal breech delivery of a low-birth-weight second twin to be more damaging than cesarean delivery. Nevertheless, because of the documented ill effects of vaginal delivery on low-birth-weight singleton breech infants, this mode of delivery was not advised for second twins weighing less than 1,500 g. On the other hand, if a second twin weighs between 1,500 and 3,500 g and the criteria for vaginal delivery of a singleton breech are met, this series suggests that vaginal breech delivery is an acceptable option.

The same group has also reported their experience with 25 external cephalic versions performed on 14 transverse and 11 breech second twins.[308] Version-to-vertex presentation was successful in 71 and 73 percent of cases, respectively. Among the 25 attempted cases, only two neonates had 5-minute Apgar scores below 7. However, in a study reported by Gocke et al.,[309] the success rate for external cephalic version of the second twin was only 46 percent. Their study analyzed 136 sets of vertex-nonvertex twins with birth weights higher than 1,500 g in whom delivery of the second twin was managed by primary cesarean delivery, external version, or primary breech extraction. No differences were noted in the incidence of neonatal mortality or morbidity among the three modes of delivery, but external version was associated with a higher failure rate than breech extraction, a higher rate of nonreassuring fetal heart rate patterns, cord prolapse, and compound presentation. Therefore, the authors, concluded that primary breech extraction of the second nonvertex twin weighing more than 1,500 g is a reasonable alternative to either cesarean delivery or external version.

Analyzing their own extensive experience along with a review of the published literature, Chervenak et al.[302] have made the following recommendations for patients presenting with twins in a vertex-nonvertex presentation. If the weight of the second twin has not been estimated sonographically within 1 to 2 weeks, this should be done during the intrapartum period. If one assumes that sonographic estimates of fetal weight are accurate to within +/− 20 percent, a cutoff of 2,000 g is unlikely to result in the birth of a neonate weighing less than 1,500 g. On the basis of the arguments cited earlier, the investigators believe that a birth weight in excess of 1,500 g is sufficient for a vaginal breech delivery, but a lower weight is not. Regardless of the estimated weight, they suggest that an attempt be made to convert the second twin to a vertex presentation by performing an external version after the first twin has been delivered. If this proves successful, a vaginal delivery can be anticipated. If the attempted version is unsuccessful and the estimated fetal weight (EFW) is between 2,000 and 3,500 g, a breech extraction can be performed if the other criteria for a singleton vaginal breech delivery are met. Reports support these recommendations and have documented the efficacy and safety of either external cephalic version[310] or total breech extraction[311,312] for the delivery of second nonvertex twins weighing more than 1,500 g. However, if the EFW of the second twin is less than 2,000 g, or the criteria for a singleton vaginal breech delivery are not met, a cesarean delivery should be performed following a failed external version.

It is interesting to note that breech vaginal delivery of a second twin has become even more controversial since Hannah et al.[313] published the results of the International Randomized Term Breech Trial. This study suggests that in singletons, planned cesarean delivery for pregnancies with breech presentation at term results in a significant reduction in adverse perinatal outcomes without increased immediate maternal morbidity. As a result of that publication, the vaginal delivery of singleton breeches has largely been abandoned. As a consequence, fewer obstetricians are obtaining or maintaining the skills needed to safely perform vaginal breech deliveries. This suggests that in the future, there will be fewer physicians capable of safely performing a second twin breech delivery.

Although vaginal delivery is an option for patients with triplets, there are no large prospective studies establishing its safety.[314] Adequate monitoring of three fetuses throughout labor and delivery is challenging. As a result, elective cesarean delivery of patients with three or more live fetuses of viable gestational age is a reasonable management strategy.

Time Interval Between Deliveries

A variable that many investigators have considered to be important in the outcome of twin pregnancies is the time interval between deliveries. After delivery of the first twin, uterine inertia may develop, the umbilical cord of the second twin can prolapse, and partial separation of its placenta may render the second twin hypoxic. In addition, the cervix can clamp down, making rapid delivery of the second twin extremely difficult if nonreassuring fetal status develops. Many reports have suggested that the interval between deliveries should ideally be within 15 minutes and certainly not more than 30 minutes.[8,66,315,316] Most of the data in support of this view, however, were obtained before the advent of intrapartum fetal monitoring.

Rayburn et al.[317] reported the outcome of 115 second twins delivered vaginally at or beyond 34 weeks' gestation after the vertex delivery of their siblings. The second twin was visually monitored with ultrasound on some occasions, and continuous monitoring of the fetal heart was performed in all cases. Oxytocin was used if uterine contractions subsided within 10 minutes after delivery of the first twin. In this series, 70 second twins delivered within 15 minutes of the first twin, 28 within 16 and 30 minutes, and 17 more than 30 minutes later. The longest interval between deliveries was 134 minutes. All of these infants survived, and none of them had traumatic deliveries. All 17 of the neonates delivering beyond 30 minutes had 5-minute Apgar scores of 8 and 10. In those cases with delivery intervals in excess of 15 minutes, the birth weight differential was not in excess of +/− 200g when first and second twins were compared. In the series reported by Chervenak et al.,[308] the fetal heart rate of the second twin was monitored with ultrasound visualization throughout the period between twin deliveries, and no difference in the occurrence of low 5-minute Apgar scores was noted in relationship to the length of the interdelivery interval.

Therefore, it seems apparent that although some second twins may require rapid delivery, others can be safely followed with fetal heart rate surveillance and remain undelivered for substantial periods of time. This less hurried approach when the second twin is not demonstrating signs of nonreassuring fetal status may reduce the incidence of both maternal and fetal trauma associated with difficult deliveries performed to meet arbitrary deadlines.

Delayed-Interval Delivery

Delayed-interval delivery, also known as asynchronous delivery, refers to the delivery of one fetus in a multiple gestation that is not followed by the immediate birth of the others. For example, Mashiach et al.[318] reported a case of a woman with a triplet pregnancy in a uterus didelphys, with fetuses A and B in the right uterine horn and fetus C in the left. Fetal demise of triplet A was noted at 22 weeks. At 27 weeks, the right horn began to contract and a macerated fetus was delivered vaginally, but the passage of fetus B was obstructed by the vertex of fetus C. A cesarean was then performed on the right uterine horn, and a 1,080g infant was delivered who died in 2 weeks. Because the left horn was not contracting, it was left intact. At 37 weeks, 72 days after the first two deliveries, an elective cesarean was performed, and a 2,490g healthy infant was delivered, who went home with the mother on the 7th postpartum day. These authors cite several other examples of significant delays in the delivery of twins who were located in separate uterine horns.

It must be recognized that many of the published case reports represent spectacular successes.[318–320] Delayed-interval delivery may be associated with perinatal death and maternal complications secondary to infection.[321] In a recent report, it was noted that when the first twin delivered between 22 and 23 weeks, delayed-interval delivery *was* associated with reduced perinatal and infant mortality in the second twin provided that delivery occurred within 3 weeks. Delayed-interval delivery was of no benefit if the first twin delivered after 24 weeks.[322]

This type of management should be reserved for patients with pregnancies complicated by extreme prematurity. The management protocol for these patients includes high ligation of the umbilical cord of the delivered twin with an absorbable suture, bed rest, ongoing monitoring of the mother for evidence of infection or coagulation disorders, and serial monitoring for growth and well-being of the viable fetuses. In the management of these pregnancies, areas that remain controversial are the routine use of cervical cerclage, prophylactic tocolytics, prophylactic antibiotics, and corticosteriods for enhancement of fetal lung maturity of the viable fetuses. Asynchronous delivery is contraindicated in women with monochorionic pregnancies, intra-amniotic infection, placental abruption, and preeclampsia. If an individual case is considered for such a treatment protocol, the potential risks, which may be considerable, along with the benefits must be discussed in detail. Fully informed consent must be obtained from the patient and her partner.

Ultrasound and the Intrapartum Management of Multiple Gestations

Ultrasound is important in the management of multiple gestations during the intrapartum period. On admission to the delivery floor, the position of each twin can be quickly and accurately assessed, and viability of both fetuses confirmed by direct visualization of their hearts. Knowledge of the presentation of each twin permits the establishment of a management protocol regarding the anticipated route of delivery. If a vaginal delivery is to be attempted, the weights of both twins can be rapidly estimated. This information is particularly important for the second twin because if it is thought to weigh less than 1,500g or more than 3,500g, a vaginal breech delivery might not be attempted. It is also possible to rule out extension of the head when a fetus is in breech presentation with an ultrasound examination. Ballas et al.[323] cited an incidence of more than 70 percent for spinal cord transection when 11 breeches with extended heads were delivered vaginally compared with no cord injuries when nine infants with deflexed heads were delivered by cesarean. Although these data were derived from singleton breeches, there is no reason to believe that they could not apply to twins as well.

Both fetuses must be monitored electronically throughout labor in order to ensure their well-being. When membranes are already ruptured, a scalp electrode can easily be attached to the head of twin A, and the second twin can be monitored with an external Doppler transducer. In practice, however, it is sometimes difficult to find the optimal spot from which to monitor the second twin. By using real-time ultrasound, the heart of twin B can be precisely located and the Doppler transducer placed accordingly. If movement of the second twin results in loss of a readable tracing, the transducer can be repositioned after real-time ultrasound has revealed the new position of twin B's heart. When a patient with twins or triplets is taken to the delivery room, the real-time ultrasound unit should accompany her. After delivery of the first infant, real-time examination immediately and precisely establishes the position of the second fetus. Visualization of the fetal heart allows the second fetus to be monitored for evidence of bradycardia until the fetus settles into the pelvis, membranes are ruptured, and a scalp electrode can be applied. Although visual monitoring of the heart does not provide subtle information such as a loss of baseline variability, it does permit early detection of significant deviations from the normal fetal heart rate range.

In addition to monitoring heart rate, visualization of the second twin permits both external and internal manipulations to be performed in a more controlled fashion. Externally, it is often possible to guide the vertex over the inlet by directing pressure from the ultrasound transducer over the fetal head while pushing the buttocks toward the fundus with the other hand. If this is unsuccessful, an internal version can be made less difficult by visualizing the operator's hand within the uterus and directing it toward the fetal feet. This technique can reduce the confusion often experienced when a small fetal part is blindly caught, and it is unclear whether it belongs to an upper or lower extremity.

CONCLUSION

The patient carrying more than one fetus presents a formidable challenge to the obstetrician. The high perinatal morbidity and mortality rates traditionally associated with multiple gestations are due to a variety of factors, some of which can not be currently altered. However, extraordinary technologic advances during the past 25 years have given us new insights into problems peculiar to multifetal pregnancies as well as tools with which to detect and treat those problems. Early diagnosis of multiple gestations and serial follow-up studies offer the potential for administering specialized regimens to selected patients, which hopefully will lead to a beneficial impact on the outcome of those pregnancies.

KEY POINTS

- Perinatal and neonatal morbidity and mortality are significantly higher in multiple gestations than singleton pregnancies.
- Preterm labor and delivery are major risks for patients with a multiple gestation.
- Any patient with a multiple gestation should be clinically managed as a high-risk pregnancy.
- The incidence of congenital structural malformations is higher in fetuses of multiple gestations than in singletons.
- Ultrasound evaluation is the single most important diagnostic test in multiple gestations.
- All patients with multiple gestations should have detailed first- and second trimester ultrasound examinations to assess for chorionicity, amnionicity, individual fetal growth, and congenital malformations.
- Twin-to-twin transfusion syndrome is a serious potential complication in monochorionic twins, and is associated with a high fetal mortality rate.
- Prophylactic cerclage, prophylactic tocolytics, routine bed rest, and home uterine activity monitoring do not provide any proven advantage in the management of multiple gestations.
- The presentation of each fetus must be sonographically verified as soon as a patient with a twin pregnancy presents in labor.
- Mode of delivery should take into account gestational age, fetal position, and the experience of the obstetrician. Vaginal delivery is an option when both twins are vertex. The mode of delivery should be individualized for vertex-nonvertex twins. Cesarean delivery is optimal when the first twin is nonvertex. For triplets and high-order multiples, vaginal delivery should be attempted only by experienced obstetricians who are continuously monitoring each of the fetuses.

REFERENCES

1. Hrubec Z, Robinette CD: The study of human twins in medical research. N Engl J Med 310:435, 1984.
2. Marivate M, Norman RJ: Twins. Clin Obstet Gynaecol 9:723, 1982.
3. Dickey RP, Taylor SN, Lu PY, et al: Risk factors for high-order multiple pregnancy and multiple birth after controlled ovarian hyperstimulation: results of 4,062 intrauterine insemination cycles. Fertil Steril 83:671, 2005.
4. Fauser BC, Devroey P, Macklon NS: Multiple birth resulting from ovarian stimulation for subfertility treatment. Lancet 365:1807, 2005.
5. Martin JA, Hamilton BE, Sutton PD, et al: Births final data 2002. National Vital Statistics Reports, Vol. 42, No. 10. Hyattsville, MD, National Center for Health Statistics 2003.

6. American Society for Reproductive Medicine: Guidelines on the number of embryos transferred. Fertil Steril 82:773, 2004.
7. Jain T, Missmer SA, Hornstein MD: Trends in embryo-transfer practices and in outcomes of the use of assisted reproductive technology in the United States. N Engl J Med 350:1639, 2004
8. Benirschke K, Kim CK: Multiple pregnancy [first of two parts]. N Engl J Med 288:1276, 1973.
9. Derom C, Derom R, Vlietnik R, et al: Increased monozygotic twinning rate after ovulation induction. Lancet 2:1236, 1987.
10. Blickstein I, Verhoeven HC, Keith LG: Zygotic splitting after assisted reproduction. N Engl J Med 340:738, 1999.
11. Blickstein I, Jones C, Keith LG: Zygotic-splitting rates after single-embryo transfers in in vitro fertilization. N Engl J Med 348:2366, 2003.
12. Hankins GV, Saade GR: Factors influencing twins and zygosity. Paediatr Perinat Epidemiol 19 Suppl 1:8, 2005.
13. Blickstein I: Estimation of iatrogenic monozygotic twinning rate following assisted reproduction: Pitfalls and caveats. Am J Obstet Gynecol 19:365, 2005.
14. Ananth CV, Joseph KS K, Smulian JC: Trends in twin neonatal mortality rates in the United States, 1989 through 1999: influence of birth registration and obstetric intervention. Am J Obstet Gynecol 190:1313, 2004.
15. Luke B: The changing pattern of multiple births in the United States: maternal and infant characteristics, 1973 and 1990. Obstet Gynecol 84:101, 1994.
16. Devine PC, Malone FD, Athanassiou A, et al: Maternal and neonatal outcome of 100 consecutive triplet pregnancies. Am J Perintol 18:225, 2001.
17. Rydhstroem H, Heraib F: Gestational duration, and fetal and infant mortality for twins vs singletons. Twin Res 4:227, 2001.
18. Matthews TJ, Menacker F, MacDorman MF: Infant mortality statistics from the 2001 period linked birth/infant death data set. National Vital Statistics Reports; Vol 52, no 2. Hyattsville, Maryland: National Center for Health Statistics, 2003.
19. Blickstein I, Keith LG: Outcome of triplets and high-order multiple pregnancies: Curr Opin Obstet Gynecol 15:113, 2003.
20. Newman RB, Hamer C, Clinton Miller M: Outpatient triplet management: a contemporary review. Am J Obstet Gynecol 161:547, 1989.
21. Skrablin S, Kuvacic I, Kalafatic D, et al: Prenatal care improves the outcome of triplets. Eur J Obstet Gynecol Reprod Biol 104:26, 2002.
22. Geipel A, Berg C, Katalinic A, et al: Prenatal diagnosis and obstetric outcomes in triplet pregnancies in relation to chorionicity. Br J Obstet Gynaecol 112:554, 2005.
23. Collins MS, Bleyl JA: Seventy-one quadruplet pregnancies: management and outcome. Am J Obstet Gynecol 162:1384, 1990.
24. Elliott JP, Radin TG: Quadruplet pregnancy: contemporary management and outcome. Obstet Gynecol 80:421, 1992.
25. Salihu HM, Aliyu MH, Kirby RS, Alexander GR: Effect of advanced maternal age on early mortality among quadruplets and quintuplets. Am J Obstet Gynecol 190:383, 2004.
26. Donovan EF, Ehrenkrang RA, Shankaran S, et al: Outcomes of very low birth weight twins cared for in the National Institute of Child Health and Human Development Neonatal Research Network's intensive care units. Am J Obstet Gynecol 179:742, 1998.
27. Blickstein I: Cerebral palsy in multifetal pregnancies: Dev Med Child Neurol 44:352, 2002.
28. Topp M, Huusom LD, Langhoff Roos J, et al: Multiple birth and cerebral palsy in Europe: a multicenter study. Acta Obstet Gynecol Scand 83:548, 2004.
29. Nielson HC, Harvey-Wilkes K, MacKinnon B, et al: Neonatal outcome of very premature infants from multiple gestation. Am J Obstet Gynecol 177:653, 1997.
30. Kaufman GE, Malone FD, Harvey-Wilkes K, et al: Neonatal morbidity and mortality associated with triplet pregnancy. Obstet Gynecol 91:342, 1998.
31. Arlettaz R, Paraskevopoulos E, Bucher HU: Triplets and quadruplets in Switzerland: comparison with singletons, evolution over the last decade. J Perinat Med 31:242, 2003.
32. Garite TJ, Clark RH, Elliott JP, Thorp JA: Twins and triplets: the effect of plurality and growth on neonatal outcome compared with singleton infants. Am J Obstet Gynecol 191: 700, 2004.
33. McDonald S, Murphy K, Beyene J, Ohlsson A: Perinatal outcomes of invitro fertilization twins: a systematic review and meta-analyses. Am J Obstet Gynecol 193:141, 2005.
34. Helmerhorst FM, Perquin DA, Donker D, Keirse MJ: Perinatal outcome of singletons and twins after assisted conception: a systematic review of controlled studies. BMJ 328:261, 2004.
35. Luke B, Brown MB, Nugent C, et al: Risk factors for adverse outcomes in spontaneous versus assisted conception twin pregnancies. Fertil Steril 81:315, 2004.
36. Lukassen HG, Schonbeck Y, Adang EM: Cost analysis of singleton versus twin pregnancies after in vitro fertilization. Fertil Steril 81:1240, 2004.
37. Malone FD, Chelmow D, Athanassiou A, D'Alton ME: Impact of gestational age at delivery of economics of triplet pregnancy. J Matern Fetal Med 8:256, 1999.
38. Henderson J, Hockley C, Petrou S, et al: Economic implications of multiple births: inpatient hospital costs in the first 5 years of life. Arch Dis Child Fetal Neonatal Ed 89:F542, 2004.
39. Barth RA, Crowe HC: Ultrasound evaluation of multifetal gestations. *In* Callen PW (ed): Ultrasonography in Obstetrics and Gynecology, ed 4, Philadelphia, WB Saunders, 2000, p 171.
40. Cetrulo CL, Ingardia CJ, Sbarra AJ: Management of multiple gestation. Clin Obstet Gynecol 23:533, 1980.
41. Persson PH, Kullander S: Long-term experience of general ultrasound screening in pregnancy. Am J Obstet Gynecol 146:942, 1983.
42. LeFevre ML, Bain RP, Ewigman BG, et al: A randomized trial of prenatal ultrasonographic screening: impact on maternal management and outcome. Am J Obstet Gynecol 169:483, 1993.
43. Souter VL, Kapur RP, Nyholt DR, et al: Brief report: A report of dizygous monochorionic twins. N Engl J Med 349:154, 2003.
44. Miura K, Niikawa NJ: Do monochorionic dizygotic twins increase after pregnancy by assisted reproductive technology? Hum Genet 50:1, 2005.
45. Cameron AH: The Birmingham twin survey. Proc R Soc Med 61:229, 1968.
46. Norton ME, D'Alton ME, Bianchi DW: Molecular zygosity studies aid the management of discordant multiple gestations. J Perinatol 17:302, 1997.
47. Monteagudo A, Roman AS: Ultrasound in multiple gestations: twins and other multifetal pregnancies. Clin Perinatol 32:329, 2005.
48. Bessis R, Papiernik E: Echographic imagery of amniotic membranes in twin pregnancies. *In* Gedda L, Parisi P (eds): Twin Research 3: Twin Biology and Multiple Pregnancy. New York, Alan R Liss, 1981, p 183.
49. Finberg HJ: The "twin peak" sign: Reliable evidence of dichorionic twinning. J Ultrasound Med 11:571, 1992.
50. Monteagudo A, Timor-Tritsch IE, Sharma S: Early and simple determination of chorionic and amniotic type in multifetal gestations in the first fourteen weeks by high-frequency transvaginal ultrasonography. Am J Obstet Gynecol 170:824, 1994.
51. Sepulveda W, Seibre NJ, Hughes K, et al: The lambda sign at 10–14 weeks of gestation as a predictor of chorionicity in twin pregnancies. Ultrasound Obstet Gynecol 7:421, 1996.
52. Bromley B, Benacerraf B: Using the number of yolk sacs to determine amnionicity in early first trimester monochorionic twins. J Ultrasound Med 14:415, 1995.
53. Weiss JL, Devine PV: False positive diagnosis of conjoined twins in the first trimester. Ultrasound Obstet Gynecol 20:516, 2002.
54. Mahony BS, Filly RA, Callen PW: Amnionicity and chorionicity in twin pregnancies: prediction using ultrasound. Radiology 155:205, 1985.
55. Hertzberg BS, Kurtz AB, Choi HY, et al: Significance of membrane thickness in the sonographic evaluation of twin gestations. AJR Am J Roentgenol 148:151, 1987.
56. Townsend RR, Simpson GF, Filly RA: Membrane thickness in ultrasound prediction of chorionicity of twin gestations. J Ultrasound Med 7:327, 1988.
57. Winn HN, Gabrielli S, Reece EA, et al: Ultrasonographic criteria for the prenatal diagnosis of placental chorionicity in twin gestations. Am J Obstet Gynecol 161:1540, 1989.
58. D'Alton ME, Dudley DK: Ultrasound in the antenatal management of twin gestation. Semin Perinatol 10:30, 1986.

59. D'Alton ME, Dudley DK: The ultrasonographic prediction of chorionicity in twin gestation. Am J Obstet Gynecol 160:557, 1989.
60. Nyberg DA, Filly RA, Golbus MS, et al: Entangled umbilical cords: a sign of monoamniotic twins. J Ultrasound Med 3:29, 1984.
61. McKeown T, Record RG: Observations on foetal growth in multiple pregnancy in man. J Endocrinol 8:386, 1952.
62. Daw E, Walker J: Growth differences in twin pregnancy. Br J Clin Pract 29:150, 1975.
63. Iffy L, Lavenhar MA, Jakobovits A, Kaminetzky HA: The rate of early intrauterine growth in twin gestation. Am J Obstet Gynecol 146:970, 1983.
64. Fenner A, Malm T, Kusserow U: Intrauterine growth of twins. Eur J Pediatr 133:119, 1980.
65. Winick M, Brasel JA, Velasco EG: Effects of prenatal nutrition upon pregnancy risk. Clin Obstet Gynecol 16:184, 1973.
66. Kohl SG, Casey G: Twin gestation. Mt Sinai J Med 42:523, 1975.
67. Leveno KJ, Santos-Ramos R, Duenhoelter JH, et al: Sonar cephalometry in twins: a table of biparietal diameters for normal twin fetuses and a comparison with singletons. Am J Obstet Gynecol 135:727, 1979.
68. Bleker OP, Kloosterman GJ, Huldekoper BL, Breur W: Intrauterine growth of twins as estimated from birthweight and the fetal biparietal diameter. Eur J Obstet Reprod Biol 7:85, 1977.
69. Schneider L, Bessis R, Tabaste JL, et al: Echographic survey of twin foetal growth: a plea for specific charts for twins. *In* Nance WE (ed): Twin Research: Clinical Studies. New York, Alan R Liss, 1977, p 137.
70. Grumbach K, Coleman BG, Arger PH, et al: Twin and singleton growth patterns compared using ultrasound. Radiology 158:237, 1986.
71. Socol ML, Tamura RK, Sabbagha RE, et al: Diminished biparietal diameter and abdominal circumference growth in twins. Obstet Gynecol 64:235, 1984.
72. Scheer K: Ultrasound in twin gestations. J Clin Ultrasound 2:197, 1975.
73. Crane JP, Tomich PG, Kopta M: Ultrasonic growth patterns in normal and discordant twins. Obstet Gynecol 55:678, 1980.
74. Graham D, Shah Y, Moodley S, et al: Biparietal diameter femoral length growth in normal twin pregnancies [abstract 112]. Society of Perinatal Obstetricians. Annual Meeting, February 1984.
75. Shah YG, Graham D, Stinson SK, et al: Biparietal diameter growth in uncomplicated twin gestation. Am J Perinatol 4:229, 1987.
76. Haines CJ, Langlois SL, Jones WR: Ultrasonic measurement of fetal femoral length in singleton and twin pregnancies. Am J Obstet Gynecol 155:838, 1986.
77. Dorros G: The prenatal diagnosis of intrauterine growth retardation in one fetus of a twin gestation. Obstet Gynecol 48(Suppl):46, 1976.
78. Leveno KJ, Santos-Ramos R, Duenhoelter JH, et al: Sonar cephalometry in twin pregnancy: discordancy of the biparietal diameter after 28 weeks' gestation. Am J Obstet Gynecol 138:615, 1980.
79. Houlton MCC: Divergent biparietal diameter growth rates in twin pregnancies. Obstet Gynecol 49:542, 1977.
80. Chitkara U, Berkowitz GS, Levine R, et al: Twin pregnancy: routine use of ultrasound examinations in the prenatal diagnosis of IUGR and discordant growth. Am J Perinatol 2:49, 1985.
81. Hill LM, Guzick D, Chenevey P, et al: The sonographic assessment of twin growth discordancy. Obstet Gynecol 84:501, 1994.
82. Neilson JP: Detection of the small-for-dates twin fetus by ultrasound. Br J Obstet Gynaecol 88:27, 1981.
83. Yarkouni S, Reece EA, Holford T, et al: Estimated fetal weight in the evaluation of growth in twin gestations: a prospective longitudinal study. Obstet Gynecol 69:636, 1987.
84. Brown CEL, Guzick DS, Leveno KJ, et al: Prediction of discordant twins using ultrasound measurement of biparietal diameter and abdominal perimeter. Obstet Gynecol 70:677, 1987.
85. Storlazzi E, Vintzileos AM, Campbell WA, et al: Ultrasonic diagnosis of discordant fetal growth in twin gestations. Obstet Gynecol 69:363, 1987.
86. Benirschke K, Kim CK: Multiple pregnancy [second of two parts]. N Engl J Med 288:1329, 1973.
87. Rogers JG, Voullaire L, Gold H: Monozygotic twins discordant for trisomy 21. Am J Med Genet 11:143, 1982.
88. Dallapiccola B, Stomeo C, Ferranti B, et al: Discordant sex in one of three monozygotic triplets. J Med Genet 22:6, 1985.
89. American College of Obstetricians and Gynecologists. Multiple gestation: complicated twin, triplet, and high-order multifetal pregnancy. ACOG Practice Bulletin No. 56. Washington DC: American College of Obstetricians and Gynecologists; October 2004.
90. Meyers C, Adam R, Dungan J, Prenger V: Aneuploidy in twin gestations: when is maternal age advanced? Obstet Gynecol 89:248, 1997.
91. Odibo AO, Elkousy MH, Ural SH, et al: Screening for aneuploidy in twin pregnancies: maternal age- and race-specific risk assessment between 9–14 weeks. Twin Res 6:251, 2003.
92. Wald NJ, Huttly WJ, Hackshaw AK: Antenatal screening for Down's syndrome with the quadruple test. Lancet 361:835, 2003.
93. Graham G, Simpson LL: Diagnosis and management of obstetrical complications unique to multiple gestations. Clin Obstetr Gynecol 47:163, 2004.
94. Maymon R, Jauniaux E, Herman A: Down's syndrome screening in twin pregnancies by nuchal translucency measurement. Current concept. Minerva Ginecol 54:211, 2002.
95. Pandyaa PP, Snijders RJM, Johnson SP, et al: Screening for fetal trisomies by maternal age and fetal nuchal translucency thickness at 10–14 weeks of gestation. Br J Obstet Gynaecol 102:957, 1995.
96. Odibo AO, Lawrence-Cleary K, Macones GA: Screening for aneuploidy in twins and higher-order multiples: is first-trimester nuchal translucency the solution? Obstet Gynecol Surv 58:609, 2003.
97. Sebire NJ, D'Ercole C, Hughes K, et al: Increased nuchal translucency thickness at 10–14 weeks of gestation as a predictor of severe twin-to-twin transfusion syndrome. Ultrasound Obstet Gynecol 10:86, 1997.
98. Malone FD, D'Alton ME, Society for Maternal Fetal Medicine: First-trimester sonographic screening for Down syndrome. Obstet Gynecol 102:1066, 2003.
99. Spencer K, Nicolaides KH: Screening for trisomy 21 in twins using first trimester ultrasound and maternal serum biochemistry in a one stop clinic: a review of three years experience. Br J Obstet Gynaecol 110:276, 2003.
100. Spencer K: Screening for trisomy 21 in twin pregnancies in the first trimester: does chorionicity impact on maternal serum free B-hCG or PAPP-A levels? Prenat Diagn 21:715, 2001.
101. Wapner RJ: Genetic diagnosis in multiple pregnancies. Semin Perinatol 19:351, 1995.
102. Edwards MS, Ellings JM, Newman RB, et al: Predictive value of antepartum ultrasound examination for anomalies in twin gestations. Ultrasound Obstet Gynecol 6:43, 1995.
103. Jenkins TM, Wapner RJ: The challenge of prenatal diagnosis in twin pregnancies. Curr Opin Obstet Gynecol 12:87, 2000.
104. Beischer NA, Pepperell RJ, Barrie JU: Twin pregnancy and erythroblastosis. Obstet Gynecol 34:22, 1969.
105. Ellis MI, Coxon A, Noble C: Intrauterine transfusion of twins. BMJ 1:609, 1970.
106. Elias S, Gerbie AB, Simpson JL, et al: Genetic amniocentesis in twin gestations. Am J Obstet Gynecol 138:169, 1980.
107. Sebire NJ, Noble PL, Odibo A, et al: Single uterine entry for genetic amniocentesis in twin pregnancies. Ultrasound Obstet Gynecol 7:26, 1996.
108. McEnerney JK, McEnerney LN: Unfavorable neonatal outcome after intraamniotic injection of methylene blue. Obstet Gynecol 61(Suppl):35, 1983.
109. Nicolini U, Monni G: Intestinal obstruction in babies exposed in utero to methylene blue. Lancet 336:1258, 1990.
110. Van Der Pol JG, Wolf H, Boer K, et al: Jejunal atresia related to the use of methylene blue in genetic amniocentesis in twins. Br J Obstet Gynaecol 99:141, 1992.
111. McFadyen I: The dangers of intraamniotic methylene blue. Br J Obstet Gynaecol 99:89, 1992.

112. Tabsh K: Genetic amniocentesis in multiple gestation. A new technique to diagnose monoamniotic twins. Obstet Gynecol 75:296, 1990.
113. Palle C, Andersen JW, Tabor A, et al: Increased risk of abortion after genetic amniocentesis in twin pregnancies. Prenat Diagn 3:83, 1983.
114. Pijpers L, Jahoda MGJ, Vosters RPL, et al: Genetic amniocentesis in twin pregnancies. Br J Obstet Gynaecol 95:323, 1988.
115. Anderson RL, Goldberg JD, Golbus MS: Prenatal diagnosis in multiple gestation: 20 years' experience with amniocentesis. Prenat Diagn 11:263, 1991.
116. Ghidini A, Lynch L, Hicks C, et al: The risk of second-trimester amniocentesis in twin gestations: A case-control study. Am J Obstet Gynecol 169:1013, 1994.
117. Yukobowitch E, Anteby EY, Cohen SM, et al: Risk of fetal loss in twin pregnancies undergoing second trimester amniocentesis. Obstet Gynecol 98: 231, 2001.
118. Toth-Pal E, Papp C, Beke A, et al: Genetic amniocentesis in multiple pregnancies. Fetal Diagn Ther 19:138, 2004
119. Wapner RJ, Johnson A, Davis G: Prenatal diagnosis in twin gestations: A comparison between second trimester amniocentesis and first trimester chorionic villus sampling. Obstet Gynecol 82: 49, 1993.
120. DeCatte L, Liebaers I, Foulon W: Outcome of twin gestations after first trimester chorionic villus sampling. Obstet Gynecol 96: 714, 2000.
121. Brambati B, Tului L, Guercilena S, Alberti E: Outcome of first-trimester chorionic villus sampling for genetic investigation in multiple pregnancy. Ultrasound Obstet Gynecol 17:209, 2001.
122. Landy HJ, Keith L, Keith D: The vanishing twin. Acta Genet Med Gemellol 31:179, 1982.
123. Robinson HP, Caines JS: Sonar evidence of early pregnancy failure in patients with twin conceptions. Br J Obstet Gynaecol 84:22, 1977.
124. Finberg HJ, Birnholz JC: Ultrasound observations in multiple gestation with first trimester bleeding. The blighted twin. Radiology 132:137, 1979.
125. Varma TR: Ultrasound evidence of early pregnancy failure in patients with multiple conceptions. Br J Obstet Gynaecol 86:290, 1979.
126. Dickey RP, Olar TT, Taylor SN, et al: Incidence and significance of unequal gestational sac diameter or embryo crown-rump length in twin pregnancy. Hum Reprod 7:1170, 1992.
127. Landy HJ, Weiner S, Corson SL, et al: The "vanishing twin": Ultrasonographic assessment of fetal disappearance in the first trimester. Am J Obstet Gynecol 155:14, 1986.
128. Robinson LK, Jones KL, Benirschke K: The nature of structural defects associated with velamentous and marginal insertion of the umbilical cord. Am J Obstet Gynecol 146:191, 1983.
129. Simpson LL, Marx GR, Elkadry EA, D'Alton ME: Cardiac dysfunction in twin-twin transfusion syndrome: a prospective, longitudinal study. Obstet Gynecol 92:557, 1998.
130. Bajoria R, Ward S, Chatterjee R: Natriuretic peptides in the pathogenesis of cardiac dysfunction in the recipient fetus of twin-twin transfusion syndrome. Am J Obstet Gynecol 186:121, 2002.
131. Malone FD, D'Alton ME: Anomalies peculiar to multiple gestations. Clin Perinatol 27:1033, 2000.
132. D'Alton ME, Simpson LL: Syndromes in twins. Semin Perinatol 19:375, 1995.
133. Denbow M, Fogliani R, Kyle P, et al: Hematological indices at fetal blood sampling in monochorionic pregnancies complicated by feto-fetal transfusion syndrome. Prenat Diagn 18:941, 1998.
134. Jain V, Fisk NM: The twin-twin transfusion syndrome. Clin Obstet Gynecol 47:181, 2004.
135. Gonsoulin W, Moise KJ Jr, Kirshon B, et al: Outcome of twin-twin transfusion diagnosed before 28 weeks of gestation. Obstet Gynecol 75:214, 1990.
136. Chescheir NC, Seeds JW: Polyhydramnios and oligohydramnios in twin gestations. Obstet Gynecol 71:882, 1988.
137. Duncombe GJ, Dickinson JE, Evans SF: Perinatal characteristics and outcomes of pregnancies complicated by twin twin transfusion syndrome. Obstet Gynecol 101:1190, 2003.
138. Reisner DP, Mahony BS, Petty CN, et al: Stuck twin syndrome: outcome in thirty-seven consecutive cases. Am J Obstet Gynecol 169:991, 1993.
139. Mari G, Detti L, Oz U, Abuhamad A: Long-term outcome in twin-twin transfusion syndrome treated with serial aggressive amnioreduction. Am J Obstet Gynecol 183:211, 2000.
140. Seng YC, Rajadurai VS: Twin-twin transfusion syndrome: a five year review. Arch Dis Child Fetal Neonatal Ed 83:F168, 2000.
141. Cincotta RB, Gray PH, Phythian G, et al: Long term outcome of twin-twin transfusion syndrome. Arch Dis Child Fetal Neonatal Ed 83:F171, 2000.
142. Dickinson JE, Evans S: Obstetric and perinatal outcomes from The Australian and New Zealand Twin-Twin Transfusion Syndrome Registry. Am J Obstet Gynecol 182:706, 2000.
143. Mari G, Roberts A, Detti L, et al: Perinatal morbidity and mortality rates in severe twin-twin transfusion syndrome: results of the International Amnioreduction Registry. Am J Obstet Gynecol 185:708, 2001.
144. Sutcliffe AG, Sebire NJ, Pigott AJ, et al: Outcome for children born after in utero laser ablation therapy for severe twin-to-twin transfusion syndrome. Br J Obstet Gynaecol 108:1246, 2001.
145. Lopriore E, Nagel HTC, Vandenbussche FPHA, Walther FJ: Long-term neurodevelopmental outcome in twin-to-twin transfusion syndrome. Am J Obstet Gynecol 189:1314, 2003.
146. Dickinson JE, Duncombe GJ, Evans SF, et al: The long term neurologic outcome of children from pregnancies complicated by twin-to-twin transfusion syndrome. Br J Obstet Gynaecol 112:63, 2005.
147. Banek CS, Hecher K, Hackeloer BJ, Bartmann P: Long-term neurodevelopmental outcome after intrauterine laser treatment for severe twin-twin transfusion syndrome. Am J Obstet Gyenecol 188: 876, 2003.
148. Bajoria R, Wigglesworth J, Fisk NM: Angioarchitecture of monochorionic placentas in relation to the twin-twin transfusion syndrome. Am J Obstet Gynecol 172:856, 1995.
149. Quintero RA, Morales WJ, Allen MH, et al: Staging of twin-twin transfusion syndrome. J Perinatol 19:550, 1999.
150. Farmakides G, Schulman H, Saldana LR, et al: Surveillance of twin pregnancy with umbilical arterial velocimetry. Am J Obstet Gynecol 153:789, 1985.
151. Giles WB, Trudinger BJ, Cook CM: Fetal umbilical artery flow velocity-time waveforms in twin pregnancies. Br J Obstet Gynaecol 92:490, 1985.
152. Pretorius DH, Manchester D, Barkin S, et al: Doppler ultrasound of twin transfusion syndrome. J Ultrasound Med 7:117, 1988.
153. Dickinson JE, Evans SF: Obstetrics and perinatal outcomes from The Australian and New Zealand Twin-Twin Transfusion Syndrome Registry. Am J Obstet Gynecol 182:706, 2000.
154. Ishimatsu J, Yoshimura O, Manabe A, et al: Ultrasonography and Doppler studies in twin-to-twin transfusion syndrome. Asia Oceania J Obstet Gynecol 18:325, 1992.
155. Fox C, Kilby MD, Khan KS: Contemporary treatments for twin-twin transfusion syndrome. Obstet Gynecol 105:1469, 2005.
156. De Lia J, Emery MG, Sheafor SA, Jennison TA: Twin transfusion syndrome: successful in utero treatment with digoxin. Int J Gynaecol Obstet 23:197, 1985.
157. Jones JM, Sbarra AJ, Dilillo L, et al: Indomethacin in severe twin-to-twin transfusion syndrome. Am J Perinatol 10:24, 1993.
158. Johnsen SL, Albrechtsen S, Pirhonen J: Twin-twin transfusion syndrome treated with serial amniocentesis. Acta Obstetricia et Gynecologica Scandinavica 83:326, 2004.
159. Johnson JR, Rossi KQ, O'Shaughnessy RW: Amnioreduction versus septostomy in twin-twin transfusion syndrome. Am J Obstet Gynecol 185:1044, 2001.
160. Saade GR, Belfort MA, Berry DL, et al: Amniotic septostomy for the treatment of twin oligohydramnios- polyhydramnios sequence. Fetal Diagn Ther 13:86, 1998.
161. Pistorius LR, Howarth GR: Failure of amniotic septostomy in the management of 3 subsequent cases of severe previable twin-twin transfusion syndrome. Fetal Diagn Ther 14:337, 1999.
162. Saade G, Moise K, Dorman K, et al: A randomized trial of septostomy versus amnioreduction in the treatment of twin oligohydramnios polyhydramnios sequence (TOPS). Am J Obstet Gynecol 187:S54, 2002.

163. Senat M, Deprest J, Boulvain M, et al: Endoscopic laser surgery versus serial amnioreduction for severe twin-to-twin transfusion syndrome. N Engl J Med 351:136, 2004.
164. Delia J, Fisk N, Hecher K, et al: Twin-to-twin transfusion syndrome-debates on the etiology, natural history and management. Ultrasound Obstet Gynecol 16:210, 2000.
165. Fisk NM, Galea P: Twin-twin transfusions-as good as it gets? N Engl J Med 351:182, 2004.
166. Demissie K, Ananth CV, Martin J, et al: Fetal and neonatal mortality among twin gestations in the United States: the role of intrapair birth discordance. Obstet Gynecol 100:474; 2002.
167. Gonzalez-Quintero VH, Luke B, O'Sullivan MJ, et al: Antenatal factors associated with significant birth weight discordancy in twin gestations. Am J Obstet Gynecol 189:813, 2003.
168. Blickstein I, Keith LG: Neonatal mortality rates among growth-discordant twins, classified according to the birth weight of the smaller twin. Am J Obstet Gynecol 190:170, 2004.
169. Amaru RC, Bush MC, Berkowitz RL, et al: Is discordant growth in twins an independent risk factor for adverse neonatal outcome? Obstet Gynecol 103:71, 2004.
170. Quigley JK: Monoamniotic twin pregnancy: a case record with review of the literature. Am J Obstet Gynecol 29:354, 1935.
171. Raphael SI: Monoamniotic twin pregnancy—a review of the literature and a report of 5 new cases. Am J Obstet Gynecol 81:323, 1961.
172. Salerno LJ: Monoamniotic twinning—a survey of the American literature since 1935 with a report of four new cases. Obstet Gynecol 14:205, 1959.
173. Simonsen M: Monoamniotic twins. Acta Obstet Gynecol Scand 45:43, 1966.
174. Rodis JF, McIlveen PF, Egan JFX, et al: Monoamniotic twins: improved perinatal survival with accurate prenatal diagnosis and antenatal fetal surveillance. Am J Obstet Gynecol 177:1046, 1997.
175. Allen VM, Windrim R, Barrett J, Ohlsson A: Management of monoamniotic twin pregnancies: a case series and systemic review of the literature. Br J Obstet Gynaecol 108:931, 2001.
176. House M, Harney K, D'Alton ME, et al: Intensive management of monoamniotic twin pregnancies improves perinatal outcome. Am J Obstet Gynecol 185:S113, 2001.
177. Roque H, Gillen-Goldstein J, Funai E, et al: Perinatal outcomes in monoamniotic gestations. J Matern Fetal Neonatal Med 13:414, 2003.
178. Demaria F, Goffinet F, Kayem G, et al: Monoamniotic twin pregnancies: antenatal management and perinatal results of 19 consecutive cases. Br J Obstet Gynaecol 111:22, 2004.
179. Heyborne KD, Porreco RP, Garite TJ, et al: Improved perinatal survival of monamniotic twins with intensive inpatient monitoring. Am J Obstet Gynecol 192:96, 2005.
180. Sherer DM, Sokolovski M, Haratz-Rubinstein N: Diagnosis of umbilical cord entanglement of monoamniotic twins by first-trimester color Doppler imaging. J Ultrasound Med 21:1307, 2002.
181. Lavery J, Gadwood KA: Amniography for confirming the diagnosis of monoamniotic twinning: a case report. J Reprod Med 35:911, 1990.
182. Pederson MH, Larsen T: Three-dimensional ultrasonography of monoamniotic twins. Ugeskr Laeger 163:618, 2001.
183. Gilbert WM, Davis SE, Kaplan C, et al: Morbidity associated with prenatal disruption of the dividing membrane in twin gestations. Obstet Gynecol 78:623, 1991.
184. Beasley E, Megerian G, Gerson A, Roberts NS: Monoamniotic twins: case series and proposal for antenatal management. Obstet Gynecol 93:130, 1999.
185. Peek MJ, McCarthy A, Kyle P, et al: Medical amnioreduction with sulindac to reduce cord complications in monoamniotic twins. Am J Obstet Gynecol 176:334, 1997.
186. Abuhamad AZ, Mari G, Copel JA, et al: Umbilical artery flow velocity waveforms in monoamniotic twins with cord entanglement. Obstet Gynecol 86:674, 1995.
187. Su LL: Monoamniotic twins: diagnosis and management. Acta Obstet Gynecol Scand 81:995, 2002.
188. Kassam SH, Tompkins MG: Monoamniotic twin pregnancy and modern obstetrics: report of a case with a peculiar cord complication. Diagn Gynecol Obstet 2:213, 1980.
189. Carr SR, Aronson MP, Coustan DR: Survival rates of monoamniotic twins do not decrease after 30 weeks' gestation. Am J Obstet Gynecol 163:719, 1990.
190. Tessen JA, Zlatnik FJ: Monoamniotic twins: a retrospective controlled study. Obstet Gynecol 77:832, 1991.
191. Kantanka KS, Buchman EJ: Vaginal delivery of monoamniotic twins with umbilical cord entanglement. A case report. J Reprod Med 46:275, 2001.
192. McLeod FN, McCoy DR: Monoamniotic twin swith an unusual cord complication. Br J Obstet Gynaecol 88:774, 1981.
193. Kaplan C, Benirschke K: The acardiac anomaly: New case reports and current status. Acta Genet Med Gemellol 28:51, 1979.
194. Pretorius DH, Leopold GR, Moore TR, et al: Acardiac twin: Report of Doppler sonography. J Ultrasound Med 7:413, 1988.
195. Benson CB, Bieber FR, Genest DR, Doubilet PM: Doppler demonstration of reversed umbilical blood flow in an acardiac twin. J Clin Ultrasound 17:291, 1989.
196. Nance WE: Malformations unique to the twinning process. Prog Clin Biol Res 69A:123, 1981.
197. Van Allen MI, Smith DW, Shepard TH: Twin reversed arterial perfusion (TRAP) sequence: A study of 14 twin pregnancies with acardius. Semin Perinatol 7:285, 1983.
198. Moore TR, Gale S, Benirschke K: Perinatal outcome of forty-nine pregnancies complicated by acardiac twinning. Am J Obstet Gynecol 163:907, 1990.
199. Robie GF, Payne GG Jr, Morgan MA: Selective delivery of an acardiac, acephalic twin. N Engl J Med 320:512, 1989.
200. Rodeck C, Deans A, Jauniaux E: Thermocoagulation for the early treatment of pregnancy with an acardiac twin. N Engl J Med. 339:1293, 1998.
201. Jolly M, Taylor M, Rose G, et al: Interstitial laser: a new surgical technique for twin reversed arterial perfusion sequence in early pregnancy. Br J Obstet Gyncaecol 108:1098, 2001.
202. Holmes A, Jauniaux E, Rodeck C: Monopolar thermocoagulation in acardiac twinning. Br J Obstet Gyncecol 108:1000, 2001.
203. Tsao K, Feldstein VA, Albanese CT, et al: Selective reduction of acardiac twin by radiofrequency ablation. Am J Obstet Gynecol 187:635, 2002.
204. Tan TY, Sepulveda W: Acardiac twin: a systematic review of minimally invasive treatment modalities. Ultrasound Obstet Gynecol 22:409, 2003.
205. Hill LM: The sonographic detection of early first-trimester conjoined twins. Prenat Diagn 17:961, 1997.
206. Durin L, Hars Y, Jeanne-Pasquier C, et al. Prenatal diagnosis of an extremely rare type of conjoined twins: cranio-rachi-pygopagus twins. Fetal Diagn Ther 20:158, 2005.
207. Tongsong T, Khunamornpong S, Piyamongkol W, Chanprapaph P: Prenatal sonographic delineation of the complex cardiac anatomy of thoraco-omphalopagus twins. Ultrasound Obstet Gynecol 25:189, 2005.
208. Zoppini C, Vanzulli A, Kustermann A, et al: Prenatal diagnosis of anatomical connections in conjoined twins by use of contrast magnetic resonance imaging. Prenat Diagn 13:995, 1993.
209. Fang KH, Wu JL, Yep GP, et al: Ischiopagus conjoined twins at 9 weeks of gestation: three dimensional ultrasound and power Doppler findings. Ultrasound Obstet Gynecol 25:309, 2005.
210. Filler RM: Conjoined twins and their separation. Semin Perinatol 10:82, 1986.
211. Mackenzie TC, Crombleholme TM, Johnson MP, et al: The natural history of prenatally diagnosed conjoined twins. J Pediatr Surg 37:303, 2002.
212. Votteler TP, Lipsky K: Long-term results of 10 conjoined twin separations. J Pediatr Surg 40:618, 2005.
213. Rosemeier F, Shumway JB, Schallen EH, et al: Successful pregnancy and cesarean delivery 22 years after separation of an ischiopagus tetrapus conjoined twin. Anesthesiology 100:1601, 2004.
214. Benirschke K: Twin placenta in perinatal mortality. NY State J Med 61:1499, 1961.

215. Litschgi M, Stucki D: Course of twin pregnancies after fetal death in utero. Z Geburtshilfe Perinatol 184:227, 1980.
216. Hanna JH, Hill JM: Single intrauterine fetal demise in multiple gestation. Obstet Gynecol 63:126, 1984.
217. D'Alton ME, Newton ER, Cetrulo CL: Intrauterine fetal demise in multiple gestation. Acta Genet Med Gemellol 33:43, 1984.
218. Enbom JA: Twin pregnancy with intrauterine death of one twin. Am J Obstet Gynecol 152:424, 1985.
219. Carlson NJ, Towers CV: Multiple gestation complicated by the death of one fetus. Obstet Gynecol 73:685, 1989.
220. Fusi L, Gordon H: Multiple pregnancy complicated by single intrauterine death: problems and outcome with conservative management. Br J Obstet Gynaecol 97:511, 1990.
221. Kilby MD, Govind A, O'Brien PM: Outcome of twin pregnancies complicated by a single intrauterine death: a comparison with viable twin pregnancies. Obstet Gynecol 84:107, 1994.
222. Johnson CD, Zhang J: Survival of other fetuses after a fetal death in twin and triplet pregnancies. Obstet Gynecol 99:698, 2002.
223. Burke MS: Single fetal demise in twin gestation. Clin Obstet Gynecol 33:69, 1990.
224. Rydhstroem H: Pregnancy with stillbirth of both twins. Br J Obstet Gynaecol 103:25, 1996.
225. Borlum KG: Third-trimester fetal death in triplet pregnancies. Obstet Gynecol 77:6, 1991.
226. Gonen R, Heyman E, Asztalos E, et al: The outcome of triplet gestations complicated by fetal death. Obstet Gynecol 75:175, 1990.
227. Cleary-Goldman J, D'Alton ME: Management of single intrauterine fetal demise in a multiple gestation. Obstet Gynecol Surv 59:285, 2004.
228. Santema JG, Swaak AM, Wallenburg HCS: Expectant management of twin pregnancy with single fetal death. Br J Obstet Gynaecol 102:26, 1995.
229. Eglowstein M, D'Alton ME: Intrauterine demise in multiple gestation: theory and management. J Matern Fetal Med 2:272, 1993.
230. Pharoah PO, Adi Y: Consequences of in-utero death in a twin pregnancy. Lancet 355:1597, 2000.
231. Pharoah PO, Cooke RW: A hypothesis for the aetiology of spastic cerebral palsy—the vanishing twin. Dev Med Child Neurol 39:292, 1997.
232. Fusi L, McParland P, Fisk N, Wigglesworth J: Acute twin-twin transfusion: a possible mechanism for brain-damaged survivors after intrauterine death of a monochorionic twin. Obstet Gynecol 78:517, 1991.
233. Okamura KO, Murotsuki J, Tanigawara S, et al: Funipuncture for evaluation of hematologic and coagulation indices in the surviving twin following co-twin's death. Obstet Gynecol 83:975, 1994.
234. Karageyim Karsidag AY, Kars B, Dansuk R: Brain damage to the survivor within 30 minutes of co-twin demise in monochorionic twins. Fetal Diagn Ther 20:91, 2005.
235. Weiss JL, Cleary-Goldman J, Budorick N, et al: Multicystic encephalomalacia after first trimester intrauterine fetal demise in monochorionic twins. Am J Obstet Gynecol 190:563, 2004.
236. Landy HJ, Weingold AB: Management of a multiple gestation complicated by an antepartum fetal demise. Obstet Gynecol Surv 44:171, 1989.
237. Anderson RL, Golbus MS, Curry CJR, et al: Central nervous system damage and other anomalies in surviving fetus following second trimester antenatal death of co-twin. Prenat Diagn 10:513, 1990.
238. Peterson IR, Nyholm H: Multiple pregnancies with single intrauterine demise description of 28 cases. Acta Obstet Gynecol Scand 78:202, 1999.
239. Aslan H, Gul A, Cebeci A, Polat I, Ceylan Y: The outcome of twin pregnancies complicated by single fetal death after 20 weeks of gestation. Twin Res 7:1, 2004.
240. Bryan E: Loss in higher multiple pregnancy and multifetal pregnancy reduction. Twin Research 5:169, 2002.
241. Onyskowova A, Dolezal A, Jedlicka V: The frequency and the character of malformations in multiple birth (a preliminary report). Teratology 4:496, 1971.
242. Hendricks CH: Twinning in relation to birth weight, mortality, and congenital anomalies. Obstet Gynecol 27:47, 1966.
243. Windham GC, Bjerkedal T, Sever LE: The association of twinning and neural tube defects: Studies in Los Angeles, California, and Norway. Acta Genet Med Gemellol 31:165, 1982.
244. Malone FD, Craigo SD, Chelmow D, D'Alton ME: Outcome of twin gestations complicated by a single anomalous fetus. Obstet Gynecol 88:1, 1996.
245. Sebire NJ, Sepulveda W, Hughes KS, et al: Management of twin pregnancies discordant for anencephaly. Br J Obstet Gynaecol 107:216, 1997.
246. Gul A, Cebecia A, Aslan H, et al: Perinatal outcomes of twin pregnancies discordant for major fetal anomalies. Fetal Diagn Ther 20:244, 2005.
247. Aberg A, Mitelman F, Cantz M, Gehler J: Cardiac puncture of fetus with Hurler's disease avoiding abortion of unaffected co-twin. Lancet 2:990, 1978.
248. Kerenyi TD, Chitkara U: Selective birth in twin pregnancy with discordancy for Down's syndrome. N Engl J Med 304:1525, 1981.
249. Beck L, Terinde R, Rohrborn G, et al: Twin pregnancy, abortion of one fetus with Down's syndrome by sectioparva, the other delivered mature and healthy. Eur J Obstet Gynaecol Reprod Biol 12:267, 1981.
250. Antsaklis A, Politis J, Karagiannopoulos C, Kaskarelis D: Selective survival of only the healthy fetus following prenatal diagnosis of thalassaemia major in binovular twin gestation. Prenat Diagn 4:289, 1984.
251. Rodeck CH, Mibeshan RS, Abramowicz J, Campbell S: Selective fetocide of the affected twin by fetoscopic air embolism. Prenat Diagn 2:189, 1982.
252. Chitkara U, Berkowitz RL, Wilkins IA, et al: Selective second-trimester termination of the anomalous fetus in twin pregnancies. Obstet Gynecol 73:690, 1989.
253. Evans MI, Goldberg JD, Horenstein J, et al: Selective termination for structural, chromosomal, and mendelian anomalies: international experience. Am J Obstet Gynecol 181:893, 1999.
254. Eddleman K, Stone J, Lynch L, Berkowitz RL: Selective termination of anomalous fetuses in multiple pregnancies: 200 cases at a single center. Am J Obstet Gynecol 187:1168, 2002.
255. Golbus MS, Cunningham N, Goldberg JD, et al: Selective termination of multiple gestations. Am J Med Genet 34:339, 1988.
256. Urig MA, Simpson GF, Elliott JP, Clewell WH: Twin-twin transfusion syndrome: The surgical removal of one twin as a treatment option. Fetal Ther 3:185, 1988.
257. Bebbington MW, Wilson RD, Machan L, Wittmann BK: Selective feticide in twin transfusion syndrome using ultrasound-guided insertion of thrombogenic coils. Fetal Diagn Ther 10:32, 1995.
258. Challis D, Gratacos E, Deprest JA: Cord occlusion techniques for selective termination in monochorionic twins. J Perinat Med 27: 327, 1999.
259. Deprest JA, Audibert F, Van Schoubroeck D, et al: Bipolar coagulation of the umbilical cord in complicated monochorionic twin pregnancy. Am J Obstet Gynecol 182:340, 2000.
260. Nicolini U, Poblete A, Boschetto C, et al: Complicated monochorionic twin pregnancies: experience with bipolar cord coagulation. Am J Obstet Gynecol 185:703, 2001.
261. Shevell T, Malone FD, Weintraub J, et al: Radiofrequency ablation in a monochorionic twin discordant for fetal anomalies. Am J Obstet Gyencol 190:575, 2004.
262. Dumez Y, Oury JF: Method for first trimester selective abortion in multiple pregnancy. Contrib Gynecol Obstet 15:50, 1986.
263. Timor-Tritsch IE, Bashiri A, Monteagudo A, et al: Two hundred ninety consecutive cases of multifetal pregnancy reduction: comparison of the transabdominal versus transvaginal approach. Am J Obstet Gynecol 191:2085, 2004.
264. Evans MI, Berkowitz RL, Wapner RJ, et al: Improvement in outcomes of multifetal pregnancy reduction with increased experience. Am J Obstet Gynecol 184:1041, 2001.
265. Stone J, Eddleman K, Lynch L, Berowitz R: A single center experience with 1000 consecutive cases of multifetal pregnancy reduction. Am J Obstet Gynecol 187:1163, 2002.
266. Bush MC, Eddleman KA: Multifetal pregnancy reduction and selective termination. Clin Perinatol 30:623, 2003.

267. Antsaklis A, Souka AP, Daskalakis G, et al: Pregnancy outcome after multifetal pregnancy reduction. J Matern Fetal Neonatal Med 16:27, 2004.
268. Lynch L, Berkowitz RL: Maternal serum alpha-fetoprotein and coagulation profiles after multifetal pregnancy reduction. Am J Obstet Gynecol 169:987, 1993.
269. Depp R, Macone GA, Rosenn MF, et al: Multifetal pregnancy reduction: evaluation of fetal growth in the remaining twins. Am J Obstet Gynecol 174:1233, 1996.
270. Schreiner-Engel P, Walther VN, Mindes J, et al: First-trimester multifetal pregnancy reduction: acute and persistent psychological reactions. Am J Obstet Gynecol 172: 541, 1995.
271. Hartikainen-Sorri AL, Jouppila P: Is routine hospitalization needed in antenatal care of twin pregnancy? J Perinat Med 12:31, 1984.
272. Saunders MC, Dick JS, Brown IM: The effects of hospital admission for bed rest on the duration of twin pregnancy: A randomized trial. Lancet 2:793, 1985.
273. Hawrylyshyn PA, Barkin M, Bernstein A, Papsin FR: Twin pregnancies-a continuing perinatal challenge. Obstet Gynecol 59:463, 1982.
274. Chervenak FA, Youcha S, Johnson RE, et al: Antenatal diagnosis and perinatal outcome in a series of 385 consecutive twin pregnancies. J Reprod Med 29:727, 1984.
275. MacLennan AH, Green RC, O'Shea R, et al: Routine hospital admission in twin pregnancy between 26 and 30 weeks' gestation. Lancet 335:267, 1990.
276. Leveno KJ, Andrews WW, Gilstrap LC, et al: Impact of elective hospitalization on outcome of twin pregnancy. Presented at the Tenth Annual Meeting, Society of Perinatal Obstetricians, Houston, Texas, January 1990.
277. Katz M, Robertson PA, Creasy RK: Cardiovascular complications associated with terbutaline treatment for preterm labor. Am J Obstet Gynecol 139:605, 1981.
278. Newman RB, Krombach RS, Myers MC, et al: Effect of cerclage on obstetric outcome in twin gestations with a shortened cervical length. Am J Obstet Gynecol 186:634, 2002.
279. Elimian A, Figueroa R, Nigam S, et al: Perinatal outcome of triplet gestation: Does prophylactic cerclage make a difference? J Maternal Fetal Med 8:119, 1999.
280. Colton T, Kayne HL, Zhang Y, et al: A meta-analysis of home uterine activity monitoring. Am J Obstet Gynecol 173:1499, 1995.
281. Dyson DC, Danbe KH, Bamber JA, et al: Monitoring women at risk for preterm labor. N Engl J Med 338:15, 1998.
282. Houlton MCC, Marivate M, Philpott RH: Factors associated with preterm labour and changes in the cervix before labour in twin pregnancy. Br J Obstet Gynaecol 89:190, 1982.
283. Neilson JP, Verkuyl AA, Crowther CA, Bannerman C: Preterm labor in twin pregnancies. Prediction by cervical assessment. Obstet Gynecol 72:719, 1988.
284. O'Connor MC, Arias E, Royston JP, Dalrymple IJ: The merits of special antenatal care for twin pregnancies. Br J Obstet Gynaecol 88:222, 1981.
285. Goldenberg RL, Iams JD, Miodovnik M, et al: The preterm prediction study: risk factors in twin gestations. National Institute of Child Health and Human Development Maternal-Fetal Medicine Units Network. Am J Obstet Gynecol 175:1047, 1996.
286. Imseis HM, Albert TA, Iams JD: Identifying twin gestations at low risk for preterm birth with a transvaginal ultrasonographic cervical measurement at 24 to 26 weeks' gestation. Am J Obstet Gynecol 177:1149, 1997.
287. Ramin KD, Ogburn PL Jr, Mulholland TA, et al: Ultrasonographic assessment of cervical length in triplet pregnancies. Am J Obstet Gynecol 180:1442, 1999.
288. Gibson JL, Macara LM, Owen P, et al: Prediction of preterm delivery in twin pregnancy: a prospective, observational study of cervical length and fetal fibronectin testing. Ultrasound Obstet Gynecol 23:561, 2004.
289. Meis PJ, Klebanoff M, Thom E et al: Prevention of recurrent preterm delivery by 17 Alpha-hydroxyprogesterone caproate. N Engl J Med 348:2379, 2003.
289a. Caritis S, Rouse D: A randomized controlled trial of 17-hydroxyprogesterone caproate (17-OHPC) for the prevention of preterm birth in twins. Abstract #1, Am J Obstet Gynecol 195:S2, 2006.
290. Luke B, Brown MB, Misiunas R, et al: Specialized prenatal care and maternal and infant outcomes in twin pregnancy. Am J Obstet Gynecol 189:934, 2003.
291. Sibai BM, Hauth J, Caritis S, et al: Hypertensive disorders in twins versus singleton gestations. National Institute of Child Health and Human Development Network of Maternal-Fetal Medicine Units. Am J Obstet Gynecol 182:938, 2000.
292. Maxwell CV, Lieberman E, Norton M, et al: Relationship of twin zygosity and risk of preeclampsia. Am J Obstet Gynecol 185:819, 2001.
293. Campbell DM, Templeton A: Maternal complications of twin pregnancy. In J Gynecol Obstet 84:71, 2004.
294. Davidson KM, Simpson LL, Knox TA, et al: Acute faty liver of pregnancy in triplet gestation. Obstet Gynecol 91:806, 1998.
295. DeVoe LD, Azor H: Simultaneous nonstress fetal heart rate testing in twin pregnancy. Obstet Gynecol 58:450, 1981.
296. Blake GD, Knuppel RA, Ingardia CJ, et al: Evaluation of nonstress fetal heart rate testing in multiple gestations. Obstet Gynecol 63:528, 1984.
297. Elliott JP, Finberg HJ: Biophysical profile testing as an indicator of fetal well-being in high-order multiple gestations. Am J Obstet Gynecol 172:508, 1995.
298. Geipel A, Berg C, Germer U, et al: Doppler assessment in the uterine circulation in the second trimester in twin pregnancies: prediction of pre-eclampsia, fetal growth restriction and birth weight discordance. Ultrasound Obstet Gynecol 20:541, 2002.
299. Giles W, Bisits A, O'Callahan S, Gill A, DAMP Study Group: The Doppler assessment in multiple pregnancy randomised controlled trial of ultrasound biometry versus umbilical artery Doppler ultrasound and biometry in twin pregnancy. Br J Obstet Gynaecol 110:593, 2003.
300. McElrath TF, Norwitz ER, Robinson JN, et al: Differences in TDx fetal lung maturity assay values between twin and singleton gestations. Am J Obstet Gynecol 182:1110, 2000.
301. Whitworth NS, Magann EF, Morrison JC: Evaluation of fetal lung maturity in diamniotic twins. Am J Obstet Gynecol 180:1438, 1999.
302. Chervenak FA, Johnson RE, Youcha S: Intrapartum management of twin gestation. Obstet Gynecol 65:119, 1985.
303. Khunda S: Locked twins. Obstet Gynecol 39:453, 1972.
304. Sevitz H, Merrell DA: The use of a beta-sympathomimetic drug in locked twins. Br J Obstet Gynaecol 88:76, 1981.
305. Nissen ED: Twins: collision, impaction, compaction, and interlocking. Obstet Gynecol 11:514, 1958.
306. Acker D, Lieberman M, Holbrook H, et al: Delivery of the second twin. Obstet Gynecol 59:710, 1982.
307. Chervenak FA, Johnson RE, Berkowitz RI, et al: Is routine cesarean section necessary for vertex-breech and vertex-transverse twin gestations? Am J Obstet Gynecol 148:1, 1984.
308. Chervenak FA, Johnson RE, Berkowitz RL, Hobbins JC: Intrapartum external version of the second twin. Obstet Gynecol 62:160, 1983.
309. Gocke SE, Nageotte MP, Garite T, et al: Management of the nonvertex second twin: primary cesarean section, external version, or primary breech extraction. Am J Obstet Gynecol 161:111, 1989.
310. Tchabo JG, Tomai T: Selected intrapartum external cephalic version of the second twin. Obstet Gynecol 79:421, 1992.
311. Fishman A, Grubb DK, Kovacs BW: Vaginal delivery of the nonvertex second twin. Am J Obstet Gynecol 168:861, 1993.
312. Greig PC, Veille JC, Morgan T, et al: The effect of presentation and mode of delivery on neonatal outcome in the second twin. Am J Obstet Gynecol 167:901, 1992.
313. Hannah ME, Hannah WJ, Hewson S, et al, for the Term Breech Trial Collaborative Group: Planned caesarean section versus planned vaginal birth for breech presentation at term: a randomized multicentre trial. Lancet 356:1375, 2000.
314. Alamia V Jr, Royck AB, Jackle RK, et al: Preliminary experience with a prospective protocol for planned vaginal delivery of triplet gestations. Am J Obstet Gynecol 179:1133, 1998.

315. Spurway JH: The fate and management of the second twin. Am J Obstet Gynecol 83:1377, 1962.
316. Ferguson WF: Perinatal mortality in multiple gestations. A review of perinatal deaths from 1609 multiple gestations. Obstet Gynecol 23:861, 1964.
317. Rayburn WF, Lavin JP, Miodovnik M, Varner MW: Multiple gestation: Time interval between delivery of the first and second twins. Obstet Gynecol 63:502, 1984.
318. Mashiach S, Ben-Rafael Z, Dor J, Serr DM: Triplet pregnancy in uterus didelphys with delivery interval of 72 days. Obstet Gynecol 58:519, 1981.
319. Woolfson J, Fay T, Bates A: Twins with 54 days between deliveries. Case report. Br J Obstet Gynaecol 90:685, 1983.
320. Farkouh LJ, Sabin ED, Heyborne KD, et al: Delayed-interval delivery: Extended series from a single maternal-fetal medicine practice. Am J Obstet Gynecol 183:1499, 2000.
321. Livingston JC, Livingston LW, Ramsey R, Sibai BM: Second-trimester asynchronous multifetal delivery results in poor perinatal outcome. Obstet Gynecol 103:77, 2004.
322. Oyelese Y, Ananth CV, Smulian JC, Vintzileos AM: Delayed interval delivery in twin pregnancies in the United States: impact on perinatal mortality and morbidity. Am J Obstet Gynecol 192:439, 2005.
323. Ballas S, Toaff R, Jaffa AJ: Deflexion of the fetal head in breech presentation. Obstet Gynecol 52:653, 1978.

Intrauterine Growth Restriction

AHMET ALEXANDER BASCHAT, HENRY L. GALAN,
MICHAEL G. ROSS, AND STEVEN G. GABBE

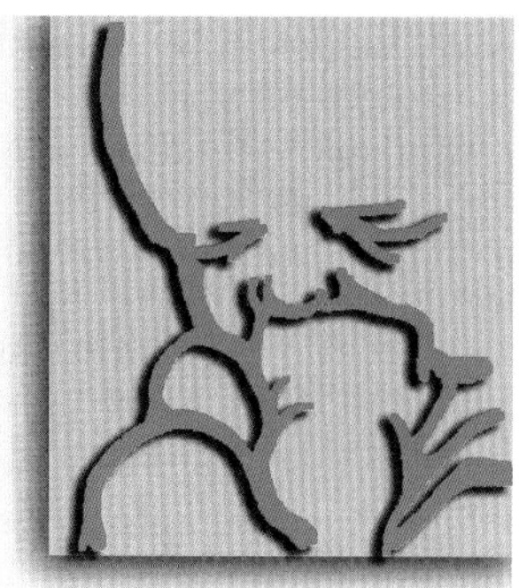

CHAPTER 29

KEY ABBREVIATIONS

Abdominal circumference	AC
Absent end-diastolic velocity	AEDV
Amniotic fluid index	AFI
Amniotic fluid volume	AFV
Appropriate for gestational age	AGA
Biophysical profile	BPS
Biparietal diameter	BPD
Cerebroplacental Doppler ratio	CPR
Computerized cardiotocography	cCTG
Contraction stress test	CST
Femur length	FL
Head circumference	HC
Humerus length	HL
Intrauterine growth restriction	IUGR
Low birth weight	LBW
Neonatal intensive care unit	NICU
Nonstress test	NST
Respiratory distress syndrome	RDS
Reversed end diastolic velocity	REDV
Small for gestational age	SGA
Sonographically estimated fetal weight	SEFW
Systolic/diastolic ratio	S/D

INTRODUCTION

The identification of pregnancies at risk for preventable perinatal handicap is a primary goal of the obstetric care provider. Pregnancies in which adverse intrauterine conditions result in failure of the fetus to reach its growth potential constitute such a high risk group. Next to prematurity, intrauterine growth restriction (IUGR) is the second leading cause of perinatal mortality.[1] Compared with appropriately grown counterparts, perinatal mortality rates in growth restricted neonates are 6 to 10 times greater; perinatal mortality rates as high as 120 per 1,000 for all cases of IUGR and 80 per 1,000 after exclusion of anomalous infants have been reported. As many as 53 percent of preterm stillbirths and 26 percent of term stillbirths are growth restricted.[2] In survivors, the incidence of intrapartum asphyxia may be as high as 50 percent.[2] Prevention of some perinatal complications that lead to adverse outcomes in growth restricted fetuses is possible with appropriate prenatal identification and management. This chapter reviews normal and disturbed fetal growth, the definition of abnormal fetal growth, the impact of fetal growth restriction, and the incorporation of this knowledge into screening, diagnosis, and management of these high-risk pregnancies.

REGULATION OF FETAL GROWTH

Fetal growth is regulated at multiple levels and requires successful development of the placental interface between maternal and fetal compartments. In the early first trimester, anchoring villi originating from the cytotrophoblast connect the decidua to the uterus and thereby establish placental adherence. This allows formation of vascular connections between the maternal circulation and the intervillous space so that increasing quantities of placental secretory products can reach the maternal circulation. Endocrine and paracrine signaling between the placenta and maternal compartment promotes maternal metabolic and cardiovascular adaptations to pregnancy that result in greater substrate availability and enhanced placental perfusion, thereby supporting placental growth. The development of placental mass is critical for its synthetic capacity, whereas vascular development permits nutrient and oxygen delivery to the growing trophoblast beyond the capacity of simple diffusion.

The villous trophoblast now becomes the primary placental site of maternal-fetal exchange. By 16 weeks' gestation, the maternal microvillous and fetal basal layer are only 4 microns apart, posing little resistance to passive diffusion. Elaboration of active transport mechanisms for three major nutrient classes (glucose, amino acids, and free fatty acids) and an increase in the villous surface area raise the capacity and efficiency of active transplacental transport. Vascular throughput across the placenta also increases in the maternal and fetal compartments. Extravillous cytotrophoblast invasion of the maternal spiral arteries results in progressive loss of the musculoelastic media, a process paralleled on the fetal side by continuous villous vascular branching. This results in significant reduction of blood flow resistance in the uterine and umbilical vessels, converting both circulations into low-resistance, high-capacitance vascular beds. The decrease in vascular resistance is related to two waves of angiogenesis within the placenta. The first is branching angiogenesis occurring at the end of the first and beginning of the second trimester, which increases the number of vascular branches. The second wave is nonbranching angiogenesis, which does not create additional branches but rather results in elongation of the existing placental vascular tree. This latter process occurs at the end of the second and beginning of the third trimester.[3] Owing to these developments, a minimum of 600 ml/min of the maternal cardiac output reaches a placental exchange area of up to 12 m^2 at term. In the fetal compartment, this is matched with a blood flow volume of 200 to 300 ml/kg/min throughout gestation. This magnitude of maternal blood flow is necessary to ensure maintenance of placental function that is energy intensive and consumes as much as 40 percent of the oxygen and 70 percent of the glucose supplied. Optimal fetal growth and development depends on a magnitude of maternal nutrient and oxygen delivery to the uterus that leaves sufficient surplus for fetal substrate utilization.

Of the actively transported primary nutrients, glucose is the predominant oxidative fuel, whereas amino acids are major contributors to protein synthesis and muscle bulk. Glucose and, to a lesser, extent amino acids drive the insulin-like growth factors axis and, therefore, stimulate longitudinal fetal growth. Fatty acids are necessary for the maintenance of cell membrane fluidity and permeability, and also act as precursors for important bioactive compounds such as prostaglandins, thromoboxanes, and leukotrienes. Long-chain polyunsaturated fatty acids such as arachidonic acid and docosahexanoic acid are essential for normal brain and retinal development. Leptin is the hormone that coregulates transplacental amino acid and fatty acid transport, and thereby modulates fetal body fat content and proportions.

Concurrent development and maturation of the fetal circulation as a conduit for nutrient and waste delivery allows preferential partitioning of nutrients in the fetus. Nutrient- and oxygen-rich blood from the primitive villous circulation enters the fetus through the umbilical vein. The ductus venosus is the first vascular partitioning shunt encountered. Through modulation in ductus venosus shunting, the proportion of umbilical venous blood that is distributed to the liver and heart changes with advancing gestation. Near term, 18 to 25 percent of umbilical venous flow shunt through the ductus venosus to reach the right atrium in this high velocity stream, wheras 55 percent reach the dominant left hepatic lobe and 20 percent reach the right liver lobes[4,5] (Fig. 29-1). The differences in direction and velocity of blood streams entering the right atrium ensures that nutrient-rich blood is distributed to the left ventricle, myocardium, and brain while low-nutrient venous return is distributed to the placenta for reoxygenation and waste exchange. This process of blood distribution is referred to as "preferential streaming."[6] In addition to this overall distribution of left- and right-sided cardiac output, several organs can modify local blood flow to meet oxygen and nutrient demands by autoregulation.

When the milestones in maternal, placental, and fetal development are met, placental and fetal growth progress normally. The metabolic and vascular maternal adaptations promote a steady and enhanced nutrient delivery to the uterus, and placental transport mechanisms allow for efficient bidirectional exchange of nutrient and waste. Placental and fetal growths across the three trimesters are characterized by sequential cellular hyperplasia, hyperplasia plus hypertrophy, and lastly, hypertrophy alone. Placental growth follows a sigmoid curve that plateaus in midgestation preceding exponential third-trimester growth of the fetus. During this exponential fetal growth phase of 1.5 percent/day, initial weight gain is due to longitudinal growth and muscle bulk and, therefore, correlates with glucose and amino acid transport. Eighty percent of fetal fat gain is accrued after 28 weeks' gestation providing essential body stores in preparation to extrauterine life. From 32 weeks onward, fat stores increase from 3.2 percent of fetal body weight to 16 percent, accounting for the significant reduction in body water content.[7]

The ultimate growth potential of the placenta and the fetus are genetically predetermined, as indicated by their relationship with the maternal body mass index and ethnicity.[8,9] This genetically predetermined growth potential is probably further modified by other maternal, placental, and fetal factors that finally determine the size

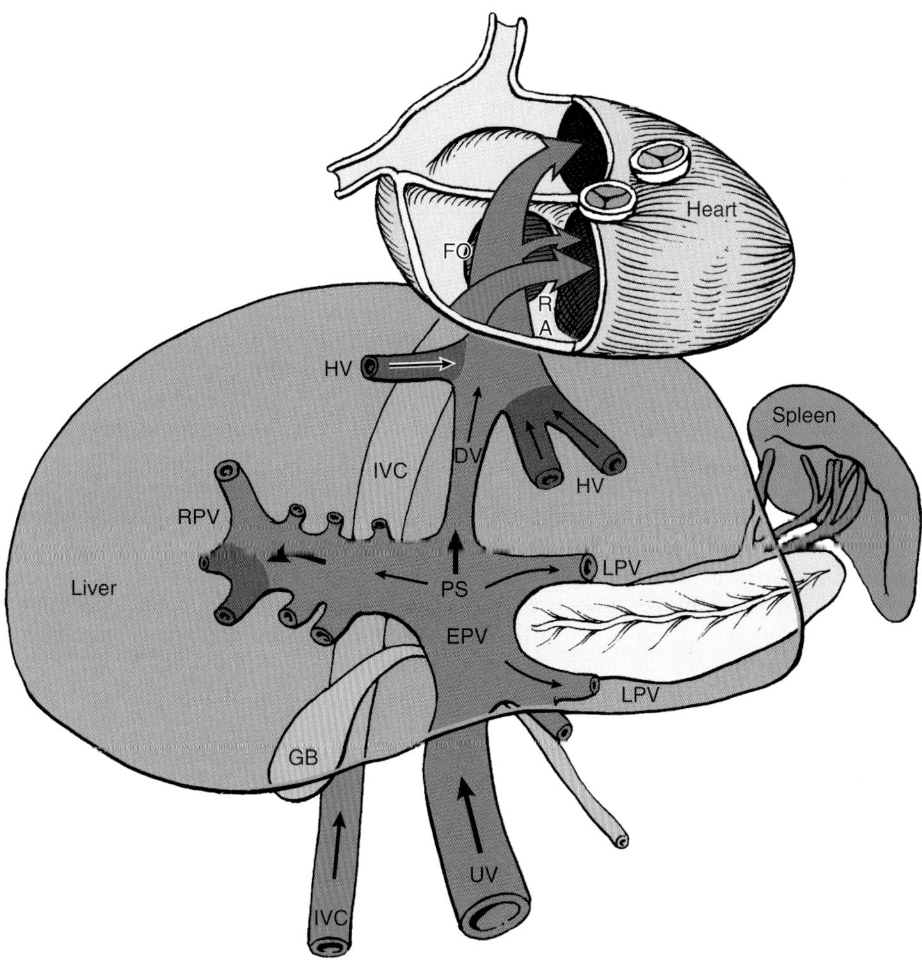

Figure 29-1. Fetal umbilical and hepatic venous circulation. The arrows indicate the direction of blood flow and the color, the degree of oxygen content (red, high; purple, medium; blue, low). The arrows indicate the direction of blood flow. DV, ductus venosus; EPV, extrahepatic portal vein; FO, foramen ovale; GB, gall bladder; HV, hepatic veins; IVC, inferior vena cava; LPV, left portal vein; PS, portal sinus; RA, right atrium; RPV, right portal vein; UV, umbilical vein. (Reproduced with permission from Mavrides E, Moscoso G, Carvalho JS, et al: The anatomy of the umbilical, portal and hepatic venous systems in the human fetus at 14–19 weeks of gestation. Ultrasound Obstet Gynecol 18:598, 2001.)

of the individual at birth. Several possible mechanisms may challenge compensatory capacity of the maternal-placental-fetal unit to such an extent that failure to reach the growth potential may be the end result.

DEFINITION AND PATTERNS OF FETAL GROWTH RESTRICTION

Normal fetal growth involves hyperplasia and hypertrophy on a cellular level. Disturbance of fetal growth dynamics can lead to a reduced cell number, cell size, or both, ultimately resulting in abnormal weight, body mass, or body proportion at birth. The classification of abnormal growth has evolved significantly over the last century. From its modern origins in 1919 when Ylppo[10] was the first to label neonates with a birth weight below 2,500 g as premature to the description of individualized growth potential, the recognition of the growth-restricted neonate has advanced significantly. With the advent of ultrasound, the recognition and study of fetal growth abnormalities now extends into the prenatal period. It is important to note that several definitions describing abnormal growth are used interchangeably in the obstetric and pediatric literature, but that they do not necessarily describe the same population.

The terminology for classifying fetal growth disorders has specifically expanded over the past 4 decades, which has led to confusion among the various terms used. From the 1960s, growth has been classified by the absolute birth weight value as low birth weight (LBW <2,500 g), very low birth weight (<1,500 g), extremely low birth weight (<1,000 g), or macrosomia (>4,000 g).[11] Subsequently, Lubchenco and Usher and McLean among others, demonstrated that only the comparison of the actual birth weight to the expected weight in a population at the same gestational age identified small neonates at risk for adverse outcome.[12–16] Adopting this concept of "light" and "heavy" for gestational age served as an introduction of population based reference ranges for birth weight in the 1970s and allowed classification of growth by the birth-weight percentile. This resulted in the currently accepted classification of birth weight as very small for gestational age (<3rd percentile), small for gestational age (SGA, <10th percentile), appropriate for gestational age (AGA, 10th to 90th percentile) or large for gestational age (>90th percentile).[17,18] Although birthweight percentiles are superior in identifying the small neonate, they fail to account for proportionality of growth and the growth potential of the individual. Therefore, neonates that have a normal birth-weight percentile but abnormal body proportion as a result of differential growth delay may be missed. Similarly, birth-weight percentiles do not distinguish between the small neonate who is normally grown given his genetic potential, and the neonate who is growth restricted owing to a disease process.

The detection of abnormal body mass, or proportions is based on anthropometric measurements and ratios that are relatively independent of gender, race, and to a certain extent, gestational age, and therefore also, the traditional birth-weight percentiles.[19] The ponderal index [(birthweight (g) /crown-to-heel length^3) × 100][20] has a high accuracy for the identification of IUGR[21] and macrosomia.[22] This index correlates more closely with perinatal morbidity and mortality than traditional birth-weight percentiles but may miss the proportionally small and lean, growth-restricted neonate.[23,24] The classification of abnormal growth is also enhanced by adjusting birth-weight reference limits for first-trimester maternal height, race, birth order and fetal/neonatal sex[8] (growth potential). The birth-weight percentile that is based on this individualized growth potential accounts for these possible sources of errors and is superior in the prediction of adverse perinatal outcome to conventional reference ranges.[9,25] It is anticipated that growth potential type curves will eventually become the primary tool in identifying the growth-restricted fetus antenatally.

The classification of abnormal growth during fetal life marks a significant advance because it opens the possibility of prenatal detection that leads to preventive or therapeutic management. The concept of percentiles has been adopted to the ultrasound biometry of the fetus. Accordingly parameters of head, abdominal, and skeletal growth are related to population-based reference ranges. The prenatal diagnosis of fetal growth restriction based on ultrasound biometry is described in detail later.

In addition to the detection of smaller individual measurements and lower weight, two principal patterns of disturbed fetal growth have been described: asymmetric and symmetric. In the asymmetric growth pattern, the abdominal circumference and lower body shows a significant growth delay, whereas there is relative or absolute sparing of head growth. In the symmetric form, body and head growth are similarly affected.[26,27] Asymmetric growth patterns result from two processes. First, liver volume is reduced owing to depletion of glycogen stores as the result of limited nutrient supply, which leads to a decrease in AC. Second, elevations in placental blood flow resistance increase right cardiac afterload and promote diversion of the cardiac output toward the left ventricle owing to the parallel arrangement of the fetal circulation and the presence of central shunts. Blood and nutrient supply to the upper part of the body thus increase presumably resulting in relative head sparing. Symmetrically restricted fetal growth typically results when interference with the growth process results in decreased cell numbers and cell size typically resulting from a first-trimester insult. As a result, all parts of the body are equally affected, producing uniformly small growth.

The pattern of fetal growth depends on the underlying cause of growth delay and the duration of the insult. Uteroplacental insufficiency is typically associated with asymmetric fetal growth delay owing to the aforementioned mechanisms. Aneuploidy, nonaneuploid syndromes, and viral infections disrupt either the regulation of growth processes or interfere with growth at the stage of cell hyperplasia. This problem typically results in a symmetric growth delay.[28] Specific conditions, such as skeletal dysplasia, may produce distinct growth patterns by their differential impacts on axial and peripheral skeletal growth. Since growth is dynamic, the pattern of growth restriction may evolve in the course of gestation. Placental disease may initially present with relative head sparing but eventually progresses to symmetric growth delay as placental insufficiency worsens. Alternatively, the acute course of a fetal viral illness may temporarily result in arrested growth with subsequent resumption of a normal growth pattern.

Although the definition and classification of fetal growth restriction has evolved significantly, research is still ongoing. Small fetal or neonatal size have to be considered as a physical sign rather than a specific disease warranting further investigation of underlying causes. For the purpose of this chapter, fetal growth restriction or IUGR only refers to fetuses with underlying placental pathology. SGA refers to neonates in whom no causative pathology for the small size is evident. From the perspective of the managing perinatologist prenatal identification of IUGR is most relevant because it allows appropriate prospective fetal management. To formulate a uniform approach to prenatal detection and perinatal management an understanding of the maternal and fetal impact of placental insufficiency is essential.

ETIOLOGIES OF INTRAUTERINE GROWTH RESTRICTION

The precise mechanisms by which various conditions interfere with normal placentation and culminate in either pregnancy loss or IUGR are of great importance. Conditions that result in fetal growth restriction broadly consist of maternal, uterine, placental, and fetal disorders. These conditions result in growth delay by affecting nutrient and oxygen delivery to the placenta (maternal causes), nutrient and oxygen transfer across the placenta (placental causes), and fetal nutrient uptake or regulation of growth processes (fetal causes). In clinical practice, there may be considerable overlap between the conditions that determine manifestation, progression, and outcome.

Maternal causes of fetal growth restriction include vascular disease such as hypertensive disorders of pregnancy, diabetic vasculopathy, chronic renal disease, collagen vascular disease, and thrombophilia. The associated decrease in uteroplacental blood flow is responsible for the majority of clinically recognized cases of IUGR. Poor maternal volume expansion, as may be observed in hypertensive disorders or genetic conditions such as angiotensinogen gene mutations,[29] or living at high altitude have also been reported to compromise placental blood flow by reducing the circulating blood volume, hyperviscosity, and sludging.[30–33] In addition, reduction of maternal oxygenation found in women living at high altitude, or with cyanotic heart disease, parenchymal lung disease, or reduced oxygen carrying capacity, as observed with certain hemoglobinopathies and anemias, may be responsible for the cases of IUGR described in these conditions.

Poor maternal weight gain is a long recognized risk factor for IUGR. Studies of the offspring of pregnant women with dietary restrictions suggest that limited protein intake, especially before 26 weeks' gestation, can result in symmetric IUGR, whereas caloric restriction (maternal intake of 600 to 900 calories daily for 6 months) has only moderate effects on birthweight.[34,35] The degree of malnourishment observed in the studies of Guatemalan women or during the Dutch famine would not ordinarily be found in the United States. Nevertheless, maternal prepregnancy weight and weight gain in pregnancy are two of the most important variables contributing to birth weight. It is conceivable that malnutrition due to gastrointestinal syndromes such as Crohn's disease, ulcerative colitis or bypass surgery can result in lower birth weight. However, an association with IUGR is infrequent in these conditions.

Glucose is a critical fetal nutrient driving longitudinal fetal growth. Reduced glucose supply to the fetoplacental unit can result in fetal growth restriction. This was suspected by Economides and Nicolaides[36] who observed significantly lower maternal and fetal glucose levels in growth-restricted fetuses. Khouzami et al.[37] documented a significant association between relative maternal hypoglycemia on a 3-hour oral glucose tolerance test and subsequent birth of non–LBW, but growth-restricted babies. Sokol et al.[38] and Langer et al.[39] have confirmed that a flat maternal response to glucose loading increased the risk for poor fetal growth as much as 20-fold.

Maternal drug ingestion may result in IUGR by a direct effect on fetal growth as well as through inadequate dietary intake. Smoking produces a symmetrically smaller fetus through reduced uterine blood flow and impaired fetal oxygenation, and is a major cause of growth restriction in developed countries. The consumption of alcohol and the use of coumadin or hydantoin derivatives are now well known to produce particular dysmorphic features in association with impaired fetal growth. Mills et al.[40] have demonstrated a significant increase in the risk of IUGR with the consumption of one to two drinks daily, in the absence of fetal alcohol syndrome. Maternal use of cocaine has been associated with not only IUGR but also reduced head circumference growth.[41]

In 1971, Lobi et al.[42] reported that advanced maternal age was a factor in the etiology of IUGR. Berkowitz et al.[43] found no evidence that the first births of women between 30 and 34 years or those older than 35 years were at increased risk for growth restriction. Chronic medical conditions of the mother do increase the risk of IUGR. However, if one controls for underlying medical complications, maternal age is not related to restricted fetal growth.

Multiple risk factors can act synergistically on fetal growth. For example, the adverse impact of smoking is doubled in thin white women and further potentiated by poor maternal weight gain.[44] Similarly, the possible benefits of low-dose aspirin and the detrimental effects of excessive blood pressure reduction are also more apparent in this group of women.[45,46]

Fetoplacental causes can result in fetal growth restriction due to abnormalities of the fetus or placenta, or both. Chromosomal abnormalities, congenital malformations and genetic syndromes have been associated with less than 10 percent of cases of IUGR.[47] Similarly, intrauterine infection, although long recognized as a cause of growth restriction, also accounts for less than 10 percent of all cases. However, genetic and infectious etiologies are of special importance because perinatal and long-term outcome are ultimately determined by the underlying condition with little potential impact through perinatal interventions.

Growth restriction has been observed in 53 percent of cases of trisomy 13, and 64 percent of cases of trisomy 18,[48] and may be manifest as early as the first trimester.[49] Other conditions that may present with fetal growth restriction include skeletal dysplasia and Cornelia De Lange syndrome. The online database of inheritance in humans lists more than 100 genetic syndromes that may be associated with fetal growth restriction. Of the infectious agents, herpes, cytomegalovirus, rubella, and toxoplasma gondii are well-documented causes of symmetric IUGR.

Abnormal placental development with subsequent placental insufficiency is a relatively common problem affecting about one third of patients with IUGR or about 3 percent of all pregnancies. Placental insufficiency accounts for the vast majority of IUGR in singleton pregnancies.[49–51] An absolute or relative decrease in placental mass affects the quantity of substrate the fetus receives and antedates the development of IUGR. Thus, abnormal placental vascular development, circumvallate placenta, partial placental abruption, placenta accreta, placental infarction, or hemangioma may result in growth restriction. Intrinsic placental pathology such as a single umbilical artery and placental mosaicism has been identified in some cases of growth restriction.[52] Placental implantation in the lower uterine segment in placenta previa is considered suboptimal for nutrient exchange and, therefore, may result in IUGR even in the absence of chronic hemorrhage.[53]

Twin gestation is often associated with IUGR (see Chapter 28). In 1966, Gruenwald[54] observed that the growth curve of twins deviated from that of singletons, with a progressive fall of growth after 32 weeks. This finding implies relative placental insufficiency as opposed to intrinsic fetal compromise and suggests that the longer the twin pregnancy continues, the greater the delay in intrauterine growth, with "catch-up" growth observed after birth. Thus, twins and higher order multiples represent a group of fetuses at high risk for IUGR, as confirmed by an incidence of 17.5 percent in one study.[55] The appropriate growth standard to apply to twin fetuses would appear to be the same as that for singletons. Two trials demonstrate that the morbidity and mortality of fetuses from twin gestations are equivalent, or elevated when the twins are monochorionic, when compared with birth weight– and gestational age–matched singletons.[56,57]

MATERNAL AND FETAL MANIFESTATIONS OF INTRAUTERINE GROWTH RESTRICTION

The impact of placental insufficiency depends on the gestational age at onset and the severity of the placental disease. Early interference with normal placentation affects all levels of placental and fetal development, and culminates in the most severe clinical picture, which may result in miscarriage or early stillbirth. If sufficient supply to the placental mass can be established, further placental differentiation may be possible, but suboptimal maternal adaptation to pregnancy and deficient nutrient delivery pose limitations. If adaptive mechanisms permit ongoing fetal survival, early-onset growth restriction with its many fetal manifestations develops. If placental disease is mild or if successful compensation has occurred, the consequences of nutrient shortage may remain largely subclinical, only to be unmasked through its restrictive effect on exponential fetal growth in the second to third trimester. In these cases, late onset growth delay, a decrease in adipose tissue, or abnormal body proportions at birth may be the consequence.

Maternal Impacts

Placental dysfunction affects several aspects of maternal adaptation to pregnancy. Associations between poor placentation with suboptimal maternal volume expansion, increased vascular reactivity and a "flat" glucose tolerance have been described. Abnormalities of placental vascular development are of special interest because they can be detected by Doppler ultrasound of the uterine arteries and frequently predate clinical disease. When trophoblast invasion remains confined to the decidual portion of the myometrium, maternal spiral and radial arteries fail to undergo the physiologic transformation into low resistance vessels, which is generally expected by 22 to 24 weeks.[58,59] Normal and abnormal spiral artery adaptation can be detected with maternal uterine artery Doppler studies, as shown in Figure 29-2. Maternal placental floor infarcts, fetal villous obliteration, and fibrosis increase placental blood flow resistance, producing maternal-fetal placental perfusion mismatch that decreases the effective exchange area.[60–63] With progressive vascular occlusion, fetoplacental flow resistance is increased throughout the vascular bed and eventually metabolically active placental mass is reduced. The diagnostic and screening utility of ultrasound findings that are suggestive of such pathology is discussed later.

Fetal Impacts

When placental dysfunction compromises nutrient delivery triggering fetal mobilization of hepatic glycogen stores, physical manifestation of growth delay becomes clinically apparent. In addition to the cardinal sign of fetal growth restriction, metabolic, endocrine, hematologic, cardiovascular, and behavioral manifestations of placental insufficiency have been described that relate to the severity and duration of placental dysfunction. Of these, cardiovascular and central nervous system (CNS) responses are best studied because their noninvasive assessment is readily achieved by multivessel Doppler, grey scale ultrasound, and fetal heart rate (FHR) analysis and therefore can be utilized for fetal surveillance. Appreciating the variety of fetal manifestations helps to understand the potential limitations of antenatal surveillance and provides a basis to appreciate the possible short- and long-term impacts of placental insufficiency.

Metabolic manifestations occur early in growth-restricted fetuses. This is because with mild to moderate decline in uterine nutrient delivery, fetal supply is compromised first, whereas placental nutrition is preferentially maintained. With progression of placental insufficiency, nutrient deficits become universal and result in decreased fetal and placental size. Accordingly, with mild restrictions in oxygen and glucose supply, fetal demands are still met by increased fractional extraction. When uterine oxygen

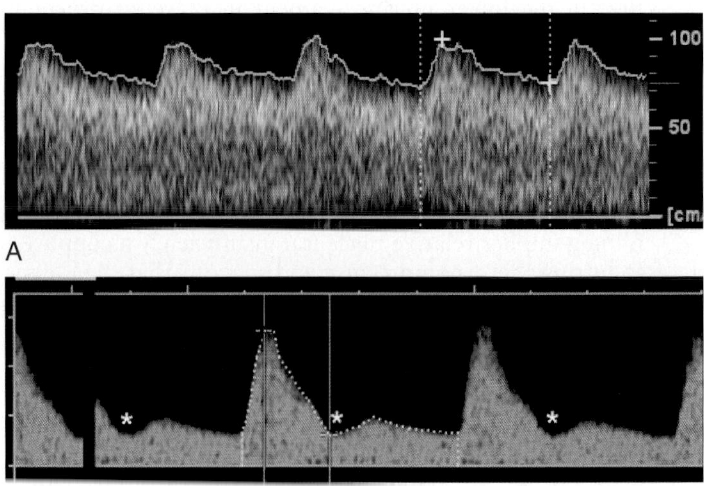

Figure 29-2. Uterine artery flow velocity waveforms. Normal trophoblast invasion results in a low-resistance, high-capacitance placental vascular circulation that can be documented with uterine artery Doppler velocimetry. The flow velocity waveform in panel *A* was obtained at 24 weeks' gestation and shows high diastolic flow velocities. Such a flow pattern indicates successful trophoblast invasion. On the other hand, the second waveform *(B)* shows lower diastolic velocities and an early diastolic notch (*). This flow pattern is reflective of increased blood flow resistance in the spiral arteries and the downstream placental vascular bed. Persistence of notching beyond 24 weeks' gestation is associated with an increased risk of fetal growth restriction and hypertensive disorders of pregnancy.

delivery falls below a critical value (0.6 mmol/min/Kg fetal body weight in sheep), fetal oxygenation begins to fall and is eventually accompanied by fetal hypoglycemia.[64] The initially mild hypoglycemia results in a blunted fetal pancreatic insulin response, allowing glycogenolysis from hepatic glycogen stores.[65–67] The minimal hepatic glycogen stores in the fetus are quickly depleted as glucose and lactate are preferentially diverted to the placenta. An increasing nutrient deficit leads to worsening fetal hypoglycemia, decreasing the maintenance of fetal oxidative metabolism and placental nutrition. With a more significant limitation of oxidative metabolism, associated with downregulation of placental transport mechanisms and intensifying hypoglycemia, the use of other fetal energy sources becomes necessary, and more widespread metabolic consequences ensue. Limitation of amino acid transfer and breakdown of endogenous muscle protein to obtain gluconeogenic amino acids depletes branched-chain and other essential amino acids.[68–71] Simultaneously, lactate accumulates owing to the limited capacity for oxidative metabolism. Placental transfer of fatty acids loses its selectivity particularly for essential fatty acids. Reduced utilization leads to increased fetal free fatty acid and triglyceride levels with a subsequent failure to accumulate adipose stores. In this setting of advancing malnutrition, cerebral and cardiac metabolism of lactate and ketones is upregulated to remove these accumulating products of anaerobic metabolism.[72–74] Acid-base balance can be maintained as long as acid production is met by sufficient buffering capacity of fetal hemoglobin and an equal disposition by these organs. Thus, metabolic compromise progresses from simple hypoglycemia, hypoxemia, and decreased levels of essential amino acids to overt hypoaminoacidemia, hypercapnia, hypertriglyceridemia, and hyperlacticemia. The lactate production is exponentially correlated to the degree of acidemia that generally results from this metabolic state.[70,75,76] A summary of metabolic responses is provided in Table 29-1.

Fetal endocrine manifestations of placental insufficiency are of relevance because they are responsible for the downregulation of growth and developmental processes. Decrease in fetal glucose and amino acids indirectly downregulates insulin and insulin-like growth factors I and II as the principal endocrine regulators of longitudinal growth. Leptin-coordinated deposition of fat stores is similarly affected.[77,78] In addition, pancreatic cellular dysfunction becomes evident through a decreased insulin/glucose ratio and impaired fetal glucose tolerance.[70,79] Significant elevations of corticotrophin-releasing hormone, adrenocorticotrophic hormone, and cortisol, as well as a decline in active vitamin D and osteocalcin, correlate with the severity of placental dysfunction.[80–83] These hormonal imbalances are believed to have additional negative impacts on linear growth, skeletal growth, bone mineralization, and the potential for postpartum catch-up growth.[84,85]

In growth-restricted fetuses, declining function at all levels of the thyroid axis correlate to the degree of hypoxemia.[86,87] Thyroid gland dysfunction may develop, as indicated by low levels of thyroxine and triiodothyronine despite elevated thyroid-stimulating hormone levels. In other instances, central underproduction of thyroid-stimulating hormone may be responsible for fetal hypothyroidism.[88] Finally, downregulation of thyroid hormone receptors may limit the biologic activity of circulating thyroid hormones in specific target tissues such as the developing brain.[89]

Table 29-1. Summary of Metabolic Responses to Placental Insufficiency

SUBSTRATE	CHANGE
Glucose	Decreased proportional to the degree of fetal hypoxemia.
Amino acids	Significant decrease in branched-chain amino acids (valine, leucine, isoleucine) as well as lysine and serine. In contrast, hydroxyproline is elevated. The decrease in essential amino acids is proportional to the degree of hypoxemia. Elevated amniotic fluid glycine–to–valine ratio. Elevations in amniotic fluid ammonia, with a significant positive correlation with the fetal ponderal index.
Fatty acids and triglycerides	Decrease in long-chain polyunsaturated fatty acids (docosahexanoic and arachidonic acids). Decrease in overall fatty acid transfer only with significant loss of placental substance. Hypertriglyceridemia due to decreased utilization. Lower cholesterol esters.
Oxygen and CO_2	Degree of hypoxemia proportional to villous damage and correlates significantly with hypercapnia, acidemia and hypoglycemia and hyperlacticemia.

Elevations in serum glucagon, adrenaline, noradrenaline, and stimulation of the fetal glucocorticoid axis have immediate effects in fetal life promoting the mobilization of hepatic glycogen stores and peripheral glycogenolysis.[66,90–92] However, persistent alterations of these hormones may have a causative relationship with the development of diabetes and vascular complications in adult life.

Fetal hematologic responses to placental insufficiency are important because they initially provide a compensatory mechanism for hypoxemia and acidemia but eventually may become contributory to the escalation of placental vascular dysfunction. Fetal hypoxemia is a trigger for erythropoietin release and stimulation of red blood cell production through both medullary and extramedullary sites resulting in polycythemia.[93–96] Oxygen-carrying capacity and the buffering capacity are thus increased through the elevation in hemoglobin count. If extramedullary hematopoiesis is increasingly induced by prolonged tissue hypoxemia or acidosis, the nucleated red blood cell count rises owing to the escape of these cells from these sites. Thus, elevated nucleated red blood cell counts correlate with metabolic and cardiovascular status and are independent markers for poor perinatal outcome.[97–100] In advanced placental insufficiency, more complex hematologic abnormalities supervene that may result from dysfunctional erythropoiesis, placental consumption, and vitamin and iron deficiency.[101–104] Subsequently, fetal anemia and thrombocytopenia are observed, particularly in fetuses with marked elevation of placental blood flow resistance and evidence of intraplacental thrombosis suggesting a causative relationship.[105–108] An increase in whole blood viscosity,[109,110] a decrease in red blood cell membrane fluidity,[111] and platelet aggregation may be important precursors for accelerating placental vascular occlusion and dysfunction.

Growth-restricted fetuses also show evidence of immune dysfunction at the cellular and humoral level. Decreases in immunoglobulin, absolute B-cell counts,[112] total white blood cell counts, neutrophil, monocyte and lymphocyte subpopulations,[113] as well as selective suppression of T-helper and cytotoxic T cells[114] are related to the degree of acidemia. These immune deficiencies explain the higher susceptibility of growth-restricted neonates to infection after delivery.

Fetal cardiovascular responses to placental insufficiency can be subdivided into early and late based on the degree of deterioration of cardiovascular status and the associated derangement of fetal acid-base balance (see later).[115] Early responses are typically adaptive in nature and result in preferential nutrient streaming to essential organs. The combination of elevated placental blood flow resistance and impaired transplacental gas transfer has several effects on the fetal circulation. Normally, nutrient-rich oxygenated blood enters the fetus through the umbilical vein, reaching the liver as the first major organ. One of the earliest cardiovascular signs of placental insufficiency is a decrease in the magnitude of umbilical venous volume flow.[116] In response to these changes in umbilical venous nutrition content and blood flow volume, the proportion of umbilical venous blood that is diverted through the ductus venosus toward the fetal heart increases.[117] This change in venous shunting across the ductus venosus increases the proportion of nutrient-rich umbilical venous blood that bypasses the liver and reaches the left side of the heart through the foramen ovale.[118] Because of the presence of central shunts at the level of the foramen ovale and ductus arteriosus, differential changes in downstream blood flow resistance can affect the proportion of cardiac output delivered through each ventricle (Fig. 29-3). Elevation of blood flow resistance in the pulmonary vascular bed and subdiaphragmatic circulation (lower body and placenta) increase right ventricular afterload.[119–121] A drop in cerebral blood flow resistance decreases left ventricular afterload.[122,123] As a consequence shunting of nutrient-rich blood from the ductus venosus through the foramen ovale to the left side of the heart increases and left ventricular output rises in relation to the right cardiac output.[124,125] At the aortic isthmus, blood coming from the right ventricle through the ductus arteriosus is diverted toward the aortic arch, therefore supplementing this central shift in cardiac output from right to left.[126] This relative shift in cardiac output toward the left ventricle that results in increased blood flow to the myocardium and brachiocephalic circulation has been termed redistribution, indicating a compensatory mechanism in response to placental insufficiency.

Late circulatory responses are associated with deterioration of cardiovascular status. Redistribution is effective only as long as adequate forward cardiac function is maintained. Marked elevations in placental blood flow resistance and progressive placental insufficiency can lead to an impairment of cardiac function. When this occurs, several aspects of cardiovascular homeostasis can be affected. Redistribution may become ineffective, there may be a measurable decline in cardiac output, and a decline in cardiac forward function may collectively lead to ineffective preload handling and elevations of central venous pressure.[127–130] The hallmark of this advancing deterioration in cardiovascular state is loss of diastolic forward flow in the umbilical circulation and a marked decline of forward flow in the venous system.[131] Finally, myocardial dysfunction and cardiac dilatation may result in holosystolic tricuspid insufficiency and spontaneous FHR decelerations and subsequent fetal demise.[132]

In addition to the central circulatory changes that affect the distribution of cardiac output, fetal organs have the ability to regulate their individual blood flow through autoregulation. Such autoregulatory mechanisms have been identified in the myocardium,[133] adrenal glands,[134] spleen,[135] liver,[136] celiac axis,[137] mesenteric vessels,[138,139] and kidneys.[140,141] These autoregulatory mechanisms are evoked at different levels of compromise, and their effect is typically complementary to central blood flow redistribution by enhancing perfusion of vital organs as long as cardiovascular homeostasis is maintained. Doppler ultrasound is the fetal assessment tool to assess these cardiovascular responses to placental insufficiency (see below). A summary of Doppler findings and their physiologic significance in the context of placental insufficiency is provided in Table 29-2.

Fetal behavioral responses to placental insufficiency and characteristics of the FHR reflect developmental status and undergo significant changes with advancing gestation. Progressive sophistication of fetal behavior and increasing variation of the FHR reflect differentiation of central regulatory centers and expansion of central processing capability. Normally, behavioral milestones progress from the initiation of gross body movements and fetal breathing in the first trimester to coupling of fetal behavior (e.g., heart rate reactivity) and integration of rest-activity cycles into stable behavioral states (states 1–4 F) by 28 to 32 weeks' gestation[142] (see Chapter 11). A steady decrease in baseline heart rate reflecting increasing vagal tone accompanies these developments. In addition, short- and long-term variability and variation, as well as the amplitude of accelerations, increase with advancing gestation that reflects increasing central processing. With the completion of these milestones, heart rate reactivity by traditional criteria is present in 80 percent of fetuses by 32 weeks' gestation. Differences in maturational and behavioral states, disruption of neural pathways, and declining oxygen tension may modulate or even abolish fetal behavior or heart rate characteristics.

Because variations of fetal behavior and the FHR may be due to several factors, observation of several variables over a sufficient length of time is necessary to separate physiologic from pathologic variation. Biophysical profile scoring (BPS) quantifies fetal behavior by assessing tone, movement, breathing activity, and FHR reactivity in an observation period of at least 30 minutes. Amniotic fluid

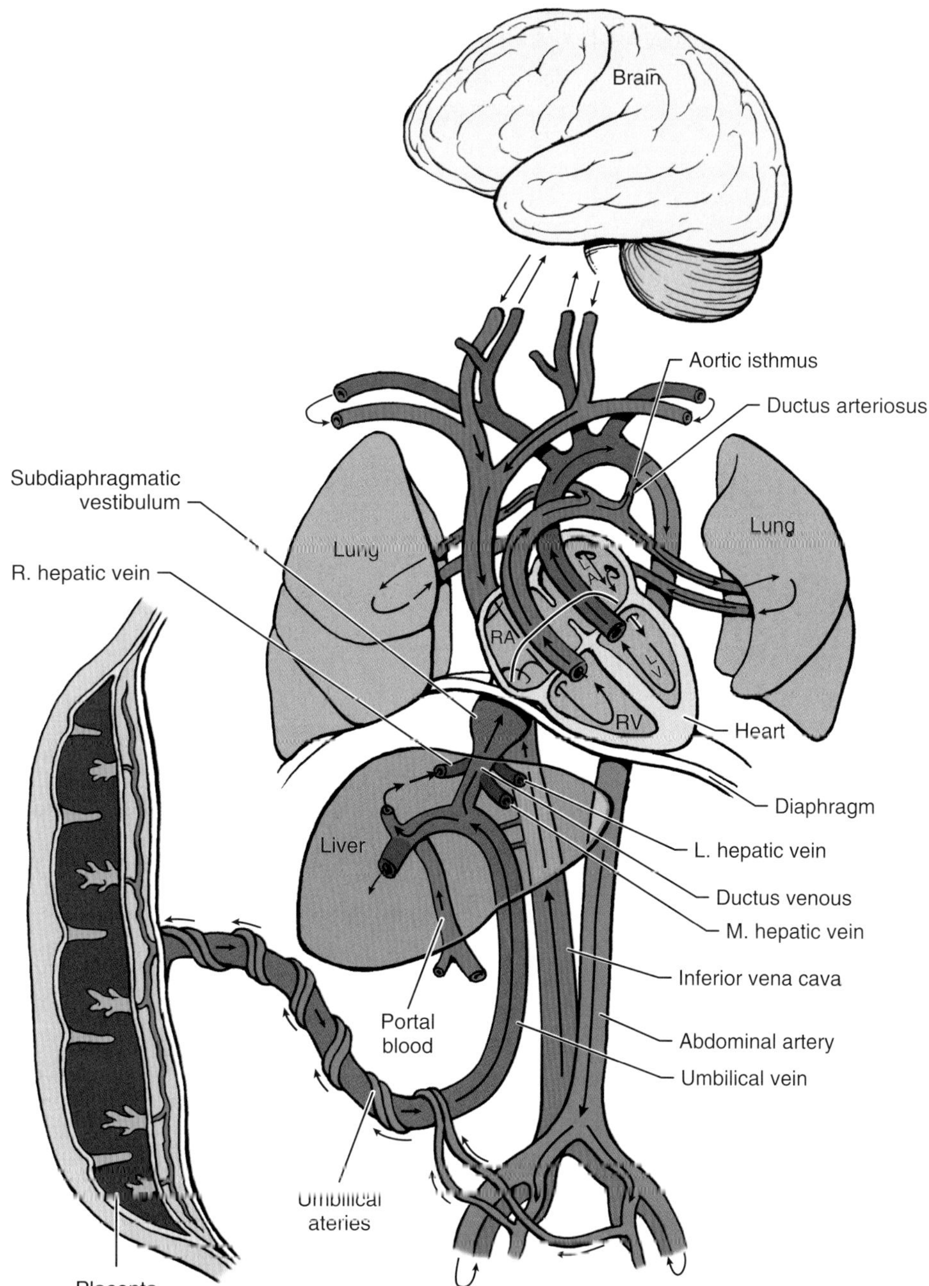

Figure 29-3. The fetal circulation. This figure illustrates the serial partitioning of nutrient and oxygen-rich blood reaching the fetus through the umbilical vein. The first partition at the level of the ductus venosus distributes the majority of umbilical venous blood to the liver. Umbilical venous blood that continues toward the heart is partitioned toward the left ventricle (LV) at the foramen ovale. This blood supplies the brain and upper part of the body through the brachiocephalic circulation and the myocardium through the coronary circulation. A minor proportion of blood from the right ventricle (RV) supplies the lungs, whereas the remainder continues through the ductus arteriosus (DA) toward the aorta. At the aortic isthmus, the blood stream coming from the aorta is partitioned based on the relationship of blood flow resistance in the brachiocephalic and subdiaphragmatic circulations. Although net forward flow is maintained under physiologic conditions, diastolic flow reversal occurs when brachiocephalic resistance falls or subdiaphragmatic (placental) resistance rises. Finally, the major proportion of descending aortic blood is partitioned at the umbilical arteries to return to the placenta for respiratory and nutrient exchange. (Reproduced with permission from Baschat AA: The fetal circulation and essential organs—a new twist to an old tale. Ultrasound Obstet Gynecol 27:349, 2006.)

volume (AFV) assessment has traditionally been a part of the BPS. From the second trimester onward, AFV is primarily related to fetal urine production and, therefore, renal perfusion. Thus, AFV assessment provides an indirect assessment of renal/vascular status and constitutes the main longitudinal monitoring component of the BPS (see Amniotic Fluid Assessment below). Visual FHR analysis has traditionally been the method of choice, which generates the problems of inter- and intraobserver variability. These problems are circumvented by computerized analysis of the FHR (cCTG). The cCTG assesses short-term, long-term, and mean minute variation and

Table 29-2. Summary of Vascular Responses in Fetuses with IUGR

DOPPLER FINDING	PHYSIOLOGIC SIGNIFICANCE
Uterine artery notching	Trophoblast invasion remains limited to the myometrial portion of the spiral arteries. Subsequent failure to fully transform into a low resistance, high capacitance vascular bed increases risk for subsequent IUGR or preeclampsia
Decreased, absent, or reversed umbilical artery end-diastolic velocity	Abnormal terminal villi and stem arteries result in increased placental vascular resistance and a proportional decrease in the umbilical artery end-diastolic velocity. Associated placental perfusion defects are responsible for impaired feto-maternal gas and nutrient exchange.
Elevation of blood flow resistance in the thoracic aorta and iliac artery	*Hind limb reflex:* Diversion of blood flow away from the carcass at the expense of the lower body. Achieved through increase in right ventricular afterload proximal to the umbilical arteries as well as increased blood flow resistance distally. In addition to centralization (see later), descending aortic blood flow is also preferentially distributed to the placenta.
1. Decrease in the cerebroplacental Doppler ratio. 2. Direct measurement of cardiac output. 3. Reversal of end-diastolic velocity in the aortic isthmus. 4. Absence or reversal of umbilical artery end-diastolic velocity.	*Centralization:* A measurable shift in the relationship between right and left ventricular afterload resulting in redistribution of cardiac output in favor of the left ventricle (i.e., the heart and brain). This can be passively mediated purely by an increase in placental blood flow resistance and therefore right ventricular afterload.
Decrease in the carotid, or middle cerebral artery Doppler index.	*Brain sparing:* Cerebral vasodilatation in response to perceived hypoxemia.
Increased superior mesenteric artery Doppler resistance	During perceived hypoxemia or redistribution of cardiac output blood flow to the gut as a nonessential organ in utero is compromised
Decrease in the splenic artery Doppler index	Splenic artery vasodilatation enhances perfusion of this important hematopoietic organ possibly facilitating an increase in red cell mass
Decreased Doppler resistance in the celiac axis	This may be a reflection of blood flow augmentation in the hepatic and splenic arteries which are the main branches of this axis
Increased Doppler resistance in peripheral pulmonary arteries	As nonessential organs in fetal life, lung perfusion may be further compromised by increased vascular resistance in the pulmonary circulation ensuring that a greater proportion of right ventricular output bypasses the lungs to reach the placenta.
Increased Doppler resistance in the renal arteries	Redistribution and increased renal vascular tone may be the mediators of oliguria and oligohydramnios observed with chronic and/or progressive hypoxemia.
Measured dilation of the ductus venosus with elevated Doppler index accompanied by a decreased hepatic artery Doppler index.	*Liver sparing:* Preferential arterial blood supply to the fetal liver invoked when increased diversion of umbilical venous blood through the ductus venosus jeopardizes hepatic perfusion.
Decreased Doppler index in the adrenal artery flow velocity waveforms.	*Adrenal sparing:* Enhanced adrenal perfusion is triggered as part of the fetal stress response to chronic malnutrition or an acute worsening imposed on the chronic state.
Umbilical venous pulsations in association with elevated venous Doppler indices	Evidence of inefficient forward delivery of cardiac output with subsequent elevation of central venous pressure that is transmitted all the way back into the umbilical vein
Normalization of cerebral Doppler indices after a period of "brain sparing"	With advanced cardiovascular deterioration, brain autoregulation may become abnormal. Probably in association with a decrease in cardiac function, the interval between systolic and diastolic velocities widens, resulting in an increase (thus normalization) of the Doppler index.
Sudden ability to visualize and measure coronary blood flow in a setting of deteriorating venous Doppler indices in a premature fetus with IUGR.	*Heart sparing:* Marked augmentation of coronary blood flow in situations of acute or chronic hypoxemia that is achieved through upregulation of coronary vascular reserve and vasodilatation.

IUGR, intrauterine growth restriction.
Rowlands DJ, Vyas SK: Longitudinal study of fetal middle cerebral artery flow velocity waveforms preceding fetal death. Br J Obstet Gynaecol 102:888, 1995.

periods of high variation in addition to traditional FHR parameters that also allow longitudinal observations. However, cCTG has not yet gained popularity in the United States as it has in Europe.

In growth-restricted fetuses with chronic hypoxemia and mild placental dysfunction, the primary CNS response is a delay in all aspects of CNS maturation.[143–146] With the help of computerized research tools, a delay of behavioral development has been documented under such circumstances. The combination of delayed central integration of FHR control, decreased fetal activity, and chronic hypoxemia results in a higher baseline heart rate with lower short- and long-term variation (on computerized analysis) and delayed development of heart rate reactivity.[147–150] These maturational differences in FHR parameters are particularly evident between 28 to 32 weeks.

Despite the maturational delay of some aspects of CNS function, several centrally regulated responses to acid-base status are still preserved.[151] Therefore, the growth-restricted fetus still maintains behavioral responses to a decline in acid-base status that are determined by the central effects of hypoxemia and acidemia independently of the cardiovascular status.[152–154] In contrast, the declining AFV that commonly accompanies the sequential loss of biophysical variables appears to be related to renal blood flow and the degree of vascular redistribution.[155,156]

With worsening fetal hypoxemia, a decline in global fetal activity initiates the cascade of late behavioral responses characteristic of placental insufficiency.[157] With further deepening hypoxemia, fetal breathing movement ceases. Gross body movements and tone decrease further until they are no longer observed in the traditional examination period.[158,159] Traditional FHR variables are frequently abnormal by this time. Reduction of global fetal activity and loss of fetal coupling (absence of heart rate reactivity and fetal breathing movements) are typically observed at a mean pH between 7.10 and 7.20. Loss of tone and movement is characteristic as the pH drops further. Late decelerations of the FHR may develop owing to a relative drop in oxygen tension that exceeds 8 mm Hg (see Chapter 15). Spontaneous decelerations due to direct depression of cardiac contractility or "cardiac" late decelerations typically herald fetal demise.

DIAGNOSTIC TOOLS IN FETAL GROWTH RESTRICTION

Fetal growth restriction is a syndrome that is marked by failure of the fetus to reach its growth potential with consequences that are related to the underlying disorder as well as the severity of fetal disease. Because a SGA fetus may be the consequence of many underlying etiologies, the differential diagnosis always includes maternal disease, placental insufficiency, aneuploidy, nonaneuploid syndromes, and viral infection. For appropriate patient counseling and choice of management options, comprehensive prenatal evaluation needs to go beyond the assessment of fetal size, using a diagnostic approach aimed at identifying the underlying causes. After confirming small fetal size, stratification into three patient groups is of particular importance. The first group consists of constitutionally small but otherwise normal fetuses. These patients will not usually require any intervention and, therefore, do not need antenatal surveillance. The second group consists of fetuses with aneuploidy, nonaneuploid syndromes, or viral infection. In these conditions, prognosis is largely determined by the underlying disease and timing of insult, with little potential for impact by perinatal interventions. Sensitive and knowledgeable counseling of the parents about the high likelihood of a poor prognosis is especially important in such cases. The third group consists of fetuses with placental disease. In these fetuses, progressive deterioration of the fetal condition worsens the prognosis. This subset of patients is most likely to benefit from fetal surveillance and subsequent intervention. Although grey-scale ultrasound provides important clues to the presence of IUGR, the liability of preterm delivery and iatrogenic complications is great if the diagnosis is based solely on biometry.[160] Although maternal disease is readily apparent through a history and physical examination, the accurate evaluation of the possible fetal disorder and stratification of risk requires the integration of several diagnostic modalities that evaluate fetal, placental, and amniotic fluid characteristics.[161–165]

Fetal Biometry

Ultrasound criteria have emerged as the diagnostic standard used in the identification of fetal growth restriction. For this purpose sonographic measurements of fetal bony and soft structures are related to reference ranges for gestation. In 1964, Wilcocks et al.[26] first demonstrated the correlation between ultrasound measurement of the fetal head and birth weight. Campbell and Dewhurst[11] published the first sonographic descriptions of fetal growth restriction with their analysis of the changes in biparietal diameter (BPD) over time. Two patterns of altered head growth were described: In "late flattening" (type 1, asymmetric type), the BPD increases normally until late pregnancy and then lags behind. In the "low-profile" or symmetric type, impaired head growth occurs much earlier in gestation (type 2). The asymmetric type represents approximately two thirds of cases of fetal growth restriction. The fetal AC is related to hepatic glycogen storage and liver size, therefore correlating closely with the nutritional state. Campbell and Wilkin[166] were the first to relate combined measurements of the BPD and AC to birth weight. Additional direct measurements that are primarily used in clinical practice today include the head circumference (HC) and femur length (FL). Secondary direct measurements include the transverse cerebellar diameter and the humerus length (HL). The most important calculated ultrasound variable of fetal growth is the sonographically estimated fetal weight (SEFW). Numerous investigators have identified distinct fetal ultrasound parameters that are useful in the calculation of the SEFW.[167–169] All of the techniques incorporate an index of abdominal size as a variable contributing to the estimation of fetal weight. Population-specific formulas have been derived to generate reference limits that generally have 95-percent confidence limits deviating approximately 15 percent from the actual value.[170]

Accurate estimation of fetal growth from these fetal measurements requires knowledge of the gestational age as a reference point to calculate percentile ranks. An estimated date of confinement should be based on the last menstrual period when the sonographic estimate of gestational age is within the predictive error (5 days in the first and 10 days in the second trimester, and 21 days in the third trimester). Once the estimated date of confinement is set by this method or a first-trimester ultrasound, it should not be changed because such practice interferes with the ability to diagnose IUGR.

Measurement of the BPD alone is a poor tool for the detection of IUGR. The physiologic variation in size inherent with advancing gestation is high. The majority of growth-restricted fetuses presenting with asymmetric growth restriction and delayed flattening of the cranial growth curve would be detected relatively late. Factors that interfere with a technically adequate measurement of the BPD include alterations of the cranial shape by external forces (oligohydramnios, breech presentation) and direct anteroposterior position of the fetal head.[171]

The HC is not subject to the same extrinsic variability as the BPD. The measurement technique is important because calculated HC measurements are systematically smaller than those directly measured. Thus, the nomogram selected should be based on measurements obtained using the same methodology. As a screening tool for IUGR, the HC poses a similar problem because the BPD in that two thirds of IUGR fetuses with asymmetric growth pattern would be detected late.

The transcerebellar diameter is one of the few soft tissue measurements that correlate well with gestational age,[172] being relatively spared from the effects of mild to moderate uteroplacental dysfunction. Whether its measurement offers any advantage over bony measurements in the assessment of compromised fetal growth is controversial.[173,174]

The AC is the single best measurement for the detection of IUGR.[170,175,176] The most accurate AC is the smallest directly measured circumference obtained in a perpendicular plane of the upper abdomen at the level of the hepatic vein between fetal respirations.[177] The AC percentile has both the highest sensitivity and negative predictive value for the sonographic diagnosis of IUGR whether defined postnatally by birth-weight percentile or ponderal Index. Using the 10th percentiles as cutoffs, the AC has a higher sensitivity (98 percent versus 85 percent) but lower positive predictive value than the SEFW (36 versus 51 percent). Its sensitivity is further enhanced by serial measurements at least 14 days apart.[178] Because of its high sensitivity, some type of abdominal measurement should be part of every sonographic growth evaluation. But because the AC reflects fetal nutrition, it should be excluded from the calculation of the composite gestational age after the early second trimester.

Calculation of the ratio between the head circumference and AC (HC/AC ratio) has been proposed as a tool to increase detection of the fetus with asymmetric growth restriction (Figs. 29-4 and 29-5).[179,180] In the normally growing fetus, the HC/AC ratio exceeds 1.0 before 32 weeks' gestation, is approximately 1.0 at 32 to 34 weeks' gestation, and falls below 1.0 after 34 weeks' gestation. In fetuses with asymmetric growth restriction, the HC remains larger than that of the body, resulting in an elevated HC/AC ratio,[181] whereas the ratio remains normal in symmetric IUGR in which both direct measurements are equally affected (see Figs. 29-4 and 29-5). Using the HC/AC ratio, 70 to 85 percent of growth-restricted fetuses are detected, with a reduction in false-negative diagnoses. Thus, a single set of measurements, even when determined in the latter part of pregnancy, can be very helpful in evaluating the status of intrauterine growth. However, both the sensitivity and the positive predictive value of this ratio for growth restriction do not equal either the AC percentile, or the SEFW.[182]

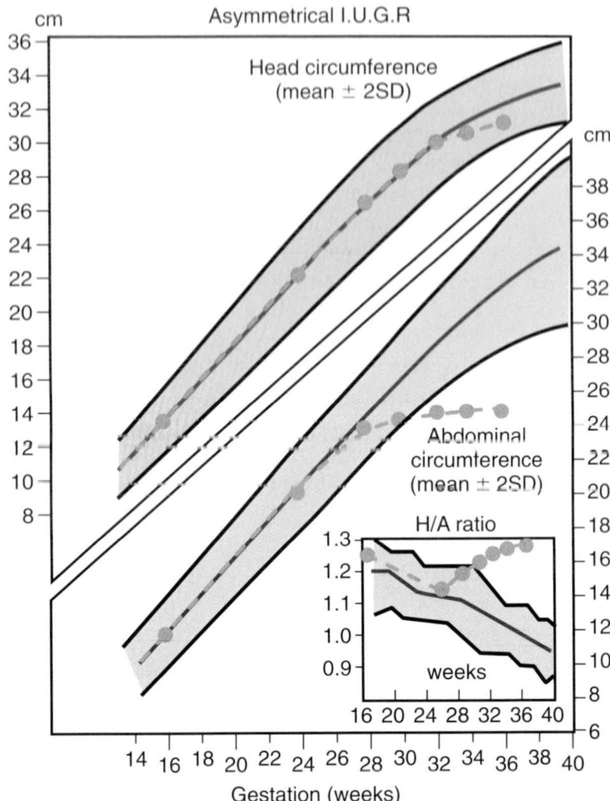

Figure 29-4. Growth chart in a case of asymmetric IUGR. Although head circumference is preserved, AC growth falls off early in the third trimester. For this reason, the H/A ratio shown in the lower right corner of the graph becomes elevated. IUGR, intrauterine growth restriction. (From Chudleigh P, Pearce JM: Obstetric Ultrasound. Edinburgh, Churchill Livingstone, 1986, with permission.)

In some cases, measurement of the HC may be difficult as a result of fetal position. One can then compare the FL, which is relatively spared in asymmetric IUGR, to the AC.[183] The FL/AC ratio is 22 at all gestational ages from 21 weeks to term and so can be applied without knowledge of the gestational age. An FL/AC ratio greater than 23.5 suggests IUGR.

Several formulae have been devised to calculate a SEFW. Using a multifactorial equation and a measurement of abdominal size, a weight can be predicted and related to gestational age. Formulas that incorporate the FL may increase the accuracy of in utero weight estimation for the fetus with IUGR. Since the SEFW cannot be measured directly, but is calculated from a combination of directly measured parameters, the error in the estimate is increased. The accuracy of most formulas (±2 standard deviations [SDs]) is ±10 percent, and none has proven superior to the first devised by Warsof and reported by Sheppard. As noted earlier, the SEFW has a lower sensitivity but higher positive predictive value than the AC and does not add to the AC percentile for the diagnosis of IUGR. However, an SEFW below the 10th percentile provides a graphic image easy for both patient and referring physician to conceptualize. Therefore, use of the estimated fetal weight has become the most common

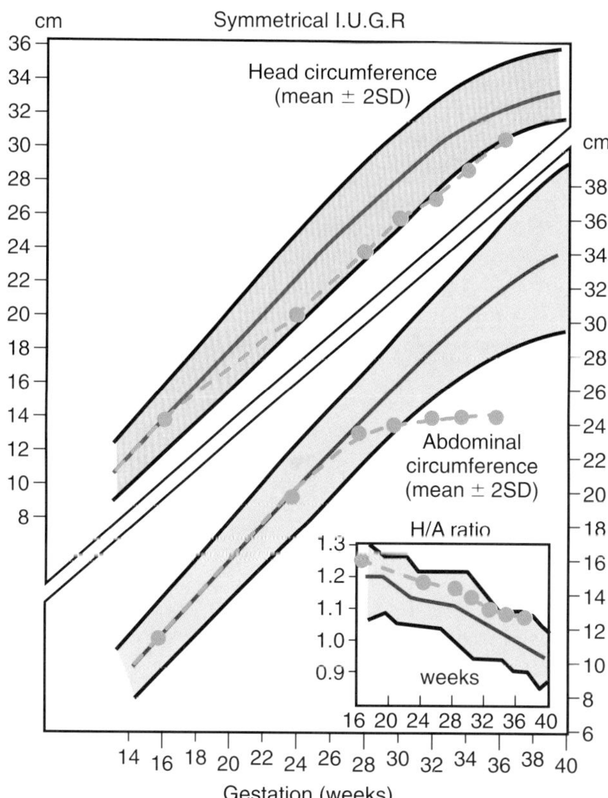

Figure 29-5. Growth chart in a case of symmetric IUGR. Note the early onset of both HC and AC growth restriction. For this reason, the H/A ratio shown in the lower right corner remains normal. IUGR, intrauterine growth restriction. (From Chudleigh P, Pearce JM: Obstetric Ultrasound. Edinburgh, Churchill Livingstone, 1986, with permission.)

method for characterizing fetal size and thereby growth abnormalities.[170]

Fetal Body Composition

The ponderal index was first described by Rohrer in 1921 as an index of corpulence.[184] This index of neonatal size (weight/length^3) that is normally distributed accurately reflected the nutritional state of the neonate. When compared with birth-weight percentile, the ponderal index demonstrates superior ability to predict neonatal asphyxia, acidosis, hypoglycemia, and hypothermia.[185] The ponderal index also correlates with direct measures of neonatal fat as estimated by skinfold thickness.[186] Attempts to translate the ponderal index directly to the fetus have been hampered by the difficulty in accurately assessing fetal length. Attempts to modify the ponderal index for fetal sonographic estimation have been made. Yagel et al.[187] demonstrated that the addition of a fetal ponderal index improved the prediction of perinatal morbidity in fetuses already suspected of having IUGR. Alternative methods for the characterization of fetal growth by physiologic compartments have recently been attempted. Several studies have examined fetal subcutaneous fat content using ultrasound examination. Subcutaneous fat deposition has been examined in the face, abdomen, arm, and thigh.[188-192] Reduction in facial fat stores has been strongly associated with being SGA. Using ultrasound, Padoan et al.[193] showed that both subcutaneous mass (fat mass) and lean mass (bone and muscle mass) are reduced in growth-restricted fetuses but that proportionately the subcutaneous mass is reduced to a greater extent than lean mass. This reduction in fat content is consistent with observations made in the growth-restricted neonate and may prove to be a sensitive indicator of the small fetus at increased risk for perinatal complications. The optimal method of in utero assessment of fetal fat has not yet been determined.

Reference Ranges Defining Fetal Growth

An absolute threshold used for the definition of IUGR can be applied to any of the fetal biometric parameters evaluated. These criteria have been defined statistically rather than outcome based and use either a threshold percentile ranking (non-normative data), or a number of standard deviations below the mean (normative data) as cutoffs. SGA is defined as a birth weight below the population 10th percentile, corrected for gestational age. However, this cutoff has also been the most widely used criterion for defining growth restriction at birth. This definition has also been adopted for the prenatal period by using a SEFW below the 10th percentile as an indicator of IUGR. Because such an approach is based purely on a weight threshold, it can serve only as a screen for the identification of the small fetus at risk for adverse outcome. Approximately 70 percent of infants with a birth weight below the 10th percentile are normally grown, that is constitutionally small and not at risk for adverse outcome as they present one end of the normal spectrum for neonatal size.[194] The remaining 30 percent consist of infants who are truly growth restricted and are at risk for increased perinatal morbidity and mortality. When the cutoff for an abnormal birthweight is adjusted to the 3rd percentile as suggested by Usher and McLean,[8,13] the proportion of truly growth-restricted infants identified increases while some with milder forms of IUGR will be missed. However, other authors have demonstrated increased mortality for birth weights through the 15th percentile with an odds ratio of 1.9 for mortality in newborns with birth weights between the 10th and 15th percentiles.[195] As the percentile cutoffs to define abnormal growth continue to be a matter of debate, risk assessment based on weight alone is further hampered by discrepancies between the SEFW and the actual birth weight. Live birth-weight criteria do not appropriately describe SEFWs, because there is a significant association of preterm birth with fetal growth restriction.[196] The weights of preterm infants are not normally distributed as they are at term, producing a significant discrepancy between birth weight–defined growth curves and SEFW-defined growth curves in preterm gestation.[197-199] SEFW growth curves are generated from patient samples representing the entire obstetric population at any gestational age. In contrast, preterm live birth normative data tables reflect only those individuals who have delivered under abnormal circumstances. Thus, the SEFW consistently demonstrate higher fetal weights over the range of preterm gestation than do birth weight–generated growth curves. Therefore, use of a SEFW cutoff below the 10th percentile is more appropriate to define abnormal fetal growth as the ability to identify fetuses at increased perinatal risk is enhanced.[200] For the AC, a 2.5th percentile cutoff is appropriate because reference ranges are based on a cross section of small, appropriately grown, preterm, and term newborns. However, because reference limits are based on healthy women delivering appropriately nourished neonates at term, the less-than-10th-percentile cutoff is consistent with IUGR.

Because of the limitation of a population-based reference range to assess fetal growth, individualized growth models have been proposed by several investigators.[201,202] The obvious advantage is the lack of dependency on population-based normative data and the ability to detect a true singularly defined growth restriction even with estimated fetal weights above the 10th percentile for the population. Some of these models require three sequential sonograms. This includes baseline biometry in the second trimester, a second sonogram to establish growth potential for an individual morphometric parameter, and a third scan to identify a growth abnormality. Because this approach is cumbersome in clinical practice, other models have been developed that account for variables that contribute the majority of the variance to newborn size. These include early pregnancy weight, maternal height, ethnic group, parity, and sex.[2] Using these variables and fetal growth patterns, the estimated size of a fetus of a given mother can be projected at term and estimated at any specific point in gestation. Deviations from this projected growth pattern can then be recognized. Overall, the diagnostic advantages of these individualized growth models has been questioned when compared with the sequential comparison of the percentile ranking of individual or composite growth parameters to population-based growth curves.[203]

Fetal growth as opposed to fetal size is a dynamic process and requires more than a single evaluation for its estimation. The appropriate observation interval for the evaluation of fetal growth has been based on the assumptions that growth is continuous rather than sporadic and that the identification of growth is limited by the technical capability of the ultrasound equipment used to measure the fetus. The recommended interval between ultrasound evaluations of fetal growth is 3 weeks, because shorter intervals increase the likelihood of a false-positive diagnosis.[204,205]

In summary, the ability to correctly identify growth-restricted fetuses at risk for adverse outcome by weight estimates alone is limited. Individualized or sequential growth assessment performs better than a single measurement of fetal size. Improved stratification of risk requires the integration of additional diagnostic possibilities.

Fetal Anatomic Survey

Although the sonographic survey of fetal anatomy does not provide an assessment of fetal growth, it is the first step toward the investigation of an underlying etiology. The anatomic survey should focus on the detection of markers of aneuploidy, nonaneuploid syndromes, and fetal infection, as well as any anatomic defects. The relationship between aneuploidy and fetal anomalies such as gastroschisis, omphalocele, diaphragmatic hernia, congenital heart defects, and sonographic markers such as echogenic bowel, nuchal thickening, and abnormal hand positioning are discussed in Chapter 9. Abnormalities of skull contour, thoracic shape, or disproportional shortening of the long bones may be indications of skeletal dysplasia or thanatophoric dwarfism. Markers for viral infection may be nonspecific but include echogenicity and calcification in organs such as the brain and liver.[206] Identification of any of these abnormalities on ultrasound significantly affects the differential diagnosis and frequently has a decisive impact on outcome.

Amniotic Fluid Assessment

The regulation of AFV by the late second and third trimester is primarily dependent on fetal urine output, production of pulmonary fluid, and fetal swallowing. Placental dysfunction and fetal hypoxemia both may result in decreased perfusion of the fetal kidneys with subsequent oliguria and decreasing AFV.[207] Although the accuracy of ultrasound in the assessment of actual AFV is poor, two techniques are used that can provide important diagnostic and prognostic information.[208] In an early study, Manning et al.[209] reported that a vertical pocket of amniotic fluid measuring 1 cm or more reflected an adequate fluid volume. Criteria for AFV assessment were subsequently broadened. A 2-cm vertical pocket was considered normal, 1 to 2 cm marginal, and less than 1 cm decreased.[210] Alternatively, AFV may be assessed by the sum of vertical pockets from four quadrants of the uterine cavity. This four-quadrant amniotic fluid index (AFI) is compared with reference ranges that require knowledge of the gestational age (see Chapter 31). Despite the availability of these numeric methods for semiquantification of AFV, an overall clinical impression of reduced amniotic fluid may be most important. Ultrasound criteria for a subjectively reduced AFV include a maximum vertical pocket below 3 cm, the fetus in a flexion attitude with limited room for movement, a small or empty bladder and stomach, and molding of the uterus around the fetal body. Movement of the transducer frequently generates uterine contractions, which may be associated with variable decelerations.

Overall, estimation of AFV in itself is a poor screening method for IUGR or fetal acidemia.[211,212] However, in clinical practice, it is an important diagnostic and prognostic tool. Oligohydramnios may be the first sign of fetal growth restriction detected on ultrasonography preceding an assessment for lagging fetal growth. If gestational age is known, ultrasound assessment of fetal growth based on the HC, AC, FL, and SEFW can be performed. If gestational age is unknown, measurements of the FL/AC ratio and single amniotic fluid pocket have to be used because they are independent of gestational age. Up to 96 percent of fetuses with fluid pockets less than 1 cm may be growth restricted.[209] In patients in whom growth delay is already suspected, AFV can be an important differential diagnostic marker. In the setting of small fetal size, abundant AFV suggests aneuploidy or fetal infection,[213] whereas normal or decreased amniotic fluid is compatible with placental insufficiency. The volume of amniotic fluid also has prognostic significance for the course of labor. Groome et al.[214] demonstrated that oligohydramnios associated with fetal oliguria is associated with a higher rate of intrapartum complications that may be attributed to reduced placental reserve.

Doppler Velocimetry

Similar to the assessment of AFV, the role of Doppler velocimetry in the management of fetal growth restriction is unique because it serves as a diagnostic as well as a monitoring tool. Doppler flow velocity waveforms may be obtained from arterial and venous vascular beds in the fetus. Arterial Doppler waveforms provide information on downstream vascular resistance, which may be altered owing to structural changes in the vasculature or regulatory changes in vascular tone. The systolic/diastolic ratio, resistance index, and the pulsatility index are the three Doppler indices most widely used to analyze arterial blood flow resistance (Table 29-3). An increase in blood flow resistance manifests itself with a relative decrease in end-diastolic velocity resulting in an increase in all three Doppler indices. Of these indices, the pulsatility index has the smallest measurement error and narrower reference limits.[215] With extreme increase in blood flow resistance, end-diastolic forward velocity may be absent (AEDV) or reversed (REDV) (Fig. 29-6).

Venous Doppler parameters complement evaluation of fetal cardiovascular status by providing an assessment of cardiac forward function. Forward blood flow in the venous system is determined by cardiac compliance, contractility, and afterload, and it is characterized by a triphasic flow pattern that reflects pressure volume changes in the atria throughout the cardiac cycle.[216] The descent of the AV ring during ventricular systole and passive diastolic ventricular filling generates the systolic and diastolic peaks, respectively (the S- and D-wave). The sudden increase in right atrial pressure with atrial contraction in late diastole causes a variable amount of reverse flow, producing a second trough after the D wave (the a-wave) (Fig. 29-7). The magnitude of forward flow during the atrial systole varies considerably in individual veins: Reversal may be physiologic in the inferior vena cava and hepatic veins but it is always abnormal in the ductus venosus. Multiple venous Doppler indices have been described to characterize this complex waveform without any clear advantages of individual indices[217] (see Table 29-3).

Table 29-3. Arterial and Venous Doppler Indices

Arterial Doppler Indices

INDEX	CALCULATION
S/D ratio	$\frac{\text{systolic peak velocity}}{\text{diastolic peak velocity}}$
Resistance index (RI)	$\frac{\text{systolic} - \text{end-diastolic peak velocity}}{\text{systolic peak velocity}}$
Pulsatility index (PI)	$\frac{\text{systolic} - \text{end-diastolic peak velocity}}{\text{time averaged maximum velocity}}$

Venous Doppler Indices

INDEX	CALCULATION
Inferior vena cava preload index	$\frac{\text{peak velocity during atrial contraction}}{\text{systolic peak velocity}}$
Ductus venosus preload index	$\frac{\text{systolic} - \text{diastolic peak velocity}}{\text{systolic peak velocity}}$
Inferior vena cava and ductus venosus pulsatility index for veins (PIV)	$\frac{\text{systolic} - \text{diastolic peak velocity}}{\text{time averaged maximum velocity}}$
Inferior vena cava and ductus venosus peak velocity index for veins (PVIV)	$\frac{\text{systolic} - \text{atrial contraction peak velocity}}{\text{diastolic peak velocity}}$
Percentage reverse flow	$\frac{\text{systolic time averaged velocity}}{\text{diastolic time averaged velocity}} \times 100$

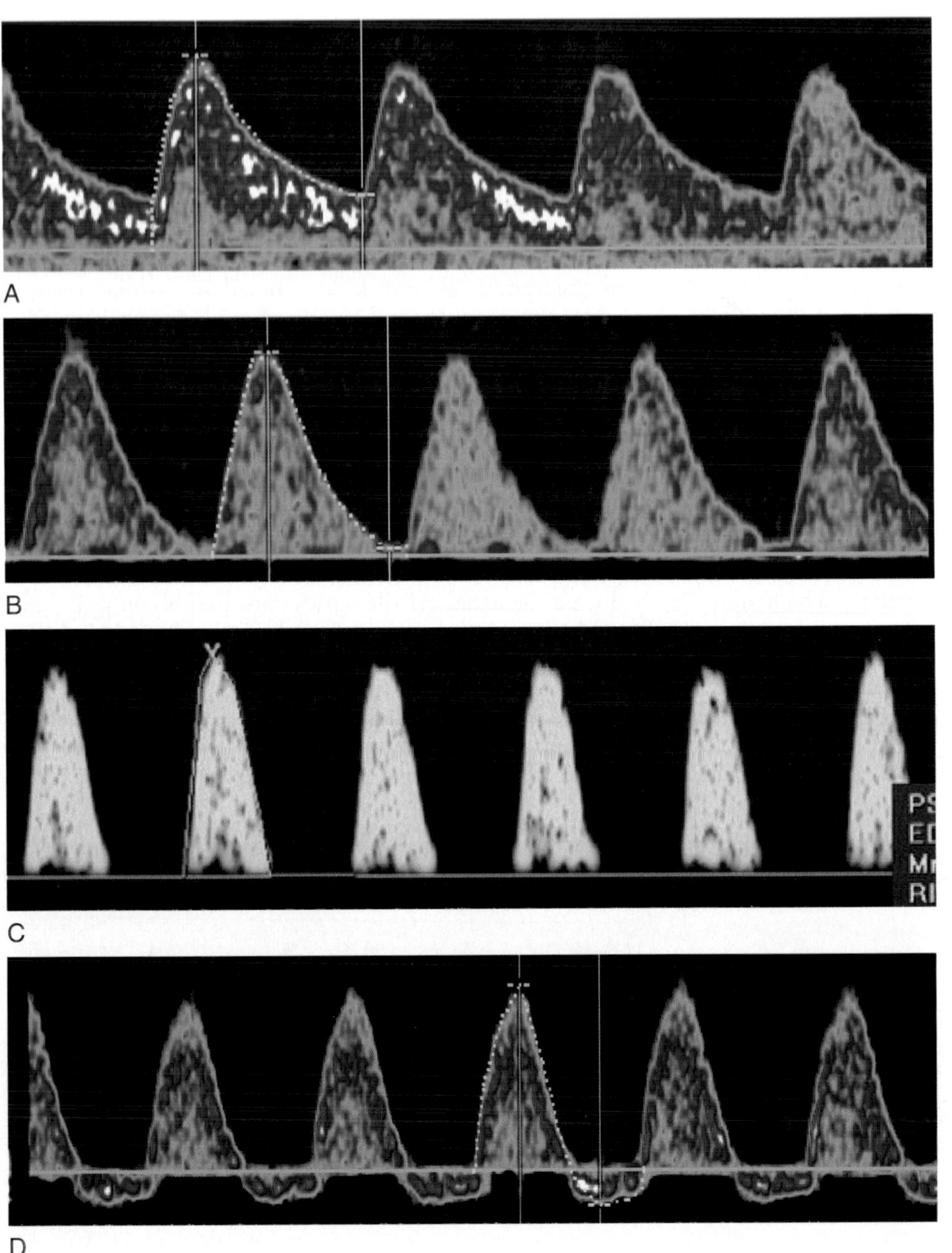

Figure 29-6. Umbilical artery flow velocity waveforms. The normal umbilical artery flow velocity waveform has positive end-diastolic velocities that increase toward term reflecting a falling blood flow resistance in the villous vascular tree *(A)*. Moderate abnormalities in the villous vascular structure raise the blood flow resistance and are associated with a decline in end-diastolic velocities *(B)*. When a significant proportion of the villous vascular tree is abnormal, end-diastolic velocities may be absent *(C)* or even reversed *(D)*.

In the diagnostic assessment of the small fetus, examination of umbilical and middle cerebral artery Doppler studies are the most important to evaluate for placental dysfunction as the underlying etiology. Randomized trials and meta-analyses confirm that the combined use of fetal biometry and umbilical artery Doppler significantly reduces perinatal mortality and iatrogenic intervention because documentation of placental vascular insufficiency effectively separates growth-restricted fetuses that require surveillance and possible intervention from constitutionally small fetuses.[218–220]

A free umbilical cord loop is examined with continuous or pulsed Doppler ultrasound far from the fetal and placental insertions (e.g., midcord segment). Most current ultrasound equipment allows concurrent use of color and pulsed Doppler with improved reproducibility of measurements. Vascular damage affecting approximately 30 percent of the placenta produces elevations in the Doppler index. More marked abnormalities result in umbilical artery AEDV or REDV. Milder forms of placental vascular dysfunction, especially near term, may not produce elevation of umbilical artery blood flow resistance sufficiently to be detectable by traditional Doppler methods.[221] If placental gas exchange is sufficiently impaired to result in perceived fetal hypoxemia, a decrease in middle cerebral artery Doppler resistance may occur (Fig. 29-8). Another Doppler index frequently used clinically to detect this condition is the ratio between umbilical artery pulsatility as index of vasoconstriction in the placenta and middle cerebral artery pulsatility as index of vasodilation in the fetal brain. In milder forms of placental disease with near-minimal increase in umbilical artery blood flow resistance the cerebroplacental Doppler ratio (CPR) may decrease. Grammellini

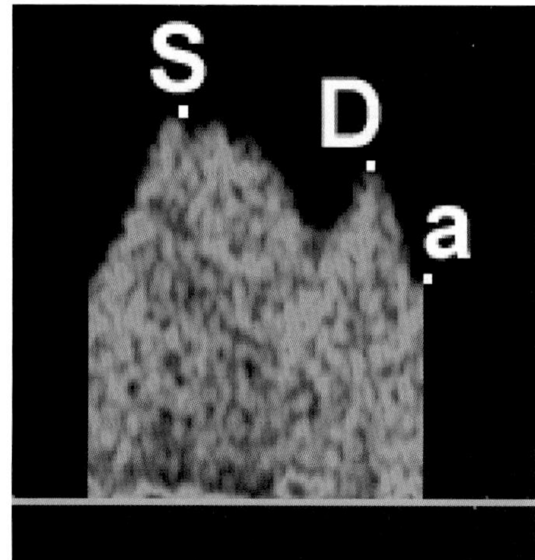

Figure 29-7. Venous flow velocity waveform. A typical venous flow velocity waveform is shown. The triphasic waveform (S, systole; D, diastole; a, atrial contraction) reflects volume flow changes during the cardiac cycle. With descent of the atrioventricular valves during ventricular systole, intraatrial pressures fall and increased forward flow during the S wave is observed. A temporary decrease in forward flow occurs when the atrioventricular valve ring ascends at the end of ventricular systole, producing the first trough in the flow velocity waveform. When atrial pressures exceed intraventricular pressures, the atrioventricular valves open, resulting in the rapid influx of blood into the ventricles. The associated increase in venous flow results in the D wave. With initiation of a new cardiac cycle, atrial contraction results in a sharp rise in intra-atrial pressure and decline in venous forward flow. This second trough is called the a-wave because it is produced by atrial contraction.

and coworkers demonstrated that a value below 1.08 identified small fetuses at risk for adverse outcome.[222] Subsequently Bahado-Singh and coworkers[223] indicated that this predictive accuracy of the CPR decreased after 34 weeks' gestation. This is presumably attributable to an increasing number of growth-restricted fetuses that may have normal umbilical artery blood flow resistance near term but demonstrate isolated "brain sparing" as the only sign of placental insufficiency of oxygen transfer.[162] These fetuses are at risk for adverse outcome.[163,164]

Because of the variable presentation across gestation, comprehensive Doppler assessment of placental function should include umbilical and middle cerebral arteries. For the umbilical artery, an abnormal test result is defined as a Doppler index measurement of greater than 2 SDs above the gestational age mean and/or a loss of end-diastolic velocity. Like growth curves, it is best to use nomograms developed from a local or comparable population. For the CPR and also for the middle cerebral artery, a greater than 2 SD decrease of the index is considered abnormal.[223,224] In a setting of small fetal size, these findings identify those fetuses at greatest risk for adverse outcome (Figs. 29-9 through 29-12).

Invasive Testing

Several invasive tests for the evaluation of the fetus with suspected growth restriction have been described. From a clinical standpoint, there are only few studies of critical importance. These include maternal TORCH serology and invasive fetal testing to obtain amniotic fluid or fetal blood for karyotyping to rule out a chromosomal abnormality such as trisomy 13, 18, or 21 (Table 29-4).

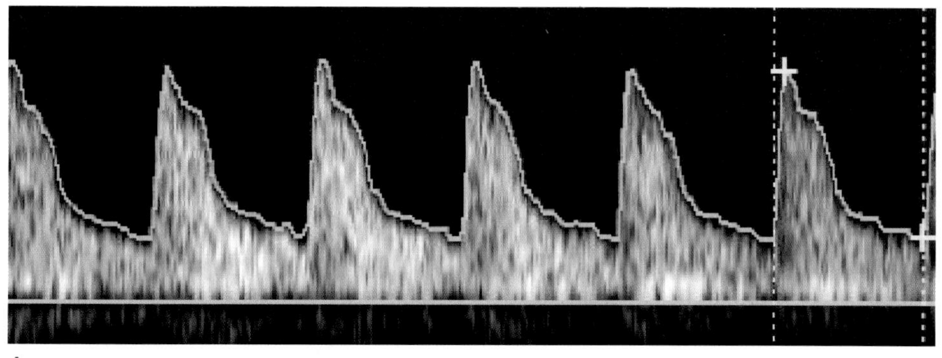

A

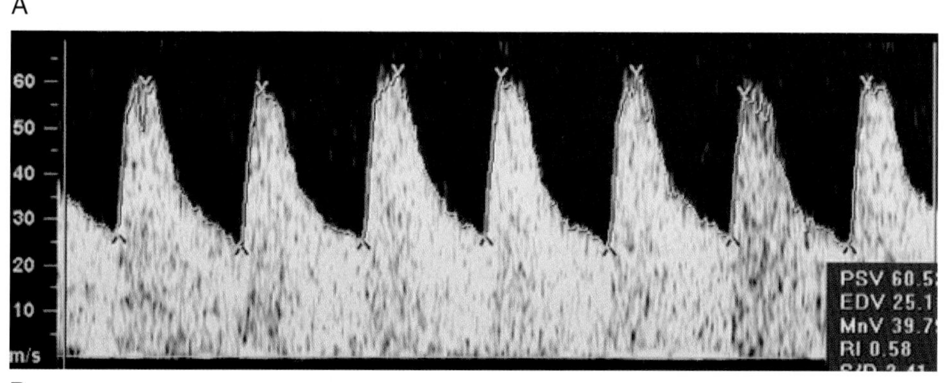

B

Figure 29-8. Middle cerebral artery flow velocity waveform. The normal middle cerebral artery flow pattern has relatively little diastolic flow *(A)*. With progressive placental dysfunction, there may be an increase in the diastolic velocity, resulting in a decrease in the Doppler index (Brain sparing, *B*). With brain sparing, the systolic down slope of the waveform becomes smoother so that the waveform almost resembles that of the umbilical artery. The associated rise in the mean velocity results in a marked decline in the Doppler index.

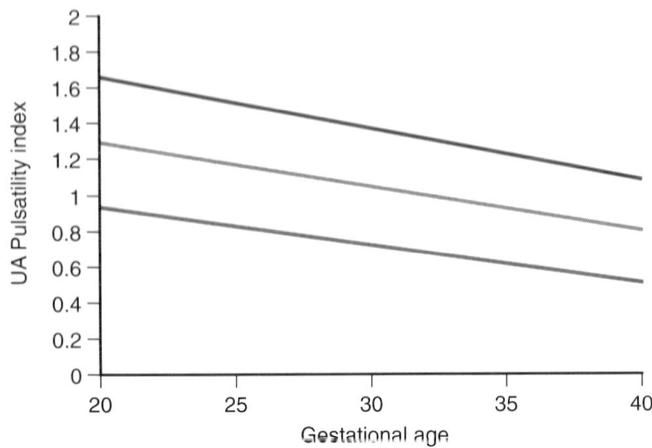

Figure 29-9. Umbilical artery pulsatility index with advancing gestational age. Displayed are the reference ranges (mean and 95-percent confidence interval) of the umbilical artery (UA) pulsatility index.

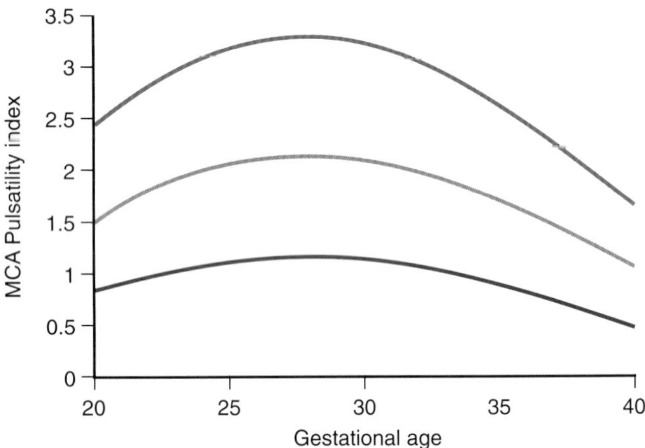

Figure 29-10. Middle cerebral artery pulsatility index with advancing gestational age. The graph shows the mean and 95 percent confidence interval of the middle cerebral artery (MCA) pulsatility index.

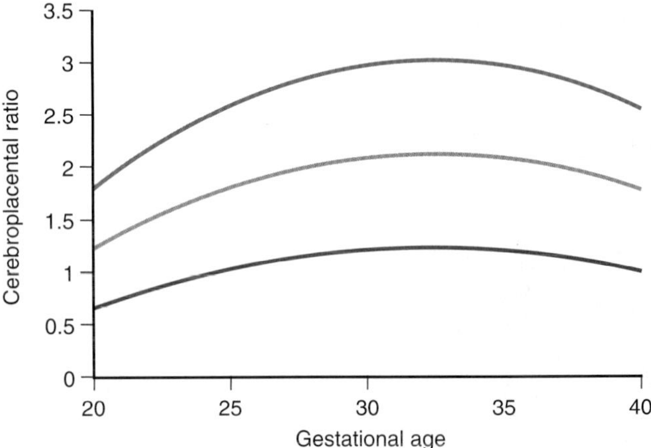

Figure 29-11. Cerebroplacental Doppler ratio with advancing gestational age. This graph displays the gestational reference range (mean and 95-percent confidence interval) of the cerebroplacental ratio based on paired measurements of the middle cerebral and umbilical artery pulsatility index.

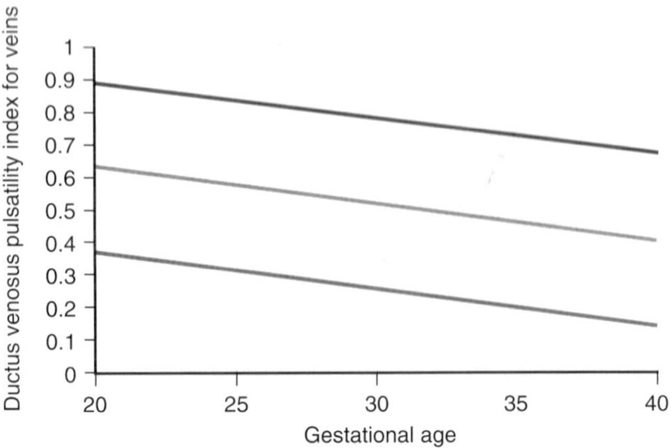

Figure 29-12. Ductus venosus pulsatility index for veins with advancing gestational age. This graph displays the gestational reference range (mean and 95-percent confidence interval) of the ductus venosus pulsatility index for veins calculated from cross-sectional data in 232 normal singleton fetuses.

Table 29-4. Chromosomal Abnormalities and IUGR

ULTRASOUND FINDINGS PRESENT			
IUGR	ANOMALY	HYDRAMNIOS	ABNORMAL KARYOTYPE
X			12/180 (7%)
X	X		18/57 (32%)
X		X	6/22 (27%)
X	X	X	7/15 (47%)

From Eydoux P, Choiset A, LePorrier N, et al: Chromosomal prenatal diagnosis: study of 936 cases of intrauterine abnormalities after ultrasound assessment. Prenat Diagn 9:255, 1989, with permission.

Trisomy 18 may present with the unusual combination of growth restriction and polyhydramnios. If the diagnosis of a lethal anomaly can be made with certainty, cesarean delivery for fetal distress is unnecessary and may be prevented. Viral polymerase chain reaction studies can be performed if there is a clinical suspicion based on the ultrasound examination or in the maternal history.

Evaluation of fetal erythropoietin and amino acid concentrations are also markers for fetal compromise with prognostic impact. Erythropoietin production in the fetus, as in the adult, is stimulated by the presence of anemia or hypoxia, and may be associated with increased red blood cell production depending on erythropoietic reserve.[225,226] Elevated blood or amniotic fluid erythropoietin levels may be of help in identifying growth-restricted fetuses at risk for long-term morbidity.[96,227,228] Ruth et al.[229] identified an association between cord blood erythropoietin levels and developmental outcome including cerebral palsy and death at 2 years in offspring with evidence of acute asphyxia at birth. None of these patients had preeclampsia. Neonates from pregnancies complicated by preeclampsia had elevated cord erythropoietin levels regardless of outcome.

An increase in the cord blood glycine/valine ratio is a specific response to intrauterine starvation resulting

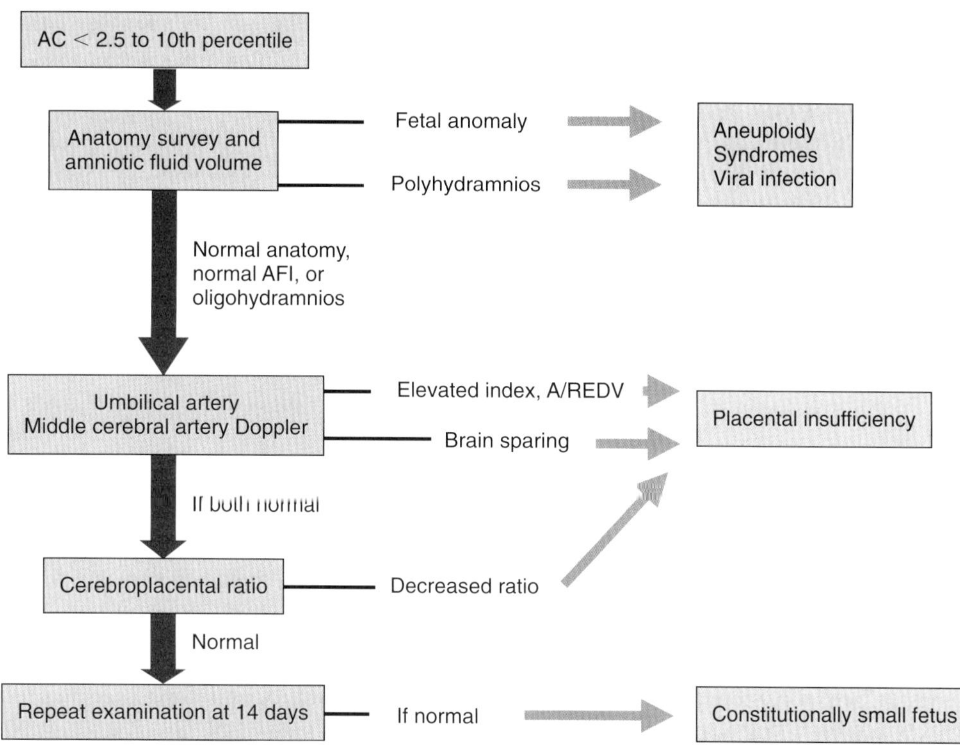

Figure 29-13. An integrated diagnostic approach to the fetus with suspected fetal growth restriction. This figure displays a decision tree following the evaluation of fetal anatomy, amniotic fluid volume, umbilical and middle cerebral artery Doppler. The most likely clinical diagnosis based on the test results is presented on the right-hand side. A high index of suspicion for aneuploidy, viral, and non-aneuploid syndromes needs to be maintained at all times.

from reduction in phosphoenolpyruvate carboxykinase activity, a rate-limiting enzyme for gluconeogenesis.[230] Elevations of the glycine/valine ratio are observed in fetal life and have been shown to be inversely proportional to fetal arterial oxygen content.[231] However, in contrast to the neonate in whom such an increased ratio is predictive of specific neonatal risks including hypoglycemia and death,[232] such a relationship has not been demonstrated for elevations demonstrated in fetal life.[233] Although fetal erythropoietin and amino acid levels are of academic interest, they currently add little to the contemporary clinical management of the IUGR fetus.

In summary, ultrasound examination is the primary diagnostic tool for the evaluation of fetal growth. In the presence of risk factors and clinical conditions that are associated with IUGR, a comprehensive gray-scale ultrasound examination of fetal anatomy, biometry, and amniotic fluid characteristics is required. In the absence of routine clinical indications, ultrasound screening of these high-risk pregnancies should be performed at 16 to 18 weeks for dating (if not otherwise established) and again at 30 to 36 weeks. If small fetal size is documented, Doppler ultrasound of the umbilical and middle cerebral arteries, and invasive tests are of critical importance to identify fetuses most likely to benefit from antenatal surveillance and perinatal interventions. A diagnostic algorithm that uses this combination of test parameters is depicted in Figure 29-13.

SCREENING AND PREVENTION OF FETAL GROWTH RESTRICTION

Fetal growth restriction as a disease entity fulfills several criteria, potentially justifying a screening program; it is a common clinical problem with an identifiable predisease state that leaves enough time for potential interventions. Although treatment options in utero are limited (see later), interventions that improve outcome exist. The various screening methods that have been proposed include identification of risk factors, as well as serum and ultrasound tests.

Maternal History

A history of poor pregnancy outcome is clearly correlated with the subsequent delivery of a growth-restricted infant. Galbraith et al.[234] and Tejani[235] have shown that prior birth of a growth-restricted infant is the obstetric factor most often associated with the subsequent birth of another growth-restricted infant. These study populations did include women with underlying medical problems. In a retrospective study of 83 multigravidas who had delivered growth-restricted infants, Tejani and Mann[236] noted that the perinatal wastage from their 200 prior pregnancies was 41 percent. This striking figure, which includes spontaneous abortions as well as neonatal and intrauterine deaths, points to the significance of poor obstetric history as a risk factor for IUGR. The history of delivery of a growth-restricted infant in the first pregnancy is associated with a 25-percent risk of delivering a second infant below the 10th percentile. After two pregnancies complicated by IUGR, there is a fourfold increase in the risk of a subsequent growth-restricted infant. When all indices of risk have been applied, the one third of patients considered at highest risk for delivering a growth restricted infant actually deliver over 60 percent of infants identified as growth restricted. The two thirds of women not considered at risk for delivering a growth-restricted infant contribute to one third of deliveries with a birth weight below the 10th percentile. The majority of these babies are considered constitutionally small.

Maternal Serum Analytes

At least four hormone/protein markers measured in the maternal sera during the early second trimester are associated with subsequent IUGR. These include serum estriol, human placental lactogen, human chorionic gonadotrophin and alpha-fetoprotein. An elevated maternal serum alpha-fetoprotein or human chorionic gonadotropin level in the second trimester are considered as markers of abnormal placentation and have been associated with an increased risk for IUGR.[237–240] Most studies conclude that a single, unexplained elevated value of 2 to 2.5 multiples of the median raises the risk of growth restriction five- to 10-fold.

Clinical Examination

From the early second trimester on, each antenatal visit includes the measurement of the distance between the maternal uterine fundus and the symphysis pubis. After 20 weeks' gestation, the normal symphyseal-fundal height in centimeters approximates the weeks of gestation after allowances for maternal height and fetal station. Belizan et al.[241] observed that after 20 weeks' gestation, a lag of the symphyseal-fundal height of 4 cm or more suggests growth restriction. The reported sensitivities of symphyseal-fundal height screening for IUGR range from 27 to 85 percent, and the positive predictive values of 18 to 50 percent.[242] Although the measurement of the symphyseal-fundal height is a poor screening tool for the detection of IUGR, the accuracy of subsequent ultrasound prediction of IUGR is enhanced if there is a clinical suspicion of IUGR based on a lagging fundal height.

Maternal Doppler Velocimetry

Abnormal uterine artery flow velocity waveforms are a manifestation of delayed trophoblast invasion that are highly associated with gestational hypertensive disorders, IUGR and fetal demise.[243–246] Therefore, Doppler velocimetry of the uterine arteries has been examined for its usefulness in predicting pregnancies destined to produce a growth-restricted fetus. Schulman[76] found that in women with hypertensive disorders, the presence of an elevated uterine artery systolic/diastolic (S/D) ratio (>2.6) and diastolic notching increased the risk for IUGR and stillbirth (see Fig. 29-2). He noted that the changes in uterine artery flow patterns precede those observed in the umbilical artery and antedate fetal growth restriction. Subsequent studies used various cutoffs to define an abnormal test result. These include S/D ratios above 2.18 at 18 weeks, resistance index above 0.58 at 18 to 24 weeks, pulsatility index above the 95th percentile (1.45) at 22 to 24 weeks, or the presence of notches have been used as abnormal results. The screen positive rate ranges between 5 and 13 percent according to the gestational age and the criterion used to define an abnormal test result. In low-risk patients, a uterine artery Doppler resistance profile that is high, persistently notched, or both, identifies women at high-risk for preeclampsia and IUGR with sensitivities and positive predictive values as high as 72 percent and 35 percent[247–249] when performed between 22 and 23 weeks' gestation.[250] Uterine artery Doppler is better at predicting severe rather than mild disease.[251] The likelihood ratio of abnormal uterine artery impedance for the development of IUGR was 3.7 with higher sensitivity for severe early onset forms. Meta-analysis of the utility of uterine artery Doppler in the prediction of intrauterine death yields a likelihood ratio of 2.4 for patients with an abnormal result. Combining uterine artery Doppler velocimetry with other tests can improve screening sensitivities. Valensise and Romanini[252] have demonstrated that the combination of abnormal second-trimester maternal uterine artery Doppler velocimetry and maternal glucose tolerance testing demonstrating a "flat" response results in a positive predictive value of 94 percent and a sensitivity of 54 percent for the detection of fetal growth restriction. The presence of a normal uterine artery flow velocity waveform bears a high negative predictive value with a likelihood ratio of 0.5 and 0.8 for the development of preeclampsia and IUGR respectively.

Preventive Strategies

Efforts to prevent fetal growth restriction have been disappointing. Low-dose aspirin has been extensively evaluated as a possible preventive agent for improving placental vascular development by virtue of its inhibitory action on platelet aggregation. However, although the use of aspirin in the second trimester has been found to be safe, initiation of therapy in the second trimester improves neither placental function nor long-term outcome.[253,254] Because subsets of patients with poor obstetric history appear to derive a benefit from aspirin, the utility of first trimester uterine artery screening with subsequent aspirin therapy has been investigated. The choice of target population profoundly affects the utility of this approach. Although low-risk patients derive little benefit, high-risk patients (e.g., those with thrombophilia, hypertension, or a past history of either preeclampsia or IUGR) given low-dose aspirin because of bilateral uterine artery notching at 12 to 14 weeks experience an 80 percent reduction of placental disease compared with placebo-matched controls.[255]

In summary, the utility of screening for fetal growth restriction has not been established. Although maternal uterine artery Doppler velocimetry identifies patients at risk, efficacy of prophylactic interventions has not been established.[256] At present, it appears prudent to regard poor obstetric history, unexplained elevations in second trimester maternal serum alpha-fetoprotein, "flat" oral glucose tolerance, and abnormal second-trimester uterine artery Doppler velocimetry as important risk factors for IUGR that warrant further investigation when the clinical suspicion of IUGR arises or maternal pre-eclampsia develops. Such patients should undergo ultrasound estimation of fetal size and a full diagnostic workup if this is confirmed.

MANAGEMENT IN CLINICAL PRACTICE

Before developing a management plan, it is important that the major underlying etiologies have been addressed by a comprehensive diagnostic workup, as described earlier. It is worth stressing that the majority of fetuses thought to be growth restricted are constitutionally small and require no intervention. Approximately 15 percent exhibit symmetric growth restriction attributable to an early fetal insult for which there is no effective therapy. Here, an accurate diagnosis is essential. Finally, approximately 15 percent of small fetuses have growth restriction owing to placental disease or reduced uteroplacental blood flow. Once the diagnosis of placental insufficiency has been made, appropriate therapeutic options may be explored. However, ongoing assessment of fetal growth and parameters of fetal well-being is a more critical component of clinical management in defining the intervention thresholds when the balance of fetal versus neonatal risks favors delivery.

Therapeutic Options

Elimination of contributors such as stress, smoking, and alcohol and drug use is advocated. Tobacco smoke contains a number of substances that are vasoactive and can cause vasoconstriction. Anecdotally, the authors have observed IUGR cases with absent end-diastolic flow in the umbilical artery in which diastolic flow returned on cessation of maternal smoking. Nonspecific therapies include bed rest in the left lateral decubitus position to increase placental blood flow. Although an inadequate diet has not been clearly established as a cause of growth restriction in this country, dietary supplementation may be helpful in those with poor weight gain or low pre-pregnancy weight. In patients with chronic malnutrition improved fetal growth has been reported with total parenteral nutrition.[257] Consideration should be given to hospitalized bed rest, which has the advantages of positive enforcement of rest and facilitation of daily fetal testing. The decision for inpatient versus outpatient management is based on the severity of the maternal and fetal condition, and the local standard of care.

Maternal hyperoxygenation has been examined in several studies for potential benefits in the treatment of the compromised growth-restricted fetus. Studies by several groups confirm that maternal hyperoxygenation can raise the fetal cord blood Po_2.[258–260] Techniques used included administration of 55-percent oxygen by face mask or 2.5 L/min by nasal prong. Prolongation of pregnancy from the first recognition of the fetal condition ranged from 9 days to 5 weeks. However, fetal growth velocity was not improved. In addition, fetuses subjected to oxygen therapy had more hypoglycemia, thrombocytopenia, and disseminated intravascular coagulation compared with controls.[260] The primary role of maternal hyperoxygenation lies in the safe short-term prolongation of pregnancy to allow the administration of corticosteroids to reduce the risk of neonatal respiratory distress syndrome and intraventricular hemorrhage in anticipation of a preterm delivery.

Maternal hyperalimentation as a means of intrauterine feeding of the growth-restricted fetus is an attractive therapeutic concept. Increasing the maternal concentration of amino acids leads to an increased umbilical uptake of some amino acids to the fetus, whereas there is no change in the three essential amino acids: lysine, histidine, and threonine.[261] These data further support that total parenteral nutrition can reverse abnormal fetal growth secondary to maternal nutritional deprivation. However, it does not overcome abnormal placental function. Outcomes are neither improved in animal models nor in human pregnancies.[262,263] Therefore, maternal hyperalimentation primarily plays a role in patients in whom malnutrition has been established as the underlying cause of growth delay.

Maternal volume expansion as a therapeutic concept is based on the observation that poor maternal blood volume status is associated with adverse pregnancy outcome, Karsdorp and coworkers studied the effects of volume expansion on feto- and uteroplacental blood flow and neonatal outcome,[264] In a small group of centrally monitored women with abnormal placental Doppler studies, they noted that volume expansion was associated with reappearance of umbilical artery end-diastolic velocities and a significant improvement of neonatal survival. With further randomized studies pending, these data suggest that inpatient correction of maternal volume status is important in improving placental perfusion.

Low-dose aspirin in combination with dipyridamole administered from 16 weeks' gestation was first reported in 1987 by Wallenburg and Rotmans to significantly reduce the incidence of fetal growth restriction in women with a history of recurrent IUGR.[265] Women receiving therapy had a rate of fetal growth restriction of 13 percent compared with 61 percent in an untreated control group. No treated woman had a child with severe growth restriction (birth weight <2.3 percentile) compared with 27 percent in the untreated group. Recently, a meta-analysis of the efficacy of low-dose aspirin (50 to 100 mg/day) has demonstrated a significant reduction in the frequency of IUGR when low-dose aspirin is used.[266] There is a dose-dependent relationship in that higher doses (100 to 150 mg/day) were significantly more effective in preventing IUGR than were lower doses (50 to 80 mg/day).

Two recent randomized trials illustrate important considerations regarding the use of aspirin to prevent pre-eclampsia or IUGR, or both. In a study of patients who were randomized at 24 weeks' gestation based on the uterine artery flow velocity waveform, low-dose aspirin was not associated with any improvement in placental function or perinatal outcome. Conversely, in patients with a poor obstetric history (thrombophilia, hypertension, past history of either preeclampsia or IUGR) randomized at 12 to 14 weeks based on the uterine artery flow velocity waveforms, those receiving aspirin experienced an 80-percent reduction in placental disease (e.g., abruptio placenta, IUGR, preeclampsia) compared with placebo-matched controls. Therefore, it appears that aspirin works best in patients with significant risk factors for IUGR and that the therapeutic optimal window to commence aspirin therapy lies between 12 to 16 weeks' gestation when branching angiogenesis of the placenta is ongoing.

Although the overall safety of aspirin has been documented in a large patient population, concerns about a possible association with abdominal wall defects have been raised with administration in the early first trimester.[267] Therefore, we suggest deferral of indicated therapy until completion of organogenesis at 12 weeks' gestation. Selected patients presenting in the second trimester may still derive benefit from aspirin, and patients should be counseled on an individualized basis.[268,269] Aspirin prophylaxis can be discontinued at any point after 34 weeks' gestation because bleeding risks at delivery and during regional anesthesia outweigh the benefits of prolonging gestation.

Corticosteroids are a universally available antenatal therapeutic option that positively affects outcome by enhancing lung maturation and preventing intraventricular hemorrhage. The impact of prenatal glucocorticoid administration on neonatal complication rate in the growth-restricted newborn has recently been examined by Bernstein and coworkers in a study of 19,759 newborns between 500 and 1,500 g. After controlling for a different set of confounding variables, this study demonstrated a significant reduction in neonatal respiratory distress syndrome (RDS), intraventricular hemorrhage, and death when prenatal glucocorticoids were administered. These benefits were not qualitatively different from those observed in appropriately sized newborns. Other studies have also refuted that the "stress" of the intrauterine condition enhances maturation and protects against prematurity.[270] In contrast, a smaller study by Elimian et al.[271] demonstrated no benefits to neonatal outcome when perinatal glucocorticoids were used. Although these studies indicate the need for randomized comparison of management, they also clearly show no benefit from the omission of antenatal corticosteroids. We recommend administration of a complete 48-hour course of antenatal steroids to any growth restricted fetus when delivery is anticipated before 34 weeks' gestation, if this can be safely accomplished.

When corticosteroids are administered, it is important to account for their effect on fetal testing parameters when interpreting antenatal surveillance results. Betamethasone, for example, temporarily reduces FHR variation on day 2 and 3 after the first injection, together with a 50-percent decrease in fetal body movements and an almost complete cessation of fetal breathing movements.[272] Subsequently, the number of fetuses with an abnormal BPS increases significantly by 48 hours after steroid administration with a return to the preadministration state at 72 hours.[273] In contrast, maternal and fetal Doppler findings are not affected to the same degree during this period.[274] A transient decrease in the middle cerebral artery blood flow resistance has been reported following 48 hours after betamethasone administration.[275]

ASSESSMENT OF FETAL WELL-BEING

Once the diagnosis of fetal growth restriction has been made and the differential diagnostic options have been explored, fetal assessment is instituted (see Chapter 11). Serial ultrasound evaluations of fetal growth are continued every 3 to 4 weeks and should include determinations of the BPD, HC/AC, fetal weight, and AFV. The institution of antenatal surveillance is a critical component in the management of the growth restricted fetus. Relationships between fetal testing parameters and subsequent outcome determine the balance between fetal and neonatal risks and, therefore, define intervention thresholds. Growth-restricted fetuses are at risk for worsening placental function, subsequent deterioration of acid-base status, decompensation, stillbirth and adverse health effects into adult life. Although prevention of long-term morbidity is an attractive goal, there is insufficient information on its relationships with prenatal variables to direct management. Of the many short-term outcomes that have been related to fetal status, only a few are presently of clinical relevance. Fetal acidemia and major neonatal complications have a significant impact on subsequent neurodevelopment, whereas the combination of fetal and neonatal deaths determines the overall perinatal mortality.[276] Therefore, the likelihood of fetal acidemia and stillbirth is the strongest fetal criterion for intervention. In contrast, gestational age–specific expectations for neonatal complications and survival force conservative management. Although neonatal complications are typically multifactorial in nature and not accurately predicted prenatally, anticipation of fetal risks remains as the primary goal. Therefore, antenatal surveillance tests need to predict fetal acid-base status, rate of anticipated progression, and the resulting risk for deterioration and stillbirth. The monitoring tools that are available to achieve this include the traditional nonstress test (NST), contraction stress testing (CST), BPS, and Doppler sonography.

Maternal Monitoring of Fetal Activity

Maternal monitoring of fetal activity has been used extensively in Great Britain, Scandinavia, and Israel for the assessment of pregnancies complicated by IUGR. In a study of 50 cases, Matthews[277] clearly showed the predictive value of fetal activity charting for growth-restricted fetuses subsequently demonstrating distress in labor. A simple technique for monitoring fetal movement is the minimum requirement of 10 movements in a 2-hour period. If this criterion is not met, additional testing is warranted. In an outpatient setting, maternal kick counts or fetal activity counts supplement medically administered antenatal surveillance. In the compliant patients with an appropriate level of awareness of fetal movements, it may also be helpful in modifying monitoring intervals as fetal deterioration occurs.

Fetal Heart Rate Analysis

The traditional NST is a visually analyzed record of the FHR baseline, variability, and episodic changes. Normal FHR characteristics are determined by gestational age, maturational and functional status of central regulatory centers, and oxygen tension.[278–280] A reactive NST exhibits two accelerations peaking at 15 bpm above baseline with each acceleration lasting 15 seconds (from baseline to baseline) within a 20 minute period. An additional 20 minutes may be given (total of 40 minutes) for the tracing to become reactive. When the NST is analyzed as part of the five-component BPS, reactivity criteria that account for gestational age are applied (see later). Irrespective of the context a "reactive" NST indicates absence of fetal hypoxemia at the moment of the FHR recording.[281–283] Many growth-restricted fetuses with a normal heart rate tracing can have low-normal Po_2 values, but acidemia is virtually excluded by a reactive NST. Heart rate reactivity also correlates highly with a fetus that is not in immediate danger of intrauterine demise.[283] On the other hand, nonreactive NST results are often falsely positive and require further evaluation. The development of repetitive decelerations may reflect fetal hypoxemia or cord compression due to the development of oligohydramnios and has been associated with a high perinatal mortality rate.[284]

The CST is an additional option for testing placental respiratory reserve.[285] Positive CST results have been reported in 30 percent of pregnancies complicated by proven growth restriction. In a study by Lin et al.,[286] 30 percent of growth-restricted infants had nonreactive NST results and 40 percent had positive CST results. Ninety-two percent of IUGR infants with a nonreactive/positive pattern exhibited perinatal morbidity. However, a 25- to 50-percent false-positive rate has been associated with the CST by some investigators. A possible role for the CST may be evaluation of placental reserve before induction in IUGR fetuses in whom vaginal delivery is attempted.

Marked intra- and interobserver variability of visual FHR analysis has been identified as a potential factor affecting the prediction of fetal status.[287] Currently, traditional FHR parameters as well as short- and long-term variation of the heart rate in milliseconds, length of episodes with low and high variation, and the rate of signal loss can be assessed by computerized analysis. The objective assessment of these variables circumvents the issue of observer variability and a direct correlation between FHR variation and Po_2 in the umbilical vein as assessed at cordocentesis before the onset of labor has been documented.[148,150] A computerized documentation of a mean minute variation below 3.5 milliseconds has been reported to predict an umbilical artery cord pH <7.20 with greater than 90-percent sensitivity. In addition, FHR variation usually decreases gradually in the weeks preceding the appearance of late decelerations and fetal hypoxemia, and therefore, is the most useful computerized FHR parameter for longitudinal assessment in IUGR.[288] As with the traditional NST, gestational age, time of the day, and presence of fetal rest-activity cycles also need to be taken into account in the interpretation of computerized results. There are wide normal ranges for FHR patterns and their variations, but the individual fetus shows a certain intrafetal consistency throughout gestation. Therefore, for monitoring of trends, each fetus should serve as its own control, using recordings of standardized duration and appropriate reference ranges.

In summary, a visually reactive FHR provides assurance of fetal well-being at the time of analysis. Although the traditional NST is most sensitive in the prediction of fetal normoxemia, computerized analysis appears superior in the prediction of hypoxemia and acidemia. Once traditional reactivity is lost, computerized analysis of heart rate variation is a potential tool available for ongoing longitudinal analysis. Computerized FHR analysis is more widely used in Europe, and an ongoing randomized trial will evaluate its use in timing delivery in growth-restricted fetuses. FHR analysis itself does not assess the severity of disease and most importantly does not anticipate the rate of deterioration. To address these issues additional fetal tests are available.

Amniotic Fluid Volume

In the context of fetal surveillance, assessment of AFV provides an indirect measure of vascular status. A relationship between oligohydramnios and progressive deterioration of arterial and venous Doppler studies has been documented in growth-restricted fetuses and prolonged pregnancies.[289,290] Therefore, declining AFV is suggestive of ineffective downstream delivery of cardiac output, allowing some form of longitudinal monitoring even in the absence of Doppler studies. If the NST is reactive, a concurrent assessment of the AFV constitutes the "modified BPS" and provides assurance of fetal well-being if both parameters are normal. Interventions based on twice-weekly modified BPS result in similar perinatal outcomes as with weekly CST and, therefore, have largely replaced CST.[291] When the FHR is nonreactive, relying on a normal AFV assessment alone is inadequate and a full BPS that incorporates multiple parameters of fetal well-being should be performed because of its superior performance in identifying jeopardized fetuses.

Biophysical Parameters

The five-component fetal BPS was developed by Manning et al.[292] and has been widely used in the surveillance of growth-restricted fetuses. A graded system is applied to categorize fetal tone, movement, breathing movement, heart rate reactivity and a maximum amniotic fluid pocket as normal (2 points) or abnormal (0 points). If used in the context of the BPS, FHR reactivity criteria that account for gestational age are used. Before 32 weeks, greater than 10 beats/minute accelerations sustained for more than 10 seconds; between 32 and 36 weeks, greater than 15 beats/minute accelerations sustained for more than 15 seconds, and after 36 weeks' gestation, greater than 20 beats/minute accelerations sustained for more than 20 seconds define reactivity. In anatomically normal fetuses, the presence of the dynamic variables is related to physiologic variations in maturation, behavioral state, and acid-base status. Vintzileos and coworkers have demonstrated that four components of the BPS are affected at different levels of hypoxemia and acidemia.[158] The earliest manifestations of abnormal fetal biophysical activity consist of the loss of heat rate reactivity, along with the absence of fetal breathing. This is followed by decreased fetal tone and movement in association with more advanced acidemia, hypoxemia, and hypercapnia. Through its relationship with vascular status, amniotic fluid assessment provides the only marker of chronic hypoxemia and is the only longitudinal monitoring component of the BPS.

Growth-restricted fetuses preserve acute central responses to acid-base status despite their maturational delay and are at risk for oligohydramnios. The five-component BPS accounts best for physiologic and individual variations in behavior and, therefore, remains closely related to arterial pH in IUGR fetuses without anomalies from 20 weeks onward.[159,293] An abnormal score of 4 or less is associated with a mean pH less than 7.20 and sensitivity in the prediction of acidemia is 100 percent for a score of 2 or less. A normal score and normal AFV indicate the absence of fetal hypoxemia at the time of testing. Longitudinal observations in growth-restricted fetuses have shown that the BPS deteriorates late and often rapidly.[156,294] Although an abnormal BPS is associated with escalating risks for stillbirth and perinatal mortality, a normal score allows no anticipation of fetal deterioration and stillbirth.

In summary, assessment of fetal biophysical variables provides an accurate measure of fetal status at the time of testing. In the patient with a nonreactive NST, a full five-component BPS needs to be performed. As a backup test for nonreactive FHR testing, the BPS leads to lower rates of intervention when compared with the CST without jeopardizing perinatal outcome. In the presence of normal AFV, a normal BPS of 8 (minus 2 for a nonreactive NST) or 10 is reassuring of fetal well-being. Nevertheless, in the absence of knowledge about placental vascular status, the rate of progression cannot be anticipated and may require even daily testing in severe IUGR. The development of oligohydramnios is concerning and frequently requires modification of management or delivery. The knowledge of fetal Doppler status is complementary to BPS because it improves the anticipation of fetal deterioration and provides an additional means to assess fetal state.[290]

Doppler Ultrasound

Doppler parameters are influenced by several variables including vascular histology, vascular tone, and fetal blood pressure. Placental respiratory function is related to the integrity of the villous vasculature and a decrease in arterial Po_2 can trigger autoregulatory adjustments of vascular smooth muscle tone. As diagnostic tools, elevated umbilical artery blood flow resistance and middle cerebral artery brain sparing provide evidence of placental dysfunction. The utility of Doppler ultrasound in the assessment of fetal well-being is based on the relationship between Doppler parameters with metabolic status, rate of disease progression, and the risk for stillbirth. In this context, distinction between early and late fetal vascular responses to placental insufficiency provides a useful framework to estimate these risks.

"Early" responses to placental insufficiency are observed in mild placental vascular disease when umbilical artery end-diastolic velocity is still present. A decrease in the cerebral/placental Doppler ratio provides an early and sensitive marker of redistribution of cardiac output often preceding overt growth delay by up to 2 weeks. The reduction of fetal growth velocity generally mirrors the elevation in umbilical artery blood flow resistance and is followed by decreasing middle cerebral artery impedance (brain sparing). The nadir of cerebral blood flow resistance is typically reached after a median of 2 weeks and is followed by an increase in aortic blood flow impedance.[295] Early cardiovascular responses are considered compensatory because they occur at a time when cardiac function is normal and are typically accompanied by preferential perfusion of vital organs and the placenta. Although the fetus may be hypoxemic, the risk for acidemia is low.

"Late" responses to placental insufficiency are observed when accelerating placental disease results in loss, or reversal of umbilical artery end-diastolic velocity and fetal deterioration becomes evident through parallel elevations in placental blood flow resistance and venous Doppler indices. Although the development of abnormal venous blood flows has been documented in many veins, the precordial veins including the ductus venosus, inferior vena cava, and the umbilical vein are typically used in clinical practice (Figs. 29-14 and 29-15).[296–300] When fetal compromise accelerates, there is a further steady rise in umbilical blood flow resistance while venous Doppler indices escalate over a wide range. Also, the development of oligohydramnios and metabolic acidemia is characteristic with ineffective downstream delivery of cardiac output.[301] The final stages of compromise are chacterized by cardiac dilatation with holosystolic tricuspid insufficiency, complete fetal inactivity, short-term variation below 3.5 msec, and spontaneous "cardiac" late decelerations of the FHR (Fig. 29-16).[302]

In the past, the major focus of Doppler studies for the assessment of fetal health has been the umbilical circulation.[303] The association between an elevation in Doppler blood flow indices in the umbilical artery, increased disturbance of placental perfusion, and the deterioration of fetal acid-base status that is proportional to the degree of the Doppler abnormality has been demonstrated by several investigators. In the fetal compartment, elevation of the umbilical artery Doppler index is observed when approximately 30 percent of the fetal villous vessels are abnormal.[304] Absence or even reversal of umbilical artery end-diastolic velocity can occur when 60 to 70 percent of the villous vascular tree is damaged.[305] Incidences of intrauterine hypoxia ranging from 50 to 80 percent in fetuses with absent end-diastolic flow have been reported.[306,307] The benefit of umbilical artery Doppler in management has been documented in randomized controlled trials and meta-analyses. In these studies, umbilical artery Doppler, when used in conjunction with standard antepartum

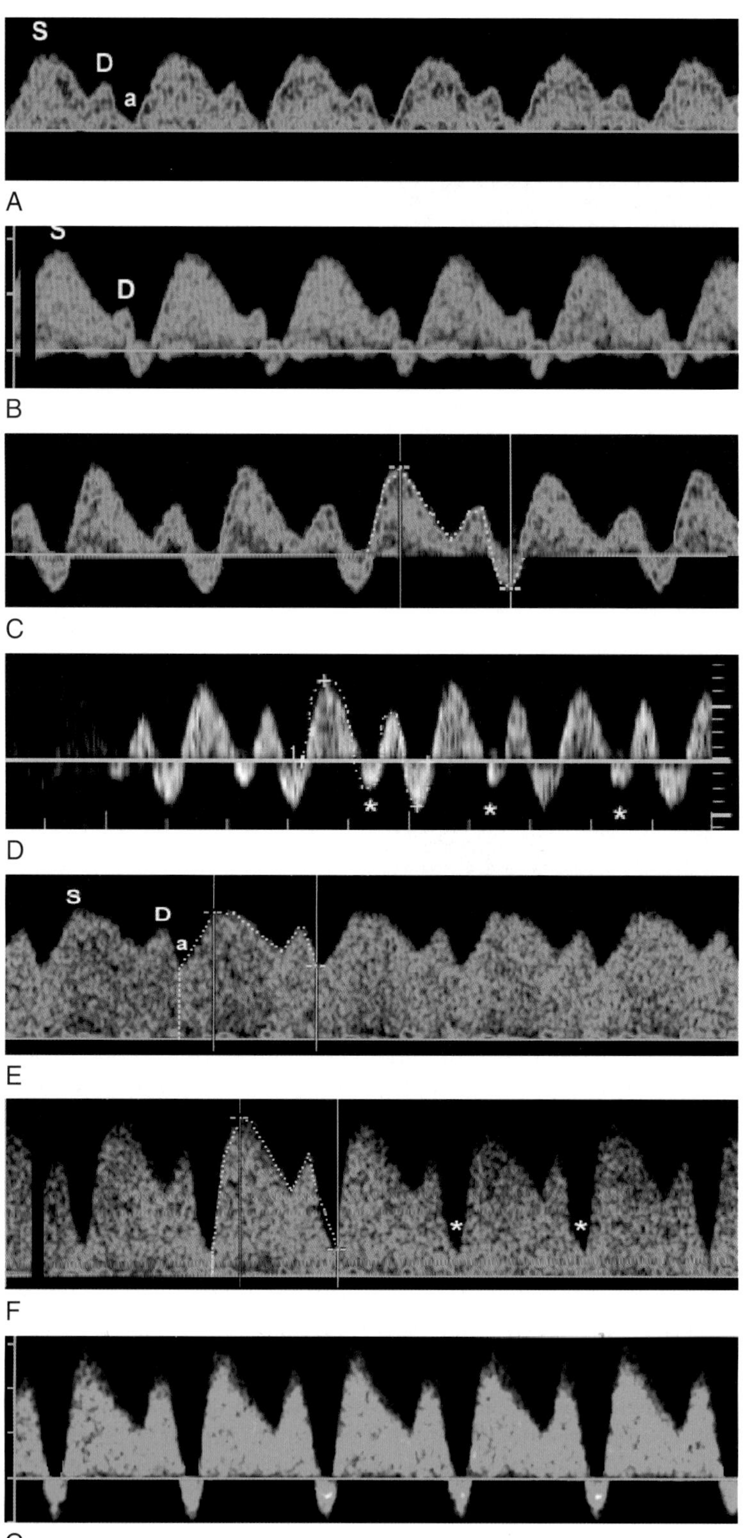

Figure 29-14. Normal and abnormal precordial venous flow velocity waveforms. The inferior vena cava and ductus venosus are the most commonly evaluated precordial veins, whereas the umbilical venous flow velocity waveform is predominantly assessed qualitatively. The inferior vena cava shows the typical triphasic pattern with systolic and diastolic peaks (S, D respectively) *(A)*. The a-wave may be reversed under physiologic conditions *(B)*. An abnormal inferior vena cava flow velocity waveform shows a relative decrease in forward flow during the first trough, the D-wave and a wave *(C)*. Under extreme circumstances there may be reversed flow during the first trough (*) *(D)*. In contrast to the inferior vena cava, the ductus venosus has antegrade blood flow throughout the cardiac cycle, with forward velocities during the S, D, and a waves *(E)*. A decrease in atrial systolic forward velocities (*) is the first sign of an abnormality and results in an increased Doppler index *(F)*. With marked elevation of central venous pressure, blood flow may reverse during atrial systole *(G)*.

testing, was associated with a decrease of up to 38 percent in perinatal mortality, antenatal admissions, inductions of labor, and cesarean deliveries for fetal distress in labor in women considered at high risk.[219,308] However, several studies that have examined the cerebral and especially the venous circulation have provided greater insight into the relationships between Doppler abnormality and outcome. Indik and coworkers[309] reported that development of umbilical venous pulsations in fetuses with AEDV in the umbilical artery were associated with a fivefold increase in mortality. Arduini et al. demonstrated that gestational age at onset, maternal hypertension, and the development of pulsations in the umbilical venous velocities were significantly correlated with the interval of time between diagnosis and delivery for late decelerations of the FHR.[310,311] Subsequently, several studies have confirmed that fetuses with abnormal arterial velocities who also developed abnormal precordial venous velocities had higher mor-

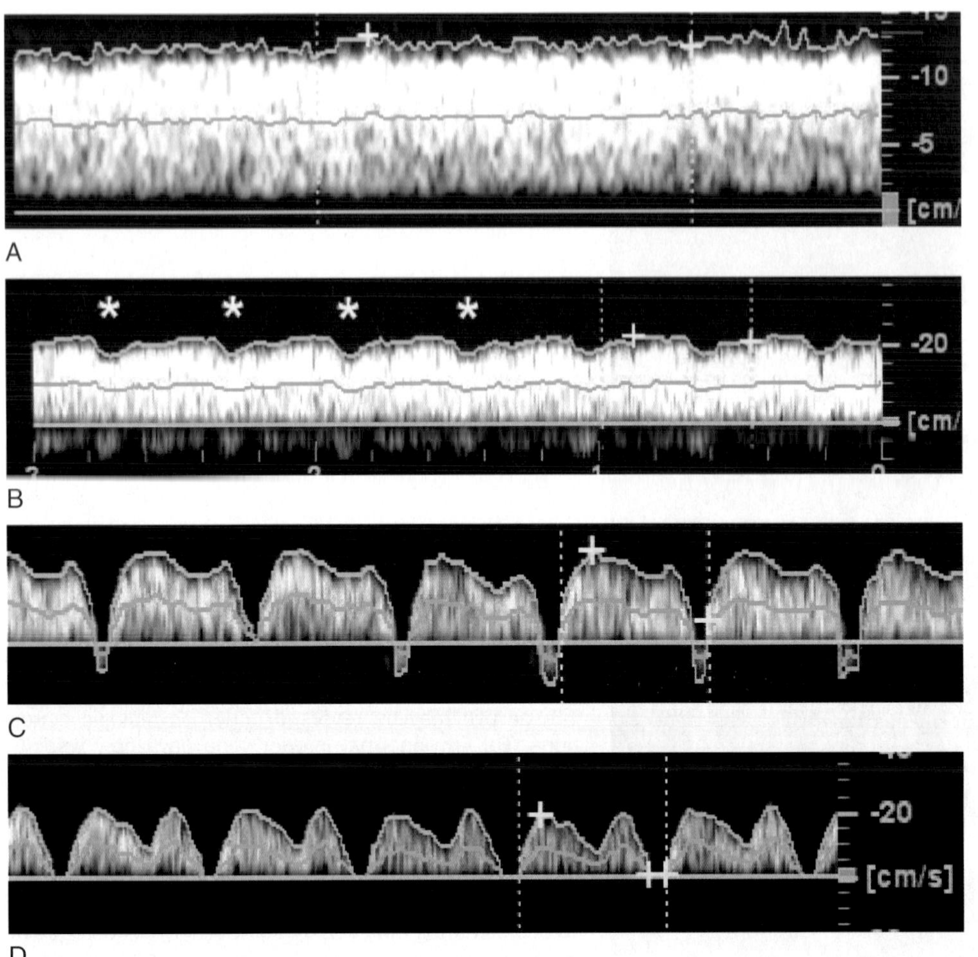

Figure 29-15. Normal and abnormal umbilical venous flow velocity. Umbilical venous blood flow is usually constant *(A)*. Monophasic umbilical venous pulsations (*) may be observed with moderate elevations of placental blood flow resistance or oligohydramnios *(B)*. Retrograde propagation of increased central venous pressure first results in biphasic and then triphasic pulsations (*C* and *D*, respectively).

bidity and mortality rates than fetuses without abnormal venous flow.[115,312] These studies and subsequent analyses confirm that fetal Doppler assessment that is based on the umbilical artery alone is not sufficient, particularly in the setting of early onset IUGR before 34 weeks. Incorporation of middle cerebral artery and venous Doppler provide the best prediction of acid-base status, risk of stillbirth, and the anticipated rate of progression.

In growth-restricted fetuses with an elevated Doppler index in the umbilical artery, brain sparing in the presence of normal venous Doppler parameters is typically associated with hypoxemia but a normal pH.[306,307] Elevation of venous Doppler indices, either alone or in combination with umbilical venous pulsations, increases the risk for fetal acidemia. This association is strengthened by serial elevations of the ductus venosus Doppler index. Dependent on the cutoff (2 versus 3 SD) and the combinations of precordial veins examined, sensitivity for prediction of acidemia ranges from 70 to 90 percent and specificity from 70 to 80 percent.[217,296]

Abnormal venous Doppler parameters are the strongest Doppler predictors of stillbirth. Even among fetuses with severe arterial Doppler abnormalities (e.g., AEDV/REDV), the risk of stillbirth is largely confined to those fetuses that have abnormal venous Dopplers.[312] The likelihood of stillbirth increases with the degree of venous Doppler abnormality. Venous Doppler findings that are particularly ominous are absence or reversal of the ductus venous a-wave and biphasic/triphasic umbilical venous pulsations. In the setting of a 25-percent stillbirth rate in a preterm severe IUGR population, these Doppler findings have a 65-percent sensitivity and 95-percent specificity.[301,313]

Although neonatal morbidity is primarily determined by gestational age at delivery and neonatal mortality is the product of several factors, both of these outcomes are also related to fetal Doppler studies. Arterial redistribution and brain sparing are not associated with a significant rise in major neonatal complications. A 2-SD elevation of the ductus venosus Doppler index is associated with a threefold increase in neonatal morbidity; further escalation of ductus venosus Doppler indices increases this relative risk to 11-fold. The neonatal mortality rate in fetuses with absent or reverse umbilical artery end-diastolic velocity ranges from 5 to 18 percent when the venous Doppler indices are normal. Elevation of the ductus venosus Doppler index greater than 2 SD doubles this mortality rate, although predictive sensitivity is only 38 percent with a specificity of 98 percent.[301,313]

In summary, Doppler evaluation of the umbilical, cerebral, and precordial vessels of the growth-restricted fetus provides important diagnostic and prognostic information. Fetal acidemia and the risk of stillbirth are high with progressive elevation of venous Doppler indices. Advanc-

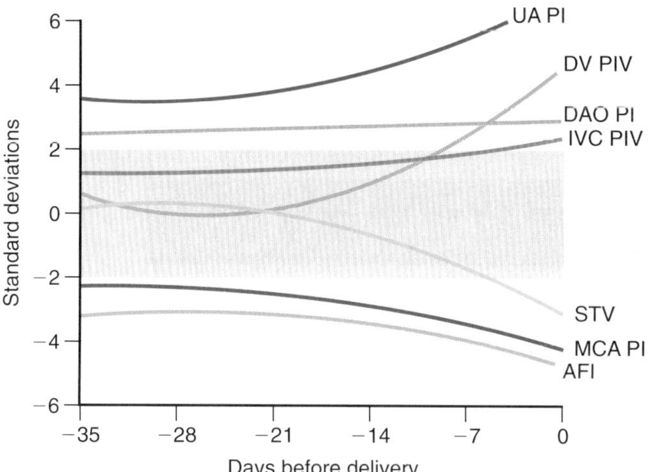

Figure 29-16. Longitudinal progression of antenatal testing variables. This figure displays trends in arterial and venous Doppler parameters (DAO, descending aorta; DV, ductus venosus; IVC, inferior vena cava; MCA, middle cerebral artery; PI, pulsatility index; PIV, PI for veins, UA, umbilical artery), amniotic fluid index (AFI), and computerized fetal heart rate short-term variation (STV) in relation to delivery expressed as standard deviation for growth restricted fetuses delivered before 32 weeks gestation. The graph demonstrates that arterial Doppler parameters may be abnormal for more than 5 weeks before delivery, whereas venous Doppler parameters and the short-term variation deteriorate in the week before delivery for fetal indications. (Reproduced with permission from Hecher K, Bilardo CM, Stigter RH, et al: Monitoring of fetuses with intrauterine growth restriction: a longitudinal study. Ultrasound Obstet Gynecol 18:564, 2001.)

ing Doppler abnormalities indicate acceleration of disease and require increased frequency of fetal monitoring. In growth-restricted fetuses, Doppler evaluation is complementary to all other surveillance modalities.

Invasive Fetal Testing

Direct determination of fetal acid base status by cordocentesis was previously frequently performed during invasive karyotyping. Nicolini et al.[314] examined 58 growth-restricted fetuses, using cordocentesis for acid-base evaluation in addition to karyotyping. They found significant differences in pH, Pco_2, Po_2, and the base equivalent in fetuses that had no evidence of end-diastolic flow by umbilical artery Doppler velocimetry. However, they observed no relationship between acid-base determination and perinatal outcome. Pardi et al.[315] examined umbilical blood acid-base status in 56 growth-restricted fetuses and demonstrated an association between acid-base status and the results of cardiotocographic and umbilical artery Doppler waveform analysis. If both FHR and Doppler studies were normal, neither hypoxemia nor acidemia was noted. When both tests were abnormal, 64 percent of the growth-restricted fetuses demonstrated abnormal acid-base analysis. The prognostic significance of these abnormalities remains uncertain. The lack of benefit, complication rate, accuracy of noninvasive assessment of fetal acid-base status, and finally, the availability for rapid karyotyping techniques from amniocytes rarely necessitates cordocentesis today.

Anticipating the Progression to Fetal Compromise

The anticipation of clinical progression is a critical component in the management of IUGR fetuses because it determines fetal surveillance intervals as well as the timing for intervention. Although deterioration of fetal status is manifested in all surveillance modalities, accelerating disease is best anticipated by AFV status and arterial and venous Doppler parameters (Fig. 29-17). Umbilical artery Doppler alone provides inaccurate prediction because progression to abnormal FHR parameters is highly variable and may range between 0 and 49 days as reported in a study by Farine and coworkers.[316] In general, early-onset IUGR presenting before 28 weeks is associated with more marked placental vascular problems producing marked Doppler changes. In contrast, IUGR presenting near term is typically associated with milder placental disease and, therefore, more subtle Doppler findings. Decreasing AFV and behavioral responses are preserved throughout gestation irrespective of Doppler status. Accordingly, longitudinal progression and clinical findings may vary based on gestational age and may be further modulated by maternal disease.[317–319] Beyond 34 weeks when the umbilical artery waveform may be normal or near-normal, assessment of the middle cerebral artery flow velocity waveform and the cerebroplacental Doppler ratio may be necessary to provide an estimate of placental disease and direct the frequency of testing.[223]

In fetuses with elevated placental blood flow resistance, onset of middle cerebral artery brain sparing and a decline in the AFI indicate accelerating disease.[155] Once brain sparing is established, the next level of deterioration occurs when umbilical artery end-diastolic velocity is lost and parallel elevations in placental blood flow resistance and precordial venous Doppler indices are observed. Although this may happen after several weeks, the anticipation of such deterioration may require twice-weekly, rather than weekly testing. When accelerating fetal compromise occurs, it is associated with a further rise in umbilical blood flow resistance (leading to REDV) whereas venous Doppler indices escalate over a wide range of distribution. Studies by Baschat, Ferrazzi, Hecher, and Bilardo indicate that 40 percent of preterm growth-restricted fetuses that deteriorate in utero have an increased ductus venosus Doppler index the week before delivery (Fig. 29-18). On the day of delivery, an additional 20 percent deteriorated further. Elevations of precordial venous Doppler indices also precede sudden deterioration of the BPS by a median of 1 week in fetuses with elevated umbilical artery blood flow resistance. These findings have important impact on testing frequency. For example, in a preterm growth-restricted fetus in whom venous Doppler indices are elevated a BPS of 10 does not provide assurance that fetal status will remain stable for the following week. In fact, a sizeable proportion of these fetuses may have a BPS of less than six after a median time of just 1 day (Fig. 29-19).[156]

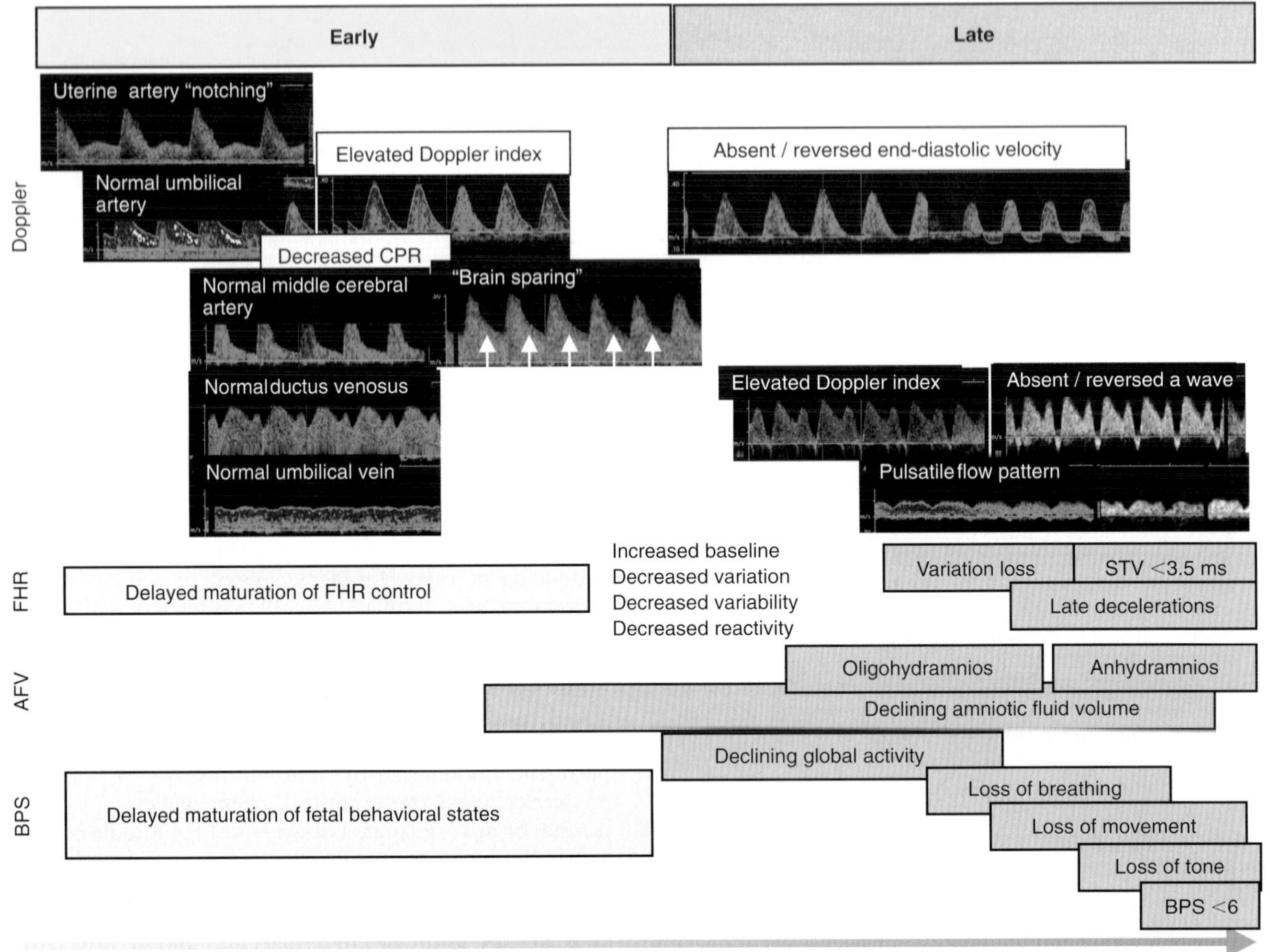

Figure 29-17. Progression of compromise in various monitoring systems. This figure summarizes the early and late responses to placental insufficiency. Doppler variables in the placental circulation precede abnormalities in the cerebral circulation. Fetal heart rate (FHR), amniotic fluid volume (AFV) and biophysical parameters (BPS) are still normal at this time, and computerized analysis of fetal behavioral patterns is necessary to document a developmental delay. With progression to late responses, venous Doppler abnormality in the fetal circulation is characteristic, often preceding the sequential loss of fetal dynamic variables and frequently accompanying the decline in amniotic fluid volume. The * in the ductus venosus flow velocity waveform marks reversal of blood flow during atrial systole (a-wave). The decline in biophysical variables shows a reproducible relationship with acid-base status. Because the BPS is a composite score of five variables, an abnormal BPS less than 6 often develops late and may be sudden. Absence or reversal of the ductus venosus a-wave, decrease of the short-term variation (STV) of the computerized fetal heart rate analysis, spontaneous late decelerations, and an abnormal BPS are the most advanced testing abnormalities. If adaptation mechanisms fail and the fetus remains undelivered, stillbirth ensues.

Therefore, three-times weekly or even daily testing may be necessary in such fetuses. This is illustrated in a study by Divon and coworkers, who performed daily BPS in fetuses with absent umbilical artery end-diastolic velocity. Delivery was indicated for maternal reasons, a BPS below 6, oligohydramnios, documented lung maturity, or a gestational age beyond 36 weeks. There were no stillbirths and no cord artery pH below 7.20, using this intensive monitoring approach.[294]

The clinical progression in Doppler and biophysical abnormalities are observed in approximately 70 to 80 percent of growth-restricted fetuses before 34 weeks' gestation.[115] Beyond this gestational age, several other presentations are possible. Umbilical artery blood flow resistance may be normal and brain sparing may be observed as the only Doppler sign of perceived hypoxemia. Alternatively, Doppler findings may be normal, and oligohydramnios and/or a decline of biophysical variables may be the only signs of placental insufficiency. On a similar note, the speed of progression may vary significantly in these different clinical scenarios. In recognition of these variable time scales and patterns of deterioration, it is evident that the combination of several testing modalities is more likely to provide evidence of deterioration. If BPS is used, particular attention needs to be placed to the amniotic fluid, because this is the only component reflecting longitudinal progression. The most comprehensive approach that addresses cardiovascular and behavioral responses in IUGR fetuses across all gestational ages has been described as "integrated fetal testing."

Integrated fetal testing uses a surveillance approach to pregnancies with IUGR that requires familiarity with the

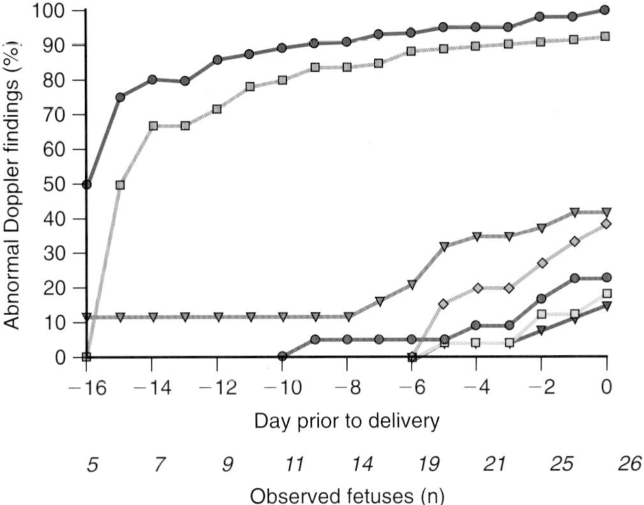

Figure 29-18. Early and late Doppler findings in growth restricted fetuses. This figure displays cumulative onset time curves of Doppler abnormalities for each fetal vessel examined. Middle cerebral artery brain sparing (▽) and absent umbilical artery end-diastolic velocity (□) are observed up to 16 days before delivery. The ductus venosus Doppler index (O), reversal of umbilical artery end-diastolic velocity (◇), reversal of the ductus venosus a-wave (▽), and declining blood flow velocities in the aorta (□) and pulmonary arteries (O) are late cardiovascular abnormalities in growth restricted fetuses. (Reproduced with permission from Ferrazzi E, Bozzo M, Rigano S, et al: Temporal sequence of abnormal Doppler changes in the peripheral and central circulatory systems of the severely growth-restricted fetus. Ultrasound Obstet Gynecol 19:140, 2002.)

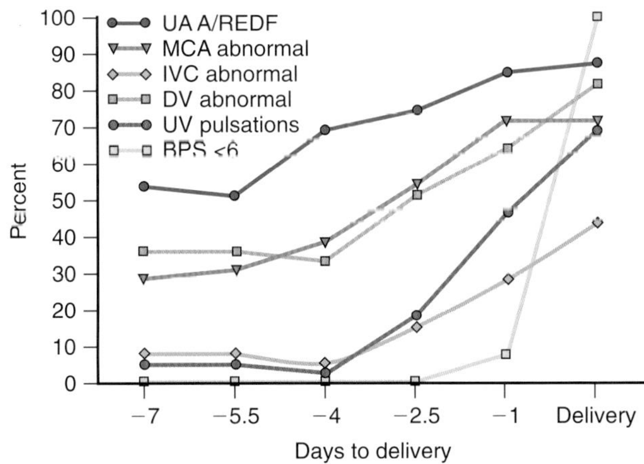

Figure 29-19. Sequential deterioration of Doppler and biophysical parameters. This figure shows the percentage of abnormal Doppler findings in individual vessels and the incidence of a biophysical profile score below 6 (BPS <6) in the last week before delivery represented by the lines. (A/REDF, absent or reversed end-diastolic flow; DV, ductus venosus; IVC, inferior vena cava; MCA, middle cerebral artery; UA, umbilical artery; UV, umbilical vein). Deterioration of Doppler findings precedes decline in biophysical profile score. (Reproduced with permission from Baschat AA, Gembruch U, Harman CR: The sequence of changes in Doppler and biophysical parameters as severe fetal growth restriction worsens. Ultrasound Obstet Gynecol 18:571, 2001.)

combined assessment of the five-component BPS and arterial and venous Doppler studies.[320] Doppler examination includes evaluation of the umbilical artery, middle cerebral artery, ductus venosus, and free umbilical vein flow velocity waveform. The testing is always supplemented with maternal assessment of fetal movement ("kick counts"). Surveillance is initiated no earlier than 24.0 weeks' gestation. In fetuses with elevated umbilical artery pulsatility and positive end-diastolic flow and absence of any additional abnormality, weekly BPS and multivessel Doppler monitoring every two weeks is performed. With the onset of brain sparing, Doppler monitoring intervals are shortened to weekly visits. In fetuses with an amniotic fluid index <5 cm or AEDV in the umbilical artery, surveillance intervals are shortened to every 3–4 days. With elevation of the ductus venosus Doppler index to >2 SD, testing frequency is increased to every 2–3 days. Further escalation of the ductus venosus Doppler index may require daily testing, and inpatient admission may be prudent based on local practice. Any change in maternal condition, especially the development of preeclampsia calls for reassessment of fetal status irrespective of the last examination result (Fig. 29-20).

THE TIMING OF DELIVERY

In the absence of definitive fetal therapy, proper timing of delivery is often the critical management issue when dealing with the growth-restricted fetus. In principle, the decision for delivery always weighs fetal risks against risks that can be anticipated as a result of preterm delivery. The risks of prematurity are of primary concern and make the management of the preterm growth restricted fetus particularly challenging. Typically, the decline in neonatal mortality is greatest between 24 to 28 weeks. whereas morbidity declines progressively thereafter toward 32 weeks. Although there are surprisingly few randomized management studies that address the issue of delivery timing in IUGR, the Growth Restriction Intervention Trial clarifies several important points.[321,322] This prospective multicenter study randomized more than 500 women with complicating fetal growth restriction into immediate versus delayed delivery when their managing physicians were unsure about the timing of delivery. In the conservatively managed group, delivery was delayed until a point when their managing obstetricians were no longer unsure about the need to deliver or when fetal testing became overtly normal. With a median delay of 4.5 days, no significant differences in short-term outcome were identified between the two groups (Table 29-5). The perinatal mortality with early delivery was associated with a higher rate of neonatal deaths, whereas delaying delivery increased the risk for stillbirth. Delivery timing also had little effects on neurodevelopment at 2 years of age. However, in the subset of fetuses delivered before 32 weeks, a trend toward poor neurodevelopment was primarily attributable to neonatal complications that occurred as a result of prematurity. Other observational studies also address the impact of gestational age on perinatal morbidity. In prenatally identified growth-restricted fetuses, the effect of gestational age overshadows all other perinatal variables. After 27.0 weeks, when

IUGR UNLIKELY		
Normal AC, AC growth rate and HC/AC ratio UA, MCA Doppler, BPS and AFV normal	Asphyxia extremely rare low risk for intrapartum distress	Deliver for obstetric, or maternal factors only, follow growth
IUGR		
AC $<$ 5th, low AC growth rate, high HC/AC ratio abnormal UA +/or CPR; normal MCA and veins BPS $\geq$ 8/10, AFV normal	Asphyxia extremely rare Increased risk for intrapartum distress	Deliver for obstetric, or maternal factors only, Every 2 weeks Doppler Weekly BPS
with blood flow redistribution		
IUGR diagnosed based on above criteria low MCA, normal veins BPS $\geq$ 8/10, AFV normal	Hypoxemia possible, asphyxia rare Increased risk for intrapartum distress	Deliver for obstetric, or maternal factors only weekly Doppler BPS 2 times/week
with significant blood flow redistribution		
UA A/REDV normal veins BPS $\geq$ 6/10, Oligohydramnios	Hypoxemia common, acidemia or asphyxia possible Onset of fetal compromise	$>$ 34 weeks: deliver $<$ 32 weeks: antenatal steroids repeat all testing daily
with proven fetal compromise		
Significant redistribution present Increased DV pulsatility BPS $\geq$ 6/10, Oligohydramnios	Hypoxemia common, acidemia or asphyxia likely	$>$ 32 weeks: deliver $<$ 32 weeks: admit, Steroids, individualize testing daily vs. tid.
with fetal decompensation		
Compromise by above criteria Absent or reversed DV a-wave, pulsatile UV BPS $<$ 6/10, Oligohydramnios	Cardiovascular instability, metabolic compromise, stillbirth imminent, high perinatal mortality irrespective of intervention	Deliver at tertiary care center with the highest level of NICU care.

Figure 29-20. Integrated fetal testing and management protocol. The management algorithm for pregnancies complicated by fetal growth restriction is based on the ability to perform arterial and venous Doppler, as well as a full five-component biophysical profile score. AC, abdominal circumference; AFV, amniotic fluid volume; A/REDV, absent/reversed end-diastolic velocity; BPS, biophysical profile score; CPR, cerebroplacental ratio; DV, ductus venosus; HC, head circumference; MCA, middle cerebral artery; NICU, neonatal intensive care unit; tid, three times daily; UA, umbilical artery. (From Baschat AA, Hecher K: Fetal growth restriction due to placental disease. Semin Perinatol 28:67, 2004.)

survival and intact survival first exceed 50 percent, a birth weight less than 550 g is associated with a high risk for neonatal death.[323,324] Gestational age is also an important factor affecting perinatal mortality in patients who remain undelivered. Frigoletto[148,325] has previously emphasized that the majority of fetal deaths in IUGR occur after the 36th week of gestation and before the onset of labor.

These studies illustrate several points that are of critical importance in the management of pregnancies complicated by IUGR today. Patients need to be aware that growth-restricted fetuses have different viability thresholds and neonatal risk statistics than their appropriately grown counterparts. The major risk for the growth-restricted fetus that remains undelivered is progression of hypoxemia to acidemia and stillbirth. Therefore, delivery is typically indicated when the risk for these complications is high, or there is no added benefit from prolongation of pregnancy. The risk for acidemia and stillbirth is highest when repetitive late decelerations are observed in association with oligohydramnios and anhydramnios, when the BPS is below 6, when the ductus venosus Doppler index elevation escalates beyond 3 standard deviations, and reversal of the ductus venosus a-wave is observed with accompanying umbilical venous pulsations. In addition, it is helpful to consider the delivery indications according to gestational epochs.

Between 24 and 27 weeks' gestation, a growth-restricted fetus is periviable, and interventions are typically undertaken for maternal conditions such as severe preeclampsia. Thresholds for fetal indications should be high, requiring strong evidence of fetal compromise and risk of stillbirth.

Table 29-5. Outcomes in the Growth Restriction Intervention Trial (GRIT)

	IMMEDIATE (n = 296)	DELAYED (n = 291)
Gestational age at entry (weeks)	32 (30–34)	32 (29–34)
Steroids already given	191 (70 percent)	189 (69 percent)
Days gained in utero	0.9 (0.4–1.2)	4.9 (2–10.8)
Birth weight (g)	1200 (875–1705)	1400 (930–1940)
Apgar <7 at 5 minutes	25 (9 percent)	17 (6 percent)
Cord pH <7.0	2 (1 percent)	4 (2 percent)
Death before discharge	29 (10 percent)	27 (9 percent)
Stillbirth	2	9
Neonatal death	23	12
Death >28 days	4	6
Survivors after 2 years	256	251
Developmental delay at age 2 years for patients delivered between 24 and 31 weeks	14 (13 percent)	5 (5 percent)

Data are reproduced from 321 and 322.

Management is frequently individualized, and a multidisciplinary approach is helpful in stressing that outcome may be poor, even with maximal support in the neonatal intensive care unit. Parents need to be aware that despite maximum management effort, perinatal mortality is in excess of 50 percent.[323,324]

Between 27 and 34 weeks gestation, fetal indications for delivery should be based on firm evidence of fetal compromise with an attempt to complete a course of antenatal corticosteroids whenever possible.

Beyond 34 weeks' gestation, lower delivery thresholds are acceptable and may include absent fetal growth, in particular arrested head growth, documented lung maturity on amniocentesis, and Doppler evidence of accelerating disease.

In summary, surveillance and management considerations are most challenging in preterm pregnancies, placing the highest demand on the accuracy of fetal testing before 34 weeks' gestation. Once fetal growth restriction is suspected or anticipated, appropriate fetal testing and daily maternal assessment of fetal activity should be instituted. Ultrasound examinations to assess fetal growth should be scheduled every 3 to 4 weeks. As long as studies show continued fetal head growth and test results remain reassuring, no intervention is required. An understanding of the strengths and limitations of individual surveillance tests in this context is important. The NST and fetal dynamic variables (fetal breathing, movement and tone) provide assurance of fetal well-being at the time of testing. Because the traditional NST is frequently nonreactive in preterm fetuses, it is inadequate as a stand alone test of fetal well-being. Umbilical artery Doppler and the five-component BPS are the surveillance tests of choice in preterm growth-restricted fetuses that circumvent this limitation of the NST. In the presence of umbilical artery end-diastolic velocity, normal AFV, and a normal BPS, weekly testing is sufficient. Testing frequency is adjusted according to fetal status with strict criteria for delivery, as indicated earlier. In preterm growth-restricted fetuses for which timing of delivery is most critical, the combination of multiple modalities, including arterial and venous Doppler, offers the most comprehensive approach to assess fetal well-being.[290,326] Such "integrated fetal testing" is suggested for centers experienced with the performance of these studies. In the preterm growth-restricted fetus presenting before 34 weeks' gestation, consideration should always be given to administration of steroids, if necessary, with continuous FHR monitoring and oxygen supplementation. Beyond 34 weeks; gestation amniocentesis for lung maturity to direct timing of delivery should be considered. It is of note that even with optimal management, there may be a yet undefined background morbidity that is predetermined by the condition and not amenable to treatment.

DELIVERY

The premature growth-restricted fetus requires the highest level of neonatal intensive care, and therefore, intrauterine transport to an appropriate institution is recommended in all cases of early-onset IUGR. Because a large proportion of growth-restricted infants suffer intrapartum asphyxia, intrapartum management demands continuous FHR monitoring. In principle, the route of delivery is determined by the severity of the fetal and maternal condition, along with other obstetric factors. Cesarean delivery without a trial of labor is indicated when the risks of vaginal delivery are unacceptable to the mother and fetus. These circumstances include prelabor evidence of fetal acidemia, spontaneous late decelerations, or late decelerations with minimal uterine activity. In addition, absent and reversed end-diastolic flow in the umbilical artery is associated with a high incidence of fetal intolerance of labor, thus cesarean delivery is often required and should be considered for these severely growth restricted fetuses. In the instance of less abnormal fetal testing typically in the setting of a more advanced gestational age, selection of the route of delivery is based on the difficulty anticipated in inducing labor, the Bishop score, and AFV. The presence of IUGR has been considered a relative contraindication to the use of prostaglandin for cervical preparation by some authors.[327] If cervical ripening is considered, preinduction oxytocin challenge testing may be helpful in determining the likelihood and safety of vaginal delivery. Pharmacologic or mechanical ripening of the cervix coupled with labor in the left lateral decubitus position with supplemental oxygen increases the likelihood of a successful vaginal delivery. During labor, a tracing without late decelerations is predictive of a good outcome in cases complicated by IUGR. However, with late decelerations, the incidence of asphyxia in growth-restricted infants is far greater than in normally grown infants.[150]

OUTCOME

IUGR can transiently or permanently impair neonatal well-being. The potential effects of this condition at birth and from complications occurring in the neonatal period have been most extensively studied. However, additional effects of this perinatal period on intermediate and long-term health are starting to emerge. Recently, a new area of research into the fetal origin of maternal diseases has also pointed out how exposure to a hostile intrauterine environment can be a predisposing factor for the development in adulthood of cardiovascular diseases and endocrine disturbances. An understanding of these problems will become important when the focus of management strategies shift from the prevention of fetal and neonatal morbidity to the improvement of intermediate and long-term development. Therefore, studies that examine the relationship between fetal growth restriction and postdelivery outcomes are best separated into those that focus on short-term and long-term outcomes.

Short-Term Outcomes

Initial reports that evaluated the association between fetal growth restriction and neonatal morbidity suggested the possibility of a protective effect of IUGR with reduced occurrence of RDS and intraventricular hemorrhage.[328] Subsequent studies do not support these early assumptions. Piper and Langer[329] found no difference in indices of fetal lung maturity comparing gestational age-matched SGA and AGA fetuses. Similarly, Thompson et al.[330] found no difference in the frequency of ventilator support when growth-restricted and AGA infants were matched for gestational age and mode of delivery. Most recently, several large trials suggest that RDS is significantly more likely to occur in growth-restricted neonates.[331,332] Bernstein has also demonstrated a significant increase in the risk for necrotizing enterocolitis and no difference in the rates of intraventricular hemorrhage when growth-restricted newborns are evaluated. Dashe[332a] noted a significant increase in RDS in infants with asymmetric IUGR when compared with neonates with symmetric IUGR (9 versus 4 percent). Other investigators have also demonstrated increased risks of multiorgan failure, intracranial hemorrhage, bronchopulmonary dysplasia, clotting disorders. and disturbed endocrine homeostasis.[333,334] Mortality rates are uniformly higher when IUGR is present. These data should put to rest the notion that fetal growth restriction is associated with any reduction in newborn illness. Additional neonatal morbidities that must be anticipated include meconium aspiration, hypoglycemia and electrolyte abnormalities.

Meconium aspiration occurs more frequently in infants with IUGR than with appropriately grown infants and is largely a problem observed after 34 weeks. Gasping in utero in response to asphyxia appears to contribute to this problem. At delivery, careful suctioning of the nasopharynx and oropharynx with the DeLee catheter has been employed to decrease the incidence of this complication.[335] Further clearing of the airway can be accomplished at delivery by direct laryngoscopy and aspiration by an experienced pediatrician. To provide immediate attention to the many potential neonatal problems, appropriate pediatric support should be present in the delivery room when an infant suspected of being growth restricted is to be delivered.

Hypoglycemia is frequently observed in growth-restricted infants owing to their inadequate glycogen reserves and a gluconeogenic pathway that is less sensitive to hypoglycemia than that of the normally grown infant.[336] In anticipation of this risk for hypoglycemia, frequent blood glucose monitoring should be instituted in all growth-restricted infants. Hypocalcemia, another well-recognized problem in IUGR, may be the result of relative hypoparathyroidism, a result of intrauterine acidosis.[337] Hyperphosphatemia secondary to tissue breakdown may also contribute. Frequent calcium monitoring is essential, because symptoms are nonspecific and similar to those associated with hypoglycemia.

Hyponatremia resulting from impaired renal function is also frequently reported in growth-restricted infants. The renal complications associated with IUGR may be attributed to asphyxia, which can produce CNS injury leading to inappropriate antidiuretic hormone (ADH) secretion.[336]

Neonates with growth restriction are at risk for polycythemia, anemia, thrombocytopenia, and complex hematologic derangements that may be problematic well beyond delivery.[101,108,338,339] Polycythemia is observed three to four times more frequently in the growth-restricted infant than in weight-matched controls. Polycythemia results from hypoxia-stimulated production of red blood cells and from transfer of blood volume from the placental to the fetal circulation in the face of intrauterine asphyxia. Thus, these infants produce more red blood cells that are shunted to them if hypoxia occurs during labor. Polycythemia leads to increased red blood cell breakdown, accounting in part for the high incidence of hyperbilirubinemia in these infants. Polycythemia is a criterion for, but does not necessarily lead to, hyperviscosity, which can result in capillary bed sludging and thrombosis. Multiple organ systems can be affected, leading to pulmonary hypertension, cerebral infarction, and necrotizing enterocolitis. Anemia can be observed in preterm IUGR fetuses with markedly abnormal placental blood flow studies. Thrombocytopenia frequently accompanies the anemia. The risk for thrombocytopenia is increased more than 10-fold if umbilical AEDV is absent. The cause for these abnormalities could involve a combination of dysfunctional erythropoiesis coupled with placental consumption of platelets and red blood cells. Neonates with such complex hematologic abnormalities are frequently unable to sustain their blood cell counts despite repeated substitution of blood products.

Hypothermia is another common problem for the growth-restricted infant and results from decreased body fat stores secondary to intrauterine malnourishment.[336] Hypothermia, if unrecognized and untreated, can contribute to the metabolic deterioration of an already unstable growth-restricted infant.

Finally, growth-restricted neonates are at increased risk for perinatal death in light of the multiple complications that may arise in the fetal and neonatal periods. The range of reported perinatal mortality is variable but depends clearly on the level of perinatal management received: Infants who received optimal intrapartum and neonatal management have a lower perinatal mortality rate than age-matched controls who did not have such intensive care.[340]

Long-Term Outcomes

The ultimate growth potential for growth-restricted infants appears to be good. The degree of catch-up growth observed in several longitudinal studies suggests that these infants can be expected to have normal growth curves and normal albeit slightly reduced size as adults. In an 8-year follow-up of children weighing less than 1,500 g at birth by Kitchen et al.,[341] 75 percent of growth-restricted infants achieved a height and weight above the 10th percentile. Of infants whose birth weight fell below the 3rd percentile, 60 percent had reached the 25th percentile for weight at 8 years. In Kitchen and associates' study,[163] however, 50 percent of the children with small head circumferences still had head circumferences below the 10th percentile at the 8-year follow-up visit in spite of their growth in height and weight. Hediger observed that growth-restricted infants experienced a period of catch-up growth in early infancy but remained near the 25th percentile through age 47 months.[342] Kumar et al.[343] noted that in infants at 1 year of age whose birth weights were less than 1,250 g, 46 percent of the growth-restricted infants remained less than the 3rd percentile for weight and 38 percent remained less than the 3rd percentile for height. In general, those infants suffering growth restriction near the time of delivery do tend to catch up. However, those neonates with earlier onset and more long-standing growth restriction in utero continue to lag behind.

The issue of long-term neurologic sequelae remains unresolved. In 1972, Fitzhardinge and Steven,[344] evaluating a group of 96 growth-restricted infants, noted that 50 percent of males and 36 percent of females had poor school performance and, overall, 25 percent had minimal cerebral dysfunction. Major neurologic deficits were much less frequent. Other studies have shown LBW and short gestation to be risk factors for cerebral palsy. However, the vast majority of children with cerebral palsy are not growth restricted.

The positive effect of intrapartum surveillance for the growth-restricted fetus is reflected in the data of Low et al.[345] In a study of 88 growth-restricted infants, they reported no severe neurologic sequelae. They did detect a lag in mental development that was significant in the growth-restricted babies when compared with appropriately grown controls, especially in the group with birth weights less than 2,300 g. This study correlates well with the data of Lipper et al.[346] on LBW babies. They observed that growth-restricted infants with a head circumference below the 10th percentile have two to three times the number of serious neurologic sequelae of their normocephalic counterparts. Strauss and Dietz found that term infants with IUGR and a head circumference less than 2 SD below the mean had significantly poorer performance on intelligence and visual motor development testing at age 7 when compared with their control siblings.[347] In an examination of 7-year-olds who suffered no perinatal complications despite IUGR and who were matched for social class with a control group, Walther[348] showed an increase in teacher-identified hyperactivity, poor concentration, and clumsiness. In a study of school performance in 8-year-olds matched for socioeconomic status, Robertson et al.[349] demonstrated a tendency toward hyperactivity in preterm growth-restricted children compared with control groups. Low et al.[350] have shown that in 9- to 11-year-olds only fetal growth restriction and socioeconomic status contributed independently to the presence of learning deficits. Intrapartum fetal asphyxia, assessed by umbilical artery base deficit, was not associated with learning deficits in this group of children.

The pattern that emerges from evaluation of these data emphasizes that neurologic outcome depends on the degree of growth restriction, especially the impact on head growth, its time of onset, the gestational age of the infant at birth, and the postnatal environment. An early intrauterine insult, between 10 and 17 weeks' gestation, could limit neuronal cellular multiplication and would obviously have a profound effect on neurologic function.[172] In the third trimester, brain development is characterized by glial multiplication, dendritic arborization, establishment of synaptic connections, and myelinization, all of which continue during the first 2 years of life. Therefore, recovery after a period of impaired growth in the third trimester is more likely to occur. Thus, the preterm appropriately grown infant has more normal neurologic development and fewer severe neurologic deficits than its preterm growth-restricted counterpart. Developmental milestones and neurologic development of mature infants with IUGR and mature infants of normal birth weight are similar. Presumably, this also reflects heightened physician awareness of the growth-restricted infant that allows detection, appropriate antepartum management, intrapartum therapy, and early pediatric intervention. The premature growth-restricted infant suffers from increased susceptibility to intrauterine asphyxia and all of the neonatal complications of the premature infant, as well as those of the infant with IUGR. If growth restriction is associated with lagging head growth before 26 weeks, even mature infants have significant developmental delay at 4 years of age.[351]

Gestational Programming of Growth-Restricted Offspring

Whereas clinicians are aware of the significant in utero and newborn consequences of IUGR, the potential long-term consequences of LBW, both for the individual and the population, have only recently been recognized. Paradoxically, infants born growth restricted or LBW have an increased risk of metabolic syndrome, including obesity, hypertension, and diabetes, a result of a programmed "thrifty phenotype."

Throughout evolution and development, humans and animals have been exposed to environmental stresses, with drought and famine representing two of the most frequent conditions. Should drought or famine occur during the gestational period, specific offspring genotypes or phenotypes may be of value in adapting the offspring to survival under these environmental conditions. It is well recognized that genetic mutations within species populations may provide a survival advantage, either to promote population growth under static environmental conditions or to ensure survival under a long-term environmental alteration. However, genetic mutations generally require prolonged, evolutionary time periods to influence the species population. Furthermore, mutations are not likely to be reversible or rapidly adaptable to altering environmental conditions. Conversely, perinatal programming may provide a species survival benefit, facilitating offspring phenotypes that are adaptable to environmental condition changes that may resolve or reverse frequently. Thus, the "thrifty phenotype" offspring[349,350] may be better able to acquire and use nutrients, resulting in a survival advantage in a environment of continual relative famine.

Whereas gestational programming may have evolved for species survival benefit, the etiology of the "thrifty phenotype" has shifted dramatically in recent eras, such that growth-restricted offspring now result from factors other than environmental nutrient restriction. Maternal disease states that did not permit fecundity or even survival before 20th-century medical treatment (e.g., autoimmune disease) and advances in medical technology (e.g., placental insufficiency associated with prior cesarean delivery[351]; higher order multiple gestations associated with in vitro fertilization) have resulted in additional cohorts of LBW infants. Furthermore, environmental exposures (e.g., cigarettes, cocaine) contribute importantly to the incidence of LBW infants. Thus the incidence of LBW and prematurity continues to increase. The percent of infants delivered preterm rose to 12.3 percent in 2003, up 16 percent since 1990. The percentage of children born at LBW rose slightly in 2003 to the highest level reported since 1970 (7.9 percent), whrereas multiple births accounted for 3.3 percent of all births in 2002.[352] Advances in neonatal care have dramatically increased the survival of growth-restricted and LBW infants to levels unimaginable 50 years ago. The postnatal environment has been further altered such that the need for calorie expenditure is markedly reduced, with an often limitless availability of food and a high-fat percentage diet. Thus, the etiologies of the thrifty phenotype have changed. Whereas, ancestral environmental conditions no longer exist in Western society, gestational programming mechanisms continue to produce what may be described as an "inadvertent thrifty phenotype"; these offspring demonstrate a markedly increased risk of obesity, hypertension, and diabetes as adults.[349]

Currently, greater than 55 percent of adults in the United States are overweight and one in five are obese (BMI >30 kg/m^2), representing a modern health crisis.[353] Obesity and its related diseases are the leading cause of death in Western society, with associated risks of hypertension, coronary heart disease (CHD), stroke, diabetes, and breast, prostate, and colon cancer. Perhaps of even greater importance, childhood obesity is now observed in greater than 20 percent of the population.[354] In conjunction with the rates of obesity, the incidence of hypertension is increasing. Among adults in the United States, nearly 30 percent of the population is hypertensive. Similarly, type 2 diabetes mellitus has dramatically increased in Western society. The World Health Organization predicts a rise in the prevalence of type 2 diabetes mellitus from 1995 to 2025 of 170 percent (84–228 million) in the industrializing world. Recent human studies indicate that a striking 25 to 63 percent of adult diabetes, hypertension, and CHD can be attributed to LBW/IUGR, with accelerated newborn-to-adolescent weight gain.[355] Thus, there is increasing evidence that the in utero environment impacts fetal development and alters a diversity of adult regulatory mechanisms,[356,359] contributing to the expression of the metabolic syndrome (see reference[360] for review). The neonatal/postnatal periods also contribute to programming, as excess intake[361] or feeding infant formula feeding is associated with increased obesity.[362]

"Programming" is a process whereby a stimulus or stress at a critical or sensitive period of development has lasting or life-long significance. One principle of gestational programming is the observation that physiologic effects of an in utero permutation may vary depending on the developmental period of the fetus or neonate, and on the species. Programming may result in altered cell number, organ structure, hormonal set points, and gene expression (Fig. 29-21). Effects may be permanent or expressed only at select offspring ages (e.g., newborn, adult) and may be dependent on the specific in utero environmental stress (e.g., undernutrition, glucocorticoid exposure). Furthermore, expression of physiologic abnormalities in the offspring may be present during basal conditions or exhibited only in response to stress or disease states.

The association of LBW and cardiovascular disease and stroke among a cohort of men and women in England was first reported by Barker et al.[350,363] Subsequent epidemiologic studies from both industrial and developing countries have confirmed this finding in many[363–369] but not all[370] studies. Although LBW alone increases the risk of cardiovascular disease, the rate and time course of infant growth among this cohort markedly alters the relative risk.[371] Rapid newborn weight gain in LBW infants has been associated with an increased risk of adult cardiovascular disease as well as obesity.[367,372–374] Our studies and others indicate that LBW offspring have altered orexigenic mechanisms that result in enhanced appetite and reduced satiety.[375] Furthermore, adipose development is altered, with tissue demonstrating a propensity to fat accumulation; increased preadipocyte differentiation and reduced lipolytic enzymes both serve to augment the accretion of adipose tissue.[376] Thus, the association of LBW and cardiovascular disease may be secondary, in part, to obesity and/or hypertension developing in this cohort. Furthermore, the relation-

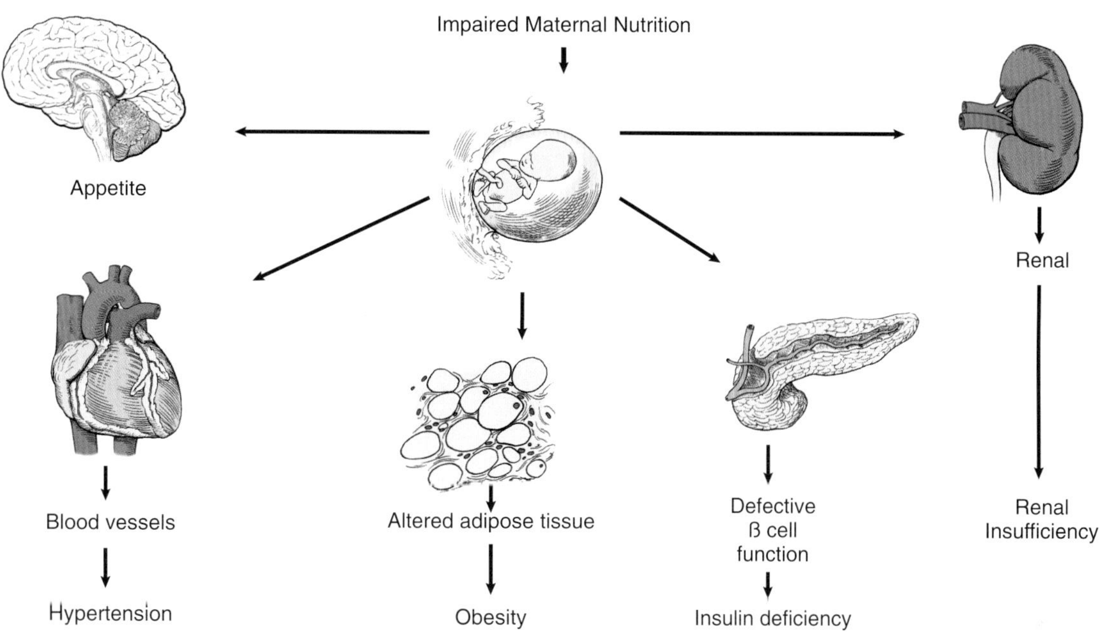

Figure 29-21. Current studies of molecular signaling. The consequences of impaired maternal nutrition may vary depending on the developmental period of the fetus or neonate, and on the species.

ship between LBW and systolic,[377–380] and diastolic[381] hypertension in both adolescence and adulthood may be confounded by the increased rate of obesity among the population.[382] However, intrinsic vascular endothelial relaxation is likely impaired in LBW offspring during infancy, childhood, or adult life,[383–386] indicating a primary vascular mechanism. Recent studies indicate abnormalities in the vascular tissue of LBW offspring, including significantly elevated endothelin-1 in conjunction with elevated systolic blood pressure, alterations in aortic elastin/collagen, and reduced expression of angiogenic proteins.[387,388]

In addition to obesity, hypertension, and enhanced vasoconstrictive properties, the permanent reduction in renal glomeruli among LBW infants contributes to the association with cardiovascular disease.[389,390] Nephron number in stillborn growth-restricted human fetuses is significantly lower than in their normally grown counterparts,[391,392] and there is a correlation between nephron number and increased glomerular volume with birth weight.[392,393] The reduction in nephron number contributes to the well-recognized renal vascular hypertension and subsequent cardiovascular dysfunction.[394–396] Because human nephrogenesis is complete by 32 to 34 weeks, a nephron deficit present at birth will persist throughout life. Thus, the late second and early third trimesters may be the critical period for interventions to optimize fetal growth-related renal development. Recent animal studies confirm a marked reduction in glomerular number among LBW offspring, with significantly higher expression of transforming growth factor-β receptor 1; these results suggest that an upregulation of fetal transforming growth factor-β signaling serves as the 'stop' signal for kidney tubule formation.

It is likely that the epidemic of obesity is due in large part to gestational programming effects, as follows (Fig. 29-22): Obese mothers produce an increased incidence of macrosomic offspring, themselves at risk for adult obesity and thus serving to perpetuate this population (lower cycle, see Fig. 29-21). Alternatively, normal weight mothers produce predominantly normal weight infants who generally develop into normal weight adults. However, growth-restricted infants resulting from normal weight mothers are now at increased risk of obesity, contributing to the population pool of obesity, and resulting in the present population shift.

In summary, gestational programming appears to have contributed to species adaptation and population survival. These developmental responses and processes are still functional in humans and have likely contributed to the current epidemic of hypertension, obesity, and diabetes. The potential exists to modify the pregnancy and newborn environment so as to optimize the benefits, and avoid the detrimental effects of gestational programming (see Fig. 29-22).

SUMMARY

An increased awareness of the fetal growth restriction and an improved ability to observe intrauterine growth and evaluate fetal well-being in utero continue to improve, along with our understanding of this multisystem fetal syndrome. Continued assessment of the underlying physiology, the efficacy of therapy, and the relationship of fetal status to specific short- and long-term developmental outcome are necessary to continue decreasing overall morbidity and mortality.

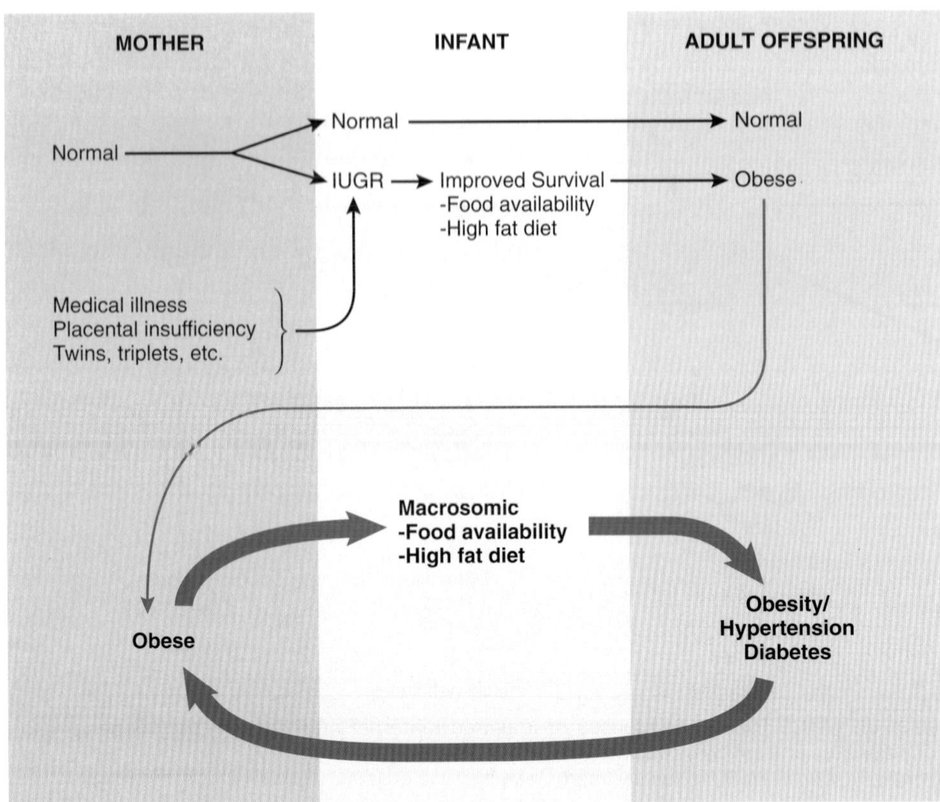

Figure 29-22. Factors contributing to the metabolic syndrome. Growth-restricted infants resulting from normal weight mothers are now at increased risk for obesity.

KEY POINTS

- Fetal growth restriction is a major cause of perinatal morbidity, perinatal mortality, and both short- and long-term morbidities.
- Although, IUGR is currently defined by fetal size alone, the four primary underlying etiologies (aneuploidy, viral infection, syndromes and placental insufficiency) produce different outcomes.
- Identification of growth restriction due to placental insufficiency requires a comprehensive diagnostic workup including measurement of the fetal AC in combination with umbilical artery Doppler studies, exclusion of fetal anomalies, and possibly invasive testing to detect aneuploidy and viral infection.
- The combination of a small AC, normal anatomy, low or normal AFV, and abnormal umbilical artery Doppler is strongly suggestive of placental insufficiency.
- Because mortality resulting from fetal growth restriction can be reduced with appropriate antenatal surveillance, all pregnancies at risk for IUGR should be carefully monitored.
- Deterioration of fetal biophysical and cardiovascular parameters follows a relatively predictable pattern, progressing from early to late changes that can be used for the prediction of fetal acid-base balance and the risk for stillbirth.
- Antenatal surveillance in preterm IUGR requires the combination of several testing modalities to provide fetal assessment of sufficient precision to guide intervention.
- In preterm gestations complicated by IUGR, the threshold for delivery is critically influenced by gestational age.

REFERENCES

1. Wolfe HM, Gross TL, Sokol RJ: Recurrent small for gestational age birth: perinatal risks and outcomes. Am J Obstet Gynecol 157:288, 1987.
2. Gardosi J, Mul T, Mongelli M, Fagan D: Analysis of birthweight and gestational age in antepartum stillbirths. Br J Obstet Gynaecol 105:524, 1998.
3. Kingdom JC, Kaufmann P: Oxygen and placental vascular development. Adv Exp Med Biol 474:259, 1999.
4. Kiserud T, Rasmussen S, Skulstad S: Blood flow and the degree of shunting through the ductus venosus in the human fetus. Am J Obstet Gynecol 182:147, 2000.
5. Haugen G, Kiserud T, Godfrey K, et al: Portal and umbilical venous blood supply to the liver in the human fetus near term. Ultrasound Obstet Gynecol 24:599, 2004.
6. Mavrides E, Moscoso G, Carvalho JS, et al: The anatomy of the umbilical, portal and hepatic venous systems in the human fetus at 14–19 weeks of gestation. Ultrasound Obstet Gynecol 18:598, 2001.
7. Sparks JW, Girard JR, Battaglia FC: An estimate of the caloric requirements of the human fetus. Biol Neonate 38:113, 1980.
8. Gardosi J, Chang A, Kalyan B, et al: Customised antenatal growth charts. Lancet 339:283, 1992.

9. Bukowski R, Burgett AD, Gei A, et al: Impairment of fetal growth potential and neonatal encephalopathy. Am J Obstet Gynecol 188:1011, 2003.
10. Ylppo A: Zur Physiologie, Klinik und zum Schicksal der Fruhgeborenen. Ztschr Kinderh 24:1, 1920.
11. Dunn PM: The search for perinatal definitions and standards. Acta Paediatr Scand 319:7, 1985.
12. Lubchenco LO, Hansman C, Boyd E: Intrauterine growth as estimated from live born birth-weight data at 24–42 weeks of gestation. Pediatrics 32:793, 1963.
13. Usher R, McLean F: Intrauterine growth of live-born Caucasian infants at sea level: standards obtained from measurements in 7 dimensions of infants born between 25 and 44 weeks of gestation. J Pediatr 74:901, 1969.
14. Battaglia FC, Lubchenco LO: A practical classification of newborn infants by weight and gestational age. J Pediatr 71:159, 1967.
15. Bernstein IM, Horbar JD, Badger GJ, et al: Morbidity and mortality among very-low-birth-weight neonates with intrauterine growth restriction. The Vermont Oxford Network. Am J Obstet Gynecol 182:198, 2000.
16. Barker DJ: Fetal growth and adult disease. Br J Obstet Gynaecol 99:275, 1992.
17. World Health Organization: Report of a Scientific Group on Health Statistics Methodology Related to Perinatal Events, Document ICD/PE/74.4:1, 1974.
18. Hoffman HJ, Stark CR, Lundin FE, Ashbrook JD: Analysis of birthweight, gestational age, and fetal viability, U. S. births, 1968. Obstet Gynecol Surv 29:651, 1974.
19. Owen P, Farrell T, Hardwick JC, Khan KS: Relationship between customised birthweight centiles and neonatal anthropometric features of growth restriction. BJOG 109:658, 2002.
20. Miller HC: Fetal growth and neonatal mortality. Pediatrics 49:392, 1972.
21. Weiner CP, Robinson D: The sonographic diagnosis of intrauterine growth retardation using the postnatal ponderal index and the crown heel length as standards of diagnosis, Am J Perinatol 6:380, 1989.
22. Lepercq J, Lahlou N, Timsit J, et al: Macrosomia revisited: ponderal index and leptin delineate subtypes of fetal overgrowth. Am J Obstet Gynecol 181:621, 1999.
23. Walther FJ, Ramaekers LHJ: The Ponderal Index as a measure of the nutritional status at birth and its relation to some aspects of neonatal morbidity. J Perinat Med 10:42, 1982.
24. Ballard JL, Rosenn B, Khoury JC, Miodovnik M: Diabetic fetal macrosomia: significance of disproportionate growth. Pediatr 122:115, 1993.
25. Clausson B, Gardosi J, Francis A, Cnattingius S: Perinatal outcome in SGA births defined by customised versus population-based birthweight standards. BJOG 108:830, 2001.
26. Wilcocks J, Donald J, Duggan TC, Day N: Fetal cephalometry by ultrasound. J Obstet Gynaecol Br Commonw 71:11, 1964.
27. Campbell S, Dewhurst CJ: Diagnosis of the small-for-dates fetus by serial ultrasonic cephalometry. Lancet 2:1002, 1971.
28. Weiner CP: Pathogenesis, evaluation, and potential treatments for severe, early onset growth retardation. Semin Perinatol 13:320, 1989.
29. Ward K, Hata A, Jeunemaitre X, et al: A molecular variant of angiotensinogen associated with preeclampsia. Nat Genet 4:59, 1993.
30. Silver HM, Seebeck M, Carlson R: Comparison of total blood volume in normal, preeclamptic and nonproteinuric gestational hypertensive pregnancy by simultaneous measurement of red blood cell and plasma volumes. Am J Obstet Gynecol 179:87, 1998.
31. Bernstein IM, Ziegler W, Stirewalt WS, et al: Angiotensinogen genotype and plasma volume in nulligravid women. Obstet Gynecol 92:171, 1998.
32. Croall J, Sherrif S, Matthews J: Non-pregnant plasma volume and fetal growth retardation. Br J Obstet Gynaecol 85:90, 1978.
33. Duvekot JJ, Cheriex EC, Pieters FAA, et al: Maternal volume homeostasis in early pregnancy in relation to fetal growth restriction. Obstet Gynecol 85:361, 1995.
34. Smith CA: Effects of maternal undernutrition upon the newborn infant in Holland (1944–1945). Am J Obstet Gynecol 30:229, 1947.
35. Lechtig A, Yarbrough C, Delgado H, et al: Effect of moderate maternal malnutrition on the placenta. Am J Obstet Gynecol 123:191, 1975.
36. Economides DL, Nicolaides KH: Blood glucose and oxygen tension levels in small-for-gestational-age fetuses. Am J Obstet Gynecol 160:385, 1989.
37. Khouzami VA, Ginsburg DS, Daikoku NH, et al: The glucose tolerance test as a means of identifying intrauterine growth retardation. Am J Obstet Gynecol 139:423, 1981.
38. Sokol RJ, Kazzi GM, Kalhan SC, Pillay SK: Identifying the pregnancy at risk for intrauterine growth retardation: possible usefulness of the intravenous glucose tolerance test. Am J Obstet Gynecol 143:220, 1983.
39. Langer O, Damus K, Maiman M, et al: A link between relative hypoglycemia-hypoinsulinemia during oral glucose tolerance tests and intrauterine growth retardation. Am J Obstet Gynecol 155:711, 1986.
40. Mills JL, Graubard BI, Harley EE, et al: Maternal alcohol consumption and birth weight. How much drinking during pregnancy is safe? JAMA 252:1875, 1984.
41. Little BB, Snell LM, Klein VR, et al: Cocaine abuse during pregnancy: maternal and fetal implications. Obstet Gynecol 74:157, 1989.
42. Lobi M, Welcher DW, Mellits ED: Maternal age and intellectual function of offspring. Johns Hopkins Med J 128:347, 1971.
43. Berkowitz GS, Skovron ML, Lapinski RH, et al: Delayed childbearing and the outcome of pregnancy. N Engl J Med 322:659, 1990.
44. Cliver SP, Goldenberg RL, Cutter GR, et al: The effect of cigarette smoking on neonatal anthropometric measurements. Obstet Gynecol 85:625, 1995.
45. Goldenberg RL, Hauth J, Cutter GR, et al: Fetal growth in women using low-dose aspirin for the prevention of pre-eclampsia: effect of maternal size. J Matern Fetal Med 4:218, 1995.
46. Goldenberg RL, Cliver SP, Cutter GR, et al: Blood Pressure, growth retardation and preterm delivery. In J Tech Asess Health Care 8:82, 1992.
47. Khoury MJ, Erickson D, Cordero JE, McCarthy BJ: Congenital malformations and intrauterine growth retardation: A population study. Pediatrics 82:83–90, 1988.
48. Eydoux P, Choiset A, LePorrier N, et al: Chromosomal prenatal diagnosis: study of 936 cases of intrauterine abnormalities after ultrasound assessment. Prenat Diagn 9:255, 1989.
49. Dugan A, Johnnson MP, Isada I, et al: The smaller than expected first trimester fetus is at increased risk for chromosomal anomalies. Am J Obstet Gynecol 167:1525, 1992.
50. Odegard RA, Vatten LJ, Nilsen ST, et al: Preeclampsia and fetal growth. Obstet Gynecol 96:950, 2000.
51. Kupferminc MJ, Peri H, Zwang E, et al: High prevalence of the prothrombin gene mutation in women with intrauterine growth retardation, abruptio placentae and second trimester loss. Acta Obstet Gynecol Scand 79:963, 2000.
52. Cowles T, Tatlor S, Zneimer S, Elder F: Association of confined placental mosaicism with intrauterine growth restriction [abstract]. Am J Obstet Gynecol 170:273, 1994.
53. Chapman MG, Furness ET, Jones WR, et al: Significance of the ultrasound location of placental site in early pregnancy. Br J Obstet Gynaecol 86:846, 1979.
54. Gruenwald P: Growth of the human fetus. II: Abnormal growth in twins and infants of mothers with diabetes, hypertension, or isoimmunization. Am J Obstet Gynecol 94:1120, 1966.
55. Houlton MCC, Marivate M, Philpott RH: The prediction of fetal growth retardation in twin pregnancy. Br J Obstet Gynaecol 88:264, 1981.
56. Baker ER, Beach ML, Craigo SD, et al: A comparison of neonatal outcomes of age-matched, growth restricted twins and growth restricted singletons. Am J Perinatol 14:499, 1997.
57. Hamilton EF, Platt RW, Morin L, et al: How small is too small in a twin pregnancy? Am J Obstet Gynecol 179:682, 1998.
58. Brosens I, Dixon HG, Robertson WB: Fetal growth retardation and the arteries of the placental bed. Br J Obstet Gynaecol 84:656, 1977.

59. Meekins JW, Pijnenborg R, Hanssens M, et al: A study of placental bed spiral arteries and trophoblast invasion in normal and severe pre-eclamptic pregnancies. Br J Obstet Gynaecol 101:669, 1994.
60. DeWolf F, Brosens I, Renaer M: Fetal growth retardation and the maternal arterial supply of the human placenta in the absence of sustained hypertension. Br J Obstet Gynaecol 87:678, 1980.
61. Aardema MW, Oosterhof H, Timmer A, et al: Uterine artery Doppler flow and uteroplacental vascular pathology in normal pregnancies and pregnancies complicated by pre-eclampsia and small for gestational age fetuses. Placenta 22:405, 2001.
62. Ferrazzi E, Bulfamante G, Mezzopane R, et al: Uterine Doppler velocimetry and placental hypoxic-ischaemic lesion in pregnancies with fetal intrauterine growth restriction. Placenta 20:389, 1999.
63. Sebire NJ, Talbert D: The role of intraplacental vascular smooth muscle in the dynamic placenta: a conceptual framework for understanding uteroplacental disease. Med Hypotheses 58:347, 2002.
64. Jones CT, Ritchie JW, Walker D: The effects of hypoxia on glucose turnover in the fetal sheep. J Dev Physiol 5:223, 1983.
65. Nicolini U, Hubinont C, Santolaya J, et al: Maternal-fetal glucose gradient in normal pregnancies and in pregnancies complicated by alloimmunization and fetal growth retardation. Am J Obstet Gynecol 161:924, 1989.
66. Hubinont C, Nicolini U, Fisk NM, et al: Endocrine pancreatic function in growth-retarded fetuses. Obstet Gynecol 77:541, 1991.
67. Van Assche FA, Aerts L, DePrins FA: The fetal endocrine pancreas. Eur J Obstet Gynecol Reprod Biol 18:267, 1984.
68. Cetin I, Marconi AM, Corbetta C, et al: Fetal amino acids in normal pregnancies and in pregnancies complicated by intrauterine growth retardation. Early Hum Dev 29:183, 1992.
69. Cetin I, Corbetta C, Sereni LP, et al: Umbilical amino acid concentrations in normal and growth-retarded fetuses sampled in utero by cordocentesis. Am J Obstet Gynecol 162:253, 1990.
70. Economides DL, Nicolaides KH, Campbell S: Metabolic and endocrine findings in appropriate and small for gestational age fetuses. J Perinat Med 19:97, 1991.
71. Paolini CL, Marconi AM, Ronzoni S, et al: Placental transport of leucine, phenylalanine, glycine, and proline in intrauterine growth-restricted pregnancies. J Clin Endocrinol Metab 86:5427, 2001.
72. Vannucci RC, Vannucci SJ: Glucose metabolism in the developing brain. Semin Perinatol 24:107, 2000.
73. Fisher DJ, Heymann MA, Rudolph AM: Fetal myocardial oxygen and carbohydrate consumption during acutely induced hypoxemia. Am J Physiol 242:H657, 1982.
74. Spahr R, Probst I, Piper HM: Substrate utilization of adult cardiac myocytes. Basic Res Cardiol 80(Suppl 1):53, 1985.
75. Soothill PW, Nicolaides KH, Campbell S: Prenatal asphyxia, hyperlacticaemia, hypoglycaemia, and erythroblastosis in growth retarded fetuses. Br Med J 294:1051, 1987.
76. Owens JA, Falconer J, Robinsin JS: Effect of restriction of placental growth on fetal uteroplacental metabolism. J Dev Physiol 9:225, 1987.
77. Fant ME, Weisoly D: Insulin and insulin-like growth factors in human development: implications for the perinatal period. Semin Perinatol 25:426, 2001.
78. Ostlund E, Tally M, Fried G: Transforming growth factor-beta1 in fetal serum correlates with insulin-like growth factor-I and fetal growth. Obstet Gynecol 100:567, 2002.
79. Nicolini U, Hubinont C, Santolaya J, et al: Effects of fetal intravenous glucose challenge in normal and growth retarded fetuses. Horm Metab Res 22:426, 1990.
80. Goland RS, Jozak S, Warren WB, et al: Elevated levels of umbilical cord plasma corticotropin-releasing hormone in growth-retarded fetuses. J Clin Endocrinol Metab 77:1174, 1993.
81. Giles WB, McLean M, Davies JJ, Smith R: Abnormal umbilical artery Doppler waveforms and cord blood corticotropin-releasing hormone. Obstet Gynecol 87:107, 1996.
82. Verhaeghe J, Van Herck E, Bouillon R: Umbilical cord osteocalcin in normal pregnancies and pregnancies complicated by fetal growth retardation or diabetes mellitus. Biol Neonate 68:377, 1995.
83. Namgung R, Tsang RC, Specker BL, et al: Reduced serum osteocalcin and 1,25-dihydroxyvitamin D concentrations and low bone mineral content in small for gestational age infants: evidence of decreased bone formation rates. J Pediatr 122:269, 1993.
84. Cianfarani S, Germani D, Rossi L, et al: IGF-I and IGF-binding protein-1 are related to cortisol in human cord blood. Eur J Endocrinol 138:524, 1998.
85. Spencer JA, Chang TC, Jones J, et al: Third trimester fetal growth and umbilical venous blood concentrations of IGF-1, IGFBP-1, and growth hormone at term. Arch Dis Child Fetal Neonatal Ed 73:F87, 1995.
86. Thorpe-Beeston JG, Nicolaides KH: Fetal thyroid function. Fetal Diagn Ther 8:60–72, 1993.
87. Thorpe-Beeston JG, Nicolaides KH, Snijders RJ, et al: Relations between the fetal circulation and pituitary-thyroid function. Br J Obstet Gynaecol 98:1163, 1991.
88. Nieto-Diaz A, Villar J, Matorras-Weinig R, Valenzuela-Ruiz P: Intrauterine growth retardation at term: association between anthropometric and endocrine parameters. Acta Obstet Gynecol Scand 75:127, 1996.
89. Kilby MD, Gittoes N, McCabe C, et al: Expression of thyroid receptor isoforms in the human fetal central nervous system and the effects of intrauterine growth restriction. Clin Endocrinol (Oxf) 53:469, 2000.
90. Weiner CP, Robillard JE: Atrial natriuretic factor, digoxin-like immunoreactive substance, norepinephrine, epinephrine, and plasma are in activity in human fetuses and their alteration by fetal disease. Am J Obstet Gynecol 159:1353, 1988.
91. Greenough A, Nicolaides KH, Lagercrantz H: Human fetal sympathoadrenal responsiveness. Early Hum Dev 23:9, 1990.
92. Ville Y, Proudler A, Kuhn P, Nicolaides KH: Aldosterone concentration in normal, growth-retarded, anemic, and hydropic fetuses. Obstet Gynecol 84:511, 1994.
93. Weiner CP, Williamson RA: Evaluation of severe growth retardation using cordocentesis—hematologic and metabolic alterations by etiology. Obstet Gynecol 73:225, 1989.
94. Thilaganathan B, Athanasiou S, Ozmen S, et al: Umbilical cord blood erythroblast count as an index of intrauterine hypoxia. Arch Dis Child Fetal Neonatal Ed 70:F192, 1994.
95. Maier RF, Gunther A, Vogel M, et al: Umbilical venous erythropoietin and umbilical arterial pH in relation to morphologic placental abnormalities. Obstet Gynecol 84: 81, 1994.
96. Snijders RJM, Abbas A, Melby O, et al: Fetal plasma erythropoetin concentration in severe growth retardation. Am J Obstet Gynecol 168:615, 1993.
97. Thilaganathan B, Nicolaides KH: Erythroblastosis in birth asphyxia. Ultrasound Obstet Gynecol 2:15, 1992.
98. Bernstein PS, Minior VK, Divon MY: Nucleated red blood cell counts in small for gestational age fetuses with abnormal umbilical artery Doppler studies. Am J Obstet Gynecol 177:1079, 1997.
99. Baschat AA, Gembruch U, Reiss I, et al: Neonatal nucleated red blood cell counts in growth-restricted fetuses: relationship to arterial and venous Doppler studies. Am J Obstet Gynecol 181:190, 1999.
100. Baschat AA, Gembruch U, Reiss I, et al: Neonatal nucleated red blood cell count and postpartum complications in growth restricted fetuses. J Perinat Med 31:323, 2003.
101. Stallmach T, Karolyi L, Lichtlen P, et al: Fetuses from preeclamptic mothers show reduced hepatic erythropoiesis. Pediatr Res 43:349, 1998.
102. Hiett AK, Britton KA, Hague NL, et al: Comparison of hematopoietic progenitor cells in human umbilical cord blood collected from neonatal infants who are small and appropriate for gestational age. Transfusion 35:587, 1995.
103. Rondo PH, Abbott R, Rodrigues LC, Tomkins AM: Vitamin A, folate, and iron concentrations in cord and maternal blood of intra-uterine growth retarded and appropriate birth weight babies. Eur J Clin Nutr 49:391, 1995.
104. Abbas A, Snijders RJ, Nicolaides KH: Serum ferritin and cobalamin in growth retarded fetuses. Br J Obstet Gynaecol 101:215, 1994.
105. Van den Hof MC, Nicolaides KH: Platelet count in normal, small, and anemic fetuses. Am J Obstet Gynecol 162:735, 1990.

106. Ohshige A, Yoshimura T, Maeda T, et al: Increased platelet-activating factor-acetylhydrolase activity in the umbilical venous plasma of growth-restricted fetuses. Obstet Gynecol 93:180, 1999.
107. Trudinger B, Song JZ, Wu ZH, Wang J: Placental insufficiency is characterized by platelet activation in the fetus. Obstet Gynecol 101:975, 2003.
108. Baschat AA, Gembruch U, Reiss I, et al: Absent umbilical artery end-diastolic velocity in growth-restricted fetuses: a risk factor for neonatal thrombocytopenia. Obstet Gynecol 96:162, 2000.
109. Drew JH, Guaran RL, Grauer S, Hobbs JB: Cord whole blood hyperviscosity: measurement, definition, incidence and clinical features. J Paediatr Child Health 27:363, 1991.
110. Steel SA, Pearce JM, Nash G, et al: Correlation between Doppler flow velocity waveforms and cord blood viscosity. Br J Obstet Gynaecol 96:1168, 1989.
111. Lemery DJ, Beal V, Vanlieferinghen P, Motta C: Fetal blood cell membrane fluidity in small for gestational age fetuses. Biol Neonate 64:7, 1993.
112. Singh M, Manerikar S, Malaviya AN, et al: Immune status of low birth weight babies. Indian Pediatr 15:563, 1978.
113. Davies N, Snijders R, Nicolaides KH: Intra-uterine starvation and fetal leucocyte count. Fetal Diagn Ther 6:107, 1991.
114. Thilaganathan B, Plachouras N, Makrydimas G, Nicolaides KH: Fetal immunodeficiency: a consequence of placental insufficiency. Br J Obstet Gynaecol 100:1000, 1993.
115. Ferrazzi E, Bozzo M, Rigano S, et al: Temporal sequence of abnormal Doppler changes in the peripheral and central circulatory systems of the severely growth-restricted fetus. Ultrasound Obstet Gynecol 19:140, 2002.
116. Rigano S, Bozzo M, Ferrazzi E, et al: Early and persistent reduction in umbilical vein blood flow in the growth-restricted fetus: a longitudinal study. Am J Obstet Gynecol 185:834, 2001.
117. Bellotti M, Pennati G, De Gasperi C, et al: Simultaneous measurements of umbilical venous, fetal hepatic, and ductus venosus blood flow in growth-restricted human fetuses. Am J Obstet Gynecol 190:1347, 2004.
118. Kiserud T: The ductus venosus. Semin Perinatol 25:11, 2001.
119. Rizzo G, Capponi A, Chaoui R, et al: Blood flow velocity waveforms from peripheral pulmonary arteries in normally grown and growth-retarded fetuses. Ultrasound Obstet Gynecol 8:87, 1996.
120. Griffin D, Bilardo K, Masini L, et al: Doppler blood flow waveforms in the descending thoracic aorta of the human fetus. Br J Obstet Gynaecol 91:997, 1984.
121. Akalin-Sel T, Nicolaides KH, Peacock J, Campbell S: Doppler dynamics and their complex interrelation with fetal oxygen pressure, carbon dioxide pressure, and pH in growth-retarded fetuses. Obstet Gynecol 84:439, 1994.
122. Wladimiroff JW, Tonge HM, Stewart PA: Doppler ultrasound assessment of cerebral blood flow in the human fetus. Br J Obstet Gynaecol 93:471, 1986.
123. Arbeille P, Maulik D, Fignon A, et al: Assessment of the fetal PO_2 changes by cerebral and umbilical Doppler on lamb fetuses during acute hypoxia. Ultrasound Med Biol 21:861, 1995.
124. Reed KL, Anderson CF, Shenker L: Changes in intracardiac Doppler flow velocities in fetuses with absent umbilical artery diastolic flow. Am J Obstet Gynecol 157:774, 1987.
125. Al Ghazali W, Chita SK, Chapman MG, Allan LD: Evidence of redistribution of cardiac output in asymmetrical growth retardation. Br J Obstet Gynaecol 96:697, 1987.
126. Fouron JC, Skoll A, Sonesson SE, et al: Relationship between flow through the fetal aortic isthmus and cerebral oxygenation during acute placental circulatory insufficiency in ovine fetuses. Am J Obstet Gynecol 181:1102, 1999.
127. Makikallio K, Jouppila P, Rasanen J: Retrograde net blood flow in the aortic isthmus in relation to human fetal arterial and venous circulations. Ultrasound Obstet Gynecol 19:147, 2002.
128. Rizzo G, Arduini D: Fetal cardiac function in intrauterine growth retardation. Am J Obstet Gynecol 165:876, 1991.
129. Rizzo G, Capponi A, Rinaldo D, et al: Ventricular ejection force in growth-retarded fetuses. Ultrasound Obstet Gynecol 5:247, 1995.
130. Gudmundsson S, Tulzer G, Huhta JC, Marsal K: Venous Doppler in the fetus with absent end-diastolic flow in the umbilical artery. Ultrasound Obstet Gynecol 7:262, 1996.
131. Hecher K, Campbell S, Doyle P, et al: Assessment of fetal compromise by Doppler ultrasound investigation of the fetal circulation. Arterial, intracardiac, and venous blood flow velocity studies. Circulation 91:129, 1995.
132. Rizzo G, Capponi A, Pietropolli A, et al: Fetal cardiac and extracardiac flows preceding intrauterine death. Ultrasound Obstet Gynecol 4:139, 1994.
133. Baschat AA, Gembruch U, Reiss I, et al: Demonstration of fetal coronary blood flow by Doppler ultrasound in relation to arterial and venous flow velocity waveforms and perinatal outcome—the 'heart-sparing effect'. Ultrasound Obstet Gynecol 9:162, 1997.
134. Tekay A, Jouppila P: Fetal adrenal artery velocimetry measurements in appropriate-for-gestational age and intrauterine growth-restricted fetuses. Ultrasound Obstet Gynecol 16:4194, 2000.
135. Abuhamad AZ, Mari G, Bogdan D: Evans AT 3rd: Doppler flow velocimetry of the splenic artery in the human fetus: is it a marker of chronic hypoxia? Am J Obstet Gynecol 172:820, 1995.
136. Kilavuz O, Vetter K: Is the liver of the fetus the 4th preferential organ for arterial blood supply besides brain, heart, and adrenal glands? J Perinat Med 27:103, 1999.
137. Gamsu HR, Vyas S, Nicolaides K: Effects of intrauterine growth retardation on postnatal visceral and cerebral blood flow velocity. Arch Dis Child 66:1115, 1991.
138. Mari G, Abuhamad AZ, Uerpairojkit B, et al: Blood flow velocity waveforms of the abdominal arteries in appropriate- and small-for-gestational-age fetuses. Ultrasound Obstet Gynecol 6:15, 1995.
139. Rhee E, Detti L, Mari G: Superior mesenteric artery flow velocity waveforms in small for gestational age fetuses. J Matern Fetal Med 7:120, 1998.
140. Veille JC, Kanaan C: Duplex Doppler ultrasonographic evaluation of the fetal renal artery in normal and abnormal fetuses. Am J Obstet Gynecol 161:1502, 1989.
141. Arduini D, Rizzo G: Fetal renal artery velocity waveforms and amniotic fluid volume in growth-retarded and post-term fetuses. Obstet Gynecol 77:370, 1991.
142. Manning FA: Fetal biophysical profile. Obstet Gynecol Clin North Am 26:557, 1999.
143. Arduini D, Rizzo G, Romanini C, Mancuso S: Computerized analysis of behavioural states in asymmetrical growth retarded fetuses. J Perinat Med 16:357, 1988.
144. Arduini D, Rizzo G, Caforio L, et al: Behavioural state transitions in healthy and growth retarded fetuses. Early Hum Dev 19:155, 1989.
145. Nijhuis IJ, ten Hof J, Nijhuis JG, et al: Temporal organisation of fetal behaviour from 24-weeks gestation onwards in normal and complicated pregnancies. Dev Psychobiol 34:257, 1999.
146. Vindla S, James D, Sahota D: Computerised analysis of unstimulated and stimulated behaviour in fetuses with intrauterine growth restriction. Eur J Obstet Gynecol Reprod Biol 83:37, 1999.
147. Henson G, Dawes GS, Redman CW: Characterization of the reduced heart rate variation in growth-retarded fetuses. Br J Obstet Gynaecol 91:751, 1984.
148. Smith JH, Anand KJ, Cotes PM, et al: Antenatal fetal heart rate variation in relation to the respiratory and metabolic status of the compromised human fetus. Br J Obstet Gynaecol 95:980, 1988.
149. Nijhuis IJ, ten Hof J, Mulder EJ, et al: Fetal heart rate in relation to its variation in normal and growth retarded fetuses. Eur J Obstet Gynecol Reprod Biol 89:27, 2000.
150. Ribbert LS, Snijders RJ, Nicolaides KH, Visser GH: Relation of fetal blood gases and data from computer-assisted analysis of fetal heart rate patterns in small for gestation fetuses. Br J Obstet Gynaecol 98:820, 1991.
151. Pillai M, James D: Continuation of normal neurobehavioural development in fetuses with absent umbilical arterial end-diastolic velocities. Br J Obstet Gynaecol 98:277, 1991.
152. Ribbert LS, Visser GH, Mulder EJ, et al: Changes with time in fetal heart rate variation, movement incidences and haemodynamics in intrauterine growth retarded fetuses: a longitudinal approach to the assessment of fetal well being. Early Hum Dev 31:195, 1993.

153. Rizzo G, Arduini D, Pennestri F, et al: Fetal behaviour in growth retardation: its relationship to fetal blood flow. Prenat Diagn 7:229, 1987.
154. Arduini D, Rizzo G, Capponi A, et al: Fetal pH value determined by cordocentesis: an independent predictor of the development of antepartum fetal heart rate decelerations in growth retarded fetuses with absent end-diastolic velocity in umbilical artery. J Perinat Med 24:601, 1996.
155. James DK, Parker MJ, Smoleniec JS: Comprehensive fetal assessment with three ultrasonographic characteristics. Am J Obstet Gynecol 166:1486, 1992.
156. Baschat AA, Gembruch U, Harman CR: The sequence of changes in Doppler and biophysical parameters as severe fetal growth restriction worsens. Ultrasound Obstet Gynecol 18:571, 2001.
157. Ribbert LS, Nicolaides KH, Visser GH: Prediction of fetal acidaemia in intrauterine growth retardation: comparison of quantified fetal activity with biophysical profile score. Br J Obstet Gynaecol 100:653, 1993.
158. Vintzileos AM, Fleming AD, Scorza WE, et al: Relationship between fetal biophysical activities and umbilical cord blood gas values. Am J Obstet Gynecol 165:707, 1991.
159. Manning FA, Snijders R, Harman CR, et al: Fetal biophysical profile score. VI. Correlation with antepartum umbilical venous fetal pH. Am J Obstet Gynecol 169:755, 1993.
160. Zeitlin J, Ancel PY, Saurel-Cubizolles MJ, Papiernik E: The relationship between intrauterine growth restriction and preterm delivery: an empirical approach using data from a European case-control study. BJOG 107:750, 2000.
161. Ott WJ: Intrauterine growth restriction and Doppler ultrasonography. J Ultrasound Med 19:661, 2000.
162. Strigini FA, De Luca G, Lencioni G, et al: Middle cerebral artery velocimetry: different clinical relevance depending on umbilical velocimetry. Obstet Gynecol 90:953, 1997.
163. Hecher K, Spernol R, Stettner H, Szalay S: Potential for diagnosing imminent risk for appropriate- and small for gestational fetuses by Doppler examination of umbilical and cerebral arterial blood flow. Ultrasound Obstet Gynecol 5:247, 1995.
164. Severi FM, Bocchi C, Visentin A, et al: Uterine and fetal cerebral Doppler predict the outcome of third-trimester small-for-gestational age fetuses with normal umbilical artery Doppler. Ultrasound Obstet Gynecol 19:225 2002.
165. Baschat AA: Pathophysiology of fetal growth restriction: implications for diagnosis and surveillance. Obstet Gynecol Surv 59: 617, 2004.
166. Campbell S, Wilkin D: Ultrasonic measurement of fetal abdomen circumference in the estimation of fetal weight. Br J Obstet Gynaecol 82:689, 1975.
167. Hadlock FP, Harrist RB, Sharman RS, et al: Estimation of fetal weight with the use of head, body, and femur measurements-a prospective study. Am J Obstet Gynecol 151:333, 1985.
168. Vintzileos AM, Campbell WA, Rodis JF, et al: Fetal weight estimation formulas with head, abdominal, femur and thigh circumference measurements. Am J Obstet Gynecol 157:410, 1987.
169. Combs CA, Jaekle RK, Rosenn B, et al: Sonographic estimation of fetal weight based on a model of fetal volume. Obstet Gynecol 82:365, 1993.
170. Sabbagha RE, Minogue J, Tamura RK, Hungerford SA: Estimation of birth weight by use of ultrasonographic formulas targeted to large-, appropriate-, and small-for-gestational age fetuses. Am J Obstet Gynecol 160:854, 1989.
171. Hadlock FP, Deter RL, Carpenter RJ, Park SK: Estimating fetal age: Effect of head shape on BPD. Am J Roentgenol 137:83, 1981.
172. Smith PA, Johansson D, Tzannatos C, Campbell S: Prenatal measurement of the fetal cerebellum and cisterna cerebellomedullaris by ultrasound. Prenat Diagn 6:133, 1986.
173. Reece EA, Goldstein I, Pilu G, Hobbins JC: Fetal cerebellar growth unaffected by intrauterine growth retardation: a new parameter for prenatal diagnosis. Am J Obstet Gynecol 157:632, 1987.
174. Hill LM, Guzick D, Rivello D, et al: The transverse cerebellar diameter cannot be used to assess gestational age in the small for gestational age fetus. Obstet Gynecol 75:329, 1990.
175. Tamura RK, Sabbagha RE: Percentile ranks of sonar fetal abdominal circumference measurements. Am J Obstet Gynecol 138:475, 1980.
176. Baschat AA, Weiner CP: Umbilical artery Doppler screening for detection of the small fetus in need of antepartum surveillance. Am J Obstet Gynecol 182:154, 2000.
177. Tamura RK, Sabbagha RE, Pan WH, Vaisrub N: Ultrasonic fetal abdominal circumference: Comparison of direct versus calculated measurement. Obstet Gynecol 67:833, 1986.
178. Divon MY, Chamberlain PF, Sipos L, et al: Identification of the small for gestational age fetus with the use of gestational age-independent indices of fetal growth. Am J Obstet Gynecol 155:1197, 1986.
179. Crane JP, Kopta MM: Prediction of intrauterine growth retardation via ultrasonically measured head/abdominal circumference ratios. Obstet Gynecol 54:597, 1979.
180. Seeds JW: Impaired fetal growth: ultrasonic evaluation and clinical management. Obstet Gynecol 64:577, 1984.
181. Campbell S, Thoms A: Ultrasound measurement of the fetal head to abdomen circumference ratio in the assessment of growth retardation. Br J Obstet Gynaecol 84:165, 1977.
182. Warsof SL, Cooper DJ, Little D, Campbell S: Routine ultrasound screening for antenatal detection of intrauterine growth retardation, Obstet Gynecol 67:33, 1986.
183. Hadlock FP, Deter RL, Harrist RB, et al: A date-independent predictor of intrauterine growth retardation: femur length/abdominal circumference ratio. AJR Am J Roentgenol 141:979, 1983.
184. Rohrer VF: Der index der Körperfülle als Mass des Ernährungszustandes. Münch Med Wochenschr 19:580, 1921.
185. Walther FJ, Ramaekers LHJ: The ponderal index as a measure of the nutritional status at birth and its relation to some aspects of neonatal morbidity. J Perinat Med 10:42, 1982.
186. Miller HC, Hassanein K: Diagnosis of impaired fetal growth in newborn infants. Pediatrics 48:511, 1971.
187. Yagel S, Zacut D, Igelstein S, et al: In utero ponderal index as a prognostic factor in the evaluation of intrauterine growth retardation. Am J Obstet Gynecol 157:415, 1987.
188. Bernstein IM, Catalano PM: Ultrasonographic estimation of fetal body composition for children of diabetic mothers. Invest Radiol 26:722, 1991.
189. Landon MB, Sonek J, Foy P, et al: Sonographic measurement of fetal humeral soft tissue thickness in pregnancy complicated by GDM. Diabetes 40(Suppl 2):66, 1991.
190. Abramowicz JS, Sherer DM, Woods JR: Ultrasonographic measurement of cheek-to-cheek diameter in fetal growth disturbances. Am J Obstet Gynecol 169:405, 1993.
191. Gardeil F, Greene R, Stuart B, Turner MJ: Subcutaneous fat in the fetal abdomen as a predictor of growth restriction. Obstet Gynecol 94:209, 1999.
192. Chauhan S, West DJ, Scardo JA, et al: Antepartum detection of macrosomic fetus: clinical versus sonographic, including soft-tissue measurements. Obstet Gynecol 95:639, 2000.
193. Padoan A, Rigano S, Ferrazzi E, et al: Differences in fat and lean mass proportions in normal and growth restricted fetuses. Am J Obstet Gynecol 191:1459, 2004.
194. Ott WJ: The diagnosis of altered fetal growth. Obstet Gynecol Clin North Am 15:237, 1988.
195. Seeds JW, Peng T: Impaired fetal growth and risk of fetal death: is the tenth percentile the appropriate standard. Am J Obstet Gynecol 178:658, 1998.
196. Weiner CP, Sabbagha RE, Vaisrub N, Depp R: A hypothetical model suggesting suboptimal intra-uterine growth in infants delivered preterm. Obstet Gynecol 65:323, 1985.
197. Ott WJ: Intrauterine growth retardation and preterm delivery. Am J Obstet Gynecol 168:1710, 1993.
198. Bernstein IM, Meyer MC, Capeless EL: "Fetal growth charts": comparison of cross-sectional ultrasound examinations with birthweight. Maternal Fetal Med 3:182, 1994.
199. Hadlock FP, Harrist RB, Martinez-Poyer J: In utero analysis of fetal growth: a sonographic weight standard. Radiology 181:129, 1991.
200. Lackman F, Capewell V, Richardson B, et al: Fetal or neonatal growth curve: which is more appropriate in predicting the impact of fetal growth on the risk of perinatal mortality? Am J Obstet Gynecol 180:S145, 1999.
201. Eik-Nes SH, Grottum P, Persson PH, Marsal K: Prediction of fetal growth by ultrasound biometry. I. Methodology. Acta Obstet Gynecol Scand 61:53, 1982.

202. Rossavik IK, Deter RL: Mathematical modeling of fetal growth. I. Basic principles. J Clin Ultrasound 12:529, 1984.
203. Shields LE, Huff RW, Jackson GM, et al: Fetal growth: a comparison of growth curves with mathematical modeling. J Ultrasound Med 5:271, 1993.
204. Mongelli M, Sverker EK, Tambyrajia R: Screening for fetal growth restriction: a mathematical model of the effect of time interval and ultrasound error. Obstet Gynecol 92:908, 1998.
205. Bobrow CS, Soothill P: Fetal growth velocity: a cautionary tale. Lancet 353:1460, 1999.
206. Baschat AA, Towbin J, Bowles NE, et al: Is adenovirus a fetal pathogen? Am J Obstet Gynecol 189:758, 2003.
207. Veille JC, Kanaan C: Duplex Doppler ultrasonographic evaluation of the fetal renal artery in normal and abnormal fetuses. Am J Obstet Gynecol 161:1502, 1989.
208. Magann EF, Chauhan SP, Barrilleaux PS, et al: Amniotic fluid index and single deepest pocket: weak indicators of abnormal amniotic volumes. Obstet Gynecol 96:737, 2000.
209. Manning FA, Hill LM, Platt LD: Qualitative amniotic fluid volume determination by ultrasound: antepartum detection of intrauterine growth retardation. Am J Obstet Gynecol 193:254, 1981.
210. Manning FA, Lange IR, Morrison I, Harman CR: Determination of fetal health: methods for antepartum and intrapartum fetal assessment. Curr Probl Obstet Gynecol 7:1, 1983.
211. Chamberlain PF, Manning FA, Morrison I, et al: Ultrasound evaluation of amniotic fluid volume. I. The relationship of marginal and decreased amniotic fluid volumes to perinatal outcome. Am J Obstet Gynecol 150:245, 1984.
212. Chauhan SP, Sanderson M, Hendrix NW, et al: Perinatal outcome and amniotic fluid index in the antepartum and intrapartum periods: A meta-analysis. Am J Obstet Gynecol 181:1473, 1999.
213. Sickler GK, Nyberg DA, Sohaey R, Luthy DA: Polyhydramnios and fetal intrauterine growth restriction: Ominous combination. J Ultrasound Med 16:609, 1997.
214. Groome LJ, Owen J, Neely CL, Hauth JC: Oligohydramics: antepartum fetal urine production and intrapertum fetal distress. Am J Obstet Gynecol 165:1077, 1991.
215. Thompson RS, Trudinger BJ, Cook CM: Doppler ultrasound waveform indices: A/B ratio, pulsatility index and Pourcelot ratio. Br J Obstet Gynaecol 95:581, 1988.
216. Hecher K, Campbell S: Characteristics of fetal venous blood flow under normal circumstances and during fetal disease. Ultrasound Obstet Gynecol 7:68, 1996.
217. Baschat AA, Guclu S, Kush ML, et al: Venous Doppler in the prediction of acid-base status of growth-restricted fetuses with elevated placental blood flow resistance. Am J Obstet Gynecol 191:277, 2004.
218. McGowan LM, Harding JE, Roberts AB, et al: A pilot randomized controlled trial of two regimens of fetal surveillance for small-for-gestational age fetuses with normal results of umbilical artery Doppler velocimetry. Am J Obstet Gynecol 182:81, 2000.
219. Neilson JP, Alfirevic Z: Doppler ultrasound for fetal assessment in high risk pregnancies (Cochrane review). In: The Cochrane Library, Issue 1, 2002. Oxford: Update Software.
220. Westergaard HB, Langhoff-Roos J, Lingman G, et al: A critical appraisal of the use of umbilical artery Doppler ultrasound in high-risk pregnancies: use of meta-analyses in evidence-based obstetrics. Ultrasound Obstet Gynecol 17:466, 2001.
221. Yagel S, Anteby EY, Shen O, et al: Simultaneous multigate spectral Doppler imaging of the umbilical artery and placental vessels: novel ultrasound technology. Ultrasound Obstet Gynecol 14:256, 1999.
222. Gramellini D, Folli MC, Raboni S, et al: Cerebral-umbilical Doppler ratio as a predictor of adverse perinatal outcome. Obstet Gynecol 79:416, 1992.
223. Bahado-Singh RO, Kovanci E, Jeffres A, et al: The Doppler cerebroplacental ratio and perinatal outcome in intrauterine growth restriction. Am J Obstet Gynecol 180:750, 1999.
224. Baschat AA, Gembruch U: The cerebroplacental Doppler ratio revisited. Ultrasound Obstet Gynecol 21:124, 2003.
225. Cox WL, Daffos F, Forestier F, et al: Physiology and management of intrauterine growth retardation. A biologic approach with fetal blood sampling. Am J Obstet Gynecol 159:36, 1988.
226. Fisher JW: Control of erythropoietin production. Proc Soc Exp Biol Med 173:289, 1983.
227. Maier RF, Bohme K, Dudenhausen JW, Obladen M: Cord blood erythropoietin in relation to different markers of fetal hypoxia. Obstet Gynecol 81:575, 1993.
228. Teramo KA, Widness JA, Clemons GK, et al: Amniotic fluid eyrthropoietin correlates with umbilical plasma erythropoietin in normal and abnormal pregnancy. Obstet Gynecol 69:710, 1987.
229. Ruth V, Autti-Ramo I, Granstrom ML, et al: Prediction of perinatal brain damage by cord plasma vasopressin, erythropoietin, and hypoxanthine values. J Pediatr 113:880, 1988.
230. Pollack A, Susa JB, Stonestreet BS, et al: Phosphoenolpyruvate carboxykinase in experimental intrauterine growth retardation in rats. Pediatr Res 13:175, 1979.
231. Economides DL, Nicolaides KH, Gahl WA, et al: Cordocentesis in the diagnosis of intrauterine starvation. Am J Obstet Gynecol 161:1004, 1989.
232. Mestyan J, Soltesz G, Schultz K, Horvath M: Hyperaminoacidemia due to the accumulation of gluconeogenic amino acid precursors in hypoglycemic small for gestational age infants. J Pediatr 87:409, 1975.
233. Bernstein IM, Silver R, Nair KS, Stirewalt WS: Amniotic fluid glycine-valine ratio and neonatal morbidity in fetal growth restriction. Obstet Gynecol 90:933, 1997.
234. Galbraith RS, Karchman EJ, Piercy WN, et al: The clinical prediction of intrauterine growth retardation. Am J Obstet Gynecol 133:231, 1979.
235. Tejani NA: Recurrence of intrauterine growth retardation. Obstet Gynecol 59:329, 1982.
236. Tejani N, Mann LI: Diagnosis and management of the small for gestational age fetus. *In* Frigoletto FD (ed): Clinical Obstetrics and Gynecology. Hagerstown, MD, Harper & Row, 1977, p 943.
237. Yaron Y, Cherry M, Kramer RL, et al: Second-trimester maternal serum marker screening: maternal serum alpha-fetoprotein, beta-human chorionic gonadotropin, estriol, and their various combinations as predictors for pregnancy outcome. Am J Obstet Gynecol 181:968, 1999.
238. Onderoglu LS, Kabukcu A: Elevated second trimester human chorionic gonadotropin level associated with adverse pregnancy outcome. Int J Gynaecol Obstet 56:245, 1997.
239. Cusick W, Rodis JF, Vintzileos AM, et al: Predicting pregnancy outcome from the degree of maternal serum alpha-fetoprotein elevation. J Reprod Med 5:327, 1996.
240. Waller DK, Lustig LS, Cunningham GC, et al: The association between maternal serum alpha-fetoprotein and preterm birth, small for gestational age infants, preeclampsia, and placental complication. Obstet Gynecol 88:816, 1996.
241. Belizan JM, Villar J, Nardin JC, et al: Diagnosis of intrauterine growth retardation by a simple clinical method: measurement of uterine height. Am J Obstet Gynecol 131:643, 1978.
242. Persson B, Stangenberg M, Lunell NO, et al: Prediction of size of infants at birth by measurement of symphysis fundus height. Br J Obstet Gynaecol 93:206, 1986.
243. Papageorghiou AT, Yu CK, Cicero S, et al: Second-trimester uterine artery Doppler screening in unselected populations: a review. J Matern Fetal Neonatal Med 12:78, 2002.
244. Soregaroli M, Valcamonico A, Scalvi L, et al: Late normalization of uterine artery velocimetry in high risk pregnancy. Eur J Obstet Gynecol Reprod Biol 95:42, 2001.
245. Harrington K, Carpenter RG, Goldfrad C, Campbell S: Transvaginal Doppler ultrasound of the uteroplacental circulation in the early prediction of pre-eclampsia and intrauterine growth retardation. Br J Obstet Gynaecol 104:674, 1997.
246. Bower S, Kingdom J, Campbell S: Objective and subjective assessment of abnormal uterine artery Doppler flow velocity waveforms. Ultrasound Obstet Gynecol 12:260, 1998.
247. North RA, Ferrier C, Long D, et al: Uterine artery Doppler velocity waveforms in the second trimester for the prediction of preeclampsia and fetal growth retardation. Obstet Gynecol 83:378, 1994.
248. Bewley S, Cooper D, Campbell S: Doppler investigation of uteroplacental blood flow resistance in the second trimester: a screening study for preeclampsia and intrauterine growth retardation. Br J Obstet Gynaecol 98:871, 1991.

249. Steele SA, Pearce JM, McParland PM, Chamberlain GVP: Early Doppler ultrasound screening in prediction of hypertensive disorders of pregnancy. Lancet 335:1548, 1990.
250. Coleman MA, McCowan LM, North RA: Mid-trimester uterine artery Doppler screening as a predictor of adverse pregnancy outcome in high-risk women. Ultrasound Obstet Gynecol 15:7, 2000.
251. Papageorghiou A, Yu CKH, Bindra R, et al: Multicenter screening for pre-eclampsia and fetal growth restriction by transvaginal uterine Doppler artery at 23 weeks of gestation. Ultrasound Obstet Gynecol 18:441, 2001.
252. Valensise H, Romanini C: Second-trimester uterine artery flow velocity waveform and oral glucose tolerance test as a means of predicting intrauterine growth retardation. Ultrasound Obstet Gynecol 3:412, 1993.
253. Yu CK, Papageorghiou AT, Parra M, et al: Fetal Medicine Foundation Second Trimester Screening Group: Randomized controlled trial using low-dose aspirin in the prevention of pre-eclampsia in women with abnormal uterine artery Doppler at 23 weeks' gestation. Ultrasound Obstet Gynecol 22:233, 2003.
254. CLASP: A randomised trial of low-dose aspirin for the prevention and treatment of pre-eclampsia among 9364 pregnant women. CLASP (Collaborative Low-dose Aspirin Study in Pregnancy) Collaborative Group. Lancet 343:619, 1994.
255. Vainio M, Kujansuu E, Iso-Mustajarvi M, Maenpaa J: Low dose acetylsalicylic acid in prevention of pregnancy-induced hypertension and intrauterine growth retardation in women with bilateral uterine artery notches. Br J Obstet Gynaecol 109:161, 2002.
256. Martin AM, Bindra R, Curcio P, et al: Screening for pre-eclampsia and fetal growth restriction by uterine artery Doppler at 11–14 wekkes of gestation. Ultrasound Obstet Gynecol 18:583, 2001.
257. Herbert WN, Seeds JW, Bowes WA, Sweeney CA: Fetal growth response to total parenteral nutrition in pregnancy. A case report. J Reprod Med 31:263, 1986.
258. Nicolaides KH, Campbell S, Bradley RJ, et al: Maternal oxygen therapy for intrauterine growth retardation, Lancet 8539:942, 1987.
259. Battaglia C, Artini PG, D'Ambrogio G, et al: Maternal hyperoxygenation in the treatment of intrauterine growth retardation. Am J Obstet Gynecol 167:430, 1992.
260. Ribbert LSM, van Lingen RA, Visser GHA: Continuous maternal hyperoxygenation in the treatment of early fetal growth retardation. Ultrasound Obstet Gynecol 1:331, 1991.
261. Ronzoni S, Marconi AM, Paolini CL, et al: The effect of a maternal infusion of amino acids on umbilical uptake in pregnancies complicated by intrauterine growth restriction. Am J Obstet Gynecol 187:741, 2002.
262. Harding J, Liu L, Evans P, et al: Intrauterine feeding of the growth retarded fetus: can we help? Early Hum Dev 29:193, 1992.
263. De Prins F, Hill DJ, Milner RD, Van Assche A: Effect of maternal hyperalimentation on intrauterine growth retardation. Arch Dis Child 63(7 Spec No):733, 1988.
264. Karsdorp VH, van Vugt JM, Dekker GA, van Geijn HP: Reappearance of end-diastolic velocities in the umbilical artery following maternal volume expansion: a preliminary study. Obstet Gynecol 80:679, 1992.
265. Wallenburg HCS, Rotmans N: Prevention of recurrent idiopathic fetal growth retardation by low-dose aspirin and dipyridamole. Am J Obstet Gynecol 157:1230, 1987.
266. Leitich H, Egarter C, Husslein P, et al: A meta-analysis of low dose aspirin for the prevention of intrauterine growth retardation. Br J Obstet Gynaecol 104:450, 1997.
267. Kozer E, Nikfar S, Costei A, et al: Aspirin consumption during the first trimester of pregnancy and congenital anomalies: a meta-analysis. Am J Obstet Gynecol 187:1623, 2002.
268. Trudinger BJ, Cook CM, Thompson RS, et al: Low-dose aspirin therapy improves fetal weight in umbilical placental insufficiency. Am J Obstet Gynecol 159:681, 1988.
269. Newnham JP, Godfrey M, Walters BJ, et al: Low dose aspirin for the treatment of fetal growth restriction: a randomized controlled trial. Aust N Z J Obstet Gynaecol 35:370, 1995.
270. Ley D, Wide-Swensson D, Lindroth M, et al: Respiratory distress syndrome in infants with impaired intrauterine growth. Acta Paediatr 86:1090, 1997.
271. Elimian A, Verma U, Canterino J, et al: Effectiveness of antenatal steroids in obstetric subgroups. Obstet Gynecol 93:174, 1999.
272. Derks JB, Mulder EJ, Visser GH: The effects of maternal betamethasone administration on the fetus. Br J Obstet Gynaecol 102:40, 1995.
273. Deren O, Karaer C, Onderoglu L, et al: The effect of steroids on the biophysical profile and Doppler indices of umbilical and middle cerebral arteries in healthy preterm fetuses. Eur J Obstet Gynecol Reprod Biol 99:72, 2001.
274. Cohlen BJ, Stigter RH, Derks JB, et al: Absence of significant hemodynamic changes in the fetus following maternal betamethasone administration. Ultrasound Obstet Gynecol 8:252, 1996.
275. Piazze JJ, Anceschi MM, La Torre R, et al: Effect of antenatal betamethasone therapy on maternal-fetal Doppler velocimetry. Early Hum Dev 60:225, 2001.
276. Soothill PW, Ajayi RA, Campbell S, et al: Relationship between fetal acidemia at cordocentesis and subsequent neurodevelopment. Ultrasound Obstet Gynecol 2:80, 1992.
277. Matthews DD: Maternal assessment of fetal activity in small-for-dates infants. Obstet Gynecol 45:488, 1975.
278. Wheeler T, Murrills A: Patterns of fetal heart rate during normal pregnancy. Br J Obstet Gynaecol 85:18, 1978.
279. Dawes GS, Houghton CRS, Redman CWG, Visser GHA: Patterns of normal fetal heart rate. Br J Obstet Gynaecol 89:276, 1982.
280. Visser GHA, Dawes GS, Redman CWG: Numerical analysis of the normal human antenatal fetal heart rate. Br J Obstet Gynaecol 88:792, 1981.
281. Nicolaides KH, Sadovsky G, Visser GHA: Heart rate patterns in normoxemic, hypoxemic, and anemic second-trimester fetuses. Am J Obstet Gynecol 160:1034, 1989.
282. Gagnon R, Campbell K, Hunse C, Patrick J: Patterns of human fetal heart rate accelerations from 26 weeks to term. Am J Obstet Gynecol 157:743 1987.
283. Visser GHA, Sadovsky G, Nicolaides KH: Antepartum heart rate patterns in small-for gestational age third trimester fetuses: Correlations with blood gases obtained at cordocentesis. Am J Obstet Gynecol 162:698, 1990.
284. Pazos R, Vuolo K, Aladjem S, et al: Association of spontaneous fetal heart rate decelerations during antepartum nonstress testing and intrauterine growth retardation. Am J Obstet Gynecol 144:574, 1982.
285. Gabbe SG, Freeman RD, Goebelsmann U: Evaluation of the contraction stress test before 33 weeks' gestation. Obstet Gynecol 52:649, 1978.
286. Lin CC, Devoe LD, River P, et al: Oxytocin challenge test and intrauterine growth retardation. Am J Obstet Gynecol 140:282, 1981.
287. Devoe L, Golde S, Kilman Y, et al: A comparison of visual analyses of intrapartum fetal heart rate tracings according to the new national institute of child health and human development guidelines with computer analyses by an automated fetal heart rate monitoring system. Am J Obstet Gynecol 183:361, 2000.
288. Visser GHA, Redman CWG, Huisjes HJ, Turnbull AC: Nonstressed antepartum heart rate monitoring: implications of decelerations after spontaneous contractions. Am J Obstet Gynecol 138:429, 1980.
289. Selam B, Koksal R, Ozcan T: Fetal arterial and venous Doppler parameters in the interpretation of oligohydramnios in postterm pregnancies. Ultrasound Obstet Gynecol 15:403, 2000.
290. Baschat AA, Galan HL, Bhide A, et al: Doppler and biophysical assessment in growth restricted fetuses: distribution of test results. Ultrasound Obstet Gynecol 27:41, 2006.
291. Nageotte MP, Towers CV, Asrat A, Freeman RK: Perinatal outcome with the modified biophysical profile. Am J Obstet Gynecol 170:1672, 1994.
292. Manning FA, Platt FA, Sipos L: Antepartum fetal evaluation: development of a fetal biophysical profile. Am J Obstet Gynecol 136:787, 1980.
293. Ribbert LS, Snijders RJ, Nicolaides KH, Visser GH: Relationship of fetal biophysical profile and blood gas values at cordocente-

sis in severely growth-retarded fetuses. Am J Obstet Gynecol 163:569, 1990.

294. Divon MY, Girz BA, Lieblich R, Langer O: Clinical management of the fetus with markedly diminished umbilical artery end-diastolic flow. Am J Obstet Gynecol 161:1523, 1989.

295. Harrington K, Thompson MO, Carpenter RG, et al: Doppler fetal circulation in pregnancies complicated by pre-eclampsia or delivery of a small for gestational age baby: 2. Longitudinal analysis. Br J Obstet Gynaecol 106:453, 1999.

296. Rizzo G, Capponi A, Talone PE, et al: Doppler indices from inferior vena cava and ductus venosus in predicting pH and oxygen tension in umbilical blood at cordocentesis in growth-retarded fetuses. Ultrasound Obstet Gynecol 7:401, 1996.

297. Fouron JC, Absi F, Skoll A, et al: Changes in flow velocity patterns of the superior and inferior venae cavae during placental circulatory insufficiency. Ultrasound Obstet Gynecol 21:53, 2003.

298. Hofstaetter C, Gudmundsson S, Hansmann M: Venous Doppler velocimetry in the surveillance of severely compromised fetuses. Ultrasound Obstet Gynecol 20:233, 2002.

299. Weiner Z, Goldberg Y, Shalev E: Internal jugular vein blood flow in normal and growth-restricted fetuses. Obstet Gynecol 96:167, 2000.

300. Senat MV, Schwarzler P, Alcais A, Ville Y: Longitudinal changes in the ductus venosus, cerebral transverse sinus and cardiotocogram in fetal growth restriction. Ultrasound Obstet Gynecol 16:19, 2000.

301. Bilardo CM, Wolf H, Stigter RH, et al: Relationship between monitoring parameters and perinatal outcome in severe, early intrauterine growth restriction. Ultrasound Obstet Gynecol 23:119, 2004.

302. Guzman ER, Vintzileos AM, Martins M, et al: The efficacy of individual computer heart rate indices in detecting acidemia at birth in growth-restricted fetuses. Obstet Gynecol 87:969, 1996.

303. Karsdorp VH, van Vugt JM, van Geijn HP, et al: Clinical significance of absent or reversed end diastolic velocity waveforms in umbilical artery. Lancet 344:1664, 1994.

304. Giles WB, Trudinger BJ, Baird PJ: Fetal umbilical artery flow velocity waveforms and placental resistance: pathological correlation. Br J Obstet Gynaecol 92:31, 1985.

305. Morrow RJ, Adamson SL, Bull SB, Ritchie JW: Effect of placental embolization on the umbilical artery velocity waveform in fetal sheep. Am J Obstet Gynecol 161:1055, 1989.

306. Nicolaides KH, Bilardo CM, Soothill P, Campbell S: Absence of end diastolic frequencies in umbilical artery: a sign of fetal hypoxia and acidosis. BMJ 209:1026, 1988.

307. Bilardo CM, Nicolaides KH, Campbell S: Doppler measurements of fetal and uteroplacental circulations: Relationship with umbilical venous blood gases measured at cordocentesis. Am J Obstet Gynecol 162:115, 1990.

308. Giles WB, Bisits A: Clinical use of Doppler in pregnancy: Information from six randomized trials. Fetal Diagn Ther 8:247, 1993.

309. Indik JH, Chen V, Reed KL: Association of umbilical venous with inferior vena cava blood flow velocities. Obstet Gynecol 77:551, 1991.

310. Arduini D, Rizzo G, Romanini C: Changes of pulsatility index from fetal vessels preceding the onset of late decelerations in growth-retarded fetuses. Obstet Gynecol 79:605, 1992.

311. Arduini D, Rizzo G, Romanini C: The development of abnormal heart rate patterns after absent end-diastolic velocity in umbilical artery: Analysis of risk factors. Am J Obstet Gynecol 168:50, 1993.

312. Baschat AA: Doppler application in the delivery timing of the preterm growth-restricted fetus: another step in the right direction. Ultrasound Obstet Gynecol 23:111, 2004.

313. Baschat AA, Gembruch U, Weiner CP, Harman CR: Qualitative venous Doppler waveform analysis improves prediction of critical perinatal outcomes in premature growth-restricted fetuses. Ultrasound Obstet Gynecol 22:240, 2003.

314. Nicolini U, Nicolaidis P, Fisk NM, et al: Limited role of fetal blood sampling in prediction of outcome in intrauterine growth retardation. Lancet 336:768, 1990.

315. Pardi G, Cetin I, Marconi AM, et al: Diagnostic value of blood sampling in fetuses with growth retardation. N Engl J Med 328:692, 1993.

316. Farine D, Kelly EN, Ryan G, et al: Absent and reversed umbilical artery end-diastolic velocity. *In* Copel JA, Reed KL (eds): Doppler Ultrasound in Obstetrics and Gynecology. New York, Raven Press, 1995, p 187.

317. Hecher K, Bilardo CM, Stigter RH, et al: Monitoring of fetuses with intrauterine growth restriction: a longitudinal study. Ultrasound Obstet Gynecol 18:564, 2001.

318. Baschat AA, Gembruch U, Reiss I, et al: Relationship between arterial and venous Doppler and perinatal outcome in fetal growth restriction. Ultrasound Obstet Gynecol 16:4073, 2000.

319. Hershkovitz R, Kingdom JC, Geary M, Rodeck CH: Fetal cerebral blood flow redistribution in late gestation: identification of compromise in small fetuses with normal umbilical artery Doppler. Ultrasound Obstet Gynecol 15:209, 2000.

320. Baschat AA: Integrated fetal testing in growth restriction: combining multi-vessel Doppler and biophysical parameters. Ultrasound Obstet Gynecol 21:1, 2003.

321. The GRIT study group: A randomised trial of timed delivery for the compromised preterm fetus: short term outcomes and Bayesian interpretation. BJOG 110:27, 2003.

322. The GRIT study group: Infant well-being at 2 years of age in the Growth Restriction Intervention Trial (GRIT): multicentred randomized trial. Lancet 364:513, 2004.

323. Baschat AA, Cosmi E, Bilardo C, et al: Predictors of neonatal outcome in early onset placental dysfunction. Obstet Gynecol 109:253, 2007.

324. Garite TJ, Clark R, Thorp JA: Intrauterine growth restriction increases morbidity and mortality among premature neonates. Am J Obstet Gynecol 191:481, 2004.

325. Frigoletto FD: Evaluation and management of deferred-fetal growth. *In* Frigoletto FD (ed): Clinical Obstetrics and Gynecology. Hagerstown, MD, Harper & Row, 1977, p 922.

326. Baschat AA, Gembruch U, Weiner CP, Harman CR: Combining Doppler and biophysical assessment improves prediction of critical perinatal outcomes. Am J Obstet Gynecol 187:S147, 2002.

327. Sawai SK, Williams MC, O'Brien WF, et al: Sequential outpatient application of intravaginal prostaglandin E_2 gel in the management of postdates pregnancies. Obstet Gynecol 78:19, 1991.

328. Procianoy RS, Garcia-Prats FA, Adams JM, et al: Hyaline membrane disease and intraventricular haemorrhage in small for gestational age infants. Arch Dis Child 55:502, 1980.

329. Piper JM, Langer O: Is lung maturation related to fetal growth in diabetic or hypertensive pregnancies? Eur J Obstet Gynecol Reprod Biol 51:15, 1993.

330. Thompson PJ, Greenough A, Gamsu HR, Nicolaides KH: Ventilatory requirements for respiratory distress syndrome in small-for-gestational-age infants. Eur J Pediatr 151:528, 1992.

331. McIntire DD, Bloom SL, Casey BM, Leveno MJ: Birth weight in relation to morbidity and mortality among newborn infants. N Engl J Med 340:1234, 1999.

332. Ley D, Wide-Swensson D, Lindroth M, et al: Respiratory distress syndrome in infants with impaired intrauterine growth. Acta Paediatr 10:1090, 1997.

332a. Dashe DS, McIntire DD, Lucas MJ, Leveno KJ: Effect of symmetric and asymmetric fetal growth on pregnancy outcomes. Obstet Gynecol 96:321, 2007.

333. Spinillo A, Capuzzo E, Piazzi G, et al: Significance of low birthweight for gestational age among very preterm infants. Br J Obstet Gynaecol 104:668, 1997.

334. Aucott SW, Donohue PK, Northington FJ: Increased morbidity in severe early intrauterine growth restriction. J Perinatol 24:435, 2004.

335. Carson BS, Losey RW, Bowes WA Jr, et al: Combined obstetric and pediatric approach to prevent meconium aspiration syndrome. Am J Obstet Gynecol 126:712, 1976.

336. Oh W: Considerations in neonates with intrauterine growth retardation. *In* Frigoletto FD (ed): Clinical Obstetrics and Gynecology. Hagerstown, MD, Harper & Row, 1977, p 989.

337. Tsang RC, Oh W: Neonatal hypocalcemia in low birth-weight infants. Pediatrics 45:773, 1970.
338. Baschat AA, Gembruch U, Harman CR: Haematologic consequences of placental insufficiency. Arch Dis Child Fetal Neonatal Ed 89:F94, 2004.
339. Kush M, Gortner L, Harman CR, Baschat AA: Sustained hematological consequences in the first week of neonatal life secondary to placental dysfunction. Early Hum Dev 82:67, 2006.
340. Kitchen WH, Richards A, Ryan MM, et al: A longitudinal study of very low-birthweight infants. II: Results of controlled trial of intensive care and incidence of handicaps. Dev Med Child Neurol 21:582, 1979.
341. Kitchen WH, McDougass AB, Naylor FD: A longitudinal study of very low-birthweight infants. III: Distance growth at eight years of age. Dev Med Child Neurol 22:1633, 1980.
342. Hediger ML, Overpeck MD, Maurer KR, et al: Growth of infants and young children born small or large for gestational age: findings from the Third National Health and Nutrition Examination Survey. Arch Pediatr Adolesc Med 152:1225, 1998.
343. Kumar SP, Anday EK, Sacks LM, et al: Follow-up studies of very low birthweight infants (1,250 grams or less) born and treated within a perinatal center. Pediatrics 66:438, 1980.
344. Fitzhardinge PM, Steven EM: The small-for-dates infant. II: Neurological and intellectual sequelae. Pediatrics 50:50, 1972.
345. Low JA, Galbraith RS, Muir D, et al: Intrauterine growth retardation: a preliminary report of long-term morbidity. Am J Obstet Gynecol 130:534, 1978.
346. Lipper E, Lee K-S, Gartner LM, et al: Determinants of neurobehavioral outcome in low birthweight infants. Pediatrics 67:502, 1981.
347. Strauss R, Dietz WH: Growth and development of term children born with low birth weight: effects of genetic and environmental factors. J Pediatr 133:67, 1998.
348. Walther FJ: Growth and development of term disproportionate small-for-gestational age infants at the age of 7 years. Early Hum Dev 18:1, 1988.
349. Robertson CMT, Etches PC, Kyle JM: Eight-year school performance and growth of preterm, small for gestational age infants: a comparative study with subjects matched for birth weight or for gestational age. J Pediatr 116:19, 1990.
350. Low JA, Handley Derry MH, Burke SO, et al: Association of intrauterine fetal growth retardation and learning deficits at age 9 to 11 years. Am J Obstet Gynecol 167:1499, 1992.
351. Dobbing J: The later development of the brain and its vulnerability. *In* Davis JA, Dobbing J (eds): Scientific Foundations of Paediatrics. Philadelphia, WB Saunders Company, 1974, p 565.

Red Cell Alloimmunization

KENNETH J. MOISE, JR.

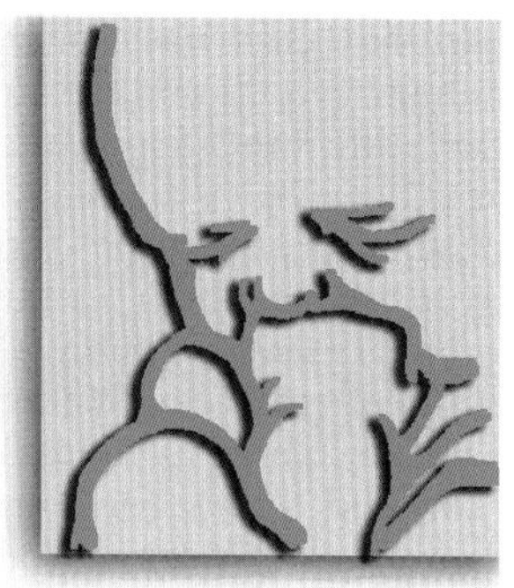

CHAPTER 30

KEY ABBREVIATIONS

American Association of Blood Banks	AABB
American College of Obstetrics and Gynecology	ACOG
Cytomegalovirus	CMV
Deoxyribonucleic acid	DNA
Diphosphotidylglycerol	DPG
Fetal blood sampling	FBS
Fetomaternal hemorrhage	FMH
Hemolytic disease of the fetus and newborn	HDFN
Hemolytic disease of the newborn	HDN
International units	IU
Intraperitoneal transfusion	IPT
Intrauterine transfusion	IUT
Intravascular transfusion	IVT
Intravenous immune globulin	IVIG
Kleihauer-Betke	KB
Middle cerebral artery	MCA
Microgram	μg
Polymerase chain reaction	PCR
Rhesus immune globulin	RhIG

NOMENCLATURE

Exposure to foreign red cell antigens invariably results in the production of anti–red cell antibodies in a process known as *red cell alloimmunization* (formerly termed *isoimmunization*). The expression *sensitization* can be used interchangeably. The active transport of these antibodies across the placenta during pregnancy results in fetal anemia, hyperbilirubinemia, and ultimately, hydrops fetalis. Before the advent of obstetric ultrasound, the perinatal effects of maternal red cell alloimmunization could be recognized only after birth in the affected neonate. Thus, the neonatal consequences of maternal red cell alloimmunization came to be known as *hemolytic disease of the newborn* (HDN). Because the peripheral blood smear of these infants demonstrated a large percentage of circulating immature red cells known as erythroblasts, the newborn entity was also known as *erythroblastosis fetalis*. Today, ultrasound and fetal blood sampling make the detection of the severely anemic fetus a reality. For this reason, the term *hemolytic disease of the fetus and newborn (HDFN)* would appear more appropriate to describe this disorder.

HISTORICAL PERSPECTIVES

The first case of HDFN was probably described in 1609 by a midwife in the French literature.[1] The case was a twin gestation in which the first fetus was stillborn and the second twin developed jaundiced and succumbed soon after birth. In 1932, Diamond[2] proposed that the clinical entities of erythroblastosis fetalis, icterus gravis neonatorum, and hydrops fetalis represented different manifestations of the same disease. Seven years later, Levine and Stetson[3] described an antibody in a woman who gave birth to a stillborn fetus. The patient experienced a severe hemolytic transfusion reaction after later receiving her husband's blood. In 1940, Landsteiner and Weiner[4] injected red cells from rhesus monkeys into rabbits. The antibody that was isolated from these was used to test human blood samples from whites, and agglutination was noted in 85 percent of individuals. The following year, Levine et al.[5] were able to demonstrate a causal relationship between RhD antibodies in RhD-negative women and HDFN in their offspring.

The advent of therapy for HDFN began in 1945 with the description by Wallerstein[6] of the technique of neonatal exchange transfusion. Later Bevis[7] and then Liley[8] proposed the use of amniotic fluid bilirubin assessment as an indirect measure of the degree of fetal hemolysis. Sir William Liley's major contribution to the story of Rhesus disease was the introduction of the intraperitoneal fetal transfusion (IPT).[9] He learned from a visiting fellow who had returned from Africa that the infusion of red cells into the peritoneal cavity of children with sickle cell disease produced normal-appearing red blood cells on peripheral blood smear. Liley realized that he had previously inadvertently entered the peritoneal cavity of fetuses at the time of amniocentesis, based on the marked contrast in the yellow hue of the ascitic fluid as compared with amniotic fluid. He postulated that purposeful entry into the fetal peritoneal cavity could be accomplished. After three unsuccessful attempts that resulted in fetal demises, the fourth fetus was delivered at 34 4/7 weeks' gestation after undergoing two successful IPTs.[9] Early attempts at IPT used fluoroscopy for needle guidance. With the introduction of real-time ultrasound in the early 1980's, IPTs became a safer procedure as fluoroscopy was abandoned. Rodeck[10] is credited with the first intravascular fetal transfusion (IVT) using a fetoscope to guide the transfusion needle into a placental plate vessel. Just 1 year later, investigators in Denmark performed the first ultrasound-guided IVT using the intrahepatic portion of the umbilical vein.[11]

The 1990's saw the introduction of genetic techniques using amniocentesis to determine fetal red cell typing.[12] The turn of the century brought the noninvasive detection of fetal anemia through Doppler ultrasound of the fetal middle cerebral artery (MCA) and the use of fetal typing through cell free DNA in maternal plasma.[13,14]

INCIDENCE

The advent of the routine administration of antenatal and postpartum Rhesus immune globulin (RhIG) has resulted in a marked reduction in cases of red cell alloimmunization secondary to the RhD antigen. A report from surveillance hospitals of the Centers for Disease Control noted in 1991 that one in every 1,000 liveborn infants exhibited some effect from Rhesus hemolytic disease.[15]

Clearly, a shift to other red cell antibodies associated with HDFN has occurred as a result of the decreasing incidence of RhD alloimmunization. In one large series of women of childbearing age, a positive screen for an antibody associated with HDFN was found in 1 percent of samples.[16] Rhesus antibodies were the most common, accounting for more than half of significant antibodies, and with the RhD antibody accounting for almost one fourth. Kell antibodies were next most frequent, followed by Duffy, MNS, Kidd, and anti-U. In another series of

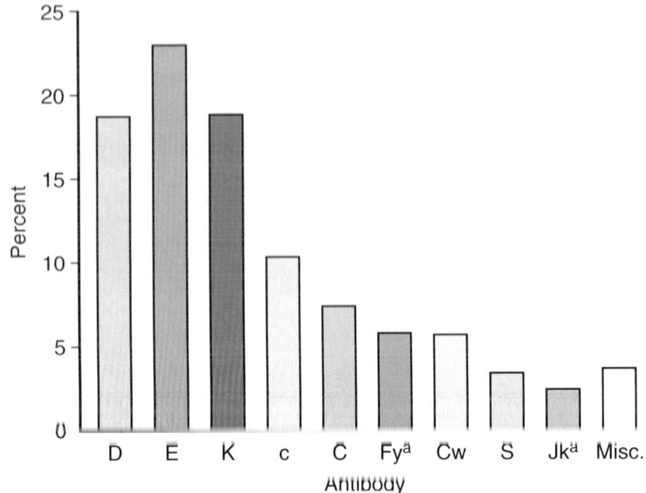

Figure 30-1. Incidence of maternal anti–red cell antibodies associated with hemolytic disease of the fetus and newborn (HDFN) in a Dutch population of pregnant women. (From van der Schoot CE, Tax GH, Rijnders RJP, et al: Prenatal typing of Rh and Kell blood group system antigens: The edge of the watershed. Trans Med Rev 17:31, 2003.)

more than 1,000 Dutch women who screened positive for antibodies at 12 weeks of gestation, anti-E was the most common antibody that was found.[17] This was followed by anti-K then anti-D (Fig. 30-1). Current birth certificate data from the Centers for Disease Control would indicate that in 2002, approximately 6.7 cases of Rhesus alloimmunization occurred per 1,000 live births in the United States.[18]

PATHOPHYSIOLOGY

Once thought to be an absolute barrier to the transfer of cells between the maternal and fetal compartments, we now appreciate that the placental interface allows for the bidirectional movement of both intact cells and free DNA. The putative "grandmother theory" of Rhesus red cell alloimmunization probably occurs more commonly than first thought. In this paradigm, maternal RhD-positive red cells gain access to the circulation of the RhD-negative fetus at the time of delivery. As many as one fourth of RhD-negative babies have been shown to be immunized in early life as a result of their delivery.[19] The immune response of an Rh-negative individual to RhD-positive red cells has been characterized into one of three groups.[20] Sixty to seventy percent of individuals are *responders* and develop an antibody to relatively small volumes of red cells. In these individuals, the probability of immunization increases with escalating volumes of cells. A small percent of this group can be called *hyper-responders* in that they will be immunized by very small quantities of red cells. The second group of individuals (10 to 20 percent) can be immunized only by exposure to very large volumes of cells. Finally, the 10 to 20 percent of individuals who remain appear to be nonresponders.

In most cases of red cell alloimmunization, a fetomaternal hemorrhage (FMH) occurs in the antenatal period or more commonly at the time of delivery. If a maternal ABO incompatibility exists between the mother and her fetus, anti-A and or anti-B antibodies lyse the fetal cells in the maternal circulation and destroy the RhD antigen.[21] Even if this protective effect is not present, only 13 percent of deliveries of RhD-positive fetuses result in RhD alloimmunization in RhD-negative women that do not receive RhIG.[22] The vast majority of RhD alloimmunized women produce an IgG response as their initial antibody. *Responders* may represent a group of individuals who had their initial exposure to the RhD antigen at birth due to maternofetal hemorrhage.[20] After a sensitizing event, the human antiglobulin anti-D titer can usually be detected after 5 to 16 weeks. However, approximately half of alloimmunized patients are *sensibilized*. In this scenario, an antibody screen will be negative, but memory B lymphocytes are present that can create an anti-D antibody response. When faced with the challenge of a subsequent pregnancy involving an RhD-positive fetus, the anti-D titer becomes detectable.

The anti-D immune response is the best characterized of the anti–red cell antibodies associated with HDFN. In one third of cases, only subclass IgG1 is produced; in the remainder of cases, a combination of IgG1 and IgG3 subclasses is found.[23] Anti-D IgG is a nonagglutinating antibody that does not bind complement. This results in a lack of intravascular hemolysis; sequestration and subsequent destruction of antibody-coated red cells in the fetal liver and spleen are the mechanism of fetal anemia. Most studies have not detected a relationship between a specific maternal human leukocyte antigen type and susceptibility to become alloimmunized to RhD.[24] However, sensitized women with high titers of anti-D are more likely to exhibit the DQB1*0201 and DR17 alleles as compared with women with low titers.[25] Fetal sex may also play a significant role in the fetal response to maternal antibodies. RhD-positive male fetuses are 13 times more likely than their female counterparts to become hydropic and three times more likely to die from their disease.[26]

Anemia results in several important physiologic changes in the fetus. Reticulocytosis from the bone marrow can be detected by fetal blood sampling once the hemoglobin deficit exceeds 2 g/dl as compared to norms for gestational age; erythroblasts are released from the fetal liver once the hemoglobin deficit reaches 7 g/dl or greater.[27] In an effort to increase oxygen delivery to peripheral tissues, fetal cardiac output increases and 2–3 diphosphotidylglycerol (DPG) levels are enhanced.[28,29] Tissue hypoxia appears as anemia progresses despite these physiologic changes. An increased umbilical artery lactate level is noted when the fetal hemoglobin falls below 8 g/dl and increased venous lactate can be detected when the hemoglobin level falls below 4 g/dl.[30] Hydrops fetalis (the accumulation of extracellular fluid in at least two body compartments) is a late finding in cases of fetal anemia. Its exact pathophysiology is unknown. Enhanced hepatic erythropoietic function with subsequent depressed synthesis of serum proteins has been proposed as the explanation for the lower serum albumin levels that have been detected.[31] Colloid osmotic pressure appears decreased.[32] However, congenital analbuminemia is not associated with hydrops fetalis, and experimental animal models in which fetal plasma proteins have been replaced with saline did not produce hydrops.[33,34] An alternative hypothesis is that tissue hypoxia due to anemia enhances capillary permeability. In addition, iron overload due to ongoing hemolysis may contribute to free radical formation and endothelial cell dysfunction.[35] Central venous pressures do appear elevated in the hydropic fetus with HDFN.[32] This may cause a functional blockage of the lymphatic system at the level of the thoracic duct as it empties into the left brachiocephalic vein. This theory is supported by reports of poor absorption of donor red cells infused into the intraperitoneal cavity in cases of hydrops.[36]

RHESUS ALLOIMMUNIZATION AND FETAL/NEONATAL HEMOLYTIC DISEASE OF THE NEWBORN

Genetics

Initial concepts on the genetics of the Rh antigens proposed the presence of three distinct genes.[37] Newer DNA techniques allowed for the localization of the Rh locus to the short arm of chromosome one.[38] Only two genes were identified—an RhD gene and an RhCE gene. Each gene is 10 exons in length, with 96 percent homology. These genes presumably represent a duplication of a common ancestral gene. Production of two distinct proteins from the RhCE gene probably occurs as a result of alternative splicing of messenger RNA.[39] One nucleotide difference, cytosine to thymine, in exon 2 of the RhCE gene results in a single amnio acid change of a serine to proline. This causes the expression of the *C* antigen as opposed to the *c* antigen.[40] A single cytosine to guanine change in exon 5 of the RhCE gene, producing a single amnio acid change of a proline to alanine, results in formation of the *e* antigen instead of the *E* antigen.[41]

The gene frequency found in different ethnic groups can be traced to the Spanish colonization in the 15th and 16th centuries. Native populations to certain land masses have less than a 1 percent incidence of RhD negativity: Eskimos, native Americans, and Japanese, and Chinese individuals. The Basque tribe in Spain is noted to have a 30 percent incidence of Rh negativity. This may well be the origin of the RhD gene deletion that is the most common genetic basis of the RhD-negative state in whites (Fig. 30-2). Whites of European descent exhibit a 15 percent incidence of RhD negativity, whereas an 8 percent incidence occurs in blacks and Hispanics of Mexico and Central America. This latter incidence probably reflects ethnic diversity secondary to Spanish colonization of the New World.

Further study of the RhD gene has revealed significant heterogeneity. Several of these genetic modifications result in a lack of expression of the RhD phenotype. Although these individuals may have an aberrant RhD gene present, serologic methods do not detect the RhD antigen on the surface of the red cells. One such example is the RhD pseudogene, which has been found in 69 percent of South African blacks and 24 percent of American blacks[42] (Fig. 30-2). In this situation, all 10 exons of the RhD gene are

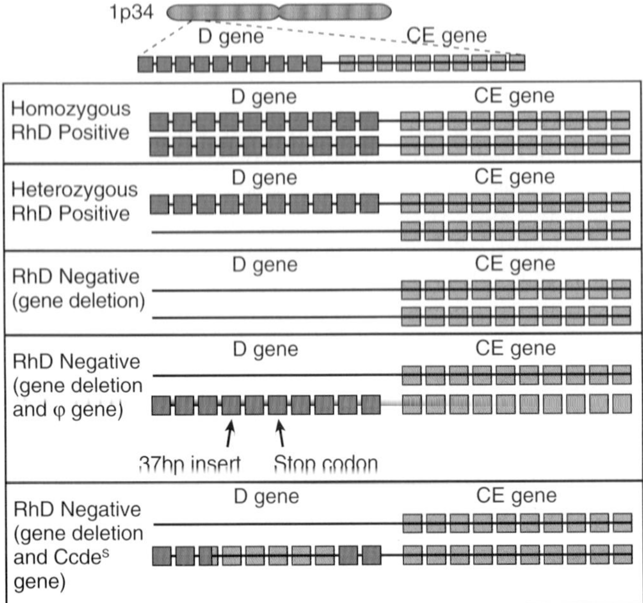

Figure 30-2. Schematic of Rh gene locus on chromosome 1. The homozygous RhD-positive state, heterozygous RhD-positive state, RhD-negative with heterozygosity for the RhD pseudogene, and RhD-negative with heterozygosity for the Ccde^s gene are demonstrated. (Reproduced with permission and modified from Moise KJ: Hemolytic disease of the fetus and newborn. *In* Creasy RK, Resnik R, Iams J [eds]: Maternal-Fetal Medicine. Principles and Practice, 5th ed. Philadelphia, Elsevier Inc, Copyright © 2004).

present. However, translation of the gene into a messenger RNA product does not occur owing to the presence of a stop codon in the intron between exons 3 and 4. Thus, no RhD protein is synthesized and the patient is serologically RhD negative. Similarly, the Ccde^s has been detected in 22 percent of American blacks. It appears to contain exons 1, 2, 9, and 10 as well as a portion of exon 3 of the original RhD gene, with other exons being duplicated from the RhCE gene. In the Taiwanese population of RhD-negative individuals, five different exons of the RhD gene were evaluated.[43] Seventeen percent of individuals had all five exons detected, and an additional 135 demonstrated the presence of at least one of the five exons tested. The presence of these genes in an RhD-negative pregnant patient has important implications for the prenatal diagnosis of the fetal blood type (see later).

PREVENTION OF RHD HEMOLYTIC DISEASE OF THE FETUS AND NEWBORN

History

The history of Rhesus prophylaxis can be traced to three unique individuals.[44] Vincent Freda was an obstetric resident who developed an interest in HDFN. He was allowed to spend part of his fourth year of his residency at Columbia-Presbyterian Medical Center in the laboratory of Alexander Weiner, one of the first investigators to identify the "Rh factor." When he returned to Columbia, he went on to establish a serology laboratory and later organized the Rh Antepartum Clinic in 1960.[45] A seat on the hospital transfusion committee became vacant, and in an unprecedented move based on his interest, the chairman of Obstetrics and Gynecology, Howard C. Taylor Jr, appointed Freda to this position even though he had not completed his residency.[46] The chairman of Pathology responded with the appointment of John Gorman to the committee, a resident in pathology with an interest in blood banking. It is here that these two individuals met and developed the collaboration that would one day end in the introduction of RhIG. In 1906, Theobald Smith[47] found that guinea pigs given excess passive antibody, failed to become immunized to diphtheria toxin. Freda and Gorman proposed that anti-D could be used in a similar fashion to prevent alloimmunization after delivery. They enlisted the aid of William Pollack, a senior protein chemist at Ortho Diagnostics, who developed an IgG globulin fraction from high titered donor plasma. An initial grant application to the National Institutes of Health was rejected. Funding was secured from the New York City Health Research Council on a second attempt. This was followed by a year's negotiations with lawyers in the state capitol to allow the investigators to perform their clinical trials at the Sing Sing prison in New York beginning in 1961 (personal communication: John Gorman). Nine RhD-negative male volunteers were injected monthly with RhD-positive cells for five successive months.[48] Four of the men were immunized with intramuscular RhIG 24 hours before the injection of the red cells. Four of the five controls became alloimmunized to RhD, whereas none of the treated individuals developed anti-RhD antibodies. Their second experiment involved 27 inmates at Sing Sing, 13 controls and 14 treated. Red cells were given intravenously. However, the warden of Sing Sing would not allow the investigators to return on any fixed schedule that would enable the prisoners to know the time and day of their revisit. He was concerned that this exact foreknowledge could involve the prisoners in an escape plan. The investigators gladly accepted this limitation as they reasoned that pregnant women who delivered over a weekend would probably not receive RhIG until Monday, up to 72 hours after delivery, owing to the closure of blood banks on weekends, as was commonly practiced at the time. None of the men receiving RhIG were alloimmunized, whereas eight of 13 controls developed anti-RhD antibodies. After two additional experiments at Sing Sing in this second group of individuals, Freda and Gorman went on to conduct a clinical trial in postpartum women at Columbia Presbyterian Medical Center starting in March of 1964.[48] In the 100 patients that received RhIG, none became sensitized as compared with a rate of 12 percent sensitization to RhD in the control group. In a follow-up study in these patients in their next pregnancy, none of the treated patients developed antibodies; five of 10 controls were alloimmunized and delivered infants affected by HDFN.

A parallel track of investigation was being undertaken by a group of British researchers in Liverpool. This group reasoned that the natural protective effect of ABO incompatibility between a mother and her fetus in preventing the formation of anti-D antibody could be used as a preventative strategy.[49] A preparation of plasma containing anti-D IgM was formulated and administered intravenously to male volunteers.[50] Although initial short-term antibody studies were promising, eventually eight of 13 treated men became immunized to RhD as compared with only one of 11 controls. After the publication of the initial work of Freda et al.[51] describing the use of a gamma globulin fraction of the plasma, the British group visited the New York investigators and obtained a sample of their gamma globulin preparation. The Liverpool group began their clinical trial in postpartum women with evidence of FMH by Kleihauer-Betke (KB) stain in April, 1964.[52] They are subsequently credited with the first publication of a successful clinical trial in women.

An observational trial in Canada was initiated and determined that the baseline rate of antenatal sensitization to RhD was 1.8 percent.[53] Between 1968 and 1974, a trial of antenatal prophylaxis using injections of 300 μg of RhIG at 28 and 34 weeks' gestation followed.[54] As compared with the previous observational study, none of the women demonstrated the development of anti-D antibodies. In a subsequent investigation involving RhIG administered only at 28 weeks' gestation, only 0.18 percent of women became sensitized.

RhIG was approved by the Division of Biologics Standards of the National Institutes of Health for general clinical use in the United States as RhoGAM (Ortho-Clinical Diagnostics, Inc., Raritan, NJ) in 1968. Recommendations for use during the immediate postpartum period were set forth by the American College of Obstetricians and Gynecologists (ACOG) in 1970.[55] The Food and Drug Administration approved the use of antenatal RhIG in 1981. Routine antenatal prophylaxis at 28 to 29 weeks' gestation was proposed by ACOG later that same year.[56]

Preparations

Four polyclonal products are currently available in the United States for the prevention of RhD alloimmunization. Two of the products (RhoGAM, Ortho-Clinical Diagnostics, Inc., Raritan, NJ, and HyperRho S/D, Talecris Biothorgenetics, Raleigh, NC) can only be given intramuscularly as they are derived from human plasma through Cohn cold ethanol fractionation—a process that results in contamination with IgA and other plasma proteins. The remaining two products (WinRho-SDF, Cangene Corporation, Winnipeg, Manitoba, and Rhophlac, ZLB Behring, King of Prussia, Penn.) are prepared through sepharose column and ion-exchange chromatography, respectively. At present, all available products are subject to solvent detergent treatment to inactivate enveloped viruses; many manufacturers also employ an additional micropore filtration step to further reduce the chance for viral contamination. Additionally, thimerosal, a mercury preservative used to prevent bacterial and fungal contamination, has been removed from all RhIG products used in the United States.

The dwindling resource of plasma donors for RhIG manufacture has led to the search for a synthetic product. Several monoclonal anti-D antibodies are now under study in large clinical trials and may soon replace the current polyclonal products.[24,57]

Indications

All pregnant patients should undergo determination of blood type and an antibody screen at the first prenatal visit. Patients found to be *weak Rh positive* (previously termed *Du-positive*) should be considered RhD-negative because their RhD gene encodes for an altered D protein associated with reduced expression of the RhD antigen on the red cell membrane. Therefore, these patients are not at risk for Rhesus alloimmunization and do not require RhIG. If there is no evidence of anti-D alloimmunization in the RhD-negative woman, the patient should receive 300 μg of RhIG at 28 weeks of gestation.[58] The 2 percent background incidence of RhD alloimmunization in the antenatal period can be expected to decline to 0.1 percent.[59] In the United Kingdom, an antenatal protocol of administering 100 μg (500 international units [IU]) of RhIG at 28 and 34 weeks is used in primigravida women.[60] Limited resources have not allowed for extension of this protocol to all subsequent pregnancies. The issue of repeating an antibody screen at 28 weeks before the administration of RhIG is controversial. The low incidence of a positive screen after a negative test at entry into prenatal care has resulted in the ACOG questioning the cost effectiveness of this practice.[58] Although ACOG leaves the decision to repeat the antibody screen up to the obstetrician, the American Association of Blood Banks (AABB) recommends that a repeat screen be obtained before antenatal RhIG.[61] If a repeat antibody screen is to be undertaken, a maternal blood sample can be drawn at the same office visit as the RhIG injection. Although the administration of the exogenous anti-D will eventually result in a weakly positive titer, this will not occur in the short interval of several hours due to the slow absorption from the intramuscular site. Some experts recommend that a second dose of RhIG be given if the patient has not delivered by 40 weeks' gestation.

Although not well studied, Level A scientific evidence has been cited by ACOG[58] to address additional indications for the antepartum administration of RhIG. These include spontaneous abortion, elective abortion, ectopic pregnancy, genetic amniocentesis, chorion villous sampling and fetal blood sampling (Table 30-1).[58] A dose of 50 μg of RhIG is effective until 13 weeks' gestation owing to the small volume of red cells in the fetoplacental circulation.[58] However most hospitals and offices do not stock this dose of RhIG because the cost is equivalent to the standard dose of 300 μg.

The use of RhIG in other scenarios involving the possibility of FMH are lacking. However most experts (Level C scientific evidence; Table 30-1) agree that such events as hydatidiform mole, threatened abortion, fetal death in the second or third trimester, blunt trauma to the abdomen, and external cephalic version warrant strong consideration for the use of RhIG.

The practice of evaluating a persistent maternal anti-D titer as an indication that additional RhIG is not required after an antenatal event is to be discouraged. Although

Table 30-1. Indications for Administration of Rhesus Immune Globulin
Spontaneous abortion*
Elective abortion*
Threatened abortion
Ectopic pregnancy*
Hydatidiform mole†
Genetic amniocentesis*
Chorion villus sampling*
Fetal blood sampling*
Placenta previa with bleeding‡
Suspected abruption‡
Intrauterine fetal demise‡
Blunt trauma to the abdomen (includes motor vehicle accidents)‡
At 28 weeks' gestation, unless father of fetus is RhD-negative
Amniocentesis for fetal lung maturity*
External cephalic version‡
Within 72 hours of delivery of an RhD-positive infant*
After administration of RhD-positive blood components‡

*Level A evidence (good and consistent scientific evidence).[58]
†Level B evidence (at least fair scientific evidence).
‡Level C evidence (consensus and expert opinion).[58]

the precise mechanism for the protective effect of RhIG is unknown, an excess amount of exogenous antibody in relation to the volume of RhD-positive red cells in the maternal circulation is essential for effective prophylaxis. Both animal and human studies have demonstrated that a low level of RhIG can actually enhance the chance for alloimmunization.[21] In the words of Vincent Freda, "the rule of thumb should be to administer Rh-immune globulin when in doubt, rather than to withhold it."[45]

Because the half-life of RhIG is approximately 16 days, 15 to 20 percent of patients receiving it at 28 weeks have a very low anti-D titer (usually 2 or 4) at the time of admission for labor at term.[62] In North America, the current recommendation is to administer 300 μg of RhIG within 72 hours of delivery if umbilical cord blood typing reveals a RhD-positive infant.[58] This is sufficient to protect from sensitization due to a FMH of 30 ml of fetal whole blood. In the United Kingdom, 100 μg is given at delivery.[60] Approximately 1 in 1,000 deliveries will be associated with an excessive FMH; risk factors identify only 50 percent of these cases.[63,64] Both ACOG and AABB now recommend routine screening of all women at the time of delivery for excessive FMH. A qualitative yet sensitive test for FMH, the rosette test, is first performed. Results return as positive or negative. A negative result warrants administration of a standard 300 μg dose of RhIG. If the rosette is positive, a KB stain or fetal cell stain using flow cytometry is undertaken to quantitate the amount of the FMH. The percentage of fetal blood cells is multiplied by a factor of 50 (to account for an estimated maternal blood volume of 5,000 ml) in order to calculate the volume of the FMH. This volume is divided by 30 to determine the number of vials of RhIG to be administered. A decimal point is rounded up or down for values of greater than 0.5 or less than 0.5, respectively. Because this calculation includes an inaccurate estimation of the maternal blood volume, one additional vial of RhIG is added to the calculation.[61] As an example, a 3 percent KB stain is calculated to indicate a 150-ml FMH. Dividing this number by 30 yields five vials of RhIG with one additional vial added; therefore, the blood bank would prescribe six vials of RhIG (a total of 1,800 μg) for this patient. No more than five units of RhIG should be administered by the intramuscular route in one 24-hour period. Should a large dose of RhIG be necessary, an alternative method would be to give the calculated dose using one of the intravenous preparations of RhIG that are now available. Doses of up to 600 μg (3,000 IU) should be administered every 8 hours until the total dose has been achieved. Should RhIG be inadvertently omitted after delivery, some protection has been proven with administration within 13 days; recommendations have been made to administer it as late as 28 days after delivery.[65] If delivery is planned within 48 hours of amniocentesis for fetal lung maturity, RhIG can be deferred until after delivery. If delivery occurs less than 3 weeks from the administration of RhIG used for antenatal indications such as external cephalic version, a repeat dose is unnecessary unless a large FMH is detected at the time of delivery.[58]

Failed prophylaxis after the appropriate dose of RhIG is employed is rare. However, once postpartum administration is undertaken, the anti-D antibody screen may remain positive for up to 6 months. Anti-D persisting after this time is likely the result of sensitization.

If a patient is undergoing her first determination of blood type in pregnancy when she presents for delivery, a *weak Rh positive* result should be viewed with caution. The patient in this scenario may in fact be RhD-negative, whereas RhD-positive fetal cells secondary to a large FMH may cause a mixed field agglutination reaction and a false interpretation of the maternal blood type. Standard testing for FMH should be carefully reviewed. If a FMH has not occurred, then the *weak Rh positive* type can be considered valid and RhIG is not required.

Administration of RhIG after a postpartum tubal ligation is controversial. The possibility of a new partner in conjunction with the availability of in vitro fertilization would seem to make the use of RhIG in these situations prudent. In some cases, RhD-negative red cells may be in short supply if the patient presents after major trauma such as a motor vehicle accident with the need for massive transfusion. In these cases, RhD-positive blood could not be used as a life-saving alternative if the patient is alloimmunized to RhD through her previous delivery. RhIG is not effective once alloimmunization to the RhD antigen has occurred. At present, prophylactic immune globulin preparations to prevent other forms of red cell alloimmunization such as anti-K1 do not exist.

Diagnostic Methods

Maternal Antibody Determination

Once a maternal antibody screen reveals the presence of an anti-D antibody, a titer is the first step in the evaluation of the RhD-sensitized patient during the first affected pregnancy. Previous titer methodologies using albumin or saline should no longer be employed because they detect varying levels of IgM antibody. The pentamer structure of this class of antibody does not allow for transplacental passage; therefore, the contribution of IgM to the titer quantitation has no clinical relevance. The human antiglobulin titer (indirect Coombs' test) is used to determine the degree of alloimmunization as it measures the maternal IgG response. Most titer values in the obstetric literature are reported as dilutions (i.e., 1:32). By blood banking convention, however, titer values should be reported as the reciprocal of the last tube dilution that demonstrates a positive agglutination reaction, that is, a final dilution of 1:16 is equivalent to a titer of 16. Variation in results between laboratories is not uncommon because many commercial laboratories use enzymatic treatment of red cells to prevent failed detection of low titer samples.

This method causes a marked elevation in titer as compared with the use of nonenzymatic treated cells. Because standard tube methodology uses red cell agglutination as the indicator reaction, subjective interpretation of endpoints by the laboratory technologist accounts for the variation in results. In addition, inherent subtle differences in the indicator red cell preparations may play a role because their shelf life is only 1 month and serial titers may require the use of different reagent lots. For these reasons, serial titers should be run in tandem using stored sera from the previous draw.

In the same laboratory, the titer should not vary by more than one dilution if the two samples are run in tandem. Thus an initial titer of 8 that returns at 16 does not represent a true increase in the amount of antibody in the maternal circulation. In addition, the clinician should be aware that newer gel microcolumn assays will result in higher titers than conventional tube testing. In one study, the mean titer was 3.4-fold increased with gel technology.[65] A critical titer is defined as the anti–red cell titer associated with a significant risk for hydrops fetalis. When this is present, further fetal surveillance is warranted. This value will vary with institution and methodologies; however, in most centers, a critical titer for anti-D between 8 and 32 is usually used.

In the United Kingdom, quantitation of anti-D is undertaken through the use of an automated technique using a device known as the AutoAnalyzer. Red cell samples are mixed with agents to enhance agglutination by the anti-D antibodies. Agglutinated cells are separated from non-agglutinated cells and then lysed. The amount of released hemoglobin is then compared with an international standard; results are reported as international units per milliliter. Levels of less than 4 IU/ml are rarely associated with HDFN; a maternal anti-D level of less than 15 IU/ml has been associated with only mild fetal anemia.[66]

Fetal Blood Typing

Several techniques have been employed to determine the fetal blood type if the patient's partner is determined to be heterozygous for the involved red cell antigen. In 50 percent of cases in which the fetus is found to be antigen negative, further maternal and fetal testing is unnecessary. Historically, initial attempts at fetal testing in these cases employed serology on blood obtained by ultrasound-directed fetal blood sampling. Unfortunately, this technique placed half of the antigen-negative fetuses at a 1- to 2-percent chance of procedure-related loss (see Chapter 7). Investigators went on to use chorion villus sampling to obtain genetic material for detection of the RhD gene. However, the major disadvantage of this method is that disruption of the chorion villi during the procedure can result in FMH and a rise in maternal titer, thereby worsening the fetal disease.[67] Therefore, this procedure should be discouraged unless the patient plans to terminate all antigen-positive fetuses that are detected. In 1990, amniocentesis was described as a reliable method for assessing the fetal blood type through DNA testing.[12] This method continues to be widely employed in North America. In England and Europe, the use of free DNA in maternal plasma has replaced amniocentesis for determination of the fetal blood type in cases of a heterozygous paternal phenotype.

The initial step in this evaluation is to determine the paternal zygosity. Because the RhC/c and E/e antigens are inherited in a closely linked fashion to RhD, antisera for these antigens can be used with gene frequency tables. Ethnicity must be taken into account when calculating the likelihood of being heterozygous because very disparate results can be noted with similar serologic findings. In addition, bayesian analysis can be employed to modify the incidence of heterozyosity based on the paternal history of previous RhD-positive offspring (Table 30-2).[68] As an example, a white partner who undergoes serologic testing with the results anti-D: positive, anti-C: negative, anti-c: positive, anti-E: negative, and anti-e:

Table 30-2. Incidence of Paternal Heterozygosity (%) Based on Serology, Ethnic Background, and Number of Previous RhD-Positive Offspring

NO OF RHD+ INFANTS	WHITE						BLACK						HISPANIC					
	0	1	2	3	4	5	0	1	2	3	4	5	0	1	2	3	4	5
DCce	90	82	69	53	36	22	41	26	15	8	4	2	85	74	59	42	26	15
DCe	9	5	2	1	0.6	0.3	19	11	6	3	1	0.7	5	2	1	0.6	0.3	0.1
DcEe	90	82	69	53	36	22	37	23	13	7	4	2	85	74	59	42	26	15
DcE	13	7	4	2	0.9	0.5	1	0.5	0.3	0.1	0.1	0	2	0.9	0.5	0.2	0.1	0.1
DCcEe	11	6	3	2	0.8	0.4	10	5	3	1	0.7	0.3	12	6	3	2	0.8	0.4
Dce	94	89	80	66	50	33	54	37	23	13	7	4	92	85	74	59	42	26

Reproduced with permission from Moise KJ: Modern management of Rhesus alloimmunization in pregnancy. Obstet Gynecol 100:600, 2002.

positive would be considered to have the genotype *Dce*. If there was no history of an RhD-positive progeny, then his chance of being heterozygous is 94 percent.[69] A history of repeated RhD-positive offspring would markedly decrease the chance of an individual being heterozygous.

As the lines of ethnicity become murky, the use of serology and historic population studies will become less reliable as a means of determining paternal zygosity. Quantitative polymerase chain reaction (PCR) has been used with some accuracy to compare the number of copies of the RhD gene in a particular individual with a baseline control gene such as human albumin.[70] In addition, it has now been recognized that in the majority of individuals with a gene deletion as the etiology of their RhD-negative status, there are two silent gene segments that flank the main RhD gene. The loss of the RhD gene results in a combined hybrid of these two *Rhesus boxes*, which can be detected through restriction fragment length polymorphism analysis.[17] Although not currently commercially available, this assay will probably be used in the near future for the determination of paternal zygosity for RhD.

Extensive experience with the use of amniocentesis for determining fetal blood type has revealed rare discrepancies. A false-negative result occurs when the amniotic fluid analysis reveals an RhD-negative fetus that is confirmed to be RhD-positive by serology after birth. In this case, the usual fetal surveillance techniques would not be employed, and there would be the potential for perinatal loss. In one series of 500 amniocenteses, false-negative results occurred in 1.5 percent of cases.[71] The most likely etiology for this inconsistency is either erroneous paternity or a rearrangement at the paternal RhD gene locus. Such rearrangements have been documented in approximately 2 percent of individuals.[72] Checking paternal blood, the source of the fetal RhD gene, with the same PCR primers used on the amniotic fluid verifies that a gene rearrangement is not a potential source of error. For this reason, most laboratories offering fetal red cell typing on amniotic fluid require an accompanying paternal blood sample. In addition, multiplex PCR that targets at least two different exons of the RhD gene is used by many centers to decrease the chance of non-detection for a gene rearrangement.

In situations in which paternity is not assured or there is no partner available to contribute a blood sample for confirmation of PCR primers, one must consider the result of a RhD-negative fetal blood type from amniotic fluid to be suspect. Hopkins[73] assessed serial titers in patients with RhD alloimmunization who subsequently delivered RhD-negative offspring and noted that serial maternal titers rose by fourfold in less than 2 percent of cases. In situations of questionable paternity or lack of availability of a paternal blood sample, a repeat maternal antiglobulin titer should be obtained 4 to 6 weeks after the results of the amniocentesis as a confirmatory strategy (see Fig. 30-7). If a fourfold or greater rise in maternal antibody titer is noted (e.g., 32 to 128), then an RhD-negative result on amniotic fluid should be questioned. Repeat amniocentesis to evaluate the ΔOD_{450} or fetal blood sampling to determine the fetal RhD status using serologic techniques should be considered.

If the maternal race is black, then the presence of a maternal pseudogene or Ccde[s] gene should be considered in the scheme of fetal testing. The presence of one of these genes in the fetus could lead to a false-positive diagnosis. The amniotic fluid result would be RhD positive, yet the fetus would be found to be RhD negative by serology after birth. This could lead to unnecessary fetal interventions with their inherent risks. For this reason, a maternal blood sample should always accompany the amniotic fluid aliquot sent for fetal RhD testing in an effort to rule out the presence of a maternal RhD pseudogene or Ccde[s] gene. If the maternal sample is positive for one of these variants, then fetal testing for the gene should also be undertaken.

Fetal RhD determination through noninvasive testing is now routine in Europe.[74] Free fetal DNA in the maternal serum has been used to detect RhD sequences in the case of a RhD-positive fetus.[75] Free fetal DNA is cleared from the maternal plasma within minutes after delivery, thereby eliminating the possibility of contamination from a previous gestation. In two large published series, free DNA testing was accurate in 99.5 and 100 percent of cases, respectively.[14,76] Once the issue of paternal rearrangement in the RhD gene has been addressed, RhD-positive results on free DNA testing can be considered reliable because RhD-positive genetic material cannot be from a maternal source. A fetal RhD-negative result is more problematic. If fetal DNA fails to amplify in a background of overwhelming maternal DNA in plasma, an RhD-negative result will be obtained. One internal control that can be used is the detection of the SRY gene found in male fetuses. The presence of this gene in free DNA indicates that fetal DNA is present, and an RhD-negative result is reliable.[74] In the case of a female fetus, presence of DNA polymorphisms not found in the maternal white cells can be used as an internal control.[74] If different polymorphisms than those found in the mother are noted in the plasma sample, one can be assured that these are of paternal origin; thus, fetal DNA is present. Again in this situation, the finding of an RhD-negative fetus can be considered reliable. In the present system,[14] DNA polymorphisms are not informative in 4 percent of cases. In these cases, a repeat maternal sample could be submitted or amniocentesis undertaken to determine the fetal RhD type.

Amniocentesis to Follow the Severity of Hemolytic Disease of the Fetus and Newborn

Because it was first introduced to clinical practice, the spectral analysis of amniotic fluid has been used in alloimmunized pregnancies to determine the level of bilirubin, an indirect indicator of the degree of fetal hemolysis.[7] The peak value at 450 nm is subtracted from the baseline (a line drawn between data points at 550 and 365 nm) to determine the delta OD450 (ΔOD_{450}). A proposed management scheme using three zones based on gestational age was later introduced in 1963.[8] The "Liley" curve has proven extremely useful in monitoring the alloimmunized pregnancy. Unfortunately, the original data were

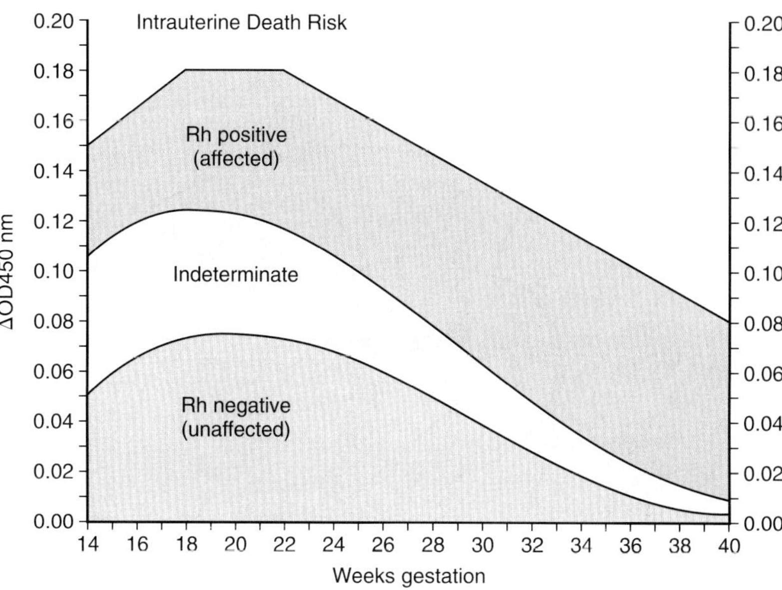

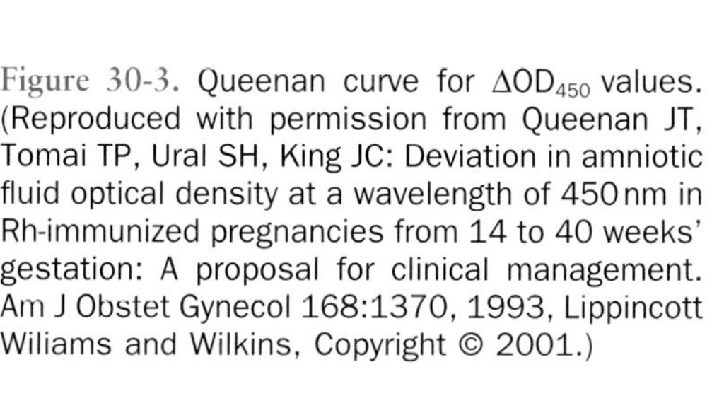
Figure 30-3. Queenan curve for ΔOD_{450} values. (Reproduced with permission from Queenan JT, Tomai TP, Ural SH, King JC: Deviation in amniotic fluid optical density at a wavelength of 450 nm in Rh-immunized pregnancies from 14 to 40 weeks' gestation: A proposal for clinical management. Am J Obstet Gynecol 168:1370, 1993, Lippincott Wiliams and Wilkins, Copyright © 2001.)

limited to 27 weeks' gestation. Despite the lack of data, later publications included extrapolated curves to earlier gestational ages.[77] The advent of fetal blood sampling to determine the actual fetal hematocrit revealed that an extrapolated Liley curve back to 18 weeks' gestation failed to predict fetal anemia in as many as 70 percent of cases in the early second trimester.[78] For a brief period after this report, many centers used fetal blood sampling exclusively in cases of severe red cell alloimmunization if fetal assessment was indicated before 27 weeks' gestation. A modified ΔOD_{450} curve (Queenan curve) for such situations was subsequently published using data from the early second trimester (Fig. 30-3).[79]

If amniocentesis is used to monitor fetal disease, serial procedures are undertaken at 10-day to 2-week intervals and continued until delivery to follow trends in the ΔOD_{450} values. All attempts should be made to avoid transplacental passage of the needle because this can lead to FMH and a rise in maternal antibody titer. A rising or plateauing ΔOD_{450} value that reaches the 80th percentile of zone two of the Liley curve or a value that enters the upper portion of the *Rh-positive, affected zone* of the Queenan curve necessitates investigation by fetal blood sampling.

Fetal Blood Sampling

Ultrasound-directed fetal blood sampling (FBS; also *percutaneous umbilical blood sampling, cordocentesis,* and *funipuncture*) allows direct access to the fetal circulation to obtain important laboratory values such as fetal blood type, hematocrit, direct Coombs' test, reticulocyte count, and total bilirubin. Although serial FBS was once proposed as a primary method of fetal surveillance after a maternal critical titer is reached, it has been associated with a 1- to 2-percent rate of fetal loss, as well up to a 50-percent risk for FMH with subsequent worsening of the alloimmunization.[80,81] For these reasons, FBS is reserved for patients with elevated ΔOD_{450} values or elevated peak MCA Doppler velocities (see later).

Ultrasound

Perhaps the greatest advance in the management of the alloimmunized pregnancy has been the use of ultrasound. Gestational age can be accurately established in order to evaluate fetal parameters that vary with gestational age including hemoglobin, ΔOD_{450} levels, and peak MCA Doppler velocities. Hydrops fetalis is defined as the presence of extracellular fluid in at least two fetal compartments. Often, ascites is the first sign of impending hydrops, with scalp edema and pleural effusions noted with worsening anemia. When hydrops is present, fetal hemoglobin deficits of 7 to 10 g/dl from the mean hemoglobin value for the corresponding gestational age can be expected.[82] Unfortunately, this represents the end-stage state of fetal anemia. Survival with intrauterine transfusion is markedly reduced in these cases. Therefore, many investigators have sought alternative ultrasound parameters that could predict the early onset of anemia.[83] In one large series, fetal abdominal circumference, head-to-abdomen circumference ratio, intraperitoneal volume, intrahepatic and extrahepatic umbilical venous diameter, and placental thickness failed to accurately predict a fetal hemoglobin deficit of greater than 5 g/dl from the mean.[84] Because the fetal liver and spleen represent sites of extramedullary hematopoiesis and the destruction and sequestration of sensitized red cells in cases of severe HDFN, enlargement of these organs has been evaluated. Both splenic perimeter and hepatic length correlate with the degree of fetal anemia. However, neither has gained widespread acceptance for noninvasive fetal surveillance in red cell alloimmunization.[85,86]

The severely anemic fetus exhibits an increased cardiac output in an effort to enhance oxygen delivery to peripheral tissues.[29] In addition, fetal anemia is associated with a lower blood viscosity that produces less shearing forces in blood vessels; this results in increased blood velocities. Using these principles, Doppler ultrasound has been employed to study the peak velocity in the fetal MCA to predict fetal anemia.[13] A value of greater than 1.5 multiples of the median (MoMs) for the corresponding

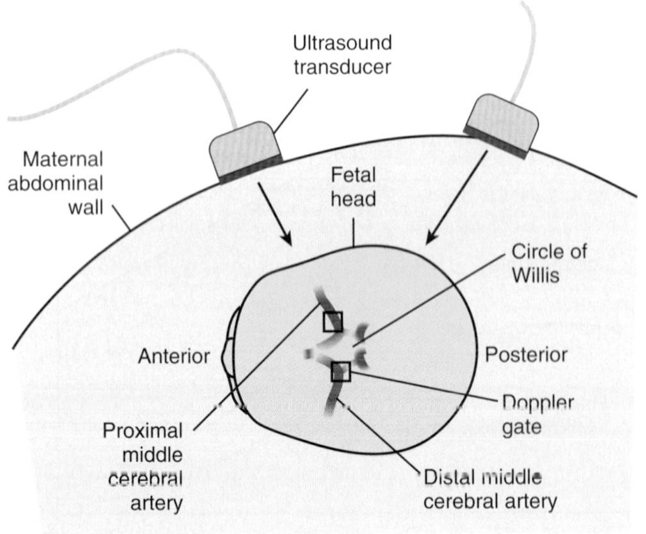

Figure 30-4. Correct determination of the fetal peak middle cerebral artery Doppler velocity.

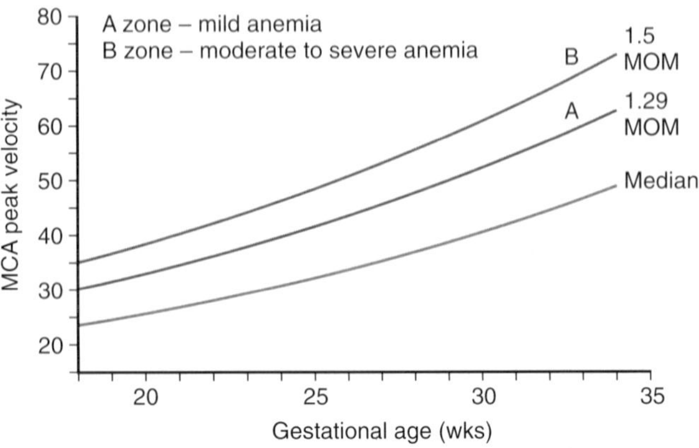

Figure 30-5. MCA Doppler peak velocities based on gestational age. Zone A = mild anemia; Zone B = moderate to severe anemia. MCA, middle cerebral artery. (Reproduced with permission from Moise KJ: Modern management of Rhesus alloimmunization in pregnancy. Obstet Gynecol 100:600, 2002, Elsevier Science Company, Copyright © 2002.)

gestational age predicts moderate to severe fetal anemia with a sensitivity of 88 percent and a negative predictive rate of 89 percent.[87]

Many centers have now replaced serial amniocenteses for ΔOD_{450} with serial MCA Doppler studies. Careful attention to technique is paramount in using this method of surveillance. Centers first employing MCA studies should undertake these in parallel to ΔOD_{450} measurements until confidence and reproducibility are achieved. Because the anteroposterior axis of the fetal head typically lies in a transverse plane, the examiner can use either fetal MCA vessel for interrogation. One must first locate the anterior wing of the sphenoid bone at the base of the skull. Color or power Doppler is then used to locate the MCA. The angle of insonation is maintained as close to zero as possible by positioning the ultrasound transducer on the maternal abdomen (Fig. 30-4). The MCA vessel closer to the maternal abdominal wall is usually studied, although the posterior vessel will give equivalent results.[88] Angle correction software is not employed. The Doppler gate is then placed in the proximal MCA because the vessel arises from the carotid siphon. Measurements in the more distal aspect of the vessel will be inaccurate as reduced peak velocities will be obtained.[88] Finally, the fetus should be in a quiescent state during the Doppler examination because accelerations of the fetal heart rate can result in a false elevation in the peak velocity, especially late in the third trimester.[89]

MCA measurements can be obtained reliably as early as 18 weeks' gestation. Studies are repeated every 1 to 2 weeks depending on the trend (Figs. 30-5 and 30-6). Values can be plotted on standard curves or converted to MoMs using internet-based calculators (*www.perinatology.com*). Values after 35 weeks' gestation are associated with a higher rate of false-positive results.

CLINICAL MANAGEMENT

The approach using the available diagnostic tools is based on the patient's past history of fetal or neonatal

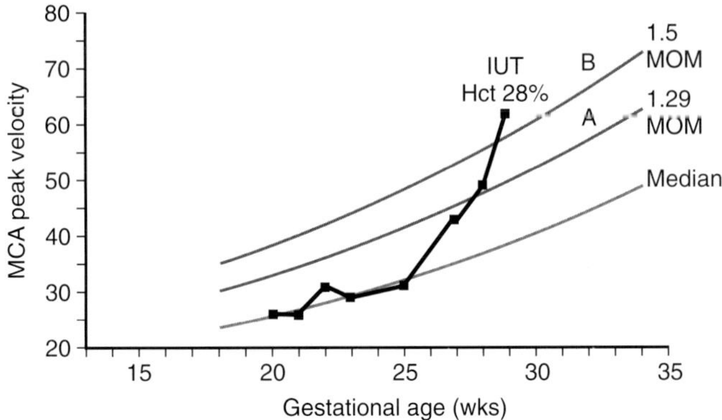

Figure 30-6. Serial MCA Doppler studies in one patient who required intrauterine transfusion. IUT, intrauterine transfusion; MCA, middle cerebral artery; MoM, multiples of the median.

manifestations of HDFN. As a general rule, the patient's first RhD-sensitized pregnancy involves minimal fetal/neonatal disease; but subsequent gestations are associated with a worsening degree of anemia.

First Affected Pregnancy

Once sensitization to the RhD antigen is detected, maternal titers are repeated every month until approximately 24 weeks; titers are repeated every 2 weeks thereafter (Fig. 30-7). Paternal blood is drawn to determine RhD status and zygosity through serologic testing. Once a critical maternal titer is reached (usually 32), serial MCA Doppler studiess are initiated at approximately 24 weeks' gestation. These are then repeated every 1 to 2 weeks depending on their trend. In remote geographic areas where availability to a referral center for MCA Doppler studies is impractical, serial amniocenteses for ΔOD_{450} starting at 24 weeks is an acceptable alternative. All efforts should be undertaken to avoid

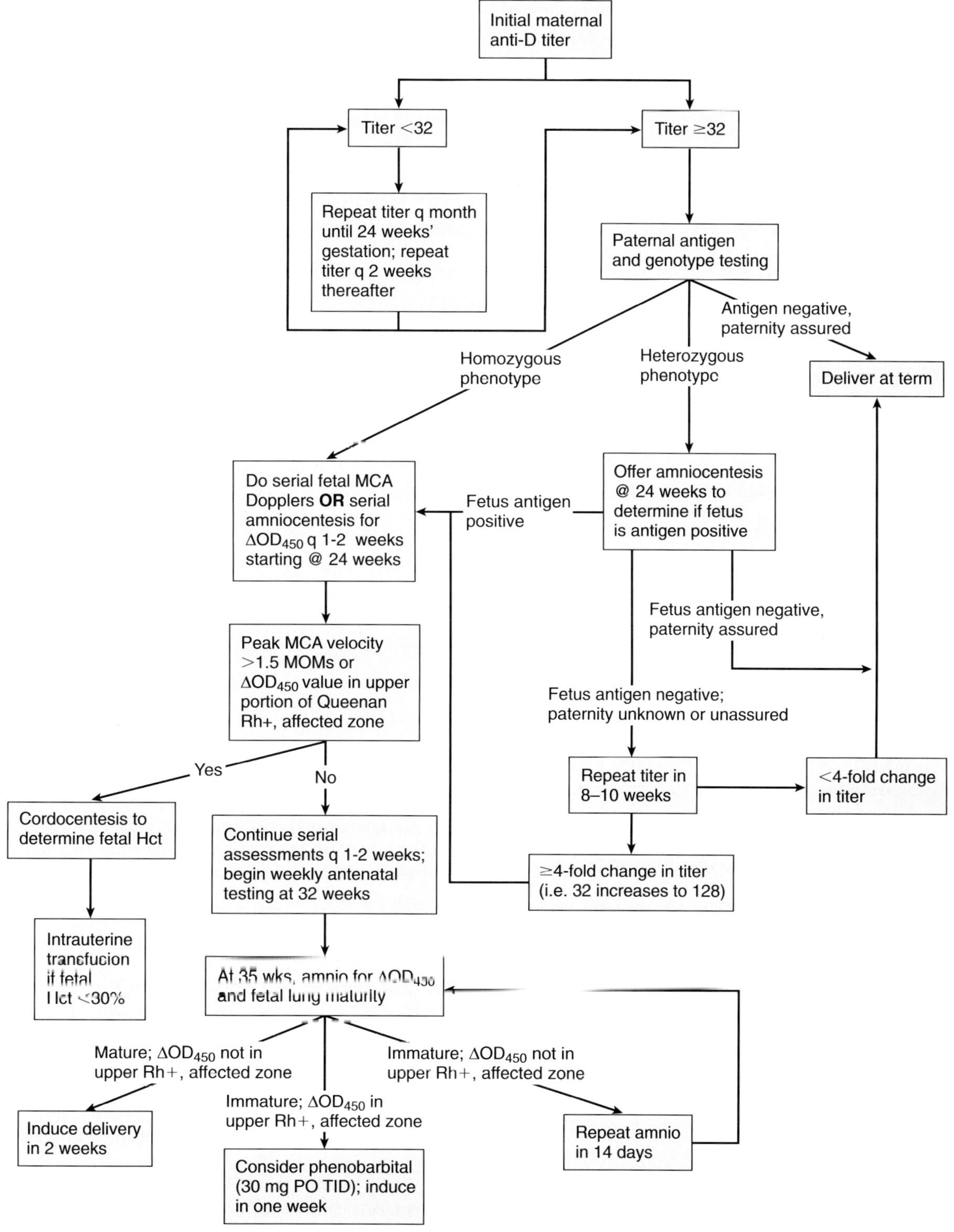

Figure 30-7. Algorithm for clinical management of a patient with red cell sensitization in the first affected pregnancy. TID, three times daily.

a transplacental entry so as to minimize the chance for a rise in the maternal titer. Amniocentesis surveillance usually involves repeat procedures at 10-day to 2-week intervals. In cases of a heterozygous paternal phenotype, an amniotic fluid sample obtained at the time of the initial amniocentesis accompanied by a maternal and paternal blood sample should be sent to a DNA reference laboratory to determine the fetal RhD status. In the case of an RhD-negative paternal blood type or a fetal RhD-negative genotype on amniotic fluid analysis, further maternal and fetal monitoring is unwarranted as long as paternity is assured.

If there is evidence of an RhD-positive fetus (homozygous paternal phenotype or RhD-positive fetus by PCR testing on amniotic fluid), serial fetal surveillance is indicated. If an MCA Doppler returns at greater than 1.5 MoMs, cordocentesis should be undertaken at an experienced referral center, with blood readied for intrauterine transfusion if the fetal hematocrit is less than 30 percent. Alternatively, if a rising or plateauing ΔOD_{450} trend into the upper portion of the *Rh-positive, affected* zone of Queenan curve or the 80th percentile of the Liley curve is noted, fetal blood sampling should be planned.

If the peak MCA value remains at less than 1.5 MoMs, amniocentesis at 35 weeks' gestation should be considered. If fetal pulmonary maturity is present and the ΔOD_{450} is not in the upper portion of the *Rh-positive, affected* zone of the Queenan curve, delivery should be induced in 2 weeks. This will enable time for fetal hepatic maturity to occur, thereby limiting the need for exchange transfusion secondary to neonatal hyperbilirubinemia. If the fetal pulmonary immaturity is noted at the time of the 35-week amniocentesis and the ΔOD_{450} is in the *Rh-positive, affected* zone of the Queenan curve, then administration of maternal phenobarbital (30 mg orally TID) with induction one week later will decrease the chance for neonatal exchange transfusion.[90] Finally, if results indicate fetal lung immaturity with a ΔOD_{450} that is not in the *Rh-positive, affected* zone of the Queenan curve, a repeat amniocentesis should be undertaken in 2 weeks. Surveillance with serial amniocentesis for ΔOD_{450} would follow this same management plan in the late third trimester.

Previously Affected Fetus or Infant

If there is a history of a previous perinatal loss related to HDFN, a previous need for intrauterine transfusion, or a previous need for neonatal exchange transfusion, the patient should be referred to a tertiary care center with experience in the management of the severely alloimmunized pregnancy (Fig. 30-8). In these cases, maternal titers are *not* predictive of the degree of fetal anemia. In the case of a heterozygous paternal phenotype, an amniocentesis at 15 weeks' gestation to determine the fetal RhD status is indicated. Serial MCA Doppler measurements should begin at 18 weeks' gestation and be repeated every 1 to 2 weeks. Alternatively, serial amniocenteses for measurement of ΔOD_{450} can be used with the Queenan curve for reference values beginning at 18 weeks. Subsequent surveillance is much the same as for the first affected pregnancy.

INTRAUTERINE TRANSFUSION

Technique

Intrauterine transfusions today are performed under continuous ultrasound guidance with direct infusions of red blood cells into the umbilical cord vessels or into the intrahepatic portion of the umbilical vein of the fetus.[91] Some centers continue to use the intraperitoneal approach as part of a combined technique with an intravascular transfusion (IVT) in an effort to create a reservoir of red cells between procedures.[92]

Typically, a freshly donated, CMV-negative unit of type O, RhD-negative red blood cells is cross-matched to a maternal blood sample. The unit is leukoreduced and irradiated with 25 Gy to prevent graft-vs-host reaction. It is then washed and packed to a final hematocrit of approximately 75 to 80 percent to prevent volume overload in the fetus.

The patient is admitted to the Labor and Delivery unit as an outpatient. The procedure is typically performed in the operating room, especially when a viable gestational age had been reached should an emergency delivery be necessary. The skin is prepped with povidine-iodine and sterile drapes applied. A long-acting local anesthetic is administered; conscious sedation may also be employed for the anxious patient. A 20- or 22-gauge procedure needle is introduced into the amniotic cavity and then into the umbilical vein under continuous ultrasound guidance. In the case of an anterior placenta, the needle is passed through the placental mass into the cord root. With a posterior placentation, the cord insertion into the placenta is preferred because this represents a site of immobility as compared with a "floating" loop of cord. A sample of fetal blood is obtained for an initial hematocrit. Optimally, the sample is processed as a spun hematocrit or through the use of an automated hemocytometer located in the operating room. A short-term paralytic agent such as vecuronium or atracurium is administered into the umbilical vein, causing cessation of fetal movement.[93,94] Paralysis is almost immediate and lasts 2 to 3 hours. The amount of packed red blood cells to be infused is based on the estimated fetal weight determined by ultrasound and standardized formulas.[95] Red cells are actively infused through the use of a syringe and sterile tubing connected to the donor unit. Once the predetermined volume of blood is infused, a small aliquot of blood is obtained to measure the hematocrit as well as the percentage of fetal versus adult hemoglobin-containing red cells through either a KB stain or fetal flow cytometry. A final fetal hematocrit of 40 percent is targeted. After the first intrauterine transfusion (IUT), subsequent procedures can be empirically scheduled at 14-day intervals until suppression of fetal erythropoiesis is noted. This usually occurs by the third IUT. Thereafter, the interval for repeat procedures can be determined based on the decline in hematocrit for the individual fetus, usually a 3- to 4-week interval. The final procedure is usually not performed past 35 weeks' gestation. The patient is scheduled for delivery approximately 3 weeks later.

Severely anemic fetuses in the early second trimester do not tolerate the acute correction of their hematocrit to normal values.[96] In these situations, the initial hematocrit should not be increased by more than fourfold at the time of the first procedure.[97] A repeat IVT is then performed within 48 hours to correct the fetal hematocrit into the normal range.

Complications and Outcome

Complications from IUT are uncommon. The total procedure-related perinatal loss was 4.7 percent of fetuses

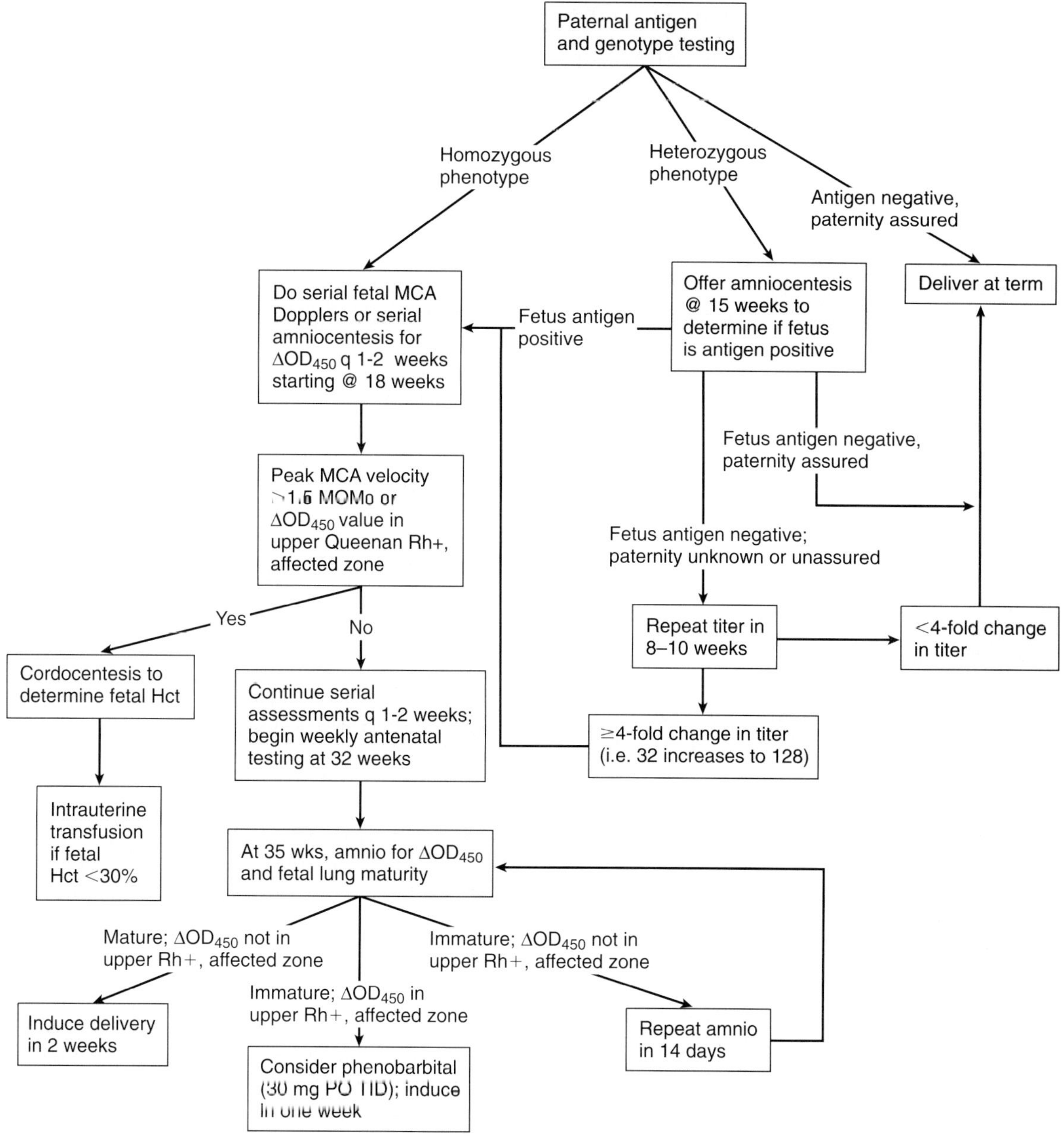

Figure 30-8. Algorithm for clinical management of a patient with red cell sensitization and a previously affected fetus or infant. TID, three times daily.

and 1.6 percent of procedures in one large series.[98] Survival after intrauterine transfusion varies with the center, its experience, and the presence of hydrops fetalis. An overall survival of 85 to 90 percent has been reported.[98,99] The presence of fetal hydrops, particularly if this does not resolve after several IUTs, has been associated with a lower rate of perinatal survival.[83] Preterm premature rupture of the membranes and chorioamnionitis occur rarely. Fetal bradycardia, particularly when there is inadvertent puncture of the umbilical artery, is usually transient and responds to removal of the procedure needle. Progression to fetal distress with the need for emergency delivery increases with advancing gestation and may complicate as many as 5 percent of procedures after 32 weeks' gestation.[100]

Neonatal Transfusions

The practice of prolonging the gestation of the treated fetus with HDFN until near term has resulted in a virtual absence of the need for neonatal exchange transfusions. Typically, these infants are born with a virtual absence of reticulocytes with a red cell population consisting mainly of transfused red cells. The blood bank may be confused if cord blood at delivery is submitted for neonatal red cell typing—the neonate will be typed as O, RhD-negative, reflecting the antigen status of the donor blood used for the IUTs. Elevated levels of circulating maternal antibodies in the neonatal circulation in conjunction with suppression of the fetal bone marrow production of red cells often results in the need for neonatal red cell *top-up* transfusions after discharge from the nursery in approximately 50 percent of infants near 1 month of age.[101] Therefore, these children should be followed weekly with hematocrits and reticulocyte counts until there is evidence of recovery of hematopoietic function. Typically, only one neonatal transfusion is required, although a maximum of up to three has been reported. Supplemental iron therapy in these infants is unnecessary because they have excess levels of stored iron due to previous hemolysis in utero and lysis of red cells from the IUTs. Supplemental folate therapy (0.5 mg/day) should be considered.

Neurologic Outcome

Only limited data are available for counseling the patient regarding long-term outcome because fetuses with severe anemia and hydrops are likely to survive today secondary to the use of IVT's. Short-term studies at up to 2 years of age have revealed that more than 90 percent of infants are neurologically normal even in the face of hydrops fetalis.[102,103]

Elevated levels of bilirubin have been associated with hearing loss in the neonate. Therefore, newborn screening for hearing loss would appear warranted in children with HDFN. Follow-up screening at 1 and 2 years of age should be considered.

OTHER TREATMENT MODALITIES

Before the advent of the IUT, plasmapheresis represented one of the few therapeutic modalities for severe HDFN. Most literature reports include single cases or relatively small case series. Despite these limitations, a review of the published cases reveals a perinatal survival of 69 percent.[104] Intravenous immune globulin (IVIG) has been used effectively as the sole antenatal treatment for HDFN.[105] Hydrops fetalis was less likely to occur and the onset of anemia occurred later in pregnancies treated with IVIG. Some experts have proposed a combined approach in patients with a previous perinatal loss in the early second trimester when technical limitations make the success of IUT unlikely.[69] Plasmapheresis is started at 12 weeks' gestation and repeated three times in that week. The maternal titer should be expected to be reduced by 50 percent. IVIG is then given to replace the globulin fraction removed by plasmapheresis in the form of a 2 g/kg loading dose after the third plasmapheresis; this is followed by 1 g/kg/week of IVIG until 20 weeks' gestation.

FUTURE THERAPEUTIC OPTIONS

Patients with high anti–red cell titers and recurrent perinatal loss in the second trimester have few options other than artificial insemination with red cell antigen-negative donor semen, surrogate pregnancy or preimplantation diagnosis (if the father is heterozygous).[106] Future avenues for therapy will probably involve selective manipulation of the maternal immune system. In vitro data and clinical case reports suggest that maternal alloantibodies to paternal leukocytes may result in an Fc blockade, thereby protecting the fetal red cells from hemolysis in cases of RhD alloimmunization.[107] Experimental sensitization to paternal leukocytes in a rabbit model of HDFN resulted in fetal hemoglobin levels that approached normal in doses that have been previously sensitized to red cells.[108] As an alternative strategy, peptides associated with the proliferation of T helper cells in the development of antibody to the RhD antigen could be used to ameliorate an established anti-D response, thereby preventing severe HDFN in a subsequent pregnancy.[109]

HEMOLYTIC DISEASE OF THE FETUS AND NEWBORN DUE TO NON-RHD ANTIBODIES

Antibodies to the red cell antigens Lewis, I and P are often encountered through antibody screening during prenatal care. Because these antibodies are typically of the IgM class, they are not associated with HDFN.[61]

However, antibodies to more than 50 other red cell antigens have been reported to be associated with HDFN (Table 30-3). More importantly, only three antibodies cause significant enough fetal hemolysis that treatment with IUT is considered necessary—anti-RhD, anti-Rhc and anti-Kell (K1). In one series from a tertiary care center for IUT in the Netherlands, 85 percent of cases involved anti-D; 10 percent, anti-K1; and 3.5 percent, anti-c. There was also one case each of anti-E, anti-e, and anti-Fy^a.[98]

Rhc

Anti-c antibody should be considered equivalent to anti-D regarding its potential to cause HDFN. In one report, 25 percent of antigen-positive fetuses were noted to have severe HDFN, 7 percent were hydropic, and 17 percent required IUTs for therapy.[110]

RhC, RhE, and Rhe

These antibodies are often found in low titer in the alloimmunized patient with anti-D. Their presence may be additive to the fetal hemolytic effect of anti-D.[111] When they occur alone, mild HDFN is usually the clinical course. Only a handful of case reports have indicated the need for treatment with IUT with each of these antibodies.[98,112,113]

M

Anti-M is a naturally occurring IgM antibody that typically presents as a cold agglutinin. Rarely, an IgG variety has been reported to cause mild HDFN. Blood bank consultation should be undertaken to determine the

Table 30-3. Non-RhD Antibodies and Associated HDFN

ANTIGEN SYSTEM	SPECIFIC ANTIGEN	ANTIGEN SYSTEM	SPECIFIC ANTIGEN	ANTIGEN SYSTEM	SPECIFIC ANTIGEN
		Frequently Associated with Severe Disease			
Kell	-K (K1)				
Rhesus	-c				
		Infrequently Associated with Severe Disease			
Colton	-Co^a	MNS	-Mur	Scianna	-Sc2
	-Co3		-M^V		-Rd
Diego	-ELO		-s	Other Ags	-Bi
	-Di^a		-s^D		-Good
	-Di^b		-S		-Heibel
	-Wr^a		-U		-HJK
	-Wr^b		-Vw		-Ht^a
Duffy	-Fy^a	Rhesus	-Be^a		-Jones
Kell	-Js^b		-C		-Joslin
	-k (K2)		-Ce		-Kg
	-Kp^a		-C^w		-Kuhn
	-Kp^b		-ce		-Li^a
	-K11		-E		-MAM
	-K22		-E^w		-Niemetz
	-Ku		-Evans		-REIT
	-Ul^a		-G		-Reiter
Kidd	-Jk^a		-Go^a		-Rd
MNS	-En^a		-Hr		-Sharp
	-Far		-Hr$_o$		-Vel
	-Hil		-JAL		-Zd
	-Hut		-Rh32		
	-M		-Rh42		
	-Mi^a		-Rh46		
	-Mt^a		-STEM		
	-MUT		-Tar		
		Associated with Mild Disease			
Duffy	-Fy^b	Kidd	-Jk^b	Rhesus	-Riv
	-Fy^3		-Jk^3		-RH29
Gerbich	-Ge^2	MNS	-Mit	Other	-At^a
	-Ge^3	Rhesus	-C^X		-JFV
	-Ge^4		-D^w		-Jr^a
	-Ls^a		-e		-Lan
Kell	-Js^a		HOFM		
			-LOCR		

HDFN, hemolytic disease of the fetus and newborn.

Reproduced with permission from Moise KJ: Hemolytic disease of the fetus and newborn. *In* Creasy RK, Resnik R, Iams J (eds): Maternal-Fetal Medicine, Principles and Practice, 5th ed. Philadelphia, Elsevier Inc, Copyright © 2004.

class of antibody present when anti-M is detected in the pregnant woman.

Duffy

The Duffy antigen system consists of two antigens, Fy^a and Fy^b. Only anti-Fy^a has been associated with mild HDFN.

Kidd

The Kidd system antigen system consists of two antigens, Jk^a and Jk^b. Rare cases of mild HDFN have been reported.

Kell

The Kell antigen system includes 23 different members. Antibodies to at least nine of the Kell antigens have been associated with HDFN. The most common of these is Kell (also designated *K, K1*) and cellano (*k, K2*). Additional antibodies that have been reported to be causative for HDFN include -Penny (*Kp^a, K3*), -Rautenberg (*Kp^b, K4*), -Peltz (*Ku, K5*), -Sutter (*Js^a,K6*), -Matthews (*Js^b, K7*), -Karhula (*Ul^a, K10*) and -K22.[114] Unlike the case of other hemolytic antibodies, fetal anemia due to Kell (anti-K1) sensitization is thought to be secondary to not only hemolysis but also to suppression of fetal erythropoiesis.[115]

The majority of cases of K1 sensitization are secondary to previous maternal blood transfusion, usually as a result of postpartum hemorrhage in a previous pregnancy.

Table 30-4. Gene Frequencies (%) and Zygosity (%) for other Red Cell Antigens Associated with HDN

	WHITE		BLACK		HISPANIC	
	ANTIGEN +	HETEROZYGOUS	ANTIGEN +	HETEROZYGOUS	ANTIGEN +	HETEROZYGOUS
C	70	50	30	32	81	51
c	80	50	96	32	76	51
E	32	29	23	21	41	36
e	97	29	98	21	95	36
K (K1)	9	97.8	2	100		
k (K2)	99.8	8.8	100	2		
M	78	64	70	63		
N	77	65	74	60		
S	55	80	31	90		
s	89	50	97	29		
U	100	—	99	—		
Fy^a	66	26	10	90		
Fy^b	83	41	23	96		
Jk^a	77	36	91	63		
Jk^b	72	32	43	21		

Reproduced with permission and modified from Moise KJ: Hemolytic disease of the fetus and newborn. *In* Creasy RK, Resnik R, Iams J (eds): Maternal-Fetal Medicine, 5th ed. Philadelphia, Elsevier Inc, Copyright © 2004.

Because 92 percent of individuals are Kell negative, the initial management of the K1-sensitized pregnancy should entail paternal red cell typing and genotype testing. If the paternal typing returns K1-negative (kk) and paternity is assured, no further maternal testing is undertaken. The majority of Kell-positive individuals will be heterozygous (Table 30-4). Amniocentesis can be used to determine the fetal genotype in these cases.[116] A lower maternal critical antibody value of 8 has been proposed to begin fetal surviellance.[117] The use of serial amniocenteses for ΔOD_{450} is less predictive for fetal anemia than in case of anti-D alloimmunization. Some authors have proposed a lower threshold of the 65 percent of zone 2 of the Liley curve to proceed to cordocentesis.[117] Others advocate serial MCA Doppler studies as a superior method for detecting fetal anemia.[118]

KEY POINTS

- Alloimmunization to the RhD, Kell (K1), and Rhc red cell antigens is the main cause for severe HDFN.
- Despite the widespread use of RhIG, approximately six cases of RhD alloimmunization occur per 1,000 livebirths in the United States.
- Hydrops fetalis is defined as extracellular fluid in two fetal compartments; it represents the end-stage of fetal anemia in HDFN.
- The Rh D, C, c, E, and e antigens are coded by two genes located on the short arm of chromosome one.
- The rule of thumb should be to administer RhIG when in doubt, rather than to withhold it.
- A critical maternal antibody titer can be used in the first affected pregnancy to decide when to begin further fetal testing.
- The fetal peak MCA Doppler velocity can be used to determine the onset of fetal anemia; it will soon replace amniocentesis for ΔOD_{450} for determining the severity of HDFN.
- In the case of a heterozygous paternal phenotype for a particular red cell antigen, fetal typing can be undertaken through amniocentesis or free fetal DNA in maternal plasma.
- Intravascular fetal intrauterine transfusions are the mainstay of fetal therapy with an overall perinatal survival of greater than 85 percent.
- Except in cases of alloimmunization to Kell antigens, irregular red cell antibodies in pregnancy should be managed in a similar fashion to RhD.

REFERENCES

1. Bowman JM: RhD hemolytic disease of the newborn. N Engl J Med 339:1775, 1998.
2. Diamond LE, Balkfan KD, Baty JM: Erythroblastosis fetalis and its association with universal edema of the fetus, icterus gravis neonatorium and anemia of the newborn. J Pediatr 1:269, 1932.
3. Levine P, Stetson R: An usual case of intragroup agglutination. JAMA 113:126, 1939.
4. Landsteiner K, Weiner AS: An agglutinable factor in human blood recognized by immune sera for rhesus blood. Proc Soc Exper Biol Med 43:223, 1940.
5. Levine P, Katzin EM, Burham L: Isoimmunzation in pregnancy: its possible bearing on etiology of erythroblastosis foetalis. JAMA 116:825, 1941.
6. Wallerstein H: Treatment of severe erythroblastosis by simultaneous removal and replacement of blood of the newborn infant. Science 103:583, 1946.

7. Bevis DC: Blood pigments in haemolytic disease of newborn. J Obstet Gynaecol Br Emp 63:68, 1956.
8. Liley AW: Liquor amnii analysis in the management of pregnancy complicated by rhesus sensitization. Am J Obstet Gynecol 82:1359, 1961.
9. Liley AW: Intrauterine transfusion of foetus in haemolytic disease. BMJ 2:1107, 1963.
10. Rodeck CH, Kemp JR, Holman CA, et al: Direct intravascular fetal blood transfusion by fetoscopy in severe Rhesus isoimmunisation. Lancet 1:625, 1981.
11. Bang J, Bock JE, Trolle D: Ultrasound-guided fetal intravenous transfusion for severe rhesus haemolytic disease. Br Med J (Clin Res Ed) 284:373, 1982.
12. Bennett PR, Le Van Kim C, Colin Y, et al: Prenatal determination of fetal RhD type by DNA amplification. N Engl J Med 329:607, 1993.
13. Mari G, for the Collaborative Group for Doppler Assesment of the Blood Velocity of Anemic Fetuses: Noninvasive diagnosis by Doppler ultrasonography of fetal anemia due to maternal red-cell alloimmunization. N Engl J Med 342:9, 2000.
14. Finning KM, Martin PG, Soothill PW, Avent ND: Prediction of fetal D status from maternal plasma: introduction of a new noninvasive fetal RHD genotyping service. Transfusion 42:1079, 2002.
15. Chavez GF, Mulinare J, Edmonds LD: Epidemiology of Rh hemolytic disease of the newborn in the United States. JAMA 265:3270, 1991.
16. Geifman-Holtzman O, Bernstein IM, Berry SM, et al: Fetal RhD genotyping in fetal cells flow sorted from maternal blood. Am J Obstet Gynecol 174:818, 1996.
17. van der Schoot CE, Tax GH, Rijnders RJ, et al: Prenatal typing of Rh and Kell blood group system antigens: the edge of a watershed. Transfus Med Rev 17:31, 2003.
18. Martin JA, Hamilton BE, Sutton PD, et al: Births: Final data for 2002. National Vital Statistics Reports 52:1, 2002.
19. Carapella-de Luca E, Casadei AM, Pascone R, et al: Maternofetal transfusion during delivery and sensitization of the newborn against the rhesus D-antigen. Vox Sang 34:241, 1978.
20. Pollack W: Rh hemolytic disease of the newborn: its cause and prevention. Prog Clin Biol Res 70:185, 1981.
21. Pollack W, Gorman JG, Hager HJ, et al: Antibody-mediated immune suppression to the Rh factor: animal models suggesting mechanism of action. Transfusion 8:134, 1968.
22. Pollack W, Gorman JG, Freda VJ, et al: Results of clinical trials of RhoGAM in women. Transfusion 8:151, 1968.
23. Pollock JM, Bowman JM: Anti-Rh(D) IgG subclasses and severity of Rh hemolytic disease of the newborn. Vox Sang 59:176, 1990.
24. Kumpel BM: Monoclonal anti-D development programme. Transpl Immunol 10:199, 2002.
25. Hilden JO, Gottvall T, Lindblom B: HLA phenotypes and severe Rh(D) immunization. Tissue Antigens 46:313, 1995.
26. Ulm B, Svolba G, Ulm MR, et al: Male fetuses are particularly affected by maternal alloimmunization to D antigen. Transfusion 39:169, 1999.
27. Nicolaides KH, Thilaganathan B, Rodeck CH, Mibashan RS: Erythroblastosis and reticulocytosis in anemic fetuses. Am J Obstet Gynecol 159:1063, 1988.
28. Lestas AN, Bellingham AJ, Nicolaides KH: Red cell glycolytic intermediates in normal, anaemic and transfused human fetuses. Br J Haematol 73:387, 1989.
29. Copel JA, Grannum PA, Green JJ, et al: Fetal cardiac output in the isoimmunized pregnancy: a pulsed Doppler—echocardiographic study of patients undergoing intravascular intrauterine transfusion. Am J Obstet Gynecol 161:361, 1989.
30. Soothill PW, Nicolaides KH, Rodeck CH, et al: Relationship of fetal hemoglobin and oxygen content to lactate concentration in Rh isoimmunized pregnancies. Obstet Gynecol 69:268, 1987.
31. Nicolaides KH, Warenski JC, Rodeck CH: The relationship of fetal plasma protein concentration and hemoglobin level to the development of hydrops in rhesus isoimmunization. Am J Obstet Gynecol 152:341, 1985.
32. Moise KJ, Jr, Carpenter RJ Jr, Hesketh DE: Do abnormal Starling forces cause fetal hydrops in red blood cell alloimmunization? Am J Obstet Gynecol 167:907, 1992.
33. Cormode EJ, Lyster DM, Israels S: Analbuminemia in a neonate. J Pediatr 86:862, 1975.
34. Moise AA, Gest AL, Weickmann PH, McMicken HW: Reduction in plasma protein does not affect body water content in fetal sheep. Pediatr Res 29:623, 1991.
35. Berger HM, Lindeman JH, van Zoeren-Grobben D, et al: Iron overload, free radical damage, and rhesus haemolytic disease. Lancet 335:933, 1990.
36. Lewis M, Bowman JM, Pollock J, Lowen B: Absorption of red cells from the peritoneal cavity of an hydropic twin. Transfusion 13:37, 1973.
37. Fischer RA, Race RR: Rh gene frequencies in Britain. Nature 157:48, 1946.
38. Cherif-Zahar B, Mattei MG, Le Van Kim C, et al: Localization of the human Rh blood group gene structure to chromosome region 1p34.3–1p36.1 by in situ hybridization. Hum Genet 86:398, 1991.
39. Le Van Kim C, Cherif-Zahar B, Raynal V, et al: Multiple Rh messenger RNA isoforms are produced by alternative splicing. Blood 80:1074, 1992.
40. Carritt B, Kemp TJ, Poulter M: Evolution of the human RH (rhesus) blood group genes: a 50 year old prediction (partially) fulfilled. Hum Mol Genet 6:843, 1997.
41. Avent ND: Antenatal therapy for haemolytic disease of the fetus and newborn. *In* Hadley A, Soothill P (eds): Alloimmune Disorders in Pregnancy. Anaemia, Thrombocytopenia, and Neutropenia in the Fetus and Newborn, Cambridge, UK, Cambridge University Press, 2002, p 121.
42. Singleton BK, Green CA, Avent ND, et al: The presence of an RHD pseudogene containing a 37 base pair duplication and a nonsense mutation in africans with the Rh D-negative blood group phenotype. Blood 95:12, 2000.
43. Lee YL, Chiou HL, Hu SN, Wang L: Analysis of RHD genes in Taiwanese RhD-negative donors by the multiplex PCR method. J Clin Lab Anal 17:80, 2003.
44. Dunn LJ: Prevention of isoimmunization in pregnancy developed by Freda and Gorman. Obstet Gynecol Surv 54:S1, 1999.
45. Freda VJ, Gorman JG, Pollack W: Prevention of Rh-hemolytic disease with Rh-immune globulin. Am J Obstet Gynecol 128:456, 1977.
46. Mittendorf R, Williams MA: Rho(D) immunoglobulin (RhoGAM): how it came into being. Obstet Gynecol 77:301, 1991.
47. Smith T: Active immunity produced by so-called balanced or neutral mixtures of diptheria toxin and anti-toxin. J Exp Med 11:241, 1909.
48. Freda VJ, Gorman JG, Pollack W, et al: Prevention of Rh isoimmunization. Progress report of the clinical trial in mothers. JAMA 199:390, 1967.
49. Chamberlain EN: Liverpool Medical Institution: Role of inheritance in common diseases. Lancet 1:526, 1960.
50. Finn R, Clarke CA, Donohoe WT, et al: Experimental studies on the prevention of Rh haemolytic disease. Br Med J 5238:1486, 1961.
51. Freda VJ, Gorman JG: Antepartum management of Rh hemolytic disease. Bull Sloane Hosp Women Columbia Presbyt Med 8:147, 1962.
52. Clarke CA, Sheppard PM: Prevention of rhesus haemolytic disease. Lancet 19:343, 1965.
53. Bowman JM, Chown B, Lewis M, Pollock JM: Rh isoimmunization during pregnancy: antenatal prophylaxis. Can Med Assoc J 118:623, 1978.
54. Bowman JM, Pollock JM: Antenatal prophylaxis of Rh isoimmunization: 28-weeks'-gestation service program. Can Med Assoc J 118:627, 1978.
55. Prenatal antibody screening and use of Rho (D) immune globulin (human). American College of Obstetricians and Gynecologists Technical Bulletin 13, 1970.
56. The selective use of Rho(D) immune globulin (RhIG). American College of Obstetricians and Gynecologists Technical Bulletin Update 61, 1981.
57. Bichler J, Spycher MO, Amstutz HP, et al: Pharmacokinetics and safety of recombinant anti-RhD in healthy RhD-negative male volunteers. Transfus Med 14:165, 2004.
58. Prevention of RhD alloimmunization. American College of Obstetricians and Gynecologists Practice Bulletin 4, 1999.
59. Bowman JM: The prevention of Rh immunization. Transfus Med Rev 2:129, 1988.

60. Urbaniak SJ: Consensus conference on anti-D prophylaxis, April 7 & 8, 1997: final consensus statement. Royal College of Physicians of Edinburgh/Royal College of Obstetricians and Gynaecologists. Transfusion 38:97, 1998.
61. Brecher ME (ed): Technical Manual of the American Association of Blood Banks, ed 14. Bethesda, MD, American Association of Blood Banks, 2002, p 825.
62. Goodrick J, Kumpel B, Pamphilon D, et al: Plasma half-lives and bioavailability of human monoclonal Rh D antibodies BRAD-3 and BRAD-5 following intramuscular injection into Rh D-negative volunteers. Clin Exp Immunol 98:17, 1994.
63. Bowman JM: Controversies in Rh prophylaxis. Who needs Rh immune globulin and when should it be given? Am J Obstet Gynecol 151:289, 1985.
64. Ness PM, Baldwin ML, Niebyl JR: Clinical high-risk designation does not predict excess fetal-maternal hemorrhage. Am J Obstet Gynecol 156:154, 1987.
65. Novaretti MC, Jens E, Pagliarini T, et al: Comparison of conventional tube test with diamed gel microcolumn assay for anti-D titration. Clin Lab Haematol 25:311, 2003.
66. Nicolaides KH, Rodeck CH: Maternal serum anti-D antibody concentration and assessment of rhesus isoimmunisation. BMJ 304:1155, 1992.
67. Moise KJ Jr, Carpenter RJ Jr: Chorionic villus sampling for Rh typing: clinical implications [letter; comment]. Am J Obstet Gynecol 168:1002, 1993.
68. Kanter MH: Derivation of new mathematic formulas for determining whether a D- positive father is heterozygous or homozygous for the D antigen. Am J Obstet Gynecol 166:61, 1992.
69. Moise KJ: Management of rhesus alloimmunization in pregnancy. Obstet Gynecol 100:600, 2002.
70. Chiu RW, Murphy MF, Fidler C, et al: Determination of RhD zygosity: comparison of a double amplification refractory mutation system approach and a multiplex real-time quantitative PCR approach. Clin Chem 47:667, 2001.
71. Van den Veyver IB, Moise KJ Jr: Fetal RhD typing by polymerase chain reaction in pregnancies complicated by rhesus alloimmunization. Obstet Gynecol 88:1061, 1996.
72. Simsek S, Faas BH, Bleeker PM, et al: Rapid Rh D genotyping by polymerase chain reaction-based amplification of DNA. Blood 85:2975, 1995.
73. Hopkins DF: Maternal anti-Rh(D) and the D-negative fetus. Am J Obstet Gynecol 108:268, 1970.
74. Daniels G, Finning K, Martin P, Soothill P: Fetal blood group genotyping from DNA from maternal plasma: an important advance in the management and prevention of haemolytic disease of the fetus and newborn. Vox Sang 87:225, 2004.
75. Lo YM, Hjelm NM, Fidler C, et al: Prenatal diagnosis of fetal RhD status by molecular analysis of maternal plasma. N Engl J Med 339:1734, 1998.
76. Rouillac-Le Sciellour C, Puillandre P, Gillot R, et al: Large-scale pre-diagnosis study of fetal RHD genotyping by PCR on plasma DNA from RhD-negative pregnant women. Mol Diagn 8:23, 2004.
77. Management of Isoimmunization in Pregnancy. American College of Obstetricians and Gynecologists Technical Bulletin 90:1986.
78. Nicolaides KH, Rodeck CH, Mibashan RS, Kemp JR: Have Liley charts outlived their usefulness? Am J Obstet Gynecol 155:90, 1986.
79. Queenan JT, Tomai TP, Ural SH, King JC: Deviation in amniotic fluid optical density at a wavelength of 450 nm in Rh-immunized pregnancies from 14 to 40 weeks' gestation: a proposal for clinical management. Am J Obstet Gynecol 168:1370, 1993.
80. Weiner CP, Williamson RA, Wenstrom KD, et al: Management of fetal hemolytic disease by cordocentesis. I. Prediction of fetal anemia [see comments]. Am J Obstet Gynecol 165:546, 1991.
81. Weiner CP, Williamson RA, Wenstrom KD, et al: Management of fetal hemolytic disease by cordocentesis. II. Outcome of treatment. Am J Obstet Gynecol 165:1302, 1991.
82. Nicolaides KH, Soothill PW, Clewell WH, et al: Fetal haemoglobin measurement in the assessment of red cell isoimmunisation. Lancet 1:1073, 1988.
83. van Kamp IL, Klumper FJ, Bakkum RS, et al: The severity of immune fetal hydrops is predictive of fetal outcome after intrauterine treatment. Am J Obstet Gynecol 185:668, 2001.
84. Nicolaides KH, Fontanarosa M, Gabbe SG, Rodeck CH: Failure of ultrasonographic parameters to predict the severity of fetal anemia in rhesus isoimmunization. Am J Obstet Gynecol 158:920, 1988.
85. Vintzileos AM, Campbell WA, Storlazzi E, et al: Fetal liver ultrasound measurements in isoimmunized pregnancies. Obstet Gynecol 68:162, 1986.
86. Roberts AB, Mitchell JM, Lake Y, Pattison NS: Ultrasonographic surveillance in red blood cell alloimmunization. Am J Obstet Gynecol 184:1251, 2001.
87. Opekes D, Seward G, Vandenbussche F, et al: Minimally invasive management of Rh alloimmunization: can amniotic fluid delta OD450 be replaced by Doppler studies? A prospective study multicenter trial. Am J Obstet Gynecol 191:S3, 2004.
88. Abel DE, Grambow SC, Brancazio LR, Hertzberg BS: Ultrasound assessment of the fetal middle cerebral artery peak systolic velocity: A comparison of the near-field versus far-field vessel. Am J Obstet Gynecol 189:986, 2003.
89. Sallout BI, Fung KF, Wen SW, et al: The effect of fetal behavioral states on middle cerebral artery peak systolic velocity. Am J Obstet Gynecol 191:1283, 2004.
90. Trevett T, Dorman K, Lamvu G, Moise KJ: Does antenatal maternal administration of phenobarbital prevent exchange transfusion in neonates with alloimmune hemolytic disease? Am J Obstet Gynecol 192:478, 2005.
91. Nicolini U, Nicolaidis P, Fisk NM, et al: Fetal blood sampling from the intrahepatic vein: analysis of safety and clinical experience with 214 procedures. Obstet Gynecol 76:47, 1990.
92. Moise KJ Jr, Carpenter RJ Jr, Kirshon B, et al: Comparison of four types of intrauterine transfusion: effect on fetal hematocrit. Fetal Ther 4:126, 1989.
93. Daffos F, Forestier F, Mac Aleese J, et al: Fetal curarization for prenatal magnetic resonance imaging. Prenat Diagn 8:312, 1988.
94. Bernstein HH, Chitkara U, Plosker H, et al: Use of atracurium besylate to arrest fetal activity during intrauterine intravascular transfusions. Obstet Gynecol 72:813, 1988.
95. Giannina G, Moise KJ Jr, Dorman K: A simple method to estimate the volume for fetal intravascular transfusion. Fetal Diagn Ther 13:94, 1998.
96. RaMoise KJ Jr, Mari G, Fisher DJ, et al: Acute fetal hemodynamic alterations after intrauterine transfusion for treatment of severe red blood cell alloimmunization. Am J Obstet Gynecol 163:776, 1990.
97. Radunovic N, Lockwood CJ, Alvarez M, et al: The severely anemic and hydropic isoimmune fetus: changes in fetal hematocrit associated with intrauterine death. Obstet Gynecol 79:390, 1992.
98. van Kamp IL, Klumper FJ, Oepkes D, et al: Complications of intrauterine intravascular transfusion for fetal anemia due to maternal red-cell alloimmunization. Am J Obstet Gynecol 192:171, 2005.
99. Schumacher B, Moise KJ Jr: Fetal transfusion for red blood cell alloimmunization in pregnancy. Obstet Gynecol 88:137, 1996.
100. Klumper FJ, van Kamp IL, Vandenbussche FP, et al.: Benefits and risks of fetal red-cell transfusion after 32 weeks gestation. Eur J Obstet Gynecol Reprod Biol 92:91, 2000.
101. Saade GR, Moise KJ, Belfort MA, et al: Fetal and neonatal hematologic parameters in red cell alloimmunization: predicting the need for late neonatal transfusions. Fetal Diagn Ther 8:161, 1993.
102. Janssens HM, de Haan MJ, van Kamp IL, et al: Outcome for children treated with fetal intravascular transfusions because of severe blood group antagonism. J Pediatr 131:373, 1997.
103. Hudon L, Moise KJ Jr, Hegemier SE, et al: Long-term neurodevelopmental outcome after intrauterine transfusion for the treatment of fetal hemolytic disease. Am J Obstet Gynecol 179:858, 1998.
104. Moise KJ, Whitecar PW: Antenatal therapy for alloimmune haemolytic anemia. *In* Hadley A, Soothill P (eds): Alloimmune Disorders in Pregnancy. Anaemia, Thrombocytopenia and Neutropenia in the Fetus and Newborn. 1, Cambridge, UK, Cambridge University Press, 2002, p 173.
105. Voto LS, Mathet ER, Zapaterio JL, et al: High-dose gammaglobulin (IVIG) followed by intrauterine transfusions (IUTs): a new alternative for the treatment of severe fetal hemolytic disease. J Perinat Med 25:85, 1997.

106. Seeho SK, Burton G, Leigh D, et al: The role of preimplantation genetic diagnosis in the management of severe rhesus alloimmunization: first unaffected pregnancy: Case report. Hum Reprod 20:697, 2005.
107. Neppert J, v Witzleben-Schurholz E, Zupanska B, et al: High incidence of maternal HLA A, B and C antibodies associated with a mild course of haemolytic disease of the newborn. Group for the Study of Protective Maternal HLA Antibodies in the Clinical Course of HDN. Eur J Haematol 63:120, 1999.
108. Whitecar P, Farb R, Subramany L, et al: Paternal leukocyte alloimmunization as a treatment for hemolytic disease of the newborn/fetus in the rabbit model. Am J Obstet Gynecol 185: S235, 2001.
109. Hall AM, Cairns LS, Altmann DM, et al: Immune responses and tolerance to the RhD blood group protein in HLA-transgenic mice. Blood 105:2175, 2005.
110. Hackney DN, Knudtson EJ, Rossi KQ, et al: Management of pregnancies complicated by anti-c isoimmunization. Obstet Gynecol 103:24, 2004.
111. Spong CY, Porter AE, Queenan JT: Management of isoimmunization in the presence of multiple maternal antibodies. Am J Obstet Gynecol 185:481, 2001.
112. Bowman JM, Pollock JM, Manning FA, Harman CR: Severe anti-C hemolytic disease of the newborn. Am J Obstet Gynecol 166:1239, 1992.
113. Joy SD, Rossi KQ, Krugh D, O'Shaughnessy RW: Management of pregnancies complicated by anti-E alloimmunization. Obstet Gynecol 105:24, 2005.
114. Daniels G: Blood group antibodies in hemolytic disease of the fetus and newborn. *In* Hadley A, Soothill P (eds): Alloimmune Disorders in Pregnancy. Anaemia, Thrombocytopenia, and Neutropenia in the Fetus and Newborn, Cambridge, UK, Cambridge University Press, 2002, p 21.
115. Vaughan JI, Manning M, Warwick RM, et al: Inhibition of erythroid progenitor cells by anti-Kell antibodies in fetal alloimmune anemia. N Engl J Med 338:798, 1998.
116. Spence WC, Maddalena A, Demers DB, Bick DP: Prenatal determination of genotypes Kell and Cellano in at-risk pregnancies. J Reprod Med 42:353, 1997.
117. Bowman JM, Pollock JM, Manning FA, et al: Maternal Kell blood group alloimmunization. Obstet Gynecol 79:239, 1992.
118. van Dongen H, Klumper FJ, Sikkel E, et al: Non-invasive tests to predict fetal anemia in Kell-alloimmunized pregnancies. Ultrasound Obstet Gynecol 25:341, 2005.

Amniotic Fluid Disorders

WILLIAM M. GILBERT

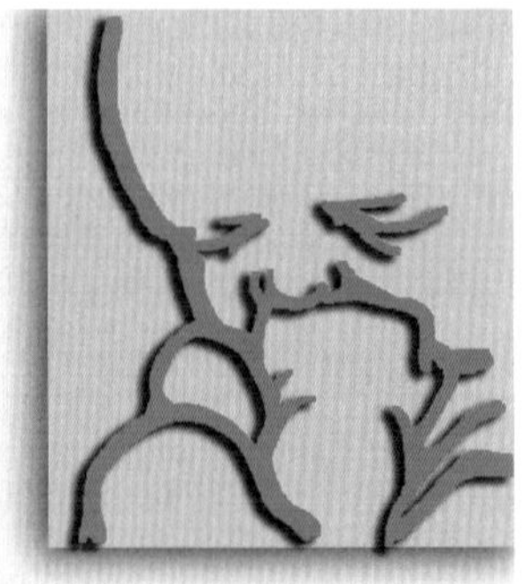

CHAPTER 31

KEY ABBREVIATIONS

Amniotic fluid	AF
Amniotic fluid index	AFI
Amniotic fluid volume	AFV
Intrauterine fetal death	IUFD
Intrauterine growth restriction	IUGR
Largest vertical pocket	LVP
Neonatal intensive care unit	NICU
Perinatal mortality rate	PMR
Premature rupture of the membranes	PROM
Twin-to-twin transfusion syndrome	TTS

INTRODUCTION

For most pregnant women and their health care providers, amniotic fluid (AF) is an unimportant byproduct of the delivery. With a normal pregnancy, little attention is paid to the AF unless meconium staining occurs in labor. It is only when certain complications of pregnancy present, compromising fetal well-being, that any interest is taken in the AF. The conditions of polyhydramnios (too much AF) or oligohydramnios (too little AF) create the greatest concern to patients and health care providers. As an example, with significant oligohydramnios in the second trimester, the perinatal mortality rate (PMR) approaches 90 to 100 percent.[1–3] Likewise, with marked polyhydramnios in midpregnancy, PMR can be higher than 50 percent.[4,5] Although these two extreme conditions are rare, other less drastic examples are much more common. Efforts to study abnormalities of AF are complicated by the fact that little is known about the processes involved in normal amniotic fluid volume (AFV) regulation. Rarely in modern medical research are the processes that underlie normal physiology so poorly understood. In studying a particular disease state, knowledge of normal physiology usually assists the researcher in determining the pathophysiology of a particular disease. However, many of the disease states associated with the extremes of AFV are better understood than is the normal physiology of AF.

In this chapter, we explore what is known about the normal mechanisms effecting the formation and removal of AF, including fetal urination, swallowing, lung liquid, and intramembranous absorption.[6–8] In addition, we examine the changes in AFV and composition across gestation, in order to help us understand its normal regulation. We then review the abnormalities of AFV, including oligohydramnios and polyhydramnios, and the possible underlying causes. Finally, we examine the various treatment options available for AFV abnormalities. The goal of the chapter is to offer the reader a complete understanding of the known mechanisms and functioning of AFV regulation, and their connection with disease states.

NORMAL AMNIOTIC FLUID VOLUME

As a result of various limitations, attempts to measure actual AFV are difficult. It is not easy to get near, or into, the amniotic compartment. To enter the amniotic cavity, an invasive procedure such as an amniocentesis must be performed. To measure the volume of AF, an inert dye must be injected, which dilutes to fill the amniotic cavity. Follow-up samples of amniotic fluid are then obtained to determine a dilution curve.[9–15] Obviously, an amniocentesis has a small but real risk of interrupting the pregnancy, and any substance injected into the uterus can cause infection despite every precaution being taken. The dye injection technique is considered the "gold standard" for determining actual AFV and is compared with

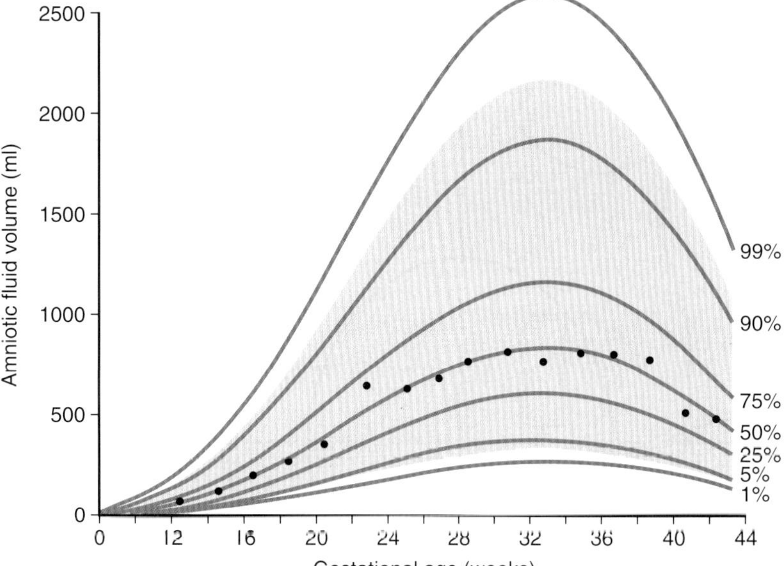

Figure 31-1. Nomogram showing amniotic fluid volume as a function of gestational age. The black dots are the mean for each 2-week interval. Percentiles calculated from polynomial regression equation and standard deviation of residuals. (Reproduced with permission from Brace RA, Wolf EJ: Normal amniotic fluid volume throughout pregnancy. Am J Obstet Gynecol 161:382, 1989.)

other methods of estimating AFV, such as ultrasound, discussed later in this chapter.

Despite these measurement limitations, Brace and Wolf identified all published measurements of AFV in 12 studies with 705 individual AFV measurements.[16] Their findings are demonstrated in Figure 31-1. From this figure, it can be seen that for each week of gestation, there can be widely varying amounts of AF, which increase with advancing gestational age. The largest variation occurs at 32 to 33 weeks of gestation. At this time, the normal range (5th to 95th percent) is from 400 to 2100 ml. This represents a wide "normal range." One of the most interesting findings of the Brace and Wolf study is that from 22 weeks through 39 weeks of gestation, the average volume of AF (black dots on Fig. 31-1) remained unchanged. At a time when the fetus weighed, on average, about 500 g at 22 weeks, up to term gestation when it weighed 3,500 g, a 7-fold increase in weight, the mean AFV was the same. This would suggest that AFV was being carefully regulated. This concept of fluid regulation is discussed later.

ULTRASOUND MEASUREMENTS OF AMNIOTIC FLUID VOLUME

Measuring true AFV is not only difficult but clinically impractical as well. Initial clinical assessments of AFV were through Leopold's abdominal measurements, or measurement of the fundal height of the pregnant uterus. If the maternal uterus was large for gestational age, and the fetus could not be easily palpated, or was ballotable, it was believed that AFV was increased. More commonly, the diagnosis of polyhydramnios was made at the time of delivery when large volumes of AF rained down on the delivery room floor. The diagnosis of oligohydramnios was considered when the fundal height was small for gestational age or the fetus could be easily palpated. Clearly, palpation as a method for determining AFV has its place, but the advent of ultrasound has afforded us the ability of looking, noninvasively, into the human uterus to examine both the fetus and AFV. Early ultrasound estimations of AFV were made by measuring the largest vertical pocket (LVP) of AF.[17] Other researchers have examined the LVP, and then considered the horizontal plain, if the LVP was less than 1 cm.[18] Chamberlain et al.[18] and Mercer et al.[19] found that with the LVP of AF less than 1 cm or 0.5 cm, respectively, perinatal morbidity and the PMR were increased. These lower values of the LVP certainly identified at-risk fetuses, but the sensitivity for identifying the majority of pregnancy complications associated with oligohydramnios, was not as strong, causing others to choose higher values as a cutoff point.

As the quality of ultrasound improved, investigators expanded their measurements to include the LVP in each of the four quadrants of the uterus throughout gestation. The uterus at any gestational age beyond 20 weeks is divided into four equal quadrants, as shown in Figure 31-2. The deepest clear pocket of AF is then measured, making sure that the ultrasound transducer is perpendicular to the floor. This four-quadrant measurement was termed the Amniotic Fluid Index (AFI) by Phelan et al. and has been described by others as well.[20–22] The clearest graphic presentation of the AFI (Fig. 31-3) is that of Moore and Cayle, who described their population of 791 normal pregnant women.[22] Their cross-sectional study obtained only one AFI measurement from each pregnancy with a normal outcome.[22] The 5th and 95th percentile of the AFI varied for each gestational age, suggesting that what may be normal for one gestational age period, may be abnormal for another. The 95th percentile for 35 to 36 weeks of gestation was a value of 24.9 cm, whereas the 95th percentile for 41 weeks of gestation was 19.4 cm. The variation in the AFI at the 5th percentile was less than that of the 95th percentile, but it still varied by as much as 2.5 cm. Finally, the investigators reported the interobserver and intraobserver variation to be 3.1 percent and 6.7 percent, respectively, which is acceptable

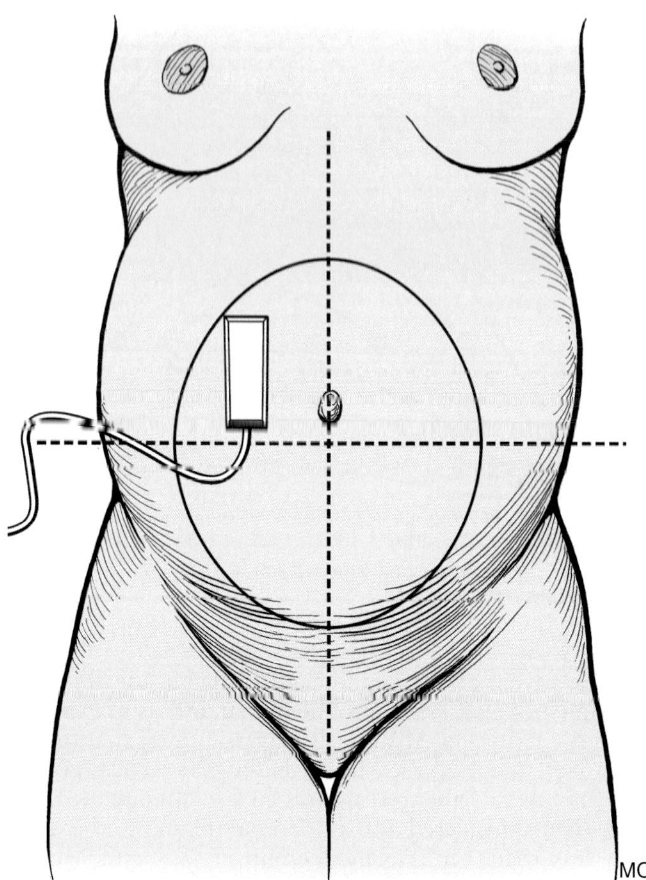

Figure 31-2. Schematic diagram of the technique for measuring the four-quadrant amniotic fluid index (AFI). (Reproduced with permission from Gilbert WM: Disorders of Amniotic Fluid. *In* Creasy RK, Resnik R [eds]: Maternal Fetal Medicine, 3rd ed. Philadelphia, W.B. Saunders, 1994, p 620.)

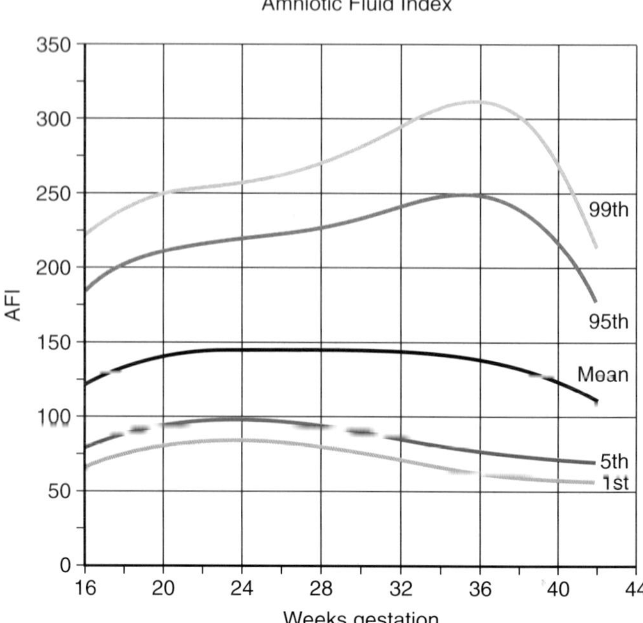

Figure 31-3. Amniotic fluid index (in millimeters) plotted with gestational age (weeks). The solid line denotes the 50th percentile; dashed lines, the 5th and 95th percentiles; and the dotted lines, + 2 standard deviations (2.5th and 97.5th percentiles). (Reproduced with permission from Moore TR, Cayle JE: The amniotic fluid index in normal human pregnancy. Am J Obstet Gynecol 62:1168, 1990.)

for this commonly performed procedure.[22] Comparing the ultrasound estimation of the AFV by the AFI (see Fig. 31-3) with the actual measured volume (see Fig. 31-1) demonstrates very similar-appearing curves.

Several authors have attempted to compare estimates of AFV by ultrasound (the LVP and the AFI) with actual measurement by the dye dilution technique, and report that the AFI does not predict actual AFV that well.[9–25] Dildy et al.[23] found that the AFI overestimated the actual volume in 88 percent of cases at lower volumes, and underestimated the actual volume in 54 percent of cases at higher volumes. The researchers went on to conclude that the difference between actual volume and estimated volume by the AFI should not change clinical practice.[23] Magann et al. have published several studies comparing the LVP with the AFI and dye dilution techniques, to determine which test is superior for predicting actual AFV, or perinatal morbidity or mortality.[9,11–15,24,25] Consistently, they reported that both ultrasound methods (LVP and AFI) poorly predicted actual AFV. In addition, they found an observed sensitivity for an AFI measurement of less than 5 cm of 10 percent (specificity of 96 percent), whereas the LVP was worse (sensitivity 5 percent, specificity 98 percent).[25] When examining cases of suspected polyhydramnios, an AFI greater than 20 cm had a sensitivity of 29 percent (specificity 97 percent), which was equal to the LVP method (sensitivity of 29 percent, specificity of 94 percent). When the LVP method was compared with the AFI method, the former had fewer false-positive tests than the latter, suggesting the LVP was the superior method.[25] In comparison, Moore[26] found the AFI superior to the LVP for identifying cases of oligohydramnios but found the two methods similar at predicting polyhydramnios.

Measurement of the AFI can also vary widely depending upon the technique used. Flack et al.[27] reported that they could increase the AFI (13 percent) by using low pressure with the ultrasound transducer on the maternal abdomen, as compared with moderate pressure, or decrease the AFI (21 percent) with high pressure on the maternal abdomen. Clearly technique is important to prevent overestimating or underestimating the ultrasound measurement of the AFI. Despite the fact that the actual measurement of AFV by Brace and Wolf[16] (see Fig. 31-1) roughly superimposes upon the graph of the normal AFI of Moore and Cayle[22] (see Fig. 31-3), it does not mean that they will necessarily correlate well with each other.

For many years, investigators have tried, with mixed success, to demonstrate the utility and applicability of ultrasound estimation of AFV in relation to perinatal outcome. Early work by Chamberlain et al.[18] found that with the LVP smaller than 1 cm, there was a marked increase in perinatal morbidity and mortality, which persisted even after correcting for birth defects. Despite overwhelming evidence that any ultrasound method for predicting AFV is poor at best, clinical practice continues to include the use of weekly or biweekly AFV estimation by ultrasound.

AMNIOTIC FLUID FORMATION

Fetal Urine

The main source of AF is fetal urination. In the human, the fetal kidneys begin to make urine before the end of the first trimester, and production of urine continues from this point, ever increasing, until term gestation. Many different animal models have been used to study fetal urine production, with the fetal sheep being the most common.[28–32] The fetal sheep provides an excellent model for comparative human study owing to its similar fetal weight at term, its sufficient size allowing catheter placement, and the fact that the sheep fetus has a low risk of premature labor after catheter placement. In the fetal sheep, urine production has been reported to be approximately 200 to 1200 ml/day in the last third of pregnancy.[28,32,33] Efforts to measure human fetal urine production have been accomplished by ultrasound measuring the change in fetal bladder volume over time. Wladimiroff and Campbell[34] initially measured three dimensions of the fetal bladder every 15 minutes and reported a human fetal urine production rate of 230 ml/day at 36 weeks of gestation, which increased to 655 ml/day at term. Others found similar volumes using the same technique.[35–38] More recently, Rabinowitz et al.,[39] using the same technique as Wladimiroff and Campbell but measuring the change in volume every 2 to 5 minutes, found fetal urine production to be much greater than previously predicted, 1,224 ml/day. In Figure 31-4, the fetal urine production rates of several studies are shown, with the greatest volume being that of Rabinowitz et al., who measured at the most frequent intervals.[34–39] Clearly, the human fetal urine production rate can be seen to be approximately 1,000 to 1,200 ml/day at term, suggesting that the entire AFV is replaced more frequently than every 24 hours.

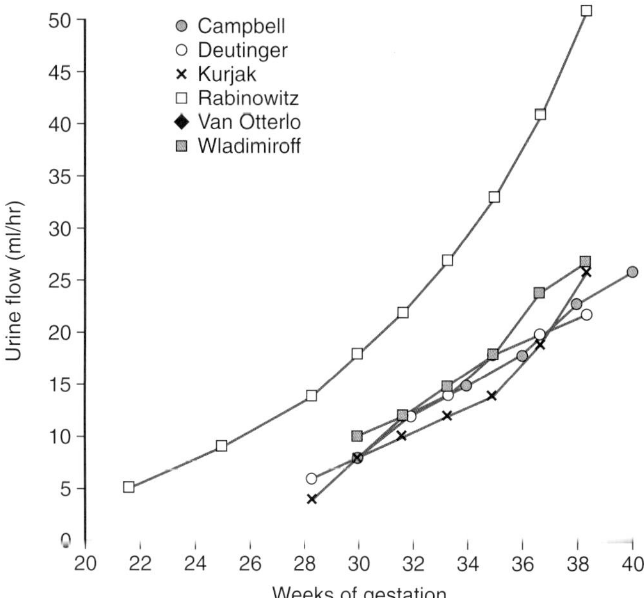

Figure 31-4. Normal changes in fetal urine flow rates across gestation. Lines represent mean values for six studies in the literature.[34–39] The individual first authors are shown in the figure itself. The highest line is data from Rabinowitz et al and represents bladder volume measurements every 5 minutes instead of every 15 minutes, as is the case for the other five studies. (Reproduced with permission from Gilbert WM, Brace RA: Amniotic fluid volume and normal flows to and from the amniotic cavity. Semin Perinatol 7:150, 1993.)

Lung Liquid

Although rarely even contemplated by the practicing clinician, fetal lung liquid plays an important role in AF formation. For years, it was presumed that there was actual movement of AF into the fetal lungs under normal conditions; however, recent data offer no support for this concept.[40,41] In fact, there is normally an outward rather than inward movement of fluid from the lungs. Throughout gestation, the fetal lungs produce fluid that exits the trachea and is either swallowed, or leaves the mouth, and enters the amniotic compartment. Although never directly measured in humans, lung liquid values from the fetal sheep have provided some valuable data. In the fetal sheep, the lungs have been reported to produce volumes of up to 400 ml/day, with 50% being swallowed and 50% exiting via the mouth.[31,42–45] In humans, we know that fetal lung liquid enters the amniotic compartment owing to the presence of surfactant within the AF, both near and at term, as measured by amniocentesis for lung maturity. During normal fetal life, the fetus performs breathing movements that provide a "to-and-fro" movement of AF into and out of the trachea, upper lungs and mouth.[46] Although AF may move back and forth, there is a net outward movement of fetal lung liquid. Clearly, the fetal lungs provide a volume of liquid to the AF, which adds to that of the fetal urine.

AMNIOTIC FLUID REMOVAL

Fetal Swallowing

In the human, fetal swallowing begins early in gestation. In the fetal sheep, swallowing has mostly been measured in the latter half of pregnancy and appears to increase with increasing gestational age. Sherman et al.[47] have reported that the ovine fetus swallows in episodes lasting 2 minutes and at volumes of 100 to 300 ml/kg/day. In the term ovine fetus, that volume represents a daily swallowing rate of 350 to 1,000 ml/day for a 3.5 kg fetus. This is obviously more than the adult sheep, which drinks 40 to 60 ml/kg daily.[47]

Many different techniques have been used to determine swallowing rates in the animal model, including repetitive sampling of injected dye and actual flow probe measurements.[28,47] For obvious reasons, actual measurement of human fetal swallowing is much more difficult. In spite of this limitation, early studies in humans in the

1960s used fetuses that underwent injection of substances into the amniotic compartment to measure swallowing. Initial work was done by Pritchard in normal and anencephalic fetuses, and later by others in his laboratory.[40,48] Human fetal swallowing was studied by injecting radioactive chromium–labeled erythrocytes and hypaque into the amniotic compartment, and swallowing rates of 72 to 262 ml/kg/day were found.[40,48] Abramovich[49] injected colloidal gold into the human amniotic compartment and found that fetal swallowing increased with advancing gestational age. He also found similar swallowing rates to those reported by Pritchard.[49] Obviously similar studies could not be performed today, but the information is helpful in our understanding of human fetal swallowing. Clearly, fetal swallowing could not remove the entire volume of fluids entering the amniotic compartment from fetal urine production and lung liquid, and therefore, other mechanisms for AF removal must occur.

Intramembranous Absorption

One major stumbling block to the understanding of AFV regulation was the discrepancy between fetal urine and lung liquid production, and its removal by swallowing. Clearly something was missing in the equation. If the measurements and estimates of AF production and removal were accurate, there would be at least 500 to 750 ml/day entering the amniotic compartment, without leaving, which would result in acute polyhydramnios. This does not occur under normal conditions (see Fig. 31-1), clearly demonstrating the presence of other mechanisms that remove AF in order to maintain a normal volume. A second route for AF removal has been suggested, namely the intramembranous pathway.[6–8,50,51] This process describes the movement of water and solutes between the amniotic compartment and the fetal blood, which circulates through the fetal surface of the placenta. The large osmotic gradient (Fig. 31-5) between AF and fetal blood provides a substantial driving force for the movement of AF into the fetal blood. This intramembranous absorption has been described in detail in the fetal sheep and also demonstrated to be present in the rhesus monkey fetus.[6–8,50,51] Several anecdotal studies suggest that intramembranous absorption also occurs in humans. In separate publications, Heller[52] and Renaud et al.[53] each injected labeled amnio acids into the amniotic compartments of women, who were shortly thereafter delivered by cesarean section. Both groups found high levels of the amino acids concentrated in the placenta within 45 minutes of injection. They concluded that the amino acids had to be absorbed by some route other than swallowing in order to explain the rapid absorption into the fetal circulation within the placenta. Intramembranous absorption could easily explain this movement. This route of absorption is now being actively investigated, and researchers have noted that 200 to 500 ml/day leaves the amniotic compartment under normal physiologic conditions.[6,7,54] In addition, it has been reported that absorption through the intramembranous pathway can increase almost 10-fold under experimental conditions in sheep.[55] Figure 31-6 demonstrates the summation of all currently identified avenues for fluid entry and exit from the amniotic compartment, along with their measured or estimated values. With the identification of intramembranous absorption as a significant route for the removal of amniotic water and solutes, it appears that all routes of entry and removal from the amniotic compartment have possibly been identified, and the equation of input and outflow has finally been balanced (Fig. 31-6). Recent work on the mechanisms associated with

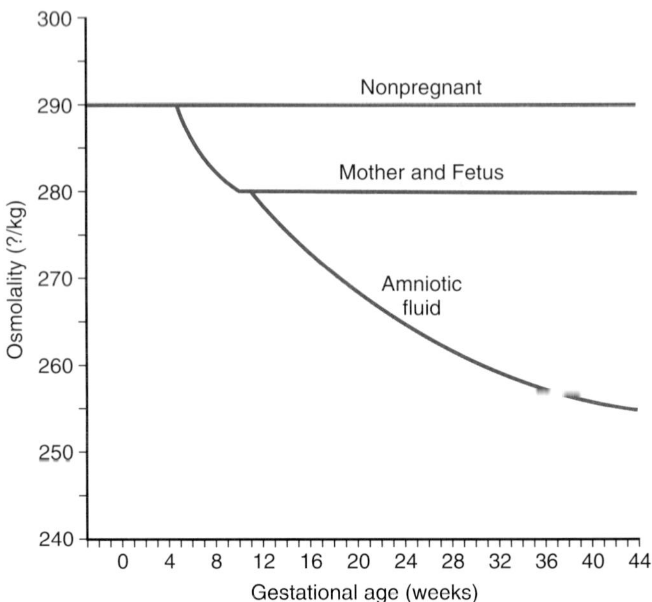

Figure 31-5. Change in maternal and fetal plasma and in amniotic fluid osmolality across gestation. (Reproduced with permission from Gilbert WM, Moore TR, Brace RA: Amniotic fluid volume dynamics. Fetal Med Review 3:89, 1991.)

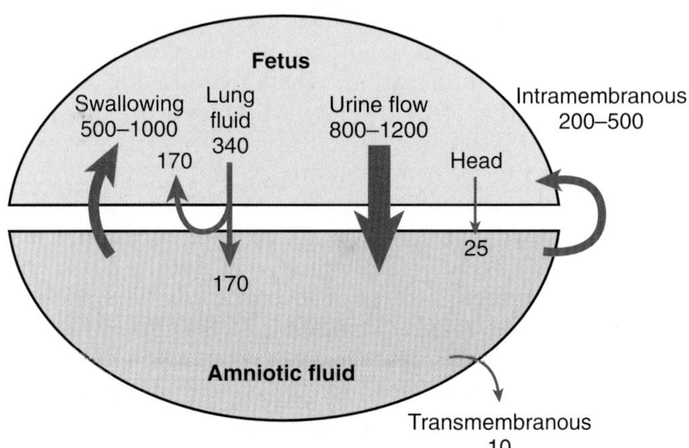

Figure 31-6. All known pathways for fluid and solute entry and exit from the amniotic fluid in the fetus near term. Arrow size is relative to associated flow rate. The solid red arrows represent directly measured flows, whereas the blue arrows represent estimated flows. The numbers represent volume flow in milliliters per day. The curved portion of the double arrow represents lung fluid that is directly swallowed after leaving the trachea, whereas the straight portion represents lung fluid that enters the amniotic cavity from the mouth and nose. (Reproduced with permission from Gilbert WM, Moore TR, Brace RA: Amniotic fluid volume dynamics. Fetal Med Review 3:89, 1991.)

intramembranous absorption should help clarify this final chapter in our understanding of the normal physiology associated with AFV regulation.

OLIGOHYDRAMNIOS

In this section, we examine the association of oligohydramnios and perinatal outcome. The incidence of oligohydramnios varies depending on which definition is used, with a general reporting rate between 1 and 3 percent.[56] When women undergoing antepartum testing for high-risk pregnancy conditions are examined, the incidence of oligohydramnios is much higher (19 to 20 percent), as would be expected. This is primarily due to the underlying maternal or fetal indication for the antepartum testing.[25] Three studies have reported actual measured AFV but have reported somewhat different values for oligohydramnios: Brace and Wolf, less than 318 ml; Magann et al., less than 500 ml; and Horsager et al., less than 200 ml.[9,10,16] With the advent of ultrasound estimation of AFV, multiple thresholds have been reported.[3,17,57–59] An early publication by Chamberlain et al.[18] reported a 50-fold increase in PMR for pregnancies with a LVP of less than 1 cm. This report was instrumental in raising concern about the risk of stillbirth and neonatal mortality in the presence of oligohydramnios. A second, less-often reported finding of that study was that 40 percent of the cases with oligohydramnios also had other confounding factors such as intrauterine growth restriction (IUGR), maternal hypertensive disorders, and congenital malformations.[18] Clearly, oligohydramnios in the presence of IUGR, or preeclampsia, has markedly worse perinatal outcomes, but what are the risks in the cases of isolated oligohydramnios? Other investigators have reported that oligohydramnios in the prolonged pregnancy has an increased risk of meconium staining of the AF, fetal distress in labor, and low 1-minute Apgar scores.[56] A common clinical finding is the existence of a low AFI in an otherwise normal pregnancy, when an ultrasound is obtained for some other reason. Because the diagnosis of oligohydramnios has been associated with poor perinatal outcomes, many women, who are at or near term are sent to labor and delivery to be considered for induction, solely due to the low AFI. Frequently, their cervical examination is unfavorable for induction, and in spite of this, an induction is attempted. This can often result in a cesarean delivery for failed induction. Although the evidence for induction in the prolonged pregnancy is solid, the term or preterm patient with isolated oligohydramnios may not need immediate delivery.

Legrew et al.[60] reported that 41 percent of women with oligohydramnios, as determined by the AFI, had a normal AFI 3 to 4 days later. They also found that a normal AFI measurement was valid for 1 week, suggesting that the test need not be repeated more often than that, except in certain high-risk cases. Other studies have considered the question of isolated oligohydramnios and perinatal outcome. Magann et al.[25] examined 1,001 high-risk women undergoing antepartum testing. They found that those with an AFI of less than 5 cm (19 percent of cases) had similar outcomes to those with normal AFIs, and concluded that an AFI less than 5 cm was not an indication for delivery.[25] Rainford et al.[61] examined 232 women who were greater than 37 weeks of gestation and who had an AFI less than 5 cms (19 percent). They found outcomes to be no worse when compared with those with a normal AFI. In fact, the risk of meconium staining of the AF was found to be increased (35 versus 16 percent) in the normal group.[61] Finally, Casey et al.,[56] examining 6,423 women at greater than 34 weeks' gestation with an AFI less than 5 cm, found increases in intrauterine fetal death (IUFD), admissions to the neonatal intensive care unit (NICU), neonatal death, low birth weight, and meconium aspiration syndrome as compared with women with an AFI greater than 5 cm. If the birth defects and IUGR were removed, there was no difference in admissions to the NICU, neonatal death, or respiratory distress syndrome. This suggests that the IUGR and birth defects contributed to the increased morbidity and mortality, and not the oligohydramnios itself.

There is increasing evidence that patients with isolated oligohydramnios with a normally grown fetus, good fetal movement, and an unfavorable cervix may be candidates for observation or possible therapeutic intervention, or both, to increase the AF level. In subsequent sections of this chapter, we examine efforts to increase AFV.

Midgestation Oligohydramnios

It has been clearly established that when the AFV is greatly decreased, especially in midpregnancy, the perinatal mortality rate approaches 100 percent.[1–3] The cause of the decrease or absence of AF largely determines the perinatal outcome (Table 31-1). With renal agenesis, virtually 100 percent of newborns die due to pulmonary hypoplasia. AF is required during certain periods of early and midgestation for fetal lung development, and without it, the lungs do not develop. If premature rupture of the membranes (PROM) results in a loss of all AF, perinatal outcome will vary based on during which period of gestation the membrane rupture occurred, and whether or not intraamniotic infection was the cause of the

Table 31-1. Fetal and Maternal Causes of Oligohydramnios

Fetal conditions
Renal agenesis
Obstructed uropathy
Spontaneous rupture of the membranes (SROM)
Premature rupture of the membranes (PROM)
Abnormal placentation—elevated MSAFP/MSHCG
Prolonged pregnancy
Maternal conditions
Dehydration-hypovolemia
Hypertensive disorders
Uteroplacental insufficiency
Antiphospholipid syndrome
Idiopathic

MSAFP, maternal serum alpha fetoprotein; MSHCG, maternal serum human chorionic gonadotropin.

membrane rupture.[62] Oligohydramnios can occur with hypertensive disorders or the antiphospholipid syndrome. In these cases, if the fetus is large enough for survival outside of the uterus, there may be little impact on perinatal outcome other than the consequences of prematurity.[62]

Evaluation and Work-Up of Midgestation Oligohydramnios

When the diagnosis of oligohydramnios is made in the second trimester, it is vitally important to obtain a complete history and physical from the patient, as well as a targeted ultrasound. The patient should be questioned for any history consistent with rupture of the membranes, leakage of bloody fluid, or wetness of her underwear. If there is a question of the possible rupture of the membranes, a sterile speculum examination should be performed in an attempt to obtain fluid that can be examined for evidence of rupture. Specific tests include examining for microscopic ferning, checking for a neutral pH on nitrazine paper, and looking for pooling in the posterior vagina. When ferning is present, the sodium chloride concentration is high enough for crystallization or ferning to occur. The sodium chloride concentration of the AF is sufficient to cause ferning, whereas vaginal secretions usually do not fern. Determining the pH of the vaginal fluid can identify the neutral pH of AF as different from the acidic pH of normal vaginal secretions. Next, a targeted ultrasound should be performed to examine for the amount of AF present, the presence of normal anatomy including fetal kidneys and bladder, and finally, for appropriate interval growth. If the fetus is normally grown with kidneys and bladder visualized, more often than not, the fetal membranes have been prematurely ruptured. If kidneys and bladder cannot be seen, then the diagnosis is most likely renal agenesis. The difference between the prognosis of these two entities is dramatic. Renal agenesis is uniformly fatal, whereas PROM can have a reasonable prognosis if it occurs after fetal viability and if infection is not present.

Third-Trimester Oligohydramnios

Although severe oligohydramnios has an increased PMR later in the third trimester, it is still not as high as earlier in pregnancy.[3,56,63] Chamberlain et al.[18] reported a 50-fold increase in PMR when the LVP of AF was less than 1 cm. This data has led many clinicians to induce or deliver women with oligohydramnios, even when there were no other indications for delivery (see discussion above). The Chamberlain et al. study was problematic in that approximately 40 percent of the patients also had IUGR or hypertensive disorders, or both.[18] This could easily explain the increase in mortality.[18] Other studies have reported similar increases in perinatal mortality associated with oligohydramnios, but most have not corrected for other underlying medical conditions.[17] When oligohydramnios is diagnosed in the prolonged pregnancy, there is an increased risk of meconium staining of the AF, meconium aspiration syndrome, fetal distress in labor, and increased cesarean delivery rates.[59,64,65] For these reasons, induction of labor is indicated with oligohydramnios in the prolonged pregnancy. An important question currently under investigation is whether or not a patient with isolated oligohydramnios will have a worse pregnancy outcome if decreased AFV is the only finding. Because induction is indicated for oligohydramnios in the post-date period, many clinicians believe that induction is indicated for oligohydramnios at or close to term.

POLYHYDRAMNIOS

With the increasing use of real-time ultrasound, the diagnosis of polyhydramnios has been on the rise. Previously, the diagnosis of polyhydramnios was made when the uterus was large for gestational age or the fetus could not be easily palpated by Leopold's maneuvers. The diagnosis was often not made until the time of delivery, when large gushes of AF preceded or followed the delivery of the newborn. Polyhydramnios has an impact on perinatal morbidity and mortality based largely on the amount of fluid present, and when in gestation it presents. The earlier in gestation it occurs and the greater the amount of fluid, the higher the morbidity and mortality.[4] The incidence of polyhydramnios has been reported to be about 1 percent in large population-based studies.[66–69] The most common cause for severe polyhydramnios in midgestation is congenital malformations, with or without aneuploidy, and monozygotic twins.[68] Table 31-2 lists maternal and fetal causes of polyhydramnios, including congenital anomalies.

Early ultrasound studies examining polyhydramnios used the LVP method for measuring AFV. Most authors report an LVP of greater than 8 cm to define polyhydramnios.[68] Hill et al. divided their patients with polyhydramnios into three groups: mild (LVP 8 to 11 cm, 79 percent of cases), moderate (LVP 12 to 15 cm, 16.5 percent cases), and severe (LVP 16+cm, 5 percent of cases). Overall the perinatal mortality rate was 127.5/1,000, which corrected to 58.8/1,000 when lethal malformations were removed.[68] This value is markedly increased

Table 31-2. Fetal and Maternal Causes of Polyhydramnios

Fetal conditions
Congenital anomalies
Gastrointestinal obstruction
CNS abnormalities
Cystic hygromas
Nonimmune hydrops
Sacrococcygeal teratoma
Aneuploidy
Twin-to-twin transfusion syndrome
Muscular dystrophy syndromes
Maternal conditions
Idiopathic
Poorly controlled diabetes mellitus

CNS, central nervous system.

over the background rate. Hill et al. found that with mild polyhydramnios, a specific diagnosis for the cause of polyhydramnios could only be found 16 percent of the time.[68] This diagnosis increased to a rate of 90 percent for moderate polyhydramnios, and 100 percent for severe polyhydramnios.[68] In a follow-up study, Many et al.[70] examined 275 women with polyhydramnios to determine if the degree of polyhydramnios had an impact on the rate of prematurity. Although excessive amniotic fluid did not impact the rate of prematurity, the presence of anomalies or diabetes mellitus was associated with an increased risk of preterm delivery.[70]

Later in pregnancy, with milder degrees of polyhydramnios, the cause is usually idiopathic or related to diabetes.[68–72] At present, there are no uniformly accepted criteria for making the diagnosis of polyhydramnios. Brace and Wolf[16] defined polyhydramnios as being present when the actual fluid volume was greater than 2,100 ml (2.5 percent incidence), but an actual measurement of AFV is difficult and clinically impractical.

Using the four-quadrant AFI, Moore and Cayle[22] reported the AFI for varying gestational ages (see Fig. 31-3) and concluded that one value for the AFI cannot be used throughout gestation but must be referenced to gestational age. The study found the 97.5 percentile at 35 weeks of gestation to be 27.9 cm, which represents the upper limits of normal for that gestational age. This value would clearly be abnormally increased for earlier and later measurements in gestation (see Fig. 31-3).

Midgestation Polyhydramnios

The pregnant woman who presents with a rapidly enlarging uterus in midpregnancy, or who presents in preterm labor, will most likely have a fetus with a congenital malformation or aneuploidy, or both.[68] Severe polyhydramnios in the second trimester has a significant PMR, which is most commonly due to prematurity or aneuploidy.[73,74] The more common congenital malformations associated with severe polyhydramnios include the host of defects associated with gastrointestinal obstruction. Esophageal atresia with or without tracheoesophageal fistula can present with early-onset severe polyhydramnios owing to the blockage of fetal swallowing. With certain malformations, AFV may still be normal because a tracheoesophageal fistula, for example, provides for the movement of fluid into the stomach, and thus, polyhydramnios may not develop.[75] Other gastrointestinal obstructions such as duodenal atresia may result in polyhydramnios.[68] Whenever a structural defect is seen in a fetus, consideration should be given to performing a karyotype owing to the dramatic increase in aneuploidy seen with one or more structural defects. Knowing the karyotype of the fetus with a defect may allow for further treatment options, or possible pregnancy termination. The fetus with polyhydramnios and trisomy 18 would be a candidate for pregnancy termination at any point in the pregnancy owing to the lethal nature of trisomy 18.

Another common cause of acute, severe, polyhydramnios in the second trimester is the condition associated with the twin-to-twin transfusion syndrome (TTS). This may be found in single placenta, monozygotic twin pregnancies. With identical twins who share a single placenta, 90 percent of the fetuses will have vascular connections between the arteries and veins on the surface of the placenta.[76] The most common connection is the artery-to-artery connection, followed by the vein-to-vein connection. The least common connection is the artery of one twin connecting to the vein of the other. This can lead to oligohydramnios of the twin with the arterial connection, and polyhydramnios in the twin with the venous connection. If the polyhydramnios/oligohydramnios is severe enough, the PMR can approach 100 percent without treatment. However, survival improves to 50 to 70 percent with intervention.[4,5] Intervention in TTS is discussed later in the chapter under therapies for polyhydramnios and in Chapter 28.

Third-Trimester Polyhydramnios

When polyhydramnios occurs in the third trimester of pregnancy, it is usually mild and not associated with a structural defect.[68] Table 31-2 lists many of the causes of polyhydramnios. Despite the fact that a diagnosis can be determined for the majority of early-onset cases, for the vast majority of cases in the third trimester, a diagnosis cannot be found. Thus, these cases are given the diagnosis of idiopathic. Despite this, however, the other causes of polyhydramnios must be ruled out before the idiopathic label can be applied.

In many cases, polyhydramnios may be transient. Golan et al.[69] examined 113 cases of polyhydramnios. On repeated examination, patients separated into two groups: Those cases in which the polyhydramnios worsened or the AFV remained markedly elevated, and those whose AFV returned to normal, or decreased to mild polyhydramnios.[69] In the former group, all complications of pregnancy were greater, including preterm delivery (2.7-fold increase), preeclampsia (2.7-fold increase), IUFD (7.7-fold increase), and neonatal demise (7.7-fold increase). In the latter group in which the polyhydramnios improved or AFV returned to normal, the most common diagnosis was idiopathic and showed a favorable outcome.[69] This study would suggest that if polyhydramnios is persistent, the fetus should be examined closely for congenital malformations and aneuploidy, and monitored to prevent an IUFD. In addition, the mother should be watched closely for other medical complications of pregnancy.[69]

Treatment of Oligohydramnios

Because of the increase in perinatal morbidity and mortality associated with oligohydramnios in the prolonged pregnancy, most authors recommend delivery in these cases. As discussed earlier, however, the patient who presents with isolated oligohydramnios in the third trimester may be a candidate for continued observation.[25,56,61] Several investigators have attempted to treat oligohydramnios with the oral administration of water in the hope of "hydrating" the fetus through the mother. Animal studies have demonstrated that there is a close relationship between the hydration or dehydration of the mother and the fetus.[77,78] Attempts to dehydrate the mother have resulted in dehydration of the fetus, and in some cases vice versa. In human pregnancies, Goodlin et al.[79] found that the maternal intravascular volume was low in cases of idiopathic oligohydramnios, and that by increasing the intravascular volume, the oligohydramnios resolved. In their initial study of the use of oral hydration as a treatment for women with a low AFI, Kilpatrick et al.[80] randomized women into two groups: The treatment group was told to drink 2 liters of water within 4 hours of a repeat AFI, and a control group that did not drink the 2 liters of water.

The treatment group had a significantly greater increase in AFI on repeat testing (6.3 cm) than the control group (5.1 cm).[80] They concluded that the oral administration of water could increase the AFI in women with oligohydramnios.[80] A follow-up study by the same group observed that women with normal AFV could increase or decrease their AFI depending upon the amount of water the mothers drank.[81] As demonstrated in Table 31-3, the AFI significantly increased in the oral hydration group as compared with the control group. The control group was given what was thought to be a "normal" volume of water to drink, but as can be seen from Table 31-3, the AFI actually decreased and urine osmolality increased. This suggests that the mothers were actually dehydrated during the control portion of the study. Both groups demonstrated that the AFI can be influenced by increasing or decreasing water intake orally.

Many other studies have shown a similar improvement in AFV with either oral or intravenous administration of water and/or crystalloids.[82,83] Several researchers have reported success in improving AFV in women with oligohydramnios by the injection of a crystalloid solution into the amniotic compartment during an amniocentesis.[84] The injection of fluid also allows for a more complete ultrasound examination of the fetus, which previously was not available owing to the lack of AF. Most of these studies, however, have been case reports, and because no large prospective studies have been performed, the routine use of amniocentesis for cases of marked oligohydramnios in midgestation cannot be justified by the literature.

Table 31-3. Change in Amniotic Fluid Index 4–6 hours After Oral Water Hydration

	CONTROL (N = 20)	HYDRATION (N = 20)
Pretreatment		
AFI (cm)	17.7 ± 5.0	18.4 ± 4.7
USG	1.013 + 0.007	1.015 + 0.008
Post treatment		
AFI (cm)	16.2 ± 4.5*	21.4 ± 4.5#
USG	1.019 ± 0.009#	1.006 ± 0.006#
Delta AFI (cm)	−1.5 ± 2.7	3.0 ± 2.4
Intake (ml)	1576 + 607	1596 + 465

AFI, Amniotic fluid index; USG, urine specific gravity; Delta AFI, change in AFI form pre- to posttreatment. *, P < 0.02, paired t test, pre vs post treatment, #, P < 0.0001, paired t test pre vs post treatment. Intake, amount of fluid intake over the previous 24 hours other than the 2 liters.

From Kilpatrick SJ, Safford KL: Maternal hydration increases amniotic fluid index in women with normal amniotic fluid. Obstet Gynecol 81:50, 1993.

Oligohydramnios in Labor

Almost 30 years ago, Gabbe et al.[85] working with fetal monkeys, noted that when AF was removed from the amniotic compartment, variable decelerations in the fetal heart rate developed. These decelerations resolved when the AF was replaced, suggesting that cord compression was the cause of the decelerations. Since that time, multiple investigators have studied amnioinfusion as a technique by which to treat variable decelerations in labor. Although most report a decrease in the frequency of variable decelerations, few have demonstrated any decrease in perinatal morbidity or mortality, or the cesarean delivery rate.[86–90] Amnioinfusion has been studied as a possible therapy in the case of thick meconium. In several prospective studies, it has been shown to improve neonatal outcomes, including meconium visualized below the newborn vocal cords, and meconium aspiration syndrome.[91–94] Sadovsky et al.[94] found that with the randomization of women with greater than light meconium to a control or amnioinfusion treatment group, 29 percent of control newborns had meconium below the umbilical cords, whereas none of the treated newborns did. Two meta-analyses that examined the therapeutic use of amnioinfusion for thick meconium demonstrated between a 75 and 84 percent reduction in meconium below the vocal cords at delivery, confirming that it should be offered to women who present with thick meconium.[95,96] Of note, a recent, multicenter, randomized trial of 1,998 women in labor at 36 weeks' gestation or later with thick meconium did not find that amnioinfusion reduced the risk of moderate or severe meconium aspiration syndrome or perinatal death.[97] The authors concluded that amnioinfusion should not be recommended to prevent meconium aspiration syndrome.

Treatment of Polyhydramnios

Treatment options for patients with polyhydramnios are usually tailored to the underlying cause of the polyhydramnios. With mild idiopathic polyhydramnios, in which the work-up is negative, and follow-up ultrasound demonstrates persistent polyhydramnios, the only possible intervention might be antepartum testing with fetal kick counts, or nonstress tests. When poorly controlled diabetes mellitus is the cause of the polyhydramnios, proper glycemic control may be beneficial as a treatment option.[71,72] With the current aggressive management of diabetes in pregnancy, it is rare to see severe polyhydramnios associated with diabetes. Usually, if the diabetes is not well controlled, then the mother will undergo antepartum testing to assess fetal well-being.

Polyhydramnios associated with a fetal structural abnormality such as an obstruction to swallowing, usually requires invasive testing by amniocentesis to rule out aneuploidy. Often, the degree of polyhydramnios in these cases is severe and the resulting overdistention of the uterus causes preterm labor long before the due date. In these cases, one medical treatment option involves the administration of a prostaglandin inhibitor such as indomethacin, which works by decreasing fetal urine production.[98–100] Prostaglandin inhibitors have been shown to decrease fetal urine output significantly. This effect occurs within 5 hours of starting the medication and decreases AFV within 24 hours.[98,99] Although indomethacin has been shown to be relatively safe when given over a short period of time, such as 72 hours, prolonged usage may be associated with risks to the fetus. Prolonged use has been shown to cause premature closure, or narrowing, of the ductus venosus within the fetal heart and renal abnormalities in the newborn period.[97,100] Complications related to indomethacin use worsen with advancing gestational age, and such treatment beyond 31 to 32 weeks of gestation should be avoided.[101] Because of the adverse effects on the fetus associated with the long-term use of indomethacin, it probably has limited use in pregnancy for the treatment of severe polyhydramnios.

For those pregnancies complicated by the TTS, or for the fetus with obstructed swallowing, repetitive amnioreductions may be required to reduce the AFV until the fetus reaches viability.[5,101,102] Severe cases of TTS, if left untreated, can have a PMR approaching 100 percent. Repetitive amnioreductions, in which an amniocentesis is performed and AF is withdrawn until the AFI is normal, can reduce the PMR from 100 percent to about 50 percent.[5,102,103] Further options for the treatment of the TTS include the ablation of the connecting blood vessels by laser photocoagulation via fetoscopy.[104] A recent large prospective trial found that the laser ablation of the connecting blood vessels resulted in better outcomes for the twin pregnancy as compared with amnioreduction alone.[105] A major problem with laser ablation is that only certain centers perform the procedure, and most insurance companies will not pay for the procedure. This is not the case with amnioreductions, which can be performed anywhere and, therefore, are usually covered by insurance. Although laser ablation treatment may "cure" the cause of the TTS, amnioreduction only treats the symptoms. As a result, the amnioreduction method of treatment may require repeated procedures every 1 to 2 weeks for the remainder of the pregnancy.

KEY POINTS

- Amniotic fluid is seldom considered important until polyhydramnios or oligohydramnios occurs, either of which may significantly impact perinatal survival.
- Amniotic fluid is dynamic, with large volume flows into and out of the amniotic compartment each day.
- Clinical estimates of actual amniotic fluid volume through ultrasound measurements of the AFI or LVP are not very accurate at predicting true volume.
- Oligohydramnios, in the presence of IUGR or a prolonged gestation, is associated with significant increases in perinatal morbidity and mortality.
- Preterm or term isolated oligohydramnios, with an otherwise normal fetus, is not associated with an increase in perinatal morbidity or mortality.
- Early-onset or severe polyhydramnios is associated with a significant increase in aneuploidy, congenital malformations, preterm delivery, and perinatal mortality.
- The cause of mild polyhydramnios, especially in the latter part of the third trimester, is usually idiopathic, or related to diabetes mellitus, and has little positive or negative impact on perinatal survival.
- Amniotic fluid volume as estimated by the amniotic fluid index, can be increased or decreased by the amount of water ingested orally.
- Indomethacin, which decreases fetal renal and possibly pulmonary fluid production, can decrease AFV over time when taken orally.
- Absorption of amniotic fluid directly from the amniotic compartment into the blood vessels on the fetal surface of the placenta can explain the large differences between fetal swallowing and urine production.

REFERENCES

1. Hackett GA, Nicolaides KH, Campbell S. The value of Doppler ultrasound assessment of fetal and uteroplacental circulations when severe oligohydramnios complicates the second trimester of pregnancy. Br J Obstet Gynaecol 94:1074, 1987.
2. Barss VA, Benacerraf BR, Frigoletto FD: Second trimester oligohydramnios, a predictor of poor fetal outcome. Obstet Gynecol 64:608, 1984.
3. Mercer LJ, Brown LG: Fetal outcome with oligohydramnios in the second trimester. Obstet Gynecol 67:840, 1986.
4. Wier PE, Raten G, Beisher N: Acute polyhydramnios- a complication of monozygous twin pregnancy. Br J Obstet Gynaecol 86: 849, 1979.
5. Reisner DP, Mahony BS, Petty CN, et al: Stuck twin syndrome: outcome in thirty-seven consecutive cases. Am J Obstet Gynecol 169:991, 1993.
6. Gilbert WM, Brace RA: The missing link in amniotic fluid volume regulation: Intramembranous absorption. Obstet Gynecol 74:748, 1989.
7. Gilbert WM, Brace RA: Novel determination of filtration coefficient of ovine placenta and intramembranous pathway. Am J Physiol 259:R1281, 1990.
8. Gilbert WM, Cheung CY, Brace RA: Rapid intramembranous absorption into the fetal circulation of arginine vasopressin injected intraamniotically. Am J Obstet Gynecol 164:1013, 1991.
9. Magann EF, Nolan TE, Hess LW, et al: Measurement of amniotic fluid volume: accuracy of ultrasonography techniques. Am J Obstet Gynecol 167:1533, 1992.

10. Horsager R, Nathan L, Leveno KJ: Correlation of measured amniotic fluid volume and sonographic predictions of oligohydramnios. Obstet Gynecol 83:955, 1994.
11. Magann EF, Bass JD, Chauhan SP, et al: Amniotic fluid volume in normal singleton pregnancies. Obstet Gynecol 90:524, 1997.
12. Magann EF, Doherty DA, Field K, et al: Biophysical profile with amniotic fluid volume assessments. Obstet Gynecol. 104:5, 2004. Comment in: Obstet Gynecol 104:3, 2004.
13. Magann EF, Doherty DA, Chauhan SP, et al: Dye-determined amniotic fluid volume and intrapartum/neonatal outcome. J Perinatol 24:423, 2004.
14. Magann EF, Doherty DA, Chauhan SP, et al: How well do the amniotic fluid index and single deepest pocket indices (below the 3rd and 5th and above the 95th and 97th percentiles) predict oligohydramnios and hydramnios? Am J Obstet Gynecol 190:164, 2004.
15. Magann EF, Doherty DA, Chauhan SP, et al: Is there a relationship to dye determined or ultrasound estimated amniotic fluid volume adjusted percentiles and fetal weight adjusted percentiles? Am J Obstet Gynecol 190:1610, 2004.
16. Brace RA, Wolf EJ: Characterization of normal gestational changes amniotic fluid volume. Am J Obstet Gynecol 161:382, 1989.
17. Manning FA, Hill LM, Platt LD: Qualitative amniotic fluid volume determination by ultrasound: antepartum detection of intrauterine growth retardation. Am J Obstet Gynecol 139:254, 1981.
18. Chamberlain PF, Manning FA, Morrison I, et al: Ultrasound evaluation of amniotic fluid volume. I: The relationship of marginal and decreased amniotic fluid volumes to perinatal outcome. Am J Obstet Gynecol 150:245, 1984.
19. Mercer LJ, Brown LG, Petres RE, et al: A survey of pregnancies complicated by decreased amniotic fluid. Am J Obstet Gynecol 149:355, 1984.
20. Phelan JP, Ohn MO, Smith CV, et al: Amniotic fluid index measurements during pregnancy. J Reprod Med 32:603, 1987.
21. Rutherford SE, Phelan JP, Smith CV, et al: The four quadrant assessment of amniotic fluid volume: an adjunct to antepartum fetal heart rate testing. Obstet Gynecol 70:353, 1987.
22. Moore TR, Cayle JE: The amniotic fluid index in normal human pregnancy. Am J Obstet Gynecol 162:1168, 1990.
23. Dildy GA III, Lira N, Moise KJ, et al: Amniotic fluid volume assessment: comparison of ultrasonographic estimates versus direct measurements with a dye-dilution technique in human pregnancies. Am J Obstet Gynecol 167:986, 1992.
24. Magann EF, Doherty DA, Chauhan SP, et al: Effect of maternal hydration on amniotic fluid volume. Obstet Gynecol 101:1261, 2003.
25. Magann EF, Chauhan SP, Barrilleaux PS, et al: Amniotic fluid index and single deepest pocket: Weak indicators of abnormal amniotic volumes. Obstet Gynecol 96:737, 2000.
26. Moore TR: Superiority of the four-quadrant sum over the single-deepest-pocket technique in ultrasonographic identification of abnormal amniotic fluid volumes. Am J Obstet Gynecol 163:762, 1990.
27. Flack NJ, Dore C, Southwell D, et al: The influence of operator transducer pressure on ultrasonographic measurements of amniotic fluid volume. Am J Obstet Gynecol 171:218, 1994.
28. Tomoda S, Brace RA, Longo L: Amniotic fluid volume and fetal swallowing rate in sheep. Am J Physiol 249:R133, 1985.
29. Alexander DP, Nixon DA, Widdas WF, et al: Gestational variations in the composition in the foetal fluids and foetal urine in the sheep. J Physiol 140:1, 1958
30. Mellor DJ, Slater JS: Daily changes in foetal urine and relationships with amniotic and allantoic fluid and maternal plasma during the last two months of pregnancy in conscious, unstressed ewes with chronically implanted catheters. J Physiol 227:503, 1972
31. Adamson TM, Brodecky V, Lambert TF, et al: The production and composition of lung liquids in the in-utero foetal lamb. *In* Comline RS, Cross KW, Dawes GS, Nathaniel PW (eds): Foetal and Neonatal Physiology. Cambridge, UK, Cambridge University Press, 1973, p 208.
32. Gresham EL, Rankin JHG, Makowski EL, et al: An evaluation of fetal renal function in a chronic sheep preparation. J Clin Invest 51:149, 1972.
33. Wintour EM, Barnes A, Brown EH, et al: Regulation of amniotic fluid volume and composition on the ovine fetus. Obstet Gynecol 52:689, 1978.
34. Wladimiroff JW, Campbell S: Fetal urine-production rates in normal and complicated pregnancy. Lancet 1:151, 1974.
35. Campbell S, Wladimiroff JW, Dewhurst CJ: The antenatal measurement of fetal urine production. J Obstet Gynaecol Br Commonw 80:680, 1973.
36. Van Otterlo LC, Wladimiroff JW, Wallenburg HCS: Relationship between fetal urine production and amniotic fluid volume in normal pregnancy and pregnancy complicated by diabetes. Br J Obstet Gynaecol 84:205, 1977.
37. Kurjak A, Kirkinsen P, Latin V, et al: Ultrasonic assessment of fetal kidney function in normal and complicated pregnancies. Am J Obstet Gynecol 141:266, 1981.
38. Deutinger J, Bartl W, Pfersmann C, et al: Fetal kidney volume and urine production in cases of fetal growth retardation. J Perinat Med 15:307, 1987.
39. Rabinowitz R, Peters MT, Vyas S, et al: Measurement of fetal urine production in normal pregnancy by real-time ultrasonography. Am J Obstet Gynecol 161:1264, 1989.
40. Duenhoelter JH, Pritchard JA: Fetal respiration: quantitative measurements of amniotic fluid inspired near term by human and rhesus fetuses. Am J Obstet Gynecol 125:306, 1976.
41. Seeds AE: Current concepts of amniotic fluid dynamics. Am J Obstet Gynecol 138:575, 1980.
42. Mescher EJ, Platzker A, Ballard PL, et al: Ontogeny of tracheal fluid, pulmonary surfactant, and plasma corticoids in the fetal lamb. J Appl Physiol 39:1017, 1975.
43. Olver RE, Strang LB: Ion fluxes across the pulmonary epithelium and the secretion of lung liquid in the foetal lamb. J Physiol 241:327, 1974.
44. Lawson EE, Brown ER, Torday JS, et al: The effect of epinephrine on tracheal fluid flow and surfactant efflux in fetal sheep. Am Rev Respir Dis 118:1023, 1978.
45. Brace RA, Wlodek ME, Cook ML, et al: Swallowing of lung liquid and amniotic fluid by the ovine fetus under normoxic and hypoxic conditions. Am J Obstet Gynecol 171:764, 1994.
46. Patrick J, Campbell K, Carmichael L, et al: Patterns of human fetal breathing at 30–31 and 38–39 weeks' gestational age. Obstet Gynecol 56:24, 1980.
47. Sherman DJ, Ross MG, Day L, et al: Fetal Swallowing: correlation of electromyography and esophageal fluid flow. Am J Physiol 258:R1386, 1990.
48. Prichard JA: Deglutition by normal and anencephalic fetuses. Obstet Gynecol 25:289, 1965.
49. Abramovich DR: Fetal factors influencing the volume and composition of liquor amnii. J Obstet Gynaecol Britt Commw 77:865, 1970.
50. Gilbert WM, Moore TR, Brace RA: Amniotic fluid volume dynamics. Fetal Med Rev 3:89, 1991.
51. Gilbert WM, Eby-Wilkens EM, Tarantal AF: The missing-link in Rhesus monkey amniotic fluid volume regulation: Intramembranous absorption. Obstet Gynecol 892:462, 1997.
52. Heller L: Intrauterine amino acid feeding of the fetus. *In* Bode H, Warshaw J (eds): Parenternal Nutrition in Infancy and Childhood. New York, NY, Plenum Press, 1974, p 206.
53. Renaud R, Kirschtetter L, Koehl D, et al: Amino-acid intra-amniotic injections. *In* Persianinov LS, Chervakova TV, Presl J (eds): Recent Progress in Obstetrics and Gynaecology. Amsterdam, Excerpta Medica, 1974, p 234.
54. Jang PR, Brace RA: Amniotic fluid composition changes during urine drainage and tracheoesophageal occlusion in fetal sheep. Am J Obstet Gynecol 167:1732, 1992.
55. Faber JJ, Anderson DF: Absorption of amniotic fluid by amniochorion in sheep. Am J Physiol 282:H850, 2002.
56. Casey BM, McIntire DD, Bloom SL, et al: Pregnancy outcomes after anterpartum diagnosis of oligohydramnios at or beyond 34 weeks' gestation. Am J Obstet Gynecol 182:909, 2000.
57. Manning FA, Harmon CR, Morrison I, et al: Fetal assessment based on fetal biophysical profile scoring. IV. An analysis of perinatal morbidity and mortality. Am J Obstet Gynecol 162:703, 1990.
58. Halperin ME, Fong KW, Zalev AH, et al: Reliability of amniotic fluid volume estimation from ultrasonograms: intraobserver and

interobserver variation before and after the establishment of criteria. Am J Obstet Gynecol 153:264, 1985.
59. Crowley P, O'Herlihy C, Boylan P: The value of ultrasound measurement of amniotic fluid volume in the management of prolonged pregnancies. Br J Obstet Gynaecol 91:444, 1984.
60. Lagrew DC, Pircon RA, Nageotte M, et al: How frequently should the amniotic fluid index be repeated? Am J Obstet Gynecol 167:1129, 1992.
61. Rainford M, Adair R, Scialli AR, et al: Amniotic fluid index in the uncomplicated term pregnancy. Prediction of outcome. J Repro Med 46:589, 2001.
62. Hill MH: Oligohydramnios: Sonographic Diagnosis and Clinical Implications. Clin Obstet Gynecol 40:314, 1997.
63. Jeng CJ, Lee JF, Wang KG, et al: Decreased amniotic fluid index in term pregnancy. Clinical significance. J Reprod Med 37:789, 1992.
64. Chauhan SP: Amniotic fluid index before and after amnioinfusion of a fixed volume of normal saline. J Reprod Med 36:801, 1991.
65. Grubb DK, Paul RH: Amniotic fluid index and prolonged antepartum fetal heart rate decelerations. Obstet Gynecol 9:558, 1992.
66. Chamberlain PF, Manning FA, Morrison I, et al: Ultrasound evaluation of amniotic fluid volume II: The relationship of increased amniotic fluid volume to perinatal outcome. Am J Obstet Gynecol 150:250, 1984.
67. Biggio JR Jr, Wenstrom KD, Dubard MB, et al: Hydramnios prediction of adverse perinatal outcome. Obstet Gynecol 94:773, 1999.
68. Hill LM, Breckle R, Thomas ML, et al: Polyhydramnios: Ultrasonically detected prevalence and neonatal outcome. Obstet Gynecol 69:21, 1987.
69. Golan A, Wolman I, Sagi J, et al: Persistence of polyhydramnios during pregnancy-its significance and correlation with maternal and fetal complications. Gynecol Obstet Invest 37:18, 1994.
70. Many A, Hill LM, Lazebnik N, et al: The association between polyhydramnios and preterm delivery. Obstet Gynecol 86:389, 1995.
71. Bartha JL, Martinez-Del-Fresno P, Comino-Delgado R: Early diagnosis of gestational diabetes mellitus and prevention of diabetes-related complications. Eur J Obstet Gynecol Reprod Biol 109:41, 2003.
72. Thomas A, Kaur S, Somville T: Abnormal glucose screening test followed by normal glucose tolerance test and pregnancy outcome. Saudi Med J 23:814, 2002.
73. Pauer HU, Viereck V, Krauss V, et al: Incidence of fetal malformations in pregnancies complicated by oligo- and polyhydramnios. Arch Gynecol Obstet 268:52, 2003.
74. Desmedt EJ, Henry OA, Beischer NA: Polyhydramnios and associated maternal and fetal complications in singleton pregnancies. Br J Obstet Gynaecol 97:1115, 1990.
75. Lloyd JR, Clatworthy HW: Hydramnios as aid to the early diagnosis of congenital obstruction of the alimentary tract: A Study of the maternal and fetal factors. Pediatrics June:903, 1958.
76. Benirschke K: Twin placenta in perinatal mortality. NY State J Med 61:1499, 1961.
77. Ross MG, Ervin MG, Leake RD, et al: Bulk flow of amniotic fluid water in response to maternal osmotic challenge. Am J Obstet Gynecol 147:697, 1983.
78. Woods LL: Fetal renal contribution to amniotic fluid osmolality during maternal hypertonicity. Am J Physiol 250:R235, 1986.
79. Goodlin RC, Anderson JC, Gallagher TF: Relationship between amniotic fluid volume and maternal plasma volume expansion. Am J Obstet Gynecol 146:505, 1983.
80. Kilpatrick SJ, Safford K, Pomeroy T, et al: Maternal hydration affects amniotic fluid index (AFI). Am J Obstet Gynecol 164:361, 1991.
81. Kilpatrick SJ, Safford KL: Maternal hydration increases amniotic fluid index in women with normal amniotic fluid volumes. Obstet Gynecol 81:49,1993.
82. Flack NJ, Sepulveda W, Bower S, et al: Acute maternal hydration in third-trimester oligohydramnios: effects on amniotic fluid volume, uteroplacental perfusion, and fetal blood flow and urine output. Am J Obstet Gynecol 173:1186, 1996.
83. Doi S, Osada H, Seki K, et al: Effect of maternal hydration on oligohydramnios: a comparison of three volume expansion methods. Obstet Gynecol 92:525, 1998.
84. Sepulveda W, Flack NJ, Fisk NM: Direct volume measurement at midtrimester amnioinfusion in relation to ultrasonographic indexes of amniotic fluid volume. Am J Obstet Gynecol 170:1160, 1994.
85. Gabbe SG, Ettinger BB, Freeman RK, et al: Umbilical cord compression associated with amniotomy: laboratory observations. Am J Obstet Gynecol 126:353, 1976.
86. Nageotte MP, Bertucci L, Towers CV, et al: Prophylactic amnioinfusion in pregnancies complicated by oligohydramnios: a prospective study. Obstet Gynecol 77:677, 1991.
87. Ogundipe OA, Spong CY, Ross MG: Prophylactic amnioinfusion for oligohydramnios: A reevaluation. Obstet Gynecol 84:544, 1994.
88. Schrimmer DB, Macri CJ, Paul RH: Prophylactic amnioinfusion as a treatment for oligohydramnios I laboring patients: a prospective randomized trial. Am J Obstet Gynecol 165:972, 1991.
89. Miyazaki FS, Taylor NA: Saline amnioinfusion for relief of variable or prolonged decelerations. Am J Obstet Gynecol 146:670, 1983.
90. Chanhan SP, Rutherford SE, Hess LW, et al: Prophylactic intrapartum amnioinfusion for patients with oligohydramnios. J Reprod Med 37:817, 1992.
91. Wenstrom KD, Parsons MT: The prevention of meconium aspiration in labor using amnioinfusion. Obstet Gynecol 73:647, 1989.
92. Eriksen NL, Hostetter M, Parisi VM: Prophylactic amnioinfusion in pregnancies complicated by thick meconium. Am J Obstet Gynecol 171:1026, 1994.
93. Macri CJ, Schrimmer DB, Leung A, et al: Prophylactic amnioinfusion improves outcome of pregnancy complicated by thick meconium and oligohydramnios. Am J Obstet Gynecol 167:117, 1992.
94. Sadovsky Y, Amon E, Bade ME, et al: Prophylactic amnioinfusion during labor complicated by meconium: A preliminary report. Am J Obstet Gynecol 161:613, 1989.
95. Glantz JC, Letteney DL: Pumps and warmers during amnioinfusion: Is either necessary? Obstet Gynecol 87:150, 1996.
96. Pierce J, Gaudier FL, Sanchez-Ramos L: Intrapartum amnioinfusion for meconium-stained fluid: Meta-analysis of prospective trials. Obstet Gynecol 95:1051, 2000.
97. Fraser WD, Hofmeyr J, Lede R, et al: Amnioinfusion for the prevention of the meconium aspiration syndrome. N Engl J Med 353:909, 2005.
98. Stevenson KM, Lumbers ER: Effects of indomethacin on fetal renal function, renal and umbilicoplacental blood flow and lung liquid production. J Dev Physiol 17:257, 1992.
99. Kirshon B, Moise KJ, Wasserstrum N, et al: Influence of short-term indomethacin therapy on fetal urine output. Obstet Gynecol 72:51, 1988.
100. Mamopoulos M, Assimakopoulos E, Reece EA, et al: Maternal indomethacin therapy in the treatment of polyhydramnios. Am J Obstet Gynecol 162:1225, 1990.
101. Moise KJ: Polyhydramnios. Clin Obstet Gynecol 40:266, 1997.
102. Elliott JP, Urig MA, Clewell WH: Aggressive therapeutic amniocentesis for treatment of twin- twin transfusion syndrome. Obstet Gynecol 77:537, 1991.
103. Dickinson JE: Severe twin-twin transfusion syndrome: Current management concepts. Aust NZ J Obstet Gynaecol 35:16, 1995.
104. De Lia JE, Cruikshank DP, Keye WR: Fetoscopic neodymium: yag laser occlusion of placental vessels in severe twin-twin transfusion syndrome. Obstet Gynecol 75:1046, 1990.
105. Senat MV, Deprest J, Boulvain M, et al: Endoscopic laser surgery versus serial amnioreduction for severe twin-to-twin transfusion syndrome. N Engl J Med 351:136, 2004.

Prolonged Pregnancy

MICHAEL Y. DIVON

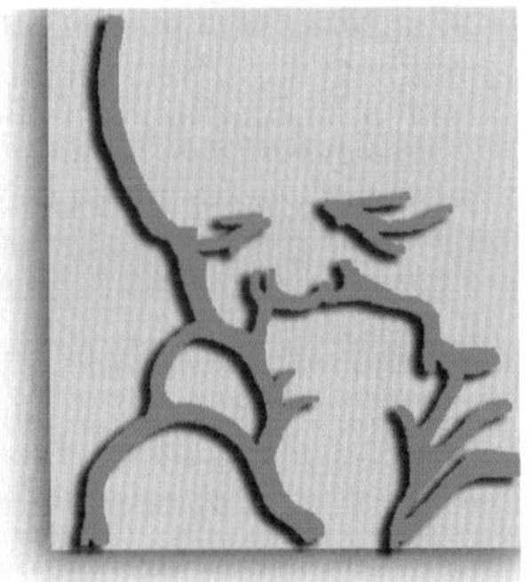

CHAPTER 32

KEY ABBREVIATIONS

American College of Obstetricians and Gynecologists	ACOG
Amniotic fluid index	AFI
Appropriate for gestational age	AGA
Central nervous system	CNS
Confidence interval	CI
Corticotropin-releasing hormone	CRH
Estimated fetal weight	EFW
Fetal heart rate	FHR
Gestational age	GA
Large for gestational age	LGA
Last menstrual period	LMP
Neonatal intensive care unit	NICU
Nucleated red blood cell	NRBC
Nonstress test	NST
Odds ratio	OR
Prostaglandin	PG
Relative risk	RR
Small for gestational age	SGA

In 1902, Ballantyne questioned the ability of the placenta to support the fetus that "has stayed too long in intrauterine surroundings."[1] Ballantyne further stated that the postmature infant "has remained so long in utero that his difficulty is to be born with safety to himself and his mother." For the better part of the 20th century, most authors recognized that prolonged pregnancy was associated with an increased risk for fetal macrosomia and its related morbidity but believed that the risk of adverse perinatal outcome was small relative to the risks related to induction of labor in the presence of an unfavorable uterine cervix. In 1954, Clifford recognized that prolonged pregnancy could result in fetal growth restriction when he described the "postmaturity with placental dysfunction syndrome."[2] Clifford suggested that these neonates appeared malnourished due to recent weight loss, with loose, peeling skin and meconium staining. Birth asphyxia, meconium aspiration, and perinatal death were reported in severe cases.

It was only in the 1970s that it became apparent that perinatal mortality was significantly increased in prolonged pregnancies, and that fetal surveillance combined with selective use of induction of labor might result in improved perinatal outcome.

DEFINITION

Different terms are used loosely to describe pregnancies whose duration has exceeded the upper limit of a normal term gestation. The lack of consensus regarding definitions of terms such as "postmaturity," "postdates," "postterm" or "prolonged pregnancy," combined with the absence of a precise definition of the upper limit of a normal term gestation, result in a wide range of pregnancies reported as "prolonged pregnancy."

The definition of the upper limit of a normal pregnancy is somewhat arbitrary and certainly imprecise. The standard definition of a prolonged pregnancy is 42 completed weeks of gestation (i.e., 294 days after the first day of the last menstrual period [LMP]) or more. This definition is endorsed by the American College of Obstetricians

Clinical Features Associated with Prolonged Pregnancy

1. Incorrect dates
2. Biologic variability
3. Maternal factors: previous prolonged pregnancy, primiparity
4. Fetal factors: congenital anomalies (e.g., adrenal hypoplasia, anencephaly)
5. Placental factors: sulfatase deficiency

and Gynecologists (ACOG), The World Health Organization, and the International Federation of Gynecology and Obstetrics.[3–5] It is based on data derived before the widespread use of fetal surveillance modalities and the use of ultrasound for pregnancy dating. In view of more recent perinatal mortality data that were derived from accurately dated pregnancies, it would be reasonable to conclude that prolonged pregnancy should be defined as a gestational age at birth of greater than or equal to 41 weeks of gestation (see section Perinatal Morbidity and Mortality, later).

The incidence of prolonged pregnancy varies depending on the criteria used to define gestational age at birth. It is estimated that 4 to 19 percent of pregnancies reach or exceed 42 weeks' gestation and 2 to 7 percent complete 43 weeks' gestation. Ventura and colleagues estimated that approximately 520,000 of the 4 million neonates born in the United States during 1993 were born at 41 weeks' gestation, whereas approximately 360,000 were born at or beyond 42 weeks' gestation.[6] Prolonged pregnancy is not only a common clinical entity, it is also associated with an increased financial burden (primarily due to increased utilization of sonography, fetal testing, induction of labor, and cesarean delivery).[7]

ETIOLOGY

Labor is a poorly defined biologic process involving fetal, placental, and maternal signals.[8,9] Recent data suggest that human parturition is determined by placental release of corticotropin-releasing hormone (CRH) and that women who have low levels of this hormone are more likely to deliver beyond their due date.[10] Although the details of these physiologic processes await further definition, it is clear that the most common cause of prolonged gestation is an error in determining the patient's due date. Using the LMP for the determination of gestational age is fraught with inaccuracy. Patients' failure to recall accurately the date of the first day of their LMP combined with the varying duration of the luteal and follicular phases of the menstrual cycle may result in an overestimation of gestational age. When prolongation of pregnancy is adequately documented, its cause is often undetermined and the most likely etiology is biologic variability of the duration of pregnancy.

Various fetal and placental abnormalities may predispose to prolongation of pregnancy. The increase in the incidence of fetal anomalies among women who deliver beyond their due date is generally explained by abnormalities of the fetal hypothalamic-pituitary-adrenal axis.[9] Indeed, major central nervous system (CNS) abnormalities (such as anencephaly) have long been associated with loss of the normal mechanisms that initiate labor at term. The role of the fetal adrenal gland in the initiation of labor was highlighted by Naeye, who documented marked adrenal hypoplasia in 10 of 19 postterm fetuses with lethal congenital anomalies.[11]

Additional evidence regarding the complexity of the mechanisms involved with initiation of labor is provided by the X-linked recessive deficiency of placental sulfatase, which leads to abnormally low estrogen production in affected male fetuses with a subsequent prolongation of pregnancy and difficulties in both cervical ripening and labor induction.[12]

The role of primary prostaglandins (such as PGE_2 and PGF_2) as uterine stimulants is well established. Nonsteroidal anti-inflammatory drugs inhibit the synthesis of these prostaglandins, and therefore, their use is thought to possibly prolong gestation. Nonetheless, the extent to which the chronic use of these drugs (such as aspirin) results in actual prolongation of pregnancy is unknown.

Various maternal conditions have been suggested as risk factors for the development of prolonged pregnancy. A recent regression analysis performed on a large data set evaluated maternal age, parity, and marital status as well as maternal health before and during pregnancy. Primiparity was identified as the only maternal variable, which had a small but significant association with prolonged pregnancies of greater than or equal to 294 days (relative risk [RR] of 1.06 and 95 percent confidence interval [CI], 1.05 to 1.07).[13] Interestingly, maternal age of 35 years or older and the use of medicines during pregnancy were associated with a small but significant protective effect (odds ratios [OR] of 0.93 and 0.93, respectively), probably suggesting that older women and those on chronic medications were delivered before 42 weeks' gestation. Zweidling suggested that women who have previously delivered beyond term have a 50 percent chance of experiencing a subsequent prolonged pregnancy.[14] Thus, history of a previous delivery beyond term is a strong predictor of a subsequent late delivery.

The significance of overestimation of the duration of gestation with the use of the LMP should not be overlooked. Congenital anomalies such as anencephaly are easily diagnosed by ultrasound, and their presence mandates management options that may not be related to the gestational age at the time of delivery. The contributions attributable to primiparity or to the presence of a male fetus are so minimal that they are unlikely to result in any clinically useful information. In contrast, the fact that 50 percent of women who previously had a prolonged pregnancy would have a similar occurrence with their subsequent pregnancy could be used in counseling the patient and outlining potential management schemes long before the patient reaches her estimated due date.

DIAGNOSIS

The term "prolonged pregnancy" represents a diagnosis that is based on the best available estimation of the duration of gestation at the time of delivery. Optimal diagnosis of gestational age at the time of delivery is hindered by inaccuracy in pregnancy dating. Recently, it has become apparent that clinical methods for estimation of gestational age are inferior to sonographic measurements obtained early in pregnancy.[15] Several studies have demonstrated that the use of more accurate estimates of gestational age based on early ultrasound or known conception dates results in a significantly lower frequency of prolonged pregnancies. Boyd et al. showed that the incidence of patients whose pregnancy exceeded 293 days was 7.5 percent by menstrual dating and fell to

2.6 percent when dates were based on early sonographic examination. This incidence fell to 1.1 percent when the diagnosis was limited to patients whose gestational age exceeded 293 days by both menstrual dates and sonographic dates.[16] A similar conclusion was reached by Gardosi et al.,[15] who evaluated 24,675 spontaneous, singleton, nonanomalous deliveries and showed a drop in the postterm (>294 days) pregnancy rate from 7.5 percent when these pregnancies were dated by LMP to 1.5 percent when ultrasound dating was used. These authors also found that 71.5 percent of routine labor inductions at 42 weeks' gestation were actually not indicated because they were performed before the patients reached 42 weeks by scan dates. Similarly, Nguyen et al.[17] evaluated 14,805 spontaneous deliveries with a reliable LMP and showed that ultrasound dating reduced the proportion of deliveries beyond 294 days of gestation by 39 percent (from 7.5 to 5.2 percent). Recently, a prospective and randomized study of 218 women by Bennett et al.[18] confirmed these results and concluded that those whose dates were established by first-trimester sonography have significantly fewer inductions of labor for postterm pregnancy when compared with women whose dates were established by second trimester sonography. Furthermore, when scan and LMP dates were compared with known dates in patients who had undergone assisted reproduction, it was shown that the 95 percent CI for scan dates was ±8.3 days. In contrast, the 95 percent CI of menstrual dating was −9 to +27 days.[19,20] These results suggest that the LMP is more likely to overestimate, rather than underestimate, the gestational age at delivery.

The error in gestational dating by the LMP is mainly due to poor recall by the patient. It is, however, important to recognize that even when the LMP is recalled with certainty, it is not a good predictor of ovulation and that physiologic variations in the duration of the follicular phase result in an error that favors an overestimation of the true gestational age. In fact, similar considerations have led to the conclusion that when both early ultrasound and a reliable LMP are available, gestational dating should be based solely on the ultrasound measurements.[21]

Because the true date of conception is seldom known, there is a possibility that any adjustment of gestational age may increase the risk of adverse perinatal outcome by failing to identify pregnancies that are actually beyond term but are misclassified as being at term. Therefore, Tunon et al.[22] have evaluated fetal outcome in pregnancies defined as postterm according to the LMP but whose scan dates indicated that they were less than 295 days at the time of delivery. A total of 11,510 singleton pregnancies with reliable LMP were studied. An Apgar score of less than 7 at 5 minutes and admission to the neonatal intensive care unit (NICU) were used as outcome variables. The authors concluded that there was no increase in perinatal morbidity when scan dates were used as the sole predictor of gestational age at delivery.

PERINATAL MORTALITY AND MORBIDITY

Several studies that have used very large computerized databases of well-dated pregnancies provide insights into the incidence and nature of adverse perinatal outcome in prolonged pregnancy. Divon et al.[23] evaluated fetal and neonatal mortality rates in 181,524 accurately dated term and prolonged pregnancies. A significant increase in fetal mortality was detected from 41 weeks' gestation onward (OR of 1.5, 1.8, and 2.9 at 41, 42, and 43 weeks, respectively). The ORs for neonatal mortality did not demonstrate a significant gestational age dependency. Fetal growth restriction (i.e., birth weight of <2 standard deviations (SDs) below the mean for gestational age) was associated with significantly higher odds ratios for both fetal and neonatal mortality rates at every gestational age examined with ORs ranging from 7.1 to 10.0 for fetal death and from 3.4 to 9.4 for neonatal death. Thus, this study documented a small but significant increase in fetal mortality in accurately dated pregnancies that extend beyond 41 weeks' gestation and demonstrated that fetal growth restriction is independently associated with a large increase in perinatal mortality in these pregnancies. These results were confirmed by other investigators.[24,25] Clausson et al.[25] studied perinatal mortality rates among 458,744 term appropriate-for-gestational-age (AGA) infants, 10,312 term small-for-gestational-age (SGA) infants, 39,415 postterm (≥294 days) AGA infants and 1,558 postterm SGA infants. ORs for perinatal death in the postterm AGA infant were not significantly different when compared with AGA term deliveries. In contrast, SGA fetuses had an OR of 10.5 (95 percent CI, 6.9 to 16.0) and 5.0 (95 percent CI, 3.0 to 8.2) for stillbirth and neonatal death, respectively. The stillbirth rate did not change significantly when fetuses with congenital malformations were excluded. However, an 80-percent drop in neonatal deaths occurred when malformed neonates were excluded from the analysis. Further support for the concept that the "small and old" fetus suffers from increased perinatal mortality was provided by Campbell et al.,[13] who performed a multivariate analysis of factors associated with perinatal death among 65,796 singleton postterm (≥294 days) births. Three variables were identified as independent predictors of perinatal mortality: (1) SGA status (i.e., birth weight <10th percentile for gestational age) had an RR of 5.7 and 95 percent CI, 4.4 to 7.4; (2) maternal age equal or greater than 35 years had an RR of 1.88 and 95 percent CI, 1.2 to 2.9; (3) interestingly, LGA status (i.e., birth weight ≥90th percentile for gestational age) was associated with a modest protective effect for perinatal death (RR of 0.51 with 95 percent CI, 0.26 to 1.0). The independent impact of an increasing gestational age on these mortality rates was minimal.

Several recent publications have questioned the traditional method used to calculate fetal mortality.[26–31] As stated by Smith,[26] "estimating the probability of an event requires that the number of events (numerator) be divided by the number of subjects at risk for that event (denominator)." Therefore, it seems logical to calculate fetal mortality as fetal deaths per 1,000 on-going pregnancies (rather than per 1,000 deliveries), whereas the probability of neonatal mortality should be calculated as the number of neonatal deaths per 1,000 live births. A similar conclusion was reached by Caughey et al.[32] Indeed, as early as 1987, Yudkin et al.,[27] argued that the risk of stillbirth would be better measured as "the number of impending stillbirths divided by the total number of undelivered fetuses." With this measure and a database of 40,635 deliveries (1978 to 1985), the authors showed an exponential increase in the risk of stillbirth, from 0.3/1000 at 29 weeks' gestation to 1.8/1,000 at 42 weeks' gestation. Hilder et al.[29] reported similar results in 1998. In both of these studies, the authors calculated the weekly risk of fetal demise conditional on fetal survival until that gestational week.[27,29] One should not, however, ignore the fact that the fetus is exposed to the risk of intrauterine demise not only during the week of delivery but also during the period leading to the week of delivery. The traditional conditional probability for stillbirth at a given gestational age fails to take into account the risks of death in all the preceding weeks. Therefore, Smith[26] applied life-table analysis techniques and calculated the week-to-week cumulative probabilities of stillbirth. This risk increased from approximately 0.4/1,000 at 37 weeks' gestation to 11.5/1,000 at 43 weeks' gestation.

It is intuitively clear that the rate of fetal death and the rate of neonatal death can be viewed as two independent phenomena acting in opposite directions. For example, early in the third trimester of pregnancy, the risk of neonatal death (per 1,000 live births) is very high, whereas the cumulative risk of fetal death (per 1,000 on-going pregnancies) is extremely low. At some gestational age, the risk of remaining unborn may be greater that the risk of dying following a live birth. Kahn et al.[33] suggested that delivery should be considered when the prospective risk of fetal death exceeds the risk of neonatal death.

Divon et al.[34] have recently suggested a functional definition of prolonged pregnancy based on daily fetal and neonatal mortality rates. Their results indicate that as gestational age advances beyond 37 weeks, the cumulative rate of fetal death increases continuously. In contrast, the rate of neonatal death initially demonstrates a slight decrease and then remains relatively low. The rate of fetal demise is significantly higher than is that of neonatal death at any time beyond 282 days' (40 + 2 weeks') gestation. Thus, beyond this gestational age, the fetus assumes an unnecessary risk of fetal demise without benefiting from any further decrease in the rate of neonatal death if it remains unborn. Therefore, it would be reasonable to consider any gestational age beyond 282 days as a functional definition of prolonged pregnancy. They conclude by stating that the overall clinical implications of their proposed functional definition of prolonged pregnancy are yet to be determined. In their study, 268,068 (40.9 percent) pregnancies were undelivered by 283 days' gestation. The relative effectiveness (i.e., benefits, risks and costs) of routine, elective and early induction of labor or early initiation of intensive fetal surveillance of a large percentage of the pregnant population requires further study. Clearly, such a study should include an analysis of the potential increase in maternal morbidity and mortality caused by the expected increase in cesarean deliveries subsequent to failed inductions of labor.

Several studies evaluated the association of perinatal morbidity with prolonged pregnancy. Campbell et al.[13] compared 65,796 Norwegian pregnancies at greater than or equal to 42 weeks with 379,445 term births (37 to 41 weeks) and concluded that prolongation of pregnancy was associated with a significant increase in adverse outcome (Table 32-1). Fetal compromise was more common in the SGA fetuses, whereas shoulder dystocia, labor dysfunction, obstetric trauma, and maternal hemorrhage were more common in the LGA fetus.

Clausson et al.[25] evaluated a large Swedish database of term and postterm (defined as ≥294 days) singleton, normally formed neonates, and showed that prolonged pregnancies were associated with an increased frequency of neonatal convulsions, meconium aspiration syndrome, and Apgar scores of less than 4 at 5 minutes (Table 32-2). Again, morbidity in post term SGA infants was higher than in post term AGA infants.

Tunon et al. compared neonatal intensive care unit (NICU) admission rates among 10,048 term pregnancies and 246 prolonged pregnancies (≥296 days by both scan and LMP dates).[22] Prolonged pregnancy was associated with a significant increase in NICU admissions (OR of 2.05, 95 percent CI, 1.35 to 3.12).

Several maternal and fetal complications were evaluated in a large (n = 45,673) retrospective, cohort study by Caughey and Musci.[35] These authors documented a significant and progressive increase in the rate of meconium staining and macrosomia (beginning at 38 weeks), operative vaginal deliveries, chorioamnionitis and endometritis (beyond 40 weeks), cesarean deliveries, and intrauterine fetal deaths (beyond 41 weeks). They concluded that risks to both mother and infant increase as pregnancy progresses beyond 40 weeks' gestation, that antenatal fetal testing should begin sooner than the current recommendation of 42 weeks of gestation, and that the optimal gestational age to initiate delivery requires further investigation. Olesen et al.[36] evaluated a large computerized Danish database of singleton, liveborn term and postterm (>42 weeks) deliveries to quantify the maternal and fetal

Table 32-1. Complication Rates in Term and Postterm Births

COMPLICATION	PREVALENCE (%) IN TERM BIRTHS	IN POSTTERM BIRTHS	RELATIVE RISK (95% CI) POSTTERM VS. TERM
Fetal distress	5.0	8.4	1.68 (1.62–1.72)
Shoulder dystocia	0.5	0.7	1.31 (1.21–1.42)
Labor dysfunction	9.4	11.9	1.26 (1.23–1.29)
Obstetric trauma	2.6	3.3	1.25 (1.20–1.31)
Hemorrhage	9.1	10.0	1.09 (1.06–1.12)

CI, confidence interval.

Adapted from Campbell MK, Ostbye T, Irgens LM: Post-term birth: risk factors and outcomes in a 10-year cohort of Norwegian births. Obstet Gynecol 89:543, 1997. Copyright 1997 American College of Obstetricians and Gynecologists, with permission.

Table 32-2. Neonatal Morbidity in Postterm AGA and SGA Infants

COMPLICATIONS	ODDS RATIOS AND 95% CI VERSUS TERM AGA NEONATES	
Convulsions		
Term SGA	2.3	(1.6–3.4)
Postterm AGA	1.5	(1.2–2.0)
Postterm SGA	3.4	(1.5–7.6)
Meconium aspiration		
Term SGA	2.4	(1.6–3.4)
Postterm AGA	3.0	(2.6–3.7)
Postterm SGA	1.6	(0.5–5.0)
Apgar score <4 at 5 min		
Term SGA	2.2	(1.4–3.4)
Postterm AGA	2.0	(1.5–2.5)
Postterm SGA	3.6	(1.5–8.7)

AGA, appropriate for gestational age; CI, confidence interval; SGA, small for gestational age.

Adapted from Clausson B, Cnattinguis S, Axelsson O: Outcomes of post-term births: the role of fetal growth restriction and malformations. Obstet Gynecol 94:758, 1999. Copyright 1999 American College of Obstetricians and Gynecologists, with permission.

risks associated with postterm delivery. Both perinatal and maternal complications were increased significantly in postterm deliveries. Small but significant increases were seen in meconium aspiration, cord complications, asphyxia before or during delivery, Apgar score <7 at 5 minutes, pneumonia, septicemia, convulsions, persistent fetal circulation, CNS trauma, bone fractures, peripheral nerve paralysis, and perinatal death (adjusted odds ratio ranged from 1.36 to 2.0). There were no significant differences in the rate of respiratory distress syndrome, CNS, and cardiac malformations or the overall rate of deaths within the first year of life. Various measures of maternal complications were also significantly increased in patients who delivered at or beyond 42 weeks' gestation. These included puerperal infection, postpartum hemorrhage, cephalopelvic disproportion, vulvar, vaginal or cervical lacerations, vaginal or vulvar hematomas, and intrapartum emergency cesarean delivery (with adjusted ORs ranging from 1.21 to 3.58). The authors made no specific recommendations based on the increased estimates of risk to mother and fetus they detected in postterm pregnancies.

LONG-TERM OUTCOME

Small study populations and the lack of appropriate controls hinder evaluation of long-term developmental outcome in children born after a prolonged gestation. Additional difficulties are introduced by inconsistent definitions of prolonged pregnancy, inaccuracy in pregnancy dating, and the fact that these studies do not differentiate between the apparently normal newborn and those suffering from perinatal asphyxia, severe growth restriction, or meconium aspiration. An uncontrolled study of 106 infants revealed a relatively large frequency of abnormal neurologic signs, sleep disorders, and inadequate social competence during the first year of life.[37] In contrast, Ting et al.[38] suggested that there are no physical or mental deficiencies in surviving dysmature infants. These results were confirmed by a prospective study of 129 well-dated children born after a prolonged pregnancy and 184 controls. This report did not demonstrate any significant differences in either intelligence scores or physical milestones at 1 and 2 years of age.[39] Thus, until large-scale prospective studies are available, it is reasonable to conclude that in the absence of perinatal asphyxia, growth restriction, or meconium aspiration, prolonged pregnancy is associated with normal, long-term neonatal developmental outcome.

ABERRANT FETAL GROWTH

In 1954, Clifford pointed out that prolongation of pregnancy is associated with placental dysfunction and neonatal dysmaturity.[2] Typically, the affected neonates would appear malnourished, with wasting of subcutaneous tissue, meconium staining, and peeling of skin. More recently, Campbell et al. identified birth weight less than or equal to the 10th percentile for gestational age as the risk factor with the largest effect on perinatal mortality (RR of 5.68; 95 percent CI, 4.37 to 7.38) in patients at greater than or equal to 42 weeks' gestation.[13] These authors also showed that macrosomia was associated with a protective effect. The RR for perinatal death in the presence of fetal macrosomia was only 0.51 (95 percent CI, 0.26 to 1.00). However, macrosomia was associated with a higher incidence of labor dysfunction, obstetric trauma, shoulder dystocia, and maternal hemorrhage.

The incidence of fetal macrosomia increases with advancing gestational age.[40] For example, a gradual increase in both birth weight and head circumference was documented by McLean et al.,[41] who studied 7,000 pregnancies between 39 and 43 weeks' gestation. Similarly, Nahum et al.[42] showed that fetal growth is a linear function of gestational age between 37 and 42 weeks' gestation with a daily fetal weight gain of 12.7 ± 1.4 g (mean ± SD). Thus, it should come as no surprise that Pollack et al.,[43] who evaluated 519 singleton pregnancies at greater than or equal to 41 weeks' gestation, detected a 23 percent incidence of infants whose birth weight was greater than 4,000 g and a 4 percent incidence of birth weights greater than 4,500 g. Chervenak et al.[44] have shown that prolonged pregnancy is not only associated with an increased incidence of macrosomia but that this increase also results in doubling the cesarean delivery rate for protraction or descent disorders.

The accurate and timely prediction of macrosomia may well influence delivery management decisions. However, one should note that the accurate estimation of fetal weight must be viewed in its broad clinical context of fetopelvic disproportion. Thus, the crucial factor is the relationship of the fetal size to the maternal pelvis rather than the common clinical preoccupation with macrosomia alone. Focusing on either one of these factors in isolation represents a conceptual error.[45] For example, despite an increase in the RR of birth trauma in infants weighing more than 4,000 g, most are delivered vaginally without complications. Likewise, a birth weight of less than 4,000 g does not preclude the possibility of shoulder dystocia. In fact, most infants with brachial plexus injury weigh less than 4,000 g at birth.

Traditionally, obstetricians have predicted fetal weight by abdominal palpation or symphysial-fundal height measurement. When ultrasound was first used to estimate fetal weight, there was widespread expectation that it would provide a more useful tool than the traditional clinical methods. Chervenak et al. evaluated 317 patients at greater than or equal to 41 weeks' gestation and reported that a sonographic estimate of fetal weight (EFW) of greater than 4,000 g had a sensitivity, specificity, positive predictive value, and negative predictive value of 61, 91, 70, and 87 percent, respectively, in the diagnosis of a birthweight greater than 4,000 g.[44] In a subsequent study of 519 pregnancies of greater than or equal to 41 weeks' gestation, Pollack et al.[43] reported that sonographic estimates of fetal weight that were obtained within 1 week of delivery in pregnancies of greater than or equal to 41 weeks were associated with a mean absolute error of 7.7 percent and a wide range of actual birth weights. For example, the 95 percent CI of an EFW of 4,000 g ranged from 3,142 g to 4,665 g, and the 95 percent CI for an EFW of 4,500 g ranged from 3,465 g to 4,993 g. The positive predictive value of an EFW greater than or equal to 4,000 g in the prediction of a birth weight greater than or equal to 4,000 g was only 64 percent and, therefore, the authors concluded that routine sonographic screening for macrosomia in prolonged pregnancies is associated with relatively low accuracy.

In an attempt to improve the accuracy of sonographic estimates of fetal weight, O'Reilly-Green and Divon used receiver operating characteristic curve analysis to identify optimal cutoff values of EFW in the prediction of macrosomia in prolonged pregnancies.[46] At the inflection point cutoff level of 3,711 g, sensitivity, specificity, and positive and negative predictive values for predicting birth weight of greater than or equal to 4,000 g were 85, 72, 49, and 94 percent, respectively. At the inflection point cutoff level of 4,192 g for predicting birth weight of greater than or equal to 4,500 g, these values were 83, 92, 30, and 99 percent. The authors concluded that cutoff values derived from their analysis resulted in reasonable sensitivities but disappointingly low positive predictive values. The ACOG Practice Bulletin on fetal macrosomia correctly states that "the diagnosis of fetal macrosomia is imprecise" and that "an accurate diagnosis of macrosomia can be made only by weighing the newborn after delivery."[47] It goes on to suggest that "labor and vaginal delivery are not contraindicated for women with estimated fetal weights up to 5,000 g in the absence of maternal diabetes," that "with an estimated fetal weight greater than 4,500 g, a prolonged second stage of labor or arrest of descent in the second stage is an indication for cesarean delivery," and that "prophylactic cesarean delivery may be considered for suspected fetal macrosomia with estimated fetal weights greater than 5,000 g in women without diabetes."

The practical implications of the low predictive value of ultrasonography have been highlighted by Rouse et al.[48,49] These authors have shown that in pregnancies not complicated by diabetes mellitus, the level of intervention and the economic costs of prophylactic cesarean delivery for fetal macrosomia diagnosed by means of ultrasonography would be excessive. The inaccuracy of sonographic estimates of fetal weight combined with the rarity of permanent brachial plexus injury led these authors to conclude that "a prophylactic cesarean policy with either a 4,000 g or 4,500 g macrosomia threshold would require more than 1,000 cesarean deliveries and millions of dollars to avert a single permanent brachial plexus injury." Even more striking is their suggestion that a policy of prophylactic cesarean delivery would result in one maternal death for every 3.2 brachial plexus injuries that would be prevented.

Despite many years of research and debate, the management of suspected fetal macrosomia is still controversial. The increased incidence of maternal and fetal morbidity associated with macrosomia has prompted some authors to recommend a proactive approach including either a cesarean delivery for cases of "established" macrosomia or a prophylactic induction of labor for "impending" macrosomia. It would seem reasonable that as fetal weight continues to increase with advancing gestational age, delivery of those pregnancies with a potential for macrosomia might prevent some cases of shoulder dystocia and a subsequent brachial plexus injury. However, this intervention could be achieved only by increasing the rate of inductions of labor or by an increased use of cesarean deliveries, both of which would subject the patient to added morbidity or even unnecessary mortality. Furthermore, preliminary evidence suggesting that such interventions would be beneficial is lacking.

Leaphart et al.[50] evaluated the practice of labor induction when fetal macrosomia is suspected. Similar to many other studies, they showed that induction of labor resulted in doubling of their baseline rate of cesarean delivery (from 17 to 36 percent), a more frequent use of regional analgesia (from 53 to 83 percent), and no difference in the incidence of shoulder dystocia relative to matched controls who were managed by awaiting spontaneous onset of labor. The authors concluded that induction of labor following a prenatal diagnosis of macrosomia results in unnecessary cesarean deliveries and emphasized that their data support a plan of expectant management when fetal macrosomia is suspected. In a prospective randomized study of 273 patients with suspected macrosomia at term, Gonen et al.[51] could not demonstrate that induction of labor resulted in reduced neonatal morbidity. The authors concluded that "ultrasonic estimation of fetal weight between 4,000 g and 4,500 g should not be considered an indication for induction of labor."

Some authors have gone as far as to suggest that the availability of a sonographic EFW indicating macrosomia is in and of itself responsible for an increased cesarean delivery rate and have questioned the logic of obtaining these EFWs if their availability does not improve perinatal outcome.[52]

Although the recommendation for proactive management of the macrosomic fetus is well intentioned, evidence-based research does not support the practice of either induction of labor or a cesarean delivery for fetal macrosomia in the absence of other indications for these interventions. A more reasonable policy for management of macrosomia would entail a conservative approach awaiting the onset of spontaneous labor in the absence of a favorable uterine cervix, adequate intrapartum management such as assessment of the adequacy of the maternal pelvis, assessment of the progress of labor and careful use of oxytocin, avoidance of vaginal operative deliveries, and avoidance of excessive traction on the impacted shoulder in favor of the maneuvers described for the management of shoulder dystocia (see Chapter 17).

FETAL SURVEILLANCE

It is widely believed that fetal surveillance may be used in an attempt to observe the prolonged pregnancy safely while awaiting either the spontaneous onset of labor or spontaneous ripening of the cervix before elective induction. The pitfalls of the use of antenatal testing in this setting are 2-fold. On the one hand, false-positive tests commonly lead to unnecessary interventions that are potentially hazardous to the gravida. On the other hand, to date, no program of fetal testing has been shown to completely eliminate the risk of stillbirth. Current research on the use of fetal testing has focused on the refinement of testing protocols and the application of new technology to address these issues.

Data presented earlier in this chapter indicate that perinatal mortality is significantly increased beginning at 41 weeks' gestation and possibly even earlier. The optimal gestational age for the initiation of fetal testing has not been established. Guidetti et al.[53] reported an increased incidence of perinatal morbidity at greater than or equal to 41 weeks' gestation. Jazayeri et al., provided physiologic evidence by demonstrating elevated plasma erythropoietin levels, as an indirect evidence of altered fetal oxygenation, in patients at greater than or equal to 41 weeks.[54] Thus, it would seem prudent to initiate fetal testing no later than 41 weeks of gestation.

Extensive experience with biophysical profile testing in high-risk populations indicates a perinatal mortality rate of 0.73 per 1,000 tested pregnancies within 1 week of a normal test, provided that the amniotic fluid volume is normal.[55] Twice-weekly testing with the biophysical profile in a series of 293 patients followed beyond 42 weeks of gestation has been reported. No stillbirths were observed in this small series.[56]

The primary disadvantages of biophysical profile scoring are the time required to perform the test and the need for an experienced sonographer. Recently, investigators have examined the efficacy of using the nonstress test (NST) as a primary testing modality with the addition of a sonographic assessment of amniotic fluid volume. Measurement of the amniotic fluid index (AFI) requires minimal sonographic experience,[57] and vibroacoustic stimulation may be used to shorten the duration of the NST.[58] Results of the use of such a protocol in the antepartum management of 5,973 high-risk pregnancies have been described by Clark et al.[59] Amniotic fluid volume assessment was performed by measurement of the AFI, with induction of labor reserved for an AFI of 5 cm or less. Twice-weekly testing was performed in a subset of 279 prolonged pregnancies. No stillbirths were recorded.

More recently, Miller et al.[60] reported the use of a similar protocol in 15,482 high-risk pregnancies for which 54,617 tests were performed. The false-negative rate of this test was 0.8 per 1,000 women tested–a rate that favorably compares with those reported for the contraction stress test or the complete biophysical profile.[55,61] Of note, 6,390 patients were assessed in this study for prolonged pregnancy. These patients were first evaluated in the 41st week of gestation, and twice-weekly testing was initiated after 42 weeks of gestation. Five stillbirths were reported in this subpopulation. An analysis of all false-positive tests showed that the routine use of NST combined with the AFI resulted in a 60-percent false-positive rate in the prediction of intrapartum fetal compromise compared with a 40-percent false-positive rate using the complete biophysical profile. This increase in false-positive tests was believed to be partly a result of poor specificity of the AFI in predicting fetal compromise.

Sylvestre et al.[62] evaluated the incidence of abnormal testing (NST and AFI) as a function of birth weight in 792 uncomplicated prolonged pregnancies (>41 weeks). They showed an inverse relationship between abnormal testing and birth weight category (36 percent, 14 percent, and 9 percent for small, average size, and large fetuses, respectively, $P < 0.001$). In addition, small fetuses were more likely to require a cesarean delivery for nonreassuring fetal status during labor than were all other fetuses (12.3 percent versus 5.3 percent, $P > 0.024$). Thus, it is reasonable to conclude that the small, postterm fetus is not only more likely to die in utero (as discussed previously) but is also more likely to fail antepartum fetal testing and to be delivered by a nonelective cesarean section for an intrapartum diagnosis of nonreassuring fetal status.

The implicit assumption in the expectant management strategy is that the presence of an abnormal fetal test (such as oligohydramnios, low biophysical profile score, or spontaneous fetal heart rate decelerations) represents a change in fetal status that requires intervention in the form of prompt delivery. A novel view of the regulation of fetal homeostasis during late gestation was offered by Onyeije and Divon.[63] These authors studied the incidence of maternal ketonuria (as a reflection of maternal starvation and dehydration) and its association with abnormal fetal surveillance tests. One thousand eight hundred and ninety five patients were managed expectantly with semiweekly fetal testing. Beginning at 41 weeks' gestation, clinically detectable ketonuria occurred in 10.9 percent of patients studied. Patients with ketonuria were at increased risk for abnormal test results, including the presence of oligohydramnios (24 versus 9.3 percent, $P < 0.0001$), nonreactive NST (6.2 verdus 2.15 percent, $P < 0.0001$), and the presence of fetal heart rate decelerations (14 versus 9.2 percent, $P > 0.0039$). The authors suggested that reversible maternal ketonuria contributes to the false-positive test results often encountered in fetal testing, and that such patients might benefit from treatment of ketonuria rather than be delivered in response to abnormal test results.

Oligohydramnios

The formation of amniotic fluid is a complex and poorly understood process. Many authors have demonstrated that amniotic fluid volume decreases as gestational age advances beyond 32 or 34 weeks' gestation. Marks and Divon evaluated the AFI in 511 well-dated prolonged pregnancies.[64] Gestational age at the time of the study ranged from 41 to 43 weeks and 6 days. AFI measurements ranged from 1.7 to 24.6 cm, with a mean and standard deviation of 12.4 cm ± 4.2 cm at 41 weeks. Oligohydramnios (AFI < 5.0 cm) was detected in 11.5 percent of the study population. Longitudinal data were available from 121 patients. These patients demonstrated a mean decrease in AFI of 25 percent per week. Thus, the authors concluded that the majority of pregnancies at greater than or equal to 41 weeks' gestation have a normal volume of amniotic fluid.

Numerous hypotheses have been offered to explain the pathophysiology of oligohydramnios. Oligohydramnios, when defined as an AFI less than or equal to 5.0 cm, has an incidence of 8.5 to 15.5 percent. In the absence of ruptured membranes or fetal urinary tract abnormalities, diminishing levels of amniotic fluid volume may be related to poor placental function.[65] Nicolaides et al.[66] hypothesized that fetal hypoxemia may result in redistribution of blood flow with decreased renal perfusion and diminished urine production, which, in turn, may cause oligohydramnios. A vicious circle could develop with oligohydramnios causing cord compression, resulting in further hypoxemia, oligohydramnios, and fetal heart rate (FHR) abnormalities. Under these circumstances, fetal hypoxemia may induce relaxation of the rectal sphincters and hence meconium staining resulting in meconium aspiration syndrome. In fact, meconium-stained amniotic fluid is found in up to 50 percent of pregnancies at 42 weeks' gestation upon rupture of the membranes. Trimmer et al.[67] detected diminished urine production in pregnancies of 42 weeks or more with oligohydramnios and suggested that decreased fetal urine production was the result of preexisting oligohydramnios, which limited fetal swallowing of amniotic fluid rather than a decrease in renal perfusion. Bar-Hava et al.[68] used pulsed wave Doppler to evaluate resistance index values in the fetal middle cerebral artery, renal, and umbilical arteries in 57 pregnancies at greater than or equal to 41 weeks' gestation. Oligohydramnios (AFI < 5 cm) was detected in 15 patients. The various resistance index values and the ratios among them were not significantly different in patients with or without oligohydramnios. Interestingly, the mean birth weight in patients with oligohydramnios was significantly lower than the mean birth weight in patients with a normal AFI (3,297 ± 438 g versus 3,742 ± 448 g, respectively). The author concluded that oligohydramnios in these patients is not associated with a noticeable redistribution of blood flow and suggested that the cause of oligohydramnios is probably unrelated to renal perfusion.

Sylvestre et al.[62] evaluated the association between birth weight and the AFI in 792 patients who were at or beyond 41 weeks' gestation. They documented a significant inverse relationship between the incidence of oligohydramnios and birth weight (27, 8.5, and 6.5 percent for small, average and large fetuses, respectively, $P < 0.001$). The fact that oligohydramnios was found more often in the smaller fetuses is intriguing. It suggests that the appearance of oligohydramnios is a pathologic rather than a physiologic process. It may indicate that the pathophysiology of oligohydramnios in prolonged pregnancy is similar to that involved with the formation of oligohydramnios in the growth-restricted fetus, and overall, it is consistent with the concept that it is the small and "older" fetus who is more prone to complications arising from asphyxia. Other causes of oligohydramnios include spontaneous rupture of membranes, genitourinary anomalies, and an abnormal karyotype. It is important to rule out these other causes of oligohydramnios before attributing reduced amniotic fluid levels to fetal hypoxemia.

Regardless of the exact cause of oligohydramnios, its presence has been used by Leveno et al.[69] to explain the increased incidence of abnormal antepartum and intrapartum FHR abnormalities seen in prolonged pregnancies. These authors suggested that prolonged FHR decelerations representing cord compression preceded 75 percent of cesarean deliveries for fetal jeopardy. The association between a reduced AFI and variable decelerations is well documented.[70,71] As suggested by Gabbe et al.[70] and Lee and Hon,[72] variable FHR decelerations detected in patients with oligohydramnios are probably related to increased umbilical cord compression. This concept is further supported by reports of intrapartum amnioinfusion in mothers with oligohydramnios. This procedure was shown to reduce the incidence of variable FHR decelerations, meconium staining below the vocal cords, and operative delivery for fetal distress.[73,74] A similar mechanism is probably functional in the antepartum period. Both Phelan et al. and Divon et al. found that the frequency of NSTs demonstrating FHR decelerations or bradycardia increased as the ultrasonographic estimates of the amniotic fluid declined.[75–78]

Quantifying amniotic fluid volume presents significant problems (see Chapter 31). Various sonographic semiquantitative estimates such as the 1-cm pocket, the 2-cm pocket, or the 3-cm pocket have been proposed as definitions of oligohydramnios.[79–81] The use of an AFI of less than or equal to 5.0 cm to define oligohydramnios was first suggested by Phelan et al. in 1987, as an arbitrary cut-off value based on retrospective studies.[75,77] Nevertheless, it has since gained popular appeal. A meta-analysis evaluated the risk of cesarean delivery for fetal distress, 5-minute Apgar score of less than 7, and umbilical artery pH less than 7.00 in patients with antepartum or intrapartum AFI or less than 5.0 cm.[82] Eighteen reports describing 10,551 patients at various gestational ages were included in the analysis. The overall incidence of oligohydramnios was 15.2 percent. The authors concluded that an AFI of less than or equal to 5.0 cm is associated with an increased risk of cesarean delivery for fetal distress (RR of 2.2; 95 percent CI, 1.5 to 3.4) and an Apgar score of less than 7 at 5 minutes (RR of 5.2; 95 percent CI, 2.4 to 11.3). However, no association was demonstrated between oligohydramnios and severe fetal acidosis. A prospective, blinded observational study of the usefulness of ultrasound assessment of amniotic fluid in the prediction of adverse outcome in the prolonged pregnancy was reported by Morris et al. [83] Fifteen hundred and eighty four pregnancies were evaluated; 72 percent delivered within 7 days of their sonographic assessment and 87.2 percent delivered at or beyond 41 weeks' gestation. The authors demonstrated that an AFI of < 5 cm (but not a single deepest vertical pocket < 2 cm) was significantly associated with birth asphyxia or meconium aspiration. In addition, there was a significant association between an AFI < 5 cm and fetal distress in labor, cord arterial pH <7.0 and low Apgar scores. Despite these statistically significant associations with adverse perinatal outcomes, the sensitivity of an AFI < 5.0 cm was very low at 28.6, 12, and 11.5 percent for major adverse outcome, fetal distress in labor, or admission to the NICU, respectively. They concluded that because of this poor sensitivity, "routine use is likely to lead to increased obstetric intervention without improvement in perinatal outcome," and that large clinical trials are necessary to assess the effectiveness of delivery based on sonographically diagnosed oligohydramnios (as well as the need to detect fetuses who are at risk of having adverse outcome but do not have oligohydramnios).

The presence of sonographically diagnosed oligohydramnios is often used as an indication for delivery of pregnancies that reach term gestation or extend beyond term. One should realize, however, that up to 50 percent of patients who are diagnosed as having oligohydramnios by ultrasound have a normal volume of amniotic fluid upon artificial rupture of the membranes.[84] In addition, there are no large-scale, prospective, randomized studies documenting the benefits of delivery once oligohydramnios has been detected. In the absence of such studies, it would seem prudent to deliver patients at or beyond term gestation who demonstrate oligohydramnios primarily because of the large body of data that documents an association between diminished amniotic fluid volume and adverse perinatal outcome.

Doppler Ultrasound

The use of umbilical artery Doppler velocimetry is not associated with an improvement of the positive predictive value of fetal testing in prolonged pregnancy.[85–87] Doppler ultrasound has been applied to investigations of the fetal circulation in an attempt to identify perturbations that might be associated with adverse outcomes. Bar-Hava et al.[68] analyzed renal artery and middle cerebral blood velocity waveforms in 57 pregnancies prolonged beyond 287 days' gestation. Findings in pregnancies complicated by oligohydramnios were compared with those found in pregnancies with normal amniotic fluid volume. It was expected that, with hypoxia, impedance in the cerebral circulation might decrease as impedance increased in the renal circulation. However, no differences were seen. These results were confirmed in a larger, prospective investigation undertaken by Zimmermann et al.[88] In this cross-sectional, prospective study, 153 pregnancies were examined beyond 287 days of gestation and 36 percent were followed beyond 42 weeks of gestation. The resistance indices of umbilical artery and middle cerebral artery waveforms were studied every 2 days until delivery. All velocities fell within the known 95 percent CIs for normal term fetuses. Doppler measurements were unable to predict adverse fetal outcomes, such as abnormal fetal heart rate tracings, thick meconium, the need for urgent operative delivery, acidemia at delivery, or neonatal encephalopathy. In contrast, Selam et al.[89] who studied 10 patients with oligohydramnios and 28 patients with a normal AFI (all patients were >41 weeks) concluded that oligohydramnios in post-term pregnancies was associated with the typical brain-sparing redistribution of blood flow (i.e., decreased resistance in the middle cerebral artery as well as increased resistance in the renal arteries).

Weiner et al.[90] used Doppler ultrasound to study fetal cardiac function in prolonged pregnancy. The velocity time integral of blood flow across each valve was multiplied by the fetal heart rate to obtain a measure of fetal ventricular function. Results were compared with measurements obtained from a control group of patients studied between 38 and 41 weeks of gestation. No differences were seen between controls and prolonged pregnancies with an AFI of 6 cm or greater. Prolonged pregnancies with abnormal amniotic fluid volumes had statistically significant differences in fetal left cardiac function. The authors concluded that an abnormality of cardiac function may be present before or coincident with the development of oligohydramnios. At present, there are no data to suggest that the use of Doppler velocimetry improves the positive predictive value of fetal testing in prolonged pregnancy.

NUCLEATED RED BLOOD CELLS

Recent publications have described a significant association between nucleated red blood cell (NRBC) counts and adverse perinatal outcome. Nucleated red blood cells are immature erythrocytes found in the peripheral blood of newborn infants. It has been suggested that elevated umbilical cord NRBC counts are associated with either acute or chronic hypoxic fetal environment.[91–94] Elevated NRBC counts have also been suggested as a possible predictor of adverse perinatal outcome, such as low Apgar scores and pH values, fetal growth restriction, perinatal brain damage, early-onset neonatal seizures, and cerebral palsy.[95–99]

Hence, both elevated NRBC counts and prolonged pregnancies are associated with adverse perinatal outcome. However, the association between these variables has received limited attention. Jazayeri et al.[54] studied a small cohort of pregnancies delivering at or beyond 41 weeks of gestation. Cord plasma erythropoietin levels were significantly increased compared with pregnancies delivered at 37 to 40 weeks of gestation. Decreased PO_2 is a known stimulator of erythropoietin production, which, in turn, increases erythroid production and results in an increased NRBC count in the fetal peripheral circulation. Therefore, it is reasonable to assume that if prolonged pregnancy is associated with fetal hypoxia, the fetal NRBC count would also be elevated. This hypothesis has been studied by Axt et al.,[100] who concluded that fetal NRBC counts are elevated in prolonged pregnancies. However, a detailed analysis of their results showed that it was an increased incidence of fetal acidosis, rather that prolongation of pregnancy, that resulted in an increased NRBC count. Similar results were reported by Perri et al.[101] who studied 75 low-risk pregnancies at 287 days and concluded that "elevated NRBC counts are associated with specific pregnancy complications rather than uncomplicated prolonged pregnancies in general."

The association between meconium staining and erythropoietin was evaluated by Manchandra et al.[102] These authors have shown that the concentration of erythropoietin was significantly increased in pregnancies beyond 41 weeks' gestation (even though cord blood pH values or base deficit values were within the normal range) and that regardless of gestational age, meconium-stained amniotic fluid was associated with a significant rise in erythropoietin. An interesting observation was made by Dolberg et al. who compared the number of NRBCs in 32 healthy infants, 45 infants with asymptomatic meconium aspiration and 11 infants with respiratory symptoms due to meconium aspiration.[103] Infants with symptomatic meconium aspiration had the highest number of NRBCs.

MANAGEMENT

In spite of many years of research, the optimal management of the prolonged pregnancy is still controversial. These pregnancies have traditionally been considered to be at elevated risk for adverse perinatal outcome. Thus, it is generally accepted that these patients should undergo some form of fetal testing. Although most authors agree that induction of labor is indicated in women with an "inducible" uterine cervix, there is lack of agreement as to the management of the patient whose cervix is deemed "unfavorable." Antenatal testing may be used in an attempt to observe the prolonged pregnancy safely while awaiting the spontaneous onset of labor or for ripening of the cervix prior to labor induction. Other opinions argue in favor of induction of labor regardless of the cervical status.

Fibronectin

Approximately 50 percent of patients who are undelivered by 41 weeks' gestation present in spontaneous labor within 7 days, and more than 90 percent do so by 44 weeks.[104] Attempts to evaluate the role of a fetal fibronectin in cervical secretions as a predictor of the onset of spontaneous labor have been inconclusive. Goffeng et al.[105] studied 80 women at 42 weeks' gestation and found that the presence of fetal fibronectin was not significantly correlated with either the Bishop score or the time interval between cervical sampling and delivery. In contrast, Mouw et al.[106] concluded that the sensitivity and specificity of fetal fibronectin concentration of at least 50 ng/ml in the prediction of spontaneous onset of labor within 3 days of examination were 71 and 64 percent, respectively. With a sensitivity of only 71 percent and a relatively low specificity, it is unlikely that this test would have any practical clinical application in the management of the prolonged pregnancy. In fact, Rozenberg et al.[107] have recently shown that the spontaneous onset of labor within 7 days of evaluation is predicted by a Bishop score >7 and a cervical length <25 mm but not with a positive fetal fibronectin.

Sweeping the Membranes

Membrane sweeping or stripping is an age-old method of inducing labor that is still in common use. This intervention results in a local increase in prostaglandin production and is believed to hasten the onset of labor. A meta-analysis of the use of sweeping of the membranes to induce labor or to prevent prolonged pregnancy has recently been published.[108] The analysis showed that sweeping of the membranes in term pregnancies shortens the duration of pregnancy by a mean of 4 days. Consequently, it decreases the frequency of patients reaching 41 or 42 weeks' gestation. Eight women need to be treated at term in order to avoid one pregnancy continuing beyond 41 weeks, and 25 women need to be treated to avoid one pregnancy continuing beyond 42 weeks' gestation. The intervention had no significant impact on mode of delivery or the incidence of maternal or neonatal infections. Vaginal bleeding, painful uterine contractions not leading to delivery, and discomfort during vaginal examination were significantly more common in women allocated to sweeping of the membranes.

Cervical Length

Second-trimester transvaginal sonographic assessment of the cervical length has gained popularity as a predictor of preterm delivery.[109] Not surprisingly, several studies have reported that a third-trimester measurement of the cervical length is a useful predictor of the likelihood of a successful induction of labor. Pandis et al.[110] evaluated the preinduction cervical length in 240 women with singleton pregnancy at 37 to 42 weeks' gestation. Both Bishop score and sonographic cervical length were obtained. Their results indicated that cervical length was a better predictor of a successful induction than the Bishop score (with a sensitivity and specificity of 87 and 71 percent versus 58 and 27 percent respectively). The best cut-off level in the prediction of a successful induction was a cervical length of less than 28 mm.

More recently, Rane et al.[111] examined the effect of parity on the relationship between pre-induction cervical length and the induction-to-delivery interval in 382 post term pregnancies undergoing induction of labor between 290 days' gestation to 295 days' gestation. They showed that 67 percent of their patients had a successful vaginal delivery within 24 hours of induction and that the preinduction cervical length was significantly associated with the induction to delivery interval. Given the same cervical length, the induction to delivery interval in multiparous patients was 37 percent lower. In a subsequent study from the same institution, Ramanathan et al.[112] studied the cervical length at 37 weeks' gestation in 1571 low risk patients in the prediction of gestational age at spontaneous versus post date delivery and mode of delivery. The incidence of spontaneous delivery by 40 weeks and 10 days was 81.2 percent, and the likelihood increased in a linear fashion with decreasing cervical length at 37 weeks, from an incidence of 0 percent with a cervix measuring >40 mm, to an incidence of 68 percent when the cervix measured <20 mm. Likewise, the incidence of cesarean delivery increased in direct proportion to the cervical length. This was true for both spontaneous labor and induction of labor. The authors concluded that "measurement of cervical length at 37 weeks can define the likelihood of spontaneous delivery before 40 weeks and 10 days and the risk of cesarean section in those requiring induction for prolonged pregnancy."

Induction of Labor

A major concern in the management of the prolonged pregnancy is the balance between the likelihood of a successful induction of labor and the risks of expectant management. The October 2000 ACOG Practice Patterns states that there is insufficient information to determine whether either labor induction or expectant management result in the best outcome in women with a prolonged pregnancy and a favorable cervix.[3] This publication does state that "according to current obstetric practice, labor is induced in most of these women." Accordingly, most practitioners feel that if the likelihood of a successful vaginal delivery is sufficiently high, there is no reason to expose the patient to the added risks associated with prolongation of pregnancy. Thus, in the absence of randomized controlled trials, induction of labor in women with prolonged pregnancy and a favorable cervix is a reasonable approach.

The management of the patient who presents with an unfavorable cervix is much more controversial. It consists of either expectant management (i.e., antenatal surveillance until there are signs of fetal jeopardy, or until the patient presents in either spontaneous labor or with a favorable cervix) or induction of labor any time after 41 weeks' gestation.

Magann et al.[113] showed that daily membrane stripping or daily placement of prostaglandin gel (0.15 mg of PGE_2) beginning at 41 weeks resulted in fewer inductions at 42 weeks. Other attempts at outpatient management have been inconclusive. Lien et al.[114] randomized patients to either PGE_2 gel or placebo gel at the time of scheduled NST and showed that there was no decrease in the induction rate or cesarean delivery rate in patients with prolonged pregnancy who received intracervical PGE_2 gel. In contrast, Ohel et al.[115] randomized patients at 40 to 41 weeks into either outpatient administration of 3 mg of vaginal PGE_2 or expectant management, and they observed that the average number of days to delivery was significantly lower in the induction group (1.6 versus 5.2 days), with no difference in the cesarean section rates between groups.

Several other investigators have evaluated the use of PGE_2 gel for inducing labor in patients with a prolonged pregnancy and an unfavorable cervix. Shaw et al.[116] studied PGE_2 gel in a double-blind, placebo-controlled trial and showed that it was associated with an improvement in cervical ripeness, shorter duration of labor, reduced need for high-dose oxytocin, and a lower rate of cesarean deliveries. A study by Papageorgiou et al.[117] confirmed these findings, because PGE_2 gel was associated with a higher success rate and a lower cesarean delivery rate when compared with oxytocin. In contrast, a large and well-designed multicenter, randomized, controlled trial of expectant management versus induction of labor reported no reduction in the induction-delivery interval or in the cesarean delivery rate in the PGE_2 group relative to placebo.[118]

Other medical and mechanical methods for induction of labor have been described such as misoprostol, relaxin, balloon catheters, nipple stimulation, and hygroscopic tents.[119] Unfortunately, the ideal mode of induction of labor has yet to be determined. Oxytocin in combination with amniotomy remains the method of choice for inducing labor in women with a favorable cervix. The use of cervical ripening agents in patients with an unfavorable cervix certainly results in a significant increase in cervical dilation and effacement. However, the use of these agents is still associated with a high cesarean delivery rate subsequent to a failed induction of labor. Relative to women who present in spontaneous labor, the cesarean delivery rate is approximately doubled when induction of labor is attempted in nulliparous women at term.[120] Overall, induction of labor at 42 weeks has been associated with a significant increase in cesarean deliveries when compared with patients in spontaneous labor (19 versus 14 percent, respectively, $P < 0.001$).[121] Independent risk factors for cesarean deliveries included nulliparity, a closed cervix, and the use of epidural anesthesia.

Induction of Labor Versus Expectant Management

Although most authors agree that induction of labor is indicated in women with an "inducible" uterine cervix, there is lack of agreement as to the management of the patient whose cervix is deemed "unfavorable." Induction of labor in all women at 42 weeks' gestation is one option. Another option is serial fetal surveillance to assess fetal well-being in women with an unfavorable cervix. These surveillance programs have focused on the detection of fetal hypoxia associated with uteroplacental insufficiency. To this end, fetal heart rate monitoring, biophysical profile, and ultrasonographic assessment of amniotic fluid volume have been used. Delivery is undertaken when signs of fetal compromise are detected. In 1992, Hannah et al.[122] randomized 3,407 women with uncomplicated pregnancies of 41 or more weeks' gestation to two management protocols: induction of labor or serial fetal monitoring. They concluded that the rates of perinatal morbidity and mortality were the same with the two approaches; however, the rate of cesarean delivery was lower in the induction group. In contrast, Almstrom et al.,[123] who also randomized patients into active and conservative management protocols, concluded that serial fetal monitoring resulted in a lower cesarean section rate. A recent meta-analysis of 11 prospective studies demonstrated that induction of labor resulted in a slightly lower cesarean section rate compared with expectant management.[124] The randomized controlled trial (n = 440) conducted by the National Institute of Child Health and Human Development Network of Maternal-Fetal Medicine Units reported no fetal or maternal advantages to elective induction of labor at 41 weeks of gestation relative to serial fetal monitoring and indicated that either management approach was acceptable.[83] Adverse fetal outcome was defined by the presence of neonatal seizures, intracranial hemorrhage, need for mechanical ventilation, or nerve injury. The incidence of adverse fetal outcome was 1.5 percent in the induction group and 1 percent in the expectant management group. The cesarean delivery rate was 18 percent in the expectant group, 23 percent in the PGE_2 gel group, and 18 percent in the placebo gel group. The authors concluded that there is good evidence that no approach is superior, thus suggesting that either induction of labor or serial monitoring would be equally reasonable.

A recent meta-analysis of 16 studies concluded that induction of labor resulted in a slightly lower cesarean section rate compared with expectant management (20.1 versus 22 percent [or 0.88; 95 percent CI 0.78, 0.99]).[125] Subjects whose labor was induced had a nonsignificantly lower perinatal mortality rate (0.09 versus 0.33 percent). In addition, there were no significant differences in the rates of meconium aspiration, meconium below the vocal cords, low Apgar scores, or NICU admissions. In contrast, the meta-analysis published in the Cochrane Review (19 studies) concluded that induction of labor after 41 weeks' gestation was associated with a significantly lower perinatal mortality rate (OR 0.2; 95 percent CI 0.06, 0.7) without an increase in the rate of cesarean delivery (OR 1.02; 95 percent CI 0.7, 1.38).[126] Thus, it would be reasonable to conclude that induction of labor at 41 weeks is not associated with an increased rate of cesarean deliveries and, in view of the fact that fetal mortality significantly increases past 41 weeks, a routine delivery is likely to result in a lower perinatal mortality rate.

SUMMARY AND RECOMMENDATION

Management of the prolonged pregnancy is primarily determined by the interplay of three factors: certainty of gestational dating, the risks associated with expectant management, and the likelihood of spontaneous vaginal delivery following an induction of labor. A detailed discussion of the risks, benefits, and alternatives should be initiated long before the patient reaches 41 weeks' gestation.

KEY POINTS

- Whenever possible, gestational age should be established by a first or an early second-trimester ultrasound examination.
- Perinatal morbidity and mortality are significantly increased when gestational age at birth is 41 weeks or more. It is more pronounced when the fetal weight is below the 10th percentile for gestational age.
- Prolonged pregnancy is associated with a significant increase in maternal morbidity, including perineal injury and cesarean delivery.
- Sweeping of the membranes at term decreases slightly the number of pregnancies reaching either 41 or 42 weeks' gestation.
- Induction of labor may be considered at or beyond 41 weeks' gestation in patients with a favorable cervix.
- Timely delivery prevents the risk of stillbirth but may result in increased maternal morbidity for patients who either undergo cesarean delivery following a failed induction of labor or, opt for an elective cesarean delivery.
- Conservative management (i.e., twice weekly fetal testing) or active management (i.e., induction of labor) is an equally reasonable option for patients with an unfavorable cervix.
- For patients managed conservatively, twice weekly fetal testing should be initiated at 41 weeks' gestation.

REFERENCES

1. Ballantyne JW: The problem of the postmature infant. J Obstet Gynaecol Br Emp 2:521, 1902.
2. Clifford SH: Postmaturity with placental dysfunction, clinical syndrome and pathologic findings. J Pediatr 44:1, 1954.
3. American College of Obstetricians and Gynecologists Practice bulletin: Management of Postterm pregnancy, September 2004.
4. World Health Organization (WHO): Recommended definition terminology and format for statistical tables related to the perinatal period and rise of a new certification for cause of perinatal deaths. Modifications recommended by FIGO as amended, October 14, 1976. Acta Obstet Gynecol Scand 56:347, 1977.
5. Federation of Gynecology and Obstetrics (FIGO): Report of the FIGO subcommittee on Perinatal Epidemiology and Health Statistics following a workshop in Cairo, November 11–18, 1984. London, International Federation of Gynecology and Obstetrics, 1986, p 54.
6. Ventura SJ, Martin JA, Taffel M: Advance report of final mortality statistics, 1993. Monthly Vital Statistics Report (Suppl). Vol 44, No 3. Hyattsville, MD, National Center for Health Statistics, 1995.
7. Fonseca L, Monga M, Silva J: Postdates pregnancy in an indigent population: The financial burden. Am J Obstet Gynecol 188:1214, 2003.

8. Norwitz ER, Robinson JN, Challis JR: The control of labor. N Engl J Med 341:660, 1999.
9. Liggins GC: The role of the hypothalamic-pituitary-adrenal axis in preparing the fetus for birth. Am J Obstet Gynecol 182:475, 2000.
10. Smith R: The timing of birth. Sci Am 280:68, 1999.
11. Naeye RL: Causes of perinatal mortality excess in prolonged gestation. Am J Epidemiol 108:429, 1978.
12. Rabe T, Hosch R, Runnebaum B: Sulfatase deficiency in the human placenta: clinical findings. Biol Res Pregnancy Perinatol 4:95, 1983.
13. Campbell MK, Ostbye T, Irgens LM: Post-term birth: risk factors and outcomes in a 10-year cohort of Norwegian births. Obstet Gynecol 89:543, 1997.
14. Zweidling MA: Factors pertaining to prolonged pregnancy and its outcome. Pediatrics 40:202, 1967.
15. Gardosi J, Vanner T, Francis A: Gestational age and induction of labor for prolonged pregnancy. Br J Obstet Gynaecol 104:792, 1997.
16. Boyd ME, Usher RH, McLean FH, Kramer MS: Obstetric consequences of postmaturity. Am J Obstet Gynecol 158:334, 1988.
17. Nguyen TH, Larsen T, Engholm G, Moller H: Evaluation of ultrasound-estimated date of delivery in 17,450 spontaneous singleton births: do we need to modify Naegele's rule? Ultrasound Obstet Gynecol 14:23, 1999.
18. Bennett KA, Crane JMG, O'Shea B, et al: First trimester ultrasound screening is effective in reducing postterm labor induction rates: a randomized controlled trial. Am J Obstet Gynecol 190:1077, 2004.
19. Mul T, Mongelli M, Gardosi J: A comparative analysis of second-trimester ultrasound dating formulae in pregnancies conceived with artificial reproductive techniques. Ultrasound Obstet Gynecol 8:397, 1996.
20. Gardosi J, Mongelli M: Risk assessment adjusted for gestational age in maternal serum screening for Down's syndrome. BMJ 306:1509, 1993.
21. Gardosi J: Dating of pregnancy: time to forget the last menstrual period. Ultrasound Obstet Gynecol 9:367, 1997.
22. Tunon K, Eik-Nes SH, Grottum P: Fetal outcome in pregnancies defined as post-term according to the last menstrual period estimate, but not according to the ultrasound estimate. Ultrasound Obstet Gynecol 14:12, 1999.
23. Divon MY, Haglund B, Nisell H, et al: Fetal and neonatal mortality in the post-term pregnancy: the impact of gestational age and fetal growth restriction. Am J Obstet Gynecol 178:726, 1998.
24. Ingemarsson I, Kallen K: Stillbirths and rate of neonatal deaths in 76,761 postterm pregnancies in Sweden, 1982–1991: a register study. Acta Obstet Gynecol Scand 76:658, 1997.
25. Clausson B, Cnattingius S, Axelsson O: Outcomes of post-term births: the role of fetal growth restriction and malformations. Obstet Gynecol 94:758, 1999.
26. Smith GCS: Estimating risks of perinatal death. Am J Obstet Gynecol 192:17, 2005.
27. Yudkin PL, Wood L, Redman CW: Risk of unexplained stillbirth at different gestational ages. Lancet 1:1192, 1987.
28. Feldman GB: Prospective risk of stillbirth. Obstet Gynecol 79:547, 1992.
29. Hilder L, Costeloe K, Thilaganathan B: Prolonged pregnancy: evaluating gestation-specific risks of fetal and infant mortality. Br J Obstet Gynaecol 105:169, 1998.
30. Cotzias CS, Paterson-Brown S, Fisk NM: Prospective risk of unexplained stillbirth in singleton pregnancies at term: population based analysis. BMJ 319:287, 1999.
31. Huang DY, Usher RH, Kramer MS, et al: Determinants of unexplained antepartum fetal deaths. Obstet Gynecol 95; 215, 2000.
32. Caughey AB, Stotland NE, Escobar GJ: What is the best measure of maternal complications of term pregnancy: ongoing pregnancies or pregnancies delivered? Am J Obstet Gynecol 189:1047, 2003.
33. Kahn B, Lumey LH, Zybert PA, et al: Prospective risk of fetal death in singleton, twin, and triplet gestations: implications for practice. Obstet Gynecol 102:685, 2003.
34. Divon MY, Ferber A, Sanderson M, et al: A functional definition of prolonged pregnancy based on daily fetal and neonatal mortality rates. Ultasound Obstet Gynecol 23:423, 2004.
35. Caughey AB, Musci TJ: Complications of term pregnancies beyond 37 weeks of gestation. Obstet Gynecol 103:57, 2004.
36. Olesen AW, Westergaard JG, Olsen J: Perinatal and maternal complications related to postterm delivery: A national register-base study, 1978–1993. Am J Obstet Gynecol 189:222, 2003.
37. Lovell KE: The effect of postmaturity on the developing child. Med J Aust 1:131, 1973.
38. Ting RV, Wang MH, Scott TF: The dysmature infant. Associated factors and outcome at 7 years of age. J Pediatr 90:943, 1977.
39. Shime J, Librach CL, Gare DJ, Cook CJ: The influence of prolonged pregnancy on infant development at one and two years of age: a prospective controlled study. Am J Obstet Gynecol 154:341, 1986.
40. Boyd ME, Usher RH, McLean FH: Fetal macrosomia: prediction, risks, proposed management. Obstet Gynecol 61:715, 1983.
41. McLean FH, Boyd ME, Usher RH, Kramer MS: Post-term infants: too big or too small? Am J Obstet Gynecol 164:619, 1991.
42. Nahum GG, Stanislaw H, Huffaker BJ: Fetal weight gain at term: linear with minimal dependence on maternal obesity. Am J Obstet Gynecol 172:1387, 1995.
43. Pollack RN, Hauer-Pollack G, Divon MY: Macrosomia in postdates pregnancies: the accuracy of routine ultrasonographic screening. Am J Obstet Gynecol 167:7, 1992.
44. Chervenak LJ, Divon MY, Hirsch J, et al: Macrosomia in the post-date pregnancy: is routine sonography screening indicated? Am J Obstet Gynecol 161:753, 1989.
45. Pollack RN, Divon MY: Problems in detecting fetal macrosomia. Contemp Ob/Gyn, p. 39–43, October, 1991.
46. O'Reilly-Green CP, Divon MY: Receiver operating characteristic curves of sonographic estimated fetal weight for prediction macrosomia in prolonged pregnancies. Ultrasound Obstet Gynecol 9:403, 1997.
47. ACOG Practice Bulletin Fetal Macrosomia. No. 22 Nov. 2000.
48. Rouse DJ, Owen J: Prophylactic cesarean delivery for fetal macrosomia diagnosed by means of ultrasonography—a faustian bargain? Am J Obstet Gynecol 181:332, 1999.
49. Rouse DJ, Owen J, Goldenberg RL, Cliver SP: The effectiveness and costs of elective cesarean delivery for fetal macrosomia diagnosed by ultrasound. JAMA 276:1480, 1996.
50. Leaphart WL, Meyer MC, Capeless EL: Labor induction with a prenatal diagnosis of fetal macrosomia. J Matern Fetal Med 6:99, 1997.
51. Gonen O, Rosen DJ, Dolfin Z, et al: Induction of labor versus expectant management in macrosomia: a randomized study. Obstet Gynecol 89:913, 1997.
52. Levine AB, Lockwood CJ, Brown B, et al: Sonographic diagnosis of the large for gestational age fetus at term: does it make a difference? Obstet Gynecol 79:55, 1992.
53. Guidetti DA, Divon MY, Langer O: Postdate fetal surveillance: is 41 weeks too early? Am J Obstet Gynecol 161:91, 1989.
54. Jazayeri A, Tsibris JCM, Spellacy WN: Elevated umbilical cord plasma erythropoietin levels in prolonged pregnancies. Obstet Gynecol 92:63, 1998.
55. Manning FA, Morrison I, Harman CR, et al: Fetal assessment based on fetal biophysical profile scoring: experience in 19,221 referred high-risk pregnancies. II. An analysis of false-negative fetal deaths. Am J Obstet Gynecol 157:880, 1987.
56. John JM, Harman CR, Lange IR, Manning FA: Biophysical profile scoring in the management of the post term pregnancy: an analysis of 307 patients. Am J Obstet Gynecol 154:269, 1986.
57. Phelan JP, Ahn MO, Smith CV, et al: Amniotic fluid index measurements during pregnancy. J Reprod Med 32:601, 1987.
58. Smith CV, Phelan JP, Platt LD, et al: Fetal acoustic stimulation testing (the Fas test). II. A randomized clinical comparison with the nonstress test. Am J Obstet Gynecol 155:131, 1986.
59. Clark SL, Sabey P, Jolley K: Nonstress testing with acoustic stimulation and amniotic fluid volume assessment: 5973 tests without unexpected fetal death Am J Obstet Gynecol 160:694, 1989.
60. Miller DA, Rabello YA, Paul RH: The modified biophysical profile: antepartum testing in the 1990's. Am J Obstet Gynecol 174:812, 1996.
61. Freeman RK, Anderson G, Dorcester W: A prospective multicenter multiinstitutional study of antepartum fetal heart rate monitoring. II. Contraction stress test versus nonstress

test for primary surveillance. Am J Obstet Gynecol 143:778, 1982.
62. Sylvestre G, Fisher M, Westgren M, Divon MY: Non-reassuring fetal status in the prolonged pregnancy: the impact of fetal weight. Ultrasound Obstet Gynecol 18:244, 2001.
63. Onyeije CI, Divon MY: The impact of maternal ketonuria on fetal test results in the setting of postterm pregnancy. Am J Obstet Gynecol 184:713, 2001.
64. Marks AD, Divon MY: Longitudinal study of the amniotic fluid index in postdates pregnancy. Obstet Gynecol 79:229, 1992.
65. Gresham EL, Rankin JHG, Makowski EL, et al: An evaluation of fetal renal function in chronic sheep preparation. J Clin Invest 51:149, 1972.
66. Nicolaides KH, Peters MT, Vyas S, et al: Relation of rate of urine production to oxygen tension in small for gestational age fetuses. Am J Obstet Gynecol 162:387, 1990.
67. Trimmer KJ, Leveno KJ, Peters MT, Kelly MA: Observations on the cause of oligohydramnios in prolonged pregnancy. Am J Obstet Gynecol 163:1900, 1990.
68. Bar-Hava I, Divon MY, Sardo M, Barnhard Y: Is oligohydramnios in post-term pregnancy associated with redistribution of fetal blood flow? Am J Obstet Gynecol 173:519, 1995.
69. Leveno KJ, Quirk JG Jr, Cunningham FG, et al. Prolonged pregnancy. I. Observations concerning the causes of fetal distress. Am J Obstet Gynecol 150:465, 1984.
70. Gabbe SG, Ettinger BB, Freeman RK, Martin CB: Umbilical cord compression associated with amniotomy: laboratory observations. Am J Obstet Gynecol 126:353, 1976.
71. Miyazaki FS, Taylor NA: Saline amnioinfusion for relief of variable or prolonged decelerations. A preliminary report. Am J Obstet Gynecol 146:670, 1983.
72. Lee ST, Hon EH: Fetal hemodynamic response to umbilical cord compression. Obstet Gynecol 22:553, 1963.
73. Strong TH, Hetzler G, Sarno AP, Paul RH: Prophylactic intrapartum amnioinfusion: a randomized clinical trial. Am J Obstet Gynecol 162:1370, 1990.
74. Wenstrom KD, Parsons MT: The prevention of meconium aspiration in labor using amnioinfusion Obstet Gynecol 73:647, 1989.
75. Phelan JP, Smith CV, Broussard P, Small M: Amniotic fluid volume assessment with the four-quadrant technique at 36–42 weeks' gestation. J Reprod Med 32:540, 1987.
76. Phelan JP, Platt LD, Yeh SY, et al: The role of ultrasound assessment of amniotic fluid volume in the management of the postdate pregnancy. Am J Obstet Gynecol 151:304, 1985.
77. Phelan JP, Ahn MO, Smith CV, et al: Amniotic fluid index measurements during pregnancy. J Reprod Med 32:601, 1987.
78. Divon MY, Marks AD, Henderson CE: Longitudinal measurement of amniotic fluid index in postterm pregnancies and its association with fetal outcome. Am J Obstet Gynecol 172:142, 1995.
79. Manning FA, Platt LD, Sipos L: Antepartum fetal evaluation: development of a fetal biophysical profile. Am J Obstet Gynecol 136;787, 1980.
80. Chamberlain PF, Manning FA, Morrison I, et al: Ultrasound evaluation of amniotic fluid volume. I. The relationship of marginal and decreased amniotic fluid volumes to perinatal outcome. Am J Obstet Gynecol 150:245, 1984.
81. Crowley P, O'Herlihey C, Boylan P: The value of ultrasound measurement of amniotic fluid volume on the management of prolonged pregnancies. Br J Obstet Gynaecol 91:444, 1984.
82. Chauhan SP, Sanderson M, Hendrix N, et al: Perinatal outcome and amniotic fluid index in the antepartum and intrapartum periods: a meta-analysis. Am J Obstet Gynecol 181:1473, 1999.
83. Morris JM Thompson K, Smithey J, et al: The usefulness of ultrasound assessment of amniotic fluid in predicting adverse outcome in prolonged pregnancy: a prospective blinded observational study. Br J Obstet Gynecol 110:989, 2003
84. O'Reilly-Green CP, Divon MY: Predictive value of amniotic fluid index for oligohydramnios in patients with prolonged pregnancies. J Matern Fetal Med 5:218, 1996.
85. Strokes HJ, Roberts RV, Newnham JP: Doppler flow velocity waveform analysis in postdate pregnancies. Aust N Z J Obstet Gynecol 31:27, 1991.
86. Guidetti DA, Divon MY, Cavalieri RL, et al: Fetal umbilical artery flow velocimetry in postdate pregnancies. Am J Obstet Gynecol 157:1521, 1987.
87. Farmakides G, Schulman H, Ducey J, et al: Uterine and umbilical Doppler velocimetry in post term pregnancy. J Reprod Med 33:259, 1988.
88. Zimmermann P, Alback T, Koskinen J, et al: Doppler flow velocimetry of the umbilical artery, uteroplacental arteries and fetal middle cerebral artery in prolonged pregnancy. Ultrasound Obstet Gynecol 5:189, 1995.
89. Selam B, Korsal R, Ozcan T: Fetal arterial and venous Doppler parameters in the interpretation of oligohydramnios in postterm pregnancies. Ultrasound Obstet Gynecol 15:403, 2000.
90. Weiner Z, Farmakides G, Schulman H, et al: Central and peripheral haemodynamic changes in post-term fetuses: correlation with oligohydramnios and abnormal fetal heart rate pattern. Br J Obstet Gynaecol 103:541, 1996.
91. Lim FT, Scherjon SA, van Beckhoven, et al: Association of stress during delivery with increased numbers of nucleated cells and hematopoietic progenitor cells in umbilical cord blood. Am J Obstet Gynecol 183:1144, 2000.
92. Ferber A, Grassi A, Akyol D, et al: The association of fetal heart rate patterns with nucleated red blood cell counts at birth. Am J Obstet Gynecol 188:1228, 2003.
93. Yeruchimovich M, Mimouni FB, Green DW, Dollberg S: Nucleated red blood cells in healthy infants of women with gestational diabetes. Obstet Gynecol 95:84, 2000.
94. Yeruchimovich M, Dollberg S, Green DW, Mimouni FB: Nucleated red blood cells in infants of smoking mothers. Obstet Gynecol 93:403, 1999.
95. Hanlon-Lundberg KM, Kirby RS: Nucleated red blood cells as a marker of acidemia in term neonates. Am J Obstet Gynecol 181:196, 1999.
96. Axt-Fliedner R, Hendrik HJ, Schmidt W: Nucleated red blood cell counts in growth-restricted neonates with absent or reversed-end diastolic umbilical artery velocity. Clin Exp Obstet Gynecol 29:242, 2002.
97. Buonocore G, Perrone S, Gioia D, et al: Nucleated red blood cell count at birth as an index of perinatal brain damage. Am J Obstet Gynecol 181:1500, 1999.
98. Blackwell SC, Refuerzo JS, Wolfe HW, et al: The relationship between nucleated red blood cell count and early onset neonatal seizures. Am J Obstet Gynecol 182:1452, 2000.
99. Korst LM, Phelan JP, Ahn MO, Martin GI: Nucleated red blood cells: an update on the marker for fetal asphyxia. Am J Obstet Gynecol 175:843, 1996.
100. Axt R, Ertan K, Hendrik J, et al: Nucleated red blood cells in cord blood of singleton term and post-term neonates. J Perinat Med 27:376, 1999.
101. Perri T, Ferber A, Digli A, et al: Nucleated red blood cells in uncomplicated prolonged pregnancy. Obstet Gynecol 104:372, 2004.
102. Manchandra R, Vora M, Gruslin A: Influence of postdatism and meconium on fetal erythropoietin. J Perinatal 19:479, 1999.
103. Dollberg S, Livny S, Mordechcyev N, Mimouni FB: Nucleated red blood cells in meconium aspiration syndrome. Obstet Gynecol 97:593, 2001.
104. Roach VJ, Rogers MS: Pregnancy outcome beyond 41 weeks' gestation. Int J Gynaecol Obstet 59:19, 1997.
105. Goffeng AR, Milsom I, Lindstedt G, et al: Fetal fibronectin in vaginal fluid of women in prolonged pregnancy. Gynecol Obstet Invest 44:224, 1997.
106. Mouw RJ, Egberts J, Kragt H, van Roosmalen J: Cervicovaginal fetal fibronectin concentrations: predictive value of impending birth in post-term pregnancies. Eur J Obstet Gynecol Reprod Biol 80:67, 1998.
107. Rozenberg P, Goffinet F, Hessabi M: Comparison of the Bishop score ultrasonographically measured cervical length, and fetal fibronectin assay in predicating time until delivery and type of delivery at term. Am J Obstet Gynecol 182: 108, 2000.
108. Boulvain M, Irion O: Stripping/sweeping of the membranes to induce labour or to prevent post-term pregnancy (Cochrane Review). *In* The Cochrane Library, Issue 4. Oxford, Update Software, 1998
109. Sonek J, Shellhaas C: Cervical sonography: a review. Ultrasound Obstet Gynecol 11:71, 1998.

110. Pandis GK, Papageorghiou AT, Ramanathan VG, et al: Preinduction sonographic measurement of cervical length in the prediction of successful induction. Ultrasound Obstet Gynecol 18:623, 2001.
111. Rane SM, Pandis GR, Guirgis RR, et al: Pre-induction sonographic measurement of cervical length in prolonged pregnancy: the effect of parity in the prediction of induction-to-delivery interval. Ultrasound Obstet Gynecol 22:40, 2003.
112. Ramanathan G, Yu C, Osei E, Nicolaides KH: Ultrasound examination at 37 weeks' gestation in the prediction of pregnancy outcome: the value of cervical assessment. Ultrasound Obstet Gynecol 22:598, 2003.
113. Magann EF, Chauhan SP, Nevils BG, et al: Management of pregnancies beyond forty-one weeks' gestation with an unfavorable cervix. Am J Obstet Gynecol 178:1279, 1998.
114. Lien JM, Morgan MA, Garite TJ, et al: Antepartum cervical ripening: applying prostaglandin E_2 gel in conjunction with scheduled non-stress tests in postdates pregnancies. Am J Obstet Gynecol 79:453, 1998.
115. Obel G, Rabay D, Rothbard H, Rauch M: Randomized trial of outpatient induction of labor with vaginal PGE_2 at 40–41 weeks of gestation versus expectant management. Arch Gynecol Obstet 258:109, 1996.
116. Shaw KJ, Medearis AL, Horenstein J, et al: Selective labor induction in post-term patients. Observations and outcomes. J Reprod Med 37:157, 1992.
117. Papageorgiou I, Tsionou C, Minaretzis D, et al: Labor characteristics of uncomplicated prolonged pregnancies after induction with intracervical prostaglandin E_2 gel versus intravenous oxytocin. Gynecol Obstet Invest 34:92, 1992.
118. The National Institute of Child Health and Human Development Network of Maternal Fetal Medicine Units: A clinical trial of induction of labor versus expectant management in post term pregnancy. Am J Obstet Gynecol 170:716, 1994.
119. Reichler A, Romem Y, Divon MY: Induction of labor. Curr Opin Obstet Gynecol 7:432, 1995.
120. Seyb ST, Berka RJ, Socol ML, Dooley SL: Risk of cesarean delivery with elective induction of labor at term in nulliparous women. Obstet Gynecol 94:600, 1999.
121. Alexander JM, McIntire DD, Leveno KJ: Prolonged pregnancy: induction of labor and cesarean births. Obstet Gynecol 97:911, 2001.
122. Hannah ME, Hannah WJ, Hellman J, et al: Induction of labor as compared with serial antenatal monitoring in post-term pregnancies. A randomized controlled trial. The Canadian Multicenter Post-term Pregnancy Trial Group. N Engl J Med 327:1587, 1992.
123. Almstrom H, Granstrom L, Ekman G: Serial antenatal monitoring compared with labor induction in post-term pregnancies. Acta Obstet Gynecol Scand 74:599, 1995.
124. Grant JM: Induction of labour confers benefits in prolonged pregnancy. Br J Obstet Gynecol 101:99, 1994.
125. Sanchez-Ramos L, Olivier F, Delke I, Kaunitz AM: Labor induction versus expectant management for postterm pregnancies; a systematic review with meta-analysis. Obstet Gynecol 101:1312, 2003.
126. Crowly P: Interventions for preventing or improving the outcome of delivery at or beyond term (Cochrane Review). *In* The Cochrane Library, Issue 2 Chicester, UK, John Wiley and sons Ltd, 2000.

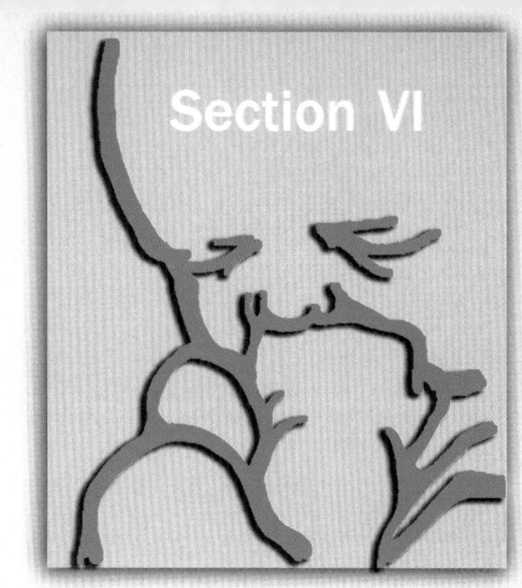

Pregnancy and Coexisting Disease

Hypertension

BAHA M. SIBAI

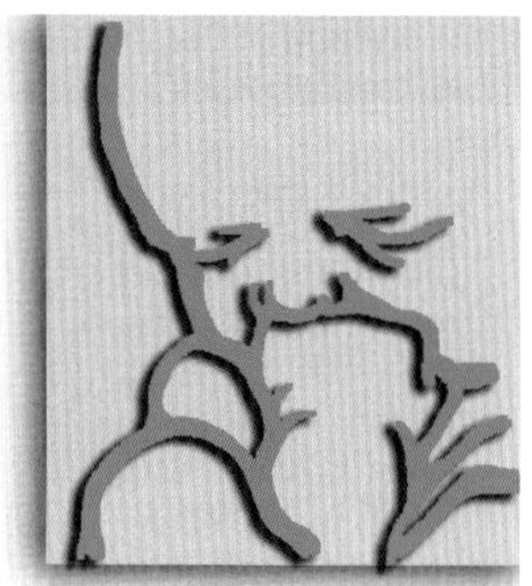

CHAPTER 33

KEY ABBREVIATIONS

Acute fatty liver of pregnancy	AFLP
Adult respiratory distress syndrome	ARDS
Alanine transaminase	ALT
Angiotensin converting enzyme inhibitor	ACE
Aspartate transaminase	AST
Blood pressure	BP
Central venous pressure	CVP
Computed axial tomography	CAT
Computed tomography	CT
Confidence interval	CI
Disseminated intravascular coagulopathy	DIC
Electrocardiogram	ECG
Electroencephalography	EEG
Glomerular filtration rate	GFR
Hemolysis, elevated liver enzymes, or low platelets syndrome	HELLP
Hemolytic uremic syndrome	HUS
Immune thrombocytopenic purpura	ITP
Intrauterine growth restriction	IUGR
Lactate dehydrogenase	LDH
Magnetic resonance imaging	MRI
Nonstress test	NST
Number needed to treat	NTT
Placental-like growth factor	PLGF
Prostaglandin I_2	PGI_2
Pulmonary capillary wedge pressure	PCWP
Small for gestational age	SGA
Soluble fms-like tyrosine kinase 1	sFlt-1
Thrombotic thrombocytopenic purpura	TTP
Thromboxane A_2	TXA_2
Tumor necrosis factor-α	TNFα
Vascular endothelial growth factor	VEGF

Hypertensive disorders represent the most common medical complications of pregnancy, with a reported incidence between 5 and 10 percent.[1] The incidence varies among different hospitals, regions, and countries. These disorders are a major cause of maternal and perinatal mortality and morbidity worldwide.[2] The term *hypertension in pregnancy* is commonly used to describe a wide spectrum of patients who may have only mild elevations in blood pressure (BP) or severe hypertension with various organ dysfunctions. The manifestations in these

Table 33-1. Hypertensive Disorders of Pregnancy

CLINICAL FINDINGS	CHRONIC HYPERTENSION	GESTATIONAL HYPERTENSION*	PREECLAMPSIA
Time of onset of hypertension	<20 weeks	Usually in third trimester	≥20 weeks
Degree of hypertension	Mild or severe	Mild	Mild or severe
Proteinuria*	Absent	Absent	Usually present
Serum urate >5.5 mg/dl (0.33 mmol/L)	Rare	Absent	Present in almost all cases
Hemoconcentration	Absent	Absent	Severe disease
Thrombocytopenia	Absent	Absent	Severe disease
Hepatic dysfunction	Absent	Absent	Severe disease

*Defined as ≥1+ by dipstick testing on two occasions or ≥300 mg in a 24-hour urine collection.
From Sibai BM: Drug therapy: treatment of hypertension in pregnant women. Drug Therapy Series. N Engl J Med 335:257, 1996. Copyright 1996 Massachusetts Medical Society, with permission.

Table 33-2. Criteria for Mild Gestational Hypertension in Healthy Pregnant Women

Systolic blood pressure <160 mm Hg and diastolic blood pressure <110 mm Hg
Proteinuria <300 mg/24 hour collection
Platelet count >100,000/mm^3
Normal liver enzymes
Absent maternal symptoms
Absent IUGR and oligohydraminos by ultrasound

IUGR, intrauterine growth restriction.

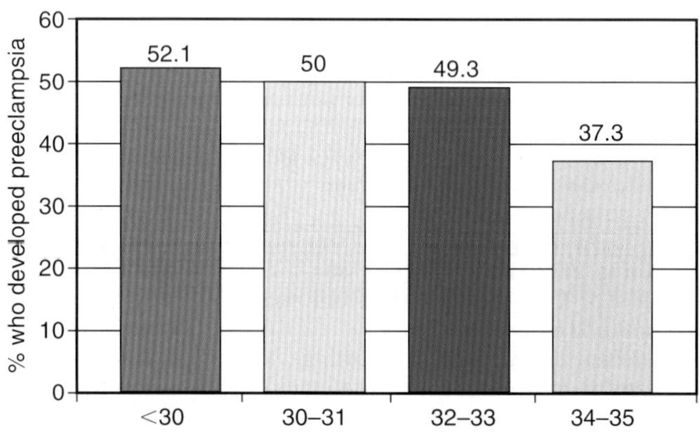

Figure 33-1. Rate of progression from gestational hypertension to preeclampsia by gestational age at diagnosis. (From Barton JR, O'Brien JM, Bergauer NK, et al: Mild gestational hypertension remote from term: progression and outcome. Am J Obstet Gynecol 184:979, 2001.)

patients may be clinically similar (e.g., hypertension, proteinuria); however, they may result from different underlying causes such as chronic hypertension, renal disease, or pure preeclampsia. The three most common forms of hypertension are acute gestational hypertension, preeclampsia, and chronic essential hypertension.

DEFINITIONS

Hypertension may be present before pregnancy, or it may be diagnosed for the first time during pregnancy. In addition, in some women, hypertension may become evident only intrapartum or during the postpartum period. For clinical purposes, women with hypertension may be classified into one of three categories (Table 33-1).[3]

Gestational Hypertension

Gestational hypertension is the development of an elevated BP during pregnancy or in the first 24 hours postpartum without other signs or symptoms of preeclampsia or preexisting hypertension. The BP must return to normal within 6 weeks after delivery. Hypertension is defined as a BP greater than or equal to 140 mm Hg systolic or 90 mm Hg diastolic (Table 33-2). The hypertension should be present on at least two occasions, at least 4 hours apart, but within a maximum of a 1-week period.[4] It is recognized that some women with gestational hypertension may have undiagnosed chronic hypertension, whereas others will subsequently progress to develop the clinical syndrome of preeclampsia.[5] In general, the likelihood of progression to preeclampsia depends on gestational age at time of diagnosis, with higher rates if the onset of hypertension is before 35 weeks' gestation[5] (Fig. 33-1).

Preeclampsia and Eclampsia

The classic triad of preeclampsia includes hypertension, proteinuria, and edema. However, there is now universal agreement that edema should not be considered as part of the diagnosis of preeclampsia.[1–8] Indeed, edema is neither sufficient nor necessary to confirm the diagnosis of preeclampsia, because edema is a common finding in normal pregnancy and approximately one third of eclamptic women never demonstrate edema.[9] In general, preeclampsia is primarily defined as gestational hypertension plus proteinuria. Proteinuria is defined as a concentration of 0.1 g/L or more in at least two random urine specimens collected 4 hours or more apart or 0.3 g (300 mg) in a 24-hour period. In the absence of proteinuria, the syndrome of preeclampsia should be considered when gestational hypertension is present in association with persistent cerebral symptoms, epigastric or right upper quadrant pain plus nausea or vomiting, fetal growth restriction, or with abnormal laboratory tests such as thrombocytopenia and elevated liver enzymes.[2,7] In mild preeclampsia, the diastolic BP remains below 110 mm Hg and the systolic BP remains below 160 mm Hg (see the box "Criteria for Severe Preeclampsia").[2,8] Eclampsia is the occurrence of seizures not attributable to other causes.[9]

Chronic Hypertension

Chronic hypertension is defined as hypertension present before the pregnancy or that is diagnosed before the 20th week of gestation. Hypertension that persists for more than 42 days postpartum is also classified as chronic hypertension.

Chronic Hypertension with Superimposed Preeclampsia

Women with chronic hypertension may develop superimposed preeclampsia, which increases morbidity for both the mother and fetus. The diagnosis of superimposed preeclampsia is based on one or more of the following findings: development of new-onset proteinuria is defined as the urinary excretion of 0.5 g protein or greater in a 24-hour specimen in women with hypertension and no proteinuria before 20 weeks' gestation or in women with hypertension and proteinuria before 20 weeks, the diagnosis requires severe exacerbation in hypertension plus development of symptoms or thrombocytopenia and abnormal liver enzymes in women with hypertension and proteinuria before 20 weeks (Table 33-3).[10,11]

Criteria for Severe Preeclampsia

1. Blood pressure of ≥160 mm Hg systolic or ≥110 mm Hg diastolic, recorded on at least two occasions at least 6 hours apart with patient at bed rest
2. Proteinuria of ≥5 g in 24 hours
3. Oliguria (≤400 ml in 24 hours)
4. Cerebral visual disturbances
5. Epigastric pain, nausea, and vomiting
6. Pulmonary edema
7. Impaired liver function of unclear etiology
8. Thrombocytopenia

Gestational Hypertension

Gestational hypertension is the most frequent cause of hypertension during pregnancy. The incidence ranges between 6 and 17 percent in nulliparous women[4,12,13] and between 2 and 4 percent in multiparous women.[2] The incidence is markedly increased in patients with multiple gestation.[14,15] In general, the majority of cases of gestational hypertension develop at or beyond 37 weeks' gestation, and thus, the overall pregnancy outcome is usually similar or even superior to that seen in women with normotensive pregnancies (Table 33-4).[4,5,12,13] Both gestational age at delivery and birth weight in these pregnancies are significantly higher than that in normotensive pregnancies.[4,12] However, women with mild gestational hypertension have higher rates of induction of labor and thus higher rates of cesarean delivery as compared with women with normotensive gestation.[4]

On the other hand, maternal and perinatal morbidities are substantially increased in women with severe gestational hypertension.[2,4,16] Indeed, these women have higher morbidities than women with mild preeclampsia. The rates of abruptio placentae, preterm delivery (at less than 37 and 35 weeks), and rates of small for gestational age

Table 33-3. Recommended Criteria to Diagnose Preeclampsia in Women with Preexisting Medical Conditions

CONDITION	CRITERIA NEEDED
Hypertension only	Proteinuria ≥500 mg/24 hours or thrombocytopenia
Proteinuria only	New-onset hypertension plus symptoms or thrombocytopenia or elevated liver enzymes
Hypertension plus proteinuria (renal disease or class F diabetes)	Worsening severe hypertension plus either new onset of symptoms, thrombocytopenia, or elevated liver enzymes

Table 33-4. Pregnancy Outcome in Women with Mild Gestational Hypertension

	KNUIST ET AL.[13] N = 396	HAUTH ET AL.[4] N = 715	BARTON ET AL.[5] N = 405	SIBAI ET AL.[12] N = 186
Gestation at delivery (wk)*	N/R	39.7	37.4†	39.1
<37 wk (%)	5.3	7.0	17.3	5.9
<34 wk (%)	1.3	1.0	4.9	1.6
Birth weight (g)*	N/R	3303	3038	3217
SGA (%)	1.5‡	6.9	13.8	7.0
<2,500 g (%)	7.1	7.7	23.5	N/R
Abruptio placentae (%)	0.5	0.3	0.5	0.5
Perinatal deaths (%)	0.8	0.5	0	0

N/R, not reported; SGA, Small for gestational age.
*Mean values.
†Women who developed hypertension at 24–35 weeks.
‡<3rd percentile.
Adapted from Sibai BM: Diagnosis and management of gestational hypertension and preeclampsia. Obstet Gynecol 102:181, 2003.

(SGA) infants in these women are similar to those seen in women with severe preeclampsia.[2,16] Therefore, these women should be managed as if they had severe preeclampsia. It is unclear whether this increase in preterm delivery is secondary to scheduled early delivery according to physician preference or because the disease process itself remains unknown.

PREECLAMPSIA

Preeclampsia is a form of hypertension that is unique to human pregnancy. The clinical findings of preeclampsia can manifest as either a maternal syndrome (hypertension and proteinuria with or without other multisystem abnormalities) or as a fetal syndrome (fetal growth restriction, reduced amniotic fluid, and abnormal oxygenation).[17] In practice, the maternal syndrome of preeclampsia represents a clinical spectrum with major differences between near-term preeclampsia without demonstrable fetal involvement versus preeclampsia that is associated with low birth weight and preterm delivery.[18] Preeclampsia is clearly a heterogeneous condition for which the pathogenesis could be different in women with various risk factors.[17,18] The pathogenesis of preeclampsia in nulliparous women may be different than that in women with preexisting vascular disease, in multifetal gestation, in diabetes mellitus, or previous preeclampsia. In addition, the pathophysiology of preeclampsia with early onset may be different than that of preeclampsia developing at term, during labor, or in the postpartum period.[17]

The incidence of preeclampsia ranges between 2 and 7 percent in healthy nulliparous women.[2,4,10] In these women, preeclampsia is generally mild, with the onset near term or intrapartum (75 percent of cases), and the condition conveys only a minimally increased risk for adverse pregnancy outcome.[2,4,10] In contrast, the incidence and severity of preeclampsia are substantially higher in women with multifetal gestation,[15,19] chronic hypertension,[10,11] previous preeclampsia,[10,20] pregestational diabetes mellitus,[10] and in those with preexisting thrombophilias.[21–23]

Several risk factors have been identified with increased risk of preeclampsia (see the box "Risk Factors for Preeclampsia"). Generally, preeclampsia is considered a disease of primigravid women. The risk increases in those who have limited sperm exposure with the same partner before conception.[17,24,25] The protective effects of long-term sperm exposure with the same partner might provide an explanation for the high risk of preeclampsia in women younger than 20 years old. A previous abortion (spontaneous and induced) or a previous normal pregnancy with the same partner is associated with a lower risk of preeclampsia. However, this protective effect is lost with a change of partner.[26] Both Scandinavian and studies in this country have confirmed the importance of paternal factors, that is, the so-called dangerous father.[27,28] Using whole population data, Lie et al.[28] demonstrated that men who fathered one preeclamptic pregnancy were nearly twice as likely to father a preeclamptic pregnancy in a different woman (1.8; 95 percent confidence interval [CI] 1.2 to 2.6; after adjustment for parity), regardless of whether the new partner had a preeclamptic pregnancy in the past or not. Thus, mothers had a substantially increased risk in their second pregnancy (2.9 percent) if they were impregnated by a man who had fathered a preeclamptic first pregnancy with another woman. This risk was nearly as high as the average risk among first pregnancies.[28]

Risk Factors for Preeclampsia

- Nulliparity
- Family history of preeclampsia
- Obesity
- Multifetal gestation
- Preeclampsia in previous pregnancy
- Poor outcome in previous pregnancy
  - Intrauterine growth retardation, abruptio, fetal death
- Preexisting medical—genetic conditions
  - Chronic hypertension
  - Renal disease
  - Type 1 (insulin-dependent) diabetes mellitus
  - Thrombophilias
    - Antiphospholipid antibody syndrome
    - Protein C, S, antithrombin deficiency
- Factor V Leiden

The recent advances in assisted reproductive technology have introduced several challenges for the maternal immune system that also increase the risk of preeclampsia. These include women older than 40 years, infertile women during their first gestation or obese women with polycystic ovary syndrome, and women who become pregnant with donated gametes, that is, donor insemination or oocyte donation, or embryo donation. The use of donated gametes can influence the maternal-fetal immune interaction. In addition, many of these women have multifetal gestations.[17,19,29]

Obesity is a definite risk for preeclampsia. Risk increases with increased body mass index.[30] The worldwide increase in obesity is thus likely to lead to a rise in the frequency of preeclampsia.[31] Obesity has a strong link with insulin resistance, which is a risk factor for preeclampsia. The exact mechanism by which obesity/insulin resistance is associated with preeclampsia is not well understood.

Two systematic reviews[21,22] found an overall higher rate of thrombophilia in women with preeclampsia compared to controls. Recently, a number of reports have failed to reproduce these findings.[32,33] The disparity in results can be seen to reflect the heterogeneity of the women being studied. Most negative studies included primarily (late) third-trimester cases. The Mello et al. study,[23] which included the largest series of preeclamptic patients so far, clearly showed the differential presence of thrombophilias in women with very early-onset severe disease (delivery <28 weeks) versus women requiring delivery during the third trimester.

Pathophysiology

The etiology of preeclampsia is unknown. Many theories have been suggested, but most of them have not withstood the test of time. Some of the theories that are

Theories Associated with the Etiology of Preeclampsia

Abnormal trophoblast invasion
Coagulation abnormalities
Vascular endothelial damage
Cardiovascular maladaptation
Immunologic phenomena
Genetic predisposition
Dietary deficiencies or excesses

still under consideration are listed in the box "Theories Associated with the Etiology of Preeclampsia."[17]

During normal pregnancy, impressive physiologic changes occur in the uteroplacental vasculature in general and in the cardiovascular system in particular. These changes are most likely induced by the interaction of the fetal (parental) allograft with maternal tissue. The development of mutual immunologic tolerance in the first trimester is thought to lead to important morphologic and biochemical changes in the systemic and uteroplacental maternal circulation.

Uterine Vascular Changes

The human placenta receives its blood supply from numerous uteroplacental arteries that are developed by the action of migratory interstitial and endovascular trophoblast into the walls of the spiral arterioles. This transforms the uteroplacental arterial bed into a low-resistance, low-pressure, high-flow system. The conversion of the spiral arterioles of the nonpregnant uterus into the uteroplacental arteries has been termed *physiologic changes*.[34] In a normal pregnancy, these trophoblast-induced vascular changes extend all the way from the intervillous space to the origin of the spiral arterioles from the radial arteries in the inner one third of the myometrium. It is suggested that these vascular changes are effected in two stages: "the conversion of the decidual segments of the spiral arterioles by a wave of endovascular trophoblast migration in the first trimester and the myometrial segments by a subsequent wave in the second trimester."[34] This process is reportedly associated with extensive fibrinoid formation and degeneration of the muscular layer in the arterial wall. These vascular changes result in the conversion of approximately 100 to 150 spiral arterioles into distended, tortuous, and funnel-shaped vessels that communicate through multiple openings into the intervillous space.

In contrast, pregnancies complicated by preeclampsia or by fetal growth restriction demonstrate inadequate maternal vascular response to placentation. In these pregnancies, the above-mentioned vascular changes are usually found only in the decidual segments of the uteroplacental arteries. Hence, the myometrial segments of the spiral arterioles are left with their musculoelastic architecture, thereby leaving them responsive to hormonal influences.[34] Additionally, the number of well-developed arterioles is smaller than that found in normotensive pregnancies. Kong and colleagues have postulated that this defective vascular response to placentation is due to inhibition of the second wave of endovascular trophoblast migration that normally occurs from about 16 weeks' gestation onward. These pathologic changes may have the effect of curtailing the increased blood supply required by the fetoplacental unit in the later stages of pregnancy, and correlate with decreased uteroplacental blood flow seen in most cases of preeclampsia. Frusca and associates studied placental bed biopsies obtained during cesarean delivery from normal pregnancies ($n = 14$), preeclamptic pregnancies ($n = 24$), and chronic hypertensive pregnancies only ($n = 5$).[35] Biopsies from the preeclamptic group demonstrated abnormal vascular changes in every case, with 18 having acute atherosclerotic changes. In contrast, 13 of the 14 biopsies from normotensive pregnancies had normal vascular physiologic changes, whereas biopsies from hypertensive patients showed all three types of physiologic changes. In addition, they found that the mean birth weight was significantly lower in the group with atherosclerosis than it was in the other group without such findings. It is important to note that these vascular changes may also be demonstrated in a significant proportion of normotensive pregnancies complicated by fetal growth restriction.[34,35] Meekins and associates[36] have found that endovascular trophoblast invasion is not an all-or-none phenomenon in normal and preeclamptic pregnancies. These authors observed that morphologic features in one spiral artery may not be representative of all vessels in a placental bed.

Using electron microscopy, Shanklin and Sibai[37] studied the ultrastructural changes in placental bed and uterine boundary vessels in 33 preeclamptic and 12 normotensive pregnancies. They found extensive ultrastructural endothelial injury in both placental site and nonplacental site vessels in all the specimens from preeclamptic women, which was absent in biopsies from normotensive women. The injury appeared to affect the endothelial mitochondria, which suggests a possible metabolic process. The endothelial injury ranged from swelling to complete erosion, and the swelling was associated with enlargement of endothelial nuclei resulting in reduction of the lumen. In some cases, the erosion was complete with associated deposition of heavy fibrin (Fig. 33-2). In addition, there was no correlation between the type or degree of endothelial damage and the level of maternal hypertension.

Vascular Endothelial Activation and Inflammation

The mechanism by which placental ischemia leads to the clinical syndrome of preeclampsia is thought to be related to the production of placental factors that enter the maternal circulation resulting in endothelial cell dysfunction. Soluble fms-like tyrosine kinase 1 (sFlt-1) is a protein that is produced by the placenta. It acts by binding to the receptor binding domains of vascular endothelial growth factor (VEGF), and it also binds to placental like growth factor (PLGF). Increased levels of this protein in the maternal circulation results in reduced levels of free VEGF and free PLFG, with resultant endothelial cell dysfunction.[38]

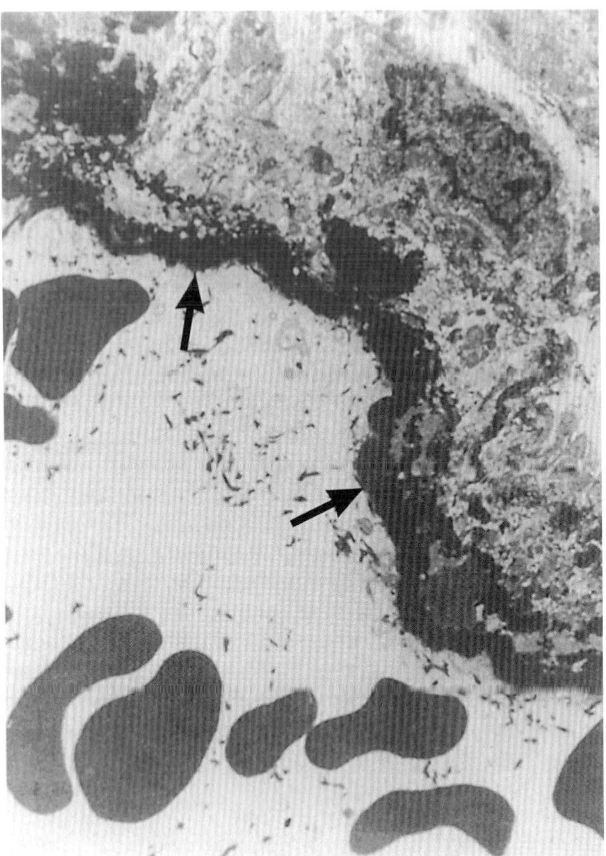

Figure 33-2. Compacted heavy fibrin deposition *(arrows)* and loose lamina fibrin replacing extensively eroded endothelium, nonplacental site region, uterine boundary zone, preeclampsia. (Original electron microscopic magnification, ×2,500.) (From Shanklin DR, Sibai BM: Ultrastructural aspects of preeclampsia. I. Placental bed and uterine boundary vessels. Am J Obstet Gynecol 161:735, 1989, with permission.)

Maternal serum and placental levels of sFlt-1 are increased in pregnancies complicated by preeclampsia above values seen during normal pregnancies. Maynard et al.[39] demonstrated that soluble placenta-derived VEGF receptor (sFlt1), an antagonist of VEGF and PLGF, is unregulated in preeclampsia, leading to increased systemic levels of sFlt1 that fall after delivery. Increased circulating sFlt1 in preeclampsia is associated with decreased circulating levels of free VEGF and PLGF, resulting in endothelial dysfunction. The magnitude of increase in sFlt levels correlates with disease severity[40,41] lending further support that the VEGF-soluble Flt balance represents one of the final common pathophysiologic pathways.

First-trimester PLGF levels are decreased in future preeclamptic and in pregnancies complicated by fetal growth restriction, whereas sFlt levels do not differ from controls.[42] Again, these data are compatible with decidual angiogenic growth factors, in particular PLGF, as being essential for early placental development (PLGF is low in both fetal growth restriction and preeclampsia) with a later involvement of sFlt as a fetal rescue signal steering the maternal response, that is, the degree of maternal systemic hypertension. This hypothesis is supported by Levine et al.,[41] who have demonstrated that during the last 2 months of pregnancy in normotensive controls, the level of sFlt-1 increased and the level of PLGF decreased.

Recently, Levine and associates[43] investigated urinary PLGF levels in pregnant women with and without preeclampsia. They found that among normotensive pregnant women, urinary PLGF increased during the first two trimesters, peaked at 29 to 32 weeks, and decreased thereafter. Among women who ultimately developed preeclampsia, the pattern of urinary PLGF was similar, but levels were significantly reduced beginning at 25 to 28 weeks. There were particularly large differences among those who subsequently developed early onset preeclampsia or in those delivering small for gestational age infants.[43]

During the past decade, our understanding of the molecular basis for the pathophysiologic abnormalities in preeclampsia has reached an unprecedented level. There is now clear appreciation for the role of cell adhesion molecules, angiogenic proteins, and activation of the inflammatory system in the pathogenesis of microvascular dysfunction in patients with preeclampsia.[44] There is clear evidence for an exaggerated inflammatory response (abnormal cytokine production and neutrophil activation) in women with the clinical findings of preeclampsia.[45,46] However, this enhanced inflammatory response is absent before the development of preeclampsia.

Faas et al.[47] developed an experimental animal model for preeclampsia by administering a very low dose of endotoxin infusion (1 mg/kg body weight) into pregnant rats. In this rat model, low-dose endotoxin produced pathologic findings similar to those seen in preeclampsia (increased BP, proteinuria, thrombocytopenia, and renal histology changes). These changes were not observed when low-dose endotoxin was infused in control nonpregnant rats. They also measured the functional activity of monocytes using the rat model for preeclampsia. They found that monocyte tumor necrosis factor-α (TNFα) production was persistently decreased, whereas total white blood cell count and granulocyte count were persistently increased in the endotoxin-treated rats as compared with saline-treated rats.[47] Because the activated monocytes produced less TNFα in this animal model for preeclampsia, they suggested that these monocytes were endotoxin tolerant and, therefore, activated. The results of this study are consistent with observations of increased granulocyte counts and increased levels of TNFα in some women with preeclampsia. However, it remains unclear whether endoxin tolerance in monocytes is a feature of women with preeclampsia.[44]

Recent studies confirming increased levels of asymmetric dimethylarginine at 23 to 25 weeks in pregnant women who develop preeclampsia have emphasized the importance of the nitric oxide–cyclic guanosine monophosphate pathway.[48] Endothelial dysfunction/inappropriate endothelial cell activation associated with alterations in nitric oxide levels in preeclampsia explain most typical clinical manifestations, including the increased endothelial cell permeability and increased platelet aggregation.[49]

Genetics and Genetic Imprinting

According to the genetic conflict theory,[17] fetal genes are selected to increase the transfer of nutrients to the fetus, whereas maternal genes are selected to limit transfer in excess of some optimal level. The phenomenon of genomic imprinting means that a similar conflict exists within fetal cells between genes that are maternally derived and genes that are paternally derived. The conflict hypothesis suggests that placental factors (fetal genes) act to increase maternal BP, whereas maternal factors act to reduce BP.[17] Endothelial cell dysfunction may have evolved as a fetal rescue strategy to increase nonplacental resistance when the uteroplacental blood supply is inadequate.[17]

Nilsson et al.[50] published a model suggesting a heritability estimate of 31 percent for preeclampsia, and 20 percent for gestational hypertension. It is unlikely that there will be one major preeclampsia gene because such a gene would be selected against through evolution, unless it also carried a major reproductive advantage. It is more likely that a rapidly growing number of susceptibility genes will be uncovered; many of these interacting with the maternal cardiovascular/hemostatic system or the regulation of maternal inflammatory responses. Genome-wide linkage studies have identified at least three preeclampsia loci showing significant linkage: 2p12 (lod 4.77, 94.05 cM, D2S286, Iceland), 2p25 (nonparametric linkage score 3, 77, 21.70 cM D2S168),[51] and 9p13 (NPL 3.74, 3890 cM, D9169).[51] These loci segregate with different populations.[52] It should be noted that these loci only explain a relatively small percentage of the overall cases of preeclampsia. In addition, although these linkage studies indicate maternal susceptibility, they do not exclude the additional involvement of fetal genes. Another important consideration regarding the genetics of preeclampsia is the confounding effect of the so-called fetal origins of adult disease hypothesis suggesting that a hostile intrauterine environment for a female fetus would form the basis for the insulin resistance syndrome with its associated endothelial dysfunction, and as such, an increased risk of preeclampsia.[17]

Epigenetic features or imprinting is also involved in the pathogenesis of preeclampsia.[53] A direct proof of the role of imprinting was recently published by Oudejans et al.[52] Oudejans et al.[52] confirmed the susceptibility locus on chromosome 10q22.1. Haplotype analysis showed a parent-of-origin effect: maximal allele sharing in the affected sibs was found for maternally derived alleles in all families but not for the paternally derived alleles.

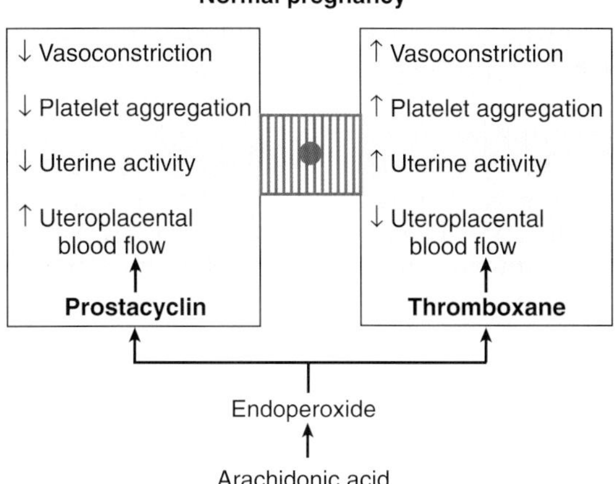

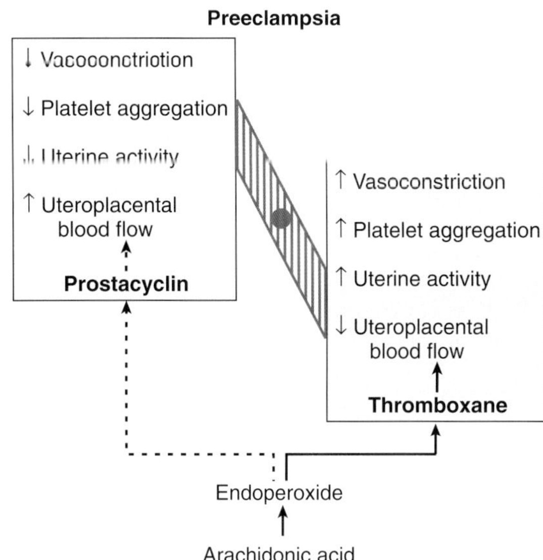

Figure 33-3. Comparison of the balance in the biologic actions of prostacyclin and thromboxane in normal pregnancy with the imbalance of increased thromboxane and decreased prostacyclin in preclamptic pregnancy. The heavy type and box for thromboxane suggest an exacerbation of its actions in preeclampsia, whereas the lighter type and box for prostacyclin suggest a diminution of its actions. (From Walsh SW: Preeclampsia: an imbalance in placenta prostacyclin and thromboxane production. Am J Obstet Gynecol 152:335, 1985, with permission.)

Changes in Prostanoids

Several investigators have described the various prostaglandins and their metabolites throughout pregnancy. They have measured the concentrations of these substances in plasma, serum, amniotic fluid, placental tissues, urine, or cord blood. The data have been inconsistent, reflecting differences in methodology.

During pregnancy, prostanoid production increases in both maternal and fetoplacental tissues.[35] Prostacyclin is produced by the vascular endothelium as well as in the renal cortex. It is a potent vasodilator and inhibitor of platelet aggregation. Thromboxane A_2 (TXA_2) is produced by the platelets and trophoblasts. It is a potent vasoconstrictor and platelet aggregator. Hence, these eicosanoids have opposite effects and play a major role in regulating vascular tone and vascular blood flow (Fig. 33-3).

Changes in prostaglandin production or catabolism in uteroplacental and umbilical tissues have been reportedly associated with the development of preeclampsia, although the reports have been inconsistent.[36–38] These discrepancies may reflect some of the inherent problems in the measurement of prostaglandins and the criteria employed for the diagnosis of preeclampsia. An imbalance in prostanoid production or catabolism has been suggested as responsible for the pathophysiologic changes in preeclampsia.[35] However, the precise role by which prostaglandins are involved in the etiology of preeclampsia remains unclear.[38,54–56]

Mills and associates[57] investigated the excretion of urinary metabolites of prostaglandin I_2 (PGI_2) and TXA_2 as measured prospectively before 22 weeks', between 26 and 29 weeks', and at 36 weeks' gestation among 134 women who ultimately developed preeclampsia and 134 matched women who remained normotensive. The authors found that reduced PGI_2 production, but no increase in TXA_2 production, occurs as early as 13 to 16 weeks in women who ultimately developed preeclampsia. In addition, the ratio of TXA_2 metabolite to PGI_2 metabolite was 24 percent higher throughout pregnancy in preeclamptic women.[57]

Lipid Peroxide, Free Radicals, and Antioxidants

Evidence is accumulating that lipid peroxides and free radicals may be important in the pathogenesis of preeclampsia.[58–60] Superoxide ions may be cytotoxic to the cell by changing the characteristics of the cellular membrane and producing membrane lipid peroxidation. Elevated plasma concentrations of free radical oxidation products precede the development of preeclampsia. In addition, some studies reported lower serum antioxidant activity in patients with preeclampsia than in normotensive pregnancies.[61]

Much of the controversy about oxidative stress is related to the nonspecificity of the markers. A recent study by Moretti et al.[60] measured oxidative stress "on-line" in exhaled breath (not subjective to in vitro artefacts) and confirmed greater oxidative stress in women with preeclampsia compared with uncomplicated pregnancies and nonpregnant controls.

Diagnosis

Preeclampsia is a clinical syndrome that embraces a wide spectrum of signs and symptoms that have been clinically observed to develop alone or in combination. Elevated BP is the traditional hallmark for diagnosis of the disease. However, recent evidence suggests that in some patients, the disease may manifest itself in the form of either a capillary leak (ascites, proteinuria) or a spectrum of abnormal hemostasis with multiple organ dysfunction. These latter patients usually present with clinical manifestations that are not typical of preeclampsia (i.e., hypertension is absent).[2,7]

The diagnosis of preeclampsia and the severity of the disease process are generally based on maternal BP. There are many factors that may influence measurement of BP with a sphygmomanometer, including the accuracy of the equipment used, size of the cuff, duration of the rest period before recording, the posture of the patient, and the Korotkoff phase used (phase IV or phase V for diastolic BP measurement). Steer recommends that all BP values be recorded with the woman in a sitting position for ambulatory patients or in a semi-reclining position for hospitalized patients.[62] The right arm should be used consistently, with the arm being in a roughly horizontal position at heart level. For diastolic BP measurements, both phases (muffling sound and disappearance sound) should be recorded. This is very important, because the level measured at phase IV is about 5 to 10 mm Hg higher than that measured at phase V.[63] Lopez et al.[63] compared Korotkoff phases IV and V in a cohort of 1,194 nulliparous pregnant women who were followed prospectively from the 20th week of pregnancy until delivery. BP measurements were obtained with random-zero sphygmomanometers and were recorded in supine, lateral, and seated positions. Lopez et al.[63] found that the prevalence of hypertension (diastolic BP 90 mm Hg or higher measured 6 hours apart) when phase IV was used was double that when phase V was used.

A rise in BP has been used by several authors as a criterion for the diagnosis of hypertension in pregnancy. This definition is usually unreliable, because a gradual increase in BP from second to third trimester is seen in most normotensive pregnancies. In a study of 16,211 singleton pregnancies, Redman and Jeffries[64] analyzed different cutoffs for diastolic BP used in the diagnosis of preeclampsia. These authors as well as Perry and Deevers have found that an elevation in diastolic BP of at least 25 mm Hg and a reading of at least 90 mm Hg were the best criteria.[65]

Villar and Sibai[66] prospectively studied BP changes during the course of pregnancy in 700 young primigravidas. One hundred thirty-seven patients (19.6 percent) had preeclampsia. The sensitivity and positive predictive values for preeclampsia of a threshold increase in diastolic BP of at least 15 mm Hg on two occasions were 39 and 32 percent, respectively. The respective values for a threshold increase in systolic pressures were 22 and 33 percent. Three recent studies from New Zealand,[67] the United States,[68] and Turkey[69] investigated pregnancy outcome in women with a rise in diastolic BP of more than 15 mm Hg but an absolute diastolic level below 90 mmHg as compared with gravidas who remained normotensive.[67–69] The New Zealand report[67] and Turkish study[69] included women with elevated BPs without proteinuria, whereas the American investigation[68] included women with an increased diastolic pressure 15 mm Hg or more plus proteinuria (≥ 300 mg/24 h). Overall, pregnancy outcomes were similar among women who remained normotensive and those who demonstrated a rise in diastolic pressure of 15 mm Hg or higher but did not reach 90 mm Hg. The use of an increase in BP as a diagnostic criterion is principally influenced by two factors: gestational age at time of first observation and frequency of BP measurements. Thus, these criteria are unreliable to diagnose preeclampsia as such.

The diagnosis of preeclampsia requires the presence of an elevated BP with proteinuria.[2] The presence of proteinuria is usually determined by the use of either dipstick or protein/creatinine ratio in random urine samples. The concentration of urinary protein is highly variable.[70] It is influenced by several factors, including contamination, urine specific gravity, pH, exercise, and posture.[71] In addition, urinary protein/creatinine excretion is highly variable in patients with preeclampsia.[72,73] Moreover, urinary dipstick determinations as well as total protein-to-creatinine ratio correlate poorly with the amount of proteinuria found in 24-hour urine determinations in women with gestational hypertension.[72–76] Therefore, the definitive test for diagnosing proteinuria should be quantitative measurement of total protein excretion over a 24-hour period. The diagnosis of severe preeclampsia requires that proteinuria of more than 5 g/24 h be documented. Using urine dipstick measurements (≥ 3+) is not adequate.[77]

The traditional criteria to confirm a diagnosis of preeclampsia (new onset of hypertension and proteinuria after 20 weeks' gestation) are appropriate to use in the majority of healthy nulliparous women. However, in some women, the development of severe gestational hypertension (without proteinuria) is associated with higher maternal and perinatal morbidities than in women with mild preeclampsia.[2,4,16] In addition, hypertension or proteinuria may be absent in 10 to 15 percent of women who develop the syndrome of hemolysis, elevated liver enzymes, and low platelets (HELLP syndrome),[78] and in 20 to 25 percent of those who develop eclampsia.[79]

The above-mentioned criteria are not reliable in women who have either hypertension or proteinuria before 20 weeks' gestation, particularly those receiving antihypertensive medications.[7,10,11,17] Because of the physiologic changes leading toward increased maternal BP and increased protein excretion with advanced gestation in such women, it is recommended that more stringent criteria be used to diagnose preeclampsia in women with preexisting microvascular disease.[17]

Prediction of Preeclampsia

A review of the world literature reveals that more than 100 clinical, biophysical, and biochemical tests have been recommended to predict or identify the patient at risk for the future development of the disease.[80–83] The results of the pooled data for the various tests and the lack of agreement between serial tests suggest that none of these clinical tests is sufficiently reliable for use as a screening test in clinical practice.[80–82]

Numerous biochemical markers have been proposed to predict which women are destined to develop preeclampsia. These biochemical markers were generally chosen on the basis of specific pathophysiologic abnormalities that have been reported in association with preeclampsia.[80–83] Thus, these markers have included markers of placental dysfunction,[45,81] endothelial and coagulation activation,[48,49,80–82] angiogenesis,[83] and markers of systemic inflammation.[45,81] However, the results of various studies evaluating the reliability of these markers in predicting preeclampsia have been inconsistent, and many of these markers suffer from poor specificity and predictive values for routine use in clinical practice.[80–83]

Doppler ultrasound is a useful method to assess uterine artery blood flow velocity in the second trimester. An abnormal uterine artery velocity wave form is characterized by a high resistance index or by the presence of an early diastolic notch (unilateral or bilateral).[84] Pregnancies complicated by abnormal uterine artery Doppler findings in the second trimester are associated with more than six-fold increase in rate of preeclampsia.[84] However, the sensitivity of an abnormal uterine artery Doppler for predicting preeclampsia ranges from 20 to 60 percent, with a positive predictive value of 6 to 40 percent.[85–87] A systemic review by Chien and colleagues[84] that included 27 studies and 12,994 patients concluded that uterine artery Doppler assessment has limited value as a screening test for preeclampsia. Current data do not support this test for routine screening of pregnant women for preeclampsia,[82] but uterine artery Doppler could be beneficial as a screening test in women at very high risk for preeclampsia if an effective preventive treatment becomes available.[17]

Prevention of Preeclampsia

There are numerous clinical trials describing the use of various methods to prevent or reduce the incidence of preeclampsia.[88] Because the etiology of the disease is unknown, these interventions have been used in an attempt to correct theoretical abnormalities in preeclampsia. A detailed review of these trials is beyond the scope of this chapter; however, the results of these studies have been the subject of several recent systemic reviews.[17,88–93] In short, randomized trials have evaluated protein or salt restriction, zinc, magnesium, fish oil, or vitamins C and E supplementation, the use of diuretics and other antihypertensive agents, as well as heparin to prevent preeclampsia in women with various risk factors.[61,88–90,94] These trials have had limited sample size, and results have revealed minimal to no benefit.[61,88–90] There is some suggestion from observational studies that heparin reduces recurrent preeclampsia in women with thrombophilias.[95] Some of the methods used are summarized in the box, "Methods Used to Prevent Preeclampsia."[89]

Calcium Supplementation

The relationship between dietary calcium intake and hypertension has been the subject of several experimental and observational studies.[96] Epidemiologic studies have documented an inverse association between calcium intake and maternal BP, and the incidences of preeclampsia and eclampsia.[97] The BP-lowering effect of calcium is thought to be mediated by alterations in plasma renin activity and parathyroid hormone. In addition, calcium

Methods Used to Prevent Preeclampsia

High-protein and low-salt diet
Nutritional supplementation (protein)
Calcium
Magnesium
Zinc
Fish and evening primrose oil
Antihypertensive drugs including diuretics
Antithrombotic agents
Low-dose aspirin
Dipyridamole
Heparin
Vitamins E and C

supplementation during pregnancy has been shown to reduce vascular sensitivity to angiotensin II.[98]

There are nine clinical studies comparing the use of calcium versus no treatment or a placebo in pregnancy.[98–107] These trials differ in the populations studied (low-risk or high-risk for hypertensive disorders of pregnancy), study design (randomization, double-blind, or use of a placebo), gestational age at enrollment (20 to 32 weeks' gestation), sample size in each group (range, 22 to 588), dose of elemental calcium used (156 to 2,000 mg/day), and the definition of hypertensive disorders of pregnancy used.

Eight of the studies were randomized and placebo controlled.[98–106] The dose of elemental calcium used was 600 to 2,000 mg/day. Five of these trials studied healthy pregnant women (low risk), and the other three studied pregnant women who had either a positive rollover test or both a positive rollover test and increased sensitivity to angiotensin II infusion.[98] Results of the nine studies are summarized in Table 33-5.

In the Cochrane review, calcium supplementation was associated with reduced hypertension; reduced preeclampsia, particularly for those at high risk and with low baseline dietary calcium intake (for those with adequate calcium intake, the difference was not statistically significant). No side effects of calcium supplementation have been recorded in the trials reviewed.[92] However, the reduction was not reflected in any overall reduction in stillbirths or neonatal death. In the largest trial to date,[104] of 4,589 women in developed countries, no reduction in the rate of preeclampsia or severity of preeclampsia or in timing of its onset was observed with calcium supplementation.[104] At present, the benefit of calcium supplementation for preeclampsia prevention in women with low dietary calcium intake remains unclear.[17,88]

Antithrombic Agents

Preeclampsia is associated with vasospasm and activation of the coagulation-hemostasis systems. Enhanced platelet activation plays a central role in the above-mentioned process and reflects abnormalities in the thromboxane/prostacyclin balance. Hence, several authors have used pharmacologic manipulation to alter the above-mentioned ratio in an attempt to prevent or ameliorate the course of preeclampsia.[93]

Aspirin inhibits the synthesis of prostaglandins by irreversibly acetylating and inactivating cyclooxygenase. In vitro, platelet cyclooxygenase is more sensitive to inhibition by low doses of aspirin (<80 mg) than vascular endothelial cyclooxygenase. This biochemical selectivity of low-dose aspirin appears to be related to its unusual kinetics that result in presystemic acetylation of platelets exposed to higher concentrations of aspirin in the portal circulation.

The majority of randomized trials for the prevention of preeclampsia have used low-doses of aspirin (50 to 150 mg/dl).[93] The rationale for recommending low-dose aspirin prophylaxis is the theory that the vasospasm and coagulation abnormalities in preeclampsia are caused partly by an imbalance in the thromboxane A_2–to–prostacyclin ratio.[17]

Recently, the Cochrane library updated the systematic review of the effectiveness and safety of antiplatelet agents (predominantly aspirin) for the prevention of preeclampsia.[93] Fifty-one trials involving 36,500 women are included in this review. There was a 19 percent reduction in the risk of preeclampsia associated with the use of antiplatelet agents (43 trials, 33,439 women; relative risk (RR) 0.81, 95 percent CI 0.75 to 0.88); number needed to treat (NNT) 69 [51, 109]). Twenty-eight trials (31,845 women) reported preterm birth. There was a small (7 percent) reduction in the risk of delivery before 37 completed weeks ([RR 0.93, 95 percent CI 0.89 to 0.98]; NNT 83 [50, 238]). Fetal or neonatal deaths were reported in 38 trials (34,010 women). Overall there was a 16-percent reduction in perinatal deaths in the antiplatelet group ([RR 0.84, 95 percent CI 0.74 to 0.96]; NNT 227 [128, 909]). SGA babies were reported in 32 trials (24,310 women), with an 8-percent reduction in risk (RR 0.92, 95 percent CI 0.85 to 1.00).[93] There were no significant differences between treatment and control groups in any other measures of outcome. The reviewers concluded that antiplatelet agents, largely low-dose aspirin, have small to moderate benefits when used

Table 33-5. Randomized Trials of Calcium Supplementation to Prevent Preeclampsia

STUDY	ENROLLMENT GA (WK)	NO. OF PATIENTS		PREECLAMPSIA (%)	
		CALCIUM	PLACEBO	CALCIUM	PLACEBO
Lopez-Jaramillo et al.[99]*	124	55	51	3.6	23.5
Lopez-Jaramillo et al.[102]†	24–32	22	34	0.0	23.5
Villar and Repke[100]*	24	90	88	0.0	3.4
Belizan et al.[101]*	20	579	588	2.6	3.9
Sanchez-Ramos et al.[98]†	24–28	29	34	13.8	44.1
Levine et al.[104]*	13–21	2,296	2,294	6.9	7.3
Lopez-Jaramillo et al.[103]*	20	125	135	3.2	15.5
Hererra et al.[105]†	28–32	43	43	9.4	37.2
Crowther et al.[106]*	13–24	227	224	4.4	10.0
Rogers et al.[107]	22–32	144	75	5.6	9.3

*Nulliparas.
†Positive rollover test or angiotensin II.

for prevention of preeclampsia. Low-dose aspirin was also found to be safe.[91,93] However, more information is clearly required to assess which women are most likely to benefit from this therapy as well as when treatment is optimally started, and what dose to use.[93] Several studies evaluated the efficacy of aspirin in the prevention of preeclampsia in high-risk pregnancies as determined by Doppler ultrasound.[85,87,108] A meta-analysis suggested that low-dose aspirin improves pregnancy outcome in women with persistent elevations in the uterine Doppler resistance index at both 18 and 24 weeks' gestation.[108] In other studies however, with abnormal uterine artery Doppler studies at 22 to 24 weeks' gestation, administration of aspirin after 23 weeks' gestation did not prevent the subsequent development of preeclampsia.[85,87] A large multicenter National Institute of Child Health and Human Development–sponsored study that included 2,539 women with pregestational insulin-treated diabetes mellitus, chronic hypertension, multifetal gestation, or preeclampsia in a previous pregnancy showed no beneficial effect from low-dose aspirin in such high-risk women (Table 33-6).[10] A major flaw in almost all studies on aspirin prophylaxis for preeclampsia published so far is both the focus on prevention as well as poor definition in several of the studies.[17,88] Some authors recommend that aspirin use should be based on individualized risk assessment for preeclampsia.[91,109] However, the available data do not support such a recommendation.

Vitamin C and E

One recent study has suggested a beneficial effect from pharmacologic doses of vitamins E and C in women identified as being at-risk for preeclampsia by means of abnormal uterine Doppler flow velocimetry.[61] However, the study had limited sample size and must be confirmed in other populations. In contrast, another randomized trial with limited sample size in women at very high risk for preeclampsia found no reduction in the rate of preeclampsia with vitamin C and E supplementation.[110]

Finally, it is important to emphasize that most of the positive trials found a benefit in the prevention of preeclampsia as defined, but not in pregnancy outcome.[17]

Table 33-6. Low-dose Aspirin in High-risk Women: NICHD Trial

ENTRY CRITERIA	NUMBER OF WOMEN	PREECLAMPSIA (%)	
		ASPIRIN*	PLACEBO*
Normotensive and no proteinuria	1,613	14.5	17.7
Proteinuria and hypertension	119	31.7	22.0
Proteinuria only	48	25.0	33.3
Hypertension only	723	24.8	25.0
Insulin-dependent diabetes	462	18.3	21.6
Chronic hypertension	763	26.0	24.6
Multifetal gestation	678	11.5	15.9
Previous preeclampsia	600	16.7	19.0

NICHD, National Institute of Child Health and Human Development.

*No difference for any of the groups.

Data from Caritis SN, Sibai BM, Hauth J, et al, for the National Institute of Child Health and Human Development: Low-dose aspirin therapy to prevent preeclampsia in women at high risk. N Engl J Med 338:701, 1998.

Laboratory Abnormalities in Preeclampsia

Women with preeclampsia may exhibit a symptom complex ranging from minimal BP elevation to derangements of multiple organ systems. The renal, hematologic, and hepatic systems are most likely to be involved.

Renal Function

Renal plasma flow and glomerular filtration rate (GFR) increase during normal pregnancy. These changes are responsible for a fall in serum creatinine, urea, and uric acid concentrations. In preeclampsia, vasospasm and glomerular capillary endothelial swelling (glomerular endotheliosis) lead to an average reduction in GFR of 25 percent below the rate for normal pregnancy.[111] Serum creatinine is rarely elevated in preeclampsia, but uric acid is commonly increased.[112] In a study of 200 women with mild preeclampsia remote from term, Sibai et al.[112] found the mean serum creatinine to be 0.80 mg/dl, mean uric acid 6.1 mg/dl, and mean creatinine clearance 112 ml/min. In a subsequent study of 95 women with severe preeclampsia, Sibai and associates[113] reported a mean serum creatinine of 0.91 mg/dl, a mean uric acid of 6.6 mg/dl, and a mean creatinine clearance of 100 ml/min.

The clinical significance of elevated uric acid levels in preeclampsia/eclampsia has been confusing. Hyperuricemia is associated with renal dysfunction, especially decreased renal tubular secretion, and has been consistently associated with glomerular endotheliosis. In addition, it has been linked with increased oxidative stress in preeclampsia.[114] Despite the fact that uric acid levels are elevated in women with preeclampsia, this test is not sensitive or specific for the diagnosis of preeclampsia. Lim and colleagues[115] studied uric acid findings in 344 women with hypertensive disorders of pregnancy. There was considerable overlap of values among the groups. A cutoff of 5.5 mg/dl is only 69 percent sensitive and 51 percent specific for the diagnosis of preeclampsia.[115]

Elevated uric acid levels above 6 mg/dl are often found in women with normotensive multifetal pregnancies.[116] As a result, some authors suggested that to secure a diagnosis of preeclampsia based upon elevated uric acid values, the upper limit should be adjusted for those with multiple gestation.[116] Elevated uric acid values are also found in women with acute fatty liver of pregnancy and underlying renal disease. It is suggested that uric acid values not be used as an indication for delivery in women with preeclampsia.[117]

Hepatic Function

The liver is not primarily involved in preeclampsia, and hepatic involvement is observed in only 10 percent of women with severe preeclampsia.[118] Fibrin deposition has been found along the walls of hepatic sinusoids in preeclamptic patients with no laboratory or histologic evidence of liver involvement.[119] When liver dysfunction does occur in preeclampsia, mild elevation of serum transaminase is most common. Bilirubin is rarely increased in preeclampsia, but when elevated, the indirect fraction predominates. Elevated liver enzymes are part of the of HELLP syndrome, a variant of severe preeclampsia.[78,118]

Hematologic Changes

Many studies have evaluated the hematologic abnormalities in women with preeclampsia.[120,121] Plasma fibrinopeptide-A, D-dimer levels, and circulating thrombin-antithrombin complexes are higher in women with preeclampsia than in normotensive gravidas. In contrast, plasma antithrombin III activity is decreased. These findings indicate enhanced thrombin generation.[120,121]

Plasma fibrinogen rises progressively during normal pregnancy. When a group of 50 severe preeclamptic women were compared with 50 normotensive women matched by gestational age, no differences in mean plasma fibrinogen levels were found between the two groups.[122] In general, plasma fibrinogen levels are rarely reduced in women with preeclampsia in the absence of abruptio placentae.

Thrombocytopenia is the most common hematologic abnormality in women with preeclampsia. It is correlated with the severity of the disease process and the presence or absence of abruptio placentae. A platelet count of less than 150,000/mm^3 has been reported in 32 to 50 percent of women with severe preeclampsia.[122,123] In a study of 1,414 women with hypertension during pregnancy, Burrows and Kelton[124] found a platelet count of less than 150,000/mm^3 in 15 percent of cases.

Leduc and associates[123] studied the coagulation profile (platelet count, fibrinogen, prothrombin time, and partial thromboplastin time) in 100 consecutive women with severe preeclampsia. A platelet count less than 150,000/mm^3 was found in 50 percent and a count of less than 100,000/mm^3 in 36 percent of the women. Thirteen women had a fibrinogen level of less than 300 mg/dl, and two had prolonged prothrombin and partial thromboplastin times, as well as thrombocytopenia on admission. They found the admission platelet count to be an excellent predictor of subsequent thrombocytopenia, and concluded that fibrinogen levels, prothrombin time, and partial thromboplastin time should be obtained only in women with a platelet count of less than 100,000/mm^3. A recent study by Barron confirmed these observations in over 800 women with hypertension in pregnancy.[125]

The HELLP Syndrome

Recent reports have described the HELLP syndrome in severe preeclampsia. There is considerable debate regarding the definition, diagnosis, incidence, etiology, and management of this syndrome.[78] Patients with such findings were previously described by many investigators. Weinstein[118] considered it a unique variant of preeclampsia and coined the term HELLP syndrome for this entity, whereas MacKenna and colleagues[126] considered it to be misdiagnosed preeclampsia. Barton and associates[127] performed liver biopsies in patients with preeclampsia and HELLP syndrome. Periportal necrosis and hemorrhage were the most common histopathologic findings. In addition, they found that the extent of the laboratory abnormalities in HELLP syndrome including the platelet count and liver enzymes did not correlate with hepatic histopathologic findings.

Laboratory Criteria for Diagnosis

The diagnostic criteria used for HELLP syndrome are variable and inconsistent. Hemolysis, defined as the presence of microangiopathic hemolytic anemia, is the hallmark of the triad of HELLP syndrome.[78] The classical findings of microangiopathic hemolysis include abnormal peripheral smear (schistocytes, burr cells, echinocytes), elevated serum bilirubin (indirect form), low serum haptoglobin levels, elevated lactate dehydrogenase (LDH) levels, and significant drop in hemoglobin levels. A significant percentage of published reports included patients who had no evidence of hemolysis; hence, these patients will fit the criteria for HELLP syndrome.[128–133] In some studies where hemolysis is described, the diagnosis is suspect as it has been based on the presence of an abnormal peripheral smear (no description of type or degree of abnormalities)[118,126] or elevated LDH levels (threshold of 180–600 U/L).[134–140]

There is no consensus in the literature regarding the liver function test to be used or the degree of elevation in these tests to diagnose elevated liver enzymes (EL).[78] In the original report by Weinstein, he mentioned abnormal serum levels of aspartate transaminase (AST), abnormal alanine transaminase (ALT), and abnormal bilirubin values; however, specific levels were not suggested.[118] In subsequent studies in which elevated liver enzymes were described (either AST or ALT), the values considered to be abnormal ranged from 17 to 72 U/L.[78] In clinical practice, many of these values are considered normal or slightly elevated. In essence, some of these studies included women with thrombocytopenia. Some of these women may have had either severe preeclampsia, gestational thrombocytopenia, or immune thrombocytopenic purpura.

Low platelet count is the third abnormality required to establish the diagnosis of HELLP syndrome. There is no consensus among various published reports regarding the diagnosis of thrombocytopenia. The reported cutoff values have ranged from 75,000/mm^3 to 279,000/mm^3.[78]

Many authors[131–140] have used elevated total lactate dehydrogenase (LDH) (usually >600 U/L) as a diagnostic criteria for hemolysis. There are five different isoforms of LDH, and only two of them, LDH_1 and LDH_2 are released from ruptured red blood cells. In the majority of women with severe preeclampsia-eclampsia, the elevation in total LDH is probably caused mostly by liver ischemia. Therefore, many authors advocate that elevated bilirubin values (indirect form), abnormal peripheral smear and/or a low serum haptoglobin level should be part of the diagnostic criteria for hemolysis.

Based on a retrospective review of 302 cases of HELLP syndrome, Martin et al.[141] devised the following classification based on the nadir of the platelet count. Class I HELLP syndrome was defined as a platelet nadir below 50,000/mm^3, class 2 a platelet nadir between 50,000 and 100,000/mm^3, and class 3 a platelet nadir between 100,000 and 150,000/mm^3. These classes have been used to predict the rapidity of recovery postpartum, maternal-perinatal outcome, and the need for plasmapheresis.

Hemolysis, defined as the presence of microangiopathic hemolytic anemia, is the hallmark of the HELLP syndrome. The role of disseminated intravascular coagulation (DIC) in preeclampsia is controversial. Most authors do not regard HELLP syndrome to be a variant of DIC, because coagulation parameters such as prothrombin time, partial thromboplastin time, and serum fibrinogen are normal.[78] However, the diagnosis of DIC can be difficult to establish in clinical practice. When sensitive determinants of this condition are used such as antithrombin III, fibrinopeptide-A, fibrin monomer, D dimer, α_2-antiplasmin, plasminogen, prekallikrein, and fibronectin, many patients have laboratory values consistent with DIC.[142,143] Unfortunately, these tests are time consuming and not suitable for routine monitoring. Consequently, less sensitive parameters are often employed. Sibai et al.[144] defined DIC as the presence of thrombocytopenia, low fibrinogen levels (plasma fibrinogen <300 mg/dl), and fibrin split products above 40 mg/ml. These authors noted the presence of DIC in 21 percent of 442 patients with HELLP syndrome. They also found that the majority of cases occurred in women who had antecedent abruptio placentae or peripartum hemorrhage and in all four women who had subcapsular liver hematomas. In the absence of these complications, the frequency of DIC was only 5 percent.[144] Aarnoudse et al.[145] diagnosed DIC in HELLP syndrome by light microscopic and immunofluorescence findings in tissue biopsies, and laboratory findings of thrombocytopenia, elevated fibrinogen degradation products, reduced antithrombin III levels, and fragmented red blood cells.

In view of the above-mentioned diagnostic problems, Sibai[78] recommended that uniform and standardized laboratory values be used to diagnose HELLP syndrome. He suggested that plasma haptoglobin and bilirubin values be included in the diagnosis of hemolysis. In addition, the degree of abnormality of liver enzymes should be defined as a certain number of standard deviations from the normal value for each hospital population. Our laboratory criteria to establish the diagnosis are presented in the box "Criteria to Establish the Diagnosis of HELLP Syndrome."

Clinical Findings

The reported incidence of HELLP syndrome in preeclampsia has been variable, reflecting the differences in diagnostic criteria. The syndrome appears to be more common in white women and is also higher in preeclamptic patients who have been managed conservatively.[78]

Early detection of HELLP syndrome can be a challenge in that many women present with nonspecific symptoms or subtle signs of preeclampsia. The various signs and symptoms reported are not diagnostic of preeclampsia and may also be found in women with severe preeclampsia-eclampsia without HELLP syndrome.[37,78,118,145] Right upper quadrant or epigastric pain and nausea or vomiting have been reported with a frequency ranging from 30 to 90 percent (Table 33-7).[137,144,146,148] Most patients give a history of malaise for several days before presentation, and some have a nonspecific viral like syndrome,[78] which led one investigator to suggest performing laboratory investigations (completed blood count and liver enzymes) in all pregnant women with suspected preeclampsia having these symptoms during the third trimester.[78] Headaches are reported by 33 to 61 percent[137,144,147] of the patients, whereas visual changes are reported in approximately 17 percent.[147] A small subset of patients with HELLP syndrome may present with symptoms related to thrombocytopenia, such as bleeding from mucosal surfaces, hematuria, petechial hemorrhages, or ecchymosis.

Although the majority of patients have hypertension (82 to 88 percent, see Table 33-7), it may be only mild in 15

Criteria to Establish the Diagnosis of HELLP Syndrome

Hemolysis
- Abnormal peripheral blood smear
- Increased bilirubin >1.2 mg/dl
- Increased lactic dehydrogenase >600 IU/L

Elevated liver enzymes
- Increased SGOT ≥72 IU/L
- Increased lactic dehydrogenase >600 IU/L

Thrombocytopenia
- Platelet count <100,000/mm^3

HELLP, hemolysis, elevated liver enzymes, or low platelets syndrome.

Table 33-7. Signs and Symptoms in Women with HELLP Syndrome

	WEINSTEIN[146] N = 57 (%)	SIBAI ET AL.[144,147] N = 509 (%)	MARTIN ET AL.[137] N = 501 (%)	RATH ET AL.[148] N = 50 (%)
RUQ/epigastric pain	86	63	40	90
Nausea/Vomiting	84	36	29	52
Headache	N/R	33	61	N/R
Hypertension	N/R	85	82	88
Proteinuria	96	87	86	100

HELLP, hemolysis, elevated liver enzymes, or low platelets syndrome; N/R, not reported; RUQ, right upper quadrant.
Adapted from Sibai BM: Diagnosis, controversies, and management of HELLP syndrome. Obstet Gynecol 103:981, 2004.

to 50 percent of the cases, and absent in 12 to 18 percent. The majority of the patients (86 to 100 percent) have proteinuria by dipstick examination. However, it has been reported to be absent in 13 percent of cases.[137,144,147]

Differential Diagnosis

The presenting symptoms, clinical findings, and many of the laboratory findings in women with HELLP syndrome overlap with a number of medical syndromes, surgical conditions, and obstetric complications. Therefore, the differential diagnosis of HELLP syndrome should include any of the conditions listed (see the box, "Medical and Surgical Disorders Confused with the HELLP Syndrome"). Because some patients with HELLP syndrome may present with gastrointestinal, respiratory, or hematologic symptoms in association with elevated liver enzymes or low platelets in the absence of hypertension or proteinuria, many initially are misdiagnosed as having other conditions such as upper respiratory infection, hepatitis, cholecystitis, pancreatitis, acute fatty liver of pregnancy (AFLP), or immune thrombocytopenic purpura (ITP).[78] Conversely, some patients with other conditions such as thrombotic thrombocytopenic purpura (TTP), hemolytic uremic syndrome (HUS), systemic lupus erythematosus, sepsis or catastrophic antiphospholipid antibody syndrome may be erroneously diagnosed as having the HELLP syndrome. In addition, in some patients, preeclampsia may be superimposed on one of these disorders, further contributing to the diagnostic difficulty. Because of the remarkably similar clinical and laboratory findings of these disease processes, even the most experienced physician can face a difficult diagnostic challenge. Therefore, efforts should be made to attempt to identify an accurate diagnosis, given that management strategy may be different among these conditions. It is important to emphasize that these patients may have a variety of unusual signs and symptoms, none of which are diagnostic of severe preeclampsia. Pregnant women with probable preeclampsia presenting with atypical symptoms should have a complete blood count, a platelet count, and liver enzyme determinations irrespective of maternal BP.

Occasionally, the presence of this syndrome is associated with hypoglycemia, leading to coma, severe hyponatremia, and cortical blindness. A rare but interesting complication of HELLP syndrome is transient nephrogenic diabetes insipidus. Unlike central diabetes insipidus, which occurs due to the diminished or absent secretion of arginine vasopressin by the hypothalamus, transient nephrogenic diabetes insipidus is characterized by a resistance to arginine vasopressin mediated by excessive vasopressinase. It is postulated that elevated circulating vasopressinase may result from impaired hepatic metabolism of the enzyme.

Management of HELLP Syndrome

Management of preeclamptic patients presenting with the HELLP syndrome is highly controversial.[78] Consequently, there are several therapeutic modalities described in the literature to treat or reverse the HELLP syndrome. Most of these modalities are similar to those used in the management of severe preeclampsia remote from term (see the box, "Therapeutic Modalities Used to Treat or Reverse HELLP Syndrome").

The clinical course of women with true HELLP syndrome is usually characterized by progressive and sometimes sudden deterioration in the maternal condition.[137,144] Because the presence of this syndrome has been associated with increased rates of maternal morbidity and mortality, many authors consider its presence to be an indication for immediate delivery.[118,148] There is also a consensus of opinion that prompt delivery is indicated if the syndrome develops beyond 34 weeks' gestation or earlier if there is multiorgan dysfunction, DIC, liver infarction or hemorrhage, renal failure, suspected abruptio placentae or nonreassuring fetal status.[78,144,149]

On the other hand, there is considerable disagreement about the management of women with HELLP syndrome

Medical and Surgical Disorders Confused with the HELLP Syndrome

Acute fatty liver of pregnancy
Appendicitis
Diabetes mellitus
Gallbladder disease
Gastroenteritis
Glomerulonephritis
Hemolytic uremic syndrome
Hepatic encephalopathy
Hyperemesis gravidarum
Idiopathic thrombocytopenia
Kidney stones
Peptic ulcer
Pyelonephritis
Systemic lupus erythematosus
Thrombotic thrombocytopenic purpura
Viral hepatitis

HELLP, hemolysis, elevated liver enzymes, or low platelets syndrome.

Therapeutic Modalities Used to Treat or Reverse HELLP Syndrome

- Plasma volume expansion
  - Bed rest
  - Crystalloids
  - Albumin 5 to 25 percent
- Antithrombotic agents
  - Low-dose aspirin
  - Dipyridamole
  - Heparin
  - Antithrombin III
  - Prostacyclin infusions
- Immunosuppressive agents
  - Steroids
- Miscellaneous
  - Fresh frozen plasma infusions
  - Exchange plasmapheresis
  - Dialysis

HELLP, hemolysis, elevated liver enzymes, or low platelets syndrome.

From Sibai BM: The HELLP Syndrome (hemolysis, elevated liver enzymes, and low platelets): much ado about nothing? Am J Obstet Gynecol 162:311, 1990, with permission.

at or before 34 weeks of gestation in whom maternal condition is stable except for mild to moderate abnormalities in blood tests and fetal condition is reassuring. In such patients, some authors recommend the administration of corticosteroids to accelerate fetal lung maturity followed by delivery after 24 hours,[78,131,132,135] whereas others recommend prolonging pregnancy until the development of maternal or fetal indications for delivery or until achievement of fetal lung maturity or 34 weeks' gestation.[126,129,130,150–152] Some of the measures used in these latter cases have included one or more of the following: bed rest, antihypertensive agents, chronic parenteral magnesium sulfate, antithrombotic agents (low-dose aspirin, dipyridamole), plasma volume expanders (crystalloids, albumin, fresh frozen plasma), and steroids (prednisone, dexamethasone, or betamethasone).

There are few case reports and few large case series describing expectant management of women with true HELLP, partial HELLP, or severe preeclampsia with elevated liver enzymes only.[126,128–130,150–152] In general, these reports suggest that transient improvement in laboratory values or pregnancy prolongation from a few days to a few weeks is possible in a select group of women with HELLP syndrome. It is important to note that most of the patients included in these studies were ultimately delivered within a week of expectant management.[78]

Investigators from the Netherlands have reported their experience with expectant management in women with HELLP syndrome below 34 weeks' gestation. Visser and Wallenburg[150] reported the use of plasma volume expansion using invasive hemodynamic monitoring and vasodilators in 128 women with HELLP syndrome before 34 weeks' gestation. Magnesium sulfate and steroids were not used in such women. Twenty-two of the 128 patients were delivered within 48 hours; the remaining 102 patients had pregnancy prolongation for a median of 15 days (range 3 to 62 days). Fifty-five of these 102 women had antepartum resolution of HELLP syndrome with a median pregnancy prolongation in these women of 21 days (range, 7 to 62 days). There were no maternal deaths or serious maternal morbidity. However, 11 (8.6 percent) resulted in fetal death at 25 to 34.4 weeks, and there were 7 (5.5 percent) neonatal deaths at 27 to 32 weeks' gestation.[150]

Van Pampus et al.[151,152] reported the use of bed rest, antihypertensive medication and salt restriction in 41 women with HELLP syndrome before 35 weeks' gestation. Fourteen women (34 percent) were delivered within 24 hours; in the remaining 27 women pregnancy was prolonged a median of 3 days (range, 0 to 59 days). Fifteen of these 27 women showed complete normalization of the laboratory abnormalities. There were no serious maternal morbidities. However, there were 10 fetal deaths at 27 to 35.7 weeks' gestation.

The results of the above-mentioned studies suggest that expectant management is possible in a very select group of patients with alleged HELLP syndrome before 34 weeks' gestation. However, despite pregnancy prolongation in some of these cases, the overall perinatal outcome was not improved compared with cases at a similar gestational age who were delivered within 48 hours after the diagnosis of HELLP syndrome.[153]

Two reports by Magann and associates[134,136] suggest that the use of corticosteroids either antepartum or postpartum results in transient improvement in laboratory values and urine output in some patients diagnosed with HELLP syndrome. It is important to note that in the antepartum group delivery was delayed by an average of only 41 hours and the study was not placebo controlled.[134] Recently, the same authors expanded on their experience with the use of high-dose dexamethasone in the management of women with HELLP syndrome. They observed improved outcomes, shorter hospital stays, and fewer blood transfusions.[139] A transient beneficial effect on hematologic findings with steroids was also reported by Tompkins and Thiagarajah.[131] However, these observations require testing in a randomized trial before routine use of steroids in the setting of HELLP syndrome can be recommended.

Confounding variables make it difficult to evaluate any treatment modality proposed for this syndrome. Occasionally, some patients without true HELLP syndrome may demonstrate antepartum reversal of hematologic abnormalities following bed rest, the use of steroids, or plasma volume expansion. However, the majority of these patients experience deterioration in either maternal or fetal condition within 1 to 10 days after conservative management. It is doubtful that such limited pregnancy prolongation will result in improved perinatal outcome, and maternal and fetal risks are substantial.[78]

Corticosteroids to Improve Pregnancy Outcome in Women with HELLP Syndrome?

It is well established that antenatal glucocorticoid therapy reduces neonatal complications and neonatal mortality in women with severe preeclampsia at 34 weeks' gestation or less.[154] The recommended regimens of corticosteroids for the enhancement of fetal maturity are betamethasone (12 mg intramuscularly every 24 hours, two doses) or dexamethasone (6 mg intramuscularly every 12 hours, four doses).[155] These regimens have been identified as the most appropriate for this purpose because they readily cross the placenta and have minimal mineralocorticoid activity. However, it is unclear whether the same or different regimens are beneficial in women with HELLP syndrome.

Corticosteroids have been suggested as safe and effective drugs for improving maternal and neonatal outcome in women with HELLP or partial HELLP syndrome.[134–139] A review of the literature reveals substantial differences in methodology, time of administration, and drug selection among investigators who advocate the use of corticosteroids in women with HELLP syndrome. Different regimens of steroids have been suggested for preventing respiratory distress syndrome (RDS) as well as to accelerate maternal recovery in the postpartum period.[78] The regimens of steroids used included intramuscular betamethasone (12 mg/12 hours or 24 hours apart on two occasions) or intravenous dexamethasone (various doses at various time intervals) or a combination of the two.[131–139] Some studies used steroids only in the antepartum period (for 24 hours, 48 hours, repeat regimens, or chronically for weeks until delivery).[129,133–135] Those who used steroids for long intervals recommend tapering them over 4 to 6 weeks.[129,130] In other studies, steroids were given for 48 hours before delivery and then continued for 24 to 48 hours postpartum,[38,132,133,139] whereas others recommend their administration only in the postpartum period.

There are five randomized trials comparing the use of high-dose dexamethasone to either no treatment[135,136,156,157] or to betamethasone[158] in women with presumed HELLP syndrome. The results of these studies demonstrated improved laboratory values and urine output in patients receiving dexamethasone but no differences in serious maternal morbidity. In addition, the number of patients studied was limited, and neither of these studies used a placebo.[78]

Maternal and Perinatal Outcome

The presence of HELLP syndrome is associated with an increased risk of maternal death (1 percent)[78] and increased rates of maternal morbidities such as pulmonary edema (8 percent),[144,147,159] acute renal failure (3 percent),[144,159] DIC (15 percent),[144] abruptio placentae (9 percent),[144] liver hemorrhage or failure (1 percent), adult respiratory distress syndrome (ARDS), sepsis, and stroke (<1 percent).[139,144] Pregnancies complicated by HELLP syndrome are also associated with increased rates of wound hematomas and the need for transfusion of blood and blood products.[78,137,139] The rate of these complications depends on the population studied, the laboratory criteria used to establish the diagnosis, and on the presence of associated preexisting medical conditions (chronic hypertension, lupus), or obstetric complications (abruptio placentae, peripartum hemorrhage, fetal demise, eclampsia). The development of HELLP syndrome in the postpartum period also increases the risk of renal failure and pulmonary edema.[159,160] The presence of abruptio placentae increases the risk of DIC, need for blood transfusions, pulmonary edema, and renal failure.[144,149,159,160] Patients who have large volume of ascites appear to have a high rate of cardiopulmonary complications.[161] Finally, women who meet all the criteria suggested for diagnosis will have higher rates of maternal complications than those who have partial HELLP or elevated liver enzymes only[147] (Table 33-8).

There is general agreement that perinatal mortality and morbidities are substantially increased in pregnancies complicated by the HELLP syndrome. The reported perinatal death rate in recent series ranged from 7.4 to 20.4 percent.[39–41,78] This high perinatal death rate is mainly experienced at very early gestational age (<28 weeks), in association with severe fetal growth restriction or abruptio placentae.[151–153] It is important to emphasize that neonatal morbidities in these pregnancies are dependent on gestational age at time of delivery and they are similar when corrected for gestational age to those in preeclamptic pregnancies without the HELLP syndrome.[150–153] The rate of preterm delivery is approximately 70 percent, with 15 percent occurring below 28 weeks' gestation.[144,150–153] As a result, these infants have a high rate of acute neonatal complications.[153]

The HELLP syndrome may develop antepartum or postpartum. Analysis of 442 cases studied by Sibai and associates[144] revealed that 309 (70 percent) had evidence of the syndrome antepartum, and 133 (30 percent) developed the manifestations postpartum. There were four maternal deaths, and morbidity was frequent (Table 33-9).

In the postpartum period, the time of onset of the manifestations may range from a few hours to 7 days, the majority developing within 48 hours postpartum. Thus, laboratory assessment for potential HELLP syndrome should be considered during the first 48 hours

Table 33-8. Maternal Complications in 316 Pregnancies with HELLP Syndrome, Partial HELLP Syndrome, or Severe Preeclampsia with Normal Laboratory Values

	HELLP (N = 67)	PARTIAL HELLP (N = 71)	SEVERE (N = 178)
Blood products transfusion (%)	25*	4	3
DIC (%)	15*	0	0
Wound hematoma/ infection (%)†	14‡	11§	2§
Pleural effusion (%)	6‡	0	1
Acute renal failure (%)	3‡	0	0
Eclampsia (%)	9	7	9
Abruptio placentae (%)	9	4	5
Pulmonary edema (%)	8	4	3
Subcapsular liver hematoma (%)	1.5	0	0
Intracerebral hemorrhage (%)	1.5	0	0
Death (%)	1.5	0	0

HELLP, hemolysis, elevated liver enzymes, or low platelets syndrome.
*$p < 0.001$, HELLP vs. partial HELLP and severe.
†Percentages of women who had cesarean delivery.
‡$p < 0.05$, HELLP vs. severe.
§$p < 0.05$, partial HELLP vs. severe.
From Audibert F, Friedman SA, Frangieh AY, Sibai BM: Clinical utility of strict diagnostic criteria for the HELLP (hemolysis, elevated liver enzymes, and low platelets) syndrome. Am J Obstet Gynecol 175:460, 1996, with permission.

Table 33-9. Serious Maternal Complications in 442 Patients with HELLP Syndrome

COMPLICATION	NO.	%
Disseminated intravascular coagulopathy	92	21
Abruptio placentae	69	16
Acute renal failure	33	8
Severe ascites	32	8
Pulmonary edema	26	6
Pleural effusions	26	6
Cerebral edema	4	1
Retinal detachment	4	1
Laryngeal edema	4	1
Subcapsular liver hematoma	4	1
Adult respiratory distress syndrome	3	1
Death, maternal	4	1

HELLP, hemolysis, elevated liver enzymes, or low platelets syndrome.
From Sibai BM, Ramadan MK, Usta I, et al: Maternal morbidity and mortality in 442 pregnancies with hemolysis, elevated liver enzymes, and low platelets (HELLP syndrome). Am J Obstet Gynecol 169:1000, 1993, with permission.

postpartum in women with significant hypertension or symptoms of severe preeclampsia. Eighty percent of the women who develop HELLP syndrome postpartum have had preeclampsia before delivery, whereas 20 percent had no evidence of either preeclampsia either antepartum or intrapartum. It is the author's experience that patients in this group are at increased risk for the development of pulmonary edema and acute renal failure (Table 33-10). The differential diagnosis should include exacerbation of systemic lupus erythematosus, thrombotic thrombocytopenic purpura, and hemolytic uremic syndrome.

Recommended Management

The clinical course of women with HELLP syndrome is usually characterized by progressive and sometimes sudden deterioration in maternal and fetal condition. Therefore, patients with a suspected diagnosis of HELLP syndrome should be hospitalized immediately and observed in a labor and delivery unit (Fig. 33-4). Such patients should be managed as if they had severe preeclampsia and should initially receive intravenous magnesium sulfate as prophylaxis against convulsions and antihypertensive medications to keep systolic BP below 160 mmHg or diastolic BP below 105 mm Hg.[78] This can be achieved with a 5-mg bolus dose of hydralazine, to be repeated as needed every 15 to 20 minutes for a maximum dose of 20 mg per hour. BP is recorded every 15 minutes during therapy and every hour once the desired values are achieved. If hydralazine does not lower BP adequately or if maternal side effects such as tachycardia or headaches develop, another drug such as labetalol or nifedipine can be used.

The recommended dose of labetalol is 20 to 40 mg IV every 10–15 minutes for a maximum of 220 mg, and the dose of nifedipine is 10 to 20 mg orally every 30 minutes for a maximum dose of 50 mg. During the observation period, maternal and fetal conditions should be followed carefully.

The recommended regimen of magnesium sulfate is a loading dose of 6 g given over 20 minutes, followed by a maintenance dose of 2 g per hour as a continuous intra-

Table 33-10. Outcome and Complications of HELLP Syndrome in Relation to Time of Onset

	ANTEPARTUM ONSET (*N* = 309) (%)	POSTPARTUM ONSET (*N* = 133) (%)	RELATIVE RISK	95% CONFIDENCE INTERVAL
Delivery at <27 weeks*	15	3	4.84	2.0–11.6
Delivery at 37–42 weeks†	15	25	0.61	0.41–0.91
Pulmonary edema	5	9	0.50	0.24–1.05
Acute renal failure†	5	12	0.46	0.24–0.87
Eclampsia	7	10	0.73	0.38–1.40
Abruptio placentae	16	15	1.05	0.65–1.70
DIC	21	20	1.09	0.73–1.64

HELLP, hemolysis, elevated liver enzymes, or low platelets syndrome.
*$p < 0.0007$.
†$p < 0.002$.
DIC, disseminated intravascular coagulopathy.
From Sibai BM, Ramadan MK, Usta I, et al: Maternal morbidity and mortality in 442 pregnancies with hemolysis, elevated liver enzymes, and low platelets (HELLP syndrome). Am J Obstet Gynecol 169:1000, 1993, with permission.

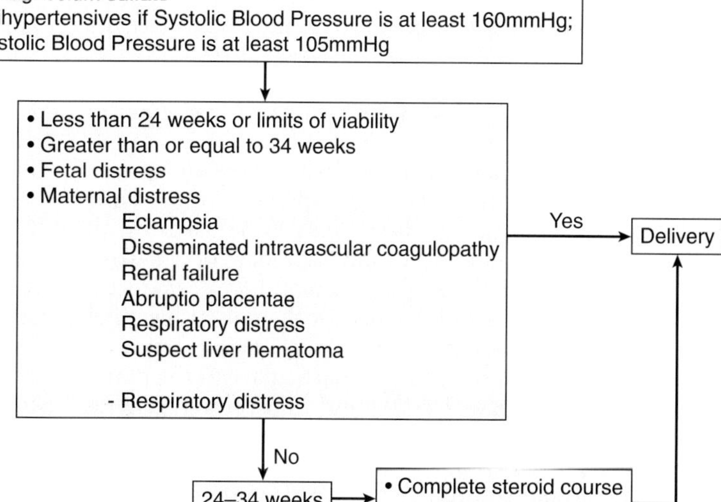

Figure 33-4. An algorithm for the management of HELLP syndrome.

venous solution. Magnesium sulfate is initiated at the beginning of the observation period and then continued during labor and for at least 24 hours postpartum.

Once the diagnosis of HELLP syndrome is confirmed, a decision must be made regarding the need for delivery (see Fig. 33-4). Women with HELLP syndrome who are less than 35 weeks' gestation should be referred to a tertiary care facility if maternal condition is stable. The first priority is to assess and stabilize the maternal condition, particularly BP and coagulation abnormalities. The next step is to evaluate fetal status with the use of fetal heart rate monitoring, biophysical profile, or Doppler assessment of fetal vessels. Finally, a decision must be made as to whether delivery should be initiated or delivery could be delayed for 48 hours to allow the full benefit of corticosteroids. Thus, in practice, delivery is undertaken in all patients with true HELLP syndrome except in those with a gestational age between 24 to 34 weeks with stable maternal and fetal conditions. These latter patients are given betamethasone and are generally then delivered within 24 hours after the last dose of corticosteroids. Maternal and fetal conditions are assessed continuously during this time period. In some of these patients, there may be transient improvement in maternal laboratory tests. However, delivery is still recommended despite such improvement.[78]

Intrapartum Management

The presence of HELLP syndrome is not an indication for immediate cesarean delivery. Such an approach might prove detrimental for both mother and fetus. The decision to perform a cesarean delivery should be based on gestational age, fetal condition, the presence of labor, and the cervical Bishop score. Elective cesarean delivery is recommended for all women with HELLP syndrome below 30 weeks' gestation not in labor and with a Bishop score less than five. Elective cesarean delivery is also undertaken for those with HELLP syndrome complicated by fetal growth restriction or oligohydramnios, particularly if the gestational age is below 32 weeks in the presence of an unfavorable cervical Bishop score (Table 33-11).

Patients having labor or rupture of membranes are allowed to deliver vaginally in the absence of obstetric complications. When induction is indicated, it is initiated with either oxytocin infusion or prostaglandins in patients with a gestational age at above 30 weeks, irrespective of the amount of cervical dilatation or effacement. A similar approach is used for those at ≤ 30 weeks if the cervical Bishop score is at least five.

Maternal pain relief during labor and delivery can be provided by intermittent use of small doses of systemic opioids. Local infiltration anesthesia can be used for all vaginal deliveries if an episiotomy or repair of a laceration is necessary. The use of a pudendal block is contraindicated in these patients because of the risk of bleeding and hematoma formation into this area. Epidural anesthesia is also contraindicated particularly if the platelet count is less than 75,000/mm^3. Therefore, general anesthesia is the method of choice for cesarean delivery in such patients. O'Brien et al.[133] assessed the impact of glucocorticoid administration on the use of epidural anesthesia in 37 women with partial HELLP syndrome who had a platelet count of less than 90,000/mm^3 before steroid administration. The authors found that administration of corticosteroids in these patients increased the use of epidural anesthesia, particularly in those who achieved a latency period of 24 hours before delivery (8/14 in steroid group vs. 0/10 in without steroids, $p = 0.006$).[133]

Table 33-11. Indications and Management During Cesarean Delivery in HELLP Syndrome

Indications for cesarean delivery
Nonreassuring fetal status
Abnormal fetal presentation
<30 weeks and Bishop score <5
<32 weeks with IUGR or oligohydramnios and Bishop score <5
Known subcapsular liver hematoma
Suspected abruptio placentae
Management during cesarean delivery
General anesthesia for platelet count <75,000/mm^3
Transfuse 6 units of platelets if count <40,000/mm^3
Insert subfascial drain
Secondary skin closure or leave subcutaneous drain
Observe for bleeding from upper abdomen before closure

HELLP, hemolysis, elevated liver enzymes, or low platelets syndrome; IUGR, intrauterine growth restriction.

Platelet transfusions are indicated either before or after delivery in all patients with HELLP syndrome in the presence of significant bleeding (ecchymosis, bleeding from gums, oozing from puncture sites, wound, intraperitoneal, and so on), and in all those with a platelet count of less than 20,000/mm^3 (see Table 33-11). However, repeated platelet transfusions are not necessary because of the short half life of the transfused platelets in such patients. Correction of thrombocytopenia is also important before any surgery. Administration of 6 units of platelets is recommended in all patients with a platelet count less than 40,000/mm^3 before intubation if cesarean delivery is needed. Generalized oozing from the incision site can occur during surgery or in the immediate postpartum period because of the continued drop in platelet count in some of these patients. The risk of hematoma formation at these sites is approximately 20 percent. Some individuals prefer to use a vertical skin incision, whereas others employ a subfascial drain and keep the skin incision open for at least 48 hours in patients requiring cesarean delivery (Fig. 33-5).[78]

Postpartum Management

Following delivery, patients with HELLP syndrome should receive close monitoring of vital signs, fluid intake and output, laboratory values, and pulse oximetry for at least 48 hours. Intravenous magnesium sulfate prophylaxis is generally continued for 48 hours, and antihypertensive drugs are employed if the systolic BP is at least 155 mm Hg or if the diastolic BP is at least 105 mm Hg. In general, the majority of patients will show evidence of resolution of the disease process within 48 hours after delivery. However, some patients, especially those with abruptio placentae plus DIC, those with severe thrombo-

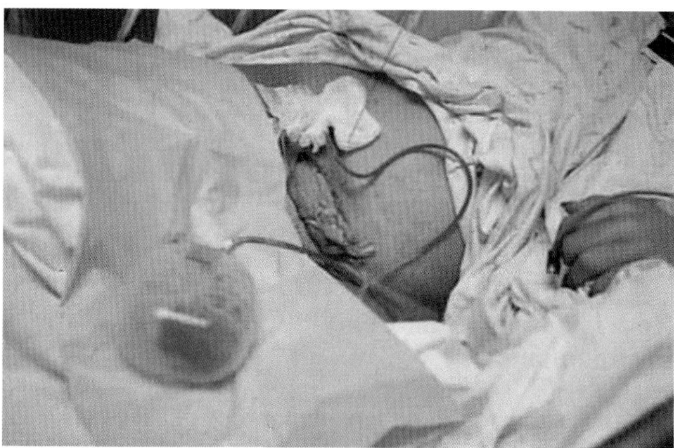

Figure 33-5. Subfascial drains used at time of cesarean section.

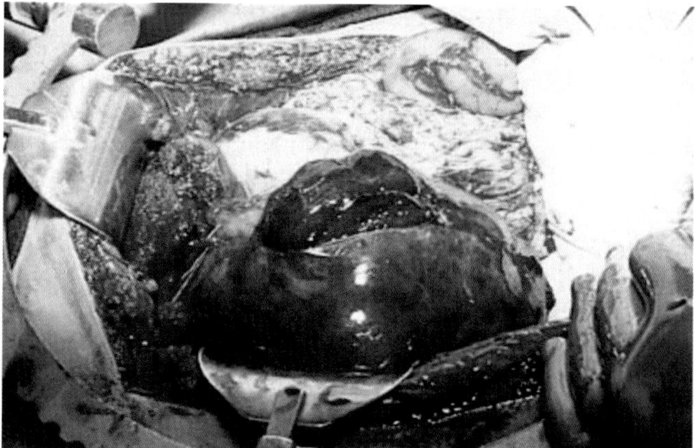

Figure 33-6. Subcapsular hematoma in patient with HELLP syndrome.

cytopenia (platelet count <20,000/mm^3), and those with severe ascites or significant renal dysfunction may show delayed resolution or even deterioration in their clinical condition.[159–161] Such patients are at risk for the development of pulmonary edema from transfusion of blood and blood products, fluid mobilization, and compromised renal function. These patients are also at risk for acute tubular necrosis and may need dialysis[159,160] and require intensive monitoring for several days. Some authors have suggested that such patients might benefit from plasmapheresis or plasma transfusions.[162] In practice, most of these patients will recover with supportive therapy only.

The clinical and laboratory findings of HELLP syndrome may develop for the first time in the postpartum period.[138,139,144] In these patients, the time of onset of the manifestations ranges from a few hours to 7 days, with the majority developing within 48 hours postpartum.[144] Hence, all postpartum women and their health care providers should be educated and be aware of the signs and symptoms of HELLP syndrome. Management of patients with postpartum HELLP syndrome should be similar to that in the antepartum period, including the use of magnesium sulfate.

Subcapsular Hematoma of the Liver in HELLP Syndrome

Because it occurs so rarely, the diagnosis of a subcapsular hematoma of the liver in pregnancy is often overlooked. Indeed, in four cases described from the University of Tennessee, the initial clinical impression was placental abruption with DIC in three cases and a complication of a postpartum tubal ligation in the fourth patient.[144] The differential diagnosis of an unruptured subcapsular hematoma of the liver in pregnancy should include acute fatty liver of pregnancy, ruptured uterus, placental abruption with DIC, and TTP. Most patients present in the third or late second trimester of pregnancy, although cases have been reported in the immediate postpartum period. In addition to the signs and symptoms of preeclampsia, physical findings consistent with peritoneal irritation and hepatomegaly may be present. Profound hypovolemic shock with hypotension in a previously hypertensive patient is a hallmark of rupture of the hematoma.

Laboratory evaluation is often consistent with DIC, including low platelet count, low fibrinogen, and prolonged prothrombin and partial thromboplastin times. As a result of hemolysis, total bilirubin and serum lactate dehydrogenase are markedly elevated. Other liver function tests such as AST and ALT are also significantly elevated.[144,162]

Rupture of a subcapsular hematoma of the liver is a life-threatening complication of HELLP syndrome[163] (Fig. 33-6). In most instances, rupture involves the right lobe and is preceded by the development of a parenchymal hematoma. The condition usually presents with severe epigastric pain that may persist for several hours before circulatory collapse. Patients frequently present with shoulder pain, shock, or evidence of massive ascites, respiratory difficulty, or pleural effusions, and often with a dead fetus. An ultrasound, computed axial tomographic (CAT) scan, or magnetic resonance imaging (MRI) of the liver should be performed to rule out subcapsular hematoma and detect the presence of intraperitoneal bleeding.[162] Paracentesis can confirm intraperitoneal hemorrhage suspected by radiographic imaging.

The presence of a ruptured subcapsular liver hematoma resulting in shock is a surgical emergency requiring acute multidisciplinary treatment.[163] Resuscitation should consist of massive transfusions of blood, correction of the coagulopathy with fresh frozen plasma and platelets, and immediate laparotomy. Options at laparotomy include packing and drainage, the preferred approach, surgical ligation of the hemorrhaging hepatic segments, embolization of the hepatic artery to the involved liver segment, and loosely suturing omentum or surgical mesh to the liver to improve integrity. Even with appropriate treatment, maternal and fetal mortality is over 50 percent. Mortality is most commonly associated with exsanguination and coagulopathy. Initial survivors are at increased risk for developing ARDS, pulmonary edema, and acute renal failure in the postoperative period.[144,163]

Surgical repair has been recommended for hepatic hemorrhage without liver rupture. More recent experience suggests, however, that this complication may be preferably managed conservatively in patients who remain hemodynamically stable.[164–166] Management should include close monitoring of hemodynamics and coagulation status. Serial assessment of the subcapsular hematoma with ultrasound or computed tomographic (CT) scan is necessary with immediate intervention for rupture or worsening maternal status. It is important with conservative management to avoid exogenous sources of trauma to the liver such as abdominal palpation, convulsions, or emesis and to use care in transportation of the patient. Indeed, any sudden increase in intraabdominal pressure could potentially lead to rupture of the subcapsular hematoma.

Smith et al.[167] reviewed their management of seven cases of spontaneous rupture of the liver occurring during pregnancy. Of the four survivors, the mean gestational age was 32.8 weeks and the mean duration of hospitalization was 16 days. All of the survivors were managed with packing and drainage of the liver, whereas the three patients treated with hepatic lobectomy died. The authors also extracted 28 cases from the literature reported since 1976. In 35 cases, there was an 82-percent overall survival for the 27 patients managed by packing and drainage, whereas only 25 percent of eight gravidas undergoing hepatic lobectomy survived. The authors emphasized that hepatic hemorrhage with persistent hypotension unresponsive to transfusion of blood products may be managed surgically with laparotomy, evaluation of the hematoma, packing the damaged liver, and draining the operative site. In certain cases in which the patient is stable enough to undergo angiography, transcatheter embolotherapy is a reasonable alternative to surgery.[168]

Any algorithm for the management of a subcapsular hematoma of the liver in pregnancy must emphasize the potential need for large amounts of blood products and the need for aggressive intervention if rupture of the hematoma is suspected. This author's experience is in agreement with the recent observations of Smith et al.,[167] in that a stable patient with an unruptured subcapsular hematoma may be managed conservatively. Constant monitoring must continue during this management, however, because patients can rapidly become unstable following rupture of the hematoma.

Survival depends on rapid diagnosis and medical and surgical stabilization. The coagulopathy must be aggressively reversed, because failure to do so is associated with an increased incidence of renal failure. In addition, these patients should be managed in an intensive care unit with close hemodynamic monitoring to avoid pulmonary edema, and respiratory compromise. Postpartum follow-up for patients with subcapsular hematoma of the liver should include serial imaging studies until the defect resolves.[166]

Hemodynamic Monitoring in Preeclampsia

The cardiovascular hemodynamics of preeclampsia have been investigated over the years by many authors using various techniques for measurement of BP, cardiac output, pulmonary capillary wedge pressure (PCWP), and central venous pressure (CVP).[169]

The true hemodynamic findings in patients with preeclampsia are controversial. A review of the English literature demonstrates considerable disagreement regarding one or more of the hemodynamic parameters studied. This lack of agreement has been attributed to differences in the definition of preeclampsia, variable severity and duration of the disease process, presence of underlying cardiac or renal disease, the techniques used to measure cardiac output and BP, and the therapeutic interventions applied before obtaining the various measurements. In addition, the dynamic minute-to-minute fluctuation of the cardiovascular parameters studied makes it difficult to standardize the conditions under which these observations are made, limiting the value of a single measurement.

Invasive techniques have been used by many authors to study the hemodynamic findings in untreated women with severe preeclampsia.[170–174] The reported cardiac index ranged from a low of 2.8 to a high of 4.8 L/min/m², and the reported PCWP from a low of 3.3 to a high of 12 mm Hg. The findings suggest that cardiac index and PCWP are either low or normal in severe preeclampsia. The reported CVP values also ranged from 2 to 6 mm Hg.

Table 33-12 compares the invasive hemodynamic findings in treated patients with severe preeclampsia.[172,175,176]

Table 33-12. Invasive Hemodynamic Findings in Treated Patients with Severe Preeclampsia/Eclampsia: Comparison of Three Large Series

	WALLENBURG[172] (*N* = 22)*	COTTON ET AL.[175] (*N* = 45)†	MABIE ET AL.[176] (*N* = 22)‡
Diastolic pressure (mm Hg)	110	110 ± 2	106 ± 2
Pulmonary artery pressure (mm Hg)	19	17 ± 1	15 ± 0.5
Cardiac index (L/min/m²)	3.8	4.1 ± 0.1	4.4 ± 0.1
SVRI (dynes · sec · cm⁻⁵, m²)	2,475	2,726 ± 1	2,293 ± 65
PWCP (mm Hg)	8	10 ± 1	8.3 ± 0.3
Central venous pressure (mm Hg)	2	4 ± 1	4.8 ± 0.4

*Values expressed as median.
†Values as mean ± SEM; includes two patients with pulmonary edema.
‡Values as mean ± SEM; excludes eight patients with pulmonary edema.
SVRI, systemic vascular resistance index; PWCP, pulmonary capillary wedge pressure; SEM, standard error of the mean.

The data for the various parameters are similar among the three studies. The findings demonstrate that treated patients with preeclampsia have normal to high cardiac index, normal to high systemic vascular resistance index, and normal to high PCWP.

In summary, the true hemodynamic findings of preeclampsia remain unknown. Moreover, the clinical utility of invasive hemodynamic monitoring in preeclampsia is debatable. The majority of the invasive monitoring data indicate that both cardiac output and systemic vascular resistance appear to be elevated in women with severe preeclampsia. This finding suggests that the problem in preeclampsia is a systemic vascular resistance that is inappropriately high for the level of cardiac output. Both the PCWP and the CVP appear to be in the low to normal range; however, there is no correlation between the two values.

Antepartum Management of Mild Hypertension-Preeclampsia

Gestational Hypertension

Women with gestational hypertension are at risk for progression to either severe hypertension, preeclampsia, or eclampsia.[2,5] The risks are increased with a lower gestational age at the time of diagnosis.[5] Therefore, these patients require close observation of maternal and fetal conditions. Maternal evaluations require weekly prenatal visits, education about reporting preeclamptic symptoms, evaluation of complete blood count, platelet count, and liver enzymes.[1,2] Fetal evaluation includes ultrasound examination of fluid and estimated fetal weight at the time of diagnosis and weekly nonstress testing.[1,2] Restriction of dietary salt as well as physical activity has not proven beneficial in the management of these patients.[2,17] Additionally, the results of several randomized trials reveal that control of maternal BP with antihypertensive drugs does not improve pregnancy outcome in women with gestational hypertension.[90,177]

In the absence of progression to severe hypertension or preeclampsia, women with gestational hypertension can continue pregnancy until term. During labor and immediately postpartum, they do not require seizure prophylaxis because the rate of eclampsia in these women is less than 1 in 500.[2]

The optimal management of women with mild gestational hypertension or preeclampsia before 37 weeks' gestation is controversial. There is disagreement regarding the benefits of hospitalization, complete bed rest and use of antihypertensive medications.

Hospitalization

In the past, management of these women has involved bed rest in the hospital for the duration of pregnancy with the belief that such management diminishes the frequency of progression to severe disease and allows rapid intervention in case of sudden disease progression including the development of abruptio placentae, eclampsia, or hypertensive crisis.[1] However, these complications are extremely rare among compliant women with mild hypertension or mild preeclampsia and absent symptoms. In addition, the results of two randomized trials in women with gestational hypertension and several observational studies in women with mild hypertension and mild preeclampsia suggest that most of these women can be safely managed at home or in a day-care facility provided they undergo frequent maternal and fetal evaluation.[178] It must be emphasized that many women included in these studies had gestational hypertension only.[178]

Bed Rest

Complete or partial bed rest for the duration of pregnancy is often recommended for women with mild hypertension-preeclampsia. There is no evidence to date suggesting that this practice improves pregnancy outcome. In addition, there are no published randomized trials comparing complete bed rest versus restricted activity in the management of women with mild preeclampsia. On the other hand, prolonged bed rest for the duration of pregnancy increases the risk of thromboembolism.[179]

Blood Pressure Medications

There are several randomized trials describing the use of antihypertensive drugs versus no treatment or a placebo in the management of women with mild hypertension or preeclampsia remote from term. Overall, these trials revealed lower rates of progression to severe disease with no improvement in perinatal outcome.[3,90,177] Of note, the sample size of these trials is inadequate to evaluate differences in fetal growth restriction, abruptio placentae, perinatal death, or maternal outcome.[90,177]

Fetal and Maternal Surveillance

There is universal agreement that fetal testing is indicated during expectant management of women with gestational hypertension or preeclampsia.[1–8] However, there is disagreement regarding which test to be used as well as the frequency of testing. Most authorities in the United States recommend daily fetal movement counts in association with either nonstress testing (NST) or biophysical profile to be performed at the time of diagnosis and serially thereafter until delivery (1 to 2 times/wk).[1,2,8] Because uteroplacental blood flow may be reduced in some of these women, ultrasound estimation of fetal weight as well as amniotic fluid status is also recommended at the time of diagnosis and serially thereafter with the frequency depending upon findings. Doppler flow velocimetry has been recommended by authorities outside the United States, particularly in the presence of suspected intrauterine growth restriction (IUGR).[6,7,180,181] The frequency of these tests is usually dependent on the severity of hypertension or preeclampsia, gestational age at the time of diagnosis, as well as fetal growth findings. Most clinical series suggest testing once weekly in women with mild gestational hypertension or preeclampsia, twice weekly if there is suspected fetal growth delay, and daily during expectant management of women with severe preeclampsia at less than 32 weeks' gestation.[1,2] However, there are no large prospective studies assessing outcomes of these monitoring techniques in women with gestational hypertension or preeclampsia.

Maternal surveillance is indicated in all women with gestational hypertension and preeclampsia. The goal of monitoring in women with mild gestational hypertension is to observe progression of the condition to severe hypertension or to preeclampsia.[1-8] In women with mild preeclampsia, the goal is early detection of severe preeclampsia. In those with severe preeclampsia, the goal is to detect the development of organ dysfunction. Therefore, all such women should be evaluated for symptoms of organ dysfunction, such as severe headaches, visual changes, altered mentation, right upper quadrant or epigastric pain, nausea or vomiting, shortness of breath, and decreased urine output.[1,2,7] In addition, they should undergo laboratory testing for 24-hour urine protein, serum creatinine, platelet count, and liver enzymes. Coagulation function tests are not necessary in the presence of a normal platelet count and liver enzymes.[123,125] The frequency of subsequent testing will depend on the initial findings, the severity of the maternal condition, and the ensuing clinical progression. Most authorities recommend evaluation and testing of platelet count, liver enzymes, and serum creatinine once weekly for women with mild gestational hypertension or mild preeclampsia, and performing these tests daily during expectant management of women with severe preeclampsia or HELLP syndrome remote from term.[1,2,78]

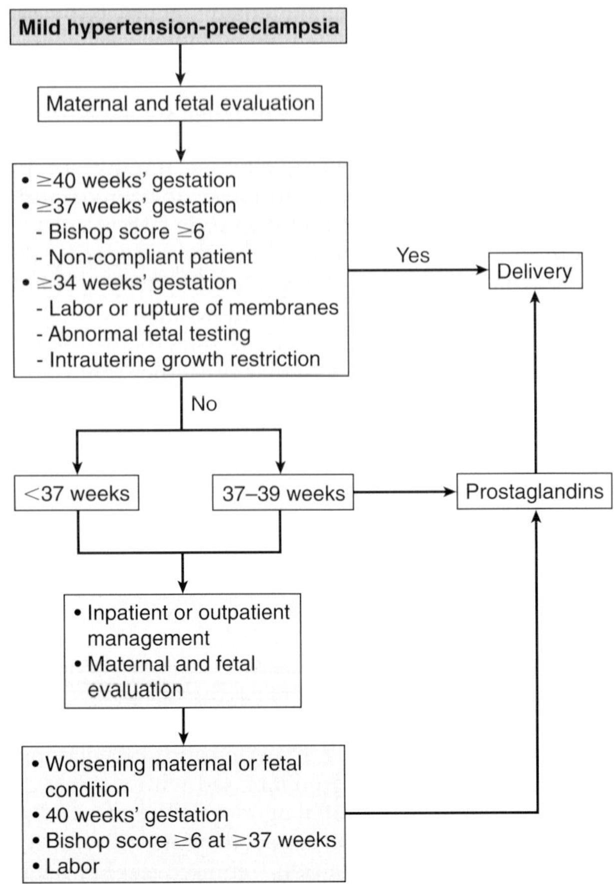

Figure 33-7. Management plan for patients with mild preeclampsia.

Recommended Management

The primary objective of management in women with gestational hypertension-preeclampsia must always be safety of the mother and then delivery of a mature newborn that will not require intensive and prolonged neonatal care. This objective can be achieved by formulating a management plan that takes into consideration one or more of the following: the severity of the disease process, fetal gestational age, maternal and fetal status at time of initial evaluation, presence of labor, cervical Bishop score, and the wishes of the mother.

Mild Hypertension or Preeclampsia

Once the diagnosis of mild gestational hypertension or mild preeclampsia is made, subsequent therapy will depend on the results of maternal and fetal evaluation (Fig. 33-7). In general, women with mild disease developing at 37 weeks' gestation or later have pregnancy outcomes similar to those found in normotensive pregnancies. Thus, at or near term in women with a favorable cervix and in those patients who are considered noncompliant, induction of labor is recommended. In addition, cervical ripening with prostaglandins and induction of labor can be used in women with mild preeclampsia and an unfavorable cervix at 37 weeks or later because of the slight increased risk for development of abruptio placentae and progression to severe disease.

In women who remain undelivered, close maternal and fetal evaluation are essential. These women are instructed to eat a regular diet with no salt restriction, and to restrict their activity but not to complete bed rest. Diuretics or antihypertensive medication are not used because of the potential to mask the diagnosis of severe disease.[2] In addition, the current data suggest that antihypertensive therapy in women with mild gestational hypertension or preeclampsia does not improve perinatal outcome. At the time of initial and subsequent visits, the women are educated and instructed about reporting symptoms of severe preeclampsia. They are also advised to come to the hospital or outpatient facility immediately if they develop abdominal pain, uterine contractions, vaginal spotting, or decreased fetal movement.

In women with mild gestational hypertension, fetal evaluation should include a non-stress test (NST) and an ultrasound examination of estimated fetal weight and amniotic fluid index. If the results are normal, then no repeat testing is undertaken as previously described.

Maternal evaluation includes measurements of hematocrit, platelet count, liver function tests, and a 24-hour urine protein once weekly. The women are usually seen twice a week for evaluation of maternal BP, urine protein by dipstick, and symptoms of impending eclampsia. This evaluation is extremely important for early detection of progression to preeclampsia or severe hypertension. The onset of maternal symptoms or a sudden increase in BP to severe values or development of proteinuria (≥2+ on dipstick) requires prompt hospitalization for close evaluation.

In women with mild preeclampsia at less than 37 weeks' gestation but at > 32 weeks, outpatient management can be considered in those with systolic BP at ≤150 mmHg and/or diastolic BP at ≤100 mmHg and a urine protein of ≤1000 mg/24 hours if they have no symptoms and if they have normal liver enzymes and a normal platelet count (>100,000/mm^3). Women who do not satisfy these criteria are hospitalized, particularly those with mild preeclampsia before 32 weeks. During ambulatory management, women are instructed to rest at home and perform BP measurements and urine dipstick daily, and are given instructions about prompt reporting of symptoms of severe disease. These women are then seen twice weekly, at which time a platelet count and liver enzymes are performed. Fetal evaluation includes daily fetal movement count, NST, and serial ultrasound evaluation of fetal growth and amniotic fluid. If there is evidence of disease progression (significant increase in BP or proteinuria to levels above the threshold mentioned previously or if they have new onset of symptoms or if there is evidence of abnormal blood tests or abnormal fetal growth), these women are then hospitalized for the duration of pregnancy. Women managed in the hospital receive similar maternal and fetal evaluation. Obstetric management is summarized in Figure 33-7.

Expectant Management of Severe Preeclampsia

The clinical course of severe preeclampsia may be characterized by progressive deterioration in both maternal and fetal conditions. Because these pregnancies have been associated with increased rates of maternal morbidity and mortality and with significant risks for the fetus (growth restriction, hypoxemia, and death), there is universal agreement that all such patients should be delivered if the disease develops after 34 weeks' gestation. Prompt delivery is also clearly indicated when there is imminent eclampsia (persistent severe symptoms), multiorgan dysfunction, severe IUGR (<5th percentile), suspected abruptio placentae, or nonreassuring fetal testing before 34 weeks' gestation.[182,183]

There is disagreement about management of patients with severe preeclampsia before 34 weeks' gestation when the maternal condition is stable and fetal condition is reassuring. In such patients, some authors consider delivery as the definitive treatment regardless of gestational age, whereas others recommend prolonging pregnancy until development of maternal or fetal indications for delivery or until achievement of fetal lung maturity or 34 weeks' gestation.[182,183]

Although delivery is always appropriate for the mother, it may not be optimal for the fetus that is extremely premature. In the past, it was believed that infants born prematurely to severely preeclamptic women had lower rates of neonatal mortality and morbidity as compared with infants of similar gestational age born to nonpreeclamptic women. This belief was based on the clinical impression that fetuses of preeclamptic women have accelerated lung and neurologic maturation as a result of stress in utero. This phenomenon, however, has never been documented in case-control studies.[182] In contrast, several recent case-control investigations have demonstrated that premature infants born after severe preeclampsia have similar neonatal complications and mortality and have higher rates of admission to neonatal intensive care units as compared with other premature infants of similar gestational age. In addition, the results of case-controlled studies reveal that fetuses of preeclamptic women do not exhibit accelerated lung or neurologic maturation.[182]

During expectant management, patients should be aware that the decision to continue such management will be made on a daily basis and that the median days of pregnancy prolongation is 7 days (range, 2 to 35 days). It is important to mention that there are only two randomized trials (133 women) that compared a policy of early elective delivery with a policy of delayed delivery.[183] Nevertheless, the results of retrospective and observational studies (more than 700 women) suggest that expectant management is associated with reduced short-term neonatal morbidity.[184,185]

In the past, there was uncertainty regarding the efficacy and safety of corticosteroids in women with severe preeclampsia before 34 weeks' gestation. A prospective double-blind randomized trial of 218 women with severe preeclampsia with a gestational age between 26 and 34 weeks receiving either betamethasone (n = 110) or placebo (n = 108) reported a significant reduction in the rate of respiratory distress syndrome (RR, 0.53; 95 percent CI, 0.35 to 0.82) in the steroids group.[154] Corticosteroids use also was associated with a reduction in the risks of neonatal intraventricular hemorrhage (RR, 0.35; 95 percent CI, 0.15 to 0.86), neonatal infection (RR, 0.39; 95 percent CI, 0.39 to 0.97), and neonatal death (RR, 0.5; 95 percent CI, 0.28 to 0.89). However, there were no differences in maternal complications between the two groups. Thus, the data support the use of steroids to reduce neonatal complications in women with severe preeclampsia at 34 weeks' gestation or less.[154]

Severe Preeclampsia

The presence of severe disease mandates immediate hospitalization in labor and delivery. Intravenous magnesium sulfate is begun to prevent convulsions, and antihypertensive medications are administered to lower severe levels of hypertension (systolic pressure ≥160 mm Hg and/or diastolic pressure ≥110 mm Hg). The aim of antihypertensive therapy is to keep systolic pressure between 140 and 155 mm Hg and diastolic pressure between 90 and 105 mm Hg. During the observation period, maternal and fetal conditions are assessed, and a decision is made regarding the need for delivery (Fig. 33-8). Those with a gestational age at 24 to 34 weeks are given corticosteroids to accelerate fetal lung maturity. Maternal evaluation includes monitoring of BP, urine output, cerebral status,

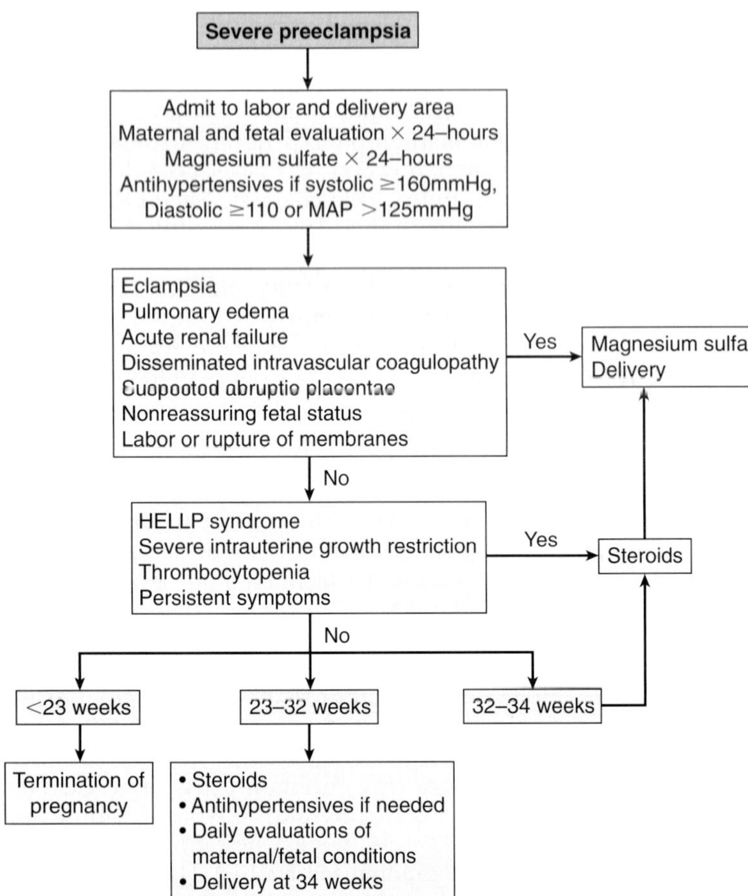

Figure 33-8. Management plan for patients with severe preeclampsia.

and the presence of epigastric pain, tenderness, labor or vaginal bleeding. Laboratory evaluation includes a platelet count, liver enzymes, and serum creatinine. Fetal evaluation includes continuous fetal heart monitoring, a biophysical profile, and ultrasonographic assessment of fetal growth and amniotic fluid. Patients with resistant severe hypertension despite maximum doses of intravenous labetalol (220 mg) plus oral nifedipine (50 mg) or persistent cerebral symptoms while on magnesium sulfate are delivered within 24 to 48 hours irrespective of fetal gestational age. In addition, patients with either thrombocytopenia (platelet count <100,000/mm^3) or elevated liver enzymes with epigastric pain and tenderness, or with serum creatinine of 2.0 mg/dl or more are also delivered within 48 hours.[78]

Women with a gestational age of 23 to 34 weeks are given corticosteroids and then delivered after 48 hours. Patients with a gestational age below 23 weeks are offered termination of pregnancy. Women at 23 to 32 weeks' gestation receive individualized management based on their clinical response during the 24-hour observation period. If BP is adequately controlled, and there is reassuring fetal assessment, magnesium sulfate is discontinued, and these women are then followed closely on the antepartum high-risk ward until 34 weeks' gestation or until development of a maternal or fetal indication for delivery. During hospitalization, they receive antihypertensive drugs, if needed, usually oral nifedipine (40 to 120 mg/day) plus labetalol (600 to 2400 mg/day), to keep systolic BP between 140 and 155 mm Hg and diastolic pressure between 90 and 105 mm Hg. Daily assessment of fetal well-being is also undertaken. In general, most patients will require delivery within 2 weeks, but some patients may continue their pregnancies for several weeks. It is important to emphasize that this therapy is appropriate only in a select group of patients and should be practiced in a tertiary care center with adequate maternal and neonatal intensive care facilities. Once the decision is made for delivery, the patients should receive magnesium sulfate in labor and for at least 24 hours postpartum.

Intrapartum Management

The goals of management of women with gestational hypertension-preeclampsia are early detection of fetal heart rate abnormalities and progression from mild to severe disease, and the prevention of maternal complications. Pregnancies complicated by preeclampsia, particularly those with severe disease or fetal growth restriction, are at risk for reduced fetal reserve and abruptio placentae.[2] Therefore, women with preeclampsia should receive continuous monitoring of fetal heart rate and uterine activity, with special attention to hyperstimulation and development of vaginal bleeding during labor. The presence of uterine irritability or recurrent fetal heart rate decelerations may be the first sign of abruptio placentae in these women.

Some women with mild hypertension-preeclampsia progress to severe disease as a result of changes in cardiac output and stress hormones during labor. Therefore, women with gestational hypertension-preeclampsia should have BP recordings every hour and should be assessed for symptoms suggestive of severe disease. Those who develop severe hypertension or symptoms should be managed as patients with severe preeclampsia.

Maternal pain relief during labor and delivery can be provided by either systemic opioids or segmental epidural anesthesia. Epidural analgesia is considered to be the preferred method of pain relief in women with mild gestational hypertension and mild preeclampsia. Although there is no unanimity of opinion regarding the use of epidural anesthesia in women with severe preeclampsia, a significant body of evidence indicates that epidural anesthesia is safe in these women.[186,187] A randomized trial of 116 women with severe preeclampsia receiving either epidural analgesia or patient-controlled analgesia reported no differences in cesarean delivery rates, and the group receiving epidural had significantly better pain relief during labor.[187]

The use of either epidural, spinal, or combined techniques of regional anesthesia is considered by most obstetric anesthesiologists to be the method of choice during cesarean delivery. In women with severe preeclampsia, general anesthesia carries the risk of aspiration and failed intubation owing to airway edema, and is associated with marked increases in systemic and cerebral pressures during intubation and extubation.[1] Women with airway or laryngeal edema may require awake intubation under fiber-optic observation with the availability of immediate tracheostomy. Changes in systemic and cerebral pressures may be attenuated by pretreatment with labetalol or nitroglycerine injections. It is important to recognize that regional anesthesia is contraindicated in the presence of coagulopathy or severe thrombocytopenia (platelet count <50,000/mm^3).

Prevention of Convulsions

Magnesium sulfate is the drug of choice to prevent convulsions in women with preeclampsia.[188] The results of 4 recent randomized trials revealed that magnesium sulfate is superior to placebo or no treatment for prevention of convulsions in women with severe preeclampsia.[189–192] The overall results of the four trials demonstrate that magnesium sulfate prophylaxis, compared with placebo (two trials, 10,795 women), nimodipine (one trial, 1,750 women), and with no treatment (one trial 228 women) in severe preeclampsia, is associated with a significantly lower rate of eclampsia (RR 0.39; 95 percent CI 0.28 to 0.55).[193] Results from one of the largest randomized trials to date, that of 10,141 women with preeclampsia in 33 nations (largely in the third world), has been recently reported.[190] Almost all of the enrolled patients had severe disease by United States standards: 50 percent received antihypertensives before randomization, 75 percent received antihypertensives after randomization, and the remainder had severe preeclampsia or imminent eclampsia. Among all enrolled women, the rate of eclampsia was significantly lower in those assigned to magnesium sulfate (0.8 percent versus 1.9 percent, RR; 0.42; 95 percent CI, 0.29 to 0.60). However, among the 1,560 women enrolled in the Western world, the rates of eclampsia were 0.5 percent in the magnesium group versus 0.8 percent in the placebo, a difference that was not significant (RR 0.67; 95 percent CI 1.19 to 2.37).[190]

There are two randomized placebo-controlled trials evaluating the efficacy and safety of magnesium sulfate in women with mild preeclampsia.[194,195] One of these trials included 135 women[194] and the other included only 222 women.[195] There were no instances of eclampsia in either group in both of these trials. In addition, the findings of both studies revealed that magnesium sulfate does not affect the duration of labor, and it does not affect the rate of cesarean delivery. However, neither of these studies had adequate sample size to address the efficacy of magnesium sulfate to prevent convulsions.[193] Therefore, whether there is a benefit of magnesium sulfate treatment in women with mild preeclampsia remains unclear. Intravenous magnesium sulfate should be administered during labor and postpartum for all women with severe preeclampsia. This author does not routinely use this therapy in women with mild gestational hypertension or preeclampsia in the absence of symptoms. In women having an elective cesarean delivery, magnesium sulfate is given at least 2 hours before the procedure and continued during surgery and for at least 12 hours postpartum.[193]

Control of Severe Hypertension

The objective of treating acute severe hypertension is to prevent potential cerebrovascular and cardiovascular complications such as encephalopathy, hemorrhage, and congestive heart failure.[2] For ethical reasons, there are no randomized trials to determine the level of hypertension to treat in order to prevent these complications. Antihypertensive therapy is recommended by some for sustained systolic BP values of 180 mm Hg or more, and for sustained diastolic values of 110 mm Hg or more. Some experts recommend treating systolic levels of 160 mm Hg or more, whereas others recommend treating diastolic levels of 105 mm Hg, and still others use a mean arterial BP of 130 mm Hg or more.[1,2,7] The definition of sustained hypertension is not clear, and ranges from 30 minutes to 2 hours.

The most commonly used and advocated agent for the treatment of severe hypertension in pregnancy is intravenous hydralazine given as bolus injections of 5 to 10 mg every 15 to 20 minutes for a maximum dose of 20 mg. Recently, several drugs have been compared with hydralazine in small, randomized trials. Magee and colleagues[196] performed a meta-analysis of 21 trials (893 women); eight trials compared hydralazine with nifedipine, and five compared hydralazine to labetalol. The results of these trials were the subject of a recent systemic review that suggested that intravenous labetalol or oral nifedipine are as effective and have fewer side effects than intravenous hydralazine.[196] The recommended dose of labetalol is 20 to 40 mg intravenously every 10 to 15 minutes for a maximum of 220 mg, and the dose of nifedipine is 10 to 20 mg orally every 30 minutes for a maximum dose of 50 mg.[1] Sustained BP values of 170 mm Hg systolic or more, or 110 mm Hg diastolic or more require therapy intrapartum. For women with thrombocytopenia and those in the postpartum period systolic values of 160 mm Hg or more, or diastolic readings of 105 mm Hg or more are the recommended thresholds for therapy.[2] For this author, the first-line agent is intravenous labetalol, and if maximum doses are ineffective, oral nifedipine is added.

Mode of Delivery

There are no randomized trials comparing the optimal method of delivery in women with gestational hypertension-preeclampsia. A plan for vaginal delivery should be attempted in all women with mild disease without other indications for cesarean delivery, and in the majority of women with severe disease, particularly those beyond 30 weeks' gestation.[1,2,17] The decision to perform cesarean delivery should be based on gestational age, fetal condition, presence of labor, and cervical Bishop score. In general, the presence of severe preeclampsia is not per se an indication for cesarean delivery.

Postpartum Management

During the immediate postpartum period, women with preeclampsia should receive close monitoring of BP, of symptoms consistent with severe disease, and accurate measurements of fluid intake and urinary output.

These women usually receive large amounts of intravenous fluids during labor as a result of prehydration before the administration of epidural analgesia, and intravenous fluids given during the administration of oxytocin and magnesium sulfate in labor and postpartum. In addition, during the postpartum period, there is mobilization of extracellular fluid leading to increased intravascular volume. As a result, women with severe preeclampsia, particularly those with abnormal renal function, those with capillary leak, and those with early onset disease are at increased risk for pulmonary edema and exacerbation of severe hypertension postpartum. These women should receive careful evaluation of the amount of intravenous fluids, oral intake, blood products, and urine output, as well as monitoring by pulse oximetry and chest auscultation.[2]

In general, most women with gestational hypertension become normotensive during the first week postpartum.[197] In contrast, in women with preeclampsia, hypertension often takes longer to resolve.[198] In addition, in some of the women with preeclampsia, there is an initial decrease in BP immediately postpartum, followed by development of hypertension again between days 3 and 6.[198] Antihypertensive drug treatment should be undertaken if the systolic BP is at least 155 mm Hg or if the diastolic is at least 105 mm Hg, with oral nifedipine 10 mg every 6 hours or long-acting nifedipine.[199] If the BP is well controlled and maternal symptoms are absent, the woman is then discharged home with instructions for daily BP measurements by a home visiting nurse for the first week postpartum or longer as necessary. Antihypertensive medications are discontinued if the BP remains below the hypertensive levels for at least 48 hours. Recently, some authors have suggested that 5 days of oral furosemide therapy (20 mg/dl) enhances recovery and reduces the need for antihypertensive therapy in women with severe preeclampsia.[200]

Severe hypertension or severe preeclampsia may develop for the first time in the postpartum period.[201] Hence, all postpartum women should be educated about the signs and symptoms of severe hypertension or preeclampsia. These women are at increased risk for eclampsia, pulmonary edema, stroke, and thromboembolism. Therefore, medical providers as well as personnel who respond to patient phone calls should be educated and instructed about important information to report to physicians.[200,201] In addition, women who have persistent severe headaches, visual changes, and epigastric pain with nausea or vomiting, and those with severe hypertension require immediate evaluation and potential hospitalization. These women often require magnesium sulfate for at least 24 hours and antihypertensive therapy. If neurologic symptoms exist, brain imaging is undertaken to rule out the presence of cerebral pathology.[201,202]

Maternal and Perinatal Outcome with Preeclampsia

Maternal and perinatal morbidities are substantially increased in women with severe gestational hypertension. Indeed, these women have higher morbidities than women with mild preeclampsia.[4,16] In addition, the rates of abruptio placentae, preterm delivery (at less than 37 and 35 weeks), and rates of SGA infants in these women are similar to those seen in women with severe preeclampsia. However, whether or not this increase in rate of preterm delivery is a result of early delivery chosen by the physician or because of the disease process itself remains unknown. Therefore, these women should be managed as if they had severe preeclampsia.[2,16]

Maternal and perinatal outcomes in preeclampsia are usually dependent on one or more of the following: gestational age at onset of preeclampsia as well as at time of delivery, the severity of the disease process, the presence of multifetal gestation, and the presence of preexisting medical conditions such as pregestational diabetes, renal disease or thrombophilias. In women with mild preeclampsia, the perinatal death rate, rates of preterm delivery, SGA infants, and abruptio placentae are similar to those of normotensive pregnancies (Table 33-13). The rate of eclampsia is less than 1 percent, but the rate of cesarean delivery is higher because of increased use of induction of labor.[2]

In contrast, perinatal mortality and morbidities as well as the rates of abruptio placentae are substantially greater in women with severe preeclampsia (see Table 33-13). The rate of neonatal complications is markedly increased in those who develop severe preeclampsia in the second trimester, whereas it is minimal in those with severe preeclampsia beyond 35 weeks' gestation.

Table 33-13. Pregnancy Outcome in Women with Mild and Severe Preeclampsia

	HAUTH ET AL.[4]		BUCHBINDER ET AL.[16]		HNAT ET AL.[20]	
	MILD ($N = 217$)	SEVERE ($N = 109$)	MILD* ($N = 62$)	SEVERE* ($N = 45$)	MILD ($N = 86$)	SEVERE ($N = 70$)
Delivery (wk)*						
<37 (%)	NR	NR	25.8	66.7	14.0	33.0
<35 (%)	1.9†	18.5†	9.7	35.6	2.3	18.6
SGA infant (%)*	10.2	18.5	4.8	11.4	NR	NR
Abruptio placentae (%)	0.5	3.7	3.2	6.7	0	1.4
Perinatal death (%)	1.0	1.8	0	8.9	0	1.4

*This study included women with previous preeclampsia. The other studies included only nulliparous women.
†These rates are for delivery at less than 34 weeks.

Severe preeclampsia is also associated with an increased risk of maternal mortality (0.2 percent) and increased rates of maternal morbidity (5 percent) such as convulsions, pulmonary edema, acute renal or liver failure, liver hemorrhage, DIC, and stroke. These complications are usually seen in women who develop preeclampsia before 32 weeks' gestation and in those with preexisting medical conditions.[204]

Counseling Women Who Have Had Preeclampsia in Prior Pregnancies

We have examined the pregnancy outcomes and incidences of preeclampsia in subsequent pregnancies, as well as the frequency of chronic hypertension and diabetes mellitus in women who had severe preeclampsia (287 women) or eclampsia (119 women) in their first pregnancies (aged 11 to 25 years) compared with 409 women (aged 12 to 25 years) who remained normotensive during their first pregnancies. Each woman had at least one subsequent pregnancy (range, 1 to 11) and was followed for a minimum of 2 years (range, 2 to 24). There was no significant difference in the incidences of diabetes mellitus in the two groups (1.3 versus 1.5 percent). The incidence of chronic hypertension was significantly higher in the preeclampsia patients (14.8 versus 5.6 percent; $p < 0.001$). This difference became even greater for those women followed for more than 10 years (51 versus 14 percent; $p < 0.001$). The incidence of severe preeclampsia was also significantly higher in the second pregnancies (25.9 to 4.6 percent) as well as in the subsequent pregnancies (12.2 to 5.0 percent) of women with preeclampsia.[205]

In a later report, subsequent pregnancy outcome and long-term prognosis were studied in 108 women who had severe preeclampsia in the second trimester.[206] These women were followed for a minimum of 2 years (range, 2 to 12 years) and had a total of 169 subsequent pregnancies. Fifty-nine (35 percent) subsequent pregnancies were normotensive, and 110 (65 percent) were complicated by preeclampsia. Overall, 21 percent of all subsequent pregnancies were complicated by severe preeclampsia in the second trimester. In addition, these women had a high rate of chronic hypertension on follow-up, with the highest incidence being in those who had recurrent severe preeclampsia in the second trimester (55 percent).

Hnat et al.[20] reported subsequent pregnancy outcome in women with previous preeclampsia enrolled in a multicenter trial. The rate of recurrent preeclampsia was 17 percent. The authors also noted that these women had a high rate of severe preeclampsia and poor perinatal outcome. In addition, even in those who remained normotensive in their subsequent pregnancy, there was a greater likelihood of adverse pregnancy outcome (preterm delivery, SGA infants, and perinatal death).

Some women with preeclampsia remote from term may have abruptio placentae. The risk of this complication is increased significantly in those with severe preeclampsia before 34 weeks' gestation and particularly in those who have severe preeclampsia in the second trimester.[207] For patients with preeclampsia complicated by abruptio placentae, the risk of subsequent abruptio ranges from 5 to 20 percent. In addition, these women are at increased risk for subsequent chronic hypertension.[207]

Pregnancy outcome and long-term prognosis were studied in 37 women with severe preeclampsia complicated by pulmonary edema, and 18 of these women had subsequent pregnancies.[207] Ten of the 18 were normotensive, four were complicated by chronic hypertension, and four by preeclampsia; one of the latter women also had pulmonary edema.

Pregnancy outcome and remote prognosis were also studied in 18 women with severe preeclampsia complicated by acute renal failure.[208] All 18 had acute tubular necrosis, nine required dialysis, and two died within 8 weeks after birth. All patients had serial evaluation of renal function, urine microscopic testing, and electrolyte studies at the onset of acute renal failure and during follow-up. All 16 surviving patients had normal renal function on long-term follow-up (average, 4 years). Four of the 16 women had seven subsequent pregnancies: one ended in miscarriage, one was complicated by preeclampsia at 35 weeks, and five were term pregnancies without complications.[208]

Pregnancies complicated by HELLP syndrome may be associated with life-threatening complications for both the mother and her infant. Therefore, clinicians should be able to answer questions regarding subsequent pregnancy outcome and long-term prognosis. Women with a history of HELLP syndrome are at increased risk of all forms of preeclampsia in subsequent pregnancies (Table 33-14).[209–212] In general, the rate of preeclampsia

Table 33-14. Pregnancy Outcome after HELLP Syndrome

	NUMBER OF WOMEN	NUMBER OF PREGNANCIES	HELLP %	PREECLAMPSIA %
Sibai et al.[209]	139	192	3	19
Sullivan et al.[210]	122	161	19	23
Van Pampus et al.[211]	77	92	2	16
Chames et al.*[212]	40	42	6	52

*HELLP ≤28 weeks in previous pregnancy.
Adapted from Sibai BM: Diagnosis, controversies, and management of HELLP syndrome. Obstet Gynecol 103:981, 2004.

in subsequent pregnancies is approximately 20 percent, with significantly higher rates if the onset of HELLP syndrome was in the second trimester. The rate of recurrent HELLP syndrome ranges from 2 to 19 percent, with the most reliable data suggesting a recurrence risk of less than 5 percent. Because of the above-mentioned risks, these women are informed that they are at increased risk for adverse pregnancy outcome (preterm delivery, fetal growth restriction, abruptio placentae and fetal death) in subsequent pregnancies. Therefore, they require close monitoring during subsequent gestations. At present, there is no preventive therapy for recurrent HELLP syndrome. There are case series describing subsequent pregnancy outcome in women with previous ruptured liver hematomas.[209,213,214] We have followed three women with previous ruptured liver hematomas through four subsequent pregnancies without complications. Other authors reviewed the literature and reported on several such women who had subsequent uneventful pregnancies under close maternal and fetal observation.[214]

Liver function tests were studied in 54 women at a median of 31 months (range, 3 to 101 months) after pregnancies complicated by the HELLP syndrome.[215] Serum levels of AST, LDH, and conjugated bilirubin were found to be normal. However, total bilirubin levels were elevated in 11 (20 percent) of the studied women. The authors of this report suggested the possibility that a dysfunction of the bilirubin-conjugating mechanism represents a risk factor for the development of this syndrome.[215]

There are 2 reports describing long-term renal function after HELLP syndrome.[159,216] One of the reports included 23 patients whose pregnancies were complicated by HELLP syndrome and acute renal failure: eight of these women had 11 subsequent pregnancies, with nine resulting in term gestation.[159] All 23 women also had normal BPs and renal function at an average follow-up of 4.6 years (range, 0.5 to 11 years). The other study compared renal function after at least 5 years following HELLP syndrome in 10 patients to the respective findings in 22 patients with previous normotensive gestation.[216] There were no differences in renal function tests between the two groups. These findings suggest that the development of HELLP syndrome with or without renal failure does not affect long-term renal function.

Remote Prognosis

Patients with preeclampsia should also be counseled regarding future cardiovascular risks and risks for underlying renal disease. There is evidence that women with preeclampsia remote from term are at increased risk for chronic hypertension later in life.[206] In addition, these patients, particularly those with recurrent preeclampsia, are more likely to have underlying renal disease.[217] In a recent report, 86 Japanese women who had severe hypertension, severe proteinuria, or both during pregnancy had a postpartum renal biopsy.[218] The authors found that women who had gestational proteinuria or preeclampsia before 30 weeks' gestation were more likely to have had underlying renal disease.[218]

Several recent studies suggested that women who develop preeclampsia may be at increased risk for coronary artery disease later in life.[219-222] Indeed, many of the risk factors and pathophysiologic abnormalities of preeclampsia are similar to those of coronary artery disease. Ramsey et al.[219] demonstrated for the first time, using laser Doppler imaging in vivo, impaired microvascular function in women 15 to 25 years of age following a pregnancy complicated by preeclampsia. Thus, microvascular dysfunction, which is associated with insulin resistance, may be a predisposing vascular mechanism for both coronary heart disease and preeclampsia. Therefore, pregnancies complicated by preeclampsia may identify women at risk of vascular disease in later life and may provide the opportunity for life style and risk factor modification to alter maternal vascular disease risk.[222]

ECLAMPSIA

Eclampsia is the occurrence of convulsions or coma unrelated to other cerebral conditions with signs and symptoms of preeclampsia. Early writings of both the Egyptians and Chinese warned of the dangers of convulsions encountered during pregnancy.[223] Hippocrates noted that headaches, convulsions, and drowsiness were ominous signs associated with pregnancy. The term *eclampsia* appeared in a treatise on gynecology written by Varandaeus in 1619. Clonic spasms in association with pregnancy were described by Pew in 1694. In 1772, De la Motte recognized that prompt delivery of pregnant women with convulsions favored their recovery.

Eclampsia is defined as the development of convulsions or unexplained coma during pregnancy or postpartum in patients with signs and symptoms of preeclampsia. In the Western world, the reported incidence of eclampsia ranges from 1 in 2,000 to 1 in 3,448 pregnancies.[224-227] The reported incidence is usually higher in tertiary referral centers, in multifetal gestation, and in populations with no prenatal care.[228-230]

Pathophysiology

The pathogenesis of eclamptic convulsions continues to be the subject of extensive investigation and speculation. Several theories and pathologic mechanisms have been implicated as possible etiologic factors, but none of these have been conclusively proven. It is not clear whether the pathologic features in eclampsia are a cause or an effect of the convulsions.[79]

Diagnosis

The diagnosis of eclampsia is secure in the presence of generalized edema, hypertension, proteinuria, and convulsions. However, women in whom eclampsia develops exhibit a wide spectrum of signs, ranging from severe hypertension, severe proteinuria, and generalized edema, to absent or minimal hypertension, no proteinuria, and no edema.[231] Hypertension is considered the hallmark for the diagnosis of eclampsia. The hypertension can be severe (at least 160 mm Hg systolic or at least 110 mm Hg diastolic) in 20 to 54 percent of cases[9,225] or mild (systolic BP between 140 and 160 mm Hg or diastolic BP between 90 and 110 mm Hg) in 30 to 60 percent of cases.[9,225] However, in 16 percent of the cases, hypertension may be absent.[9] In addition, severe hypertension is more common in patients who develop antepartum eclampsia (58 percent) and in those who develop eclampsia at ≥ 32 weeks' gestation (71 percent).[9] Moreover, hypertension is absent in only 10 percent of women who develop eclampsia at or before 32 weeks' gestation.[9]

The diagnosis of eclampsia is usually associated with proteinuria (at least 1+ on dipstick).[9,231] In a series of 399 women with eclampsia studied by the author, substantial proteinuria (≥ 3+ on dipstick) was present in only 48 percent of the cases, whereas proteinuria was absent in 14 percent of the cases.[9] Abnormal weight gain (with or without clinical edema) in excess of 2 pounds per week during the third trimester might be the first sign prior the onset of eclampsia. However, edema was absent in 26 percent of 399 eclamptic women studied by the author.[9]

Several clinical symptoms are potentially helpful in establishing the diagnosis of eclampsia. These include persistent occipital or frontal headaches, blurred vision, photophobia, epigastric and/or right upper quadrant pain, and altered mental status. Patients have at least one of these symptoms in 59 to 75 pecent of the cases (Table 33-15).[201,225,232] Headaches are reported by 50 to 75 percent of the patients, whereas visual changes are reported in 19 to 32 percent of the patients.[79] These symptoms may occur before or after the onset of convulsions.[79]

Time of Onset of Eclampsia

The onset of eclamptic convulsions can be during the antepartum, intrapartum, or postpartum periods. The reported frequency of antepartum convulsions among recent series has ranged from 38 to 53 percent (Table 33-16),[79] whereas the frequency of postpartum eclampsia has ranged from 11 to 44 percent.[79] Although most cases of postpartum eclampsia occur within the first 48 hours, some cases can develop beyond 48 hours postpartum and

Table 33-15. Symptoms in Women with Eclampsia

	DOUGLAS & REDMAN[225] N = 325	KATZ ET AL[232] N = 53	CHAMES ET AL[201] N = 89
Headache	50	64	70
Visual changes	19	32	30
RUQ/epigastric pain	19	Not reported	12
At least one	59	Not reported	75

RUQ, Right upper quadrant.
Data presented as percentage.
From Sibai BM: Diagnosis, differential diagnosis and management of eclampsia. Obstet Gynecol 105:402, 2005.

Table 33-16. Time of Onset of Eclampsia in Relation to Delivery

	DOUGLAS & REDMAN[225] N = 383	KATZ ET AL[232] N = 53	MATTAR & SIBAI[9] N = 399	CHAMES ET AL[201] N = 89
Antepartum	38	53	53	67*
Intrapartum	18	36	19	—
Postpartum	44	11	28	33
≤48 hours	39	5	11	7
>48 hours	5	6	17	26

*Includes antepartum and intrapartum cases.
Data presented as percentage.
Adapted from Sibai BM: Diagnosis, differential diagnosis and management of eclampsia. Obstet Gynecol 105:402, 2005.

have been reported as late as 23 days postpartum.[9,201,233] In the latter cases, an extensive neurologic evaluation may be needed to rule out the presence of other cerebral pathology.[9,201,233]

Almost all cases (91 percent) of eclampsia develop in the third trimester (≥ 28 weeks).[9] The remaining cases occur between 21 to 27 weeks' gestation (7.5 percent), or at or before 20 weeks' gestation (1.5 percent).[9] Eclampsia occurring before the 20th week of gestation is generally associated with molar or hydropic degeneration of the placenta with or without a coexistent fetus.[234,235] Although rare, eclampsia can occur during the first half of pregnancy without molar degeneration of the placenta.[9,234] These women may be misdiagnosed as having hypertensive encephalopathy, a seizure disorder, or TTP. Women in whom convulsions develop in association with hypertension and proteinuria during the first half of pregnancy should be considered to have eclampsia until proven otherwise.[79] These women should have an ultrasound examination of the uterus to rule out molar pregnancy or hydropic or cystic degeneration of the placenta. They also should have an extensive neurologic and medical evaluation to rule out another pathologic process.

Late postpartum eclampsia is defined as eclampsia that occurs more than 48 hours but less than 4 weeks after delivery.[233] Historically, eclampsia was believed not to occur more than 48 hours after delivery. However, several recent reports have confirmed the existence of late postpartum eclampsia.[201,225,233] These women have signs and symptoms consistent with preeclampsia in association with convulsions.[7,9] Some of these women will demonstrate a clinical picture of preeclampsia during labor or immediately postpartum (56 percent), whereas others demonstrate these clinical findings for the first time more than 48 hours after delivery (44 percent).[233] Of interest is the fact that late-postpartum eclampsia developed despite the use of prophylactic magnesium sulfate during labor and for at least 24 hours postpartum in previously diagnosed preeclamptic women.[201,233] Therefore, women in whom convulsions develop in association with hypertension or proteinuria or with headaches or blurred vision after 48 hours of delivery should be considered to have eclampsia and initially treated as such.[233]

Cerebral Pathology of Eclampsia

Autoregulation of the cerebral circulation is a mechanism for the maintenance of constant cerebral blood flow during changes in BP and may be altered in eclampsia. Through active changes in cerebrovascular resistance at the arteriolar level, cerebral blood flow normally remains relatively constant when cerebral perfusion pressure ranges between 60 and 120 mm Hg. In this normal range, vasoconstriction of cerebral vessels occurs in response to elevations in BP, whereas vasodilation occurs as BP is lowered. Once cerebral perfusion pressure exceeds 130 to 150 mm Hg, however, the autoregulatory mechanism fails. In extreme hypertension, the normal compensatory vasoconstriction may become defective and cerebral blood flow increases. As a result, segments of the vessels become dilated, ischemic, and increasingly permeable. Thus, exudation of plasma occurs, giving rise to focal cerebral edema and compression of vessels, resulting in a decreased cerebral blood flow.[236] Hypertensive encephalopathy, a possible model for eclampsia, is an acute clinical condition that results from abrupt severe hypertension and subsequent significant increases in intracranial pressure. Because this is an acute disturbance in the hemodynamics of cerebral arterioles, morphologic changes in anatomy may not be uniformly evident in pathologic material. Several autopsy findings that are relatively constant include cerebral swelling and fibrinoid necrosis of vessel walls.

The cause of eclampsia is unknown, and there are many unanswered questions regarding the pathogenesis of its cerebral manifestations. Cerebral pathology in cortical and subcortical white matter in the form of edema, infarction, and hemorrhage (microhemorrhage and intracerebral parenchymal hemorrhage) is a common autopsy finding in patients who die from eclampsia.[237–239] However, although autopsy series provide information regarding the central nervous system abnormality in patients dying of eclampsia, this information is not necessarily indicative of the central nervous system abnormality present in the majority of patients who survive this condition.[240] The diagnosis of eclampsia is not dependent on any single clinical or diagnostic neurologic findings. Focal neurologic signs such as hemiparesis or an unconscious state are rare in cases of eclampsia reported from countries in the developed world.[9,225,241] Although eclamptic patients may initially manifest a variety of neurologic abnormalities, including cortical blindness, focal motor deficits, and coma, most of them have no permanent neurologic deficits.[242–246] These neurologic abnormalities are probably due to a transient insult, such as hypoxia, ischemia, or edema.[247,248]

Several neurodiagnostic tests such as electroencephalography (EEG), CAT, cerebral Doppler velocimetry, MRI, and cerebral angiography (both traditional and MRI angiography) have been studied in women with eclampsia. In general, the EEG is acutely abnormal in the majority of eclamptic patients; however, these abnormalities are not pathognomonic of eclampsia. In addition, the abnormal EEG findings are not affected by the use of magnesium sulfate.[236] Moreover, lumbar puncture is not helpful in the diagnosis and management of eclamptic women. The results of CAT and MRI reveal the presence of edema and infarction within the subcortical white matter and adjacent gray matter mostly in the parieto-occipital lobes.[240,246–248] (See the box "Reported CT Scan Findings in Complicated Eclampsia.") Cerebral angiography and Doppler velocimetry suggest the presence of vasospasm.[249,250]

On the basis of cerebral imaging findings, attention has been directed to hypertensive encephalopathy as a model for the central nervous system abnormalities in eclampsia. The two conditions share many clinical, radiologic, and pathologic features.[240,247,248] There is failure of normal cerebral blood flow autoregulation in patients with hypertensive encephalopathy and in some patients with eclampsia.[240,250–252] Two theories have been proposed to explain these cerebral abnormalities: forced

Reported CT Scan Findings in Complicated Eclampsia

Cerebral edema
- Diffuse white matter low-density areas
- Patchy areas of low density
- Occipital white matter edema
- Loss of normal cortical sulci
- Reduced ventricular size
- Acute hydrocephalus

Cerebral hemorrhage
- Intraventricular hemorrhage
- Parenchymal hemorrhage (high density)

Cerebral infarction
- Low-attenuation areas
- Basal ganglia infarctions

CT, computed tomography.
From Barton JR, Sibai BM: Cerebral pathology in eclampsia. *In* Sibai BM (ed): Clinics Perinatology, Vol. 18. Philadelphia, WB Saunders Company, 1991, p 891, with permission.

Differential Diagnosis of Eclampsia

- Hypertensive encephalopathy
- Seizure disorder
- Hypoglycemia, hyponatremia
- Posterior leukoencephalopathy
- TTP
- Postdural puncture syndrome
- Vasculitis/angiopathy
- AFE
- Cerebrovascular accidents
  - Hemorrhage
  - Ruptured aneurysm or malformation
  - Arterial embolism, thrombosis
  - Venous thrombosis
  - Hypoxic ischemic encephalopathy
  - Angiomas

AFE, amniotic fluid embolism.

dilation and vasospasm.[240] The forced dilation theory suggests that the lesions in eclampsia are caused by loss of cerebrovascular autoregulation. At increased arterial pressures, normal cerebral vasoconstriction initially occurs. However, when the upper limit of autoregulation is reached, cerebral vasodilation begins, allowing local hyperperfusion with subsequent interstitial or vasogenic edema.[240,246] According to the vasospasm theory, cerebral overregulation occurs in response to acute severe hypertension, with resultant ischemia, cytotoxic edema, and infarction.[240,250–252]

Recently, magnetic resonance diffusion–weighted imaging and apparent diffusion coefficient mapping were used to characterize the relative frequency of vasogenic and cytotoxic edema in two small series of eclamptic women.[251,252] Cerebral edema (mostly vasogenic) was present in up to 93 to 100 percent of these women.[251,252] However, concurrent foci of infarction evidenced by reduced apparent diffusion coefficient (restricted diffusion) were present in 6 of 27 eclamptic women studied by Zeeman et al.[251] and in three of 17 eclamptic and preeclamptic women studied by Loureiro et al.[252] In addition, five of these six women reported by Zeeman et al. had persistent abnormalities on repeat MRI testing 6 to 8 weeks later, suggesting that these lesions might not be reversible.[251] Moreover, four of the 17 women reported by Loureira et al. had persistent MRI abnormalities at a median of 8 weeks follow-up.[252]

In summary, cerebral imaging findings in eclampsia are similar to those found in patients with hypertensive encephalopathy. Cerebral imaging is not necessary for the diagnosis and management of most women with eclampsia. Cerebral imaging is indicated for patients with focal neurologic deficits or prolonged coma. In these patients, hemorrhage and other serious abnormalities requiring specific pharmacologic therapy or surgery must be excluded. Cerebral imaging may also be helpful in patients who have an atypical presentation for eclampsia (onset before 20 weeks' gestation or more than 48 hours after delivery, and eclampsia refractory to adequate magnesium sulfate therapy). Advances in MRI and MR angiography as well as in cerebral vascular Doppler velocimetry may aid our understanding regarding the pathogenesis and improving long-term outcome of this condition.[79]

Differential Diagnosis of Eclampsia

The presenting symptoms, clinical findings, and many of the laboratory findings overlap with a number of medical and surgical conditions.[79,253–255] The most common cause of convulsions developing in association with hypertension or proteinuria during pregnancy or immediately postpartum is eclampsia. Rarely, other etiologies producing convulsions in pregnancy or postpartum may mimic eclampsia.[79]

These diagnoses are particularly important in the presence of focal neurologic deficits, prolonged coma, or in the presence of atypical eclampsia. In addition, in some patients, gestational hypertension or preeclampsia may develop in association with these disorders (connective tissue disease, thrombophilias, seizure disorder, hypertensive encephalopathy), further contributing to the diagnostic difficulty.[253] Therefore, an effort should be made to identify an accurate diagnosis given that management strategies may differ among these conditions.

Maternal and Perinatal Outcome

Eclampsia is associated with a slightly increased risk of maternal death in developed countries (0 to 1.8 percent),[9,79,226,227,257] but the maternal mortality rate is as high as 14 percent in developing countries.[229,230,238,257] The high maternal mortality reported from developing countries occurs primarily among patients who have had multiple seizures outside the hospital and those without prenatal care.[229,230,257] In addition, this high mortality rate could be attributed to the lack of resources and intensive care facilities needed to manage maternal complications from eclampsia. A review of all reported pregnancy-related deaths in the United States for the years 1979 to 1992 identified 4,024 pregnancy-related deaths.[258] A total of 790 (19.6 percent) were considered due to preeclampsia-eclampsia, with 49 percent of these

790 considered related to eclampsia. The authors found that the risk of death from preeclampsia or eclampsia was higher for women older than 30 years, those without prenatal care, and black women; the greatest risk of death was found among women with pregnancies at or before 28 weeks' gestation.[258]

Pregnancies complicated by eclampsia are also associated with increased rates of maternal morbidities such as abruptio placentae (7 to 10 percent),[9,79] DIC (7 to 11 percent),[9,225,258] pulmonary edema (3 to 5 percent), acute renal failure (5 to 9 percent), aspiration pneumonia (2 to 3 percent), and cardiopulmonary arrest (2 to 5 percent).[79] Adult respiratory distress syndrome (ARDS) and intracerebral hemorrhage are rare complications in series of eclamptic patients reported from the developed world.[9,225,240,256] It is important to note that maternal complications are significantly higher among women who develop antepartum eclampsia, particularly among those who develop eclampsia remote from term.[79]

Perinatal mortality and morbidities remain high in eclamptic pregnancies. The reported perinatal death rate in recent series ranged from 5.6 to 11.8 percent.[79,256] This high perinatal death rate is related to prematurity, abruptio placentae, and severe fetal growth restriction.[79] The rate of preterm delivery is approximately 50 percent, with approximately 25 percent occurring before 32 weeks' gestation.[79,225,231]

Is Eclampsia Preventable?

Prevention of eclampsia requires knowledge of its etiology and pathophysiology, as well as methods to predict patients at high risk for development of convulsions. However, as discussed earlier, the pathogenesis of eclampsia is largely unknown. Prevention of eclampsia can be primary by preventing the development of preeclampsia or secondary by using pharmacologic agents that prevent convulsions in women with established preeclampsia. Prevention can also be tertiary by preventing subsequent convulsions in women with established eclampsia. At present, there is no effective preventive therapy for preeclampsia.

Current management schemes designed to prevent eclampsia are based on early detection of gestational hypertension or preeclampsia and subsequent use of preventive therapy in such women.[256,259,260] Some of the recommended preventive therapies have included close monitoring (in-hospital or outpatient), use of antihypertensive therapy to keep maternal BP below a certain level (less than severe range or to normal values), timely delivery, and prophylactic use of magnesium sulfate during labor and immediately postpartum in those considered to have preeclampsia.[2] These management schemes assume that the clinical course in the development of eclampsia is characterized by a gradual process that begins with progressive weight gain, followed by hypertension (mild to severe), and proteinuria, with the subsequent onset of premonitory symptoms, and ending with the onset of generalized convulsions or coma.[232,260] This clinical course may be true in some women who develop eclampsia in developed countries. However, recent data from large series of eclamptic women from the United States and Europe indicate that approximately 20 percent of eclamptic women do not have any premonitory signs or symptoms before the onset of convulsions.[79,259,260] In many of these women, the onset of convulsions is abrupt and does not follow an indolent progression from mild to severe disease prior to the onset of eclampsia.[79]

It is also assumed that appropriate and timely standard preventive therapy will avoid eclampsia in virtually all patients with gestational hypertension-preeclampsia.[79,259,260] The efficacy of in-hospital management of patients with gestational hypertension or preeclampsia for the prevention of eclampsia has not been evaluated in randomized trials. Moreover, data from retrospective studies from the developed countries indicate that approximately 50 percent of eclamptic women develop their first convulsion while in the hospital under "close medical supervision."[225,231,259,260] Thus, it is doubtful that early and prolonged hospitalization of women with mild hypertension or preeclampsia will prevent the majority of cases of eclampsia.

There are several randomized trials describing the use of antihypertensive drugs versus no treatment or a placebo in the treatment of women with mild hypertension or preeclampsia. Overall, these trials revealed lower rates of progression to severe disease. However, the study design and the sample size of these trials is inadequate to evaluate potential benefits regarding prevention of eclampsia.[90]

Prophylactic magnesium sulfate is recommended only for women who are hospitalized with the established diagnosis of preeclampsia.[2] Its use is recommended only during labor and for 12 to 24 hours' postpartum.[2] Therefore, it can be expected to have a potential effect in preventing eclampsia that develops only during this time period (40 percent of total).[193]

There are several randomized trials comparing the efficacy of magnesium sulfate with other anticonvulsive agents for the prevention of recurrent seizures in women with eclampsia.[261] In these trials, magnesium sulfate was compared with diazepam, phenytoin, and a lytic cocktail. Overall, these trials revealed that magnesium sulfate was associated with a significantly lower rate of recurrent seizures (9.4 percent versus 23.1 percent; RR 0.41; 95 percent CI 0.32 to 0.51) and a lower rate of maternal death (3.0 percent versus 4.8 percent; RR 0.62; 95 percent CI 0.39 to 0.99) than that observed with other agents.[261]

The low incidence of eclampsia in developed countries is probably related to prevention of cases of eclampsia in women with a classic presentation and with a classic progression from mild to severe preeclampsia.[79] As a result, the majority of eclamptic cases described in reported series from the United States and Europe were found to have an atypical presentation (abrupt onset, development of convulsions while receiving prophylactic magnesium sulfate, or onset of convulsions beyond 48 hours after delivery).[79] Indeed, most eclamptic convulsions in these series developed in hospitalized women, and in some of these women, the onset of convulsions was not preceded by warning signs or symptoms.[79] Overall, the percentage of eclampsia considered unpreventable in these series ranges from 31 to 87 percent.[79]

Maternal Transport of the Eclamptic Patient

During the past 20 years, there has been a marked reduction in the number of eclamptic patients. Consequently, most obstetricians have little or no experience in the management of eclampsia. A recent survey of a random sample of obstetricians from all 50 states indicated that about 50 percent of obstetricians in private practice had not seen an eclamptic patient during the past year.

Because management of the eclamptic patient requires the availability of neonatal and obstetric intensive care units and personnel with special expertise, it is recommended that eclamptic patients with term gestations be cared for only at Level II or III hospitals with adequate facilities and with consultants from other specialties. For those eclamptic patients who are remote from term, referral should be made to a tertiary care center. The following steps should be taken before transfer of these critically ill patients:

1. The referring physician or nurse should consult with the physician at the perinatal center regarding the referral and appropriate treatment. All maternal records including prenatal data and a detailed summary of the patient's condition should be sent with the patient.
2. BP should be stabilized and convulsions controlled.
3. Adequate prophylactic anticonvulsive medications should be given. An accepted regimen is 4 g intravenous magnesium sulfate as a loading dose, with a simultaneous intramuscular dose of 10 g.
4. Maternal laboratory assessment (complete blood count with platelet count, liver enzymes) and fetal monitoring should be undertaken.
5. Such patients should be sent in an ambulance with medical personnel in attendance for proper management in case of subsequent convulsions.

Treatment of Eclamptic Convulsions

Eclamptic convulsions are a life-threatening emergency and require proper care in order to minimize morbidity and mortality. The development of an eclamptic convulsion is frightening to observe. Initially, the patient's face becomes distorted with protrusion of her eyes. This is followed by a congested facial expression. Foam often exudes from the mouth. The woman usually bites her tongue unless it is protected. Respirations are absent throughout the seizure. Typically, the convulsion, which can be divided into two phases, will continue for 60 to 75 seconds. The first phase, which lasts 15 to 20 seconds, begins with facial twitching, proceeding to the body becoming rigid with generalized muscular contractions. The second phase lasts approximately 60 seconds and consists of the muscles of the body alternately contracting and relaxing in rapid succession. This phase begins with the muscles of the jaw and rapidly involves the eyelids, other facial muscles, and then all the muscles of the body. Coma follows the convulsion, and the woman usually remembers nothing of the recent events. If she has repeated convulsions, some degree of consciousness returns after each convulsion. She may enter a combative state, and be agitated and difficult to control. Rapid and deep respirations usually begin as soon as the convulsions end. Maintenance of oxygenation is usually not a problem after a single convulsion; the risk of aspiration is low in the well-managed patient.

Because eclampsia is so frightening, the natural tendency is to attempt to abolish the convulsion. Drugs such as diazepam should not be given in an attempt to stop or shorten the convulsion, especially if the patient does not have an intravenous line in place and someone skilled in intubation is not immediately available. If diazepam is used, no more than 5 mg should be given over a 60-second period. Rapid administration of diazepam may lead to apnea or cardiac arrest, or both.

Prevent Maternal Injury During the Convulsions

The first priority in the management of eclampsia is to prevent maternal injury and to support cardiovascular functions. During or immediately after the acute convulsive episode, supportive care should be given to prevent serious maternal injury and aspiration, assess and establish airway potency, and ensure maternal oxygenation. During this time, the bed's side rails should be elevated and padded, and a padded tongue blade is inserted between the teeth (avoid inducing gag reflex), and physical restraints may be needed. To minimize the risk of aspiration, the patient should lie in the lateral decubitus position, and vomitus and oral secretions are suctioned as needed.[79] Aspiration may be caused by forcing the padded tongue blade to the back of the throat, stimulating the gag reflex with resultant vomiting.

Maintain adequate oxygenation during the convulsive episode, because hypoventilation and respiratory acidosis often occur. Although the initial seizure lasts only a few minutes, it is important to maintain oxygenation by supplemental oxygen administration through a face mask with or without an oxygen reservoir at 8 to 10 L/min.[79] After the convulsion has ceased, the patient begins to breathe again, and oxygenation is rarely a problem. However, maternal hypoxemia and acidosis may develop in women who have had repetitive convulsions, in those with aspiration pneumonia, with pulmonary edema, or a combination of these factors. It is the author's policy to use transcutaneous pulse oximetry to monitor oxygenation in all eclamptic patients. Arterial blood gas analysis is required if the pulse oximetry results are abnormal (oxygen saturation at or below 92 percent). Sodium bicarbonate is not given unless the pH is below 7.10.

Fortunately, magnesium toxicity resulting in maternal death is rare. However, in Pritchard's series of eclamptic women, magnesium sulfate was responsible for the only death reported[241] and nearly led to a maternal death at the University of Tennessee, Memphis.[262] In both cases, the patients received an overdose of magnesium sulfate because of an error in preparing the drug.

Prevention of Recurrent Convulsions

The next step in the management of eclampsia is to prevent recurrent convulsions. Magnesium sulfate is the drug of choice to treat and prevent subsequent convulsions in women with eclampsia.[257,261] A loading dose of 6 g over 15 to 20 minutes is recommended, followed by a maintenance dose of 2 g per hour as a continuous intravenous solution. Approximately 10 percent of eclamptic women have a second convulsion after receiving magnesium sulfate.[257,261] In these women, another bolus of 2 g magnesium sulfate can be given intravenously over 3 to 5 minutes. An occasional patient will have recurrent convulsions while receiving adequate and therapeutic doses of magnesium sulfate. In this patient, recurrent seizures can be treated with sodium amobarbital, 250 mg intravenously over 3 to 5 minutes.[79]

Rarely, a woman may experience an eclamptic seizure, lapse into a coma, and die. Magnesium toxicity should be considered in those women who do not regain consciousness. A case report of magnesium sulfate toxicity details the features of this serious complication.[262] Within a few minutes of starting what was supposed to be a magnesium loading dose, 4 g magnesium sulfate in 250 ml saline, the patient went into cardiorespiratory arrest. Immediate resuscitation including intubation was performed. Approximately one half of the loading dose had been given. An intracerebral accident or eclampsia was thought to be the cause of the coma; the loading dose was continued and maintenance therapy started. Initial blood gases were normal, and the electrocardiogram (ECG) was normal 15 minutes after the arrest. Mechanical ventilatory support was required. The patient's vital signs were stable; however, her pupils were nonreactive. Serum electrolytes, glucose, blood urea nitrogen, and creatinine were normal. CT scan of the head and cerebral angiograms were normal. A magnesium level of 35 mg/dl was reported 3.5 hours later from a blood sample taken through femoral venipuncture at the time of arrest. The magnesium sulfate infusion was stopped immediately. During the first 5 hours after the cardiorespiratory arrest, 1,344 mg of magnesium were excreted in the urine. Twelve hours after the arrest, an uncomplicated low vertical cesarean delivery was done for a breech presentation. The 3,160-g male infant had Apgar scores of 8 and 9 at 1 and 5 minutes, respectively. Maternal and cord blood magnesium levels at delivery were 5.8 mg/dl. Both mother and baby were discharged from the hospital with no apparent sequelae. Of interest, the patient reported she could hear and see what was occurring around her, but she could not make any movements while she was intubated. Figure 33-9 presents the maternal magnesium levels in this case.[262]

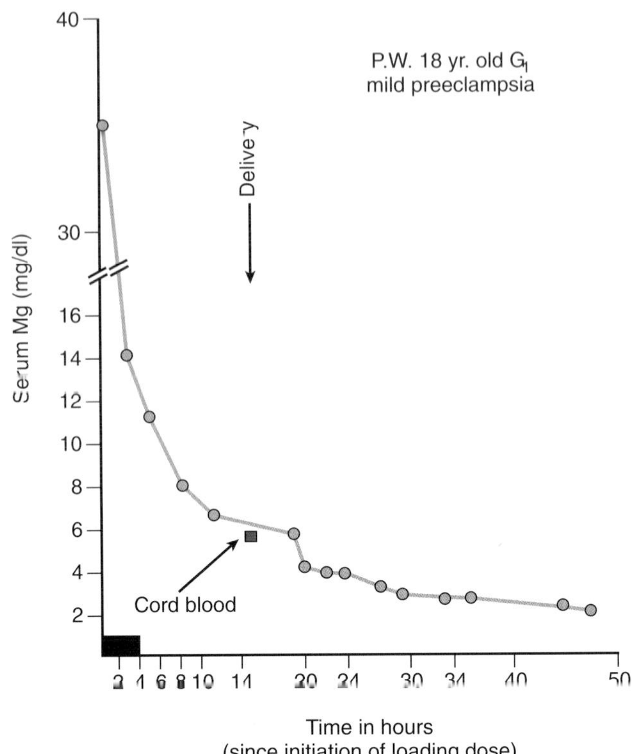

Figure 33-9. A patient with magnesium toxicity. (From McCubbin JH, Sibai BM, Abdella TN, et al: Cardiopulmonary arrest due to acute maternal hypermagnesemia, letter. Lancet 1:1058, 1981, with permission.)

Control of Severe Hypertension

The next step in the management of eclampsia is to reduce the BP to a safe range. The objective of treating severe hypertension is to avoid loss of cerebral autoregulation and to prevent congestive heart failure without compromising cerebral perfusion or jeopardizing uteroplacental blood flow that is already reduced in many women with eclampsia.[79] Thus, maintaining systolic BP between 140 and 160 mm Hg and diastolic BP between 90 and 110 mm Hg is a reasonable goal. This can be achieved with bolus 5 to 10 mg doses of hydralazine or labetalol (20 to 40 mg intravenously) every 15 minutes as needed.[2] Other potent antihypertensive medications such as sodium nitroprusside or nitroglycerine are rarely needed in eclampsia. Diuretics are not used except in the presence of pulmonary edema.

Intrapartum Management

Maternal hypoxemia and hypercarbia cause fetal heart rate and uterine activity changes during and immediately following a convulsion. The fetal heart rate tracing may reveal bradycardia, transient late decelerations, decreased beat-to-beat variability, and compensatory tachycardia. Uterine contractions can increase in frequency and tone.[263] These changes usually resolve spontaneously within 3 to 10 minutes following the termination of convulsions and the correction of maternal hypoxemia. The patient should not be rushed to have an emergency cesarean delivery based on these findings, especially if the maternal condition is not stable.

In a review of 10 women who had undergone electronic internal fetal monitoring during an eclamptic convulsion, six had fetal bradycardia (fetal heart rate <120 beats/min) that varied in duration from 30 seconds to 9 minutes.[263] The interval from onset of the seizure to the fall in fetal heart rate was 5 minutes. Transitory fetal tachycardia occurred frequently after the prolonged bradycardia. In addition, loss of beat-to-beat variability with transitory late decelerations occurred during the recovery phase. Uterine hyperactivity demonstrated by both increased uterine tone and increased frequency of uterine contractions occurs during an eclamptic seizure. The duration of the increased uterine activity varies from 2 to 14 minutes.

Fetal outcome is generally good after an eclamptic convulsion. The mechanism for the transitory fetal bradycardia may be a decrease in uterine blood flow caused by intense vasospasm and uterine hyperactivity. The absence of maternal respiration during the convulsion may also result in fetal hypoxia and heart rate changes. Because the fetal heart rate pattern usually returns to normal after a convulsion, other conditions should be considered if an abnormal pattern persists. It may take longer for the heart rate pattern to return to baseline in an eclamptic woman whose fetus is preterm with growth restriction. Placental abruption may occur after the convulsion and should be considered if uterine hyperactivity remains or the bradycardia persists.

It is advantageous to the fetus to allow in utero recovery from the maternal convulsion, hypoxia, and hypercarbia before delivery. However, if the bradycardia and/or recurrent late decelerations persist beyond 10–15 minutes despite all resuscitive efforts, then a diagnosis of abruptio placentae or persistent nonreassuring fetal status should be considered.[79]

The presence of eclampsia is not an indication for cesarean delivery. The decision to perform a cesarean delivery should be based on gestational age, fetal condition, presence of labor, and cervical Bishop score.[2] Cesarean delivery is recommended for those with eclampsia before 30 weeks' gestation who are not in labor with an unfavorable cervix (Bishop score is below 5). Patients having labor or rupture of membranes are allowed to deliver vaginally in the absence of obstetric complications. When labor is indicated, it is initiated with either oxytocin infusions or prostaglandins in all patients with a gestational age at or above 30 weeks, irrespective of the Bishop score. A similar approach is used for those before 30 weeks' gestation if the cervical Bishop score is at least 5.

Maternal pain relief during labor and delivery can be provided by either systemic opioids or epidural anesthesia as recommended for women with severe preeclampsia.[2] Either epidural, spinal, or combined techniques of regional anesthesia can be used for cesarean delivery. Regional anesthesia is contraindicated in the presence of coagulopathy or severe thrombocytopenia (platelet count less than 50,000/mm^3). In women with eclampsia, general anesthesia increases the risk of aspiration and failed intubation due to airway edema and is associated with marked increases in systemic and cerebral pressures during intubation and extubation.[2] Women with airway or laryngeal edema may require awake intubation under fiber-optic observation with the availability of immediate tracheostomy. Changes in systemic or cerebral pressures may be attenuated by pretreatment with labetalol or nitroglycerine injections.[2]

Postpartum Management

After delivery, patients with eclampsia should receive close monitoring of vital signs, fluid intake and output, and symptoms for at least 48 hours. These women usually receive large amounts of intravenous fluids during labor, delivery, and postpartum. In addition, during the postpartum period, there is mobilization of extracellular fluid leading to increased intravascular volume. As a result, women with eclampsia, particularly those with abnormal renal function, those with abruptio placentae, and those with preexisting chronic hypertension are at increased risk for pulmonary edema and exacerbation of severe hypertension postpartum.[9] Careful attention to fluid status is essential.

Parenteral magnesium sulfate should be continued for at least 24 hours after delivery or for at least 24 hours after the last convulsion. If the patient has oliguria (less than 100 ml/4 hours), the rate of both fluid administration and the dose of magnesium sulfate should be reduced. Once delivery has occurred, other oral antihypertensive agents such as labetalol or nifedipine can be used to keep systolic BP below 155 mm Hg and diastolic BP below 105 mm Hg. Nifedipine offers the benefit of improved diuresis in the postpartum period.

Subsequent Pregnancy Outcome and Remote Prognosis

Pregnancies complicated by eclampsia may be associated with life-threatening complications for both the mother and infant. Therefore, clinicians should be prepared to answer questions regarding subsequent pregnancy outcome and long-term prognosis. Women with a history of eclampsia are at increased risk for all forms of preeclampsia in subsequent pregnancies (Table 33-17).[264–267] In general, the rate of preeclampsia in subsequent pregnancies is approximately 25 percent, with substantially higher rates if the onset of eclampsia was in the second trimester. The rate of recurrent eclampsia is approximately 2 percent. Because of these risks, these women should be informed that they are at increased risk for adverse pregnancy outcome in subsequent pregnancies.[264] At present, there is no preventive therapy for recurrent antepartum eclampsia.

The long-term effects of eclampsia on maternal BP and neurologic outcome have been the subject of few reports.[264,265,269] The findings of these studies revealed that eclampsia did not cause hypertension in women who were normotensive before the eclamptic pregnancy. Two of these studies found that the rate of chronic hypertension on follow-up was significantly higher in those who had

Table 33-17. Recurrent Preeclampsia-Eclampsia in Women with Eclampsia

	CHESLEY[265]	LOPEZ-LLERA & HORTON[266]	ADELUSI & OJENGBEDE[267]	SIBAI ET AL[264]
Number of women	171	110	64	182
Number of pregnancies	398	110	64	366
Eclampsia (%)	1.0	—	15.6	1.9
Preeclampsia (%)	23	35	27	22

From Sibai BM: Diagnosis, differential diagnosis and management of eclampsia. Obstet Gynecol 105:402, 2005.

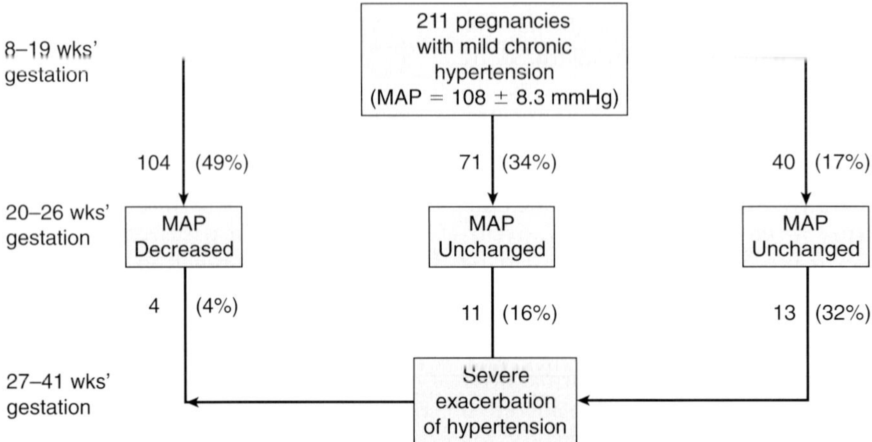

Figure 33-10. Mean arterial blood pressure (MAP) during pregnancy. (Modified from Sibai BM, Abdella TN, Anderson GD: Pregnancy outcome in 211 patients with mild chronic hypertension. Obstet Gynecol 61:571, 1983.)

eclampsia remote from term as compared with those who had eclampsia at or beyond 37 weeks of gestation.[264,265] In addition, one of these reports revealed that women who had eclampsia as multiparas were at increased risk of death from cardiovascular renal disease.[264] Moreover, these investigations revealed no evidence of neurologic deficit during the follow-up period.[264]

INCIDENCE OF CHRONIC HYPERTENSION

According to data derived from the National Health and Nutrition Examination Survey, 1988–1991, the prevalence of chronic hypertension among women of childbearing age increases from 0.6 to 2.0 percent for women 18 to 29 years old to 4.6 to 22.3 percent for women 30 to 39 years old. Racial differences in prevalence are noteworthy because higher prevalence is observed in blacks.[270] Because of the current trend of child bearing at an older age, it is expected that the incidence of chronic hypertension in pregnancy will continue to rise. During the new millennium, and estimating a prevalence of chronic hypertension during pregnancy of 3 percent, at least 120,000 pregnant women (3 percent of 4 million pregnancies) with chronic hypertension per year will be seen in the United States.[271]

Definition and Diagnosis

In pregnant women, chronic hypertension is defined as elevated BP that is present and documented before pregnancy. In women whose prepregnancy BP is unknown, the diagnosis is based on the presence of sustained hypertension before 20 weeks of gestation, defined as either systolic BP of at least 140 mm Hg or diastolic BP of at least 90 mm Hg on at least two occasions measured at least 4 hours apart.[271]

The diagnosis may be difficult in women with previously undiagnosed chronic hypertension who begin prenatal care after 16 weeks' gestation because a physiologic decrease in BP usually begins at that time. An analysis of pregnancy outcome in 211 patients with mild chronic hypertension suggests that the use of antihypertensive drugs is not necessary to achieve a good pregnancy outcome.[272] The changes in average mean arterial pressure throughout the course of pregnancy are summarized in Figure 33-10. This decrease may result in normal BP findings in the second trimester that will eventually increase again during the third trimester. These women are more likely to be erroneously diagnosed as having gestational hypertension.[272]

Women with chronic hypertension are at increased risk of superimposed preeclampsia. The development of superimposed preeclampsia is associated with high rates of adverse maternal and perinatal outcomes.[273] The diagnosis of superimposed preeclampsia should be made as described in Table 33-3.

Etiology and Classification

The etiology as well as the severity of chronic hypertension is an important consideration in the management of pregnancy. Chronic hypertension is subdivided into primary (essential) and secondary. Primary hypertension is by far the most common cause of chronic hypertension seen during pregnancy (90 percent). In 10 percent of the cases, chronic hypertension is secondary to one or more underlying disorders such as renal disease (glomerulonephritis, interstitial nephritis, polycystic kidneys, renal artery stenosis), collagen vascular disease (lupus, scleroderma), endocrine disorders (diabetes mellitus with vascular involvement, pheochromocytoma, thyrotoxicosis, Cushing's disease, hyperaldosteronism), or coarctation of the aorta.[1,274,276]

Chronic hypertension during pregnancy can be subclassified as either mild or severe, depending on the systolic and diastolic BP readings. Systolic and diastolic (Korotkoff phase V) BPs of at least 180 mm Hg or 110 mm Hg, respectively, constitute severe hypertension.[274,275]

For management and counseling purposes, chronic hypertension in pregnancy is also categorized as either low risk or high risk as described in Figure 33-11. The patient is considered to be at low risk when she has mild essential hypertension without any organ involvement. The BP criteria are based on BP measurements at the initial visit irrespective of treatment with antihypertensive medications. For example, if the patient has a BP of 140/80 mm Hg on antihypertensive drugs, she is still classified as low risk. It is important to note that a patient initially classified as low risk early in pregnancy may become high risk if she later develops severe hypertension or if she develops preeclampsia.[275]

Maternal-Perinatal Risks

Pregnancies complicated by chronic hypertension are at increased risk for the development of superimposed preeclampsia and abruptio placentae. The reported rates of preeclampsia in the literature in mild hypertension range from 10 to 25 percent (Table 33-18).[272,273,277,278] The rate of preeclampsia in women with severe chronic hypertension ranges from 50 to 79 percent.[278–280] Sibai and associates[273] studied the rate of superimposed preeclampsia among 763 women with chronic hypertension followed prospectively at several tertiary medical centers in the United States. The overall rate of superimposed preeclampsia was 25 percent. The rate was not affected by maternal age, race, or presence of proteinuria early in pregnancy. However, the rate was significantly greater in women who had hypertension for at least 4 years (31 percent versus 22 percent), in those who had had preeclampsia during a previous pregnancy (32 percent versus 23 percent), and in those whose diastolic BP was 100 to 110 mm Hg when compared with those whose diastolic BP was below 100 mm Hg at baseline (42 percent versus 24 percent).[273]

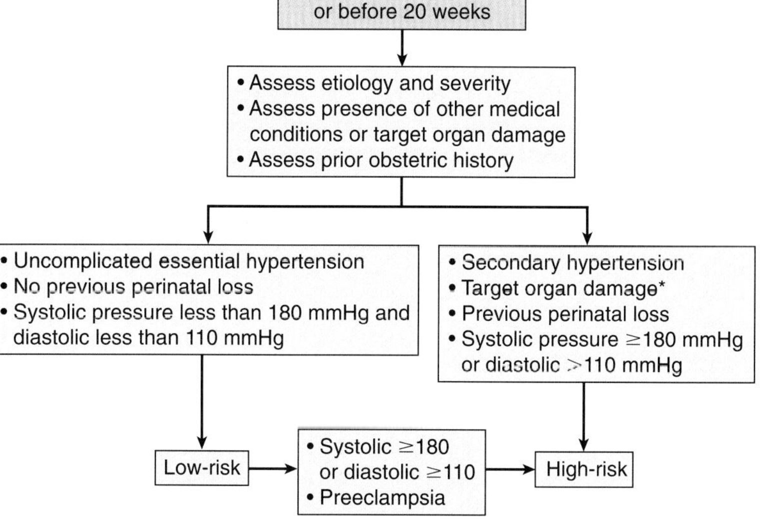

Figure 33-11. Initial evaluation of women with chronic hypertension. (From Sibai BM: Chronic hypertension in pregnancy. Obstet Gynecol 100:369, 2002.)

Table 33-18. Rates of Adverse Pregnancy Outcome in Observational Studies Describing Mild Chronic Hypertension in Pregnancy

	PREECLAMPSIA %	ABRUPTIO PLACENTAE %	DELIVERY AT <37 WK %	SGA %
Sibai et al. (n = 211)[272]	10	1.4	12.0	8.0
Rey & Couturier (n = 337)[278]	21	0.7	34.4	15.5
McCowan et al. (n = 142)[277]	14	NR	16	11.0
Sibai et al. (n = 763)[273]	25	1.5	33.3	11.1

NR, not reported; SGA, small for gestational age.
From Sibai BM: Chronic hypertension in pregnancy. Obstet Gynecol 100:369, 2002. With permission.

The reported rate of abruptio placentae, in women with mild chronic hypertension, has ranged from 0.7 to 1.5 percent (Table 33-18). The rate in those with severe or high-risk hypertension may be 5 to 10 percent.[278,279] In a recent multicenter study that included 763 women with chronic hypertension, the overall rate of abruptio placentae was reported at 1.5 percent and the rate was significantly higher in those who developed superimposed preeclampsia than in those without this complication (3 percent versus 1 percent, P = .04).[273] However, the rate was not influenced by either maternal age, race, or duration of hypertension.[273] In addition, the results of a systematic review of nine observational studies revealed that the rate of abruptio placentae is doubled (odds ratio [OR], 2.1; 95 percent CI, 1.1 to 3.9) in women with chronic hypertension compared with either normotensive patients or the general obstetric population.[271]

In addition to preeclampsia and abruptio placentae, women with high-risk chronic hypertension are at increased risk for life-threatening maternal complications such as pulmonary edema, hypertensive encephalopathy, retinopathy, cerebral hemorrhage, and acute renal failure.[275] These risks are particularly increased in women with uncontrolled severe hypertension, significant renal disease early in pregnancy, and in those with left ventricular dysfunction before conception.[279,281]

Fetal and neonatal complications are also increased in women with chronic hypertension. The risk of perinatal mortality is 3 to 4 times greater compared with the general obstetric population (OR, 3.4; 95 percent CI 3.0 to 3.7).[271] The likelihood of premature delivery and SGA infants is also increased in women with chronic hypertension (see Table 33-18). In women with severe chronic hypertension in the first trimester, the reported rates of preterm deliveries were 62 to 70 percent and the rates of SGA infants were 31 to 40 percent.[278,279] Recently, Sibai et al.[273] reported risk factors for adverse perinatal outcome in a secondary analysis of 763 women with mild chronic hypertension who were enrolled in a multicenter trial comparing low-dose aspirin to a placebo for the prevention of preeclampsia. They found that the development of superimposed preeclampsia was associated with higher rates of preterm delivery (OR, 3.9; 95 percent CI, 2.7 to 5.4), neonatal intraventricular hemorrhage (OR, 4.5; 95 percent CI, 1.5 to 14.2) and perinatal death (OR, 2.3; 95 percent CI, 1.4 to 4.8). In addition, the presence of proteinuria early in pregnancy was an independent risk factor associated with higher rates of preterm delivery (OR, 3.1; 95 percent CI, 1.8 to 5.3), SGA infants (OR, 2.8; 95 percent CI, 1.6 to 5.0), and neonatal intraventricular hemorrhage (OR, 3.9; 95 percent CI, 1.3 to 11.6).[273]

Goals of Antihypertensive Therapy in Pregnancy

In nonpregnant individuals, long-term BP control can lead to significant reductions in the rates of stroke and cardiovascular morbidity and mortality.[276] In those with mild to moderate hypertension, the benefit is achieved after at least 5 years of treatment.[276] The side effects of therapy are, of course, restricted to the treated individual. In contrast to hypertension in pregnancy, the duration of therapy is shorter, the benefits to the mother may not be obvious during the short time of treatment, and the exposure to medication will include both mother and fetus.[282] In this respect, one must balance the potential short-term maternal benefits against possible short-term and long-term benefits and risks to the fetus and infant.[271,275,282]

Most women with chronic hypertension during pregnancy have mild essential uncomplicated hypertension and are at minimal risk for cardiovascular complications within the short time frame of pregnancy.[275,282] Several retrospective[272,273,277–280] and prospective[283–286] studies have been conducted to determine whether antihypertensive therapy in these women improves pregnancy outcome. An overall summary of these studies revealed that, regardless of the antihypertensive therapy used, maternal cardiovascular and renal complications were minimal or absent.[275,282] Based on the available data, there is no compelling evidence that short-term antihypertensive therapy is beneficial for the mother in women with low-risk hypertension except for a reduction in the rate of exacerbation of hypertension.[90,275]

There are no placebo-controlled trials examining the benefits of antihypertensive therapy in women with severe hypertension in pregnancy, and none are likely to be performed. Antihypertensive therapy is necessary in these women to reduce the acute risk of stroke, congestive heart failure or renal failure.[276] In addition, control of severe hypertension may also permit pregnancy prolongation and thereby improve perinatal outcome. However, there is no available evidence that control of severe hypertension reduces the rates of either superimposed preeclampsia or abruptio placentae.[272–279]

There are no trials examining the treatment of women with chronic hypertension and other risk factors, such as preexisting renal disease, diabetes mellitus, or cardiac disease.[271] On the other hand, there is evidence from retrospective and observational studies that uncontrolled mild-to-moderate hypertension may exacerbate target organ damage during pregnancy in women with renal disease, diabetes mellitus with vascular disease, and women with left ventricular dysfunction.[287,288] Therefore, some authors recommend aggressive treatment of mild hypertension in these women because of the belief that such management may reduce both short-term and long-term cardiovascular complications.

There are many retrospective and prospective studies examining the potential fetal-neonatal benefits of pharmacologic therapy in women with mild essential uncomplicated hypertension (low risk).[90,271] Some have compared treatment with no treatment or with a placebo, others compared two different antihypertensive drugs, and others used a combination of drugs. The gestational age at the time of treatment, the level of BP achieved during treatment, and the duration of therapy in these studies is highly variable. Only four of these studies were randomized trials that included women enrolled before 20 weeks' gestation.[282–286] Only two of the trials had a moderate sample size to evaluate the risks of superimposed preeclampsia and abruptio placentae.[285,286] The findings of these two trials revealed contradictory results regarding the effects of antihypertensive therapy on the rates of superimposed preeclampsia (a significant reduction in the study by Steyn and Odendaal[286]) and abruptio placentae (a moderate, but not significant reduction in the study by Steyn and Odendaal). Antihypertensive therapy did not affect gestational age at time of delivery in any of the four trials; only the small trial by Butters et al.[284] demonstrated a significantly lower average birth weight and significantly higher rate of SGA infants in the atenolol treated group. It is important to note that the total number of women enrolled in these trials was only 450 and the largest trial included 263 women.[285] In addition, there was imbalance in the number of women with risk factors for preeclampsia and abruptio placentae between the study groups in the trial by Steyn and Odendaal.[286] This imbalance favored the treated arm of the study. Therefore, none of these trials had a sample size with adequate power sufficient enough to detect moderate (20 to 30 percent) reductions or increase in the rates of preeclampsia, SGA infants, or abruptio placentae.[275]

The Safety of Antihypertensive Drugs in Pregnancy

The potential adverse effects for most commonly prescribed antihypertensive agents are either poorly established or unclearly quantified.[271] Most of the evidence on harm associated with antihypertensives in pregnancy is limited to case reports. The interpretation of these reports is difficult because it is impossible to ascertain the exact number of women exposed to antihypertensive drugs during pregnancy.[271] Also, it is likely that the number of published case reports is an underestimate of the actual number of women experiencing the reported adverse reaction. This limitation is amplified by the fact that information related to previous exposure during pregnancy is nonexistent. Furthermore, the condition for which pregnant women are treated with antihypertensive drugs can be partially responsible for the adverse fetal and neonatal outcomes.

In general, available information about teratogenecity except in laboratory animals is limited and selective. All available data have been obtained from registries such as State Medicaid registry data.[289] Because of absent multicenter randomized trials in women with chronic hypertension, there are no placebo-controlled evaluations regarding the safety of these drugs when used at the time of conception and throughout pregnancy. At the present time, there are minimal data to help the clinician evaluate the benefits or risks of most antihypertensive drugs when used in pregnancy. Nevertheless, the limited data in the literature suggest that there are potential adverse fetal effects such as oligohydramnios and fetal-neonatal renal failure when angiotensin converting enzyme (ACE) inhibitors are used in the second or third trimester.[271,289] Similar effects are to be expected with the use of angiotensin II receptor blockers. Therefore, these agents should be avoided once pregnancy is established[271,289] (see Chapter 8).

The use of atenolol during the first and second trimester has been associated with significantly reduced fetal growth along with decreased placental growth and weight.[284,290] On the other hand, no such effects on fetal or placental growth were reported with other β-blockers, such as metoprolol, pindolol, and oxprenolol, but data on the use of these agents in early pregnancy are very scarce.[271]

Prospective trials examining the effect of either methyldopa or labetalol in women with mild chronic hypertension revealed no adverse maternal or fetal outcome with the use of these medications.[271,282] In a large and unique trial in which methyldopa or labetalol was started between 6 and 13 weeks' gestation in patients with chronic hypertension, none of the exposed newborns had major congenital anomalies.[285]

There is a large clinical experience with the use of thiazide diuretics during pregnancy. The available data suggest that treatment with diuretics in the first trimester and throughout gestation is not associated with an increased risk of major fetal anomalies or adverse fetal-neonatal events.[271,282] However, their use did reduce plasma volume expansion. There is little information regarding the use of calcium channel blockers in women with mild chronic hypertension. The available evidence suggest that the use of calcium channel blockers, particularly nifedipine in the first trimester was not associated with increased rates of major birth defects.[289,291] The effects of nifedipine on fetal-neonatal outcome were evaluated in a prospective randomized trial of 283 women with mild to moderate hypertension in pregnancy in which 47 percent of the participants had chronic hypertension.[292] Sixty-six of these women were enrolled between 12 and 20 weeks' gestation. In this study, the use of slow-release nifedipine was not associated with adverse fetal-neonatal outcomes.[292]

The long-term effects on children of mothers exposed to antihypertensive drugs during pregnancy are lacking except for limited information concerning the use of methyldopa and nifedipine.[293,294] A follow-up study of infants after 7.5 years showed no long-term adverse effects on development among those exposed to methyldopa in utero as compared with infants not exposed to such treatment.[293] A similar study examined the effects of slow-release nifedipine after 1.5 years of follow-up demonstrated no adverse effects on development.[294]

Recommended Management of Chronic Hypertension in Pregnancy

The primary objective in the management of pregnancies complicated by chronic hypertension is to reduce maternal risks and achieve optimal perinatal survival. This objective can be achieved by formulating a rational approach that includes preconceptual evaluation and counseling, early antenatal care, frequent antepartum visits to monitor both maternal and fetal well-being, timely delivery with intensive intrapartum monitoring, and proper postpartum management.

Evaluation and Classification

Management of patients with chronic hypertension should ideally begin before pregnancy, whereby extensive evaluation and complete workup is undertaken to assess the etiology, the severity, as well as the coexistence of other medical illnesses, and to rule out the presence of target organ damage resulting from longstanding hypertension. An in-depth history should delineate in particular the duration of hypertension, the use of antihypertensive medications, their type, and the response to these medications. Also, attention should be given to the presence of cardiac or renal disease, diabetes mellitus, thyroid disease, and a history of cerebrovascular accident, or congestive heart failure. A detailed obstetric history should include maternal and neonatal outcomes of previous pregnancies stressing a history of the development of abruptio placentae, superimposed preeclampsia, preterm delivery, SGA infants, intrauterine fetal death, and neonatal morbidity and mortality.[275]

Laboratory evaluation is obtained to assess the function of different organ systems that are likely to be affected by chronic hypertension, and as a baseline for future assessments. These should include the following for all patients: urinalysis, urine culture and sensitivity, 24-hour urine evaluations for protein, electrolytes, complete blood count, and a glucose tolerance test.[276]

Women with long-standing hypertension for several years, particularly those with a history of poor compliance or poor BP control, should be evaluated for target organ damage, including left ventricular hypertrophy, retinopathy, and renal injury. These women should undergo an ECG examination and echocardiography if the ECG is abnormal, ophthalmologic evaluation, and creatinine clearance.[275]

Selectively, certain tests should be obtained to identify secondary causes of hypertension such as pheochromocytoma, primary hyperaldosteronism, or renal artery stenosis. These conditions require selective biochemical testing and are amenable to diagnosis with either CT or MRI.[1,274] Pheochromocytoma should be suspected in women with paroxysmal severe hypertension, hyperglycemia, and sweating. Primary aldosteronism is extremely rare in pregnancy and should be considered in women with severe hypertension and marked hypokalemia. Based on this evaluation, the patient is then classified as having low-risk or high-risk chronic hypertension and managed accordingly (Fig. 33-12).[275]

Low-Risk Hypertension

Women with low-risk chronic hypertension without superimposed preeclampsia usually have a pregnancy outcome similar to that of the general obstetric population.[272,275,285] In addition, discontinuation of antihypertensive therapy early in pregnancy does not affect the rate of preeclampsia, abruptio placentae, or preterm delivery in these women.[272,285] Many clinicians chose to discontinue antihypertensive treatment at the first prenatal visit because the majority of these women will have good pregnancy outcome without such therapy.[285] Although many of these women will not require subsequent pharmacologic therapy, careful management is still essential (see Fig. 33-11). At the time of initial and subsequent visits, the patient is educated about nutritional requirements, weight gain, and sodium intake (maximum of 2.4 g of sodium per day). They are also counseled that consumption of alcohol and smoking during pregnancy can aggravate maternal hypertension and are associated with adverse effects on the fetus such as fetal growth restriction and abruptio placentae. During each subsequent visit, they are observed very closely for early signs of preeclampsia and fetal growth restriction.[275]

Fetal evaluation should include an ultrasound examination at 16 to 20 weeks' gestation, to be repeated at 30

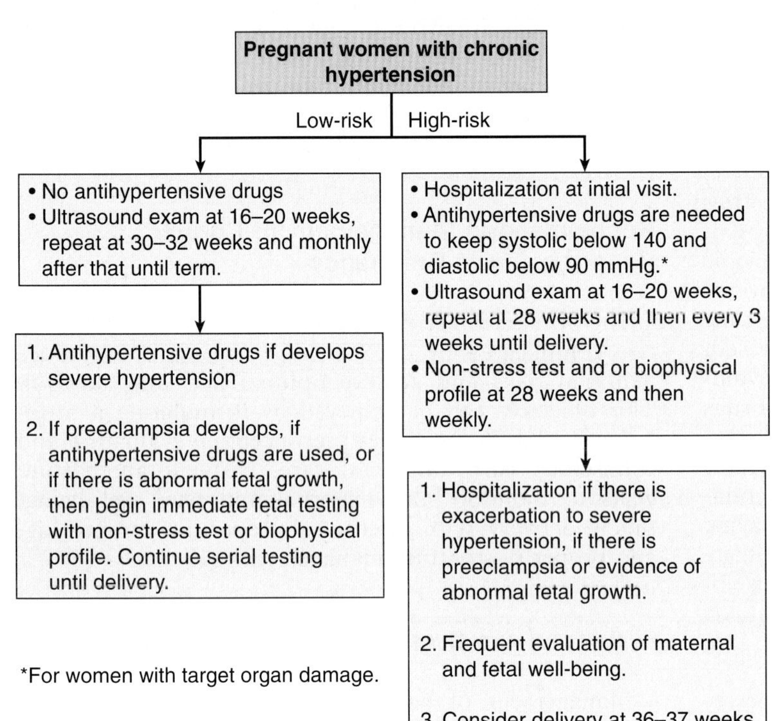

Figure 33-12. Antepartum management of chronic hypertension. (From Sibai BM: Chronic hypertension in pregnancy. Obstet Gynecol 100:369, 2002.)

to 32 weeks', and monthly thereafter until term. Antihypertensive treatment with either nifedipine or labetalol is initiated if the patient develops severe hypertension before term. The development of either severe hypertension, preeclampsia, or abnormal fetal growth requires immediate fetal testing with a NST or biophysical profile. Women who develop severe hypertension, and those with documented fetal growth restriction by ultrasound examination, require hospitalization and often delivery. If superimposed preeclampsia is diagnosed at or beyond 37 weeks, delivery is undertaken as well. In the absence of these complications, the pregnancy may be continued until 40 weeks' gestation.

HIGH-RISK HYPERTENSION

Women with high-risk chronic hypertension are at increased risk for adverse maternal and perinatal complications. The likelihood and impact of these complications will depend on the etiology of the hypertension as well as the degree of target organ damage. Women with significant renal insufficiency (serum creatinine >1.4 mg/dl), diabetes mellitus with vascular involvement (class R/F), severe collagen vascular disease, cardiomyopathy, or coarctation of the aorta should receive thorough counseling regarding the adverse effects of pregnancy before conception. These women should be advised that pregnancy may exacerbate their condition with the potential for congestive heart failure, acute renal failure requiring dialysis, and even death. In addition, perinatal loss and neonatal complications are markedly increased in these women. All such patients should be managed by or in consultation with a subspecialist in maternal-fetal medicine, as well as in association with other medical specialists as needed. In addition, these women must be observed and delivered at a tertiary care center with the appropriate resources for maternal and neonatal care.[275]

Hospitalization of women with high-risk hypertension at the time of the first prenatal visit is recommended. This facilitates evaluation of cardiovascular and renal status and regulation of antihypertensive medications, as well as other prescribed treatments (insulin, cardiac drugs, thyroid medications, and so on), if needed. Women receiving ACE inhibitors, or angiotensin II receptor antagonists should have these medications discontinued under close observation. Antihypertensive therapy with one or more of the drugs listed in Table 33-19 is subsequently used in all women with systolic BP of 180 mm Hg or more, or diastolic BP of 110 mm Hg or more. In women without target organ damage, the aim of antihypertensive therapy is to keep systolic BP between 140 and 150 mm Hg and diastolic BP between 90 and 100 mm Hg. In addition, antihypertensive therapy is indicated in women with mild hypertension plus target organ damage because there are short-term maternal benefits from lowering BP in such women. In these women, maintaining systolic BP below 140 mm Hg and diastolic BP below 90 mm Hg is advised. In some women, BP may be difficult to control initially demanding the use of intravenous therapy with hydralazine or labetalol or oral short acting nifedipine with doses as described in Table 33-19.[275] For maintenance therapy, one may choose either oral methyldopa, labetalol, slow-release nifedipine, or a diuretic. Methyldopa is the drug most commonly recommended to treat hypertension during pregnancy.[1,274] However, it is rarely used in nonpregnant hypertensive women. Therefore, it is not practical to switch medications to methyldopa because of pregnancy. In addition, methyldopa is associated with dry mouth and drowsiness in many pregnant women. Other side effects include liver function abnormalities. The recommended first drug of choice for control of hypertension in pregnancy is labetalol starting at 100 mg twice daily, to be increased to a maximum of 2,400 mg/d. If maternal BP is not controlled with maximum doses of labetalol, a second drug such as a thiazide diuretic or nifedipine may be added. For women with diabetes mellitus and vascular disease, oral nifedipine is recommended.[13] Oral nifedipine or a thiazide diuretic is the drug of choice for young black women with hypertension because these women often manifest a low-renin type hypertension or salt-sensitive hypertension.[282] If maternal BP is adequately controlled with these medications, the patient can continue with the same drug after delivery.

Table 33-19. Drugs Used to Treat Hypertension in Pregnancy

DRUG	STARTING DOSE	MAXIMUM DOSE
Acute treatment of severe hypertension		
Hydralazine	5–10 mg IV every 20 min	20 mg*
Labetalol†	20–40 mg IV every 10–15 min	220 mg*
Nifedipine	10–20 mg oral every 30 min	50 mg*
Long term treatment of hypertension		
Methyldopa	250 mg BID	4 gram/day
Labetalol	100 mg BID	2400 mg/day
Nifedipine	10 mg BID	120 mg/day
Thiazide diuretic	12.5 mg BID	50 mg/day

BID, twice a day; IV, intravenously.
*If desired blood pressure levels are not achieved, switch to another drug.
†Avoid labetalol in women with asthma or congestive heart failure.

Diuretics are commonly prescribed in women with essential hypertension before conception.[276,282] The use of diuretics throughout pregnancy is controversial. Of concern, women who use diuretics from early in pregnancy do not have an increase in plasma volume to the degree expected in normal pregnancy.[283] However, this reduction in plasma volume has not been shown to be associated with an adverse effect on fetal outcome.[283,295] Therefore, it is appropriate to start diuretics as a single agent during pregnancy or to use them in combination with other agents, particularly in women with excessive salt retention.[275] However, diuretics should be discontinued immediately if superimposed preeclampsia develops or if there is evidence of suspected fetal growth restriction because of the potential of reduced uteroplacental blood flow secondary to reduced plasma volume in women with these complications.[283]

Early and frequent prenatal visits are the key for successful pregnancy outcome in women with high-risk chronic hypertension. These women need close observation throughout pregnancy and may require serial evaluation of 24-hour urine protein excretion and a complete blood count with a metabolic profile at least once every trimester. Further laboratory testing can be performed depending on the clinical progress of the pregnancy. During each visit, the woman should be advised about the adverse effects of smoking and alcohol abuse, and should receive nutritional advice regarding diet and salt intake.[275]

Fetal evaluation should include an ultrasound examination at 16 to 20 weeks' gestation, to be repeated at 28 weeks and subsequently every three weeks till delivery. NST or biophysical profile testing is usually started at 28 weeks and then repeated weekly. The development of uncontrolled severe hypertension, preeclampsia, or evidence of fetal growth restriction requires maternal hospitalization for more frequent evaluation of maternal and fetal well-being. The development of any of these complications at or beyond 34 weeks' gestation should be considered an indication for delivery. In all other women, delivery should be considered at 36 to 37 weeks' gestation after documentation of fetal lung maturity.[275]

Postpartum Management

Women with high-risk chronic hypertension are at risk for postpartum complications such as pulmonary edema, hypertensive encephalopathy, and renal failure.[208,281] These risks are particularly increased in women with target organ involvement, superimposed preeclampsia, or abruptio placentae.[208] In these patients, BP must be closely controlled for at least 48 hours after delivery. Intravenous labetalol or hydralazine can be used as needed, and diuretics may be appropriate in women with circulatory congestion and pulmonary edema.[281] This therapy is usually required in those who develop exaggerated and sustained severe hypertension in the first week postpartum.

Oral therapy may be needed to control BP after delivery. In some women, it is often necessary to switch to a new agent such as an ACE inhibitor particularly in those with pregestational diabetes mellitus and those with cardiomyopathy. Some patients may wish to breast-feed their infants. All antihypertensive drugs are found in the breast milk, although differences are found in the milk-plasma ratio of these drugs. Additionally, the long-term effect of maternal antihypertensive drugs on breast-feeding infants has not been specifically studied. Milk concentrations of methyldopa appear to be low and are considered to be safe. The β-blocking agents (atenolol and metoprolol) are concentrated in breast milk, whereas labetalol or propanolol have low concentrations.[289,296] Concentrations of diuretic agents in breast milk are low; however, they may induce a decrease in milk production.[289]

There is little information about the transfer of calcium channel blockers to breast milk, but there are no apparent side effects. ACE inhibitors and angiotensin II receptor antagonists should be avoided because of their effects on neonatal renal function, even though their concentrations appear to be low in breast milk (see Chapter 8).

Finally, in breast-feeding women, the use of methyldopa as a first-line oral therapy is a reasonable choice. If methyldopa is contraindicated, labetalol may be used.

HYPERTENSIVE EMERGENCIES IN CHRONIC HYPERTENSION

On rare occasions, pregnant women may present with life-threatening clinical conditions that require immediate control of BP, such as hypertensive encephalopathy, acute left ventricular failure, acute aortic dissection, or increased circulating catecholamines (pheochromocytoma, clonidine withdrawal, cocaine ingestion).[297,298] Patients at highest risk for these complications include those with underlying cardiac disease, chronic glomerular renal disease, multiple drugs to control their hypertension, superimposed preeclampsia in the second trimester, and abruptio placentae complicated by DIC. Although a diastolic BP of 115 mm Hg or greater is usually considered a hypertensive emergency, this level is actually arbitrary, and the rate of change of BP may be more important than its absolute level.[297] The association of elevated BP with evidence of new or progressive end-organ damage determines the seriousness of the clinical situation.[299]

Hypertensive Encephalopathy

Untreated essential hypertension progresses to a hypertensive crisis in up to 1 to 2 percent of cases for unknown reasons. Hypertensive encephalopathy is usually seen in patients with a systolic BP above 250 mm Hg or a diastolic BP above 150 mm Hg.[299] Patients with the acute onset of hypertension may develop encephalopathy at pressure levels that are generally tolerated by those with chronic hypertension. Normally, cerebral blood flow is approximately 50 ml/100 g tissue per minute. When the BP falls, cerebral arterioles normally dilate, whereas when BP increases, they constrict to maintain constant cerebral blood flow.[299] This mechanism usually remains operative between 60 and 120 mm Hg diastolic BP. Hypertensive encephalopathy is currently considered to be a derangement of the autoregulation of cerebral arterioles, which occurs when the upper limit of autoregulation is exceeded. With severe hypertension (130 to 150 mm Hg cerebral perfusion pressure), cerebral blood vessels constrict as much as possible and then reflex cerebral vasodilatation occurs. This results in overperfusion, damage to small blood vessels, cerebral edema, and increased intracranial pressure (breakthrough theory). Others believe that hypertensive encephalopathy results from an exaggerated vasoconstrictive response of the arterioles resulting in cerebral ischemia (overregulation theory). Patients who have impaired autoregulation involving the cerebral arterioles may experience necrotizing arteriolitis, microinfarcts, petechial hemorrhages, multiple small thrombi, or cerebral edema.[298] Typically, hypertensive encephalopathy has a subacute onset over 24 to 72 hours.[299]

During a hypertensive crisis, other evidence for end-organ damage may be present: cardiac, renal, or retinal dysfunction secondary to impaired organ perfusion and loss of autoregulation of blood flow.[298] Ischemia of the retina (with flame-shaped retinal hemorrhages, retinal infarcts, or papilledema) may occur, causing decreased visual acuity. Impaired regulation of coronary blood flow and marked increase in ventricular wall stress may result in angina, myocardial infarction, congestive heart failure, malignant ventricular arrhythmia, pulmonary edema, or dissecting aortic aneurysm. Necrosis of the afferent arterioles of the glomerulus results in hemorrhages of the cortex and medulla, fibrinoid necrosis, and proliferative endarteritis resulting in elevated serum creatinine (>3 mg/dl), proteinuria, oliguria, hematuria, hyaline or red blood cell casts, and progressive azotemia.[359] Severe hypertension may result in abruptio placentae with resultant DIC. In addition, high levels of angiotensin II, norepinephrine, and vasopressin accompany ongoing vascular damage. These circulating hormones increase relative efferent arteriolar tone, resulting in sodium diuresis and hypovolemia. Because levels of renin and angiotensin II are increased, the aldosterone level is also elevated. The impact of these endocrine changes may be important in maintaining the hypertensive crisis.

Treatment of Hypertensive Encephalopathy

The ultimate goal of therapy is to prevent the occurrence of a hypertensive emergency. Patients at risk for a hypertensive crisis should receive intensive management during labor and for a minimum of 48 hours after delivery. Although pregnancy may complicate the diagnosis, once the life-threatening conditions are recognized, pregnancy should not in any way slow or alter the mode of therapy. The only reliable clinical criterion to confirm the diagnosis of hypertensive encephalopathy is prompt response of the patient to antihypertensive therapy. The headache and sensorium often clear dramatically—sometimes within 1 to 2 hours after the treatment. The overall recovery may be somewhat slower in patients with uremia and those in whom the symptoms have been present for a prolonged period before the therapy is given. Sustained cerebrovascular deficits should suggest other diagnoses.

Patients with hypertensive encephalopathy or other hypertensive crisis should be hospitalized for bed rest. Intravenous lines should be inserted for fluids and medications. Although there is a tendency to restrict sodium intake in patients with a hypertensive emergency, volume contraction from sodium diuresis may be present. A marked drop in diastolic BP with a rise in heart rate on standing from the supine position is evidence of volume contraction. Infusion of normal saline solution during the first 24 to 48 hours to achieve volume expansion should be considered. Saline infusion may help decrease the activity of the renin-angiotensin-aldosterone axis and result in better BP control. Simultaneous repletion of potassium losses and continuous monitoring of BP, volume status, urinary output, electrocardiographic readings, and mental status is mandatory. An intra-arterial line provides the most accurate BP information. Laboratory studies include a complete blood count with differential, reticulocyte count, platelets, and blood chemistries. A urinalysis should be obtained for protein, glucose, blood, cells, casts, and bacteria. Assessment for end-organ damage in the central nervous system, retina, kidneys, and cardiovascular system should be done periodically. Antepartum patients should have continuous fetal monitoring.[297,300]

Lowering Blood Pressure

There are risks associated with too rapid or excessive reduction of elevated BP. The aim of therapy is to lower mean BP by no more than 15 to 25 percent. Small reductions in BP in the first 60 minutes, working toward a diastolic level of 100 to 110 mm Hg, have been recommended.[297,298] Although cerebral blood flow is maintained constantly over a wide range of BPs, there is a lower as well as an upper limit to autoregulation. In chronic hypertensive women who have a rightward shift of the cerebral autoregulation curve secondary to medial hypertrophy of the cerebral vasculature, lowering BP too rapidly may produce cerebral ischemia, stroke, or coma. Coronary blood flow, renal perfusion, and uteroplacental blood flow also may deteriorate, resulting in acute renal failure, myocardial infarction, fetal distress, or death. Hypertension that proves increasingly difficult to control is an indication to terminate the pregnancy. If the patient's outcome appears to be grave, consideration of perimortem cesarean delivery should be made.[297]

The drug of choice in a hypertensive crisis is sodium nitroprusside. Other agents such as nitroglycerin, nifedipine, trimetaphan, labetalol, and hydralazine can also be used.

Sodium Nitroprusside

Sodium nitroprusside causes arterial and venous relaxation by interfering with both influx and the intracellular activation of calcium. It is given as an intravenous infusion of 0.25 to 8.0 µg/kg/min. The onset of action is immediate, and its effect may last 3 to 5 minutes after discontinuing the infusion. Hypotension caused by nitroprusside should resolve within a few minutes of stopping the infusion, because the drug's half life is so short. If it does not resolve, other causes for hypotension should be suspected. The effect of nitroprusside on uterine blood flow is controversial. Nitroprusside is metabolized into thiocyanate, which is excreted in the urine. Cyanide can accumulate if there is either increased production due to large doses (>10 µg/kg/min) or prolonged administration (>48 hours), or if there is renal insufficiency or decreased metabolism in the liver. Signs of toxicity include anorexia, disorientation, headache, fatigue, restlessness, tinnitus, delirium, hallucinations, nausea, vomiting, and metabolic acidosis. When it is infused at less than 2 mg/kg/min, cyanide toxicity is unlikely. At a maximum dose rate of 10 mg/kg/min, infusion should never last more than 10 minutes. Animal experiments and the few reported cases of nitroprusside use in pregnancy have revealed that thiocyanate toxicity to mother and fetus rarely occur if it is used in a regular pharmacologic dose. Tachyphylaxis to nitroprusside usually develops before toxicity occurs. Whenever toxicity is suspected, therapy should be initiated with 3 percent sodium nitrite at a rate not exceeding 5 ml/min, up to a total dose of 15 ml. Then, infusion of 12.5 g of sodium thiosulfate in 50 ml of 5 percent dextrose in water over a 10-minute period should be started.[301]

NITROGLYCERIN

Nitroglycerin is an arterial but mostly venous dilator. It is given as an intravenous infusion of 5 µg/min that is gradually increased every 3 to 5 minutes to titrate BP up to a maximum dose of 100 mg/min. It is the drug of choice in preeclampsia associated with pulmonary edema and for control of hypertension associated with tracheal manipulation. Side effects such as headache, tachycardia, and methemoglobinemia may develop. It is contraindicated in hypertensive encephalopathy because it increases cerebral blood flow and intracranial pressure.[299]

KEY POINTS

- Hypertension is the most common medical complication during pregnancy.
- Preeclampsia is a leading cause of maternal mortality and morbidity worldwide.
- The pathophysiologic abnormalities of preeclampsia are numerous, but the etiology is unknown.
- At present, there is no proven method to prevent preeclampsia.
- The HELLP syndrome may develop in the absence of maternal hypertension.
- Expectant management improves perinatal outcome in a select group of women with severe preeclampsia before 32 weeks' gestation.
- Magnesium sulfate is the ideal agent to prevent or treat eclamptic convulsions.
- Rare cases of eclampsia can develop before 20 weeks' gestation and beyond 48 hours postpartum.
- Antihypertensive agents do not improve pregnancy outcome in women with mild uncomplicated chronic hypertension.
- Labetalol is the drug of choice for the treatment of chronic hypertension; ACE inhibitors should be avoided.

REFERENCES

1. Report of the National High Blood Pressure Education Program. Working Group Report on High Blood Pressure in Pregnancy. Am J Obstet Gynecol 183:S1, 2000.
2. Sibai BM: Diagnosis and management of gestational hypertension and preeclampsia. Obstet Gynecol 102:181, 2003.
3. Sibai BM: Drug therapy: treatment of hypertension in pregnant women. N Engl J Med 335:257, 1996.
4. Hauth JC, Ewell MG, Levine RL, et al: Pregnancy outcomes in healthy nulliparas women who subsequently developed hypertension. Calcium for preeclampsia prevention study group. Obstet Gynecol 95:24 2000.
5. Barton JR, O'Brien JM, Bergauer NK, et al: Mild gestational hypertension remote from term: progression and outcome. Am J Obstet Gynecol 184:979, 2001.
6. Helewa ME, Burrows RF, Smith J, et al: Report of the Canadian Hypertension Society Consensus Conference: 1. Definitions, evaluation and classification of hypertensive disorders in pregnancy. Can Med Assoc J 157:715, 1997.
7. Brown MA, Hague WM, Higgins J, et al: The detection, investigation, and management of hypertension in pregnancy. Full consensus statement of recommendations from the Council of the Australian Society for the Study of Hypertension in pregnancy. Aust N Z J Obstet Gynaecol 40:139, 2000.
8. ACOG Committee on Practice Bulletins—Obstetrics. Diagnosis and Management of Preeclampsia and Eclampsia. Obstet Gynecol 99:159, 2002.
9. Mattar F, Sibai BM: Eclampsia VIII risk factors for maternal morbidity. Am J Obstet Gynecol 182:307, 2000.
10. Caritis S, Sibai B, Hauth J, et al: Low-dose aspirin to prevent preeclampsia in women at high risk. N Engl J Med 338:701, 1998.
11. Sibai BM, Lindheimer M, Hauth J, et al, and the National Institute of Child Health and Human Development Network of Maternal-Fetal Medicine Units: Risk factors for preeclampsia, abruptio, and adverse neonatal outcome in women with chronic hypertension. N Engl J Med 339:667, 1998.
12. Sibai BM, Caritis SN, Thom E, et al, and the National Institute of Child Health and Human Development Network of Maternal-Fetal Medicine Units: Prevention of preeclampsia with low-dose aspirin in healthy nulliparous pregnant women. N Engl J Med 329:1213, 1993.
13. Knuist M, Bonsel GJ, Zondervan HA, Treffers PE: Intensification of fetal and maternal surveillance in pregnant women with hypertensive disorders. Int J Gynecol Obstet 61:127, 1998.
14. Campbell DM, MacGillivray I: Preeclampsia in twin pregnancies: Incidence and outcome. Hypertens Pregnancy 18:197, 1999.
15. Sibai BM, Hauth J, Caritis S, et al, for the Network of Maternal-Fetal Medicine Units of the National Institute of Child Health and Human Development: Hypertensive disorders in twin versus singleton pregnancies. Am J Obstet Gynecol 182:938, 2000.
16. Buchbinder A, Sibai BM, Caritis S, et al: Adverse perinatal outcomes are significantly higher in severe gestational hypertension than in mild preeclampsia. Am J Obstet Gynecol 186:66, 2002.
17. Sibai BM, Dekker G, Kupferminc M: Pre-eclampsia. Lancet 365: 785, 2005.
18. Vatten LJ, Skjaerven R: Is pre-eclampsia more than one disease? Br J Obstet Gynaecol 111:298, 2004.
19. Wen SW, Demissie K, Yang Q, Walker MC: Maternal morbidity and obstetric complications in triplet pregnancies and quadruplet and higher-order multiple pregnancies. Am J Obstet Gynecol 191:254, 2004.
20. Hnat MD, Sibai BM, Caritis S, et al: Perinatal outcome in women with recurrent preeclampsia compared with women who develop preeclampsia as nulliparas. Am J Obstet Gynecol 186:422, 2002.
21. Lin L, August P: Genetic thrombophilias and preeclampsia: a meta-analysis. Obstet Gynecol 105:182, 2005.
22. Kupferminc MJ: Thrombophilia and pregnancy. Reprod Biol Endocrinol 1:111, 2003.
23. Mello G, Parretti E, Marozio L: Thrombophilia is significantly associated with severe preeclampsia: results of a large scale case-controlled study. Hypertension 46:1270, 2005.
24. Einarsson JI, Sangi-Haghpeykar H, Gardner NO: Sperm exposure and development of preeclampsia. Am J Obstet Gynecol 191:254, 2004.
25. Dekker G, Robillard PY: The birth interval hypothesis—Does it really indicate the end of the primipaternity hypothesis. J Reprod Immunol 59:245, 2003.
26. Saftlas AF, Levine RJ, Klebanoff MA, et al: Abortion, changed paternity, and the risk of preeclampsia in nulliparous women. Am J Epidemiol 157:1108, 2003.
27. Esplin MS, Fausett MB, Fraser A, et al: Paternal and maternal components of the predisposition to preeclampsia. N Engl J Med 344:867, 2001.
28. Lie RT, Rasmussen, S, Brunborg H, et al: Fetal and maternal contributions to risk of pre-eclampsia: a population based study. Br Med J 316:1343, 1998.

29. Wang JX, Knottnerus AM, Schuit G, et al: Surgically obtained sperm and risk of gestational hypertension and pre-eclampsia. Lancet 359:673, 2002.
30. O'Brien TE, Ray JG, Chan WS: Maternal body mass index and the risk of preeclampsia: a systematic overview. Epidemiology 14:368, 2003.
31. Cedergren MI: Maternal morbid obesity and the risk of adverse pregnancy outcome. Obstet Gynecol 103:219, 2004.
32. Livingston JC, Barton JR, Park V, et al: Maternal and fetal inherited thrombophilias are not related to the development of severe preeclampsia. Am J Obstet Gynecol 185:153, 2001.
33. Morrison ER, Miedzybrodzka ZH, Campbell DM, et al: Prothrombotic genotypes are not associated with preeclampsia and gestatinal hypertension: results from a large population-based study and systematic review. Thromb Haemost 87:779, 2002.
34. Kong TY, DeWolf F, Robertson WB, Brosens I: Inadequate maternal vascular response to placentation in pregnancies complicated by preeclampsia and by small-for-gestational age infants. Br J Obstet Gynaecol 93:1049, 1986.
35. Frusca T, Morassi L, Pecorell S, et al: Histological features of uteroplacental vessels in normal and hypertensive patients in relation to birthweight. Br J Obstet Gynaecol 96:835, 1989.
36. Meekins JW, Pijneborg R, Hanssens M, et al: A study of placental bed spiral arteries and trophoblast invasion in normal and severe preeclamptic pregnancies. Br J Obstet Gynaecol 101:669, 1994.
37. Shanklin DR, Sibai BM: Ultrastructural aspects of preeclampsia. I. Placental bed and uterine boundary vessels. Am J Obstet Gynecol 161:735, 1989.
38. Sibai BM: Discussion. Evidence supporting a role for blockade of the vascular endothelial growth factor system in the pathophysiology of preeclampsia. Am J Obstet Gynecol 190:1547, 2004.
39. Maynard SE, Min JY, Merchan J, et al: Excess placental soluble fms-like tyrosine kinase 1 (sFlt1) may contribute to endothelial dysfunction, hypertension, and proteinuria in preeclampsia. Clin Invest 111:649, 2003.
40. Chaiworapongsa T, Romero R, Espionza J, et al: Evidence supporting a role for blockade of the vascular endothelial growth factor system in the pathophysiology of preeclampsia. Am J Obstet Gynecol 190:1541, 2004.
41. Levine RJ, Maynard SE, Qian C, et al: Circulating angiogenic factors and the risk of preeclampsia. N Engl J Med 350:672, 2004.
42. Thadhani R, Ecker JL, Mutter WP, et al: Insulin resistance and alterations in angiogenesis: additive insults that may lead to preeclampsia. Hypertension 43:988, 2004.
43. Levine RJ, Thadhani R, Qian C, et al: Urinary placental growth factor and risk of preeclampsia. JAMA 293:77, 2005.
44. Sibai BM: Preeclampsia: An inflammatory syndrome? Am J Obstet Gynecol 191:1061, 2004.
45. Sargent IL, Germain SJ, Sacks GP, et al: Trophoblast deportation and the maternal inflammatory response in pre-eclampsia. J Reprod Immunol 59:153, 2003.
46. von Ddelszen P, Magee LA: Could an infectious tripper explain the differential maternal response to the shared placental pathology of preeclampsia and normotensive intrauterine growth restriction? Acta Obstet Gynecol Scand 81:642, 2002.
47. Faas MM, Brockema M, Moes H, et al: Altered monocyte function in experimental preeclampsia in the rat. Am J Obstet Gynecol 191:1192, 2004.
48. Savvidou MD, Hingorani AD, Tsikas D, et al: Endothelial dysfunction and raised plasma concentrations of asymmetric dimethylarginine in pregnant women who subsequently develop pre-eclampsia. Lancet 361:1151, 2003.
49. Wang Y, Gu Y, Zhang Y, Lewis DF: Evidence of endothelial dysfunction in preeclampsia: decreased endothelial nitric oxide synthase expression is associated with increased cell permeability in endothelial cells from preeclampsia. Am J Obstet Gynecol 190:817, 2004.
50. Nilsson E, Salonen RH, Cnattingius S, Lichtenstein P: The importance of genetic and environmental effects for pre-eclampsia and gestational hypertension: a family study. Br J Obstet Gynaecol 111:200, 2004.
51. Laivuori H, Lahermo P, Ollikainen V, et al: Susceptibility loci for preeclampsia on chromosomes 2p25 and 9p13 in Finnish families. Am J Hum Genet 72:168, 2001.
52. Oudejans CB, Mulders J, Lachmeijer AM, et al: The parent-of-origin effect of 10q22 in pre-eclamptic females coincides with two regions clustered for genes with down-regulated expression in adrogenetic placentas. Mol Hum Reprod 10:589, 2004.
53. Cross JC: The genetics of pre-eclampsia: A feto-placental or maternal problem? Clin Genet 64:96, 2003.
54. Walsh SW, Parisi VM: The role of arachidonic acid metabolites in preeclampsia. Semin Perinatol 10:335, 1986.
55. Paarlberg KM, deJong CLD, Van Geijn HP, et al: Vasoactive mediators in pregnancy-induced hypertensive disorders: a longitudinal study. Am J Obstet Gynecol 179:1559, 1998.
56. Smith AJ, Waiters WA, Buckley NA, et al: Hypertensive and normal pregnancy: a longitudinal study of blood pressure, distensibility of dorsal hand veins and the ratio of the stable metabolites of thromboxane A_2 and prostacyclin in plasma. Br J Obstet Gynaecol 102:900, 1995.
57. Mills JL, DerSimonian R, Raymond E, et al: Prostacyclin and thromboxane changes predating clinical onset of preeclampsia: a multicenter prospective study. JAMA 282:356, 1999.
58. Roberts JM, Lain KY: Recent insights into the pathogenesis of pre-eclampsia. Placenta 233:59–72, 2002.
59. Aly AS, Khandelwal M, Zhao J, et al: Neutrophils are stimulated by syncytiotrophoblast microvillous membranes to generate superoxide radicals in women with preeclampsia. Am J Obstet Gynecol 190:252, 2004.
60. Moretti M, Phillips M, Abouzeid A, et al: Increased breath markers of oxidative stress in normal pregnancy and in preeclampsia. Am J Obstet Gynecol 190:1184, 2004.
61. Chappell LC, Seed PT, Briley AL, et al: Effect of antioxidants on the occurrence of pre-eclampsia in women at increased risk: a randomized trial. Lancet 354:810, 1999.
62. Steer PJ: The definition of pre-eclampsia. Br J Obstet Gynaecol 106:753, 1999.
63. Lopez MC, Belizan JM, Villar J, Bergel E: The measurement of diastolic blood pressure during pregnancy: which Korotkoff phase should be used? Am J Obstet Gynecol 170:574, 1992.
64. Redman CWG, Jeffries M: Revised definition of preeclampsia. Lancet 1:809, 1988.
65. Perry IJ, Beevers DG: The definition of pre-eclampsia. Br J Obstet Gynaecol 101:587, 1994.
66. Villar MA, Sibai BM: Clinical significance of elevated mean arterial blood in second trimester and threshold increase in systolic or diastolic pressure during third trimester. Am J Obstet Gynecol 60:419, 1989.
67. North RA, Taylor RS, Schellenberg J-C: Evaluation of a definition of pre-eclampsia. Br J Obstet Gynaecol 106:767, 1999.
68. Levine RJ, Ewell MG, Hauth JC, et al: Should the definition of preeclampsia include a rise in diastolic blood pressure of ≥ 15 mmHg to a level < 90 mmHg in association with proteinuria? Am J Obstet Gynecol 183:787, 2000.
69. Ohkuchi A, Iwasaki R, Ojima T, et al: Increase in systolic blood pressure of $>$ or $=30$ mmHg and/or diastolic blood pressure of $>$ or $=15$ mmHg during pregnancy: Is it pathologic? Hypertension in pregnancy 22:275, 2003.
70. Halligan AWF, Bell SC, Taylor DJ: Dipstick proteinuria: caveat emptor. Br J Obstet Gynaecol 106:1113, 1999.
71. Bell SC, Halligan AWF, Martin J, et al: The role of observer error in antenatal dipstick proteinuria analysis. Br J Obstet Gynaecol 106:1177, 1999.
72. Kieler H, Zettergen T, Svensson H, et al: Assessing urinary albumin excretion in pre-eclamptic women: which sample to use? BJOG 110:12, 2003.
73. Wikstrom A-K, Wikstrom J, Larsson A, Olovsson M: Random albumin/creatinine ratio for quantitation of proteinuria in manifest pre-eclampsia. BJOG 113:930, 2006.
74. Durnwald C, Mercer B: A prospective comparison of total protein/creatinine ration versus 24-hour urine protein in women with suspected preeclampsia. Am J Obstet Gynecol 189:848, 2003.
75. Ragip AAL, Baykal C, Karacay O, et al: Random urine protein-creatinine ratio to predict proteinuria in new-onset mild hypertension in late pregnancy. Obstet Gynecol 104:367, 2004.
76. Waugh JJS, Clark TJ, Khan KS, Kilby MD: Accuracy of urinanalysis dipstick techniques in predicting significant proteinuria in pregnancy. Obstet Gynecol 103:769, 2004.

77. Meyer NL, Mercer BM, Friedman SA, Sibai BM: Urinary dipstick protein: a poor predictor of absent or severe proteinuria. Am J Obstet Gynecol 170:137, 1994.
78. Sibai BM: Diagnosis, controversies, and management of HELLP syndrome. Obstet Gynecol 103:981, 2004.
79. Sibai BM: Diagnosis, differential diagnosis, and management of eclampsia. Obstet Gynecol 105:402, 2005.
80. Friedman SA, Lindheimer MD: Prediction and differential diagnosis. *In* Lindheimer MD, Roberts JM, Cunningham GF (eds): Chesley's Hypertensive Disorders in Pregnancy. Stamford, CT, Appleton & Lange, 1999, p 201.
81. Tjoa ML, Qudejans CBM, Van Vugt JMG, et al: Markers for presymptomatic prediction of preeclampsia and intrauterine growth restriction. Hyperten Pregnancy 23:171, 2004.
82. Conde-Agudelo A, Villar J, Lindheimer M: World Health Organization Systematic Review of Screening Tests for Preeclampsia. Obstet Gynecol 104:1367, 2004.
83. Widmer M, Villar J, Benigni A, et al: Mapping the theories of preeclampsia and the role of angiogenic factors. Obstet Gynecol 109:168, 2007.
84. Chien PE, Arnott N, Gordon A, et al: How useful is uterine artery Doppler flow velocimetry in the prediction of pre-eclampsia, intrauterine growth retardation and perinatal death? An overview. Br J Obstet Gynaecol 107:196, 2000.
85. Yu CKH, Papageorghiou AT, Parra M, et al: Randomized controlled trial using low-dose aspirin in the prevention of pre-eclampsia in women with abnormal uterine artery Doppler at 23 weeks' gestation. Ultrasound Obstet Gynecol 22:233, 2003.
86. Yu CKH, Papageorghiou AT, Boli A, et al: Screening for pre-eclampsia and fetal growth restriction in twin pregnancies at 23 weeks of gestation by transvaginal uerine artery Doppler ultrasound. Obstet Gynecol 20:535, 2002.
87. Subtil D, Goeusse P, Houfflin-Debarge V, et al and theEssai Regional Aspirine Mere-Enfant (ERASME) Collaborative Group: Randomised comparison of uterine artery Doppler and aspirin (100 mg) with placebo in nulliparous women: The Essai Regional Aspirine Mere-Enfant study (Part 2). Br J Obstet Gynecol 110:485, 2003.
88. Sibai BM: Prevention of preeclampsia: A big disappointment. Am J Obstet Gynecol 179:1275, 1998.
89. Makrides M, Duley L, Olsen SF: Fish oil and other prostaglandin precursor supplementation during pregnancy to improve outcomes in pre-eclampsia, preterm birth, low birth weight and small for gestational age. *In* The Cochrane Library, Issue 1. Oxford, UK, Update Software, 2003.
90. Abalos E, Duley L, Steyn DW, Henderson-Smart DJ: Antihypertensive drug therapy for mild to moderate hypertension during pregnancy. *In* The Cochrane Library, Issue 12. Oxford: Update Software, 2003.
91. Coomarasamy A, Honest H, Papaioannou S, et al: Aspirin for prevention of preeclampsia in women with historical risk factors: A systemic review. Obstet Gynecol 10–1:1319, 2003.
92. Atallah AN, Hofmeyr GJ, Duley L: Calcium supplementation during pregnancy for preventing hypertensive disorders and related problems (Cochrane Review). *In* The Cochrane Library, Issue 1. Oxford, UK, Update Software, 2003.
93. Knight M, Duley L, Henderson-Smart DJ, King JF: Antiplatelet agents for preventing and treating pre-eclampsia. *In* The Cochrane Library, Issue 1. Oxford, UK, Update Software, 2003.
94. North RA, Ferrier C, Gamble G, et al: Prevention of preeclampsia with heparin and antiplatelet drugs in women with renal disease. Aust N Z J Obstet Gynaecol 35:357, 1995.
95. Kupferminc MJ, Fait G, Many A, et al: Low molecular weight heparin for the prevention of obstetric complications in women with thrombophilia. Hypertens Pregnancy 20:35, 2001.
96. Hatton DC, McCarron DA: Dietary calcium and blood pressure in experimental models of hypertension: a review. Hypertension 23:513, 1994.
97. Belizan JM, Villar J, Repke J: The relationship between calcium intake and pregnancy induced hypertension: up to date evidence. Am J Obstet Gynecol 158:898, 1988.
98. Sanchez-Ramos L, Briones DK, Kaunitz AM, et al: Prevention of pregnancy-induced hypertension by calcium supplementation in angiotensin-II sensitive patients. Obstet Gynecol 84:349, 1994.
99. Lopez-Jaramillo P, Narvaez M, Weigel RM, et al: Calcium supplementation reduces the risk of pregnancy-induced hypertension in an Andes population. Br J Obstet Gynaecol 96:648, 1987.
100. Villar J, Repke JT: Calcium supplementation during pregnancy may reduce preterm delivery in high-risk populations. Am J Obstet Gynecol 163:1124, 1990.
101. Belizan JM, Villar J, Gonzalez L, et al: Calcium supplementation to prevent hypertensive disorders of pregnancy. N Engl J Med 325:1399, 1991.
102. Lopez-Jaramillo P, Narvaez M, Felix C, Lopez A: Dietary calcium supplementation and prevention of pregnancy hypertension. Lancet 335:293, 1990.
103. Lopez-Jaramillo P, Delgado F, Jacoine P, et al: Calcium supplementation and the risk of preeclampsia in Ecuadorian pregnant teenagers. Obstet Gynecol 90:162, 1997.
104. Levine RJ, Hauth JC, Curet LB, et al: Trial of calcium to prevent preeclampsia. N Engl J Med 337:69, 1997.
105. Herrera JA, Arevalo-Herrara M, Herrara S: Prevention of preeclampsia by linoleic acid and calcium supplementation: a randomized controlled trial. Obstet Gynecol 91:585, 1998.
106. Crowther CA, Hiller JE, Pridmore B, et al: Calcium supplementation in nulliparous women for the prevention of pregnancy-induced hypertension, preeclampsia and preterm birth: an Australian randomized trial. Aust N Z J Obstet Gynaecol 39:12, 1999.
107. Rogers MS, Fung HYM, Hung CY: Calcium and low-dose aspirin prophylaxis in women at high risk of pregnancy-induced hypertension. Hypertens Pregnancy 18:165, 1999.
108. Coomarasamy A, Papaioannou S, Gee H, Khan KS: Aspirin for the prevention of preeclampsia in women with abnormal Uterine Artery Doppler: A meta-analysis. Obstet Gynecol 98:861, 2001.
109. Coomarasamy A, Braunholtz D, Song F, et al: Individualising use of aspirin to prevent preeclampsia: A frame work for clinical decision making. Br J Obstet Gynaecol 110:882, 2003.
110. Beazley D, Ahokas R, Livingston J, et al: Vitamin C and E supplementation in women at high risk for preeclampsia: A double-blind, placebo-controlled trial. Am J Obstet Gynecol 192:520, 2005.
111. Cunningham FG, Lindheimer MD: Hypertension in pregnancy. N Engl J Med 326:927, 1992.
112. Sibai BM, Barton JR, Akl S, et al: A randomized prospective comparison of nifedipine and bed rest versus bed rest alone in the management of preeclampsia remote from term. Am J Obstet Gynecol 167:879, 1992.
113. Sibai BM, Mercer BM, Schiff E, Friedman SA: Aggressive versus expectant management of severe preeclampsia at 28 to 32 weeks' gestation: a randomized controlled trial. Am J Obstet Gynecol 171:818, 1994.
114. Bowen RS, Moodley J, Dutton MF, Theron AJ: Oxidative stress in preeclampsia. Acta Obstet Gynecol Scand 80:719, 2001.
115. Lim KH, Friedman SA, Ecker JK, et al: The clinical utility of serum uric acid measurements in hypertensive diseases of pregnancy. Am J Obstet Gynecol 178:1067, 1998.
116. Hsu CD, Chung YK, Lee IS, et al: Maternal serum uric acid levels in preeclamptic women with multiple gestations. Am J Perinatal 14:613, 1997.
117. Odendaal HJ: Severe preeclampsia and eclampsia. *In* Sibai BM (ed): Hypertensive Disorders in Women. Philadelphia, Saunders, 2001, p 14.
118. Weinstein L: Syndrome of hemolysis, elevated liver enzymes, and low platelet count; a severe consequence of hypertension in pregnancy. Am J Obstet Gynecol 142:159, 1982.
119. Arias F, Mancill-Jimenez R: Hepatic fibrinogen deposits in pre-eclampsia-immunofluorescent evidence. N Engl J Med 11:294, 1976.
120. Weiner C: Preeclampsia-eclampsia syndrome and coagulation. Clin Perinatol 18:713, 1992.
121. Perry KG Jr, Martin JN Jr: Abnormal hemostasis and coagulopathy in preeclampsia and eclampsia. Clin Obstet Gynecol 35:338, 1992.
122. Sibai BM, Watson DL, Hill GA, et al: Maternal-fetal correlations in patients with severe preeclampsia-eclampsia. Obstet Gynecol 62:745, 1983.
123. Leduc L, Wheeler JM, Kirshon B, et al: Coagulation profile in severe preeclampsia. Obstet Gynecol 79:14, 1992.

124. Burrows F, Kelton JG: Fetal thrombocytopenia in relation to maternal thrombocytopenia. N Engl J Med 329:1463, 1993.
125. Barron WM, Heckerling P, Hibbard JU, Fisher S: Reducing unnecessary coagulation testing in hypertensive disorders of pregnancy. Obstet Gynecol 94:364, 1999.
126. MacKenna J, Dover NL, Brame RG: Preeclampsia associated with hemolysis, elevated liver enzymes and low platelets-an obstetric emergency? Obstet Gynecol 62:751, 1983.
127. Barton JR, Riely CA, Adamec TA, et al: Hepatic histopathologic condition does not correlate with laboratory abnormalities in HELLP syndrome. Am J Obstet Gynecol 167:1538, 1992.
128. Clark SL, Phelan JR, Allen SH, Golde SR: Antepartum reversal of hematologic abnormalities associated with the HELLP syndrome. J Reprod Med 32:781, 1987.
129. Heyborne KD, Burke MS, Porreco RP: Prolongation of premature gestation in women with hemolysis, elevated liver enzyme, and low platelets. A report of 5 cases. J Reprod Med 35:53, 1990.
130. Heller CS, Elliott JP: High-order multiple pregnancies complicated by HELLP syndrome. A report of four cases with corticosteroid therapy to prolong gestation. J Reprod Med 42:743, 1997.
131. Tompkins MJ, Thiagarajah S: HELLP syndrome: the benefit of corticosteroids. Am J Obstet Gynecol 181:304, 1999.
132. O'Brien JM, Milligan DA, Barton JR: Impact of high-dose corticosteroid therapy for patients with HELLP syndrome. Am J Obstet Gynecol 183:921, 2000.
133. O'Brien JM, Shumate SA, Satchwell SL, et al: Maternal benefit to corticosteroid therapy in patients with HELLP (hemolysis, elevated liver enzymes, and low platelets) syndrome: impact on the rate of regional anesthesia. Am J Obstet Gynecol 186:475, 2002.
134. Crane JMG, Tabarsi B, Hutchens D: The maternal benefits of corticosteroids with HELLP syndrome. J Obstet Gynaecol Can 25:650, 2003.
135. Magann EF, Bass D, Chauhan SP, et al: Antepartum corticosteroids: disease stabilization in patients with the syndrome of hemolysis, elevated liver enzymes, and low platelets (HELLP). Am J Obstet Gynecol 171:1148, 1994.
136. Magann EF, Perry KO Jr, Meydrech EF, et al: Postpartum corticosteroids: accelerated recovery from the syndrome of hemolysis, elevated liver enzymes, and low platelets (HELLP). Am J Obstet Gynecol 171:1154, 1994.
137. Martin JN Jr, Rinehart B, May WL, et al: The spectrum of severe preeclampsia: Comparative analysis by HELLP syndrome classification. Am J Obstet Gynecol 180:1373, 1999.
138. Martin JN Jr, Perry KG, Blake PG, et al: Better maternal outcomes are achieved with dexamethasone therapy for postpartum HELLP syndrome. Am J Obstet Gynecol 177:1011, 1997.
139. Martin JN Jr, Thigsen BD, Rose CH, et al. Maternal benefit of high-dose intravenous corticosteroid therapy for HELLP. Am J Obstet Gynecol 189:830, 2003.
140. Rose CH, Thigpen BD, Bofill JA, et al: Obstetric implications of antepartum corticoid therapy for HELLP syndrome. Obstet Gynecol 104:1011, 2004
141. Martin JN Jr, Blake PG, Lowry SL, et al: Pregnancy complicated by preeclampsia-eclampsia with the syndrome of hemolysis, elevated liver enzymes, and low platelet count: how rapid is postpartum recovery? Obstet Gynecol 76:737, 1990.
142. Van Dam PA, Reiner M, Baeklandt M, et al: Disseminated intravascular coagulation and the syndrome of hemolysis, elevated liver enzymes, and low platelets in severe preeclampsia. Obstet Gynecol 73:97, 1989.
143. de Boer K, Buller HR, ten Cate JW, Treffers PE: Coagulation studies in the syndrome of haemolysis, elevated liver enzymes, and low platelets. Br J Obstet Gynaecol 98:42, 1991.
144. Sibai BM, Ramadan MK, Usta I, et al: Maternal morbidity and mortality in 442 pregnancies with hemolysis, elevated liver enzymes, and low platelets (HELLP syndrome). Am J Obstet Gynecol 169:1000, 1993.
145. Aarnoudse JG, Houthoff HF, Weits J, et al: A syndrome of liver damage and intravascular coagulation in the last trimester of normotensive pregnancy. A clinical and histopathological study. Br J Obstet Gynaecol 93:145, 1986.
146. Weinstein L: Preeclampsia/eclampsia with hemolysis, elevated liver enzymes and thrombocytopenia. Obstet Gynecol 66:657, 1985.
147. Audibert F, Friedman SA, Frangieh AY, Sibai BM: Clinical utility of strict diagnostic criteria for the HELLP (hemolysis, elevated liver enzymes, and low platelets) syndrome. Am J Obstet Gynecol 175:460, 1996.
148. Rath W, Loos W, Kuhn W, Graeff H: The importance of early laboratory screening methods for maternal and fetal outcome in cases of HELLP syndrome. Eur J Obstet Gynecol Reprod Biol 36:43, 1990.
149. Haddad B, Barton JR, Livingston JC, et al: Risk factors for adverse maternal outcomes among women with HELLP (hemolysis, elevated liver enzymes, and low platelet count) syndrome. Am J Obstet Gynecol 183:444, 2000.
150. Visser W, Wallenburg HCS: Temporising management of severe pre-eclampsia with and without the HELLP syndrome. Br J Obstet Gynaecol 102:111, 1995.
151. Van Pampus MG, Wolf H, Westenberg SM, et al: Maternal and perinatal outcome after expectant management of the HELLP syndrome compared with preeclampsia without HELLP syndrome. Eur J Obstet Gynecol Reprod Biol 76:31,1998.
152. Van Pampus MG, Wolf H, Ilsen A, Treffers PE: Maternal outcome following temporizing management of the (H)ELLP syndrome. Hypertens Pregnancy 19:211, 2000.
153. Abramovici D, Friedman SA, Mercer BM, et al: Neonatal outcome in severe preeclampsia at 24 to 36 weeks' gestation. Does HELLP (hemolysis, elevated liver enzymes, and low platelet count) syndrome matter? Am J Obstet Gynecol 180:221, 1999.
154. Amorium MMR, Santas LC, Faundes A: Corticosteroid therapy for prevention of respiratory distress syndrome in severe preeclampsia. Am J Obstet Gynecol 180:1283, 1999.
155. Anonymous: Effect of corticosteroids for fetal maturation on perinatal outcomes. NIH Consensus Development Panel on the Effect of Corticosteroids for Fetal Maturation on Perinatal Outcomes. JAMA 273:413, 1995.
156. Vigil-DeGracia P, Garcia-Caceres E: Dexamethasone in the postpartum treatment of HELLP syndrome. Int J Gynaecol Obstet 59:217, 1997.
157. Yalcin OT, Sener T, Hassa H, et al: Effects of postpartum corticosteroids in patients with HELLP syndrome. Int J Gynaecol Obstet 61:141, 1998.
158. Isler CM, Barrilleaux PS, Magann EF, et al: A prospective, randomized trial comparing the efficacy of dexamethasone and betamethasone for the treatment of antepartum HELLP syndrome. Am J Obstet Gynecol 184:1332, 2001.
159. Sibai BM, Ramadan MK: Acute renal failure in pregnancies complicated by hemolysis, elevated liver enzymes, and low platelets. Am J Obstet Gynecol 168:1682, 1993.
160. Drakeley AJ, LeRoux PA, Anthony J, Penny J: Acute renal failure complicating severe preeclampsia requiring admission to an obstetric intensive care unit. Am J Obstet Gynecol 186:253, 2002.
161. Woods JB, Blake PG, Perry KG Jr, et al: Ascites: a portent of cardiopulmonary complications in the preeclamptic patient with the syndrome of hemolysis, elevated liver enzymes, and low platelets. Obstet Gynecol 80:87, 1992.
162. Martin JN Jr, Files JC, Blake PG, et al: Postpartum plasma exchange for atypical preeclampsia-eclampsia as HELLP syndrome. Am J Obstet Gynecol 172:1107, 1995.
163. Onrust S, Santema JG, Aarnoudse JG: Pre-eclampsia and the HELLP syndrome still cause maternal mortality in the Netherlands and other developed countries. Can we reduce it? Eur J Obstet Gynecol Reprod Biol 82:41, 1999.
164. Goodlin RC, Anderson JC, Hodgson PE: Conservative treatment of liver hematoma in the postpartum period. J Reprod Med 30:368, 1985.
165. Manas KJ, Welsh JD, Rankin RA: Hepatic haemorrhage without rupture in preeclampsia. N Engl J Med 312:424, 1985.
166. Barton JR, Sibai BM: Diagnosis and management of HELLP syndrome. Clin Perinatol 31:807, 2004.
167. Smith JG Jr, Moise KJ Jr, Dildy GA, et al: Spontaneous rupture of the liver during pregnancy: current therapy. Obstet Gynecol 77:171, 1991.
168. Reinehart BK, Terrone DA, Magann EF, et al: Preeclampsia-associated hepatic hemorrhage and rupture: mode of management related to maternal and perinatal outcome. Obstet Gynecol Surv 54:196, 1999.

169. Sibai BM, Mabie WC: Hemodynamics of preeclampsia. Clin Perinatol 18:727, 1991.
170. Groenendijk R, Trimbos JBMJ, Wallenburg HCS: Hemodynamic measurements in preeclampsia. Preliminary observations. Am J Obstet Gynecol 150:812, 1985.
171. Cotton DB, Jones MM, Longmire S, et al: Role of intravenous nitroglycerin in the treatment of severe pregnancy-induced hypertension complicated by pulmonary edema. Am J Obstet Gynecol 143:91, 1986.
172. Wallenburg HS: Hemodynamics in hypertensive pregnancy. *In* Rubin PC (ed): Handbook of Hypertension-Hypertension in Pregnancy, Vol. 10. Elsevier, Amsterdam, 1988, p 66.
173. Belfort MA, Anthony J, Buccimmazza L, et al: Hemodynamic changes associated with intravenous infusion of the calcium antagonist verapamil in the treatment of severe gestational proteinuric hypertension. Obstet Gynecol 75:970, 1990.
174. Belfort MA, Uys P, Dommisse J, et al: Hemodynamic changes in gestational proteinuric hypertension: the effects of rapid volume expansion and vasodilator therapy. Br J Obstet Gynaecol 96:634, 1989.
175. Cotton DB, Lee W, Huhta JC, Dorman K: Hemodynamic profile of severe pregnancy-induced hypertension. Am J Obstet Gynecol 158:523, 1988.
176. Mabie WE, Ratts TE, Sibai BM: The hemodynamic profile of severe preeclamptic patients requiring delivery. Am J Obstet Gynecol 161:1443, 1989.
177. Magee LA, Ornstein MP, Von Dadelszen P: Fortnightly review: management of hypertension in pregnancy. BMJ 318:1332, 1999.
178. Barton JR, Witlin AG, Sibai BM: Management of mild preeclampsia. Clin Obstet Gynecol 42:465, 1999.
179. Goldenberg RL, Cliver SP, Bronstein J, et al: Bedrest in pregnancy. Obstet Gynecol 84:131, 1994.
180. Yoon BH, Lee CM, Kim SW: An abnormal umbilical artery waveform: a strong and independent predictor of adverse perinatal outcome in patients with preeclampsia. Am J Obstet Gynecol 171:713, 1994.
181. Pattinson RC, Norman K, Odendaal HJ: The role of Doppler velocimetry in the management of high risk pregnancies. Br J Obstet Gynaecol 101:114, 1994.
182. Friedman SA, Lubarsky S, Schiff E: Expectant management of severe preeclampsia remote from term. Clin Obstet Gynecol 42:470, 1999.
183. Churchill D, Duley L: Interventionist versus expectant care for severe pre-eclampsia before term (Cochrane Review). *In* The Cochrane Library, Issue 3, 2004. Chichester, UK: John Wiley & Sons, Ltd.
184. Vigil-DeGracia P, Montufar-Rueda C, Ruiz J: Expectant management of severe preeclampsia and preeclampsia superimposed on chronic hypertension between 24 and 34 weeks' gestation. Eur J Obstet Gynecol Reprod Biol 107:24, 2003.
185. Haddad B, Deis S, Goffinet F, et al: Maternal and perinatal outcomes during expectant management of 239 severe preeclamptic women between 24 and 33 weeks' gestation. Am J Obstet Gynecol 190:1590, 2004.
186. Lucas MJ, Sharma SK, McIntire DD, et al: A randomized trial of labor analgesia in women wih pregnancy-induced hypertension. Am J Obstet Gynecol 185:970, 2001.
187. Head BB, Owen J, Vincent RD Jr, et al: A randomized trial of intrapartum analgesia in women with severe preeclampsia. Obstet Gynaecol 99:452, 2002.
188. Duley L, Galmezoglu AM, Henderson-Smart DJ: Magnesium sulfate and other anticonvulsants for women with preeclampsia. *In* The Cochrane Library, Issue 2. Oxford, UK, Update Software, 2003.
189. Coetzee EJ, Dommisse J, Anthony J: A randomized controlled trial of intravenous magnesium sulfate versus placebo in the management of women with severe preeclampsia. Br J Obstet Gynaecol 105:300, 1998.
190. The Magpie Trial Group: Do women with pre-eclampsia, and their babies, benefit from magnesium sulfate? The Magpie Trial: a randomised, placebo-controlled trial. Lancet 359:1877, 2002.
191. Moodley J, Moodley VV: Prophylactic anticonvulsant therapy in hypertensive crises of pregnancy—the need for a large, randomized trial. Hypertens Pregnancy 13:245, 1994.
192. Belfort MA, Anthony J, Saade GR, Allen JC, for the Nimodipine Study Group: A comparison of magnesium sulfate and nimodipine for the prevention of eclampsia. N Engl J Med 348:304,2003.
193. Sibai BM: Magnesium sulfate prophylaxis in preeclampsia. Lessons learned from recent trials. Am J Obstet Gynecol 190:1520, 2004.
194. Witlin AG, Friedman SA, Sibai BM: The effect of magnesium sulfate therapy on the duration of labor in women with mild preeclampsia at term: a randomized, double-blind, placebo-controlled trial. Am J Obstet Gynecol 176:623. 1997.
195. Livingston JC, Livingston LW, Ramsey R, et al: Magnesium sulfate in women with mild preeclampsia: A randomized, double blinded, placebo-controlled trial. Obstet Gynecol 101:217, 2003.
196. Magee LA, Cham C, Waterman EJ, et al: Hydralazine for treatment of severe hypertension in pregnancy: Meta-analysis. BMJ 327:1, 2003.
197. Ferrazani S, DeCarolis S, Pomini F, et al: The duration of hypertension in the puerperium of preeclamptic women: relationship with renal impairment and week of delivery. Am J Obstet Gynecol 17:506, 1994.
198. Walters BNJ, Walters T: Hypertension in the puerperium. Lancet 2:330, 1987.
199. Barton JR, Hiett AK, Conover WB: The use of nifedipine during the postpartum period in patients with severe preeclampsia. Am J Obstet Gynecol 162:788, 1990.
200. Ascarelli MH, Johnson V, McCreasy H, et al: Postpartum preeclampsia management with furosemide: A randomized clinical trial. Obstet Gynecol 105:29, 2005.
201. Chames MC, Livingston JC, Ivester TS, et al: Late postpartum eclampsia: A preventable disease? Am J Obstet Gynecol 186:1174, 2002.
202. Mathys LA, Coppage KH, Lambers DS, et al: Delayed postpartum preeclampsia: An experience of 151 cases. Am J Obstet Gynecol 190:1464, 2004.
203. Sibai BM, Coppage KH: Diagnosis and management of stroke during pregnancy/postpartum. Clin Perinatol 31:853, 2004.
204. Zhang J, Meikle S, Trumble A: Severe maternal morbidity associated with hypertensive disorders in pregnancy in the United States. Hypertens Pregnancy 22:203, 2003.
205. Sibai BM, El-Nazer A, Gonzalez-Ruiz AR: Severe preeclampsia-eclampsia in young primigravid women: subsequent pregnancy outcome and remote prognosis. Am J Obstet Gynecol 155:1011, 1986.
206. Sibai BM, Mercer B, Sarinoglu C: Severe preeclampsia in the second trimester: recurrence risk and long-term prognosis. Am J Obstet Gynecol 165:1408, 1991.
207. Sibai BM: Management and counseling of patients with preeclampsia remote from term. Clin Obstet Gynecol 2:426, 1992.
208. Sibai BM, Villar MA, Mabie BC: Acute renal failure in hypertensive disorders of pregnancy: pregnancy outcome and remote prognosis in thirty-one consecutive cases. Am J Obstet Gynecol 62:777, 1990.
209. Sibai BM, Ramadan MK, Chari RS, Friedman SA: Pregnancies complicated by hemolysis, elevated liver enzymes, and low platelets (HELLP): subsequent pregnancy outcome and long-term prognosis. Am J Obstet Gynecol 172:125, 1995.
210. Sullivan CA, Magann EF, Perry KG, et al: The recurrence risk of the syndrome of hemolysis, elevated liver enzymes, and low platelets (HELLP) in subsequent gestations. Am J Obstet Gynecol 171:940, 1994.
211. Van Pampus MG, Wolf H, Mayruhu G, et al: Long-term followup in patients with a history of (H)ELLP syndrome. Hypertens. Pregnancy 20:15, 2001.
212. Chames MC, Haddad B, Barton JR, et al: Subsequent pregnancy outcome in women with a history of HELLP syndrome at < or =28 weeks of gestation. Am J Obstet Gynecol 188:1504, 2003.
213. Greenstein D, Henderson JM, Boyer TB: Liver hemorrhage: recurrent episodes during pregnancy complicated by preeclampsia. Gastroenterology 106:1668, 1994.
214. Wust MD, Bolte AC, deVries JI, et al: Pregnancy outcome after previous pregnancy complicated by hepatic rupture. Hypertens Pregnancy 23:29, 2004.
215. Knapen M, VanAltena A, Peters WHM, et al. Liver function following pregnancy complicated by the HELLP syndrome. Br J Obstet Gynaecol 105:1208, 1998.

216. Jacquemyn Y, Jochems L, Duiker E, et al: Long-term renal function after HELLP syndrome. Gynecol Obstet Invest 57:117, 2004.
217. Ihle BU, Long P, Oats J: Early onset preeclampsia: Recognition of underlying renal disease. BMJ 294, 1987.
218. Murakami S, Saitoh M, Kubo T, et al: Renal disease in women with severe preeclampsia or gestational proteinuria. Obstet Gynecol 96:945, 2000.
219. Ramsay JE, Stewart F, Green IA, Sattar N: Microvascular dysfunction: A link between pre-eclampsia and maternal coronary heart disease. Br J Obstet Gynaecol 110:1029, 2003.
220. Wilson BJ, Watson MS, Prescott GJ, et al: Hypertensive diseases of pregnancy and risk of hypertension and stroke in later life: results from cohort study. BMJ 326:1, 2003.
221. Haukkamaa L, Salminen M, Laivuori H, et al: Risk for subsequent coronary artery disease after preeclampsia. Am J Cardiol 93:805, 2004.
222. Sattar N, Greer IA: Pregnancy complications and maternal cardiovascular risk: opportunities for intervention and screening? Review. BMJ 20;325:157, 2002.
223. Chesley LC: History. *In* Chesley LC (ed): Hypertensive Disorders in Pregnancy, 2nd ed. New York, Appleton-Century-Crofts, 1978, p 17.
224. Saftlas AF, Olson DR, Franks AC, et al: Epidemiology of preeclampsia and eclampsia in the United States. 1979–1986. Am J Obstet Gynecol 163:460, 1990.
225. Douglas KA, Redman CW: Eclampsia in the United Kingdom. BMJ 309:1395, 1994.
226. Lee W, O'Connell CM, Baskett TF: Maternal and perinatal outcomes of eclampsia: Nova Scotia 1981–2000. J Obstet Gynaecol Can 26:119, 2004.
227. Rugard O, Carling MS, Berg G: Eclampsia at a tertiary hospital 1973–99. Acta Obstet Gynecol Scand 83:240, 2004.
228. Makhseed M, Musimi VM: Eclampsia in Kuwait 1981–1993. Aust NZJ Obstet Gynaecol 36:258, 1996.
229. Moodley J: Maternal deaths associated with hypertensive disorders of pregnancy: a population-based study. Hypertens Pregnancy 23:247, 2004.
230. Koum K, Hy S, Tir S, et al: Characteristics of antepartum and intrapartum eclampsia in the National Maternal and Child health Center in Cambodia. J Obstet Gynaecol Res 130:74, 2004.
231. Sibai BM. Eclampsia VI: Maternal-perinatal outcome in 254 consecutive cases. Am J Obstet Gynecol 163:1049, 1990.
232. Katz VL, Farmer R, Kuller J: Preeclampsia into eclampsia: toward a new paradigm. Am J Obstet Gynecol 182:1389, 2000.
233. Lubarsky SL, Barton JR, Friedman SA, et al: Late postpartum eclampsia revisited. Obstet Gynaecol 83:502, 1994.
234. Sibai BM, Abdella TH, Taylor HA: Eclampsia in the first half of pregnancy. A report of three cases and review of the literature. J Reprod Med 27:706, 1982.
235. Newman RB, Eddly GL: Association of eclampsia and hydatidiform mole: case report and review of the literature. Obstet Gynecol Surv 43:185, 1988.
236. Barton JR, Sibai BM: Cerebral pathology in eclampsia. *In* Sibai BM (ed): Clinics Perinatology, Vol. 18. Philadelphia, WB Saunders Company, 1991, p 891.
237. Sheehan JL, Lynch JB: Pathology of toxemia of pregnancy. New York, Churchill Livingstone, 1973.
238. Richards AM, Moodley J, Graham DI, Bullock MRR: Active management of the unconscious eclamptic patient. Br J Obstet Gynaecol 93:554, 1986.
239. Lopez-Llera M: Main clinical types and subtypes of eclampsia. Am J Obstet Gynecol 166:4, 1992.
240. Dahmus MA, Barton JR, Sibai BM: Cerebral imaging in eclampsia: magnetic resonance imaging versus computed tomography. Am J Obstet Gynecol 167:935, 1992.
241. Pritchard JA, Cunningham FG, Pritchard SA: The Parkland Memorial hospital protocol for treatment of eclampsia: Evaluation of 245 cases. Am J Obstet Gynecol 148:951, 1984.
242. Bryans CI, Southerland WL, Zuspem FP: Eclampsia: a follow-up study of eclamptic women. Obstet Gynecol 21:71, 1963.
243. Moodley J, Bobat SM, Hoffman M, Bill PLA: Electroencephalogram and computerized cerebral tomography findings in eclampsia. Br J Obstet Gynaecol 100:984, 1993.
244. Drislane FW, Wang AM: Multifocal cerebral hemorrhage in eclampsia and severe preeclampsia. J Neurol 244:194, 1997.
245. Sanders TG, Clayman DA, Sanchez-Ramos L, et al: Brain in eclampsia: MR imaging with clinical correlation. Radiology 180:475, 1991.
246. Morriss MC, Twickler DM, Hatab MR, et al: Cerebral blood flow and cranial magnetic resonance imaging in eclampsia and severe preeclampsia. Obstet Gynecol 89:561, 1997.
247. Cunningham FG, Twickler DM: Cerebral edema complicating eclampsia. Am J Obstet Gynecol 182:94, 2000.
248. Schwartz RB, Feske SK, Polak JF, et al: Preeclampsia-eclampsia: Clinical and neuroradiographic correlates and insights into the pathogenesis of hypertensive encephalopathy. Radiology 217:371, 2000.
249. Williams KP, Wilson S: Persistence of cerebral hemodynamic changes in patients with eclampsia: a report of three cases. Am J Obstet Gynecol 181:1162, 1999.
250. Belfort MA. Kennedy A, Rassner UA: Novel techniques for cerebral evaluation in preeclampsia and eclampsia. Clin Obstet Gynecol 48:387, 2005.
251. Zeeman GG, Fleckenstein JL, Twickler DM, Cunningham FG: Cerebral infarction in eclampsia. Am J Obstet Gynecol 190:714, 2004.
252. Loureiro R, Leite CC, Kahhale S, et al: Diffusion imaging may predict reversible brain lesions in eclampsia and severe preeclampsia: Initial experience. Am J Obstet Gynecol 189:1350, 2003.
253. Witlin AG, Friedman SA, Egerman RS, et al: Cerebrovascular disorders complicating pregnancy. Beyond eclampsia. Am J Obstet Gynecol 176:139, 1997.
254. Shearer VE, Harish SJ, Cunningham FG: Puerperal seizures after post-dural puncture headache. Obstet Gynecol 85:255, 1995.
255. Hinchey J, Chaves C, Appignani B, et al: A reversible posterior leukoencephalopathy syndrome. N Engl J Med 334:494, 1996.
256. Leitch CR, Cameron AD, Walker JJ: The changing pattern of eclampsia over a 60-year period. Br J Obstet Gynaecol 104:917, 1997.
257. The Clampsia Trial Collaborative Group: Which anticonvulsant for women with eclampsia? Evidence from the Collaborative Eclampsia Trial [published erratum appears in Lancet 1995;346:258]. Lancet 345:1455, 1995.
258. MacKay AP, Berg CJ, Atrash HK: Pregnancy-related mortality from preeclampsia and eclampsia. Obstet Gynecol 97:533, 2001.
259. Sibai BM, Abdella TN, Spinnato JA, Anderson GA: Eclampsia V. The incidence of nonpreventable eclampsia. Am J Obstet Gynecol 154:581, 1986.
260. Campbell DM, Templeton AA: Is eclampsia preventable? *In* Bonnar J, MacGillivray I, Symonds EM (eds): Pregnancy hypertension. Baltimore; University Park Press, 1980, p 483.
261. Witlin AG, Sibai BM: Magnesium sulfate in preeclampsia and eclampsia. Obstet Gynecol 92:883, 1998.
262. McCubbin JH, Sibai BM, Abdella TN, et al: Cardiopulmonary arrest due to acute maternal hypermagnesemia [Letter]. Lancet 1:1058, 1981.
263. Paul RH, Kee SK, Bernstein SG: Changes in fetal heart rate and uterine contraction pattern associated with eclampsia. Am J Obstet Gynecol 130:165, 1978.
264. Sibai BM, Sarinoglu C, Mercer BM: Eclampsia VII. Pregnancy outcome after eclampsia and long-term prognosis. Am J Obstet Gynecol 166:1757, 1992.
265. Chesley LC: Remote prognosis. *In* Chesley LC (ed): Hypertensive disorders of pregnancy. New York; Appleton-Century-Crafts, 1976, p 421.
266. Lopez-Llera M, Horton JLH: Pregnancy after eclampsia. Am J Obstet Gynecol 119:193, 1974.
267. Adelusi B, Ojengbede OA: Reproductive performance after eclampsia. Int J Gynecol Obstet 24:183, 1986.
268. Lopez-Llera M: Recurrent eclampsia Clinical data, morbidity and pathogenic considerations. Eur J Obstet Gynaecol Reprod Biol 50:39, 1993.
269. Bryans CI, Southerland WL, Zuspan FP: Eclampsia: A follow-up study of eclamptic women. Obstet Gynecol 21:701, 1963.
270. Burt VL, Whetton P, Rochella EJ, et al: Prevalence of hypertension in the US adult population: Results from the third national

health and nutrition examination survey, 1988–1991. Hypertension 23:305, 1995.
271. Ferrer RL, Sibai BM, Murlow CD, et al: Management of mild chronic hypertension during pregnancy: A review. Obstet Gynecol 96:849, 2000.
272. Sibai BM, Abdella TN, Anderson GD: Pregnancy outcome in 211 patients with mild chronic hypertension. Obstet Gynecol 61:571, 1983.
273. Sibai BM, Lindheimer M, Hauth J, et al: Risk factors for preeclampsia, abruptio placentae, and adverse neonatal outcomes among women with chronic hypertension. N Engl J Med 339:667, 1998.
274. American College of Obstetricians and Gynecologists: Chronic hypertension in pregnancy. ACOG Practice Bulletin No. 29. Obstet Gynecol 98:177, 2001.
275. Sibai BM: Chronic hypertension in pregnancy. Obstet Gynecol 100:369, 2002.
276. Chobanian AV, Bakris GL, Black HR, et al: The Seventh Report of the Joint National Committee on Prevention, Detection, Evaluation, and Treatment of High Blood Pressure: the JNC 7 report. JAMA (United States) 289:2560, 2003.
277. McCowan LM, Buist RG, North RA, Gamble G: Perinatal morbidity in chronic hypertension. Br J Obstet Gynaecol 103:123, 1996.
278. Rey E, Couturier A: The prognosis of pregnancy in women with chronic hypertension. Am J Obstet Gynecol 171:410, 1994.
279. Sibai BM, Anderson GD: Pregnancy outcome of intensive therapy in severe hypertension in first trimester. Obstet Gynecol 67:517, 1986.
280. Vigil-DeGarcia P, Montufar-Rueda C, Smith A: Hypertension in pregnancy 23:289, 2004.
281. Mabie WC, Ratts TE, Ramanathan KB, Sibai BM: Circulatory congestion in obese hypertensive women: A subset of pulmonary edema in pregnancy. Obstet Gynecol 72:553, 1988.
282. Umans JG, Lindheimer MD: Antihypertensive treatment. *In* Lindheimer MD, Roberts JM, Cunningham FG (eds): Chesley's Hypertensive Disorders in Pregnancy, 2nd ed. Norwalk CT, Appleton and Lange, 1998, p 581.
283. Sibai BM, Grossman RA, Grossman HG: Effects of diuretics on plasma volume in pregnancies with long-term hypertension. Am J Obstet Gynecol 150:831, 1984.
284. Butters L, Kennedy S, Rubin PC: Atenolol in essential hypertension during pregnancy. BMJ 301:587, 1990.
285. Sibai BM, Mabie WC, Shamsa F, et al: A comparison of no medication versus methyldopa or labetalol in chronic hypertension during pregnancy. Am J Obstet Gynecol 162:960, 1990.
286. Steyn DW, Odendaal HJ: Randomized controlled trial of ketanserin and aspirin in prevention of pre-eclampsia. Lancet 350:1267, 1997.
287. Jones DC, Hayslett JP: Outcome of pregnancy in women with moderate or severe renal insufficiency. N Engl J Med 335:226, 1996.
288. Easterling TR, Carr DB, Brateng D, et al: Treatment of hypertension in pregnancy: Effect of atenolol on maternal disease, preterm delivery and fetal growth. Obstet Gynecol 98:427, 2001.
289. Briggs GG, Freeman RK, Yaffee SJ: Drugs in Pregnancy and Lactation: A Reference Guide to Fetal and Neonatal Risk, 5th ed. Baltimore, Williams & Wilkins, 1998.
290. Easterling TR, Brateng D, Schmucker B, et al: Prevention of preeclampsia: A randomized trial of atenolol in hyperdynamic patients before onset of hypertension. Obstet Gynecol 93:725, 1999.
291. Magee LA, Schick B, Donnenfeld AE, et al: The safety of calcium channel blockers in human pregnancy: A preospective, multicenter cohort study. Am J Obstet Gynecol 174:823, 1996.
292. Gruppo di Studio Ipertensione in Gravidanza: Nifedipine versus expectant management in mild to moderate hypertension in pregnancy. Br J Obstet Gynaecol 105:718, 1998.
293. Cockburn J, Moar VA, Ounsted M, Redman LW: Final report of study on hypertension during pregnancy: the effect of specific treatment on the growth and development of the children. Lancet 1:647, 1982.
294. Bartolus R, Ricci E, Chatenoud L, Parazzini F: Nifedipine administration in pregnancy: Effect on the development of children at 18 months. Br J Obstet Gynaecol 107:792, 2000.
295. Collins R, Yusuf S, Peto R: Overview of randomized trials of diuretics in pregnancy. Br Med J 290:17, 1985.
296. White WB: Management of hypertension during lactation. Hypertension 6:297, 1984.
297. Barton JR, Sibai BM: Acute life-threatening emergencies in preeclampsia-eclampsia. Clin Obstet Gynecol 35:402, 1992.
298. Blumenfeld JD, Laragh JH: Management of hypertensive crises: The scientific basis for treatment decisions: Review. Am J Hypertens 14:1154, 2001.
299. Coppage KH, Sibai BM: Hypertensive Emergencies. Obstetric Intensive Care Manual, 2nd ed. New York, McGraw-Hill, 2004, p 51.
300. Silver HM: Acute hypertensive crisis in pregnancy. Med Clin North Am 73:623, 1989.
301. Gifford R Jr: Management of hypertensive crisis. JAMA 266:829, 1991.

Heart Disease

THOMAS R. EASTERLING AND KAREN STOUT

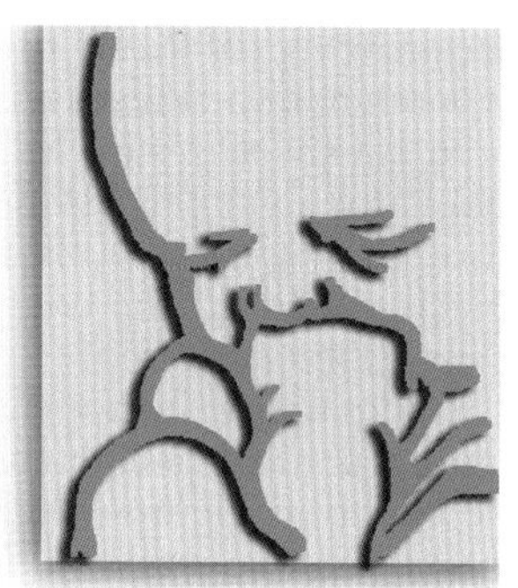

CHAPTER 34

KEY ABBREVIATIONS

Activated partial thromboplastin time	aPTT
Adult respiratory distress syndrome	ARDS
Aortic diameter	AD
Body surface area	BSA
Cardiac index	CI
Cardiac output	CO
Central venous pressure	CVP
Electrocardiogram	ECG
Heart rate	HR
Mean arterial pressure	MAP
New York Heart Association	NYHA
Patent ductus arteriosus	PDA
Positive end-expiratory pressure	PEEP
Pulmonary artery wedge pressure	PAWP
Pulmonary flow	Q_p
Pulmonary vascular resistance	PVR
Relative risk	RR
Right ventricle	RV
Stroke volume	SV
Systemic flow	Q_s
Systemic vascular resistance	SVR
Total peripheral resistance	TPR
Transposition of the great vessels	TGV
Ventricular septal defect	VSD

Cardiovascular adaptations to pregnancy are well tolerated by healthy young women. However, these adaptations are of such magnitude that they can significantly compromise women with abnormal or damaged hearts. Without accurate diagnosis and appropriate care, heart disease in pregnancy can be a significant cause of maternal mortality and morbidity. Under more optimal conditions, many women with significant disease can experience good outcomes and should not necessarily be discouraged from becoming pregnant. This chapter develops an understanding of cardiovascular physiology as a basis for care of the pregnant woman with heart disease. Although published experience with more common conditions can be used to support these principles, information regarding many other conditions is limited to case reports. Data from case reports may, however be biased toward more complicated cases with more adverse outcomes. The best care for women with heart disease is usually achieved from a thorough understanding of maternal cardiovascular physiology, knowledge of existing literature, and extensive clinical experience brought by a multidisciplinary team of clinicians.

MATERNAL HEMODYNAMICS

Hemodynamics refers to the relationship between blood pressure, cardiac output, and vascular resistance. Blood pressure is measured by auscultation, use of an automated cuff, or directly with an intra-arterial catheter. Cardiac output is measured by dilutional techniques requiring central venous access, by Doppler or two-dimensional echocardiographic techniques, or by electrical impedance. Peripheral resistance is calculated using Ohm's law:

$$TPR = MAP \times 80/CO$$

where TPR is total peripheral resistance ($\text{dyne} \cdot \text{sec} \cdot \text{cm}^{-5}$), MAP is mean arterial pressure (millimeters of mercury [mm Hg]), and CO is cardiac output (L/min).

Pregnancy and events unique to pregnancy, such as labor and delivery, are associated with significant and frequently predictable changes in these parameters. The hemodynamic changes of pregnancy, although well tolerated by an otherwise healthy women, may be tolerated poorly by a woman with significant cardiac disease. Therefore, the importance of understanding these changes and placing them in the context of a specific cardiac lesion cannot be overstated.

The maternal hemodynamics of 89 nulliparous women who remained normotensive throughout pregnancy are described in Figure 34-1.[1] MAP falls sharply in the first trimester, reaching a nadir by midpregnancy. Thereafter, blood pressure increases slowly, reaching near nonpregnant levels by term. CO rises throughout the first and second trimesters, reaching a maximum by the middle of the third trimester. In the supine position, a pregnant woman in the third trimester may experience significant hypotension due to venocaval occlusion by the gravid uterus. In normal pregnancy, venocaval occlusions may produce symptoms such as diaphoresis, tachycardia, or nausea but will rarely result in significant complications. Fetal heart rate decelerations may be observed but usually resolve when the mother, often spontaneously, shifts to a more comfortable position. Women with significant right or left ventricular outflow obstruction, such as aortic stenosis, may seriously decompensate in the supine position due to poor ventricular filling.

CO is the product of heart rate (HR) and stroke volume (SV):

$$CO = HR \times SV.$$

HR and SV increase as pregnancy progresses to the third trimester. After 32 weeks, SV falls, with the maintenance of CO becoming more and more dependent on HR. Vascular resistance falls in the first and early second trimesters. The magnitude of the fall is sufficient to offset the rise in CO, resulting in a net decrease in blood pressure.

Labor, delivery, and the postpartum period are times of acute hemodynamic changes that may result in maternal decompensation. Labor itself is associated with pain and anxiety. Tachycardia is a normal response. Significant catecholamine release increases afterload. Each uterine contraction acutely redistributes 400 to 500 ml of blood from the uterus to the central circulation. In Figure 34-2, Robson et al.[2] describe the hemodynamic changes associated with unmedicated labor. HR, blood pressure, and CO all increase with uterine contractions, with the magnitude of the change increasing as labor advances. Obstructive cardiac lesions impede the flow of blood through the heart, blunting the expected rise in CO at the expense of increasing pulmonary pressures and pulmonary congestion. In Figure 34-3, intrapartum hemodynamic changes of a patient with aortic stenosis and a peak gradient of 160 mm Hg are shown.[3] In this individual, pulmonary pressures rise in parallel with uterine contractions.

Immediately after delivery, blood from the uterus is returned to the central circulation. In normal pregnancy, this compensatory mechanism protects against the hemodynamic effects that may accompany postpartum hemorrhage. In the context of cardiac disease, this acute centralization of blood may increase pulmonary pressures

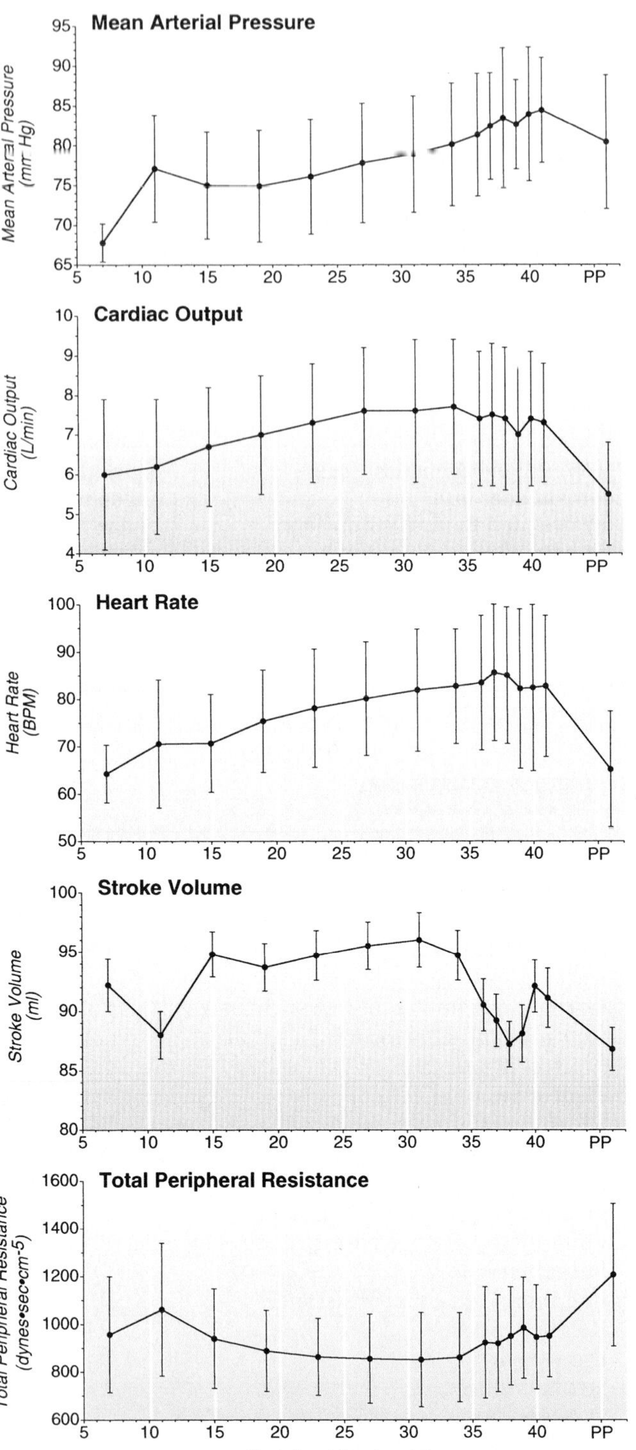

Figure 34-1. Changes in hemodynamic parameters throughout pregnancy (mean ± SD). SD, standard deviation.

and pulmonary congestion.[4] During the first 2 postpartum weeks, extravascular fluid is mobilized, diuresis ensues, and vascular resistance increases returning to nonpregnant norms. Decompensation during postpartum fluid mobilization is common in women with mitral stenosis. Volume loading coupled with vasconstriction may also unmask maternal cardiomyopathy. Unsuspected cardiac disease may be diagnosed when a woman returns to the

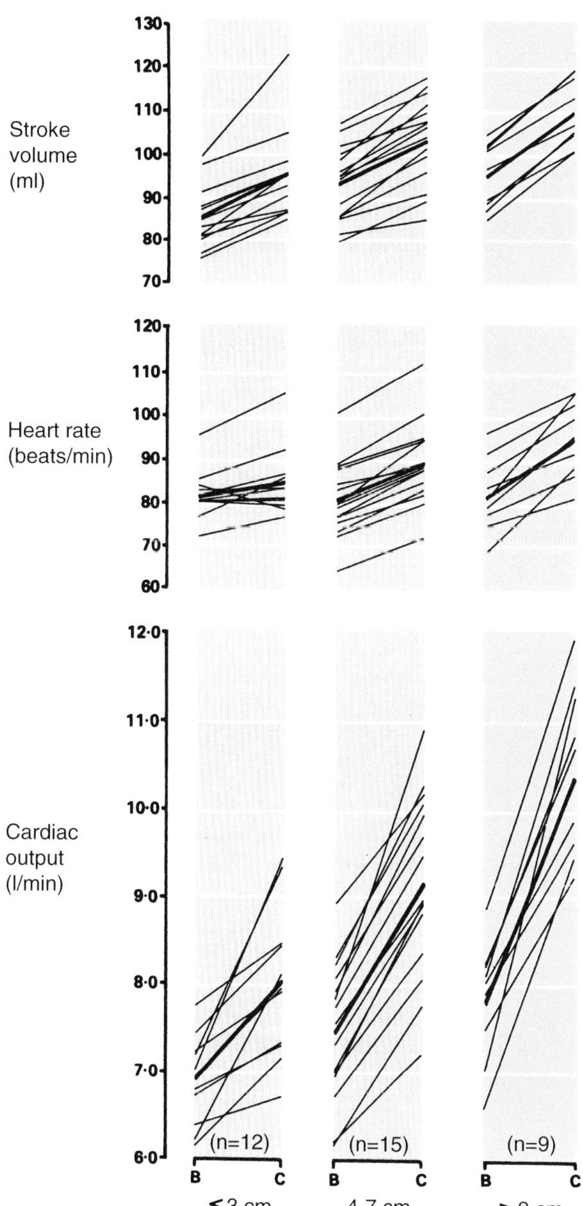

Figure 34-2. Changes in hemodynamic parameters at three different points during labor (≤3 cm, 4 to 7 cm, and ≥8 cm). Each line represents the change in an individual subject. *B*, before contraction; *C*, during contraction. (From Robson S, Dunlop W, Boys R, Hunter S: Cardiac output during labour. BMJ 295:1169, 1987, with permission.)

emergency room several days postpartum with dyspnea and oxygen desaturation. Maternal CO usually normalizes by 2 weeks postpartum.[5]

Three key features of the maternal hemodynamic changes in pregnancy are particularly relevant to the management of women with cardiac disease: (1) increased CO, (2) increased HR, and (3) reduced vascular resistance. In conditions such as mitral stenosis, in which CO is relatively fixed, the drive to achieve an elevated CO may result in pulmonary congestion. If a patient has an atrial septal defect, the incremental increase in systemic flow associated with pregnancy will be magnified in the pulmonary circulation to the extent that pulmonary flow exceeds systemic flow. If, for example, a shunt ratio of 3:1 is maintained in pregnancy, pulmonary flow may be as high as 20 L/min and may be associated with increasing dyspnea and potential desaturation.

Many cardiac conditions are HR dependent. Flow across a stenotic mitral valve is dependent on the proportion of time in diastole. Tachycardia reduces left ventricular filling and CO. Coronary blood flow is also dependent on the length of diastole. Patients with aortic stenosis have increased wall tension and, therefore, increased myocardial oxygen requirements. Tachycardia reduces coronary perfusion time in diastole while simultaneously further increasing myocardial oxygen requirements. The resulting imbalance between oxygen demand and supply may precipitate myocardial ischemia. Patients with complex congenital heart disease can experience significant tachyarrhythmias. The increasing HR in pregnancy may be associated with a worsening of tachyarrhythmias.

Reduction in vascular resistance may be beneficial to some patients; afterload reduction reduces cardiac work. Cardiomyopathy, aortic regurgitation, and mitral regurgitation all benefit from reduced afterload. Alternatively, patients with intracardiac shunts, in which right and left ventricular pressures are nearly equal when not pregnant, may reverse their shunt during pregnancy and desaturate due to right to left shunting.

BLOOD VOLUME

Very early in the first trimester, pregnant women experience an expansion of renal blood flow and glomerular filtration rate. Filtered sodium increases by approximately 50 percent. Despite physiologic changes that would promote loss of salt and water and contraction of blood volume, the pregnant woman will expand her blood volume by 40 to 50 percent. In part, the stimulation to retain fluid may be a response to the fall in vascular resistance and reduction in blood pressure. The renin-angiotensin system is activated, and the plasma concentration of aldosterone is elevated. Although the simplicity of this explanation is attractive, the actual process is probably much more complicated.[6]

As plasma volume expands, the hematocrit falls, and hematopoiesis is stimulated. Red cell mass will expand from 18 to 25 percent depending on the status of individual iron stores. Physiologic anemia with a maternal hematocrit between 30 percent and 35 percent does not usually complicate pregnancy in the context of maternal heart disease. More significant anemia, however, may increase cardiac work and induce tachycardia. Microcytosis due to iron deficiency may impair perfusion of the microcirculation of patients who are polycythemic due to cyanotic heart disease, because microcytic red blood cells are less deformable. Iron and folate supplementation may be appropriate.

In a similar fashion, serum albumin concentration falls by 22 percent despite an expansion of intravascular albumin mass by 20 percent. As a result, serum oncotic pressure falls in parallel by 20 percent to approximately 19 mm Hg.[7] In normal pregnancy, intravascular fluid

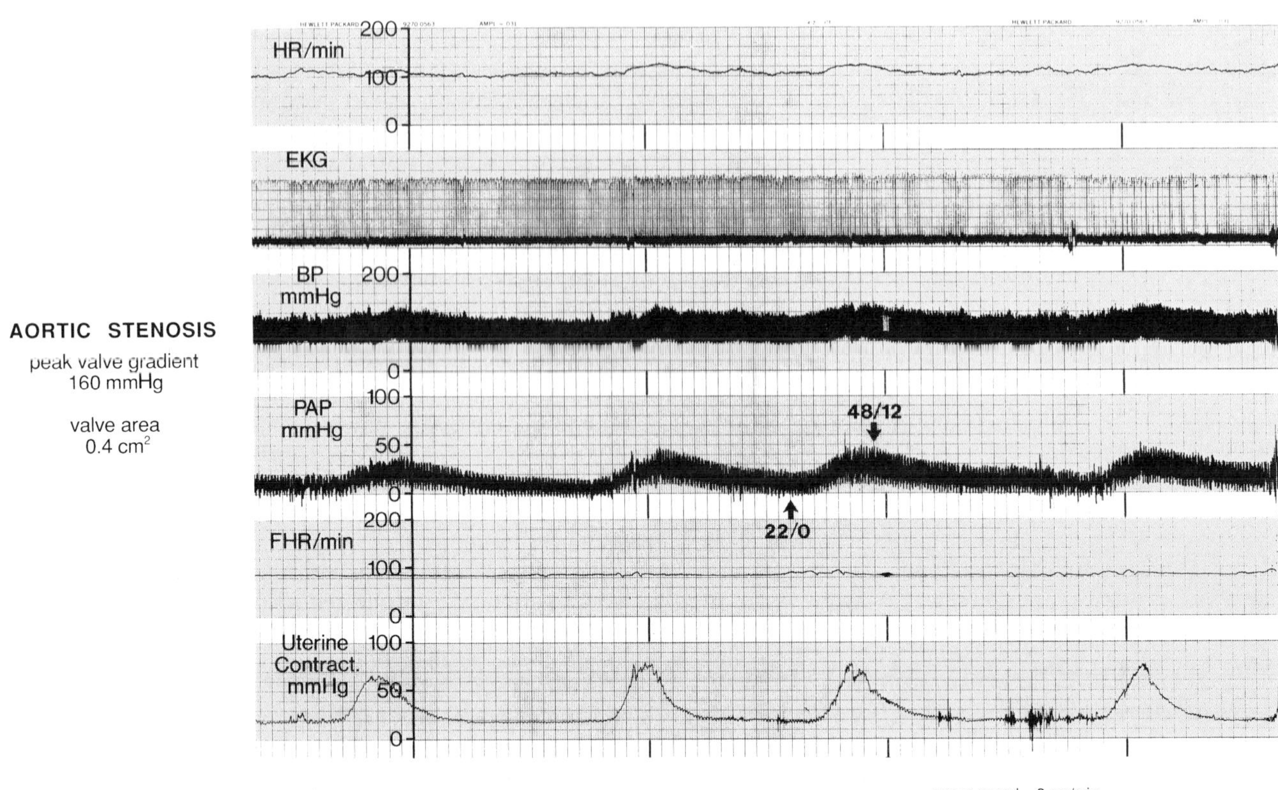

Figure 34-3. Hemodynamic monitoring of a patient with severe aortic stenosis in labor. (From Easterling T, Chadwick H, Otto C, Benedetti T: Aortic stenosis in pregnancy. Obstet Gynecol 72:113, 1988. Reprinted with permission from American College of Obstetricians and Gynecologists.)

balance is maintained by a fall in interstitial oncotic pressure. However, if left ventricular filling pressure becomes elevated or if pulmonary vascular integrity is disrupted, pulmonary edema will develop earlier in the disease process than in nonpregnant women.

DIAGNOSIS AND EVALUATION OF HEART DISEASE

Many women with heart disease have been diagnosed and treated before pregnancy. For example, in women with prior surgery for congenital heart disease, detailed historical information may be available. Others report only that they have a murmur or a "hole in my heart." Alternatively, heart disease may be diagnosed for the first time during pregnancy owing to symptoms precipitated by increased cardiac demands.

The classic symptoms of cardiac disease are palpitations, shortness of breath with exertion, and chest pain. Because these symptoms also may accompany normal pregnancy, a careful history is needed to determine if the symptoms are out of proportion to the stage of pregnancy. Symptoms are of particular concern in a patient with other reasons to suspect underlying cardiac disease, such as being native to an area where rheumatic heart disease is prevalent.

A systolic flow murmur is present in 80 percent of pregnant women, most likely due to the increased flow volume in the aorta and pulmonary artery.[8] Typically, a flow murmur is grade 1 or 2, midsystolic, loudest at the cardiac base, and not associated with any other abnormal physical examination findings. A normal physiologic split second heart sound is heard in patients with a flow murmur. Any diastolic murmur and any systolic murmur that is loud (≥grade 3/6) or radiates to the carotids should be considered pathologic. Careful evaluation for elevation of the jugular venous pulse, for peripheral cyanosis or clubbing, and for pulmonary crackles is needed in women with suspected cardiac disease.

Indications for further cardiac diagnostic testing in pregnant women include a history of known cardiac disease, symptoms in excess of those expected in a normal pregnancy, a pathologic murmur, evidence of heart failure on physical examination, or arterial oxygen desaturation in the absence of known pulmonary disease. The preferred next step in evaluation of pregnant women with suspected heart disease is transthoracic echocardiography. A chest radiograph is helpful only if congestive heart failure is suspected. An electrocardiogram (ECG) may be nonspecific, but could have changes suggestive of the underlying heart disease such as right ventricular hypertrophy and biatrial enlargement seen in patients with significant mitral stenosis. If symptoms are consistent with a cardiac arrhythmia, an event monitor or 24-hour ECG monitor may be indicated. Rarely, cardiac catheterization is needed for full diagnosis of valvular or congenital heart disease. The exception is an acute coronary syndrome during pregnancy in which the risk of radiation exposure with cardiac catheterization is small compared with the benefit of early diagnosis and early revascularization to prevent myocardial infarction.

Echocardiography provides detailed information on cardiac anatomy and physiology that allows optimal management of women with heart disease. Basic data obtained on echocardiography include left ventricular ejection fraction, pulmonary artery systolic pressure, qualitative evaluation of right ventricular systolic function, and evaluation of valve anatomy and function. When valvular stenosis is present, the pressure gradient (ΔP) across the valve is calculated from the Doppler-derived velocity (v) of flow across the valve: $\Delta P = 4v^2$. Similarly, pulmonary artery systolic pressure can be calculated from the maximal Doppler velocity obtained across a tricuspid regurgitant jet.

Aortic valve area is calculated using the continuity equation. SV is calculated from the product of the cross-sectional area of the left ventricular outflow tract and the time-velocity integral derived from Doppler evaluation of the outflow tract. A time-velocity integral is then derived from the stenotic valve. Because the left ventricular outflow tract and the aortic valve are in continuity, SVs across each are equal. Therefore, valve area can be derived by dividing the stroke volume by the aortic valve time-velocity integral. Mitral valve area is measured directly by two-dimensional planimetry or by the Doppler pressure half-time method.[9] In patients with congenital disease, detailed evaluation of anatomy and previous surgical repair is possible. When complex congenital heart disease is present or when image quality is suboptimal, transesophageal imaging provides improved image quality. Cardiac magnetic resonance imaging may be used to define complex anatomy that is not well evaluated by echocardiography, but caution must be taken with magnetic resonance contrast agents such as gadolinium.

GENERAL CARE

Management of cardiac disease in pregnancy is frequently complicated by unique social and psychological concerns. Children with congenital heart disease may have experienced multiple hospitalizations and be fearful of the medical environment. Some have been cautioned against pregnancy and, therefore, have never expected to bear children. Women with rheumatic heart disease have frequently lived outside the traditional medical care system owing to conditions of poverty, immigration, and cultural differences. Care must be exercised to facilitate their access to care and their comfort with the environment of care. Their practitioner must be patient but persistent in the face of deviations from more traditional standards of compliance and medical care.

Deterioration in cardiac status during pregnancy is frequently insidious. Continuity of care with a single provider facilitates early intervention before overt decompensation. Regular visits should include particular attention to HR, weight gain, and oxygen saturation. An unexpected increase in weight may indicate the need for more aggressive outpatient therapy. A fall in oxygen saturation often precedes a clearly abnormal chest examination or radiograph. Regular use of a structured history of symptoms (see the box "Structured Review of Cardiac Symptoms") alerts the physician to a change in condition. Regular review educates the patient and reinforces his or her role as a "partners in care."

The physiologic changes of pregnancy are usually continuous and, therefore, offer adequate time for maternal compensation despite cardiac disease. Intercurrent events superimposed on pregnancy in the context of maternal heart disease are usually responsible for acute decompensation. The most common significant intercurrent events during the antepartum period are febrile episodes. Screening for bacteriuria and vaccination against influenza and pneumococcus are appropriate. Patients should be instructed to report symptoms of upper respiratory infection, particularly fever. Many women with heart disease (adolescents, recent immigrants, and those living in poverty) are also at risk for iron deficiency. Prophylaxis against anemia with iron and folate supplementation may decrease cardiac work.

A strategy of standard cardiac care for labor and delivery is described in the box. The general principles for care are similar for most cardiac diagnoses. Physiologically, the ideal labor for a woman with heart disease is short

Structured Review of Cardiac Symptoms

"How many flights of stairs can you walk up with ease?"—"Two? One? None?"
"Can you walk a level block?"
"Can you sleep flat in bed?" "How many pillows?"
"Dose your heart race?"
"Do you have chest pain?"
 "with exercise?"
 "when your heart races?"

Standard Cardiac Care for Labor and Delivery

1. Accurate diagnosis
2. Mode of delivery based on obstetric indications
3. Medical management initiated early in labor
   - Prolonged labor avoided.
   - Induction with a *favorable* cervix
4. Maintenance of hemodynamic stability
   - Invasive hemodynamic monitoring when required
   - Initial, compensated hemodynamic reference point
   - Specific emphasis based on particular cardiac condition
5. Avoidance of pain and hemodynamic responses
   - Epidural analgesia with narcotic/low-dose local technique
6. Prophylactic antibiotics when at risk for endocarditis
7. Avoidance of maternal pushing
   - Caudal for dense perineal anesthesia
   - Low forceps or vacuum delivery
8. Avoidance of maternal blood loss
   - Proactive management of the third stage
   - Early but appropriate fluid replacement
9. Early volume management postpartum
   - Often careful but aggressive diuresis

Table 34-1. Prophylactic Regimens for Labor and Delivery

PATIENTS	REGIMENS
High-risk patients	
Prosthetic valves—both bioprosthetic and homografts Complex cyanotic congenital heart disease (CHD) Surgically constructed systemic pulmonic shunts or conduits Previous bacterial endocarditis	Ampicillin + gentamicin Ampicillin 2.0 g IM or IV Gentamicin 1.5 mg/kg (not to exceed 120 mg) in active labor; 6 h later, ampicillin 1 g IM/IV or amoxicillin 1 g PO
High-risk patients allergic to ampicillin/amoxicillin	Vancomycin + gentamicin Vancomycin 1.0 g IV over 1–2 h + gentamicin as above in active labor
Moderate-risk patients Most other CHD Acquired valvular dysfunction (e.g., rheumatic heart disease) Hypertrophic cardiac myopathy Mitral valve prolapse with regurgitation	Amoxicillin or ampicillin Amoxicillin 2.0 g orally or ampicillin 2.0 g IM/IV in active labor
Moderate-risk patients allergic to ampicillin/amoxicillin	Vancomycin Vancomycin 1.0 g IV over 1–2 h in active labor

IM, intramuscular; IV, intravenous; PO, by mouth.

Adapted from Dajani AS, Taubert KA, Wilson W, et al: Prevention of bacterial endocarditis: recommendations by the American Heart Association. JAMA 277:1794, 1997.

and pain free. Although induction of labor facilitates organization of care and early pain control, shortening the duration of pregnancy by 1 or 2 weeks at the cost of a 2- or 3-day induction of labor is not worthwhile. Induction of labor with a favorable cervix is therefore preferred. Some patients with severe cardiac disease benefit from invasive hemodynamic monitoring with an arterial catheter and a pulmonary artery catheter. These methods are discussed in detail later. Cesarean delivery is usually reserved for obstetric indications. The American Heart Association does not recommend routine antibiotic prophylaxis for the prevention of endocarditis, although it is optional in high-risk patients having a vaginal delivery (Table 34-1). Because bacteremia is common at the time of vaginal delivery and cesarean delivery,[10,11] many practitioners will provide antibiotic prophylaxis in all patients at risk.

Women with significant heart disease should be counseled before pregnancy regarding the risk of pregnancy, interventions that may be required and potential risks to the fetus. However, women with significant uncorrected disease often present with an ongoing established pregnancy. In this situation, the risks and benefits of termination of pregnancy versus those of continuing a pregnancy should be addressed. The decision to become pregnant or carry a pregnancy in the context of maternal disease is a balance of two forces: (1) the objective medical risk, including the uncertainty of that estimate; and (2) the value of the birth of a child to an individual woman and her partner. The first goal of counseling is to educate the patient. Only a few cardiac diseases represent an overwhelming risk of maternal mortality: Eisenmenger's syndrome, pulmonary hypertension with right ventricular dysfunction, and Marfan's syndrome with significant aortic dilation and severe left ventricular dysfunction. Most other conditions require aggressive management and significant disruption in lifestyle. Intercurrent events such as antepartum pneumonia or obstetric hemorrhage pose the greatest risk of initiating life-threatening events. Fastidious care can reduce but not eliminate the risk of these events. Maternal congenital heart disease increases the risk of congenital heart disease in the fetus from 1 percent to approximately 4 to 6 percent.[12–14] Marfan's syndrome and some forms of hypertrophic cardiomyopathy are inherited as autosomal dominant conditions; the offspring of these women carry a 50 percent chance of inheriting the disease. The second goal of counseling is to help each woman integrate the medical information into her individual value system and her individual desire to become a mother. Many women with significant but manageable heart disease choose to carry a pregnancy. The basis for their decisions should be individualized.

VALVULAR DISEASE

The American College of Cardiology and the American Heart Association have published guidelines for the management of valvular heart disease including some guidelines for management during pregnancy.[15] These guidelines create a general framework for preconceptional care and care during pregnancy, realizing that treatment of a specific patient must be individualized.

MITRAL STENOSIS

Mitral stenosis is nearly always due to rheumatic heart disease. Valvular dysfunction progresses continuously throughout life. Deterioration may be accelerated by recurrent episodes of rheumatic fever. Rheumatic fever itself is an immunologic response to group A β-hemolytic streptococcus infections. The incidence of rheumatic fever in a population is heavily influenced by conditions of poverty and crowding. These same individuals are at risk to have reduced access and utilization of health care resources and may present undiagnosed or untreated.

Patients with asymptomatic mitral stenosis have a 10-year survival of greater than 80 percent. Once a patient is significantly symptomatic, 10-year survival without treatment is less than 15 percent. In the presence of pulmonary hypertension, mean survival falls to less than 3 years. Death is due to progressive pulmonary edema, right-sided heart failure, systemic embolization, or pulmonary embolism.[15]

Stenosis of the mitral valve impedes the flow of blood from the left atrium to the left ventricle during diastole. The normal mitral valve area is 4.0 to 5.0 cm^2. Symptoms with exercise can be expected with valve areas less than or equal to 2.5 cm^2. Symptoms at rest are expected at less than or equal to 1.5 cm^2. The left ventricle responds with Starling mechanisms to increased venous return with increased performance, elevating CO in response to demand. The left atrium is limited in its capacity to respond. Therefore, CO is limited by the relatively passive flow of blood through the valve during diastole; increased venous return results in pulmonary congestion rather than increased CO. Thus, the drive for increased CO in pregnancy cannot be achieved, resulting in increased pulmonary congestion. The relative tachycardia experienced in pregnancy shortens diastole, decreases left ventricular filling, and therefore, further compromises CO and increases pulmonary congestion.

The diagnosis of mitral stenosis in pregnancy before maternal decompensation is uncommon. Tiredness and dyspnea on exertion are characteristic symptoms of mitral stenosis but are also ubiquitous among pregnant women. Although the presence of a diastolic rumble or jugular venous distention may suggest mitral stenosis, these findings are subtle and may be overlooked or not appreciated. Not uncommonly, an intercurrent event such as a febrile episode will result in exaggerated symptoms and the diagnosis of pulmonary edema or oxygen desaturation. Under these circumstances, particularly in the context of a patient from an at-risk group, an echocardiogram should be performed to rule out mitral-valvular disease.

Echocardiographic diagnosis of mitral stenosis is based on the characteristic appearance of the stenotic, frequently calcified valve. Calculation of valve area from pressure half-time of the Doppler wave or by two-dimensional planimetry provides an objective measure of severity. Valve areas of 1.0 cm^2 or less will usually require pharmacologic management during pregnancy and invasive hemodynamic monitoring during labor. Valve areas of 1.4 cm^2 or less usually require careful expectant management. Left atrial enlargement identifies a patient at risk for atrial fibrillation, subsequent atrial thrombus, and the potential for systemic embolization. Pulmonary hypertension, a complication of worsening mitral disease, can be diagnosed and quantified with Doppler evaluation of the regurgitant jet across the tricuspid valve. Elevated pulmonary pressures may be due to hydrostatic forces associated with elevated left atrial pressures or, in more advanced disease, due to pathologic elevations of pulmonary vascular resistance (PVR). Hydrostatic pulmonary hypertension may respond to therapy that lowers left atrial pressure. Pulmonary hypertension due to elevated PVR is life threatening in pregnancy and may precipitate right-sided heart failure in the postpartum period.

Pregnancy itself does not negatively affect the natural history of mitral stenosis. Chesley[16] reviewed the medical histories of 134 women with functionally severe mitral stenosis who survived pregnancies between 1931 and 1943. These women lived before modern management of mitral stenosis and, therefore, represent the natural history of the disease. By 1974, only nine of the cohort remained alive. Their death rate was exponential; during each year of follow-up, the rate for the remaining cohort was 6.3 percent. Women with subsequent pregnancies had comparable survival to those who did not again become pregnant, allowing the authors to conclude that pregnancy itself did not negatively affect long-term outcome.

The goal of antepartum care in the context of mitral stenosis is to achieve a balance between the drive to increase CO and the limitations of flow across the stenotic valve. Most women with significant disease require diuresis with a drug such as furosemide. In addition, β-blockade reduces HR, improves diastolic flow across the valve, and relieves pulmonary congestion. Al Kasab et al.[17] evaluated the impact of β-blockade on 25 pregnant women with significant mitral stenosis. Figure 34-4 describes the functional status of women before pregnancy, during pregnancy before β-blockade, and after β-blockade. The deterioration associated with pregnancy and the improvement with treatment is evident. Fastidious antepartum care as described earlier should supplement pharmacologic management.

Women with a history of rheumatic valvular disease who are at risk for contact with populations with a high prevalence of streptococcal infection should receive prophylaxis with daily oral penicillin G or monthly benzathine penicillin.[15] Most pregnant women live in close contact with groups of children and usually are considered at risk. Atrial fibrillation is a complication associated with mitral stenosis due to left atrial enlargement. Rapid ventricular response to atrial fibrillation may result in sudden decompensation. Digoxin, β-blockers, or calcium channel blockers can be used to control ventricular response. In the context of hemodynamic decompensation, electrical cardioversion may be necessary. Anticoagulation with

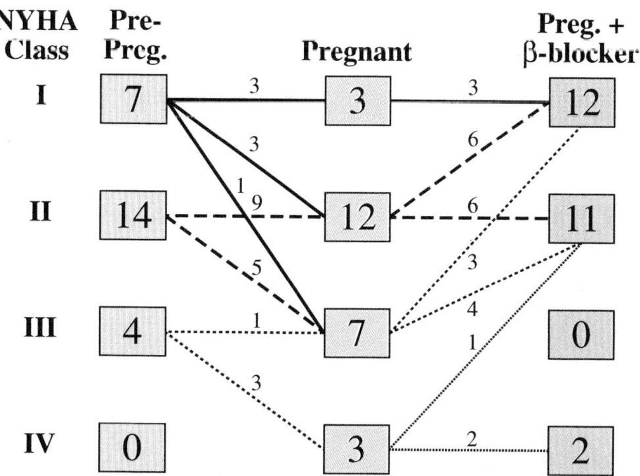

Figure 34-4. The effects of β-blockade on functional status of women with mitral stenosis. (From Al Kasab S, Sabag T, Al Zaibag M, et al: Beta-adrenergic receptor blockade in the management of pregnant women with mitral stenosis. Am J Obstet Gynecol 163:37, 1990, with permission.)

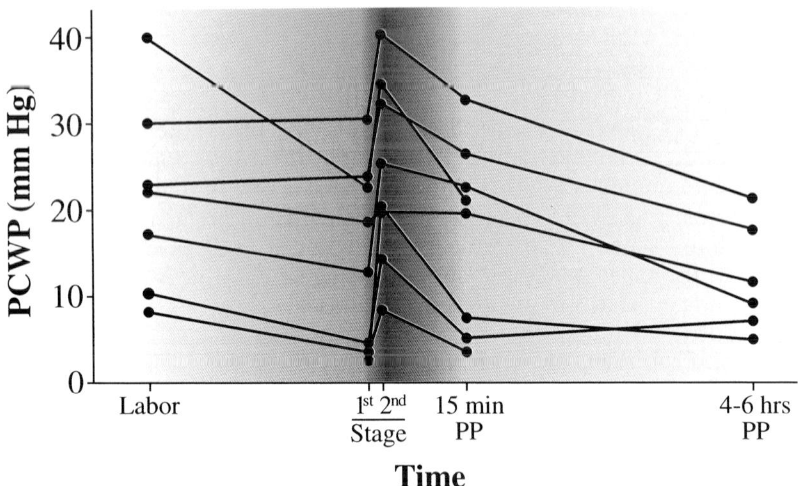

Figure 34-5. The changes in pulmonary capillary wedge pressure associated with delivery and subsequent diuresis in women with mitral stenosis. (From Clark S, Phelan J, Greenspoon J, et al: Labor and delivery in the presence of mitral stenosis: central hemodynamic observations. Am J Obstet Gynecol 152:384, 1985, with permission.)

heparin should be used before and after cardioversion to prevent systemic embolization. Patients with chronic atrial fibrillation and a history of an embolic event should also be anticoagulated.[15]

Labor and delivery can frequently precipitate decompensation in patients with critical mitral stenosis. Pain induces tachycardia. Uterine contractions increase venous return and, therefore, pulmonary congestion. Women frequently cannot tolerate the work of pushing in the second stage. Clark et al.[4] described the abrupt elevation in pulmonary artery pressures in the immediate postpartum period associated with return of uterine blood to the general circulation (Fig. 34-5). Aggressive, anticipatory diuresis will reduce pulmonary congestion and the potential for oxygen desaturation.

The hemodynamics of women with symptomatic stenosis or a valve area of 1 cm^2 or less should be managed with the aid of a pulmonary artery catheter. Ideally, hemodynamic parameters are assessed when the patient is well compensated, early in labor. These findings serve as a reference point to guide subsequent therapy. Pain control is best achieved with an epidural. HR control is maintained through pain control and β-blockade. To avoid pushing, the second stage is shortened with low forceps or vacuum delivery. Aggressive diuresis is initiated immediately postpartum. Cesarean delivery is reserved for obstetric indications.

Aggressive medical management including hospital bed rest in selected cases is sufficient to manage most women with mitral stenosis. The woman with uncommonly severe disease may require surgical intervention. Although successful valve replacement and open commissurotomy have been reported in pregnancy,[18,19] they are now rarely needed. Two centers have reported successful balloon valvotomy in a series of 40 and 44 women with minimal complications.[20,21] Complications of balloon valvuloplasty outside of pregnancy occur at the following rates: mortality (0.5 percent), cerebrovascular accident (1 percent), and mitral regurgitation requiring surgery (2 percent).[15] Medical management should be clearly exhausted before assuming these risks during pregnancy, when emergent intervention such as valve replacement is more complicated and carries a significant risk to the fetus.

Rheumatic disease can also affect the aortic valve. Management of significant mitral stenosis, which limits ventricular filling, in the context of aortic stenosis that is critically dependent on ventricular filling, is particularly complicated.

MITRAL REGURGITATION

Mitral regurgitation may be due to a chronic progressive process such as rheumatic valve disease or myxomatous mitral valve disease, frequently associated with mitral valve prolapse. As regurgitation increases over time, forward flow is maintained at the expense of left ventricular dilation with eventual impaired contractility. Left atrial enlargement may be associated with atrial fibrillation that should be managed with ventricular rate control and anticoagulation. The patient with chronic mitral regurgitation may remain asymptomatic even with exercise. Preconceptional counseling should include consideration of valve replacement in consultation with a cardiologist. In general, valve replacement is recommended for (1) symptomatic patients, (2) atrial fibrillation, (3) ejection fraction less than 50 to 60 percent, (4) left ventricular end-diastolic dimension greater than 45 to 50 mm, or (5) pulmonary systolic pressure greater than 50 to 60 mm Hg.[15] As discussed later, the benefits of valve replacement before pregnancy must be balanced against the risks associated with a prosthetic valve in pregnancy and the potential for prosthetic valve deterioration in pregnancy. If surgery is required, valve repair rather than replacement is preferred when possible to avoid the need for anticoagulation.

Acute mitral regurgitation in young patients is uncommon and may be associated with ruptured chordae tendineae due to endocarditis or myxomatous valve disease. Without time for left ventricular compensation, forward flow may be severely compromised. Urgent valve surgery is usually required. Inotropic left ventricular support and systemic afterload reduction can be used to stabilize the patient.

The hemodynamic changes associated with pregnancy can be expected to have mixed effects. A reduction in systemic vascular resistance (SVR) tends to promote forward flow. The drive to increase CO will exacerbate left ventricular volume overload. Increased atrial dilation may initiate atrial fibrillation. Pulmonary congestion can be managed by careful diuresis with the knowledge that adequate forward flow is usually dependent on a high preload to achieve adequate left ventricular filling. Atrial fibrillation should be managed as in the nonpregnant state. An increase in SVR due to progressive hypertension secondary to advancing preeclampsia may significantly impair forward flow and should be treated. Labor and delivery should be managed with standard cardiac care. Catecholamine release due to pain or stress impairs forward flow. Particular attention should be paid to left ventricular filling. Excessive preload results in pulmonary congestion. Insufficient preload will not fill the enlarged left ventricle and will result in insufficient forward flow. A pulmonary artery catheter can be used to determine appropriate filling pressure in early labor or before induction. Although a large v wave may complicate the interpretation of pulmonary artery wedge pressure, the pulmonary artery diastolic pressure can be used as a reference point. Diuresis in the early postpartum period may be required.

Myxomatous mitral valve disease or mitral valve prolapse is a common condition, affecting as many as 12 percent of young women.[22] In the absence of conditions of abnormal connective tissue such as Marfan's or Ehler-Danlos syndromes and clinically significant mitral regurgitation, women with mitral prolapse can be expected to have uncomplicated pregnancies. They may experience an increase in tachyarrhythmias that can be treated with β-blockers. Prophylactic antibiotics are usually used at the time of delivery.

AORTIC STENOSIS

Most patients who develop calcific stenotic tricuspid aortic valves do so outside their childbearing years (age 70 to 80). Patients with bicuspid valves develop significant stenosis after the age of 50 to 60 years. Rheumatic disease can also affect the aortic valve, usually after the development of significant mitral disease. The majority of pregnant women with significant aortic stenosis have congenitally stenotic valves: bicuspid valves with congenitally fused leaflets, unicuspid valves, or tricuspid valves with fused leaflets.[23]

The natural history of aortic stenosis is characterized by a long, asymptomatic period. With increasing outflow obstruction, patients develop angina, syncope, and left ventricular failure. Without valve replacement, only 50 percent of patients will survive 5 years after the development of angina; 3 years after the development of syncope; and 2 years after the development of left ventricular failure.[24] Although valve replacement is the only definitive treatment for calcific aortic stenosis, valvuloplasty may prove beneficial in some young adults whose valves are not calcified. Medical management of symptomatic patients is not generally efficacious. Mechanical valve replacement requires anticoagulation, complicating subsequent pregnancies.

Young women with aortic stenosis are usually asymptomatic. Although they may develop increasing exercise intolerance in pregnancy, the progression is insidious and not easily distinguished from the effects of normal pregnancy. The diagnosis is usually made by the auscultation of a harsh systolic murmur. The murmur can easily be distinguished from a physiologic murmur of pregnancy by its harshness and radiation into the carotid arteries. Diagnosis is confirmed by echocardiography where the gradient across the valve can be measured by Doppler, and the valve area can be calculated with the continuity equation. Many women with significant aortic stenosis experience the expected increase in CO associated with pregnancy.[3] Increased flow across the fixed, stenotic valve results in a proportionately increased gradient across the valve. Although the pressure gradient during pregnancy may be higher than that observed postpartum, these differences are not significant.

Four series of patients with aortic stenosis in pregnancy have been reported.[3,25–27] The reports summarize experiences with wide ranges in severity of disease and management ranging from the 1960s and 1970s to the present. Arias[25] described a series of 23 cases managed before 1978 with a maternal mortality of 17 percent. More recent series, however, do not demonstrate this high level of maternal risk.[3,26,27] The potential for serious adverse outcomes reported by Arias should, however, serve as an indication for intensive management. The rate of mortality should not necessarily be used as an indication for termination or surgical intervention. Pregnant patients have been successfully managed with aortic gradients in excess of 160 mm Hg.[3] In general, patients with a peak aortic gradient of 60 mm Hg or less have had uncomplicated courses. Those with higher gradients require increasingly intensive management.

Aortic valve replacement and balloon valvotomy have been reported during pregnancy. Balloon valvotomy in a young patient without valve calcification can provide significant long-term palliation. Valvotomy before pregnancy may provide an interval of hemodynamic stability sufficient to complete a pregnancy without the complications associated with a mechanical prosthetic valve. Consideration for valve replacement or valvotomy during pregnancy should be reserved for patients who remain clinically symptomatic despite hospital care. In general, intervention should not be based solely on a pressure gradient or valve area.

Aortic stenosis is a condition of excess left ventricular afterload. Ventricular hypertrophy increases cardiac oxygen requirement, whereas increased diastolic ventricular pressure impairs diastolic coronary perfusion. Each increases the potential for myocardial ischemia. The left ventricle requires adequate filling to generate sufficient systolic pressure to produce flow across the stenotic valve. Given a hypertrophied ventricle and some degree of diastolic dysfunction, the volume-pressure relationship is very steep. A small loss of left ventricular filling results in a proportionately large fall in left ventricular pressure and, therefore, a large fall in forward flow, CO. The pregnant patient with significant aortic stenosis is very sensitive to loss of preload associated with hemorrhage or epidural induced hypotension. The window of appropriate filling pressure is narrow. Excess fluid may result in pulmonary edema; insufficient fluid may result in hypotension and coronary ischemia.

In general, pulmonary edema associated with excess preload is much easier to manage than hypotension due to hypovolemia.

Appropriate antepartum care is described earlier. Given that most aortic stenosis in young women is congenital in origin, fetal echocardiography is indicated. Although some controversy persists, cesarean delivery is generally reserved for obstetric indications. Pain during labor and delivery can be safely managed with regional analgesia using a low-dose bupivacaine and narcotic technique. Dense anesthesia during the second stage can be obtained with minimal hemodynamic complications using a caudal. Patients with gradients above 60 to 80 mm Hg benefit from the use of a pulmonary artery and an arterial catheter during labor. Hospital admission one day before planned induction of labor with a favorable cervix is preferred. A prolonged induction should be avoided. Pulmonary artery and radial artery catheters as well as epidural and caudal catheters are placed. The patient should be gently hydrated overnight to achieve a pulmonary artery wedge pressure (PAWP) of 12 to 15 mm Hg. Some patients with milder disease spontaneously diurese in the face of a volume load such that an elevation in PAWP cannot be achieved. An elevated PAWP serves as a buffer against a loss of preload. If with bleeding or the onset of anesthesia PAWP falls, volume can be administered before a reduction in forward flow. In general, pushing is minimized, and the second stage is shortened with operative vaginal delivery. Antibiotics are administered for the prevention of endocarditis.

Postpartum, patients should be monitored hemodynamically for 24 to 48 hours. Diuresis is usually spontaneous; the patient can be allowed to find her predelivery compensated state. When diuresis must be induced to treat pulmonary edema, it should be done gently and carefully. Predelivery hemodynamic parameters should be used as an endpoint. Some have found that a significant delay in valve replacement after the postpartum period is associated with maternal complications.[3] These observations may be the result of accelerated valve deterioration due to pregnancy. For this reason, valve replacement within weeks of delivery may be indicated.

AORTIC REGURGITATION

Aortic regurgitation is most often due to a congenitally abnormal valve. Other causes include Marfan's syndrome, endocarditis, and rheumatic disease. As with mitral regurgitation, the left ventricle compensates for a loss in forward flow with an increase in left ventricular end-diastolic volume. Afterload reduction prevents progressive left ventricular dilation and is recommended for patients with left ventricular dysfunction or dilation. Valve replacement is generally recommended for (1) New York Heart Association (NYHA) functional class III and class IV symptoms, (2) an ejection fraction less than 50 percent, or (3) left ventricular end-systolic dimension greater than 55 mm.[15] Acute regurgitation may be due to aortic root dissection or endocarditis and usually represents a medical emergency requiring urgent valve replacement.

The reduction in vascular resistance associated with pregnancy tends to improve cardiac performance. If afterload reduction has been achieved with an angiotensin-converting inhibitor before pregnancy, hydralazine or a calcium channel blocker such as nifedipine should be substituted. Modest elevations of HR should be tolerated. Bradycardia may be associated with increased regurgitation due to prolongation of diastole. Labor and delivery is managed with standard cardiac care. Pulmonary artery catheterization is not usually required. As the hemodynamic changes associated with pregnancy resolve, a rise in vascular resistance should be anticipated and afterload reduction maintained.

PROSTHETIC VALVES

Definitive therapy for significant valvular disease requires surgical repair, or more commonly replacement. Mechanical valves are durable but require anticoagulation. Porcine tissue valves, when used in a young woman, usually require replacement during her lifetime. Reports of pregnancies associated with prosthetic valves suggest significant variability in outcomes. Table 34-2 summarizes a review of 151 pregnancies complicated by a prosthetic valve.[28] Mechanical valves and anticoagulation were associated with a moderate increase in miscarriage and thromboembolic events. A report from France of 55 pregnancies suggests a less favorable prognosis.[29] Mechanical valves were associated with a maternal mortality rate of 3.7 percent and a thromboembolic rate of 14.8 percent. Thromboembolism was increased fourfold with heparin use rather than warfarin. Mitral valves accounted for 81 percent of thrombotic complications.

The impact of pregnancy on the life of a porcine valve has been studied.[28] Ten-year graft survival following two pregnancies was 16.7 percent compared with 54.8 percent following a single pregnancy. Therefore, pregnancy seems to adversely affect the life of a porcine valve.

Decisions surrounding the timing and choice of valve replacement for a woman of reproductive age are complex. Managing a pregnancy with moderate valve disease may be less complicated than managing a pregnancy with a prosthetic valve. The durability of a mechanical valve has considerable advantages for a young person, but it is associated with more adverse outcomes in pregnancy. Delay in valve replacement until childbearing is completed is appropriate when the severity of heart disease is believed to be manageable in pregnancy.

Anticoagulation is required with a mechanical valve. Oral anticoagulation with warfarin in the first trimester

Table 34-2. Pregnancy Outcomes with Prosthetic Valves

	MECHANICAL	PORCINE
Women	31	57
Pregnancies	56	95
Fetal loss	27.7%	12.3%
Premature birth	5.9%	7.7%
Valve deterioration	5.3%	7.0%
Thromboembolic event	5.3%	—

is associated with congenital anomalies; and potentially serious fetal bleeding may be encountered with use during the second and third trimesters. The American College of Cardiology/American Heart Association guidelines recommend consideration of heparin in the first trimester to avoid warfarin embryopathy, and the use of warfarin until 36 weeks, when subcutaneous heparin is substituted until after delivery.[15] These recommendations remain controversial in that they may underestimate the risk of fetal intracerebral bleeding in the absence of labor.[30] The fetus exposed to warfarin in the second and third trimesters is at risk for developmental toxicity. Individual patients should be counseled regarding the risks of either strategy and participate actively in a final choice of therapy. If heparinization is chosen, the activated partial thromboplastin time (aPTT) should be increased to two to three times control at middosing interval. Intravenous heparin can be administered on an ambulatory basis and should be considered for mitral valves, which are more likely to clot, and for patients who may be noncompliant with subcutaneous administration. Women treated for prolonged periods with heparin should be counseled regarding the risk of osteoporosis. Maternal platelet counts should be followed to screen for the development of HIT, heparin induced thrombocytopenia. If HIT is diagnosed, heparin must be discontinued immediately and anticoagulation maintained with other agents.

Successful thrombolytic therapy of a clotted valve in pregnancy has been reported.[31,32] Although significant uterine bleeding has been occasionally encountered, fibrinolysis is safer for the fetus than emergent valve replacement, However, thrombolytics carry a risk of maternal thromboembolic events.

CONGENITAL HEART DISEASE

Congenital heart disease is present in 0.7 to 1 percent of live births, accounting for as many as 30 percent of infants with birth anomalies. Before the development of corrective surgery, many children died shortly after birth or in childhood. In 1939, the first patent ductus arteriosus (PDA) was ligated. In 1945, the first Blalock Taussig shunt was performed for palliation of cyanotic heart disease. In 1953, cardiac bypass was introduced. Introduction of surgery under hypothermia in the late 1960s permitted longer and more complex repairs.[33,34] Of children who survived surgery to correct tetralogy of Fallot between 1955 and 1960, the 23-year survival is 86 percent, approaching the expected survival rate of 96 percent for normal children.[35] Before the 1960s, rheumatic heart disease was more common in pregnancy than congenital heart disease by a ratio of 4:1. By the 1980s, the ratio was 1:1.[27] Currently, congenital disease is now estimated to exceed rheumatic disease by 4:1. Although most enter pregnancy with known heart disease, some women have their disease first recognized due to the hemodynamic demands of pregnancy.

Increased survival of children with congenital disease has created a population of young women with complex medical and psychosocial conditions entering their child bearing years. Those whose congenital heart disease was diagnosed in infancy have frequently experienced multiple cardiothoracic surgeries and extended hospitalizations. They have lived with continued concerns from parents and health care professionals regarding their ongoing health problem. Their childhoods have been restricted. At an early age, they faced the possibility of their own death. The psychosocial impact of this experience has been described as "growing up heart sick."[36] These young women describe a childhood of overprotectiveness and "being watched." They also describe a lack of information regarding childbearing and contraception. They "seemed to believe that someone else could and would decide whether they should become pregnant."[36] Body image disorders over eternal skinniness, scars from surgery, and delayed development of secondary sex characteristics are common. Health care providers should strive to (1) objectively share information regarding reproductive health care, (2) direct decision making toward the patient rather than toward parents and health care professionals, and (3) improve self-esteem and body image. As stated by Murphy et al.,[36] "Women with congenital heart disease want some way of being normal in their lives. Helping them to gain knowledge so that they can make responsible choices concerning contraception, pregnancy, and childbearing may be a way of assisting them to regain normalcy through feelings that they have control of their own bodies and lives." When treating congenital heart disease during pregnancy, one must be willing to acknowledge and address the impact of the patient's disease on her life.

Table 34-3 summarizes the distribution of congenital heart disease in childhood and in pregnancy.[27,34] The spontaneous closure of lesions such as ventricular septal defect (VSD) and correction of patent ductus are reflected by reduced reporting in pregnancy. The increased reporting of aortic stenosis in pregnancy is probably due to a worsening of disease with age and the ease of recognition during pregnancy. The complexity and diversity of congenital heart disease confounds our ability to describe the prognosis or a management plan for the breadth of conditions. Major risks in pregnancy include (1) cyanosis, (2) left (or systemic) ventricular dysfunction, and (3) pulmonary hypertension, particularly with right ventricular dysfunction.

Outcomes have been most clearly described based on the presence or absence of maternal cyanosis.

Table 34-3. Incidence of Congenital Heart Defects in Childhood and in Pregnancy

	CHILDHOOD (%)	PREGNANCY (%)
Ventricular septal defect	35	13
Atrial septal defect	9	9
Patent ductus arteriosus	8	2.7
Pulmonary stenosis	8	8
Aortic stenosis	6	20
Coarctation of the aorta	6	8
Tetralogy of Fallot	5	12
Transposition of the great vessels	4	5.4

Table 34-4. Neonatal Outcome with Congenital Heart Disease: Liveborn Versus Termination

	LIVEBORN INFANT (%)	TERMINATION (%)
Noncyanotic	86	5
Cyanotic	85	26
Corrected	95	17
Palliative	87	17
Uncorrected	71	42

$$\text{Termination rate} = \frac{\text{No. of terminations}}{\text{No. of pregnancies}}$$

$$\text{Live-born rate} = \frac{\text{No. of live-born infants}}{\text{No. of pregnancies} - \text{No. of terminations}}$$

Table 34-5. Neonatal Outcome with Congenital Heart Disease by SAB, SGA, Preterm, and Birth Weight

	SAB (%)	SGA (%)	PRETERM (%)	BIRTH WEIGHT
Noncyanotic	12	6	9	3,300 ± 600
Cyanotic	21	52	35	2,400 ± 800
Corrected	11	25	0	
Uncorrected/ palliative	25	67	53	

Preterm, preterm birth; SAB, spontaneous abortion; SGA, small for gestational age.

Table 34-4 is derived from a report of 482 pregnancies from 233 women with congenital heart disease who delivered between 1968 and 1982.[13] The rate of terminations was higher in the group of women with cyanotic heart disease and particularly high (42 percent) in those with uncorrected lesions. This reflects the anticipated poor neonatal outcome and maternal risks associated with uncorrected cyanotic disease. It is likely that patients with more severe disease are overly represented in the group of women who chose to terminate, which would bias the group who continued pregnancy toward a better outcome. Eighty-six to 90 percent of pregnancies without cyanosis ended in a live birth compared with 71 percent an uncorrected lesion. Given an expected baseline rate of miscarriage, these outcomes are good. Corrected cyanotic disease was associated with outcomes comparable to noncyanotic disease. Table 34-5 is derived from a report of 144 pregnancies from women with congenital heart disease delivered between 1976 and 1986.[27] Adverse outcomes are again concentrated among women with uncorrected cyanotic heart disease.

Common maternal complications include congestive heart failure and pulmonary edema (4 percent), arrhythmia (4 percent), and hypertension (6 percent). Congestive heart failure and hypertension were commonly associated with uncorrected left ventricular outflow obstruction.[13,27] Arrhythmias were observed after surgery in and around atrial or ventricular septa. Maternal death was uncommon, 0 per 482 pregnancies in one series[13] and 1 per 144 pregnancies in a second.[27] Maternal deaths are most commonly reported in association with Eisenmenger's syndrome, which is discussed more fully later.

Men and women with congenital heart disease are at increased risk for having children with congenital heart disease. In a prospective study with aggressive pediatric evaluation, Whittemore[13] estimated the incidence to be as high as 14.2 percent. In a retrospective study, Rose found the risk to be 8.8 percent.[12] The rate of congenital heart disease associated with an affected mother is 2 to 3.5 times that observed with an affected father. Specific parental defects are not generally associated with the same defect in the child. The risk for cardiac maldevelopment is inherited rather than the risk for a specific defect. The risk of congenital heart disease and the character of the risk should be discussed with an affected mother. In Whittemore's report, 58 of 60 affected infants were diagnosed with relatively benign correctable lesions (atrial septal defect, VSD, pulmonary stenosis, aortic stenosis, patent ductus arteriosis, or mitral valve prolapse). Only two infants from 372 pregnancies (0.5 percent) were diagnosed with complex congenital heart disease.[13] Gill et al.[14] examined the recurrence pattern of congenital heart disease in 6640 pregnancies for whom fetal echocardiography was obtained due to a family history of congenital heart disease. The recurrence rate was 2.9 percent (95 percent confidence interval (CI), 2 to 4 percent) for mothers with congenital heart disease, a rate lower than reported by others. However, the study is limited to diagnoses established by fetal echocardiography and, therefore, may underrepresent the true incidence of abnormalities. The type and severity of cardiac defect seen in the mother did not predict the type or severity of cardiac defect in the offspring, with a few exceptions. Atrioventricular canal defects, especially those associated with situs abnormalities had a highly concordant recurrence rate.[14] All women who have congenital heart disease should undergo fetal echocardiographic examination at midpregnancy.

Contraceptive counseling should be offered to all women with congenital heart disease. Given the problems experienced growing up with heart disease, contraceptive education should probably be initiated as part of general health care education, before the overt need for birth control. In the context of congenital heart disease, complications associated with pregnancy are usually greater than those associated with any form of birth control. Cyanosis, pulmonary hypertension, low CO, dilated cardiac chambers, sluggish venous conduits (e.g., Fontan), and atrial fibrillation place patients at risk for thrombosis. This small group of women should probably avoid combined estrogen/progestin oral contraceptives. Progestin-only pills are not associated with risk for thrombosis but require regular dosing to achieve optimal efficacy. Parenteral progestins are safe for women with cardiac disease and are extremely effective. They do cause irregular bleeding, which may be significant if the patient is anticoagulated. The intrauterine device may be a suitable choice for some women with congenital heart lesions. It does carry a risk for pelvic inflammatory disease and therefore a theoretical risk of bacteremia and endocarditis. However, the actual risk has been estimated to be 1 per 1 million patient-years.[37]

ISOLATED SEPTAL DEFECTS

Ventricular and atrial septal defects represent greater than 40 percent of congenital heart disease identified in childhood. Many defects identified in children close with advancing age. In adulthood, 50 percent of large VSDs (>1.5 cm) lead to the development of Eisenmenger's syndrome. Ten percent of uncorrected atrial septal defects also develop pulmonary hypertension. The management of Eisenmenger's syndrome in pregnancy is discussed later.

A harsh systolic murmur that radiates to the left sternal border but not to the carotids suggests the presence of a VSD. The diagnosis can be confirmed by color flow Doppler echocardiography demonstrating a small, high-velocity lesion. The peak velocity of the jet across the septum can be used to assess the pressure gradient between the ventricles. A high velocity between ventricles indicates a large pressure gradient and low pressure in the right ventricle (RV), and the absence of pulmonary hypertension. In the absence of associated cardiac lesions and pulmonary hypertension, the presence of a VSD does not usually complicate pregnancy. Small defects create loud murmurs but are not usually hemodynamically significant. The high-velocity jet of a small lesion does create a risk for endocarditis.

Atrial septal defects are more difficult to diagnose by auscultation. The characteristic finding, a split S_2 that is fixed with respiration, is subtle and usually not appreciated without specific attention. Increased right-sided flow secondary to shunting across the defect may create a flow murmur that will be augmented in pregnancy. Other endocardial cushion defects may be associated with ostium primum defects. In the absence of other anomalies, the significance of the atrial septal defect is related to its size rather than to its etiology. Hemodynamically significant defects result in significant shunting from the systemic circulation to the pulmonary circulation. As with the VSD, Eisenmenger's syndrome may develop but usually at an older age. Increased pulmonary blood flow may result in dyspnea on exertion and restriction of activity. Atrial arrhythmias are commonly associated with atrial enlargement or intrinsic conduction abnormalities in the case of ostium primum defects.

Piesiewicz et al.[38] reported 54 pregnancies from women with secundum atrial septal defect. Impaired functional status (NHYA class III or IV) increased from 5.5 percent in the second trimester to 11.1 percent in the third trimester. Although left-to-right shunting was present in all patients in the second trimester, three patients (5.5 percent) developed bidirectional shunting in the third trimester. One additional patient reversed her shunt. Right ventricular (RV) diameter and systolic pulmonary artery pressure increased from the second to third trimester (34.1 ± 8.4 mm Hg to 39.1 ± 12.2 mm Hg). Over the same time frame, pulmonary flow (Q_p)/systemic flow (Q_s) decreased. Increased flow associated with pregnancy seems to adversely affect right ventricular function and pulmonary pressures. The fall in Q_p/Q_s suggests that the rise in pulmonary pressure is due to increased pulmonary vascular resistance. The authors also reported supraventricular arrythmias in 50 percent of women in the third trimester.

The patient with a significant pulmonary/systemic shunt ratio can be expected to normally expand her CO during pregnancy. However, the price of a normal systemic CO is a high pulmonary flow. The pregnant patient may begin to experience symptoms at rest that she previously noted with exercise. She may also experience an increase in tachyarrhythmias. HR control with a β-blocker may provide symptomatic relief. Early diuresis may benefit the patient postpartum. Elevated pulmonary blood flow associated with pregnancy could accelerate the progression of pulmonary vascular disease. In the absence of associated anomalies, arrhythmias, and pulmonary hypertension, the presence of an atrial septal defect does not usually complicate pregnancy.

PATENT DUCTUS ARTERIOSIS

The diagnosis of a patent ductus arteriosis is suggested by the characteristic continuous murmur at the upper left sternal border. Most are identified and ligated in childhood. Of patients with an uncorrected patent ductus, as many as 50 percent develop Eisenmenger's syndrome, the majority in childhood. In adults with a small patent ductus, the major risk is endocarditis. In the absence of Eisenmenger's syndrome, pregnancy is not usually complicated. As with the atrial septal defect, the increase in pulmonary blood flow associated with the increase in CO in pregnancy may result in increased dyspnea with exertion and at rest. Early diuresis may benefit the patient postpartum.

TETRALOGY OF FALLOT

Tetralogy of Fallot is a syndrome of abnormalities due to maldevelopment of the truncus arteriosus characterized by (1) right ventricular outflow tract obstruction, (2) VSD, (3) overriding aorta, and (4) right ventricular hypertrophy. Tetralogy of Fallot is the most common cyanotic congenital heart disease, and it was among the first to be successfully surgically palliated by Blalock and Taussig in 1945 and subsequently physiologically repaired. Therefore, a significant number of adults with congenital heart disease have repaired Tetralogy of Fallot. The severity of the clinical presentation in infancy is dependent on the degree of outflow tract obstruction. More severe obstruction leads to more significant cyanosis and right-to-left shunting. Surgical repair generally includes closure of a VSD and relief of right ventricular outflow tract obstruction. Some patients with repaired Tetralogy of Fallot have near-normal cardiac physiology, but many have residual lesions that may complicate pregnancy.

Patients with significant cyanosis at birth often had palliative Blalock-Taussig shunts in infancy using the subclavian artery to connect the systemic circulation with the pulmonary circulation, thus increasing pulmonary blood flow and reducing cyanosis. As a consequence, blood pressures in the arm supplied by the transected artery may not be reflective of aortic pressure. Patients should be asked if one arm is unreliable for blood pressure measurements, or examined to look for evidence of a thoracotomy scar resulting from the Blalock-Taussig shunt.

Efforts to correct the right ventricular outflow tract obstruction may result in incomplete relief and persistent pulmonary stenosis. More often, significant pulmonary insufficiency is a consequence of the transannular patch approach used to enlarge the outflow tract and valve. Several studies have demonstrated that women with severe pulmonary insufficiency and right ventricular dysfunction are more likely to have complications with pregnancy. Veldtman and colleagues[39] reported a series of 43 women with Tetralogy of Fallot who had 112 pregnancies. Five percent experienced cardiac complications: supraventricular tachycardia (two), heart failure (two), pulmonary embolism associated with pulmonary hypertension (one), and progressive RV dilation (one).

Tetralogy of Fallot is often well tolerated during pregnancy. Preconceptual evaluation should include assessment of right and left ventricular function, severity of pulmonary insufficiency, and stenosis, with consideration for repair of severe pulmonary insufficiency before pregnancy, if appropriate.

TRANSPOSITION OF THE GREAT VESSELS

Transposition of the great vessels (TGV) is present in only 5 percent of pregnant women with congenital heart disease but is overrepresented in the publication of case reports and case series. In complete TGV, systemic venous blood returns to the right atrium, and passes through the tricuspid valve, into the RV, and directly into the transposed aorta. Although an adequate circulation for fetal life, infants decompensate at birth owing to an inadequate pulmonary circulation. Some will have a sufficiently large VSD to achieve adequate pulmonary blood flow and oxygenation; others will require an immediate palliative procedure, an atrial septostomy.

TGV was first definitively corrected in 1964 with the Mustard operation.[40] A baffle is constructed through the left and right atriums so that systemic venous return is channeled through the mitral valve into the left ventricle, and pulmonary venous return is directed through the tricuspid valve into the RV. With a modest surgical intervention, the right and left pumps are placed in series with physiologic flow of systemic venous return through the pulmonary circulation. The RV, as the systemic ventricle, must work against systemic resistance, and the tricuspid valve is exposed to systemic pressures. Long-term complications are associated with failure of the systemic ventricle and arrhythmia. Of patients surviving the first 30 days after repair, 90 percent will be alive in 10 years and 87 percent will be alive in 20 years. After 13 years, only 5 percent suffer significant disability (NYHA class II to IV).[41] A more physiologic repair can be achieved when transposition is accompanied by a VSD. The ventricular septum is reconstructed so that the aortic outflow tract lies within the left ventricle and a conduit is constructed to connect the RV to the pulmonary artery (Rastelli repair).[42] The pulmonary conduit is prone to stenosis and deterioration of the transplanted valve. More recently, a direct surgical switch between the pulmonary artery and the aorta has been performed. Given the time when these operations were introduced, fewer young women entering pregnancy will have a Mustard repair. Increasing numbers will have a great vessel switch.

The hemodynamic changes of pregnancy will have a mixed impact on a patient with a Mustard repair. Increased CO increases the volume load on the right heart. Decreased vascular resistance reduces afterload on the right side of the heart. The box "Pregnancy Outcomes with Transposition of the Great Vessels" summarizes nine papers reporting a total of 49 pregnancies in 36 women.[27,41,43–49] No maternal mortality was reported. Neonatal outcomes were generally good. Two women entered pregnancy with disability due to their heart disease (NYHA class III to IV). One delivered at 26 weeks due to preterm labor. The other developed severe congestive heart failure near term and died 19 months postpartum. Congestive heart failure was frequently associated with uncontrolled tachyarrhythmias.

Guedes et al.[50] have reported echocardiographic findings of 16 women with a Mustard repair completing 28 pregnancies. Mean gestational age at delivery was 38.1 ± 1.5 weeks, with a mean birth weight of 3,040 ± 540 g. In four of 21 pregnancies, right ventricular function deteriorated. In three of the four patients, function did not return to baseline conditions. Although concerning, the authors noted that the rate of deterioration was not clearly different than a cohort who did not get pregnant.

Congenitally corrected TGV (ventricular inversion) is characterized by the passage of systemic venous blood into the right atrium, directly into the left ventricle, and out through the transposed pulmonary artery. Pulmonary venous return passes directly from the left atrium into the RV and out through the aorta. The RV again serves as the systemic ventricle. Congenitally corrected TGV may be an isolated anomaly but may also be associated with other anomalies that result in cyanosis. See box for summary of two series of pregnancies with congenitally corrected TGV.[51,52] Again, maternal and neonatal outcomes are good. Consistent with outcomes associated with other cyanotic forms of congenial heart disease, miscarriage and premature birth are concentrated among the cyanotic lesions.

Young women with surgically or congenitally corrected TGV can be expected to successfully complete pregnancy. Women who are functionally impaired or who

Pregnancy Outcomes with Transposition of the Great Vessels

Women	36
Pregnancies	49
Live births	41 (84%)
Miscarriages	5
Terminations	2
Fetal deaths	1
Premature birth <35 weeks	5 (12%)
Congenital heart disease	0 (0%)
Congestive heart failure	6 (15%)
Arrhythmia	8 (20%)

Pregnancy Outcomes with Congenitally Corrected Transposition of the Great Vessels

Women	41
Cyanotic	4 (10%)
Pregnancies	105
Cyanotic	13 (12%)
Live births	77 (73%)
Miscarriages*	22
Terminations	6
Fetal deaths	1
Premature birth <35 weeks*	6 (8%)
Congenital heart disease	1 (1%)
Congestive heart failure	5 (6%)
Cerebrovascular accident	1 (1%)

*Miscarriages and premature births concentrated among cyanotic mothers.

are cyanotic before pregnancy can expect more adverse outcomes and may deteriorate postpartum. Evaluation before pregnancy should include assessment of functional status; evaluation of right, systemic, heart function; and confirmation of normal oxygenation. When the right side of the heart is the systemic heart, pharmacologic afterload reduction should be maintained until pregnancy is confirmed. Angiotensin-converting enzyme inhibitors should be discontinued early in the first trimester.

The reported experience with TGV is to date the most extensive for any complex defect. The conclusions drawn from this experience are probably applicable to other less common conditions. Functional status and cyanosis are the most reliable predictors of complicated pregnancies. Arrhythmia is common and is frequently the cause of cardiac decompensation.

FONTAN REPAIR

The Fontan repair was initially performed to achieve a physiologic correction of tricuspid atresia by connecting the right atrium directly to the pulmonary artery.[53] The Fontan repair and subsequent modifications are currently used to correct a variety of complex congenital heart conditions characterized by a single functional ventricle. The repair achieves a noncyanotic, functional flow of systemic venous return through the lungs and a functionally systemic ventricle. Without a pulmonary pump, the cardiac price for this result is intolerance of increased intrathoracic pressure and elevated systemic and right atrial pressure if left ventricular end-diastolic or left atrial pressures increase.

Experience with pregnancy in women with the Fontan repair is limited. Young women have been discouraged from attempting pregnancy because of concerns regarding the ability of a single ventricle system to adapt to the demands of pregnancy. In a survey of 76 women of reproductive age, Canobbio et al.[54] reported that 66 percent were counseled not to become pregnant despite a stable surgical outcome and a strong desire to have children. The remaining 34 percent were not counseled regarding pregnancy. Contraceptive usage, despite counseling against pregnancy, was inconsistent. The box "Pregnancy Outcomes with Fontan Repair" summarizes the outcomes of 33 pregnancies from 21 women reported by this group. Although the miscarriage rate was higher than the general population, the preterm birth rate was low. Maternal complications were limited to arrhythmia, usually atrial, and congestive heart failure in the postpartum period. Although not reported in these small series, sluggish flow through the right atrial and pulmonary circulation may increase the risk for thrombosis. The incidence of pulmonary emboli in nonpregnant patients with Fontan circulation may be as high as 17 percent.

Pregnancy Outcomes with Fontan Repair

Women	21
Pregnancies	33
Live births	15 (45%)
Miscarriages	13
Terminations	5
Fetal deaths	0
Premature birth <35 weeks	1 (7%)
Congenital heart disease	1 (7%)
Congestive heart failure	1 (7%)
Arrhythmia	2 (15%)

EISENMENGER'S SYNDROME

The pathophysiology known as Eisenmenger's syndrome was first described in 1897. Vicktor Eisenmenger described a 32-year-old patient who was short of breath and cyanotic from childhood and died from hemoptysis. Autopsy revealed a VSD and severe pulmonary vascular disease.[55] The term is now used to describe pulmonary-to-systemic shunting associated with cyanosis and increased pulmonary pressures secondary to pulmonary vascular disease. Eisenmenger's syndrome may develop from any intracardiac shunt resulting in blood from the high-pressure systemic circulation being directed into the pulmonary circulation. Systemic pressure and excessive flow lead to microvascular injury, obliteration of pulmonary arterioles and capillaries, and in the end, elevated pulmonary vascular resistance. The time to onset of shunt reversal is variable, but most patients who have a large VSD or large patent ductus arteriosus develop shunt reversal in infancy. Those who have an atrial septal defect are delayed until early adulthood. Survival at 10 years from diagnosis is 80 percent; at 25 years, it is 42 percent.[55]

Patients with Eisenmenger's syndrome are at risk for congestive heart failure, hemoptysis due to pulmonary hemorrhage, sudden death due to arrhythmia, cerebrovascular accident, and hyperviscosity syndrome. The diagnosis should be considered in any cyanotic patient and is confirmed by echocardiography with the demonstration of increased pulmonary pressure and an intracardiac shunt. If the shunt is due to an atrial septal defect or a PDA, transesophageal examination may be necessary to establish the diagnosis. Treatment is nonspecific, and includes supportive care and avoidance of destabilizing events such as surgery and unnecessary medications. Symptomatic hyperviscosity syndrome due to an elevated hematocrit can be treated with hydration and, if necessary, phlebotomy. Iron deficiency, preexisting or secondary to phlebotomy, can exacerbate hyperviscosity; microcytic cells are less deformable and therefore more prone to occlude the microcirculation. Definitive therapy can be achieved only with heart/lung or lung transplantation. However, the 4-year survival with lung transplantation is less than 50 percent, a less favorable prognosis than that for many patients with Eisenmenger's syndrome.

VSD, atrial septal defect, and PDA are responsible for 89 percent of reported cases of Eisenmenger's syndrome in pregnancy.[56] Each lesion is initially associated with shunting from the systemic, oxygenated circulation to the pulmonary circulation. As pulmonary vascular resistance and pulmonary pressures increase over time and approach systemic pressures, the characteristic murmurs of a VSD or PDA diminish. Reversal of flow from the right to the left, the development of hypoxemia, and increasing hematocrit herald the development of Eisenmenger's syndrome. The fall in SVR associated with pregnancy may initiate shunt reversal in a patient not previously cyanotic.

In 1979, Gleicher reviewed published cases of Eisenmenger's syndrome in pregnancy.[57] Seventy pregnancies from 44 women were evaluated. Fifty-two percent of the women died during pregnancy. Thirty percent of the pregnancies resulted in maternal death. The risk of death associated with first, second, and third pregnancies were 36 percent, 27 percent, and 33 percent, respectively. A first successful pregnancy did not confirm the safety of subsequent pregnancies. Most deaths (70 percent) occurred at the time of delivery or within 1 week postpartum. Excessive blood loss was associated with 35 percent of deaths, whereas thromboembolic conditions were responsible for 44 percent. Maternal mortality associated with cesarean delivery (80 percent) exceeded that associated with vaginal delivery (34 percent). Maternal death was not reported with first-trimester termination of pregnancy. Only 26 percent of pregnancies resulted in a term birth. Fifty-five percent of newborns were delivered preterm, and 32 percent were small for gestational age.

A more modern review of cases in the United Kingdom between 1991 and 1995 confirms the poor prognosis for pregnant women with Eisenmenger's syndrome despite considerable advancement in the management of cardiac disease in pregnancy.[58] Mortality remains extremely high; 40 percent of the women died. In addition, 85 percent of the births were preterm. A review of published cases from 1978 to 1996 again confirmed a mortality rate of 36 percent.[58] The majority of deaths (96 percent) occurred within the first 35 days postpartum. Late diagnosis (relative risk [RR], 5.4) and delayed hospitalization significantly increased maternal mortality.[58]

Although the risks associated with Eisenmenger's syndrome in pregnancy are clear, appropriate management is controversial. Decreased activity, hospital observation, and oxygen supplementation are usually employed. Reduction of pulmonary pressures and improved systemic oxygen saturation after oxygen supplementation indicate that pulmonary vascular resistance is not fixed and suggest a better prognosis. Intercurrent antepartum events such as pneumonia or urinary tract infection are poorly tolerated. Preventing microcytosis with iron supplementation may decrease the risk of microvascular slugging.

Cesarean delivery is reserved for obstetric indications and is avoided whenever possible. Hemodynamic stability must be maintained during labor and the postpartum period. When pulmonary vascular resistance is not fixed, oxygen supplementation may decrease pulmonary pressures. Systemic hypotension from hemorrhage or sympathectomy from epidural analgesia results in increased right-to-left shunting, increasing hypoxemia, increasing pulmonary vascular resistance, and worsening shunt. Volume overload or excessive systemic resistance, particularly postpartum, may further tax the failing right side of the heart. A pulmonary artery catheter and a peripheral arterial catheter are usually used to guide hemodynamic management. Narcotic-based regional analgesia provides adequate pain relief without excessive hemodynamic instability. Anticoagulation remains controversial. If patients are anticoagulated, caution should be exercised to avoid excessive treatment and associated hemorrhage.

Although use of a selective pulmonary vasodilator, inhaled nitric oxide, has been reported to reduce pulmonary pressures, increase CO, and improve systemic oxygenation, maternal death was not averted.[59] Use of sildenafil and L-arginine has been reported with apparent hemodynamic benefit and the survival of a single patient.[60] Unlike many cardiac conditions in pregnancy, meticulous care frequently fails to prevent maternal death.

COARCTATION OF THE AORTA

Coarctation of the aorta results from a constriction of the aorta at or about the level of the ductus arteriosus or left subclavian artery. Patients have a characteristic discrepancy in blood pressure between their right arm and lower extremities. Complications include dissection at the site of coarctation, rupture of associated berry aneurysms, and cerebrovascular accidents, heart failure, and ischemic heart disease associated with cephalic hypertension.

Modern reports of coarctation in pregnancy are limited. Historically, pregnancy was associated with a maternal mortality of 9 percent owing to aortic rupture, congestive heart failure, cerebrovascular accidents, and endocarditis.[61] β-Blockade may serve to protect against dissection and promote diastolic flow through the aortic narrowing.

Pediatric screening identifies most significant coarctations leading to repair. After repair, systemic hypertension may persist and require treatment. In a series of 18 patients and 36 pregnancies, the prematurity rate was not elevated. Preeclampsia was diagnosed in 14 percent of all pregnancies and 17 percent of nulliparous pregnancies. One infant in 36 was diagnosed with congenital heart disease.[62]

An increasing cohort of young women with corrected congenital heart disease will be presenting to their obstetricians pregnant and desiring to bear children. Some basic conclusions can be drawn from our experience with congenital heart disease to date. First, Eisenmenger's syndrome and pregnancy remain a lethal combination. New, effective strategies for therapy are not anticipated. Second, cyanotic heart disease in the absence of pulmonary hypertension is associated with increased rates of miscarriage and preterm birth. Third, mothers with cardiac disability (NYHA class III to IV) or with evidence of right heart dilation have a more complicated course in pregnancy. Fourth, arrhythmias may become worse in pregnancy and precipitate cardiac decompensation. Aggressive pharmacologic treatment is appropriate. Finally, many young women who are initially well compensated and acyanotic can have successful pregnancies.

CARDIOMYOPATHY

Dilated cardiomyopathy is characterized by the development of pulmonary edema in the context of left ventricular dysfunction and dilation. Patients usually present with signs and symptoms of pulmonary edema: dyspnea, cough, orthopnea, tachycardia, and occasionally, hemoptysis. These symptoms of pulmonary edema, although characteristic of heart failure, may also be due to previously undiagnosed congenital or rheumatic heart disease, preeclampsia, embolic disease, intrinsic pulmonary disease, tocolytic use, or sepsis. The diagnosis of cardiomyopathy is made in the clinical circumstances of characteristic signs and symptoms and findings of left ventricular dysfunction and dilation on echocardiographic examination. Ventricular dysfunction may be due to conditions extrinsic to the heart such as thyrotoxicosis or hypertension or due to intrinsic myocardial dysfunction. Accurate diagnosis directs appropriate therapy and permit assessment of long-term prognosis.

Peripartum cardiomyopathy is a rare syndrome of heart failure presenting in late pregnancy or postpartum. The diagnosis is made after excluding other causes of pulmonary edema and heart failure. Failure to adhere to a rigorous definition of disease in the literature confounds conclusions regarding etiology and prognosis. A definition based on criteria for idiopathic dilated cardiomyopathy has been suggested (see the box "Diagnostic Criteria for Peripartum Cardiomyopathy").[63] The incidence is estimated to be between 1 in 1,300 and 1 in 15,000.[64] Although some of the variability in reported incidence is due to regional and ethnic differences, much is due to the imprecise definition of the disease. The cause of peripartum cardiomyopathy is unknown. Nutritional and immunologic mechanisms have been proposed. The prevalence of antibodies to echovirus and coxsackievirus is not higher among women with cardiomyopathy compared with controls.[65]

The mortality rate for peripartum cardiomyopathy is reported to be 25 to 50 percent. Death is usually due to progressive congestive heart failure, arrhythmia, or thromboembolism.[65] Within 6 months, half of patients demonstrate resolution of left ventricular dilation. Their prognosis is very good. Of those who do not, an 85 percent mortality rate can be expected within the next 4 to 5 years.[65] The magnitude of risk for subsequent pregnancies after peripartum cardiomyopathy is unclear. A recent survey of 67 pregnancies in 63 women suggests a mortality rate of 8 percent when left ventricular dysfunction has not resolved, and 2 percent in patients with normal function.[66]

Acute treatment of cardiomyopathy is directed at improving cardiac function and, when present, treating the inciting event. Diuretics are used to decrease preload and relieve pulmonary congestion. Digoxin may improve myocardial contractility and facilitate rate control when atrial fibrillation is present. Afterload reduction is achieved with angiotensin-converting enzyme inhibitors[67,68] postpartum, or hydralazine before delivery. β-Blockade in stable, euvolemic patients has been clearly demonstrated to improve cardiac function and survival outside of pregnancy,[69–71] and should not be withheld from pregnant women. Significantly dilated and hypokinetic cardiac chambers pose a risk for clot formation. Anticoagulation with heparin antepartum or warfarin postpartum should be considered. Implanted defibrillators have been used in pregnancy without significant complications.[72] Hemodynamic management during labor and delivery is frequently directed by a pulmonary artery catheter. Pain control decreases cardiac work and reduces tachycardia. A carefully dosed epidural is appropriate. Cesarean delivery is reserved for obstetric indications.

Diagnostic Criteria for Peripartum Cardiomyopathy

1. Heart failure within the last month of pregnancy or 5 months postpartum
2. Absence of prior heart disease
3. No determinable cause
4. Echocardiographic indication of left ventricular dysfunction
   - Ejection fraction <45 percent or fractional shortening <30 percent
   - Left ventricular end-diastolic dimension >2.7 cm/m²

MYOCARDIAL INFARCTION

Myocardial infarction is a rare event among women of reproductive age. From a population base of 3.6 million women-years, Petitti et al.[73] identified 186 cases (5.0 per 100,000 women-years). The incidence was very low before 35 years of age, (1 per 100,000 women-years) but increased to 5.3 for ages 35 to 39 and to 18.4 for ages 40 to 44. The risk for myocardial infarction in pregnancy from this population was 1.5 per 100,000 deliveries. Based on a 9-month exposure per pregnancy, the incidence is comparable to nonpregnant women younger than 35 years old.[73] Earlier estimates have been as high as 10 per 100,000 pregnancies.[74]

Owing to the rarity of the event, information regarding myocardial infarction in pregnancy is derived from case reports and, therefore, is subject to considerable reporting bias. Roth and Elkayam have summarized information from reports of 123 pregnancies (see the box "Myocardial Infarction in Pregnancy").[75] Coronary dissection and normal coronary arteries are observed in almost 50 percent of cases. Delivery within 2 weeks of infarction

Myocardial Infarction in Pregnancy	
Pregnancies	123
Mean age ± SD	32 ± 6 years
Age range	16–45 years
Anterior infarction	73%
Multiparous	84%
Hypertension	19%
Diabetes mellitus	5%
Smoking	26%
Family history of MI	8%
Hyperlipidemia	2%
Preeclampsia	11%
CHF after MI	19%
Coronary anatomy	
Stenosis	43%
Thrombus	21%
Dissection	16%
Aneurysm	4%
Spasm	1%
Normal	29%
Death	
Maternal	21%
Infant	13%*

CHF, congestive heart failure; MI, myocardial infarction; SD, standard deviation.
*62% of infant deaths associated with mother's death.

may be associated with maternal mortality as high as 50 percent. Myocardial infarction has been reported in association with diabetes mellitus, pheochromocytoma, Ehlers-Danlos type IV, antiphospholipid syndrome, multiple gestation, and sickle cell anemia.[75] Medications such as ergot alkaloids given for bleeding, bromcriptine for lactation suppression, ritodrine and nifedipine for tocolysis, and prostaglandin E_2 in conjunction with severe hypertension have also been associated with myocardial infarction.[76–83]

The diagnosis of myocardial infarction in pregnancy is often delayed due to the rarity of the event and due to common symptoms of pregnancy. During normal pregnancy, most women experience some increase in exercise intolerance and dyspnea. Chest pain due to reflux is common. Electrocardiographic changes that suggest ischemia have been reported in as many as 37 percent of women having a repeat cesarean delivery.[75] However, ST-segment elevation is not a normal finding and, in the context of ongoing chest pain, should markedly increase the suspicion of acute myocardial infarction. The MB fraction of creatinine kinase isoenzymes may be elevated at cesarean delivery as well.[84] Troponin I levels are not elevated during labor and delivery.[85] If confusion regarding the appropriate diagnosis exists in the context of a constellation of findings suggestive of myocardial infarction, an echocardiogram can be used to confirm abnormal wall motion in the ischemic region.

Acute therapy is based on rapid coronary reperfusion. Coronary angioplasty and stenting have been reported in pregnancy and should not be withheld when appropriate for the mother's condition.[86–89] Thrombolytic therapy has also been used in pregnancy.[75] Although effective, there may be a small but real incidence of associated maternal bleeding, preterm delivery, or fetal loss. Surgery after thrombolytic therapy is associated with significant risk for hemorrhage.

Medications commonly used in the management of myocardial infarction such as morphine, organic nitrates, lidocaine, β-blockers, aspirin, magnesium sulfate, and calcium antagonists may be used in appropriate doses in pregnancy. Care should be taken to avoid the supine position and maternal hypotension during procedures. The fetus, if viable, should be monitored.

Elective delivery within 2 weeks of infarction should be avoided because it is associated with an increased risk for maternal death. Cesarean delivery is reserved for obstetric indications. Labor and delivery is managed with standard cardiac care. Pain is controlled, usually with carefully administered regional analgesia. Tachycardia is prevented with pain control and treated with β-blockers as needed. Hemodynamic stability is maintained frequently using information from pulmonary and peripheral arterial catheters. Maternal pushing is avoided, and the second stage of labor is shortened with low forceps or vacuum. Diuresis is gently initiated postpartum with diuretics.

The experience with pregnancy after a remote myocardial infarction is limited. Of 33 reported cases, recurrent infarction and significant complications have not been reported.[90]

MARFAN'S SYNDROME

Marfan's syndrome is an autosomal dominant genetic disorder caused by an abnormal gene for fibrillin on chromosome 15.[91] Disease prevalence is estimated to be four to six per 10,000. Sporadic cases represent 15 percent of those diagnosed. The production of abnormal connective tissue results in the characteristic feature of the disease: aortic root dilation, dislocation of the optic lens, deformity of the anterior thorax, scoliosis, long limbs, joint laxity, and arachnodactyly. Diagnosis is usually based on family history, and physical examination, including ocular, cardiovascular, and skeletal features.

Untreated, life expectancy is reduced by a third, with the majority of deaths due to aortic dissection and rupture. Elective aortic repair is associated with a low mortality (1.5 percent), whereas emergent repair results in a much higher mortality (11.7 percent).[92] Therefore, elective repair has been recommended when the aortic root diameter measures 5.5 to 6.0 cm. Using an absolute aortic diameter (AD) as an indication for surgery ignores relevant differences in aortic size associated with patients of different stature.[93] These considerations are particularly important when caring for young women. An aortic ratio between measured and predicted AD can be calculated. The predicted diameter for young adults can be calculated: $AD_{predicted} = 1.02 + (0.98 \times \text{body surface area [BSA]})$. A ratio of less than 1.3 with a dilation rate of less than 5 percent/y suggests a low risk for a cardiovascular event.[93]

The risk for aortic dissection is associated with the rate of change of blood pressure in the aorta over time in systole. Although simple reduction in blood pressure does not reduce the risk for dissection, β-blockade lowers

Marfan's Syndrome in Pregnancy

Women	84
Pregnancies	241
Live births	181 (75%)
Miscarriages	38 (16%)
Terminations	17 (7%)
Fetal deaths	2 (0.8%)
Aortic events	8 (4.3%)
Dissection	6 (3.3%)*
Rapid dilation	2 (1.1%)*
Death	2 (1.1%)*

*Observed in patients with an aortic root diameter less than 4 cm.

the risk of reaching a clinical cardiac endpoint at 10 years from approximately 20 percent to 10 percent.[94]

Literature surveys of case reports suggest a maternal mortality rate associated with Marfan's syndrome in pregnancy in excess of 50 percent.[95] These case reports likely represent bias of reporting more severely affected pregnancies. Three population-based studies are summarized in the box "Marfan's Syndrome in Pregnancy."[96–98] Aortic events, dissection or rapid dilation, occurred in 8 percent of cases. In seven of nine, the AD was known to be greater than 4.0 cm. Of the remaining two, one died due to aortic dissection and rupture without a diagnosis and without a measurement of AD; the other had a prior graft replacement. A second death was due to endocarditis associated with mitral valve prolapse.

These studies suggest that women with mild disease, an AD less than 4.0 cm, can attempt pregnancy with only modest risk. The risk associated with more advanced disease is certainly greater. Given the data available, a precise risk of death from aortic dissection or rupture cannot be quantified. Women with ADs greater than 5.5 cm should certainly be counseled to have graft and valve replacement before pregnancy. They will then assume the risk associated with an artificial valve and the risk associated with the remaining aorta. These risks may be significant, however, adequate data do not exist to quantify the risk. Women with aortic roots greater than 4.0 cm but less than or equal to 5.5 cm are at significant risk, but aortic replacement may be premature. Fifty percent of the offspring of women with Marfan's syndrome should be expected to have the disease.

Management of pregnancies affected by Marfan's syndrome should begin with an accurate assessment of the aortic root. An absolute diameter or preferably an aortic ratio can be used to assess specific risk. The aortic root should be protected from hemodynamic forces with β-blockade. A resting HR of approximately 70 beats per minute can usually be achieved. Although β-blockade may potentially contribute to impaired fetal growth, this risk is outweighed by the maternal risk without such treatment.

Labor and delivery is managed with standard cardiac care, with particular emphasis on the prevention of tachycardia. Patients with aortic roots less than 4.0 cm can be delivered vaginally, reserving cesarean delivery for obstetric indications. Some authors have recommended cesarean delivery for women with larger roots based on concerns about increased pressure in the aorta during labor.[98] Data do not exist to make this a firm recommendation.

PULMONARY HYPERTENSION

Although pulmonary hypertension is fundamentally a pulmonary disease, the major pathologic impact is on the right side of the heart. The incidence of primary pulmonary hypertension is 1 to 2 per 1 million, with women affected more commonly than men.[99] Secondary pulmonary hypertension may develop as a complication of cardiac disease such as mitral stenosis or secondary to intrinsic pulmonary disease. Drugs such as cocaine or appetite suppressants may also be associated with pulmonary hypertension.[99] If left untreated, the median survival after diagnosis is 2.5 years.[100] Pulmonary vasodilator therapy with oral nifedipine or intravenous prostacyclin have improved this prognosis. Of those who initially respond to nifedipine, the 5-year survival is 95 percent.[101] The 5-year survival for those who require treatment with prostacyclin is 54 percent.[102] The maternal mortality with severe pulmonary hypertension is reported to be as high as 50 percent.[103–105] Sudden, irreversible deterioration in the postpartum period is common.[103,104,106]

The symptoms of pulmonary hypertension are nonspecific. Increasing fatigue and shortness of breath are associated with progressive right-sided heart failure but are also ubiquitous in pregnancy. They can easily be attributed to a presumed upper respiratory infection. Hoarseness may be present due to impingement on the laryngeal nerve by an enlarged pulmonary artery. Patients may exhibit disproportionate lower extremity edema or oxygen desaturation out of proportion for a presumed illness. The diagnosis can be confirmed with echocardiography, in which the velocity of the regurgitant jet across the tricuspid valve can estimate pulmonary systolic pressure. A dilated, hypokinetic RV with displacement of the intraventricular septum into the left ventricle suggests right-sided heart failure.

Pulmonary hypertension with right ventricular dysfunction is poorly tolerated in pregnancy. A mortality rate approaching 50 percent should be expected. Antepartum management often requires hospitalization. Oxygen therapy may reduce pulmonary vascular resistance and improve right ventricular performance. Pharmacologic treatment with nifedipine or intravenous prostacyclin may also be effective.[107] Anticoagulation with heparin should be considered. Worsening disease will usually be manifest by falling CO rather than rising right ventricular pressure. Labor and delivery should be managed with standard cardiac care, with particular attention to right ventricular filling as assessed by measurement of central venous pressure (CVP). Although the RV requires adequate filling to generate forward flow against an elevated pulmonary vascular resistance, modest elevations in CVP may precipitate increasing right ventricular dysfunction. Given fluid mobilization postpartum and the potential need to treat volume loss associated with delivery, appropriate filling may be difficult to achieve. Gentle diuresis may be required. Modest underloading or overloading of the RV can result in rapid decompensation and death.

Women with pulmonary hypertension and right ventricular dysfunction should be strongly discouraged from becoming pregnant. Because pulmonary artery pressures fall as the RV fails, the condition of the RV may be a more important consideration than an absolute systolic pulmonary pressure. Some women may consider pregnancy after a favorable response to treatment with nifedipine or prostacyclin. In a small series, two women whose pulmonary pressures and right ventricular function had normalized carried three pregnancies successfully while being treated with nifedipine or prostacyclin.[107] Neither experienced deterioration in their condition during the first year postpartum.

OTHER CONDITIONS

Young women may experience malignant ventricular arrhythmias due to idiopathic ventricular fibrillation, cardiomyopathy, long-QT syndrome, congenital heart disease, or hypertrophic cardiomyopathy. Implantable defibrillators can effectively protect them from sudden death. In a report of 44 pregnancies, no women experienced generator erosion or lead fractures due to the expanding pregnancy. Twenty-five percent experienced discharges during pregnancy without complication.[67]

Hypertrophic cardiomyopathy is a genetic condition usually inherited in an autosomal dominant pattern with variable penetrance. Although the condition can be subclassified, the physiologic impact of different forms is similar. Patients are at risk for failure and ischemia due to ventricular obstruction and arrhythmia. The ventricular septum hypertrophies such that the left ventricular outflow tracts is increasingly obstructed during systole. Although the impact of obstruction is similar to aortic valvular disease, the degree of obstruction is variable under different physiologic conditions. Reduced ventricular filling associated with blood loss, dehydration, or tachycardia increases the functional obstruction. Reviews of case reports suggest a maternal mortality rate of 1 to 2 percent in these cases.[108–110] Given the biases associated with case report-derived data, this estimate probably sets an upper limit of expected mortality. Thaman et al.[111] have reported 271 pregnancies in 127 women with hypertrophic cardiomyopathy, which were only complicated by two cases of pulmonary edema postpartum that resolved with appropriate therapy. In pregnancy, increased blood volume and left ventricular dimension will tend to benefit the patient. Increased HR will not. β-Blockers are generally used to manage tachycardia and some arrhythmias. Implantable defibrillators may also be used. Labor and delivery is managed with standard cardiac care, with particular emphasis to ensure generous left ventricular filling. Excessive volume loading may reveal a stiff ventricle and diastolic dysfunction. In some patients, a relatively small increase in vascular volume results in a substantial increase in pulmonary pressure, pulmonary congestion, and desaturation. Although diastolic dysfunction may be difficult to diagnose by echocardiography, careful attention to an O_2 saturation monitor during labor and postpartum can reveal the need for augmented diuresis. Supine hypotension must be carefully avoided, and obstetric bleeding should be treated early and aggressively with volume replacement.

CRITICAL CARE—HEMODYNAMIC MONITORING AND MANAGEMENT

Diseases unique to pregnancy, the physiologic stresses of pregnancy, and the special conditions surrounding labor and delivery operate to create circumstances in which intensive care may be necessary more frequently than would be required among young nonpregnant individuals. Specialists in intensive care may not be familiar with the physiology of pregnancy and associated unique conditions such as preeclampsia or amniotic fluid embolus. They may also be unfamiliar with maternal-fetal physiologic relationships and decision making that must balance the needs of the mother and the fetus. Therefore, obstetricians must be familiar with basic principles and techniques of critical care medicine in order to primarily manage critically ill pregnant women or to serve as valuable consultants to a critical care team.

Acute indications for invasive hemodynamic monitoring can be broadly categorized based on questions of physiology (see the box "Indications for Hemodynamic Monitoring"). Severe preeclampsia, sepsis, adult respiratory distress syndrome (ARDS), pneumonia, previously undiagnosed heart disease, and fluid management after resuscitation from obstetric hemorrhage are the most common conditions that require hemodynamic monitoring. Certain conditions, particularly maternal heart disease as discussed earlier, require a planned, prospective decision for invasive monitoring. In these cases, the

Indications for Hemodynamic Monitoring

1. **Why is the patient hypoxic?**
   - Are pulmonary capillary pressures high due to relative volume overload? (e.g., mitral stenosis postpartum)
   - Are pulmonary capillary pressures high due to depressed cardiac function? (e.g., cardiomyopathy)
   - Is capillary membrane integrity intact? (e.g., ARDS, pneumonia)
2. **Why is the patient persistently hypertensive?**
   - Is vascular resistance elevated?
   - Is cardiac output elevated?
3. **Why is the patient hypotensive?**
   - Is left ventricular filling pressure low? (e.g., after hemorrhage)
   - Is vascular resistance low? (e.g., septic shock)
4. **Why is the patient's urine output low?**
   - Is left ventricular filling pressure low resulting in low cardiac output?
5. **Is the patient expected to be unstable in labor?**
   - Is the window of left ventricular filling narrow? (e.g., aortic stenosis)
   - Will normal physiologic changes associated with delivery be tolerated poorly? (e.g., volume loading postpartum—mitral stenosis, pulmonary hypertension)

therapeutic window for hemodynamic management is narrow and knowledge of the patient's baseline, compensated hemodynamic status can serve as a goal for intrapartum management.

In many cases, initial therapy can and should be made empirically based on an understanding of the patient's pathophysiology. If subsequent interventions are needed, specific data obtained from hemodynamic monitoring may be required. Physicians with a large experience treating a particular disease may rely less on invasive monitoring as an improved understanding makes the clinical course more predictable. In contrast, physicians with less experience may have a lower threshold for using invasive hemodynamic monitoring. Therefore, understanding principles of management is particularly important for obstetricians who do not necessarily anticipate critically ill patients in their practice.

Hemodynamic Monitoring

The objective of hemodynamic monitoring is to provide continuous assessment of systemic and intracardiac pressures and to provide the means to determine CO and, therefore, to calculate systemic and pulmonary resistances. An arterial catheter is usually placed in the radial artery to measure systemic pressure. The diastolic pressure obtained usually correlates well with noninvasive measurements. Systolic pressure may be significantly higher than noninvasive measurements due to a very brief peak in pressure in early systole. (The spike in pressure contributes little to MAP.) The noninvasive measurement is usually more clinically relevant to the patient's condition. The arterial catheter permits easy access to arterial blood sampling and relieves the patient from the discomfort of frequent blood draws.

Measurement of intracardiac pressures and CO are obtained through the insertion of a catheter into the central venous circulation and advancement into and through the right side of the heart. Venous access is most commonly obtained through the right internal jugular vein; a subclavian approach may also be employed. Traditionally, insertion is guided by using the sternocleidomastoid muscle and the clavicle as landmarks. The higher frequency ultrasound transducer found on a vaginal probe can also be used to facilitate insertion under direct visualization. Once central venous access has been obtained and confirmed, a pulmonary artery catheter can be "floated" into the right side of the heart and pulmonary artery. Figure 34-6 demonstrates the waveforms and normal pressure values found as the catheter passes through the heart. Success in "floating" the catheter is initially confirmed by observation of characteristic waveforms in the RV, pulmonary artery, and wedged position, and subsequently with a radiograph. In experienced hands, complications from pulmonary artery catheterization are uncommon: pneumothorax (<0.1 percent), pulmonary infarction (0 to 1.3 percent), pulmonary artery rupture (<0.1 percent), and septicemia (0.5 to 2.0 percent).[112] Arrhythmias are usually transient and associated with passage of the catheter through the RV. If the patient has significant pulmonary hypertension, difficulty may

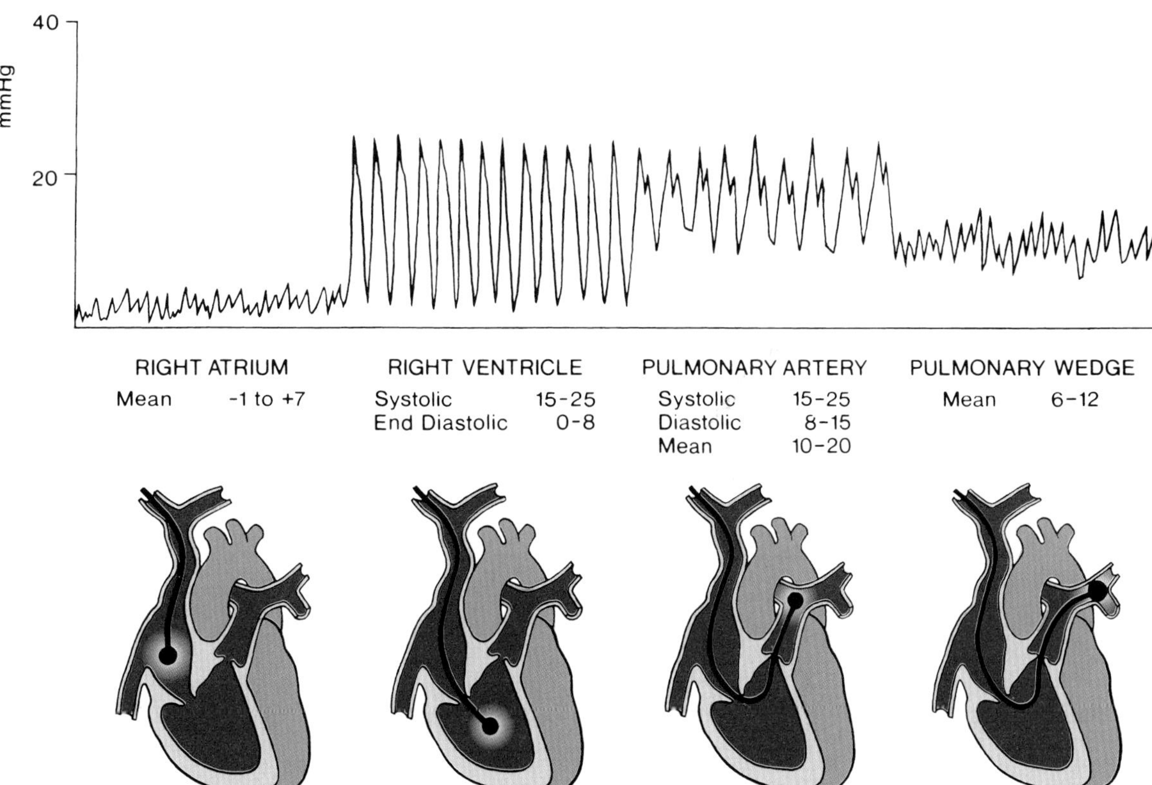

Figure 34-6. Hemodynamic waveforms and normal pressure values associated with catheter positions during advancement of a pulmonary artery catheter.

be encountered maintaining placement in the pulmonary artery.

Once the catheter has been successfully placed, continuous readings of CVP and pulmonary artery pressures can be obtained. By inflating the balloon at the catheter tip, the catheter can be wedged in the pulmonary artery to obtain a PAWP. PAWP reflects the filling pressure, preload, in the left ventricle. CVP measured in the right atrium is a measure of right ventricular filling pressure. In pregnant women, CVP cannot be assumed to accurately reflect left ventricular filling. Right atrial pressures and systolic pulmonary pressures can be measured noninvasively by echocardiography.

CO is measured by thermodilution. A bolus of cold fluid is injected into the right atrium, and a curve of temperature change over time is recorded as the bolus passes through the pulmonary artery. From the shape of the curve, CO can be calculated; when the CO is higher, the dilutional curve is shorter in time and greater in maximum temperature change. More recently, catheters have been equipped with a heating element in the right atrial segment so that continuous measurement of CO can be performed. CO can be measured noninvasively with Doppler and impedance techniques. Doppler technique has been validated under a wide range of clinical circumstances.[113–116] Impedance technique tends to underestimate CO in pregnancy but accurately reflects changes in hemodynamics in many conditions. In conditions of pathologically high flow, impedance may significantly underestimate CO.[117–119] Cardiac index (CI) can be derived from CO in order to adjust for maternal size: CI = CO/BSA. However, BSA does not seem to be related to CO in pregnancy; therefore, CO is usually preferred.[115] When CO is measured noninvasively and CVP is not available, resistance is expressed as TPR rather than SVR. In most clinical conditions, the differences between the two are not important.

Table 34-6 summarizes formulas used to calculate hemodynamic parameters not directly measured. Normal values for CO, MAP, HR, SV, and TPR are summarized in Figure 34-1. In a study of 10 normal pregnant women at term, Clark et al. determined that CVP, pulmonary artery pressure, PAWP, and left ventricular work index were not different from nonpregnant measurements made approximately 3 months postpartum.[120] The relationship between PAWP and left ventricular work index fell within the normal range for nonpregnant individuals, suggesting normal contractility in pregnancy. Pulmonary vascular resistance was 34 percent lower, and colloid osmotic pressure was reduced by 14 percent.

Hemodynamic Management

Strategies of hemodynamic therapy that may be applicable to a variety of clinical circumstances are discussed in this section. As outlined earlier, the use of hemodynamic monitoring should be directed at answering specific questions of maternal pathophysiology. Table 34-7 summarizes the most common clinical goals of therapy. To achieve each goal, a number of physiologic interventions are possible. Each of these interventions will precipitate a secondary or compensatory response. The secondary response, if excessive, may adversely affect the patient. The choice of intervention from available options will often be determined by the potential for and magnitude of adverse effect. Hemodynamic monitoring permits the physician to choose an intervention and subsequently assess the positive and negative effect.

Disruption of alveolar capillary fluid dynamics is frequently associated with acute oxygen desaturation due to excess alveolar fluid. Pulmonary edema is usually due to excess hydrostatic capillary pressure (e.g., cardiomyopathy, mitral stenosis) or to a disruption of alveolar capillary membrane integrity (e.g., pneumonia, ARDS). Although a reduction in serum oncotic pressure is rarely a primary cause of pulmonary edema, the reduced serum albumin level in normal pregnancy can act in synergy with other forces, resulting in earlier or more severe pulmonary edema than would normally occur.

The use of pulse oximetry facilitates the early detection of maternal desaturation. Oxygen supplementation improves maternal saturation but does not correct the underlying cause. If desaturation is progressive, further intervention will be required. In the normal heart, diuresis to reduce preload works to decrease alveolar water in patients with elevated PAWP and in patients with capillary leak. A reduction in capillary pressure from high normal to low normal will reduce the egress of water across damaged membranes. In many circumstances,

Table 34-6. Calculated Hemodynamic Variables

		CALCULATION	UNITS
Mean arterial pressure	MAP	$\frac{sBP + 2\ dBP}{3}$	mm Hg
Stroke volume	SV	$\frac{CO \cdot 1000}{HR}$	ml
Systemic vascular resistance	SVR	$\frac{(MAP - CVP) \cdot 80}{CO}$	dyne·sec·cm^{-5}
Total peripheral resistance	TPR	$\frac{MAP \cdot 80}{CO}$	dyne·sec·cm^{-5}
Pulmonary vascular resistance	PVR	$\frac{mPAP - PAWP}{CO}$	dyne·sec·cm^{-5}

CO, cardiac output; CVP, central venous pressure; dBP, diastolic blood pressure; mPAP, mean pulmonary artery pressure; PAWP, pulmonary artery wedge pressure; sBP, systolic blood pressure.

Table 34-7. Hemodynamic Interventions

CLINICAL GOAL	PHYSIOLOGICAL INTERVENTIONS	AGENTS	COMPENSATORY RESPONSE
↑ Oxygenation	↑ F_{IO_2}	O_2	
	↓ capillary pressure	Diuretic	↓ BP, ↓ CO
	↑ airway pressure	PEEP	↓ CO
	↓ resistance	Vasodilator	↑ CO
↓ Blood pressure	↓ cardiac output		
	↓ HR	β-Blocker	↓ CO
	↓ SV	Diuretic	↓ CO
	↑ resistance	α-Agonist	↓ CO
↑ Blood pressure	↑ cardiac output	Ionotropic	↑ CO
		Volume	↑ CO, ↓ O_2 saturation
	↑ cardiac output		
	↑ contractility	Ionotropic	↑ HR
↑ Perfusion	↑ preload	Volume	↓ O_2 saturation
	↓ resistance	Vasodilator	↓ BP

these interventions are made empirically based on a diagnosis and an understanding of maternal physiology. For example, tocolysis with β-mimetic agents can induce pulmonary edema. Timely diagnosis, discontinuation of the offending agent, oxygen supplementation, and a single diuretic dose will usually be sufficient therapy. When initial interventions do not achieve an adequate effect, invasive monitoring may be required to direct subsequent care. Maternal diuresis to improve oxygen saturation, when excessive, may lead to a reduction in CO. Fetal decompensation is usually encountered before a significant reduction in maternal perfusion and hypotension. The maternal PAWP and CO can be used to direct maternal diuresis. If desaturation continues despite hemodynamic management, intubation may be required. Positive end-expiratory pressure (PEEP) can be used to increase intra-alveolar pressure to impede the forces driving water into alveolar spaces. PEEP may impede venous return and decrease CO due to the effects of the associated increase in extracardiac intrathoracic pressure. A PAWP in excess of PEEP is required for adequate ventricular filling. Only in the sickest of pregnant women will PEEP have a clinically significant impact on CO.

Disorders of blood pressure and perfusion can be managed with the knowledge of maternal hemodynamics. Figure 34-7 describes the relationships between MAP, CO, and vascular resistance. CO and MAP are represented on the x- and y-axes, respectively. Resistance is represented by diagonal isometric lines. Vasodilators or vasopressors that act on resistance produce vectors of change that run perpendicular to lines of resistance. Interventions that decrease CO (β-blockers, diuresis) or increase CO (dopamine, volume) produce vectors of change that run roughly parallel to lines of resistance. The region labeled "normal" represents the goal of therapy. Plotting patient data on the chart allows one to visually determine the vector or combination of vectors that could return hemodynamics to normal.

Patient A represents a patient who is hypotensive with a low CO as might be expected after hemorrhage or in heart failure. Given a low PAWP associated with hemorrhage, volume administration would be expected to create a vector that would return hemodynamics to normal. Alternatively, the patient could have a normal or high PAWP associated with heart failure and would need an inotropic agent such as dopamine. Patient B has a normal blood pressure but a high vascular resistance and low CO such as might be expected with a cardiomyopathy. Afterload reduction with a medication such as hydralazine will produce a vector of vasodilation and return hemodynamics to normal. Patient C is hypertensive with a mixed hemodynamic pattern. She will need a combination of vectors to approach normal hemodynamics (e.g., hydralazine and β-blocker). Patient D is hypotensive and hyperdynamic with a low vascular resistance. The hemodynamics might be found in a patient with early sepsis. Treatment with volume could increase pressure but at the

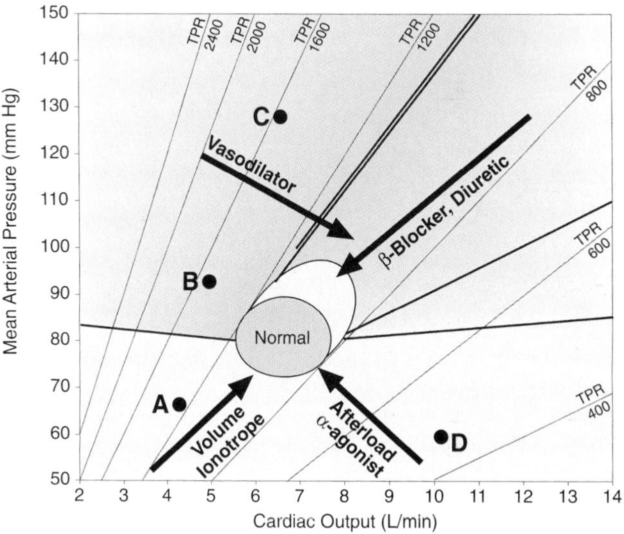

Figure 34-7. Hemodynamic flow chart. Cardiac output and mean arterial pressure are plotted on the x- and y-axes, respectively. Diagonal lines are isometric lines of vascular resistance. Anticipated vectors of change can be used to predict patient response to intervention.

expense of high filling pressures and a potentially negative impact on developing ARDS. Alternatively, a small dose of an α-adrenergic agent such as neosynephrine would create a vector perpendicular to lines of resistance that return hemodynamics to normal. Figure 34-7 allows one to see that vasoconstriction would achieve a normal blood pressure before adversely affecting CO.

Key Points

- Hemodynamic changes in pregnancy may adversely affect maternal cardiac performance.
- Intercurrent events such as infection during pregnancy are usually the cause of decompensation.
- Women with heart disease in pregnancy frequently have unique psychosocial needs.
- Labor, delivery, and postpartum are periods of hemodynamic instability.
- Invasive hemodynamic monitoring should be used to address specific clinical questions.
- Many maternal heart conditions can be medically managed during pregnancy. A few conditions such as Eisenmenger's syndrome are associated with a very high risk of maternal mortality.
- Many women with congenital heart disease can successfully complete a pregnancy.
- Preconceptual counseling is based on achieving a balance between medical information and the patient's value system.

REFERENCES

1. Easterling T, Benedetti T, Schmucker B, Millard S: Maternal hemodynamics in normal and preeclamptic pregnancies: a longitudinal study. Obstet Gynecol 76:1061, 1990.
2. Robson S, Dunlop W, Boys R, Hunter S: Cardiac output during labour. BMJ 295:1169, 1987.
3. Easterling T, Chadwick H, Otto C, Benedetti T: Aortic stenosis in pregnancy. Obstet Gynecol 72:113, 1988.
4. Clark S, Phelan J, Greenspoon J, et al: Labor and delivery in the presence of mitral stenosis: central hemodynamic observations. Am J Obstet Gynecol 152:384, 1985.
5. Robson S, Boys R, Hunter S, Dunlop W: Maternal hemodynamics after normal delivery and delivery complicated by postpartum hemorrhage. Obstet Gynecol 74:234, 1989.
6. Davison J, Lindheimer M: Volume homeostasis and osmoregulation in human pregnancy. Baillieres Clin Endocrinol Metab 3:451, 1989.
7. Whittaker P, Lind T: The intravascular mass of albumin during pregnancy: a serial study in normal and diabetic women. Br J Obstet Gynaecol 100:587, 1993.
8. Mishra M, Chambers J, Jackson G: Murmurs in pregnancy: an audit of echocardiography. BMJ 304:1413, 1989.
9. Otto C (ed): Valvular stenosis: diagnosis, quantification, and clinical approach. *In* Textbook of Clinical Echocardiography. Philadelphia, WB Saunders Company, 2000, p 229.
10. Lamey J, Eschenbach D, Mitchell S, et al: Isolation of mycoplasmas and bacteria from blood of postpartum women. Am J Obstet Gynecol 143:104, 1982.
11. Boggess K, Watts D, Hillier S, et al: Bacteremia shortly after placental separation during cesarean section. Obstet Gynecol 87:779, 1996.
12. Rose V, Gold R, Lindsay G, Allen M: A possible increase in the incidence of congenital heart defects among the offspring of affected patients. J Am Coll Cardiol 6:376, 1985.
13. Whittemore R, Hobbins J, Engle M: Pregnancy and its outcome in women with and without surgical treatment of congenital heart disease. Am J Cardiol 50:641, 1982.
14. Gill H, Splitt M, Sharland G, Simpson J: Patterns of recurrence of congenital heart disease: An analysis of 6,640 consecutive pregnancies evaluated by detailed fetal echocardiography. J Am Coll Cardiol, 42:923, 2003.
15. Bonow R, Carabello B, de Leon A, et al: ACC/AGA guidelines for the management of patients with valvular heart disease. Executive summary: a report of the American College of Cardiology/American Heart Association Task Force on practice guidelines (committee on management of patients with valvular heart disease). J Heart Valve Dis 7:672, 1998.
16. Chesley L: Severe rheumatic cardiac disease and pregnancy: the ultimate prognosis. Am J Obstet Gynecol 136:552, 1980.
17. Al Kasab S, Sabag T, Al Zaibag M, et al: Beta-adrenergic receptor blockade in the management of pregnant women with mitral stenosis. Am J Obstet Gynecol 163:37, 1990.
18. Becker R: Intracardiac surgery in pregnant women. Ann Thorac Surg 36:463, 1983.
19. Szekely P, Snaith L: Heart Disease and Pregnancy. Edinburgh, Churchill Livingstone, 1974.
20. Farhat M, Gamra H, Betbout F, et al: Percutaneous balloon mitral commissurotomy during pregnancy. Heart 77:564, 1997.
21. Gupta A, Lokhandwala Y, Satoskaar P, Salvi V: Balloon mitral valvotomy in pregnancy: maternal and fetal outcomes. J Am Coll Surg 187:409, 1998.
22. Devereuz R, Kramer-Fox R, Kligfield P: Mitral valve prolapse: causes, clinical manifestations, and management. Ann Intern Med 111:305, 1989.
23. Selzer A: Changing aspects of the natural history of valvular aortic stenosis. N Engl J Med 317:91, 1998.
24. Carabello B, Crawford F: Valvular heart disease. N Engl J Med 337:32, 1997.
25. Arias F, Pineda J: Aortic stenosis and pregnancy. J Reprod Med 20:229, 1978.
26. Lao T, Sermer M, MaGee L, et al: Congenital aortic stenosis and pregnancy: a reappraisal. Am J Obstet Gynecol 169:540, 1993.
27. Shime J, Mocarski E, Hastings D, et al: Congenital heart disease in pregnancy: short- and long-term implications. Am J Obstet Gynecol 156:313, 1987.
28. Lee C, Wu C, Lin P, et al: Pregnancy following cardiac prosthetic valve replacement. Obstet Gynecol 83:353, 1994.
29. Hanania G, Thomas D, Michel P, et al: Pregnancy in patients with heart valves. A French retrospective study (155) cases. Arch Mal Coeur Vaiss 87:429, 1994.
30. Ville Y, Jenkins E, Shearer M: Fetal intraventricular haemorrhagia and maternal warfarin. Lancet 341:1211, 1993.
31. Azzano O, French P, Robin J, et al: Thrombolytic therapy with rt-PA for thrombosis of a tricuspid valve prosthesis during pregnancy. Arch Mal Coeur Vaiss 88:267, 1995.
32. Rinaldi J, Yassine M, Aboujaoude F, et al: Successful thrombolysis on an aortic valve prosthesis by plasminogen tissue activator during pregnancy. Arch Mal Coeur Vaiss 92:427, 1999.
33. Wilson N, Neutze J: Adult congenital heart disease: principles and management guidelines—part I. Aust N Z J Med 23:498, 1993.
34. Findlow D, Doyle E: Congenital heart disease in adults. Br J Anaesth 78:416, 1997.
35. Murphy J, Gersh B, Mair D, et al: Long-term outcome in patients undergoing surgical repair of tetralogy of Fallot. N Engl J Med 329:593, 1993.
36. Gantt L: Growing up heartsick: the experiences of young women with congenital heart disease. Health Care Women Int 13:241, 1992.
37. Swan L, Hillis W, Cameron A: Family planning requirements of adults with congenital heart disease. Heart 78:9, 1997.
38. Piesiewicz W, Goch A, Binokowski Z, et al: Changes in the cardiovascular system during pregnancy in females with secundum atrial septal defect. Polish Heart J 60:218, 2004.

39. Veldtman G, Connolly H, Grogan M, et al: Outcomes of pregnancy in women with tetralogy of Fallot. J Am Coll Cardiol 44:174, 2004.
40. Mustard W: Successful two-stage correction of transposition of the great vessels. Pediatr Surg 55:469, 1964.
41. Genoni M, Jenni R, Hoerstrup S, et al: Pregnancy after atrial repair for transposition of the great arteries. Heart 81:276, 1999.
42. Rastelli G, Wallace R, Ongley P: Complete repair of transposition of the great vessels with pulmonary stenosis: a review and report of a case corrected by using a new technique. Circulation 39:83, 1969.
43. Nwosu U: Pregnancy following Mustard operation for transposition of great arteries. J Tenn Med Assoc 85:509, 1992.
44. Neukermans K, Sullivan T, Pitlick D: Successful pregnancy after the Mustard operation for transposition of the great arteries. Am J Cardiol 57:838, 1988.
45. Megerian G, Bell E, Huhta J, et al: Pregnancy outcome following Mustard procedure for transposition of the great arteries: a report of five cases and review of the literature. Obstet Gynecol 83:512, 1994.
46. Lynch-Salamond D, Maze S, Combs C: Pregnancy after Mustard repair for transposition of the great arteries. Obstet Gynecol 82:676, 1993.
47. Lao T, Sermer M Colman J: Pregnancy following surgical correction for transposition of the great arteries. Obstet Gynecol 83:665, 1994.
48. Dellinger E, Hadi H: Maternal transposition of the great arteries in pregnancy: a case report. J Reprod Med 39:324, 1994.
49. Clarkson P, Wilson N, Neutze J, et al: Outcome of pregancy after the Mustard operation for transposition of the great arteries with intact ventricle septum. Am Coll Cardiol 24:190, 1994.
50. Guedes A, Mercier L, Leduc L, et al: Impact of pregnancy on the systemic right ventricle after a Mustard operation for transposition of the great arteries. J Am Coll Cardiol 44:433, 2004.
51. Therrien J, Barnes I, Somerville J: Outcome of pregnancy in patients with congenitally corrected transposition of the great arteries. Am J Cardiol 84:820, 1999.
52. Connolly H, Grogan M, Warnes C: Pregnancy among women with congenitally corrected transposition of great arteries. J Am Coll Cardiol 33:1692, 1999.
53. Fontan F, Baudet E: Surgical repair for tricuspid atresia. Thorax 26:240, 1971.
54. Canobbio M, Mair D, Van der Velde M, Koos B: Pregnancy outcomes after the Fontan repair. J Am Coll Cardiol 28:763, 1996.
55. Vongpatanasin W, Brickner E, Hillis L, Lange R: The Eisenmenger syndrome in adults. Ann Intern Med 128:745, 1998.
56. Weiss B, Zemp L, Burkhardt S, Heiss O: Outcome of pulmonary vascular disease in pregnancy: a systematic overview from 1978 through 1996. J Am Coll Cardiol 31:1650, 1998.
57. Gleicher N, Midwall J, Hochberger D, Jaffin H: Eisenmenger's syndrome and pregnancy. Obstet Gynecol Surv 34:721, 1979.
58. Yentis S, Steer P, Plaat F: Eisenmenger's syndrome in pregnancy: maternal and fetal mortality in the 1990's. Br J Obstet Gynaecol 105:921, 1998.
59. Lust K, Boots R, Dooris M, Wilson J: Management of labor in Eisenmenger syndrome with inhaled nitric oxide. Am J Obstet Gynecol 181:419, 1999.
60. Lacassie H, Germain A, Valdes G, et al: Management of Eisenmenger syndrome in pregnancy with sildenafil and L-arginine. Obstet Gynecol 103:1118, 2004.
61. Deal K, Wooley C: Coarctation of the aorta and pregnancy. Ann Intern Med 78:706, 1973.
62. Saidi A, Bezold L, Altman C, et al: Outcome of pregnancy following intervention for coarctation of the aorta. Am J Cardiol 82:786, 1988.
63. Hibbard J, Lindheimer M, Lang R: A modified definition for peripartum cardiomyopathy and prognosis based on echocardiography. Obstet Gynecol 94:311, 1999.
64. Lampert M, Lang R: Peripartum cardiomyopathy. Am Heart J 130:860, 1995.
65. Heider A, Kuller J, Strauss R, Wells S: Peripartum cardiomyopathy: a review of the literature. Obstet Gynecol Sur 54:526, 1999.
66. Ostrzega E, Elkayam U: Risk of subsequent pregnancy in women with a history of peripartum cardiomyopathy: results of a survey. Circulation 92(Suppl I):1, 1995.
67. The SOLVD Investigators: Effect of enalapril on survival in patients with reduced left ventricular ejection fractions and congestive heart failure. N Engl J Med 325:293, 1991.
68. The CONSENSUS Trial Study Group: Effects of enalapril on mortality in severe congestive heart failure. N Engl J Med 316:1429, 1987.
69. Waagstein F, Caidahl K, Wallentin I, et al: Long-term β-blockade in dilated cardiomyopathy. Circulation 80:551, 1989.
70. MERIT-HF Study Group: Effect of metoprolol CR/XL in chronic heart failure: metoprololCR/XL randomised intervention trial in congestive heart failure (MERIT-HF). Lancet 353:2001, 1999.
71. CIBIS Investigators and Committees: A randomized trial of β-blockade in heart failure. Circulation 90:1765, 1994.
72. Natale A, Davidson T, Geiger M, Newby K: Implantable cardioverter-defibrillators and pregnancy. Circulation 96:2808, 1997.
73. Petitti D, Sidney S, Queesenberry C, Bernstein A: Incidence of stroke and myocardial infarction in women of reproductive age. Stroke 28:280, 1997.
74. Ginz B: Myocardial infarction in pregnancy. J Obstet Gynaecol Br Commonw 77:610, 1970.
75. Roth A, Elkayam U: Acute myocardial infarction associated with pregnancy. Ann Intern Med 125:751, 1996.
76. Fujiwara Y, Yamanaka O, Nakamura T, et al: Acute myocardial infarction induced by ergonovine administration for artificially induced abortion. Jpn Heart J 34:803, 1993.
77. Hopp L, Weisse A, Iffy L: Acute myocardial infarction in a healthy mother using bromocriptine for milk suppression. Can J Cardiol 12:415, 1996.
78. Liao J, Cockrill B, Yurchak P: Acute myocardial infarction after ergonovine administration for uterine bleeding. Am J Cardiol 68:823, 1991.
79. Meyer W, Benton S, Hoon T, et al: Acute myocardial infarction associated with prostaglandin E2. Am J Obstet Gynecol 165:359, 1991.
80. Oei S, Oei S, Brolmann H: Myocardial infarction during nifedipine therapy for preterm labor. N Engl J Med 340:154, 1999.
81. Ottman E, Hall S: Myocardial infarction in the third trimester of pregnancy secondary to an aortic valve thrombus. Obstet Gynecol 81:804, 1993.
82. Ruch A, Duhring J: Postpartum myocardial infarction in a patient receiving bromocriptine. Obstet Gynecol 74:448, 1989.
83. Yaegashi N, Miura M, Okamura K: Acute myocardial infarction associated with postpartum ergot alkaloid administration. Int J Gynecol Obstet 64:67, 1999.
84. Tsung S: Several conditions causing elevation of serum CK-MB and C-BB. Am J Clin Pathol 75:711, 1981.
85. Shivvers S, Wians F, Keffer J, Ramin S: Maternal cardiac troponin I levels during normal labor and delivery. Am J Obstet Gynecol 180:122, 1999.
86. Sebastian C, Scherlag M, Kugelmass A, Schechter E: Primary stent implantation for acute myocardial infarction during pregnancy: use of abciximab, ticlopidine, and aspirin. Cathet Cardiovasc Diagn 45:275, 1998.
87. Giudici M, Artis A, Webel R, Alpert M: Postpartum myocardial infarction treated with percutaneous transluminal coronary angioplasty. Am Heart J 118:614, 1999.
88. Eickman F: Acute coronary artery angioplasty during pregnancy. Cathet Cardiovasc Diagn 38:369, 1996.
89. Ascarelli M, Grider A, Hsu H: Acute myocardial infarction during pregnancy managed with immediate percutaneous transluminal coronary angioplasty. Obstet Gynecol 88:655, 1996.
90. Dufour P, Occelli B, Puech F: Brief communication: pregnancy after myocardial infarction. Int J Obstet Gynecol 59:251, 1997.
91. Kainulainen K, Pulkkinin L, Savolainen A, et al: Location on chromosome 15 of the gene defect causing Marfan syndrome. N Engl J Med 323:935, 1990.
92. Gott V, Greene P, Alejo D, et al: Replacement of the aortic root in patients with Marfan's syndrome. N Engl J Med 340:1307, 1999.
93. Leggert M, Unger T, O'Sullivan C, et al: Aortic root complications in Marfan's syndrome: Indentification of a lower risk group. Heart 75:389, 1996.
94. Shores J, Berger K, Murphy E, Pyeritz R: Progression of aortic dilatation and the benefit of long-term B-adrenergic blockade in Marfan's syndrome. N Engl J Med 330:1335, 1994.

95. Elkayam U, Ostrzega E, Shotan A, Mehra A: Cardiovascular problems in pregnant women with the Marfan syndrome. Ann Intern Med 123:117, 1995.
96. Lipscomb K, Smith J, Clarke B, et al: Outcome of pregnancy in women with Marfan's syndrome. Br J Obstet Gynecol 104:201, 1997.
97. Pyeritz R: Maternal and fetal complications of pregnancy in the Marfan syndrome. Am J Med 71:784, 1981.
98. Rossiter J, Repke J, Morales A, et al: A prospective longitudinal evaluation of pregnancy in the Marfan syndrome. Am J Obstet Gynecol 173:1599, 1995.
99. Rubin L: ACCP consensus statement: primary pulmonary hypertension. Chest 104:236, 1993.
100. D'Alonzo GE, Barst R, Ayres S, et al: Survival in patients with primary pulmonary hypertension. Ann Intern Med 115:343, 1991.
101. Rich S, Kaufmann E, Levy P: The effect of high doses of calcium-channel blockers on survival in primary pulmonary hypertension. N Engl J Med 327:76, 1992.
102. Rubin L, Mendoza J, Hood M, et al: Treatment of primary pulmonary hypertension with continuous intravenous prostacyclin. Ann Intern Med 112:485, 1990.
103. Metcalfe J, McAnulty J, Ueland K (eds): Pulmonary artery hypertension. *In* Heart Disease and Pregnancy: Physiology and Management. Boston/Toronto, Little, Brown & Co., 1986, p 265.
104. McCaffrey R, Dunn L: Primary pulmonary hypertension in pregnancy. Obstet Gynecol Surv 19:567, 1964.
105. Martinez J, Comas C, Sala X, et al: Maternal primary pulmonary hypertension associated with pregnancy. Eur J Obstet Gynaecol Reprod Biol 54:143, 1994.
106. Nelson D, Main E, Crafford W, Ahumada G: Peripartum heart failure due to primary pulmonary hypertension. Obstet Gynecol 62:58S, 1983.
107. Easterling T, Ralph D, Schmucker B: Pulmonary hypertension in pregnancy: treatment with pulmonary vasodilators. Obstet Gynecol 93:494, 1999.
108. Shah D, Sunderji S: Hypertrophic cardiomyopathy and pregnancy: report of a maternal mortality and review of the literature. Obstet Gynecol Surv 40:444, 1985.
109. Piacenza J, Kirkorian G, Audra P, Mellier G: Hypertrophic cardiomyopathy and pregnancy. Eur J Obstet Gynaecol Reprod Biol 80:17, 1998.
110. Varnava R, Hamid M, Sachdev B, et al: Pregnancy related complications in women with hypertrophic cardiomyopathy. Heart 89:752, 2003.
111. Thaman R, Varnava A, Hamid MS, et al: Pregnancy related complications in women with hypertrophic cardiomyopathy. Heart 89:752, 2003.
112. Matthay M, Chatterjee K: Bedside catheterization of the pulmonary artery: risks compared with benefits. Ann Intern Med 109:826, 1988.
113. Robson S, Dunlop W, Moore M, Hunter S: Combined Doppler and echocardiographic measurement of cardiac output: theory and application in pregnancy. Br J Obstet Gynaecol 94:1014, 1987.
114. Lee W, Rokey R, Cotton D: Noninvasive maternal stroke volume and cardiac output determinations by pulsed Doppler echocardiography. Am J Obstet Gynecol 158:505, 1988.
115. Easterling T, Carlson K, Schmucker B, et al: Measurement of cardiac output in pregnancy by Doppler technique. Am J Perinatol 7:220, 1990.
116. Easterling T, Watts D, Schmucker B, Benedetti T: Measurement of cardiac output during pregnancy: validation of Doppler technique and clinical observations in preeclampsia. Obstet Gynecol 69:845, 1987.
117. de Swiet M, Talbert D: The measurement of cardiac output by electrical impedance plethysmography in pregnancy: are the assumptions valid? Br J Obstet Gynaecol 93:721, 1986.
118. Easterling T, Benedetti T, Carlson K, Watts D: Measurement of cardiac output in pregnancy: impedance versus thermodilution techniques. Br J Obstet Gynaecol 96:67, 1989.
119. Masaki D, Greenspoon J, Ouzounian J: Measurement of cardiac output in pregnancy by thoracic electrical bioimpedance and thermodilution. Am J Obstet Gynecol 161:680, 1989.
120. Clark S, Cotton D, Lee W, et al: Central hemodynamic assessment of normal pregnancy. Am J Obstet Gynecol 161:1439, 1989.

Respiratory Diseases in Pregnancy

JANICE E. WHITTY AND MITCHELL P. DOMBROWSKI

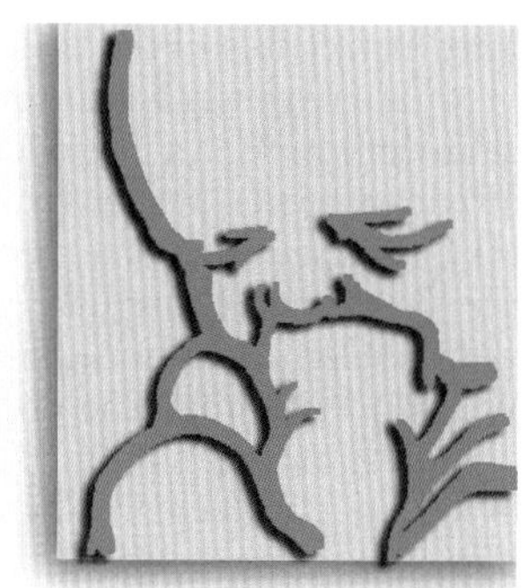

CHAPTER 35

KEY ABBREVIATIONS

Acquired immunodeficiency syndrome	AIDS
Amniotic fluid index	AFI
Bacille Calmette-Guerrin	BCG
Confidence interval	CI
Direct amplification tests	DATs
Dry powder inhaler	DPI
Food and Drug Administration	FDA
Forced expiratory volume in one second	FEV_1
Forced vital capacity	FVC
Highly active antiretroviral therapy	HAART
Human immunodeficiency virus	HIV
Isoniazid	INH
Latent tuberculosis infection	LTBI
Metered-dose inhaler	MDI
National Asthma Education and Prevention Program	NAEPP
Odds ratio	OR
Peak expiratory flow rate	PEFR
Percutaneous needle aspiration	PTNA
Pneumocystis carinii pneumonia	PCP
Positive end-expiratory pressure	PEEP
Purified protein derivative	PPD
Rifampin	RIF
Tuberculosis	TB

Pulmonary diseases are among the most common medical complications of pregnancy. The occurrence of pulmonary disease during gestation may result in increased morbidity or mortality for both the mother and her fetus. Pregnancy may have an adverse or positive impact on the pulmonary function of the gravida depending on the particular complication that is being encountered. The cardiorespiratory changes that occur in pregnancy are reviewed in Chapter 3, and the obstetrician and medical consultants should have a thorough understanding of these changes and their potential impact on the respiratory disease in question. It is also extremely important to realize that the majority of diagnostic tests used to evaluate pulmonary function are not harmful to the fetus and, if indicated, should be performed during gestation. In this section, we discuss some of the respiratory complications that may be encountered during gestation, the impact of pregnancy on the disease, and the potential impact of the disease on pregnancy.

PNEUMONIA IN PREGNANCY

Pneumonia is an uncommon complication of pregnancy, observed in 1 per 118 deliveries to 1 per 2,288 deliveries.[1,2] However, pneumonia contributes to considerable maternal mortality and is reportedly the most common nonobstetric infection to cause maternal mortality in the peripartum period.[3] Before the introduction of antibiotic therapy, maternal mortality was as high as 24 percent.[4] However, with modern management and antibiotic therapy, maternal mortality ranges from 0 to 4 percent.[2,5,6] Preterm delivery is another significant complication of pneumonia and, even with antibiotic therapy and modern management, continues to occur in 4 to 43 percent of affected pregnancies.[2,5,6]

The incidence of pneumonia in pregnancy may be increasing primarily as a reflection of the declining health status of certain segments of the childbearing population.[6] In addition, the epidemic of human immunodeficiency virus (HIV) infection has increased the number of potential mothers who are at risk for opportunistic lung infections. HIV infection further predisposes the pregnant woman to the infectious complications of the acquired immunodeficiency syndrome (AIDS).[7] Reported incidence rates range from 97 to 290 cases per 1,000 HIV-infected persons per year.[8] HIV-infected persons are 7.8 times more likely to develop pneumonia than non-HIV-infected individuals with similar risk factors.[8] Women with medical conditions that increase the risk of pulmonary infection, such as cystic fibrosis, are now living to childbearing age more frequently than in the past. This disorder also contributes to the increased incidence of pneumonia in pregnancy.

Pneumonia can complicate pregnancy at any time during gestation and may be associated with preterm birth, poor fetal growth, and perinatal loss. In an early report by Hopwood,[9] 17 of the 23 patients developed pneumonia between 25 and 36 weeks' gestation. In that series, seven gravidas delivered during the course of their acute illness, and there were two maternal deaths. Benedetti et al.[5] described 39 cases of pneumonia in pregnancy. Sixteen gravidas presented before 24 weeks' gestation, 15 between 25 and 36 weeks' gestation, and eight after 36 weeks' gestation. Twenty-seven patients in this series were followed to completion of pregnancy; only two required delivery during the acute phase of pneumonia. Of these 27 patients, three suffered a fetal loss and 24 delivered live fetuses, although there was one neonatal death due to prematurity.[5] Madinger et al.[2] reported 25 cases of pneumonia occurring among 32,179 deliveries and observed that fetal and obstetric complications were much more common than in earlier studies. Preterm labor occurred in 11 of 21 patients who had complete follow-up data. Pneumonia was present at the time of delivery in 11 patients, particularly in those women who experienced bacteremia, required mechanical ventilation, or in those with a serious underlying maternal disease. In addition to the complication of preterm labor, there were three perinatal deaths in this series. In Berkowitz and La Sala's report[6] of 25 patients with pneumonia complicating pregnancy, full-term delivery of normally grown infants occurred in 14 women, one delivered preterm, three had a voluntary termination of pregnancy, three had term deliveries of growth-restricted babies, and four were lost to follow-up. Birth weight was significantly lower in the study group (2,770 ± 224 g versus 3,173 ± 99 g in the control group, $p < 0.01$). In this series, pneumonia complicated 1 in 367 deliveries, and Berkowitz and La Sala attributed the increase in the incidence of pneumonia in this population to a decline in general health status, including anemia and a significant incidence of cocaine use in the study group (52 versus 10 percent in the general population), as well as HIV positivity in the study group (24 versus 2 percent in controls).

BACTERIOLOGY

Most series describing pneumonia complicating pregnancy have used incomplete methodologies to diagnose the etiologic pathogens involved, relying primarily on cultures of blood and sputum. In the majority of cases, no identifiable pathogen is reported; however, pneumococcus and *Haemophilus influenzae* remain the most common identifiable causes of pneumonia in pregnancy.[2,5,6] Because comprehensive serologic testing has rarely been undertaken, the true incidence of viral pneumonia, *Legionella,* and *Mycoplasma* pneumonia in pregnancy is difficult to estimate. The data presented in three series all supported pneumococcus as the predominant pathogen causing pneumonia in pregnancy, with *H. influenzae* being the second most common organism.[2,5,6] In Berkowitz and La Sala's series, one patient had *Legionella* species.[6] Several unusual pathogens have been reported to cause pneumonia in pregnancy, including mumps, infectious mononucleosis, swine influenza, influenza A, varicella, coccidioidomycosis, and other fungi.[10] Varicella pneumonia complicates primary varicella infections in 9 percent of infections in pregnancy, as compared with 0.3 to 1.8 percent in the nonpregnant population.[11] Influenza A has a higher mortality in pregnant than in nonpregnant patients.[12] The increase in virulence of viral infections reported in pregnancy may be secondary to the alterations in maternal immune status that characterize pregnancy, including reduced lymphocyte proliferative response, reduced cell-mediated cytotoxicity, and a decrease in the number of T-helper lymphocytes (see Chapter 4).[12,13] Viral pneumonias can also be complicated by superimposed bacterial infection, particularly with pneumococcus.

Chemical pneumonitis results after the aspiration of gastric contents. Chemical pneumonitis can be superinfected with pathogens present in the oropharynx and gastric juices, primarily anaerobes and gram-negative bacteria.[10]

Heterosexual transmission of HIV has become an increasingly important mode of transmission. Many of these women are of childbearing age. They are at risk for developing *Pneumoncystis carinii* pneumonia (PCP) during pregnancy. The reported maternal mortality from PCP is as high as 50 percent.[14] Although the risk of maternal mortality is high with PCP infection, the majority of HIV-infected pregnant women in the United States today are receiving prophylaxis. This may actually lead to a decrease in the incidence and mortality from PCP pneumonia in pregnancy.

BACTERIAL PNEUMONIA

Streptococcus pneumoniae (pneumococcus) is the most common bacterial pathogen to cause pneumonia in pregnancy, with *H. influenzae* being the next most common. These pneumonias typically present as an acute illness accompanied by fever, chills, purulent productive cough, and a lobar pattern on chest radiograph (Fig. 35-1). Streptococcal pneumonia produces a "rusty" sputum, with gram-positive diplococci on Gram's stain and asymmetric consolidation with air bronchograms on chest radiograph.[13] *H. influenzae* is a gram-negative coccobacillus that produces consolidation with air bronchograms, often in the upper lobes.[13] Less frequent bacterial pathogens include *Klebsiella pneumoniae,* which is a gram-negative rod that causes extensive tissue destruction, with air bronchograms, pleural effusion, and cavitation noted

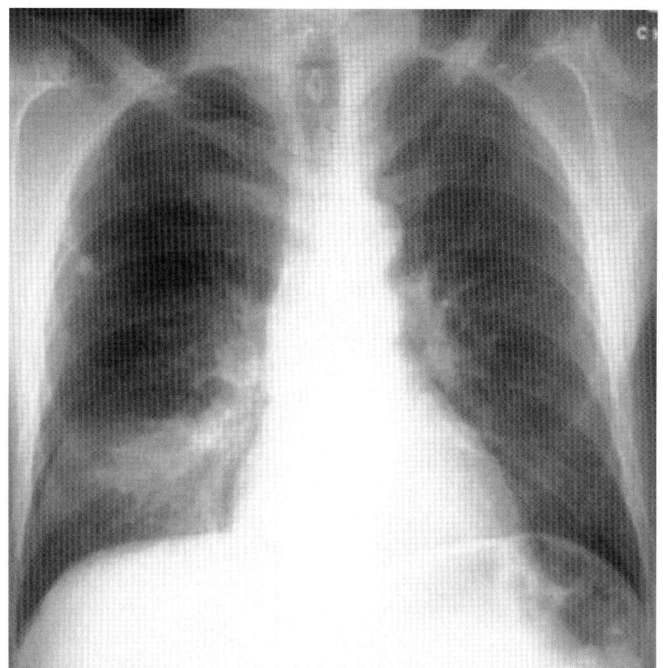

Figure 35-1. Right lower lobe pneumonia.

on chest radiograph. Patients with *Staphylococcus aureus* pneumonia present with pleuritis, chest pain, purulent sputum, and consolidation without air bronchograms noted on chest radiograph.[13]

Patients with atypical pneumonia pathogens, such as *Mycoplasma pneumoniae, Legionella pneumophila,* and *Chlamydia pneumoniae* (TWAR agent), present with gradual onset and a lower fever, appear less ill, and have a mucoid sputum and a patchy or interstitial infiltrate on chest radiograph. The severity of the findings on chest radiograph is usually out of proportion to the mild clinical symptoms. *M. pneumoniae* is the most common organism responsible for atypical pneumonia and is best detected by the presence of cold agglutinins, which are present in 70 percent of cases.

The normal physiologic changes in the respiratory system associated with pregnancy result in a loss of ventilatory reserve. This, coupled with the relative immunosuppression that accompanies pregnancy, puts the mother and fetus at great risk from respiratory infection. Therefore, any gravida suspected of having pneumonia should be managed aggressively. Hospital admission is generally recommended, and an investigation should be undertaken to determine the pathologic etiology. A recent study examined 133 women admitted with pneumonia during pregnancy using protocols based on the British and American Thoracic Society admission guidelines for management in non-pregnant individuals.[15] The authors reported that if the American Thoracic Society guidelines were utilized, 25 percent of the pregnant women with pneumonia could have avoided admission.[16] Using the American criteria, none of the gravidas who would have been managed as an outpatient had any complications.[17] If the British Thoracic Society guidelines had been used, 66 percent of the pregnant women in this group would have been assigned to outpatient therapy. However, of those, 14 percent would have required readmission for complications. Of note, the majority of the 133 women who were hospitalized with pneumonia in this study did not receive a chest radiograph for confirmation of diagnosis. This limits the value of the study for use in guiding admission criteria for pneumonia in pregnancy. Therefore, until additional information is available, admission for all pregnant women with pneumonia is prudent.

Work-up should include physical examination, arterial blood gases, chest radiograph, sputum for Gram's stain and culture, as well as blood cultures. Several recently published studies have called into question the use of cultures to identify the microbiology of community-acquired pneumonia. The successful identification of the bacterial etiology with cultures ranges from 2.1 percent to approximately 50 percent.[18–20] Review of available clinical data reflects an overall reliance on clinical judgment and the patient response to treatment to guide therapy.[17,21,22] There are other tests available to identify the etiology of pneumonia that do not require culture and are more sensitive and specific. An assay approved by the Food and Drug Administration (FDA) for pneumococcal urinary antigen has been assessed in several studies.[23] The sensitivity for identifying pneumococcal disease in adults is reportedly 60 to 90 percent, with specificity close to 100 percent.[23] In one study, the pneumococcal antigen was detected in 26 percent of patients in whom no pathogens had been identified.[24] This suggests that cases that are undiagnosed by standard testing can be identified with the assay. In this study, 10 percent of samples from patients with pneumonia caused by other agents were positive for the pneumococcal assay, indicating a potential problem with specificity.[9] Therefore, if the response to therapy directed at pneumococcus is inadequate, coverage for other potential pathogens should be added. There is a test for Legionella urinary antigen as well[25] with a sensitivity of 70 percent and specificity of 90 percent for serogroup 1. This is especially useful in the United States and Europe because about 85 percent of Legionella isolates are serogroup 1.[25] Legionella is a common cause of severe community-acquired pneumonia. Therefore, the urinary antigen for serogroup 1 should be considered for any patient requiring admission into an intensive care unit for pneumonia.

Percutaneous transthoracic needle aspiration (PTNA) has been advocated as a valuable and safe method to increase the chance of establishing a causative agent in pneumonia. This test should be reserved for use in compromised individuals, suspected tuberculosis (TB) in the absence of a productive cough, selected cases of chronic pneumonia, pneumonia associated with neoplasm, or foreign body, suspected PCP pneumonia, and suspected conditions that necessitate lung biopsy.[17]

When admission for pneumonia is required, there is evidence that inpatient and 30-day mortality has been reduced when antibiotics are administered in less than 8 hours.[19,26] Therefore, current U.S. federal standards require that the first dose of antibiotics be administered within 4 hours of arrival to the hospital.[27] Empiric antibiotic coverage should be started, usually with a third-generation cephalosporin such as ceftriaxone or cefotaxime. *Legionella* pneumonia has a high mortality rate and sometimes presents with consolidation, mimicking pneumococcal pneumonia. Therefore, it is recommended that a macrolide, such as azithromycin, be added to the empiric therapeutic regimen. Dual coverage has been demonstrated to improve response to therapy even for abbreviated macrolide regimens.[17] This is theoretically because of an added anti-inflammatory effect of the macrolides.[20] Azithromycin administration has been shown to be an independent predictor of positive outcome and reduced length of hospital stay in mild to moderate community-acquired pneumonia.[17] However, the use of macrolides to treat community-acquired pneumonia should be limited when possible, because their use has also been associated with increased penicillin resistance among *S. pneumoniae*.[28]

Once the results of the antigen, sputum culture, blood cultures, Gram's stain, and serum studies are obtained and a pathogen has been identified, antibiotic therapy should be directed toward the identifiable pathogen. The quinolones as a class should be avoided in pregnancy because they may damage developing fetal cartilage. However, with the emergence of highly resistant bacterial pneumonia, their use may be life saving and therefore justified in specific circumstances. The respiratory quinolones are not only effective against highly penicillin-resistant *S. pneumoniae* strains, but their use reportedly does not increase resistance.[28] The respiratory quinolones include levofloxacin, gatifloxacin, and moxifloxacin. These are ideal agents for community acquired pneumonia because they are highly active against penicillin-resistant strains of *S. pneumoniae*. They are also active against Legionella and the other atypical pulmonary pathogens. Another advantage is a favorable pharmacokinetic profile, such that blood/lung levels are the same whether the drug is administered orally or intravenously.[28] Arguments against more extensive respiratory quinolone use are based on concerns about the potential for developing resistance, the variable incidence of Legionella, and cost. An additional caveat is that the respiratory quiolones are partially effective against m. TB. Therefore, evaluation for this infection should be done when considering the use of quinolones for pneumonia. The third-generation cephalosporins are effective agents for the majority of pathogens causing a community-acquired pneumonia. They are also effective against penicillin-resistant *S. pneumoniae*.

In addition to antibiotic therapy, oxygen supplementation should be given. Frequent arterial blood gas measurements should be obtained. Arterial saturation should be monitored with pulse oximetry. with a goal of maintaining the PO_2 at 70 mm Hg, a level necessary to ensure adequate fetal oxygenation. When the gravida is afebrile for 48 hours and has signs of clinical improvement, an oral cephalosporin can be initiated and intravenous therapy discontinued. A total of 10 to 14 days of treatment should be completed.

Pneumococcal polysaccharide vaccination prevents pneumococcal pneumonia in otherwise healthy populations, with an efficacy of 65 percent to 84 percent.[17] The vaccine is safe in pregnancy and should be administered to high-risk gravidas. Those at high-risk include individuals with sickle cell disease secondary to autosplenectomy, patients who have had a surgical splenectomy, and individuals who are immunosuppressed. An additional advantage to maternal immunization with the pneumococcal vaccine is that several studies have demonstrated that there is a significant transplacental transmission of vaccine-specific antibodies.[29] After in utero exposure to the vaccine, there are significantly high concentrations of pneumococcal antibodies in infants at birth and at 2 months of age.[29] In addition colostrum and breast milk antibodies are also significantly increased in women who have received the pneumococcal vaccine.[30,31]

Pneumonia in pregnancy can be complicated by respiratory failure requiring mechanical ventilation. In such cases, team management should include the obstetrician, maternal-fetal medicine specialist, and intensivist. In addition to meticulous management of the gravida's respiratory status, maintenance of the left lateral recumbent position is advocated to improve uteroplacental perfusion. The potentially viable fetus should be monitored with continuous fetal monitoring. Serial ultrasound examinations for amniotic fluid index (AFI) and growth will help to guide clinical management. If positive end-expiratory pressure (PEEP) greater than 10 cm H_2O is required to maintain oxygenation, central monitoring with a pulmonary artery catheter should be instituted to adequately monitor volume status and maintain maternal and uteroplacental perfusion. There is no evidence that elective delivery results in an overall improvement in respiratory function.[32] Therefore, elective delivery should be undertaken with caution. However, if there is clear evidence of fetal compromise or profound maternal compromise and impending demise, delivery should be accomplished.

VIRAL PNEUMONIAS

Influenza Virus

There are an estimated 4 million cases of pneumonia complicating influenza annually in the United States, and this is the sixth leading cause of death in this country.[33] Although three types of influenza virus can cause human disease (types A, B, and C), most epidemic infections are due to influenza A.[10] Influenza A typically has an acute onset after a 1- to 4-day incubation period and first manifests as high fever, coryza, headache, malaise, and cough. In uncomplicated cases, the chest examination and chest radiograph remain clear.[10] If symptoms persist longer than 5 days, especially in a pregnancy, complications should be suspected. Pneumonia may complicate influenza as the result of either secondary bacterial infection or primary viral infection of the lung parenchyma.[10] In the epidemic of 1957, autopsies demonstrated that pregnant women died from fulminant viral pneumonia most commonly, whereas nonpregnant patients died most often from secondary bacterial infection.[34] A large nested case-control study evaluated the rate of influenza-related complications over 17 influenza seasons in women enrolled in the Tennessee Medicaid system.[35] This study demonstrated a high risk for hospitalization for influenza-related reasons in low-risk pregnant women during the last trimester of pregnancy. The authors predicted that 25 of 10,000 women in the third trimester during the influenza season will be hospitalized with influenza-related complications.[35] A more recent matched cohort study using the administrative database of pregnant women enrolled in the Tennessee Medicaid population examined pregnant women age 25 to 44 years with respiratory hospitalization during influenza seasons 1985 to 1993.[36] In this population of pregnant women, those with asthma accounted for half of all respiratory hospitalizations during influenza season. Of pregnant women with the diagnosis of asthma, 6 percent required respiratory hospitalization during the influenza season (odds ratio [OR] 10.63, 95 percent confidence interval [CI], 8.61 to 13.83) as compared with women without a medical comorbidity. This study detected no significant increases in adverse perinatal outcome associated with respiratory hospitalization during flu season.[36]

Primary influenza pneumonia is characterized by rapid progression from a unilateral infiltrate to diffuse bilateral disease. The gravida may develop fulminant respiratory failure requiring mechanical ventilation and PEEP. When pneumonia complicates influenza in pregnancy, antibiotics should be started, directed at the likely pathogens that can cause secondary infection, including *Staphylococcus aureus,* pneumococcus, *H. influenza,* and certain enteric gram-negative bacteria. Antiviral agents, such as amantadine and ribavirin, can be considered.[37] It has been recommended that the influenza vaccine be given routinely to gravidas in the second and third trimesters of pregnancy during the flu season (October to March). Women at high risk for pulmonary complications, such as those with asthma, chronic obstructive pulmonary disease, cystic fibrosis, and splenectomy, should be vaccinated regardless of the trimester in order to prevent the occurrence of influenza and the development of secondary pneumonia. In addition to maternal protection, prospective studies have demonstrated higher cord blood antibody levels to influenza in babies born to mothers who were immunized during pregnancy. There is a delay in the onset and decrease in severity of influenza in infants who have higher antibody levels.[38]

Varicella

Varicella zoster is a DNA virus that usually causes a benign self-limited illness in children but may infect up to 2 percent of all adults.[39] Varicella infection occurs in 0.7 of every 1,000 pregnancies.[40] Pregnancy may increase the likelihood of varicella pneumonia complicating the primary infection.[11,40,41] Varicella pneumonia occurs most often in the third trimester, and the infection is likely to be severe.[11,40,41] The maternal mortality from varicella pneumonia may be as high as 35 percent to 40 percent as compared with 11 to 17 percent in nonpregnant individuals.[11,40] Although one review reported a decreased mortality with only three deaths in 28 women with varicella pneumonia,[40] another study documented a maternal mortality rate of 35 percent.[11] A recent paper described 347 pregnant women with varicella-zoster viral infection. Of these 18 (5.2 percent) had pneumonia treated with acyclovir. None of these women died. The authors also noted that women with varicella-zoster viral pneumonia were significantly more likely to be current smokers (OR, 5.1; 95 percent CI, 1.6 to 16), and to have 100 or more skin lesions.[42]

Varicella pneumonia usually presents 2 to 5 days after the onset of fever, rash, and malaise and is heralded by the onset of pulmonary symptoms including cough, dyspnea, pruritic chest pain, and hemoptysis.[11] The severity of the illness may vary from asymptomatic radiographic abnormalities to fulminant pneumonitis and respiratory failure[11,43] (Fig. 35-2). All gravidas with varicella pneumonia should be aggressively treated with antiviral therapy and admitted to the intensive care unit for close observation or intubation, if indicated. Acyclovir, a DNA polymerase inhibitor, should be started. The early use of acyclovir has been associated with an improved hospital course after the fifth day and a lower mean temperature, lower respiratory rate, and improved oxygenation and survival.[11,43,44] The use of acyclovir is associated with improved survival as well.[43,44] Treatment with acyclovir is safe in pregnancy. Among 312 exposed pregnancies, there was no increase in the number of birth defects and no consistent pattern of congenital abnormalities.[45] A dose of 7.5 mg/kg intravenously every 8 hours has been recommended.[46]

Varicella vaccine is a live attenuated vaccine. It is the first vaccine against the herpesvirus. Extensive prelicensure studies have demonstrated that the vaccine is safe

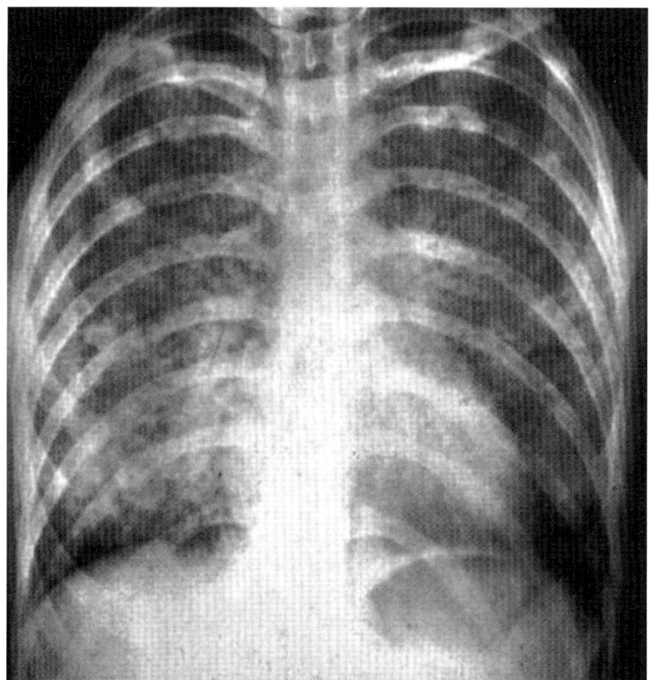

Figure 35-2. This chest radiograph demonstrates bilateral nodular and interstitial pneumonia characteristic of varicella pneumonia. The patient, a 27-year-old gravida 6, para 2, abortus 3 woman, was exposed to varicella infection in her two children. Characteristic skin vesicles of varicella occurred several days before the development of pulmonary symptoms. She required endotracheal intubation and mechanical ventilation for 6 days. She was treated with intravenous acyclovir and ceftazidime for possible superimposed infection. The patient recovered fully and delivered a healthy infant at term.

and efficacious against varicella. Varicella vaccine was added to the universal childhood immunization schedule in the United States in 1995.[47] The program of universal childhood vaccination against varicella in the United States has resulted in a sharp decline in the rate of death due to varicella.[48] This vaccine is not recommended for use in pregnancy. However, the overall decline in the incidence of varicella secondary to vaccination will likely result in a decreased incidence of varicella infection and varicella pneumonia in pregnancy. A recent study assessed the risk of congenital varicella syndrome and other birth defects in offspring of women who inadvertently received varicella vaccine during pregnancy or within 3 months of conception.[49] Fifty-eight women received their first dose of varicella vaccine during the first or second trimester. No cases of congenital varicella syndrome were identified among fifty-six live births (rate 0 percent, 95 percent CI, 0, 15.6). Among the prospective reports of live births, five congenital anomalies were reported. No specific pattern of anomalies was identified in either the susceptible cohort or the sample population as a whole. Although the numbers in the study are small, the results should provide some reassurance to health care providers and women with inadvertent exposure before or during pregnancy.[49]

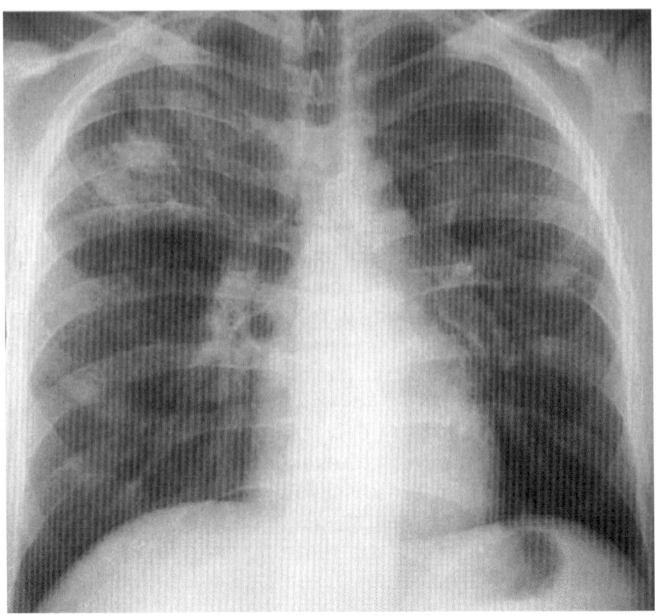

Figure 35-3. *Pneumocystis carinii* pneumonia with mixed interstitial and alveolar opacities, ground-glass appearance.

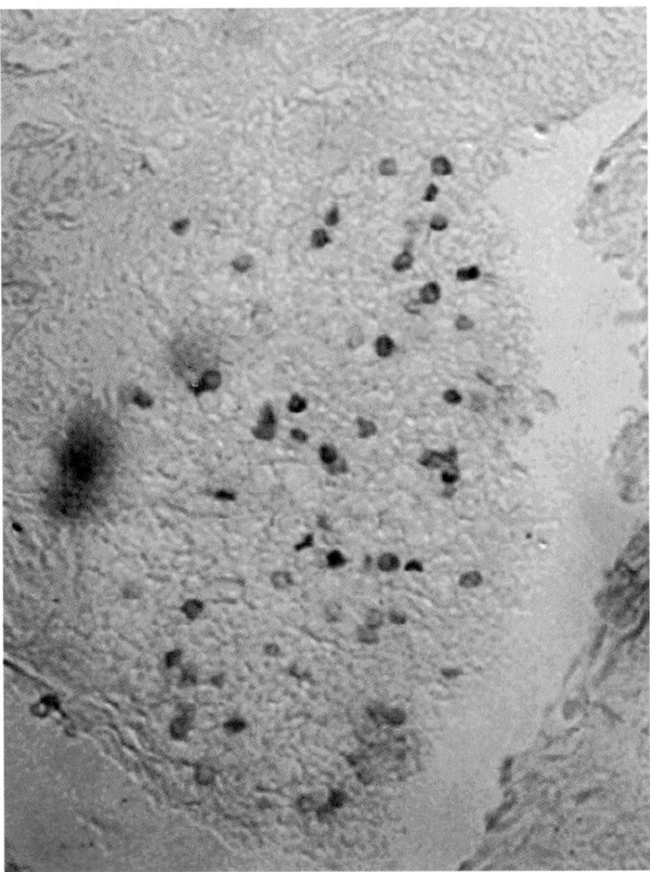

Figure 35-4. Wright-Giemsa stain of *Pneumocystis carinii* pneumonia.

Pneumocystis Carinii Pneumonia

PCP remains the most prevalent opportunistic infection in patients infected with the HIV.[50] PCP, an AIDS-defining illness, occurs more frequently when the T-helper cell count (CD4+) is less than 200 cells per cubic millimeter.[50] When AIDS is complicated by PCP, the mortality rate is 10 to 20 percent during the initial infection, but this rate can increase substantially with the need for mechanical ventilation.[51] The transmission of pneumocystis is not fully understood. There is some evidence that person-to-person transmission is the most likely mode; however, acquisition from environmental sources may also occur.[50]

The symptoms of PCP are nonspecific, and therefore, it may be difficult to diagnose. Typical radiographic features of PCP are bilateral perihilar interstitial infiltrates that become increasingly homogeneous and diffuse as the disease progresses[52] (Fig. 35-3). The diagnosis of PCP requires microscopical examination in order to identify pneumocystis from a clinical source such as sputum, bronchoalveolar fluid, or lung tissue (Fig. 35-4). Pneumocystis cannot be propagated in culture. The fungus has trophic forms as well as a cyst state. These can be detected with a modified Papanicolaou, Wright-Giemsa or Gram-Weigert stains.[50] Monoclonal antibodies are useful for detecting pneumocystis as well.[39,40] The application of polymerase chain reaction (PCR) to detect pneumocystis has been an area of active research and may be valuable for detection in sputum and bronchoalveolar-lavage fluid.[50] Trimethoprim-sulfamethoxazole is the preferred treatment for PCP. Thus far, resistance to this therapeutic agent has not been identified.[50]

A significant number of new infections with HIV are occurring in women of childbearing age. As of 1995, greater than 80 percent of women with AIDS were of reproductive age.[55] PCP pneumonia is the most common cause of AIDS-related death in the United States. Literature on PCP in pregnancy is scarce. A report describes five cases of PCP in pregnancy and also reviews the literature.[11] In this series of 22 pregnant women with PCP,

11 patients (50 percent) died of pneumonia.[11] The incidence of respiratory failure in this series was 59 percent. In individuals who required mechanical ventilation, the survival rate was 31 percent. The average gestational age was 25 weeks, with a range of 6 weeks' gestation up to 1 week postpartum.[1] Fifteen of the 22 patients had CD4+ counts performed, and the mean was 93 cells per cubic millimeter. The patients in this series were treated with a variety of regimens including trimethoprim-sulfamethoxazole alone, trimethoprim-sulfamethoxazole and steroids, and pentamidine. Six patients received trimethoprim-sulfamethoxazole alone and six were given trimethoprim-sulfamethoxazole and steroids; four patients (66 percent) survived in each group. Only 12 babies survived; there were five stillbirths, and four neonates died shortly after birth. In this series, PCP pneumonia complicating pregnancy in the third trimester had a better maternal and fetal outcome as compared with disease in the first or second trimester. There was also a suggestion that treatment with trimethoprim-sulfamethoxazole with or without steroids was associated with an increased survival rate.

The high mortality rate in this series may be skewed by the fact that this is a retrospective review, and severe cases are more likely to be reported than mild ones.[11] In addition all the women in this series were unaware of their HIV infection until the diagnosis of PCP was made. Therefore, none had received PCP prophylaxis.

In summary, PCP pneumonia remains a dreaded complication of HIV infection and an AIDS-defining illness. There is a very high maternal and fetal mortality rate when PCP complicates pregnancy. Primary prophylaxis against PCP with trimethoprim-sulfamethoxazole in HIV-infected adults, including pregnant women and patients receiving highly active antiretroviral therapy, should begin when the CD4+ count is less than 200 cells per cubic millimeter or there is a history of oropharyngeal candidiasis[56] (see Chapter 48). Prophylaxis should be discontinued when the CD4+ cells count increases to more than 200 cells per cubic millimeter for a period of 3 months.[50] The use of highly active antiretroviral therapy (HAART) as well as prophylaxis with trimethoprim-sulfamethoxazole may decrease incidence of PCP pneumonia in developed countries. However, many countries worldwide do not have the resources for HAART and, therefore, remain a reservoir for infection with PCP.

TUBERCULOSIS IN PREGNANCY

The incidence of TB in the United States began to decline in the early part of the 20th century and fell steadily until 1953, when the introduction of isoniazid led to a dramatic decrease in the number of cases, from 84,000 cases in 1953 to 22,255 cases in 1984.[57] However, since 1984, there have been significant changes in TB morbidity trends. From 1985 through 1991, reported cases of TB increased by 18 percent, representing approximately 39,000 more cases than expected had the previous downward trend continued. This increase is due to many factors, including the HIV epidemic, deterioration in the health care infrastructure, and significantly more cases among immigrants.[57] The emergence of drug-resistant TB has also become a serious concern. In New York City, in 1991, 33 percent of TB cases were resistant to at least one drug, and 19 percent were resistant to both isoniazid (INH) and rifampin (RIF).[58] Between 1985 and 1992, the number of TB cases in women of childbearing age increased by 40 percent.[59] One report noted TB-complicated pregnancies in 94.8 cases per 100,000 deliveries between 1991 and 1992.[60]

Diagnosis

The majority of gravidas diagnosed with TB in pregnancy are asymptomatic. Recently, the American Thoracic Society and the Centers for Disease Control issued a statement on targeted tuberculin testing for Latent Tuberculosis Infection (LTBI).[61] This is a strategic component of TB control that identifies persons at high risk for developing TB who would benefit by treatment of LTBI, if detected. Persons at risk include those who have had recent infection with mycobacterium TB and those who have clinical conditions that are associated with an increased risk for progression of LTBI to active TB (Tables 35-1 and 35-2).

All gravidas at high risk for TB should be screened with subcutaneous administration of intermediate-strength purified protein derivative (PPD). If anergy is suspected, control antigens such as candida, mumps, or tetanus toxoids should also be placed.[62] The sensitivity of the PPD is 90 to 99 percent for exposure to TB. The tine

Table 35-1. High-Risk Factors for Tuberculosis

Close contact with persons known or suspected to have tuberculosis
Medical risk factors known to increase risk of disease if infected
Birth in a country with high tuberculosis prevalence
Medically underserved status
Low income
Alcohol addiction
Intravenous drug use
Residency in a long-term care facility (e.g., correctional institutions, mental institutions, nursing homes and facilities)
Health professionals working in high-risk health care facilities

Table 35-2. Clinical Risk Factors for Developing Active Tuberculosis

HIV infection
Recent tuberculosis infection
Injection drug use
Silicosis
Solid Organ Transplant
Chronic renal failure
Jejunoileal bypass
Diabetes mellitus
Carcinoma of head or neck
Underweight by ≥ 15%

HIV, human immunodeficiency virus.

test is not recommended for screening because of its low sensitivity.

The onset of the recent TB epidemic stimulated the need for rapid diagnostic tests using molecular biology methods to detect *M. tuberculosis* in clinical specimens. Two direct amplification tests (DATs) have been approved by the Food and Drug Administration (FDA), the *Mycobacterium tuberculosis* Direct test (MTD) (Gen-Probe, San Diego, CA), and the Amplicor *Mycobacterium tuberculosis* (Amplicor MTB) test (Roche Diagnostic Systems, Inc., Branchburg, NJ). Both tests amplify and detect *M. tuberculosis* 16S ribosomal DNA.[63] When testing acid-fast stain smear-negative respiratory specimens, the specificity remains greater than 95 percent, but the sensitivity ranges from 40 to 77 percent.[64,65] To date, these tests are FDA approved only for testing acid-fast stain smear-positive respiratory specimens obtained from untreated patients or those who have received no more than 7 days of anti-TB therapy. The PPD remains the most commonly used screening test for TB. Three cutoff levels have been recommended for defining a positive tuberculin reaction: greater than 5 mm, greater than 10 mm, and 15 mm or more induration (Fig. 35-5). Induration of greater than 5 mm is a positive reaction in individuals with highest risk for conversion to active TB. That includes individuals who are HIV positive, recent contacts with persons infected with TB, fibrotic changes on chest radiograph consistent with prior TB, and the individual with organ transplants and other immunosuppressed persons[61] (see Table 35-2).

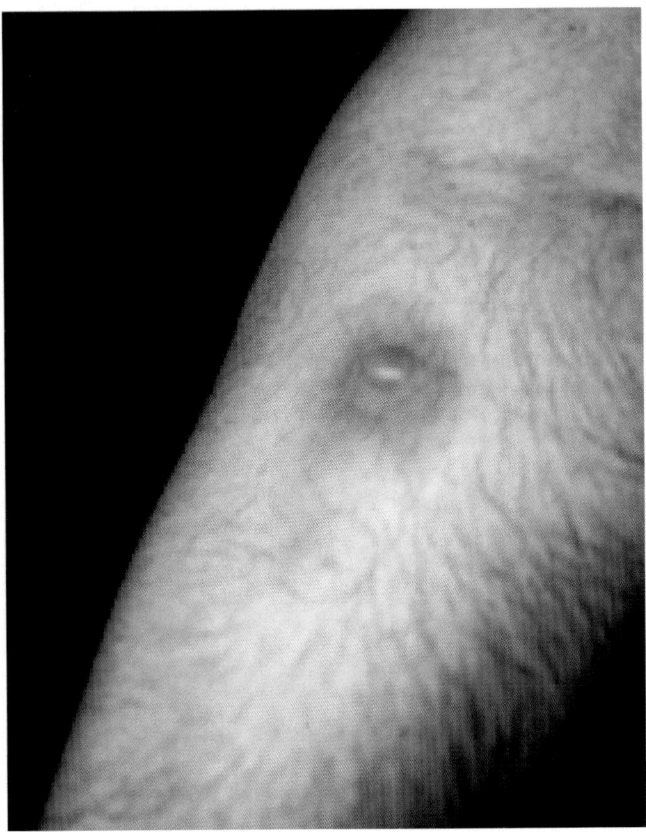

Figure 35-5. Positive PPD, induration greater than 10 mm. PPD, purified protein derivative.

Immigrants from areas where TB is endemic may have received the Bacille Calmette-Guérin (BCG) vaccine. Such individuals likely have a positive response to the PPD. However, this reactivity should wane over time. Therefore, the PPD should be used to screen these patients for TB unless their skin tests are known to be positive.[66] If the BCG vaccine was given 10 years earlier and the PPD is positive with a skin test reaction of 10 mm or more, that individual should be considered infected with TB and managed accordingly.[66]

Women with a positive PPD skin test must be evaluated for active TB with a thorough physical examination for extrapulmonary disease and a chest radiograph once they are beyond the first trimester.[13] Symptoms of active TB include cough (74 percent), weight loss (41 percent), fever (30 percent), malaise and fatigue (30 percent), and hemoptysis (19 percent).[67] Individuals with active pulmonary TB may have radiographic findings including adenopathy, multinodular infiltrates, cavitation, loss of volume in the upper lobes, and upper medial retraction of hilar markings (Fig. 35-6). The finding of acid-fast bacilli in early morning sputum specimens confirms the diagnosis of pulmonary TB. At least three first-morning sputum samples should be examined for the presence of acid-fast bacilli. If sputum cannot be produced, sputum-induction, gastric washings, diagnostic bronchoscopy, or PTNA may be indicated.

Extrapulmonary TB occurs in up to 16 percent of cases in the United States; however, in patients with AIDS the pattern may occur in 60 percent to 70 percent of all patients.[68] Extrapulmonary sites include lymph nodes, bone, kidneys, and breasts. Extrapulmonary TB appears to be rare in pregnancy.[69] Extrapulmonary TB that is confined to the lymph nodes has no effect on obstetric outcomes, but TB at other extrapulmonary sites does adversely affect the outcome of pregnancy.[70] Rarely, mycobacteria invade the uteroplacental circulation, and congenital TB results.[9,59,71] The diagnosis of congenital TB is based on one of the following factors: (1) dem-

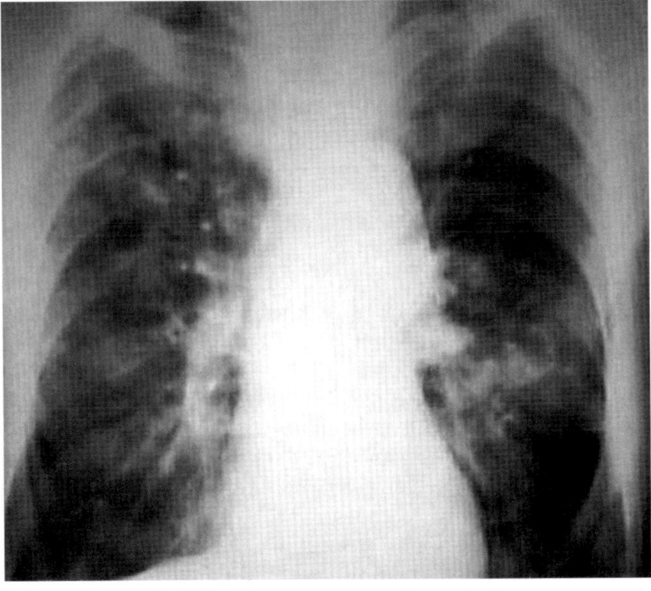

Figure 35-6. Pulmonary tuberculosis.

onstration of primary hepatic complex or cavitating hepatic granuloma by percutaneous liver biopsy at birth; (2) infection of the maternal genital tract or placenta; (3) lesions noted in the first week of life; and (4) exclusion of the possibility of postnatal transmission by a thorough investigation of all contacts, including attendants.[59]

Prevention

The majority of gravidas with a positive PPD in pregnancy are asymptomatic with no evidence of active disease and, therefore, are classified as having LTBI. The risk of progression to active disease is highest in the first 2 years of conversion. It is important to prevent the onset of active disease while minimizing maternal and fetal risk. An algorithm for management of the positive PPD is presented in Figure 35-7.[72] In women with a known recent conversion (2 years) to a positive PPD and no evidence of active disease, the recommended prophylaxis is isoniazid (INH), 300 mg/day, starting after the first trimester and continuing for 6 to 9 months.[13] INH should be accompanied by pyridoxine (vitamin B_6) supplementation, 50 mg/day, in order to prevent the peripheral neuropathy that is associated with INH treatment. Women with an unknown or prolonged duration of PPD positivity (>2 years) should receive INH, 300 mg/day for 6 to 9 months after delivery. INH prophylaxis is not recommended for women older than 35 years of age who have an unknown or prolonged PPD positivity in the absence of active disease. The use of INH is discouraged in this group because of an increased risk of hepatotoxicity. INH is associated with hepatitis in both pregnant and nonpregnant adults. The risk of liver inflammation in pregnancy from INH use is rare, and therefore, this therapy should be instituted when the risk of conversion to active disease is high.[64,65] Monthly monitoring of liver function tests may prevent this adverse outcome. Among individuals receiving INH, 10 to 20 percent develop mildly elevated liver function tests. These changes resolve once the drug is discontinued.[73]

Treatment

The gravida with active TB should be treated initially with INH, 300 mg/day, combined with RIF, 600 mg/day (Table 35-3).[74] Resistant disease results from initial infection with resistant strains (33 percent) or can develop during therapy.[75] If resistance to isoniazid is identified or anticipated, ethambutol 2.5 g/day should be added and the treatment period should be extended to 18 months.[74] Ethambutol is teratogenic in animals; however, this has not been demonstrated in humans. The most common side effect of ethambutol therapy is optic neuritis. Streptomycin should be avoided during pregnancy because it is associated with eighth nerve damage in neonates.[76] Antituberculous agents not recommended for use in pregnancy include ethionamide, streptomycin, capreomycin, kanamycin, cycloserine, and pyrazinamide.[13] However, recent case reports documenting use of the above-mentioned antituberculous agents in pregnancy have revealed no adverse fetal or neonatal effects. There were no congenital abnormalities, and pregnancy outcome in the individuals treated was good.[77,78] Untreated TB has been associated with higher morbidity and mortality among pregnant women.[79] Therefore, the management of the gravida with multi-drug resistant TB should be individualized. The patient should be counseled about the small risk of teratogenicity, and the increased risk of maternal and fetal morbidity and mortality from progression of disease

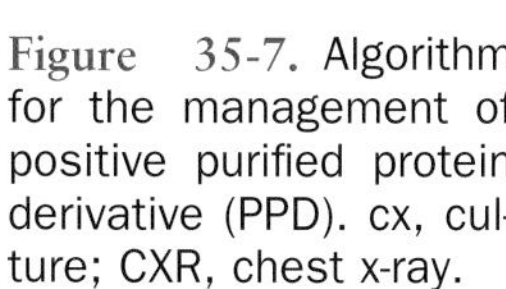
Figure 35-7. Algorithm for the management of positive purified protein derivative (PPD). cx, culture; CXR, chest x-ray.

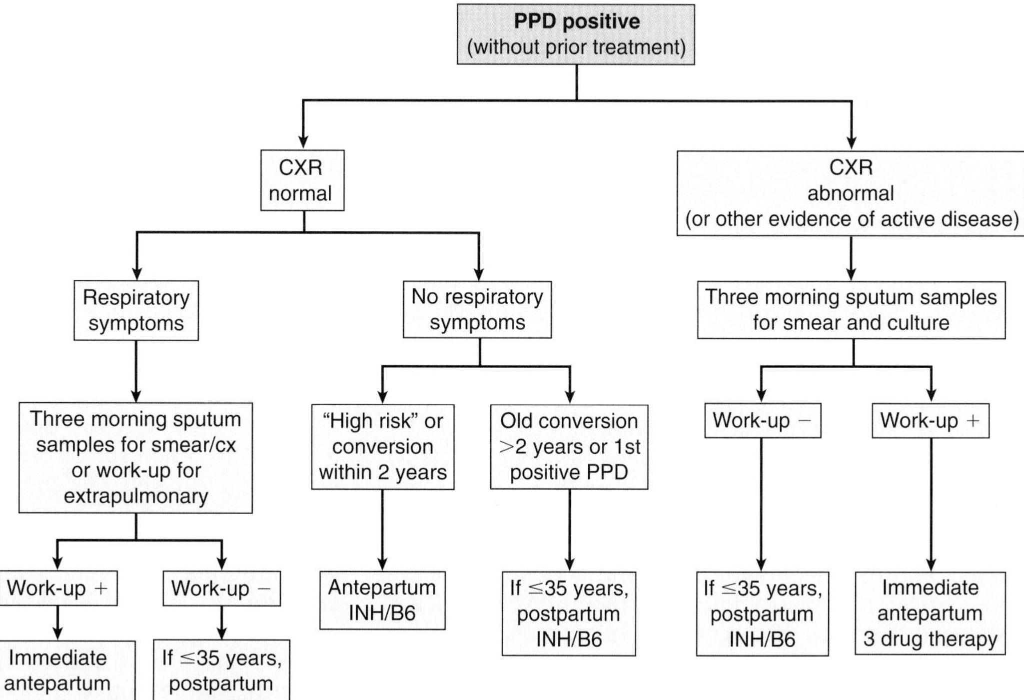

Table 35-3. Antituberculosis Drugs

DRUG	DOSAGE FORM	DAILY DOSE	WEEKLY DOSE	MAJOR ADVERSE REACTIONS
First-Line Drugs (for Initial Treatment):				
Isoniazid	PO, IM	10 mg/kg up to 300 mg	15 mg/kg up to 900 mg	Hepatic enzyme elevation, peripheral neuropathy hepatitis, hypersensitivity
Rifampin	PO	10 mg/kg up to 600 mg	10 mg/kg up to 600 mg	Orange discoloration of secretions and urine, nausea, vomiting, hepatitis, febrile reaction, purpura (rare)
Pyrazinamide	PO	15–30 mg/kg up to 2 g	50–70 mg/kg	Hepatotoxicity, hyperuricemia, arthralgias, skin rash, gastrointestinal upset
Ethambutol	PO	15 mg/kg up to 2.5 g	50 mg/kg	Optic neuritis (decreased red-green color discrimination, decreased visual acuity), skin rash
Streptomycin	IM	15 mg/kg up to 1 g	25–30 mg/kg up to 1 g	Ototoxicity, nephrotoxicity
Second-Line Drugs (Daily Therapy):				
Capreomycin	IM	15–30 mg/kg up to 1 g		Auditory, vestibular, and renal toxicity
Kanamycin	IM	15–30 mg/kg up to 1 g		Auditory and renal toxicity, rare vestibular toxicity
Ethionamide	PO	15–20 mg/kg up to 1 g		Gastrointestinal disturbance, hepatotoxicity, hypersensitivity
Para-aminosalycylic acid	PO	150 mg/kg up to 1 g		Gastrointestinal disturbance, hypersensitivity, hepatotoxicity, sodium load
Cycloserine	PO	15–20 mg/kg up to 1 g		Psychosis, convulsions, rash

IM, intramuscular; PO, by mouth.

when treatment is delayed. The risk of postpartum transmission of TB to the baby may be higher among those born to patients with drug-resistant TB.[78] Therefore, in patients with active disease at time of delivery, separation of the mother and newborn should be accomplished in order to prevent infection of the newborn.

Women who are being treated with antituberculous drugs may breast-feed. Only 0.75 to 2.3 percent of INH and 0.05 percent of RIF are excreted into breast milk. Ethambutol excretion into breast milk is also minimal. However, if the infant is concurrently taking oral antituberculous therapy, excessive drug levels may be reached in the neonate, and breast-feeding should be avoided. Breast-fed infants of women taking INH therapy should receive a multivitamin supplement, including pyridoxine.[13] Neonates of women taking antituberculous therapy should have a PPD skin test at birth and again at 3 months of age. Infants born to women with active TB at the time of delivery should receive INH prophylaxis (10 mg/kg/day) until maternal disease has been inactive for 3 months, as evidenced by negative maternal sputum cultures.[13] Active TB in the neonate should be treated appropriately with INH and RIF immediately upon diagnosis or with multiagent therapy should drug-resistant organisms be identified. Infants and children who are at high risk of intimate and prolonged exposure to untreated or ineffectively treated persons should receive the BCG vaccine.[79]

Summary

In summary, high-risk gravidas should be screened for TB and treated appropriately with INH prophylaxis for infection without overt disease and with dual antituberculous therapy for active disease. In addition, the newborn should be screened for evidence of TB as well. Proper screening and therapy will result in a good outcome for mother and fetus in the majority of cases.

ASTHMA DURING PREGNANCY

Asthma, which may be the most common potentially serious complication of pregnancy, is characterized by chronic airway inflammation with increased airway responsiveness to a variety of stimuli, and airway obstruction that is partially or completely reversible.[81] Approximately 4 to 8 percent of pregnancies are complicated by asthma.[82,83] In general, the prevalence, morbidity, and morality from asthma are increasing.

In 2004, the National Asthma Education and Prevention Program[84] (NAEPP) Working Group on Asthma and Pregnancy defined mild intermittent, mild persistent, moderate persistent, and severe persistent asthma according to symptomatic exacerbations (wheezing, cough, or dyspnea) and objective tests of pulmonary function. The most commonly used parameters are the peak expiratory

Table 35-4. Modified NAEPP Asthma Severity Classification

Mild intermittent
- Symptoms ≤ twice/week
- Nocturnal symptoms ≤ twice/month
- PEFR or FEV_1 ≥80% predicted, variability <20%

Mild persistent
- Symptoms > twice/week but not daily
- Nocturnal symptoms > twice/month
- PEFR or FEV_1 ≥80% predicted, variability 20–30%

Moderate persistent asthma
- Daily symptoms
- Nocturnal symptoms > once/week
- PEFR or FEV_1 >60% to <80% predicted, variability >30%
- Regular medications necessary to control symptoms

Severe asthma
- Continuous symptoms/frequent exacerbations
- Frequent nocturnal symptoms
- PEFR or FEV_1 ≤60% predicted, variability >30%
- Regular oral corticosteroids necessary to control symptoms

FEV_1, forced expiratory volume in one second; NAEPP, National Asthma Education and Prevention Program; PEFR, peak expiratory flow rate.

flow rate (PEFR) and the forced expiratory volume in one second (FEV_1). The NAEPP guidelines did not list the need for regular medication to be a factor for classifying asthma severity during pregnancy. However, in a recent prospective observational study of 1,739 pregnant women with asthma, patients with mild asthma, but who required regular medications to control their asthma, were similar to subjects with moderate asthma in respect to asthma exacerbations.[85] Pregnant patients requiring regular systemic corticosteroids to control asthma symptoms were similar to severe asthmatics in respect to exacerbations. Modified NAEPP asthma severity criteria are presented in Table 35-4.

Insight into the pathogenesis of asthma has changed with the recognition that airway inflammation is present in nearly all cases. The effects of pregnancy on asthma are variable, with 23 percent improving and 30 percent becoming worse during pregnancy.[85] Asthma has been associated with considerable maternal morbidity; 2.3 percent with mild, 19.3 percent with moderate, and 26.9 percent with severe asthma required hospitalization during pregnancy for asthma exacerbations.[83]

Gravidas with asthma have increased frequency of chronic hypertension[86] and maternal smoking,[87] which may also complicate the effects of other influences. Ethnicity may be a particularly important confounding factor in assessing the relationship between asthma and pregnancy outcomes, since American blacks (ages 15 to 44) are five times more likely to die from asthma and are twice as likely to be hospitalized from asthma compared with whites.[88]

Earlier studies on the effects of asthma on pregnancy have had inconsistent findings in regard to perinatal mortality, preeclampsia, preterm birth, hemorrhage, and low birth weight[82,86,95] (see Box). Asthma medications and poor asthma control leading to hypoxia have been hypothesized to explain these observations.[96] There are some data to support a correlation with poor asthma control indicated by increased hospitalization for exacerbations and decreased FEV_1 values to low birth weight and ponderal index.[92,96,97] Studies have repeatedly shown that patients with more severe asthma may have the greatest risk for complications during pregnancy, whereas better controlled asthma is associated with decreased risks.[86,91,93,94,96,98,99]

Two recently published, large, multicenter, prospective cohort studies evaluating the effects of maternal asthma on perinatal outcomes are in considerable agreement. In 2003, Bracken et al.[98] described 1,333 women with no asthma history and 873 pregnant women with asthma. Preterm delivery was not associated with asthma diagnosis or severity. However, oral corticosteroid use was associated with a reduction of gestation of 2.22 weeks (P = .001) and theophylline use was associated with a reduction of 1.11 weeks (P = .002). Birth weight less than 10th percentile was associated with moderate persistent severity (OR = 2.01, 95 percent CI 1.11 to 3.65). In 2004, Dombrowski et al.[99] reported 873 subjects with mild asthma, 866 with moderate or severe asthma, and 881 nonasthmatic controls. There were no significant differences in the rates of preterm delivery less than 32 weeks' or less than 37 weeks' gestation. There were no significant differences for neonatal outcomes except for the discharge diagnosis of neonatal sepsis among the group with mild asthma, a finding that may be related to type 1 error. No significant differences for maternal complications were observed except for an increase in overall cesarean delivery rate among the moderate-severe group odds ratio (OR) = 1.4 (95 percent CI 1.1–1.8). In a secondary analysis of this cohort, Schatz et al.[100] reported that oral corticosteroid use was significantly associated with both preterm delivery less than 37 weeks, OR = 1.54 (95 percent CI 1.02 to 2.33) and birth weight less than 2,500 g, OR = 1.80 (95 percent CI 1.13 to 2.88). Both of these studies suggest that if possible, asthma should be controlled without oral corticosteroids. Most importantly, these studies demonstrate that classification of asthma severity with therapy tailored according to asthma severity can result in excellent perinatal and maternal outcomes.

Asthma Management

The ultimate goal of asthma therapy is maintaining adequate oxygenation of the fetus by prevention of hypoxic episodes in the mother. The effective management of asthma during pregnancy relies on four integral components outlined below:

Objective Measures for Assessment and Monitoring

Subjective measures of lung function by the patient and physician provide an insensitive and inaccurate assessment of airway hyperresponsiveness, airway inflammation, and asthma severity. The FEV_1 following a maximal inspiration is the single best measure of pulmonary function. However, repeated measurement of FEV_1 is impractical because it requires a spirometer. The PEFR correlates well with the FEV_1, and has the advantages that it can be measured reliably with inexpensive, disposable, portable peak flow meters. Patient self-monitoring of PEFR provides valuable insight to the course of asthma throughout the day, assesses circadian variation in pulmonary function, and helps detect early signs of deterioration so that timely therapy can be instituted.

Avoid or Control Asthma Triggers

Limiting adverse environmental exposures during pregnancy is important for controlling asthma. Irritants and allergens that provoke acute symptoms also increase airway inflammation and hyperresponsiveness. Avoiding or controlling such triggers can reduce asthma symptoms, airway hyperresponsiveness, and the need for medical therapy. Association of asthma with allergies is common; 75 to 85 percent of patients with asthma have positive skin tests to common allergens including animal dander, house dust mites, cockroach antigens, pollens, and molds. Other common nonimmunologic triggers include tobacco smoke, strong odors, air pollutants, food additives such as sulfites, and certain drugs including aspirin and β-blockers. Another trigger can be strenuous physical activity. For some patients, exercise-induced asthma can be avoided with inhalation of albuterol, 5 to 60 minutes before exercise. Specific measures for avoiding asthma triggers are listed in Table 35-5.

Patient Education

Women should be made aware that controlling asthma during pregnancy is especially important for the well-being of the fetus. Education should emphasize reduction of asthma triggers. The patient should have a basic understanding of the medical management during pregnancy, including self-monitoring of PEFRs and the correct use of inhalers.

Pharmacologic Therapy

The goal of asthma therapy is multiphasic: (1) relieve bronchospasm, (2) protect the airways from irritant stimuli, (3) prevent the pulmonary and inflammatory response to an allergen exposure, and (4) resolve the inflammatory process in the airways, leading to improved pulmonary function with reduced airway hyperresponsiveness. The step care therapeutic approach includes increasing the number and frequency of medications with increasing asthma severity.

Table 35-5. Limiting Exposure to Asthma Triggers

Use allergen-impermeable mattress and pillow covers
Weekly washing of bedding in hot water
Animal dander control
  Weekly bathing of the pet
  Keeping pets out of the bedroom
  Remove the pet from the home
Cockroach control using poison traps
Avoid tobacco smoke
Inhibit mite and mold growth by reducing humidity
Do not be present when home is being vacuumed

Asthma Pharmacotherapy

It is safer for pregnant women with asthma to be treated with asthma medications than it is for them to have asthma symptoms and exacerbations.[84] Current medical treatment for asthma emphasizes treatment of airway inflammation in order to decrease airway hyperresponsiveness and prevent asthma symptoms. Although it is assumed that asthma medications are as effective in pregnant as in nonpregnant patients, differences in maternal physiology and pharmacokinetics may affect the absorption, distribution, metabolism, and clearance of medications during pregnancy. Endocrinologic and immunologic changes during pregnancy include elevations in free plasma cortisol, possible tissue refractoriness to cortisol,[101] and changes in cellular immunity.[102]

Typical dosages of commonly used asthma medications and inhaled corticosteroid for low, medium, and high doses are listed in Tables 35-6 and 35-7, respectively.

Inhaled Corticosteroids

Inhaled corticosteroids are the preferred treatment for the management of all levels of persistent asthma during pregnancy.[84] Airway inflammation is present in nearly all cases; therefore, inhaled corticosteroids have even been advocated as first-line therapy for patients with mild asthma.[103] The use of inhaled corticosteroids among non-pregnant asthmatics has been associated with a marked reduction in fatal and near-fatal asthma.[104] Inhaled corticosteroids produce clinically important improvements in bronchial hyperresponsiveness that appear to be dose related,[104] can occur as early as a few weeks but take months to attain maximal effect,[106] and include prevention of increased bronchial hyperresponsiveness after

Table 35-6. Typical Dosages of Asthma Medications

Cromolyn MDI	2–4 puffs tid–qid
Albuterol MDI	2–8 puffs as needed
Salmeterol MDI	2 puffs bid
Fluticasone/salmeterol (Advair) DPI	1 inhalation bid, dose depends on severity of asthma
Ipatropium MDI	4–8 puffs as needed
Montelukast	10 mg tablet at night
Zafirlukast	40 mg at night
Theophylline	Maintain serum levels of 5–12 mcg/ml (decrease dosage by half if treated with erythromycin or cimetidine)
Prednisone	20–60 mg/day burst for active symptoms

bid, twice a day; DPI, dry powder inhaler; MDI, metered-dose inhaler; qid, four times a day; tid, three times a day.

Table 35-7. Comparative Daily Doses for Inhaled Corticosteroids

		LOW DOSE	MEDIUM DOSE	HIGH DOSE
Beclomethasone MDI	42 mcg/puff	4–12 puffs	12–20 puffs	>20 puffs
	84 mcg/puff	2–6 puffs	6–10 puffs	>10 puffs
Triamcinolone MDI	100 mcg/puff	4–10 puffs	10–20 puffs	>20 puffs
Budesonide DPI	200 mcg/puff	1–2 puffs	2–3 puffs	>3 puffs
Fluticasone MDI	44 mcg/puff	2–6 puffs		
	110 mcg/puff	2 puffs	2–6 puffs	>6 puffs
	220 mcg/puff		1–3 puffs	>3 puffs
Flunisolide MDI	250 mcg/puff	2–4 puffs	4–8 puffs	>8 puffs

Note that total daily puffs is usually divided as a bid or tid regimen.
DPI, dry powder inhaler; MDI, metered-dose inhaler.

seasonal exposure to allergens.[107,108] Continued administration is also effective in reducing the immediate pulmonary response to an allergen challenge. In a prospective observational study of 504 pregnant subjects with asthma, 177 patients were not initially treated with either inhaled budesonide or inhaled beclomethasone.[109] This cohort had a 17 percent acute exacerbation rate compared with only a 4-percent rate among those treated with inhaled corticosteroids from the start of pregnancy.

The NAEPP Working Group reviewed 10 studies including 6,113 patients who took inhaled corticosteroids during pregnancy for asthma. Based on these studies, there was no evidence of inhaled corticosteroid use and any increases in congenital malformations or adverse perinatal outcomes.[84] Included among these studies was the Swedish Medical Birth Registry, which included 2,014 infants whose mothers had used inhaled budesonide in early pregnancy.[110] Therefore, there are more data describing budesonide use during pregnancy than other inhaled corticosteroids. Budesonide may be considered a preferred medication, but if a woman is well-controlled by a different inhaled corticosteroid before pregnancy, it seems reasonable to continue that medication during pregnancy. All inhaled corticosteroids are currently labeled FDA pregnancy class C, except budesonide, which is class B.

Cromolyn

Cromolyn, which is virtually devoid of significant side effects, blocks both the early- and late-phase pulmonary response to allergen challenge as well as preventing the development of airway hyperresponsiveness.[111] Cromolyn sodium does not have any intrinsic bronchodilator or antihistaminic activity. Compared with inhaled corticosteroids, the time to maximal clinical benefit is longer for cromolyn sodium (4 weeks versus 2 weeks). Cromolyn sodium appears to be less effective than inhaled corticosteroids in reducing objective and subjective manifestations of asthma. Cromolyn appears to be safe during pregnancy.[100]

Theophylline

New dosing guidelines have recommended that serum theophylline concentrations be maintained at 5 to 12 mcg/ml during pregnancy.[84] Subjective symptoms of adverse theophylline effects including insomnia, heartburn, palpitations, and nausea, may be difficult to differentiate from typical pregnancy symptoms. High doses have been observed to cause jitteriness, tachycardia, and vomiting in mothers and neonates.[112,113] Theophylline can have significant interactions with other drugs causing decreased clearance and resultant toxicity. Two commonly used drugs, cimetidine and erythromycin, may increase theophylline serum levels[114] 70 percent and 35 percent, respectively.

The main advantage of theophylline is the long duration of action, 10 to 12 hours with the use of sustained-release preparations, which is especially helpful in the management of nocturnal asthma.[115] Theophylline may be employed as an alternate treatment when β_2-agonists and inhaled anti-inflammatory agents do not adequately control symptoms. Theophylline is indicated only for chronic therapy and is not effective for the treatment of acute exacerbations during pregnancy.[116] Theophylline has anti-inflammatory actions[117] that may be mediated from inhibition of leukotriene production and its capacity to stimulate PGE_2 production.[118] Theophylline may potentiate the efficacy of inhaled corticosteroids.[119]

Eight human studies had a total of 660 women with asthma who took theophylline during pregnancy.[84] These studies and clinical experience confirm the safety of theophylline at a serum concentration of 5 to 12 mcg/ml during pregnancy. In a recent randomized controlled trial, there were no differences in asthma exacerbations or perinatal outcomes in a cohort receiving theophylline compared with the cohort receiving inhaled beclomethasone.[99] However, the theophylline cohort had significantly more reported side effects, discontinuation of study medication, and an increased proportion of those with an FEV_1 less than 80 percent predicted.

Inhaled β_2-Agonists

Beta$_2$-agonists are currently recommended for use with all degrees of asthma during pregnancy.[84,120] Albuterol has the advantage of a rapid onset of effect in the relief of acute bronchospasm through smooth muscle relaxation. Albuterol is an excellent bronchoprotective agent for pretreatment before exercise. This group also includes long-acting β_2-agonists salmeterol and formoterol. β_2-agonists are associated with tremor, tachycardia, and palpitations, and have been associated with an increased risk of death with chronic use.[121,122] They do not block the development of airway hyperresponsiveness.[111] Indeed, a comparison of an inhaled glucocorticoid, budesonide, with the inhaled terbutaline, raised the question whether routine use of this medication could result in increased airway hyperresponsiveness.[103] An increased frequency of bronchodilator use could be an indicator of the need for additional anti-inflammatory therapy.

Beta$_2$-agonists appear to be safe based on a review of six published studies with 1,599 women with asthma who took β_2-agonists during pregnancy.[84] Additionally, in a large prospective study, no significant relationship was found between the use of inhaled β_2-agonists (n = 1,828) and adverse pregnancy outcomes.[100]

Leukotriene Moderators

Leukotrienes are arachidonic acid metabolites that have been implicated in transducing bronchospasm, mucous secretion, and increased vascular permeability.[123] Bronchoconstriction associated with aspirin ingestion can be blocked by leukotriene receptor antagonists.[124] Treatment with the leukotriene receptor antagonist montelukast (Singulair) has been shown to significantly improve pulmonary function as measured by FEV_1.[122] The leukotriene receptor antagonists zafirlukast (Accolate), and montelukast (Singulair) are both pregnancy category B. It should be noted that there are minimal data regarding the efficacy or safety of these agents during human pregnancy.

Oral (Systemic) Corticosteroids

The NAEPP Working Group reviewed eight human studies including one report of two meta-analyses.[84] The majority of subjects in these studies did not take oral corticosteroids for asthma. The panel concluded that findings from the current evidence review are conflicting. Oral corticosteroid use during the first trimester of pregnancy is associated with a three-fold increased risk for isolated cleft lip with or without cleft palate, with a background incidence of about 0.1 percent, the excess risk attributable to oral steroids would be 0.25 to 0.3 percent.[125] However, very few pregnant women who had oral steroid–dependent asthma were included in the studies, and the length, timing, and dose of exposure to the drug were not well described.

Oral corticosteroid use during pregnancy in patients who have asthma has been associated with an increased incidence of preeclampsia, preterm delivery, and low birth weight.[86,91,98,100,125] However, it is difficult to separate the effects of the oral corticosteroids on these outcomes from the effects of severe or uncontrolled asthma, which has been associated with maternal and fetal mortality. Because of the uncertainties in these data and the definite risks of severe uncontrolled asthma to the mother and fetus, the Working Group recommends the use of oral corticosteroids when indicated for the long-term management of severe asthma or severe exacerbations during pregnancy.

Management of Allergic Rhinitis

Rhinitis, sinusitis and gastroesophageal reflux may exacerbate asthma symptoms, and their management should be considered an integral aspect of asthma care. Intranasal corticosteroids are the most effective medications for control of allergic rhinitis. Loratadine (Claritin) or cetirizine (Zyrtec) are recommended second-generation antihistamines. Oral decongestants have been associated with gastroschisis; therefore, inhaled decongestants or inhaled corticosteroids should be considered before use of oral decongestants.[84]

Step Therapy

The step-care therapeutic approach increases the number and frequency of medications with increasing asthma severity (Table 35-8). A burst of oral corticosteroids is indicated for exacerbations not responding to initial β_2 agonist therapy regardless of asthma severity. Additionally, patients who require increasing inhaled albuterol therapy to control their symptoms may benefit from oral corticosteroids. In such cases, a short course of oral prednisone, 40 to 60 mg per day for 1 week, followed by 7 to 14 days of tapering, may be effective.

Table 35-8. Step Therapy-Medical Management of Asthma

Mild Intermittent
No daily medications needed
Mild Persistent
Preferred:
Low-dose inhaled corticosteroid
Alternative:
Cromolyn, leukotriene receptor antagonist, or theophylline (serum level 5–12 mcg/ml)
Moderate Persistent
Preferred:
Low- to medium-dose inhaled corticosteroid and salmeterol or Medium-dose inhaled corticosteroid
Alternative:
Low to medium-dose inhaled corticosteroid and leukotriene receptor antagonist or
Low to medium-dose inhaled corticosteroid and theophylline (serum level 5–12 mcg/ml)
Severe Persistent
Preferred:
High-dose inhaled corticosteroid and salmeterol and oral corticosteroid if needed
Alternative:
High-dose inhaled corticosteroid and theophylline (serum level 5–12 mcg/ml) and oral corticosteroid if needed
Albuterol 2–4 puffs as needed for PEFR or $FEV_1 < 80$ percent, asthma exacerbations, or exposure to exercise or allergens; oral corticosteroid burst if inadequate response to albuterol regardless of asthma severity (NAEPP 04)

FEV_1, forced expiratory volume in one second; NAEPP, National Asthma Education and Prevention Program; PEFR, peak expiratory flow rate.

Antenatal Management

Patients with moderate and severe asthma should be considered to be at risk for pregnancy complications. Adverse outcomes can be increased by underestimation of asthma severity and undertreatment of asthma exacerbations. The first prenatal visit should include a detailed medical history with attention to medical conditions that could complicate the management of asthma, including: diabetes mellitis, hypertension, cardiac disease, adrenal disease, hyperthyroidism, HIV, hemoglobinopathies, hepatic disease, and active pulmonary disease (cystic fibrosis, bronchiectasis, TB, sarcoidosis, recurrent sinus and pulmonary infections, bronchitis). The patient should be questioned about the presence and severity of symptoms, episodes of nocturnal asthma, the number of days of work missed due to asthma exacerbations, history of acute asthma emergency care visits, and smoking history. The type and amount of asthma medications, including the number of puffs of β_2-agonists used each day, should be recorded. Asthma severity can then be determined (see Table 35-8).

Gravidas with moderate or severe asthma should have scheduling of prenatal visits based on clinical judgment. In addition to routine care, monthly or more frequent evaluations of asthma history (emergency visits, hospital admissions, symptom frequency, severity, nocturnal symptoms, medications, dosages and compliance) and pulmonary function (FEV_1 or PEFR) are recommended. Those with mild well-controlled asthma may receive routine prenatal care. Patients should be instructed on proper dosing and administration of their asthma medications. Step-care therapeutic approach includes increasing the number and frequency of medications with increasing asthma severity (see Table 35-8). The least number of medications needed to control asthma symptoms should be used.

Patients should be instructed on proper PEFR technique. Measurements should be recorded while standing, taking a maximum inspiration and noting the reading on the peak flow meter. Personal best PEFR should be determined and personalized green, yellow, and red zones should be established and explained (Table 35-9). Those with moderate to severe asthma should be instructed to maintain an asthma diary containing daily assessment of asthma symptoms including: morning and evening peak flow measurements, symptoms and activity limitations, indication of any medical contacts initiated, and a record of regular and as-needed medications taken. They should determine PEFR before medications, in the morning and after dinner.

Table 35-9. Individualized PEFR Zones

Establish "personal best" PEFR, then calculate:
1. Green Zone >80 percent of personal best PEFR
2. Yellow Zone 50 to 80 percent of personal best PEFR
3. Red Zone <50 percent of personal best PEFR

(Typical PEFR = 380–550 L/minute)

PEFR, peak expiratory flow rate.

As previously discussed, avoidance and control of asthma triggers (see Table 35-5) are particularly important in pregnancy because pharmacologic control of asthma potentially has adverse fetal effects. Specific recommendations should be made for appropriate environmental controls, based upon the patient's history of exposure and, when available, demonstrated skin test reactivity.

Moderate and severe asthmatics should have additional fetal surveillance in the form of ultrasound examinations and antenatal fetal surveillance. Because asthma has been associated with intrauterine growth restriction and preterm birth, it is necessary to accurately establish pregnancy dating. Ultrasound examinations also are needed to evaluate fetal viability, anatomy, amniotic fluid volume, placental location, and interval fetal growth. Repeat ultrasound examinations are recommended for patients with suboptimally controlled asthma, and following asthma exacerbations to evaluate fetal activity, growth, and amniotic fluid volume. The intensity of antenatal fetal surveillance should be based upon the severity of the asthma. All patients should be instructed to be attentive to fetal activity. In most cases, women with moderate and severe asthma should undergo fetal testing by 32 weeks' gestation.

Home Management of Asthma Exacerbations

An asthma exacerbation that causes minimal problems for the mother may have severe sequelae for the fetus. Indeed, an abnormal fetal heart rate tracing may be the initial manifestation of an asthmatic exacerbation. A maternal Po_2 less than 60 or hemoglobin saturation less than 90 percent may be associated with profound fetal hypoxia. Therefore, asthma exacerbations in pregnancy must be aggressively managed. Patients should be given an individualized guide for decision-making and rescue management.

Patients should be educated to recognize signs and symptoms of early asthma exacerbations such as coughing, chest tightness, dyspnea, or wheezing, or by a 20-percent decrease in their PEFR. This is important so that prompt home rescue treatment may be instituted in order to avoid maternal and fetal hypoxia. In general, patients should use inhaled albuterol 2 to 4 puffs every 20 minutes up to 1 hour. A good response is considered if symptoms are resolved or become subjectively mild, normal activities can be resumed, and the PEFR is greater than 70 percent of personal best. The patient should seek further medical attention if the response is incomplete or if fetal activity is decreased (Table 35-10).

Hospital and Clinic Management

The principal goal should be the prevention of hypoxia. Continuous electronic fetal monitoring should be initiated if gestation has advanced to the point of potential fetal viability. Albuterol (2.5 to 5 mg every 20 minutes for three doses, then 2.5 to 10 mg every 1 to 4 hours as needed, or 10 to 15 mg/hour continuously) should

Table 35-10. Home Management of Acute Asthma Exacerbations

Use albuterol MDI 2–4 puffs and measure PEFR

Poor response:
PEFR <50% predicted or symptoms are severe, repeat albuterol 2–4 puffs by MDI and obtain emergency care.

Incomplete response:
PEFR is 50–80% predicted or if persistent wheezing and shortness of breath, then repeat albuterol treatment 2–4 puffs MDI at 20 minute intervals up to 2 more times. If PEFR 50–80% predicted or if decreased fetal movement, contact care giver or go for emergency care.

Good response:
PEFR >80 percent predicted, no wheezing or shortness of breath and fetus is moving normally. May continue inhaled albuterol 2–4 puffs MDI every 3–4 hrs as needed

PEFR, peak expiratory flow rate; MDI, metered-dose inhaler.

be delivered by nebulizer driven with oxygen.[84] Occasionally, nebulized treatment is not effective because the patient is moving air poorly, in such cases, terbutaline 0.25 mg can be administered subcutaneously every 15 minutes for three doses. The patient should be assessed for general level of activity, color, pulse rate, use of accessory muscles and airflow obstruction determined by auscultation and FEV_1 or PEFR before and after each bronchodilator treatment. Measurement of oxygenation through pulse oximeter or arterial blood gases is essential. Arterial blood gases should be obtained if oxygen saturation remains less than 95 percent; chest radiographs are not commonly needed. Guidelines for the management of moderate asthma exacerbations are presented in Table 35-11 and those for severe exacerbations in Table 35-12.

Labor and Delivery Management

Asthma medications should not be discontinued during labor and delivery. Although asthma is usually quiescent during labor, consideration should be given to assessing PEFRs upon admission and at 12-hour intervals. The patient should be kept hydrated and should receive adequate analgesia in order to decrease the risk of bronchospasm. If systemic corticosteroids have been used in the previous 4 weeks, then intravenous corticosteroids (hydrocortisone 100 mg q 8 hours) should be administered during labor and for the 24-hour period following delivery to prevent adrenal crisis.[84]

It is rarely necessary to perform a cesarean delivery for an acute asthma exacerbation. Usually, maternal and fetal compromise will respond to aggressive medical management. Occasionally, delivery may improve the respiratory status of a patient with unstable asthma who has a mature fetus. Prostaglandin (PG) E_2 or E_1 can be used for cervical ripening, the management of spontaneous or induced abortions, or postpartum hemorrhage. Carboprost (15-methyl PGF_2-alpha) and methylergonovine can cause bronchospasm. Magnesium sulfate, which is

Table 35-11. Emergency Department and Hospital-Based Management of Moderate Asthma Exacerbations*

Initial Assessment and Treatment
History, physical examination (auscultation, use of accessory muscles, heart rate, respiratory rate), PEFR or EFV_1, oxygen saturation, and other tests as indicated.
- Initiate fetal assessment (consider continuous electronic fetal monitoring and/or biophysical profile if pregnancy has reached fetal viability)
- Albuterol by MDI or nebulizer, up to three doses in first hour
- Oral systemic corticosteroid if no immediate response or if patient recently took oral systemic corticosteroid
- Oxygen to maintain O_2 saturation >95%
- Repeat assessment: symptoms, physical examination, PEFR, O_2 saturation
- Continue albuterol every 60 minutes for 1–3 hours provided there is improvement

Good Response
- FEV_1 or PEFR 70%
- Response sustained 60 minutes after last treatment
- No distress
- Physical examination: normal
- Reassuring fetal status
- Discharge home

Incomplete Response
- FEV_1 or PEFR 50% but <70%
- Mild or moderate symptoms
- Continue fetal assessment until patient stabilized
- Monitor FEV_1 or PEFR, O_2 saturation, pulse
- Continue inhaled albuterol and oxygen
- Inhaled ipratropium bromide
- Systemic (oral or intravenous) corticosteroid
- Individualize decision for hospitalization

Poor Response
- FEV_1 or PEFR <50%
- Pco_2 >42 mm Hg
- Physical exam: symptoms severe, drowsiness, confusion
- Admit to Hospital Intensive Care
- Continue fetal assessment
- See Table 35-12

Discharge Home
- Continue treatment with albuterol
- Oral systemic corticosteroid, if indicated
- Initiate or continue inhaled corticosteroid until review at medical follow-up
- Patient education
  - Review medicine use
  - Review/initiate action plan
  - Recommend close medical follow-up

FEV_1, forced expiratory volume in one second; MDI, metered-dose inhaler; NAEPP, National Asthma Education and Prevention Program; Pco_2, carbon dioxide partial pressure; PEFR, peak expiratory flow rate.
*FEV_1 or PEFR 50%–80% predicted/personal best with moderate symptoms.
Adapted from NAEPP 2004.

a bronchodilator, is a safe choice for treating preterm labor. Indomethacin can induce bronchospasm in the aspirin-sensitive patient. There are no reports of the use of calcium channel blockers for tocolysis among women with asthma.

Table 35-12. Emergency Department and Hospital-Based Management of Severe Asthma Exacerbations*

Impending or Actual Respiratory Arrest
- Admit to hospital intensive care
- Intubation and mechanical ventilation with 100% O_2
- Nebulized albuterol plus inhaled ipratropium bromide
- Intravenous corticosteroid

Initial Assessment and Treatment
Physical examination: accessory muscle use, chest retraction
History: high-risk patient
- Initiate assessment (consider continuous electronic fetal monitoring and/or biophysical profile if pregnancy has reached fetal viability)
- High-dose albuterol by nebulization every 20 minutes or continuously for 1 hour plus inhaled ipratropium bromide
- Oxygen to achieve O_2 saturation >95%
- Systemic corticosteroid

Repeat Assessment
Symptoms, physical examination, PEF, O_2 saturation, other tests as needed
Continue fetal assessment

Good Response
- FEV_1 or PEFR >70%
- Response sustained 60 minutes after last treatment
- No distress
- Physical examination: normal
- Reassuring fetal status
- Discharge home

Incomplete Response
- FEV_1 or PEFR 50% but <70%
- Mild or moderate symptoms
- Continue fetal assessment until patient stabilized
- Monitor FEV_1 or PEFR, O_2 saturation, pulse
- Continue inhaled albuterol and oxygen
- Inhaled ipratropium bromide
- Systemic (oral or intravenous) corticosteroid
- Admit to Hospital Ward

Poor Response
- FEV_1 or PEFR <50%
- PCO_2 >42 mm Hg
- Physical examination: symptoms severe, drowsiness, confusion
- Admit to hospital intensive care
- Continue fetal assessment

Hospital Intensive Care
- Inhaled albuterol hourly or continuously plus inhaled ipratropium bromide
- Intravenous corticosteroid
- Oxygen
- Possible intubation and mechanical ventilation
- Continue fetal assessment until patient stabilized

FEV_1, forced expiratory volume in one second; NAEPP, National Asthma Education and Prevention Program; PCO_2, carbon dioxide partial pressure; PEFR, peak expiratory flow rate.
*FEV_1 or PEFR <50% predicted/personal best with severe symptoms at rest.
Adapted from NAEPP 2004.

Lumbar epidural anesthesia has the benefit of reducing oxygen consumption and minute ventilation during labor.[126] Fentanyl may be a better analgesic than meperidine, which causes histamine release, but meperidine is rarely associated with the onset of bronchospasm during labor. A 2-percent incidence of bronchospasm has been reported with regional anesthesia.[127] Ketamine is useful for induction of general anesthesia because it can prevent bronchospasm.[128] Communication between the obstetric, anesthetic, and pediatric caregivers is important for optimal care.

Breast-Feeding

In general, only small amounts of asthma medications enter breast milk.[129] Prednisone, theophylline, antihistamines, beclomethasone, β_2 agonists, and cromolyn are not considered to be contraindications for breast feeding.[4,51] However, among sensitive individuals, theophylline may cause toxic effects in the neonate including vomiting, feeding difficulties, jitteriness, and cardiac arrhythmias.

RESTRICTIVE LUNG DISEASE

Restrictive ventilatory defects occur when lung expansion is limited because of alterations in the lung parenchyma or because of abnormalities in the pleura, chest wall, or the neuromuscular apparatus.[130] These conditions are characterized by a reduction in lung volumes and an increase in the ratio of FEV_1 to forced vital capacity (FVC).[131] The interstitial lung diseases include idiopathic pulmonary fibrosis, sarcoidosis, hypersensitivity pneumonitis, pneumoconiosis, drug-induced lung disease, and connective tissue disease. Additional conditions that cause a restrictive ventilatory defect include pleural and chest wall diseases, and extrathoracic conditions such as obesity, peritonitis, and ascites.[131] Restrictive lung disease in pregnancy has not been well studied. Consequently, little is known about the effects of restrictive lung disease on the outcome of pregnancy or the effects of pregnancy on the disease process itself. A recent study presented data on nine pregnant women who were prospectively managed with interstitial and restrictive lung disease.[132] Diagnoses included idiopathic pulmonary fibrosis, hypersensitivity pneumonitis, sarcoidosis, kyphoscoliosis, and multiple pulmonary emboli. Three of the gravidas presented in this paper had severe disease characterized by a vital capacity of 1.5 L or less (50 percent predicted) or a diffusing capacity less than or equal to 50 percent predicted. Five of the patients had exercise-induced oxygen desaturation, and four patients required supplemental oxygen. Of the group, one patient had an adverse outcome and was delivered at 31 weeks. She subsequently required mechanical ventilation for 72 hours. All other patients were delivered at or beyond 36 weeks, with no adverse intrapartum or postpartum complications. All infants were at or above the 30th percentile for growth.[132] The authors concluded that restrictive lung disease was well tolerated in pregnancy. However, exercise intolerance was common, and early oxygen supplementation may be required.[132]

Sarcoidosis

Sarcoidosis is a systemic granulomatosis disease of undetermined etiology that often affects young adults. Pregnancy outcome for the majority of women with sarcoidosis is good.[133,134] In a study of 35 pregnancies in 18 patients with sarcoidosis, disease activity remained stable in nine patients. During pregnancy, improvement was demonstrated in six patients, and in three, there was a worsening of the disease.[133] During the postpartum period, 15 patients remained stable; however, in three women, a progression of the disease continued. Another retrospective study presented 15 pregnancies complicated by maternal sarcoidosis over a 10-year period.[134] Eleven of these patients remained stable, two experienced disease progression, and two died due to severe complications of severe sarcoidosis. In this group, factors indicating a poor prognosis reportedly included parenchymal lesions on chest radiograph, advanced radiographic staging, advanced maternal age, low inflammatory activity, requirement for drugs other than steroids, and the presence of extrapulmonary sarcoidosis.[134] Both of the patients who succumbed during gestation had severe disease at the onset of pregnancy. The overall rate of cesarean delivery rate was 40 percent and, in addition, 4 of 15 infants (27 percent) weighed less than 2,500 g. None of the patients developed preeclampsia. One possible explanation for the commonly observed improvement in sarcoidosis may be the increased concentration of cortisol during pregnancy. However, because sarcoidosis improves spontaneously in many nonpregnant patients, the improvement may be coincident with but not due to pregnancy.

Maycock et al.[135] described 16 pregnancies in 10 patients with sarcoidosis. Eight of the 10 patients showed improvement in at least some of the manifestations of sarcoidosis during the antepartum period. In two patients, no effect was noted. A recurrence of the abnormal findings was observed in the postpartum period within several months after delivery in approximately half of the patients. In addition, some had new manifestations of sarcoidosis not previously noted. Another study examined 17 pregnancies in 10 patients and concluded that pregnancy had no consistent effect on the course of the disease.[136] Scadding[137] separated patients into three categories based on characteristic patterns of their chest radiographs. When the chest radiograph had resolved before pregnancy, the normal radiograph persisted throughout gestation. In women with resolving radiographic changes before pregnancy, resolution continued throughout the prenatal period. Patients with inactive fibrotic residual disease had stable chest radiographs, and those with active disease tended to have partial or complete resolution of those changes during pregnancy. Most patients in this latter group, however, experienced exacerbation of the disease within 3 to 6 months after delivery.[137]

Patients with pulmonary hypertension complicating restrictive lung disease may suffer a mortality rate as high as 50 percent during gestation. These patients need close monitoring during labor, delivery, and the postpartum period. Invasive monitoring with a pulmonary artery catheter may be indicated to optimize cardiorespiratory function. Gravidas with restrictive lung disease including pulmonary sarcoidosis may benefit from early institution of steroid therapy for evidence of worsening pulmonary status. Individuals with evidence of severe disease need close monitoring and may require supplemental oxygen therapy during gestation as well.

During labor, consideration should be given to early use of epidural anesthesia, if it is not contraindicated. The early institution of pain management in this population will minimize pain, decrease sympathetic response, and therefore, decrease oxygen consumption during labor and delivery. The use of general anesthesia should be avoided, if possible, because these patients may develop pulmonary complications after general anesthesia including pneumonia and difficulty weaning from the ventilator. In addition, close fetal surveillance throughout gestation is warranted, because impaired oxygenation may compromise fetal growth.

An additional consideration is the need to counsel all women with restrictive lung disease about the potential for continued impairment of their respiratory status during pregnancy, particularly if their respiratory disease is deteriorating at the time of conception. The individual with clinical signs consistent with pulmonary hypertension or severe restrictive disease should be cautioned about the possibility of maternal mortality resulting from worsening pulmonary function during gestation.

In summary, although the literature on restrictive lung disease in pregnancy is limited, it supports the conclusion that the majority of patients with restrictive lung disease complicating pregnancy including those with pulmonary sarcoidosis will have a favorable pregnancy outcome. However, the clinician should keep in mind that a subgroup of women with restrictive lung disease can have significant worsening of their clinical condition during gestation.

Cystic Fibrosis

Cystic fibrosis involves the exocrine glands and epithelial tissues of the pancreas, sweat glands, and mucous glands in the respiratory, digestive, and reproductive tracts. Chronic obstructive pulmonary disease, pancreatic exocrine insufficiency, and elevated sweat electrolytes are present in most patients with cystic fibrosis.[138] The disease is genetically transmitted with an autosomal recessive pattern of inheritance. The cystic fibrosis gene was identified and cloned in 1989. The gene is localized to chromosome 7, and the molecular defect accounting for the majority of cases has been identified.[139–141] In the United States, approximately 4 percent of the white population are heterozygous carriers of the cystic fibrosis gene. The disease occurs in one in 3,000 live white births.[142] Morbidity and mortality in cystic fibrosis is usually secondary to progressive chronic bronchial pulmonary disease. Pregnancy and the attendant physiologic changes can stress the pulmonary, cardiovascular, and nutritional status of women with cystic fibrosis. The purpose of this section is to familiarize the obstetrician with the physiologic effects of this complex disease and the impact of the disease on pregnancy and the impact of pregnancy on the disease. Additional factors that need to be addressed are the genetics of this disorder (see Chapter 6) and the implications for the newborn, as well as social issues including who will raise the child should the mother succumb to her disease.

Survival for patients with cystic fibrosis has increased dramatically since 1940. According to the Cystic Fibrosis Foundation's Patient Registry, mean survival in 1992 had increased to 29.6 years.[138] Women had a slightly lower median age of survival (27.3 years) as compared with men (29.6 years). The reasons for sex differences in mortality are unclear. This increase in survival of patients with cystic fibrosis is likely secondary to earlier diagnosis and intervention, and also to advances in antibiotic therapy and nutritional support. Therefore, more women with cystic fibrosis are now entering reproductive age. In contrast to men with cystic fibrosis who, for the most part are infertile, women with cystic fibrosis are more often fertile. Infertility in women with cystic fibrosis may occasionally be due to anovulatory cycles and secondary amenorrhea, which result from significant malnutrition, associated with advanced disease. A more common reason for infertility appears to result from alteration in the physiologic properties of cervical mucus.[143]

The first case of cystic fibrosis complicating pregnancy was reported in 1960, and a total of 13 pregnancies in 10 patients with cystic fibrosis were reported in 1966.[144,145] Cohen[146] conducted a survey of 119 cystic fibrosis centers in the United States and Canada, and identified a total of 129 pregnancies in 100 women by 1976. Hillman surveyed 127 cystic fibrosis centers in the United States, between 1976 and 1982.[138] A total of 191 pregnancies were reported during this period in women with cystic fibrosis, ranging in age from 16 to 36 years, with a mean age of 22.6 years.[138] The annual number of cystic fibrosis pregnancies reported to the Cystic Fibrosis Foundation's Patient Registry doubled between 1986 and 1990, with 52 pregnancies reported in 1986, compared with 111 pregnancies reported in 1990. This same registry recently reported on a total of 680 pregnancies in 8,136 women between 1985 and 1997.[147] This documents a dramatic increase in pregnancy complicated by cystic fibrosis. Increasing numbers are reported in other countries as well.[148–151] Because the number of women with cystic fibrosis achieving pregnancy is steadily increasing, it is important that the obstetrician is familiar with the disease.

The Effect of Pregnancy on Cystic Fibrosis

The physiologic changes associated with pregnancy (see Chapter 3) are well tolerated by healthy gravidas; however, those with cystic fibrosis may adapt poorly. During pregnancy, there is an increase in resting minute ventilation that at term may approach 150 percent of control values.[152] This increase in minute ventilation is due to the increased oxygen consumption and increased carbon dioxide burden that occur during pregnancy. In addition, increased levels of circulating progesterone stimulates the respiratory drive. Enlargement of the abdominal contents and upward displacement of the diaphragm lead to a decrease in functional residual volume and a decrease in residual volume.[152] Pregnancy is also accompanied by subtle alterations in gas exchange with widening of the alveolar-arterial oxygen gradient that is most pronounced in the supine position.[152] These alterations in pulmonary function are of little consequence to the normal pregnant woman. However, in the gravida with cystic fibrosis, these changes may contribute to respiratory decompensation that can lead to an increase in morbidity and mortality for the mother and the fetus as well.

During normal pregnancy, blood volume increases by an average of 50 percent. Cardiac output increases as well, reaching a plateau in midpregnancy.[153] During labor, blood volume rises acutely, in large part due to the release of blood from the contracting uterus and is additionally increased after delivery, secondary to augmented venous return with the release of caval obstruction. Women with cystic fibrosis and advanced lung disease may suffer from pulmonary hypertension with high pulmonary artery pressures. Regardless of the etiology, pulmonary hypertension is associated with unacceptable maternal risk during pregnancy and is considered to be a contraindication to pregnancy.[153] Women with significant pulmonary hypertension may develop cardiovascular collapse at the time of labor and delivery, with a maternal mortality exceeding 25 percent.[154] Additionally, women with pulmonary hypertension may not be able to adequately increase cardiac output during pregnancy and, therefore, suffer uteroplacental insufficiency, leading to intrauterine growth restriction and stillbirth.[142]

Nutritional requirements are increased during pregnancy, with approximately 300 kcal/day in additional fuel being needed to meet the requirements of mother and fetus.[155] Most patients with cystic fibrosis have pancreatic exocrine insufficiency. As a result, digestive enzymes and bicarbonate ions are diminished, resulting in maldigestion, malabsorption, and malnutrition.[155]

The 1966 report by Grand et al.[145] included 13 pregnancies in 10 women with cystic fibrosis. Of these, five women had a progressive decline in their pulmonary function, two of whom died of cor pulmonale in the immediate postpartum period. Pregnancy was well tolerated in 5 of 10 women, two of whom went on to have subsequent pregnancies that were similarly well tolerated. In this study, the pregravid pulmonary status of the patient was the most important predictor of outcome. However, there was no quantification of pulmonary function. A case report by Novy and colleagues in 1967 described in detail the pulmonary function and gas exchange in a pregnant woman with cystic fibrosis.[156] The patient had severe disease, as evidenced by a vital capacity of only 0.72 L and an arterial Po_2 of 50 mm Hg at presentation. The patient suffered a progressive increase in residual volume and a decline in vital capacity that was accompanied by worsening hypoxemia and hypercapnia, resulting in respiratory distress and right-sided heart failure in the early postpartum period.[156] Based on the experience with this patient and a review of the literature, the authors recommended therapeutic abortion in any patient demonstrating progressive pulmonary deterioration and hypoxemia despite maximal medical management.[156] In 1980, Cohen et al.[146] described 100 patients and a total of 129 pregnancies. Ninety-seven of 129 (75 percent) pregnancies were completed, and 89 percent delivered viable infants. Twenty-seven percent of these fetuses were delivered preterm. There were 11 perinatal deaths and no congenital anomalies. In this study, 65 percent of patients required antibiotic therapy before delivery. In 1983, Palmer et al.[157] retrospectively reviewed the pre-pregnancy status of eight women with cystic fibrosis who subsequently completed 11 pregnancies. She found that five women tolerated pregnancy without difficulty but three had irreversible deterioration in their clinical status. She identified four maternal factors that were predictive of outcome: clinical status (Shwachman score), nutritional status (percentage of predicted weight for height), the extent of chest radiographic abnormalities (assessed by the Brasfield chest radiograph score), and the magnitude of pulmonary function impairment.[157] Women with good clinical studies, good nutritional status (within 15 percent of their predicted ideal body weight for height), with nearly normal chest radiographs and only mild obstructive lung disease, tolerated pregnancy well without deterioration.[157]

There are several reports suggesting that patients with mild cystic fibrosis, good nutritional status, and less impairment of lung function tolerate pregnancy well. However, those with poor clinical status, malnutrition, hepatic dysfunction, or advanced lung disease are at increased risk from pregnancy.[158–160] Kent and Farquharson[160] reviewed the literature and reported 217 pregnancies. In this series, the frequency of preterm delivery was 24.3 percent and the perinatal death rate was 7.9 percent. Poor outcomes were associated with a maternal weight gain of less than 4.5 kg and an FVC of less than 50 percent of that predicted. Edenborough et al.[161] also reported on pregnancies in women with cystic fibrosis. There were 18 live births (81.8 percent), one third of which were preterm deliveries, and 18.2 percent of patients had abortions. There were four maternal deaths within 3.2 years after delivery. In this series, lung function was available before delivery, immediately after delivery, and after pregnancy. Although the patients demonstrated a decline of 13 percent in FEV_1 and 11 percent in FVC during pregnancy, most returned to baseline pulmonary function after pregnancy. Although most of the women in this series tolerated pregnancy well, those with moderate to severe lung disease, an FEV_1 of less than 60 percent of predicted, more often had preterm infants and had increased loss of lung function compared with those with milder disease.[161] In two series, prepregnancy FEV_1 was found to be the most useful predictor of outcome in pregnant women with cystic fibrosis.[161,162] In addition, there was also a positive correlation of prepregnancy FEV_1 and maternal survival. Another study examined the outcome of 72 pregnancies in 55 women with cystic fibrosis in the United Kingdom between 1977 and 1996. The outcomes of pregnancies were known for 69 of the 72 pregnancies. There were 48 live births (70 percent), of which 22 were premature (46 percent); there were 14 therapeutic abortions (20 percent) and seven miscarriages (10 percent). In this cohort, there were no stillbirths, neonatal losses, or early maternal deaths. Percent FEV_1 in this cohort ranged from 60 percent to 94 percent.[149]

A more recent report examined survival in 8,136 women enrolled in the U.S. Cystic Fibrosis Foundation National Patient Registry from 1985 to 1997.[147] Six hundred and eighty of these women became pregnant. The author matched the 680 women in an index year to 3,327 control women with cystic fibrosis. Women who reported a pregnancy were more likely to have had a higher percent of predicted FEV_1 (67.5 percent predicted versus 67.1 percent predicted, respectively; $p < 0.001$) and a higher weight (52.9 versus 46.4 kg, respectively; $p < 0.001$). The 10-year survival rate in pregnant women (77 percent; 95 percent CI, 71 to 82 percent) was higher than in those women who did not become pregnant. A separate analysis, matching pregnant patient's FEV_1 percent predicted, age, *P. aeruginosa* colonization, and pancreatic function obtained similar results. In this cohort, pregnancy was not harmful in any subgroup including patients with an FEV_1 40 percent of predicted or diabetes mellitus.[147] The author concluded women with cystic fibrosis who became pregnant were initially healthier and had better 10-year survival rates than women with cystic fibrosis who did not become pregnant.

Pulmonary involvement in cystic fibrosis includes chronic infection of the airways and bronchiectasis. There is selective infection with certain microorganisms, such as *S. aureus, H. influenzae, P. aeruginosa,* and *Berkholderia cepacia. P. aeruginosa* is the most frequent pathogen.[138] Parenteral antibiotics are the mainstays of treatment of these acute infections. However, pregnancy and cystic fibrosis–associated alterations in pharmacokinetics can have grave consequences for these patients. It is well known that pregnant subjects have lower serum levels and higher urine levels of antibiotics than nonpregnant subjects. The lower levels in plasma are attributed to the increase in volume of distribution and an increase in glomerular filtration and renal clearance of the drugs.[163] Cloxacillin, dicloxacillin, ticarcillin, and methicillin are cleared more rapidly in patients with cystic fibrosis.[164–166] Plasma ceftazidime and gentamicin levels are likewise decreased in patients with cystic fibrosis.[167,168] Therefore, monitoring drug levels is indicated when therapeutic response is less than optimal.

Counseling Patients with Cystic Fibrosis in Pregnancy

There are several factors that must be considered when counseling a woman who has cystic fibrosis and is considering pregnancy, including the possibility that her fetus will have cystic fibrosis (see Chapter 6). Approximately 4 percent of the white population in the United States are heterozygous carriers of the cystic fibrosis gene. The disease occurs in 1 in 3,000 white births. When the mother has cystic fibrosis and the proposed father is a white individual of unknown genotype, the risk of the fetus having cystic fibrosis is 1 in 50, as compared with 1 in 3,000 in the general white population. If the prospective father is a known carrier of a cystic fibrosis mutation, the risk to the fetus increases to 1 in 2. If, however, DNA testing does not identify a cystic fibrosis mutation in the prospective father, it is still possible that the father is a carrier of an unidentified cystic fibrosis mutation, making the risk of cystic fibrosis to the offspring 1 in 492.[169]

It is important that the woman with cystic fibrosis be advised about the potential adverse affects of pregnancy on maternal health status. Factors that may predict poor outcome include prepregnancy evidence of poor nutritional status, significant pulmonary disease with hypoxemia, and pulmonary hypertension. Liver disease and diabetes mellitus are also poor prognostic factors. Gravidas with poor nutritional status, pulmonary hypertension (cor pulmonale), and deteriorating pulmonary function early in gestation should consider therapeutic abortion, because the risk of maternal mortality may be unacceptably high.

The woman with cystic fibrosis who is considering pregnancy should also give consideration to the need for strong psychosocial and physical support after delivery. The rigors of child-rearing may add to the risk of maternal deterioration during this period. Family members should also be willing to provide physical and emotional support, and should be aware of the potential for deterioration in the mother's health and the potential for maternal mortality. In addition, the need for care of a potentially preterm growth–restricted neonate with all of its attendant morbidities and potential mortality should be discussed. Over the long term, the woman and her family should also consider the fact that her life expectancy may be shortened by cystic fibrosis, Overall 20 percent of mothers with cystic fibrosis succumb to the disease before the child's 10th birthday, and this number increases to 40 percent if the FEV_1 is less than 40 percent of predicted.[149] Plans should be made for rearing of the child in the event of maternal death.

Management of the Pregnancy Complicated by Cystic Fibrosis

Care of the gravida with cystic fibrosis should be a coordinated, team effort. Physicians familiar with cystic fibrosis, its complications, and management should be included, as well as a maternal-fetal medicine specialist and neonatal team. The gravida should be assessed for potential risk factors such as severe lung disease, pulmonary hypertension, poor nutritional status, pancreatic failure, and liver disease, preferably before attempting gestation, but certainly during the early months of pregnancy. Gravidas should be advised to be 90 percent of ideal body weight before conception if possible. A weight gain in pregnancy of 11 to 12 kg is recommended.[138] Frequent monitoring of weight, blood glucose, hemoglobin, total protein, serum albumin, prothrombin time, and fat-soluble vitamins A and E is suggested.[138] At each visit, the history of caloric intake and symptoms of maldigestion and malabsorption should be taken, and pancreatic enzymes should be adjusted if needed. Patients who are unable to achieve adequate weight gain through oral nutritional supplements may be given nocturnal enteral nasogastric tube feeding. In this situation, the risk of aspiration should be considered, especially in patients with a history of gastroesophageal reflux, which is common in cystic fibrosis.[138] If malnutrition is severe, parenteral hyperalimentation may be necessary for successful completion of the pregnancy.[170] Baseline pulmonary function should be assessed, preferably before conception. Assessment should include FVC, FEV_1, lung volumes, pulse oximetry, and arterial blood gases, if indicated. These values should be serially monitored during gestation and deterioration in pulmonary function addressed immediately. An echocardiogram can assess the patient for pulmonary hypertension and cor pulmonale. If pulmonary hypertension (cor pulmonale) is diagnosed, the gravida should be advised of the high maternal risk.

Early recognition and prompt treatment of pulmonary infections are important in the management of the pregnant woman with cystic fibrosis. Treatment includes intravenous antibiotics in the appropriate dose, keeping in mind the increased clearance of these drugs secondary to pregnancy and cystic fibrosis. Plasma levels of aminoglycosides should be monitored and adjusted as indicated. Chest physical therapy and bronchial drainage are also important components of the management of pulmonary infections in cystic fibrosis. Because *P. aeruginosa* is the most frequently isolated bacteria associated with chronic endobronchitis and bronchiectasis, antibiotic regimens should include coverage for this organism.

If the patient with cystic fibrosis has pancreatic insufficiency and diabetes mellitus, careful monitoring of blood glucose and insulin therapy is indicated. As previously mentioned, pancreatic enzymes may need to be replaced in order to optimize the patient's nutritional status. Because of malabsorption of fats and frequent use of antibiotics, the patient with cystic fibrosis is prone to vitamin K deficiency. Therefore, prothrombin time should be checked regularly, and parenteral vitamin K should be administered if the prothrombin time is elevated.

It is imperative when managing pregnancy in a woman with cystic fibrosis to recognize that the fetus is at risk for uteroplacental insufficiency and intrauterine growth restriction. The maternal nutritional status and weight gain during pregnancy will likewise impact fetal growth. Therefore, fundal height should be measured routinely, and serial ultrasound evaluations of fetal growth and amniotic fluid volume should be made. Maternal kick counts may be useful for monitoring fetal status starting at 28 weeks. Nonstress testing should be started at 32 weeks or sooner, if there is evidence of fetal compromise. If there is evidence of severe fetal compromise such as no interval fetal growth, persistent decelerations, or poor biophysical profile scoring, delivery should be accomplished. Likewise, evidence of profound maternal deterioration such as a marked and sustained decline in pulmonary function, development of right-sided heart failure, refractory hypoxemia, and progressive hypercapnia and respiratory acidosis may be maternal indications for early delivery. If the fetus is potentially viable, the administration of betamethasone may be beneficial. Vaginal delivery should be attempted when possible.

Labor, delivery, and the postpartum period can be particularly dangerous for the patient with cystic fibrosis. The augmentation in cardiac output stresses the cardiovascular system and can lead to cardiopulmonary failure in the patient with pulmonary hypertension and cor pulmonale. These patients are also more likely to develop right-sided heart failure. Heart failure should be treated with aggressive diuresis and supplemental oxygen. Management may be optimized by insertion of a pulmonary artery catheter to monitor right- and left-sided filling pressures. Pain control will reduce the sympathetic response to labor and tachycardia. This will benefit the patient who is demonstrating pulmonary or cardiac compromise. In the patient with a normal PTT, insertion of an epidural catheter for continuous epidural analgesia may be beneficial. This is also useful in the event a cesarean delivery is indicated, because general anesthesia and its possible effects on pulmonary function can be avoided. If general anesthesia is needed, preoperative anticholinergic agents should be avoided because they tend to promote drying and inspissation of airway secretions. Close fetal surveillance is also extremely important, because the fetus who may have been suffering from uteroplacental insufficiency during gestation is more prone to develop evidence of fetal compromise during labor. Delivery by cesarean section should be reserved for the usual obstetric indications.

In summary, more women with cystic fibrosis are living to childbearing age and are capable of conceiving. Clinical experience thus far has demonstrated that pregnancy in women with cystic fibrosis and mild disease is well tolerated. Women with severe disease have an associated increase in maternal and fetal morbidity and mortality. The potential risk to any individual with cystic fibrosis desirous of pregnancy should be assessed and discussed with the patient and her family in detail.

Key Points

- Pneumonia is the most common nonobstetric infection to cause maternal mortality. Preterm delivery complicates pneumonia in up to 43 percent of cases. *S. pneumoniae* is the most common bacterial pathogen to cause pneumonia. Empiric antibiotic coverage should be started, including a third-generation cephalosporin and a macrolide, such as azithromycin, to cover atypical pathogens.

- The HIV-infected gravida with a CD4+ count less than 200 cells per cubic millimeter should receive prophylaxsis with trimethoprim-sulfamethoxazole in order to prevent PCP pneumonia as well as HAART.

- High-risk gravidas should be screened for TB and treated appropriately with INH prophylaxis for infection without overt disease and with dual anti-TB therapy for active disease. If resistant TB is identified, ethambutol 2.5 g/day should be added to therapy and the treatment period should be extended to 18 months.

- Asthma treatment should be tailored according to asthma severity. Inhaled corticosteroids are the preferred treatment for persistent asthma. Excellent perinatal outcomes can be obtained in most cases. PEFR and FEV_1 should be used to evaluate and manage persistent asthma.

- The interstitial lung diseases include idiopathic pulmonary fibrosis, sarcoidosis, hypersensitivity pneumonitis, drug-induced lung disease, and connective tissue disease. Restrictive lung disease is generally well tolerated in pregnancy; however, exercise intolerance and need for oxygen supplementation may develop. Gravidas with pulmonary hypertension complicating restrictive lung disease may suffer a high mortality rate.

- An increasing number of women with cystic fibrosis are surviving to the reproductive years and usually maintain their fertility with meticulous management of pulmonary function, including pulmonary toilet and aggressive surveillance for signs of pulmonary infection and treatment of antibiotics in adequate doses. Close attention to nutrition is required secondary to maldigestion, malabsorption, and malnutrition, which can complicate cystic fibrosis. Gravidas with good clinical studies, good nutritional status, nearly normal chest radiographs, and only mild obstructive lung disease will tolerate pregnancy well. Fetal growth should be monitored closely.

REFERENCES

1. Oxorn H: The changing aspects of pneumonia complicating pregnancy. Am J Obstet Gynecol 70:1057, 1955.
2. Madinger NE, Greenspoon JS, Gray-Ellrodt A: Pneumonia during pregnancy: has modern technology improved maternal and fetal outcome? Am J Obstet Gynecol 161:657, 1989.
3. Kaunitz AM, Hughes JM, Grimes DA, et al: Causes of maternal mortality in the United States. Obstet Gynecol 65:605, 1985.
4. Finland M, Dublin TD: Pneumococcic pneumonias complicating pregnancy and the puerperium. JAMA 112:1027, 1939.
5. Benedetti TJ, Valle R, Ledger W: Antepartum pneumonia in pregnancy. Am J Obstet Gynecol 144:413, 1982.
6. Berkowitz K, LaSala A: Risk factors associated with the increasing prevalence of pneumonia during pregnancy. Am J Obstet Gynecol 163:981, 1990.
7. Koonin LM, Ellerbrock TV, Atrash HK, et al: Pregnancy-associated deaths due to AIDS in the United States. JAMA 261:1306, 1989.
8. Dinsmoor MJ: HIV infection and pregnancy. Med Clin North Am 73:701, 1989.
9. Hopwood HG: Pneumonia in pregnancy. Obstet Gynecol 25:875, 1965.
10. Rodrigues J, Niederman MS: Pneumonia complicating pregnancy. Clin Chest Med 13:679, 1992.
11. Haake DA, Zakowski PC, Haake DL, et al: Early treatment with acyclovir for varicella pneumonia in otherwise healthy adults: retrospective controlled study and review. Rev Infect Dis 12:788, 1990.
12. McKinney WP, Volkert P, Kaufman J: Fatal swine influenza pneumonia during late pregnancy. Arch Intern Med 150:213, 1990.
13. American College of Obstetricians and Gynecologists: Pulmonary disease in pregnancy. ACOG Technical Bulletin 224. Washington, DC, ACOG, 1996.
14. Ahmad H, Mehta NJ, Manikal VM, et al: *Pneumocystis carinii* pneumonia in pregnancy: division of infectious disease. Chest 120:666, 2001.

15. Yost P, Bloom S, Richey S, et al: Appraisal of treatment guidelines of antepartum community acquired pneumonia: Am J Obstet Gynecol 183:131, 2000.
16. American Thoracic Society: Guidelines for the initial management of adults with community-acquired pneumonia: diagnosis assessment of severity, and initial antimicrobial therapy. Am Rev Respir Dis 148:1418, 1993
17. Harrison BDW, Farr BM, Connolly CK, et al: The hospital management of community-acquired pneumonia: Recommendation of the British Thoracic Society. J R Coll Phys 21:267, 1987.
18. Merchant S, Mullins CD, Shih YT: Factors associated with hospitalization cost for patients with community-acquired pneumonia. Clin Ther 25:593, 2003.
19. Campbell SG, Marrie TJ, Anstey R, et al: Utility of blood cultures in management of adults with community acquired pneumonia discharged from the emergency department. Emerg Med J 20:521, 2003.
20. Pimentel LP, McPherson SJ: Community-acquired pneumonia in the emergency department: a practical approach to diagnosis and management. Emerg Med Clin North Am 21: 395, 2003.
21. Garbino J, Sommer R, Gerber A, et al: Prospective epidemiologic survey of patients with community-acquired pneumonia requiring hospitalization in Switzerland. Int J Infect Dis 6:288, 2002.
22. Mandell LA, Marrie TJ, Grossman RE, et al: Canadian guidelines for the initial management of community-acquired pneumonia: an evidence-based update by the Canadian infectious diseases society and the Canadian thoracic society. Clin Infect Dis 1:383, 2000.
23. Murdoch DR, Laing RT, Mills GD, et al: Evaluation of a rapid immunochromatographic test for detection of *Streptococcus pneumoniae* antigen in urine samples from adults with community-acquired pneumonia. J Clin Microbiol 39:3495, 2001
24. Gutierrez F, Rodriequez JC, Ayelo A, et al: Evaluation of the immunochromatographic Binax NOW assay for detection of *Streptococcus pneumoniae* urinary antigen in a prospective study of community-acquired pneumonia in Spain. Clin Infect Dis 36:286, 1996.
25. Waterer GW, Baselski VS, Wunderink RG: Legionella and community-acquired pneumonia: a review of current diagnostic test from a clinician's viewpoint. Am J Med 110:41, 2001.
26. Niederman MS, Ahmed OA: Community-acquired pneumonia in elderly patients. Clin Geriatr Med 19:101, 2003
27. Golden WE, Brown P, Godsey N: CMS release new standards for community acquired pneumonia. J Ark Med Soc 99:288, 2003.
28. Cunha BA: Empiric therapy of community-acquired pneumonia. Chest 125:1913, 2004.
29. Munoz FM, Englund JA, Cheesman CC, et al: Maternal immunization with pneumococcal polysaccharide vaccine in the third trimester of gestation. Vaccine 20:826, 2001.
30. Shahid NS, Steinhoff MC, Hoque SS, et al: Serum, breast milk, and infant antibody after maternal immunization with pneumococcal vaccine. Lancet 346:1252, 1995.
31. Deubzer HE, Obaro SK, Newman VO, et al: Colostrum obtained from women vaccinated with pneumococcal vaccine during pregnancy inhibits epithelial adhesion of *Streptococcus pneumoniae*. J Infect Dis 190:1758, 2004.
32. Tomlinson MW, Caruthers TJ, Whitty JE, Gonik B: Does delivery improve maternal condition in the respiratory-compromised gravida? Obstet Gynecol 91:108, 1998.
33. National Center for Health Statistics: National hospital discharge survey: annual summary 1990. Vital Health Stat 13:1, 1992.
34. Hollingsworth HM, Pratter MR, Irwin RS: Acute respiratory failure in pregnancy. J Intensive Care Med 4:11, 1989.
35. Neuzil KM, Reed GW, Mitchel EF, et al: Impact of influenza on acute cardiopulmonary hospitalizations in pregnant women. Am J Epidemiol 148:1094, 1998.
36. Hartert TV, Neuzil KM, Shintani AK, et al: Maternal morbidity and perinatal outcome among pregnant women with respiratory hospitalizations during influenza season. Am J Obstet Gynecol 189:1705, 2003.
37. Kirshon B, Faro S, Zurawin RK, et al: Favorable outcome after treatment with amantadine and ribavirin in a pregnancy complicated by influenza pneumonia: a case report. J Reprod Med 33:399, 1988.
38. Harper SA, Fukuda K, Uyeka TM, et al: Prevention and Control of Influenza. Recommendations of the Advisory Committee on Immunization Practice (ACIP). MMWR 52 No. RR-8:1–34, 2003.
39. Cox SM, Cunningham FG, Luby J: Management of varicella pneumonia complicating pregnancy. Am J Perinatol 7:300, 1990.
40. Esmonde TG, Herdman G, Anderson G: Chickenpox pneumonia: an association with pregnancy. Thorax 44:812, 1989.
41. Smego RA, Asperilla MO: Use of acyclovir for varicella pneumonia during pregnancy. Obstet Gynecol 78:1112, 1991.
42. Harger JH, Ernest JM, Thurnau GR, et al: Risk factors and outcome of varicella-zoster virus pneumonia in pregnant women. J Infect Dis 185:422, 2002.
43. Harris RE, Rhades ER: Varicella pneumonia complicating pregnancy: report of a case and review of literature. Obstet Gynecol 25:734, 1965.
44. Jones AM, Thomas N, Wilkins EG: Outcome of varicella pneumonitis in immunocompetent adults requiring treatment in a high dependency unit. J Infect 43:135, 2001.
45. Andrews EB, Yankaskas BC, Cordero JF, et al: Acyclovir in pregnancy registry: six years' experience. Obstet Gynecol 79:7, 1992.
46. Brown ZA, Baker DA: Acyclovir therapy during pregnancy. Obstet Gynecol 73:526, 1989.
47. Hambleton S, Gershon AA: The impact of varicella vaccination in the United States. Semin Pediatr Infect Dis 16:38, 2005.
48. Nguyen HQ, Jumaan AO, Seward JF: Decline in mortality due to varicella after implementation of varicella vaccination in the United States. N Engl J Med 352:450, 2005.
49. Shields KE, Galil K, Seward J, et al: Varicella vaccine exposure during pregnancy: Data from the first 5 years of the pregnancy registry. Obstet Gynecol 98:14, 2001.
50. Thomas CF Jr, Limper AH: Pneumocystis pneumonia. N Engl J Med 350:2487, 2004.
51. Randall CJ, Yarnold PR, Schwartz DN, et al: Improvements in outcomes of acute respiratory failure for patients with human immunodeficiency virus-related *Pneumocystis carinii* pneumonia. Am J Respir Crit Care Med 162:393, 2000.
52. DeLorenzo LJ, Huang CT, Maguire GP, Stone DJ: Roentgenographic patterns of *Pneumocystis carinii* pneumonia in 104 patients with AIDS. Chest 91:323, 1987.
53. Ambruster C, Pokieser L, Hassl A: Diagnosis of *Pneumocystis carinii* pneumonia by bronchoalveolar lavage in AIDS patients: Comparison of Diff-Quik, fungifluor stain, direct immunofluorescence test and polymerase chain reaction. Acta Cytol 39:1089, 1995
54. Kovacs JA, Ng VL, Masur H, et al: Diagnosis of *Pneumocystis carinii* pneumonia: improved detection in sputum with use of monoclonal antibodies. N Engl J Med 318:589, 1988.
55. Wortley PM, Fleming PL: AIDS in women in the United States: recent trends. JAMA 278:911, 1997.
56. Masur H, Kaplan JE, Holmes KK: Guidelines for preventing opportunistic infections among HIV-infected persons—2002; recommendations of the U.S. Public Health Service and the Infectious Disease Society of America. Am Intern Med 137:435, 2002.
57. Centers for Disease Control and Prevention: Initial therapy for tuberculosis in the era of multidrug resistance-recommendations of the advisory council for the elimination of tuberculosis. MMWR 42(RR-7):1, 1993.
58. Frieden TR, Sterling T, Pablos-Mendez A, et al: The emergence of drug-resistant tuberculosis in New York City. N Engl J Med 328:521, 1993.
59. Cantwell MF, Shehab AM, Costello AM: Brief report: congenital tuberculosis. N Engl J Med 330:1051, 1994.
60. Margono F, Mroveh J, Garely A, et al: Resurgence of active tuberculosis among pregnant women. Obstet Gynecol 83:911, 1994.
61. Centers for Disease Control and Prevention: The use of preventive therapy for tuberculosis infection in the United States. MMWR 39:9, 1990.
62. Good JT Jr, Isemen PT, Lakshnminarayan S, Sahn SA: Tuberculosis is association with pregnancy. Am J Obstet Gynecol 140:492, 1998.
63. Griffith DE: Mycobacteria as pathogens of respiratory infection. Infect Dis Clin North Am 12:593, 1998.

64. American Thoracic Society Workshop: Rapid diagnostic tests for tuberculosis—what is the appropriate use? Am J Respir Crit Care Med 155:1804, 1997.
65. Barnes PF: Rapid diagnostic tests for tuberculosis, progress but no gold standard. Am J Respir Crit Care Med 155:1497, 1997.
66. Centers for Disease Control and Prevention: The role of BCG vaccine in the prevention and control of tuberculosis in the United States: a joint statement by the Advisory Council for the Elimination of Tuberculosis and the Advisory Committee on Immunization Practices. MMWR 45:1, 1996.
67. Good JT, Iseman MD, Davidson PT, et al: Tuberculosis in association with pregnancy. Am J Obstet Gynecol 140:492, 1081.
68. American Thoracic Society: Mycobacteriosis and the acquired immunodeficiency syndrome. Am Rev Respir Dis 136:492, 1987.
69. Hamadeh MA, Glassroth J: Tuberculosis and pregnancy. Chest 101:1114, 1992.
70. Jana N, Vasishta K, Saha SC, Ghosh K: Obstetrical outcomes among women with extrapulmonary tuberculosis. N Engl J Med 341:645, 1999.
71. Vallejo JC, Starke JR: Tuberculosis and pregnancy. Clin Chest Med 13:693, 1992.
72. Riley L: Pneumonia and tuberculosis in pregnancy. Infect Dis Clin North Am 11:119, 1997.
73. Robinson CA, Rose NC: Tuberculosis: current implications and management in obstetrics. Obstet Gynecol Surv 51:115, 1999.
74. Fox CW, George RB: Current concepts in the management and prevention of tuberculosis in adults. J La State Med Soc 144:363, 1992.
75. Van Rie A, Warren R, Richardson M, et al: Classification of drug-resistant tuberculosis in an epidemic area. Lancet 356:22, 2000.
76. Robinson GC, Cambion K: Hearing loss in infants of tuberculosis mothers treated with streptomycin during pregnancy. N Engl J Med 271:949, 1964.
77. Lessnau KL, Qarah S: Multidrug-resistant tuberculosis in pregnancy: Case report and review of the literature. Chest 123:953, 2003
78. Shin S, Guerra D, Rich M, et al: Treatment of multidrug-resistant tuberculosis during pregnancy: A report of 7 cases. Clin Infect Dis 36:996, 2003.
79. Rendig EK Jr: The place of BCG vaccine in the management of infants born to tuberculosis mothers. N Engl J Med 281:520, 1969.
80. Mitnick C, Bayona J, Palacios E, et al: Community-based therapy for multidrug-resistant tuberculosis in Lima, Peru. N Engl J Med 348:119, 2003.
81. Schatz M, Zeiger RS, Hoffman CP: Intrauterine growth is related to gestational pulmonary function in pregnant asthmatic women. Kaiser-Permanente Asthma and Pregnancy Study Grp. Chest 98:389, 1990.
82. Alexander S, Dodds L, Armson BA: Perinatal outcomes in women with asthma during pregnancy. Obstet Gynecol 92:435, 1998
83. Kwon HL, Belanger K, Bracken M: Asthma prevalence among pregnant and childbearing-aged women in the United States: estimates from national health surveys. Ann Epidemiol 13:317, 2003.
84. NAEPP expert panel report managing asthma during pregnancy: Recommendations for pharmacologic treatment—2004 update. NHLBI, NIH Publication No 05–3279. *http://www.nhlbi.nih.gov/health/prof/lung/asthma/astpreg.htm*
85. Schatz M., Dombrowski MP, Wise R, et al for The NICHD Maternal-Fetal Medicine Units Network, and NHLBI: Asthma morbidity during pregnancy can be predicted by severity classification. J Allergy Clin Immunol 112:283, 2003.
86. Schatz M, Zeiger R, Hoffman C, et al: Perinatal outcomes in the pregnancies of asthmatic women: A prospective controlled analysis. Am J Respir Crti Care Med 151:1170, 1995
87. Dombrowski MP, Bottoms SF, Boike GM, et al: Incidence of preeclampsia among asthmatic patients lower with theophylline. Am J Obstet Gynecol 155:265,1986.
88. Liu S, Wen SW, Demissie K, et al: Maternal asthma and pregnancy outcomes: a retrospective cohort study. Am J Obstet Gynecol 184:90, 2001.
89. Bahna SL, Bjerkedal T: The course and outcome of pregnancy in women with bronchial asthma. Acta Allergologica 27:397, 1972
90. Doucette JT, Bracken MB: Possible role of asthma in the risk of preterm labor and delivery. Epidemiology 4:143, 1993.
91. Perlow JH, Montgomery D, Morgan MA, et al: Severity of asthma and perinatal outcome. Am J Obstet Gynecol 167:963,1992.
92. Jana N, Vasishta K, Saha SC, Khunnu B: Effect of bronchial asthma on the course of pregnancy, labour and perinatal outcome. J Obstet Gynaecol 21:227,1995.
93. Demisse K, Breckenridge MB, Rhoads GG: Infant and maternal outcomes in the pregnancies of asthmatic women. Am J Respir Crit Care Med 158:1091;1998.
94. Kallen B, Rydhstroem H, Aberg A: Asthma during pregnancy—a population based study. Eur J Epidemiol 16:167;2000.
95. Stenius-Aarniala BS, Teramo PK: Asthma and pregnancy: a prospective study of 198 pregnancies. Thorax 43:12, 1988.
96. Schatz M, Dombrowski M: Asthma and allergy during pregnancy: Outcomes of pregnancy in asthmatic women. Immunol Asthma Clin N Am 20:1, 2000.
97. Fitzsimons R, Greenberger PA, Patterson R: Outcome of pregnancy in women requiring corticosteroids for severe asthma. J Allergy Clin Immunol 78:349, 1986.
98. Bracken MB, Triche EW, Belanger K, et al: Asthma symptoms, severity, and drug therapy: a prospective study of effects on 2205 pregnancies. Obstet Gynecol 1024:739, 2003.
99. Dombrowski MP, Schatz M, Wise R, et al for The NICHD Maternal-Fetal Medicine Units Network, and The NHLBI: Asthma during pregnancy. Obstet Gynecol 103:5, 2004.
100. Schatz M, Dombrowski MP, Wise R, et al for The NICHD Maternal-Fetal Medicine Units Network, and The NHLBI: The relationship of asthma medication use to perinatal outcomes. J Allergy Clin Immunol 113:1040, 2004.
101. Nolten W, Rueckert P: Elevated free cortisol index in pregnancy: Possible regulatory mechanisms. Am J Obstet Gynecol 139:492, 1981.
102. Bailey K, Herrod H, Younger R, et al: Functional aspects of T-lymphocyte subsets in pregnancy. Obstet Gynecol 66:211, 1985.
103. Haahtela T, Jarvinen M, Kava T, et al: Comparison of β_2-agonist, terbutalline, with an inhaled corticosteroid, budesonide, in newly detected asthma. N Engl J Med 325:338,1991.
104. Ernst P, Spetzer WO, Suissa S, et al: Risk of fatal and near-fatal asthma in relation to inhaled coriticosteroid use. JAMA 268:3462, 1992.
105. Kraan J, Koeter GH, Van Der Mark THW, et al: Dosage and time effects of inhaled budesonide on bronchial hyperactivity. Am Rev Respir Dis 137:44, 1988.
106. Woolcock AJ, Yan K, Salome CM: Effects of therapy on bronchial hyperresponsiveness in the long-term management of asthma. Clin Allergy 18:165, 1988.
107. Lowhagen O, Rak S: Modification of bronchial hyperreactivity after treatment with sodium cromoglycate during pollen season. J Allergy Clin Immunol 75:460, 1985.
108. Woolcock AJ, Jenkins C: Corticosteroids in the modulation of bronchial hyperresponsiveness. Immunol Allergy Clin North Am 10:543, 1990.
109. Stenius-Aarniala BSM, Hedman J, Teramo KA: Acute asthma during pregnancy. Thorax 51:411, 1996.
110. Kallen B, Rydhstroem H, Aberg A: Congenital malformations after use of inhaled budesonide in early pregnancy. Obstet Gynecol 93:392, 1999.
111. Cockcroft DW, Murdock KY: Comparative effects of inhaled salbutamol, sodium cromoglycate, and beclomethasone dipropionate on allergen-induced early asthmatic responses, last asthmatic responses, and increased bronchial responsiveness to histamine. J Allergy Clin Immunol 79:734, 1987.
112. Arwood LL, Dasta JF, Friedman C: Placental transfer of theophylline: two case reports. Pediatrics 63:844, 1979.
113. Yeh TF, Pildes RS: Transplacental aminophylline toxicity in a neonate [letter]. Lancet 1:910, 1977.
114. Hendeles L, Jenkins J, Temple R: Revised FDA Labeling Guideline for Theophylline Oral Dosage Forms. Pharmacotherapy 15:409, 1995.

115. Joad JP, Ahrens RC, Lindgren SD, et al: Relative efficacy of maintenance therapy with theophylline, inhaled albuterol, and the combination for chronic asthma. J Allergy Clin Immunol 79:78, 1987.
116. Wendel PJ, Ramin SM, Barnett-Hamm C, et al: Asthma treatment in pregnancy: A randomized controlled study. Am J Obstet Gynecol 175:150, 1996.
117. Pauwels R, Van Renterghem D, Van Der Straeten M, et al: The effect of theophylline and enprofylline on allergen-induced bronchoconstriction. J Allergy Clin Immunol 76:583, 1985.
118. Juergens UR, Degenhardt V, Stober M, Vetter H: New insights in the bronchodilatory and anti-inflammatory mechanisms of action of theophylline. Arzneimittelforschung 49:694, 1999.
119. Evans DJ, Taylor DA, Zetterstrom O, et al: A comparison of low-dose inhaled budesonide plus theophylline and high-dose inhaled budesonide for moderate asthma. N Engl J Med 337:1412, 1997.
120. Schatz M, Zeiger RS, Harden KM, et al: The safety of inhaled β-agonist bronchodilators during pregnancy. J Allergy Clin Immunol 82:686, 1988.
121. Sears MR, Taylor DR. Print CG, et al: Regular inhaled β-agonist treatment in bronchial asthma. Lancet 336:1391, 1990.
122. Spitzer WO, Suissa S, Ernst P, et al: The use of β-agonists and the risk of death and near death from asthma. N Engl J Med 326:501, 1992.
123. Knorr B, Matz J, Bernstein JA, et al: Montelukast for chronic asthma in 6 to 14 year old children. JAMA 279:1181, 1998.
124. Wenzel SE: New approaches to anti-inflammatory therapy for asthma. Am J Med 104:287, 1998.
125. Park Wyllie L, Mazzotta P, Pastuszak A, et al: Birth defects after maternal exposure to corticosteroids: prospective cohort study and meta-analysis of epidemiological studies. Teratology 62:385, 2000.
126. Hägerdal M, Morgan CW, Sumner AE, et al: Minute ventilation and oxygen consumption during labor with epidural analgesia. Anesthesiology 59:425, 1983.
127. Fung DL: Emergency anesthesia for asthma patients. Cliv Rev Allergy 3:127, 1985.
128. Hirshman CA, Downes H, Farbood A, et al: Ketamine block of bronchospasm in experimental canine asthma. Br J Anaesth 51:713, 1979.
129. American Academy of Pediatrics Committee on Drugs: Transfer of drugs and other chemicals into human milk. Pediatrics 84:924, 1989.
130. West JB (ed): Pulmonary pathophysiology. *In* Pulmonary Pathophysiology. Baltimore, Williams & Wilkins, 1978, p 92.
131. King TE Jr: Restrictive lung disease in pregnancy. Clin Chest Med 13:607, 1992.
132. Boggess KA, Easterling TR, Raghu G: Management and outcome of pregnant women with interstitial and restrictive lung disease. Am J Obstet Gynecol 173:1007, 1995.
133. Agha FP, Vade A, Amendola MA, Cooper RF: Effects of pregnancy on sarcoidosis. Surg Gynecol Obstet 155:817, 1982.
134. Haynes de Regt R: Sarcoidosis and pregnancy. Obstet Gynecol 70:369, 1987.
135. Maycock RL, Sullivan RD, Greening RR, et al: Sarcoidosis and pregnancy. JAMA 164:158, 1957.
136. Reisfield DR: Boeck's sarcoid and pregnancy. Am J Obstet Gynecol 75:795, 1958.
137. Scadding JG: Sarcoidosis. London, Eyre & Spottiswoode, 1967, p 519.
138. Hilman BC, Aitken ML, Constantinescu M: Pregnancy in patients with cystic fibrosis. Clin Obstet Gynecol 39:70, 1996.
139. Kerem B, Rommens JM, Buchanan JA, et al: Identification of the cystic fibrosis gene: genetic analysis. Science 245:1073, 1989.
140. Riordan JR, Rommens JM, Kerem B, et al: Identification of the cystic fibrosis gene: cloning and characterization of complementary DNA. Science 245:1066, 1989.
141. Rommens JM, Iannuzzi MC, Kerem B, et al: Identification of the cystic fibrosis gene: chromosome walking and jumping. Science 245:1059, 1989.
142. Kotloff RM, FitzSimmons SC, Fiel SB: Fertility and pregnancy in patients with cystic fibrosis. Clin Chest Med 13:623, 1992.
143. Kopito LE, Kosasky HJ, Shwachman H: Water and electrolytes in cervical mucus from patients with cystic fibrosis. Fertil Steril 24:512, 1973.
144. Siegel B, Siegel S: Pregnancy and delivery in a patient with CF of the pancreas; report of a case. Obstet Gynecol 16:439, 1960.
145. Grand RJ, Talamo RC, di Sant' Agnese PA, et al: Pregnancy in cystic fibrosis of the pancreas. JAMA 195:993, 1966.
146. Cohen LF, di Sant' Agnese PA, Friedlander J: Cystic fibrosis and pregnancy: a national survey. Lancet 2:842, 1980.
147. Goss CH, Rubenfel GD, Otto K, Aitken ML: The effect of pregnancy on survival in women with cystic fibrosis. Chest 124:1460, 2003.
148. Gilljam M, Antoniou M, Shin J, et al: Pregnancy in cystic fibrosis: Fetal and maternal outcome. Chest 118:85, 2000
149. Edenborough FP, Mackenzie WE, Stableforth DE: The outcome of 72 pregnancies in 55 women with cystic fibrosis in the United Kingdom 1977–1996. Br J Obstet Gynaecol 107:254, 2000
150. Odegaard I, Stray-Pedersen B, Hallberg K, et al: Prevalence and outcome of pregnancies in Norwegian and Swedish women with cystic fibrosis. Acta Obstet Gynecol Scand 81:693, 2002.
151. Odegaard I, Stray-Pedersen B, Hallberg K, et al: Maternal and fetal morbidity in pregnancies of Norwegian and Swedish women with cystic fibrosis. Acta Obstet Gynecol Scand 81:698, 2002.
152. Weinberger SE, Weiss ST, Cohen WR, et al: Pregnancy and the lung. Am Rev Respir Dis 121:559, 1980.
153. McAnulty JH, Metcalfe J, Ueland K: Cardiovascular disease. *In* Burrow GN, Ferris TF (eds): Medical Complications During Pregnancy, 3rd ed. Philadelphia, WB Saunders Company, 1988.
154. Gleicher N, Midwall J, Hochberger D, et al: Eisenmenger's syndrome and pregnancy. Obstet Gynecol Surv 34:721, 1979.
155. Rush D, Johnstone FD, King JC: Nutrition and pregnancy. *In* Burrows GN, Ferris TF (eds): Medical Complications During Pregnancy, 3rd ed. Philadelphia, WB Saunders Company, 1988.
156. Novy MJ, Tyler JM, Shwachman H, et al: Cystic fibrosis and pregnancy. Report of a case with a study of pulmonary function and arterial blood gases. Obstet Gynecol 30:530, 1967.
157. Palmer J, Dillon-Baker C, Tecklin JS, et al: Pregnancy in patients with cystic fibrosis. Ann Intern Med 99:596, 1983.
158. Corkey CWB, Newth CJL, Corey M, et al: Pregnancy in cystic fibrosis: a better prognosis in patients with pancreatic function. Am J Obstet Gynecol 140:737, 1981.
159. Canny GJ, Corey M, Livingstone RA, et al: Pregnancy and cystic fibrosis. Obstet Gynecol 77:850, 1991.
160. Kent NE, Farquharson DF: Cystic fibrosis in pregnancy. Can Med Assoc J 149:809, 1993.
161. Edenborough FP, Stableforth DE, Webb AK, et al: Outcome of pregnancy in women with cystic fibrosis. Thorax 50:170, 1995.
162. Olson GL: Cystic fibrosis in pregnancy. Semin Perinatol 21:307, 1997.
163. Heikkila A, Erkkola R: Review of β-lactam antibiotics in pregnancy: the need for adjustment of dosage schedules. Clin Pharmacokinet 27:49, 1994.
164. Jusko WJ, Mosovich LL, Gerbracht LM, et al: Enhanced renal excretion of dicloxacillin in patients with cystic fibrosis. Pediatrics 56:1038, 1975.
165. Yaffe SJ, Gerbracht LM, Mosovich LL, et al: Pharmacokinetics of methicillin in patients with cystic fibrosis. J Infect Dis 135:828, 1977.
166. Spino M, Chai RP, Isles AF, et al: Cloxacillin absorption and disposition in cystic fibrosis. J Pediatr 105:829, 1984.
167. De Groot R, Smith AL: Antibiotic pharmacokinetics in cystic fibrosis: differences and clinical significance. Clin Pharmacokinet 13:228, 1987.
168. MacDonald NE, Anas NG, Peterson RG, et al: Renal clearance of gentamicin in cystic fibrosis. J Pediatr 103:985, 1983.
169. Lemna WK, Feldman GL, Kerem B, et al: Mutation analysis for heterozygote detection and the prenatal diagnosis of cystic fibrosis. N Engl J Med 322:291, 1990.
170. Cole BN, Seltzer MH, Kassabian J, et al: Parenteral nutrition in a pregnant cystic fibrosis patient. JPEN J Parenter Enteral Nutr 11:205, 1987.

Renal Disease

David F. Colombo and Philip Samuels

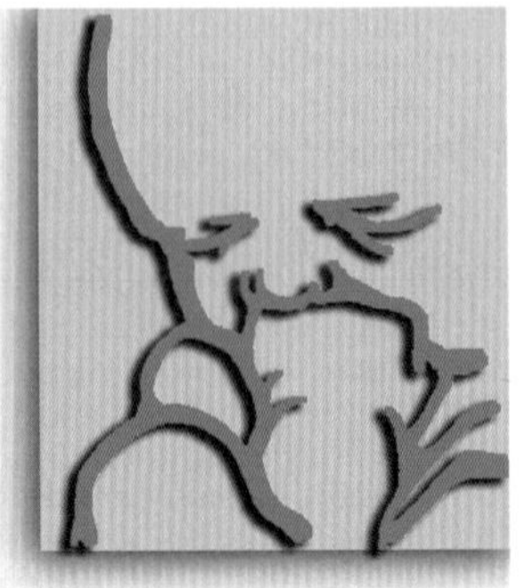

CHAPTER 36

Key Abbreviations

Acute renal failure	ARF
Adult respiratory distress syndrome	ARDS
Asymptomatic bacteruria	ASB
Blood urea nitrogen	BUN
Glomerular filtration rate	GFR
Intrauterine growth restriction	IUGR
Red blood cell	RBC
Urinary tract infection	UTI
White blood cell	WBC

INTRODUCTION

Of all the organ systems, one could argue that none is altered more by pregnancy than the kidney and urinary collecting system. Before the 1970s, women with preexisting renal disease were strongly discouraged from attempting pregnancy secondary to the expectation of poor perinatal outcome and the likelihood of renal disease progression. At present, through better understanding of the prognosis of kidney disease during pregnancy, women with most renal diseases are no longer discouraged from attempting conception. This even holds true for women who have undergone renal transplantation.

This chapter first reviews the normal changes in the kidney and urinary collecting system in pregnancy and follows with the basic evaluation of the renal status, acute and chronic renal disorders in pregnancy, and the treatment of the postrenal transplant patient.

ALTERED RENAL PHYSIOLOGY IN PREGNANCY

Pregnancy is associated with significant anatomic changes in the kidney and its collecting system (see Chapter 3). These changes begin shortly after conception and may persist for several months postpartum.[1,2] The kidney is noted to increase in size and weight during the course of a pregnancy. Of more clinical significance is the marked dilatation of the collecting system including both the renal pelves and ureters. This dilatation is most pronounced on the right side. This change is likely due to hormonal changes (i.e., progesterone, endothelin, relaxin) and the mechanical obstruction of the uterus itself.[3–5] Figure 36-1, an intravenous pyelogram of a gravid patient, is representative of the normal anatomic changes in the urinary tract during pregnancy.

Renal plasma flow increases greatly during pregnancy.[6] It peaks in the first trimester and, although it decreases near term, remains higher than in the nonpregnant patient. This change is due in part to increased cardiac output and decreased renal vascular resistance. The glomerular filtration rate (GFR) increases by 50 percent during a normal gestation.[7] It rises early in pregnancy and remains elevated throughout gestation. The percentage increase in GFR is greater than the percentage increase in renal plasma flow. This elevation of the filtration fraction leads to a fall in the serum urea nitrogen (BUN) and serum creatinine values.

Because GFR increases to such a great degree, electrolytes, glucose, and other filtered substances reach the renal tubules in greater amounts. The kidney handles sodium efficiently, reabsorbing most of the filtered load in the proximal convoluted tubule. Glucose reabsorp-

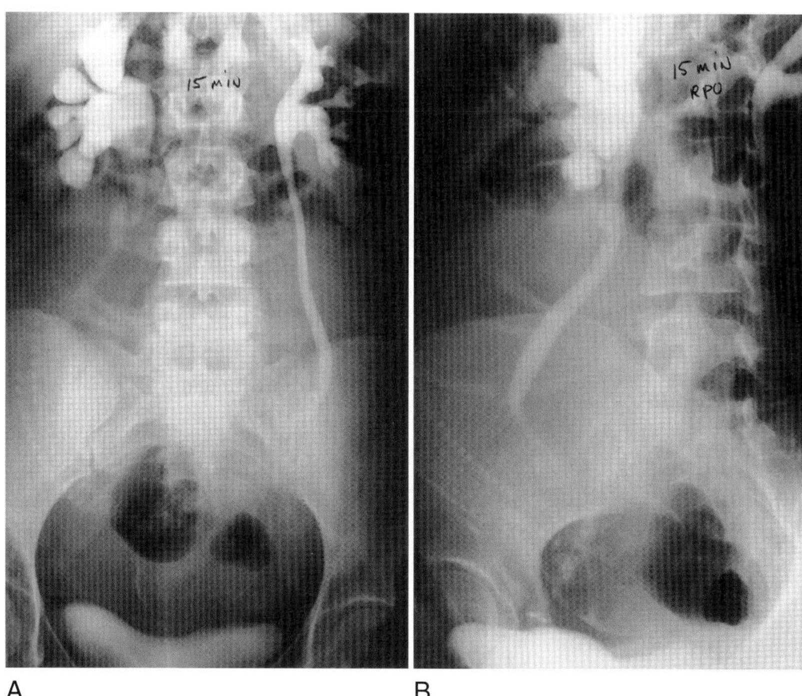

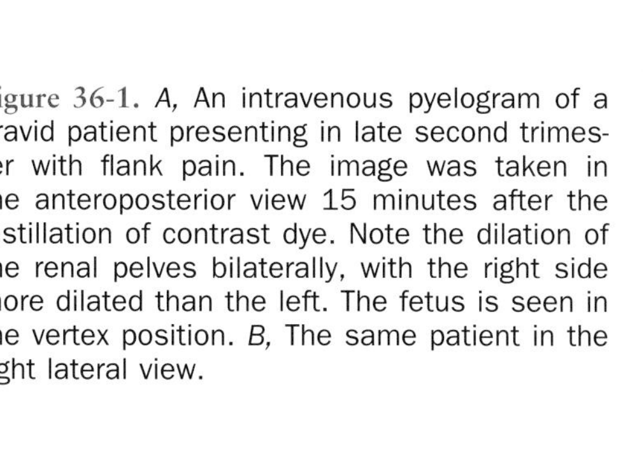
Figure 36-1. *A,* An intravenous pyelogram of a gravid patient presenting in late second trimester with flank pain. The image was taken in the anteroposterior view 15 minutes after the instillation of contrast dye. Note the dilation of the renal pelves bilaterally, with the right side more dilated than the left. The fetus is seen in the vertex position. *B,* The same patient in the right lateral view.

Table 36-1. Summary of Renal Changes in Normal Pregnancy

ALTERATION	MANIFESTATION	CLINICAL RELEVANCE
Increased renal size	Renal length about 1 cm greater on radiographs	• Postpartum decreases in size should not be mistaken for parenchymal loss
Dilatation of pelves, calyces, and ureters	Resembles hydronephrosis on ultrasound or IVP. (usually more prominent on the right)	• Not to be mistaken for obstructive uropathy. • Upper urinary tract infections are more virulent.
Changes in acid-base metabolism	Renal bicarbonate reabsorption threshold decreases	• Serum bicarbonate is 4–5 mM/L lower in pregnancy. • PCO_2 is 10 mm Hg lower in normal pregnancy • PCO_2 of 40 mm Hg actually represents retention in pregnancy.
Renal water-handling	Osmoregulation altered as the osmotic thresholds for AVP release decreased.	• Serum osmolarity decreased by approximately 10 mOsm/L.

AVP, vasopressin; IVP, intravenous pyelography; PCO_2, carbon dioxide tension.

Adapted with permission from Lindheimer M, Grünfeld JP, Davison JM: Renal disorders. *In* Barron WM, Lindheimer M (eds): Medical Disorders During Pregnancy, 3rd ed. St Louis, Mosby, Inc, 2000, p 39.

tion, however, does not increase proportionately during pregnancy. The average renal threshold for glucose is reduced to 155 mg/dl from 194 mg/dl in the nonpregnant individual.[8] Therefore, glycosuria can be seen in normal pregnancy.

Urate is handled by filtration and secretion. Its clearance increases early in pregnancy, leading to lower serum levels of uric acid. In late pregnancy, urate clearance and serum urate levels return to their prepregnancy values. Serum urate levels are elevated in patients with preeclampsia. Whether this is due to decreased renal plasma flow, hemoconcentration, renal tubular dysfunction, or other renal circulatory changes continues to remain uncertain. A summary of the renal changes in normal pregnancy is shown in Table 36-1.

ASYMPTOMATIC BACTERIURIA

The prevalence of asymptomatic bacteriuria (ASB) in sexually active woman has been reported to be as high as 5 to 6 percent (see Chapter 49).[9,10] The diagnosis of ASB is based on a clean-catch voided urine culture revealing greater than 100,000 colonies/ml of a single organism.[11] Some investigators have suggested that two consecutively voided specimens should contain the same organism before making the diagnosis of bacteriuria.[12,13] If a urine culture is negative for bacteria at the first prenatal visit, the risk of developing acute cystitis is less than 1 percent.[10,14]

It is important to diagnose and treat ASB in pregnancy. If left untreated, a symptomatic urinary tract infection (UTI) will develop in up to 40 percent of these patients.[10,15] Recognition and therapy for ASB can eliminate 70 percent of acute UTIs in pregnancy. Nonetheless, 2 percent of pregnant women with negative urine cultures develop symptomatic cystitis or pyelonephritis. This group accounts for 30 percent of the cases of acute UTI that develop during gestation. The American College of Obstetricians and Gynecologists advocates routine screening of all women for ASB at their first prenatal visit.[16] Other than progression to more serious infection, there is little evidence that ASB has an effect on pregnancy outcome.[9,17]

Escherichia coli is the organism responsible for most cases of ASB. Therefore, patients can be safely treated with nitrofurantoin, ampicillin, cephalosporins, and short-acting sulfa drugs. Table 36-2 lists choices of antibiotic therapy for the pregnant patient with ASB. Sulfa compounds should be avoided near term, because they compete for bilirubin-binding sites on albumin in the fetus and newborn and pose a risk for kernicterus. Nitrofurantoin should not be used in patients with glucose-6-phosphate dehydrogenase deficiency, because there is a risk for hemolytic crisis. If the fetus has this enzyme deficiency, it may also experience hemolysis. Therapy for ASB should be continued for 10 to 14 days, with a follow-up culture performed 1 to 2 weeks after discontinuing therapy. Approximately 15 percent of women experience a reinfection or do not respond to initial therapy. Therapy should be reinstituted after careful microbial sensitivity testing. Women with recurrent UTI during pregnancy and those with a history of pyelonephritis should undergo imaging of the upper urinary tract. This procedure should be delayed until the patient is 3 months postpartum so that the anatomic and physiologic changes of pregnancy can regress.

Occasionally, it is difficult to distinguish severe cystitis from pyelonephritis. Although the drugs used for treatment are similar, treatment of the pyelonephritis during pregnancy generally requires intravenous antibiotics. Sandberg and coinvestigators[18] studied symptomatic UTIs in 174 women. They reported that C-reactive protein was elevated in 91 percent of pregnant women with acute pyelonephritis but only 5 percent of women with cystitis. They also noted that the urine-concentrating ability was lower in women with acute pyelonephritis. Because the erythrocyte sedimentation rate is normally elevated in pregnancy, they found that this was not a useful parameter for distinguishing pyelonephritis from cystitis.

Table 36-2. Antimicrobial Treatment for the Pregnant Patient with Bacteriuria

Amoxicillin 500 mg three times a day
Ampicillin 250 mg four times a day
Cephalosporin 250 mg four times a day
Nitrofurantoin 100 mg four times a day
Sustained-release nitrofurantoin 100 mg two times a day
Trimethoprim (160 mg)/Sulfamethoxazole (800 mg) two times a day

The agent of choice should be given for a 7-day course. A repeat urine culture is recommended 2 weeks after the treatment has been completed.

PYELONEPHRITIS

Pyelonephritis complicates 1 to 2 percent of all pregnancies, and importantly contributes substantially to maternal morbidity. It is the most common nonobstetric cause of hospitalization during pregnancy (see Chapter 49).[19] Recurrent pyelonephritis has been implicated as a cause of fetal death and intrauterine growth restriction (IUGR). There appears to be an association between acute pyelonephritis and preterm labor.[20,21] Fan and coworkers,[22] however, have shown that if pyelonephritis is aggressively treated, it does not increase the likelihood of preterm labor, premature delivery, or low-birth-weight infants. Hill et al.,[23] described 440 cases of acute pyelonephritis over a 2-year period. He found the disease to be more prevalent in younger primagravid women. The majority of cases (53 percent) presented during the second trimester. There was no difference in clinical outcome between different ethnic groups. The most common pathogen was *Escherichia coli*, accounting for 83 percent of cases, with gram-positive organisms isolated in another 11.6 percent.[23]

Acute pyelonephritis during pregnancy is most often treated on an inpatient basis, using intravenous antibiotics. Empiric therapy should begin as soon as the presumptive diagnosis is made. Therapy can be tailored to the specific organism after sensitivities have been obtained approximately 48 hours later. Because septicemia may occasionally result from pyelonephritis, blood cultures should be obtained if patients do not respond rapidly to initial antibiotic therapy. Generally, a broad-spectrum first-generation cephalosporin is the initial therapy of choice. Fan and coinvestigators[22] reviewed 107 cases of pyelonephritis in 103 pregnancies. The authors noted that 33 percent of the cases a decade ago were resistant to ampicillin and 13 percent to first-generation cephalosporins. It is likely that current rates of resistance to ampicillin and first-generation cephalosporins are even higher. Thus, it is important to treat affected women initially as inpatients. If resistance to more common therapies are encountered, a later generation cephalosporin or an aminoglycoside can be safely administered. Peak and trough aminoglycoside levels are advised when using these agents. Serum creatinine and BUN levels should be followed as well. During the febrile period, acetaminophen should be employed to keep the temperature below 38°C. Small doses of acetaminophen should not mask fever and symptoms in a patient who is unresponsive to treatment.

Intravenous antibiotic therapy should be continued for 24 to 48 hours after the patient becomes afebrile and costovertebral angle tenderness disappears. After the cessation of intravenous therapy, treatment with appropriate oral antibiotics should be continued for 10 to 14 days. On termination of therapy, urine cultures should be obtained in each trimester for the remainder of gestation. After an episode of acute pyelonephritis, antibiotic suppression should also be implemented and continued for the remainder of the pregnancy. Nitrofurantoin 50 mg once or twice daily is an acceptable regimen for suppression. In a study by van Dorsten and colleagues,[25] the overall frequency of positive urine cultures following hospitalization for pyelonephritis was 38 percent. Nitrofurantoin suppression reduced this rate to 8 percent. Nitrofurantoin did not lower the rate of positive cultures if the antibiotic chosen for inpatient therapy was inappropriate or if the urine culture was positive at time of discharge.[24]

The most common maternal complications associated with pyelonephritis are anemia (23 percent), septicemia (17 percent), transient renal dysfunction (2 percent), and pulmonary insufficiency (7 percent).[24] Cunningham and coworkers[25] point out that pulmonary injury resembling adult respiratory distress syndrome (ARDS) can occur in pregnant women with acute pyelonephritis. Clinical manifestations of this complication usually occur 24 to 48 hours after the patient is admitted.[25,26] Some of these patients require endotracheal intubation, mechanical ventilation,[27] and positive end expiratory pressure. In Cunningham's series, there was no evidence that pulmonary edema was caused by excessive amounts of intravenous fluid.[25] This presentation of ARDS probably results from endotoxin-induced alveolar capillary membrane injury. Towers et al. found evidence of pulmonary injury in 11 of 130 patients with pyelonephritis. A fever of greater than 103°F, a maternal heart rate above 110 bpm, and gestational age beyond 20 weeks were factors associated with an increased risk for pulmonary injury. The most predictive factors were fluid overload and tocolytic therapy.[28]

Austenfeld and Snow[29] reported 64 pregnancies in 30 women who had previously undergone ureteral reimplantation for vesicoureteral reflux. During pregnancy, 57 percent of these women experienced one or more UTIs, and 17 percent had more than one UTI or an episode of pyelonephritis.[29] More frequent urine cultures and aggressive therapy during pregnancy are recommended for this group of high risk of parturients.

ACUTE RENAL DISEASE IN PREGNANCY

Urolithiasis

Urolithiasis affects 0.03 percent of all pregnancies, the same frequency as observed in the general population.[30] Colicky abdominal pain, recurrent UTI, and hematuria suggest urolithiasis. If the diagnosis is suspected, intravenous pyelography should be undertaken, limiting this study to the minimum number of exposures necessary to make the diagnosis. Ultrasound can often be used to establish the diagnosis without radiation exposure. Newer ultrasound flow studies can actually follow flow from the ureter to the bladder and detect obstruction without the use of ionizing radiation. Urine microscopy may detect crystals and help distinguish the type of stone before it is passed. For any women suspected or proved to have renal stones, serum calcium and phosphorous levels should be assayed to rule out hyperparathyroidism. Serum urate should also be determined.

Because of the physiologic hydroureter of pregnancy, many women with symptomatic urolithiasis spontaneously pass their stones. Treatment should be conservative, consisting of hydration and narcotic analgesia.[31] Epidural anesthesia has been advocated to establish a segmental block from T11 to L2. It is unknown whether this promotes passage of the stone. For that reason, this approach remains controversial. Lithotripsy is contraindicated during pregnancy.

Recurrent UTI with urease-containing organisms causes precipitation of calcium phosphate in the kidney that may lead to the development of staghorn calculi. Surgery is rarely indicated in these patients during gestation. Patients with staghorn calculi should have frequent urine cultures, and bacteriuria should be treated aggressively. Recurrent infections can pose a risk for chronic pyelonephritis with resultant loss of kidney function.

Glomerulonephritis

Acute glomerulonephritis is an uncommon complication of pregnancy, with an estimated incidence of 1 per 40,000 pregnancies.[32] Poststreptococcal glomerulonephritis is rarely observed in the adult population. In this disorder, renal function tends to deteriorate during the acute phase of the disease but usually recovers later.[33] Acute glomerulonephritis can be difficult to distinguish from preeclampsia. Periorbital edema, a striking clinical feature of acute glomerulonephritis, is often seen in preeclampsia. Hematuria, red blood cell (RBC) casts in the urine sediment, and depressed serum complement levels indicate glomerular disease. The rise in antistreptolysin O titers may help establish the diagnosis of poststreptococcal glomerulonephritis.

Treatment of acute glomerulonephritis in pregnancy is similar to that for the nonpregnant individual. Blood pressure control is essential, and careful attention to fluid balance is imperative. Sodium intake should be restricted to 500 mg/day during the acute disease. Serum potassium levels must also be carefully monitored.

Packham and coworkers[34] extensively reviewed 395 pregnancies in 238 women with primary glomerulonephritis. Only 51 percent of infants were born after 36 weeks' gestation. Excluding therapeutic abortion, 20 percent of fetuses were lost, 15 percent after 20 weeks' gestation. IUGR was noted in 15 percent of cases. Maternal renal function deteriorated in 15 percent of pregnancies and failed to resolve postpartum in 5 percent.[34] Hypertension was recorded in 52 percent of the pregnancies and developed before 32 weeks' gestation in 26 percent of cases. In most cases, this blood pressure elevation was not an exacerbation of chronic hypertension, because only 12 percent of pregnancies carried this diagnosis. Eighteen percent of the women who developed de novo hypertension in pregnancy remained hypertensive postpartum. Increased proteinuria was recorded in 59 percent of these pregnancies and was irreversible in 15 percent.[34]

The highest incidence of fetal and maternal complications occurred in patients with primary focal and segmental hyalinosis and sclerosis. The lowest incidence of complications was observed in non-immunoglobulin A (IgA)–diffuse mesangial proliferative glomerulonephritis.[34] The presence of severe vessel lesions on renal biopsy was associated with a significantly higher rate of fetal loss after 20 weeks' gestation. Packham and coworkers[35] also studied 33 pregnancies in 24 patients with biopsy-proven membranous glomerulonephritis. Fetal loss occurred in 24 percent of pregnancies, preterm delivery in 43 percent, and a term live-born infant in only 33 percent of patients. Hypertension was noted in 46 percent of these pregnant women. Thirty percent of patients had proteinuria in the nephrotic range during the first trimester.[35] The presence of significant proteinuria during the first trimester correlated with poor fetal and maternal outcome.[35]

Jungers et al.[36] described 69 pregnancies in 34 patients with IgA glomerulonephritis. The fetal loss rate in this group was 15 percent. Preexisting hypertension was associated with poor fetal outcome. Hypertension at the time of conception also correlated with a deterioration of maternal renal function during pregnancy. Hypertension in the first pregnancy was highly predictive of recurrence of hypertension in a subsequent pregnancy.[36] Kincaide-Smith and Fairley[37] analyzed 102 pregnancies in 65 women with IgA glomerulonephritis. They noted that hypertension occurred in 63 percent of pregnancies, with 18 percent being severe. In this subset of women, a decline in renal function was observed in 22 percent.[37]

Abe[38] reported 240 pregnancies in 166 women with preexisting glomerular disease. Eight percent of the pregnancies resulted in a spontaneous abortion, 6 percent in a stillbirth, and 86 percent were live born. Most losses occurred in women with a GFR less than 70 ml/min and preexisting hypertension. Even though the majority of women with significant renal insufficiency had good pregnancy outcomes, the long-term prognosis for these cases was worse if the GFR was less than 50 ml/min and the serum creatinine was more than 1.5 mg/dl.[39] The histopathogenic diagnosis of membranoproliferative glomerulonephritis seemed to carry the worst prognosis, with 29 percent developing hypertension and 33 percent exhibiting a long-term decrease in renal function.

Imbasciati and Ponticelli[39] summarized six studies containing a total of 906 pregnancies in 558 women with preexisting glomerular disease. The overall perinatal mortality was 13 percent. Hypertension, renal insufficiency, and nephrotic range proteinuria were the strongest predictive factors for a poor pregnancy outcome. In this report, the histologic type of glomerulonephritis had little correlation with pregnancy outcome. Hypertension persisted in 3 to 12 percent of patients who developed hypertension for the first time during pregnancy. In 25 percent of patients, hypertension worsened during pregnancy and then normalized postpartum.[39] Some of these cases might represent superimposed preeclampsia. However, that diagnosis is very difficult to establish in a patient with baseline hypertension and proteinuria. Remarkably, only 3 percent of these 166 women experienced an acceleration of their glomerular disease after pregnancy.

Acute Renal Failure in Pregnancy

Acute renal failure (ARF) is defined as a urine output of less than 400 ml in 24 hours. To establish the diagnosis, ureteral and urethral obstruction must be excluded. The incidence of ARF during pregnancy is approximately 1 per 10,000. It is seen most frequently following septic first trimester abortions and in cases of sudden severe volume depletion resulting from hemorrhage.[40] It may also be observed with marked volume contraction associated with severe preeclampsia[41] and with acute fatty liver of pregnancy.[41,42]

The incidence of ARF in pregnancy has decreased over the years. Stratta and colleagues[43] reported 81 cases of pregnancy-related ARF between 1958 and 1987, accounting for 9 percent of the total number of ARF cases needing dialysis during that interval. In three successive 10-year periods (1958 to 1967, 1968 to 1977, and 1978 to 1987), the incidence of pregnancy-related ARF fell from 43 to 2.8 percent of the total number of cases of ARF. The incidence changed from 1 in 3,000 to 1 in 15,000 pregnancies over the study period.[43] In these 81 ARF cases, 11.6 percent experienced irreversible renal damage with the majority occurring in the setting of severe preeclampsia/eclampsia.[43]

Renal ischemia is the common denominator in cases of ARF. With mild ischemia, quickly reversible prerenal failure results. With more prolonged ischemia, acute tubular necrosis occurs. This process is also reversible, because glomeruli are not affected. Severe ischemia, however, may produce acute cortical necrosis. This pathology is irreversible, although on occasion, a small amount of renal function is preserved.[44] Stratta and colleagues[45] have reported 17 cases of ARF complicating pregnancies over 15 years, and all were due to preeclampsia/eclampsia. Cortical necrosis occurred in 29.5 percent of these women.[45] Whether or not ARF was associated with cortical necrosis did not appear to be related to maternal age, parity, gestational age, duration of preeclampsia before delivery, or eclamptic seizures. The only significant factor associated with cortical necrosis was placental abruption.[45] Turney and coworkers[46] demonstrated that acute cortical necrosis, which occurred in 12.7 percent of their patients with ARF, carried a 100-percent mortality rate within 6 years.

Sibai and colleagues[47] studied the remote prognosis in 31 consecutive cases of ARF in patients with hypertensive disorders of pregnancy. Eighteen of the 31 patients had "pure" preeclampsia, whereas 13 pregnancies had other hypertensive disorders and renal disease. Five percent of the 18 patients with pure preeclampsia required dialysis during hospitalization, and all 18 patients had acute tubular necrosis. Of the other 13 women, 42 percent required dialysis and three patients had bilateral cortical necrosis. The majority of pregnancies in both groups were complicated by placental abruption and hemorrhage.[47] All 16 surviving patients in the pure preeclampsia group recovered normal renal function on long-term follow-up. Conversely, nine of the 11 surviving patients in the nonpreeclamptic group required long-term dialysis, and four ultimately died of end-stage renal disease.[47] Turney and colleagues[47] also performed follow-up examinations of their patients. They found that maternal survival was adversely affected by increasing age. Their 1-year maternal survival rate was 78.6 percent. Follow-up of survivors showed normal renal function up to 31 years after ARF.[46]

Individuals with reversible ARF first experience a period of oliguria of variable duration. Polyuria, or a high output phase, then occurs. It is important to recognize that BUN and serum creatinine levels continue to rise early in the polyuric phase. During the recovery phase, urine output approach is normal. In these patients, it is important to monitor electrolytes frequently and to treat any imbalance carefully. The urine to plasma osmolality ratio should be determined early in the course of the disease. If the ratio is 1.5 or greater, prerenal pathology is likely, and the disorder tends to be of shorter duration and less severity. A ratio near 1.0 suggests acute tubular necrosis.

The main goal of treatment is the elimination of the underlying cause. Volume and electrolyte balance must receive constant scrutiny. To assess volume requirements, invasive hemodynamic monitoring is useful and lessens the need for clinical guesswork. This is especially true during the polyuric phase. Central hyperalimentation may also be required if renal failure is prolonged.

Acidosis frequently occurs in cases of ARF. Therefore, arterial blood gases should be followed regularly. Acidosis must be treated promptly as it may exacerbate hyperkalemia, which may develop rapidly and can be fatal. If hyperkalemia occurs, potassium restriction should be instituted immediately. Sodium bicarbonate, used to treat acidosis, may overload the patient with sodium and water. In this case, peritoneal or hemodialysis may be necessary. The main indications for dialysis in ARF of pregnancy are hypernatremia, hyperkalemia, severe acidosis, volume overload, and worsening uremia. There is a single report of a successful kidney transplant during pregnancy in the first trimester. The patient received a kidney from her father at approximately 13 weeks gestation and experienced a successful pregnancy.[48]

Hemolytic Uremic Syndrome

The postpartum hemolytic uremic syndrome is a rare idiopathic disorder that must be considered when a patient exhibits signs of hemolysis and decreasing renal function particularly during the postpartum period. This idiopathic syndrome was first described in 1968 and may occur as early as the first trimester and up to 2 months postpartum.[49–52] In fact, it has even been reported following an ectopic pregnancy.[53] Most individuals have no predisposing factors. Prodromal symptoms include vomiting, diarrhea, and a flulike illness. A report of 49 cases documented a 61 percent mortality rate.[51] With improved intensive care monitoring and treatment, the prognosis is likely much better.

Disseminated intravascular coagulation with hemolysis usually accompanies the renal failure. However, disseminated intravascular coagulation is not the cause of the syndrome. Microscopically, the kidney shows thrombotic microangiopathy. The glomerular capillary wall is thick, and biopsy specimens taken later in the course of the disease show severe nephrosclerosis and deposition of complement.

Some researchers believe that this syndrome is due to decreased production of prostacyclin in the kidneys.[54,55] Prostacyclin infusions have been used to treat patients, but this therapy still remains experimental. One observer noted a decrease in antithrombin III in a patient with postpartum hemolytic uremic syndrome. This patient was successfully treated with an infusion of antithrombin III,[56] which is readily available today.

Coratelli and coworkers[50] reported a case of hemolytic uremic syndrome diagnosed at 13 weeks' gestation and confirmed by renal biopsy. Circulating endotoxin was detected and was progressively reduced by hemodialysis performed daily from the third to the ninth days of the disease. Complete normalization of renal function occurred by day 34. These investigators suggest that initiation of early dialysis may play an important role in supporting patients through the disease process. They also propose that endotoxins are key pathogenic factors in the disorder.[49] Conversely, Li and coworkers[57] discovered hemolytic uremic syndrome in a women recovering from an uncomplicated cesarean delivery. Endotoxins could not be isolated in the patient's serum, stool, or renal biopsy material. This patient eventually underwent dialysis and recovered.[57] Conte and coworkers[58] suggest that plasma exchange in cases of ARF caused by the postpartum hemolytic uremic syndrome can be vital. Plasma exchange continues to play a key role in the therapy of this disorder.

Polycystic Kidney Disease

Adult polycystic kidney disease is an autosomal dominant disorder that usually begins to manifest itself in the fifth decade of life. Women of reproductive age may occasionally display symptoms including hypertension, a key part of this disorder. If a patient with adult polycystic kidney disease becomes pregnant, hypertension may be exacerbated and may not improve postpartum.[39] The overall prognosis for the disorder does not appear to worsen with an increasing number of pregnancies.

Vesicoureteral Reflux

Vesicoureteral reflux increases with pregnancy. It usually does not cause problems unless the reflux is severe. If the condition is severe enough to warrant corrective surgery, this procedure should be performed before pregnancy. Even with surgical correction, women with ureterovesical reflux are at increased risk for pyelonephritis and should have urine cultures performed frequently.[39] Antibiotic prophylaxis if indicated prior to pregnancy should be continued. For individuals not receiving prophylaxis, such therapy should be considered.

Brandes and Fritsche[60] reported a case of ARF due to obstruction of the ureters by a gravid uterus. This case was complicated by a twin gestation with polyhydramnios at 34 weeks' gestation. The serum creatinine level peaked at 12.2 mg/dl, but resolved immediately after amniotomy.[59] In cases remote from term, ureteral stenting or dialysis may be necessary if obstruction or reflux is present.

Renal Artery Stenosis

Renal artery stenosis is an extremely rare complication of pregnancy. Heyborne et al.[60] have reviewed the literature on this subject. This disorder may present as chronic hypertension with superimposed preeclampsia or as recurrent isolated preeclampsia. Although Doppler flow studies may be suggestive, renal angiography is the most specific and sensitive diagnostic procedure. Percutaneous transluminal angioplasty can be carried out at the time of angiography. Heyborne et al.[60] present a case in which this procedure was successfully accomplished at 26 weeks' gestation.

Nephrotic Syndrome

The nephrotic syndrome was initially characterized by the following findings: a 24-hour urine protein excretion of 3.5 g or more, reduced serum albumin, edema, and hyperlipidemia.[62] At present, the syndrome is defined by massive proteinuria alone, which is often the result of damage to the glomeruli.[61] The most common etiology of nephrotic syndrome in pregnancy, especially the third trimester, is preeclampsia. Other etiologies include membranous and membranoproliferative glomerulopathy, minimal change disease, lupus nephropathy, hereditary nephritis, diabetic nephropathy, renal vein thrombosis, and amyloidosis.[62]

Women with newly diagnosed or persistent nephrotic syndrome need to be monitored closely in pregnancy. Whenever possible, the etiology of the proteinuria should be determined. In some cases, steroid therapy may be employed to treat this condition; however, its use can actually aggravate the underlying disease process.[62] One common complication of nephrotic syndrome in pregnancy is profound edema secondary to protein excretion, which is further complicated by the normal decline in serum albumin associated with pregnancy.[62] A second area of concern is a possible hypercoagulable state precipitated by urinary losses of antithrombin III, reduced levels of protein C and S, hyperfibrinogenemia, and enhanced platelet aggregation.[63]

CHRONIC RENAL DISEASE IN PREGNANCY

Chronic renal disease can be silent until its advanced stages. Because obstetricians routinely test a women's urine for the presence of protein, glucose, and ketones, they may be the first to detect chronic renal disease.

Any gravida with more than trace proteinuria should collect a 24-hour urine specimen for creatinine clearance and total protein excretion. Before pregnancy, 24-hour urinary protein excretion should not exceed 0.2 g. During gestation, quantities up to 0.3 g per day may be normal. Moderate proteinuria (less than 2 g/day) is seen in glomerular disease.

Microscopic examination of the urine can reveal much about renal status. If renal disease is suspected, a catheterized specimen should be obtained. More RBCs than one to two per high-power field or RBC casts are indicative of renal disease. RBCs usually indicate glomerular disease or collagen vascular disease. Less frequently, they suggest trauma or malignant hypertension. Increased numbers of white blood cells (WBCs) (more than one to two per high-power field) or the appearance of WBC casts are usually indicative of acute or chronic infection. Cellular casts are found in the presence of renal tubular dysfunction, and hyaline casts are associated with significant proteinuria.

The obstetrician can easily be misled when relying solely on BUN and serum creatinine levels to assess renal function. A 70-percent decline in creatinine clearance, an indirect measure of GFR, can be seen before a significant rise in serum BUN or serum creatinine occurs. Little change in serum creatinine or the BUN may be observed until the creatinine clearance falls to 50 ml/min. Below that level, small decrements in creatinine clearance can lead to large increases in the BUN and creatinine. A single creatinine clearance value less than 100 ml/min is not diagnostic of renal disease. An incomplete 24-hour urine collection is the most frequent cause of this finding. Therefore, an abnormal clearance rate should prompt a repeat assay.

Serum urate is an often overlooked but helpful parameter in detecting renal dysfunction. Excretion of uric acid is dependent not only on glomerular filtration but also on tubular secretion. Therefore, an elevated serum urate in the presence of a normal BUN and serum creatinine may implicate tubular disease. A solitary increase in uric acid may also signify impending or early preeclampsia.

Effect of Pregnancy on Renal Function

Although baseline creatinine clearance is decreased in women with chronic renal insufficiency, a physiologic rise will still occur in most pregnancies. A moderate fall in creatinine clearance may then be observed during late gestation in patients with renal disease. This decline is typically more severe in women with diffuse glomerular disease and reverses after delivery.

The long-term effect of pregnancy on renal disease remains controversial. If the serum creatinine is less than 1.5 mg/dl, pregnancy should have little effect on the long-term prognosis. Pregnancy, however, is associated with an increased incidence of pyelonephritis in patients with chronic renal disease. There are few data concerning the long-term effect of pregnancy on renal disease in women with significant azotemia. Occasionally, some women with a baseline serum creatinine of more than 1.5 mg/dl experience a significant decrease in renal function during gestation that does not improve during the postpartum period.[39,64] This deterioration occurs more frequently in women with diffuse glomerulonephritis. It is not possible, however, to predict which women with renal insufficiency will experience a permanent reduction in renal function. If renal function significantly deteriorates during gestation, termination of the pregnancy may not reverse the process. Therefore, termination cannot be routinely recommended for patients who become pregnant and whose baseline serum creatinine level exceeds 1.5 mg/dl. Ideally, women with chronic renal disease should be counseled before conception about the possible deterioration in their renal function.

Severe hypertension remains the greatest threat to a pregnant patient with chronic renal disease. Left uncontrolled, hypertension can lead to intracerebral hemorrhage as well as deteriorating renal function. Most pregnant women with chronic renal dysfunction also have preexisting hypertension.[65,66] Approximately 50 percent of these patients have worsening hypertension as pregnancy progresses, and diastolic blood pressures of 110 mm Hg or greater develop in about 20 percent of cases.[67] Those women with diffuse proliferative glomerulonephritis and nephrosclerosis are at greatest risk for the development of severe hypertension. Blood pressure control is the cornerstone of successful treatment of chronic renal disease in pregnancy.

Worsening proteinuria is common during pregnancy complicated by chronic renal disease and often reaches the nephrotic range.[67] In general, massive proteinuria alone does not indicate an increased risk for mother or fetus.[68] Low serum albumin, however, has been correlated with low birth weight.[69] The development of massive proteinuria is not necessarily a harbinger of preeclampsia, although such women are clearly at risk for this complication. In late pregnancy, it is often difficult to differentiate preeclampsia from worsening chronic renal disease. For this reason first trimester 24-hour urine collections for creatinine clearance and total protein are essential.

Effect of Chronic Renal Disease on Pregnancy

More than 85 percent of women with chronic renal disease will have a surviving infant if renal function is well preserved. Earlier reports were more pessimistic, citing a 5.8-percent incidence of stillbirth, a 4.9-percent incidence of neonatal deaths, and an increase in second-trimester losses.[67] If hypertension is not controlled and if renal function is not well preserved, there is still a high likelihood of pregnancy loss.[35] Antepartum fetal surveillance and advances in neonatal care have contributed to an improved perinatal outcome in these patients. One study reported a total fetal loss rate of 13.8 percent, including miscarriage, stillbirths, and neonatal deaths.[66]

The outlook for women with severe renal insufficiency whose baseline serum creatinine level is more than 1.5 mg/dl is less clear. This is due in part to the limited number of pregnancies in such patients as well as to the large number who undergo elective termination. One study reported no surviving infants when the maternal BUN was greater than 60 mg/dl.[68] Other investigations, however, have found that about 80 percent of such pregnancies resulted in surviving infants.[66,70] Preterm birth and IUGR remain important complications in these pregnancies. The reported incidence of preterm birth ranges from 20 to 50 percent.[67,71]

Imbasciati and Ponticelli[29] summarized three studies containing 81 pregnancies in 78 women with serum creatinine concentrations greater than 1.4 mg/dl.[39] The perinatal loss rate was only 9 percent. However, 33 percent of the infants were growth restricted, and 50 percent were born preterm secondary to either maternal or fetal indications. Disturbingly, 33 percent of the women showed acceleration of their renal disease after delivery. Some individuals believe that growth restriction may be due to the lack of plasma volume increase as the pregnancy progresses. Cunningham et al.[72] demonstrated that women with moderate renal dysfunction did exhibit increased creatinine clearance and plasma volume expansion during gestation, whereas women with severe renal dysfunction did not.[72]

Management of Chronic Renal Disease in Pregnancy

A 24-hour urine collection for creatinine clearance and total protein excretion should be obtained as soon as the pregnancy is confirmed. These parameters should be monitored periodically. The patient should be seen once every 2 weeks until 32 weeks' gestation and weekly thereafter. These are general guidelines, and more frequent visits may be necessary in individual cases.

Control of hypertension is critical in managing patients with chronic renal disease. Home blood pressure monitoring is advised for women with underlying hypertension. β-blockers, calcium channel blockers, and hydralazine can be used to treat blood pressure effectively as long as the dosages are monitored carefully. Clonidine is occasionally useful in refractory patients. Doxazosin and prazosin may be used if necessary. Angiotensin-converting enzyme (ACE) inhibitors are contraindicated. These drugs have been associated with fetal and neonatal oliguria/anuria[73,74] as well as malformations.[75] In one study, one of 19 infants had anuria and required dialysis,[73] whereas in another report, an infant required peritoneal dialysis.[74] Furthermore, congenital anomalies, including microcephaly and encephalocele,[73] have been associated with the use of ACE inhibitors.

The use of diuretics in pregnancy is controversial.[76,77] For massive debilitating edema, a short course of diuretics can be helpful. Electrolytes must be monitored carefully. Salt restriction does not appear to be beneficial once edema has developed. Salt restriction, however, should be instituted without hesitation in pregnant women with true renal insufficiency.

Fetal growth should be assessed with serial ultrasonography, because growth restriction is common in women with chronic renal disease. Antepartum fetal heart rate testing should be initiated at 28 to 32 weeks' gestation.[78]

Obstetricians should have a low threshold for hospitalizing women with chronic renal disease. Increasing hypertension and decreasing renal function warrant immediate hospitalization. A sudden deterioration of renal function may be due to infection, dehydration, electrolyte imbalance, or obstruction.

The timing of delivery should be individualized. Maternal indications for delivery include uncontrollable hypertension, the development of superimposed preeclampsia, and decreasing renal function after fetal viability has been reached. Fetal indications are dictated by assessment of fetal growth and biophysical testing.

Renal biopsy is rarely indicated during pregnancy. It is never indicated after 34 weeks' gestation, when delivery of the fetus and subsequent biopsy would prove a safer alternative. Excessive bleeding secondary to the greatly increased renal blood flow has been reported by some[79] but not all[80] observers. If coagulation indices are normal and blood pressure is well controlled, morbidity should be no greater than that observed in the nonpregnant patient.[81] Packham and Fairley[82] report a series of 111 renal biopsies performed in 104 pregnant women over 20 years. The complication rate was 4.5 percent. The most likely clinical dilemma necessitating renal biopsy in a pregnant woman would be the development of nephrotic syndrome and increasing hypertension between 22 and 32 weeks' gestation. In this case, renal biopsy may distinguish chronic renal disease from preeclampsia, and the findings may have a significant impact on the treatment plan.

Hemodialysis in Pregnancy

Women with chronic hemodialysis can have successful pregnancies.[83–89] Many women with chronic renal failure, however, experience oligomenorrhea, and their fertility is often impaired.[90] These women commonly fail to use a method of contraception. Therefore, it is important that testing be undertaken if pregnancy is suspected.

As in all patients with impaired renal function, the most important aspect of care is meticulous control of blood pressure. During dialysis, wide fluctuations in blood pressure often occur. One case report describes a nonreassuring fetal heart rate pattern associated with hypotension during dialysis.[91] Therefore, sudden volume shifts should be avoided.[89] In late pregnancy, continuous fetal heart rate monitoring should be carried out during dialysis. If possible, positioning of the patient on her left side with uterine displacement off the vena cava is preferred. During dialysis, careful attention to electrolyte balance is advised. Pregnant patients are in a state of chronic compensated respiratory alkalosis, and large drops in serum bicarbonate should be prevented. Dialysates containing glucose and bicarbonate are preferred, and those containing citrates should be avoided.[89]

Women should be counseled that a successful pregnancy requires longer and more frequent periods of dialysis.[84,89,91,92] Patients must also follow a careful diet, ingesting at least 70 g of protein and 1.5 g of calcium daily. Weight gain should be limited to 0.5 kg between dialysis sessions. Chronic anemia is often a problem in hemodialysis patients. The hematocrit should be kept above 25 percent, and transfusion with packed RBCs or erythropoietin therapy may be necessary to accomplish this objective.[84]

The criteria for initiating hemodialysis during pregnancy are controversial. Cohen and coinvestigators[86] believe that beginning regular hemodialysis in patients with moderate renal insufficiency may improve pregnancy outcome. In two cases, when regular hemodialysis was commenced in the second trimester, both patients carried to term, although these infants were growth restricted.[86] Redrow and coworkers[87] report 14 pregnancies in 13 women undergoing dialysis. Ten of those pregnancies were successful. Five of eight pregnancies managed with chronic ambulatory peritoneal dialysis or chronic cycling peritoneal dialysis were successful. The investigators hypothesize several advantages for peritoneal dialysis. These include a more constant chemical and extracellular environment for the fetus, higher hematocrit levels, infrequent episodes of hypotension, and no requirement for heparin. They also postulate that intraperitoneal insulin facilitates the management of blood glucose in diabetic patients and that intraperitoneal magnesium used in the dialysate reduces the likelihood of preterm labor.

Preterm birth does occur more frequently in patients undergoing dialysis.[93] Progesterone is removed during dialysis and at least one group has advocated that parenteral progesterone therapy should be administered to the patient undergoing such treatment.[94] In their review, Yasin and Doun[89] report a 40.7-percent incidence of premature contractions.

Renal Transplant

Pregnancy following renal transplantation has become increasingly common. Many previously anovulatory patients begin ovulating postoperatively and regain fertility as renal function normalizes.[95] As in the case of women on hemodialysis, many transplant recipients do not recognize that they are pregnant until well into the second trimester.

Many transplant recipients stop taking all medications on discovering that they are pregnant. The importance of continuing immunosuppressive therapy cannot be emphasized strongly enough to renal allograft recipients. Glucocorticoids, especially prednisone, are metabolized in the placenta by 11 β-ol-dehydrogenase, with only limited amounts reaching the fetus. Adrenocortical insufficiency has been rarely reported in infants born to mothers taking glucocorticoids.[96] Nevertheless, a pediatrician should be present at the delivery and should be aware of this possibility.

Azathioprine cannot be activated in the fetus because of its lack of inosinate pyrophosphorylase.[97] Azathioprine has been shown to cause decreased levels of IgG and IgM as well as a smaller thymic shadow on chest x-ray study in these neonates.[98] Chromosomal aberrations, which cleared within 20 to 32 months, have also been demonstrated in lymphocytes of infants exposed to azathioprine in utero.[99] The long-term implications of this treatment are not yet known. IUGR has been reported in infants born to mothers receiving azathioprine.[100] These risks are outweighed, however, by the disastrous consequences of allograft rejection that may occur if the patient stops her medication.

Cyclosporin A appears to be relatively safe for use during gestation but does hold some risks. Women may develop arterial hypertension secondary to its interference with the normal hemodynamic adaptation to pregnancy.[101] Although cyclosporin crosses the placenta, there is no evidence of teratogenesis.[102,103] Intrauterine growth restriction, in the absence of maternal hypertension, has been reported in a patient taking cyclosporin A during pregnancy.[104] Overall, most women receiving cyclosporin have had no complications attributable to the drug, and the risk of allograft rejection certainly outweighs the fetal risk of the medication.

Davison[105] reviewed 1,569 renal transplants in 1,009 women. He found that 22 percent of the women elected to abort their pregnancies, 16 percent had a spontaneous abortion, and 8 percent experienced perinatal deaths. Furthermore, he observed that 45 percent of the surviving pregnancies were delivered preterm and 22 percent were complicated by IUGR.[105] Three percent of the infants were born with major malformations, a rate no different from that expected in the background population. Preeclampsia complicated 30 percent of the pregnancies, but as previously noted, the diagnosis is difficult to make in a patient who may already have hypertension and proteinuria. The allograft rejection rate in these women was 9 percent, a rate no different from that expected in a nonpregnant population.[105] The long-term rejection rate was also the same as for women who had not experienced a pregnancy.

During pregnancy, renal allograft recipients must be carefully watched for signs of rejection. As previously mentioned, significant episodes of rejection may occur in as many as 9 percent of transplant recipients during gestation. Unfortunately, the clinical hallmarks of rejection, such as fever, oliguria, tenderness, and decreasing renal function, are not always exhibited by the pregnant patient. Occasionally, rejection may mimic pyelonephritis or preeclampsia, which occurs in approximately one third of renal transplant patients. In these cases, renal biopsy is indicated to distinguish rejection from preeclampsia. Rejection has been known to occur during the puerperium, when maternal immune competence returns to its prepregnancy level.[106] Therefore, it may be advisable to increase the dose of immunosuppressive medications in the immediate postpartum period.

Infection can be disastrous for the renal allograft. Therefore, urine cultures should be obtained at least monthly during pregnancy, and any bacteriuria should be aggressively treated. It is crucial to remember that the allograft is denervated, and pain may not accompany the pyelonephritis. The only symptoms may be fever and nausea.

Renal function, as determined by 24-hour creatinine clearance and protein excretion, should be assessed monthly. Approximately 15 percent of transplant recipients exhibit a significant decrease in renal function in late pregnancy.[62] This condition usually, but not always, reverses after pregnancy. Proteinuria develops in about 40 percent of patients near term, but most often disappears soon after delivery unless significant hypertension is present.

As for patients with chronic renal disease, serial ultrasonography should be used to assess fetal growth, and antepartum fetal heart rate testing should be started at 28 to 32 weeks' gestation. Approximately 50 percent of renal allograft recipients deliver preterm. Preterm labor, preterm rupture of membranes, and IUGR are common. Vaginal delivery should be accomplished when possible, with cesarean delivery reserved for obstetric indications. Allograft recipients may have an increased frequency of cephalopelvic disproportion from pelvic osteodystrophy,[107] resulting from prolonged renal disease with hypercalcemia or extended steroid use. The transplanted kidney, however, rarely obstructs vaginal delivery despite its pelvic location.

Although there have been many successful pregnancies in renal allograft recipients, there is no consensus as to when it is safe to attempt pregnancy after transplantation. Lindheimer and Katz[108,109] have suggested guidelines, which are summarized in Table 36-3.

Table 36-3. Guidelines for Renal Allograft Recipients Who Wish to Conceive

Wait 2 years after cadaver transplant or 1 year after graft from living donor
Immunosuppression should be at maintenance levels
Plasma creatinine <1.5 mg/dl
Absent or easily controlled hypertension
No or minimal proteinuria
No evidence of active graft rejection
No pelvicalyceal distention on a recent ultrasound or intravenous pyelogram
Prednisone dose 15 mg/day
Azathioprine dose 2 mg/kg/day
Cyclosporin A dose 2–4 mg/kg (available data on the use of this drug in pregnancy includes <150 patients)

Lindheimer M, Katz A: Pregnancy in the renal transplant patient. Am J Kidney Dis 19:173, 2000.

Key Points

- Asymptomatic bacteriuria complicates 10 percent of pregnancies, and if the condition is left untreated, it will result in symptomatic urinary tract infections in 40 percent of patients.
- Pyelonephritis complicates 1 to 2 percent of pregnancies, making it the most frequent nonobstetric cause of hospitalization during pregnancy.
- Patients with glomerulonephritis can have successful pregnancies, but pregnancy loss rates increase greatly if the patient has preexisting hypertension.
- Creatinine clearance can decline 70 percent before significant increases are seen in the BUN or serum creatinine level. Therefore, a 24-hour urine specimen for creatinine clearance should be collected from any patient in whom renal disease is suspected.
- The chance of successful pregnancy is reduced if the creatinine clearance is less than 50 ml/min or if the serum creatinine level is more than 1.5 mg/dl.
- Severe hypertension is the greatest threat to the pregnant woman with chronic renal disease.
- Growth restriction and preeclampsia are common in women with chronic renal disease. These patients should have frequent sonograms and begin antepartum fetal surveillance at 28 weeks' gestation.

❑ Patients with chronic renal disease are often anovulatory. Following transplantation, as renal function returns, they ovulate and may become pregnant unexpectedly.

❑ Patients should wait 2 years after receiving a cadaver renal allograft and 1 year after receiving a living allograft before contemplating pregnancy. Furthermore, there should be no signs of allograft rejection.

❑ Renal transplant patients should remain on their immunosuppressive medications throughout gestation.

REFERENCES

1. Cietak KA, Newton JR: Serial quantitative maternal nephrosonography in pregnancy. Br J Radiol 58:405, 1985.
2. Cietak KA, Newton JR: Serial qualitative maternal nephrosonography in pregnancy. Br J Radiol 58:399, 1985.
3. Rassmussen PE, Nielson FR: Hydronephrosis during pregnancy: A literature survey. Eur J Obstet Gynecol Reprod Biol 27:249, 1988.
4. Danielson LA, Sherwood OD, Conrad KP: Relaxin is a potent vasodilator in conscious rats. J Clin Invest 103:525, 1999.
5. Conrad KP, Gandley RE, Ogawa T, et al: Endothelin mediates renal vasodilitation and hyperfiltration during pregnancy in chronically instrumented conscious rats. Am J Physiol 276:767, 1999.
6. DeAlvarez R: Renal glomerulotubular mechanisms during normal pregnancy: Glomerular filtration rate, renal plasma flow, and creatinine clearance. Am J Obstet Gynecol 75:931, 1958.
7. Davidson J: Changes in renal function and other aspects of homeostasis in early pregnancy. J Obstet Gynaecol Br Commonw 81:1003, 1974.
8. Christensen P: Tubular reabsorbtion of glucose during pregnancy. Scand J Clin Lab Invest 10:364, 1958.
9. Sheffield JSM, Cunningham FGM: Urinary tract infection in women. Obstetr Gynecol; 106:1085, 2005.
10. Hooton TM, Scholes D, Stapleton AE, et al: A prospective study of asymptomatic bacteriuria in sexually active young women. N Engl J Med 343:992, 2000.
11. Kass E: Asymptomatic infections of the urinary tract. Trans Assoc Am Physicians 60:56, 1956.
12. Norden C, Kass E: Bacteriuria of pregnancy—a critical reappraisal. Annu Rev Med 19:431, 1968.
13. McFadyen I, Eykryn S, Gardner N: Bacteriuria of pregnancy. J Obstet Gynaecol Br Commonw 1973; 80:385.
14. Whalley P: Bacteriuria of pregnancy. Am J Obstet Gynecol 97:723, 1967.
15. Savage W, Hajj S, Kass E: Demographic and prognostic characteristics of bacteriuria in pregnancy. Medicine (Balt) 46:385, 1967.
16. American Academy of Pediatrics and American College of Obstetricians and Gynecologists. Guidelines for Prenatal Care, 5th ed. Elk Grove Village, IL, American Academy of Pediatrics and American College of Obstetricians and Gynecologists, 2002.
17. Smaill F: Antibiotics for asymptomatic bacteriuria in pregnancy (Cochrane Review). Oxford, editor. The Cochrane Library 2, 2001.
18. Sandberg T, Likin-Janson G, Eden CS: Host response in women with symptomatic urinary tract infection. Scand J Infect Dis 21:67, 1989.
19. Plattner MS: Pyelonephritis in pregnancy. J Perinatol Neonat Nurs 8:20, 1994.
20. Brumfitt W: The significance of symptomatic and asymptomatic infection in pregnancy. Contrib Nephrol 25:23, 1981.
21. Gilstrap L, Leveno K, Cunningham F, et al: Renal infections and pregnancy outcome. Am J Obstet Gynecol 141:709, 1981.
22. Fan YD, Pastorek JG II, Miller JM, Mulvey J: Acute pyelonephritis in pregnancy. Am J Perinatol 4:324, 1987.
23. Hill JBM, Sheffield JSM, McIntire DDP, Wendel GDJ: Acute pyelonephritis in pregnancy. Obstet Gynecol 105:18, 2005.
24. Van Dorsten JP, Lenke RR, Schifrin BS: Pyelonephritis in pregnancy: the role of in-hospital management and nitrofurantoin suppression. J Reprod Med 32:895, 1987.
25. Cunningham FG, Lucas MJ, Hankins GD: Pulmonary injury complicating antepartum pyelonephritis. Am J Obstet Gynecol 156:797, 1987.
26. Pruett K, Faro S: Pyelonephritis associated with respiratory distress. Obstet Gynecol 69:444, 1987.
27. Goorman G, Schlaeffer E, Kopernic G: Adult respiratory distress syndrome as a complication of acute pyelonephritis during pregnancy. Eur J Obstet Gynecol Reprod Biol 36:75, 1990.
28. Towers CV, Kaminskas CM, Garite CM, et al: Pulmonary injury associated with antepartum pyelonephritis: Can at risk patients be identified? Am J Obstet Gynecol 164:974, 1991.
29. Austenfeld MS, Snow BW: Complications of pregnancy in women after reimplantation for vesicoureteral reflux. J Urol 140:1103, 1988.
30. Harris R, Dunnihoo D: The incidence and significance of urinary calculi in pregnancy. Am J Obstet Gynecol 99:237, 1967.
31. Strong D, Murchison R, Lynch D: The management of ureteral calculi during pregnancy. Obstet Gynecol Surv 146:604, 1978.
32. Nadler N, Salinas-Madrigal L, Charles A, Pollack V: Acute glomerulonephritis during late pregnancy. Obstet Gynecol 34:277, 1969.
33. Wilson C: Changes in renal function. *In* Morris N, Browne J (eds): Nontoxemic Hypertension in Pregnancy. Boston, Little Brown, 1958, p 177.
34. Packham DK, North RA, Fairly KF, et al: Primary glomerulonephtiris and pregnancy. Q J Med 71:537, 1989.
35. Packham DK, North RA, Fairly KF, et al: Membranous glomerulonephritis and pregnancy. Clin Nephrol 30:487, 1988.
36. Jungers P, Forget D, Houillier P, et al: Pregnancy in IgA nephropathy, reflux nephropathy, and focal glomerular sclerosis. Am J Kidney Dis 9:334, 1987.
37. Kincaid-Smith P, Fairley KF: Renal disease in pregnancy: three controversial areas: mesangial IgA nephropathy, focal glomerular sclerosis (focal and segmental hyalinosis and sclerosis), and reflux nephropathy. Am J Kidney Dis 9:328, 1987.
38. Abe S: An overview of pregnancy in women with underlying renal disease. Am J Kidney Dis 17:112, 1991.
39. Imbasciati E, Ponticello C: Pregnancy and renal disease: predictors for fetal and maternal outcome. Am J Nephrol 11:353, 1991.
40. Davison J: Renal disease. *In* deSwiet M (ed): Medical Disorders in Obstetric Practice. Oxford, Blackwell, 1984, p 236.
41. Pertuiset N, Grunfeld JP: Acute renal failure in pregnancy. Baillieres Clin Obstet Gynaecol 1:873, 1987.
42. Grunfeld JP, Pertuiset N: Acute renal failure in pregnancy. Am J Kidney Dis 9:359, 1987.
43. Stratta P, Canavese C, Dogliani M, et al: Pregnancy related acute renal failure. Clin Nephrol 32:14, 1989.
44. Grunfeld JP, Ganeval D, Bournerias F: Acute renal failure in pregnancy. Kidney Int 18:179, 1980.
45. Stratta P, Canavese C, Colla L, et al: Acute renal failure in preeclampsia-eclampsia. Gynecol Obstet Invest; 27:225, 1987.
46. Turney JH, Ellis CM, Parsons FM: Obstetric acute renal failure 1956–1987. Br J Obstet Gynaecol 96:679, 1989.
47. Sibai B, Villar MA, Mabie BC: Acute renal failure in hypertensive disorders of pregnancy: pregnancy outcome and remote prognosis in thirty-one consecutive cases. Am J Obstet Gynecol 162:777, 1990.
48. Hold P, Wong C, Dhanda R, et al: Successful renal transplantation during pregnancy. Am J Transplant 5:2315, 2005.
49. Coratelli P, Buongiorno E, Passavanti G: Endotoxemia in hemolytic uremic syndrome. Nephron 50:365, 1988.
50. Robson J, Martin A, Burkley V: Irreversible postpartum renal failure: a new syndrome. Q J Med 37:423, 1968.
51. Seconds A, Louradour N, Suc J, Orfila C: Postpartum hemolytic uremic syndrome: a study of three cases with a review of the literature. Clin Nephrol 12:229, 1979.
52. Wagoner R, Holley K, Johnson W: Accelerated nephrosclerosis and postpartum acute renal failure in normotensive patients. Ann Intern Med 69:237, 1968.

53. Creasey GW, Morgan J: Hemolytic uremic syndrome after ectopic pregnancy: postectopic nephrosclerosis. Obstet Gynecol 69:448, 1987.
54. Remuzzi G, Misiani R, Marchesi D, et al: Treatment of hemolytic uremic syndrome with plasma. Clin Nephrol 12:279, 1979.
55. Webster J, Rees A, Lewis P, Hensby C: Prostacyclin deficiency in haemolytic uraemic syndrome. Br Med J 281:271, 1980.
56. Brandt P, Jesperson J, Gregerson G: Postpartum haemolytic-uremic syndrome successfully treated with antithrombin III. Br Med J 281:449, 1980.
57. Li PK, Lai FM, Tam JS, Lai KN: Acute renal failure due to post-partum haemolytic uremic syndrome. Aust N Z J Obstet Gynaecol 28:228, 1988.
58. Conte F, Mewroni M, Battini G, et al: Plasma exchange in acute renal failure due to postpartum hemolytic-uremic syndrome: report of a case. Nephron 50:167, 1988.
59. Brandes JC, Fritsche C: Obstructive acute renal failure by a gravid uterus: a case report and review. Am J Kidney Dis 18:398, 1991.
60. Hayborn KD, Schultz MF, Goodlin RC, Durham JD: Renal artery stenosis during pregnancy: a review. Obstet Gynecol Surv 46:509. 1991.
61. Coe FL, Brenner BM: Approach to the patient with diseases of the kidney and urinary tract. *In* Fauci AS, Braunwald E, Isselbacher KJ, et al (eds): Principles of Internal Medicine, 14th ed. New York, McGraw-Hill, 1998, p 1495.
62. Davison J, Lindheimer M: Pregnancy in women with renal allografts. Semin Nephrol 4:240, 1984.
63. Denker BM, Brenner BM: Cardinal manifestations of renal disease. *In* Fauci AS, Braunwald E, Isselbacher KJ, et al (eds): Principles of Internal Medicine, 14th ed. New York, McGraw-Hill, 1998 p 258.
64. Hou S: Pregnancy in women with chronic renal disease. N Engl J Med 312:839, 1985.
65. Bear R: Pregnancy in patients with renal disease: a study of 44 cases. Obstet Gynecol 48:13, 1976.
66. Hou S, Grossman S, Madias N: Pregnancy in women with renal disease and moderate renal insufficiency. Am J Med 78:185, 1985.
67. Katz A, Davison J, Hayslett J, et al: Pregnancy in women with kidney disease. Kidney Int 18:192, 1980.
68. Mackay E: Pregnancy and renal disease: a ten-year study. Aust N Z J Obstet Gynaecol 3:21, 1963.
69. Studd J, Blainey J: Pregnancy and the nephrotic syndrome. Br Med J 1:276, 1969.
70. Kincaid-Smith P, Fairley K, Bullen M: Kidney disease and pregnancy. Med J Aust 11:1155, 1967.
71. Surian M, Imbasciati E, Banfi G, et al: Glomerular disease and pregnancy. Nephron 36:101, 1984.
72. Cunningham FG, Cox SG, Harstad TW, et al: Chronic renal disease and pregnancy outcome. Am J Obstet Gynecol 163:453, 1990.
73. Piper JM, Ray WA, Rosa FW: Pregnancy outcome following exposure to angiotensin-converting enzyme inhibitors. Obstet Gynecol 80:429, 1992.
74. Hulton SA, Thompson PD, Cooper PA, Rothberg AD: Angiotensin-converting enzyme inhibitors in pregnancy may result in neonatal renal failure. S Afr Med J 78:673, 1990.
75. Cooper WO, Hernandez-Diaz S, Arbogast PG, et al: Major Congenital Malformations after First-Trimester Exposure to ACE Inhibitors. N Engl J Med 354:2443, 2006.
76. Sibai B, Grossman R, Grossman H: Effects of diuretics on plasma volume in pregnancy with long term hypertension. Am J Obstet Gynecol 150:831, 1984.
77. Rodriquez S, Leikin S, Hillar M: Neonatal thrombocytopenia associated with antepartum administration of thiazide drugs. N Engl J Med 270:881, 1964.
78. Sanchez-Casajuz A, Famos I, Santos M: Monitorization fetal en el transcurso de hemodialissi durante el embarazo. Rev Clin Esp 149:187, 1978.
79. Schewitz L, Friedman E, Pollak V: Bleeding with renal biopsy in pregnancy. Obstet Gynecol 26:1965, 1965.
80. Lindheimer M, Spargo B, Katz A: Renal biopsy in pregnancy-induced hypertension. J Reprod Med 15:189, 1975.
81. Lindheimer M, Fisher K, Spargo B, Katz A: Hypertension in pregnancy: a biopsy with long term follow-up. Contrib Nephrol 25:71, 1981.
82. Packham DK, Fairley K: Renal biopsy: indications and complications in pregnancy. Br J Obstet Gynaecol 94:935, 1987.
83. Ackrill P, Goodwin F, Marsh F, et al: Successful pregnancy in patient on regular dialysis. Br Med J 2:172, 1975.
84. Kobayashi H, Matsumoto Y, Otsubo O, et al: Successful pregnancy in a patient undergoing chronic hemodialysis. Obstet Gynecol 57:382, 1981.
85. Savdie E, Caterson R, Mahony J, Clifton-Bligh P: Successful pregnancies treated by haemodialysis. Med J Aust 2:9, 1982.
86. Cohen D, Frenkel Y, Maschiach S, Eliahou HE: Dialysis during pregnancy in advanced chronic renal failure patients: outcome and progression. Clin Nephrol 29:144, 1988.
87. Redrow M, Cherem L, Elliott J, et al: Dialysis in the management of pregnant patients with renal insufficiency. Medicine 67:199, 1988.
88. Hou S: Pregnancy in women requiring dialysis for renal failure. Am J Kidney Dis 9:368, 1987.
89. Yasin SY, Doun SWB: Hemodialysis in pregnancy. Obstet Gynecol Surv 43:655, 1988.
90. Lim V, Henriquez C, Sievertsen G, Prohman L: Ovarian function in chronic renal failure in chronic renal failure: evidence suggesting hypothalamic anovulation. Ann Intern Med 57:7, 1980.
91. Nageotte MP, Grundy HO: Pregnancy outcome in women requiring chronic hemodialysis. Obstet Gynecol 72:456, 1988.
92. EDTA Registration Committee: Successful pregnancies in women treated by dialysis and kidney tranplantation. Br J Obstet Gynaecol 87:839, 1980.
93. Fine L, Barnett E, Danovitch G, et al: Systemic lupus erythematosus in pregnancy. Ann Intern Med 94:667, 1981.
94. Johnson T, Lorenz R, Menon K, Nolan G: Successful outcome of a pregnancy requiring dialysis: effects on serum progesterone and estrogens. J Reprod Med 22:217, 1979.
95. Merkatz I, Schwartz G, David D, et al: Resumption of female reproductive function following renal transplantation. JAMA 216:1749, 1971.
96. Penn I, Markowski E, Harris P: Parenthood following renal transplantation. Kidney Int 18:221, 1980.
97. Saarikoski S, Sappala M: Immunosuppression during pregnancy: transmission of azathioprine and its metabolities from mother to fetus. Am J Obstet Gynecol 115:1100, 1973.
98. Cote C, Meuwissen H, Pickering R: Effects on the neonate of prednisone and azathioprine administered to the mother during pregnancy. J Pediatr 85:324, 1974.
99. Price H, Salaman J, Laurence K, Langmaid H: Immunosuppressive drugs and the fetus. Transplantation 21:294, 1976.
100. Scott J: Fetal growth retardation associated with maternal administration of immunosuppressive drugs. Am J Obstet Gynecol 128:668, 1977.
101. Ponticelli C, Montagnino G: Causes of arterial hypertension in kidney transplantation. Contrib Nephrol 54:226, 1987.
102. Derfler K, Schuller A, Herold C, et al: Successful outcome of a complicated pregnancy in a renal transplant recipient taking cyclosporin A. Clin Nephrol 29:96, 1988.
103. Salamalekis EE, Mortakis AE, Phocas I, et al: Successful pregnancy in a renal transplant recipient taking cyclosporin A: hormonal and immunological studies. Int J Gynaecol Obstet 30:267, 1989.
104. Pickerell MD, Sawers R, Michael J: Pregnancy after renal transplantation: severe intrauterine growth retardation during treatment with cyclosporin A. Br Med J 1:825, 1988.
105. Davison J: Renal transplantation and pregnancy. Am J Kidney Dis 9:374, 1987.
106. Parsons V, Bewick M, Elias J, et al: Pregnancy following renal transplantation. J R Soc Med 72:815, 1979.
107. Huffer W, Kuzela D, Popovtzer M: Metabolic bone disease in chronic renal failure in renal transplant patients. Am J Pathol 78:385, 1975.
108. Lindheimer M, Katz A: Pregnancy in the renal transplant patient. Am J Kidney Dis 19:173, 2000.
109. Lindheimer M, Grünfeld JP, Davison JM: Renal disorders. *In* Barron WM, Lindheimer M (eds): Medical Disorders During Pregnancy, 3rd ed. St Louis, MO, Mosby, Inc., 2000, p 39.

Diabetes Mellitus Complicating Pregnancy

MARK B. LANDON, PATRICK M. CATALANO, AND STEVEN G. GABBE

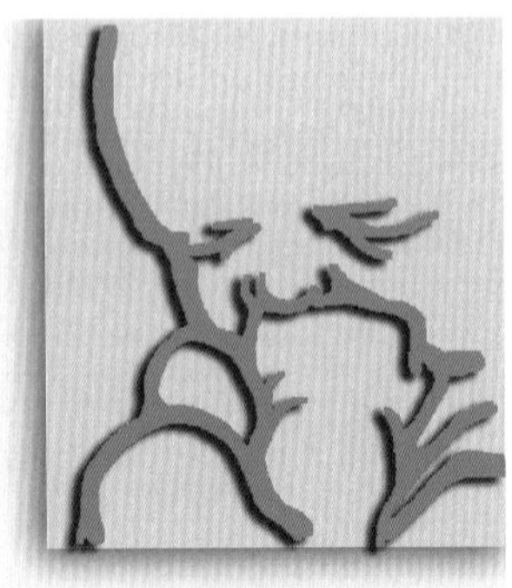

CHAPTER 37

KEY ABBREVIATIONS

American College of Obstetricians and Gynecologists	ACOG
Biophysical profile	BPP
Continuous subcutaneous insulin infusion (pump therapy)	CSII
Depomedroxyprogesterone acetate	DMPA
Diabetic ketoacidosis	DKA
Disposition index	DI
Gestational diabetes mellitus	GDM
Glucose tolerance test	GTT
Glucose transporter	GLUT
Hemoglobin A_{1c}	HbA_{1c}
High-density lipoprotein	HDL
Hyaline membrane disease	HMD
Infant of the diabetic mother	IDM
Insulin-dependent diabetes mellitus	IDDM
Insulin-like growth factor	IGF
Low-density lipoprotein	LDL
Maternal serum alpha-fetoprotein	MSAFP
Maturity onset diabetes of youth	MODY
Nonstress test	NST
Oral contraceptive	OC
Phosphatidylglycerol	PG
Respiratory distress syndrome	RDS
Total urinary protein excretion	TPE
Tumor necrosis factor-α	TNF-α
Urinary albumin excretion	UAE
Very-low-density lipoprotein	VLDL

The introduction of insulin therapy 85 years ago remains an important landmark in the care of pregnancy for the diabetic woman. Before insulin became available, pregnancy was not advised because it was likely to be accompanied by fetal mortality and a substantial risk for maternal death. Over the past 35 years, management techniques have been developed which can prevent many complications of diabetic pregnancy. These advances, based on understanding of pathophysiology, now result in perinatal mortality rates in optimally managed cases that approach that of the normal population. This dramatic improvement in perinatal outcome can be largely attributed to clinical efforts to establish improved maternal glycemic control both before conception and during gestation (Fig. 37-1). Excluding major congenital malformations, which continue to plague pregnancies in women with type 1 and type 2 diabetes mellitus, perinatal loss for the diabetic woman has fortunately become an uncommon event.

Although the benefit of careful regulation of maternal glucose levels is well accepted, failure to establish optimal glycemic control as well as other factors continue to result in significant perinatal morbidity. For this reason, both clinical and basic laboratory research efforts continue to focus on the etiology of congenital malformations and fetal growth disorders. Clinical experience has also resulted in a more realistic appreciation of the impact that vascular complications can have on pregnancy and the manner in which pregnancy may impact these disease processes. With modern management techniques and an organized team approach, successful pregnancies have

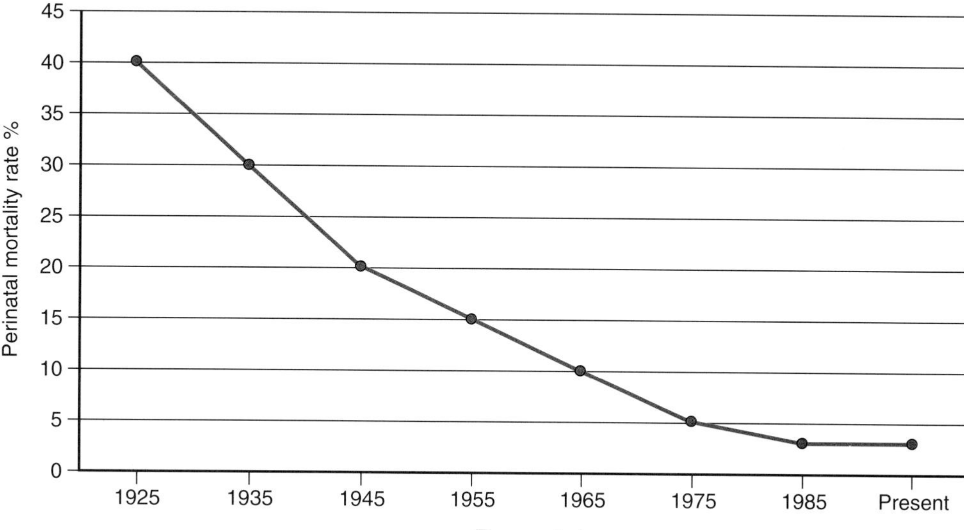

Figure 37-1. Perinatal mortality rate in pregnancy complicated by insulin-dependent diabetes mellitus.

become the norm even for women with the most complicated diabetes.

Gestational diabetes mellitus (GDM), the most common type of diabetes found in pregnancy, represents a continuing challenge for both clinicians and investigators. After 40 years since the concept of GDM was introduced, the clinical significance of this disorder, particularly in its mildest variety, sparks great debate. Controversy also remains concerning screening techniques, diagnostic criteria, thresholds for insulin initiation, and whether oral hypoglycemic agents are suitable treatment.

Before considering these clinical issues, it is important to understand the metabolic effects of pregnancy in relation to the pathophysiology of diabetes mellitus.

PATHOPHYSIOLOGY

Normal Glucose Tolerance

There are significant alterations in maternal metabolism during pregnancy, which provide for adequate maternal nutritional stores in early gestation in order to meet the increased maternal and fetal demands of late gestation and lactation. Although we are apt to think of diabetes mellitus as a disorder exclusively of maternal glucose metabolism, in fact, diabetes mellitus affects all aspects of nutrient metabolism. In this section, we will consider maternal glucose metabolism as it relates to pancreatic β-cell production of insulin and insulin clearance, endogenous (i.e., primarily hepatic) glucose production and suppression with insulin and peripheral glucose insulin sensitivity. We also address maternal protein and lipid insulin metabolism. Finally, the impact of these alternations on maternal metabolism are examined as they relate to maternal energy expenditure and fetal growth.

Glucose Metabolism

Normal pregnancy has been characterized as a diabetogenic state because of the progressive increase in postprandial glucose levels and increased insulin response in late gestation. However, early gestation can be viewed as an anabolic state because of the increases in maternal fat stores and decrease in free fatty acid concentration. Weiss et al.[1] have described significant decreases in maternal insulin requirements in early gestation. The mechanism for this decrease in insulin requirements have been ascribed to various factors including increased insulin sensitivity, decreased substrate availability secondary to factors such as nausea, the fetus acting as a glucose sink, or enhanced maternal insulin secretion. Longitudinal studies in women with normal glucose tolerance have shown significant alterations in all aspects of glucose metabolism as early as the end of the first trimester.[2]

There are progressive increases in insulin secretion in response to an intravenous glucose challenge with advancing gestation (Fig. 37-2*A* and *B*). The increases in insulin concentration are more pronounced in lean as compared to obese women, most probably as a response to the greater decreases in insulin sensitivity in lean women as will be described later. Data regarding insulin clearance in pregnancy are limited. In separate studies Bellman,[3] Lind et al.,[4] and Burt and Davidson[5] reported no difference in insulin disappearance rate when insulin was infused intravenously in late gestation in comparison with nongravid subjects. In contrast, Goodner and Freinkel,[6] using a radiolabeled insulin described a 25-percent increase in insulin turnover in a pregnant as compared with a nonpregnant rat model. Catalano et al.[7] using the euglycemic-clamp model reported a 20-percent increase in insulin clearance in lean women and 30-percent increase in insulin clearance in obese women by late pregnancy (Fig. 37-3). Although the placenta is rich in insulinase, the exact mechanism for the increased insulin clearance in pregnancy remains speculative.

Although there is a progressive decrease in fasting glucose with advancing gestation, the decrease is most probably a result of the increase in plasma volume in early gestation and increase in fetoplacental glucose use in late gestation. Kalhan and Cowett,[8,9] using various stable isotope methodologies in cross-sectional study designs, were the first to describe increased fasting hepatic glucose production

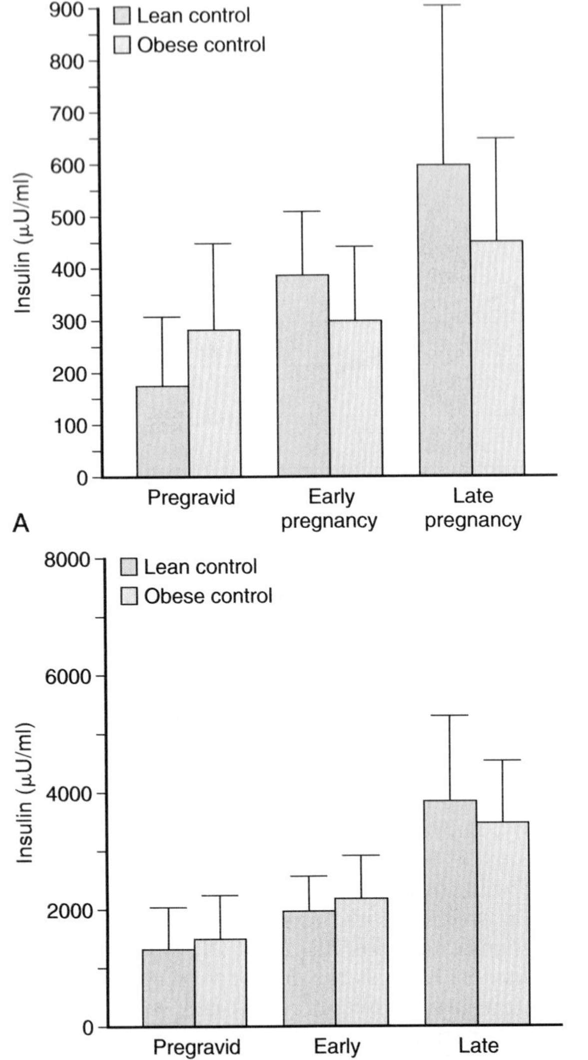

Figure 37-2. Longitudinal increase in insulin response to an intravenous glucose challenge in lean and obese women with normal glucose tolerance, pregravid, and early and late pregnancy. *A,* First phase: Area under the curve from 0 to 5 minutes. *B,* Second phase: Area under the curve from 5 to 60 minutes.

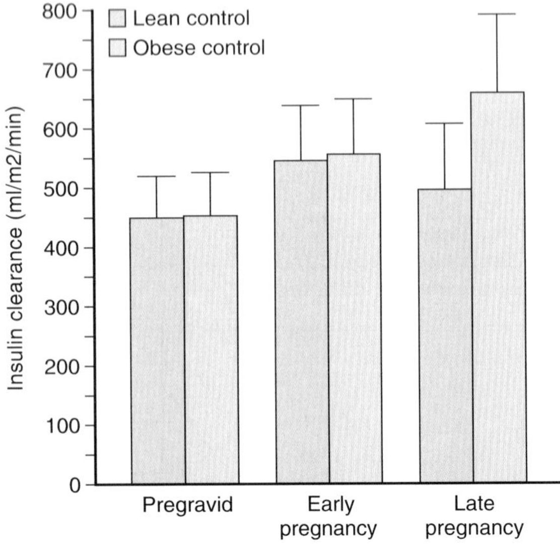

Figure 37-3. Longitudinal increases in metabolic clearance rate of insulin (ml/m^2/min) in lean and obese women with normal glucose tolerance; pregravid, and early and late pregnancy.

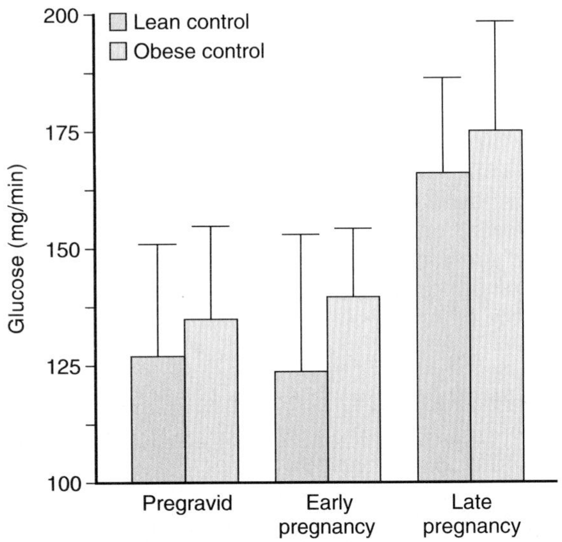

Figure 37-4. Longitudinal increase in basal endogenous (primarily hepatic) glucose production (mg/min) in lean and obese women with normal glucose tolerance; pregravid, early and late pregnancy.

in late pregnancy. Additionally, Catalano et al.,[10] using a stable isotope of glucose in a prospective longitudinal study design reported a 30-percent increase in maternal fasting hepatic glucose production with advancing gestation (Fig. 37-4), which remained significant even when adjusted for maternal weight gain. Tissue sensitivity to insulin involves both liver and peripheral tissues, primarily skeletal muscle. The increase in fasting maternal hepatic glucose production occurred despite a significant increase in fasting insulin concentration, thereby indicating a decrease in maternal hepatic glucose sensitivity in women with normal glucose tolerance. Additionally, in obese women, there was a decreased ability of infused insulin to suppress hepatic glucose production in late gestation as compared with pregravid and early pregnancy measurements, thereby indicating a further decrease in hepatic insulin sensitivity[11] in obese women.

Estimates of peripheral insulin sensitivity in pregnancy have included the measurement of insulin response to a fixed oral or intravenous glucose challenge or the ratio of insulin to glucose under a variety of experimental conditions. In recent years, newer methodologies such as the minimal model[12] and the euglycemic-hyperinsulinemic[13] clamp have improved our ability to quantify peripheral insulin sensitivity. In lean women in early gestation, Catalano et al.[14] reported a 40-percent decrease in maternal peripheral insulin sensitivity using the euglycemic-hyperinsulinemic clamp. However, when adjusted for changes in insulin concentrations during the clamp and residual hepatic glucose production (i.e., the insulin sensitivity index), insulin sensitivity *decreased* only 10 percent (Fig. 37-5). In contrast there was a 15-percent

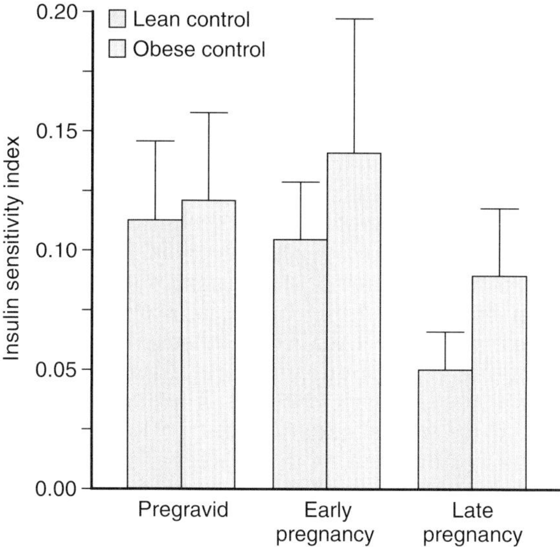

Figure 37-5. Longitudinal changes in the insulin sensitivity index (glucose infusion rate adjusted for residual endogenous glucose production and insulin concentrations achieved during the glucose clamp) in lean and obese women with normal glucose tolerance, pregravid, and early and late gestation.

increase in the insulin sensitivity index in obese women in early pregnancy as compared with pregravid estimates.[15] Hence, the decrease in insulin requirements in early gestation observed in some women requiring insulin may be a consequence of an increase in insulin sensitivity, particularly in women with decreased insulin sensitivity prior to conception.

As compared with the metabolic alterations in early pregnancy, there is a uniformity of opinion regarding the decrease in peripheral insulin sensitivity in late gestation. Spellacy and Goetz[16] were among the first investigators to report an increase in insulin response to a glucose challenge in late gestation. Additionally, Burt[17] demonstrated that pregnant women experienced less hypoglycemia in response to exogenous insulin in comparison with nonpregnant subjects. Later research by Fisher et al.[18] using a high-dose glucose infusion test, Buchanan et al.[19] using the Bergman minimal model, and Ryan et al.[20] and Catalano et al.[2] using the euglycemic-hyperinsulinemic clamp have demonstrated a decrease in insulin sensitivity ranging from 33 percent to 78 percent. It should be noted, however, that all these quantitative estimates of insulin sensitivity are very likely overestimates due to non–insulin-mediated glucose disposal by the fetus and placenta. Hay et al.[21] reported that in the pregnant ewe model, approximately one third of maternal glucose utilization was accounted for by uterine, placental, and fetal tissue. Additionally, Marconi et al.[22] reported that based on human fetal blood sampling, fetal glucose concentration was a function of fetal size and gestational age in addition to maternal glucose concentration.

Historically, the decrease in insulin sensitivity during pregnancy has been ascribed to an increased production of various placental and maternal hormones, such as human placental lactogen, progesterone, estrogen, cortisol, and prolactin. However, more recent evidence has focused on the role of several new mediators of insulin resistance such as leptin, tumor necrosis factor-α (TNF-α), and resistin. Among these factors, TNF-α and leptin are known to be produced in the placenta and, therefore, could play a central role in the development of insulin resistance. A recent study by Kirwan et al.[23] reported that TNF-α was inversely correlated with the changes in insulin sensitivity before conception through late gestation. In combination with other placental hormones, multivariate stepwise regression analysis revealed that TNF-α was the strongest independent predictor of insulin sensitivity in pregnancy, accounting for approximately half of the variance in the decrease in insulin sensitivity during gestation.

Placenta glucose transport is a nonenergy requiring process and takes place through facilitated diffusion. Glucose transport is dependent on a family of glucose transporters referred to as GLUT glucose transporter family. The principal glucose transporter in the placenta is GLUT 1, which is located in the syncytiotrophoblast.[24] GLUT 1 is located on both the microvillus and basal membranes. Basal membrane GLUT 1 may be the rate-limiting step in placental glucose transport. There is a two- to threefold increase in the expression of syncytiotrophoblast glucose transporters with advancing gestation.[25] Although GLUT 3 and GLUT 4 expression have been identified in placental endothelial cells and intervillous nontrophoblastic cells, respectively, the role they may play in placental glucose transport remains speculative.[26,27]

DIABETES MELLITUS

Diabetes mellitus is a chronic metabolic disorder characterized by either absolute or relative insulin deficiency, resulting in increased glucose concentrations. Although glucose intolerance is the common outcome of diabetes mellitus, the pathophysiology remains heterogeneous. The two major classifications of diabetes mellitus are type 1, formerly referred to as insulin-dependent diabetes or juvenile onset diabetes, and type 2, formerly referred to as non–insulin-dependent or adult-onset diabetes. During pregnancy, classification of women with diabetes has often relied on the White classification,[28] first proposed in the 1940s. This classification is based on factors such as the age of onset of diabetes and duration, as well as end organ involvement, primarily retinal and renal (Table 37-1).

All forms of diabetes can occur during pregnancy. In addition to type 1 and type 2 diabetes, there are genetic causes of diabetes, the most common of which is maturity onset diabetes of the young (MODY). MODY is characterized by β-cell dysfunction and is an autosomal dominant mode of inheritance, usually becoming manifest in young adulthood. Mutations in the glucokinase gene are a frequent cause of MODY. Various mutations have been described, and each mutation is associated with varying degrees of disease severity. The most common of these mutations (MODY2) occurs in the European population and involves the glucokinase gene. Because the age of onset of diabetes in women with MODY coincides with the reproductive years, it may be difficult to distin-

Table 37-1. Modified White Classification of Pregnant Diabetic Women

CLASS	DIABETES ONSET AGE (Y)		DURATION (Y)	VASCULAR DISEASE	INSULIN NEED
Gestational diabetes					
A_1	Any		Any	0	0
A_2	Any		Any	0	+
Pregestational diabetes					
B	>20		<10	0	+
C	10–19	or	10–19	0	+
D	<10	or	>20	+	+
F	Any		Any	+	+
R	Any		Any	+	+
T	Any		Any	+	+
H	Any		Any	+	+

Modified from White P: Pregnancy complicating diabetes. Am J Med 7:609, 1949.

guish between the two. The glucokinase gene acts as a sensor in the β-cell, which leads to a secretory defect in insulin response. Ellard et al.[29] reported that 2.5 percent of women with GDM in the United Kingdom have the glucokinase mutation, whereas Stoffel[30] in a small population in the United States reported that 5 percent of patients had a glucokinase mutation. The implication is that if the mother has the mutation, the fetus is at an increased risk for macrosomia. The implications for the fetus, if the mutation is inherited from the father, are a significant decrease in growth secondary to relative insulinopenia.

Type 1 Diabetes Mellitus

Type 1 diabetes mellitus is usually characterized by an abrupt onset at a young age and absolute insulinopenia with life-long requirements for insulin replacement, although depending on the population, the onset of type 1 diabetes may occur in individuals in their third or fourth decades of life. Patients with diabetes mellitus may have a genetic predisposition for antibodies directed against their pancreatic islet cells. The degree of concordance for the development of type 1 diabetes in monozygotic twins is 33 percent, suggesting that the events subsequent to the development of autoantibodies and appearance of glucose intolerance are also related to environmental factors. Because of the complete dependence on exogenous insulin, pregnant women with type 1 diabetes are at increased risk for the development of diabetic ketoacidosis (DKA). Additionally, because intensive insulin therapy is used in women with type 1 diabetes to decrease the risk for spontaneous abortion and congenital anomalies in early gestation, these women are at increased risk for hypoglycemic reactions. Studies by Diamond et al.[31] and Rosenn et al.[32] have shown that women with type 1 diabetes are at increased risk for hypoglycemic reactions during pregnancy because of diminished counterregulatory epinephrine and glucagon response to hypoglycemia. The deficiency in this counterregulatory response may be in part due to an independent effect of pregnancy.

The alterations in glucose metabolism in women with type 1 diabetes are not well characterized. Because of maternal insulinopenia, insulin response during gestation can only be estimated relative to pregravid requirements. Estimates of the change in insulin requirements are complicated by the degree of preconceptual glucose control and potential presence of insulin antibodies. Weiss and Hofman[1] reported on the change in insulin requirements in women with type 1 diabetes and strict glucose control either before conception or before 10 weeks' gestation. There was a 12-percent *decrease* in insulin requirements from 10 to 17 weeks' gestation and a 50-percent *increase* in insulin requirement from 17 weeks' until delivery as compared with pregravid requirements. After 36 weeks' gestation, there was a decrease in insulin requirements. A 5-percent decrease in insulin requirements after 36 weeks' gestation was also noted by McManus and Ryan.[33] The decrease in insulin requirements was associated with a longer duration of diabetes mellitus but not with adverse perinatal outcome. The fall in insulin requirements in early pregnancy in women with type 1 diabetes may be a reflection of increased pregravid insulin sensitivity as was described previously.

Schmitz et al.[34] have evaluated the longitudinal changes in insulin sensitivity in women with type 1 diabetes in early and late pregnancy as well as postpartum in comparison with nonpregnant women with type 1 diabetes. In the pregnant women with type 1 diabetes, there was a 50-percent decrease in insulin sensitivity only in late gestation. There was no significant difference in insulin sensitivity in pregnant women with type 1 diabetes in early pregnancy or within 1 week of delivery as compared with the nonpregnant women with type 1 diabetes. Therefore, based on the available data women with type 1 diabetes appear to have a similar decrease in insulin sensitivity when compared with women with normal glucose tolerance.

Relative to the issue of placental transporters (GLUT 1), there is a report by Jansson and Powell[35] describing an increase in both basal GLUT 1 expression and glucose transport activity from placental tissue in women with White class D pregnancies.

Type 2 Diabetes/Gestational Diabetes

The pathophysiology of type 2 diabetes involves abnormalities of both insulin sensitive tissue (i.e., both a decrease in skeletal muscle and hepatic sensitivity to insulin) and β-cell response as manifested by an inadequate insulin response for a given degree of glycemia. Initially in the course of development of type 2 diabetes, the insulin response to a glucose challenge may be increased relative to that of individuals with normal glucose tolerance but is inadequate to maintain normoglycemia. Whether or not decreased insulin sensitivity precedes β-cell dysfunction in the development of type 2 diabetes continues to be debated. Arguments and experimental data support both hypotheses. As noted by Sims and Calles-Escadon,[36] heterogeneity of metabolic abnormalities exists in any classification of diabetes mellitus.

Despite the limitations of any classification system, certain generalizations can be made regarding women with type 2 or GDM. These individuals are typically older and more often heavier compared with individuals with type 1 diabetes or normal glucose tolerance. The onset of the disorder is usually insidious, with few patients complaining of classical triad of polydipsia, polyphagia, and polyuria. Individuals with type 2 diabetes are often initially recommended to lose weight, increase their activity (i.e., exercise), and follow a diet that is low in fats and high in complex carbohydrates. Oral agents are often used to either increase insulin response or, with newer drugs, enhance insulin sensitivity. Individuals with type 2 diabetes may eventually require insulin therapy in order to maintain euglycemia but are at significantly less risk for DKA. Data from monozygotic twin studies have reported a lifetime risk of both twins developing type 2 diabetes that ranges between 58 percent and almost 100 percent, suggesting that the disorder has a strong genetic component.

Women with type 2 pregestational diabetes are usually classified as class B diabetes according to the White classification system. Women developing GDM (i.e., glucose intolerance first recognized during pregnancy) share many of the metabolic characteristics of women with type 2 diabetes. Although earlier studies reported a 10- to 35-percent incidence of islet cell antibodies in women with GDM as measured by immunofluorescence techniques,[37,38] more recent data using specific monoclonal antibodies have described a much lower incidence, on the order of 1 to 2 percent,[39] suggesting a low risk of type 1 diabetes in women with GDM. Furthermore, postpartum studies of women with GDM have demonstrated defects in insulin secretory response[40] and decreased insulin sensitivity,[41] indicating that typical type 2 abnormalities in glucose metabolism are present in women with GDM. Of interest, the alterations in insulin secretory response and insulin resistance in women with a previous history of GDM as compared with a weight-matched control group may differ depending on whether or not the women with previous GDM are lean or obese.[42] Thus, in women with GDM, the hormonal events of pregnancy may represent an unmasking of a genetic susceptibility to type 2 diabetes.

There are significant alterations in glucose metabolism in women who develop GDM relative to the changes in glucose metabolism in women with normal glucose tolerance. Decreased insulin response to a glucose challenge has been demonstrated by Yen et al.,[43] Fisher et al.,[44] and Buchanan et al.[19] in women with GDM in late gestation. In prospective longitudinal studies of both lean and obese women with GDM, Catalano et al.[14] also showed a progressive decrease in first-phase insulin response in late gestation in lean women developing GDM as compared with a weight-matched control group (Fig. 37-6*A*). In contrast, in obese women developing GDM, there was no difference in first-phase insulin response but rather a significant increase in second-phase insulin response to an intravenous glucose challenge as compared with a weight-matched control group (see Fig. 37-6*B*). These

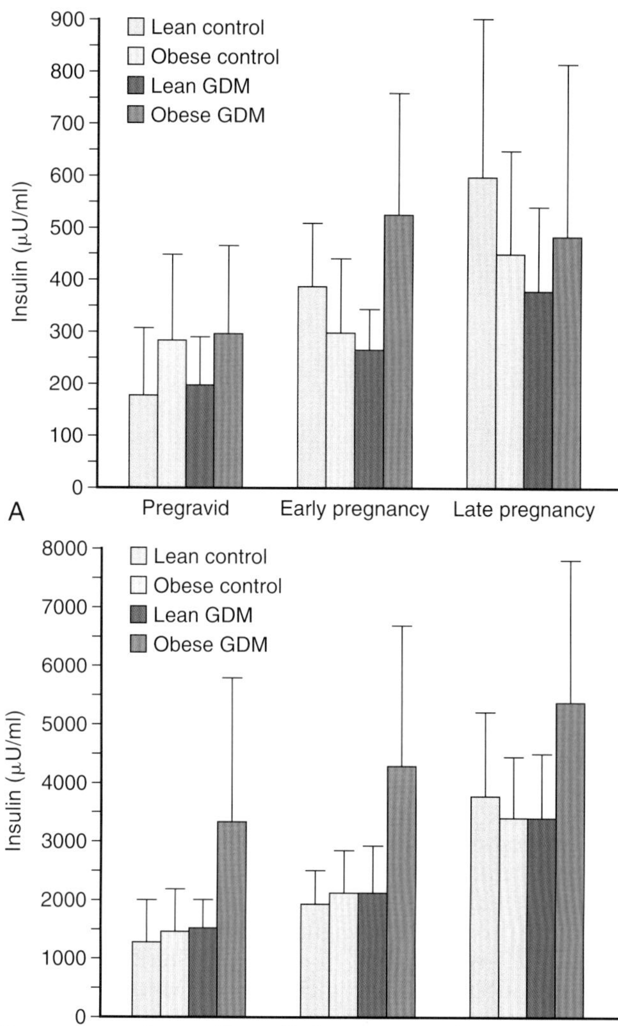

Figure 37-6. *A* and *B*, Longitudinal increase in insulin response to an intravenous glucose challenge in lean and obese women with normal glucose tolerance and gestational diabetes; pregravid, early and late pregnancy. *A*, First phase: Area under the curve from 0 to 5 min. *B*, Second phase: Area under the curve from 5 to 60 min.

differences in insulin response may be related to the ethnicity of the various study groups. Although there is an increase in the metabolic clearance rate of insulin with advancing gestation, there is no evidence that there is a significant difference between women with normal glucose tolerance and GDM.[15]

There is a significant decrease in fasting glucose concentration with advancing gestation in women developing GDM. In late pregnancy, glucose and hepatic glucose production increase in women with GDM in comparison with a control group.[45] Whereas there was no significant difference in either fasting glucose concentration or hepatic glucose production in the longitudinal studies of Catalano et al.,[14,15] these differences may again be population specific or related to the degree of fasting hypoglycemia. However, to date all reports indicate that in late gestation, women with GDM have increased fasting insulin concentrations (Fig. 37-7) and less suppression of hepatic glucose production during insulin infusion,

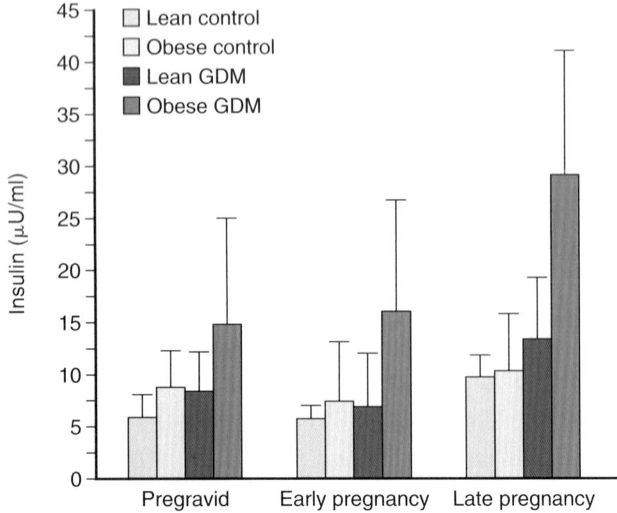

Figure 37-7. Longitudinal increase in basal or fasting insulin (μ/ml) in lean and obese women with normal glucose tolerance and gestational diabetes; pregravid, and early and later pregnancy.

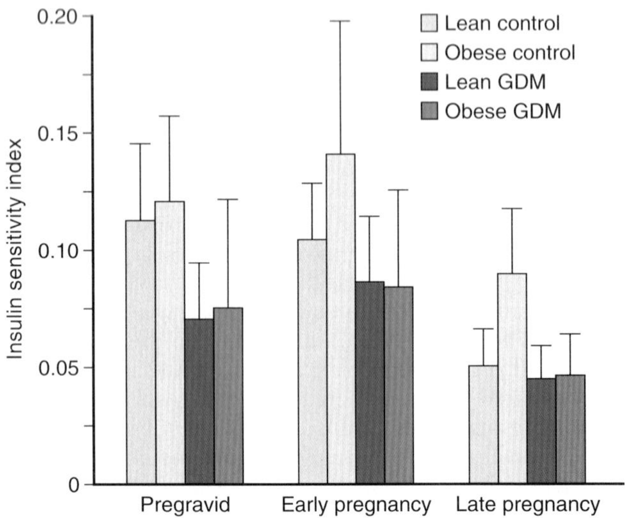

Figure 37-8. Longitudinal changes in the insulin sensitivity index (glucose infusion rate adjusted for residual endogenous glucose production and insulin concentrations achieved during the glucose clamp) in lean and obese women with normal glucose tolerance and gestational diabetes; pregravid, early and late pregnancy.

thereby indicating decreased hepatic glucose insulin sensitivity in women with GDM as compared with a weight-matched control group.[14,15,45] In the studies of Xiang et al.,[45] there was significant correlation between fasting free fatty acid concentrations and hepatic glucose production, suggesting that increased free fatty acid concentrations may contribute to hepatic insulin resistance.

Women with GDM have decreased insulin sensitivity in comparison with weight-matched control groups. Ryan et al.[20] was the first to report a 40-percent decrease in insulin sensitivity in women with GDM in comparison with a pregnant control group in late pregnancy using a hyperinsulinemic-euglycemic clamp. Xiang et al.,[45] found that women with GDM who had normal glucose tolerance within 6 months of delivery had significantly decreased insulin sensitivity as estimated by the glucose clearance rate during a hyperinsulinemic-euglycemic clamp, as compared with a matched control group. Catalano et al.,[14,15] using similar techniques, described the longitudinal changes in insulin sensitivity in both lean and obese women developing GDM in comparison with a matched control group. Women developing GDM had decreased insulin sensitivity as compared with the matched control group (Fig. 37-8). The differences in insulin sensitivity were greatest before and during early gestation, and by late gestation, the differences in insulin sensitivity between the groups were less pronounced but still significant. Of interest, there was an increase in insulin sensitivity from the time prior to conception through early pregnancy (12 to 14 weeks), particularly in those women with greatest decreases in insulin sensitivity prior to conception. The changes in insulin sensitivity from the time before conception through early pregnancy were significantly correlated with changes in maternal weight gain and energy expenditure.[46] The relationship between these alterations in maternal glucose insulin sensitivity and weight gain and energy expenditure may help explain the decrease in maternal weight gain and insulin requirements in women with diabetes in early gestation.[1]

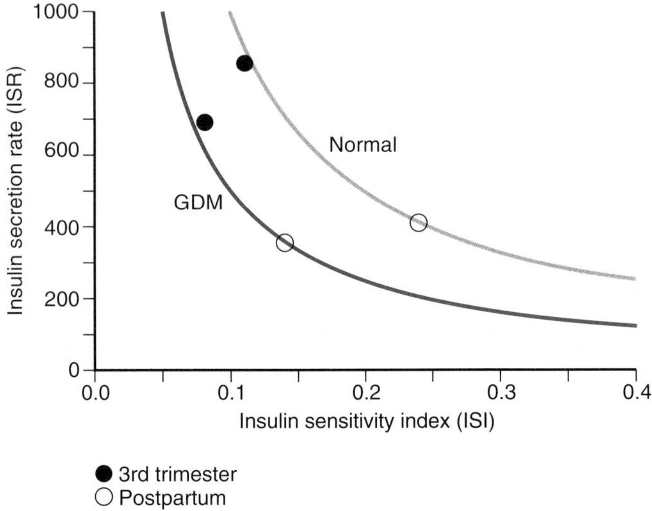

Figure 37-9. Insulin sensitivity index.

The interactions of β-cell response and insulin sensitivity are hallmarks of the metabolic adaptations of pregnancy. As described by Bergman,[47] there is a fixed relationship between insulin response and insulin resistance in nonpregnant individuals following a hyperbolic curve, i.e., the disposition index. Buchanan[48] described a similar relationship between insulin response and insulin action during pregnancy. Indeed, when the disposition index has been compared between women with normal glucose tolerance and GDM both during and after pregnancy, the failure of the β-cell to compensate for insulin resistance in GDM has been similar to the hyperbolic changes in the control group (Fig. 37-9). This relationship between insulin sensitivity and insulin resistance, however, may not hold in early pregnancy when there is both an increase in insulin sensitivity and insulin response.

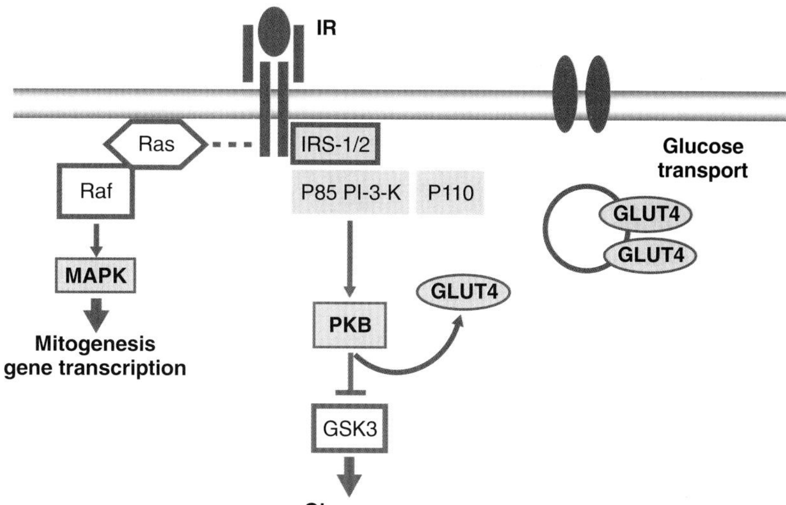

Figure 37-10. Schematic model of insulin signaling cascade in skeletal muscle. GLUT, glucose transporter; IR, insulin receptor; IRS, insulin receptor substrate.

Studies in human skeletal muscle and adipose tissue have demonstrated that postreceptor defects in the insulin signaling cascade are related to decreased insulin sensitivity in pregnancy. Garvey et al.[49] were the first to demonstrate that there were no significant differences in the glucose transporter (GLUT 4) responsible for insulin action and skeletal muscle in pregnant as compared with nonpregnant women. Based on the studies of Friedman et al.[50] in both pregnant women with normal glucose tolerance and GDM as well as weight-matched nonpregnant control subjects, there appeared to be defects in the insulin-signaling cascade relating to pregnancy as well as what may be additional abnormalities in women with GDM. All pregnant women appeared to have a decrease in insulin receptor substrate-1 (IRS-1) expression. The down-regulation of the IRS-1 protein closely parallels the decreased ability of insulin to induce additional steps in the insulin signaling cascade, resulting in movement of the GLUT 4 to the cell surface membrane and to facilitate glucose transport into the cell. The downregulation of IRS-1 protein closely parallels the ability of insulin to stimulate 2-deoxyglucose uptake in vitro. In addition to the above-mentioned mechanisms, women with GDM demonstrate a distinct decrease in the ability of the insulin receptor β (that component of the insulin receptor not on the cell surface) to undergo tyrosine phosphorylation. The additional defect in the insulin signaling cascade results in a 25-percent lower glucose transport activity (Fig. 37-10).

Amino Acid Metabolism

Although glucose is the primary source of energy for the fetus and placenta, there are no appreciable amounts of glucose stored as glycogen in the fetus or placenta. However, accretion of protein is essential for growth of fetoplacental tissue. There is increased nitrogen retention in pregnancy in both maternal and fetal compartments. There is an increase of approximately 0.9 kg of maternal fat-free mass by 27 weeks.[51] There is a significant decrease in most fasting maternal amino acid concentrations in early pregnancy prior to the accretion of significant maternal or fetal tissue.[52] These anticipatory changes in fasting amino acid metabolism occur after a shorter period of fasting in comparison with nonpregnant women, and may be another example of the accelerated starvation of pregnancy as described by Freinkel.[53] Furthermore, amino acid concentrations such as serine correlate significantly with fetal growth in both early and late gestation.[54] Maternal amino acid concentrations were significantly decreased in mothers of small-for-gestational-age neonates in comparison with maternal concentration in appropriately grown neonates.[55]

Based on a review of various studies, Duggleby and Jackson[56] have estimated that during the first trimester of a pregnancy, protein synthesis is similar to that of nonpregnant. However, there is a 15-percent increase in protein synthesis during the second trimester and a further increase in the third trimester by about 25 percent. Additionally, there are marked interindividual differences at each time point. These differences have a strong relationship with fetal growth, that is, mothers who had increased protein turnover in midpregnancy had babies who had increased lean body mass after adjustment for significant covariables.[57]

Amino acids can be used either for protein accrual or oxidized as an energy source. Urea synthesis has been estimated in a number of studies using stable isotopes. In general, there is a modest shift in oxidation in early pregnancy, with an accrual of amino acids for protein synthesis in late gestation.[56] Furthermore, Kalhan et al.[58] reported that there are significant pregnancy-related adaptations in maternal protein metabolism early in gestation before any significant increase in fetal protein accretion. Preliminary studies by Catalano et al.[59] have reported that there is decreased insulin sensitivity as manifested by a decreased suppression of leucine turnover during insulin infusion in late gestation in all pregnant women. There is evidence for an increase in basal leucine turnover in women with GDM as compared with a matched control group. Whether these decreases in amino acid insulin sensitivity are related to decreased whole body/

liver protein synthesis or increased breakdown are not known at this time.

Recently, Cetin et al.[60] reported that placental amino acid exchange is altered in pregnancies complicated by GDM. Ornithine concentrations were significantly increased in women with GDM as compared with controls, and in the cord blood of infants of women with GDM, there were significant increases in multiple amino acids including phenylalanine and leucine but decreases in glutamate. The investigators speculate that in infants of women with GDM, the altered in utero fetal milieu impacts fetal growth through multiple mechanisms, affecting various nutrient compartments.

Amino acids are actively transported across the placenta from mother to fetus through energy-requiring amino acid transporters. These transporters are highly stereospecific, but they have low substrate specificity. Additionally, they may vary with location between the microvillus and basal membranes.[61] Decreased amino acid concentrations have been reported in growth restricted neonates in comparison with appropriately grown neonates. Decreased amino acid transporter activity has been implicated as a possible mechanism. However, the potential role, if any, of placental amino acid transporters in the development of fetal macrosomia in women with diabetes is currently unknown.[62]

Lipid Metabolism

Although there is ample literature regarding the changes in glucose metabolism during gestation, the data regarding the alterations in lipid metabolism are meager by comparison. Darmady and Postle measured serum cholesterol and triglyceride before, during, and after pregnancy in 34 normal women.[63] There was a decrease in both cholesterol and triglyceride at approximately 7 weeks' gestation. Both of the levels increased progressively until term. There was then a decrease in serum triglyceride postpartum. The decrease was more rapid in women who breast-fed compared with those women who bottle fed their infants.[63] Additionally, Knopp et al.[64] have reported that there is a two- to fourfold increase in total triglyceride concentration and a 25- to 50-percent increase in total cholesterol concentration during gestation. There is a 50-percent increase in low-density lipoprotein (LDL) cholesterol and a 30-percent increase in high-density lipoprotein (HDL) cholesterol by midgestation, which decreases slightly in the third trimester. Maternal triglyceride and very-low-density lipoprotein (VLDL) levels in late gestation are positively correlated with maternal estriol and insulin concentrations.

Free fatty acids have been associated with fetal overgrowth, particularly of fetal adipose tissue. There is a significant difference in the arteriovenous free fatty acid concentration at birth much as there is with arteriovenous glucose concentration. Knopp et al.[64] reported that neonatal birth weight was positively correlated with triglyceride and free fatty acid concentration in late pregnancy. Similar conclusions were reached by Ogburn et al.,[61] who showed that higher insulin concentrations decrease free fatty acid concentrations, inhibit lipolysis and result in increased fat deposition. Last, Kleigman[62] reported that infants of obese women had an increased birth weight and skinfold thickness, and higher free fatty acid levels when compared with infants of lean women.

Lipid metabolism in women with diabetes mellitus is influenced by whether the woman has type 1 or type 2 diabetes. This also applies when these women become pregnant. In women with type 2 diabetes and GDM, Knopp et al.[64] reported an increase in triglyceride and a decrease in HDL concentration. However, Montelongo et al.[65] reported little change in free fatty acid concentrations through all three trimesters after a 12-hour fast. Koukkou et al.[66] noted an increase in total triglyceride but a lower LDL cholesterol in women with GDM. In women with type 1 diabetes, there was no change in total triglyceride but a lower cholesterol concentration, secondary to a decrease in HDL. This is of interest because HDL acts as plasma antioxidant and thus may be related to the increase in congenital malformations in women with type 1 diabetes. Oxidative stress has been implicated as a potential factor in the incidence of anomalies in women with type 1 diabetes.

Hyperinsulinemic-euglycemic clamp studies in pregnant women with normal glucose tolerance and GDM revealed a decreased ability of insulin to suppress plasma free fatty acids with advancing gestation. Insulin's ability to suppress plasma free fatty acid was lower in women with GDM as compared to women with normal glucose tolerance.[67]

Taken together, these studies demonstrate that there is decreased nutrient insulin sensitivity in all women with advancing gestation. These decreases in insulin sensitivity are further exacerbated by the presence of decreased pregravid maternal insulin sensitivity, which becomes manifest in later pregnancy as GDM, resulting in greater nutrient availability and higher ambient insulin concentrations for the developing fetoplacental unit, which may eventually result in fetal overgrowth.

Maternal Weight Gain and Energy Expenditure

Estimates of the energy cost of pregnancy range from a cost of 80,000 kcal to a net saving of up to 10,000 kcal.[66] As a result, the recommendations for nutritional intake in pregnancy differ and depend upon the population being evaluated. Furthermore, based on more recent data, recommendations for individuals within a population may be more varied than previously believed, making general guidelines for nutritional intake difficult.[68,69]

The theoretical energy cost of pregnancy was originally estimated by Hytten[51] using a factorial method. The additional cost of pregnancy consisted of (1) the additional maternal and fetoplacental tissue accrued during pregnancy and (2) the additional "running cost" of pregnancy (e.g., the work of increased cardiac output). In Hytten's model, the greatest increases in maternal energy expenditure occur between 10 and 30 weeks' gestation, primarily because of maternal accretion of adipose tissue. However, the mean increases in maternal adipose tissue vary considerably among various ethnic groups. Forsum et al.[70] reported a mean increase of more than 5 kg of adipose tissue in Swedish women, whereas Lawrence et al.[71] found no increase in adipose tissue stores in women from the Gambia.

Basal metabolic rate accounts for 60 to 70 percent of total energy expenditure in individuals not engaged in competitive physical activity and correlates well with total energy expenditure. As with the changes in maternal accretion of adipose tissue, there are wide variations in the change in maternal basal metabolic rate during gestation, not only in different populations but again within relatively homogeneous groups. The cumulative energy changes in basal metabolic rate range from a high of 52,000 kcal in Swedish women[72] to a net savings of 10,700 kcal in women from the Gambia[71] without nutritional supplementation. The mean increase in basal metabolic rate in Western women relative to a nonpregnant, nonlactating control group averages approximately 20 percent.[71] However, the coefficient of variation of basal metabolic rate in these populations during gestation ranges from 93 percent in women in the United Kingdom[72] to more than 200 percent in Swedish women.[70] When assessing energy intake in relation to energy expenditure, however, estimated energy intake remains lower than the estimates of total energy expenditure. These discrepancies have usually been examined by factors such as (1) increased metabolic efficiency during gestation,[73] (2) decreased maternal activity,[74] and (3) unreliable assessment of food intake.[75]

Data in nonpregnant subjects may help explain some of the wide variations in metabolic parameters during human gestation, even with homogeneous populations. Swinburn et al.[76] reported that in the Pima Indian population, subjects with decreased insulin sensitivity gained less weight as compared with more insulin-sensitive subjects (3.1 versus 7.6 kg) over a period of 4 years. Furthermore, the percentage weight change per year was highly correlated with glucose disposal as estimated from clamp studies. Catalano et al.[77] conducted a prospective longitudinal study in early pregnancy of the changes in maternal accretion of body fat and basal metabolic rate in lean and obese women with normal GDM. Women with GDM had decreased insulin sensitivity for glucose in early gestation as compared with the control group and had significantly smaller increases in body fat than women with normal glucose tolerance. In these lean women, there was a significant inverse correlation between the changes in fat accretion and insulin sensitivity (i.e., women with decreased pregravid insulin sensitivity had less accretion of body fat as compared with women with increased pregravid insulin sensitivity). These results are consistent with a previous report showing that total weight gain in women with GDM was 2.5 kg less as compared with a weight-matched control group.[77]

In the basal state, lean women increase the use of carbohydrate as a metabolic fuel, whereas in obese women, there is an increased use of lipids for oxidative needs. However, with the decrease in insulin sensitivity in late gestation, all women lean or obese with normal glucose tolerance or GDM have an increase in fat oxidation and a decrease in nonoxidative glucose metabolism (storage). Of interest, these increases in lipid oxidation in pregnancy are positively correlated with the increases in maternal leptin concentrations, possibly accounting for a role of leptin in human pregnancy. The results of these studies show that there is a relationship between the changes in maternal insulin sensitivity and accretion of adipose tissue in early gestation.[78] The ability of women with decreased pregravid glucose insulin sensitivity (obese women and women with GDM) to conserve energy, not significantly increase body fat, and make sufficient nutrients available to produce a healthy fetus, supports the hypothesis that decreased maternal insulin sensitivity may have a reproductive metabolic advantage in women when food availability is marginal. In contrast, decreased maternal insulin sensitivity before conception in areas where food is plentiful and a sedentary lifestyle is more common may manifest itself as GDM and increase the long-term risk for both diabetes and obesity in the woman and her offspring.[79]

PERINATAL MORBIDITY AND MORTALITY

Fetal Death

In the past, sudden and unexplained stillbirth occurred in 10 to 30 percent of pregnancies complicated by type 1 diabetes mellitus insulin-dependent diabetes mellitus, (IDDM).[80,81] Although relatively uncommon today, such losses still plague the pregnancies of patients who do not receive optimal care. Stillbirths have been observed most often after the 36th week of pregnancy in patients with vascular disease, poor glycemic control, hydramnios, fetal macrosomia, or preeclampsia. Women with vascular complications may develop fetal growth restriction and intrauterine demise as early as the second trimester. In the past, prevention of intrauterine death led to a strategy of scheduled preterm deliveries for type 1 diabetic women. This empiric approach reduced the number of stillbirths, but errors in estimation of fetal size and gestational age as well as the functional immaturity characteristic of the infant of the diabetic mother (IDM) contributed to many neonatal deaths from hyaline membrane disease (HMD).

The precise cause of the excessive stillbirth rate in pregnancies complicated by diabetes remains unknown. Because extramedullary hematopoiesis is frequently observed in stillborn IDMs, chronic intrauterine hypoxia has been cited as a likely cause of these intrauterine fetal deaths. Studies of fetal umbilical cord blood samples in pregnant women with type 1 diabetes have demonstrated "relative fetal erythremia and lactic acidemia."[82] Maternal diabetes may also produce alterations in red blood cell oxygen release and placental blood flow.[83]

Reduced uterine blood flow is thought to contribute to the increased incidence of intrauterine growth restriction observed in pregnancies complicated by diabetic vasculopathy. Investigations using radioactive tracers have also suggested a relationship between poor maternal metabolic control and reduced uteroplacental blood flow.[84] Ketoacidosis and preeclampsia, two factors known to be associated with an increased incidence of intrauterine deaths, may further decrease uterine blood flow. In DKA, hypovolemia and hypotension caused by dehydration may reduce flow through the intervillous space, whereas in preeclampsia, narrowing and vasospasm of spiral arterioles may result.

Alterations in fetal carbohydrate metabolism also may contribute to intrauterine asphyxia.[85,86] There is considerable evidence linking hyperinsulinemia and fetal hypoxia. Hyperinsulinemia induced in fetal lambs by an infusion of exogenous insulin produces an increase in oxygen consumption and a decrease in arterial oxygen content.[85,86] Persistent maternal-fetal hyperglycemia occurs independent of maternal uterine blood flow, which may not be increased enough to allow for enhanced oxygen delivery in the face of increased metabolic demands. Thus, hyperinsulinemia in the fetus of the diabetic mother appears to increase fetal metabolic rate and oxygen requirement in the face of several factors such as hyperglycemia, ketoacidosis, preeclampsia, and maternal vasculopathy, which can reduce placental blood flow and fetal oxygenation.

Congenital Malformations

With the reduction in intrauterine deaths and a marked decrease in neonatal mortality related to HMD and traumatic delivery, congenital malformations have emerged as the most important cause of perinatal loss in pregnancies complicated by type 1 and type 2 diabetes mellitus. In the past, these anomalies were responsible for only 10 percent of all perinatal deaths. At present, however, malformations account for 30 to 50 percent of perinatal mortality.[81] Neonatal deaths now exceed stillbirths in pregnancies complicated by pregestational diabetes mellitus, and fatal congenital malformations account for this changing pattern.

Most studies have documented a two- to sixfold increase in major malformations in infants of type 1 and type 2 diabetic mothers. At The Ohio State University Diabetes in Pregnancy Program, we observed 29 congenital anomalies in 289 (10 percent) diabetic woman enrolled over a 10-year period.[87] In a prospective analysis, Simpson et al. observed an 8.5 percent incidence of major anomalies in the diabetic population, whereas the malformation rate in a small group of concurrently gathered control subjects was 2.4 percent.[88] Similar figures were obtained in the Diabetes in Early Pregnancy Study in the United States.[89] The incidence of major anomalies was 2.1 percent in 389 control patients and 9.0 percent in 279 diabetic women. In general, the incidence of major malformations in worldwide studies of offspring of diabetic mothers has ranged from 5 to 10 percent (Table 37-2).

The insult that causes malformations in IDM impacts on most organ systems and must act before the seventh week of gestation.[90] Central nervous system malformations, particularly anencephaly, open spina bifida, and, possibly, holoprosencephaly, are increased 10-fold.[90,91] Cardiac anomalies, especially ventricular septal defects and complex lesions such as transposition of the great vessels, are increased fivefold. The congenital defect thought to be most characteristic of diabetic embryopathy is sacral agenesis or caudal dysplasia, an anomaly found 200 to 400 times more often in offspring of diabetic women (Fig. 37-11). However, this defect is not pathognomonic for diabetes, since it occurs in nondiabetic pregnancies.

Impaired glycemic control and associated derangements in maternal metabolism appear to contribute to abnormal embryogenesis. The notion of excess glucose as the single teratogenic agent in diabetic pregnancy has thus been replaced with the view of a multifactorial etiology[90] (see the box "Proposed Factors Associated with Teratogenesis in Pregnancy Complicated by Diabetes Mellitus").

Maternal hyperglycemia has been proposed by most investigators as the primary teratogenic factor, but hyperketonemia, hypoglycemia, somatomedin inhibitor excess, and excess free oxygen radicals have also been suggested.[90] The profile of a woman most likely to produce an anomalous infant would include a patient with poor periconceptional control, long-standing diabetes, and

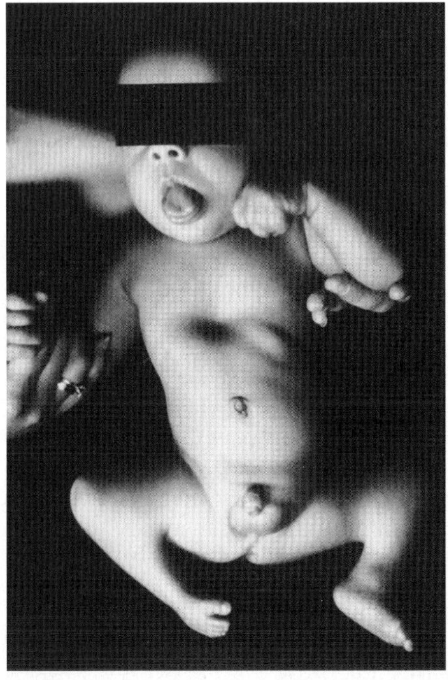

Figure 37-11. Infant of a diabetic mother.

Table 37-2. Frequency of Congenital Malformations in Infants of Diabetic Mothers

Mills[90]	25/279	9.0
Greene[262]	35/451	7.7
Steel and Duncan[264]	12/239	7.8
Fuhrmann et al[259]	22/292	7.5
Simpson et al[99]	9/106	8.5
Albert et al[89]	29/289	10.0

Proposed Factors Associated with Teratogenesis in Pregnancy Complicated By Diabetes Mellitus

- Hyperglycemia
- Ketone body excess
- Somatomedin inhibition
- Arachidonic acid deficiency
- Free oxygen radical excess

vascular disease.[91] Genetic susceptibility to the teratogenic influence of diabetes may be a factor. Koppe and Smoremberg-Schoorl as well as Simpson and colleagues have suggested that certain maternal HLA types may be more often associated with anomalies.[92,93]

Several mechanisms have been proposed by which the above-mentioned teratogenic factors produce malformations. Freinkel et al.[94] suggested that anomalies might arise from inhibition of glycolysis, the key energy-producing process during embryogenesis. He found that D-mannose added to the culture medium of rat embryos inhibited glycolysis and produced growth restriction and derangement of neural tube closure.[94] Freinkel et al.[94] stressed the sensitivity of normal embryogenesis to alterations in these key energy-producing pathways, a process he labeled "fuel-mediated" teratogenesis. Goldman and Baker[95] suggested that the mechanism responsible for the increased incidence of neural tube defects in embryos cultured in a hyperglycemic medium may involve a functional deficiency of arachidonic acid, because supplementation with arachidonic acid or myoinositol will reduce the frequency of neural tube defects in this experimental model.[95] Pinter and Reece,[96] and Pinter et al.[97] have confirmed these studies and demonstrated that hyperglycemia-induced alterations in neural tube closure include disordered cells, decreased mitoses, and changes indicating premature maturation. These authors have further demonstrated that hyperglycemia during organogenesis has a primary deleterious effect on yolk sac function with resultant embryopathy.

Altered oxidative metabolism from maternal diabetes may cause increased production of free oxygen radicals in the developing embryo, which are likely teratogenic. Supplementation of oxygen radical–scavenging enzymes, such as superoxide dismutase to the culture medium of rat embryos protects against growth delay and excess malformations.[98] It has been suggested that excess free oxygen radicals may have a direct effect on embryonic prostaglandin biosynthesis. Free oxygen radical excess may enhance lipid peroxidation, and in turn, generated hydroperoxides might stimulate thromboxane biosynthesis and inhibit prostacyclin production, an imbalance that could have profound effects on embryonic development.[90]

Fetal Macrosomia

Macrosomia has been variously defined as birth weight greater than 4,000 to 4,500 g as well as large for gestational age, in which birth weight is above the 90th percentile for population and sex-specific growth curves. Fetal macrosomia complicates as many as 50 percent of pregnancies in women with GDM and 40 percent of pregnancies complicated by type 1 and type 2 diabetes, including some women treated with intensive glycemic control (Fig. 37-12). Delivery of an infant weighing greater than 4,500 g occurs 10 times more often in women with diabetes as compared with a population of women with normal glucose tolerance.[99]

According to the Pedersen hypothesis, maternal hyperglycemia results in fetal hyperglycemia and hyperinsulinemia, resulting in excessive fetal growth. Increased fetal β-cell mass may be identified as early as the second trimester.[100] Evidence supporting the Pedersen hypothesis has come from the studies of amniotic fluid and cord blood insulin and C-peptide concentrations. Both are increased in the amniotic fluid of insulin-treated women with diabetes at term[101] and correlate with neonatal fat mass.[102] Lipids and amino acids, which are elevated in pregnancies complicated by GDM, may also play a role in excessive fetal growth by stimulating the release of insulin and other growth factors from the fetal pancreatic β cells and placenta. Infants of mothers with GDM have an increase in fat mass compared with fat-free mass.[103] Additionally, the growth is disproportionate, with chest/head and shoulder/head ratios larger than those of infants of women with normal glucose tolerance. This factor may contribute to the higher rate of shoulder dystocia and birth trauma observed in these infants.[104]

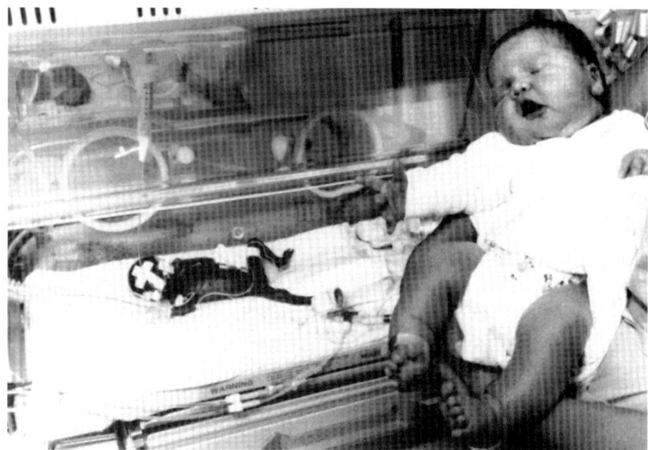

Figure 37-12. Two extremes of growth abnormalities.

The results of several clinical series have validated the Pedersen hypothesis inasmuch as tight maternal glycemic control has been associated with a decline in the incidence of macrosomia. In a series of 260 insulin-dependent women achieving fasting plasma glucose concentrations between 109 and 140 mg/dl, Gabbe et al.[105] observed 58 (22 percent) macrosomic infants. Kitzmiller and Cloherty[106] reported that 11 percent of 134 women achieving fasting glucose concentrations between 105 and 121 mg/dl were delivered of an infant with a birth weight in excess of 4,000 g. A more dramatic reduction in the rate of macrosomia has been reported when more physiologic control has been achieved. Roversi and Gargiulo[107] instituted a program of "maximally tolerated" insulin administration and observed macrosomia in only 6 percent of cases. Jovanovic and coworkers[108] eliminated macrosomia in 52 women who achieved mean glucose level of 80 to 87 mg/dl throughout gestation. Landon and colleagues,[109] using daily capillary glucose values obtained during the second and third trimester in women requiring insulin, reported a rate of 9 percent macrosomia when mean values were below 110 mg/dl compared with 34 percent when less optimal control was achieved. Jovanovic et al.[110] have suggested that 1-hour postprandial glucose measurements correlate best with the frequency of macrosomia. After controlling for other factors, these authors noted that the strongest prediction for birth weight was third-trimester nonfasting glucose measurements.

In a series of metabolic studies, Catalano et al.[111] estimated body composition in 186 neonates using anthropometry. Fat-free mass, which comprised 86 percent of mean birth weight, accounted for 83 percent of the variance in birth weight, and fat mass, which comprised only 14 percent of birth weight, accounted for 46 percent of the variance in birth weight. There was also significantly greater fat-free mass in male as compared with female infants. Using independent variables such as maternal height, pregravid weight, weight gain during pregnancy, parity, paternal height and weight, neonatal sex and gestational age, the authors accounted for 29 percent of the variance in birth weight, 30 percent of the variance in fat-free mass and 17 percent of the variance in fat mass.[112] Including estimates of maternal insulin sensitivity in 16 additional subjects, they were able to explain 48 percent of the variance in birth weight, 53 percent in fat-free mass and 46 percent in fat mass.[113] Studies by Caruso et al.[114] have corroborated these findings, reporting that women with unexplained fetal growth restriction had greater insulin sensitivity as compared with a control group of women whose infants were appropriate weight for gestational age. The potential mechanisms for this relate to the possibility that maternal circulating nutrients for glucose, free fatty acids, and amino acids available for placental transport to the fetus are decreased because of the relative increase in maternal insulin sensitivity. A positive correlation between birth weight and weight gain has been observed in women with normal glucose tolerance. The correlation was strongest in women who were lean before conception and became progressively weaker as pregravid weight for height increased.[77] In women with GDM, there were no significant correlations between maternal weight gain and birth weight, irrespective of pregravid weight for height. These studies emphasize the role of the maternal metabolic environment and fetal growth.

Normalization of birth weight in infants of women with GDM, however, may in itself not achieve optimal growth. In a study of approximately 400 infants of women with normal glucose tolerance and GDM, Catalano et al.,[79] showed that the infants of women with GDM had increased fat mass but not lean body mass or weight as compared with a control group even after adjustment for potential confounding variables (Table 37-3). Similarly, when only infants who were appropriate-for-gestational age (i.e., between the 10th and 80th percentiles) were examined, the infants of the women with GDM had significantly greater fat mass and percent body fat but had less lean mass as compared with the control group but no difference in birth weight. Of note, in the infants of the women with GDM, the strongest correlates with fat mass were fasting glucose and gestational age. This accounted for 17 percent of the variance in infant fat mass.

In addition to the perinatal association with fetal macrosomia in the infants of women with abnormal glucose tolerance, there are significant long-term risks. The increase in birth weight of these infants tends to normalize by 1 year of age before increasing again in early childhood.[115] There is an increase in the risk of obesity in these children at age 1 to 9 years and in adolescents aged 14 to 16 years. Silverman and colleagues[115] have reported that there is a strong correlation between amniotic fluid insulin levels and increased body mass index (wt/ht^2) in 14- to 17-year-old children, indicating an association between islet cell activation in utero and development of childhood obesity. This obesity present in childhood then predisposes to obesity in the adult. Pettitt and colleagues[116] have shown that infants born to Pima Indian women with impaired glucose tolerance were more obese as children than infants of women with normal glucose tolerance, even when they developed diabetes later in life. These data suggest that there are both in utero maternal metabolic factors as well as genetic factors in the later development of type 2 diabetes and obesity.

Table 37-3. Neonatal Body Composition

	GDM (n = 195)	NGT (n = 220)	P value
Weight (g)	3,398 ± 550	3,337 ± 549	0.26
FFM (g)	2,962 ± 405	2,975 ± 408	.74
Fat mass (g)	436 ± 206	362 ± 198	.0002
Body fat	12.4 ± 4.6	10.4 ± 4.6	.0001

FFM, fat-free mass; GDM, gestational diabetes mellitus; NGT, normal glucose tolerance.

Hypoglycemia

Neonatal hypoglycemia, a blood glucose less than 35 to 40 mg/dl during the first 12 hours of life, results from a rapid drop in plasma glucose concentrations following clamping of the umbilical cord. Hypoglycemia is particularly common in macrosomic newborns, in which rates exceed 50 percent. With near-physiologic control of maternal glucose levels during pregnancy, overall rates of 5 to 15 percent have been reported.[108,109] The degree of hypoglycemia may be influenced by at least two factors: (1) maternal glucose control during the latter half of pregnancy, and (2) control of maternal glycemia control during labor and delivery.[117] Prior poor maternal glucose control can result in fetal β-cell hyperplasia, leading to exaggerated insulin release following delivery. IDMs exhibiting hypoglycemia have elevated cord C-peptide and free insulin levels at birth and an exaggerated pancreatic response to glucose loading.[118]

Respiratory Distress Syndrome

The precise mechanism by which maternal diabetes effect pulmonary development remains unknown. Experimental animal studies have focused primarily on the effects of hyperglycemia and hyperinsulinemia on pulmonary surfactant biosynthesis. An extensive review of the literature confirms that both of these factors are involved in delayed pulmonary maturation in the IDM.[119]

In vitro studies have documented that insulin can interfere with substrate availability for surfactant biosynthesis.[120,121] Smith[121] has postulated that insulin interferes with the normal timing of glucocorticoid-induced pulmonary maturation in the fetus. Cortisol apparently acts on pulmonary fibroblasts to induce synthesis of fibroblast-pneumocyte factor, which then acts on type II cells to stimulate phospholipid synthesis.[122] Carlson and coworkers[123] demonstrated that insulin blocks cortisol action at the level of the fibroblast by reducing the production of fibroblast-pneumocyte factor.

Clinical studies investigating the effect of maternal diabetes on fetal lung maturation have produced conflicting data. The role of amniocentesis in determining fetal lung maturity is discussed with timing and mode of delivery. With the introduction of protocols that have emphasized glucose control and antepartum surveillance until lung maturity has been established, respiratory distress syndrome (RDS) has become a less common occurrence in the IDM. Several studies agree that in well-controlled diabetic women delivered at term, the risk of RDS is no higher than that observed in the general population.[124,125] Kjos et al.[125] studied the outcome of 526 diabetic gestations delivered within 5 days of amniotic fluid fetal lung maturation testing and reported HMD in five neonates (0.95 percent), all of whom were delivered before 34 weeks' gestation. Mimouni et al.[126] compared outcomes of 127 IDMs with matched controls and have concluded that diabetes in pregnancy as currently managed is not a direct risk factor for the development of RDS. Yet, cesarean delivery not preceded by labor and prematurity, both of which are increased in diabetic pregnancies, clearly increase the likelihood of neonatal respiratory disease. With cesarean delivery, most of these cases represent retained lung fluid or transient tachypnea of the newborn, which usually resolves within the first days of life.

Calcium and Magnesium Metabolism

Neonatal hypocalcemia, with serum levels below 7 mg per dl, occurs at an increased rate in the IDM when one controls for predisposing factors such as prematurity and birth asphyxia.[127] With modern management, the frequency of neonatal hypocalcemia is less than 5 percent in the infants of diabetic women.[127] Hypocalcemia in the IDM has been associated with a failure to increase parathyroid hormone synthesis following birth.[128] Decreased serum magnesium levels have also been documented in pregnant diabetic women as well as their infants. Mimouni et al.[128] described reduced amniotic fluid magnesium concentrations in women with type 1 diabetes mellitus. These findings may be explained by a drop in fetal urinary magnesium excretion, which would accompany a relative magnesium deficient state. Magnesium deficiency paradoxically then may inhibit fetal parathyroid hormone secretion.

Hyperbilirubinemia and Polycythemia

Hyperbilirubinemia is frequently observed in the IDM. Neonatal jaundice has been reported in as many as 25 to 53 percent of pregnancies complicated by pregestational diabetes mellitus and 38 percent of pregnancies with GDM.[127,129,130] Although several mechanisms have been proposed to explain these clinical findings, the pathogenesis of hyperbilirubinemia remains uncertain. In the past, the jaundice observed in the IDM often was attributed to prematurity. Studies that have analyzed morbidity carefully, according to gestational age, however, have rejected this concept.[131]

Although severe hyperbilirubinemia may be observed independent of polycythemia, a common pathway for these complications most likely involves increased red blood cell production, which is stimulated by increased erythropoietin in the IDM. Presumably, the major stimulus for red cell production is a state of relative hypoxia in utero, as described previously. Although cord erythropoietin levels generally are normal in IDMs whose mothers demonstrate good glycemic control during gestation, Shannon and colleagues found that hemoglobin A_{1c} (HbA_{1c}) values in late pregnancy were significantly elevated in mothers of hyperbilirubinemic infants.[130,132]

MATERNAL CLASSIFICATION AND RISK ASSESSMENT

Priscilla White[133] first noted that the patient's age at onset of diabetes, the duration of the disease, and the presence of vasculopathy significantly influenced perinatal outcome. Her pioneering work led to a classification system that has been widely applied to pregnant women with diabetes.[133] A modification of this scheme is presented in Table 37-1. Counseling a patient and formulating a plan of management requires assessment of both maternal and fetal risk. The White classification facilitates this evaluation.

Class A_1 diabetes mellitus includes those patients who have demonstrated carbohydrate intolerance during a 100-g 3-hour oral glucose tolerance test (GTT); however, their fasting and 2-hour postprandial glucose levels are maintained within physiologic range by dietary regulation alone. Class A_2 includes gestational diabetic women who require insulin or oral hypoglycemic therapy in response to repetitive elevations of fasting or postpartum glucose levels following dietary intervention.

The Second and Third International Workshop Conferences on Gestational Diabetes sponsored by the American Diabetes Association in cooperation with the American College of Obstetricians and Gynecologists (ACOG) recommended that the term gestational diabetes rather than Class A diabetes be used to describe women with carbohydrate intolerance of variable severity with onset or recognition during the present pregnancy.[134,135] The definition applies whether insulin or only diet modification is used for treatment and whether or not the condition persists after pregnancy. It does not exclude the possibility that unrecognized glucose intolerance may have antedates or begun with pregnancy. The term gestational diabetes fails to specify whether the patient requires dietary adjustment alone or treatment with diet and insulin. This distinction is important because those patients who are normoglycemic while fasting appear to have a significantly lower perinatal mortality rate.[136] Women with GDM who require insulin are at greater risk for a poor perinatal outcome than those whose diabetes is controlled by diet alone.

Patients requiring insulin are designated by the letters B, C, D, R, F, and T. Class B patients are those whose onset of disease occurs after age 20. They have had diabetes for less than 10 years and have no vascular complications. Included in this subgroup of patients are those who have been previously treated with oral hypoglycemic agents.

Class C diabetes includes patients who have the onset of their disease between the ages of 10 and 19 or have had the disease for 10 to 19 years. Vascular disease is not present.

Class D represents women whose disease is of 20 years duration or more, or whose onset occurred before age 10, or who have benign retinopathy. The latter includes microaneurysms, exudates, and venous dilation.

Nephropathy

Renal disease develops in 25 to 30 percent of women with insulin-dependent diabetes mellitus with a peak incidence after approximately 16 years of diabetes.[137] Overt diabetic nephropathy is diagnosed in women with both type 1 or type 2 diabetes mellitus when persistent proteinuria exists in the absence of infection or other urinary tract disease. The criteria for diagnosis in the nonpregnancy state including a total urinary protein excretion (TPE) of greater than 500 mg/24 h or greater than 300 mg/24 h of urinary albumin excretion (UAE).

Before the development of overt diabetic nephropathy, some individuals develop incipient diabetic nephropathy defined by repetitive increases in UAE known as microalbuminuria. The diagnosis is established from a 24-hour urine collection exhibiting UAE of 20 to 199 μgm/min or 30 to 299 mg/24 h. Without specific interventions, approximately 80 percent of individuals with type 1 diabetes who develop sustained microalbuminuria will have their UAE increase at 10 to 20 percent/year to the stage of overt nephropathy. In the nonpregnant individual, improvement of glycemic and blood pressure control have been demonstrated to reduce the risk or slow the progression of diabetic nephropathy.[138,139] Renoprotective or antihypertensive therapy consisting of either angiotensin converting enzyme inhibitors or angiotensin II receptor blockers are indicated prior to pregnancy in women with microalbuminuria or overt nephropathy.[140–143] These agents should, however, be discontinued once pregnancy is established because they are associated with fetal proximal tubular dysgenesis and oligohydramnios. It is important to note that women who exhibit microalbuminuria in early pregnancy have a 35- to 60-percent risk for superimposed preeclampsia.[144,145]

Women with diabetic nephropathy have a significantly reduced life expectancy. Disease progression is characterized by hypertension, declining glomerular filtration rate and eventual end-stage renal disease requiring dialysis or transplantation. In women with overt nephropathy, end-stage renal disease occurs in 50 percent by 10 years and in greater than 75 percent of cases by 20 years. Class F describes the 5 to 10 percent of pregnant patients with underlying renal disease. This includes those with reduced creatinine clearance and/or proteinuria of at least 400 mg in 24 hours measured during the first twenty weeks of gestation. Two factors present before 20 weeks' gestation appear to be predictive of perinatal outcome in these women (e.g., preterm delivery, low birthweight, or preeclampsia). These are

1. Proteinuria greater than 3.0 g/24 h.
2. Serum creatinine greater than 1.5 mg/dl.

In our series of 45 class F women, 12 women had such risk factors.[146] Preeclampsia developed in 92 percent with a mean gestational age at delivery of 34 weeks compared with an incidence of preeclampsia of 36 percent in 33 women without these risk factors who reached an average gestational age of 36 weeks. Remarkably, perinatal survival was 100 percent in this series, and no deliveries occurred prior to 30 weeks' gestation. Comparable series detailing perinatal outcomes in Class F patients are presented in Table 37-4.

The management of the diabetic women with nephropathy requires great expertise. Limitation of dietary protein, which may reduce protein excretion in nonpregnant patients, has not been adequately studied during pregnancy. Although the method is controversial, some nephrologists recommend a modified reduction in protein

Table 37-4. Comparative Studies of Outcomes in Class F Diabetes Mellitus

	KITZMILLER[147]	GRENFEL[276]	REECE[148]	GORDON[146]	ROSENN[150]
(n)	26	20	31	45	61
Chronic HTN	31%	27%	22%	26%	47%
Initial Creat >1.9 mg/dl	38%	10%	22%	11%	—
Initial proteinuria >3.0 gm/24 hr	8.3%	—	22%	13%	—
Preeclampsia	15%	55%	35%	53%	51%
Cesarean delivery	—	72%	70%	80%	82%
Perinatal survival (%)	88.9	100	93.5	100	94%
Major anomalies	3 (11.1%)	1 (4.3%)	3 (9.7%)	2 (4%)	4 (6%)
IUGR (%)	20.8	NA	19.4	11.0	11%
Delivery					
<34 weeks (%)	30.8	27	22.5	15.5	25%
34–36 weeks (%)	40.7	23	32.3	35.5	28%
>36 weeks (%)	28.5	50	45.2	49	47%

Creat, creatinine; HTN, hypertension; IUGR, intrauterine growth restriction.

intake for pregnant women with nephropathy. Control of hypertension in pregnant women with diabetic nephropathy is crucial to prevent further deterioration of kidney function and to optimize pregnancy outcome. Although debatable, some cautiously use diuretics when patients are extremely nephrotic because this group may be prone to volume-dependent forms of hypertension. Again, ACE inhibitors and receptor blockers, which reduce intraglomerular pressure and improve proteinuria in nonpregnant diabetic patients, should be discontinued during pregnancy.

Several studies have failed to demonstrate a permanent worsening of diabetic renal disease as a result of pregnancy.[146–148] Furthermore, it has been suggested that pregnancy itself does not increase the risk of developing nephropathy, although development of proteinuria and poor glycemic control are markers for subsequent renal disease. Kitzmiller and colleagues[147] reviewed 35 pregnancies complicated by diabetic nephropathy. Proteinuria increased in 69 percent and hypertension developed in 73 percent. After delivery, proteinuria declined in 65 percent of cases. In only two patients did protein excretion increase after gestation. In Gordon's series, 26 women (58 percent) had more than a 1-g increase in proteinuria, and by the third trimester, 25 (56 percent) excreted more than 3.0 g/24 h.[146] In the vast majority of cases, protein excretion returned to baseline levels following gestation.

Changes in creatinine clearance during pregnancy are variable in class F patients. Kitzmiller,[149] in reviewing 44 patients from the literature, noted that about one third of women had an expected rise in creatinine clearance during gestation, compared with one third who had a decline of more than 15 percent by the third trimester. In Gordon's series, 12 of 16 women in this category developed preeclampsia. Of interest, most patients with a severe reduction in creatinine clearance (<50 ml/min) in the first trimester do not demonstrate a further reduction in clearance during pregnancy.[146] However, a decline in renal function can be anticipated in 20 to 30 percent of cases. Several authors have suggested that any deterioration of renal function after pregnancy is probably consistent with the natural course of diabetic nephropathy and is not related to pregnancy per se.[150] This finding has been confirmed by Rossing and colleagues[151] who conducted an observational study of women who developed diabetic nephropathy between 1984 and 1989 who were followed to 2000. Over the 10 years postpartum, the mean decline in creatinine clearance was 3.2 + 3.4 ml/min/year in 17 parous women compared with 3.2 + 5.1 ml/min/year in 42 women who never became pregnant.

With improved survival of diabetic patients after renal transplantation, a growing number of kidney recipients have now achieved pregnancy (class T). Armenti of the United States National Transplant Registry has described 28 pregnancies in diabetic renal transplant recipients.[152] The majority of patients had underlying hypertension, although preeclampsia was diagnosed in only 17 percent of cases. Allograft rejection occurred in one case. Overall, despite an increase in deliveries before 37 weeks, perinatal survival was 100 percent. These excellent results have resulted from improvements in both perinatal management and newer immunosuppressive regimens. Earlier reports of pregnancies after renal transplantation documented a significant risk for perinatal loss (22 percent) and preeclampsia (67 percent).[153]

Presently, many transplant centers strive to perform combined kidney-pancreas transplants in diabetic individuals with end stage renal disease. McCrory and colleagues[154] reported 23 pregnancies following combined transplantation in which 25 percent of women developed preeclampsia and 70 percent of pregnancies resulted in preterm birth. A report from the International Pancreas Transplant Registry of 19 pregnancies after combined transplantation documented a 100-percent live-birth rate. One woman each developed pancreas graft rejection and kidney graft rejection following pregnancy.[155]

Retinopathy

Class R diabetes designates patients with proliferative retinopathy, representing neovascularization or growth of new retinal capillaries. These vessels may cause vitreous hemorrhage with scarring and retinal detachment, resulting in vision loss. As with nephropathy, prevalence of retinal disease is highly related to the duration of diabetes. At 20 years, nearly 80 percent of diabetic individuals have some element of diabetic retinopathy. Excellent glycemic control prevents retinopathy and may slow its progression. Parity is not associated with a risk for subsequent retinopathy.[156] However, pregnancy does convey a greater than a twofold independent risk for progression of existing retinopathy.[157] Progression of diabetic retinopathy during pregnancy is associated with hypertensive disease.[158] Retinopathy may worsen significantly during pregnancy in spite of the major advances that have been made in diagnosis and treatment of existing retinopathy. Ideally, women planning a pregnancy should have a comprehensive eye examination and treatment before conception. For those discovered to have proliferative changes during pregnancy, laser photocoagulation therapy with careful follow-up has helped maintain many pregnancies to a gestational age at which neonatal survival is likely.

In a large series of 172 patients, including 40 cases with background retinopathy and 11 with proliferative changes, only one patient developed new onset proliferative retinopathy during pregnancy.[159] A review of the literature by Kitzmiller[160] confirms the observation that progression to proliferative retinopathy during pregnancy rarely occurs in women with background retinopathy or those without any eye ground changes. Of the 561 women in these two categories, only 17 (3.0 percent) developed neovascularization during gestation.[160] In contrast, 23 of 26 (88.5 percent) with untreated proliferative disease experienced worsening retinopathy during pregnancy.

Pregnancy may increase the prevalence of some background retinal changes.[161] Characteristic streak-blob hemorrhages and soft exudates have been noted, and such retinopathy may progress despite strict metabolic control. At least two studies have related worsening retinal disease to plasma glucose at the first prenatal visit as well as the magnitude of improvement in glycemia during early pregnancy.[162,163] In a subset of 140 women without proliferative retinopathy at baseline followed in the Diabetes in Early Pregnancy Study, progression of retinopathy was seen in 10.3, 21.1, 18.8, and 54.8 percent of patients with no retinopathy, microaneurysms only, mild nonproliferative retinopathy, and moderate-to-severe nonproliferative retinopathy at baseline, respectively. Elevated glycosylated hemoglobin at baseline and the magnitude of improvement of glucose control through week 14 were associated with a higher risk of progression of retinopathy.[163] Women with an initial glycohemoglobin greater than 6 SD above the control mean were nearly three times as likely to experience worsening retinopathy compared with those within 2 SD of the mean. Whether improving control or simply suboptimal control itself contributes to a deterioration of background retinopathy remains uncertain. Hypertension may also be a significant risk factor for the progression of retinopathy during pregnancy.[158] Rosenn and colleagues[158] reported that worsening of retinopathy occurred in 55 percent of women with a hypertensive disorder of pregnancy compared to 25 percent of women without chronic hypertension or preeclampsia. Hypertension was associated with the progression of retinopathy after controlling for changes in glycemic status.

For women with proliferative changes, laser photocoagulation is indicated and most will respond to this therapy. However, those women who demonstrate severe florid disc neovascularization that is unresponsive to laser therapy during early pregnancy may be at great risk for deterioration of their vision. Termination of pregnancy should be considered in this group of patients.

In addition to background and proliferative eye disease, vaso-occlusive lesions associated with the development of macular edema have been described during pregnancy.[164] Cystic macular edema is most often found in patients with proteinuric nephropathy and hypertensive disease leading to retinal edema. Macular capillary permeability is a feature of this process. The degree of macular edema is directly related to the fall in plasma oncotic pressure present in these women. In Sinclair's series, seven women with minimal or no retinopathy before becoming pregnant developed severe macular edema associated with pre-proliferative or proliferative retinopathy during the course of their pregnancies. Although proliferation was controlled with photocoagulation, the macular edema worsened until delivery in all cases and was often aggravated by photocoagulation.[164] Although both macular edema and retinopathy regressed after delivery in some patients, in others, these pathologic processes persisted, resulting in significant visual loss.

Coronary Artery Disease

Class H diabetes refers to the presence of diabetes of any duration associated with ischemic myocardial disease. There is concern that the small number of women who have coronary artery disease are at an increased risk for mortality during gestation. This is particularly true for women who suffer an infarction during pregnancy.[165] The maternal mortality rate exceeded 50 percent for cases of infarction during pregnancy in cases reported prior to 1980.[157] A high index of suspicion for ischemic heart disease should be maintained in women with long-standing diabetes because anginal symptoms may be minimal and infarction may thus present as congestive heart failure.[166] Although there are in excess of one dozen reports of successful pregnancies following myocardial infarction in diabetic women, cardiac status should be carefully assessed early in gestation or preferably before pregnancy. If electrocardiographic abnormalities are encountered, echocardiography may be employed to assess ventricular function or modified stress testing may be performed. The decision to undertake a pregnancy in a woman with type 1 or type 2 diabetes mellitus and coronary artery disease needs to be made only after serious consideration. The potential for morbidity and mortality must be thoroughly reviewed with the patient and her family. The management of myocardial infarction during pregnancy is discussed in Chapter 34.

DETECTION AND SIGNIFICANCE OF GESTATIONAL DIABETES MELLITUS

It has been estimated that 2 to 3 percent of pregnancies are complicated by diabetes mellitus and that ninety percent of the cases represent women with GDM.[167] An increased prevalence of GDM is found in women of ethnic groups which have high frequencies of type 2 diabetes. These include women of Hispanic, African, Native American, Asian, and/or Pacific Island ancestry.[168] Women with GDM represent a group with significant risk for developing glucose intolerance later in life. Whereas, O'Sullivan projected that 50 percent of GDM would become diabetic in follow-up study of 22 to 28 years, Kjos and colleagues have reported that 60 percent of Latina women will develop type 2 diabetes, and this level of risk may actually be manifest by 5 years after the GDM index pregnancy.[169–171] The likelihood for subsequent diabetes apparently increases when GDM is diagnosed in early pregnancy, and is accompanied by impaired β-cell function and obesity.

As noted earlier, GDM is a state restricted to pregnant women whose impaired glucose tolerance is discovered during pregnancy. Because, in most cases, patients with GDM have normal fasting glucose levels, some challenge of glucose tolerance must be undertaken. Traditionally, obstetricians relied upon historical and clinical risk factors to select those patients most likely to develop GDM. This group included patients with a family history of diabetes, or those whose past pregnancies were marked by an unexplained stillbirth, or the delivery of a malformed or macrosomic infant. Obesity, hypertension, glycosuria, and maternal age older than 25 were other indications for screening. Interestingly, more than half of all patients who exhibit an abnormal GTT lack the risk factors mentioned earlier. Coustan and colleagues[172] have reported that in a series of 6,214 women, using historic risk factors and an arbitrary age cutoff of 30 years for screening would miss 35 percent of cases of GDM.

In the summary and recommendations of the Second and Third International Workshop-Conference on GDM, screening was recommended for all pregnant

Table 37-5. Screening Strategy for Detecting GDM

Risk assessment for GDM should be ascertained at the first prenatal visit.
- Low risk
  - Blood glucose testing is not routinely required if all of the following characteristics are present:
    - Member of an ethnic group with a low prevalence of GDM
    - No known diabetes in first-degree relatives
    - Age <25 years
    - Weight normal before pregnancy
    - No history of abnormal glucose metabolism
    - No history of poor obstetric outcome
- Average risk
  - Perform blood glucose screening at 24–28 weeks using one of the following:
    - Two-step procedure: 50 g GCT followed by a diagnostic OGTT in those meeting the threshold value in the GCT
    - One-step procedure: diagnostic OGTT performed on all subjects
- High risk
  - Perform blood glucose testing as soon as feasible, using the procedures described above.
    - If GDM is not diagnosed, blood glucose testing should be repeated at 24–28 weeks or at any time a patient has symptoms or signs suggestive of hyperglycemia

GCT, glucose challenge test; GDM, gestational diabetes mellitus; OGTT, oral glucose tolerance test.
Adapted from Fourth International Workshop Conference on GDM, Diabetes Care, Volume 21, Supplement 2, August 1998.

women. Following the Fourth International Workshop-Conference in 1997, universal screening was recommended for women in ethnic groups with relatively high rates of carbohydrate intolerance during pregnancy and of diabetes later in life.[173] It was recognized that certain features place women at low risk for GDM (Table 37-5), and it may not be cost-effective to screen this subgroup of women. Those at low risk include women who are not members of ethnic groups at increased risk for developing adult-onset diabetes, who have no previous history of abnormal glucose tolerance or poor obstetric outcomes usually associated with GDM and who have all of the following characteristics: age younger than 25 years, normal body weight, and no family history of diabetes. Danilenko-Dixon and colleagues have reported that such low risk women represent only 10 percent of their population and this identifying such women may add complexity to screening in a busy clinic or office practice.[174] The ACOG recognizes that while universal screening is the most sensitive approach, selective screening may be employed with the criteria cited earlier.[175]

Despite the widespread acceptance of screening for and treating GDM in the United States, some expert panels have questioned the benefit of GDM screening programs altogether.[176] The criteria for the diagnosis of GDM originally designated a population at increased risk for the development of type 2 diabetes in later life. The fact that O'Sullivan's original work establishing the criteria used for the diagnosis of GDM failed to evaluate an association between mild carbohydrate tolerance and perinatal outcome has led many to question the overall significance of this diagnosis. Because of the lack of high-quality evidence concerning the benefit of treatment of milder cases of GDM, it is difficult to determine the extent to which screening impacts maternal and neonatal health outcomes.[177] It has been suggested that the criteria for the diagnosis of GDM are conceptually flawed in that they represent a dichotomous definition of normal and abnormal gestational glucose tolerance, when the risk of adverse maternal-fetal outcomes and later diabetes should be logically graded upward with higher values on the oral GTT and with the degree of fasting hyperglycemia.[178] Two studies have in fact addressed the relationship between mild degrees of carbohydrate tolerance and rates of neonatal macrosomia. In a study of 3,637 women without GDM, Sermer and colleagues[179] demonstrated a graded increase in adverse outcomes (including large infants) with increasing maternal carbohydrate intolerance. Similarly, Sacks identified fasting and 2-hour glucose values as independent risk factors for macrosomia in a multivariate analysis of more than 3,500 pregnant women. However, because no clinically meaningful glucose threshold could be identified, Sacks[180] concluded that the criteria for GDM will likely be established by consensus.

Both a recent large-scale retrospective cohort study and a randomized clinical trial have both suggested a benefit to treatment of GDM in reducing the risk of perinatal complications. Langer and colleagues[181] compared perinatal outcomes in 555 GDM women diagnosed after 37 weeks with 1,110 subjects treated for GDM as well as 1,110 subjects matched for demographic features and gestational age at delivery. A single feature of a composite adverse outcome (stillbirth, macrosomia, neonatal hypoglycemia, erythrocytosis, and hyperbilirubinemia) was present in 50 percent of untreated subjects, 18 percent of treated subjects, and 11 percent of nondiabetic subjects. These significant differences were present when untreated GDM were stratified according to disease severity (fasting plasma glucose level on the diagnostic oral GTT).

Crowther and colleagues have conducted the only large scale multicenter randomized trial to determine whether treatment of GDM improves perinatal outcome.[182] Over a 10-year period, 1,000 women were randomly assigned between 24 to 34 weeks' gestation to receive dietary advice, blood glucose monitoring, and insulin therapy as needed versus routine care. The authors found the composite rate of serious complications was lower in the intervention group than in the routine care group (1 versus 4 percent). However, none of the individual components of the composite reached statistical significance. Among the components of the composite, only the rate of shoulder dystocia (16 versus 7 cases) was significantly different among comparison groups. Thus, the differences in serious perinatal complications reported in this study should be interpreted with caution.

An international blinded observational study is currently in progress to assess the association between maternal hyperglycemia and perinatal outcomes as well as a Maternal-Fetal Medicine Networks Unit randomized trial addressing the efficacy of treatment of mild GDM.[183,184] Together, these studies should help guide thresholds for intervention in women with carbohydrate intolerance during pregnancy.[185]

The 50-g glucose challenge may be performed in the fasting or fed state. Sensitivity is improved if the test is performed in the fasting state.[186,187] A plasma value between 130–140 mg/dl is commonly used as a threshold for performing a 3-hour oral GTT. Coustan et al.[186] have demonstrated that 10 percent of GDM women have screening test values between 130 and 139 mg/dl. This study indicated that the sensitivity of screening would be increased from 90 percent to nearly 100 percent if universal screening were employed using a threshold of 130 mg/dl. The prevalence of positive screening tests requiring further diagnostic testing increases from 14 percent (140 mg/dl) to 23 percent (130 mg/dl), which is accompanied by an approximately 12-percent increase in the overall cost to diagnose each case of GDM.

Whereas most women can be screened for GDM at approximately 24 to 28 weeks' gestation, it is advisable to screen earlier in pregnancy those with strong risk factors such as morbid obesity, a strong family history, previous GDM, prior macrosomic stillbirth, or an infant weighing more than 4,500 g.[188] If initial screening is negative, repeat testing is performed at 24 to 28 weeks. Using the plasma cutoff of 135 to 140 mg/dl, one can expect approximately 15 to 20 percent of patients with an abnormal screening value to have an abnormal 3-hour oral GTT. Patients whose 1-hour screening value exceeds 190 mg/dl (10.5 mmol/L) will exhibit an abnormal oral GTT in 90 percent of cases.[189] In women with a screening value between 190 and 215 mg/dl, it is preferable to check a fasting blood glucose level before administering a 100-g carbohydrate load.[190] If the fasting glucose is greater than 95 mg/dl, the patient is treated for GDM.

The criteria for establishing the diagnosis of gestational diabetes are listed in Table 37-6. The U.S. National Diabetes Data Group criteria represent a theoretic conversion of O'Sullivan's thresholds in whole blood. Carpenter and Coustan[189] prefer to use another modification of these data, which is supported by a comparison of the old Somogyi-Nelson method and current plasma glucose oxidase assays. These criteria have been modified by the Fourth International Workshop Conference on GDM. Several studies have confirmed that patients diagnosed using the less stringent Carpenter criteria experience as much perinatal morbidity (macrosomia and cesarean delivery) as subjects diagnosed by the National Diabetes Data Group Criteria.[191–193] Using either criteria, the patient must have at least two abnormal glucose determinations to be diagnosed with GDM.

Table 37-6. Detection of Gestational Diabetes—Upper Limits of Normal

SCREENING TEST 50-G, 1-HOUR	**PLASMA (MG/DL) 130–140**	
Oral GTT*	NDDG[192]	Carpenter[189]
Fasting	105	95
1-hour	190	180
2-hour	165	155
3-hour	145	140

GTT, glucose tolerance test; NDDG, National Diabetes Data Group.

*Diagnosis of gestational diabetes is made when any two values are met or exceeded.

National Institutes of Health Diabetes Data Group: Classification and diagnosis of diabetes mellitus and other categories of glucose intolerance. Diabetes 28:1039, 1979.

Treatment of the Patient with Type 1 or Type 2 Diabetes Mellitus

Because fetal glucose levels reflect those of the mother, it is not surprising that clinical efforts aimed at optimizing maternal control are considered the key component responsible for the decline in perinatal death in pregnancies complicated by diabetes mellitus over the last few decades. Self–blood glucose monitoring combined with intensive insulin therapy has resulted in improved glycemia for many pregnant diabetic women (Table 37-7). Women with pregestational diabetes should monitor their glucose control 5 to 7 times daily using glucose-oxidase impregnated reagent strips and a glucose reflectance meter.[194]

To achieve the best glycemic control possible for each patient, during pregnancy conventional insulin therapy is abandoned in favor of intensive therapy. An attempt is made to stimulate physiologic insulin requirements by providing basal and prandial insulin needs through three or four daily injections or continuous insulin infusion (pump therapy) (CSII). Insulin regimens have classically included multiple injections of insulin usually prior to breakfast, the evening meal, and often bedtime complimented by self–blood glucose monitoring and adjustment of insulin dose according to glucose profiles. Patients are instructed on dietary composition, insulin action, recognition and treatment of hypoglycemia, adjusting insulin dosage for exercise and sick days, as well as monitoring for hyperglycemia and potential ketosis. These principles form the foundation for intensive insulin therapy in which an attempt is made to simulate physiologic insulin requirements. Insulin administration is provided for both basal needs and meals, and rapid adjustments are made in response to glucose measurements. The treatment regimen generally involves three to four daily injections or the use of CSII devices. With either approach, frequent self–blood glucose monitoring is fundamental to achieve the therapeutic objective of physiologic glucose control. Glucose determinations are made in the fasting state and before lunch, dinner, and bedtime. Postprandial and nocturnal values are also helpful. Patients are instructed on an insulin dose for each meal and at bedtime, if nec-

Table 37-7. Target Plasma Glucose Levels in Pregnancy

TIME	MG/DL
Before breakfast	60–90
Before lunch, supper, bedtime snack	60–105
Two hours after meals	≤120
2 a.m. to 6 a.m.	>60

essary. Mealtime insulin needs are determined by the composition of the meal, the premeal glucose measurement, and the level of activity anticipated following the meal. Basal or intermediate acting insulin requirements are determined by periodic 2-a.m. to 4-a.m. glucose measurements, as well as late afternoon values, which reflect morning intermediate-acting insulin action. During pregnancy, diabetic women should develop the self-management skills that are essential to an intensive insulin therapy regimen.

In patients in whom diabetes is not well controlled, a brief period of hospitalization is often necessary for the initiation of therapy. Individual adjustments to the regimens implemented can then be made. It is gratifying for many patients to feel that they can take charge of their own diabetic control. Women who have previously followed a prescribed dosage regimen for years gain confidence in making adjustments in their insulin dosage after a short period of time. Patients are encouraged to contact their physician at any time if questions should arise concerning the management of their diabetes. During early pregnancy, patients are instructed to report their glucose values by telephone, fax, or email at least weekly.

Insulin therapy must be individualized, with dosage determinations tailored to diet and exercise. Semisynthetic human insulin preparations and newer insulin analogues (Table 37-8) are used during pregnancy. Insulin lispro and insulin aspart are rapid-acting insulin preparations that have considerable advantages over regular insulin. Insulin lispro features reversal of proline and lysine at positions B28 and B29, and remains in monomeric form and is thus rapidly absorbed. Its duration of action is shorter than that of regular insulin so that unexpected hypoglycemia hours after injection is avoided. Insulin lispro appears to be safe for use during pregnancy, and it is a category B drug. An early report raised some question regarding a possible association with progression of retinopathy. However, recent experience suggests this is not the case.[195–197]

Insulin aspart has been studied in a limited number of women with GDM during the third trimester.[198] Pettit et al.[198] assessed the short-term efficacy of insulin aspart in comparison with human regular insulin in 16 women with GDM. Glycemic excursions were significantly lower with insulin aspart.

The long-acting insulin analogues glargine and detemir have been designed to more accurately mimic basal insulin secretion, yet neither has been adequately evaluated for safety or efficacy during pregnancy. Insulin glargine has a flat profile when compared with NPH so that when administered with short-acting insulin, unpredictable spikes in insulin levels with resulting hypoglycemia appear to be less common.[194,199] A concern with insulin glargine is its high affinity for insulin-like growth factor (IGF) receptors. Theoretically, this might increase the progression of retinopathy in certain women. Further studies are needed to establish both the safety and efficacy of insulin glargine and detemir during pregnancy.

Insulin is generally administered in two to three injections. We prefer a three-injection regimen, although most patients present taking a combination of intermediate-acting and short-acting insulin before dinner and breakfast. As a general rule, the amount of intermediate-acting insulin will exceed the short-acting component by a two-to-one ratio. Patients usually receive two thirds of their total dose with breakfast and the remaining third in the evening as a combined dose with dinner or split into components with short-acting or rapid-acting insulin at dinner and intermediate-acting insulin at bedtime in an effort to minimize periods of nocturnal hypoglycemia. These episodes frequently occur when the mother is in a relative fasting state, whereas placental and fetal glucose consumption continue. Finally, some women may require a small dose of short-acting or rapid-acting insulin before lunch, thus constituting a four-injection regimen.

Open-loop CSII pump therapy is preferred by many IDDM women during pregnancy. The pump is a battery powered unit, which may be worn during most daily activities like a beeper. These systems provide continuous short-acting insulin therapy through a subcutaneous infusion. The basal infusion rate and bolus doses to cover meals are determined by frequent self-monitoring of blood glucose. The basal infusion rate is generally close to 1 unit per hour.

Table 37-8. Type of Human Insulin and Insulin Analogues

	SOURCE	ONSET (H)	PEAK (H)	DURATION (H)
Short acting				
Humulin R (Lilly)	Human	0.5	2–4	5–7
Velosulin-H (Novo Nordisk)	Human	0.5	1–3	8
Novolin R (Novo Nordisk)	Human	0.5	2.5–5	6–8
Lispro	Analogue	0.25	0.5–1.5	4–5
Aspart	Analogue	0.25	1–3	3–5
Intermediate acting				
Humulin Lente (Lilly)	Human	1–3	6–12	18–24
Humulin NPH (Lilly)	Human	1–2	6–12	18–24
Novolin L (Novo Nordisk)	Human	2.5	7–15	22
Novolin N (Novo Nordisk)	Human	1.5	4–20	24
Long acting				
Humulin Ultralente (Lilly)	Human	4–6	8–20	>36
Glargine	Analogue	1	—	24
Determir	Analogue	1–2	—	24

Pregnant patients may require hospitalization before initiation of pump therapy. Women must be educated regarding the strategy of continuous infusion and have their glucose stabilized over several days. This requires that multiple blood glucose determinations be made for the prevention of periods of hyperglycemia and hypoglycemia. Glucose values may become normalized with minimal amplitude of daily excursions in most patients.

Episodes of hypoglycemia are often reduced with pump therapy. When they do occur, they are usually secondary to errors in dose selection or failure to adhere to the required diet. The risk of nocturnal hypoglycemia, which is increased in the pregnant state, necessitates that great care be undertaken in selecting patients for CSII. Patients using the pump who fail to exhibit normal counterregulatory responses to hypoglycemia should probably check their glucose values at 2 to 3 a.m. to detect nocturnal hypoglycemia.

The mechanics of the CSII systems are relatively simple. A fine-gauge butterfly needle device is attached by connecting tubing to the pump. This cannula is reimplanted every 2 to 3 days at a different site in the anterior abdominal wall. Rapid-acting insulin (usually insulin lispro) is stored in the pump syringe. Infusion occurs at a basal rate, which can be fixed or altered for specific time of day by a computer program. For example, the basal rate can be programmed for a lower dose at night. Preprandial boluses can be adjusted manually before each meal and snack. Half of the total daily insulin is usually given as the basal rate and the remainder as premeal boluses infused before each meal. The largest bolus (30 to 35 percent) is administered with breakfast, followed by 25 percent before dinner and 15 to 20 percent before snacks.

Patients without any pancreatic reserve may have rapid elevations of blood glucose if there is pump failure or intercurrent infection. Since the advent of buffered insulin, insulin aggregation leading to occlusion of the silastic infusion tubing is uncommon. Failure of the pump is associated with a steady rise in ketonemia in the nonpregnant patient.

It is unclear whether CSII is superior to multiple injection regimens. Coustan and colleagues[200] randomized 22 patients to intensive conventional therapy with multiple injections versus pump therapy. There were no differences between the two treatment groups with respect to outpatient mean glucose levels, glycosylated hemoglobin levels, or glycemic excursions. More recently, Gabbe and colleagues[201] reported a large retrospective cohort study of women who began pump therapy during gestation as compared with a group treated with multiple injection regimens. Women using pumps, most with insulin lispro, had fewer hypoglycemic reactions and comparable glucose control and pregnancy outcomes.[201] Studies in nonpregnant individuals employing CSII comparing new insulin analogues to regular insulin indicate fewer hypoglycemic episodes and improved postprandial control.[202]

Diet therapy is critical to successful regulation of maternal diabetes. A program consisting of three meals and several snacks is employed for most patients. Dietary composition should be 50 to 60 percent carbohydrate, 20 percent protein, and 25 to 30 percent fat with less than 10 percent saturated fats, up to 10 percent polyunsaturated fatty acids, and the remainder derived from monosaturated sources.[203] Caloric intake is established based on prepregnancy weight and weight gain during gestation. Weight reduction is not advised. Patients should consume approximately 35 Kcal/kg ideal body weight. Obese women may be managed with an intake as low as 25 Kcal/kg actual weight. Any further caloric restriction resulting in ketonuria requires an increase in caloric consumption.

The presence of maternal vasculopathy should be thoroughly assessed early in pregnancy. The patient should be evaluated by an ophthalmologist familiar with diabetic retinopathy. Ophthalmologic examinations are performed during each trimester and repeated more often if retinopathy is defected. Baseline renal function is established by assaying a 24-hour urine collection for creatinine clearance and protein. An electrocardiogram and urine culture are also obtained.

Most patients with type 1 and type 2 diabetes mellitus are followed with outpatient visits at 1-to 2-week intervals. At each visit, control is assessed and adjustments in insulin dosage are made. However, patients should be instructed to call at any time if periods of hypoglycemia (<50 mg/dl) or hyperglycemia (>200 mg/dl) occur. The increased risk of hypoglycemia in pregnant individuals may be related to defective glucose counterregulatory hormone mechanisms.[204,205] Both epinephrine and glucagon appear to be suppressed in pregnant diabetic women during hypoglycemia. For these reasons, patients should test glucose levels frequently, and family members should be instructed on the technique of glucagon injection for the treatment of severe reactions.

Ketoacidosis

With the implementation of antenatal care, programs stressing strict metabolic control of blood glucose levels for women requiring insulin, DKA has fortunately become a less common occurrence. Kilvert and colleagues[206] reported 11 cases of ketoacidosis in 635 insulin treated pregnancies between 1971 and 1990. One fetal loss and one spontaneous miscarriage complicated the pregnancies affected by DKA.

DKA can occur in the newly diagnosed diabetic patient, and the hormonal milieu of pregnancy may become the background for this phenomenon. Because pregnancy is a state of relative insulin resistance marked by enhanced lipolysis and ketogenesis, DKA may develop in a pregnant woman with glucose levels barely exceeding 200 mg/dl (11.1 mmol/L). Thus, DKA may be diagnosed during pregnancy with minimal hyperglycemia accompanied by a fall in plasma bicarbonate and a pH value less than 7.30. Serum acetone is positive at a 1:2 dilution.

Early recognition of signs and symptoms of DKA improves both maternal and fetal outcome. As in the nonpregnant state, clinical signs of volume depletion follow the symptoms of hyperglycemia, which include polydipsia and polyuria. Malaise, headache, nausea, and vomiting are common complaints. A pregnant woman with poor fluid intake and persistent vomiting over 8 to 12 hours should be evaluated for potential DKA. A low

Table 37-9. Management of Diabetic Ketoacidosis During Pregnancy

1. Laboratory assessment
   Obtain arterial blood gases to document degree of acidosis present; measure glucose, ketones, electrolytes, at 1–2 h intervals
2. Insulin
   Low-dose, intravenous (IV)
   Loading dose: 0.2–0.4 units/kg
   Maintenance: 2.0–10.0 units/hr
3. Fluids
   Isotonic Sodium Chloride
   Total replacement in first 12 h = 4–6 L
   1 L in first hr
   500–1,000 mL/hr for 2–4 h
   250 ml/h until 80% replaced
4. Glucose
   Begin 5% D/NS when plasma level reaches 250 mg/dl (14 mmol/L)
5. Potassium
   If initially normal or reduced, an infusion rate up to 15–20 mEq/h may be required; if elevated, wait until levels decline into the normal range, then add to IV solution in a concentration of 20–30 mEq/L
6. Bicarbonate
   Add one ampule (44 mEq) to 1 L of 0.45 NS if pH is <7.10

D/NS, dextrose in normal saline.

serum bicarbonate level prompts an arterial blood gas determination to rule out this diagnosis. Occasionally, DKA may present in a woman with undiagnosed diabetes receiving β-mimetic agents to arrest preterm labor. Because of the risk of hyperglycemia and DKA in women requiring insulin who then receive intravenous β-mimetic medications such as a ritodrine, magnesium sulfate has become the preferred tocolytic for cases of preterm labor in these cases.

Once the diagnosis of DKA is established and the patient is stabilized, she should be transported to a facility where tertiary care in both perinatology and neonatology is available. Therapy hinges on the meticulous correction of metabolic and fluid abnormalities. An attempt at treatment of any underlying cause for DKA, such as infection, should be instituted as well. The general management of DKA in pregnancy is outlined in Table 37-9. Fluid resuscitation and insulin infusion should be maintained even in the face of normoglycemia until bicarbonate levels return to normal, indicating that acidemia has cleared. DKA does represent a substantial risk for fetal compromise. However, successful fetal resuscitation often accompanies correction of maternal acidosis. Therefore, every effort should be made to correct maternal condition before intervening and delivering a preterm infant.

ANTEPARTUM FETAL EVALUATION

Maternal diabetes may result in fetal hyperglycemia and hyperinsulinemia, and thereby increase the risk for fetal hypoxia. Thus, protocols for antepartum fetal assessment in pregnancies complicated by diabetes mellitus have been incorporated into the care plan for outpatient monitoring during the third trimester. During this time period, when the risk of sudden intrauterine death increases, a program of fetal surveillance is initiated. Because improvement in maternal control has played a major role in reducing perinatal mortality in diabetic pregnancies, antepartum fetal monitoring tests are now used primarily to reassure the obstetrician and avoid unnecessary premature intervention. These techniques have few false-negatives results, and in a patient in whom diabetes is well controlled and who exhibits no vasculopathy or significant hypertension, reassuring antepartum testing allows the fetus to benefit from further maturation in utero.

Maternal assessment of fetal activity serves as a simple screening technique in a program of fetal surveillance. During the third trimester, women are instructed to perform daily fetal movement counting. To date, few studies have applied this method to a large number of women with diabetes mellitus. Patients with a variety of high-risk antepartum conditions including diabetes appear to have an increased incidence of alarming fetal activity patterns.[207] Although the false-negative rate with maternal monitoring of fetal activity is low (~1 percent), the false-positive rate may be as high as 60 percent. Maternal hypoglycemia, although generally believed to be associated with decreased fetal movement, may actually stimulate fetal activity.[208]

Sadovsky and coworkers[209] reported that fetal movement at 25 to 33 weeks' gestation in 67 diabetic pregnancies was lower than in controls, whereas in the final two months of pregnancy, activity levels were similar to the nondiabetic population. In this series, there were four cases of cessation of fetal movement. Two fetuses died in utero 10 and 11 hours after maternal perception that activity had stopped, an interval shorter than that seen in other complications of pregnancy.

The nonstress test (NST) remains the preferred method to assess antepartum fetal well-being in the patient with diabetes mellitus.[210] If the NST is nonreactive, a biophysical profile (BPP) or contraction stress test is then performed (Fig. 37-13). Heart rate monitoring is begun early in the third trimester, usually by 32 weeks' gestation. Two studies have also demonstrated an increased fetal death rate within 1 week of a reactive NST in pregnancies complicated by IDDM when compared with other high-risk gestations.[211,212] If the NST is to be used as the primary method of antepartum heart rate testing, we prefer that it be done at least twice weekly once the patient reaches 32 weeks' gestation. In patients with vascular disease or poor control, in whom the incidence of abnormal tests and intrauterine deaths is greater, testing is often performed earlier and more frequently.

Doppler umbilical artery velocimetry has been proposed as a clinical tool for antepartum fetal surveillance in pregnancies at risk for placental vascular disease. We have found that Doppler studies of the umbilical artery may be predictive of fetal outcome in diabetic pregnancies complicated by vascular disease.[213] Elevated placental resistance as evidenced by an increased systolic/diastolic ratio is associated with fetal growth restriction and

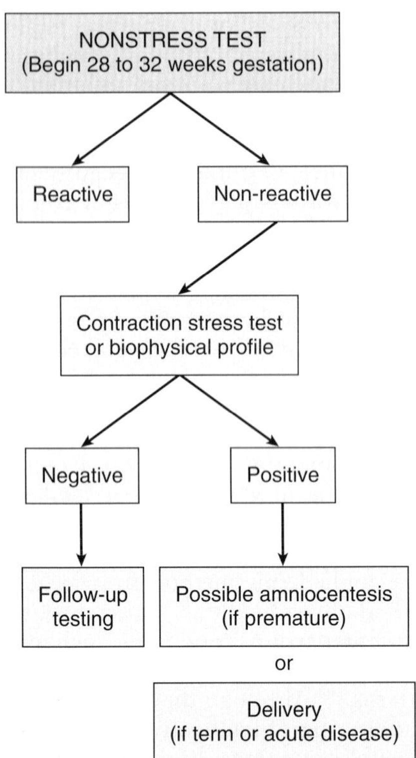

Figure 37-13. Scheme for antepartum fetal testing.

Table 37-10. Antepartum Fetal Surveillance in Low-Risk Insulin Dependent Diabetes Mellitus*

STUDY	
Ultrasonography at 4–6 week intervals	Yes
Maternal assessment of fetal activity, daily at 28 weeks	Yes
Nonstress test (NST) weekly at 28 weeks	Yes Twice weekly at 34 weeks
Contraction stress test or biophysical profile if NST nonreactive; L/S, lung profile	Yes, if elective delivery planned prior to 39 weeks

*Low-risk IDDM: excellent control (160–120 mg/dl), no vasculopathy (classes B, C), no stillbirth.
L/S, lecithin/sphingomyelin ratio.

Table 37-11. Antepartum Fetal Surveillance in High-Risk Insulin Dependent Diabetes Mellitus*

STUDY	
Ultrasonography at 4–6 week intervals	Yes
Maternal assessment of fetal activity, daily at 28 weeks	Yes
Nonstress test (NST)	Minimum twice weekly
Contraction stress test or biophysical profile if NST nonreactive; L/S, lung profile at 37–38 weeks	Yes

*High-risk IDDM: poor control (macrosomia, hydramnios), vasculopathy (classes D, F, R), prior stillbirth.
L/S, lecithin/sphingomyelin ratio.

preeclampsia in these high-risk patients.[213] In contrast, patients with well-controlled diabetes without vascular disease rarely demonstrate abnormal fetal umbilical artery waveforms.

Johnstone and colleagues[214] have reported the largest experience with serial Doppler umbilical waveforms in pregnancies complicated by diabetes. In their study of 128 women, significant abnormal flow patterns were observed in nine cases. Three of these women had nephropathy, and three had preeclampsia. All of these pregnancies had normal outcomes. Importantly, several cases of fetal distress as defined by abnormal biophysical testing were accompanied by normal Doppler studies. Therefore, it appears that undue reliance should *not* be placed on normal waveform values in the diabetic pregnancy.[214]

It is important to include not only the results of antepartum fetal testing but to weigh all of the clinical features involving mother and fetus before a decision is made to intervene for suspected fetal distress, especially if this decision may result in a preterm delivery (Tables 37-10 and 37-11). In reviewing nine series involving 993 diabetic patients, an abnormal test of fetal condition led to delivery 5 percent of the time.[215] It appears that outpatient testing protocols work well in diabetic patients requiring insulin. Whether such testing is required for all women with diabetes mellitus remains controversial.[216] In a study of 114 women with well-controlled IDDM, 10 patients were delivered for abnormal fetal testing. Eight of these 10 women had nephropathy or hypertension. Nephropathy or hypertension was associated with intervention for fetal well-being in 8 of 20 women with these risk factors in comparison with 2 of 94 without these complications. Thus, it appears that women whose diabetes is poorly controlled, who have hypertension, or who have significant vasculopathy that may be associated with fetal growth restriction are at increased risk for fetal compromise and probably benefit most from a program of antepartum fetal surveillance.[217]

Ultrasound is a valuable tool in evaluating fetal growth, estimating fetal weight, and detecting hydramnios and malformations. A determination of maternal serum alpha-fetoprotein (MSAFP) at 16 weeks' gestation is often employed in association with a detailed ultrasound study during the midtrimester in an attempt to detect neural tube defects and other anomalies. Normal values of MSAFP for diabetic women are lower than in the nondiabetic population.[218] A lower threshold for the upper limit of normal, 1.5 multiples of the median, thus may be preferable in pregnancies complicated by diabetes mellitus in order to help detect spina bifida and other major malformations that are increased in this population. A comprehensive ultrasound examination including fetal echocardiography is performed at 20 to 22 weeks' gestation for the investigation of possible cardiac anomalies. Using such an approach, Greene and Benacerraf[219] detected 18 of 32 malformations in a series of 432 diabetic pregnancies. The specificity was in excess of 99 percent, and the negative predictive value was 97 percent. Spina bifida was identified in all cases; however, ventricular septal defects, limb abnormalities, and facial clefts were missed. A review of the prenatal diagnosis experience in 289 women with IDDM in The Ohio State University Diabetes in Pregnancy Program revealed 29 anomalies in which 12 were cardiac, 14 were noncardiac, and 3 were combined.[87] Twelve of fifteen (80 percent) cardiac and 10 of 17 (59 percent) noncardiac lesions were identified prenatally. When considering cardiac defects alone, we could not identify a glycosylated hemoglobin cutoff for these anomalies. Therefore, we believe detailed cardiac imaging should be offered to all patients with type 1 and type 2 diabetes mellitus to assist in the detection of cardiac lesions, especially those of the great vessels and cardiac septum.

Ultrasound examinations should be performed during the third trimester to assess fetal growth. The detection of fetal macrosomia, the leading risk factor for shoulder dystocia, is important in the selection of patients who are best delivered by cesarean section. An increased rate of cephalopelvic disproportion and shoulder dystocia accompanied by significant risk of traumatic birth injury and asphyxia have been consistently associated with the vaginal delivery of large infants. The risk of such complications rises exponentially when birth weight exceeds 4 kg and is greater for the fetus of a diabetic mother when compared with a fetus with similar weight whose mother does not have diabetes.[220] Sonographic measurements of the fetal abdominal circumference have proved most helpful in predicting fetal macrosomia.[221] The abdomen is likely to be large because of increased glycogen deposition in the fetal liver and subcutaneous fat deposition. Using serial sonographic examinations, accelerated abdominal growth can often be identified by 32 weeks' gestation.[222]

TIMING AND MODE OF DELIVERY

Delivery should be delayed until fetal maturation has taken place, provided that the patient's diabetes is well controlled and antepartum surveillance remains normal. In our practice, elective induction of labor is often planned at 38 1/2 to 40 weeks' gestation in well-controlled patients without vascular disease. Patients with vascular disease are delivered before term only if hypertension worsens, if significant fetal growth restriction is present, or if biophysical testing mandates early delivery. Before elective delivery prior to 39 weeks' gestation, an amniocentesis may be performed to document fetal pulmonary maturity. There is much evidence that tests of fetal lung maturity have the same predictive value in diabetic pregnancies as they do in the normal population.[125]

The presence of the acidic phospholipid phosphatidylglycerol (PG) is the final marker of fetal pulmonary maturation. Several authors have suggested that fetal hyperinsulinemia may be associated with delayed appearance of PG and an increased incidence of RDS. Landon et al.[109] have correlated the appearance of PG in amniotic fluid with maternal glycemic control during gestation. RDS may occur in the IDM with a mature L/S ratio or fetal lung maturity index but absent PG. Moore and colleagues[223] compared PG production in amniotic fluid specimens from 295 diabetic women and 590 matched controls. These authors reported that the onset of PG production was delayed in GDM from 35.9 ± 1.1 weeks to 37.3 ± 1.0 weeks and to 38.7 ± 0.9 weeks in pregestational diabetic pregnancies.[223] In this study, delayed appearance of PG was not associated with level of glycemic control. It follows that the clinician must be familiar with the laboratory analysis of amniotic fluid in his or her institution and the neonatal outcome associated with various tests of fetal lung maturity.

When antepartum testing suggests fetal compromise, delivery must be considered. If amniotic fluid analysis yields a mature test result, delivery should be accomplished promptly. In the presence of presumed lung immaturity, the decision to proceed with delivery should be based on confirmation of deteriorating fetal condition by several abnormal tests. For example, if the NST as well as the BPP indicates fetal compromise, delivery is indicated. Finally, there are several maternal indications for delivery including significant preeclampsia, worsening renal function, or deteriorating vision secondary to proliferative retinopathy. If a patient reaches term gestation with a mature fetal lung profile and is at significant risk for intrauterine demise because of poor control or a history of a prior stillbirth, delivery is planned.

Choosing the route of delivery for the diabetic patient remains controversial. Cesarean delivery rates as high as 50 percent are common in series of pregestational diabetic women. This figure is likely to represent the practice trends of most U.S. obstetricians and perinatologists.[210] Delivery by cesarean section usually is favored when fetal distress has been suggested by antepartum heart rate monitoring.

The increased rate of shoulder dystocia and brachial plexus injury in the offspring of diabetic women has prompted adoption of early induction strategies as well as selection of patients for cesarean section based on ultrasound estimation of fetal size. Such approaches are limited by the relative inaccuracy of ultrasound prediction of birth weight. Despite the limitations, Kjos and colleagues demonstrated that induction at 38 weeks in a population of women with GDM was associated with a lower frequency of large-for-gestational age infants and shoulder dystocia without an increased rate of cesarean delivery.[224] This is in contrast to studies of induction in nondiabetic women in which suspected macrosomia is apparently associated with an increased rate of cesarean delivery. In a sophisticated *decision tree* analysis of cost effectiveness, Rouse and colleagues found that whereas elective cesarean delivery for macrosomia to prevent permanent brachial plexus injury was prohibitively expensive in the non-diabetic woman at a cost of several million dollars per permanent brachial plexus injury prevented, 489 cesarean deliveries at a cost/avoided birth injury of $880,000 per case for those diabetic pregnancies with an estimated fetal size greater than 4,000 g seemed to be at least tenable.[225]

Acker et al.[226] have reported that the overall risk for shoulder dystocia in the macrosomic IDM is greater than for the large, normal infant. In their series of diabetic women, the risk for shoulder dystocia with a fetal weight greater than 4,000 g was approximately 30 percent. Somewhat less impressive, yet significantly greater fre-

Table 37-12. Rate of Shoulder Dystocia Related to Birth Weight and Diabetic Status

BIRTH WEIGHT (G)	WITHOUT DIABETES (%)	WITH DIABETES (%)
<4,000	0.1–1.1	0.6–3.7
4,000–4,449	1.1–10.0	4.9–23.1
≥4,500	4.1–22.6	20.0–50.0

Adapted from ACOG Practice Patterns No. 7. October 1997.

quencies of shoulder dystocia for delivery of macrosomic IDMs versus non-IDMs have been reported by Nesbitt and colleagues (Table 37-12).[220] At present, ACOG recommends consideration of cesarean delivery in diabetic women when estimated fetal weight exceeds 4,500 g.[227] Our approach is to consider elective cesarean when the estimated weight is 4,000 to 4,500 g, taking into consideration obstetric history and clinical pelvimetry. Despite attempts to select patients with obvious fetal macrosomia for elective cesarean delivery, arrest of dilatation or descent despite adequate labor should alert the physician to the possibility of cephalopelvic disproportion. About 25 percent of macrosomic infants (>4,000 g) delivered after a prolonged second stage have shoulder dystocia.[228] It follows that cesarean delivery should be considered in a patient who demonstrates significant protracted labor or failure of descent.

GLUCOREGULATION DURING LABOR AND DELIVERY

Because neonatal hypoglycemia is in part related to maternal glucose levels during labor, it is important to maintain maternal plasma glucose levels within the physiologic normal range. The patient is given nothing by mouth after midnight of the evening before induction or elective cesarean delivery. The usual bedtime dose of insulin is administered, or for women receiving pump therapy, the infusion is continued overnight. Upon arrival to the labor and delivery department, early in the morning, the patient's capillary glucose level is assessed with a bedside reflectance meter. Continuous infusion of both insulin and glucose are then administered based on maternal glucose levels (Table 37-13). Ten units of short acting insulin may be added to 1,000 ml of solution containing 5 percent dextrose. An infusion rate of 100 to 125 ml/h (1 unit/h), in most cases, will result in good glucose control. Insulin may also be infused from a syringe pump at a dose of 0.25 to 2.0 units/h and adjusted to maintain normal glucose values. Glucose levels are recorded hourly, and the infusion rate is adjusted accordingly. Well-controlled patients are often euglycemic once active labor begins and then require glucose at an infusion rate of 2.5 mg/kg/min.[229] It may be necessary to increase the insulin infusion during the second stage of labor in response to hyperglycemia associated with increased catecholamine secretion.

When cesarean delivery is to be performed, it should be scheduled for early morning. This simplifies intrapartum glucose control and allows the neonatal team to prepare for the care of the newborn. The patient is given nothing by mouth, and her usual morning insulin dose is withheld. If her surgery is not performed early in the day, one third to one half of the patient's intermediate-acting dose of insulin may be administered. Regional anesthesia is employed because an awake patient permits earlier detection of hypoglycemia. Following surgery, glucose levels are monitored every 2 hours and an intravenous solution of 5 percent dextrose is administered.

Table 37-13. Insulin Management During Labor and Delivery

Usual dose of intermediate-acting insulin is given at bedtime.
Morning dose of insulin is withheld
Intravenous infusion of normal saline is begun
Once active labor begins or glucose levels fall below 70 mg/dl, the infusion is changed from saline to 5% dextrose and delivered at a rate of 2.5 mg/kg/min.
Glucose levels are checked hourly using a portable reflectance meter allowing for adjustment in the infusion rate.
Regular (short-acting) insulin is administered by intravenous infusion if glucose levels exceed 140 mg/dl.

From Jovanovic L, Peterson CM: Management of the pregnant, insulin-dependent diabetic woman. Diabetes Care 3:63, 1980.

Following delivery, insulin requirements are usually significantly lower than were pregnancy or prepregnancy needs. The objective of tight control used in the antepartum period is relaxed for the first 24 to 48 hours. Patients delivered vaginally, who are able to eat a regular diet, are given one third to one half of their end of pregnancy dose of neutral protamine Hagedorn (NPH) insulin and short-acting or rapid-acting insulin the morning of the first postpartum day. Frequent glucose determinations are used to guide insulin dosage. Most patients are stabilized on this regimen within a few days after delivery.

Women with diabetes are encouraged to breast-feed. The additional 500 kcal required daily are given as approximately 100 g of carbohydrate and 20 g of protein.[230] The insulin dose may be somewhat lower in lactating diabetic women. Hypoglycemia appears to be common in the first week following delivery and immediately after nursing.

MANAGEMENT OF THE PATIENT WITH GESTATIONAL DIABETES

The mainstay of treatment of GDM is nutritional counseling and dietary intervention. The optimal diet should provide caloric and nutrient needs to sustain pregnancy without resulting in significant postprandial hyperglycemia.[231] Women with GDM generally do not need hospitalization for dietary instruction and management. Once the diagnosis is established, patients are begun on a dietary program of 2,000 to 2,500 kcal daily.[231] This represents approximately 35 kcal/kg of present pregnancy weight. Jovanovic-Peterson and Peterson[232] have noted that such a diet composed of 50 to 60 percent carbohydrate will cause excessive weight gain and postprandial hyperglycemia, and require insulin therapy in 50 percent of patients. For this reason, several groups have studied the use of calorie restricted diets.[233] Algert and colleagues[233] have reported that obese women with GDM may be managed on as little as 1,700 to 1,800 kcal/day with less weight gain and no apparent reduction in fetal size. Magee et al.[234] designed a study to evaluate strict caloric restriction as a treatment for obese subjects with GDM. They randomized patients to a 2,400 kcal/d diet compared with a 1,200 kcal/d group. Average glucose levels and fasting glucose were reduced in the hypocaloric group. However, fasting glucose levels and postchallenge glucose levels were not significantly different. Significant ketonuria did develop in the calorie-restricted group, which may have a detrimental effect on fetal neurologic development.[235] Thus, the authors went on to study a 1,800 kcal diet, which improved glycemia and did not increase serum ketone levels.[236] Similar results have been reported by Jovanovic-Peterson and Peterson, who recommend 30 kcal/kg present pregnant weight for normal weight women, 24 kcal/kg for overweight women, and 12 kcal/kg for morbidly obese women.[237] These authors indicate that mild caloric restriction with modification of the carbohydrate component may be advised in obese GDM women.[238]

Once the patient with GDM is placed on an appropriate diet, surveillance of blood glucose levels is necessary to be certain that glycemic control has been established. At a minimum, practitioners have performed weekly assessment of fasting or postprandial glucose levels or both at clinic or office visits. Some clinicians prefer to have patients perform daily self–blood glucose monitoring, which in two retrospective studies has been associated with a decline in macrosomia at the expense of nearly half of all women requiring insulin therapy.[239,240] A practical approach may be to provide women with GDM with a reflectance meter; however, if after a few weeks, both fasting and postprandial measurements are within the normal range, the frequency of testing can be reduced and tailored accordingly.

Whereas the ACOG have recommended that fasting plasma glucose levels be maintained below 105 mg/dl and 2-hour postprandial values be less than 120 mg/dl in women with GDM, thresholds of a fasting glucose less than 95 mg/dl and 1-hour postprandial glucose less than 140 mg/dl, as well as 2-hour postprandial glucose less than 120 mg/dl have been suggested by the Fourth International Workshop Conference.[241] If a patient repetitively exceeds these thresholds, then insulin therapy is suggested. The use of the above-mentioned cutoffs for initiating insulin are based on data regarding increased perinatal morbidity when such values are exceeded in women with preexisting diabetes. At present, there are no data from controlled trials to identify ideal glycemic targets for prevention of fetal risk for women with GDM.

Langer and colleagues[242] have critically evaluated thresholds for insulin therapy in patients with GDM and concluded that to evaluate the effect of therapy, appropriate endpoints should include fetal macrosomia or LGA infants, and neonatal metabolic complications. Langer and colleagues[242] evaluated insulin secretion patterns in women with GDM and non-GDM during an oral GTT. Patients with a fasting plasma glucose less than 95 mg/dl had significantly greater insulin production than those with a glucose level of 95 mg/dl. To test whether the assignment to insulin therapy for a patient with a fasting value of 95 mg/dl or higher was appropriate, Langer et al.[242] compared rates of delivery of LGA infants among women with GDM grouped according to their fasting plasma glucose levels and whether diet or diet and insulin were used. They found that patients with a fasting glucose between 96 and 105 mg/dl had a greater incidence of LGA infants (28.6 percent) when receiving diet therapy alone versus obese women with GDM receiving both diet and insulin. In women with an initial fasting glucose between 95 and 104 mg/dl, 70 percent required insulin therapy to achieve optimal control.[243]

Whereas Langer and coworkers[240] have documented a relationship between maternal glycemia and macrosomia in GDM, which would establish guidelines for insulin therapy, some authors have suggested that estimation of glycemia alone may not be sufficient to optimally prescribe insulin therapy in these cases. Buchanan and colleagues[244] have reviewed the utility of fetal ultrasound measurements to guide insulin therapy in women with GDM. In their study of diet-treated patients with GDM, ultrasound preformed at 29 to 33 weeks was used to identify pregnancies with fetuses having a large abdominal circumference (>75th percentile). These patients were then randomized to diet versus diet and insulin treatment. The insulin-treated group ultimately had a frequency of LGA infants of 13 percent, which was far below the 45 percent present in the diet-treated group. The cost-effectiveness of this approach needs to be compared with administration of insulin to women with fasting hyperglycemia on diet therapy, because approximately two thirds of women require insulin therapy for a large fetal abdominal circumference on ultrasound examination in this range of maternal glycemia.

Finally, oral hypoglycemic therapy has emerged as a suitable alternative to insulin treatment in women with GDM.[245] In 2000, Langer and colleagues reported a randomized trial of 404 women receiving insulin versus glyburide and reported similar improvement in glycemia with both regimens. The frequency of macrosomia and neonatal hypoglycemia was similar in the two study groups. Only 4 percent of women failed glyburide therapy, requiring a change to insulin. Cord blood analysis revealed no detectable glyburide in exposed pregnancies. Subsequently, several smaller studies reported success in achieving good glycemic control with glyburide, but with slightly higher failure rates (15 to 20 percent).[225,246–248] Jacobson and colleagues[249] recently reported on the implementation of glyburide as an alternative to insulin in a large managed care organization. These authors noted a similar frequency of LGA infants and macrosomia among 268 women treated with insulin compared with 236 receiving glyburide. In this nonrandomized study, more women in the glyburide group achieved lower mean fasting and postprandial glucose levels compared with insulin-treated subjects. Importantly, the authors noted an increased rate of preeclampsia, need for neonatal phototherapy, and birth injury in the "glyburide group," all of which point to the need for further study concerning safety.[250] Along with such studies, it is likely that other oral agents will also be evaluated for use during pregnancy.

Bung and colleagues[251] conducted a prospective study of the utility of exercise in the treatment of GDM. These authors randomized 41 women with GDM who manifested elevated fasting glucose levels and would normally require insulin therapy. In the final analysis, 17 women completed a supervised bicycle ergometry training program compared with 17 women receiving insulin treatment. No statistical differences were observed in weekly blood glucose determinations between study groups. All fetal heart rate patterns were reactive before and after exercise. Thus, regular exercise may be an effective treatment for GDM. Brisk walking for 30 minutes at least three times each week may be recommended. Because the total number of women with GDM studied in randomized trials is limited, the role of exercise as a primary therapy in GDM is unknown.[252]

Patients with GDM who are well controlled are at low risk for an intrauterine death. For this reason, we do not routinely institute antepartum fetal heart rate testing in uncomplicated diet-controlled GDM patients unless the patient has a hypertensive disorder, a history of a prior stillbirth, or suspected macrosomia.[253] Women in these categories as well as those who require insulin treatment of GDM undergo twice-weekly heart rate testing at 32 weeks' gestation. Women with uncomplicated GDM do undergo fetal heart rate testing at 40 weeks' gestation. Using such a protocol at The Ohio State University Hospital Diabetes in Pregnancy Program, only three intrauterine deaths in more than 2,000 patients with uncomplicated GDM have been observed in the last 16 years. Thus, it appears that the third-trimester stillbirth rate in these patients is no higher than that of the general obstetric population. A study of 389 women with GDM documented an antepartum stillbirth rate of 7.7 per 10,000, which was not significantly different from the rate of 4.8 per 1,000 observed in nondiabetic low-risk patients.[254] In this study, because 7 percent of fetuses were delivered on the basis of a low BPP score, the benefit of testing all GDM pregnancies remains in question. At present, without a large prospective study comparing outcomes in monitored and nonmonitored women with GDM without other risk factors, it is not possible to determine if any benefits exist to antepartum fetal surveillance in this seemingly low-risk population.

For pregnancies determined to be at sufficient risk to undergo testing, a biweekly regimen appears to be preferable to weekly testing. In a series of 1,390 women with GDM, there were no antepartum stillbirths within 4 days of a reassuring test, whereas two fetal deaths occurred at 28 and 36 weeks, respectively, in insulin-requiring women 1 week after negative testing.[255]

Because many obstetricians have extrapolated the increased risk for stillbirth in women with type 1 and type 2 diabetes to those with GDM, a remarkable number of these pregnancies are subject to scheduled delivery at term. If glycemic control is suboptimal, or maternal hypertension or a previous stillbirth exists, such an approach seems warranted. The use of amniocentesis to document fetal lung maturity in such cases should be based on clinical circumstances. As with antepartum fetal testing, in the otherwise uncomplicated group, should elective induction be the standard approach for these pregnancies complicated by GDM? Lurie and coworkers[256] have in part addressed this issue by retrospectively examining the outcomes of 124 women with GDM delivered beyond 40 weeks' gestation compared with the same number of women with GDM delivered before their expected date of confinement. Antepartum fetal surveillance was not routinely begun until 40 weeks' gestation. No significant differences in perinatal outcome, rates of cesarean delivery, or shoulder dystocia were found between study groups. A vaginal delivery rate of 75.8 percent was achieved in women with GDM delivering beyond 40 weeks' gestation. These authors concluded that elective induction before 40 weeks' gestation should be avoided and every attempt should be made to allow women with GDM, both diet and insulin treated, to proceed to spontaneous labor. In contrast, a follow-up prospective study from the same institution of 96 insulin-requiring patients with GDM demonstrated that induction at 38 to 39 weeks was associated with a 1.4 percent shoulder dystocia rate versus 10.2 percent in historic controls.[257]

Kjos and colleagues[224] conducted a prospective randomized trial of active induction of labor at 38 weeks' gestation versus expectant management in a series which included 187 insulin-requiring women with GDM. The cesarean delivery rate was not significantly different in the expectant-management group (31 percent) from the active-induction group (25 percent). However, an increased prevalence of LGA infants (23 percent versus 10 percent) was observed in the expectant management group. Moreover, the frequency of shoulder dystocia was 3 percent in this group, with no cases reported in those undergoing induction at 38 weeks' gestation. These data led the authors to conclude that scheduled elective induction be considered in insulin-requiring patients with GDM because it does not increase the risk of cesarean delivery and lowers the risk for fetal death. In patients managed expectantly, careful monitoring of fetal growth should be performed because of an apparent increasing risk for macrosomia with advancing gestational age in this population.

COUNSELING THE DIABETIC PATIENT

Anomalies of the cardiac, renal, and central nervous systems arise during the first 7 weeks of gestation, a time when it is most unusual for patients to seek prenatal care. Therefore, the management and counseling of women with diabetes in the reproductive age group should begin before conception. Unfortunately, it has been estimated that less than 20 percent of diabetic women in the United States obtain prepregnancy counseling.[210] Prepregnancy counseling includes an assessment of vascular status and glycemic control. Physicians who care for young women with diabetes must be aware of the importance of such counseling. At this time, the nonpregnant patient may learn techniques for self glucose monitoring as well as the

Table 37-14. Comparative Rates of Major Malformations in Offspring of Diabetic Women Receiving Preconceptional Counseling

STUDY	WITH PRECONCEPTIONAL COUNSELING	WITHOUT PRECONCEPTIONAL COUNSELING
Fuhrmann et al[259]	1/128 (0.8%)	22/292 (7.5%)
Steel et al[275]	2/143 (1.4%)	10/96 (10.4%)
Kitzmiller et al[260]	1/84 (1.2%)	12/110 (10.9%)
Whillhoite et al[264]	1/62 (1.6%)	8/123 (6.5%)

need for proper dietary management. Folic acid dietary supplementation at a dose of at least 0.4 mg daily should be prescribed because there is increasing evidence that this vitamin may reduce the frequency of neural tube defects although it has not specifically been studied in the diabetic population. During counseling, questions may be answered regarding risk factors for complications and the plan for general management of diabetes in pregnancy. Planning for pregnancy should optimally be accomplished over several months. Glycosylated hemoglobin measurements are performed to aid in the timing of conception.

A reduced rate of major congenital malformation in patients optimally managed before conception is observed with special diabetes clinics (Table 37-14). In Copenhagen, the rate of malformations fell from 19.4 percent to 8.5 percent in class D and F patients who attended a prepregnancy clinic.[258] Fuhrmann et al.[259] found that intensive treatment begun before conception in 307 East German diabetic women reduced the malformation rate to 1 percent. Nearly 90 percent of women in this study maintained mean glucose levels less than 100 mg/dl (5.6 mmol/L). In contrast, the incidence of anomalies in the offspring of 593 diabetic women who registered for care after 8 weeks' gestation was 8.0 percent (47/593). Only 205 of those women had mean daily glucose levels of less than 100 mg/dl (5.6 mmol/L). Mills et al.[97] have reported that diabetic women registered before pregnancy had fewer infants with anomalies when compared with late registrants (4.9 versus 9.0 percent). Although the incidence of 4.9 percent remains higher than that in a normal control population (2 percent), normalization of glycemia was not established in the early entry group.

Kitzmiller and colleagues[260] studied 84 women with pregestational diabetes mellitus who were recruited for preconception education and management during a 7-year period. A group of 110 pregnancies in women with IDDM presenting in the first trimester without preconceptional counseling served as controls in this study. One anomaly (1.2 percent) occurred in the preconception group versus 12 (10.9 percent) malformations in the control population.

Glycosylated hemoglobin levels obtained during the first trimester may be used to counsel diabetic women regarding the risk for an anomalous infant. In a retrospective study of 116 women at the Joslin Clinic, Miller and colleagues[261] observed that elevated hemoglobin A_{1c} concentrations early in pregnancy correlated with an increased incidence of malformations. In 58 patients with elevated glycosylated hemoglobin levels, 13 (22 percent) malformed infants were noted. This is in contrast to a 3.4-percent incidence of major malformations in 58 women whose glycosylated hemoglobin levels were in the normal range. Overall, the risk of a major fetal anomaly may be as high as 25 percent when the glycosylated hemoglobin level is several percent above normal values. Greene[262] has reported that 14 of 35 pregnancies with a glycosylated hemoglobin exceeding 12.8 percent were complicated by major malformations. In his series from the Joslin Clinic, the risk for major anomalies did not become evident until glycosylated hemoglobin values exceed 6 SD above the mean. In contrast to the investigations cited above is the DIEP (Diabetes in Early Pregnancy) study,[89] in which malformation rates in IDMs were not correlated with first trimester maternal glycosylated hemoglobin levels. The authors suggested that more sensitive measures are needed to identify teratogenic mechanisms or that not all malformations can be prevented by good glycemic control. Further review of these data, which included glycosylated hemoglobin levels only in the early entry patients, demonstrates that these women were a relatively homogeneous group with respect to glycemic control; 93 percent had glycosylated hemoglobin levels less than 7 SD below the mean, a level of control which barely increases the risk for anomalies according to Greene's data.[262] Regardless of the glycosylated hemoglobin value obtained, all patients require a careful program of surveillance, as outlined earlier, to detect fetal malformations. The risk for spontaneous abortion also appears to be increased with marked elevations in glycosylated hemoglobin. However, for diabetic women in good control, there appears to be no greater likelihood of miscarriage.[263] In summary, women with type 1 and type 2 diabetes mellitus should be advised to achieve a HbA1c level less than 1 percent above the upper limit of the normal range before conceiving to reduce the risk for a major fetal malformation or miscarriage.

CONTRACEPTION

There is no evidence that diabetes mellitus impairs fertility. Thus, family planning is an important consideration for the diabetic woman. A careful history and complete gynecologic examination and counseling are required before selecting a method of contraception. Barrier methods continue to be a safe and inexpensive method of birth control. The diaphragm, used correctly with a spermicide, has a failure rate of less than 10 percent. Because there are no inherent risks to the diaphragm and other barrier methods, these have become the preferred interim method of contraception for women with diabetes mellitus. The intrauterine device may also be used by diabetic women without concerns about an increased risk of infection.[265]

Combined oral contraceptives (OCs) are the most effective reversible method of contraception with failure rates generally less than 1 percent. There is, however, continued controversy regarding their use in the diabetic woman. The serious side effects of pill use, including thromboembolic disease and myocardial infarction, may be increased in diabetic women using combined OCs. In a retrospective study, Steel and Duncan[266] observed five cardiovascular complications in 136 diabetic women using primary low-dose pills. Three patients had cerebrovascular accidents, one had a myocardial infarction, and one an axillary vein thrombosis. In a recent retrospective case-control study, despite diabetes increasing the risk for cerebral thromboembolism fivefold compared with controls, this risk was not enhanced by use of combined oral contraceptives.[267]

In Steel and Duncan's report, several women exhibited rapid progression of retinopathy. Klein and colleagues[268] studied OC use in a cross-sectional study of 384 insulin dependent women and reported no association between OCs and progression of vascular complications. For physicians who prescribe low-dose OCs to diabetic women, their use should probably be restricted to patients without serious vascular complications or additional risk factors such as a strong family history of myocardial disease or smoking. In these women, a monophasic preparation (progestin only) may be considered. In women receiving oral contraceptives, the lowest dose of estrogen and progesterone should be employed. Patients should have blood pressure monitoring after the first cycle and quarterly with baseline and follow-up lipid levels as well.

Women using OCs may demonstrate increased resistance to insulin as a result of a diminished concentration of insulin receptors.[269] Despite the fact that carbohydrate metabolism may be affected by the progestin component of the pill, disturbances in diabetic control are actually uncommon with its use. In Steel and Duncan's study,[270] 81 percent of patients using the pill did not require a change in insulin dose. Triphasic OCs may also be used safely in former GDM women without other risk factors. Skouby et al.[271] have demonstrated that normal glucose tolerance and lipid levels can be expected in non-obese former GDM women followed after 6 months of therapy. Kjos and colleagues[272] performed a prospective randomized study of 230 women with recent GDM. OC users were randomized to low-dose norethindrone or levonorgestrel preparations in combination with ethinyl estradiol. The rate of subsequent diabetes in OC users was 15 to 20 percent, after one year follow-up. This rate was not significantly different from non-OC users (17 percent). Importantly, no adverse effects on total cholesterol, LDL, HDL, or triglycerides were found with OC use.

At present, there is little information available concerning long-acting progestins in women with diabetes or previous GDM. A statistically significant, yet clinically limited deterioration in carbohydrate tolerance has been reported in healthy depomedroxyprogesterone acetate (Depo-Provera; DMPA) users.[273] As observed with other progestins, DMPA may lower serum triglyceride and HDL-C levels but not total cholesterol or LDL-C.[274] For this reason, DMPA is not recommended as a first line method of contraception for women with diabetes. The progestin-only OC would be preferred because it does not produce significant metabolic effects in diabetic women.

Key Points

- Pregnancy has been characterized as a diabetogenic state because of increased postprandial glucose levels in a late gestation.
- Both hepatic and peripheral (tissue) insulin sensitivity are reduced in normal pregnancy. As a result, a progressive increase in insulin secretion follows a glucose challenge.
- In women with GDM, the hormonal milieu of pregnancy may represent an unmasking of a susceptibility to the development of type 2 diabetes mellitus.
- According to the Pedersen hypothesis, maternal hyperglycemia results in fetal hyperglycemia and hyperinsulinemia, resulting in excessive fetal growth. Tight maternal glycemic control is associated with a reduced risk for fetal macrosomia.
- Congenital malformations occur with a two- to sixfold increased rate in offspring of women with pregestational diabetes compared with the normal population. Impaired glycemic control and associated derangement in maternal metabolism appear to contribute to abnormal embryogenesis.
- Women with class F (nephropathy) diabetes have an increased risk for preeclampsia and preterm delivery that correlates with their degree of renal impairment.
- Diabetes retinopathy may worsen during pregnancy, yet for women optimally treated with laser photocoagulation *before* pregnancy, significant deterioration of vision is uncommon.
- Screening for GDM is generally performed between 24 and 28 weeks' gestation. Screening strategies include universal screening or limiting screening to women over age 25 with risk factors for developing adult-onset diabetes mellitus.
- Treatment of women with type 1 and type 2 diabetes mellitus during pregnancy requires intensive therapy consisting of frequent self–blood glucose monitoring and aggressive insulin dosing by multiple injections or CSII (insulin pump).

❑ The cornerstone of treatment for GDM is dietary therapy. Insulin or glyburide are reserved for individuals who manifest significant fasting hyperglycemia or postprandial glucose elevations despite dietary intervention.

❑ Antepartum fetal assessment for women with both pregestational diabetes or GDM is based on the degree of risk believed to be present in each case. Glycemic control, prior obstetric history, and the presence of vascular disease or hypertension are important considerations.

❑ Delivery should be delayed until fetal maturation has occurred, provided that diabetes is well controlled and fetal surveillance remains normal. The mode of delivery for the suspected large fetus remains controversial. In cases of suspected macrosomia, a low threshold for cesarean delivery has been recommended to prevent a traumatic birth.

❑ Women with type 1 and type 2 diabetes mellitus should seek prepregnancy consultation. Efforts to improve glycemic control before conception have been associated with a significant reduction in the rate of congenital malformations in the offspring of such women.

REFERENCES

1. Weiss PAM, Hoffman H: Intensified conventional insulin therapy for the pregnant diabetic patient. Obstet Gynecol 64:629, 1984.
2. Catalano PM, Tyzbir ED, Roman NM, et al: Longitudinal changes in insulin release and insulin resistance in non-obese pregnant women. Am J Obstet Gynecol 165:1667, 1991.
3. Bellman O, Hartman E: Influence of pregnancy on the kinetics of insulin. Am J Obstet Gynecol 122:829, 1975.
4. Lind T, Bell S, Gilmore E: Insulin disappearance rate in pregnant and non-pregnant women and in non-pregnant women given GHRH. Eur J Clin Invest 7:47, 1977.
5. Burt RL, Davidson IWF: Insulin half-life and utilization in normal pregnancy. Obstet Gynecol 43:161, 1974.
6. Goodner CJ, Freinkel N: Carbohydrate metabolism in pregnancy: The degradation of insulin by extracts of maternal and fetal structures in the pregnant rat. Endocrinology 65:957, 1959.
7. Catalano PM, Drago NM, Amini SB: Longitudinal changes in pancreatic b cell function and metabolic clearance rate of insulin in pregnant women with normal and abnormal glucose tolerance. Diabetes Care 21:403, 1998.
8. Kalhan SC, D'Angelo LJ, Savin SM, et al: Glucose production in pregnant women at term gestation: Sources of glucose for human fetus. J Clin Invest 63:388, 1979.
9. Cowett RA, Susa JB, Kahn CB, et al: Glucose kinetics in nondiabetic and diabetic women during the third trimester of pregnancy. Am J Obstet Gynecol 146:773, 1983.
10. Catalano PM, Tyzbir ED, Wolfe RR, et al: Longitudinal changes in basal hepatic glucose production and suppression during insulin infusion in normal pregnant women. Am J Obstet Gynecol 167:913, 1992.
11. Sivan E, Chen X, Hombo CJ, et al: Longitudinal study of carbohydrate metabolism in healthy obese women. Diabetes Care 20:1470, 1997.
12. Pacini G, Bergman RN: MINMOD: A computer program to calculate insulin sensitivity and pancreatic responsitivity from the frequently sampled intravenous glucose tolerance test. Comput Methods Programs Biomed 23:113, 986.
13. DeFronzo RA, Tobin JD, Andres R: Glucose clamp technique: A method for quantifying insulin secretion and resistance. Am J Physiol 237:E214, 1979.
14. Catalano PM, Tyzbir ED, Wolfe RR, et al: Carbohydrate metabolism during pregnancy in control subjects and women with gestational diabetes. Am J Physiol 264:E60, 1993.
15. Catalano PM, Huston L, Amini SB, Kalhan SC: Longitudinal changes in glucose metabolism during pregnancy in obese women with normal glucose tolerance and gestational diabetes. Am J Obstet Gynecol 180:903, 1999.
16. Spellacy WN, Goetz FC, Greenberg BZ, et al: Plasma insulin normal "early" pregnancy. Obstet Gynecol 25:862, 1965.
17. Burt RL: Peripheral utilization of glucose in pregnancy. III Insulin intolerance. Obstet Gynecol 2:558, 1956.
18. Fisher PM, Sutherland HW, Bewsher PD: The insulin response to glucose infusion in normal human pregnancy. Diabetologia 19:15, 1980.
19. Buchanan TZ, Metzger BE, Freinkel N, et al: Insulin sensitivity and β-cell responsiveness to glucose during late pregnancy in lean and moderately obese women with normal glucose tolerance or mild gestational diabetes. Am J Obstet Gynecol 162:1008, 1990.
20. Ryan EA, O'Sullivan MJ, Skyler JS: Insulin action during pregnancy. Studies with the euglycemic clamp technique. Diabetes 34:380, 1985.
21. Hay WW, Sparks JW, Wilkening RB, et al: Partition of maternal glucose production between conceptus and maternal tissue in sheep. Am J Physiol 234:E347, 1983.
22. Marconi AM, Paolini C, Buscaglia M, et al: The impact of gestational age and fetal growth on the maternal-fetal glucose concentration difference. Obstet Gynecol 87:937, 1996.
23. Kirwan JP, Hauguel-de Mouzon S, Lepercq J, et al: TNFα is a predictor of insulin resistance in human pregnancy. Diabetes 51:2207, 2002.
24. Barros LF, Yudilevich DL, Jarvis SM, et al: Quantitation and immunolocalization of glucose transporters in the human placenta. Placenta 16:623, 1995.
25. Jansson T, Wennergren M, Illsley NP: Glucose transporter expression and distribution in the human placenta throughout gestation and in intrauterine growth retardation. J Clin Endocrinol Metab 77:1554, 1993.
26. Hauguel-de Mouzon S, Challier J, Kacemi A, et al: The GLUT3 glucose transporter isoform is differentially expressed with the human placental cell types. J Clin Endocrinol Metab 82:2689, 1997.
27. Xing A, Cauzac M, Challier J, et al: Unexpected expression of GLUT 4 glucose transporter in villous stromal cells of human placenta. J Clin Endocrinol Metab 83:4097, 1999.
28. White P: Pregnancy complicating diabetes. Am J Med 7:609, 1949.
29. Ellard S, Beards F, Allen LIS, et al: A high prevalence of the glucokinase mutation in gestational diabetic subjects selected by dual criteria. Diabetalogia 43:250, 2000.
30. Stoffel M, Bell MK, Blackburn CC, et al: Identification of glucokinase mutations in subjects with gestational diabetes mellitus. Diabetes 42:937, 1993.
31. Diamond MP, Reece EA, Caprios L, et al: Impairment of counter regulatory hormone responses to hypoglycemia in pregnant women with insulin-dependent diabetes mellitus. Am J Obstet Gynecol 166:70, 1992.
32. Rosenn BM, Miodovnik M, Khoury JC, et al: Counter regulatory hormonal responses to hypoglycemic during pregnancy. Obstet Gynecol 87:568, 1996.
33. McManus RM, Ryan EA: Insulin requirements in insulin-dependent and insulin-requiring GDM women during the final month of pregnancy. Diabetes Care 15:1323, 1992.
34. Schmitz O, Klebe J, Moller, J, et al: In vivo insulin action in type 1 (insulin-dependent) diabetic pregnant women as assessed by the insulin clamp technique. J Clin Endocrinol Metab 61:877, 1985.
35. Jansson T, Powell TL: Glucose transport and GLUT1 expression are upregulated in placentas from pregnancies complicated by severe diabetes (abstract). Placenta 18:A30, 1997.
36. Sims EAH, Calles-Escadon J: Classification of diabetes: A fresh look for the 1990s? Diabetes Care 13:1123, 1990.
37. Steel JM, Irvine WJ, Clark BJ: The significance of pancreatic islet cell antibody and abnormal glucose tolerance during pregnancy. J Clin Lab Immunol 4:83, 1980.

38. Ginsberg-Fellner F, Mark EM, Nechemias C, et al: Autoantibodies to islet cells: Comparison of methods. (Letter.). Lancet 2:1218, 1982.
39. Catalano PM, Tyzbir ED, Sims EAH: Incidence and significance of islet cell antibodies in women with previous gestational diabetes mellitus. Diabetes Care 13:478, 1990.
40. Ward WK, Johnson CLW, Beard JC, et al: Abnormalities of islet β-cell function, insulin action and fat distribution in women with histories of gestational diabetes: Relationship to obesity. J Clin Endocrinol Metab 61:1039, 1985.
41. Catalano PM, Bernstein IM, Wolfe RR, et al: Subclinical abnormalities of glucose metabolism in subjects with previous gestational diabetes. Am J Obstet Gynecol 166:1255, 1986.
42. Ryan EA, Imes S, Liu D, et al: Defects in insulin secretion and action in women with a history of gestational diabetes. Diabetes 44:506, 1995.
43. Yen SCC, Tsai CC, Vela P: Gestational diabetogenesis: Quantitative analysis of glucose-insulin interrelationship between normal pregnancy and pregnancy with gestational diabetes. Am J Obstet Gynecol 111:792, 1971.
44. Fisher PM, Sutherland HW, Bewsher PD: The insulin response to glucose infusion in gestational diabetes. Diabetologia 19:14, 1980.
45. Xiang AH, Peters RH, Trigo E, et al: Multiple metabolic defects during late pregnancy in women at high risk for type 2 diabetes. Diabetes 48:848, 1999.
46. Catalano PM, Roman-Drago N, Amini SB, Sims EAH: Longitudinal changes in body composition and energy balance in lean women with normal and abnormal glucose tolerance during pregnancy. Am J Obstet Gynecol 179:156, 1998.
47. Bergman RN, Philips LS, Cobelli C: Physiologic evaluation of factors controlling glucose disposition in man. Measurement of insulin sensitivity and β-cell sensitivity from the response to intravenous glucose. J Clin Invest 68:1457, 1981.
48. Buchanan TA: Pancreatic β-cell defects in gestational diabetes: Implications for the pathogenesis and prevention of type 2 diabetes. J Clin Endocrinol Metab 86:898, 2001.
49. Garvey WT, Maianu L, Hancock JA, et al: Gene expression of GLUT4 in skeletal muscle from insulin-resistance patients with obesity, IGT, GDM, and NIDDM. Diabetes 41:465, 1992.
50. Friedman JE, Ishizuka T, Shao J, et al: Impaired glucose transport and insulin receptor tyrosine phosphorylation in skeletal muscle from obese women with gestational diabetes. Diabetes 48:1807, 1999.
51. Hytten FE, Leitch I: The gross composition of the components of weight gain. In Landis EM, Pappenheimer JR (eds): The Physiology of Human Pregnancy, 2nd ed. London, Blackwell Scientific, 1971, p 371.
52. Metzger BD, Unger RH, Freinkel N: Carbohydrate metabolism in pregnancy. XIV. Relationships between circulation glucagon, insulin, glucose and amino acids in response to a "mixed meal" in late pregnancy. Metabolism 26:151, 1977.
53. Freinkel N, Metzger BE, Nitzan M, et al: "Accelerated starvation" and mechanisms for the conservation of maternal nitrogen during pregnancy. Israel J Med Sci 8:426, 1972.
54. Kalkhoff RK, Kandaraki E, Morrow PG, et al: Relationship between neonatal birth weight and maternal plasma amino acids profiles in lean and obese nondiabetic women with type 1 diabetic pregnant women. Metabolism 37:234, 1988.
55. Ogata ES: The small for gestational age neonate. *In* Consell RM (ed): Principles of Perinatal-Neonatal Metabolism, 2nd ed. New York, Springer-Verlag, 1998, p 1097.
56. Duggleby SC, Jackson AA: Protein, amino acid and nitrogen metabolism during pregnancy: How might the mother meet the needs of her fetus? Curr Opin Clin Nutr Metab Care 5:503, 2002.
57. Duggleby SC, Jackson AA: Relationship of maternal protein turnover and lean body mass during pregnancy and birthweight. Clin Sci (Lond) 101:65, 2001.
58. Kalhan SC, Rossi KQ, Gruca LL, et al: Relation between transamination of brached-chain amino acids and urea synthesis: Evidence from human pregnancy. Am J Physiol 275:E423, 1998.
59. Catalano P, Drago N, Highman T, et al: Longitudinal changes in amino acid insulin sensitivity during pregnancy. J Soc Gynecol Invest 145:131A, 1996.
60. Cetin I, Nobile de Santis MS, Taricco E, et al: Maternal and fetal amino acid concentrations in normal pregnancies and in pregnancies with gestational diabetes mellitus. Am J Obstet Gynecol 192:610, 2005.
61. Ogburn PL, Goldstein M, Walker J, Stonestreet BS: Prolonged hyperinsulinemia reduces plasma fatty acid levels in the major lipid groups in fetal sheep. Am J Obstet Gynecol 161:728, 1989.
62. Kliegman R, Gross T, Morton S, Dunnington R: Intrauterine growth and post natal fasting metabolism in infants of obese mothers. J Pediatr 104:601, 1984.
63. Darmady JM, Postle AD: Lipid metabolism in pregnancy. Br J Obstet Gynaecol 82:211, 1982.
64. Knopp RH, Chapman M, Bergeline RO, et al: Relationship of lipoprotein lipids to mild fasting hyperglycemia and diabetes in pregnancy. Diabetes Care 3:416, 1980.
65. Montelongo A, Lasuncion MA, Pallardo LF, et al: Longitudinal study of plasma lipoproteins and hormones during pregnancy in normal and diabetic women. Diabetes 41:1651, 1992.
66. Koukkou E, Watts GF, Lowy C: Serum lipid, lipoprotein and apolipoprotein changes in gestational diabetes mellitus: a cross-sectional and prospective study. J Clin Pathol 49:634, 1996.
67. Catalano PM, Nizielski SE, Shao J, et al: Down regulation of IRS-1 and PPARgamma in obese women with gestational diabetes: Relationship to free fatty acids during pregnancy. Am J Physiol Endocrinol 282:E522–33, 2002.
68. Catalano PM, Hollenbeck C: Energy requirements in pregnancy: A review. Obstet Gynecol Surv 47:368, 1992.
69. Goldberg GR, Prentice AM, Coward WA, et al: Longitudinal assessment of energy expenditure in pregnancy by the doubly labels water method. Am J Clin Nutr 57:494, 1993.
70. Forsum E, Sadurskis A, Wager J: Resting metabolic rate and Boyd composition of healthy Swedish women during pregnancy. Am J Clin Nutr 47:94, 1988.
71. Lawrence M, Lawrence F, Coward WA, et al: Energy requirements of pregnancy in the Gambia. Lancet ii:1072, 1987.
72. Forsum E, Kabir N, Sadurskis A: Westerp: Total energy expenditure of healthy Swedish women during pregnancy and lactation. Am J Cline Nutr 56:334, 1992.
73. Butte NF, Wong WW, Treuth MS, et al: Energy requirements during pregnancy ased on otal energy expenditure and energy disposition. Am J Clin Nutr 79:1078, 2004.
74. King JC, Butte NF, Bronstein MN, et al: Energy metabolism during pregnancy: Influence of maternal energy status. Am J Cline Nutr 59:4395, 1994.
75. Prentice AM, Poppitt SD, Goldberg CR, et al: Energy balance in pregnancy and lactation. *In* Allen L, King J, Lonnerdal B (eds): Nutrient Regulation During Pregnancy, Lactation and Infant Growth, New York, Plenum Press, 1994, p 11.
76. Swinburn BA, Myomba BC, Saad MF, et al: Insulin resistance associated with lower rates of weight gain in PIMA Indians. J Clin Invest 88:168, 1991.
77. Catalano PM, Roma NM, Tyzbir ED, et al: Weight gain in women with gestational diabetes. Obstet Gynecol 81:523, 1993.
78. Okereke NC, Huston-Presley L, Amini SB, et al: Longitudinal changes in energy expenditure and body composition in obese women with normal and impaired glucose tolerance. Am J Physiol Endocrinol Metab 287:E472, 2004.
79. Catalano PM, Thomas A, Huston-Presley L, et al: Increased fetal adiposity: A very sensitive marker of abnormal in utero development. Am J Obstet Gynecol 189:1698, 2003.
80. Landon MB, Gabbe SG: Fetal surveillance in the pregnancy complicated by diabetes mellitus. Clin Perinatol 20:549, 1993.
81. Centers for Disease Control and Prevention: Perinatal mortality and congenital malformations in infants born to women with insulin dependent diabetes. MMWR Morb Mortal Wkly Rep 39:363, 1990.
82. Salversen DR, Brudenell MJ, Nicholaides KH: Fetal polycythemia and thrombocytopenia in pregnancies complicated by maternal diabetes. Am J Obstet Gynecol 166:1987, 1992.
83. Madsen H: Fetal oxygenation in diabetic pregnancy. Dan Med Bull 33:64, 1986.
84. Nylund L, Lunell NO, Lewander R, et al: Uteroplacental blood flow in diabetic pregnancy: Measurements with indium 113m and a computer linked gamma camera. Am J Obstet Gynecol 144:298, 1982.

85. Kitzmiller JL, Phillippe M, von Oeyen P, et al: Hyperglycemia hypoxia, and fetal acidosis in Rhesus monkeys (abstract). Presented in 28th Annual Meeting of The Society for Gynecologic Investigation, St. Louis, MO, March, 1981.
86. Phillips AF, Dubin JW, Matty PJ, et al: Arterial hypoxemia and hyperinsulinemia in the chronically hyperglycemia fetal lamb. Pediatr Res 16:653, 1982.
87. Albert TJ, Landon MB, Wheller JJ, et al: Prenatal detection of fetal anomalies in pregnancies complicated by insulin-dependent diabetes mellitus. Am J Obstet Gynecol (in press).
88. Simpson JL, Elias S, Martin O, et al: Diabetes in pregnancy, Northwestern University Series (1977–1981). I. Prospective study of anomalies in offspring of mothers with diabetes mellitus. Am J Obstet Gynecol 146:263, 1983.
89. Mills JL, Knopp RH, Simpson JP, et al: Lack of relation of increased malformation rates in infants of diabetic mothers to glycemic control during organogenesis. N Engl J Med 318:671, 1988.
90. Eriksson U: The pathogenesis of congenital malformations in diabetic pregnancy. Diabetes Metab Rev 11:63, 1995.
91. Reece EA, Hobbins JC: Diabetic embryopathy: pathogenesis, prenatal diagnosis and prevention. Obstet Gynecol Surv 41:325, 1986.
92. Koppe J, Smoremberg-School M: Diabetes, congenital malformations and HLA types. *In* Listen E, Band H, Frus-Hansen B (eds): Intensive Care in the Newborn, Vol. 4. Newark, Masson Publishing, 1983, pp 15.
93. Simpson JL, Mills J, Ober C, et al: DR3+ and DR4+ diabetes women have increased risk for anomalies. Presented at the 37th Annual Meeting of the Society for Gynecologic Investigation. Abstract 3901, St. Louis, Missouri, 1990.
94. Freinkel N, Lewis NJ, Akazawa S, et al: The honeybee syndrome: Implication of the teratogenicity of mannose in rat-embryo culture. N Engl J Med 310:223, 1984.
95. Goldman AS, Baker L, Piddington R, et al: Hyperglycemia-induced teratogenesis is mediated by a functional deficiency of arachidonic acid. Proc Natl Acad Sci 82:8227, 1985.
96. Pinter E, Reece EA: Arachidonic acid prevents hyperglycemia-associated yolk sac damage and embryopathy. Am J Obstet Gynecol 166:691, 1986.
97. Pinter E, Reece EA, Leranth CZ, et al: Yolk sac failure in embryopathy due to hyperglycemia ultrastructural analysis of yolk sac differentiation associated with embryopathy in rat conceptuses under hyperglycemic conditions. Teratology 33:73, 1986.
98. Eriksson NJ: Protection by free oxygen radical scavenging enzymes against glucose-induced embryonic malformations in vitro. Diabetologia 34:325, 1991.
99. Spellacy WN, Miller S, Winegar A, Peterson PQ: Macrosomia-maternal characteristics and infant complications. Obstet Gynecol 66:185, 1985.
100. Reiher H, Fuhrmann K, Noack S, et al: Age-dependent insulin secretion of the endocrine pancreas in vitro from fetuses of diabetic and nondiabetic patients. Diabetes Care 6:446, 1983.
101. Fallucca F, Garguilo P, Troili F, et al: Amniotic fluid insulin, C-peptide concentrations and fetal morbidity in infants of diabetic mothers. Am J Obstet Gynecol 153:534, 1985.
102. Krew MA, Kehl RJ, Thomas A, Catalano PM: Relationship of amniotic fluid C-peptide levels to neonatal body composition. Obstet Gynecol 84:96, 1994.
103. Brans YW, Shannon DL, Hunter MA, et al: Maternal diabetes and neonatal macrosomia, II Neonatal anthropometric measurements. Early Hum Dev 8:297, 1983.
104. Modanlou HD, Komatsu G, Dorchester W, et al: Large-for-gestational age neonates: Anthropometric reasons for shoulder dystocia. Obstet Gynecol 60:417, 1982.
105. Gabbe SG, Mestman JH, Freeman RK, et al: Management and outcome of pregnancy in diabetes mellitus, class B-R. Am J Obstet Gyencol 129:723, 1977.
106. Kitzmiller JL, Gloherty JP: Diabetic pregnancy and perinatal morbidity. Am J Obstet Gynecol 131:560, 1978.
107. Roversi GD, Gargiulo M: A new approach to the treatment of diabetic pregnant women. Am J Obstet Gynecol 135:567, 1979.
108. Jovanovic L, Druzin M, Peterson CM: Effect of euglycemia on the outcome of pregnancy in insulin-dependent diabetic women as compared with normal control subjects. Am J Med 72:921, 1981.
109. Landon MB, Gabbe SG, Piana R, et al: Neonatal morbidity in pregnancy complicated by diabetes mellitus predictive value of maternal glycemic profiles. Am J Obstet Gynecol 156:1089, 1987.
110. Jovanovic-Peterson L, Peterson CM, Reed CF, et al: Maternal postprandial glucose levels and infant birthweight: The Diabetes in Early Pregnancy Study. Am J Obstet Gynecol 164:103, 1991.
111. Catalano PM, Tyzbir ED, Allen SR, et al: Evaluation of fetal growth by estimation of body composition. Obstet Gynecol 79:46, 1992.
112. Catalano PM, Drago NM, Amini SB: Factors affecting fetal growth and body composition. Am J Obstet Gynecol 172:1459, 1995.
113. Catalano PM, Drago NM, Amini SB: Maternal carbohydrate metabolism and its relationship to fetal growth and body composition. Am J Obstet Gynecol 172:1464, 1995.
114. Caruso A, Paradisi G, Ferrazzani S, et al: Effect of maternal carbohydrate metabolism in fetal growth. Obstet Gynecol 8, 1998.
115. Silverman BL, Rizzo TA, Cho NH, Metzger BE: Long-term effects of the intrauterine environment. Diabetes, 21:142, 1998.
116. Pettit DJ, Nelson RG, Saad MF, et al: Diabetes and obesity in the offspring of Pima Indian women with diabetes during pregnancy. Diabetes Care 16:310, 1993.
117. Taylor R, Lee C, Kyne-Grzebalski D, et al: Clinical outcomes of pregnancy in women with type I diabetes. Obstet Gynecol 99:537, 2002.
118. Hertel J, Anderson GE, Brandt NJ, et al: Metabolic events in infants of diabetic mothers during first 24 hours after birth. Acta Paediart Scand 71:19, 1982.
119. Bourbon JR, Farrell PM: Fetal lung development in the diabetic pregnancy. Pediatr Res 19:253, 1985.
120. Smith BT, Giroud CJP, Robert M, Avery ME: Insulin antagonism of cortisol action on lecithin synthesis by cultures of fetal lung cells. J Pediatr 87:953, 1975.
121. Smith BT: Pulmonary surfactant during fetal development and neonatal adaptation: Hormonal control. *In* Robertson B, Van Golde LMB, Batenburg JJ (eds): Pulmonary Surfactant. Amsterdam, Elsevier, 1985, p 357.
122. Post M, Barsoumian A, Smith BT: The cellular mechanisms of glucocorticoid acceleration of fetal lung maturation. J Biol Chem 261:2179, 1986.
123. Carlson KS, Smith BT, Post M: Insulin acts on the fibroblast to inhibit glucocorticoid stimulation of lung maturation. J Appl Physiol 57:1577, 1984.
124. Dudley DKL, Black DM: Reliability of lecithin/sphingomyelin ratios in diabetic pregnancy. Obstet Gynecol 66:521, 1985.
125. Kjos SL, Walther F: Prevalence and etiology of respiratory distress in infants of diabetic mothers: predictive value of lung maturation tests. Am J Obstet Gynecol 163:898, 1990.
126. Mimouni F, Miodovnik M, Whittset J, et al: Respiratory distress syndrome in infants of diabetic mothers in the 1980s: no direct adverse effect of maternal diabetes with modern management. Obstet Gynecol 69:191, 1987.
127. Cordero L, Treuer SH, Landon MB, Gabbe SG: Management of infants of diabetic mother. Arch Pediatr Adolesc Med 152:249, 1998.
128. Mimouni F, Miodovnik M, Tsang RC, et al: Decreased amniotic fluid magnesium concentration in diabetic pregnancy. Obstet Gynecol 69:12, 1987.
129. Widness JA, Cowett RM, Coustan DR, et al: Neonatal morbidities in infants of mothers with glucose intolerance in pregnancy. Diabetes 34:61, 1985.
130. Ylinen K, Raivio K, Teramo K: Haemoglobin A1c predicts the perinatal outcome in insulin-dependent diabetic pregnancies. Br J Obstet Gynaecol 88:961, 1981.
131. Stevenson DK, Bartoletti AL, Ostrander CR, Johnson JD: Pulmonary excretion of carbon monoxide in the human infants as an index of bilirubin production. II. Infants of diabetic mothers. J Pediatr 94:956, 1979.
132. Shannon K, Davis JC, Kitzmiller JL, et al: Erythropoiesis in infants of diabetic mothers. Pediatr Res 30:161, 1986.
133. White P: Pregnancy complicating diabetes. Am J Med 7:609, 1949.

134. Summary and Recommendations of the Second International Workshop-Conference on Gestational Diabetes, Diabetes 34:123, 1985.
135. Summary and Recommendations of the Third Int'l Workshop Conference, Diabetes 40:197, 1991.
136. Gabbe SG, Mestman JH, Freeman RK, et al: Management and outcome of Class A diabetes mellitus. Am J Obstet Gynecol 127:465, 1977.
137. Selby JV, Fitzsimmons SC, Newman JM, et al: The natural history and epidemiology of diabetic nephropathy. JAMA 263:1954, 1990.
138. Rossing P: Promotion, prediction and prevention of progression of nephropathy in type 1 diabetes mellitus [Review]. Diabet Med 15:900, 1998.
139. Parving H-H, Hovind P, Rossing K, et al: Evolving strategies for renoprotection: diabetic nephropathy [Review]. Curr Opin Nephrol Hypertens 10:515, 2001.
140. Lip GYH, Churchill D, Beevers M, et al: Angiotensin-converting enzyme inhibitors in early pregnancy. Lancet 350:1446, 1997.
141. Burrows RF, Burrows EA: Assessing the teratogenic potential of angiotensin-converting enzyme inhibitors in pregnancy. Aust NZ J Obstet Gynaecol 38:306, 1998.
142. Cox RM, Anderson JM, Cox P: Defective embryogenesis with angiotensin II receptor antagonists in pregnany. Br J Obstet Gynaecol 110:1038, 2003.
143. Hod M, van Dijk DJ, Karp M, et al: Diabetic nephropathy and pregnancy: the effect of ACE inhibitors prior to pregnancy on maternal outcome. Nephrol Dial Transplant 10:2328, 1995.
144. Combs CA, Rosenn B, Kitzmiller JL, et al: Early-pregnancy proteinuria in diabetes related to preeclampsia. Obstet Gynecol 82:802, 1993.
145. Ekbom P, Damn P, Feldt-Rasmussen B, et al: Pregnancy outcome in type 1 diabetic women with microalbuminuria. Diabetes Care 24:1739, 2001.
146. Gordon M, Landon MB, Samuels P, et al: Perinatal outcome and long-term follow-up associated with modern management of diabetic nephropathy (Class F). Obstet Gynecol 87:401, 1996.
147. Kitzmiller JL, Brown ER, Phillippe M, et al: Diabetic nephropathy and perinatal outcome. Am J Obstet Gynecol 141:741, 1981.
148. Reece EA, Coustan DR, Hayslett JP, et al: Diabetic nephropathy: Pregnancy performance and fetomaternal outcome. Am J Obstet Gynecol 159:56, 1988.
149. Kitzmiller JL: Diabetic nephropathy. *In* Reece EA, Coustan DR, Gabbe SG (eds): Diabetes in pregnancy. Philadelphia, Lippincott Williams Wilkins, 2004, p 383.
150. Rosenn BM, Miodovnik M, Khoury JC, et al: Outcome of pregnancy in women with diabetic nephropathy. Am J Obstet Gynecol 176:S631, 1997.
151. Rossing K, Jacobsen P, Hommel E, et al: Pregnancy and progression of diabetic nephropathy. Diabetologia 45:36, 2002.
152. Armenti VT, McGrory CH, Cater J, et al: The national transplantatin registry: comparision between pregnancy outcomes in diabetic cyclosporine-treated female kidney recipients and CyA-treated female pancreas-kidney recipients. Transplant Proc 29:669, 1997.
153. Ogburn PL Jr, Kitzmiller JL, Hare JW, et al: Pregnancy following renal transplantation in Class T diabetes mellitus. JAMA 255:911, 1986.
154. McCrory CH, Grosheck MA, Sollinger HW, et al: Pregnancy outcomes in female pancreas-kidney transplants. Transplant Proc 31:652, 1999.
155. Barrou BM, Gruessner AC, Sutherland DE, et al: Pregnancy after pancreas transplantation in the cyclosporine era: report from the International Pancreas Transplant Registry. Transplantation 65:524, 1998.
156. Carstensen LL, Frost-Lansen K, Fulgeberg S, Nerup J: Does pregnancy influence the prognosis of uncomplicated insulin-dependent diabetes? Diabetes Care 5:1, 1982.
157. Klein BEK, Moss SE, Klein R: Effect of pregnancy on the progression of diabetic retinopathy. Diabetes Care 13:34, 1990.
158. Rosenn B, Miodovnik KM, Kranias G, et al: Progression of diabetic retinopathy in pregnancy: association with hypertension in pregnancy. Am J Obstet Gynecol 166:1214, 1992.
159. Horvat M, Maclear H, Goldberg L, Crock CW: Diabetic retinopathy in pregnancy: A 12 year prospective study. Br J Ophthalmol 64:398, 1980.
160. Kitzmiller JL, Gavin LA, Gin GD, et al: Managing diabetes and pregnancy. Curr Probl Obstet Gynecol Fertil 11:113, 1988.
161. Moloney JBM, Drury MI: The effect of pregnancy on the natural course of diabetic retinopathy. Am J Ophthalmol 93:745, 1982.
162. Phelps RL, Sakol P, Metzger BE, et al: Changes in diabetic retinopathy during pregnancy, correlations with regulation of hyperglycemia. Arch Ophthalmol 104:1806, 1986.
163. Chew EY, Mills JL, Metzger BE, et al: Metabolic control and progression of retinopathy. The diabetes in early pregnancy study. Diabetes Care 18:631, 1995.
164. Sinclair SH, Nesler C, Foxman B, et al: Macular edema and pregnancy in insulin dependent diabetes. Am J Ophthalmol 97:154, 1984.
165. Gordon MC, Landon MB, Boyle J, et al: Myocardial infarction during pregnancy in a patient with Class R/F diabetes mellitus: A case report and review of literature on Class H IDDM. Obstet Gynecol Surv 51:437, 1996.
166. Hare JW: Maternal complications. *In* Hare JW (ed): Diabetes complicating pregnancy. The Joslin Clinic Method. New York, Alan R Liss, 1989, p 96.
167. Stephenson MJ: Screening for gestational diabetes mellitus: a critical review. J Fam Prac 37:277, 1993.
168. Solomon CG, Willett WC, Carey VJ, et al: A prospective study of pregravid determinants of gestational diabetes mellitus. JAMA 278:1078, 1997.
169. O'Sullivan JB: Body weight and subsequent diabetes mellitus. JAMA 248:949, 1982.
170. Dornhorst A, Rossi M: Risk and prevention of type 2 diabetes in women with gestational diabetes. Diabetes Care 21:B43, 1998.
171. Kjos SL, Peters RK, Xiang A, et al: Predicting future diabetes in Latino women with gestational diabetes. Utility of early postpartum glucose tolerance testing. Diabetes 44:586, 1995.
172. Coustan DR, Nelson C, Carpenter NW, et al: Maternal age and screening for gestational diabetes: a population based study. Obstet Gynecol 73:557, 1989.
173. Metzger BE, Coustan DR: and the Organizing Committee: Summary and recommendations of the Fourth International Workshop-Conference on Gestational Diabetes Mellitus. Diabetes Care 21:B161, 1998.
174. Danilenko-Dixon DR, VanWinter JT, Nelson RL, et al: Universal versus selective gestational diabetes screening: Application of the 1997 American Diabetes Association recommendations. Am J Obstet Gynecol 181:79, 1999.
175. ACOG Practice Bulletin Number 30. Gestational Diabetes, September 2001.
176. Periodic health examination, 1992 update: 1. Screening for gestational diabetes mellitus. Can Med Assoc J 147:435, 1992.
177. Brody SC, Harris R, Lohr K: Screening for gestational diabetes: A summary of the evidence for the U.S. Preventive Services Task Force. Obstet Gynecol 101:380, 2003.
178. Naylor CD: Diagnosing gestational diabetes mellitus: Is the gold standard valid? Diabetes Care 12:565, 1989.
179. Sermer M, Naylor CD, Gore DJ, et al: Impact of increasing carbohydrate intolerance on maternal-fetal outcomes in 3637 women without gestational diabetes. Am J Obstet Gynecol 173:146, 1995.
180. Sacks DA, Greenspoon JS, Abu-Fadil S, et al: Toward universal criteria for gestational diabetes: The 75-gram glucose tolerance test in pregnancy. Am J Obstet Gynecol 172:607, 1995.
181. Langer O, Yogev Y, Most O, Xenakis EM: Gestational diabetes: The consequences of not treating. Am J Obstet Gynecol 192:989, 2005.
182. Crowther CA, Hiller JE, Moss JR, et al: Effect of treatment of gestational diabetes mellitus on pregnancy outcomes. N Engl J Med 352:2477, 2005.
183. HAPO Study cooperative Research Group: The Hyperglycemia and Adverse Pregnancy Outcome (HAPO) Study. Int J Gynaecol Obstet 78:69, 2002.
184. Landon MB, Thom E, Spong CY, et al: A planned randomized clinical trial of treatment for mild gestational diabetes. J. Matern Fetal Neonatal Med 11:226, 2002.
185. Greene MF, Solomon CG: Gestational diabetes mellitus—time to treat. N Engl J Med 352:24, 2005.
186. Coustan DR, Widness JA, Carpenter NW, et al: Should the fifty-gram, one-hour plasma glucose screening test be adminis-

tered in the fasting or fed state? Am J Obstet Gynecol 154:1031, 1986.
187. Sermer M, Naylor CD, Gare DJ, et al: Impact of time since last meal on the gestational glucose challenge test. Am J Obstet Gynecol 171:607, 1994.
188. Landon MB: Gestational diabetes mellitus: Screening and diagnosis. Laboratory Medicine 21:527, 1990.
189. Carpenter MW, Coustan DR: Criteria for screening tests of gestational diabetes. Am J Obstet Gynecol 144:768, 1982.
190. Bobrowski RA, Bottoms SF, Michallef JA, et al: Is the 50-gram glucose screening test ever diagnostic? J Matern Fetal Med 5:317, 1996.
191. Sacks DA, Abu-Fadil S, Greenspoon J, et al: Do the current standards for glucose tolerance testing in pregnancy represent a valid conversion of O'Sullivan's original criteria? Am J Obstet Gynecol 161:638, 1989.
192. National Institutes of Health Diabetes Data Group: Classification and diagnosis of diabetes mellitus and other categories of glucose intolerance. Diabetes 20:139, 1979.
193. Naylor CD, Sermer M, Chen E, et al: Cesarean delivery in relation to birth weight and gestational glucose intolerance: Pathophysiology or practice style? Toronto Tri-Hospital Gestational Diabetes Investigators. JAMA 275:1165, 1996.
194. Landon MB, Gabbe SG: Insulin treatment of the pregnant patient with diabetes mellitus. *In* Reece EA, Coustan DR, Gabbe SG (ed): Diabetes Mellitus in Women. Philadelphia, Lippincott, Williams, and Wilkins. 2004.
195. Kitzmiller JL, Main EK, Ward B, et al: Insulin lispro and the development of proliferative retinopathy during pregnancy. Diabetes Care 22:873, 1999.
196. Buchbinder A, Miodovnik M, McElvy S, et al: Is insulin lispro a culprit in the progression of diabetic retinopathy during pregnancy? Am J Obstet Gynecol 182:S79, 2000.
197. Loukovaara S, Immonen I, Teramo KA, Kaaja R: Progression of retinopathy during pregnancy in type 1 diabetic women treated with insulin lispro. Diab Care 26:1193, 2003.
198. Pettitt DJ, Kolaczynski JW, Ospina P, et al: Comparision of an insulin analog, insulin aspart and regular human insulin with no insulin in gestational diabetes mellitus. Diabetes Care 26:183, 2003.
199. Devlin JT, Hothersall L, Wilkis JL: Use of insulin glargine during pregnancy in type 1 diabetic women. Diabetes Care 25:1095, 2002.
200. Coustan DR, Reece EA, Sherwin RS, et al: A randomized clinical trial of the insulin pump versus intensive conventional therapy in diabetic pregnancy. JAMA 255:631, 1986.
201. Gabbe SG, Holing E, Temple P: Benefits, risks, costs, and patient satisfaction associated with insulin pump therapy for the pregnancy complicated by type 1 diabetes mellitus. Am J Obstet Gynecol 182:1283, 2000.
202. Bode BW, Weinstein R, Bell D, et al: Comparision of insulin aspart with buffered regular insulin and insulin lispro of continous subcutaneous insulin infusion: a randomized study in type 1 diabetes. Diabetes Care 25:439, 2002.
203. American Diabetes Association: Gestational diabetes mellitus position statement. Diabetes Care 25:S94, 2002.
204. Diamond MP, Reece EA, Caprio S, et al: Impairment of counterregulatory hormone responses to hypoglycemia in pregnant women with insulin-dependent diabetes mellitus. Am J Obstet Gynecol 166:70, 1992.
205. Rosenn BM, Miodovnik M, Khourty JC, et al: Courterregulatory hormonal responses to hypoglycemia during pregnancy. Obstet Gynecol 87:568, 1996.
206. Kilvert JA, Nicholson HO, Wright AD: Ketoacidosis in diabetic pregnancy. Diabetic Medicine 10:278, 1993.
207. Rayburn WF, McKean HE: Maternal perception of fetal movement and perinatal outcome. Obstet Gynecol 56:161, 1980.
208. Holden KP, Jovanovic L, Druzin M, et al: Increased fetal activity with low maternal blood glucose levels in pregnancies complicated by diabetes. Am J Perinatol 1:161, 1984.
209. Sadovsky E, Brjejinski A, Mor-Yosef S, et al: Fetal activity in diabetic pregnancy. J Fetal Med 3:1, 1983.
210. Landon MB, Gabbe SG, Sachs L: Management of diabetes mellitus and pregnancy: A survey of obstetricians and maternal-fetal specialists. Obstet Gynecol 75:635, 1990.
211. Barret JM, Salyer SL, Boehm FH: The non-stress test: An evaluation of 1000 patients. Am J Obstet Gynecol 141:153, 1981.
212. Miller JM, Horger EO: Antepartum heart rate testing in diabetic pregnancy. J Repro Med 30:515, 1985.
213. Landon MB, Gabbe SG, Bruner JP, Ludmir J: Doppler umbilical artery velocimetry in pregnancy complicated by insulin dependent diabetes mellitus. Obstet Gynecol 73:961, 1989.
214. Johnstone FD, Steel JM, Haddad NG, et al: Doppler umbilical artery flow velocity waveforms in diabetic pregnancy. Br J Obstet Gynecol 99:135, 1992.
215. Landon MB, Gabbe SG: Fetal surveillance in the pregnancy complicated by diabetes mellitus. Clin Perinatol 20:549, 1993.
216. Landon MB, Langer O, Gabbe SG, et al: Fetal surveillance in pregnancies complicated by insulin dependent diabetes mellitus. Am J Obstet Gynecol 167:617, 1992.
217. Landon MB, Vickers S: Fetal surveillance in pregnancy complicated by diabetes mellitus: is it necessary? J Matern Fetal Neonatal Med 12:413, 2002.
218. Milunsky A, Alpert E, Kitzmiller JL, et al: Prenatal diagnosis of neural tube defects VIII. The importance of serum alpha-fetoprotein screening in diabetic pregnant women. Am J Obstet Gynecol 142:1030, 1982.
219. Greene MF, Benacerraf B: Prenatal diagnosis in diabetic gravidas: utility of ultrasound and MSAFP screening. Obstet Gynecol 77:420, 1991.
220. Nesbitt TS, Gilbert WM, Herrchen B: Shoulder dystocia and associated risk factors with macrosomic infants born in California. Am J Obstet Gynecol 179:476, 1998.
221. Tamura RK, Shabbagha RE, Depp R, et al: Diabetic macrosomia: accuracy of third trimester ultrasound. Obstet Gynecol 67:828, 1986.
222. Landon MB, Mintz MG, Gabbe SG: Sonographic evaluation of fetal abdominal growth: predictor of the large-for-gestational age infant in pregnancies. Am J Obstet Gynecol 160:115, 1989
223. Moore TR: A comparison of amniotic fluid pulmonary phospholipids in normal and diabetic pregnancy. Am J Obstet Gynecol 186:641, 2002.
224. Kjos S, Henry O, Montoro M, et al: Insulin-requiring diabetes in pregnancy: A randomized trial of active induction of labor and expectant management. Am J Obstet Gynecol 169:611, 1993.
225. Rouse DJ, Owen J, Goldenberg RL, et al: The effectiveness and costs of elective cesarean delivery for fetal macrosomia diagnosed by ultrasound. JAMA 276:1480, 1996.
226. Acker DB, Sachs BP, Friedman EA: Risk factors for shoulder dystocia. Obstet Gynecol 6:762, 1985.
227. ACOG practice bulletin: Shoulder dystocia. Number 40, November 2002.
228. Benedetti TJ, Gabbe SG: Shoulder dystocia: A complication of fetal macrosomia and prolonged second stage of labor with midpelvic delivery. Obstet Gynecol 52:526, 1978.
229. Jovanovic L, Peterson CM: Management of the pregnant, insulin-dependent diabetic woman. Diabetes Care 3:63, 1980.
230. Hollingsworth DR, Ney DM: Dietary management of diabetes during pregnancy. *In* Reece EA, Coustan DR (eds): Diabetes Mellitus in Pregnancy: Principles and Practice. New York, Churchill Livingstone, 1988, p 285.
231. Mumford MI, Jovanovic-Peterson L, Peterson CM: Alternative therapies for the management of gestational diabetes. Clin Perinatol 20:619, 1993.
232. Jovanovic-Peterson L, Peterson CM: Nutritional management of the obese gestational diabetic pregnant women. J Am Coll Nutr 11:246, 1992.
233. Algert S, Shragg P, Hollingsworth DR: Moderate caloric restriction in obese women with gestational diabetes. Obstet Gynecol 65:487, 1985.
234. Magee MS, Knopp RH, Benedetti TJ: Metabolic effects of 1200 kcal diet in obese pregnant women with gestational diabetes. Diabetes 39:324, 1990.
235. Rizzo T, Metzger BE, Burns WJ, et al: Correlations between antepartum maternal metabolism and intelligence of offspring. N Engl J Med 325:911, 1991.
236. Knopp RH, Magee MS, Raisys V, et al: Hypocaloric diets and ketogenesis in the management of obese gestational diabetic women. J Am Coll Nutr 10:649, 1991.

237. Peterson CM, Jovanovic-Peterson L: Percentage of carbohydrate and glycemia response to breakfast, lunch, and dinner in women with gestational diabetes. Diabetes 40:172, 1991.
238. Jovanovic L: American Diabetes Association's Fourth International Workshop Conference on Gestational Diabetes Mellitus: Summary and Discussion. Therapeutic Interventions. Diabetes Care 2):B131, 1998.
239. Goldberg J, Franklin B, Lasser L, et al: Gestational diabetes: Impact of home glucose monitoring on neonatal birth weight. Am J Obstet Gynecol 154:546, 1986.
240. Langer O, Rodriguez DA, Xenakis EMJ, et al: Intensified versus conventional management of gestational diabetes. Am J Obstet Gynecol 170:1036, 1994.
241. Metzger BE, Coustan DR: Summary and recommendations of the Fourth International Workshop Conference on Gestational Diabetes Mellitus. Diabetes Care 21:B161, 1998.
242. Langer O, Brustman L, Anyaegbunam A, et al: Glycemic control in gestational diabetes mellitus - how tight is tight enough; small for gestational age versus large for gestational age? Am J Obstet Gynecol 161:645, 1989.
243. Langer O, Berkus M, Brustman L, et al: Rationale for insulin management in gestational diabetes mellitus. Diabetes 40:186, 1991.
244. Buchanan TA, Kjos S, Schafer U, et al: Utility of fetal measurements in the management of GDM. Diabetes Care 21:B99, 1998.
245. Langer O, Conway DL, Berkus MD, et al: A comparison of glyburide and insulin in women with gestational diabetes mellitus. N Engl J Med 343:1134, 2000.
246. Conway DL, Gonzales O, Skiver D: Use of glyburide for the treatment of gestational diabetes: the San Antonio experience. J Matern Fetal Neonatal Med 15:51, 2004.
247. Kremer CJ, Duff P: Glyburide for the treatment of gestational diabetes. Am J Obstet Gynecol 190:1438, 2004.
248. Chmait R, Dinise T, Moore T: Prospective observational study to establish predictors of glyburide success in women with gestational diabetes mellitus. J Perinatol 24:617, 2004.
249. Jacobson GF, Ramos GA, Ching JY, et al: Comparison of glyburide and insulin for the management of gestational diabetes in a large managed care organization. Am J Obstet Gynecol 193:118, 2005.
250. Durnwald C, Landon MB: Glyburide: The new alternative for treating gestational diabetes? Am J Obstet Gynecol 193:1, 2005.
251. Bung P, Artal R, Khodiguian N, Kjos S: Exercise in gestational diabetes: an optional therapeutic approach? Diabetes 40:182, 1991.
252. Avery MD, Leon AS, Kopher RA: Effects of a partially home-based exercise program for women with gestational diabetes. Obstet Gynecol 89:10, 1997.
253. Landon MB, Gabbe SG: Antepartum fetal surveillance in gestational diabetes mellitus. Diabetes 34:50, 1985.
254. Girz BA, Divon MY, Merkatz IR: Sudden fetal death in women with well controlled, intensively monitored gestational diabetes. J Perinatol 12:229, 1992.
255. Kjos S, Leung A, Henry OA, et al: Antepartum surveillance in diabetic pregnancies: predictors of fetal distress in labor. Am J Obstet Gynecol 173:1532, 1995.
256. Lurie S, Matzkel A, Weissman A, et al: Outcome of pregnancy in Class A1 and A2 gestational diabetic patients delivered beyond 40 weeks gestation. Am J Perinatal 9:484, 1992.
257. Lurie S, Insler V, Hagay Z: Induction of labor at 38 to 39 weeks of gestation reduces the incidence of shoulder dystocia in gestational diabetic patient Class A2. Am J Perinatol 13:293, 1996.
258. Molsted-Pedersen L: Pregnancy and diabetes, a survey. Acta Endocrinol 238:13, 1980.
259. Fuhrmann K, Reiher H, Semmler K, et al: Prevention of congenital malformations in infants of insulin-dependent diabetic mothers. Diabetes Care 6:219, 1983.
260. Kitzmiller JL, Gavin LA, Gin GD, et al: Preconception management of diabetes continued through early pregnancy prevents the excess frequency of major congenital anomalies in infants of diabetic mothers. JAMA 265:731, 1991.
261. Miller E, Hare JW, Cloherty JP, et al: Elevated maternal HbA_1 in early pregnancy and major congenital anomalies in infants of diabetic mothers. N Engl J Med 304:1331, 1981.
262. Greene MF: Prevention and diagnosis of congenital anomalies in diabetic pregnancies. Clin Perinatol 20:533, 1993.
263. Mills J, Simpson JL, Drisoll SG, et al: Incidence of spontaneous abortion among normal and insulin-dependent diabetic women whose pregnancies were identified within 21 days of conception. N Engl J Med 319:1617, 1988.
264. Whillhoite MB, Bennert HW, Palomaki GE, et al: The impact of preconception counseling on pregnancy outcomes. The experience of the Maine Diabetes in Pregnancy Program. Diabetes Care 16:450, 1993.
265. Kjos SL, Ballagh SA, LaCour M, et al: The copper T380A intrauterine device in women with type II diabetes mellitus. Obstet Gynecol 84:1006, 1994.
266. Steel JM, Duncan LJP: Serious complications of oral contraceptives in insulin-dependent diabetes. Contraception 17:291, 1978.
267. Lidegard O: Oral contraceptives, pregnancy, and the risk of cerebral thromboembolism: The influence of diabetes, hypertension, migraine and previous thrombotic disease. Br J Obstet Gynecol 102:153, 1995.
268. Klein BEK, Moss SE, Klein R: Oral contraceptives in women with diabetes. Diabetes Care 13:895, 1990.
269. DePiaro R, Forte F, Bertoli A, et al: Changes in insulin receptors during oral contraception. J Clin Endocrinol Metab 52:29, 1981.
270. Steel JM, Duncan LJP: The effect of oral contraceptives on insulin requirements in diabetes. Br J Fam Plan 3:77, 1978.
271. Skouby S, Kuhl C, Molsted-Pederson L, et al: Triphasic oral contraception: Metabolic effects in normal women and those with previous gestational diabetes. Am J Obstet Gynecol 163:495, 1985.
272. Kjos SL, Shoupe D, Dougan S, et al: Effect of low-dose oral contraceptives on carbohydrate and lipid metabolism in women with recent gestational diabetes: results of a controlled randomized prospective study. Am J Obstet Gynecol 163:1822, 1990.
273. Liew DFM, Ng CSA, Yong YM, et al: Long term effects of Depo-Provera on carbohydrate and lipid metabolism. Contraception 31:51, 1985.
274. DeSlypere JP, Thiery N, Vermeulen A: Effect of long-term hormonal contraception on plasma lipids. Contraception 31:633, 1985.
275. Steel JM, Duncan LJP: The effect of oral contraceptives on insulin requirements in diabetes. Br J Fam Plan 3:77, 1978.
276. Grenfel A, Brudnell JM, Doddridge MC, Watkins PJ: Pregnancy in diabetic women who have proteinuria. Q J Med 59:379, 1986.

Thyroid and Parathyroid Diseases in Pregnancy

JORGE H. MESTMAN

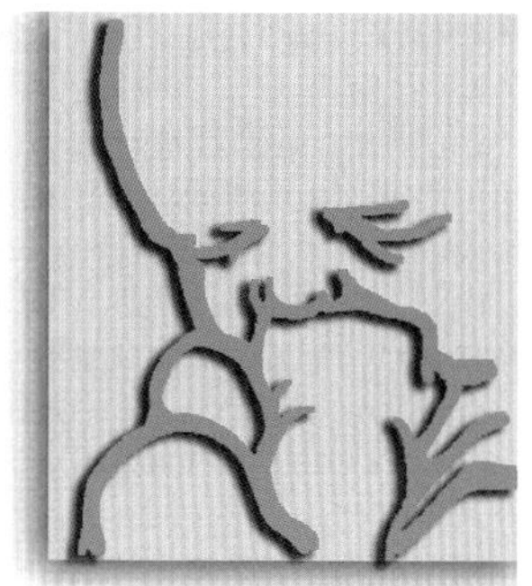

CHAPTER 38

KEY ABBREVIATIONS

1,25-dihydroxyvitamin D	$1,25(OH)_2D_3$
American Association of Clinical Endocrinologists	AACE
American College of Obstetricians and Gynecologists	ACOG
American Thyroid Association	ATA
Antithyroglubulin antibodies	TgAb
Endocrine Society	ES
Familial hypocalciuric hypercalcemia	FHH
Fine-needle aspiration biopsy	FNAB
Free thyroxine	FT_4
Free thyroxine index	FT_4I
Free triiodothyronine	FT_3
Free triiodothyronine index	FT_3I
Human chorionic gonadotropin	hCG
Hyperemesis gravidarum	HG
Immunoglobulin G	IgG
Intelligence quotient	IQ
Intrauterine growth restriction	IUGR
Levothyroxine	L-thyroxine
Methimazole	MM
Parathyroid hormone	PTH
Parathyroid hormone–related protein	PTHrP
Postpartum thyroiditis	PPT
Primary hyperparathyroidism	PHP
Propylthiouracil	PTU
Resin triiodothyronine uptake	RT_3U
Thyroid-blocking antibodies	TRBAb
Thyroid function tests	TFTs
Thyroid hormone–binding ratio	THBR
Thyroid peroxidase	TPO
Thyroid-stimulating hormone	TSH
Thyroid-stimulating immunoglobulins	TSI
Thyrotropin-releasing hormone	TRH
Thyroxine	T_4
Thyroxine-binding globulin	TBG
Total triiodothyronine	TT_3
Total thyroxine	TT_4
Triiodothyronine	T_3
TSH receptor antibodies	TRAb or TSHRBAb

Thyroid diseases and diabetes mellitus are the most frequent endocrine pathologies seen in pregnancy; parathyroid diseases on the other hand are rare, but may present a diagnostic and therapeutic challenge to the obstetrician. The obstetrician should be aware of the symptoms and signs of the particular disease, the effect of pregnancy on the interpretation of endocrine tests, and the transfer of hormones and medications across the placenta with the potential complications for the fetus and neonate. In this chapter, we present a brief description of the disease, its etiology, and the interpretation of functional endocrine tests, appropriate therapy, and the potential effects of both the disease and drug therapy on the concepts. It is imperative that a team approach be used in the management of these conditions; the close cooperation of the obstetrician, endocrinologist, pediatrician, and anesthesiologist offers the patient the best maternal and perinatal outcomes.

PARATHYROID DISEASES

Parathyroid diseases, uncommon in pregnancy, may produce significant perinatal and maternal morbidity and mortality if not diagnosed and properly managed. After a brief review of calcium homeostasis during pregnancy, primary hyperparathyroidism, hypoparathyroidism, and osteoporosis are discussed. Several reviews on these topics have recently been published.[1–3]

Calcium Homeostasis During Pregnancy

Parathyroid hormone (PTH) and 1,25-dihydroxyvitamin D (1,25[OH]$_2$D$_3$) are responsible for maintaining calcium homeostasis. Approximately 50 percent of serum calcium is protein bound, mostly to albumin; 10 percent is complexed to anions; and 40 percent circulates free as ionized calcium. During pregnancy, there is an active transfer of maternal calcium to the fetus. A full-term infant requires 25 to 30 g of calcium during the course of pregnancy for new bone mineralization.

Total serum calcium during gestation is 8 percent below postpartum levels.[4] The upper limit of normal is 9.5 mg/dl. This decrease in total serum calcium is due to the physiologic hypoalbuminemia secondary to the normal expansion of the intravascular volume observed early in pregnancy. Ionized calcium levels, however, remain unchanged throughout gestation. Serum phosphate and renal tubular reabsorption of phosphorus also remain normal throughout pregnancy. Maternal serum PTH levels, when measured by a sensitive assay that accurately measures the levels of intact PTH, are slightly decreased in the first half of pregnancy (about 20 percent of the mean nonpregnant values) and return to normal by midgestation.[5]

Blood levels of 1,25(OH)$_2$D$_3$ (calcitriol) increase early in gestation as a result of stimulation of renal 1α-hydroxylase activity by estrogen, placental lactogen, and PTH, as well as synthesis of calcitriol by the placenta.[6] Both free and total 1,25(OH)$_2$D$_3$ are increased in pregnancy, the total because of an increase in vitamin D–binding protein.[7]

Twenty-four–hour urinary calcium excretion also increases with each trimester of gestation and falls in the postpartum period[5,8] reflecting the increased intestinal calcium absorption induced by higher levels of 1,25(OH)$_2$D$_3$ during gestation. Pregnancy-induced hypertension is characterized by decreased urinary calcium excretion probably explained by a decrease in serum 1,25-dihydroxyvitamin D serum levels.[9]

Parathyroid hormone–related protein (PTHrP), a peptide responsible for the hypercalcemia found in many malignant tumors, increases in early pregnancy. Hirota et al.[10] measured PTHrP in each trimester of human pregnancy, in umbilical venous blood, and postpartum. A steady increase in plasma values was observed throughout pregnancy, with a peak in the third trimester and high values in cord blood. The plasma concentration in the postpartum period was directly related to the degree of breast-feeding. The source of maternal serum PTHrP is multiple; both fetal and maternal sites have been postulated (placenta, amnion, decidua, fetal parathyroid glands, breast, umbilical cord). PTHrP plays a role in placental calcium transport and also may have a role in protecting the maternal skeleton during pregnancy because the carboxyl-terminal portion of PTHrP ("osteocalcin") has been shown to inhibit osteoclastic bone resorption.[3,11] PTHrP may be involved in the transfer of maternal calcium into breast milk.[12–14]

Serum calcitonin levels are higher during pregnancy and in the postpartum period when compared with those of nonpregnant controls. In 20 percent of patients, the values exceed the normal nonpregnant range.[15] The origin of calcitonin is thyroidal C cells, breast, and placenta. Its role in pregnancy has not been elucidated, although it may protect the maternal skeleton from excessive resorption of calcium.[1]

Osteocalcin is a bone-specific protein released by osteoblasts into the circulation proportional to the rate of new bone formation. It is slightly decreased during the second trimester of pregnancy, with an increase in the postpartum period.[5,16] Markers of bone resorption increase during pregnancy, reaching values in the last trimester of pregnancy up to twice normal. These changes are consistent with the increase in bone turnover at the time of maximal transfer of maternal calcium to the fetus.

Following delivery, urinary calcium excretion is reduced; ionized serum calcium remains within normal limits; and total calcium, 1,25(OH)$_2$D$_3$, and serum PTH return to prepregnancy levels. Intestinal absorption of calcium decreases to the nonpregnnat rate due to the above-mentioned return to normal levels of vitamin 1,25(OH)$_2$D$_3$.[3] Early concern of calcium loss in lactating mothers, with the development of osteopenia, has not been confirmed; and extra calcium supplementation during breast-feeding appears to be unnecessary, because calcium supplementation above normal does not significantly reduce the amount of bone loss during gestation.[17] The alteration in calcium and bone metabolism that accompanies human lactation represents a physiologic response that is independent of calcium intake.[2,18]

Hyperparathyroidism

Primary hyperparathyroidism (PHP) is an uncommon disease in women of childbearing age. The incidence of the disease in pregnancy is unknown, but it is definitely rare; and most of the reported cases have been single ones complemented with a review of the literature. More than 150 cases have been documented in the English literature until 1999,[19] and since then, isolated cases have been reported. With the introduction of routine automated diagnostic techniques in clinical medicine, the majority of patients with PHP are asymptomatic, and their serum calcium elevations are mild. There are few clinical indications for ordering a serum calcium level in pregnancy.

The first case of PHP during pregnancy was reported in 1931.[20] Shortly thereafter, the first case of neonatal hypocalcemia causing tetany in a mother with undiagnosed hypercalcemia due to hyperparathyroidism was described by Friderichsen.[21] The most common cause of PHP in pregnancy is a single parathyroid adenoma, present in about 80 percent of all cases. Primary hyperplasia of the four parathyroid glands accounts for about 15 percent of the cases reported, 3 percent are due to multiple adenomas, and only a few cases due to parathyroid carcinoma have been reported in the English literature.[22] In 1962, Ludwig[23] reviewed the literature on the subject, describing 21 women with 40 pregnancies. The incidence of fetal wastage was 27.5 percent. Neonatal tetany due to hypocalcemia representing the first indication of maternal hyperparathyroidism occurred in 19 percent of these cases. In 1972, Johnstone and coworkers[24] confirmed a perinatal mortality of 25 percent, with a high incidence of neonatal hypocalcemia. Most of the patients reported in early years had significant metabolic complications of hyperparathyroidism, the two most common being renal and bone disease. In contrast to the previous high neonatal morbidity and mortality Kelly,[25] reviewing the literature from 1976 to 1990, found only two perinatal deaths (5 percent) among 37 infants born of hyperparathyroid mothers. Two additional cases of perinatal deaths were reported in mothers with hypercalcemic crises.[26,27]

Today, almost 70 percent of patients are asymptomatic in the nonpregnant state, and the diagnosis is made through the routine use of biochemical screening.[28] In pregnancy, because routine calcium determinations are not performed, manifestations of the disease are present in almost 70 percent of the diagnosed patients. In a review of 70 pregnant women, gastrointestinal symptoms such as nausea, vomiting, and anorexia were present in 36 percent of patients, whereas 34 percent presented with weakness and fatigue. In 26 percent, mental symptoms, including headaches, lethargy, agitation, emotional lability, confusion, and inappropriate behavior, were reported. Nephrolithiasis was detected in 36 percent, bone disease in 19 percent, acute pancreatitis in 13 percent, and hypertension in 10 percent. Only 24 percent of these patients were asymptomatic.[29]

Parathyroid cancer is a rare cause of hyperparathyroidism, with four cases documented in pregnancy. Serum calcium levels are significantly higher than in other causes of PHP.[21,30–32] Perinatal mortality and morbidity were significant. Hypercalcemia with values higher than 13 mg/dl in the presence of a palpable neck mass should raise a strong suspicion of parathyroid carcinoma. On the contrary, in the presence of mild hypercalcemia and a neck mass, the most common cause of the neck lesion is a thyroid nodule. One other characteristic clinical feature of parathyroid carcinoma is the patient's poor response to the usual clinical therapeutic measures such as intensive hydration and loop diuretics. Surgery is the only effective therapy.

Hyperparathyroidism should be considered in the differential diagnosis of acute pancreatitis during pregnancy. Acute pancreatitis has been reported in 13 percent of women with primary hyperparathyroidism. The incidence in nonpregnant hyperparathyroid women is about 1.5 percent, and is less than 1 percent in normal pregnancy.[33] This complication is associated with significant rates of neonatal and maternal morbidity.[34] It is more common in the primipara than in women who have had multiple pregnancies. Acute pancreatitis with PHP is mostly likely to occur during the last trimester of pregnancy or the postpartum period, but has also been reported in the first trimester of pregnancy, mimicking hyperemesis gravidarum (HG). Indeed, in two cases, hyperthyroidism was also present, which most likely represents the syndrome of transient hyperthyroidism of HG (see section on Thyroid Diseases, later). Serum calcium should be obtained in any pregnant woman with persistent significant nausea, vomiting, and abdominal pain.

Hyperparathyroid crisis, a serious complication of PHP, has been reported during gestation and the postpartum period, and is characterized by severe nausea and vomiting, generalized weakness, changes in mental status, and severe dehydration. Hypertension may be present and should be differentiated from preeclampsia. The serum calcium is frequently higher than 14 mg/dl; hypokalemia and elevation in serum creatinine are routinely seen. If not recognized and treated promptly, hyperparathyroid crisis may progress to uremia, coma, and death. Of the 12 cases reported in the literature, four occurred in the postpartum period. Patients presented with severe nausea, vomiting, and elevation in serum creatinine due to dehydration. Serum calcium levels higher than 20 mg/dl were reported in three cases,[19,35,36] and three patients died.[35,37,38] Six cases have been associated with pancreatitis. Four fetal deaths have also been reported.

Bone disease in patients with PHP is now unusual. However, in early series, it was a common complication.[24] Radiologic evaluation of the bones showed diffuse demineralization, subperiosteal resorption of the phalanges, and in severe cases, single or multiple cystic lesions and generalized osteoporosis. A 27-year-old woman was described with generalized musculoskeletal pain and radiographic evidence of advanced bone disease at 34 weeks' gestation.[39]

The two most common causes of neonatal morbidity are prematurity and neonatal hypocalcemia, the latter related to levels of maternal hypercalcemia. In early reports, it was frequently the only clue of maternal hyperparathyroidism. Neonatal hypocalcemia develops between the 2nd and 14th day of life, and lasts for a few days.[21,24]

The diagnosis of PHP is based on persistent hypercalcemia in the presence of increased serum PTH levels.[28,40] A persistent serum calcium value higher than 9.5 mg/dl should make the examiner suspicious of hypercalcemia. Serum phosphorus is decreased in about 50 percent of pregnant women with PHP. A determination of 24-hour urinary calcium excretion is helpful in the diagnosis, because most women with PHP have an increase in urinary calcium excretion that is higher than the usual hypercalciuria of normal pregnancy. Urinary calcium excretion is low or low normal in the syndrome of familial hypocalciuric hypercalcemia (FHH), another cause of hypercalcemia that needs to be included in the differential diagnosis. The serum alkaline phosphatase level may be increased in PHP. However, it is also increased in normal pregnancy. High-resolution ultrasonography of the neck is not useful, because it seldom differentiates a parathyroid lesion from nodular thyroid disease. Parathyroid imaging studies are contraindicated in pregnancy.

Differential Diagnosis of Hypercalcemia

Although most young women with hypercalcemia have PHP, other unusual causes should be ruled out, mainly endocrine disorders, vitamin D or A overdose, the use

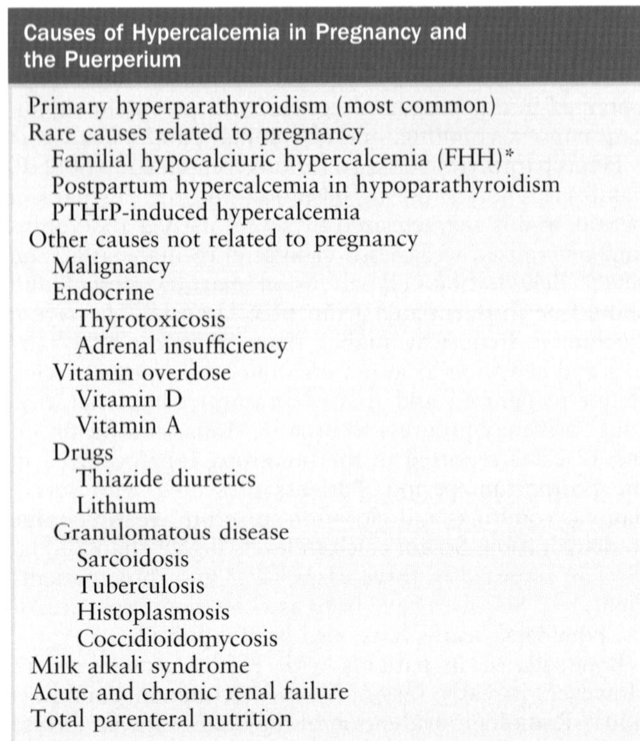

Causes of Hypercalcemia in Pregnancy and the Puerperium

Primary hyperparathyroidism (most common)
Rare causes related to pregnancy
- Familial hypocalciuric hypercalcemia (FHH)*
- Postpartum hypercalcemia in hypoparathyroidism
- PTHrP-induced hypercalcemia

Other causes not related to pregnancy
- Malignancy
- Endocrine
  - Thyrotoxicosis
  - Adrenal insufficiency
- Vitamin overdose
  - Vitamin D
  - Vitamin A
- Drugs
  - Thiazide diuretics
  - Lithium
- Granulomatous disease
  - Sarcoidosis
  - Tuberculosis
  - Histoplasmosis
  - Coccidioidomycosis

Milk alkali syndrome
Acute and chronic renal failure
Total parenteral nutrition

*Different expression with significant neonatal manifestations.
From Mestman JH: Endocrine diseases in pregnancy. *In* Sciarra JJ (ed): Gynecology and Obstetrics. Philadelphia, Lippincott-Raven, 1997, p 11, with permission.

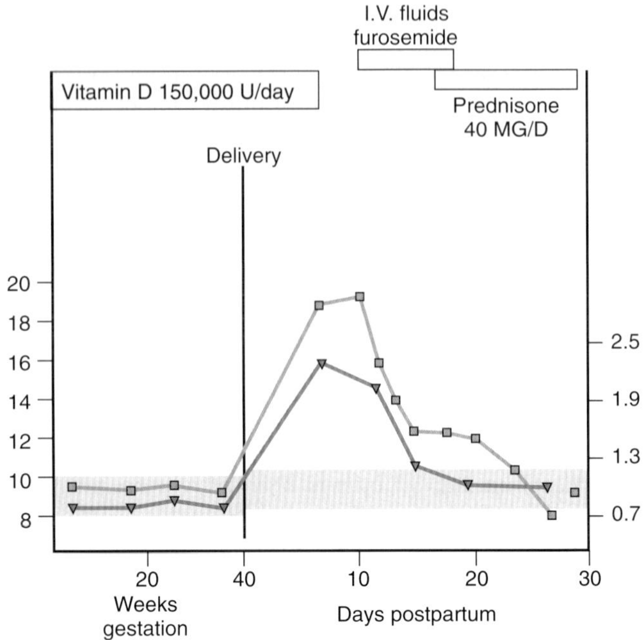

Figure 38-1. Serum calcium *(closed squares)* and creatinine *(closed triangles)* levels during pregnancy and 1 month after delivery in a woman with hypoparathyroidism who was treated with vitamin D and calcium. IV, intravenously administered; stippled area, normal range.

of thiazide diuretics, or granulomatous diseases (see the box "Causes of Hypercalcemia in Pregnancy and the Puerperium"). A brief discussion of three uncommon syndromes associated with hypercalcemia during pregnancy follows.

1. FHH is an autosomal dominant condition with a high penetrance for hypercalcemia. The disorder is associated with an inactivating mutation in the gene for the calcium-sensor receptor.[41] The main function of the receptor is in the regulation of calcium balance through changes in the parathyroid and kidneys. Mild hypercalcemia, slight elevation in serum PTH, mild hypermagnesemia, and low urinary calcium excretion are the typical findings. There is moderate hyperplasia of the four parathyroid glands. Total parathyroidectomy is seldom indicated owing to the benign course of the disease.[42] Infants born to mothers with FHH may present with different clinical manifestations. First, asymptomatic hypercalcemia can develop in an affected offspring if the mother is a carrier for FHH. In a second situation, severe neonatal hypocalcemia can occur in a mother with FHH syndrome. Although neonatal hypocalcemia could be severe, neonatal parathyroid function returns to normal a few weeks after delivery.[43] In the third situation, severe neonatal hypercalcemia, also called neonatal severe hyperparathyroidism,[44] occurs in infants homozygous for the FHH gene defect. Some infants require parathyroidectomy soon after birth.
2. Postpartum hypercalcemia may occur in women with treated hypoparathyroidism.[45,46] The mechanism for hypercalcemia is not well understood. Nausea and vomiting develop a few days after delivery, dehydration ensues, and other manifestations of hypercalcemia develop, mainly mental changes. Serum calcium may be significantly elevated. Patients with treated hypoparathyroidism should be followed postpartum with serum calcium determinations, and vitamin D should be discontinued if hypercalcemia occurs. In severe cases, intravenous fluids and glucocorticoid therapy are required[47] (Fig. 38-1).
3. A few cases of hypercalcemia, mediated by PTHrP, during pregnancy and in the postpartum period have been reported.[48,49] In one case, hypercalcemia developed in two successive pregnancies. In the second pregnancy, serum PTHrP levels were elevated three times normal and the infant was born with mild hypercalcemia that returned to normal within 24 hours after delivery.[48] In the other case,[49] a 25-year-old woman had massive bilateral breast enlargement at 24 weeks' gestation. Her serum calcium level was 14.3 mg/dl, but her serum PTH level was undetectable. She underwent bilateral mastectomy during pregnancy. The immunohistochemical studies demonstrated PTHrP antigenic activity in breast tissue.

Therapy

Surgery is the only effective treatment for PHP. A novel oral agent that acts directly on the calcium sensor is being investigated. It has not been approved for clinical use in pregnancy.[50] Surgery is a safe procedure when performed by a surgeon with extensive experience in neck surgery. Complications due to surgery, particularly in the presence of a single lesion, are low and the cure rate is excellent. In nonpregnant individuals without symptoms or complications and with serum calcium below 12 mg/dl, the conservative approach is an alternative therapeutic choice.

Guidelines for the management of PHP in nonpregnant individuals have been suggested.[51] The proper management of PHP in pregnancy has not been uniformly agreed upon. For asymptomatic pregnant women in whom serum calcium is below 11 mg/dl, close follow-up with proper hydration and avoidance of medications that could elevate calcium such as thiazide diuretics is reasonable, although there are no studies in the literature supporting this or any other approach. Because most of the neonatal complications have been reported in patients with symptomatic disease, a surgical approach is indicated in such patients, as well as those with complications such as nephrolithiasis and bone disease, as well as those with persistent hypercalcemia (>11 mg/dl). It is preferable to perform the surgery in the second trimester of pregnancy. In the series reported by Carella and Gossain,[29] 38 women underwent parathyroidectomy during pregnancy, seven during the first trimester and the other 18 in the second trimester. In the total group of 25, there was only 1 fetal loss. In 12 women in whom surgery was performed during the third trimester of pregnancy, the incidence of perinatal complications was 58 percent.

For women with PHP first diagnosed after 28 weeks' gestation, the optimal treatment strategy is unclear, and the decision in such a situation should be based on general patient condition, severity of hypercalcemia, and other complicating circumstances. A significant lower incidence of complications, both maternal and fetal were reported in a review of 16 published cases operated on after 27 weeks gestation.[52]

Medical therapy is reserved for those patients with significant hypercalcemia who are not surgical candidates. Oral phosphate therapy as inorganic phosphorus in doses of 1.5 to 2.5 g/day has been shown to be effective in controlling hypercalcemia.[53] Side effects of oral phosphate therapy include nausea, vomiting, and hypokalemia. These problems can be easily avoided by decreasing the dose of the medication. In patients in whom surgery is not advisable, it is important to prevent elevations in serum calcium. Good hydration, early treatment of urinary tract infections, and avoiding medications known to cause elevations in serum calcium such as vitamin D, vitamin A, aminophylline, and thiazide diuretics are all important therapeutic measures. Serum calcium should be determined on a regular basis.

In patients undergoing surgical treatment, hypocalcemia, albeit transient, may occur after surgery in some cases. Serum calcium should be checked every 6 hours, and if the patient develops hypocalcemic symptoms, intravenous calcium in the form of calcium gluconate, 10 to 20 ml of a 10 percent solution, should be given over a period of 5 to 10 minutes. Intermittent infusions may be repeated or calcium gluconate can be diluted in 5-percent dextrose or isotonic saline and infused continuously at 1 mg/kg body weight per hour. In patients with bone disease, postsurgical hypocalcemia may be profound, and aggressive treatment is needed. These patients may benefit from vitamin D supplementation in the form of calcitriol 0.25 to 0.5 µg/day for a few days before operative intervention.[54]

Hypoparathyroidism

The most common etiology of hypoparathyroidism is damage to or removal of the parathyroid glands in the course of surgery for disorders of the thyroid gland. The incidence of permanent hypoparathyroidism following thyroid surgery has been estimated to be between 0.2 and 3.5 percent. In many cases, hypocalcemia in the immediate postoperative period is only transitory. Idiopathic hypoparathyroidism is a much less common cause of the disease, frequently associated with other autoimmune endocrinopathies, as part of the polyglandular autoimmune syndrome type 1. Antibodies directed against parathyroid calcium–sensing receptor have been detected in 56 percent of patients with idiopathic hypoparathyroidism.[55]

The requirement for calcium supplementation and vitamin D may decrease in some but not all women with hypoparathyroidism during the second half of pregnancy and lactation. In a few cases, hypocalcemic symptoms ameliorate with progression of pregnancy. The explanation for the above-mentioned findings is not clear. It may be related to the increased intestinal absorption of calcium or the production of vitamin D by the placenta.

Clinical clues for the diagnosis of hypoparathyroidism include a previous history of thyroid surgery, and clinical, radiologic, and laboratory information. Typical symptoms of hypocalcemia are numbness and tingling of the fingers and toes and around the lips. Patients may complain of carpopedal spasm, laryngeal stridor, and dyspnea. Convulsions may be a manifestation of severe hypocalcemia. Symptoms of irritability, emotional lability, impairment of memory, and depression are common. On physical examination, patients with idiopathic hypoparathyroidism demonstrate changes in the teeth, skin, nails, and hair as well as papilledema and cataracts. Chvostek's sign, a twitch of the facial muscles, notably those of the upper lip, when a sharp tap is given over the facial nerve, is seen in many patients with hypocalcemia. Chvostek's sign has also been described in 10 percent of normal adults. Trousseau's sign, the induction of carpopedal spasm by reducing the circulation in the arm with a blood pressure cuff, is another sign of hypocalcemia. The constriction should be maintained above the systolic blood pressure for 2 minutes before the test is considered negative.

The diagnosis of hypoparathyroidism is confirmed by the presence of persistent low serum calcium and high serum phosphate levels. Plasma alkaline phosphatase is usually normal. The differential diagnosis of hypocalcemia includes rickets, osteomalacia, and hypomagnesemia.

Marked hypocalcemia may occur in severely ill patients. The etiology is unclear, and a return to normal serum calcium is the rule following recovery from the acute event.[56]

In 1942, Anderson and Musselman[57] published a review of the literature on hypoparathyroidism and tetany in pregnancy, collecting 240 cases. Twenty-six of the cases were due to post–thyroid surgery, and 140 were the so-called idiopathic type. It is likely that in some of these cases tetany was not due to hypoparathyroidism. Therapeutic abortion was recommended because of the high fetal and maternal mortality rate. Other reports have confirmed that hypoparathyroidism, if not properly treated, may increase perinatal loss, including spontaneous abortions, stillbirths, and neonatal deaths.[58,59] Radiologic bone changes may be present in the newborn as a consequence of intrauterine hyperparathyroidism. They are characterized by generalized skeletal demineralization, subperiosteal bone resorption, bowing of the long bones, osteitis fibrosa cystica, and rib and limb deformities. Loughead et al.[60] described 16 infants of hypoparathyroid mothers. Secondary hyperparathyroidism in the infants resolved by 1 month of age.

Vitamin D deficiency in the mother has been associated with decreased fetal growth. Maternal serum calcium may be normal or slightly decreased. Brunvand et al.[61] followed 30 Pakistani women during pregnancy, 13 with elevated serum PTH levels at the time of delivery, and 29 with serum levels of $1,25(OH)_2D_3$ below normal. There was a positive correlation between serum maternal ionized calcium levels and the crown-heel length of the newborn. The authors suggested that vitamin D deficiency could interfere with fetal growth through an effect on maternal calcium homeostasis.

Treatment of hypoparathyroidism in pregnancy does not differ from the nonpregnant state, including a normal high-calcium diet and vitamin D supplementation. The normal calcium supplementation of pregnancy is about 1.2 g/day. Vitamin D requirements may decrease in some patients by the second half of gestation. Calcitriol 1 to 3 μg/day is used almost routinely in most patients affected with hypoparathyroidism.[47,62,63] Calcitriol must be given in single or divided doses, because its half life is much shorter than vitamin D. If vitamin D is used, the dose is in the range of 50,000 to 150,000 IU/weekly. The importance of compliance with medications should be strongly emphasized, particularly when calcitriol is prescribed, in view of its short half life. The major problem in the treatment of hypoparathyroidism is the recurrence of hypercalcemia and hypocalcemia. Therefore, serum calcium determinations should be performed at regular intervals. The most common symptoms of vitamin D intoxication are nausea, constipation, fatigue, headaches, and in more severe cases, vomiting and dehydration. It is important to assess serum calcium and phosphorous during pregnancy, particularly in the postpartum period, to detect the early onset of hypercalcemia (see earlier).[53,64]

Lactation in mothers taking vitamin D may be contraindicated, because a metabolite of vitamin D, $1,25(OH)_2D_3$, has been detected in breast milk in high concentration in a mother taking 50,000 IU of vitamin D daily.[65] Regardless of the form of vitamin D prescribed, serum calcium determinations should be conducted in the postpartum period, particularly in breast-feeding mothers.

Pseudohypoparathyroidism

Pseudohypoparathyroidism encompasses several different disorders having as a common feature varying degrees of target organ resistance to PTH. Somatic changes are present in some forms of the syndrome, including short stature, obesity, round face, brachydactyly, and mental retardation, with brain calcifications. This variant is known as Albright's syndrome type 1a. Most patients suffer from hypocalcemia, due to a derangement of renal 1α-hydroxylase and production of calcitriol. A few cases have been reported during pregnancy. Spontaneous normocalcemia occurred in two patients during four pregnancies. The authors provided evidence of placental synthesis of calcitriol to account for the normocalcemia. In both patients, serum PTH, which was significantly increased before pregnancy, was reduced by 50 percent during gestation. Serum cord calcium, phosphorus, and calcitriol concentrations were within normal limits.[66,67] These infants are at risk for intrauterine fetal hyperparathyroidism, perhaps because of the relative maternal hypocalcemia during pregnancy.[68]

Osteoporosis

The condition of idiopathic osteoporosis related to pregnancy was recognized in the 1950s.[69] In the last few years, there has been an increased interest in several clinical aspects of osteoporosis in pregnancy and lactation.[70–74] In general, osteoporosis is suspected in pregnancy when the patient presents with severe, persistent back or hip pain and radiologic examination shows signs of osteopenia. Studies measuring calcitrophic hormones and biochemical markers of bone reabsorption in each trimester in pregnancy and in the postpartum period showed a slight decrease in bone mass in the third trimester,[73] followed by recovery within the first 6 months postpartum. In a study of a group of white, upper middle class, postmenopausal women, there was no association between the number of pregnancies and lactation as predictors of decreased bone mineral density.[75]

Osteoporosis may be diagnosed during pregnancy or in the postpartum period. Whether these are two different syndromes or represent the same clinical entity is unclear, because the symptoms may begin during pregnancy, but the diagnosis is made for the first time after delivery. Osteoporosis diagnosed during pregnancy may be localized in the hips, lumbar spine, or both. Pain in one hip or back pain is the presenting symptom in most cases, usually in the second half of gestation. Spontaneous recovery is the usual course a few months postpartum.[76] A case has been reported of onset in the first trimester, with recovery following abortion.[77]

Although osteoporosis has been diagnosed during pregnancy, pregnancy unmasks rather than causes low bone mass. As suggested by Rizzoli and Bonjour and others,[72,78,79] postural changes during pregnancy, including increased lordosis, when superimposed on a small and transient decrease in bone mass, may lead to pain and even fractures. In a study of 24 women with symptoms of bone pain for many years, 18 of them complained of back pain, five reported hip pain, and one noted ankle pain in late pregnancy and up to 8 months after delivery.[71] Radiologic examination of the spine showed vertebral deformities in 17. Bone mass was measured in 21, and seven women had evidence of osteoporosis and 13 were osteopenic. The authors conclude that bone mass was probably low before pregnancy and that a transient and slight decrease in bone mass during pregnancy could have weakened the bone further. Radiologic examination of the localized painful area and studies of bone density following delivery are indicated. In some cases, a short course of calcitonin or bisphosphonate plus calcium supplementation may be needed.

The impact of lactation on the progression of osteoporosis is controversial. The study by Kritz-Silverstein et al.[75] revealed that lactation by itself was not a determinant of bone mineral density. Although one investigation reported that lactation for more than 8 months was associated with greater bone mineral at both the femoral neck and shaft,[80] another study found that nursing for longer than 9 months produced a greater decrease in bone mass than that observed during the first 6- to 9-month period of nursing.[81] Given this controversy, the health care provider must decide if cessation of lactation is advisable in the management of osteoporosis.

Heparin-associated osteoporosis has been reported in several cases during pregnancy.[82] It may be related to the total dose of heparin. Treatment with calcium supplementation or calcitriol, although not proven, may be helpful in those patients receiving heparin therapy. Barbour et al.[83] followed 14 pregnant women requiring heparin therapy. Five of the 14 patients experienced a 10-percent decrease from baseline proximal femur bone density measurements as compared with none in a matched control group. They concluded that heparin adversely affected bone density in about one third of exposed patients.

THYROID DISEASES

Thyroid disorders in pregnancy present a unique opportunity for health care professionals to use a similar "team approach" that has successfully improved the care of women with diabetes mellitus. Because of changes in thyroid economy occurring early in pregnancy, it is imperative to advise women with chronic thyroid diseases to plan their pregnancies and contact their health care professionals as soon as the diagnosis of pregnancy is made. Autoimmune thyroid disease occurs five to eight times more often in women than in men, and its course could be affected by the immunologic changes occurring in pregnancy and in the postpartum period.[84–86]

In early pregnancy, the maternal thyroid gland is challenged with an increased demand for thyroid hormone secretion, due mainly to three different factors: (1) the increase in thyroxine-binding globulin (TBG) due to the effect of estrogen on the liver, (2) the stimulatory effect of human chorionic gonadotropin (hCG) on the thyroid-stimulating hormone (TSH) thyroid receptor, and (3) the supply of iodine available to the thyroid gland. This last factor is of importance in areas of iodine deficiency. In the United States, the iodine content in the diet, although decreased in the last decades, appears to be insufficient in only about 10 percent of pregnancies.[86] The suggested total daily iodine ingestion for pregnant women is 229 μg a day and for lactating women 289 μg daily; prenatal vitamins should contain at least 150 μg of iodine.[87]

The normal thyroid gland is able to compensate for the increase in thyroid hormones demands by increasing their secretion and maintaining the serum levels of free hormones within normal limits. However, in those situations in which there is a subtle pathologic abnormality of the thyroid gland, such as chronic autoimmune thyroiditis, the normal increase in the production of thyroid hormones is not met. As a consequence, the pregnant woman could develop biochemical markers of hypothyroidism (i.e., an elevation in serum TSH, and an increase in the size of the thyroid gland).

Active secretion of thyroid hormones by the fetal thyroid gland commences at about 18 weeks' gestation, although iodine uptake occurs between 10 and 14 weeks.[88] Transfer of thyroxine from the mother to the embryo occurs from early pregnancy. Maternal thyroxine has been demonstrated in coelomic fluid at 6 weeks[89] and in the fetal brain at 9 weeks.[90] This maternal transfer continues until delivery, but only in significant amounts in the presence of fetal hypothyroidism.[91] Thyroid hormone receptor gene expression has been shown in the human fetal brain by 8 weeks' gestation, supporting the important role of maternal thyroid hormone during the first trimester of human pregnancy in fetal brain development.[92] Recent studies, that need to be confirmed, suggest that mild maternal thyroid deficiency in the first trimester could result in long-term neuropsychological damage to the offspring.[93,94]

The levels of maternal thyroid hormone concentrations, both total thyroxine (TT_4) and total triiodothyronine (TT_3) increase from early pregnancy as the result of an elevation in TBG and a reduced peripheral TBG degradation rate.[93] TBG reaches a plateau by 20 weeks' gestation and remains unchanged until delivery.[94] In spite of these acute changes in total hormone concentration, the serum free fractions of both T_4 and T_3 remain within normal limits, unless there is a decreased supply of iodine to the mother or in the presence of abnormalities of the thyroid gland.[95]

hCG is a weak thyroid stimulator, acting on the thyroid TSH receptor. It is estimated that a 10,000 IU/L increment in circulating hCG corresponds to a mean T_4 increment in serum of 0.1 ng/dl and, in turn, to a lowering of TSH of 0.1 mU/L. In situations in which there is a high production of hCG, such as in cases of multiple pregnancies, hydatidiform mole, and HG, serum T_4 concentrations rise to levels seen in thyrotoxicosis with a transient suppression in serum TSH values. Low TSH values may be seen in 15 percent of uncomplicated pregnancies, returning to normal with progression of pregnancy.[96]

Thyroid Function Tests

Measurement of serum TSH is the most practical, simple, and economic screening test for thyroid dysfunction.[97] Normal TSH concentrations are dependent on gestational age and whether there is a singleton or twin pregnancy[98]; it is lower in the first trimester as compared with the second and third trimester of pregnancy There are significant clinical data at the present time to support an upper limit of serum TSH for first trimester of pregnancy as a value of 2.5 mU/L.[99,100] There is a fairly good inverse correlation between TSH and hCG concentrations. An elevated serum TSH value is consistent with the diagnosis of primary hypothyroidism, whereas a suppressed one, with few exceptions, is suggestive of hyperthyroidism (Fig. 38-2). As mentioned earlier, low or suppressed TSH values are present in about 15 percent of pregnant women in the first trimester of gestation, most of them without active thyroid pathology; in the vast majority of them, the TSH returned to normal with progression of pregnancy.[96] In one study, 9 percent had low values (between 0.05 and 0.4 mU/L) and in another 9 percent the values were suppressed less than 0.05 mU/L.[101] In the presence of an abnormal serum TSH value, the determination of FT_4 or its equivalent free thyroxine index (FT_4I) is necessary for the proper assessment of thyroid function. A word of caution regarding the determination of free thyroxine levels in the different trimester of pregnancy.[100] Although discrepant findings have been reported, in most studies, FT_4 concentrations increase slightly in the first trimester of pregnancy and decline with progression of pregnancy. There is a significant inconsistency among the different assay of FT_4 reported by commercial laboratories because of methodology used and also because of variation in dietary iodine intake among the different populations studied. At present, none of the manufacturers of the automated FT_4 assays has provided trimester-specific reference ranges.[100] Values in the lowered limits of normal and even in the hypothyroid range are not uncommonly seen in daily clinical practice, particularly in the third trimester of pregnancy.

Because the determination of FT_4 by the dialysis method, the gold standard for FT_4 assessment, is not routinely available because it is a cumbersome and time-consuming procedure, and is very expensive, the determination of TT_4 adjusted by a factor of 1.5 for pregnant patients has been suggested.[99,100] A better alternative is to estimate the FT_4, using the so-called FT_4I, calculated using the TT_4 value and an indirect determination of serum TBG concentration. The interpretation and the significance of the FT_4I may be confusing to physicians. In a recent survey of obstetrician-gynecologists by the American College of Obstetricians and Gynecologists (ACOG), about 50 percent of the respondents were uncertain of the meaning of the FT_4I.[102]

Before the commercial use of the automated determination of free thyroxine, the traditional method used to assess or estimate free thyroxine levels was measuring unoccupied binding sites in the TBG molecule by the resin T_3 uptake test (RT_3U), also reported as thyroid hormone–binding ratio (THBR). The results of such tests are reported as percent, as in the case of RT_3U, or as an index, which is simply a normalized RT_3U value, reported as a value of 0.85 to 1.1. The value then is multiplied by the serum TT_4 or TT_3 concentration to obtain the FT_4I or FT_3I. These tests have been applied in situations, such as pregnancy or estrogen therapy, in which the TT_4 and TT_3 are elevated owing to an increase in serum TBG concentrations secondary to the effect of estrogen. With the recent concerns about discrepancies in FT_4 determination in different commercial laboratories, and the consistent decline in serum concentrations with progression of pregnancy, the FT_4I appears to be the most reliable test for assessing indirectly the FT_4 and FT_3 concentration

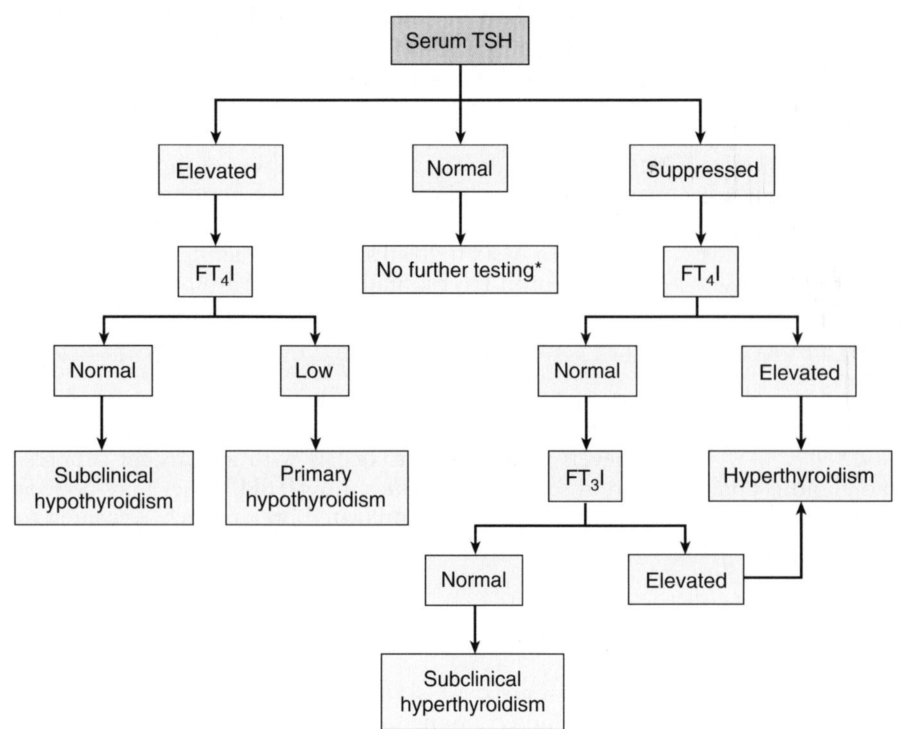

Figure 38-2. Algorithm for the diagnosis of thyroid disease. *If there is clinical suspicion of secondary hypothyroidism, a determination of FT_4I is indicated. In this situation, the serum TSH is normal in the presence of low FT_4I. FT_3I, free triiodothyronine index or its equivalent, free triiodothyronine; FT_4I, free thryoxine index or its equivalent, free thyroxine; TSH, thyroid-stimulating hormone.

Indications for Determination of Maternal TSI or TRAb

Graves' disease (TSI)
- Fetal or neonatal hyperthyroidism in previous pregnancies
- Active disease, on treatment with antithyroid drugs
- Euthyroid, postablation, in the presence of:
  - Fetal tachycardia
  - Intrauterine growth restriction
  - Incidental fetal goiter on ultrasound

Chronic thyroiditis without goiter (TRAb)
Incidental fetal goiter on ultrasound (TRAb)
Infant born with congenital hypothyroidism (TRAb)

TSI, TSH stimulating immunoglobulin; TRAb, TSH receptor antibodies.
From Mestman JH: Endocrine diseases in pregnancy. *In* Sciarra JJ (ed): Gynecology and Obstetrics. Philadelphia, Lippincott-Raven, 1997, p 27, with permission.

Therefore, it is imperative for the practicing physician to be familiar with the interpretation and significance of thyroid tests as reported by a given commercial laboratory. The use of a limited number of thyroid function tests (TFTs), properly ordered and interpreted, allow the physician to assess thyroid function and make the proper therapeutic decisions.

A suppressed TSH value and high concentrations of FT_4 or FT_4I are diagnostic of hyperthyroidism. There are special situations in which hyperthyroidism may occur in the presence of low TSH and normal concentrations of FT_4. In such cases, a serum FT_3 or FT_3I determination should be obtained. High values are diagnostic of hyperthyroidism, the so-called T_3-toxicosis syndrome, sometimes seen in patients with an autonomous or "hot" thyroid nodule.

The determination of TSH receptor antibodies (TSHRBAb or TRAb) is indicated in very special circumstances (see the box "Indications for Determination of Maternal TSI or TRAb"), in order to predict the possibility of fetal or neonatal thyroid dysfunction. These antibodies are immunoglobulins, usually of the immunoglobulin G (IgG) subclass, having different functional activity: stimulating (in most patients with Graves' disease) or blocking (in some patients with Hashimoto's thyroiditis, particularly in those without goiter) the TSH receptor of the thyroid gland. They do cross the placental barrier and may affect fetal thyroid function. The determination of TSH receptor antibodies (TSRAb) is commercially available using *binding assays*. These assays do not discriminate between stimulating and blocking antibodies. However, a *specific bioassay* is commercially available for the determination of stimulating antibodies (thyroid-stimulating immunoglobulins [TSIs]). In the majority of cases, detected TRAb in the serum of patients with Graves' disease indicates a stimulating effect, and in the serum of patients with chronic or Hashimoto's thyroiditis suggests a blocking or inhibitory effect. TSIs, formerly known as long-acting thyroid-stimulating antibody, when present in high concentrations in the maternal serum may cause fetal or neonatal hyperthyroidism.[103] Thyroid-blocking antibodies (TRAb) in high titers in the mother may produce neonatal hypothyroidism, a condition that is transient owing to the short half life of these

Indications for Thyroid Testing in Pregnancy

Family history of autoimmune thyroid disease
Women on thyroid therapy
Presence of goiter
Previous history of:
- High-dose neck radiation
- Therapy for hyperthyroidism
- Postpartum thyroid dysfunction
- Previous birth of an infant with thyroid disease

Type 1 diabetes mellitus

From Mestman JH: Thyroid diseases in pregnancy other than Graves' disease and postpartum thyroid dysfunction. Endocrinologist 9:924, 1999, with permission.

antibodies.[104] Both antibodies may be present in patients with Graves' disease, and could explain the spontaneous improvement or aggravation of the disease with progression of pregnancy and in the postpartum period, respectively. The chances for the offspring to be affected by these maternal antibodies are very low, up to 2 percent of mothers with autoimmune thyroid disease. However, if mothers with high titers are not properly identified, the consequences for the infant could be irreversible neurologic and metabolic sequelae. Titers of these antibodies decrease with the progression of pregnancy. This could explain, in the case of Graves' disease, the tendency to spontaneous clinical improvement and the decrease in antithyroid drug requirement in the second half of pregnancy. A value of TRAb or TSI three to five times greater than normal is considered predictive of fetal or neonatal thyroid dysfunction.

Goiter is commonly seen in pregnancy in areas of iodine deficiency. However, in the United States and other areas of the world with sufficient iodine intake, the thyroid gland does not clinically increase in size during pregnancy. Therefore, the detection of a goiter in pregnancy is an abnormal finding that needs careful evaluation. The most common cause of diffuse goiter is chronic autoimmune thyroiditis or Hashimoto's thyroiditis. Most patients are euthyroid and the diagnosis is made by the determination of thyroid antibodies, mainly thyroid peroxidase (TPO). Antibody concentration decreases during pregnancy and increases in the postpartum period. High values in the first trimester of pregnancy are predictors of the syndrome of postpartum thyroid dysfunction.[105]

The indications for requesting TFTs are represented in the box "Indications for Thyroid Testing in Pregnancy." Whether routine thyroid screening in pregnant women is necessary remains a controversial issue, which is to be decided in the next few years.[106–108]

Prepregnancy Counseling

The physician may be faced with different clinical situations when counseling a woman contemplating pregnancy. With the advent of available information in the electronic media, it is important for the health care professional to offer the patient and her family objective and scientific data, supported by medical literature published in recognized peer-reviewed medical journals. The clinical situations may be summarized as follows:

1. *Hyperthyroidism under antithyroid drug treatment:* A choice of the three classic therapeutic options for hyperthyroidism treatment should be given: (1) long-term antithyroid drug therapy, (2) radioactive ^{131}I ablation, and (3) near-total thyroidectomy. Potential side effects of antithyroid drugs on the fetus should be discussed. If the patient opts for ablation therapy, there is no long-term effect of ^{131}I given to the future mother or the offspring. However, it is customary to wait 6 months after the therapeutic dose is administered before pregnancy is contemplated. Surgery is another option, selected by some physicians and patients concerned about the potential side effects of antithyroid drugs or radioactive treatment. Regardless of the form of therapy chosen, it is important for the patient to be euthyroid at the time of conception. In a large series of hyperthyroid pregnant women, a doubling in congenital malformations was reported when hyperthyroidism was not controlled in the first trimester of pregnancy as compared with women who were euthyroid early in gestation.[109]
   In 42 women with a previous history of Graves' disease, treated with antithyroid drugs, with no detectable anti-TSH receptor antibodies and normal thyroid function tests, pregnancy outcome was compared with 102 pregnant control women. None of the women with Graves' disease developed thyroid dysfunction during gestation, and the perinatal outcome was comparable to the control group.[110]
2. *Previous ablation treatment for Graves' disease:* Two points are important: (1) the dose of thyroid replacement therapy needs to be increased in most women soon after conception[111,112]; and (2) although the mother may be euthyroid, high maternal titers for TSI or TSHRAb may be present, with the fetus being at risk of developing hyperthyroidism.[113] Close follow-up during pregnancy and communication between the obstetrician and endocrinologist are essential.
3. *Previous treatment with radioactive iodine ^{131}I for thyroid carcinoma:* Pregnancy does not affect the natural history of women previously treated for thyroid cancer. Spontaneous miscarriages have been reported to be as high as 40 percent in the first year after radiation treatment as compared with 18 percent in women who have received no radiation.[114] Therefore, it appears reasonable for patients with thyroid carcinoma to wait 1 year after completion of radioactive treatment before conception. Adjustment of the thyroid dose should be done early in pregnancy and in each trimester; serum TSH should be kept in the low normal range or undetectable.
   No adverse effect on fertility or genetic risk to the offspring was reported in 50 pregnancies of 40 women treated with high-dose ^{131}I.[115]
4. *Treated hypothyroidism:* Women who are under treatment with thyroid hormone may require higher doses soon after conception.[111,112,116] As shown by Kaplan,[112] the dose of thyroid hormone needed increases according to the etiology of hypothyroidism, with higher doses necessary for those women post thyroid ablation. The increase in requirements is observed in the first 6 to 8 weeks of gestation.[94] As soon as the diagnosis of pregnancy is made, thyroid tests should be performed, and thyroid doses adjusted accordingly. Following delivery, the dose should be reduced to prepregnancy levels. Common medications may affect the absorption of levothyroxine (L-thyroxine), such as ferrous sulfate[117] and calcium[118] among others. Patients should take L-thyroxine at least 2 hours apart from other medications.
5. *Euthyroid chronic thyroiditis:* Patients with Hashimoto's thyroiditis are at greater risk for spontaneous abortion and the development of postpartum thyroiditis.[119–122] Thyroid tests are indicated in early pregnancy to detect elevations in TSH and assess the need for treatment with thyroid hormones in prepregnancy euthyroid women or to adjust the dose in patients already on thyroid therapy.

Maternal-Placental-Fetal Interactions

Studies in the past 2 decades have shown an important role of maternal thyroid hormones in embryogenesis.[123,124] It is known that maternal thyroxine crosses the placenta in the first half of pregnancy, at a time when the fetal thyroid gland is not functional. Several studies have suggested an adverse effect on the intellectual development of children of mothers with mild thyroid deficiency in the first 20 weeks of gestation.[93,94]

Maternal TSH does not cross the placenta. Thyrotropin-releasing hormone (TRH) does cross the placental barrier, but its physiologic significance is unknown. TRH has been given to mothers to accelerate fetal lung maturation in premature infants.[124]

Methimazole (MM) and propylthiouracil (PTU), drugs used for the treatment of hyperthyroidism, cross the placenta and, if given in inappropriate doses, may produce fetal goiter and hypothyroidism.[125] Preparations containing iodine given in large doses or for prolonged periods of time are contraindicated in pregnancy, because accumulation by the fetal thyroid may induce goiter and hypothyroidism.[126,127]

Hyperthyroidism

Hyperthyroidism affects pregnancy in about 0.1 to 0.4 percent of patients.[128,129] Classically, it has been stated that Graves' disease is the most common cause of hyperthyroxinemia in pregnancy, with other etiologies being uncommon (see the box "Etiologies of Hyperthyroidism

Etiologies of Hyperthyroidism in Pregnancy

Graves' disease
Nodular thyroid disease
Subacute thyroiditis
Iatrogenic
Hyperemesis gravidarum
Molar disease
Rare:
- Iodine induced
- TSH-producing pituitary tumor

in Pregnancy"). As is discussed subsequently, transient hyperthyroidism due to inappropriate secretion or action of hCG is becoming recognized as the most common cause of hyperthyroidism in pregnancy.[96,130] In our experience, single toxic adenoma and multinodular toxic goiter are found in less than 10 percent of cases. Subacute thyroiditis is rarely seen during gestation.

Transient Hyperthyroidism of Hyperemesis Gravidarum

This disorder is characterized by severe nausea and vomiting, with onset between 4 to 8 weeks' gestation, requiring frequent visits to the emergency room and sometimes repeated hospitalizations for intravenous hydration. Weight loss of at least 5 kg, ketonuria, abnormal liver function tests, and hypokalemia are common findings, depending on the severity of vomiting and dehydration. FT_4 levels are elevated, sometimes up to four to six times normal, whereas FT_3 is elevated in up to 40 percent of affected women, although FT_3 values are not as high as serum FT_4. The T_3/T_4 ratio is less than 20, as compared with Graves' hyperthyroidism, in which the ratio is higher than 20. Serum TSH measured by a sensitive assay is consistently very low or suppressed. In spite of the significant biochemical hyperthyroidism, signs and symptoms of hypermetabolism are minimal or absent. Patients may complain of mild palpitations and heat intolerance, but perspiration, proximal muscle weakness, and frequent bowel movements are rare. On physical examination, ophthalmopathy and goiter are absent, a mild tremor of the outstretched fingers is occasionally seen, and tachycardia may be present due in part to dehydration. Significant in the medical history is the lack of hyperthyroid symptoms before conception, because patients with Graves' disease diagnosed for the first time during gestation give the history of hypermetabolic symptoms several months before pregnancy. Spontaneous normalization of hyperthyroxinemia parallels the improvement in vomiting and weight gain, with most of the cases resolving spontaneously between 14 and 20 weeks' gestation, although persistence of hyperthyroidism beyond 20 weeks' gestation has been reported in 15 to 25 percent of cases.[131,132] Suppressed serum TSH may lag for a few more weeks after normalization of FT_4 hormone levels (Fig. 38-3).

Antithyroid medications are not needed. In one series in which antithyroid medication was used, pregnancy outcome was not significantly different from a similar group of patients receiving no therapy.[133] Furthermore, a case has been reported in which normalization of serum thyroid levels with antithyroid medications did not resolve severe vomiting that was controlled only after first-trimester termination of pregnancy.[134] Occasionally, severe vomiting and hyperthyroidism may require parenteral nutrition.

The degree of thyroid abnormalities is directly related to the severity of vomiting and weight loss. In 67 patients studied by Goodwin et al.[129,135] liver and electrolyte abnormalities were routinely found in women with more symptoms, including severe vomiting, weight loss of at least 5 kg, and significant dehydration. They also presented with more significant elevations in FT_4 levels and

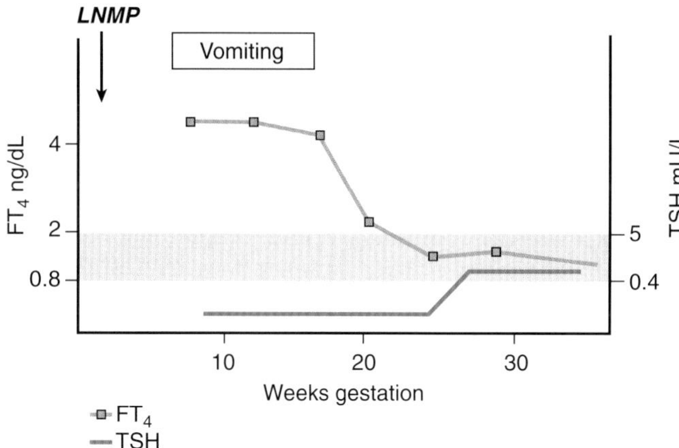

Figure 38-3. Clinical course of transient hyperthyroidism of hyperemesis gravidarum. FT_4, free thyroxine; LNMP, last normal menstrual period; TSH, thyroid-stimulating hormone.

suppression of serum TSH values. Those with a lesser degree of HG had a less severe disorder of thyroid function. Transient hyperthyroidism due to HG should be suspected in women who present in the first few weeks after conception with the sudden onset of severe nausea and vomiting and thyroid tests in the hyperthyroid range. These patients do not complain of hypermetabolic symptoms antedating pregnancy, a goiter is not detected by palpation, and symptoms or signs of tissue thyrotoxicosis are mild or absent. In addition, thyroid anti-TPO antibodies, markers of autoimmune thyroid disease, are negative. The differential diagnosis may also be difficult, because vomiting may also be a presenting symptom of hyperthyroidism of Graves' disease.[136]

The cause for the elevations of thyroid hormones in patients with HG remains controversial.[96,137] Most likely, high levels of hCG, a known stimulator of the TSH receptor, play an important role, as well as prolongation in its biologic activity as seen in twin pregnancies.[138] There is a significant, albeit weak correlation between the degree of thyroid stimulation and total hCG levels in normal women and those with HG.[135] It seems likely, however, that certain hCG fractions may be more important than the total hCG as thyroid stimulators. The thyroid-stimulating activity of hCG in early pregnancy and in molar gestations correlates best with the percentage of basic, partially desialated hCG in serum.[96] A case has been reported in a mother and daughter with recurrent HG, in whom hCG levels were not elevated. Both were heterozygous for a missense mutation in the extracellular domain of the thyrotropin receptor. The mutant receptor was more sensitive than the wild-type receptor to hCG, thus accounting for the occurrence of hyperthyroidism despite the presence of normal hCG levels.[139]

The diagnosis of transient hyperthyroidism of HG should be considered in women with severe vomiting, no clinical manifestations of Graves' disease, and biochemical evidence of hyperthyroidism in early pregnancy. Vomiting should be persistent and severe with a significant weight loss, because most women with morning sickness of pregnancy have normal thyroid function tests.[140] The syndrome may repeat in future pregnancies.

Gestational trophoblastic diseases, partial and complete hydatidiform moles, and choriocarcinoma are other causes of hyperthyroidism early in pregnancy.[130] Patients may present without symptoms in spite of chemical hyperthyroidism, or with various degrees of severity, including congestive heart failure. Evacuation of the mole eliminates the source of the excessive hCG and reverses the clinical and biochemical features of hyperthyroidism. Treatment with β-adrenergic blocking agents is effective in controlling the symptoms. Sodium iopanoate has been used to reduce the release of hormones by the thyroid gland and block peripheral conversion of T_4 to T_3.

Graves' Disease

The natural course of hyperthyroidism due to Graves' disease in pregnancy is characterized by an exacerbation of symptoms in the first trimester and during the postpartum period, and an amelioration of symptoms in the second half of pregnancy. Stimulation of the thyroid gland by hCG in the first trimester has been suggested as the cause of exacerbation.[141] Immunologic responses caused by changes in lymphocyte subsets could explain spontaneous improvement in the second half of pregnancy and recurrences in the postpartum period.[142] Kung and Jones,[143] in a study comparing Graves' disease in pregnant and nonpregnant women, postulated that the amelioration of symptoms seen with progression of pregnancy was due to a decrease in the titers of TSRAb with stimulating activity and an increase in TSRBAb with thyroid-blocking activity. The reverse was true in the postpartum period, when aggravation of Graves' hyperthyroidism usually occurs. In another study, it was suggested that the amelioration of Graves' disease in the last half of pregnancy is induced by a decrease of TSHRAb (TSI) but not by the appearance of thyroid stimulation–blocking antibodies.[144]

When hyperthyroidism is properly managed throughout pregnancy, the outcome for mother and fetus is good; however, maternal and neonatal complications for untreated or poorly controlled mothers are significantly increased (Table 38-1).[145–148]

In the vast majority of patients in whom the diagnosis is made for the first time during pregnancy, hyperthyroid symptoms antedate conception. The clinical diagnosis of thyrotoxicosis may present difficulties during gestation, because many symptoms and signs are commonly seen in normal pregnancy, such as mild palpitations, heart rate between 90 and 100 beats/min, mild heat intolerance, shortness of breath on exercise, and warm skin. There are some clinical clues that increase the likelihood of the diagnosis of hyperthyroidism: presence of goiter, ophthalmopathy, proximal muscle weakness, tachycardia with a pulse rate over 100 beats/min, and weight loss or inability to gain weight in spite of a good appetite. Occasionally, the patient may be seen for the first time in congestive heart failure, and the etiologic diagnosis is difficult, because many of the physical findings are suggestive of cardiac valvular disease, particularly mitral insufficiency or stenosis. Hyperthyroidism under poor control is frequently complicated by preeclampsia. The physician should suspect hyperthyroidism in the presence of systolic hypertension with an inappropriately low diastolic blood pressure and a wide pulse pressure, also seen in other conditions such as aortic insufficiency.

Classic symptoms of hyperthyroidism include nervousness, increased sweating, increased appetite, heat intolerance, insomnia, proximal muscle weakness, irritability, changes in personality, frequent bowel movements, decreased tolerance to exercise (sometimes manifested as shortness of breath), eye irritation, frequent lacrimation, pruritus, and weight loss. Not all symptoms are present in a given patient. The physician should be aware of subtle complaints, particularly in the presence of weight loss or inability to gain weight. As mentioned earlier, in the first trimester of pregnancy, the differential diagnosis from transient hyperthyroidism of HG presents a real challenge for the health care professional.

On physical examination, the thyroid gland is enlarged in almost every patient with Graves' disease. Indeed, the absence of a goiter makes the diagnosis unlikely. The gland is diffusely enlarged, between two and six times the normal size, varies from soft to firm, sometimes being irregular to palpation, and with one lobe being more prominent than the other one. A thrill may be felt or a bruit may be heard, indications of a hyperdynamic circulation. Examination of the eyes may reveal obvious ophthalmopathy, but in the majority of cases exophthalmos is absent or mild, with one eye slightly more prominent than the other. Extraocular movements may be impaired on careful eye examination. Stare is common, as well as injection or edema of the conjunctiva. Although severe ophthalmopathy is rare in pregnancy, corticosteroids and surgical orbital wall decompression may be required to restore visual activity in these patients.[149] Pretibial myxedema is rare, seen in less than 10 percent of women. A hyperdynamic heart with a loud systolic murmur is a common finding. Proximal muscle weakness, fine tremor of the outstretched fingers, and hyperkinetic symptoms are seen frequently. The skin is warm and moist, and palmar erythema is accentuated.

As discussed earlier (see section on thyroid function tests), an FT_4 determination or the calculation of the FT_4I (using total thyroxine levels and a test for assessment of TBG, such as RT_3U) are standard tests in most clinical laboratories, with the result available in 24 to 48 hours. Almost every patient with Graves' disease will have an elevated FT_4 concentration. A suppressed TSH value in the presence of a high FT_4 or FT_4 index confirms

Table 38-1. Potential Maternal and Fetal Complications in Uncontrolled Hyperthyroidism

MATERNAL	FETAL
Pregnancy-induced hypertension	Hyperthyroidism
Preterm delivery	Neonatal hyperthyroidism
Congestive heart failure	Intrauterine growth restriction
Thyroid storm	Small for gestational age
Miscarriage	Prematurity
Placental abruption	Stillbirth
Infection	Central hypothyroidism

After Mestman JH: Hyperthyroidism in pregnancy. Endocrinol Metab Clin North Am 27:138, 1998, with permission.

the diagnosis of hyperthyroidism.[97,150] It must be kept in mind, however, that a suppressed serum TSH is present in about 15 percent of normal pregnant women in the first trimester of pregnancy.[151] In some unusual situations, the serum FT_4 may be at the upper limit of normal or be slightly elevated, in which case the determination of FT_3 or the FT_3I will confirm the diagnosis of hyperthyroidism. Thyroid peroxidase antibodies (anti-TPO) or thyroid antimicrosomal antibodies, markers of thyroid autoimmune disease, are elevated in most patients with Graves' disease; this test is indicated in patients in whom the etiology of the hyperthyroidism is in doubt.

Significant maternal and perinatal morbidity and mortality were reported in early studies of pregnancies complicated by hyperthyroidism.[151,152] In the past 20 years, however, there has been a significant decrease in the incidence of maternal and fetal complications directly related to improved control of maternal hyperthyroidism.[146,148,153–156] The most common maternal complication is preeclampsia. In women with uncontrolled hyperthyroidism, the risk of severe preeclampsia was five times greater than in those patients with controlled disease.[148] Other complications include preterm delivery, placental abruption, and miscarriage. Congestive heart failure may occur in women untreated or treated for a short period of time in the presence of preeclampsia or operative delivery.[157,158] Left ventricular dysfunction is usually detected by echocardiography in women with cardiovascular manifestations. Although these changes are reversible, they may persist for several weeks after achieving a euthyroid state. In one study,[159] reduction in peripheral vascular resistance and higher cardiac output were still present in spite of normalization of thyroxine levels. This is an important finding with significant clinical implications. Left ventricular decompensation in hyperthyroid pregnant women may develop in the presence of superimposed preeclampsia, at the time of delivery or with undercurrent complications such as anemia or infection. We have seen congestive heart failure in the first half of pregnancy in women with long-standing hyperthyroidism. It is likely that the aggravation of hyperthyroidism seen in the first part of pregnancy played an important role in the development of this complication. Careful monitoring of fluid administration is imperative in these situations. Thyroid storm has been rarely reported in pregnancy.[160,161]

Fetal and neonatal complications are also related to maternal control of hyperthyroidism. Intrauterine growth restriction (IUGR), prematurity, stillbirth, and neonatal morbidity are the most common complications. Millar et al.[148] demonstrated that hyperthyroidism uncontrolled during the entire gestation was associated with a ninefold greater incidence of low-birth-weight infants as compared with the control population. It was almost 2.5 times greater in those whose hyperthyroidism was treated during pregnancy and became euthyroid at some time during gestation. In those mothers achieving a euthyroid state before or early in pregnancy, the incidence of low-birth-weight infants was no different from that in the control population. Mitzuda et al.[147] correlated the risk of delivering a small-for-gestational-age infant, with the presence of maternal thyrotoxicosis lasting more than 30 weeks of pregnancy, a duration of Graves' disease for most of 10 years, and onset of Graves' disease before age 20. Momotani and Ito[156] reported an incidence of spontaneous abortions (25.7 percent) and premature delivery (14.9 percent) in mothers hyperthyroid at the time of conception, as compared with 12.8 percent and 9.5 percent, respectively, in euthyroid mothers.

The use of ultrasonography to monitor the size of the fetal thyroid gland as an indicator to guide maternal therapy in women with Graves' disease was evaluated by Luton et al.[162] in France. In a group of women considered high risk owing to the presence of TRAb (TSH Receptor Antibodies) and on antithyroid therapy, fetal goiter was detected in 11 of 41 patients. Four fetuses were hyperthyroid and seven were hypothyroid. All of them benefited from adjusting drug therapy. The authors concluded that ultrasonography of the fetal thyroid gland by an experienced ultrasonographer is an excellent diagnostic tool, in conjunction with close teamwork, to ensure normal fetal thyroid function.

Treatment of hyperthyroidism is essential to prevent maternal, fetal, and neonatal complications (see Table 38-1). The goal of treatment is normalization of thyroid tests as soon as possible and to maintain euthyroidism with the minimum amount of antithyroid medication. Excessive amounts of antithyroid drugs crossing the placenta may affect the fetal thyroid, with the development of fetal hypothyroidism with or without goiter. Patients should be monitored at regular intervals and the dose of their medications adjusted to keep the FT_4 or, preferably, the FT_4I in the upper one third of the range of normal.[153] For this purpose, thyroid tests should be performed every 2 weeks at the beginning of treatment and every 2 to 4 weeks when euthyroidism is achieved. Patients with small goiters, short duration of symptoms, and on minimal amounts of antithyroid medication will be able to discontinue antithyroid drugs by 34 weeks' gestation or beyond. It is not recommended that antithyroid therapy be discontinued before 32 weeks' gestation, because in our experience, relapses may occur in a significant number of patients.[163]

In this country, the two antithyroid drugs available are PTU and MM (Tapazole). Both drugs are effective in controlling symptoms. To our knowledge, no studies have shown PTU to be superior to MM, both drugs having similar placental transfer kinetics.[164] Furthermore, when the efficacies of both drugs have been compared, euthyroidism was achieved with equivalent amounts of drugs and in the same period of time.[165,166] Neonatal outcomes were no different in both groups. Aplasia cutis, an unusual scalp lesion, has occurred in a small group of fetuses of patients taking MM,[167–169] but this is not a contraindication for its use in pregnancy. Several reports have described a specific embryopathy in infants of mothers treated with MM in the first trimester of pregnancy.[170–172] This has been called "methimazole embryopathy" and includes cloanal atresia and esophageal atresia, minor dysmorphic features, and developmental delay. Very few cases have been reported, but none with the use of PTU. The prevalence of these malformations in the general population is 1:2,500 for esophageal atresia and 1:1,000 for cloanal atresia. The doses of methimazole were 5 to 50 mg/day in one study, and in the second study booth affected mothers took over 20 mg/day.[173] Although these complications have not been reported in a relatively large series of pregnant women treated with MM or carbimazole, it appears prudent to avoid MM in the first trimester of pregnancy if PTU is available.

The initial recommended dose of PTU is 100 to 450 mg/day, and for MM, 10 to 40 mg/day divided in two daily doses.[174] Methimazole is given once or twice daily, allowing for improvement in patient compliance. Owing to its shorter half-life, PTU should be given every 8 hours. In our experience, 20 mg of MM daily or 100 to 150 mg of PTU three times a day is an effective initial dose in most patients. Those with large goiters and longer duration of the disease may need larger doses at the initiation of therapy. In patients with minimal symptoms, an initial dose of 10 mg of MM daily or PTU 50 mg two or three times a day may be initiated. In most patients, clinical improvement is seen in 2 to 6 weeks, and improvement in thyroid tests occurs within the first 2 weeks of therapy, with normalization to chemical euthyroidism in 3 to 7 weeks.[165] Resistance to drug therapy is unusual and is most likely due to poor patient compliance.[175] Once clinical improvement occurs, mainly weight gain and a reduction in tachycardia, the dose of antithyroid medication may be reduced by half of the initial dose. The daily dose is adjusted every few weeks according to the clinical response and the results of thyroid function tests. Serum TSH remains suppressed despite the normalization of thyroid hormone levels (Fig. 38-4). Normalization of serum TSH is an indicator to reduce the dose of medication. We do not recommend adding thyroxine to antithyroid drug therapy in the management of Graves' disease in pregnancy. If there is an exacerbation of symptoms or worsening of the thyroid tests, the amount of antithyroid medication is doubled.

The main concern of maternal drug therapy is the potential impact on the fetus; mainly, goiter and hypothyroidism. In most studies, these problems have been prevented by using doses no greater than 200 mg of PTU or 20 mg of MM in the last few weeks of gestation.[176]

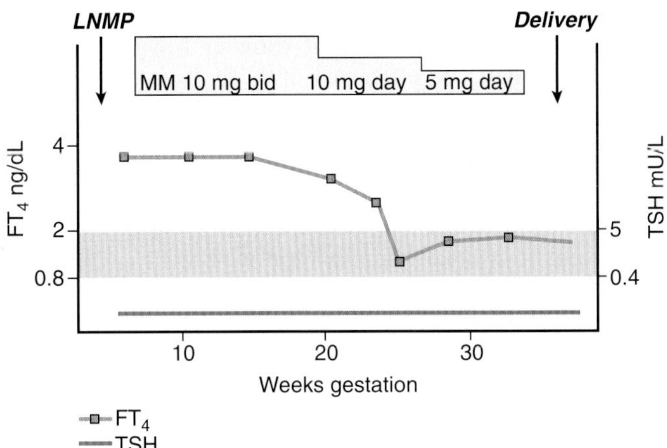

Figure 38-4. Management of hyperthyroidism. bid, twice daily; FT_4, free thyroxine; LNMP, last normal menstrual period; MM, methimazole; TSH, thyroid-stimulating horomone.

However, small elevations in serum TSH in the neonate have been reported, even with lower doses of antithyroid medication.[177] Furthermore, in one study, cord blood FT_4 values were not correlated to the antithyroid dose at term.[153]

Side effects of antithyroid drugs occur in 3 to 5 percent of treated patients.[174] The most common complications of both drugs are pruritus and skin rash. They usually resolve by switching to the other antithyroid medication. In general, the rash occurs 2 to 6 weeks after initiation of therapy. Because pruritus may be an initial symptom of hyperthyroidism, it is customary to ask the patient during the first visit if she has been bothered by this. Other complications that are much less common are migratory polyarthritis, a lupus-like syndrome, and cholestatic jaundice. Agranulocytosis, a serious but unusual complication, has been reported in 1 in 300 patients receiving the drug.[178] It is manifested by fever, malaise, gingivitis, and sore throat. Agranulocytosis occurs in the first 12 weeks of therapy and appears to be related to the dose of the medication.[179] Women should be made aware of the symptoms at the time the prescription is given, and advised to discontinue the drug at once. In this setting, a leukocyte count should be obtained immediately. Although some have recommended routine white blood counts in patients on antithyroid therapy, such testing is not indicated, because granulocytopenia or agranulocytosis may appear without warning symptoms.

β-Adrenergic blocking agents (propranolol 20 to 40 mg every 6 hours or atenolol 25 to 50 mg/day) are very effective in controlling hyperdynamic symptoms and are indicated for the first few weeks in symptomatic patients.[128] One situation in which β-adrenergic blocking agents may be very effective is in the treatment of severe hyperthyroidism during labor. In a case reported in which both mother and fetus were affected, labetalol was infused at a rate of 2 mg/min, controlling maternal and fetal tachycardia within 45 minutes.[180]

Subtotal thyroidectomy in pregnancy is effective in managing the disease. However, nowadays, indications for surgical treatment are few and include an allergy to both antithyroid drugs,[181] very large goiters, patient preference, and the exceptional case of resistance to drug therapy.

^{131}I therapy is contraindicated in pregnancy because, when given after 10 weeks' gestation, it produces fetal hypothyroidism.[182,183] A pregnancy test is mandatory in any woman of childbearing age before a therapeutic dose of ^{131}I is administered.

Iodine crosses the placenta. If given in large amounts and for prolonged periods, it may produce a fetal goiter and hypothyroidism.[126,184] Therefore, its therapeutic use is not recommended in pregnancy. However, iodine has been used in small amounts, 6 to 40 mg/day in a study of pregnant Japanese women with mild hyperthyroidism.[185] Elevation in serum TSH was observed in 2 of 35 newborns, and the mothers were slightly hyperthyroid at the time of delivery. In spite of this observation, iodine therapy is not routinely indicated in the treatment of hyperthyroidism in pregnancy.

Excessive amounts of antithyroid drugs have induced fetal hypothyroidism and goiter. The diagnosis of goiter is made by ultrasonography, which shows hyperextension of the neck and a neck mass. Few cases of hypothyroidism have been confirmed by measuring serum thyroxine and TSH in fetal blood obtained by cordocentesis.[186] Treatment with intraamniotic injection of L-thyroxine has resulted in resolution of the goiter.

Breast-feeding should be permitted if the daily dose of PTU or MM is less than 200 or 20 mg/day, respectively. It is prudent to give the total dose in divided doses after each feeding. The infant should be followed with thyroid function tests.[174] In a very provocative study, PTU was given to lactating hyperthyroid mothers whose infants were born with elevated serum TSH levels. Infant TSH levels normalized even with continuation of PTU therapy by the mothers.[187] In another report, thyroid tests were done at regular intervals in breast-fed infants of mothers taking up to 20 mg of MM daily, showing no evidence of hypothyroidism.[188] The children were followed up to 74 months of age. There was no evidence of physical or intellectual developmental deficits as compared with 176 controls.

Assessment of fetal well-being with the use of ultrasonography, the nonstress test, and a biophysical profile is indicated for cases in poor metabolic control, in the presence of fetal tachycardia and IUGR, in pregnancies complicated by preeclampsia or any other obstetric or medical complications.

Treatment of Thyroid Storm

Thyroid storm is a clinical diagnosis based on severe signs of thyrotoxicosis, with significant hyperpyrexia (>103°F) and neuropsychiatric symptoms that are essential for the clinical diagnosis. Tachycardia with a pulse rate exceeding 140 beats/min is not uncommon, and congestive heart failure is a frequent complication. Gastrointestinal symptoms such as nausea and vomiting, accompanied by liver compromise, have been reported. Laboratory tests show the classic hyperthyroid changes, although the actual elevation in FT_4 values does not help in the diagnosis.[161]

Management includes the following:

1. Admission to the intensive care unit for supportive therapy such as fluids and correction of electrolyte abnormalities, oxygen therapy as needed, and control of hyperpyrexia. Acetaminophen is the drug of choice, because aspirin may increase FT_4 hormones.
2. Management of congestive heart failure, which may require large doses of digoxin.
3. Proper antibiotic therapy in case of infection.
4. β-Adrenergic blocker therapy such as propranolol 60 to 80 mg every 4 hours orally or 1 mg/min intravenously to control hyperadrenergic symptoms. Esmolol, a short-acting β-acting antagonist given intravenously with a loading dose of 250 to 500 μg/kg of body weight followed by a continuous infusion at 50 to 100 μg/kg/min may also be used.
5. MM 30 mg or PTU 300 mg every 6 hours (if unable to take oral medications a nasogastric tube may be needed); thionamides block the synthesis of thyroid hormones in a few hours.
6. One hour after the administration of thionamides, iodine is administered in the form of Lugol's solution, 10 drops three times a day or, if available, sodium iodide, given intravenously 1 g every 12 hours.
7. Glucocorticoids in the form of hydrocortisone every 8 hours or equivalent amounts of other glucocorticoids are also helpful, because they reduce the peripheral conversion of serum T_4 to T_3.

In summary, thyroid storm is a life-threatening condition, requiring early recognition and aggressive therapy in an intensive care unit setting.

Neonatal Hyperthyroidism

Neonatal hyperthyroidism is infrequent, with an incidence of less than 1 percent of infants born to mothers with Graves' disease, therefore affecting 1 in 50,000 neonates. In the vast majority of cases, the disease is caused by the transfer of maternal immunoglobulin antibodies to the fetus. These stimulating thyroid antibodies to the TSH receptor (TSIs), when present in high concentrations in maternal serum, cross the placental barrier, stimulate the fetal thyroid gland, and may produce fetal or neonatal hyperthyroidism.[189] When the mother is treated with antithyroid medications, the fetus benefits from maternal therapy, remaining euthyroid during pregnancy. However, the protective effect of the antithyroid drug is lost after delivery, and neonatal hyperthyroidism may develop within a few days after birth. High titers of TSI receptor antibodies, a three- to fivefold increase over baseline, in the third trimester of pregnancy are predictors of neonatal hyperthyroidism.[147,190] If neonatal hyperthyroidism is not recognized and treated properly, neonatal mortality may be as high as 30 percent. Because the half-life of the antibodies is only a few weeks, complete resolution of neonatal hyperthyroidism is the rule.[190]

A few cases of familial neonatal Graves' disease[191] have been reported. The pathogenesis is not clearly understood. This condition may persist for several years.

Sporadic cases of neonatal hyperthyroidism without evidence of the presence of circulating TSI in mother or infant have recently been published.[192,193] Activation of mutations in the TSH receptor molecule are the cause of this entity. It is inherited as an autosomal dominant trait, and in contrast to Graves' neonatal hyperthyroidism, the condition persists indefinitely. Treatment with antithyroid medications followed by thyroid ablation therapy are eventually needed.

Fetal Hyperthyroidism

In mothers with a history of Graves' disease previously treated with ablation therapy, either surgery or ^{131}I, concentrations of TSI may remain elevated, in spite of maternal euthyroidism. The concentration of these IgG immunoglobulins is low early in normal pregnancy, reaching a level in the fetus similar to that of the mother around 30 weeks' gestation. Therefore, the symptoms of fetal hyperthyroidism are not evident until 22 to 24 weeks of gestation. When TSI levels are present in high concentrations, fetal hyperthyroidism may result, characterized by fetal tachycardia, IUGR, oligohydramnios, and occasionally, a goiter identified on ultrasonography.[113,162,194–196] The diagnosis may be confirmed by measuring thyroid hormone levels in cord blood obtained by cordocentesis.[197,198] Serial cordocentesis for monitoring drug therapy has been proposed, but its value has been questioned.[199,200] Heckel et al.[113] reviewed nine cases of fetal hyperthyroidism treated by maternal administration of antithyroid medications. Fetal tachycardia was the most frequent sign, whereas oligohydramnios and IUGR were reported in only two cases. Fetal goiter was detected by ultrasonography in three cases. Treatment consisted of antithyroid medication given to the mother, PTU 100 to 400 mg/day or MM 10 to 20 mg/day. The dose is guided by the improvement and resolution of fetal tachycardia and normalization of fetal growth, both of which are indicators of good therapeutic response.

In summary, the diagnosis of fetal hyperthyroidism should be suspected in the presence of fetal tachycardia with or without fetal goiter in mothers with a history of Graves' disease treated by ablation therapy and with high titers of serum TSI antibodies. Fetal ultrasonography in experts hands may be a valuable diagnostic tool.[162] The diagnosis may be confirmed by the determination of fetal thyroid hormones by cordocentesis.[190]

Neonatal Central Hypothyroidism

Infants of untreated hyperthyroid mothers may be born with transient central hypothyroidism of pituitary or hypothalamic origin. High levels of maternal thyroxine cross the placental barrier, and feed back to the fetal pituitary, resulting in suppression of fetal pituitary TSH. The diagnosis is made in the presence of a low FT_4 and normal or low TSH in cord blood. This complication should be easily avoidable with proper management of maternal hyperthyroidism.[201–203]

Hypothyroidism

Until a few years ago, very few series of hypothyroidism in pregnancy were published[204–208] despite the fact that the incidence of hypothyroidism, defined as any elevation in serum TSH above 5 mIU/l, is between 0.19 and 2.5 percent.[209–213] In these studies, serum TSH was measured in the first half of pregnancy. Subclinical hypothyroidism, defined as an elevation of serum TSH with normal FT_4 levels, is more often encountered than clinical hypothyroidism. Mild elevations in serum TSH are frequently detected in hypothyroid women on thyroid replacement therapy soon after conception because of the increased demand for thyroid hormones in the first weeks of gestation.[111,112,214] In a recent study, serum TSH and FT_4 were measured in 17,298 women tested before 20 weeks' gestation who delivered singleton infants on the obstetric service at Parkland Memorial Hospital in Dallas; 404 (2.3 percent) women were diagnosed with subclinical hypothyroidism. Preterm birth, defined as delivery at or before 34 weeks' gestation, was almost twofold higher in women with subclinical hypothyroidism, and their pregnancies were 3 times more likely to be complicated by placental abruption. The authors concluded that the reduction in intelligence quotient (IQ) of offspring of women with subclinical hyprothyroidism may be related to the effects of prematurity.[215]

The two most common etiologies of primary hypothyroidism are autoimmune thyroiditis (Hashimoto's thyroiditis) and postthyroid ablation therapy, either surgical or ^{131}I induced. Original studies reported a high incidence of congenital malformations, perinatal mortality, and impaired mental and somatic development in infants of hypothyroid women.[216] One retrospective study reported an 8.1 percent rate of fetal death.[217] In contrast, recent reports have shown no increase in the incidence of congenital malformations but did note an increase in perinatal morbidity, particularly associated with prematurity. Preeclampsia was increased in patients with poorly controlled hypothyroidism.[204–206]

Regardless of the etiology, primary hypothyroidism is classified as subclinical hypothyroidism (normal FT_4 and elevated TSH) and overt hypothyroidism (low FT_4 and elevated TSH). The spectrum of women with hypothyroidism in pregnancy includes (1) women with subclinical and overt hypothyroidism diagnosed for the first time during pregnancy; (2) hypothyroid women who discontinue thyroid therapy at the time of conception because of poor medical advice or because of the misconception that thyroid medications affect the fetus; (3) those women on thyroid therapy requiring larger doses in pregnancy; (4) those women previously diagnosed but not compliant with their medication; (5) hyperthyroid patients on excessive amounts of antithyroid drug therapy; and (6) some patients on lithium or amiodarone therapy, because both drugs may affect thyroid function, particularly in women affected by chronic thyroiditis.[218,219]

In contrast to patients with subclinical hypothyroidism who are asymptomatic, patients with overt hypothyroidism may complain of tiredness, cold intolerance, fatigue, muscle cramps, constipation, and deepening of the voice. On physical examination, the skin is dry and cold, deep tendon reflexes are delayed, and bradycardia may be detected as well as periorbital edema. A goiter is present in almost 80 percent of patients with chronic thyroiditis. The characteristic of the goiter is a diffuse enlargement, about two to three times the normal size, firm to palpation, painless, and with a rubbery consistency. In the other 20 percent, no goiter is found (atrophic thyroiditis, also known as primary myxedema or chronic thyroiditis without goiter).

The diagnosis of hypothyroidism is confirmed by the determination of serum TSH and FT_4 or FT_4I. As mentioned in the section on thyroid tests, recent studies suggested lower TSH values during pregnancy, with upper limits of normal of 2.5 to 3 mU/L in the first trimester. All previously reported studies had used a TSH of more than 5 to 6 mU/L for diagnostic purposes The degree of severity of the clinical symptoms varies with the thyroid abnormalities on laboratory testing, although there is not always a good correlation between clinical and chemical parameters. In our own series,[206] the mean TSH value at the time of diagnosis of overt hypothyroidism was 89.7 ± 86.2 mU/ml (normal, 0.4 to 5.0), with a mean FT_4I of 2.1 ± 1.5 (normal, 4.5 to 12). In the group with subclinical hypothyroidism, the mean serum TSH value was 28.4 ± 47.1 mU/ml, with a mean FT_4I of 8.7 ± 3.6. Serum thyroid antibodies or thyroid peroxidase antibodies (anti-TPO) also known as antimicrosomal antibodies, are elevated in almost 90 percent of patients with autoimmune thyroiditis. Serum antithyroglobulin antibodies (TgAb) are elevated in about 60 percent of patients with chronic thyroiditis; in some patients, TgAb is the only antibody present. The titer of antibodies does not correlate with the size of the goiter or the clinical severity of hypothyroidism.

As in the case of hyperthyroidism, the most common complication in hypothyroid pregnant women is pregnancy-induced hypertension, with an incidence of 21 percent in 60 patients with overt hypothyroidism (Table 38-2). Low birth weight was reported in 16.6 percent of infants. In one series,[203] two of 12 women with subclinical hypothyroidism developed postpartum hemorrhage. In our series of 23 women who conceived while being hypothyroid and completed their pregnancy in our institution, 10 presented with subclinical and 13 with overt hypothyroidism. In 13 of 23, the diagnosis of hypothyroidism was made for the first time during pregnancy, and the other 10 women had discontinued thyroid medication at least 3 months before conception. The incidence of complications was much less than in previous reports. No problems were seen in those women who were euthyroid before 24 weeks' gestation. The results of this study suggest that achieving euthyroidism early in pregnancy prevents late complications, even in women with severe hypothyroidism. In our series, the mean serum TSH in the overt hypothyroid patients at presentation (16.1 weeks) was 90.4 IU/ml and the FT_4I was 1.4 (normal, 4.5 to 12).[220]

The impact of maternal hypothyroidism on the intellectual development of the offspring has been the subject of several studies.[93,94,221,222] In the report from Haddow et al.,[93] children born of mothers with mild elevations of serum TSH measured between 16 and 18 weeks' gestation, were studied at age 7 to 9. They reported a 4-point decrease in IQ score on the Wechsler Intelligence Scale for Children. In another study from Japan, Lui et al.[222] examined a group of eight children at age 4 and 10. IQs were compared in these children, whose mothers were hypothyroid in the first trimester, with their siblings. In the latter group, the mothers were euthyroid throughout gestation. There was no difference in the IQs of both groups of children. Man et al.[221] had reported lower IQs in children from a group of mothers considered hypothyroxinemic in pregnancy (serum TSH was not available at the time of the study). When they were studied at age 7, 5 of 21 (24 percent) had an IQ of less than 80, as compared with 10 percent of control children. These preliminary studies appear to support earlier animal research[223] showing the importance of maternal transfer of thyroxine in the first trimester of pregnancy, at a time when the fetal thyroid has not yet developed. From a practical point of view, these studies emphasize the importance of adjusting the dose of thyroxine in women under treatment for hypothyroidism soon after conception.

When and how to screen for thyroid disease in pregnant and nonpregnant individuals is still controversial, with different positions adapted by several medical organizations. A Consensus Development Conference regarding subclinical thyroid disease was sponsored by the American Association of Clinical Endocrinologists (AACE), the American Thyroid Association (ATA), and the Endocrine Society (ES). Their recommendation, based on an extensive review of the published literature available at that time, limited thyroid tests to women at high risk for thyroid disease.[106] The ACOG, stated that "there is insufficient data to warrant routine screening of asymptomatic pregnant women for hypothyroidism."[107] In a joint statement by the AACE, ATA and ES,[108] based of the risk of mild hypothyroidism on brain development and "infant survival," a TSH level and a determination of FT_4 in the presence of an abnormal TSH value, should be performed routinely during a prepregnancy evaluation or as soon as pregnancy is diagnosed. It is my personal opinion and recommendation to assess thyroid function early in pregnancy in

Table 38-2. Maternal and Neonatal Complications of Hypothyroidism in Pregnancy

	NO. OF PATIENTS WITH OVERT HYPOTHYROIDISM				NO. OF PATIENTS WITH SUBCLINICAL HYPOTHYROIDISM		
	16	23	11	TOTAL 50 (%)	12	45	TOTAL 57 (%)
Pregnancy-induced hypertension	7	5	1	13 (26)	2	7	9 (15)
Placental abruption	3	0	0	3 (6)	0	0	0
Postpartum hemorrhage	3	1	0	4 (8)	2	0	2 (3.5)
Stillbirths	2	1	1	4 (8)	1	0	1 (1.7)
Congenital malformations	0	1	1	2 (3)	0	0	
Low birth weight	5	5	0	10 (20)	1	4	5 (8.7)
Anemia (Hct <26%)	5	0	0	5 (10)	0	1	1 (1.7)

Hct, hematocrit.

From Mestman JH: Endocrine diseases in pregnancy. *In* Sciarra JJ (ed): Gynecology and Obstetrics. Philadelphia, Lippincott-Raven, 1997, p 33, with permission.

those women at high risk for developing hypothyroidism (see the box "Indications for Thyroid Testing in Pregnancy"). At least a serum TSH and anti-TPO antibodies should be measured; those with positive antibodies and a serum TSH greater than 2.5 mU/L should be treated with L-thyroxine, to keep the serum TSH within present normal levels for pregnancy, between 0.3 and 2.5 mU/L. These recommendations are based on our existing literature and should be reviewed and modified according to new studies, now in progress in several institutions.

L-thyroxine is the drug of choice for the treatment of hypothyroidism. In view of the complications mentioned earlier, it is important to normalize thyroid tests as soon as possible. An initial dose of 0.150 mg of L-thyroxine is well tolerated by the majority of young hypothyroid patients. In those with severe hypothyroidism, there is a delay in the normalization of serum TSH, but normal serum FT_4 or FT_4I values are achieved in the first 2 weeks of therapy. The maintenance dose required for most patients is between 0.125 and 0.250 mg of levothyroxine per day. Higher doses may be required for patients after total thyroidectomy for thyroid carcinoma, since the goal in these cases is suppression of serum TSH.[116]

Patients on thyroid therapy before conception should have their TSH checked at 4–6 weeks of gestation and the amount of L-thyroxine adjusted accordingly. The serum TSH should be repeated every 4 to 6 weeks during the first 20 weeks, at 24 to 28 weeks and at 32–34 weeks' gestation. An increase in thyroid requirements is seen in about 20 to 30 percent of patients in the second half of pregnancy. Immediately after delivery, they should return to prepregnancy dosage. Interference in the absorption of thyroxine was previously discussed.[117,118]

Single Nodule of the Thyroid Gland

It is estimated that nodular thyroid disease is clinically detectable in 10 percent of pregnant women. In most cases, it is discovered during the first routine clinical examination or is detected by the patient herself. The chances for a single or solitary thyroid nodule to be malignant are between 5 and 10 percent,[223] depending on risk factors such as previous radiation therapy to the upper body, rapid growth of a painless nodule, patient age, and family history of thyroid cancer. Papillary carcinoma accounts for almost 75 to 80 percent of malignant tumors, and a follicular neoplasm for 15 to 20 percent; a few percent are represented by medullary thyroid carcinoma. Undifferentiated thyroid carcinoma is extremely rare in patients younger than 50 years of age. There is a paucity of information in the literature regarding the management and timing of the work-up in the presence of thyroid nodularity.[224–228] It is generally agreed that elective surgery should be avoided in the first trimester and after 24 weeks' gestation because of the potential risks of spontaneous abortion and premature delivery, respectively. In a selective group of patients operated on during or in the few months after delivery, the incidence of thyroid cancer was reported to be near 40 percent.[227,228] In both studies, fine-needle aspiration biopsy (FNAB) of the thyroid nodule was obtained before surgery, with findings consistent with papillary carcinoma or highly suspicious lesions.

Careful examination of the neck enables the physician to define and characterize the thyroid lesion. In addition to the size of the nodule, the consistency, tenderness, fixation to the skin, and presence of metastasis should be noted. A hard, painless nodule, measuring more than 2 cm in diameter, is suspicious of malignancy. High-resolution real-time ultrasound is very helpful in defining the size of the lesion, characterizing the dominant one, in the presence of a multinodular gland, and identifying microcalcifications suspicious for either papillary or medullary thyroid carcinoma. FNAB is routinely used for diagnostic purposes.

In a retrospective study, a conservative approach to the management of a single thyroid nodule was recommended.[229] In this study, 61 women were pregnant at the time of the diagnosis of a differentiated thyroid carcinoma. The diagnosis was papillary cancer in 87 percent of them and follicular cancer in 13 percent. Fourteen women were operated on during pregnancy, whereas the other 47 women underwent surgical treatment 1 to 84 months after delivery. The outcome was compared with a group of 598 nonpregnant women matched for age. The median follow-up was 22.4 years as compared with 19.5 years in the nonpregnant group. Treatment and outcome were similar in both groups, those operated on during pregnancy and those in whom thyroidectomy was performed postpartum. The authors concluded that both diagnostic studies and initial therapy might be delayed until after delivery in most patients.

In the presence of a single thyroid nodule detected on physical examination, the following approach is recommended in our institution (Fig. 38-5)[228]:

1. *Serum TSH:* a suppressed serum TSH may indicate the presence of an autonomous nodule, which rarely is malignant.[230] In such cases, FT_4 and FT_3 are measured to rule out hyperthyroidism. It should be kept in mind that in normal first-trimester pregnancies, serum TSH level may be transiently low or undetected.[95]
2. If the serum TSH is within normal limits, the next step is *ultrasonography*, which will distinguish a solid from a cystic lesion. In addition, it may show a multinodular gland not detected by palpation.
3. In the presence of a *solid lesion less than 2 cm or a cystic lesion less than 4 cm* in diameter, observation with or without thyroxine suppression therapy is recommended. If clinically indicated, such as in the presence of cervical adenopathy or an increase in the size of the lesion with progression of pregnancy, FNAB of the lesion is considered. It is important to point out the rarity of enlargement of these small nodules in the course of a few months of follow-up.
4. In patients with a *solid or mixed lesion on ultrasound greater than 2 cm or a cystic nodule greater than 4 cm,* the diagnostic approach differs according to gestational age: (a) *Before 20 weeks' gestation,* FNAB is done. The most important component of the FNAB is the cytopathologist's interpretation. A specific diagnosis is required: malignant, benign, fol-

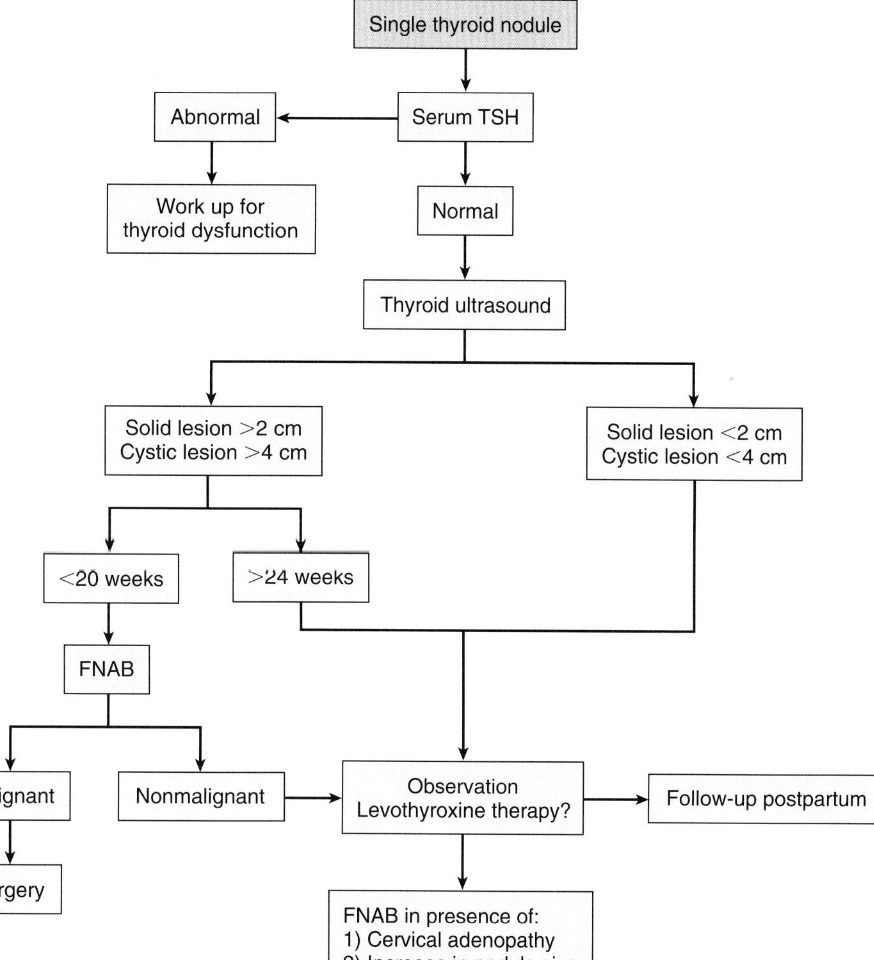

Figure 38-5. Evaluation of single thyroid nodules in pregnancy. FNAB, fine-needle aspiration biopsy.

licular lesion, or inadequate specimen. With an inadequate specimen, a repeat FNAB is recommended. (b) *For lesions diagnosed after 24 weeks' gestation,* FNAB may be postponed until after delivery, unless there is a strong suspicion of malignancy. Suppressive therapy with thyroxine to prevent further growth of the lesion, although considered controversial by some,[223] may be considered. If there is further growth of the lesion in spite of suppressive therapy, FNAB is recommended. (c) *For lesions diagnosed between 20 and 24 weeks' gestation,* the decision to wait until after delivery or to complete the work-up is made by the patient and her physician. The patient's anxiety and fear of having a potential malignant lesion should be considered when advice is given. Most malignant lesions of the thyroid gland are slow growing, and the long-term prognosis is good in the majority of patients.

5. *If the lesion is papillary carcinoma,* surgery is recommended before 24 weeks' gestation, although long-term follow-up of patients diagnosed in pregnancy indicates that postponement of surgery until after delivery does not affect morbidity or mortality.[229]
6. *For follicular lesions,* the decision about surgery is a personal one, because the chance for the lesion to be malignant is only between 15 and 20 percent. A similar approach is followed with Hürthle cell lesions.

The above-mentioned protocol has been used in our institution for many years. In view of a recent publication discussed previously,[229] it is imperative for the physician to discuss the different therapeutic options with the patient and her family. If the lesion is diagnosed before 24 weeks' gestation, patients should be informed of the recent data showing no deleterious effect in postponing therapy until after delivery. The anxiety of the patient and her family, and their wishes should be considered in making the final decision. The long-term prognosis of most thyroid cancers is exceptionally good, but patients should be followed for many years. General principles of care include the determination of the serum thyroglobulin level, a good indicator of tumor activity, before surgery and at regular intervals thereafter; the decision to use radioactive iodine, which is indicated for completeness of thyroid ablation; and the importance of thyroid suppression therapy to keep the serum TSH suppressed in order to prevent possible recurrence of the lesion.[231]

In a retrospective study from the California Cancer Registry from 1991 to 1999, 129 cases of thyroid cancer diagnosed during pregnancy were compared with 466 identified in the postpartum period; the author's conclusion was that thyroid cancer diagnosed during pregnancy "does not appear to have a significant impact on the prognosis of the disease."[232]

Chronic Autoimmune Thyroiditis (Hashimoto's Thyroiditis)

Chronic or Hashimoto's thyroiditis[233,234] is an inflammatory disorder of the thyroid gland, the incidence depending on the population's age, gender, iodine intake, and geographical area. For example, in a long-term follow-up study in the Whickham survey,[235] there was an incidence in women of 3.5 cases per 1,000 per year, as contrasted with an incidence in men of 0.8 case per 1,000 per year. Chronic autoimmune thyroid disease is more common in women with other autoimmune diseases, particularly type 1 diabetes mellitus.[236] In our own unpublished studies from Los Angeles County-University of Southern California Womens' Hospital, positive anti-TPO antibodies were detected in 21 percent of unselected women in the first trimester of pregnancy, in whom the mean TSH value was higher than the group of women with negative antibodies.[237]

The classic clinical picture is characterized by the presence of a goiter, moderate in size; bilateral in most cases; with one lobe larger than the other; a firm, rubbery consistency; and moving freely on swallowing. It is painless, although rapid growth of the gland may elicit some tenderness on palpation. Absence of a goiter (atrophic thyroiditis) may be present in 30 percent of patients.

On presentation, most patients have no symptoms. The discovery of the goiter is made on routine physical examination, or detected by the patient or a family member. Occasionally, the patient may complain of mild to severe hypothyroid symptoms. The diagnosis may be suggested by a hyperechoic pattern on ultrasound of the thyroid.[238] The diagnosis is confirmed by the presence of thyroid autoantibodies (anti-TPO or antithyroglobulin autoantibodies [TgAb]). The actual antibody titer is not correlated with the size of the goiter, symptoms, or severity of the disease. From a practical point of view, there is no need to perform a determination of TgAb if anti-TPO antibodies are positive; in those patients suspected to have chronic thyroiditis with negative anti-TPO antibodies, about 5 to 10 percent of them will have only positive TgAb. Serum TSH should be ordered to rule out thyroid dysfunction. If the serum TSH is elevated, a serum FT_4 will define if the patient suffers from subclinical or clinical hypothyroidism (see section on hypothyroidism, earlier). Patients with euthyroid chronic thyroiditis may develop hypothyroidism over time. The odds ratio was 8 over 20 years in those women with a normal serum TSH and positive antibodies.[235]

The importance of diagnosing chronic thyroiditis in women of childbearing age relates to the potential consequences in pregnancy and the postpartum period. Women with chronic thyroiditis are at higher risk for spontaneous abortion, premature delivery,[242–244] pregnancy induced hypertension, development of hypothyroidism for the first time in pregnancy, and postpartum thyroiditis (PPT).[121]

Several investigators[239–241] have reported an association between thyroid autoantibodies and spontaneous miscarriages. Determination of serum TSH and anti-TPO antibodies should be performed in women with recurrent miscarriages. In the presence of normal TSH values, whether thyroid therapy is beneficial in preventing fetal loss in future pregnancies has not been systematically evaluated.

In a recent publication, 115 euthyroid women with positive TPO antibodies at the time of conception, were divided in 2 groups; one of them received treatment with levo-thyroxine. In the treated group, the incidence of spontaneous abortions and premature delivery was comparable to a control population. In the untreated group the incidence of spontaneous abortions was 13.8% vs. 3.5% of the treated women and premature delivery 22.4% vs. 7% respectively.[244a]

In a subset of women with chronic thyroiditis, particularly those without a goiter (atrophic form), antibodies to the TSH receptor with blocking capabilities are present (TSHRBAb).[245] These antibodies cross the placenta and, at high titers, may block the action of TSH in the fetal thyroid, causing transient congenital hypothyroidism.[246,247] The neonatal disease resolves spontaneously over 3 to 6 months as the maternal antibody is degraded.[248] In a population of 1,614,166 patients screened in New York, nine mothers and their infants out of 788 infants with suspected congenital hypothyroidism had these antibodies.[249] Therefore, in mothers who have given birth to infants with congenital hypothyroidism, thyroid tests including TSHRBAb should be determined.

As is discussed in the following section, the presence of thyroid antibodies, particularly high titers in the first trimester of pregnancy, predicts the development of the syndrome of PPT.

Postpartum Thyroid Dysfunction

Thyroid dysfunction, hyper- and hypothyroidism, is recognized with increasing frequency in the 12 months following delivery, or following spontaneous or medically induced abortions. Most of the cases are due to intrinsic thyroid disease, with a few due to hypothalamic or pituitary lesions (see the box "Postpartum Thyroid Dysfunction"). Patients with autoimmune thyroid disease, chronic thyroiditis and Graves' disease are most frequently affected.

PPT, a variant of Hashimoto's or chronic thyroiditis, is the most common cause of thyroid dysfunction in

Postpartum Thyroid Dysfunction

Chronic thyroiditis
- Transient hyperthyroidism (low RAIU)
- Transient hypothyroidism
- Permanent hypothyroidism

Graves' disease
- Exacerbation of hyperthyroidism (high RAIU)
- Transient hyperthyroidism of chronic thyroiditis (low RAIU)

Hypothalamic pituitary disease
- Sheehan's syndrome
- Lymphocytic hypophysitis

RAIU, radioactive iodine uptake.

From Mestman JH: Endocrine diseases in pregnancy. *In* Sciarra JJ (ed): Gynecology and Obstetrics. Philadelphia, Lippincott-Raven, 1997, p 34, with permission.

the postpartum period. The prevalence is between 1.1 and 16.7 percent of all women,[121,240,250–253] the difference between studies depending on the design of the study, the definition of PPT, the time of postpartum testing and other factors.[121] In women with type 1 diabetes mellitus, the incidence is close to 30 percent.[254] The clinical diagnosis is not always obvious and the clinician should be concerned about nonspecific symptoms such as tiredness, fatigue, depression, palpitations, and irritability in women following the birth of their child or a miscarriage or abortion. Fatigue is the most common complaint.[250] In some cases, the clinical symptoms resemble the syndrome of postpartum depression. Indeed, thyroid antibodies have been found more frequently in euthyroid women with postpartum depression, but this is still a controversial issue.[255] Because the clinical symptoms are mild, and many times are confused with the usual tiredness of women in the months following delivery, an argument can be made for routine screening in the postpartum period. This controversial issue has been reviewed.[256] It is the author's opinion that a careful history and physical examination will allow the physician to decide if thyroid tests are indicated in a given situation. Recognizing the mild degree of the symptoms, the presence of a goiter, history of similar symptoms in previous pregnancies, family history of thyroid disease, and type 1 diabetes mellitus, among other features, will prompt the health care professional to order serum TSH with anti-TPO antibodies. Those patients at risk should be evaluated in the first year postpartum because of the different manifestations of the disease.

PPT may also develop in women with negative antibodies. In a study from The Netherlands, the authors suggested two forms of PPT: (1) an autoimmune form, which is most common and eventually will develop into chronic hypothyroidism, and (2) a nonautoimmune form, without antibodies, that appears to be transient without progressing to permanent hypothyroidism.[257]

The clinical course is not uniform in the majority of patients. In about one third of the cases, mild symptoms of hyperthyroidism develop between 2 and 4 months postpartum. On physical examination, a goiter is felt in the majority of cases, which is firm and nontender to palpation. Tachycardia may be detected. The goiter may be discovered for the first time, or the patient may have noticed an increase in the size of a previously diagnosed goiter. Thyroid tests are in the hyperthyroid range and thyroid antibodies, anti-TPO antibody titers, are elevated in most cases. Spontaneously, without specific therapy, hypothyroidism develops in a few months, with spontaneous recovery and return to a euthyroid state by 7 to 12 months following delivery. Antibody titers have a tendency to increase during this process, and a change in the size of the goiter is usually noted. In a few patients, permanent hypothyroidism may develop. About 50 percent of patients, however, will develop permanent hypothyroidism within 5 years of the diagnosis of PPT.[258,259]

In one third of patients, the course of PPT is different, characterized by an initial episode of hypothyroidism between 3 and 7 months postpartum without the initial hyperthyroid phase. In the other one third of patients, the initial episode of hyperthyroidism is followed by a return to normal thyroid function. It has been suggested that some ultrasonographic changes of the thyroid gland, such as hypoechogenicity, are typical of PPT and may aid in the diagnosis of the syndrome.[260]

Postpartum thyroid dysfunction may also occur in patients with a known history of Graves' disease. It is common for women with Graves' disease to have an exacerbation of their symptoms in the first 2 months postpartum.[261] The symptoms of hyperthyroidism are more severe than those in patients with PPT. They may present with ophthalmopathy and hypermetabolic findings. Therapy with antithyroid medications is needed in these cases. On the other hand, patients with Graves' disease may have a bout of hyperthyroidism secondary to a concomitant episode of PPT.[262,263] The differential diagnosis in this situation is important, because the treatment is different. If not contraindicated, as in breast-feeding mothers, a 4- or 24-hour thyroid radioactive iodine uptake is helpful. It will be very low in patients with PPT, whereas it is high normal or elevated in patients with recurrent hyperthyroidism due to Graves' disease. When it is due to recurrent Graves' disease, treatment with antithyroid medications is indicated, or the physician may advise ablation therapy with ^{131}I.

Therefore, PPT is characterized by symptoms of thyroid dysfunction, that present in four different forms: (1) an episode of hyperthyroidism (2 to 4 months), followed by hypothyroidism (4 to 6 months) and reverting to euthyroidism (after the seventh month); (2) an episode of hyperthyroidism (3 to 4 months) reverting to euthyroidism; (3) an episode of hypothyroidism (4 to 6 months) reverting to a euthyroid state; and (4) permanent hypothyroidism after the hypothyroid phase (Fig. 38-6). However, there are exceptions to these chronologic phases. It is recommended that a diagnosis of PPT be considered for any thyroid abnormality occurring within 1 year after delivery or miscarriages.

Because most cases of postpartum thyroid dysfunction recover spontaneously, treatment is indicated for symptomatic patients. In the presence of hyperthyroid symptoms, β-adrenergic–blocking drugs (propranolol 20 to 40 mg every 6 hours or atenolol 25 to 50 mg every 24 hours) are effective in controlling the symptoms. Antithyroid medications are not effective, because the hyperthyroxinemia is secondary to the release of thyroid hormones due to the acute injury to the gland (destructive hyperthyroidism). There is no new hormone produc-

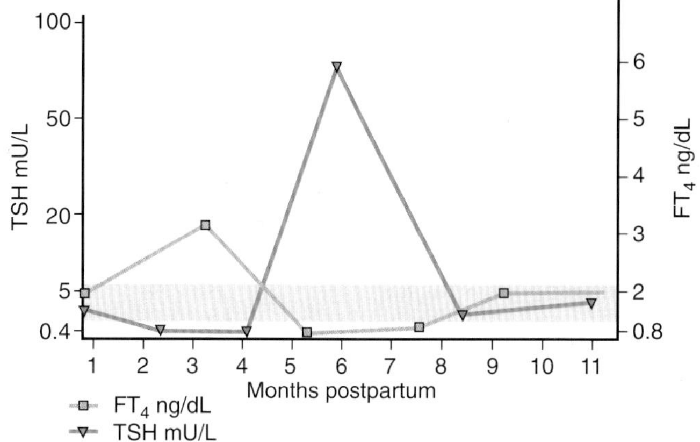

Figure 38-6. Clinical course of postpartum thyroiditis.

tion, and therefore, medications that work by blocking new thyroid hormone formation are ineffective. For hypothyroid symptoms, small amounts of levothyroxine 0.050 mg/day will control symptoms, allowing for a spontaneous recovery of thyroid function after discontinuation of the drug.

There are some features that may predict the development of PPT: presence of a goiter and high titers of thyroid antibodies in the first half of pregnancy, episodes of PPT in previous pregnancies, hypothyroidism antedating pregnancy,[264] and a strong family history of autoimmune thyroid disease.[265] Women with type 1 diabetes mellitus are at high risk for developing PPT. PPT may recur in future pregnancies, with a recurrence rate between 30 and 70 percent.[266–268] PPT has been reported to be associated with other autoimmune endocrine disorders, such as adrenal insufficiency and lymphocytic hypophysitis.[269]

An increased risk of developing Graves' hyperthyroidism in the postpartum period was recently reported, particularly in women from 35 to 39 years of age. The risk was estimated to be 5.6 times greater when compared with nulliparous women.[270]

KEY POINTS

- Hyperthyroidism due to Graves' disease needs to be differentiated in the first trimester of pregnancy from the syndrome of transient hyperthyroidism of HG.
- Transient hyperthyroidism of HG is the most common cause of hyperthyroxinemia in pregnancy; the cause is high or inappropriate levels of hCG.
- Both MM and PTU are used for the management of Graves' hyperthyroidism. The dosage should be adjusted frequently, aiming to use the minimum amount of drug that will keep the FT_4 at the upper limits of normal. PTU is preferable in the first trimester, because a few cases of "methimazole embryopathy" have been reported.
- Breast-feeding is not contraindicated in women on either MM or PTU, provided that the maximum daily dose is 200 mg of PTU and 20 mg of MM.
- Hypothyroid women should have their thyroid tests checked early in pregnancy. An increase in dosage is needed in more than 50 percent of patients.
- Women with risk factors for thyroid disease, such as a family history of thyroid disease, presence of goiter, and a previous history of postpartum thyroiditis (PPT), should be studied before or early in pregnancy. A determination of serum TSH, FT_4 or FT_4I, and anti-TPO antibodies is recommended in such women.
- PPT affects up to 16.7 percent of all women in the postpartum period. Women with chronic thyroiditis are at higher risk to develop this syndrome.

Acknowledgment

The author wishes to thank Elsa C. Ahumada for her secretarial assistance.

REFERENCES

1. Kovacs CS, Kronenberg HM: Maternal fetal calcium and bone metabolism during pregnancy, puerperium and lactation. Endocr Rev 18:832, 1997.
2. Mestman JH: Parathyroid disorders in pregnancy. Semin Perinatol 22:485, 1998.
3. Kovacs CS, Fulethan G: Calcium and bone disorders during pregnancy and lactation. Endocrinol Metab Clin North Am 35:21, 2006.
4. Pitkin RM: Calcium metabolism in pregnancy and perinatal period: A review. Am J Obstet Gynecol 151:99, 1985.
5. Dahlman T, Sjoberg HE, Bucht E: Calcium homeostasis in normal pregnancy and puerperium: A longitudinal study. Acta Obstet Gynecol Scand 73:393, 1994.
6. Seki K, Makimura N, Mitsui C, et al: Calcium regulating hormones and osteocalcin levels during pregnancy: A longitudinal study. Am J Obstet Gynecol 164:1248, 1991.
7. Seely EW, Brown EM, DeMaggio DM, et al: A prospective study of calciotrophic hormones in pregnancy and postpartum reciprocal changes in serum intact parathyroid hormone and 1,25 dihydroxyvitamin D. Am J Obstet Gynecol 176:214, 1997.
8. Gertner JM, Coustan DR, Kliger AS, et al: Pregnancy as a state of physiologic absorptive hypercalciuria. Am J Med 81:451, 1986.
9. Frenkl Y, Barkai G, Mashiach S, et al: Hypocalciuria of preeclampsia is independent of parathyroid hormone level. Obstet Gynecol 77:689, 1991.
10. Hirota Y, Anai T, Miyakawa I: Parathyroid hormone related protein levels in maternal and cord blood. Am J Obstet Gynecol 177:702, 1997.
11. Cornish J, Callon KE, Nicholson GC, Reid JR: Parathyroid hormone-related protein (107–139) inhibits bone resorption in vivo. Endocrinology 138:1299, 1997.
12. Grill V, Hillary J, Ho PMW, et al: Parathyroid hormone related protein: A possible endocrine function in lactation. Clin Endocrinol 37:405, 1992.
13. VanHouten JN, Dann P, Stewart AF, et al: Mammary-specific deletion of parathyroid hormone–related protein preserves bone mass during lactation. J Clin Invest 112:1429, 2003.
14. VanHouten J, Dan P, McGeoch G, et al: The calcium-sensing receptor regulates mammary gland parathyroid hormone-related protein production and calcium transport. J Clin Invest 113:5998, 2004.
15. Samaan NA, Anderson GD, Adam-Mayne ME: Immunoreactive calcitonin in the mother, neonate, child and adult. Am J Obstet Gynecol 121:622, 1975.
16. Gallacher SJ, Fraser WD, Owens OJ, et al: Changes in calciotrophic hormones and biochemical markers of bone turnover in normal human pregnancy. Eur J Endocrinol 131:369, 1994.
17. Kalkwarf HJ, Specker BL, Bianchi DC, et al: The effect of calcium supplementation on bone density during lactation and after weaning. N Engl J Med 337:523, 1997.
18. Abrams SA: Bone turnover during lactation—can calcium supplementation make a difference? (Editorial) J Clin Endocrinol Metab 83:1056, 1998.
19. Iqbal N, Aldasouqi S, Peacock M, et al: Life threatening hypercalcemia associated with primary hyperparathyroidism during pregnancy: Case report and review of the literature. Endocr Pract 5:337, 1999.
20. Hunter D, Turnbull H: Hyperparathyroidism: generalized osteitis fibrosa with observations upon bones, parathyroid tumors and the normal parathyroid glands. Br J Surg 19:203, 1931.
21. Friderichsen D: Tetany in a suckling with latent osteitis fibrois in the mother. Lancet 1:85, 1939.
22. Montoro MN, Paler RJ, Goodwin JM, et al: Parathyroid carcinoma during pregnancy. Obstet Gynecol 96:841, 2000.

23. Ludwing GD: Hyperparathyroidism in relation to pregnancy. N Engl J Med 267:637, 1962.
24. Johnstone RE II, Kreindler T, Johnstone RE: Hyperparathyroidism during pregnancy. Obstet Gynecol 40:580, 1972.
25. Kelly T: Primary hyperparathyroidism during pregnancy. Surgery 110:1028, 1991.
26. Croom RD III, Thomas CG Jr: Primary hyperparathyroidism during pregnancy. Am J Surg 131:328, 1976.
27. Clark D, Seeds JW, Cefalo R: Hyperparathyroid crisis in pregnancy. Am J Obstet Gynecol 140:841, 1981.
28. Silverberg SJ, Bilezikian JP: Evaluation and management of primary hyperparathyroidism. J Clin Endocrinol Metab 81:2036, 1996.
29. Carella M, Gossain V: Hyperparathyroidism and pregnancy: case report and review. J Gen Intern Med 7:448, 1992.
30. Hess HM, Dickson J, Fox HE: Hyperfunctioning parathyroid carcinoma presenting an acute pancreatitis in pregnancy. J Reprod Med 25:83, 1980.
31. Parham GP, Orr JW: Hyperparathyroidism secondary to parathyroid carcinoma in pregnancy: A case report. J Reprod Med 32:123, 1987.
32. Palmueri-Sevier A, Palmueri GMA, Baumgartner CJ, et al: Case report: Long term remission of parathyroid cancer. Possible relation to Vitamin D and calcitriol therapy. Am J Med Sci 306:309, 1993.
33. Corlett RC, Mishell DR: Pancreatitis in pregnancy. Am J Obstet Gynecol 113:281, 1972.
34. Dahan M, Chang RJ: Pancreatitis secondary to hyperparathyroidism during pregnancy. Obstet Gynecol 98:923, 2001.
35. Matthias GSH, Helliwell TR, Williams A: Postpartum hyperthyroid crisis: Case report. Br J Obstet Gynecol 94:807, 1987.
36. Stander JH, Ahern RE: The parathyroids in pregnancy. J Mount Sinai Hosp 14:629, 1947.
37. Schenker JG, Kallner B: Fatal postpartum hyperparathyroidism crisis due to primary chief cell hyperplasia of parathyroids: Report of a case. Obstet Gynecol 25:705, 1965.
38. Soyannowo MA, McGeown MG, Bell M, et al: A case of acute hyperparathyroidism with thyrotoxicosis and pancreatitis presenting as hyperemesis gravidarum. Postgrad Med J 44:861, 1968.
39. Subrayen KT, Moodley SC, Jialal I, et al: Hyperparathyroidism in twin pregnancy: A case report. S Afr Med J 72:287, 1987.
40. Ficinski M, Mestman JH: Primary hyperparathyroidism during pregnancy. Endocr Pract 2:362, 1996.
41. Marx S: Familial hypocalciuric hypercalcemia. *In* Coe F, Favus MJ (eds): Primer on the Metabolic Bone Diseases and Disorders of Mineral Metabolism. New York, Raven Press, 1993, p 166.
42. Pratt EI, Beren BB, Neuhauser EBD, et al: Hypercalcemia and idiopathic hyperplasia of the parathyroid glands in infant. J Pediatr 30:388, 1947.
43. Thomas BR, Bennett JD: Symptomatic hypocalcemia and hypoparathyroidism in infants of mothers with hyperparathyroidism and familial benign hypercalcemia. J Perinatol 15:23, 1995.
44. Pollak M. Chou YH, Marx S, et al: Familial hypocalciuric hypercalcemia and neonatal severe hyperparathryoidism: The effect of mutant gene dosage on phenotype. J Clin Invest 93:1108, 1994.
45. Wright AD, Joplin GF, Dixon HG: Postpartum hypercalcemia in treated hypoparathyroidism. BMJ 1969;1:23–25.
46. Cundy T, Haining SA, Builland-Cumming DF: Remission of hypoparathyroidism during lactation: Evidence for a physiological role for prolactin in the regulation of Vitamin D metabolism. Clin Endocrinol (Oxf) 26:667, 1987.
47. Caplan Rh, Beguin EA: Hypercalcemia in a calcitriol treated hypoparathyroid woman during lactation. Obstet Gynecol 76:485, 1990.
48. Lepre F, Grill V, Martin TJ: Hypercalcemia in pregnancy and lactation associated with parathyroid hormone-related protein. N Engl J Med 328:666, 1993.
49. Khosla S,VanHeerden JA, Gharib H, et al: Parathyroid hormone related protein and hypercalcemia secondary to massive mammary hyperplasia. N Engl J Med 322:1157, 1990.
50. Silverberg SJ, Bone HG, Marriott TB, et al: Short term inhibition of parathyroid hormone secretions by a calcium receptor agonist in patients with primary hyperparathyroidism. N Engl J Med 337:1506, 1997.
51. Bilezikian JP, Potts JT, Fulehan GH, et al: Summary statement from a workshop on asymptomatic primary hyperthyroidism: a perspective for the 21st century. J Bone Miner Res Suppl 2:N2, 2002.
52. Schnatz PF: Parathyroidectomy in the third trimester of pregnancy. Obstet Gynecol Surv 60:672, 2005.
53. Montoro M, Collea JU, Mestman JH: Management of hyperparathyroidism in pregnancy with oral phosphate therapy. Obstet Gynecol 55:431, 1980.
54. Prendville S, Burman KD, Wartofsky L, et al: Evaluation and treatment of post thyroidectomy hypocalcemia. The Endocrinologist 8:34, 1998.
55. Li Y, Song YH, Rais N, et al: Autoantibodies to the extracellular domain of the calcium sensing receptor in patients with acquired hypoparathyroidism. J Clin Invest 5:601, 1996.
56. Zaloga GP, Cerhnow B: The multifactorial basis for hypocalcemia during sepsis: Studies of the PTH-vitamin D axis. Ann Intern Med 107:36, 1987.
57. Anderson GW, Musselman L: The treatment of tetany in pregnancy. Am J Obstet Gynecol 43:547, 1942.
58. Graham WP, Gordon GS, Loken HF, et al: Effect of pregnancy and of the menstrual cycle on hypoparathyroidism. J Clin Endocrinol Metab 24:512, 1964.
59. Bronsky D, Kiamko RT, Moncada R: Intrauterine hyperparathyroidism secondary to maternal hypoparathyroidism. Pediatrics 42:606, 1968.
60. Loughead JL, Mughal Z, Mimouni F, et al: Spectrum and natural history of congenital hyperparathyroidism secondary to maternal hypocalcemia. Am J Perinatol 7:350, 1990.
61. Brunvand L, Quistad E, Urdal P, et al: Vitamin D deficiency and fetal growth. Early Hum Dev 45:27, 1996.
62. Sadeghi-Nejad A, Wolfsdorf JI, Senior B: Hypoparathyroidism and pregnancy. Treatment with calcitrol. JAMA 243:254, 1980.
63. Salle BL, Berthezene F, Glorieux GH: Hypoparathyroidism during pregnancy: Treatment with calcitriol. J Clin Endocrinol Metab 52:810, 1981.
64. Rude RK, Haussler MR, Singer FR: Postpartum resolution of hypocalcemia in a lactating hypoparathyroid patient. Endocrinol Jpn 31:227, 1984.
65. Goldberg LD: Transmission of a vitamin D metabolite in breast milk. Lancet 2:1258, 1972.
66. Zerwekh JE, Breslau NA: Human placental production of 1α,25-dihydroxy-vitamin D: Biochemical characterization and production in normal subjects and patients with pseudohypoparathyroidism. J Clin Endocrinol Metab 62:192, 1986.
67. Breslau NA, Zerwekh JE: Relationship of estrogen and pregnancy to calcium homeostasis in pseudohypoparathyroidism. J Clin Endocrinol Metab 62:45, 1986.
68. Glass EJ, Barr DG: Transient neonatal hyperparathyroidism secondary to maternal pseudohypoparathyroidism. Arch Dis Child 56:565, 1981.
69. Nordin BEC, Roper A: Post pregnancy osteoporosis: A syndrome? Lancet 1:431, 1955.
70. Carbone LD, Palmieri GM, Graves SC, Smull K: Osteoporosis of pregnancy: Long term follow up of patients and their offspring. Obstet Gynecol 86:664, 1995.
71. Dunne F, Walters B, Marshall T, Heath DA: Pregnancy associated osteoporosis. Clin Endocrinol 39:487, 1993.
72. Rizzoli R, Bonjour JP: Pregnancy associated osteoporosis. Lancet 347:1274, 1996.
73. Drinkwater BL, Chesnut CH III: Bone density changes during pregnancy and lactation in active women: A longitudinal study. Bone Miner 14:153, 1991.
74. Wisser J, Florio I, Neff M, et al: Changes in bone density and metabolism in pregnancy. Acta Obstet Gynecol Scand 84:349, 2005.
75. Kritz-Silverstein, D, Barrett-Connor E, Hollenbach KA: Pregnancy and lactation as determinants of bone mineral density in postmenopausal women. Am J Epidemiol 136:1052, 1992.
76. Beaulieu J, Razzano C, Levine R: Transient osteoporosis of the hip in pregnancy. Clin Orthop 115:165, 1976.
77. Chigira M, Watanabe H, Udagawa E: Transient osteoporosis of the hip in the first trimester of pregnancy: A case report and review of the Japanese literature. Arch Orthop Trauma Surg 107:178, 1988.

78. Smith R, Athanasou NA, Ostlere SJ, Vipond SE: Pregnancy associated osteoporosis. Q J Med 88:865, 1995.
79. Goldman GA, Friedman S, Hod M, Ovadia J: Idiopathic transient osteoporosis of the hip in pregnancy. Int J Gynaecol Obstet 46:317, 1994.
80. Melton L, Bryant S, Wahner H, et al: Influence of breastfeeding and other reproductive factors on bone mass later in life. Osteopor Int 3:76, 1993.
81. Sowers M, Crutchfield M, Jannausch M, et al: A prospective evaluation of bone mineral changes in pregnancy. Obstet Gynecol 77:841, 1991.
82. Dahlman T, Sjoberg H, Heligren M, et al: Calcium homeostasis in pregnancy during long term heparin treatment. Br J Obstet Gynecol 99:412, 1992.
83. Barbour LA, Kick SD, Steiner JF, LoVerde ME: A prospective study of heparin induced osteoporosis in pregnancy using bone densitometry. Am J Obstet Gynecol 170:862, 1994.
84. Mestman JH: Thyroid diseases in pregnancy. Clin Obstet Gynecol 40:45, 1997.
85. Smallridge R: Symposium on thyroid disease in pregnancy and the postpartum period. Thyroid 9:629, 1999.
86. Glinoer D: Thyroid disease and pregnancy. *In* Holly JMP (ed): Clinical Endocrinology and Metabolism. Philadelphia, Elsevier Publishing, p 1.
87. American Thyroid Association: Statement on early maternal thyroidal insufficiency: recognition, Clinical manangement and research directions. Thyroid 15:77, 2006.
88. Thorpe-Beeston JG, Nicolaides KH, Felton CV, et al: Maturation of the secretion of thyroid hormone and thyroid stimulating hormone in the fetus. N Engl J Med 324:532, 1991.
89. Contempre B, Jauniaux E, Calvo R, et al: Detection of thyroid hormones in human embryonic cavities during the first trimester of pregnancy. J Clin Endocrinol Metab 77:1719, 1993.
90. Bernal J, Pekonen F: Ontogenesis of the nuclear 3,5,3′-triidothyronine receptor in the human fetal brain. Endocrinology 114:677, 1984.
91. Vulsma T, Gons MH, DeVijlder JJM: Maternal fetal transfer of thyroxine in congenital hypothyroidism due to a total organification defect or thyroid agenesis. N Engl J Med 13:321, 1989.
92. Iskaros J, Pickard M, Evans I, et al: Thyroid hormone receptor gene expression in first trimester human fetus brain. J Clin Endocrinol Metab 85:2620, 2000.
93. Haddow JE, Palomaki GE, Allan WC, et al: Maternal thyroid deficiency during pregnancy and subsequent neurophyschological development of the child. N Engl J Med 341:549, 1999.
94. Alexander EK, Marqusee E, Lawrence J, et al: Timing and magnitude of increases in levothyroxine requirements during pregnancy in women with hypothyroidism. N Engl J Med 351:241, 2004.
95. Glinoer D: The regulation of thyroid function during normal pregnancy: importance of the iodine nutrition status. *In* Glineor D (ed): Clinical Endocrinology and Metabolism. Philadelphia, Elsevier Publishing, p 133.
96. Hershman JM: Physiological and pathological aspects of the effect of human chorionic gonadotropin on the thyroid. *In* Glineor D (ed): Clinical Endocrinology and Metabolism. Philadelphia, Elsevier Publishing, p 249.
97. Brent GA, Mestman JH: Physiology and tests of thyroid function. *In* Sciarra J (ed): Gynecology and Obstetrics, Vol 5. Philadelphia, Lippincott-Raven, 1999, p 1.
98. Dashe JS, Casey BM, Wells CE, et al: Thyroid stimulating hormone in singleton and twin pregnancy: importance of gestational age-specific reference ranges. Obstet Gynecol 106:753, 2005.
99. Demers LM, Spencer CA: Laboaratory medicine practice guidelines: Laboratory support for the diagnosis and monitoring of thyroid disease. Clin Endocrinol (Oxf) 58:138, 2003.
100. Mandel SJ, Spencer CA, Hollowell JG: Are detection and treatment of thyroid insufficiency in pregnancy feasible? Thyroid 15:44, 2005.
101. Glinoer D: Maternal and fetal impact of chronic iodine deficiency. Clin Obstet Gynecol 40:102, 1997.
102. Power MI, Kilpatrick S, Schulkin J: Diagnosing and managing thyroid disorders during pregnancy: a survey of obstetricians-gynecologists. J Reprod Med 49:79, 2004.
103. Zakarija M, McKenzie JM, Hoffman WH: Predications and therapy of intrauterine and late onset neonatal hyperthyroidism. J Clin Endocriol Metab 62:368, 1986.
104. Iseki M, Shimizu M, Oikawa T, et al: Sequential serum measurements of thyrotropin binding inhibitor immunoglobulin G in transient familial neonatal hypothyroidism. J Clin Endocrinol Metab 57:384, 1983.
105. Stagnaro-Green A, Roman SH, Cobin RH, et al: A prospective study of lymphcyte-initiated immunosuppression in normal pregnancy: Evidence of a T cell etiology for postpartum thyroid dysfunction. J Clin Endocrinol Metab 74:645, 1992.
106. Surks MI, Ortiz E, Daniels GH, et al: Subclinical thyroid disease: Scientific review and guidelines for diagnosis and management. JAMA 291:228, 2004.
107. American College of Obstetricians and Gynecologists: ACOG practice bulletin. Clinical management guidelines for obstetricians-gynecologists. Obstet Gynecol 100:387, 2002.
108. Gharib H, Tuttle RM, Baskin HJ, et al: Subclinical thyroid dysfunction: a joint statement on management from the American Association of Clinical Endocrinologists, the American Thyroid Association, and the Endocrine Society. J Clin Endocrinol Metab 90:581, 2005.
109. Momotani N, Ito K, Hamada N, et al: Maternal hyperthyroidism and congenital malformation of the offspring. Clin Endocrinol 20:695, 1984.
110. Luton D, LeGac I, Noel M, et al: Thyroid function during pregnancy in women with past Graves' disease. Br J Obstet Gynecol 112:1565, 2005.
111. Mandel SL, Larsen PR, Seely EW, et al: Increased need for thyroxine during pregnancy in women with primary hypothyroidism. N Engl J Med 323:91, 1990.
112. Kaplan MM: Management of women on thyroxine therapy during pregnancy. Endocr Pract 2:281, 1996.
113. Heckel S, Favre R, Schlienger JL, et al: Diagnosis and successful in utero treatment of a fetal goitrous hyperthyroidism caused by maternal Graves' disease. Fetal Diagn Ther 12:54, 1997.
114. Schlumberger M, Vathaire F, Ceccarelli C, et al: Exposure to radioactive iodine 131 for scintigraphy or therapy does not preclude pregnancy in thyroid cancer patients. J Nucl Med 37:606, 1996.
115. Bal C, Kumar A, Tripathi M, et al: High-dose radioiodine treatment for differentiated thyroid carcinoma is not associated with change in female fertility or any genetic risk to the offspring. Int J Radiat Oncol Biol Phys 63:449, 2005.
116. Mestman JH: Thyroid hormone replacement during pregnancy. *In* Meikle AW (ed): Hormone Replacement Therapy. Philadelphia, Humana Press, 1997, p 119.
117. Campbell NRC, Hasinoff BB, Stalts H, et al: Ferrous sulfate reduces thyroxine efficacy in patients with hypothyroidism. Ann Intern Med 117:1010, 1992.
118. Singh N, Singh P, Hershman JM: Effect of calcium carbonate on the absorption of levothyroxine. JAMA 283:2822, 2000.
119. Amino N, Tada H, Hidaka Y: Postpartum autoimmune thyroid syndrome: A model of aggravation of autoimmune disease. Thyroid 9:705, 1999.
120. Caixas A, Albareda M, Garcia-Patterson A, et al: Postpatum thyroiditis in women with hypothyroidism antedating pregnancy? J Clin Endocrinol Metab 84:4000, 1999.
121. Stagnaro-Green A: Postpartum thyroiditis. *In* Glineor D (ed): Clinical Endocrinology and Metabolism. Philadelphia, Elsevier Publishing, p 303.
122. Premawardhama LD, Parkes AB, John R, et al: Thyroid peroxidase antibodies in early pregnancy: utility for prediction of postpartum thyroid dysfunction and implications for screening. Thyroid 14:610, 2004.
123. Porterfield SP, Hendrich CE: The role of thyroid hormones in prenatal and neonatal neurological development: Current perspectives. Endocr Rev 14:94–106, 1993.
124. DeZegher F, Spitz B, Devlieger H: Prenatal treatment with thyrotropin releasing hormone to prevent neonatal respiratory distress. Arch Dis Child 67:450, 1992.
125. Burrow GN: Neonatal goiter after maternal propylithiouracil therapy. J Clin Endocrinol Metab 25:403, 1965.
126. Galina MP, Avnet NL, Einhorn A: Iodines during pregnancy: An apparent cause of neonatal death. N Engl J Med 267:1124, 1962.

127. Serreau R, Polack M, Leger J, et al: Fetal thyroid goiter after massive iodine exposure. Prenat Diagn 24:751, 2004.
128. Mestman JH: Hyperthyroidism in pregnancy. Endocrinol Metab Clin N Am 27:127, 1998.
129. Masiukiewicz U, Burrow GN: Hyperthyroidism in pregnancy. Diagnosis and treatment. Thyroid 9:647, 1999.
130. Goodwin TM, Montoro MN, Mestman JH: Transient hyperthyroidism and hyperemesis gravidarum: Clinical aspects. Am J Obstet Gynecol 167:648, 1992.
131. Bouillon R, Maesens M, Van Assche A, et al: Thyroid function in patients with hyperemesis gravidarum. Am J Obstet Gynecol 143:922, 1982.
132. Lao TT, Chin RKH, Chang AMZ: The outcome of hypermetic pregnancies complicated by transient hyperthyroidism. Aust NZ J Obstet Gynecol 27:99, 1987.
133. Bober SA, McGill AC, Tunbridge WM: Thyroid function in hyperemesis gravidarum. Acta Endocrinol 111:404, 1986.
134. Kirshon B, Lee W, Cotton DB: Prompt resolution of hyperthyroidism and hyperemesis gravidarum after delivery. Obstet Gynecol 71:1032, 1988.
135. Goodwin TM, Montoro M, Mestman J, et al: The role of chorionic gonadotropin in transient hyperthyroidism of hyperemesis gravidarum. J Clin Endocrinol Metab 75:1333, 1992.
136. Rosenthal FD, Jones C, Lewis SI: Thyrotoxic vomiting. Br Med J 2:209, 1976.
137. Goodwin TM, Hershman JM: Hyperthyroidism due to inappropriate production of human chorionic gonadotropin. Clin Obstet Gynecol 40:32, 1997.
138. Grun JP, Meuris S, De Nayer P, et al: The thyrootrophic role of human chorionic gonadotropin (hCG) in the early stages of twin (versus single) pregnancies. Clin Endocrinol 46:719, 1997.
139. Rodien P, Bremont C, Raffin-Sanson ML: Familial gestational hyperthyroidism caused by a mutant thyrotropin receptor hypersensitive to human chorionic gonadotropin. N Engl J Med 339:1823, 1998.
140. Mori M, Amino N, Tamaki H, et al: Morning sickness and thyroid function in normal pregnancy. Obstet Gynecol 72:355, 1988.
141. Tamaki H, Itoh E, Kaneda T, et al: Crucial role of serum human chorionic gonadotropin for the aggravation of thyrotoxicosis in early pregnancy in Graves' disease. Thyroid 3:189, 1993.
142. Weetman AP: The immunology of pregnancy. Thyroid 9:543, 1999.
143. Kung AWC, Jones BM: A change from stimulatory to blocking antibody activity in Graves' disease during pregnancy. J Clin Endocrinol Metab 83:514, 1998.
144. Amino N, Izumi Y, Hidaka Y, et al: No increase of blocking type anti-thyrotropin receptor antibodies during pregnancy in patients with Graves' disease. J Clin Endocrinol Metab 88:5871, 2003.
145. Mestman JH, Manning PR, Hodgman J: Hyperthyroidism and pregnancy. Arch Intern Med 134:434, 1974.
146. Davis LE, Lucas MJ, Hankins GDV, et al: Thyrotoxicosis complicating pregnancy. Am J Obstet Gynecol 160:63, 1988.
147. Mitsuda N, Tamaki H, Amino N, et al: Risk factors for developmental disorders in infants born to women with Graves disease. Obstet Gynecol 80:359, 1992.
148. Millar LK, Wing DA, Leung AS, et al: Low birth weight and preeclampsia in pregnancies complicated byyperthyroidism. Obstet Gynecol 84:946, 1994.
149. Stafford IP, Dildy GA, Miller JM: Severe Graves' ophthalmopathy in pregnancy. Obstet Gynecol 105:1221, 2005.
150. Mestman JH: Hyperthyroidism in pregnancy. *In* Glineor D (ed): Clinical Endocrinology and Metabolism. Philadelphia, Elsevier Publishing, p 267.
151. Bell GO, Hall J: Hyperthyroidism in pregnancy. Med Clin N Am 44:363, 1960.
152. Hawe P: The management of thyrotoxicosis during pregnancy. Br J Surg 52:731, 1965.
153. Momotani N, Noh J, Oyangi H, et al: Antithyroid drug therapy for Graves' disease during pregnancy: Optimal regimen for fetal thyroid status. N Engl J Med 315:24, 1986.
154. Surgue D, Druury MI: Hyperthyroidism complicating pregnancy results of treatment by antithyroid drugs in 77 pregnancies. B J Obstet Gynecol 87:970, 1980.
155. Sherif IH, Dyan WT, Basairi S, et al: Treatment of hyperthyroidism in pregnancy. Acta Obstet Gynecol Scand 70:461, 1991.
156. Momatani N, Ito K: Treatment of pregnant patients with Basedow's disease. Exp Clin Endocrinol 97:268, 1991.
157. Clark SL, Phelan JP, Montoro MN, et al: Transient ventricular dysfunction associated with cesarean section in a patient with hyperthyroidism. Am J Obstet Gynecol 151;384, 1985.
158. Mestman JH: Severe hyperthyroidism in pregnancy. *In* Clark SL, Cotton DB, Hankins GDV, Phelan JP (eds): Critical Care Obstetrics, 2nd ed. London, Blackwell Scientific Publications, 1991, p 307.
159. Easterline TR, Schumacker BC, Carlson KL, et al: Maternal hemodynamics in pregnancies complicated by hyperthyroidism. Obstet Gynecol 78:348, 1991.
160. Guenter KE, Friedland GA: Thyroid storm and placenta previa in a primigravida. Obstet Gynecol 44:403, 1965.
161. Mestman JH, Singer PA: Thyroid storm need not be lethal. Contemp Obstet Gynecol 22:135, 1983.
162. Luton D, Le Gac I, Vuillard E, et al: Management of Graves' disease during pregnancy: the key role of fetal thyroid gland monitoring. J Clin Endocrinol Metab 90:6093, 2005.
163. Mestman JH: Disorder of the thyroid gland. *In* Sciarra JJ (ed): Gynecology and Obstetrics. Philadelphia, Lippincott-Raven Publishers, 1996, p 1.
164. Mortimer RH, Cannell GR, Addison RS, et al: Methimazole and prophylthiouracil equally cross the perfused human term placental lobule. J Clin Endocrinol Metab 82:3099, 1997.
165. Wing DA, Miller LK, Koonings PP: A comparision of propylthiouracil versus methimazole in the treatment of hyperthyroidism in pregnnacy. Am J Obstet Gynecol 170:90, 1994.
166. Momotani N, Noh JY, Ishikawa N, et al: Effects of prophylthiouracil and methimazole on fetal thyroid status in mothers with Graves' hyperthyroidism. J Clin Endocrinol Metab 82:3633, 1997.
167. Milham S: Scalp defects in infants of mothers treated for hyperthyroidism with methimazole or carbimazole during pregnancy. Teratology 32:321, 1985.
168. Van Dikje CP, Heydendael RJ, De Kleine MJ: Methimazole, carbimazole and congenital skin defects. Ann Intern Med 106:60, 1987.
169. Mandel SK, Brent GA, Larsen PR: Review of antithyroid drug use during pregnancy and report of a case of aplasia cutis. Thyroid 4:129, 1994.
170. Ramirez A, Espinoza de los Monteros A, Parra A, et al: Esophageal atresia and trachoesophageal fistula in two infants born to hyperthyroid women receiving methimazole (Tapazole) during pregnancy. Am J Med Genet 44:200, 1992.
171. Johnsson E, Larsson G, Ljunggren M: Severe malformations in infants born to hyperthyroid mothers on methimazole. Lancet 350:1520, 1997.
172. Greenberg F: Choanal atresia and athelia: Methimazole teratgenicity or a new syndrome? Am J Med Gene 28:931, 1987.
173. Karlsson FA: Severe embryopathy and exposure to methimazole in early pregnancy. J Clin Endocrinol Metab 87:947, 2002.
174. Mandel SJ, Cooper DS: The use of antithyroid drugs in pregnancy and lactation. J Clin Endocrinol Metab 86:2354, 2001.
175. Cooper DS: Propylithiouracil levels in hyperthyroid patients unresponsive to large doses. Ann Intern Med 192:328, 1985.
176. Burrow GN: Thyroid function and hyperfunction during gestation. Endocr Rev 14:194, 1993.
177. Cheron RG, Kaplan MM, Larsen PR, et al: Neonatal thyroid function after propylthiouracil therapy for maternal Graves' disease. N Engl J Med 304:525, 1981.
178. Rosove MH: Agranulocytosis and antithyroid drugs. West J Med 126:339, 1977.
179. Cooper DS, Golminz D, Levin AA, et al: Agranulocytosis associated with antithyroid drugs: Effects of patient's age and drug dose. Ann Intern Med 98:26, 1983.
180. Bowman MI, Bergmann M, Smith JF: Intrapartum labetalol for the treatment of maternal and fetal thyrotoxicosis. Thyroid 8:795, 1988.
181. Bruner J, Landon MB, Gabbe SG: Diabetes mellitus and Graves' disease in pregnancy complicated by materal allergies to antithyroid medication. Obstet Gynecol 72:443, 1988.

182. Stoffer SS, Hamburger JI: Inadvent 131I therapy for hyperthyroidism in the first trimester of pregnancy. J Nucl Med 17:146, 1976.
183. Berg GE, Nystrom EH, Jacobson L, et al: Radioiodine treatment of hyperthyroidism in a pregnancy woman. J Nucl Med 39:357, 1998.
184. Vicens-Calvet E, Potau N, Carreras E, et al: Diagnosis and treatment in utero of goiter with hypothyroidism caused by iodide overload. J Pediatr 133:147, 1998.
185. Momotani N, Hisaoka T, Noh J, et al: Effects of iodine on thyroid status of fetus versus mother in treatment of Graves' disease complicated by pregnancy. J Clin Endocrinol Metab 75:738, 1992.
186. Perelman AH, Johnson RL, Clemons RD, et al: Intrauterine diagnosis and treatment of fetal goitrous hypothyroidism. J Clin Endocinrol Metab 71:618, 1990.
187. Momotani N, Yamashita R, Yoshimoto M, et al: Recovery from fetal hypothyroidism: Evidence for the safety of breastfeeding while taking propylthiouracil. Clin Endocrinol (Oxf) 31:591, 1989.
188. Azizi F, Khoshniat M, Bahrainian M, Hedayati M: Thyroid function and intellectual development of infants nursed by mothers taking methimazole. J Clin Endocrnol Metab 85:3233, 2000.
189. McKenzieJM, Zakarija M: Fetal and neonatal hyperthyroidism and hypothyroidism due to maternal TSH receptor antibodies. Thyroid 2:155, 1992.
190. Polak M, Le Gac I, Yuillard E, et al: Fetal and neonatal thyroid function in relation to maternal Graves' disease. *In* Glineor D (ed): Clinical Endocrinology and Metabolism. Philadelphia, Elsevier Publishing, p 289.
191. Hollingsworth DR, Mabry CC: Congential Graves' disase. Four familial cases with long term follow up and perspective. Am J Dis Child 130:148, 1976.
192. Kopp P, Van Sande J, Parma J, et al: Brief report: Congenital hyperthyroidism caused by a mutation in the thyrotropin receptor gene. N Engl J Med 322:150, 1995.
193. De Roux N, Polak M, Coet J: A neomutation of thyroid stimulating hormone receptor in severe neonatal hyperthyroidism. J Clin Endocrinol Metab 81:2023, 1996.
194. Cove DH, Johnston P: Fetal hyperthyroidism: Experience of treatment in four siblings. Lancet 1:430, 1985.
195. Perelman AH, Clemons RD: The fetus in maternal hyperthyroidism. Thyroid 2:225, 1992.
196. Wanstrom KD, Weiner CP, Williamson I, et al: Prenatal diagnosis of fetal hyperthyroidism using funipuncture. Obstet Gynecol 76:513, 1990.
197. Bruinse HW, Vermuelen-Weiner C, Wit JM: Fetal treatment for thyrotoxicosis in nonthyrotoxic pregnant women. Fetal Ther 3:152, 1988.
198. Porreco RP, Bloch CA: Fetal blood sampling in the management of intrauterine thyrotoxicosis. Obstet Gynecol 76:509, 1990.
199. Heckel S, Favre R, Schlienger JL, et al: Diagnosis and successful in utero treatment of a fetal goitrous hyperthyroidism caused by maternal Graves' disease. Fetal Diagn Ther 12:54, 1997.
200. Kilpatrick S: Umbilical cord sampling in women with thyroid disease in pregnancy: is it necessary? Obstet Gynecol 198:1, 2003.
201. Mandel SH, Hanna CE, LaFranci SH: Neonatal hypopituitary hypothyroidism associated with maternal thyrotoxicosis. Journal of Pediatric Endocrinology 3:189, 1989.
202. Kempers MJE, van Tijn DA, van Trotsenburg ASP, et al: Central congenital hypothyroidism due to gestational hyperthyroidism: detection where prevention failed. J Clin Endocrinol Metab 88:5851, 2003.
203. Higuchi R, Miyawaki M, Kumagai T, et al: Central hypothyroidism in infants who were born to mothers with thyrotoxicosis before 32 weeks gestation: 3 cases. Pediatrics 115:623, 2005.
204. Montoro MN, Collea JV, Frasier SD, et al: Successful outcome of pregnancy in women with hypothyroidism. Ann Intern Med 94:31, 1981.
205. Davis LE, Leveno KJ, Cunningham FG: Hypothyroidism complicating pregnancy. Obstet Gynecol 72:108, 1988.
206. Leung AS, Millar LK, Koonings PP, et al: Perinatal outcome in hypothyroid pregnancies. Obstet Gynecol 81:349, 1993.
207. Wasserstrom N, Anania CA: Perinatal consequences of maternal hypothyroidism in early pregnancy and inadequate treatment. Clin Endocrinol 42:353, 1995.
208. Abalovich M, Gutierrez S, Alcaraz G, et al: Overt and subclinical hypothyroidism complicating pregnancy. Thyroid 12;63, 2002.
209. Klein RZ, Haddow JE, Faix JD, et al: Prevalence of thyroid deficiency in pregnant women. Clin Endocrinol (Oxf) 35:41, 1991.
210. Kamijo K, Saito T, Sato M, et al: Transient subclinical hypothyroidism in early pregnancy. Endorcinol Jpn 37:397, 1990.
211. Lejeune B, Leomone M, Kinchac J, et al: The epidemiology of autoimmune and functional thyroid disorders in pregnancy. (Abstract.) Endocrinol Invest 15(Suppl):77, 1992.
212. Dussault JH, Fisher DA: Thyroid function in mothers of hypothyroid newborns. Obstet Gynecol 93:15, 1999.
213. Fukushi M, Honma K, Fujita K: Maternal thyroid deficiency during pregnancy and subsequent neurophysiological development of the child (letter) N Engl J Med 341;2016, 1999.
214. Tamaki H, Amino N, Takeoka K, et al: Thyroxine requirements during pregnancy for replacement therapy of hypothyroidism. Obstet Gynecol 76:230, 1990.
215. Casey BM, Dashe JS, Wells CE, et al: Subclinical hypothyroidism and pregnancy outcome. Obstet Gynecol 105:239, 2005.
216. Man EB: Maternal hypothyroxinemia, development of 4 and 7 years old offspring. *In* Fisher DA, Burrows GN (eds): Perinatal Thyroid Physiology and Disease. New York, Raven Press, 1975, p 177.
217. Allan WC, Haddow JE, Palomaki GE, et al: Maternal thyroid deficiency and pregnancy complications: implications for population screening. J Med Screen 7:127, 2000.
218. Harjai KJ, Licata AA: Effects of amiodarone on thyroid function. Ann Intern Med 126:63, 1997.
219. Wilson R, McKillop KH, Crocket GT, et al: The effect of lithium therapy on parameters thought to be involved in the development of autoimmune thyroid disease. Clin Endocrinol (Oxf) 34:357, 1991.
220. Zograbyan A, Goodwin TM, Montoro MN, et al: What are the risk factors for perinatal complications in hypothyroidism. Abstract 142 presented at the 71st Annual Meeting of the American Thyroid Association, September 16, 1998, Portland, Oregon.
221. Man EB, Brown JF, Serunian SA: Maternal hypothyroxinemia: Psychoneurological defects of progency. Ann Clin Lab Sci 21:227, 1991.
222. Liu H, Momotani N, Yoshimura J, et al: Maternal hypothyroidism during early pregnancy and intellectual development of the progeny. Arch Intern Med 154:785, 1994.
223. Singer PA, Cooper DS, Daniels G: Guidelines for the diagnosis and management of thyroid nodules and well differentiated thyroid cancer. Arch Intern Med 156:2165, 1996.
224. Hamberger JI: Thyroid nodules in pregnancy. Thyroid 2:165, 1992.
225. Hay ID: Nodular thyroid disease diagnosed during pregnancy: How and when to treat. Thyroid 9:667, 1999.
226. Tan GH, Gharib H, Goeliner JR, et al: Management of thyroid nodules in pregnancy. Arch Intern Med 156:2317, 1996.
227. Rosen JB, Walfish PG, Nikore V: Pregnancy and surgical thyroid disease. Surgery 98:1135, 1985.
228. Doherty CM, Shindo ML, Rice DH, et al: Management of thyroid nodules during pregnancy. Laryngoscope 105:251, 1995.
229. Moosa M, Mazzaferri EL: Outcome of differentiated thyroid cancer diagnosed in pregnancy women. J Clin Endocrinol Metab 82:2862 , 1997.
230. Cortelazzi D, Castagnone D, Tassis B, et al: Resolution of hyperthyroidism in a pregnant woman with toxic thyroid nodule by percutaneous ethanol injection. Thyroid 5:473, 1995.
231. Kamei N, Gullu S, Dagci Ilgin S, et al: Degree of thyrotropin suppression in differentiated thyroid cancer wihtout recurrence of metastases. Thyroid 9:1245, 1999.
232. Yasmeen S, Cress R, Romano PS, et al: Tyroid cancer in pregnancy. Int J Gynaecol Obstet 9:15, 2005.
233. Singer PA: Thyroiditis: Acute, subacute, and chronic. Med Clin N Am 75:61, 1991.
234. Pearce EN, Farwell AP, Braverman LE: Current concepts: Thyroiditis. N Engl J Med 3348:2646, 2003.

235. Vanderpump MPJ, Tunbridge WMG, French JM, et al: The incidence of thyroid disorders in the community: A twenty year follow up of the Whickham Survey. Clin Endocrinol 43:55, 1995.
236. McCanlies E, O'Leary LA, Foley TP, et al: Hashimoto's thyroiditis and insulin dependent diabetes mellitus: Differences among individuals with and without abnormal thyroid function. J Clin Endocrinol Metab 83:1548, 1998.
237. Spencer C, Lee R, Kazarosyan M, et al: Thyroid reference ranges in pregnancy: studies on an iodine sufficient cohort. Abstract 043 13th International Thyroid Congress, Buenos Aires, Argentina, October 30–November 4, 2005. Thyroid 15:S16, 2005.
238. Gutekunst R, Hafermann W, Mansky T, et al: Ultrasonography related to clinical and laboratory findings in lymphocytic thyroiditis. Acta Endocrinol (Copenh) 121:129, 1989.
239. Stagnaro-Green A, Roman SH, Cobin RH, et al: Detection of at risk pregnancy by means of highly sensative assays for thyroid autoantibodies. JAMA 264:1422, 1990.
240. Glineor D, Fernandez-Soto M, Bourdoux P, et al: Pregnancy in patients with mild thyroid abnormalities: Maternal and fetal repercussions. J Clin Endocrinol Metab 73:421, 1991.
241. Singh A, Danta ZN, Stone S, et al: Presence of thyroid antibodies in early reproductive failure. Biochemical versus clinical pregnancies. Fertil Steril 63:277, 1995.
242. Glineor D, Riahi M, Grun JP, et al: Risk of subclinical hypothyroidism in pregnancy women with asymptomatic autoimmune thyroid disorders. J Clin Endocrinol Metab 79:197, 1994.
243. Stagnaro-Green A, Chen X, Bogden JD, et al: The thyroid and pregnancy: a novel risk factor for very preterm delivery. Thyroid 15:351, 2005.
244. Spong CY: Maternal thyroid disorders and preterm birth: another piece of the puzzle? Thyroid 15349, 2005.
244a. Negro R, Formoso G, Mangieri T, et al: Levothyroxine treatment in euthyroid pregnant women with autoimmune thyroid diseases: Effects on obstetrical complications. J Clin Endocrinol Metab 91:2587, 2006.
245. Arikawa K, Ichikawa Y, Yoshida T, et al: Blocking type antithyrotropin receptor antibody in patients with nongoitrous hypothyroidism: Its incidence and characteristics of action. J Clin Endocrinol Metab 60:953, 1985.
246. Matsuura N, Yamada Y, Nohara Y, et al: Familial neonatal transient hypothyroidism due to maternal TSH binding inhibitor immunoglobulins. N Engl J Med 303:738, 1980.
247. Ginsberg J, Walfish PG, Rafter DJ, et al: Thyrotropin blocking antibodies in the sera of mothers with congenitally hypothyroid infants. Clin Endocrinol 25:189, 1986.
248. LaFranchi S: Congenital hypothyroidism: Etiologies, diagnosis, and management. Thyroid 9:735, 1999.
249. Brown RS, Bellasario RL, Botero D, et al: Incidence of transient congenital hypothyroidism due to maternal thyrotropin antibodies in over one million babies. J Clin Endocrinol Metab 81:1147, 1996.
250. Amino N, Mori H, Iwatani O, Tanizawa O, et al: High prevalence of transient postpartum thyrotoxicosis and hypothyroidism. N Engl J Med 306:849, 1982.
251. Roti E, Emerson SH: Postpartum thyroiditis. J Clin Endocrinol Metab 74:3, 1992.
252. Smallridge RC: Postpartum thyroid diseases through the ages: A historical view. Thyroid 9:671, 1999.
253. Gerstein HC: How common is postpartum thyroiditis? A methodolgic overview of the literature. Arch Intern Med 150:1397, 1990.
254. Alvarez-Marfany M, Roman SH, Drexler AJ, et al: Long term prospective study of postpartum thyroid dysfunction in women with insulin dependent diabetes mellitus. J Clin Endocrinol Metab 79:10, 1994.
255. Kent GN, Stucky BG, Allen JR, et al: Postpartum thyroid dysfunction: Clinical assessment and relationship to psychiatric affective morbidity. Clin Endocrinol (Oxf) 51:429, 1999.
256. Amino N, Tada H, Hidaka Y, et al: Therapeutic Controversey: Screening for postpartum thyroiditis. J Clin Endocrinol Metab 84:1813, 1999.
257. Kuijpens JL, Pop VJ, Vader HL, et al: Prediction of postpartum thyroid dysfunction: Can it be improved? Eur J Endocrinol 139:36, 1998.
258. Othman S, Phillips DIW, Parkes AB, et al: A long term follow up of postpartum thyroiditis. Clin Endocrinol (Oxf) 32:559, 1990.
259. Tachi J, Amino N, Tamaki H, et al: Long term follow up and HLA association in patients with postpartum hypothyroidism. J Clin Endorcinol Metab 66:480, 1988.
260. Premawardhana LDKE, Parkes AB, Ammari F, et al: Postpartum thyroiditis and long term thyroid status prognostic influence of thyroid peroxidase antibodies and ultrasound echogenicity. J Clin Endocrinol Metabl 85:71, 2000.
261. Amino N, Miyai K, Yamamoto T, et al: Transient recurrence of hyperthyroidism after delivery in Graves' disease. J Clin Endocrinol Metab 44:130, 1977.
262. Eckel Rh, Green WL: Postpartum thyrotoxicosis in a patient with Graves'disease associated with low radioactive iodine uptake. JAMA 243:1545, 1980.
263. Momotani N, Noh J, Ishikawa N, et al: Relationship between silent thyroiditis and recurrent Graves' disease in the postpartum period. J Clin Endocrinol Metab 79:285–289, 1994.
264. Lazarus JH: Clinical manifestations of postpartum thyroid disease. Thyroid 9:685, 1999.
265. Jansson R, Bernander S, Karlsson A, et al: Autoimmune thyroid dysfunction in the postpartum period. J Clin Endocrinol Metab 58:681, 1984.
266. Amino N, Miyai K, Kuro P, et al: Transient postpartum hypothyroidism: Fourteen cases with autoimmune thyroiditis. Ann Intern Med 87:155, 1977.
267. Dahlberg PA, Jansson R: Different aetiologies in postpartum thyroiditis. Acta Endocrinol 104:195, 1983.
268. Lazarus JH, Ammari F, Oretti R, et al: Clinical aspects of recurrent postpartum thyroiditis. J R Coll Gen Pract 47:305, 1996.
269. Mehta H, Badenhoop K, Walfish PG: Adrenal insufficiency after recurrent postpartum thyroiditis (postpartum Schmidt syndrome): A case report. Thyroid 8:269, 1998.
270. Benhaim Rochester D, Davies TF: Increased risk of Graves' disease after pregnancy. Thyroid 11:1287, 2005.

Pituitary and Adrenal Disorders in Pregnancy

MAUREEN P. MALEE

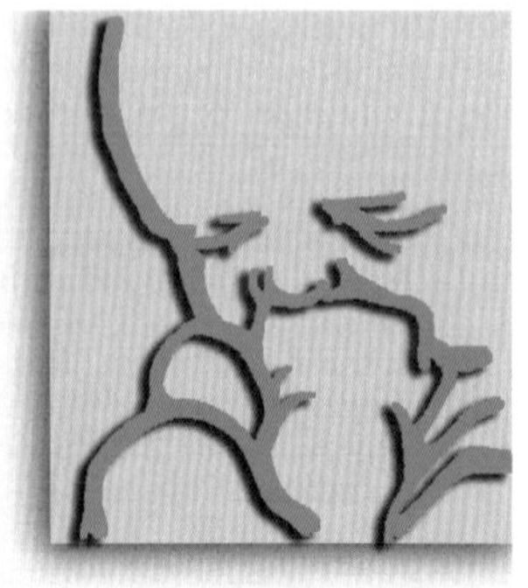

CHAPTER 39

KEY ABBREVIATIONS

Adrenocorticotrophic hormone	ACTH
Arginine vasopressin	AVP
Computerized tomography scan	CT
Corticotropin-releasing hormone	CRH
Desmopressin	dDAVP
Diabetes insipidus	DI
Intravenously	IV
Magnetic resonance imaging	MRI

PITUITARY DISEASE IN PREGNANCY

The pituitary gland typically enlarges during pregnancy due to lactotroph hyperplasia. Pituitary secretions are altered, and the enlargement is typically accompanied by a parallel increase in prolactin levels.[1] Magnetic resonance imaging (MRI) studies reveal an enlarged pituitary without evidence of tumor.[2] This physiologic enlargement may rarely result in compression of the optic chiasm with bitemporal hemianopsia.

Pituitary Adenomas

Pituitary adenomas are benign neoplasms of anterior pituitary cells. Functional adenomas can secrete hormones, and may also be the cause of headaches. They are classified by size as micro- or macroadenomas, with microadenomas being smaller than 10 mm. The diagnosis is usually confirmed by MRI or computed tomography (CT) scan, and baseline visual field studies are recommended. Adenomas can also be classified by the hormone they secrete, with prolactin-secreting adenomas being the most prevalent, representing 25 percent of cases.

Hyperprolactinemia can manifest as galactorrhea, menstrual disorders, infertility, hirsutism, headache and visual field defects. Correction of hyperprolactinemia restores ovulation in 80 to 90 percent of women and usually restores fertility.[3]

Medical treatment with dopamine agonists is standard treatment for microadenomas. The medications in use in the United States include bromocriptine and cabergoline. These agents decrease prolactin levels in up to 90 percent of patients and reduce the size of the adenoma by 50 percent in more than half of treated patients.[4] Although cabergoline is perhaps more effective and better tolerated, bromocriptine remains the drug of choice as it is not teratogenic and is not associated with untoward effects in later pregnancy.[5] Therapy is generally discontinued once pregnancy is achieved.[6]

As the normal pituitary enlarges during pregnancy, the potential exists for expansion of adenomas during pregnancy. This occurs infrequently with microadenomas, with only 1.3 percent of women experiencing symptomatic tumor enlargement in contrast to 23.2 percent in those with macroadenomas.[7] Bromocriptine has been used successfully during pregnancy for symptomatic tumor enlargement and is the preferred first-line approach.[8] Previously, such women were offered surgical intervention, which carries with it risks of hypopituitarism, hemorrhage, and transient diabetes insipidus.[7]

The asymptomatic patient is followed clinically. MRI studies and visual field studies are not repeated unless there is clinical suspicion of tumor enlargement. Serial prolactin levels are not useful, because they typically increase during pregnancy and are not necessarily elevated with tumor enlargement.[9] In those in whom the macroadenoma extends into the suprasellar region abutting the optic chiasm or into the cavernous sinus, the risk of tumor enlargement is greater. This population is followed more rigorously, with visual field testing every trimester. In the event that symptomatic tumor enlargement occurs during pregnancy, bromocriptine treatment is reinstated. The typical starting dose is 2.5 mg/day, and it is increased as tolerated. Surgery is reserved for cases that fail to respond to medical intervention. Transsphenoidal resection is the recommended therapy, although surgery may lead to hypopituitarism in 20 percent of cases.[10]

Breastfeeding is unaffected by hyperprolactinemia and does not effect tumor growth. Following delivery, radiologic assessment of tumor size and a prolactin level are obtained after the first postpartum visit. Because serum levels of prolactin remain elevated with lactation, caution should be used in interpreting these results. Bromocriptine is typically reinstituted upon completion of breastfeeding.[11]

Diabetes Insipidus

Diabetes insipidus (DI) involves water loss secondary to inadequate tubular reabsorption. Polyuria, polydipsia, and excessive thirst are characteristic findings. There are three types of DI, which are classified according to etiology. Hypothalamic or central DI involves inadequate arginine vasopressin (AVP) secretion to stimuli; causes are genetic (rare) or acquired. Acquired central DI can result from tumor, surgery, trauma, infection, Sheehan's syndrome or autoimmune destruction of the posterior pituitary gland. Nephrogenic DI is characterized by decreased renal sensitivity to normal or elevated AVP levels, and it can be familial or acquired. Primary polydipsia, which is typically psychogenic in origin, results from excessive fluid intake and AVP suppression.[12,13]

Pregnancy is associated with alterations in water balance and AVP metabolism. There is lowering of the osmostat, the setpoint at which AVP is secreted, and the placenta produces vasopressinase, which inactivates AVP and results in a threefold increase in its clearance.[12] In women with DI who become pregnant, the AVP analog, desmopressin (dDAVP) is resistant to placental vasopressinase and remains the treatment of choice.[13] The drug is given intranasally in doses of approximately 0.1 mg, given up to three times daily. When monitoring for the clinical response to dDAVP, it is important to remember that both sodium and osmolality are reduced.[13] Use of dDAVP throughout pregnancy has not been associated with adverse fetal outcomes.[14,15] Furthermore, there is minimal transfer into breast milk and poor gastrointestinal absorption. Thus, no untoward effect upon neonatal water metabolism is observed with breastfeeding.[13]

Sheehan's Syndrome

Sheehan's syndrome refers to the development of pituitary necrosis postpartum, typically precipitated by obstetric hemorrhage with severe hypotension.[16] Depending on the extent of infarction, an acute or chronic form can result.[12] The acute form, associated with approximately 90-percent glandular infarction, can be lethal if unrecognized and treated promptly. A CT scan may reveal an empty sella, and the patient may present with hemodynamic instability, tachycardia and hypotension, unresponsive to routine aggressive fluid resuscitation. Hypoglycemia and failure to lactate may be presenting signs of this diagnosis. Such a presentation in a patient with a history of obstetric hemorrhage should provoke a work-up, measuring ACTH, cortisol, thyroxine, prolactin, and growth hormone, and prompt treatment with stress doses of glucocorticoids necessary for survival.[12]

In the chronic form, the degree of infarction is less, as are the physiologic consequences. The patient may present with signs and symptoms consistent with chronic Sheehan's syndrome months to years after the insult. The patient may experience amenorrhea, loss of libido, and symptoms consistent with adrenal insufficiency; partial diabetes insipidus has been described in up to 50 percent of cases of chronic Sheehan's syndrome. Basal hormone levels are indicated, and stimulation tests may be necessary to confirm the diagnosis, after which appropriate replacement treatment can be instituted.[12,16,17]

ADRENAL DISEASE IN PREGNANCY

Adrenal disease rarely complicates pregnancy. The principal disorders described include Cushing's syndrome, Addison's disease, primary hypoaldosteronism, and pheochromocytoma.

Cushing's Syndrome

Cushing's syndrome is the term used to describe the symptom complex caused by excessive circulating glucocorticoids.[18,19] The term Cushing's syndrome encompasses pituitary hypersecretion of adrenocorticotropic hormone (ACTH), Cushing's disease, which accounts for the majority of nonpregnant patients with Cushing's syndrome; patients with adrenal adenomas or carcinomas; and patients with ectopic ACTH or corticotropin-releasing hormone (CRH) syndrome. Pregnancy is rare in untreated patients with Cushing's syndrome, with amenorrhea and oligomenorrhea being present in 70 to 85 percent of untreated patients.[20] In the pregnant population, Cushing's syndrome results from an adrenal adenoma in about 50 percent of cases, followed by a pituitary adenoma (30 percent), adrenal carcinoma (10 percent), and ectopic ACTH syndrome (5 percent).[20–22] The relatively high percentages of adrenal adenomas and carcinomas in the pregnant population with Cushing's syndrome is unexplained, although primary pituitary disease is more likely to be associated with infertility. The low percentage of cases as a result of ectopic ACTH production (e.g., oat/small cell lung carcinoma) reflects the mean age for ectopic ACTH syndrome,[23] which is 53 years old, and the male-to-female ratio of 10:1.

Cushing's syndrome adversely affects both maternal and fetal outcomes. Maternal morbidity includes hypertension (67 percent), congestive heart failure secondary to severe hypertension (10 percent), preeclampsia (10 percent), and gestational diabetes (30 percent).[24] Maternal mortality has been reported from complications of hypertension associated with the diagnosis of Cushing's syndrome.[20] Fetal outcomes are also compromised when Cushing's syndrome complicates pregnancy. High rates of preterm labor and delivery are common (30 to 60 percent), as is fetal growth restriction (26 percent of cases). Fetal demise has been reported in 7 to 17 percent of cases.[20,25]

The diagnosis of Cushing's syndrome can be particularly challenging during pregnancy. Some of the typical features overlap those of normal pregnancy, such as striae, hypertension and edema. Bruisability, proximal muscle weakness, and pigmentation of the striae should raise the index of suspicion for coexistent disease.[26]

The diagnosis of Cushing's syndrome in pregnancy is established as in the nonpregnant state. Initially, one confirms the presence of hypercortisolemia without diurnal variation. Occasional circadian rhythmicity is preserved. Norms for pregnancy should be used as a reference because urinary free cortisol is increased in pregnancy, and serum levels are elevated as well owing to the increase in cortisol-binding globulin. Thus, dexamethasone suppression testing is helpful and a 50-percent suppression of the midnight cortisol level relative to the morning cortisol level supports the diagnosis.[27,28] If suppression fails, an adrenal tumor, autonomous adrenal nodule, or ectopic ACTH production may be present. One typically follows determination of serum cortisol with serum ACTH levels. However, Cushing's syndrome in pregnancy is accompanied by elevated ACTH levels secondary to placental production or from placental CRH-stimulated ACTH production.[20,22] Thus ACTH levels cannot be used in pregnancy to distinguish between pituitary and adrenal etiologies.[29,30] Inferior petrosal sinus sampling for ACTH has been accomplished successfully in the pregnant patient,[29] but imaging studies, typically MRI, more often delineate the etiology of the hypersecretion.[31]

Once the diagnosis of Cushing's syndrome is established, prompt treatment is indicated. Treatment of the hypercortisolemia is associated with decreased maternal and fetal morbidity and mortality.[20,32,33] Treatments include adrenalectomy, pituitary adenomectomy, and pharmacologic therapy. The associated risks and benefits, as well as gestational age guide appropriate therapy.[34,35] In a patient with mild hypercortisolism close to term, close surveillance of blood pressure, glucose homeostasis, and fetal well-being can be entertained, with definitive therapy delayed until the postpartum period.[36,37] In two different series, several women underwent adrenalectomy for a unilateral adenoma. No surgical complications were reported, including use of a laparoscopic retroperitoneal approach,[38,39] and maternal and fetal outcomes appeared to improve.[21,40] Four reported cases of transsphenoidal surgery for Cushing's disease in pregnancy have been associated with generally favorable outcomes.[41] Surgical management is apparently preferable for both Cushing's syndrome and Cushing's disease in pregnancy. Surgery is typically scheduled for the second trimester.[21] If the diagnosis is established during the third trimester, definitive treatment is typically delayed until after delivery. Medical therapy is available until definitive treatment is achieved. Metyrapone, which inhibits the conversion of 11-deoxycortisol to cortisol has been successfully employed in select cases. In response to the blockade, there is an accumulation of androgenic precursors, but in the small number of patients so treated, there has not been virilization of female fetuses, postdelivery hypoadrenalism, or teratogenicity.[42–45] Reports indicate that careful monitoring of the response to metyrapone yields control of hypercortisolemia in more than 90 percent of patients.[46]

In all patients who undergo surgical treatment during pregnancy, exogenous cortisol replacement is necessary until the hypothalamic-pituitary-adrenal axis returns to normal, which typically occurs postpartum. Stress doses of steroids are indicated for delivery and intercurrent illnesses.[20]

Primary Hyperaldosteronism

Primary hyperaldosteronism has been rarely diagnosed during pregnancy. Most cases occur secondary to an adrenal adenoma. Pregnancy complicates the diagnosis because elevated aldosterone levels are present in normal fasting pregnancy. However, in cases of primary hyperaldosteronism, plasma renin activity is suppressed.[47–50] Salt loading also shows failure to suppress aldosterone. In the event that baseline and suppression testing results are equivocal, or imaging does not suggest unilateral disease, medical treatment can be considered during pregnancy, and more definitive investigation pursued following delivery.[49] Spironolactone, typically used for medical management in the nonpregnant patient with hyperaldosteronism should be avoided during pregnancy because it possesses significant antiandrogen activity.[50] Blood pressure control is achieved with standard medications such as labetalol and methyldopa. In the event that blood pressure cannot be controlled medically, and the lesion is obvious on imaging studies, surgery may be considered. The hypokalemia that typically accompanies hyperaldosteronism is diminished by the antikaliuretic effect of progesterone. Following delivery, hypertension and hypokalemia may be exacerbated as progesterone levels decline.[51,52]

Adrenocortical Insufficiency

The inadequate production of adrenal corticosteroids can be either acute or chronic. Although most cases of adrenal insufficiency are diagnosed outside of pregnancy, the disease may first present in pregnancy and present a diagnostic challenge. The chronic form may present with numerous nonspecific signs and symptoms, whereas the acute form may present as cardiovascular collapse.

The signs and symptoms of chronic adrenocortical insufficiency in both pregnant and nonpregnant patients include fatigue, hypotension, hyperpigmentation, weakness, syncope, nausea, vomiting, anorexia, and weight loss. Although some or all of these findings can be encountered in an otherwise uncomplicated early pregnancy, their persistence should raise suspicion. Primary adrenal insufficiency, or Addison's disease, is a rare condition, and is typically due to autoimmune phenomenon.[53] 21-Hydroxylase autoantibodies have been detected in more than 80 percent of patients with idiopathic Addison's disease, and they are positively correlated with the severity of adrenal dysfunction.[54,55] Infiltrative (tuberculosis, histoplasmosis) and hemorrhagic causes (coagulation disorders, sepsis) of primary adrenal insufficiency are less frequent. Secondary adrenal insufficiency is most often due to exogenous glucocorticoid; ACTH suppression may persist up to a year after steroid use is discontinued. Addison's disease is an infrequent complication of pregnancy associated with a risk for maternal and fetal mortality in the absence of diagnosis and treatment. From case reports, it appears that the most critical periods are during the first trimester and the first 2 weeks postpartum.[56,57] A risk for fetal growth restriction appears in offspring of untreated mothers.[57] However, newborns do not require additional glucocorticoid supplementation, because their hypothalamic-pituitary-adrenal axis functions autonomously.[57]

The diagnosis of primary adrenal failure is most challenging.[53] The finding of a nonpregnant "normal" cortisol level should increase suspicion as cortisol levels increase with gestation. Circadian rhythmicity is preserved, so attention must be paid to time of day of sampling and the increase in cortisol binding globulin that accompanies pregnancy. The combination of a greatly elevated ACTH with a low or normal cortisol drawn coincidentally is most revealing of the diagnosis. In the absence of ACTH determination, an ACTH stimulation test (250 ug intravenously [IV]) unaccompanied by a brisk cortisol response measured 30 minutes after administration confirms the diagnosis. Aldosterone levels are also typically reduced in primary adrenal insufficiency, and renin values are elevated.[58] Hyponatremia and hyperkalemia may be observed, accompanied by hypotension, decreased extracellular fluid volume, decreased glomerular filtration rate and increased blood urea nitrogen.

Before the introduction of glucocorticoid replacement therapy in women with primary adrenal failure, pregnancy was accompanied by a significant risk of maternal death. With routine oral glucocorticoid and mineraloco rticoid replacement, pregnancy and labor and delivery are typically uneventful.[53] Labor and delivery should be considered stressful events, with additional parenteral glucocorticoid therapy provided during the second stage. In the event of an operative delivery, additional glucocorticoid (e.g., 100 mg hydrocortisone IV every 6 hours) should be provided and continued for 24 to 48 hours after delivery, with return to routine oral dosages by postoperative day 3. In the event of a presumptive addisonian crisis, recommendations are for 100 to 200 mg hydrocortisone IV, for a total amount of 400 mg over a 6-hour period, together with 3 to 4 liters of normal saline IV fluids. Hypoglycemia and hypokalemia should be corrected with glucose and potassium. Mineralocorticoid replacement is indicated in cases of hypotension or refractory hypokalemia.

Pheochromocytoma

Pheochromocytoma is a rare tumor of chromaffin cells and an unusual cause of secondary hypertension.[59] It infrequently complicates a pregnancy (0.007 percent).[60] However, if unrecognized and untreated, its presence can be accompanied by lethal consequences.[61] Maternal mortality has declined significantly over the past 40 years. In a series reported in 1971, the overall mortality was 48 percent, declining to 6 percent in a consolidation of case reports from the late 1980s to 2000. A postpartum diagnosis carries the greatest risk for mortality; 19 percent even in the most recent reported series.[62] Similarly, significant fetal risk continues to accompany this maternal diagnosis, although overall mortality has declined from 55 percent in the 1971 report to 15 percent in the reports consolidated from 1988 to 2000.[62]

Maternal mortality is typically a consequence of abrupt catecholamine release, and it can be induced by uterine contractions, uterine position, fetal movement, and inappropriate pharmacologic interventions for unrelated complaints.[63] Such catecholamine release can provoke myocardial infarction, cerebral hemorrhage, or other lethal events. Fetal death is not due to catecholamine release, as the placental enzyme catechol-O-methyltransferase metabolizes maternal catecholamines. However, the catecholamines provoke severe hypertension, with consequences such as hypoxemia, growth restriction, and fetal death.[64,65]

The presentation of a pheochromocytoma in a pregnant woman is similar to that in a nonpregnant individual.[66] Hypertensive crisis symptoms and signs such as palpitations, nausea, sweating, anxiety, and headache are common.[67] The index of suspicion must be high, particularly if paroxysmal hypertension develops before 20 weeks' gestation. Once suspected, confirmation of the diagnosis is not altered by pregnancy or other coincidental diseases. Measurement of plasma or urine metanephrines is the most sensitive assay for the diagnosis of pheochromocytoma.[68] Once confirmed, the tumor is localized by MRI[68] and typically is found in the adrenal gland in over 90 percent of cases. Ten to 15 percent of tumors are bilateral, and 10 percent are found in other locations such as the renal hilus, the organ of Zuckerkrandl, or elsewhere along periaortic sympathetic chain.

The treatment for pheochromocytoma is primary surgical resection, whether the patient is pregnant or not. Medical therapy with α-blockers, such as phenoxybenzamine, is instituted as soon as the diagnosis is made[69] to maintain blood pressure control and is well tolerated during pregnancy.[70] Side effects such as nasal congestion and tachycardia may be treated with selective $beta_1$ antagonists. In the first and second trimester, surgery is performed once adequate blood pressure control is achieved.[68] Surgery may be delayed until postpartum if the diagnosis is made in the third trimester. Laparoscopic adrenalectomy can be performed safely for tumors less than 7 cm in size.[71] Elective cesarean delivery is the preferred mode of delivery because labor may be associated with unpredictable catecholamine surges.[72] Vaginal delivery is associated with a higher maternal mortality rate (31 percent) compared with cesarean delivery (19 percent).[73] The management of a pregnant woman with the pheochromocytoma necessitates multidisciplinary planning to optimize outcome.

KEY POINTS

- Pituitary adenomas are classified by size and hormonal production. Prolactinomas are the most common pituitary tumors. Medical management is usually effective, visual field disturbances are infrequent, and the pregnancy is rarely affected.
- Diabetes insipidus has several etiologies. During pregnancy, dDAVP is the primary therapy.
- Sheehan's syndrome can result from an obstetric hemorrhage, and present in either an acute or chronic form. The acute form can result in cardiovascular collapse. Treatment involves fluid resuscitation and replacement therapy of affected hormones.
- Cushing's syndrome is caused by excessive glucocorticoids, and usually results from an adrenal adenoma when it complicates pregnancy. If undiagnosed and untreated, Cushing's syndrome can adversely affect maternal and fetal outcomes.
- Both medical and surgical therapy are options for treatment of Cushing's syndrome during pregnancy. If surgical intervention is warranted, glucocorticoid replacement is necessary.
- Primary aldosteronism is rarely diagnosed in pregnancy and typically results from an adrenal adenoma. Primary medical management can be attempted, and if this fails, surgery is recommended.
- Addison's disease is usually an autoimmune phenomenon. It occurs in both acute and chronic forms. Signs and symptoms of Addison's disease often overlap those of normal pregnancy.
- The diagnosis of Addison's disease can be difficult. Once diagnosed, glucocorticoid replacement therapy is instituted. Addisonian crisis, if unrecognized, is associated with considerable mortality.
- Pheochromocytomas are secondary to adrenal tumors in more than 90 percent of cases. Lack of recognition and treatment results in considerable maternal and fetal morbidity and mortality. Diagnosis is established by measurement of metanephrines.
- The definitive treatment for pheochromocytoma is surgical, following blood pressure control with α-blockers.

REFERENCES

1. Goluboff LG, Ezrin C: Effect of pregnancy on the somatotroph and the prolactin cell of the human adenohypophysis. J Clin Endocrinol Metab 29:1533, 1969.
2. Elster AD, Sanders TG, Vines FS, et al: Size and shape of the pituitary gland during pregnancy and post partum: measurement with MR imaging. Radiology 181:531, 1991.
3. Molitch ME: Prolactin. *In* Melmed S (ed): The Pituitary, ed 2, Cambridge: Blackwell Publishing, 2002, p 77.
4. Molitch ME, Elton RL, Balackwell RE, et al: Bromocriptine as primary therapy for prolactin-secreting macroadenomas: results of a prospective multicenter study. J Clin Endocrinol Metab 60:698, 1985.
5. Raymond JP, Goldstein E, Konopka P, et al: Follow-up of children born of bromocriptine-treated mothers. Horm Res 22:239, 1985.
6. Bigazzi M, Ronga R, Lancranjan I, et al: A pregnancy in an acromegalic woman during bromocriptine treatment: effects on growth hormone and prolactin in the maternal, fetal, and amniotic compartments. J Clin Endocrinol Metab 48:9, 1979.
7. Molitch ME: Management of prolactinomas during pregnancy. J Reprod Med 44:1121, 1999.
8. Kupersmith MJ, Rosenberg C, Kleinberg D: Visual loss in pregnant women with pituitary adenomas. Ann Intern Med 121:473, 1994.
9. Divers WAJ, Yen SS: Prolactin-producing microadenomas in pregnancy. Obstet Gynecol 4:425, 1983.
10. Tominaga A, Uozumi T, Arita K: Effects of surgery on testosterone secretion in male patients with pituitary adenomas. Endocr J 43:307, 1996.
11. Holmgren U, Bergstrand G, Hagenfeldt K, et al: Women with prolactinoma–effect of pregnancy and lactation on serum prolactin and on tumour growth. Acta Endocrinol (Copenh) 111:452, 1986.
12. Molitch ME: Pituitary diseases in pregnancy. Semin Perinatol 22:457, 1998.
13. Durr JA: Diabetes insipidus in pregnancy. Am J Kidney Dis 9:276, 1987.
14. Kaellen BAJ, Carlsson SS, Bengtsson BKA: Diabetes insipidus and use of desmopressin (Minirin) during pregnancy. Eur J Endocrinol 132:144, 1995.
15. Ray JG: DDAVP use during pregnancy: an analysis of its safety for mother and child. Obstet Gynecol Surv 53:450, 1998.
16. Sheehan HL, Davis JC: Pituitary necrosis. Br Med Bull 24:59, 1968.
17. Iwasaki Y, Oiso Y, Yamauchi K, et al: Neurohypophyseal function in postpartum hypopituitarism: Impaired plasma vasopressin response to osmotic stimuli. J Clin Endocrinol Metab 68:560, 1989.
18. Orth DN: Cushing's syndrome. N Engl J Med 32:791, 1995.
19. Plotz CM, Knowlton AI, Ragan C: The natural history of Cushing's syndrome. Am J Med 3:597, 1952.
20. Buesher MA, McClamrock HD, Adashi EY: Cushing's syndrome in pregnancy. Obstet Gynecol 79:130, 1992.
21. Pricolo VE, Monchik JM, Prinz RA, et al: Management of Cushing's syndrome secondary to adrenal adenoma during pregnancy. Surgery 108:1072, 1990.
22. Aron DC, Schnall AD, Sheeler LR: Cushing's syndrome and pregnancy. Am J Obstet Gynecol 162:244, 1990.
23. Orth DN, Liddle GW: Results of treatment with 108 patients with Cushing's syndrome. N Engl J Med 285:243, 1971.
24. Hadden DR: Arenal disorders of pregnancy. Endocrinol Metab Clin N Amer 24:139, 1995.
25. Pickard J, Jochen AL, Sadur CN, et al: Cushing's syndrome in pregnancy. Obstet Gynecol Surg 45:87, 1990.
26. Ross E, Linch D: Cushing's syndrome-killing disease: discriminatory value of signs and symptoms aiding early diagnosis. Lancet 1:646, 1982.
27. Sheeler LR: Cushing's syndrome and pregnancy. Endocrinol Metab Clin N Am 23:619, 1994.
28. Invitti C, Pecori Giraldi F, De Martin M, Cavagnini F: The Study Group of the Italian Society of Endocrinology on the Pathophysiology of the Hypothalamic-Pituitary-Adrenal Axis. Diagnosis and management of Cushing's syndrome: results of an Italian multicentre study. J Clin Endocrinol Metab 84:440, 1999.
29. Mellor A, Harvey RD, Pobereskin LH, Sneyd JR: Cushing's disease treated by trans-sphenoidal selective adenomectomy in mid-pregnancy. Br J Anaesth 80:850, 1998.
30. Ross RJM, Chew SL, Perry L, et al: Diagnosis and selective cure of Cushing's disease during pregnancy by transsphenoidal surgery. Eur J Endocrinol 132:722, 1995.
31. Keely E: Endocrine causes of hypertension in pregnancy-when to start looking for Zebras. Sem Perinatology 22:471, 1998.
32. Mulder WJ, Berghout A, Wiersinga WM: Cushing's syndrome during pregnancy. Neth J Med 36:234, 1990.
33. Lo KWK, Lau TK: Cushing's syndrome in pregnancy secondary to adrenal adenoma. Gynecol Obstet Invest 45:209, 1998.

34. Guilhaume B, Sanson ML, Billaud L, et al: Cushing's syndrome and pregnancy: aetiologies and prognosis in twenty-two patients. Eur J Med 1:83, 1992.
35. Aron DC, Schnall AM, Sheeler LR: Cushing's syndrome and pregnancy. Am J Obst Gynecol 162:244, 1990.
36. Sheeler LR: Cushing's syndrome and pregnancy. Endocrinol Metab Clin North Am 23:619, 1994.
37. Martin RW, Lucas JA, Martin JN, et al: Conservative management of Cushing's syndrome in pregnancy. J Reprod Med 34:493, 1989.
38. Bevan JS, Gough MH, Gillmer MDG, Burke CW: Cushing's syndrome in pregnancy: The timing of definitive treatment. Clin Endocrinol (Oxf) 27:225, 1987.
39. Ashima M, Tanaka M, Haraoka M, Nalto S: Retroperitoneal laparoscopic adrenalectomy in a pregnant woman with Cushing's syndrome. J Urol 164:770, 2000.
40. Lo KW, Lau T: Cushing's syndrome in pregnancy secondary to adrenal adenoma. Gynecol Obstet Invest 45:209, 1998.
41. Mellor A, Harvey RD, Pobereskin J, et al: Cushing's disease treated by trans-sphenoidal selective adenomectomy. Br J Anaesth 80:850, 1982.
42. Gormley MJ, Hadden DR, Kennedy TL, et al: Cushing's syndrome in pregnancy: treatment with metyrapone. Clin Endocrinol 16:283, 1982.
43. Close CF, Mann MC, Watts JF, Taylor KG: ACTH-independent Cushing's syndrome in pregnancy with spontaneous resolution after delivery: control of the hypercortisolism with metyrapone. Clin Endocrinol (Oxf) 39:375, 1993.
44. Wallace C, Toth EL, Lewanczuk RZ, Siminoski K: Pregnancy-induced Cushing's syndrome in multiple pregnancies. J Clin Endocrinol Metab 81:15, 1996.
45. Hana V, Dokoupilova M, Marek J, Plavka R: Recurrent ACTH-independent Cushing's syndrome in multiple pregnancies and its treatment with metyrapone. Clin Endocrinol (Oxf) 54:277, 2001.
46. Verhelst JA, Trainer PJ, Howlett TA, et al: Short and long-term responses to metyrapone in the medical management of 91 patients with Cushing's syndrome. Clin Endocrinol 35:169, 1991.
47. Baron F, Sprauve ME, Huddleston JF, et al: Diagnosis and surgical treatment of primary aldosteronism in pregnancy: a case report Obstet Gyenecol 86:644, 1995.
48. Solomon CG, Thiet M, Moore FJ, et al: Primary hyperaldosteronism in pregnancy. A case report. J Reprod Med 41:255, 1996.
49. Webb JC, Bayliss P: Pregnancy complicated by primary aldosteronism. South Med J 90:243, 1997.
50. Robar CA, Poremba JA, Pelton JJ, et al: Current diagnosis and management of aldosterone-producing adenomas during pregnancy. The Endocrinologist 8:403, 1998.
51. Nezo M, Miura Y, Noshiro T, et al: Primary aldosteronism as a cause of severe postpartum hypertension in two women. Am J Obstet Gynecol 182:745, 2000.
52. Murakami T, Watanabe Ogura E, Tanaka Y, et al: High blood pressure lowered by pregnancy. Lancet 356:1980, 2000.
53. Ambrosi B, Barbetta L, Morricone L: Diagnosis and management of Addison's disease during pregnancy. J Endocrinol Invest 26:698, 2003.
54. Falorni A, Laureti S: Adrenal autoimmunity and correlation with adrenal dysfunction. The Endocrinologist 10:145, 2000.
55. Betterle C, Volpato M, Smith BR, et al: Adrenal cortex and steroid 21 hydroxylase autoantibodies in adult patients with organ-specific autoimmune disease: markers of low progression to clinical Addison's disease. Clin Endocrinol Metab 82:932, 1997.
56. Brent F: Addison's disease and pregnancy. Am J Surg 79:645, 1950.
57. Osler M: Addison's disease and pregnancy. Acta Endocrinol (Copenh) 41:67, 1962.
58. Symonds EM, Craven DJ: Plasma renin and aldosterone in pregnancy complicated by adrenal insufficiency. Brit J Obstet Gynaec 83:191, 1977.
59. Manger WM, Gifford RWJ: *In* Phaechromocytoma. Springer-Verlag, New York, 1977, p 1.
60. Harrington JL, Farley DR, van Heerden JA, Ramin KD: Adrenal tumors and pregnancy. World J Surg 23:182, 1999.
61. Brunt LM: Phaeochromocytoma in pregnancy. Br J Surg 88:481, 2001.
62. Mannelli M, Bemporad D: Diagnosis and management of pheochromocytoma during pregnancy. J Endocrinol Invest 25:567, 2002.
63. Schenker JG, Chowers I: Pheochromocytoma and pregnancy. Review of 89 cases. Obstet Gynaecol Surv 26:739, 1971.
64. Barzel US, Barllan Z, Runmery G, et al: Pheochromocytoma and pregnancy. Am J Obstet Gynecol 89:519, 1964.
65. Greiss FC Jr, Anderson SC, King LC: Uterine vascular bed: effect of acute hypoxia. Am J Obstet Gynecol 113:1057, 1972.
66. Schenker JG, Granat M: Pheochromocytoma and pregnancy. An updated appraisal. Aust N Z J Obstet Gynaecol 22:1, 1982.
67. Mannelli M, Lanni L, Cilotti A, Conti A: Pheochromocytoma in Italy: a multicentric retrospective study. Eur J Endocrinol 141:619, 1999.
68. Freier DT, Thomson NW: Pheochromocytoma and pregnancy: the epitome of high risk. Surgery 114:1148, 1993.
69. Wheeler MH, Chare MJB, Austin TR, Lazarus JH: The management of the patient with catecholamines excess. World J Surg 6:735, 1982.
70. Ahlawat SK, Jain S, Kumari S, et al: Pheochromocytoma associated with pregnancy: case report and review of the literature. Obstet Gynecol Surv 54:728, 1999.
71. Janetschek G, Neumann HP: Laparoscopic surgery for pheochromocytoma. Urol Clin North Am 28:97, 2001.
72. Almog B, Kupferminc MJ, Many A, Lessing JB: Pheochromocytoma in pregnancy—a case report and review of the literature. Acta Obstet Gynecol Scand 79:709, 2000.
73. Schenker JG, Granat M: Phaeochromocytoma and pregnancy—an updated appraisal. Aust N Z J Obstet Gynaecol 22:1, 1982.

Hematologic Complications of Pregnancy

PHILIP SAMUELS

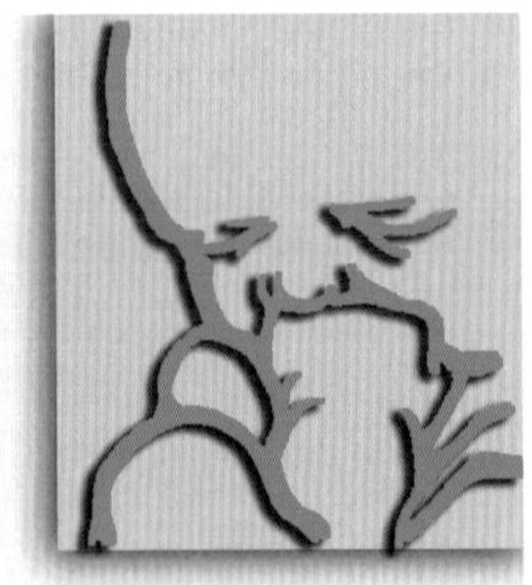

CHAPTER 40

KEY ABBREVIATIONS

Hemolysis, elevated liver enzymes, low platelets	HELLP
Hemolytic uremic syndrome	HUS
Immune thrombocytopenic purpura	ITP
Immunoglobulin G	IgG
Intravenous immunoglobulin	IVIG
Polymerase chain reaction	PCR
Red blood cell	RBC
Thrombotic thrombocytopenic purpura	TTP
Unusually large multimers of von Willebrand's factor	ULVWf
Urinary tract infection	UTI
von Willebrand's cleaving enzyme	ADAMTS-13
von Willebrand's disease	vWD
von Willebrand's factor	vWF

PREGNANCY-ASSOCIATED THROMBOCYTOPENIA

Affecting approximately 4 percent of pregnancies, thrombocytopenia is the most frequent hematologic complication of pregnancy resulting in consultation. Hospital laboratories vary on their lower limit of a normal platelet count, but it is usually between 135,000 and 150,000/mm^3. Platelet counts generally fall slightly, owing to hemodilution and increased destruction, as gestation progresses. Platelet counts, however, should not fall below the normal range. In pregnancy, the vast majority of cases of mild to moderate thrombocytopenia are caused by gestational thrombocytopenia.[1] This form of thrombocytopenia has little likelihood of causing maternal or neonatal complications.[2] The obstetrician, however, is obliged to rule out other forms of thrombocytopenia that are associated with severe maternal or perinatal morbidity. The common and rare causes of thrombocytopenia in the gravida at term are shown in the box "Causes of Thrombocytopenia During Pregnancy." Until the late 1980s, it was assumed that all patients with an unexplained low platelet count carried a diagnosis of immune thrombocytopenic purpura (ITP), a recognized cause of neonatal thrombocytopenia. Platelet antibody testing cannot distinguish among ITP, thrombocytopenia accompanying preeclampsia, and gestational thrombocytopenia.[3,4] The distinction between these disorders is important because each of these diagnoses carries distinct maternal and neonatal implications.

Gestational Thrombocytopenia

Patients with gestational thrombocytopenia generally present with mild (platelet count = 100,000 to 149,000/mm^3) to moderate (platelet count = 50,000 to 99,000/mm^3) thrombocytopenia.[5] These patients usually require no therapy, and the fetus appears to be at little, if any, risk of being born with profound thrombocytopenia (platelet count < 50,000/mm^3) or a bleeding diathesis. This distinct entity was first suggested but not specifically defined in a study published in 1986 by Hart et al.[6] In this study, 28 of 116 pregnant women (24 percent) who were evaluated prospectively during an 8-month period had platelet counts less than 150,000/mm^3 at least once during pregnancy. In all 17 patients who were followed after delivery, platelet counts returned to normal.

Causes of Thrombocytopenia During Pregnancy

Common causes
- Gestational thrombocytopenia
- Severe preeclampsia
- HELLP syndrome
- Immune thrombocytopenic purpura
- Disseminated intravascular coagulation

Rare causes
- Lupus anticoagulant/antiphospholipid antibody syndrome
- Systemic lupus erythematosus
- Thrombotic thrombocytopenic purpura
- Hemolytic uremic syndrome
- Type 2b von Willebrand's syndrome
- Folic acid deficiency
- Human immunodeficiency virus infection
- Hematologic malignancies
- May-Hegglin syndrome (congenital thrombocytopenia)

Platelet-associated immunoglobulin G (IgG) was present in 79 percent of these 28 women, and 61 percent had serum antiplatelet IgG. None of these women had positive antibodies after delivery. Hart et al.[6] were actually describing gestational thrombocytopenia before the condition had been recognized as a distinct entity. Furthermore, they were the first to demonstrate that conventional platelet antibody testing cannot distinguish gestational thrombocytopenia from ITP.[6] Samuels et al.[3] also investigated 74 mothers with gestational thrombocytopenia. Forty-six (62 percent) of these patients had circulating antiplatelet IgG in their plasma (a positive indirect test); these women gave birth to two neonates with thrombocytopenia, both having platelet counts greater then 50,000/mm^3. Burrows and Kelton[5,7,8] have further shown, in several large series, that there is little risk to the mother or neonate in cases of gestational thrombocytopenia. In one study no mother or infant, in a group of 334 women with gestational thrombocytopenia, experienced bleeding complications.[8] In their earlier study of 1,357 healthy, pregnant women, 112 (8.3 percent) had platelet counts less than 150,000/mm^3.[5] The lowest platelet count was 97,000/mm^3. The incidence of thrombocytopenia (platelet count <150,000/mm^3) in the infants of these 112 women was 4.3 percent, not statistically significantly different from infants born to healthy pregnant women without thrombocytopenia (1.5 percent). None of these infants had platelet counts less than 100,000/mm^3. Indeed, the reports by Samuels et al.[3] and Burrows and Kelton[5,7] have convincingly demonstrated that gestational thrombocytopenia is an entity distinct from ITP.

The decrease in platelet count, occurring in gestational thrombocytopenia, is not merely due to dilution of platelets with increasing blood volume. It appears to be due to an acceleration of the normal increase in platelet destruction that occurs during pregnancy.[1] This is demonstrated by the fact that the mean platelet volume is increased in patients with gestational thrombocytopenia. The increase in platelet-associated IgG seen in these patients may merely reflect immune complexes adhering to the platelet surface rather than specific antiplatelet antibodies. Pregnant women who have gestational thrombocytopenia do not require any special therapy during the puerperium unless their platelet counts fall below 20,000/mm^3 or if there is clinical bleeding. These complications, however, are rare, and it is difficult to determine whether these patients with profound thrombocytopenia, have gestational thrombocytopenia, the new onset of ITP or a blood dyscrasia.

Immune Thrombocytopenic Purpura

Although it affects only 1 to 3 per 1,000 pregnancies, ITP has received attention in the obstetrics literature because of the potential for profound neonatal thrombocytopenia in infants born to mothers with this condition.

In 1954, Peterson and Larson[9] were the first to recognize that profound thrombocytopenia (platelet count <50,000/mm^3) may develop in infants born to women with ITP. A subsequent report confirmed this observation.[10] In 1973, Territo et al.[11] made the first effort to predict which infants were at increased risk of being born with profound thrombocytopenia. They demonstrated, in a small number of patients, that neonates born to mothers with platelet counts less than 100,000/mm^3 were at highest risk. Many larger studies have since shown that this arbitrary cutoff, although generally true, is not useful in individual cases. Subsequently, a number of efforts have been made to use historic and noninvasive parameters to assess the risk for severe neonatal thrombocytopenia, including the use of maternal glucocorticoids, whether or not the mother had undergone splenectomy, and the presence of maternal antiplatelet antibodies. None of these, however, has shown the desired positive or negative predictive value.[12–16]

In general, pregnancy has not been determined to cause ITP or to change its severity. Other studies, however, have demonstrated that in individual patients exacerbations of ITP often occur during pregnancy and improve postpartum.[3,17,18] Harrington et al.[19] were the first to demonstrate that ITP was humorally mediated. Shulman et al.[20] showed that the mediator of this disorder was IgG. These findings were confirmed when Cines and Schreiber[21] developed the first platelet antiglobulin test, a radioimmunoassay, in 1979. Today, this test is usually performed using enzyme-linked immunosorbent assay or flow cytometry. New assays have shown that these autoantibodies may be directed against specific platelet surface glycoproteins, including the IIb/IIIa and Ib/IX complexes.[22] After the platelets are coated with antibody, they are removed from circulation by binding to the Fc receptors of macrophages in the reticuloendothelial system, especially the spleen. Approximately 90 percent of women with ITP have platelet-associated IgG.[21] Unfortunately, this is not specific for ITP, because studies have shown that these tests are also positive in women with gestational thrombocytopenia and preeclampsia.[3,4]

To make the issue more confusing, the pathogenesis of ITP in children and adults usually differs. Childhood ITP most often follows a viral infection and clinically presents with petechiae and bleeding.[23] This form of ITP is generally self-limited and disappears over time. Conversely, adults have milder bleeding and easy bruisability, and are often diagnosed after a prolonged period of subtle symptoms. Adult ITP usually runs a chronic course, and long-term therapy is often eventually needed. Many pregnancies occur in women in their late teens and early twenties. In these women, with a history of ITP, it may be difficult to ascertain whether the patient has childhood ITP or adult ITP. Also, no study has shown whether the risk of neonatal thrombocytopenia is similar in both forms of ITP.

ITP has a predisposition for women aged 18 to 40, with an overall female-male ratio of 1.7.[24] It is a diagnosis of exclusion. The patient must have isolated thrombocytopenia with an unremarkable peripheral smear. She must have only bleeding clinically consistent with a depressed platelet count, and she must not be taking any medication, herbal compound, or illicit drug that may cause thrombocytopenia. Finally, the patient must have no other disease process than can cause thrombocytopenia.[24,25]

ITP is different from other causes of thrombocytopenia in pregnancy because of the aforementioned risk of profound neonatal thrombocytopenia. This has further been confounded by the fact that before 1990, it was assumed that all patients with unexplained thrombocytopenia during gestation had ITP. It was only after 1990 that gestational thrombocytopenia became recognized as a distinct entity.[2,3] The inclusion of cases of gestational thrombocytopenia in many studies has made it difficult to determine the true incidence of neonatal thrombocytopenia in women with ITP.

Table 40-1 lists several studies in which all patients had true ITP and delineates the rates of profound neonatal thrombocytopenia. Even these carefully performed investigations show wide ranges in the rates of profound neonatal thrombocytopenia.

In 1980, Scott et al.[26] were the first to institute direct fetal platelet determinations by using fetal scalp sampling in a series of women with ITP. This procedure, however, requires operator skill, an engaged fetal vertex, a dilated cervix, ruptured membranes, and the ability to obtain a pure sample of fetal blood without any contamination with maternal blood or amniotic fluid. For these reasons as well as the development of cordocentesis, this procedure was abandoned.

With the development and increased use of ultrasound-guided cordocentesis in the mid-1980s, accurate in utero sampling of fetal platelets became feasible. Some authors initially advocated routine use of this technique in mothers with ITP.[27–29]

However, like fetal scalp sampling, cordocentesis to establish fetal platelet counts in women with ITP has been largely abandoned. The information obtained does not affect the clinical management of the pregnancy. Although profound neonatal thrombocytopenia is not uncommon in pregnancies complicated by ITP, immediate neonatal complications are unusual. The mode of delivery has never been shown to affect neonatal outcome and should be based on obstetric indications.

In a meta-analysis by Burrows and Kelton,[30] a 14.6-percent incidence of profound thrombocytopenia in infants born to mothers with ITP was reported. This meta-analysis did not, however, take into account that many of the studies included in the analysis did not exclude patients with gestational thrombocytopenia. Therefore, the risks of profound thrombocytopenia may very well be greater than this reported incidence. These authors also noted a neonatal morbidity rate of 24 per 1,000 with few serious complications. This figure may be low as well for the reasons mentioned above.

Samuels et al.[3] reported a neonatal morbidity rate of 278 per 1,000 infants born to mothers with true ITP. The sample size, however, was too small to determine if mode of delivery or degree of neonatal thrombocytopenia had an impact on this morbidity. This rate may be overly high, because these were patients referred to two large tertiary care centers. Nonetheless, this study does point out that ITP does not always carry a benign course for the neonate. The neonatal morbidities included intraventricular hemorrhage, hemopericardium, gastrointestinal bleeding and extensive cutaneous manifestations of bleeding.[3] Regardless of the complication rates in profoundly thrombocytopenic neonates, cordocentesis is rarely indicated in patients with ITP as it does not provide information that will change clinical management.

Thrombotic Thrombocytopenic Purpura and Hemolytic Uremic Syndrome

These two conditions are characterized by microangiopathic hemolytic anemia and severe thrombocytopenia. Pregnancy does not predispose a patient to these conditions, but they should be considered when evaluating the gravida with severe thrombocytopenia. Thrombotic thrombocytopenic purpura (TTP) is characterized by a pentad of findings, which are shown in the box "Pentad of Findings in TTP."[31,32] The complete pentad occurs only in approximately 40 percent of patients, but approximately 75 percent present with a triad of

Table 40-1. Incidence of Profound Neonatal Thrombocytopenia in Mothers Known to Have Immune Thrombocytopenic Purpura

REPORTS	TOTAL PATIENTS WITH ITP	INFANTS WITH PLATELET COUNT <50,000/MM^3	95% CONFIDENCE INTERVAL
Karapatkin et al.[15]	19	6 (31.6%)	20.9%–52.5%
Burrows and Kelton[8]	60	3 (5%)	0%–10.5%
Noriega-Guerra et al.[13]	21	8 (38.1%)	17.3%–58.9%
Samuels et al.[3]	88	18 (20.5%)	12.0%–28.9%
Pooled (Crude)	188	35 (18.6%)	13%–24%

ITP, immune thrombocytopenic purpura.

Pentad of Findings in Thrombotic Thrombocytopenic Purpura (TTP)*

+Microangiopathic hemolytic anemia
+Thrombocytopenia
+Neurologic abnormalities including confusion, headache, paresis, visual hallucinations, seizures
Fever
Renal dysfunction

*The classic pentad is only found in 40% of patients.
+These three findings are present in 74% of patients.[32]

microangiopathic hemolytic anemia, thrombocytopenia, and neurologic changes.[33] Pathologically, these patients have thrombotic occlusions of arterioles and capillaries.[31] These occur in multiple organs, and there is no specific clinical manifestation for the disease. The clinical picture reflects the organs that are involved.

TTP/HUS may mimic preeclampsia. Because preeclampsia is much more common than this disorder, it should be considered first. However, delay in diagnosing TTP/HUS can have fatal consequences.

To diagnose the hemolytic anemia associated with TTP, the indirect antiglobulin test or Coombs' test must be negative. This rules out an immune-mediated cause for the anemia. Lactic dehydrogenase should be elevated, the indirect bilirubin should be increased, and haptoglobin should be decreased. Schistocytes are usually seen on the peripheral smear, if it is carefully reviewed. To be classified as TTP, the platelet count should be less than 100,000/mm^3. In renal insufficiency associated with TTP, the urine sediment is usually normal with an occasional red blood cell (RBC). This finding helps distinguish this disorder from a lupus flare, which more often has associated hematuria (see Chapter 42). The serum creatinine is usually greater than 2 mg/dl. This degree of renal dysfunction is unusual, but not rare, in preeclampsia. There is usually 1+ to 2+ proteinuria on urine dipstick.

The neurologic findings in TTP are usually nonspecific. They include headache, confusion and lethargy. Infrequently tonic-clonic seizures occur, and rarely lateralizing signs are noted.

Terrell and coworkers[34] examined the epidemiology of TTP/HUS occurring in Oklahoma between 1996 and 2004. In 206 reported cases, they found that 37 percent were idiopathic. However, 13 percent were associated with an autoimmune disease, and 7 percent occurred in pregnancy and the postpartum period. These researchers were able to project that the incidence of suspected TTP/HUS is 11 cases/million population/year, whereas the incidence of proven cases is 4.5 cases/million population/year.[34] If this disease is so rare, why include it in a text on obstetrics? If untreated, TTP carries a 90 percent mortality rate, whereas treatment with plasma exchange decreases the mortality rate to 20 percent.[35] Therefore, obstetricians must be aware of this disease process, so it can be quickly and aggressively treated.

Much progress has been made in determining the pathophysiology of TTP. Tsai and colleagues have found that a deficiency of ADAMTS-13 activity is strongly associated with TTP.[36,37] This metalloprotease, also known as von Willebrand's cleaving enzyme, cleaves unusually large multimers of von Willebrand factor (ULVWf). If there is a deficiency in the activity or concentration of ADAMTS-13, ULVWf circulate in increased amounts, leading to increased platelet aggregation and the initiation of TTP. ADAMTS-13 can be assayed in commercial laboratories.

Weiner[38] has published the most extensive literature review concerning TTP. In this series of 45 patients, 40 developed the disease antepartum, with 50 percent occurring before 24 weeks' gestation. The mean gestational age at onset of symptoms was 23.4 weeks. This finding may be helpful when trying to distinguish TTP from other causes of thrombocytopenia and microangiopathic hemolytic anemia occurring during gestation.

However, TTP may be confused with rarely occurring early-onset severe preeclampsia. In preeclampsia, antithrombin III levels are frequently low, and this is not the case with TTP.[29] This test, therefore, may be a useful discriminator between these two disorders. In Weiner's review, the fetal and maternal mortality rates were 84 and 44 percent, respectively. These mortality rates are overly pessimistic, because this series included many patients who contracted the disease before plasma infusion/exchange therapy was utilized to treat TTP.

Although the hemolytic uremic syndrome (HUS) has many features in common with TTP, it usually has its onset in the postpartum period. Patients with HUS display a triad of microangiopathic hemolytic anemia, acute nephropathy, and thrombocytopenia. HUS is rare in adults, and the thrombocytopenia is usually milder than that seen in TTP, with only 50 percent of patients having a platelet count less than 100,000/mm^3 at the time of diagnosis. The thrombocytopenia worsens as the disease progresses.[40] A major difference between TTP and HUS is that 15 to 25 percent of patients with the latter develop chronic renal disease.[32] HUS often follows infections with verotoxin-producing enteric bacteria. Cyclosporine therapy, cytotoxic drugs, and oral contraceptives may predispose adults to develop HUS.[38–40] The majority of cases of HUS occurring in pregnancy develop at least 2 days after delivery.[32] In fact, in one series, only nine of 62 cases (6.9 percent) of pregnancy-associated HUS occurred antepartum.[38] Four of these nine patients developed symptoms on the day of delivery. The mean time from delivery to development of HUS in patients in this series was 26.6 days. The maternal mortality rate may exceed 50 percent in postpartum HUS. However, this mortality rate is based on old data. With plasmapheresis and dialysis, the likelihood of maternal death is probably much less. It is not important to make the distinction between TTP and HUS, because the initial therapy for both disorders is plasmapheresis.

EVALUATION OF THROMBOCYTOPENIA DURING PREGANCY AND THE PUERPERIUM

Before deciding on a course to follow in treating the patient with thrombocytopenia, the obstetrician must evaluate the patient and attempt to ascertain the etiology of her low platelet count. Important management decisions are dependent on arriving at an accurate diagnosis.

A complete medical history, although time consuming, is critically important. It is essential to learn whether the patient has previously had a depressed platelet count or bleeding diathesis. It is also important to know whether these clinical conditions occur coincidentally with pregnancy. A complete medication history should be elicited, because certain medications, such as heparin, can result in profound maternal thrombocytopenia. The obstetric history should focus on whether there have been any maternal or neonatal bleeding problems in the past. Excessive bleeding from an episiotomy site or cesarean delivery incision site, or bleeding from intravenous sites during labor should alert the physician to the possibility of thrombocytopenia in the previous pregnancy. The obstetrician should also question whether the infant had any bleeding diathesis or if there was any problem following a circumcision. The obstetrician should also ask pertinent questions to determine whether severe preeclampsia or HELLP (Hemolysis, Elevated Liver Enzymes, Low Platelets) syndrome is the cause of her thrombocytopenia. The treatment of preeclampsia and HELLP are discussed in Chapter 33. Importantly, all thrombocytopenic pregnant women should be carefully evaluated for the presence of risk factors for human immunodeficiency virus infection, because this infection can cause an ITP-like syndrome. Also, a family history should be elicited, as there are familial forms of thrombocytopenia.

An accurate assessment of gestational age should also be carried out. This is important, because some of the etiologies of thrombocytopenia in pregnancy are dependent on the gestational age. A thorough physical examination of the patient should be performed. The physician should look for the presence of ecchymoses or petechiae. The conjunctivae often show petechiae, as do the nail beds. Blood pressure should be determined to ascertain whether the patient has impending preeclampsia. If the patient is developing HELLP syndrome, scleral icterus may be present. The eye grounds should be examined for evidence of arteriolar spasm or hemorrhage.

It is imperative that a peripheral blood smear be examined by an experienced hematologist or pathologist whenever a case of pregnancy-associated thrombocytopenia is diagnosed. The presence or absence of evidence of microangiopathic hemolysis on the smear will help in establishing a diagnosis. This specialist can also rule out platelet clumping, which will result in a factitious thrombocytopenia. Platelet clumping in EDTA, a lavender top tube, occurs in about 3 per 1,000 individuals and may lead to a spurious diagnosis of thrombocytopenia. If platelet clumping is suspected, the physician should ask the laboratory to perform a platelet count on citrate collected blood, a blue top tube. If the count is normal, then there is probably platelet clumping, and the patient is not thrombocytopenic. Other laboratory evaluation should be performed as necessary to rule out preeclampsia and HELLP syndrome, as well as disseminated intravascular coagulopathy. If a diagnosis of ITP is entertained, appropriate platelet antibody testing may aid in the diagnosis but is of limited utility during pregnancy.

After determining the etiology of thrombocytopenia, the physician can better determine whether imminent delivery is necessary, if the thrombocytopenia should be treated before initiating delivery, or if the low platelet count should be watched.

THERAPY OF THROMBOCYTOPENIA DURING PREGNANCY

Gestational Thrombocytopenia

Gestational thrombocytopenia, the most common form of thrombocytopenia encountered in the third trimester, requires no special intervention or therapy. The most important therapeutic issue is to refrain from treatment and testing that may lead to unnecessary intervention or iatrogenic preterm delivery. In patients with mild to moderate thrombocytopenia and no antenatal or antecedent history of thrombocytopenia, the patient should be treated as a normal pregnant patient. If the maternal platelet count drops below 50,000/mm^3, the patient may still have gestational thrombocytopenia, but there are not enough data on mothers with counts this low to determine if there are any maternal or fetal risks. These patients, therefore, should be treated as if they have de novo ITP. Although approximately 4 percent of patients have gestational thrombocytopenia, less than 1 percent of uncomplicated pregnant women have gestational thrombocytopenia with platelet counts less than 100,000/mm^3.[8]

Immune Thrombocytopenic Purpura

Treatment of the gravida with ITP during pregnancy and the puerperium requires attention to both mother and fetus. As in other cases of thrombocytopenia, maternal therapy needs to be instituted only if there is evidence of a bleeding diathesis or to prevent a bleeding complication if surgery is anticipated. There is usually no spontaneous bleeding unless the platelet count falls below 20,000/mm^3.[41] In a meta-analysis of 17 studies, the risk of fatal hemorrhage in an individual younger than 40 years of age with a platelet count less than 30,000/mm^3 was 0.4 percent. The predicted 5-year mortality rate in this setting was 2.2 percent.[42] Surgical bleeding does not usually occur until the platelet count is less than 50,000/mm^3.

The conventional forms of raising the platelet count in the patient with ITP include glucocorticoid therapy, intravenous gammaglobulins, platelet transfusions, and splenectomy. If the patient is having a bleeding diathesis or if the platelet count is below 20,000/mm^3, there is usually a need to raise the platelet count in a relatively short period of time. Although oral glucocorticoids can be used, intravenous glucocorticoids may work more rapidly. Any steroid with a glucocorticoid effect can be used. However, hematologists have had the most experience with methylprednisolone. This medication can be given intravenously and has very little mineralocorticoid effect. It is important to avoid steroids with strong mineralocorticoid effects because these agents can disturb electrolyte balance, cause fluid retention, and result in hypertension. The usual dose of methylprednisolone is 1.0 to 1.5 mg/kg of *total body weight* intravenously daily in divided doses. It usually takes approximately 2 days for a response, but it may take up to 10 days for a maximum response. Even though methylprednisolone has very little mineralocorticoid effect, some may be observed because of the large dose that is being administered. Therefore, it is important to follow the patient's electrolytes. There is little likelihood that methylprednisolone will cause neonatal adrenal suppression because little crosses the placenta. It is metabolized by placental 11-β-ol-dehydrogenase to an inactive 11-keto metabolite. Park-Wylie et al. performed a meta-analysis, which confirmed the general safety of glucocorticoids during pregnancy.[43] They did, however, find a 3.4-fold increased risk of cleft lip and palate with first trimester exposure (see Chapter 8). The risk/benefit ratio should be discussed with the patient prior to initiation of therapy.

After the platelet count has risen satisfactorily using intravenous methylprednisolone, the patient can be switched to oral prednisone. The usual dose is 60 to 100 mg/day. Prednisone can be given in a single dose, but there is less gastrointestinal upset with divided doses. The physician can rapidly taper the dose to 30 to 40 mg/day and decrease it slowly thereafter. The dose should be titrated to keep the platelet count at approximately 100,000/mm^3. If therapy is initiated with oral prednisone, the usual daily dose is 1 mg/kg total body weight.

The likelihood of a favorable response to glucocorticoids is about 70 percent. It is important to realize that if the patient has been taking glucocorticoids for a period of at least 2 to 3 weeks, she may have adrenal suppression and should undergo increased doses of steroids during labor and delivery in order to avoid an adrenal crisis. Tapering should be slowly thereafter. Also, if the patient has been on glucocorticoids for some time, she may experience significant side effects, including fluid retention, hirsutism, acne, striae, poor wound healing, and monilia vaginitis. In rare circumstances, patients on long-term steroids during gestation can develop osteopenia or cataract formation. The chance of any fetal or neonatal side effects from the glucocorticoids, however, is remote.

Although glucocorticoids are the mainstays of treating maternal thrombocytopenia, up to 30 percent of patients do not respond to these medications. In such cases, intravenous immunoglobulin (IVIG) is used. This agent probably works by binding to the IgG Fc receptors on reticuloendothelial cells and preventing destruction of platelets. It may also adhere to receptors on platelets and prevent antiplatelet antibodies from binding to these sites. The usual dose is 0.4 g/kg/day for 3 to 5 days. However, it may be necessary to use as much as 1 g/kg/day. The response usually begins in 2 to 3 days and peaks in 5 days. An alternate regimen is to give 1 g/kg once and observe the patient. Often this single dose will result in an adequate increase in platelets. The length of this response is variable, and the timing of the dose is extremely important. If the obstetrician wants a peak platelet count for delivery, therapy should be instituted about 5 to 8 days before the planned delivery. The most frequent adverse reaction is postinfusion headache. This may be lessened by slowing the infusion rate.

IVIG is a blood product from many pooled donors. Early in its use, there were concerns about hepatitis C transmission. These cases resulted from the product of a single manufacturer. Since 1994, there have been no cases of viral transmission associated with the infusion of IVIG.[44] This is due to careful donor screening,[45] as well as an intensive purification process. These steps include ethanol fractionation and polyethylene glycol precipitation,[46] as well as solvent/detergent treatments. These techniques have been tested against hepatitis B, hepatitis C, human immunodeficiency virus, mumps, vaccinia, vesicular somatitis, and ECHO viruses. There has been no evidence that these viruses survive the purification process.

Intravenous immune globulin should be used before seriously contemplating splenectomy, because some patients experience remission with IVIG or postpartum. In severe life-threatening hemorrhage, recombinant factor VIIa can be used in conjunction with other therapies.[47]

Intravenous anti-D has been used in emergent settings in Rh+, direct antiglobulin–negative patients. However, this should generally be avoided in pregnant women. In life-threatening situations, when other methods fail, one could consider this option. The usual dose is 50 to 75 μg/kg.[25] Anti-D binds to IgG Fc receptors different than those bound by IVIG.

In midtrimester, splenectomy can also be used to raise the maternal platelet count. This procedure is reserved for those who do not respond to medical management, with the platelet count remaining below 20,000/mm^3. It can also be performed postpartum if the patient does not respond to medical management. In extremely emergent cases of life-threatening bleeding or nonresponse, splenectomy can be safely performed at the time of cesarean delivery after extending a midline incision cephalad.

Platelet transfusions are indicated when there is clinically significant bleeding and while awaiting other therapies to become effective. Platelets can be given if the maternal platelet count is less than 50,000/mm^3 during splenectomy, or during cesarean delivery if significant clinical bleeding is evident. They can be transfused before a vaginal delivery if the mother's platelet count is less than 20,000/mm^3. Each "pack" of platelets increases the platelet count by approximately 10,000/mm^3. The half life of these platelets is extremely short because the same antibodies and reticuloendothelial cell clearance rates that affect the mother's endogenous platelets also affect the transfused platelets. However, if platelets are transfused at the time the skin incision is made, hemostasis adequate to carry out the surgical procedure will be provided.

If the patient with profound thrombocytopenia undergoes cesarean delivery, certain surgical precautions should be taken. The bladder flap may be left open to avoid hematoma formation. If the parietal peritoneum is closed, subfascial drains are helpful if hemostasis is imperfect. If severe, life-threatening hemorrhage occurs, recombinant factor VIIa and platelet transfusion can be used.

In summary, the treatment of thrombocytopenia during gestation is dependent on its etiology. The obstetrician need not act on the mother's platelet count unless it is below 30,000/mm^3,[25] if it is below 50,000/mm^3 with evidence of clinical bleeding, or if surgery is anticipated. In these cases, the treatment depends on the diagnosis. Furthermore, whether delivery needs to be expedited or can be delayed is also dependent on the etiology of thrombocytopenia. The possibility of profound fetal/neonatal thrombocytopenia need be considered only if the mother carries a true diagnosis of ITP or, in the case of presumed gestational thrombocytopenia, when the platelet count is less than 50,000/mm^3, as this may actually be de novo ITP.[48] The key to managing these patients is to arrive at an accurate etiology for the thrombocytopenia and to approach the patient and her fetus rationally, realizing that therapy needs to be individualized.

MANAGEMENT OF THROMBOTIC THROMBOCYTOPENIC PURPURA AND HEMOLYTIC UREMIC SYNDROME

Before the use of plasma exchange, maternal and fetal outcomes in pregnancies complicated by TTP were uniformly poor.[35] The first cases treated with plasma exchange for TTP during pregnancy were reported in 1984.[49] One paper described a patient who had previous fetal deaths from chronic TTP and experienced a successful pregnancy when treated with aspirin, dipyridamole, and plasma infusion.[50] Others have found that dipyridamole and aspirin are not helpful.[51] There are no large series of patients with TTP in pregnancy. A review of 11 patients described in case reports reveals that the prognosis has improved greatly with plasma infusion and plasma exchange.[52] These researchers also demonstrated that cyclosporin may increase the duration of remission.

HUS has been more difficult to treat. Only a few case reports have appeared. Supportive therapy remains the mainstay in cases of HUS.[38,49] Dialysis is often necessary with close attention to fluid management. Platelet function inhibitors were used in two cases during pregnancy.[53,54] Plasma infusion and plasma exchange can be attempted, but the results have not been as good as observed in cases of TTP.[54] Vincristine has been administered with some success in non-pregnant patients, but has not been tried in pregnancy.[55] Prostacyclin infusion has been effective in children but has not been used during pregnancy.[54,56]

NEONATAL ALLOIMMUNE THROMBOCYTOPENIA

In neonatal alloimmune thrombocytopenia, a rare disorder, the mother lacks a specific platelet antigen and develops antibodies to this antigen. The disease is somewhat analogous to Rh isoimmunization, but involves platelets. If the fetus inherits an antigen from its father and the mother lacks the antigen, maternal antibody can develop and cross the placenta. This results in severe neonatal thrombocytopenia. The mother, however, will have a normal platelet count. Deaver and coinvestigators[57] reviewed 58 cases of neonatal alloimmune thrombocytopenia. The overall mortality rate was 9 percent, and the total incidence of suspected intracranial hemorrhage was 28 percent. The mortality rate was 24 percent for the firstborn infant and only 5 percent for subsequent offspring. The improved outcome in the latter group appeared to be related to more frequent use of cesarean delivery and to earlier use of corticosteroids in these children because obstetricians and pediatricians were expecting the disease.[57] The most common antibodies noted in these patients is anti-PLA 1 antibodies.[58] Several other antibodies have been identified. If this disorder is suspected, the mother's blood should be sent to a reference laboratory with experience in diagnosing neonatal alloimmune thrombocytopenia. Transfusion of maternal platelets into the neonate also improved outcome in these cases. After birth or in utero, the child can be transfused with the mother's platelet because she lacks the antigen that would lead to platelet destruction by circulating antibodies. Bussel and colleagues[59] have demonstrated that the antenatal use of intravenous immunoglobulin may help to prevent thrombocytopenia in infants at risk for neonatal alloimmune thrombocytopenia. These investigators administrated 1 g/kg per week to at-risk mothers and observed no toxicity. The concomitant use of glucocorticoids has not necessarily been shown to boost the effect of the intravenous immunoglobulin.[60] Because of the frequency with which very low platelet counts are encountered in these fetuses, there is a risk of fetal exsanguination with cordocentesis.[61] These patients should be managed in a tertiary care center where there has been experience caring for mothers and infants with this rare disorder.

IRON DEFICIENCY ANEMIA

During a singleton pregnancy, maternal plasma volume gradually expands by approximately 50 percent (1,000 ml) (see Chapter 3). The total red blood cell (RBC) mass also increases, but only by approximately 300 mg (25 percent), and this starts later in pregnancy.[61] It is not surprising, therefore, that hemoglobin and hematocrit levels usually fall during gestation. These changes are not necessarily pathologic but usually represent a physiologic alteration of pregnancy. By 6 weeks postpartum, in the absence of excessive blood loss during the puerperium, hemoglobin and hematocrit levels have returned to normal, if the mother has adequate iron stores.

Most researchers and clinicians diagnose anemia when the hemoglobin concentration is less than 11 g/dl or the hematocrit is less than 32 percent. Using these criteria, 50 percent of pregnant women are anemic. The incidence of anemia changes depending on the population studied. It is unfortunate that this problem is often ignored. In the developing nations, iron deficiency is an overwhelming problem. Worldwide there are many maternal deaths because of excessive blood loss in women who were already anemic. The previously cited arbitrary cutoff for hemoglobin/hematocrit may need to be adjusted. Beaton[62] suggests that these numbers should be adjusted downward and different targets should be established for different times in pregnancy. As pregnancy progresses, hemoglobin levels are often in the range of 10 to 10.5 g/dl in the late second and early third trimesters. These patients, if iron stores are present, do regain their normal hemoglobin/hematocrit postpartum. Causes of anemia in pregnancy are shown in the box "Causes of Anemia During Pregnancy."

Causes of Anemia During Pregnancy

- Common causes—85% of anemia
  - Physiologic anemia
  - Iron deficiency
- Uncommon causes
  - Folic acid deficiency
  - Hemoglobinopathies
    - Sickle cell disease
    - Hemoglonin SC
    - β-Thalassemia minor
  - Bariatric surgery
  - Gastrointestinal bleeding
- Rare causes
  - Hemoglobinpathies
    - β-Thalassemia major
    - α-Thalassemia
  - Vitamin B-12 deficiency
  - Syndromes of chronic hemolysis
    - Hereditary spherocytosis
    - Paroxysmal nocturnal hemoglobinuria
  - Hematologic malignancy

Approximately 75 percent of anemias that occur during pregnancy are secondary to iron deficiency.[63] Ho and co-investigators[64] performed elaborate hematologic evaluations of 221 gravidas at term in Taiwan. None of the studied patients received an added iron preparation during gestation. Of the previously nonanemic patients, 10.4 percent developed clinical anemia after a full-term delivery. Of these 23 patients, 11 (47.8 percent) developed florid iron deficiency anemia, and another 11 demonstrated moderate iron depletion.[65] The other anemic patient in the group had folate deficiency. Of the 198 non-anemic gravidas at term, 46.5 percent showed evidence of iron depletion even though they had a normal hematocrit. [64]

To distinguish the normal physiologic changes of pregnancy from those of pathologic iron deficiency, one must understand the normal iron requirements of pregnancy (Table 40-2) and the proper use of hematologic laboratory parameters. In adult women, iron stores are located in the bone marrow, liver and spleen in the form of ferritin. Ferritin constitutes approximately 25 percent (500mg) of the 2-g of iron stores found in the normal woman. Approximately 65 percent of stored iron is located in the circulating RBCs.[63,65–67] If the dietary iron intake is poor, the interval between pregnancies is short, or the delivery is complicated by hemorrhage, iron deficiency anemia readily and rapidly develops.

The first pathologic change to occur in iron deficiency anemia is the depletion of bone marrow, liver, and spleen iron stores. The serum iron level falls, as does the percentage saturation of transferrin. The total iron-binding capacity rises, because this is a reflection of unbound transferrin. A falling hemoglobin and hematocrit follow. Microcytic hypochromic RBCs are released into the circulation. If iron deficiency is combined with folate or vitamin B_{12} deficiency, normocytic and normochromic RBCs are observed on the peripheral blood smear.

Care must be taken when using laboratory parameters to establish the diagnosis of iron deficiency anemia during

Table 40-2. Iron Requirements for Pregnancy and the Puerperium

FUNCTION	REQUIREMENT
Increased red blood cell mass	450 mg
Fetus and placenta	360 mg
Vaginal delivery	190 mg
Lactation	1 mg/day

gestation. A serum iron concentration less than 60 mg/dl with less than 16 percent saturation of transferrin is suggestive of iron deficiency. Conversely, a single normal serum iron concentration does not rule out iron deficiency. For example, a patient may take iron for several days, and this may result in a transiently normal serum iron concentration while iron stores are still negligible. An increase in iron-binding capacity is not reliable, because 15 percent of pregnant women without iron deficiency show an increase in this parameter.[68] If a patient has been iron deficient for an extended period of time, her serum iron level can rise before she has depleted her iron stores. The ferritin level indicates the total status of her iron stores. Serum ferritin levels normally decrease minimally during pregnancy. However, a significantly reduced ferritin concentration is indicative of iron deficiency anemia and is the best parameter to judge the degree of iron deficiency. Ferritin levels are variable and can change 25 percent from one day to the next.[69] Harthoorn-Lasthuizen et al.[70] examined erythrocyte zinc protoporphyrin testing in pregnancy. They found that serum ferritin levels did not predict the development of iron-deficient erythropoiesis. However, erythrocyte zinc protoporphyrin measurements did help determine which patients were developing iron deficiency before they developed frank anemia, and these patients benefited from iron therapy.[70] Van de Broek et al.[71] believed that the erythrocyte zinc protoporphyrin level was not particularly helpful and that a serum ferritin of less than 30 μg/L was more than adequate to determine iron deficiency.

Ahluwalia[72] believes that measuring serum transferrin receptors can give a better index of true iron status. Ferritin can be elevated in acute and chronic infections, whereas transferrin receptors do not change in response to an infection. This is important in countries where chronic infection is common in pregnant women. Also receptor concentrations are not confounded by the hemodynamic changes of pregnancy. This test is not yet readily available but may help us in the future to detect iron-deficient patients.[72]

Finally, when hematologic parameters remain confusing, bone marrow aspiration usually provides the definitive diagnosis. The procedure, however, is rarely necessary.

Whether all women should receive prophylactic iron in addition to that contained in prenatal vitamins during pregnancy remains controversial. Long[73] believes that the physiologic changes of pregnancy are responsible for much of the decrease in hematocrit and, unless the patient is symptomatic or the hematocrit is very low, iron supplementation is unnecessary. In reviewing the Cochrane database, Millman et al.[74] found that 20 percent of fertile women have iron stores greater than 500 mg, which is the required minimum for pregnancy. They also noted that 40 percent of women have iron stores between 100 and 500 mg, and 40 percent have virtually no iron stores. Based on this data, most women do need some iron supplementation.[74] There is no consensus, however, on how much iron supplementation may be needed in patients with iron deficiency.

In pregnancy, iron absorption from the duodenum increases, providing 1.3 to 2.6 mg of elemental iron daily.[75,76] An acid environment in the duodenum helps this absorption. Therefore, the frequent ingestion of antacid medications, commonly used by many patients, decreases the absorption of iron. Chronic use of H_2 blockers and proton pump inhibitors also diminishes iron absorption. Vitamin C, in addition to the iron, may increase the acid environment of the stomach and increase absorption. In patients who do not show clear signs of iron deficiency, it is uncertain whether prophylactic iron, in addition to what is in prenatal vitamins, leads to an increased hemoglobin concentration at term. Iron prophylaxis, however, is safe as only amounts that can be used are absorbed. With the exception of dyspepsia and constipation, side effects are few. One 325-mg tablet of ferrous sulfate daily provides adequate prophylaxis. It contains 60 mg of elemental iron, 10 percent of which is absorbed. If the iron is not needed, it will not be absorbed and will be excreted in the feces. The standard generic iron tablets and the amount of elemental iron they provide are listed in Table 40-3.

In iron-deficient patients, one iron tablet three times daily has been recommended, although the evidence-based source of this recommendation is difficult to ascertain. Most individuals can absorb as much iron as they need taking iron twice daily. Iron should be taken 30 minutes before meals to allow maximum absorption. However, when taken in this manner, dyspepsia and nausea are more common. Therapy, therefore, must be individualized to maximize patient compliance.

Zavaleta et al.[77] examined the use of zinc in addition to iron, because it is thought that zinc may enhance hematopoiesis. However, they found that zinc, in addition to iron, did not increase the hemoglobin concentration in patients. Young et al.[78] studied the effectiveness of weekly iron supplementation. They found that weekly iron supplementation was almost as effective as daily supplementation in raising the hemoglobin concentration in iron deficient patients. This approach can be used in patients with less than optimal compliance.

For those patients who are noncompliant or are unable to take oral iron and are severely anemic, intravenous iron can be given. Singh et al.[79] found that parenteral iron can be safely given and significantly raises the hematocrit in patients. It also raises the serum ferritin. There were no adverse effects in their study of patients.[79] Hallak et al.[80] examined the safety and efficacy of parenteral iron administration. Of 26 patients receiving parenteral iron, only one developed signs of mild allergy during the test dose and was excluded from the study. The remaining 21 pregnant patients completed the course of therapy and received a mean of 1,000 mg of elemental iron. Their hemoglobin increased an average of 1.6 g/dl from the beginning to the end of therapy and rose another 0.8 g/dl during the following 2 weeks. Ferritin levels increased from 2.9 ng/ml at the beginning of therapy to 122.8 ng/dl by the end of treatment.[80] Ferritin levels decreased to a mean of 109.4 ng/ml 2 weeks later. Only mild transient side effects were noted. The authors concluded that parenteral iron therapy can be used safely during pregnancy.[80]

Parenteral iron is indicated in those who cannot or will not take oral iron therapy and are not anemic enough to require transfusion. In fact, by building iron stores in the patients before delivery, we may be able to prevent a need for transfusion postpartum in the severely anemic patient. Iron dextran comes in a concentration of 50 mg/ml. It can be given intramuscularly or intravenously, although intramuscular injection is very painful. Iron dextran can result in anaphylaxis, which is caused by dissociation of the iron component and carbohydrate component. The reaction may be immediate or delayed. Therefore, a 0.5-ml test dose should be given, and epinephrine should be readily available. Anaphylaxis usually occurs within several minutes but may take 2 days to develop. In the past 3 years, our group has given iron dextran to 14 patients. Two developed a severe reaction within minutes of the test dose. Although neither patient developed shortness of breath, both exhibited severe bone pain and myalgias. The dosage for iron dextran therapy is shown in Table 40-4.

In addition to iron dextran, there are two newer parenteral iron preparations. Both of these compounds have the disadvantage of requiring multiple doses to accomplish what can be done with one dose of iron dextran. However, they have the advantage of less likelihood of a severe adverse reaction. Iron sucrose complex is given

Table 40-3. Elemental Iron Available from Common Generic Iron Preparations

PREPARATION		ELEMENTAL IRON (MG)
Ferrous gluconate	325 mg	37–39
Ferrous sulfate	325 mg	60–65
Ferrous fumarate	325 mg	107

Table 40-4. Parenteral Iron Administration

MEDICATION	DOSE	PREPARATION
Iron dextran	Total dose (ml) = 0.0442 (Desired hgb − Observed hgb) × LBW + (0.26 × LBW). 100 mg/dose maximun	50 mg elemental iron/ml
Iron sucrose	100 mg/dose, usually 1 dose/day, usually 10 doses needed	20 mg elemental iron/ml
Sodium ferric gluconate complex	125 mg/dose, usually 1 dose/day, usually 8 doses needed	12.5 mg of elemental iron/ml

hgb, hemoglobin; LBW, lean body weight.

intravenously with a maximum dose of 100 g. It is usually given daily. Patients generally require 10 doses (1 g) to obtain the rise in ferritin and subsequent rise in hemoglobin concentration that are desired. Sodium ferric gluconate complex can be used similarly. The maximum dose is 125 mg. It is usually given daily, and eight doses (1 g) are most often required to obtain the desired results. Sodium ferric gluconate appears to have the least risk of adverse side effects. If the patient has concomitant renal insufficiency, subcutaneous erythropoietin can be given to help raise the hemoglobin concentration if iron stores have already been raised. These agents should be used only in patients with severe iron deficiency who cannot absorb iron or who will not or cannot take oral iron. A parenteral iron overdose can lead to hemosiderosis.

It is still not certain whether anemia results in an increased risk for poor pregnancy outcome. In their literature review, Scholl and Hediger[81] concluded that anemia diagnosed in early pregnancy is associated with preterm delivery and low birth weight. In this study, women with iron deficiency anemia had twice the risk of preterm delivery and three times the risk of delivering a low-birth-weight infant.[81] Preterm labor, however, is a multifactorial problem, and there were many confounders in this study. Yip[82] reviewed the literature concerning pregnancy outcome with anemia. He found through epidemiologic studies that there is an association between moderate anemia and poor perinatal outcome, yet he was unable to determine whether this relationship was causal.[82] Sifakis and Pharmakides[83] observed that hemoglobin concentrations less than 6 g/dl are associated with preterm birth, spontaneous abortion, low birth weight, and fetal deaths. Nevertheless, a mild to moderate anemia did not appear to have any significant effect on fetal outcomes.[83] Hemminki and Starfield[84] reviewed controlled trials, concluding that routine iron administration did not decrease preterm labor or raise birth weight. Conversely, Stephansson et al.[85] found an increased risk of stillbirth and growth-restricted infants in women with hemoglobin concentrations greater than 14.6 g/dl at their prenatal visit.

In summary, iron deficiency is very prevalent in the general pregnant population. In developing nations, severe anemia is alarmingly common and is a major cause of maternal morbidity and mortality. Routine iron administration like that found in prenatal vitamins should be used unless it is certain that the patient is iron replete. Iron prophylaxis can be taken as one iron tablet daily, or as one study showed, can be given on a weekly basis. There appears to be an association between poor pregnancy outcome and maternal anemia, especially severe anemia. It is uncertain, however, if this is a causal relationship.

MEGALOBLASTIC ANEMIA

Folic acid, a water-soluble vitamin, is found in green vegetables, peanuts, and liver. Folate stores are located primarily in the liver and are usually sufficient for 6 weeks. After 3 weeks of a diet deficient in folate, the serum folate level falls. Two weeks later, hypersegmentation of neutrophils occurs. After 17 weeks without folic ingestion, RBC folate levels drop. In the next week a megaloblastic bone marrow develops. During pregnancy, folate deficiency is the most common cause of megaloblastic anemia. The daily folate requirement in the nonpregnant state is approximately 50 μg, but this rises at least fourfold during gestation.[86] Fetal demands increase the requirement, as does the decrease in the gastrointestinal absorption of folate during pregnancy.[86]

Clinical megaloblastic anemia seldom occurs before the third trimester of pregnancy. If the patient is at risk for folate deficiency or has mild anemia, an attempt should be made to detect this disorder before megaloblastosis occurs. Serum folate and RBC folate levels are the best tests for folate deficiency.[87,88]

Folate deficiency rarely occurs in the fetus and is not a cause of significant perinatal morbidity. There is some evidence that fetuses that are homozygous for the C677T variant of the gene encoding for 5, 10 methylene tetrahydrofolate reductase have a 20-percent lower folate level and may be at risk for a neural tube defect.[89] Because infants born to mothers with type 1 and type 2 diabetes mellitus have an increased incidence of neural tube defects, Kaplan et al.[90] studied 31 pregnant diabetic women and 54 controls to determine if there are aberrations in folate metabolism in patients with diabetes. They found that there were no differences in how ingested folate is processed in the pregnant patient with diabetes.[90] Prenatal vitamins that require physician prescription contain 1-mg of folic acid. Most nonprescription prenatal vitamins contain 0.8 mg of folic acid. These amounts are more than adequate to prevent and treat folate deficiency. Women with significant hemoglobinopathies, patients taking anticonvulsant medications, women carrying a multiple gestation, and women with frequent conception may require more than 1-mg supplemental folate daily. If the patient is folic acid deficient, her reticulocyte count will be depressed. Within 3 days after the administration of sufficient folic acid, reticulocytosis usually occurs. In fact, folic acid deficiency should be considered when a patient has unexplained thrombocytopenia. The leukopenia and thrombocytopenia, which accompany megaloblastosis, are rapidly reversed. The hematocrit level may rise as much as 1 percent per day after 1 week of folate replacement.

Vollsett et al.[91] performed a retrospective analysis of 14,492 pregnancies in 5,883 women in Norway to determine if elevated homocysteine levels were associated with pregnancy complications. An elevated homocysteine level is often found with depressed folate levels. They compared those in the upper quartile of homocysteine levels with those in the lower quartile. They noted a 32-percent (odds ratio: 1.32) higher risk for preeclampsia, 38 percent (odds ratio: 1.38) higher risk for prematurity, and a 10 percent (odds ratio, 2.01) higher risk for very low birth weight. All trends were statistically significant, but the limitations inherent in retrospective epidemiologic studies apply here.[91] Nelen et al.[92] found a relation between recurrent early pregnancy loss and genetically related disturbances in folate and homocysteine metabolism.

Iron deficiency is frequently observed in association with folic acid deficiency. If a patient with folate defi-

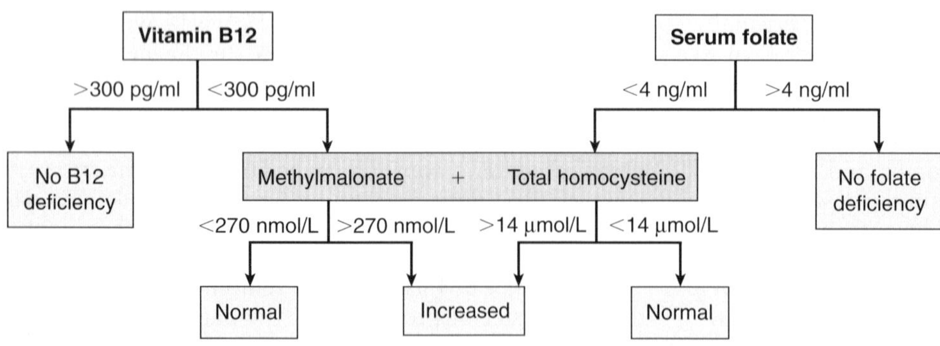

Increased methylmalonate and folate levels indicate vitamin B12 deficiency.
Normal methylmalonate and increased homocysteine levels indicate folate deficiency.

Figure 40-1. Use of methylmalonate and homocysteine levels in the workup of megaloblastic anemia.

ciency does not develop a significant reticulocytosis within 1 week after administration of sufficient replacement therapy, appropriate tests for iron deficiency should be performed.[87]

Until recently, vitamin B_{12} deficiency in pregnancy was either very rare or not recognized. However, bariatric surgery has become increasingly common. Individuals who were morbidly obese and not ovulating, suddenly ovulate and become pregnant. In the past 6 months, we have encountered 6 patients who have had gastric bypass surgery for obesity. We have found laboratory evidence of a cobalamin (vitamin B_{12}) deficiency in four of these patients. Cobalamin is found only in animal products, and the daily minimum required intake is 6 to 9 μg. Total body stores are 2 to 5 mg, and one half of this is stored in the liver.[93] For cobalamin to be absorbed, an individual needs the following: (1) acid-pepsin in the stomach; (2) intrinsic factor secreted by parietal cells in the stomach; (3) pancreatic proteases; and (4) an intact ileum with receptors to bind the cobalamin-intrinsic factor complex.[94] Because of the abundant vitamin B_{12} stores in the body, it takes several years for a clinical vitamin B_{12} deficiency to develop.[94] Prolonged vitamin B_{12} deficiency can result in subacute combined degeneration, which involves the dorsal horns and lateral columns of the spinal cord. This can result in sensory and proprioception deficits, which can progress and cause serious disabilities. Fortunately, these changes are reversible when detected early.

In addition to bariatric surgery, gastrointestinal diseases such as Crohn's disease may lead to an inability to absorb vitamin B_{12}. Because of advances in medical care, more individuals with these chronic disorders are becoming pregnant. As primary care physicians for women, we must be prepared to diagnose and coordinate care in these complex patients. Furthermore, we are encountering more patients taking metformin, which is being prescribed for polycystic ovarian syndrome. It is important to note that this medication can also result in vitamin B_{12} deficiency.[95] Approximately 10 to 30 percent of patients taking metformin may have depressed vitamin B_{12} levels. This can be reversed with increased calcium intake.[95] The major causes of vitamin B_{12} deficiency are listed in the box "Causes of Vitamin B_{12} Deficiency that May be Encountered in Pregnancy."

Megaloblastic anemia usually leads to a suspicion of folate or vitamin B_{12} deficiency. As noted earlier, if there is an associated iron deficiency, the RBC indices may portray a normocytic, normochromic picture. Therefore, it is important to look at more specific tests for vitamin B_{12} and folate deficiencies. Vitamin B_{12} levels may fall during pregnancy, but this finding may not represent a pathologic process.[96] Also, serum vitamin B_{12} levels may be normal in up to 5 percent of individuals with a true deficiency.[97,98]

Causes of Vitamin B_{12} Deficiency that May be Encountered in Pregnancy

Strict vegetarian diet
Use of proton pump inhibitors
Metformin
Gastritis
Gastrectomy
Ileal bypass
Crohn's disease
Sprue
Helicobacter pylori infection

Evaluation of methylmalonate and homocysteine levels can be used to distinguish folate deficiency from Vitamin B_{12} deficiency. Vitamin B_{12} is a cofactor in the metabolism of both methylmalonic acid and homocysteine. A deficiency in vitamin B_{12}, therefore, will lead to an increased concentration of both of these compounds.[99] Folic acid is a cofactor in the metabolism of homocysteine. A folate deficiency, therefore, will lead to an elevated homocysteine level. Savage[99] found elevated methylmalonic acid levels in 98 percent of individuals with a vitamin B_{12} deficiency but in only 12 percent of individuals with a folate deficiency. He also found elevated homocysteine levels in 96 percent of individuals with a vitamin B_{12} deficiency and 91 percent of individuals with a folate deficiency.[99] Figure 40-1 schematically shows how to incorporate methylmalonic acid and homocysteine testing into the evaluation of megaloblastic anemia.

HEMOGLOBINOPATHIES

Hemoglobin is a tetrameric protein composed of two pairs of polypeptide chains with a heme group attached to each chain.[100] The normal adult hemoglobin A_1 comprises

Table 40-5. Frequency of Common Hemoglobinopathies in Black Adults in the United States

HEMOGLOBIN TYPE	FREQUENCY
Hemoglobin AS	1 in 12
Hemoglobin SS	1 in 708
Hemoglobin AC	1 in 41
Hemoglobin CC	1 in 4,790
Hemoglobin SC	1 in 757
Hemoglobin S/β-thalassemia	1 in 1,672

95 percent of hemoglobin. It consists of two α-chains and two β-chains. The remaining 5 percent of hemoglobin usually consists of hemoglobin A_2 (containing two α-chains and two δ-chains) and hemoglobin F (with two α-chains and two γ-chains). In the fetus, hemoglobin F (fetal hemoglobin) declines during the third trimester of pregnancy, reaching its permanent nadir several months after birth. Hemoglobinopathies arise when there is a change in the structure of a peptide chain or a defect in the ability to synthesize a specific polypeptide chain. The patterns of inheritance are often straightforward. The prevalences of the most common hemoglobinopathies are listed in Table 40-5.

Hemoglobin S

Hemoglobin S, an aberrant hemoglobin, is present in patients with sickle cell disease (hemoglobin SS) and sickle cell trait (hemoglobin AS). A single substitution of valine for glutamic acid at the sixth position in the β-polypeptide chain causes a significant change in the physical characteristics of this hemoglobin. At low oxygen tensions, RBCs containing hemoglobin S assume a sickle shape. Sludging in small vessels occurs, resulting in microinfarction of the affected organs. Sickle cells have a life span of 5 to 10 days, compared with 120 days for a normal RBC. Sickling is triggered by dehydration, hypoxia, or acidosis. Infants with sickle cell anemia show no signs of the disease until the concentration of hemoglobin F falls to adult levels. Some patients do not experience symptoms until adolescence.

Approximately 1 of 12 black adults in the United States is heterozygous for hemoglobin S and, therefore, sickle cell trait (hemoglobin AS) and carries the affected gene. These individuals generally have 35 to 45 percent hemoglobin S and are asymptomatic. The child of two individuals with sickle cell trait has a 50-percent probability of inheriting the trait and a 25-percent probability of actually having sickle cell disease. One of every 625 black children born in the United States is homozygous for hemoglobin S, and the frequency of sickle cell disease among blacks is 1 in 708.[101] All at-risk patients should undergo hemoglobin electrophoresis. Although it is more expensive, it will identify all patients with aberrant hemoglobin types.

The traditional teaching is that women with sickle cell trait are not at increased risk for maternal and perinatal morbidity. A report by Larrabee and Monga[102] questions this. In their study, 162 women with hemoglobin AS had a 24.7 percent incidence of preeclampsia compared with 10.3 percent of controls. Furthermore, the mean birth weight of infants born to women with hemoglobin AS was 3,082 g compared with 3,369 g for controls ($p < 0.0001$). The rate of postpartum endometritis was 12.3 percent for sickle trait patients compared with 5.1 percent for controls ($p < 0.001$) despite similar rates of cesarean delivery.[102] This study indicates that our surveillance should be higher in patients with hemoglobin AS.

If a patient has hemoglobin AS, the spouse/partner should be tested, and if both are carriers of a hemoglobinopathy, prenatal diagnosis should be offered. Prenatal diagnosis can be performed rapidly by DNA analysis with polymerase chain reaction (PCR) amplification of DNA fragments.[103] This test can be performed on amniocytes at commercial and medical center–based laboratories.

Painful vaso-occlusive episodes involving multiple organs are the clinical hallmark of sickle cell disease. The most common sites for these episodes are the extremities, joints and abdomen. Vaso-occlusive episodes can also occur in the lung, resulting in pulmonary infarction. Analgesia, oxygen, and hydration are the clinical foundations for treating these painful crises.

Sickle cell disease can affect virtually all organ systems. Osteomyelitis is common, and osteomyelitis caused by Salmonella is found almost exclusively in these patterns. The risk of pyelonephritis is increased, especially during pregnancy. Sickling may also occur in the renal medulla, in which oxygen tension is reduced, resulting in papillary necrosis. These patients also exhibit renal tubular dysfunction and hyposthenuria. Because of chronic hemolysis and decreased RBC survival, patients with sickle cell anemia often demonstrate some degree of jaundice. Biliary stasis commonly occurs during crises, and cholelithiasis is seen in about 30 percent of cases.[104,105] Because of chronic anemia, high-output cardiac failure can occur. Left ventricular hypertrophy, and cardiomegaly are common.

Pregnancies complicated by sickle cell disease are at risk for poor perinatal outcomes. The rate of spontaneous abortion may be as high as 25 percent.[106–108] The perinatal mortality rate is approximately 15 percent.[107–112] Powars and coworkers[113] studied 156 pregnancies in 79 women with sickle cell anemia. In this group, the perinatal mortality rate was 52.7 percent before 1972, and 22.7 percent after that time. In a report by Seoud and coworkers,[114] the perinatal mortality rate was 10.5 percent. Much of this poor perinatal outcome is related to preterm birth. Approximately 30 percent of infants born to mothers with sickle cell disease have birth weights less than 2,500 g.[112] In the report by Seoud et al.,[114] the mean birth weight was 2,443 g. In a multicenter study, Smith et al.[115] reported that 21 percent of infants born to mothers with sickle cell disease were small for gestational age. It has been hypothesized that sickling in the uterine vessels may lead to decreased fetal oxygenation and intrauterine growth restriction.[112] Persistent hemoglobin F in the mother decreases episodes of painful crises during pregnancy and may also have a protective effect on the neonate. However, in a study by Anyaegbunam and colleagues,[117] hemoglobin F levels were inversely correlated with birth weight percentile. In contrast, Morris et al.[118] studied 270 singleton pregnancies in 175 women with sickle cell disease. The overall rate of fetal wastage was

32.2 percent. Mothers with high hemoglobin F levels had a significantly lower perinatal mortality rate. Ohne-Frempong and Smith-Whitley[119] reviewed the use of hydroxyurea in children with sickle cell disease. This drug reduces the incidence of painful crises and increases hemoglobin F concentration.[119] The safety of hydroxyurea in pregnancy has not been established. If an individual becomes pregnant while using hydroxyurea, it should be discontinued, but pregnancy termination is not justified. Parvovirus B-19 infection is usually asymptomatic in pregnant women but can cause fetal hydrops. In women with sickle cell disease, parvovirus B-19 can cause an aplastic crisis.[120]

Stillbirth rates of 8 to 10 percent have been described in patients with sickle cell disease.[107] These fetal deaths happen not only during crises but also unexpectedly. Therefore, careful antepartum fetal testing must be used, including serial ultrasonography to assess fetal growth. In another study, Anyaegbynam and coworkers[121] examined Doppler flow velocimetry in patients with hemoglobinopathies. They showed abnormal systolic/diastolic ratios for the uterine or umbilical arteries in 88 percent of patients with hemoglobin SS compared with 7 percent with hemoglobin AS and 4 percent with hemoglobin AA. Howard et al.[122] observed that maternal exchange transfusions did not change uteroplacental Doppler blood flow velocimetry in these patients. These findings suggest that although maternal well-being may be improved, there is no change in uteroplacental pathology.

Although maternal mortality is rare in patients with sickle cell anemia, maternal morbidity is significant. Infections are common, occurring in 50 to 67 percent of women with hemoglobin SS. Most are urinary tract infections (UTIs), which can be detected by frequent urine cultures. Common infecting organisms for the bladder, kidneys, lungs and other sites include *Streptococcus pneumoniae, Haemophilis influenzae* type B, *Escherichia coli,* Salmonella, and Klebsiella.[123] Patients with hemoglobin AS are at greater risk for a UTI and should be screened as well. Pulmonary infection and infarction are also common. Patients with sickle cell anemia should receive pneumococcal vaccine before pregnancy. Maternal deaths have been reported in association with pulmonary complications in sickle cell disease.[124] Any infection demands prompt attention, because fever, dehydration, and acidosis results in further sickling and painful crises. The incidence of pregnancy-induced hypertension is increased in patients with sickle cell anemia and may complicate almost one third of pregnancies in these patients.[110,115] Although painful crises appear to be more common during gestation,[125–127] this was not observed in one study.[115]

The care of the pregnant patient with sickle cell anemia must be individualized and meticulous. These patients benefit from care in a medical center experienced in treating the multitude of problems that can complicate such pregnancies. From early gestation, good dietary habits should be promoted. A folate supplement of at least 1 mg/day should be administered as soon as pregnancy is confirmed. Although hemoglobin and hematocrit levels are decreased, iron supplements need not be routinely given. Serum iron and ferritin levels should be checked monthly and iron supplementation started only when these levels are diminished. Abudu and co-workers[128] found that serum ferritin values were significantly higher in pregnant women with hemoglobin SS disease than in those with hemoglobin AA. They concluded that the physiologic changes of pregnancy in patients with hemoglobin SS did not result in an iron deficiency state and that the use of prophylactic iron supplementation in these patients appears to be unjustified. Aken'Ova et al.[129] found that ferritin and iron levels decreased in pregnant patients with sickle cell disease in Nigeria. This points out that iron and ferritin levels should be checked during pregnancy. It must be emphasized that routine iron supplementation, even that in prenatal vitamins, should not be given, because iron overload may lead to hemosiderosis and possibly hemochromatosis.

The role of prophylactic transfusions in the gravida with sickle cell anemia is controversial. This therapy, which replaces the patient's sickle cells with normal RBCs, can both improve oxygen-carrying capacity and suppress the synthesis of sickle hemoglobin. A previous study showed a sevenfold reduction in perinatal mortality in patients receiving prophylactic transfusions.[130] In the same group of patients, there was a significant decrease in fetal growth restriction and preterm births. Morrison and coworkers[131] have also previously reported reduced perinatal wastage and maternal morbidity using a regimen of exchange transfusion. In contrast, workers at Johns Hopkins believe that meticulous prenatal care gives results as favorable as those obtained with prophylactic transfusion.[106] Many patients in that series, however, did require transfusion for painful crises and anemia. Koshy and coinvestigators[132] followed 72 pregnant patients with sickle cell anemia, one half of whom received prophylactic transfusions and one half transfusions only for medical or obstetric emergencies. There was no significant difference in perinatal outcome between the offspring of mothers who received prophylactic transfusions and those who did not. Two risk factors were identified as harbingers of an unfavorable outcome: (1) the occurrence of a perinatal death in a previous pregnancy and (2) twins in the present pregnancy. Even though there was no difference in perinatal morbidity and mortality, prophylactic transfusion did appear to decrease significantly the incidence of painful crises. The investigators concluded that the omission of prophylactic RBC transfusion will not harm the pregnant patients with sickle cell disease or their offspring.[124]

Tuck and co-workers[133] have delineated the risks involved with exchange transfusion. In a study of 51 pregnancies transfused between 1978 and 1984, 22 percent developed atypical RBC antibodies and 14 percent had immediate minor transfusion reactions. These data showed no significant difference in maternal or fetal outcomes among patients who were transfused prophylactically and those who were not.[133] Mahomed[134] reviewed the Cochrane database and found there was not enough evidence to make any conclusions about the use of prophylactic RBC transfusion in patients with sickle cell disease. Many of the cited studies did not show evidence of benefit to the fetus from exchange transfusion. A recent review by Hassell[135] summarizes the various

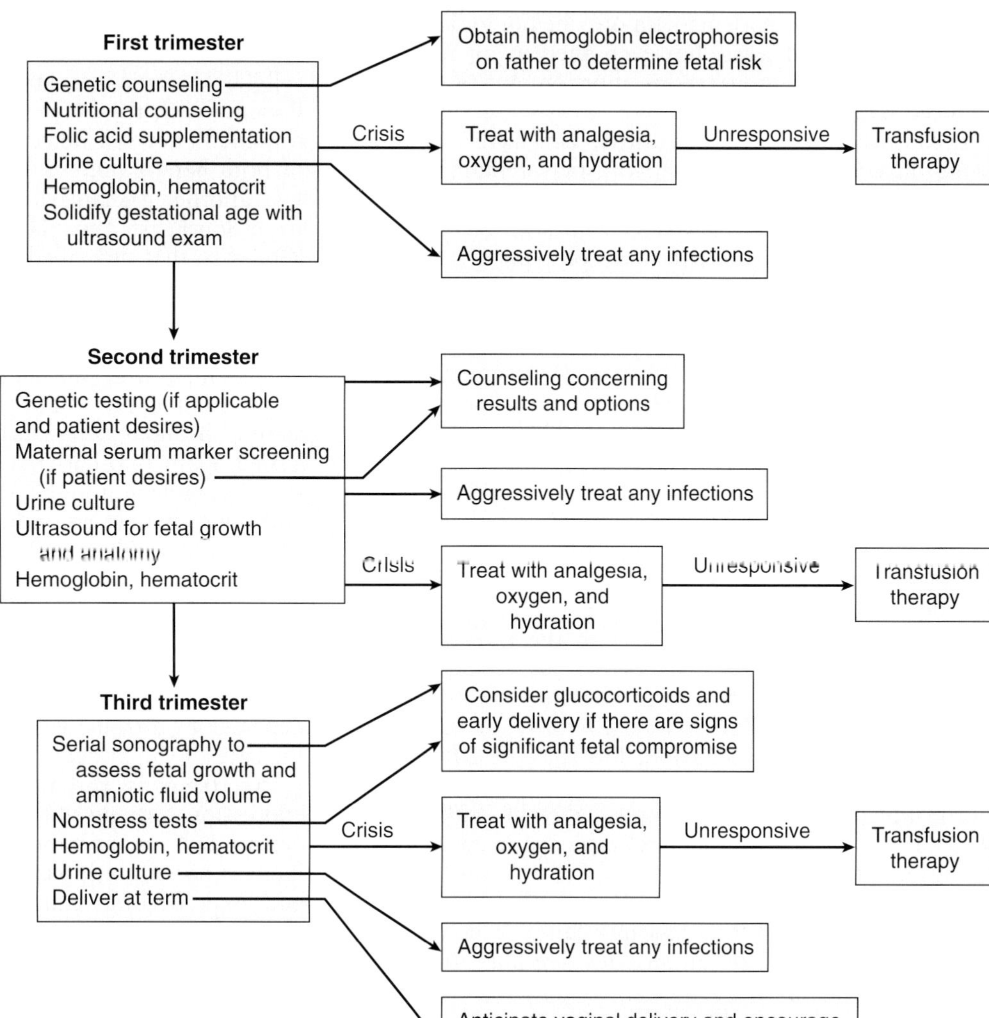

Figure 40-2. Schematic presentation of the care of patients with sickle cell anemia.

small studies and concludes that prophylactic transfusion does not improve fetal and neonatal outcome. He did not, however, attempt to quantify changes in maternal well-being. This needs to be carefully evaluated before stating that prophylactic transfusions should be eliminated from the care of the pregnant patient with sickle cell disease.

If one chooses to perform prophylactic transfusion, the goal is to maintain a percentage of hemoglobin A above 20 percent at all times and preferably above 40 percent, as well as to maintain the hematocrit above 25 percent. Morrison et al.[131] recommend that prophylactic transfusion begin at 28 weeks' gestation. Buffy-coat–poor washed RBCs are used to reduce the risk of isosensitization. Other risks of transfusion therapy include viral infection, transfusion reactions and hemochromatosis.

Either booster or exchange transfusions can be used. Exchange transfusions are preferable because they result in less stress on the cardiovascular system, thus decreasing the possibility of congestive heart failure. Exchange transfusions also raise the percentage of hemoglobin A more efficiently. These are usually carried out by erythrocytapheresis. If only booster transfusions are used, diuretics should probably be administered to prevent fluid overload. The patient should be positioned on her left side during the transfusion procedure to maximize uterine blood flow.

Vaginal delivery is preferred for patients with sickle cell disease, and cesarean delivery should be reserved for obstetric indications. Patients should labor in the left lateral recumbent position and receive supplemental oxygen. Although adequate hydration should be maintained, fluid overload must be avoided. Conduction anesthesia is recommended, because it provides excellent pain relief and can be used for cesarean delivery, if necessary. Figure 40-2 provides a schematic presentation of the care of patients with sickle cell anemia. It can also be adapted to patients with other hemoglobinopathies.

Hemoglobin SC Disease

Hemoglobin C is another β-chain variant. It results from a G to A point mutation in the first nucleotide of codon 6. The gene is present is 2 percent of blacks.[136] Clinically significant hemoglobin SC disease occurs in 1 in 833 black adults in the United States.[101] Women with both S and C hemoglobin suffer less morbidity in pregnancy than do patients with only hemoglobin S.[106,108] As in sickle cell disease, however, there is an increased incidence of early spontaneous abortion and pregnancy-induced hypertension.[106–109]

Because patients with SC disease can have only mild symptoms, this hemoglobinopathy may remain undiagnosed until a crisis occurs during pregnancy.

These crises may be marked by sequestration of a large volume of RBCs in the spleen accompanied by a dramatic fall in hematocrit.[137,138] Patients may have enlarged, tender spleen. Because these patients have increased splenic activity, they may be mildly thrombocytopenic throughout pregnancy. During gestation, patients with hemoglobin SC should receive the same program of prenatal care outlined for women with hemoglobin SS (see Fig. 40-2).

Thalassemia

Thalassemia is due to a defect in the rate of globin chain synthesis. Any of the polypeptide chains can be affected. As a result, there is production and accumulation of abnormal globin subunits, leading to ineffective erythropoiesis and a decreased life span of RBCs. The disease may range from minimal suppression of synthesis of the affected chain to its complete absence. Either α- or β-thalassemia can occur. Heterozygous patients are often asymptomatic.

Thalassemia can be detected by prenatal diagnosis. Prenatal diagnosis of β-thalassemia can be accomplished by DNA from villi or amniocytes. Because there are many beta globin mutations, it is important to report the patient's ethnicity and the geographic region of the family when submitting specimens. The laboratory can then test for specific mutations based upon this information and will be able to identify β-thalassemia in 90 percent of cases.[136] α-Thalassemia is also amenable to prenatal diagnosis using quantitative PCR or Southern blot analysis.[136]

Homozygous α-thalassemia results in the formation of tetramers of β-chains known as hemoglobin Bart. This hemoglobinopathy can result in hydrops fetalis. Ghosh and coinvestigators[139] reported their experience caring for 26 Chinese women who were at risk to deliver a fetus with homozygous α-thalassemia. Six of the 26 fetuses were affected. In two of the six cases, progressive fetal ascites appeared before 24 weeks' gestation. These pregnancies were terminated and the diagnoses confirmed. In the remaining four patients, there was evidence of intrauterine growth restriction by 28 weeks' gestation. At later gestational ages, an increase in the transverse cardiac diameter was seen in the affected fetuses.[132] Woo and colleagues[140] reported that umbilical artery velocimetry reveals a hyperdynamic circulatory state in fetuses that are hydropic because of α-thalassemia. In a study from Taiwan, Hsieh et al.[141] demonstrated that umbilical vein blood flow measurements can help to distinguish hydrops fetalis caused by hemoglobin Bart from hydrops fetalis having other causes. The umbilical vein diameter, blood velocity, and blood flow in fetuses with hemoglobin Bart were usually higher than those in fetuses with hydrops fetalis due to other etiologies.

β-Thalassemia is the most common form of thalassemia. Patients with the heterozygous state are usually asymptomatic. They are detected by an increase in their level of both hemoglobin A_2 and hemoglobin F. Hemoglobin E is another β-chain variant found generally in patients from Southeast Asia. The clinical course is variable and similar to that described for β-thalassemia. In the homozygous state of β-thalassemia, synthesis of hemoglobin A_1 may be completely suppressed. Hemoglobin A_2 levels of >50 percent are found in 40 percent of patients with β-thalassemia, and an elevated hemoglobin F level is observed in 50 percent of these patients. The homozygous state of β-thalassemia is known as thalassemia major, or Cooley's anemia. Patients with this disorder are transfusion dependent and have marked hepatosplenomegaly and bone changes secondary to increased hematopoiesis. These individuals usually die of infectious or cardiovascular complications before they reach childbearing age. They also have a high rate of infertility, although successful full-term pregnancies have been reported.[135] The few patients who do become pregnant generally exhibit severe anemia and congestive heart failure.[142] Prenatal care is dependent on transfusion therapy similar to that used in the care of the patient with sickle cell disease.

Heterozygous β-thalassemia has different forms of expression. Patients with thalassemia minima have microcytosis but are asymptomatic. Those with thalassemia intermedia exhibit splenomegaly and significant anemia and may become transfusion dependent during pregnancy. Their anemia can be significant enough to produce high-output cardiac failure.[143] If these patients have not undergone splenectomy, they are at risk for a hypersplenic crisis.[144] Also, extramedullary hematopoiesis may impinge upon the spine, resulting in neurologic symptoms.[145]

These patients should be managed with a treatment program similar to that followed for patients with sickle cell disease (see Fig. 40-2). As in the case of sickle hemoglobinopathies, iron supplementation should be given only if necessary, because indiscriminate use of iron can lead to hemosiderosis and hemochromatosis. White and coworkers[146] have shown that patients with a β-thalassemia usually have a much higher ferritin concentration than normal patients and those who are α-thalassemia carriers. In β-thalassemia carriers, the incidence of iron deficiency anemia is four times less common than it is in α-thalassemia carriers and normal patients.[146] Although iron is not necessary, folic acid supplementation appears important in β-thalassemia carriers. Leung and coinvestigators[147] showed that the daily administration of folate significantly increased the predelivery hemoglobin concentration in both nulliparous and multiparous patients.

As in the case of sickle cell disease, antepartum fetal evaluation is essential in patients with thalassemia who are anemic. Patients with thalassemia should undergo frequent ultrasonography to assess fetal growth, as well as nonstress testing to evaluate fetal well-being. Asymptomatic thalassemia carriers need no special testing.

Occasionally, individuals will inherit two hemoglobinopathies, such as sickle cell thalassemia (hemoglobin S

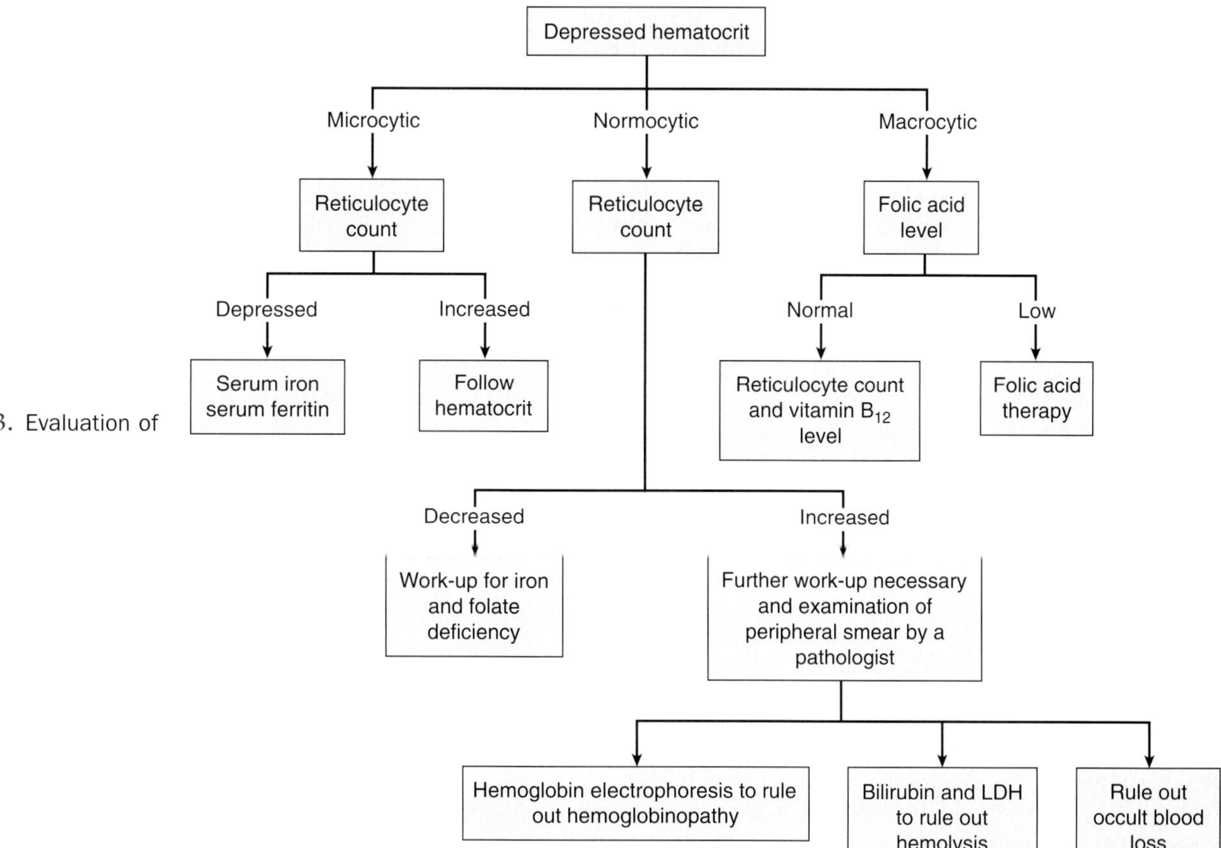

Figure 40-3. Evaluation of anemia.

thal). The prevalence of this disorder among adult blacks in the United States is 1 in 1,672.[148] The clinical course is variable. If minimal suppression of β-chains occurs, patients may be free of symptoms. However, with total suppression of β-chain synthesis, a clinical picture similar to that of sickle cell disease will develop. The course of these patients during pregnancy is quite variable, and their therapy must be individualized.

In summary, Figure 40-3 presents a stepwise approach to the workup of anemia and the diagnosis of the conditions discussed in this chapter.

VON WILLEBRAND'S DISEASE

Von Willebrand's disease (vWD) is the most common congenital bleeding disorder in humans, and up to 1 percent of the population may have some form of the disorder.[149] Type 1 is an autosomal dominant disorder, whereas type 3 and occasionally type 2 are autosomal recessive.[150] vWD is related to quantitative or qualitative abnormalities of von Willebrand's (vWF). This multimeric glycoprotein serves as carrier protein of factor VIII, prolonging its life span in plasma. It also promotes platelet adhesion to the damaged vessel and platelet aggregation. Distinct abnormalities of vWF are responsible for the three types of vWD. Types 1 and 3 are characterized by a quantitative defect of vWF, whereas type 2, comprising subtypes 2A, 2B, 2M, and 2N, refers to molecular variants with a qualitative defect of vWF. The knowledge of the structure of the vWF gene and the use of PCR have led to the identification of the molecular basis of vWD in a significant number of patients.[151] In type 2B, the only clinical symptom in pregnancy may be thrombocytopenia.[152] Therefore, this diagnosis should be considered in the gravida presenting with isolated thrombocytopenia during pregnancy.[150,152,153]

The clinical severity of vWD is variable. Menorrhagia, easy bruising, gingival bleeding, and epistaxis are common. Menorrhagia is most severe in patients with type 2 and 3 vWD and most common in patients with type 1 disease.[154] In a compilation of two studies, 17 percent of women presenting with severe menorrhagia had a form of vWD.[154] Some patients may be entirely asymptomatic until they have severe bleeding after surgery or trauma. Von Willebrand's disease does not appear to affect fetal growth or development.

Classically, the bleeding time is prolonged in patients with vWD as a result of diminished platelet aggregation. Occasionally, the activated partial thromboplastin time is also abnormal. In pregnancy, clotting factors including the factor VIII complex increase, and the patient's bleeding time may improve as gestation progresses.[154,155] This is especially true for type 1A vWD. In type 1B, the patient may not correct her bleeding time.[156] In type 2B, the platelet count decreases. There will, however, be an improvement in the vWF multimeric pattern.[157]

Heavy bleeding may be encountered in patients with vWD undergoing elective or spontaneous first-trimester abortion because the levels of factor VIII have not yet risen.[158] Most importantly, postpartum hemorrhage may be a serious problem. The concentration of factor VIII appears to determine the risk of hemorrhage. If the level is greater than 50 percent of normal and the patient has a normal bleeding time, excessive bleeding should not occur at vaginal delivery.[156,159–161] In a study by Kadir et al.,[158] 18.5 percent of patients with vWD experienced a significant postpartum hemorrhage, and 6 of 31 patients required transfusion. The clinical course during labor is variable. In a study by Chediak and co-workers,[162] bleeding complications were seen in six of eight (75 percent) pregnancies. Five of the newborns had vWD, one of whom was born with a scalp hematoma. Conti and associates,[163] conversely, reported no bleeding complications during the puerperium in five women with vWD. Ieko and colleagues[164] demonstrated that factor VIII concentrate could raise the platelet levels in patients with type 2B vWD. Ito et al.[165] followed six women with type 1 vWD in 10 term pregnancies, three induced abortions, and one spontaneous abortion. They found that bleeding complications occurred within 1 week after term delivery and immediately after both spontaneous and induced abortions.

As noted earlier, bleeding during pregnancy is rare because levels of factor VIII and vWF increase during pregnancy. However, shortly after delivery, they drop. If the factor VIII level is less than 50 percent, treatment during labor and delivery should be initiated. Hemorrhage can also occur several days postpartum. Therefore, factor VIII levels should be checked before the patient goes home after delivery. Desmopressin is the treatment of choice for type 1 vWD.[166] It elicits the release of vWF from endothelial cells. Intranasal preparations of 300 μg are usually employed. In emergent or preoperative situations, 0.3 μg/kg of desmopressin can be given intravenously over 30 minutes.[150] This agent can rarely cause hyponatremia and fluid retention. For those patients who do not respond to desmopressin or for those with vWD types other than 1A, Humate-P or Alphanate should be employed. These commercially available concentrates of antihemophiliac factor have been tested extensively in clinical studies. They contain 2 to 3 times more vWF than they do factor VIII concentrate.[167] The usual dose of Humate-P or Alphanate is 40 to 50 units/kg. This can be given daily to keep factor VIII levels at least 50 percent of normal.[167] These compounds have been heated at high temperature and treated with solvents and detergents to inactivate blood-borne viruses. It is important to note that products containing highly purified factor VIII, obtained by recombinant DNA should not be used. They contain very little vWF and are ineffective in vWD. Therefore, The infused factor VIII has a very short half-life.[166]

Bleeding during pregnancy is rare. Patients with classic type 1 vWD usually need no treatment owing to the increase in factor VIII levels during pregnancy. Those with a history of postpartum hemorrhage should be given an intravenous dose of desmopressin immediately after delivery, and the dose should be repeated 24 hours later. For those with types 2 and 3 disease, factor VIII/vWF concentrates are occasionally needed. Before a cesarean delivery, bleeding time should be measured. If it is prolonged, patients with type 1 vWD should be given desmopressin and patients with vWD type 2 or 3 should receive factor VIII/vWF concentrate.

Key Points

- Four percent of pregnancies will be complicated by maternal platelet counts of less than 150,000/mm^3. The vast majority of these patients have gestational thrombocytopenia with a benign course and need no intervention.
- Surgical bleeding occurs if the platelet count falls below 50,000/mm^3 and spontaneous bleeding occurs if the platelet count falls below 20,000/mm^3.
- Glucocorticoids are the first-line medication used to raise a low platelet count.
- Iron deficiency anemia is the most common cause of anemia in pregnancy, and serum ferritin is the single best test to diagnose it.
- If a patient with presumed iron deficiency does not increase her reticulocyte count with iron therapy, she may also have a concomitant folic acid deficiency.
- Patients pregnant with twins, those on anticonvulsant therapy, those with a hemoglobinopathy, and those who conceive frequently need supplemental folic acid during gestation.
- Most hereditary hemoglobinopathies can be detected in utero, and prenatal diagnosis should be offered to the patient early in pregnancy.
- As in the nonpregnant patient, analgesia, hydration, and oxygen are the key factors in treating pregnant women with sickle cell crisis.
- Patients with sickle cell disease are at high risk of having a fetus with growth restriction and adverse fetal outcomes. Therefore, they warrant frequent sonography and antepartum fetal evaluation.
- In the pregnant patient with vWD, the normal increase in the factor VIII clotting complex reduces the risk of bleeding.

REFERENCES

1. McRae KR, Samuels P, Schreiber AD: Pregnancy-associated thrombocytopenia: pathogenesis and management. Blood 80:2697, 1992.
2. Aster RH: Gestational thrombocytopenia. A plea for conservative management. N Engl J Med 323:264, 1990.
3. Samuels P, Bussel JB, Braitman LE, et al: Estimation of the risk of thrombocytopenia in the offspring of pregnant women with presumed immune thrombocytopenia purpura. N Engl J Med 323:229, 1990.
4. Samuels P, Main EK, Tomaski A, et al: Abnormalities in platelet antiglobulin tests in preeclamptic mothers and their neonates. Am J Obstet Gynecol 107:109, 1987.
5. Burrows RF, Kelton JG: Incidentally detected thrombocytopenia in healthy mothers and their infants. N Engl J Med 319:142, 1988.
6. Hart D, Dunetz C, Nardi M, et al: An epidemic of maternal thrombocytopenia associated with elevated antiplatelet antibody in 116 consecutive pregnancies: relationship to neonatal platelet count. Am J Obstet Gynecol 154:878, 1986.

7. Burrows RF, Kelton JG: Fetal thrombocytopenia and its relationship to maternal thrombocytopenia. N Engl J Med 329:1463, 1993.
8. Burrows RF, Kelton JG: Low fetal risks in pregnancies associated with idiopathic thrombocytopenia purpura. Am J Obstet Gynecol 163:1147, 1990.
9. Peterson OH Jr, Larson P: Thrombocytopenia purpura in pregnancy. Obstet Gynecol 4:454, 1954.
10. Tancer ML: Idiopathic thrombocytopenic purpura and pregnancy: report on 5 new cases and review of the literature. Am J Obstet Gynecol 79:148, 1960.
11. Territo J, Finklestein J, Oh W, et al: Management of autoimmune thrombocytopenia in pregnancy and in the neonate. Obstet Gynecol 51:590, 1973.
12. Carloss HW, MacMillan R, Crosby WH: Management of pregnancy in women with immune thrombocytopenic purpura. JAMA 244:2756, 1980.
13. Noriega-Guerra L, Aviles-Miranda A, de la Cadena OA, et al: Pregnancy in patients with autoimmune thrombocytopenic purpura. Am J Obstet Gynecol 133:439, 1979.
14. Heys RFI: Child bearing and idiopathic thrombocytopenic purpura. J Obstet Gyneacol Br Commonw 73:205, 1966.
15. Karapatkin M, Porges RF, Karapatkin S: Platelet counts in infants of women with autoimmune thrombocytopenia: effects of steroid administration to the mother. N Engl J Med 305:936, 1981.
16. Cines DB, Dusak B, Tomaski A, et al: Immune thrombocytopenic purpura and pregnancy. N Engl J Med 306:826, 1982.
17. Cines DB: Idiopathic thrombocytopenia purpura complicating pregnancy. Medical Grand Rounds 3:344, 1984.
18. Kelton JG, Inwood MJ, Narr RM, et al: The prenatal prediction of thrombocytopenia in infants of mothers with clinically diagnosed immune thrombocytopenia. Am J Obstet Gynecol 144:449, 1982.
19. Harrington WI, Minnich V, Arimura G: The autoimmune thrombocytopenias. *In* Tascantins LM (ed): Progress in Hematology. New York, Grune Stratton, 1956, p 166.
20. Shulman MR, Marder VJ, Weinrach RS: Similarities between thrombocytopenia in idiopathic purpura. Ann N Y Acad Sci 124:449, 1965.
21. Cines DB, Schreiber AD: Immune thrombocytopenia: use of a Coombs antiglobulin test to detect IgG and C3 on platelets. N Engl J Med 300:106, 1979.
22. He R, Reid DM, Jones CE, Shulman NR: Spectrum of Ig classes, specificities, and titers of serum anti glycoproteins in chronic idiopathic thrombocytopenia purpura. Blood 83:1024, 1994.
23. Yeager AM, Zinkham WH: Varicella-associated thrombocytopenic: clues to the etiology of childhood idiopathic thrombocytopenic purpura. Johns Hopkins Med J 146:270, 1980.
24. Stasi R, Stipa E, Masi M, et al: Long-term observation of 208 adults with chronic idiopathic thrombocytopenic purpura. Am J Med 98:4536, 1995.
25. Cines DB, Bussell JB: How I treat idiopathic thrombocytopenic purpura (ITP). Blood 106:2244, 2005.
26. Scott JR, Cruikshank DR, Kochenour NK, et al: Fetal platelet counts in the obstetric management of immunologic thrombocytopenia purpura. Am J Obstet Gynecol 136:495, 1980.
27. Moise KJ, Carpenter RJ, Cotton DB, et al: Percutaneous umbilical cord blood sampling in the evaluation of fetal platelet counts in pregnant patients with autoimmune thrombocytopenic purpura. Obstet Gynecol 160:427, 1989.
28. Kaplan C, Daffos F, Forstier F, et al: Fetal platelet counts in thrombocytopenic pregnancy. Lancet 336:979, 1990.
29. Sciosia AL, Grannum PA, Copel JA, Hobbins JC: The use of percutaneous umbilical blood sampling in immune thrombocytopenic purpura. Am J Obstet Gynecol 159:1066, 1988.
30. Burrows RF, Kelton JG: Pregnancy in patients with idiopathic thrombocytopenic purpura: assessing the risks for the infant at delivery. Obstet Gynecol Surv 458:781, 1993.
31. Moschcowitz E: Hyaline thrombosis of the terminal arterioles and capillaries: a hitherto undescribed disease. Proc N Y Pathol Soc 24:21, 1924.
32. Miller JM, Pastorek JG: Thrombotic thrombocytopenic purpura and the hemolytic uremic syndrome in pregnancy. Clin Obstet Gynecol 34:64, 1991.
33. Ridolfi RL, Bell WR: Thrombotic thrombocytopenic purpura: report of 25 cases and a review of the literature. Medicine 60:413, 1981.
34. Terrell DR, Williams LA, Vesely SK, et al: The incidence of thrombotic thrombocytopenic purpura-hemolytic uremic syndrome: All patients, idiopathic patients, and patients with severe ADAMTS-13 deficiency. J Thrombo Haemost 3:1432–1436, 2005.
35. Ruggenenti P, Noris M, Remuzzi G: Thrombotic microangiopathy, hemolytic uremic syndrome, and thrombotic thrombocytopenic purpura. Kidney Int 60:831, 2001.
36. Tsai HM, Rice L, Sarode R, et al: Antibody inhibitors to von Willebrand factor metalloproteinase and increased binding of von Willebrand factor to platelets in ticlopidine-associated thrombotic thrombocytopenic purpura. Ann Intern Med 132:794, 2000.
37. Tsai HM: Advances in the pathogenesis, diagnosis and treatment of thrombotic thrombocytopenic purpura. J Am Soc Nephrol 14:1072, 2003.
38. Weiner CP: Thrombotic microangiopathy in pregnancy and the postpartum period. Semin Hematol 24:119, 1987.
39. Weiner CP, Kwaan HC, Xu C, et al: Antithrombin III activity in women with hypertension during pregnancy. Obstet Gynecol 65:301, 1985.
40. Neild GH: Haemolytic uraemic syndrome. Nephron 59:194, 1991.
41. Cortlazzo S, Finazzi G, Buelli M, et al: High risk of severe bleeding in aged patients with chronic idiopathic thrombocytopenic purpura. Blood 77:31, 1991.
42. Cohen YC, Dbulbegovic B, Shamai-Lubovitz O, Mozes B: The bleeding risk and natural history of idiopathic thrombocytopenic purpura in patients with persistent low platelet counts. Arch Intern Med 160:1630, 2000.
43. Parks-wylie L, Mazzotta P, Pastuszak A, et al: Birth defects after maternal exposure to corticosteroids: prospective cohort study and meta-analysis of epidemiological studies. Teratology 62:385, 2000.
44. Tabor E: the epidemiology of virus transmission by plasma derivatives: clinical studies verifying the lack of transmission of hepatitis B and C viruses and HIV type 1. Transfusion 39:1160, 1999.
45. Dodd RY: Infectious risk of plasma donations: relationship to safety of intravenous immune globulins. Clin Exp Immunol 104(Suppl 1):31, 1996.
46. Uemura Y, Yang YH, Heldebrant CM, et al: Inactivation and elimination of viruses during preparation of human intravenous immunoglobulin. Vox Sang 67:246, 1994.
47. Culic S: Recombinant factor VIIa for refractory haemorrhage in autoimmune idiopathic thrombocytopenic purpura. Br J Haematol 120:909, 2003.
48. Cooke RL, Miller RC, Katz VL, et al: Immune thrombocytopenic purpura in pregnancy: a reappraisal of management. Obstet Gynecol 78:578, 1991.
49. Lian ECY, Byrnes JJ, Harkness DR: Two successful pregnancies in a woman with chronic thrombotic thrombocytopenic purpura. Int J Obstet Gynecol 29:359, 1989.
50. Ezra Y, Mordel N, Sadovsky E, et al: Successful pregnancies of two patients with relapsing thrombotic thrombocytopenic purpura. Int J Obstet Gynecol 29:359, 1989.
51. Rosove MH, Ho WG, Goldinfer D: Ineffectiveness of aspirin and dipyridamole in the treatment of thrombotic thrombocytopenic purpura. Ann Intern Med 96:27, 1982.
52. Egerman RS, Witlin AG, Friedman SA, Sibai BM: Thrombotic thrombocytopenic purpura and hemolytic uremic syndrome in pregnancy: review of 11 cases. Am J Obstet Gynecol 175:950, 1996.
53. Ponticelli C, Rivolta E, Imbasciatti E, et al: Hemolytic uremic syndrome in adults. Arch Int Med 140:353, 1980.
54. Beattie TJ, Murphy AV, Willoughby MLN, Belch JJF: Prostacyclin infusion in haemolytic-uraemic syndrome of children. BMJ 283:470, 1981.
55. Olah KS, Gee H: Postpartum haemolytic uraemic syndrome precipitated by antibiotics. Br J Obstet Gynaecol 97:83, 1990.
56. Gutterman LA, Levin DM, George BS, Sharma HM: The hemolytic-uremic syndrome: recovery after treatment with vincristine. Ann Intern Med 98:612, 1983.
57. Deaver JE, Leppert PC, Zaroulis CG: Neonatal alloimmune thrombocytopenic purpura. Am J Perinatol 3:127, 1986.

58. Okada N, Oda M, Sano T, et al: Intracranial hemorrhage in utero due to fetomaternal Bak(a) incompatibility. Nippon Ketsueki Gakkai Zasshi 51:1086, 1988.
59. Bussel JB, McFarland JG, Berkowitz R: Antenatal treatment of fetal alloimmune cytopenias. Blut 59:136, 1989.
60. Menell JS, Bussel JB: Antenatal management of thrombocytopenias. Clin Perinatol 21:591, 1994.
61. Paidas AH, Berkowitz RL, Lynch L, et al: Alloimmune thrombocytopenia: fetal and neonatal losses related to cordocentesis. Am J Obstet Gynecol 172:475, 1995.
62. Beaton GH: Iron needs during pregnancy: do we need to rethink our targets? Am J Clin Nutr 72(Suppl):265S, 2000.
63. Pitkin RM: Nutritional influences during pregnancy. Med Clin North Am 61:3, 1977.
64. Ho CH, Yuan CC, Yeh SH: Serum ferritin, folate and cobalamin levels and their correlation with anemia in normal full-term pregnant women. Eur J Obstet Gynecol Reprod Biol 26:7, 1987.
65. Chopa J, Noe E, Matthew J, et al: Anemia in pregnancy. Am J Public Health 57:857, 1967.
66. DeLeeuw NKM, Lowenstein L, Hsieh YS: Iron deficiency and hydremia of normal pregnancy. Medicine 45:291, 1966.
67. Holly RG: Dynamics of iron metabolism in pregnancy. Am J Obstet Gynecol 93:370, 1965.
68. Carr MC: Serum iron/TIBC in the diagnosis of iron deficiency anemia during pregnancy. Obstet Gynecol 38:602, 1971.
69. Boued JL: Iron deficiency: assessment during pregnancy and its importance in pregnant adolescents. Am J Clin Nutr 59:5025, 1994.
70. Harthoorn-Lasthuizen EJ, Lindemans J, Langenhuijsen MM: Erythrocyte zinc protoporphyrin testing in pregnancy. Acta Obstet Gynecol Scand 79:660, 2000.
71. van den Broek NR, Letsky EA, White SA, Shenkin A: Iron status in pregnant women; which measurements are valid? Br J Haematol 103:817, 1998.
72. Ahluwalia N: Diagnostic utility of serum transferrin receptors measurement in assessing iron status. Nutr Rev 56:133, 1998.
73. Long PJ: Rethinking iron supplementation during pregnancy. J Nurse Midwifery 40:36, 1995.
74. Milman N, Bergholt T, Byg KE, et al: Iron status and iron balance during pregnancy. A critical reappraisal of iron supplementation. Acta Obstet Gynecol Scand 78:749, 1999.
75. Zuspan FP, Long WN, Russell JK, et al: Anemia in pregnancy. J Reprod Med 6:13, 1971.
76. Pritchard JA: Changes in the blood volume during pregnancy and delivery. Anesthesiology 26:393, 1965.
77. Zavaleta N, Caulfield LE, Garcia T: Changes in iron status during pregnancy in Peruvian women receiving prenatal iron and folic acid supplements with or without zinc. Am J Clin Nutr 71:956, 2000.
78. Young MW, Lupafya E, Kapenda E, Bobrow EA: The effectiveness of weekly iron supplementation in pregnant women of rural northern Malawi. Trop Doct 30:84, 2000.
79. Singh K, Fong YF, Kuperan P: A comparison between intravenous iron polymaltose complex (Ferrum Hausmann) and oral ferrous fumarate in the treatment of iron deficiency anaemia in pregnancy. Eur J Haematol 60:119, 1998.
80. Hallak M, Sharon AS, Diukman R, et al: Supplementing iron intravenously in pregnancy: a way to avoid blood transfusions. J Reprod Med 42:99, 1997.
81. Scholl TO, Hediger ML: Anemia and iron-deficiency anemia: compilation of data on pregnancy outcome. Am J Clin Nutr 59:4925, 1994.
82. Yip R: Significance of abnormally low or high hemoglobin concentration during pregnancy: special consideration of iron nutrition. Am J Clin Nutr 72:272S, 2000.
83. Sifakis S, Pharmakides G: Anemia in pregnancy. Ann N Y Acad Sci 900:125, 2000.
84. Hemminki E, Starfield B: Routine administration of iron and vitamins during pregnancy: review of controlled clinical trials. Br J Obstet Gynaecol 85:404, 1978.
85. Stephansson O, Dickman PW, Johansson A, Cnattingius S: Maternal hemoglobin concentration during pregnancy and risk of stillbirth. JAMA 284:2611, 2000.
86. Rothman D: Folic acid in pregnancy. Am J Obstet Gynecol 108:49, 1970.
87. Giles C, Ball EW: Iron and folic acid deficiency in pregnancy. BMJ 1:656, 1965.
88. Ek J: Plasma and red cell folate values in newborn infants and their mothers in relation to gestational age. J Pediatr 97:288, 1980.
89. Molloy AM, Mills JL, Kirke PN, et al: Folate status and neural tube defects. Biofactors 10:291, 1999.
90. Kaplan JS, Iqbal S, England BG, et al: Is pregnancy in diabetic women associated with folate deficiency? Diabetes Care 22:1017, 1999.
91. Vollsett SE, Refsum H, Irgens LM, et al: Plasma total homocysteine, pregnancy complications, and adverse pregnancy outcomes: the Hordaland homocysteine study. Am J Clin Nutr 71:962, 2000.
92. Nelen WL, van der Molen EF, Blom HJ, et al: Recurrent early pregnancy loss and genetic-related disturbances in folate and homocysteine metabolism. Br J Hosp Med 58:511, 1997.
93. Green R, Kinsella LJ: Editorial: Current concepts in the diagnosis of cobalamin deficiency. Neurology 45:1435, 1995.
94. Tefferi A, Pruthi RK: The biochemical basis of cobalamin deficiency. Mayo Clin Proc 69:181, 1994.
95. Bauman WA, Shaw S, Jayatilleke E, et al: Increased intake of calcium reverses vitamin B-12 malabsorption induced by metformin. Diabetes Care 23:1227, 2000.
96. Metz J, McGrath K, Bennett M, et al: Biochemical indices of vitamin B_{12} nutrition in pregnant patients with subnormal serum vitamin B_{12} level. Am J Hematol 48:251, 1995.
97. Lindenbaum J, Savage DG, Stabler SP, Allen RH: Diagnosis of cobalamin deficiency: II. Relative sensitivities of serum cobalamin, methylmalonic acid and total homocysteine concentrations. Am J Hematol 34:99, 1990.
98. Naurath HJ, Joosten E, Riezler R, et al: Effects of vitamin B_{12}, folate, and vitamin B_6 supplements in elderly people with normal serum vitamin concentrations. Lancet 346:85, 1995.
99. Savage DG, Lindenbaum J, Stabler SP, Allen RH: Sensitivity of serum methylmalonic acid and total homocysteine determinations for diagnosing cobalamin and folate deficiencies. Am J Med 96:238, 1994.
100. Lambert EK, Bloom RN, Kosby M: Pregnancy in patients with hemoglobinopathies and thalassemias. J Reprod Med 19:193, 1977.
101. Motulsky AG: Frequency of sickling disorders in US blacks. N Engl J Med 288:31, 1973.
102. Larrabee KD, Monga M: Women with sickle cell trait are at increased risk for preeclampsia. Am J Obstet Gynecol 177:425, 1997.
103. Lynch JR, Brown JM: The polymerase chain reaction: current and future clinical applications. J Med Genet 27:2, 1990.
104. Barret-Connor E: Cholelithiasis in sickle cell anemia. Am J Med 45:889, 1968.
105. Cameron JL, Moddrey WC, Ziridema GD, et al: Biliary tract disease in sickle cell anemia: surgical considerations. Ann Surg 174:702, 1971.
106. Charache S, Scott J, Niebyl J, Bonds D: Management of sickle cell disease in pregnant patients. Obstet Gynecol 55:407, 1980.
107. Fort AT, Morrison JC, Berreras L, et al: Counseling the patient with sickle cell disease about reproduction: pregnancy outcome does not justify the maternal risk. Am J Obstet Gynecol 111:391, 1971.
108. Freeman MG, Ruth GJ: SS disease and SC disease-obstetric considerations and treatment. Clin Obstet Gynecol 12:134, 1969.
109. Curtis EM: Pregnancy in sickle cell anemia, sickle cell–hemoglobin C disease, and variants thereof. Am J Obstet Gynecol 77:1312, 1959.
110. Horger EO III: Sickle cell and sickle cell-hemoglobin disease during pregnancy. Obstet Gynecol 39:873, 1972.
111. Milner PF, Jones BR, Dobler J: Outcome of pregnancy in sickle cell anemia and sickle cell–hemoglobin C disease. Am J Obstet Gynecol 138:239, 1980.
112. Fessas P, Loukopoulos D: Beta thalassaemias. Clin Hematol 3:411, 1974.
113. Powars DR, Sandhu M, Niland-Weiss J, et al: Pregnancy in sickle cell disease. Obstet Gynecol 67:217, 1986.
114. Seoud MA, Cantwell C, Nobles G, Levy OL: Outcome of pregnancies complicated by sickle cell disease and sickle-c hemoglobinopathies. Am J Perinatol 11:187, 1994.

115. Smith JA, England M, Bellevue R, et al: Pregnancy in sickle cell disease: experience of the cooperative study of sickle cell disease. Obstet Gynecol 87:199, 1996.
116. Fiakpui EF, Moron EM: Pregnancy in sickle hemoglobins. J Reprod Med 11:28, 1973.
117. Anyaegbunam A, Billet HH, Langer O, et al: Maternal hemoglobin F levels may have an adverse effect on neonatal birth weight in pregnancies with sickle cell disease. Am J Obstet Gynecol 161:654, 1989.
118. Morris JS, Dunn DT, Poddorr D, Serjeant GR: Hematological risk factors for pregnancy outcome in Jamaican women with homozygous sickle cell disease. Br J Obstet Gynaecol 101:770, 1994.
119. Ohne-Frempong K, Smith-Whitley K: Use of hydroxyurea in children with sickle cell disease: what comes next? Semin Hematol 34:30, 1997.
120. Miller ST, Sleeper LA, Pegelow CH et al: Prediction of adverse outcomes in children with sickle cell disease. N Engl J Med 342:8, 2000.
121. Anyaegbunam A, Langer O, Brustman L, et al: The application of uterine and umbilical artery velocimetry to the antenatal supervision of pregnancies complicated by maternal sickle hemoglobinopathies. Am J Obstet Gynecol 159:544, 1988.
122. Howard RJ, Tuck SM, Pearson TC: Blood transfusion in pregnancy complicated by sickle cell disease: effects on blood rheology and uteroplacental Doppler velocimetry. Clin Lab Haematol 16:253, 1994.
123. Smith JA, Espeland M, Bellevue R, et al: Pregnancy in sickle cell disease: experience of the Cooperative Study of Sickle Cell Disease. Obstet Gynecol 87:199, 1996.
124. Van Eric A, Visschers G, Jansen W, et al: Maternal death due to sickle cell chronic lung disease. Am J Obstet Gynecol 99:162, 1992.
125. Perkins RP: Inherited disorders of hemoglobin synthesis and pregnancy. Am J Obstet Gynecol 111:130, 1971.
126. Baum KF, Dunn DT, Maude GH, Serjeant GR: The painful crisis of homozygous sickle cell disease: a study of the risk factors. Arch Intern Med 147:1231, 1987.
127. Claster S, Vichinsky EP: Managing sickle cell disease. BMJ 327:1151, 2003.
128. Abudu OO, Macaulay K, Oluboyede OA: Serial evaluation of iron stores in pregnant Nigerians with hemoglobin SS or SC. J Natl Med Assoc 82:41, 1990.
129. Aken'Ova YA, Adeyefa I, Okunade M: Ferritin and serum iron levels in adult patients with sickle cell anaemia at Ibadan, Nigeria. Afr J Med Med Sci 26:39, 1997.
130. Cunningham FG, Pritchard JA, Mason R: Pregnancy and sickle cell hemoglobinopathies: results with and without prophylactic transfusions. Obstet Gynecol 62:419, 1983.
131. Morrison JC, Schneider JM, Whybrew WD, et al: Prophylactic transfusions in pregnant patients with sickle hemoglobinopathies: benefit versus risk. Obstet Gynecol 56:274, 1980.
132. Koshy M, Burd L, Wallace D, et al: Prophylactic red cell transfusions in pregnant patients with sickle cell disease: a randomized cooperative study. N Engl J Med 319:1447, 1988.
133. Tuck SM, James CE, Brewster EM, et al: Prophylactic blood transfusion in maternal sickle cell syndromes. Br J Obstet Gynaecol 94:121, 1987.
134. Mahomed K: Prophylactic versus selective blood transfusion for sickle cell anaemia during pregnancy. Cochrane Database Syst Rev 2:2000.
135. Hassell K: Pregnancy and sickle cell disease. Hematol Oncol Clin N Am 19:903, 2005.
136. Rappaport VJ, Velazquez M, Williams K: Hemoglobinopathies in pregnancy. Obstet Gynecol Clin N Am 31:287, 2004.
137. Fullerton WT, Hendrickse J, Williams W, et al: Hemoglobin SC: clinical course. *In* Jonxis JHP (ed): Abnormal hemoglobins in Africa: A Symposium. Oxford, Blackwell Scientific Publications, 1965, p 215.
138. Solanki DL, Kletter GG, Castro O: Acute splenic sequestration crises in adults with sickle cell disease. Am J Med 80:985, 1986.
139. Ghosh A, Tan MH, Liang ST, et al: Ultrasound evaluation of pregnancies at risk for homozygous alpha-thalassaemia-1. Prenat Diagn 7:307, 1987.
140. Woo JS, Liang ST, Lo RL, Chan FY: Doppler blood flow velocity waveforms in alpha-thalassemia hydrops fetalis. J Ultrasound Med 6:679, 1987.
141. Hsieh FJ, Chang FM, Huang HC, et al: Umbilical vein blood flow measurement in nonimmune hydrops fetalis. Obstet Gynecol 71:188, 1988.
142. Mordel N, Birkenfeld A, Goldfarb AN, Rachmilewitz EA: Successful full-term pregnancy in homozygous beta-thalassemia major: case report and review of the literature. Obstet Gynecol 73:837, 1989.
143. Necheles T: Obstetric complications associated with haemoglobinopathies. Clin Hematol 2:497, 1973.
144. Savona-Ventura C, Bonello F: Betathalassemia syndromes in pregnancy. Obstet Gynecol Survey 49:129, 1994.
145. Singounas EG, Sakas DE, Hadley OM: Paraplegia in a pregnant thalassemic woman due to extramedullary hematopoiesis: Successful management with transfusions. Surg Neurol 36:210, 1991.
146. White JM, Richards R, Jelenski G, et al: Iron state in alpha and beta thalassaemia trait. J Clin Pathol 39:256, 1986.
147. Leung CF, Lao TT, Chang AM: Effect of folate supplement on pregnant women with beta-thalassaemia minor. Eur J Obstet Gynecol Reprod Biol 33:209, 1989.
148. Schmidt RM: Laboratory diagnosis of hemoglobinopathies. JAMA 224:1276, 1973.
149. Phillips MD, Santhouse A: von Willebrand disease: recent advances in pathophysiology and treatment. Am J Med Sci 316:77, 1998.
150. Castaman G, Rodeghiero F: Current management of von Willebrand's disease. Drugs 50:602, 1995.
151. Mazurier C, Ribba AS, Gaucher C, Meyer D: Molecular genetics of von Willebrand disease. Ann Genet 41:34, 1998.
152. Giles AR, Hoogendoorn H, Benford K: Type IIB von Willebrand's disease presenting as thrombocytopenia during pregnancy. Br J Haematol 67:349, 1987.
153. Rick ME, Williams SB, Sacher RA, McKeown LP: Thrombocytopenia associated with pregnancy in a patient with type IIB von Willebrand's disease. Blood 69:786, 1987.
154. Kouides PA: Females with von Willebrand disease: 72 years as the silent majority. Haemophilia 4:665, 1998.
155. Kasper CK, Hoags MS, Aggeler PM, Stone S: Blood clotting factors in pregnancy: factor VIII concentrations in normal and AHF-deficient women. Obstet Gynecol 24:242, 1984.
156. Takahashi H, Hayashi N, Shibata A: Type IB von Willebrand's disease and pregnancy: comparison of analytical methods of von Willebrand factor for classification of von Willebrand's disease subtypes. Thromb Res 50:409, 1988.
157. Casonato A, Sarrori MT, Bertomoro A, et al: Pregnancy-induced worsening of thrombocytopenia in a patient with type IIB von Willebrand's disease. Blood Coagul Fibrinolysis 2:33, 1991.
158. Kadir RA, Lee CA, Sabin CA, et al: Pregnancy in women with von Willebrand's disease or factor XI deficiency. Br J Obstet Gynaecol 105:314, 1998.
159. Noller KL, Bowie EJW, Kempers RD, Owen CA: von Willebrand's disease in pregnancy. Obstet Gynecol 41:865, 1973.
160. Evans P: Obstetric and gynecologic patients with von Willebrand's disease. Obstet Gynecol 38:37, 1971.
161. Lipton RA, Ayromlooi J, Coller BS: Severe von Willebrand's disease during labor and delivery. JAMA 248:1355, 1982.
162. Chediak JR, Alban GM, Maxey B: von Willebrand's disease and pregnancy: management during delivery and outcome of offspring. Am J Obstet Gynecol 155:618, 1986.
163. Conti M, Mari D, Conti E, et al: Pregnancy in women with different types of von Willebrand disease. Obstet Gynecol 68:282, 1986.
164. Ieko M, Sakurama S, Sagan A, et al: Effect of factor VIII concentrate on type IIB von Willebrand's disease-associated thrombocytopenia presenting during pregnancy in identical twin mothers. Am J Hematol 35:26, 1990.
165. Ito M, Yoshimura K, Toyoda N, Wada H: Pregnancy and delivery in patient with von Willebrand's disease. J Obstet Gynaecol Res 23:37, 1997.
166. Mannucci PM: Treatment of von Willebrand's disease. J Intern Med Suppl 740:129, 1997.
167. Mannucci PM: Treatment of von Willebrand's disease. N Engl J Med 351:683, 2004.

Thromboembolic Disorders

Christian M. Pettker and Charles J. Lockwood

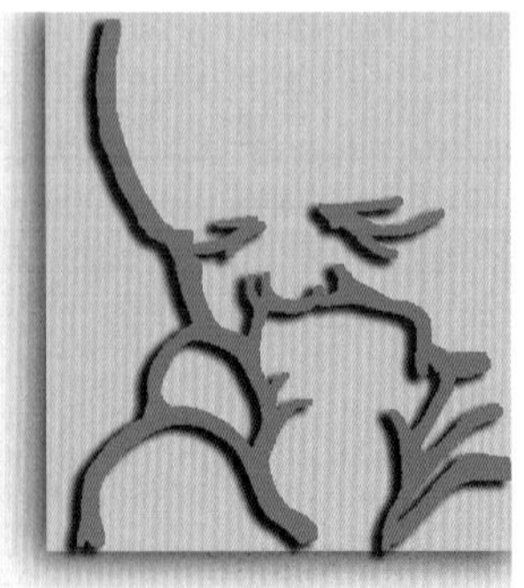

CHAPTER 41

KEY ABBREVIATIONS

Activated partial thromboplastin time	aPTT
Activated protein C	APC
Acute pulmonary embolus	APE
Adenosine disphosphate	ADP
Antiphospholipid antibodies	APAs
Antiphospholipid antibody syndrome	APAS
Computerized tomography	CT
Deep vein thrombosis	DVT
Enzyme-linked immunosorbent assay	ELISA
Heparin-induced thrombocytopenia	HIT
Inferior vena cava	IVC
International normalized ratio	INR
Low-molecular-weight heparin	LMWH
Magnetic resonance angiography	MRA
Magnetic resonance imaging	MRI
Prospective Investigation of Pulmonary Embolism Diagnosis	PIOPED
Protein Z–dependent protease inhibitor	ZPI
Pulmonary embolus	PE
Systemic lupus erythematosus	SLE
Thrombin-activatable fibrinolysis inhibitor	TAFI
Thromboxane A2	TXA2
Tissue factor	TF
Tissue factor pathway inhibitor	TFPI
Type-1 plasminogen activator inhibitor	PAI-1
Venous thromboembolism	VTE
Venous ultrasonography	VUS
Ventilation perfusion scan	V/Q

INTRODUCTION

Pregnancy, childbirth, and the puerperium pose serious challenges to a woman's vascular and hemostatic systems. The development of the elaborate high-capacity, low-resistance uteroplacental circulation requires a delicate balance between the maintenance of blood fluidity in the intervillous space and a greatly enhanced hemostatic response to avoid hemorrhage. This essential adaptation of the mother's hemostatic system to pregnancy is generally protective but contributes to an increased risk of superficial and deep vein thrombosis (DVT) as well as pulmonary embolus (PE). Mothers with underlying acquired or inherited thrombophilias are at greatest risk. The prompt identification and appropriate treatment of the thromboembolic and diagnosis of the thrombophilic disorders in pregnancy, although challenging and complex, is critical in avoiding potentially catastrophic thromboembolic sequelae.

EPIDEMIOLOGY

Occurring in approximately 1/1000 to 1/2000 pregnancies, venous thromboembolism (VTE) is a rare disorder but a leading cause of mortality and serious morbidity in pregnant women.[1–9] This risk represents a nearly 10-fold increase compared with nonpregnant women of childbearing age. According to the most recent U.S vital statistics, PE is the leading cause of maternal mortality, contributing to 19.6 percent of maternal deaths, or 2.3 pregnancy-related deaths per 100,000 live births.[10]

Classic teaching considered the postpartum period to be the time of maximal thrombotic occurrence. However, management styles of prior eras (e.g., bed rest in the postpartum period and estrogen to suppress lactation) likely inflated this risk.[6] More recent studies have shown that a majority of thromboembolic events happen in the antepartum period, with a nearly equal distribution across each trimester.[1,3,11–13] However, given the shorter duration of the postpartum period (6 versus 13 weeks) and after adjusting for duration of exposure, the risk of VTE is approximately three- to eightfold higher in the period following delivery.[9]

RISK FACTORS

Virchow's triad—vascular stasis, hypercoagulability, and vascular trauma—describes the three classic antecedents to thrombosis, and many of the physiologic changes of pregnancy contribute to these criteria. Other pregnancy-specific risk factors for thrombosis include increased parity, postpartum endomyometritis, operative vaginal delivery, and cesarean delivery. Cesarean delivery in particular is associated with a ninefold increase in the risk of thromboembolism compared with vaginal delivery.[11] Risk factors not unique to pregnancy include age greater than 35 years, obesity, trauma, immobility, infection, smoking, nephrotic syndrome, hyperviscosity syndromes, cancer, surgery (particularly orthopedic procedures), and a prior history of DVT or PE.[14]

PHYSIOLOGY OF HEMOSTASIS

Vasoconstriction and Platelet Action

Vasoconstriction and platelet activity play a primary role in the initial restoration of the circulatory system following vascular disruption and endothelial damage. Vasoconstriction limits blood flow as well as the size of thrombus necessary to repair the defect. Platelet adherence to damaged vessels is mediated by the formation of von Willebrand factor bridges anchored at one end to subendothelial collagen and at the other to the platelet GPIb/IX/V receptor.[15] Platelet adhesion stimulates release of α-granules containing von Willebrand factor, thrombospondin, platelet factor 4, fibrinogen, beta-thromboglobulin, and platelet-derived growth factor, as well as dense-granules containing adenosine diphosphate (ADP) and serotonin. These latter molecules, when combined with the release of thromboxane A2 (TxA2) contribute to further vasoconstriction (serotonin, TxA2) and platelet activation (TxA2, ADP, thrombin). ADP release, which causes a conformational change in the GPIIb/IIIa receptor on platelets, promotes aggregation by forming interplatelet fibrinogen, fibronectin, and vitronectin bridges,[16] as all three molecules bind to the GPIIb/IIIa receptor.

The Coagulation Cascade

Tissue factor (TF), a cell membrane-bound glycoprotein, is the primary initiator of hemostasis and the coagulation cascade.[17] TF is expressed constitutively by epithelial, stromal, and perivascular cells throughout the body, and in reference to pregnancy in particular, endometrial stromal cells and uterine decidua.[17,18] TF is present in low concentrations in blood, on activated platelets, and in high levels, in amniotic fluid, accounting for the coagulopathy seen in amniotic fluid embolism.[19] It is also interesting to note that although intrauterine survival is possible in the absence of platelets or fibrinogen, it is not possible in the absence of tissue factor.[20] Clotting is initiated by the binding of TF to factor VII (Fig. 41-1).

Although tissue factor is the initiator of hemostasis, thrombin is the ultimate arbiter of clotting, because it not only activates platelets and generates fibrin but also

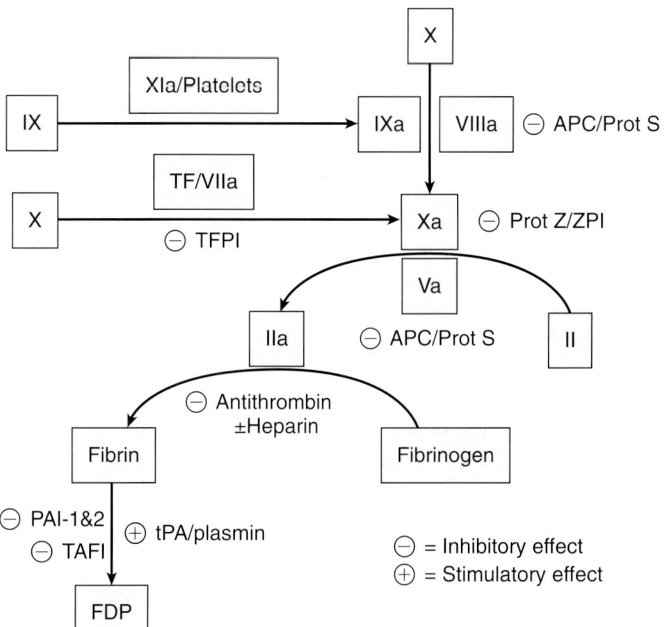

Figure 41-1. Hemostatic, thrombotic, and fibrinolytic pathways.

activates critical clotting factors and cofactors (V, VII, VIII, and XIII).

Following endothelial injury and in the presence of ionized calcium, perivascular cell- or platelet-bound TF comes into contact with factor VII on anionic cell membrane phospholipids. Factor VII has low intrinsic clotting activity but can be autoactivated after binding to TF or can be activated by thrombin or factors IXa, Xa, or XIIa.[17] The TF/FVIIa complex initiates the coagulation cascade by activating both factors X and IX. The latter (IXa) complexes with its cofactor, factor VIIIa, to indirectly activate factor X. Once generated, factor Xa binds with its cofactor Va to convert prothrombin (factor II) to thrombin (IIa). The cofactors V and VIII can each be activated by either thrombin or factor Xa. Activated factor XII activates factor XI on the surface of activated platelets which provides an alternative route to factor IX activation. Factor XII can be activated by kallikrein/kininogen as well as by plasmin. Figure 41-1 provides a diagram of the interaction of the various components of the coagulation cascade. The key event of hemostasis occurs when thrombin cleaves fibrinogen to produce fibrin. Fibrin monomers self-polymerize and are cross-linked by thrombin-activated factor XIIIa.

The Anticoagulant System

Inappropriate activation of the hemostatic system, that is, thrombosis, is prevented by the anticoagulant system (see Fig. 41-1). Tissue factor pathway inhibitor (TFPI) binds to the prothrombinase complex (factor Xa/TF/VIIa) to stop TF-mediated clotting.[21] However, factor XIa generation can bypass this block and, furthermore, in the 10 to 15 seconds before TFPI-mediated prothrombinase inhibition, a sufficient amount of factor Va, VIIIa, IXa, Xa, and thrombin can be generated to sustain clotting for some time. As a result, additional physiologic anticoagulant molecules are required to maintain blood fluidity.

Paradoxically, thrombin also plays a pivotal role in the anticoagulant system by binding to thrombomodulin, allowing it to activate protein C (APC). APC binds to anionic endothelial cell membrane phospholipids or to the endothelial cell protein C receptor to inactivate factors Va and VIIIa.[22] Protein S is an important cofactor in this process, enhancing APC activity. Factor Va is also a cofactor in APC-mediated factor VIIIa inactivation.

Factor Xa can also be inhibited by the protein Z–dependent protease inhibitor (ZPI). When ZPI forms a complex with its cofactor, protein Z, its inhibitory activity is enhanced 1000-fold, although ZPI can also inhibit factor XIa independent of protein Z.[23] Deficiencies of protein Z can promote both bleeding and thrombosis, athough the latter predominates, particularly in the presence of other thrombophilias.

Thrombin activity is modulated by a number of serine protease inhibitors (e.g., heparin cofactor II, α-2 macroglobulin, antithrombin), which serve to inactivate thrombin and Xa. The most active inhibitor within this group is antithrombin (also known as antithrombin III). Antithrombin binds to either thrombin or factor Xa and then to heparin or other glycosaminoglycans, augmenting antithrombin's rate of thrombin inactivation 1000-fold.[24,25] The other two inhibitors work in a similar fashion.

Fibrinolysis

Fibrinolysis is a further critical element in preventing overwhelming thrombosis (see Fig. 41-1). Tissue-type plasminogen activator, embedded in fibrin, cleaves plasminogen to generate plasmin, which, in turn, cleaves fibrin into fibrin degradation products. The latter are indirect measures of fibrinolysis. These fibrin degradation products can also inhibit thrombin action, a favorable result when limited, but contributing to disseminated intravascular coagulation when occurring in excess. A second plasminogen activator, urokinase-type plasminogen activator, is produced by endothelial cells. There is also a series of fibrinolysis inhibitors that prevent hemorrhage from premature breakdown of the fibrin clot. The α-2-plasmin inhibitor is bound to the fibrin clot, where it prevents premature fibrinolysis. Platelets and endothelial cells release type 1 plasminogen activator inhibitor (PAI-1), an inactivator of tissue-type plasminogen activator. In pregnancy, the decidua is also a rich source of PAI-1, whereas the placenta produces mostly PAI-2.[26] The thrombin-activatable fibrinolysis inhibitor (TAFI) is another fibrinolytic inhibitor that is also activated by the thrombin-thrombomodulin complex.[27] Thrombin-activatable fibrinolysis inhibitor cleaves fibrin, rendering it resistant to inactivation by plasmin.

PATHOPHYSIOLOGY OF THROMBOSIS IN PREGNANCY

Characteristic physiologic changes in the local decidual and systemic hemostatic systems occur in pregnancy in preparation for the hemostatic challenges of implantation, placentation, and childbirth. Decidual TF and PAI-1 expression are greatly increased in response to progesterone, and levels of PAI-2, which are negligible prior to pregnancy, increase until term.[26,27] Pregnancy is associated with systemic changes that enhance hemostatic capability but promote thrombosis. For example, there is a doubling in circulating concentrations of fibrinogen and 20- to 1,000-percent increases in factors VII, VIII, IX, X, and XII, all of which peak at term in preparation for delivery.[28,29] Levels of von Willebrand factor also increase up to 400 percent at term.[28] In contrast, levels of prothrombin and factor V remain unchanged, whereas levels of factor XIII and XI decline modestly. Concomitantly, there is a 40-percent decrease in the levels of free protein S, conferring an overall resistance to activated protein C.[28] Further reductions in free protein S concentrations are caused by cesarean delivery and infection, accounting for the high rate of PE in such patients. Coagulation parameters may be normalized as early as 3 weeks postpartum, but they generally return to baseline at 6 weeks postpartum.

The risk of thrombosis in pregnancy is also related to physical changes in the gravid woman. Venous stasis in the lower extremities results from compression of the inferior vena cava and pelvic veins by the enlarging uterus.[30,31] Despite the presence of the sigmoid colon promoting uterine dextrorotation, ultrasound findings indicate lower flow velocities in the left leg veins throughout pregnancy.[32] This would explain why multiple studies have confirmed that the incidence of thrombosis is much greater in the left leg than in the right leg.[1,12,33] Hormone-mediated increases in deep vein capacitance secondary to increased circulating levels of estrogen and local production of prostacyclin and nitric oxide also contribute to the increased risk of thrombosis.

Antiphospholipid Antibody Syndrome

Overall, antiphospholipid antibody syndrome (APAS) is responsible for approximately 14 percent of thromboembolic disease in pregnancy.[14,34] The diagnosis of APAS requires the presence of prior or current vascular thrombosis, or characteristic obstetric complications, together with at least one laboratory criterion (e.g., anticardiolipin antibodies or lupus anticoagulant).[35] The antiphospholipid antibodies (APAs) are a class of self-recognition immunoglobulins directed against proteins bound to negatively charged (anionic) phospholipids. Anticardiolipin antibodies and the lupus anticoagulants represent the two most widely employed end points, but other applicable tests include anti-β2 glycoprotein antibodies, and anti-prothrombin and anti-annexin antibodies.[36] These antibodies must be present on two or more occasions at least 6 weeks apart for diagnosis.[35] APAs are present in 2.2 percent of the general obstetric population, and most of these patients have uncomplicated pregnancies.[37] Thus, providers should use caution when ordering and interpreting tests in the absence of APAS-qualifying clinical criteria.

APAS has been associated with both venous (DVT, PE) and arterial (stroke) vascular events. A meta-analysis of 18 studies has shown an elevated risk of DVT, PE, and recurrent venous thromboembolism among patients with systemic lupus erythematous (SLE) who test positive for the APAs. Overall, when compared with those SLE patients do not test positive for either test, those with lupus anticoagulants and anticardiolipin antibodies have a six- and twofold increased risk of venous thrombosis, respectively.[38] These antibodies pose a risk to patients without SLE as well. The lifetime prevalence of arterial or venous thrombosis in affected non-SLE patients is approximately 30 percent, with an event rate of 1 percent per year.[39,40] The risks of thromboembolic events are highly dependent on the presence of other predisposing factors, including pregnancy, estrogen exposure, immobility, surgery, and infection. APAS has also been associated with adverse pregnancy outcome and accounts for 14 percent of VTE in pregnancy.[14,34] In fact, there is a 5-percent risk of a thrombotic event in pregnancy, even with prophylaxis.[41]

Inherited Thrombophilias

The inherited thrombophilias are a heterogeneous group of genetic disorders associated with arterial and venous thrombosis as well as fetal loss. As with APAS, the occurrence of a thromboembolic event is highly dependent on other predisposing factors such as pregnancy, exogenous estrogens, immobility, obesity, surgery, infection, trauma, and the presence of other thrombophilias. However, the most important risk modifier is a personal or family history of venous thrombosis.[42] Table 41-1 presents the prevalence and risk of venous thrombosis among pregnant patients with and without a personal or family history of venous thrombosis. As noted earlier, the thrombophilias are divided into high and low risks based on the overall risk of VTE.

DIAGNOSIS OF VENOUS THROMBOEMBOLISM

Deep Venous Thrombosis

Clinical Signs and Symptoms

The clinical findings typical of DVT include erythema, warmth, pain, edema, and tenderness localized to the area of the embolus. Occasionally, a palpable cord may correspond to a thrombosed vein, and Homans' sign is the pain and tenderness elicited on compression of the calf muscles by squeezing the muscles or dorsiflexion of the foot. These are rather nonspecific signs and symptoms that involve a broad differential diagnosis, including cellulitis, ruptured or strained muscle or tendon, trauma, ruptured popliteal (Baker's) cyst, cutaneous vasculitis, superficial thrombophlebitis, and lymphedema. In fact, evidence suggests that the specificities of these manifestations are less than 50 percent, and among patients with these signs and symptoms, the diagnosis of DVT is confirmed by objective testing in only approximately one-third of the group.[55,56]

Risk Scoring System

Because the positive predictive value of a test increases with the prevalence of the disease to be detected, the key to accurate diagnosis of either DVT or PE is the initial assessment of patient risk. This concept directs the diagnostic paradigm outlined in Figure 41-2. Wells and associates have proposed a risk model based on a patient's clinical history and signs and symptoms of DVT (Table 41-2).[57,58] The pretest probability using this method is divided into three categories of DVT risk (high, 3; moderate, 1 to 2; low, 0).

Patients with a high prediagnostic test probability have a prevalence of DVT of 85 percent, with 96 percent involving the more morbid proximal leg vein. Those in the moderate and low pretest probability categories have DVT prevalences of 33 and 5 percent, and proximal leg vein involvement in 72 and 62 percent cases, respectively.

Table 41-1. Inherited Thrombophilias and the Associations with Venous Thromboembolism (VTE) in Pregnancy

RISK GROUP	THROMBOPHILIA TYPE	INHERITANCE	PREVALENCE IN THE EUROPEAN POPULATION (%)	PREVALENCE IN PREGNANT PATIENTS WITH VTE (%)	RR OR OR OF VTE IN PREGNANCY [95% CI]	PROBABILITY OF VTE IN PREGNANCY (PTS WITH PERSONAL OR FAMILY (%))	PROBABILITY OF VTE IN PREGNANCY (PTS WITHOUT PERSONAL OR FAMILY (%))	REFERENCES
High risk	Factor V Leiden homozygous	Autosomal dominant	0.07*	<1[+]	25.4 [8.8–66]	>>10	1.5	42–46
	Prothrombin gene G20210A mutation homozygous	Autosomal dominant	0.02*	<1[+]	N/A	>>10	2.8	47, 48
	Antithrombin III deficiency	Autosomal dominant	0.02–1.1	1–8	119	11–40	3.0–7.2	43, 46, 47
	Compound heterozygous (FVL/prothrombin G20210A)	Autosomal dominant Autosomal dominant	0.17*	<1*	84 [19–369]	4.7 (overall probability of VTE in pregnancy)		42, 43, 49
Low risk	Factor V Leiden heterozygous	Autosomal dominant	5.3	44	6.9 [3.3–15.2]	>10	0.26	42–45, 50
	Prothrombin G20210A mutation heterozygous	Autosomal dominant	2.9	17	9.5 [2.1–66.7]	>10	0.37–0.5	42, 43, 48, 49
	Protein C deficiency	Autosomal dominant	0.2–0.3	<14	13.0 [1.4–123]	∞	0.8–1.7	43, 46, 47 51
	Protein S deficiency	Autosomal dominant	0.03–0.13	12.4	∞	∞	<1–6.6	42, 43, 47 52
	Hyperhomocysteinemia	Autosomal recessive	<5	∞	6.1 [1.3–28.4][†]	∞	∞	46, 53, 54

OR, odds ratio; RR, relative risk.
*Calculated based on a Hardy-Weinberg equilibrium.
[†]OR adjusted for renal disease, folate, and B_{12} deficiency, while odds ratios are adjusted for these confounders.
∞, Data not available.

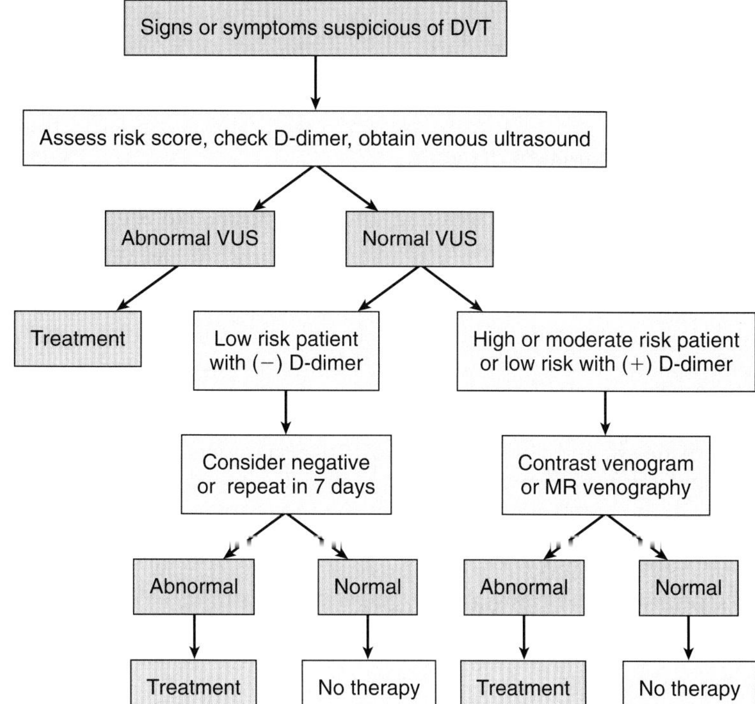

Figure 41-2. Diagnostic algorithm for deep vein thrombosis.

Table 41-2. Deep Venous Thrombosis Clinical Characteristic Score

RISK OR SIGN	POINTS
Active cancer	+1
Immobilization (cast, paralysis, paresis)	+1
Bed rest >3 days or surgery within 12 weeks	+1
Local tenderness along deep venous system	+1
Entire leg swollen	+1
Asymmetric calf swelling >3 cm (10 cm below tibial tuberosity)	+1
Pitting edema only in symptomatic leg	+1
Collateral nonvaricose superficial veins	+1
Prior deep vein thrombosis	+1
Alternative diagnosis at least as likely as deep venous thrombosis	−2

Adapted from Wells P, Hirsh J, Anderson D, et al: A simple clinical model for the diagnosis of deep-vein thrombosis combined with impedance plethysmography: potential for an improvement in the diagnostic process. J Intern Med 243:15, 1998; Wells P, Anderson D, Rodger M, et al: Evaluation of D-Dimer in the diagnosis of suspected deep-vein thrombosis. N Engl J Med 349:1227, 2003.

A recent review of clinical prediction rules verified the Wells score as the most frequently evaluated in the literature and demonstrated high negative predictive values (median 96 percent, range 87 to 100 percent).[59] This highlights the fact that the determination of prediagnostic study risk is critical before proceeding to the selection and interpretation of diagnostic tests, regardless of the pretest model used.

Contrast Venography

Contrast venography is an invasive technique that involves the injection of dye into a vein distal to the site of suspected thrombosis, followed by imaging of multiple views of the lower extremity with x-ray study. DVTs are characterized by intraluminal filling defects seen on two or more views or an abrupt termination of contrast material. Traditionally considered the gold standard diagnostic test for DVT, venography has been assigned an arbitrary sensitivity and specificity of 100 percent.[60] However, given the limitations of patient intolerance and technical difficulty, this test cannot be performed in up to 20 percent of patients.[61] Moreover, the risks of radiation and contrast allergy (up to 5 percent) preclude its universal use, particularly in pregnancy.[62]

Venous Ultrasonography

The most common diagnostic modality employed in the evaluation of patients with suspected DVT is venous ultrasonography (VUS), with or without color Doppler. This modality has virtually replaced the cumbersome and less accurate impedance plethysmography technique. The ultrasound transducer is placed over the common femoral vein beginning at the inguinal ligament and then sequentially moved to image the greater saphenous vein, the superficial femoral vein, and the popliteal vein to its trifurcation with the deep veins of the calf. Compression VUS involves the application of pressure with the probe to determine whether the vein under investigation is compressible. The most accurate ultrasonic criterion for diagnosing venous thrombosis is noncompressibility of the venous lumen in a transverse plane under gentle probe pressure using duplex and color flow Doppler imaging.[55] The overall sensitivity and specificity of VUS has been reported at 90 to 100 percent for proximal vein thromboses but traditionally has been considered lower for the detection of calf vein thromboses.[63] However, a recent meta-analysis demonstrated that VUS identified isolated calf vein DVTs with a sensitivity of 92.5 percent, specificity of 98.7 percent, and accuracy of 97.2 percent.[64]

MAGNETIC RESONANCE IMAGING

Magnetic resonance imaging (MRI) appears to be superior to VUS and equivalent to contrast venography in diagnosing DVT. For the diagnosis of acute lower extremity DVT, MRI is reported to have a sensitivity of 100 percent (range 87 to 100 percent), a specificity of 100 percent (range 92 to 100 percent), and accuracy of 96 percent (range 89 to 99).[65] Furthermore, MRI is even more sensitive and accurate than VUS in the detection of pelvic and calf DVTs. In a prospective trial, MR venography performed as well as contrast venography.[66] Overall, the literature suggests that the ranges of sensitivity and specificity for MRI in the diagnosis of DVT are 80 to 100 percent and 90 to 100 percent, respectively, with median published rates of 100 percent for both.[60]

D-DIMER ASSAYS

Laboratory evaluation of serum concentrations of D-dimer, a product of the degradation of fibrin by plasmin, has been increasingly advocated as a helpful test in the diagnosis of DVT. Testing relies on the use of monoclonal antibodies to D-dimer fragments. The test is limited by factors that may contribute to false-positive testing, including pregnancy, the postpartum and postoperative periods, and superficial thrombophlebitis.[67,68] A meta-analysis in 2004 by Heim et al.[69] compared the accuracy of D-dimer testing with lower extremity VUS or contrast venography in symptomatic patients. A major limitation of this study consisted of the inclusion of 23 studies using 21 different D-dimer assays, and not surprisingly, the results demonstrated a wide variation in assay sensitivity, specificity, and negative predictive values, generally below 90 percent. The authors conclude that the use of the D-dimer assay as the sole screening test in the diagnosis of DVT is not supported by the literature. This work is supported by another meta-analysis from 1994 of studies evaluating patients with suspected DVT, demonstrating a sensitivity of 96.8 percent but a specificity of 35 to 45 percent.[70] In contrast, a recent prospective, randomized study by Wells et al. suggests that the use of more accurate D-dimer testing methods, when coupled with the Wells risk assessment scoring system (see Table 41-2), is an effective "rule-out" test. In this study, follow-up with lower extremity VUS was not necessary in patients with low pretest likelihood scores and negative D-dimer results, and moreover, these patients had a very low incidence of subsequent thrombosis.[58] It is unclear whether this simple paradigm is applicable in pregnancy because the Wells assessment system was not designed for, or tested in, pregnant patients and one could make an argument that pregnancy itself should be assigned a point within the scoring system because its thrombotic potential approaches that of a patient with active cancer. Conversely, D-dimer testing in pregnancy is likely to have a higher negative predictive value given the higher rate of false-positive D-dimer results. The most accurate and reliable tests for D-dimers appear to be two rapid enzyme-linked immunosorbent assays (ELISAs) (Instant-IA D-dimer, Stago, Asniéres, France and VIDAS DD, bioMérieux, Marcy-l'Etoile, France) and a rapid whole blood assay (SimpliRED D-dimer, Agen Biomedical, Brisbane, Australia).

WORKUP OF PATIENTS WITH SUSPECTED DEEP VEIN THROMBOSIS

The diagnostic paradigm outlined in Figure 41-2 can be employed to diagnose DVT in pregnant patients with maximal sensitivity and specificity. A major assumption of this strategy is the availability of a sensitive assay for D-dimer. When a D-dimer test is unavailable or inappropriate, the testing algorithm should begin with lower extremity compression sonography.

Pulmonary Embolus

CLINICAL SIGNS AND SYMPTOMS

Tachypnea (>20 breaths per minute) and tachycardia (>100 bpm) are present in 90 percent of patients with acute PE, but these findings lack specificity and generate a broad differential diagnosis.[71] Presyncope and syncope are rarer symptoms and indicate a massive embolus.[72] Scoring systems, similar to that for DVT, can be used to stratify high-risk and low-risk populations to modify the pretest probability and improve the accuracy of subsequent diagnostic tests. Table 41-3 presents one such system that stratifies patients into three risk groups: low (cumulative score <2), intermediate (score 2 to 6), and high (score >6). The prevalence of PE in each group is <10 percent, approximately 30 percent, and >70 percent, respectively.[72] More recently, a simplified adaptation of this risk scoring system has been proposed and validated.[73] In this paradigm, patients are categorized as either "PE unlikely" if their risk score is ≤4, which includes two thirds of all patients, or "PE likely" if their risk score was greater than 4. Caution should be used when applying any of these risk scoring systems in preg-

Table 41-3. APE Clinical Characteristic Score

RISK OR SIGN	POINTS
Clinical signs and symptoms of DVT	+3
Alternative diagnosis deemed less likely than PE	+3
Heart rate > 100 bpm	+1.5
Immobilization or surgery in previous 4 weeks	+1.5
Prior VTE	+1.5
Hemoptysis	+1
Active cancer	+1

APE, acute pulmonary embolus; DVT, deep vein thrombosis; VTE, venous thromboembolism.

Adapted from Fedullo P, Tapson V: The evaluation of suspected pulmonary embolism. N Engl J Med 349:1247, 2003.

nancy, because they have not been validated in pregnant patients. Furthermore, as is the case with DVT, given the thrombogenic nature of pregnancy, all pregnant patients could conceivably be considered high risk for thrombotic events.

NONSPECIFIC STUDIES

The classic electrocardiographic changes associated with PE are the S1, Q3, and inverted T3. Other findings include nonspecific ST changes, right bundle branch block, or right axis deviation. These findings are usually associated with cor pulmonale and right-sided heart strain or overload, reflective of more serious cardiopulmonary compromise. About 26 to 32 percent of patients with massive PE had the above-mentioned electrocardiographic changes.[74] Arterial blood gases and oxygen saturation have limited value in the assessment for acute PE (APE), particularly in a pregnant population. Measurements of Po_2 are greater than 80 mm Hg in 29 percent of PE patients younger than 40 years of age.[75] In another study, up to 18 percent of patients with APE had Po_2 measurements of more than 85 mm Hg.[71] The chest radiograph may be abnormal in up to 84 percent of affected patients.[71] The common findings on x-ray study are pleural effusion, pulmonary infiltrates, atelectasis, and elevated hemidiaphragm. The eponymous findings of pulmonary infarction such as a wedge-shaped infiltrate (Hampton's hump) or decreased vascularity (Westermark's sign) are rare.[60] Although a normal chest X-ray in the setting of dyspnea, tachypnea, and hypoxemia in a patient without known preexistent pulmonary or cardiovascular disease is suggestive of PE, a chest radiograph cannot be used to confirm the diagnosis.[60]

An acute, large PE can create changes consistent with cor pulmonale and right-sided heart strain. Large emboli in the main pulmonary artery and its primary branches can result in acute right-sided heart failure, which is the ultimate cause of death in most patients with APE. Between 30 and 80 percent of patients with PE display echocardiographic abnormalities in right ventricular size or function.[76–78] Typical findings include a dilated and hypokinetic right ventricle, tricuspid regurgitation, and absence of preexisting pulmonary arterial or left-sided heart pathology. Transesophageal echocardiography with or without contrast appears to improve the imaging of main or right pulmonary artery emboli and, occasionally, of left pulmonary artery clots.[79]

PULMONARY ARTERIOGRAPHY

Until the advent of sensitive multidetector-row computerized tomographic (CT) pulmonary angiography (spiral CT), intravenous contrast pulmonary arteriography or angiography was considered the gold standard for diagnosis of PE, and as such, has a sensitivity and specificity of 100 percent.[60] However, the sensitivity and interobserver agreement of traditional pulmonary angiography for smaller peripheral lesions decreases from 98 percent for lobar emboli, to 90 percent for segmental, and to 66 percent for subsegmental emboli.[80] This technique involves venous catheterization, typically through the right femoral vein, although the basilic and right internal jugular veins can also be used. An intraluminal filling defect on two views of a pulmonary artery confirms the diagnosis of PE. Of all diagnostic modalities, this technique involves the highest risk, including a 0.5 percent mortality risk and a 3 percent complication rate, primarily due to the risks of contrast injection and catheter placement, including respiratory failure (0.4 percent), renal failure (0.3 percent), cardiac perforation (1 percent), and groin hematoma requiring transfusion (0.2 percent).[72,80–82] Relative contraindications to the procedure include renal insufficiency and settings of significant hemorrhage risk (e.g., disseminated intravascular coagulation or thrombocytopenia). Patients with evidence of cardiopulmonary compromise do pose a higher complication risk. Left bundle branch block should be treated with a temporary pacemaker during the procedure to avoid induction of complete heart block.[60]

VENTILATION-PERFUSION SCANNING

Until the advent of spiral CT, the ventilation-perfusion (V/Q) scan played a critical role in the diagnosis of PE for many decades. This test used comparative imaging of the pulmonary vascular bed and airspace.[55] Perfusion scanning employed intravenously injected radioisotope-labeled albumin macroaggregates that deposited in the pulmonary capillary bed. Ventilation scanning involved the inhalation of radiolabeled aerosols whose distribution was evaluated by gamma camera. The comparison of these two images allowed for interpretation of characteristic patterns that were then used to assign diagnostic probabilities (high, intermediate, or low). The interpretation of this testing often relied on factoring for the level of pretest clinical suspicion based on the patient's signs, symptoms, and other nondiagnostic test results. Greater than 90 percent of high risk patients with high probability V/Q scans had PE, whereas less than 6 percent of low-risk patients with low probability scans had a PE.

The Prospective Investigation of Pulmonary Embolism Diagnosis (PIOPED) study was a multicenter effort designed to evaluate the accuracy of V/Q scanning in nearly 1,000 patients with suspected PE.[83] Overall, patients with high-probability V/Q scans had a PE in 87.2 percent of cases; however, only 41 percent of patients with a PE had high probability scans, demonstrating a sensitivity of 41 percent and specificity of 97 percent. When the patients were stratified according to pretest risk, high-probability V/Q results were associated with PE in 95 percent, 86 percent, and 56 percent of high, moderate, and low risk patients, respectively. Intermediate-probability, low-probability, and normal scans were associated each with 33.3 percent, 13.5 percent, and 3.9 percent risks of PE, respectively.

The results of PIOPED indicate that PE can be present in a substantial proportion of patients with low and intermediate scans if the clinical suspicion is high, and that 44 percent of low-risk patients with a high-probability scan do not have PE. This emphasizes the importance of pretest risk stratification of the patient undergoing workup for PE but also points out the limitations of the V/Q scan as a diagnostic modality. In cases of nondiagnostic V/Q results, further testing is critical to avoid catastrophic consequences of undiagnosed PE or the hazards and inconveniences of unnecessary anticoagulation.

Spiral Computed Tomographic Pulmonary Angiography (Spiral Computed Tomography)

Spiral CT scanning has rapidly evolved into the preferred screening and diagnostic modality for PE. It requires injection of intravenous contrast while simultaneously imaging the distribution of contrast in the pulmonary vasculature with a CT scanner.[60] Although this can be an effective judge of large, segmental, and central emboli, CT is of more limited value with small subsegmental vessels and horizontally oriented vessels in the right middle lobe. Cross et al. initially compared spiral CT with V/Q scanning for initial assessment of patients with suspected PE and showed that the rate of definitive positive or negative diagnosis was significantly higher for spiral CT than for V/Q scans (90 percent versus 54 percent), although the rate of detection of PE in each group was not different.[84] Furthermore, CT could demonstrate nonembolic reasons for the patients' symptoms (e.g., pneumonia) more often, adding more information to aid in clinical management.

A meta-analysis in 2004 of 23 studies demonstrated a very low 3-month rate of subsequent thromboembolic events and fatal PE after a negative spiral CT (1.4 percent and 0.51 percent respectively), results that are comparable to a negative pulmonary angiogram or a normal or near-normal V/Q scan.[85] Newer technology and thinner CT sections appear to improve the accuracy of spiral CT for diagnosing small vessel emboli and may reduce overall false-negative results to 5 percent.[86]

Magnetic Resonance Angiography

Magnetic resonance angiography (MRA) may be performed using MRI of a patient during intravenous injection of gadolinium. Faster image acquisition rates and improved image timing to respiratory and cardiac motion have allowed this technique to develop. Preliminary experience by Meaney and colleagues suggested a sensitivity of 100 percent, specificity of 95 percent, and positive and negative predictive values of 87 percent and 100 percent, respectively, for MRA in 30 patients also assessed by classic pulmonary angiography.[87] Another prospective study involving 141 patients showed an overall sensitivity of only 77 percent in comparison to pulmonary angiography, with the sensitivity broken down to 40 percent, 84 percent, and 100 percent for isolated subsegmental, segmental and central pulmonary emboli, respectively.[88] Because MRA does not involve ionizing radiation, it is an appealing alternative to CT scanning and angiography for pregnancy, and further assessment in large trials are needed to prove its ultimate utility as a primary diagnostic modality.

D-Dimer Assays

As with evaluation of DVT, D-dimer is a very sensitive, but not specific, test for PE. A negative D-dimer concentration (<500 ng/mL), measured by sensitive ELISA, is associated with a 95-percent negative predictive value but only a 25-percent specificity for the diagnosis of PE in nonpregnant patients.[60] A meta-analysis of studies examining the accuracy of D-dimer concentrations in the diagnosis of PE showed a sensitivity of 95 percent (88 to 100 percent), specificity of 45 percent (38 to 53 percent), and positive and negative likelihood ratios of 1.74 (1.55 to 1.91) and 0.11 (0.03 to 0.39), respectively.[89] Again, however, the accuracy of D-dimer testing depends on the particular assay used. A quantitative rapid ELISA assay demonstrated a sensitivity of 98 percent, specificity of 40 percent, and positive and negative likelihood ratios of 1.62 and 0.05, respectively, whereas the whole blood D-dimer assay yielded a lower sensitivity (82 percent) but higher specificity (63 percent) with positive and negative likelihood ratios of 2.21 and 0.28, respectively.[89] The authors of that study conclude that a negative result on the quantitative rapid ELISA assay is as reliable as a normal lung scan in ruling out PE. Because of physiologic increases in D-dimer in pregnancy and after surgery, the specificity for diagnosis of PE in antepartum and postpartum patients is probably lower, although the negative predictive value is probably higher. Thus, a negative D-dimer in a pregnant patient may effectively rule out PE in pregnancy.

Lower Extremity Evaluation

Most (90 percent) PEs arise from lower extremity DVTs, and among patients with the diagnosis of PE, half will be found to harbor a lower extremity DVT, including up to 20 percent of PE patients without signs or symptoms of lower extremity DVT.[72] Thus, in stable high-risk patients in whom V/Q scanning or other noninvasive testing is not diagnostic, or even negative, evaluation of the leg veins for DVT can establish the need for anticoagulation if a DVT is diagnosed. In such cases, however, a negative venous ultrasound study is still associated with a 25-percent risk of PE, suggesting that further studies are generally needed.[90]

Workup of Patients with Suspected Pulmonary Embolus

Evaluation of patients with suspected PE must begin with a pretest risk determination (see Table 41-3). D-dimer testing may be useful, given its strong negative predictive value particularly in antepartum, postpartum, and postoperative patients, depending on the availability of a sensitive ELISA or whole blood assay. If a patient presents with concomitant symptoms of DVT, noninvasive lower extremity venous assessment should be performed first, because a diagnosis of DVT will mandate treatment irrespective of the pulmonary findings. There is an emerging consensus that spiral CT scanning should be the first-line diagnostic modality.

Figure 41-3 outlines a traditional testing paradigm for patients with suspected PE. Evaluation begins with either a spiral CT or V/Q scan. If results return positive or high probability for CT or V/Q, respectively, a PE is "ruled in" and treatment initiated. If the V/Q returns normal or near normal, a PE is "ruled out" and no treatment begun. If the patient has a negative spiral CT or her V/Q scan returns low or intermediate probability, additional tests are ordered, beginning with VUS. If the results of this test are positive, she is treated as if she has a PE. If this test returns negative, an intravenous contrast pulmonary angiogram is initiated. If the results of this "definitive" test are negative, a PE is "ruled out" whereas a positive result, per force, mandates treatment.

An alternative approach is suggested by the work of van Belle and colleagues.[73] They conducted a large, prospective, observational study involving more than 3,000 nonpregnant patients with signs and symptoms suggestive of PE in order to assess the diagnostic value of a combination of risk scoring, D-dimer assay and spiral CT. As described earlier, this simplified paradigm classified risk as either "PE unlikely" (see Table 41-3 score ≤4) or "PE likely" (Table 41-3 score >4). Those classified as "unlikely" had D-dimer testing, and PE was ruled out if the D-dimer test result was normal. All other patients (i.e., "PE likely," and "PE unlikely" with positive D-dimer) underwent spiral CT, most with the more sensitive multidetector-row methodology. A PE was considered present or excluded based on the CT results. The combination of "PE unlikely" and a normal D-dimer test result occurred in about one third of patients, a group who avoided additional testing and in whom subsequent nonfatal thrombotic events occurred in 0.5 percent within 3 months. In the other two thirds of patients requiring spiral CT, a PE was detected in 20.1 percent, and these patients received treatment. Of the remaining 45.5 percent of patients in whom the CT angiogram was negative, 95 percent were not treated and the prevalence of subsequent fatal PE was less than 1 percent, a risk that is comparable to the rate of fatal PE after a negative intravenous contrast pulmonary angiogram. Thus, this very simple diagnostic paradigm employing a simple clinical decision tree, D-dimer testing, and CT angiography may be the optimal screening approach. However, this approach has not been validated in pregnancy. Caveats include the lack of precise applicability of Table 41-3's scoring system to pregnancy, the availability of sensitive D-dimer testing, and sensitive multidetector-row spiral CT methodology.

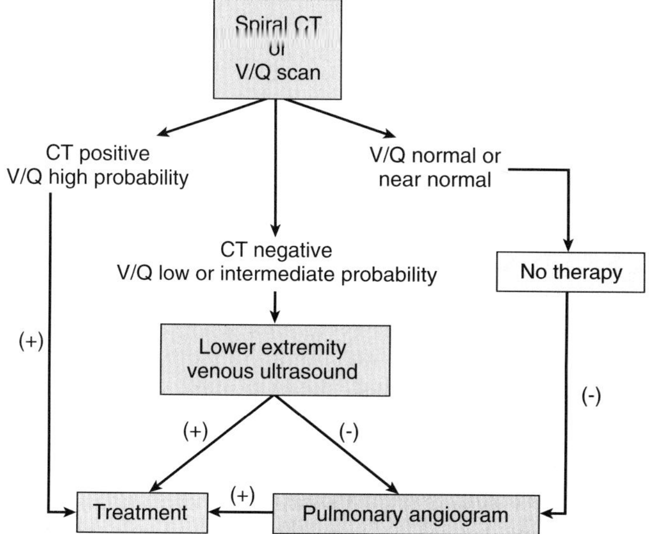

Figure 41-3. Traditional diagnostic algorithm for pulmonary embolism.

Figure 41-4 presents our adaptation of this simplified diagnostic paradigm to pregnancy. Patients with an "unlikely" risk score receive D-dimer testing. If negative, VUS is performed, and if VUS is negative, PE is ruled out. If the VUS is positive, the patient is presumptively treated

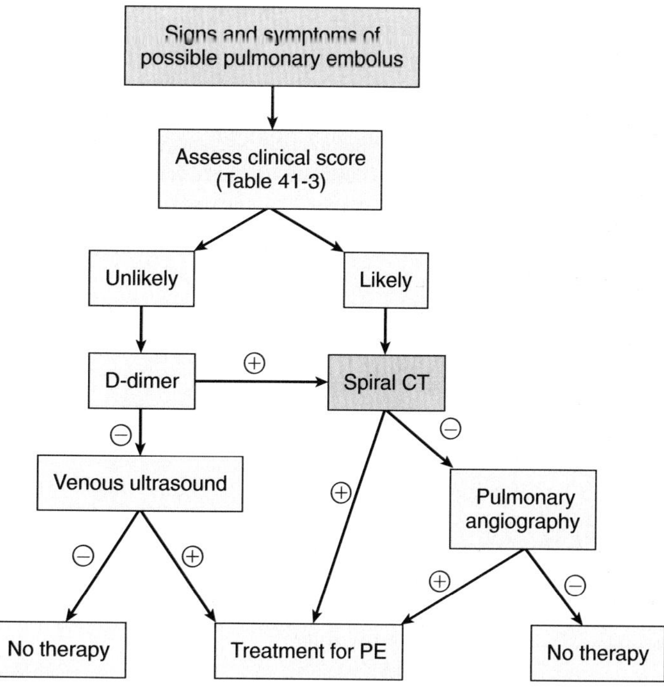

Figure 41-4. Alternative diagnostic approach of suspected pulmonary embolism.

for a PE. For patients whose risk score falls in the "likely" category or for "unlikely" patients who are D-dimer positive, a spiral CT is performed. If this is positive, treatment is begun. If this is negative, and the index of suspicion remains high, an intravenous contrast pulmonary angiogram is obtained. If this is negative, the diagnosis is ruled out. If positive, the patient is treated for a PE. It should be stressed that this diagnostic algorithm has not been tested in a prospective fashion. Moreover, MR pulmonary angiography may replace intravenous contrast pulmonary angiography in some centers. Finally, some radiology departments may have sufficient confidence in their spiral CT sensitivity to forgo contrast pulmonary angiography.

Radiation Exposure in Pregnancy

The diagnosis of DVT and PE in pregnant patients poses unique challenges because of concerns of fetal radiation exposure. The American College of Obstetricians and Gynecologists advises that exposure to less than 5 rads has not been associated with increases in pregnancy loss or fetal anomalies.[91] Exposure to ionizing radiation doses above 1 rad, however, may create a marginally increased risk of childhood leukemia (from 1/3,000 baseline to 1/2,000).[92,93] Table 41-4 outlines the radiation exposure of different radiation modalities. A combination of chest radiograph, V/Q scan, and pulmonary angiography exposes the fetus to less than 0.5 rads.[6] Although the concern for possible adverse effects should not prevent a medically important test from being performed, judicious use and selection of tests is advised.

MRI and ultrasonography have not been associated with any adverse fetal effects, and teratogenic effects have not been described after administration of gadolinium contrast media.[94] Concerns about fetal goiter following maternal radiographic contrast exposure suggest that fetal heart rates should be assessed to rule out hypothyroidism and neonatal thyroid function should be tested during the first week of life.[94]

Table 41-4. Fetal Radiation Exposure of Various Ionizing Modalities

RADIOLOGIC MODALITY	FETAL RADIATION EXPOSURE (RADS)
Chest X-Ray Study	<0.01
Venography	
Limited, shielded	<0.05
Full (unilateral), unshielded	0.31
Pulmonary Angiography	
Brachial vein	0.05
Femoral vein	0.22–0.37
V/Q Scan	
Ventilation scan	0.001–0.019
Perfusion scan	0.006–0.012
Spiral CT	0.013

CT, computed tomography; V/Q, ventilation perfusion scan.
Adapted from Toglia M, Weg J: Venous thromboembolism during pregnancy. N Engl J Med 335:108, 1996.

TREATMENT OF THROMBOEMBOLISM IN PREGNANCY

Unfractionated Heparin

Unfractionated heparin effects anticoagulation by enhancing antithrombin activity, increasing factor Xa inhibitor activity, and inhibiting platelet aggregation.[95] Unfractionated heparin (FDA category C) does not cross the placenta and is not teratogenic.[96] Heparin also does not enter breast milk and is considered safe for breastfeeding. The chief side effects of heparin include hemorrhage, osteoporosis and thrombocytopenia. The former is more common with treatment coinciding with surgery or liver disease or concomitant aspirin use. Heparin-associated bone loss is usually reversible, and correlates more with therapy exceeding 15,000 units/day for more than 6 months and can be opposed by supplemental calcium use (1,500 mg/day).[97,98] Heparin-induced thrombocytopenia (HIT) occurs in 3 percent of patients. Type I HIT is the most common form, occurs within days of exposure, is self-limited, and is not associated with a significant risk of hemorrhage or thrombosis. Immunoglobulin-mediated type II HIT, on the other hand, is rare, usually occurs 5 to 14 days following initiation of therapy, and paradoxically increases the risk of thrombosis. Monitoring for HIT should include serial platelet counts until day 14, or until heparin is stopped, whichever occurs first.[99] A 50-percent decline in platelet count from its pretreatment maximum suggests the immune-mediated HIT type II and should prompt cessation of all heparin exposure, including that in intravenous flushes. The diagnosis of HIT type II can be confirmed by serotonin release assays, heparin-induced platelet aggregation assays, flow cytometry, or solid-phase immunoassays.[100]

Protamine sulfate reverses the effect of intravenously administered unfractionated heparin. It is given by low intravenous infusion of less than 20 mg/min, with no more than 50 mg given over 10 minutes. The total dose of protamine required is calculated based on the residual amount of circulating heparin, with a ratio of 1 mg of protamine sulfate necessary for every 100 units of residual circulating heparin. Residual heparin is calculated by assuming a half-life of 30 to 60 minutes of intravenous heparin. However, repeated serial administrations of lower doses of protamine, coinciding with serial measurements of the activated partial thromboplastin time (aPTT), are required when the heparin is dosed subcutaneously.

Low-Molecular-Weight Heparin

The low-molecular-weight heparins (LMWHs; dalteparin, enoxaparin, and tinzaparin) are reliable and safe alternatives to unfractionated heparin and have fewer side effects. Enzymatic manipulation of standard heparin produces lower molecular weight molecules with equivalent antifactor Xa, but little or no antithrombin effects. The LMWHs have longer half lives, and a closer correlation between antifactor Xa activity and body weight than subcutaneously administered unfractionated heparin. However, we follow antifactor Xa levels in pregnant patients because there is far greater variability in binding, distribution, metabolism, and excretion. The LMWHs (pregnancy category B) do not cross the placenta and do not enter breast milk. There is a lower risk of hemorrhage associated with LMWH. However, regional anesthesia is contraindicated within 18 to 24 hours of therapeutic LMWH administration. Accordingly, we recommend switching to unfractionated heparin at 36 weeks or earlier if preterm delivery is expected. Protamine is not as effective in fully reversing the antifactor Xa activity of LMWH, although it may reduce bleeding. Dosing of 1 mg of protamine for every 100 antifactor Xa units of LMWH can normalize aPTT values, but antifactor Xa levels can only be reversed by 80 percent.[101,102] The risk of HIT type II is also lower in patients receiving LMWH; however, platelet counts should still be checked every 2 to 3 days from day 4 to day 14.[99,103,104]

Fondaparinux

Fondaparinux is a synthetic heparin pentasaccharide that complexes with the antithrombin binding site for heparin to permit the selective inactivation of factor Xa, but not thrombin. A major advantage of this medication is that there does not appear to be a risk of HIT type II. It has comparable efficacy to both LMWH and unfractionated heparin in nonpregnant patients.[105,106] Although it has been used in a small number of pregnant patients without complication, umbilical cord plasma concentrations at 10 percent of those of maternal plasma have been demonstrated, suggesting limited transplacental passage.[107] Use of fondaparinux should be limited to women without other therapeutic alternatives, such as those with a history of HIT type II or heparin allergies.

Coumarin

The coumarins are vitamin K antagonists that block the vitamin K dependent, function-enhancing posttranslational modifications of prothrombin and factors VII, IX, and X, as well as the anticlotting agents protein C and S. Coumadin (Warfarin) has been shown to be effective for both the primary and secondary prevention of VTE, stroke, myocardial infarction, and systemic embolism due to artificial valves and atrial fibrillation.[108] Coumadin is a pregnancy category X medication because fetal exposure can cause nasal and midface hypoplasia, microphthalmia, mental retardation, and other ocular, skeletal, and central nervous system malformations (see Chapter 8). Teratogenic potential is greatest between the 6th and 12th weeks of pregnancy. The risk of warfarin also includes fetal hemorrhage. As a result, warfarin is rarely employed, although the exceptional case of a patient requiring therapeutic anticoagulation, who cannot be sufficiently treated with the heparins, may require its use. Warfarin is also a favored drug for the postpartum period because it is safe to use during lactation.

Therapy is started at a dose of 5 to 10 mg for 2 days, with subsequent doses titrated to achieve an international normalized ratio (INR) of 2.0 to 3.0. Peak effects occur within 72 hours, and its half life is from 36 to 42 hours.[108] Because of protein C's shorter half life relative to the other vitamin K–dependent clotting factors, warfarin may initially create a prothrombotic state, particularly in pregnancy. Thus, patients who are initiated on warfarin should be on therapeutic doses of unfractionated or LMWH for 5 days and until the INR is therapeutic for 48 hours. Coumadin effects can be reversed by vitamin K.[109] The INR generally normalizes within 6 hours of a 5 mg dose of vitamin K and within 4 days with cessation of warfarin therapy. Fresh-frozen plasma can be used to achieve immediate reversal of effects.

Treatment of Acute Deep Vein Thrombosis or Pulmonary Embolus

Women with new-onset VTE diagnosed during pregnancy should receive therapeutic anticoagulation. Therapeutic anticoagulation should be continued for at least 20 weeks. If this period of time expires before the end of the postpartum period, prophylactic anticoagulation should be initiated in patients without highly thrombogenic thrombophilias and continued for 6 weeks to 6 months postpartum, depending on the severity of the thrombotic event and the underlying risk factors. During pregnancy, unfractionated heparin and the LMWHs are the drugs of choice, given their efficacy and safety profile. Therapeutic doses of the LMWH enoxaparin may start at 1 mg/kg, subcutaneously, twice daily. Dosing should be titrated to achieve antifactor Xa levels of 0.6 to 1.0 U/mL when tested 4 hours after injection because of inconsistent efficacy of this weight based regimen in pregnant patients.[110] Unfractionated heparin for acute DVT or PE is initially given intravenously and titrated to keep the activated partial thromboplastin time (aPTT) 1.5 to 2.5 times control (checked every 4 to 6 hours during the titration period), usually according to weight-based protocols (Table 41-5).[111] Intravenous heparin should be continued for 5 to 10 days or until clinical improvement is noted. This can be changed to subcutaneous injections every 8 to 12 hours to keep the aPTT 1.5 to 2.0 times control, when tested 6 hours after injection.

As noted earlier, the major concerns of therapeutic anticoagulation in pregnancy are regional anesthesia use and hemorrhage risk. Regional anesthesia is contraindicated within 18 to 24 hours of therapeutic LMWH use; thus LMWH should be converted to unfractionated heparin at 36 weeks or earlier if clinically indicated. Vaginal or cesarean delivery greater than 24 hours after therapeutic LMWH dosing should not pose a risk of hemorrhage, although protamine sulfate may be necessary to partially reverse anticoagulation. Protamine sulfate may also be used to normalize completely an elevated aPTT in patients on therapeutic unfractionated heparin near the time of delivery. Heparin anticoagulation may be restarted 3 to 6 hours after vaginal delivery and 6 to 8 hours after cesarean delivery. Coumadin anticoagulation may be started on the first postpartum or postoperative day. As noted earlier, because of the paradoxical increase in activated protein C resistance and factor VIII

Table 41-5. Weight-based Nomogram for Unfractionated Heparin

Give a bolus of 80 U per kg, followed by a maintenance dosage of 18 U/kg/h following aPTT values every 6 hours and with following adjustments for aPTT values obtained:

APTT VALUE	ADJUSTMENT
<35 seconds (<1.2 X control value)	Repeat full bolus (80 U/kg), then increase infusion rate by 4 U/kg/h
35–45 seconds (1.2–1.5 X control)	Repeat half bolus (40 U/kg), then increase infusion rate by 2 U/kg/h
46–70 seconds (1.6–2.3 X control)	No change in infusion rate
71–90 seconds (2.4–3 X control)	Decrease infusion rate by 2 U/kg/h
>90 seconds (>3 X control)	Stop infusion for one hour, then decrease to 3 U/kg/h

aPTT, activated partial thromboplastin time.

Adapted from Raschke R, Reilly B, Guidry J, et al: The weight-based heparin dosing nomogram compared with a "standard care" nomogram. A randomized controlled trial. Ann Intern Med 119:874, 1993.

after starting coumadin, therapeutic doses of the heparins should be continued for 5 days and until the INR reaches therapeutic range (2.0 to 3.0) for 2 successive days.

Prophylactic Applications and Dosing

We recommend prophylactic *antepartum* and postpartum anticoagulation in patients with high-risk thrombophilias and no personal or family history of venous thrombosis, and in patients with low-risk thrombophilias but with family (first-degree relative) or personal history of venous thrombosis. Prophylactic postpartum therapy is warranted in all patients with low-risk thrombophilias without a personal or family history of thrombosis after a cesarean delivery. Prophylactic doses of the LMWH enoxaparin may start at 40 mg subcutaneously daily. Weight-based dosing in pregnant patients may be unreliable, and we suggest titrating doses to achieve anti-factor Xa levels of 0.1 to 0.2 U/mL 4 hours after injection. Unfractionated heparin prophylaxis may range from 5,000 to 10,000 units subcutaneously every 12 hours. Because of inconsistent efficacy in pregnant patients, this dosing should be titrated to achieve heparin levels (by protamine titration assay) of 0.1 to 0.2 U/mL.[112]

The risk of hemorrhage or complication from regional anesthesia is minimal greater than 12 hours after prophylactic LMWH. Again, given the difficulty of timing administration with the onset of labor, we recommend converting from LMWH to unfractionated heparin at 36 weeks or earlier as clinically indicated. As with therapeutic use, anticoagulation may be restarted 3 to 6 hours and 6 to 8 hours after vaginal and cesarean delivery respectively.

Other Considerations of Therapy and Prevention

Perioperative Prevention

There is very limited evidence regarding the value of perioperative thromboprophylaxis with cesarean delivery.[113,114] Perioperative administration of low-dose unfractionated heparin may be appropriate in patients undergoing cesarean delivery with clear risk factors such as obesity, malignancy, immobility, or a high-risk chronic medical disease. As noted, patients with low thrombogenic thrombophilias require postoperative prophylaxis.

Nonpharmacologic interventions aimed at preventing VTE include graduated elastic compression stockings and pneumatic compression devices. In pregnancy, a cohort study suggested that the use of graduated compression stockings reduced the prevalence of postpartum VTE from 4.3 to 0.9 percent.[115] Because these stockings and pneumatic compression devices pose no hemorrhagic risk and little harm, they should be strongly considered for thromboprophylaxis in all pregnant patients. The left lateral decubitus position in the third trimester may also reduce the risk of VTE.

Inferior Vena Cava Filters

The use of inferior vena cava (IVC) filters is primarily restricted to patients with absolute contraindications to medical anticoagulation or those who have failed therapeutic anticoagulation. Pregnant patients with a history of HIT type II or with true heparin or LMWH allergies in need of prophylaxis are potential candidates for IVC filters. However, the introduction of fondaparinux may eliminate this need. The use of IVC filters is discouraged in younger patients, but newer retrievable filters may be appropriate.[116]

Key Points

- Pregnancy, childbirth, and the puerperium pose serious hemorrhagic challenges that are met by increased decidual and systemic clotting potential.
- VTE is a leading cause of mortality and serious morbidity in pregnant women, having a prevalence of 1/1,000 to 1/2,000 pregnancies with the greatest risk of fatal PE occurring following caesarean deliveries.
- Inherited and acquired thrombophilias account for most VTEs in pregnancy.
- Because the positive predictive value of a test increases with the prevalence of the disease to be detected, the key to accurate diagnosis of either DVT or PE is the initial assessment of patient risk.

- D-dimer testing is used in the evaluation of low-risk patients with suspected VTE because of its high negative predictive value; pregnancy likely confers an even higher negative predictive value given the higher rate of false-positive D-dimer results.

- Venous compression ultrasonography is the most common diagnostic modality employed in the evaluation of patients with suspected DVT, with an overall sensitivity and specificity of 90 to 100 percent for proximal vein thromboses.

- Spiral computed tomographic pulmonary angiography (spiral CT) is now the preferred screening and diagnostic modality for PE with a very low 3-month rate of subsequent VTE after a negative spiral CT.

- Heparin remains the mainstay of therapy for VTE, with its most serious but rare complication being immunoglobulin-mediated HIT type II which usually occurs 5 to 14 days following initiation of therapy and paradoxically increases the risk of thrombosis.

- Protamine sulfate can entirely reverse the anticoagulant effect of unfractionated heparin and partially (80 percent) reverse the effect of low-molecular-weight heparin.

- Graduated elastic compression stockings and pneumatic compression devices appear to reduce the likelihood of VTE in pregnancy and, at a minimum, should be used in all high-risk patients undergoing cesarean delivery.

REFERENCES

1. Ginsberg J, Brill-Edwards P, Burrows R, et al: Venous thrombosis during pregnancy: leg and trimester of presentation. Thromb Haemost 67:519, 1992.
2. Kierkegaard A: Incidence and diagnosis of deep vein thrombosis associated with pregnancy. Acta Obstet Gynecol Scand 62:239, 1983.
3. Rutherford S, Montoro M, McGehee W, Strong T: Thromboembolic disease associated with pregnancy: an 11-year review (SPO Abstract). Obstetr Gynecol 164:286 1991.
4. Simpson E, Lawrenson R, Nightingale A, Farmer R: Venous thromboembolism in pregnancy and the puerperium: incidence and additional risk factors from a London perinatal database. BJOG 108:56, 2001.
5. Stein P, Hull R, Jayali F, et al: Venous thromboembolism in pregnancy: 21-year trends. Am J Med 117:121, 2004.
6. Toglia M, Weg J: Venous thromboembolism during pregnancy. N Engl J Med 335:108, 1996.
7. Treffers P, Huidekoper B, Weenink G, Kloosterman G: Epidemiological observations of thrombo-embolic disease during pregnancy and the puerperium, in 56,022 women. Int J Gynaecol Obstet 21:327, 1983.
8. James K, Lohr J, Deshmukh R, Cranley J: Venous thrombotic complications of pregnancy. Cardiovasc Surg 4:777, 1996.
9. McColl M, Ramsay J, Tait R, et al: Risk factors for pregnancy associated venous thromboembolism. Thromb Haemost 78:1183, 1997.
10. Chang J, Elam-Evans L, Berg C, et al: Pregnancy-related mortality surveillance—United States, 1991–1999. MMWR Surveillance Studies 52:1, 2003.
11. Macklon N, Greer I: Venous thromboembolic disease in obstetrics and gynecology: the Scottish experience. Scott Med J 41:83, 1996.
12. Bergqvist D, Hedner U: Pregnancy and venous thrombo-embolism. Acta Obstet Gynecol Scand 62:449, 1983.
13. Bergqvist A, Bergqvist D, Hallbrook T: Deep vein thrombosis during pregnancy: a prospective study. Acta Obstet Gynecol Scand 62:443, 1983.
14. Girling J, de Swiet M: Inherited thrombophilia and pregnancy. Curr Opin Obstet Gynecol 10:135,1998.
15. Ruggeri Z, Dent J, Saldivar E: Contribution of distinct adhesive interactions to platelet aggregation in flowing blood. Blood 94:172, 1999.
16. Pytela R, Pierschbacher M, Ginsberg M, et al: Platelet membrane glycoprotein IIb/IIIa: member of a family of Arg-Gly-Asp-specific adhesion receptors. Science 231:1559, 1986.
17. Nemerson Y: Tissue factor and hemostasis. Blood 71:1, 1988.
18. Preissner K, de Boer H, Pannekoek H, de Groot P: Thrombin regulation by physiological inhibitors: the role of vitronectin. Semin Thromb Hemost 165:1335, 1996.
19. Lockwood C, Bach R, Guha A, et al: Amniotic fluid contains tissue factor, a potent initiator of coagulation. Am J Obstet Gynecol 165:1335, 1991.
20. Mackman N: Role of tissue factor in hemostasis, thrombosis, and vascular development. Arterioscler Thromb Vasc Biol 24:1015, 2004.
21. Broze G: The rediscovery and isolation of TFPI. J Thromb Haemost 1:1671, 2003.
22. Dahlback B: Progress in the understanding of the protein C anticoagulant pathway. Int J Hematol 79:109, 2004.
23. Broze G: Protein Z–dependent regulation of coagulation. Thromb Haemost 86:8, 2001.
24. Preissner K, Zwicker L, Muller-Berghaus G: Formation, characterization and detection of a ternary complex between protein S, thrombin and antithrombin III in serum. Biochem J 243:105, 1987.
25. Bouma B, Meijers J: New insights into factors affecting clot stability: a role for thrombin activatable fibrinolysis inhibitor. Semin Hematol 41:13, 2004.
26. Schatz F, Lockwood C: Progestin regulation of plasminogen activator inhibitor type-1 in primary cultures of endometrial stromal and decidual cells. J Clin Endocrinol Metab 77:621, 1993.
27. Lockwood C, Krikun G, Schatz F: The decidua regulates hemostasis in the human endometrium. Semin Reprod Endocrinol 17:45, 1999.
28. Bremme K: Haemostatic changes in pregnancy. Baillieres Clin Haematol 16:153, 2003.
29. Hellgren M, Blomback M: Studies on blood coagulation and fibrinolysis in pregnancy, during delivery and in the puerperium. Gynecol Obstet Invest 12:141, 1981.
30. Wright H, Osborn S, Edmunds D: Changes in the rate of flow of venous blood in the leg during pregnancy, measured with radioactive sodium. Surg Gynecol Obstet 90:481, 1950.
31. Goodrich S, Wood J: Peripheral venous distensibility and velocity of venous blood flow during pregnancy or during oral contraceptive therapy. Am J Obstet Gynecol 90:740, 1964.
32. Macklon N, Greer I, Bowman A: An ultrasound study of gestational and postural changes in the deep venous system of the leg in pregnancy. BJOG 104:191–7, 1997.
33. Hull R, Raskob G, Carter C: Serial impedance plethysmography in pregnant patients with clinically suspected deep-vein thrombosis: clinical validity of negative findings. Ann Intern Med 112:663, 1990.
34. Ginsberg J, Wells P, Brill-Edwards P, et al: Antiphospholipid antibodies and venous thromboembolism. Blood 86:3685, 1995.
35. Wilson W, Gharavi A, Kolke T, et al: International consensus statement on preliminary classification criteria for definite antiphospholipid syndrome: report of an international workshop. Arthritis Rheum 42:1309, 1999.
36. Galli M, Barbui T: Antiphospholipid antibodies and thrombosis: strength of association. Hematol J 4:180, 2003.
37. Lockwood C, Romero R, Feinberg R, et al: The prevalence and biologic significance of lupus anticoagulant and anticardiolipin antibodies in the general obstetric population. Am J Obstet Gynecol 161:369, 1989.

38. Wahl D, Guillemin F, de Maistre E, et al: Risk for venous thrombosis related to antiphospholipid antibodies in systemic lupus erythematous—a meta-analysis. Lupus 6:646, 1997.
39. Galli M, Luciani D, Bertolini G, Barbui T: Anti-beta 2-glycoprotein I, antiprothrombin antibodies, and the risk of thrombosis in the antiphospholipid syndrome. Blood 102:2717, 2003.
40. Garcia-Fuster M, Fernandez C, Forner M, Vaya A: Risk factors and clinical characteristics of thromboembolic venous disease in young patients: a prospective study. Med Clin (Barc) 123:217, 2004.
41. Branch D, Silver R, Blackwell J, et al: Outcome of treated pregnancies in women with antiphospholipid syndrome: an update of the Utah experience. Obstet Gynecol 80:612, 1992.
42. Zotz R, Gerhardt A, Scharf R: Inherited thrombophilia and gestational venous thromboembolism. Baillieres Clini Haematol 16:243, 2003.
43. Gerhardt A, Scharf R, Beckmann M, et al: Prothrombin and factor V mutations in women with a history of thrombosis during pregnancy and the puerperium. N Engl J Med 342:374, 2000.
44. Juul K, Tybjaerg-Hansen A, Steffensen R, et al: Factor V Leiden: The Copenhagen City Heart Study and 2 meta-analyses. Blood 100:3, 2002.
45. Price D, Ridker P: Factor V Leiden mutation and the risks for thromboembolic disease: a clinical perspective. Ann Intern Med 127:895, 1997.
46. Franco R, Reitsma P: Genetic risk factors of venous thrombosis. Hum Genet 109:369, 2001.
47. Friedrich P, Sanson B, Simioni P, et al: Frequency of pregnancy-related venous thromboembolism in anticoagulant factor–deficient women: implications for prophylaxis. Ann Intern Med 125:955, 1996.
48. Aznar J, Vaya A, Estelles A, et al: Risk of venous thrombosis in carriers of the prothrombin G20210A variant and factor V Leiden and their interaction with oral contraceptives. Hematologica 85:1271, 2000.
49. Emmerich J, Rosendaal F, Cattaneo M, et al: Combined effect of factor V Leiden and prothrombin 20210A on the risk of venous thromboembolism-pooled analysis of 8 case-control studies including 2310 cases and 3204 controls. Study Group for Pooled-Analysis in Venous Thromboembolism. Thromb Haemost 86:809, 2001.
50. Ridker P, Miletich J, Hennekins C, Buring J: Ethnic distribution of factor V Leiden in 4047 men and women. Implications for venous thromboembolism screening. JAMA 277:1305, 1997.
51. Vossen C, Conard J, Fontcuberta J, et al: Familial thrombophilia and lifetime risk of venous thrombosis. J Thromb Haemos 2:1526, 2004.
52. Goodwin A, Rosendaal F, Kottke-Marchant K, Bovill E: A review of the technical, diagnostic, and epidemiologic considerations for protein S assays. Arch Pathol Lab Med 126:1349, 2002.
53. Langman L, Ray J, Evrovski J, et al: Hyperhomocysteinemia and the increased risk of venous thromboembolism: more evidence from a case-control study. Arch Intern Med 160:961, 2000.
54. Morelli V, Lourenco D, D'Almeida V, et al: Hyperhomocyteinemia increases the risk of venous thrombosis independent of the C677T mutation of the methylenetetrahydrofolate reductase gene in selected Brazilian patients. Blood Coagul Fibrinol 13:271, 2002.
55. Hirsh J, Hoak J: Management of Deep Vein Thrombosis and Pulmonary Embolism: A Statement for Healthcare Professionals From the Council on Thrombosis (in Consultation with the Council on Cardiovascular Radiology), American Heart Association. Circulation 93:2212, 1996.
56. Sandler D, Martin J, Duncan J, et al: Diagnosis of deep-vein thrombosis: comparison of clinical evaluation, ultrasound, plethysmography, and venoscan with X-ray venogram. Lancet 8405:716, 1984.
57. Wells P, Hirsh J, Anderson D, et al: A simple clinical model for the diagnosis of deep-vein thrombosis combined with impedance plethysmography: potential for an improvement in the diagnostic process. J Intern Med 243:15, 1998.
58. Wells P, Anderson D, Rodger M, et al: Evaluation of D-dimer in the diagnosis of suspected deep-vein thrombosis. N Engl J Med 349:1227, 2003.
59. Tamariz L, Eng J, Segal J, et al: Usefulness of clinical prediction rules for the diagnosis of venous thromboembolism: a systematic review. Am J Med 117:676, 2004.
60. Tapson V, Carroll B, Davidson B, et al. The diagnostic approach to acute venous thromboembolism. Clinical practice guideline. American Thoracic Society. American Journal of Respiratory and Clinical Care Medicine 160:1043, 1999.
61. Heijboer H, Cogo A, Buller H, et al: Detection of deep vein thrombosis with impedance plethysmography and real-time compression ultrasonography in hospitalized patients. Arch Intern Med 152:1901, 1992.
62. Bockenstedt P: D-dimer in venous thromboembolism. N Engl J Med 349:1203, 2003.
63. Kassai B, Boissel J, Cucherat M, et al: A systematic review of the accuracy of ultrasound in the diagnosis of deep venous thrombosis in asymptomatic patients. Thromb Haemost 91:655, 2004.
64. Gottlieb R, Widjaja J, Tian L, et al: Calf sonography for detecting deep venous thrombosis in symptomatic patients: experience and review of the literature. J Clin Ultrasound 27:415, 1999.
65. Evans A, Sostman H, Witty L, et al: Detection of deep venous thrombosis: prospective comparison of MR imaging and sonography. J Magn Reson Imaging 6:44, 1996.
66. Carpenter J, Holland G, Baum R, et al: Magnetic resonance venography for the detection of deep venous thrombosis: comparison with contrast venography and duplex Doppler ultrasonography. J Vasc Surg 1993;18:734–41.
67. Epiney M, Boehlen F, Boulvain M, et al: D-dimer levels during delivery and the postpartum. J Thromb Haemost 3:268, 2005.
68. Koh S, Pua H, Tay D, Ratnam S: The effects of gynaecological surgery on coagulation activation, fibrinolysis, and fibrinolytic inhibitor in patients with and without ketorolac infusion. Thromb Res 79:501, 1995.
69. Heim S, Schectman J, Siadaty M, Philbrick J: D-dimer testing for deep venous thrombosis: a meta-analysis. Clin Chem 50:1136, 2004.
70. Bounameaux H, de Moerloose P, Perrrier A, Reber G: Plasma measurement of D-dimer as a diagnostic aid in suspected venous thromboembolism: an overview. Thromb Haemost 71:1, 1994.
71. Stein P, Terrin M, Hales C, et al: Clinical, laboratory, roentgenographic, and electrocardiographic findings in patients with acute pulmonary embolism and no pre-existing cardiac or pulmonary disease. Chest 100:598, 1991.
72. Fedullo P, Tapson V: The evaluation of suspected pulmonary embolism. N Engl J Med 349:1247, 2003.
73. van Belle A, Buller H, Huisman M, et al: Effectiveness of managing suspected pulmonary embolism using an algorithm combining clinical probability, D-dimer testing, and computed tomography. JAMA 295:172, 2006.
74. The Urokinase Pulmonary Embolism Trial: a national cooperative study. Circulation 47(Suppl II):1, 1973.
75. Green R, Meyer T, Dunn M, Glassroth J: Pulmonary embolism in younger adults. Chest 101:1507, 1992.
76. Come P: Echocardiographic evaluation of pulmonary embolism and its response to therapeutic interventions. Chest 101:151S, 1992.
77. Kasper W, Meinertz T, Kersting F, et al: Echocardiography in assessing acute pulmonary hypertension due to pulmonary embolism. Am J Cardiol 45:567, 1980.
78. Gibson N, Sohne M, Buller H: Prognostic value of echocardiography and spiral computed tomography in patients with pulmonary embolism. Curr Opin Pulmon Med 11:380, 2005.
79. Pruszczyk P, Torbicki A, Pacho R, et al: Noninvasive diagnosis of suspected severe pulmonary embolism: transesophageal echocardiography vs spiral CT. Chest 112:722, 1997.
80. Stein P, Athanasoulis C, Alavi A, et al: Complications and validity of pulmonary angiography in acute pulmonary embolism. Circulation 85:462, 1992.
81. Mills S, Jackson D, Older R, et al: The incidence, etiologies, and avoidance of complications of pulmonary angiography in a large series. Radiology 136:295, 1980.
82. Dalen J, Brooks H, Johnson L, et al: Pulmonary angiography in acute pulmonary embolism: indications, techniques, and results in 367 patients. Am Heart J 81:175, 1971.
83. Value of the ventilation/perfusion scan in acute pulmonary embolism. Results of the prospective investigation of pulmonary

embolism diagnosis (PIOPED). The PIOPED Investigators. JAMA 263:2653, 1990.

84. Cross J, Kemp P, Walsh C, et al: A randomized trial of spiral CT and ventilation perfusion scintigraphy for the diagnosis of pulmonary embolism. Clin Radiol 53:177, 1998.
85. Moores L, Jackson WJ, Shorr A, Jackson J: Meta-analysis: outcomes in patients with suspected pulmonary embolism managed with computed tomographic pulmonary angiography. Ann Intern Med 141:866, 2004.
86. Remy-Jardin M, Remy J, Baghaie F, et al: Clinical value of thin collimation in the diagnostic workup of pulmonary embolism. Am J Roentgenol 175:407, 2000.
87. Meaney J, Weg J, Chenevert T, et al: Diagnosis of pulmonary embolism with magnetic resonance angiography. N Engl J Med 336:1422, 1997.
88. Oudkerk M, van Beek E, Wielopolski P, et al: Comparison of contrast-enhanced magnetic resonance angiography and conventional pulmonary angiography for the diagnosis of pulmonary embolism: a prospective study. Lancet 359:1643, 2002.
89. Stein P, Hull R, Patel K, et al: D-dimer for the exclusion of acute venous thrombosis and pulmonary embolism: a systematic review. Ann Intern Med 140:589, 2004.
90. Stein P, Hull R, Saltzman H, Pineo G: Strategy for diagnosis of patients with suspected pulmonary embolism. Chest 103:1553, 1993.
91. American College of Obstetricians and Gynecologists: Guidelines for diagnostic imaging during pregnancy. ACOG Committee Opinion No. 299. Obstet Gynecol 104:647, 2004.
92. Brent R: The effect of embryonic and fetal exposure to x-ray, microwaves, and ultrasound: counseling the pregnant and nonpregnant patient about these risks. Semin Oncol 16:347, 1989.
93. Stewart A, Kneale G: Radiation dose effects in relation to obstetric x-rays and childhood cancers. Lancet 1:1185, 1970.
94. Webb J, Thomson H, Morcos S, Members of Contrast Media Safety Committee of European Society of Urogenital Radiology (ESUR): The use of iodinated and gadolinium contrast media during pregnancy and lactation. Eur Radiol 15:1234, 2005.
95. Hirsh J: Heparin. N Engl J Med 324:1565, 1991.
96. Ginsberg J, Hirsh J, Turner D, et al: Risks to the fetus of anticoagulant therapy during pregnancy. Thromb Haemost 61:197, 1989.
97. Griffith G, Nichols GJ, Asher J, Flanagan B: Heparin osteoporosis. JAMA 193:85, 1965.
98. Dahlman T: Osteoporotic fractures and the recurrence of thromboembolism during pregnancy and the puerperium in 184 women undergoing thromboprophylaxis with heparin. Am J Obstet Gynecol 168:1265, 1993.
99. Warkentin T, Greinacher A: Heparin-Induced Thrombocytopenia: Recognition, Treatment, and Prevention. The Seventh ACCP Conference on Antithrombotic and Thrombolytic Therapy. Chest 126:311S, 2004.
100. Walenga J, Jeske W, Fasanella A, et al: Laboratory diagnosis of heparin-induced thrombocytopenia. Clinical and Applied Thrombosis and Hemostasis 5(Suppl 1):S21, 999.
101. Hirsh J, Raschke R: Heparin and low-molecular-weight heparin: the Seventh ACCP Conference on Antithrombotic and Thrombolytic Therapy. Chest 126(3 Suppl):188S, 2004.
102. Holst J, Lindblad B, Bergqvist D, et al: Protamine neutralization of intravenous and subcutaneous low-molecular-weight heparin (tinzaparin, Logiparin). An experimental investigation in healthy volunteers. Blood Coagul Fibrinol 5:795–803, 1994.
103. Fausett M, Vogtlander M, Lee R, et al: Heparin-induced thrombocytopenia is rare in pregnancy. Am J Obstet Gynecol 185:148, 2001.
104. Lepercq J, Conard J, Borel-Derlon A, et al. Venous thromboembolism during pregnancy: a retrospective study of enoxaparin safety in 624 pregnancies. BJOG 108:1134, 2001.
105. Buller H, Davidson B, Decousus H, et al: Fondaparinux or enoxaparin for the initial treatment of symptomatic deep venous thrombosis: a randomized trial. Ann Intern Med 140:867, 2004.
106. Buller H, Davidson B, Decousus H, et al: Subcutaneous fondaparinux versus intravenous unfractionated heparin in the initial treatment of pulmonary embolism. N Engl J Med 349:1695, 2003.
107. Dempfle C: Minor transplacental passage of fondaparinux in vivo. N Engl J Med 350:1914, 2004.
108. Hirsh J, Dalen J, Anderson D, et al: Oral anticoagulants: mechanism of action, clinical effectiveness, and optimal therapeutic range. Chest 119(1 Suppl):8S, 2001.
109. Ansell J, Hirsh J, Poller L, et al: The Pharmacology and Management of the Vitamin K Antagonists. The Seventh ACCP Conference on Antithrombotic and Thrombolytic Therapy. Chest 126:204S, 2004.
110. Barbour L, Oja J, Schultz L: A prospective trial that demonstrates that dalteparin requirements increase in pregnancy to maintain therapeutic levels of anticoagulation. Am J Obstet Gynecol 191:1024, 2004.
111. Raschke R, Reilly B, Guidry J, et al: The weight-based heparin dosing nomogram compared with a "standard care" nomogram. A randomized controlled trial. Ann Intern Med 119:874, 1993.
112. Barbour L, Smith J, Marlar R: Heparin levels to guide thromboembolism prophylaxis during pregnancy. Am J Obstet Gynecol 173:1869, 1995.
113. Burrows R, Gan E, Gallus A, et al: A randomized double-blind placebo controlled trial of low molecular weight heparin as prophylaxis in preventing venous thrombotic events after cesarean section. BJOG 108:835, 2001.
114. Gates S, Brocklehurst P, Ayers S, Bowler U: Thromboprophylaxis and pregnancy: two randomized controlled pilot trials that used low-molecular-weight heparin. Am J Obstet Gynecol 191:1296, 2004.
115. Zaccoletti R, Zardini E: Efficacy of elastic compression stockings and administration of calcium heparin in the prevention of puerperal thromboembolic complications. Minerva Ginecologica 44:263, 1992.
116. Ferraro F, D'Ignazio N, Matarazzo A, et al: Thromboembolism in pregnancy: a new temporary caval filter. Minerva Anestesiol 67:381, 2001.

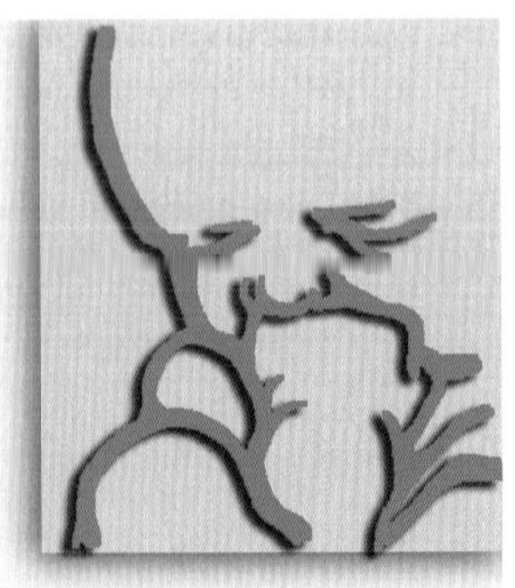

Collagen Vascular Diseases

CALLA HOLMGREN AND D. WARE BRANCH

CHAPTER 42

KEY ABBREVIATIONS

Anti-double-stranded DNA	Anti-ds DNA
Antinuclear antibodies	ANA
Antiphospholipid antibodies	aPL
Antiphospholipid syndrome	APS
Congenital complete heart block	CCHB
Diffuse proliferative glumerulonephritis	DPGN
Food and Drug Administration	FDA
Gestational hypertension	GH
Human leukocyte antigen	HLA
Interleukin-1	IL-1
Intrauterine growth restriction	IUGR
Intravenous immune globulin	IVIG
Juvenile rheumatoid arthritis	JRA
Lupus anticoagulant	LA
Lupus nephritis	LN
Mycophenolate mofentil	MMF
Neonatal lupus erythematosus	NLE
Non-steroidal anti-inflammatory drugs	NSAIDs
Nuclear ribonucleoprotein	nRNP
Preterm birth	PTB
Preterm premature rupture of the membranes	PPROM
Recurrent pregnancy loss	RPL
Rheumatoid arthritis	RA
Rheumatoid factor	RF
Single-stranded DNA	ssDNA
Systemic lupus erythematosus	SLE
Systemic sclerosis	SSc
Transforming growth factor-β	TGF-β
Tumor necrosis factor-α	TNF-α

SYSTEMIC LUPUS ERYTHEMATOSUS

Introduction

Systemic lupus erythematosus (SLE) is the most common serious autoimmune disease affecting women of reproductive age. It is an idiopathic chronic inflammatory disease that affects skin, joints, kidneys, lungs, serous membranes, nervous system, liver, and other organs of the body. Like other autoimmune diseases, its course is characterized by periods of remission and relapse. Frequent presenting symptoms include extreme fatigue, weight loss, myalgia, arthralgia, and fever (Table 42-1).

Epidemiology

The annual incidence of SLE is 5 to 10 per 100,000 individuals, depending on the population studied. The overall prevalence is 1 in 2,500 to 1 in 6,500. The incidence and prevalence vary among populations; SLE is approximately two to four times more frequent in blacks and Hispanics.[1] The disease is at least five to 10 times more common among adult women than adult men,[2] and the prevalence in women is 1 in 245 (black women) to 1 in 2,400. The lifetime risk of developing SLE for a white woman is one in 700.[1] The peak age of onset is between 15 and 25 years, and the mean age of time of diagnosis is 30 years. Although pediatric SLE occurs, most cases of SLE are associated with adolescence or young adulthood.

Approximately 10 percent of patients with SLE also have an affected relative.[3] In addition to this, concordance between twins is reportedly greater than 50 percent.[4]

Several alterations in the human leukocyte antigen (HLA) system have been linked to the development of SLE, and homozygous carriers of mutations responsible for complement deficiency disorders also appear to be predisposed to development of the disease.

Table 42-1. Approximate Frequency of Clinical Symptoms in SLE

SYMPTOMS	PATIENTS (%)
Fatigue	80–100
Fever	80–100
Arthralgia, arthritis	95
Myalgia	70
Weight loss	>60
Skin	
butterfly rash	50
photosensitivity	60
mucous membrane lesions	35
Renal involvement	50
Pulmonary	
Pleurisy	50
Effusion	25
Pneumonitis	5–10
Cardiac (pericarditis)	10–50
Lymphadenopathy	50
CNS	
Seizures	15–20
Psychosis	<25

CNS, central nervous system; SLE, systemic lupus erythematosus.

Clinical Manifestations

Diagnostic Criteria

In 1971, the American Rheumatism Association devised criteria for SLE, primarily to facilitate clinical studies. These criteria were revised in 1982[5] and in 1997[6] (Table 42-2). An individual must have at least four of 11 clinical and laboratory criteria at one time or serially to be classified as having SLE. These criteria are very sensitive and specific for SLE, but were never intended to be the only basis for the diagnosis of SLE. Frequently, individual patients will present with less than four clinical or laboratory features of SLE, thus not meeting strict diagnostic criteria. Some experts use the terms such as probable lupus or lupus-like disease in reference to these cases. Individuals with lupus-like disease may benefit from therapies for SLE and require special care during pregnancy.

Clinical Features

The most common presenting complaints in women diagnosed with SLE include fatigue, weight loss, arthralgias, arthritis, and myalgias. Pleurisy and pericarditis are also seen. The joints most commonly involved are the proximal interphalangeal, knee, wrist, and metacarpophalangeal. Morning stiffness that improves as the day evolves is typical. The migratory nature of the joints involved can be striking. Deforming, erosive arthritis is uncommon.

Table 42-2. Revised ARA Classification Criteria for SLE (1982 and 1997)

CRITERION	DEFINITION
Malar rash	Fixed erythema, flat or raised, over the malar eminences, tending to spare the nasolabial folds
Discoid rash	Erythematous raised patches with adherent keratotic scaling and follicular plugging; atrophic scarring may occur in older lesions
Photosensitivity	Skin rash as a result of unusual reaction to sunlight, by patient history or physician observation
Oral ulcers	Oral or nasopharyngeal ulceration, usually painless
Arthritis	Nonerosive arthritis involving two or more peripheral joints, characterized by tenderness, swelling, or effusion
Serositis	a. Pleuritis—convincing history of pleuritic pain or rubbing heard by a physician or evidence of pleural effusion b. Pericarditis documented by ECG or rub or evidence of effusion
Renal	a. Persistent proteinuria greater than 0.5 g/day or greater than 3+ if quantitation not performed b. Cellular casts—red cell, hemoglobin, granular, tubular, or mixed
Neurologic	a. Seizures—in the absence of offending drugs or known metabolic derangements; e.g., uremia, ketoacidosis, or electrolyte imbalance b. Psychosis—in the absence of drugs or metabolic derangements
Hematologic	a. Hemolytic anemia–with reticulocytosis b. Leukopenia—less than 4,000/mm on two or more occasions c. Lymphopenia—less than 1,500/mm on two or more occasions d. Thrombocytopenia—less than 100,000/mm in absence of drugs
Immunologic	a. Anti-DNA: antibody to native DNA in abnormal titer b. Anti-Sm: presence of antibody to Sm nuclear antigen c. Positive finding of antiphospholipid antibodies based on (1) an abnormal serum level of IgG or IgM anticardiolipin antibodies, (2) a positive test result for lupus anticoagulant using a standard method, or (3) a false-positive serologic test for syphilis for 6 months
Antinuclear antibody	An abnormal titer of antinuclear antibody by immunofluorescence or an equivalent assay at any point in time and in the absence of drugs known to be associated with drug-induced lupus syndrome

ARA, American Rheumatism Association; ECG, electrocardiogram.

The sun-sensitive, erythematous butterfly rash along the malar eminences and across the upper nose occurs in about 50 percent of patients. Patients also may have a pruritic, maculopapular eruption, particularly in sun-exposed areas. Two distinct forms of cutaneous lupus are discoid and subacute. The lesions of discoid lupus mature to clearly outlined papules and plaques, with a central area eventually becoming atrophied and depressed. Scarring is the result. In contrast, subacute lesions appear as distinctly defined erythematous plaques that do not undergo central atrophy and scarring. Subacute lesions are usually more widespread than discoid lesions, with the latter tending to be confined to the face, neck, scalp, and upper arms or shoulders.

Clinically obvious renal disease eventually occurs in about 50 percent of patients with SLE. Lupus nephritis (LN) is likely a result of immune complex deposition leading to complement activation and inflammatory tissue damage in the kidney. The most common presenting sign of renal involvement is proteinuria; about 40 percent of patients with SLE renal disease have hematuria or pyuria, and about a third have urinary casts.

Confirming the diagnosis of LN requires a renal biopsy. This verification is an important factor in determining prognosis and providing appropriate treatment. Renal biopsy findings are used to group LN into four basic histologic and clinical categories. Of the four, diffuse proliferative glomerulonephritis (DPGN) is the most common (40 percent) and most severe. DPGN has a 10-year survival rate of approximately 60 percent. Patients with DPGN typically present with hypertension, moderate-to-heavy proteinuria and nephrotic syndrome, hematuria, pyuria, casts, hypocomplementemia and circulating immune complexes. Another category is focal proliferative glomerulonephritis, which is usually associated with mild hypertension and proteinuria. Serious renal insufficiency with focal proliferative glomerulonephritis is uncommon. Membranous glomerulonephritis typically presents with moderate to heavy proteinuria but lacks the active urinary sediment and does not cause renal insufficiency. Mesangial glomerulonephritis appears to be the least clinically severe lesion and carries the best long-term prognosis.

Laboratory Tests

The diagnosis of SLE, suspected based upon the clinical presentation, is confirmed by demonstrating the presence of pertinent circulating autoantibodies. Most clinicians initially test for autoantibodies directed against nuclear antigens, most commonly using immunofluorescent assays for antinuclear antibodies (ANA). Positive test results are typically reported in terms of the antibody titer and the pattern of antibody binding. A homogeneous pattern is found most commonly in patients with SLE (65 percent), although its specificity is low. A peripheral pattern is the most specific for SLE, but is not very sensitive. The speckled and nucleolar patterns are more specific for other autoimmune diseases.

Immunoflourescent assays that identify specific nuclear antigen-antibody reactions are better for confirming the diagnosis of SLE, monitoring disease activity, and guiding immunotherapy. Particularly useful are anti–double-stranded DNA (anti-dsDNA) antibodies, present in 80 to 90 percent of patients with newly diagnosed SLE. When elevated, these antibodies have been associated with a symptomatic flare in 80 percent of SLE patients followed prospectively.[7,8] In pregnancy, anti-dsDNA antibodies correlate with flare and preterm delivery.[8,9] Antibodies to single-stranded DNA (ssDNA) are also found in a large proportion of untreated SLE patients but are less specific for SLE than anti-dsDNA. Patients with SLE may have antibodies to RNA-protein conjugates, often referred to as soluble or extractable antigens, because they can be separated from tissue extracts. These antigens include the Sm antigen, nuclear ribonucleoprotein, and the Ro/SSA and La/SSB antigens. The Sm and nuclear ribonucleoprotein antigens are nuclear in origin, and the presence of anti-Sm, found in about 30 to 40 percent of patients with SLE, is highly specific for the disease. Anti-Ro/SS-A and La/SS-B, found in the sera of both SLE patients and patients with Sjögren's syndrome, are of particular importance to obstetricians because they are associated with neonatal lupus.

Systemic Lupus Erythematosus and Pregnancy

Preexisting SLE or onset during pregnancy carries important implications for the mother and the fetus. For the mother, the primary concerns are SLE exacerbation, nephritis and preeclampsia, possible need for preterm delivery, and an increased rate of cesarean delivery. Fetal-neonatal concerns include miscarriage and fetal death, preeclampsia, placental insufficiency and intrauterine growth restriction (IUGR), preterm birth (PTB) and complications thereof, and neonatal lupus.

The Risk of Systemic Lupus Erythematosus Exacerbation (Flare)

Whether or not pregnancy is associated with a higher rate of SLE exacerbation is a matter of considerable debate. Early studies were hampered by poor study design and difficulties differentiating between SLE and obstetric disorders, for example, severe hypertension due to preeclampsia. The small, retrospective series published during the 1960s and 1970s suggested that pregnancy in women with SLE was associated with substantial risk for severe maternal morbidity and mortality and that this risk was related to SLE activity.[10] Given this concern, many practitioners held the opinion that patients with SLE should not become pregnant.

Studies since 1980 have done much to clarify the relationship of pregnancy to the rate and nature of SLE exacerbations. Overall, 15 to 60 percent of women with SLE have a flare during pregnancy or the postpartum period.[3,11–23] Several prospective studies deserve special consideration. Using a previously published scoring system to define SLE exacerbations, Lockshin et al.[11] matched non-pregnant SLE patients with 28 SLE patients undertaking 33 pregnancies. There was no difference in the flare score between the cases and controls, and a similar number in either group required a change in their medication. When only signs or symptoms specific for SLE were included, exacerbations occurred in only 13 percent of cases. Mintz et al.[13] prospectively studied 92 pregnancies in women with SLE and used a similar group of nonpregnant SLE patients on oral contraceptives derived from a previous study as controls. Exacerbations were defined by criteria different from those used by Lockshin et al.[11] As a matter of policy, all pregnant women were started on 10 mg prednisone daily, even if there was no evidence of SLE activity. The rate of SLE flares per month at risk was similar in both groups. Most of the exacerbations tended to be easily controlled with low to moderate doses of glucocorticoids, but seven patients (8 percent) had severe exacerbations requiring more aggressive therapies. Interestingly, the majority (54 percent) of the exacerbations occurred in the first trimester. Urowitz et al.[15] reported their experience comparing 79 pregnancies in patients with active SLE with a matched control group of 59 nonpregnant active SLE women. They also compared these women with 216 women with inactive disease. Using a previously defined SLE exacerbation score, they found no significant difference in disease activity between the three groups. Georgiou et al.[22] prospectively evaluated the frequency of SLE exacerbation during 59 pregnancies in 47 women with SLE and 59 nonpregnant women matched for parameters other than disease activity and duration. Using accepted clinical criteria, they reported an SLE exacerbation in 8 (13.5 percent) of the pregnant patients compared with 13 (22 percent) of the nonpregnant group. More than half of the exacerbations in the pregnant women occurred during the first trimester; all exacerbations were mild and easily treated with glucocorticoids.

In contrast to the negative findings discussed above, two prospective series suggest that pregnant women with SLE have higher rates of exacerbation. Petri et al.[3] found SLE flares (flares per person years) to be more common among pregnant women than among controls. Fortunately, more than three quarters of the flares were mild to moderate in nature. Only inactive patients at the onset of pregnancy showed a significant reduction in SLE activity (41 percent). Ruiz-Irastorza et al.[16] analyzed the course of SLE in 78 pregnancies in 68 patients and a matched control group of 50 nonpregnant women. Sixty-five percent of the patients experienced an exacerbation of SLE during pregnancy, for a flare rate of 0.082 per patient-month. In the control group, 42 percent of the patients flared, with a flare rate of 0.039 per patient-month, representing a statistically significant difference.

Without a doubt, preexisting disease activity, plays a large role in the risk of SLE flare during pregnancy. Derksen et al.[19] reported that SLE exacerbation occurred in fewer than 20 percent of women with sustained remission prior to pregnancy. More recently, Cortez-Hernandez and colleagues[23] studied 60 women with 103 pregnancies and found that SLE exacerbations during pregnancy were more likely in women who discontinued maintenance therapy before pregnancy or had a history of more than three severe flares before pregnancy. The findings of several other studies support the notion that women with active disease should postpone pregnancy until sustained remission can be achieved.[20–22]

Thus, from the available literature one can surmise that if pregnancy predisposes to a lupus flare, it does so only modestly. A majority of studies of pregnant women with SLE indicate that most flares are mild to moderate in nature and easily treated with glucocorticoids.[11,13,15,16,20–22] The routine or prophylactic use of glucocorticoids in all pregnant SLE patients, as suggested by some investigators, seems unnecessary in view of the excellent results achieved by others without the routine prophylactic immunosuppression.

To ensure timely and accurate detection of an SLE exacerbation, thorough and frequent clinical assessment remains essential. The criteria for measuring an SLE flare during pregnancy have been recently tested and found valid.[24] Commonly presenting symptoms of flare during pregnancy are extreme fatigue, skin lesions (>90 percent), and arthritis/arthralgias (>80 percent).[22,25]

Serologic evaluation of SLE disease activity may be beneficial in confirming a flare in confusing cases. As mentioned earlier, elevations in anti-dsDNA titers that precede or accompany a lupus flare in more than 80 percent of patients are a specific indicator.[7,8] In addition, some reports suggest that the serial serologic evaluation of complement components and activation products is beneficial in predicting an SLE flare during pregnancy. In two studies, Devoe and colleagues found that an SLE exacerbation was signaled by a decline of C3 and C4 into the subnormal range.[26,27] Buyon et al.[28] found that an SLE exacerbation was associated with an absence of the usual increase in C3 and C4 levels during normal pregnancies. However, the practical utility of serial determinations of complement components or their activation products during pregnancy remains unproven. Lockshin et al.[29] reported that low-grade activation of the classic pathway may be attributed to pregnancy alone. Wong et al.[30] prospectively studied 19 continuing pregnancies complicated by SLE and found that neither ANA nor C3 or C4 levels predicted which patients were going to have a flare, whereas Nossent and Swaak[31] observed that fewer than half of the pregnancies with decreased serum C3 levels were associated with a clinical SLE flare. Last, although some have found that hypocomplementemia correlates with poor pregnancy outcomes,[32–34] hypocomplementemia may occur in pregnant patients without SLE or adverse pregnancy outcomes.[35]

Lupus Nephritis Exacerbation

Women with LN face several challenges during pregnancy. Pregnancy may worsen renal function. Moreover, underlying renal disease is associated with increased risks of maternal and fetal complications. Those with chronic renal disease are likely to experience worsening proteinuria during gestation as renal perfusion increases. In turn, this inevitably poses the diagnostic dilemma as to whether the increased proteinuria represents an exacerbation of underlying renal disease, preeclampsia, or both.

As with an SLE exacerbation in general, whether or not renal flares are more common in pregnant women with SLE remains controversial. Two studies have reported high frequencies of renal flares (43 to 46 percent) during pregnancy,[25,30] but others have reported lower figures (9 to 28 percent).[13,16,31,36] Three studies assessed the patients' status during pregnancy in regard to whether the SLE was active or in remission prior to conception.[37–39] In all three, the rate of SLE exacerbation was lower in pregnancies in which the patient was in remission before conception.

Studies of pregnancy outcome in women with past or current LN are limited. This may be explained, in part, by (1) the reduced fertility associated with long-term cyclophosphamide or impaired renal function, or both, and (2) the traditional assumption that pregnancy should be discouraged in women with a history of LN. The earliest reports suggest that LN was a major contributor to serious maternal morbidity or death.[40–42] More recent series suggest that the outlook of pregnancy for women with LN is usually favorable if the disease is well controlled and renal function preserved.[43] Oviasu et al.[44] reviewed eight studies (151 pregnancies) published between 1973 and 1991 to determine the effect of completed pregnancy on maternal renal function in established LN and reported transient deterioration of renal function in 17 percent and permanent deterioration in 8 percent of the pregnancies.[44]

Better outcomes were reported in three studies published in the 1990s.[43–45] Out of 143 patients with LN, only one developed irreversible loss of renal function after pregnancy. It is important to note that the majority of women in these studies had normal renal function, mild proteinuria, and well-controlled hypertension *before* conception. Petri and colleagues at the Hopkins Lupus Pregnancy Center reported that only women who began pregnancy with nephrotic syndrome went on to renal failure after delivery.[25] Hayslett and Lynn[37] and Bobrie et al.[39] found that the rate of renal deterioration was somewhat lower among pregnancies in which the patient was in remission before conception. In a recent study, Moroni and colleagues[46] reported that renal flare occurred in 5 percent (1/20) of pregnancies in women with inactive LN before conception compared with 39 percent (12/31) in women with active LN before conception. The sole predictors for renal flare were a plasma creatinine greater than 1.2 mg/dL or proteinuria equal to 500 mg in 24-hour collection. Permanent deterioration occurred in two women with active LN before conception, one of whom eventually died.

A troublesome clinical situation is differentiating between renal exacerbation and preeclampsia, because both may present with proteinuria, hypertension, and evidence of multiorgan dysfunction. Some of the features that may prove helpful in the distinction between the two conditions are listed in Table 42-3. Preeclampsia is more likely in women with decreased levels of antithrombin III.[47,48] Complement concentrations are not always helpful because activation may also occur in women with preeclampsia.[49] In the most severe and confusing cases, the correct diagnosis is possible only by renal biopsy. In reality, situations involving either the more severe cases of SLE flare or preeclampsia inevitably raise concerns about maternal and fetal well-being and often prompt delivery, thus rendering the distinction between the two clinically moot.

Women with active LN (especially DPGN), nephritic syndrome, and severe hypertension are at considerable risk of preeclampsia and early delivery. Moderate renal insufficiency (creatinine 1.5 to 2.0 mg/dl) is a relative contraindication to pregnancy and advanced renal insufficiency (creatinine greater than 2.0 mg/dl) should be considered an absolute contraindication to pregnancy.

Table 42-3. Distinguishing Between Preeclampsia and SLE/LN Flare

TEST	PREECLAMPSIA	SLE
Serologic		
Decreased complement	++	+++
Elevated Ba or Bb fragments with low CH50	±	++
Elevated anti-dsDNA	–	+++
Antithrombin III deficiency	++	±
Hematologic		
Microangiopathic hemolytic anemia	++	–
Coombs' positive hemolytic anemia	–	++
Thrombocytopenia	++	++
Leukopenia	–	++
Renal		
Hematuria	+	+++
Cellular casts	–	+++
Elevated serum creatinine	±	++
Elevated ratio of serum blood urea nitrogen/creatinine	++	±
Hypocalciuria	++	±
Liver Transaminases	++	±

+++, present; ++, occasionally present; ±, may or may not be present; –, not present; LN, lupus nephritis; SLE, systemic lupus erythematosus.

Pregnancy Loss

In most retrospective studies, the rate of pregnancy loss appears to be higher in women with SLE than in the general obstetric population, ranging between 8 and 41 percent, with a median of 22 percent.[10,12,37,38,50–55] A large case-controlled study compared obstetric outcomes in 481 pregnancies in 203 lupus patients with those of 566 pregnancies in 177 healthy relatives and 356 pregnancies in 166 healthy unrelated women.[55a] The investigators found that pregnancy loss occurred significantly more often in women with SLE (21 percent) than in either their healthy relatives (8 percent) or unrelated healthy controls (14 percent). However, the pregnancy loss rates observed in most prospective trials of lupus pregnancies have been better than those of their retrospective counterparts, possibly because of careful monitoring of SLE activity and routine antenatal surveillance. In the most recent, well-detailed, prospective trials, fetal deaths in the second or third trimester accounted for between 10 to 40 percent of the total losses.[22,23]

Control of disease activity appears to have a helpful effect on the rate of pregnancy loss,[56] with one early study reporting live births in 64 percent of women with active disease within 6 months of conception, compared with 88 percent in women with quiescent disease.[37] In a more recent, prospective study, pregnancy loss occurred in 75 percent of women with active disease compared with 14 percent of women with inactive disease.[22] Not surprisingly, pregnancy loss is more likely if SLE is diagnosed during the index pregnancy.[38,52,57]

Preexisting renal disease appears to increase the rate of pregnancy loss in women with SLE, but loss rates vary widely among studies, likely because of variations in the degree of renal impairment of patients included. Also, the degree of renal impairment is a factor in the rate of pregnancy loss in women with LN. In a recent study of LN in pregnancy that included only women with inactive disease and normal renal function (serum creatinine less than 0.8 mg/dl), the overall fetal survival rate was greater 90 percent, after exclusion of embryonic losses (losses less than 10 weeks' gestation).[20] These results contrast markedly to those of another study in which the rate of fetal loss was 50 percent in pregnant women with LN and moderate-to-severe renal insufficiency (serum creatinine = 1.5 mg/dl).[37] In another study comparing obstetric outcomes according to the degree of renal impairment in women with LN, spontaneous abortion occurred in 26 percent of women with minimally impaired renal function (serum creatinine less than 1 mg/dl, clearance greater than 80 ml/min, and proteinuria less than 1 g/day) and 36 percent in women with "mild" impairment (clearance 50 to 80 ml/min, proteinuria 1 to 3 g/day).[50]

Fetal death (greater than 10 weeks' gestation) among SLE pregnancies is tied to the presence of antiphospholipid antibodies (aPL) (see the section on Antiphospholipid Syndrome). In several studies, the existence of aPL has been the single most sensitive predictor of fetal death,[58] with a positive predictive value of more than 50 percent.[59] For women with SLE and a prior fetal death, the predictive value is more than 85 percent.[60] In the most recent prospective trial, the presence of any aPL was the single strongest predictor of subsequent pregnancy loss, even in women with active disease and underlying renal impairment.[23]

Preeclampsia

It is difficult to estimate the exact incidence of pregnancy-related hypertension associated with SLE. This is in large part due to inconsistencies in the definition and classification of these disorders, as well as the inclusion of patients with LN in the various studies. Nevertheless, it appears that between 20 to 30 percent of women with SLE develop either gestational hypertension (GH) or preeclampsia (GH with proteinuria) sometime during pregnancy.[37,58,61–63] Women with LN are most susceptible, probably owing to the known association between preeclampsia and underlying renal disease of any origin. In one prospective series, preeclampsia occurred in 7 of 19 (37 percent) women with LN, compared with 15 of 106 (14 percent) without. Other factors that likely predispose SLE patients to GH or preeclampsia include chronic hypertension, secondary antiphospholipid syndrome (APS), and chronic steroid use[17,37,45,50,62,63a] (see Table 42-3).

Fetal Growth Restriction

Uteroplacental insufficiency resulting in IUGR and small-for-gestational-age neonates has been reported in between 12 and 40 percent of pregnancies complicated by SLE.[16,21,23,45,56,64] It would seem likely that factors such as underlying renal insufficiency and chronic hypertension play a role.[23,62,65] Medications, such as glucocorticoids, might also be related to IUGR. In a recent prospective trial Georgiou and colleagues reported no significant differences in the rate of IUGR between SLE pregnancies and healthy controls.[22] In this study, glucocorticoids were given only for symptomatic SLE flare.

Preterm Birth

PTB has been reported in as few as 3 percent and as many as 73 percent of pregnancies complicated by SLE.[13,30,37,38,50,52,57,58,60,66,67] aPLs, chronic hypertension, and disease activity have all been reported to increase the likelihood of PTB in women with SLE.[22,23] Only a few studies have included controls for comparison. PTB was more common in a group of women with SLE than in a group of matched controls (12 percent vs 4 percent) in one retrospective case-control study.[55a] In a recent prospective trial, PTB in women with SLE and healthy controls was statistically similar (8 percent versus 15 percent),[22] although PTB was more common among women with active SLE compared with those with inactive disease (12.5 percent versus 4 percent).

A substantial proportion of PTB associated with SLE is without a doubt the result of iatrogenic delivery for obstetric and medical indications. Data from the few studies that provide sufficient detail suggest that between 28 to 66 percent of preterm deliveries are indicated because of preeclampsia and another 12 to 33 percent because of suspected or confirmed fetal compromise.[23,52,55a,60,66] An association between SLE and preterm premature rupture of membranes (PPROM) has also been reported, occurring in 39 percent of pregnancies delivered at 24 to 36 weeks' gestation.[66]

Neonatal Lupus Erythematosus

Neonatal lupus erythematosus (NLE) is an infrequent condition of the fetus and neonate, occurring in 1 of 15,000 of all live births and in a relatively small percentage of lupus pregnancies. It is a result of passively acquired immunity in pregnant women with circulating antibodies directed against Ro/SSA and La/SSB ribonucleoprotein antigens.[69–73] These antibodies can cross the placenta as early as 11 weeks' gestation, and they are associated with congenital complete atrioventricular heart block (CCHB), a neonatal lupus rash, and hepatic and blood cell abnormalities.

Anti-Ro/SSA antibodies are found in 75 to 95 percent mothers who deliver babies with NLE.[70,72,73] A smaller percentage has only anti-La/SSB. Dermatologic NLE has also been associated with anti-U1RNP without anti-Ro/SSA or anti-La/SSB.[70,74] Fortunately, of mothers with SLE who are serologically positive for anti-Ro/SSA antibodies, no more than 15 percent to 20 percent deliver an infant affected with evidence of NLE. The most common manifestation is dermatologic NLE. Of all women with anti-Ro/SSA or anti-La/SSB, 1 to 5 percent deliver an infant with CCHB. It is important to note, however, that once a woman with SLE and anti-Ro/SSA antibodies delivers one infant with CCHB, the risk for recurrence is at least two- to threefold higher than in women with anti-Ro/SSA-La/SSB antibodies who has never had an affected child.[73] Recurrence of dermatologic NLE is approximately 25 percent.[72,76]

The skin lesions of NLE are erythematous, scaling annular, or elliptical plaques occurring on the face or scalp. They are analogous to the subacute cutaneous lesions in adults. They typically appear in the first weeks of life, probably induced by exposure of the skin to ultraviolet light, and may last for up to 6 months.[77] Hypopigmentation may persist for up to 2 years. Hematologic NLE is rare and may be manifest as autoimmune hemolytic anemia, leukopenia, thrombocytopenia and hepatosplenomegaly.

Cardiac NLE lesions include CCHB and the less frequently reported endocardial fibroelastosis. CCHB is due to disruption of the cardiac conduction system, especially in the area of the atrioventricular node. The diagnosis of CCHB is typically made around 23 weeks' gestation[73] when a fixed bradycardia of 60 to 80 beats per minute is detected during a routine prenatal visit. Fetal echocardiography reveals complete atrioventricular dissociation with a structurally normal heart. CCHB is irreversible, and greater than 65 percent of surviving infants will require a pacemaker, 50 percent of them at birth. In the more severely affected fetus, more widespread endomyocardial damage leads to fibroelastosis and markedly diminished cardiac pump function, hydrops fetalis, and fetal death. In the largest series of prenatally diagnosed CCHB, the 3-year survival was 79 percent; the majority of deaths occurred before 90 days of life.[73]

Suspected cases of CCHB in utero should be evaluated by fetal echocardiography and maternal tests for anti-Ro/SSA and anti-La/SSB antibodies. If the diagnosis of CCHB due to NLE is made, some experts currently recommend administration of a glucocorticoid that crosses the placenta to limit further damage to the fetal heart. Maternal plasmapheresis, to reduce the antibody load, or invasive fetal pacing to increase the fetal ventricular rate also have been used. None of these treatments have been shown to be effective.[78] In addition, all of the aforementioned maternal treatments have known potential and real side effects. The efficacy of prenatal treatments is being examined in a registry of cases collected by Dr. J.P. Buyon, Hospital for Joint Disease, New York University, New York City (jill.buyon@med.nyu.edu).

Although of unproven efficacy, many experts recommend screening fetuses of antibody-positive mothers who have *previously* delivered an infant with CCHB using echocardiographic-Doppler techniques to measure the mechanical PR interval[79] from 16 weeks' forward. Because of the grave nature of CCHB, the finding of any conduction disturbance would prompt attempts at preventing further or ongoing damage using glucocorticoids or intravenous immune globulin (IVIG). Again, this approach is of unproven efficacy.

The apparent success of IVIG in the treatment of fetal-neonatal alloimmune thrombocytopenia has led to speculation that IVIG might be effective in preventing or treating autoantibody-mediated CCHB. An international, multicenter trial has been suggested.

OBSTETRIC MANAGEMENT

Women with SLE who are contemplating pregnancy should be counseled before conception about potential obstetric problems including pregnancy loss, gestational hypertensive disorders, IUGR, and PTB. They should also be informed of the risk of SLE flare and special concerns related to APS and NLE. Laboratory evaluation before pregnancy should include an assessment for anemia and thrombocytopenia, underlying renal disease (urinalysis, serum creatinine and 24-hour urine for creatinine clearance and total protein), and aPL (lupus anticoagulant, anticardiolipin and anti-β_2-glycoprotein I antibodies). Many experts routinely obtain anti-Ro/SSA and anti-La/SSB antibodies in patients with SLE; however, the cost-effectiveness of these tests is not proven.

Women with active SLE should be discouraged from becoming pregnant until they are in remission. Cytotoxic drugs should be stopped before conception, and every effort should be made to reduce or eliminate long-term treatment with nonsteroidal anti-inflammatory drug (NSAID). However, maintenance therapy with hydroxychloroquine or low doses of glucocorticoids need not be discontinued.

The prenatal care of the patient with SLE should be guided by the potential risks to the mother and fetus. Prenatal visits should occur every 1 to 2 weeks in the first and second trimesters and every week thereafter. A primary goal of the antenatal visits after 20 weeks' gestation is the detection of hypertension, proteinuria, or suspicion of IUGR. Because of the risk of uteroplacental insufficiency, fetal ultrasonography should be performed every 4 to 6 weeks starting at 18 to 20 weeks' gestation. In the usual case, fetal surveillance (daily fetal movement counts and periodic nonstress tests and amniotic fluid volume measurements) should be instituted at 30 to 32 weeks' gestation. More frequent ultrasonography and fetal testing may be indicated in patients with SLE flare, hypertension, proteinuria, clinical evidence of IUGR, or APS. Fetal surveillance as early as 24 to 25 weeks may be necessary in patients with APS.[80]

Management of SLE during labor and delivery is a continuation of antenatal care. Exacerbations of SLE can occur during labor and may require the acute administration of steroids. Regardless, stress doses of glucocorticoids should be given during labor or at the time of cesarean delivery to all patients who have been treated with chronic steroids within the year. Intravenous hydrocortisone, given in doses of 100 mg every 9 hours for three doses, is an acceptable regimen. Obstetric complications, such as preeclampsia and IUGR, should be managed in the usual fashion, and not specifically altered because of the SLE. Neonatology support may be needed at delivery for problems associated with CCHB and other manifestations of NLE.

It is uncertain which patients, if any, are at risk for SLE flare following delivery, and it probably best to maintain frequent contact with SLE patients in the postpartum period. Maintenance medications discontinued during labor and delivery should be restarted immediately following delivery, at similar doses as during the pregnancy. Dose adjustments can be handled in the outpatient setting.

Treatment of Systemic Lupus Erythematosus in Pregnancy

Glucocorticoids

Glucocorticoids are often used to treat SLE during pregnancy. These medications can be given as maintenance therapy or in "bursts" to treat SLE flares. The doses used in pregnancy are the same as those in nonpregnant patients. Tapering to the lowest dose required to manage the disease is prudent because glucocorticoids are associated with preeclampsia, gestational diabetes mellitus, and PPROM.

Some experts have recommended the use of prophylactic glucocorticoids during pregnancy.[13,36,81] However, this practice is not evidence based, and comparable maternal and fetal outcomes have been documented in patients without prophylactic treatment in the presence of stable disease.[82]

Despite the fact that glucocorticoids have a low potential for teratogenesis,[83] they are not without risk during pregnancy. Patients requiring long-term therapy are best treated with prednisolone or methylprednisolone because of their conversion to relatively inactive forms by the abundant 11-β-ol dehydrogenase found in the human placenta. Glucocorticoids such as dexamethasone and betamethasone with fluorine at the 9-a position are poorly metabolized by the placenta, and long-term use during pregnancy should be avoided. Recent analyses suggest a very slight increased risk of cleft lip and palate associated with glucocorticoid exposure in the early first trimester.[84-86] Maternal side effects may be significant and include weight gain, striae, acne, hirsutism, immunosuppression, osteonecrosis and gastrointestinal ulceration. Long-term glucocorticoid therapy during pregnancy has been associated with an increased risk of preeclampsia,[58,87,88] PPROM, uteroplacental insufficiency, and IUGR.[89] Because of the increased risk of glucose intolerance,[87,88] women treated over the long term with glucocorticoids should be screened for gestational diabetes mellitus somewhat earlier and more than once, probably at 22 to 24, 28 to 30, and 32 to 34 weeks' of gestation.

Antimalarial Medications

In the past, many patients and their physicians have discontinued antimalarials before or during pregnancy because of concerns about teratogenicity, specifically otic[90] and ocular damage.[91] Considerable clinical experience, in cases with malaria prophylaxis, failed to confirm rare reports of these adverse fetal effects. And recent case series suggest hydroxychloroquine is relatively safe during pregnancy.[92-95] The findings of a recent case-controlled trial, which compared the effects of in utero exposure to hydroxychloroquine, were confirmatory.[96] No differences were noted between the 122 infants with in utero exposure to hydroxychloroquine and the 70 control infants regarding the number and type of defects identified at birth. There was also no difference in the percentages of infants affected with visual, hearing, growth, or developmental abnormalities at follow-up (median follow-up, 24 months).

Just as importantly, hydroxychloroquine may be emerging as the best overall agent for maintenance SLE therapy during pregnancy. In a recent randomized controlled trial, women who continued hydroxychloroquine during pregnancy experienced a significant reduction in SLE disease activity compared with women who changed to glucocorticoid therapy.[97] Many experts now recommend continuing hydroxychloroquine during pregnancy in patients being treated with this agent.

Cytotoxic Agents

Cytotoxic agents, including azathioprine, methotrexate, and cyclophosphamide, are used to treat only the most severely affected patients with SLE. Limited data suggest that azathioprine, a derivative of 6-mercaptopurine, is not teratogenic in humans but is associated with IUGR[98,99] and impaired neonatal immunity.[100] Thus, in women requiring chronic azathioprine, consideration of pregnancy demands that the patient and physician have carefully weighed potential fetal risks against the benefits of the medication.

Cyclophosphamide has been reported to be teratogenic in both animal[101] and human studies[102,103]; it should be avoided during the first trimester. Thereafter, cyclophosphamide should be used only in special circumstances, such as in women with severe, progressive proliferative glomerulonephritis.[104]

Methotrexate is toxic to actively dividing trophoblast and causes miscarriage and early fetal death. Moreover, methotrexate is documented to cause malformations in up to 30 percent of surviving pregnancies when using doses greater than 10 mg per week in the first trimester. These malformations include cranial dysostosis with delayed ossification, hypertelorism, wide nasal bridge, micrognathia, and ear anomalies.[105] Case reports have also described cleft palate and deformities of the toes and fingers when methotrexate is used in early pregnancy.[106] Principles underlying teratogenicity of a drug are discussed in Chapter 8.

Nonsteroidal Anti-inflammatory Drugs

NSAIDs are the most common type of analgesics used in the treatment of SLE outside of pregnancy. Although effective, they readily cross the placenta and can block prostaglandin synthesis in a wide variety of fetal tissues. Maternal ingestion of normal adult doses of aspirin in the week before delivery has been associated with intracranial hemorrhage in preterm neonates.[107,108] Although short-term (less than 72 hours) tocolytic therapy with indomethacin appears to be safe,[109,110] long-term use has been associated with a number of untoward fetal effects. After 32 weeks' gestation, indomethacin can cause constriction or closure of the fetal ductus arteriosus.[111] Long-term use of any NSAID has been associated with decreased fetal urinary output, oligohydramnios, and neonatal renal insufficiency.[112] Given these risks, long-term use of adult dosages of aspirin and other NSAIDs should be avoided during pregnancy, especially after the first trimester. Acetaminophen and narcotic-containing preparations are reasonable alternatives if analgesia is needed during pregnancy.

OTHER IMMUNOSUPPRESSIVE AGENTS

Several other treatments, including cyclosporin, high-dose IVIG, mycophenolate mofetil (MMF), and thalidomide, are sometimes used in SLE patients.[104] Only IVIG has been used during pregnancy without reports of adverse fetal effects. MMF is a reversible inhibitor of inosine monophosphate dehydrogenase. It works by blocking de novo purine synthesis. MMF is an Food and Drug Administration (FDA) Category C drug, but teratogenic risks are a concern because experiments in animals revealed developmental toxicity, malformations, and intrauterine death at dosages that coincide with recommended clinical dosages.[98] Given this information, there is a possibility of increased risk in humans, and therefore, MMF is contraindicated in pregnancy. Thalidomide is strictly contraindicated during pregnancy because of its known potent teratogenicity.

ANTIPHOSPHOLIPID SYNDROME

Introduction

aPL are a family of autoantibodies that bind to epitopes associated with negatively charged phospholipids or proteins that bind to negatively charged phospholipids. Clinicians first recognized that aPL were associated with hypercoagulability 50 years ago, and an association with pregnancy loss was established in the mid-1970s. The term APS was introduced in 1986 to formalize the association of aPL with these clinical features. Over a decade of subsequent international laboratory and clinical experience led to the development of an international consensus statement on preliminary criteria for definite APS, published in 1999 and revised in 2005 (Table 42-4) [113,114] Clinicians should recognize that the diagnosis of APS rests first and foremost on clinical features and is confirmed by demonstrating repeatedly positive tests for aPL.

Epidemiology

The actual prevalence and incidence of APS is unknown. APS may exist as an isolated immunologic derangement (primary APS) or in combination with other autoimmune diseases (secondary APS), most commonly SLE. aPL are found in up to 5 percent of apparently healthy controls and in up to 35 percent of patients with SLE.[115] The prospective risks associated with a positive test for aPL antibodies in otherwise healthy subjects are unknown (Table 42-5).

Pathophysiology

Whether aPL per se are the cause of adverse obstetric outcomes associated with the antibodies remains a

Table 42-4. Preliminary Classification Criteria for APS*

Clinical criteria
- Vascular thrombosis
  - a. One or more clinical episodes of arterial, venous, or small-vessel thrombosis in any tissue or organ, AND
  - b. Thrombosis confirmed by imaging or Doppler studies or histopathology, with the exception of superficial venous thrombosis, AND
  - c. For histopathologic confirmation, thrombosis should be present without significant evidence of inflammation in the vessel wall.
- Pregnancy morbidity
  - a. One or more unexplained deaths of a morphologically normal fetus at or beyond the 10th week of gestation, with normal fetal morphology documented by ultrasound or by direct examination of the fetus, OR
  - b. One or more premature births of a morphologically normal neonate at or before the 34th week of gestation because of severe preeclampsia or severe placental insufficiency, OR
  - c. Three or more unexplained consecutive spontaneous abortions before the 10th week of gestation, with maternal anatomic or hormonal abnormalities and paternal and maternal chromosomal causes excluded.

Laboratory criteria
- a. Anticardiolipin antibody of IgG and/or IgM isotype in blood, present in medium or high titer, on at least 2 occasions at least 6 weeks apart, measured by standard enzyme-linked immunosorbent assay for β_2-glycoprotein I-dependent anticardiolipin antibodies, OR
- b. Lupus anticoagulant present in plasma, on 2 or more occasions at least 6 weeks apart, detected according to the guidelines of the International Society on Thrombosis and Hemostasis.

*Definite antiphospholipid syndrome (APS) is considered to be present if at least 1 of the clinical and 1 of the laboratory criteria are met.

Table 42-5. Nonautoimmune Causes for Positive Antiphospholipid Antibody Tests

ASSAY TYPE	ANTIBODY TYPE	CAUSES
ELISA	β_2-glycoprotein independent	Infection: syphilis, Lyme disease, leptospirosis, pinta, HIV
	β_2-glycoprotein dependent	Advanced age
		Drugs
	Either	Lymphoproliferative disease
		Hyperimmunoglobulin M
Lupus anticoagulant	—	Infection; HIV, drugs

ELISA, enzyme-linked immunosorbent assay; HIV, human immunodeficiency virus.

subject of debate, although mounting evidence supports a direct antibody-mediated effect. Working with mice, some investigators found administration of human aPL results in clinical manifestations of APS, including fetal loss.[116,117] Rodent venous thrombosis models have also been developed.[118]

A variety of mechanisms by which aPL may cause pregnancy loss (and thrombosis) have been suggested. Considerable work has focused on aPL interfering with the normal in vivo function of phospholipids or phospholipid-binding proteins crucial to the regulation of coagulation. Candidate molecules or pathways that might be adversely affected include β_2-glycoprotein I (which has anticoagulant properties), prostacyclin, prothrombin, protein C, annexin V, and tissue factor. aPL may activate endothelial cells, as indicated by increased expression of adhesion molecules, secretion of cytokines, and production of arachidonic acid metabolites. Other evidence suggests that aPL cross-react with oxidized low-density lipoprotein and bind only to oxidized cardiolipin,[119] implying that aPL may participate in oxidant-mediated injury of the vascular endothelium. These abnormalities may result in thrombosis during the development of the normal maternoplacental circulation, perhaps through interference with trophoblastic annexin V,[120] which is abundant in the human placenta, or by impairing trophoblastic hormone production or invasion.[121]

The in vivo targets of aPL remain uncertain. Normal living cells do not express phospholipids bound by aPL on their surface. The antibodies do, however, bind to phospholipids expressed by perturbed cells, such as activated platelets or apoptotic cells. Recent work points to the complement system as having a primary role in APS-related pregnancy loss, showing that C3 activation is required for fetal loss in a mouse model.[122] Moreover, the beneficial effect of heparin seen in this model appears to be linked to heparin's anticomplement, not anticoagulant activity. Anticoagulants other than heparin do not prevent fetal loss in this murine system,[123] suggesting that thrombosis may not be the immediate cause of pregnancy morbidity and mortality in this syndrome.

Regardless of the primary mechanism, the negative effect of APS on human pregnancy appears to be tied to abnormal maternal-fetal circulation. Some investigators have found narrowing of the spiral arterioles, intimal thickening, acute atherosis, and fibrinoid necrosis in cases of fetal loss associated with APS. Others have found extensive placental necrosis, infarction, and thrombosis.

Diagnosis

Clinical Manifestation

The International Consensus Statement provides simplified criteria for the diagnosis of APS.[113,124] Patients with bona fide APS must manifest at least one of two clinical criteria (vascular thrombosis or pregnancy morbidity). Thrombosis may be either arterial or venous and must be confirmed by an imaging or Doppler study or by histopathology. Pregnancy morbidity is divided into three categories: (1) otherwise unexplained fetal death (10 weeks' gestation or older), (2) PTB (less than 34 weeks' gestation) for severe preeclampsia or placental insufficiency, or (3) otherwise unexplained recurrent preembryonic or embryonic pregnancy loss. Other clinical features, such as autoimmune thrombocytopenia, are associated with aPL but are not considered specific enough to be diagnostic criteria.

Obstetric features of APS, which include events of both the preembryonic-embryonic and the fetal-neonatal periods, are divided into three categories—one encompassing early pregnancy loss, and the other two relating primarily to complications in the second or third trimester (see Table 42-5). In the original description of APS, the single obstetric criterion for diagnosis was fetal loss.[125,126] Recently, APS-related pregnancy loss has been extended to include women with early recurrent pregnancy loss [RPL] including those occurring in the preembryonic (less than 6 menstrual weeks of gestation) and embryonic periods (6 through 9 menstrual weeks of gestation).[114] In serologic evaluation of women with RPL, 10 to 20 percent have detectable aPL.[127–132]

Complications occurring in the fetal-neonatal period of pregnancies affected by APS can be serious. At least 40 percent of pregnancy losses reported by women with lupus anticoagulant (LA) or medium-to-high positive IgG aCL occur in the fetal period.[133–137] For those pregnancies complicated by APS with fetal survival past 20 weeks' gestation, the median rate of gestational hypertension-preeclampsia is 32 percent, ranging up to 50 percent.[134–140] Indeed, preeclampsia may develop as early as 15 to 17 weeks' gestation,[134] and two groups of investigators have reported that women with early-onset, severe preeclampsia are more likely to test positive for aPL antibodies compared to healthy controls.[141,142] Several investigators have relatively high rates of IUGR in association with aPL antibodies.[134,138,141,143,144] Even with currently used treatment protocols, the rate of IUGR approaches 30 percent.[134,138] Pregnancies complicated by APS are also more likely to exhibit nonreassuring fetal heart rate patterns during antenatal tests of fetal well being and intrapartum monitoring.[59,134,135] Not surprisingly, the rate of PTB in these series ranges from 32 to 65 percent.[134,138,140]

LABORATORY FEATURES

Laboratory testing for aPL is necessary to confirm or refute the diagnosis of APS. As indicated in Table 42-5, a patient with APS should manifest at least one of three laboratory criteria: (1) presence of LA, or (2) medium-to-high titers of β_2-glycoprotein I-dependent IgG or IgM isotype anticardiolipin antibodies, or (3) medium to high titers of IgG or IgM isotype anti-β_2-glycoprotein I antibodies. Very importantly, positive tests must be confirmed on two separate occasions, at least 12 weeks apart.

LA is identified by in vitro coagulation assays and named as such because the antibodies present prolong clotting times. It is important that published laboratory criteria for the diagnosis of LA be followed. Anticardiolipin antibodies are detected by a standardized enzyme-linked immunosorbent assay that measures β_2-glycoprotein I-dependent IgG and IgM anticardiolipin antibodies. The standard anticardiolipin antibody assay detects β_2-glycoprotein I-dependent anticardiolipin antibodies because β_2-glycoprotein I is present in the diluted patient serum and in the bovine serum typically used in the assay buffer-diluent. There is the possibility that the use of bovine serum biases the standard anticardiolipin antibody assay to detect antibodies that react with both bovine and human β_2-glycoprotein I and explains differences in reactivity between anticardiolipin antibodies and anti-β_2-glycoprotein I assays.

Recent work in the field of aPL has emphasized assays that specifically detect the antibody that binds to β_2-glycoprotein I itself. Most experts now believe that positive tests for this antibody or group of antibodies, referred to as anti-β_2-glycoprotein I, are relatively specific for APS. Thus, anti–β_2-glycoprotein I antibodies are now included as one of three antibodies diagnostic of the condition.

Whereas LA is reported as being positive or negative, anticardiolipin and anti–β_2-glycoprotein I antibodies are reported in terms of international units (designated GPL for IgG binding and MPL for IgM binding). In most laboratories, there is substantial concordance between LA activity and anticardiolipin and anti–β_2-glycoprotein I antibodies, with approximately 70 percent of patients with definite APS having both LA and anticardiolipin or anti–β_2-glycoprotein I antibodies. However, the antibodies detected in three assays are likely not to be identical. As a general rule, LA and IgG anti–β_2-glycoprotein I antibodies are more specific for APS, and anticardiolipin antibody detected in the standard enzyme-linked immunosorbent assay is the more sensitive test for APS. For both anticardiolipin and anti-β_2-glycoprotein I antibodies, specificity is highest for the IgG isotype and for medium-to-high titers. Low positive results should be viewed with suspicion because they may be found in up to 5 percent of normal individuals and should not be used to make the diagnosis of APS. When they occur alone, IgM results are widely considered to have reduced specificity for APS. In spite of well-intentioned efforts at standardization and the availability of positive standard sera, substantial interlaboratory variation when testing the same sera remains a serious problem for both anticardiolipin and anti–β_2-glycoprotein I antibodies. This is due in part to the large number of commercial kits and homemade assays used worldwide.

Clinicians should recognize that the international consensus criteria were developed primarily for research purposes to ensure more uniform characterization, as well as subcategorization, of patients included in studies. This objective is crucial for credible investigative efforts and for appreciation of subtleties of treatment. The consensus criteria also serve to emphasize standardization of laboratory testing, an area of proven concern in aPL. As with other autoimmune conditions, such as SLE, there are individuals who present with one or more clinical or laboratory features suggestive of APS but in whom the diagnosis cannot be made by the relatively strict international consensus criteria. In such cases, experienced clinical judgment is required for best care.

Pregnancy in Women with Antiphospholipid Syndrome

Even with treatment, the potential complications of pregnancy in women with APS include RPL (including fetal death), preeclampsia, placental insufficiency, maternal thrombosis (including stroke), and complications due to treatment. In women with SLE, the potential complications also include lupus exacerbation.

It is perhaps obvious that pregnancy-related risks vary depending on the population in which the diagnosis of APS is made. Women diagnosed because of recurrent preembryonic or embryonic loss, who appear to be typically healthy, are not at high risk for maternal thrombosis, fetal death, preeclampsia, or placenta insufficiency requiring PTB.[14,145–149]

These low-risk patients contrast with those patients that have a history of medical problems (see discussion under Clinical Manifestations earlier). In a case series of APS pregnancies that included women with SLE and prior thrombosis, the median rate of gestational hypertension–preeclampsia was 32 percent, ranging up to 50 percent.[134,139–141,143,150] Placental insufficiency requiring delivery is also relatively frequent in some of these case series.[134,139,143] In contrast to the high rate of preeclampsia observed in some case series of women previously diagnosed with APS, aPL are not found in a statistically significant proportion of a general obstetric population presenting with preeclampsia[151] or in women at moderate risk to develop preeclampsia because of conditions such as underlying chronic hypertension or preeclampsia in a prior pregnancy.[152]

Management

Given the array of potential complications in APS pregnancy, appropriate obstetric care calls for frequent prenatal visits, at least every 2 weeks before midgestation and every week thereafter. The objectives are close observation for maternal thrombosis, hypertension, and other features of preeclampsia, periodic patient evaluation and obstetric ultrasound to assess fetal growth and amniotic fluid volume, and appropriate fetal surveillance testing. The latter should begin at 32 weeks' gestation, or earlier if the clinical situation is suspicious for placental insufficiency, and continue at least weekly until delivery. Frequent rheumatologic consultation every 2 to 4 weeks during pregnancy is recommended, especially in women with SLE.

The ideal treatment for APS during pregnancy would (1) improve maternal and fetal-neonatal outcome by preventing pregnancy loss, preeclampsia, placental insufficiency, and PTB; and (2) reduce or eliminate the maternal thrombotic risk of APS during pregnancy. Treatment of APS in pregnancy to improve fetal outcome has evolved considerably. Enthusiasm for glucocorticoids waned when a small, randomized trial found maternally administered heparin to be as effective as prednisone.[153] Maternally administered heparin is widely considered the treatment of choice at present (Table 42-6), usually initiated in the early first trimester after ultrasonographic demonstration of a live embryo. The dose of heparin required for safe and effective treatment is debated, however. In one trial of nearly 100 women, two thirds of whom had recurrent preembryonic and embryonic pregnancy loss and none of whom had a history of thromboembolic disease, a heparin dose of 5000 U twice daily was associated with a 71-percent live-birth rate.[148] Another study of women with aPL and predominantly preembryonic and embryonic pregnancy loss, none of whom had a history of thromboembolic disease, with heparin administered in a twice daily regimen and adjusted to keep the mid-interval activated partial thromboplastin time approximately 1.5 times the control mean, was associated with an 80-percent live-birth rate.[146] In most case series and trials, daily low-dose aspirin is included in the treatment regimen. A paradigm for the management of APS in pregnancy is shown in Figure 42-1.

It is important that clinicians be aware that the heparin doses recommended for APS patients with prior thrombosis are considerably higher than the 5000 U twice daily used by Rai and colleagues.[148] Indeed, full anticoagulation is urged by some experts.[154] The optimal dose of heparin for women with APS diagnosed because of prior fetal loss or neonatal death after delivery at less than 34 weeks' gestation, for severe preeclampsia or placental insufficiency, but who do not have a history of thromboembolism, is controversial. These women are at risk for thromboembolic disease,[155] and it seems reasonable that these cases receive sufficient thromboprophylaxis (see Table 42-6).

Low-molecular-weight heparins are an acceptable option for the treatment of APS pregnancy. Cost considerations limit the use of low-molecular-weight heparins in the United States, and there is little reason to suspect that one preparation would be better than the other if used in regimens that provide equivalent anticoagulant effects over 24 hours. A direct comparison of standard heparin versus low molecular-weight-heparin in pregnancy is lacking. The potential complications of heparin treatment during pregnancy include hemorrhage, osteoporosis with fracture, and heparin-induced thrombocytopenia. Fortunately, the reported rate of osteoporosis and associated fracture is low, although cases have occurred, even with low-molecular-weight heparin.[139] However, it is likely that the risk is higher in women with underlying autoimmune disease who have required glucocorticosteroid treatment. Heparin-induced thrombocytopenia, which may be lethal, is also fortunately infrequent in pregnant women.[156]

Women with particularly serious thrombotic histories, such as recurrent thrombotic events or cerebral thrombotic events, are understandably viewed as being at very high risk for thrombosis during pregnancy. In selected such cases, we recommend the judicious use of warfarin anticoagulation rather than heparin.

Table 42-6. Subcutaneous Heparin Regimens Used in the Treatment of Antiphospholipid Syndrome During Pregnancy

Prophylactic Regimens	
Recurrent Preembryonic and Embryonic Loss; No History of Thrombotic Events	
Standard heparin	1. 5,000–7,500 U every 12 hours in the first trimester, 5,000–10,000 U every 12 hours in the second and third trimesters
Low-molecular-weight heparin	1. Enoxaparin 40 mg once daily or dalteparin 5,000 U once daily, OR 2. Enoxaparin 30 mg every 12 hours or dalteparin 5,000 U every 12 hours
Prior Fetal Death or Early Delivery Because of Severe Preeclampsia or Severe Placental Insufficiency; No History of Thrombotic Events	
Standard heparin	1. 7,500–10,000 U every 12 hours in the first trimester, 10,000 U every 12 hours in the second and third trimesters
Low-molecular-weight heparin	1. Enoxaparin 40 mg once daily or dalteparin 5,000 U once daily, OR 2. Enoxaparin 30 mg every 12 hours or dalteparin 5,000 U every 12 hours
Anticoagulation Regimens—Recommended in Women with A History of Thrombotic Events	
Standard heparin	1. 7,500 U every 8–12 hours adjusted to maintain the mid-interval heparin levels in the therapeutic range
Low-molecular-weight heparin	1. Weight-adjusted (e.g., enoxaparin 1 mg/kg every 12 hours or dalteparin 200 U/kg every 12 hours)

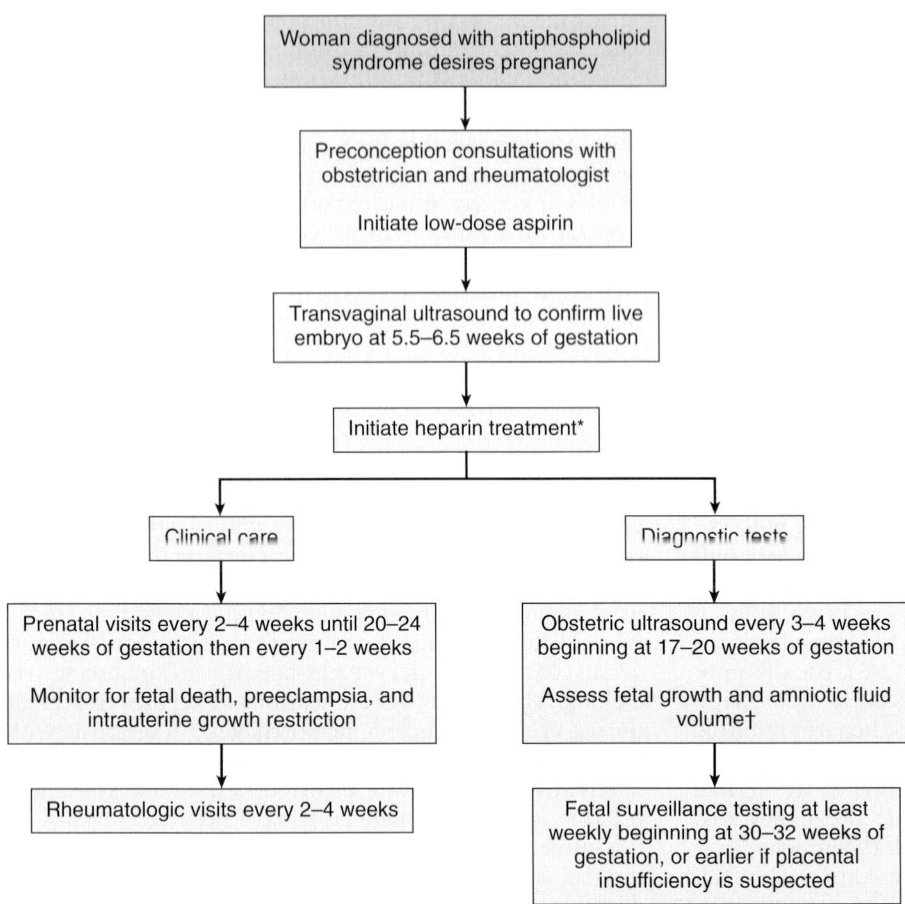

Figure 42-1. Suggested algorithm for the management of antiphospholipid syndrome in pregnancy. See Table 42-6 for dosing. In the United Kingdom, Doppler assessment of the uterine arteries is commonly used at 20–24 weeks' gestation for the prediction of preeclampsia and placental insufficiency risks. This is not commonly done in the United States.

IVIG has also been used during pregnancy, usually in conjunction with heparin and low-dose aspirin, especially in women with particularly poor histories or RPL during heparin treatment.[157] However, a randomized, controlled, pilot study of IVIG treatment during pregnancy in unselected APS cases found no benefit to this expensive therapy relative to heparin and low-dose aspirin.[158]

Clinicians should realize that otherwise healthy women with RPL and low titers of aPL do not require treatment. The controlled trial of Pattison and colleagues[159] included a majority of such women and found no difference in live-birth rates using either low-dose aspirin or a placebo.

Anticoagulant coverage of the postpartum period in women with APS and prior thrombosis is critical.[160] We prefer switching the patient to warfarin thromboprophylaxis as soon as she is clinically stable after delivery. In most cases, an international normalized ratio of 2.0 to 3.0 is desirable. There is no international consensus regarding the postpartum management of those women without prior thrombosis in whom APS is diagnosed because of a prior fetal loss, or neonatal death after delivery at or before 34 weeks' gestation, or for severe preeclampsia or placental insufficiency, although all agree there is an increased risk of thrombosis. The recommendation in the United States is anticoagulant therapy for 6 weeks following delivery. The need for postpartum anticoagulation in women with APS diagnosed solely on the basis of recurrent preembryonic or embryonic losses is uncertain but may be unnecessary. Both heparin and warfarin are safe to use in patients who are breast-feeding.

RHEUMATOID ARTHRITIS

Introduction

Rheumatoid arthritis (RA) is a debilitating disease involving chronic symmetric inflammatory arthritis of the synovial joints with an incidence of 2.5 to 7 per 10,000 per year and a prevalence of approximately 1 percent in the adult U.S. population. RA is usually diagnosed between ages 40 and 50 years, but can appear at any age of life and the prevalence increases with age into the 60s or 70s in both women and men. Although found in virtually all populations, it is more common in some (Native American) and less common in others (Native African). As with most autoimmune conditions, RA is more common in women than in men, with a ratio of 2 to 3 female cases to one male.[161]

Juvenile rheumatoid arthritis (JRA) is diagnosed in children before age 16 years and can be clinically indistinguishable from RA at time of presentation. However, JRA tends to have a milder clinical course and typically resolves without serious disability in 70 to 90 percent of children diagnosed.

Pathophysiology

The histologic features of RA include symmetric inflammatory synovitis marked by cellular hyperplasia, accumulation of inflammatory leukocytes, and angiogenesis with membrane thickening, edema, and fibrin deposition as common early findings. Inflammatory damage at the synovium eventually leads to typical joint erosion involving a locally invasive synovial tissue called pannus.

The inflammatory damage in RA appears to be primarily mediated by CD4+ T cells. The CD4+ T cells recognize unknown endogenous or exogenous antigens, are activated by these antigens, and stimulate monocytes, macrophages, and synovial fibroblasts to produce cytokines interleukin-1 (IL-1), IL-6, and tumor necrosis factor-α (TNF-α), which, in turn, are key contributors to inflammation in RA. CD4+ T cells also express osteoprotegerin ligands that stimulate osteoclastogenesis, as confirmed in animal models of RA.[162] Activated CD4+ T cells also stimulate B cells to produce immunoglobulins, one of which is rheumatoid factor (RF), the characteristic autoantibody in patients with RA. RF is present in the peripheral circulation and synovium of RA patients. Whether or not RF autoantibodies are substantially involved in tissue damage remains controversial. There is some evidence that RF autoantibodies form aggregates in synovial fluid, resulting in complement activation and local inflammation, and eventual joint erosion.

Concordance for RA is found in approximately 15 percent of monozygotic twins and 5 percent of dizygotic twins. It is estimated that heritable factors account for approximately 60 percent of the predisposition to RA.[163] The HLA region (HLA class II gene locus DRB1, encoding HLA-DR), is of primary importance in RA susceptibility. Variant forms of DRB1 have been identified in association with RA including DRB1*0401, *0404, *0405, *0101, *1402, and *1001. These alleles encode for similar amino acid sequences (so-called shared epitopes) that are suspected of bestowing susceptibility to RA. Other suspect HLA complex genes are located on chromosomes 1p and 1q, 9, 12 p, 16 cen, and 18q.[164,165]

Clinical Manifestations and Laboratory Findings

RA typically has an insidious onset over several months; less commonly, the disease onset is acute and somewhat rapid. Twice as many patients present during winter months compared with the summer months, and trauma (including surgery) may be a precursor. The most common initial features of RA are morning stiffness, pain, and swelling of peripheral joints. Fatigue, weakness, weight loss, and malaise can also be common findings. The disease tends to involve primarily the joints of the wrists, knees, shoulders, and metacarpophalangeal joints in an erosive arthritis that usually follows a slowly progressive course marked by exacerbations and remissions. Eventually, joint deformities may occur; these are especially obvious at the metacarpophalangeal joint and proximal and distal interphalangeal joints of the hands.

Rheumatoid nodules, composed of a local proliferation of small vessels, histiocytes, fibroblasts, and other cells, present in 20 to 30 percent of affected patients and are usually located in the subcutaneous tissues of the extensor surfaces of the forearm. Although uncommon, extra-articular tissues may also be affected. These extra-articular tissues include the lung (pleuritis, pleural effusions, interstitial fibrosis, pulmonary nodules, pneumonitis, and airway disease) and heart (pericarditis, effusion, myocarditis, endocardial inflammation, conduction defects, and arteritis leading to myocardial infarction).

The classification criteria published by the American College of Rheumatology are shown in Table 42-7. Physical examination should reveal evidence of joint inflammation including joint tenderness, synovial thickening, joint effusion, erythema, and decreased range of motion. Symmetric involvement should be noted. Radiographic evidence of RA includes joint space narrowing and erosion

Table 42-7 Classification Criteria for the Diagnosis of Rheumatoid Arthritis (1987, ACR)

CRITERIA*	DEFINITION
Morning stiffness	Morning stiffness in and around the joints, lasting at least 1 hour before maximal improvement
Arthritis of three joint areas	At least 3 joint areas simultaneously have had soft tissue swelling or fluid (not bony overgrowth alone) observed by a physician. The 14 possible areas are right or left PIP, MCP, wrist, elbow, knee, ankle, and MTP joints
Arthritis of hand joints	At least 1 area swollen (as defined above) in a wrist, MCP, or PIP joint
Symmetric arthritis	Simultaneous involvement of the same joint areas (as defined in 2) on both sides of the body (bilateral involvement of PIPs, MCPs, or MTPs is acceptable without absolute symmetry)
Rheumatoid nodules	Subcutaneous nodules, over bony prominences, or extensor surfaces, or in juxtaarticular regions, observed by a physician
Serum rheumatoid	Demonstration of abnormal amounts of serum rheumatoid factor by any method for which the result has been positive in less than 5% of normal control subjects
Radiographic changes	Radiographic changes typical of rheumatoid arthritis on posteroanterior hand and wrist radiographs, which must include erosions or unequivocal bony decalcification localized in or most marked adjacent to the involved joints (osteoarthritis changes alone do not qualify)

*For classification purposes, a patient shall be said to have rheumatoid arthritis if he/she has satisfied at least four of these seven criteria. Criteria one through four must have been present for at least 6 weeks. Patients with two clinical diagnoses are not excluded. Designation as classic, definite, or probable rheumatoid arthritis is *not* to be made.

MCP, metacarpophalangeal joint; MTP, metatarsophalangeal joint; PIP, proximal interphalangeal joint.

Arnett FC, Edworthy SM, Bloch DA, et al: The American Rheumatism Association 1987 revised criteria for the classification of rheumatoid arthritis. Arthritis Rheum 31:315, 1988.

and, though too expensive for routine use, magnetic resonance imaging may detect synovial hypertrophy, edema, and early erosive changes.

Of those patients with clinical features of RA, 70 percent are also seropositive for RF. In addition, some of those who are initially seronegative eventually convert, leaving only 10 percent of patients with RA without a positive RF. Approximately 5 percent of people in the general population test positive for RF, as do many patients with viral infections, parasitic infections, chronic bacterial infections, irradiation or chemotherapy, or other autoimmune conditions, for example, SLE, scleroderma, and mixed connective tissue disease.

Pregnancy and Rheumatoid Arthritis

Clinical Course of Rheumatoid Arthritis During Pregnancy

Numerous studies (Table 42-8) show that at least 50 percent, and maybe as much as 75 percent, of patients with RA demonstrate improvement in their disease in at least 50 percent of their pregnancies.[166–173] For a majority of patients, the improvement in RA starts in the first trimester heralded by a reduction in joint stiffness and pain.[169] The peak improvement in symptoms generally occurs in the second or third trimester. Other aspects of the disease may also improve during pregnancy, including subcutaneous nodules associated with RA.[171] In addition, Hazes and colleagues reported a protective effect of pregnancy in development of RA.[174]

Even with the overall improvement in symptoms, the clinical course of RA during pregnancy is characterized by short-term fluctuations in symptoms. Most but not all patients who experience an improvement in RA during pregnancy have a similar improvement in subsequent pregnancies. At present, there is no laboratory or clinical feature that predicts improvement of RA in pregnancy, and in a few patients, the disease worsens. Nearly three quarters of patients whose disease has improved during pregnancy will suffer a relapse in the first several postpartum months.[169,171] The level of disease during the first year after delivery generally returns to that of a year before conception, but it may be worse.[173] There are few studies of JRA, but one found that only one case in 20 had a worsening or reactivation of the disease associated with pregnancy.[176]

There are no data to suggest that RA in remission is likely to have a better course during pregnancy than active RA. The long-term prognosis for RA patients undertaking pregnancy appears to be similar to those that avoid pregnancy. Oka and Vainio[173] compared 100 consecutive pregnant RA patients with age- and disease-matched controls, and found no significant differences between the groups in terms of the severity of their disease.

The mechanisms by which pregnancy favorably affects RA is unknown. Plasma cortisol, which rises during pregnancy to peak at term, was initially thought to be important in the amelioration of RA.[166] However, there is no correlation between cortisol concentrations and disease state.[176] Some studies suggest that estrogens or estrogens and progestagens favorably affect arthritis,[177] but there are conflicting studies,[178] and a double-blind crossover trial found that estrogen did not benefit patients with RA.[179] Sex hormones may interfere with immunoregulation and interactions with the cytokine system.[180] Promising data suggest that certain proteins circulating in higher concentrations during pregnancy or unique to pregnancy are associated with improvement of RA. These include pregnancy-associated a_2-glycoprotein[181] and gamma globulins eluted from placenta.[182] Other investigators believe that the placenta may modify RA by clearing immune complexes[183] or that modification of immune globulins during pregnancy alters their inflammatory activity.[184]

In 1993, Nelson and coworkers[185] reported that amelioration of RA during pregnancy is associated with a maternal-fetal disparity in HLA class II antigens. Maternal-fetal HLA class II disparity was noted in 26 of the 34 pregnancies (75 percent) described as having remission or improvement in their arthritis, compared with only three of 12 whose condition remained unchanged or worsened. The authors suggested that the maternal immune response to paternal HLA antigens may have a role in pregnancy-induced remission of RA.[185]

Obstetric Complications

About 15 to 25 percent of pregnancies in women with RA end in miscarriage,[186,187] a figure that may or may not be slightly higher than in normal women. One controlled study found that women with RA have a significantly higher frequency of miscarriage than normal women, even before the onset of their disease (25 versus 17 percent before disease, 27 versus 17 percent after

Table 42-8. Improvement of Rheumatoid Arthritis in Pregnancy

AUTHOR	PATIENTS	PATIENTS WITH IMPROVEMENT (%)	PREGNANCIES	PREGNANCIES WITH IMPROVEMENT (%)
Hench[161]	22	20 (91)	37	33 (89)
Oka[168]	93	73 (78)	114	88 (77)
Betson[164]	21	13 (62)	21	13 (62)
Ostensen[171]	10	8 (90)	10	9 (90)
Ostensen[175]*	51	NA	76	35 (46)

*Study of patients with juvenile rheumatoid arthritis.

disease).[186] However, another controlled study did not find that women with RA have a higher proportion of miscarriage before the onset of disease,[161] although the frequency of fetal death was higher in patients who later develop RA than in nonaffected relatives. There are scant data available, but women with RA do not appear to be at significant risk for PTB, preeclampsia, fetal growth impairment, or stillbirth.

Management

Ideally, a woman with RA should have a preconception visit to discuss the present state of her disease to reduce and or change maintenance medications so as to avoid fetal risks (see later). Given that a majority of patients experience improvement in RA during pregnancy, routine prenatal care is usually sufficient. Those patients with persistent symptoms may require more attention and care by a rheumatologist. Rest is an important part of the management of RA, and the patient should be counseled to plan adequately for this. Physical therapy can be helpful in patients whose disease does not improve with pregnancy. In an otherwise uncomplicated pregnancy, antepartum fetal testing, including serial ultrasound, nonstress testing, or use of the biophysical profile, is not necessary in a patient with RA.

Antirheumatic Medications

Within the last decade, there have been dramatic advancements in the pharmacologic management of RA (Table 42-9). Whereas in the past, patients would frequently be maintained on glucocorticoids and NSAIDs, modern day treatment often involves new disease modifying antirheumatic drugs (DMARDs) along with NSAIDs. Older agents, such as penicillamine and gold salts, are now rarely used and are not discussed. Use of glucocorticoids in pregnancy, including maternal and fetal risk, is discussed in the section covering SLE.

If at all possible, an attempt should be made to manage RA with acetaminophen, because it is a FDA pregnancy category A, and low-dose glucocorticoids (5 to 10 mg prednisone/day). However, because of changes in the pharmacotherapy used to treat RA, many patients present to their obstetrician having taken other medications. DMARDs are one such group. This classification of medications includes leflunomide, an isoxazole derivative that competitively inhibits dihydroorotate dehydrogenase, the rate-limiting enzyme required for the de novo synthesis of pyrimidines. Activated lymphocytes are dependent on this pyrimidine synthesis pathway, and by instituting a blockade, antiproliferative effects are noted. Leflunomide is teratogenic and is associated with fetal death. Thus, it is contraindicated in pregnancy. Importantly, this medication has an extremely long half life of 15 to 18 days, such that merely discontinuing the medication before pregnancy may not be sufficient to spare a embryonic exposure. An elimination protocol using oral cholestyramine and measuring plasma levels of leflunomide should be followed. Methotrexate is also included in the DMARDs group and is contraindicated in pregnancy or in those attempting to conceive.

TNF antagonists include medications like etanercept, infliximab, and adalimumab. As the category implies, these drugs work by antagonizing TNF-α, a key inflammatory cytokine in RA released by activated monocytes, macrophages, and T lymphocytes. The most common side effect seen is an increase in the number of serious bacterial infections seen in patients on these medications. The effect of TNF antagonists in pregnancy has been

Table 42-9. Drugs Used for Rheumatoid Arthritis

DRUG	MECHANISM OF ACTION	DOSAGE	MONITORING REQUIRED
NSAIDs	Anti-inflammatory	600 mg–800 mg PO q 6–8 hours	Gastrointestinal upset
Glucocorticoids	Anti-inflammatory/ immunosuppressive	Varies based on medication used	
Acetaminophen	Analgesic	650 mg PO q 4–6 h, not to exceed 3–4 g/day	None
DMARDs			
Leflunomide	Inhibits pyrimidine synthesis	Loading dose of 100 mg daily for 3 days, then 20 mg daily	Not for use in pregnancy. Extensive washout procedure recommended
Methotrexate	Inhibits dihydrofolate reductase	7.5–25 mg once a week	CBC, ALT q month
TNF antagonists			
Etanercept	Binds TNF-α and TNF-β	25 mg twice/week or 50 mg once/week 3 mg/kg of body weight at 0, 2, 6 wks then every 8 wk	Alert for infectious processes, specifically TB, histoplasmosis
Infliximab	Chimeric anti–TNF-α antibody	40 mg every second week	
Adalimumab	Human anti–TNF-α antibody	20–40 mg once a week	
Anakinra	Interleukin-1 receptor antagonist	100 mg daily	CBC monthly × 3 months then q 3 months

ALT, alanine transaminase; CBC, complete blood count; DMARDs, disease-modifying antirheumatic drugs; NSAIDs, nonsteroidal anti-inflammatory drugs; TNF-α, tumor necrosis factor-α; TNF-β, tumor necrosis factor-β.

evaluated by Katz et al.[188] In this study, they followed 96 pregnancies in women taking infliximab. Of those patients, 67 percent had a normal live birth, 15 percent ended in miscarriage, and 19 percent of the pregnancies were electively terminated. One of the infants had tetralogy of Fallot, another demonstrated an intestinal malrotation, and one twin had hypothyroidism. The authors concluded that outcomes were similar to that of the general population. It is too early, however, to suggest that TNF antagonists are safe in pregnancy. Anakinra, a relatively newly introduced DMARD, blocks the IL-1 receptor. The use of anakinra in pregnancy has not been evaluated and, therefore, is not recommended.

The use of NSAIDs in pregnancy, also covered in the section dealing with SLE, should be avoided except in specific instances and, if used, restricted to a limited time period. Chronic use of these medications is contraindicated.

SYSTEMIC SCLEROSIS

Introduction

Systemic sclerosis (SSc) is a multisystem disorder affecting the skin and internal organs. It is characterized histologically by a marked increase in collagen, mostly in the dermis with hyalinization and often obliteration of small blood vessels. The term scleroderma most specifically refers to the skin fibrosis most noticeable to the patient but is frequently used interchangeably with term systemic sclerosis. SSc is uncommon, occurring in no more than 10 to 15 individuals per million per year. The ratio of women to men is 10:1 in the 15- to 44-year age group. However, the mean age of onset is in the range from 30 to 50 years, a time when many affected women may potentially become pregnant.[189]

Pathogenesis

The pathophysiologic changes of SSc include vascular abnormalities, immunologic abnormalities, and disordered collagen synthesis. The initial event most likely occurs in small blood vessels, with early proliferation of intimal layer endothelial cells that produce cytokines, growth factors, adhesion proteins, vasoactive proteins, coagulation factors, and extracellular matrix. Aberrant production of substances such as von Willebrand's factor may also occur. A hallmark feature of SSc is increased fibroblast activity with an accelerated rate of fibroblast collagen synthesis.

Early in the disease process, the dermis contains mononuclear cell infiltrates and sometimes calcium, owing to the deposition of calcium hydroxyapatite. Thinning of the epidermis and loss of normal dermal appendages are other pathologic changes seen in SSc. Small arteries and arterioles exhibit characteristic endothelial cell proliferation and intimal thickening, as well as increased amounts of fibrinogen and fibrin with lumina often occluded by fibrosis. Remaining vessels become dilated and are visible through the skin as telangiectasias.

Internal organs have similar histologic changes. Fibromucoid intimal thickening in the kidney results in narrowing and thinning of the lumen. Cortical glomerular involvement is typically focal in nature and includes endothelial cell proliferation and thickening of the basement membrane. In the lung, the most common finding is interstitial fibrosis with increased numbers of fibroblasts, capillary congestion, and thickening and occlusion of alveolar walls and arteriolar intima. Densely hyalinized fibrosis is found in the gastrointestinal tract and random focal fibrosis in the myocardium.

An association between an increase of HLA-DR11 (whites) and DR15 (Asians) in patients with SSc has been described. Associations have also been described with the SSc-associated autoantibodies, topo-isomerase I, and anticentromere antibody, although results have varied in ethnic and racial groups.[190]

A number of different non-HLA genes have recently been identified with SSc. Genes encoding extracellular matrix proteins have been identified, notably C0L1A1 and C0L1A2, genes encoding type I collagen. Analysis of a Native American population with a particularly high prevalence of SSc identified a candidate gene near the fibrillin 1 gene on chromosome 15q. Polymorphisms in transforming growth factor-β (TGF-β) 1, 2, and 3 genes have also been identified in association with SSc, as have polymorphisms in TNF-α, tumor necrosis factor-β (TNF-β), CXC chemokine receptor 2 (CXCR2), tissue inhibitor of metalloproteinase 1 (TIMP-1), and interleukin-4R (IL-4R) alpha.[191]

Clinical Manifestations and Diagnosis

Classification

The American College of Rheumatology has suggested preliminary criteria for the classification of SSc based on clinical and laboratory assessments of patients[192] (Table 42-10). The major criterion for classification was sclerodermatous skin change in any location proximal of the metacarpophalangeal joints. This feature had a sensitivity of 91 percent and a specificity of greater than 99 percent in establishing the diagnosis. Minor criteria were also established and consisted of the presence of sclerodactyly, digital pitting scars on the fingertips, loss of digital finger pad substance, and bibasilar pulmonary fibrosis.

Within the diagnosis of SSc, there are several recognized subgroups. These subgroups have been established based on clinical features and have clinical and prognostic importance. *Diffuse* cutaneous scleroderma refers to skin thickening present on the trunk in addition to face and proximal and distal extremities. *Limited* cutaneous SSc refers to skin thickening limited to sites distal to the elbow and knee but also involving the face and neck. CREST syndrome, sometimes referred to as a form of limited cutaneous SSc, involves calcinosis of involved skin, Raynaud's phenomenon, esophageal dysmotility, sclerodactyly and telangiectasias. Subgroup classification also extends to include disease duration. Measured from the time of the first symptom attributable to SSc, the clas-

Table 42-10. Classification of Systemic Sclerosis

	SKIN FEATURES	SYSTEMIC FEATURES
Diffuse cutaneous	Above the elbows or knees and/or on trunk	
Limited cutaneous	Distal to the elbow, knees and above the clavicles	
CREST syndrome (3 of 5 present)	Subcutaneous calcinosis, Raynaud's phenomenon, Esophageal dysfunction sclerodactyly, telangiectasia	
Systemic sclerosis sine	No skin involvement	Presence of internal organ manifestations, vascular and serologic abnormalities
Localized scleroderma	Asymmetric plaques of fibrotic skin	No systemic disease

CREST syndrome, calcinosis of involved skin, Raynaud's phenomenon, esophageal dysmotility, sclerodactyly, and telangiectasias.

Table 42-11. Subsets of Systemic Sclerosis

Diffuse Cutaneous SSc (dSSc)

- Onset of Raynaud's within 1 year of onset of skin changes
- Truncal and acral skin involvement
- Presence of tendon friction rubs
- Early and significant incidence of interstitial lung disease, oliguric renal failure, diffuse gastrointestinal disease, and myocardial involvement
- Absence of anticentromere antibodies (ACA)
- Nailfold capillary dilantation and capillary destruction
- Antitopoisomerase antibodies (30% of patients)

Limited Cutaneous SSc (lSSc)

- Raynaud's phenomenon for years (occasionally decades)
- Skin involvement limited to hands, face, feet and forearms (acral) or absent
- A significant late incidence of pulmonary hypertension, with or without interstitial lung disease, trigeminal neuralgia, skin calcifications, telangiectaisa
- A high incidence of ACA (70–80%)
- Dilated nailfold capillary loops, usually without capillary dropout

From LeRoy EC, Black C, Fleischmgjer R, et al: Scleroderma (systemic sclerosis): classification, subsets and pathogenesis. J Rheumatol 15:202, 1988.

sification varies but one definition includes early as being less than 3 years' duration and late as 6 or more years' duration (Table 42-11).

Patients who develop early diffuse disease are more likely to present with arthritis, finger and hand swelling, and skin thickening. The skin thickening, which usually starts on the fingers and hands, may eventually involve the neck and face. Marked deformities of the hands and fingers may occur and is attributed to fibrosis of arterioles and small arteries. In these circumstances, the normal vasoconstrictor response to various stimuli, including cold, causes near-complete obliteration of the vessel, and as a result, digital ischemia may occur. Internal organ involvement and dysfunction is a common finding in early diffuse disease and probably results from the same vasculopathy seen in the extremities. Lower esophageal dysfunction is most common, but other portions of the gastrointestinal tract may be involved, producing malabsorption, diarrhea, and constipation.

Patients with SSc develop a variety of pulmonary lesions, with the most common being progression interstitial fibrosis. Pulmonary hypertension, a problem of special interest to the obstetrician, may also occur in long-standing disease. Nearly half of the patients with well-established SSc have evidence of myocardial involvement, specifically dysrhythmias. Renal disease occurs to some extent in many patients and is a major cause of mortality among patients with SSc. Severely involved cases may present with proteinuria and renal insufficiency, hypertension, or both. Sudden onset of severe hypertension and progressive renal insufficiency with microangiopathic hemolysis is known as scleroderma renal crisis. These crises usually occur in cold weather, suggesting that the pathophysiology is similar to that of Raynaud's phenomenon.

Diagnosis

The diagnosis of SSc is primarily clinical. ANA are present in most patients with SSc, but anti-DNA antibodies are not. About half of patients have serum cryoglobulins. Antibodies to centromere detected by indirect immunofluorescence are common among patients with limited cutaneous SSc (CREST syndrome), but not among those with diffuse cutaneous disease. Up to 40 percent of patients have antibody to an extractable nuclear antigen designated ScI, although the biologic significance of these autoantibodies is unclear.

Pregnancy

Effects of Pregnancy on Systemic Sclerosis

Whether or not pregnancy plays a *causative* role in the genesis of SSc is a subject of controversy. One recent report[193] noted an increased risk of SSc related to nulliparity and that the risk of developing SSc decreased with increasing number of births, an association possibly due to subfecundity. In contrast, a considerable literature has grown around the concept that fetal microchimerism is a cause of SSc, or at least contributes to the pathogenesis of SSc.[193] Numerous studies have evaluated the effect of fetal cells on maternal disease. Bianchi et al.,[194] in 1996, reported that fetal cells remain in maternal circulation up to 27 years after childbirth, and Nelson et al.[195] questioned whether microchimerism arising from pregnancy could imitate graft-versus-host disease. Using these studies as a basis, Nelson et al.[195] evaluated the presence of fetal microchimerism in women with SSc compared with matched healthy controls. Semiquantitative PCR assays were used to detect Y chromosome–specific sequences in the maternal blood. Y—specific DNA was detected in 25 percent of the control patients and 59 percent of the SSC patients. In addition, the total cell number was significantly increased in the SSc patients, with a mean number of male cell DNA equivalents among controls of 0.38 cells per 16 ml of whole blood and 11.1 among scleroderma patients.[196] Another group of investigators, however, did not find increased Y chromosome DNA in skin biopsies of women with SSc, although they also found an increased number of male cells present in the patients with SSc when compared with healthy controls.[197] Lambert et al.[200] recently quantified the maternal microchimeric HLA specific DNA in patients with SSc and controls using real-time PCR assays. Maternal microchimerism was present more often in women with SSc (72 percent) than in healthy controls (22 percent); however, the levels of microchimeric cells were not significantly different.[193] Thus, these and several other studies[198,199] have yielded contradictory results, possibly from using different detection methods or from quantitative variations.[200] At this time, the impact of maternal microchimerism on SSC is not yet known.

The largest and most recent case series suggest that overall maternal outcomes in women with SSc are generally good, with worsening of disease in pregnancy in no more than 20 percent of cases. In most pregnancies (60 to 80 percent), the disease remains clinically stable.[189,201,202] Esophageal manifestations may worsen, which is most likely a result of a decreased tone in the lower esophageal sphincter.[184]

Pregnancy is probably safest in SSc patients without obvious renal, cardiac, or pulmonary disease. Although data are scant, women with SSc patients with moderate-to-severe cardiac or pulmonary involvement likely face increased risks of substantial morbidity or mortality and should not undertake pregnancy. In addition, SSc patients with moderate to severe renal disease and hypertension probably face a substantial risk for preeclampsia, and perhaps for mortality due to renal crisis. Pregnancy should be discouraged in these women as well. Finally, there may be an increased risk of renal crisis in patients with early diffuse SSc,[202] and it may be prudent to delay pregnancy in these patients.

Postpartum, about one third of women with SSc have exacerbations of Raynaud's phenomenon, arthritis, and skin thickening.[202]

Effects of Systemic Sclerosis on Pregnancy

Pregnancy in women with SSc is uncommon, with no more than a few hundred cases reported in the published literature. Early reports that fertility was impaired in women with SSc may have been due to factors such as maternal age or a desire to avoid pregnancy or children.[189]

Fetal Outcomes

As with many other autoimmune conditions, early case reports and small series focused on poor pregnancy outcomes. In addition, one group of investigators found that a predisposition to miscarriage might predate the onset of SSC in some women. Of 154 patients who eventually developed SSc and 115 matched controls, a significantly greater number of cases had a history of miscarriage (29 versus 17 percent).[203]

However, reports and case series of women with preexisting SSc do not point to SSc being associated with pregnancy loss. For example, among the 29 pregnancies accumulated in case reports, there were two miscarriages (7 percent), two fetal deaths (7 percent), and one neonatal death attributable to prematurity; two other infants died because of multiple anomalies. Among 103 pregnancies in several small series,[204–207] there were 24 miscarriages (23 percent), three fetal deaths (3 percent), and two neonatal deaths due to prematurity. Taken together, noncontrolled reports suggest that 72 to 83 percent of pregnancies among women with SSc are successful, excluding perinatal deaths due to anomalies.

Case-control studies provide a slightly different view. In the case-controlled study by Giordano et al.,[208] 80 SSc patients had 299 pregnancies. Of these, 50 ended in miscarriage (17 percent), a rate significantly higher than the rate of miscarriage in the matched controls (10 percent). There was no difference in the miscarriage rate between patients with diffuse cutaneous versus limited cutaneous SSc. The retrospective study of Steen et al.[201] included 86 pregnancies after the onset of SSc. Of these, 15 percent ended in miscarriage and 2 percent in midtrimester fetal deaths, percentages similar to those in RA controls or neighborhood controls. A later prospective study found that 16 percent of 80 SSc pregnancies ended in miscarriage compared with 14 percent in a control group.[202] With these studies, the available data suggest that the rate of miscarriages and fetal deaths in patients with SSc might be slightly increased compared with controls. It is worth emphasizing that in the prospective study by Steen (1999) women with late, diffuse SSc demonstrated an increased risk for miscarriage, 42 percent compared with 13 percent for all other subjects.

Of ongoing pregnancies, about one third of SSc pregnancies are delivered preterm. In Steen's[202] series, 15 percent of pregnancies in women with SSc delivered early secondary to preterm labor or PPROM. In other reports and case series, at least 25 percent of ongoing pregnancies in SSc patients were delivered prematurely.[172,201,204–209] PTB is particularly prominent in women with early, diffuse cutaneous disease.[202]

Given the microvascular pathology of the condition and the relative frequency of renal involvement in SSc, one might speculate that preeclampsia and IUGR occur significantly more often in SSc pregnancies. This is supported by high rates of preeclampsia in case reports, although this is not so apparent in case series. In one case series, 10 percent of pregnancies were complicated by IUGR,[201] but the same authors found a lower rate of IUGR in subsequent pregnancies.[202]

Neonatal manifestations of skin sclerosis, perhaps secondary to SSc, have been reported in a few cases. The risks of this condition, as well as its relationship to SSc itself, however, remain unclear.

MANAGEMENT

Preconception counseling is important in patients with scleroderma. Those with early diffuse scleroderma or patients with significant cardiopulmonary involvement or severe renal disease should be counseled regarding risks associated with pregnancy. Special attention should be given to the evaluation of possible renal or cardiopulmonary involvement. The option of pregnancy termination should be entertained in patients with diffuse SSc, cardiopulmonary involvement or moderate-to-severe renal involvement.

Even in the nonpregnant state, there is no satisfactory therapy for SSc. Patients with limited cutaneous SSc are usually managed with vasodilators and anti-inflammatory agents. As discussed earlier, use of NSAIDs should be limited or avoided if at all possible during pregnancy. Oral vasodilators for the prevention and treatment of Raynaud's phenomenon may be continued, although definitive proof of fetal safely is lacking. Patients with early, diffuse cutaneous SSc may be taking glucocorticoids. Other immunosuppressive or cytotoxic agents should be avoided.

The use of angiotensin-converting enzyme inhibitors appears to be particularly effective in treating SSc-related hypertension and renal crises. However, the use of these drugs in pregnancy is associated with fetoneonatal renal insufficiency and, as a general rule, should be avoided. In the case of SSc-related hypertension, the practitioner must evaluate whether the benefits of these medications outweigh the risks of discontinuing them.[210]

Given the rarity of this illness, evidenced-based recommendations regarding prenatal care are lacking. It would seem reasonable that SSc patients with continuing pregnancies should be seen by a physician every 1 to 2 weeks in the first half of pregnancy and once weekly thereafter. Although serial laboratory testing is not necessary, laboratory assessment of unusual or suspicious symptoms or signs may be helpful. Pregnancies should be monitored for evidence of preeclampsia, because this complication may be more likely with scleroderma.[202] The possible risk of IUGR and fetal death suggest that serial examination of the fetus by sonography might be beneficial. Most experts would suggest fetal surveillance be instituted by 30 or 32 weeks' gestation, or sooner if the clinical situation demands.

In patients with mild-to-moderate disease, few additional precautions are needed during the labor and delivery process. Wound healing may be a problem in patients with advanced disease or those on steroids. In patients with significant pulmonary, cardiac or renal impairment, intensive care management may be needed.

Postpartum resumption of prepregnancy management should be implemented. Most often, reinstitution of maintenance medication is all that is required.

KEY POINTS

- SLE is the most common serious autoimmune disease affecting women of reproductive age. The most common presenting complaints in women diagnosed with SLE include fatigue, weight loss, arthralgias, arthritis, and myalgias. SLE is associated with an increase in poor pregnancy outcomes including IUGR, stillbirth, and spontaneous abortion.
- Renal disease, LN, eventually occurs in about 50 percent of patients with SLE. Confirmation of the diagnosis requires a renal biopsy. SLE complicated by active LN with advanced renal insufficiency (creatinine greater than 2.0 mg/dl) should be considered an absolute contraindication to pregnancy.
- Immunoflourescent assays, such as the anti-dsDNA antibodies that identify specific nuclear antigen-antibody reactions are better for confirming the diagnosis of SLE, monitoring disease activity, and guiding immunotherapy.
- Overall, 15 to 60 percent of women with SLE have a flare during pregnancy or the postpartum period. The level of preexisting disease activity plays a large role in the risk of SLE flare during pregnancy. Women with active SLE should be discouraged from becoming pregnant until they are in remission. If pregnancy predisposes to a lupus flare, it does so only modestly.
- Once a woman with SLE and anti-Ro/SSA antibodies delivers an infant with CCHB, the risk for recurrence is at least two- to threefold higher than in women with anti-Ro/SSa or anti-La/SSB antibodies who have never had an affected child.
- Hydroxychloroquine may be safely continued during pregnancy and is a highly effective agent for maintenance SLE therapy.
- aPL are found in up to 5 percent of apparently healthy controls and in up to 35 percent of patients with SLE. Patients with APS are at increased risk for RPL, hypertension complicating pregnancy, particularly with its onset early in gestation, IUGR, nonreassuring fetal heart rate patterns, and PTB.
- Low-dose heparin and low-dose aspirin are the therapies of choice for patients with APS. Women with APS who have had a prior thrombosis will require doses of heparin that are considerably higher.
- RA tends to improve during pregnancy but may relapse in the postpartum period. RA does not appear to have a deleterious effect on pregnancy.

REFERENCES

1. Kotzin BL: Systemic lupus erythematosus. Cell 85:303, 1996.
2. Beeson PB: Age and sex associations of 40 autoimmune diseases. Am J Med 96:457, 1994.

3. Petri M, Howard D, Repke J: Frequency of lupus flare in pregnancy: The Hopkins lupus pregnancy center experience. Arthritis Rhem 34:1538, 1991.
4. Hayslett JP: The effect of systemic lupus erythematosus on pregnancy and pregnancy outcome. Am J Reprod Immunol 28:199, 1992.
5. Tan EM, Cohen AS, Fries JF, et al: The 1982 revised criteria for the classification of systemic lupus erythematosus. Arthritis Rheum 25:1271, 1982.
6. Hochberg MC: Updating the American College of Rheumatology revised criteria for the classification of systemic lupus erythematosus. Arthritis Rheum 40:1725, 1997.
7. Ter Borg EJ, Hurst G, Hummel EJ, et al: Measurements of increases in anti-double stranded DNA antibody levels as a predictor of disease exacerbation in SLE: A long term, prospective study. Arthritis Rheum 33:634, 1990.
8. Bootsma H, Spronk PE, Derksen R, et al: Prevention of relapses in systemic lupus erythematosus. Lancet 345:1595, 1995.
9. Tomer Y, Viegas OAC, Swissa M, et al: Levels of lupus autoantibodies in pregnant SLE patients: correlations with disease activity and pregnancy outcome. Clin Exp Rheumatol 14:275, 1996.
10. Garsenstein M, Pollach VE, Kark RM: Systemic lupus erythematosus and pregnancy. N Engl J Med 267:165, 1962.
11. Lockshin MD, Reinitz E, Druzin ML, et al: Case-control prospective study demonstrating absence of lupus exacerbation during or after pregnancy. Am J Med 77:893, 1984.
12. Meehan RT, Dorsey JK: Pregnancy among patients with systemic lupus erythematosus receiving immunosuppressive therapy. J Rheumatol 14:252, 1987.
13. Mintz R, Niz J, Gutierrez G, et al: Prospective study of pregnancy in systemic lupus erythematosus: Results of a multidisciplinary approach. J Rheumatol 13:732, 1986.
14. Lockshin MD: Pregnancy does not cause systemic lupus erythematosus to worsen. Arthritis Rheum 32:665, 1989.
15. Urowitz MB, Gladman DD, Farewell VT, et al: Lupus and pregnancy studies. Arthritis Rheum 36:1392, 1993.
16. Ruiz-Irastorza G, Lima F, Alves J, et al: Increased rate of lupus flare during pregnancy and the puerperium: a prospective study of 78 pregnancies. Br J Rheumatol 35:133, 1996.
17. Kleinman D, Katz VL, Kuller JA: Perinatal outcomes in women with systemic lupus erythematosus. J Perinatol 18:178, 1998.
18. Johns KR, Morand EF, Littlejohn GO: Pregnancy outcome in systemic lupus erythematosus (SLE): a review of 54 cases. Aust N Z J Med 28:18, 1998.
19. Derksen RH, Bruinse HW, de Groot PG, Kater L: Pregnancy in systemic lupus erythematosus: a prospective study. Lupus 3:149, 1994.
20. Huong DL, Wechsler B, Vauthier-Brouzes D, et al: Pregnancy in past or present lupus nephritis: a study of 32 pregnancies from a single centre. Ann Rheum Dis 60:599, 2001.
21. Aggarwal N, Sawhney H, Vasishta K, et al: Pregnancy in patients with systemic lupus erythematosus. Aust N Z J Obstet Gynaecol 39:28, 1999.
22. Georgiou PE, Politi EN, Katsimbri P, et al: Outcome of lupus pregnancy: a controlled study. Rheumatology 39:1014, 2000.
23. Cortes-Hernandez J, Ordi-Ros J, Labrador M, et al: Predictors of poor renal outcome in patients with lupus nephritis treated with combined pulses of cyclophosphamide and methylprednisolone. Lupus 12:287, 2003.
24. Ruiz-Irastorza G, Khamashta MA, Gordon C, et al: Measuring systemic lupus erythematosus activity during pregnancy: Validation of the lupus activity index in pregnancy scale. Arthritis Rheum 51:78, 2004.
25. Petri, M: Hopkins Lupus Pregnancy Center: 1987 to 1996. Rheum Dis Clin North Am 23:1, 1997.
26. Devoe LD, Taylor RL: Systemic lupus erythematosus in pregnancy. Am J Obstet Gynecol 135:473, 1979.
27. Devoe LD, Loy GL: Serum complement levels and perinatal outcome in pregnancies complicated by systemic lupus erythematosus. Obstetr Gynecol 63:796, 1984.
28. Buyon JP, Cronstein BN, Morris M, et al: Serum complement values (C3 and C4) to differentiate between systemic lupus activity and preeclampsia. Am J Med 81:194, 1986.
29. Lockshin MD, Qamar T, Redecha P, Harpel PC: Hypocomplementemia with low C1s-C1 inhibitor complex in systemic lupus erythematosus. Arthritis Rheum 12:1467, 1986.
30. Wong KL, Chan FY, Lee CP: Outcome of pregnancy in patients with systemic lupus erythematosus. A prospective study. Arch Intern Med 151:269, 1991.
31. Nossent HC, Swaak TJ: Systemic lupus erythematosus. VI. Analysis of the interrelationship with pregnancy. J Rheumatol 17:771, 1990.
32. Shibata S, Sasaki T, Hirabayashi Y, et al: Risk factors in the pregnancy of patients with systemic lupus erythematosus: association of hypocomplementaemia with poor prognosis. Ann Rheum Dis 51:619, 1992.
33. Rubbert A, Pirner K, Wildt L, et al: Pregnancy course and complications in patients with systemic lupus erythematosus. Am J Reprod Immunol 28:205, 1992.
34. Girardi G, Salmon JB: The role of complement in pregnancy and fetal loss. Autoimmunity 36:19, 2003.
35. Adelsberg BR: The complement system in pregnancy. Am J Reprod Immunol 4:38, 1983.
36. Tincani A, Faden D, Tarantini M, et al: Systemic lupus erythematosus and pregnancy: a prospective study. Clin Exp Rheumatol 10:439, 1992.
37. Hayslett JP, Lynn RI: Effect of pregnancy in patients with lupus nephropathy. Kidney Int 18:207, 1980.
38. Jungers P, Dougados M, Pelissier C, et al: Lupus nephropathy and pregnancy. Arch Intern Med 142:771, 1982.
39. Bobrie G, Liote F, Houillier P, et al: Pregnancy in lupus nephritis and related disorders. Am J Kidney Dis 9:339, 1987.
40. Garenstein M, Pollach VE, Kark RM: Systemic lupus erythematosus and pregnancy. N Engl J Med 267:165, 1962
41. Estes D, Larson DL: Systemic lupus erythematosus and pregnancy. Clin Obstet Gynecol 8:307, 1965.
42. Bear R: Pregnancy and lupus nephritis: A detailed report of six cases with a review of the literature. Obstet Gynecol 47:715, 1976.
43. Julkunen H: Pregnancy and lupus nephritis. Scand J Urol Nephrol 35:319, 2001.
44. Oviasu E, Hicks J, Cameron JS: The outcome of pregnancy in women with lupus nephritis. Lupus 1:19–25, 1999.
45. Packham DK, Lam SS, Nichols K, et al: Lupus nephritis and pregnancy. QJM 83:315, 1992.
46. Moroni G, Quaglini S, Banfi G, et al: Pregnancy in lupus nephritis. Am J Kidney Dis 40:713, 2002.
47. Weiner CP, Brandt J: Plasma antithrombin III activity: an aid in the diagnosis of preeclampsia-eclampsia. Am J Obstet Gynecol 142:275, 1982.
48. Weiner CP, Kwaan HC, Xu C, et al: Antithrombin III activity in women with hypertension during pregnancy. Obstet Gynecol 65:301, 1985.
49. Mellembakken JR, Hogasen K, Mollnes TE, et al: Increased systemic activation of neutrophils but not complement in preeclampsia. Obstet Gynecol 97:371, 2001.
50. Fine LG, Barnett EV, Danovitch GM, et al: Systemic lupus erythematosus in pregnancy. Arch Intern Med 94:667, 1981.
51. Fraga A, Mintz G, Orozco J, et al: Sterility and fertility rates, fetal wastage and maternal morbidity in systemic lupus erythematosus. J Rheumatol 1:293, 1974.
52. Gimovsky, ML, Montoro M, Paul RH: Pregnancy outcome in women with systemic lupus erythematosus. Obstet Gynecol 63:686, 1984.
53. McHugh NJ, Reilly PA, McHugh LA: Pregnancy outcome and autoantibodies in connective tissue disease. J Rheumatol 16:42, 1989.
54. Zulman JI, Talal N, Hoffman GS, et al: Problems associated with the management of pregnancies in patients with systemic lupus erythematosus. J Rheumatol 7:37, 1979.
55. Siampoulou-Marridou A, Manoussakis MN, Mavridis AK, et al: Outcome of pregnancy in patients with autoimmune rheumatic disease before the disease onset. Ann Rheum Dis 47:982, 1988.
55a. Petri M, Albritton J: Fetal outcome of lupus pregnancy: a retrospective case-control study of the Hopkins Lupus Cohort. J Rheumatol 20:650, 1993.
56. Johns KR, Morand EF, Littlejohn GO: Pregnancy outcome in systemic lupus erythematosus (SLE): a review of 54 cases. Aust N Z J Med 28:18, 1998.
57. Imbasciati E, Surian M, Bottino W et al: Lupus nephropathy and pregnancy. Nephron 36:46, 1984.

58. Lockshin MD, Qamar T, Druzin ML: Hazards of lupus pregnancy. J Rheumatol 14:214, 1987.
59. Lockshin MD, Druzin ML, Goei S, et al: Antibody to cardiolipin as a predictor of fetal distress or death in pregnant patients with systemic lupus erythematosus. N Engl J Med 313:152, 1985.
60. Englert HJ, Derue GM, Loizou S, et al: Pregnancy and lupus: Prognostic indicators and response to treatment. QJMed 66:125, 1988.
61. Nicklin JL: Systemic lupus erythematosus and pregnancy at the Royal Women's Hospital, Brisbane 1979–1989. Aust N Z J Obstet Gynaecol 31:128, 1991.
62. Julkunen H, Kaaja R, Palosuo T, et al: Pregnancy in lupus nephropathy. Acta Obstet Gynecol Scand 72:258, 1993.
63. Kleinman D, Katz VL, Kuller JA: Perinatal outcomes in women with systemic lupus erythematosus. J Perinatol 18:178, 1998.
63a. Ramsey-Goldman R, Kutzer JE, Kuller LH, et al: Pregnancy outcome and anticardiolipin antibody in women with systemic lupus erythematosus. Am J Epidemiol 138:1057, 1993.
64. Yasmeen S, Wilkins EE, Field NT, et al: Pregnancy outcomes in women with systemic lupus erythematosus. J Matern Fetal Med 10:91, 2001.
65. Rahman P, Gladman DD, Urowitz MB: Clinical predictors of fetal outcome in systemic lupus erythematosus. J Rheumatol 25:1526, 1998.
66. Varner MW, Meehan RT, Syrop CH, et al: Pregnancy in patients with systemic lupus erythematosus. Am J Obstet Gynecol 145:1025, 1983.
67. Houser MT, Fish AJ, Tagatz GE, et al: Pregnancy and systemic lupus erythematosus. Am J Obstet Gynecol 138:409, 1980.
68. Johnson MJ, Petri M, Witter FR, et al: Evaluation of preterm delivery in a systemic lupus erythematosus pregnancy clinic. Obstet Gynecol 86:396, 1985.
69. Scott JS, Maddison PJ, Taylor MV, et al: Connective tissue disease, antibodies to ribonucleoprotein and congenital heart disease. N Engl J Med 309:209, 1983.
70. Lee LA: Neonatal lupus erythematosus. J Invest Dermatol 100:9S, 1993.
71. Reed BR, Lee LA, Harmon C, et al: Autoantibodies to SS-A/Ro in infants with congenital heart block. Pediatrics 103:889, 1983.
72. Buyon JP, Clancy RM: Neonatal lupus syndromes. Curr Opin Rheumatol 15:535, 2003.
73. Buyon JP, Hiebert R, Copel J, et al: Autoimmune-associated congenital heart block: demographics, mortality, morbidity and recurrence rates obtained from a national neonatal lupus registry. J Am Coll Cardiol 31:1658, 1998.
74. Provost TT, Watson R, Gaither KK, et al: The neonatal lupus erythematosus syndrome. J Rheumatol Suppl 14(Suppl 13):199, 1987.
75. Julkunen H, Kurki P, Kaaja R, et al: Isolated congenital heart block. Long term outcome of mothers and characterization of the immune response to SS-A/Ro and to SS-B/La. Arthritis Rheum 36:1588, 1993.
76. Waltuck J, Buyon JP: Autoantibody associated complete heart block: Outcome in mothers and children. Ann Intern Med 120:544, 1994.
77. Neiman AR, Lee LA, Weston WL, Buyon JP: Cutaneous manifestations of neonatal lupus without heart block: characteristics of mothers and children enrolled in a national registry. J Pediatr 137:674, 2000.
78. Breur JM, Visser GH, Kruize AA, et al: Treatment of fetal heart block with maternal steroid therapy: case report and review of the literature. Ultrasound Obstet Gynecol 24:467, 2004.
79. Glickstein JS, Buyon J, Friedman D: Pulsed Doppler echocardiographic assessment of the fetal PR interval. Am J Cardiol 86:236, 2000.
80. Druzin ML, Locksrun M, Edersheim TG, et al: Second trimester fetal monitoring and preterm delivery in pregnancies with systemic lupus erythematosus and/or circulating anticoagulant Am J Obstet Gynecol 157:1503, 1987.
81. Le Huong D, Wechsler B, Vauthier-Brouzes D, et al: Outcome of planned pregnancies in systemic lupus erythematosus: a prospective study on 62 pregnancies. Br J Rheumatol 36:772, 1997.
82. Derksen RH, Bruinse HW, de Groot PG, Kater L: Pregnancy in systemic lupus erythematosus: a prospective study. Lupus 3:149, 1994.
83. Brooks PM, Needs CJ: Antirheumatic drugs in pregnancy and lactation. Baillieres Clin Rheumatol 4:157, 1990.
84. Kallen B, Rydhstraem H, Aberg A: Congenital malformations after the use of inhaled budesonide in early pregnancy. Obstet Gynecol 93:392, 1999.
85. Robert E, Vollset SE, Botto L, et al: Malformation surveillance and maternal drug exposure: the madre project. Int J Risk Safety Ed 6:75, 1994.
86. Carmichael SL, Shaw GM: Maternal corticosteroid use and risk of selected congenital anomalies. Am J Med Genet 86:242, 1999.
87. Laskin CA, Bombardier C, Hannah ME, et al: Prednisone and aspirin in women with autoantibodies and unexplained recurrent fetal loss. N Engl J Med 337:148, 1997.
88. Vaquero E, Lazzarin N, Valensise H, et al: Pregnancy outcome in recurrent spontaneous abortion associated with antiphospholipid antibodies: a comparative study of intravenous immunoglobulin versus prednisone plus low-dose aspirin. Am J Reprod Immunol 45:174, 2001.
89. Rahman P, Gladman DD, Urowitz MB: Clinical predictors of fetal outcome in systemic lupus erythematosus. J Rheumatol 25:1526, 1998.
90. Hart C, Naughton RF: The ototoxicity of chloroquine phosphate. Arch Otolaryngol 80:407, 1964.
91. Nylander U: Ocular damage in chloroquine therapy. Acta Ophthalmol 45(Suppl 92):5, 1967.
92. Buchanan NM, Toubi E, Khamashta MA, et al: Hydroxychloroquine and lupus pregnancy: review of a series of 36 cases. Ann Rheum Dis 55:486, 1996.
93. Khamashta MA, Buchanan NM, Hughes GR: The use of hydroxychloroquine in lupus pregnancy: the British experience. Lupus 5:S65, 1996.
94. Klinger G, Morad Y, Westall CA, et al: Ocular toxicity and antenatal exposure to chloroquine or hydroxychloroquine for rheumatic diseases. Lancet 358:813, 2001.
95. Motta M, Tincani A, Faden D, et al: Antimalarial agents in pregnancy. Lancet 359:524, 2002.
96. Costedoat-Chalumeau N, Amoura Z, Duhaut P, et al: Safety of hydroxychloroquine in pregnant patients with connective tissue diseases: a study of one hundred thirty-three cases compared with a control group. Arthritis Rheum 48:3207, 2003.
97. Levy RA, Vilela VS, Cataldo MJ, et al: Hydroxychloroquine (HCQ) in lupus pregnancy: double-blind and placebo-controlled study. Lupus 10:401, 2001.
98. Armenti VT, Ahlswede KM, Ahlswede BA, et al: National transplantation pregnancy registry: outcomes of 154 pregnancies in cyclosporine-treated female kidney transplant recipients. Transplantation 57:502, 1994.
99. Armenti VT, Moritz MJ, Davison JM: Drug safety issues in pregnancy following transplantation and immunosuppression: effects and outcomes. Drug Saf 19:219, 1998.
100. Cote CJ, Meuwissen HJ, Pickering RJ: Effects on the neonate of prednisone and azathioprine administered to the mother during pregnancy. J Pediatr 85:324, 1974.
101. Ujhazy E, Balonova T, Durisova M, et al: Teratogenicity of cyclophosphamide in New Zealand white rabbits. Neoplasma 40:45, 1993.
102. Kirshon B, Wasserstrum N, Willis R, et al: Teratogenic effects of first-trimester cyclophosphamide therapy. Obstet Gynecol 72:462, 1988.
103. Enns GM, Roeder E, Chan RT, et al: Apparent cyclophosphamide (cytoxan) embryopathy: a distinct phenotype? Am J Med Genet 86:237, 1999.
104. Ruiz-Irastorza G, Khamashta MA, Castellino G, Hughes GR: Systemic lupus erythematosus. Lancet 357:1027, 2001.
105. Cardonick E, Moritz M, Armenti V: Pregnancy in patients with organ transplantation: a review. Obstet Gynecol Surv 59:214, 2004.
106. Granzow JW, Thaller SR, Panthaki Z: Cleft palate and toe malformations in a child with fetal methotrexate exposure. J Craniofac Surg 14:747, 2003.
107. Stuart JJ, Gross SJ, Elrad H, et al: Effects of acetylsalicylic acid ingestion on maternal and neonatal hemostasis. N Engl J Med 307:909, 1982.
108. Rumack CM, Guggenheim MA, Rumack BH, et al: Neonatal intracranial hemorrhage and maternal use of aspirin. Obstet Gynecol 58:52S, 1981.

109. Macones GA, Robinson CA: Is there justification for using indomethacin in preterm labor? An analysis of neonatal risks and benefits. Am J Obstet Gynecol 177:819, 1997.
110. Vermillion ST, Newman RB: Recent indomethacin tocolysis is not associated with neonatal complications in preterm infants. Am J Obstet Gynecol 181:1083, 1999.
111. Pryde PG, Besinger RE, Gianopoulos JG, Mittendorf R: Adverse and beneficial effects of tocolytic therapy. Semin Perinatol 25:316, 2001.
112. Ostensen M, Villiger PM: Nonsteroidal anti-inflammatory drugs in systemic lupus erythematosus. Lupus 10:135, 2001.
113. Sydney Criteria.
114. Wilson WA, Gharavi AE, Koike T, et al: International consensus statement on preliminary classification criteria for definite antiphospholipid syndrome. Report of an international workshop. Arthritis Rheum 42:1309, 1999.
115. Levine JS, Rauch J, Branch DW: Antiphospholipid syndrome. N Engl J Med 346:752, 2002.
116. Branch DW, Dudley DJ, Mitchell MD, et al: Immunoglobulin G fractions from patients with antiphospholipid antibodies cause fetal death in BALB/c mice: A model for autoimmune fetal loss. Am J Obstet Gynecol 163:210, 1990.
117. Blank M, Cohen J, Toder V, Shoenfeld Y: Induction of antiphospholipid syndrome in naive mice with mouse lupus monoclonal and human polyclonal anticardiolipin antibodies. Proc Natl Acad Sci U S A 88:3069, 1991.
118. Pierangeli SS, Gharavi AE, Harris EN: Experimental thrombosis and antiphospholipid antibodies: New insights. J Autoimmun 15:241, 2000.
119. Hörkkö S, Miller E, Dudl E, et al: Antiphospholipid antibodies are directed against epitopes of oxidized phospholipids: Recognition of cardiolipin by monoclonal antibodies to epitopes of oxidized low density lipoprotein. J Clin Invest 98:815, 1996.
120. Rand JH, Wu S, Andree HAM, et al: Pregnancy loss in the antiphospholipid antibody syndrome—a possible thrombogenic mechanism. N Engl J Med 337:154, 1997.
121. di Simone N, Meroni PL, Del Papa N, et al: Antiphospholipid antibodies affect trophoblast gonadotropin secretion and invasiveness by binding directly and through adhered beta$_2$-glycoprotein I. Arthritis Rheum 43:140, 2000.
122. Holers VM, Girardi G, Mo L, et al: Complement C3 activation is required for antiphospholipid antibody-induced fetal loss. J Exp Med 195:211, 2002.
123. Girardi G, Salmon JB: The role of complement in pregnancy and fetal loss. Autoimmunity 36:19, 2003.
124. Wilson WA, Gharavi AE, Koike T, et al: International consensus statement on preliminary classification criteria for definite antiphospholipid syndrome: report of an international workshop. Arthritis Rheum 42:1309, 1999.
125. Harris EN: Syndrome of the black swan. Br J Rheumatol 26:324, 1987.
126. Asherson RA, Cervera R, de Groot PG, et al: Catastrophic Antiphospholipid Syndrome Registry Project Group. Catastrophic antiphospholipid syndrome: international consensus statement on classification criteria and treatment guidelines. Lupus 12:530, 2003.
127. Kutteh WH: Antiphospholipid antibody-associated recurrent pregnancy loss: treatment with heparin and low-dose aspirin is superior to low-dose aspirin alone. Am J Obstet Gynecol 174:1584, 1996.
128. Rai R, Cohen H, Dave M, Regan L: Randomised controlled trial of aspirin and aspirin plus heparin in pregnant women with recurrent miscarriage associated with phospholipid antibodies (or antiphospholipid antibodies). BMJ 314:253, 1997.
129. Pattison NS, Chamley LW, Birdsall M, et al: Does aspirin have a role in improving pregnancy outcome for women with the antiphospholipid syndrome? A randomized controlled trial. Am J Obstet Gynecol 183:1008, 2000.
130. Clifford K, Rai R, Watson H, Regan L: An informative protocol for the investigation of recurrent miscarriage: preliminary experience of 500 consecutive cases. Hum Reprod 9:1328, 1994.
131. Yetman DL, Kutteh WH: Antiphospholipid antibody panels and recurrent pregnancy loss: prevalence of anticardiolipin antibodies compared with other antiphospholipid antibodies. Fertil Steril 66:540, 1996.
132. Branch DW, Silver R, Pierangeli S, et al: Antiphospholipid antibodies other than lupus anticoagulant and anticardiolipin antibodies in women with recurrent pregnancy loss, fertile controls, and antiphospholipid syndrome. Obstet Gynecol 89:549, 1997.
133. Branch DW, Rote NS, Dostal DA, Scott JR: Association of lupus anticoagulant with antibody against phosphatidylserine. Clin Immunol Immunopathol 42:63, 1987.
134. Branch DW, Silver RM, Blackwell JL, et al: Outcome of treated pregnancies in women with antiphospholipid syndrome: An update of the Utah experience. Obstet Gynecol 80:614, 1992.
135. Oshiro BT, Silver RM, Scott JR, et al: Antiphospholipid antibodies and fetal death. Obstet Gynecol 87:489, 1996.
136. Lockwood CJ, Romero R, Feinberg RF, et al: The prevalence and biologic significance of lupus anticoagulant and anticardiolipin antibodies in a general obstetric population. Am J Obstet Gynecol 161:369, 1989.
137. Pattison NS, Charnley LW, McKay EJ, et al: Antiphospholipid antibodies in pregnancy: Prevalence and clinical associations. Br J Obstet Gynaecol 100:909, 1993.
138. Lima F, Khamashta MA, Buchanan NM, et al: A study of sixty pregnancies in patients with the antiphospholipid syndrome. Clin Exp Rheumatol 14:131, 1996.
129. Pauzner R, Dulitzki M, Langevitz P, et al: Low molecular weight heparin and warfarin in the treatment of patients with antiphospholipid syndrome during pregnancy. Thromb Haemost 86:1379, 2001.
140. Huong DLT, Wechsler B, Bletry O, et al: A study of 75 pregnancies in patients with antiphospholipid syndrome. J Rheumatol 28:2025, 2001.
141. Branch DW, Dudley DJ, Mitchell MD, et al: Immunoglobulin G fractions from patients with antiphospholipid antibodies cause fetal death in BALB/c mice: A model for autoimmune fetal loss. Am J Obstet Gynecol 163:210, 1990.
142. Moodley J, Bhoola V, Duursma J, et al: The association of antiphospholipid antibodies with severe early onset preeclampsia. S Afr Med J 85:105, 1995.
143. Lockshin MD, Druzin ML, Qamar T: Prednisone does not prevent recurrent fetal death in women with antiphospholipid antibody. Am J Obstet Gynecol 160:439, 1989.
144. Polzin WJ, Kopelman IN, Robinson RD, et al: The association of antiphospholipid antibodies with pregnancy complicated by fetal growth restriction. Obstet Gynecol 78:1108, 1991.
145. Miyakis S, Lockshin MD, Atsumi T, et al: International consensus statement on an update of the classification criteria for definite antiphospholipid syndrome (APS). J Thromb Haemost 4:295, 2006.
146. Kutteh WH: Antiphospholipid antibody-associated recurrent pregnancy loss: treatment with heparin and low-dose aspirin is superior to low-dose aspirin alone. Am J Obstet Gynecol 174:1584, 1996.
147. Silver RM, Porter TF, van Leeuwen I, et al: Anticardiolipin antibodies: Clinical consequences of "low titers." Obstet Gynecol 87:494, 1996.
148. Rai R, Cohen H, Dave M, Regan L: Randomised controlled trial of aspirin and aspirin plus heparin in pregnant women with recurrent miscarriage associated with phospholipid antibodies (or antiphospholipid antibodies). BMJ 314:253, 1997.
149. Farquharson RG, Quenby S, Greaves M: Antiphospholipid syndrome in pregnancy: a randomized, controlled trial of treatment. Obstet Gynecol 100:408, 2002.
150. Caruso A, de Carolis S, Ferrazzani S, et al: Pregnancy outcome in relation to uterine artery flow velocity waveforms and clinical characteristics in women with antiphospholipid syndrome. Obstet Gynecol 82:970, 1993.
151. Dreyfus M, Hedelin G, Kutnahorsky R, et al: Antiphospholipid antibodies and preeclampsia: A case-control study. Obstet Gynecol 97:29, 2001.
152. Branch DW, Porter TF, Rittenhouse L, et al: Antiphospholipid antibodies in women at risk for preeclampsia. Am J Obstet Gynecol 184:825, 2001.
153. Cowchock FS, Reece EA, Balaban D, et al: Repeated fetal losses associated with antiphospholipid antibodies: A collaborative randomized trial comparing prednisone with low-dose heparin treatment. Am J Obstet Gynecol 166:1318, 1992.
154. Ginsberg JS, Greer I, Hirsh J: Use of antithrombotic agents during pregnancy. Chest 119:122S, 2001.
155. Erkan D, Merrill JT, Yazici Y, et al: High thrombosis rate after fetal loss in antiphospholipid syndrome: Effective prophylaxis with aspirin. Arthritis Rheum 44:1466, 2001.

156. Fausett MB, Vogtlander M, Lee RM, et al: Heparin-induced thrombocytopenia is rare in pregnancy. Am J Obstet Gynecol 185:148, 2001.
157. Clark AL, Branch DW, Silver RM, et al: Pregnancy complicated by the antiphospholipid syndrome: Outcomes with intravenous immunoglobulin therapy. Obstet Gynecol 93:437, 1999.
158. Branch DW, Peaceman AM, Druzin M, et al: A multicenter, placebo-controlled pilot study of intravenous immune globulin treatment of antiphospholipid syndrome during pregnancy. The Pregnancy Loss Study Group. Am J Obstet Gynecol 182:122, 2000.
159. Pattison NS, Chamley LW, Birdsall M, et al: Does aspirin have a role in improving pregnancy outcome for women with the antiphospholipid syndrome? A randomized controlled trial. Am J Obstet Gynecol 183:1008, 2000.
160. Ginsberg JS, Greer I, Hirsh J: Use of antithrombotic agents during pregnancy. Chest 119:122S, 2001.
161. Silman AJ, Hochberg MC (eds): Epidemiology of the Rheumatic Diseases, 2nd ed. Oxford University Press, 2001.
162. Kong YY, Yoshida H, Sarosi I, et al: OPGL is a key regulator of osteoclastogenesis, lymphocyte development and lymph-node organogenesis. Nature 397:315, 1999.
163. MacGregor AJ, Snieder H, Rigby AS, et al: Characterizing the quantitative genetic contribution to rheumatoid arthritis using data from twins. Arthritis Rheum 43:30, 2000.
164. Jawaheer D, Seldin JM, Anoms, CI, et al: Screening the genome for rheumatoid arthritis susceptibility genes. Arthritis Rheum 48:906, 2003.
165. Fisher SA, Lanchbury JS, Lewis CM: Meta-analysis of four rheumatoid arthritis genome-wide linkage studies: Confirmation of a susceptibility locus on chromosome 16. Arthritis Rheum 48:1200, 2003.
166. Hench PS: The ameliorating effect of pregnancy on chronic atrophic (infectious) rheumatoid arthritis, fibrositis, and intermittent hydrarthritis. Proc Mayo Clin 13:161, 1938.
167. Oka M: Activity of rheumatoid arthritis and plasma 17-hydroxycorticosteroids during pregnancy and following parturition. Acta Rheumatol Scand 4:243, 1958.
168. Oka M: Effect of pregnancy on onset and course of rheumatoid arthritis. Ann Rheum Dis 12:227, 1953.
169. Persellini RH: The effect of pregnancy on rheumatoid arthritis. Bull Rheum Dis 27:922, 1977.
170. Betson JR, Dorn RV: Forty cases of arthritis and pregnancy. J Int Coll Surg 42:521, 1964.
171. Ostensen M, Husby G: A prospective clinical study of the effect of pregnancy on rheumatoid arthritis and ankylosing spondylitis. Arthritis Rheum 26:1155, 1983.
172. Silman AJ, Roman E, Beral V, Brown A: Adverse reproductive outcomes in women who subsequently develop rheumatoid arthritis. Ann Rheum Dis 47:979, 1988.
173. Oka M, Vainio V: Effect of pregnancy on the prognosis and serology of rheumatoid arthritis. Acta Rheumatologica Scandinavica 12:47, 1966.
174. Hazes JM, Dijkmans BAC, Vandenbroucke JP, et al: Pregnancy and the risk of developing rheumaoid arthritis. Arthritis Rheum 33:1770, 1990.
175. Ostensen M: Pregnancy in patients with a history of juvenile rheumatoid arthritis. Arthritis Rheum 34:881, 1991.
176. Ostensen M: Glucocorticosteroids in pregnant patients with rheumatoid arthritis. Z Rheumatol 59:II70, 2000.
177. Royal College of General Practitioners: Oral Contraceptives and Health: Interim Report. London, Pitman, 1974.
178. Gilbert M, Rotstein J, Cunningham C: Norethynodrel with mestranol in the treatment of rheumatoid arthritis. JAMA 190:235, 1964.
179. Bijlsma WJ, Huger-Bruning O, Thijssen JHH: Effect of estrogen treatment on clinical and laboratory manifestations of rheumatoid arthritis. Ann Rheum Dis 46:777, 1987.
180. DaSilva JA, Hall GM: The effects of gender and sex hormones on outcome in rheumatoid arthritis. Bailliers Clin Rheumatol 6:196, 1992.
181. Kasukawa R, Ohara M, Yoshida H, Yoshida T: Pregnancy-associated a_2-glycoprotein in rheumatoid arthritis. Intern Arch Allergy Applied Immunol 58:67, 1979.
182. Sany J, Clot J, Borneau M, Ardary M: Immunomodulating effect of human placenta-eluted gamma globulins in rheumatoid arthritis. Arthritis Rheum 25:17, 1982.
183. Klippel GL, Cerere FA: Rheumatoid arthritis and pregnancy. Rheum Dis Clin North Am 15:213, 1989.
184. Mannik M, Nardella FA: IgG rheumatoid factor and self-association of these antibodies. Clin Rheum Dis 11:551, 1985.
185. Nelson JL, Voigt LF, Koepsell TD, et al: Pregnancy outcome in women with rheumatoid arthritis before disease onset. J Rheumatol 19:18, 1993.
186. Kaplan D: Fetal wastage in patients with rheumatoid arthritis. J Rheumatol 13:857, 1986.
187. Morris WIC: Pregnancy in rheumatoid arthritis and systemic lupus erythematosus. Aust N Z J Obstet Gynaecol 9:136, 1969.
188. Katz, JA, Antoni C, Keenan GF, et al: Outcome of pregnancy in women receiving infliximab for the treatment of Crohn's disease and rheumatoid arthritis. Am J Gastroenterol 99:2385, 2004.
189. Steen VD: Scleroderma and pregnancy. Rheum Dis Clin North Am 23:133, 1997.
190. Morrow J, Nelson JL, Watts R, Isenberg DA (eds): Autoimmune Rheumatic Diseases, 2nd ed. Oxford, UK, Oxford University Press, 1999.
191. Johnson RW, [illegible], Arnett FC: The genetics of systemic sclerosis. Curr Rheumatol Reports 4:99, 2002.
192. LeRoy EC, Black C, Fleischmajer R, et al: Scleroderma (systemic sclerosis): classification, subsets and pathogenesis. J Rheumatol 15:202, 1988.
193. Lambert NC: HLA-DQA1 as a risk factor for microchimerism: comment on the article by Artlett et al. Arthritis Rheum 50:2713, 2004.
194. Bianchi DW, Zickwolf GK, Weil GJ, et al: Male fetal progenitor cells persist in maternal blood for as long as 27 years postpartum. Proc Natl Acad Sci U S A 93:705, 1996.
195. Nelson JL: Maternal-fetal immunology and autoimmune disease: is some autoimmune disease auto-alloimmune or allo-autoimmune? Arthritis Rheum 39:191, 1996.
196. Nelson JL: Microchimerism and the causation of scleroderma. Scand J Rheumatol Suppl 107:10, 1998.
197. Ohtsuka T, Miyamoto Y, Yamakage A, Yamazaki S: Quantitative analysis of microchimerism in systemic sclerosis skin tissue. Arch Dermatol Res 293:387, 2001.
198. Murata H, Nakauchi H, Sumida T: Microchimerism in Japanese women patients with systemic sclerosis. Lancet 354:220, 1999.
199. Selva-O'Callaghan A, Mijares-Boeckh-Behrens T, Prades EB, et al: Lack of evidence of foetal microchimerism in female Spanish patients with systemic sclerosis. Lupus 12:15, 2003.
200. Lambert NC, Stevens AM, Tylee TS, et al: From the simple detection of microchimerism in patients with autoimmune diseases to its implication in pathogenesis. Ann N Y Acad Sci 945:164, 2001.
201. Steen VD, Conte C, Day N, et al: Pregnancy in women with systemic sclerosis. Arthritis Rheum 32:151, 1989.
202. Steen VD: Pregnancy in women with systemic sclerosis. Obstet Gynecol 94:15, 1999.
203. Silman AJ, Black C: Increased incidence of spontaneous abortion and infertility in women with scleroderma before disease onset: A controlled study. Ann Rheum Dis 47:441, 1988.
205. Black CM: Systemic sclerosis and pregnancy. Bailliere's Clin Rheumatol 4:105, 1990.
206. Johnson TR, Banner EA, Winkelmann RK: Scleroderma and pregnancy. Obstet Gynecol 23:467, 1964.
206. Slate WG, Graham AR: Scleroderma and pregnancy. Am J Obstet Gynecol 101:335, 1968.
207. Weiner RS, Brinkman CR, Paulus HE: Scleroderma, CREST syndrome and pregnancy. Arthritis Rheum 29:51, 1986.
208. Giordano M, Valentini G, Lupoli S: Pregnancy and systemic sclerosis. Arthritis and Rheumatism 28:237, 1985.
209. Englert H, Brennan P, McNeil D, et al: Reproductive function prior to disease onset in women with scleroderma. J Rheumatol 19:1575, 1992.
210. Baethge BA, Wolf RE: Successful pregnancy with scleroderma renal disease and pulmonary hypertension in a patient using angiotensin converting enzyme inhibitors. Ann Rheum Dis 48: 776, 1989.

Hepatic and Gastrointestinal Diseases

MITCHELL S. CAPPELL

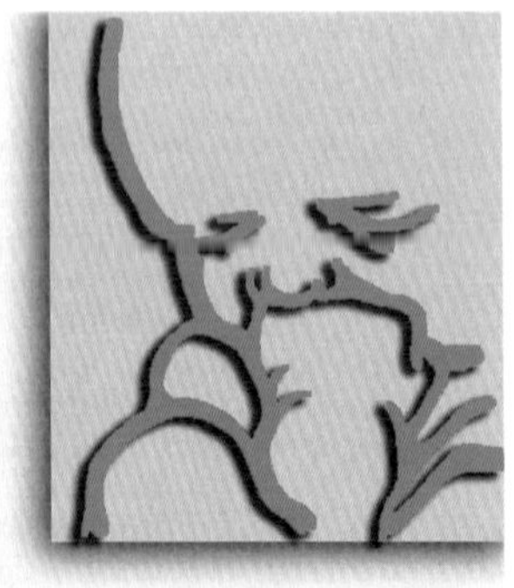

CHAPTER 43

Hepatic Disorders

KEY ABBREVIATIONS

Acute fatty liver of pregnancy	AFLP
Acute intermittent porphyria	AIP
Computed tomography	CT
Disseminated intravascular coagulation	DIC
Endoscopic retrograde cholangiopancreatography	ERCP
Esophagogastroduodenoscopy	EGD
Hemolysis, elevated liver enzymes, and low platelet count syndrome	HELLP
Hepatocellular cancer	HCC
Intrahepatic cholestasis of pregnancy	ICP
long-chain 3-hydroxyacyl coenzymeA dehydrogenase	LCHAD
Magnetic resonance imaging	MRI

Hepatic, biliary, and pancreatic disorders are relatively uncommon but not rare during pregnancy. For example, about 3 per 100 women develop serum liver function test abnormalities during pregnancy,[1] and about 1 per 500 women develop potentially life-threatening hepatic diseases during pregnancy that endanger fetal viability.[2,3]

Hepatic, biliary, and pancreatic disorders are often complex and clinically challenging problems during pregnancy. First, the differential diagnosis during pregnancy is extensive. It includes both disorders related to pregnancy as well as disorders unrelated to pregnancy. Second, the clinical presentation and natural history of these disorders may be altered during pregnancy. Indeed, some disorders, such as intrahepatic cholestasis of pregnancy, are unique to pregnancy. Third, the diagnostic evaluation is altered and constrained by the pregnancy. For example, radiologic tests raise concern about fetal safety during pregnancy. Fourth, the interests of both the mother and the fetus must be considered in therapeutic decisions during pregnancy. Usually, these interests do not conflict, because generally what is good for the mother is good for the fetus. Sometimes, however, maternal therapy must be modified to substitute alternative but safer therapy because of concerns about drug teratogenicity.[4] Rarely, the maternal and fetal interests are diametrically opposed, as in the use of chemotherapy for maternal cancer, a therapy that is potentially life-saving to the mother but life-threatening to the fetus.[5] These conflicts raise significant medical, legal, and ethical issues.

Obstetricians, hepatologists, surgeons, and internists should be familiar with hepatic, biliary, and pancreatic disorders that can present in pregnancy and how these conditions affect and are affected by pregnancy. This chapter reviews hepatic, biliary, and pancreatic disorders during pregnancy, with a focus on features unique to pregnancy.

PHYSIOLOGIC EFFECTS OF PREGNANCY ON THE ABDOMEN AND LIVER

Abdominal assessment is modified during pregnancy. The expanding gravid uterus can displace abdominal viscera and may conceal an abdominal mass on physical examination.[5] During pregnancy the blood pressure normally declines modestly. A rise in blood pressure during pregnancy may, therefore, portend preeclampsia or eclampsia. Physiologic alterations of laboratory values during pregnancy include mild leukocytosis, physiologic anemia of pregnancy, and electrolyte changes, particularly mild hyponatremia.[6] The risk of thromboembolic phenomena is increased during pregnancy owing to mild hypercoagulopathy from hyperestrogenemia and vascular stasis from vascular compression by the enlarged gravid uterus.[7] The changes in serum glucose levels during pregnancy are complex. Normal pregnancy is characterized by fasting hypoglycemia, postprandial hyperglycemia, and hyperinsulinemia.[8] Tight control of the serum glucose level is important in diabetic patients for proper fetal development.

Pregnancy does not affect the liver span. The liver may be pushed cephalad by the gravid uterus, but a liver span greater than 12 cm, when appreciated, remains a valid indicator of hepatomegaly. Spider angiomata and palmar erythema, cutaneous lesions often associated with chronic liver disease, may appear transiently during normal pregnancy without underlying liver disease.[9] During pregnancy, the serum alkaline phosphatase level normally increases mildly owing to placental production. The serum albumin level declines during pregnancy primarily from hemodilution and secondarily from decreased hepatic synthesis. Serum bilirubin levels tend to change little during pregnancy owing to the effect of mildly impaired hepatic excretion balanced by the opposing effects of hemodilution and hypoalbuminemia.[10] Serum bile acids tend to progressively increase during pregnancy owing to impaired hepatic transport and biliary secretion. Serum levels of cholesterol, triglycerides, and phospholipids increase moderately during pregnancy owing to increased hepatic synthesis.[11] The serum aminotransferase levels are largely unaffected by pregnancy.

DIFFERENTIAL DIAGNOSIS OF HEPATOBILIARY SYMPTOMS AND CONDITIONS DURING PREGNANCY AND IN THE NEONATE

Jaundice

As in the general population, acute viral hepatitis is the most common cause of jaundice during pregnancy.[2,3] The differential diagnosis of jaundice during the first and second trimesters of pregnancy also includes drug hepatotoxicity and gallstone disease such as acute cholecystitis, choledocholithiasis, ascending cholangitis, and gallstone pancreatitis. In addition to these disorders, the differential diagnosis of jaundice during the third trimester includes the following pregnancy-related causes: intrahepatic cholestasis of pregnancy, acute fatty liver of pregnancy, and HELLP (hemolysis, elevated liver function tests and low platelet count) syndrome. Moderate direct hyperbilirubinemia without jaundice during the third trimester may also be due to preeclampsia, eclampsia, and Budd-Chiari syndrome. Predominantly indirect hyperbilirubinemia during pregnancy is usually due to hemolysis (including the HELLP syndrome), or Gilbert's syndrome.

Right Upper Quadrant Abdominal Pain

The differential diagnosis of right upper quadrant abdominal pain is extensive during pregnancy (Table 43-1).

Table 43-1. Differential Diagnosis of Right Upper Quadrant Abdominal Pain During Pregnancy

Hepatic disorders
- Hepatitis
- Hepatic vascular engorgement
- Hepatic hematoma
- Hepatic malignancy

Biliary tract disease
- Biliary colic
- Choledocholithiasis
- Cholangitis
- Cholecystitis

Diseases related to pregnancy
- Preeclampsia or eclampsia
- Hemolysis, elevated liver enzymes, and low platelet count (HELLP) syndrome

Renal disorders
- Pyelonephritis
- Nephrolithiasis

Gastrointestinal disorders
- Peptic ulcer disease
- Perforated duodenal ulcer

Other conditions in the right upper quadrant
- Rib fracture
- Shingles

Referred pain from other organ disease
- Pneumonia
- Pulmonary embolus or infarct
- Pleural effusion
- Radiculopathy
- Inferior wall myocardial infarction
- Colon cancer

In the medical history, the pain intensity, nature, temporal pattern, radiation pattern, exacerbating factors, and alleviating factors help narrow the differential diagnosis. Biliary colic produces a waxing and waning intensity of pain. Acute cholecystitis is associated with right upper quadrant pain, as well as pain referred to the right shoulder. The pain of acute pancreatitis is often boring in quality, located in the abdominal midline and radiating to the back. Careful physical examination of the abdomen including inspection, palpation, and auscultation can further pinpoint the cause of the pain. Laboratory evaluation of significant abdominal pain routinely includes a hemogram, serum electrolytes, and liver function tests, and often includes a leukocyte differential, coagulation profile, and serum amylase determination. In evaluating the laboratory results, gestational changes in normative values, as aforementioned, must be considered. Radiologic tests may be extremely helpful diagnostically, but the choice of radiologic imaging is constrained by the pregnancy, as discussed later.

Occasionally, the pregnancy is not known by the patient or is not revealed to the physician, particularly in early pregnancy, when physical findings are absent. The physician should be vigilant for possible pregnancy in a fertile woman with abdominal pain, particularly in the setting of missed menses, because pregnancy affects the differential diagnosis, clinical evaluation, and mode of therapy. Pregnancy tests should be performed early in the evaluation of acute abdominal pain in a fertile woman.

Nausea and Vomiting

Nausea and vomiting are frequently observed during pregnancy. Nausea and vomiting of pregnancy is the most common cause. It is caused by the physiologic effects of the pregnancy without demonstrable mucosal or mural disease. Hyperemesis gravidarum is a serious and potentially life-threatening form of nausea and vomiting of pregnancy associated with loss of more than 5 percent of the pregravid weight. The differential diagnosis of nausea and vomiting during pregnancy also includes hepatic and pancreatobiliary diseases such as pancreatitis, viral hepatitis, symptomatic cholelithiasis, acute cholecystitis, acute fatty liver of pregnancy, and occasionally, intrahepatic cholestasis of pregnancy. Gastrointestinal causes include gastroesophageal reflux disease, peptic ulcer disease, viral gastroenteritis, appendicitis, gastroparesis diabeticorum, and gastrointestinal obstruction. Other causes include adnexal torsion, pyelonephritis, urolithiasis, and Addison's disease (glucocorticoid deficiency).

Pruritus

The differential of pruritus during pregnancy includes intrahepatic cholestasis of pregnancy, cholestatic viral hepatitis, primary sclerosing cholangitis, primary biliary cirrhosis, and mechanical choledochal obstruction from benign or malignant strictures.

Hepatic Lesions

Hepatic lesions identified on abdominal imaging studies are classified as cystic or solid. The differential diagnosis of cystic hepatic lesions includes simple hepatic cysts, hepatic cysts associated with polycystic kidney disease, Caroli's disease (congenital dilatation of the intrahepatic bile ducts), bacterial abscesses, amebic abscesses, intraparenchymal hemorrhage, hemangiomas, ecchinococcal cysts, and rarely hepatic malignancies. The differential of a solid hepatic mass includes hepatic adenoma, focal nodular hyperplasia, hepatocellular carcinoma, and hepatic metastases.

Ascites

Hepatic causes of ascites during pregnancy include cirrhosis, acute fatty liver of pregnancy, Budd-Chiari syndrome, portal vein thrombosis, hepatic fibrosis, and hepatocellular carcinoma. Other causes of ascites during pregnancy include ovarian cancer, abdominal tuberculosis, cardiac failure, protein-losing nephropathy, and severe protein malnutrition (kwashiorkor).

Neonatal Cholestasis

Neonatal cholestasis is characterized by conjugated hyperbilirubinemia, pale stools, and dark urine. The differential includes prematurity; anatomic anomalies such as biliary atresia; infections such as cytomegalovirus, or toxoplasmosis; and metabolic defects such as cystic fibrosis, alpha$_1$-antitrypsin deficiency, or bile acid synthetic defects.

ABDOMINAL IMAGING DURING PREGNANCY

Fetal safety of diagnostic imaging is a concern for pregnant patients. Ultrasonography is considered safe and is the preferred abdominal imaging modality during pregnancy.[12] Unfortunately, the test sensitivity depends on operator technique, patient cooperation, and patient anatomy. For example, test sensitivity is decreased by abdominal fat and intestinal gas.[12] Magnetic resonance imaging (MRI) is preferable to computerized tomography (CT) scanning during pregnancy to avoid ionizing radiation, but gadolinium administration should be avoided during MRI in the first trimester.[13] Rapid-sequence MRI is preferable to conventional MRI because the rapid-sequence method entails briefer exposure.

Radiation can cause fetal growth restriction, chromosomal mutations, and neurologic abnormalities including mental retardation, and it also increases the risk of childhood leukemia.[14] Radiation dosage is the most important risk factor, but fetal age at exposure is also important. Fetal mortality is greatest from radiation exposure during the first week after conception, before oocyte implantation, and the risk of neurologic malformations is greatest during the first trimester, when organogenesis occurs.[14]

The patient should undergo counseling before diagnostic roentgenography. Exposure to more than 15 rads during the second and third trimesters or more than 5 rads during the first trimester should prompt consideration of elective termination of pregnancy.[14] Diagnostic studies with high radiation exposure, such as abdominal CT, typically expose the fetus to less than 1 rad and can be considered when extremely strongly indicated.[13] A medical physicist can estimate the fetal exposure from the roentgenographic study. Fetal radiation exposure should be minimized by shielding, collimation, and rapid-sequence studies.

THERAPEUTIC ENDOSCOPY DURING PREGNANCY

Therapeutic Endoscopic Retrograde Cholangiopancreatography

Choledocholithiasis usually requires urgent therapy because of potentially life-threatening ascending cholangitis or gallstone pancreatitis. Symptomatic choledocholithiasis is best managed by therapeutic endoscopic retrograde cholangiopancreatogrpahy (ERCP) in the nonpregnant patient to avoid complex biliary surgery during cholecystectomy. In experienced hands, therapeutic ERCP in the general population has an acceptable morbidity rate of about 5 percent and a low mortality of about 0.5 percent.[15] Therapeutic ERCP is theoretically more attractive than biliary surgery for choledocholithiasis during pregnancy because surgery entails a significant risk of fetal wastage.[16] Aside from maternal risks, therapeutic ERCP during pregnancy entails theoretical risks to the fetus from induction of premature labor, teratogenicity of medications, cardiac arrhythmias, systemic hypotension, and transient hypoxia.[15] Jamidar and colleagues[17] analyzed 29 ERCPs performed on 23 pregnant patients, including 15 performed in the first trimester. ERCP findings included choledocholithiasis in 15, bile leaks after open or laparoscopic cholecystectomy in three, primary sclerosing cholangitis in two, and other abnormalities in three. Therapy at ERCP included sphincterotomy with stone extraction for choledocholithiasis in 14 and biliary stent placement in three. Excluding two unknown pregnancy outcomes and two elective abortions, 17 of the 19 pregnancies (89 percent) resulted in healthy infants, including 16 born at term. One pregnant patient spontaneously aborted 3 months after ERCP, but the abortion did not seem to be temporally or etiologically related to the procedure. One pregnant patient who suffered pancreatitis after therapeutic ERCP, performed for a pancreatic stricture, delivered an infant who died soon after birth. This was the only documented maternal or fetal procedure-related complication. Numerous case reports and several other small clinical series have reported similar results on fetal safety of this procedure.[15]

The accumulated data suggest that therapeutic ERCP can be performed during pregnancy for strong indications to avoid complex biliary surgery or to postpone cholecystectomy until after parturition. Special precautions to minimize fetal risks of ERCP during pregnancy include consultation with a neonatologist, radiation physicist, and anesthesiologist before ERCP; referral to a tertiary medical center for management by a team of experts; lead shielding of the mother's abdomen except for the region of the proximal pancreas and biliary tree; use of a modern fluoroscope to minimize radiation leakage; avoidance of spot radiographs for documentation because they require considerable radiation energy; and, if possible, delaying ERCP until the second trimester to reduce radiation teratogenicity.[15]

Endoscopic Variceal Sclerotherapy or Banding

Pregnancy appears to increase the risk of variceal bleeding from portal hypertension because of the gestational increase in plasma volume.[18] Endoscopic sclerotherapy and banding are particularly attractive therapies for variceal bleeding during pregnancy because the radiologic alternative of transjugular intrahepatic portosystemic shunt requires radiation, and the surgical alternatives can cause fetal wastage. Esophagogastroduodenoscopy (EGD) can be performed during pregnancy with relatively low fetal risks, and the technique should be considered when indicated, such as for acute upper gastrointestinal hemorrhage.[15,19] Endoscopic sclerotherapy raises concerns beyond that of diagnostic EGD from the additional procedure time, the typically severe underlying maternal illness, and the therapy itself. In one clinical series, 10 patients underwent a mean of three endoscopic sclerotherapy sessions during pregnancy for active variceal bleeding in five and for prophylaxis in five.[20] Hemostasis was achieved in all actively bleeding patients. One patient suffered a complication from sclerotherapy of an esophageal stricture, which was successfully treated using peroral esophageal dilators. All patients had a normal vaginal delivery at term.[20] Nine other patients successfully underwent endoscopic sclerotherapy for actively or recently bleeding esophageal varices with delivery of healthy infants in all cases.[15] One study reported less favorable pregnancy outcomes after endoscopic sclerotherapy, which is attributable to the underlying maternal disease. Four of 17 pregnant patients undergoing endoscopic sclerotherapy for variceal bleeding due to noncirrhotic portal hypertension had a stillbirth or neonatal death.[21] Still, the available data should justify endoscopic sclerotherapy (or banding) during pregnancy for actively bleeding esophageal varices, after informed consent, owing to the poor outcomes of the alternative available therapies.

Team Approach and Informed Consent

A team approach with consultation and referral helps optimize the management of complex diseases during pregnancy that affect both the mother and the fetus and that require disparate areas of expertise. The obstetrician may consult with the hepatologist regarding timing of delivery in patients with obstetric-related hepatic disease. The gastroenterologist contemplating therapeutic ERCP for symptomatic choledocholithiasis may consult with the obstetrician about the optimal procedure timing and with the anesthesiologist about analgesia during endoscopy. The internist may discuss with the radiologist the benefits versus risks of radiologic tests, and the radiologist may, in turn, consult with a physicist about methods to monitor and reduce fetal radiation exposure. Complex hepatic problems during pregnancy are best handled at a tertiary hospital with the requisite experience and expertise.

The patient should be informed about the consequences to both herself and her fetus of diagnostic tests and therapy, and should be actively involved in medical decisions. The patient makes the decision, under the vigilant guidance of the experts, and with advice from the father, family, and friends. When an intervention, such as roentgenographic tests, entails significant potential fetal risk, a signed, witnessed, and informed consent is, of course, recommended.

PANCREATICOBILIARY DISEASE

Acute Pancreatitis

Acute pancreatitis occurs in 0.1 to 1 percent of pregnancies, most commonly during the third trimester.[22] Gallstones cause more than 70 percent of cases, because alcoholism is relatively uncommon during pregnancy.[22,23] Other causes include drugs, abdominal surgery, trauma, hyperlipidemia, hyperparathyroidism, vasculitis, and infections such as mumps and mononucleosis.[22] Some cases are idiopathic.

Pregnancy does not significantly alter the clinical presentation of acute pancreatitis.[22,23] Epigastric pain is the most common symptom. The pain commonly radiates to the back. Nausea, emesis, and pyrexia frequently occur. Signs include midabdominal tenderness, abdominal guarding, hypoactive bowel sounds, abdominal distention, and increased tympany. Severe cases are associated with shock and pancreatic ascites. Grey-Turner's sign or Cullen's sign suggest retroperitoneal bleeding.[22,23]

Acute pancreatitis is diagnosed by the clinical presentation, laboratory tests, and radiologic examinations. Serum amylase and lipase are reliable markers of acute pancreatitis during pregnancy. The lipase level is unchanged during a normal pregnancy, and the amylase level rises only mildly during a normal pregnancy.[24] Hyperamylasemia may also occur in diabetic ketoacidosis, renal failure, bowel perforation, or bowel obstruction, but the serum lipase and amylase-to-creatinine clearance ratio are normal in these conditions and are elevated in acute pancreatitis. Hypertrigylceridemia can falsely lower the serum amylase level in pancreatitis, but the lipase level remains elevated.[4] Abdominal ultrasonography is useful in gauging pancreatic inflammation in thin patients with mild to moderate acute pancreatitis, but CT scanning is better at delineating areas of pancreatic necrosis in patients with severe pancreatitis.[23] Abdominal ultrasonography is also useful to detect cholelithiasis and bile duct dilatation, but endoscopic ultrasonography is required to reliably detect choledocholithiasis.

Acute pancreatitis during pregnancy is usually mild and responds to medical therapy including discontinuing oral intake, intravenous fluid administration, gastric acid suppression, analgesia, and sometimes nasogastric suction. Meperidine is the traditional choice for analgesia because it does not cause contraction of the sphincter of Oddi. Short term administration of meperidine appears to be relatively safe during pregnancy.[25] Pancreatitis complicated by a pancreatic phlegmon, abscess, sepsis, or hemorrhage necessitates antibiotic therapy, total parenteral nutrition, and possible radiologic aspiration or surgical debridement, with monitoring of the patient in an intensive care unit.[23] Large and persistent pancreatic pseudocysts require endoscopic or radiologic drainage or surgery.[23] Endoscopic sphincterotomy can be performed for gallstone pancreatitis during pregnancy with minimal fetal radiation exposure.[26] The pregnancy should not cause delay of these therapies. The maternal mortality rate is low in uncomplicated pancreatitis, but exceeds 10 percent in complicated pancreatitis.[23] Pancreatitis is associated with fetal wastage during the first trimester, and it is associated with premature labor in the third trimester.[27]

Cholelithiasis and Cholecystitis

Pregnancy promotes bile lithogenicity and sludge formation because estrogen increases cholesterol synthesis and progesterone impairs gallbladder motility.[28] In a large study in Chile, 12 percent of pregnant women had cholelithiasis detected by abdominal ultrasonography.[29] Most gallstones are asymptomatic during pregnancy.[30] Complications of cholelithiasis include biliary colic, cholecystitis, choledocholithiasis, jaundice, ascending cholangitis, hepatic abscess, and gallstone pancreatitis. Pregnancy does not increase the frequency or severity of these complications.[30] Symptoms of gallstone disease during pregnancy are the same as in other patients.[29,30] The usual initial symptom is biliary colic that is located in the epigastrium or right upper quadrant and may radiate to the back or shoulders. The pain can occur spontaneously or be induced by eating a fatty meal. The pain typically lasts for several hours. Diaphoresis, nausea, and emesis are common. Physical examination is unremarkable, other than occasional right upper quadrant tenderness. About two thirds of patients with biliary colic experience recurrent attacks during the following 2 years.[4]

Acute cholecystitis is a chemical inflammation usually caused by cystic duct obstruction by a gallstone. It is the third most common nonobstetric surgical emergency during pregnancy, with an incidence of about 4 cases per 10,000 pregnancies.[23] As in biliary colic, the pain is located in the epigastrium and right upper quadrant, but the pain is usually more severe and prolonged. Other clinical findings include nausea, emesis, pyrexia, tachycardia, right-sided subcostal tenderness, Murphy's sign, and leukocytosis.[31] Serum biochemical parameters of liver function and serum levels of amylase may be mildly abnormal. Jaundice suggests choledocholithiasis, and pronounced hyperamylasemia suggests gallstone pancreatitis.

Patients with recurrent biliary colic or with acute cholecystitis usually undergo cholecystectomy.[29,31,32] Preoperative management includes discontinuing oral intake, administration of intravenous fluids, analgesia, and usually, antibiotics.[28] Ampicillin, cephalosporins, and clindamycin are relatively safe antibiotics during pregnancy.[31,33] Cholecystectomy is best performed during the second trimester; cholecystectomy during the first trimester is associated with fetal wastage, and cholecystectomy during the third trimester is associated with premature labor.[31,32] Cholecystectomy has, however, become increasingly accepted during the first and third trimesters because of improved surgical outcomes.[32] Tocolysis may be necessary during cholecystectomy performed in the third trimester. Intraoperative cholangiography is performed only during pregnancy for strong indications to avoid radiation teratogenicity. Laparoscopic cholecystectomy is safe during pregnancy[4] (see Chapter 23). Both maternal and fetal mortality rates from acute cholecystitis are less than 5 percent during pregnancy.[30]

Choledocholithiasis

Symptomatic choledocholithiasis is uncommon during pregnancy. Choledocholithiasis can produce gallstone pancreatitis, manifested by pyrexia, nausea, and severe abdominal pain; or ascending cholangitis manifested by pyrexia, right upper quadrant pain, and jaundice (Charcot's triad).[23] Endoscopic ultrasound is relatively safe in pregnancy and is sensitive in detecting choledocholithiasis.[34] Patients with choledocholithiasis and gallstone pancreatitis should undergo endoscopic retrograde cholangiography and sphincterotomy with stone extraction, as previously described. Pancreatography can be avoided to minimize fetal radiation exposure.[26] These patients then usually undergo cholecystectomy postpartum but can undergo cholecystectomy antepartum with an acceptable rate of maternal and fetal mortality.[23]

Choledochal Cysts

Choledochal cysts are rare. They typically produce a diagnostic triad of abdominal pain, jaundice, and a palpable abdominal mass in nonpregnant patients. Pregnancy can exacerbate the abdominal pain and can increase the jaundice because of choledochal compression by the enlarged gravid uterus. However, pregnancy can mask the palpable abdominal mass due to the enlarged gravid uterus.[35,36] Severe pain suggests cyst rupture or concomitant pancreatitis.[35] A choledochal cyst can be diagnosed by abdominal ultrasound, although cholangiography is sometimes required. Surgical management is generally recommended because of the risk of recurrent cholangitis and malignant degeneration. The standard surgery is cystectomy, cholecystectomy, and reconstitution of biliary-intestinal flow by either a Roux-en-Y hepaticojejunostomy or choledochojejunostomy.[36] Medical management, including antibiotics and temporary percutaneous or endoscopic drainage, may sometimes suffice until delivery.[35,36]

COMMON LIVER DISEASES INCIDENTAL TO PREGNANCY

Acute Viral Hepatitis A, B, and C

Acute viral hepatitis A, B, and C present similarly in pregnancy as in the nonpregnant state. For example, acute hepatitis B is usually self-limited and mild during pregnancy. Typical symptoms of acute viral hepatitis include anorexia, nausea, malaise, and right upper quadrant discomfort. Patients with acute hepatitis A or hepatitis B typically have highly elevated serum aminotransferase levels. Jaundice may occur. Acute hepatitis C is frequently subclinical and typically causes only mild serum aminotransferase level elevations. Maternal mortality is rare from acute hepatitis A, B, or C during pregnancy. Fetal mortality and neonatal morbidity are increased by acute hepatitis A or B but remain relatively low.

Wilson's Disease

Noncirrhotic women treated for early Wilson's disease have relatively intact fertility and, therefore, may become pregnant. Their serum levels of copper and ceruloplasmin increase during pregnancy.[37] They require maintenance therapy during pregnancy to prevent a flare of disease that can increase maternal morbidity and fetal mortality. Although the data are limited, trientine (triethylene tetramine dihydrochloride) or zinc therapy for Wilson's disease may be maintained during pregnancy without significant fetal toxicity.[38] D-penicillamine is potentially teratogenic, and its use during pregnancy should be discouraged when alternatives are available.

Autoimmune Hepatitis

Women with autoimmune hepatitis should be maintained on immunosuppressive therapy during pregnancy. Patients with well-compensated and well-controlled autoimmune hepatitis tolerate pregnancy well while maintained on this therapy, with only a moderately increased rate of fetal mortality and perinatal complications.[39] These patients typically have a reversible mild deterioration of serum parameters of liver function during pregnancy, particularly of the serum bilirubin and alkaline phosphatase, attributed to the cholestatic effects of pregnancy. Patients who discontinue the immunosuppressive therapy can develop severe acute flares during pregnancy.

Hepatic Hemangiomas, Cysts, and Abscesses

Hepatic hemangiomas and focal nodular hyperplasia are usually asymptomatic during pregnancy and are detected incidentally during obstetric ultrasound.[12,34] These hepatic lesions sometimes grow during pregnancy, possibly because of estrogen stimulation and can occasionally cause hepatic hemorrhage or biliary obstruction due to compression by the enlarged gravid uterus.[40,41] Clinical findings may include abdominal pain, jaundice, or hypotension. Surgical intervention may be necessary.[40,41] Giant hepatic hemangiomas may cause hemolysis.

Hepatic cysts may be isolated or associated with polycystic kidney disease, malignancy, or amebic or echinococcal infection.[40,42] Pyogenic liver abscesses during pregnancy arise from ascending cholangitis, appendicitis, or diverticulitis.[40,41] Both antibiotics and percutaneous drainage are usually indicated.

Hepatocellular Carcinoma and Hepatic Metastases

Hepatocellular carcinoma (HCC) usually occurs in the setting of cirrhosis secondary to chronic viral hepatitis, hemochromatosis, or alcoholism. It is rarely diagnosed during pregnancy.[40,41] The poor prognosis during pregnancy may result from delayed diagnosis. Screening high-risk patients by serum alpha-fetoprotein determination and abdominal ultrasonography can detect HCC earlier.[40,43] The fibromellar variant of HCC, typically found in younger women, has a better prognosis. Hepatic metastases from colon cancer can occur during pregnancy.[5]

LIVER DISEASES SIGNIFICANTLY AFFECTED BY PREGNANCY

Hepatitis E

Hepatitis E, although rare and sporadic in industrialized countries, is the most common epidemic water-born form of hepatitis in developing countries. It is usually transmitted by fecal-oral transmission through a contaminated water supply. Infected patients typically have a prodrome with malaise and pyrexia, followed by an acute illness with anorexia, nausea, vomiting, abdominal pain, and jaundice. Patients often have hepatomegaly and usually have significant elevations of the serum aminotransferase levels. The infection is typically mild and self-limited without chronicity or clinical sequelae.

Pregnant patients have a more severe illness, with frequent fulminant hepatitis. The mortality rate rises progressively with the term of pregnancy, up to a 20 percent mortality for acute infection in the third trimester.[44] Maternal infection is likewise associated with a high risk of fetal or neonatal mortality. Fulminant hepatitis may require liver transplantation. The cause of the increased severity of this hepatitis during pregnancy is unknown but may relate to attenuated cellular immunity during pregnancy.

In the United States, this infection is rare and not routinely tested for in the evaluation of acute hepatitis, but it should be tested for when patients with an acute hepatitis have recently traveled to an endemic area and have had hepatitis A, B, and C excluded by serologic tests. The infection is diagnosed by detecting anti-hepatitis E virus (HEV) antibodies in the serum. Acute infection is diagnosed by detection of immunoglobulin M antibodies, whereas prior infection is diagnosed by detection of immunoglobulin G antibodies. The infection is largely prevented by public health measures, such as a clean water supply. Pregnant women should avoid travel in endemic areas and should not drink water from the municipal water supply in endemic areas.

Chronic Hepatitis B

Pregnancy does not appear to significantly affect the progression of chronic hepatitis B. Maternal chronic hepatitis B infection may, however, be transmitted to the neonate, usually during delivery.[45] The risk of vertical transmission is about 90 percent in mothers who are hepatitis B-e antigen positive but is only about 25 percent in mothers who are hepatitis B-e antigen negative.[46] Perinatal infection is clinically important because infected neonates tend to become chronic carriers and then have a markedly increased risk of developing hepatocellular carcinoma in adulthood. Infants born to infected mothers should be passively immunized with hepatitis B hyperimmune globulin and actively immunized with hepatitis B vaccine immediately after birth to prevent neonatal infection from intrapartum exposure.[47]

Chronic Viral Hepatitis C

Women with chronic hepatitis C may exhibit transient normalization of their serum aminotransferase levels associated with an increase in the serum viral load during pregnancy, possibly due to mildly attenuated immunity.[48] The clinical significance of this phenomenon in terms of progression of the liver disease is unclear, but chronically infected patients may develop mild progression of their liver disease, as evidenced by increased hepatic fibrosis, during pregnancy.

The risk of vertical transmission of hepatitis C from a chronically infected mother with viremia to the neonate is about 5 percent.[49] Infants born to mothers with hepatitis C infection should undergo periodic testing for hepatitis C during the first eighteen months of life to detect persistent infection.

Hepatocellular Adenomas

Hepatocellular adenomas are benign hepatic tumors that are promoted by hyperestrogenemia. Pregnancy is associated with accelerated adenoma growth and consequent development of symptoms, such as nausea, vomiting, and right upper quadrant pain. Hepatic adenomas that are symptomatic or larger than 5 cm in diameter should be considered for surgical excision before conception in women contemplating pregnancy.

Acute Intermittent Porphyria

The porphyrias are rare diseases caused by deficiency of various heme biosynthetic enzymes that result in accumulation of toxic porphyrin precursors. Acute intermittent porphyria (AIP), due to porphobilinogen deaminase deficiency, is the most common hepatic porphyria, with a frequency of about 1 per 10,000 people. Acute intermittent porphyria is transmitted as an autosomal trait with incomplete penetrance[50] and is strongly affected by environmental factors, including female sex hormone levels. Women have more severe symptoms than men, and their symptoms are exacerbated by oral contraceptive administration or during menstruation and pregnancy.[50,51] About one third of female patients first present during pregnancy or immediately postpartum. Hyperemesis gravidarum is a common precipitant. Diffuse abdominal pain is common. Other symptoms include vomiting, constipation, and neuropsychiatric abnormalities.[50] Autonomic abnormalities can cause tachycardia, hypertension, or ileus. Unlike other porphyrias, AIP lacks dermatologic manifestations.

AIP should be considered in any pregnant patient with abdominal pain and a puzzling diagnostic evaluation. Increased urinary levels of porphobilinogen and delta-aminolevulinic acid are diagnostic.[50] Management includes avoidance of precipitating drugs, avoidance of fasting, and possible administration of hematin or parenteral glucose.[50] The maternal mortality is less than 10 percent, with a fetal wastage rate of 13 percent and frequent low-birth-weight infants.[50,51] Genetic counseling is recommended.

Sickle Cell Hemoglobinopathies

Crises in patients with sickle hemoglobinopathies, including hemoglobin SS, hemoglobin SC, and hemoglobin S/β-thalassemia, can present with intense abdominal pain. These hematologic disorders occur primarily in blacks. Patients with these hemoglobinopathies are prone to develop preeclampsia, eclampsia, or sickle crisis during pregnancy.[52,53] They can develop ischemia and microinfarction of multiple organs including extremities, joints, and abdominal viscera.[53] The abdominal pain in sickle crisis can be excruciating. Hemoglobin SS patients have an increased risk of acute cholecystitis during pregnancy.[30,53] These maternal hemoglobinopathies significantly increase fetal mortality.[52]

Portal Hypertension

The plasma volume gradually increases during pregnancy to a maximum of about 40 percent above baseline.[54] The primary contributing factor is sodium retention mediated by increased serum aldosterone, estrogen, and rennin levels, but water retention is a secondary factor.[54] The maternal cardiac output increases in proportion with the plasma volume. Portal pressure appears to physiologically increase during pregnancy owing to these increases in plasma volume and cardiac output, as well as increased vascular resistance due to external compression of the inferior vena cava by the gravid uterus. Therefore, pregnancy can exacerbate preexisting portal hypertension; cause shunting of blood into portosystemic collaterals, particularly esophageal varices; increase intravariceal pressure; and increase the risk of variceal hemorrhage. About 30 percent of pregnant patients with portal hypertension develop variceal hemorrhage, and about 75 percent of pregnant patients with preexisting esophageal varices develop variceal hemorrhage.[54] The risk of variceal hemorrhage is highest during the second trimester, when the portal hypertension peaks, and during labor, when venous collateral resistance abruptly increases from use of the Valsalva maneuver to push the fetus through the birth canal.

Portal hypertension without cirrhosis is usually due to portal vein obstruction or hepatic fibrosis. Female fertility is much better preserved in portal hypertension without cirrhosis than with cirrhosis. Pregnant patients, therefore, more frequently have portal hypertension without cirrhosis than with cirrhosis. Noncirrhotic patients with portal hypertension have a much lower mortality rate from each episode of variceal hemorrhage than cirrhotic patients due to better preserved liver function, a lower incidence of coagulopathy or thrombocytopenia, and a much lower risk of hepatic failure precipitated by variceal hemorrhage. Indeed, about 25 percent of cirrhotics experience hepatic failure during pregnancy.

Women with prior variceal hemorrhage or with borderline liver function contemplating pregnancy should be advised of the high risks of maternal hepatic decompensation or variceal hemorrhage during pregnancy and of the poor fetal prognosis. They should also be advised of the risk of transmitting genetic hepatic diseases, such as alpha$_1$-antitrypsin deficiency, or of transmitting hepatotropic viral infections, such as hepatitis B, to their offspring. Women with well-compensated chronic liver disease without prior variceal hemorrhage should undergo EGD before conception for risk stratification. Patients with silent esophageal varices are at high risk of variceal hemorrhage during pregnancy, whereas patients without esophageal varices are at low risk of this complication. Patients with esophageal varices should be informed of the benefits of beta-adrenergic receptor antagonists during pregnancy to reduce portal pressure, but they should also be advised of the fetal risks of these medications, which may include fetal bradycardia and growth restriction.

About 2.5 percent of cirrhotics experience splenic artery rupture during pregnancy. Pregnant patients with portal hypertension should undergo an ultrasound examination with Doppler studies of the upper abdomen to screen for splenic artery aneurysms at the time of their routine antenatal pelvic ultrasound. Administration of iron is contraindicated in pregnant patients with hemochromatosis and is inadvisable in pregnant patients with several other types of chronic liver disease, such as chronic hepatitis C. Routine serum parameters of liver function, including a coagulation profile, should be serially monitored during pregnancy. Variceal hemorrhage during pregnancy is managed as it would be in nonpregnant patients, initially with endoscopic variceal banding or sclerotherapy, as described earlier. Octreotide therapy is normally administered before endoscopic therapy and maintained for several days after endoscopic therapy in nonpregnant patients. Several cases of prolonged administration of octreotide for pituitary tumors have been reported in pregnant patients with good pregnancy outcomes.[55] During parturition, the second stage of labor should be shortened to minimize portal hypertension, intravenous fluids should be administered cautiously to avoid volume overload, and any coagulopathy should be corrected to minimize the risk of intrapartum variceal hemorrhage.[54]

Budd-Chiari Syndrome

The Budd-Chiari syndrome refers to hepatic vein thrombosis or occlusion that increases the hepatic sinusoidal pressure and can lead to portal hypertension or hepatic necrosis.[56] Many cases are secondary to congenital vascular anomalies or hypercoagulopathies. This syndrome is rare in general and is consequently rare in pregnancy even though pregnancy tends to promote this syndrome owing to pregnancy-related increases in the serum level of estrogen and pregnancy-related decreases in the serum level of antithrombin III.[57,58] This syndrome usually presents in the last trimester or the puerperium. The characteristic clinical triad is abdominal pain, hepatomegaly, and ascites.[57,58] Acute and chronic presentations occur. The serum bilirubin and alkaline phosphatase levels are typically moderately elevated, with normal to mildly elevated serum aminotransferase levels. This syndrome is diagnosed by pulsed Doppler ultrasound, hepatic venography, or magnetic resonance angiography.[57–59] Without therapy, death usually occurs within 1 decade after diagnosis. The definitive therapy is liver transplantation. Selective thrombolytic therapy and surgical or radiologic remedy of portal hypertension for intractable ascites or variceal bleeding have also been described.[57,58] Patients have had subsequent successful pregnancies after undergoing liver transplantation for Budd-Chiari syndrome presenting during the puerperium.[59]

Pregnancy After Liver Transplantation

Although cirrhotic women are often infertile, women often regain fertility after successful liver transplantation for cirrhosis with restoration of liver function. Immunosuppressive therapy should be maintained during pregnancy after liver transplantation even though the fetal safety of most immunosuppressive therapies is inadequately analyzed. Pregnancy appears to be relatively well tolerated after liver transplantation, provided the transplanted liver has demonstrated good function in the recipient before conception. Maternal complications during pregnancy include hypertension, preeclampsia, infections associated with immunosuppression, and occasionally, acute hepatic rejection.[60]

Fetal outcome is variable, with a large increase in fetal or neonatal mortality and a moderate increase in neonatal complications, particularly prematurity and low birth weight. However, about 70 percent of live-born babies do well without congenital anomalies or neonatal complications.[60]

LIVER DISEASE STRONGLY RELATED OR UNIQUE TO PREGNANCY

Alcoholism During Pregnancy

Alcoholism during pregnancy can result in the fetal alcohol syndrome characterized by facial abnormalities such as an absent philtrum, growth restriction, and neurodevelopmental deficits. Affected infants occasionally develop hepatic dysfunction, manifested by hepatomegaly or elevations of serum aminotransferase or alkaline phosphatase levels.[61]

Hepatic Involvement in Hyperemesis Gravidarum

About 15 percent of patients with hyperemesis gravidarum experience liver dysfunction, including severalfold elevations of the serum aminotransferase levels, jaundice, or pruritus. The hepatic dysfunction may be related to dehydration, malnutrition, and electrolyte abnormalities. This dysfunction is typically mild and resolves with control and reversal of the underlying abnormalities.

Herpes Simplex Hepatitis

Herpes simplex hepatitis is uncommon during pregnancy. However, about half of all cases of this hepatitis in immunocompetent adults occur during pregnancy, possibly due to attenuated immunity during pregnancy. Herpes simplex hepatitis has a high mortality rate during pregnancy owing to a propensity for viral dissemination and delayed diagnosis.[62] Patients typically present with right upper quadrant pain, very high serum aminotransferase levels, and moderate hyperbilirubinemia after a brief viral prodrome. The diagnosis may be made by viral culture or histologic analysis of infected tissue. Acyclovir therapy is recommended.

Intrahepatic Cholestasis of Pregnancy (Prepared by George Kroumpouzos)

Generalized pruritus occurs secondary to intrahepatic cholestasis of pregnancy (ICP), the most common pregnancy-induced liver disorder. The condition manifests itself with jaundice (intrahepatic jaundice of pregnancy or obstetric cholestasis) or without (pruritus gravidarum). ICP is common in Chile, Bolivia, and Scandinavia[63] and less prevalent in Europe (0.1 to 1.5 percent) and United States (<0.1 percent). It can recur in subsequent pregnancies or with oral contraceptives.[64] There is a family history in half of the cases and associations with multiple gestation pregnancy[63] and hepatitis C.[65] ICP may be preceded by a urinary tract infection.

Itching may precede the laboratory abnormalities of the condition, affecting the palms and soles and extending to the legs and abdomen. Excorations due to scratching are invariably seen but no primary skin lesions. Mild nausea and discomfort in the upper right quadrant may accompany the pruritus. Mild jaundice (20 percent) can develop 2 to 4 weeks of the onset of pruritus and may be associated with subclinical steatorrhea and increased risk of hemorrhage.[64] Up to 50 percent of patients develop darker urine and light-colored stools. Elevation of serum bile acids is the most sensitive marker of ICP,[64,65] and correlates with the severity of pruritus. Mild abnormalities of the liver function tests are found, such as elevation of transaminases, alkaline phosphatase, cholesterol and triglycerides; the conjugated bilirubin is elevated (2 to 5 mg/dl) in jaundiced patients. Malabsorption of fat may cause vitamin K deficiency and a prolonged prothrombin time. The symptoms and laboratory abnormalities of ICP typically resolve within 2 to 4 weeks postpartum.

Hormonal, immunologic, genetic, environmental, and alimentary factors have been implicated in the etiology of ICP.[63] Estrogens interfere with bile acid secretion. Progestins inhibit hepatic glucuronyltransferase, and the increased sulfated progesterone metabolites, especially the 3a, 5a -isomers, may saturate the maximal transport capacity of the hepatocyte. An immunologic study[66] showed a Th1 cytokine response and decreased maternal-fetal lymphocyte reaction in ICP. Genetic factors have been suggested by the existence of familial cases, geographic variation and a higher prevalence of ICP in mothers of patients with progressive familial intrahepatic cholestasis or benign recurrent intrahepatic cholestasis. Several studies showed a heterozygous MDR3 missense mutation associated with ICP.[67]

Fetal risks in ICP include stillbirth and preterm delivery. Antepartum testing may be unreliable and a negative antepartum test is not reassuring. Malabsorption of vitamin K increases the risk of intracranial hemorrhage. These complications are related to decreased fetal elimination of toxic bile acids that can cause vasoconstriction of human placental chorionic veins. The risk of serious fetal complications makes intensive fetal surveillance mandatory. Most authors recommend fetal surveillance and cardiotocographic monitoring from the 34th week of gestation.[68] If gestational age is less than 36 weeks, one should monitor liver function tests and bile acids, and consider treatment with ursodeoxycholic acid as well as delivery at 36 to 37 weeks with fetal maturity or continue surveillance if liver function tests improve. If gestational age is more than 36 weeks, amniocentesis and delivery should be considered if the cervix is favorable and fetal lung maturity is satisfactory.

Treatment with topical antipruritics, emollients, and oral antihistamines is rarely effective. Epomediol, silymarine, S-adenosylmethionine, activated charcoal, and phenobarbital have met limited success.[63,69] Anecdotal reports show some response to ultraviolet light B. Dexamethasone suppression of fetoplacental estrogen production was effective in an uncontrolled study.[70] Cholestyramine (up to 18 g/day) can be effective only mild to moderate ICP.[63] It needs to be administered for several days before a clear benefit for pruritus can be obtained and it does not improve the biochemical abnormalities of ICP.[69] Furthermore, it can precipitate vitamin K and should be administered in conjunction with weekly vitamin K supplementation.[63] Recurrence of itching is common after the first week of treatment.

Ursodeoxycholic acid reduces bile acid levels in cord blood, colostrums, and amniotic fluid. A meta-analysis[64] of randomized controlled trials demonstrated that ursodeoxycholic acid (450 to 1200 mg/day) is highly effective in controlling the pruritus and laboratory abnormalities associated with ICP[65,71,72] and may have a synergistic effect with S-adenosylmethionine.[71] Ursodeoxycholic acid has been safe for both mother and fetus, and it may decrease the fetal risks associated with ICP.[73] Compared to cholestyramine, ursodeoxycholic acid is definitely safer, works faster, has a more sustained effect on pruritus, and shows higher efficacy in improving the liver function abnormalities of ICP.[63]

Preeclampsia and Eclampsia (See Chapter 33)

Preeclampsia (see Chapter 33), characterized by hypertension and proteinuria, complicates 3 to 6 percent of pregnancies.[74] The preeclampsia is severe when the proteinuria exceeds 5 g/24 hours or when the blood pressure is more than 160/110 mm Hg.[75] Severe preeclampsia may cause oliguria, jaundice, thrombocytopenia, pulmonary edema, and neurologic abnormalities of headaches or visual disturbances.[2,74] Risk factors for preeclampsia include diabetes mellitus, antiphospholipid antibody syndrome, hydatiform mole, and fetal hydrops.[74,75] Preeclampsia usually presents later in pregnancy.

About 10 percent of patients with severe preeclampsia develop hepatic dysfunction.[76,77] Symptoms include nausea, emesis, and right upper quadrant pain that may radiate to the right shoulder.[2] Severe pain may herald hepatic infarction, hemorrhage, or rupture.[3] Right upper quadrant tenderness is common. Mild hyperbilirubinemia and marked serum aminotransferase elevations often occur.[2,74] Pathologic examination of a liver biopsy usually demonstrates sinusoidal fibrin deposition and periportal hemorrhage, and occasionally demonstrates hepatocellular necrosis.[74] Hepatic involvement is often accompanied by hemolysis, thrombocytopenia, renal dysfunction, altered sensorium, eclampsia, or hepatic decompensation.[56]

Patients who present near term with mild preeclampsia have minimally increased mortality rates.[56,74] Eclampsia is a severe, life-threatening form of preeclampsia characterized by seizures.[2,74] More than 20 percent of women without prenatal care die, but less than 1 percent managed in tertiary hospitals during pregnancy die.[56,74] About 15 percent of the maternal mortality from eclampsia is attributable to hepatic complications including hepatic failure, hemorrhage, and infarction.[3,74] Fetal mortality is less than 5 percent in deliveries performed later than 34 weeks of gestation[74] but is much higher in deliveries occurring during the second trimester.[56]

Hemolysis, Elevated Liver Function Tests, and Low Platelet Count Syndrome

The hemolysis, elevated liver function tests, and low platelet count (HELLP) syndrome occurs in about 3 per 1000 pregnancies.[2,3,77] Patients typically present in the third trimester or occasionally present postpartum.[78,79] Typical clinical findings include hemolytic anemia, thrombocytopenia, and abnormal results of serum liver function tests.[77] Laboratory criteria for this syndrome include microangiopathic hemolysis with schistocytes present on the peripheral blood smear, platelet count less than 50,000/mm^3, serum total bilirubin higher than 1.2 mg/100 mL, serum lactate dehydrogenase higher than 600 U/L, and serum aspartate aminotransferase higher than 70 U/L.

Patients usually have epigastric or right upper quadrant pain. Other symptoms include right shoulder pain, nausea, emesis, malaise, headache, visual disturbances, mucocutaneous bleeding, and jaundice.[77–79] Physical examination may reveal right upper quadrant tenderness and peripheral edema. Patients usually have hypertension and proteinuria. Hepatic pathologic abnormalities include periportal hemorrhage, focal parenchymal necrosis with hyaline deposition, fibrin microthrombi, and steatosis.[54]

This syndrome is a medical emergency, with a maternal mortality rate of 1 to 2 percent and a fetal mortality rate of 10 to 35 percent that depends on the gestational age at delivery.[3,70,79] This syndrome is also associated with intrauterine growth restriction and premature delivery.[3,78]

MANAGEMENT OF PREECLAMPSIA, ECLAMPSIA, AND HELLP SYNDROME

Preeclampsia, eclampsia, and HELLP syndrome are related disorders with shared pathogenic, pathologic, and clinical features (see Chapter 33).[2] Indeed, about 20 percent of patients with preeclampsia or eclampsia develop the HELLP syndrome.[3,77,78] Hypertension is universal with preeclampsia or eclampsia, as are hemolytic anemia and thrombocytopenia with HELLP, but these features may occur in either syndrome. The management is tailored to the clinical manifestations as well as the clinical diagnosis. Patients with mild preeclampsia can be managed at home, but patients with severe preeclampsia, eclampsia, or HELLP syndrome should be managed in an intensive care unit, preferably at a tertiary medical center.

Delivery is the definitive therapy.[3,56] If these disorders manifest after 34 weeks of gestation and after documentation of fetal lung maturity, the fetus should be promptly delivered.[3,78] Vaginal delivery can usually be performed, but cesarean delivery is sometimes necessary, with use of general anesthesia and preoperative transfusion of platelets. Laboratory abnormalities usually peak during the first 48 hours postpartum. During this time period, the patient should remain in an intensive care unit and receive transfusions of platelets or clotting factors as necessary for disseminated intravascular coagulation (DIC). Hypertension is managed aggressively, with parenteral agents, if necessary. Magnesium is administered to prevent seizures. Specific treatment is administered for renal insufficiency or pulmonary edema. Plasmapheresis has been used for persistence of the HELLP syndrome beyond 72 hours postpartum. The platelet count normalizes within 1 week after delivery. Management of these syndromes before 34 weeks of gestation is problematic. Delivery can be deferred for several days if neither maternal complications nor fetal distress supervenes. Corticosteroids may be administered to accelerate fetal lung maturity.

Hepatic Hemorrhage and Rupture

One percent or more of patients with the HELLP syndrome have a subcapsular hepatic hematoma.[80] Other causes of hepatic hematomas include eclampsia or preeclampsia complicated by DIC, hepatic trauma, and hepatocellular carcinoma.[81,82] Pain commonly occurs in the right upper quadrant, epigastrium, or right shoulder.[80,82,83] Signs include hypotension, hepatomegaly, hepatic tenderness, and rebound tenderness with peritonitis.[78,83] Laboratory findings may reflect HELLP or DIC if they are present but are otherwise nonspecific. Pathologic examination of the liver reveals sinusoidal fibrin deposition and extensive, primarily periportal, hepatic hemorrhage.[3,56,78] Hepatic subcapsular hematoma can be diagnosed by ultrasonography or MRI, but CT scanning is the most sensitive and specific imaging test.[80,82]

Both the maternal and perinatal mortality from hepatic hemorrhage exceeds 30 percent.[70,75,76] The patient should be hemodynamically stabilized, and any coagulopathy should be corrected preoperatively.[70,75,76] An unruptured subcapsular hematoma may sometimes be managed medically and expectantly, with frequent serial CT scans and close clinical monitoring.[70] Invasive therapies include evacuation of the hematoma, with packing and drainage, angiographic embolization, hepatic artery ligation, or hepatic resection. The mortality rate is highest with hepatic lobectomy and lowest with transarterial embolization of a bleeding hepatic artery identified at angiography.[78,83,84]

Hepatic rupture is a rare but catastrophic complication of pregnancy resulting from progressive hepatic bleeding and stretch of Glisson's capsule.[81] Patients are usually multiparous and older.[80,82,83] The rupture usually involves the right hepatic lobe and usually occurs just before or just after delivery. Hepatic rupture is a medical emergency because the fetus poorly tolerates concomitant shock. The fetus should be rapidly delivered and the liver surgically repaired. Patients with hepatic hemorrhage rarely have recurrence during subsequent pregnancies.[84]

Acute Fatty Liver of Pregnancy

Acute fatty liver of pregnancy (AFLP) is a rare but severe disease characterized by hepatic microvesicular steatosis associated with mitochondrial dysfunction. It is related to an autosomally inherited mutation that causes deficiency of the long-chain 3-hydroxyacyl coenzymeA dehydrogenase (LCHAD), a fatty acid beta-oxidation enzyme.[4] It usually manifests in the third trimester and rarely manifests immediately postpartum.[56,85] It occurs in about 1 per 10,000 pregnancies.[2,3] It is more common in primiparas, twin pregnancies, and patients with preeclampsia.[85–87]

The initial symptoms, including anorexia, nausea, emesis, malaise, fatigue, and headache, are nonspecific.[56,85] About half of the patients have epigastric or right upper quadrant pain, and about half have hypertension.[86,87] Physical examination may reveal hepatic tenderness, usually without hepatomegaly. Serum aminotransferase and bilirubin levels are variably elevated. Jaundice usually manifests later in the course of the illness or after delivery. Characteristic laboratory abnormalities include a prolonged prothrombin time, hypofibrinogenemia, and increased serum levels of fibrin-split products. Other laboratory abnormalities include increased serum levels of ammonia, uric acid, blood urea nitrogen, and creatinine.[56,86,87] Hepatic imaging studies primarily help to exclude other disorders or to detect hepatic hemorrhage.[85]

Liver biopsy is usually diagnostic but is not indicated for suspected AFLP unless the presentation is atypical or the postpartum jaundice is prolonged.[2,86] Hepatic pathology reveals intracytoplasmic microsteatosis in hepatocytes, preservation of hepatic architecture, and isolated foci of inflammatory and necrotic cells.[86,87] Sinusoidal deposition of fibrin is usually not present in AFLP but is usually present in preeclampsia and eclampsia. AFLP differs from severe acute viral hepatitis in that the serum aminotransferase levels in AFLP rarely exceed 1,000 U/L, the viral serologic tests are negative, and hepatic pathologic analysis reveals much less inflammatory infiltration and hepatocytic necrosis.[56,74,86,87] AFLP may be difficult to distinguish from HELLP syndrome and preeclampsia or eclampsia with DIC.[78,87] Fortunately, the definitive treatment for all of these disorders is prompt fetal delivery. Most patients improve clinically and biochemically within several days after delivery.[85]

Complications include pulmonary edema; pancreatitis, diabetes insipidus, DIC, seizures, coma, and hepatic failure manifested by jaundice, encephalopathy, [illegible] or variceal bleeding.[85,87] The complications may require specific therapy: hepatic encephalopathy with lactulose, renal failure with hemodialysis, gastrointestinal bleeding with blood transfusions and endoscopic therapy, DIC with blood products, and diabetes insipidus with desmopressin. The maternal mortality is very low with early diagnosis, appropriate supportive therapy, and early delivery. The fetal mortality rate associated with AFLP is less than 15 percent.[3,86,88] The mother, neonate, and father should be tested for LCHAD mutations. AFLP rarely recurs in a subsequent pregnancy.[86]

SUMMARY

Although relatively uncommon, hepatic, biliary, and pancreatic disorders are clinically important owing to their potentially severe effects on the mother and fetus. These disorders are often complex and clinically challenging problems during pregnancy. The differential diagnosis of these disorders is particularly extensive during pregnancy because it includes pregnancy-related as well as unrelated conditions. The patient history, physical examination, laboratory data, and radiologic findings usually provide the diagnosis. Abdominal ultrasound is generally the recommended radiologic imaging modality; roentgenograms are generally contraindicated during pregnancy because of radiation teratogenicity. Concerns about the fetus limit the pharmacotherapy. Maternal and fetal survival have recently increased in many of these life-threatening conditions, such as liver disease during pregnancy, because of improved diagnostic technology, better maternal and fetal monitoring, earlier diagnosis, and improved therapy.

KEY POINTS

- The differential diagnosis of hepatobiliary conditions is extensive in pregnancy in that it includes pregnancy-related as well as pregnancy-unrelated disorders. Indeed, several clinical syndromes, such as intrahepatic cholestasis of pregnancy and acute fatty liver of pregnancy, are unique to pregnancy.
- Pregnancy affects the normative values of serum parameters of liver function and pancreatic injury. During pregnancy the serum level of albumin declines, whereas the serum levels of amylase, alkaline phosphatase, bile acids, cholesterol, and triglycerides rise. Yet these serum parameters are still clinically important measures of liver function and pancreatic injury during pregnancy, provided the changes in normative values are appreciated.
- Many causes of significant-to-severe liver dysfunction during pregnancy—including preeclampsia, eclampsia, HELLP syndrome, and acute fatty liver of pregnancy—are rapidly relieved and completely reversed by delivery of the baby. Early delivery of the baby after fetal lung maturity is documented is generally the definitive therapy for these disorders.
- Pregnancy aggravates preexisting portal hypertension and increases the risk of variceal hemorrhage. As in nonpregnant patients, endoscopic sclerotherapy or banding appear to be first-line therapies for esophageal variceal bleeding in pregnant patients.
- Pregnancy greatly aggravates acute hepatitis E infection, hepatocellular adenomas, acute intermittent porphyria, and herpes simplex hepatitis.
- Neonates born to mothers who have acute or chronic hepatitis B are at high risk of vertical transmission of infection during delivery. Such infants should be passively immunized with hepatitis B hyperimmune globulin and actively immunized with hepatitis B vaccine at birth to prevent this infection.

REFERENCES

1. Ch'ng CL, Morgan M, Hainsworth I, Kingham JG: Prospective study of liver dysfunction in pregnancy in Southwest Wales. Gut 51:876, 2002.
2. Knox TA, Olans LB: Liver disease in pregnancy. N Engl J Med 335:569, 1996.
3. Riely CA: Liver disease in the pregnant patient; American College of Gastroenterology. Am J Gastroenterol 94:1728, 1999.
4. Cappell MS, Friedel D: Abdominal pain during pregnancy. Gastroenterol Clin North Am 32:1, 2003.
5. Cappell MS: Colon cancer during pregnancy. Gastroenterol Clin North Am 32:341, 2003.
6. Delgado I, Neubert R, Dudenhauseu JW: Changes in white blood cells during parturition in mothers and newborns. Gynecol Obstet Invest 38:227, 1994.
7. Stirling Y, Woolf L, North WR, et al: Haemostasis in normal pregnancy. Thromb Haemost 52:176, 1984.
8. Phelps RL, Metzger BE, Freinkel N: Carbohydrate metabolism in pregnancy. XVII. Diurnal profiles of plasma glucose, insulin, free fatty acids, triglycerides, cholesterol, and individual amino acids in late normal pregnancy. Am J Obstet Gynecol 140:730, 1981.
9. Bean WB, Cogswell R, Dexter M: Vascular changes of the skin in pregnancy. Surg Obstet Gynecol 88:739, 1949.
10. Bacq Y, Zarka O, Brechot JF, et al: Liver function tests in normal pregnancy: a prospective study of 103 pregnant women and 103 matched controls. Hepatology 23:1030, 1996.
11. Knopp RH, Warth MR, Carrol CJ: Lipid metabolism in pregnancy. I. Changes in lipoprotein triglyceride and cholesterol in normal pregnancy and the effects of diabetes mellitus. J Reprod Med 10:95, 1973.
12. Derchi LE, Serafini G, Gandolfo N, et al: Ultrasound in gynecology. Eur Radiol 11:2137, 2001.
13. Osei EK, Faulkner K: Fetal doses from radiological examinations. Br J Radiol 72:773, 1999.
14. Toppenberg KS, Hill DA, Miller DP: Safety of radiographic imaging during pregnancy. Am Fam Physician 59:1813, 1999.
15. Cappell MS: The fetal safety and clinical efficacy of gastrointestinal endoscopy during pregnancy. Gastroenterol Clin North Am 32:123, 2003.
16. Dixon NP, Faddis DM, Silberman H: Aggressive management of cholecystitis during pregnancy. Am J Surg 154:292, 1987.
17. Jamidar PA, Beck GJ, Hoffman BJ, et al: F. Endoscopic retrograde cholangiopancreatography in pregnancy. Am J Gastroenterol 90:1263, 1995.
18. Pritchard JA: Changes in the blood volume during pregnancy and delivery. Anesthesiology 26:393, 1965.
19. Cappell MS, Colon VJ, Sidhom OA: A study of eight medical centers of the safety and clinical efficacy of esophagogastroduodenoscopy in 83 pregnant females with follow-up of fetal outcome with comparison control groups. Am J Gastroenterol 91:348, 1996.
20. Kochhar R, Kumar S, Goel RC, et al: Pregnancy and its outcome in patients with noncirrhotic portal hypertension. Dig Dis Sci 44:1356, 1999.
21. Aggarwal N, Sawhney H, Vasishta K, et al: Non-cirrhotic portal hypertension in pregnancy. Int J Gynaecol Obstet 72:1, 2001.
22. Laraki M, Harti A, Bouderka MA, et al: Acute pancreatitis and pregnancy. Rev Fr Gynecol Obstet 88:514, 1993.
23. Ramin KD, Ramsey PS: Disease of the gallbladder and pancreas in pregnancy. Obstet Gynecol Clin North Am 28:571, 2001.
24. Karsenti D, Bacq Y, Brechot JF, et al: Serum amylase and lipase activities in normal pregnancy: a prospective case-control study. Am J Gastroenterol 96:697, 2001.
25. Briggs GG, Freeman RK, Yaffe SJ: Drugs in Pregnancy and Lactation: A Reference Guide to Fetal and Neonatal Risk. Philadelphia, Lippincott Williams & Wilkins; 2002, p 859.
26. Barthel JS, Chowdhury T, Miedema BW: Endoscopic sphincterotomy for the treatment of gallstone pancreatitis during pregnancy. Surg Endosc 12:394, 1998.
27. Legro RS, Laifer SA: First-trimester pancreatitis: maternal and neonatal outcome. J Reprod Med 40:689, 1995.
28. Van Bodegraven AA, Bohmer CJ, Manoliu RA, et al: Gallbladder contents and fasting gallbladder volumes during and after pregnancy. Scand J Gastroenterol 33:993, 1998.
29. Valdivieso V, Covarrubias C, Siegel F, et al: Pregnancy and cholelithiasis: pathogenesis and natural course of gallstones diagnosed in early puerperium. Hepatology 17:1, 1993.
30. Davis A, Katz VL, Cox R: Gallbladder disease in pregnancy. J Reprod Med 40:759, 1995.
31. Ghumman E, Barry M, Grace PA: Management of gallstones in pregnancy. Br J Surg 84:1645, 1997.
32. Glasgow RE, Visser BC, Harris HW, et al: Changing management of gallstone disease during pregnancy. Surg Endosc 12:241, 1998.
33. Dashe JS, Gilstrap III LC: Antibiotic use in pregnancy. Obstet Gynecol Clin North Am 24:617, 1997.
34. Snady H: Endoscopic ultrasonography in benign pancreatic disease. Surg Clin North Am 81:329, 2001.
35. Hewitt PM, Krige JE, Bornman PC, Terblanche J: Choledochal cyst in pregnancy: a therapeutic dilemma. J Am Coll Surg 181:237, 1995.
36. Nassar AH, Chakhtoura N, Martin D, et al: Choledochal cysts diagnosed in pregnancy: a case report and review of treatment options. J Matern Fetal Med 10:363, 2001.
37. Walshe JM: The management of pregnancy in Wilson's disease treated with trientine. Q J Med 58:81, 1986.
38. Brewer GJ, Johnson VD, Dick RD, et al: Treatment of Wilson's disease with zinc. XVII: treatment during pregnancy. Hepatology 31:364, 2000.
39. Heneghan MA, Norris SM, O'Grady JG, et al: Management and outcome of pregnancy in autoimmune hepatitis. Gut 48:97, 2001.
40. Athanassiou AM, Craigo SD: Liver masses in pregnancy. Semin Perinatol 22:166, 1998.
41. Maged DA, Keating HJ 3rd: Noncystic liver mass in the pregnant patient. South Med J 83:51, 1990.
42. Kesby GJ: Pregnancy complicated by symptomatic adult polycystic liver disease. Am J Obstet Gynecol 179:266, 1998.
43. Entezami M, Hardt W, Ebert A, et al: Hepatocellular carcinoma as a rare cause of excessive rise in alpha-fetoprotein in pregnancy. Zentralbl Gynakol 121:503, 1999.
44. Kumar A, Beniwal B, Kar P, et al: Hepatitis e: In pregnancy. Obstet Gynecol Surv 60:7, 2005.
45. Arevalo JA: Hepatitis B in pregnancy. West J Med 150:668, 1989.
46. Tong MJ, Thursby M, Rakela J, et al: Studies on the maternal-infant transmission of the viruses which cause acute hepatitis. Gastroenterology 80:999, 1981.
47. Vranckx R, Alisjahbana A, Meheus A: Hepatitis B virus vaccination and antenatal transmission of HBV markers to neonates. J Viral Hepat 6:135, 1999.
48. Conte D, Fraquelli M, Prati D, et al: Prevalence and clinical course of chronic hepatitis C virus (HCV) infection and rate of HCV vertical transmission in a cohort of 15,250 pregnant women. Hepatology 31:751, 2000.
49. Su GL: Hepatitis C in pregnancy. Curr Gastroenterol Rep 7:45, 2005.
50. Jeans JB, Savik K, Gross CR, et al: Mortality in patients with acute intermittent porphyria requiring hospitalization: a United States case series. Am J Med Genet 65:269, 1996.
51. Milo R, Neuman M, Klein C, et al: Acute intermittent porphyria in pregnancy. Obstet Gynecol 73:450, 1989.
52. Smith JA, Espeland M, Bellevue R, et al: Pregnancy in sickle cell disease: experience of the Cooperative Study of Sickle Cell Disease. Obstet Gynecol 87:199, 1996.
53. Seoud MA, Cantwell C, Nobles G, et al: Outcome of pregnancies complicated by sickle cell and sickle-C hemoglobinopathies. Am J Perinatol 11:187, 1994.
54. Sandhu BS, Sanyal AJ: Pregnancy and liver disease. Gastroenterol Clin North Am 32:407, 2003.
55. Chandraharan E, Arulkumaran S: Pituitary and adrenal disorders complicating pregnancy. Curr Opin Obstet Gynecol 15:101, 2003.
56. Wolf JL: Liver disease in pregnancy. Med Clin North Am 80:1167, 1996.
57. Singh V, Sinha SK, Nain CK, et al: Budd-Chiari syndrome: our experience of 71 patients. J Gastroenterol Hepatol 15:550, 2000.
58. Slakey DP, Klein AS, Venbrux AC, Cameron JL: Budd-Chiari syndrome: current management options. Ann Surg 233:522, 2001.
59. Salha O, Campbell DJ, Pollard S: Budd-Chiari syndrome in pregnancy treated by caesarean section and liver transplant. Br J Obstet Gynaecol 103:1254, 1996.

60. Armenti VT, Herrine SK, Radomski JS, Moritz MJ: Pregnancy after liver transplantation. Liver Transpl 6:671, 2000.
61. Habbick BF, Zaleski WA, Casey R, Murphy F: Liver abnormalities in three patients with fetal alcohol syndrome. Lancet i:580, 1979.
62. Kang AH, Graves CR: Herpes simplex hepatitis in pregnancy: a case report and review of the literature. Obstet Gynecol Surv 54:463, 1999.
63. Kroumpouzos G: Intrahepatic cholestasis of pregnancy: what's new (editorial). J Eur Acad Dermatol Venereol 16:316, 2002.
64. Kroumpouzos G, Cohen LM. Specific dermatoses of pregnancy: an evidence-based systematic review. Am J Obstet Gynecol 188:1083, 2003.
65. Laifer SA, Stiller RJ, Siddiqui DS et al: Ursodeoxycholic acid for the treatment of intrahepatic cholestasis of pregnancy. J Maternal -fetal Med 10:131, 2001.
66. Peng B, Liu S: [Study of relationship between T helper cell type-1 and type-2 cytokines and intrahepatic cholestasis of pregnancy]. Chung-Hua Fu Chan Ko Tsa Chih [Chinese Journal of Obstetrics and Gynecology] 37:516, 2002.
67. Dixon PH, Weerasekera N, Linton KJ, et al: Heterozygous MDR3 missense mutation associated with intrahepatic cholestasis of pregnancy: evidence for a defect in protein trafficking. Hum Mol Genetics 9:1209, 2000.
68. Kroumpouzos G, Cohen LM: Skin Disease. *In* James DK, Steer PJ, Weiner CP, Gonik B (eds): High-Risk Pregnancy: Management Options, 3rd ed. Philadelphia, Elsevier, 2005 (in press).
69. Laatikainen T: Effect of cholestyramine and Phenobarbital on pruritus and serum bile acid levels in cholestasis of pregnancy. Am J Obstet Gynecol 132:501, 1978.
70. Hirvioja M-L, Tuimala R: The treatment of intrahepatic cholestasis of pregnancy by dexamethasone. Br J Obstet Gynaecol 99:109, 1992.
71. Nicastri PL, Diaferia A, Tartagni M, et al: A randomized placebo-controlled trial of ursodeoxycholic acid and S-adenosylmethionine in the treatment of intrahepatic cholestasis of pregnancy. Br J Obstet Gynaecol 105:1205, 1998.
72. Palma J, Reyes H, Ribalta J, et al: Ursodeoxycholic acid in the treatment of cholestasis of pregnancy: a randomized, double-blind study controlled with placebo. J Hepatol 27:1022, 1997.
73. Davies MH, da Silva RCMA, Jones SR, et al: Fetal mortality associated with cholestasis of pregnancy and the potential benefit of therapy with ursodeoxycholic acid. Gut 37:580, 1995.
74. Walker JJ: Pre-eclampsia. Lancet 356:1260, 2000.
75. Odegard RA, Vatten LJ, Nilsen ST, et al: Risk factors and clinical manifestations of pre-eclampsia. Br J Obstet Gynaecol 107:1410, 2000.
76. Rolfes DB, Ishak KG: Liver disease in toxemia of pregnancy. Am J Gastroenterol 81:1138, 1986.
77. Weinstein L: Syndrome of hemolysis, elevated liver enzymes, and low platelet count: a severe consequence of hypertension in pregnancy. Am J Obstet Gynecol 142:159, 1982.
78. Barton JR, Sibai BM: Care of the pregnancy complicated by HELLP syndrome. Gastroenterol Clin North Am 21:937, 1992.
79. Sibai BM: The HELLP syndrome (hemolysis, elevated liver enzymes, and low platelets): much ado about nothing? Am J Obstet Gynecol 162:311, 1990.
80. Barton JR, Sibai BM: Hepatic imaging in HELLP syndrome (hemolysis, elevated liver enzymes, low platelet count). Am J Obstet Gynecol 174:1820, 1996.
81. Sheikh RA, Yasmeen S, Pauly MP, et al: Spontaneous intrahepatic hemorrhage and hepatic rupture in the HELLP syndrome: four cases and a review. J Clin Gastroenterol 28:323, 1999.
82. Coelho T, Braga J, Sequeira M: Hepatic hematomas in pregnancy. Acta Obstet Gynecol Scand 79:331, 2000.
83. Sibai BM, Ramadan MK, Usta I, et al: Maternal morbidity and mortality in 442 pregnancies with hemolysis, elevated liver enzymes, and low platelets (HELLP syndrome). Am J Obstet Gynecol 169:1000, 1993.
84. Rinehart BK, Terrone DA, Magann EF, et al: Preeclampsia-associated hepatic hemorrhage and rupture: mode of management related to maternal and perinatal outcome. Obstet Gynecol Surv 54:196, 1999.
85. Monga M, Katz AR: Acute fatty liver in the second trimester. Obstet Gynecol 93:811, 1999.
86. Castro MA, Fassett MJ, Reynolds TB, et al: Reversible peripartum liver failure: a new perspective on the diagnosis, treatment, and cause of acute fatty liver of pregnancy, based on 28 consecutive cases. Am J Obstet Gynecol 181:389, 1999.
87. Mabie WC: Acute fatty liver of pregnancy. Gastroenterol Clin North Am 21:951, 1992.
88. Pereira SP, O'Donohue J, Wendon J, Williams R: Maternal and perinatal outcome in severe pregnancy-related liver disease. Hepatology 26:1258, 1997.

Gastrointestinal Disorders

KEY ABBREVIATIONS

Computerized tomography	CT
Crohn's disease	CD
Ectopic pregnancy	EP
Esophagogastroduodenoscopy	EGD
Gastroesophageal reflux disease	GERD
Hyperemesis gravidarum	HG
Inflammatory bowel disease	IBD
Irritable bowel syndrome	IBS
Lower esophageal sphincter	LES
Magnetic resonance imaging	MRI
Nonsteroidal anti-inflammatory drugs	NSAIDs
Pelvic inflammatory disease	PID
Peptic ulcer disease	PUD
Small bowel obstruction	SBO
Ulcerative colitis	UC

Gastrointestinal complaints and disorders are common in women of all ages,[1] including women during their childbearing years, and thus often occur during pregnancy. These complaints and disorders present unique clinical challenges during pregnancy. First, the differential diagnosis during pregnancy is extensive. Aside from gastrointestinal disorders unrelated to pregnancy, their complaints may be caused by obstetric or gynecologic disorders related to pregnancy or other intraabdominal diseases incidental to pregnancy. Moreover, some gastrointestinal conditions, such as hyperemesis gravidarum, are unique to pregnancy. Second, the clinical presentation and natural history of gastrointestinal disorders can be altered during pregnancy, as described later for appendicitis. Third, the diagnostic evaluation is altered and constrained by pregnancy. For example, radiologic tests and invasive examinations raise concern about their fetal safety during pregnancy. Fourth, the interests of both the mother and the fetus must be considered in therapeutic decisions during pregnancy. Usually, these interests do not conflict, because what is good for the mother is generally good for the fetus. Sometimes, however, maternal therapy must be modified to substitute alternative but safer therapy because of concerns about drug teratogenicity (e.g., substituting a histamine$_2$ receptor antagonist for misoprostol, an abortifacient that is contraindicated during pregnancy).[2,3] Rarely, the maternal and fetal interests are diametrically opposed, as in the use of chemotherapy for maternal cancer, a therapy that can be life-saving to the mother but life-threatening to the fetus.[4] These conflicts raise significant medical, legal, and ethical issues.

The obstetrician and gynecologist, as well as the gastroenterologist and surgeon, should be familiar with the medical and surgical gastrointestinal conditions that can present in pregnancy and how these conditions affect and are affected by pregnancy. This chapter reviews gastrointestinal symptoms and disorders during pregnancy, with a focus on aspects of these disorders unique to pregnancy.

PHYSIOLOGIC EFFECTS OF PREGNANCY ON ABDOMINAL DISORDERS

Abdominal assessment during pregnancy is modified by displacement of abdominal viscera by the expanding gravid uterus. For example, the location of maximal abdominal pain and tenderness from acute appendicitis migrates superiorly and laterally as the appendix is displaced by the growing gravid uterus.[5] A rigid abdomen with rebound tenderness remains a valid indicator of peritonitis during pregnancy, but abdominal wall laxity in late pregnancy might mask the classic signs of peritonitis.[6] An abdominal mass may be missed on physical examination owing to an enlarged gravid uterus.[4]

Many extraintestinal abdominal conditions or disorders are promoted by pregnancy. Mild hydronephrosis and hydroureter are common during pregnancy, particularly during the early third trimester, owing to diminished muscle tone in the urinary tract from elevated progesterone levels and mechanical obstruction from fetal compression. Hydronephrosis in pregnancy is usually asymptomatic but can cause positional abdominal discomfort.[7] Mucosal immunity may be attenuated during pregnancy as part of physiologic immunologic tolerance of the foreign fetal antigens in the uterus.[8] This phenomenon, as well as urinary stasis during pregnancy, contributes to an increased rate of cystitis and pyelonephritis during pregnancy. Pregnancy also promotes cholelithiasis because of increased cholesterol synthesis and gallbladder hypomotility related to gestational hormones.

Physiologic alterations of laboratory values during pregnancy include mild leukocytosis, physiologic anemia of pregnancy, mild dilutional hypoalbuminemia, mildly increased alkaline phosphatase level, and electrolyte changes, particularly mild hyponatremia.[5,9] The erythrocyte sedimentation rate is physiologically elevated and is a less reliable monitor of inflammatory activity during pregnancy.[10] Gestational hormones, particularly estrogen, contribute to a mild hypercoagulopathy during pregnancy by increasing the synthesis of clotting factors. Thromboembolic phenomena are also promoted by intraabdominal vascular stasis from vascular compression by the enlarged gravid uterus.

The fetus poorly tolerates maternal hypotension, hypovolemia, anemia, and hypoxia. This intolerance affects the type and timing of therapy for abdominal disorders during pregnancy. The gravid uterus can compress the inferior vena cava in the supine position and thereby compromise venous return, aggravating systemic hypoperfusion from hypovolemia or gastrointestinal bleeding. Simply turning the patient to the left side to displace the uterus may relieve this compression, improve venous return, and normalize the blood pressure.[9] The blood pressure normally declines modestly during pregnancy. A rise in blood pressure during pregnancy may, therefore, portend preeclampsia or eclampsia.

DIFFERENTIAL DIAGNOSIS AND EVALUATION OF GASTROINTESTINAL SYMPTOMS DURING PREGNANCY

Physiologic changes during pregnancy may cause abdominal symptoms, including nausea, emesis, early satiety, bloating, pyrosis, and abdominal discomfort. Serious disorders that produce these symptoms may, therefore, be difficult to distinguish from physiologic changes during pregnancy. Significant symptoms should not be dismissed as normal during pregnancy without a careful history, physical examination, and appropriate evaluation.

Occasionally, the pregnancy is not known by the patient or is not revealed to the physician, particularly in early pregnancy, when physical findings are absent. The physician should be vigilant for possible pregnancy in a fertile woman with abdominal symptoms, particularly in the setting of missed menses, because pregnancy affects the differential diagnosis, clinical evaluation, and mode of therapy. Pregnancy tests should be performed early in the evaluation of significant abdominal symptoms in this situation.

Abdominal Pain

The differential diagnosis of abdominal pain during pregnancy is extensive.[5] The abdominal pain is typically localized to the abdominal quadrant in which the afflicted organ is located, as illustrated for pain in the right lower quadrant in Table 43-2. This general rule has exceptions in nonpregnant patients due to referred pain from other nearby regions but is even less reliable during pregnancy owing to displacement of viscera by the growing gravid uterus and owing to referred or poorly localized pain from obstetric conditions.

In the medical history, the pain intensity, nature, temporal pattern, radiation, exacerbating factors, and alleviating factors help narrow the differential diagnosis. The abdominal pain is progressively increasing in appendicitis but is nonprogressive in viral gastroenteritis. The pain from small intestinal obstruction may be intermittent but is severe. Renal and biliary colic also produce a waxing and waning intensity of pain. Acute cholecystitis is associated with right upper quadrant pain, as well as pain referred to the right shoulder. The pain of acute pancreatitis is often boring in quality, located in the abdominal midline, and radiating to the back. Careful physical examination of the abdomen including inspection, palpation, and auscultation can further pinpoint the etiology. Laboratory evaluation of significant abdominal pain routinely includes a hemogram, serum electrolytes, and liver function tests; and often includes a leukocyte differential, coagulation profile, and serum amylase determination. In evaluating the laboratory results, gestational changes in normative values, as mentioned earlier, must be considered. Radiologic tests may be extremely helpful diagnostically, but the choice of radiologic imaging is constrained by the pregnancy, as discussed later.

When the diagnosis is uncertain, close and vigilant monitoring by a surgical team, with frequent abdominal examination and regular laboratory tests, can often clarify the diagnosis. The character, severity, localization, or instigating factors of abdominal pain often change with time. For example, acute appendicitis typically changes from a dull, poorly localized, moderate pain to an intense and focal pain as the inflammation extends from the appendiceal wall to the surrounding peritoneum. The differential diagnosis of severe abdominal pain is described in Table 43-3.

Gastrointestinal causes of abdominal pain are discussed later under their individual headings in this chapter, and hepatobiliary causes are discussed in the previous section of this chapter. Obstetric causes of abdominal pain are also prominent during pregnancy. Ectopic pregnancy (EP) classically presents with abdominopelvic pain and vaginal bleeding after a period of amenorrhea. The pain initially may be diffuse and vague but later becomes

Table 43-2. Differential Diagnosis of Right Lower Quadrant Abdominal Pain

Gastrointestinal disorders
- Appendicitis
- Crohn's disease
- Ruptured Meckel's diverticulum
- Intestinal intussusception
- Cecal perforation
- Colon cancer
- Ischemic colitis
- Irritable bowel syndrome

Renal disease
- Nephrolithiasis
- Cystitis
- Pyelonephritis

Obstetric and gynecologic diseases
- Ruptured ectopic pregnancy
- Ovarian tumors
- Ovarian cyst rupture
- Ovarian torsion
- Endometriosis
- Uterine leiomyomas

Other
- Trochanteric bursitis

Table 43-3. Common Causes of Acute, Severe Abdominal Pain During Pregnancy: Pain Characteristics and Diagnostic Tests

CONDITION	LOCATION	CHARACTER	RADIATION	DIAGNOSTIC TESTS
Ruptured ectopic pregnancy	Lower abdominal or pelvic	Localized, severe	None	Serum βhCG and abdominal ultrasound
Pelvic inflammatory disease	Lower abdominal or pelvic	Gradual in onset, localized	Flanks and thighs	Abdominal ultrasound
Appendicitis	First periumbilical, later RLQ (RUQ in late pregnancy)	Gradual in onset, becomes focal	Back or flank	Abdominal ultrasound in appropriate clinical setting
Acute cholecystitis	RUQ	Focal	Right scapula, shoulder or back	Abdominal ultrasound & serum liver function tests
Pancreatitis	Epigastric	Localized, boring	Middle of back	Serum amylase & lipase, abdominal ultrasound
Perforated peptic ulcer	Epigastric or RUQ	Burning, boring	Right back	Abdominal ultrasound, laparotomy
Urolithiasis	Abdomen or flanks	Varies from intermittent and aching to severe and unremitting	Groin	Urinalysis, abdominal ultrasound, and occasionally fluoroscopy with contrast urography

βhCG, beta human chorionic gonadotropin; RUQ, right upper quadrant; RLQ, right lower quadrant.

focal and severe. Physical signs include mild uteromegaly, cervical tenderness, and an adnexal mass. EP is often differentiated from a viable intrauterine pregnancy by serial βhCG determinations,[11] but it is best differentiated from intrauterine pregnancy by transabdominal or transvaginal pelvic ultrasonography with simultaneous βhCG determination.[12] Rupture of an EP often presents with abdominal pain, rebound tenderness, and hypotension.[11]

In abdominal pregnancy, the abdominal pain is associated with signs of abdominal tenderness, a closed noneffaced cervix, and a palpable mass distinct from the uterus.[5] Sonography and other radiologic modalities, as well as serial βhCG determinations, are used to detect and localize the pregnancy. Abdominal pain is the most common symptom of heterotopic pregnancy. Abdominal ultrasound is sometimes diagnostic, but laparotomy may be required for the diagnosis.

The lower abdominal pain associated with preterm labor is characteristically associated with vaginal discharge or spotting. Back pain, urinary urgency, and vaginal pressure commonly occur. The diagnosis is made by cervical examination, external and internal fetal monitoring, and high-resolution sonography. The abdominal pain from spontaneous abortion—whether threatened, incomplete, or complete—tends to be mild to moderate, crampy, and diffuse, and is typically associated with vaginal bleeding. Placenta previa sometimes presents with abdominal pain or painful uterine contractions in late pregnancy. Vaginal hemorrhage is, however, the predominant symptom. Sonography is usually diagnostic.[12] Although placental abruption commonly causes abdominal pain, it is typically distinguished from gastrointestinal disorders by the presence of vaginal bleeding. Patients typically exhibit uterine tenderness and frequent uterine contractions. Sonography may be diagnostic.[12]

Choriocarcinoma, a malignant trophoblastic proliferation, typically presents with an abdominal mass and vaginal bleeding but may cause abdominal pain. The symptoms usually occur after term pregnancy, abortion, or incomplete evacuation of a hydatiform mole. The diagnosis is suggested by persistently elevated βhCG levels in the absence of pregnancy.

Gynecologic disorders are also in the differential dignosis of abdominal pain during pregnancy. The lower abdominal pain from pelvic inflammatory disease (PID) is typically associated with pyrexia and vaginal discharge.[13] Hemorrhagic infarction of large uterine leiomyomas (fibroids), called the painful myoma syndrome, is characterized by severe abdominal pain, nausea, emesis, pyrexia, and uterine bleeding. Ultrasonography or magnetic resonance imaging (MRI) is usually diagnostic. The abdominal pain of a tubo-ovarian abscess is frequently associated with a palpable lower abdominal mass, pyrexia, and leukocytosis. Patients often have risk factors such as prior pelvic surgery, assisted reproduction, or PID.[14] MRI or sonography is helpful in the diagnosis, but laparoscopy is often required for confirmation.

Adnexal torsion typically causes lower abdominal pain that is sharp and sudden in onset. Signs include unilateral lower quadrant tenderness, a palpable adnexal mass, cervical tenderness, or rebound tenderness from peritonitis. Ultrasonography, including duplex scanning, is valuable in the detection of adnexal masses, particularly cysts. The abdominal pain from early ovarian cancer tends to be vague and diffuse. Patients may also complain of abdominal distention and urinary frequency. Abdominal sonography is highly sensitive at mass detection but is insufficiently accurate at distinguishing malignant from benign ovarian lesions.[12] Surgery may be required for confirming the diagnosis and for definitive therapy.

The differential of abdominal pain during pregnancy includes renal disorders. Symptoms from cystitis may include suprapubic discomfort, without frank abdominal pain, but patients usually have urinary frequency, urgency, or dysuria.[15] The diagnosis is made by urinalysis and urine culture in the appropriate clinical setting. Symptoms from acute pyelonephritis include pyrexia, chills, nausea, emesis, and flank pain. The pain may radiate to the abdomen or pelvis and cause costovertebral tenderness. Patients often have risk factors such as nephrolithiasis, recurrent lower urinary tract infection, diabetes mellitus, or congenital ureteral abnormalities.[8] The diagnosis is usually made by urine and blood cultures in the appropriate clinical setting. Renal ultrasound is performed in patients who fail to respond clinically within 3 days of instituting therapy or who have recurrent infection. The abdominal pain from urolithiasis typically radiates from the back or abdomen to the groin. Other symptoms include gross hematuria, nausea, emesis, urinary urgency, and urinary frequency.[16] Ultrasonography is the standard initial diagnostic test during pregnancy.[16]

Patients with sickle cell hemoglobinopathies, including hemoglobin SS, hemoglobin SC, and hemoglobin S/βthalassemia, are prone to sickle crises during pregnancy. The patients are usually black. The abdominal pain in sickle crisis can be excruciating.

Upper Gastrointestinal Symptoms

Nausea and Vomiting

Nausea and vomiting during pregnancy is most commonly due to hyperemesis gravidarum or nausea and vomiting of pregnancy, idiopathic disorders without demonstrable mucosal or mural disease. The differential of nausea and vomiting includes many other conditions (Table 43-4). Nausea and vomiting of pregnancy should be diagnosed only after exclusion of organic disorders by the history, physical findings, bloods tests, and appropriate diagnostic studies.

Dyspepsia or Pyrosis

The differential diagnosis of dyspepsia or pyrosis during pregnancy is listed in Table 43-5. During pregnancy, gastroesophageal reflux disease (GERD) is extremely common,[17] whereas peptic ulcer disease (PUD) is relatively uncommon. The diagnosis of GERD rather than PUD is suggested by pain radiating substernally, pain exacerbated by drinking acidic citrus drinks and by recumbency; symptoms of water brash or regurgitation; and the presence of extraintestinal manifestations, including nocturnal asthma, hoarseness, laryngitis, or periodontal disease.

Table 43-4. Differential Diagnosis of Nausea and Vomiting During Pregnancy

Nausea and vomiting of pregnancy
Hyperemesis gravidarum
Pancreatitis
Symptomatic cholelithiasis
Viral hepatitis
Peptic ulcer disease
Gastric cancer
Intestinal obstruction
Intestinal pseudoobstruction
Gastroparesis diabeticorum
Gastritis
Gastroesophageal reflux disease
Acute pyelonephritis
Drug toxicity
Vagotomy
Preeclampsia/eclampsia
Acute fatty liver of pregnancy
Hemolysis, elevated liver enzymes, and low platelets (HELLP) syndrome
Anorexia nervosa/bulimia
Other neuropsychiatric disorders

Table 43-5. Differential Diagnosis of Dyspepsia or Pyrosis During Pregnancy

Gastroesophageal reflux disease
Peptic ulcer disease
Nausea and vomiting of pregnancy
Hyperemesis gravidarum
Pancreatitis
Biliary colic
Acute cholecystitis
Viral hepatitis
Appendicitis
Acute fatty liver of pregnancy (in late pregnancy)
Irritable bowel syndrome/nonulcer dyspepsia

Hematemesis

Upper gastrointestinal bleeding is uncommon, but not rare, during pregnancy. The most common causes during pregnancy are GERD, gastritis, and ulcers.[18,19] Bleeding from a Mallory-Weiss tear may result from nausea and vomiting of pregnancy. Unusual causes of bleeding include esophageal varices, and gastric cancer. Patients with upper gastrointestinal bleeding that causes hemodynamic instability are approached like nonpregnant patients, with the following differences. In the general population the hematocrit is not a reliable indicator of bleeding severity because of the lag between blood loss and hematocrit decline. The hematocrit is an even less reliable indicator of bleeding severity during pregnancy because of the conflicting effects of intravascular fluid accumulation and increased erythrocyte mass during normal pregnancy. Maternal blood pressure is not a reliable indicator of fetal well-being. Fluid, including transfusions of packed erythrocytes when indicated, should be aggressively administered to pregnant patients with acute gastrointestinal bleeding because of the extraordinary fetal sensitivity to hypoperfusion, the difficulty in assessing volume status during pregnancy, and the usually satisfactory cardiac function of pregnant patients.

Dysphagia

The differential of dysphagia during pregnancy is similar to that in the general adult population, except that esophageal cancers are relatively rare in these patients because these cancers predominantly occur in the elderly. Pregnant patients with acquired immunodeficiency syndrome can have dysphagia or odynophagia from esophageal candidiasis or esophageal lymphoma. Dysphagia from a peptic stricture is uncommon in pregnant patients, despite their high frequency of GERD, because they typically have short term and uncomplicated GERD.

Definitive therapy for severe dysphagia is best performed before rather than during pregnancy to ensure adequate nutrition during pregnancy, a paramount concern for normal fetal development. Thus, surgery for severe achalasia or other benign esophageal diseases should be performed before a contemplated pregnancy.

Lower Gastrointestinal Symptoms

Diarrhea

The pathogenesis and differential diagnosis of diarrhea in pregnant women is similar to that in the nonpregnant population.[20] Acute diarrhea is usually caused by viral, bacterial, or parasitic enteropathogens. Viral agents, such as rotavirus and Norwalk virus, typically cause an acute self-limited diarrhea, with upper gastrointestinal symptoms, and rare long-term sequelae. Bacterial causes of diarrhea include Campylobacter, Shigella, pathogenic *Escherichia coli,* and Salmonella. Pseudomembranous colitis due to *Clostridium difficile* must be considered in the differential diagnosis when the diarrhea starts after antibiotic administration. Bacterial pathogens tend to produce frequent small-volume stools, abdominal pain, and pyrexia. Inflammation of intestinal mucosa may produce fecal blood or leukocytes. Bacterial colitis is usually diagnosed by stool analysis and stool cultures. Pregnant patients with advanced human immunodeficiency virus infection are prone to opportunistic enteric bacterial, fungal, parasitic, and viral infections, which often cause diarrhea. Noninfectious causes of diarrhea include medications, functional causes, food intolerances, and inflammatory bowel disease. Hyperthyroidism can cause hyperdefecation.

Constipation

Pregnancy tends to promote constipation from poor fluid intake due to nausea and vomiting; iron supplementation; decreased patient mobility; slowed gastrointestinal transit due to the effects of progesterone and estrogen; and gastrointestinal compression by the enlarged gravid uterus.[20] General measures can reverse these constipating factors during pregnancy. Adequate fluid intake and moderate exercise are important. Increased fiber intake—

either by increasing dietary fiber, such as wheat bran, or by administering medications, such as methylcellulose—is recommended to promote stool bulk and stool softness. Patients should be advised to defecate in the morning or after meals when colonic motor activity is stimulated through the gastrocolonic reflex. Sorbitol and lactulose, poorly absorbed sugars that cause an osmotic diarrhea, may be effective for constipation during pregnancy. However, they may cause abdominal bloating and flatulence; they should be used with caution in diabetic patients; and they should be avoided in pregnant patients with nausea because they can exacerbate this symptom. Stimulant laxatives, such as senna or bisacodyl, may be considered in patients with severe constipation who fail to respond to conservative measures, bulk laxatives, or osmotic laxatives. Laxatives to be avoided during pregnancy include castor oil because it may initiate premature uterine contractions, and hypertonic saline laxatives, such as phosphosoda, because they promote sodium and water retention, which is inadvisable during pregnancy.[20]

RED BLOOD PER RECTUM

Hemorrhoids are the most common cause of rectal bleeding during pregnancy. Other causes in the differential diagnosis of rectal bleeding during pregnancy include ulcerative colitis, Crohn's disease (CD), rectal fissure, and infectious colitis, as well as uncommon diagnoses during pregnancy, such as diverticular bleeding, ischemic bowel disease, and colon cancer.

DIAGNOSTIC TESTING DURING PREGNANCY

Radiologic Imaging

Fetal safety during diagnostic imaging is a concern for pregnant patients and pregnant medical personnel. Ultrasonography is considered safe during pregnancy and is the preferred imaging modality for abdominal pain during pregnancy.[12] Unfortunately, the test sensitivity depends on operator technique, patient cooperation, and patient anatomy, in that sensitivity is decreased by abdominal fat and intestinal gas.[12] MRI is preferable to computed tomography (CT) during pregnancy to avoid ionizing radiation, but gadolinium administration should be avoided during the first trimester.[21] Rapid-sequence MRI imaging is preferable to conventional MRI because of briefer exposure. The patient should undergo counseling before diagnostic roentgenography.

Data concerning fetal malformations, growth restriction, and mortality from ionizing radiation are derived from past experience, especially from Japanese atomic bomb survivors. Radiation can cause chromosomal mutations and neurologic abnormalities, including mental retardation, and moderately increases the risk of childhood leukemia.[22] Radiation dosage is the most important risk factor, but fetal age at exposure and proximity to the radiation source are also important factors. Fetal mortality is greatest from radiation exposure during the first week after conception, before oocyte implantation.[21,22] Exposure to more than 15 rads during the second and third trimesters or more than 5 rads during the first trimester, when the risk of neurologic malformations is greatest, should prompt consideration of elective termination of pregnancy.[21,22] Diagnostic studies with the most radiation exposure, such as intravenous pyelography or barium enema, typically expose the fetus to less than 1 rad.[21] Thus, one diagnostic fluoroscopic procedure is relatively safe in pregnancy. Fetal radiation exposure should be minimized by shielding, collimation, and rapid-sequence studies.

Endoscopy During Pregnancy

Endoscopy is often performed in the evaluation of abdominal symptoms in nonpregnant patients. Flexible sigmoidoscopy is performed to evaluate minor lower gastrointestinal complaints including rectal symptoms, whereas esophagogastroduodenoscopy (EGD) is performed to evaluate epigastric pain, dyspepsia, or pyrosis. Although endoscopy is extremely safe in the general population, endoscopy during pregnancy raises the unique issue of fetal safety. Endoscopy could potentially cause fetal complications from teratogenicity of medications, cardiac arrhythmias, systemic hypotension or hypertension, and transient hypoxia. Teratogenicity is of particular concern during the first trimester during organogenesis.

Sigmoidoscopy seems to be relatively safe during pregnancy. No woman suffered endoscopic complications in a study of 46 patients undergoing sigmoidoscopy during pregnancy.[23] Excluding one unknown pregnancy outcome and four voluntary abortions, 38 of 41 pregnant women delivered healthy infants, including 27 at full term. Their mean Apgar scores were not significantly different from the mean national Apgar scores. Moreover, study patients did not have a worse outcome than pregnant controls matched for sigmoidoscopy indications who did not undergo sigmoidoscopy, in terms of mean infant Apgar scores at birth and in terms of the rates of fetal or neonatal demise, premature delivery, low birth weight, and delivery by cesarean section. Additionally, no endoscopic complications were reported in 13 flexible sigmoidoscopies during pregnancy analyzed by a mailed survey of 3,300 gastroenterologists.[19] All pregnancies resulted in delivery of healthy infants at term.

These studies, in addition to scattered case reports, strongly suggest that sigmoidoscopy during pregnancy does not induce labor or cause adverse perinatal outcome, is not contraindicated, and should be strongly considered in medically stable patients with strong indications. Sigmoidoscopy is not recommended during pregnancy for routine cancer screening or surveillance, which can be deferred until at least 6 weeks postpartum. Sigmoidoscopy should be performed with maternal monitoring by electrocardiography, sphygmomanometry, and pulse oximetry, after obstetric consultation and medical stabilization. Analgesic medication should be minimized during sigmoidoscopy, especially during the first trimester. Colonoscopy is currently considered experimental during pregnancy owing to insufficient data but should be considered for extremely strong indications, such as suspected colon cancer, after obtaining informed consent that includes the theoretical but unsubstantiated fetal risks of colonoscopy.

EGD is relatively safe for the fetus and the pregnant mother. In a case-controlled study of 83 EGDs during pregnancy, the mean week of gestation was 20 weeks. Indications for EGD included gastrointestinal bleeding in 37, abdominal pain in 28, vomiting in 14, and other indications in four.[18] EGD did not cause any maternal complications. EGD did not induce labor. Excluding six voluntary abortions and three unknown pregnancy outcomes, 70 (95 percent) of 74 patients delivered healthy infants. In this study, the four poor pregnancy outcomes, including three stillbirths or deaths from severe prematurity and one involuntary abortion, occurred in high-risk pregnancies and were unrelated to EGD temporally or etiologically. No live-born infant had a congenital malformation noted in the neonatal nursery. The pregnancy outcome in study patients—including the mean Apgar scores at 1 and 5 minutes postpartum and the frequency of low birth weight, infant deaths, congenital defects, and delivery by cesarean section—was not statistically significantly different from the mean scores or rates in a group of 48 pregnant controls matched for EGD indications who did not undergo EGD because of the pregnancy. The two patient groups had similar pregnancy outcomes, even though the study patients generally were sicker and had a stronger indication for EGD than the controls. This study suggested that EGD is at least as safe as not performing EGD in pregnant patients with a strong indication for EGD. Similar results were reported in a study of 73 pregnant patients undergoing EGD, analyzed by a mailed survey of 3,300 gastroenterologists.[19]

EGD is recommended during pregnancy for hemodynamically significant upper gastrointestinal bleeding. EGD is rarely helpful and rarely necessary for nausea and vomiting, or even hyperemesis gravidarum, during pregnancy. EGD is reserved for atypical situations, such as severe and refractory nausea and vomiting accompanied by significant abdominal pain, hematemesis, or signs of gastroduodenal obstruction. EGD is neither necessary nor indicated to evaluate typical symptoms of gastroesophageal reflux during pregnancy. EGD should be reserved for cases when the presentation is atypical and severe, when the condition is refractory to intense pharmacologic therapy, when esophageal surgery is contemplated, and when complications such as gastrointestinal bleeding or dysphagia, supervene. EGD is useful in diagnosing complicated PUD, including gastric outlet obstruction, malignant gastric ulcer, refractory ulcer, and persistently bleeding ulcer. EGD should be performed in relatively stable patients with electrocardiographic monitoring after obstetric consultation and after normalization of vital signs, which may require transfusion of packed erythrocytes and supplemental oxygenation. Fetal monitoring should be performed, if available, once the fetal heart sounds become detectable. Informed consent is particularly important during pregnancy. The patient should be informed of the benefits and apparent safety of endoscopy, but the patient should be cautioned that the potential fetal risks are incompletely characterized.

Team Approach and Informed Consent

A team approach with consultation and referral helps optimize the management of complex diseases during pregnancy that affect both the mother and the fetus and that require disparate areas of expertise. The gastroenterologist contemplating endoscopy may consult with the obstetrician about the optimal procedure timing and with the anesthesiologist about analgesia during endoscopy. The internist may discuss with the radiologist the benefits versus risks of radiologic tests, and the radiologist may, in turn, consult with a physicist about methods to monitor and reduce fetal radiation exposure. The surgeon may consult with the obstetrician about the timing of abdominal surgery in relation to the pregnancy and about performing simultaneous cesarean delivery and abdominal surgery. These complex problems during pregnancy are best handled at a tertiary hospital, where the requisite experience and expertise is available.

The patient should be informed about the consequences for both herself and her fetus of diagnostic tests and therapy, and should be actively involved in medical decisions. The patient makes the decision, under the vigilant guidance of the medical experts, and with advice from her partner, family, and friends. When an intervention, such as roentgenographic tests, entails significant potential fetal risk, a signed, witnessed, and informed consent is recommended.

GASTROINTESTINAL DISORDERS

Predominantly Upper Gastrointestinal Disorders

Hyperemesis Gravidarum

Nausea and vomiting of pregnancy and hyperemesis gravidarum (HG) are diagnoses of exclusion. They should not be diagnosed until other conditions are excluded by appropriate tests. Patients with epigastric or right upper quadrant pain should undergo an abdominal ultrasound, serum tests of liver function, serum amylase, and serum lipase to exclude gallbladder and pancreatic disease. Patients with nausea and vomiting complicated by dysphagia or hematemesis may require EGD. Patients with nausea and vomiting during pregnancy associated with heartburn and regurgitation should be instructed about antireflux measures of diet and lifestyle modifications, and should receive mild antireflux medications, as described later.

HG occurs in about 0.5 percent of pregnancies.[24] Risk factors include primigravidas, multiple gestation, molar pregnancy, prior unsuccessful pregnancy, and prior HG.[25] HG typically begins early in pregnancy; severe vomiting beginning after the first trimester is unlikely to be due to HG. The pathophysiology is unknown but is believed to be multifactorial. Postulated etiologic factors include gestational hyperestrogenemia, gastric dysrhythmias, and hyperthyroidism.[24] Aside from nausea and vomiting, symptoms include xerostomia, sialorrhea, and dysgeusia. Despite the typical weight gain during a normal pregnancy, patients with HG lose more than 5 percent of their pregravid weight.[25] Complications from HG include inadequate caloric intake, nutritional deficiencies, dehydration, and electrolyte derangements. Physical findings reflective of hypovolemia include dry mucous membranes, poor skin turgor, and hypotension. Serum electrolyte abnormalities include hyponatremia, hypocalcemia, and hypokalemia. Ketonuria may occur. Chronic vomiting of gastric contents may cause a hypochloremic metabolic acidosis. Inadequate nutrition can lead to vitamin or micronutrient deficiencies.

The initial therapy is focused on aggressive intravenous rehydration and restoration of electrolyte deficiencies. Thiamine should be administered before administering dextrose to avoid Wernicke's encephalopathy. After intravenous repletion, the diet is gradually advanced, initially to salty fluids and then to a bland diet as tolerated. Nasoenteral or nasogastric feedings are useful alternatives in patients who do not tolerate oral feedings. TPN is rarely necessary for adequate nutrition. Experimental therapies for HG include ginger, methylprednisone, and erythromycin.

Nausea and vomiting of pregnancy is an exceedingly common mild condition that is diagnosed after exclusion of other causes of nausea and vomiting. It differs from HG by less severe symptoms, absence of weight loss, and lack of dehydration, vitamin deficiencies, or other nutritional deficiencies. Although previously called morning sickness, most patients experience symptoms throughout the day.[26] Nausea and vomiting was classically associated with a favorable pregnancy outcome, although it has been associated with possible physical and psychosocial disorders later in childhood after delivery, as well as psychological stress on the expectant mother.[27]

Patients with mild nausea during pregnancy typically require counseling and reassurance without treatment. Patients may benefit from a diet that emphasizes salty liquids, soups, starches, and chicken, and avoids fatty foods, vegetables, and fibrous foods.[24] Bendectin (doxylamine-vitamin B_6) was commonly administered for nausea and vomiting of pregnancy, but was withdrawn in 1983 because of unproven allegations of teratogenicity.[24] Several of the individual components of Bendectin, such as vitamin B_6 (pyridoxine), have been used to treat this condition with some success.[28] A delayed release form of doxylamine-pyridoxine (Diclectin) is currently approved in Canada for the treatment of nausea and vomiting of pregnancy.

Gastroesophageal Reflux and Peptic Ulcer Disease

Gastroesophageal reflux disease (GERD) is manifested by pyrosis, regurgitation, water brash, dyspepsia, hypersalivation, or rarely, pulmonary symptoms. The incidence of pyrosis approaches 80 perecent during pregnancy.[5] The incidence of GERD is likewise high during pregnancy.[29] This high incidence may relate to a hypotonic lower esophageal sphincter (LES) and gastrointestinal dysmotility, attributed to gestational hormones, and to gastric compression by the gravid uterus.

Symptomatic PUD is uncommon during pregnancy, and antecedent PUD often improves during pregnancy.[30] Nausea, emesis, dyspepsia, and anorexia are so frequent during pregnancy that it may be difficult to diagnose PUD when these symptoms occur.[31] Nonsteroidal anti-inflammatory drugs (NSAIDs), including aspirin, can cause gastric or intestinal ulceration. These ulcers more commonly cause gastrointestinal bleeding than abdominal pain, possibly because of the analgesic properties of NSAIDs.[32]

Although the efficacy of modern acid-suppressive drugs has rendered life style modifications less important in the nonpregnant patient with PUD, these modifications remain important in the pregnant patient because of concern about drug teratogenicity.[31,33] Pregnant patients with PUD should avoid caffeine, alcohol, and NSAIDs, although acetaminophen is safe and the cyclo-oxygenase II inhibitors are less gastrotoxic than the nonselective NSAIDs.[32] Patients with GERD should keep the head of the bed elevated at night. They should avoid wearing tight belts, recumbency after eating, drinking caffeinated or alcoholic beverages, eating chocolate or fatty foods, taking NSAIDs, and smoking tobacco. Antacids are generally safe for the fetus, but those containing magnesium should be avoided near delivery because they can retard labor and possibly cause neurologic depression in the newborn, and those containing sodium bicarbonate should be avoided throughout pregnancy because they may cause fluid overload or metabolic alkalosis.[34] Antacids and dietary measures often suffice during the first trimester for minimally symptomatic disease.[2] Antacids must be administered frequently because of low potency, and frequent administration can cause diarrhea or constipation and electrolyte or mineral abnormalities. Sucralfate has minimal systemic absorption, but its aluminum content is of concern to the fetus in mothers with renal insufficiency.[35] Misoprostol is an abortifacient and is contraindicated during pregnancy.[3] Histamine$_2$ receptor antagonists are useful in treating GERD and PUD when symptoms are more severe or occur later in pregnancy.[2,35] Ranitidine and famotidine are preferable because nizatidine is possibly toxic to the fetus,[36] and cimetidine has antiandrogenic effects.[37] Proton-pump inhibitors were initially reserved for refractory, severe, or complicated GERD and PUD during pregnancy but have recently been increasingly used due to accumulating evidence of relative fetal safety. Lansoprazole, rabeprazole, and pantoprazole (Food and Drug Administration [FDA] pregnancy category B) appear to be safer than omeprazole (FDA category C), and are therefore recommended during pregnancy.[38,39] Metoclopamide is probably not teratogenic, but frequently causes maternal side effects. *Helicobacter pylori* eradication should be deferred until after parturition and lactation because of concern about the fetal safety of administered antibiotics such as clarithromycin and metronidazole.[40]

Surgery for GERD is best performed either before or after pregnancy.[2,35] EGD is the initial intervention for bleeding from GERD or PUD,[30,41] but a hemodynamically unstable patient refractory to endoscopic therapy requires expeditious surgery, because the fetus poorly tolerates maternal hypotension.[42,43] Pregnant PUD patients may also require surgery for gastric outlet obstruction, refractory ulcer, or malignant ulcer.[44] Patients in advanced pregnancy should undergo cesarean delivery just before gastric surgery for gastrointestinal bleeding.[42,43]

DIAPHRAGMATIC HERNIA

A congenital or traumatic diaphragmatic hernia is a potentially catastrophic event during pregnancy, with both maternal and fetal mortality rates from strangulation exceeding 40 percent.[45] The increased intraabdominal pressure from the enlarged gravid uterus increases the risk of strangulation. Herniorrhaphy is recommended during the first 2 trimesters, even for asymptomatic hernias incidentally discovered at surgery.[45,46] Expectant management is recommended for asymptomatic patients during the third trimester, with cesarean delivery and herniorrhaphy performed when the fetus is sufficiently mature. Cesarean delivery is performed to avoid increased abdominal pressure during active labor, which can cause bowel strangulation.[46]

Predominantly Lower Gastrointestinal Disorders

ACUTE APPENDICITIS

Acute appendicitis is the most common nonobstetric surgical emergency during pregnancy, with an incidence of about 1 per 1,000 pregnancies.[6,47] Appendiceal obstruction, usually from an appendicolith, is the primary pathophysiologic event, although stasis and other factors are also implicated. As the appendiceal lumen distends, the patient initially experiences poorly localized pain. Severe luminal distention, mural inflammation and edema, and bacterial translocation produce somatic pain that becomes severe and well localized at McBurney's point in the right lower quadrant. Displacement of the appendix by the gravid uterus during late pregnancy may cause the point of maximal abdominal pain and tenderness to migrate superiorly and laterally from McBurney's point.[5] Rectal or pelvic tenderness may occur in early pregnancy but is unusual in late pregnancy because the appendix migrates from its pelvic location. Other clinical findings include anorexia, nausea, emesis, pyrexia, tachycardia, and abdominal tenderness.[48] Periappendiceal inflammation or peritonitis causes involuntary guarding and rebound tenderness. Involuntary guarding and rebound tenderness are less reliable signs of peritonitis in late pregnancy because of abdominal wall laxity.[6] Patients may have significant leukocytosis and a predominance of neutrophils in the leukocyte differential.[49]

The diagnosis is made clinically without overreliance on radiologic imaging. Sonography may demonstrate appendiceal mural thickening and periappendiceal fluid, but the sonographic findings are usually nonspecific and mostly help to exclude other pathology, such as an adnexal mass.[12] CT is more accurate but exposes the fetus to radiation.

The diagnosis may be missed in pregnant patients because (1) leukocytosis, a classic sign of acute appendicitis, occurs physiologically during pregnancy; (2) nausea and emesis, common symptoms of acute appendicitis, are also common during pregnancy; and (3) the abdominal pain is sometimes atypically located.[49] Other diseases are often confused with appendicitis. The differential diagnosis of appendicitis in pregnancy is shown in Table 43-6.

Up to one quarter of pregnant women with appendicitis develop appendiceal perforation.[5] Appendiceal displacement predisposes to rapid development of generalized peritonitis after perforation because the omentum is not nearby to contain the infection.

Appendicitis during pregnancy mandates surgery, after intravenous hydration and correction of electrolyte abnormalities. Antibiotics are usually administered for uncomplicated appendicitis and are absolutely required for appendicitis complicated by perforation, abscess, or peritonitis.[5] Penicillins (including ampicillin/sulbactam), cephalosporins, clindamycin, and gentamicin are considered safe during pregnancy.[5] Quinolones are not recom-

Table 43-6. Differential Diagnosis of Appendicitis During Pregnancy

Gynecologic conditions
Ruptured ovarian cyst
Adnexal torsion
Pelvic inflammatory disease or salpingitis
Endometriosis
Ovarian cancer
Obstetric causes
Abruptio placenta
Chorioamnionitis
Endometritis
Uterine fibroid degeneration
Labor (preterm or term)
Viscus perforation after abortion
Ruptured ectopic pregnancy
Gastrointestinal causes
Crohn's disease
Colonic diverticulitis (right side)
Cholecystitis
Pancreatitis
Mesenteric lymphadenitis
Gastroenteritis
Colon cancer
Intestinal obstruction
Hernia (incarcerated inguinal or internal)
Colonic intussusception
Ruptured Meckel's diverticulum
Colonic perforation
Acute mesenteric ischemia
Other causes
Pyelonephritis
Urolithiasis

mended. Clindamycin is preferred to metronidazole for anaerobic coverage, even though both are category B drugs in pregnancy.[40] Clindamycin and gentamicin is a relatively inexpensive, effective, and safe antibiotic combination. Laparoscopy may be considered during the first two trimesters for nonperforated appendicitis or when the diagnosis is uncertain[50] (see Chapter 23). Appendectomy is recommended even if appendicitis is not evident at surgery.[48,49] The maternal mortality rate from appendicitis is about 0.1 percent without perforation but exceeds 4 percent with perforation.[47] The fetal mortality rate is approximately 2 percent without perforation but exceeds 30 percent with perforation.[47]

Intestinal Obstruction

Acute intestinal obstruction is the second most common nonobstetric abdominal emergency, with an incidence of 1 per 1,500 pregnancies.[51,52] It may be incidental or secondary to pregnancy. The obstruction most commonly occurs in the third trimester because of the mechanical effects of the enlarged gravid uterus.[53] In particular, some cases occur at term because of the mechanical effects of fetal head descent and of the abrupt decrease in uterine size at delivery.[51,52] Adhesions, particularly from prior gynecologic surgery or appendectomy, cause 60 to 70 percent of small bowel obstruction (SBO) during pregnancy.[52,54] Other causes of SBO include neoplasms, particularly ovarian, endometrial, or cervical malignancy; CD; external or internal hernias; volvulus; intussusception; EP; prior radiotherapy; and intraluminal gallstones, fecoliths, or other concretions.[51,52] Colonic obstruction is caused by adhesions, colon cancer, other neoplasms, diverticulitis, and volvulus.[51,52]

Intestinal obstruction classically presents with a symptomatic triad of abdominal pain, emesis, and obstipation.[51,52] The pain may be constant or periodic. Small bowel obstruction is more painful than colonic obstruction. The pain with SBO may be diffuse and poorly localized, and may radiate to the back, flanks, or perineum.[55] Abdominal pain is milder with volvulus and intussusception. Intestinal malrotation may produce nonspecific symptoms of mild, crampy, abdominal pain and nonbilious emesis.[56] Intestinal strangulation may be heralded by guarding and rebound tenderness. Emesis occurs more frequently and earlier in small bowel than colonic obstruction.[51,52] Constipation from complete intestinal obstruction is usually severe and unremitting, and is associated with abdominal pain.[52] The abdomen is typically distended and tympanitic to percussion. Bowel sounds are high pitched, hypoactive, and tinkling in early intestinal obstruction and are absent in late obstruction.

The approach to intestinal obstruction is the same in pregnancy as in the general population except that the decisions are more urgently required because both the fetus and the maternal intestine are at risk. Fetal exposure to radiation is a concern, but supine and upright radiographs are needed to diagnose and monitor intestinal obstruction.[52] Volvulus is suspected when a single bowel loop is grossly dilated. Surgery is recommended for unremitting and complete intestinal obstruction, whereas medical management is advisable for intermittent or partial obstruction.[51] Parenteral fluids are aggressively administered to reverse the fluid and electrolyte deficits caused by emesis and fluid sequestration. Nasogastric suction helps decompress the bowel. Morbidity and mortality from intestinal obstruction are related to diagnostic delays. The maternal mortality rate is typically less than 6 percent, whereas the fetal mortality ranges from 20 to 30 percent.[51,54]

Intestinal Pseudoobstruction

Intestinal pseudoobstruction (adynamic ileus) is characterized by severe abdominal distention detected on physical examination and diffuse intestinal dilatation noted on abdominal roentgenogram. Intestinal pseudoobstruction is diagnosed only after exclusion of (mechanical) intestinal obstruction by the clinical presentation, laboratory studies, and early clinical evolution. Patients with mechanical obstruction tend to be much sicker than those with pseudoobstruction for the degree of intestinal dilatation detected by abdominal imaging and tend to progress more rapidly. Intestinal pseudoobstruction is a well-described but uncommon complication of cesarean section or vaginal delivery.[57,58] Patients with pseudoobstruction have nausea, emesis, obstipation, and diffuse abdominal pain that typically develops over several days.[57] Patients often have hypoperistalsis. Pyrexia, leukocytosis, and increasing abdominal tenderness may herald gastrointestinal ischemia. Treatment includes nasogastric aspiration, parenteral fluid administration, electrolyte repletion, and rectal tube decompression. The pseudoobstruction usually spontaneously resolves.[57] Therapeutic options for severe colonic dilatation, manifested by a colonic luminal diameter greater than 10 cm on abdominal roentgenogram, include colonoscopic decompression; or surgical therapies including cecostomy, cecectomy with diverting ileostomy, or colonic resection when intestinal necrosis supervenes.[59] Parenteral neostigmine is often administered in nonpregnant patients but is contraindicated during pregnancy.[57] The mortality rate approaches 10 percent with impending perforation but reaches 70 percent after cecal perforation.[59]

Colon Cancer

Colon cancer is uncommon during pregnancy, with an estimated incidence of 1 per 13,000 to 1 per 50,000 pregnancies.[4,60] With approximately 4 million pregnancies per annum in the United States, these incidence estimates translate into 80 to 300 colon cancers during pregnancy per annum in the United States.

The clinical presentation and evaluation of colon cancer in pregnant patients is similar to that in other patients, with notable exceptions. Common symptoms of colon cancer in pregnant patients include abdominal pain, rectal bleeding, nausea and vomiting, and abdominal distention.[4,61] Colon cancer tends not to produce signs until advanced. Rectal examination is essential in the evaluation of suspected colon cancer during pregnancy.

The cancer often arises in the rectum during pregnancy and may be palpable by digital rectal examination. Stool should be tested for the presence of occult blood, even though the finding of occult blood has a low positive predictive value for colon cancer or adenomas during pregnancy because of the low disease prevalence in this rather young patient population. Iron deficiency anemia is common during pregnancy owing to increased gestational demands. Iron deficiency anemia, therefore, is not nearly as strongly associated with colon cancer in the pregnant patient as it is in the elderly patient.[4] About one fifth of colon cancers occur in the rectum in the general population, whereas about two thirds of colon cancers occur in the rectum during pregnancy.[62] The predominance of rectal cancer during pregnancy may artifactually result from increased self-referral owing to increased patient attention to rectal symptoms because of rectal compression by the gravid uterus or from increased physician detection due to frequent pelvic and rectal examinations during pregnancy.[1]

During pregnancy colon cancer often presents at an advanced pathologic stage attributed to delayed diagnosis.[62] Advanced pathologic stage is highly correlated with a poor prognosis. The incidence of ovarian metastases in women is only about 5 percent, but rises to about 25 percent in women younger than 40 years old.[63] Pregnant patients are typically younger than 40 years old and seem to have a similarly high incidence of ovarian metastases.[4] Although abdominal CT is the imaging modality of choice for detection of hepatic metastases from colon cancer in the general population, CT is relatively contraindicated during pregnancy and abdominal ultrasound is substituted for hepatic evaluation during pregnancy. This test is highly sensitive for metastatic lesions greater than 2 cm in diameter, but is poorly sensitive for metastatic lesions smaller than 1 cm in diameter. Hepatic metastases typically produce discrete echogenic masses. Complete colonoscopy is indicated preoperatively in nonpregnant patients for pathologic diagnosis and for excluding synchronous colonic lesions. Colonoscopy during pregnancy is currently experimental, but partial colonoscopy may be necessary before colon cancer surgery to obtain a pathologic diagnosis and to exclude synchronous lesions. Colonoscopy may be technically difficult during late pregnancy because of colonic compression by the enlarged gravid uterus. If the gestation is advanced, and the fetus is viable, it may be preferable to proceed with delivery and then perform colonoscopy and cancer surgery.

Surgery is the primary curative therapy for colon cancer. In the absence of distant metastases, the primary tumor is resected with wide surgical margins that are at least 5 cm beyond the edge of gross tumor together with resection of regional mesenteric lymph nodes. In the presence of widespread distant metastases, only palliative surgery is considered. The timing and type of surgery during pregnancy depends on gestational age, maternal cancer prognosis, and intraoperative findings, as well as maternal desires. When the cancer is diagnosed during the first half of pregnancy, cancer surgery should be promptly performed to minimize the risk of metastases.[4] Such surgery can often be performed without removing the gravid uterus and disturbing the pregnancy.[62] Total abdominal hysterectomy is recommended to facilitate access to the rectum when needed for intraoperative exposure; when the mother's life expectancy is less than the time needed for the fetus to become viable; or when the cancer extends into the uterus. Otherwise, when the cancer appears resectable, curative surgery should be performed, leaving the pregnancy intact.[4] When the cancer is diagnosed during the second half of pregnancy, cancer surgery should ideally be delayed until, but not beyond, the time that fetal viability is normally expected because further delay permits cancer growth and metastasis.[61] Bilateral salpingo-oophorectomy is indicated for ovarian metastases. Colon cancer surgery is associated with a moderately increased, but still acceptable, rate of fetal death, but it is associated with a high risk of preterm delivery and low birth weight.[64]

Pregnant patients considering adjuvant chemotherapy should be counseled about the potential fetal risks as well as the potential maternal benefits. Chemotherapy is generally contraindicated during the first trimester and should be strictly restricted during this trimester to patients with Dukes stage C cancer who accept a significant teratogenic risk after informed and written consent. Chemotherapy is much less teratogenic during the second and third trimesters, after organogenesis is completed. Patients who refused preoperative chemotherapy during the first trimester because of fetal teratogenicity should consider receiving postoperative chemotherapy during the second trimester when the risk of teratogenicity is much less. Although pelvic radiotherapy is often performed for rectal cancer with local extramural extension, this therapy is perilous to the fetus, and it is contraindicated during pregnancy. Radiotherapy is possible only after delivery or termination of pregnancy.

Patients younger than 40 years old generally have a poor prognosis from colon cancer, attributed to a delayed diagnosis and an advanced pathologic stage at diagnosis.[65] Likewise, the maternal prognosis from colon cancer, whether colonic or rectal, diagnosed during pregnancy is poor. Fetal prognosis depends on the pathologic stage of the maternal cancer, gestational age at diagnosis, and type and timing of therapy. Fetal viability is endangered by severe maternal debility and malnourishment from advanced cancer because the fetus depends on maternal homeostasis and nutrition for normal development. A few healthy infants have been born after colorectal surgery, including abdominoperineal resection, early in pregnancy.[4] When the cancer is diagnosed late in pregnancy, the fetus is less affected by maternal illness because it can be delivered. The overall fetal prognosis from maternal colon cancer is generally relatively favorable because the colon cancer is usually diagnosed near term. Infant survival is about 80 percent.[4] Live-born infants are, however, often born prematurely and often have a low birth weight, factors associated with an increased risk of pulmonary complications and subsequent neurodevelopmental handicaps.

Exciting novel diagnostic modalities for colon cancer diagnosis with promising applications in pregnancy include capsule endoscopy in which the colon may be imaged by a microcamera placed within a pill-sized device swallowed by the patient, and a large array of genetic markers to detect genetic abnormalities associated with colon cancer in minute quantities of DNA in stool shed from colonic mucosa.[66]

Inflammatory Bowel Disease

The inflammatory bowel diseases (IBD), including ulcerative colitis (UC) and CD, are idiopathic, immunologically mediated disorders that peak in incidence during a woman's reproductive period. The incidence of UC in women younger than 40 years of age is 40 to 100 per 100,000 and of CD is 2 to 4 per 100,000.[5] Ulcerative colitis is a colonic disease manifested by bloody diarrhea, crampy abdominal pain, and pyrexia. CD can involve any part of the gastrointestinal tract but most commonly involves the terminal ileum. It is characterized by diarrhea, abdominal pain, anorexia, pyrexia, and malnutrition. Patients with CD may have fistulas and anorectal disease. Extraintestinal manifestations of IBD include arthritis, uveitis, sclerosing cholangitis, and cutaneous lesions.

Ulcerative colitis does not significantly affect fertility.[67] CD, however, decreases fertility because of extension of ileal inflammation to the nearby oviducts or ovaries and the systemic effects of malnutrition.[68] Inflammatory bowel disease activity is mostly independent of pregnancy. Patients with inactive or mild disease before conception tend to have the same disease activity during pregnancy. Active disease at conception increases the likelihood of active disease during pregnancy and of a poor pregnancy outcome, including spontaneous abortion, miscarriage, or stillbirth.[69,70] The onset of CD, and to a lesser extent UC, during pregnancy is associated with increased fetal loss.[70] Fetal growth may be impaired in active CD because of maternal malabsorption and malnutrition.

Differentiating the signs and symptoms of IBD from physiologic changes related to pregnancy or from other obstetric, gynecologic, or surgical conditions may be difficult. Nausea, emesis, abdominal discomfort, and constipation may be noted during any pregnancy but may also signal a flare of IBD. The differential diagnosis of acute right lower quadrant abdominal pain in a pregnant woman with CD includes disease exacerbation, EP, appendicitis, or adnexal disease. Pyrexia, bloody diarrhea, and weight loss suggest CD exacerbation.

The diagnostic evaluation is influenced by the pregnancy, but indicated tests should be performed. Laboratory evaluation includes a hemogram, serum chemistry profile, and electrolyte determinations, taking into account the physiologic alterations of late pregnancy including anemia, leukocytosis, and hypoalbuminemia. Flexible sigmoidoscopy is well tolerated during pregnancy without maternal complications or fetal toxicity,[41] but diagnostic roentgenographic tests are best deferred until after delivery.[69]

The beneficial effects of IBD therapy on the mother and the pregnancy must be weighed against the potential of fetal toxicity and teratogenicity (Table 43-7). Active disease poses greater risk to the fetus than most therapies.[71] Sulfasalazine, 5-aminosalicylates, and corticosteroids seem to be safe,[67,69] but methotrexate is not.[72] Azathioprine or 6-mercaptopurine can be continued during pregnancy to maintain remission.[69,73] These drugs appear to be safe during pregnancy. Metronidazole is probably best avoided during the first trimester.[74] Diphenoxylate should be avoided.[5] Emergency surgery for toxic megacolon, intestinal obstruction, or massive bleeding should be done expeditiously, whereas elective surgery, such as fistulectomy, should be performed during the second trimester or postpartum.[70,75] Severe perianal CD may necessitate cesarean delivery, because an episiotomy during vaginal delivery can exacerbate perianal disease.[76]

Hemorrhoids

Hemorrhoids are common in adults and are particularly common during pregnancy. Contributing factors during pregnancy include increased constipation, resulting in

Table 43-7. Pharmacologic Therapy for Inflammatory Bowel Disease During Pregnancy

DRUG	FDA CATEGORY DURING PREGNANCY	RECOMMENDATION DURING PREGNANCY
Sulfasalazine	B	Relatively safe. Concern about sulfa moiety causing neonatal jaundice.
Mesalamine	B	Relatively safe.
Remicaide (anti-TNF)	B	Not teratogenic in mice exposed to an analogous antibody. Insufficient clinical data.
Loperamide	B	Relatively safe.
Metronidazole	B	Avoid if possible since carcinogenic in rodents.
Corticosteroids	C	Relatively safe. Concern regarding fetal adrenal function and maternal hyperglycemia. Monitor the neonates of mothers who received substantial doses of corticosteroids during pregnancy.
Ciprofloxacin	C	Use with caution, small studies show no significant risk during pregnancy.
Diphenoxylate	C	Avoid, possible teratogen.
Cyclosporine	C	Embryotoxic and fetotoxic at very high doses in rats and rabbits.
6-mercaptopurine	D	Avoid starting after conception. Might cause IUGR.
Azathioprine	D	Avoid starting after conception. Might cause IUGR. Teratogenic in laboratory animals.
Methotrexate	X	Contraindicated. Teratogen and abortifacient.

FDA, Food and Drug Administration; IUGR, intrauterine growth retardation.

increased straining at defecation; gestational increases in the circulating blood volume, resulting in venous dilatation and engorgement; and vascular compression from the enlarging gravid uterus resulting in venous stasis.[20] Hemorrhoids above the dentate line are internal, whereas those below the dentate line are external.

Hemorrhoids characteristically produce a clinical triad of very bright red blood per rectum, resembling the color of arterial blood; blood coating rather than admixed with stool; and postdefecatory bleeding, most commonly noted on the toilet paper.[77] Other clinical manifestations include anorectal discomfort, pruritus, or pain associated with prolapse, thrombosis, or incarceration of hemorrhoids.

When the pain from external hemorrhoids is mild to moderate, conservative treatment including stool softeners, mild analgesics, and warm sitz baths are recommended.[20] Surgical excision under local anesthesia can be performed safely during pregnancy for severely painful or acutely thrombosed external hemorrhoids. General measures for internal hemorrhoids include fiber supplements, fluids, and a high-fiber diet to decrease constipation; switching to a slow-release iron supplement to mitigate the constipating effects of iron; topical local anesthetics for rectoanal discomfort; and skin protectants applied after defecation to reduce anal pruritus.[20] Therapies for severe or refractory symptoms from internal hemorrhoids include band ligation, injection, sclerotherapy, and coagulation. These therapies are generally safe and effective during pregnancy.[78]

Mesenteric Ischemia and Infarction

Bowel infarction can occur during pregnancy secondary to intestinal obstruction or mesenteric venous thrombosis.[79] Digoxin, ergot alkaloids, cocaine, and other vasoconstrictors are also associated with mesenteric ischemia.[81] Patients with mesenteric venous thrombosis typically have an insidious onset of poorly localized abdominal pain, with a relatively unremarkable physical examination.[80] The thrombosis is diagnosed by the noninvasive modalities of MR imaging or CT scanning, and by the invasive modality of the venous phase of angiography. Hematologic evaluation for hypercoagulopathy is recommended.[79]

Irritable Bowel Syndrome

The irritable bowel syndrome (IBS) is most common in younger women. The pathogenesis is poorly defined. Both intestinal motor and sensory abnormalities, particularly hyperalgesia, have been described.[82] IBS is diagnosed, according to the Rome II criteria, by the presence of both abdominal pain and disordered defecation for at least 3 months, not necessarily continuous, during the past year in the absence of demonstrable organic disease.[83] Endoscopic, radiologic, and histologic intestinal studies reveal no evident organic disease. Young women typically have diarrhea-predominant IBS but sometimes have predominantly constipation or alternating diarrhea and constipation. Abdominal bloating and distention are common symptoms.

Little data exist concerning the effect of pregnancy on IBS.[84] Gestational hormones, particularly progesterone, may exacerbate the symptoms of IBS.[85] Presumed IBS in the absence of warning signs or symptoms, such as rectal bleeding, should not require invasive tests, such as sigmoidoscopy, during pregnancy. Contrariwise, signs and symptoms of organic disease, such as rectal bleeding or involuntary weight loss, should not be attributed to IBS without proper evaluation. In particular, sigmoidoscopy is indicated for nonhemorrhoidal rectal bleeding during pregnancy.[23] IBS is best treated during pregnancy by dietary modification and behavioral therapy for severe symptoms rather than by systemic drugs.[86] Patients with diarrhea-predominant IBS may benefit from elimination of foods from the diet that precipitate diarrhea, such as alcohol, caffeinated beverages, poorly digestible sugars, and fatty foods. Pregnant patients usually require a large amount of dairy products in their diet to ensure adequate calcium intake. Patients may benefit from lactase supplements when ingesting dairy products. Dietary fiber and fluid ingestion may improve constipation-predominant IBS. IBS is not believed to affect fertility and pregnancy outcome in the absence of nutritional deficiencies or concomitant disorders.[84]

Splenic Artery Aneurysm Rupture

Splenic artery aneurysm rupture is associated with pregnancy, possibly because of the effects of gestational hormones on the elastic properties of the arterial wall. Patients present in shock with left upper quadrant abdominal pain. The diagnosis is suggested by demonstration of a rim of calcification from the aneurysm on plain abdominal roentgenogram and is confirmed by abdominal CT scanning or angiography. Treatment consists of fluid resuscitation and prompt surgery, with hemostasis and possible splenectomy. The maternal mortality rate exceeds 75 percent, and the fetal mortality exceeds 90 percent.[87] Splenic artery aneurysms should therefore be surgically corrected even if asymptomatic.[87,88] Abdominal aortic and renal aneurysms can also rupture during pregnancy.

SUMMARY

The differential diagnosis of abdominal symptoms and signs is particularly extensive in pregnancy. The differential includes gastrointestinal, obstetric, gynecologic, and other disorders, that are related or unrelated to the pregnancy. The patient history, physical examination, laboratory data, and radiologic findings usually provide the diagnosis of abdominal disorders during pregnancy. The pregnant woman has physiologic alterations that affect the clinical presentation, including atypical normative laboratory values. Abdominal ultrasound is generally the recommended radiologic imaging modality; roentgenograms are generally contraindicated during pregnancy because of radiation teratogenicity. Flexible sigmoidoscopy and EGD can be performed during pregnancy when strongly indicated. Concerns about the fetus limit the pharmacotherapy during pregnancy. Maternal and fetal survival have recently improved for many life-threatening gastrointestinal conditions, such as appendicitis, because of improved diagnostic technology, better maternal and fetal monitoring, improved laparoscopic technology, and earlier and better therapy.

KEY POINTS

- The differential diagnosis of gastrointestinal symptoms and signs, such as abdominal pain, is particularly extensive during pregnancy. Aside from gastrointestinal and other intraabdominal disorders incidental to pregnancy, the differential diagnosis includes obstetric, gynecologic, and gastrointestinal disorders related to pregnancy.

- Pregnancy can affect the clinical presentation, frequency, or severity of gastrointestinal diseases. For example, GERD markedly increases in frequency, whereas PUD markedly decreases in frequency (or becomes inactive) during pregnancy.

- Abdominal ultrasound is the most useful abdominal imaging modality to evaluate gastrointestinal conditions during pregnancy. Other imaging modalities, such as CT, may raise concerns about fetal safety.

- EGD and flexible sigmoidoscopy can be performed when strongly indicated during pregnancy, for example, for significant acute upper and lower gastrointestinal bleeding, respectively.

- Most gastrointestinal drugs appear to be relatively safe to the fetus and can be used with caution when strongly indicated during pregnancy, especially during the second and third trimesters after organogenesis has occurred (FDA category B and C). Gastrointestinal drugs to be avoided during pregnancy include misoprostol, which is an abortifacient (category X), methotrexate (category X), 6-mercaptopurine (category D), azathioprine (category D), most chemotherapeutic agents, and certain antibiotics.

REFERENCES

1. Powers RD, Guertter AT: Abdominal pain in the ED (emergency department): stability and change over 20 years. Am J Emerg Med 13:301, 1995.
2. Broussard CN, Richter JE: Treating gastro-esophageal reflux disease during pregnancy and lactation: what are the safest therapy options. Drug Saf 19:325, 1998.
3. Costa SH, Vessey MP: Misoprostol and illegal abortion in Rio de Janeiro, Brazil. Lancet 341:1258, 1993.
4. Cappell MS: Colon cancer during pregnancy. Gastroenterol Clin North Am 32:341, 2003.
5. Cappell MS, Friedel D: Abdominal pain during pregnancy. Gastroenterol Clin North Am 32:1, 2003.
6. Tracey M, Fletcher HS: Appendicitis in pregnancy. Am Surg 66:555, 2000.
7. Puskar D, Balagovic I, Filipovic A, et al: Symptomatic physiologic hydronephrosis in pregnancy: incidence, complications and treatment. Eur Urol 39:260, 2001.
8. Petersson C, Hedges S, Stenqvist K, et al: Suppressed antibody and interleukin-6 responses to acute pyelonephritis in pregnancy. Kidney Int 45:571, 1994.
9. Martin C, Varner MW: Physiologic changes in pregnancy: surgical implications. Clin Obstet Gynecol 37:241, 1994.
10. Van den Broe NR, Letsky EA: Pregnancy and the erythrocyte sedimentation rate. Br J Obstet Gynaecol 108:1164, 2001.
11. Wong E, Suat SO: Ectopic pregnancy: a diagnostic challenge in the emergency department. Eur J Emerg Med 7:189, 2000.
12. Derchi LE, Serafini G. Gandolfo N, et al: Ultrasound in gynecology. Eur Radiol 11:2137, 2001.
13. Blanchard AC, Pastorek II JG, Weeks T: Pelvic inflammatory disease during pregnancy. South Med J 80:1363, 1987.
14. Friedler S, Ben-Shachar I, Abramov Y, et al: Ruptured tubo-ovarian abscess complicating transcervical cryopreserved embryo transfer. Fertil Steril 65:1065, 1996.
15. Millar LK, Cox SM: Urinary tract infections complicating pregnancy. Infect Dis Clin North Am 11:13, 1997.
16. Evans HJ, Wollin TA: The management of urinary calculi in pregnancy. Curr Opin Urol 11:379, 2001.
17. Marrero JM, Goggin PM, de Caestecker JS, et al: Determinants of pregnancy heartburn. Br J Obstet Gynaecol 99:731, 1992.
18. Cappell MS, Colon VJ, Sidhom OA: A study at eight medical centers of the safety and clinical efficacy of esophagogastroduodenoscopy in 83 pregnant females with follow-up of fetal outcome and with comparison to control groups. Am J Gastroenterol 91:348, 1996.
19. Frank B: Endoscopy in pregnancy. *In* Karlstadt RG, Surawicz CM, Croitoru R (eds): Gastrointestinal disorders during pregnancy. Arlington, VA, American College of Gastroenterology, 1994, p 24.
20. Wald A: Constipation, diarrhea, and symptomatic hemorrhoids during pregnancy. Gastroenterol Clin North Am 32:309, 2003.
21. Karam PA: Determining and reporting fetal radiation exposure from diagnostic radiation. Health Phys 79(Suppl 5):S85, 2000.
22. Toppenberg KS, Hill DA, Miller DP: Safety of radiographic imaging during pregnancy. Am Fam Physician 59:1813, 1999.
23. Cappell MS, Colon VJ, Sidhom OA: A study at 10 medical centers of the safety and efficacy of 48 flexible sigmoidoscopies and 8 colonoscopies during pregnancy with followup of fetal outcome and with comparison to control groups. Dig Dis Sci 41:2353, 1996.
24. Koch KL, Frissora CL: Nausea and vomiting during pregnancy. Gastroenterol Clin North Am 32:201, 2003.
25. Hamaoui E, Hamaoui M: Nutritional assessment and support during pregnancy. Gastroenterol Clin North Am 32:59, 2003.
26. Lacroix R, Eason E, Melzack R: Nausea and vomiting during pregnancy: A prospective study of its frequency, intensity, and patterns of change. Am J Obstet Gynecol 182:931, 2000.
27. Martin RP, Wisenbaker J, Huttunen MO: Nausea during pregnancy: relation to early childhood temperament and behavior problems at twelve years. J Abnorm Child Psychol 27:323, 1999.
28. Sahakian V, Rouse D, Sipes S, et al: Vitamin B_6 is effective therapy for nausea and vomiting of pregnancy: a randomized, double-blind placebo-controlled study. Obstet Gynecol 78:33, 1991.
29. Castro L de P: Reflux esophagitis as the cause of heartburn in pregnancy. Am J Obstet Gynecol 98:1, 1967.
30. Cappell MS: Gastric and duodenal ulcers during pregnancy. Gastroenterol Clin North Am 32:263, 2003.
31. Winbery SL, Blaho KE: Dyspepsia in pregnancy. Obstet Gynecol Clin North Am 28:333, 2001.
32. Cappell MS, Schein JR: Diagnosis and treatment of nonsteroidal anti-inflammatory drug-associated upper gastrointestinal toxicity. Gastroenterol Clin North Am 29:97, 2000.
33. Lalkin A, Magee L, Addis A, et al: Acid-suppressing drugs during pregnancy. Can Fam Physician 43:1923, 1997.
34. Nakatsuka T, Fujikake N, Hasebe M, et al: Effects of sodium bicarbonate and ammonium chloride on the incidence of furosemide-induced fetal skeletal anomaly, wavy rib, in rats. Teratology 48:139, 1993.
35. Charan M, Katz PO: Gastroesophageal reflux disease in pregnancy. Curr Treat Options Gastroenterol 4:73, 2001.

36. Morton DM: Pharmacology and toxicity of nizatidine. Scand J Gastroenterol 22(Suppl 136):1, 1987.
37. Koren G, Zemlickis DM: Outcome of pregnancy after first trimester exposure to H-2 receptor antagonists. Am J Perinatol 8:37, 1991.
38. Physicians Desk Reference, 59th edition. Montvale, NJ, Thomson Healthcare, 2005.
39. Briggs GG, Freeman RK, Yaffe SJ: Drugs in Pregnancy and Lactation: A Reference Guide to Fetal and Neonatal Risk, 6th ed. Philadelphia, Lippincott Williams & Wilkins, 2002.
40. Dashe JS, Gilstrap III LC: Antibiotic use in pregnancy. Obstet Gynecol Clin North Am 24:617, 1997.
41. Cappell MS: The fetal safety and clinical efficacy of gastrointestinal endoscopy during pregnancy. Gastroenterol Clin North Am 32:123, 2003.
42. Aston A, Kalaichandran S, Can IV: Duodenal ulcer hemorrhage in the puerperium. Can J Surg 34:482, 1991.
43. Schein M: Choice of emergency operative procedure for bleeding duodenal ulcer. Br J Surg 78:633, 1991.
44. Chan YM, Ngai SW, Lao TT: Gastric adenocarcinoma presenting with persistent, mild gastrointestinal symptoms in pregnancy: a case report. J Reprod Med [illegible]:906, 1999.
45. Dumont M: Diaphragmatic hernia and pregnancy. J Gynecol Obstet Biol Reprod [illegible]
46. Kurzel RE, Naunheim KS, Schwartz RA: Repair of symptomatic diaphragmatic hernia during pregnancy. Obstet Gynecol 71:869, 1988.
47. Mazze RI, Kallen B: Appendectomy during pregnancy: a Swedish registry of 778 cases. Obstet Gynecol 77:835, 1991.
48. Tamir IL, Bongard FS, Klein SR: Acute appendicitis in the pregnant patient. Am J Surg 160:571, 1990.
49. Mourad J, Elliott JP, Erickson L, et al: Appendicitis in pregnancy: new information that contradicts long-held clinical beliefs. Am J Obstet Gynecol 182:1027, 2000.
50. De Perrot M, Jenny A, Morales M, et al: Laparoscopic appendectomy during pregnancy. Surg Laparosc Endosc Percutan Tech 10:368, 2000.
51. Connolly MM, Unti JA, Nom PF: Bowel obstruction in pregnancy. Surg Clin North Am 75:101, 1995.
52. Perdue PW, Johnson HW Jr, Stafford PW: Intestinal obstruction complicating pregnancy. Am J Surg 164.384, 1992.
53. Davis MR, Bohon CJ: Intestinal obstruction in pregnancy. Clin Obstet Gynecol 26:832, 1983.
54. Meyerson S, Holtz T, Ehrinpreis M, et al: Small bowel obstruction in pregnancy. Am J Gastroenterol 90:299, 1995.
55. Dufour P, Haentjens-Verbeke K, Vinatier D, et al: Intestinal obstruction and pregnancy. J Gynecol Obstet Biol Reprod 25:297, 1996.
56. Rothstein RD, Rombeau JL: Intestinal malrotation during pregnancy. Obstet Gynecol 81:817, 1993.
57. Fielding LP, Schultz SM: Treatment of acute colonic pseudo-obstruction. J Am Coll Surg 192:[illegible], 2001.
58. Roberts CA: Ogilvie's syndrome after cesarean delivery. J Obstet Gynecol Neonatal Nurs 29:239, 2000.
59. Sharp HT: Gastrointestinal surgical conditions during pregnancy. Clin Obstet Gynecol 37:306, 1994.
60. Woods JB, Martin JN Jr, Ingram FH, et al: Pregnancy complicated by carcinoma of the colon above the rectum. Am J Perinatol 9:102, 1992.
61. Nesbitt JC, Moise KJ, Sawyers JL: Colorectal carcinoma in pregnancy. Arch Surg 120:636, 1985.
62. Bernstein MA, Madoff RD, Caushaj PF: Colon and rectal cancer in pregnancy. Dis Colon Rectum 36:172, 1993.
63. Tsukamoto N, Uchino H, Matsukuma K, Kamura T: Carcinoma of the colon presenting as bilateral ovarian tumors during pregnancy. Gynecol Oncol 24:386, 1986.
64. Kort B, Katz VL, Watson WJ: The effect of nonobstetric operation during pregnancy. Surg Gynecol Obstet 177:371, 1993.
65. Smith C, Butler JA: Colorectal cancer in patients younger than 40 years of age. Dis Colon Rectum 32:843, 1989.
66. Imperiale TF, Ransohoff DF, Itzkowitz SH, et al, the Colorectal Cancer Study Group: Fecal DNA versus fecal occult blood for colorectal-cancer screening in an average-risk population. N Engl J Med 351:2704, 2004.
67. Jospe ES, Peppercorn MA: Inflammatory bowel disease and pregnancy: a review. Dig Dis 17:201, 1999.
68. Woolfson K, Cohen Z, McLeod RS: Crohn's disease and pregnancy. Dis Colon Rectum 33:869, 1990.
69. Friedman S: Management of inflammatory bowel disease during pregnancy and nursing. Semin Gastrointest Dis 12:245, 2001.
70. Rajapakse R, Korelitz BI: Inflammatory bowel disease during pregnancy. Curr Treat Options Gastroenterol 4:245, 2001.
71. Sachar D: Exposure to mesalamine during pregnancy increased preterm deliveries (but not birth defects) and decreased birth weight. Gut 43:316, 1998.
72. Hausknecht RU: Methotrexate and misoprostol to terminate early pregnancy. N Engl J Med 333:537, 1995.
73. Alstead EM, Ritchie JK, Lennard-Jones JE, et al: Safety of azathioprine in pregnancy in inflammatory bowel disease. Gastroenterology 99:443, 1990.
74. [illegible] No. 245. Washington, DC, American College of Obstetricians and Gynecologists, March 1998.
75. Hill J, Clark A, Scott NA: Surgical treatment of acute manifestations of Crohn's disease during pregnancy. J R Soc Med 90:64, 1997.
76. Ilnyckyji A, Blanchard JF, Rawsthorne P, Bernstein CN: Perianal Crohn's disease and pregnancy: role of the mode of delivery. Am J Gastroenterol 94:3274, 1999.
77. Cappell MS, Friedel D: The role of sigmoidoscopy and colonoscopy in the diagnosis and management of lower gastrointestinal disorders: endoscopic findings, therapy, and complications. Med Clin North Am 86:1253, 2002.
78. Medich DS, Fazio VW: Hemorrhoids, anal fissure, and carcinoma of the colon, rectum, and anus during pregnancy. Surg Clin North Am 75:77, 1995.
79. Engelhardt TC, Kerstein MD: Pregnancy and mesenteric venous thrombosis. South J Med 82:1441, 1989.
80. Cappell MS: Intestinal (mesenteric) vasculopathy: I. acute superior mesenteric arteriopathy and venopathy. Gastroenterol Clin North Am 27:783, 1998.
81. Cappell MS: Colonic toxicity of administered drugs and chemicals. Am J Gastroenterol 99:1175, 2004.
82. Verne GN, Robinson ME, Price DD: Hypersensitivity to visceral and cutaneous pain in the irritable bowel syndrome. Pain 93:7, 2001.
83. Thompson WG, Longstreth GF, Drossman DA, et al: Functional bowel disorders and functional abdominal pain. Gut 45(Suppl 2):II43, 1999.
84. Kane SV, Sable K, Hanauer SB: The menstrual cycle and its effect on inflammatory bowel disease and irritable bowel syndrome: a prevalence study. Am J Gastroenterol 93:1867, 1998.
85. Mathias JR, Clench MH: Relationship of reproductive hormones and neuromuscular disease of the gastrointestinal tract. Dig Dis 16:3, 1998.
86. West L, Warren J, Cutts T: Diagnosis and management of irritable bowel syndrome, constipation, and diarrhea in pregnancy. Gastroenterol Clin North Am 21:793, 1992.
87. Stanley JC, Wakefield TW, Graham LM, et al: Clinical importance and management of splanchnic artery aneurysms. J Vasc Surg 3:836, 1986.
88. Hallet JW Jr: Splenic artery aneurysms. Semin Vasc Surg 8:321, 1995.

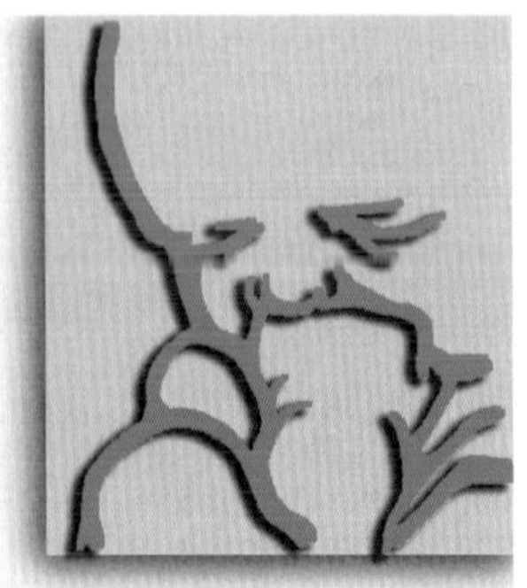

Neurologic Disorders

PHILIP SAMUELS AND JENNIFER R. NIEBYL

CHAPTER 44

KEY ABBREVIATIONS

Arteriovenous	AV
Blood pressure	BP
Central nervous system	CNS
Cerebrospinal fluid	CSF
Computerized tomographic scan	CT
Electroencephalogram	EEG
Hemolysis, elevated liver enzymes, and low platelet count	HELLP
Idiopathic intracranial hypertension	ICH
Intelligence quotient	IQ
Intramuscular	IM
Intrauterine growth restriction	IUGR
Magnetic resonance imaging	MRI
Multiple sclerosis	MS
Neural tube defect	NTD
Thymus helper	Th

SEIZURE DISORDERS

Because they affect approximately 1 percent of the general population, seizure disorders are the most frequent major neurologic complication encountered in pregnancy. Seizure disorders may be divided into those that are acquired and those that are idiopathic. Acquired seizure disorders, which account for less than 15 percent of all seizures, may result from trauma, infection, space-occupying lesions, or metabolic disorders. More than 85 percent of seizure disorders are classified as idiopathic, meaning that no etiologic agent or inciting incident can be identified. Idiopathic seizures can be divided into types such as tonic-clonic, partial complex with or without generalization, myoclonic, focal, or absence.

In general, initial therapy is based on the type of seizure disorder experienced by the patient. There are, however, many crossovers, and patients may respond differently to each medication despite their seizure type. Therefore, it is not unusual to encounter a patient with any seizure type who may be taking any of the major antiepileptic medications. Furthermore, patients may be placed on a certain medication because they did not tolerate the side effect profile of another anticonvulsant (Table 44-1). Many patients with epilepsy have done very well on their medications, and so they have not been evaluated by a neurologist in many years. Some patients have been seizure free for many years and have stopped their medications, or may stop them when they are pregnant.[1] Still others have poorly controlled seizures, and it is unclear whether this is due to noncompliance with or ineffectiveness of their medication regimen. Other patients may be taking two medications when they may need only one. The obstetrician and neurologist must work closely together to guide the patient through her pregnancy and find the safest and most effective medical therapy for the patient. Through this cooperation, the majority of pregnant women with seizure disorders can have a successful pregnancy with minimal risk to mother and fetus.

Effects of Epilepsy on Reproductive Function

Women with seizure disorders should seek care from an obstetrician/gynecologist as soon as they become sexually active. Contraception may present a challenge to women with epilepsy, and the use of oral contraceptives may require special adjustments. Certain antiepileptic medications have been associated with contraceptive failure. Carbamazepine, phenobarbital, and phenytoin

Table 44-1. Common Side Effects of Anticonvulsants

DRUG	MATERNAL EFFECTS	FETAL EFFECTS
Phenytoin	Nystagmus, ataxia, hirsutism, gingival hyperplasia, megaloblastic anemia	Possible teratogenesis and carcinogenesis, coagulopathy, hypocalcemia
Phenobarbital	Drowsiness, ataxia	Possible teratogenesis, coagulopathy, neonatal depression, withdrawal
Primidone	Drowsiness, ataxia, nausea	Possible teratogenesis, coagulopathy, neonatal depression
Carbamazepine	Drowsiness, leukopenia, ataxia, mild hepatotoxicity	Possible craniofacial and neural tube defects
Valproic acid	Ataxia, drowsiness, alopecia, hepatotoxicity, thrombocytopenia	Neural tube defects and craniofacial and skeletal defects
Ethosuximide	Nausea, hepatotoxicity, leukopenia, thrombocytopenia	Possible teratogenesis
Lamotrigine	Rash, headache, ataxia, diplopia, blurred vision, dizziness	Possible increase in oral clefts

enhance the activities of hepatic microsomal oxidative enzymes.[2] The cytochrome P450 system is shared by these medications and the steroid hormones. This increased enzymatic activity may lead to rapid clearance of these hormones, which may allow ovulation to occur. Therefore, medicated patients taking low-dose oral contraceptives may have more breakthrough bleeding[3] and may be at increased risk for unplanned pregnancy.[4,5] This rapid clearance does not appear to be induced by valproate, benzodiazepines,[2] or lamotrigine.[6]

Fertility rates may be lower in patients with epilepsy. A retrospective study by Webber and colleagues[7] reviewed fertility rates in individuals with epilepsy over a 50-year period. They found that fertility rates were significantly lower in both men and women with epilepsy, and that this could not be explained solely by the rate of marriage in these patients. Men appeared to be more adversely affected than women. Women with epilepsy had fertility rates 85 percent of the expected rate. Furthermore, in this retrospective review, women with partial seizures seemed to have lower fertility rates than those with generalized seizures. In a study by Dansky et al.,[8] fertility rates appeared to be lower in those women with early onset epilepsy than those with late-onset disease. Cramer and Jones[2] also investigated the fertility rate in 263 unselected patients with epilepsy. They found that the fertility rate was half that of the general population, and 25 percent of married patients had no children.[2] In Finland, the birth rate was lower in patients with epilepsy than in the referenced cohort.[9] The hazard ratio, a type of relative risk, was 0.58 in men and 0.88 in women. Yet, even in these studies, the majority of patients with epilepsy were able to conceive without difficulty.

Effect of Pregnancy on Epilepsy

It has been taught that between 30 percent and 50 percent of patients show an increase in seizure frequency during pregnancy. This was confirmed in the classic study of Knight and Rhind[10] of 153 pregnancies in 59 patients between 1953 and 1973. In that study, 45 percent of patients showed an increase in seizure frequency during pregnancy, whereas 50 percent had no change and 4.8 percent experienced a decrease. Anticonvulsant levels could not be readily measured until the mid 1970s. When this study was performed, anticonvulsant doses were usually only increased by physicians when patients had breakthrough seizures. An important finding from that study, however, was that patients with more frequent seizures tended to have exacerbations during pregnancy.[11] In fact, virtually all patients who had more than one seizure each month experienced worsening of their epilepsy during pregnancy, whereas only about 25 percent of patients who had not had a seizure in over 9 months experienced exacerbation of epilepsy during pregnancy.

With the introduction of new medications and the ability to monitor anticonvulsant levels, these absolute numbers are no longer true. The relationship, however, does remain. Patients with more frequent seizures tend to have exacerbations of seizures during pregnancy. In a large study by Schmidt et al.,[11] 63 percent of patients had no change or a decrease in seizure frequency during pregnancy, whereas only 37 percent of patients had an increase of seizures during pregnancy. Importantly, in 34 of the 50 patients who showed an increase in seizure frequency during pregnancy, the increase was associated with noncompliance with their drug regimen or sleep deprivation. Conversely, in seven of the 18 pregnancies in which improvement of seizure frequency was shown, this was related to improved compliance with the drug regimen or a correction of sleep deprivation for the 9 months preceding pregnancy. In a study by Tanganelli and Regesta,[12] seizure frequency did not change or improved in 82.6 percent of pregnancies. As has been shown in other studies, increases in seizure frequency were often due to noncompliance with medication regimens as well as frequent seizures in the preconception period. In contrast, Sabers et al.[13] summarized 151 pregnancies in 124 women with epilepsy between 1978 and 1992. They found that 21 percent of patients had exacerbations of their seizures during pregnancy and 71 percent were taking only one medication.[13]

In summary, we now have the means to monitor anticonvulsant levels in patients when necessary, and we have the medications to control seizures. We also understand that sleep deprivation can be a catalyst for seizures. With patient cooperation and close surveillance, seizure frequency should remain the same or even improve in most epileptic patients during pregnancy.

Effects of Pregnancy on the Disposition of Anticonvulsant Medications

It is well known that the levels of anticonvulsant medications can change dramatically during pregnancy. They usually decrease in total concentration as pregnancy progresses. Many factors including altered protein binding, delayed gastric emptying, nausea and vomiting, changes in plasma volume, and changes in the volume of distribution can affect the levels of anticonvulsant medications.

Because phenytoin is one of the most widely prescribed anticonvulsant medications, its metabolism and elimination are discussed. Landon and Kirkley[14] and Kochenour et al.[15] showed that the serum concentration of phenytoin tends to fall during pregnancy and rise again during the puerperium and postpartum periods. Several factors can account for this. In early gestation, patients often have nausea and vomiting. Phenytoin is usually administered on a once-daily basis. If the patient vomits the medication, the drug levels will be highly variable. Furthermore, an increase in calcium intake during pregnancy, as well as the use of antacids, leads to the formation of insoluble complexes with phenytoin, resulting in lower total drug levels. Also, with delayed gastric emptying in pregnancy, the time to peak drug level is lengthened. Phenytoin is inactivated in the liver. Its rate of conversion may increase greatly during pregnancy, because the activity of oxidative enzymes increases. This is due to increased progesterone levels, which induce enzyme activity. This may also be enhanced by increased folic acid, which serves as a cofactor in these metabolic processes. Outside of pregnancy, approximately 90 percent of phenytoin is protein bound. Plasma albumin levels decrease during pregnancy, whereas other protein levels may rise. This process causes changes in the total phenytoin level that do not necessarily reflect the free, active phenytoin concentrations. This effect is also enhanced by free fatty acids displacing phenytoin from albumin. In a study by Yerby et al.,[16] free levels of phenobarbital, carbamazepine, and phenytoin rose significantly throughout pregnancy while total levels fell. Therefore, the relationship observed in nonpregnant women between total drug and free or active drug is not maintained. Free phenytoin levels, therefore, should be measured. If free levels are unavailable, drug doses should be adjusted according to the total serum level and the clinical picture. If the patient has increased seizure activity, medication doses should be increased as long as the patient is not showing signs of toxicity. Likewise, if the medication level is low but the patient is seizure free, no adjustment in dosing is necessary.

Similar pharmacokinetic changes occur with the administration of phenobarbital and carbamazepine but to different degrees. Both of these drugs also show changes in protein binding and increased hepatic clearance during pregnancy. With phenobarbital, the protein binding is considerably less than phenytoin, and changes in plasma protein are less likely to be clinically significant. Primidone is an occasionally used anticonvulsant medication that is metabolized to phenobarbital and another active metabolite, phenylethylmalonic acid diamide. When checking primidone levels, one must also check levels of phenobarbital. Infants born to mothers who have been taking barbiturates during pregnancy may exhibit some withdrawal symptoms that begin about 1 week after birth and usually last 1 to 2 weeks.[17] These symptoms usually involve minor irritability but may occasionally be more serious.

Carbamazepine also has an active metabolite, carbamazepine 10,11-epoxide. This metabolite can be measured, and this measurement can be clinically useful in many instances. Carbamazepine is not as highly protein bound as phenytoin and, therefore, is not subject to as wide a fluctuation due to changes in protein levels. Carbamazepine also induces its own metabolic enzymes in the liver, so the half life changes as the dose increases.[15]

Lamotrigine (Lamictal) clearance increases more than 50 percent during pregnancy.[18] This effect occurs early in pregnancy and reverts quickly after delivery. Most patients require a higher dose to maintain therapeutic levels during pregnancy.[18] Concomitant use of carbamazepine may also increase lamotrigine requirements.

All anticonvulsants interfere with folic acid metabolism. Patients on anticonvulsants may actually become folic acid deficient and develop macrocytic anemia. Folic acid deficiency has been associated with neural tube defects (NTDs) and other congenital malformations.[19,20] Because organogenesis occurs during the first weeks after conception, folic acid supplementation should be begun before pregnancy if possible. A dose of 4 mg daily is recommended. As previously stated, increasing folic acid ingestion may increase the activity of hepatic microsomal enzymes and thus the clearance of anticonvulsant medications. Levels should be checked frequently, therefore, after folic acid therapy is implemented. Furthermore, therapy with phenytoin may result in increased metabolism of vitamin D, leading to decreased vitamin D levels. The patient should be reminded to take her prenatal vitamins, which include an adequate amount of vitamin D.

Neonatal hemorrhage, due to decreased vitamin K–dependent clotting factors (II, VII, IX, X), has been seen in infants born to mothers taking phenobarbital, phenytoin, and primidone.[21] In one series,[21] eight of 16 infants exposed to these medications had a cord blood coagulation pattern similar to that of a vitamin K deficiency. This occurred earlier than the customary hemorrhagic disease of the newborn. These infants responded to vitamin K infusion. Bleyer and Skinner[22] reviewed a case of their own and 21 other cases of hemorrhagic disease following anticonvulsant therapy that have appeared in the literature. They reached similar conclusions that these cases are vitamin K–dependent clotting factor deficiencies and that, at birth, infants should be given 1 mg of vitamin K intramuscularly. A more recent study did not find any increased risk of bleeding in the neonate if the infant received 1 mg of vitamin K intramuscularly (IM) at birth.[23]

Effect of Epilepsy on Pregnancy

The majority of women with seizure disorders who become pregnant have an uneventful pregnancy with an excellent outcome. There appear, however, to be several pregnancy complications that are more prevalent in the mother with epilepsy than in the general population. In a review of all birth certificates for infants born in the state of Washington from 1980 to 1981, Yerby and coworkers[24] identified 200 births to mothers with seizure disorders. Although birth certificate studies are often limited, these researchers controlled for many variables including previous adverse pregnancy outcome and socioeconomic status.[24] They found that mothers with seizure disorders were 2.66 times more likely to have had a previous fetal death after 20 weeks' gestation than the control population. Because of the retrospective nature of this study, the authors were unable to correlate this with intrauterine growth restriction (IUGR) or other fetal problems. This increased incidence of stillbirth is confirmed in other investigations.[10,25,26] It is unclear in any of these studies what type of fetal surveillance was used and if there were any predictors that these fetuses were at risk. With the increased use of ultrasound to identify IUGR, malformations, and oligohydramnios, many of the stillborn fetuses may have been identified as being at risk and might have undergone antepartum fetal testing and intervention before the fetal demise occurred. These studies also were not stratified by medications taken, dosages, drug levels, or seizure activity during pregnancy.

Hiilesmaa et al.,[27] in a study of 150 pregnant women with seizure disorders, found no difference in perinatal mortality between patients and controls. However, there were three third-trimester stillbirths in the epileptic group and two in the control group. Yerby and colleagues[24] also found an increased incidence of preeclampsia in women with seizure disorders. This finding has also been identified in other large retrospective studies.[10,25] However, Hiilesmaa et al.[27] found no difference in the rate of preeclampsia between pregnant women with epilepsy and controls. Yerby et al.[24] also showed a 2.79-fold increase in low-birth-weight infants. In a carefully performed study in Italy, Mastroiacovo and coworkers[28] found that the mean birth weight in neonates born to women with epilepsy was 107 g lower than controls. The mean birth weight in the epilepsy group, however, still fell within the normal range for gestational age. The clinical significance of this finding, therefore, is questionable. When considering all commonly used anticonvulsants, this decrease in neonatal weight appeared to be more common in infants exposed in utero to phenobarbital.

Mastroiacovo et al.[28] also found a decrease in head circumference in infants of mothers with epilepsy. This effect was seen in both untreated women with epilepsy and those receiving medications. Although this change was statistically significant, the mean head circumferences of both study and control infants still fell within the normal range. These authors found no difference in neonatal length comparing groups of mothers with epilepsy and control populations. Hiilesmaa et al.[29] also found a decrease in head circumference in neonates born to women with epilepsy. This decrease was most marked in women taking carbamazepine both alone or in combination with phenobarbital. Again, the mean head circumferences, however, were still within the expected normal range.[29] In the follow-up of this study, head circumferences were still smaller at 18 months of age.

Along similar lines, Hvas et al.[30] compared pregnancy outcomes in 193 women with epilepsy with those of 24,094 women without epilepsy delivering between 1989 and 1997. They found that birth weight of infants born to women with epilepsy was 208 g less than those born to women without a seizure disorder. The odds ratio that a woman treated with epilepsy would give birth to an infant with IUGR was 1.9. Head circumference and body length were also diminished in the infants born to women taking antiepileptic drugs. When smokers with and without epilepsy were compared, there was an increased risk of preterm birth in those who smoked. Battine et al.[31] examined anthropometrics in children born to women with epilepsy in Canada, Japan, and Italy. They found some distinct geographic differences in risk for decreased head circumference that may or may not be related to the drug regimen. The relative risk for small head circumference in infants exposed to more than one medication (polytherapy) was 2.7. A dose-dependent response for both head circumference and body weight was seen with the use of phenobarbital and primidone. The authors state that in addition to drug regimen, genetic, ethnic, and environmental effects should be taken into account when considering explanations for decreased head circumference and birth weight in infants born to women treated for epilepsy.

Hiilesmaa et al.[27,29] found no increase in pregnancy complications in women with epilepsy. They also observed no increase in preterm labor, bleeding, pregnancy-induced hypertension, operative vaginal delivery, or cesarean delivery rates.

Richmond et al.[32] showed increased rates of nonproteinuric hypertension, induction of labor, and fetal cardiovascular malformations in 414 women with epilepsy. Rates of other antenatal, intrapartum, and neonatal complications were similar to controls. They concluded that women with epilepsy are not at increased risk for obstetric complications providing appropriate care is available.

Viinikainen[33] reviewed 179 pregnancies in women with epilepsy compared to controls. There were no significant differences in the incidences of preeclampsia, preterm labor, perinatal mortality or low birth weight. The rate of small for gestational age infants was significantly higher, and neonatal head circumferences were significantly smaller in women with epilepsy.

In summary, women with seizure disorders are at increased risk of IUGR and stillbirth. It also appears that infants born to mothers with seizure disorders, on average, are smaller than their control counterparts. Furthermore, the incidence of preeclampsia may be higher in mothers with seizure disorders. The vast majority of pregnancies, however, are uncomplicated with no increase in complications over the expected rate. Nonetheless, because of these few potential problems, the obstetrician should be more surveillant for pregnancy-related complications in pregnant women with seizure disorders.

Effects of Anticonvulsant Medications on the Fetus

There is little doubt that anticonvulsant medications are associated with an increase in congenital malformations, but the magnitude of this risk and the association of certain anomalies with specific drugs remain debatable (see Chapter 8). Although there was some evidence for teratogenicity related to phenytoin in the 1960s, Hanson and Smith[34] identified a specific fetal hydantoin syndrome in 1975. They noted growth and performance delays, craniofacial abnormalities (including clefting), and limb anomalies (including hypoplasia of nails and distal phalanges). They first described this syndrome in five infants exposed to phenytoin in utero. Hanson et al.[35] later reported that 7 to 11 percent of infants exposed to phenytoin had this recognizable pattern of malformations. They furthermore found that 31 percent of exposed fetuses had some aspects of the syndrome. Yet in 1988 Gaily et al.[36] reported no evidence of the hydantoin syndrome in 82 women exposed in utero to phenytoin. Some of the patients had hypertelorism and hypoplasia of the distal phalanges, but none had the full hydantoin syndrome.

Since the original reports by Hanson and colleagues, many studies have reported congenital malformations in infants born to mothers taking anticonvulsant medications, particularly cleft lip and palate, congenital heart disease, and for valproic acid and carbamazepine, NTDs. The overall rate of anomalies is doubled, but the rate of NTDs with valproic acid is increased 10-fold, from 1–2/1,000 to 1 to 2 percent.[37] It remains of prime importance, however, to treat the patient with the medication that best controls her seizures.

Nakane and colleagues[38] published the first major, multi-institutional study investigating the teratogenicity of antiepileptic medications. This study, carried out between 1974 and 1977, examined 902 pregnancies in mothers with idiopathic epilepsy. The overall rate of congenital malformations was 7.2 percent. This included 8.7 percent in the mothers who received anticonvulsant medications during pregnancy and 1.9 percent in nonmedicated mothers. Looking only at live-born infants, 9.9 percent had malformations (11.5 percent in the medicated group and 2.3 percent in the nonmedicated group). Therefore, the incidence of malformations in mothers receiving anticonvulsant therapy was about five times that of the nonmedicated group. Interestingly, Canger et al.[39] began collecting data in Italy at the time Nakane's group completed their data collection. Canger and coworkers studied 517 women with epilepsy throughout pregnancy. They found a 9.7-percent rate of malformations, a proportion strikingly similar to that of Nakane.[38]

In Nakane's study,[38] the predominant malformations were cleft lip and palate (3.14 percent) and cardiovascular malformations (2.95 percent). Nakane et al. also noted that as the number of anticonvulsant medications used in combination during pregnancy increased, the incidence of fetal malformations rose dramatically.[38] The malformation rate was less than 5 percent when one medication (monotherapy) was used and was greater than 20 percent when four medications were used. Of note, 537 patients were taking two or more medications, whereas 93 patients were taking only one medication. Congenital heart disease was significantly higher in infants born to mothers taking phenobarbital, and cleft lip and palate was more common in infants born to women taking primidone.

Kaneko and colleagues[40] performed a prospective study to determine primary factors responsible for the increased incidence of malformations in infants born to mothers being treated with anticonvulsants. They specifically looked at various drug combinations. The overall malformation rate was 14 percent. In the 16.1 percent of patients who were receiving a single medication, the malformation rate was 6.5 percent.[40] The malformation rate for those treated with multiple medications was 15.6 percent.

Kaneko et al.[41] subsequently published a follow-up study to detect malformations in infants exposed in utero to anticonvulsant medications. They compared these results with their previous investigation.[40] The first study examined infants born between 1978 and 1984, whereas the later study evaluated infants born between 1985 and 1989. Whereas 14 percent of infants had some malformation in the previous study, the malformation rate was only 6.3 percent in the second group.[41] Again, there was no relationship between the medication taken and the type of malformation found.[41] The lower rate of malformations may be attributable to the increase in patients receiving monotherapy. In the earlier study, 16.1 percent of patients received a single medication, whereas 63.4 percent received a single medication in the later study. Jick and Terris[42] matched two nonexposed pregnant women to each of 297 pregnant women exposed to antiepileptic medication. The rate of anomalies in infants born to women with epilepsy was 3.4 percent,[42] a rate even lower than that found by Kaneko et al. in their 1992 study.[41] Nonetheless, Jick and Terris found the relative risk for a woman on antiepileptic medications to give birth to an infant with an anomaly was 3.3.[42]

Most neurologists are treating patients with a single agent. Now that blood levels of anticonvulsant medications can be easily measured, single medications can be given at higher doses to make certain that therapeutic levels are achieved. This approach has lessened the need for multiple medications.

The same concept was verified in a study by Lindhout et al.[43] They compared the pattern of malformations in the offspring of two cohorts of women with seizure disorders, one from 1972 to 1979 and one from 1980 to 1985. In the earlier cohort, 15 of 151 (10 percent) of live-born infants had at least one congenital anomaly. The most common anomalies were those most frequently reported for anticonvulsant medications: congenital heart defects, facial clefts, facial dysmorphism, and developmental delays. In the latter cohort, 13 of 172 infants (7.6 percent) exposed in utero to anticonvulsant medications had congenital malformations. The most frequent anomalies in this group were spinal defects and hypospadias. All of these anomalies were associated with maternal therapy with valproate, carbamazepine, or both. In the earlier cohort of patients, the mean number of drugs used during gestation was 2.2 compared with 1.7 in the later cohort. Whereas only 28 percent of women in the earlier cohort received only one medication, 47 percent of the women received monotherapy in the second group of patients. The lower overall rate of malformations in the latter cohort appeared to be due to the reduction in the number of pregnancies during which a combination of medications was used. It is also apparent in this study that neither the duration of maternal epilepsy nor maternal age was associated with malformations in the infants born to these mothers.

Dravet et al.[44] described the risk for malformations in the infants of 227 women participating in a prospective study between 1984 and 1988. There was a 7-percent malformation rate among infants born to mothers taking antiepileptic medications compared with 1.36 percent in the control group. Therefore, fetuses exposed in utero to anticonvulsants had a relative risk of 6.9 of being born with a congenital malformation. This is double the risk demonstrated by Jick and Terris.[42] In this study, the frequency of spina bifida was 17 times more than would be expected in the general population, and heart defects were 9.6 times greater than expected. Cleft lip with or without cleft palate was 8.4 times more frequent than expected in the general population. Using logistic regression, these authors concluded that valproate and phenytoin were the two most teratogenic medications.[44] Also in this study, there was a high correlation with congenital heart defects and maternal ingestion of phenobarbital. The cases of NTDs and congenital heart defect were studied carefully and could not be related to a familial disposition for these defects. As other studies have shown, there was a higher incidence of malformations in infants born to mothers receiving polytherapy (16 percent) than in those receiving monotherapy (6 percent).

A study by Koch et al.[45] however, showed no difference between the rate of malformations in mothers receiving polytherapy and mothers receiving a single medication. Furthermore, they found that the infants born to mothers with epilepsy, regardless of therapy, had only twice as many major malformations as infants born to the control population. The number of minor anomalies, however, was approximately three times greater in infants born to mothers receiving anticonvulsant medication than in the control group. In the mothers receiving monotherapy, those taking valproate had the highest rate of minor malformations.[45] In this study, there appeared to be a link between the dose of valproate and the rate of malformations.

Gaily and Granstrom[46] also investigated minor anomalies in children of mothers with epilepsy. These authors point out that many of the supposedly specific syndromes resulting from intrauterine exposure to certain medications have many common features. They argue that specific syndromes and their association with specific drugs, as well as the frequencies of these syndromes, have not been confirmed in epidemiologic studies. They found that many of the minor anomalies that are thought to be specific features of a medication appear to be genetically linked with epilepsy.[46] Indeed, this is in contrast to many of the other published studies. In this study only distal digital hypoplasia appeared to be a specific marker for phenytoin teratogenicity.

Yerby and colleagues[47] also looked prospectively at malformations in infants born to mothers with epilepsy. They further investigated whether pure folate deficiency might be responsible for the malformations. None of the women in their study had deficient folate levels. There was no difference in major malformations between patients and controls in this study.[47] The infants born to mothers taking anticonvulsant medications, however, had a higher mean number of minor anomalies. They found no difference in the number of minor anomalies whether the child was exposed in utero to one anticonvulsant medication or to several.[47] The authors also confirm the great overlap in minor anomalies and various medications, further casting doubt on whether individual medications cause specific syndromes.[47]

Nulman and colleagues[48] examined 36 mother-child pairs exposed to carbamazepine, 34 pairs exposed to phenytoin, nine pairs of nonmedicated epileptic women, and matched each to nine mother-child pairs not exposed to teratogens. Minor anomalies were more common in offspring of mothers receiving either carbamazepine or phenytoin (relative risk 2.1).[48]

Teenagers are often treated with valproate as the anticonvulsant of choice because of its low side effect profile in this age group. It has, however, been reported to be associated with specific anomalies. DiLiberti et al.[49] in 1984, reported a specific fetal valproate syndrome. This was based on seven infants. They found a consistent facial phenotype in all seven children and other birth defects in four. This syndrome phenotype was confirmed by Ardinger and colleagues[50] in 1988. Jager-Roman et al.,[51] in 1986, reported fetal distress in 50 percent of 14 infants receiving valproate. Furthermore, 28 percent had low Apgar scores. They also found the same craniofacial defects as reported by DiLiberti et al.[49] Lindhout and Schmidt[52] confirmed the association between NTDs and valproate exposure in utero. They contend that there is a 1.5-percent risk of an infant being born with a NTD if the mothers took valproate in the first trimester. Lindhout et al.[53] also studied 34 cases of NTDs in mothers taking anticonvulsant medications. In 33 of the 34 cases, mothers were exposed to either valproate or carbamazepine. Most of the cases of NTDs were lumbosacral. There was only one case of anencephaly. This implies that these medications have a predisposition to cause lumbosacral defects, because in the general population, spina bifida and anencephaly are equally distributed. In only two cases were other major malformations found. The development of NTDs in these infants of mothers taking valproate also appeared to be a dose-dependent phenomenon. Wegner and Nau[54] have shown, in a mouse model, that valproate alters folic acid metabolism in embryos. This could account for the increased risk of NTDs in infants born to mothers who have taken valproate.

The U.K. registry[55] has reported a higher malformation rate with valproate, 5.9 percent, than with carbamazepine, 2.3 percent, and lamotrigine, 2.1 percent. In the North American registry, the relative risk of having an affected offspring for the valproate-exposed woman was 7.3.[56] Valproate is associated with major malformations other than NTDs (relative risk 3.77). The risk is dose dependent, beginning at 600 mg/day and becomes more prominent at 1,000 mg/day.[57] Polytherapy including valproate carries more risk than any other polytherapy.[58–60] In summary, the pattern of physical abnormalities is related to the use of anticonvulsant drugs, rather than to epilepsy itself.[61]

In 1989, Jones et al.[62] reported a pattern of minor craniofacial defects, fingernail hypoplasia, and developmental delay in infants exposed in utero to carbamazepine. Rosa[63] has also shown that there is a 1-percent risk of spina bifida in infants of mothers taking carbamazepine. Carbamazepine increases the incidence of NTDs, cardiovascular, and urinary tract anomalies, and cleft palate.[64] Because this spectrum of defects (except spina bifida) is similar to that in the fetal hydantoin syndrome, Jones et al.[61] hypothesized that, because both drugs are metabolized through an arene oxide pathway, perhaps an epoxide intermediary is the teratogenic agent. Those fetuses with low levels of epoxide hydrolase are exposed to higher levels of epoxide intermediaries, and this may lead to an increase in malformations. Conversely, fetuses with high enzyme levels clear epoxides rapidly, minimizing exposure to the potential teratogens. Phenytoin, phenobarbital, and to a lesser extent, carbamazepine are metabolized through this pathway.[65] Much work in this area is being performed by Finnell et al., who believe that low levels of epoxide hydrolase activity may be the common link explaining why only certain fetuses exposed to anticonvulsant medications in utero develop congenital malformations.

New antiepileptic drugs have been approved and have been rapidly incorporated into clinical practice in the last decade. There is a need for these medications because 25 to 30 percent of epileptic patients are not adequately controlled by conventional therapies.[66] These newer medications work at the level of neurotransmitters such as gamma-aminobutyric acid and also by blockade of sodium channels. Table 44-2 lists these drugs, with their dosages, and describes other considerations in their use. Gabapentin is also used in chronic pain, mood stabilization, and neuropathies. Therefore, the obstetrician may encounter patients other than those with epilepsy on gabapentin. At present, there are limited data on its fetal effects in pregnancy. Patients should be warned that we do not yet know enough about the effects of the drug on the developing fetus to appropriately counsel them. Nonetheless, if this medication is necessary to keep seizures under control, it should be used.

Lamotrigine is an adjunctive therapy for the treatment of simple and complex seizures with and without secondary generalization. Approximately 10 percent of patients discontinue the medication because of a rash.[67] Severe rashes such as Stevens-Johnson syndrome and toxic epidermal necrolysis have been reported. The severe rashes have occurred with more frequency in pediatric patients. In a more recent study, rash necessitating discontinuation of therapy was found in only 2 percent of 11,316 treated patients.[68] Ohman et al.[69] report a successful pregnancy and noted that the cord blood levels of lamotrigine were equal to those of maternal serum. Also, the median milk/maternal plasma concentration ratio of 0.61 indicates that there are significant milk levels. In the lamotrigine pregnancy registry, of 595 exposures to date, 17 had major defects, (2.9 percent), not significantly increased over the expected rate.[70] One report showed an increased risk of oral clefts.[70a] Lamotrigine is also commonly used as a mood stabilizer.

Topiramate and tiagabine are also used as adjunctive therapies for epilepsy. Both are effective, but there is little information on the use of these medications in pregnancy. In summary, the neurologist and obstetrician should work together and use whichever medications work best for the patient.

There has been much debate over whether epilepsy itself and the use of antiepileptic medications are associated with psychomotor delays or mental retardation. In the landmark study by Nelson and Ellenberg,[25] an intelligence quotient (IQ) below 70 was seen in 65.2 per 1,000 7-year-old children in the seizure group compared with 34 per 1,000 in the age-matched control group, a statistically significant difference. Before generalizations can be made, many confounding factors must be evaluated including other anomalies and social environment. In a review by Granstrom and Gaily,[71] none of the major antiepileptic medications appeared to carry special risk for mental retardation. They suggest, however, that polytherapy and inherited deviations in antiepileptic medication metabolism in the fetus increase the risk for mental retardation. This study is important because these researchers stress that other factors associated with maternal epilepsy such as seizures during pregnancy, inherited brain disorders, and a nonoptimal psychosocial environment can also affect a child's psychomotor development.[71] These factors are hard to control in any study. In a report by

Table 44-2. Newer Antiepileptic Agents

MEDICATION	USUAL DOSE (MG/DAY)	DOSES/DAY	SPECIAL NOTES
Gabapentin	900–3,600	3	Not enzyme inducer Antacids interfere
Lamotrigine	300–500	1 or 2	Rash in 11.2% Not enzyme inducer Half-life affected by meds
Topiramate	100–400	2	May interfere with O.C.s Moderate enzyme inducer
Tiagabine	8–56	2 to 4	Does not interfere with O.C.s Not enzyme inducer
Oxcarbazepine	600–2,400	2	Moderate enzyme inducer
Levetiracetam	1,000–3,000	2	Not enzyme inducer
Zonisamide	400–600	2	Not enzyme inducer

OC, oral contraceptive.

Gaily et al.,[72] two of 48 (4.1 percent) infants of mothers with epilepsy had mental retardation, and two additional infants had borderline intelligence. The mean IQ of the infants exposed in utero to anticonvulsant medications was statistically lower than the control group. When these four children were excluded from the analysis, the difference in mean IQ disappeared.[72] There was no increased risk of low intelligence attributable to fetal exposure either to antiepileptic medications below toxic levels or to brief maternal convulsions. No particular medication appeared to be associated with a lower IQ. Social class also appeared to play a role in the differences in IQs in these patients.

Moore et al.[73] reviewed 57 infants with fetal anticonvulsant syndromes. Eighty-one percent reported behavioral problems, with hyperactivity being the most common (34 percent). Two or more autistic features were found in 34 (60 percent) of the 57 children. Four were diagnosed with autism and two with Asperberger's syndrome. Learning difficulties were found in 77 percent; and speech delay in 81 percent. Gross and fine motor delays were identified in 60 percent and 42 percent, respectively.[73] These percentages seem high, but it is important to remember that all of these children had already been identified as having an anticonvulsant syndrome.

In summary, there appears to be a small, undefined risk of a slightly lower IQ, psychomotor delay, and an increase in behavior problems in infants born to mothers with epilepsy.[74–76] It does not appear that any particular medication results in a higher risk of this outcome.

Preconceptional Counseling for the Reproductive Age Woman with a Seizure Disorder

Although it is not always possible, it is preferable to counsel the patient with epilepsy before she becomes pregnant. A detailed history should be taken to determine if there are any seizure disorders or congenital malformations in the family. The obstetrician must stress that the patient has greater than a 90-percent chance of having a successful pregnancy resulting in a normal newborn. A detailed history of medication use and seizure frequency should be obtained. The patient must be informed that if she has frequent seizures before conception, this pattern will probably continue. Furthermore, if she has frequent seizures, she should be encouraged to delay conception until control is better, even if this entails a change or an additional medication. The obstetrician must stress that controlling seizures is of primary importance and that the patient will need to take whatever medication or medications are necessary to achieve this goal throughout her pregnancy. If the patient has had no seizures during the past 2 to 5 years, an attempt may be made to withdraw her from anticonvulsant medications. This is usually done over a 1- to 3-month period, slowly reducing the medication. Up to 50 percent of patients relapse and need to start their medications again. This withdrawal should be attempted only if the patient is completely seizure free for 2 years, has a normal electroencephalogram (EEG), and only with the help of a neurologist. During the period of withdrawal from medications, patients should refrain from driving.

Furthermore, as previously shown, it is best to have the patient taking a single medication during pregnancy. If the patient is on multiple medications, the patient can be changed to monotherapy over several months. The drug of choice for the specific type of epilepsy should be the one chosen for monotherapy. As the other medications are gradually withdrawn, levels of the remaining medication should be monitored to make certain that the level remains therapeutic. When other medications are withdrawn, the level of the primary medication often increases without a dose increment. If it does not, however, the dose of the primary medication may need to be increased. The patient should refrain from conceiving until seizures have been well controlled for several months on the single medication. The patient must also be counseled that she should get adequate rest and sleep during pregnancy, because sleep deprivation is associated with increased seizure frequency.

The choice of antiepileptic medication depends on the seizure type. The most important point is to control maternal seizures. There may be some additional concern for using valproate in pregnancy due to the reported increased incidence of fetal distress[51] and malformations including NTDs.[57] However, if valproate is the anticonvulsant that works best for the patient, it should be used with appropriate counseling and, in pregnancy, ultrasound to detect possible fetal anomalies should be performed at the appropriate time. If valproate is selected, the total dose should be divided into three to four administrations daily to avoid high peak plasma levels. As described earlier, malformations also occur with the use of carbamazepine.[62–64]

There is less information concerning the newer antiepileptic drugs and teratogenesis. If they need to be used for good seizure control, they should be implemented as part of the patient's therapy.

Folic acid supplementation should be begun before or early in pregnancy. Folic acid supplementation may help to prevent NTDs, which have been seen most commonly with carbamazepine and valproate treatment but have been reported in women taking other anticonvulsants as well. Studies have shown that folic acid may decrease the incidence of NTDs in at-risk women.[16] It is important that this be implemented early in pregnancy, because open NTDs occur by the end of the fifth week of gestation. Furthermore, low folate levels have been associated with an increase in adverse pregnancy outcomes in women taking anticonvulsants.[77] Anticonvulsant levels should be checked frequently after implementing or increasing folic acid administration, because folate leads to lower anticonvulsant levels.[77] A daily dose of folic acid of 4 mg/day should be more than ample. Patients should also be encouraged to take their prenatal vitamins, which contain vitamin D. This is because anticonvulsants may interfere with the conversion of 25-hydroxycholecalciferol to 1-25-dihydroxycholecalciferol, the active form of vitamin D.

Mothers with idiopathic epilepsy often ask if their child will develop epilepsy. There is a surprising paucity of studies in this area. Children of parents without seizures have a 0.5- to 1-percent risk of developing epilepsy. It appears that the infant born to a mother with a seizure disorder of unknown etiology has a four times greater chance of developing idiopathic epilepsy than the general population.[78] Furthermore, it appears that epilepsy in the father does not increase a child's risk of developing a seizure disorder. Many of the rare seizure disorders have a stronger genetic component.[79]

Care of the Patient During Pregnancy

Once the patient becomes pregnant, it is of the utmost importance to establish accurate gestational dating. This procedure will prevent any confusion over fetal growth in later gestation. The patient's anticonvulsant level should be followed as needed and dosages adjusted accordingly to keep the patient seizure free. It is a common pitfall to monitor levels too frequently and adjust dosages in a likewise frequent manner. It is important to remember that it takes several half-lives for a medication to reach a steady state (Table 44-3). Drugs like phenobarbital have extremely long half-lives, and the levels should not be checked too frequently. If levels are measured before the drug reaches a steady state and the dosage is increased, the patient will eventually become toxic from the medication. Drug levels should be drawn immediately before the next dose (trough levels) in order to assess if dosing is adequate. If the patient is showing signs of toxicity, a peak level may be obtained.

At approximately 16 weeks' gestation, the patient should undergo blood testing for maternal serum marker screening in an attempt to detect a NTD. This, coupled with ultrasonography, gives a more than 90-percent detection rate for open NTDs. If the patient is difficult to scan or if she wants to be even more certain that there is no NTD, amniocentesis can be undertaken. This should be considered if the patient is taking valproate or carbamazepine, because these medications appear to carry almost the same risk as if the patient had a family history of a NTD.[52,53,63] At 18 to 22 weeks, the patient should undergo a comprehensive, targeted, ultrasound examination by an experienced obstetric sonographer to look for congenital malformations. A fetal echocardiogram can be obtained at 20 to 22 weeks to look for cardiac malformations, which are among the more common malformations in women taking any antiepileptic medications. If fetal echocardiography is not readily available, it is reassuring to remember that an adequate four-chamber view of the heart on ultrasound will identify 68 to 95 percent of major cardiac anomalies.[80,81]

As previously noted, there appears to be an increased risk for IUGR for fetuses exposed in utero to anticonvulsant medications. If the patient's weight gain and fundal growth appear appropriate, regular ultrasound examinations for fetal weight assessment are probably unnecessary. If, however, there is a question of poor fundal growth or if the patient's habitus precludes adequate assessment of this clinical parameter, serial ultrasonography for fetal weight can be performed.

In older and retrospective studies, there appears to be an increased risk of stillbirth in mothers taking anticonvulsant medications.[10,24–26] In a prospective study, however, this complication was not seen.[27] As previously noted, in the studies that showed an increase in still births, factors such as IUGR or oligohydramnios were not prenatally identified. With modern surveillance and the more common use of ultrasonography, many of these risk factors can be detected before the fetus faces imminent risk. Nonstress testing, therefore, is not necessary in all mothers with seizure disorders. It should be limited to those who have other medical or obstetric complications that place the patient at an increased risk for a stillbirth.

The key to managing anticonvulsants in pregnancy is individualization of therapy. If at all possible, the patient should be maintained on a single medication, and drug levels should be drawn at appropriate intervals to make certain that the patient is receiving an adequate dose. If the patient is taking phenytoin, free levels should be obtained. A drug dosage should not be increased solely because the total level of drug is falling. The free level of drug may still be therapeutic. However, if the patient develops any seizure activity, dosages should then be adjusted upward. A brief seizure during pregnancy does not appear to be deleterious to the fetus.[28] It is best to use the lowest dose of a single medication possible that will keep the patient seizure free. This, however, must be individualized. For instance, if the patient usually experiences seizures during the day and drives, it is important to make certain that the patient remains seizure free. For this type of patient, drug dosages should be increased if levels fall. If, on the other hand, the patient only has brief partial complex seizures that do not generalize and occur

Table 44-3. Anticonvulsants Commonly Used During Pregnancy

DRUG	THERAPEUTIC LEVEL (MG/L)	USUAL NONPREGNANT DOSAGE	HALF-LIFE
Carbamazepine	4–10	600–1,200 mg/day in three or divided doses (Two doses if extended-release forms are used)	Initially 36 h, chronic therapy 16 h
Phenobarbital	15–40	90–180 mg/day in two or three divided doses	100 h
Phenytoin	10–20, total; 1–2, free	300–500 mg/day in single or divided doses*	Avg 24 h
Primidone	5–15	750–1,500 mg/day in three divided doses	8 h
Valproic acid	50–100	550–2,000 mg/day in three or divided doses	Avg 13 h
Ethosuximide	40–120	1,000–2,000 mg/day in two divided doses	60 h

*If a total dose of more than 300 mg is needed, dividing the dose will result in a more stable serum concentration.

only during her sleep, it is optimal to keep the medications at the lowest serum concentration that will keep her seizure free. An occasional seizure of this type would not harm either the patient or her fetus. Early hemorrhagic disease of the newborn can occur in infants exposed to anticonvulsants in utero, and this appears to be due to a deficiency of the vitamin K–dependent clotting factors II, VII, IX, and X. The use of vitamin K in the third trimester to prevent hemorrhagic disease is somewhat controversial. Although some advocate administering 10 to 20 mg of vitamin K orally, daily, to mothers during the final few weeks of pregnancy, this is certainly not the standard of care. Very little hemorrhagic disease of the newborn is seen today, and this is probably because most infants receive 1 mg of vitamin K intramuscularly at birth.[23]

Labor and Delivery

Vaginal delivery is the route of choice for the mother with a seizure disorder. If the mother has frequent seizures brought on by the stress of labor, she may undergo cesarean delivery after stabilization. Furthermore, seizures during labor may cause transient fetal bradycardia.[27] The fetal heart rate should be given time to recover. If it does not, then one must assume fetal compromise or placental abruption and proceed with cesarean delivery. Because stress often exacerbates seizure disorders, an epidural anesthetic can benefit many laboring patients with epilepsy.

Management of anticonvulsant medications during a prolonged labor presents a challenge. During labor, oral absorption of medications is erratic and, if the patient vomits, almost negligible. If the patient is taking phenytoin or phenobarbital, these medications may be administered parenterally. An anticonvulsant level should be obtained first to help ascertain the appropriate dosage. Phenobarbital may be given IM, and phenytoin may be given intravenously. Fosphenytoin, although expensive, is available and makes the administration of intravenous phenytoin much easier. If the patient's phenytoin level is normal, the usual daily dose may be administered intravenously. The medication should only be mixed in normal saline and must be administered at a rate no faster than 50 mg/min. Fosphenytoin is easier to use. Because of the long half-life of phenobarbital, if the patient's serum level is therapeutic, a 60- to 90-mg intramuscular dose is probably sufficient to maintain the patient throughout labor and delivery. The main problem arises if the patient is taking carbamazepine. This medication is not manufactured in a parenteral form, although extended-release forms now exist. Oral administration may be attempted, but if the patient has seizures or a preseizure aura, she may be loaded with a therapeutic dose of phenytoin to carry her through labor. The usual loading dose is 10 to 15 mg/kg administered intravenously at a rate no faster than 50 mg/min. This should be effective in controlling seizures. Benzodiazepines may also be used for acute seizures, but one must remember that they can cause early neonatal depression as well as maternal apnea.[82] Prenatal diagnostic techniques cannot be expected to detect all malformations. Even if the infant appears to have no anomalies, an experienced clinician should be present at the delivery of the infant born to a mother taking anticonvulsant medications.

New Onset of Seizures in Pregnancy and the Puerperium

Occasionally, seizures are diagnosed for the first time during pregnancy. This may present a diagnostic dilemma (Table 44-4). If the seizures occur in the third trimester, they are eclampsia until proven otherwise and should be treated as such until the attending physician can perform a proper evaluation. The treatment of eclampsia is delivery, but the patient must first be stabilized. It is often difficult, however, to distinguish eclampsia from an epileptic seizure. The patient may be hypertensive initially after an epileptic seizure and may exhibit some myoglobinuria secondary to muscle breakdown. The diagnosis becomes clearer over time, but in either case, rapid, thoughtful action must be undertaken. The first physician to attend a patient after a seizure may not be an obstetrician/gynecologist, and magnesium sulfate may not be started acutely. This should be remedied as soon as possible.

If the patient develops seizures for the first time at an earlier gestational age, she should be evaluated and started on the proper medication. The physician must look for acquired causes of seizures including trauma, infection, metabolic disorders, space-occupying lesions, central nervous system (CNS) bleeding, and ingestion of drugs such as cocaine and amphetamines. When a seizure occurs, the patient must be stabilized, and the physician must make certain that an adequate airway is established for the protection of both mother and fetus. The physician should also seek focal signs that may be more suggestive of a space-occupying lesion, CNS bleeding, or an abscess. Blood samples should be obtained for electrolytes, glucose, calcium, magnesium, renal function studies, and toxicologic studies while intravenous access is being established. If the patient had a tonic-clonic seizure, and the attending physician believes that this is probably new-onset epilepsy, she should be started on the appropriate anticonvulsant medication while awaiting results of laboratory studies. If she is not in status epilepticus, this medication may be given orally.

If the patient presents with recurrent generalized seizures, status epilepticus, immediate therapeutic action must be taken. The drug of choice is intravenous phenytoin, because it is highly effective, and has a long duration of action and a low incidence of serious side effects. This medication should be administered in a loading dose of 15 to 20 mg/kg at a rate not exceeding 50 mg/min. Rapid infusion may cause transient hypotension and heart block. If possible, the patient should be placed on a cardiac monitor while receiving a loading dose of phenytoin. Also, this medication must be given in a glucose-free solution to avoid precipitation.[83] Fosphenytoin, if available, can be given more rapidly with fewer side effects. If phenytoin is unavailable, a benzodiazepine may be used as a first-line drug for status epilepticus. These drugs, however, cause respiratory depression, and the physician must have the ability to intubate the patient, if necessary,

Table 44-4. Differential Diagnosis of Peripartum Seizures

	BLOOD PRESSURE	PROTEINURIA	SEIZURES	TIMING	CSF	OTHER FEATURES
Eclampsia	+++	+++	+++	Third trimester	Early: RBC, 0–1,000, protein, 50–150 mg/dl Late: grossly bloody	Platelets normal or ↓ RBC normal
Epilepsy	Normal	Normal to +	+++	Any trimester	Normal	Low anticonvulsant levels
Subarachnoid hemorrhage	+ to +++ (labile)	0 to +	+	Any trimester	Grossly bloody	
Thrombotic thrombocytopenic purpura	Normal to +++	++	++	Third trimester	RBC 0–100	Platelets ↓↓ RBC fragmented
Amniotic fluid embolus	Shock		+	Intrapartum	Normal	Hypoxia, cyanosis Platelets ↓↓ RBC normal
Cerebral vein thrombosis	+	–	++	Postpartum	Normal (early)	Headache Occasional pelvic phlebitis
Water intoxication	Normal	–	++	Intrapartum	Normal	Oxytocin infusion rate >45 mU/min Serum NA <124 mEq/L
Pheochromocytoma	+++ (labile)	+	+	Any trimester	Normal	Neurofibromatosis
Autonomic stress syndrome of high paraplegics	+++ with labor pains	–	–	Intrapartum	Normal	Cardiac arrhythmia
Toxicity of local anesthetics	Variable	–	++	Intrapartum	Normal	

Modified from Donaldson JO: Peripartum convulsion. In Donaldson JO (ed): Neurology of Pregnancy. Philadelphia, WB Saunders, 1989, p 312.

when these medications are used. If these measures are ineffective, an anesthesiologist and neurologist should be immediately consulted if they are not already involved in the patient's care.

Any patient experiencing seizures for the first time during pregnancy without a known cause should undergo an EEG and intracranial imaging. In looking only at eclamptic patients, Sibai et al.[84] found that EEGs were initially abnormal in 75 percent of patients but normalized within 6 months in all women studied. Although this group found no uniform abnormalities on computed tomography (CT) in this series of eclamptic patients, they did find that 46 and 33 percent had some abnormal findings on magnetic resonance imaging (MRI) and CT, respectively. Most of the findings were nonspecific and were not helpful in diagnosis or treatment. If the physician is not certain that the patient has eclampsia, an imaging study should be part of the evaluation described above.

Postpartum Period

The levels of anticonvulsant medications must be monitored frequently during the first few weeks postpartum, because they can rise rapidly. If the patient's medication dosages were increased during pregnancy, they will need to be decreased rather rapidly after delivery to prepregnancy levels. All of the major anticonvulsant medications cross into breast milk. The levels vary in breast milk from 18 to 79 percent of the plasma levels.[82,85] The use of these medications, however, is not a contraindication to breastfeeding. Primidone, phenobarbital, and benzodiazepines may have a sedative effect on the fetus with later withdrawal symptoms in the nursery. Topiramine has been associated with neonatal weight loss and probably should not be used if the mother is breast-feeding.

All methods of contraception are available to women with idiopathic seizure disorders. The majority of women are able to take oral contraceptives without any adverse side effects.[86] Oral contraceptive failures are more common in women taking certain anticonvulsants, because some of the major anticonvulsant medications induce hepatic enzymes (cytochrome P 450), which metabolize estrogen faster.[86,87] The enzyme-inducing drugs are phenytoin, carbamazepine, phenobarbital, primidone, and felbamate. With topiramate and oxcarbazepine, the enzyme-inducing effects occur at higher doses, 200 mg and 1200 mg, respectively. This enzyme-inducing effect is not seen with lamotrigine, zonisamide, gabapentin, tiagabine, valproate,[87] ethosuximide, or levetiracetam (see Table 44-2).

In conclusion, the majority of women with idiopathic epilepsy have an uneventful pregnancy with an excellent outcome. To optimize neonatal outcome, the patient should take only one medication and, when possible, use the lowest dose effective in keeping her free of seizures. It is important, however, for the patient to realize that prevention of seizures is the most important goal during pregnancy. Simple interventions such as taking folic acid before conception, taking prenatal vitamins containing vitamin D, and giving the infant vitamin K at birth will help to optimize the outcome. There is an increase in congenital malformations in infants exposed to anticonvulsant medications in utero. The majority of infants exposed to these medications, however, will have no malformations. With modern techniques for prenatal diagnosis, including ultrasound and quadruple screening, many of these malformations can be detected early. The majority of women with epilepsy labor normally and have spontaneous vaginal deliveries. In short, with close cooperation and excellent communication among the obstetrician, neurologist, and pediatrician, the vast majority of these patients will have a safe pregnancy with an excellent outcome.

MIGRAINE

Headaches are extremely common in women, and the majority of migraine headaches occur in women of childbearing age. Migraines can be classified as those with aura (other neurologic signs and symptoms) and those without aura. Maggioni and colleagues[88] surveyed 430 women 3 days postpartum about their headache histories, and 126 (29.3 percent) were found to be primary headache sufferers. Of these patients, 81 suffered from migraine without aura, 12 suffered from migraine with aura, and 33 had tension-type headaches. Migraines are associated with vasodilation of the cerebral vasculature and last a variable amount of time. They are often accompanied by photosensitivity and nausea. Migraines with aura may be accompanied by sensations in the extremities and other lateralizing signs, sometimes making them difficult to distinguish from transient ischemic attacks.

Migraine symptoms tend to improve during pregnancy.[88-89] Maggioni et al.[88] found that 80 percent of patients experienced either complete remission or a 50 percent reduction in headaches during pregnancy. Improvement was more common after the first trimester. Granella and coworkers[89] found that migraines disappeared during pregnancy in 67 percent of cases. Aube found that 60 to 70 percent of women either go into remission or improve significantly, usually in the second and third trimesters.[90] The migraine type did not seem to be a prognostic factor. Those with menstrual migraines showed the most improvement. In this study, however, 4 to 8 percent showed significant worsening during pregnancy. Chen and coworkers[91] identified 508 women with a history of migraine from the Collaborative Perinatal Project. They found that patients with migraines smoke more heavily and had a longer smoking history than did their headache-free peers. They also found that in nonsmokers, migraine was often associated with allergies.[91] In the recent study by Ertresveg,[92] 58 percent of subjects with migraine reported having no headache during pregnancy. Transient neurologic symptoms were more common in patients with a history of migraine.

Chancellor and colleagues[93] followed nine patients whose migraines first occurred during pregnancy at various gestational ages. They were followed for more than 4 years after pregnancy, and the prognosis for headache was excellent. Four of the nine patients developed complications of pregnancy, including preeclampsia in two. Maggioni found no increase in pregnancy complications in patients with migraine.[88] It is unknown if the headaches were caused by developing preeclampsia. It is important to rule out other significant complications of pregnancy before assigning a new diagnosis of migraine to a pregnant patient. Jacobson and Redman[94] reported a patient who actually lost consciousness during pregnancy because of a basilar migraine.

Supportive therapy is recommended for patients who experience migraine attacks during gestation. Acetaminophen[95] is initially recommended, and narcotic analgesics can be used as necessary. The use of nonsteroidal anti-inflammatory agents should be avoided, if possible, after 24 weeks' gestation, because when used for more than 48 hours, they can cause premature closure of the ductus arteriosus and/or oligohydramnios. Nonetheless, they can be used up to 48 hours under physician supervision (see Chapter 8). When pain is severe, parenteral narcotics, prochlorperazine and other antiemetic therapy may be used. β-blockers may be safely administered during pregnancy for prophylaxis, and propranolol is probably safest.[96] The calcium channel blockers used in the treatment of migraine can also be safely administered during gestation.[97] Tricyclic antidepressants are occasionally used for migrane prophylaxis (see Chapter 8).

Ergotamine should be avoided during pregnancy. Previous reports have suggested that it may cause birth defects that have a vascular disruptive etiology. Hughes and Goldstein[98] report a case in which an infant showed evidence of early arrested cerebral maturation and paraplegia. They hypothesize that ergotamine, acting either alone or in synergy with propranolol and caffeine, produced fetal vasoconstriction, resulting in tissue ischemia and subsequent malformation. It is important to note that this etiology is strictly theoretical. In addition, ergots are uterotonic and have an abortifacient potential. These drugs, therefore, should be avoided during pregnancy.

Sumatriptan, a serotonin receptor agonist, is very successful in treating migraines. In a review by O'Quinn and colleagues, there were no untoward effects in 76 first-trimester exposures to sumatriptan.[99] Using logistic regression, Olesen and colleagues[100] compared 34 sumatriptan exposures with 89 migraine controls and 15,995 healthy women. They found the risk of preterm birth was elevated (odds ratio 6.3), as was the risk of IUGR.[100] They do state that they did not control for disease severity. A larger study by Kallen et al.[101] has not confirmed these findings. In 658 infants whose mothers had used sumatriptan during pregnancy, there was no significant difference in prematurity, or low birth weight.[101] Hilaire et al.[102] found birth defects in 3 to 5 percent of infants exposed to sumatriptan in the first trimester, a rate not greater than expected. Table 44-5 lists some medications that can be used for treating migraines.

Dietary factors may precipitate migraine attacks. Careful history may uncover foods that should be avoided, including foods containing monosodium glutamate, red

Table 44-5. Drug Therapy for Migraine Headaches in Pregnancy

MEDICATION	CLASS	USE	DOSAGE	ROUTE OF ADMINISTRATION	SAFE FOR PREGNANCY
Acetaminophen	Pain reliever	Acute pain	4 g/day maximum	PO or PR	Yes
Codeine	Narcotic	Acute pain	30–90 mg q3–4 h	PO	Yes
Meperidine	Narcotic	Acute pain	25–100 mg q3–6 h	PO, IM, or IV	Yes
Ibuprofen	Nonsteroidal	Acute pain	2,400 mg/day in divided doses	PO	Use <48 h in late pregnancy
Prochloroperazine	Phenothiazine	Nausea	5–25 mg q2–8 h depending on route	PO, PR, IM, IV	Yes
Promethazine	Phenothiazine	Nausea	12.5–50 mg q2–8 h depending on route	PO, PR, IM, IV	Yes
Butalbital (50 mg) acetaminophen 325 mg, caffeine 40 mg	Sedative, pain reliever, vasoconstrictor	Acute migraine	2 tablets q4 h, not to exceed 6 tablets daily	PO	Yes
Isometheptene mucate (65 mg), Dichloralphenazone (100 mg), Acetaminophen (325 mg)	Vasoconstrictor, sedative, pain reliever	Acute migraine	2 capsules immediately followed by 1 hourly for no more than 5 capsules in 12 hours	PO	Yes
Caffeine	Vasoconstrictor	Acute pain	500 mg in 50 ml IV solution—may repeat	PO or IV	Yes
Sumatriptan	Vasoconstrictor	Acute pain relief	300 mg/day PO max 6 mg SQ × 2/day max	PO or SQ	Yes
Nortriptyline	TCA	Prophylaxis	25–100 mg qhs	PO	Yes
Amitriptyline	TCA	Prophylaxis	50–150 mg qhs	PO	Yes
Propranolol	Beta-blocker	Prophylaxis	80–120 mg bid	PO	Small risk for IUGR
Nadolol	Beta-blocker	Prophylaxis	20–80 mg qd	PO	Caution for IUGR
Atenolol	Beta-blocker	Prophylaxis	25–100 mg qd	PO	Caution for IUGR
Carbamazepine	Membrane stabilizer	Prophylaxis	Up to 1,200 mg/day in three divided doses	PO	Risk of NTD, other anomalies

bid, twice daily; hs, bedtime; IM, intramuscularly; IUGR, intrauterine growth restriction; IV, intravenously; NTD, neural tube defect; PO, orally; PR, per rectum; qd, daily; SQ, subcutaneous; TCA, tricyclic antidepressant.

wine, cured meats, and strong cheeses containing tyramine. Relative hypoglycemia and alcohol can also trigger migraine attacks.

CEREBROVASCULAR DISEASES

Stroke is diagnosed in 34 per 100,000 deliveries, with 1.4 deaths per 100,000. The risk of stroke increases with age older than 35 years and in African American women.[103] It can be categorized as ischemic (arterial occlusion), cerebral venous thrombosis, intracerebral hemorrhage, and subarachnoid hemorrhage.[104]

Arterial Occlusion

Twelve percent of arterial occlusions occur in women between the ages of 15 and 45 years, and approximately one third of these patients may be pregnant.[105] In a study from India, 37 percent of patients affected with cerebrovascular disease were younger than 40 years of age, with a significant number of thromboses occurring during pregnancy and the puerperium.[106] Overall, the incidence of cerebral arterial occlusion in pregnancy is approximately 1 per 20,000 live births.[105,107] The mortality rate for pregnant women with cerebral arterial occlusion is twice that of men and three times that of nonpregnant women. According to Jennett and Cross,[107] middle cerebral artery occlusion is most common during pregnancy, whereas internal carotid artery occlusion is observed most often in the puerperium. Hemiplegia and dysphasia are frequent findings.[107] Predisposing factors such as preeclampsia, chronic hypertension, or hypotensive episodes can be demonstrated in about one third of these patients. Cancer has been reported as an underlying etiology.[108] Brick and Riggs[109] have shown that oral contraceptives also raise the risk of ischemic cerebral vascular disease. Perhaps because of their relative frequency in the general population, the factor V Leiden mutation and other hereditary thrombophilias may be a predisposing factor in many of these patients. One half of the pregnancy-related cases occur during the immediate postpartum period and the remainder during the second and third trimesters. Lidegaard[110] concluded that pregnancy was associated with an elevated odds ratio of only 1.3 for cerebral thromboembolism. Brick[111] reported the case of a woman who had a documented partial obstruction of the left middle cerebral artery during the third trimester of pregnancy. Following delivery, her symptoms abated, and angiography 11 weeks later revealed complete resolution of the obstruction. Embolic stroke should also be considered. In one postpartum patient, a patent foramen ovale was discovered in association with anticardiolipin antibodies.[112]

In cases of cerebral arterial occlusion, care must be taken to avoid increased intracranial pressure. If signs of increased intracranial pressure develop, parenteral dexamethasone should be administered. Osmotic diuresis can be used if needed. Supportive measures are also necessary, including close monitoring of electrolytes to detect inappropriate secretion of antidiuretic hormone. Successful thrombolytic therapy has been reported.[113] Physical and rehabilitative therapy should be started as soon as possible. These patients can progress normally through pregnancy and deliver vaginally.

A case of maternal death from carotid artery thrombosis associated with the HELLP syndrome (hemolysis, elevated liver enzymes, and low platelet count) has been reported by Katz and Cefalo,[114] and a case of cerebellar infarction by Soh et al.[115] They proposed that the infarction occurred because the patient experienced a rebound thrombocytosis leading to a hypercoagulable state. They stress the importance of closely following patients with HELLP syndrome so that those who develop a reactive thrombocytosis can be monitored for signs and symptoms of CNS thrombosis.

Cortical Vein Thrombosis

The chief symptoms in patients with cortical vein thrombosis are headache, lethargy, and vomiting. Hemiplegia has a gradual onset, and seizure activity is common (see Table 44-4).[116,117] This disorder occurs most frequently during the immediate postpartum period and may be attributed to a hypercoagulable state.[118] An incidence of 1 in 10,000 pregnancies was suggested in one study.[119] With the availability of CT and MRI, accurate diagnosis is possible. In one case in which a blood patch failed to relieve an apparent spinal headache, the ultimate diagnosis was a cortical vein thrombosis.[120]

Many patients with cortical vein thrombosis show signs of seizure activity, and prophylactic anticonvulsants were once routinely given.[114] The drug of choice is phenytoin. The patient should be given an intravenous loading dose of 10 mg/kg followed by 300 to 500 mg orally each day. Phenytoin levels should be checked frequently to make certain that they are therapeutic and that the patient does not develop phenytoin toxicity. Some neurosurgeons have advocated expectant management and do not routinely utilize anticonvulsants.

Subarachnoid Hemorrhage

The rate of subarachnoid hemorrhage complicating pregnancy is approximately 1 per 10,400.[121] With cocaine abuse increasing, the incidence may rise, as the associated increase in vasospasm associated with this drug causes bleeding from preexisting berry aneurysms and arteriovenous (AV) malformations.[122] Most berry aneurysms are thought to be due to a congenital defect in the elastic and smooth muscle layers of cerebral blood vessels. They are usually located in the vessels of the circle of Willis or those arising from it. Robinson and coworkers[123] evaluated 26 patients with spontaneous subarachnoid hemorrhage during pregnancy and found that approximately one half were caused by berry aneurysms and one half by AV malformations. They observed that AV malformations are more common in patients younger than 25 years of age and usually bleed before 20 weeks' gestation. Conversely, berry aneurysms occur in patients older than 30 years of age and usually bleed in the third trimester. Pregnancy appears to increase the risk of bleeding from an AV malformation.

In a study of women with severe preeclampsia,[124] stroke was hemorrhagic-arterial in 25 of 27 patients and thrombotic-arterial in two others. In the 24 patients being treated immediately before the stroke, systolic blood pressure (BP) was 160 mm Hg or higher in 96 percent and more than 155 mm Hg in 100 percent. In contrast, only 13 percent exhibited prestroke diastolic pressures of 110 mm Hg or higher. Only three patients received prestroke antihypertensive medications.

Diagnosis and Treatment

Any patient with localized signs of cerebral or meningeal irritation must be thoroughly evaluated. If the clinical examination dictates that further evaluation is necessary, MRI/magnetic resonance angiography or a CT scan should be performed. If necessary, contrast dyes may be used. Cerebral angiography can be safely used to pinpoint the origin of cerebral bleeding. Subarachnoid hemorrhages, whether caused by AV malformations or berry aneurysms, should be treated surgically, when possible. Surgery under hypothermia or hypotension appears to cause no adverse fetal effects. The fetal heart rate should be monitored. If fetal bradycardia occurs, BP should be raised sufficiently to normalize the fetal heart rate.[125] Kawasaki and colleagues[126] report a case of cerebellar hemorrhage in a 32-week primigravida. She was treated conservatively until term and was delivered by elective cesarean section. Her surgery, which was delayed until after delivery, was successful. D'Haese et al.[127] have reported a case of combined cesarean delivery and clipping of an aneurysm.

If the patient has undergone corrective surgery for an aneurysm or AV malformation, she should be allowed to deliver vaginally. Because the Valsalva maneuver can increase intracranial pressure,[120] epidural anesthesia is recommended. Interestingly, Szabo and colleagues[128] have reported that moderate increases in BP do not cause spontaneous hemorrhage in nonpregnant patients with intracranial AV malformations. If the aneurysm or AV malformation has not been surgically corrected, Robinson et al.[123] recommend elective cesarean delivery. However, there are no data on which to base this decision. Therefore, the mode of delivery should be determined by the obstetrician after discussion about the individual case with neurologists, neurosurgeons, and anesthesiologists. Laidler and colleagues[129] discussed the advantages of regional anesthesia in these patients. Buckley and coworkers[130] have described a case of simultaneous cesarean delivery and ablation of a cerebral AV malformation. Levy and Jaspan have reviewed the anesthetic and obstetric management of an untreated vascular anomaly that had bled earlier in pregnancy in a patient who developed severe preeclampsia.[131]

Because pregnancy has a deleterious effect on AV malformations, those patients with inoperable lesions should be counseled about the dangers of future childbearing. The patient should be thoroughly evaluated before any recommendations are made for permanent sterilization.

Venous-venous (VV) malformations are low-pressure phenomena. Patients should progress to term and deliver vaginally without any hemorrhagic event or complications.

Women with a history of stroke have a low risk of recurrence during subsequent pregnancies, although the puerperium carries increased risk.[132,133] A previous ischemic stroke is not a contraindication to a subsequent pregnancy. Studies have not addressed the role of prophylactic anticoagulation.[133]

MULTIPLE SCLEROSIS

Multiple sclerosis (MS) is a demyelinating disease that attacks men and women equally. The onset of symptoms usually occurs between the ages of 20 and 40 years. In the United States, the disease is more common in those residing above 40 degrees north latitude. The prevalence for those living in the southern United States is 10 per 100,000, whereas it is approximately 50 per 100,000 in those living in the northern states.[134] MS has no clear genetic predisposition.

The diagnosis of MS is often made years after the initial onset of sensory symptoms. The onset is usually subtle. Common presenting symptoms include weakness of one or both lower extremities, visual complaints, and loss of coordination. Because the disease primarily affects the white matter of the CNS, symptoms attributable to disruption of gray matter are uncommon. The disease is characterized by exacerbations and remissions. Less than one third of patients show steady progression of their disease after its onset.

It is impossible to predict the long-range prognosis of a patient with MS. About one half of patients are still able to work at their usual profession 10 years after the onset of the illness. After 20 years, however, only about one third remain employed. In a study of 185 women with MS, Weinshenker and colleagues[135] showed that there was no association between long-term disability and (1) total number of term pregnancies, (2) the timing of pregnancy relative to the onset of MS, or (3) the worsening of MS in relation to a pregnancy. The average life expectancy in patients with MS is also impossible to predict. Patients may live with the disease for more than 25 years.

Runmanker and Andersen[136] demonstrated that the risk of onset of MS is reduced during gestation. whereas the risk of onset during the postpartum period was no different than for the nonpregnant state. Furthermore, these investigators demonstrated a lower risk of onset of MS in parous than in nulliparous patients. Of 170 pregnant patients with MS studied by Millar and coworkers,[137] relapses occurred in only 45, the majority during the postpartum period. Birk and coinvestigators[138] carefully followed pregnancies in eight women with MS. None worsened during pregnancy. Six of the eight women, however, experienced relapses within the first 7 weeks after delivery. They also reported that there were differences in suppressor T-cell levels during pregnancy, but these were not predictive of changes in clinical disease. The lower rate of progression and exacerbation during pregnancy may be attributable to a pregnancy-induced shift from thymus helper (Th) 1 cytokines to Th 2 cytokines, which is reversed after delivery.[139]

Frith and McLeod[140] studied 85 pregnancies and found no increased risk of relapse during pregnancy. They noted that most of the relapses that did occur during pregnancy took place in the third trimester. In another series, Frith and McLeod[141] reported that relapses occur most frequently in the last trimester and also in the first 3 months postpartum. Nelson and colleagues[142] analyzed 191 pregnancies in women with nonprogressive MS. The exacerbation rate during the 9-month postpartum period was 34 percent, three times that of the 9 months during pregnancy. The rate was highest in the 3 months immediately following delivery and stabilized after 6 months postpartum. The exacerbation rates were the same in breast-feeding and non–breast-feeding women. The average time to flare was also similar in both groups. This study verifies that it is safe for women with MS to breast-feed their newborns.

Bernardi and colleagues[143] showed a decreased risk of relapse during the 9 months of pregnancy and the first 6 months postpartum. In this study of 52 women, these researchers concluded that pregnancy, as a whole, is a protective event. Worthington et al.,[144] however, found more frequent relapses in the first 6 months postpartum, but not after that. Long-term prognosis was unaffected by pregnancy. Vendru et al.[145] demonstrated that pregnancy delays the onset of long-term disability. As an index of progression, they used the length of time from onset of disease until wheelchair dependence. In patients with at least one pregnancy after onset, the mean time to wheelchair dependence was 18.6 years compared with 12.5 years for other women. In a study encompassing 12 European countries, Confavreux and colleagues[146] studied 269 pregnancies in 254 women with MS. They determined the relapse rate in each trimester using the Kuntzke Expanded Disability Status Scale with 0 as good function and 10 as very disabled. They found the rate of relapse declined during pregnancy, especially in the third trimester. Relapses increased in the first 3 months postpartum before returning to prepregnancy rates. Neither breast-feeding nor epidural analgesia had an adverse effect on the rate of relapse or on the progression of disability.

Paraplegic patients with MS are more susceptible to urinary tract infections during pregnancy but may feel no symptoms. Therefore, they should be screened routinely. If the patient has become paraplegic or has lumbosacral lesions as a result of MS, there may be little pain associated with labor. It might be difficult therefore for the patient to discern when labor begins. Uterine contractions occur normally, but voluntary expulsive efforts may be hindered in the second stage of labor. Delivery by forceps or vacuum extraction therefore may be indicated. Dahl et al.[147] found more frequent inductions and operative interventions in women with MS, as well as a higher proportion of neonates that were small for gestational age. Mueller et al.,[148] however, found no increased risk of low birth weight or prematurity. Bader and colleagues[149] report that women with MS who receive epidural anesthesia for vaginal delivery do not have a significantly higher incidence of postpartum exacerbation of their MS than those receiving only local anesthesia.

Corticosteroids and immunosuppressive agents are occasionally used to treat MS. In one case report, plasmapheresis was instituted with dramatic improvement in a woman with rapidly progressive MS.[150] Orvieto et al.[151] report using intravenous immunoglobulins to successfully prevent MS relapses for 6 months postpartum in 14 patients. There are several new drugs and biopharmaceuticals available for the treatment of MS. There is virtually no pregnancy experience with many of these agents. Therefore, they should be used only if the neurologist and obstetrician feel that the benefits outweigh the potential risks.

CARPAL TUNNEL SYNDROME

The medial border of the carpal tunnel consists of the pisiform and hamate bones, and its lateral border consists of the scaphoid and trapezium bones. They are covered on the palmar surface by the flexor retinaculum. The median nerve and flexor tendons pass through this carpal tunnel, which has little room for expansion. If the wrist is extremely flexed or extended, the volume of the carpal tunnel is reduced. In pregnancy, weight gain and edema can produce the carpal tunnel syndrome that results from compression of the median nerve. Wallace and Cook[152] first reported the association between carpal tunnel syndrome and pregnancy in 1957. Although 20 percent of pregnant women complain of pain on the palmar surface of the hand, few actually have the true carpal tunnel syndrome.[153] Stolp-Smith et al.[154] found 50 of 14,579 (0.34 percent) pregnant patients presenting between 1987 and 1992 actually met criteria for carpal tunnel syndrome. Commonly, the syndrome consists of pain, numbness, and tingling in the distribution of the median nerve in the hand and wrist. This includes the thumb, index finger, long finger, and radial side of the ring finger on the palmar aspect. Compressing the median nerve and percussing the wrist and forearm with a reflex hammer, the Tinel maneuver, often exacerbates the pain. In severe cases, weakness and decreased motor function can occur. The definitive diagnosis is made by electromyography, but this test is often unnecessary.

McLennan and coworkers[155] studied 1,216 consecutive pregnancies. Of these patients, 427 (35 percent) reported hand symptoms. Fewer than 20 percent of these 427 affected women described the classic carpal tunnel syndrome. No patient required operative intervention. Most symptoms were bilateral and commenced in the third trimester of pregnancy. Ekman-Ordeberg et al.[156] found a 2.3-percent incidence of carpal tunnel syndrome in a prospective study of 2,358 pregnancies. The syndrome appeared to be more common in primigravidas with generalized edema. Increased weight gain during pregnancy also raises the risk.[157] Conservative therapy with splinting of the wrist at night completely relieved symptoms in 46 of 56 patients.[156] Of the remaining 10 women, three required surgery before delivery. In Stolp-Smith's study, symptoms began with equal frequency in all trimesters, but diagnosis was delayed until the third trimester in 50 percent of the patients.[154] Only four patients required surgical intervention during gestation, and three additional patients required surgery postpartum. Wand[158] retrospectively studied 40 women with carpal tunnel syndrome developing in pregnancy and 18 women with carpal tunnel syndrome that occurred in the puerperium. He confirmed that the syndrome occurs most frequently in primigravidas older than 30 years of age. All cases that developed before delivery occurred during the third trimester and resolved within 2 weeks after delivery. In those cases developing during the puerperium in women who breastfed their infants, the symptoms lasted longer, a mean of 5.8 months. In another series, Wand[159] studied 27 women who developed carpal tunnel syndrome during the puerperium. The condition was associated with breast-feeding in 24 of these women. Symptoms lasted an average of 6.5 months in the breast-feeding women. Only two of these patients required surgical decompression.

Supportive and conservative therapies are usually adequate for the treatment of carpal tunnel syndrome. Symptoms usually subside in the postpartum period as total body water returns to normal. Pain scores fall by one half during the first week after delivery and by half again during the next week.[160] The reduction in score is strongly correlated with loss of the weight gained during pregnancy. However, about half of the women with carpal tunnel syndrome during pregnancy still have some symptoms one year later,[161,162] more commonly in those whose symptoms started early in pregnancy.

Splints placed on the dorsum of the hand, which keep the wrist in a neutral position and maximize the capacity of the carpal tunnel, often provide dramatic relief. Local injections of glucocorticoids may also be used in severe cases. Although diuretics may help to control the symptoms of carpal tunnel syndrome over a short period of time, their use is not recommended because the symptoms return rather rapidly after the cessation of treatment. In an uncontrolled series, Ellis[163] reported that pyridoxine in a dose of 100 to 200 mg daily for 12 weeks provided relief in a large percentage of patients with carpal tunnel syndrome. Before this can be recommended, controlled trials need to be undertaken.

Surgical correction of this syndrome should not be delayed in patients with deteriorating muscle tone and motor function. Even small changes can be documented by EMG which can be carried out safely during pregnancy. Decompression surgery for carpal tunnel syndrome is a simple procedure that can be safely carried out during pregnancy using local anesthesia, an axillary block, or a Bier block. With new endoscopic procedures, the procedure is even less invasive. Assmus and Hashemi[164] report 314 hands surgically treated during pregnancy or the puerperium for carpal tunnel syndrome. One hundred thirty-three cases were performed during pregnancy, most in the last trimester including four who had both hands treated simultaneously. Of the patients, 98 percent reported good or excellent results.[164] There were no complications, and local anesthesia was used in all cases. These authors recommend surgery if sensory loss is present or if motor latency is more than 5 msec. It is important to warn patients that carpal tunnel syndrome can recur in future pregnancies.[165]

PSEUDOTUMOR CEREBRI AND IDIOPATHIC INTRACRANIAL HYPERTENSION

Pseudotumor cerebri is an older term, which encompasses known causes of the syndrome such as vitamin A toxicity, as well as the idiopathic form. Idiopathic intracranial hypertension (ICH) describes the majority of cases, which typically occur in obese women.

ICH may complicate as many as 1 in 870 births.[166] It has been thought to be seen more frequently in pregnant women, particularly those who are obese.[167–169] However, in a study by Ireland and colleagues[170] the incidences in pregnant women and in oral contraceptive users were no higher than in control groups. More than 95 percent of these patients present with headaches, and 15 percent have diplopia. Papilledema is found in virtually all patients.[167,169] To establish the diagnosis, one must demonstrate elevated cerebrospinal fluid (CSF) pressure, normal CSF composition, and the absence of an intracranial mass on MRI or CT scan.[171]

The pathogenesis of this disorder is unknown. Bates and colleagues[172] found CSF prolactin to be markedly elevated in cases of ICH. Prolactin appears to have an affinity for receptors in the choroid plexus, where CSF is produced. Prolactin has osmoregulatory functions and, therefore, may have a role in the increased CSF production found in ICH.[167] Some believe that reduced CSF reabsorption is the etiology. Ahlskog and O'Neill[173] noted an association between the occurrence of ICH and the following conditions: corticosteroid therapy and its withdrawal, nalidixic acid therapy, nitrofurantoin therapy, tetracycline therapy, hypoparathyroidism, deficiencies or excesses of vitamin A, and iron deficiency anemia.

Pregnancy outcome appears to be unaffected by the illness.[167,171] There is no increase in fetal wastage or congenital anomalies.[167] Koppel and colleagues[174] reported a case of ICH that presented in a 15-year-old primigravida following eclampsia. It lasted for 3 weeks. Wheatley and colleagues[175] noted a case of ICH occurring in a pregnancy complicated by diabetes mellitus. They caution that it is important to make the distinction between symptoms of ICH and visual impairment caused by diabetic retinopathy, because the treatments are different. Thomas[176] described a case of ICH occurring in two consecutive pregnancies in a woman with hemoglobin SC. In both instances, symptoms resolved following delivery and both infants were born at term.

Most patients respond well to conservative management.[177] The main objectives of treatment are relief of pain and preservation of vision. The patient should be followed closely with visual acuity and visual field determinations at intervals indicated by the clinical condition. In patients with mild disease, analgesics may be adequate. If pain persists, diuretics may be used. Acetazolamide, a carbonic anhydrase inhibitor, will reduce CSF production in many patients,[177] and no adverse effects have been found with its use in pregnancy.[178] The usual dose is 500 mg twice daily. In more difficult cases, prednisone in doses of 40 to 60 mg daily usually provides good results.[166] Patients may be treated for 2 weeks, with the dose being tapered over the next month.[167] Serial lumbar punctures to reduce CSF pressure are rarely necessary today. Surgical approaches are reserved for refractory patients in whom rapid visual deterioration occurs.

ICH is not an indication for cesarean delivery. A review of the literature reveals that 73 percent of the reported patients delivered vaginally.[167] Cesarean delivery should be undertaken only for obstetric indications. Both epidural and spinal anesthesia, when expertly administered, can be safely used in patients with ICH.[179] Bearing down, which can increase CSF pressure, should be avoided when possible. Therefore, the second stage of labor should be shortened by outlet forceps or by vacuum extraction when possible.

The recurrence rate for ICH appears to be between 10 and 12.3 percent in nonpregnant patients.[168,169] Pregnancy does not appear to predispose to a recurrence.[167]

KEY POINTS

- Idiopathic seizures affect approximately 1 percent of the general population and are the most frequent neurologic complication of pregnancy.
- Prepregnancy counseling is imperative in the patient with a seizure disorder, and preconceptional folic acid therapy, 4 mg daily, should be implemented in patients receiving anticonvulsants under the direction of an obstetrician and a neurologist.
- Those women with seizures occurring less than once each month will most likely have the best control of seizures during pregnancy.
- The anticonvulsant medication that best controls the patient's seizures should be used during pregnancy.
- Because of the changes in plasma volume, drug distribution, and metabolism that occur during pregnancy, anticonvulsant levels should be checked and dosages adjusted when clinically indicated.
- Patients taking anticonvulsants have an increased risk of giving birth to an infant with both major and

minor anomalies, but this risk is less than 10 percent. Therefore, the majority of patients with epilepsy give birth to healthy infants.

❑ Carbamazepine and valproate are associated with an increased risk of NTDs, as well as other anomalies.

❑ The pattern of physical abnormalities observed in the infants of patients taking anticonvulsants is related to the dose, type, and number of anticonvulsant drugs, rather than the epilepsy itself.

❑ Pregnancy does not hasten the onset of MS, nor does it hasten the onset of disability from MS. Exacerbations are decreased during pregnancy.

❑ Carpal tunnel syndrome is common in pregnancy and usually responds to conservative splinting, glucocorticoid injection, or both. Surgery can be safely undertaken if indicated during pregnancy.

REFERENCES

1. Williams J, Myson V, Steward S, et al: Self-discontinuation of antiepileptic medication in pregnancy: Detection by hair analysis. Epilepsia 43:824, 2002.
2. Cramer JA, Jones EE: Reproductive function in epilepsy. Epilepsia 32(Suppl 6):S19, 1991.
3. Back DJ, Bates M, Bowden A, et al: The interaction of phenobarbital and other anticonvulsants with oral contraceptive steroid therapy. Contraception 22:495, 1980.
4. Coulam CB, Annegers JF: Do anticonvulsants reduce the efficacy of oral contraceptives? Epilepsia 20:519, 1979.
5. Janz D, Schmidt D: Anti-epileptic drugs and failure of oral contraceptives. Lancet 1:1113, 1974.
6. Richens A: Safety of lamotrigine. Epilepsia 35 (Suppl 5):S37, 1994.
7. Webber MP, Hauser WA, Ottman R, Annegers JF: Fertility in persons with epilepsy: 1935–1974. Epilepsia 27:746, 1986.
8. Dansky LV, Anderman E, Anderman F: Marriage and fertility in epileptic patients. Epilepsia 21:261, 1980.
9. Artama M, Isojarvi JI, Raitanen J, et al: Birth rate among patients with epilepsy: A nationwide population-based cohort study in Finland. Am J Epidemiol 159:1057, 2004.
10. Knight AH, Rhind EG: Epilepsy and pregnancy: a study of 153 pregnancies in 59 patients. Epilepsia 16:99, 1975.
11. Schmidt D, Canger R, Avanzini G, et al: Change of seizure frequency in pregnant epileptic women. J Neurol Neurosurg Psychiatry 46:751, 1983.
12. Tanganelli P, Regesta G: Epilepsy, pregnancy, and major birth anomalies: an Italian prospective, controlled study. Neurology 42(Suppl 5):89, 1992.
13. Sabers A, Rogvi-Hansen B, Dam M, et al: Pregnancy and epilepsy: a retrospective study of 151 pregnancies. Acta Neurol Scand 97:164, 1998.
14. Landon MJ, Kirkley M: Metabolism of diphenylhydantoin (phenytoin) during pregnancy. Br J Obstet Gynaecol 86:125, 1979.
15. Kochenour NK, Emery MG, Sawohuck RJ: Phenytoin metabolism in pregnancy. Obstet Gynecol 56:577, 1980.
16. Yerby MS, Friel PN, McCormick K, et al: Pharmacokinetics of anticonvulsants in pregnancy: alterations in plasma protein binding. Epilepsy Res 5:223, 1990.
17. Desmond MM, Schwanecke RP, Wilson GS, et al: Maternal barbiturate utilization and neonatal withdrawal symptomatology. J Pediatr 80:190, 1972.
18. Tran TA, Leppik IE, Blesi K, et al: Lamotrigine clearance during pregnancy. Neurology 59:251, 2002.
19. Ogawa Y, Kaneko S, Otani K, Fukushima Y: Serum folic acid in epileptic mothers and their relationship to congenital malformations. Epilepsy Res 8:75, 1991.
20. Milunsky A, Jick H, Jick SS, et al: Multivitamin/folic acid supplementation in early pregnancy reduces the prevalence of neural tube defects. JAMA 262:2847, 1989.
21. Mountain KR, Hirsh J, Gallus AS: Neonatal coagulation defect due to anticonvulsant drug treatment in pregnancy. Lancet 1:265, 1970.
22. Bleyer WA, Skinner AL: Fatal neonatal hemorrhage after maternal anticonvulsant therapy. JAMA 235:626, 1976.
23. Kaaja E, Kaaja R, Matila R, et al: Enzyme-inducing antiepileptic drugs in pregnancy and the risk of bleeding in the neonate. Neurology 58:549, 2002.
24. Yerby M, Koepsell T, Daling J: Pregnancy complications and outcomes in a cohort of women with epilepsy. Epilepsia 26:631, 1985.
25. Nelson KB, Ellenberg JH: Maternal seizure disorder, outcome of pregnancy, and neurologic abnormalities in the children. Neurology 32:1247, 1982.
26. Kallen B: A register study of maternal epilepsy and delivery outcome with special reference to drug use. Acta Neurol Scand 73:253, 1986.
27. Hiilesmaa VK, Bardy A, Teramo K: Obstetric outcome in women with epilepsy. Am J Obstet Gynecol 152:499, 1985.
28. Mastroiacovo P, Bertollini R, Licata D: Fetal growth in the offspring of epileptic women: results of an Italian multicentric cohort study. Acta Neurol Scand 78:110, 1988.
29. Hiilesmaa VK, Teramo K, Granstrom ML: Fetal head growth retardation associated with maternal antiepileptic drugs. Lancet 1:165, 1981.
30. Hvas CL, Henriksen TB, Ostergaard JR, Dam M: Epilepsy and pregnancy: effect of antiepileptic drugs and lifestyle on birthweight. Br J Obstet Gynaecol 107:896, 2000.
31. Battine D, Keneko S, Andermann E, et al: Intrauterine growth in the offspring of epileptic women: a prospective multicenter study. Epilepsy Res 36:53, 1999.
32. Richmond JR, Krishnamoorthy P, Andermann E, et al: Epilepsy and pregnancy: A obstetric perspective. Am J Obstet Gynecol 190:371, 2004.
33. Viinikainen K, Heinonen S, Eriksson K, et al: Community-based, prospective, controlled study of obstetric and neonatal outcome of 179 pregnancies in women with epilepsy. Epilepsia 47:186, 2006.
34. Hanson JW, Smith DW: The fetal hydantoin syndrome. J Pediatr 87:285, 1975.
35. Hanson JW, Myrianthopoulos NC, Sedgwick Harvey MA, Smith DW: Risks to the offspring of women treated with hydantoin anticonvulsants, with emphasis on the fetal hydantoin syndrome. J Pediatr 89:662, 1976.
36. Gaily E, Granstrom ML, Hiilesmaa V, Bardy A: Minor anomalies in offspring of epileptic mothers. J Pediatr 112:520, 1988.
37. Rosa FW: Spina bifida in infants of women treated with carbamazepine during pregnancy. N Engl J Med 324:674, 1991.
38. Nakane Y, Okuma T, Takahashi R, et al: Multi-institutional study on the teratogenicity and fetal toxicity of antiepileptic drugs: a report of a collaborative study group in Japan. Epilepsia 21:663, 1980.
39. Canger R, Battine D, Canevini MP, et al: Malformations in offspring of women with epilepsy: a prospective study. Epilepsia 40:1231, 1999.
40. Kaneko S, Otani K, Fukushima Y, et al: Teratogenicity of antiepileptic drugs: analysis of possible risk factors. Epilepsia 29:459, 1988.
41. Kaneko S, Otani K, Kondo T, et al: Malformation in infants of mothers with epilepsy receiving antiepileptic drugs. Neurology 42(Suppl 5):68, 1992.
42. Jick SS, Terris BZ: Anticonvulsants and congenital malformations. Pharmacotherapy 17:561, 1997.
43. Lindhout D, Meinardi H, Meijer JWA, Nau H: Antiepileptic drugs and teratogenesis in two consecutive cohorts: changes in prescription policy paralleled by changes in pattern of malformations. Neurology 42(Suppl 5):94, 1992.

44. Dravet C, Julian C, Legras C, et al: Epilepsy, antiepileptic drugs, and malformations in children of women with epilepsy: a French prospective cohort study. Neurology 42(Suppl 5):75, 1992.
45. Koch S, Losche G, Jager-Roman E, et al: Major and minor birth malformations and antiepileptic drugs. Neurology 42(Suppl 5):83, 1992.
46. Gaily E, Granstrom ML: Minor anomalies in children of mothers with epilepsy. Neurology 42(Suppl 5):128, 1992.
47. Yerby MS, Leavitt A, Erickson M, et al: Antiepileptics and the development of congenital anomalies. Neurology 42(Suppl 5):132, 1992.
48. Nulman I, Scolnik D, Chitayat D, et al: Findings in children exposed in utero to phenytoin and carbamazepine monotherapy: independent effects of epilepsy and medications. Am J Med Genet 68:18, 1997.
49. DiLiberti JH, Farndon PA, Dennis NR, Curry CJR: The fetal valproate syndrome. Am J Med Genet 19:473, 1984.
50. Ardinger HH, Atkin JF, Blackston RD, et al: Verification of the fetal valproate syndrome phenotype. Am J Med Genet 29:171, 1988.
51. Jager-Roman E, Deichl A, Jakob S, et al: Fetal growth, major malformations, and minor anomalies in infants born to women receiving valproic acid. J Pediatr 108:997, 1986.
52. Lindhout D, Schmidt D: In-utero exposure to valproate and neural tube defects. Lancet 2:1392, 1986.
53. Lindhout D, Omtzigt JGC, Cornel MC: Spectrum of neural-tube defects in 34 infants prenatally exposed to antiepileptic drugs. Neurology 42(Suppl 5):111, 1992.
54. Wegner C, Nau H: Alteration of embryonic folate metabolism by valproic acid during organogenesis: implications for mechanism of teratogenesis. Neurology 42(Suppl 5):17, 1992.
55. Tomson T, Perucca E, Battino D: Navigating toward fetal and maternal health: The challenge of treating epilepsy in pregnancy. Epilepsia 45:1171, 2004.
56. Wyszynski DF, Nambisan M, Surve T, et al: Increased rate of major malformations in offspring exposed to valproate during pregnancy. Neurology 64:961, 2005.
57. Koren G, Nava-Ocampo AA, Moretti ME, et al: Major malformations with valproic acid. Can Fam Physician 52:441, 2006.
58. Artama M, Auvinen A, Raudaskoski T, et al: Antiepileptic drug use of women with epilepsy and congenital malformations in offspring. Neurology 64:1874, 2005.
59. Wide K, Winbladh B, Kallen B: Major malformations in infants exposed to antiepileptic drugs in utero, with emphasis on carbamazepine and valproic acid: A nation-wide, population-based register study. Acta Paediatrica 93:174, 2004.
60. Morrow J, Russell A, Guthrie E, et al: Malformation risks of antiepileptic drugs in pregnancy: A prospective study from the UK Epilepsy and Pregnancy Register. J Neurol Neurosurg Psychiatry 77:193, 2006.
61. Holmes LB, Harvey EA, Coull BA, et al: The teratogenicity of anticonvulsant drugs. N Engl J Med 344:1132, 2001.
62. Jones KL, Lacro RV, Johnson KA, Adams J: Pattern of malformations in the children of women treated with carbamazepine during pregnancy. N Engl J Med 320:1661, 1989.
63. Rosa FW: Spina bifida in infants of women treated with carbamazepine during pregnancy. N Engl J Med 324:674, 1991.
64. Matalon S, Schechtman S, Goldzweig G, et al: The teratogenic effect of carbamazepine: A meta-analysis of 1255 exposures. Reprod Toxicol 16:9, 2002.
65. Finnell RH, Buehler BA, Kerr BM, et al: Clinical and experimental studies linking oxidative metabolism to phenytoininduced teratogenesis. Neurology 42(Suppl 5):25, 1992.
66. Dichter MA, Brodie MJ: New antiepileptic drugs. N Engl J Med 334:1583, 1996.
67. Gilman JT: Lamotrigine: an antiepileptic agent for the treatment of partial seizures. Ann Pharmacother 29:144, 1995.
68. Mackay FJ, Wilton LV, Pearce GL, et al: Safety of long-term lamotrigine in epilepsy. Epilepsia 38:881, 1997.
69. Ohman I, Vitols S, Tomson T: Lamotrigine in pregnancy: pharmacokinetics during delivery, in the neonate, and during lactation. Epilepsia 41:709, 2000.
70. GlaxoSmithKline International, Lamotrigine Pregnancy Registry, Interim Report, 1/2005.
70a. Holmes LB, Wyszynski DF, Baldwin EJ, et al: Increased risk for non-syndromic cleft palate among infants exposed to lamotrigine during pregnancy. Birth Defects Res 76:5, 2006.
71. Granstrom ML, Gaily E: Psychomotor development in children of mothers with epilepsy. Neurology 42(Suppl 5):144, 1992.
72. Gaily E, Kantola-Sorsa E, Granstrom ML: Intelligence of children of epileptic mothers. J Pediatr 113:677, 1988.
73. Moore SJ, Turnpenny P, Quinn A, et al: A clinical study of 57 children with fetal anticonvulsant syndromes. J Med Genet 37:489, 2000.
74. Dean JC, Hailey H, Moore SJ, et al: Long term health and neurodevelopment in children exposed to antiepileptic drugs before birth. J Med Genetics 39:251, 2002.
75. Parisi P, Francia A, Vanacore N, et al: Psychomotor development and general movements in offspring of women with epilepsy and anticonvulsant therapy. Early Hum Dev 74:97, 2003.
76. Adab N, Kini U, Vinten J, et al: The longer term outcome of children born to mothers with epilepsy. J Neurology Neurosurg Psychiatry 75:1575, 2004.
77. Dansky LV, Andermann E, Rosenblatt D, et al: Anticonvulsants, folate levels, and pregnancy outcome: a prospective study. Ann Neurol 21:176, 1987.
78. Annegers JF, Hauser WA, Elveback LR, et al: Seizure disorders in offspring of patients with a history of seizures a maternal paternal difference? Epilepsia 17:1, 1976.
79. Blandfort M, Tsuboi T, Vogel F: Genetic counseling in the epileptics. Hum Genet 76:303, 1987.
80. Bronshtein M, Zimmer EZ, Gerlis LM, et al: Early ultrasound diagnosis of fetal congenital heart defects in high-risk and low-risk pregnancies. Obstet Gynecol 82:225, 1993.
81. Wigton TR, Sabbagha RE, Tamura RK, et al: Sonographic diagnosis of congenital heart disease: comparison between the four-chamber view and multiple cardiac views. Obstet Gynecol 82:219, 1993.
82. Yerby MS: Problems and management of the pregnant woman with epilepsy. Epilepsia 28(Suppl 3):S29, 1987.
83. Orland MJ, Saltman RJ: Seizures. Washington Manual of Medical Therapeutics, 25th ed. 1986.
84. Sibai BM, Spinnato JA, Watson DL, et al: Eclampsia IV. Neurological findings and future outcome. Am J Obstet Gynecol 152:184, 1985.
85. Kaneko S, Sato T, Suzuki K: The levels of anticonvulsants in breast milk. Br J Clin Pharmacol 7:624, 1974.
86. Mattson RH, Cramer JA, Darney PD, Naftolin F: Use of oral contraceptives by women with epilepsy. JAMA 256:238, 1986.
87. ACOG Committee on Practice Bulletins: Use of hormonal contraception in women with coexisting medical conditions. Obstet Gynecol 107:1453, 2006.
88. Maggioni F, Alessi C, Maggino T, Zanchin G: Headache during pregnancy. Cephalalgia 17:765, 1997.
89. Granella F, Sances G, Zanferrar C, et al: Migraine without aura and reproductive life events: a clinical epidemiological study of 1300 women. Headache 33:385, 1993.
90. Aube M: Migraine in pregnancy. Neurology 53(Suppl):S26, 1999.
91. Chen TC, Leviton A, Edelstein S, Ellenberg JH: Migraine and other diseases in women of reproductive age: the influence of smoking on observed associations. Arch Neurol 44:1024, 1987.
92. Ertresvag JM, Zwart JA, Helde G, et al: Headache and transient focal neurological symptoms during pregnancy, a prospective cohort. Acta Neurol Scand 111:223, 2005.
93. Chancellor AM, Wroe SJ, Cull RE: Migraine occurring for the first time in pregnancy. Headache 30:224, 1990.
94. Jacobson SL, Redman CW: Basilar migraine with loss of consciousness in pregnancy: case report. Br J Obstet Gynaecol 96:494, 1989.
95. Silberstein SD: Headaches in pregnancy. J Headache Pain 6:172, 2005.
96. Fox AW, Diamond ML, Spierings EL: Migraine during pregnancy: Options for therapy. CNS Drugs 19:465, 2005.
97. Dey R, Khan S, Akhouri V, et al: Labetalol for prophylactic treatment of intractable migraine during pregnancy. Headache 42:642, 2002.

98. Hughes HE, Goldstein DA: Birth defects following maternal exposure to ergotamine, beta blocker, and caffeine. J Med Genet 25:396, 1988.
99. O'Quinn S, Ephross SA, Williams V, et al: Pregnancy and perinatal outcomes in migraineurs using sumatriptan: a prospective study. Arch Gynecol Obstet 263:7, 1999.
100. Olesen C, Steffensen FH, Sorensen HT, et al: Pregnancy outcome following prescription for sumatriptan. Headache 40:20, 2000.
101. Kallen B, Lygner PE: Delivery outcome in women who used drugs for migraine during pregnancy with special reference to sumatriptan. Headache 41:351, 2001.
102. Hilaire ML, Cross LB, Eichner SF: Treatment of migraine headaches with sumatriptan in pregnancy. Ann Pharmacother 38:1726, 2004.
103. James AH, Bushnell CD, Jamison MG, et al: Incidence and risk factors for stroke in pregnancy and the puerperium. Obstet Gynecol 106:509, 2005.
104. Jeng JS, Tang SC, Yip PK: Incidence and etiologies of stroke during pregnancy and puerperium as evidenced in Taiwanese women. Cerebrovascular Diseases 18:290, 2004.
105. Jennett WB, Cross JN: Influence of pregnancy and oral contraception on the incidence of strokes in women of childbearing age Lancet 1:1019, 1967.
106. Banerjee AK, Varma M, Vasista RK, Chopra JS: Cerebrovascular disease in north-west India: a study of necropsy material. J Neurol Neurosurg Psychiatry 52:512, 1989.
107. Cross JN, Castro PO, Jennett WB: Cerebral strokes associated with pregnancy in the puerperium. BMJ 3:214, 1968.
108. Berghella V, Broth RE, Chapman AE, et al: Metastatic unknown primary tumor presenting in pregnancy as multiple cerebral infarcts. Obstet Gynecol 101(5 P 2):1060, 2003.
109. Brick JF, Riggs JE: Ischemic cerebrovascular disease in the young adult: emergence of oral contraceptive use and pregnancy as the major risk factors in the 1980s. W V Med J 85:7, 1989.
110. Lidegaard O: Oral contraceptives, pregnancy and the risk of cerebral thromboembolism: the influence of diabetes, hypertension, migraine, and previous thrombotic disease. Br J Obstet Gynaecol 102:153, 1995.
111. Brick JF: Vanishing cerebrovascular disease of pregnancy. Neurology 38:804, 1988.
112. Giberti L, Bino G, Tanganelli P: Pregnancy, patent foramen ovale and stroke: A case of pseudoperipheral facial palsy. Neurological Sciences 26:43, 2005.
113. Johnson DM, Kramer DC, Cohen E, et al: Thrombolytic therapy for acute stroke in late pregnancy with intra-arterial recombinant tissue plasminogen activator. Stroke 36:53, 2005.
114. Katz VL, Cefalo RC: Maternal death from carotid artery thrombosis associated with the syndrome of hemolysis, elevated liver function, and low platelets. Am J Perinatol 6:360, 1989
115. Soh Y, Yasuhi I, Nakayama D, et al: A case of postpartum cerebellar infarction with hemolysis, elevated liver enzymes, low platelets (HELLP) syndrome. Gynecol Obstet Invest 53:240, 2002.
116. Estanol B, Rodriguez A, Counte G, et al: Intracranial venous thrombosis in young women. Stroke 10:680, 1979.
117. Krayenbuhl HA: Cerebral venous and sinus thrombosis. Clin Neurosurg 14:1, 1967.
118. Bansal BC, Prakash C, Gupta RR, Brahmanandam KRV: Study of serum lipid and blood fibrinolytic activity in cases of cerebral venous/venous sinus thrombosis during the puerperium. Am J Obstet Gynecol 119:1079, 1974.
119. Abraham J, Rios PS, Inbaraj SG, et al: An epidemiological study of hemiplegia due to stroke in south India. Stroke 1:477, 1970.
120. Stocks GM, Wooller DJ, Young JM, et al: Postpartum headache after epidural blood patch: Investigation and diagnosis. Brit J Anaesth 84:407, 2000.
121. Miller HJ, Hinkley CM: Berry aneurysms in pregnancy: a ten year report. South Med J 63:279, 1970.
122. Henderson CE, Torbey M: Rupture of intracranial aneurysm associated with cocaine use during pregnancy. Am J Perinatol 5:142, 1988.
123. Robinson JL, Hall CJ, Sevzimer CB: Arterial venous malformations, aneurysms, and pregnancy. J Neurosurg 41:63, 1974.
124. Martin JN Jr, Thigpen BD, Moore RC, et al: Stroke and severe preeclampsia and eclampsia: A paradigm shift focusing on systolic blood pressure. Obstet Gynecol 105:246, 2005.
125. Minielly R, Yuzpe AA, Drake CC: Subarachnoid hemorrhage secondary to ruptured cerebral aneurysm in pregnancy. Obstet Gynecol 53:64, 1979.
126. Kawasaki N, Uchida T, Yamada M, et al: Conservative management of cerebellar hemorrhage in pregnancy. Int J Gynaecol Obstet 31:365, 1990.
127. D'Haese J, Christiaens F, d'Haens J, Camu F: Combined cesarean section and clipping of a ruptured cerebral aneurysm: a case report. J Neurosurg Anesthesiol 9:341, 1997.
128. Szabo MD, Crosby C, Sundaram P, et al: Hypertension does not cause spontaneous hemorrhage of intracranial arteriovenous malformations. Anesthesiology 70:761, 1989.
129. Laidler JA, Jackson IJ, Redfern N: The management of caesarean section in a patient with an intracranial arteriovenous malformation. Anaesthesia 44:490, 1989.
130. Buckley TA, Yau GH, Poon WS, Oh T: Caesarean section and ablation of a cerebral arteriovenous malformation. Anaesth Intensive Care 18:248, 1990.
131. Levy DM, Jaspan T: Anaesthesia for caesarean section in a patient with recent subarachnoid haemorrhage and severe pre-eclampsia. Anaesthesia 54:994, 1999.
132. Lanska DJ, Kryscio RJ: Risk factors for peripartum and postpartum stroke and intracranial venous thrombosis. Stroke 31(6):1274–82, 2000.
133. Coppage KH, Hinton AC, Moldenhauer J, et al: Maternal and perinatal outcome in women with a history of stroke. Am J Obstet Gynecol 190:1331, 2004.
134. McAlpine D, Lumsden CE, Acheson ED: Multiple Sclerosis, a Reappraisal, 2nd ed. Baltimore, Williams & Wilkins, 1972.
135. Weinshenker BG, Hader W, Carriere W, et al: The influence of pregnancy on disability from multiple sclerosis: a population-based study in Middlesex County, Ontario. Neurology 39:1438, 1989.
136. Runmanker B, Andersen O: Pregnancy is associated with a lower risk of onset and a better prognosis in multiple sclerosis. Brain 118:253, 1995.
137. Millar JHD, Allison RS, Cheeseman EA: Pregnancy as a factor influencing relapse in disseminated sclerosis. Brain 82:417, 1959.
138. Birk K, Ford C, Smeltzer S, et al: The clinical course of multiple sclerosis during pregnancy and the puerperium. Arch Neurol 47:738, 1990.
139. Al-Shammri S, Rawoot P, Azizieh F, et al: Th1/Th2 cytokine patterns and clinical profiles during and after pregnancy in women with multiple sclerosis. J Neurol Sci 222:21, 2004.
140. Frith JA, McLeod JC: Pregnancy and multiple sclerosis. J Neurol Neurosurg Psychiatry 51:495, 1988.
141. Frith JA, McLeod JG: Pregnancy and multiple sclerosis: an Australian perspective. Clin Exp Neurol 24:1, 1987.
142. Nelson LM, Franklin GM, Jones MC: Risk of multiple sclerosis exacerbation during pregnancy and breast-feeding. JAMA 259:3441, 1988.
143. Bernardi S, Grasso MG, Bertollini R, et al: The influences of pregnancy on relapses of multiple sclerosis: a cohort study. Acta Neurol Scand 84:403, 1991.
144. Worthington J, Jones R, Crawford M, Forti A: Pregnancy and multiple sclerosis-a 3-year prospective study. J Neurol 241:228, 1994.
145. Verdru P, Theys P, D'Hooghe MB, Carton H: Pregnancy and multiple sclerosis: the influence on longterm disability. Clin Neurol Neurosurg 96:38, 1994.
146. Confavreux C, Hutchinson M, Hours MM, et al: Rate of pregnancy-related relapse in multiple sclerosis. Pregnancy in Multiple Sclerosis Group. N Engl J Med 339:285, 1998.
147. Dahl J, Myhr KM, Daltveit AK, et al: Pregnancy, delivery, and birth outcome in women with multiple sclerosis. Neurology 65:1961, 2005.
148. Mueller Ba, Zhang J, Critchlow CW: Birth outcomes and need for hospitalization after delivery among women with multiple sclerosis. Am J Obstet Gynecol 186:446, 2002.
149. Bader AM, Hunt CO, Datta S, et al: Anesthesia for the obstetric patient with multiple sclerosis. J Clin Anesth 1:21, 1988.

150. Khatri BO, D'Cruz O, Preissler G, et al: Plasmaphoresis in a pregnant patient with multiple sclerosis. Arch Neurol 47:11, 1990.
151. Orvieto R, Achiron R, Rotstein Z, et al: Pregnancy and multiple sclerosis: a 2-year experience. Eur J Obstet Gynecol Reprod Biol 82:191, 1999.
152. Wallace JT, Cook AW: Carpal tunnel syndrome in pregnancy. Am J Obstet Gynecol 73:1333, 1957.
153. Nicholas CG, Noone RB, Graham WP: Carpal tunnel syndrome in pregnancy. Hand 3:80, 1971.
154. Stolp-Smith KA, Pascoe MK, Ogburn PL Jr: Carpal tunnel syndrome in pregnancy: frequency severity and prognosis. Arch Phys Med Rehabil 79:1285, 1998.
155. McLennan HG, Oats JN, Walstab JE: Survey of hand symptoms in pregnancy. Med J Aust 147:542, 1987.
156. Ekman-Ordeberg G, Salgeback S, Ordeberg G: Carpal tunnel syndrome in pregnancy: a prospective study. Acta Obstet Gynecol Scand 66:233, 1987.
157. Turgut F, Cetinsahinahin M, Turgut M, et al: The management of carpal tunnel syndrome in pregnancy J Clin Neurosci 8:332, 2001.
158. Wand JS: Carpal tunnel syndrome in pregnancy and lactation. J Hand Surg 15:93, 1990.
159. Wand JS: The natural history of carpal tunnel syndrome in lactation. J R Soc Med 82:349, 1989.
160. Finsen V, Zeitlmann H: Carpal tunnel syndrome during pregnancy. Scand J Plas Recons Surg Hand Surg 40:41, 2006.
161. Pazzaglia C, Caliandro P, Aprile I, et al: Multicenter study on carpal tunnel syndrome and pregnancy incidence and natural course. Acta Neurochir 92:35, 2005.
162. Padua L, Aprile I, Caliandro P, et al: Carpal tunnel syndrome in pregnancy: Multiperspective follow-up of untreated cases. Neurology 59:1643, 2002.
163. Ellis JM: Treatment of carpal tunnel syndrome with vitamin B_6. South Med J 80:882, 1987.
164. Assmus H, Hashemi B: Surgical treatment of carpal tunnel syndrome in pregnancy: results from 314 cases. Nervenarzt 71:470, 2000.
165. Tobin SM: Carpal tunnel syndrome in pregnancy. Am J Obstet Gynecol 97:493, 1967.
166. Katz VL, Peterson R, Cefalo RC: Pseudotumor cerebri and pregnancy. Am J Perinatol 6:442, 1989.
167. Peterson CM, Kelly JV: Pseudotumor cerebri in pregnancy: case reports and literature reviewed. Obstet Gynecol Surv 40:323, 1985.
168. Weisberg LA: Benign intracranial hypertension. Medicine (Baltimore) 54:197, 1975.
169. Johnston I, Paterson A: Benign intracranial hypertension. II. CSF pressures and the circulation. Brain 97:301, 1974.
170. Ireland B, Corbett JJ, Wallace RB: The search for causes of idiopathic intracranial hypertension: a preliminary case-control study. Arch Neurol 47:315, 1990.
171. Koontz WL, Herbert WNP, Cefalo R: Pseudotumor cerebri in pregnancy. Obstet Gynecol 62:325, 1983.
172. Bates GW, Whiteworth NS, Parker JL, et al: Elevated cerebrospinal fluid prolactin concentration in women with pseudotumor cerebri. South Med J 75:807, 1982.
173. Ahlskog JE, O'Neill BP: Pseudotumor cerebri. Ann Intern Med 97:249, 1982.
174. Koppel BS, Kaunitz AM, Tuchman AJ: Pseudotumor cerebri following eclampsia. Eur Neurol 30:6, 1990.
175. Wheatley T, Clark JD, Edwards OM, Jordan K: Retinal haemorrhages and papilloedema due to benign intracranial hypertension in a pregnant diabetic. Diabetic Med 3:482, 1986.
176. Thomas E: Recurrent benign intracranial hypertension associated with hemoglobin SC disease in pregnancy. Obstet Gynecol 67:7S, 1986.
177. Rubin RC, Henderson ES, Ommaya AK, et al: The production of cerebrospinal fluid in man and its modification by acetazolamide. J Neurosurg 25:430, 1966.
178. Lee AG, Pless M, Falardeau J, et al: The use of acetazolamide in idiopathic intracranial hypertension during pregnancy. Am J Ophthal 139:855, 2005.
179. Palop R, Choed-Amphai E, Miller R: Epidural anesthesia for delivery complicated by benign intracranial hypertension. Anesthesiology 50:159, 1979.

Malignant Diseases and Pregnancy

LARRY J. COPELAND AND MARK B. LANDON

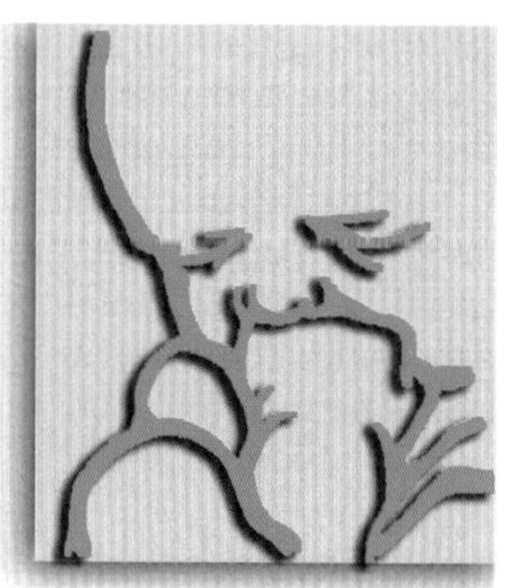

CHAPTER 45

KEY ABBREVIATIONS

Acute lymphoblastic leukemia	ALL
Acute nonlymphocytic leukemia	ANLL
β-human chorionic gonadotropin	β-hCG
Carcinoembryonic antigen	CEA
Chronic myelocytic leukemia	CML
Computed tomography	CT
Federal Drug Administration	FDA
Fine-needle aspiration	FNA
Gestational trophoblastic disease	GTD
Interferon	IFN
Magnetic resonance imaging	MRI
Nitrogen mustard, vincristine, procarbazine, prednisone chemotherapy regimen	MOPP
Transverse rectus abdominis myocutaneous flap	TRAM
World Health Organization	WHO

The juxtaposition of life and death can present numerous emotional and ethical conflicts to the patient, her family, and her physicians. The diagnosis of cancer for anyone is understandably frightening. To deal with cancer in the context of pregnancy is particularly burdensome, because the patient may have to balance competing maternal and fetal interests. On occasion, a pregnant woman may be required to make decisions affecting her life or longevity versus the life or well-being of her unborn. Cancer in pregnancy complicates the management of both the cancer and the pregnancy. Diagnostic and therapeutic interventions must carefully address the associated risks to both the patient and the fetus. Informed decisions require evaluation of a number of factors, and with counseling, these considerations are the foundation on which treatment decisions are made. There has been an evolution in the philosophy of care from one of total disregard of the pregnancy with frequent immediate termination to a more thoughtful approach in which management decisions consider both maternal and fetal outcomes so as to limit risk of death or morbidity to both.

Although cancer is the second most common cause of death for women in their reproductive years, only about 1 in 1,000 pregnancies[1] is complicated by cancer. Because there are no large prospective studies that address cancer treatment in pregnancy, physicians tend to base treatment strategies on small retrospective studies or anecdotal reports that occasionally present conflicting information.[2]

A successful outcome is dependent on a cooperative multidisciplinary approach. The management plan must be formulated within a medical, moral, ethical, legal, and religious framework that is acceptable to the patient and guided by communication and educational resources of the health care team.

The malignancies most commonly encountered in the pregnant patient are, in descending order, breast cancer, cervical cancer, melanoma, ovarian cancer, thyroid cancer, leukemia, lymphoma, and colorectal cancer.[3] The frequencies of these diseases complicating pregnancy may increase secondary to the trend to delay childbearing, and age is the most potent predictor of cancer. Before specific malignancies are discussed, some general principles are reviewed.

CHEMOTHERAPY DURING PREGNANCY

Pharmacology of Chemotherapy During Pregnancy

Because pregnancy alters physiology, there is potential for altered pharmacokinetics associated with chemotherapy. Orally administered medications are subjected to altered gastrointestinal motility. Peak drug concentrations are decreased owing to the 50-percent expansion in plasma volume, producing a longer drug half-life unless there is a concurrent increase in metabolism or excretion. The increase in plasma proteins and fall in albumin may alter drug availability, and amniotic fluid may act as a pharmacologic third space, potentially increasing toxicity due to delayed metabolism and excretion. Hepatic oxidation and renal blood flow are both elevated during pregnancy and may influence the metabolism and excretion of most drugs.[4] However, because pharmacologic studies in the pregnant woman are lacking, we currently assume that initial drug dosages are similar to that given to the nonpregnant woman and adjustments to dose are based on toxicity on a course-by-course basis.

Because most antineoplastic agents can be found in breast milk, breast-feeding is contraindicated.[5]

Drug Effects on the Fetus

ACUTE EFFECTS

Because antineoplastic agents are targeted for the rapidly dividing malignant cell, one would expect the exposed fetus to be particularly susceptible to serious toxicity. Clear documentation of such is not the case. Spontaneous abortions, fetal organ toxicity, premature birth, and low birth weight are potential risks in the pregnant patient receiving chemotherapy. Excluding the intentional use of abortifacients, it is difficult to clearly demonstrate that the use of chemotherapy results in an increase in the clinically recognized spontaneous abortion rate over the expected 15 to 20 percent. Fetal organ toxicity has not been reported as a major problem, although neonatal myelosuppression[6] and hearing loss in a 1-year-old child[7] have been reported. Because early induction of labor or surgical delivery is often a component of the overall treatment plan, it has been difficult to identify premature birth as a specific result of the chemotherapy. On the other hand, it appears that low birth weight is associated with the administration of chemotherapy in the second and third trimesters.[8]

TERATOGENICITY

All drugs undergo animal teratogenicity testing, and based on these results, the drugs are assigned risk categories (Table 45-1) by the U.S. Food and Drug Administration (FDA).[9] Based on this system, most chemotherapeutic agents are rated as C, D, or X.[9] However, animal teratogenicity testing cannot always be reliably extrapolated to humans. For example, a drug (e.g., aspirin) may show teratogenic effects in animals and not affect humans. The opposite is also true and, as such, has serious potential to do harm; for example, a drug may show no animal teratogenicity (e.g., thalidomide) but cause serious human anomalies (see Chapter 8). Because detailed ultrasonography may fail to identify subtle anatomic but serious functional abnormalities before 20 weeks' gestation, patients should be appropriately counseled and may want to consider the option of pregnancy termination if first-trimester chemotherapy is planned or administered. The risk of teratogenicity during the second and third trimesters is significantly reduced and is likely no different from that for pregnant woman who are not exposed to chemotherapy.[4]

Although the literature addressing chemotherapy administration during pregnancy is somewhat limited and dated, reviews by Nicholson[10] and Doll and col-

Table 45-1. FDA Risk Categories for Drug Use During Pregnancy

CATEGORY	DEFINITION
A	Controlled studies have demonstrated no risk, and the possibility of fetal harm appears remote.
B	*Either* animal studies have failed to identify a risk but there are no controlled studies in women, *or* animal studies have shown an adverse effect that was not confirmed in controlled studies in women.
C	*Either* animal studies have revealed adverse effects and there are no controlled studies in women, *or* studies in women and animals are not available. Use drugs only if the potential benefit justifies the potential risk to the fetus.
D	There is evidence of fetal risk, but the benefits may be acceptable despite the risk in either a life-threatening situation or a serious disease for which safer drugs are ineffective.
X	Studies in animals or humans have demonstrated fetal abnormalities, and the risk of the drug in pregnant women clearly outweighs any possible benefit.

Adapted from Briggs GG, Freeman RK, Yaffe SJ: Instructions for use of the reference guide. *In* Briggs GG, Freeman RK, Yaffe SJ (eds): A Reference Guide to Fetal and Neonatal Risk: Drugs in Pregnancy and Lactation. 5th ed. Baltimore, Williams & Wilkins, 1998, p xxii.

leagues[4] provide us with some information regarding the frequency of affected offspring. Nicholson reported that first-trimester exposure resulted in about a 10-percent frequency of major fetal malformations. For a similar situation, Doll and colleagues reported 17- and 25-percent frequencies for single-agent chemotherapy and combination chemotherapy, respectively. However, some of the patients from the latter study also received irradiation, and exclusion of these cases reduces the malformation rate to 6 percent. The risk of fetal malformation varies with the drug classification and specific drug. In general, antimetabolites and the alkylating agents appear to carry the highest risk.[11]

ANTIMETABOLITES

Historically, aminopterin was used as an abortifacient, and in cases of failed abortion, the risk of fetal malformation was about 50 percent. Methotrexate has replaced aminopterin for chemotherapeutic purposes, and although similar types of anomalies occur, a lower overall frequency of 7 percent has been reported.[11] The use of low-dose methotrexate for systemic diseases (e.g., rheumatic disease and psoriasis) does not appear to produce teratogenicity.[12]

ALKYLATING AGENTS

The alkylating agents are a commonly used group of drugs for the management of malignancies. Unfortunately, most of the alkylating agents have demonstrated some teratogenic potential. Because these drugs are frequently given in combination with other nonalkylating agents, it is often difficult to identify the risk specific to the alkylating agent.

ANTITUMOR ANTIBIOTICS

Even when administered in early pregnancy, antitumor antibiotics appear to be associated with a low risk of teratogenicity. There is conflicting information in the literature as to whether the anthracyclines cross the placenta.[13–15] There is no evidence of bleomycin or dactinomycin teratogenicity.[16–18]

VINCA ALKALOIDS

Vincristine and vinblastine, although potent teratogens in animals, do not appear to be as teratogenic in humans.[19]

MISCELLANEOUS

Cisplatin has been used in at least 10 pregnancies[7,16–26] without fetal malformation or toxicity, other than the possible abnormality reported by Elit and colleagues.[20] Henderson and colleagues[7] reported bilateral sensorineural hearing loss at age 1 following in utero second-trimester exposure to carboplatin. However, other potential causes of the hearing loss existed in this infant, including prematurity, prior cisplatin exposure, and neonatal gentamicin. Procarbazine and asparginase have both been associated with subsequent fetal malformations.[4,10,27]

Taxane chemotherapy is employed in the treatment of malignant tumors of multiple sites, and experience with this class of drugs remains limited, although a few reports to date are favorable.[28,29]

COMBINATION CHEMOTHERAPY

There is no convincing evidence that there is a synergistic effect on the rate of malformations with the use of multiple-agent regimens when compared with single-agent therapy.[4,10]

NATIONAL REGISTRY

In 1984, the National Cancer Institute established a national registry for in utero exposure to chemotherapy.[30–32] The registry is currently located at the University of Oklahoma, under the direction of Dr. John J. Mulvihill (jmulvihill@ouhsc.edu). Through September 2006, the registry had summaries of 720 pregnancies. The rate of anomalies following first-trimester exposure was 19 percent, versus 6 percent after later exposure (and 3 percent in the general population). Of 422 pregnancies with third-trimester exposure, 66 (16 percent) of newborns had a functional abnormality, which was primarily myelosuppression occurring in a frequency related to time between last chemotherapy and delivery.

DELAYED EFFECTS

Although second malignancies, impaired growth and development, intellectual impairment, and infertility have been reported after chemotherapy administration to children, the delayed effects of in utero exposure are less well documented.[6,33,34]

In summary, the risks of exposing a fetus to chemotherapy correlate highly with the gestational age at the time of the exposure. Most organogenesis occurs between 3 and 8 weeks of embryonic life, and it is during this time that major structural abnormalities are most likely to occur from exposure to chemotherapeutic agents. Second- and third-trimester chemotherapy exposure does not appear to carry a significantly increased risk of major fetal anomalies.

RADIATION, DIAGNOSTIC AND THERAPEUTIC

The potential for fetal injury arises from exposure to ionizing radiation, both the low-dose diagnostic procedures and the more intense doses associated with radiation therapy. This subject is discussed in Chapter 8. In general, magnetic resonance imaging (MRI) is probably the safest, most useful imaging technique in the pregnant patient.[35]

SURGERY AND ANESTHESIA, GENERAL FACTORS

Although aspects of surgery are addressed later under the specific cancer sites, some general principles should be considered. Although complications of surgery can threaten the fetus, extraperitoneal surgery is not related to spontaneous abortion or preterm labor. Abdominal or pelvic surgery, if flexibility in timing exists, is best performed in the second trimester to limit the risk of first-trimester spontaneous abortion or preterm labor. In the first trimester, progesterone therapy is indicated (weeks 7 to 12) following a bilateral oophorectomy. Perioperative cautions include attention to the relative safety of all drugs administered. Fever secondary to either infection or atelectasis should be treated promptly, because it may be associated with fetal abnormalities.

There is no evidence that there are significant risks of anesthesia independent of coexisting disease.[36] In the second and third trimesters, careful attention to positioning is required so as to avoid compression of the vena cava from the enlarged uterus. Finally, continuous or intermittent fetal monitoring should be employed in cases in which extrauterine survival is possible.

PREGNANCY FOLLOWING CANCER TREATMENT

With improved survival rates for many childhood and adolescent malignancies, one must be prepared to offer prenatal counseling to the young woman who presents with a cancer history.[37] Issues worthy of review and in need of clarification for the obstetrician and the patient are listed in the box "Counseling Issues for Pregnancy Following Cancer Treatment."

Previous abdominal irradiation for a Wilms' tumor appears to adversely affect the risk of pregnancy complications, including increased perinatal mortality, low birth weight, and abnormal pregnancy. In contrast, a review of pregnancies following treatment for Hodgkin's lymphoma revealed no increase in poor pregnancy outcome.[38] However, the rate of ovarian failure following the multiple drug combinations is greater than 50 percent in some reports.[39] Also, a combination of pelvic irradiation and chemotherapy for Hodgkin's disease results in an even higher rate of ovarian failure. Over recent years, a number of women with early cervical cancer have received fertility preservation surgery with radical trachelectomy and regional lymphadenectomy. The preliminary fertility and pregnancy outcomes have been favorable.[40,41]

Will pregnancy increase the risk of recurrence or accelerate recurrence? Even in women with estrogen receptor–positive breast cancer, there is no evidence that subsequent pregnancy adversely affects survival. In addition to the altered hormonal milieu, concern is also directed toward the potential for accelerated tumor activity associated with alterations in the pregnant patient's immune system. There are no data to support this concern. Long-term follow-up studies of children with in utero exposure to antineoplastic agents have not demonstrated any impairment in growth, despite an increased frequency of intrauterine growth restriction.[6,33] In those children who have been tested for intellectual development, no impairment has been identified.[42]

Counseling Issues for Pregnancy Following Cancer Treatment

1. What is the risk of recurrence of the malignancy?
2. If a recurrence was diagnosed, depending on the most likely sites, what would be the nature of the probable treatment? How would such treatment compromise both the patient and the fetus?
3. Will prior treatments—pelvic surgery, radiation to pelvis or abdomen, or chemotherapy—affect fertility or reproductive outcome?
4. Will the hormonal milieu of pregnancy adversely affect an estrogen-receptor—positive tumor?

CANCER DURING PREGNANCY

General Considerations

The risk of having a coincident malignant tumor with pregnancy is approximately 0.1 percent. Approximately one third of recorded maternal deaths are secondary to a coexisting malignancy. Delays in diagnosis of the cancer during pregnancy are common for a number of reasons: (1) many of the presenting symptoms of cancer are often attributed to the pregnancy; (2) many of the physiologic and anatomic alterations of pregnancy can compromise physical examination; (3) many serum tumor markers (β-human chorionic gonadotropin [β-hCG], alpha-fetoprotein, CA 125, and others) are increased during pregnancy; and (4) our ability to optimally perform either imaging studies or invasive diagnostic procedures may be altered during pregnancy.

Because the gestational age is significant when evaluating the risks of treatments, it is important to determine gestational age accurately. An early ultrasound evaluation may be useful to assure accurate dating.

BREAST CANCER

The predicted number of breast cancer cases in women in the United States for the year 2005 is 212,930, and the predicted number of related deaths is 40,870.[43] Approximately 2 to 3 percent of all breast cancers in women younger than age 40 occur with pregnancy or lactation, and approximately 1 in 1,360 to 3,330 pregnancies is complicated by breast cancer.[44] Although it has been predicted that there may be an increase in the frequency of breast cancer complicating pregnancy due to delayed childbearing, recent publications are consistent with a frequency of breast cancer concurrent with pregnancy of 1.3 per 10,000 live births.[45]

In general, the risk of breast cancer is directly related to the duration of ovarian function. Therefore, both early menarche and late menopause appear to increase the likelihood of developing breast cancer. However, interruption of the normal cyclic ovarian function by pregnancy appears protective. This apparent protective effect may be secondary to the normal hormonal milieu of pregnancy that produces epithelial proliferation, followed by marked differentiation and mitotic rest. Multiparous women and in particular multiparous patients who breast-feed have a lower risk of developing breast cancer than do nulliparous women. However, based on one study of almost 90,000 women, breast-feeding may not be an independent protective factor.[46] Paradoxically, carriers of BRCA1 and BRCA2 mutations may have an increased risk of developing breast cancer by having children.[47]

Diagnosis and Staging

Breast abnormalities should be evaluated in the same manner as if the patient were not pregnant. The most common presentation of breast cancer in pregnancy is a painless lump discovered by the patient. Despite the striking physiologic breast changes of pregnancy, including nipple enlargement and increases in glandular tissue resulting in engorgement and tenderness, breast cancer should be screened for during pregnancy. Because the breast changes become more pronounced in later pregnancy, it is important to perform a thorough breast examination at the initial visit. Diagnostic delays are often attributed to physician reluctance to evaluate breast complaints or abnormal findings in pregnancy. Although bilateral serosanguinous discharge may be normal in late pregnancy, masses require prompt and definitive evaluation. The lengths of delays in diagnosis of breast cancer in pregnancy are commonly 3 to 7 months or longer.[48] A case-control study from Princess Margaret Hospital suggested that pregnant patients are at higher risk of presenting with advanced disease because pregnancy impedes early detection.[49] Mammography in pregnancy is controversial. Although the radiation exposure to the fetus is negligible,[50] the hyperplastic breast of pregnancy is characterized by increased tissue density, making interpretation more difficult.[51]

Fine-needle aspiration (FNA) of a mass for cytologic study is recommended. FNA is reliable for a diagnosis of carcinoma (false-positive results are rare), but if a solid mass is negative for tumor it should be evaluated by excisional biopsy. Similar to the nonpregnant patient, approximately 20 percent of breast biopsies performed in pregnancy reveal cancer.

Before proceeding with treatment, staging should be undertaken. All draining lymph nodes should be evaluated. The contralateral breast must be carefully assessed. Laboratory tests should include baseline liver function tests and serum tumor markers, carcinoembryonic antigen (CEA), and CA 15-3. CA 15-3 appears to be a useful tumor marker for monitoring breast cancer in pregnancy.[52] A chest radiograph is indicated, and if the liver function tests are abnormal, the liver can be evaluated by ultrasound. With precautions of good hydration and insertion of a urinary bladder catheter, a bone scan can be performed in pregnancy. However, in an asymptomatic patient with normal blood tests, because the yield is low, bone scanning is usually not performed in those circumstances. In a symptomatic patient, radiographs of the specific symptomatic bones are advised. Sentinel lymph node biopsy techniques appear safe in pregnancy.[53,54]

Although one report suggests an increased incidence of inflammatory breast cancer in pregnancy,[55] other reviews have not confirmed this observation. It is generally thought that breast cancers in pregnancy are histologically identical to the nonpregnant patient of similar age. Because inflammatory breast cancer can be mistaken for mastitis, a biopsy of breast tissue should be performed when a suspected breast abscess is incised and drained.

Treatment

The treatment of breast carcinoma at any time is often overshadowed by psychological and emotional factors. Because of potential risks to the developing fetus, treatment decisions carry an additional burden. Therapy must be individualized in accordance with present knowledge and with the specific desires of the patient.

LOCAL THERAPY

The usual criteria for breast-preserving therapy versus modified radical mastectomy pertain to the patient with breast cancer, stages I to III.[56] However, the option of lumpectomy, axillary node dissection, and irradiation is complicated by the presence of the pregnancy.[57] One publication presents a mathematical model suggesting that the risk of axillary metastases due to treatment delay is minimal and may be acceptable to some third-trimester patients with early breast cancer who prefer lumpectomy with radiation postpartum.[58] Consideration should be given to the delay of irradiation until after delivery. Experimental calculations suggest that a tumor dose of 5,000 cGy will expose the fetus to 10 to 15 cGy while the fetus is within the true pelvis. Later in pregnancy, parts of the fetus may receive as much as 200 cGy.[59] Brent[60] has suggested that 5 cGy is a relatively safe upper limit of fetal exposure. Although the potential for teratogenesis is reduced later in pregnancy, radiation can affect fetal growth and may carry a potential risk for future carcinogenesis.

PREGNANCY TERMINATION

Because early studies suggested more unfavorable outcomes in pregnant women, it was assumed that the hormonal changes of pregnancy contributed to rapid tumor growth. Therefore, therapeutic abortion was frequently advised. At present, a harmful effect of continuing pregnancy has not been demonstrated in most published series (Table 45-2).[61] However, it is difficult to evaluate potential selection bias toward performing an abortion in patients with advanced disease. Because young women tend to have hormone receptor–negative tumors,[62] it is difficult to make an argument, based on hormonal concerns, for either termination of pregnancy or oophorectomy as an adjunct to therapy.[63–65]

CHEMOTHERAPY

Women who present with either metastatic breast carcinoma or rapidly progressive inflammatory carcinoma

Table 45-2. Survival from Breast Cancer in Patients Undergoing Therapeutic Abortion Compared with Those not Undergoing Abortion

	DELIVERED		THERAPEUTIC ABORTION		
AUTHORS	NO. OF PATIENTS	5-YR SURVIVAL	NO. OF PATIENTS	5-YR SURVIVAL	COMMENTS
Adair (1953)	36	44	23	70	25 pregnant at diagnosis, 34 pregnant after treatment for cancer. Only node-positive patients benefited from abortion
Holleb and Farrow (1962)	12	33	12	17	Surgery during first trimester
Rissanen (1968)	20	50	7	43	4 patients (1 aborted; 3 delivered) were stage IV
Clark and Reid (1978)	93	29	13	15	12% spontaneous abortion; 1 stillbirth. Abortion was not biased for more advanced disease
King et al. (1985)	35	67	18	53	For stage I patients: delivery vs. abortion: 18 vs. 4 patients; 5-yr survival is 88% vs. 33%

Modified from Holmes FA: Breast cancer during pregnancy. Cancer Bull 46:405, 1994.

Table 45-3. 5- and 10-Year Survival Rates, by Nodal Status, of Pregnant or Lactating Patients Treated for Breast Cancer

		OVERALL		NODE NEGATIVE		NODE POSITIVE	
INVESTIGATORS	NO. OF PATIENTS	5-YR (%)	10-YR (%)	5-YR (%)	10-YR (%)	5-YR (%)	10-YR (%)
White and White[71]	806	13	9	21	13	7	6
Holleb and Farrow[63]	117	31	—	65	—	17	—
Byrd et al.[70]	29	55	—	100	80	28	6
Applewhite et al.[48]	48	25	15	56	22	18	13
Riberio and Palmer[73]	59	31	24	90	90	37	21
Clark and Reid[74]							
Pregnant	121	—	22	—	35	—	22
Lactating	80	—	32	—	69	—	18
King et al.[55]	63	53	49	82	71	36	36
Petrek et al.[75]	56	61	45	82	77	47	25

frequently elect pregnancy termination. In general, delay of therapy should be avoided, especially for the patient with inflammatory breast cancer. Immediate initiation of chemotherapy is critical to providing the patient with inflammatory carcinoma with any chance for long-term survival. In the patient with a clinical indication for adjuvant chemotherapy other than inflammatory carcinoma, the delay of instituting chemotherapy and awaiting fetal pulmonary maturity should be considered in select third-trimester situations. A French study reported that 17 of 20 pregnancies, in patients treated with chemotherapy for breast carcinoma, resulted in live births.[66] Others concur with the use of chemotherapy in the second and third trimesters in the management of breast cancer.[67–69] Pregnancy is a contraindication to the use of tamoxifen due to the risk of adverse fetal outcomes.[34] Data regarding the safety of trastuzumab (Herceptin) in pregnancy are lacking.

Prognosis

As with any malignant disease, prognosis best correlates with the anatomic extent of disease at the time of diagnosis. The presence and extent of nodal involvement is especially predictive of prognosis in both nonpregnant and pregnant patients. Table 45-3 provides 5- and 10-year survival data by nodal status.[55,63,70–75] Although nodal status is of prognostic significance, the number of positive nodes is also important. In the pregnant patient, the 5-year survival rate is 82 percent for patients with three or fewer positive nodes and 27 percent if greater than three nodes contain tumor.[55] Pregnancy, probably due to the associated delays in diagnosis, appears to increase the frequency of nodal disease, with 60 to 85 percent of patients exhibiting axillary nodal disease at diagnosis.[55,76]

When controlled for age and stage, pregnancy does not seem to affect prognosis adversely.[49,75,77,78] Some have suggested a worse prognosis if the cancer is diagnosed in the second trimester.[77]

Subsequent Pregnancy

The risk of pregnancy after breast cancer has been a focus of a number of studies.[79–81] Although the consensus is that subsequent pregnancies do not adversely affect survival, there are recommendations regarding the timing of a subsequent pregnancy.[82,83] It is generally advised that women with node-negative disease wait for 2 to 3 years, and this interval should be extended to 5 years for patients with positive nodes. Others have advised that no delay is indicated for the patient with good prognostic disease who does not receive postoperative adjuvant chemotherapy.[84] It has been advised that patients should undergo a complete metastatic work up before a subsequent pregnancy.

Although no studies indicate that subsequent pregnancy adversely affects survival, the retrospective reports that suggest a potential favorable affect of subsequent pregnancy are too small to draw firm conclusions.[77,85] A trend toward better survival is also noted in patients who received adjuvant chemotherapy and subsequently became pregnant.[78,86]

LACTATION AND BREAST RECONSTRUCTION

Lactation is possible in a small percentage of patients after breast-conserving therapy for early stage breast cancer.[87,88] Lumpectomy using a radial incision rather than the cosmetically preferred circumareolar incision is less likely to disrupt ductal anatomy. Disruption of the ductal system may increase the rate of mastitis. Breast-feeding is contraindicated in women receiving chemotherapy, because significant levels of the drug can be found in breast milk.

Breast reconstruction with the use of autologous tissue has increased secondary to questions about the use of silicone-filled implants. The transverse rectus abdominis myocutaneous flap (TRAM) is one popular method of breast reconstruction. Because the donor site is a portion of the anterior abdominal wall, there is potential concern when the patient develops abdominal distention from pregnancy. In one case report and review of the literature, nine cases of pregnancy following breast reconstruction experienced no problem with anterior abdominal wall integrity.[89]

HODGKIN'S DISEASE AND NON-HODGKIN'S LYMPHOMA

Hodgkin's Disease

Approximately 31,800 cases of lymphoma will be diagnosed in women in the United States in the year 2006, and only about 11 percent of these will be Hodgkin's disease.[43] Hodgkin's disease, commonly encountered in patients in their late teens and twenties, occurs at a mean age of 32 years. Non-Hodgkin's lymphomas occur at a mean age of 42 and, therefore, are reported less frequently in association with pregnancy. Lymphomas complicate approximately 1 in 6,000 pregnancies. Spontaneous abortion, stillbirth rates, and preterm births do not appear to be increased.[90,91] Pregnancy does not appear to affect adversely the course of the disease.[92,93] Routine termination of pregnancy should not be advised. Although some advocate therapeutic abortion for the patient with a first-trimester pregnancy and Hodgkin's disease to allow complete staging, others, probably more appropriately, have limited the role of therapeutic abortion to those women requiring infradiaphragmatic irradiation or those with systemic symptoms or visceral disease, which are best managed with multiagent chemotherapy.

Hodgkin's disease frequently presents with enlarged cervical or axillary lymph nodes. The diagnosis is established by biopsy of the suspicious nodes. The presence of systemic symptoms such as night sweats, pruritus, or weight loss suggests more extensive disease. Two histologic variants, nodular sclerosis and lymphocyte predominant, have a better prognosis than mixed-cellularity and lymphocyte-depleted tumors.

Clinical staging for lymphoma necessitates the systemic evaluation by history, laboratory findings, bone marrow, and radiographic imaging. Clinical treatment and staging should be individualized. Pathologic staging for Hodgkin's disease may involve laparotomy and splenectomy; however, this is not usually necessary for non-Hodgkin's lymphoma, because disseminated disease can usually be documented without surgery. The minimal staging for Hodgkin's disease during pregnancy includes radiographic examination of the chest, liver function tests, bone marrow biopsy, complete blood count, and urinalysis. Chest tomography or computed tomographic (CT) scan of the mediastinum may be necessary to evaluate nodal enlargement in the chest. Evaluation of the abdomen is compromised by the gravid uterus, and MRI may be the safest technique for demonstrating intraabdominal adenopathy. Isotope scans of the liver and bone are best avoided during pregnancy. A single-shot lymphangiogram results in an exposure of less than 1 rad to the fetus and is probably safe after the first trimester.[94] Ultrasonography is safe and may provide useful information.

Disease stage (Table 45-4) is the most important factor in treatment planning and prognosis. The survival rate for early-stage Hodgkin's disease exceeds 90 percent, whereas patients with disseminated nodal disease have a 5-year survival rate of about 50 percent. As expected, patients with stage IV disease have poor survival rates. Although radiation therapy is the mainstay of treatment for early-stage Hodgkin's disease, combination chemotherapy is employed for the treatment of advanced-stage disease with organ involvement. The nitrogen mustard, vincristine, procarbazine, and prednisone (MOPP) regimen in combination with radiation is often used to treat patients with bulky, large mediastinal masses or disseminated nodal disease. Most investigators agree that treatment should not be withheld during pregnancy except in early-

Table 45-4. Staging Classification of Hodgkin's Disease*

STAGE	DESCRIPTION
I	Involvement of a single lymph node region (I) or of a single extralymphatic organ site (I_E)
II	Involvement of two or more lymph node regions on the same side of the diaphragm (II) or localized involvement of an extralymphatic organ site and of one or more lymph node regions on the same side of the diaphragm (II_E)
III	Involvement of lymph node regions on both sides of the diaphragm (III), which also may be accompanied by localized involvement of an extralymphatic organ or site (III_E), of the spleen (III_S), or of both (III_{SE})
IV	Diffuse or disseminated involvement of an extralymphatic organ with or without localized lymph node involvement (liver, bone marrow, lung, skin)

*Symptoms of unexplained fever, night sweats, and unexplained weight loss of 10 percent of normal body weight result in classification of patients as B; absence of these symptoms is denoted as A.

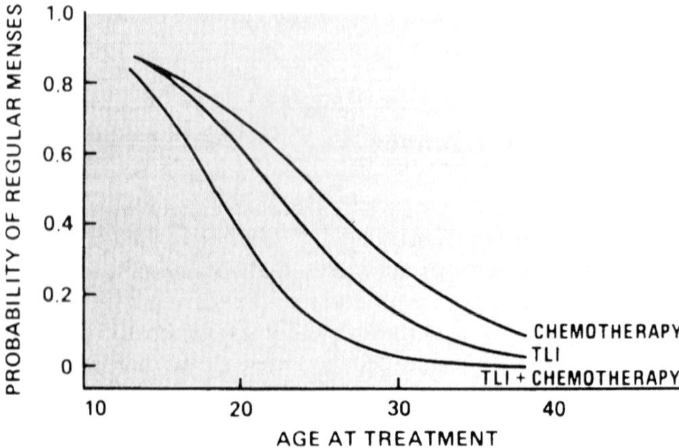

Figure 45-1. Probability of regular menses after chemotherapy, total lymphoid irradiation (TLI), and TLI and chemotherapy in patients with Hodgkin's disease. The synergistic effect is more apparent in younger women. (From Horning SJ, Hoppe RT, Kaplan HS: Female reproduction after treatment for Hodgkin's disease. N Engl J Med 304:1377, 1981, with permission.)

stage disease, particularly if the diagnosis is made in late gestation. Radiotherapy to the supradiaphragmatic regions may be performed with abdominal shielding after the first trimester. Thomas and Peckham[94] reported three cases of mantle field irradiation with abdominal shielding for supradiaphragmatic disease. The estimated radiation exposures to the fetus for these patients at 10, 15, and 16 weeks were 2.5, 4.4, and 10.4 rad, respectively. Although these pregnancies went to term with apparent normal outcomes, long-term follow-up on these infants was not presented. Spontaneous abortion has been reported with an estimated first-trimester fetal dose of 9 rad secondary to scatter from delivering 4,400 rad to the chest of a patient receiving treatment for a recurrence.[95] Another patient in the same report received 3,300 rad to a mantle field at 16 weeks' gestation, and no adverse affects were noted. In general, if the estimated exposure to a first-trimester fetus is expected to exceed 10 rad or if combination chemotherapy is planned for the first trimester, therapeutic abortion should be considered because of an increased risk of fetal malformations.[96] Asymptomatic early-stage disease presenting in the second half of pregnancy may be followed closely while preparations are made for early delivery.[95] The use of corticosteroids and single-agent chemotherapy has been proposed for the patient with systemic symptoms.

Subdiaphragmatic or advanced disease requires chemotherapy. Because many of the most commonly used chemotherapeutic agents are known teratogens, such treatment is best avoided in the first trimester. Similar treatments should also be approached with caution later in pregnancy, although most case reports have documented only intrauterine growth restriction and neonatal neutropenia as complications. Long-term follow-up toxicity studies are lacking.

Following therapy for Hodgkin's disease, it has been suggested that pregnancy planning should take into consideration that about 80 percent of recurrences manifest within 2 years. Treatments for Hodgkin's disease may compromise the reproductive potential of young patients.[39,97] As reflected in Figure 45-1, ovarian failure is more likely to occur in older patients, even if treated with fewer courses of chemotherapy.[97] Some studies have reported a rate of only 12 percent of normal ovarian function following therapy for Hodgkin's disease.[98] Combined treatment with irradiation and chemotherapy provides the highest risk of ovarian failure.

Bilateral midline oophoropexy at staging laparotomy has been advocated for the patient requiring pelvic node irradiation.[99] Even with this technique the ovaries may be exposed to a significant dose of irradiation, ranging from 600 to 3,500 rad.[94] Additionally, there are concerns of adhesions interfering with ovum pick-up and transport. Whereas combined oral contraceptives have been advocated to preserve ovarian function, there is no evidence of efficacy.[100] Depending on their availability, new reproductive technologies, including oocyte donation and embryo cryopreservation, can be considered for select situations.[101]

Patients who become pregnant after treatment for Hodgkin's lymphoma do not demonstrate increased adverse perinatal outcomes such as fetal wastage, preterm birth, and birth defects when compared with sibling controls.[102,103] Although fetal anomalies have occurred after treatment for Hodgkin's disease,[104] chromosomal abnormalities or a new gene mutation have not been diagnosed.[97] The absence of a repetitive pattern of malformations makes it difficult to imply a casual relationship between any birth defects observed and previous therapy for Hodgkin's disease.

Non-Hodgkin's Lymphoma

Non-Hodgkin's lymphoma occurs at a mean age of 42 years and, therefore, is reported less frequently than Hodgkin's disease in association with pregnancy. In general, non-Hodgkin's disease is more likely to affect a pregnancy adversely because patients usually have an aggressive histology and advanced-stage disease. Burkitt's lymphoma is usually rapidly progressive and may involve the breast and ovary. Lymphoma of the breast has a particularly poor prognosis, and it has been speculated that there may be a hormonal influence on this malignancy in pregnant patients.[105] In a report by Ward and Weiss,[106] about 60 percent (12 of 21) of second- and third-trimester cases of non-Hodgkin's lymphoma resulted in surviving infants. The perinatal mortality rate associated with patients who were either not treated or treated by surgery was almost 40 percent (5 of 13), whereas almost 90 percent (seven of eight) of infants of mothers treated by chemotherapy survived. Of the mothers treated with chemotherapy, 50 percent of the infants (four of eight) survived. Of the 13 patients who were not treated or who were treated with surgical resection, five of their babies (38 percent) survived. The nature of the presenting disease probably played a predilection role regarding the treatments. Including additional, more recent, reports, it is evident that about 60 to 70 percent of patients and about 75 percent of infants survive.

Adult T-cell leukemia/lymphoma, caused by the human T-cell lymphotropic virus type I, is found in Japan, the Caribbean, and the southern United States. The virus is present in familial clusters and is transmitted by sexual intercourse, blood transfusions, and breast milk. Infants seroconvert between 12 and 19 months of age at a rate of 20 to 25 percent.[107,108]

ACUTE LEUKEMIA

Although the incidence of leukemia in pregnancy is not specifically known, it is estimated to occur in less than 1 in 75,000 pregnancies. Acute leukemia represents about 90 percent of leukemias coexisting with pregnancy. Acute myeloid leukemia accounts for about 60 percent and acute lymphoblastic leukemia (ALL) for about 30 percent of cases. More three fourths of the cases are diagnosed after the first trimester.[6,109]

The prognosis for acute leukemia in pregnancy is guarded.[6,109–112] In adults, acute leukemia in the non pregnant patient, if untreated, has a median survival time of about 2 months.[113] In the treated patient, the median survival time is between 1 and 2 years. Immediate and aggressive therapeutic intervention will yield complete remission rates of about 75 percent, and 40 percent of these are sustained. Although there is no evidence that pregnancy adversely affects the prognosis of acute leukemia,[114] a 1987 report identified a median survival time of 16 months in the pregnant patient,[6] and another study in 1988 reported a median survival of 27.5 months in a nonpregnant population.[115] However, the differences in patient populations (the latter study was a report on the more favorable ALL) and the varied treatments precludes any reliable comparison.[113] Optimal care of the pregnant patient with acute leukemia necessitates a team effort and is best achieved in a cancer referral center.

The diagnosis of acute leukemia is rarely difficult. The signs and symptoms of anemia, granulocytopenia, and thrombocytopenia, including fatigue, fever, infection, and easy bleeding or petechiae, usually prompt a complete blood count. A normal or elevated white blood cell count is present in up to 90 percent of patients with ALL. Counts in excess of 50,000 are found in only one fourth of patients. In contrast, patients with acute nonlymphocytic leukemia (ANLL) may present with markedly elevated white blood cell counts, although one third present with leukopenia.[116] The diagnosis of leukemia should be confirmed by bone marrow biopsy and aspirate. The biopsy material is usually hypercellular with leukemic cells. The smear of the aspirate reveals decreased erythocyte and granulocytic precursors as well as megakaryocytes. Leukemic cells comprise greater than one half of the marrow's cellular elements in most patients. The morphology of the marrow and the peripheral leukemic cells help to distinguish between lymphocytic and nonlymphocytic leukemias. This latter group includes acute myelocytic (granulocytic), promyelocytic, monocytic, and myelomonocytic leukemias, and erythroleukemia. Acute myelocytic leukemia is the most common form of ANLL. Patients who develop ANLL as a result of previous chemotherapy have a particularly poor response to treatment.

There are numerous reports of successful pregnancies in patients aggressively treated with combination chemotherapy for acute leukemia. Acute leukemia and its therapy are associated with an increase in stillbirths (approximately 15 percent), prematurity (approximately 50 percent), and fetal growth restriction.[110,113] In 1988 and 1991, reports by Aviles and colleagues,[42,117] no serious long-term effects of in utero exposure to chemotherapy were reported. The first report included 17 children, aged 4 to 22, whose mothers received treatment for acute leukemia.[117] In the second report, 43 children who were born to mothers with a variety of hematologic malignancies were examined at 3 to 19 years of age.[42] In both studies, greater than 40 percent of the cases involved exposure during the first trimester.

If the mother is exposed to cytotoxic drugs within 1 month of delivery, the newborn should be monitored closely for evidence of granulocytopenia or thrombocytopenia.

CHRONIC LEUKEMIA

Chronic leukemia accounts for approximately 10 percent of cases of leukemia during pregnancy, with the majority of these being patients with chronic myelocytic leukemia (CML).[113] Chronic lymphocytic leukemia has a median age of onset of about 60 years, making cases during pregnancy rare. The median age of patients with CML is 35 years. CML is characterized by excessive production of mature myeloid cell elements, with granulocyte counts averaging 200,000/dl. Most patients have thrombocytosis and a mild normochromic normocytic anemia. Platelet function is often abnormal, although hemorrhage is usually limited to patients with marked thrombocytopenia. CML tends to be indolent, and normal hematopoiesis is only mildly affected in the early stages of disease. Therefore, delay of aggressive treatment is a more feasible option than with acute leukemia. Unless complications such as severe systemic symptoms, autoimmune hemolytic anemia, recurrent infection, or symptomatic lymphatic enlargement occur, treatment for chronic leukemia should be withheld until after delivery. Therapy, when necessary, usually includes prednisone and an alkylating agent such as chlorambucil or cyclophosphamide. High-dose steroids alone may be used to treat autoimmune hemolytic anemia. Currently, the median survival time for CML is more than 60 months, with survivals up to 10 years common.

Often, the diagnosis of CML antedates the pregnancy. Although pregnancy does not appear to affect CML adversely, therapy does increase the frequency of preterm birth and low birth weight. Information about contemporary management and prognosis is scarce secondary to the fact that few recent cases of CML during pregnancy have been reported. There are reports of CML treatment with leukapheresis during pregnancy. This treatment appears to be both safe and effective. Leukapheresis results in improvement of blood counts, systemic symptoms, and splenomegaly. Also, this treatment, although costly and involved, offers less risk of teratogenesis than cytotoxic treatments.[109,118] Although allogeneic stem cell transplants offer the highest cure rates, such therapy is hazardous during pregnancy. Interferon (IFN) therapy has been reported in a limited number of pregnancies with good outcomes. In 2001, the FDA gave accelerated approval to imatinib mesylate (Gleevec), a synthetic inhibitor of the BCR/ABL kinase, STI571, for (1) treatment of patients in the chronic phase after failure of IFN-α therapy; (2) accelerated phase; and, (3) blast crisis. This drug carries a category D warning in pregnancy.[119–123]

Hairy cell leukemia during pregnancy is rare, with only six reported cases. A predilection for men and the older age groups is the reason for the infrequency. IFN-α treatment has been used in two cases with no adverse fetal effects.[119]

MELANOMA

The incidence of malignant melanoma is increasing in the childbearing years, and it is estimated that 1 percent of the population will develop this disease.[124] However, one study reported malignant melanoma in 2.8 per 1,000 deliveries.[125] The understanding of the natural history of melanoma has been advanced by the identification of prognostic variables.[126] Prognostic features of the primary tumor include tumor thickness, Clark's level of invasion, Breslow's modifications, and Chung's modifications (Fig. 45-2),[127] ulceration, and body location.

A topic of continued debate is whether pregnancy exerts a negative effect on the course of malignant melanoma. Reports from the 1950s suggested that melanoma arising during pregnancy is associated with an aggressive clinical course.[128,129] Subsequent reports, some being controlled studies, suggest melanoma diagnosed during pregnancy is more likely to be diagnosed at an advanced stage.[130–132] More recent studies have been largely limited to patients with stage I disease and thus do not address this issue.[133,134] Although many studies suggest that melanoma developing during pregnancy is more likely to appear in locations associated with a poor prognosis,[130–134] others show no increase in poor prognostic location of lesions in the pregnant patient.[135–136] A recent retrospective cohort study conducted in Sweden concluded that pregnant women with melanoma have survival times similar to that of their nonpregnant counterparts.[137]

The World Health Organization (WHO) 1991 study examined the relevant prognostic features of melanoma in the childbearing years and in pregnancy.[134] This report

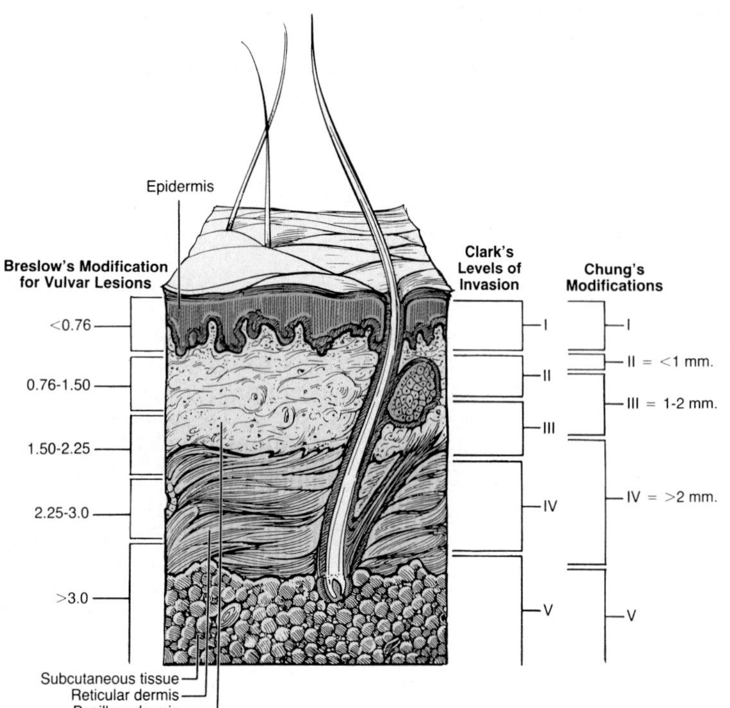

Figure 45-2. Schematic comparison of the different levels of invasion for melanoma. (From Gordon AN: Vulvar tumors. *In* Copeland LJ [ed]: Textbook of Gynecology, 2nd ed. Philadelphia, WB Saunders Company, 2000, p 1202, with permission.)

Table 45-5. WHO Stages I and II Study of Malignant Melanoma

RELATIONSHIP TO TIME OF PREGNANCY	NO. OF PATIENTS	MEAN TUMOR THICKNESS (mm)
Before	85	1.29
During	92	2.38*
After all	143	1.96
Between	68	1.78

*$p < 0.004$. When corrected for tumor thickness, survival rates were not different. Multivariate analysis identified tumor thickness as an independent prognostic variable, not pregnancy.

From MacKie RM, Bufalino R, Morabito A, et al: Lack of effect on pregnancy outcome of melanoma. Lancet 337:653, 1991, with permission.

Table 45-6. Primary Melanoma Tumor Thickness in Pregnant and Nonpregnant Patients

	TUMOR THICKNESS (mm)		
STUDY	PREGNANT	NONPREGNANT	*P* VALUE
Slingluft et al.[136]	2.7	1.5	0.052
Mackie et al.[134]	2.3	1.7	0.002
Travers et al.[139]	2.3	1.2	0.0001

suggested that patients who were diagnosed during pregnancy had tumors demonstrating significantly greater tumor thickness (Table 45-5). However, after correcting for tumor thickness, survival rates were similar. Additional studies from Massachusetts General Hospital and Duke University have supported the observation of greater tumor thickness in patients diagnosed during pregnancy (Table 45-6). Other investigators have found no difference in lesion thickness in pregnancy.[138] The issue remains unsettled, and explanations for the increased tumor thickness include hormonal stimulation, growth factor stimulation, immunologic alterations of pregnancy, and delays in diagnosis.[139] Delays in diagnosis are understandable because it is not uncommon for pigmentation changes to take place during pregnancy. Therefore, tissue sampling is often delayed secondary to abnormalities being dismissed as a normal change of pregnancy.

Surgery remains the most effective modality for the treatment of melanoma. For patients with stage I or II tumors, the standard surgical excision with margins appropriate for tumor thickness should be performed. Regional lymph node dissection is undertaken in the patient with regional disease. Because adjuvant chemotherapy is experimental and has not demonstrated improved survival, it is not recommended for the pregnant patient because of the potential risk to the fetus. Adjuvant IFN and vaccines for the nonpregnant patient are also under evaluation. These treatments hold more promise for the pregnant patient, based on fetal considerations. Advanced metastatic disease carries a poor prognosis. Because chemotherapy with dacarbazine results in a clinical response, usually of short duration, in no more than 30 percent of patients, it is usually most appropriate to plan for early delivery in cases of disseminated disease presenting late in pregnancy.

Is there a role for therapeutic abortion? Despite rare reports of regression after delivery, no studies support any therapeutic benefit associated with therapeutic abortion.[140,141] However, given the aggressive nature of the current therapies available for metastatic disease, it is appropriate to consider termination when managing advanced disease presenting in the first trimester.[141]

The patient who has undergone apparent successful treatment for a malignant melanoma may express concern about the safety of a future pregnancy. No adverse impact on recurrence or survival has been identified in most studies addressing this issue.[131,134,135] However, the timing of subsequent pregnancy deserves some consideration. The probability of survival of a specific cancer should be evaluated based on the known prognostic variables. The 5-year survival rate for the patient with a melanoma less than 1.5 mm thick is 90 percent. For a tumor of intermediate thickness (1.5 to 4 mm), the 5-year survival rate is 50 to 75 percent, and for a more deeply invasive tumor, survival is less than 50 percent. Although some report that approximately 60 to 70 percent of patients develop their recurrence within 2 years and 80 to 90 percent within 5 years, the WHO study claimed that 83 percent of recurrences develop within the first 2 years.[141] Based on this information, it is generally recommended that patients wait 2 to 3 years before attempting another pregnancy, especially with nodal disease.[134] There are insufficient data on the select group of patients who develop their initial melanoma during pregnancy to make recommendations regarding the safety of a subsequent pregnancy.

Another issue of concern is which form of birth control should be used. The use of oral contraceptives has not been demonstrated to affect adversely the natural history of a previously treated melanoma.[142,143]

CERVICAL CANCER

Approximately 3 percent of all invasive cervical cancers occur during pregnancy. Cervical cancer is the most common gynecologic malignancy associated with pregnancy, occurring in approximately 1 per 2,200 pregnancies.[144–146]

However, the true incidence is difficult to ascertain due to the reporting biases associated with the reports originating from large referral centers. Also, various reports may include patients who have preinvasive lesions as well as patients who are diagnosed postpartum.

All pregnant women should be evaluated on their initial obstetric visit with visualization of the cervix and cervical cytology, including an endocervical brush. The general principles of screening for cervical neoplasia apply during pregnancy. The Papanicolaou smear is used to screen the normal-appearing cervix. If the cervix appears friable, cervical cytology alone may not be sufficient to alert the physician to the presence of a malignant tumor. False-negative cervical cytology is at increased risk in pregnancy owing to excess mucus and bleeding from cervical eversion. Therefore, it is necessary to obtain a biopsy to ensure that tissue friability is not secondary to tumor.

Also, an ulcerative or exophytic lesion must have histologic sampling performed. Although approximately one third of pregnant patients with cervical cancer are asymptomatic at the time of diagnosis, the most common symptoms are vaginal bleeding or discharge. Evaluation for the possibility of neoplastic disease of the lower genital tract is required in the evaluation of vaginal bleeding in the pregnant as well as the nonpregnant patient.

Considering the routine practice of performing cervical cytology in early pregnancy, one would expect there to be a preponderance of early-stage disease diagnosed in the first trimester. Surprisingly, this is not the situation. The diagnosis of cervical cancer is commonly made postpartum rather than during pregnancy, and although stage IB disease is the most common stage found, all stages are represented in significant numbers. Both patient and physician factors, including lack of prenatal care, failure to obtain cervical cytology or to biopsy gross cervical abnormalities, false-negative cytology, and failure to evaluate abnormal cytology or vaginal bleeding properly, contribute to the delays in diagnosis. Unfortunately, the complaint of spotting or bleeding during pregnancy is common and usually secondary to pregnancy-related conditions.

Cervical cytology suggestive of a squamous intraepithelial lesion or a report of atypical glandular cells during pregnancy requires appropriate clinical evaluation (Fig. 45-3). Colposcopy during pregnancy is usually enhanced by the physiologic eversion of the lower endocervical canal. However, vascular changes and redundant vagina may alter or obscure normal visualization, rendering interpretation difficult, and referral to a gynecologic oncologist may be appropriate. During pregnancy, failure to visualize the entire transformation zone and squamocolumnar junction is uncommon. Although endocervical curettage is not generally recommended during pregnancy, lesions involving the lower endocervical canal can often be directly visualized and biopsied. Whereas the pregnant cervix is hypervascular, serious hemorrhage from an outpatient biopsy is uncommon, and the risk of bleeding is offset by the risk of missing an early invasive cancer. Following a coloposcopic evaluation with appropriate tissue sampling, most patients with preinvasive lesions can be followed with repeat colposcopy at 6- to 8-week intervals to delivery.[147,148]

Patients require a careful and complete colposcopic evaluation 6 weeks' postpartum. Cone biopsy during pregnancy, when necessary, should ideally be performed

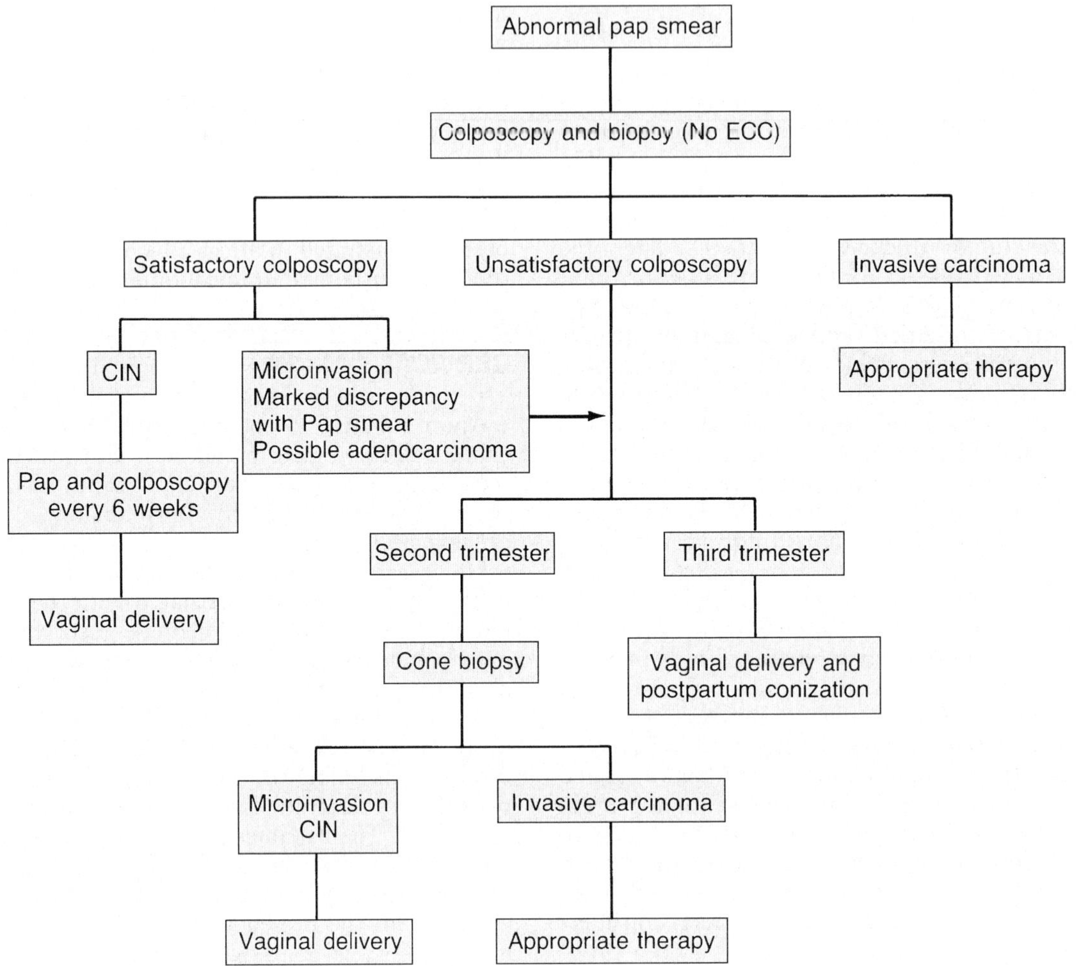

Figure 45-3. Suggested protocol for evaluation of abnormal cervical cytology in pregnancy. ECC, endocervical curettage; CIN, cervical intraepithelial neoplasia. (From Hacker NF, Berek JS, Lagasse LD, et al: Carcinoma of the cervix associated with pregnancy. Obstet Gynecol 59:735, 1982, with permission.)

during the second trimester to reduce the risks of first-trimester abortion and rupture of membranes or premature labor in the third trimester.[149–151] Complications from conization of the pregnant cervix are common. Therapeutic conization for intraepithelial squamous lesions is contraindicated during pregnancy. Diagnostic cone biopsy in pregnancy is reserved for patients whose colposcopic-directed biopsy has shown superficial invasion (suspect microinvasion) or in other situations in which an invasive lesion is suspected but cannot be confirmed by biopsy. When a cone biopsy is necessary during pregnancy, one should keep in mind the anatomic alteration of the cervix secondary to pregnancy. A shallow disk-like cone is usually satisfactory to clarify the diagnosis with a minimum of morbidity. It should be kept in mind that patients who have had a conization during pregnancy are at higher risk for residual disease. Therefore, close follow up is essential.

Following the diagnosis of invasive cervical cancer, a staging evaluation is indicated. The standard cervical staging is clinical and usually based on the results of physical examination, cystoscopy, proctoscopy, chest radiograph, and intravenous pyelogram. A CT scan or, in some centers, lymphangiography is often performed to identify lymph node metastasis. In the pregnant patient, the standard staging evaluation is modified. The chest radiograph is performed with abdominal shielding. Sonography is used to detect hydronephrosis and, if additional retroperitoneal imaging is desired for the evaluation of lymphadenopathy, consideration should be given to employing MRI because it does not involve ionizing radiation.

Microinvasion

In patients with a microinvasive squamous carcinoma with negative margins on cone biopsy, consideration can be given to conservative management until delivery. The risk of occult metastatic disease is predominantly dependent on two pathologic features: (1) the depth of invasion and (2) the presence or absence of lymph-vascular space involvement.[152] Whether the cone biopsy can be considered sufficient long-term therapy or whether a postpartum hysterectomy with or without lymphadenectomy should be performed is also based on the detailed analysis of the pathologic features of the cone biopsy. In these cases, consultation with a gynecologic oncologist is appropriate.

Invasive, Early-Stage Disease

Because the definitive treatment of invasive cervical cancer is not compatible with continuation of pregnancy, the clinical question that must be addressed is when to proceed with delivery so that therapy can be completed. Considering this requirement, treatment options will be influenced by gestational age, tumor stage and metastatic evaluation, and maternal desires and expectations regarding the pregnancy. The management of early invasive cervical cancer (stages IB and IIA) in the young patient is usually by radical hysterectomy, pelvic lymphadenectomy, and aortic lymph node sampling.[153] The primary advantage over radiation therapy for these patients is preservation of ovarian function. For the woman with a high probability of having a poor prognostic lesion and, therefore, requiring postoperative irradiation, consideration can be given to performing a unilateral or bilateral oophoropexy at the time of the hysterectomy. The ovarian suspension should be intraperitoneal, because retroperitoneal placement seems to predispose to subsequent ovarian cyst formation. In the first trimester, this surgery is usually carried out with the fetus in utero. In the third trimester, the radical hysterectomy and pelvic lymphadenectomy are performed after completion of a high classic cesarean delivery. Delays in therapeutic intervention have not been reported to increase recurrence rates for patients with small-volume stage I disease.[154] Although the pelvic vessels are large, the dissection is enhanced by more easily defined tissue planes.[155–157]

Second trimester situations are more problematic. Serious consideration should be given to administering one to three cycles of platinum-based chemotherapy and thereby allowing an additional 7 to 15 weeks of fetal maturation. In one study, maturation from 26 to 27 weeks' gestation compared with 34 to 35 weeks increased neonatal survival from 67 percent to 97 percent.[158] The neoadjuvant chemotherapy approach (chemotherapy before either surgery or irradiation) would unlikely compromise and may enhance the overall efficacy of treatment. Also, having passed the primary interval of organogenesis, it is unlikely that serious fetal sequelae will occur secondary to the chemotherapy. Certainly in terms of general fetal salvage and outcome, the risk of extreme prematurity would far outweigh the risk of the chemotherapy exposure. Although this management of second-trimester cervical cancer presentations seems logical, there is scant information about this treatment approach. However, neoadjuvant chemotherapy with vincristine and platinum-based chemotherapy for ovarian cancers has been reported with no fetal sequelae identified.[19]

Invasive, Locally Advanced Disease

The management of the patient with more advanced local disease is based on treatment with chemotherapy and irradiation, both external beam to treat the regional nodes and shrink the central tumor and brachytherapy to complete the delivery of a tumoricidal dose to the cervix and adjacent tissues.[153] Coordinating a chemoradiation treatment plan for pregnant patients with stage IIB, stage III, and stage IVA is challenging. The patient with a first-trimester pregnancy can usually be treated in the standard fashion with initiation of chemotherapy and external therapy to the pelvis or extended field, as dictated by standard treatment guidelines. Most of these patients proceed to abort spontaneously within 2 to 5 weeks of initiating the radiation. Patients in the late first trimester are least likely to abort spontaneously, and it may be necessary to perform a uterine evacuation on the completion of external therapy in some patients. Following either spontaneous abortion or uterine evacuation, the brachytherapy component of the radiation therapy can proceed in the standard fashion. Patients in either their second or third trimester should have a high classic cesarean delivery before starting standard chemotherapy and irradiation. Again, it would seem appropriate to strongly consider neoadjuvant chemotherapy for this group of patients, especially the patient with a second-trimester or early third-trimester presentation, when the opportunity for further fetal maturation can be provided.

Invasive, Distant Metastasis

Metastatic disease to extrapelvic sites carries a poor prognosis. Although a select few patients with aortic node metastasis may receive curative therapy, it is unlikely for the patient with pulmonary metastasis, bone metastasis, or supraclavicular lymph node metastasis to be cured. Personal patient choices and ethical considerations are the major factors guiding treatment in these situations.

Small cell neuroendocrine tumors of the cervix associated with pregnancy are rare. Neoadjuvant or adjuvant chemotherapy with cisplatin, etoposide, and doxorubicin is recommended, and long-term survivors have been reported.[159,160]

Method of Delivery

Controversy continues to surround the issue of the method of delivery for the term patient with cervical cancer. It seems heroic and unjustifiably risky to encourage vaginal delivery of a patient with a large, firm, barrel-shaped tumor or a large friable and hemorrhagic exophytic tumor. However, many small-volume stage IB, IIA, and early IIB tumors are potential candidates for vaginal delivery. Whether vaginal delivery promotes systemic dissemination of tumor cells is unknown. Although the general opinion is that survival rates are not influenced by the mode of delivery,[144,161] a recent multivariate analysis "showed a possible trend ($p = 0.08$) toward worse outcomes after vaginal delivery."[146]

Although systemic tumor dissemination secondary to vaginal delivery has not been documented, there are reports of episiotomy implants for both squamous carcinoma and adenocarcinoma following vaginal delivery.[162–164] Episiotomy implants are sufficiently rare that the risk should not be a determining factor for a given patient. However, the episiotomy should be carefully followed in a cervical cancer patient who delivers vaginally. Episiotomy nodules in these patients must be promptly evaluated by biopsy, because an early diagnosis may permit curative therapy.[149] Diagnostic delays secondary to suspicion of the nodules representing stitch abscess should be avoided.

Survival

Although some authors have suggested that the survival of patients with cervical cancer associated with pregnancy is compromised,[152] most reports indicate that the prognosis is not altered.[144–146,165–167]

OVARIAN CANCER

With the increased use of diagnostic ultrasound, ovarian cysts and neoplasms are more frequently encountered in early pregnancy.[168] Although adnexal masses are often observed in pregnancy, only 2 to 5 percent are malignant ovarian tumors.[169,170] Ovarian cancer occurs in approximately 1 in 18,000 to 1 in 47,000 pregnancies.[171,172]

Whereas the three major categories of ovarian tumors, epithelial, germ cell, and stromal, occur during pregnancy, there is a disproportionate number of patients with germ cell tumors compared with the nonpregnant patient. A review of the literature since 1984 reveals 40 patients having malignant primary ovarian tumors during pregnancy. Germ cell tumors account for 45 percent (Fig. 45-4)[173]; 37.5 percent are epithelial tumors, 10 percent are stromal tumors, and 7.5 percent are categorized as miscellaneous. This distribution is undoubtedly skewed by the reporting bias associated with rare tumors. Characteristic of epithelial tumors in young patients who are not pregnant, the majority of epithelial ovarian tumors complicating pregnancy are of low grade (grade 1 or low malignant potential) or early stage, not uncommonly both low grade and stage I.

Management of the adnexal mass in pregnancy is controversial. The risks of surgical intervention may favor a conservative approach.[174,175] Serial sonograms may be of some value in determining the nature and biologic potential of the tumor. If the clinical presentation is consistent with torsion, rupture, or hemorrhage, immediate surgical intervention is indicated. Prompt

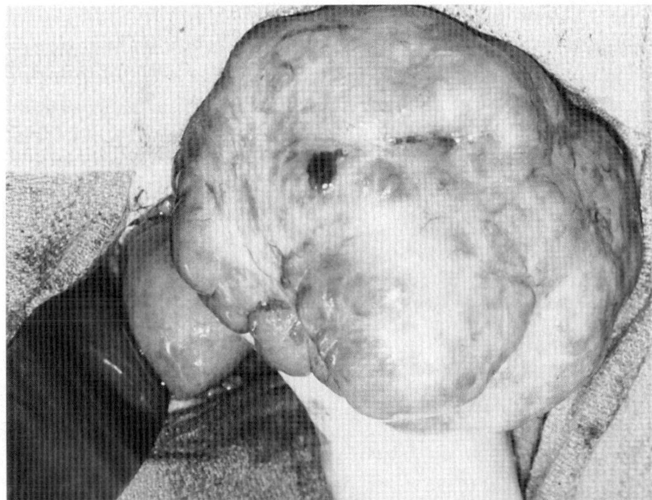

Figure 45-4. Dysgerminoma, the most common malignant ovarian neoplasm found in pregnancy, characterized by a lobulated solid gross appearance. (From Copeland LJ: Gestational trophoblastic neoplasia. *In* Copeland LJ [ed]: Textbook of Gynecology, 2nd ed. Philadelphia, WB Saunders Company, 2000, p 1391, with permission.)

surgical exploration is also performed for the mass associated with ascites or when there is evidence of metastatic disease. Because surgical exploration during pregnancy is associated with an increase in pregnancy loss and neonatal morbidity, it is ideal to delay surgical intervention until term or after delivery. A number of opposing risks require consideration before following a conservative approach. The risk of greatest concern is that a delay of surgical intervention could permit a malignant ovarian tumor to spread, resulting in a decreased opportunity for cure. However, considering the rarity of advanced-stage poorly differentiated epithelial tumors in this age group, this risk is relatively small. There does appear to be an increased probability that an adnexal mass during pregnancy will undergo torsion or rupture,[176–177] and surgical intervention for these events is associated with higher fetal loss than an elective procedure.[177–178] Although ovarian tumors may be the cause of obstructed labor,[178] this is uncommon. Skilled sonographic examination is essential to determining the potential for malignancy based on size and imaging characteristics. Serial sonographic evaluations will also identify the rare tumor that remains pelvic as the gestation progresses. Because most ovarian masses relocate to the abdomen as the pregnancy advances, other explanations should be considered for persistent pelvic masses, including pelvic kidney, uterine fibroids, and colorectal or bladder tumors.

When a malignant ovarian tumor is encountered at laparotomy, surgical intervention should be similar to that for the nonpregnant patient. If the patient is preterm and the tumor appears confined to one ovary, consideration should be given to limiting the staging to removal of the ovary, cytologic washings, and a thorough manual exploration of the abdomen and pelvis. The potential benefit of more extensive staging, including aortic node sampling, may be offset by higher pregnancy loss or neonatal morbidity. Before surgery, a comprehensive discussion with the patient should guide the extent of surgery if metastatic disease, especially a high-grade epithelial lesion, is encountered. Depending on the gestational age and the patient's desires, limited surgery followed by chemotherapy and additional extirpative surgery following delivery must be offered in select cases.[179]

Preoperative serum tumor markers are of limited value during pregnancy secondary to the physiologic increases in hCG, alpha-fetoprotein, and CA 125. Kobayashi and colleagues[180] have reported the mean CA 125 levels during pregnancy. CA 125 increases during the first trimester (mean, 72 U/ml) and then normalizes during the second trimester. CA 125 values tend to be significantly elevated following second-trimester abortion (mean, 447 U/ml) and term delivery (mean, 204 U/ml). Following diagnostic confirmation of a malignant ovarian tumor, the appropriate serum markers are useful to monitor the course of the disease.

Virilizing ovarian tumors during pregnancy are most commonly secondary to theca-lutein cysts, and their evaluation and management should be conservative. These benign exaggerated physiologic "tumors" may redevelop with subsequent pregnancies.[181]

Postoperative Adjuvant Therapy

Postoperative adjuvant therapy should follow the treatment guidelines for the nonpregnant patient. Following tumor debulking, patients with advanced epithelial tumors should receive combination chemotherapy. Until 1995, the standard therapy was a platinum and alkylating combination. However, with the demonstration of the superior effectiveness of the combination of cisplatin and paclitaxel,[182] these agents offer the patient a better survival. Unfortunately, there is limited information available regarding the potential toxic effects of paclitaxel on a developing fetus.[28] There are favorable case reports on the treatment of stage III serous ovarian carcinoma with postoperative platinum-based chemotherapy.[183–185] There are also a number of favorable treatment outcomes reported in patients with malignant germ cell tumors and pregnancy.[186–196]

Young and colleagues[197] reviewed their collective experience with stromal ovarian tumors in pregnancy. One third of the patients presented with tumor rupture. Because the role of adjuvant chemotherapy for stromal tumors is complex and controversial, consultation with a gynecologic oncologist is recommended.

Vulvar and Vaginal Cancer

Because vulvar and vaginal cancers usually occur after age 40, the diagnosis of either disease concurrent with pregnancy is rare. Fewer than 30 cases of vulvar carcinoma diagnosed and treated during pregnancy have been reported.[198–202]

Vulvar carcinoma in pregnancy is usually stage I or II disease. The diagnosis is based on biopsy, and neither pregnancy nor the young age of a patient should discourage the biopsy of a vulvar mass. Because verrucous squamous carcinoma tends to be misdiagnosed as condyloma, it is important to inform the pathologist of the clinical characteristics of unusually large or aggressive condyloma-like lesions. Surgical management is similar to that used in the nonpregnant patient, with the preference being to perform surgery in the second trimester to avoid the fetal risks of exposure to anesthesia in the first trimester and the maternal risks associated with operating on the hypervascular vulva in the third trimester. The surgical management of vulvar carcinoma is trending to more conservative procedures.[203] Vaginal delivery has been reported following surgical resection of vulvar cancers during pregnancy.[198,199]

Vaginal carcinoma is less common than vulvar carcinoma. The same limitations apply to vaginal cancer as apply to locally advanced cervical cancer in pregnancy. The cornerstone of treatment is irradiation therapy. Clear cell adenocarcinoma of the vagina has been reported in 16 pregnant patients, and 13 were long-term survivors.[204]

ENDOMETRIAL CANCER

Approximately 30 cases of endometrial cancer associated with pregnancy have been reported. Although many of these cases are diagnosed in the first trimester, abnormal bleeding later in pregnancy or postpartum may be the presenting symptom of this tumor. Only about 30 percent of these cases are associated with a viable fetus.[205–208]

GASTROINTESTINAL CANCERS

Upper Gastrointestinal Cancers

The diagnostic delay in detecting upper gastrointestinal cancers is often attributable to the frequency and duration of gastrointestinal symptoms in pregnancy. In the United States, stomach cancer is rarely diagnosed in women during the reproductive years. During pregnancy, persistent severe upper gastrointestinal symptoms are best evaluated by gastroduodenoscopy rather than radiologic studies. Because curative resection of localized stomach cancer is possible in only approximately 30 percent of patients, it is imperative that treatment not be delayed.

Malignant hepatic tumors are rare during the reproductive years. Hepatocellular tumors detected during pregnancy should be resected, because the maternal and fetal mortality associated with subcapsular hemorrhage and liver rupture during pregnancy is high. Elevated steroid levels may predispose the tumor to rupture during pregnancy. There is no increase in the vascularity of the liver during pregnancy. In patients with unresectable hepatomas, therapeutic abortion may be considered to decrease the risk of subsequent rupture and bleeding.

Colon and Rectal Cancer

The incidence of colon cancer during pregnancy is about 1 in 13,000 live-born deliveries.[209] Colorectal carcinoma is usually found in women beyond childbearing age, with only 8 percent of patients diagnosed before age 40. Over 200 cases of colorectal cancer in pregnancy have been reported.[210]

Since pregnancy is often accompanied by constipation and exacerbations of hemorrhoids and anal fissures, the symptoms of colorectal carcinoma, namely, rectal bleeding, constipation, pain, and backache, tend to be attributed to the pregnancy, and diagnostic delay is common. The majority of colorectal carcinomas during pregnancy are rectal and palpable on rectal examination, in contrast to more proximal lesions found in the nonpregnant patient (Table 45-7).[211] Patients with unexplained hypochromic microcytic anemia should be evaluated with stool guaiac testing. If a colorectal lesion is suspected, endoscopic methods of evaluation are preferred to radiologic imaging studies. Unfortunately, most cases of colorectal cancer are not diagnosed until late pregnancy or at the time of delivery. Delays in diagnosis are probably responsible for a higher likelihood of advanced stage colorectal cancer in pregnancy and an associated poor prognosis. The hormonal effect of pregnancy on tumor development is unknown.[210] A report by Woods and colleagues[209] suggests that colorectal carcinoma in pregnancy adversely affects the pregnancy. Only 78 percent of their cases resulted in healthy live-born infants.[209]

Table 45-7. Distribution of Colon and Rectal Carcinomas in Nonpregnant and Pregnant Populations

PATIENT GROUP	TOTAL	COLON	RECTUM
General population	1,704	1,244 (73%)	460 (27%)
Age under 40 years	186	127 (68%)	59 (32%)
Pregnant	244	41 (17%)	203 (83%)

From Medich DS, Fazio VW: Hemorrhoids, anal fissure, and carcinoma of the colon, rectum, and anus during pregnancy. Surg Clin North Am 75:77, 1995, with permission.

Management of colon cancer is determined by gestational age at diagnosis and tumor stage. During the first half of pregnancy, colon resection with anastomosis is indicated for colon or appendiceal cancers.[212,213] Abdominoperineal resection or low anterior resection has been accomplished up to 20 weeks' gestation without disturbing the gravid uterus. In some cases, access to the rectum may not be possible without a hysterectomy or uterine evacuation.

In late pregnancy, a diverting colostomy may be necessary to relieve a colonic obstruction and allow the development of fetal maturity before instituting definitive therapy. Some patients with a diagnosis after 20 weeks may opt to continue the pregnancy to fetal viability. Vaginal delivery is planned unless the tumor is obstructing the pelvis or is located on the anterior rectum. If cesarean delivery is performed, tumor resection can be accomplished immediately. Neoadjuvant chemotherapy or radiation therapy for colorectal carcinoma in the pregnant patient has not demonstrated sufficient response to risk fetal exposure.

In one report, the stage-specific survival rates for pregnant patients with rectal cancer were 83, 27, and 0 percent for stages B, C, and D, respectively.[210] The corresponding survival rates for the same stages of colon cancer were 75, 33, and 0 percent.[210] No Dukes' A classification rectal or colon cancer was reported, consistent with the frequency of diagnostic delays.[210]

URINARY TRACT CANCERS

Fewer than 50 cases of renal cell carcinoma and less than 10 cases of bladder cancer have been reported during pregnancy. Urethral carcinoma during pregnancy is also rare. The hallmark of urinary tract cancers is hematuria. The initial evaluation of hematuria in pregnancy should be urethrocystoscopy, urinary cytology, and renal ultrasonography. The primary therapy for renal cell carcinoma is surgery, and the survival rate for localized disease may exceed 50 percent. Although preoperative arterial embolization may facilitate surgery on hypervascular tumors, improved survival rates have not been conclusively demonstrated. Adjuvant radiotherapy or chemotherapy tends to have minimal impact on long-term outcomes.

Transitional carcinoma of the bladder can be managed by local fulguration or resection if it is well differentiated and superficial. Less differentiated, deeply invasive, and recurrent tumors may require a partial or complete cystectomy. Treatment of urethral carcinoma varies with the size and location. Distal urethral tumors are usually treated with excision and interstitial brachytherapy implants.

CENTRAL NERVOUS SYSTEM TUMORS

The spectrum of central nervous system tumors found in pregnant patients is similar to that of the nonpregnant patient.[214] In pregnancy, 32 percent of brain tumors are gliomas, 29 percent meningiomas, 15 percent acoustic neuromas, and the other 24 percent are divided among other more rare subtypes. Spinal tumors account for only about one eighth of the central nervous system tumors. Vertebral hemangiomas comprise 61 percent of the spinal tumors and 18 percent of meningiomas. Unfortunately, the presenting symptoms of headache and nausea and vomiting are often attributed to normal complaints of pregnancy, and delays in diagnosis result. Meningiomas, pituitary adenomas, acoustic neuromas, and vertebral hemangiomas may demonstrate rapid enlargement during pregnancy. This may be secondary to fluid retention, increase in blood volume, or hormonal stimulation.[215] MRI is the preferred imaging technique used to diagnose intracranial neoplasms.

Because painful contractions and pushing increase intracranial pressure, it is recommended that labor be as pain free as possible, and the second stage of labor should be assisted with forceps to reduce the risk of herniation.[215] The anesthetic management of labor and delivery for patients with intracranial neoplasms has been reviewed by Finfer.[216]

Whereas high-grade glial tumors should undergo prompt diagnosis and treatment, low-grade glial tumors such as astrocytomas and oligodendrogliomas do not usually require immediate intervention. Adjuvant cranial radiotherapy with abdominal shielding should be considered for patients with high-grade tumors. Adjuvant chemotherapy is not usually effective and, therefore, should probably be delayed until after delivery.

Successful surgical removal of a variety of central nervous system tumors has been reported.[214,216–220] Corticosteroids are recommended to reduce the surrounding edema of intracranial masses.

Bromocriptine may be used during pregnancy if a prolactin secreting adenoma enlarges, causing symptoms. The safety of this medication is supported by a report of no adverse fetal effects in more than 1,400 pregnancies following first trimester exposure.

MISCELLANEOUS TUMORS

Similar to the management for small cell neuroendocrine tumors of the cervix,[159] neuroendocrine tumors or neuroblastomas of other primary sites tend to demonstrate excellent response to surgery[221] or chemotherapy.[222] Pheochromocytoma during pregnancy is rare and may mimic hypertensive disorders of pregnancy[223] (see Chapter 39).

FETAL-PLACENTAL METASTASIS

Metastatic spread of a maternal primary tumor to the placenta or fetus is rare. In general, the biologically aggressive spectrum of malignancies seem to carry the highest risk for fetal metastases. One review identified 45 cases of placental metastases and seven cases of fetal metastases.[224] Malignant melanoma is the most frequently reported tumor metastatic to the placenta. Hematologic malignancies are the second most common tumor to spread to the placenta. Placental and fetal dissemination of lymphomas have been reported.[225–229] One case of vertical transmission of a mother's leukemia cell line was demonstrated through identification of a leukemia clone.[230] There is one case report of a central nervous system tumor metastatic to the placenta.[231] A fetal intracranial metastasis has been reported as a vertical transmission from a maternal small cell lung cancer.[illegible] Choriocarcinoma metastatic to a fetus usually results in death within a few months of age.[illegible]

GESTATIONAL TROPHOBLASTIC DISEASE AND PREGNANCY-RELATED ISSUES

It is uncommon for a normal viable pregnancy to be complicated by gestational trophoblastic disease (GTD). A comprehensive summary of the evaluation and management of the complete spectrum of GTD is beyond the scope of this chapter. However, the aspects of GTD related to the general obstetric and postpartum care are reviewed.

Hydatidiform Mole (Complete Mole)

The incidence of hydatidiform mole has great geographic variability. In the United States it occurs in approximately 1 in 1,000 to 1 in 1,500 pregnancies. The two clinical risk factors that carry the highest risk of a molar pregnancy are (1) the extremes of the reproductive years (age 50 or older carries a relative risk of over 500)[235] and (2) the history of a prior hydatidiform mole (the risk for development of a second molar pregnancy is 1 to 2 percent,[236–238] and the risk of a third after two is approximately 25 percent).[239] Patients with these risk factors should have an ultrasound evaluation of uterine contents in the first trimester. Although historically approximately 50 percent of patients were not diagnosed with a molar pregnancy beforee vaginal expulsion of molar tissue, currently in developed countries, most patients are diagnosed either by ultrasound while asymptomatic or by ultrasound for the evaluation of vaginal spotting or cramping symptoms. Approximately 95 percent of complete hydatidiform moles have a 46,XX paternal homologous chromosomal pattern.

The safest technique of evacuating a hydatidiform mole is with the suction aspiration technique. Oxytocin should not be initiated until the patient is in the operating room and evacuation is imminent in order to minimize the risk of embolization of trophoblastic tissue. The alterna-

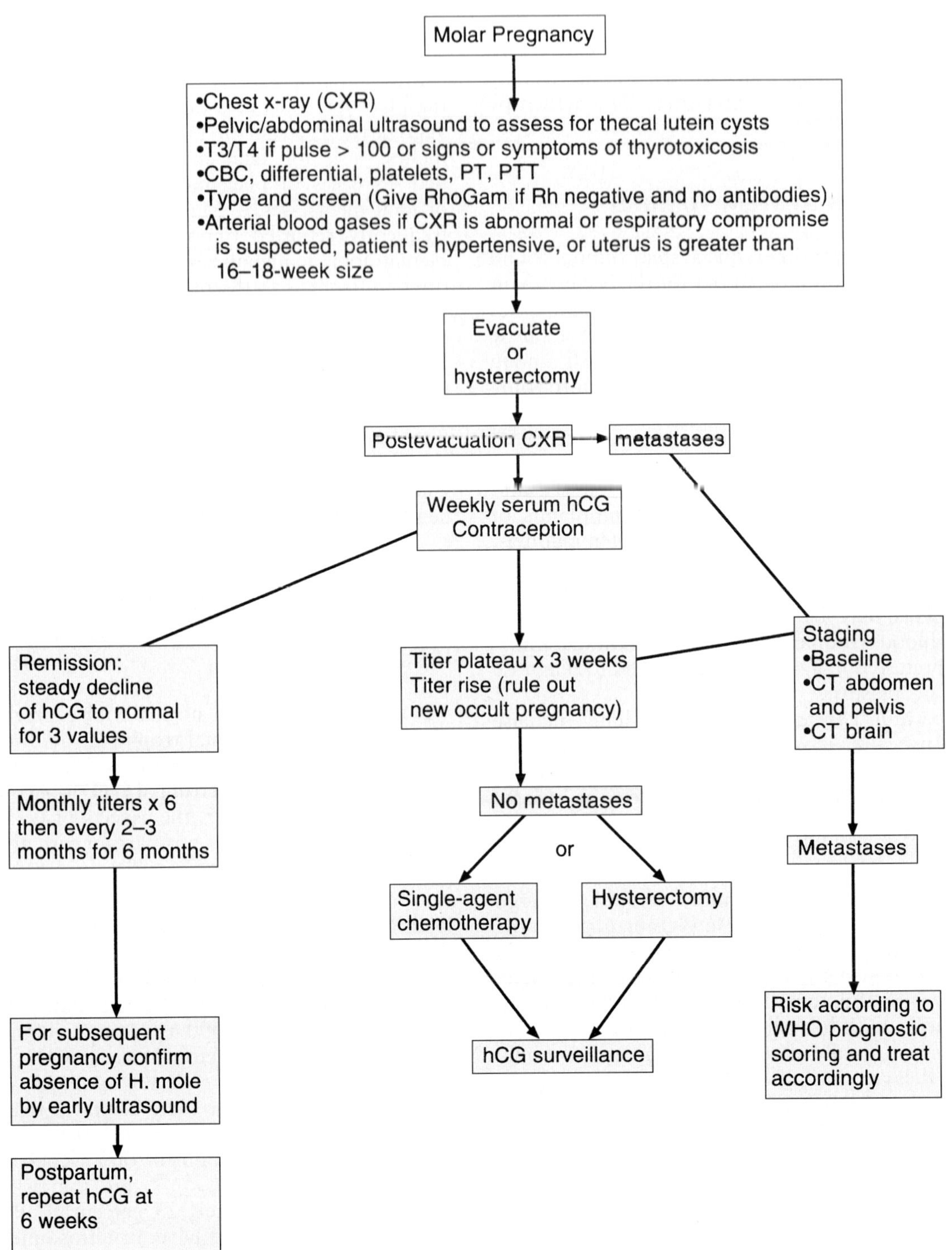

Figure 45-5. Algorithm for the management of molar pregnancy. (From Copeland LJ: Gestational trophoblastic neoplasia. *In* Copeland LJ [ed]: Textbook of Gynecology, 2nd ed. Philadelphia, WB Saunders Company, 2000, p 1414, with permission.)

tive management for the elderly patient who requests concurrent sterilization is hysterectomy. Following either evacuation or hysterectomy, weekly β-hCG is drawn until the hCG titer is within normal limits for 3 weeks. The titers are then observed at monthly intervals for 6 to 12 months. Figure 45-5 illustrates an algorithm for molar pregnancy management.[240]

For the patient with a complete molar pregnancy, the risk of requiring chemotherapy for persistent GTD is approximately 20 percent. Clinical features that increase this risk include delayed hemorrhage, excessive uterine enlargement, theca-lutein cysts, serum hCG greater than 100,000 mIU/ml, and maternal age older than 40. It is obviously particularly important not to misinterpret a rising β-hCG due to a new intervening pregnancy as persistent GTD, because intervention with chemotherapy would be a significant risk to a new gestation, inducing either abortion or possible teratogenic defects.

Invasive Mole (Chorioadenoma Destruens)

Because invasion of the myometrium by molar tissue is clinically occult, it is difficult to assess the true incidence, estimated to be between 5 and 10 percent. The clinical hallmark of invasive mole is hemorrhage, often severe, either vaginal or intraperitoneal.

Partial Hydatidiform Mole

Most partial moles have a triploid (paternally inherited, diandric, triploidies) karyotype, and the next most common are tetraploidies. A minority of partial moles exhibit a mosaic or partially diploid karyotype.[241–243] Karyotype analysis of the accompanying fetus is important in planning therapeutic intervention. A partial mole associated with a nonviable fetal chromosomal abnormality requires either mechanical or medically induced uterine evacuation (Fig. 45-6).[244] In the presence of an abundance of hydropic tissue, there is always the concern that trophoblastic tissue embolization may occur during uterine contractions induced to evacuate molar tissue. The management of a patient with sonographic findings suggestive of a diagnosis of a partial mole is particularly challenging if the karyotype analysis of the fetus is diploid, especially if the diagnosis is made in the second or third trimester. When a normal karyotype exists, it is appropriate to consider diagnostic possibilities other than partial mole, such as a twin gestation—one normal developing fetus and one molar pregnancy. Also, degenerative changes (hydropic villi), retroplacental hematomas, placental abnormalities (chorioangiomas), degenerative uterine myomas, and aborted tissue, sometimes referred to as a "transitional mole," may lead to imaging abnormalities that are difficult to interpret.

Approximately 2 to 6 percent of patients develop persistent GTD after a partial molar pregnancy.[245,246] Therefore, because choriocarcinoma can follow a true partial mole, these patients require the same postevacuation surveillance and management as the patient with a complete mole, with a follow-up of at least 6 months.[247]

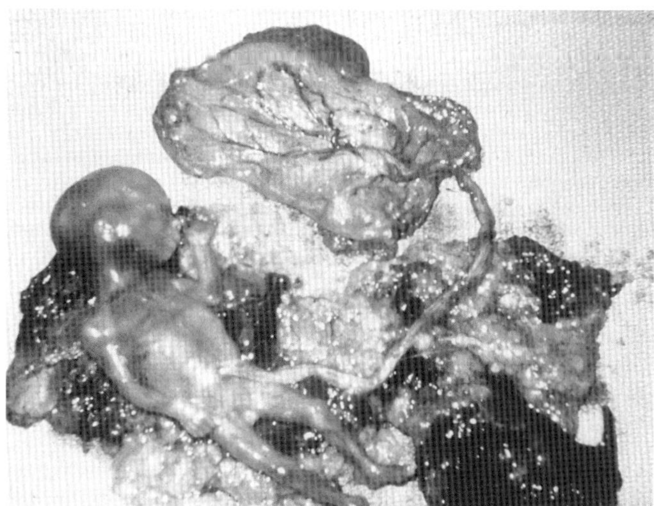

Figure 45-6. Partial mole with dead fetus of abnormal karyotype. (From Copeland LJ: Gestational trophoblastic neoplasia. *In* Copeland LJ [ed]: Textbook of Gynecology, 2nd ed. Philadelphia, WB Saunders Company, 2000, p 1416, with permission.)

Placental Site Trophoblastic Tumor

Less than 1 percent of all patients with GTD have placental site trophoblastic tumor. Although this tumor usually presents with abnormal vaginal bleeding following a term pregnancy, it can also be a sequela to a molar pregnancy or abortion. The postpartum presentation is characterized by a slightly enlarged uterus, persistent bleeding or, occasionally, amenorrhea, and a slightly elevated β-hCG level. The hCG may not reliably reflect disease progression. The histologic diagnosis may be obtained by uterine curettage, possibly hysteroscopically directed. Because this disease tends to metastasize late and be somewhat resistant to chemotherapy, surgical excision (hysterectomy) should be considered.[248] If the patient is desirous of future childbearing, management considerations that have been reported with some success include systemic chemotherapy, regional infusion chemotherapy, uterine curettage, and local excision of tumor by hysterotomy and uterine reconstruction.[249]

Choriocarcinoma

Choriocarcinoma develops in approximately 1 in every 40,000 term pregnancies and this clinical presentation represents about one fourth of all cases of choriocarcinoma. The other cases follow molar disease or an abortion (spontaneous, therapeutic, or ectopic). GTD following a term pregnancy is always either choriocarcinoma or a placental site trophoblastic tumor, assuming a singleton pregnancy.

Choriocarcinoma is notorious for masquerading as other diseases. This is secondary to hemorrhagic metastases producing symptoms such as hematuria, hemoptysis, hematemesis, hematochezia, stroke, or vaginal bleeding. The common sites for metastatic disease are listed in Table 45-8. The diagnosis of choriocarcinoma is based on history, imaging studies, and a serum β-hCG level. Histo-

Table 45-8. Common Sites for Metastatic Choriocarcinoma*

SITE	PERCENT
Lung	60–95
Vagina	40–50
Vulva/cervix	10–15
Brain	5–15
Liver	5–15
Kidney	0–5
Spleen	0–5
Gastrointestinal	0–5

*Frequencies vary, depending on whether data are based on autopsy studies or are obtained from pretreatment imaging.

From Copeland LJ: Gestational trophoblastic neoplasia. *In* Copeland LJ (ed): Textbook of Gynecology, 2nd ed. Philadelphia, WB Saunders Company, 2000, p 1391, with permission.

logic confirmation is neither necessary for the diagnosis nor a prerequisite to initiate therapy. Again, it is necessary to exclude the presence of a new gestation as the source of a rising β-hCG level before extensive diagnostic imaging or therapeutic intervention. It is also important to rule out phantom hCG production if the clinical scenario warrants, such as situations with low titers and no histologic or convincing imaging evidence of GTD.

The complexities of the general treatment approach or treatment for special situations is beyond the scope of this chapter. It is recommended that the reader refer to a gynecology or gynecologic oncology resource for discussions of the therapeutic subtleties and pitfalls. Choriocarcinoma should be managed by a gynecologic oncologist, preferably one with a special interest in the disease.

Key Points

- Because many of the common complaints of pregnancy are also early symptoms of metastatic cancer, pregnant women with cancer are at risk for delays in diagnosis and therapeutic intervention.
- The safest interval for most cancer therapies in pregnancy is the second and third trimesters, thereby avoiding induction of teratogenic risks or miscarriage in the first trimester. For most malignancies diagnosed during the second trimester, chemotherapy should be undertaken as indicated because fetal risk is generally lower than the risk of delaying treatment or proceeding with preterm delivery.
- Antimetabolites and alkylating agents present the greatest hazard to the developing fetus.
- Diagnostic delays of breast cancer in pregnancy are often attributed to physician reluctance to properly evaluate breast complaints or abnormal findings in pregnancy.
- Treatment for Hodgkin's disease may compromise the reproductive potential, and combined treatment with irradiation and chemotherapy provides the highest risk of ovarian failure.
- If a mother is exposed to cytotoxic drugs within 1 month of delivery, the newborn should be monitored closely for evidence of granulocytopenia or thrombocytopenia.
- The effect of pregnancy on the clinical course of melanoma has been the subject of debate. When corrected for tumor thickness, pregnancy does not appear to be an independent prognostic variable for survival.
- After stratifying for stage and age, patients with pregnancy-associated cervical carcinoma have survival rates similar to the nonpregnant patient.
- Because most malignant ovarian tumors found in pregnancy are either germ cell tumors or low-grade, early-stage epithelial tumors, the therapeutic plan will usually permit continuation of the pregnancy and preservation of fertility.
- Although rare, most colorectal carcinomas in pregnancy are detectable on rectal examination, underscoring the need for a rectal examination at the patient's first prenatal visit.
- Phantom hCG should be ruled out in patients suspected of having gestational trophoblastic disease when not documented by other clear clinical evidence (histology, imaging and clinical history), especially when hCG titers are low.

REFERENCES

1. Donnegan WL: Cancer and pregnancy. Cancer 33:194, 1983.
2. Koren G, Weiner L, Lishner M, et al: Cancer in pregnancy: identification of unanswered questions on maternal and fetal risks. Obstet Gynecol Surv 45:509, 1990.
3. Doll DC, Ringenberg QS, Yarbro JW: Management of cancer during pregnancy. Arch Intern Med 148:2058, 1988.
4. Doll DC, Ringenberg QS, Yarbro JW: Antineoplastic agents and pregnancy. Semin Oncol 16:337, 1989.
5. Ben-Baruch G, Menczer J, Goshen R, et al: Cisplatin excretion in human milk. J Natl Cancer Inst 84:451, 1992.
6. Reynoso EE, Shepherd FA, Messner HA, et al: Acute leukemia during pregnancy: the Toronto leukemia study group experience with long term follow-up in children exposed in utero to chemotherapeutic agents. J Clin Oncol 5:1098, 1987.
7. Henderson CE, Elia G, Garfinkel D, et al: Platinum chemotherapy during pregnancy for serous cystadenocarcinoma of the ovary. Gynecol Oncol 49:92, 1993.
8. Zemlickis D, Lishner M, Degendorfer P, et al: Fetal outcome after in utero exposure to cancer chemotherapy. Arch Intern Med 152:573, 1992.
9. Briggs GG, Freeman RK, Yaffe SJ: Instructions for use of the reference guide. *In* Briggs GG, Freeman RK, Yaffe SJ (eds): A Reference Guide to Fetal and Neonatal Risk: Drugs in Pregnancy and Lactation, 7th ed. Philadelphia, Lippincott, Williams & Wilkins, 2005, p xxi.
10. Nicholson HO: Cytotoxic drugs in pregnancy. J Obstet Gynaecol Br Commonw 75:307, 1968.
11. Schardein JL: Cancer chemotherapeutic agents. *In* Schardein JL (ed): Chemically Induced Birth Defects, 2nd ed. New York, Marcel Dekker, 1993.
12. Kozlowski RD, Steinbrunner JV, Mackenzie AH, et al: Outcome of first-trimester exposure to low-dose methotrexate in eight patients with rheumatic disease. Am J Med 88:589, 1990.
13. Roboz J, Gleichner N, Wu K, et al: Does doxorubicin cross the placenta? Lancet 2:2691, 1979.
14. Barni S, Ardizzola A, Zanetta G, et al: Weekly doxorubicin chemotherapy for breast cancer in pregnancy: a case report. Tumori 78:349, 1992.
15. Karp GI, Von Oeyen P, Valone F, et al: Doxorubicin in pregnancy: possible transplacental passage. Cancer Treat Rep 67:773, 1983.
16. Malone JM, Gershenson DM, Creasy RK, et al: Endodermal sinus tumor of the ovary associated with pregnancy. Obstet Gynecol 68:86, 1986.
17. Kim DS, Park MI: Maternal and fetal survival following surgery and chemotherapy of endodermal sinus tumor of the ovary during pregnancy: a case report. Obstet Gynecol 73:503, 1989.
18. Christman JE, Teng NNH, Lebovic GS, Sikic BI: Case report: delivery of a normal infant following cisplatin, vinblastine, and bleomycin chemotherapy for malignant teratoma of the ovary during pregnancy. Gynecol Oncol 37:292, 1990.
19. Tewari K, Cappuccini F, Gamkino A, et al: Neoadjuvant chemotherapy in the treatment of locally advanced cervical carcinoma in pregnancy. Cancer 82:1529, 1998.

20. Elit L, Bocking A, Kenyon C, Natale R: An endodermal sinus tumor diagnosed in pregnancy: case report and review of the literature. Gynecol Oncol 72:123, 1999.
21. Metz SA, Day TG, Pursell SH: Adjuvant chemotherapy in a pregnant patient with endodermal sinus tumor. Gynecol Oncol 32:371, 1989.
22. Malfetano JH, Goldkrand JW: Cisplatinum combination chemotherapy during pregnancy for advanced epithelial ovarian carcinoma. Obstet Gynecol 75:545, 1990.
23. King LA, Nevin PC, Williams PP, et al: Treatment of advanced epithelial ovarian carcinoma in pregnancy with cisplatin-based chemotherapy. Gynecol Oncol 41:78, 1991.
24. van der Zee AGJ, de Bruijn HWA, Bouma J, et al: Endodermal sinus tumor of the ovary during pregnancy: a case report. Am J Obstet Gynecol 164:504, 1991.
25. Farahmand SH, Marchetti DL, Asirwatham JE, Dewey MR: Case report: ovarian endodermal sinus tumor associated with pregnancy: review of the literature. Gynecol Oncol 41:156, 1991.
26. Horbelt D, Delmore J, Meisel R, et al: Mixed germ cell malignancy of the ovary concurrent with pregnancy. Obstet Gynecol 84:662, 1994.
27. [illegible] J, [illegible] L: The effects of cancer chemotherapeutic agents on the developing fetus. Obstet Gynecol Surv 38:6, 1983.
28. Sood AK, Shahin MS, Sorosky JI: Paclitaxel and platinum chemotherapy for ovarian carcinoma during pregnancy. Gynecol Oncol 83:599, 2001.
29. Gonzalez-Angula AM, Walters RS, Carpenter RJ Jr, et al: Paclitaxel chemotherapy in a pregnant patient with bilateral breast cancer. Clin Breast Cancer 5:317, 2004.
30. Beidler N: Cancer treatment during pregnancy: there's strength in numbers for researchers. J Natl Cancer Inst 92:372, 2000.
31. Mulvihill JJ, Stewart KR: A registry of pregnancies exposed to chemotherapeutic agents. Teratology 33:80, 1986.
32. Hassed S, Mumm C, Reed A, et al: Registry of pregnancies exposed to chemotherapeutic agents. Am J Hum Genet 73:190, 2003.
33. Garber JE: Long-term follow-up of children exposed in utero to antineoplastic agents. Semin Oncol 16:437, 1989.
34. Partridge AH, Garber JE: Long-term outcomes of children exposed to antineoplastic agents in utero. Semin Oncol 27:712, 2000.
35. Leyendecker JR, Gorengaut V, Brown JJ: MR imaging of maternal diseases of the abdomen and pelvis during pregnancy and the immediate postpartum period. Radiographics 24:1301, 2004.
36. Mazze RI, Kallen B: Reproductive outcome after anesthesia and operation during pregnancy: a registry study of 5405 cases. Am J Obstet Gynecol 161:1178, 1989.
37. Nagarajan R, Robison LL: Pregnancy outcomes in survivors of childhood cancer. J Natl Cancer Inst Monogr 34:72, 2005.
38. Aisner J, Wiernik PH, Pearl P: Pregnancy outcome in patients treated for Hodgkin's disease. J Clin Oncol 11:507, 1993.
39. Clark ST, Radford JA, Crowther D, et al: Gonadal function following chemotherapy for Hodgkin disease: a comparative study of MVPP and a seven-drug hybrid regimen. J Clin Oncol 13:134, 1995.
40. Plante M, Renaud MC, Francoid H, Roy M: Vaginal radical trachelectomy: an oncologically safe fertility-preserving surgery. An updated series of 72 cases and review of the literature. Gynecol Oncol 94:614, 2004.
41. Bernardini M, Barrett J, Seaward G, Coven A: Pregnancy outcomes in patients after radical trachelectomy. Am J Obstet Gynecol 189:1378, 2004.
42. Aviles A, Diaz-Maqueo JC, Talavera A, et al: Growth and development of children and mothers treated with chemotherapy during pregnancy; current status of 43 children. Am J Hematol 36:243, 1991.
43. Jemal A, Siegel R, Ward E, et al: Cancer statistics, 2006. CA Cancer J Clin 56:106, 2006.
44. Lewison EF: Breast cancer and pregnancy or lactation. Surg Gynecol Obstet 99:417, 1954.
45. Smith LH, Dalrymple JL, Leiserowitz GS, et al: Obstetrical deliveries associated with maternal malignancy in California, 1992 through 1997. Am J Obstet Gynecol 184:1504, 2001.
46. Michels KB, Willett WC, Rosner BA, et al: Prospective assessment of breastfeeding and breast cancer incidence among 89,877 women. Lancet 347:431, 1996.
47. Jernstrom H, Lerman C, Ghadirian P, et al: Pregnancy and risk of early breast cancer in carriers of BRCA1 and BRCA2. Lancet 354:1846, 1999.
48. Applewhite RR, Smith LR, DiVincenti F: Carcinoma of the breast associated with pregnancy and lactation. Ann Surg 39:101, 1973.
49. Zemlickis D, Lishner M, Degendorfer P, et al: Maternal and fetal outcomes after breast cancer in pregnancy. Am J Obstet Gynecol 166:781, 1992.
50. Parente JT, Amsel M, Lerner R, Chinea F: Breast cancer associated with pregnancy. Obstet Gynecol 71:861, 1988.
51. Max MH, Lamer TW: Breast cancer in 120 women under 35 years old. Ann Surg 50:23, 1984.
52. Botsis D, Sarandakou A, Kassanos D, et al: Breast cancer markers during normal pregnancy. Anticancer Res 19:3539, 1999.
53. Gentilini O, Cremonesi M, Trifiro G, et al: Safety of sentinel node biopsy in pregnant patients with breast cancer. Ann Oncol 15:1348, 2004.
54. Keleher A, Wendt R III, Delpassand E, et al: The safety of lymphatic mapping in pregnant breast cancer patients using Tc-99m sulfur colloid. Breast J 10:492, 2004.
55. King RM, Welch JS, [illegible] JK Jr, [illegible]: Carcinoma of the breast associated with pregnancy. Surg Gynecol Obstet [illegible], [illegible]
56. Petrek JA, Theriault RL: Pregnancy-associated breast cancer and subsequent pregnancy in breast cancer survivors. *In* Harris JR, Lippman ME, Morrow M, Osborne CK (eds): Diseases of the Breast, 3rd ed. Philadelphia, Lippincott, Williams & Wilkins, 2004, p. 1037.
57. Kuerer HM, Gwyn K, Ames FC, et al: Conservative surgery and chemotherapy for breast carcinoma during pregnancy. Surgery 131:108, 2002.
58. Nettleton J, Long J, Kuban D, et al: Breast cancer during pregnancy: quantifying the risk of treatment delay. Obstet Gynecol 87:414, 1996.
59. van der Vange N, van Donegan JA: Breast cancer and pregnancy. Eur J Surg Oncol 17:1, 1991.
60. Brent RL: The effect of embryonic and fetal exposure to x-ray, microwaves, and ultrasound: counseling the pregnant and nonpregnant patient about these risks. Semin Oncol 16:347, 1989.
61. Holmes FA: Breast cancer during pregnancy. Cancer Bull 46:405, 1994.
62. Elledge RM, Ciocca DR, Langione DR, et al: Estrogen receptor, progesterone receptor, and HER-2/neu protein in breast cancers from pregnant patients. Cancer 71:2499, 1993.
63. Holleb AI, Farrow JH: The relationship of carcinoma of the breast and pregnancy in 283 patients. Surg Gynecol Obstet 115:65, 1962.
64. Lee TN, Horz JM: Significance of ovarian metastases in therapeutic oophorectomy for advanced breast cancer. Cancer 27:1374, 1971.
65. Ravdin RG, Lewison EF, Slack NH: The results of a clinical trial concerning the worth of prophylactic oophorectomy for breast cancer. Surg Gynecol Obstet 131:1055, 1970.
66. Giacolone PL, Laffargue F, Benos P: Chemotherapy for breast carcinoma during pregnancy: a French national survey. Cancer 86:2266, 1999.
67. Bernik SF, Bernik TR, Whooley BP, et al: Carcinoma of the breast during pregnancy: a review and update on treatment options. Surg Oncol 7:45, 1999.
68. Berry DL, Theriault RL, Holmes FA, et al: Management of breast cancer during pregnancy using a standardized protocol. J Clin Oncol 17:855, 1999.
69. Ring AE, Smith IE, Jones A, et al: Chemotherapy for breast cancer during pregnancy: 18-year experience from five London teaching hospitals. J Clin Oncol 23:4192, 2005.
70. Byrd BF Jr, Bayer DS, Robertson JC, Stephenson SE: Treatment of breast tumors associated with pregnancy and lactation. Ann Surg 155:940, 1962.
71. White TT, White WC: Breast cancer and pregnancy: report of 49 cases followed five years. Ann Surg 144:384, 1956.
72. Applewhite RR, Smith LR, DiVincenti F: Carcinoma of the breast associated with pregnancy and lactation. Ann Surg 39:101, 1973.
73. Riberio GG, Palmer MK: Breast carcinoma associated with pregnancy: a clinician's dilemma. BMJ 2:1524, 1977.

74. Clark RM, Reid J: Carcinoma of the breast in pregnancy and lactation. Int Radiat Oncol Biol Phys 4:693, 1978.
75. Petrek JA, Dukoff R, Rogatko A: Prognosis of pregnancy-associated breast cancer. Cancer 67:869, 1991.
76. Donegan WL: Breast cancer and pregnancy. Obstet Gynecol 50:244, 1977.
77. Peters MV: The effect of pregnancy in breast cancer. *In* Forrest APM, Kunkler PB (eds): Prognostic Factors in Breast Cancer. Baltimore, Williams & Wilkins, 1968, p 120.
78. Reed W, Hannisdal E, Skovlund E, et al: Pregnancy and breast cancer: A population-based study. Virchows Arch 443:44, 2003.
79. Gelber S, Coates AS, Goldhirsch A, et al: Effect of pregnancy on overall survival after the diagnosis of early-stage breast cancer. J Clin Oncol 19:1671, 2001.
80. Mueller BA, Simon MS, Deapen D, et al: Childbearing and survival after breast carcinoma in young women. Cancer 98:1131, 2003.
81. Blakely LJ, Buzdar AU, Lozada JA, et al: Effects of pregnancy after treatment for breast carcinoma on survival and risk of recurrence. Cancer 100:465, 2004.
82. Danforth DN Jr: How subsequent pregnancy affects outcome in women with a prior breast cancer. Oncology 11:21, 1991
83. Velentgas P, Daling JR, Malone KE, et al: Pregnancy after breast carcinoma: outcomes and influence on mortality. Cancer 85:2424, 1999.
84. Epstein RJ, Henderson IC: The Danforth article reviewed: the jury is in. Oncology 11:30, 1991.
85. Partridge A, Schapira L: Pregnancy and breast cancer: Epidemiology, treatment, and safety issues. Oncology 19:693, 2005.
86. Sutton R, Buzdar AU, Hortobagyi GN: Pregnancy and offspring after adjuvant chemotherapy in breast cancer patients. Cancer 71:2499, 1990.
87. Higgins S, Haffty B: Pregnancy and lactation after breast-conserving therapy for early-stage breast cancer. Cancer 73:2175, 1994.
88. Tralins A: Is lactation possible after breast irradiation? Proc Am Soc Clin Oncol 12:77, 1993.
89. Miller MJ, Ross ME: Case report: pregnancy following breast reconstruction with autologous tissue. Cancer Bull 45:546, 1993.
90. Barry RM, Diamond HD, Craver LF: Influence of pregnancy on the course of Hodgkin's disease. Am J Obstet Gynecol 84:445, 1962.
91. Sweet DL Jr: Malignant lymphoma: implications during the reproductive years and pregnancy. J Reprod Med 17:198, 1976.
92. Lishner M, Zemlickis D, Degendorfer P, et al: Maternal and fetal outcome following Hodgkin's disease in pregnancy. Br J Cancer 65:114, 1992.
93. Gelb AB, van de Rijn M, Warnke RA: Pregnancy-associated lymphomas. A clinicopathologic study. Cancer 78:304, 1996.
94. Thomas PRM, Peckham MJ: The investigation and management of Hodgkin's disease in the pregnant patient. Cancer 38:1443, 1976.
95. Jacobs C, Donaldson SS, Rosenberg SA, Kaplan HS: Management of the pregnant patient with Hodgkin's disease. Ann Intern Med 95:649, 1981.
96. Friedman E, Jones GW: Fetal outcome after maternal radiation treatment of supradiaphragmatic Hodgkin's disease. Can Med Assoc J 149:1281, 1993.
97. Dein RA, Mennuti MT, Kovach P, Gabbe SG: The reproductive potential of young men and women with Hodgkin's disease. Obstet Gynecol Surv 39:474, 1984.
98. Horning SJ, Hoppe RT, Kaplan HS: Female reproduction after treatment for Hodgkin's disease. N Engl J Med 304:1377, 1981.
99. Chapman RM, Sutcliffe SB, Malpas JS: Cytotoxic induced ovarian failure in women with Hodgkin's disease. I. Hormone function. JAMA 242:1877, 1979.
100. Chapman RM, Sutcliffe SB, Lees LH: Cyclical combination chemotherapy and gonadal function. Lancet 1:285, 1979.
101. Jarrell JJ: Reproductive toxicology. *In* Copeland LJ (ed): Textbook of Gynecology. Philadelphia, WB Saunders Company, 2000, p 453.
102. Holmes GE, Holmes FF: Pregnancy outcome of patients treated for Hodgkin's disease. Cancer 41:1317, 1978.
103. Janov AJ, Anderson J, Cella DF, et al: Pregnancy outcome in survivors of advanced Hodgkin's disease. Cancer 70:688, 1992.
104. McKeen EA, Mulvihill JJ, Rosner F, Zarrari MH: Pregnancy outcome in Hodgkin's disease. Lancet 2:590, 1979.
105. Selvais PL, Mazy G, Gosseye S, et al: Breast infiltration by acute lymphoblastic leukemia during pregnancy. Am J Obstet Gynecol 169:1619, 1993.
106. Ward FT, Weiss RB: Lymphoma and pregnancy. Semin Oncol 16:397, 1989.
107. Ohba T, Matusuo I, Katabuchi H, et al: Adult T-cell leukemia/lymphoma in pregnancy. Obstet Gynecol 72:445, 1988.
108. Manns A, Blattner WA: The epidemiology of the human T-cell lymphotropic virus type I and type II: etiologic role in human disease. Transfusion 31:67, 1991.
109. Caligiuri MA, Mayer RJ: Pregnancy and leukemia. Semin Oncol 16:338, 1989.
110. Catanzarite VA, Ferguson JE: Acute leukemia and pregnancy: a review of management and outcome, 1972–1982. Obstet Gynecol Surv 39:663, 1984.
111. Juarez S, Cuadrado JM, Feliu J, et al: Association of leukemia and pregnancy: clinical and obstetric aspects. Am J Clin Oncol 11:159, 1988.
112. Zuazu J, Julia A, Sierra J, et al: Pregnancy outcome in hematologic malignancies. Cancer 67:703, 1991.
113. Antonelli NM, Dotters DJ, Katz VL, Kuller JA: Cancer in pregnancy: a review of the literature. Part II. Obstet Gynecol Surv 51:135, 1996.
114. Chelghoum Y, Vey N, Raffoux E, et al: Acute leukemia during pregnancy: a report on 37 patients and a review of the literature. Cancer 104(l):110, 2005.
115. Hoelzer D, Thiel E, Loffler H, et al: Prognostic factors in a multicenter study for treatment of acute lymphoblastic leukemia in adults. Blood 71:123, 1988.
116. Wiernik PH: Acute leukemias of adults. *In* DeVita VT Jr, Hellman S, Rosenberg SA (eds): Cancer: Principles and Practice of Oncology. Philadelphia, JB Lippincott, 1982, p 302.
117. Aviles A, Niz J: Long term follow-up of children born to mothers with acute leukemia during pregnancy. Med Pediatr Oncol 16:3, 1988.
118. Bazarbashi MS, Smith MR, Karanes C, et al: Successful management of Ph chromosome chronic myelogenous leukemia with leukapheresis during pregnancy. Am J Hematol 38:235, 1991.
119. Baer MR, Ozer H, Foon KA: Interferon-alpha therapy during pregnancy in chronic myelogenous leukemia and hairy cell leukemia. Br J Haematol 81:167, 1992.
120. Delmer A, Rio B, Baudner F, et al: Pregnancy during myelosuppressive treatment for chronic myelogenous leukemia. Br J Haematol 82:783, 1992.
121. Cohen MH, Johnson JR, Pazdur R: U.S. Food and Drug Administration Approval Summary: conversion of imatinib mesylate (STI571; Gleevec) tablets from accelerated approval to full approval. Clin Cancer Res 11:12, 2005.
122. Kantarjian H, Sawyers C, Hochhous A, et al: International STI571 CML Study Group. Hematologic and cytogenetic responses to imatinib mesylate in chronic myelogenous leukemia. N Engl J Med 346:645, 2002.
123. Tertian G, Tchernia G, Papiernik E, et al: Hydroxyurea and pregnancy. Am J Obstet Gynecol 166:1868, 1992.
124. Friedman RJ, Rigel DS, Kopf AW: Early detection of malignant melanoma: the role of the physician examination and self examination of the skin. CA Cancer J Clin 35:130, 1985.
125. Smith RS, Randall P: Melanoma during pregnancy. Obstet Gynecol 34:825, 1969.
126. Balch CM, Soong SJ, Milton GW, et al: A comparison of prognostic factors and surgical results in 1,786 patients with localized (stage I) melanoma treated in Alabama, USA, and New South Wales, Australia. Ann Surg 146:677, 1982.
127. Gordon AN: Vulvar tumors. *In* Copeland LJ (ed): Textbook of Gynecology. Philadelphia, WB Saunders Company, 2000, p 1202.
128. Pack GT, Scharnagel IM: The prognosis for malignant melanoma in the pregnant woman. Cancer 4:324, 1951.
129. Byrd BF, McGanty WJ: The effect of pregnancy on the normal course of malignant melanoma. South Med 47:324, 1951.
130. George PA, Fortner JG, Pack GT: Melanoma with pregnancy: a report of 115 cases. Cancer 13:854, 1960.

131. Shiu MH, Schottenfeld D, Maclean B, Fortner JG: Adverse effect of pregnancy on melanoma. Cancer 37:181, 1976.
132. Houghton AN, Flannery J, Viola MV: Malignant melanoma of the skin occurring during pregnancy. Cancer 48:407, 1981.
133. Wong DJ, Stassner HT: Melanoma in pregnancy. Clin Obstet Gynecol 33:782, 1990.
134. MacKie RM, Bufalino R, Morabito A, et al: Lack of effect on pregnancy outcome of melanoma. Lancet 337:653, 1991.
135. McManamny DS, Moss ALH, Pocock PV, et al: Melanoma and pregnancy: a long-term follow-up. Br J Obstet Gynaecol 96:1419, 1989.
136. Slingluff CL Jr, Reintgen D, Vollmer RT, et al: Malignant melanoma arising during pregnancy: a study of 100 patients. Ann Surg 211:552, 1990.
137. Lens MB, Rosdahl I, Ahlbom A, et al: Effect of pregnancy on survival in women with cutaneous malignant melanoma. J Clin Oncol 22:4369, 2004.
138. Lederman JS, Sober AJ: Effect of prior pregnancy on melanoma survival. Arch Dermatol 121:716, 1985.
139. Travers R, Sober A, Barnhill R, et al: Increased thickness of pregnancy-associated melanoma: a study of the MGH pigmented lesion clinic. Melanoma Res 3(Suppl):44, 1993.
140. Colburn DS, Nathanson L, Belilos E: Pregnancy and malignant melanoma. Semin Oncol 16:377, 1989.
141. Ross MI: Melanoma and pregnancy: prognostic and therapeutic considerations. Cancer Bull 46:412, 1994.
142. Ostelind A, Tucker MA, Stone BJ, et al: The Danish case control study of cutaneous malignant melanoma III: hormonal and reproductive factors in women. Int J Cancer 42:821, 1988.
143. Lederman JS, Lew RA, Koh HK, Sober AJ: Influence of estrogen administration on tumor characteristics and survival in women with cutaneous melanoma. J Natl Cancer Inst 74:981, 1985.
144. Hacker NF, Berek JS, Lagasse LD, et al: Carcinoma of the cervix associated with pregnancy. Obstet Gynecol 59:735, 1982.
145. Zemlickis D, Lishner M, Degendorfer P, et al: Maternal and fetal outcome after invasive cervical cancer in pregnancy. J Clin Oncol 9:1956, 1991.
146. Nevin D, Soeters R, Dehaeck K, et al: Cervical carcinoma associated with pregnancy. Obstet Gynecol Surv 50:228, 1995.
147. Benedet JL, Selke PA, Nickerson KG: Colposcopic evaluation of abnormal Papanicolaou smears in pregnancy. Am J Obstet Gynecol 157:932, 1987.
148. Economos K, Perez Veridiano N, Delke I, et al: Abnormal cervical cytology in pregnancy: a 17-year experience. Obstet Gynecol 81:915, 1993.
149. Averette HE, Nasser N, Yankow SL: Cervical conization in pregnancy. Am J Obstet Gynecol 106:543, 1970.
150. Hannigan EV, Whitehouse HH III, Atkinson WD, et al: Cone biopsy during pregnancy. Obstet Gynecol 60:450, 1982.
151. Hannigan EV: Cervical cancer in pregnancy. Clin Obstet Gynecol 33:837, 1990.
152. Copeland LJ, Silva EG, Gershenson DM, et al: Superficially invasive squamous cell carcinoma of the cervix. Gynecol Oncol 45:307, 1992.
153. Lewandowski GS, Copeland LJ, Vaccarello L: Surgical issues in the management of carcinoma of the cervix in pregnancy. Surg Clin North Am 75:89, 1995.
154. Duggan B, Muderspach LI, Roman LD, et al: Cervical cancer in pregnancy: reporting on planned delay in therapy. Obstet Gynecol 82:598, 1993.
155. Sood AK, Sorosky JL, Krogman S, et al: Surgical management of cervical cancer complicating pregnancy: a case-control study. Gynecol Oncol 63:294, 1996.
156. Monk BJ, Montz FJ: Invasive cervical cancer complicating intrauterine pregnancy. Treatment with hysterectomy. Obstet Gynecol 80:199, 1992.
157. Sivanesaratnam V, Javalakshmi P, Loo C: Surgical management of early invasive cancer of the uterine cervix associated with pregnancy. Gynecol Oncol 48:68, 1993.
158. Greer BE, Easterling TR, McLennan DA, et al: Fetal and maternal considerations in the management of stage IB cervical during pregnancy. Gynecol Oncol 34:61, 1989.
159. Lewandowski GS, Copeland LJ: A potential role for invasive chemotherapy in the treatment of small cell neuroendocrine tumors of the cervix. Gynecol Oncol 48:127, 1993.
160. Balderston KD, Tewari K, Gregory WT, et al: Neuroendocrine small cell cervix cancer in pregnancy: long-term survivor following combined therapy. Gynecol Oncol 71:128, 1998.
161. Shingleton HM, Orr JW: Cervical cancer complicating pregnancy. *In* Cancer of the Cervix. Edinburgh, Churchill Livingstone, 1983, p 284.
162. Copeland LJ, Saul PB, Sneige N: Cervical adenocarcinoma: tumor implantation in the episiotomy sites of two patients. Gynecol Oncol 28:230, 1987.
163. Gordon AN, Jensen R, Jones HW III: Squamous carcinoma of the cervix complicating pregnancy: recurrence in episiotomy after vaginal delivery. Obstet Gynecol 73:850, 1989.
164. Cliby WA, Dodson WA, Podratz KC: Cervical cancer complicated by pregnancy: episiotomy site recurrences following vaginal delivery. Obstet Gynecol 84:179, 1994.
165. Hopkins MP, Morley GW: The prognosis and management of cervical cancer associated with pregnancy. Obstet Gynecol 80:9, 1992.
166. Jones WB, Shingleton HM, Russell A, et al: Cervical carcinoma and pregnancy. A national pattern of care study of the American College of Surgeons. Cancer 77:1479, 1996.
167. Germann N, Haie-Meder C, Morice P, et al: Management and clinical outcomes of pregnant patients with invasive cervical cancer. Ann Oncol 16:397, 2005.
168. Fleischer AC, Shah DM, Entman SS: Sonographic evaluation of maternal disorders during pregnancy. Radiol Clin North Am 28:51, 1990.
169. Hess LW, Peaceman A, O'Brien W, et al: Adnexal mass occurring with intrauterine pregnancy: a report of 54 patients requiring laparotomy for definitive management. Am J Obstet Gynecol 158:1029, 1988.
170. El Yahia AR, Rahman J, Rahman MS, et al: Ovarian tumors in pregnancy. Aust N Z J Obstet Gynaecol 31:327, 1991.
171. Munnell EW: Primary ovarian cancer associated with pregnancy. Clin Obstet Gynecol 6:983, 1963.
172. Dgani R, Shoham Z, Atar E, et al: Ovarian carcinoma during pregnancy: a study of 23 cases in Israel between the years of 1960 and 1984. Gynecol Oncol 33:326, 1989.
173. Copeland LJ: Gestational trophoblastic neoplasia. *In* Copeland LJ (ed): Textbook of Gynecology. Philadelphia, WB Saunders Company, 2000, p 1391.
174. Platek DN, Henderson CE, Goldberg GL: The management of a persistent adnexal mass in pregnancy. Am J Obstet Gynecol 173:12236, 1995.
175. Schmeler KM, Mayo-Smith WW, Peipert JF, et al: Adnexal masses in pregnancy: Surgery compared with observation. Obstet Gynecol 105:1098–1103, 2005.
176. Jacob JH, Stringer CA: Diagnosis and management of cancer during pregnancy. Semin Perinatol 14:79, 1990.
177. Jolles CJ: Gynecologic cancer associated with pregnancy. Semin Oncol 16:417, 1989.
178. Katz VL, Watson WJ, Hansen WF, et al: Massive ovarian tumor complicating pregnancy: a case report. J Reprod Med 38:907, 1993.
179. Ferrandina G, DiStefano M, Testa A, et al: Management of an advanced ovarian cancer at 15 weeks of gestation. Case report and literature review. Gynecol Oncol 97:693, 2005.
180. Kobayashi F, Sagawa N, Nakamura K, et al: Mechanism and clinical significance of elevated CA 125 levels in the sera of pregnant women. Am J Obstet Gynecol 160:563, 1989.
181. VanSlooten AJ, Rechner SF, Dods WG: Recurrent maternal virilization during pregnancy caused by benign androgen-producing ovarian lesions. Am J Obstet Gynecol 167:1342, 1992.
182. McGuire WP, Hoskins WJ, Brady MF, et al: Cyclophosphamide and cisplatin compared with paclitaxel and cisplatin in patients with stage III and stage IV ovarian cancer. N Engl J Med 334:1, 1996.
183. Malfetano JH, Goldkrand JW: Cisplatinum combination chemotherapy during pregnancy for advanced epithelial ovarian carcinoma. Obstet Gynecol 75:545, 1990.
184. King LA, Nevin PC, Williams PP, Carson LF: Case report of treatment of advanced epithelial ovarian carcinoma in pregnancy with cisplatin-based chemotherapy. Gynecol Oncol 41:78, 1991.

185. Henderson CE, Giovanni E, Garfinkel D, et al: Case report: platinum chemotherapy during pregnancy for serous cystadenocarcinoma of the ovary. Gynecol Oncol 49:92, 1993.
186. Buller RE, Darrow V, Manetta A, et al: Conservative surgical management of dysgerminoma concomitant with pregnancy. Obstet Gynecol 79:887, 1992.
187. Weed JC, Roh RA, Mendenhall HW: Recurrent endodermal sinus tumor during pregnancy. Obstet Gynecol 54:653, 1979.
188. Petrucha RA, Ruffolo E, Messina AM, et al: Endodermal sinus tumor: report of a case associated with pregnancy. Obstet Gynecol 55(Suppl):90, 1980.
189. Schwartz RP, Chatwani AJ, Strimel W, Putong PB: Endodermal sinus tumors in pregnancy: report of a case and review of the literature. Gynecol Oncol 15:434, 1983.
190. Ito K, Teshima K, Suzuki H, Noda K: A case of ovarian endodermal sinus tumor associated with pregnancy. Tohoku J Exp Med 142:183, 1984.
191. Malone JM, Gershenson DM, Creasy RK, et al: Endodermal sinus tumor associated with pregnancy. Obstet Gynecol 68:86, 1984.
192. Kim DS, Park MI: Maternal and fetal survival following surgery and chemotherapy of endodermal sinus tumor of the ovary during pregnancy: a case report. Obstet Gynecol 73:503, 1989.
193. Metz SA, Day TG, Pursell SH: Adjuvant chemotherapy in a pregnant patient with endodermal sinus tumor. Gynecol Oncol 32:371, 1989.
194. van der Zee AGL, de Bruijn HWA, Bouma J, et al: Endodermal sinus tumor of the ovary during pregnancy: a case report. Am J Obstet Gynecol 164:504, 1991.
195. Farahmand SH, Marchetti DL, Asirwatham JE, Dewey MR: Case report: ovarian endodermal sinus tumor associated with pregnancy: review of the literature. Gynecol Oncol 41:156, 1991.
196. Horbelt D, Delmore J, Meisel R, et al: Mixed germ cell malignancy of the ovary concurrent with pregnancy. Obstet Gynecol 84:662, 1994.
197. Young RH, Dudley AG, Scully RE: Granulosa cell, Sertoli-Leydig cell and unclassified sex-cord stromal tumors associated with pregnancy: a clinical pathological analysis of 36 cases. Gynecol Oncol 18:181, 1984.
198. Collins CG, Barclay DL: Cancer of the vulva and cancer of the vagina in pregnancy. Clin Obstet Gynecol 6:927, 1973.
199. Lutz MH, Underwood PB, Rozier JC, et al: Genital malignancy in pregnancy. Am J Obstet Gynecol 129:536, 1977.
200. Moore DH, Fowler WC, Currie JL, Walton LA: Squamous cell carcinoma of the vulva in pregnancy. Gynecol Oncol 41:74, 1991.
201. Heller DS, Cracchiolo B, Hameed M, et al: Pregnancy-associated invasive squamous cell carcinoma of the vulva in a 28-year-old, HIV-negative woman. A case report. J Reprod Med 45:659–661, 2000.
202. Bakour SH, Jaleel H, Weaver JB, et al: Vulvar carcinoma presenting during pregnancy, associated with recurrent bone marrow hypoplasia: a case report and literature review. Gynecol Oncol 87:207–209, 2002.
203. Burke TW, Stringer CA, Gershenson DM, et al: Radical wide excision and selective inguinal node dissection for squamous cell carcinoma of the vulva. Gynecol Oncol 38:328, 1990.
204. Senekjian EK, Hubby M, Bell DA, et al: Clear cell adenocarcinoma of the vagina and cervix in association with pregnancy. Gynecol Oncol 24:207, 1986.
205. Schneller JG, Nicastri AD: Intrauterine pregnancy coincident with endometrial carcinoma: a case study and review of the literature. Gynecol Oncol 54:87, 1994.
206. Fine BA, Baker TR, Hempling RE, et al: Pregnancy coexisting with serous papillary adenocarcinoma involving both uterus and ovary. Gynecol Oncol 53:369, 1994.
207. Vaccarello L, Apte SM, Copeland LJ, et al: Endometrial carcinoma associated with pregnancy: a report of three cases and review of the literature. Gynecol Oncol 74:118, 1999.
208. Ayhan A, Gunalp S, Karaer C, et al: Endometrial adenocarcinoma in pregnancy. Gynecol Oncol 75:298, 1999.
209. Woods JB, Martin JN Jr, Ingram FH, et al: Pregnancy complicated by carcinoma of the colon above the rectum. Am J Perinatol 9:102, 1992.
210. Bernstein MA, Madoff RD, Caushaj PF: Colon and rectal cancer in pregnancy. Dis Colon Rectum 36:172, 1993.
211. Medich DS, Fazio VW: Hemorrhoids, anal fissure, and carcinoma of the colon, rectum, and anus during pregnancy. Surg Clin North Am 75:77, 1995.
212. Nesbitt JC, Moise KJ, Sawyers JL: Colorectal carcinoma in pregnancy. Arch Surg 120:636, 1985.
213. Morgan DR, Fernandez CO, DeSarno C, et al: Adenocarcinoma of the appendix in pregnancy: A case report. J Reprod Med 49:753, 2004.
214. Roelvink NCA, Kamphorst W, van Alphen HAM, et al: Pregnancy-related primary brain and spinal tumors. Arch Neurol 44:209, 1987.
215. DeAngelis LM: Central nervous system neoplasms in pregnancy. Adv Neurol 64:139, 1994.
216. Finfer SR: Management of labor and delivery in patients with intracranial neoplasms. Br J Anaesth 67:784, 1991.
217. Lunardi P, Rizzo A, Missori P, et al: Pituitary apoplexy in an acromegalic woman operated on during pregnancy by transsphenoidal approach. Int J Gynecol Obstet 34:71, 1990.
218. Coyne TJ, Atkinson RL, Prins JB: Adrenocorticotropic hormone-secreting pituitary tumor associated with pregnancy. Case report. Neurosurgery 31:953, 1992.
219. Johnson RJ Jr, Voorhies RM, Witkin M, et al: Fertility following excision of a symptomatic craniopharyngioma during pregnancy: case report. Surg Neurol 39:257, 1993.
220. Tokuda Y, Hatayama T, Sakoda K: Metastasis of malignant struma ovarii to the cranial vault during pregnancy. Neurosurgery 33:515, 1993.
221. Doyle KJ, Luxford WM: Acoustic neuroma in pregnancy. Am J Otol 15:111, 1994.
222. Arango HA, Kalter CS, Decesare SL, et al: Management of chemotherapy in a pregnancy complicated by a large neuroblastoma. Obstet Gynecol 84:665, 1994.
223. Harper MA, Murnaghan GA, Kennedy L, et al: Pheochromocytoma in pregnancy. Five cases and a review of the literature. Br J Obstet Gynaecol 96:594, 1989.
224. Dildy GA III, Moise KJ Jr, Carpenter RJ Jr, et al: Maternal malignancy metastatic to the products of conception: a review. Obstet Gynecol Surv 44:535, 1989.
225. Rothman LA, Cohen CJ, Astarola J: Placental and fetal involvement by maternal malignancy: a report of rectal carcinoma and a review of the literature. Am J Obstet Gynecol 116:1023, 1973.
226. Kurtin PJ, Gaffney TA, Haberman TM: Peripheral T cell lymphoma involving the placenta. Cancer 70:2963, 1992.
227. Pollack RN, Sklarin NT, Rao S, et al: Metastatic placental lymphoma associated with maternal human immunodeficiency virus infection. Obstet Gynecol 81:856, 1993.
228. Tsujimura T, Matsumoto K, Aozasa K: Placental involvement by maternal non-Hodgkin's lymphoma. Arch Pathol Lab Med 117:325, 1993.
229. Catlin EA, Roberts JD Jr, Evana R, et al: Transplacental transmission of natural-killer cell lymphoma. N Engl J Med 341:85, 1999.
230. Osada S, Horibe K, Oiwa K, et al: A case of infantile acute monocytic leukemia caused by vertical transmission of the mother's leukemic cells. Cancer 65:1146, 1990.
231. Pollack RN, Pollak M, Rochon L: Pregnancy complicated by medulloblastoma with metastases to the placenta. Obstet Gynecol 81:858, 1993.
232. Teksam M, McKinney A, Short J, Casey SO, et al: Intracranial metastasis via transplacental (vertical) transmission of maternal small cell lung cancer to fetus: CT and MRI findings. Acta Radiol 45:577, 2004.
233. Andreitchouk AE, Takahashi O, Kedama H, et al: Choriocarcinoma in infant and mother: a case report. J Obstet Gynaecol Res 22:585, 1996.
234. Kishkurno S, Ishida A, Takahashi Y, et al: A case of neonatal choriocarcinoma. Am J Perinatol 14:79, 1993.
235. Bandy LC, Clarke-Pearson DL, Hammond CB: Malignant potential of gestational trophoblastic disease at the extreme age of reproductive life. Obstet Gynecol 64:395, 1984.
236. Matalon M, Modan B: Epidemiologic aspects of hydatidiform mole in Israel. Am J Obstet Gynecol 112:107, 1972.

237. Lurain JR, Brewer JI, Turok EE, Halpern B: Gestational trophoblastic disease: treatment results at the Brewer Trophoblastic Disease Center. Obstet Gynecol 60:354, 1982.
238. Berkowitz RS, Goldstein DP, Bernstein MR, Sablinska B: Subsequent pregnancy outcomes in patients with molar pregnancies and gestational trophoblastic tumors. J Reprod Med 32:680, 1987.
239. Sand PK, Lurain JR, Brewer JI: Repeat gestational trophoblastic disease. Obstet Gynecol 63:140, 1984.
240. Copeland LJ: Gestational trophoblastic neoplasia. *In* Copeland LJ (ed): Textbook of Gynecology, 2nd ed. Philadelphia, WB Saunders Company, 2000, p 1414.
241. Jacobs PA, Szulman AE, Funkhouser J, et al: Human triploidy: relationship between parental origin of the additional haploid complement and development of partial hydatidiform mole. Ann Hum Genet 46:223, 1982.
242. McFadden DE, Kwong LC, Yam IY, Langlois S: Parental origin of triploidy in human fetuses: evidence for genomic imprinting. Hum Genet 92:465, 1993.
243. Jauniaux E: Partial moles: from postnatal to prenatal diagnosis. Placenta 20:379, 1999.
244. Copeland LJ: Gestational trophoblastic neoplasia. *In* Copeland LJ (ed): Textbook of Gynecology, 2nd ed. Philadelphia, WB Saunders Company, 2000, p 1416.
245. Rice LW, Berkowitz RS, Lage JM, Goldstein DP: Persistent gestational trophoblastic tumor after partial molar pregnancy. Gynecol Oncol 48:165, 1993.
246. Goto S, Yamada A, Ishizuka T, Tomoda Y: Development of post molar trophoblastic disease after partial molar pregnancy. Gynecol Oncol 48:165, 1993.
247. Seckl MH, Fisher RA, Salerno G, et al: Choriocarcinoma and partial hydatidiform moles. Lancet 356:36, 2000.
248. Chang YL, Chang TC, Hsueh S, et al: Prognostic factors and treatment for placental site trophoblastic tumor-report of 3 cases and analysis of 88 cases. Gynecol Oncol 73:216, 1999.
249. Leiserowitz GS, Webb MJ: Treatment of placental site trophoblastic tumor with hysterotomy and uterine reconstruction. Obstet Gynecol 88:696, 1996.

Dermatologic Disorders of Pregnancy

JOHN PAPOUTSIS AND GEORGE KROUMPOUZOS

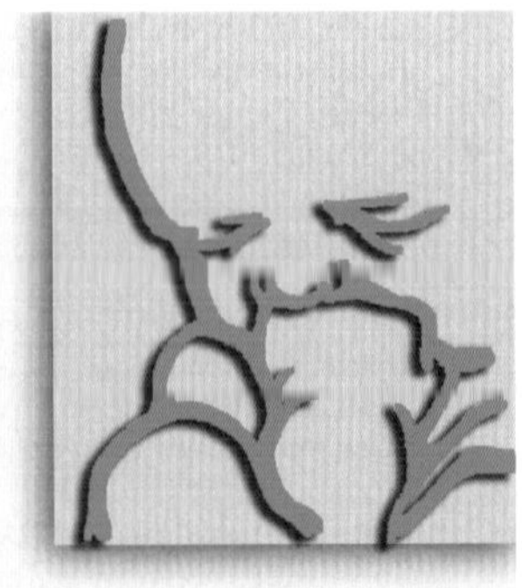

CHAPTER 46

KEY ABBREVIATIONS

Herpes gestationis	HG
Intrahepatic cholestasis of pregnancy	ICP
Prurigo of pregnancy	PP
Pruritic folliculitis of pregnancy	PFP
Pruritic urticarial papules and plaques of pregnancy	PUPPP
Psoralen with ultraviolet light A	PUVA
Ultraviolet light B	UVB

INTRODUCTION

This chapter reviews both the physiologic skin changes induced by pregnancy and the following categories of skin problems that can occur during pregnancy:

- Preexisting skin diseases and tumors
- Diagnosis and treatment of melanoma
- Pruritus
- Specific dermatoses of pregnancy

Some of the common skin changes and diseases that are discussed in the text are defined (Table 46-1).

PHYSIOLOGIC SKIN CHANGES INDUCED BY PREGNANCY

The human skin undergoes substantial changes during pregnancy induced by the combined effect of endocrine, metabolic, mechanical, and blood flow alterations. Physiologic changes, although they may prompt cosmetic complaints, are not associated with risks to the mother or fetus and can be expected to resolve or improve postpartum (Table 46-2).[1–3]

Pigmentary Changes

Mild forms of localized or generalized hyperpigmentation occur to some extent in up to 90 percent of pregnant women and are most noticeable in the areolae, nipples, genital skin, axillae, and inner thighs. Familiar examples include the darkening of the linea alba (linea nigra) and periareolar skin. Melasma (chloasma or "mask of pregnancy") refers to the diffuse macular facial hyperpigmentation reported in up to 70 percent of pregnant women.[2] Hyperpigmented, symmetric, poorly demarcated patches are commonly seen on the malar areas (malar pattern) and are often distributed over the entire central face (centrofacial pattern) (Fig. 46-1). In less than 10 percent of cases, hyperpigmentation occurs on the ramus of the mandible (mandibular pattern).[4,5] Melasma results from melanin deposition in the epidermis (70 percent, enhancement under Wood's light), dermal macrophages (10 to 15 percent, no enhancement under Wood's light) or both (20 percent). It is likely secondary to the hormonal changes of gestation with increased expression of alpha-melanocyte–stimulating hormone. Melasma typically is exacerbated by exposure to ultraviolet and visible light.[5,6] Hyperpigmentation is often more pronounced in brunettes and women with more melanocytes than in women with lighter baseline skin tone; the use of a high factor sun block during pregnancy may decrease the severity of hyperpigmentation.

Table 46-1. Common Skin Changes and Diseases with Brief Descriptions

Pseudoacanthosis nigricans	Hyperpigmentation of the skin folds and neck mimicking acanthosis nigricans
Dermal melanocytosis	Clusters of melanocytes abnormally located in the dermis and resulting in ill-defined bluish/grey patches
Vulvar melanosis	Irregularly distributed patches of pigmentation on the vulva
Verrucous areolar hyperpigmentation	Pigmented wart-like papules on the areolae
Miliaria	Sweat retention reflecting obstruction of eccrine sweat ducts
Hyperhidrosis	Skin disorder characterized by increased sweat secretion
Dyshidrosis	Recurrent vesicular eruption of palms and soles
Fox-Fordyce disease	Chronic pruritic disorder of the apocrine glands characterized by blockage of the apocrine duct and sweat retention
Onycholysis	The detachment of nail plate from nail bed
Subungual hyperkeratosis	Deposition of keratinous material on the distal nail beds
Palmoplantar pompholyx eczema	See dyshidrosis above (synonyms)
Acne conglobata	Variant of acne vulgaris characterized by severe eruptive nodulocystic lesions without systemic manifestations
Pemphigus vulgaris	Autoimmune bullous disorder of the skin and oral mucosa produced by anti-desmoglein 3 antibodies that cause intraepidermal acantholysis
Pemphigus vegetans	Variant of pemphigus vulgaris characterized by pustules that form fungoid vegetations or papillomatous proliferations
Pemphigus foliaceus	Autoimmune bullous disorder of the skin produced by anti-desmoglein 3 antibodies that cause subcorneal acantholysis
Spitz nevi	Seen predominantly in children or young adults and characterized by prominent epithelioid and/or spindled melanocytes that can have atypical features

Table 46-2. Physiologic Skin Changes in Pregnancy

PIGMENTARY
Common:
Hyperpigmentation
Melasma
Uncommon:
Jaundice
Pseudoacanthotic changes
Dermal melanocytosis
Verrucous areolar pigmentation
Vulvar melanosis
HAIR CYCLE AND GROWTH
Hirsutism
Postpartum *telogen effluvium*
Postpartum male pattern alopecia
Diffuse hair thinning (late pregnancy)
NAIL
Subungual hyperkeratosis
Distal onycholysis
Transverse grooving
Brittleness and softening
GLANDULAR
Increased eccrine function
Increased sebaceous function
Decreased apocrine function
CONNECTIVE TISSUE
Striae
Skin tags (molluscum fibrosum gravidarum)
VASCULAR
Spider telangiectasias
Pyogenic granuloma (granuloma gravidarum)
Palmar erythema
Nonpitting edema
Severe labial edema
Varicosities
Vasomotor instability
Gingival hyperemia
Hemorrhoids

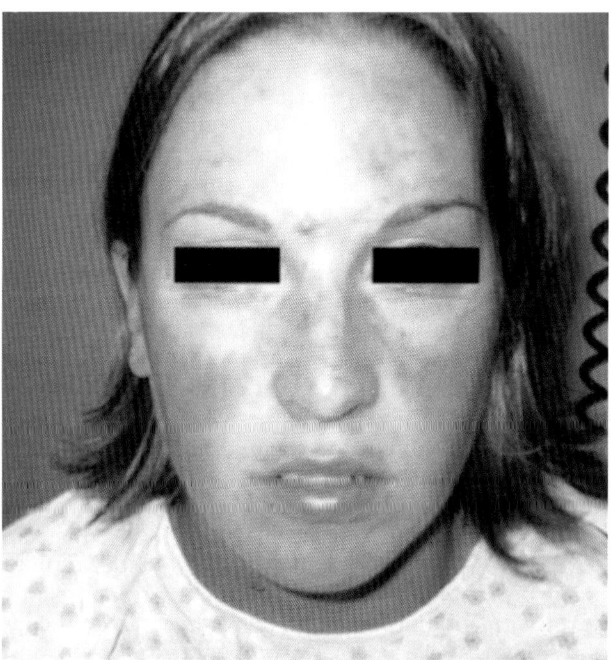

Figure 46-1. Centrofacial type of melasma involving the cheeks, nose, upper lip, and forehead.

Melasma usually resolves postpartum but may recur in subsequent pregnancies or with the use of oral contraceptives.[4] Troublesome persistent melasma can be treated postpartum with topical hydroquinone 2 to 4 percent and sunscreen, with or without a topical retinoid and mild topical steroid.[7] Despite treatment postpartum melasma persists in approximately 30 percent of patients, especially in women with the dermal or mixed subtypes in whom the deeper level of pigmentation results in decreased efficacy of topical agents. Combination therapies including laser treatment[8,9] and chemical peels[10] may be effective in resistant cases. There have been no reports of adverse fetal effects from laser skin treatment during pregnancy. Most laser experts agree that laser radiation does not penetrate through the skin into deeper soft tissues and, therefore, should not affect the fetus or the placenta. Still, because of liability issues, most dermatologists and plastic surgeons prefer not to perform laser procedures during gestation.

Uncommon pigmentary patterns, such as pseudoacanthosis nigricans,[11] dermal melanocytosis, vulvar melanosis and verrucous areolar hyperpigmentation can also be seen (see Table 46-2).[12] Postinflammatory hyperpigmentation secondary to specific dermatoses of pregnancy (see the section entitled "Specific Dermatoses of Pregnancy") is also common in women with darker skin types.

Vascular Changes

As a result of the combination of rising estrogen levels and increased blood volume (plasma volume increases to 149 percent of normal levels by the end of gestation), blood flow to the skin increases (four to 16 times in the first 2 months of pregnancy and doubles again during the third month) resulting in significant vascular sequelae (see Table 46-2). Spider nevi (spider angiomas) and telangiectasias develop in approximately two thirds of white women and 10 percent of black women between the second and fifth months of pregnancy, and usually resolve within 3 months postpartum.[1,4] Approximately 10 percent of women have persistent spider nevi; treatment with electrodessication or pulsed-dye laser is effective in women who find these cosmetically troubling.

Palmar erythema, likely secondary to capillary engorgement, is also very common, occurring in up to 70 percent of white and 30 percent of black women. Although varicosities of the distal leg veins and hemorrhodial veins develop in more than 40 percent of women, thrombosis within these superficial varicosities occurs infrequently (<10 percent). Nonpitting edema can be seen on the ankles (70 percent) and face (50 percent) and is most pronounced in the early months of gestation. Hormonal factors are primarily responsible for venous dilatation in pregnancy. Varicosities may regress postpartum but usually not completely; women should be counseled to delay treatment until they have completed their childbearing because varicosities are likely to recur in subsequent pregnancies.

Gum hyperemia and gingivitis are common and frequently result in mild bleeding from the gums during routine oral hygiene. This is most prominent during the third trimester and resolves postpartum. Good dental hygiene minimizes symptoms. Periodontal disease has been associated with adverse pregnancy outcomes, and so women without a recent dental examination should be referred.[13]

The pyogenic granuloma of pregnancy (granuloma gravidarum or pregnancy epulis) is a benign proliferation of capillaries that usually occurs in the gingiva but can occasionally be identified on the lip or other extramucosal sites (Fig. 46-2). Pyogenic granulomas commonly appear between the second and fifth months of pregnancy and affect up to 2 percent of pregnancies.[4] Presenting as a vascular deep-red or purple, exuberant, often pedunculated nodule between the teeth or on the buccal or lingual surface of the marginal gingival, a pyogenic granuloma may be more likely after mucosal trauma. Typical histopathologic features on biopsy can be used to differentiate this lesion from other conditions in atypical cases. Spontaneous shrinkage of the tumor usually occurs postpartum, and most cases do not require treatment. Surgical excision or electrosurgical destruction should be reserved for cases complicated by excessive bleeding or severe discomfort.

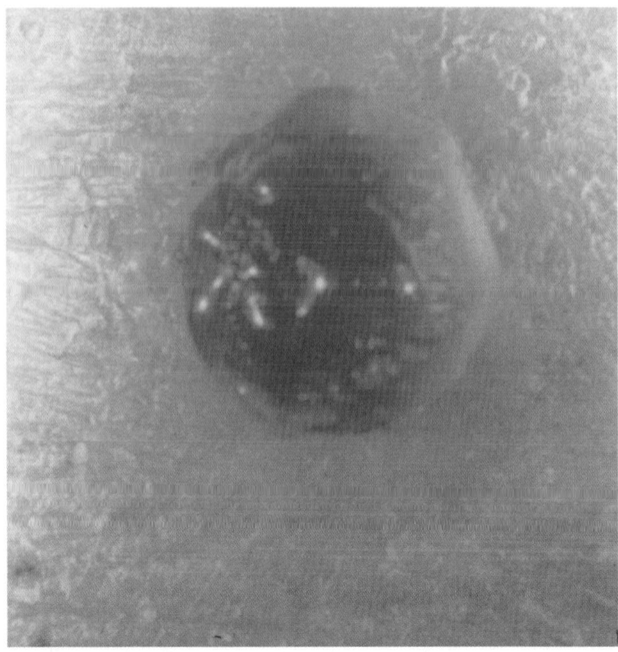

Figure 46-2. Pyogenic granuloma of pregnancy (granuloma gravidarum), a benign vascular proliferation, is typically seen as a nodule on the gingivae and is shown here at a less common extramucosal site.

Connective Tissue Changes

Striae gravidarum (striae distensae or "stretch marks") develop in up to 90 percent of whites between the sixth and seventh months of gestation and less commonly in Asians and blacks.[4] Risk factors include younger maternal age, increased pregnancy weight gain, and concomitant use of corticosteroids; however, genetic susceptibility likely plays a key role. Striae are most prominent on the abdomen, breasts, buttocks, groin, and axillae; although they are usually asymptomatic, a proportion of patients complain of mild to moderate pruritus. The treatment of striae gravidarum is a challenge; at present, there is no optimal treatment. The erythema (red color) of early striae responds well to various pulsed-dye lasers or intense pulsed light. The red color tends to become pale over time (with or without treatment), but the atrophic lines never disappear completely and do not respond to laser treatment. Topical tretinoin 0.1 percent cream has been shown to improve the appearance of the striae (decreased their length by 20 percent) and is occasionally used in combination with topical glycolic acid (up to 20 percent) in an effort to increase elastin content of the affected areas.[11] Nevertheless, tretinoin can be very irritating to the skin and does not make striae completely disappear. No topical therapy prevents or affects the course of striae. They are less apparent postpartum but may never disappear.

Skin tags (molluscum fibrosum gravidarum) present as 1- to 5-mm fleshy pedunculated exophytic growths on the neck, axillae, inframammary areas, or groin, and usually appear during the later months of gestation. Treatment can be postponed until completion of the pregnancy because lesions may regress postpartum. Cryotherapy with liquid nitrogen or snipping or shave removal is effective for persistent or enlarging lesions. Skin tags do not have malignant potential, and treatment is unnecessary unless inflammation or ulceration develops.

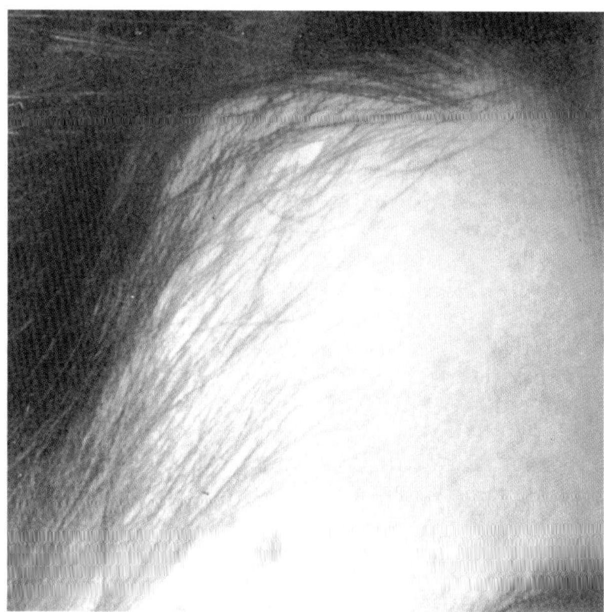

Figure 46-3. Telogen effluvium that develops within 5 months postpartum typically presents with temporal recession and hair thinning.

Glandular Changes

Increased eccrine function has been reported during pregnancy and may account for the increased prevalence of miliaria, hyperhidrosis and dyshidrosis.[4,12] Conversely, apocrine activity may decrease during gestation contributing to the decreased prevalence of Fox-Fordyce disease and possibly hidradenitis suppurativa in pregnancy.[2] Changes in sebaceous function are variable, and the effects of pregnancy on acne vulgaris are unpredictable. Treatment for acne vulgaris during pregnancy is discussed later. During pregnancy, the sebaceous glands on the areolae enlarge (Montgomery's glands or tubercles).

Hair and Nail Changes

Most pregnant women develop mild hirsutism affecting their face, sexual skin areas, trunk, and extremities that commonly regresses within 6 months postpartum. In addition, postpartum hair shedding (telogen effluvium) may be noted as a greater proportion of hairs enter the telogen phase. Most authors have found a progressive increase in the percentage of anagen scalp hairs during pregnancy. Thinning from postpartum hair shedding (telogen effluvium) may cause distress (Fig. 46-3). The severity of telogen effluvium varies considerably, and the hair loss becomes noticeable when more than 40 to 50 percent of hairs become affected. Recovery is spontaneous, and there are no effective treatments. Patients can be counseled that hair thinning usually resolves within 1 to 5 months but that complete resolution may occasionally take up to 15 months.[1,4] Frontoparietal hair recession and diffuse hair thinning in the later months of pregnancy have been noted in some women. Nail changes can be seen as early as the first trimester of gestation. These changes include brittleness, onycholysis, subungual hyperkeratosis, and transverse grooving (see Table 46-1). There is no specific treatment for nail changes during pregnancy, and most are expected to resolve postpartum. An attempt should be made to eliminate external sensitizers (nail polish, nail polish removers) and infections. The nails should be kept short if they are brittle or prone to onycholysis.[6]

PREEXISTING SKIN DISEASES AND TUMORS AFFECTED BY PREGNANCY

Pregnancy can aggravate or, less often, improve many skin conditions and primary skin tumors.[15] Diseases that may improve during pregnancy include atopic eczema, acne, some subtypes of psoriasis, Fox-Fordyce disease, hidradenitis suppurativa, linear IgA dermatosis, sarcoidosis, and autoimmune progesterone dermatitis (see Table 46-1).

Atopic Dermatitis

Atopic dermatitis (atopic eczema) is the most common pregnancy dermatosis and is often exacerbated by pregnancy, although remission has been noted in up to 24 percent of cases.[16] Often, a history of prior atopy (27 percent), family history of atopy (50 percent), or prior infant with eczema (19 percent) can be contributory. Other risk factors for eczema include black or Asian race and tobacco use.[17,18] Most patients present with eczema in the flexural surfaces of their extremities, occasionally with concomitant lesions on the trunk. Less common presentations are palmoplantar pompholyx eczema, follicular truncal, and facial eczema. Eczematous lesions can develop bacterial or viral (e.g., herpetic eczema) superinfection in pregnancy; treatment with dicloxacillin or a first-generation cephalosporin should be used as necessary in these cases.

Atopic dermatitis is not associated with an increased risk of adverse fetal outcomes. The effect of breast-feeding and maternal food antigen avoidance during pregnancy on atopic eczema in the offspring is controversial. Treatment for gestational exacerbations of atopic dermatitis is largely symptomatic. Topical application of a moisturizer and low- to mid-potent topical steroid cream or ointment is the first-line treatment. Systemic antihistamines, such as diphenhydramine, can also be used as necessary for relief of pruritus. A short course of oral steroids may be required for severe eczema. Ultraviolet light B (UVB) is a safe adjunct in treating eczema in pregnancy. There is less experience with the newer topical immunomodulators (pimecrolimus, tacrolimus).[19] No pattern of anomalies has been reported after exposure to these drugs *in utero*, but several infants have had neonatal hyperkalemia.[20] For the time being, these agents should be avoided in pregnancy because of the recent "black box" warning about a potential cancer risk that was added to these drugs' labels by the Food and Drug Administration.

Irritant hand dermatitis and nipple eczema are often seen postpartum.[1] Irritant hand dermatitis is treated with emollients and hand protection. Resistant cases should resolve readily after treatment with mid-potent topical steroids. Nipple eczema can evolve into painful fissures and be complicated with bacterial superinfection, most commonly with *Staphylococcus aureus*. Superinfected nipple eczema should be treated with a topical steroid combined with a topical or systemic antibiotic.

Acne Vulgaris

The effects of pregnancy on acne vulgaris are unpredictable. In one study, pregnancy affected acne in approximately 70 percent of women, with 41 percent reporting improvement and 29 percent worsening with pregnancy.[21] Two patients had improvement and exacerbations with two different pregnancies. Some patients may develop acne for the first time during pregnancy or in the postpartum period, which is called postgestational acne. Comedonal acne should be treated with topical keratolytic agents, such as benzoyl peroxide, whereas inflammatory acne should be treated with azelaic acid, topical erythromycin, topical clindamycin, or oral erythromycin base. Although first trimester use of topical tretinoin has not been associated with an increased rate of fetal malformations in controlled studies, the number of reported exposures is too small to exclude a small increased risk. Percutaneous absorption is 5 to 30 percent; therefore, a theoretical concern remains and the use of topical tretinoin is not recommended during pregnancy (see Chapter 8).

Other Inflammatory Skin Diseases

Recurrent flares of urticaria may worsen in pregnancy. Of interest, these recurrent flares show common features with hereditary angioedema and may have been exacerbated in the past by oral contraceptive use or prior to menses. Chronic plaque psoriasis may develop for the first time during pregnancy. Women with existing chronic psoriasis can be counseled that between 40 and 63 percent of women have symptomatic improvement, compared with only 14 percent of women with symptomatic deterioration; postpartum flares are common (80 percent).[22] Topical steroids and topical calcipotriene are relatively safe treatment options for localized psoriasis in pregnancy.[23] For severe psoriasis that has not responded to topical medications, UVB or a short course of cyclosporine are considered second-line treatment options.

Autoimmune Progesterone Dermatitis

Autoimmune progesterone dermatitis is caused by hypersensitivity to progesterone through autoimmune or nonimmune mechanisms. Although this rare dermatosis can take various forms (urticarial, papular, vesicular, or pustular) the hallmark is recurrent cyclic lesions that usually appear during the luteal phase of the menstrual cycle. Limited information is available regarding the effects of pregnancy on autoimmune progesterone dermatitis. Case series report instances of both improvement and exacerbation.[24] Increased cortisol levels and the gradual increase in the sex hormone levels during pregnancy with subsequent hormonal desensitization in some patients are both possible mechanisms for observed improvement. Diagnosis is based on either an immediate local urticarial reaction or more frequently a delayed hypersensitivity reaction following intradermal challenge with synthetic progesterone. Intramuscular administration of progesterone should be avoided in these patients because it has been associated with angioedema. Circulating antibodies to progesterone or the corpus luteum have been detected by indirect immunofluorescence in several patients. However, the exact sensitivity of this test is unknown but seems to be lower than the intradermal progesterone challenge; therefore, these antibodies are not widely used to confirm this diagnosis. No specific therapy for the condition during pregnancy has been proposed. Autoimmune estrogen dermatitis has also been reported in a patient presenting with urticaria in early pregnancy.[26]

Impetigo Herpetiformis

Impetigo herpetiformis is a rare variant of generalized pustular psoriasis that develops primarily during pregnancy, often in association with hypocalcemia[27] or low serum levels of vitamin D.[28] Although familial occurrences have been reported, more commonly, a personal or family history of psoriasis is absent. The eruption usually develops in the third trimester but can also be seen in earlier trimesters and for the first time postpartum. Although the overwhelming majority of cases resolve postpartum, persistent cases have been reported, and can be associated with oral contraceptive use.[29] Impetigo herpetiformis is considered a type of severe pustular psoriasis probably elicited by a metabolic milieu, such as pregnancy or hypocalcemia.[1,12] Various infections during pregnancy may also trigger a flare of pustular psoriasis in a genetically predisposed individual.[30]

Impetigo herpetiformis is characterized by numerous grouped discrete sterile pustules at the periphery of erythematous patches (Fig. 46-4*A*). Lesions typically originate in the major flexures (axillae, inframammary areas, groin, and gluteal fold) and progress onto the trunk, usually sparing the face, hands, and feet. Painful mucosal erosions may also develop. Onycholysis or complete nail shedding secondary to subungual lesions has been reported. Constitutional symptoms are common including fever, malaise, diarrhea, and vomiting with resultant dehydration. Rarely, patients develop complications secondary to hypocalcemia including tetany, convulsions, and delirium. Common laboratory findings are leukocytosis and elevated erythrocyte sedimentation rate; rarer perturbations include hypocalcemia, decreased serum vitamin D levels, and signs of hypoparathyroid-

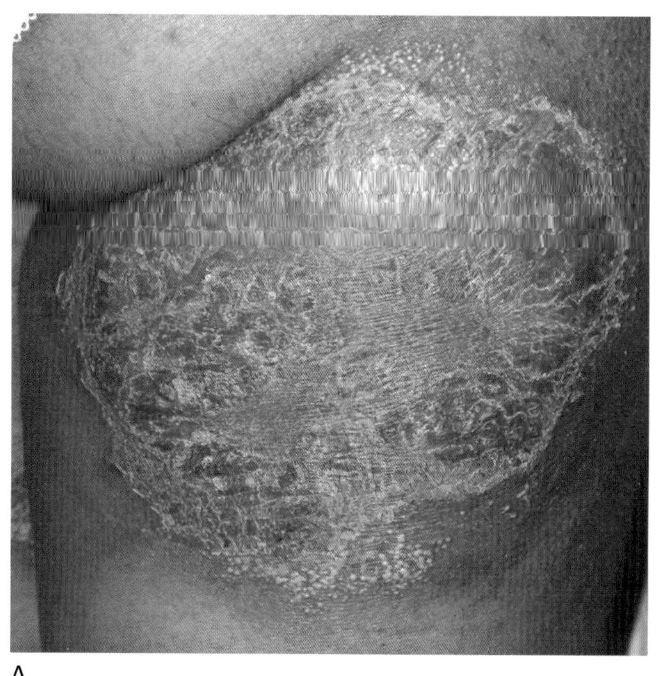

A

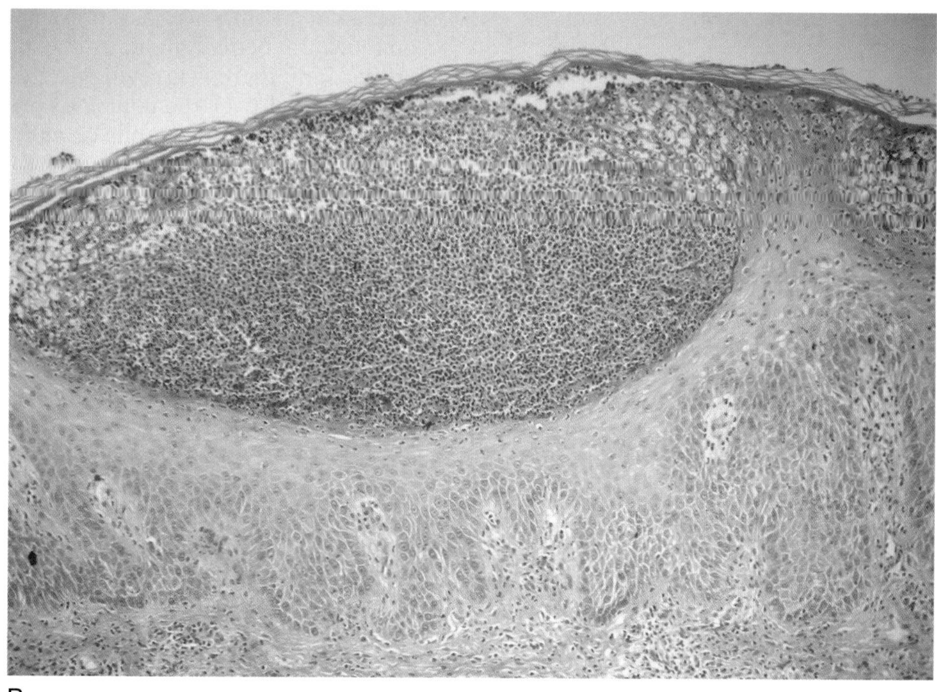

B

Figure 46-4. *A*, Impetigo herpetiformis: discrete grouped sterile pustules at the periphery of an erythematous crusted plaque. *B*, Histopathology of impetigo herpetiformis shows the characteristic spongiform pustule of Kogoj, which is formed of neutrophils in the uppermost portion of the spinous layer (hematoxylin-eosin stain). (Photographs courtesy of Aleksandr Itkin, MD.)

ism. Although maternal prognosis is excellent with early diagnosis, aggressive treatment, and supportive care, an increased risk of perinatal mortality may persist despite maternal treatment.[31] The risk is difficult to quantify because it is based on sparse case reports that span decades; death from cardiac or renal failure or septicemia have been reported but are currently uncommon. Intensive fetal monitoring has been recommended by most authors because fetal adverse effects (stillbirth, neonatal death, fetal abnormalities secondary to placental insufficiency) were reported even when the disease was well controlled. After acute treatment, the appropriate level of fetal surveillance is not known, however periodic assessment of fetal well-being is likely prudent after viability.

Definite diagnosis of impetigo herpetiformis is based on histopathology with characteristic features of pustular psoriasis (Fig. 46-4*B*). Direct and indirect skin immunofluorescence is negative. Systemic steroids are first-line therapy for impetigo herpetiformis; 20 to 40 mg/day of prednisone is usually effective. One case of pustular psoriasis exacerbated by pregnancy has been treated with cyclosporine.[32] Calcium and vitamin D replacement therapy should be undertaken, if necessary, and can lead to remission of the eruption.[25] Systemic antibiotics should be administered if bacterial superinfection is suspected. Postinflammatory hyperpigmentation may develop, but scarring is usually absent. Impetigo herpetiformis has been treated postpartum with systemic steroids, oral retinoids[33] or photochemotherapy (PUVA; psoralen with ultraviolet light A)[34] as single agents or in combination. Resistant cases can be treated postpartum with a combination of PUVA and clofazimine or methotrexate.

Cutaneous Manifestations of Autoimmune Diseases

Cutaneous lesions may be prominent in some individuals affected by autoimmune disorders, and these patients often have questions regarding how pregnancy will affect the appearance of these lesions. The cutaneous manifestations of chronic discoid lupus are not affected by pregnancy. Cutaneous flares of systemic lupus erythematosus can usually be managed with oral steroid treatment. Dermatomyositis/polymyositis may show exacerbation of the characteristic heliotrope rash in approximately half of the affected individuals.[34] The cutaneous progression of scleroderma is not significantly altered by pregnancy, and symptoms of Raynaud's phenomenon may improve. Pregnant women with limited skin disease do significantly better than those with diffuse scleroderma.[35] The medical and obstetric management of pregnancies complicated by collagen vascular disease is discussed in detail in Chapter 42.

Bullous Diseases

Bullous diseases develop secondary to autoantibodies that target constituents of the skin and/or oral mucosa. They are uncommon during pregnancy and run a variable course. Pemphigus vulgaris,[36] vegetans, or foliaceus may develop or worsen during pregnancy while linear IgA disease may improve.[37] In more than 50 percent of cases of pemphigus vulgaris, lesions may initially appear within the oral cavity. Diffuse skin involvement with multiple flaccid vesicles follows, with confluence of vesicles forming large eroded areas. Skin biopsy with immunofluorescence studies are needed for a definitive diagnosis. These studies are indicated in patients with new-onset lesions, most critically to differentiate pemphigus from herpes gestationis (see the section entitled "Specific Dermatoses of Pregnancy"). In cases of pemphigus, fetal and neonatal skin lesions can occur secondary to transplacental transfer of IgG antibodies but resolve spontaneously within 2 to 3 weeks after birth. Pemphigus should be treated with oral corticosteroids, and high doses may be required. The fetal effects of pemphigus are not well understood. A few reports link pemphigus to cases of preterm labor or stillbirth often in cases in which the fetus had characteristic skin lesions. Increased fetal surveillance is prudent in pregnancies affected by active pemphigus, although the effectiveness of this surveillance in preventing morbidity and fetal loss is not known.

Acrodermatitis enteropathica is a rare autosomal recessive disorder of zinc deficiency characterized by dermatitis, diarrhea, and alopecia. Vesiculobullous or eczematous skin lesions can develop on the extremities and periorificial sites, such as the mouth, perianal, and genital areas. The disease usually flares early in gestation[38] as serum zinc levels decrease but may also flare with the use of oral contraceptives.

Skin Tumors

Most skin neoplasms that present or enlarge during pregnancy are benign in nature. Contrary to conventional wisdom, there is no evidence that melanocytic nevi typically darken over the course of pregnancy. Pennoyer et al.[39] compared photographs of moles taken during the first trimester and again in the third trimester. Only 3 percent of nevi enlarged during pregnancy, and another 3 percent regressed; therefore, enlarging moles during pregnancy should be considered abnormal. In contrast, dysplastic nevi in women with familial dysplastic nevus syndrome do have a tendency to increase in size and undergo color change during pregnancy.[40] Spitz nevi, a type of melanocytic nevi, may also increase in size or erupt during pregnancy.[41] Although pigmented lesions may exhibit a mild degree of histopathologic atypia during pregnancy, pregnancy itself does not directly induce malignant transformation. Any suspicious pigmented skin lesion should prompt a dermatologic referral, especially when accompanied by with symptoms of pruritus. The ABCD clinical criteria may be helpful to obstetricians in determining which pigmented lesions are of higher malignant potential: *A*symmetry, *B*order irregularity, *C*olor variation, and *D*iameter greater than 6 mm, especially in an otherwise enlarging or changing lesion.[42] Seborrheic keratoses are also common and may enlarge or darken during gestation. None of these benign lesions require treatment during pregnancy; patients can be reassured that the majority of these lesions will revert back to their pre-pregnancy appearance.

Malignant Melanoma

Malignant melanoma accounts for approximately 8 percent of malignant tumors during pregnancy, with an overall incidence of approximately 2.8 cases per 1000 births.[43] Melanomas that develop during pregnancy are thicker than melanomas in nonpregnant women,[44] possibly due to a delayed diagnosis because of a shared misconception by the patient and her physician that darkening and changing of a nevus is normal in pregnancy.[39] Despite initial concerns, several epidemiologic studies evaluating the effect of pregnancy status at diagnosis suggest that the 5-year survival rate is similar after controlling for other factors.[45,46] In the largest study to date, Lens[47] compared 185 women diagnosed with melanoma during pregnancy with more than 5,000 women of childbearing age who developed melanoma while not pregnant. Pregnancy status at the time of diagnosis was associated with a hazard ratio for death of 1.08 (95 percent confidence interval [CI] 0.0 to 1.9). The major prognostic determinants of survival in pregnant women with localized melanoma are tumor thickness (Breslow's scale) and ulceration status,[48] with level of invasion only significant in women with tumors smaller than 1-mm in thickness.

Surgery is the treatment of choice in patients with early melanoma in pregnancy.[49] Sentinel lymph node biopsy using a combination of isosulfan blue dye and tenetium should be performed as indicated and is not contraindicated in pregnancy.[50] For pregnant women with advanced disease, the prognosis, risks, and benefits of systemic therapy should be discussed. The decision to administer systemic therapy should be determined based on the gestational age at presentation with consideration given to the potential consequence of delayed treatment on ultimate survival. In early gestation, the option of termination of pregnancy should also be considered. Melanoma is the most common type of malignancy to metastasize to the placenta and fetus, representing 31 percent of such metastases.[51] However, it should be emphasized that placental and fetal metastases are extraordinarily rare (27 cases) and that even in the setting of placental metastasis, fetal metastasis only occurs in 17 percent of cases. However because of the association between melanoma and placental metastasis, histologic evaluation of the placenta should be performed. Not surprisingly, the presence of placental metastases is associated with widespread disease and dismal maternal survival rates. The role of systemic therapy in preventing metastases to the placenta and fetus has not been adequately studied.

In the past, women with a history of melanoma had been counseled to delay pregnancy secondary to concerns that pregnancy might worsen their prognosis. In fact, pregnancy subsequent to a diagnosis of melanoma is associated with nonsignificant decrease in mortality (hazard ratio 0.58; 95 percent CI 0.32 to 1.05).[47] Similarly, there is no evidence to support an increased risk of melanoma recurrence with oral contraceptive use.[52,53] In most cases, melanoma cell lines lack type I estrogen receptors[54,55]; in contrast there appears to be some evidence for an inhibitory effect of estrogens on melanoma cell lines through type II estrogen receptors.[53] These findings may indicate a protective effect of female gender on the prognosis of melanoma.[56,57] The primary reason to delay pregnancy following a recent diagnosis of melanoma is the time-dependent risk of tumor recurrence and subsequent maternal mortality. Patients should be counseled based on their risk of recurrence, taking into account the thickness of their original tumor and other prognostic factors. Women with a significant risk of recurrence may want to delay pregnancy until they can be assured of a low recurrence risk. In women with a thin tumor with a low risk of recurrence, no delay may be necessary.

PRURITUS IN PREGNANCY

Itching is the most common dermatologic symptom of pregnancy. Mild pruritus attributed to pregnancy (pruritus gravidarum) is common, occurring most frequently over the abdomen with or without the presence of striae. Pruritus has been reported in 3 to 14 percent of pregnancies,[58] but a more recent report suggests that significant pruritus requiring a more thorough evaluation occurs in only 1.6 percent of patients.[59] A broad differential diagnosis needs to be considered; often, the specific constellation of clinical and laboratory findings establishes a diagnosis and guides management decisions. Pruritic skin diseases that are not specifically related to pregnancy, such as atopic dermatitis and scabies, should be considered. In cases of pruritus without eruption, systemic diseases are more likely: intrahepatic cholestasis of pregnancy is a common etiology (see Chapter 43 for diagnosis and management). However, other diseases such as lymphoma, liver, renal, and thyroid disease should be considered.[12] In the patient with pruritus and skin lesions other than excoriations, referral to a dermatologist for evaluation of a specific dermatosis of pregnancy (see the section entitled "Specific Dermatoses of Pregnancy") is appropriate unless a clear etiologic agent for a systemic or topical allergic reaction can be elucidated.

SPECIFIC DERMATOSES OF PREGNANCY

Specific dermatoses of pregnancy refer to a group of skin diseases that are encountered predominantly during or immediately following pregnancy and include only those skin diseases that result directly from the state of gestation or the products of conception.[16] Included in this definition are: herpes gestationis (HG), pruritic urticarial papules and plaques of pregnancy (PUPPP), prurigo of pregnancy (PP), and pruritic folliculitis of pregnancy (PFP) (Table 46-3).

Herpes Gestationis

HG, also known as pemphigoid gestationis, is a rare autoimmune skin disease accounting for only 1 in

Table 46-3. Overview of Specific Dermatoses of Pregnancy

	PREVALENCE (UNITED STATES)	CLINICAL DATA	LESION MORPHOLOGY AND DISTRIBUTION	IMPORTANT LABORATORY FINDINGS	FETAL RISKS
Herpes gestationis (HG)	1:50,000	• Second or third trimester or postpartum • Flare at delivery (75%) • Resolution postpartum • +++ recurrence in future pregnancies	• Abdominal urticarial lesions progress into a generalized bullous eruption	Biopsy: immunofluorescence shows linear deposition of C3 along basement membrane	• Neonatal HG • Small-for-gestational age infants • Preterm delivery
Pruritic urticarial papules and plaques of pregnancy (PUPPP)	1:130 to 1:300	• Third trimester or postpartum • Primigravidas • Resolution postpartum • Association with multiple gestation • No recurrence in future pregnancies	• Polymorphous eruption starts in the abdominal striae and shows periumbilical sparing	• None	• None
Prurigo of pregnancy (PP)	1:300 to 1:450	• Second or third trimester • Resolution postpartum • + recurrence in future pregnancies	• Grouped excoriated papules over the extremities and occasionally abdomen	• None	• None
Pruritic folliculitis of pregnancy (PFP)	Approximately 30 cases	• Second or third trimester • Resolution postpartum • +/– recurrence in future pregnancies	• Follicular papules and pustules	• Biopsy: sterile folliculitis	• None

Table modified from Kroumpouzos G, Gohen LM: Specific dermatoses of pregnancy: an evidence-based systematic review. Am J Obstet Gynecol 18:1083, 2003.

1,700 cases of significant pruritus during pregnancy.[59] Although HG shares many features with bullous pemphigoid, including autoantibodies to a 180-kD basement membrane antigen,[60] HG is confined to pregnant women or women affected by gestational trophoblastic disease. Some authors have suggested that exposure to paternal antigens may play a critical role in disease initiation, but "skip pregnancies" while having the same partner have also been reported and would argue against this association.[61] Of interest, expression of the HG antigen in the placenta begins in the midtrimester, correlating with the timing of clinical symptoms. HG primarily affects whites, with only scattered case reports in blacks[62]; this observation is consistent with the association between HG and the human leukocyte antigens DR3 (61 to 80 percent), DR4 (52 percent) or both (43 to 50 percent), which are less frequent in the black population. The antibody that incites the pathology in HG belongs to the IgG1 subclass and recognizes the NC16A2 (MCW-1) epitope in the noncollagenous domain (NC16A) of the transmembrane 180-kd antigen.

Clinically, HG usually presents in the second or third trimester of pregnancy, with extremely pruritic urticarial lesions that typically begin on the abdomen and trunk, commonly involving the umbilicus (Fig. 46-5*A*). These urticarial plaques rapidly progress to widespread bullous lesions (Fig. 46-5*B*) that may affect the palms and soles but rarely the face and mucous membranes. Tense bullous lesions arise in both inflamed and clinically normal skin, and they usually heal without scarring. Up to 25 percent of cases can present in the postpartum period, although these may represent recrudescences of previously undiagnosed mild HG. The most important clinical and laboratory features of HG are summarized in Table 46-3.

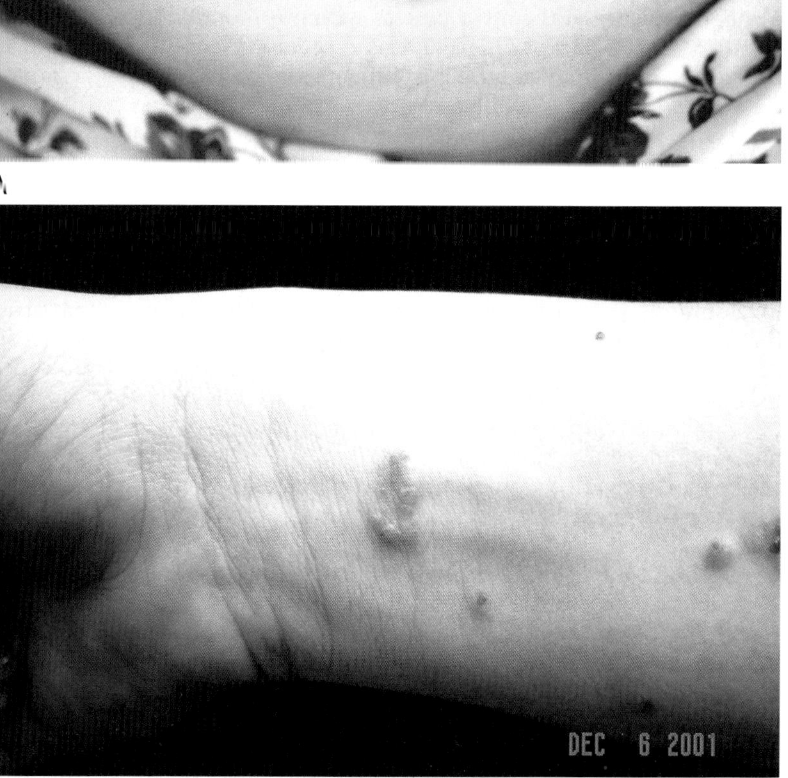

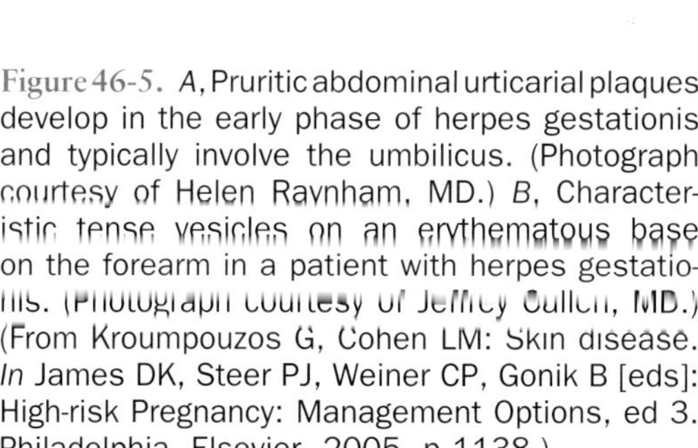
Figure 46-5. *A*, Pruritic abdominal urticarial plaques develop in the early phase of herpes gestationis and typically involve the umbilicus. (Photograph courtesy of Helen Raynham, MD.) *B*, Characteristic tense vesicles on an erythematous base on the forearm in a patient with herpes gestationis. (Photograph courtesy of Jeffrey Callen, MD.) (From Kroumpouzos G, Cohen LM: Skin disease. *In* James DK, Steer PJ, Weiner CP, Gonik B [eds]: High-risk Pregnancy: Management Options, ed 3. Philadelphia, Elsevier, 2005, p 1138.)

Although the differential diagnosis of HG includes drug eruption, erythema multiforme, and allergic contact dermatitis, the most common diagnosis to exclude is the far more common pruritic papules and plaques of pregnancy (PUPPP, see later). PUPPP can manifest with urticarial and vesicular lesions that are almost indistinguishable from those of HG, although PUPPP classically begins in the abdominal striae and spares the umbilicus. Definitive diagnosis is based on immunofluorescence of perilesional skin demonstrating the hallmark finding of HG, linear C3 deposition along the basement membrane zone.[1] In addition, skin histopathology shows a spongiotic epidermis, marked papillary dermal edema, and an eosinophilic infiltrate. Although serum IgG levels to the HG antigen can be measured, they do not consistently correlate with the severity of disease.

Oral corticosteroids remain the cornerstone of treatment in HG. The majority of patients respond rapidly to relatively low-dose treatment with prednisone (20 to 40 mg/day). In resistant cases, higher doses of prednisone (80 mg/day or more) can be effective. Once new blister formation has been suppressed, prednisone should be tapered to 5 to 10 mg/day. Typically, up to 75 percent of patients spontaneously resolve or improve in the late third trimester, and steroid treatment can often be discontinued during these weeks. However, immediate postpartum flares are common within the days following delivery, and steroid doses can be increased in anticipation. A subset of patients will have persistent HG or recurrent flares lasting weeks or months. Patients at risk for prolonged or chronic HG tend to be older with higher parity, more widespread lesions and a history of HG in prior pregnancies.[63] Oral contraceptive use has been implicated in postpartum flares; 20 to 50 percent of patients using oral contraceptives within 6 months of delivery have associated flares. This association should be considered when counseling patients on their contraceptive options. In contrast, breast-feeding has been associated with a significantly shorter duration of active lesions: 5 versus 24 weeks for bullous lesions and 24 versus 68 weeks for urticarial lesions; however, it should be noted that this observation was based on a cohort of 25 patients.[64] HG recurs in 95 percent of future pregnancies, and lesions may be more severe, appear earlier in gestation, and persist longer postpartum. Treatment for chronic, recalcitrant HG is generally unsatisfactory, although case reports have described the use of plasmapheresis, high-dose intravenous immunoglobulin combined with cyclosporine, and minocycline with nicotinamide.

The maternal effects of HG are largely limited to symptomatic pruritus and a small risk of lesion superinfection. An association between HG and Grave's disease has been reported and HG[65] is an indication for performing both immediate and periodic screening tests of thyroid function. An association with small-for-gestational age infants and preterm delivery has been reported but the effect of HG on the fetus remains difficult to estimate from the small study cohorts that result from the rarity of the disease. The largest cohort to date compared fetal outcome between the affected and unaffected pregnancies of 74 women; a 16 percent versus 2 percent rate of delivery at less than 32 weeks complicated pregnancies with active HG.[66] Mild placental insufficiency has been postulated as a mechanism. Therefore, sonographic evaluation of fetal interval growth and periodic assessment of fetal well-being in the third trimester is appropriate. Finally, approximately 5 to 10 percent of neonates manifest bullous skin lesions secondary to passive transplacental transfer of HG antibody.[67] Parents should be reassured that these lesions resolve spontaneously without scarring over the period of a few weeks as the maternal antibodies clear from the infant's blood. However, parents should be counseled regarding the signs and symptoms of bacterial superinfection so that timely treatment can prevent progression to systemic infection.

Pruritic Urticarial Papules and Plaques of Pregnancy

Pruritic urticarial papules and plaques of pregnancy (PUPPP, or "polymorphic eruption of pregnancy") is the most common specific dermatosis of pregnancy, occurring classically in primigravidas in the mid to late third trimester.[68,69] Typically lesions begin in the abdominal striae and spare the periumbilical region (Fig. 46-6*A*).[1,70] PUPPP can be difficult to characterize because the eruption is polymorphous and can include urticarial and occasionally vesicular, purpuric, polycyclic, or targetoid lesions.[69] Although lesions can spread over the trunk and extremities, they usually spare the palms and soles, and involvement of the face is very unusual. Generalized PUPPP may resemble a toxic erythema or atopic dermatitis (Fig. 46-6*B*).

Skin histopathology shows spongiotic dermatitis with variable numbers of eosinophils but can often be nonspecific. In contrast to HG, immunofluorescence studies are negative. The pathogenesis of PUPPP has not been established, but the immunohistologic profile (T-helper lymphocytes, dermal dendritic cells, and epidermal Langerhans cells)[71] suggests a delayed hypersensitivity reaction to an unknown antigen. Other authors have proposed that rapid abdominal wall distention in primigravidas may trigger an inflammatory process; this theory has been supported by the association between PUPPP and multiple-gestation pregnancy, excess maternal weight gain, and fetal macrosomia.[72,73] A recent meta-analysis[70] revealed a 10-fold higher prevalence of multiple gestation in pregnancies affected by PUPPP. Progesterone receptors are increased in PUPPP lesions, and progesterone has been shown to aggravate the inflammatory process at the tissue level.[74] Finally, fetal DNA has been detected in PUPPP lesions[75]; further studies are necessary to clarify the importance of microchimerism in the pathogenesis of PUPPP.

PUPPP is not associated with adverse maternal or fetal outcomes. Therefore, the goal of therapy is the relief of maternal discomfort. Mild PUPPP can be treated with antipruritic topical medications, topical steroids, and oral antihistamines. In cases of severe bothersome itching, a

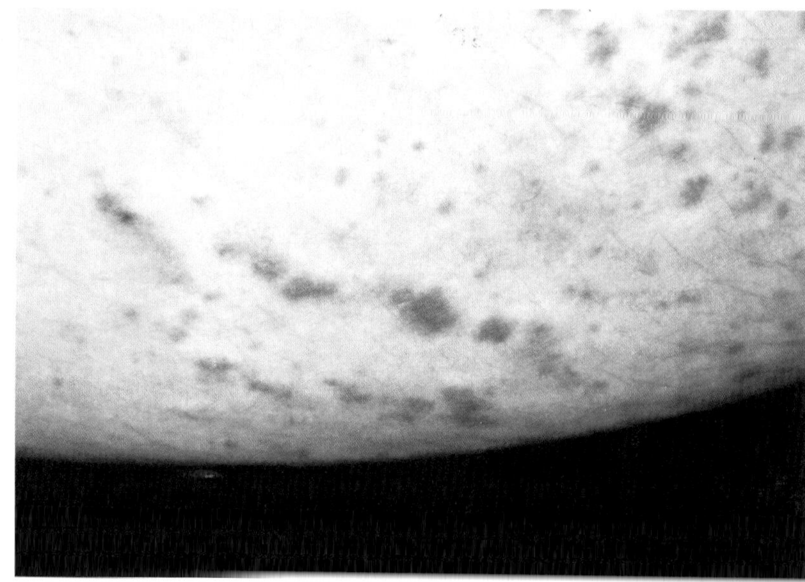

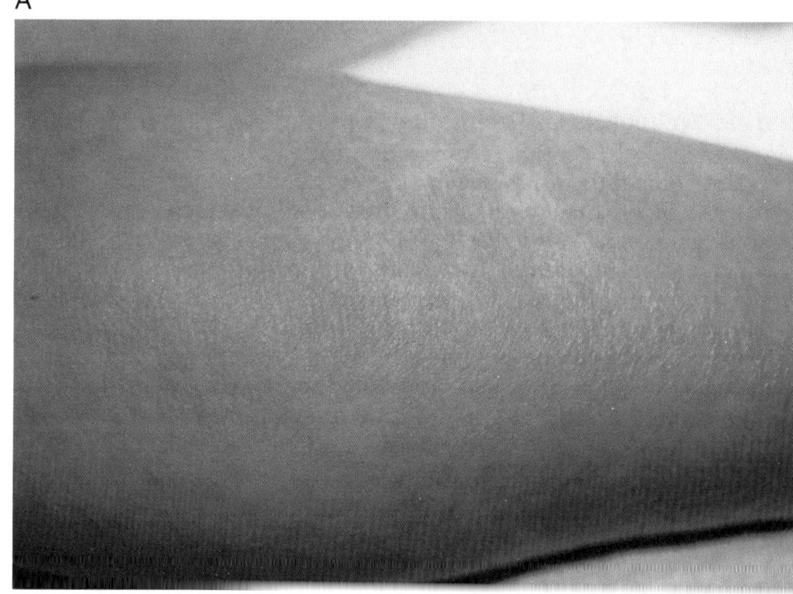

Figure 46-[illegible] *A*, PUPPP shows urticarial lesions that typically start in the abdominal striae. *B*, Widespread PUPPP may resemble a toxic erythema or atopic dermatitis. (Photograph courtesy of Helen Raynham, MD.)

short course of oral prednisone may be necessary. UVB has been used anecdotally with some success.[70]

Prurigo of Pregnancy

Prurigo of pregnancy (PP) manifests itself with grouped excoriated or crusted pruritic papules over the extensor surfaces of the extremities, and occasionally on the trunk and elsewhere[1] (see Table 46-3). The condition lacks pathognomonic histopathologic features, and skin immunofluorescence is negative. Serologic tests may show elevated IgE levels.[15] Early reports[76] of a dismal fetal outcome in patients with PP have not been confirmed by subsequent studies, and PP has not been associated with increased maternal risk. PP should be differentiated from pruritic dermatoses unrelated to pregnancy, other specific dermatoses of pregnancy, drug eruptions, arthropod bites, and infestations such as scabies. PP is treated with moderately potent topical steroids, if necessary intralesional or under occlusion, and oral antihistamines.[70] A short course of oral steroid is rarely required.

PP has been associated with a family history of intrahepatic cholestasis of pregnancy (ICP) (see Chapter 43). It has been proposed that PP and ICP are closely related conditions, distinguished only by the absence of primary lesions in ICP.[16] These authors reported an association with a personal or family history of atopic dermatitis and elevation of serum IgE, and suggested that PP may be the result of ICP in women with an atopic predisposition. Yet, the association with atopy was not corroborated by other studies. PP remains the least defined of the specific dermatoses of pregnancy.

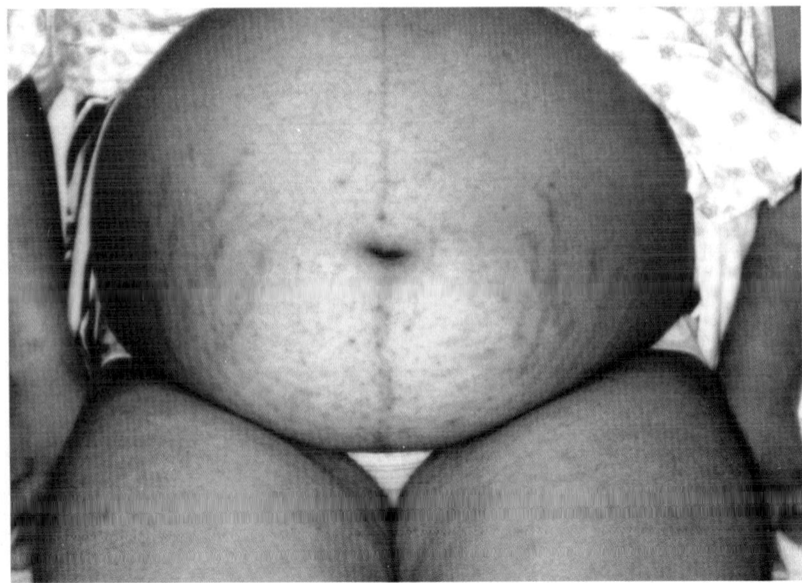

Figure 46-7. Pruritic folliculitis of pregnancy: discrete follicular erythematous or pigmented papules on the abdomen.

Pruritic Folliculitis of Pregnancy

Pruritic folliculitis of pregnancy (PFP) is a rare specific dermatosis of pregnancy, the exact prevalence of which remains unknown (see Table 46-3). Approximately 30 cases have been reported.[70] It presents with pruritic follicular erythematous papules and pustules that affect primarily the trunk (Fig. 46-7).[77] PFP resolves spontaneously at delivery or postpartum but may recur in subsequent pregnancies.[78] The histopathology is that of folliculitis, and special stains for microorganisms are negative. Skin immunofluorescence studies and serology are negative. The differential diagnosis of PFP includes an infectious folliculitis and specific dermatoses of pregnancy. An infectious folliculitis can be ruled out with stains for microorganisms and cultures from the pustular lesions. PFP was associated with decreased birth weight and a male-to-female ratio of 2 : 1 in one study.[16] Preterm delivery was reported in one case, but no other maternal or fetal risks have been noted.

The pregnant female should be reassured that PFP resolves postpartum and has not been associated with substantial risks for the fetus. PFP has been treated with low- or mid-potent topical steroids, benzoyl peroxide, and UVB.[79] The etiology of PFP remains unknown. Increased serum androgen levels in PFP or association with ICP have been reported but were probably coincidental. It has been postulated that PFP may be a form of hormonally induced acne, based on clinical similarities with the acne that develops after the administration of systemic steroids or progestogens. Other authors[59] have considered PFP to be a variant of PUPPP based on reports of follicular lesions in some PUPPP patients. Nevertheless, the clinical presentation and histopathology of PFP differ overall from those of PUPPP. An association with *Pityrosporum* has been debated.[80] Further studies are required to define whether PFP is a distinct specific dermatosis of pregnancy.

Key Points

- With the physiologic skin changes of pregnancy, there are no risks for the mother or fetus. The changes should be expected to resolve postpartum.
- Preexisting melanocytic nevi may show mild changes in pregnancy but no increased risk of malignant transformation.
- Preexisting skin disorders are more likely to worsen than improve in pregnancy; atopic dermatitis (eczema) is the most common dermatosis in pregnancy.
- In melanoma, the prognosis not adversely affected by pregnancy.
- Pruritus occurs in up to 3 to 14 percent of pregnancies. There is a constellation of clinical and laboratory findings to establish etiology.
- Impetigo herpetiformis (pustular psoriasis) is often a result of reduced calcium or vitamin D. There are serious maternal and fetal risks with this disease.
- In patients with herpes gestationis, there is a flare at delivery. Treatment is with oral steroids. There are several fetal risks, such as small-for-gestational age infants, preterm delivery, and neonatal herpes gestationis, associated with this disease.
- PUPPP starts in the abdominal striae and spares the periumbilical area. There is an association with multiple gestation pregnancy, but there are no maternal or fetal risks.
- Prurigo of pregnancy and pruritic folliculitis of pregnancy carry no maternal or fetal risks.

REFERENCES

1. Kroumpouzos G, Cohen LM: Dermatoses of pregnancy. J Am Acad Dermatol 45:1, 2001.
2. Winton GB, Lewis CW: Dermatoses of pregnancy. J Am Acad Dermatol 6:977, 1982.
3. McKay M: Physiologic skin changes of pregnancy. *In* Black M, McKay M, Braude P, et al (eds): Obstetric and Gynecologic Dermatology, ed 5, London, Mosby, 2002, p 17.
4. Wong RC, Ellis CN: Physiologic skin changes in pregnancy. J Am Acad Dermatol 10:929, 1984.
5. Sanchez NP, Pathak MA, Sato S, et al: Melasma: A clinical, light microscopic, ultrastructural, and immunofluorescence study. J Am Acad Dermatol 4:698, 1981.
6. Snell RS, Bischitz PG: The effects of large doses of estrogen and progesterone on melanin pigmentation. J Invest Dermatol 35:73, 1960.
7. Kligman AM, Willis I: A new formula for depigmenting human skin. Arch Dermatol 111:40, 1975.
8. Angsuwarangsee S, Polnikorn N: Combined ultrapulse CO_2 laser and Q-switched alexandrite laser compared with Q-switched alexandrite laser alone for refractory melasma: split-face design. Dermatol Surgery [illegible], 2003.
9. [illegible] of cutaneous pigmented lesions with the Q-switched ruby laser and the Q-switched neodymium:yttritium-aluminum-garnet laser. A comparative study. J Dermatol Surgery Oncol 20:795, 1994.
10. Lee GY, Kim HJ, Whang KK: The effect of combination treatment of the recalcitrant pigmentary disorders with pigmented laser and chemical peeling. Dermatol Surgery 28:1120, 2002.
11. Kroumpouzos G, Avgerinou G, Granter S: Acanthosis nigricans without diabetes during pregnancy (letter). Br J Dermatol 146:925, 2002.
12. Kroumpouzos G, Cohen LM: Skin disease. *In* James DK, Steer PJ, Weiner CP, Gonik B (eds): High-risk Pregnancy: Management Options, ed 3. Philadelphia, Elsevier, 2005, p 1138.
13. Khader YS, Ta'ani Q: Peridontal diseases and the risk of preterm birth and low birth weight: A meta-analysis. J Periodontology 76:161, 2005.
14. Rangel O, Arias I, Garcia E, Lopez-Padilla S: Topical tretinoin 0.1 percent for pregnancy-related abdominal striae: an open-label, multicenter, prospective study. Adv Ther 18:181, 2001.
15. Winton GB: Skin diseases aggravated by pregnancy. J Am Acad Dermatol 20:1, 1989.
16. Vaughan Jones SA, Hern S, Nelson-Piercy C, et al: A prospective study of 200 women with dermatoses of pregnancy correlating the clinical findings with hormonal and immunopathological profiles. Br J Dermatol 141:71, 1999.
17. Moore MM, Rifas Shiman, SL, Rich-Edwards JW, et al: Perinatal predictors of atopic dermatitis occurring in the first six months of life. Pediatr 113:468, 2004.
18. Schafer T, Dirschedl P, Kunz B: Maternal smoking during pregnancy and lactation increases the risk for atopic eczema in the offspring. J Am Acad Dermatol 36:550, 1997.
19. Hale EK, Pomeranz MK: Dermatologic agents during pregnancy and lactation: an update and clinical review. Int J Dermatol 41:197, 2002.
20. Kainz A, Harabacz I, Cowlrick IS, et al: Review of the course and outcome of 100 pregnancies in 84 women treated with tacrolimus. Transplantation 70:1718, 2000.
21. Shaw JC, White LE: Persistent acne in adult women. Arch Dermatol 137:1252, 2001.
22. Boyd AS, Morris LF, Phillips CM, et al: Psoriasis and pregnancy: hormone and immune system interaction. Int J Dermatol 35:169, 1996.
23. Tauscher AE, Fleischer AB Jr, Phelps KC, et al: Psoriasis and pregnancy. J Cutan Med Surg 6:561, 2002.
24. Bierman SM: Autoimmune progesterone dermatitis of pregnancy. Arch Dermatol 107:896, 1973.
25. Bajaj AK, Swarup V, Gupta OP, et al: Impetigo herpetiformis. Dermatologica 155:292, 1977.
26. Lee AY, Lee KH, Lim YG. Oestrogen urticaria associated with pregnancy. Br J Dermatol 141:774, 1999.
27. Ott F, Krakowski A, Tur E, et al: Impetigo herpetiformis with lowered serum level of vitamin D and its diminished intestinal absorption. Dermatologica 164:360, 1982.
28. Oumeish OY, Farraj SE, Bataineh AS: Some aspects of impetigo herpetiformis. Arch Dermatol 118:103, 1982.
29. Rackett SC, Baughman RD: Impetigo herpetiformis and *Staphylococcus aureus* lymphadenitis in a pregnant adolescent. Pediatric Dermatol 14:387, 1997.
30. Beveridge GW, Harkness RA, Livingston JRB: Impetigo herpetiformis in two successive pregnancies. Br J Dermatol 78:106, 1966.
31. Finch TM, Tan CY: Pustular psoriasis exacerbated by pregnancy and controlled by cyclosporin A (letter). Br J Dermatol 142:582, 2000.
32. Gimenez-Garcia R, Gimenez Garcia MC, Llorente de la Fuente A: Impetigo herpetiformis: response to steroids and etretinate. Int J Dermatol 28:551, 1989.
33. Breier-Maly J, Ortel B, Breier F, et al: Generalized pustular psoriasis of pregnancy (Impetigo herpetiformis). Dermatol 198:61, 1999.
34. Gutierrez G, Dagnino R, Mintz G: Polymyositis/dermatomyositis and pregnancy. Arthritis Rheum 27:291, 1984.
35. Steen VD: Scleroderma and pregnancy. Rheum Dis Clin North Am [illegible], 1997.
36. Yair D, Shenhav M, [illegible], et al: [illegible] associated with pemphigus. Br J Obstet Gynecol [illegible], [illegible]
37. Collier PM, Kelly SE, Wojnarowska FW: Linear IgA disease and pregnancy. J Am Acad Dermatol 30:407, 1994.
38. Bronson DM, Barsky R, Barsky S: Acrodermatitis enteropathica: recognition at long last during a recurrence in pregnancy. J Am Acad Dermatol 9:140, 1983.
39. Pennoyer JM, Grin CM, Driscoll MS: Changes in size of melanocytic nevi during pregnancy.J Am Acad Dermatol 36:378, 1997.
40. Ellis DL: Pregnancy and sex steroid hormone effects on nevi of patients with dysplastic nevus syndrome. J Am Acad Dermatol 25:467, 1991.
41. Onsun N, Saracoglu S, Demirkesen C, et al: Eruptive widespread Spitz nevi: Can pregnancy be a stimulating factor? J Am Acad Dermatol 40(5 Pt 2):866, 1999.
42. Brodell RT, Helms SE: The changing mole: additional warning signs of malignant melanoma. Postgrad Med 104:145, 1998.
43. Slingluff CL Jr, Reintgen DS, Vollmer RT, et al: Malignant melanoma arising during pregnancy. A study of 100 patients. Ann Surg 211:552, 1990.
44. Travers RL, Sober AJ, Berwick M, et al: Increased thickness of pregnancy-associated melanoma. Br J Dermatol 132:876, 1995.
45. Mackie RM, Bufalino R, Morabito A, et al: Lack of effect of pregnancy on outcome of melanoma. Lancet 337:653, 1991.
46. Wong JH, Sterns EE, Kopald KH, et al: Prognostic significance of pregnancy in stage I melanoma. Arch Surg 124:1227, 1989.
47. [illegible], et al. Effect of pregnancy on survival in women with cutaneous malignant melanoma. J Clin Oncol 22:4369, 2004.
48. Balch CM: Prognostic factors analysis of 17,600 melanoma patients: validation of the American Joint Committee on Cancer melanoma staging system. J Clin Onc 19:3622, 2001.
49. Schwartz JL, Mozurkewich EL, Johnson TM: Current management of patients with melanoma who are pregnant, want to get pregnant, or do not want to get pregnant (editorial). Cancer 97:2130, 2003.
50. Nicklas AH, Baker ME: Imaging strategies in the pregnant cancer patient. Semin Oncol 27:623, 2000.
51. Alexander A, Samlowski WE, Grossman D, et al: Metastatic melanoma in pregnancy; risk of transplacental metastases in the infant. J Clin Oncol 21:2179, 2003.
52. Smith M, Fine JA, Barnhill RL, Berwick M: Hormonal and reproductive influences and risk of melanoma in women. Int J Epidemiol 27:751, 1998.
53. Lama G, Angelucci C, Bruzzese N, et al: Sensitivity of human melanoma cells to oestrogens, tamoxifen and quercetin: is there any relationship with Type I and II oestrogen binding site expression? Melanoma Res 9:530, 1999.
54. Flowers JL, Seigler HF, McCarty KS, et al: Absence of estrogen receptors in human melanoma as evaluated by monoclonal antiestrogen receptor antibody. Arch Dermatol 123:764, 1987.
55. Lecavalier MA, From L, Gaid N: Absence of estrogen receptors in dysplastic nevi and malignant melanoma. J Am Acad Dermatol 23:242, 1990.

56. Thorn M, Adam HO, Ringborg U, et al: Long-term survival in malignant melanoma with special reference to age and sex as prognostic factors. J Natl Cancer Inst 79:969, 1987.
57. Ries LG, Pollack ES, Young JL: Cancer patient survival; Surveillance, epidemiology and end results program, 1973–79. J Natl Cancer Inst 70:693, 1983.
58. Furhoff A: Itching in pregnancy. Acta Med Scan 196:403, 1974.
59. Roger D, Vaillant L, Fignon A, et al: Specific pruritic diseases of pregnancy: A prospective study of 3192 pregnancy women. Arch Dermatol 130:734, 1994.
60. Morrison LH, Labib RS, Zone JJ, et al: Herpes gestationis autoantibodies recognize a 180-kd human epidermal antigen. J Clin Invest 81:2023, 1988.
61. Engineer L, Bhol K, Ahmed AR: Pemphigoid gestationis: a review. Am J Obstet Gynecol 183:483, 2000.
62. Shornick JK, Meek TJ, Nesbitt LT, Gilliam JN: Herpes gestationalis in blacks. Arch Dermatol 120:511, 1984.
63. Boulinguez S, Bedane C, Prost C, et al: Chronic pemphigoid gestationis: Comparative clinical and immunopathological study of 10 patients. Dermatology 206:113, 2003.
64. Holmes RC, Black MM, Jurecka W, et al: Clues to the etiology and pathogenesis of herpes gestationis. Br J Dermatol 109:131, 1983.
65. Shornick JK, Black MM: Secondary autoimmune diseases in herpes gestationis (pemphigoid gestationis). J Am Acad Dermatol 26:563, 1992.
66. Shornick JK, Black MM: Fetal risks in herpes gestationis. J Am Acad Dermatol 26:63, 1992.
67. Karna P, Broecker AH: Neonatal herpes gestationis. J Pediatr 119:299, 1991.
68. Lawley TJ, Hertz KC, Wade TR, et al: Pruritic urticarial papules and plaques of pregnancy. JAMA 241:1696, 1979.
69. Aronson IK, Bond S, Fiedler VC, et al: Pruritic urticarial papules and plaques of pregnancy: clinical and immunopathologic observations in 57 patients. J Am Acad Dermatol 39:933, 1998.
70. Kroumpouzos G, Cohen LM: Specific dermatoses of pregnancy: an evidence-based systematic review. Am J Obstet Gynecol 188:1083, 2003.
71. Carli P, Tarocchi S, Mello G, et al: Skin immune system activation in pruritic urticarial papules and plaques of pregnancy. Int J Dermatol 33:884, 1994.
72. Cohen LM, Capeless EL, Krusinski PA, et al: Pruritic urticarial papules and plaques of pregnancy and its relationship to maternal-fetal weight gain and twin pregnancy. Arch Dermatol 125:1534, 1989.
73. Elling SV, McKenna P, Powell FC: Pruritic urticarial papules and plaques of pregnancy in twin and triplet pregnancies. J Eur Acad Dermatol Venereol 14:378, 2000.
74. Im S, Lee E-S, Kim W, et al: Expression of progesterone receptor in human keratinocytes. J Korean Med Sci 15:647, 2000.
75. Aractingi S, Bertheau P, Le Goue C, et al: Fetal DNA in skin of polymorphic eruptions of pregnancy. Lancet 352:1898, 1998.
76. Spangler AS, Reddy W, Bardawil WA, et al: Papular dermatitis of pregnancy. A new clinical entity? JAMA 181:577, 1962.
77. Zoberman E, Farmer ER: Pruritic folliculitis of pregnancy. Arch Dermatol 117:20, 1981.
78. Roger D, Vaillant L, Fignon A, et al: Specific pruritic dermatoses of pregnancy. A prospective study of 3192 women. Arch Dermatol 130:734, 1994.
79. Kroumpouzos G, Cohen LM: Pruritic folliculitis of pregnancy. J Am Acad Dermatol 43:132, 2000.
80. Kroumpouzos G: Pityosporum folliculitis during pregnancy is not pruritic follicitus of pregnancy (letter). J Am Acad Dematol 53:1098, 2005.

Maternal and Perinatal Infection: The Sexually Transmitted Diseases Chlamydia, Gonorrhea, and Syphilis

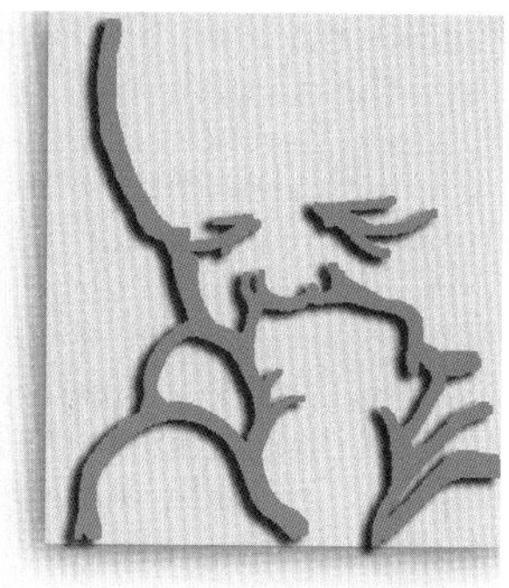

KIRK D. RAMIN AND DANIEL V. LANDERS

CHAPTER 47

KEY ABBREVIATIONS

By mouth	PO
Centers for Disease Control and Prevention	CDC
Central nervous system	CNS
Cerebrospinal fluid	CSF
Direct fluorescence assays	DFA
Elementary bodies	EB
Enzyme immunoassays	EIA
Human immunodeficiency virus	HIV
Human papillomavirus	HPV
Institute of Medicine	IOM
Intramuscular	IM
Intravenous	IV
Lipopolysaccharide	LPS
Major outer membrane protein	MOMP
Microhemagglutination *T. pallidum*	MHA-TP
Monthly Morbidity and Mortality Report	MMWR
Nucleic acid amplification tests	NAATS
Polymerase chain reaction	PCR
Rapid plasma reagin	RPR
Reticulate body	RB
Ribonucleic acid	RNA
Sexually transmitted disease	STD
Venereal Disease Research Laboratories	VDRL
World Health Organization	WHO
World War II	WWII

INTRODUCTION

Maternal and perinatal infections represent common complications of the peripartum interval. In many industrialized nations, the role of sexually transmitted pathogens is declining in its relative contribution to infections in women; however, in the United States and developing nations, the epidemic persists. Many of these pathogens are either proven or presumed to play an integral role in infectious morbidities of pregnancy and the neonatal period, and thus, understanding the social, economic, and pathophysiologic burden is essential. Indeed, as our ability to readily screen the population as a whole for the most prevalent or malignant of these infectious agents (e.g., Chlamydia, gonorrhea, and syphilis) has improved, epidemiologic statistics have provided evidence for their implied role in preterm labor, preterm premature rupture of the membranes, intrauterine growth restriction, neonatal conjunctivitis, neonatal pneumonia, and congenital syphilis. Thus, a greater understanding of the role of these prevalent pathogens in mediating disease pathogenesis has mandated that the obstetrician be well versed in the identification and management of these organisms. In this chapter, we review current trends in epidemiology, diagnosis, treatment, and prevention.

EPIDEMIOLOGY

The two most valuable sources of incidence and prevalence data on the sexually transmitted pathogens are provided by the Centers for Disease Control and Prevention (CDC) and the World Health Organization (WHO). The CDC reports sexually transmitted disease (STD) estimates for the United States using reported cases and estimates after accounting for underreporting. The Institute of Medicine (IOM) provides WHO estimates on worldwide incidences and prevalence of the four curable sexually transmitted infections (Chlamydia, gonorrhea, syphilis, and trichomonas). Overall, the WHO places annual estimates of worldwide incidence at 89.1 million new cases of Chlamydia infection, 62.6 million new cases of gonorrhea, and 12.2 million new cases of syphilis among persons aged 15 to 49 years. In addition, epidemiologic studies have revealed a number of basic truths regarding STDs: (1) sexually active adolescents have the highest rates of STDs of any age group[1]; (2) gender differences are observed in the transmission of the most prevalent STDs, with more efficient transmission from men to women; (3) curable STDs (i.e., not human immunodeficiency virus (HIV), human papillomavirus (HPV), or chronic recurrent herpes simplex virus) are associated with more serious long-term consequences in women than in men; (4) having one or more STDs predisposes an individual to acquisition and transmission of other STDs; (5) STDs in developing nations are both hyperendemic and epidemic; and (6) there exists marked racial disparity.

Chlamydia

Genital tract chlamydial infections are generally ascribed to *Chlamydia trachomatis* and account for the most prevalent reported infectious disease in the United States annually. More than 800,000 cases are reported to the CDC annually, with an actual presumed number of new cases (accounting for estimates of underreporting) of 3 million annually.[1] These infections present unique problems for public health control programs because 50 to 70 percent of infections in women are clinically silent. Unrecognized and untreated, the bacteria may remain infectious in the host for months and be readily transmitted to sex partners. Furthermore, most reported infections occur in the 15- to 24-year-old age group, individuals who do not partake in preventative health care programs. Estimates on worldwide exposure approximate 90 million new cases of *C. trachomatis* infection occur on an annual basis, and account for a rising majority of perinatal and neonatal complications.[2–5] Of note, a primary goal of *Healthy People 2010* is the elimination of racial disparities among multiple sexually transmitted pathogens. An assessment of the racial disparities of nationally notifiable disease for the year 2002 revealed a nearly 10-fold increase rate for Chlamydia in blacks when compared with whites (805.9 versus 90.2 per 100,000).[6]

The cost of treatment, prevention and management of complications of Chlamydia infections is estimated at $2.4 billion in health care costs annually.[3–5] Taken together, these factors have resulted in the endorsement of a nationwide broad-based screening program by both the CDC and IOM. Specific recommendations regarding population-based screening and prevention programs are reviewed later in this chapter.

Gonorrhea

The reported incidence of *Neisseria gonorrhoeae* infection approximates 300,000 cases in the United States annually.[1] However, the actual number of reported cases may be underrepresented by as much as 40 percent yielding a U.S. estimate of 700,000 cases annually.[7] In contrast to Chlamydia, the worldwide prevalence of gonorrhea may be significantly less than that observed in the United States, as supported by epidemiologic data from Canada and Western Europe.[8]

Historically, review of trends in incidence of reported gonorrhea in the United States from 1941 to 1997 reveal peak increases among both men and women in the interval around World War II (WWII), and again in 1975, peaking at 473 cases per 100,000.[7] The steady decline since 1975 has been accompanied by three interesting observations. First, the male-to-female ratio of reported cases has declined from a high of 3:1 to its current gender equivalence of 1:1.[7] Second, racial disparity is noted, with a 24-fold higher rate among blacks when compared with whites (570.4 versus 23.6 per 100,000).[6] Third, the single greatest determinant of gonorrhea incidence since 1975 is age: annual reported cases are twice as high in adolescents (aged 15 to 19 years) than in women aged 20 to 24 years.[8,9]

Syphilis

Historically, syphilis has long been recognized as a chronic systemic infectious process secondary to infection with the spirochete *Treponema palladum.* Throughout the centuries, epidemics of syphilis have been periodically reported. In the United States, the observed incidence of primary and secondary syphilis initially mirrored that of gonorrhea (reflecting the principle that epidemiologic synergy among the STDs occurs), with a rising peak during and shortly after WWII to 76 per 100,000 population to its reported nadir of 4 per 100,000 in 1955 to 1957.[11] Since the mid-1950s, recurrent epidemics have occurred, the most recent in 1985 to 1990, with a peak incidence of 23.5 cases per 100,000.[10]

Of concern are observations from both the WHO and CDC that the prevalence of syphilis in both the United States and developing nations has fluctuated over the past 2 decades. Again noted are elements of racial disparity, with a disproportionate number of cases in blacks when compared with whites (9.4 versus 1.1 per 100,000),[6] as well as gender disparity, with a predilection in women aged 15 to 24 years.[7]

Congenital Syphilis

As might be expected, the trend toward increasing prevalence in reproductive-aged women is accompanied by fluctuations in the incidence of congenital syphilis. Thus, there existed an epidemic of congenital syphilis from 1986 to 1992.[11] Fortunately, 2002 congenital syphilis surveillance data from the CDC report that provisional cases are at 348 per 100,000 births.[1] Of concern; however, is the observation that the rates of congenital syphilis remain disproportionately high in black and southern U.S. populations.[1,6,7] In their most recent report, the CDC summarized 2002 congenital syphilis surveillance data, which indicated that congenital syphilis rates decreased among all racial and ethnic minority populations, as well as in all regions of the United States, except the Northeast. Thus, rates of congenital syphilis per 100,000 live-born infants were determined from U.S. natality data and demonstrated a 21.1 percent decrease, from 14.2 to 11.2 cases per 100,000 live births, reflecting that primary and secondary syphilis rates among reproductive aged women declined 35.3 percent, from 1.7 to 1.1 cases per 100,000 women.[12] The rate of congenital syphilis fell 50.6 percent among American Indian/Alaska Native infants, 22.4 percent among Hispanic infants, 21.4 percent among Asian/Pacific Islander infants, and 19.8 percent among non-Hispanic black infants; the rate remained unchanged among non-Hispanic white infants.[12]

Review of the data involved in recent trends in congenital syphilis demonstrate one of the successes of sexually transmitted disease prevention and therapy, and is worth mentioning at this juncture. To summarize the report of the CDC,[12] among the 451 cases of congenital syphilis reported in 2002, a total of 333 (73.8 percent) occurred because the mother had no documented treatment or received inadequate treatment of syphilis before or during pregnancy; many of these cases occurred among infants born to women who had no prenatal care or no documented prenatal care. In 63 (14.0 percent) cases, the mother was treated adequately but did not have an adequate serologic response to therapy, and the infant was evaluated inadequately for congenital disease. In 39 (8.6 percent) cases, the mother was treated adequately but did not have an adequate serologic response to therapy, and the infant's evaluation revealed laboratory or clinical signs of congenital syphilis. A total of 16 (3.6 percent) cases were reported for other reasons. In 288 (63.9 percent) of the cases reported in 2002, the mother received prenatal care; the mother did not receive prenatal care in 130 (28.8 percent) cases, and no information on prenatal care was reported for 33 (7.3 percent) cases. When examined for trimester of pregnancy in which prenatal care occurred, in 86 instances care was initiated during the first trimester of pregnancy, 93 during the second trimester, and 59 during the third trimester. A total of 18 (30.5 percent) mothers who initiated prenatal care during the third trimester did so less than 30 days before delivery. In 2002, among those infants with congenital syphilis, 18 (4.0 percent) were stillborn, and eight (1.8 percent) died within 30 days of delivery. Taken together, these findings highlight that decreases in incidence of congenital syphilis closely parallel decreases in prevalence of primary and secondary syphilis among women, and interventions designed to prevent, detect, and treat syphilis among women of reproductive age have likely played an important role in the eventual decline of congenital disease. Indeed, following the epidemic of 1985 to 1990, efforts to eliminate syphilis were initiated with the implementation of a "National Plan to Eliminate Syphilis" in 1998.[13] Elimination efforts initially focused on syphilis among racial/ethnic minority populations and persons living in the South, and employed the following three methods: enhanced screening of women at high risk for acquiring syphilis, increased provider awareness, education, and training regarding syphilis, and increased awareness of the disease among communities with high rates of infection. However, it is important to note that although the incidence of congenital syphilis decreased with the implementation of the aforementioned initiative, the majority of congenital syphilis cases reported were preventable.[9,12,13]

PATHOGENESIS

Endocervical Infections

Chlamydia and gonorrhea are the sexually transmitted pathogens generally associated with endocervical infections, and have been noted to bear resemblance in their profile of observed maternal and perinatal clinical syndromes.[14,15] Although they are common in their association with increased cervical discharge, they are unique in almost every other aspect of their pathogenesis.

CHLAMYDIA

Species of chlamydiae were initially serotyped according to their biologic and biochemical properties, and a greater than 95 percent homology in their 16s ribosomal ribonucleic acid (RNA) sequences was observed. Subsequent molecular analyses led to the reclassification of some *Chlamydia psittaci* strains as *Chlamydia pneumoniae*, a human pathogen, and *Chlamydia pecorum*, a pathogen of ruminants. Nevertheless, of the four species of chlamydiae (*C. trachomatis, psittaci, pneumoniae,* and *pecorum*), only *C. trachomatis* and *C. pneumoniae* claim primates as their endogenous hosts. Each of the species bear multiple strains based on serotype, which, in turn, are associated with distinct clinical entities. These are as summarized in Table 47-1.

Chlamydiae are obligate intracellular bacteria that grow in eukaryotic epithelial cells, and employ a growth cycle unique to that from all other pathogens. During the 1970s, the infectivity and growth cycle of chlamydiae was initially characterized.[16–20] Known to specifically infect the cuboidal or noncilliated columnar epithelial cells common to the endocervix, urethra, and conjunctiva, this growth cycle involves infection of a susceptible host cell via a receptor-specific phagocytic process. This phagocytic process involves chlamydiae elementary bodies (EB) binding to the host cell through a heparin sulfate–like molecule to glycosamnioglycan receptors, and subsequently are phagocytosed into cytoplasmic vacuoles termed phagosomes.[21] In this fashion, chlamydiae may be considered to have a unique biphasic life cycle with dimorphic forms that are functionally and morphologically distinct. Once endocytosed, the EB differentiates into a larger pleomorphic form called the reticulate body (RB), which replicates by binary fission. The chlamydiae remain in the phagosome throughout their growth cycle, presumptively as an acquired means of escaping host lysosomes.[18–21] The endosome is transported to the distal region of the Golgi apparatus and incorporates host-derived sphingolipids into the inclusion membrane. Thus, it appears that chlamydiae are able to intercept host vesicular traffic bound for the plasma membrane to sequester lipids and possibly other host substances synthesized in the Golgi. Subversion of host vesicular traffic may represent a dual advantage for chlamydiae in obtaining materials from the host for its metabolism as well as in modifying the inclusion membrane to evade lysosomal fusion and immune detection.

Table 47-1. Spectrum of Human and Mammalian Diseases Caused by Chlamydiae Serotypes

SPECIES SEROTYPE	ACUTE DISEASES	CLINICAL SEQUELAE
C. trachomatis		
A, B, Ba, C	Conjunctivitis	Trachoma
D-K	Acute urethral syndrome cervicitis, endometritis, salpingitis, inclusion conjunctivitis, neonatal pneumonia	Proctitis, epididymitis, Reiter's Syndrome Pelvic inflammatory disease, ectopic pregnancy Tubal infertility, Fitz-Hugh Curtis Syndrome
L1, L2, L3	Lymphogranuloma venereum	
C. pneumoniae	Pharyngitis	
	Sinusitis	Reactive airway disease
	Bronchitis	
	Community-acquired Pneumonia	
C. psittaci		
Parrot	Atypical pneumonia	
Cats	Conjunctivitis	
Ewes	Abortion	

Because chlamydiae depend on their host cell for the generation of ATP, they require viable cells for survival.[22] Chlamydiae are incapable of de novo nucleotide biosynthesis and thus are dependent on host nucleotide pools. In this manner, one may consider this unique pathogen to be virus like. On the other hand, chlamydiae resemble a bacterial pathogen in that they contain both DNA and RNA, have a modified rigid cell wall with a lipopolysaccharide similar to that in the outer membrane of gram negative bacteria (albeit lacking the intervening peptidoglycan layer), and multiply by binary fission.[18-22]

Some interesting insights into the interaction of chlamydiae and its host immune system have emerged in the last decade. These new observations include the extensive but unexpected polymorphism of the major outer membrane protein (MOMP), the evidence for genetic susceptibility to disease, and the association of antibody response to the 60 kDa heat shock protein (CHSP60) with the development of adverse sequelae following ocular and genital infections. By way of summary, MOMP is a major target for protective host immune responses, such as neutralizing antibodies and possibly, protective T-cell responses.[23,24] The basis for MOMP antigenic variation is allelic polymorphism at the omp-1 locus, and immune selection appears to be occurring in host populations frequently exposed to *C. trachomatis*.[25] Combined with the observations that there appears to be a clear genetic susceptibility to disease, because only a subset of infected persons appear to have long-term complications after acute or repeated chlamydial infections, it is now believed that chronic immune activation plays a role in propagating clinical disease.[26] Thus, susceptibility to chlamydial pelvic inflammatory disease in a study of sex workers in Nairobi, Kenya, has been associated with an HLA class I allele, HLA A-31.[27,28] Similarly, allelic variation in the class II allele (DQ) have been shown to be positively associated with *C. trachomatis* tubal infertility.[29,30]

In addition to host genotype playing a role in determining the severity of Chlamydia-mediated disease, aberrations in humoral immunity also appear to modulate clinical disease. Antibody response to a 57-kDa chlamydial protein was initially observed more frequently in women with tubal infertility than in controls.[15,26] This protein was subsequently identified as a heat shock protein of the GroEL family of stress proteins. The association between antibody response to CHSP60 and pelvic inflammatory disease, ectopic pregnancy, tubal infertility, and trachoma has been subsequently observed in a number of population-based serotype studies.[15,16] Suffice it to say, although it remains unclear whether antibody to CHSP60 is causally involved in chlamydial immunopathogenesis or is merely a marker of persistent chlamydial infection, in cells persistently infected with *C. trachomatis,* the constitutive expression of CHSP60 may provide continued antigenic stimulation for the CHSP60 antibody response observed in persons with long-term sequelae. Moreover, observed immunopathology may also result from aberrations in self-tolerance mediated by shared and similar epitopes between CHSP60 and endogenous HSP60, which, in turn, results in a classic immune cascade resulting in tissue damage.

GONORRHEA

In contrast to chlamydiae species, the pathogenesis of *N. gonorrhoeae* and human disease is more straightforward, and reflects classic bacterial pathogenesis. *N. gonorrhoeae* is a gram-negative diplococcus for which humans are the only natural hosts. Like the other endocervical infectious pathogens, gonorrhea also bears a predilection for the columnar epithelium, which lines the mucous membranes of the anogenital tract.[7,31] Gonococcal pathogens adhere to these mucosal cells through attachment of pili and other surface proteins, resulting in the release of lipopolysaccharide, which likely instigates mucosal damage. Following adherence, *N. gonorrhoeae* is pinocytosed and thereby transported into epithelial cells. Unlike chlamydiae, the gonococcus does not replicate in the phagosome and, hence, evade lysosomal degradation. Rather, gonococci persist in the host by virtue of their ability to alter the host environment. In sum, multiple structures of *N. gonorrhoeae* enable pathogenesis by a variety of immune evasive mechanisms, including IgA proteases, iron-repression, and cell-adherence mechanisms.[7,31]

Systemic Infection

Syphilis is a chronic disease caused by the spirochete *Treponema* subspecies *pallidum*. *T. palladum* belongs to the order Spirochaetales; characterized by slender, nonflagellated, flexuous, tightly spiraled protozoan-like organisms. Motility is attained by the flexuous bending of this long slender body. This motility is responsible for the attainment of access through disrupted integument (mostly mucous membranous) primarily during sexual contact. This anaerobic and obligate human parasite is acquired by 50 percent of individuals having sexual contact with an infected partner.[7] Following mucosal invasion, an incubation period of approximately 1 week to 3 months ensues until the chancre appears heralding primary infection. The chancre arises at the point of entry by the spirochetes. The chancre is a broad-based, typically nontender ulcerated lesion that gives a characteristic "woody" or "rubbery" feel on palpation. It is seldom secondarily infected, and it resolves without medical treatment in 3 to 6 weeks. The organism then hematogenously spreads through the body during the period in which the immune system has responded, approximately 4 to 10 weeks.[7] Secondary syphilis is characterized by a generalized maculopapular eruption, constitutional symptoms, major organ involvement, and lymphadenopathy. Like the other major organ systems, the central nervous system (CNS) is invaded in about 40 percent of individuals during this hematogenous phase.[32,33] Secondary syphilis resolves over 2 to 6 weeks as the patient enters the latent phase of the disease.[7] The latent phase is divided into early latent (<1 year) and late latent (>1 year) disease in which no symptoms or signs of clinical disease are noted. If left untreated, progress to tertiary disease with cardiovascular, CNS, and the musculoskeletal system involvement occurs. The organism has an affinity for the arterioles, and the inflammatory response that follows results in obliterative endarteritis.[34] Subsequent end-organ destruction then occurs. In immunocompromised individuals (immune suppressive medications, HIV infection, other) the progression to tertiary disease, especially CNS, is known to occur early after the onset of disease. Congenital infection results from transplacental migration of the organism to the fetus. Congenital disease occurs with all stages of maternal infection, as well as at any gestational age.[35] Past theories of a placental impasse during the first half of gestation were disproved by pathologic examination of infected first-trimester abortuses and by the demonstration of living organisms in amniotic fluid obtained by amniocentesis in the early second trimester.[35,36] It is now believed that transplacental infection must be close to 100 percent during the early stages of maternal disease due to the known hematogenous spread with lower rates of transmission, falling to 10 percent, as bacteremia abates with the subsequent mounting of the maternal immunologic response during late latent disease.[37–39] Like Chlamydia, *T. pallidum* invades the host and evades the host defense mechanisms while being completely dependent upon the host for survival. It lacks the fundamental biosynthetic machinery to create complex molecules and fatty acids.[40,41] The ability to evade the host defense mechanisms stems from its basic construct of an inner membrane with few integral membrane proteins protruding through the surface gaining exposure through the outer membrane.[42] Berman concluded that this construct "...may provide some understanding of how the organism elicits such a vigorous inflammatory and immunological response, but manages to evade immunological clearance, although a paucity of surface proteins means that its surface presents few targets for a host immune response."[43] Of paramount importance in the pathogenesis of fetal disease is knowledge of fetal immunologic development. Disease early in gestation incites little response because the immune system functions little until midgestation. Following this period, the fetus is able to mount a vigorous response with marked endarteritis and end-organ involvement. Characteristics of subsequent fetal damage and loss are covered further in the section on diagnosis.

DIAGNOSIS

Chlamydia and Gonorrhea

In women, the gold standard for diagnosis of gonorrhea infection requires isolation of the organism by culture. Traditionally, specimens are streaked on a selective (Thayer-Martin or Martin-Lewis) or nonselective (chocolate agar) medium. Inoculated media are incubated at 35° to 36.5°C in an atmosphere supplemented with 5 percent CO_2 and examined at 24-hour intervals for 72 hours. Subsequent diagnosis is made by identification of the organism with growth on this selective media, with a Gram stain and oxidase test on colonies identifying gram-negative, oxidase-positive diplococci morphology. A confirmed laboratory diagnosis of *N. gonorrhoeae* cannot be made on the basis of these tests alone. A presumptive test result is sufficient to initiate antimicrobial therapy, but additional tests must be performed to confirm the identity of an isolate as *N. gonorrhoeae*. Culture isolation is also suitable for nongenital tract specimens. Using selective media is necessary if the anatomic source of the specimen normally contains other bacterial species. Given ongoing concerns by the CDC regarding resistant species,[44] all gonorrhea cases in the United States are confirmed by culture to allow for antimicrobial susceptibility testing. In women, a single endocervical culture on selective media detects 80 to 90 percent of uncomplicated gonorrhea.[31,44] Thus, it is recommended that for optimal yield, two consecutive endocervical specimens or a combination of an endocervical and rectal-vaginal swab should be obtained.[7]

The advantages of gonorrheal culture are high sensitivity and specificity, low cost, suitability for use with different types of specimens, and the ability to retain the isolate for additional testing. The major disadvantage of culture for *N. gonorrhoeae* is that specimens must be transported under conditions adequate to maintain the viability of organisms. Another disadvantage is that a minimum of 24 to 72 hours is required from specimen collection to the report of a presumptive culture result.[44]

Because curative antibiotic therapies for chlamydial infections are available and inexpensive, early diagnosis is an essential component of management and prevention. Historically, isolation of Chlamydia in cell culture had been the traditional method for laboratory diagnosis and has remained the gold standard in diagnoses because of its specificity. However, culture requires expensive equipment, technical expertise, and stringent transport conditions to preserve specimen viability. Thus, chlamydial culture is being replaced by antigen-detection methods, such as enzyme immunoassays (EIA) and direct fluorescence assays (DFA), which have less demanding transport requirements and can provide results on the same day. Assays are typically based on the capture of the chlamydial lipopolysaccharide using monoclonal or polyclonal antibodies linked to a solid-phase support. Early problems with low specificity because of cross-reactivity between the chlamydial lipopolysaccharide (LPS) and that of other gram-negative bacteria have been largely overcome by confirmation with DFA or a blocking antibody assay.

A substantial number of EIA tests have been marketed for detecting *C. trachomatis* infection. By contrast, the performance and cost characteristics of EIA tests for *N. gonorrhoeae* infection have not made them competitive with culture.[44] *C. trachomatis* EIA tests detect chlamydial LPS with a monoclonal or polyclonal antibody that has been labeled with an enzyme. The enzyme converts a colorless substrate into a colored product, which is detected by a spectrophotometer. Specimens can be stored and transported without refrigeration and should be processed within the time indicated by the manufacturer.

The DFA procedure identifies either the MOMP or LPS as its antigen, and staining consists of coincubation with a fluorescein-labeled monoclonal antibody that binds to *C. trachomatis* elementary bodies. DFA with a *C. trachomatis*–specific anti-MOMP monoclonal antibody is considered to be highly specific. Similar to EIAs, DFA is not appropriate as a diagnostic test for the direct detection of *N. gonorrhoeae* in clinical specimens.[44]

Nucleic acid–based hybridization probes and nucleic acid amplification tests (NAATs) based on polymerase chain reaction (PCR), ligase chain reaction, and transcription-mediated amplification technology are now commercially available.[16,44] The common characteristic among NAATs is that they are designed to amplify nucleic acid sequences that are specific for the organism being detected, and thus do not require viable organisms. The increased sensitivity of NAATs is attributable to their ability to produce a positive signal from as little as a single copy of the target DNA or RNA. The majority of commercial NAATs have been cleared by the Food and Drug Administration to detect *C. trachomatis* and *N. gonorrhoeae* in endocervical swabs from women, urethral swabs from men, and urine from both men and women.[44] The ability of NAATs to detect *C. trachomatis* and *N. gonorrhoeae* without a pelvic examination is a key advantage of NAATs, and this ability facilitates screening men and women in other nontraditional screening venues. A disadvantage of NAATs is that specimens can contain amplification inhibitors that result in false-negative results.

In addition to the NAATs, nucleic acid hybridization assays are now available to detect *C. trachomatis* or *N. gonorrhoeae*. Both the PACE and Hybrid Capture assays can detect *C. trachomatis* or *N. gonorrhoeae* in a single specimen. In the Gen-Probe hybridization assays, a DNA probe that is complementary to a specific sequence of *C. trachomatis* or *N. gonorrhoeae* rRNA hybridizes with any complementary rRNA that is present in the specimen.[44] RNA hybridization probes in the Digene assay are specific for DNA sequences of *C. trachomatis* and *N. gonorrhoeae*, including both genomic DNA and cryptic plasmid DNA.[44] One of the advantages of the nucleic acid hybridization tests is the ability to store and transport specimens for up to 7 days at ambient temperatures.

Duplex testing for the simultaneous detection of chlamydial and gonococcal DNA from a single specimen is also commercially available in some markets.[44] However, it bears mention that inherent in the increased sensitivity of these molecular techniques is the potential for false-positive results due to cross-contamination between specimens as well as contamination from equipment, reagents, and supplies.

Serology screening has no or limited value in testing for uncomplicated genital *C. trachomatis* infection and should not be used for screening because previous chlamydial infection frequently elicits long-lasting antibodies that cannot be easily distinguished from the antibodies produced in a current infection. A serologic screening or diagnostic assay is not available for *N. gonorrhoeae*.

Syphilis

The ability to diagnose infection with the organism *T. pallidum* has been problematic for two primary reasons. The first is the failure of the organism, as of yet, to be cultured on an artificial medium. The second lies in the long recognized tendency of clinical manifestations to mimic or imitate a variety of other diseases. Reports continue to surface touting the difficulty with which syphilis is recognized at any stage.[45] Although the primary genital lesion of syphilis, the chancre, is commonly recognized by affected males, women more often than not fail to identify this lesion. As reviewed earlier in this chapter, the chancre is a painless, sharply demarcated woody based (induration) 1- to 2-cm erosion of the mucosal surface at the site of the organism's entrance. It occurs typically without constitutional symptoms and is seldom secondarily infected. Examination of the serous exudates from the chancre under dark-field microscopy definitively diagnoses the condition by identification of the flexuous (spiraled) bodied organism. Unfortunately, dark-field microscopy lacks sensitivity, owing in part to specimen collection technique. The lesion must be abraded with a gauze sponge or cotton-tip application until bleeding ensues. The lesion is then squeezed to express clear serum, which is pressed onto a microscope slide. Direct fluorescent-antibody tests have the advantage that they can be performed on slides that are air dried as well as on stored paraffin-embedded tissue.[46] PCR has increased the sensitivity of detection in samples obtained from genital lesions, cerebrospinal fluid (CSF), amniotic fluid, serum, as well as paraffin-embedded tissue.[47] Great difficulty in the diagnosis of syphilis lies in the fact that primary syphilis often goes unrecognized by the infected individual as eluded to earlier.

Because most individuals infected with *T. pallidum* are in the asymptomatic latent phase of the disease, serologic testing is the primary means of diagnosis. Historically, reliance has been placed on two nonspecific antibody tests, the rapid plasma reagin (RPR) and the Venereal Disease Research Laboratories (VDRL) tests. Both pregnant and nonpregnant women are primarily screened using one of these two tests. In an effort to reduce the incidence of congenital syphilis, the WHO and the CDC recommend at a minimum screening all pregnant women in the first trimester.[48,49] It would be ideal if pregnant women were additionally screened at the start of the third trimester to enhance the detection of newly acquired infection [illegible].[10] If prenatal screening is not available, then screening at the time of delivery should be performed.[48] Once appropriately treated, most individuals (pregnant or not) lose reactivity to these nontreponemal serologic tests.[49] Confirmation that the infection is indeed due to *Treponema pallidum* is performed by the Treponema-specific microhemagglutination-*T. pallidum* (MHA-TP) and fluorescent treponemal antibody absorbed (FTA-ABS) tests. For most individuals, the MHA-TP and FTA-ABS tests remain positive lifelong.[49] False-positive reactions occur with both nonspecific antibody tests (RPR, VDRL) due to viral infections and autoimmune disease. Although most HIV-infected individuals exhibit normal serologic testing, occasionally one encounters patients with expressed lesion exudates or biopsy-proven disease, and serologic testing is negative.[51] The following recommendations for diagnosing syphilis in HIV-infected individuals have been made by the CDC.[52] First, individuals with HIV should be screened for syphilis and all sexually active individuals with syphilis should be screened for HIV. If clinical examination and findings suggest syphilis in the presence of negative serologic testing, then DFA for *T. pallidum* staining of lesion exudate/biopsy or dark field microscopic examination should be performed. In these individuals, all laboratories should titrate the nontreponemal tests (RPR/VDRL) to the exact final endpoint to better guide response to therapy. Last, neurosyphilis must be entertained as a diagnosis in the HIV-infected individuals and appropriate consultations obtained to better interpret serologic results. Neurosyphilis is diagnosed in non–HIV-infected and HIV-infected patients by examination of CSF through spinal tap.

Spinal tap and examination of CSF is not currently recommended in non–HIV-infected individuals who have early asymptomatic syphilis.[49] Individuals in whom CSF testing should be considered include those with neurologic or ophthalmologic symptoms, active tertiary disease, treatment failure, and HIV-positive individuals.[49]

Nonimmune fetal hydrops, polyhydramnios, and intrauterine fetal demise have long been associated with congenital syphilis. Recent reports confirm the constellation of nonimmune hydrops (ascites, pleural effusion, scalp/skin edema), hepatomegaly, polyhydramnios, and placentomegaly as markers for congenital syphilis.[53,54] Hollier and colleagues prospectively identified and followed 24 women with untreated syphilis to better define the pathophysiology of fetal disease.[55] Ultrasound examination with amniocentesis and funipuncture was performed. Maternal treatment was with benzathine penicillin G IM as per current CDC guidelines (Table 47-2). Six women had primary, 12 secondary, and six early latent disease. Ultrasound examination was abnormal in 16 (66 percent) of the 24 fetuses. Thirteen of these fetuses had hepatomegaly, three had hepatomegaly and ascites, and one had nonimmune hydrops. Increased placental thickness was seen in 17 (71 percent) and hydramnios in only one fetus with abnormal ultrasound. Sixteen (66 percent) of these fetuses had either congenital syphilis or *T. pallidum* identified in the amniotic fluid specimens. Maternal stage of disease (primary, secondary, early latent) correlated with fetal infection rates of 50 percent, 67 percent, and 83 percent respectively. Gamma glutamyl transpeptidase was elevated in 79 percent of fetuses compared with aspartate amniotransferase elevation in only 58 percent of cases. The authors recommend ultrasound examination as an important tool in the diagnosis and

Table 47-2. Recommended Treatment for *T. pallidum* Infections

Recommended Regimens

Primary, Secondary, Early Latent Disease

Benzathine penicillin G 2.4 million units IM as a single dose

Children: 50,000 units/kg IM (maximum 2.4 million units) as a single dose

Late Latent and Latent Disease of Unknown Duration

Benzathine penicillin G 2.4 million units IM weekly for 3 doses (7.2 million total units)

Children: 50,000 units/kg IM weekly for 3 doses (maximum 150,000 units/kg or 7.2 million units)

Penicillin Allergy (documented)

Pregnancy: Desensitization and penicillin therapy as above

*NonPregnant: Doxycycline 100 mg PO twice daily for 2 weeks or tetracycline 500 mg PO four times a day for 2 weeks

*Ceftriaxone 1 g IM or IV daily for 8–10 days

*Azithromycin 2.0 g PO as a single dose

Tertiary Disease

Neurosyphilis: Aqueous crystalline penicillin G 18–24 million units IV daily (3–4 million units every 4 hours or continuous infusion) for 10–14 days.

Alternative: Procaine penicillin 2.4 million units IM once daily with probenecid 500 mg PO four times a day for 10–14 days.

No Neurosyphilis: Benzathine penicillin G 2.4 million units IM weekly for 3 weeks (7.2 million units total).

The Centers for Disease Control and Prevention recommends penicillin as the treatment of choice in individuals with syphilis.

From Centers for Disease Control and Prevention. Sexually transmitted diseases treatment guidelines 2006. MMWR 55 (RR-11):1, 2006.

*Efficacy Data are limited.

management of the syphilis-infected gravida and her unborn child. The authors conclude that the pathophysiologic disease process begins with hepatic and placental involvement, followed by amniotic fluid infection, and the development of hematologic abnormalities. The intrauterine fetal demise of one of the 24 fetuses serves as a chilling reminder of the severity of devastation following infection with this relatively simple organism.

TREATMENT

Chlamydia

The recommended treatment regimen for uncomplicated genital Chlamydia infection has remained unchanged since 1998. The CDC recommends either azithromycin, 1 g in a single oral dose, or doxycycline, 100 mg orally twice a day for 7 days (Table 47-3). Although the results of clinical trials indicate that azithromycin and doxycycline are equally efficacious, single-dose treatment maximizes compliance.[56] To minimize transmission and reinfection, patients should be instructed to abstain from sexual intercourse for 7 days after single-dose therapy or until completion of a 7-day regimen and should also be instructed to abstain from sexual intercourse until all of their sex partners have been treated. Longitudinal studies of Chlamydia-infected adolescent female patients demonstrate a high risk for Chlamydia reinfection and other STD infections within a few months of initial diagnosis. Because of the high incidence of Chlamydia infection that can occur in the months following a treated infection, CDC guidelines suggest that providers consider the repeat screening of Chlamydia-infected female patients 3 to 4 months after treatment.

Table 47-3. Recommended Treatment for *Chlamydia Trachomatis* Infections

Recommended Regimens

Azithromycin 1 g orally in a single dose
OR
Doxycycline 100 mg orally twice a day for 7 days.

Alternative Regimens

Erythromycin base 500 mg orally four times a day for 7 days,
OR
Erythromycin ethylsuccinate 800 mg orally four times a day for 7 days,
OR
Ofloxacin 300 mg orally twice a day for 7 days,
OR
Levofloxacin 500 mg orally for 7 days.

The Centers for Disease Control and Prevention recommends treating persons with a positive sensitive nucleic acid amplification Chlamydia test. Although tetracycline and doxycycline have the greatest activity against *C. trachomatis*, these drugs should not be used in pregnancy because of their enamel effects. Owing to gastrointestinal side effects with erythromycin, azithromycin is the drug of choice in pregnancy.

Adapted from the Centers for Disease Control and Prevention: Sexually transmitted diseases treatment guidelines 2002. MMWR 51(RR-6):1, 2002.

Gonorrhea

Although uncomplicated genital gonorrhea infections can be treated with single-dose therapy, there are fewer oral treatment options when compared with efficacious therapy in chlamydial infections (Table 47-4). Moreover, recent emergence of quinolone-resistant *Neisseria gonorrhoeae* in California, Hawaii, Asia, and the Pacific islands, has led to the generalized recommendation that these agents should not be used to treat gonorrhea infections acquired in these areas or in areas with an increased prevalence of quinolone resistance.[44,56] The CDC recommendations became somewhat complicated in July 2002, when Wyeth Pharmaceuticals (Collegeville, PA) discontinued cefixime. In the absence of cefixime, the primary recommended treatment option for gonorrhea in Hawaii and California is ceftriaxone.[44] In addition, because of the risk of coinfectivity with *N. gonorrhoeae* and *Chlamydia trachomatis*, the CDC recommends empirically treating patients with positive gonorrhea test results for both gonorrhea and chlamydia.[44]

Syphilis

It was not long after the introduction of penicillin about the time of WWII that it became recognized as the primary antimicrobial for the treatment of syphilis. Penicillin has been effective in the treatment of and the prevention of disease progression in both nonpregnant and pregnant women, as well as, in the prevention and treatment of congenital syphilis (see Table 47-2).[49,56] CDC 2006 treatment guidelines recommend benzathine penicillin G 2.4 million units IM as a single dose for primary, secondary, and early latent syphilis in both pregnant and nonpregnant women.[49] Likewise, children

Table 47-4. Recommended Treatment for Uncomplicated Genital *Neisseria Gonorrhoeae* Infections

Recommended Regimens

Ceftriaxone 125 mg IM in a single dose,
OR
Ciprofloxacin 500 mg orally in a single dose,
OR
Ofloxacin 400 mg orally in a single dose,
OR
Levofloxacin 250 mg orally in a single dose,

PLUS,
(If Chlamydial infection is not ruled out)
Azithromycin 1 g orally in a single dose
OR
Doxycycline 100 mg orally twice a day for 7 days.

The Centers for Disease Control and Prevention recommends treating persons with a positive gonorrhea test result for both gonorrhea and Chlamydia unless a negative result has been obtained with a sensitive nucleic acid amplification Chlamydia test.

Adapted from the Centers for Disease Control and Prevention: Sexually transmitted diseases treatment guidelines 2002. MMWR 51(RR-6):1, 2002.

are treated with benzathine penicillin G 50,000 units/kg IM (maximum dose 2.4 million units as a single dose). Late latent syphilis and latent syphilis of unknown duration are treated with 2.4 million units IM benzathine penicillin G weekly for 3 doses (7.2 million units total).[49] Children, in turn, are treated with 50,000 units/kg weekly for 3 doses (150,000 units/kg or 7.2 million units maximum) for late latent and latent syphilis of unknown duration.

Individuals with documented allergies to penicillin present a particular treatment problem. Treatment recommendations differ as to whether the individual is pregnant or not. For early disease in nonpregnant women doxycycline 100 mg by mouth (PO) twice daily for 2 weeks (tetracycline 500 mg four times daily) has been used with little available data. Alternatively, ceftriaxone 1 g intramuscularly (IM)/intravenously (IV) daily for 8 to 10 days or azithromycin 2.0 g PO as a single dose may be effective. These alternatives should not be considered in individuals who are HIV positive, noncompliant, or pregnant. These aforementioned individuals should undergo penicillin desensitization and penicillin therapy.

Therapy for tertiary syphilis is dependent on the presence or absence of neurosyphilis. Provided CSF examination is negative, then individuals are treated with benzathine penicillin G 2.4 million units IM weekly for three weeks (7.2 million units total).[49] If neurosyphilis has been diagnosed, then aqueous crystalline penicillin G 18 to 24 million units IV daily (3 to 4 million units every 4 hours or continuous infusion) for 10 to 14 days is given. An alternative therapy in compliant individuals is procaine penicillin 2.4 million units IM once daily with probenecid 500 mg orally four times a day for 10 to 14 days. Follow-up CSF evaluation is recommended to assess response to therapy. Attempts at targeted mass treatment for syphilis in populations at risk to reduce outbreaks and ultimately congenital syphilis have met with failure.[57]

The implementation of appropriate screening and treatment of pregnant women should theoretically result in the elimination of congenital syphilis.[37,43] Unfortunately, children continue to be born with increased prematurity, low birth weight, hepatomegaly, cutaneous and bone lesions in developed as well as developing nations.[48] Almost 90 percent of stillbirths attributed to congenital syphilis occur among women who are never treated or inappropriately treated.[58] Alexander and colleagues examined the CDC guidelines for the treatment of maternal syphilis among 340 gravidas and found better than 95 percent success for all stages of clinical disease in preventing congenital disease.[59] Sheffield et al.[60] evaluated 43 women who received antepartum therapy with treatment failure. Her work revealed that preterm delivery (<36 weeks), short interval between treatment and delivery, higher VDRL titer at time of treatment and delivery, and early stage of maternal disease were associated with treatment failure. The optimal management (transplacental versus neonatal) treatment of the fetus with severe or advanced clinical disease remains unknown and requires consultation with experienced clinicians.[61]

Key Points

- Sexually active adolescents have higher rates of sexually transmitted diseases than any other age groups.
- Marked racial disparity exists in the rates of Chlamydia, gonorrhea, and syphilis, with the highest rates found among minority populations.
- Transmission and long-term sequelae of sexually transmitted diseases are greater in women than in men.
- Much of the end organ damage seen with sexually transmitted disease is a result of the host's immune response and to a lesser extent due to the invading organism itself.
- Even though *T. pallidum* and *C. trachomatis* lack the biosynthetic machinery necessary for life and thus are dependent on the host, they are masters at evading the host's immune system.
- The majority of cases of congenital syphilis in the United States should be preventable.
- *Neisseria gonorrhoeae* is a gram-negative diplococcus for which humans are the only natural hosts.
- Given concerns for antibiotic resistance, all cases of gonorrhea in the United States are confirmed by culture to allow susceptibility testing.
- Serologic testing for uncomplicated genital *C. trachomatis* infection has little or no value as previous infection elicits long lasting antibody response.
- Penicillin is the antimicrobial of choice in treating syphilis among pregnant women and reducing the incidence of congenital syphilis.

REFERENCES

1. Centers for Disease Control and Prevention. Selected Notifiable Disease Reports, July 9, 2004. MMWR 2004, p 592.
2. Hammerschlag MR, Anderka M, Semine DZ, et al: Prospective study of maternal and infantile infection with *Chlamydia trachomatis*. Pediatrics 64:142, 1979.
3. Mangione-Smith R, O'Leary J, McGlynn EA: Health and cost-benefits of Chlamydia screening in young women. Sex Transm Dis 26:309, 1999.
4. Sweet RL, Landers DV, Walker C, et al: *Chlamydia trachomatis* infection and pregnancy outcome. Am J Obstet Gynecol 156:824, 1987.
5. Schachter J, Grossman M, Sweet RL, et al: Prospective study of perinatal transmission of *Chlamydia trachomatis*. JAMA 255:3374, 1986.
6. Centers for Disease Control and Prevention: Racial Disparities in Nationally Notifiable Diseases—United States, 2002. MMWR 54:9, 2005.
7. Sweet RL, Gibbs R: Sexually Transmitted Diseases. *In* Sweet R, Gibbs R (eds): Infectious Diseases of the Female Reproductive Tract, ed 4. Philadelphia, Lippincott Williams & Wilkins, 2002, p 118.
8. Hook EW, Handsfield HA: Gonococcal infections in adults. *In* Holmes KK, Sparling PF, Mardh P-A, et al (eds): Sexually Transmitted Diseases. New York, McGraw-Hill, 1999, p 451.

9. Ickovics JR, Niccolai LM, Lewis JB, et al: High postpartum rates of sexually transmitted infections among teens: Pregnancy as a window of opportunity for prevention. Sex Trans Infect 79:469, 2003.
10. Aral SO, Holmes KK: Social and behavioral determinants of the epidemiology of stds: industrialized and developing countries. *In* Holmes KK, Sparling PF, Mardh P-A, et al (eds): Sexually Transmitted Diseases. New York, McGraw-Hill, 1999, p 39.
11. Centers for Disease Control and Prevention: Summary of Notifiable Diseases, United States 1992. MMWR 41:1, 1993.
12. Centers for Disease Control and Prevention: Primary and secondary syphilis: United States 2002. MMWR 52:1117, 2003.
13. Kaplan J: National syphilis elimination launch: Nashville, Tennessee, Oct 7, 1999: Syphilis elimination: History in the making—opening remarks (From the CDC). Sex Transm Dis 27:63, 2000.
14. Stamm WE: *Chlamydia trachomatis* infections of the adult. *In* Holmes KK, Sparling PF, Mardh P-A, et al (eds): Sexually Transmitted Diseases. New York, McGraw-Hill, 1999, p 407.
15. Sweet RS, Gibbs R: Chlamydial Infections. *In* Sweet R, Gibbs R (eds): Infectious Diseases of the Female Reproductive Tract, ed 4 Philadelphia, Lippencott Williams & Wilkins, 2002, p 57.
16. Schachter J. Chlamydial infections. N Engl J Med 298:428, 1978.
17. Sweet RS, Schachter J, Landers DV: Chlamydial infections in obstetrics and gynecology. Clin Obstet Gynecol 26:143, 1983.
18. Friis RR: Interaction of L cells and *Chlamydia psittaci:* entry of the parasite and host responses to its development. J Bacteriol 110:706, 1972.
19. Kuo CC, Wang SP, Grayson JT: Effect of polycations, polyanions, and neuraminidase on the infectivity of trachoma-inclusion conjunctivitis and LGV organisms in HeLa cells: sialic acid residues as possible receptors for trachoma-inclusion conjunctivitis. Infect Immun 8:74, 1973.
20. Nurminen M, Leinonen M, Saikku P, et al: The genus-specific antigen of chlamydias resembles to the lipopolysacchardie of enteric bacteria. Science 220:1279, 1983.
21. Bavoil PH, Ohlin A, Schachter J: Role of disulfide bonding in outer membrane structure and permeability in *Chlamydia trachomatis.* Infect Immun 44:479, 1984.
22. Schachter J: Biology of *Chlamydia trachomatis. In* Holmes KK, Sparling PF, Mardh P-A, et al (eds): Sexually Transmitted Diseases. New York, McGraw-Hill, 1999, p 391.
23. Brunham RC, Peeling RW: *Chlamydia trachomatis* antigens: role in immunity and pathogenesis. Infect Agents Dis 3:218, 1994.
24. Brunham RC, Plummer F, Stephens RS: Bacterial antigenic variation, host immune response and pathogen-host co-evolution. Infect Immun 61:2273, 1994.
25. Brunham R, Yang C, Maclean I, et al: *Chlamydia trachomatis* from individuals in a sexually transmitted disease core group exhibit frequence sequence variation in the major outer membrane protein (omp1) gene. J Clin Invest 94:458, 1994.
26. Morrison RP, Manning DS, Caldwell HD: Immunology of *Chlamydia trachomatis* infections: immunoprotective and immunopathologic responses. *In* Gallin JI, Fauci AS, Quinn TC (eds): Advances in Host Defense Mechanisms, vol 8, Sexually Transmitted Diseases. New York, Raven Press, 1992, p 57.
27. Hayes LJ, Bailey RL, Mabey DCW, et al: Genotyping of *Chlamydia trachomatis* from a trachoma endemic village in the Gambia by a nested polymerase chain reaction: identification of strain variants. J Infect Dis 166:1173, 1992.
28. Conway DJ, Holland MJ, Campbell AE, et al: HLA class I and class II polymorphism and trachomatous scarring in a *Chlamydia trachomatis*–endemic population. J Infect Dis 174:643, 1996.
29. Kimani J, Maclean IW, Bwayo JJ, et al: Risk factors for *Chlamydia trachomatis* pelvic inflammatory disease among sex workers in Nairobi, Kenya. J Infect Dis 173:1437, 1996.
30. Brunham RC, Maclean IW, Binns B, Peeling RW: *Chlamydia trachomatis:* its role in tubal infertility. J Infect Dis 152:1275, 1985.
31. Sparling PF: Biology of *Neisseria gonorrhoeae. In* Holmes KK, Sparling PF, Mardh P-A, et al (eds): Sexually Transmitted Diseases. New York, McGraw-Hill, 1999, p 433.
32. Stokes JH, Beerman H, Ingraham NR: Modern Clinical Syphilology, Diagnosis and Treatment. Case Study, 3rd ed. Philadelphia, WB Saunders, 1945.
33. Lukehart SA, Hook EW III, Baker-Zander SA, et al: Invasion of central nervous system by *Treponema pallidum:* implications for diagnosis and treatment. Ann Intern Med 109:855, 1988.
34. Tranont EC: Syphilis in adults: from Christopher Columbus to Sir Alexander Flemming to AIDS. Clin Infect Dis 21:1361, 1995.
35. Harter CA, Bernirsche K: Fetal syphilis in the first trimester. Am J Obstet Gynecol 124:705, 1976.
36. Nathan L, Bohman VR, Sanchez PJ, et al: In utero infection with *Treponema pallidum* in early pregnancy. Prenat Diagn 17:119–23, 1997.
37. Ingraham NR: The value of penicillin alone in the prevention and treatment of congenital syphilis. Acta Derm Venereol 31(Suppl 24):60, 1951.
38. Zenker PN, Berman SM: Congenital syphilis: trends and recommendations for evaluation and management. Pediatr Infect Dis J 10:516, 1991.
39. Fiumara NJ, Flemming WL, Downing JG, et al: The incidence of prenatal syphilis at the Boston City Hospital. N Engl J Med 247:48, 1952.
40. Radolf JD, Steiner B, Shevchenko D: *Treponema pallidum:* doing a remarkable job with what it's got. Trends Microbiol 7:7, 1999.
41. Pennisi E: Genome reveals wiles and weak points of syphilis. Science 281:324–5, 1998.
42. Weinstock GM, Hardham JM, McLeod MP, et al: The genome of *Treponema pallidum:* New light on the agent of syphilis. FEMS Microbiol Rev 22:323, 1998.
43. Berman SM: Maternal syphilis: Pathophysiology and treatment. Bull World Health Org 82(no.6):1, 2004.
44. Centers for Disease Control and Prevention. Screening tests to detect *Chlamydia trachomatis* and *Neiserria gonorrhea* infections—2002. MMWR 51(RR-15):1, 2002.
45. Baum EW, Bernhardt M, Sams WM Jr, et al: Secondary syphilis. Still the great imitator. JAMA 249:3069, 1983.
46. Larsen SA, Hunter EF, Creighton ET: Syphilis. *In* Holmes KK, Mardh P-A, Sparling PF, et al (eds): Sexually Transmitted Diseases. New York, McGraw-Hill, 1990, p 927.
47. Burstain JM, Grimprel E, Lukehart SA, et al: Sensitive detection of *Treponema pallidum* by using the polymerase chain reaction. J Clin Microbiol 29:62, 1991.
48. Saloojee H, Velaphi S, Goga Y, et al: The prevention and management of congenital syphilis: An overview and recommendations. Bull World Health Org 82:424, 2004.
49. Centers for Disease Control and Prevention. Sexually transmitted diseases treatment guidelines. MMWR 55(RR-11):1, 2006.
50. Lubiganon P, Piaggio G, Villar J, et al: The epidemiology of syphilis in pregnancy. Int J STD AIDS 13:486, 2002.
51. Hicks CB, Benson PM, Lupton, GP, Tramont EC: Seronegative secondary syphilis in a patient infected with the human immunodeficiency (HIV) with Kaposi sarcoma: A diagnostic dilemma. Ann Intern Med 107:492, 1987.
52. Centers for Disease Control. Current trends—Recommendations for diagnosing and treating syphilis in HIV-infected patients. MMWR 37:600, 1988.
53. Burton JR, Thorpe EM Jr, Shaver DC, et al: Nonimmune hydrops fetalis associated with maternal infection with syphilis. Am J Obstet Gynecol 167:56, 1992.
54. Jacobs A, Rotenberg O: Nonimmune hydrops fetalis due to congenital syphilis associated with negative intrapartum maternal serology screening. Am J Perinatol 15:233, 1998.
55. Hollier LM, Harstad TW, Sanchez PJ, et al: Fetal syphilis: Clinical and laboratory characteristics. Obstet Gynecol 97:947, 2001.
56. Ingraham NR: The value of penicillin alone in the prevention and treatment of congenital syphilis. Acta Derm Venereol Suppl (Stock) 31:60, 1951.
57. Rekart ML, Patrick DM, Chakraborty B, et al: Targeted mass treatment for syphilis with oral azithromycin. Lancet 361:313, 2003.
58. Gust DA, Levine WC, St Louis ME, et al: Mortality associated with congenital syphilis in the United State, 1992–1998. Pediatrics 109:E79, 2002.
59. Alexander JM, Sheffield JS, Sanchez PJ, et al: Efficacy of treatment for syphilis in pregnancy. Obstet Gynecol 93:5, 1999.
60. Sheffield JS, Sanchez PJ, Morris G, et al: Congenital syphilis after maternal treatment for syphilis during pregnancy. Am J Obstet Gynecol 186:569, 2002.
61. Wendel GD Jr, Sheffield JS, Hollier LM, et al: Treatment of syphilis in pregnancy and prevention of congenital syphilis. Clin Infect Dis 35(Suppl 2):S200, 2002.

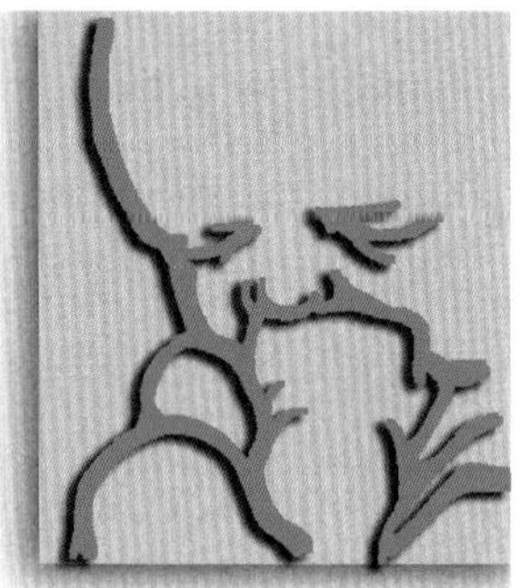

Maternal and Perinatal Infection—Viral

HELENE BERNSTEIN

CHAPTER 48

KEY ABBREVIATIONS

Acquired immunodeficiency syndrome	AIDS
AIDS Clinical Trials Group	ACTG
American College of Obstetricians and Gynecologists	ACOG
CC-chemokine receptor type 5	CCR5
Centers for Disease Control and Prevention	CDC
Central nervous system	CNS
Chorionic villous sampling	CVS
Complete blood count	CBC
Confidence interval	CI
Congenital rubella syndrome	CRS
C-X-C chemokine receptor type 4	CXCR4
Cytomegalovirus	CMV
Deoxyribonucleic acid	DNA
Enzyme-linked immunoassay	ELISA
Epstein-Barr virus	EBV
Erythema infectiosum	EI
Food and Drug Administration	FDA
Glycoprotein	gp
Hemagglutinin proteins	HA
Hepatitis A virus	HAV
Hepatitis B core antigen	HBcAg
Hepatitis B immune globulin	HBIG
Hepatitis B surface antibody	HBsAb
Hepatitis B surface antigen	HBsAg
Hepatitis B virus	HBV
Hepatitis C virus	HCV
Hepatitis delta antigen	HDAg
Hepatitis delta virus	HDV
Herpes simplex virus	HSV
Highly active antiviral therapy	HAART
Human immunodeficiency virus	HIV
Human papillomavirus	HPV
Immunoglobulin G	IgG

Intrauterine growth restriction	IUGR
Intravenous	IV
Long terminal repeat	LTR
Measles, mumps, rubella	MMR
Mycobacterium avium complex	MAC
Non-nucleoside reverse transcriptase inhibitor	NNRTI
Nucleic acid test	NAT
Nucleoside reverse transcriptase inhibitors	NRTIs
Opportunistic infection	OI
Papanicolaou smear	PAP
Peripheral blood mononuclear cells	PBMCs
Polymerase chain reaction	PCR
Protease inhibitor	PI
Purified protein derivative test	PPD
Rapid plasma reagin	RPR
Reverse transcription	RT
Recombinant immunoblot assay	RIBA
Regulator of viral expression	rev
Ribonuclease	RNase
Ribonucleic acid	RNA
Sexually transmitted diseases	STRs
Subacute sclerosing panencephalitis	SSPE
Transcriptional transactivation	tat
Tuberculin skin text	PPD
Tuberculosis	TB
Varicella zoster immune globulin	VZIG
Varicella zoster virus	VZV
Venereal disease research labs	VDRL
West Nile virus	WNV
Woman and Infants Transmission Study	WITS
Zidovudine	AZT

Viruses have been identified in virtually all living organisms. They are among the simplest of living organisms, yet they have altered history significantly in the past and continue to do so today. Viruses are obligate intracellular parasites that use the host cell's structural and functional components for replication, and they exhibit a remarkable diversity of strategies for the expression of their genes and for their replication. Viral infections can range from being asymptomatic or subclinical to overwhelming and highly lethal, with findings such as meningoencephalitis or hemorrhagic fever with shock. The duration of viral infection is also highly variable. A number of viruses are limited to acute infections, whereas others can cause chronic infections or establish latency within the host, with reactivation many years following the acute infection episode. Certain viruses can also integrate into the host cell genome; some of these viruses have demonstrated oncogenic potential.

Virus particles are known as virions, and they contain nucleic acid and structural proteins, which together are referred to as a nucleocapsid. Viral nucleic acid can be composed of DNA or RNA, which may be single or double stranded. The viral genome can be linear or circular and may exist in multiple segments or as a single segment. There is great variation in the number of genes contained within viruses ranging from two genes in parvovirus B19 to more than 200 genes in cytomegalovirus. Some viruses have lipid bilayer envelopes external to the nucleocapsid; these envelopes are derived from the host cell and contain viral proteins. Herpesviruses have an additional layer, called a tegument, between the nucleocapsid and envelope. Viruses are classified by the International Committee on Taxonomy of Viruses into Orders, Families, Subfamilies, Genera, and Species. Classification is based on morphology, nucleic acid type and characteristics, the presence or absence of an envelope, genome replication strategy, and homology to other identified viruses.

Viruses enter cells by binding to receptors present on the surface of the host cell that recognize viral proteins that are part of either the envelope or nucleocapsid of the virus. This interaction between viral proteins and cellular receptors defines, in part, the host-range of the virus and limits infection to susceptible host cells. The virus then penetrates the host cell through translocation of the entire virion across the plasma membrane, endocytosis, or fusion of the viral envelope with the cell membrane. The virus then uncoats its nucleic acid for replication. The next step in viral replication is the expression of viral genes and replication of the viral genome; this may occur in either the cytoplasm or nucleus of the cell depending on the type of virus. Assembly of progeny virions then occurs, followed by release of newly formed virions, usually by cell lysis or by budding from the cell surface in the case of enveloped viruses.

In spite of their inability to replicate independently, viruses play an important role in infectious disease. In order to initiate a productive infection, viruses must enter cells, replicate their genome, and package their genome into virions. By default most viruses alter the structure or function of the host cell, and the inability of a virus to complete any of these steps results in a nonproductive infection. Viral pathogenesis may be mediated through several mechanisms. These include direct effects on infected host cells, which may result in cell death through lysis or apoptosis. Infected cells can also be killed by antiviral antibody and complement or by cell-mediated immune mechanisms. In addition, some viral genomes encode oncogenes, which can cause transformation of infected host cells. Viral proteins can also impact the function of uninfected cells, including the host immune system. Finally, the host immune response to viral infection can cause both local and systemic effects, through the release of cytokines, chemokines, and antibodies, which contribute to the signs and symptoms of viral infections including fever, rash, arthralgias, and myalgias. The outcome of viral infection also depends on host factors including immune status, age, nutritional status, and genetic background. Genetic factors can alter susceptibility to viral infection, the immune response generated following infection, and the long-term consequences of viral infection.

This chapter discusses many of the viral infections that are relevant to pregnancy and have a significant impact on

Table 48-1. Summary of Etiology, Diagnosis, and Management of Major Perinatal Viral Infections

	COMPLICATIONS		DIAGNOSIS		MANAGEMENT*	
CONDITION	**MATERNAL**	**FETAL/ NEONATAL**	**MATERNAL**	**FETAL/NEONATAL**	**MATERNAL**	**FETAL/NEONATAL**
HIV infection	Opportunistic infection, malignancy	Primarily perinatal infection	Detection of antibody	PCR culture	HAART	HAART for prevention of vertical transmission
Parvovirus infection	Rare	Anemia hydrops	Detection of antibody	Ultrasound PCR	Supportive care	Intrauterine transfusion for severe anemia
Rubeola	Otitis media, pneumonia, encephalitis	Abortion, preterm delivery	Detection of antibody	N/A	Prevention—vaccination prior to pregnancy	N/A
Rubella	Rare	Congenital infection	Detection of antibody	Ultrasound RT-PCR or culture	Prevention—vaccination prior to pregnancy Supportive care	Pregnancy termination for affected fetus
CMV	Chorioretinitis, pneumonia in immunocompromised patient	Congenital infection	Detection of antibody, PCR	Culture PCR Ultrasound	Ganciclovir for severe infection	Consider pregnancy termination when mother has primary infection
Herpes simplex	Disseminated infection in immunocompromised patient	Neonatal infection	Clinical examination, culture, PCR	Clinical examination, culture, PCR	Acyclovir, valacyclovir, or famciclovir for severe primary infection	Cesarean delivery when mother has overt infection
Varicella	Pneumonia Encephalitis	Congenital or perinatal infection	Clinical examination, detection of antibody, PCR	Ultrasound*	VZIG, acyclovir for prophylaxis or treatment	VZIG, acyclovir for prophylaxis or treatment of neonate
Hepatitis						
A	Rare	None	Detection of antibody	N/A	Prevention—hepatitis A vaccine Supportive care	Administer immune globulin to neonate if mother acutely infected at delivery
B	Chronic liver disease	Neonatal infection	Detection of surface antigen	N/A	Prevention—HBIG+HBV for susceptible household contacts	HBIG+HBV immediately after delivery
C	Chronic liver disease	Neonatal infection	Detection of antibody	N/A	Supportive care	None
D	Chronic liver disease	Neonatal infection	Detection of antigen and antibody	N/A	Supportive care	HBIG+HBV immediately after delivery
E	Increased mortality	Neonatal infection	Detection of antibody RT-PCR	N/A	Supportive care	None

CMV, cytomegalovirus; CNS, central nervous system; HAART, highly active antiretroviral therapy; HBIG, hepatitis B immune globulin; HBV, hepatitis B vaccine; HIV, human immunodeficiency virus; PCR, polymerase chain reaction; RT-PCR, reverse transcriptase PCR; VZIG, varicella zoster immune globulin.

*See text for detailed discussion of patient management.

maternal health and/or pregnancy outcome. The virology, epidemiology, diagnosis, clinical manifestations, management during pregnancy, and impact on the fetus/neonate is detailed for the viruses listed in Table 48-1.

HUMAN IMMUNODEFICIENCY VIRUS

Virology

Human immunodeficiency virus (HIV) is a member of the *Retroviridae* family, which is characterized by spherical, enveloped viruses. The virus envelope surrounds an icosahedral capsid containing the viral genome, which consists of two identical pieces of positive sense, single-stranded RNA, about 9.2 kb long, held together noncovalently by hydrogen bonds. HIV has three main genes: *gag, pol,* and *env,* which are surrounded by long terminal repeat (LTR) regions. The *gag* gene encodes the precursor for the virion capsid proteins, which include the full-length p55 polyprotein precursor and its cleavage products: p17 matrix, p24 capsid, p9 nucleocapsid, and p7. The *pol* gene encodes the precursor polyprotein for several virion enzymes including protease, reverse transcriptase, RNase H, and integrase. The *env* gene encodes the envelope glycoprotein (gp160), which is cleaved to the surface unit (gp120) and the transmembrane protein (gp41), which is necessary for fusion. The transcriptional transactivator (*tat*) and regulator of viral expression (*rev*) genes are encoded by two overlapping exons and produce small nonvirion proteins, which are essential for replication. Nonessential accessory genes include *vif, vpr, vpu,* and *nef.* The *vpr* gene product is packaged into virions. Retroviruses are unique in that the viral genome is reverse transcribed into DNA through the viral enzyme reverse transcriptase, followed by integration into the host cell genome through the viral enzyme integrase.[1] This enables HIV to become latent within quiescent infected cells, and makes eradication of the virus thus far impossible.

The HIV envelope glycoprotein (gp120) is a ligand for the CD4 molecule; thus, HIV predominantly infects CD4+ cells, which include T cells, monocytes, and macrophages. Two primary coreceptors for HIV have also been identified, CXCR4 and CCR5. These coreceptors interact with the envelope glycoprotein and are also required for viral entry and infection.[2,3] Both adults and neonates are almost always initially infected with a strain of HIV that uses the CCR5 coreceptor,[4,5] which may reflect viral fitness. Individuals homozygous for a 32-base pair deletion within the CCR5 gene are much less likely to acquire HIV infection even following significant exposure to HIV, and some CCR5 polymorphisms have been shown to correlate with disease progression of HIV in perinatally infected children and adults.[6–8]

Epidemiology

As of the year 2000, there were an estimated 850,000 to 950,000 persons infected with HIV living in the United States; close to one third remain unaware of their infection status.[9] Between 2000 and 2003, HIV/acquired immunodeficiency syndrome (AIDS) was diagnosed in an additional 125,800 persons within 32 states participating in a Centers for Disease Control and Prevention (CDC)–sponsored study, and women accounted for 35,241 (28 percent) of these new cases. New HIV infections in women resulted largely from high-risk heterosexual contact (77.7 percent) and intravenous (IV) drug use (19.4 percent). Of new HIV infections, 68.8 percent were in black non-Hispanic women, followed by 18.6 percent in white, non-Hispanic women, and 10.8 percent in Hispanic women. Although black women comprised only 13 percent of the study population, their infection rate, which was approximately 19 times the rate of non-Hispanic whites and five times the rate of Hispanics, was disproportionate.[9] Other factors that increase the risk of HIV transmission or are associated with an increased prevalence of HIV seropositivity include high numbers of sexual contacts, high-risk sexual exposure, receptive anal intercourse, sexual contact with an uncircumcised man, IV drug and/or crack cocaine use, residing in the inner city, and the presence of other sexually transmitted diseases (STDs), particularly those that cause genital ulcers (herpes, syphilis, chancroid).[10–12]

HIV infection is limited to humans and chimpanzees, and most infections in the United States are caused by HIV-1. HIV-1 is divided into three groups: M, N, and O. More than 95 percent of HIV-1 infections are caused by group M, which is divided into subtypes (or clades) A to K. The predominant type of HIV within the United States is clade B, whereas other clades predominate in other regions of the world. HIV-2, a related strain of HIV, is endemic in Africa, Portugal, and France, and appears to have a decreased rate of vertical transmission compared with HIV-1.[13,14] Although clinicians practicing within the United States infrequently encounter patients infected with HIV-2 or a nonclade-B subtype of HIV-1, the different strains and clades of HIV can impact diagnosis and quantitation of viral load. Much less is known about the treatment of these related viruses given their prevalence in areas of the world where antiretroviral treatment is not readily available.

Clinical Manifestations

The clinical presentation of HIV infection or AIDS depends on when infection occurred and whether there is a resulting immunodeficiency. Following exposure and primary infection 50 to 70 percent of individuals infected with HIV develop the acute retroviral syndrome. At this time, patients may present with mononucleosis-like symptoms, which may include fever, rigors, arthralgias, myalgias, maculopapular rash, urticaria, abdominal cramps, diarrhea, and lymphocytic meningitis.[15] The acute phase of infection usually occurs 4 to 6 weeks following HIV exposure and can last several weeks. Following primary infection with HIV, patients enter the latent phase of illness which can last approximately 5 to 10 years. During the latent or asymptomatic phase of infection viral replication occurs predominately within lymphatic tissue. Although patients are asymptomatic, this latent phase is characterized by inappropriate chronic immune activation and progressive destruction of lymphatic tissue.[16] Acute primary infection and asymptomatic infection with HIV are described as clinical category A. After a variable period of time, HIV-infected individuals progress to clinical category B, which is characterized by the presence of clinical conditions, which are attributable to HIV infection or are complicated by HIV infection (Table 48-2). Ultimately the patient develops AIDS, which is defined as clinical category C, and includes one or more of the conditions listed in Table 48-3.[17]

Diagnosis

The principal diagnostic test for HIV infection is the identification of virus-specific antibody. The initial serologic screening test is typically an enzyme-linked immunosorbant assay (ELISA), which is highly sensitive, inexpensive, and well suited for screening large numbers of patients.[18] If the ELISA is positive, it is usually repeated, and after two positive ELISA assays, a Western blot or immunofluorescent antibody assay is performed for confirmation. The Western blot detects specific viral antigens

Table 48-2. Category B, Symptomatic Conditions in an HIV-Infected Adolescent or Adult

Bacillary angiomatosis
Candidiasis, oropharyngeal (thrush)
Candidiasis, vulvovaginal; persistent, frequent, or poorly responsive to therapy
Cervical dysplasia (moderate or severe)/cervical carcinoma in situ
Constitutional symptoms, such as fever (38.5°C) or diarrhea lasting greater than 1 month
Hairy leukoplakia, oral
Herpes zoster (shingles), involving at least two distinct episodes or more than one dermatome
Idiopathic thrombocytopenic purpura
Listeriosis
Pelvic inflammatory disease, particularly if complicated by tubo-ovarian abscess
Peripheral neuropathy

HIV, human immunodeficiency virus.

Table 48-3. Category C, Conditions Included in the 1993 AIDS Surveillance Case Definition

Candidiasis of bronchi, trachea, lungs, or esophagus
Cervical cancer, invasive*
Coccidioidomycosis, disseminated or extrapulmonary
Cryptococcosis, extrapulmonary
Cryptosporidiosis, chronic intestinal (greater than 1 month's duration)
Cytomegalovirus disease (other than liver, spleen, or nodes), including retinitis
Encephalopathy, HIV related
Herpes simplex: chronic ulcer(s) (greater than 1 month's duration); or bronchitis, pneumonitis, or esophagitis
Histoplasmosis, disseminated or extrapulmonary
Isosporiasis, chronic intestinal (greater than 1 month's duration)
Kaposi's sarcoma
Lymphoma, Burkitt's or immunoblastic (or equivalent term)
Lymphoma, primary, of brain
Mycobacterium avium complex or M. Kansasii, disseminated or extrapulmonary
Mycobacterium tuberculosis, any site (pulmonary* or extrapulmonary)
Mycobacterium, other species or unidentified species, disseminated or extrapulmonary
Pneumocystis carinii pneumonia
Pneumonia, recurrent*
Progressive multifocal leukoencephalopathy
Salmonella septicemia, recurrent
Toxoplasmosis of brain
Wasting syndrome due to HIV

AIDS, acquired immunodeficiency syndrome; HIV, human immunodeficiency virus.

*Added in the 1993 expansion of the AIDS surveillance case definition.

and is considered positive when any two of the following three antigens are identified: p24 (capsid), gp41 (envelope), and gp120/160 (envelope). Most serologic tests in use today detect antibodies specific for HIV-1 and HIV-2, and there are several salivary or rapid blood tests with similar efficacy to the ELISA assay.[19] In the patient with suspected acute HIV infection, antibody tests may be negative. Therefore, HIV nucleic acid quantitation, p24 antigen detection, or HIV isolation through viral culture should be used for diagnosis.[20]

Given the increasing prevalence of HIV infection in the United States and the finding that early identification and treatment of HIV-infected pregnant women with antiretroviral therapy is the best way to prevent perinatal HIV transmission, both the American College of Obstetricians and Gynecologists (ACOG) and the CDC recommend an "opt out" approach to ensure routine HIV screening for all pregnant women. In areas of high HIV prevalence, offering repeat HIV testing in the third trimester is appropriate. In addition, many centers are offering rapid HIV testing in labor for women with undocumented HIV status because 40 to 85 percent of infants perinatally infected with HIV in the United States are born to women whose HIV status is unknown before delivery.[21–23] Women who are found to be HIV seropositive on rapid testing are offered intrapartum and postpartum prophylaxis to limit perinatal HIV transmission without waiting for confirmatory testing.[24]

Because the fetus receives maternal immunoglobulin G (IgG) by transplacental passage, serologic tests of the HIV-exposed neonate will be positive and do not necessarily predict mother-to-child transmission of HIV. In neonates the diagnosis of HIV is typically made through polymerase chain reaction (PCR) amplification of HIV-specific DNA sequences from neonatal peripheral blood mononuclear cells (PBMCs). Diagnosis of HIV infection can also be confirmed by direct culture of virus from PBMCs or detection of p24 antigen in serum, although these methods are substantially less sensitive than PCR-based methods. Two positive specimens (excluding cord blood) are required for a definitive diagnosis; the presence of one positive test is a presumptive diagnosis. Further details on case definitions for HIV infection are available from the CDC at www.cdc.gov.[20]

Management During Pregnancy

In pregnant women with known HIV, a thorough history should be obtained including the duration of HIV infection, likely route of transmission, prior use, duration and tolerance of antiretroviral medications, immunization history, prior hospitalizations, and opportunistic infections. Laboratory evaluation should include at minimum a CD4 count and HIV viral load. If the patient is newly diagnosed or has a detectable viral load on antiretroviral therapy, an HIV genotype and phenotype should also be obtained.[25] Viral loads are usually determined using the Roche Amplicor HIV-1 Monitor, which uses reverse transcription (RT)-PCR technology, and is the only assay approved by the Food and Drug Administration (FDA). If the patient's HIV viral load is undetectable using this assay, retesting or using a different type of HIV viral load test is recommended (Bayer branched-chain DNA assay or Roche RT-PCR version 1.5 assay).[26]

Although some patients may have an undetectable viral load, in these circumstances, it is more likely that the patient has been infected with a non–clade B isolate of HIV. Consultation with an infectious disease physician with experience in the management of HIV disease can be helpful in these cases or when the woman's genotype and phenotype assay demonstrates significant resistance to antiretroviral therapy. Additional testing should include serology to evaluate: hepatitis B surface antigen (HBsAg), hepatitis B surface antibody (HBsAb), hepatitis C virus antibody, rapid plasma reagin (RPR) or Venereal Disease Research Laboratory (VDRL) test, a complete blood count (CBC) with platelet count, baseline blood chemistry, liver function tests, chlamydia and gonorrhea testing, a Papanicolaou smear (PAP), and a tuberculin skin test (PPD). If the PPD is positive, a chest radiograph should be performed to rule out active pulmonary disease. Women with abnormal PAP smears should be evaluated with colposcopy. Women with a CD4 count below 200 should also be tested for antibodies to cytomegalovirus and *Toxoplasma gondii*.

Patients should be extensively counseled about the impact of HIV infection on pregnancy, including the risk of perinatal transmission, potential methods of delivery, and treatment options. Studies have shown that pregnancy does not affect the progression of HIV disease.[27–29] Some reports have shown an increase in the risk of preterm delivery in HIV-infected pregnant women, particularly in women on combination antiretroviral therapy. However, many of the women participating in these studies had other risk factors for preterm delivery.[30–35] The Woman and Infants Transmission Study (WITS), a large observational study in the United States, and the AIDS Clinical Trials Group (ACTG) did not find an increased incidence of preterm delivery in HIV-infected women. Therefore, treatment that can limit the mother-to-child transmission of HIV should not be withheld based on this concern.[36,37] Care of the HIV-infected pregnant woman is enhanced by having a multidisciplinary team, which may include the physician, social workers, nutritionists, psychologists, and peer counselors.

Management of the HIV-infected pregnant woman should include frequent visits and counseling about the benefits of compliance with medications to reduce perinatal HIV transmission and the development of resistance to antiretroviral therapy. Viral load monitoring and CD4 counts should be obtained monthly when starting a new medication regimen or when a change in viral load is detected. Patients on stable antiretroviral regimens with undetectable viremia can have viral loads and CD4 counts checked in each trimester. Patients who are HIV-infected should receive vaccinations for hepatitis A, pneumococcus, and influenza. Hepatitis BsAg and HBsAb negative patients should also receive hepatitis B vaccination.

In patients older than 35 years of age at delivery who desire determination of the fetal karyotype, the risks and benefits of amniocentesis or chorionic villous sampling (CVS) should be discussed and a referral to a genetic counselor made. Invasive procedures to rule out aneuploidy have the potential to increase the risk of perinatal HIV transmission, and these uncertainties should be reviewed with the patient. A recent study described amniocentesis on 23 HIV-infected women on antiretroviral treatment with no incidence of perinatal HIV transmission, although several of the procedures were performed in the third trimester within days of delivery.[38] There is a recently published study of 63 women who were HIV infected and underwent amniocentesis or CVS. There was no increased risk of HIV transmission.[38a] In the United States, several recent cases of amniocentesis or CVS performed on women on highly active antiretroviral therapy with undetectable viral loads have also not resulted in perinatal transmission (H. Bernstein and B. Ross, unpublished communication). Larger studies are needed to better estimate the associated risk, if any, of HIV transmission with amniocentesis or CVS.

Treatment of Human Immunodeficiency Virus Infection During Pregnancy

Patients should receive treatment with antiretroviral therapy both to reduce mother-to-child transmission of HIV and for maternal benefit. When evaluating antiretroviral therapy for use in pregnancy, considerations should include possible changes in dosing requirements secondary to the physiologic changes associated with pregnancy; potential side effects of antiretroviral drugs; teratogenicity, mutagenicity, or carcinogenicity; and the pharmacokinetics and toxicity of transplacentally transferred drugs.

One of the first studies to show that antiretroviral therapy reduced perinatal HIV transmission was conducted by the ACTG (Protocol 076).[33] This randomized, placebo-controlled study included HIV-infected women with a CD4 count above 200/mm^3 who were treatment naïve and beyond the first trimester of pregnancy. Randomization was ethical because both the efficacy of zidovudine (AZT) in preventing perinatal HIV transmission was unknown, and the possible side effects of intrauterine AZT exposure were unknown when the study began in 1991. The treatment arm included prenatal oral AZT and intravenous AZT during labor. Following delivery, infants in the treatment arm also received oral AZT for 6 weeks (Table 48-4). The study was prematurely terminated when an interim data analysis showed a substantially reduced risk of vertical transmission (8.3 percent versus 25.5 percent in placebo arm) without deleterious side effects. Several follow-up studies have shown that oral AZT and other nucleoside analog drugs are also effective in preventing perinatal HIV transmission.

Another landmark study was the HIVNET 012 trial in which patients in Uganda were randomly assigned to treatment with nevirapine (200 mg by mouth [PO]) at the onset of labor, followed by oral treatment of the baby with a single dose of 2 mg/kg within 72 hours of birth versus treatment with AZT. Within this population, 99 percent of the infants were breast-fed. At 16 weeks' post delivery, the rates of neonatal HIV infection were 25 percent in the AZT group and 13 percent in the nevirapine group ($p = 0.0001$).[39] Although nevirapine was more effective, subsequent analysis revealed a high rate of nevirapine resistance in women treated with this regimen.[40] In the United States, a prospective placebo-controlled study, PACTG 316, examined the efficacy of adding nevirapine prophylaxis in addition to standard, ongoing antiretro-

Table 48-4. Pediatric AIDS Clinical Trials Group (PACTG) 076 Zidovudine (ZDV) Regimen

TIME OF ZDV ADMINISTRATION	REGIMEN
Antepartum	Oral administration of 100 mg AZT five times daily*, initiated at 14–34 weeks gestation and continued throughout the pregnancy.
Intrapartum	During labor, intravenous administration of AZT in a one-hour initial dose of 2 mg/kg body weight, followed by a continuous infusion of 1 mg/kg body weight/hour until delivery.
Postpartum	Oral administration of AZT to the newborn (AZT syrup at 2 mg/kg body weight/dose every six hours) for the first six weeks of life, beginning at 8–12 hours after birth.

AZT, zidovudine.
*Oral AZT administered 300 mg twice daily is currently used in general clinical practice.

viral therapy to further limit the perinatal transmission of HIV.[41] The study was discontinued, because overall perinatal transmission in both arms of the study was below 2.0 percent. Current U.S. recommendations discourage intrapartum administration of nevirapine. The potential emergence of nevirapine resistance and drug side effects (see later) could negatively impact both the current health and future treatment options of the HIV-infected woman.[42]

The standard of care in the United States is to treat pregnant HIV-infected women with highly active antiretroviral therapy (HAART) to maximally suppress viral replication, to reduce perinatal transmission of HIV, and to minimize the risk of development of drug resistant virus. HAART should include three drugs from at least two classes of antiretrovirals; the most commonly used antiretrovirals in pregnancy are shown in Table 48-5. Up to date U.S. treatment recommendations are available at *www.AIDSinfo.nih.gov*.[42] With the combination of HAART and an undetectable viral load, the risk of mother-to-child transmission of HIV is between 1 and 2 percent.[36,41,43] Combivir (AZT 300 mg/lamivudine 150 mg) and nelfinavir (1,250 mg) administered twice daily comprise what may be the most widely used antiretroviral regimen during pregnancy, particularly for antiretroviral naïve patients. Twice-daily dosing of nelfinavir is preferred because dosing three times a day (TID) results in subtherapeutic levels during pregnancy.[44] This regimen is well tolerated, and has a good safety and efficacy profile. Other regimens have been successfully used in women who are intolerant to one or more of the components of this regimen or who have inadequate suppression of viremia.

Zidovudine should be included in the treatment regimen whenever possible, because of its proven efficacy in preventing mother to child transmission of HIV. Antiretroviral treatment may be deferred or discontinued within the first trimester of pregnancy owing to nausea and the potential risk of teratogenesis. Additionally, in treatment-naive patients with a viral load of less than 1,000 copies/ml, zidovudine monotherapy may be considered in lieu of HAART. However, zidovudine monotherapy has the potential to induce zidovudine resistance and, therefore, should be used with reservation. Even HIV-infected women with an undetectable viral load should receive some antiretroviral regimen because their risk of perinatal transmission is 9.8 percent if left untreated.[43]

Side effects of antiretroviral drugs used within pregnancy have been described and will be briefly discussed (see Table 48-5). Zidovudine has been associated with clinically significant anemia. In addition, all nucleoside reverse transcriptase inhibitors (NRTIs) bind to mitochondrial DNA polymerase gamma and can cause dysfunction presenting rarely as clinically significant myopathy, cardiomyopathy, neuropathy, lactic acidosis, or fatty liver. Lactic acidosis and hepatic failure have been reported largely with long term or combination stavudine and didanosine use, and are linked to a genetic defect in mitochondrial fatty acid metabolism.[45] However, the potential for metabolic problems exists with all NRTIs; the risk in descending order is zalcitabine, didanosine, stavudine, lamivudine, zidovudine, abacavir, and tenofovir.[46–48] Stavudine and didanosine in pregnancy, especially in combination, should be avoided whenever possible, and appropriate testing should be performed on any symptomatic patient. Mitochondrial toxicity has also been observed in children born to HIV-infected mothers treated with NRTIs,[49,50] although no increase in the rate of death was observed.[51] Serial CBCs, hemoglobin levels, electrolytes and liver function tests should be performed on patients treated with NRTIs.

The non-nucleoside reverse transcriptase inhibitor (NNRTI) efavirenz has been linked with three cases of meningomyelocele and one case of Dandy-Walker malformation in exposed offspring. Therefore, its use should be avoided in the first trimester of pregnancy.[52,53] Nevirapine, another NNRTI, has been associated with increased hepatic transaminase levels, rash, and toxicity. Clinically significant hepatic perturbation occurs in approximately 4 percent of patients, with a risk of liver failure of 0.04 to 0.4 percent, and severe rash in approximately 2 percent. Liver function tests should be monitored every 2 weeks during the first 18 weeks of nevirapine therapy and then monthly, and in any patient who develops a rash. Women with CD4 counts greater than 250 have a 9.8 fold increased risk of significant hepatotoxicity when taking nevirapine, thus current recommendations are to only use this drug if the benefits outweigh the risks in HIV-infected pregnant women.[54]

Protease inhibitors are being used increasingly in pregnancy,[25,36] and they appear to have minimal transplacental passage and few adverse side effects.[55] Lower serum concentrations of some protease inhibitors have been reported in pregnant women, particularly with indinavir and, more recently, lopinavir/ritonavir.[44,56] In addition, the use of protease inhibitors is associated with hyperglycemia and exacerbation of underlying diabetes mellitus. It is not known whether the use of protease inhibitors during pregnancy increases the risks of gestational diabetes; however, an early glucose loading test followed by repeat testing after 28 weeks is reasonable.

Table 48-5. Commonly Used Antriretroviral Drugs in Pregnancy

ANTIRETROVIRAL DRUG	FDA PREGNANCY CATEGORY	PLACENTAL PASSAGE	ANIMAL STUDIES CARCINOGEN/ TERATOGEN	PHARMACOKINETICS IN PREGNANCY	CONCERNS IN PREGNANCY	RATIONALE FOR RECOMMENDED USE IN PREGNANCY
NRTIs						
Zidovudine (Retrovir) (AZT) (ZDV)	C	Yes	Positive (rodent, noninvasive vaginal epithelial tumors), teratogen at near lethal dose	Not significantly altered in pregnancy	No evidence of human teratogenicity. Well tolerated, short-term safety demonstrated for mother and infant.	Preferred NRTI for use in combination antiretroviral regimens in pregnancy based on efficacy studies and extensive experience; should be included in regimen unless significant toxicity or stavudine use.
Lamivudine (3TC) (Epivir)	C	Yes (human)	Negative (no tumors, lifetime rodent study), Negative	Pharmacokinetics not significantly altered in pregnancy; no change in dose indicated.	No evidence of human teratogenicity. Well-tolerated, short-term safety demonstrated for mother and infant.	Because of extensive experience using 3TC in pregnancy in combination with ZDV, 3TC and ZDV is the recommended dual NRTI backbone for pregnant women.
Didanosine (Videx) (ddI)	B	Yes (human)	Negative (no tumors, lifetime rodent study), Negative	Pharmacokinetics not significantly altered in pregnancy; no change in dose indicated.	Cases of lactic acidosis, some fatal, have been reported in pregnant women receiving ddI and D4T together.	Alternate NRTI for dual nucleoside backbone of combination regimens. ddI should be used with D4T only if no other alternatives are available.
Stavudine (D4T) (Zerit)	C	Yes (rhesus Monkey)	Positive (at very high dose exposure liver and bladder tumors in mice and rats), not a teratogen, but sternal bone calcium decreased in rodents	Pharmacokinetics not significantly altered in pregnancy; no change in dose indicated.	No evidence of human teratogenicity. Cases of lactic acidosis, some fatal, have been reported in pregnant women receiving ddI and D4T together	Alternate NRTI for dual nucleoside backbone of combination regimens. D4T should be used with ddI only if no other alternatives are available. Do not use with ZDV due to potential for antagonism.
Abacavir (Ziagen) (ABC)	C	Yes (rats)	Positive (tumors of liver, thyroid in female rats, and preputial and clitoral gland of mice and rats). Positive teratogen in rodents, anasarca and skeletal malformations at 35× human exposure during organogenesis	Phase I/II study in progress.	Hypersensitivity reactions occur in ~5–8% of nonpregnant persons; a much smaller percentage are fatal and are usually associated with rechallenge. Rate in pregnancy unknown. Patient should be educated regarding symptoms of hypersensitivity reaction.	Alternate NRTI for dual nucleoside backbone of combination regimens.
NNRTIs						
Nevirapine (Viramune) (NVP)	C	Yes (human)	Positive (hepatocellular adenomas and carcinomas in mice and rats). Negative teratogenicity	Pharmacokinetics not significantly altered in pregnancy; no change in dose indicated.	No evidence of human teratogenicity. Increased risk of symptomatic, often rash associated, and potentially fatal liver toxicity among women with $CD4^+$ counts >250/mm^3 when first initiating therapy; unclear if pregnancy increases risk.	Nevirapine should be initiated in pregnant women with $CD4^+$ counts >250 cells/mm^3 with caution, due to the increased risk of potentially life-threatening hepatotoxicity in women with high $CD4^+$ counts. Women who enter pregnancy on nevirapine regimens and are tolerating them well may continue therapy, regardless of $CD4^+$ count.

Table 48-5. Commonly Used Antiretroviral Drugs in Pregnancy—cont'd

Protease Inhibitors (PI)						
Nelfinavir (Viracept)	B	Minimal (humans)	Positive thyroid follicular adenomas and carcinomas in rats). Negative teratogenicity	Adequate drug levels are achieved in pregnant women with nelfinavir 1,250 mg, given twice daily.	No evidence of human teratogenicity. Well-tolerated, short-term safety demonstrated for mother and infant. Nelfinavir dosing at 750 mg three times daily produced variable and generally low levels in pregnant women, 1,250 mg BID is recommended dose	Given pharmacokinetic data and extensive experience with use in pregnancy, this is the preferred PI for combination regimens in pregnant women, particularly if HAART is being given solely for perinatal prophylaxis. In clinical trials of initial therapy in non-pregnant adults, nelfinavir-based regimens had a lower rate of viral response compared to lopinavir/ritonavir or efavirenz-based regimens, but similar viral response compared with atazanavir or nevirapine-based regimens.
Lopinavir/Ritonavir (Kaletra)	C	Unknown	Positive (hepatocellular adenomas and carcinomas in mice and rats). No teratogenicity, but delayed skeletal ossification and increase in skeletal variations in rats at maternally toxic dose.	Phase I/II safety and pharmacokinetic study in progress using twice-daily lopinavir 400 mg and ritonavir 100 mg.	Limited experience in human pregnancy.	Preliminary studies suggest increased dose may be required during pregnancy, though specific dosing recommendations not established. If used during pregnancy, monitor response to therapy closely. If expected virologic result is not observed, consult with a specialist with expertise in HIV in pregnancy.
Saquinavir/Ritonavir Used as: Saquinavir-soft gel capsule [SGC] (Fortovase)/ritonavir (Norvir)	B	Minimal (humans)	Negative	Adequate drug levels in pregnant women with saquinavir-SGC 800 mg boosted with ritonavir 100 mg, given twice daily. Recommended adult dosing of saquinavir-SGC 1,000 mg plus ritonavir 100 mg may be used. No pharmacokinetic data on saquinavir-hard gel capsule (HGC)/ritonavir in pregnancy, but better GI tolerance in non-pregnant adults.	Well-tolerated, short-term safety demonstrated for mother and infant. Inadequate drug levels observed in pregnant women with saquinavir-SGC given alone at 1,200 mg three times daily.	Given pharmacokinetic data and moderate experience with use in pregnancy, ritonavir-boosted saquinavir-SGC can be considered a preferred PI for combination regimens in pregnancy.

GI, gastrointestinal; HAART, highly active antiretroviral therapy; NNRTIs, non-nucleoside reverse transcriptase inhibitors; NRTIs, nucleoside reverse transcriptase inhibitors.

Table 48-6. Prophylactic Antibiotic Regimens for Common Opportunistic infections*

CONDITION	INDICATION FOR PROPHYLAXIS	ANTIBIOTIC REGIMEN
Pneumocystis carinii pneumonia	Prior infection or CD4 < 200/mm^3	TMP-SMX 1 DS tablet qd indefinitely
Toxoplasmic encephalitis	CD4 < 100/mm^3 + serology	TMP-SMX 1 DS tablet qd indefinitely
Tuberculosis	+PPD > 5 mm No active disease on chest x-ray	INH; 300 mg qd, plus pyridoxine, 50 mg qd × 12 mo
Disseminated infection with *Mycobacterium avium* complex (MAC)	CD4 < 50/mm^3	Azithromycin 1,200 mg weekly
Cryptococcosis	CD4 < 50/mm^3	Routine prophylaxis not recommended Patients who have been treated for an acute cryptococcal infection should receive fluconazole, 200 mg qd, indefinitely

*Recommendations in this table are based on information presented in Centers for Disease Control and Prevention.
INH, isoniazid; TMP-SMX, trimethoprim-sulfamethoxazole.

In addition to appropriate antiretroviral therapy, patients should also receive prophylaxis against opportunistic infections (OIs) if their CD4 count is below 200 cells/mm^3. Transient decreases in absolute CD4 numbers may occur secondary to the hemodilution of pregnancy. In these cases, the relative percent of CD4+ cells can be used to guide decisions regarding OI prophylaxis. Prophylaxis regimens for *Pneumocystis jiroveci* pneumonia (previously known as *Pneumocystis carinii* pneumonia), toxoplasmosis, tuberculosis, *Mycobacterium avium* complex, and cryptococcosis are listed in Table 48-6. If a patient is diagnosed with tuberculosis, *Mycobacterium avium* complex, *Pneumocystis carinii* pneumonia, or cryptococcal meningitis, treatment of the acute infection should be initiated before starting HAART. For other OIs, HAART may be started before or concurrent with treatment.[57]

Factors That Impact the Perinatal Transmission of Human Immunodeficiency Virus

Multiple factors have been identified that are associated with increased perinatal HIV transmission: low CD4 count, chorioamnionitis, preterm delivery, and illicit drug use (Table 48-7).[58–61] One of the strongest predictors of perinatal HIV transmission is viral load.[62–64] In support of this observation, two large studies reported the absence of transmission when the viral load was undetectable (in conjunction with anti-retroviral therapy)[61,65] and data from PACTG study 367 stratifies perinatal HIV transmission risk relative to the last antepartum HIV viral load prior to delivery and the type of antiretroviral therapy (Tables 48-8 and 48-9).[66,67] This data supports the concept that reducing maternal viral load and providing highly active antiretroviral therapy can effectively limit perinatal HIV transmission. Increasing duration of ruptured membranes has also been associated with perinatal HIV transmission.[59,68,69] However the incremental increased risk of transmission does not appear to be clinically significant. A large meta-analysis of 4,721 deliveries determined that the risk of HIV transmission increases by 2 percent over the baseline risk of transmission for each hour increment following the rupture of membranes.[70] Therefore, presuming a patient on HAART with an undetectable viral load has a baseline perinatal HIV transmission rate of 1 percent, the risk of transmission after 1 hour of ruptured membranes would be 1.02 percent, and after 8 hours, the risk of HIV transmission would be 1.16 percent.

Table 48-7. Factors that Increase the Risk of Perinatal HIV Transmission

History of previous child with HIV infection
Mother with AIDS
Preterm delivery
Decreased maternal CD4 count
High maternal viral load
Firstborn twin
Chorioamnionitis
Intrapartum blood exposure (e.g., episiotomy, vaginal laceration forceps delivery)

AIDS, acquired immunodeficiency syndrome; HIV, human immunodeficiency virus.

Table 48-8. Mother to Child Transmission of HIV According to Last Antenatal Viral Load

RNA (COPIES/mL)	TRANSMISSION RATE
No RNA data	17.1% (39/228)
≥10,000	5.6% (22/391)
1,000 to 9,999	2.0% (12/588)
<1,000 or undetectable	0.7% (13/1874)

Table 48-9. Mother to Child Transmission of HIV According to Antenatal ART Regimen

MATERNAL ART	TRANSMISSION RATE
None	18.5% (33/178)
Single Agent	5.1% (18/356)
2 NRTIs	1.4% (9/655)
≥3 Agents:	1.3% (25/1884)
NRTIs alone	3.4% (4/119)
NNRTI (no PI)	1.5% (7/462)
+PI(s)	1.1% (14/1303)

Several recent reports have investigated the role of elective cesarean delivery in reducing the perinatal transmission of HIV. The largest studies were performed prior to the widespread use of HAART by the European Mode of Delivery Collaboration and a meta-analysis by the International Perinatal HIV Group Study.[71,72] In women receiving either no treatment or zidovudine monotherapy, elective cesarean delivery performed before labor or spontaneous rupture of membranes was associated with a substantial reduction in perinatal transmission of HIV. In the meta-analysis, the adjusted odds ratio (OR) was 0.43 among infants delivered by cesarean delivery and the perinatal transmission rate of HIV was 1.8 percent in the European study. Cesarean delivery after the onset of labor or after spontaneous rupture of membranes did not protect against HIV transmission in either study. Current ACOG recommendations are to offer an elective cesarean delivery at 38 weeks' gestation to HIV-infected women with a viral load greater than 1,000 copies/mL.[73] Women with an undetectable viral load receiving HAART have a low risk of perinatal HIV transmission (1 to 2 percent), and it is unclear whether elective cesarean delivery is of benefit[36,41,43]; vaginal delivery is considered a safe alternative. HIV-infected women have increased morbidity and mortality following cesarean delivery.[74–76] Therefore, the patient's autonomy in decision making regarding the route of delivery should be respected and prophylactic antibiotics should be administered.[77]

Intrapartum Management of Human Immunodeficiency Virus

Every effort should be made to avoid instrumentation that would increase the neonate's exposure to infected maternal blood and secretions. Recommendations include leaving the fetal membranes intact, avoiding fetal scalp sampling and fetal scalp electrode placement, and avoiding episiotomy and assisted vaginal delivery. Intravenous zidovudine should be given to the mother with a loading dose of 2 mg/kg administered over 1 hour and a maintenance dose of 1 mg/kg/hr.[33] Other antiretrovirals should be taken with a sip of water, with the exception of stavudine, which is antagonistic to zidovudine. If spontaneous rupture of membranes has occurred, augmentation or induction of labor with oxytocin is appropriate.

For HIV-infected women who have not received antepartum antiretroviral therapy, there are four recommended intrapartum drug regimens to limit mother-to-child transmission of HIV. They include maternal zidovudine monotherapy, zidovudine and lamivudine in combination, nevirapine, and nevirapine and zidovudine in combination; specific dosage regimens are available at www.AIDSinfo.nih.gov.[42] When nevirapine is used, an zidovudine and lamivudine tail for 3 to 7 days should be strongly considered to limit maternal drug resistance.

Postpartum Care of the Woman Infected with Human Immunodeficiency Virus

The guidelines for the management of HIV infection outside pregnancy recommend treatment for individuals with a CD4 count below 350 cells/mm^3 or an HIV RNA level greater than 55,000 copies/mm^3. As such, some HIV-infected pregnant women are offered therapy primarily to limit the mother-to-child transmission of HIV. For women who do not meet the criteria for antiretroviral therapy outside of pregnancy, the option of whether to continue or discontinue antiretroviral treatment at the conclusion of pregnancy should be discussed. All drugs should be simultaneously discontinued if the patient wishes to stop therapy in the postpartum period. If the patient's regimen includes a NNRTI, consultation with an infectious disease specialist may be warranted due to the extended half life of NNRTIs. Breast-feeding is contraindicated because it is associated with an additional 15- to 20-percent risk of HIV transmission.[78–81]

PARVOVIRUS

Virology

Parvoviruses are among the smallest DNA viruses. Humans are the only known hosts of B19 parvovirus. The DNA is negative stranded, and the virus has two major genes: the REP or NS gene, which encodes functions required for transcription and DNA replication, and the CAP or S gene that encodes the coat proteins VP1 and VP2. The cellular receptor for B19 parvovirus is erythrocyte P antigen, explaining the propensity to infect erythrocytes and their precursors. P antigen is also expressed on megakaryocytes, endothelial cells, placenta, fetal liver, and fetal heart.[82] Parvovirus B19 is spread through respiratory droplets, infected blood products, perinatally, and with hand-to-mouth contact. The incubation period ranges from 4 to 20 days following exposure.

Epidemiology

Parvovirus B19 was identified in the 1970s in blood bank specimens, and was first linked to sickle cell disease patients with transient aplastic crisis. Parvovirus B19 was also associated with fifth disease, also called erythema infectiosum, and later to hydrops fetalis.[82] Although seroprevalence varies with age, roughly 65 percent of pregnant women have evidence of prior infection and are immune.[83] Conversely, susceptible women have a substantial risk of seroconversion following exposure to B19 parvovirus (50 percent). Day-care workers, teachers and parents have all been shown to be at increased risk of seroconversion.[84,85]

Clinical Manifestations

The most common presentation of B19 parvovirus infection is erythema infectiosum, which is characterized by a facial rash consistent with a "slapped-cheek" appearance and a reticulated or lace-like rash on the trunk and extremities (Fig. 48-1). The rash is immune complex–mediated and may reappear for several weeks following stimuli including changes in temperature, sunlight exposure, and emotional stress.[86] Infection can

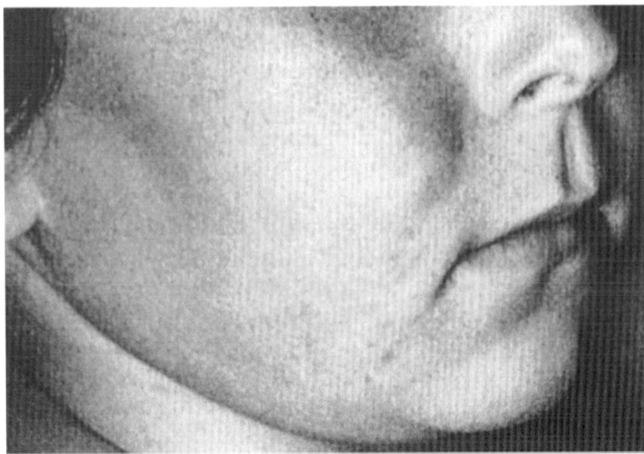

A

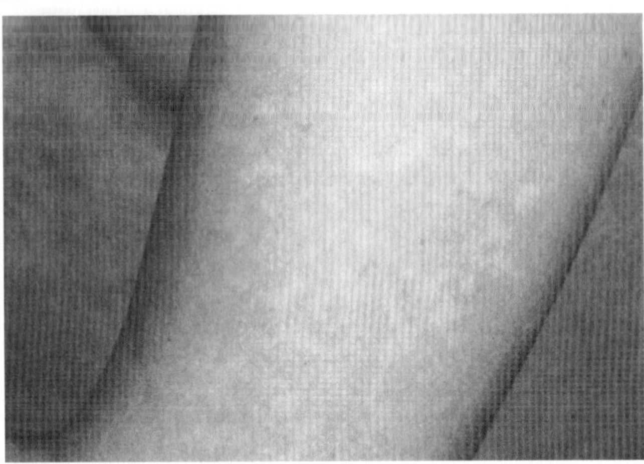

B

Figure 48-1. Characteristic "slapped cheek" rash of erythema infectiosum (*A*). Note lace-like rash on upper extremity (*B*).

also be accompanied by fever, malaise, lymphadenopathy, and a symmetric peripheral arthropathy. The hands are most frequently affected, followed by the knees and wrists. Symptoms are self-limiting but may last for several months.[87] Asymptomatic infection occurs 20 percent of the time. Persistent parvovirus infection is rare and presents clinically as pure red cell aplasia in patients who fail to mount a neutralizing antibody response.[88] Fetal infection can be asymptomatic or characterized by aplastic anemia of varying severity. Severe anemia can lead to high-output congestive heart failure and nonimmune hydrops. Fetal heart failure may also be due in part to direct infection of the myocardium.[89]

Diagnosis

Serologic testing can detect IgG and IgM antibodies to B19 parvovirus through ELISA assay; interpretation of these tests is described in Table 48-10. PCR amplification of viral DNA from fetal and maternal blood is more sensitive at confirming acute parvovirus infection than IgM antibody; thus, this approach should be considered when the diagnosis of congenital parvovirus infection is in question.[90]

Table 48-10. Interpretation of Serologic Tests for Maternal Parvovirus Infection

CONDITION	MATERNAL ANTIBODY IGM	IGG
Susceptible	–	–
Immune—infection >120 days ago	–	+
Infection within 7 days	+	–
Infection within 7–120 days	+	+

Table 48-11. Association Between Gestational Age at Time of Exposure and Risk of Fetal Parvovirus Infection

TIME OF EXPOSURE (WEEKS' GESTATION)	FREQUENCY OF SEVERELY AFFECTED FETUSES (%)
1–12	19
13–20	15
>20	6

Management of Parvovirus During Pregnancy

Following documented exposure to B19 parvovirus, serologic testing for parvovirus-specific IgG and IgM should be performed. If the woman has parvovirus-specific IgG antibody, prior exposure or infection has occurred and no further workup is needed. Susceptible women should have repeat serology performed in about 3 weeks. In cases of confirmed infection, pregnant women should be treated with supportive care because maternal B19 parvovirus infection is usually self-limited. The relationship between the gestational age at the time of exposure to B19 parvovirus and the risk of fetal parvovirus infection resulting in a severely affected fetus is shown in Table 48-11. Serial ultrasound examinations to evaluate the fetus for hydrops should be performed for 8 to 10 weeks after maternal illness. If no signs of hydrops are seen during this period, further evaluation is unnecessary. Recent studies have shown that measurement of the fetal middle cerebral artery peak systolic velocity can be useful in documenting fetal anemia before the development of hydrops in cases of congenital B19 parvovirus infection.[91,92]

Fetal infection occurs following approximately 33% of maternal infections.[93] However, the rate of fetal death secondary to intrauterine B19 parvovirus infection is dependent on the timing of the maternal infection. Fetal death is rare when maternal infection occurs after 20 weeks of gestation, but the fetal mortality rate is approximately 11 percent when maternal B19 infection occurs during the first 20 weeks of pregnancy and is associated with fetal hydrops.[94,95] Other studies have shown an overall 5-percent fetal loss rate.[96] Although 33 percent of fetal hydrops resolves without treatment,[97] there are no reliable predictors for the resolution of hydrops versus fetal death. Thus, cordocentesis and intrauterine transfusion are recommended when fetal hydrops is present.[97–99]

Most fetuses infected with B19 parvovirus have normal long-term development.[101–103] Three cases of persistent neurologic morbidity and three cases of persistent infection with severe anemia have been reported following fetal infection.[89,104] Two of these children died in the neonatal period, and these cases should be taken into account when counseling parents about the short- and long-term prognosis following intrauterine parvovirus infection.

MEASLES

Virology

Measles, or rubeola, is an enveloped, negative-stranded RNA virus that is a member of the paramyxoviridae family, which also includes respiratory syncytial virus, canine distemper virus, mumps virus, and parainfluenza viruses. Measles has virally encoded fusion and hemagglutinin proteins on its envelope. The hemagglutinin protein is thought to bind a cellular receptor protein, and penetration of measles virus into the host cell requires the fusion protein. Other gene products encoded by the measles virus include nucleoprotein; matrix protein; phosphoprotein, which regulates transcription; large protein, which includes the viral polymerase; and C and V proteins.[105]

Epidemiology

Measles is a highly infectious, acute viral illness that is limited to humans. It is spread primarily through respiratory droplets and, following exposure, 75 to 90 percent of susceptible contacts become infected. Since the 1960s, a live, attenuated vaccine has been readily available, and the incidence of measles cases has dramatically decreased.[106] This has resulted in three major patterns of measles outbreaks in the United States: unvaccinated preschoolers (including those younger than 15 months of age), previously vaccinated school-age children and college students, and persons originating from outside the United States. The incidence of outbreaks in previously vaccinated individuals has been reduced since the implementation of a two-dose vaccination strategy.[107] Between 2001 and 2003, 44 percent of the measles cases reported in the United States occurred in an immigrant population.[108]

Clinical Manifestations

Measles has an incubation period of 10 to 14 days. Infected individuals first manifest prodromal symptoms, which may include fever, malaise, myalgias, and headache. This is followed by ocular symptoms, including photophobia and a nonexudative conjunctivitis. Koplik spots, tiny white spots on a red base on the buccal mucosa lateral to the molar teeth, may appear during the prodrome and are pathognomonic for measles infection. If Koplik spots are visualized, they typically appear a day or so before the rash and disappear within 2 days of its appearance. The rash of measles appears between 2 and 7 days following the prodrome and is initially present behind the ears or on the face as a blotchy erythema. The rash then spreads to the trunk, followed by the extremities; the hands and feet may be spared. The rash is initially macular and blanches with pressure, but becomes papular and coalescent with a red, nonblanching component. The rash tends to fade after about 5 days. Fever can persist for up to 6 days and may reach 41°C; a productive cough may develop that can persist after defervescence. Lymphadenopathy accompanies the fever and can persist for several weeks.[109]

Complications can include laryngitis, bronchiolitis, pneumonia, and otitis media due to secondary bacterial infections. Rare complications include hepatitis, encephalitis, atypical measles, and acute encephalitis. Encephalitis occurs in about 1 in 1,000 cases of measles, resulting from either viral infection of the central nervous system or a hypersensitivity reaction to systemic viral infection. Symptoms include recurrence of fever and headache, vomiting, and a stiff neck, followed by stupor and convulsions. The mortality rate is 10 percent, and permanent neurologic sequelae, including mental retardation, develop in 50 percent of individuals. Atypical measles, which occurs in adults vaccinated with the formalin-inactivated measles vaccine, is characterized by high fever, pneumonia with pleural effusions, obtundation, and a hemorrhagic exanthem.[110] Patients usually have high antibody titers to measles, with the exception of a lack of antibodies to the fusion protein. Atypical measles is usually self-limiting, and patients are not contagious to others. A rare complication of measles infection is subacute sclerosing panencephalitis, which occurs in 0.5 to 2 per 1,000 cases of measles years after the acute infection. Subacute sclerosing panencephalitis is most common in children who contracted measles before 2 years of age, and is characterized by progressive neurologic debilitation and a virtually uniformly fatal outcome.

Diagnosis

Koplik spots are pathognomonic for measles infection. In their absence, diagnosis is based on a history of recent exposure or the presence of a rash. An increase in antibody titer may be detected as early as the first or second day of the rash. Assay for IgM antibodies specific for measles is available in some laboratories. Differential diagnoses include rubella, scarlet fever, infectious mononucleosis, secondary syphilis, toxic shock syndrome, Kawasaki's disease, erythema infectiosum, and drug rash. A guide to differentiating these illnesses is shown in Table 48-12.[111]

Management of Measles During Pregnancy

Pregnant women with measles infection should receive appropriate supportive care for their symptoms and be carefully observed for evidence of complications. The largest, most recently reported study of measles in pregnancy found that pregnant women were twice as likely to

Table 48-12. A Guide to the Differential Diagnosis of Measles

	CONJUNCTIVITIS	RHINITIS	SORE THROAT	ENANTHEM	LEUKOCYTOSIS	SPECIFIC LABORATORY TESTS AVAILABLE
Measles	++	++	0	+	0	+
Rubella	0	±	±	0	0	+
Exanthem subitum	0	±	0	0	0	+
Enterovirus infection	0	±	±	0	0	+
Adenovirus infection	+	+	+	0	0	+
Scarlet fever	±	±	++	0	+	+
Infectious mononucleosis	0	0	++	±	±	+
Drug rash	0	0	0	0	0	0

require hospitalization (60 percent), three times as likely to acquire pneumonia (26 percent), and six times as likely to die from complications (3 percent) compared with nonpregnant adults.[112] Given the higher rate of maternal morbidity and mortality in the setting of measles infection, secondary bacterial infections should be treated promptly with antibiotics. Ribavirin can be considered in cases of viral pneumonia.[111]

There is a 20- to 60-percent risk of spontaneous abortion and preterm delivery following measles infection during pregnancy.[112–114] If miscarriage does not occur, patients should be counseled that measles does not appear to be associated with an increased risk of fetal malformations and that the risk of congenital measles infection appears to be well below 25 percent,[113] with two recent studies assessing a total of 98 maternal measles infections showed an absence of congenital measles infections.[112,115] Detailed serial ultrasounds may be performed: Evidence of in utero infection includes microcephaly, growth restriction, and oligohydramnios. There have been conflicting reports regarding a potential association between measles infection in pregnancy and Crohn's disease in offspring.[116,117] Others have reported an association between measles exposure at the time of birth and the development of Hodgkin's disease in children.[118]

The most effective way to prevent measles infection in pregnancy is to ensure that patients are vaccinated prior to pregnancy using a two dose series which usually includes the trivalent MMR (measles, mumps, rubella) vaccine. This live, attenuated vaccine should not be given to pregnant women, and patients should practice effective contraception for three months following vaccination, although no cases of congenital measles infection have been reported as a result of the measles vaccine.[106,119,120] Although most pregnant women will have been vaccinated against measles as children, a recent study showed that between 3.2 and 20.5 percent of pregnant women have either absent or low antibody titers, which would classify them as seronegative.[119] Any pregnant women exposed to measles should have an IgG titer drawn. Seronegative (susceptible) women should be treated with 0.25 ml/kg of immune globulin intramuscularly within 6 days of exposure (maximum dose of 15 ml).[105,117,118] Neonates delivered to a parturient who developed measles within 7 to 10 days of delivery should receive intramuscular immune globulin at a dose of 0.25 mg/kg. These children should also receive the MMR vaccine at 12 to 15 months of age.[117,118]

RUBELLA

Virology

Rubella is a small, spherical, enveloped virus containing single-stranded RNA, which is part of the togavirus family. Transmission is thought to occur through respiratory droplets and close personal contact. Following infection of the respiratory mucosa, the virus is found within cervical lymph nodes and then is disseminated hematogenously.

Epidemiology

Rubella outbreaks occur primarily in school-aged children and in settings where crowded conditions exist such as military bases, religious communities, college campuses, and prisons. However, following licensure of an effective rubella vaccine in 1969, no major outbreaks have occurred in the United States. In 1999, there were 271 reported cases of rubella infection in the United States, primarily in foreign-born individuals from Mexico and Central America.[122] The epidemiology of rubella is similar in the United Kingdom, with most infections occurring in foreign-born individuals.[123]

Clinical Manifestations

The incubation period following exposure is 12 to 19 days, and acute infection with rubella is likely underdiagnosed because 20 to 50 percent of rubella infections are asymptomatic.[124]

Rubella infection is not associated with a prodromal illness. Symptomatic, infected patients present with a rash, malaise, fever, conjunctivitis, and generalized lymphadenopathy. The rash is nonpruritic, begins on the face and neck as a faint macular erythema, and spreads rapidly to the trunk and extremities (Fig. 48-2). The rash blanches with pressure and usually vanishes by the third day. Transient polyarthralgias or polyarthritis lasting 5

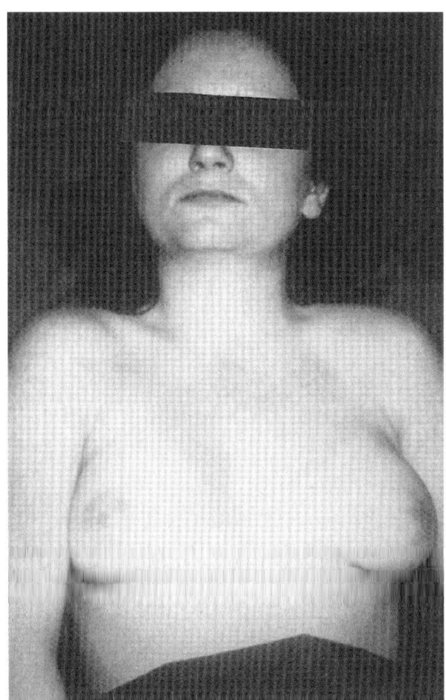

Figure 48-2. Typical erythematous, maculopapular rash of rubella.

to 10 days may appear in adolescents and adults following the rash.[124] Rare complications include thrombocytopenic purpura, encephalitis, neuritis, and orchitis.

Diagnosis

Serology is most commonly used to document exposure or infection with rubella.[125] IgM specific for rubella is detectable before the onset of the rash.[123] Isolation and culture of the virus is possible, as is detection of viral RNA by RT-PCR. In cases of suspected congenital rubella infection, RT-PCR can be used to detect rubella virus within chorionic villi, fetal blood, and amniotic fluid specimens.[126–128]

Management of Rubella Infection During Pregnancy

Maternal rubella infection is usually self-limited. However, congenital rubella infection can have significant deleterious effects on the fetus, in addition to causing miscarriage and stillbirth. Unfortunately, administration of intravenous immune globulin (IVIG) to pregnant women infected with rubella is not efficacious in preventing congenital rubella infection.[122] Therefore, vaccination before conception is recommended, and the primary purpose of the rubella vaccine is to prevent congenital rubella infection. Rubella serology is typically performed on obstetrical intake to identify women with inadequate levels of antibody. These women should receive rubella vaccine in the postpartum period.

Rubella vaccine consists of live, attenuated virus and is available as a monovalent form, bivalent form (measles-rubella), or a trivalent form (MMR). Because the vaccine contains live virus, it is contraindicated in pregnancy. The CDC has followed 324 women who received rubella vaccination within 3 months of conception.[122] None of the 324 infants born to these mothers had malformations compatible with congenital rubella syndrome (CRS), but five had evidence of subclinical rubella infection. These findings are supported by a recently published prospective study involving 94 pregnant women with exposure to rubella vaccine within 3 months of conception; none delivered an infant with CRS.[129] Based on these data, the estimated risk for serious malformations attributable to rubella vaccine ranges from zero to 1.6 percent. Therefore, therapeutic termination of pregnancy is not recommended in these cases.[122] Breast-feeding is not a contraindication to receiving MMR vaccine.

Congenital Infection

There were 28 cases of congenital rubella infection documented in the United States from 1997 to 1999, and 92 percent of these infants were born to foreign-born mothers.[121] This number is exceedingly low, secondary to nationwide efforts to immunize children against rubella infection. Several studies have established relationships between the frequency and severity of CRS and the timing of rubella infection in pregnancy. In general, infection in early pregnancy is associated with increased CRS severity. When maternal infection occurs within the first 12 weeks of pregnancy and is accompanied by a rash, more than 80 percent of fetuses become infected with rubella.[128] Of these infants, 67 percent have findings consistent with CRS.[129] First-trimester infection with rubella is also associated with miscarriage, although some of the women in these studies terminated their pregnancy secondary to exposure. As the pregnancy progresses, the risk of congenital rubella infection decreases. It is 54 percent at 13 to 14 weeks and 25 percent at the end of the second trimester.[130] The association of congenital rubella infection with CRS also decreases with increasing gestational age, with fetal defects being rare in fetuses infected beyond the 16th week of pregnancy.[130,131] Given that the association of congenital rubella infection and CRS is not absolute at any gestational age, ultrasound may be a useful adjunct in determining whether a fetus is affected, although this technique cannot detect many of the associated abnormalities.

The most common manifestation of congenital rubella infection is growth retardation. Sensorineural hearing loss is the most common single defect associated with CRS.[121] When infection occurs before 12 weeks' gestation, other common defects include cardiac lesions (13 percent), most frequently patent ductus arteriosus, and eye defects (13 percent) such as cataracts, glaucoma, and retinitis.[129] Other findings consistent with CRS include microphthalmia, microcephaly, cerebral palsy, mental retardation, and intrauterine growth restriction (IUGR). Most of these findings are seen only in fetuses infected within the first 12 weeks of gestation. Severe disease can also include thrombocytopenic purpura or hepatosplenomegaly. Fetuses infected between 13 and 16 weeks of gestation have up to a 35-percent risk of being affected by CRS[128] and typically have hearing loss as their principal manifestation of CRS. Fetuses infected at more advanced gestational ages rarely have sequelae associated with CRS.

Following congenital rubella infection, infants may shed virus for up to 1 year after birth.[130] Even in neonates who are asymptomatic at birth, up to one third can manifest long-term complications including type 1 diabetes mellitus and progressive panencephalitis in the second decade of life.[131,132]

CYTOMEGALOVIRUS INFECTION

Virology

Cytomegalovirus (CMV) is a double-stranded, DNA-enveloped virus that replicates within the nucleus of infected cells. It is part of the β herpesvirus group and has more than 200 genes and multiple strains. The complexity of the CMV genome allows this virus to cause both persistent and latent infections. Recurrent infection occurs following superinfection with a new strain or after reactivation of CMV from latently infected cells. CMV is not highly contagious. Transmission is largely through contact with infected saliva or urine, although infection can also occur through blood or by sexual contact. The incubation period is about 40 days following exposure.[133]

Epidemiology

In developed countries, the seroprevalence of CMV is dependent on age and socioeconomic status.[137] Within the United States, the primary CMV infection rate in pregnant women ranges from 0.7 to 4 percent, and the rate of recurrent infection can be as high at 13.5 percent. Young infants and children with subclinical infection are a major source of CMV infection in pregnant women. Thus day-care workers are at an increased risk. Approximately 50 percent of children attending day care have been found to actively shed CMV virus in their saliva and urine, and fomites within day-care centers are potential sources of CMV infection.[138,139] Small children also pose a risk of CMV infection to members of their own family, with annual seroconversion rates of approximately 10 percent for parents and uninfected siblings.[140] CMV seropositivity correlates with lower socioeconomic status, birth outside North America, increasing parity, older age, abnormal PAP smears, infection with Trichomonas, and the number of sex partners.[141] There is also an increased rate of CMV infection in immunocompromised patients, including those with AIDS and status post organ transplant.[136] Between 0.2 and 2.2 percent of infants born in the United States are infected with CMV in utero secondary to maternal infection, and congenital CMV is the leading cause of hearing loss in children. Another 6 to 60 percent of children become infected within the first 6 months of life secondary to intrapartum transmission or breast-feeding.[142] Fortunately, peripartum infected infants rarely have serious sequelae of CMV infection.[143]

Clinical Manifestations

Infected patients may be asymptomatic or have a mononucleosis-like syndrome with fever, malaise, myalgias, chills, and cervical lymphadenopathy. Infrequent complications include pneumonia, hepatitis, Guillain-Barré syndrome, and aseptic meningitis. Laboratory abnormalities include atypical lymphocytosis, elevated hepatic transaminases, and a negative heterophile antibody response (distinguishing CMV from Epstein-Barr virus infection).[133]

Diagnosis

Maternal CMV infection is typically diagnosed through serology by documenting the presence of CMV-specific IgM antibody and at least a four-fold increase in IgG titers when multiple specimens are compared. Both false-positive and false-negative results can occur with CMV-specific IgM. Therefore, CMV IgG results should be repeated when clinical suspicion of CMV is high, and IgM testing is negative.[144] CMV may also be diagnosed by culture or PCR of infected blood, urine, saliva, amniotic fluid, or cervical secretions. Routine screening for CMV infection during pregnancy is not recommended given the prevalence of seropositivity.

Fetal infection can be documented by culture and PCR of amniotic fluid where the sensitivity of PCR can reach 100 percent in gestations greater than 21 weeks; however false negative PCR and culture can occur at earlier gestational ages.[145] Fetal serology and CMV culture from fetal blood have a substantially lower detection rate, thus amniotic fluid is the preferred testing source. Fetal CMV infection can occur weeks to months following maternal CMV infection, thus repeat testing may be warranted at 7 week intervals.[145] Detection of CMV does not predict the severity of congenital CMV infection, however, as 80 to 90 percent of children with congenital CMV infection have no neurologic sequelae.[146,147] Ultrasound can be useful to assist in the diagnosis of a congenitally infected infant with likely impairment. Findings consistent with fetal injury include microcephaly, ventriculomegaly, intracerebral calcifications, ascites, hydrops, echogenic bowel, intrauterine growth restriction, and oligohydramnios. Unusual findings include fetal heart block and meconium peritonitis.[148,149] In the setting of confirmed fetal infection with serial normal ultrasounds, the risk of clinical symptoms of congenital CMV infection following birth is approximately 10 percent.

Management of Cytomegalovirus During Pregnancy

Pregnant women should be counseled regarding preventive measures including careful handling of potentially infected articles, such as diapers, and frequent hand washing when around young children or immunocompromised individuals. Ganciclovir has been shown in vitro to cross the placenta by diffusion but has not been effective in intrauterine treatment of congenital CMV infection. A recent study treating CMV-infected fetuses with CMV-specific hyperimmune globulin showed a decreased incidence of congenital CMV infection and an impressive decrease in the number of infants born with symptomatic CMV disease.[150] This study was small, nonrandomized, and may have had a selection bias; however, the findings support consideration of passive immunization during pregnancy to limit the occurrence of congenital CMV disease in susceptible individuals.[150]

Congenital Infection

Congenital CMV infection is diagnosed by detection of virus or viral nucleic acid within the first 2 weeks of life. The risk of intrauterine CMV transmission is highest in the third trimester, and the overall risk of transmission to the fetus is 30 to 40 percent.[148,149] Serious sequelae occur most commonly after infection in the first trimester where 24 percent of infected fetuses demonstrated sensorineural hearing loss and 32 percent had other CNS sequelae. After the second trimester 2.5 percent of infected fetuses demonstrated sensorineural hearing loss and 15 percent had CNS sequelae.[153] Congenital CMV infection may occur following primary or recurrent CMV infection of pregnant women,[142] but the incidence of serious sequelae is much lower following recurrent infection.[154,155]

Most infants congenitally infected with CMV exhibit no obvious clinical findings at birth. However, subclinical congenital CMV infection is associated with hearing loss in 15 percent of cases.[150] With increased neonatal screening, hearing loss has recently been correlated with the detection of CMV DNA by PCR at birth.[156] After primary CMV infection, approximately 5 to 18 percent of infants exhibit serious sequelae, usually when infection occurred during the first half of pregnancy. Clinical findings in these infected infants may include: jaundice, petechiae, thrombocytopenia, hepatosplenomegaly, growth restriction, and nonimmune hydrops. Long-term neurologic sequelae include developmental delays, seizure activity, and gross neurologic impairment including sensorineural hearing loss.[150,151] Unfortunately, there is no commercially available vaccine against CMV at this time.

HERPESVIRUS

Virology

Herpes simplex virus (HSV) is a large enveloped, double-stranded DNA virus that is a member of the herpesvirus family. The HSV genome is complex and encodes more than 70 polypeptides, including several glycoproteins that are present on the envelope of the virus.[157] One of the envelope proteins, glycoprotein g, allows for the distinction of two well-defined antigenic and biologic types of HSV; type 1, which is most frequently associated with oral, nongenital infection, and type 2, which is usually associated with genital infection. HSV replicates in the host cell nucleus and has the capacity to form latent infection within dorsal root ganglia. The virus persists in an apparently inactive state for varying amounts of time and then may be reactivated by various stimuli.[158]

Epidemiology

The mouth and lips are the most common sites of HSV-1 infection; and infection is more prevalent in lower socioeconomic populations in which 75 to 90 percent of individuals have antibodies against HSV-1 by 10 years of age. HSV-2 infection is usually acquired through sexual contact and is also related to socioeconomic factors. In the United States, 25 to 65 percent of individuals have antibodies to HSV-2, and the seroprevalence correlates with the number of sexual partners.[154]

Clinical Manifestations

Patients infected with HSV-1 usually present with herpes simplex labialis (cold sores). HSV-2 infection typically involves the genital area and may affect the vulva, vagina, or cervix. Painful vesicles appear 2 to 14 days after exposure, followed by spontaneous rupture, leaving lesions that appear as shallow eroded ulcers (Fig. 48-3). Later in the infection, a dry crust appears, and the lesions heal without scarring. Primary infection can be associated with fever, malaise, anorexia, and bilateral inguinal lymphadenopathy, and is infrequently associated with aseptic meningitis. Women may also have dysuria and urinary retention secondary to urethral involvement. Healing of primary infection may take several weeks and is less severe in individuals with prior HSV-1 infection. Rates of symptomatic and subclinical shedding of HSV from the cervix and vulva are increased in the first 3 months following primary infection: 2.3 percent in HSV-2 infection and 0.65 percent in women with HSV-1 infection.[155] Some individuals may have asymptomatic or subclinical primary infections with HSV.

Nonprimary, first episodes of genital HSV infection occur when patients are infected with a second strain of

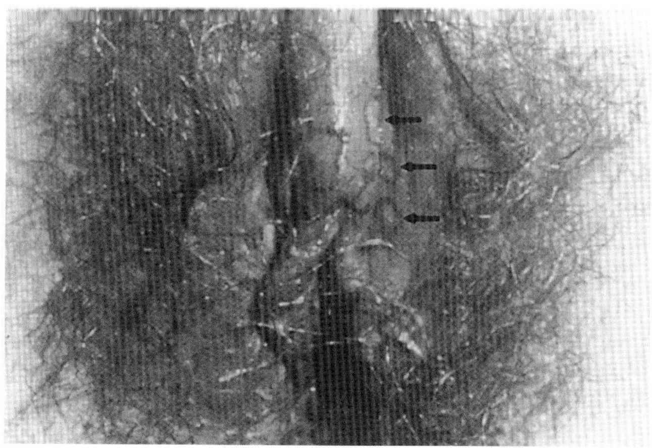

Figure 48-3. Ulcerated lesions (*arrows*) characteristic of herpes simplex infection. (From Duff P, Christian JS, Yancey MK: Infections associated with pregnancy. *In* Coulam CB, Faulk WP, McIntyre JA [eds]: Immunologic Obstetrics. New York, WW Norton & Co, 1992, p 578, with permission.)

Table 48-13. Comparison of Primary Versus Recurrent Herpes Simplex Virus Infection

STAGE OF ILLNESS	TYPE OF INFECTION PRIMARY	RECURRENT
Incubation period and/or prodrome	2–10	1–2
Vesicle, pustule (days)	6	2
Wet ulcer (days)	6	3
Dry crust (days)	8	7
Total	22–30	13–14

HSV (1 or 2) but have preexisting antibodies from prior infection at a non-genital site (usually oral). Secondary or recurrent HSV infections usually represent reactivation of virus and vary in their frequency and intensity. Recurrent infections are usually less severe than primary infection and do not occur in all individuals. One third of HSV infected individuals have no recurrences, one third have approximately three recurrences per year, and another third have more than three recurrences per year.[158] Recurrences are associated with fewer lesions and a shorter period of viral shedding. Table 48-13 compares clinical findings during primary and recurrent HSV infection.

Disseminated HSV infection is rare; it occurs primarily in immunocompromised individuals but can also occur in pregnancy. Disseminated HSV infection is characterized by skin, mucus membrane, and visceral organ involvement, and may include ocular involvement, meningitis, encephalitis and ascending myelitis. Treatment with intravenous acyclovir should be initiated promptly in suspected cases of disseminated HSV.

Diagnosis

Definitive diagnosis of active HSV infection requires culture of the virus. Culture can differentiate between HSV-1 and HSV-2 infection. Specimens should be collected from fresh vesicles or pustules, if possible, because viral recovery from crusted lesions is poor. PCR amplification of HSV DNA is also possible, and it provides a faster, more sensitive method to diagnose HSV infection.[160] Serology can be useful to assess and differentiate primary infection from secondary infection through detection of HSV IgM.[158] Cytologic preparations (Tzanck test) show characteristic multinucleated giant cells and intranuclear inclusions. However, this method is rarely used given the enhanced sensitivity and specificity of the above-mentioned methods.

Management of Herpesvirus During Pregnancy

Maternal primary infection with HSV before labor does not usually impact the fetus; increased rates of miscarriage following primary HSV infection have been reported, but a recent prospective study showed no increase in spontaneous pregnancy loss.[161] In addition, intrauterine HSV infection is rare, occurring in approximately 1 in 200,000 deliveries. Sequelae in such cases include skin vesicles or scarring, eye disease, microcephaly or hydranencephaly.[162] An association between HSV infection in the third trimester of pregnancy and IUGR has also been reported. However, this observation was based on five patients.[163] Birth weight of infants born to asymptomatic HSV-shedding mothers is lower than that of nonshedding mothers, but this effect is small and may be due to differences in gestational age at birth.[164]

For women with primary HSV infection during pregnancy, oral acyclovir dosed at 400 mg TID, valacyclovir 1,000 mg BID, or famciclovir 250 mg TID can be given for 7 to 10 days to decrease the duration of maternal symptoms. Women who have more than two HSV recurrences per year are candidates for prophylaxis to decrease the frequency and severity of recurrences using one of the following oral regimens: acyclovir 400 mg BID, valacyclovir 500 to 1,000 mg daily, or famciclovir 250 mg BID.

The greatest risk to infants perinatally exposed to HSV is the development of neonatal herpes infection. Neonatal HSV infection complicates approximately 1 in 3,500 deliveries in the United States and is associated with significant neonatal morbidity and mortality. The estimated risk of neonatal HSV during primary maternal infection is 50 percent,[165] and in cases of recurrent HSV infection, the incidence of neonatal HSV likely ranges from 0 to 3 percent.[166] Thus, neonatal HSV infection is most often caused by primary maternal HSV infection, rather than recurrent infection. ACOG recommends elective cesarean delivery for women with demonstrable genital herpes lesions or prodromal symptoms in labor to reduce the incidence of neonatal HSV infection.[166] Unfortunately, up to 85 percent of neonatal HSV infection cases occur following asymptomatic maternal infection, limiting efforts to prevent neonatal HSV infection by performing cesarean delivery. A recent cost/benefit analysis of the current guidelines for the prevention of neonatal HSV infection found that given the low risk of neonatal HSV transmission with recurrent maternal infection, it takes 1,580 elective cesarean sections to prevent one case of neonatal HSV.[167]

The risk of neonatal HSV infection in cases of nongenital, maternal HSV lesions (e.g., thigh, buttock, mouth) is low; therefore, cesarean delivery is not recommended for these women. The duration of ruptured membranes before delivery increases the risk of neonatal HSV infection. However, there is no evidence that there is a period of time beyond which cesarean delivery is no longer beneficial. In the case of premature rupture of membranes, acyclovir or other antivirals should be considered in women with active HSV lesions being managed expectantly and given steroids to enhance fetal lung maturity.[166]

Various studies have investigated strategies to limit neonatal HSV transmission. Antepartum maternal HSV cultures are not useful in predicting the infant's risk of exposure during delivery.[168,169] Several small studies have assessed the effectiveness of prophylactic acyclovir at reducing the incidence of HSV shedding during pregnancy and reducing the number of cesarean deliveries, but not all had significant results. A recent meta-analysis of these studies revealed that prophylaxis with acyclovir 400 mg three times a day beginning at 36 weeks' gestation reduced clinical HSV recurrences at the time of delivery (OR 0.25), asymptomatic HSV shedding (OR 0.09), and the cesarean section rate (OR 0.30).[170] These findings should be interpreted with care, because women can still shed virus while taking acyclovir.[171] However, this strategy may be considered for women who have experienced a recurrence of HSV at some point during their pregnancy.

Neonatal Herpes Infection

Approximately 70 percent of neonatal HSV infections are caused by HSV-2. Factors predicting neonatal HSV transmission include cervical HSV shedding, invasive monitoring, preterm delivery, maternal age less than 21 years of age,[172] and HSV viral load.[160] Neonatal HSV infection is treated with intravenous acyclovir.[173] There are three categories of neonatal HSV infections: local (skin, eye and mouth) disease, encephalitis, and disseminated infection. There is significant neonatal mortality with disseminated disease (60 percent), and a neonatal mortality rate of 15 percent with encephalitis.[171] Long-term morbidity is also associated with neonatal herpes infection. Only 40 percent of survivors are normal following encephalitis or disseminated disease.[158] Complications of neonatal HSV infection also include disseminated intravascular coagulopathy and hemorrhagic pneumonitis.

VARICELLA

Virology

Varicella, or chickenpox, is caused by the varicella zoster virus (VZV), a member of the α-herpesvirus subfamily. This enveloped virus contains double-stranded DNA and has at least 69 genes. Viral replication initially occurs within respiratory epithelial cells and is followed by systemic viremia. Long-term, latent infection occurs within the non-neuronal cells of the dorsal root ganglia. Humans are the only known host for varicella zoster viruses.[174]

Epidemiology

Varicella is a highly contagious disease transmitted by respiratory droplets or close contact. Approximately 95 percent of susceptible household contacts become infected following exposure. The incubation period is about 14 days. Patients are infectious from 1 day before the rash until lesions are crusted. Immunity is usually life long. Prior to the advent of the VZV vaccine, most natural varicella infections occurred in early childhood. Childhood VZV infection is usually self-limited. More than 50 percent of the mortality attributable to varicella infection occurs in adults, who represent less than 10 percent of all varicella infections.[175] The majority of adults (>90%) are immune to VZV, even in the absence of a clinical history of chickenpox.

Clinical Manifestations

Infected patients classically present with a centripetal rash characterized by erythematous macules, papules, and vesicles that are pruritic and appear in crops. The rash spreads to the extremities, and excoriation and scabbed lesions are typically seen. Fever is common, and infected adults frequently present with malaise, myalgias, arthralgias, and headache. Bacterial superinfection of skin lesions can occur.[177] Patients should be watched carefully for the development of varicella pneumonia because the rates of this complication are much higher in pregnancy, approaching 20 percent.[178,179] Cough and dyspnea usually occur about 3 days after the appearance of the first skin lesions. Cyanosis, hemoptysis, and pleuritic chest pain are common. Encephalitis is a rare complication of VZV infection in adults.

Reactivation of latent VZV infection can result in herpes zoster or shingles, which occurs primarily in elderly and immunocompromised patients. Shingles is characterized by a rash in a segmental distribution that correlates with specific dermatomes. Pain, itching, and paresthesias can occur as a prodrome or with the appearance of the rash. Although zoster is usually self-limited, patients are infectious and can transmit VZV to susceptible individuals.[177]

Diagnosis

Diagnosis is usually made based on a history of exposure and the presence of a rash. PCR can identify VZV-specific DNA from vesicular fluid or throat swabs. Serologic confirmation of infection can be made by ELISA, which can quantitate VZV specific IgG and IgM.[180] Although less often utilized clinically, the Tzanck stain can be used to identify multinucleated giant cells present within lesions, and varicella can also be cultured.

Management of Varicella During Pregnancy

Pregnant women infected with VZV should be offered supportive care including calamine lotion, antipyretics, and if necessary, systemic antipruritics. Oral acyclovir is safe in pregnancy and may decrease the duration of illness if instituted within 24 hours of the rash, but does not prevent congenital infection.[181] Maternal varicella pneumonia has a 14-percent mortality rate, and these patients should be treated with intravenous acyclovir in addition to appropriate supportive care.[182] If a woman develops varicella between 5 days before and 2 days after delivery, varicella zoster immune globulin (VZIG) should be given to the newborn to reduce the incidence of neonatal varicella. The infant should also be isolated from the mother until all vesicles have crusted over to prevent transmission of VZV. If possible, delivery should be delayed until 5 to 7 days after the onset of maternal illness to potentially prevent neonatal VZV, which can have a 20- to 30-percent mortality rate.[179]

Prevention includes ascertaining VZV status prior to pregnancy in women without a clinical history of infection and offering the live, attenuated VZV vaccine (Varivax, Merck) to susceptible women. Adults should receive two subcutaneous doses of vaccine 4 to 8 weeks apart. The vaccine is 70 to 80 percent effective in preventing natural infection. Because this is a live vaccine, it is contraindicated during pregnancy, and pregnancy should be deferred for 3 months following vaccination. Cases of vaccination during pregnancy have been reported with no evidence of intrauterine transmission of VZV.[183] If a pregnant woman with a negative history of VZV is exposed to varicella, serology should be performed within 96 hours of exposure. More than 90 percent of individuals with no history of VZV disease are seropositive for varicella IgG, and, thus, are not at risk for acute infection. If susceptibility to VZV is confirmed or serology is unable to be obtained in a timely fashion, VZIG should be administered within 96 hours of exposure at 1 vial per 10 kg of body weight to a maximum of five vials.[179,184] This preparation is 60 to 80 percent effective at preventing infection. Prophylactic acyclovir, given 800 mg PO five times daily for 5 to 7 days starting within 9 days of exposure has also been shown to be effective at preventing VZV infection in children with an 85 percent reduction in infection.[185] These two therapies can potentially be combined to further reduce the risk of maternal varicella infection, as a small study comparing varicella postexposure prophylaxis in children has shown that acyclovir and VZIG together are more efficacious than VZIG alone.[186] Given the time constraints following exposure, consideration to performing varicella serology at the beginning of pregnancy for women with a negative history of chickenpox should be given.

Congenital Infection

Congenital varicella infection can lead to spontaneous abortion, intrauterine fetal demise, and varicella embryopathy. Congenital varicella syndrome is characterized by cutaneous scars, limb hypoplasia, muscle atrophy, malformed digits, psychomotor retardation, microcephaly, cortical atrophy, cataracts, chorioretinitis, and microophthalmia.[179] There is a low frequency of anomalies following exposure before 13 weeks; only 0.4 percent of neonates were born with features of varicella embryopathy in a study of 472 women.[182] The highest risk occurs with maternal infection between 13 and 20 weeks' gestation, with an incidence of congenital varicella of 2 percent.[187] No congenital malformations have been observed when maternal infection occurs after 20 weeks, but neonatal skin lesions or scarring can be seen after birth. Ultrasound examination is the preferred assessment tool because serology and identification of VZV DNA do not predict degree of fetal injury.[188] Ultrasound findings suggestive of fetal varicella syndrome can include polyhydramnios, hydrops, echogenic foci within abdominal organs, cardiac malformations, limb deformities, microcephaly, and IUGR.[189–191]

HEPATITIS

Viral hepatitis comprises a spectrum of syndromes ranging from entirely subclinical and unapparent to fulminant disease. Symptoms of acute viral hepatitis infection may include jaundice, malaise, fatigue, anorexia, nausea, vomiting, and right upper quadrant pain. Hepatic transaminases and bilirubin are moderately to markedly elevated, and liver biopsy shows extensive hepatocellular injury with a prominent inflammatory infiltrate (Fig. 48-4). Most cases of viral hepatitis are self-limited and resolve without treatment, but certain viruses can cause persistent infection, leading to chronic liver disease (see Chapter 43). The majority of hepatitis cases in the United States are caused by hepatitis viruses A, B, C and D, whereas hepatitis E is endemic to Asia, Africa, and Mexico. Other viruses can cause liver infection and inflammation (hepatitis) including cytomegalovirus, herpes simplex virus, Epstein-Barr virus, rubella, and yellow fever.[192]

Hepatitis A

Hepatitis A (HAV) is a small, single-stranded RNA virus that is a member of the picornavirus family. HAV is transmitted primarily through oral-fecal contact and is responsible for approximately one third of the cases of acute hepatitis in the United States. The incubation period for this virus is approximately 28 to 30 days following exposure. Risk factors for infection with HAV include exposure to contaminated food or water, recent travel outside the United States, illicit drug use, and having a child in day care.[193] HAV infection may be complicated by cholestatic hepatitis, which is characterized by pruritus, dark urine, direct hyperbilirubinemia, and elevated alkaline phosphatase. This syndrome may last several months. Corticosteroid therapy is effective at alleviating symptoms.[192]

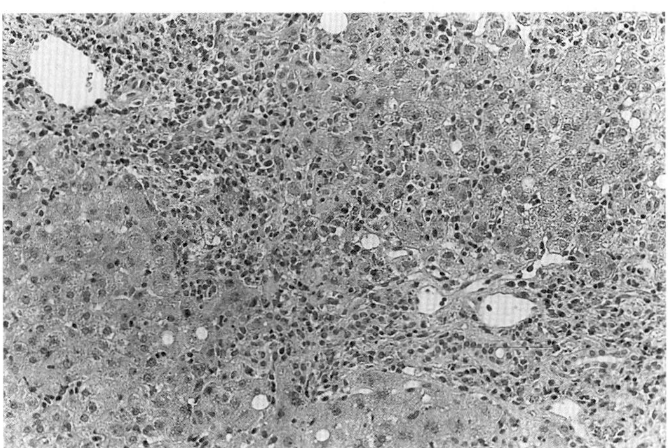

Figure 48-4. Photomicrograph of liver biopsy showing characteristic histologic changes of acute viral hepatitis. Note the intense inflammatory infiltrate.

The incidence of HAV in pregnancy is approximately 1 in 1,000, and diagnosis is made based on HAV IgM and IgG serology.[194] HAV infection is usually self-limited; fewer than 0.5 percent of patients require hospitalization. HAV does not cause chronic infection. Physical activity should be limited to prevent hepatic trauma, and drugs with potential hepatotoxicity should be avoided. Sexual and household contacts of infected individuals should receive immunoprophylaxis with a single dose of HAV immune globulin and with HAV vaccine, which is safe for use in pregnancy.[194] Perinatal transmission has not been documented. However, infants delivered to an acutely infected mother should receive HAV immune globulin to prevent horizontal transmission following delivery.[195]

Hepatitis B

Virology

Hepatitis B (HBV) is caused by a small, enveloped double-stranded DNA virus. The intact virus is called the Dane particle. There are three antigens of clinical importance associated with HBV. They are the surface antigen (HBsAg), which is the viral envelope glycoprotein; the core antigen (HBcAg), which associates with viral nucleic acid; and HBeAg, a protein, which is secreted from infected cells and is not a part of the infectious virion. HBV is transmitted primarily through parenteral routes, sexual transmission, and perinatal exposure. The incubation period is 4 weeks to 6 months following exposure.[192]

Epidemiology

HBV causes 40 to 45 percent of all cases of hepatitis in the United States, and it is estimated that 1 million individuals in the United States are chronic viral carriers. The incidence of acute HBV infection in pregnancy is 1 to 2 per 1,000, and 5 to 15 per 1,000 pregnant women are chronically infected with HBV.[196] Certain populations have an increased prevalence of HBV infection, including Asians, Eskimos, drug addicts, dialysis patients, prisoners, and residents and employees of chronic care facilities.[192]

Diagnosis

Acute HBV infection is diagnosed by detection of HBsAg and IgM to the core antigen (HBc). The long-term presence of HBsAg identifies those with chronic hepatitis. Chronic hepatitis B infection has three forms. Typical chronic hepatitis B (formerly described as chronic active) is characterized by positive HBsAg, HBeAg, an HBV DNA titer ranging from 10^7–10^{11}, and positive nuclear HBcAg in the liver. HBeAg-negative chronic hepatitis B is characterized by positive HBsAg, negative HBeAg, and HBV DNA titer ranging from 10^5–10^9, and positive cytoplasmic HBcAg in the liver. Inactive hepatitis B carrier state (formerly described as chronic persistent hepatitis) is characterized by positive HBsAg, negative HBeAg, and HBV DNA titer ranging from 10^1–10^5, and negative hepatic HBcAg.[197] Following hepatitis infection or vaccination, patients are positive for HBsAb. Antibody to the core or e antigen is present only in patients who have been infected with hepatitis.[198]

Clinical Manifestations

Eighty-five to ninety percent of patients infected with HBV have full resolution of symptoms and clear their infection. Less than 1 percent of HBV-infected patients develop fulminant hepatitis, which can be characterized by massive hepatic necrosis and may be accompanied by pancreatitis. Ten to fifteen percent of patients become chronically infected with HBV. Fifteen to thirty percent of patients with chronic HBV infection subsequently develop liver cirrhosis over their lifetime and are at substantially increased risk for hepatocellular carcinoma.[192]

Management of HBV Infection During Pregnancy

HBV infection may be prevented by vaccination. The HBV vaccine is a recombinant vaccine, is safe in pregnancy, and should be offered to patients with significant risk factors including a history of STDs, women who are health care workers, and those with infected household or sexual contacts.[199] In cases of acute hepatitis infection during pregnancy, supportive care should be offered. For women who have positive HBsAg serology in the absence of acute HBV infection, further testing is warranted to determine their level of viremia and whether they have ongoing liver injury manifested by elevated liver function tests. Amniocentesis is safe in HBV infected women.[200–202]

Infants born to mothers who are seropositive for HBsAg should receive hepatitis B immune globulin and the hepatitis B vaccine series.[197] The combination of HBV vaccine and immune globulin is 85 to 95 percent effective at preventing vertical transmission of HBV. In the United States, all newborns receive HBV vaccine, as part of the CDC's recommendations to decrease the incidence of HBV.[203] There is no contraindication to HBV-infected mothers breast-feeding, because perinatal transmission does not appear to be increased in a breast-feeding population.[204]

Similar to HIV, the rate of perinatal transmission of HBV correlates with maternal viral load.[205] It is reasonable to measure maternal viral load between 30 and 34 weeks to allow counseling regarding risk of infection. Lamivudine and HBIG have been recently shown to limit intrauterine transmission of HBV in pregnant women with virema.[206,207] These studies were small and only the HBIG study was randomized, but intervention should be considered in women with HBV viral loads in excess of 10^8 copies/ml secondary to their increased rate of vertical HBV transmission.[205,207] Lamivudine can be administered orally at a dose of 150 mg daily starting at 34 weeks. In addition, up to 80 to 90 percent of the infants of women acutely infected with HBV in the third trimester of pregnancy will be HBsAg positive at birth.[189] It is not known whether treatment with antivirals during acute HBV infection lowers this risk. Pregnant women with known hepatitis B should be vaccinated against hepatitis A to prevent further liver injury.

Hepatitis C

Virology/Epidemiology

HCV is an enveloped, single-stranded RNA virus that is part of the *flaviviridae* family. HCV is transmitted primarily parenterally and though vertical transmission. The risk of sexual transmission of HCV is substantially lower than that of HBV. Risk factors for HCV seropositivity include intravenous drug use and a history of transfusion of blood or blood products.[208] More than 50 percent of individuals infected with HCV are chronic carriers, making HCV the most common chronic blood borne pathogen in the United States.[209] The incubation period for HCV following exposure is 5 to 10 weeks, and 75 percent of acutely infected individuals are asymptomatic.

Diagnosis

The recommended initial screening test is ELISA for HCV-specific antibodies: Universal screening in pregnancy is not recommended, but individuals at risk should be tested (Table 48-14). For individuals who screen positive by ELISA, the CDC recommends a more specific supplemental assay to verify serologic evidence of HCV infection. The two tests recommended by the CDC are the recombinant immunoblot assay or a nucleic acid test.[210] HCV viral loads may be quantitated through PCR.[205,206] Patients chronically infected with HCV can have significant variation in their viral loads and hepatic transaminase levels. Thus a single negative HCV viral load or normal hepatic transaminase level does not rule out chronic carrier status.[209]

Table 48-14. Risk Factors for Hepatitis C Virus (HCV)

Definite Indications for Screening
History of injection of illegal drugs (even once, many years prior)
Known HIV Positive
Persistently abnormal liver function tests
History of long-term hemodialysis
History of blood transfusion or organ transplant before July 1992
History of clotting factor concentrates before 1987
History of exposure to blood from an individual known to have HCV
History of Incarceration
Consider Screening (Need Uncertain)
In vitro fertilization from anonymous donors
History of intranasal cocaine or other noninjectable illegal drug use
History of tattooing or body piercing
Known sexually transmitted disease or multiple partners
Steady sex-partner of known HCV-positive individual
Steady sex-partner of individual with history of injection drug use

Hepatitis C Virus in Pregnancy

There is currently no effective vaccine against HCV. Patients chronically infected with HCV can be treated with interferon and ribavirin to lower HCV viral loads, but interferon treatment of chronic HCV is contraindicated in pregnancy.[209] Therefore, pregnant women with HCV infection are managed expectantly. Perinatal transmission of HCV is correlated with a detectable maternal HCV viral load. Women with detectable HCV viremia have a 4- to 7-percent perinatal HCV transmission rate, whereas perinatal HCV transmission in women with undetectable HCV viremia is rare. Maternal drug use is another risk factor for perinatal HCV transmission,[213] as is maternal HIV coinfection.[214] Overall, these studies show that the strongest predictor of perinatal HCV transmission is maternal HCV viral load. Data from a recently published randomized study indicate that elective cesarean delivery is unlikely to substantially reduce perinatal HCV transmission.[215] However this study was significantly limited as maternal viral load was not reported. The protective effect of elective cesarean in the subset of women with high viral load has not been adequately studied. Pregnant women with a history of hepatitis C infection should be immunized against hepatitis A and B if not immune, and breastfeeding is not contraindicated in women chronically infected with HCV.

Hepatitis D

Hepatitis delta virus (HDV) is an incomplete RNA virus related to plant viruses. The hepatitis D genome encodes a single nucleocapsid protein, HDAg, which is present as two peptides. The short form is required for RNA replication and the long form is packaged with HDV RNA and the HBsAg envelope glycoprotein. Hepatitis D virus uses HBV as a helper virus. Therefore, it requires simultaneous or previous infection with HBV.[216]

HDV is present worldwide and has a high prevalence in the Mediterranean basin, Middle East, Central Asia, West Africa and Amazon basin. Risk factors include intravenous drug use and exposure to tainted blood products.[216] The chronicity rate of HDV infection is 1 to 3 percent when HDV is acquired as a coinfection with HBV and 70 to 80 percent in cases of superinfection of HDV in an individual chronically infected with HBV. Patients chronically infected with both HBV and HDV have a 70 to 80 percent risk for developing cirrhosis and portal hypertension, and 25 percent die of hepatic failure.[217]

Acute infection with HDV is characterized by HDV antigen without HDV antibody. Individuals chronically infected with HDV will have both antigen and IgG antibody against HDV. Acute hepatitis D infection is associated with an increased incidence of fulminant hepatic failure and carries a mortality rate of 2 to 20 percent.

HDV has been perinatally transmitted,[218] although prophylaxis against perinatal HBV transmission is effective at preventing perinatal HDV transmission given that HDV requires coinfection with HBV.[194]

Hepatitis E

Hepatitis E virus is an enveloped, RNA virus that is most closely related to the togavirus family, which also includes rubella.[219] Hepatitis E is transmitted by oral-fecal contact and is endemic outside of the United States in regions such as Africa, Asia and Latin America. Similar to hepatitis A, hepatitis E infection causes only acute disease. No chronic carrier status is associated with this virus. Diagnosis can be made by the presence of a specific IgM or of viral nucleic acid. (RT PCR). The mortality rate following acute hepatitis E infection in the general population is 1 percent. Significantly higher mortality (up to 20 percent) has been observed in pregnant women infected with hepatitis E, and is highest at more advanced gestational age.[194,220] In addition, a recent report showed that pregnant women infected with hepatitis E have a preterm delivery rate of 66 percent.[220] Hepatitis E virus can also be perinatally transmitted, and it has been associated with significant perinatal morbidity and mortality.[221]

INFLUENZA

Influenza virus causes an acute, febrile upper respiratory tract illness. Spread by respiratory droplets, it is highly contagious and occurs as an epidemic typically during the winter months. Influenza virus reservoirs include mammalian and avian species. "Bird flu" is a type of influenza infection. Infection is characterized by the abrupt onset of fever, chills, headache, myalgias, and malaise in addition to respiratory symptoms, including a dry cough and nasal discharge.[222] Complications include pneumonia, occurring in up to 12 percent of influenza-infected pregnant women,[223] Reye's syndrome, and disseminated intravascular coagulation. Treatment includes supportive care and antivirals including rimantidine, amantidine, zanamivir, and oseltamivir in the setting of acute and/or severe infection. The effect of antiviral therapy on the fetus is not known. Therefore its use should be restricted to cases of severe disease where the benefits outweigh the risks.

Pregnant women infected with influenza virus are at increased risk for complications and hospitalization. Thus ACOG and the CDC recommend vaccination of all pregnant women during the influenza season (October to May) using the intramuscular, inactivated vaccine.[224] Optimally women will be vaccinated in October and November to minimize their risk of acquiring influenza. However, vaccination can be performed at any time at any gestational age. A study of 2000 pregnant women receiving the inactivated vaccine demonstrated no adverse fetal effects and this vaccine is safe in breastfeeding women.[225] The intranasal vaccine contains live virus and should not be used during pregnancy.

WEST NILE VIRUS

West Nile virus (WNV) is a flavivirus transmitted by mosquitoes that infects a variety of birds and mammals, including humans. Most infections are subclinical (80%) and most symptomatic infections present with "West Nile fever" consisting of fever, headache, fatigue, rash, lymphadenopathy, and eye pain. Much less common is severe disease, which includes gastrointestinal symptoms, ataxia, extrapyramidal signs, seizures, weakness, mental status changes, and other neurological findings. Severe disease is associated with aseptic meningitis, encephalitis, and flaccid paralysis. No specific treatment is available for WNV infection; supportive care should be provided. Diagnosis of WNV infection is based on the presence of specific IgM antibody and by neutralization assays. PCR is of limited usefulness because of transient and low viremia.

The CDC has received reports of 74 cases of WNV infection in pregnancy, has an open registry to document infections, and is encouraging clinicians to report WNV infections in pregnancy.[226] A few women had severe disease, including encephalitis.[227–229] Two recent studies of pregnant women infected with WNV showed good neonatal outcome in the majority of exposed infants.[230,231] Only three infants had WNV infection; one infant whose mother acquired WNV three weeks prior to delivery developed encephalitis and died.[230] In addition, there is one additional reported case of fetal WNV infection following severe maternal disease, where the infant was born with chorioretinitis and destruction of neural tissue. Given this finding, the CDC recommends that WNV-infected pregnant women have an ultrasound of the fetus at least 2 to 4 weeks following maternal infection to assess for structural abnormalities.[226] Amniotic fluid, chorionic villi, or fetal blood may be tested to assess fetal WNV infection, but the sensitivity, specificity, and predictive value of these tests are not known.[226] If a WNV-infected pregnant woman has a miscarriage or elective pregnancy termination, testing the products of conception is advised.

There is one documented case of WNV transmission during breastfeeding. However, no adverse outcome was noted. Therefore, the CDC recommends that women infected with WNV continue breastfeeding.[226] Prevention of potential maternal WNV infection includes: avoiding the outdoors during peak mosquito feeding times, wearing protective clothing, and using insect repellants containing DEET.

COXSACKIE VIRUS

Coxsackie virus is the causative agent of hand, foot, and mouth disease, an enterovirus transmitted through the fecal-oral route. Several serotypes exist, and adult infection typically results in a self-limited febrile illness requiring no treatment.[229] There is one reported case of coxsackie B virus infection in pregnancy leading to acute liver failure which resolved following expectant management.[232] Coxsackie virus infection during pregnancy has also been associated in several studies with an increased rate of miscarriage[229,233] and an increased rate of insulin dependent diabetes in offspring,[229,234–236] although a causative relationship has not been established.

HUMAN PAPILLOMAVIRUS

Human papillomaviruses (HPV) are a group of small DNA viruses. Some types cause warts (HPV types 6, 11), while other types do not cause warts and are instead highly associated with the development of cervical and oral cancer (HPV types 16, 18, 31, 33, 52b, 58). Infections are sexually and/or vertically transmitted and the incidence of infection in college-aged women is nearly 50 percent.[237] Therefore, it is not uncommon for pregnant women to have evidence of HPV infection. A recent study found that 37 percent of pregnant women with no visible evidence of HPV infection were positive for HPV DNA in the cervix, demonstrating a high rate of HPV infection even in asymptomatic pregnant women.[238] Anogenital warts, caused by nononcogenic types of HPV, are one presentation of HPV infection. Genital warts present during pregnancy may be managed expectantly. However, the hormonal effects of pregnancy can cause rapid proliferation and growth of warts necessitating treatment. Trichloroacetic acid and/or cryotherapy are used in the management of anogenital warts in pregnancy, as podophyllin is contraindicated in pregnancy and little is known regarding the safety of imiquimod in pregnancy. Vaginal delivery is not contraindicated in women with genital warts, unless the wart burden and position would result in dystocia. Very rarely maternal HPV infection is associated with pediatric laryngeal papillomatosis, a disease caused by HPV types 6 and 11. However, given the high prevalence of maternal HPV infection and the rarity of laryngeal papillomatosis, cesarean delivery is not recommended to prevent this disease.[238,239] Cervical dysplasia is another manifestation of HPV infection[240]; testing for oncogenic HPV subtypes is warranted in the setting of an ASCUS PAP smear, independent of pregnancy.

EPSTEIN-BARR VIRUS

The causative agent of infectious mononucleosis is Epstein-Barr Virus (EBV), a member of the herpesvirus family. Clinical presentation includes malaise, headache, fever, pharyngitis, lymphadenopathy, atypical lymphocytosis, heterophile antibody, and transient mild hepatitis. Infection is typically self-limited. EBV establishes a latent infection in B lymphocytes, can be reactivated, and is associated with the development of Hodgkin's and non-Hodgkin's lymphoma.[241] Most adults (>95%) are seropositive for EBV, thus primary EBV infection in pregnancy is rare. Primary infection and/or reactivation of EBV is not associated with significant adverse pregnancy outcome.[242] There is an association between EBV reactivation in pregnancy and the development of childhood acute lymphoblastic leukemia,[243] and in utero EBV transmission has been demonstrated by detection of EBV DNA in neonatal lymphocytes.[244] However, in utero infection has not been associated with adverse outcome. Routine testing is not indicated given the extremely high prevalence of seropositivity and the lack of impact on pregnancy.

SMALLPOX

Variola virus is the causative agent of smallpox. Variola virus infection is restricted to humans and is highly transmissible via inhalation of airborne droplets or by direct contact with smallpox lesions on an infected individual.[245] Secondary to widespread vaccination, the last case of reported smallpox in the United States was in 1949 and the World Health Organization declared its global eradication in 1980. Recent concerns regarding the potential use of variola virus as a bioterrorism agent has led to renewed interest in the clinical presentation and treatment of smallpox disease.

Smallpox infection first presents with a high fever, chills, headache, backache, and vomiting, differentiating it from chickenpox (varicella virus) which has a minimal prodrome.[245] Delirium is present in 15 percent of cases and some infections progress to encephalitis. Skin lesions appear 2 to 3 days following the onset of symptoms, and progress from macule to papule to vesicle, vesicle to pustule to scabs, which then form pitted scars. Smallpox lesions appear in a centrifugal distribution and affect the soles and palms, in contrast to varicella infection which exhibits a centripetal distribution of lesions and spares the palms and soles. Diagnosis should be confirmed by PCR reaction of pustular fluid and/or scabs in a biocontainment facility.

Once symptoms develop, maternal treatment is supportive and vaccination and containment are critical. Maternal mortality is increased following variola infection, and the mortality rate of unvaccinated women is over 60 percent.[245] Death is usually secondary to viral pneumonitis, bacterial pneumonia, or cardiovascular collapse. Pregnant women are at increased risk of acquiring hemorrhagic smallpox, a more severe and lethal form of infection. If infection occurs prior to 24 weeks, 75 percent of pregnancies end in loss or premature delivery. During the latter half of pregnancy, smallpox infection is associated with a 55 percent rate of subsequent preterm delivery. Variola virus can cross the placenta leading to intrauterine infection. During epidemics of the disease, the reported incidence of congenital variola (infection) ranged from 9 percent to 60 percent.

Vaccination within 2 to 3 days of initial exposure affords almost complete protection against disease.[245,246] The currently available vaccine, Dryvax, is composed of live, attenuated vaccinia virus. However, it is associated with an increased risk of complications relative to other viral vaccines. Complications include postvaccinal encephalitis (incidence 12 per million vaccines, 40 percent mortality rate), mild generalized vaccinia, and eczema vaccinatum. Currently, smallpox vaccination is restricted to certain subpopulations, such as women in military service and researchers utilizing related viruses. Data on women vaccinated during pregnancy are being compiled in the National Smallpox Vaccine in Pregnancy

Registry.[246] Rarely fetal infection follows maternal vaccination (fetal vaccinia) and is characterized by skin lesions and internal organ involvement but is not associated with fetal malformations. Therefore, vaccination is not considered an indication for termination of pregnancy. Current CDC recommendations are to defer elective smallpox vaccination while pregnant. However, immediate vaccination is warranted following smallpox exposure, secondary to the risk of clinical smallpox infection to the mother and fetus.[246]

KEY POINTS

- Preconceptional vaccination with live attenuated viral vaccines can prevent antenatal rubeola, rubella, and varicella infection but should be avoided in pregnancy.
- Hepatitis A and B vaccination is safe in pregnancy and should be offered to susceptible women at risk. Influenza vaccine is also safe in pregnancy and should be offered to all women pregnant during winter months.
- All pregnant women should be offered HIV screening, using an "opt out" approach. In areas of high seroprevalence repeat screening in the third trimester may be warranted.
- Rapid HIV testing should be offered in early labor to women without documented HIV status.
- Treatment of HIV-infected women with HAART significantly reduces the risk of perinatal HIV transmission and prolongs maternal survival.
- Elective cesarean delivery limits HIV transmission in women with an increased viral load. HIV-infected women with a viral load below 1,000 copies/ml have a risk of perinatal HIV transmission less than 2 percent and are candidates for vaginal delivery.
- Fetal parvovirus infection may result in fetal anemia and hydrops. Women with documented infection should be screened with serial ultrasound and middle cerebral artery Doppler studies.
- Primary maternal CMV infection during pregnancy is associated with a significant risk of fetal injury. Prenatal diagnosis and prediction of the severity of sequelae are imperfect.
- Women without a history of varicella should be considered for serum testing. Susceptible women exposed to varicella should be treated with VZIG to reduce the risk of transmission.
- All pregnant women should be screened for hepatitis B infection. Infants delivered to seropositive mothers should receive both hepatitis B immune globulin (HBIG) and hepatitis B vaccine shortly after birth.

REFERENCES

1. Luciw PA: Human immunodeficiency viruses and their replication. *In* Fields B, Knipe P, Howley P, et al (eds): Fields Virology, ed 3. Philadelphia, Lippincott-Raven, 1996, Vol 1, p 1881.
2. Berger EA, Murphy PM, Farber JM: Chemokine receptors as HIV-1 coreceptors: roles in viral entry, tropism, and disease. Annu Rev Immunol 17:657, 1999.
3. Zhang YJ, Dragic T, Cao Y, et al: Use of coreceptors other than CCR5 by non-syncytium–inducing adult and pediatric isolates of human immunodeficiency virus type 1 is rare in vitro. J Virol 72:9337, 1998.
4. Casper CH, Clevestig P, Carlenor E, et al: Link between the X4 phenotype in human immunodeficiency virus type 1–infected mothers and their children, despite the early presence of R5 in the child. J Infect Dis 186:914, 2002.
5. Ometto L, Zanchetta M, Mainardi M, et al: Co-receptor usage of HIV-1 primary isolates, viral burden, and CCR5 genotype in mother-to-child HIV-1 transmission. AIDS 14:1721, 2000.
6. Bienzle D, MacDonald KS, Smaill FM, et al: Factors contributing to the lack of human immunodeficiency virus type 1 (HIV-1) transmission in HIV-1 discordant partners. J Infect Dis 182:123, 2000.
7. Mangano A, Gonzalez E, Dhanda R, et al: Concordance between the CC chemokine receptor 5 genetic determinants that alter risks of transmission and disease progression in children exposed perinatally to human immunodeficiency virus. J Infect Dis 183:1574, 2001.
8. Ometto L, Bertorelle R, Mainardi M, et al: Analysis of the CC chemokine receptor 5 m303 mutation in infants born to HIV-1-seropositive mothers. AIDS 13:871, 1999.
9. Diagnoses of HIV/AIDS—32 States, 2000–2003. MMWR Morb Mortal Wkly Rep 53:1106, 2004.
10. Alpert PL, Shuter J, DeShaw MG, et al: Factors associated with unrecognized HIV-1 infection in an inner-city emergency department. Ann Emerg Med 28:159, 1996.
11. Kelen GD, Hexter DA, Hansen KN, et al: Trends in human immunodeficiency virus (HIV) infection among a patient population of an inner-city emergency department: implications for emergency department-based screening programs for HIV infection. Clin Infect Dis 21:867, 1995.
12. Nagachinta T, Gold CR, Cheng F, et al: Unrecognized HIV-1 infection in inner-city hospital emergency department patients. Infect Control Hosp Epidemiol 17:174, 1996.
13. Cavaco-Silva P, Taveira NC, Lourenco MH, et al: Vertical transmission of HIV-2. Lancet 349:177, 1997.
14. Matheron S, Courpotin C, Simon F, et al: Vertical transmission of HIV-2. Lancet 335:1103, 1990.
15. Ho DD, Sarngadharan MG, Resnick L, et al: Primary human T lymphotropic virus type III infection. Ann Intern Med 103:880, 1985.
16. Pantaleo G, Fauci AS: New concepts in the immunopathogenesis of HIV infection. Annu Rev Immunol 13:487, 1995.
17. 1993 revised classification system for HIV infection and expanded surveillance case definition for AIDS among adolescents and adults. MMWR Recomm Rep 41:1, 1992.
18. Sloand EM, Pitt E, Chiarello RJ, et al: HIV testing. State of the art. JAMA 266:2861, 1991.
19. Martinez P, Ortiz de Lejarazu R, Eiros JM, et al: Usefulness of oral mucosal transudate for HIV antibody testing. JAMA 277:1592, 1997.
20. Guidelines for national human immunodeficiency virus case surveillance, including monitoring for human immunodeficiency virus infection and acquired immunodeficiency syndrome. Centers for Disease Control and Prevention. MMWR Recomm Rep 48:1, 1999.
21. Bulterys M, Jamieson DJ, O'Sullivan MJ, et al: Rapid HIV-1 testing during labor: a multicenter study. JAMA 292:219, 2004.
22. Paul SM, Grimes-Dennis J, Burr CK, et al: Rapid diagnostic testing for HIV. Clinical implications. N J Med 99:20, 2002.
23. Peters V, Liu KL, Dominguez K, et al: Missed opportunities for perinatal HIV prevention among HIV-exposed infants born 1996–2000, pediatric spectrum of HIV disease cohort. Pediatrics 111:1186, 2003.

24. ACOG committee opinion number 304, November 2004. Prenatal and perinatal human immunodeficiency virus testing: expanded recommendations. Obstet Gynecol 104:1119, 2004.
25. Watts DH: Management of human immunodeficiency virus infection in pregnancy. N Engl J Med 346:1879, 2002.
26. Guidelines for laboratory test result reporting of human immunodeficiency virus type 1 ribonucleic acid determination. Recommendations from a CDC working group. Centers for Disease Control. MMWR Recomm Rep 50:1, 2001.
27. Burns DN, Landesman S, Minkoff H, et al: The influence of pregnancy on human immunodeficiency virus type 1 infection: antepartum and postpartum changes in human immunodeficiency virus type 1 viral load. Am J Obstet Gynecol 178:355, 1998.
28. Saada M, Le Chenadec J, Berrebi A, et al: Pregnancy and progression to AIDS: results of the French prospective cohorts. SEROGEST and SEROCO Study Groups. AIDS 14:2355, 2000.
29. Weisser M, Rudin C, Battegay M, et al: Does pregnancy influence the course of HIV infection? Evidence from two large Swiss cohort studies. J Acquir Immune Defic Syndr Hum Retrovirol 17:404, 1998.
30. Combination antiretroviral therapy and duration of pregnancy. AIDS 14:2913, 2000.
31. Brocklehurst P, French R: The association between maternal HIV infection and perinatal outcome: a systematic review of the literature and meta-analysis. Br J Obstet Gynaecol 105:836, 1998.
32. Bucceri A, Luchini L, Rancilio L, et al: Pregnancy outcome among HIV positive and negative intravenous drug users. Eur J Obstet Gynecol Reprod Biol 72:169, 1997.
33. Connor EM, Sperling RS, Gelber R, et al: Reduction of maternal-infant transmission of human immunodeficiency virus type 1 with zidovudine treatment. Pediatric AIDS Clinical Trials Group Protocol 076 Study Group. N Engl J Med 331:1173, 1994.
34. Lambert JS, Watts DH, Mofenson L, et al: Risk factors for preterm birth, low birth weight, and intrauterine growth retardation in infants born to HIV-infected pregnant women receiving zidovudine. Pediatric AIDS Clinical Trials Group 185 Team. AIDS 14:1389, 2000.
35. Lorenzi P, Spicher VM, Laubereau B, et al: Antiretroviral therapies in pregnancy: maternal, fetal and neonatal effects. Swiss HIV Cohort Study, the Swiss Collaborative HIV and Pregnancy Study, and the Swiss Neonatal HIV Study. AIDS 12:F241, 1998.
36. Tuomala RE, Shapiro DE, Mofenson LM, et al: Antiretroviral therapy during pregnancy and the risk of an adverse outcome. N Engl J Med 346:1863, 2002.
37. Cooper ER, Charurat M, Mofenson L, et al: Combination antiretroviral strategies for the treatment of pregnant HIV-1-infected women and prevention of perinatal HIV-1 transmission. J Acquir Immune Defic Syndr 29:484, 2002.
38. Maiques V, Garcia-Tejedor A, Perales A, et al: HIV detection in amniotic fluid samples. Amniocentesis can be performed in HIV pregnant women? Eur J Obstet Gynecol Reprod Biol 108:137, 2003.
38a. Somigliana E, Bucceri AM, Tibaldi C, et al: Italian collaborative study on HIV infection in pregnancy: Early invasive diagnostic techniques in pregnant women who are infected with the HIV: a multicenter case series. Am J Obstet Gynecol 193:437, 2005.
39. Guay LA, Musoke P, Fleming T, et al: Intrapartum and neonatal single-dose nevirapine compared with zidovudine for prevention of mother-to-child transmission of HIV-1 in Kampala, Uganda: HIVNET 012 randomised trial. Lancet 354:795, 1999.
40. Eshleman SH, Guay LA, Mwatha A, et al: Characterization of nevirapine resistance mutations in women with subtype A vs. D HIV-1 6–8 weeks after single-dose nevirapine (HIVNET 012). J Acquir Immune Defic Syndr 35:126, 2004.
41. Dorenbaum A, Cunningham CK, Gelber RD, et al: Two-dose intrapartum/newborn nevirapine and standard antiretroviral therapy to reduce perinatal HIV transmission: a randomized trial. JAMA 288:189, 2002.
42. Public Health Service Task Force recommendations for the use of antiretroviral drugs in pregnant women infected with HIV-1 for maternal health and interventions to reduce perinatal HIV-1 transmission in the United States. Centers for Disease Control and Prevention. *www.AIDSinfo.nih.gov:1,* 2005.
43. Ioannidis JP, Abrams EJ, Ammann A, et al: Perinatal transmission of human immunodeficiency virus type 1 by pregnant women with RNA virus loads <1,000 copies/ml. J Infect Dis 183:539, 2001.
44. Mirochnick M, Capparelli E: Pharmacokinetics of antiretrovirals in pregnant women. Clin Pharmacokinet 40:1071, 2001.
45. Ibdah JA, Yang Z, Bennett MJ: Liver disease in pregnancy and fetal fatty acid oxidation defects. Mol Genet Metab 71:182, 2000.
46. Brinkman K, ter Hofstede HJ, Burger DM, et al: Adverse effects of reverse transcriptase inhibitors: mitochondrial toxicity as common pathway. AIDS 12:1735, 1998.
47. Fortgang IS, Belitsos PC, Chaisson RE, et al: Hepatomegaly and steatosis in HIV-infected patients receiving nucleoside analog antiretroviral therapy. Am J Gastroenterol 90:1433, 1995.
48. Gerard Y, Maulin L, Yazdanpanah Y, et al: Symptomatic hyperlactataemia: an emerging complication of antiretroviral therapy. AIDS 14:2723, 2000.
49. Blanche S, Tardieu M, Rustin P, et al: Persistent mitochondrial dysfunction and perinatal exposure to antiretroviral nucleoside analogues. Lancet 354:1084, 1999.
50. Mandelbrot L, Landreau-Mascaro A, Rekacewicz C, et al: Lamivudine-zidovudine combination for prevention of maternal-infant transmission of HIV-1. JAMA 285:2083, 2001.
51. Nucleoside exposure in the children of HIV-infected women receiving antiretroviral drugs: absence of clear evidence for mitochondrial disease in children who died before 5 years of age in five United States cohorts. J Acquir Immune Defic Syndr 25:261, 2000.
52. De Santis M, Carducci B, De Santis L, et al: Periconceptional exposure to efavirenz and neural tube defects. Arch Intern Med 162:355, 2002.
53. Fundaro C, Genovese O, Rendeli C, et al: Myelomeningocele in a child with intrauterine exposure to efavirenz. AIDS 16:299, 2002.
54. Baylor MS, Johann-Liang R: Hepatotoxicity associated with nevirapine use. J Acquir Immune Defic Syndr 35:538, 2004.
55. Mirochnick M, Dorenbaum A, Holland D, et al: Concentrations of protease inhibitors in cord blood after in utero exposure. Pediatr Infect Dis J 21:835, 2002.
56. Hayashi S, Beckerman K, Homma M, et al: Pharmacokinetics of indinavir in HIV-positive pregnant women. AIDS 14:1061, 2000.
57. Treating opportunistic infections among HIV-infected adults and adolescents: recommendations from CDC, the National Institutes of Health, and the Infectious Diseases Society of America. MMWR Recomm Rep 53:1, 2004.
58. Goldenberg RL, Vermund SH, Goepfert AR, et al: Choriodecidual inflammation: a potentially preventable cause of perinatal HIV-1 transmission? Lancet 352:1927, 1998.
59. Landesman SH, Kalish LA, Burns DN, et al: Obstetrical factors and the transmission of human immunodeficiency virus type 1 from mother to child. The Women and Infants Transmission Study. N Engl J Med 334:1617, 1996.
60. Mandelbrot L, Mayaux MJ, Bongain A, et al: Obstetric factors and mother-to-child transmission of human immunodeficiency virus type 1: the French perinatal cohorts. SEROGEST French Pediatric HIV Infection Study Group. Am J Obstet Gynecol 175:661, 1996.
61. Mofenson LM, Lambert JS, Stiehm ER, et al: Risk factors for perinatal transmission of human immunodeficiency virus type 1 in women treated with zidovudine. Pediatric AIDS Clinical Trials Group Study 185 Team. N Engl J Med 341:385, 1999.
62. Dickover RE, Garratty EM, Herman SA, et al: Identification of levels of maternal HIV-1 RNA associated with risk of perinatal transmission. Effect of maternal zidovudine treatment on viral load. JAMA 275:599, 1996.
63. Fang G, Burger H, Grimson R, et al: Maternal plasma human immunodeficiency virus type 1 RNA level: a determinant and projected threshold for mother-to-child transmission. Proc Natl Acad Sci U S A 92:12100, 1995.
64. Mayaux MJ, Dussaix E, Isopet J, et al: Maternal virus load during pregnancy and mother-to-child transmission of human immunodeficiency virus type 1: the French perinatal cohort studies. SEROGEST Cohort Group. J Infect Dis 175:172, 1997.

65. Garcia PM, Kalish LA, Pitt J, et al: Maternal levels of plasma human immunodeficiency virus type 1 RNA and the risk of perinatal transmission. Women and Infants Transmission Study Group. N Engl J Med 341:394, 1999.
66. Riley LE, Yawetz S: Case records of the Massachusetts General Hospital. Case 32-2005. A 34-year-old HIV-positive woman who desired to become pregnant. N Engl J Med 353:1725, 2005.
67. Shapiro D, Tuomala R, Pollack H, et al: Mother to Child HIV-1 Transmisssion Risk According to Antiretroviral Therapy, Mode of Delivery, and Viral Load in 3,081 U.S. Women. *In* 11th Conference on Retroviruses and Opportunistic Infections, San Francisco, 2004.
68. Minkoff H, Burns DN, Landesman S, et al: The relationship of the duration of ruptured membranes to vertical transmission of human immunodeficiency virus. Am J Obstet Gynecol 173:585, 1995.
69. Umans-Eckenhausen MA, Lafeber HN: Prolonged rupture of membranes and transmission of the human immunodeficiency virus. N Engl J Med 335:1533, 1996.
70. Duration of ruptured membranes and vertical transmission of HIV-1: a meta-analysis from 15 prospective cohort studies. AIDS 15:357, 2001.
71. Elective caesarean-section versus vaginal delivery in prevention of vertical HIV 1 transmission: a randomised clinical trial. The European Mode of Delivery Collaboration. Lancet 353:1035, 1999.
72. The mode of delivery and the risk of vertical transmission of human immunodeficiency virus type 1—a meta-analysis of 15 prospective cohort studies. The International Perinatal HIV Group. N Engl J Med 340:977, 1999.
73. ACOG committee opinion scheduled Cesarean delivery and the prevention of vertical transmission of HIV infection. Number 234, May 2000 (replaces number 219, August 1999). Int J Gynaecol Obstet 73:279, 2001.
74. Bulterys M, Chao A, Dushimimana A, et al: Fatal complications after Cesarian section in HIV-infected women. AIDS 10:923, 1996.
75. Nielsen TF, Hokegard KH: Postoperative cesarean section morbidity: a prospective study. Am J Obstet Gynecol 146:911, 1983.
76. Semprini AE, Castagna C, Ravizza M, et al: The incidence of complications after caesarean section in 156 HIV-positive women. AIDS 9:913, 1995.
77. Duff P, Robertson AW, Read JA: Single-dose cefazolin versus cefonicid for antibiotic prophylaxis in cesarean delivery. Obstet Gynecol 70:718, 1987.
78. Dunn DT, Newell ML, Ades AE, et al: Risk of human immunodeficiency virus type 1 transmission through breastfeeding. Lancet 340:585, 1992.
79. Embree JE, Njenga S, Datta P, et al: Risk factors for postnatal mother-child transmission of HIV-1. AIDS 14:2535, 2000.
80. Nduati R, John G, Mbori-Ngacha D, et al: Effect of breastfeeding and formula feeding on transmission of HIV-1: a randomized clinical trial. JAMA 283:1167, 2000.
81. Nduati R, Mbori-Ngacha D, John G, et al: Breastfeeding in women with HIV. JAMA 284:956, 2000.
82. Young NS: Parvoviruses. *In* Fields B, Knipe P, Howley P, et al (eds): Fields Virology, ed 3. Philadelphia, Lippincott-Raven, 1996, Vol 1, p 2199.
83. Valeur-Jensen AK, Pedersen CB, Westergaard T, et al: Risk factors for parvovirus B19 infection in pregnancy. JAMA 281:1099, 1999.
84. Cartter ML, Farley TA, Rosengren S, et al: Occupational risk factors for infection with parvovirus B19 among pregnant women. J Infect Dis 163:282, 1991.
85. Gillespie SM, Cartter ML, Asch S, et al: Occupational risk of human parvovirus B19 infection for school and day-care personnel during an outbreak of erythema infectiosum. JAMA 263:2061, 1990.
86. Anderson LJ: Role of parvovirus B19 in human disease. Pediatr Infect Dis J 6:711, 1987.
87. Risks associated with human parvovirus B19 infection. MMWR Morb Mortal Wkly Rep 38:81, 1989.
88. Thurn J: Human parvovirus B19: historical and clinical review. Rev Infect Dis 10:1005, 1988.
89. Brown T, Anand A, Ritchie LD, et al: Intrauterine parvovirus infection associated with hydrops fetalis. Lancet 2:1033, 1984.
90. Dieck D, Schild RL, Hansmann M, et al: Prenatal diagnosis of congenital parvovirus B19 infection: value of serological and PCR techniques in maternal and fetal serum. Prenat Diagn 19:1119, 1999.
91. Cosmi E, Mari G, Delle Chiaie L, et al: Noninvasive diagnosis by Doppler ultrasonography of fetal anemia resulting from parvovirus infection. Am J Obstet Gynecol 187:1290, 2002.
92. Hernandez-Andrade E, Scheier M, Dezerega V, et al: Fetal middle cerebral artery peak systolic velocity in the investigation of non-immune hydrops. Ultrasound Obstet Gynecol 23:442, 2004.
93. Prospective study of human parvovirus (B19) infection in pregnancy. Public Health Laboratory Service Working Party on Fifth Disease. BMJ 300:1166, 1990.
94. Enders M, Weidner A, Zoellner I, et al: Fetal morbidity and mortality after acute human parvovirus B19 infection in pregnancy: prospective evaluation of 1018 cases. Prenat Diagn 24:513, 2004.
95. Enders M, Weidner A, Zoellner I, et al: Fetal morbidity and mortality after acute human parvovirus B19 infection in pregnancy: prospective evaluation of 1018 cases. Obstet Gynecol Surv 60:83, 2005.
96. Rodis JF, Quinn DL, Gary GW, Jr, et al: Management and outcomes of pregnancies complicated by human B19 parvovirus infection: a prospective study. Am J Obstet Gynecol 163:1168, 1990.
97. Rodis JF, Borgida AF, Wilson M, et al: Management of parvovirus infection in pregnancy and outcomes of hydrops: a survey of members of the Society of Perinatal Obstetricians. Am J Obstet Gynecol 179:985, 1998.
98. Grose C, Itani O, Weiner CP: Prenatal diagnosis of fetal infection: advances from amniocentesis to cordocentesis—congenital toxoplasmosis, rubella, cytomegalovirus, varicella virus, parvovirus and human immunodeficiency virus. Pediatr Infect Dis J 8:459, 1989.
99. Naides SJ, Weiner CP: Antenatal diagnosis and palliative treatment of non-immune hydrops fetalis secondary to fetal parvovirus B19 infection. Prenat Diagn 9:105, 1989.
100. Sahakian V, Weiner CP, Naides SJ, et al: Intrauterine transfusion treatment of nonimmune hydrops fetalis secondary to human parvovirus B19 infection. Am J Obstet Gynecol 164:1090, 1991.
101. Miller E, Fairley CK, Cohen BJ, et al: Immediate and long term outcome of human parvovirus B19 infection in pregnancy. Br J Obstet Gynaecol 105:174, 1998.
102. Perkin MA, English PM: Immediate and long term outcome of human parvovirus B19 infection in pregnancy. Br J Obstet Gynaecol 105:1337, 1998.
103. Rodis JF, Rodner C, Hansen AA, et al: Long-term outcome of children following maternal human parvovirus B19 infection. Obstet Gynecol 91:125, 1998.
104. Conry J, Torok T, Andrews I: Perinatal encephalopathy secondary to in utero human parvovirus B-19 (HPV) infection. Neurology A346, 1993.
105. Griffin D, Bellini W: Measles virus. *In* Fields B, Knipe P, Howley P, et al (eds): Fields Virology, ed 3. Philadelphia, Lippincott-Raven, 1996, Vol 1, p 1267.
106. Leads from the MMWR. Measles prevention: supplementary statement. JAMA 261:827, 1989.
107. The measles epidemic. The problems, barriers, and recommendations. The National Vaccine Advisory Committee. JAMA 266:1547, 1991.
108. Tsimberidou AM, Giles F, Romaguera J, et al: Activity of interferon-alpha and isotretinoin in patients with advanced, refractory lymphoid malignancies. Cancer 100:574, 2004.
109. Giladi M, Schulman A, Kedem R, et al: Measles in adults: a prospective study of 291 consecutive cases. Br Med J (Clin Res Ed) 295:1314, 1987.
110. Annunziato D, Kaplan MH, Hall WW, et al: Atypical measles syndrome: pathologic and serologic findings. Pediatrics 70:203, 1982.
111. Brunell PA: Measles. *In* Bennett J, Plum F (eds): Cecil Textbook of Medicine, 20th ed. Philadelphia, W. B. Saunders Company, 1996, p 1758.

112. Eberhart-Phillips JE, Frederick PD, Baron RC, et al: Measles in pregnancy: a descriptive study of 58 cases. Obstet Gynecol 82:797, 1993.
113. Chiba ME, Saito M, Suzuki N, et al: Measles infection in pregnancy. J Infect 47:40, 2003.
114. Stein SJ, Greenspoon JS: Rubeola during pregnancy. Obstet Gynecol 78:925, 1991.
115. Ali ME, Albar HM: Measles in pregnancy: maternal morbidity and perinatal outcome. Int J Gynaecol Obstet 59:109, 1997.
116. Ekbom A, Wakefield AJ, Zack M, et al: Perinatal measles infection and subsequent Crohn's disease. Lancet 344:508, 1994.
117. Pardi DS, Tremaine WJ, Sandborn WJ, et al: Perinatal exposure to measles virus is not associated with the development of inflammatory bowel disease. Inflamm Bowel Dis 5:104, 1999.
118. Nyari TA, Dickinson HO, Parker L: Childhood cancer in relation to infections in the community during pregnancy and around the time of birth. Int J Cancer 104:772, 2003.
119. Measles prevention. MMWR Morb Mortal Wkly Rep 38 Suppl 9:1, 1989.
120. Measles prevention: supplementary statement. MMWR Morb Mortal Wkly Rep 38:11, 1989.
121. Neubert AG, Samuels P, Goodman DB, et al: The seroprevalence of the rubeola antibody in a prenatal screening program. Obstet Gynecol 90:507, 1997.
122. Control and prevention of rubella: evaluation and management of suspected outbreaks, rubella in pregnant women, and surveillance for congenital rubella syndrome. MMWR Recomm Rep 50:1, 2001.
123. Tookey P: Congenital rubella: down but not out. Lancet 360:803, 2002.
124. Brunell P: Rubella (German measles). *In* Bennett J, Plum F (eds): Cecil Textbook of Medicine, 20th ed. Philadelphia, W. B. Saunders Company, 1996, p 1761.
125. Mann JM, Preblud SR, Hoffman RE, et al: Assessing risks of rubella infection during pregnancy. A standardized approach. JAMA 245:1647, 1981.
126. Mace M, Cointe D, Six C, et al: Diagnostic value of reverse transcription-PCR of amniotic fluid for prenatal diagnosis of congenital rubella infection in pregnant women with confirmed primary rubella infection. J Clin Microbiol 42:4818, 2004.
127. Tanemura M, Suzumori K, Yagami Y, et al: Diagnosis of fetal rubella infection with reverse transcription and nested polymerase chain reaction: a study of 34 cases diagnosed in fetuses. Am J Obstet Gynecol 174:578, 1996.
128. Tang JW, Aarons E, Hesketh LM, et al: Prenatal diagnosis of congenital rubella infection in the second trimester of pregnancy. Prenat Diagn 23:509, 2003.
129. Bar-Oz B, Levichek Z, Moretti ME, et al: Pregnancy outcome following rubella vaccination: a prospective controlled study. Am J Med Genet A 130:52, 2004.
130. Miller E, Cradock-Watson JE, Pollock TM: Consequences of confirmed maternal rubella at successive stages of pregnancy. Lancet 2:781, 1982.
131. Munro ND, Sheppard S, Smithells RW, et al: Temporal relations between maternal rubella and congenital defects. Lancet 2:201, 1987.
132. Cherry J (ed): Textbook of Pediatric Infectious Diseases, 5th ed. Philadelphia, Saunders, 2004, Vol 2, p 2134.
133. Cooper LZ, Krugman S: Clinical manifestations of postnatal and congenital rubella. Arch Ophthalmol 77:434, 1967.
134. McIntosh ED, Menser MA: A fifty-year follow-up of congenital rubella. Lancet 340:414, 1992.
135. Townsend JJ, Baringer JR, Wolinsky JS, et al: Progressive rubella panencephalitis. Late onset after congenital rubella. N Engl J Med 292:990, 1975.
136. Britt W, Alford C: Cytomegalovirus. *In* Fields B, Knipe P, Howley P, et al (eds): Fields Virology, 3rd ed. Philadelphia, Lippincott-Raven, 1996, Vol 1, p 2493.
137. Betts RF: Cytomegalovirus infection epidemiology and biology in adults. Semin Perinatol 7:22, 1983
138. Hutto C, Little EA, Ricks R, et al: Isolation of cytomegalovirus from toys and hands in a day care center. J Infect Dis 154:527, 1986.
139. Pass RF, August AM, Dworsky M, et al: Cytomegalovirus infection in day-care center. N Engl J Med 307:477, 1982.
140. Taber LH, Frank AL, Yow MD, et al: Acquisition of cytomegaloviral infections in families with young children: a serological study. J Infect Dis 151:948, 1985.
141. Chandler SH, Alexander ER, Holmes KK: Epidemiology of cytomegaloviral infection in a heterogeneous population of pregnant women. J Infect Dis 152:249, 1985.
142. Stagno S, Reynolds DW, Huang ES, et al: Congenital cytomegalovirus infection. N Engl J Med 296:1254, 1977.
143. Stagno S, Pass RF, Dworsky ME, et al: Maternal cytomegalovirus infection and perinatal transmission. Clin Obstet Gynecol 25:563, 1982.
144. Stagno S, Tinker MK, Elrod C, et al: Immunoglobulin M antibodies detected by enzyme-linked immunosorbent assay and radioimmunoassay in the diagnosis of cytomegalovirus infections in pregnant women and newborn infants. J Clin Microbiol 21:930, 1985.
145. Stagno S, Britt W: Cytomegalovirus Infections, 6th ed. Philadelphia, Elsevier, 2006.
146. Hohlfeld P, Vial Y, Maillard-Brignon C, et al: Cytomegalovirus fetal infection: prenatal diagnosis. Obstet Gynecol 78:615, 1991.
147. Lamy ME, Mulongo KN, Gadisseux JF, et al: Prenatal diagnosis of fetal cytomegalovirus infection. Am J Obstet Gynecol 166:91, 1992.
148. Lewis PE 2nd, Cefalo RC, Zaritsky AL: Fetal heart block caused by cytomegalovirus. Am J Obstet Gynecol 136:967, 1980.
149. Pletcher BA, Williams MK, Mulivor RA, et al: Intrauterine cytomegalovirus infection presenting as fetal meconium peritonitis. Obstet Gynecol 78:903, 1991.
150. Nigro G, Adler SP, La Torre R, et al: Passive immunization during pregnancy for congenital cytomegalovirus infection. N Engl J Med 353:1350, 2005.
151. Kumar ML, Prokay SL: Experimental primary cytomegalovirus infection in pregnancy: timing and fetal outcome. Am J Obstet Gynecol 145:56, 1983.
152. Stagno S, Pass RF, Cloud G, et al: Primary cytomegalovirus infection in pregnancy. Incidence, transmission to fetus, and clinical outcome. JAMA 256:1904, 1986.
153. Pass RF, Fowler KB, Boppana SB, et al: Congenital cytomegalovirus infection following first trimester maternal infection: symptoms at birth and outcome. J Clin Virol 35:216, 2006.
154. Fowler KB, Stagno S, Pass RF, et al: The outcome of congenital cytomegalovirus infection in relation to maternal antibody status. N Engl J Med 326:663, 1992.
155. Stagno S, Pass RF, Dworsky ME, et al: Congenital cytomegalovirus infection: The relative importance of primary and recurrent maternal infection. N Engl J Med 306:945, 1982.
156. Bradford RD, Cloud G, Lakeman AD, et al: Detection of cytomegalovirus (CMV) DNA by polymerase chain reaction is associated with hearing loss in newborns with symptomatic congenital CMV infection involving the central nervous system. J Infect Dis 191:227, 2005.
157. Whitley R: Herpes simplex viruses. *In* Fields B, Knipe P, Howley P, et al (eds): Fields Virology, 3rd ed. Philadelphia, Lippincott-Raven, 1996, Vol 1, p 2297.
158. Whitley R: Herpes simplex virus infections. *In* Bennett J, Plum F (eds): Cecil Textbook of Medicine, 20th ed. Philadelphia, W. B. Saunders Company, 1996, p 1770.
159. Koelle DM, Benedetti J, Langenberg A, et al: Asymptomatic reactivation of herpes simplex virus in women after the first episode of genital herpes. Ann Intern Med 116:433, 1992.
160. Cone RW, Hobson AC, Brown Z, et al: Frequent detection of genital herpes simplex virus DNA by polymerase chain reaction among pregnant women. JAMA 272:792, 1994.
161. Brown ZA, Selke S, Zeh J, et al: The acquisition of herpes simplex virus during pregnancy. N Engl J Med 337:509, 1997.
162. Baldwin S, Whitley RJ: Intrauterine herpes simplex virus infection. Teratology 39:1, 1989..
163. Brown ZA, Vontver LA, Benedetti J, et al: Effects on infants of a first episode of genital herpes during pregnancy. N Engl J Med 317:1246, 1987.
164. Brown ZA, Benedetti J, Selke S, et al: Asymptomatic maternal shedding of herpes simplex virus at the onset of labor: relationship to preterm labor. Obstet Gynecol 87:483, 1996.

165. Prober CG, Sullender WM, Yasukawa LL, et al: Low risk of herpes simplex virus infections in neonates exposed to the virus at the time of vaginal delivery to mothers with recurrent genital herpes simplex virus infections. N Engl J Med 316:240, 1987.
166. ACOG practice bulletin. Management of herpes in pregnancy. Number 8, October 1999. Clinical management guidelines for obstetrician-gynecologists. Int J Gynaecol Obstet 68:165, 2000.
167. Randolph AG, Washington AE, Prober CG: Cesarean delivery for women presenting with genital herpes lesions. Efficacy, risks, and costs. JAMA 270:77, 1993.
168. Arvin AM, Hensleigh PA, Prober CG, et al: Failure of antepartum maternal cultures to predict the infant's risk of exposure to herpes simplex virus at delivery. N Engl J Med 315:796, 1986.
169. Prober CG, Hensleigh PA, Boucher FD, et al: Use of routine viral cultures at delivery to identify neonates exposed to herpes simplex virus. N Engl J Med 318:887, 1988.
170. Sheffield JS, Hollier LM, Hill JB, et al: Acyclovir prophylaxis to prevent herpes simplex virus recurrence at delivery: a systematic review. Obstet Gynecol 102:1396, 2003.
171. Whitley R, Arvin A, Prober C, et al: Predictors of morbidity and mortality in neonates with herpes simplex virus infections. The National Institute of Allergy and Infectious Diseases Collaborative Antiviral Study Group. N Engl J Med [illegible], 1991.
172. Brown ZA, Wald A, Morrow RA, et al: Effect of serologic status and cesarean delivery on transmission rates of herpes simplex virus from mother to infant. JAMA 289:203, 2003.
173. Whitley RJ, Gnann JW, Jr.: Acyclovir: a decade later. N Engl J Med 327:782, 1992.
174. Arvin A: Varicella-zoster virus. *In* Fields B, Knipe P, Howley P, et al (eds): Fields Virology, 3rd ed. Philadelphia, Lippincott-Raven, 1996, Vol 1, p 2547.
175. Varicella-related deaths among adults—United States, 1997. MMWR Morb Mortal Wkly Rep 46:409, 1997.
176. Wharton M: The epidemiology of varicella-zoster virus infections. Infect Dis Clin North Am 10:571, 1996.
177. Brunell PA: Varicella. *In* Bennett J, Plum F (eds): Cecil Textbook of Medicine, 20th ed. Philadelphia, W. B. Saunders Company, 1996, p 1763.
178. Brunell PA: Varicella in pregnancy, the fetus, and the newborn: problems in management. J Infect Dis 166 Suppl 1:S42, 1992.
179. Chapman S, Duff P: Varicella in pregnancy. Semin Perinatol 17:403, 1993.
180. McGregor JA, Mark S, Crawford GP, et al: Varicella zoster antibody testing in the care of pregnant women exposed to varicella. Am J Obstet Gynecol 157:281, 1987.
181. Kesson AM, Grimwood K, Burgess MA, et al: Acyclovir for the prevention and treatment of varicella zoster in children, adolescents and pregnancy. J Paediatr Child Health 32:211, 1996.
182. Smego RA, Jr, Asperilla MO: Use of acyclovir for varicella pneumonia during pregnancy. Obstet Gynecol 78:1112, 1991.
183. Wald ER: Transmission of varicella-vaccine virus: what is the risk? J Pediatr 133:310, 1998.
184. Leads from the MMWR. Varicella-zoster immune globulin for the prevention of chickenpox. JAMA 251:1401, 1984.
185. Asano Y, Yoshikawa T, Suga S, et al: Postexposure prophylaxis of varicella in family contact by oral acyclovir. Pediatrics 92:219, 1993.
186. Goldstein SL, Somers MJ, Lande MB, et al: Acyclovir prophylaxis of varicella in children with renal disease receiving steroids. Pediatr Nephrol 14:305, 2000.
187. Enders G, Miller E, Cradock-Watson J, et al: Consequences of varicella and herpes zoster in pregnancy: prospective study of 1739 cases. Lancet 343:1548, 1994.
188. Isada NB, Paar DP, Johnson MP, et al: In utero diagnosis of congenital varicella zoster virus infection by chorionic villus sampling and polymerase chain reaction. Am J Obstet Gynecol 165:1727, 1991.
189. Kustermann A, Zoppini C, Tassis B, et al: Prenatal diagnosis of congenital varicella infection. Prenat Diagn 16:71, 1996.
190. Lecuru F, Taurelle R, Bernard JP, et al: Varicella zoster virus infection during pregnancy: the limits of prenatal diagnosis. Eur J Obstet Gynecol Reprod Biol 56:67, 1994.
191. Pretorius DH, Hayward I, Jones KL, et al: Sonographic evaluation of pregnancies with maternal varicella infection. J Ultrasound Med 11:459, 1992.
192. Ockner R: Acute Viral Hepatitis. *In* Bennett J, Plum F (eds): Cecil Textbook of Medicine, 20th ed. Philadelphia, W. B. Saunders Company, 1996, p 762.
193. Shapiro CN, Coleman PJ, McQuillan GM, et al: Epidemiology of hepatitis A: seroepidemiology and risk groups in the USA. Vaccine 10 Suppl 1:S59, 1992.
194. ACOG educational bulletin. Viral hepatitis in pregnancy. Number 248, July 1998 (replaces No. 174, November 1992). American College of Obstetricians and Gynecologists. Int J Gynaecol Obstet 63:195, 1998.
195. Protection against viral hepatitis. Recommendations of the Immunization Practices Advisory Committee (ACIP). MMWR Recomm Rep 39:1, 1990.
196. Snydman DR: Hepatitis in pregnancy. N Engl J Med 313:1398, 1985.
197. Kao JH, Chen DS: Global control of hepatitis B virus infection. Lancet Infect Dis 2:395, 2002.
198. Hoofnagle J, Lindsay K: Acute viral hepatitis. *In* Goldman G, Ausiello D (eds): Cecil Textbook of Medicine, 22th ed. Philadelphia, W.B. Saunders Company, 2004, p 911.
199. Hepatitis B vaccination–United States, 1982–2002. MMWR Morb Mortal Wkly Rep 51:549, 2002.
200. Davies G, Wilson RD, Desilets V, et al: Amniocentesis and women with hepatitis B, hepatitis C, or human immunodeficiency virus. J Obstet Gynaecol Can 25:145, 2003.
201. Ko TM, Tseng LH, Chang MH, et al: Amniocentesis in mothers who are hepatitis B virus carriers does not expose the infant to an increased risk of hepatitis B virus infection. Arch Gynecol Obstet 255:25, 1994.
202. Minola E, Maccabruni A, Pacati I, et al: Amniocentesis as a possible risk factor for mother-to-infant transmission of hepatitis C virus. Hepatology 33:1341, 2001.
203. Hepatitis B virus: a comprehensive strategy for eliminating transmission in the United States through universal childhood vaccination. Recommendations of the Immunization Practices Advisory Committee (ACIP). MMWR Recomm Rep 40:1, 1991.
204. Hill JB, Sheffield JS, Kim MJ, et al: Risk of hepatitis B transmission in breast-fed infants of chronic hepatitis B carriers. Obstet Gynecol 99:1049, 2002.
205. Wang Z, Zhang J, Yang H, et al: Quantitative analysis of HBV DNA level and HBeAg titer in hepatitis B surface antigen positive mothers and their babies: HBeAg passage through the placenta and the rate of decay in babies. J Med Virol 71:360, 2003.
206. van Zonneveld M, van Nunen AB, Niesters HG, et al: Lamivudine treatment during pregnancy to prevent perinatal transmission of hepatitis B virus infection. J Viral Hepat 10:294, 2003.
207. Li XM, Shi MF, Yang YB, et al: Effect of hepatitis B immunoglobulin on interruption of HBV intrauterine infection. World J Gastroenterol 10:3215, 2004.
208. Osmond DH, Padian NS, Sheppard HW, et al: Risk factors for hepatitis C virus seropositivity in heterosexual couples. JAMA 269:361, 1993.
209. Recommendations for prevention and control of hepatitis C virus (HCV) infection and HCV-related chronic disease. Centers for Disease Control and Prevention. MMWR Recomm Rep 47:1, 1998.
210. Alter MJ, Kuhnert WL, Finelli L: Guidelines for laboratory testing and result reporting of antibody to hepatitis C virus. Centers for Disease Control and Prevention. MMWR Recomm Rep 52:1, 2003.
211. Alter HJ, Sanchez-Pescador R, Urdea MS, et al: Evaluation of branched DNA signal amplification for the detection of hepatitis C virus RNA. J Viral Hepat 2:121, 1995.
212. Jorgensen PA, Neuwald PD: Standardized hepatitis C virus RNA panels for nucleic acid testing assays. J Clin Virol 20:35, 2001.
213. Resti M, Azzari C, Galli L, et al: Maternal drug use is a preeminent risk factor for mother-to-child hepatitis C virus transmission: results from a multicenter study of 1372 mother-infant pairs. J Infect Dis 185:567, 2002.
214. Schuval S, Van Dyke RB, Lindsey JC, et al: Hepatitis C prevalence in children with perinatal human immunodeficiency virus infection enrolled in a long-term follow-up protocol. Arch Pediatr Adolesc Med 158:1007, 2004.

215. A significant sex—but not elective cesarean section—effect on mother-to-child transmission of hepatitis C virus infection. J Infect Dis 192:1872, 2005.
216. Purcell R, Gerin J: Hepatitis delta virus. *In* Fields B, Knipe P, Howley P, et al (eds): Fields Virology, 3rd ed. Philadelphia, Lippincott-Raven, 1996, Vol 1, p 2819.
217. Jacobson IM, Dienstag JL, Werner BG, et al: Epidemiology and clinical impact of hepatitis D virus (delta) infection. Hepatology 5:188, 1985.
218. Ramia S, Bahakim H: Perinatal transmission of hepatitis B virus-associated hepatitis D virus. Ann Inst Pasteur Virol 139:285, 1988.
219. Purcell R: Hepatitis E virus. *In* Fields B, Knipe P, Howley P, et al (eds): Fields Virology, 3rd ed. Philadelphia, Lippincott-Raven, 1996, Vol 1, p 2831.
220. Kumar A, Beniwal M, Kar P, et al: Hepatitis E in pregnancy. Int J Gynaecol Obstet 85:240, 2004.
221. Khuroo MS, Kamili S, Jameel S: Vertical transmission of hepatitis E virus. Lancet 345:1025, 1995.
222. Hayden F: Influenza. *In* Goldman G, Ausiello D (eds): Cecil Textbook of Medicine, 22th ed. Philadelphia, Elsevier, 2004, p 1995.
223. Goodnight WH, Soper DE: Pneumonia in pregnancy. Crit Care Med 33:S390, 2005.
224. ACOG committee opinion number 305, November 2004. Influenza vaccination and treatment during pregnancy. Obstet Gynecol 104:1125, 2004.
225. Influenza vaccination in pregnancy: practices among obstetrician-gynecologists–United States, 2003–04 influenza season. MMWR Morb Mortal Wkly Rep 54:1050, 2005.
226. Interim guidelines for the evaluation of infants born to mothers infected with West Nile virus during pregnancy. MMWR Morb Mortal Wkly Rep 53:154, 2004.
227. Bruno J, Rabito FJ, Jr., Dildy GA, 3rd: West Nile virus meningoencephalitis during pregnancy. J La State Med Soc 156:204, 2004.
228. Chapa JB, Ahn JT, DiGiovanni LM, et al: West Nile virus encephalitis during pregnancy. Obstet Gynecol 102:229, 2003.
229. Ornoy A, Tenenbaum A: Pregnancy outcome following infections by coxsackie, echo, measles, mumps, hepatitis, polio and encephalitis viruses. Reprod Toxicol 21:446, 2006.
230. O'Leary DR, Kuhn S, Kniss KL, et al: Birth outcomes following West Nile virus infection of pregnant women in the United States: 2003–2004. Pediatrics 117:e537, 2006.
231. Paisley JE, Hinckley AF, O'Leary DR, et al: West Nile virus infection among pregnant women in a northern Colorado community, 2003 to 2004. Pediatrics 117:814, 2006.
232. Archer JS: Acute liver failure in pregnancy. A case report. J Reprod Med 46:137, 2001.
233. Axelsson C, Bondestam K, Frisk G, et al: Coxsackie B virus infections in women with miscarriage. J Med Virol 39:282, 1993.
234. Dahlquist G, Frisk G, Ivarsson SA, et al: Indications that maternal coxsackie B virus infection during pregnancy is a risk factor for childhood-onset IDDM. Diabetologia 38:1371, 1995.
235. Dahlquist GG, Ivarsson S, Lindberg B, et al: Maternal enteroviral infection during pregnancy as a risk factor for childhood IDDM. A population-based case-control study. Diabetes 44:408, 1995.
236. Hyoty H, Taylor KW: The role of viruses in human diabetes. Diabetologia 45:1353, 2002.
237. Ho GY, Bierman R, Beardsley L, et al: Natural history of cervicovaginal papillomavirus infection in young women. N Engl J Med 338:423, 1998.
238. Worda C, Huber A, Hudelist G, et al: Prevalence of cervical and intrauterine human papillomavirus infection in the third trimester in asymptomatic women. J Soc Gynecol Investig 12:440, 2005.
239. Lacey CJ: Therapy for genital human papillomavirus-related disease. J Clin Virol 32 Suppl 1:S82, 2005.
240. Uberti-Foppa C, Origoni M, Maillard M, et al: Evaluation of the detection of human papillomavirus genotypes in cervical specimens by hybrid capture as screening for precancerous lesions in HIV-positive women. J Med Virol 56:133, 1998.
241. Kieff E: Infectious mononucleosis: Epstein-Barr virus infection. *In* Goldman G, Ausiello D (eds): Cecil Textbook of Medicine, 22th ed. Philadelphia, W.B. Saunders Company, 2004, p 1995.
242. Eskild A, Bruu AL, Stray-Pedersen B, et al: Epstein-Barr virus infection during pregnancy and the risk of adverse pregnancy outcome. BJOG 112:1620, 2005.
243. Lehtinen M, Koskela P, Ogmundsdottir HM, et al: Maternal herpesvirus infections and risk of acute lymphoblastic leukemia in the offspring. Am J Epidemiol 158:207, 2003.
244. Meyohas MC, Marechal V, Desire N, et al: Study of mother-to-child Epstein-Barr virus transmission by means of nested PCRs. J Virol 70:6816, 1996.
245. Suarez VR, Hankins GD: Smallpox and pregnancy: from eradicated disease to bioterrorist threat. Obstet Gynecol 100:87, 2002.
246. Women with smallpox vaccine exposure during pregnancy reported to the National Smallpox Vaccine in Pregnancy Registry–United States, 2003. MMWR Morb Mortal Wkly Rep 52:386, 2003.

Maternal and Perinatal Infection—Bacterial

PATRICK DUFF

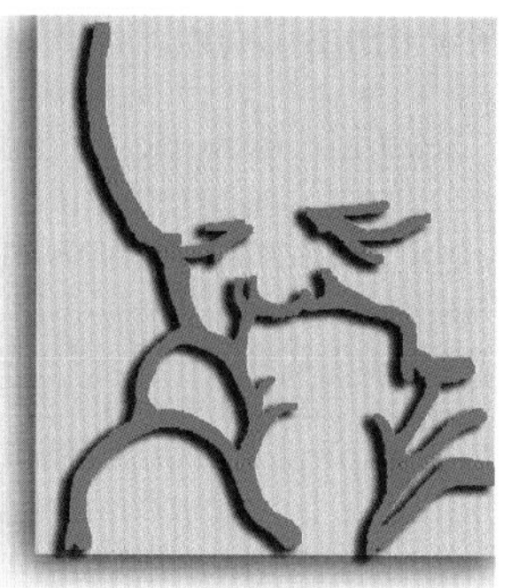

CHAPTER 49

KEY ABBREVIATIONS

Activated partial thromboplastin time	aPTT
Adult respiratory distress syndrome	ARDS
Centers for Disease Control and Prevention	CDC
Computerized tomography	CT
Group B streptococcus	GBS
Listeria monocytogenes	LM
Magnetic resonance imaging	MRI
Polymerase chain reaction	PCR
Premature rupture of the membranes	PROM

INTRODUCTION

Bacterial infections are the single most common complication encountered by the obstetrician. Some infections such as puerperal endometritis and lower urinary tract infection are of principal concern to the mother and pose little or no risk to the fetus or neonate. Others, such as group B streptococcal infection (GBS), pyelonephritis, and chorioamnionitis, may cause serious morbidity, even life-threatening complications, for both the mother and baby. The purpose of this chapter is to review in detail the major bacterial infections that the obstetrician confronts in clinical practice.

GROUP B STREPTOCOCCAL INFECTION

Epidemiology

Streptococcus agalactiae is a gram-positive encapsulated coccus that produces beta hemolysis when grown on blood agar. On average, approximately 20 to 25 percent of pregnant women harbor GBS in their lower genital tract and rectum. The GBS is one of the most important causes of early-onset neonatal infection. The prevalence of neonatal GBS infection now is approximately 0.5 per 1,000 live births, and approximately 10,000 cases of neonatal streptococcal septicemia occur each year in the United States.[1]

Neonatal GBS infection can be divided into *early-onset* and *late-onset* infection. Approximately 80 to 85 percent of cases of neonatal GBS infection are early in onset and result almost exclusively from vertical transmission from a colonized mother. Early-onset infection presents primarily as a severe pneumonia and overwhelming septicemia. In preterm infants, the mortality rate from early-onset GBS infection may approach 25 percent. In term infants, the mortality rate is lower, averaging approximately 5 percent.[1] Late-onset neonatal GBS infection occurs as a result of both vertical and horizontal transmission. It is typically manifested by bacteremia, meningitis, and pneumonia. The mortality rate from late-onset infection is approximately 5 percent for both preterm and term infants.[1]

Unfortunately, obstetric interventions have proven ineffective in preventing late-onset neonatal infection. Therefore, the remainder of this discussion focuses on early-onset infection. Major risk factors for early-onset infection include preterm labor, especially when complicated by preterm premature rupture of the membranes (PROM); intrapartum maternal fever (chorioamnionitis); prolonged rupture of membranes, defined as greater than 18 hours; previous delivery of an infected infant; young age; and black and Hispanic ethnicity.[1] Approximately 25 percent of pregnant women have at least one risk factor for GBS infection. The neonatal attack rate in colonized patients is 40 to 50 percent in the presence of a risk factor, and less than 5 percent in the absence of a risk factor. In infected infants, neonatal mortality approaches 30 to 35 percent when a maternal risk factor is present but is less than 5 percent when a risk factor is absent.[2,3]

Maternal Complications

Several obstetric complications occur with increased frequency in pregnant women who are colonized with GBS. The organism is one of the major causes of chorioamnionitis and postpartum endometritis. It also may cause postcesarean delivery wound infection, usually in conjunction with other aerobic and anaerobic bacilli and staphylococci. GBS also are responsible for approximately 2 to 3 percent of lower urinary tract infections in pregnant women.[1] GBS urinary tract infection, in turn, is a risk factor for preterm PROM and for preterm labor. Thomsen et al.[4] recently reported a study of 69 women at 27 to 31 weeks' gestation who had streptococcal urinary tract infections. Patients were assigned to treatment with either penicillin or placebo. Treated patients had a significant reduction in the frequency of both preterm PROM and preterm labor. Other investigations have confirmed the association between GBS colonization and preterm labor and preterm PROM. Women with the latter complication who are colonized with GBS tend to have a shorter latent period and higher frequency of chorioamnionitis and puerperal endometritis compared with noncolonized women.[5]

Diagnosis

The gold standard for the diagnosis of GBS infection is bacteriologic culture. Todd-Hewitt broth or selective blood agar is the preferred medium. Specimens for culture should be obtained from the lower vagina, perineum, and perianal area, using a simple cotton swab. In recent years, considerable research has been devoted to assessment of rapid diagnostic tests for the identification of colonized women. Table 49-1 summarizes the results of several investigations of rapid diagnostic tests. The information in this table is based upon the review by Yancey et al.[6] These authors noted that, although the rapid diagnostic tests had reasonable sensitivity in identifying heavily colonized patients, they had poor sensitivity in identifying lightly and moderately colonized patients.

Although the first generation of rapid diagnostic tests were not as valuable as originally hoped, Bergeron et al.[7] recently reported exceptionally favorable results with a new polymerase chain reaction (PCR) assay for GBS. In a series of 112 patients, the authors documented a sensitivity of 97 percent, specificity of 100 percent, positive predictive value of 100 percent, and negative predictive value of 99 percent. This PCR assay now is commercially available and offers clear promise as a rapid test for screening patients at the time of admission for labor.

Prevention of Group B Streptococcal Infection

In the past 20 years, several different strategies have been proposed for the prevention of neonatal GBS infection.[2,3,8–10] Each strategy has had major imperfections. In 1996, however, the Centers for Disease Control and Prevention (CDC) published a series of recommendations that incorporated the major advantages of previous protocols and minimized some of the more problematic aspects of selected strategies.[11] The initial CDC guidelines recommended either universal culturing of all patients at 35 to 37 weeks and intrapartum treatment of all colonized women or selective treatment on the basis of identified risk factors. Subsequently, in a large population-based survey, Rosenstein and Schuchat[12] assessed the theoretical impact of the CDC recommendations and showed that a strategy of universal culturing and treatment of *all* colonized patients would prevent 78 percent of cases of neonatal infection. In contrast, only 41 percent of cases were prevented when patients were targeted for prophylaxis only on the basis of risk factors. In addition, Locksmith et al.[13] confirmed that universal culturing also was of value in decreasing the rate of maternal infection compared with a strategy of only treating on the basis of risk factors.

In 2002, the CDC issued revised guidelines for prevention of early-onset GBS infection.[1] The new guidelines recommend universal cultures for all patients as the optimal method of prevention. Cultures should be performed at 35 to 37 weeks. All patients who test positive should receive intrapartum antibiotic prophylaxis with one of the regimens outlined in Table 49-2. Ideally, antibiotics should be administered at least 4 hours before delivery. DeCueto et al.[14] demonstrated that the rate of neonatal GBS infection was reduced significantly when patients were treated for at least this period of time.

Table 49-1. Reliability of Rapid Diagnostic Tests for Group B Streptococci

	TEST PERFORMANCE			
TEST	SENSITIVITY (%)	SPECIFICITY (%)	PV$^+$ (%)	PV$^-$ (%)
Gram stain	34–100	60–70	13–33	86–100
Growth in starch medium	93–98	98–99	65–98	89–99
Antigen detection (coagglutination, latex particle agglutination, enzyme immunoassay)	4–88*	92–100	15–100	76–99
DNA probe†	71	90	61	94

*Sensitivities for identification of heavily colonized women ranged from 29–100%.

†Specimens were grown in culture for 3.5 h before DNA probe was used.

Information in this table is based upon reference 6. PV$^-$, predictive value-negative; PV$^+$, predictive value-positive.

Table 49-2. Antibiotics with Activity Against Group B Streptococci

DRUG	DOSE FOR INTRAPARTUM PROPHYLAXIS
Ampicillin	2 grams initially, then 1 g Q4h
Pencillin	5 million units initially, then 2.5 million units Q4h
Cefazolin*	1 g Q8h
Clindamycin†	900 mg Q8h
Vancomycin†	1,000 mg Q12h

Recommendations based upon reference 1.

*Cefazolin should be used in patients who have a history of a non-life-threatening allergy to penicillin.

†Clindamycin or vancomycin should be used in patients who have a history of a life threatening allergy to penicillin. Clindamycin should be used only if sensitivity testing confirms that the organism is sensitive (up to 10% of strains of GBS may be resistant). Vancomycin should be used if the organism is resistant to clindamycin or sensitivity tests are not available.

The new CDC guidelines also addressed issues that previously had been imprecisely defined.[1] Colonized patients scheduled for an elective cesarean delivery do not require intrapartum prophylaxis. Patients who tested positive for GBS in a previous pregnancy should not be assumed to be colonized and should be retested in the present pregnancy. This recommendation is supported by a later report from Edwards et al.[15] These authors noted that only 59 percent of patients who were culture positive in a previous pregnancy were positive in the present pregnancy. Conversely, however, patients who have GBS bacteriuria in pregnancy, even if treated, should be considered heavily colonized and should be targeted for intrapartum prophylaxis. Moreover, patients who had a previous infant with GBS infection also should be considered colonized and treated during labor.

URINARY TRACT INFECTIONS

Acute Urethritis

Acute urethritis (acute urethral syndrome) usually is caused by one of three organisms: coliforms (principally *Escherichia coli*), *Neisseria gonorrhoeae*, and *Chlamydia trachomatis*. Coliform organisms are part of the normal vaginal and perineal flora, and may be introduced into the urethra during intercourse or when wiping after defecation. *N. gonorrhoeae* and *C. trachomatis* are sexually transmitted pathogens.[16]

Affected patients typically experience frequency, urgency, and dysuria. Hesitancy, dribbling, and a mucopurulent urethral discharge also may be present. On microscopic examination, the urine usually has white blood cells, but bacteria may not be consistently present. Urine cultures may have low colony counts of coliform organisms, and cultures of the urethral discharge may be positive for gonorrhea and chlamydia. A rapid diagnostic test, such as a nucleic acid probe, may be used in lieu of culture for these organisms.[16]

Most patients with acute urethritis warrant empiric treatment before the results of urine or urethral cultures are available. Infections caused by coliforms usually respond to the antibiotics described later for treatment of asymptomatic bacteriuria and cystitis. If gonococcal infection is suspected, the patient should be treated with intramuscular ceftriaxone (125 mg in a single dose).[17] If the patient is allergic to beta lactam antibiotics, an effective alternative is spectinomycin, administered intramuscularly in a single dose of 2 g. If chlamydial infection is suspected or confirmed, the patient should be treated with azithromycin powder (1,000 mg) in a single dose.[17]

Asymptomatic Bacteriuria and Acute Cystitis

The prevalence of asymptomatic bacteriuria in pregnancy is 5 to 10 percent, and the vast majority of cases antedate the onset of pregnancy. The frequency of acute cystitis in pregnancy is 1 to 3 percent. Some cases of cystitis arise de novo; others develop as a result of failure to identify and treat asymptomatic bacteriuria.[18]

E. coli is responsible for 80 to 90 percent of cases of *initial* infections and 70 to 80 percent of recurrent cases. *Klebsiella pneumoniae* and *Proteus* species also are important pathogens, particularly in patients who have a history of recurrent infection. Approximately 3 to 7 percent of infections are caused by gram-positive organisms such as GBS, enterococci, and staphylococci.[16,18]

All pregnant women should have a urine culture at their first prenatal appointment to detect preexisting asymptomatic bacteriuria. If the culture is negative, the likelihood of the patient subsequently developing an *asymptomatic* infection is less than 5 percent. If the culture is positive (defined as greater than 10^5 colonies/mL urine from a midstream, clean-catch specimen), prompt treatment is necessary to prevent ascending infection.

Patients with acute cystitis usually have symptoms of frequency, dysuria, urgency, suprapubic pain, hesitancy, and dribbling. Gross hematuria may be present, but high fever and systemic symptoms are uncommon. In symptomatic patients, the leukocyte esterase and nitrate tests are usually positive. When a urine culture is obtained, a catheterized sample is preferred because it minimizes the probability that urine will be contaminated by vaginal flora. With a catheterized specimen, a colony count greater than 10^2/mL is considered indicative of infection.[19]

Asymptomatic bacteriuria and acute cystitis characteristically respond well to short courses of oral antibiotics. Single-dose therapy is not as effective in pregnant women as in nonpregnant patients. However, a 3-day course of treatment appears to be comparable to a 7- to 10-day regimen for an initial infection.[16] The longer courses of therapy are most appropriate for patients with recurrent infections. Table 49-3 lists several antibiotics of value for treatment of asymptomatic bacteriuria and cystitis.

When sensitivity tests are available, for example, for patients with asymptomatic bacteriuria, they may be used

Table 49-3. Antibiotics for Treatment of Asymptomatic Bacteriuria and Acute Cystitis

DRUG	STRENGTH OF ACTIVITY	ORAL DOSE	RELATIVE COST
Amoxicillin	Some *E. coli,* most *Proteus* species, group B streptococci, enterococci, some staphylococci	875 mg bid	Low
Amoxicillin-clavulanic acid (Augmentin)	Most gram-negative aerobic bacilli and gram-positive cocci	875 mg bid	High
Ampicillin	Some *E. coli,* most *Proteus* species, group B streptococci, enterococci, some staphylococci	250 mg qid	Low
Cephalexin (Keflex)	Most *E. coli,* most *Klebsiella* and *Proteus* species, group B streptococci, staphylococci	250 mg qid	Low
Nitrofurantoin monohydrate macrocrystals–sustained release preparation (Macrobid)	Most uropathogens except enterococci and *Proteus* species	100 mg bid	Moderate
Sulfisoxazole (Gantrisin)	Most gram-negative aerobic bacilli	2 g × 1 dose, then 1 g qid	Low
Trimethoprim-sulfamethoxazole-double strength (Bactrim-DS, or Septra-DS)	Most uropathogens except some strains of *E. coli*	800 mg/160 mg bid	Low

bid, twice daily; qid, four times daily.
Modified from Duff P: Urinary tract infections. Prim Care Update Ob/Gyns 1:12, 1994, with permission.

to guide antibiotic selection. When empiric treatment is indicated, the choice of antibiotics must be based on established patterns of susceptibility. In recent years, 20 to 30 percent of strains of *E. coli* have developed resistance to ampicillin. Thus, this drug should not be used when the results of sensitivity tests are unknown unless the suspected pathogen is enterococci.[17,20]

When choosing among the drugs listed in Table 49-3, the clinician should consider the following factors. First, the sensitivity patterns of ampicillin, amoxicillin, and cephalexin are the most variable. Second, these drugs, along with amoxicillin-clavulanic acid, also have the most pronounced effect on normal bowel and vaginal flora and, thus, are the most likely to cause diarrhea or monilial vulvovaginitis. In contrast, nitrofurantoin monohydrate has only minimal effect on vaginal or bowel flora. Moreover, it is more uniformly effective against the common uropathogens, except for *Proteus* species, than trimethoprim-sulfamethoxazole. Third, amoxicillinclavulanic acid and trimethoprim-sulfamethoxazole usually are the best empiric agents for treatment of patients with suspected drug resistant pathogens.[21] In this situation, the latter drug offers a major cost advantage over the former. Finally, because of theoretical concerns about their effect on protein binding of bilirubin, sulfonamide drugs should be avoided near the time of delivery.

For patients who have an initial infection and experience a prompt response to treatment, a urine culture for test of cure is unnecessary.[16,21] Cultures during, or immediately after, treatment are indicated for patients who have a poor response to therapy or who have a history of recurrent infection. During subsequent clinic appointments, the patient's urine should be screened for nitrites and leukocyte esterase. If either of these tests is positive, repeat urine culture and retreatment are indicated.

Acute Pyelonephritis

The incidence of pyelonephritis in pregnancy is 1 to 2 percent.[18] The vast majority of cases develop as a consequence of undiagnosed or inadequately treated lower urinary tract infection. Two major physiologic changes occur during pregnancy that predispose to ascending infection of the urinary tract. First, the high concentration of progesterone secreted by the placenta has an inhibitory effect on ureteral peristalsis. Second, the enlarging gravid uterus often compresses the ureters, particularly the right, at the pelvic brim, thus creating additional stasis. Stasis, in turn, facilitates migration of bacteria from the bladder into the ureters and renal parenchyma (Fig. 49-1).

Approximately 75 to 80 percent of cases of pyelonephritis occur on the right side. Ten to 15 percent are left sided, and a slightly smaller percentage are bilateral.[18] *E. coli* is again the principal pathogen.[18,20] *Klebsiella pneumoniae* and *Proteus* species also are important causes of infection, particularly in women with recurrent episodes of pyelonephritis. Highly virulent gram-negative bacilli, such as *Pseudomonas*, *Enterobacter*, and *Serratia,* are unusual isolates except in immunocompromised patients. Gram-positive cocci do not usually cause upper tract infection. Anaerobes also are unlikely pathogens unless the patient is chronically obstructed or instrumented.

The usual clinical manifestations of acute pyelonephritis in pregnancy are fever, chills, flank pain and tenderness, frequency, urgency, hematuria, and dysuria. Patients also may have signs of preterm labor, septic shock, and adult respiratory distress syndrome (ARDS). Urinalysis usually is positive for white cell casts, red blood cells, and bacteria. Urine colony counts greater than 10^2 colonies/ml, in samples collected by catheterization, confirm the diagnosis of infection.

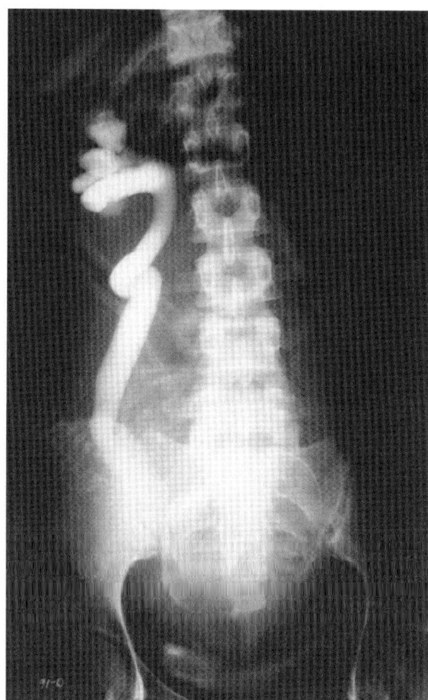

Figure 49-1. Intravenous pyelogram in a pregnant woman shows marked dilation of the right ureter and mild dilation of renal collecting system.

Pregnant patients with pyelonephritis may be considered for outpatient therapy if their disease manifestations are mild, they are hemodynamically stable, and they have no evidence of preterm labor.[22] If an outpatient approach is adopted, the patient should be treated with agents that have a high level of activity against the common uropathogens. Acceptable oral agents include amoxicillin-clavulanic acid, 875 mg twice daily, or trimethoprim-sulfamethoxazole-DS, twice daily for 7 to 10 days. Alternatively, a visiting home nurse may be contracted to administer a parenteral agent, such as ceftriaxone, 2 g intramuscularly or intravenously, once daily. Although an excellent drug for lower tract infections, nitrofurantoin monohydrate does not consistently achieve the serum and renal parenchymal concentrations necessary for successful treatment of more serious infections.

Pregnant patients who appear to be moderately to severely ill or who show any signs of preterm labor should be hospitalized for intravenous antibiotic therapy. They should receive appropriate supportive treatment and be monitored closely for complications such as sepsis, ARDS, and preterm labor. One of the best choices for empiric intravenous antibiotic therapy is cefazolin, 1 g every 8 hours.[17,20] For hospitalized patients, this drug is less expensive to administer than the newer broader spectrum cephalosporins or penicillins and has an equivalent spectrum of activity against the coliform organisms most likely to be responsible for infection. If the patient is critically ill or is at high risk for a resistant organism, a second antibiotic, such as gentamicin (1.5 mg/kg every 8 hours) or aztreonam (500 mg to 1 g every 8 to 12 hours) should be administered, along with cefazolin, until the results of susceptibility tests are available.[17]

Once antibiotic therapy is initiated, approximately 75 percent of patients defervesce within 48 hours. By the end of 72 hours, almost 95 percent of patients are afebrile and asymptomatic.[18] The two most likely causes of treatment failure are a resistant microorganism or obstruction. The latter condition is best diagnosed with computed tomography (CT) scan or renal ultrasonography and typically results from a stone or physical compression of the ureter by the gravid uterus.

Once the patient has begun to defervesce and her clinical examination has improved, she may be discharged from the hospital. Oral antibiotics should be prescribed to complete a total of 7 to 10 days of therapy. Selection of a specific oral agent should be based on considerations of efficacy, toxicity, and expense.

Approximately 20 to 30 percent of pregnant patients with acute pyelonephritis develop a recurrent urinary tract infection later in pregnancy. The most cost-effective way to reduce the frequency of recurrence is to administer a daily prophylactic dose of an antibiotic, such as sulfisoxazole, 1 g, or nitrofurantoin monohydrate macrocrystals, 100 mg. Patients receiving prophylaxis should have their urine screened for bacteria at each subsequent clinic appointment. They also should be questioned about recurrence of symptoms. If symptoms recur, or the dipstick test for nitrite or leukocyte esterase is positive, a urine culture should be obtained to determine if retreatment is necessary.

UPPER GENITAL TRACT INFECTIONS

Chorioamnionitis

Epidemiology

Chorioamnionitis (amnionitis, intraamniotic infection) occurs in approximately 1 to 5 percent of term pregnancies.[23] In patients with preterm delivery, the frequency of clinical or subclinical infection may approach 25 percent.[24] Although chorioamnionitis may result from hematogenous dissemination of microorganisms, it more commonly is an ascending infection caused by organisms that are part of the normal vaginal flora. The principal pathogens are *Bacteroides* and *Prevotella* species, *E. coli*, anaerobic streptococci, and GBS. Several clinical risk factors for chorioamnionitis have been identified. The most important are young age, low socioeconomic status, nulliparity, extended duration of labor and ruptured membranes, multiple vaginal examinations, and preexisting infections of the lower genital tract.[23]

Diagnosis

In most situations, the diagnosis of chorioamnionitis can be established on the basis of the clinical findings of maternal fever and maternal and fetal tachycardia, in the absence of other localizing signs of infection. In more severely ill patients, uterine tenderness and purulent amniotic fluid may be present. The disorders that should be considered in the differential diagnosis of chorioamnionitis include respiratory tract infection, pyelonephritis, viral syndrome, and appendicitis.[23]

Table 49-4. Diagnostic Tests for Chorioamnionitis

TEST	ABNORMAL FINDING	COMMENT
Maternal white blood cell count (WBC)	≥15,000 cells/mm^3 with preponderance of leukocytes	Labor and/or corticosteroids also may result in elevation of WBC
Amniotic fluid glucose	≤10 to 15 mg	Excellent correlation with positive amniotic fluid culture and clinical infection
Amniotic fluid interleukin-6	≥7.9 ng/mL	Excellent correlation with positive amniotic fluid culture and clinical infection
Amniotic fluid leukocyte esterase	≥1$^+$ reaction	Good correlation with positive amniotic fluid culture and clinical infection
Amniotic fluid gram stain	Any organism in an oil immersion field	Allows identification of particularly virulent organism such as group B streptococci. However, the test is very sensitive to inoculum effect. In addition, it cannot identify pathogens such as mycoplasmas.
Amniotic fluid culture	Growth of aerobic or anaerobic microorganism	Results are not immediately available for clinical management
Blood cultures	Growth of aerobic or anaerobic microorganism	Will be positive in 5–10% of patients. However, will usually not be of value in making clinical decisions unless patient is at increased risk for bacterial endocarditis, is immunocompromised, or has a poor response to initial treatment.

Laboratory confirmation of the diagnosis of chorioamnionitis is not routinely necessary in term patients who are progressing to delivery. However, in preterm patients who are being evaluated for tocolysis or corticosteroids, laboratory assessment may be of value in excluding or establishing the diagnosis of intrauterine infection. In this clinical context, amniotic fluid should be obtained by transabdominal amniocentesis. Table 49-4 summarizes the abnormal laboratory findings that may be present in infected patients.[23–28]

MANAGEMENT

Both the mother and infant may experience serious complications when chorioamnionitis is present. Bacteremia occurs in 3 to 12 percent of infected women. When cesarean delivery is required, up to 8 percent of women develop a wound infection, and approximately 1 percent develop a pelvic abscess. Fortunately, maternal death due to infection is exceedingly rare.[23]

Five to 10 percent of neonates delivered to mothers with chorioamnionitis have pneumonia or bacteremia. The predominant organisms responsible for these infections are GBS and *E. coli*. Meningitis occurs in less than 1 percent of term infants and in a slightly higher percentage of preterm infants. Mortality due to infection ranges from 1 to 4 percent in term neonates but may approach 15 percent in preterm infants because of the confounding effects of other complications such as hyaline membrane disease and intraventricular hemorrhage.[23]

In order to prevent maternal and neonatal complications, parenteral antibiotic therapy should be initiated as soon as the diagnosis of chorioamnionitis is made, unless delivery is imminent. Three separate investigations have demonstrated that mother-infant pairs who receive prompt intrapartum treatment have better outcomes than patients treated after delivery.[29–31] The principal benefits of early treatment include decreased frequency of neonatal bacteremia and pneumonia, and decreased duration of maternal fever and hospitalization.

The most extensively tested intravenous antibiotic regimen for treatment of chorioamnionitis is the combination of ampicillin (2 g every 6 hours) or penicillin (5 million units every 6 hours) plus gentamicin (1.5 mg/kg every 8 hours).[17,23] These antibiotics specifically target the two organisms most likely to cause neonatal infection: GBS and *E. coli*. With rare exceptions, gentamicin is preferred to tobramycin or amikacin because it is available in an inexpensive generic formulation. Amikacin should be reserved for immunocompromised patients who are particularly likely to be infected by highly virulent, drug-resistant aerobic gram-negative bacilli. In patients who are allergic to beta-lactam antibiotics, clindamycin (900 mg every 8 hours) should be substituted for ampicillin.

If a patient with chorioamnionitis requires cesarean delivery, a drug with activity against anaerobic organisms should be added to the antibiotic regimen. Either clindamycin (900 mg every 8 hours) or metronidazole (500 mg every 12 hours) is an excellent choice for this purpose. Failure to provide effective coverage of anaerobes may result in treatment failures in 20 to 30 percent of patients.[17]

Extended-spectrum cephalosporins, penicillins, and carbapenems also provide excellent coverage against the bacteria that cause chorioamnionitis. Dosages and dose intervals for several of these agents are listed in Table 49-5.[17] As a general rule, these drugs are more expensive than the generic combination regimens outlined above.

Antibiotics usually can be discontinued soon after delivery. Edwards and Duff[32] recently reported a randomized clinical trial in which patients were treated intrapartum with ampicillin plus gentamicin. In one group of patients, treatment was discontinued after the first postpartum dose. In the second group, patients were treated until they had been afebrile and asymptomatic for 24 hours. Patients in both groups received at least one dose of clindamycin if they delivered by cesarean. There were no

Table 49-5. Single Agents of Value in Treatment of Chorioamnionitis and Puerperal Endometritis

DRUG	DOSAGE AND DOSE INTERVAL	RELATIVE COST TO THE PHARMACY*
Extended Spectrum Cephalosporins		
Cefotaxime	2 g Q8–12h	Intermediate
Cefotetan	2 g Q12h	Low
Cefoxitin	2 g Q6h	High
Ceftizoxime	2 g Q12h	Intermediate
Extended Spectrum Penicillins		
Ampicillin-sulbactam	3 g Q6h	Low
Mezlocillin	3–4 g Q6h	Intermediate
Piperacillin	3–4 g Q6h	Intermediate
Piperacillin-tazobactam	3.375 g Q6h	Intermediate
Ticarcillin-clavulanic acid	3.1 g Q6h	Low
Carbapenem		
Ertapenem	1 g Q24h	High
Imipenem-cilastatin	500 mg Q6h	High
Meropenem	1 g Q8h	High

*Cost estimates do not include dose preparation fees and administration charges.

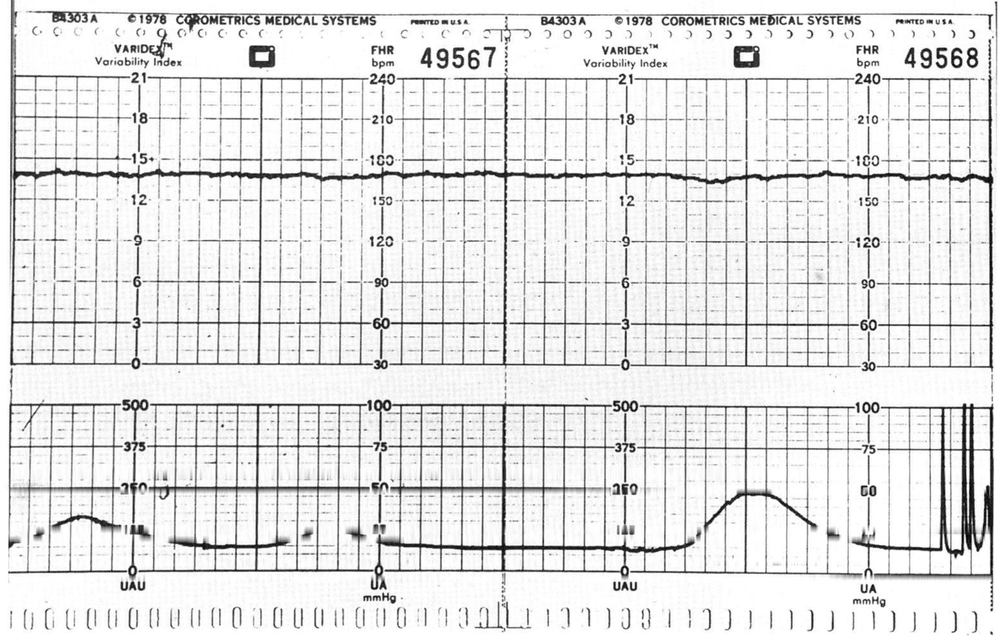

Figure 49-2. Fetal heart tracing from a patient with chorioamnionitis. Note the tachycardia of 170 bpm and the decrease in both short- and long-term variability.

significant differences in treatment outcome in the two groups.

Patients with chorioamnionitis are at increased risk for dysfunctional labor. Approximately 75 percent require oxytocin for augmentation of labor, and up to 30 to 40 percent require cesarean delivery, usually for failure to progress in labor. Although chorioamnionitis by itself should not be regarded as an indication for cesarean delivery, affected patients need close monitoring during labor to esure that uterine contractility is optimized. In addition, the fetus also needs close surveillance. Fetal heart rate abnormalities such as tachycardia and decreased variability (Fig. 49-2) occur in more than three fourths of cases, and additional tests such as vibroacoustic stimulation or scalp stimulation may be necessary to evaluate fetal well-being.[33]

Puerperal Endometritis

EPIDEMIOLOGY

The frequency of puerperal endometritis in women having vaginal delivery is approximately 1 to 3 percent. In women having a scheduled cesarean delivery before the onset of labor and rupture of membranes, the frequency of endometritis ranges from 5 to 15 percent. When cesarean delivery is performed after an extended period of labor and ruptured membranes, the incidence of infection is 30 to 35 percent without antibiotic prophylaxis and 15 to 20 percent with prophylaxis. In highly indigent patient populations, the frequency of infection may be even higher.[34]

Endometritis is a polymicrobial infection caused by microorganisms that are part of the normal vaginal flora. These bacteria gain access to the upper genital tract, peritoneal cavity, and occasionally, the bloodstream as a result of vaginal examinations during labor and manipulations during surgery. The most common pathogens are GBS, anaerobic streptococci, aerobic gram-negative bacilli (predominantly *E. coli, Klebsiella pneumoniae,* and *Proteus* species), and anaerobic gram negative bacilli (principally *Bacteroides* and *Prevotella* species). *C. trachomatis* is not a common cause of early-onset puerperal endometritis but has been implicated in late-onset infection. The genital mycoplasmas may be pathogens in some patients, but they usually are present in association with more highly virulent bacteria.[34]

The principal risk factors for endometritis are cesarean delivery, young age, low socioeconomic status, extended duration of labor and ruptured membranes, and multiple vaginal examinations. In addition, preexisting infection or colonization of the lower genital tract (gonorrhea, GBS, bacterial vaginosis) also predisposes to ascending infection.

Clinical Presentation and Diagnosis

Affected patients typically have a fever of 38°C or higher within 36 hours of delivery. Associated findings include malaise, tachycardia, lower abdominal pain and tenderness, uterine tenderness, and discolored, malodorous lochia. A small number of patients also may have a tender, indurated inflammatory mass in the broad ligament, posterior cul de sac, or retrovesical space.

The initial differential diagnosis of puerperal fever should include endometritis, atelectasis, pneumonia, viral syndrome, pyelonephritis, and appendicitis. Distinction among these disorders usually can be made on the basis of physical examination and a limited number of laboratory tests such as white blood cell count, urinalysis and culture, and in select patients, chest radiograph. Blood cultures are indicated in patients who have a poor initial response to therapy and in those who are immunocompromised or at increased risk for bacterial endocarditis.

Management

Patients who have mild to moderately severe infections, particularly after vaginal delivery, can be treated with short intravenous courses of single agents such as the extended-spectrum cephalosporins and penicillins or carbapenem antibiotics such as imipenem-cilastatin, meropenem, and ertapenem. Table 49-5 lists several antibiotics that have acceptable breadth of coverage against the polymicrobial genital tract flora. Combination antibiotic regimens should be considered for more severely ill patients, particularly those who are indigent and in poor general health and those who have had cesarean deliveries. Table 49-6 lists several antibiotic combinations of proven value in treatment of puerperal endometritis.[17]

Once antibiotics are begun, approximately 90 percent of patients defervesce within 48 to 72 hours. When the patient has been afebrile and asymptomatic for approximately 24 hours, parenteral antibiotics should be discontinued, and the patient should be discharged. As a general rule, an extended course of oral antibiotics is not necessary following discharge.[17,35] There are at least two notable exceptions to this rule. First, patients who have had a vaginal delivery and who defervesce within 24 hours are candidates for early discharge. In these individuals, a short course of an oral antibiotic such as amoxicillin-clavulanate (875 mg Q12h) may be substituted for continued parenteral therapy. Second, patients who have had staphylococcal bacteremia may require a more extended period of administration of parenteral and oral antibiotics with specific antistaphylococcal activity.[36]

Patients who fail to respond to the antibiotic therapy outlined earlier usually have one of two problems. The first is a resistant organism. Table 49-7 lists possible weaknesses in coverage of selected antibiotics and indicates the appropriate change in treatment. The second

Table 49-6. Combination Antibiotic Regimens for Treament of Puerperal Endometritis

ANTIBIOTICS	INTRAVENOUS DOSE	RELATIVE COST TO THE PHARMACY*
Regimen 1		
Clindamycin	900 mg Q8h	Intermediate
Gentamicin	1.5 mg/kg Q8h or 7 mg/kg ideal body weight Q24h†	Low
Regimen 2		
Clindamycin	900 mg Q8h	Intermediate
Aztreonam	1–2 g Q8h	High
Regimen 3		
Metronidazole	500 mg Q12h	Low
Penicillin	5 million units Q6h	Low
or		
Ampicillin	2 g Q6h	Low
Gentamicin	1.5 mg/kg Q8h or 7 mg/kg ideal body weight Q24h†	Low

*Cost estimate does not include dose preparation fees and administration charges.

†Single daily dosing of aminoglycoside antibiotics is more effective and less expensive than multidose treatment. In addition, it is less likely to cause toxicity. At present, there is little information concerning the effects of single large doses of aminoglycosides on the developing fetus. Therefore, this regimen should be reserved for postpartum patients.

Table 49-7. Treatment of Resistant Microorganisms in Patients with Puerperal Endometritis

INITIAL ANTIBIOTIC(S)	PRINCIPAL WEAKNESS IN COVERAGE	MODIFICATION OF THERAPY
Extended spectrum cephalosporins	Some aerobic and anaerobic gram negative bacilli Enterococci	Change treatment to clindamycin or metronidazole plus penicillin or ampicillin plus gentamicin
Extended-spectrum penicillins	Some aerobic and anaerobic gram-negative bacilli	As above
Clindamycin plus gentamicin or aztreonam	Enterococci Some anaerobic gram-negative bacilli	Add ampicillin or penicillin* Consider substitution of metronidazole for clindamycin

*Ampicillin alone is highly active against enterococci.
Penicillin *plus* gentamicin work synergistically to provide excellent coverage against this organism.

Table 49-8. Differential Diagnosis of Persistent Puerperal Fever

CONDITION	DIAGNOSTIC TEST(S)	TREATMENT
Resistant microorganism	Blood culture	Combination antibiotics to cover all possible pelvic pathogens
Wound infection	Physical examination Needle aspiration Ultrasound	Incision and drainage Add antibiotic to cover staphylococci
Pelvic abscess	Physical examination Ultrasound CT MRI	Drainage Combination antibiotics to cover all possible pelvic pathogens
Septic pelvic vein thrombophlebitis	Ultrasound CT MRI	Heparin anticoagulation Combination antibiotics to cover all possible pelvic pathogens
Recrudescence of connective tissue disease	Serology	Corticosteroids
Drug fever	Inspection of temperature graph WBC—identify eosinophilia	Discontinue antibiotics
Mastitis	Physical examination	Add antibiotic to cover staphylococci

CT, computed tomography; MRI, magnetic resonance imaging; WBC, white blood cells.

major cause of treatment failure is a wound infection. Infected wounds should be opened completely to provide drainage. If extensive cellulitis at the margin of the incision is present, an antibiotic with specific coverage against staphylococci, such as nafcillin (2 g IV Q6h), should be added to the treatment regimen.[17]

When changes in antibiotic therapy do not result in clinical improvement and no evidence of wound infection is present, several unusual disorders should be considered. The differential diagnosis of persistent puerperal fever is summarized in Table 49-8.[34]

Prevention of Puerperal Endometritis

Prophylactic antibiotics clearly are of value in reducing the frequency of postcesarean delivery endometritis, particularly in women having surgery after an extended period of labor and ruptured membranes.[37] The most appropriate agent for prophylaxis is a limited spectrum (first-generation) cephalosporin, such as cefazolin. Cefazolin should be administered in an intravenous dose of 1 g immediately after the neonate's umbilical cord is clamped. A second dose is indicated approximately 8 hours after the first dose in high-risk patients, especially when operating time is prolonged beyond 1 hour. Although extended-spectrum penicillins and cephalosporins are effective for prophylaxis, they offer no advantage over cefazolin and are several-fold more expensive. Moreover, widespread use of these drugs for prophylaxis ultimately may limit their usefulness for treatment of established infections.[37]

Patients who have an immediate hypersensitivity to beta-lactam antibiotics pose a special problem. The best alternative is to administer a single dose of clindamycin (900 mg) plus gentamicin (1.5 mg/kg), immediately after the cord is clamped. Although these antibiotics commonly are used for treatment of overt infections, their administration still is warranted in penicillin-allergic patients who are at high risk for postoperative infection.[17]

Serious Sequelae of Puerperal Infection

Wound Infection

Wound infection after cesarean delivery usually occurs in association with endometritis, rarely as an isolated infection. Approximately 3 to 5 percent of patients with endometritis have a concurrent wound infection.[13] The major risk factors for wound infection are listed in Table 49-9. The principal causative organisms are *Staphylococcus aureus*, aerobic streptococci, and aerobic and anaerobic bacilli.[38]

The diagnosis of wound infection always should be considered in patients who have a poor clinical response to antibiotic therapy for endometritis. Clinical examination characteristically shows erythema, induration, and tenderness at the margins of the abdominal incision. When the wound is probed with either a cotton tipped applicator or fine needle, pus usually exudes. Some patients, however, may have an extensive cellulitis without harboring frank pus in the incision. Clinical examination should be sufficient to establish the correct diagnosis. Gram's stain and culture of the wound exudate are not routinely needed because the results of these tests rarely influence selection of antibiotics or duration of antibiotic treatment.

When pus is present in the incision, the wound must be opened and drained completely. Antibiotic therapy should be modified to provide coverage against staphylococci because some regimens for endometritis may not specifically target this organism. Nafcillin, 2 grams intravenously every 6 hours, would be a suitable drug for this purpose. In a patient who is allergic to beta-lactam antibiotics, vancomycin, 1 g intravenously every 12 hours, is an acceptable alternative.[17]

Once the wound is opened, a careful inspection should be made to be certain that the fascial layer is intact. If it is disrupted, surgical intervention is necessary to reapproximate the fascia. Otherwise, the wound should be irrigated two to three times daily with a solution such as warm saline, a clean dressing should be applied, and the incision should be allowed to heal by secondary intention. Antibiotics should be continued until the base of the wound is clean and all signs of cellulitis have resolved. Patients usually can be treated at home once the acute signs of infection have subsided.

Necrotizing fasciitis is an uncommon, but extremely serious, complication of abdominal wound infection.[39] It also has been reported in association with infection of the episiotomy site.[40] This condition is most likely to occur in patients with type 1 diabetes mellitus, cancer, or an immunodeficiency disorder. Multiple bacterial pathogens, particularly anaerobes, have been isolated from patients with necrotizing fasciitis.

Necrotizing fasciitis should be suspected when the margins of the wound become discolored, cyanotic, and devoid of sensation. When the wound is opened, the subcutaneous tissue is easily dissected free of the underlying fascia, but muscle tissue is not affected. If the diagnosis is uncertain, a tissue biopsy should be performed and examined by frozen section.

Necrotizing fasciitis is a life-threatening condition and requires aggressive medical and surgical management. Broad spectrum antibiotics with activity against all potential aerobic and anaerobic pathogens should be administered. Intravascular volume should be maintained with infusions of crystalloid, and electrolyte abnormalities should be corrected. Finally, and most importantly, the wound must be debrided and all necrotic tissue removed. In many instances, the required dissection is extensive and may best be managed in consultation with an experienced general or plastic surgeon.

Table 49-9. Principal Risk Factors for Postcesarean Wound Infection

Poor surgical technique
Low socioeconomic status
Extended duration of labor and ruptured membranes
Preexisting infection such as chorioamnionitis
Obesity
Type 1 diabetes mellitus
Immunodeficiency disorder
Corticosteroid therapy
Immunosuppressive therapy

Pelvic Abscess

With the advent of modern antibiotics, pelvic abscesses after cesarean or vaginal delivery have become extremely rare. Less than 1 percent of patients with puerperal endometritis develop a pelvic abscess.[34] When present, abscesses typically are located in the anterior or posterior cul de sac, most commonly the latter, or within the broad ligament. The usual bacteria isolated from abscess cavities are coliforms and anaerobic gram-negative bacilli, particularly *Bacteroides* and *Prevotella* species.[41]

Patients with an abscess typically experience persistent fever despite initial therapy for endometritis. In addition, they usually have malaise, tachycardia, lower abdominal pain and tenderness, and a palpable pelvic mass anterior, posterior, or lateral to the uterus. The peripheral white blood cell count usually is elevated, and there is a shift toward immature cell forms. Ultrasound, CT scan, and magnetic resonance imaging (MRI) may be used to confirm the diagnosis of pelvic abscess.[42] Although CT and MRI may be slightly more sensitive, ultrasound offers the advantages of decreased expense and ready availability.

Patients with a pelvic abscess require surgical intervention to drain the purulent collection. When the abscess is in the posterior cul de sac, colpotomy drainage may be possible. For abscesses located anterior or lateral to the uterus, drainage may be accomplished by CT- or ultrasound-guided placement of a catheter drain.[43] When access is limited or the abscess is extensive, open laparotomy is indicated.

Patients with a pelvic abscess must receive antibiotics with excellent activity against coliform organisms and anaerobes.[17,41] One regimen that has been tested extensively in obstetric patients with serious infections is the combination of penicillin (5 million units IV every 6 hours) or ampicillin (2 g IV every 6 hours) plus gentamicin (1.5 mg/kg IV every 8 hours or 7 mg/kg of ideal body weight every 24 hours) plus clindamycin (900 mg IV every 8 hours) or metronidazole (500 mg IV every 12 hours). If a patient is allergic to beta-lactam antibiotics, vancomycin (500 mg IV every 6 hours or 1 g IV every 12 hours) can be substituted for penicillin or ampicillin. Aztreonam (1 g IV every 8 hours) can be used in lieu of gentamicin when the patient is at risk for nephrotoxicity. Alternatively, the single agents imipenem-cilastatin (500 mg IV every 6 hours), meropenem (1 g every 8 hours), or ertapenem (1 g every 24 hours) provide excellent coverage against the usual pathogens responsible for an abscess. Antibiotics should be continued until the patient has been afebrile and asymptomatic for a minimum of 24 to 48 hours.

Septic Pelvic Thrombophlebitis

Like pelvic abscess, septic pelvic thrombophlebitis is extremely rare, occurring in 1:2,000 pregnancies overall and in less than 1 percent of patients who have puerperal endometritis.[44] Intrauterine infection may cause seeding of pathogenic microorganisms into the venous circulation; in turn, these organisms may damage the vascular endothelium and initiate thrombosis.

Septic pelvic thrombophlebitis occurs in two distinct forms.[44] The most commonly described disorder is acute thrombosis of one (usually the right), or both, ovarian veins *(ovarian vein syndrome)*.[45] Affected patients typically develop a moderate temperature elevation in association with lower abdominal pain in the first 48 to 96 hours postpartum. Pain usually localizes to the side of the affected vein but may radiate into the groin, upper abdomen, or flank. Nausea, vomiting, and abdominal bloating may be present.

On physical examination, the patient's pulse usually is elevated. Tachypnea, stridor, and dyspnea may be evident if pulmonary embolization has occurred. The abdomen is tender, and bowel sounds often are decreased or absent. Most patients demonstrate voluntary and involuntary guarding, and 50 to 70 percent have a tender, ropelike mass originating near one cornua and extending laterally and cephalad toward the upper abdomen. The principal conditions that should be considered in the differential diagnosis of ovarian vein syndrome are pyelonephritis, nephrolithiasis, appendicitis, broad ligament hematoma, adnexal torsion, and pelvic abscess.

The second presentation of septic pelvic vein thrombophlebitis is termed *enigmatic fever*.[46] Initially, affected patients have clinical findings suggestive of endometritis and receive systemic antibiotics. Subsequently, they experience subjective improvement, with the exception of temperature instability. They do not appear to be seriously ill, and positive findings are limited to persistent fever and tachycardia. Disorders that should be considered in the differential diagnosis of enigmatic fever are drug fever, viral syndrome, collagen vascular disease, and pelvic abscess.

The diagnostic tests of greatest value in evaluating patients with suspected septic pelvic vein thrombophlebitis are CT scan and MRI (Fig. 49-3).[47] These tests are

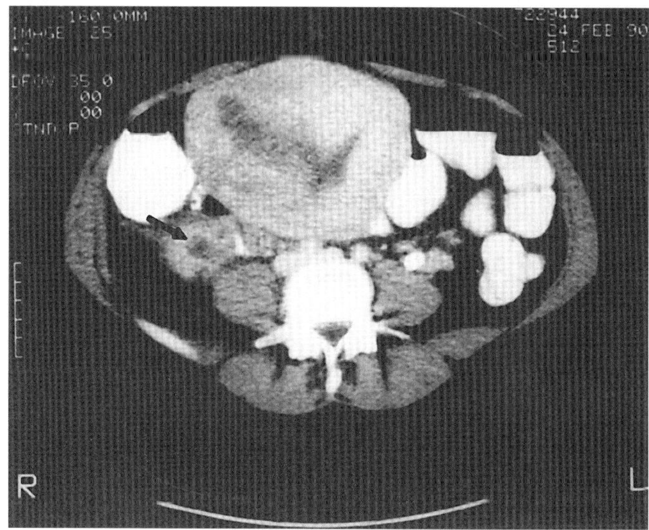

Figure 49-3. CT scan shows a thrombus *(arrow)* in right ovarian vein.

most sensitive in detecting large thrombi in the major pelvic vessels. They are not as useful in identifying thrombi in smaller vessels. In such cases, the ultimate diagnosis may depend upon the patient's response to an empiric trial of heparin.[44,48]

Patients with septic pelvic vein thrombophlebitis should be treated with therapeutic doses of intravenous heparin. The dose of heparin should be adjusted to maintain the activated partial thromboplastin time (aPTT) at approximately 2 times normal or to achieve a serum heparin concentration of 0.2 to 0.7 IU/ml. Therapy should be continued for 7 to 10 days. Long-term anticoagulation with oral agents probably is unnecessary unless the patient has massive clotting throughout the pelvic venous plexus or has sustained a pulmonary embolism. Patients should be maintained on broad-spectrum antibiotics throughout the period of heparin administration.

Once medical therapy is initiated, the patient should have objective evidence of a response within 48 to 72 hours. If no improvement is noted, surgical intervention may be necessary.[44,48] The decision to perform surgery should be based on clinical assessment and the relative certainty of the diagnosis. The surgical approach, in turn, should be tailored to the specific intraoperative findings. In most instances, treatment requires only ligation of the affected vessels. Extension of the thrombosis along the vena cava to the point of origin of the renal veins may necessitate embolectomy. Excision of the infected vessel and removal of the ipsilateral adnexa and uterus is indicated only in the presence of a well-defined abscess. Whenever any of the above-mentioned procedures are being considered, consultation with an experienced vascular surgeon is imperative.

Septic Shock

Septic shock in obstetric patients usually is associated with four specific infections: septic abortion, acute pyelonephritis, and severe chorioamnionitis or endometritis.

Fortunately, fewer than 5 percent of patients with any of these infections develop septic shock. The most common organisms responsible for septic shock are the aerobic gram-negative bacilli, principally *E. coli, Klebsiella pneumoniae*, and *Proteus* species. Highly virulent, drug-resistant coliforms such as *Pseudomonas, Enterobacter*, and *Serratia* species are uncommon except in immunosuppressed patients.[49]

Aerobic gram-negative bacilli have a complex lipopolysaccharide in their cell wall, which is termed *endotoxin*. When released into the systemic circulation, endotoxin is capable of causing a variety of immunologic, hematologic, neurohormonal, and hemodynamic derangements that ultimately result in multiorgan dysfunction.

In the early stages of septic shock, patients usually are restless, disoriented, tachycardic, and hypotensive. Although hypothermia is occasionally present, most patients have a relatively high fever (39 to 40°C). Their skin may be warm and flushed owing to an initial phase of vasodilation (*warm shock*). Subsequently, as extensive vasoconstriction occurs, the skin becomes cool and clammy. Cardiac arrhythmias may be present, and signs of myocardial ischemia may occur. Jaundice, often due to hemolysis, may be evident. Urinary output typically decreases, and frank anuria may develop. Spontaneous bleeding from the genitourinary tract or venipuncture sites may occur as a result of disseminated intramuscular coagulation. ARDS is a common complication of severe sepsis and is associated with manifestations such as dyspnea, stridor, cough, tachypnea, and bilateral rales and wheezing.[50] In addition to these systemic signs and symptoms, affected patients also may have findings related to their primary site of infection such as purulent lochia, uterine tenderness, peritonitis, or flank tenderness.

The differential diagnosis of septic shock in obstetric patients includes hypovolemic and cardiogenic shock, diabetic ketoacidosis, an anaphylactic reaction, an anesthetic reaction, and amniotic fluid or venous embolism. Distinction among these disorders usually can be made on the basis of a thorough history and physical examination, and a limited number of laboratory studies. The white blood cell count initially may be decreased but, subsequently, is elevated in the majority of patients. A large percentage of bands is usually evident. The hematocrit may be decreased if blood loss has occurred. Tests of coagulation such as platelet count, serum fibrinogen concentration, serum concentration of fibrin degradation products, prothrombin time, and aPTT are frequently abnormal. Serum concentrations of the transaminase enzymes and bilirubin often are increased. Similarly, increased concentrations of blood urea nitrogen and creatinine reflect deterioration of renal function. Chest radiograph in patients with septic shock is indicated to determine if pneumonia or ARDS is present. In addition, CT scan, MRI, and ultrasound may be of value in localizing an abscess.[42] Affected patients also require electrocardiographic monitoring to detect arrhythmias or signs of ischemic injury.

The first goal of treatment of septic shock is to correct the hemodynamic derangements precipitated by endotoxin. Two large-bore intravenous catheters and a urinary catheter should be inserted. Isotonic crystalloid such as Ringer's lactate solution or normal saline should be administered and the infusion titrated in accordance with the patient's pulse, blood pressure, and urine output. Application of the military antishock garment also may be helpful in stabilizing the patient's blood pressure, especially when bleeding is occurring.

If the initial fluid infusion is not successful in restoring hemodynamic stability, a right-sided heart catheter should be inserted to monitor pulmonary artery wedge pressure. In addition, dopamine should be administered. In low doses, this vasopressor stimulates myocardial contractility and improves perfusion of central organs. In higher doses, the drug has primarily vasoconstrictive effects and may actually compromise tissue perfusion.

Corticosteroids no longer are recommended for treatment of septic shock. Although these drugs may initially improve hemodynamic instability, they ultimately promote superinfection with resistant microorganisms and do not improve overall mortality.[51,52] In selected patients with refractory hypotension, intravenous administration of the narcotic antagonist naloxone has led to reversal of the shock state.[53] The dose and duration of administration of naloxone have not been well standardized.

The second objective of treatment is to administer broad-spectrum antibiotics targeted against the most likely pathogens.[17] For genital tract infections, the combination of penicillin (5 million units IV every 6 hours) or ampicillin (2 g IV every 6 hours) plus clindamycin (900 mg IV every 8 hours) or metronidazole (500 mg IV every 8 hours) plus gentamicin (1.5 mg/kg IV every 8 hours or 7 mg/kg ideal body weight IV every 24 hours) or aztreonam (1 to 2 g IV every 8 hours) is an appropriate regimen. Alternatively, imipenem-cilastatin (500 mg IV every 6 hours), meropenem (1 g every 8 hours), or ertapenem (1 g IV every 24 hours) can be administered as single agents. Patients also may require surgery, for example, to evacuate infected products of conception, drain a pelvic abscess, or remove badly infected pelvic organs. Indicated surgery never should be delayed because a patient is unstable, since operative intervention may be precisely the step necessary to reverse the hemodynamic derangements of septic shock.

Patients with septic shock require meticulous supportive care. Core temperature should be maintained as close to normal as possible by use of antipyretics and a cooling blanket. Coagulation abnormalities should be identified promptly and treated by infusion of platelets and coagulation factors, as indicated. Finally, patients should be given oxygen supplementation and observed closely for evidence of ARDS, one of the major causes of mortality in cases of severe sepsis.[50] Oxygenation should be monitored by means of a pulse oximeter or radial artery catheter. If evidence of respiratory failure develops, the patient should be intubated and supported with mechanical ventilation.

The prognosis in patients with septic shock clearly depends upon the severity of the patient's underlying illness. In otherwise healthy patients, mortality should not exceed 15 percent.[54] Fortunately, most obstetric patients are in the latter category. Therefore, the prognosis for complete recovery is excellent provided that the patient receives competent, timely intervention.

Toxoplasmosis

Epidemiology

Toxoplasma gondii is a protozoan that has three distinct forms: trophozoite, cyst, and oocyst. The life cycle of *T. gondii* is dependent on wild and domestic cats, which are the only host for the oocyst. The oocyst is formed in the cat intestine and subsequently excreted in the feces. Mammals, such as cows, ingest the oocyst, which is disrupted in the animal's intestine, releasing the invasive trophozoite. The trophozoite then is disseminated throughout the body, ultimately forming cysts in brain and muscle.[55]

Human infection occurs when infected meat is ingested or when food is contaminated by cat feces, via flies, cockroaches, or fingers. Infection rates are highest in areas of poor sanitation and crowded living conditions. Stray cats and domestic cats that eat raw meat are most likely to carry the parasite. The cyst is destroyed by heat.[55]

Approximately 40 to 50 percent of adults in the United States have antibody to this organism, and the prevalence of antibody is highest in lower socioeconomic populations. The frequency of seroconversion during pregnancy is 5 percent, and approximately 3 in 1,000 infants show evidence of congenital infection. Clinically significant congenital toxoplasmosis occurs in approximately 1 in 8,000 pregnancies. Toxoplasmosis is more common in western Europe, particularly France, most likely because of the practice in that country of eating rare or raw meat. More than 80 percent of women of childbearing age in Paris have antibody to *T. gondii*, and the incidence of congenital toxoplasmosis is about twice as frequent as that in the United States.[56]

Clinical Manifestations

The ingested organism invades across the intestinal epithelium and spreads hematogenously throughout the body. Intracellular replication leads to cell destruction. Clinical manifestations of infection are the result of direct organ damage and the subsequent immunologic response to parasitemia and cell death. Host immunity is mediated primarily through T-lymphocytes.[55]

Most infections in humans are asymptomatic. Even in the absence of symptoms, however, patients may have evidence of multiorgan involvement, and clinical disease can follow a long period of asymptomatic infection. Symptomatic toxoplasmosis usually presents as an illness similar to mononucleosis.

In contrast to infection in the immunocompetent host, toxoplasmosis can be a devastating infection in the immunosuppressed patient. Because immunity to *T. gondii* is cell-mediated, patients with human immunodeficiency virus infection and those treated with chronic immunosuppressive therapy after organ transplantation are particularly susceptible to new or reactivated infection. In these patients, dysfunction of the central nervous system is the most common manifestation of infection. Findings typically include encephalitis, meningoencephalitis, and intracerebral mass lesions. Pneumonitis, myocarditis, and generalized lymphadenopathy also occur commonly.[55]

Diagnosis

The diagnosis of toxoplasmosis in the mother can be confirmed by serologic and histologic methods. Serologic tests that suggest an acute infection include detection of IgM-specific antibody, demonstration of an extremely high IgG antibody titer, and documentation of IgG seroconversion from negative to positive. Clinicians should be aware that serologic assays for toxoplasmosis are not well standardized. When initial laboratory tests appear to indicate that an acute infection has occurred, repeat serology should be performed in a well-respected reference laboratory.[57]

T. gondii is most easily identified in lymphatic or brain tissue. Histologic preparations can be examined by light and electron microscopy. For light microscopy, specimens should be stained with either Giemsa's or Wright's stains.[55,57]

Congenital Toxoplasmosis

Congenital infection can occur if a woman develops acute primary toxoplasmosis during pregnancy. Chronic or latent infection is unlikely to cause fetal injury except perhaps in an immunosuppressed patient. Approximately 40 percent of neonates born to mothers with acute toxoplasmosis show evidence of infection. Congenital infection is most likely to occur when maternal infection develops in the third trimester. Less than half of affected infants are symptomatic at birth. The clinical manifestations of congenital toxoplasmosis are varied and are summarized in Table 49-10.[56–58]

The most valuable tests for antenatal diagnosis of congenital toxoplasmosis are ultrasound, cordocentesis, and amniocentesis.[56,58,59] Ultrasound findings suggestive of infection include ventriculomegaly, intracranial calcifications, microcephaly, ascites, hepatosplenomegaly, and growth restriction. Fetal blood samples can be tested for IgM-specific antibody after 20 to 22 weeks' gestation. Fetal blood and amniotic fluid can be inoculated into mice, and the organism can subsequently be recovered from the blood of infected animals. In addition, Hohlfeld et al.[59] have now identified a specific gene of *T. gondii*

Table 49-10. Clinical Manifestations of Congenital Toxoplasmosis

Rash
Hepatosplenomegaly
Ascites
Fever
Chorioretinitis
Periventricular calcifications
Ventriculomegaly
Seizures
Mental retardation
Uveitis

in amniotic fluid using PCR. In their investigation, 34 of 339 infants had congenital toxoplasmosis confirmed by serologic testing or autopsy. All amniotic fluid specimens from affected pregnancies were positive by PCR, and test results were available within 1 day of specimen collection.

In a subsequent investigation, Romand et al.[60] reported that the PCR test had an overall sensitivity of 64 percent (95 percent confidence interval, 53 to 75 percent) for diagnosing congenital toxoplasmosis. No false-positive results were noted, and the positive predictive value was 100 percent.

MANAGEMENT

Toxoplasmosis in the immunocompetent adult is usually an asymptomatic or self-limited illness and does not require treatment. Immunocompromised patients, however, should be treated, and the regimen of choice is a combination of oral sulfadiazine (4-g loading dose, then 1 g four times daily) plus pyrimethamine (50 to 100 mg initially, then 25 mg daily). In such patients, extended courses of treatment may be necessary to cure the infection.[57]

Treatment also is indicated when acute toxoplasmosis occurs during pregnancy. Treatment of the mother reduces the risk of congenital infection and decreases the late sequelae of infection.[56,58,61] Pyrimethamine is not recommended for use during the first trimester of pregnancy because of possible teratogenicity although this has not been reported to date. Sulfonamides can be used alone, but single-agent therapy appears to be less effective than combination therapy. In Europe, spiramycin has been used extensively in pregnancy with excellent success. It is available for treatment in the United States through the CDC.

Aggressive early treatment of infants with congenital toxoplasmosis is indicated and consists of combination therapy with pyrimethamine, sulfadiazine, and leucovorin for 1 year. Early treatment reduces, but does not eliminate, the late sequelae of toxoplasmosis such as chorioretinitis.[62]

In the management of the pregnant patient, *prevention* of acute toxoplasmosis is of paramount importance. Pregnant women should be advised to avoid contact with cat litter if at all possible. If they must change the litter, they should do so daily, wear gloves, and wash their hands afterward. They should always wash their hands after preparing meat for cooking and should never eat raw or rare meat. Meat should be cooked thoroughly until the juices are clear. Fruits and vegetables also should be washed carefully to remove possible contamination by oocysts.

Listeriosis

Listeria monocytogenes (LM) is a gram-positive bacillus responsible for severe infections in humans and a large variety of animal species. It is a facultative intracellular pathogen that invades macrophages and most tissue cells of infected hosts, where it can proliferate. LM can cause meningitis, encephalitis, bacteremia, and febrile gastroenteritis. In infected hosts, the bacteria cross the intestinal wall at Peyer's patches to invade the mesenteric lymph nodes and the blood. The main target organ is the liver, where the bacteria multiply inside hepatocytes. Most disease occurs in patients with impaired cell-mediated immunity, and it is an important cause of severe infections in neonates, pregnant women, the elderly, and transplant recipients. Although dramatic epidemics have received the most publicity, most cases of perinatal listeriosis are isolated.

LM is naturally widespread in nature and can be readily found in soil and vegetation. Recent seroepidemiologic studies show that the infection is food borne. Heightened surveillance and quality control by the food industry have been instituted (Table 49-11), leading to a reduction in the number of cases and deaths from this infection in the past decade. However, most parents are still not aware of the risks of listeriosis and recommended practices for listeriosis prevention; thus, they are not taking precautions during their pregnancy to prevent listeriosis.[63] Because LM can grow and multiply at temperatures as low as 0.5°C (or 32.9°F), refrigerating these foods does not always help. Cooking contaminated foods at high temperatures destroys the bacteria. LM can also be contracted through the handling of miscarried products of animals, when the miscarriage is due to listeriosis. Therefore, it is important for pregnant women working with animals not to touch these, if possible (or to wear gloves if this cannot be avoided). Owing to the ubiquity of the organism in the environment, outbreaks and sporadic disease continue to occur.[64]

Table 49-11. USDA's Food Safety and Inspection Service (FSIS) and the U.S. Food and Drug Administration (FDA) Advice for Pregnant Women to Prevent Listeriosis during Pregnancy

Do not eat hot dogs, luncheon meats, or deli meats unless they are reheated until steaming hot.

Do not eat soft cheeses such as feta, Brie, Camembert, blue-veined cheeses, and Mexican-style cheeses such as "queso blanco fresco." Hard cheeses, semi-soft cheeses such as mozzarella, pasteurized processed cheese slices and spreads, cream cheese, and cottage cheese can be safely consumed.

Do not eat refrigerated pâté or meat spreads. Canned or shelf-stable pâté and meat spreads can be eaten.

Do not eat refrigerated smoked seafood unless it is an ingredient in a cooked dish such as a casserole. Examples of refrigerated smoked seafood include salmon, trout, whitefish, cod, tuna, and mackerel which are most often labeled as "nova-style," "lox," "kippered," "smoked," or "jerky." This fish is found in the refrigerated section or sold at deli counters of grocery stores and delicatessens. Canned fish such as salmon and tuna or shelf-stable smoked seafood may be safely eaten.

Do not drink raw (unpasteurized) milk or eat foods that contain unpasteurized milk.

The incubation period of LM ranges from as little as 1 day to as long as 90 days, making identification of the food or activity that caused the listeriosis extremely difficult. Maternal symptoms can vary from "flu like" or "food poisoning" to septicemia, meningitis, or pneumonia. Because there is no reliable serologic evaluation, listeriosis is a difficult infection to test for outside the septic peak when it can be demonstrated in blood cultures. An overall perinatal mortality rate of 50 percent due to late miscarriage, premature delivery, and stillbirth was recorded before the use of modern therapies.[65] The clinical characteristics of neonatal listeriosis are similar to neonatal GBS sepsis, with early and late onset forms of disease. The mortality rate among liveborn infants is approximately 10 percent.[66]

The standard therapy for listeriosis is a combination of ampicillin and gentamicin or, for patients who are intolerant of beta-lactam agents, trimethoprim-sulfamethazole. If LM chorioamnionitis is diagnosed preterm, in contrast to other types of chorioamnionitis, in utero therapy with high-dose penicillin or trimethoprim-sulfamethoxazole is possible, and preterm delivery may be avoided.

KEY POINTS

- Overall, 85 percent of neonatal GBS infections are early in onset and result from transmission from a colonized mother.
- All pregnant women should be cultured for GBS at 35 to 37 weeks. Culture-positive patients should receive intrapartum antibiotic prophylaxis to prevent early-onset neonatal infection.
- Patients with GBS bacteriuria should be considered heavily colonized and be targeted for intrapartum prophylaxis.
- All pregnant women should have a urine culture at their first prenatal appointment to detect asymptomatic bacteriuria.
- The vast majority of cases of pyelonephritis occur as a consequence of undiagnosed or inadequately treated lower urinary tract infections.
- The organisms most likely to cause chorioamnionitis and puerperal endometritis are GBS, *E. coli*, and gram-positive and gram-negative anaerobes.
- Prophylactic antibiotics are highly effective in preventing postcesarean endometritis.
- Resistant organisms and wound infection are the most common causes of persistent fever in patients who are being treated for puerperal endometritis.
- Septic pelvic thrombophlebitis is another important cause of refractory postoperative fever. This condition is best diagnosed by CT or MRI.
- The most common causes of septic shock in obstetric patients are septic abortion, pyelonephritis, chorioamnionitis, and endometritis.

REFERENCES

1. Prevention of perinatal group B streptococcal disease. Revised guidelines from the CDC. MMWR (Suppl) 51:1, 2002.
2. Yancey MK, Duff P: An analysis of the cost-effectiveness of selected protocols for the prevention of neonatal group B streptococcal infection. Obstet Gynecol 83:367, 1994.
3. Boyer KM, Gotoff SP: Prevention of early-onset neonatal group B streptococcal disease with selective intrapartum chemoprophylaxis. N Engl J Med 314:1665, 1986.
4. Thomsen AC, Morup L, Hansen KB: Antibiotic elimination of group-B streptococci in urine in prevention of preterm labor. Lancet 1:591, 1987.
5. Newton ER, Clark M: Group B streptococcus and preterm rupture of membranes. Obstet Gynecol 71:198, 1988.
6. Yancey MK, Armer T, Clark P, Duff P: Assessment of rapid identification tests for genital carriage of group B streptococci. Obstet Gynecol 80:1038, 1992.
7. Bergeron MG, Ke D, Menard C, et al: Rapid detection of group B streptococci in pregnant women at delivery. N Engl J Med 343:175, 2000.
8. Siegel JD, McCracken GH, Threlkeld N, et al: Single dose penicillin prophylaxis against neonatal group B streptococcal infections. N Engl J Med 303:769, 1980.
9. Yow MD, Mason EO, Leeds LJ, et al: Ampicillin prevents intrapartum transmission of group B streptococcus. JAMA 241:1245 1979.
10. Boyer KM, Gadzala CA, Kelly PD, Gotoff SP: Selective intrapartum chemoprophylaxis of neonatal group B streptococcal early-onset disease. III. Interruption of mother-to-infant transmission. J Infect Dis 148:810, 1983.
11. Prevention of perinatal group B streptococcal disease: a public health perspective. MMWR 45(Suppl):1, 1996.
12. Rosenstein NE, Schuchat A: Opportunities for prevention of perinatal group B streptococcal disease: a multistate surveillance analysis. Obstet Gynecol 90:901, 1997.
13. Locksmith GJ, Clark P, Duff P: Maternal and neonatal infection rates with three different protocols for prevention of group B streptococcal disease. Am J Obstet Gynecol 180:416, 1999.
14. DeCueto M, Sanchez M-J, Sanpedro A, et al: Timing of intrapartum ampicillin and prevention of vertical transmission of group B streptococcus. Obstet Gynecol 91:112, 1998.
15. Edwards RK, Clark P, Duff P: Intrapartum antibiotic prophylaxis 2: positive predictive value of antenatal group B streptococci cultures and antibiotic susceptibility of clinical isolates. Obstet Gynecol 100:540, 2002.
16. Duff P: Urinary tract infections. Prim Care Update Ob/Gyns 1:12, 1994.
17. Duff P: Antibiotic selection in obstetrics: making cost-effective choices. Clin Obstet Gynecol 45:59, 2002.
18. Duff P: Pyelonephritis in pregnancy. Clin Obstet Gynecol 27:17, 1984.
19. Stamm WE, Counts GW, Running KR, et al: Diagnosis of coliform infection in acutely dysuric women. N Engl J Med 307:463, 1982.
20. Dunlow S, Duff P: Prevalence of antibiotic-resistant uropathogens in obstetric patients with acute pyelonephritis. Obstet Gynecol 76:241, 1990.
21. Stamm WE, Hooton TM: Management of urinary tract infections in adults. N Engl J Med 329:1328, 1993.
22. MacMillan MC, Grimes DA: The limited usefulness of urine and blood cultures in treating pyelonephritis in pregnancy. Obstet Gynecol 78:745, 1991.
23. Gibbs RS, Duff P: Progress in pathogenesis and management of clinical intraamniotic infection. Am J Obstet Gynecol 164:1317, 1991.
24. Armer TL, Duff P: Intraamniotic infection in patients with intact membranes and preterm labor. Obstet Gynecol Surv 46:589, 1991.
25. Romero R, Jimenez C, Lohda AK, et al: Amniotic fluid glucose concentration: A rapid and simple method for the detection of intraamniotic infection in preterm labor. Am J Obstet Gynecol 163:968, 1990.
26. Kirshon B, Rosenfeld B, Mari G, Belfort M: Amniotic fluid glucose and intraamniotic infection. Am J Obstet Gynecol 164:818, 1991.

27. Gauthier DW, Meyer WJ, Bieniarz A: Correlation of amniotic fluid glucose concentration and intraamniotic infection in patients with preterm labor or premature rupture of membranes. Am J Obstet Gynecol 165:1105, 1991.
28. Romero R, Yoon BH, Mazor M, et al: The diagnostic and prognostic value of amniotic fluid white blood cell count, glucose, interleukin-6, and Gram stain in patients with preterm labor and intact membranes. Am J Obstet Gynecol 169:805, 1993.
29. Sperling RS, Ramamurthy RS, Gibbs RS: A comparison of intrapartum versus immediate postpartum treatment of intra-amniotic infection. Obstet Gynecol 70:861, 1987.
30. Gilstrap LC, Leveno KJ, Cox SM, et al: Intrapartum treatment of acute chorioamnionitis: Impact on neonatal sepsis. Am J Obstet Gynecol 159:579, 1988.
31. Gibbs RS, Dinsmoor MJ, Newton ER, et al: A randomized trial of intrapartum versus immediate postpartum treatment of women with intra-amniotic infection. Obstet Gynecol 72:823, 1988.
32. Edwards RK, Duff P: Single additional dose postpartum therapy for women with chorioamnionitis. Obstet Gynecol 102:957, 2003.
33. Duff P, Sanders R, Gibbs RS: The course of labor in term patients with chorioamnionitis. Am J Obstet Gynecol 147:391, 1983.
34. Duff P: Pathophysiology and management of postcesarean endomyometritis. Obstet Gynecol 67:269, 1986.
35. Milligan DA, Brady K, Duff P: Short-term parenteral antibiotic therapy for puerperal endometritis. J Maternal Fetal Med 1:60, 1992.
36. Duff P: Staphylococcal infections. *In* Gleicher N (ed): Principles and Practice of Medical Therapy in Pregnancy, 2nd ed. New York, Appleton & Lange, 1992, p 518.
37. Duff P: Prophylactic antibiotics for cesarean delivery: A simple cost-effective strategy for prevention of postoperative morbidity. Am J Obstet Gynecol 157:794, 1987.
38. Gibbs RS, Blanco JD, St. Clair PJ: A case-control study of wound abscess after cesarean delivery. Obstet Gynecol 62:498, 1983.
39. Golde S, Ledger WJ: Necrotizing fasciitis in postpartum patients. Obstet Gynecol 50:670, 1977.
40. Shy KK, Eschenbach DA: Fatal perineal cellulitis from an episiotomy site. Obstet Gynecol 54:292, 1979.
41. Weinstein WM, Onderdonk AB, Bartlett JG, Gorbach SL: Experimental intra-abdominal abscesses in rats: Development of an experimental model. Infect Immun 10:1250, 1974.
42. Knochel JQ, Koehler PR, Lee TG, Welch DM: Diagnosis of abdominal abscesses with computed tomography, ultrasound, and ^{111}In leukocyte scans. Radiology 137:425, 1980.
43. Gerzof SG, Robbins AH, Johnson WC, et al: Percutaneous catheter drainage of abdominal abscesses. A five-year experience. N Engl J Med 305:653, 1981.
44. Duff P, Gibbs RS: Pelvic vein thrombophlebitis: Diagnostic dilemma and therapeutic challenge. Obstet Gynecol Surv 38:365, 1983.
45. Brown TK, Munsick RA: Puerperal ovarian vein thrombophlebitis: A syndrome. Am J Obstet Gynecol 109:263, 1971.
46. Dunn LJ, Van Voorhis LW: Enigmatic fever and pelvic thrombophlebitis. N Engl J Med 276:265, 1967.
47. Brown CEL, Lowe TE, Cunningham FG, Weinreb JC: Puerperal pelvic vein thrombophlebitis: Impact on diagnosis and treatment using x-ray computed tomography and magnetic resonance imaging. Obstet Gynecol 68:789, 1986.
48. Duff P: Septic pelvic-vein thrombophlebitis. *In* Pastorek JG (ed): Obstetric and Gynecologic Infectious Disease. New York, Raven Press, 1994, p 165.
49. Duff P, Gibbs RS: Maternal sepsis. *In* Berkowitz RL (ed): Critical Care of the Obstetric Patient. New York, Churchill Livingstone, 1983, P 189.
50. Kaplan RL, Sahn SA, Petty TL: Incidence and outcome of the respiratory distress syndrome in gram-negative sepsis. Arch Intern Med 139:867, 1979.
51. The Veterans Administration Systemic Sepsis Cooperative Study Group: Effect of high dose glucocorticoid therapy on mortality in patients with clinical signs of systemic sepsis. N Engl J Med 317:659, 1987.
52. Sprung CL, Caralis PV, Marcial EH, et al: The effects of high dose corticosteroids in patients with septic shock. A prospective controlled study. N Engl J Med 311:1137, 1984.
53. Holaday JW, Faden AI: Nalaxone reversal of endotoxin hypotension suggests role of endorphins in shock. Nature 275:450, 1979.
54. Freid MA, Vosti KL: The importance of underlying disease in patients with gram-negative bacteremia. Arch Intern Med 121:418, 1968.
55. Krick JA, Remington JS: Toxoplasmosis in the adult—an overview. N Engl J Med 298:550, 1978.
56. Daffos F: Prenatal management of 746 pregnancies at risk for congenital toxoplasmosis. N Engl J Med 318:271, 1988.
57. Egerman RS, Beazley D: Toxoplasmosis. Semin Perinatol 22:332, 1998.
58. Desmonts G, Couvreur J: Congenital toxoplasmosis. A prospective study of 378 pregnancies. N Engl J Med 290:1110, 1974.
59. Hohlfeld P, Daffos F, Costa JM, et al: Prenatal diagnosis of congenital toxoplasmosis with a polymerase-chain reaction test on amniotic fluid. N Engl J Med 331:695, 1994.
60. Romand S, Wallon M, Franck J, et al: Prenatal diagnosis using polymerase chain reaction on amniotic fluid for congenital toxoplasmosis. Obstet Gynecol 97:296, 2001.
61. Foulon W, Villena I, Stray-Pedersen B, et al: Treatment of toxoplasmosis during pregnancy: A multicenter study of impact on fetal transmission and children's sequelae at age 1 year. Am J Obstet Gynecol 180:410, 1999.
62. Guerina NG, Hsu HW, Meissner HC, et al: Neonatal serologic screening and early treatment for congenital *Toxoplasma gondii* infection. N Engl J Med 330:1858, 1994.
63. Cates SC, Carter-Young HL, Conley S, O'Brien B: Pregnant women and listeriosis: preferred educational messages and delivery mechanisms. J Nutr Educ Behav 36:121, 2004.
64. MacDonald PD, Whitwam RE, Boggs JD, et al: Outbreak of listeriosis among Mexican immigrants as a result of consumption of illicitly produced Mexican-style cheese. Clin Infect Dis 40:677, 2005.
65. McLauchlin J: Human listeriosis in Britain, 1967–85, a summary of 722 cases. 1. Listeriosis during pregnancy and in the newborn. Epidemiol Infect 104:181, 1990.
66. Frederiksen B, Samuelsson S: Feto-maternal listeriosis in Denmark 1981–1988. J Infect 24:277, 1992.

Psychiatric Disorders

KATHERINE L. WISNER, DOROTHY K.Y. SIT, SARAH K. REYNOLDS, MARGARET ALTEMUS, DEBRA L. BOGEN, KEERTHY R. SUNDER, DAWN MISRA, AND JAMES M. PEREL

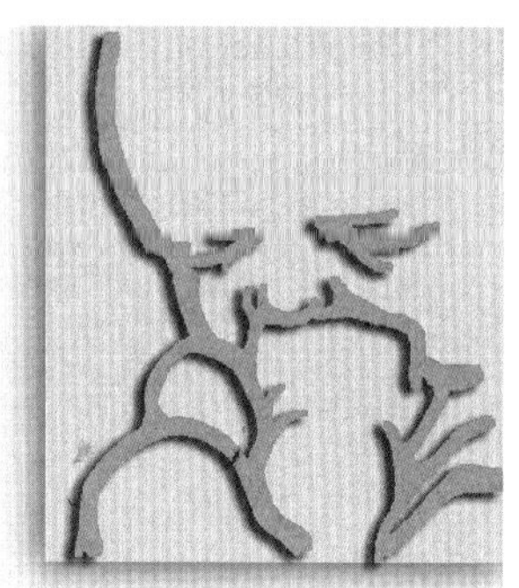

CHAPTER 50

KEY ABBREVIATIONS

American Academy of Pediatrics	AAP
Anorexia nervosa	AN
Antiepileptic drugs	AED
Bipolar disorder	BD
Body mass index	BMI
Borderline personality	BP
Bulimia nervosa	BN
Carbamazepine	CBZ
Center for Addiction and Pregnancy	CAP
Clinical antipsychotic trials of intervention effectiveness	CATIE
Cognitive behavioral therapy	CBT
Confidence interval	CI
Diagnostic and Statistical Manual of Mental Disorders	DSM-IV
Docosahexaenoic acid	DHA
Edinburgh Postnatal Depression Scale	EPDS
Electroconvulsive therapy	ECT
Food and Drug Administration	FDA
Interpersonal psychotherapy	IPT
Major depressive episode	MDE
Methadone maintenance treatment	MMT
Mood disorder questionnaire	MDQ
Neonatal abstinence syndrome	NAS
Neonatal intensive care unit	NICU
Neural tube defect	NTD
Olanzapine	OLZ
Omega-3 fatty acids	O-3 FAs
Personality disorder	PD
Selective-serotonin reuptake inhibitor	SSRI
Thyroid-stimulating hormone	TSH
Tricyclic antidepressant	TCA
Valproic acid	VPA
Verapamil	VPM

INTRODUCTION

Mental health is fundamental to health. This statement, made by Surgeon General David Satcher, emphasized the foundation that emotional well-being provides for health. In medical practice, we compartmentalize symptoms and diseases into manageable units; however, the patient comes as an integrated whole. The effect of pathology in any part of the body affects the entire patient. Psychiatric disorders are defined in the Diagnostic and Statistical Manual of Mental Disorders (DSM-IV),[1] a categorical classification that divides mental disorders into types based on criteria sets with defining features. This chapter covers the major classifications of disorders that affect women of childbearing age as well as the tragedies of suicide and infanticide. For the pregnant woman, the capacity to function optimally, enjoy relationships, manage the pregnancy, and prepare for the infant's birth is critical.

Perinatal health can be conceptualized within a model that integrates the complex social, psychological, behavioral, environmental, and biologic forces that shape pregnancy. Engel[2] described the biopsychosocial model of

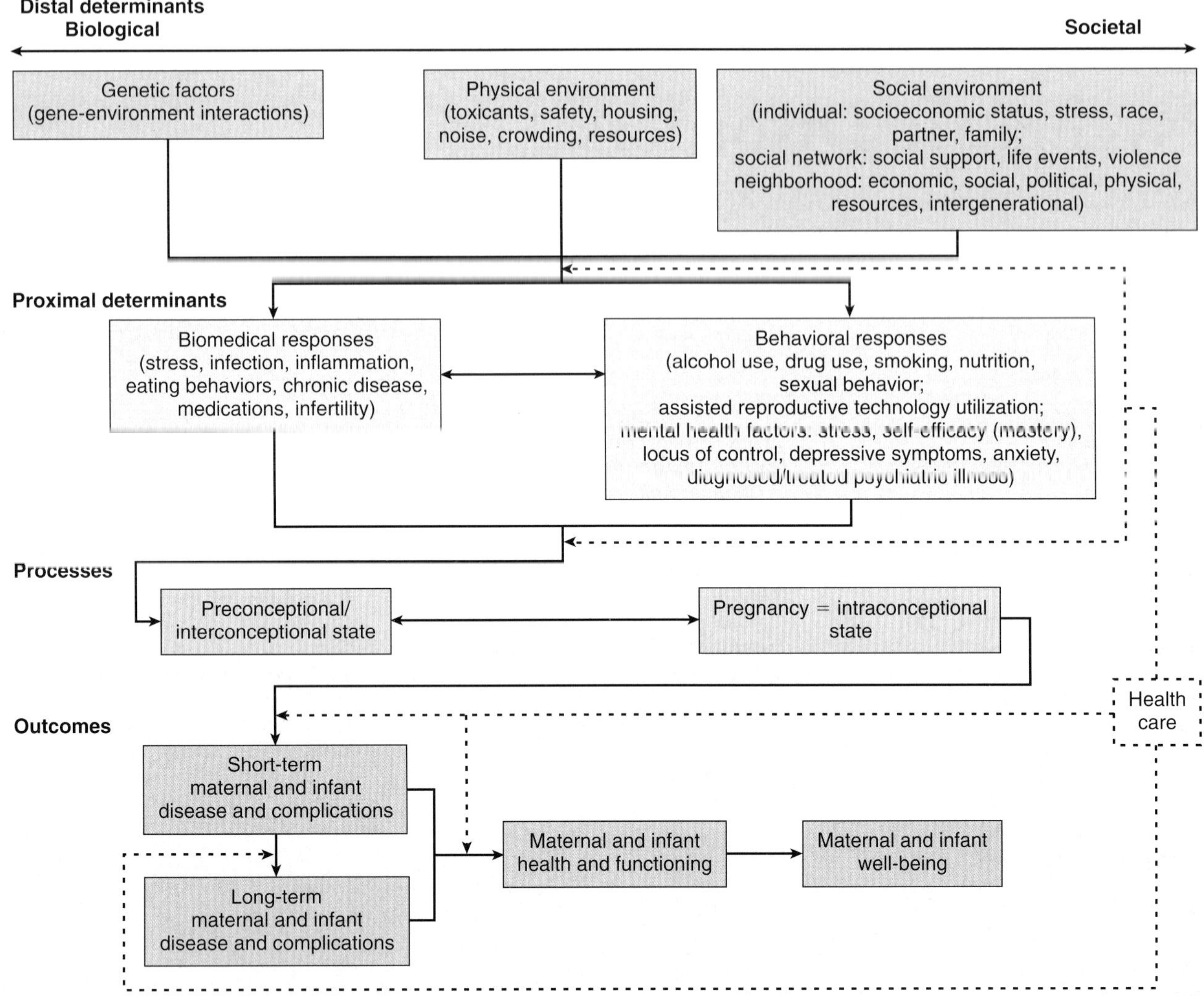

Figure 50-1. Integrated perinatal health framework: a multiple determinants model with a life span approach. (From Misra DP, Guyer B, Allston A: Integrated perinatal health framework. A multiple determinants model with a life span approach. Am J Prev Med 25:65, 2003. Included here (with adaptations) with permission from Dawn P. Misra, Ph.D. [03/07/05]. [Illustrative examples are in brackets.])

vulnerability to disease in relation to the life cycle. In each individual, the relative contributions of biologic, psychological, and social factors vary. Depression in response to stressful life situations occurs only in some women; in others, episodes occur without extraordinary stressful events. The influence of life stress on depression is moderated by gene-environment interactions. For example, Caspi et al.[3] demonstrated that the risk of an episode of major depression in response to stressful life events is directly related to carriage of various alleles of the promoter region of the serotonin transporter gene.

Misra et al.[4] presented a comprehensive perinatal framework that integrates a life span approach with a multiple determinants model (Fig. 50-1). The model contains four hierarchical levels that provide a paradigm for considering the determinants of perinatal health outcomes. The first level in the model is *Distal Determinants,* which brings focus to *distal* (in time) risk factors that place a woman at greater susceptibility to *proximal* (current) risk factors. Distal determinants derive from biologic, physical, and social domains. Although they have the potential to directly influence health status, distal factors typically increase or decrease a woman's likelihood of developing health problems, engaging in high-risk behaviors, or being exposed to potential toxins. Some of the most powerful influences on pregnancy outcome are related to these *distal* women's health factors that occur long before pregnancy. At the next level, *proximal determinants,* risk factors that have a direct impact on a woman's health status, are represented by biomedical and behavioral responses. The interaction between *distal* and *proximal* risk factors determines an individual's overall health status. It is the interrelationship between a woman's health status directly before conception and the demands of pregnancy that affect perinatal health outcomes. For example, a woman who is told that her infant has spina bifida after ultrasound (owing to long-term poor folate intake, a distal risk consolidated into a negative outcome) develops a recurrence of a major depressive episode (proximal risk) that further impacts maternal and fetal health. The third level, *processes,* is presented to emphasize the interaction of pre-, inter- and intraconceptional factors (as time variables in the women's health life course) on perinatal outcomes. At the fourth level, *outcomes*, the model includes constructs of disease, functioning, and well-being, which together provide a comprehensive assessment of health status (both short and long term). Potential opportunities for interventions to impact perinatal health are included in this model. Each patient can be understood as coming to pregnancy with sets of malleable risks and assets that shape pregnancy outcome. To the extent that biopsychosocial exposures with negative impact upon pregnancy outcome can be diminished, eliminated, or replaced with positive factors, the risk of poor pregnancy outcome can be reduced. The role of health care professionals is to impact the patient's exposures and behaviors toward more positive comprehensive outcomes at various points depicted in Figure 50-1.

OVERVIEW: PSYCHIATRIC DISORDERS IN WOMEN

Each woman brings her individual constellation of assets and vulnerabilities to pregnancy in the domains represented by the model in Figure 50-1. Why certain women develop primary mood disorders as opposed to eating disorders or schizophrenia is an active area of research inquiry. Our discussion of psychiatric disorders includes six major diagnostic categories that occur commonly in women of childbearing age: mood disorders, anxiety disorders, eating disorders, schizophrenia, substance use disorders, and personality disorders (PDs). This review focuses on the interrelationships between these disorders and the course of pregnancy, postpartum, and breast-feeding. Within the life cycle context, the impact of childbearing on existing disorders or vulnerabilities in the female patient is of primary interest, as well as episodes that are etiologically related to childbearing. Treatment considerations for psychiatric disorders during childbearing invoke special modifications of the risk-benefit decision-making process.

MOOD DISORDERS

The mood disorders are characterized by a disturbance of affective state as the most prominent feature. Major depression and bipolar disorder (BD) are the exemplars of this category.

Major Depressive Episode

DIAGNOSIS AND PREVALENCE

In the DSM-IV,[1] a major depressive episode (MDE) is defined as at least a 2-week period of either persistent depressed mood or loss of interest or pleasure in daily activities (the "gatekeeper" symptoms) plus four associated symptoms (or three if both gatekeeper symptoms are present). *Persistent* is operationalized as the symptom must be present for most of the day nearly every day. The patient also must have impairment of function in interpersonal relationships or work. Note that it is possible to have a *diagnosis* of MDE without the *symptom* of depression. A woman could have persistent loss of interest or pleasure but no depressed mood and four other symptoms from the following list: appetite disturbance or significant weight change, sleep loss/excess, psychomotor agitation/retardation, fatigue or energy loss, feelings of worthlessness or guilt, impaired thinking or concentration, and suicidal ideation. Note that appetite, sleep, and motor activity can be either decreased or increased. A fatigued woman who derives no pleasure from previously enjoyable activities, sleeps 15 hours per day, sits for long periods when awake, and is gaining weight has MDE. A guilt-ridden woman with depressed mood and 4 hours per day of sleep, weight loss of 15 pounds, and pacing at night also has MDE.[5] Another mood disorder, dysthymia, is chronic depression (for at least 2 years) that does not meet full symptomatic criteria for an MDE.

How prevalent is major depression? Data from the World Health Organization Global Burden of Disease Study[6] revealed that mental illness accounted for more than 15 percent of the disease burden in established market economies. This is more than the disease burden inflicted by all cancers, and second only to ischemic heart disease in magnitude of burden. Nearly twice as many women (12.0 percent) as men (6.6 percent) suffer from a depressive disorder each year.[7] Major depression is the leading cause of disease burden among girls ages 5 and older worldwide.[8] Women are at the greatest risk for MDE between 25 and 44 years, the primary age window for childbearing. MDE during pregnancy often is undiagnosed and untreated. In a large sample (N = 3472) of pregnant women screened in obstetric settings, 20 percent had significant symptoms and only 13.8 percent were receiving treatment.[9]

The most commonly used measure to screen for MDE during childbearing is the Edinburgh Postnatal Depression Scale (EPDS; Fig. 50-2), which has been validated for use both during and after pregnancy. This brief self-report instrument contains ten items ranked from 0 to 3. [illegible] et al.[10] suggested a cutoff score of greater than or equal to 10, at which sensitivities range from 91 percent (specificity 76 percent) to 88 percent (specificity 72 percent) for MDE. Like any screening tool, positive scores on the EPDS must be followed with further diagnostic assessment.[11] Peindl et al.[12] examined the relationship between serial postpartum EPDS scores and the development of postpartum depression (PPD). The relative risk of a diagnosis of MDE on the day of EPDS completion was 63.7 (95 percent confidence interval [CI] = 8.2 to 494.3) for women with EPDS greater than 10 compared with women with an EPDS less than 9.

TREATMENT OF MAJOR DEPRESSIVE EPISODE DURING PREGNANCY

Wisner and colleagues[13] created a model to structure risk-benefit decision-making during pregnancy. Individually tailored therapeutic interventions are considered in view of their capacity to maximize maternal wellness while minimizing toxicity for the maternal-fetal pair. The

How are you feeling?
As you have recently had a baby, we would like to know how you are feeling now. Please check the answer which comes closest to how you have felt in the past 7 days, not just how you feel today.

		Score
1.	I have been able to laugh and see the funny side of things:	
	As much as I always could	0
	Not quite so much now	1
	Definitely not so much now	2
	Not at all	3
2.	I have looked forward with enjoyment to things:	
	As much as I ever did	0
	Rather less than I used to	1
	Definitely less than I used to	2
	Hardly at all	3
3.	I have blamed myself unnecessarily when things went wrong:	
	Yes, most of the time	3
	Yes, some of the time	2
	Not very often	1
	No, never	0
4.	I have been anxious or worried for no good reason:	
	No, not at all	0
	Hardly ever	1
	Yes, sometimes	2
	Yes, very often	3
5.	I have felt scared or panicky for no very good reason:	
	Yes, quite a lot	3
	Yes, sometimes	2
	No, not much	1
	No, not at all	0
6.	Things have been getting on top of me:	
	Yes, most of the time I haven't been able to cope at all	3
	Yes, sometimes I haven't been coping as well as usual	2
	No, most of the time I have coped quite well	1
	No, I have been coping as well as ever	0
7.	I have been so unhappy that I have had difficulty sleeping:	
	Yes, most of the time	3
	Yes, sometimes	2
	Not very often	1
	No, not at all	0
8.	I have felt sad or miserable:	
	Yes, most of the time	3
	Yes, quite often	2
	Not very often	1
	No, not at all	0
9.	I have been so unhappy that I have been crying:	
	Yes, most of the time	3
	Yes, quite often	2
	Only occasionally	1
	No, never	0
10.	The thought of harming myself has occurred to me:	
	Yes, quite often	3
	Sometimes	2
	Hardly ever	1
	Never	0

Figure 50-2. Edinburgh Postnatal Depression Scale. © 1987 The Royal College of Psychiatrists. The Edinburgh Postnatal Depression Scale may be photocopied by individual researchers or clinicians for their own use without seeking permission from the publishers. The scale must be copied in full and all copies must acknowledge the following source: Cox, J.L., Holden, J.M., & Sagovsky, R. (1987). Detection of postnatal depression. Development of the 10-item Edinburgh Postnatal Depression Scale. British Journal of Psychiatry, 150, 782–786. Written permission must be obtained from the Royal College of Psychiatrists for copying and distribution to others or for republication (in print, online or by any other medium).

patient and physician each contribute expertise to the process, because the patient's assignment of her own values dictates her choice. For example, some women will not consent to pharmacotherapy during pregnancy regardless of the severity of the depressive episode. Others choose pharmacotherapy because they are not confident that other treatments will be effective, or because discontinuing medication invariably has been followed by recurrence with major psychosocial consequences. The verbal informed consent process promotes the treatment alliance, recognizes the patient's responsibility to make choices for herself and her baby, and provides an opportunity for ongoing assessment of the woman's competence to make decisions. Informed consent is a *process* that extends across pregnancy and the postpartum period.

The physiologic milieu created by MDE, with increased stress as well as sleep and appetite disruption, is not ideal for pregnancy. In a large Danish population of women, the frequency of cranial neural crest malformations was higher for pregnant women who were exposed to severe life events (unexpected death of a spouse or older child) in the first trimester than in those without such exposure.[14] These findings support the hypothesis that the physiologic sequelae of stress during early pregnancy can impact birth outcomes and may contribute to malformations that are typically attributed to drugs or radiation. Because life stress often precedes the emergence of MDE, and MDE is associated with distress by definition, it has been difficult to separate the independent contribution of MDE to teratogenic risk.[5,13]

The risk of relapse in pregnant women who discontinued antidepressant medication proximate to conception was significantly more frequent compared prospectively with those who maintained treatment.[15] Among 82 women who continued their medication, 21 (26 percent) relapsed compared with 44 (68 percent) of the 65 women who discontinued medication (hazard ratio, 5.0; 95 percent CI, 2.8 to 9.1).

Consideration of multiple domains of reproductive toxicity has improved the sophistication of risk-benefit decision-making.[13,16] These domains are intrauterine fetal death, physical malformations, growth effects, neurobehavioral teratogenicity, and neonatal toxicity. Several recent prospective controlled investigations provided information about the effects of antidepressant treatment during pregnancy for the following medications: fluoxetine, combined newer serotonin-selective reuptake inhibitors (sertraline, paroxetine and fluvoxamine [SSRI]), combined tricyclic antidepressants (TCA), and venlafaxine.[17–21] [Note: The antidepressant bupropion is discussed under substance use disorders owing to its use for smoking cessation.] Outcomes after exposure to these agents were compared with those of control subjects, who were exposed to presumed nonteratogens (such as acetaminophen, dental x-ray with shielding).

Intrauterine Fetal Death

There is no evidence that the rate of stillbirths is increased during antidepressant treatment.[17,18,20,21]

Physical Malformations

In prospective controlled studies, there is no evidence to implicate fluoxetine, newer SSRI, TCA, or venlafaxine as causes of major birth defects in humans or animals.[17,18,20,21] An increased risk for three or more minor malformations was found in one study[17] during exposure to fluoxetine. Minor malformations have no functional or cosmetic significance.

Based upon preliminary analyses of two recent unpublished epidemiologic studies, the Food and Drug Administration (FDA)[22] advised that paroxetine use during the first trimester of pregnancy may increase the risk for malformations. In a study using Swedish national registry data, women who received paroxetine in early pregnancy had a twofold increased risk for having an infant with a cardiac defect compared with the entire national registry population. The risk of a cardiac defect was 2 percent in paroxetine-exposed infants versus 1 percent among all registry infants. In another study with an American insurance claims database, the risk of a cardiac defect was about 1.5 percent in paroxetine-exposed infants versus 1 percent among infants exposed to other antidepressants. Most of the cardiac defects observed in these studies were atrial or ventricular septal defects, which are the most common type of congenital malformations.

Growth Impairment

Prenatal growth and birth weights of infants exposed to TCA, newer SSRI, and venlafaxine during the first trimester were comparable to those of infants exposed to drugs identified as nonteratogens.[17,18,20,21] Chambers et al.[17] found that fetuses exposed to fluoxetine after 25 weeks' gestation had significantly lower birth weights that were associated with decreased maternal weight gain. Chambers et al.[17] also reported an increased risk for premature birth (14.3 percent) in infants whose mothers took fluoxetine in the third trimester compared with infants whose mothers discontinued fluoxetine before the third trimester (4.1 percent). Simon et al.[23] found that exposure to SSRI during pregnancy was associated with a 0.9-week decrease in mean gestational age and a 175-g decrease in mean birth weight; however, no significant difference remained after adjustment for gestational age. The differences in gestational age and birth weights were not limited to third trimester exposure. In this study, TCA exposure was not associated with significant differences in perinatal outcomes. Poor weight gain during pregnancy may be due to decreased appetite, a criterion symptom of depression, which has not been assessed as an additional exposure in most investigations. Appetite suppression, usually concomitant with treatment initiation, is an established side effect of SSRI therapy,[24] and its occurrence during pregnancy may result in suboptimal weight gain.[24a]

Behavioral Teratogenicity

Behavioral teratogenicity refers to long-term postnatal effects on offspring behavior due to prenatal exposure to agents that affect the central nervous system. Cognitive function, temperament, and general behavior were similar in children who were exposed prenatally to tricyclics or fluoxetine compared with controls.[18,19]

SSRI treatment during pregnancy has been associated with reduced acute pain response and less favorable motor development in the infant.[25] On the Bayley Scales of Infant Development, children with first-trimester SSRI exposure were similar to unexposed children in their psychomotor development; however, infants with SSRI exposure beyond the first trimester showed lower scores for gross and fine motor movements. Infants with exposure to SSRI at any point in pregnancy did not differ in mental development compared to controls. Prospective studies are underway to clarify the extent to which the subtle motor signs at follow-up in children exposed late in pregnancy to SSRIs are related to poor neonatal adjustment problems, delayed neurobehavioral teratogenicity, the sequelae of maternal depression, or interactions between these exposures.

Neonatal Toxicity

Both direct pharmacologic effects and withdrawal symptoms can occur after prenatal exposure to any antidepressant.[26] Poor neonatal adaptation (hypotonia, difficulty feeding, desaturation on feeding) has been reported in infants whose mothers received fluoxetine in the third trimester (31.5 percent) compared with infants whose mothers discontinued fluoxetine before 26 weeks' gestation (8.9 percent).[17] The newborns of mothers who took fluoxetine during pregnancy had similar birth weights but a fourfold higher risk for tremor, restlessness, and rigid muscle tone compared with matched controls.[27] These effects were transient; after 2 weeks, there was no difference between the signs of neonates exposed to SSRIs and those of the control group. Sanz et al.[28] described the World Health Organization database, which contained 74 cases of neonatal syndrome associated with late pregnancy exposure to the following SSRIs: paroxetine (n = 51; 69% of cases), fluoxetine (n = 10), sertraline (n = 7), citalopram (n = 6), and venlafaxine (n = 6).

Based on the concept that neonatal signs are due to direct pharmacologic action, tapering and discontinuation of the antidepressant dose over 10 days to 2 weeks before the delivery date has been suggested.[28] Reintroduction of medication immediately after birth is prudent. If a woman has a history of rapid decompensation during medication taper, this strategy may carry more risk to the maternal-fetal pair than continued dosing.

Drug Treatment During Pregnancy

There has been only one publication about the management of TCA dosage across pregnancy that included serum drug levels.[29] However, doses of SSRI also may need to be increased to maintain antidepressant efficacy during pregnancy.[30] A strategy to determine the minimum *effective* dose of any antidepressant across gestation has been developed, in which dosage is titrated to symptoms.[29] The mothers selected a target depressive symptom that was most disturbing (typically insomnia or irritability toward other children). Women were asked to contact the physician each time the symptom emerged, and an incremental dose was added, for example, 10 mg of nortriptyline. The dosages increased during the second half of pregnancy and rapidly accelerated during the third trimester. The final dose achieved during gestation was an average of 1.6 times the nonpregnant dose for TCA.

Hendrick et al.[31] determined the maternal and umbilical cord blood antidepressant and metabolite concentrations in 38 mother/baby pairs. Drug and metabolite concentrations were detectable in 86.8 percent of umbilical cord samples. The mean ratios of umbilical cord to maternal serum concentrations ranged from 0.29 to 0.89. The lowest ratios were for sertraline and paroxetine; the highest were for citalopram and fluoxetine.

Guidelines for the treatment of depression based on expert consensus were published in 2001.[32] For mild cases of depression, psychotherapy was the treatment of choice as the initial intervention. For moderate to severe cases with marked functional impairment, fluoxetine was the drug of first choice due to the data available about this agent across several domains of reproductive toxicity. Sertraline and paroxetine were also identified by some experts. In the ensuing 5 years, greater attention to neonatal toxicity, which occurs most commonly in fluoxetine- and paroxetine-treated women near term, has shifted preference toward sertraline or other SSRI use during gestation for newly diagnosed women or known responders. The FDA's advisory statement about paroxetine associated malformations has resulted in decreased use during gestation; however, the relatively low absolute risk for malformations may be acceptable to some women who respond well to the drug. Again, established efficacy for any antidepressant is a strong consideration in drug choice during the risk-benefit decision making process.

Psychotherapy

Interpersonal psychotherapy (IPT) is a brief, manual-based treatment to address interpersonal problems in the context of an MDE. IPT is given across 12 to 16 weekly sessions that focus on grief, interpersonal role disputes, role transitions, or interpersonal deficits. Depressed pregnant women treated with IPT had a significant symptomatic improvement compared with a parenting education control group, and 60 percent of women who received IPT achieved recovery criteria.[33] However, IPT is not widely available outside academic settings. Other focused short-term therapies, such as cognitive behavioral therapy, are attractive options for MDE during childbearing.

Novel Treatments

Exposure to bright morning light has been established as an efficacious treatment for MDE. In a recent meta-analysis, Golden et al.[34] found that bright light therapy was efficacious for seasonal affective disorder as well as nonseasonal MDE. The responsivity of depressed pregnant women to bright light therapy was explored in two small studies. In an open trial, the mean depressive symptom reduction in 16 pregnant women was comparable to antidepressant pharmacotherapy across 5 weeks.[35] In a pilot randomized clinical trial of ten women, significant improvement of depressive symptoms was demonstrated.[36]

Manber and colleagues[37] performed a novel randomized controlled study of acupuncture treatment specific to MDE, acupuncture treatment targeted to a condition other than MDE, and a massage control group. The group who received acupuncture treatment specifically for MDE had a significantly higher rate of response compared with the other two groups (69 percent versus 47 percent and 32 percent, respectively). The response rate was comparable to other therapies for an MDE.

Omega-3 fatty acids (O-3 FAs) are long-chain polyunsaturated fatty acids recognized as critical nutrients that the body cannot make. An inverse relationship between O-3 FA consumption and depressive symptoms in general populations has been demonstrated.[38] O-3 FA intake by pregnant women in the United States is inadequate, and high requirements during pregnancy increase the risk of deficiency and potentially depression.[39] Hibbeln et al.[39] studied the relationship of postpartum depression to fish intake. Published rates of postpartum depression were compared with the docosahexaenoic acid (DHA) content in mothers' milk and to seafood consumption rates from 23 countries. Higher concentrations of DHA in mothers' milk and greater seafood consumption both predicted lower prevalence rates of postpartum depression. The efficacy of O-3 FAs as treatment for antidepressant-refractory depression in non-pregnant samples has been demonstrated in double-blind, placebo-controlled trials.[40,41] In an open flexible-dose trial, Freeman et al.[42] administered the O-3 FAs eicosapentaenoic acid and DHA to 15 pregnant women. The mean decrease in EPDS score was 40.9 percent, and the mean decrease in the Hamilton Rating Scale for Depression score was 34.1 percent. The efficacy and safety of O-3 FAs for depression during pregnancy is being evaluated in a randomized, placebo-controlled study. However, an open trial of seven women treated with nearly 3 g of fish oil in the final trimester of pregnancy failed to prevent postpartum depression in four of the seven women.[43]

Postpartum Depression

This heartbreaking description of postpartum depression was written by Marie Osmond in *Behind the Smile: My Journey Out of Postpartum Depression:*

I can hear the breathing of my sleeping newborn son in his bassinet next to the bed. . . . I feel like I am playing hide and seek from my own life, except that I just want to hide and never be found. I want to escape my body. I don't recognize it any more. I have lost my resemblance to my former self. I can't laugh, enjoy food, sleep, concentrate on work, or even carry on a conversation. I don't know how to go on feeling like this: the emptiness, the endless loneliness. Who am I? I can't go on."[44]

How is postpartum depression defined? The two major international psychiatric diagnostic systems vary in their definitions. The International Classification of Diseases permits designation as *mental and physical disorders associated with the puerperium* only if the disorders begin within the first 6 weeks after birth and do not meet criteria for disorders classified elsewhere.[45] The DSM-IV[1] allows the designation *with postpartum onset* to be made as specifier for a limited number of diagnoses that begin within the first 4 weeks postpartum. Epidemiologists have defined the duration of *postpartum* based on judgments about the break point between increased risk for psychiatric illness after birth and baseline risk for psychiatric episodes in childbearing-aged women.[45] Kendell and colleagues[46–48] and Munk-Olsen and colleagues[48a] found a significant peak in the rate of contact for mood disorders in the 90-day period after childbirth. Therefore, the definition varies; however, the negative effects of the disorder for mother and baby do not depend on time of onset. As research about the effect of childbearing upon psychiatric illness and etiological factors evolves, a consensus definition is more likely.

Gaynes and colleagues[49] found a 14.5-percent incidence of depression during pregnancy and the same rate in the first 3 postpartum months, although higher rates have been reported among inner city women,[50] mothers of preterm infants,[51] and adolescent mothers.[52] Depression persists from months to years after childbirth, with lingering limitations in physical and psychological functioning following recovery from depressive episodes.[53–55] Twenty-five to fifty percent of women who experience depression in the postpartum period have episodes that last 7 months or longer.[56] The most significant factor in the duration of the depression is delay in receiving treatment.

Etiology

Postpartum depression occurs in a distinct biologic milieu compared with depression at other times in a woman's life. Bloch et al.[57] provided direct evidence that reproductive hormones play a role in the development of postpartum depression. The withdrawal of hormones at birth was simulated by inducing a hypogonadal state in women with leuprolide, adding back supraphysiologic doses of estradiol and progesterone for 8 weeks, and then withdrawing both steroids under double-blind conditions. Five of eight women with a history of postpartum depression, compared with none of the eight women without a history of depression, developed significant mood symptoms. Symptoms developed at the end of the add-back phase (simulation of end pregnancy) and peaked in the withdrawal (postpartum simulation) phase. Women with postpartum depression appeared differentially sensitive to the mood-destabilizing effects of withdrawal from gonadal steroids compared with women with no history of depression.

To test the hypothesis that postpartum depression is related to a hypoestrogenic state, and therefore may be treatable with estrogen, Gregoire et al.[58] compared estradiol to placebo for the treatment of postpartum MDE. Estradiol was delivered as 200 μg of 17-β-estradiol per day by transdermal patches. The estradiol-treated group showed a 50-percent reduction in depression scores in the first month of treatment; however, the study has not been replicated, and estradiol treatment is not standard therapy. Although it is tempting to attribute postpartum MDE to hormonal withdrawal, this conclusion is overly simplistic. As predicted by the multiple determinants model in Figure 50-1, MDE has contributions from several risk factor domains. Evidence of this statement derives from a prospective study of 680 female twins. Kendler[55] assessed liability to depression. The strongest predictors were (in descending order) stressful life events, genetic factors, previous history of an MDE, and neuroticism. Other authors have also identified stressful life events,[59] and previous history of depression in the patient and her family[60,61] as predictors of postpartum depression. Variables that are not related to the development of postpartum depression are educational level, cultural background, infant sex, breast-feeding, and unplanned pregnancy.[61]

The emergence of an episode of mood disorder in the postpartum period dictates investigation for altered neurologic status. Women with postpartum disorders should receive a complete review of systems, medical history, and focused physical examination to assess for organic contributions to the mood disorder. The use of prescribed (particularly pain medications) and over-the-counter medication use as well as drugs and alcohol must be assessed. Thyroid studies should be obtained to rule out postpartum thyroiditis; if present, the thyroid disorder usually requires treatment in addition to depression.[61]

Treatment of Postpartum Depression

Because of the dearth of treatment studies specifically in women with postpartum depression, the assumption is that medications effective for MDE in women outside of childbearing are effective during childbearing. Clinical experience and limited research support this assumption. Appleby and colleagues[62] published the only placebo-controlled randomized trial that was double blind (in relation to drug treatment) with four treatment cells: fluoxetine (20 mg/day) or placebo each with one or six sessions of cognitive behavioral counseling. The improvement in fluoxetine-treated patients was significantly greater than in those who received placebo, and there was no additional improvement with counseling. There are four open-label trials of antidepressant for postpartum MDE, all of which demonstrated efficacy at doses used for general populations. The drugs were sertraline,[63] venlafaxine,[64] fluvoxamine,[65] and grouped TCA and SSRI antidepressants.[66]

In a randomized control trial of sertraline (n = 55) and nortriptyline (n = 54) for the treatment of postpartum major depression,[66a] the proportion of women who responded and remitted at 4, 8 and 24 weeks follow-up did not differ between the drugs (Fig. 50-3). The time to response and remission at 8 and 24 weeks follow-up were similar for both drugs. Over three-quarters of the women who remitted fully by 8 weeks achieved a ≥50% reduction in symptoms by 4 weeks. The total side effect burden for each drug was similar although the side effect profiles differed for each drug.

Intent to Treat Analyses: Primary Symptom Outcomes at Weeks 4 and 8

	Sertraline		Nortriptyline	
	N=55		N=54	
Week 4		%		%
Remitted	15	27%	16	30%
Responded	25	46%	30	56%
Week 8				
Remitted	25	46%	26	48%
Responded	31	56%	37	69%

Figure 50-3. Treatment of postpartum depression during breast-feeding.

Treatment During Breast-Feeding

The magnitude of antidepressant exposure through breast milk is substantially lower than the exposure during pregnancy. A comprehensive pooled analysis of antidepressants in maternal serum, breast milk, and infant serum has been published.[67] The general approach to studying risk to infants when lactating mothers take antidepressants has been mother and nursing infant serum level monitoring. Maternal treatment with nortriptyline, paroxetine, and sertraline usually produces nonquantifiable levels in breast-fed infants.[67] These are drugs of first choice for the breastfeeding woman; however, established efficacy of another drug for the individual woman must be considered strongly in the decision-making process (Table 50-1). Sertraline has been the subject of most study from different investigative teams among the SSRI, and no adverse effects have been reported in breast-fed infants.[63,68–72]

Weissman et al.[67] identified maternal antidepressant medications associated with reports of negative effects in the infant: citalopram (n = 1), paroxetine (n = 1), fluoxetine (n = 5) and the tricyclic doxepin (n = 2). With the SSRI medications, adverse effects consist primarily of irritability, difficulty consoling, and poor feeding. The age at report of adverse event was between birth and 8 weeks for all cases except two for fluoxetine. Adverse events were associated with elevated infant serum drug levels in all cases. Fluoxetine was associated with the highest proportion (22 percent) of elevated infant levels, although not all infants with such levels had adverse signs. Fluoxetine and its metabolite norfluoxetine have very long half lives (84 and 146 hours, respectively). Continuous dosing through breast milk (particularly after prenatal loading) creates the potential to promote infant serum level development. Chambers et al.[17] reported that breast-fed infants of fluoxetine-treated mothers had significantly less weight gain than those of breast-feeding mothers who did not take fluoxetine. All mothers in this study had taken fluoxetine during pregnancy. A wide range of drug metabolic capacity is probable among infants, as in adults. Serum level monitoring in premature and sick infants has not been described in the literature and would be a significant contribution.

Although TCA are not first-line drugs for treatment of MDE, they have some advantages in breast-feeding women. Previous response to a TCA, low cost, and serum level correlation with response may warrant use of these agents in some situations. Data for nortriptyline, the most studied of the TCA, are provided in Table 50-1. The only adverse effects in breastfed infants whose mother took a TCA was for doxepin, a sedating antidepressant with a metabolite that has a long half life.[73] Overall, the low risk to infants from breast-feeding during maternal antidepressant therapy resulted in Weissman et al.'s[67] conclusion that current data do not support monitoring breast milk or serum levels in healthy infants.

Table 50-1. Selected Antidepressant Levels In Breast-Fed Infant's Sera

	SERUM LEVEL RANGE IN BREAST-FED INFANTS, NG/ML	TYPICAL MATERNAL DOSE RANGE, MG/DAY
Drugs of First Choice for the Breastfeeding Woman		
Nortriptyline*	Nortriptyline, below limit of quantifiability to 10	50–150; therapeutic serum levels known
Nortriptyline metabolites	E-10-OH- Nortriptyline = <4–16	
	Z-10-OH- Nortriptyline = <4–17	
Sertraline	Sertraline, below limit of quantifiability to 8	50–200
Sertraline metabolites	Norsertraline, below limit of quantifiability to 26	
Paroxetine	Paroxetine, below limit of quantifiability	10–60
No active metabolites		
Other Antidepressants[†]		
Fluoxetine	Fluoxetine, below quantifiability to 340	20–60
Fluoxetine metabolite[‡]	Norfluoxetine, below quantifiability to 265	
Citalopram	Citalopram, below quantifiability to 12.7	20–40
	Desmethylcitalopram, below quantifiability to 3.1	
Venlafaxine	Venlafaxine, below quantifiability to 5	75–300
Venlafaxine metabolite	O-desmethylvenlafaxine, below quantifiability to 38	

*The most-studied tricyclic antidepressant during breast-feeding; current minimal use of this drug class.
[†]Established efficacy of an antidepressant in a woman is a strong consideration in drug selection.
[‡]As active as fluoxetine and has a longer half life than the parent drug.

Bipolar Disorder

Diagnosis and Prevalence

The diagnosis of MDE is limited to the lifetime experience of normal mood plus episodes of depression, whereas BD includes normal, depressed, and elevated mood states (mania or its less intense form, hypomania). Mania consists of a persistent, abnormally elevated, expansive or irritable mood with inflated self-esteem/grandiosity, excessive physical and/or goal-directed activity, agitation, distractibility, and poor judgment, for a minimum of 1 week. Impairment in function at work or in interpersonal relationships must be present. Hypomania is defined by a minimum of 4 days of persistent increased creativity, productivity, and sociability, or increased irritability that family or coworkers notice. During hypomania, function may be enhanced by creativity and enhanced thought fluency. Many artists, writers, and world leaders have had BD.[74] BD is divided into two major categories. BD I is characterized by the presence of depression and mania. This illness affects women and men equally,[75] and the lifetime prevalence is estimated at 1.3 percent.[76] Much higher prevalence rates (3.7 to 6.4 percent) have been reported for BD II (depression plus hypomania rather than full-blown mania) and bipolar spectrum disorders.[77] Several bipolar variants occur more commonly in women, such as BD II, mixed states in which both mania and depressive symptoms occur together, and a rapid-cycling course (four or more episodes yearly).[78]

Conditions that frequently co-occur with BD include panic disorder, agoraphobia, social phobia, marijuana use, and bulimia nervosa (BN).[79] Women more commonly have past sexual abuse, alcohol abuse/dependence, migraines, drug-induced metabolic syndrome, pain disorders, and hypothyroidism compared with men.[80–85] Despite maintenance therapy, the relapse risk within a 1 year time frame is 37 to 44 percent[86] and 87 percent at 5 years follow-up.[87] Women frequently describe a seasonal pattern of mood episodes, with winter depression[88] characterized by atypical symptoms like weight gain, hypersomnia and extremely low energy.[89] In contrast, spring and summer are associated with hypomania or mania. Depression is the predominant symptom polarity in many bipolar patients, and is mistaken for unipolar depression in 30 percent of cases.[90]

Patients who present with depression are inadequately screened for bipolarity, which contributes to the significant delay in diagnosis (about 11 years) from illness onset to the confirmation of BD.[91] In addition, antidepressant medication without an antimanic agent increases the risk for cycle acceleration, mania, or a mixed state. The mood criterion symptoms for hypomania (high mood and/or irritability) can be used as a simple screen[11]: "Have you ever had 4 continuous days in which you felt so good, high, excited, or "hyper" that other people thought you were not your usual self or you got into trouble? Have you ever had 4 continuous days when you were so irritable you found yourself shouting at people, or starting fights or arguments?" If the patient is symptomatic, inquiry about her safety risk is warranted: "Along with your mood symptoms, have you had thoughts of dying, wishing you were dead, or taking your life?" The Mood Disorder Questionnaire (MDQ)[92] is a self-report screening tool with good sensitivity and specificity in a psychiatric population; however, in the general population, the MDQ had a sensitivity of 0.28 and a specificity of 0.97.[93] Use the MDQ for screening of the general population, in which prevalence will be low and therefore the predictive value of positive tests will be very low, is not appropriate.

Natural History Across Childbearing

It is difficult to predict the course of bipolar symptoms during pregnancy. Some researchers have described a benign course or mood stabilization for women with BD during gestation,[94] whereas others have observed that pregnancy has no effect on the risk for episodes.[95] Abrupt discontinuation of lithium increases the risk of recurrence.[95,96] The overall risk of a new episode of mania was significantly greater after rapid (less than 2 weeks) than gradual (2 to 4 weeks) discontinuation (5-year hazard ratio = 2.8). The difference in risk of a new episode of depression was even greater (hazard ratio = 5.4). Women with BD have a high risk for both recurrence and first admission for bipolar illness in the immediate period after birth.[97,98] Close clinical monitoring after birth and treatment with the agent most effective for the individual patient is the most reasonable strategy. Postpartum psychosis is typically a manifestation of BD[98,99] and presents in 1 to 2 per 1000 births within 2 weeks of delivery.[100] Women develop mood lability, confusion, delusional thinking, hallucinations, poor concentration, impaired judgment and insight. Acute-onset postpartum psychosis is an emergency, and women must be screened for thoughts of harming themselves or others, especially the newborn.[98]

Treatment for Bipolar Disorder

Although medication maintenance is the mainstay of treatment for BD, psychotherapy and positive interpersonal relationships are critical adjuncts to pharmacotherapy. To optimize the care of patients with BD, a therapeutic alliance must be established. The physician has a major role in providing educational support and promoting treatment adherence.[101,102] Early treatment for low-level symptoms has resulted in lower rates of relapse, increased time to recurrence, improved medication adherence, and better functioning.[103–105] Treatment adherence is an essential component for optimal treatment outcomes and patient satisfaction with care.[106]

Several drug classes are indicated for the treatment of mania. Lithium, antiepileptic drugs (AEDs), and several newer atypical antipsychotic medications are efficacious for mania. Unfortunately, these antimanic agents result in a treatment response in only 36 to 50 percent of cases.[1,107] Therefore, patients often receive more than one drug to manage their mood symptoms. Strategies to minimize fetal exposure include (1) use the lowest *effective* dose; (2) minimize the number of drugs to achieve response, and (3) divide daily doses to avoid high peak serum concentrations.

Lithium

Lithium is the standard drug for maintenance therapy for BD. Before initiating lithium treatment, assessments of renal, thyroid, and pregnancy status are recommended.[1,107] The starting dose is 300 mg twice daily. Serum drug levels and renal function tests should be repeated after 5 days of treatment. The target serum level is 0.4 to 1.0 mEq/L at 12 hours post dose. If the woman's serum drug level falls below this range, and her mood symptoms persist and there are no major side effects, a dose increase is appropriate. The dose can be increased by 300 mg every 5 to 7 days as tolerated with re-evaluation of serum level status. Treatment response is usually achieved at 900 to 1200 mg total per day. Higher doses may be necessary for episodes of mania.

Patients are encouraged to have their lithium level monitored every 2 to 4 weeks throughout pregnancy; weekly in the last month, and every few days shortly after delivery.[98,108] Typical side effects of lithium include sedation, tremor, renal dysfunction, weight gain, nausea, and vomiting. Lithium has a relatively narrow window between therapeutic and toxic serum levels. Toxicity is associated with excessive sedation, severe tremors, acute renal dysfunction, and intractable vomiting. Women who are dehydrated from hyperemesis or sodium-depleting conditions are especially vulnerable. Lithium toxicity must be managed immediately with lithium discontinuation, rehydration therapy and vigilant monitoring of fluid/electrolyte balance and renal function. Diuretics and nonsteroidal anti-inflammatory drugs should be avoided in lithium-treated patients because these drugs interfere with the renal clearance of lithium and increase the risk for toxicity.

Lithium exposure during the first trimester was linked with Ebstein's anomaly in the years after it came into common use. Subsequent prospective studies demonstrated that the risk was overestimated due to voluntary reporting to a registry, which inflates the number of cases (numerator) while underestimating the population exposed (denominator).[98] The risk of Ebstein's anomaly after first trimester exposure is 1/1000 to 1/2000 (20 to 40 times higher than the general population (see Chapter 8).[109] Lithium-exposed neonates are at risk for large for gestational age newborns, hypotonia, feeding difficulties, depressed reflexes, cyanosis, apnea, bradycardia, hypothyroidism. and diabetes insipidus.[98,108] The neonatal symptoms appear to be temporary and may be linked with higher maternal serum concentrations at delivery (>0.64 mEq/L).[110] The suspension of lithium 24 to 48 hours before a scheduled delivery or at the onset of labor reduces the likelihood for perinatal complications.[110] Developmental milestones are normal during infancy and early childhood.[111]

Viguera et al.[112] examined 10 pairs of lithium-treated mothers and their breast-feeding babies 4 to 12 weeks after delivery. They measured maternal and infant serum, breast milk lithium concentrations, and renal or thyroid dysfunction in the infants. In 9 of 10 mother infant pairs, no adverse effects were detected. One infant had an elevated thyroid-stimulating hormone (TSH) that resolved by 2 weeks after lithium exposure was discontinued, and infant renal function remained normal. Infant serum lithium levels were 25 percent of maternal levels. The investigators recommended clinical monitoring of breastfed infants and serum levels of lithium, TSH, blood urea nitrogen and creatinine every 6 to 8 weeks while breastfeeding. In addition, mothers must be educated about the risk of lithium toxicity with neonatal dehydration and advised to seek pediatric evaluation for changes in the behavior of their infant.[90]

Valproic Acid

Valproic acid (VPA) was the first FDA-indicated AED for the treatment of BD (specifically for mania). The typical starting dose is 500 to 750 mg daily. Therapeutic levels range from 50 to 125 ug/mL. Adverse effects include nausea, weight gain, fatigue, tremor, ataxia, diarrhea, abdominal pain, alopecia, hepatitis, thrombocytopenia, and rarely pancreatitis. The European and International Registry of Antiepileptic Drugs in Pregnancy surveillance system of more than 3,000 pregnancies revealed that the rate of major congenital malformations was significantly higher in women who took VPA (6.1 percent) compared with those who took carbemazepine (CBZ) (2.3 percent) or lamotrigine (2.9 percent)[113] (see Chapter 8). Therefore, avoiding first-line use of VPA in women who are considering pregnancy is reasonable, although all AEDs except lamotrigine and oxcarbazepine have been associated with an increased risk of malformations. In unplanned pregnancies, women often seek prenatal care after neural tube closure (6 weeks from the last menstrual period),[114] which negates the major benefit of changing medication.[98] VPA is concentrated in the fetal compartment and divided doses combined with the lowest effective dose is recommended to avoid high single peak levels.[98] Neonatal complications associated with VPA use near delivery include decelerations, withdrawal symptoms of irritability, jitteriness, feeding difficulties, abnormal tone, hepatic toxicity, hypoglycemia, and a reduction in neonatal fibrinogen levels. At birth, cord blood levels of VPA can reach twice as high as maternal levels.[98]

Carbamazepine

CBZ is prescribed at doses between 400 and 1600 mg daily for BD to achieve a target range of 4 to 12 ug/mL.[115] Drug-induced toxicity is usually detectable from clinical symptoms, and the serum level provides objective evidence. The American Academy of Neurology and a British panel of neurology experts published best practice guidelines for the management of AEDs in pregnancy. They found no consensus or epidemiologic evidence to support recommendations for monitoring AED drug levels, including CBZ, in pregnancy.[116,117] During pregnancy, the total AED levels drop, but the amount of unbound (bioavailable) drug remains unchanged. Serum levels are useful in the assessment of patients who are experiencing exacerbation of mood symptoms, side effects and treatment adherence.

Hepatitis, leukopenia, thrombocytopenia, rash, sedation, ataxia are important side effects. Due to the potential for bone marrow suppression, combining CBZ and the antipsychotic clozapine is contraindicated. Maternal CBZ therapy is associated with reduction in birth weight (about 250 grams) and mean head circumference.[98] Fetal serum levels of carbamazepine are 50 percent to 80 percent of maternal levels.[118] Since adequate levels of Vitamin K are necessary for normal mid-facial growth and for the functioning of clotting factors, CBZ exposure in utero could increase the risk of neonatal bleeding.[98] Some experts recommend administering Vitamin K 20 mg daily throughout pregnancy[116,119] and 1 mg intramuscularly to neonates.[98]

Oxcarbazepine

Oxcarbazepine is a newer AED that has been used to treat mania. It is prescribed in divided doses (total dose, 600 to 1200 mg/day). The parent compound is rapidly and almost completely metabolized to an active hydroxy metabolite. The metabolite undergoes hepatic glucuronidation, and the conjugate product is excreted renally. Important adverse effects are: hyponatremia, hypersensitivity reactions, and decreased thyroxine levels (without altered triiodothyronine or TSH). Side effects include headaches, dizziness, gait disturbance, fatigue, concentration and memory changes. In 55 babies exposed in utero to oxcarbazepine (20 combination therapy, 35 monotherapy), one malformation (cardiac) was reported in an infant that was also exposed to phenobarbital.[120] The metabolite is distributed equally between the mother and placental tissue.[121] Bulau et al.[122] evaluated a breast-feeding infant whose mother took the drug during pregnancy. At 5 days after birth, the infant drug concentrations for parent drug and metabolite were only 12 percent and 7 percent, respectively, of the levels drawn shortly after birth.

Lamotrigine

Lamotrigine is indicated for bipolar depression maintenance therapy.[123] Recommended doses of lamotrigine for bipolar depression range from 50 to 200 mg/day.[123] Higher doses of lamotrigine (200 to 500 mg/day) have been used for long-term maintenance therapy of patients with BD.[124] Patients encountered side effects such as headaches, nonserious rash, dizziness, diarrhea, abnormal dreams, and pruritus,[125,126] which did not differ from the rates in placebo-treated patients.[127] The problematic rash associated with lamotrigine typically appears as maculopapular or erythematous.[128] The rash is most likely to occur with rapid dose escalation, when combined with VPA, and among adolescents.[115] The rate of lamotrigine-associated rash in patients with mood disorders was investigated in clinical trials. Calabrese et al.[126] performed a retrospective analysis of rates of lamotrigine-related rash in 12 multicenter studies. A total of 1,955 patients were treated with lamotrigine in open-label settings, 1,198 patients received lamotrigine in controlled studies, and 1,056 patients received placebo. In controlled studies, the rates of benign rash were 8.3 percent in lamotrigine-treated and 6.4 percent in placebo-treated patients. Serious rash occurred in 0 percent of lamotrigine-treated and 0.1 percent (N = 1) of placebo-treated patients. In the open-label settings, the overall rate of rash for lamotrigine was 13.1 percent (N = 257) and of serious rash, 0.1 percent (N = 2). One case of Stevens-Johnson syndrome that did not require hospitalization occurred in a patient treated with lamotrigine. There were no cases of toxic epidermal necrolysis in any setting. Although the condition is potentially life-threatening, the low risk of rash due to lamotrigine should be weighed against more common risks associated with depression in patients with BD.[126]

A greater than 65-percent increase in the apparent clearance of lamotrigine between preconception and the second and third trimesters in 12 pregnant women was observed, and 11 women experienced increased seizures that required dose increases.[129] After birth, lamotrigine metabolism reverted to the prepregnancy rate within 2 weeks of delivery. Lamotrigine undergoes hepatic glucuronidation (conjugation) and renal excretion.[130] Infant and childhood glucuronidation activity remains substantially lower than that of adults. Oxazepam, lorazepam, aspirin, acetaminophen, VPA, and olanzapine (OLZ) are other drugs metabolized by glucuronidation. These drugs have the potential to increase toxicity in breast-feeding women and their newborns.

From a pregnancy registry, Messenheimer et al.[128] observed 10 major malformations among 360 first-trimester lamotrigine monotherapy exposures (2.8 percent). The observed risk among 76 lamotrigine and VPA combined first-trimester exposures was 10.5 percent compared with 3.1 percent for lamotrigine monotherapy. No evidence of growth problems, post-birth discovery of occult malformations, neonatal seizures, or deviations in psychomotor development to 1 year of age were observed in 62 infants exposed to lamotrigine in utero.[131]

Atypical Antipsychotics

Newer antipsychotic medications were developed for the treatment of schizophrenia but also have efficacy for mania, and all are FDA-indicated for manic episodes. The usual daily maintenance dose ranges for these drugs are OLZ, 5 to 20 mg; risperidone, 1 to 6 mg; quetiapine, 400 to 800 mg in two divided doses; ziprasidone, 80 to 160 mg in two divided doses; and aripiprazole 15 to 30 mg. Initial dosing is lower, and drugs are titrated upward against tolerance. In general, extrapyramidal side effects (e.g., tremor, rigidity, akathisia, bradykinesia, tardive dyskinesia, dystonia) are less common with atypical than the older typical antipsychotics (such as haloperidol). Other side effects include somnolence, dry mouth, akathisia (internal sense of restlessness), and increased hepatic transaminases. A marked and sustained hyperprolactinemia is associated with risperidone (88 percent of patients), as compared with conventional antipsychotics like haloperidol (48 percent) or OLZ (minimal, if any).[132] The metabolic effects of atypical agents are a major public health concern. Patients are at risk for significant weight gain, elevated triglycerides, and new-onset metabolic syndrome or insulin intolerance (OLZ, in particular).[133] Significantly more women who took atypical agents were overweight (body mass index [BMI] = 25 to 29.9 kg/m^2) with a median BMI of 28.8, compared with women who took typical agents, who had a median BMI of 22.9.[134] Obese women are more likely to develop complications during pregnancy and delivery and have increased rates of cesarean delivery, induction of labor, large-for-gestational age babies, and macrosomic babies larger than 4,000 g at birth.[135] Use of an atypical antipsychotic agent should prompt a review of BMI and health risks secondary to drug use in the management of the pregnant patient.

The reproductive risks of atypical antipsychotics have received minimal research attention.[136] Women with mental illness have an overall higher risk for adverse pregnancy outcome than the general population. In Australia, Jablensky et al.[137] determined the rate of complications during pregnancy, labor, and delivery, and the neonatal characteristics of infants born to women with BD, schizophrenia, or major depression in a population-based cohort (N = 3,174 children born during from 1980 to 1992). A comparison sample of 3,129 births to women without a psychiatric diagnosis was randomly selected from women who gave birth during the same time frame. Women with schizophrenia had more than twice the risk for placental abruption compared to healthy controls (odds ratio [OR] = 2.75; 95-percent CI, 1.32 to 5.74); whereas women with bipolar illness (OR, 0.69; 95-percent CI, 0.31 to 1.54) or unipolar depression (OR, 1.34; 95-percent CI, 0.68 to 2.65) did not have elevated risk for placental complications. Compared with nonpsychiatrically ill women, the rates of antepartum hemorrhage were significantly higher in mothers with schizophrenia (OR, 1.65; 95-percent CI, 1.02 to 2.69) and bipolar illness (OR, 1.66; 95 percent CI, 1.15 to 2.39); but not unipolar depression (OR, 1.24; 95-percent CI, 0.84 to 1.84). Although genetic liability and gene-environment interactions contribute to these outcomes, maternal risk factors, substance abuse, nutritional status, and biological and behavioral concomitants of severe mental illness are major determinants of increases in reproductive pathology in this cohort (Fig. 50-1).

Alternate or Supplemental Treatment Options

Some patients do not respond, have prohibitive side effects, or have medical disorders that complicate the use of lithium, anticonvulsants, and antipsychotics. Additional therapies are being evaluated to expand the therapeutic armamentarium during childbearing. An inverse correlation between O-3 FA consumption (through per capita seafood consumption) and the population prevalence of BD has been demonstrated.[138] Increased duration of remission of bipolar episodes occurred in subjects who were randomized to fish oil versus placebo supplementation.[139] The recommended initial fish oil dose is 2 g daily, with a gradual titration to 4 g daily according to side effects (gastrointestinal discomfort, increased bleeding time).[140]

Reports of the use of calcium channel blockers for BD have been published for two decades. Verapamil (VPM) possesses clinically relevant dopamine antagonist properties, as evidenced by its ability to increase prolactin release,[141] as well as antiepileptic activity.[142] Although open case series data showed reduction of manic symptoms,[143] results of controlled studies have been less encouraging. Janicak et al.[144] did not find differences in patients treated with VPM compared with those treated with placebo in a 3-week double-blind randomized trial hospitalized patients with mania. The efficacy of VPM (or any other calcium channel blocker) has never been explored in randomized acute treatment trials with adequate power, and additional research is warranted. If it is found to be efficacious, VPM would be an attractive alternative in pregnant and breastfeeding women.[143]

Electroconvulsive therapy (ECT) is associated with a high rate of response in serious mood disorders. Women who are nonresponsive to standard treatments, those with severe depression, acute mania or mixed states are candidates for ECT.[145] ECT is an attractive alternative for severely ill pregnant patients, because the acute treatment involves only short-acting drugs used during the procedure.[98,146] Maintenance ECT can be provided instead of drug therapy after remission of illness.

Breast-Feeding for Women with Bipolar Disorder

The mother's commitment to breastfeeding is an important consideration in the postpartum management of women with mood disorders. Sleep deprivation, which is often unavoidable in the postpartum period, is a major precipitant of mania and hypomania. If a partner or support person can feed the baby at night, sleep can be preserved in vulnerable women; however, this level of support is not always available. The American Academy of Pediatrics (AAP) Committee on Drugs[147] considers carbamazepine and VPA to be usually compatible with breastfeeding, while lamotrigine is a drug for which the effect in nursing infants is unknown but may be of concern. Lithium is in the category of drugs that have been associated with significant effects on some nursing infants and should be given to nursing mothers with caution[147] (see Chapter 8).

Prevention of Bipolar Episode Recurrence Postpartum

For the woman with BD, the risk for recurrence in the puerperium is the highest at any point in her life.[100] Viguera et al.[96] retrospectively compared recurrence rates in childbearing compared with nonchildbearing women who discontinued lithium treatment. In the year before lithium discontinuation, the rate of recurrence was 21 percent. After lithium discontinuation, the rates of recurrence over the first 40 weeks were similar in pregnant (52 percent) and nonpregnant (58 percent) women. In the high-risk postpartum period, recurrences occurred at three times the rate observed in the nonpregnant women during the same time frame (70 percent versus 24 percent). Nine women who continued lithium and remained well during pregnancy were also observed, and three suffered rapid postpartum recurrences despite continued lithium treatment. VPA did not reduce the number or time to episode recurrence in postpartum women with BD compared with nonmedicated women in a prospective trial.[97] In the clinical management of these mothers, educating significant others to observe for symptoms of decompensation and to report them to the treatment team is arguably the most important strategy at this point in our knowledge of prophylactic therapies. The most prudent pharmacologic plan is to use the drug or drugs to which the individual woman has responded and prepare a plan for rapid augmentation if a breakthrough episode of either polarity occurs.[100]

ANXIETY DISORDERS

Diagnosis and Prevalence

Anxiety disorders are characterized by prominent symptoms of anxiety. Examples are panic disorder, agoraphobia, obsessive-compulsive disorder, posttraumatic stress disorder, generalized anxiety disorder, and phobias. Each of these disorders is distinct and defined by specific diagnostic criteria according to DSM-IV.[1] However, the rule rather than the exception is for multiple anxiety disorders to occur in an individual.[148–150] In a large population-based study, the National Institute of Mental Health Epidemiologic Catchment Area study, anxiety disorders were more prevalent than any other mental disorder (8.3 percent of the population).[150] In women, the 12-month prevalence of anxiety disorders is 3 to 5 percent for panic disorder, 5 percent for agoraphobia, 4 percent for generalized anxiety disorder, 2 percent for obsessive-compulsive disorder, 9 percent for social phobia, 13 percent for other specific phobias, and 1 percent for posttraumatic stress disorder.[149–152] At some point during their lives, 31 percent of women will have an anxiety disorder. Rates of obsessive-compulsive disorder are similar in men and women, but other anxiety disorders are 1.5 to 2 times more common in women. Without treatment, the course of anxiety disorders is usually chronic. In addition, women with anxiety disorders have an increased risk for development of comorbid major depression.

Panic attacks are characterized by brief (5 to 15 minutes), intense episodes of fear or discomfort. Panic attacks occur in a variety of anxiety disorders, as well as in healthy individuals exposed to acute stress. Symptoms include palpitations, sweating, shortness of breath, choking, nausea, abdominal discomfort, dizziness, unsteadiness, numbness or tingling, chills, hot flashes, or a fear of dying or losing control. Panic disorder is diagnosed if panic attacks are recurrent or associated with a continuing fear of future attacks that leads to anxiety between attacks. The most disabling consequence of panic disorder, agoraphobia, occurs in 30 to 40 percent of women with untreated panic disorder. Individuals with agoraphobia restrict their activities outside the home or insist on being accompanied by another individual due to fear of having a panic attack where help is unavailable.

Generalized anxiety disorder is characterized by excessive worrying about multiple problems. The issues of concern to persons with generalized anxiety disorder are realistic but the level of worry is much more intense than appropriate. For example, a woman might worry for hours about whether a friend received a thank you note for a baby shower gift. Individuals with generalized anxiety disorder often have physical symptoms associated with worrying, such as muscle tension, fatigue, headache, nausea, diarrhea or abdominal pain. To meet criteria for the disorder, subjects must have significant impairment of functioning and anxiety for 6 months or more.

In contrast to generalized anxiety disorder, women with obsessive-compulsive disorder focus on more idiosyncratic and often unrealistic concerns. For example, a new mother might check her healthy, full-term baby every 10 minutes throughout the night to make sure that the infant continues to breathe, or count to 30 every time she diapers the baby to prevent some harm from occurring. Obsessive-compulsive disorder is characterized by disturbing intrusive thoughts and performance of compulsions to temporarily relieve the distress generated by the intrusive thoughts. Intrusive thoughts usually center on a few key themes: contamination, causing harm, offensive violent or sexual images, religious preoccupations, and urges for symmetry or ordering. Compulsions performed to relieve these intrusive worries include cleaning or washing, checking, repeating, ordering, hoarding, and mental rituals like counting and praying. To meet criteria for the disorder, the symptoms must interfere with functioning and last at least 1 hour per day.

Exposure to trauma in which a woman experienced or witnessed an event that involved actual or threatened death or serious injury (such as military combat or rape) can result in posttraumatic stress disorder. The traumatic event is persistently re-experienced in one (or more) of the following ways: recurrent and intrusive distressing recollections of the event, recurrent distressing dreams, acting or feeling as if the event were recurring (flashbacks), and intense distress at cues that remind her of the event. Physiologic hyperarousal and exaggerated startle responses occur. Symptoms usually begin within 3 months of the trauma and they must persist for at least 1 month to meet diagnostic criteria for posttraumatic stress disorder. For some women, childbirth is experienced as an extreme traumatic event that can result in posttraumatic stress disorder. The reported prevalence of posttraumatic stress disorder after childbirth ranges from 1.5 percent to 6 percent.[153] Mothers with posttraumatic stress disorder attributable to childbirth suffer with nightmares and flashbacks of the birth, anger, and anxiety, in addition to coping with new motherhood. Surprisingly little research has been done with this clinical population.

Finally, excessive fear of a discrete object or situation constitutes a phobia. Social phobia refers to fears of speaking or eating in public and fears of humiliation in social interactions. These fears must be excessive and significantly impair an individual's social or occupational functioning for the diagnosis to be made. Other common specific phobias are body injury phobia (blood drawing or medical procedures), acrophobia (heights), arachnophobia (spiders), and claustrophobia (enclosed spaces). Even the possibility of confronting the feared object or situation stimulates anxiety, which is described as anticipatory anxiety. Anticipatory anxiety can be a feature of any anxiety disorder. Individuals with panic disorder often have fear of situations from which they could not escape if they had a panic attack, including airplanes, bridges, and subways. These fears are considered to be a feature of panic disorder and agoraphobia, and would not warrant an additional diagnosis of simple phobia.

FEAR OF LABOR AND DELIVERY

In modern obstetric practice, perinatal morbidity and mortality of mother and neonate are rare; however, some women have intense fear about childbearing. Approximately 10 to 20 percent of pregnant women develop extreme fear of delivery,[154–156] which may be considered a type of phobia. Some women request a surgical delivery to avoid labor.[148,157] Factors such as prior emotional problems, low social support, poor relationship satisfaction, unemployment, and prior complicated deliveries have been found to be risk factors for intense fear of delivery.[158–162] In Finland, 176 women who had fear of childbirth were randomly assigned at the 26th gestational week to have either intensive therapy or conventional therapy.[160] Birth-related concerns were significantly decreased in the intensive therapy group but increased in the conventional therapy group. Labor was significantly shorter in the intensive therapy group (6.8 ± 3.8 hours) compared with the conventional group (8.5 ± 4.8 hours), but there was no difference in the number of women (62 percent) who decided to have a vaginal delivery after initially requesting an elective cesarean section.

Natural History Across Childbearing

Pregnancy, delivery, and lactation produce profound changes in physiology, including changes in multiple hormonal and neurotransmitter systems that modulate anxiety symptoms. Although pregnancy and postpartum have been identified as times of increased risk for relapse of depressive disorders, the course of anxiety disorders has not been elucidated. The offspring of highly anxious women are exposed to an altered physiologic milieu during pregnancy and maternal anxiety-related behaviors postpartum. In a cohort of 8,000, more women scored above threshold on an anxiety scale during weeks 18 and 32 of pregnancy compared with 8 weeks and 8 months postpartum. Antenatal anxiety was associated with an increased risk of postpartum depression, even after controlling for antenatal depression.[163] Anxiety disorders are as common as major depression in the postpartum period.[73,164] Preliminary evidence from case reports and retrospective studies suggest that a reduction of panic attacks occurs in pregnancy but that an increase occurs postpartum.[165–170] However, subsequent reports of the effects of pregnancy on the course of panic disorder have shown no improvement during pregnancy.[169,171–174] Pregnancy may exacerbate obsessive-compulsive symptoms.[175,176] The first months after birth are a high-risk period for the first lifetime onset of anxiety disorders such as panic disorder[170,177] and obsessive-compulsive disorder.[176,178] Hyperthyroidism is associated with panic attacks and anxiety symptoms, and should be considered in the differential diagnosis of postpartum onset anxiety disorders. There is no information on the effects of pregnancy on the course of generalized anxiety disorder, phobias, or posttraumatic stress disorder.

Effect of Anxiety During Childbearing

Stress, pregnancy fears, and anxiety have been associated with obstetric complications. Anxiety and fear of delivery increase the risk of preeclampsia,[59,179] severe pain during labor, increased analgesic use,[156] oxytocin use, and surgical deliveries.[159,161,180–183] High levels of anxiety symptoms increase uterine artery resistance,[184] which limits blood supply to the fetal compartment. Fetuses of pregnant women who report greater stress have reduced heart rate variability, which has been associated with subsequent poor emotional regulation.[185–190] Low socioeconomic status, which often is accompanied by heightened levels of life stress, increases the risk for higher and less variable fetal heart rate throughout the second and third trimesters.[191]

Maternal psychological stress and anxiety are associated with shortened gestation and lower birth weight for gestational age after adjustment for the effects of medical, behavioral and demographic risk factors.[159,192–200] Reduced gestational age and low birth weight for gestational age increase the risk of behavioral and neurologic delays during childhood and multiple health problems in adulthood such as obesity and cardiovascular disease.[201–203] Maternal anxiety during pregnancy is associated with attention deficits, motor immaturity, and difficult temperament in offspring. A prospective, longitudinal study of more than 7,000 pregnant women showed that anxiety during pregnancy doubled the risk for hyperactivity in 4-year-old boys after controlling for obstetric and sociodemographic risks as well as mothers' post–natal anxiety levels.[204,205] This effect persisted through age 7 years.[206] In a prospective study in which anxiety during pregnancy and child outcomes at age 8 to 9 years old were examined, prenatal anxiety was associated with child inattention and hyperactivity symptoms, externalizing problems, and self-report anxiety scores even after controlling for gestational smoking, birth weight, postnatal anxiety, and parent education level.[207] Research to assess the effects of treatment for anxiety during pregnancy, and whether these adverse outcomes are prevented, is a critical frontier.

In cross-sectional studies, lactating women reported decreased anxiety and depression compared with bottle feeding mothers.[208–215] Decreased anxiety and depression symptoms were observed immediately after a breast-feeding episode but not following a bottle-feeding episode[216–218] or after holding the infant.[219] Women with panic disorder may experience a reduction in panic attacks during lactation but relapse during or after weaning.[165,168]

Treatment of Anxiety Disorders

The boundary between normal and pathologic anxiety cannot be drawn with great precision. When anxiety substantially impairs work, family, or social adjustment, careful assessment is indicated and treatment is appropriate. Panic disorder often responds to antidepressant medications, which are first-line therapies. Benzodiazepines are effective but are associated with abuse in a subset of patients. Cognitive therapy, a time-limited, structured psychotherapy, also is efficacious for panic disorder. In contrast, obsessive-compulsive disorder is effectively treated only with serotonin selective reuptake inhibitors. A specific behavioral therapy technique, including exposure and response prevention, is the most effective type for obsessive compulsive disorder. Generalized anxiety disorder responds to a variety of antidepressant medications and cognitive therapy. Posttraumatic stress disorder is partially responsive to antidepressant medication and cognitive therapy is a primary treatment. The first-line treatment for social phobia is SSRI. Specific phobias are most effectively treated with desensitization psychotherapy.

A risk-benefit evaluation for treatments during pregnancy must be individualized for the pregnant woman with anxiety disorder, which, like major depression, also has a negative impact on pregnancy outcome. If psychotherapy treatment is refused, not available, or ineffective, pharmacologic treatment should be considered. The use of antidepressants in pregnancy and lactation has been reviewed in the section on major depression. Because alternative treatments are available for anxiety disorders, benzodiazepines often can be avoided or used for limited time periods during pregnancy and lactation. Evidence from the available studies is conflicting about whether benzodiazepines have teratogenic effects; however, the risk, if any, is relatively small.[220,221] Less is known about the effects of benzodiazepine use during pregnancy and lactation on infant neurobehavioral development. Neonatal withdrawal symptoms, including seizures, have been reported postpartum.

EATING DISORDERS

Eating disorders are characterized by serious disturbances in eating behavior. The most familiar and well described are anorexia nervosa (AN) and bulimia nervosa (BN). Binge-eating disorder and subclinical forms of AN and BN also occur in women. Eating disorders are particularly relevant during pregnancy and lactation, when the requirement for adjustments in nutritional intake is directly affected by active eating disorders.

Diagnosis and Prevalence

AN is characterized by the woman's refusal to maintain a minimally normal body weight, defined as a body weight less than 85 percent of that expected for age and height. Amenorrhea (absence of at least three menstrual cycles) is required for the diagnosis of AN. The prevalence of AN in adolescents and young women is 0.5 to 1 percent, and the mean age of onset is 17 years of age. The course of AN is highly variable, with a range of outcomes that include recovery, residual partial symptomatology, and a fluctuating or chronic course.

BN occurs in 1 to 3 percent of young adult women. Women with BN maintain body weight at or above a minimally normal range but use binge eating plus compensatory methods to prevent weight gain. A binge is excess eating in a discrete period of time (within 2 hours) of an amount of food that is decisively larger than most people would eat during a similar period of time. The binge eating and inappropriate compensatory behaviors must occur at least twice a week for 3 months. Inappropriate compensatory behaviors that occur in both AN and BN are self-induced vomiting; laxative, diuretic, or other medication (such as ipecac) abuse; fasting; and excessive exercise. A disturbance in the perception of body shape and weight is an essential feature of both disorders. The course of BN also may be chronic or recur intermittently. In BN, menstrual irregularities are common, but they have minimal impact on later ability to achieve pregnancy.[222] Follow-up of women 11.5 years after initial evaluation for BN revealed that 74.6 percent had been able to achieve pregnancy and only 1.7 percent reported an inability to conceive.

The ratio of women to men with both AN and BN is striking at 10:1. The etiology of eating disorders has contributions from multiple domains[223]: the societal ideal of thinness and encouragement of women to define themselves by way others perceive them; families that demand conformity and high achievement; genetic susceptibility (from 50 to 80 percent of the variance in liability to AN and BN is accounted for by genetic factors); and personality traits that include low self-esteem, impulsivity, obsessionality, perfectionism, and affective dysregulation; and life events, such as chronic disease (for example, diabetes mellitus). Dieting frequently triggers the onset of eating disorder in vulnerable individuals.

Natural History Across Childbearing

Sollid et al.[224] performed a follow-up study with 302 women who were hospitalized with an eating disorder before pregnancy and their 504 children. Outcomes were compared with 900 control subjects and their 1,552 children. The risk of a low-birth weight infant was twice as high in women with a history of eating disorder compared with women without a history (odds ratio, OR, 2.2; 95-percent CI, 1.4 to 3.2). The risks for preterm delivery and a small-for-gestational-age infant also were increased. Possible contributors to the cause of impaired fetal growth are weight-controlling behaviors (such as strict dieting, vomiting, and excessive physical exercise) that lead to undernutrition. Women with past or current eating disorders were also at significantly higher risk of hyperemesis during pregnancy compared to controls.[224a]

Patients with a history of AN have a significantly higher likelihood of several adverse obstetric events than women without AN (respectively: premature birth, 20 percent versus 8 percent of controls; birth weight, mean 3,139 g versus 3,337 g; surgical births, 16 percent versus 3 percent).[225] In a retrospective case-control study of obstetric complications in 122 primigravidae who were previously treated for BN,[225a] the odds ratios for postpartum depression, miscarriage, and preterm delivery were 2.8 (95-percent CI, 1.2 to 6.2), 2.6 (95-percent CI, 1.2 to 5.6) and 3.3 (95-percent CI, 1.3 to 8.8) respectively. The risk estimates were not explained by differences in adiposity, demographics, alcohol/substance/laxative misuse, smoking, or year of birth. Women with a history of BN or binge eating disorder have three times the risk of perinatal depression compared to women without eating disorders.[226] In fact, mothers with a history of eating disorders are at equal or greater risk of developing postpartum depression than women with a history of major depression. The development of depression in women with eating disorders was partly attributable to a specific personality trait related to perfectionism, concern over mistakes, in which mistakes are perceived as failures.[226]

Pregnancy can be a stimulus that moves a woman through the continuum from subthreshold symptoms to frank eating disorder.[223] Changing body shape and loss of control of weight gain may reactivate deviant eating patterns and concerns about body shape in women with a history of an eating disorder. Crow et al.[227] examined the course specifically for BN and substance abuse during pregnancy. Body dissatisfaction was rated as improved during pregnancy by 21.4 percent, worse by 13.0 percent, and unchanged by 34.8 percent. Symptoms of binge eating and purging decreased during pregnancy; however, the number of women completely abstinent from bulimic symptoms did not change significantly. In women previously diagnosed with eating disorders, 22 percent relapsed during pregnancy and had an increased risk for hyperemesis gravidarum.[228]

Of concern, maternal dieting behaviors are associated with an increased risk of neural tube defect (NTD).[229] In an analysis of 538 cases of NTD and 539 controls who delivered from 1989 to 1991, several first-trimester behaviors were associated with increased risk of NTD: dieting to lose weight (OR, 2.1; 95-percent CI, 1.1 to 4.1) and fasting diets (OR, 5.8, 95-percent CI, 1.7 to 20.0). The dieting behaviors may increase NTD risk because of effects on intake, absorption, and metabolism of micronutrients, such as folic acid.

Treatment Principles

Specific treatment goals for patients with eating disorders include the following factors[230]: (1) Address dysfunctional attitudes about self, weight and shape, and relationships with others. Alternatives to the patient's perfectionism, low self-esteem, pursuit of thinness, mood lability and poor coping skills must be developed through psychotherapy and experience to promote recovery. (2) Establish healthy eating behaviors. Typically, chaotic eating patterns are common. Women have impairments in their social lives and interpersonal relationships. (3) Weight and nutritional stabilization are essential for recovery. Normalization of nutritional status improves physical and mental well-being. (4) Treat comorbid conditions such as depression and anxiety. Treatments targeted to these disorders may improve adherence to healthy behaviors. A nonconfrontational educational approach is used to engage the woman with an eating disorder.[230] Clinical features can be explained as consequences of physiologic changes that occur in starvation: feeling cold owing to lack of the thermogenic effects of food for calorie needs; electrolyte disturbances from starvation, vomiting, or diuretic or laxative abuse; and decreased heart rate from loss of cardiac muscle.[230] (5)

Treat acute symptoms. Although most patients with BN are treated as outpatients, patients with AN may require hospitalization because of emaciation and electrolyte disturbances.[230] Cardiac rhythm disturbances[231] are common in patients with both AN and BN, and are typically reversible with improvement in nutritional status; however, an exception is cardiomyopathy due to chronic ipecac (emetine) abuse.[232,233] Inpatient treatment during pregnancy is recommended for significant metabolic disturbances, suicidal ideation, or ongoing weight loss.

Detection of eating disorders is enhanced by an awareness of risk behaviors such as refusal of routine weight checks, multiple cosmetic surgeries, and a BMI of less than 19. In addition to routine laboratory investigations, women with eating disorders also need to be evaluated for electrolyte, blood urea nitrogen, creatinine, EKG, and thyroid abnormalities. The medical complications of AN may be life threatening (Table 50-2).[223,230,234] Electrolyte disturbances also may be responsible for the sometimes fatal syndrome that occurs during the refeeding of severely malnourished patients with AN.[235] Osteopenia and osteoporosis of the lumbar spine occurs in women with active AN (54 percent) compared with recovered women (21 percent); in contrast, patients with BN typically have bone mineral densities within the normal range.[236]

Table 50-2. Physical and Laboratory Findings in Women with Eating Disorders

Common in Women with Eating Disorders
Bradycardia
Hypotension and Orthostasis
Hypothermia
Cardiac murmur (mitral valve prolapse)
Dry skin
More Common in Anorexia Nervosa Due to Severe Calorie Restriction
Emaciated, may wear oversized clothes
Sunken cheeks, sallow skin
Lanugo (fine downy body hair)
Atrophic breasts/atrophic vaginitis
Pitting edema of extremities
Dull, thinning scalp hair
Cold extremities, acrocyanosis
Fluid retention after laxative or diuretic withdrawal
Laboratory: Anemia, ↑BUN, ↑cholesterol, ↑liver function studies, ↑amylase; ↓platelets, ↓magnesium, ↓zinc, ↓phosphates, ↓thyroid
With laxative abuse: metabolic acidosis
More Common in Women Who Purge
Parotitis
Calluses on dorsal hand surface from self-induced emesis
Oral mucosal abrasions
Dental enamel erosion, tooth chipping, extensive cosmetic dental work
Cardiac and skeletal myopathies from ipecac abuse
Laboratory: metabolic alkalosis; ↓sodium, ↓chloride, ↓potassium, ↑bicarbonate from purging

Data from American Psychiatric Association: Diagnostic and Statistical Manual of Mental Disorders, 4th ed. Washington, DC, American Psychiatric Association, 1994; Rome E, Ammerman S, Rosen D, et al: Children and adolescents with eating disorders: the state of the art. Pediatrics 111:98, 2003; Mitchell-Gieleghem A, Mittelstaedt ME, Bulik C: Eating disorders and childbearing: concealment and consequences. Birth 29:182, 2002.

Psychotherapy

The most well-studied psychotherapy for eating disorders is cognitive-behavioral therapy (CBT).[230] The therapist identifies the stimuli to thought processes and emotions that maintain the binge-purge-starve cycle. The woman develops strategies to manage the disturbed eating, change the dysfunctional cognitions, and build alternative ways to manage distress. CBT has been found to be effective in many studies for about half of patients.[230] In locations where CBT is not available, self-help manuals based upon the principles of CBT have wide appeal. *Overcoming Binge Eating*[237] is readable and provides a clear discussion of the implementation of self-help strategies.[230]

Pharmacotherapy of Anorexia Nervosa

No medications are approved by the FDA for the treatment of AN. Although few randomized clinical trials are available to guide treatment, pharmacotherapy in AN is usually instituted to treat depression, obsessive perfectionism, and cognitive disturbances; to target potential neurotransmitter disturbances; or treat psychiatric or medical comorbidities.[230] The core symptoms of AN are relatively refractory to psychotropic agents.[238] Recent studies have included haloperidol, sertraline, fluoxetine, chlorpromazine, and amisulpride.[230] All have been shown to be of some benefit in helping the patient to gain weight and improve body image. The medications currently being studied are the atypical antipsychotics, particularly OLZ.[239] Rarely, patients with AN have psychosis and require antipsychotic agents.

Relapse prevention is the most challenging clinical problem in the treatment of AN,[240] and longitudinal studies demonstrate that AN is a chronic disorder.[230,241] The 1-year relapse rate after weight restoration in an inpatient setting is 50 to 60 percent. Kaye et al.[242] found that fluoxetine was more effective than placebo in relapse prevention.

Pharmacotherapy of Bulimia Nervosa

Placebo-controlled studies with antidepressant drugs have been far more promising for treating BN than AN[238] for acute management. The first-line medication most commonly used is an SSRI, usually fluoxetine at a dose of 20 to 80 mg/day for at least 12 weeks, owing to the use of this drug in the largest number of controlled investigations. In general, switching to another antidepressant such as venlafaxine or duloxetine is appropriate if there is no improvement, whereas augmentation with another agent (topiramate, see later) is reasonable if there is a partial response.[230] Lasting symptomatic improvement and sustained remission require concomitant psychological interventions. Although antidepressant medication is useful for BN, it is less effective as a solo treatment than CBT alone, and CBT plus medication may provide additive efficacy.[243] Adding fluoxetine to the treatment of those who failed to improve with CBT was effective in reducing binge-purge episodes.[244] A combination of CBT and an antidepressant drug is a prudent clinical strategy.

Topiramate has been evaluated in short-term randomized controlled trials for efficacy in BN.[245,246] The mean weekly number of binge-purge days decreased from baseline significantly by 44.8 percent with topiramate compared to 10.7 percent with placebo. Treatment was started at 25 mg/day and titrated by 25 to 50 mg/week to a maximum of 400 mg/day (median 100 mg/day). Topiramate improved multiple behavioral dimensions of BN, such as self-esteem, eating attitudes, anxiety, and body image. In a study of obese patients with binge eating disorder, McElroy et al.[247] found that patients had fewer binge episodes and a statistically significant reduction in body weight. Topiramate treatment was associated with enduring improvement in some patients but was also characterized by a high discontinuation rate. Owing to side effects (memory impairment, paresthesias, fatigue) a low initial dose (15 mg or 25 mg) is used and the dosage is increased gradually (25 mg every 2 weeks) as tolerated.[230] Reproductive toxicity information on newer AED, such as topiramate, is limited.

SCHIZOPHRENIA

Diagnosis and Prevalence

Schizophrenia is a disabling brain disease that affects 1 percent of the population. The defining feature of schizophrenia is psychosis, which does not refer to the *severity* of the episode but to specific symptoms. Schizophrenia is characterized by the presence (for at least 6 months) of symptoms from three clusters: (1) positive symptoms (delusions or fixed false beliefs; hallucinations or distortions of reality), (2) negative symptoms (decrease or loss of normal functions: lack of pleasure, social withdrawal, minimal speech production), and (3) cognitive impairment (inattention, poor working memory, and executive function deficits).[248] The etiology of schizophrenia is unknown, but proposed mechanisms are (1) excessive dopamine transmission, (2) in utero exposure to influenza or other viral agents, which results in neurobiologic disruptions,[249,250] and (3) altered neuroplasticity or neurodevelopmental trajectories.[251,252] Schizophrenia is distinguished from mood disorders with psychotic symptoms by the persistence of hallucinations or delusions when mood symptoms have remitted. The mortality and morbidity of schizophrenia is high, and 10 percent of patients complete suicide.

Gender differences are prominent in the course and presentation of schizophrenia. Women are more likely to have a later onset, prominent mood symptoms, and a better prognosis than men. The median age of onset is in the late 20s for women. Women have lower symptom severity, fewer hospitalizations, a higher likelihood to return to work and more social support than males.[253] About 67 percent of women compared with 29 percent of men with schizophrenia are married, and women are twice as likely to have children.[253]

Natural History of Schizophrenia Across Childbearing

Women with schizophrenia have lower fertility rates compared with healthy women despite less frequent use of contraception and higher rates of irreversible causes of infertility (hysterectomy, menopause, sterilization).[254] Pregnant women with schizophrenia are less likely to obtain prenatal care and have an increased risk for interventions during labor and delivery[136] than unaffected women. Investigators have not observed exacerbations of acute psychosis during pregnancy[255] or the postpartum, except for comorbid mood disorders.[256] However, about 27 percent of women with past psychosis experience recurrence of psychosis and 38 percent develop comorbid nonpsychotic depression in the first postpartum year.[257]

The children born to women with schizophrenia may be susceptible to subtle problems in neurodevelopment but the origins (genetic, environment, psychosocial) remain a challenge to decipher. Most studies lack important data on the mothers' nutritional status, exposures to psychotropic medications, other prescription, or over-the-counter drugs that impact reproductive outcomes.[137,258] Concurrent maternal smoking, substance use, and socioeconomic problems increase the risk for less optimal outcomes.[259,260]

In assisting patients with risk-benefit decision making during pregnancy, the data on relapse risk for schizophrenia must be extrapolated to pregnant patients. A meta-analysis of 66 studies and more than 4,000 patients indicated that individuals with chronic schizophrenia who stop treatment have a cumulative relapse rate of 53 percent, compared with 16 percent among patients who remain on antipsychotic therapy over a 10-month period.[261] The highest rate of relapse occurred within the first 3 months of treatment discontinuation. Sudden cessation of antipsychotic medication,[262] younger age, early age of illness onset, need for high doses of antipsychotic therapy, and recent psychiatric admission predicted recurrent episodes.[261] Patients with severe and persistent symptoms of schizophrenia, frequent relapses, histories of dangerous behavior, poor self-care, and hospitalization often reasonably choose to remain on antipsychotic treatment throughout pregnancy. Very few women with schizophrenia achieve a sustained symptom-free period and good function without antipsychotic medications before pregnancy. If a woman chooses to remain monitored without medication, a plan should be developed for reinstituting medication rapidly if prodromal symptoms occur. The antipsychotic agent that achieved the greatest symptom reduction and the least side effects for the individual patient balanced against its side effects is the preferred drug.[263]

Treatment Interventions

Antipsychotic medication and psychosocial interventions aimed at maximizing function are the mainstays of treatment for schizophrenia. Mothers with schizophrenia often struggle with poverty, poor housing, social isolation, and difficulty obtaining basic services for their offspring. Seeman et al.[264] developed a comprehensive clinical service that offers case management, consultation, pharmacotherapy, parent education groups, family programs, job training, and stress reduction. This model is a framework for a patient-centered, multidisciplinary program to address the psychiatric and social needs of women with schizophrenia.

Patients with schizophrenia are three times more likely to smoke cigarettes than persons without mental illness. Encouragement to stop is essential because smoking increases psychotropic drug metabolism,[265] raises the risk for medical comorbid disorders (chronic bronchitis, cardiovascular disease, lung cancer), and adversely affects obstetrical outcomes.

Antipsychotic drugs that block dopamine-2 receptors reduce symptoms of schizophrenia,[266] such as hallucinations. A great variability in the response of individuals to antipsychotics is the rule. In an double-blind controlled trial of 1,500 patients with schizophrenia sponsored by the National Institute of Health, subjects were randomized to one of four atypical antipsychotics (OLZ, quetiapine, risperidone, ziprasidone) or an older typical antipsychotic (perphenazine) and followed for up to 18 months (Clinical Antipsychotic Trials of Intervention Effectiveness [CATIE] trial).[267] Few differences in outcome were observed among groups treated with the various medications. The older typical antipsychotic, perphenazine, was as well tolerated as the newer compounds and as effective as three of the four newer agents. The fourth drug, OLZ, was slightly better than all the others in terms of lower drug discontinuation and hospitalization rates but paradoxically was associated with higher rates of weight gain and metabolic side effects. Neurologic toxicity with long-term administration remains the primary concern with the older typical antipsychotics.

Although the CATIE study excluded pregnant and breast-feeding women, the results have implications for the treatment of childbearing women. Significantly more data about use during pregnancy are available for the older typical antipsychotics, and exposure for the period limited to pregnancy can be favorable in the risk-benefit analysis for some women, particularly women with insulin resistance, hypertension, and obesity. Standard clinical practice does not include serum level monitoring for drugs used to treat schizophrenia.

The independent effects of antipsychotic medications versus schizophrenia and its sequelae on pregnancy and neonatal outcomes have not been differentiated.[268] The majority of outcome data are for women with schizophrenia compared with a population without the disorder. Identification of specific illness characteristics, comorbidities, and environmental exposures in the comprehensive intervention model (Fig. 50-1) has not been achieved. Control of the disorder (which usually requires medication continuation), pregnancy education, nutritional services, treatment for substance use, and community services are paramount.

Women with schizophrenia had increased rates of preterm delivery (OR, 1.5; 95-percent CI, 1.2 to 1.7) and low birth weight (OR, 1.4; 95-percent CI, 1.1 to 1.6) (OR, 1.2; 95-percent CI, 0.8 to 1.6) compared with women without the disorder.[260] Results from ongoing cohort study in which women who were treated with a mixed group of atypical antipsychotics in pregnancy were: one (0.9 percent) major malformation occurred among 151 women who took atypical antipsychotics (OLZ, risperidone, quetiapine, and clozapine) in pregnancy.[269] Low birth weight occurred in 10% of exposed and 2% of comparison infants. Monitoring the side effects of atypical antipsychotics during pregnancy includes evaluating orthostatic blood pressure, heart rate, and weight gain.

Specific Antipsychotics

Clozapine was the first atypical agent; however, burdensome side effects (weight gain, lowered seizure threshold, tachycardia, dyslipidemia, sedation, drooling) and monitoring for agranulocytosis create significant barriers to use. Clozapine is reserved for patients whose illness is nonresponsive to treatment with less toxic drugs.[266] Clozapine use in pregnancy has been associated with gestational diabetes,[270,271] shoulder dystocia,[271,272] hypotonia,[273] and neonatal convulsions.[274,275]

The most reproductive data among the atypicals are available for OLZ, which is structurally similar to clozapine. Goldstein et al.[275] prospectively identified 37 pregnancies with OLZ exposure at doses of 5 to 25 mg daily. One woman experienced an ectopic pregnancy, and 13 women underwent elective abortions unrelated to fetal anomalies. Of the remaining 23 pregnancies, 3 (13 percent) resulted in miscarriage. No major or minor malformations were associated with the remaining 20 pregnancies, but four had adverse outcomes that included a stillbirth, gestational diabetes, premature birth and post-dates birth. Pharmacologically, OLZ is highly protein bound; 5 to 14 percent of ingested drug penetrates the fetal compartment 4 hours post-ingestion[276] and 40 to 60 percent of OLZ or its metabolites traverse the placenta.[275] In the CATIE study, OLZ treatment was linked with numerous complications (weight gain, increased glycosylated hemoglobin, cholesterol, and triglycerides) which suggested metabolic syndrome.[267]

Risperidone is another atypical agent with diverse receptor blocking activities. At doses above 6 mg daily, hyperprolactinemia and motor side effects may emerge. Two mother-infant pairs treated with risperidone throughout conception and pregnancy achieved normal delivery, healthy birth weights and age-appropriate developmental milestones at 9 and 12 months.[277] Quetiapine is an atypical antipsychotic with a wide dose range that allows for easier titration. The appeal of this drug is diminished by side effects such as sedation, weight gain, and headache. The few reports of infants exposed to quetiapine in utero showed normal intrauterine growth, full term deliveries and high Apgar scores.[278,279]

Ziprasidone is a suitable choice for managing psychosis,[266] with its neutral effects on weight, lipid and glucose metabolism[280]; however, its use may be associated with prolonged QTc syndrome.[136] Aripiprazole is the newest atypical antipsychotic agent with novel dopamine antagonist and partial agonist activity. There are no published reports on perinatal exposures with ziprasidone or aripiprazole.

Breast-Feeding

The high concentration of clozapine in breastmilk has been attributed to its lipophilicity, and breast-fed infants have been reported to develop sedation, agranulocytosis, and cardiovascular effects.[281] The excretion of OLZ, a highly protein-bound agent, in breast milk has been assessed in small case series.[282–284] The median estimated dose in infants was 1.6 to 4.0 percent of the maternal dose.[282,284] In a woman who took OLZ (10 mg) daily through childbearing, maternal plasma levels were 33.4 ng/mL at delivery; the infant level was about a third of the maternal level at 11.3 ng/mL.[283] The baby was breast-fed, and infant levels were below the limit of quantifiability (<2 ng/ml) at 2 and 6 weeks. These data show this infant's ability to metabolize the drug burden from prenatal exposure and imply minimal additional dosing through breast milk.

Three breast-fed infants of mothers who were treated with risperidone had nondetectable serum drug metabolite levels and no evidence of adverse reactions.[285] A mother who was treated with risperidone (6 mg/day) provided serial samples of plasma and breast milk every 4 hours over a 24-hour period. The infant drug intake was estimated to be 0.84 percent of the maternal dose for risperidone, 3.5 percent for its metabolite, and 4.3 percent of the weight-adjusted maternal dose.[286] A woman who was treated with quetiapine 200 mg daily provided serial milk samples. Investigators estimated that the infant would ingest 0.09 to 0.43 percent of the weight-adjusted maternal dose.[287] The infant was assessed at 4.5 months and was developing normally. There are no published data on breast-fed infants whose mothers were treated with other drugs.

SUBSTANCE-RELATED DISORDERS

Substance-related disorders among pregnant women comprise a public health problem associated with major individual and societal costs. Yet women who abuse substances rarely are identified by health care professionals. The most objective picture of pregnant women who use drugs was derived from blinded urine toxicology screens conducted at representative hospitals nationally.[288] Such studies revealed that the common perception of substance abuse as an affliction of poor, minority, and young women was erroneous. Similar rates of substance use during pregnancy occurred in women of different ages, races, and social classes. The specific substances used differed by race and social class, with black and poor women more likely to use illicit substances, particularly cocaine, and white and educated women more likely to use alcohol,[288] although polysubstance use was common.

Conducted by the National Institute of Drug Abuse in the early 1990s, the National Pregnancy and Health Survey was the first national survey of drug use among pregnant women in the United States. A representative sample of the 4 million women who delivered during 1992 was obtained. Illicit drugs (marijuana, cocaine, methamphetamine, heroin, methadone, inhalants, hallucinogens, or nonmedical use of psychotherapeutics during pregnancy) were used by 5.5 percent of pregnant women.[289] In a national survey done in 2002 to 2003 of pregnant women aged 15 to 44 years, 9.8 percent reported drinking alcohol during the past month, 4.1 percent reported binge alcohol use, and less than 1 percent reported heavy alcohol use.[290] In the year after pregnancy, women increased their substance use although not to the level of nonpregnant women who were not recent mothers[290] (Fig. 50-4).

Obstetricians are in a unique position to identify women with substance use disorders and to encourage treatment. Pregnancy is a strong motivator for change because most women want to protect their baby; however, women do not volunteer information about substance abuse unless asked. They fear stigma, being judged, or legal and custody concerns. For example, they may worry that they will be reported to a child welfare agency or that their employer might learn about their drug use. Universal screening improves detection and has the potential to improve pregnancy and infant outcomes.

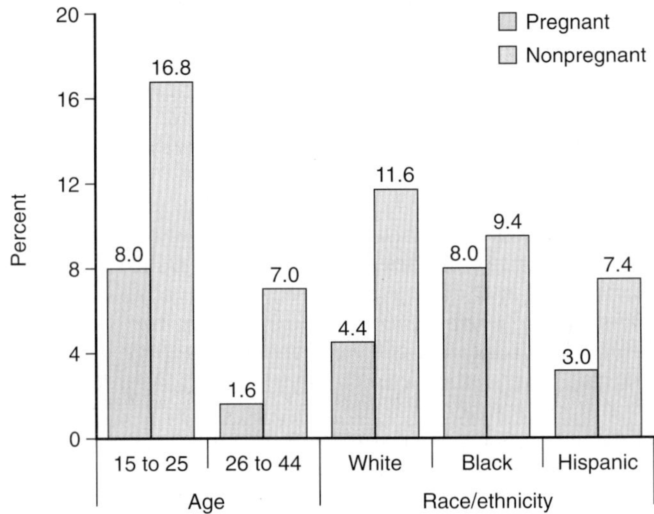

Figure 50-4. Drug and alcohol use during pregnancy. (From National Survey on Drug Abuse and Health: *Substance Use During Pregnancy: 2002 and 2003 Update.* http://oas.samhsa.gov/2k5/pregnancy/pregnancy.htm. Accessed December 19, 2006.)

In the DSM-IV, psychoactive substance use disorders are classified into two categories—abuse and dependence.[248] The diagnosis of abuse is established if at least one of the following criteria is fulfilled in the past 12 months: (1) recurrent use resulted in failure to fulfill major role obligation at work, home, or school; (2) recurrent use in physically hazardous situations; (3) legal problems result from use; and (4) continued use despite persistent or recurrent social or interpersonal problems caused or exacerbated by substance use. Substance abuse is distinguished from dependence. At least three of the following criteria must be met in the past 12 months for substance dependence: (1) tolerance (marked increase in amount; marked decrease in effect); (2) characteristic withdrawal symptoms and substance is taken to relieve withdrawal; (3) substance is taken in larger amount and for longer period than intended; (4) persistent desire or repeated unsuccessful attempt to quit; (5) significant time and activity are spent to obtain, use, and recover from use; (6) given up or reduced important social, occupational, or recreational activities; and (7) use continues despite knowledge of adverse consequences. Although physiologic tolerance and withdrawal are not essential diagnostic criteria for dependence, they often occur. Abuse is often a precursor to dependence, or a category for those who do not fulfill the criteria for dependence but use substances in maladaptive ways that are harmful to themselves or others.

Co-occurring Psychiatric Disorders

Comorbidity, or co-occurrence, of substance use with psychiatric illness is the rule rather than the exception. The neurobiologic sequelae of chronic stress may affect brain reward and other pathways to predispose or unmask vulnerability to psychiatric disorders, substance use disorders, or both.[291] In a general population of women who were seeking treatment for cocaine and alcohol abuse, the co-occurring psychiatric disorders were: any mood or anxiety disorder, 70 percent; major depression, 40 percent; [illegible], [illegible] percent; panic disorder, [illegible] percent; post traumatic stress disorder, 46 percent; and social phobia, 10 percent. In women, the co-occurring condition usually began prior the onset of substance use.[292]

Life stress is very high in substance abusing women, who have problems in multiple domains.[288] One third to one half of substance abusing women experienced sexual abuse during childhood,[288] and they are frequently involved with drug-using partners. Interpersonal violence is common in the lives of substance-abusing women.[288,292]

Obtaining a Substance Use History

Substance use history can be obtained by physician interview or with a screening tool. The overall approach and emotional tone of the clinician is more important than the precise wording or specific content. Women are more likely to divulge substance use when asked in a nonjudgmental manner by an empathetic interviewer and within the context of general health questions. Similar to obtaining a sexual history, the questions should be sequenced from least to most threatening to the patient. Questions should be open-ended as much as possible—for example, "How many cigarettes do you smoke?" as opposed to "Do you smoke?" or worse, "You don't smoke, do you?"

Physicians and other health care providers, like all people, have developed personal beliefs and biases over their lifetime, which can interfere with their approach to the issue of substance use. It is challenging but important that physicians recognize and confront their personal biases in order to keep them from interfering with the care they provide. Helping women with substance use disorders challenges physicians to go beyond the traditional medical care paradigm to an expanded model of psychosocial care, which includes assistance from social services and establishing collaboration with addictions and psychiatric professionals (see section on PDs for other management strategies).

Screening Principles

A general screening measure for substances in pregnancy is the 4Ps Plus (Table 50-3; http://www.childstudy.org/nti/4pp/), which was designed to identify obstetric patients who need in-depth assessment. The 4Ps Plus has been validated in multiple obstetric populations. This five-question screen is administered during a prenatal visit and takes less than 1 minute to complete.[293] The first *P* is for *Parents*, and the query is about their use of substances. A positive response does not predict the woman's substance use but allows the physician to introduce the issue in a non-threatening manner. The second question, about the *Partner*, pertains to the partner's substance use. The partner's use does not predict the woman's substance use in pregnancy, but it is correlated with risk for domestic violence, a common psychosocial problem in women with substance use. The third *P*, for the woman's *Past* use of alcohol, places her at risk for use during pregnancy and can be coupled with prevention education as part of prenatal care. The final two questions are related to the current time. The fourth *P*,

Table 50-3. Screening with the 4 Ps Plus

• Parents	Did either of your parents ever have a problem with alcohol or drugs?
• Partner	Does your partner have a problem with alcohol or drugs?
• Past	Have you ever had any beer or wine or liquor?
• Pregnancy	

- In the month before you knew you were pregnant, how many *cigarettes* did you smoke?
- In the mouth before you knew you were pregnant, how much *beer/wine/liquor* did you drink?

Copyright NTI, 1998, with permission. Chasnoff IJ, Hung WC: The 4 P's *Plus*. Chicago: NTI Publishing, 1999.[293]

for *Pregnancy*, contains an open-ended question about cigarette use in the month *before* pregnancy. The fifth *P* is the amount of wine/beer/liquor consumed in the month before pregnancy. The authors observed that substance use *during* pregnancy was not as effective a screen as asking about a woman's use of substances *before* pregnancy. Women often use substances at prepregnancy levels until the pregnancy is confirmed after early first-trimester exposure has occurred. They often decrease, or report less use, owing to the stigma about drug use during gestation. In administering the 4Ps Plus, it is preferable to use the terms beer and wine (and liquor) because some women do not recognize beer to be alcohol.

Laboratory screening is another approach to substance use detection but it must be negotiated with the pregnant woman. In general, laboratory measures detect current exposure but do not reflect the historic pattern of use. Because pregnant women with substance use disorders are at increased risk for a variety of infections and medical conditions, a comprehensive medical history, examination, and diagnostic studies are indicated. The studies should include a complete blood count, syphilis and hepatitis B and C serology, tuberculosis test, and confidential human immunodeficiency virus screening.[294–296]

Comprehensive Programs

Numerous barriers to care for pregnant substance users have been identified. The lack of understanding on the part of health care professionals, the attitudes and behavior of substance-abusing women, and lack of coordination between obstetric and mental health professionals are examples. Programs that navigate these barriers for opiate-dependent gravidas have a positive impact on pregnancy outcomes. Comprehensive programs, such as the Center for Addiction and Pregnancy (CAP),[297] provide treatment across the disciplines of psychiatry, obstetrics, and pediatrics to deliver patient-centered care that is preventive in focus. CAP staff provide services such as prenatal care, drug treatment, family planning, lactation support, parent education and case management by outreach workers. In the first 100 births in CAP participants, 82 percent were delivered vaginally, the mean gestational age was 38 weeks, the neonatal intensive care unit (NICU) admission rate was 10 percent, and Bayley Scales of Infant Development at 6 and 12 months were normal. Cost savings was estimated at nearly $5,000 per mother-infant pair owing to shorter length of stay and lower frequency of NICU admissions.[297]

In women on methadone maintenance treatment, Chang et al.[298] compared reproductive outcomes for women in an enhanced program (prenatal care, methadone maintenance, supervised childcare, and relapse prevention strategies) with those of women in a standard prenatal care setting. Both groups had similar demographics, parity, and daily methadone dose. Despite a greater mean number of urine toxicology screens, subjects in the enhanced program had a lower percentage of positive results. The enhanced group had significantly more prenatal visits (8.8 versus 2.7), longer gestations (38.2 wks versus 35.7 wks), and larger infants (2,943 g versus 2,280 g).

Specific Drugs of Abuse

The impact of maternal substance use on pregnancy and infant outcomes is influenced by a variety of factors, such as the specific exposures, gestational timing, duration of exposures, nutritional status, and multiple other factors. Disentangling the effects of substance use, co-occurring mental disorders and the biopsychosocial milieu on pregnancy and infant outcomes is a challenging task (see Fig. 50-1).[4] The following sections provide an overview of specific classes of drugs and their use during pregnancy.

Alcohol

Most women who drink before becoming pregnant either reduce their intake or stop drinking during pregnancy. Day et al.[299] reported that 4.6 percent of women reported drinking an average of one drink per day by the end of the third trimester of pregnancy, compared with 44 percent before pregnancy. However, the number of heavy drinkers (at least five drinks per occasion or at least seven drinks per week) was 3.5 percent in a study in women studied from 1988 to 1995.[300]

A dose at which negative outcomes do not occur for alcohol consumption has not been defined during pregnancy.[301] Women who consumed more than three drinks per week had a significantly increased risk for miscarriage.[302] Women who consumed five or more drinks per week increased their risk by two to three times for intrauterine fetal death compared with nondrinkers.[303] Consumption of one or more alcoholic drinks per day was associated with reduced birth weight and intrauterine growth retardation.[304,305]

Prenatal exposure to alcohol is probably the most common preventable cause of mental retardation in the United States.[306] Children exposed to binge drinking are 1.7 times more likely to have mental retardation and 2.5 times more likely to demonstrate delinquent behavior than unexposed children.[307] Neonatal effects of alcohol exposure can be subtle, such as slower habituation (attenuation of response to repetitive stimuli) and longer reaction times.[308,309] Moderate prenatal alcohol exposure is associated with learning problems, memory deficits and mood disorders in school-aged children.[310–312]

Fetal alcohol spectrum disorders encompass the array of physical, cognitive, and behavioral deficits found in children born to mothers who consume alcohol during pregnancy. The incidence of fetal alcohol syndrome, the most severe manifestation of exposure, is approximately 1 in 100 births.[313] The characteristic facial dysmorphology is midfacial hypoplasia, flat philtrum, low nasal bridge, epicanthal folds, shortened palpebral fissure, low-set ears, and microcephaly. Affected children may have visual, skeletal, and cardiac anomalies[314–316] (see Chapter 8).

Detecting alcohol use among pregnant women is an important step toward preventing alcohol-related birth defects. Although not currently in clinical use, biomarkers of maternal alcohol use during pregnancy are being developed and validated.[317] Several short screening tools to detect pregnancy risk drinking are available. In a critical review, Chang[318] identified the T-ACE[319] (see Fig. 8-2) as a valuable and efficient tool for identifying alcohol use specifically in pregnant women. This brief tool was developed for detection of risk drinking (defined as greater than or equal to 1 ounce of absolute alcohol per day). The four questions of the T-ACE reliably differentiated risk drinkers from nonrisk drinkers. The T-ACE questions take about 1 minute to ask. A positive screen indicates the need for education about the risks of alcohol use during pregnancy. Such brief interventions promote harm reduction, facilitate antenatal visit compliance, promote healthier choices during pregnancy, and support patients in making life-style changes. Screening is also useful to identify women who require referral to substance use treatment programs for alcohol intoxication and withdrawal during pregnancy. Oral benzodiazepines (diazepam or lorazepam) are recommended for alcohol withdrawal during pregnancy or labor.[320] Disulfiram (Antabuse) potentiates teratogenicity and, therefore, is contraindicated for aversion therapy during pregnancy.[321]

SMOKING

Women are more likely to attempt to stop smoking during pregnancy than at any other point in their lives, but only one third stop successfully[322] and many relapse after birth. An office-based intervention for pregnant smokers called the 5 As (*Ask* about tobacco use, *Advise* to quit, *Assess* willingness to make a quit attempt, *Assist* in quit attempt and *Arrange* follow-up) was endorsed by the American College of Obstetricians and Gynecologists (http://www.acog.org/departments/dept_notice.cfm?recno=13&bulletin=1863). A single copy of the manual is available without charge by emailing the College at *smoking@acog.org*. The approach involves providing patients with a brief counseling session and pregnancy specific self-help materials, and increases quit rates among pregnant smokers by a factor of 2 to 3. Web-based tools are also available for education and support for smoking cessation (http://www.cdc.gov/tobacco/how2quit.htm).

Carbon monoxide and nicotine from inhaled tobacco smoke interfere with oxygen supply to the fetus. Although it is not associated with congenital malformations,[323,324] smoking is associated with increased risk for miscarriage,[325,326] intrauterine and perinatal fetal deaths,[327] preterm birth, and intrauterine growth retardation.[328] Paradoxically, smoking appears to reduce the risk of preeclampsia, probably by inhibition of thromboxane A2 production or suppression of the immune system.[329,330] Newborns with in utero exposure to maternal smoking experienced poorer autonomic regulation and decreased auditory responsiveness compared to nonexposed infants.[331,332] Infants of smokers have more than three times the risk of sudden infant death syndrome compared with infants of nonsmokers.[333]

A dose-response relationship between maternal smoking and offspring intelligence was demonstrated and the association was evident across all social classes.[334] An analysis of nearly 3,000 subjects who participated in an 11-year community cohort study in Western Norway was performed to examine the impact of passive smoking exposure on risk of respiratory disease in adulthood.[335] After adjustment for multiple confounders, 17.3 percent of the adult incidence of asthma was attributable to maternal smoking, whereas 9.3 percent was due to exposure from other household smokers.

Behavioral therapy is the first-line choice for pregnant women; however, pharmacologic approaches may be necessary, particularly in heavy smokers.[336] Although almost 4 in 10 smokers quit at the start of pregnancy, 20 percent of pregnant women smoked at the end of the first trimester, and half smoked 10 or more cigarettes per day.[337] In a large study of nicotine replacement therapy, pregnant women who smoked 10 or more cigarettes after the first trimester were randomly assigned to receive nicotine patches 15 mg patches for 16 h/day for 8 weeks, then 10 mg patches for 3 weeks versus placebo patches. Overall, 26 percent of women stopped smoking and 14 percent were nonsmokers 1 year after delivery, although there was no significant difference between the drug and placebo groups. The mean birth weight difference was 186 g (95-percent CI 35 to 336 g) higher in the nicotine group than placebo group. There was no difference in the rate of preterm delivery between the two groups.[337] Nicotine patch use in the second and third trimesters was not associated with maternal or fetal compromise from fetal heart rate, amniotic fluid volume, umbilical blood flow activity, and birth weight.[338]

Bupropion is another pharmacologic approach to smoking cessation. The Canadian Motherisk group[339] studied 136 pregnant women who took bupropion during the first trimester of pregnancy. They reported 105 live births, 20 miscarriages, 10 elective abortions, 1 stillbirth, and 1 neonatal death. There were no major malformations. The mean birth weight was 3,450 g and gestational age was 40 weeks. Except for a higher rate of miscarriages among bupropion-exposed pregnancies, there were no other statistically significant outcome differences between exposed and comparison groups. The higher rate of miscarriages is similar to that found in several studies that have evaluated antidepressants during pregnancy. Studies of longer term outcomes for children exposed in utero have not been published.

With respect to breast-feeding, only two cases of mother-infant serum levels of bupropion during lactation are available.[340] No quantifiable levels of bupropion or its metabolite were found in lactating women treated with a low dose (150 mg/day). Motivation to breastfeed is an opportunity to urge continued cessation or reduction of smoking beyond that achieved during pregnancy. Smoking is not contraindicated during breastfeeding.[341] The most recent AAP Policy Statement from the Section on Breastfeeding concludes:

> "Tobacco smoking by mothers is not a contraindication to breastfeeding, but health care professionals should advise all tobacco-using mothers to avoid smoking within the home and to make every effort to wean themselves from tobacco as rapidly as possible."

Cocaine

About 1 percent of women used cocaine at some time during their pregnancy.[289] Cocaine can be snorted, injected or smoked. Crack cocaine is often smoked in a pipe, and inhaled and absorbed into the bloodstream. Crack and injected cocaine reach the brain quickly and bring an intense and immediate high.

The relationship between prenatal cocaine exposure and major morphologic defects is strongly affected by factors associated with cocaine use.[343] In a prospective, large-scale, blinded, systematic investigation of congenital anomalies in prenatally cocaine-exposed children, no increased number or consistent pattern of abnormalities was found,[344] although significantly more cocaine-exposed infants were premature and had lower birth weight, length, and head circumference compared with nonusing controls matched on race, parity, level of pregnancy risk, and socioeconomic status.[344]

The risk of abruptio placentae is elevated in women who use cocaine. In meta-analytic study, Hulse et al.[345] calculated a pooled odds ratio of 3.92 (95-percent confidence interval, 2.77 to 5.46). The strength and consistency of the association, its biologic plausibility, and the results of animal studies suggest that cocaine use during pregnancy is a causal factor in abruptio placentae. Premature rupture of membranes also was statistically associated with cocaine use.[343]

Frank et al.[346] reviewed outcomes in early childhood after prenatal cocaine exposure in five domains: physical growth; cognition; language skills; motor skills; and behavior, attention, affect, and neurophysiology. After controlling for confounders, there was no consistent association between prenatal cocaine exposure and physical growth, developmental test scores, or receptive or expressive language. Less optimal motor scores were found up to age 7 months but not thereafter. An association was found between prenatal cocaine exposure and decreased attentiveness and emotional expressivity, as well as differences on neurophysiologic testing. However, outcomes thought to be specific effects of in utero cocaine exposure were correlated with other factors, such as prenatal exposure to tobacco and other drugs, as well as the child's environment. Children with a history of prenatal cocaine exposure benefit from preschool programs that enhance outcomes for other low-income children.[347]

Singer et al.[348] compared 41 cocaine-exposed very low birth weight infants (<1500 g) with 41 noncocaine-exposed, very low birth weight infants of comparable race, social class, age, and incidence of bronchopulmonary dysplasia. Cocaine-exposed infants were at increased risk of intraventricular hemorrhage and had a higher incidence of developmental delay compared with controls. There are no medications currently available to treat cocaine addiction specifically.

Marijuana

During pregnancy, the most frequently used illicit drug was marijuana (2.9 percent of women).[289] Prenatal marijuana use is not associated with increased rates of major birth defects, stillbirth, or spontaneous abortions or birth defects.[349,350] Infants born to women who used marijuana during their pregnancies displayed altered responses to visual stimuli, increased tremulousness, exaggerated startle response, and high-pitched cries, which may indicate neurologic impairment.[351] Deficits in sustained attention, memory, and cognitive function (such as problem-solving skills) in both preschool and school-aged children have been demonstrated in marijuana-exposed children.[331,352]

An association between childhood cancers (nonlymphoblastic leukemia, rhabdomyosarcoma, and astrocytoma) and marijuana use in pregnancy has been reported[352–354]; however, evidence for an association is weak.[355] Three different types of childhood cancers were identified, and the studies were not designed to evaluate marijuana exposures specifically. Certainly smoking, whether tobacco or marijuana, carries risks during pregnancy and for overall health should be avoided.[355] Counseling and brief interventions that target lifestyle changes and provide support toward abstinence are primary goals of treatment.

Continued exposure to marijuana through breastfeeding was associated with decreased offspring motor capability.[356] Motor and mental development were examined in 1-year-old infants in whom prenatal and lactational exposure to marijuana, alcohol, cigarettes, and cocaine was defined by maternal interview. Marijuana exposure through breast milk was associated with significantly less optimal infant motor development. The finding persisted after adjusting for the effects of prenatal and lactational exposure to nicotine, alcohol, and cocaine. However, none of the variance in infant mental scores was explained by maternal pre- or postpartum use of marijuana. Nonetheless, the AAP lists marijuana as contraindicated during breastfeeding.[341]

Opioids

During pregnancy, 1 percent of women report opiate use and as many as 4 percent test positive for opiates.[356a,356b] The treatment of opioid dependence (on both heroin and prescription narcotics) with methadone or buprenorphine decreases opioid and other drug abuse, reduces criminal activity, improves individual functioning, and decreases human immunodeficiency infection rates.[357]

Hulse et al.[357a] studied the relationship between neonatal mortality and opiate use during pregnancy. The pooled estimate of the relative risk of neonatal mortality for heroin use was 3.27 (95-percent CI, 0.95 to 9.60) and for methadone 1.75 (95-percent CI, 0.60 to 4.59); neither is statistically significant. However, women who used heroin and converted to methadone maintenance late in pregnancy had an increased pooled relative risk estimate of 6.37 (95-percent CI, 2.57 to 14.68). These investigators[358] also conducted a meta-analysis to evaluate the effect of heroin and methadone on mean birth weight. Birth weight was reduced in the offspring of heroin ([mean reduction = 489 g [95-percent CI, 284 to

693 g]) and methadone users (279 g [95-percent CI, 229 to 328 g]). The pooled relative risk for low birth weight for maternal heroin use was 4.61 (95-percent CI, 2.78 to 7.65) and for methadone 1.36 (95-percent CI, 0.83 to 2.22). However, continued heroin use during MMT may counteract the birth weight advantage gained from methadone treatment alone. Factors such as fetal exposure to heroin plus methadone, less prenatal care, and lifestyle factors associated with the use of heroin are likely to play a role in less optimal birth weight.

Methadone maintenance treatment (MMT) is the current standard for the treatment of opioid dependence in pregnancy.[359] Methadone is a long-acting opiate agonist that reduces heroin craving, drug seeking, and other high-risk behaviors. MMT is offered as part of a comprehensive care program that includes behavior therapy and support services.[298] MMT improves perinatal outcomes such as reduction in the risk of preeclampsia and improved birth weight and head circumference.[360,361]

The methadone doses used to treat pregnant women have increased across time.[363] Women who delivered from December, 1982 to September, 1986 were compared with a group who delivered from February, 2000 to November, 2000. In the earlier cohort, women were younger (mean age 28 years) than in the later one (mean age 35; p = <0.001). The mean peak methadone dose was significantly higher in the later verus the earlier cohort (98 versus 52 mg/day); similarly, the mean dose change from conception to delivery was significantly different (later = 24-mg/day increase, earlier = 1-mg/day decrease). Higher doses of methadone were not associated with an increased risk of neonatal withdrawal but did have a positive effect on decreasing maternal drug abuse. Methadone concentrations from the cord blood of infants who required treatment for withdrawal were significantly lower than the group who did not receive treatment.[364] The majority of the infants who required treatment for withdrawal had nonquantifiable concentrations of methadone in a serum sample at 2 days, whereas the median concentration in untreated infants was 23 ng/ml ($p = 0.002$).

Methadone has direct effects upon fetal neurobehavioral functions. Women on MMT with uncomplicated pregnancies were evaluated at peak and trough methadone levels.[365] At peak methadone levels, the fetal heart rate was slower, less variable, and displayed fewer accelerations. Fetuses displayed less motor activity, and the integration between heart rate and motor activity was attenuated. Real-time ultrasound recordings at 34 to 37 weeks' gestation were obtained from methadone-treated and untreated women. Both a slower rate of fetal breathing and fewer fetal breathing movements per breathing episode were found for the methadone group regardless of time since the mothers' daily dose.[366]

Between 30 percent to 80 percent[367] of infants exposed to opioids in utero require treatment for neonatal abstinence syndrome (NAS). NAS is characterized by irritability, tremulousness, sweating, nasal stuffiness, poor suckling, diarrhea, and vomiting.[368,369] NAS can begin as early as 48 hours and as late as 14 days. Neither the incidence nor severity of NAS correlate directly with maternal methadone dose at delivery.[370] NAS can occur in infants with maternal methadone doses as low as 10 mg per day.[371] Maternal smoking affects the timing and severity of NAS[372] in prenatally exposed infants. Babies born to mothers who reported smoking 20 or more cigarettes per day had significantly higher NAS peak scores and took longer to reach peak scores than lighter smokers.

Perinatal outcomes for women who were treated with daily methadone doses of less than 60 mg, 60 to 89 mg, and 90 mg or more were assessed.[373] The methadone dose was not significantly associated with preterm birth or low birth weight. Arbitrarily limiting methadone dose as a way of minimizing the risk of NAS is not warranted. In an investigation of high-dose (>100 mg/day) and low-dose (<100 mg/day) administration, no difference in the rate of medication treatment for NAS or days of infant hospitalization between the high-dose (mean = 132 mg) and low-dose (mean = 62 mg) groups was observed. The group of mothers who received high-dose medication had less illicit drug use at delivery.[374]

To minimize the fetal load of methadone at birth, some investigators have suggested tapering the dose during pregnancy. Luty et al.[375] investigated the safety of methadone detoxification in pregnancy in a retrospective case series of 101 pregnant opiate-dependent women who underwent a 21-day methadone taper during hospitalization. One miscarriage occurred with detoxification in the first trimester. No miscarriages occurred in the second trimester and no increase in preterm births in the third trimester was observed. Similarly, in 34 women at a mean gestational age of 24 weeks, Dashe et al.[376] studied 34 women in MMT programs who tapered their daily methadone dose to 20 mg per day. In opiate-using women not on MMT, methadone was commenced at 20 mg daily and increased by 5 to 10 mg every 6 hours as needed to alleviate withdrawal symptoms. After reaching a stable dose in both groups, the methadone was tapered by 20 percent or less of the stable dose every 3 days. Each woman was observed in the hospital for several days after methadone was discontinued. Daily qualitative assessments of fetal activity were augmented with semiweekly fetal heart rate monitoring with gestations at or more than 24 weeks. Mild maternal symptoms of withdrawal that included cravings or restlessness were managed with supportive care, counseling, or both. Withdrawal signs that included nausea, vomiting, abdominal discomfort, or a concerning fetal heart rate tracing were managed with clonidine (38 percent) or methadone (62 percent). A 0.2-mg transdermal dose of clonidine was supplemented by 0.1 mg orally every 4 to 6 hours to decrease physiologic symptoms. Newborns were kept in the hospital nursery for 3 to 7 days to observe for NAS. The median time to detoxification in the mother was 12 days, and there were no observed fetal deaths, preterm births, growth restriction or other perinatal complications. Fifteen percent of neonates needed treatment for NAS.

Overall, 20 (59 percent) women successfully completed detoxification and did not relapse, while 10 (29 percent) resumed prenatal opioid use and 4 (12 percent) did not complete detoxification and elected methadone maintenance. The decision to opt for methadone detoxification compared with MMT during pregnancy involves consideration of the risks of obstetric and neonatal complications produced by methadone dependence at delivery versus the risks of relapse and continued intravenous drug use after detoxification. If a woman declines MMT, plans to move to an area where MMT is unavailable or plans to detoxify in a structured treatment program, a carefully individualized tapering regimen managed closely by a multidisciplinary team provides a viable treatment option.

Buprenorphine is a partial agonist-partial antagonist synthetic opioid with a long duration of action (72 hours) that has been used to treat opioid dependence both in Europe and the United States. Jones et al.[377] compared the rates of NAS in neonates of 30 methadone- and buprenorphine-maintained mothers in a randomized, double-blind parallel group–controlled trial. Treatment involved daily administration of either sublingual buprenorphine or oral methadone with flexible dosing of 4 to 24 mg or 20 to 100 mg, respectively. Two of 10 (20 percent) buprenorphine-exposed and 5 of 11 (45.5 percent) methadone-exposed neonates were treated for NAS ($p = 0.23$). The total amount of opioid-agonist medication administered to treat NAS in methadone-exposed neonates was three times greater than for buprenorphine-exposed neonates. The length of hospitalization was shorter for buprenorphine-exposed than for methadone-exposed neonates. The peak NAS total scores did not significantly differ between groups. Findings from this pilot study suggest that buprenorphine is similar to methadone on outcome measures of NAS and maternal and neonatal safety when administered during or after starting in the second trimester of pregnancy. A large-scale prospective investigation is being conducted to determine whether buprenorphine is an alternative to MMT during pregnancy.

The AAP recently removed methadone from the list of contraindicated medications during breast-feeding and did not define an upper limit for dose during lactation.[341] The transfer of methadone into human milk is minimal.[378] The milk-to-plasma ratio of methadone in lactating women who took methadone (40 to 105 mg/day, mean 80 mg/day) was assessed in 8 mother-infant pairs.[379] The estimated mean dosage received by infants was 2.8 percent of the maternal dose. The doses of methadone received through milk are unlikely to fully prevent NAS but may be beneficial. Breast-feeding during NAS treatment resulted in infant discharge 8 days earlier than infants who were formula fed.[380] Two infants who abruptly discontinued breastfeeding by mothers on methadone (70 mg and 130 mg/day) developed withdrawal symptoms.[381]

Infants of mothers on MMT are at risk for feeding problems, which may be due to altered sucking patterns. Opiate-exposed infants showed prolonged sucking, fewer pauses, more feeding problems and increased arousal.[382] Their mothers showed increased activity independent of their infants' feeding problems, which may result in less responsivity to infant cues. Intrauterine drug exposure may adversely impact development of brain stem respiratory and swallow centers, which dysregulate the underlying biorhythms of feeding.[383] Apnea and sudden infant death syndrome occur with increased incidence in infants born to both cocaine- and opiate-addicted mothers, which may be due to respiratory pattern abnormalities. In utero drug exposure may result in delayed in maturation of the neurorespiratory axis.[384]

Acute Pain Management for Women on Maintenance Opioids

Treatment of acute pain in labor and postdelivery is challenging in women with substance use disorders. Alford[357] identified common misconceptions about patients who receive maintenance treatment with methadone (or buprenorphine): (1) The maintenance opioid agonist provides analgesia; (2) the use of opioids for analgesia may result in addiction relapse; (3) the additive effects of opioid analgesics and maintenance opioid therapy may cause respiratory and central nervous system depression; and (4) complaints of pains demonstrate drug seeking secondary to opioid addiction.

Alford[357] also provided recommendations for acute pain management in patients who take maintenance opioids to treat addiction. Uninterrupted maintenance treatment (after verification of the daily dose) is imperative. Undertreating acute pain may lead to decreased responsiveness to opioid analgesics, which renders subsequent pain control more difficult. Multimodal analgesia (for example, nonsteroidal anti-inflammatory drugs and acetaminophen) and adjuvant analgesics that enhance opioid effects (e.g., TCAs) may be coadministered. Analgesic dosing should be continuous or scheduled, rather than as needed. Mixed agonist and antagonist opioid analgesics, such as pentazocine, nalbuphine, and butorphanol must be avoided because they may displace the maintenance opioid from the μ receptor and precipitate acute opioid withdrawal.[357]

PERSONALITY DISORDERS

Certain patients do not display obvious symptoms of disorders such as depression or psychosis; nevertheless, they seem to consistently cause difficulty in the clinic. They appear unable to conform to the clinic expectations and they frustrate and defeat their clinicians by rejecting help, making excessive demands, having emotional outbursts, and failing to adhere to treatment recommendations. A disproportionate number have PDs that underlie the behavior that results in frustration. These patients have been described variously as hateful,[385] difficult,[386] or problem patients.[387] These labels illustrate the frustration that arises in the patient-physician relationship.

PDs are a heterogeneous group of disorders that arise when an individual's personality traits are maladaptive and inflexible. The person's rigid belief systems and behaviors prevents adaptability of thinking, and limits use of problem-solving skills with effective coping strategies when confronted with new or stressful events.[388] Coping with major medical illness or a high-risk pregnancy creates a major challenge for these individuals. Most patients with PD have significant difficulty in interpersonal relationships[389,390] and are emotionally sensitive.

They may react strongly to a long clinic wait or terse office staff.

Diagnosis and Prevalence

Unlike many of the disorders described in this chapter, there is no acute stressor or even a clear onset for PDs. Such traits develop gradually in adolescence or early adulthood and persist throughout life. The authors of the DSM-IV[1] grouped the disorders into three clusters on the basis of similarities among the disorders: an *odd/eccentric cluster*; an *emotional/erratic cluster*; and an *anxious/fearful cluster*. Even within these subgroups, there is substantial variation in the form and severity of behavioral problems. Although the clinical features of a PD sound similar to characteristics that anyone could display occasionally, an actual PD is defined by exhibiting extremes on various traits and would not be diagnosed unless the patterns of behavior were chronic, pervasive, and dysfunctional.[1,248] The personality difficulty must lead to emotional distress and/or significantly impaired functioning across several domains. Within the health care system, women with a PD or PD-related traits (such as hostility or anxiety) often use medical resources extensively.[391–394]

Although we were unable to locate any epidemiologic data on PDs specifically in obstetric settings, information is available from primary care and internal medicine settings. Prevalence rates vary from 24 percent with interview-based diagnoses of PD[394] to 32 percent based on a questionnaire that indicated that the person was at high risk for PD.[393] Some investigators have suggested a much greater prevalence of PD among certain patient groups. Between 47 and 60 percent of chronic pain patients meet criteria for a PD,[395–397] and an association also has been found between PD and fibromyalgia.[398] The relationship of PD with medically unexplained symptoms is particularly strong,[399] and one investigator[400] demonstrated that an increasing number of medically unexplained symptoms among patients in primary care positively correlated with PD-relevant traits (neuroticism, harm avoidance) and with the degree of functional impairment. Patients with an Axis I disorder, such as depression, also are more likely to have a co-morbid PD, which typically interferes with their successful treatment.[391] A common clinical perception is that dependent (anxious/fearful cluster), histrionic, and borderline PDs (both from emotional/erratic cluster) are more often diagnosed in women. Although there is some empirical support for borderline PD being more common in women,[385,386] when population sex-ratios are controlled, these gender differences tend to attenuate or disappear.[387,401,402]

Clinical Implications

Mental health treatments for patients with PD tend to be long-term with slow progress, particularly in severe forms of the disorder. Available treatments include both psychotherapy and pharmacotherapy, although it is generally agreed that medication alone cannot fully treat the multi-dimensional problems associated with PD. Limited data have been published on the efficacy of different treatments; however, for severe PD, dialectical behavior therapy has the greatest amount of empirical support.[403] Obstetricians generally do not have the time or training to provide formal psychotherapy to patients with PD. However, physicians can develop rapport, feel less frustrated, and develop better clinical recognition skills. This can help the physician make the decision to refer a patient to a mental health specialist for screening and treatment recommendations if PD is suspected. Physicians also will be in a better position to develop and coordinate effective treatment strategies for other disorders in the context of a PD. There are a number of strategies that can be used to interact with persons who have PDs.

Build a Working Alliance

The first step is to use basic clinical skills. One of the most important ways to begin to develop an alliance is when introducing yourself: When you enter the room, initiate eye contact with the patient, and maintain it while shaking her hand and introducing yourself. Second, use reflective listening in which you simply restate to the patient what she has said, perhaps by paraphrasing. This conveys that you listened and understood what she was telling you, which will facilitate the communication. For example, if a patient with gestational diabetes defensively explains that she did not check her glucose levels as prescribed because she kept forgetting to take her glucometer to work, a reflective statement such as "It sounds like you've had a hard time checking it four times daily" is neutral yet communicates interest and attentiveness.

Structure the Relationship

A common feature of many patients with PD is difficulty in conforming to the expectations or "script" of their current context. In the medical setting, they may make unreasonable demands for special treatment from the physician or clinic. They may become dependent and begin calling the physician excessively at the clinic or at home. Other patients with PD are mistrustful of authority figures, and may infer dishonesty or hostile intent on the part of the physician and clinic staff when there is any minor inconsistency in clinic procedure.

For these reasons, it is useful to make clear the procedures and respective roles of the doctor-patient relationship from the outset (e.g., appointments, emergencies, prescriptions, other aspects of clinic procedure). Doing so is to the benefit of the patient because it reduces the possibility of misunderstanding and promises that cannot be kept. The rules should be presented in a frank, nonjudgmental way, and it is highly useful to try to elicit some form of verbal agreement from the patient to these rules. The rules should be presented as nonnegotiable, with the option to seek another physician or clinic if she cannot agree to them. Allowing her to air concerns and discuss any pitfalls can both heighten adherence to the rules and reduce the likelihood of future problems. An important caveat is to keep the number of such rules to the minimum necessary and avoid listing numerous potential egregious behaviors and appearing as though you have negative expectations of the patient.

On the other hand, the moment it appears that a problem behavior is arising, swift and clear communication of the unacceptability of the behavior is needed. For example, the patient who becomes angry and begins shouting in the waiting area should be calmly told, "We don't tolerate shouting in the clinic; you'll have to calm down or leave immediately and reschedule your appointment." This conveys that the behavior (not the patient) is entirely unacceptable and yet the physician-patient relationship is reparable: the patient may reschedule her appointment. Finally, to reduce the frequency and disruptiveness of unscheduled phone contacts and requests for visits, it can be useful to schedule brief, frequent visits[404] that follow a structured format.

Respect Patient Autonomy

Patients with PD may behave in a passive manner regarding their medical care and fail to adhere to the medical regimen, yet become angry when the physician cannot "fix" the problem for them. Other patients may feel very uncomfortable in a "one-down" role and may chafe at the notion that they are being "told what to do." To guard against these problems, it is advisable to encourage the most collaborative relationship possible. The most useful approach is: "How can we work this out together?"[405] A physician's willingness to take this approach can be severely tested if the patient has serious medical problems or is engaging in egregious behaviors (drug abuse, consistent nonadherence with diabetes therapy) that could produce poor birth outcomes. A useful approach is to make statements that highlight the patient's freedom to choose, such as "I can't force you to do anything; I can only tell you the consequences of your behavior, but ultimately it's up to you to make the decision." Give these patients as much choice as possible; for example, ask them about their medication preferences and allow them to regulate medication within prescribed limits.

Find Something to Validate in the Patient Response

Validation is a key technique to reduce conflict, strengthen the alliance, and promote change. Validation requires the physician to communicate to the patient, in word or action, that her response makes sense and is understandable within the current context.[406] In the face of a great deal of problematic behavior, a physician may have to search for the "kernel of truth" and reflect this back to the patient. The physician may acknowledge, "I understand how hard it has been for you to get to your appointments." Or, "A lot of women would be very stressed by all the things you have going on in your home." Or "I know you are angry about this; you have a reason to be mad" as Groves[385] suggested.

Physician Self-Regulation

When faced with a hostile, antagonistic patient, or one who is sobbing and demanding, it can be difficult for a physician to manage his or her own emotional reaction. Indeed, many physicians may disavow their strong feelings of irritation at a patient because they think they are unprofessional or uncompassionate. Managing emotional reactions requires that they be recognized and discussed with a colleague on a regular basis.[405,407] Peer support is for maintaining morale, warding off burnout, and providing an objective viewpoint. Physicians need not necessarily like the patient nor condone her behavior. Nonetheless, making a conscious effort to strive for empathy and a nonjudgmental stance toward the patient can greatly reduce physician frustration and increase effectiveness. Likewise, physicians must bear in mind that behavior change typically occurs slowly, and patience is required to develop some sense of acceptance of the patient-physician relationship.

SUICIDE

Suicide is a tragic outcome associated with psychiatric illness, particularly mood disorders. In their review of suicide in women, Chaudron and Caine[408] reported that pregnancy itself and having young children in the home had a protective effect against maternal suicide; however, an increased risk was noted among parents who experienced the death of a child or whose child had a psychiatric illness. Another exception is postpartum psychiatric illness, most commonly postpartum psychosis, which may be associated with an increased suicide risk.[409]

Suicide assessment requires direct questioning of the patient about her desire to live or die, specific thoughts about killing herself, plans for carrying out the act, and access to and lethality of means.[408] The American Psychiatric Association practice guidelines for the assessment of suicidal behaviors provide a comprehensive list of more than 40 questions that can help clinicians assess suicidal thoughts, plans and behaviors.[410,411] Initial questions address patients' feelings about living ("Have you ever thought that life was not worth living?" "Did you ever wish you could go to sleep and just not wake up?"). These are followed by questions that address specific thoughts about death, self-harm, and suicide ("Have things ever reached the point that you've thought of harming yourself?"). If thoughts of self-harm are endorsed, physicians should evaluate the details of the thoughts including the nature, intensity, frequency, timing, persistence, and circumstances. Physicians must also ask whether the patient has made a specific plan. Routinely asking about pills, household poisons, firearms, or access to dangerous settings as part of the suicide assessment is critical. Has the patient made preparations for the plan or for after her death (i.e., purchasing the means, writing a will, arranging for childcare)? Answers to each of these questions allow evaluation of the immediate safety of the patient. If screening elucidates a significant potential risk, immediate emergency psychiatric consultation or involuntary commitment to a psychiatric facility is indicated.

The practice guidelines[410] also identify situations in which a suicide assessment is clinically appropriate: emergency room evaluations, abrupt change in clinical presentation, lack of improvement or gradual worsening despite treatment, anticipation or experience of a significant interpersonal loss or stressor (divorce, loss of custody of children, financial loss, legal problems, personal humiliation) or onset of a physical illness that is associated with a threat to life, disfigurement, severe pain, or loss of function. Patients with increased risk are those with previous suicide attempts, major mood disorders, schizophrenia, and substance use.

A potential association between antidepressant use and emergent suicidal behavior has been the subject of an FDA black box warning for the use of antidepressants for children and adolescents, as well as considerable debate.[412] Although 60 percent of suicides occur in persons with mood disorders (the majority untreated), little is known about the relationship between antidepressant drug use and the rate of suicide.[413] Gibbons et al.[413] compiled data from all Americans who committed suicide between 1996 and 1998 with National Vital Statistics from the Centers for Disease Control and Prevention. They analyzed associations between prescription and suicide rate at the county level. The overall relationship between antidepressant prescription and suicide rate was not significant.

INFANTICIDE AND NEONATICIDE

Resnick[414] differentiated filicide (murder of a child) into neonaticide (killing within 24 hours of birth) and infanticide (killing after the first day). In further elaboration of this conceptual framework, Oberman[415] defined four subtypes of infanticide which provide a model for a "differential diagnosis" of infanticide (Table 50-4).

The total dependence of the newborn on the caretaker creates a number of risks for the newborn. Direct killing of an infant by poisoning, traumatic injury, or starvation has been described.[416] The serious cognitive disorganization in women with postpartum psychosis can lead to failure to provide the vulnerable newborn with life-sustaining needs, such as adequate fluid and nutritional intake, appropriate environmental temperatures, safety, and emergency medical care. Environmental factors that are correlated with parental psychiatric illness, such as violence, hostility, irritability, and involvement in parental delusions are also important predictors of poor infant outcomes.[417]

Postpartum Psychosis

The tragic case of Andrea Yates resulted in discussions about the current conceptualization of postpartum psychosis juxtaposed against legal criteria that involve only tests of the cognitive capacity to acknowledge actions.[418] Women are more vulnerable to psychosis in the post-birth period than at any other time during their lives. In the first 30 days after birth, a woman is 21.7 times more likely to develop psychosis than in the 2-year period prior to childbirth. If she has not had a child before, she is 35 times more likely to suffer psychosis than women who have children.[419] The magnitude of these relative risks demonstrates that *postpartum psychiatric morbidity is a major public health problem.*[420,420a] The reasons for the vulnerability of postpartum women to psychosis and the high risk for post-birth decompensation in women with BP have not been elucidated. Sleep deprivation and marked interference with circadian rhythms related to labor are likely contributors to mood instability.[98] Hormone elevations near the end of gestation and massive post-birth withdrawal also contribute to the risk.[57]

Specific types of delusional thoughts are related to risk for infanticide. Delusional altruistic homicide (often associated with maternal suicide) to save them both "from a fate worse than death" was described in a review of filicides.[421] This type of delusion occurred in Andrea Yates. In his classic paper, Resnick[422] was discouraged by the observation that 40 percent of the perpetrators of filicide had seen either psychiatrists or physicians shortly before the tragedy. Sensitive direct questions about thoughts of harm to the infant, as well as harm to the self, are imperative in the examination. Non-judgmental inquiry can be made as follows: "Some new mothers have thoughts such as wishing the baby were dead or about harming the baby; has this happened to you?"

The clinical picture of postpartum psychosis is characterized by rapid onset of hectic mood fluctuation, marked

Table 50-4. Major Categories of Infanticide

CATEGORY	DESCRIPTION
Neonaticide	Unaware of pregnancy, no prenatal care, unassisted birth (often into toilet), family/friends unaware of pregnancy, minimal physical signs of pregnancy
Assisted/Coerced	Killing is done in conjunction with violent, abusive, usually male partner
Neglect	Caretaker distraction results in accidental death, such as baby left in care of young siblings, limited resources, overwhelmed by economic obligations
Abuse	Chronic child abuse, poor caretaker impulse control, efforts to discipline result in unintentional death especially at meal times and bedtimes
Overt mental illness	Acute onset postpartum psychosis with altruistic homicide delusions that involve the infant; Chronic schizophrenia, social isolation, incapable of parenting without assistance

cognitive impairment suggestive of delirium, bizarre behavior, insomnia, visual and auditory hallucinations, and unusual hallucinations (tactile and olfactory). Women with acute onset psychoses related to childbearing usually had recurrence of previously undiagnosed cyclic mood disorders rather than the triggering of a new disorder.[422] As discussed in the section on BD, postpartum psychosis is frequently a manifestation of bipolar illness: mania or depression with psychotic features. In an historical cohort design, our group[423] studied mothers who presented to a psychiatric evaluation center. Half of the group (N = 118) who had at least one child under the age of 3 years presented with episodes that began during pregnancy or postpartum. Women who presented with psychoses during childbearing had symptom patterns that differed from women who presented with nonchildbearing related psychoses.[424]

Delusions must be differentiated from the far more common occurrence of obsessional thoughts in the context of depression. Many depressed women have obsessional thoughts.[177,425] Obsessions are recurrent and persistent thoughts, impulses, or images that are experienced as intrusive and inappropriate and cause marked anxiety or distress. For example, some mothers have obsessional thoughts about drowning their baby, and refuse to bathe the child. Women often have "what if" questions such as: "What if I throw the baby over the banister?" Obsessions differ from psychotic symptoms because the patient recognizes that the thoughts, impulses or images are a product of her own mind (not imposed by an external force as might occur in psychosis). Additionally, obsessional visual images also may occur but are brief and perceived as being in the "mind's eye" as opposed to an external hallucination. For example, a woman might have frightening images of her dead baby in a bath tub, but she is aware that the image was not actually present in the real world.

Prevention of infanticide involves increased *awareness* and a heightened index of suspicion by physicians, midwives, obstetric nurses, and other health care professionals, patients, and their families. Women with a previous episode of postpartum psychosis and women with BD are at high risk for the onset of postpartum psychosis. At a minimum, postpartum *monitoring* for the emergence of symptoms should be a collaborative plan between the physician and the patient's family. Because postpartum disorders are common in the general population of new mothers, *screening* (such as with the EPDS, see Fig. 50-2), to identify cases for *early intervention* is an important public health goal. Aggressive *treatment* for women who develop the disorder with a thoughtful plan for family monitoring of the infant for safety or alternative care while the mother recovers is imperative.[98,420]

NEONATICIDE

Neonaticide refers to the death of an newborn within the first 24 hours of life.[421] A striking consistency in the clinical presentations of neonaticides occurs. The adolescent or adult woman has minimal weight gain during pregnancy, perceives birth as the need to have a bowel movement, and secretly delivers into a toilet.[426,427] She puts the baby in a bag, abandons or hides it, and continues her usual activities. If not rescued, the infant may drown or die from exposure. Affected women vary in terms of age, race, and demographics, and may have other children. Family members, friends, and boyfriends were not aware of their pregnancies, and the father is rarely identified. Childhood sexual trauma, physical abuse, and emotional abuse are common in women who commit neonaticide.

A common element in these cases is the psychophysiologic denial of pregnancy; that is, the conscious awareness of the pregnancy is suppressed. This is classic denial, in that the woman behaves in a way that demonstrates failure to accept either an obvious fact (pregnancy) or its significance.[428] A fragmentation of perceptions (no pregnancy, delivery, pain), and memory (no sexual encounter, continued menses) occurs to suppress painful emotional memories. Intriguing is the physiologic denial of pregnancy, in which the woman denies somatic symptoms of pregnancy, perceives no fetal movements, claims to have menstrual cycles, and recognizes impending birth only as a bowel movement. Essentially, the pregnancy is *not there, not real* for these patients in both mind and body. Most of these patients will not be seen by an obstetrician unless they present for another problem and the pregnancy is discovered, or if the baby is recovered and the mother is presented for obstetrical examination (often by police).

Neonaticide is polar opposite of a desired but unachievable pregnancy, which in extreme cases results in pseudocyesis (see later). Psychophysiologic mechanisms are common to both states, and both have neurohormonal underpinnings but opposite somatic manifestations.

PSEUDOCYESIS

Pseudocyesis is a condition in which the woman believes that she is pregnant but no conceptus exists.[427] Pseudocyesis is characterized by an increase in body weight, enlargement of the mammary glands, and milk production. In animal models, it is associated with the abnormal persistence of the corpus luteum.[429] Spontaneous cases of pseudocyesis have been reported in a number of mammalian species, including dogs, cats, bears, rodents and humans; curiously, it occurs rarely in nonhuman primates.[429]

Women with pseudocyesis have amenorrhea, lactation, colostrum secretion, increased abdominal girth, and subjective experiences of fetal movement. Physical changes consistent with pregnancy have been detected upon examination, such as an enlarged uterus and softened congested cervix. Women with pseudocyesis present with behaviors and somatic symptoms consistent with pregnancy, and they may be admitted to the delivery suite. Psychophysiologic mechanisms are common to both pseudocyesis and denial of pregnancy, which have neurohormonal underpinnings but opposite somatic manifestations. Gentle and supportive provision of information to challenge the belief of pregnancy with referral for psychotherapy is an appropriate intervention strategy.[430] Pseudocyesis must be differentiated from psychosis, in which a fixed conviction of pregnancy persists despite evidence to the contrary and other psychotic symptoms are present. Delusions of pregnancy have been described in patients with schizophrenia.[431]

FINAL COMMENT

We ended where we began; this is, with the powerful mind-body connections that impact the entire spectrum of outcomes for childbearing women. The biopsychosocial forces that impact women at the time of pregnancy create a plethora of childbearing experiences for our patients. As health care professionals, we influence the trajectory of these forces to promote the well-being of the mother, her newborn, and her family.

ADDITIONAL RESOURCES

National Library of Medicine, free search for reproductive and developmental toxicity of drugs during pregnancy and lactation, www.toxnet.nlm.nih.gov

Patient information is available from the Organization of Teratology Information Services http://otispregnancy.org/otis_fact_sheets.asp

Specifically about paroxetine during pregnancy, http://otispregnancy.org/pdf/paxil.pdf

National Institute of Mental Health, http://www.nimh.nih.gov

Society for Women's Health Research, http://www.womenshealthresearch.org/index.htm

For information about the use and interpretation of the Mood Disorders Questionnaire, and downloadable copies, http://www.psycheducation.org/

The Depression and Bipolar Support Alliance, a patient-directed organization, www.dbsalliance.org

National Alliance for the Mentally Ill (NAMI), a nonprofit, grass roots, self-help, support, and advocacy organization of consumers, families and friends of people with severe mental illnesses such as schizophrenia, major depression, bipolar disorders, obsessive-compulsive disorder, and anxiety disorders, http://www.nami.org

The National Depressive and Manic Depressive Association is to educate patients, families, professionals and the public concerning the nature of depressive and manic-depressive illness as treatable medical diseases, http://www.ndmda.org

Anxiety Disorders Association of America, http://www.adaa.org

Suicide Prevention Resource Center, www.sprc.org

Bennett SS, Indman P. *Beyond the Blues: Prenatal and Postpartum Depression.* A Treatment Manual. Moodswings Press, 2002.

Patty Duke has bipolar disorder and an educational website, http://www.officialpattyduke.com/polar.htm

Light therapy: www.cet.org

Shields, Brooke. *Down Came the Rain: My Journey Through Postpartum Depression.* Hyperion, 2005.

National Eating Disorders Association, toll-free: 800-931-2237, http://www.NationalEatingDisorders.org

National Association of Anorexia and Associated Disorders, telephone: 847-831-3438, http://www.anad.org

National Institutes of Health- alcohol and substance use information (www.nih.niaaa.gov; www.nih.nida.gov)

National Partnership to Help Pregnant Smokers Quit (www.helppregnantsmokersquit.org)

Community based advocacy groups (www.jointogether.org) that support efforts to reduce and prevent substance abuse.

KEY POINTS

- Mental health is fundamental to health. To the extent that maternal biopsychosocial exposures with negative impact on pregnancy outcomes can be diminished, eliminated, or replaced with positive factors, the risk of poor pregnancy outcome can be reduced.
- Major depression is a treatable illness that is the leading cause of disease burden among girls age 5 years and older worldwide.
- The incidence of depression during pregnancy is 14.5 percent. Among women who continue their medication compared with those who stop their antidepressant treatment proximate to conception, the risk for depression recurrence during pregnancy is 26 percent versus 68 percent, respectively.
- The first-line medications for treatment of a breast-feeding woman are sertraline, paroxetine, and nortriptyline; however, established efficacy of another drug in the individual woman must be considered strongly in the decision-making process for drug choice.
- A brief and efficient 10-item self-report screening instrument, the Edinburgh Postnatal Depression Scale, is available to screen for perinatal depression.
- Women who present with depression should be evaluated for BD before prescribing antidepressant treatment.
- Abrupt discontinuation of psychotropic medication creates a higher risk for recurrence than does gradual tapering and discontinuation (over at least 2 weeks).
- Cognitive behavioral psychotherapy or behavioral therapy and antidepressants are the first line treatments for anxiety disorders and eating disorders.
- Antipsychotic drug maintenance treatment and psychosocial support interventions aimed at maximizing function are the mainstays of treatment for schizophrenia. Concurrent maternal smoking, substance use, and socioeconomic problems increase the risk for less optimal pregnancy outcomes.
- The perception of substance use disorders as afflictions solely of poor, minority, and young women is erroneous. Screening measures are available and easy to use, and multidisciplinary treatment intervention results in improved reproductive outcomes.

REFERENCES

1. American Psychiatric Association: American Psychiatric Association: Diagnostic and Statistical Manual for Psychiatric Disorders, 4th Edition, Text Revision. Washington, DC: American Psychiatric Association, 2000.
2. Engel GL: The need for a new medical model: a challenge for biomedicine. Science 196:129, 1977.
3. Caspi A, Sugden K, Moffitt TE, et al: Influence of life stress on depression: moderation by a polymorphism in the 5-HTT gene [see comment]. Science 301:386, 2003.
4. Misra DP, Guyer B, Allston A: Integrated perinatal health framework. A multiple determinants model with a life span approach. Am J Prev Med 25:65, 2003.
5. Pomeranz R, Wisner K: Pharmacologic and non-drug treatments for depression during pregnancy. The Female Patient OB/GYN Edition 30:23, 2005.
6. Murray C, Lopez A: The global burden of disease and injury series, volume 1: A comprehensive assessment of mortality and disability from diseases, injuries, and risk factors in 1990 and projected to 2020. *In* Cambridge M (ed): Vol 1: Harvard School of Public Health on behalf of the World Health Organization and the World Bank. Boston, Harvard University Press, 1996.
7. Regier D, Narrow W, Rae D, et al: The de facto mental and addictive disorders service system. Epidemiologic Catchment Area prospective 1-year prevalence rates of disorders and services. Arch Gen Psychiatry 50:85, 1993.
8. Narrow W: One-year prevalence of mental disorders, excluding substance use disorders, in the U.S.: NIMH ECA prospective data. Population estimates based on U.S. Census estimated residential population age 18 and over on July 1, 1998. Unpublished.
9. Marcus SM, Flynn HA, Blow FC, Barry KL: Depressive symptoms among pregnant women screened in obstetrics settings [see comment]. J Women's Health 12:373, 2003.
10. Cox J, Holden J, Sagovsky R: Detection of postnatal depression: Development of the 10-item Edinburgh Postnatal Depression Scale. Br J Psychiatry 150:782, 1987.
11. Wisner K, Parry B, Piontek C: Clinical practice: Postpartum depression. N Engl J Med 347:194, 2002.
12. Peindl K, Wisner K, Hanusa B: Identifying depression in the first postpartum year: Guidelines for office-based screening and referral. J Affect Disord 80:37, 2004.
13. Wisner K, Zarin D, Holmboe E, et al: Risk-benefit decision making for treatment of depression during pregnancy. Am J Psychiatry 157:1933, 2000.
14. Hansen D, Lou H, Olsen J: Serious life events and congenital malformations: A national study with complete follow-up. Lancet 356:875, 2000.
15. Cohen L, Altshuler LL, Harlow B, et al: Relapse of major depression during pregnancy in women who maintain or discontinue antidepressant treatment. JAMA 295:499, 2006.
16. Wisner K, Gelenberg A, Leonard H, et al: Pharmacologic treatment of depression during pregnancy. JAMA 282:1264, 1999.
17. Chambers C, Johnson K, Dick L, et al: Birth outcomes in pregnant women taking fluoxetine. N Engl J Med 335:1010, 1996.
18. Nulman I, Rovet J, Stewart D, et al: Child development following exposure to tricyclic antidepressants or fluoxetine throughout fetal life: A prospective, controlled study. Am J Psychiatry 159:1889, 2002.
19. Nulman I, Rovet J, Stewart D, et al: Neurodevelopment of children exposed in utero to antidepressant drugs. N Engl J Med 336:258, 1997.
20. Kulin N, Pastuszak A, Sage S, et al: Pregnancy outcome following maternal use of new selective serotonin reuptake inhibitors. JAMA 279:609, 1998.
21. Einarson A, Fatoye B, Sarkar M, et al: Pregnancy outcome following gestational exposure to venlafaxine: A multicenter prospective controlled study. Am J Psychiatry 158:1728, 2001.
22. U.S. Food and Drug Administration. Center for Drug Evaluation and Research. FDA Public Health Advisory. Paroxetine, December 8, 2005. http://www.fda.gov/cder/drug/advisory/paroxetine200512.htm
23. Simon G, Cunningham M, Davis R: Outcomes of prenatal antidepressant exposure. Am J Psychiatry 159:2055, 2002.
24. Sussman N, Ginsberg D, Bikoff J: Effects of nefazodone on body weight: A pooled analysis of selective serotonin reuptake inhibitor-and inipramine-controlled trials. J Clin Psychiatry 62:256, 2001.

24a. Bodnar LM, Sunder KR, Wisner KL: Clinical case conference: SSRI treatment during pregnancy: Deceleration of weight gain because of depression of drug? Am J Psychiatry 163:986, 2006.

25. Casper R, Fleischer B, Lee-Ancajas J, et al: Exposure to serotonin reuptake inhibitors (SSRIs) is associated with neonatal adjustment problems and subtle motor changes in infancy compared to early pregnancy exposure to SSRIs or not drug exposure. Neuropsychopharmacology 29(Suppl):S139, 2004.
26. Moses-Kolko E, Bogen D, Perel J, et al: Neonatal signs after late in utero exposure to serontonin reputake inhibitors: Literature review and implications for clinical applications. JAMA 293:2372, 2005.
27. Laine K, Heikkinin T, Ekblad U, Kero P: Effects of exposure to selective serotonin reuptake inhibitors during pregnancy on serotonergic symptoms in newborns and cord blood monoamine and prolactin concentrations. Arch Gen Psychiatry 60:720, 2003.
28. Sanz EI, De-las-Cuevas C, Kiuru A, et al: Selective serotonin reuptake inhibitors in pregnant women and neonatal withdrawal syndrome: a database analysis.[see comment]. Lancet 365:482, 2005.
29. Wisner K, Perel J, Wheeler S: Tricyclic dose requirements across pregnancy. Am J Psychiatry 150:1541, 1993.
30. Hostetter A, Stowe Z, Strader J Jr, et al: Dose of selective serotonin uptake inhibitors across pregnancy: Clinical implications. Depress Anxiety 11:51, 2000.
31. Hendrick V, Stowe ZN, Altshuler LL, et al: Placental passage of antidepressant medications. Am J Psychiatry 160:993, 2003.
32. Altshuler L, Cohen L, Moline M, et al: The Expert Consensus Guidline Series. Treatment of depression in women. Postgrad Med 1, 2001.
33. Spinelli M, Endicott J: Controlled clinical trial of interpersonal psychotherapy versus parenting education program for depressed pregnant women. Am J Psychiatry 160:555, 2003.
34. Golden R, Gaynes B, Ekstrom R, et al: The efficacy of phototherapy in the treatment of mood disorders: A review and meta analysis. Am J Psychiatry 162:656, 2005.
35. Oren D, Wisner K, Spinelli M, et al: An open trial of morning light therapy for treatment of antepartum depression. Am J Psychiatry 159:666, 2002.
36. Epperson C, Terman M, Terman J, et al: Randomized clinical trial of bright light therapy for antepartum depression: Preliminary findings. J Clin Psychiatry 65:421, 2004.
37. Manber R, Schnyer RN, Allen JJ, et al: Acupuncture: a promising treatment for depression during pregnancy. J Affect Disord 83:89, 2004.
38. Tanskanen A, Hibbeln J, Hintikka J, et al: Fish consumption, depression, and suicidality in a general population. Arch Gen Psychiatry 58:512, 2001.
39. Hibbeln JR: Seafood consumption, the DHA content of mothers' milk and prevalence rates of postpartum depression: a cross-national, ecological analysis. J Affect Disord 69:15, 2002.
40. Peet M, Horrobin D: A dose-ranging study of the effects of ethyl-eicosapentaenoate in patients with ongoing depression despite apparently adequate treatment with standard drugs. Arch Gen Psychiatry 59:913, 2002.
41. Nemets B, Stahl Z, Belmaker R: Addition of Omega-3 fatty acid to maintenance medication treatment for recurrent unipolar depressive disorder. Am J Psychiatry 159:477, 2002.
42. Freeman M: Omega-3 fatty acids in psychiatry: A review. Ann Clin Psychiatry 12:159, 2000.
43. Marangell LB, Martinez JM, Zboyan HA, et al: Omega-3 fatty acids for the prevention of postpartum depression: negative data from a preliminary, open-label pilot study. Depress Anxiety 19:20–23, 2004.
44. Osmond M, Wilkie M, Moore J: Behind the Smile: My Journey Out of Postpartum Depression. New York, Warner Books, Inc., 2001.
45. Elliott SA, Leverton TJ, Sanjack M, et al: Promoting mental health after childbirth: a controlled trial of primary prevention of postnatal depression. Br J Clin Psychol 39:223, 2000.

46. Kendell RE, Wainwright S, Hailey A: The influence of childbirth on psychiatric morbidity. Psychol Med 6:297, 1976.
47. Kendell RE, McGuire RJ, Connor Y, Cox JL: Mood changes in the first three weeks after childbirth. J Affect Disord 13:317, 1998.
48. Kendell RE: Diagnosis and classification of functional psychoses. Br Med Bull 43:499, 1987.
48a. Munk-Olsen T, Munk Laursen T, Pederson CB, et al: New parents and mental disorders: A population-based register study. JAMA 296:2582, 2006.
49. Gaynes BN, Gavin N, Meltzer-Brody S, et al: Perinatal depression: Prevalence, screening accuracy, and screening outcomes. Summary, Evidence Report/Technology Assessment No. 119. (Prepared by the RTI-University of North Carolina Evidence-based Practice Center under Contract No. 290-02-0016.) AHRQ Publication No. 05-E006-1. Rockville, MD: Agency for Healthcare Research and Quality. February 2005.
50. Hobfoll SE, Ritter C, Lavin J, et al: Depression prevalence and incidence among inner-city pregnant and postpartum women. J Consult Clin Psychol 63:445, 1995.
51. Logsdon MC, Davis DW, Birkimer JC, Wilkerson S: Predictors of depression in mothers of pre-term infants. J Soc Behav Per- [illegible]
52. [illegible] among adolescents. J Abnorm Psychol 99:69, 1990.
53. England R: Infant development and management of infant problems in a family setting. Aust Fam Physician 23:1877, 1994.
54. Hays RD, Wells KB, Sherbourne CD, et al: Functioning and well-being outcomes of patients with depression compared with chronic general medical illnesses. Arch Gen Psychiatry 52:11, 1995.
55. Kendler KS, Neale MC, Kessler RC, et al: The lifetime history of major depression in women. Reliability of diagnosis and heritability. Arch Gen Psychiatry 50:863, 1993.
56. O'Hara MW: Post-partum "blues," depression, and psychosis: A review. J Psychosom Obstet Gynaecol 73:205, 1987.
57. Bloch M, Schmidt P, Danaceau M, et al: Effects of gonadal steroids in women with a history of postpartum depression. Am J Psychiatry 157:924, 2000.
58. Gregoire AJ, Kumar R, Everitt B, et al: Transdermal oestrogen for treatment of severe postnatal depression [see comment]. Lancet 347:930, 1996.
59. Mazure CM, Bruce ML, Maciejewski PK, Jacobs SC: Adverse life events and cognitive-personality characteristics in the prediction of major depression and antidepressant response. Am J Psychiatry 157:896, 2000.
60. O'Hara M, Neunaber D, Zekoski E: Prospective study of postpartum depression: Prevalence, course, and predictive factors. J Abnorm Psychol 93:158, 1984.
61. Wisner K, Stowe Z: Psychobiology of postpartum mood disorders. [illegible]
62. Appleby L, Warner R, Whitton A, Faragher B: A controlled study of fluoxetine and cognitive-behavioral counselling in the treatment of postnatal depression. BMJ 314:932, 1997.
63. Stowe Z, Owens M, Landry J: Sertraline and desmethylsertraline in human breast milk and nursing infants. Am J Psychiatry 154:1255, 1997.
64. Cohen LS, Viguera AC, Bouffard SM, et al: Venlafaxine in the treatment of postpartum depression. J Clin Psychiatry 62:592, 2001.
65. Suri R, Burt V, Altshuler LL, et al: Fluvoxamine for postpartum depression. Am J Psychiatry 158:1739, 2001.
66. Wisner K, Peindl K, Gigliotti T: Tricyclics vs SSRIs for postpartum depression. Arch Women Ment Health 1:189, 1999.
66a. Wisner KL, Hanusa BH, Perel JM, et al: Postpartum depression: a randomized trial of sertraline vs nortriptyline. J Clin Psychopharmacol 26:1, 2006.
67. Weissman A, Levy B, Hartz A, et al: Pooled analysis of antidepressant levels in lactating mothers, breast milk, and nursing infants. Am J Psychiatry 161:1066, 2004.
68. Altshuler L, Burt VK, McMullen M, Hendrick V: Breastfeeding and sertraline: A twenty four hour analysis. J Clin Psychiatry 56:243, 1995.
69. Wisner K, Perel J, Blumer J: Serum sertraline and N-desmethylsertraline levels in breast-feeding mother-infant pairs. Am J Psychiatry 155:186, 1998.
70. Mammen O, Perel J, Rudolph G, et al: Sertraline and norsertraline levels in three breastfed infants. J Clin Psychiatry 58:100, 1997.
71. Kristensen J, Ilett KF, Dusci L, et al: Distribution and excretion of sertraline and N-desmethylsertraline in human milk. Br J Clin Pharmocol 45:453, 1998.
72. Dodd S, Stocky A, Buist A, et al: Sertraline in paired blood plasma and breast-milk samples from nursing mothers. Hum Psychopharmacol 15:261, 2000.
73. Wenzel A, Haugen E, Jackson LC, et al: Prevalence of generalized anxiety at eight weeks postpartum. Arch Women Ment Health 6:43, 2003.
74. Goodwin F, Jamison K: Suicide in Manic-Depressive Disorder. New York, Oxford University Press, 1990.
75. Goodwin FK, Jamison KR: Manic-Depressive Illness. Oxford, England, Oxford University Press, 1990.
76. Bebbington P, Ramana P: The epidemiology of bipolar affective disorder. Soc Psychiatry Psychiatr Epidemiol 30:279, 1995.
77. Judd L, Akiskal H: The prevalence and disability of bipolar [illegible] Disord 73:123, 2003.
78. Benazzi F: Gender differences in bipolar II and unipolar depressed outpatients: A 557-case study. Ann Clin Psychiatry 11:55, 1999.
79. McElroy S, Altshuler L, Suppes T, et al: Axis I psychiatric comorbidity and its relationship to historical illness variables in 288 patients with bipolar disorder. Am J Psychiatry 158:420, 2001.
80. Leverich G, McElroy S, Suppes T, et al: Early physical and sexual abuse associated with an adverse course of bipolar illness. Biol Psychiatry 51:288, 2002.
81. Frye M, Altshuler L, McElroy S, et al: Gender differences in prevalence, risk, and clinical correlates of alcoholism comorbity in bipolar disorder. Am J Psychiatry 160:883, 2003.
82. Robb J, Young L, Cooke R, Joffe R: Gender differences in patiens with bipolar disorder influence outcome in the medical outcomes survey (SF-20) subscale scores. J Affect Disord 49:189, 1998.
83. Kupka R, Nolen W, Post R, et al: High rate of autoimmune thyroiditis in bipolar disorder: lack of association with lithium exposure. Biol Psychiatry 51:305, 2002.
84. McIntyre R, Mancini D, McCann S, et al: Valproate, bipolar disorder and polycystic ovarian syndrome. Biopolar Disord 5:28, 2003.
85. Low N, DuFort G, Cervantes P: Prevalence, clinical correlates, and treatment of migraine in bipolar disorder. Headache 43:940, 2003.
86. Gitlin M, Swendsen J, Heller T, Hammen C: Relapse and impairment [illegible]
87. Tohen M, Waternaux C, Tsuang M: Outcome in mania: A 4-year prospective follow-up of 75 patients utilizing survival analysis. Arch Gen Psychiatry 47:1106, 1990.
88. Suhail K, Cochrane R: Seasonal variations in hospital admissions for affective disorders by gender and ethnicity. Soc Psychiatry Psychiatr Epidemiol 33:211, 1998.
89. Benazzi F: Prevalence and clinical features of atypical depression in depressed outpatients: A 467-case study. Psychiatry Res 86:259, 1999.
90. Akiskal H, Maser J, Zeller P, et al: Switching from unipolar to bipolar II. An 1 year prospective study of clinical and temperamental predictors in 559 patients. Arch Gen Psychiatry 52:114, 1995.
91. Baldessarini R, Tondo L, Hennen J: Treatment delays in bipolar disorders [Letter]. Am J Psychiatry 156:811, 1999.
92. Hirschfeld R, Williams J, Spitzer R, et al: Development and validation of a screening instrument for bipolar spectrum disorder: The Mood Disorder Questionnaire. Am J Psychiatry 157:1873, 2000.
93. Hirschfeld R, Cass A, Holt D, Carlson C: Screening for bipolar disorder in patients treated for depression in a family medicine clinic. J Am Board Fam Pract 18:233, 2005.
94. Grof P: Protective effect of pregnancy in women with lithium-repsonsive bipolar disorder. J Affect Disord 61:31, 2000.

95. Faedda G, Tondo L, Baldessarini R, et al: Outcome after rapid vs gradual discontinuation of lithium treatment in bipolar disorders. Arch Gen Psychiatry 50:448, 1993.
96. Viguera A, Nonacs R, Cohen L, et al: Risk of recurrence of bipolar disorder in pregnant and nonpregnant women. Am J Psychiatry 157:179, 2000.
97. Wisner K, Hanusa B, Peindl K, Perel J: Prevention of postpartum episodes in women with bipolar disorder. Biol Psychiatry 56:592, 2004.
98. Yonkers K, Wisner K, Stowe Z, et al: Management of bipolar disorder during pregnancy and the postpartum period. Am J Psychiatry 161:608, 2004.
99. Terp I, Mortensen P: Postpartum psychoses. Clinical diagnoses and relative risk of admission after parturition. Br J Psychiatry 172:521, 1998.
100. Kendell R, Chalmers J, Platz CL: Epidemiology of puerperal psychoses. Br J Psychiatry 150:662, 1987.
101. Gonzalez-Pinto A, Gonzalez C, Enjuto S, et al: Psychoeducation and cognitive-behavioral therapy in bipolar disorder: An update. Acta Psychiatr Scand 109:83, 2004.
102. Bauer MS, McBride L, Chase C, et al: Manual-based group psychotherapy for bipolar disorder: a feasibility study. J Clin Psychiatry 59:449, 1998.
103. Colom F, Vieta E, Martinez-Aran A, et al: A randomized trial on the efficacy of group psychoeducation in the prophylaxis of recurrences in bipolar patients whose disease is in remission. Arch Gen Psychiatry 60:402, 2003.
104. Perry A, Tarrier N, Morriss R, et al: Randomized controlled trial of efficacy of teaching patients with bipolar disorder to identify early symptoms of relapse and obtain treatment. BMJ 318:149, 1999.
105. Cochran SD: Preventing medical noncompliance in the outpatient treatment of bipolar affective disorders. J Consult Clin Psychol 52:873, 1984.
106. Katon W, Robinson P, Von Korff M, et al: A multifaceted intervention to improve treatment of depression in primary care. Arch Gen Psychiatry 53:924, 1996.
107. Zornberg G, Pope H: Treatment of depression in bipolar disorder: New directions for research. J Clin Psychopharmacol 13:397, 1993.
108. Kozma C: Neonatal toxicity and transient neurodevelopmental deficits following prenatal exposure to lithium: Another clinical report and a review of the literature. Am J Med Genet 132:441, 2005.
109. Cohen L, Freidman J, Jefferson J, et al: A reevaluation of risk of in utero exposure to lithium. JAMA 271:146, 1994.
110. Newport D, Viguera A, Beach A, et al: Lithium placental passage and obstetrical outcome: Implications for clinical management during late pregnancy. Am J Psychiatry 162:2162, 2005.
111. Jacobson S, Jones K, Johnson K, et al: Prospective multicentre study of pregnancy outcome after lithium exposure during first trimester. Lancet 339:530, 1992.
112. Viguera A, Newport D, Ritchie J, et al: Lithium and Lactation. 2004 NIMH/NCDEU Annual Meeting, Boca Raton, FL, 2004.
113. Morrow J: Getting it right for children born to mothers with epilepsy: morphology. Epilepsia 45(Suppl 3):206, 2004.
114. Lammer EJ, Sever LE, Oakley GP, Jr: Teratogen update: valproic acid. Teratology 35:465, 1987.
115. Ketter T, Frye M, Cora-Locatelli G, et al: Metabolism and excretion of mood stabilizers and new anticonvulsants. Cell Mol Neurobiol 19:511, 1999.
116. (AAN) AAoN: Practice parameter: management issues for women with epilepsy (summary statement) Report of the Quality Standard Subcommittee of the American Academy of Neurology. Neurology 51:944, 1998.
117. Crawford P: Best practice guidelines for the management of women with epilepsy. Epilepsia 46(Suppl 9):117, 2005.
118. Nau H, Kuhnz W, Egger H, et al: Anticonculsants during pregnancy and lactation. Transplacental, maternal and neonatal pharmacokinetics. Clin Pharmacokinet 6:508, 1982.
119. Delgado-Escueta A, Janz D: Consensus guidelines: Preconception counseling, management, and care of pregnant women with epilepsy. Neurology 42:149, 1992.
120. Meischenguiser R, D'Giano CH, Ferraro SM: Oxcarbazepine in pregnancy: clinical experience in Argentina. Epilepsy Behav 5:163, 2004.
121. Myllynen P, Pienimaki P, Jouppila P, Vahakangas K: Transplacental passage of oxcarbazepine and its metabolites in vivo. Epilepsia 42:1482, 2001.
122. Bulau P, Paar WD, von Unruh GE: Pharmacokinetics of oxcarbazepine and 10-hydroxy-carbazepine in the newborn child of an oxcarbazepine-treated mother. Eur J Clin Pharmacol 34:311, 1988.
123. Calabrese J, Bowden C, Sachs G, et al: A double-blind placebo-controlled study of lamotrignine monotherapy in outpatients with bipolar I depression. Lamictal 602 study group. J Clin Psychiatry 60:79, 1999.
124. McElroy S, Zarate C, Cookson J, et al: A 52-week, open-label continuation study of lamotrigine in the treatment of bipolar depression. J Clin Psychiatry 65:204, 2004.
125. Bowden C, Calabrese J, Sachs G, Group LS: A placebo-controlled 18-month trial of lamotrigine and lithium maintenance treatment in recently manic or hypomanic patients with bipolar I disorder. Arch Gen Psychiatry 60:392, 2003.
126. Calabrese J, Sullivan J, Bowden C, et al: Rash in multicenter trials of lamotrigine in mood disorders: Clinical relevance and management. J Clin Psychiatry 63:1012, 2002.
127. Bowden C, Asnis G, Ginsberg L, et al: Safety and tolerability of lamotrigine and bipolar disorder. Drug Safety 27:173, 2004.
128. Messenheimer J, Tennis P, Cunnington M: Eleven-year interim resuilts of an international observational study of pregnancy outcomes after exposure to lamotrigine. Epilepsia 45(Suppl 7):232, 2004.
129. Tran TA, Leppik IE, Blesi K, et al: Lamotrigine clearance during pregnancy. Neurology 59:251, 2002.
130. Ohman I, Vitols S, Tomson T: Lamotrigine in pregnancy: Pharmacokinetics during delivery, in the neonate, and during lactation. Epilepsia 41:709, 2000.
131. Dominguez Salgado M, Morales A, et al: Gestational lamotrigine monotherapy: Congential malformations and psychomotor development. Epilepsia 45(Suppl 7):229, 2004.
132. Kinon BJ, Gilmore JA, Liu H, Halbreich UM: Hyperprolactinemia in response to antipsychotic drugs: characterization across comparative clinical trials. Psychoneuroendocrinology 28(Suppl 2):69, 2003.
133. Nasrallah H: A review of the effect of atypical antipsychotics on weight. Psychoneuroendocrinology 28(Suppl 1):83, 2003.
134. McKenna K, Koren G, Tetelbaum M, et al: Pregnancy outcomes of women using atypical antipsychotic drugs: A prospective comparative study. Clin Psychiatry 66:444, 2005.
135. Jensen D, Damm P, Sorensen B, et al: Pregnancy outcome and prepregnancy body mass index in 2459 glucose-tolerant Danish women. Am J Obstet Gynecol 189:239, 2003.
136. Seeman M: Gender differences in the prescribing of antipsychotic drugs. Am J Psychiatry 161:1324, 2004.
137. Jablensky A, Morgan V, Zubrick S, et al: Pregnancy delivery, and neonatal complications in a population cohort of women with schizophrenia and major affective disorders. Am J Psychiatry 162:79, 2005.
138. Noaghiul S, Hibbeln J: Cross-national comparisons of seafood comsumption and rates of bipolar disorders. Am J Psychiatry 160:2222, 2003.
139. Stoll A, Severus E, Freeman M, et al: Omega-3 fatty acids in bipolar disorder: A double-blind placebo-controlled trial. Arch Gen Psychiatry 56:407, 1999.
140. Freeman M: *In* Katherine L, Wisner MD (ed): Pittsburgh, PA, 2003, personal communication.
141. Fearrington EL, Rand CH Jr, Rose JD: Hyperprolactinemia-galactorrhea induced by verapamil. Am J Cardiol 51:1466, 1983.
142. Straub H, Kohling R, Speckmann EJ: Strychnine-induced epileptiform activity in hippocampal and neocortical slice preparations: suppression by the organic calcium antagonists verapamil and flunarizine. Brain Res 773:173, 1997.
143. Wisner K, Peindl K, Perel J, et al: Verapamil treatment for women with bipolar disorder. Biol Psychiatry 51:745, 2002.
144. Janicak P: Verapamil for the treatment of acute mania: A double-blind, placebo-controlled trial. Am J Psychiatry 155:972, 1998.
145. Mukherjee S, Sackeim H, Schnur D: Electronconvulsive therapy of acute manic episodes: A review of 50 years' experience. Am J Psychiatry 151:169, 1994.

146. Miller L: Use of electroconvulsive therapy during pregnancy. Hosp Community Psychiatry 45:444, 1994.
147. Committee on Drugs AAOP: The transfer of drugs and other chemicals into human milk. Pediatrics 108:776, 2001.
148. Atiba EO, Adeghe A-H, Murphy PJ, et al: Patient's expectation and cesarean section rate. Lancet 341:246, 1993.
149. Kessler RD, McGonagle KA, Zhao S, et al: Life-time and 12-month prevalence of DSM-III-R psychiatric disorders in the United States. Arch Gen Psychiatry 51:8, 1994.
150. Myers J, Weissman M, Tischler G, et al: Six-month prevalence of psychiatric disorders in three communities, 1980–1982. Arch Gen Psychiatry 41:959, 1984.
151. Eaton W, Kessler R, Wittchen HU, et al: Panic and panic disorder in the United States. Am J Psychiatry 151:413, 1994.
152. Karno M, Golding JM, Sorenson SB, Burnam MA: The epidemiology of obsessive-compulsive disorder in five U.S. communities. Arch Gen Psychiatry 45:1094, 1988.
153. Beck C: Post-traumatic stress disorder due to childbirth: The aftermath. Nurs Res 53:216, 2004.
154. Areskog B, Uddenberg N, Kjessler B: Fear of childbirth in late pregnancy. Gynecol Obstet Invest 12:262, 1981.
155. Ryding E: Psychosocial indications for cesarean section. A ret- [illegible] 1991.
156. Sjogren B, Thomassen P: Obstetric outcome in 100 women with severe anxiety over childbirth. Acta Obstet Gynecol Scand 76:948, 1997.
157. Nielsen TF, Otterblad P, Ingemarsson I: The end of the rise. Birth 21:34, 1994.
158. Melender H: Experences of fears associated with pregnancy and childbirth: A study of 329 pregnant women. Birth 29:101, 2002.
159. Ryding EL, Wijma B, Wijma K, Rydhstrom H: Fear of childbirth during pregnancy may increase the risk of emergency cesarean section. Acta Obstet Gynecol Scand 77:542, 1998.
160. Saisto T, Salmela-Aro K, Nurmi JE, et al: A randomized controlled trial of intervention in fear of childbirth. Obstet Gynecol 98:820, 2001.
161. Sjostrom K, Valentin L, Thelin T, Marsal K: Maternal anxiety in late pregnancy and fetal hemodynamics. Eur J Obstet Gynecol Reprod Biol 74:149, 1997.
162. Zar M, Wijma K, Wijma B: Relations between anxiety disorders and fear of childbirth during late pregnancy. Clin Psychol Psychotherapy 9:122, 2002.
163. Heron J, O'Connor TG, Evans J, et al: The course of anxiety and depression through pregnancy and the postpartum in a community sample. J Affective Disord 80:65, 2004.
164. [illegible] partum depression in mothers and fathers: whatever happened to anxiety? J Affective Dis 74:139, 2003.
165. [illegible] effects of pregnancy on the course of panic disorder. Anxiety 1:227, 1995.
166. George DT, Ladenheim JA, Nutt DJ: Effect of pregnancy on panic attacks. Am J Psychiatry 144:1078, 1987.
167. Villeponteaux VA, Lydiard RB, Laraia MT, et al: The effects of pregnancy on preexisting panic disorder. J Clin Psychiatry 53:201, 1992.
168. Cowley DS, Roy-Byrne PP: Panic disorder during pregnancy. J Psychosom Obstet Gynaecol 10:193, 1989.
169. Cohen LS, Sichel DA, Faraone SV, et al: Course of panic disorder during pregnancy and the puerperium: A preliminary study. Biol Psychiatry 39:950, 1996.
170. Sholomskas DE, Wickamaratne PJ, Dogolo L, et al: Postpartum onset of panic disorder: a coincidental event? J Clin Psychiatry 54:476, 1993.
171. Cox D, Reading A: Fluctuations in state anxiety over the course of pregnancy and the relationship with outcome. J Psychosom Obstet Gynaecol 10:71, 1989.
172. DaCosta D, Larouche J, Drista M, et al: Variations in stress levels over the course of pregnancy: Factors associated with elevated hassles, state anxiety and pregnancy-specific stress. J Psychosom Res 47:609, 1999.
173. Northcott C, Stein M: Panic disorder in pregnancy. J Clin Psychiatry 55:539, 1994.
174. Wisner KL, Peindl KS, Hanusa BH: Effects of childbearing on the natural history of panic disorder with comorbid mood disorder. J Affect Disord 41:173, 1996.
175. Altemus M: Obsessive-compulsive disorder during pregnancy and postpartum. *In* Yonkers K, Little B (eds): Management of Psychiatric Disorders in Pregnancy. London, Arnold, 2001, p 149.
176. Williams K, Koran L: Obsessive-compulsive disorder in pregnancy, the puerperium, and the prementstrum. J Clin Psychiatry 58:330, 1997.
177. Wisner K, Peindl K, Gigliotti T, Hanusa B: Obsessions and compulsions in women with postpartum depression. J Clin Psychiatry 60:176, 1999.
178. Sichel DA, Cohen LS, Dimmock JA, Rosenbaum JF: Postpartum obsessive-compulsive disorder: A case series. J Clin Psychiatry 54:156, 1993.
179. Kurki T, Hiilesmaa V, Raitasalo R, et al: Depression and anxiety in early pregnancy and risk for preeclampsia. Obstet Gynecol 95:487, 2000.
180. Beck N, Siegal LJ, Davidson NP, et al: The prediction of pregnancy outcome: maternal preparation, anxiety and attitudinal sets. J Psychosom Res 24:343, 1980.
181. [illegible] J Psychosom Res 23:109, 1979.
182. DiRenzo G, Polito P, Volpe A, et al: A multicentric study of fear of childbirth in pregnant women at term. J Psychosom Obstet Gynaecol 3:155, 1984.
183. Standley K, Soule B, Copans S: Dimensions of prenatal anxiety and their influences on pregnancy outcome. Am J Obstet Gynecol 135:22, 1979.
184. Teixeira JM, Fisk NM, Glover V: Association between maternal anxiety in pregnancy and increased uterine artery resistance index: a cohort based study. Br Med J 16:153, 1999.
185. Bazhenova OV, Plonskaia O, Porges SW: Vagal reactivity and affective adjustment in infants during interaction challenges. Child Dev 72:1314, 2001.
186. Calkins SD: Cardiac vagal tone indices of terperamental reactivity and behavioral regulation in young children. Dev Psychobiol 31:125, 1997.
187. DiPietro J, Hodgson K, Costigan KA, et al: Developmental of fetal movement—fetal heart rate coupling from 20 weeks through term. Early Hum Dev 44:139, 1996.
188. Huffman L, Bryan Y, del Carmen R, et al: Infant temperament and cardiac vagal tone: Assessments at twelve weeks of age. Child Dev 69:624, 1998.
189. Porges S, Doussard-Roosevelt J, Portales A, Suess P: Cardiac vagal tone: Stability and relation to difficulties in infants and 3-year-olds. Dev Psychobiol 27:289, 1994.
190. [illegible] control and hostility in healthy subjects. Am J Cardiol [illegible], 1994.
191. [illegible] development: Associations with socioeconomic class and fetal sex. Dev Psychobiol 33:79, 1998.
192. Paarlberg KM, Hoets AJV, Passchier J, et al: Psychosocial factors and pregnancy outcome: a review with emphasis on methodological issures. J Psychosom Res 39:563, 1995.
193. Wadhwa PD, Sandman CA, Porto M, et al: The association between prenatal stress and infant birth weight and gestational age at birth: a prospective investigation. Am J Obstet Gynecol 179:1079, 1993.
194. Hedegaard M, Henriksen TB, Sabroe S, et al: Psychological distress in pregnancy and preterm delivery. BMJ 307:234, 1993.
195. Lou HC, Hansen D, Nordentoft M, et al: Prenatal stressors of human life affect fetal brain development. Dev Med Child Neurol 36:826, 1994.
196. Copper RL, Goldenberg RL, Das A, et al: The preterm prediction study: Maternal stress is associated with spontaneous preterm birth at less than thirty-five weeks gestation. Am J Obstet Gynecol 175:1286, 1994.
197. Feldman PJ, Dunkel-Schetter C, Sandman CA, Wadhwa PD: Maternal social support predicts birth weight and fetal growth in human pregnancy. Psychosom Med 62:715, 2000.
198. Ruiz RJ, Fullerton JT: The measurement of stress in pregnancy. Nurs Health Sci 1:19, 1999.

199. Berkin MR, Bland JM, Peacock JL, Anderson HR: The effect of anxiety and depression during pregnancy on obstetric complications. Br J Obstet Gynaecol 100:629, 1993.
200. Paarlberg KM, Vingerhoets JJM, Passchier J, et al: Psychosocial predictors of low birthweight. Br J Obstet Gynaecol 106:834, 1999.
201. Godfrey KM: Maternal regulation of fetal development and health in adult life. Eur J Obstet Gynecol Reprod Biol 78:141, 1998.
202. Barker DJ: The fetal origins of coronary heart disease. Acta Paediatr 422:78, 1997.
203. Strauss RS: Adult functional outcome of those born small for gestational age. JAMA 283:625, 2000.
204. O'Connor TG, Heron J, Golding J, et al: Maternal antenatal anxiety and children's behavioral/emotional problems at 4 years: Report from the Avon Longitudinal Study of Parents and Children. Br J Psychiatry 180:502, 2002.
205. O'Connor TG, Heron J, Glover V, Team TAS: Antenatal anxiety predicts child behavior/emotional problems independently of postnatal depression. J Am Acad Child Adolesc Psychiatry 41:1470, 2002.
206. O'Connor TG, Heron J, Golding J, Glover V: Maternal antenatal anxiety and behavioural/emotional problems in children: a test of a programming hypothesis. J Child Psychol Psychiatry 44:1025, 2003.
207. Van den Bergh BR, Marcoen A: High antenatal maternal anxiety is related to ADHD symptoms, externalizing problems and anxiety in 8–9 year olds. Child Dev 75:1085, 2004.
208. Yonkers K, Ramin SM, Rush AJ, et al: Onset and persistence of postpartum depression in an inner-city maternal health clinic system. Am J Psychiatry 158:1856, 2001.
209. Hannah P, Adams D, Lee A, et al: Links between early postpartum mood and post-natal depression. Br J Psychiatry 160:777, 1992.
210. Lane A, Keville R, Morris M, et al: Post-natal depression and elation among mothers and their partners: prevalence and predictors. Br J Psychiatry 171:550, 1997.
211. Virden SF: The relationship between infant feeding and maternal role adjustment. J Nurse-Midwifery 33:31, 1988.
212. Berg-Cross L, Berg-Cross G, McGeehan D: Experience and personality differences among breast- and bottle-feeding mothers. Psychol Women Q 3:344, 1979.
213. Mezzacappa ES, Guethlein W, Vaz N, Bagiella E: A preliminary study of breast-feeding and maternal symptomatology. Ann Behav Med 22:71, 2000.
214. Abou-Saleh MT, Ghubash R, Karim L, et al: Hormonal aspects of postpartum depresson. Psychoneuroendocrinology 23:465, 1998.
215. Astbury J, Brown S, Lumley J, Small R: Birth events, birth experiences and social differences in postnatal depression. Aust J Public Health 18:176, 1994.
216. Heck H, deCastro JM: The caloric demand of lactation does not alter spontaneous meal patterns, nutrient intakes, or moods of women. Physiol Behav 54:641, 1993.
217. Modahl C, Newton N: Mood state difference between breast and bottle feeding mothers. In Carenza L, Zinchella L (eds): Emotion and Reproduction: Proceedings of the Serrano Symposium, Vol 20B. New York, Academic Press, 1979, p 819.
218. Mezzacappa ES, Katkin ES: Breast-feeding is associated with reductions in perceived stress and negative mood in mothers. Health Psychol 21:187, 2002.
219. Heinrichs M, Meinlschmidt G, Neumann I, et al: Effects of suckling on hypothalamic-pituitary-adrenal axis responses to psychosocial stres in postpartum lactating women. J Clin Endocrinol Metab 86:4798, 2001.
220. Czeizel A, Rockenbauer M, Sorensen H, Olsen J: A population-based case-control study of oral chlordiazepoxide use during pregnancy and risk of congenital abnormalties. Neurotoxicol Teratol 26:593, 2004.
221. Ornoy A, Arnon J, Shechtman S, et al: Is benzodiazepine use during pregnancy really teratogenic? Reprod Toxicol 12:511, 1998.
222. Crow S, Thuras P, Keel P, Mitchell J: Long-term menstural and reproductive function in patients with bulimia nervosa. Am J Psychiatry 159:1048, 2002.
223. Mitchell-Gieleghem A, Mittelstaedt ME, Bulik C: Eating disorders and childbearing: concealment and consequences. Birth 29:182, 2002.
224. Sollid C, Wisborg K, Hjort J, Secher N: Eating disorder that was diagnosed before pregnancy and pregnancy outcome. Am J Obstet Gynecol 190:206, 2004.
224a. Kouba S, Hallstrom T, Lindholm C, Hirschberg AL: Pregnancy and neonatal outcomes in women with eating disorders. Obstet Gynecol 105:255, 2005.
225. Bulik C, Sullivan P, Fear J, et al: Fertility and reproduction in women with a history of anorexia nervosa: A controlled study. J Clin Psychiatry 60:130, 1999.
225a. Morgan JF, Lacey JH, Chung E: Risk of postnatal depression, miscarriage, and preterm birth in bulimia nervosa: retrospective controlled study. Psychosom Med 68:487, 2006.
226. Mazzeo SE, Slof-Op't Landt MC, Jones I, et al: Associations among postpartum depression, eating disorders, and perfectionism in a population-based sample of adult women. Int J Eat Disord 39:202, 2006.
227. Crow S, Keel P, Thuras P, Mitchell J: Bulimia symptoms and other risk behaviors during pregnancy in women with bulimia nervosa. Int J Eat Disord 36:220, 2004.
228. Kouba S, Hallstrom T, Lindholm C, Hirshberg A: Pregnancy and neonatal outcomes in women with eating disorders. Obstet Gynecol 105:255, 2005.
229. Carmichael S, Shaw G, Schaffer D, et al: Dieting behaviors and risk of neural tube defects. Am J Epidemiol 158:1127, 2003.
230. Hsu LK: Eating disorders: practical interventions. J Am Med Womens Assoc 59:113, 2004.
231. Mont L, Castro J, Herreros B, et al: Reversibility of cardiac abnormalities in adolescents with anorexia nervosa after weight recovery. J Am Acad Child Adolesc Psychiatry 42:808, 2003.
232. Schneider D, Perez A, Knilamus T, et al: Clinical and pathologic aspects of cardiomyopathy from ipecac administration in Munchausen's syndrome by proxy. Pediatrics 97:902, 1996.
233. Ho PC, Dweik R, Cohen MC: Rapidly reversible cardiomyopathy associated with chronic ipecac ingestion. Clin Cardiol 21:780, 1998.
234. Rome E, Ammerman S, Rosen D, et al: Children and adolescents with eating disorders: the state of the art. Pediatrics 111:98, 2003.
235. Golden NH, Meyer W: Nutritional rehabilitation of anorexia nervosa. Goals and dangers. Int J Adolesc Med Health 16:131, 2004.
236. Zipfel S, Seibel M, Lowe B, et al: Osteoporosis in eating disorders: A folllow-up study of patients with anorexia and bulimia nervosa. J Clin Endocrinol Metab 86:5227, 2001.
237. Fairburn CG: Overcoming Binge Eating. New York, The Guilford Press, 1995.
238. Casper R: How useful are pharmacological treatments in eating disorders? Psychopharm Bull 36:88, 2002.
239. Powers P, Santana C: Available pharmacological treatments for anorexia nervosa. Expert Opin Pharmacother 5:2287, 2004.
240. Hsu L: Eating Disorders. New York, Guilford, 1990.
241. Steinhausen H: The outcome of anorexia nervosa in the 20th century. Am J Psychiatry 159:1284, 2002.
242. Kaye W: Central nervous system neurotransmitter activity in anorexia nervosa and bulimia nervosa. *In* Fairburn C, Brownell K (eds): Eating Disorders and Obesity. New York, Guilford, 2002, p 272.
243. Walsh B, Wilson G, Loeb K, et al: Medication and psychotherapy in the treatment of BN. Am J Psychiatry 154:523, 1997.
244. Walsh B, Agras W, Devlin M, et al: Fluoxetine for BN following poor response to psychotherapy. Am J Psychiatry 157:1332, 2000.
245. Hoopes S, Reimherr F, Hedges D, et al: Treatment of bulimia nervosa with topiramate in randomized, double-blind, placebo-controlled trial, part 1: Improvement in binge and purge measures. J Clin Psychiatry 64:1335, 2003.
246. Hedges D, Reimherr F, Hoopes S, et al: Treatment of bulimia nervosa with topiramate in a randomized, double-blind, placebo-controlled trial, part 2: Improvement in psychiatric measures. J Clin Psychiatry 64:1449, 2003.

247. McElroy S, Shapira N, Arnold L, et al: Topiramate in the long-term treatment of binge-eating disorder associated with obesity.[erratum appears in J Clin Psychiatry 66:138, 2005]. J Clin Psychiatry 65:1463, 2004.
248. American Psychiatric Association: Diagnostic and Statistical Manual of Mental Disorders, 4th ed. Washington, DC, American Psychiatric Association, 1994.
249. Brown A, Begg M, Gravenstein S, et al: Serologic evidence of prenatal influenza in the etiology of schizophrenia. Arch Gen Psychiatry 61:774, 2004.
250. Kinney D, Levy D, Yurgelun-Todd D, et al: Season of birth obstetrical complications in schizophrenics. J Psychiat Res 28:499, 1994.
251. Frost D, Tamminga C, Medoff D, et al: Neuroplasticity and schizophrenia. Biol Psychiatry 56:540, 2004.
252. Waddington J: Developmental neuroscience and pathobiology. Lancet 341:531, 1993.
253. Hafner H: Gender differences in schizophernia. Psychoneuroendocinology 28(Suppl 2):17, 2003.
254. Howard L, Kumar C, Leese M, Thornicroft G: The general fertility rate in women with psychotic disorders. Am J Psychiatry 159:991, 2002.
255. Trixler M, Gati A, Tenyi T: Risks associated with childbearing in schizophrenia. [illegible]
256. Davies A, McIvor R, Kumar R: Impact of childbirth on a series of schizophrenic mothers: A comment on the possible influence of oestrogen on schizophrenia. Schizophrenia Res 16:25, 1995.
257. Howard L, Goss C, Leese M, et al: The psychosocial outcome of pregnancy in women with psychotic disorders. Schizophrenia Res 71:49, 2004.
258. Bennedsen BE, Mortensen PB, Olesen AV, Henriksen TB: Congenital malformations, stillbirths, and infant deaths among children of women with schizophrenia. Arch Gen Psychiatry 58:674, 2001.
259. Bennedsen B: Adverse pregnancy outcome in schizophrenic women: Occurence and risk factors. Schizophrenia Res 33:1, 1998.
260. Nilsson E, Lichtenstein P, Cnattingius S, et al: Women with schizophrenia: Pregnancy outcome and infant death among their offspring. Schizophrenia Res 58:221, 2002.
261. Gilbert PL, Harris MJ, McAdams LA, Jeste DV: Neuroleptic withdrawal in schizophrenic patients. A review of the literature. Arch Gen Psychiatry 52:173, 1995.
262. Baldessarini RJ, Viguera AC: Neuroleptic withdrawal in schizophrenic patients. Arch Gen Psychiatry 52:189, 1995.
263. Della-Giustina K, Chow G: Medications in pregnancy and lactation. Emerg Med Clin North Am 21:585, 2003.
264. Seeman M, Cohen R: Focus on women: A service for women with schizophrenia. [illegible]
265. Goff D, Henderson D, Amico E: Cigarette smoking in schizophrenia: Relationship to psychopathology and medication side effects. Am J Psychiatry 149:1189, 1992.
266. Tamminga C: Similarities and differences among antipsychotics. J Clin Psychiatry 64(Suppl 17):7, 2003.
267. Lieberman J, Stroup T, McEvoy J, et al: Effectiveness of antipsychotic drugs in patients with chronic schizophrenia. N Engl J Med 353:1209, 2005.
268. Webb R, Howard L, Abel H: Antipsychotic drugs for non-affective psychosis during pregnancy and postpartum. Cochrane Database of Systematic Reviews 2: CD004411, 2004.
269. McKenna K, Koren G, Tetelbaum M, et al: Pregnancy outcome of women using atypical antipsychotic drugs: a prospective comparative study. J Clin Psych 66:444, 2005.
270. Nguyen H, Lalonde P: Clozapine and pregnancy. Encephale 29:19, 2003.
271. Waldman M, Safferman A: Pregnancy and clozapine [Letter]. Am J Psychiatry 150:168, 1993.
272. Dickson R, Hogg L: Pregnancy of a patient treated with clozapine. Psychiatr Serv 49:1081, 1998.
273. DiMichele V, Ramenghi L, Sabatino G: Clozapine use in two full-term pregnancies [Letter]. Eur Psychiatry 11:214, 1996.
274. Stoner S, Sommi R, Marken P, et al: Clozapine use in two full-term pregnancies [Letter]. J Clin Psychiatry 58:364, 1997.
275. Goldstein D, Corbin L, Fung M: Olanazpine-exposed pregnancies and lactation: Early experience. J Clin Psychopharmacol 20:399, 2000.
276. Schenker S, Yang Y, Mattiuz E, et al: Olanzapine transfer by human placenta. Clin Exp Pharmacol Physiol 26:691, 1999.
277. Ratnayake T, Libretto S: No complications with resperidone treatment before and throughout pregnancy and during the nursing period [Letter]. J Clin Psychiatry 63:76, 2002.
278. Taylor R, O'Toole M, Ohlsen R, et al: Safety of quetiapine during pregnancy. Am J Psychiatry 160:588, 2003.
279. Tenyi T, Trixler M, Keresztes Z: Queteapine and pregnancy. Am J Psychiatry 159:674, 2002.
280. Simpson G, Glick I, Weiden P, et al: Randomized, controlled, double-blind multicenter comparison of the efficacy and tolerability of ziprasidone and olanzapine in acutely ill patients with schizophrenia disorder. Am J Psychiatry 161:1837, 2004.
281. Barnas C, Bergant A, Hummer M, et al: Clozapine concentrations in maternal and fetal plasma, amniotic fluid and breast milk [Letter]. Am J Psychiatry 151:945, 1994.
282. Croke S, Buist A, Hackett LP, et al: Olanzapine excretion in human breast milk: estimation of infant exposure. Int J Neuropsychopharmacol 5:243, 2002.
283. Kirchheiner J, Berghofer A, Bolk-Weischedel D: Healthy outcome under olanzapine treatment in a pregnant woman. Pharmacopsychiatry 33:78, 2000.
284. Ambresin G, Berney P, Schulz P, Bryois C: Olanzapine excretion into breast milk: a case report. J Clin Psychopharmacol 24:93, 2004.
285. Ilett K, Hackett L, Kreistensen J, et al: Transfer of risperidone and 9-hydroxyrisperidone into human milk. Ann Pharmacother 38:273, 2004.
286. Hill R, McIvor R, Bach B, et al: Risperidone distribution and excretion into human milk: Case report and estimated infant exposure during breastfeeding. J Clin Psychopharmacol 20:285, 2000.
287. Lee A, Giesbrecht E, Dunn E, Ito S: Excretion of quetiapine in breastmilk. Am J Psychiatry 161:1715, 2004.
288. Hans S: Demographic and psychosocial characteristics of substance-abusing pregnant women. Clin Perinatol 26:55, 1999.
289. National Institute on Drug Abuse: National Pregnancy and Health Survey: Drug use among women delivering live births. *In* National Institute on Health: Vol Publication No. BKD192: National Clearinghouse for Drug and Alcohol Information, 1992.
290. Substance Abuse and Mental Health Services Administration: National Survey on Drug Abuse and Health published Substance Use During Pregnancy, 2002 and 2003 update.
291. Brady K, Sinha R: Co-occurring mental and substance use disorders: The neurobiological effects of chronic stress. Am J Psychiatry 162:1483, 2005.
292. Brady K, Grice D, Dustan L, Randall C: Gender differences in substance use disorders. Am J Psychiatry 150:1707, 1993.
293. Chasnoff I, McGourty R, Bailey G, et al: The 4P's Plus© Screen for Subtance Use in Pregnancy: Clinical Applictions and Outcomes. J Perinatol 25:368, 2005.
294. Ellwood D, Sutherland P, Kent C, O'Connor M: Maternal narcotic addiction: Pregnancy outcomes in patients managed by a specialized drug dependency antenatal clinic. Aust N Z J Obstet Gynaecol 27:92, 1987.
295. Fiellin D, Reid M, O'Connor P: Screening for alcohol problems in primary care: A systematic review. Arch Intern Med 160:1977, 2000.
296. Minkoff H, McCalla S, Delke I, et al: The relationship of cocaine use to syphilis and human immunodeficiency virus infections among inner city parturient women. Am J Obstet Gynecol 163:521, 1990.
297. Jansson LM, Svikis D, Lee J, et al: Pregnancy and addiction. A comprehensive care model. J Subst Abuse Treat 13:321, 1996.
298. Chang G, Carroll K, Behr H, et al: Improved perinatal outcome after enhanced prenatal care for opiate addicts. Am J Gynecol 166:311, 1992.
299. Day N, Jasperse D, Richardson G, et al: Prenatal exposure to alcohol. Effect on infant growth and morphologic characteristics. Pediatrics 84:536, 1989.

300. Ebrahim S, Luman E, Floyd R, et al: Alcohol consumption by pregnant women in the United States during 1988–1995. Obstet Gynecol 92:187, 1998.
301. Stratton K, Howe C, Battaglia F (eds): Institute of Medicine Summary. Fetal Alcohol Syndrome. Washington, DC, National Academy Press, 1996.
302. Windham G, Von Behren J, Fenster L, et al: Moderate maternal alcohol consumption and the risk of spontanious abortion. Epidemiology 8:5009, 1997.
303. Kesmodel U, Wisborg K, Olsen S, et al: Moderate alcohol intake during pregancy and the risk of stillbirth and death in the first year of life. Am J Epidemiol 155:305, 2002.
304. Lundberg L, Bracken M, Saftlas A: Low-to-moderate gestational alcohol use and intrauterine growth retardation, low birthweight, and preterm delivery. Ann Epidemiol 7:498, 1997.
305. Passaro K, Little R, Savitz D, et al: The effect of maternal drinking before conception and in early pregnancy on infant birthweight. The ALSPAC Study Team. Avon Longitudinal Study of Pregnancy and Childhood. Epidemiology 7:377, 1996.
306. Abel E, Sokol R: Incidence of fetal alcohol syndrome and economic impact of FAS-related anomalies. Drug Alcohol Depend 19:51, 1987.
307. Bailey B, Delaney-Black V, Covington C, Sokol R: Prenatal exposure to binge drinking and cognitive and behavioral outcomes at age 7 years. Am J Obstet Gynecol 191:1037, 2004.
308. Jacobson S, Jacobson J, Sokol RJ: Effects of fetal alcohol exposure in infant reaction time. Alcohol Clin Exp Res 18:1125, 1994.
309. Streissguth A, Barr H, Martin D: Alcohol exposure in utero and functional deficits in children during the first four years of life. In O'Connor M (ed): Mechanisms of Alcohol Damage in Utero. London, Pittman: Ciba Foundation Symposium 105; 1984, p 176.
310. O'Connor T, Heron J, Glover V, et al: Antenatal anxiety predicts child behavior/emotional problems independently of postnatal depression. J Am Acad Child Adolesc Psychiatry 41:1470, 2002.
311. Streissguth A, Bookstein F, Sampson P, Barr H: Neurobehavioral effects of prenatal alcohol, III: PLS analyses of neuropsychologic tests. Neurotoxicol Teratol 11:493, 1989.
312. Streissguth AP, Barr HM, Sampson PD: Moderate prenatal alcohol exposure: effects on child IQ and learning problems at age 7 1/2 years. Alcohol Clin Exp Res 14:662, 1990.
313. Sampson P, Streissguth A, Bookstein F, et al: Incidence of fetal alcohol syndrome and prevalence of alcohol-related neurodevelopment disorder. Teratology 56:317, 1997.
314. Jones K, Smith D: Recognition of the fetal alcohol syndrome in early infancy. Lancet 2:989, 1973.
315. Stromland K: Ocular involvement in the fetal alcohol syndrome. Surv Ophthalmol 31:277, 1987.
316. Streissguth A, Clarren S, Jones K: Natural history of the fetal alcohol syndrome: A 10-year follow-up of 11 patients. Lancet 2:85, 1985.
317. Bearer C: Markers to detect drinking during pregnancy. Alcohol Res Health 25:210, 2001.
318. Chang G: Alcohol-screening instruments for pregnant women. Alcohol Res Health 25:204, 2001.
319. Sokol R, Martier S, Ager J: The T-ACE questions: Practical prenatal detection of risk-drinking. Am J Obstet Gynecol 160:863, 1989.
320. Miller L, Raskin V: Pharmacological therapies in pregnant women with drug and alcohol addictions. *In* Miller N, Gold M (eds): Pharmacological Therapies for Drug and Alcohol Addictions. New York, Marcel Dekker, 1995, p 265.
321. Nora A, Nora J, Blue J: Limb reduction abnormalities in infants born to disulfiram treated alcoholic mothers. Lancet 2:664, 1977.
322. Klesges L, Johnson K, Ward K, Barnard M: Smoking cessationin pregnant women. Obstet Gynecol 28:269, 2001.
323. McDonald A, Armstrong B, Sloan M: Cigarette, alcohol, and coffee consumption and congenital defects. Am J Public Health 82:91, 1992.
324. Shiono P, Klebanoff M, Berendes H: Congenital malformations and maternal smoking during pregnancy. Teratology 34:65, 1986.
325. Kline J, Stein Z, Susser M, Warburton D: Smoking: A risk factor for spontaneous abortion. N Engl J Med 297:793, 1977.
326. Ness R, Grisso J, Hirschinger N, et al: Cocaine and tobacco use and the risk of spontaneous abortion. N Engl J Med 340:333, 1999.
327. Cnattingius S, Haglund B, Meirik O: Cigarette smoking as a risk factor for late fetal and early neonatal death. BMJ 297:258, 1988.
328. Wisborg K, Henriksen T, Hedegaard M, Secher N: Smoking during pregnancy and preterm birth. Br J Obstet Gynecol 103:800, 1996.
329. Conde-Agudelo A, Althabe F, Belizan J, Kafury-Goeta A: Cigarette smoking during pregnancy and risk of pre-ecalmpsia: A systematic review. Am J Obstet Gynecol 181:1026, 1999.
330. Fergusson D, Horwood L, Shannon F: Smoking during pregnancy. N Z Med J 89:41, 1979.
331. Fried P, Makin J: Neonatal behavioral correlates of prenatal exposure to marijuana, cigarettes, and alcohol in a low risk population. Neurotoxicol Teratol 9:1, 1987.
332. Picone T, Allen L, Olsen P, Ferris M: Pregnancy outcome in North American women: II. Effects of diet, cigarette smoking, stress and weight gain on placentas, and on neonatal physical and behavioral characteristics. Am J Clin Nutr 36:1214, 1982.
333. Wisborg K, Kesmodel U, Henriksen T, et al: A prospective study of smoking during pregnancy and SIDS. Arch Dis Child 83:203, 2000.
334. Mortensen E, Michaelsen F, Sanders S, Reinisch M: A dose-response relationship between maternal smoking during late pregnancy and adult intelligence in male offspring. Paediatr Perinat Epidemiol 19:4, 2005.
335. Skorge D, Eagan T, Eide G, et al: The adult incidence of asthma and respiratory symptoms by passive smoking in utero or in childhood. Am J Resp Crit Care Med 172:61, 2005.
336. Sit D, Wisner K: Smoking cessation in pregnancy [Letter]. Arch Women's Ment Health 7:211, 2004.
337. Wisborg K, Henriksen T, Jespersen L, Secher N: Nicotine patches for pregnant smokers: A randomized controlled study. Obstet Gynecol 96:967, 2000.
338. Dempsey D, Benowitz N: Risks and benefits of nicotine to aid smoking cessation during pregnancy. Drug Saf 24:277, 2001.
339. Chun-Fai-Chan B, Koren G, Fayez I, et al: Pregnancy outcome of women exposed to bupropion during pregnancy: A prospective comparative study. Am J Obstetr Gynecol 192:932, 2005.
340. Baab S, Peindl K, Piontek C, Wisner K: Serum bupropion levels in two breastfeeding mother-infant pairs. J Clin Psychiatry 63:910, 2002.
341. American Academy of Pediatrics Committee on Drugs: The transfer of drugs and other chemicals into human milk. Pediatrics 108:776, 2001.
342. Gartner L, Morton J, Lawrence RA, et al: Breastfeeding and the use of human milk. Pediatrics 115:496, 2005.
343. Addis A, Moretti M, Ahmed SF, et al: Fetal effects of cocaine: An updated meta-analysis. Reprod Toxicol 15:341, 2001.
344. Behnke M, Eyler F, Garvan C, Wobie K: The search for congenital malformations in newborns with fetal cocaine exposure. Pediatrics 107:E74, 2001.
345. Hulse GK, Milne E, English DR, Holman CD: Assessing the relationship between maternal cocaine use and abruptio placentae. Addiction 92:1547, 1997.
346. Frank D, Augustyn M, Grant-Knight W, et al: Growth, development, and behavior in early childhood following cocaine exposure. JAMA 285:1613, 2001.
347. Frank D, Rose-Jacobs R, Beeghly M, et al: Level of prenatal cocaine exposure and 48-month IQ: Importance of preschool enrichment. Neurotoxicol Teratol 27:15, 2005.
348. Singer L, Yamashita T, Hawkins S, et al: Increased incidence of intraventricular hemorrhage and developmental delay in cocaine-exposed, very low birth weight infants. J Pediatr 124:731, 1994.
349. Kline J, Hutzler M, Levin B, et al: Marijuana and spontaneous abortion of known karyotype. Paediatr Perinat Epidemiol 5:320, 1991.
350. Tennes K, Avitable N, Blackard C, et al: Marijuana: Prenatal and postnatal exposure in the human. *In* Pinkert T (ed): Consequences of Maternal Drug Abuse: NIDA Research Monograph 59. Rockville, MD, Department of Health and Human Services, Publication No. 85–1400, 1985, p 48.

351. Lester B, Dreher M: Effects of marijuana use during pregnancy on newborn crying. Child Dev 60:764, 1989.

352. Fried P: Behavioral outcomes in preschool-aged children exposed prenatally to marijuana: A review and speculative interpretation. *In* Wetherington C, Smeriglio C, Finnegan L (eds): Behavioral Studies Of Drug Exposed Offspring: Methodological Issues In Human And Animal Research. NIDA Reserach Monograph 164. Washington, DC, US Government Printing Office, 1996, p 242.

353. Grufferman S, Schwartz A, Ruymann F, Mauer H: Parent's use of cocaine and marijuana and increased risk of rhabdomyosarcoma in their children. Cancer Causes Control 4:217, 1993.

354. Robison LL, Buckley JD, Daigle AE, et al: Maternal drug use and risk of childhood nonlymphoblastic leukemia among offspring. An epidemiologic investigation implicating marijuana (a report from the Childrens Cancer Study Group). Cancer 63:1904, 1989.

355. Hall W, MacPhee D: Cannabis use and cancer. Addiction 97:243, 2002.

356. Astley S, Little S: Maternal marijuana use during lactation and infant development at one year. Am J Epidemiol 130:804, 1989.

356a. [illegible] M: NHIS Fact Sheet. Hyattsville, MD, National Center for Health Statistics, 1999.

356b. Lester BM, Elshohly M, Wright LL, et al: The maternal lifestyle study: Drug use by meconium toxicology report. Pediatrics 170: 309, 2001.

357. Alford D, Compton P, Samet J: Acute pain management for patients recieving maintenance methadone or buprenorphine therapy. Ann Intern Med 144:127, 2006.

357a. Hulse GK, Milne E, English DR, Holman CD: Assessing the relationship between maternal opiate use and neonatal mortality. Addiction 93:1033, 1998.

358. Hulse GK, Milne E, English DR, Holman CD: The relationship between maternal use of heroin and methadone and infant birth weight. Addiction 92:1571, 1997.

359. Anonymous: National Consensus Development Panel on effective medical treatment of opiate addiction. JAMA 280:1936, 1998.

360. Finnegan L: Management of pregnant drug-dependent women. Ann N Y Acad Sci 311:146, 1978.

361. Hans S: Developmental consequences of prenatal exposure to methadone. Ann N Y Med Sci 562:195, 1989.

362. Jha R, Carrick P, Pairaudeau P, et al: Maternal opiate use: Pregnancy outcome in patients managed by a multidisiplinary approach. J Obstet Gynecol 17:331, 1997.

363. Kunins V, Shapira S, Juliana P, Gourevitch M: Dose changes during pregnancy: Evolving practice in methadone maintenance across two decades. 129th Annual Meeting of the American Public Health Association, Abstract #[illegible]. October [illegible], 2001 2001.

364. Kuschel C, Austerberry L, Cornwell M, et al: Can methadone concentrations predict the severity of withdrawal in infants at risk of neonatal abstinence syndrome? Arch Dis Child Fetal Neonatal Ed 89:F390, 2004.

365. Jansson L, DiPietro J, Elko A: Fetal response to maternal methadone administration. Am J Obstet Gynecol 193:611, 2005.

366. Wouldes T, Roberts A, Pryor J, et al: The effect of methadone treatment on the quantity and quality of human fetal movement. Neurotoxicol Teratol 26:23, 2004.

367. van Baar A, Fleury P, Soepatmi S, et al: Neonatal behavior after drug dependent pregnancy. Arch Dis Child 64:235, 1989.

368. Finnegan L, Kron R, Connaughton J, Emich J: A scoring system for evaluation and treatment of the neonatal abstinence syndrome. A new clinical tool. *In* Marcelli P, Garatlini S, Sereni F (eds): Basic and Therapeutic Aspects of Perinatal Pharmacology. New York, Raven Press, 1975.

369. Finnegan L: Neonatal abstinence. *In* Nelson N (ed): Current Therapy in Neonatal-Perinatal Medicine. Philadelphia, BC Decker, Inc., 1990, p 314.

370. Doberzak T, Kandall S, Friedman P: Relationships between maternal methadone dosage, maternal-neonatal methadone levels, and neonatal withdrawal. Obstet Gynecol 81:936, 1993.

371. Malpas T, Darlow B, Lennox R, Horwood L: Maternal methadone dosage and neonatal withdrawal. Aust NZ J Obstet Gynaecol 35:175, 1995.

372. Choo R, Heustis M, Schroeder J, et al: Neonatal abstinence syndrome in methadone-exposed infants is alterned by level of prenatal tobacco exposure. Drug Alcohol Depend 75:253, 2004.

373. Bogen D, Hanusa B, Barnhart W, Wisner K: Prenatal outcomes of methadone vs heroin exposed mother-infant dyads. Paper presented at: 2nd Annual Interdisciplinary Women's Health Research Symposium, 2005, Bethesda, MD.

374. McCarthy J, Leamon M, Parr M, Anania B: High-dose methadone maintenance in pregnancy: Maternal and neonatal outcomes. Am J Obstet Gynecol 193:606, 2005.

375. Luty J, Nikolaou V, Beran J: Is opiate detoxification unsafe in pregnancy? J Subst Abuse Treat 24:363, 2003.

376. Dashe J, Jackson G, Olscher D, et al: Opioid detoxification in pregnancy. Obstet Gynecol 92:854, 1998.

377. Jones H, Johnson R, Jasinski D, et al: Buprenorphine versus methadone in the treatment of pregnant opioid-dependent patients: Effects on the neonatal abstinence syndrome. Drug Alcohol Depend 79:1, 2005.

378. Phillip B, Merewood A, O'Brien S: Methadone and breastfeeding: New Horizons. Pediatrics 111:1429, 2003.

379. Begg E, Malpas T, Hackett LP, Ilett KF: Distribution of R- and S-methadone into human milk during multiple, medium to high oral dosing. Br J [illegible] 52:681, 2001.

380. Holland J: Shortened length of stay for neonatal abstinence syndrome. Paper presented at: Academy of Breastfeeding Medicine Annual Meeting; November, 2001, Washington, DC.

381. Malpas T, Darlow B: Neonatal abstinence syndrome following abrupt cessation of breastfeeding. N Z Med J 112:12, 1999.

382. LaGasse L, Messinger D, Lester B, et al: Prenatal drug exposure and maternal and infant feeding behaviour. Arch Dis Child Fetal Neonat Ed 88:F391, 2003.

383. Gewolb I, Fishman D, Qureshi M, Vice F: Coordination of suck-swallow-respiration in infants born to mothers with drug-abuse problems. Dev Med Child Neurol 46:700, 2004.

384. Gibson E, Evans R, Finnegan L, Spitzer A. Increased incidence of apnea in infants born to both cocaine and opiate addicted mothers. Pediatr Res 27:10A, 1990.

385. Groves J: Taking care of the hateful patient. N Engl J Med 289:883, 1978.

386. Crutcher J, Bass M: The difficult patient and the troubled physician. J Fam Pract 11:933, 1980.

387. Emerson J, Pankratz L, Joos S, Smith S: Personality disorders in problematic medical patients. Psychosomatics 35:469, 1994.

388. Trimpey M, Davidson S: Nursing care of personality disorders int he medical surgical settinhg. Nurs Clin N Am 33:173, 1998.

389. Paris J, Brown R, Nowlis D: Long term follow-up of borderline patients in a general hospital. Compr Psychiatry 28:530, 1987.

390. Shea M, Pilkonis P, Bechkham E, et al: Personality disorders and treatment outcome in the NIMH Treatment of Depression Collaborative Research Program. Am J Psychiatry 147:711, 1990.

391. Smith T, Benjamin L: The functional impairment associated with personality disorders. Curr Opin Psychiatry 15:135, 2002.

392. Dobbels F, Put D, Vanhaecke J: Personality disorders: A challenge for transplantation. Prog Transplant 10:226, 2000.

393. Hueston W, Werth J, Mainous AI: Personality disorder traits: Prevalence and effects on health status in primary care patients. Int J Psychiatry Med 29:63, 1999.

394. Rendu A, Moran P, Patel A, et al: Economic impact of personality disorders in UK primary care attenders. Br J Psychiatry 181:62, 2002.

395. Monti D, Herring C, Schwartzman R, et al: Personality assessment of patients with complex regional pain syndrome type I. Clin J Pain 14:295, 1998.

396. Polatin P, Kinney R, Gatchel R, et al: Psychiatric illness and chronic low-back pain. Spine 18:66, 1993.

397. Reich J, Tupin J, Abramowitz S: Psychiatric diagnosis of chronic pain patients. Am J Psychiatry 140:1495, 1983.

398. Epstein S, Kay G, Clauw D, et al: Psychiatric disorders in patients with fibromyalgia. Psychosomatics 40:57, 1999.

399. De Gucht V, Fischler B, Heiser W: Personality and affect as determinants of medically unexplained symptoms in primary care: A follow-up study. J Psychosomatic Res 56:279, 2004.

400. Katon W, Walker E: Medically unexplained symptoms in primary care. J Clin Psychiatry 59.15, 1998.

401. Lipsitt D: Medical and psychological characteristics of "crocks." Int J Psychiatry Med 1:15, 1970.
402. Leiderman D, Grisso J: The gomer phenomenon. J Health Soc Behav 26:222, 1985.
403. Koerner K, Dimeff D: Further data on dialectical behavior therapy. J Clin Psychol 7:104, 2002.
404. Gross R, Olfson M, Gameroff M, et al: Borderline personality disorder in primary care. Arch Intern Med 162:53, 2002.
405. Sparr L, Boehnlein J, Cooney T: The medical management of the paranoid patient. Gen Hosp Psychiatry 8:49, 1986.
406. Linehan M: Validation in psychotherapy. *In* Bohart A, Greenberg L (eds): Empathy Reconsidered: New Directions. Washington, DC, American Psychological Association, 1997, p 353.
407. Gorman M: Culture clash: Working with a difficult patient. Am J Nurs 96:58, 1996.
408. Chaudron L, Caine E: Suicide among women: A critical review. J Am Womens Assoc 59:125, 2004.
409. Appleby L, Mortensen P, Faragher E: Suicide and other causes of mortality after postpartum psychiatric admission. Br J Psychiatry 173:209, 1998.
410. American Psychiatric Association: Practice guideline for the assessment and treatment of patients with suicidal behavior. Am J Psychiatry 160(Suppl):1, 2003.
411 Association Psychiatric Assciation: Practice guidelines for the treament of psychiatric disorders. Washington, DC, America Psyciatric Press, 2000.
412. Greenhouse J, Kelleher K: Thinking outside the (black) box: Antidepressants, suicidality, and research synthesis. Pediatrics 116:231, 2005.
413. Gibbons R, Hur K, Bhaumik D, Mann J: The relationship between antidepressant medication use and rate of suicide. Arch Gen Psychiatry 62:165, 2005.
414. Resnick P: Murder of a newborn: A psychiatric review of neonaticide. Am J Psychiatry 126:1414, 1970.
415. Oberman M: A brief history of infanticide and the law. *In* Spinelli M (ed): Infanticide: Psychosocial and Legal Perspectives on Mothers Who Kill. Washington, DC, American Psychiatric Publishing, Inc., 2003, p 3.
416. Meade J, Brissie R: Infanticide by starvation: Calculation of caloric deficit to determine degree of deprivation. J Forens Sci 30:1263, 1985.
417. Rutter M, Quinton D: Parental psychiatric disorder: effects on children. Psychol Med 14:853, 1984.
418. McFarlane J: Criminal defense in cases of infanticide and neonaticide. *In* Spinelli M (ed): Infanticide: Psychosocial and Legal Perspectives on Mothers Who Kill. Washington, DC, American Psychiatric Publishing, Inc., 2003, p 133.
419. Kendell R, Chalmers J, Platz C: Epidemiology of puerperal psychoses. Br J Psychiatry 50:662, 1987.
420. Wisner K, Gracious B, Piontek C, et al: Postpartum disorders: Phenomenology, treatment approaches, and relationship to infanticide. *In* Spinelli M (ed): Psychosocial and Legal Perspectives on Mothers Who Kill. London, American Psychiatric Publishing, Inc., 2003, p 35.
420a. Wisner KL, Chambers CH, Sit DK: A major public health problem in search of a definition: Postpartum depression. JAMA 296:2616, 2006.
421. Resnick P: Child murder by parents: A psychiatric review of filicide. Am J Psychiatry 126:325, 1969.
422. Wisner K, Peindl K, Hanusa B: Symptomatology of affective and psychotic illnesses related to childbearing. J Affect Disord 30:77, 1994.
423. Wisner K, Peindl K, Hanusa B: Psychiatric episodes in women with young children. J Affect Disord 34:1, 1995.
424. Wisner K, Perel J, Wheeler S: Tricyclic dose requirements across pregnancy. Am J Psychiatry 150:1541, 1993.
425. Wisner K, Peindl K, Hanusa B: Effects of childbearing on the natural history of panic disorder with comorbid mood disorder. J Affect Dis 41:173, 1996.
426. Spinelli M: A systematic investigation of 16 cases of neonaticide. Am J Psychiatry 158:811, 2001.
427. Spinelli M: Neonaticide: A systematic investigation of 17 cases. *In* Spinelli M (ed): Infanticide: Psychosocial and Legal Perspectives on Mothers Who Kill. Washington, DC, American Psychiatric Publishing, Inc., 2003, p 105.
428. Miller L: Denial of pregnancy. *In* Spinelli M (ed): Infanticide: Psychosocial and Legal Perspectives on Mothers Who Kill. Washington, DC, American Psychiatric Publishing, Inc., 2003, p 3.
429. Guedes D, Young R: A case of pseudo-pregnancy in captive brown howler monkeys *(Alouatta guariba)*. Folia Primeatologica 75:335, 2004.
430. Bianchi-Demicheli F, Ludicke F, Chardonnens D: Imaginary pregnancy 10 years after abortion and sterilization in menopausal women: A case report. Maturitas 48:479, 2004.
431. Shiwach R, Dudley A: Delusional pregnancy with polydipsia: A case report. J Psychosom Res 42:477, 1997.

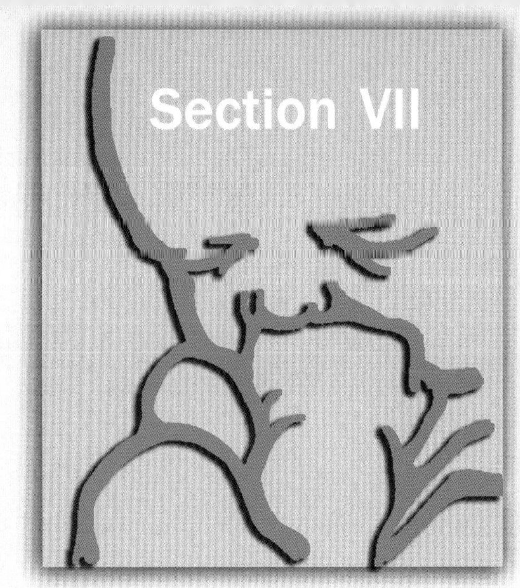

Legal and Ethical Issues in Perinatology

Legal and Ethical Issues in Obstetric Practice

GEORGE J. ANNAS AND SHERMAN ELIAS

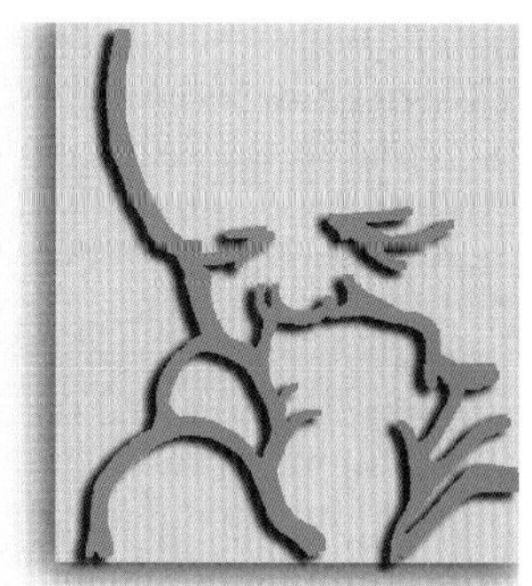

CHAPTER 51

KEY ABBREVIATIONS

American Medical Association	AMA
American College of Obstetricians and Gynecologists	ACOG
Institutional review board	IRB
U.S. Department of Health and Human Services	HHS

Society has great expectations that modern medical technologies will improve longevity and quality of human life, and nowhere are these expectations higher than in the practice of obstetrics and the desire and expectation of having a healthy child. Along with the rapidly expanding capabilities in diagnosis and treatment, physicians find themselves facing numerous ethical dilemmas while practicing in a medicolegal climate in which malpractice suits can threaten even the most competent and conscientious practitioner.

We cannot address in a single chapter the seemingly infinite ethical and legal controversies facing contemporary obstetric practice and research. Instead, we focus on several topics of particular relevance to the practicing obstetrician. We begin with abortion because the continuing debate over abortion affects all the other areas.

ABORTION*

The political debate over abortion during the past 3 decades has shifted among various dichotomous views: life versus choice, fetus versus woman, fetus versus baby, constitutional right versus states' rights, government versus physician, and physician and patient versus state legislature. Hundreds of statutes and almost two dozen Supreme Court decisions on abortion later, the core aspects of *Roe v. Wade,*[1] the most controversial health-related decision by the Court ever, remain substantially the same as they were in 1973. Attempts to overturn *Roe* in both the courtroom and the Congress have failed. Pregnant women still have a constitutional right to abortion. The fetus is still not a person under the Constitution. States still cannot make abortion a crime (either for the woman or the physician) before the fetus becomes viable. States still can outlaw abortion after the fetus becomes viable only if there is an exception that permits abortion to protect the life or health of the pregnant woman. And states still can impose restrictions on abortion before fetal viability only if those restrictions do not create a substantial obstacle to pregnancy termination.

Political tactics have shifted from the use of antiabortion rhetoric to legal activism to the use of legislative and judicial forums to change the status of abortion. The hope seems to be that more heated rhetoric will help turn the public and physicians against abortion itself, regardless of its constitutionally protected status.

Roe and Casey

More than 30 years ago, in *Roe v. Wade,* the Supreme Court held that women have a constitutional right of privacy that is "fundamental" and "broad enough to encompass a woman's decision . . . to terminate her pregnancy."[2] If a right is fundamental, the state must demonstrate a "compelling state interest" to restrict it. The Court determined that the state's interest in the life of the fetus becomes compelling only at the point of "viability," defined as the point at which the fetus can survive independent of its mother. Even after viability, the state cannot favor the life of the fetus over the life or health of the pregnant woman: physicians must be able to use their "medical judgment for the preservation of the life or health of the mother." *Roe*'s companion case,

*This section is adapted from Annas,[2] with permission.

Doe v. Bolton, specifically included mental health in this determination, saying, "The medical judgment may be exercised in the light of all factors—physical, emotional, psychological, familial, and the woman's age—relevant to the well-being of the patient. All of these factors may relate to health. This allows the attending physician the room he needs to make his best medical judgment."

When the Court heard *Planned Parenthood v. Casey*[3] in 1992, most commentators assumed that there were more than enough votes to overturn *Roe.* Instead, three seemingly anti-*Roe* Justices together wrote a joint opinion that although describing the abortion right as a liberty right (instead of a privacy right) and prohibiting the state from unduly burdening it before viability (instead of requiring the state to demonstrate a "compelling interest" in regulating abortion) nonetheless confirmed the "core holding" of *Roe:* that states could not outlaw abortion before the fetus becomes viable and could do so thereafter only when the life or health of the woman was not threatened by continuing the pregnancy.[4] Twenty-four–hour waiting periods were approved; spousal notification was ruled unconstitutional. With the loss of all hope that the Court would ever overturn *Roe,* antiabortion advocates needed a new approach to keep the abortion debate alive. They found it in so-called partial-birth abortions.

Partial-Birth Abortion in Congress

In June 1995, the first Partial-Birth Abortion Ban Bill was introduced in Congress to make it a federal crime to perform "an abortion in which the person performing the abortion partially vaginally delivers a living fetus before killing the fetus and completing the delivery." In March 1996, the House passed a revised Senate version, which provided in part:

(a) Whoever, in or affecting interstate or foreign commerce, knowingly performs a partial-birth abortion and thereby kills a human fetus shall be fined under this title or imprisoned not more than two years or both.

(b) . . . the term partial-birth abortion means an abortion in which the person performing the abortion partially vaginally delivers a living fetus before killing the fetus and completing the delivery . . . it is an affirmative defense . . . that the partial-birth abortion was performed by a physician who reasonably believed (1) the partial-birth abortion was necessary to save the life of the mother; and (2) no other procedure would suffice for that purpose.[5]

In April 1996, President Bill Clinton vetoed the bill at a White House press conference at which five women described how they made the decision to terminate their pregnancies with what could be considered a partial-birth abortion under the proposed law. He said that the debate was "not about the prochoice/prolife debate" but about the tragic circumstances of "a few hundred Americans every year who desperately want their children." The President said that he would sign a bill that was consistent with *Roe v. Wade.* In the President's words, "I will accept language that says serious, adverse health consequences to the mother [provide an exception]."[6]

When the Senate voted in September 1996 to sustain the President's veto, the leader of the fight to override it was Senator Rick Santorum (R-Pa.), who was challenged as having no personal experience or expertise in this area. A week after the vote, Santorum had his own story to tell.[7] The Senator's wife had been pregnant with their fourth child when they were informed that ultrasonography showed that their child had a "fatal defect," which turned out to be complete urinary tract obstruction. They were given three options; have an abortion, do nothing, or choose in utero surgery to insert a shunt. They chose the shunt procedure, which was successfully performed at 20 weeks' gestation. The procedure resulted in infection that put Karen Santorum in serious danger. An abortion would have removed the source of her infection, but she refused. Instead, she went into labor and gave birth to an extremely premature infant, Gabriel. Two hours later he died in his parents' arms.

To some, this personal experience makes Santorum a more credible antiabortion advocate. But his experience also illustrates at least two major problems with the legislation he supports. First, his wife's actions can be considered praiseworthy only because she had a choice that is protected by current law. Second, the distinction between premature delivery and abortion on the edges of viability has always been problematic. Santorum, for example, has been quoted as having said, in relation to this experience, that even when the life of the mother is at stake, and "you have to end a pregnancy early . . . that does not necessarily mean having an abortion. You can induce labor, using a drug like Pitocin [oxytocin]."[8] If one accepts the standard medical definition of abortion (termination of a pregnancy when the fetus is not viable), this is a distinction without a difference. Whether a planned abortion is performed or labor is induced, both are intended to terminate a nonviable pregnancy. The real issue is not the method used to terminate the pregnancy, but the justification for terminating it. It is also reasonable to argue that after a fetus is viable, abortion is simply no longer possible by definition; the only option is premature delivery.

What makes the term "partial-birth abortion" so politically powerful is its inaccurate conflation of two polar-opposite results of pregnancy, birth and abortion. Senator Daniel Patrick Moynihan (D-N.Y.) has, for example, described it as "as close to infanticide as anything I have ever come upon."[9] But close is not identical. When Virginia attorney general Mark Earley describes the procedure as a "disturbing form of infanticide,"[10] he is making a legally inaccurate political statement. An almost-born child is not yet born, and is not a person under the Constitution. And, as the Supreme Court has repeatedly held, if the viable fetus is killed for the sake of the woman's life or health, the act is not infanticide by definition.

Medical Practice and Medical Politics

In January 1997, Santorum reintroduced the Partial-Birth Abortion Ban Act in the Senate. Approximately 1 month later, the executive director of the National

Coalition of Abortion Providers told reporters that he had lied in 1995 when he claimed that partial-birth abortions were rare and were performed only in extreme situations; instead, he said that "thousands" were performed annually, and most "on healthy fetuses and healthy mothers."[11] The total number of abortions performed in the United States has been steadily declining, although there are no accurate statistics on the frequency of partial-birth abortions. There were two important differences in Congress this time around: medical organizations took conflicting positions, and substantial compromises were attempted in the Senate. The first time around, the American Medical Association (AMA) had taken no position, and the American College of Obstetricians and Gynecologists (ACOG) had urged the President to veto the bill.

In January 1997, ACOG's Executive Board issued its first and only statement on "intact dilatation and extraction." The Board wrote that it understood that the bill attempted to outlaw a procedure containing all of the following elements:

1. Deliberate dilatation of the cervix, usually over a sequence of days;
2. Instrumental conversion of the fetus to a footling breech;
3. Breech extraction of the body excepting the head; and
4. Partial evacuation of the intracranial contents of the living fetus to effect vaginal delivery of a dead but otherwise intact fetus.[12]

The Board described this as "one method of terminating a pregnancy" after 16 weeks. The Board noted that it was sometimes used to save the life or health of the mother, but that its "select panel . . . could identify no circumstances under which this procedure would be the only option to save the life or preserve the health of the woman . . . [although it] may be the best or most appropriate procedure." The Board's primary point was that only the woman's physician should make the decision about what particular procedure to use in individual circumstances, and that therefore "the intervention of legislative bodies into medical decision making is inappropriate, ill advised, and dangerous."

The AMA took a different position. On the eve of the Senate vote in May 1997, the AMA's Board of Trustees agreed to support the legislation if Santorum added two physician-friendly procedural amendments.[13] These were a requirement that the physician's action be "deliberate and intentional," and a procedure to involve the state Medical Board in the trial of an accused physician. State bans on partial-birth abortion are based on the inherent police power that states have to protect the health and safety of the public. The federal government has no such power; the federal bill is instead based on the power of Congress to regulate interstate commerce. Because the AMA endorsed the federal bill, it implicitly agreed that what physicians do with individual patients in their offices is a matter of interstate commerce, and therefore, subject to regulation by the federal government. This is a stunning concession.

Attempts to reach a real compromise that could have resulted in a bill that President Clinton could sign, and that would probably have been upheld by the courts as constitutional, were made primarily by Senator Dianne Feinstein (D-Calif.), Senator Barbara Boxer (D-Calif.), and Senator Thomas Daschle (D-S.D.). The Feinstein-Boxer amendment would have dealt specifically with the problem the President had with the original bill by adding "serious adverse health consequences to the woman" as an additional exception to the prohibition. Daschle offered to ban all abortions, by any technique, after viability. The only exception would be to save the life of the pregnant woman or to protect her from "grievous injury" to her physical health, defined as "a severely debilitating disease or impairment specifically caused by the pregnancy, or an inability to provide necessary treatment for a life-threatening condition."[14]

Daschle's bill defined the realm of the debate as the period after viability (roughly the third trimester) but nonetheless attempted to limit the reach of *Roe v. Wade* by restricting the exception regarding the health of the pregnant woman to physical (not mental) health and to the risk of "grievous" harm [illegible] ACOG endorsed the Daschle compromise but, in doing so, seemed to put politics over loyalty to patients, because the Daschle proposal limited the ability of a physician to act to protect the health of a patient after the fetus becomes viable.

In May 1997, the Senate adopted the Santorum bill by a vote of 64 to 36, and in October 1997, it was passed by the House and sent to the President. Two days later, President Clinton again vetoed the bill. He issued a three-paragraph message to the House of Representatives, in which he said he was vetoing the bill "for exactly the same reasons I returned an earlier substantially identical version . . . last year"—that is, because of its failure to include an exception for abortion to prevent "serious harm" to a woman's health.

In 2000, in *Stenberg v. Carhart,* the U.S. Supreme Court ruled, 5 to 4, that state laws outlawing "partial-birth abortions," that were worded substantially identical to the laws passed by Congress and vetoed by President Clinton, are unconstitutional.[15] The reasons are two-fold. The first is that the law is unconstitutionally vague because the procedure it purports to outlaw is described in words that could be read to outlaw other abortion procedures that everyone agrees are constitutional. This places physicians in fear of prosecution, and may thus cause them not to perform abortions they otherwise would, putting an "undue burden" on pregnant women wishing to terminate their pregnancies. Second, the act makes no exception for the "health of the woman," and *Roe v. Wade* requires that this exception exist throughout the pregnancy. Ultimately, the central question regarding abortion remains—who should make the decision: the state or women and their physicians together? The answer of the Supreme Court, as articulated in *Roe v. Wade,* and reinforced in *Stenberg,* is that the decision belongs to the woman and her physician together.[16]

Government Regulation of Medical Procedures

Both sides admit that even if the technique of intact dilatation and extraction is outlawed, it is unlikely that even one abortion will be prevented. Thus, perhaps the primary lesson of the past 30 years is that the controversy over abortion in America is not susceptible to political solution. Moreover, because neither Congress nor the states can alter the constitutional law of abortion as set forth in *Roe v. Wade* and *Casey*, if the debate about partial-birth abortion were only a debate about abortion itself, it would be of little practical consequence. The debate, however, exposes other important issues.

The chief issue is the proper role of the government in regulating medical care. Historically, prochoice forces have favored this framing of the abortion debate. When the debate about abortion is argued as a choice between having a woman and her physician make the decision versus having the state legislature or Congress make it, the woman and her physician are the overwhelming choice of Americans. The government-versus-physician framework is also uncomfortable for Republicans, who tend to argue against government interference with private decision making. And even when government regulation seems appropriate, most Republicans prefer regulation by the individual states to regulation by the federal government.

A more focused way to frame the debate is to ask whether decisions about specific medical procedures should be made by physicians or legislators. The AMA's support of the ban on partial-birth abortion seems to be a repudiation of its historic position against government interference in this realm. If the AMA believes that the federal government can outlaw a constitutionally protected procedure performed in the privacy of a physician's office on the basis of the federal government's power to regulate interstate commerce, then the AMA has conceded that the federal government can regulate all medical procedures. On the other hand, the AMA has never had a consistent position on abortion.[17]

The issue of who (the medical profession or the state—or health plans, for that matter) has the authority to determine what is and what is not a legitimate medical procedure has implications for all care provided by physicians, not just for abortions.[18] *Roe v. Wade* and *Casey* both teach that government restrictions on legitimate medical procedures that are used to perform abortions before the fetus is viable are unconstitutional (at least if the use of such procedures does not increase the risks to the woman's health). These cases also teach that the failure to make exceptions to outlawed procedures (so that they can be used to protect the life and health of the pregnant woman) also makes the bills regulating partial-birth abortion unconstitutional as passed.

The failure to allow physicians to protect the woman's health after the fetus becomes viable, the vagueness of the definition of partial-birth abortion, and the application of the ban before fetal viability has resulted in regulations from more than two dozen states being found unconstitutional.[19–24] One U.S. Circuit court, however, did approve the law if it was very narrowly interpreted, although the reasoning of the majority in this 5 to 4 opinion is deeply flawed.[25]

In the only case to reach the Supreme Court before the President's veto in March 1998, the Court refused to hear an appeal of a lower court decision that the Ohio ban on partial-birth abortion was unconstitutional. Three Justices (Clarence Thomas, Antonin Scalia, and William Rehnquist), however, voted to hear the appeal so that the Court could reopen what has become the central issue in the debate: whether the Constitution requires an exception to a ban on abortion after viability that includes the pregnant woman's mental health.[26] Although we can only guess at why none of the other six Justices voted to hear this case (it takes four Justices to agree to hear an appeal to the Court), it would appear that all of them think that a woman's mental health is as protected under the Constitution as her physical health.

President Clinton was thus on strong constitutional grounds when he based his vetoes on the failure of these bills to allow for a physician's action to preserve a pregnant woman's health. ACOG was on strong ground in asserting that the proper person to make a judgment about the health of the woman is the physician (acting, of course, in partnership with the woman). As the Court put it in *Roe v. Wade*, this "decision vindicates the right of the physician to administer medical treatment according to his professional judgment." This means that if intact dilatation and extraction is a legitimate medical procedure, it is constitutionally protected under *Roe v. Wade*. If, however, it is not such a procedure, but rather in the category of nonmedical interventions, like female genital mutilation[27] and execution by lethal injection, it has (and deserves) no such protection. Therefore, another way to frame the debate about abortion is to ask who should have the authority to determine which procedures are legitimate medical procedures.

Efforts to reframe the abortion debate have always involved a dichotomy that allows us to ignore or marginalize either women or fetuses by asking us to avert our attention from abortion itself and concentrate on something else. Often, this something else is the physician and the relation of medicine to government. At other times, it is (appropriately, we think) the pregnant woman and her life and health. Pregnancy is a unique human condition; there is nothing else like it in medicine or life, and we must therefore deal with it on its own terms and not by analogy. To do so is simply impossible in the political arena.

Professional organizations should set and follow the terms of their own specialties, and in this area, ACOG is the proper body to make this determination. When professional organizations like the AMA determine the content and scope of reasonable medical practice not on the basis of their professional skills and the health interests of their patients, but rather on the basis of their reading of the prevailing political winds, they undermine their own credibility and explicitly agree that standards for medical practice should be set by politicians rather than by the medical profession.

The appointment of two new Justices to the U.S. Supreme Court could move the Court to permit states to place additional limitations on abortion, even to permitting the federal government to outlaw so-called partial-birth abortions. This would, we believe, be undesirable not only as a matter of constitutional law—which protects not only individual women patients, but the doctor-patient relationship itself—but also as a matter of medical practice: medical standards should not be set by Congress.

GENETIC COUNSELING, SCREENING, AND PRENATAL DIAGNOSIS

Any woman who seeks prenatal care from her obstetrician should have the right to have the physician fully inform her of any reason the physician has to believe that her fetus might have a disability and to inform her further of the existence of diagnostic tests that might identify the precise genetic condition. The physician incurs this duty to disclose because it is this type of information that enables the pregnant woman to have a healthy child. Therefore, it is entirely reasonable for the pregnant woman to expect her physician to apprise her of any relevant information regarding her fetus as well as options she might have.[28]

A wrongful birth suit must allege and prove not only that the physician was negligent in the care of the pregnant woman, but also that had the negligent act not been done the child would not have been born (e.g., had the woman been properly informed that she was at risk to have a child with Down syndrome, she would have sought amniocentesis or chorionic villus sampling and had an abortion if her fetus were so affected). A related but far more controversial lawsuit is brought by the child through its parents or guardian against the physician because it was born, a so-called wrongful life suit. Until recently, most courts rejected lawsuits by the child because they thought it was impossible to put a monetary value on life in an impaired condition compared with nonexistence. The choice for these children is *never* to be born healthy, but only to be born with a disability such as Down syndrome or Tay-Sachs disease or not to be born at all. We think that future courts are likely to limit such actions to *serious* disabilities, those in which fetuses, if they could speak to us, which, of course, they can only do through their parents, would agree with an "objective societal consensus" that their own best interest would be served if they were aborted. Put another way, they would be better off *from their own perspective* if they never existed. Conditions like deafness and Down syndrome would not qualify, whereas conditions like Tay-Sachs would. Measuring damages *is* problematic, but courts are likely to award at least the added medical costs caused by the handicap itself. However, because medical costs can be recovered in a wrongful birth case directly, wrongful life cases are only likely to be brought in those rare instances in which for some reason (e.g., the child has been given up for adoption) the parents have lost the right to sue on their own behalf.[29]

Genetic Counseling and Prenatal Diagnosis

The following conclusions may be drawn regarding the legal and ethical obligations of the obstetrician in relationship to genetic counseling and prenatal diagnosis:

First, the law requires physicians to give accurate information to parents and forbids withholding material information from them. These principles are consistent with the doctrine of informed consent and the reasonable expectations of pregnant women under a physician's care. The physician does not guarantee a healthy child, but the reasonable expectation of the patient is that she will be apprised of any information the physician has that the child might be disabled and of the alternative ways to proceed so that the patient can determine what action to take.[30]

Second, no obstetrician can be required to perform chorionic villus sampling or genetic amniocentesis. Indeed, many are not qualified to perform these procedures and for them to do so may itself be malpractice, as stated by the Judicial Council of the AMA[31]: Physicians who consider the legal and ethical requirements applicable to genetic counseling to be in conflict with their moral values and conscience may choose to limit such services to preconception diagnosis and advice or not provide any genetic services. However, there are circumstances in which the physician who is so disposed is nevertheless obligated to alert prospective parents that a potential genetic problem does exist, that the physician does not offer genetic services, and that the patient should seek medical genetic counseling from another qualified specialist.

Third, genetic counseling should be morally nondirective; that is, the counselor should remain impartial and objective in providing information that will allow competent counselees to make their own informed decision. The Judicial Council of the AMA[31] has given the following opinion: Physicians, whether they oppose or do not oppose contraception, sterilization, or abortion, may decide that they can engage in genetic counseling and screening, but should avoid the imposition of their personal moral values and the substitution of their own moral judgment for that of the prospective parents. The ethical and moral decisions have to be made by the family and should not be imposed by the physician.

Fourth, to ensure the patient's interest in both autonomy and privacy, no information obtained in genetic counseling or screening should be disclosed to any third party, including insurers and employers, without the patient's informed consent.[32,33] Such strict nondisclosure policies should be maintained unless and until specific legislation is enacted that would clearly delineate the circumstance in which confidentiality must be breached, analogous to certain contagious diseases, gunshot wounds, and child abuse. On the other hand, counselors should be permitted to attempt to persuade patients to make disclosures of important information to potentially affected relatives if there is a high probability of serious harm and if the disclosure is limited to pertinent genetic information. We recommend that the genetic counselor make clear, both verbally and in writing, the policy that he or she follows so that the patient can refuse to be screened or counseled if he or she is not in agreement with the disclosure policy. Such agreements serve to heighten the public's confidence in genetic counseling and encourage people to participate voluntarily in both screening and counseling.

Genetic Screening†

Our ability to translate our expanding genetic knowledge into usable information for individual patients is becoming more difficult. Taking a family history and, when indicated, recommending certain tests to identify carriers of genetic diseases are standard in obstetric care (see Chapter 6). Today's screening tests usually focus on conditions that occur either in the family or in the racial or ethnic group of one or both prospective parents. However, as our ability to identify genes associated with particular diseases increases, a panel of screening tests to identify carriers of numerous genes will be offered more routinely. Our challenge will then become to inform those offered screening or testing for reproductive purposes about all the genetic information that can be obtained and the implications of that information.

Consent for Screening

Our current model for screening and testing requires pretest counseling.[35] Such counseling is a method of obtaining informed consent, and the obligation to counsel can be seen as inherent in the fiduciary nature of the doctor-patient relationship.[36,37] For ordinary medical procedures, the physical risks and treatment alternatives are the chief items of information that must be disclosed. There are few physical risks in genetic screening. What must be conveyed in counseling regarding genetic screening is that the tests may yield new information that may ultimately force unwelcome choices such as whether to marry, abort, or adopt. Self-determination and rational decision making are the central values protected by informed consent.[36,37] In the setting of reproductive genetics, what is at stake is the right to decide whether or not to have a genetic test, with emphasis on the right to refuse if the potential harm in terms of stigma or unacceptable choices outweighs, for the individual person or family, the potential benefit.

Generic Consent for Genetic Screening

With the completion of the Human Genome Project, tens if not hundreds of new genetic screening tests may become available in routine clinical practice. Already some researchers have suggested population-based screening to identify carriers of the genes for such conditions as the fragile X syndrome and myotonic dystrophy. Each new screening test presents the same questions: What information should be given to which patients, when should it be presented, who should present it, and how and by whom should the results be conveyed? It will soon be impossible to do meaningful prescreening counseling about all available carrier tests. Giving too much information, "information overload," can amount to misinformation and make the entire counseling process either misleading or meaningless.[38] To prevent disclosure from being pointless or counterproductive, we believe that strategies based on general or "generic" consent should be developed for genetic screening. Their aim would be to provide sufficient information to permit patients to make informed decisions about carrier screening, yet avoid the information overload that could lead to "misinformed" consent.[39]

Traditionally, goals of reproductive genetic counseling, including counseling about screening carrier status, involve helping the person or family to (1) comprehend the medical facts, including the diagnosis, the probable course of the disorder, and the available management; (2) appreciate the way heredity contributes to the disorder, and the risk of recurrence in specified relatives; (3) understand the options for dealing with the risk of recurrence; (4) choose the course of action that seems appropriate to them in view of their risk and their family goal and act in accordance with that decision; and (5) make the best possible adjustment to the disorder in an affected family member or to the risk of recurrence of that disorder.[10] These concepts are addressed in Chapter 6.

For example, in the current context of counseling a couple when at least one is of Italian ancestry, each of these issues would be discussed as it relates specifically to β-thalassemia, with an explanation of hemoglobin electrophoresis as a screening test to determine carrier status. If consideration of another prenatal test were appropriate—for example, maternal screening to detect fetal aneuploidy and neural tube defects—a separate discussion including information on their sensitivity and specificity, and of each of the possible associated fetal disorders would also be required. Even knowledgeable couples could become confused, frustrated, and anxious if faced with scores of options for genetic screening.

In contrast, an approach based on generic consent would emphasize broader concepts and common denominator issues in genetic screening. We envision a situation in which patients would be told of the availability of a panel of screening tests that can be performed on a single blood sample. They would be told that these tests could determine whether they carry genes that put them at increased risk of having a child with a birth defect that could involve serious physical abnormalities, mental disabilities, or both. Several common examples could be given to indicate the frequency and spectrum of severity of each type or category of condition for which screening was being offered. For example, prenatal screening could include tests for structural abnormalities such as neural tube defects and chromosome abnormalities. In the future, fetal blood cells or DNA may be retrieved from maternal blood for both screening and definitive diagnosis.[41]

In the course of counseling, important factors common to all genetic screening tests would be highlighted. Among these are the limitations of screening tests, especially the fact that negative results cannot guarantee a healthy infant; the possible need for additional, invasive tests such as chorionic villus sampling or amniocentesis, to establish a definitive diagnosis; the reproductive options that might have to be considered, such as prenatal diagnosis, adoption, gamete donation, abortion, or acceptance

†This section has been adapted from Elias and Annas,[34] with permission.

of risks; the costs of screening; issues of confidentiality, including potential disclosure to other family members; and the possibility of social stigmatization, including discrimination in health insurance and employment. If carrier status is detected in the woman, it must be emphasized that the partner should also be screened. As part of prenatal testing, the woman would be told that she would be advised of her options if the fetus was found to be affected with an untreatable condition.[37]

This type of generic consent to genetic screening can be compared with obtaining consent to perform a physical examination. Patients know that the purpose of the examination is to locate potential problems that are likely to require additional follow-up and that could present them with choices they would rather not have to make. The patient is not generally told, however, about all the possible abnormalities that can be detected by a routine physical examination or routine blood work, but only the general purpose of each. On the other hand, tests that may produce especially sensitive and stigmatizing information, such as screening of blood for the human immunodeficiency virus, should not be performed without specific consent. Similarly, because of its reproductive implications, genetic testing has not traditionally been carried out without specific consent. Even in a generic model, tests for untreatable fatal diseases such as Huntington's disease should not be combined with other tests or performed without specific consent.[37]

What is central in the concept of generic consent for genetic screening is not a waiver of the individual patient's right to information. Rather, it would reflect a decision by the genetics community that the most reasonable way to conduct a panel of screening tests to identify carriers of serious conditions is to provide basic, general information to obtain consent for the screening and much more detailed information on specific conditions only after they have been detected. Since, in the vast majority of cases, no such conditions will in fact be found, this method is also the most efficient and cost effective.

Limits to Generic Consent

Some people require more specific and in-depth information on which to base their decision regarding screening. Therefore, it is essential to build into the screening program ample opportunity for patients to obtain all the additional information they need to help them make decisions. Counseling could be provided in person by a physician or other health professional who can be open and responsive to the concerns and questions of patients Alternatively, audiovisual aids could be used, which would help ensure consistency in the information provided, would be more efficient, and respond to the shortage of genetic counselors.

Generic consent for genetic screening would not, however, solve what is likely to be an even more central problem in genetic screening: are there genetic conditions for which screening should not be offered to prospective parents? Examples might include genes that predispose a person to a particular disease late in life such as Alzheimer's disease, Parkinson's disease, or breast cancer.[37,42] From the perspective of the fetus, life with the possibility—or even the high probability—of developing these diseases in late adulthood is likely to be preferred to no life at all. It is unreasonable to argue that failing to provide information on testing would be tantamount to forcing a "wrongful life" on the child.[35] Because of a personal experience with a friend or family member who suffered from one of these diseases, however, the couple might see abortion as a reasonable choice under such circumstances.

We must address this question directly and publicly. Are there genetic diseases and predispositions for which screening of prospective parents and testing of fetuses should *not* be offered as a matter of good medical practice and public policy, regardless of the technical ability to screen and the wishes of the couple? Offering carrier screening to assist couples in making reproductive decisions is not a neutral activity but, rather, implies that some action should be taken on the basis of the results of the test. Thus, for example, merely offering screening for a breast cancer or colon cancer gene suggests to couples that artificial insemination, adoption, and abortion are all reasonable choices if they are found to be carriers of such a gene. We do not believe that pregnancies in women who want to have a child should be terminated for this reason, and thus we believe carrier screening for the breast cancer gene should not be offered in the context of reproductive planning. But if abortion can be obtained electively without giving a reason, is this really the choice of the physician? In the absence of an effective way to set the standard of care for carrier screening, prenatal screening tests for these and similar genes will inevitably be offered by at least some commercial companies and private physicians.

A standard of care for genetic screening and consent in the face of hundreds of available genetic tests will inevitably be set. We believe the medical profession should take the lead in setting such standards and that, with public input, the model of generic consent for genetic screening will ultimately be accepted.

FORCED CESAREAN DELIVERY

American patients have a constitutional right to refuse any medical treatment, including life-sustaining or even life-saving treatment as long as they are competent. This is the general rule, but historically some physicians have argued that this rule should not apply to pregnant patients near delivery, at least if the physician believes that treatment refusals might compromise the health of the soon-to-be child. The view that women who refuse cesarean delivery are in some way willfully abusing their fetuses seems prevalent and deeply held.[43] In 1987, for example, 46 percent of Maternal-Fetal Medicine fellowship directors indicated that women who refused medical advice and thereby endangered the life of the fetus should be detained. Although court orders are rarely sought, the conditions under which they are used are troublesome. In 1987, Kolder et al.[44] reported a U.S. national survey of 21 court orders for cesarean deliveries, hospital detentions, or intrauterine transfusion.

Among 21 cases in which court orders were sought, the orders were obtained in 86 percent; in 88 percent of those cases, the orders were received within 6 hours. The majority of the women involved were black, Asian, or Hispanic, and all were poor. Nearly one half were unmarried, and one fourth did not speak English as their primary language.

Until 1990, with the exception of one case in the Georgia State Supreme Court, all cases had been decided by lower courts and therefore had little precedential importance.[45] In the vast majority of cases, judges were called on an emergency basis and ordered interventions within hours. Without time to analyze the issues, without representation for the pregnant woman, without briefing or thoughtful reflection on the situation, in almost total ignorance of the relevant law, and in an unfamiliar setting faced by a relatively calm physician and a woman who can easily be labeled "hysterical," the judge will almost always order whatever the doctor advises. Physicians may feel better after being "blessed" by the judge, but they should not. First, the appearance of legitimacy is deceptive; the judge has acted injudiciously, and there is no opportunity for meaningful appeal. Second, the medical situation has not changed, except that more time has been lost that could have been used to continue discussion with the woman directly. And, finally, the physician has now helped transform himself or herself into an agent of the state's authority.[47]

There is nothing in *Roe v. Wade*[1] or any other appellate decision that gives either physicians or judges the right to favor the life or well-being of the fetus over that of the pregnant woman. Forcing pregnant women to follow medical advice also places unwarranted faith in that advice. Physicians often disagree about the appropriateness of obstetric interventions, and they can be mistaken.[46] In three of the first five cases in which court-ordered cesarean delivery were sought, the women ultimately delivered vaginally and uneventfully. In the face of such uncertainty—uncertainty compounded by decades of changing and conflicting expert opinion on the management of pregnancy and childbirth—the moral and legal primacy of the competent, informed pregnant woman in decision making is overwhelming.[47]

From a strictly utilitarian perspective, this marriage of the state and medicine is likely to harm more fetuses than it helps, because many women will reasonably avoid physicians altogether during pregnancy if failure to follow medical advice can result in forced treatment, involuntary confinement, or criminal charges. Extending notions of child abuse to "fetal abuse" simply brings government into pregnancy with few, if any, benefits and with great potential for invasions of privacy and deprivations of liberty. It is not helpful to use the law to convert a woman's and society's moral responsibility to her fetus into the woman's legal responsibility alone.[35] After birth, the fetus becomes a child, and can and should thereafter be treated in its own right. Before birth, however, we can obtain access to the fetus only through its mother and, in the absence of her informed consent, can do so only by treating her as a fetal container, a nonperson without rights to bodily integrity.

The ACOG has issued an opinion from its Committee on Ethics entitled "Patient Choice: Maternal Fetal Conflict"[48] that we believe provides thoughtful and useful guidance for the medical practitioner. The conclusions of this statement are as follows:

1. With advances in medical technology, the fetus has become more accessible to diagnostic and treatment modalities. The feto-maternal relationship remains a unique one, requiring a balance of maternal health, autonomy, and fetal needs. Every reasonable effort should be made to protect the fetus, but the pregnant woman's autonomy should be respected.
2. The vast majority of pregnant women are willing to assume significant risk for the welfare of the fetus. Problems arise only when this potentially beneficial advice is rejected. The role of the obstetrician should be one of an informed educator and counselor, weighing the risks and benefits to both patients as well as realizing that tests, judgments, and decisions are fallible. Consultation with others, including an institutional ethics committee, should be sought when appropriate to aid the pregnant woman and obstetrician in making decisions. The use of the courts to resolve these conflicts is almost never warranted.
3. Obstetricians should refrain from performing procedures that are unwanted by a pregnant woman. The use of judicial authority to implement treatment regimens in order to protect the fetus violates the pregnant woman's autonomy. Furthermore, inappropriate reliance on judicial authority may lead to undesirable societal consequences, such as the criminalization of noncompliance with medical recommendations.

In 1990, the District of Columbia Court of Appeals, in a strongly worded opinion, essentially adopted the ACOG's statement as law, holding that the decision of the pregnant woman must be honored in all but "extremely rare and truly exceptional" cases.[50] And in 1997, the U.S. Supreme Court ruled that all Americans have a fundamental constitutional right to refuse any medical intervention, including life-sustaining fluids and nutrition, and made no exceptions for competent pregnant women.

FETAL RESEARCH

Federal Regulations

Society has a critical stake in both the treatment of fetal disorders and the maintenance of respect for the human dignity of the fetus. Fetal research and its regulation is one of the most controversial and complex areas in the field of human experimentation. The National Commission for the Protection of Human Subjects of Biomedical and Behavioral Research, for example, spent the first year of its existence working on the subject of fetal experimentation under a congressional mandate before working on any other topic. This mandate itself was most influenced by the 1973 *Roe* decision discussed earlier. The consequence of this decision was an increase in the number of fetuses aborted; hence, the amount of fetal material available for research also increased.

Before experimentation involving human fetuses begins, current U.S. Department of Health and Human Services (HHS) regulations require that appropriate animal studies be performed, and that investigators play no role in any decision to terminate a pregnancy. The purpose of any in utero experiment must be to meet the health needs of the particular fetus, and the fetus must be placed at risk only to the minimum extent necessary to meet such needs. In the case of nontherapeutic research, the risk to the fetus must be "minimal" and the knowledge must be "important" and not obtainable by other means. The consent of both the mother and father is required, unless the father's identity is not known, he is not reasonably available, or the pregnancy resulted from rape. Fetal research protocols must be approved by an institutional review board (IRB), taking special care to review the subject selection process and the method of obtaining informed consent.

Technically, these federal regulations apply only to investigators who receive federal research funds or who are affiliated with institutions that have signed an agreement with HHS that all research performed in their institution and by their staff will be approved by an IRB under these regulations. We believe, however, the principles set forth by these regulations to be so fundamentally important to the protection of the integrity of the fetus, the potential parents, and the research enterprise itself that they provide the minimum guidelines that should be adhered to voluntarily in all institutions undertaking fetal research projects.

State Statutes

More state legislation has been enacted regarding fetal research than any other type of research, and the poor quality of the legislation adds to the complicated nature of this issue. About one half of the states currently have statutes regulating fetal research; 15 were passed soon after the *Roe* decision and in direct response to it. Most state statutes restrict both in utero and ex utero research, and the restrictions are generally more stringent than the federal regulations with the exception of New Mexico's statute, which is modeled after federal regulations. In Massachusetts, for example, it is a crime to study the fetus in utero unless the research does not "substantially jeopardize" the life or health of the fetus, and the fetus is not the subject of an elected abortion. The law was recently amended to specifically permit stem cell research that involves the destruction of a human embryo. Therapeutic research, such as shunting procedures to treat fetal urinary tract obstruction, is permissible even in this restrictive state. Utah, the only state to deal exclusively with in utero fetuses, prohibits all research on "live unborn children." Some states limit their prohibition to the living abortus and thus do not apply to fetal surgery. California restricts experimentation only on ex utero fetuses, outlawing "any type of scientific or laboratory research or any other kind of experimentation or study, except to protect or preserve the life and health of the fetus." Thus, there is little consistency or rationale among jurisdictions regarding regulations directly pertaining to fetal research. Nonetheless, one is bound by the laws of the state in which one performs fetal research, and knowledge of its provisions is advisable.[51–54]

Consent

A fundamental premise of Anglo-American law is that no one can touch or treat a competent adult without the adult's informed consent. This doctrine is based primarily on the value we place on autonomy, or self-determination, and secondarily on rational decision making. The first requires that individuals have the ultimate say concerning whether their bodies will be "invaded"; the latter requires disclosure of certain material information, including a description of the proposed procedure, risks of death and serious disability, alternatives, success rates, and problems of recuperation before one is asked to consent to an "invasion."[55]

These issues are relatively straightforward when dealing with an adult, but how do they apply when experimentation or therapy is directed toward a fetus. especially when the distinction between experimentation and therapy is often unclear? In general, therapy involves procedures performed primarily for the benefit of the patient that are considered "good and accepted practice," whereas experimentation involves new or innovative procedures not yet considered standard practice performed for the primary purpose of testing a hypothesis or gaining new knowledge.[56]

In the therapeutic setting, the consent of either one of the parents is usually sufficient for beneficial procedures to be performed on children. In the case of the fetus, however, if the proposed investigative therapeutic procedure will place the mother at any risk of death or serious disability, she alone has the right to consent and the corresponding right to withhold consent because her body will necessarily be invaded and only she—not her husband—has the right to determine if this will be done. Even after fetal viability, *Roe* and *Casey* give the woman and her physician the right to terminate the pregnancy if her life or health is endangered. This is consistent with the Court's ruling that when conflict exists between a potential father and the pregnant woman over the issue of an abortion, the woman's position should prevail because she has more at stake (e.g., her body, health risks) than the potential father.[57] The same logic applies here. Consent of the pregnant woman is a mandatory prerequisite for both investigative procedures and therapy. Her consent must be informed, and she should be told as clearly as possible about the proposed experimental procedure or therapy and its risks to herself and her fetus, as well as alternatives, success rates, and the likely problems of recuperation.[58,59]

KEY POINTS

- Any restrictions on abortion, including "partial birth" abortion are unconstitutional unless they provide an exception for the pregnant woman's life and health.

- Before fetal viability states cannot "unduly burden" a woman's decision to terminate a pregnancy.

- The legal and ethical obligations relating to genetic counseling and prenatal diagnosis can be summarized as follows: (1) the physician must give accurate information to the parents and cannot withhold vital information from them; (2) an obstetrician cannot be required to perform prenatal diagnostic procedures; (3) prenatal genetic counseling should be morally nondirective; and (4) to protect patient privacy and autonomy, no information obtained in genetic counseling or screening should be disclosed to any third party without the patient's authorization.

- Self-determination and rational decision making are the central purposes of informed consent, and information on recommended procedures, risks, benefits, and alternatives should be presented in a way that furthers these purposes.

- Consent of the pregnant woman is a mandatory prerequisite for both investigative procedures and therapy. Her consent must be informed, and she should be told as clearly as possible about the proposed experimental procedures or therapy, its risks to herself and her fetus, as well as alternatives, success rates, and the likely problems of recuperation.

- The fetomaternal relationship is a unique one that requires physicians to promote a balance of maternal health and fetal welfare while respecting maternal autonomy. Obstetricians should refrain from performing procedures that are refused by pregnant women: the decision of the competent pregnant woman must be honored in all but "extremely rare and truly exceptional" cases, although reasonable steps to persuade a woman to change her mind are appropriate.

REFERENCES

1. *Roe v. Wade,* 410 U.S. 113 (1973).
2. Annas GJ: Partial birth abortion, Congress and the Constitution. N Engl J Med 339:279, 1998.
3. *Planned Parenthood of Southeastern Pennsylvania v. Casey,* 502 U.S. 1056 (1992).
4. Annas GJ: The Supreme Court, liberty, and abortion. N Engl J Med 327:651, 1992.
5. H.R. 1833, 104th Cong.
6. Remarks on returning without approval to the House of Representatives partial birth abortion legislation Weekly Compilation of Presidential Documents. April 10, 1996;643.
7. Santorum R: A brief life that changed our lives forever. National Right to Life News. May 23, 1997;6.
8. Klein J: The senator's dilemma. New Yorker. January 5, 1998;30.
9. Vobejda B, Brown D: Harsh details shift tenor of abortion fight: both sides bend facts on late-term procedure. Washington Post. September 17, 1996;A1.
10. Hsu S: Virginia ban on certain abortions is blocked, law too vague U.S. judge says. Washington Post. June 26, 1998;C1.
11. Gianelli DM: Abortion rights leader urges end to 'half truths.' American Medical News. March 3, 1997;3, 28.
12. American College of Obstetricians and Gynecologists: Statement on intact dilatation and extraction, January 12, 1997.
13. Gianelli DM: House affirms AMA stance on abortion. American Medical News. July 7, 1997;3, 30.
14. Seelye KQ: Democratic leader proposes measure to limit abortions. New York Times. May 9, 1997;A32.
15. *Stenberg v. Carhart,* 530 U.S. 914 (2000).
16. Annas GJ: "Partial-Birth Abortion" and the Supreme Court. N Engl J Med 344:152, 2001.
17. Wolinksy H, Brune T: The Serpent on the Staff: The Unhealthy Politics of the American Medical Association. New York, GP Putnam's Sons, 1994.
18. Kassirer JP: Practicing medicine without a license-the new intrusions by Congress. N Engl J Med 336:1747, 1997.
19. *Women's Medical Professional Corp. v. Voinovich,* 130 F.3d 187 (6th Cir. 1997).
20. *Planned Parenthood of So. Arizona v. Woods,* 982 F. Supp. 1369 (D. Arizona 1997).
21. *Carhart v. Stenberg,* 972 F. Supp. 507 (D. Nebraska 1997).
22. *Summit Medical Associates v. James,* 984 F. Supp. 1404 (M.D. Alabama 1998).
23. *Evans v. Kelley,* 977 F. Supp. 1283 (E.D. Michigan 1997).
24. Massie AM: So-called "partial-birth abortion" bans: bad medicine? Maybe. Bad Law? Definitely! U P H L Rev 59:301, 1998.
25. *Hope Clinic v. Ryan,* 1999 U.S. App. LEXIS 26925.
26. *Voinovich v. Women's Medical Professional Corp.,* 523 U.S. 1036 (1998).
27. Annas CL: Irreversible error: the power and prejudice of female genital mutilation. J Contemp Health Law Policy 12:325, 1996.
28. Annas GJ, Coyne B: "Fitness" for birth and reproduction: legal implication of genetic screening. Family Law Q 9:463, 1975.
29. Annas GJ, Elias S: Legal and ethical implications of fetal diagnosis and gene therapy. Am J Med Genet 35:215, 1990.
30. Annas GJ: Medical paternity and "wrongful life." Hastings Center Rep 11:8, 1981.
31. Recent opinions of the Judicial Council of the American Medical Association. JAMA 251:278, 1984.
32. Annas GJ: Problems of informed consent and confidentiality in genetic counseling. *In* Milunsky A, Annas GJ (eds): Genetics and the Law. New York, Plenum Press, 1975.
33. President's Commissions for the Study of Ethical Problems in Medicine and Biomedical and Behavioral Research: Screening and Counseling for Genetic Conditions, February 1983. Library of Congress No. 83-600502. Washington, DC, U.S. Government Printing Office, 1983.
34. Elias S, Annas GJ: Generic consent for genetic screening. N Engl J Med 330:1611, 1994.
35. Elias S, Annas GJ: Reproductive Genetics and the Law. Chicago, Yearbook, 1987.
36. Annas GJ: The Rights of Patients, 3rd ed. New York, NYU Press, 2004.
37. Andrews LB, Fullarton JE, Holtsman NA, Motulsky AG (eds): Assessing genetic risks: implications for health and social policy. Washington, DC, National Academy Press, 1994.
38. Rodwin M: Medicine, Money and Morals. New York, Oxford University Press, 1993.
39. Social Policy Research Priorities for the Human Genome Project. *In* Annas GJ, Elias S (eds): Mapping Our Genes: Using Law and Ethics as Guides. New York, Oxford University Press, 1992, p 269.
40. Fraser FC: Genetic counseling. Am J Hum Genet 26:636, 1974.
41. Simpson JL, Elias S: Isolating fetal cells from maternal blood: advances in prenatal diagnosis through molecular technology. JAMA 270:2357, 1993.
42. Biesecker BB, Boehnke M, Calzone K, et al: Genetic counseling for families with inherited susceptibility to breast and ovarian cancer. JAMA 269:1970, 1993.
43. Lieberman JR, Mazor M, Chain W, et al: The fetal right to live. Obstet Gynecol 53:515, 1979.

44. Kolder VEB, Gallagher J, Parsons MT: Court-ordered obstetrical interventions. N Engl J Med 316:1192, 1987.
45. Nelson LJ, Milliken N: Compelled medical treatment of pregnant women. JAMA 259:1060, 1988.
46. Notzon FC, Placek PJ, Taffel SM: Comparisons of national cesarean-section rates. N Engl J Med 316:386, 1987.
47. Annas GJ: Protecting the liberty of pregnant patients. N Engl J Med 316:1213, 1987.
48. ACOG Committee Opinion: Patient Choice: Maternal-Fetal Conflict. Number 55. Washington DC, American College of Obstetricians and Gynecologist, October 1987.
49. *In Re A.C.*, 573 A 2d 1235 (DC App 1990).
50. Annas GJ: Standard of Care: The Law of American Bioethics. New York, Oxford University Press, 1993.
51. Annas GJ, Caplan A, Elias S: Stem cell politics, ethics and medical progress. Nat Med 5:13, 1999.
52. Annas GJ, Glantz LH, Katz BH: Informed Consent to Human Experimentation. Cambridge, MA, Ballinger, 1977.
53. Friedman JM: The federal fetal experimentation regulations: an establishment clause analysis. Minn Law Rev 61:961, 1977.
54. Brock EA: Fetal research: what price progress? Detroit Coll Law Rev 3:403, 1979.
55. Annas GJ, Densberger JE: Competence to refuse medical treatment: autonomy vs. paternalism. Toledo Law Rev 15:561, 1984.
56. Annas GJ, Glantz LH, Katz BF: The Rights of Doctors, Nurses and Allied Health Professionals. Cambridge, MA, Ballinger, 1981.
57. *Danforth v. Planned Parenthood,* 428 U.S. 52 (1976).
58. Elias S, Annas GJ: Perspectives on fetal surgery. Am J Obstet Gynecol 145:807, 1983.
59. Annas GJ: Waste and longing: the legal status of placental-blood banking. N Engl J Med 340:1521, 1999.

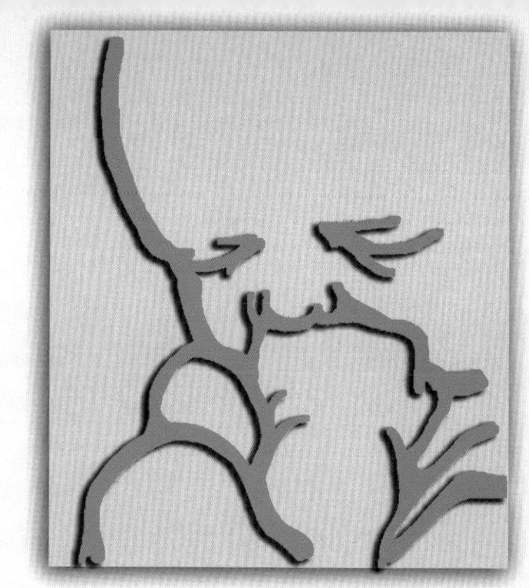

Appendices

Normal Values in Pregnancy

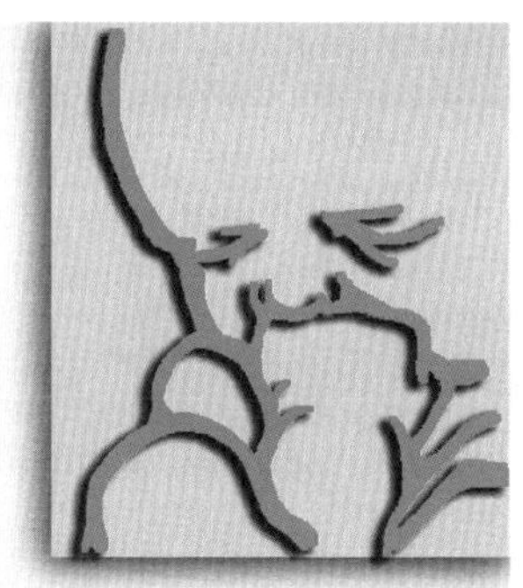

Invasive Monitoring

MEASURE	VALUE (36–38 WEEKS)	UNITS
Cardiac output	6.2 ± 1.0	liters/minute
Systemic vascular resistance	1,210 ± 266	dyne cm second^{-5}
Heart rate	83 ± 10	beats/minute
Pulmonary vascular resistance	78 ± 22	dyne cm second^{-5}
Colloid oncotic pressure	18.0 ± 1.5	mm Hg
Mean arterial pressure (MAP)	90.3 ± 5.8	mm Hg
Pulmonary capillary wedge pressure (PCWP)	7.5 ± 1.8	mm Hg
Central venous pressure (CVP)	3.6 ± 2.5	mm Hg
Left ventricular stroke work index	48 ± 6	g mm^{-2}

Cardiac output is increased in pregnancy but is essentially unchanged over the course of pregnancy.

Heart rate gradually rises 5 to 10 bpm over the course of pregnancy.

References: Clark SL, Cotton DB, Lee W, et al: Central hemodynamic assessment of normal term pregnancy. Am J Obstet Gynecol 161:1439, 1989.

Spatling L, Fallenstein F, Huch A, et al: The variability of cardiopulmonary adaptation to pregnancy at rest and during exercise. Br J Obstet Gynaecol 99(Suppl 8):1, 1992.

Noninvasive Monitoring

MEASURE	10–18 WEEKS	18–26 WEEKS	26–34 WEEKS	34–42 WEEKS
Cardiac output (L/min)	7.26 ± 1.56	7.60 ± 1.63	7.38 ± 1.63	6.37 ± 1.48
Stroke volume (mL)	85 ± 21	85 ± 21	82 ± 21	70 ± 14
SVR (dyne cm second^{-5})	966 ± 226	901 ± 224	932 ± 240	1,118 ± 325
Heart rate (beats/min)	87 ± 14	90 ± 14	92 ± 14	92 ± 7
Mean arterial pressure (mm Hg)	87 ± 7	84 ± 7	84 ± 7	86 ± 7

SVR, systemic vascular resistance.

Reference: Van Oppen CA, Van Der Tweel I, Alsbach JGP, et al: A longitudinal study of maternal hemodynamics during normal pregnancy. Obstet Gynecol 88:40, 1996.

Third-Trimester Arterial Blood Gas Values

	NORMAL ALTITUDE	MODERATE ALTITUDE (1,388 M, PROVO, UT)
Arterial pH	7.44 ± 0.04	7.46 ± 0.02
Arterial Po_2 (mm Hg)	85 ± 5	86.2 ± 7.3
O_2 Saturation (%)		96 ± 1
Arterial Pco_2 (mm Hg)	29.7 ± 2.8	26.6 ± 2.7
Sodium bicarbonate (mEq/L)	22.0 ± 2.1	18.6 ± 1.9

References: Hankins GD, Clark SL, Harvey CJ, et al: Third trimester arterial blood gas and acid base values in normal pregnancy at moderate altitude. Obstet Gynecol 88:347, 1988.

Eng M, Butler J, Bonica JJ: Respiratory function in pregnant obese women. Am J Obstet Gynecol 123:241, 1975.

Pulmonary Function Tests

	8–11 WEEKS	20–23 WEEKS	28–31 WEEKS	36–40 WEEKS
Respiratory Rate (br/min)	15 (14–20)	16 (15–18)	18 (15–20)	17 (16–18)
Tidal Volume (mL)	640 (550–710)	650 (625–725)	650 (575–720)	700 (660–755)

(Median, 25th–75th Percentile)

Adapted from Spatling L, Fallenstein F, Huch A, et al: The variability of cardiopulmonary adaptation to pregnancy at rest and during exercise. Br J Obstet Gynaecol 99:1, 1992.

Mean Values

Vital capacity		
First trimester	3.8	Liters
Second trimester	3.9	Liters
Third trimester	4.1	Liters
Inspiratory capacity		
First trimester	2.6	Liters
Second trimester	2.7	Liters
Third trimester	2.9	Liters
Expiratory reserve volume		
First trimester	1.2	Liters
Second trimester	1.2	Liters
Third trimester	1.2	Liters
Residual volume		
First trimester	1.2	Liters
Second trimester	1.1	Liters
Third trimester	1.0	Liters

References: Gazioglu K, Kaltreider NL, Rosen M, Yu PN: Pulmonary function during pregnancy in normal women and in patients with cardiopulmonary disease. Thorax 25:445, 1920.

Puranik BM, Kaore SB, Kurhade GA, et al: A longitudinal study of pulmonary function tests during pregnancy. Indian J Physiol Pharmacol 38:129, 1994.

Peak Flows (5th% Shown as Lower Limit of Normal) Stable Over Gestation

	PEAK FLOW (L/MIN)
Standing	>320
Sitting	>310
Supine	>300

Adapted from Harirah HM, Donia SE, Nasrallah FK, et al: Effect of gestational age and position on peak expiratory flow rate: a longitudinal study. Obstet Gynecol 105:372, 2005.

LIVER FUNCTION TESTS

	WEEK 12	WEEK 32	INTRAPARTUM
Total alkaline phosphatase (IU/L)	42 (17–88)	82 (46–165)	97 (48–249)
Gamma glutamyl transferase (IU/L)	7 (2–18)	6 (3–20)	9 (5–79)
Aspartate transaminase (AST, IU/L)	9 (4–18)	9 (5–21)	11 (5–103)
Alanine transaminase (ALT, IU/L)	9 (4–30)	8 (2–22)	12 (5–115)
Total bilirubin (IU/L)	4 (1–12)	4 (2–9)	4 (2–10)

Medians, Range Sixty-six women with uncomplicated pregnancies followed longitudinally.

Reference: van Buul EJA, Steegers EAP, Jongsma HW, et al: Haematological and biochemical profile of uncomplicated pregnancy in nulliparous women; a longitudinal study. Neth J Med 46:73, 1995.

ELECTROLYTES, OSMOLALITY, AND RENAL FUNCTION

	12 WEEKS	20 WEEKS	28 WEEKS	38 WEEKS
Total osmolality (mosmol/kg)	267–279	269–285	273–283	271–289
Sodium (mmol/L)	133–141	136–142	135–143	135–141
Potassium (mmol/L)	3.5–4.3	3.5–4.3	3.5–4.4	3.6–4.5
Chloride (mmol/L)	102–108	103–111	104–112	102–111
Creatinine clearance (ml/24 hours)	76–188	88–168	40–192	52–208
Blood urea nitrogen (BUN)	1.7–4.4	1.9–5.3	1.9–4.2	1.8–4.6
Serum albumin (g/L)	37–47	34–42	31–42	31–39
Urine volume (mL/24 hours)	750–2,500	850–2,400	750–2,700	550–3,900

5th–95th Percentile

Adapted from van Buul EJA, Steegers EAP, Jongsma HW, et al: Haematological and biochemical profile of uncomplicated pregnancy in nulliparous women; a longitudinal study. Neth J Med 46:73, 1995.

24-Hour Urinary Protein (mg/24 Hours)

First trimester	80.0 ± 60.6
Second trimester	116.7 ± 69.3
Third trimester	115.3 ± 69.2

Mean ± SD

Reference: Higby K, Suiter J, Phelps JY, et al: Normal values of urinary albumin and total protein excretion during pregnancy. Am J Obstet Gynecol 171:984, 1994.

METABOLIC MARKERS AND LIPIDS

	4–16 WEEKS	16–24 WEEKS	24–34 WEEKS	TERM
Uric acid (mg/dL)	3.21 ± 0.10	3.48 ± 0.13	3.49 ± 0.11	4.72 ± 0.13
Creatinine (mg/dL)	0.58 ± 0.03	0.50 ± 0.04	0.50 ± 0.03	0.57 ± 0.03
Total cholesterol (mg/dL)	153.5 ± 3.8	194.0 ± 5.2	218.3 ± 6.4	220.4 ± 8.4
Triglycerides	70.1 ± 4.5	109.6 ± 5.8	139.6 ± 6.9	159.0 ± 8.1
Free fatty acids (mEq/L)	0.42 ± 0.03	0.34 ± 0.02	0.21 ± 0.02	0.67 ± 0.04

Medians ± SD

Reference: Lain KY, Markovic N, Ness RB, Roberts JM: Effect of smoking on uric acid and other metabolic markers throughout normal pregnancy. J Clin Endocrinol Metab 90:5743, 2005.

White Blood Cell Count (10^9/L)

18 Weeks	8.8 (5.6–13.8)
32 Weeks	9.7 (6.0–15.7)
39 Weeks	9.4 (5.8–15.1)

(Mean ± 1.96 × SD)

Reference: Nils Milman, unpublished data, personal communication.

RED BLOOD CELL INDICES

Red Cell Indices In Iron-Treated Women (66 mg Elemental Iron as Fumarate)

Red blood cell count (10^{12}/L)	
First trimester (9–13 wk)	>3.45
Second trimester (19–22 wk)	>3.29
Third trimester (31–34 wk)	>3.23
Term (39–43 wk)	>3.54
Hemoglobin (g/dL)	
First trimester (9–13 wk)	>11.1
Second trimester (19–22 wk)	>10.64
Third trimester (31–34 wk)	>10.47
Term (39–43 wk)	>11.5
Hematocrit (%)	
First trimester (9–13 wk)	>33
Second trimester (19–22 wk)	>32
Third trimester (31–34 wk)	>31
Term (39–43 wk)	>34
Mean cell volume (MCV, fl, 5th–95th percentile)	
First trimester (9–13 wk)	88–101
Second trimester (19–22 wk)	89–104
Third trimester (31–34 wk)	90–104
Term (39–43 wk)	90–102
Mean corpuscular hemoglobin (MCH, pg)	
First trimester (9–13 wk)	>30.1
Second trimester (19–22 wk)	>29.9
Third trimester (31–34 wk)	>30.2
Term (39–43 wk)	>30.1
Mean cell hemoglobin concentration (MCHC, g/dL)	
First trimester (9–13 wk)	>32.6
Second trimester (19–22 wk)	>31.7
Third trimester (31–34 wk)	>32.2
Term (39–43 wk)	>31.9

<5th Percentile Shown as Lower Limit of Normal

Personal communication, N. Milman; Based on Milman N, Agger OA, Nielsen OJ: Iron supplementation during pregnancy. Effect on iron status markers, serum erythropoietin and human placental lactogen. A placebo controlled study in 207 Danish women. Dan Med Bull 38:471, 1991.

Iron, Folate, and Vitamin B_{12} Levels

Mean Ferritin (ug/L)	
First trimester (mean 12.6 wk)	46.8 ± 2.5
Third trimester (32 wk)	20.8 ± 1.3
Term (38 wk)	21.7 ± 1.6
Mean Total Iron Binding Capacity (TIBC, umol/L)	
First trimester (mean 12.6 wk)	59.3 ± 0.6
Third trimester (32 wk)	73.8 ± 0.9
Term (38 wk)	77.7 ± 0.9
Folate (umol/L)	
First trimester (mean 12.6 wk)	6.7 ± 0.3
Third trimester (32 wk)	6.4 ± 0.3
Term (38 wk)	6.9 ± 0.4
B_{12}	
First trimester (mean 12.6 wk)	345.6 ± 8.9
Third trimester (32 wk)	259.3 ± 6.0
Term (38 wk)	241.8 ± 6.5

Platelet Count (10^9/L)

First trimester (12 wk)	240 (170–310)
Third trimester (28 wk)	250 (150–360)
Term (38 wk)	240 (140–370)

Median (5th–95th percentile)

Adapted from van Buul EJA, Steegers EAP, Jongsma HW, et al: Haematological and biochemical profile of uncomplicated pregnancy in nulliparous women; a longitudinal study. Neth J Med 46:73, 1995.

Fasting Homocysteine With and Without Folic Acid Supplementation (Various Doses) (μmol/L)

	8 WEEKS	20 WEEKS	32 WEEKS
Unsupplemented	6.48 ± 1.30	5.22 ± 1.29	5.16 ± 1.32
Supplemented	6.32 ± 1.34	4.18 ± 1.32	4.42 ± 1.37

Means ± 1SD

Reference: Murphy MM, Scott JM, McPartlin JM, Fernandez-Ballart JD: The pregnancy-related decrease in fasting plasma homocysteine is not explained by folic acid supplementation, hemodilution, or a decrease in albumin in a longitudinal study. Am J Clin Nutr 76:614, 2002.

Coagulation Factors

	11–15 WEEKS	21–25 WEEKS	31–35 WEEKS	36–40 WEEKS
Factor VII	111 (60–206)	150 (80–280)	162 (84–312)	171 (87–336)
Factor X	103 (62–169)	115 (74–177)	123 (78–194)	127 (72–208)
Factor V	93 (46–188)	82 (66–185)	82 (34–195)	85 (39–184)
Factor II	125 (70–224)	125 (73–214)	115 (74–179)	115 (68–194)

(% of Standards Shown, Mean and Range)

Reference: Stirling Y, Woolf L, North WRS, et al: Haemostasis in normal pregnancy. Thromb Haemost 52:176, 1984.

COAGULATION PARAMETERS AND TESTING

Coagulation Parameters in Normal Pregnancy and Puerperium (*n* = 117)

	10 WEEKS	20 WEEKS	30 WEEKS	36 WEEKS
INR	0.97 ± 0.08	0.91 ± 0.06	0.88 ± 0.07	0.87 ± 0.07
PTT (sec)	27.0 ± 2.7	26.9 ± 2.7	27.1 ± 2.9	27.5 ± 2.8
Fibrinogen (mg%)	412.5 ± 69.5	463.9 ± 83.9	538.8 ± 107.3	556.9 ± 113.3
Antithrombin III	101.5 ± 12.7	101.4 ± 10.3	104.2 ± 12.5	102.8 ± 13.5
Protein C (%)	99.4 ± 21.3	107.5 ± 24.9	99.3 ± 26.0	94.9 ± 25.5
Protein S (%)	64.1 ± 15.8	62.1 ± 14.2	54.0 ± 13.3	51.7 ± 17.9
PAI (AU/mL)	10.3 ± 4.7	11.3 ± 5.0	20.5 ± 7.3	22.4 ± 7.5

INR, international normalized ratio; PAI, plasminogen activator inhibitor; PTT, partial thromboplastin time.

(Mean ± SD)

Reference: Cerneca F, Ricci G, Someone R, et al: Coagulation and fibrinolysis changes in normal pregnancy. Increased levels of procoagulants and reduced levels of inhibitors during pregnancy induce a hypercoagulable state, combined with a reactive fibrinolysis. Eur J Obstet Gynecol Reprod Biol 73:31, 1997

Calcium Metabolism

	13–16 WEEKS	21–24 WEEKS	29–32 WEEKS	>37 WEEKS
Total calcium (mmol/L)	2.25–2.35	2.15–2.30	2.10–2.25	2.05–2.25
Ionized calcium (mmol/L)	1.10–1.20	1.05–1.20	1.10–1.15	1.05–1.15

(± 1 SD)

Adapted from Pitkin RM, Reynolds WA, Williams GA, Hargis GK: Calcium metabolism in normal pregnancy: a longitudinal study. Am J Obstet Gynecol 133:781, 1979.

	8–11 WEEKS	20–23 WEEKS	28–31 WEEKS	>37 WEEKS
Calcitonin (ng/L)	73–101	79–108	87–113	83–109
Parathyroid hormone (ng/L)	7–15	4.5–12	5–15	10–17
1,25 Dihydroxy Vitamin D (ng/L)	58–78	94–122	98–136	94–150

Adapted from Seki K, Makimura N, Mitsui C, et al: Calcium regulating hormones and osteocalcin levels during pregnancy: a longitudinal study. Am J Obstet Gynecol 164:1248, 1991.

TSH (mIU/L) and Free T_4 (ng/dL) by Race (means, IQ range)[1]

	BLACK	WHITE
First trimester		
TSH	0.9 (0.4–1.6)	1.3 (0.8–2.0)
Free T_4	1.0 (0.9–1.1)	1.0 (0.9–1.1)
Second trimester		
TSH	1.0 (0.6–1.5)	1.6 (1.0–2.2)
Free T_4	0.9 (0.8–1.0)	0.9 (0.8–1.0)
Third trimester		
TSH	1.2 (0.9–1.9)	1.5 (1.4–2.1)
Free T_4	0.8 (0.7–0.9)	0.8 (0.7–0.9)
Delivery		
TSH	2.1 (1.3–3.1)	2.8 (2.0–4.4)
Free T_4	0.8 (0.7–0.9)	0.8 (0.7–0.9)

Screening and Diagnostic Thresholds across Pregnancy[2]
TSH >2.5 mIU/L – requires further workup for hypothyroidism
Total T_4 <100 nmol/L (7.8 µ/dL) – diagnostic of hypothyroidism
T_4, thyroxine; TSH, thyroid-stimulating hormone.

References: 1. Walker JA, Illions EH, Huddleston JF, Smallridge RC: Racial comparisons of thyroid function and autoimmunity during pregnancy and the postpartum period. Obstet Gynecol 106:1365, 2005.

2. Mandel SJ, Spencer CA, Hollowell JG: Are detection and treatment of thyroid insufficiency in pregnancy feasible? Thyroid 15:44, 2005.

Sequential Measurements of Plasma CRH, ACTH, Cortisol, Aldosterone, and Urinary Free Cortisol during Pregnancy

WEEKS OF GESTATION	CRH (PG/ML)	ACTH (PG/ML)	CORTISOL (µG/DL)	DHEAS (µG/DL)	ALDOSTERONE (PG/ML)	URINARY FREE CORTISOL (µG/24 H)
11–15	115 ± 56	8.8 ± 2.8	10.5 ± 1.4	102 ± 14	412 ± 63.6	54.8 ± 7.3
21–25	145 ± 30	9.8 ± 1.5	20.0 ± 1.1	85.1 ± 9.0	487 ± 42.8	84.4 ± 8.4
31–35	1,570 ± 349	12.1 ± 2.0	22.0 ± 1.2	62.6 ± 6.8	766 ± 94	105 ± 8.8
36–40	4,346 ± 754	18.6 ± 2.6	26.0 ± 1.1	63.8 ± 7.1	1,150 ± 170	111 ± 8.7

ACTH, adrenocorticotrophic hormone; CRH, corticotrophin-releasing hormone; DHEAS, dehydroepiandrosterone.

Reference: Goland R, Jozak S, Conwell I: Placental corticotropin-releasing hormone and the hypercortisolism of pregnancy. Am J Obstet Gynecol 171:1287, 1994.

Umbilical Cord Blood at Delivery

	ARTERY	VEIN
pH	7.06–7.36	7.14–7.45
P_{CO_2} (mm Hg)	27.8–68.3	24.0–56.3
P_{O_2} (mm Hg)	9.8–41.2	12.3–45.0
Base deficit (mmol/L)	0.5–15.3	0.7–12.6

Reference: Eskes TKAB, Jongsma HW, Houx PCW: Percentiles for gas values in human umbilical cord blood. Eur J Obstet Gynecol Reprod Biol 14:341, 1983.

White blood cell count (10^9/L)	11.1–16.2
Red cell count (10^{12}/L)	4.13–4.62
Hemoglobin (g/dL)	15.3–17.2
Hematocrit (%)	45.2–50.9
MCV (fl)	107.4–113.3
Platelet count (10^9/L)	237–321
Reticulocyte count (10^9/L)	145.8–192.6

25th–75th Percentile

Reference: Mercelina-Roumans P, Breukers R, Ubachs, J, Van Wersch J: Hematological variables in cord blood of neonates of smoking and non-smoking mothers. J Clin Epidemiol 49:449, 1996.

Anatomy of the Pelvis

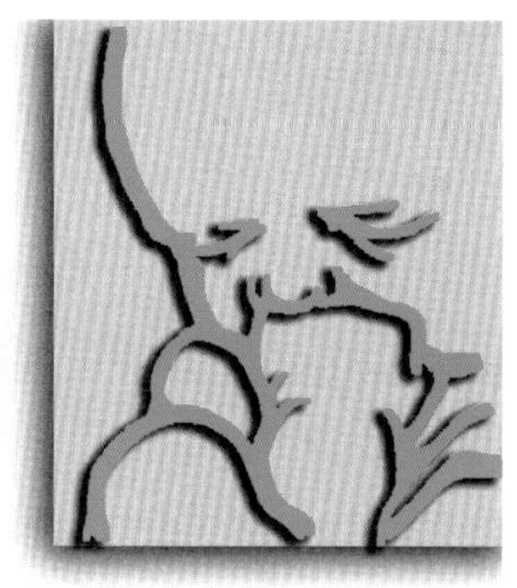

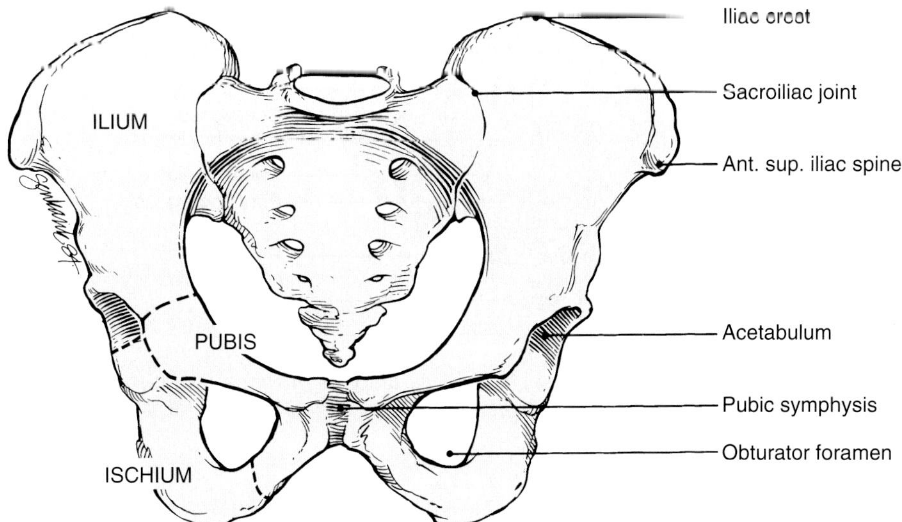

Figure A-1. Major components of the bony pelvis shown in a frontal superior view of the female pelvis. The plane of the pelvic brim faces forward and forms an angle of about 60 degrees to the horizontal. Features that most clearly distinguish the female from the male pelvis include a wider subpubic angle, wider sciatic notch, and greater distance from pubic symphysis and anterior edge of the acetabulum.

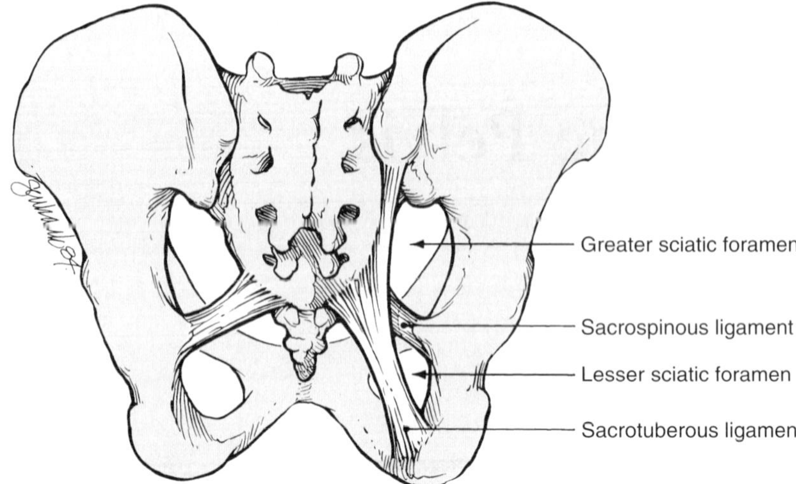

Figure A-2. Major ligaments and notches of the female pelvis, posterior view. During pregnancy, temporary changes take place in the ligaments that permit both movement of the joints and enlargement of the pelvic cavity. This becomes important during parturition.

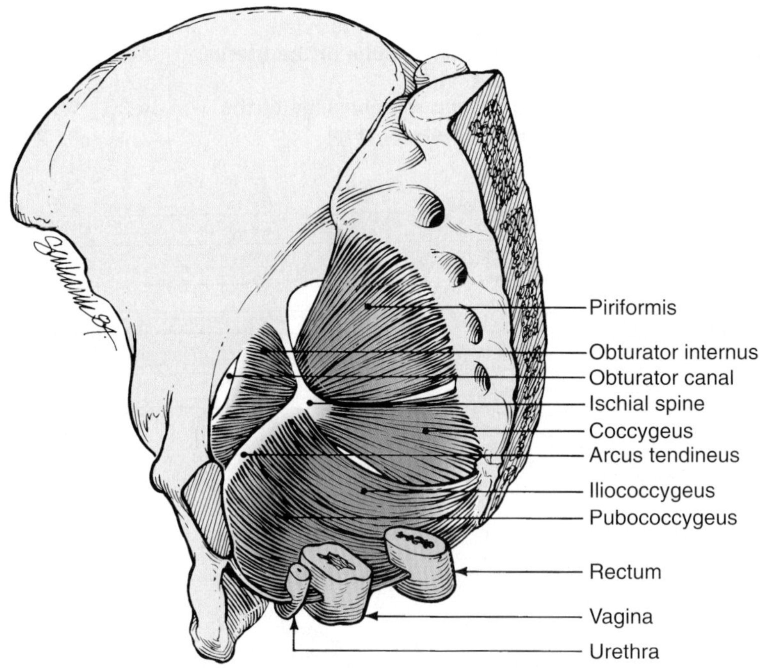

Figure A-3. Muscles of the pelvic diaphragm, oblique view. The pelvic diaphragm forms a muscular floor for the support of the pelvic organs. Note the location of the urethra, uterus, and rectum as they pierce the floor of the pelvic diaphragm.

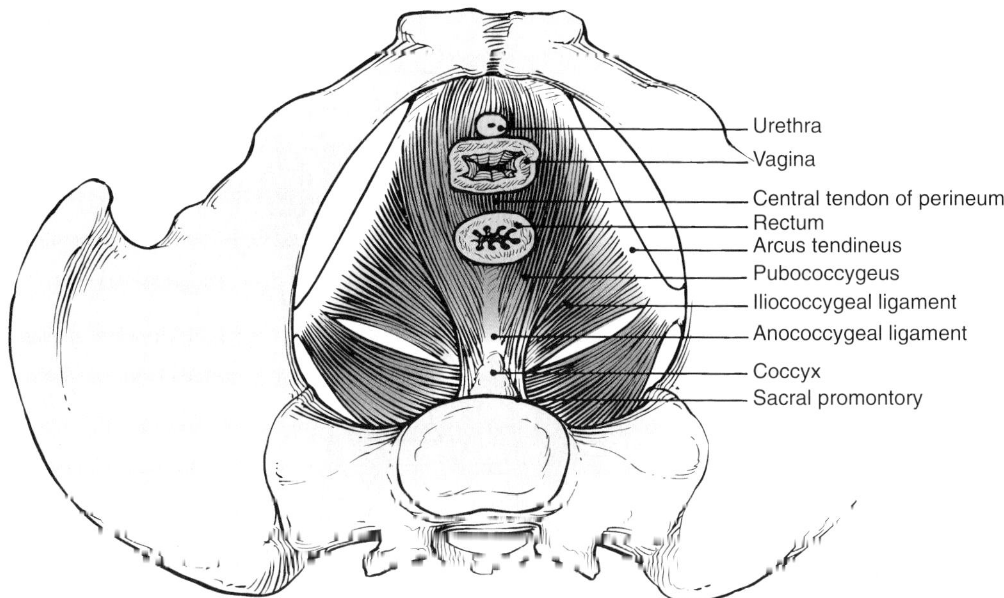

Figure A-4. Muscles of the pelvic diaphragm, superior view. As seen from above, the pelvic diaphragm consists of a number of different muscles and ligaments. The spaces between these muscles transmit a number of vessels and nerves as they leave the pelvis. Note the relationship of the central tendon of the perineum to the rectum and uterus.

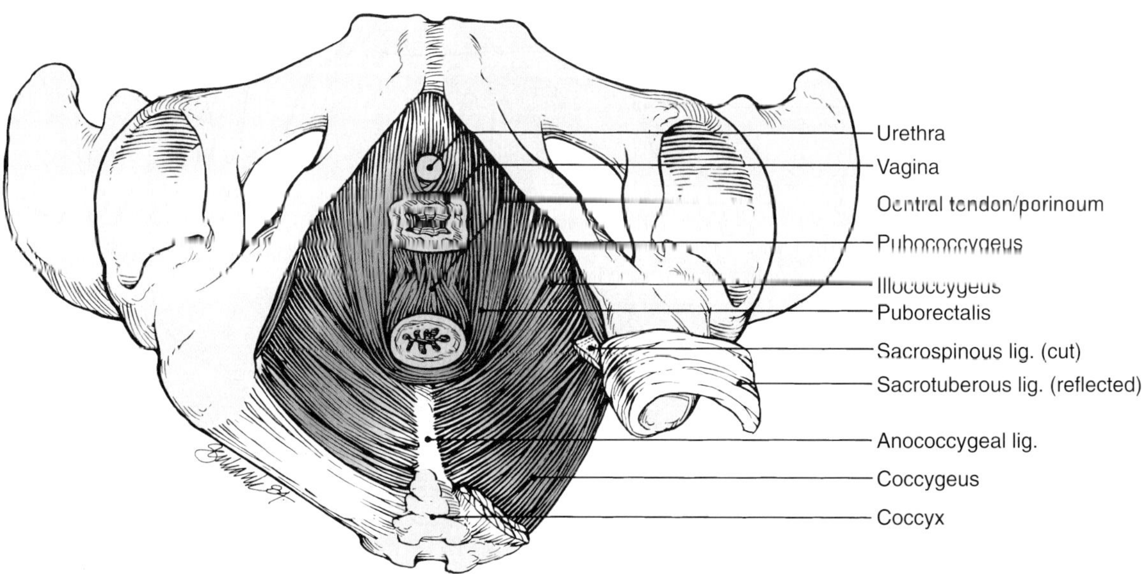

Figure A-5. Inferior view of muscles of the pelvic diaphragm. The pelvic diaphragm is bilaterally symmetric, with the perineal body (central tendon) and the anococcygeal ligament forming a strong median raphe. lig., ligament.

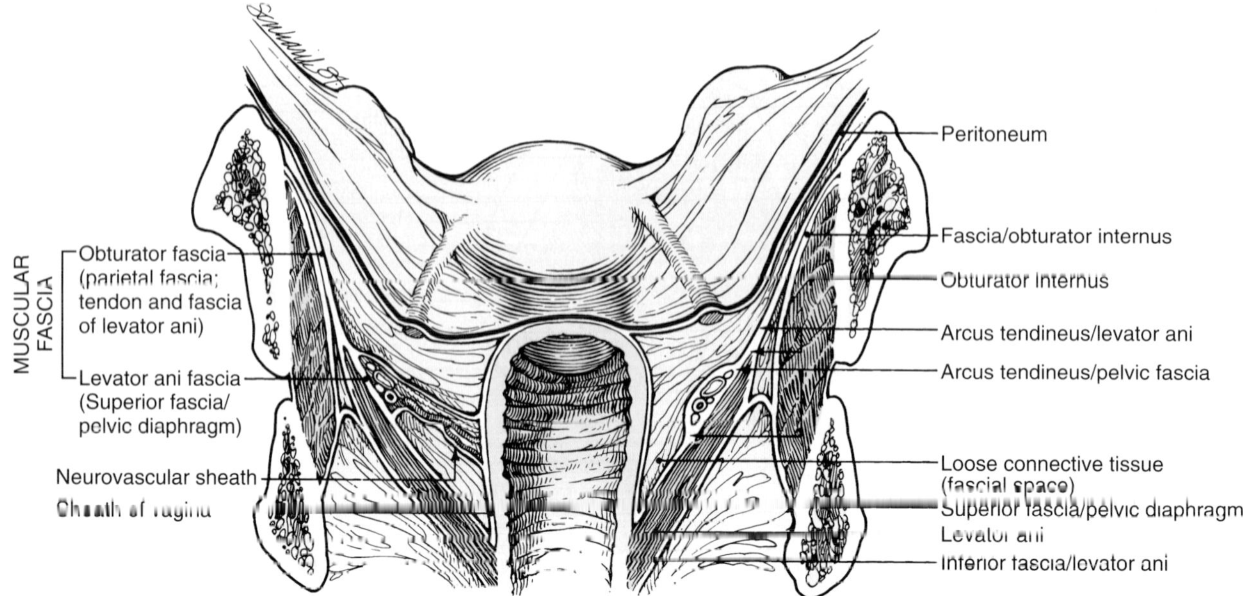

Figure A-6. Fascial and peritoneal relationships of the pelvic diaphragm. In this frontal view of the pelvis, the levator ani can be seen to slope downward and medially, surrounding the vagina. The loose connective tissue beneath the pelvic peritoneum is variable in thickness, depending on the general adiposity of the individual. Note also the continuity of the different fascias as they merge to form the neurovascular sheaths.

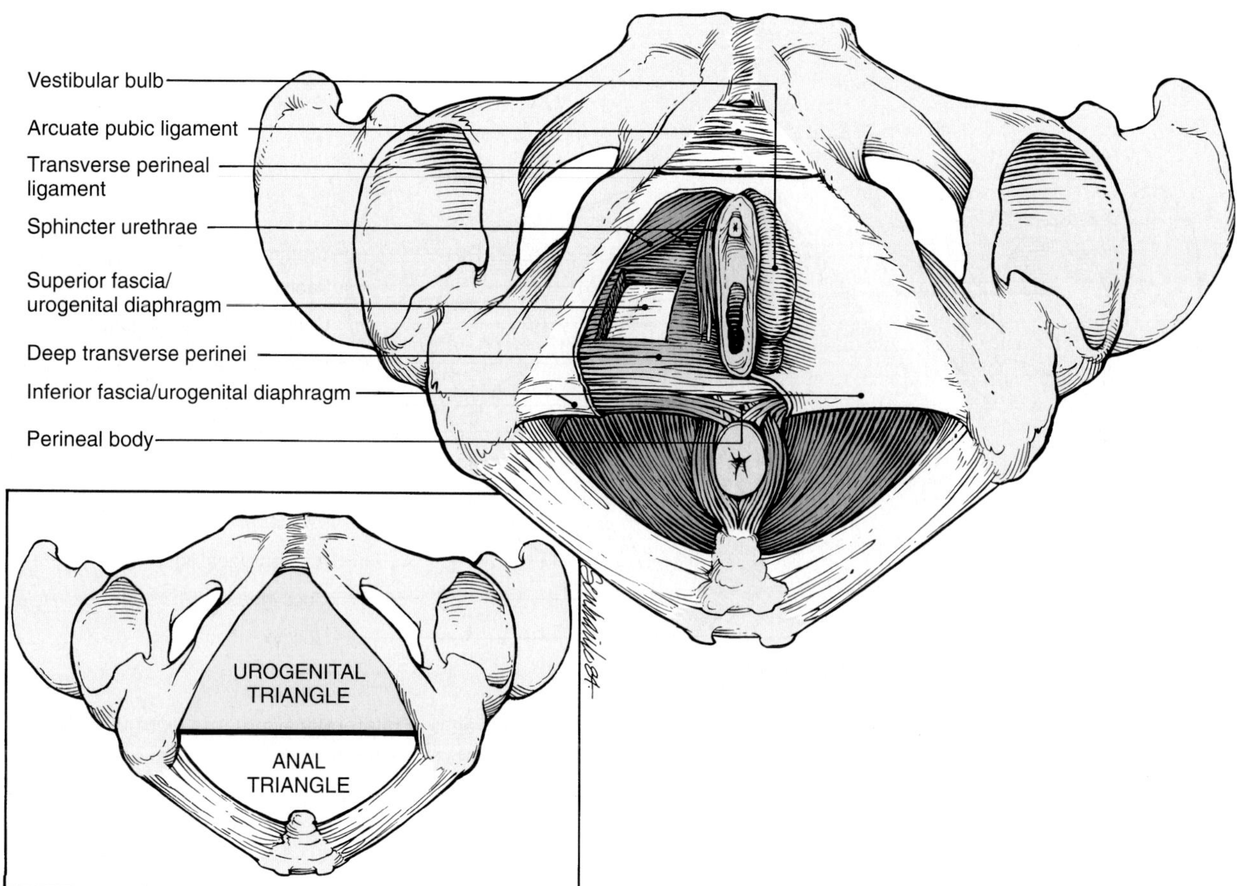

Figure A-7. Muscles of the deep perineal space, inferior view. As viewed with the patient in dorsal lithotomy position, the deep perineal space consists of smaller muscles than the superficial perineal space. Note that the vestibular bulb lies within the superficial perineal space. *Inset:* Division of the perineum into a urogenital (anterior) triangle and an anal (posterior) triangle.

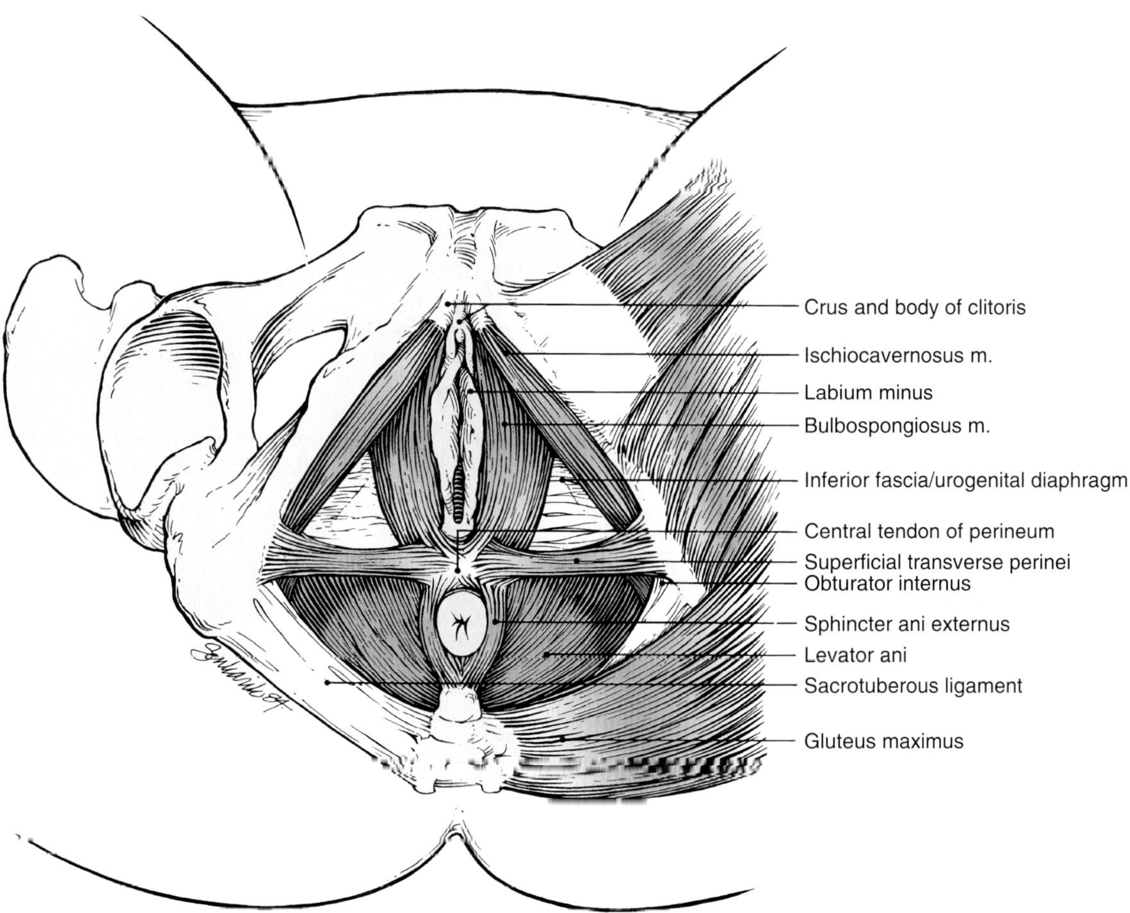

Figure A-8. Muscles of the superficial perineal space, from below. As viewed with the patient in dorsal lithotomy position, the muscles of the superficial perineal space of the urogenital triangle and the muscles of the anal triangle all converge in the midline. m., muscle.

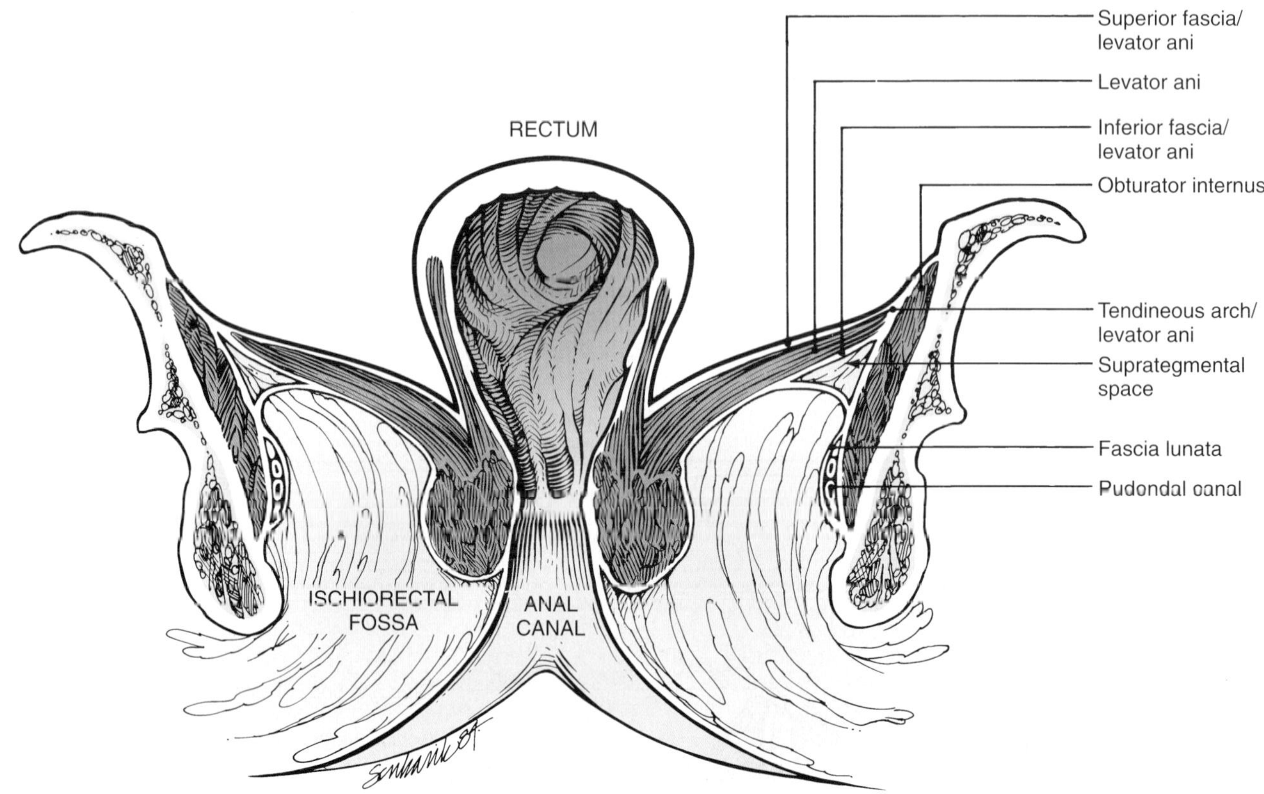

Figure A-9. Ischiorectal fossa, frontal section. The ischiorectal fossa surrounds the rectum and vagina and forms most of the potential space within the posterior triangle of the perineum. The fascia of the levator ani merges with the visceral sheath of the rectum and vagina to lend support.

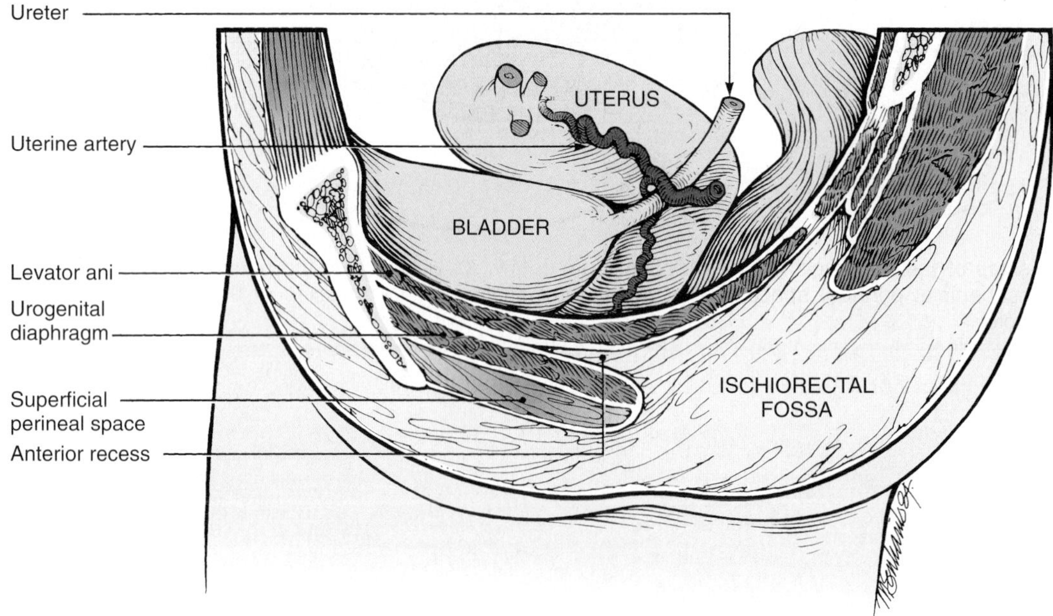

Figure A-10. Ischiorectal fossa and urogenital diaphragm, sagittal section. The ischiorectal fossa extends both forward and backward from the anal triangle. The urogenital diaphragm subdivides the urogenital triangle, with the anterior recess of the ischiorectal fossa superior to it. The subcutaneous fat between the inferior aspect of the superficial perineal space and the skin varies among individuals.

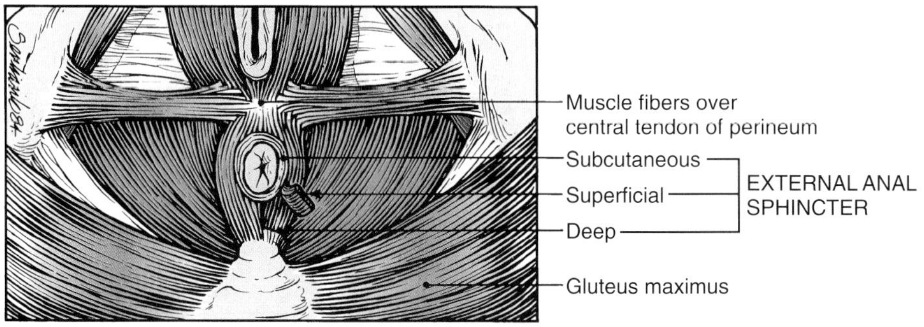

Muscle fibers over central tendon of perineum
Subcutaneous
Superficial
Deep
EXTERNAL ANAL SPHINCTER
Gluteus maximus

Figure A-11. External anal sphincter as viewed in dorsal lithotomy position. The external anal sphincter is composed of three muscles that arise from the coccyx and converge into the central tendon of the perineum. Midline or mediolateral episiotomy may damage this sphincter; proper reapproximation is essential for fecal continence.

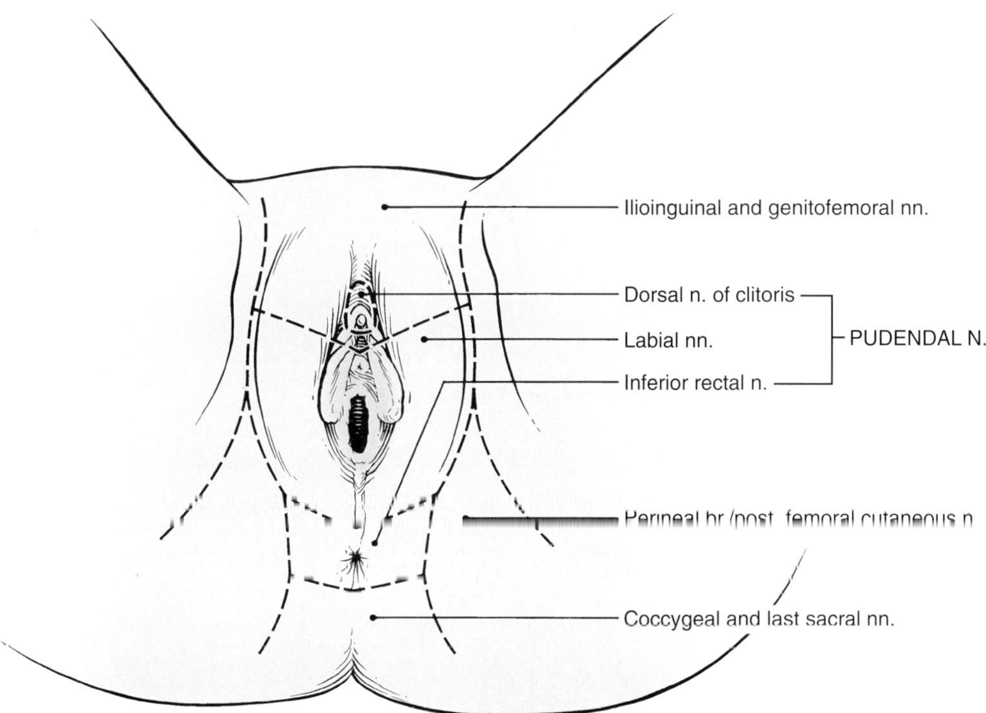

Figure A-12. Cutaneous nerve supply to the perineum. Most cutaneous innervation to the perineum comes from the pudendal nerve, but important regions are supplied by other sources. Pudendal block thus only anesthetizes a portion of the perineal surface. The exact limits of each specific nerve supply are variable. N., nerve; nn., nerves.

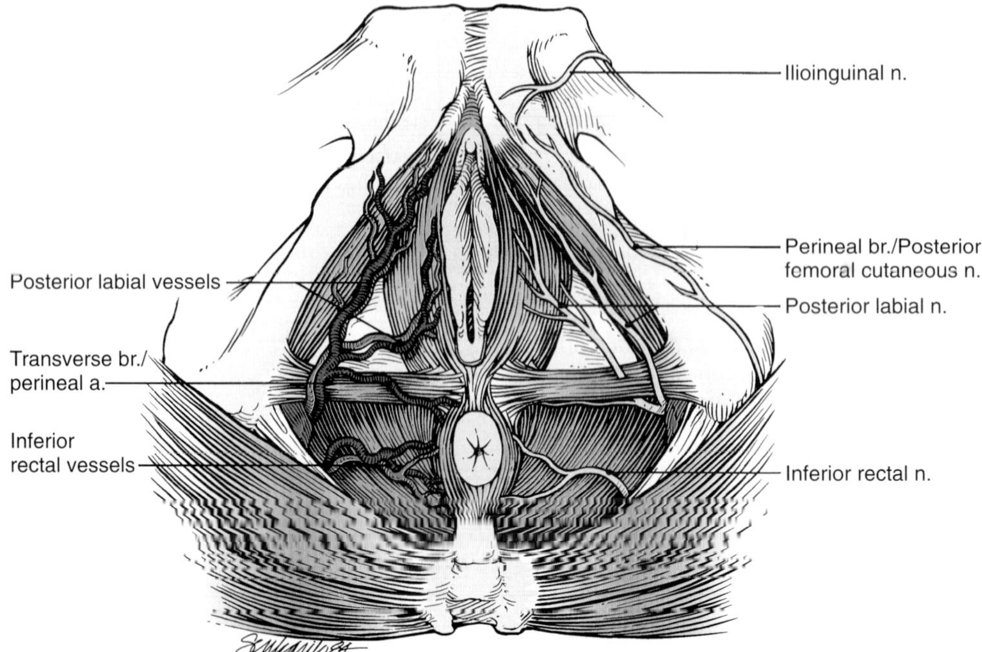

Figure A-13. Superficial perineal blood supply and nerves, as viewed with the patient in dorsal lithotomy position. The vessels and nerves to the superficial perineal space follow each other. The vasculature is markedly engorged during pregnancy, and there may be significant bleeding from these vessels because of laceration, trauma, or episiotomy. Note the transverse branch of the perineal artery, a vessel often encountered during routine midline or mediolateral episiotomy. br., branch; a., artery; n., nerve.

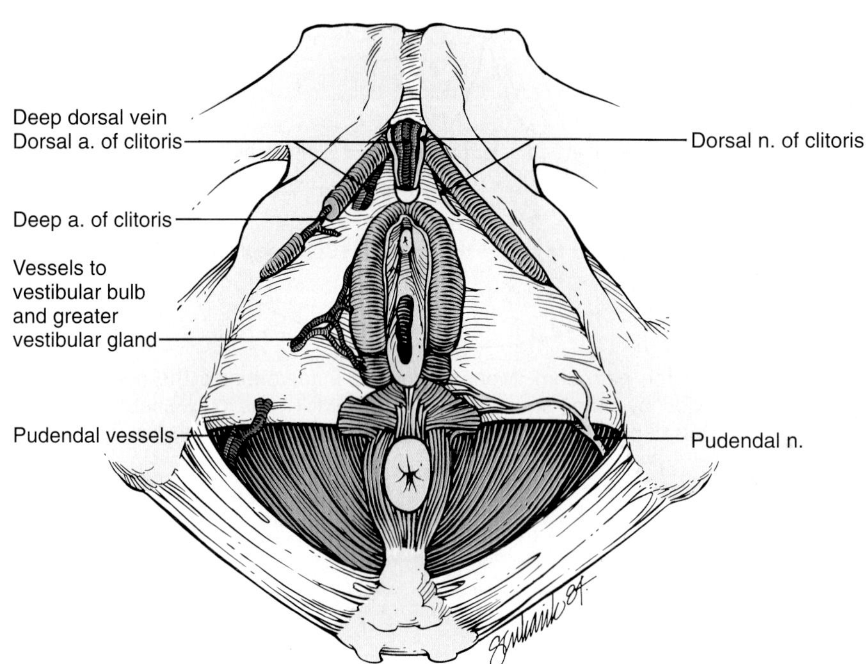

Figure A-14. Vessels and nerves of the deep perineal space. The vasculature and innervation to the deep perineal space enters the anterior triangle from superior to inferior, in contrast to the superficial perineal space vessels and nerves. Note that the blood supply and innervation to the vestibular bulb and greater vestibular gland (Bartholin's gland) are derived from the deep perineal vessels and nerves. a., artery; n., nerve.

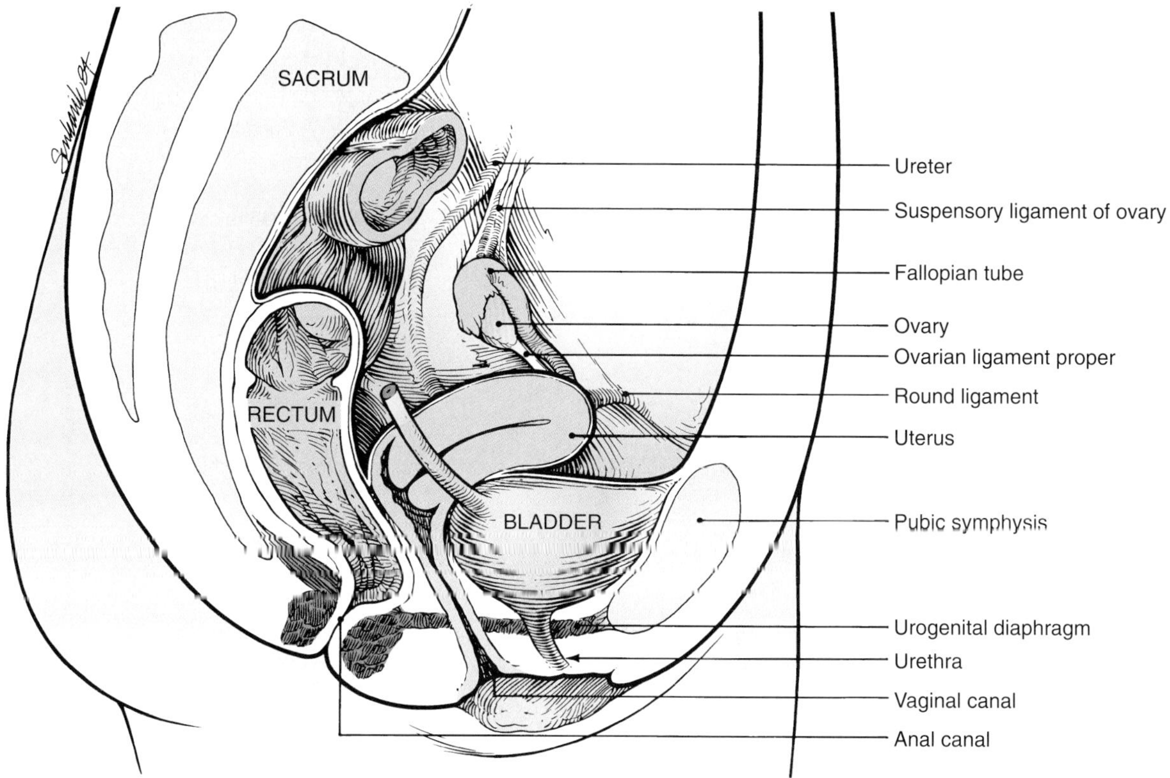

Figure A-15. Major organs of the pelvis, sagittal section. The internal organs of the pelvis are supported by the levator ani. Note how the anteverted, anteflexed uterus gains further support from both the urinary bladder and rectum. The ureter crosses the lateral aspect of the uterus at the level of the internal os on its way to the bladder. The actual position of the ovary and fimbriated end of the tube is quite variable.

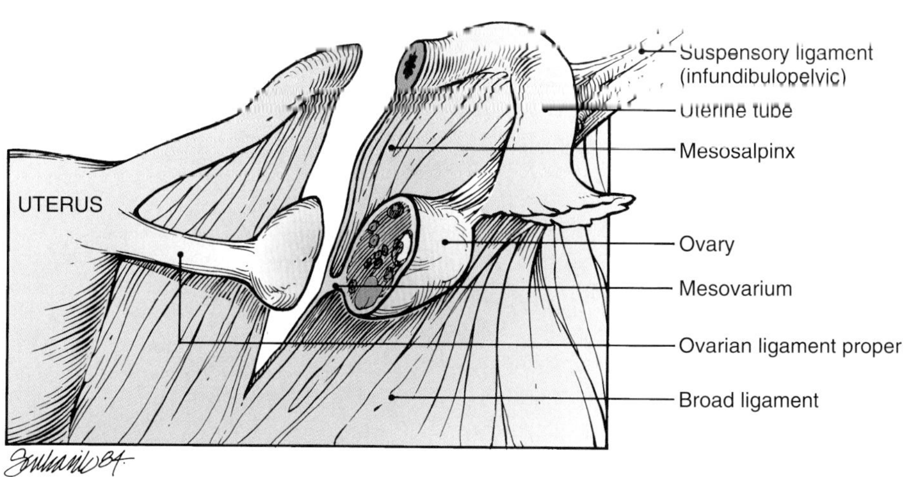

Figure A-16. Anatomy of the fallopian tube and ovary, posterior view. The ovary and tube are suspended by mesenteries derived as specialized portions of the broad ligament. The vasculature and nerves enter through the mesovarium and mesosalpinx.

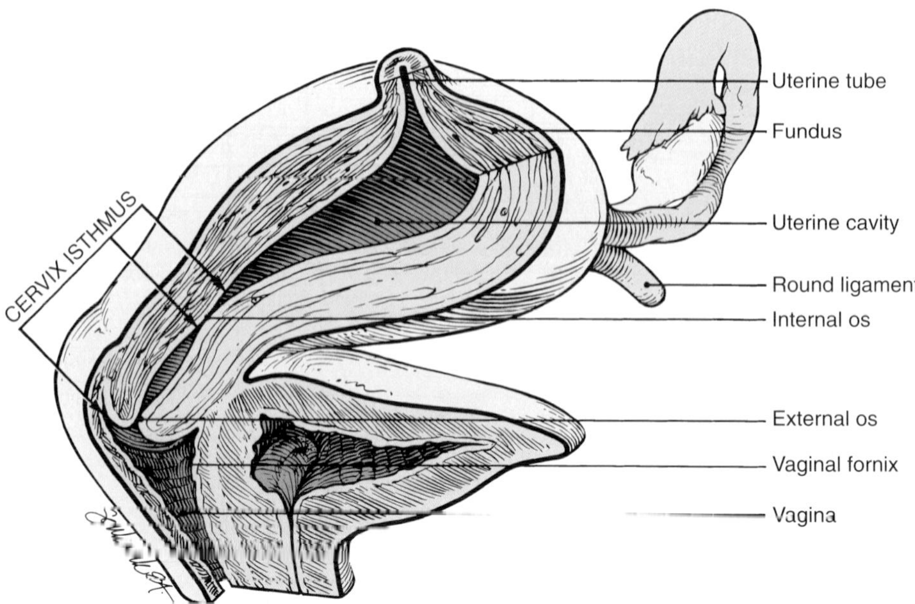

Figure A-17. Anatomic regions of the uterus, lateral view. The uterus is composed of cervix, isthmus, corpus, and fundus. Because the regions of the uterus grow at different rates during pregnancy, the distance between cornual fallopian tube and fundus increases markedly with increasing gestation. Note that the peritoneal reflection of the bladder occurs at the level of the uterine isthmus.

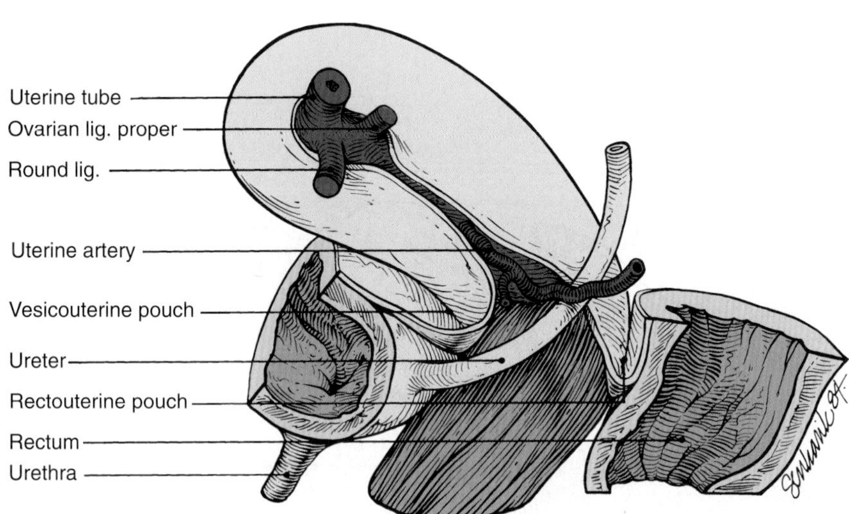

Figure A-18. Anatomic relationships of the uterus, lateral view. The broad ligament contains the uterus and forms an anterior and posterior covering. The triangular space along the lateral uterine wall lies between the leaves of the broad ligament. Note the relationship of the ureter to the uterine artery. lig., ligament.

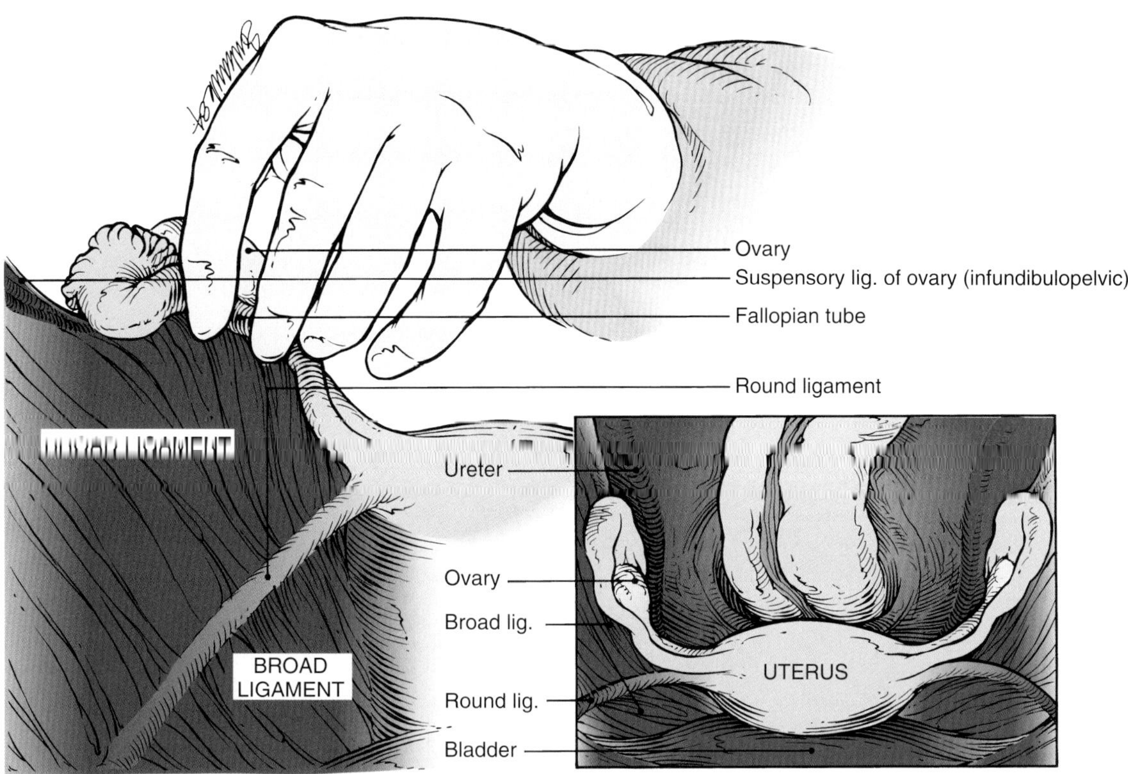

Figure A-19. Broad ligament and contained organs, frontal view. The round ligament runs within the anterior leaf of the broad ligament and inserts through the inguinal canal to the labium majus. *Inset:* The relationships as seen from an anterosuperior perspective. Note the rectovaginal pouch as seen from above and anteriorly. lig., ligament.

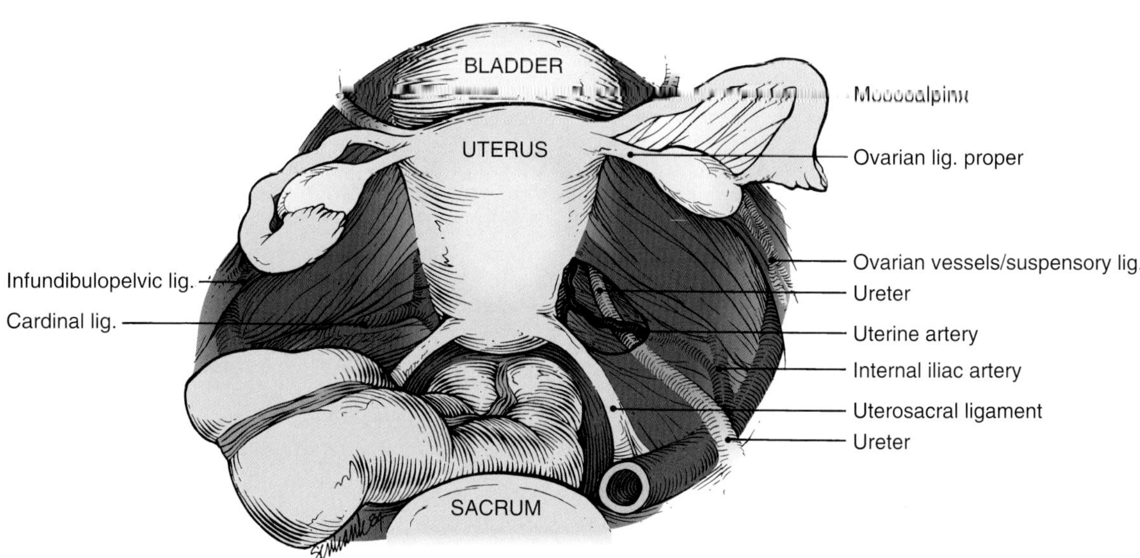

Figure A-20. Organs of the pelvis, posterior view. The rectouterine pouch is demarcated by the uterosacral ligaments. This pouch is often termed the *posterior cul-de-sac.* In this diagram, a section of the posterior leaf of the broad ligament has been removed to show the relationship of the uterine artery to the ureter. Intraligamentous tumors, infection, endometriosis, or previous surgery can often alter this relationship. lig., ligament.

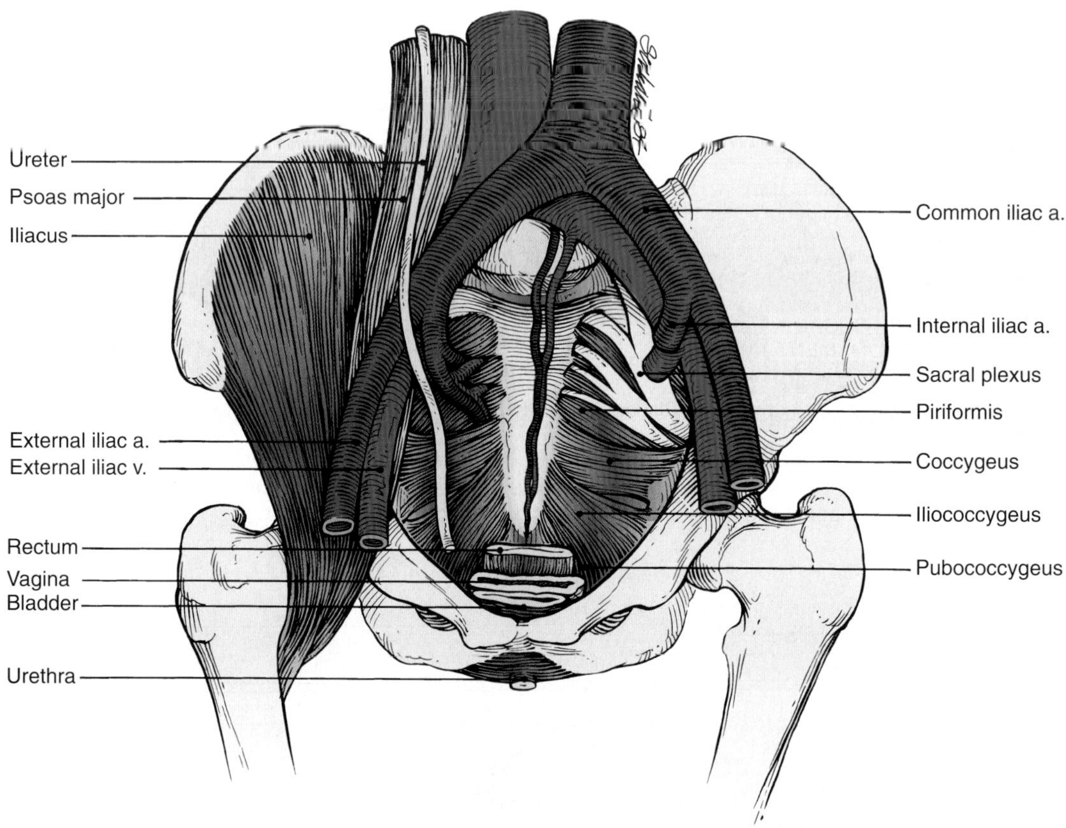

Figure A-21. Major vessels of the pelvis, frontal view. The major vasculature of the pelvis is shown in relationship to the pelvic diaphragm. The proximity of the ureter to the internal iliac (hypogastric) artery is noteworthy. Ligation of the hypogastric artery may thus jeopardize the ureter unless care is taken. Note the anterior and posterior trunks of the internal iliac artery. a., artery; v., vein.

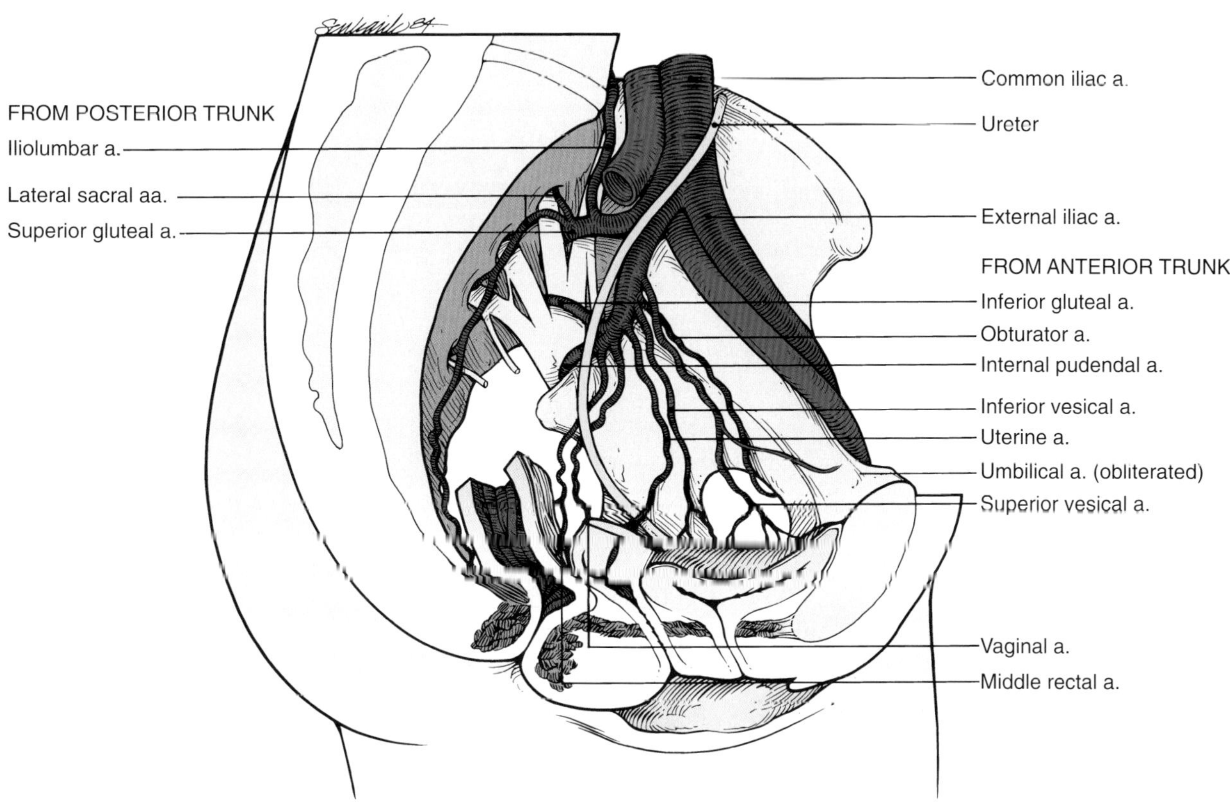

Figure A-22. Major vessels of the pelvis, lateral view. The major subdivisions of the anterior and posterior trunks are highly variable, and no singular branching pattern accounts for most patients. Note the relationship of the vessels to the sacral plexus. The uterus has been amputated at the level of the isthmus to permit a better view of the branching patterns of the anterior trunk. a., artery; aa., arteries.

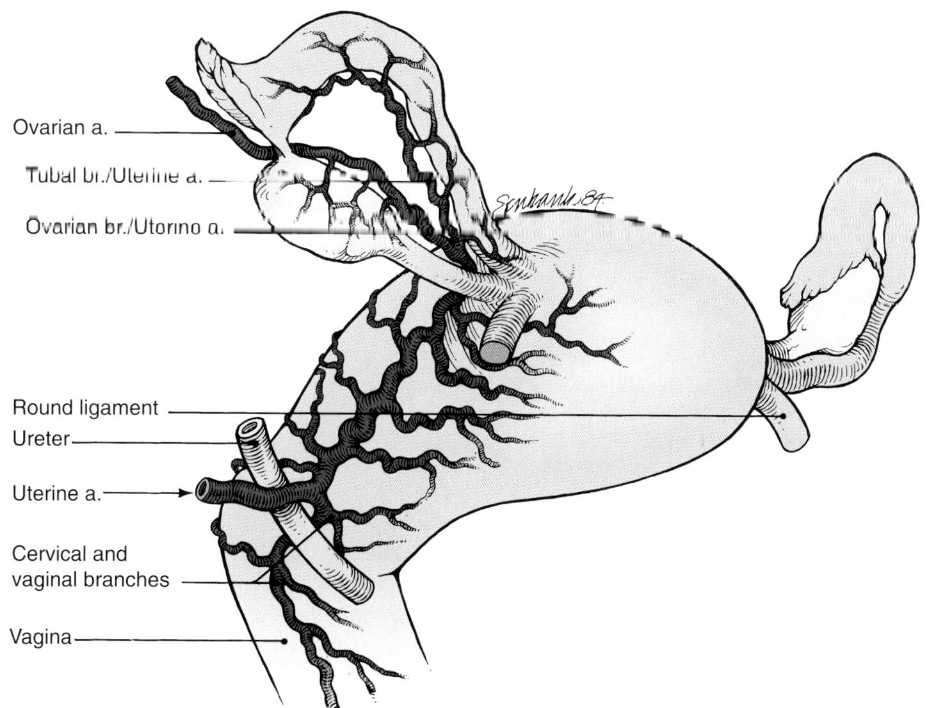

Figure A-23. Blood supply to the uterus, tube, and ovary. The vasculature supply to the major pelvic organs is derived from the internal iliac (uterine) artery and the ovarian artery. Note the anastomotic plexuses of vessels along the lateral aspect of the uterus at the region of the cornu. Descending branches from the uterine artery supply the cervix and vagina. a., artery; br., branch.

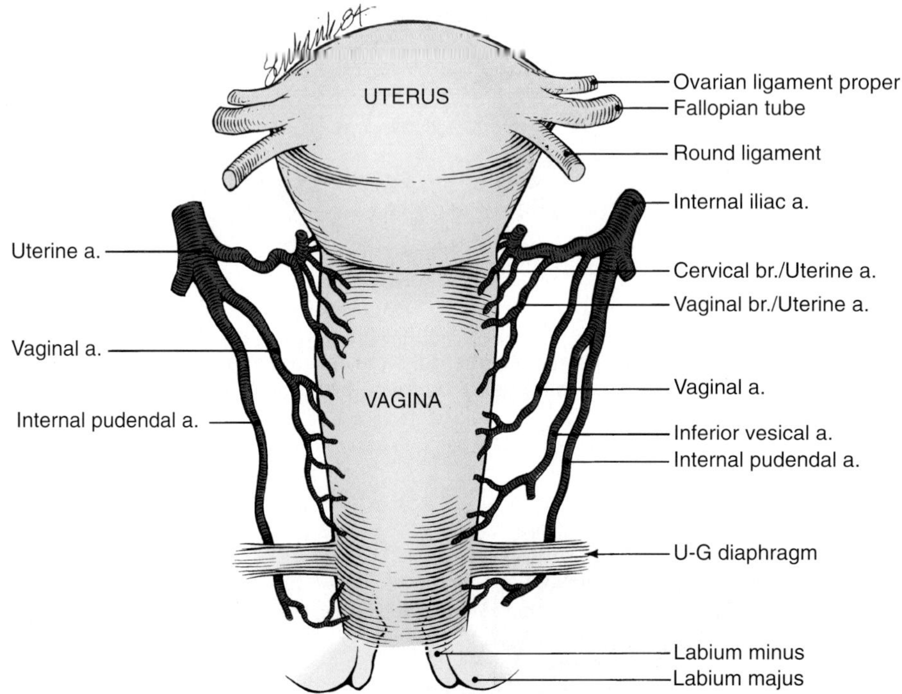

Figure A-24. Blood supply to the vagina. Like the uterus, the vagina derives its blood supply from two major sources: the uterine and pudendal arteries. The internal pudendal artery supplies the vagina from inferior to superior. The vaginal artery, often a branch from the uterine artery, and the uterine artery itself supply the superior position of the vagina. a., artery; U-G, urogenital; br., branch.

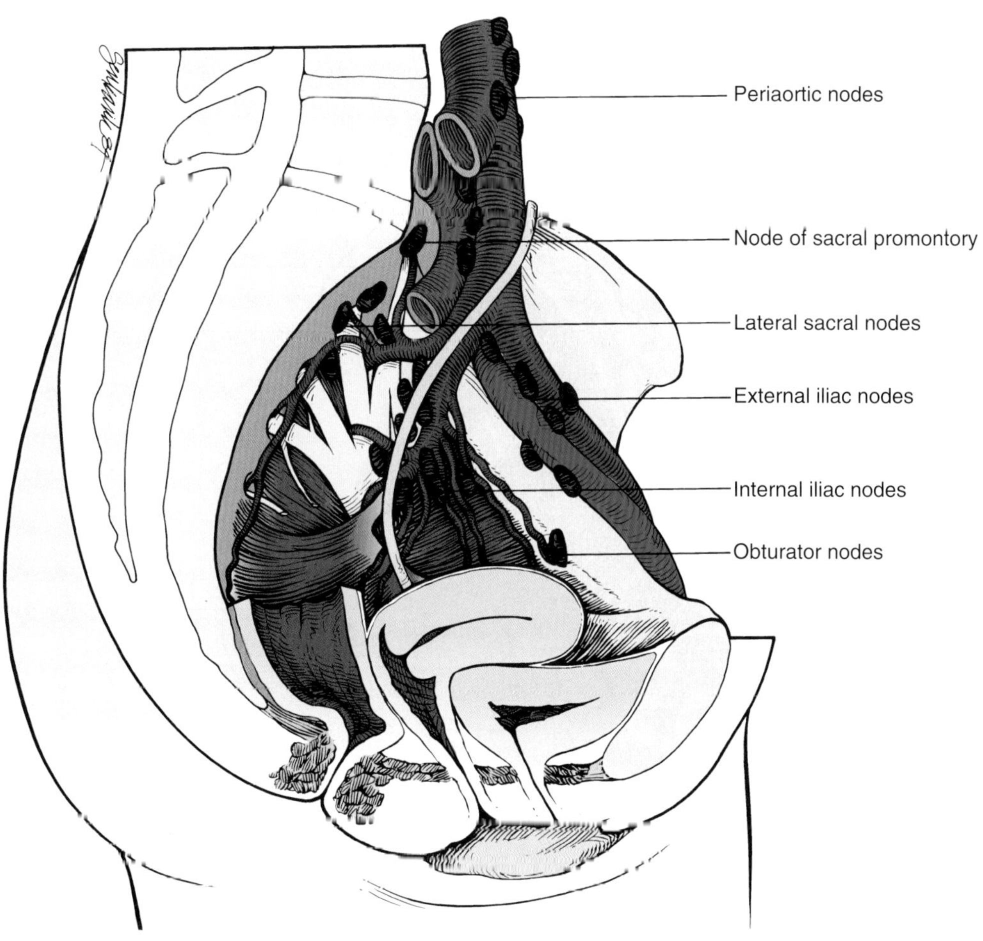

Figure A-25. Major lymphatics of the pelvis. The major lymph nodes of the pelvis follow the major vessels. Each group of nodes receives contributions from multiple organs. The groupings are somewhat arbitrary, because no distinct separation of individual node groups exists.

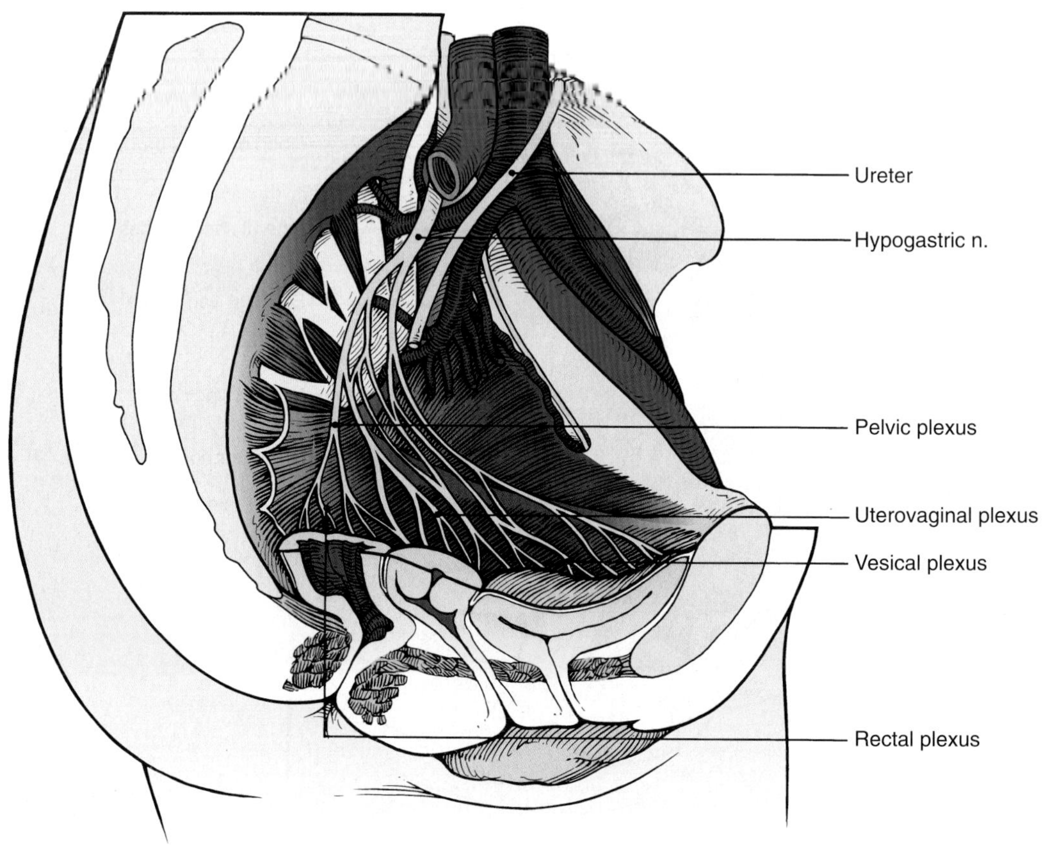

Figure A-26. Major nerves of the pelvis, lateral view. Few branches of the sacral plexus are evident, because these nerves leave the pelvis even as the branches are forming. Most of the pelvic plexus lies medial to the vasculature. n., nerve.

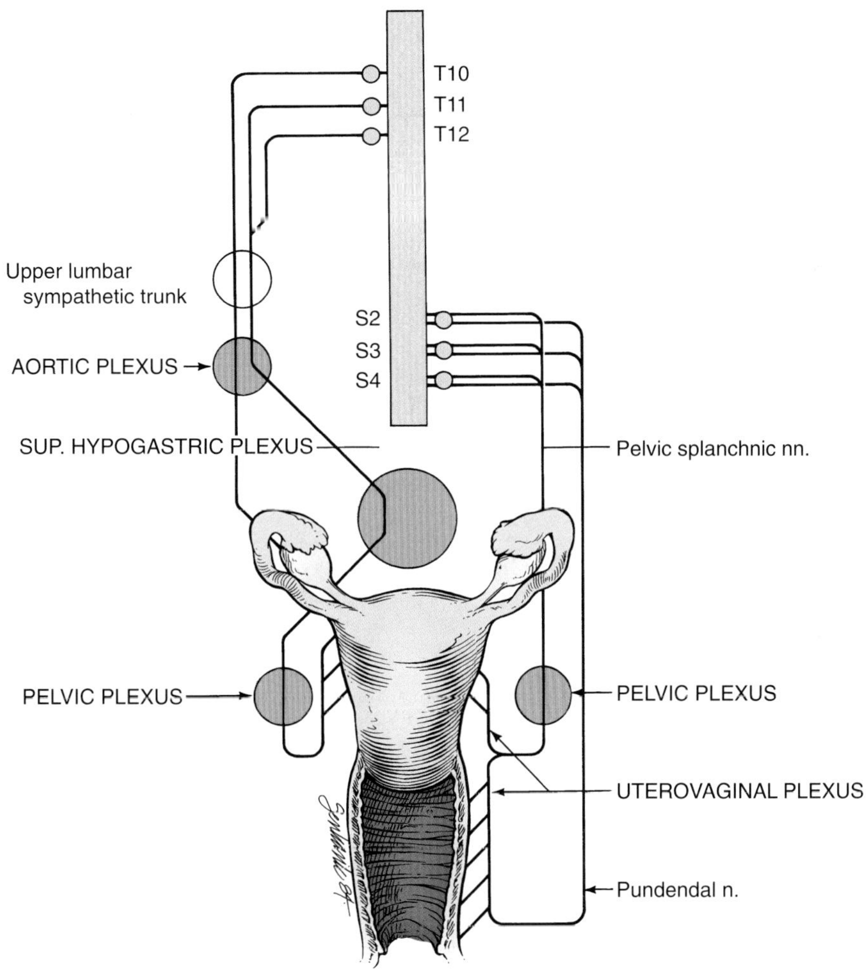

Figure A-27. Afferent innervation of the female genital tract. The left side of this diagram demonstrates the sympathetic nervous system. Fibers entering the spinal cord are illustrated on the right. The major afferent pain fibers for the uterus, tubes, and ovaries enter the cord at T10, T11, and T12. The afferent innervation of the vagina and external genitalia enter at S2, S3, and S4. sup., superior; n., nerve; nn., nerves.

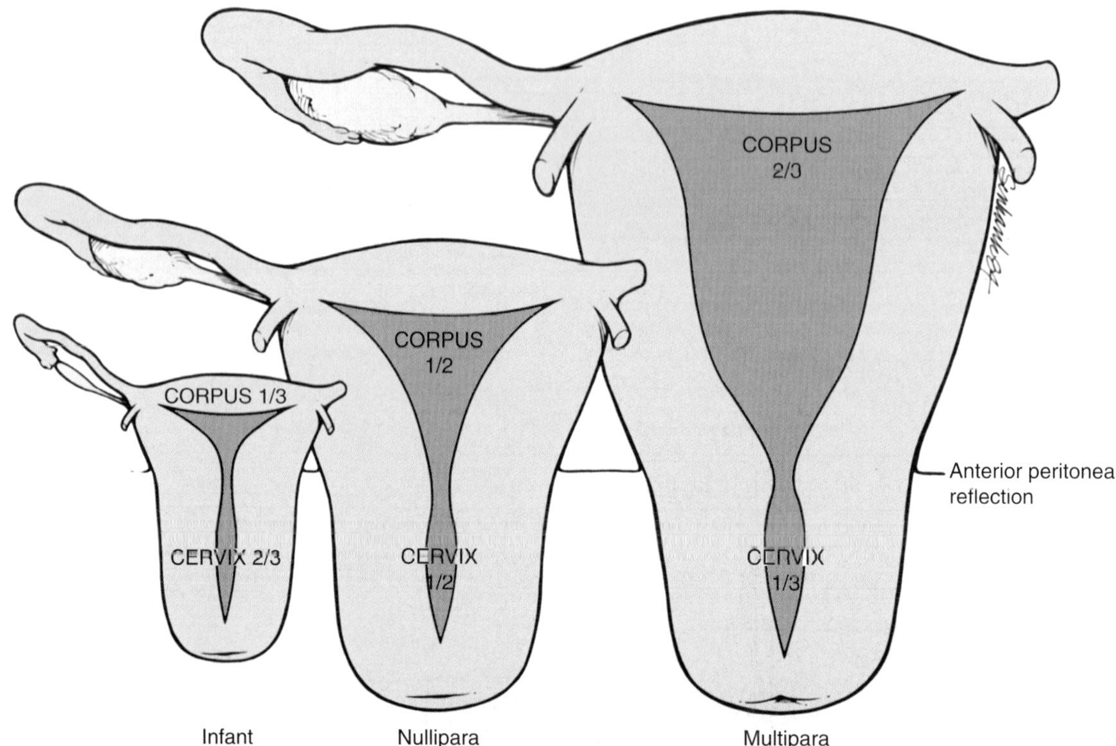

Figure A-28. Changes in the uterus with age and parity. At puberty, growth occurs primarily in the corpus and the fundus, although the cervix continues to grow as well. After menopause, the uterus regresses to a state more closely allied to that of the premenarcheal anatomy. During pregnancy, the cervical portion is relatively greater than in the nonpregnant state.

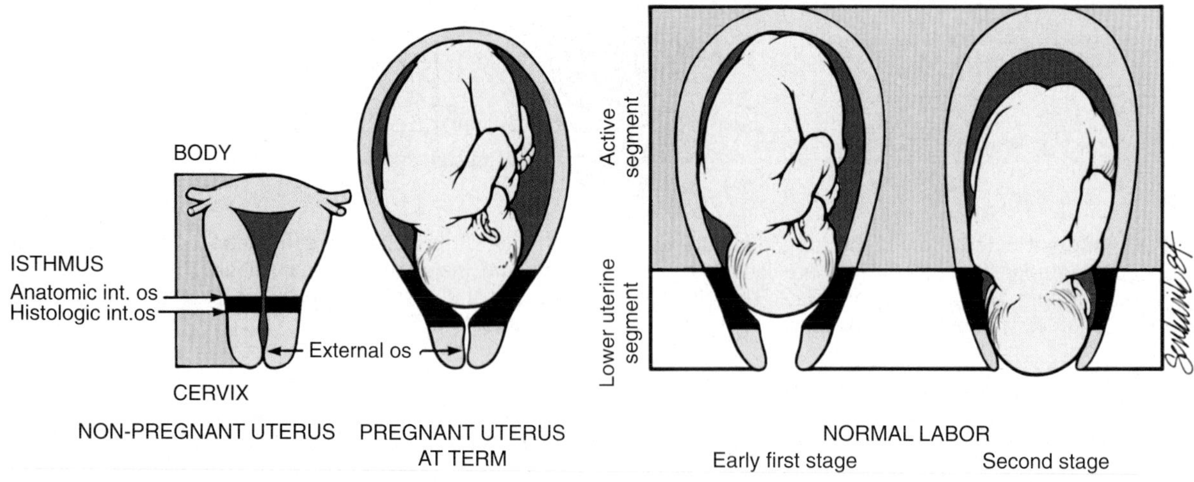

Figure A-29. Changes in the uterus caused by pregnancy and parturition. The hormonal changes of pregnancy as well as dynamic forces of labor cause the development of the lower uterine segment from the vestigial uterine isthmus. After parturition, these changes regress dramatically. Low transverse cesarean delivery incisions are performed through this thinned isthmic region, known as the *lower uterine segment.*

Key Points

- To facilitate childbearing, the female pelvis—as opposed to the male pelvis—is characterized by a wider subpubic angle, increased width of the sciatic notch, and greater distance from the symphysis pubis to the anterior edge of the acetabulum.
- The levator ani, the major supporting structure for the pelvic viscera, is a tripartite muscle mass composed of the iliococcygeus, pubococcygeus, and puborectalis; the iliococcygeus is the broadest and most posterior portion.
- Innervation of the levator ani is through the third and fourth sacral nerves.
- The major nerve supply of the perineum is derived from the pudendal. However, the ilioinguinal, genitofemoral, perineal branch of the posterior femoral cutaneous, coccygeal, and last sacral nerve also contribute; thus, a pudendal nerve block anesthetizes only a portion of the perineum.
- The internal iliac (hypogastric) artery arises at the level of lumbosacral articulation. It can be distinguished from the external iliac by its smaller size and by its more medial and more posterior position.
- The ureter lies more superficially and is either medial or slightly anterior to the internal iliac artery.
- The cardinal ligaments are located at the base of the broad ligament, are continuous with the connective tissue of the parametrium, and are attached to the pelvic diaphragm through continuity with the superficial superior fascia of the levator ani.
- Because the origin of the uterine artery is variable, its isolation and ligation for control of postpartum bleeding are often fruitless. The uterine artery usually arises as an independent vessel from the internal iliac artery, but it may also arise from the inferior gluteal, internal pudendal, umbilical, or obturator arteries.
- Afferent pain fibers for the uterus, tubes, and ovary enter the cord at T10, T11, T12; thus, spinal or epidural anesthesia must extend to these levels. Fortunately, efferent fibers to the uterus enter above these levels, thus not interfering with contractions.
- The body of the nonpregnant uterus weighs approximately 70 g, whereas at term it weighs approximately 1,100 g.

SUGGESTED READING

Moore KL, Dalley AF II: Pelvis and perineum. *In* Clinically Oriented Anatomy, 5th ed. Baltimore, Lippincott Williams & Wilkins, 2006, pp 357–476.

Index

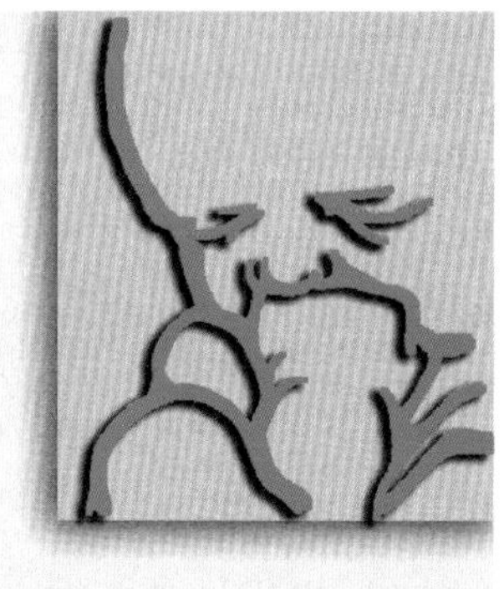

Note: Page numbers followed by f indicate figures; t tables; b box.

G

H

I

O

Q

R

T

U

V